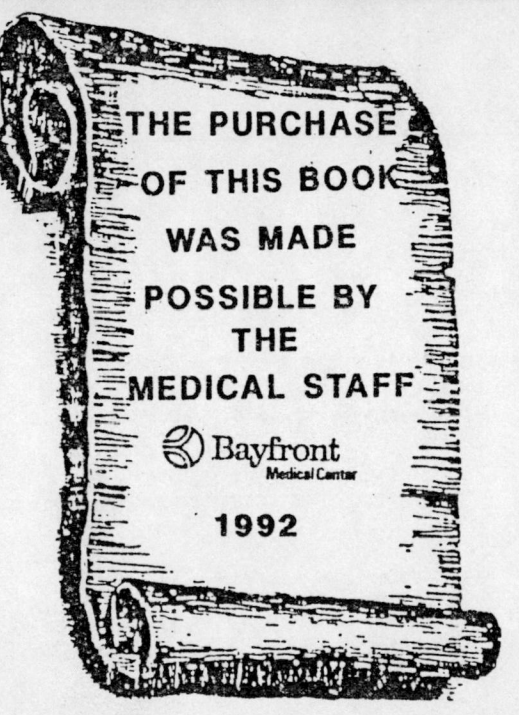

Second Edition

Principles and Practice of

Medical Therapy in Pregnancy

Second Edition

Principles and Practice of

Medical Therapy in Pregnancy

APPLETON & LANGE
Norwalk, Connecticut/San Mateo, California

EDITOR

NORBERT GLEICHER, MD

President, the Center for Human Reproduction
Chicago, Illinois
Professor of Obstetrics and Gynecology and
Microbiology/Immunology
University of Health Sciences/
Chicago Medical School
North Chicago, Illinois

SECTION EDITORS

URI ELKAYAM, MD

Chief of Cardiology, USC University Hospital
Professor of Medicine
University of Southern California School of Medicine
Los Angeles, California

ROBERT M. GALBRAITH, MD

Professor and Chairman
Department of Basic Immunology
and Clinical Microbiology
Medical University of South Carolina
Charleston, South Carolina

STANLEY A. GALL, MD

Professor and Chairman
Department of Obstetrics and Gynecology
University of Louisville School of Medicine
Louisville, Kentucky

GLORIA E. SARTO, MD, PhD

Professor and Chair
Department of Obstetrics and Gynecology
University of New Mexico School of Medicine
Albuquerque, New Mexico

BAHA M. SIBAI, MD

Professor and Chief
Maternal-Fetal Medicine Division
Department of Obstetrics and Gynecology
University of Tennessee School of Medicine
Memphis, Tennessee

Notice: The authors and the publisher of this volume have taken care to make certain that the doses of drugs and schedules of treatment are correct and compatible with the standards generally accepted at the time of publication. Nevertheless, as new information becomes available, changes in treatment and in the use of drugs become necessary. The reader is advised to carefully consult the instruction and information material included in the package insert of each drug or therapeutic agent before administration. This advice is especially important when using new or infrequently used drugs. The publisher disclaims any liability, loss, injury, or damage incurred as a consequence, directly or indirectly, of the use and application of any of the contents of this volume.

92 93 94 95 96 / 10 9 8 7 6 5 4 3 2 1

Prentice Hall International (UK) Limited, *London*
Prentice Hall of Australia Pty. Limited, *Sydney*
Prentice Hall Canada, Inc., *Toronto*
Prentice Hall Hispanoamericana, S.A., *Mexico*
Prentice Hall of India Private Limited, *New Delhi*
Prentice Hall of Japan, Inc., *Tokyo*
Simon Schuster Asia Pte. Ltd., *Singapore*
Editora Prentice Hall do Brasil Ltda., *Rio de Janeiro*
Prentice Hall, *Englewood Cliffs, New Jersey*

Library of Congress Cataloging-in-Publication Data

Principles and practice of medical therapy in pregnancy / edited by Norbert Gleicher.—2nd ed.
p. cm.
Rev. ed. of: Principles of medical therapy in pregnancy. c1985.
Includes index.
ISBN 0–8385–7979–5
1. Pregnancy, Complications of—Treatment. I. Gleicher, Norbert. II. Principles of medical therapy in pregnancy.
[DNLM: 1. Pregnancy Complications—therapy. WQ 240 P9565]
RG572.P75 1991
618.3—dc20
DNLM/DLC 91–17931
for Library of Congress CIP

Acquisitions Editor: R. Craig Percy
Production Service: Editorial Services of New England, Inc.
Production Editor: Elizabeth Ryan
Designer: Michael J. Kelly

PRINTED IN THE UNITED STATES OF AMERICA

ISBN 0-8385-7979-5

To my family, especially
my wife Birgit and
daughter Anja, my friends
and coworkers—for their
tolerance, patience, and love.

Norbert Gleicher

Contents

† Deceased

Contributors

Ernest L. Abel, PhD
Professor
Departments of Obstetrics and Gynecology and Psychology
Wayne State University School of Medicine
Detroit, Michigan

Alfred Abu-Hamad, MD
Fellow in Maternal-Fetal Medicine
Department of Obstetrics and Gynecology
University of Miami
Miami, Florida

Daniel J. Adler, MD
Program Coordinator of Education
Section of Gastroenterology
Department of Medicine
Lenox Hill Hospital
Cornell University Medical College
New York, New York

Yogi K. Ahluwalia, MD
Clinical Associate Professor
Department of Psychiatry
Chicago Medical School
Chairman
Department of Psychiatry
Mount Sinai Hospital Medical Center
Chicago, Illinois

Erol Amon, MD
Associate Professor
Division of Maternal-Fetal Medicine
Department of Obstetrics and Gynecology
St. Mary's Health Center and
St. Louis University School of Medicine
St. Louis, Missouri

Marvin S. Amstey, MD
Professor
Department of Obstetrics and Gynecology
University of Rochester School of Medicine and Dentistry
Chief
Department of Obstetrics and Gynecology
Highland Hospital
Rochester, New York

E. Everett Anderson, MD
Professor of Urology
Division of Urology
Department of Surgery
Duke University Medical Center
Durham, North Carolina

William W. Andrews, MD, PhD
Assistant Professor
Division of Maternal-Fetal Medicine
Department of Obstetrics and Gynecology
University of Alabama at Birmingham
Birmingham, Alabama

George J. Annas, JD, MPH
Chair, Health Law Department
Utley Professor of Health Law
Director, Law, Medicine and Ethics Program
Boston University Schools of Medicine and Public Health
Boston, Massachusetts

Edward L. Applebaum, MD
Francis L. Lederer Professor and Department Head
Department of Otolaryngology-Head-and-Neck Surgery
The University of Illinois College of Medicine at Chicago and
Illinois Eye and Ear Infirmary
Chicago, Illinois

Carolyn Weller Arnolds, RN, MS
Clinical Nurse Specialist
Division of Maternal-Fetal Medicine

Department of Obstetrics and Gynecology
Rush-Presbyterian-St. Luke's Medical Center
Chicago, Illinois

Efstratios A. Assimakopoulos, MD
Fellow
Department of Obstetrics and Gynecology
Yale University School of Medicine
New Haven, Connecticut

David A. Baker, MD
Associate Professor
Director, Division of Infectious Diseases
Department of Obstetrics and Gynecology
Health Sciences Center
School of Medicine
State University of New York
Stony Brook, New York

Thomas N. Balaskas, MD
Instructor
Division of Maternal-Fetal Medicine
Department of Obstetrics and Gynecology
University of Louisville School of Medicine
Louisville, Kentucky

Jamie S. Barkin, MD
Professor of Medicine
Chief, Division of Gastroenterology
Department of Medicine
University of Miami
Mt. Sinai Medical Center
Miami, Florida

Riad Barmada, MD
Professor and Head
Department of Orthopaedics
University of Illinois at Chicago
Chicago, Illinois

William M. Barron, MD
Associate Professor
Department of Medicine and Obstetrics and Gynecology
University of Chicago School of Medicine
Chicago, Illinois

Roger E. Bawdon, PhD
Associate Professor
Department of Obstetrics and Gynecology
University of Texas Southwestern Medical School
Dallas, Texas

Al B. Benson III, MD
Assistant Professor of Medicine
Division of Hematology-Oncology
Department of Medicine
Northwestern University
Associate Director
Clinical Trials
Illinois Cancer Council
Chicago, Illinois

Constance A. Benson, MD
Assistant Professor of Medicine
Section of Infectious Disease
Department of Medicine
Rush Medical College
Rush-Presbyterian-St. Luke's Medical Center
Chicago, Illinois

Jason C. Birnholz, MD
Diagnostic Ultrasound Consultants, Ltd.
Oak Brook, Illinois

Karen J. Blakemore, MD
Assistant Professor
Division of Maternal-Fetal Medicine
Department of Gynecology and Obstetrics
The Johns Hopkins University School of Mecicine
Baltimore, Maryland

Jorge D. Blanco, MD
John T. Armstrong Professor and Vice-Chairman
Division of Maternal-Fetal Medicine
Department of Obstetrics, Gynecology and Reproductive Sciences
University of Texas Medical School at Houston
Chief of Obstetrics and Gynecology
LBJ General Hospital
Houston, Texas

Leo R. Boler, Jr., MD
Attending
Department of Obstetrics and Gynecology
Mount Sinai Hospital Medical Center
Chicago, Illinois

Richard Paul Bonfiglio, MD
Assistant Professor
Physical Medicine and Rehabilitation
Chicago Medical School
Chicago, Illinois

Peter M. Brooks, MD
Professor of Rheumatology
Department of Medicine
University of Sydney
Sydney, Australia
Head, Department of Rheumatology
Royal North Shore Hospital
St. Leonards, New South Wales
Australia

W. Watson Buchanan, MD
Professor of Medicine
Division of Rheumatology
Department of Medicine
McMaster University Faculty of Health Sciences
Hamilton, Ontario
Canada

Teresa M. Castellano, MS
Co-director, Prenatal Diagnosis and Genetic Counseling Services
Division of Genetics
Department of Obstetrics and Gynecology
The University of New Mexico Medical Center
Albuquerque, New Mexico

Dinesh N. Chauhan, MD
Chief, Obstetric Anesthesia
Methodist Hospital, Central
Memphis, Tennessee

Michel Chrétien, OC, MD
Professor
Department of Medicine
University of Montreal and
McGill University
Scientific Director, Clinical Research Institute of Montreal
Hôtel-Dieu Hospital
Montreal, Quebec
Canada

Carl W. Christensen, MD, PhD
Assistant Professor
Division of Gynecologic Oncology
Department of Obstetrics and Gynecology
Wayne State University School of Medicine
Detroit, Michigan

Stefanie Schupp Christian, MD
Chief Resident
Division of Maternal-Fetal Medicine
Department of Obstetrics and Gynecology
Madigan Army Medical Center
Tacoma, Washington

David A. Clark, MD, PhD
Professor
Departments of Medicine and
Obstetrics and Gynecology
McMaster University
Hamilton, Ontario
Canada

Daniel L. Clarke-Pearson, MD
Professor
Division of Gynecologic Oncology
Department of Obstetrics and Gynecology
Duke University Medical Center
Durham, North Carolina

Melody A. Cobleigh, MD
Associate Professor of Medicine
Section of Medical Oncology
Department of Medicine
Rush-Presbyterian/St. Luke's Medical Center
Chicago, Illinois

Edmond Confino, MD
Assistant Professor
Department of Obstetrics and Gynecology
Chicago Medical School
Director of Gynecology
Mount Sinai Hospital Medical Center
Chicago, Illinois

F. Susan Cowchock, MD
Professor, Department of Medicine and Obstetrics and Gynecology
Assistant Professor, Department of Medicine and Obstetrics and Gynecology
Joint Appointment in Divisions of Genetics and Endocrinology, Department of Medicine and Division of Reproductive Endocrinology and Infertility, Department of Obstetrics and Gynecology
Thomas Jefferson University Medical College
Thomas Jefferson University Hospital
Philadelphia, Pennsylvania

William T. Creasman, MD
Sims-Hester Professor and Chairman
Department of Obstetrics and Gynecology
Medical University of South Carolina
Charleston, South Carolina

Karen C. Cummiskey, MD
Assistant Professor
Division of Maternal-Fetal Medicine
Department of Obstetrics and Gynecology
University of Louisville School of Medicine
Louisville, Kentucky

John T. Cunningham, MD
Associate Professor
Chief of Gastrointestinal Endoscopy
Division of Gastroenterology
Department of Medicine
Medical University of South Carolina
Charleston, South Carolina

Gary C. Cupit, PharmD
Product Manager
Gastrointestinal Business Group
SmithKline Beecham Pharmaceuticals
Philadelphia, Pennsylvania

John L. Currie, MD
Associate Professor, Oncology
Associate Professor, Gynecology and Obstetrics
Director, Division of Gynecologic Oncology
Department of Gynecology and Obstetrics
Johns Hopkins Medical Institutions
Baltimore, Maryland

George W. Dameron, Jr., MD†
Director, Obstetrics and Gynecology Residency
Bayfront Medical Center
Assistant Clinical Professor
University of South Florida School of Medicine
St. Petersburg, Florida

Walter E. Davis, MD
Assistant Consulting Professor of Medicine
Division of Hematology/Oncology
Department of Medicine
Duke University Medical Center
Chief, Hematology and Oncology
Durham County General Hospital
Durham, North Carolina

John M. Davison, MD
Professor of Obstetric Medicine
Department of Obstetrics and Gynaecology
University of Newcastle upon Tyne
Newcastle upon Tyne
England

Salim Daya, MBChB, MSc
Associate Professor
Department of Obstetrics and Gynaecology
McMaster University
Director
Fertility Clinic
McMaster University Medical Centre
Hamilton, Ontario
Canada

Gustaaf Albert Dekker, MD, PhD
Chef-de-Clinique
Division of Maternal-Fetal Medicine
Department of Obstetrics and Gynecology
Free University Hospital
Amsterdam
The Netherlands

Gunter Deppe, MD
Professor
Director, Division of Gynecologic Oncology
Department of Obstetrics and Gynecology
Wayne State University School of Medicine
Detroit, Michigan

Laura DiGiovanni, MD
Assistant Professor
Division of Maternal-Fetal Medicine
Department of Obstetrics and Gynecology
University of Chicago School of Medicine
Chicago, Illinois

Jay F. Dobkin, MD
Associate Professor of Clinical Medicine
Department of Medicine
College of Physicians and Surgeons of Columbia University
Director, AIDS Center
Columbia-Presbyterian Medical Center
New York, New York

Steven D. Douglas, MD
Professor of Pediatrics and Microbiology
University of Pennsylvania School of Medicine
Section Chief for Immunology
Children's Hospital of Philadelphia
Philadelphia, Pennsylvania

Arie Drugan, MD
Director
Division of Genetics
Department of Obstetrics
Rambam Medical Center
Haifa
Israel

Bruce H. Drukker, MD
Professor and Chairperson
Department of Obstetrics, Gynecology and Reproductive Biology
College of Human Medicine
Michigan State University
East Lansing, Michigan

Patrick Duff, MD
Professor
Division of Maternal-Fetal Medicine
Department of Obstetrics and Gynecology
University of Florida College of Medicine
Gainesville, Florida

Thomas R. Easterling, MD
Assistant Professor
Division of Perinatal Medicine
Department of Obstetrics and Gynecology
University of Washington Medical School
Seattle, Washington

Robert D. Eden, MD
Associate Professor
Division of Maternal-Fetal Medicine
Department of Obstetrics and Gynecology
Wayne State University School of Medicine
Detroit, Michigan

Sherman Elias, MD
Director, Division of Reproductive Genetics
Professor, Department of Obstetrics and Gynecology
University of Tennessee, Memphis
Memphis, Tennessee

Uri Elkayam, MD
Chief of Cardiology
USC University Hospital
Professor of Medicine

† Deceased

University of Southern California
School of Medicine
Los Angeles, California

Mark I. Evans, MD
Professor of Obstetrics and Gynecology and Molecular Biology and Genetics
Director, Reproductive Genetics
Hutzel Hospital/Wayne State University School of Medicine
Detroit, Michigan

Lester J. Fahrner, MD
Clinical Instructor
Department of Internal Medicine
College of Medicine
University of Illinois
Urbana, Illinois
Chief
Department of Dermatology
Christie Clinic
Champaign, Illinois

Fiona M. Fairlie, MD
Senior Registrar
Glasgow Royal Maternity Hospital
Glasgow
Scotland

Sebastian Faro, MD, PhD
Professor, Vice-Chairman and Director
Section of Infectious Disease
Department of Obstetrics and Gynecology
Baylor College of Medicine
Houston, Texas

Michael Feingold, MD
Associate Professor
Perinatologist
Division of Maternal-Fetal Medicine
Department of Obstetrics and Gynecology
Boston University School of Medicine
Boston, Massachusetts

Paula F. Feldman, MS
Genetics Counselor
Department of Pediatric Subspecialties
Geisinger Clinic
Danville, Pennsylvania

Joe C. Files, MD
Associate Professor
Division of Hematology
Department of Medicine
University of Mississippi Medical Center
Jackson, Mississippi

Stephen J. Fortunato, MD
Associate Professor and Vice Chairman
Division of Maternal-Fetal Medicine
Departments of Obstetrics and Gynecology and Microbiology
Wright State University
Miami Valley Hospital
Dayton, Ohio

Robert M. Galbraith, MD
Professor and Chairman
Department of Basic Immunology and Clinical Microbiology
Medical University of South Carolina
Charleston, South Carolina

Stanley A. Gall, MD
Professor and Chairman
Department of Obstetrics and Gynecology
University of Louisville School of Medicine
Louisville, Kentucky

Stanley A. Gall, Jr., MD
Senior Resident in Surgery
Division of General and Thoracic Surgery
Department of Surgery
Duke University School of Medicine
Durham, North Carolina

Patricia M. Garcia, MD, MPH
Fellow
Division of Maternal-Fetal Medicine
Department of Obstetrics and Gynecology
Northwestern University Medical School
Chicago, Illinois

Peter Garner, MA, MSc, MB, BChir
Professor of Obstetrics/Gynecology and Medicine
Chief, Division of Reproductive Endocrinology
Department of Obstetrics and Gynecology
University of Ottawa
Ottawa, Ontario
Canada

Christina Gianoulakis, PhD
Associate Professor
Douglas Hospital Research Center
Department of Psychiatry and Physiology
McGill University
Montreal, Quebec
Canada

Larry C. Gilstrap III, MD
Professor
Director
Maternal-Fetal Medicine Fellowship and Clinical Genetics
Department of Obstetrics and Gynecology
University of Texas Southwestern Medical Center
Dallas, Texas

Norbert Gleicher, MD
President, the Center for Human Reproduction
Chicago, Illinois
Professor of Obstetrics and Gynecology and Microbiology/Immunology
University of Health Sciences/Chicago Medical School
North Chicago, Illinois

Roberta P. Glick, MD
Assistant Professor
Department of Neurosurgery
University of Illinois and
Cook County Hospitals
Chicago, Illinois

Kathy Gookin, RN, MSN
Division of Maternal-Fetal Medicine
Department of Obstetrics and Gynecology
University of Mississippi Medical Center
Jackson, Mississippi

Leo I. Gordon, MD
Associate Professor of Medicine
Assistant Dean for Graduate and Continuing Medical Education
Division of Hematology/Oncology
Department of Medicine
Northwestern University Medical School
Chicago, Illinois

Jack M. Graham, MD
Fellow in Maternal-Fetal Medicine
Department of Obstetrics, Gynecology and Reproductive Sciences
University of Texas Medical School at Houston
Houston, Texas

Thomas L. Gross, MD
Associate Professor and Chairman
Division of Maternal-Fetal Medicine
Department of Obstetrics and Gynecology
University of Illinois College of Medicine at Peoria
Saint Francis Medical Center
Peoria, Illinois

Michael R. Harrison, MD
Professor of Surgery and Pediatrics
Chief, Division of Pediatric Surgery
Co-Director, The Fetal Treatment Program
Division of Pediatric Surgery
Department of Surgery
University of California, San Francisco
San Francisco, California

Timothy W. Harstad, MD
Fellow
Division of Maternal-Fetal Medicine
Department of Obstetrics and Gynecology
University of Texas Southwestern Medical Center
Dallas, Texas

Avery S. Hart, MD
Attending Physician
Division of General Medicine
Department of Medicine
Cook County Hospital
Chicago, Illinois

James H. Hill, MD†
Associate Professor
Department of Otolaryngology-Head-and-Neck Surgery
The University of Illinois College of Medicine at Chicago
Illinois Eye and Ear Infirmary
Chicago, Illinois

John C. Hobbins, MD
Professor of Obstetrics and Gynecology and Diagnostic Radiology
Divison of Maternal-Fetal Medicine
Department of Obstetrics and Gynecology
Yale University School of Medicine
Director of Obstetrics
Yale-New Haven Hospital
New Haven, Connecticut

William L. Holcomb, Jr., MD
Instructor
Division of Maternal-Fetal Medicine
Department of Obstetrics and Gynecology
Washington University School of Medicine
St. Louis, Missouri

Ira R. Horowitz, MD
Assistant Professor
Department of Gynecology and Obstetrics and Oncology
The Johns Hopkins University School of Medicine
Director, Gynecologic Oncology
The Union Memorial Hospital
Baltimore, Maryland

Teng-Liang Huang, MD
Associate Professor
Department of Orthopaedics
University of Illinois
Chief of Orthopaedics
West Side VA Hospital
Chicago, Illinois

Shakir A. Hyder, MD
Staff Physician, Assistant Professor
Department of Medicine

† Deceased

Olin E. Teague Veterans' Center
Texas A&M University College of Medicine
Temple, Texas

Tariq Javed, DMD, MSD, MS
Professor and Chairman
Department of Stomatology
College of Dental Medicine
Medical University of South Carolina
Charleston, South Carolina

Michael M. Kaplan, MD
Clinical Practice of Endocrinology
Southfield, Michigan

Adrian I. Katz, MD
Professor
Division of Nephrology
Department of Medicine
University of Chicago School of Medicine
Chicago, Illinois

George M. Kazzi, MD
Associate Professor
Department Chief
Division of Maternal-Fetal Medicine
Department of Obstetrics and Gynecology
Harper-Grace Hospitals
Wayne State University School of Medicine
Detroit, Michigan

Krystyna Kiel, MD
Assistant Professor
Division of Radiation Oncology
Northwestern Memorial Hospital
Chicago, Illinois

Raymond S. Koff, MD
Professor of Medicine and
Assistant Dean
Boston University School of Medicine
Chairman
Department of Medicine
Framingham Union Hospital
Framingham, Massachusetts

Norman V. Kohn, MD
Assistant Professor
Department of Neurology
Chicago Medical School
Chairman
Department of Neurology
Mount Sinai Hospital Medical Center
Chicago, Illinois

Elmer W. Koneman, MD
Professor
Department of Pathology
University of Colorado Health Sciences Center
Section Chief
Microbiology Laboratory
Veterans Administration Hospital
Denver, Colorado

Burton I. Korelitz, MD
Chief, Section of Gastroenterology
Department of Medicine
Lenox Hill Hospital
New York, New York

Anil Kumar, MD
Private Practice
Lancaster Cardiology Medical Group
Lancaster, California

Thaddeus W. Kurczynski, MD, PhD
Associate Professor
Director, Genetics Center
Department of Pediatrics
Medical College of Ohio
Toledo, Ohio

Timothy M. Kuzel, MD
Assistant Professor of Medicine
Division of Hematology/Oncology
Department of Medicine
Northwestern University Medical School
Chicago, Illinois

Patricia S. Latham, MD
Assistant Professor of Medicine and Pathology
Division of Gastroenterology
Department of Medicine
University of Maryland
Baltimore, Maryland

Renata Laxova, MD, PhD
Professor of Medicine Genetics and Pediatrics
Division of Genetics and Metabolism
Departments of Medical Genetics and Pediatrics
University of Wisconsin Medical School
Madison, Wisconsin

Richard V. Lee, MD
Professor of Medicine and Pediatrics
Adjunct Professor of Anthropology
Chief, Division of Maternal and Adolescent Medicine
Associate Director, WHO Collaborating Center for Health in Housing
Department of Medicine
Children's Hospital of Buffalo
State University of New York at Buffalo
Buffalo, New York

William M. Lee, MD
Professor
Director, Clinical Center for Liver Diseases
Department of Internal Medicine
University of Texas Southwestern Medical School
Dallas, Texas

Roger R. Lenke, MD
Vice Chairman/Chief of Obstetrics
Division of Fetal-Maternal Medicine
Department of Obstetrics and Gynecology
University of Colorado Health Sciences Center
Denver, Colorado

Yacov Levy, MD
Head, Division of Pediatric Immunology
Soroka Hospital
Lecturer, Department of Pediatrics
Ben Gurion University Medical School
Beer Sheva
Israel

Marshall D. Lindheimer, MD
Professor of Obstetrics and Gynecology and Medicine
Division of Biological Sciences
Departments of Obstetrics and Gynecology and Medicine
University of Chicago
Chicago, Illinois

Charles H. Livengood III, MD
Assistant Professor
Director, Chlamydia Laboratory
Director, Infectious Disease Unit
Division of Gynecology
Department of Obstetrics and Gynecology
Duke University Medical Center
Durham, North Carolina

David H. Lynch, PhD
Staff Scientist
Department of Immunology
Immunex Corporation
Seattle, Washington

Mark C. Maberry, MD
Assistant Professor
Division of Maternal-Fetal Medicine
Department of Obstetrics and Gynecology
University of Texas Southwestern Medical Center
Dallas, Texas

William C. Mabie, MD
Associate Professor
Division of Maternal-Fetal Medicine
Department of Obstetrics and Gynecology
University of Tennessee, Memphis
Memphis, Tennessee

John M. Malone, Jr., MD
Assistant Professor
Division of Gynecologic Oncology
Department of Obstetrics and Gynecology
Wayne State University School of Medicine
Hutzel Hospital
Detroit, Michigan

Vinay K. Malviya, MD
Vice Chief and Associate Professor
Division of Gynecologic Oncology
Department of Obstetrics and Gynecology
Wayne State University School of Medicine
Hutzel Hospital
Detroit, Michigan

Frank A. Manning, MD, MSc(Oxon)
Professor and Chairman
Department of Obstetrics and Gynecology and Reproductive Sciences
University of Manitoba Faculty of Medicine
Winnipeg, Manitoba
Canada

James N. Martin, Jr., MD
Professor
Division of Maternal-Fetal Medicine
Department of Obstetrics and Gynecology
University of Mississippi Medical Center
Jackson, Mississippi

John H. McAnulty, MD
Professor of Medicine
Division of Cardiology
Department of Medicine
Oregon Health Sciences University
Portland, Oregon

James F. McCaul IV, MD
Director of Obstetrics and Maternal-Fetal Medicine
Division of Maternal-Fetal Medicine
Department of Obstetrics and Gynecology
United States Navy
Portmouth Naval Hospital
Portsmouth, Virginia

Sterling W. McColgin, MD
Director, Maternal-Fetal Medicine
Department of Obstetrics and Gynecology
Saint Joseph Hospital
Denver, Colorado

Susan H. McDunn, MD
Fellow
Divsion of Hematology/Oncology
Department of Medicine
Northwestern University Medical Center
Chicago, Illinois

Kathryn D. McGowan, MD
Fellow in Medical Genetics and Obstetrics
Center for Medical Genetics and
Division of Maternal-Fetal Medicine
The Johns Hopkins University School of Medicine
Baltimore, Maryland

G. Rodney Meeks, MD
Associate Professor
Division of Maternal-Fetal Medicine
Department of Obstetrics and Gynecology
University of Mississippi Medical Center
Jackson, Mississippi

Anil O. Mehra, MD
Clinical Fellow
Division of Cardiology
Department of Medicine
University of Southern California School of Medicine
Los Angeles, California

Marla A. Mendelson, MD
Director, Heart Disease and Pregnancy Program
Division of Cardiology
Department of Medicine
Northwestern University Medical School
Chicago, Illinois

Brian M. Mercer, MD
Assistant Professor
Division of Maternal-Fetal Medicine
Department of Obstetrics and Gynecology
University of Tennessee, Memphis
Memphis, Tennessee

Geno J. Merli, MD
Clinical Associate Professor of Medicine
Department of Internal Medicine
Thomas Jefferson University Hospital
Jefferson Medical College
Philadelphia, Pennsylvania

Barbara E. B. Meyer, PhD
Assistant Professor, Adjunct
Department of Psychiatry and Behavorial Sciences
University of Health Sciences/The Chicago Medical School
Clinical Psychologist
Coordinator, Behavioral Medicine Clinic
Department of Psychiatry and Behavioral Sciences
Mount Sinai Hospital Medical Center
Chicago, Illinois

Joseph M. Miller, Jr., MD
Professor
Division of Maternal-Fetal Medicine
Department of Obstetrics and Gynecology
Louisiana State University Medical Center
Medical Director of Obstetrics and Nurseries
Charity Hospital
New Orleans, Louisiana

David J. Mishkin, DMD
Professor and Director
Division of Periodontics
Department of Stomatology
College of Dental Medicine
Medical University of South Carolina
Charleston, South Carolina

John C. Morrison, MD
Professor
Director of Maternal-Fetal Medicine
Departments of Obstetrics and Gynecology; Pediatrics
University of Mississippi School of Medicine
Jackson, Mississippi

Robert L. Murphy, MD
Associate Professor of Clinical Medicine
Division of Infectious Diseases
Department of Medicine
Northwestern University Medical School
Chicago, Illinois

John C. Murray, MD
Assistant Professor of Medicine
Division of Dermatology
Department of Medicine
Duke University Medical Center
Durham, North Carolina

Stephen A. Myers, DO
Associate Professor
University of Health Sciences/Chicago Medical School
Division of Maternal-Fetal Medicine
Department of Obstetrics and Gynecology
Mount Sinai Hospital Medical Center
Chicago, Illinois

Christopher J. Needs, MM, BS, BPharm
Department of Rheumatology
Royal North Shore Hospital
St. Leonards, New South Wales
Sydney
Australia

Alan M. Neuman, MD
Attending
Department of Obstetrics and Gynecology
Sacred Heart Hospital
Pensacola, Florida

Kenneth L. Noller, MD
Professor and Chairman
Department of Obstetrics and Gynecology
University of Massachusetts Medical School
Worcester, Massachusetts

José A. Nores, MD
Division of Maternal-Fetal Medicine
Department of Obstetrics and Gynecology
Yale University School of Medicine
New Haven, Connecticut

Carole Ober, PhD
Associate Professor
Division of Maternal-Fetal Medicine
Department of Obstetrics and Gynecology
University of Chicago School of Medicine
Chicago, Illinois

Patricia N. Olney, MS
Genetic Counselor
Department of Obstetrics and Gynecology
University of New Mexico School of Medicine
Albuquerque, New Mexico

Elise A. Olsen, MD
Assistant Professor of Medicine
Division of Dermatology
Department of Medicine
Duke University Medical Center
Durham, North Carolina

Enrique L. Ostrzega, MD
Visiting Assistant Professor of Clinical Medicine
Division of Cardiology
Department of Medicine
University of Southern California School of Medicine
Los Angeles, California

Mary J. O'Sullivan, MD
Professor
Director of Obstetrics
Department of Obstetrics and Gynecology
University of Miami/Jackson Memorial Hospital
Miami, Florida

Ann L. Parke, MBBS
Associate Professor of Medicine
Division of Rheumatic Diseases
Department of Medicine
University of Connecticut Health Center
Farmington, Connecticut

Michael T. Parsons, MD
Associate Professor
Division of Maternal-Fetal Medicine
Department of Obstetrics and Gynecology
University of South Florida
Tampa, Florida

Joseph G. Pastorek II, MD
Associate Professor
Chief, Section of Infectious Disease
Member, Section of Maternal-Fetal Medicine
Department of Obstetrics and Gynecology
Louisiana State University Medical Center
New Orleans, Louisiana

James T. Perkins, MD
Clinical Assistant Professor
Department of Pathology
Northwestern University
Director, Blood Bank
University of Illinois Hospital
Chicago, Illinois

Joseph K. Perloff, MD
Streisand/American Heart Association Professor of Medicine and Pediatrics
Division of Cardiology
Departments of Medicine and Pediatrics
University of California, Los Angeles, School of Medicine
Los Angeles, California

Kenneth G. Perry, Jr., MD
Instructor and Fellow
Division of Maternal-Fetal Medicine
Department of Obstetrics and Gynecology
University of Mississippi Medical Center
Jackson, Mississippi

David L. Pitrak, MD
Assistant Professor
Department of Medicine
Section of Infectious Diseases
University of Illinois College of Medicine at Chicago
Chief, Section of Infectious Diseases
West Side VA Medical Center
Chicago, Illinois

Mary Helen Quigg, MD
Assistant Professor
Department of Obstetrics and Gynecology
Wayne State University School of Medicine
Detroit, Michigan

Shahbudin H. Rahimtoola, MD
George C. Griffith Professor of Cardiology
Professor of Medicine
Chief, Division of Cardiology
Department of Medicine
University of Southern California
Los Angeles, California

Karen A. Raimer, MD
Fellow
Division of Maternal-Fetal Medicine
Department of Obstetrics and Gynecology
University of Miami
Miami, Florida

Jaya Ramanathan, MD
Associate Professor
Department of Anesthesiology
University of Tennessee, Memphis
Memphis, Tennessee

Susan M. Ramin, MD
Assistant Professor
Division of Maternal-Fetal Medicine

Department of Obstetrics and Gynecology
University of Texas Southwestern Medical Center at Dallas
Dallas, Texas

J. Scott Rankin, MD
Professor of Surgery
Chief, Division of Cardiothoracic Surgery
Department of Surgery
University of California, San Francisco, Medical Center
San Francisco, California

E. Albert Reece, MD
The Abraham Roth Professor and Chairman
Professor of Internal Medicine
Director, Division of Maternal-Fetal Medicine
Department of Obstetrics and Gynecology
Temple University School of Medicine
Philadelphia, Pennsylvania

Cheryl L. Reid, MD
Associate Professor of Medicine
Director, Interventional Echocardiography
Division of Cardiology
Department of Medicine
University of California, Irvine
UCI Medical Center
Irvine, California

John T. Repke, MD
Associate Professor of Obstetrics and Gynecology
Medical Director, Obstetrics Clinics
Division of Maternal-Fetal Medicine
Department of Gynecology and Obstetrics
The Johns Hopkins University School of Medicine
Baltimore, Maryland

William E. Roberts, MD
Assistant Professor
Division of Maternal-Fetal Medicine
Department of Obstetrics and Gynecology
University of Mississippi School of Medicine
Jackson, Mississippi

Jaime J. Rodriguez, MD
Instructor
Division of Maternal-Fetal Medicine
Department of Obstetrics and Gynecology
University of Tennessee, Memphis
Memphis, Tennessee

Joseph Rosman, MD
Assistant Professor of Medicine
Department of Medicine
University of Health Sciences
Chicago Medical School
North Chicago, Illinois
Director, Medical Intensive Care Unit
Mount Sinai Hospital
Chicago, Illinois

Heschi H. Rotmensch, MD
Senior Lecturer and Chief
Department of Medicine "E"
Sackler School of Medicine
Wolfson Medical Center
Tel Aviv, Israel

Siegfried T. Rotmensch, MD
Assistant Professor
Director, High-Risk Obstetrics Clinics
Division of Maternal-Fetal Medicine
Department of Obstetrics and Gynecology
Yale University School of Medicine
New Haven, Connecticut

Alan J. Sacks, MD
Assistant Professor
Division of Maternal-Fetal Medicine
Department of Obstetrics and Gynecology
Mount Sinai School of Medicine
New York, New York

Maura Sandrock, MS, RD
Clinical Nutrition Specialist
Home Nutritional Services
Bellevue, Washington

Gloria E. Sarto, MD, PhD
Professor and Chair
Department of Obstetrics and Gynecology
University of New Mexico School of Medicine
Albuquerque, New Mexico

Harold J. Sauer, MD
Assistant Professor
Department of Obstetrics, Gynecology and Reproductive Biology
College of Human Medicine
Michigan State University
East Lansing, Michigan

Michael Schatz, MD
Assistant Clinical Professor
Division of Allergy and Immunology
Department of Medicine
University of California, San Diego, School of Medicine
Staff Allergist
Department of Allergy
Kaiser-Permanente Medical Center
San Diego, California

Leonard Schreier, MS, MD
Clinical Assistant Professor of Medicine
Division of Allergy
Department of Medicine
Wayne State School of Medicine

Detroit, Michigan
Chairman, Section of Allergy
Department of Medicine
St. Joseph Mercy Hospital
Pontiac, Michigan

John Segreti, MD
Assistant Professor
Division of Infectious Disease
Department of Internal Medicine
Rush Medical College
Chicago, Illinois

H.F. Seigler, MD
Professor of Surgery and Immunology
Department of Surgery
Duke University Medical Center
Durham, North Carolina

David C. Shaver, MD
Associate Professor
Division of Maternal-Fetal Medicine
Department of Obstetrics and Gynecology
University of Tennessee, Memphis
Memphis, Tennessee

Avraham Shotan, MD
Fellow
Division of Cardiology
Department of Medicine
University of Southern California School of Medicine
Los Angeles, California

Baha M. Sibai, MD
Professor and Chief
Maternal-Fetal Medicine Division
Department of Obstetrics and Gynecology
University of Tennessee School of Medicine
Memphis, Tennessee

M. Amanda Skoll, MD
Assistant Professor
Division of Maternal-Fetal Medicine
Department of Obstetrics and Gynecology
University of Montreal
Sainte-Justine Hospital
Montreal, Quebec, Canada

Jay S. Skyler, MD
Professor of Medicine, Pediatrics, and Psychology
Division of Endocrinology and Behavioral Medicine Research Center
Department of Medicine
University of Miami
Miami, Florida

Ellen Blair Smith, MD
Austin Gynecological Oncology Associates
Austin, Texas

Pamela E. Smith, MD
Director, Medical Education
Department of Obstetrics and Gynecology
Mount Sinai Hospital
Chicago, Illinois

Michael L. Socol, MD
Associate Professor of Obstetrics and Gynecology
Chief of Obstetrics
Head of Section of Maternal-Fetal Medicine
Department of Obstetrics and Gynecology
Northwestern University Medical School
Chicago, Illinois

Robert J. Sokol, MD
Dean, Wayne State University School of Medicine
Professor of Obstetrics and Gynecology
Wayne State University School of Medicine
Detroit, Michigan

John A. Spratt, MD
Assistant Professor
Division of Cardiothoracic Surgery
Department of Surgery
Medical College of Virginia
Richmond, Virginia

Howard T. Strassner, MD
Assistant Professor
Director, Division of Maternal-Fetal Medicine
Department of Obstetrics and Gynecology
Rush-Presbyterian-St. Luke's Medical Center
Rush Medical College
Chicago, Illinois

Martin S. Tallman, MD
Assistant Professor
Division of Hematology-Oncology
Department of Medicine
Northwestern University Medical School
Chicago, Illinois

Steven A. Teich, MD
Assistant Clinical Professor
Department of Ophthalmology
Mount Sinai School of Medicine
New York, New York

James A. Tiesi, MD
Department of Neurosurgery
University of Illinois and
Cook County Hospitals
Chicago, Illinois

Kenneth F. Trofatter, Jr., MD, PhD
Associate Professor
Director, Division of Maternal-Fetal Medicine
Department of Obstetrics and Gynecology

University of Tennessee Memorial Hospital
Knoxville, Tennessee

Kwong-Yok Tsang, PhD
Associate Professor
Department of Microbiology and Immunology
Medical University of South Carolina
Charleston, South Carolina

Ruth E. Tuomala, MD
Assistant Professor
Department of Obstetrics and Gynecology
Harvard Medical School
Obstetrician/Gynecologist and Director of OB/GYN Infectious Diseases
Division of Perinatology
Department of Obstetrics and Gynecology
Brigham and Women's Hospital
Boston, Massachusetts

Ilan Tur-Kaspa, MD
Research Assistant Professor
Department of Physiology and Biophysics
The University of Illinois at Chicago
Department of Obstetrics and Gynecology
Mount Sinai Hospital Medical Center
Chicago, Illinois

Michael Vermesh, MD
Assistant Professor
Division of Reproductive Endocrinology and Infertility
Department of Obstetrics and Gynecology
University of Southern California School of Medicine
Los Angeles, California

Marion S. Verp, MD
Associate Professor
Director, Medical Genetic Services
Department of Obstetrics and Gynecology
University of Chicago School of Medicine
Chicago, Illinois

José Villar, MD, MPH, MSc
Medical Officer
Manager, Region of the Americas
Special Programme of Research, Development and Research Training in Human Reproduction (HRP)
World Health Organization
Geneva
Switzerland

Camille J. Wahbeh, MD
Assistant Professor
Duke/FAHEC Obstetrics and Gynecology Program
Department of Obstetrics and Gynecology
Duke University Medical Center
Fayetteville, North Carolina

Kevin S. Weibel, DO
Fellow
Division of Hematology/Oncology
Department of Internal Medicine
Northwestern University Medical School
Chicago, Illinois

Paul J. Weinbaum, MD
Associate Professor
Head, Division of Maternal-Fetal Medicine
Department of Obstetrics and Gynecology
Albany Medical College
Albany, New York

Carl P. Weiner, MD
Professor
Division of Maternal-Fetal Medicine
Department of Obstetrics and Gynecology
University of Iowa
Iowa City, Iowa

Robert A. Welch, MD
Assistant Professor
Division of Maternal-Fetal Medicine
Department of Obstetrics and Gynecology
Wayne State University School of Medicine
Detroit, Michigan

George D. Wendel, Jr., MD
Associate Professor
Division of Maternal-Fetal Medicine
Department of Obstetrics and Gynecology
University of Texas Southwestern Medical Center
Dallas, Texas

Katharine D. Wenstrom, MD
Assistant Professor
Division of Maternal-Fetal Medicine
Department of Obstetrics and Gynecology
University of Iowa
Iowa City, Iowa

Arie L. M. Widerhorn, MD
Department of Medicine
Tel Aviv-Elias Sourasky Medical Center
Sackler Faculty of Medicine
Tel Aviv University
Tel Aviv
Israel

Joseph Widerhorn, MD
Assistant Professor of Clinical Medicine
Assistant Director
Electrophysiology Laboratory/Arrhythmia Service
Division of Cardiology
Department of Medicine
University of Southern California School of Medicine
Los Angeles, California

Jane N. Winter, MD
Associate Professor
Division of Hematology/Medical Oncology
Department of Medicine
Northwestern University Medical School
Chicago, Illinois

Thomas R. Witt, MD
Associate Professor
Department of General Surgery
Rush Medical College
Chicago, Illinois

Honor M. Wolfe, MD
Assistant Professor
Division of Maternal-Fetal Medicine
Department of Obstetrics and Gynecology
Wayne State University School of Medicine
Detroit, Michigan

Edward A. Zbella, MD
Director
Fertility Institute of West Florida
Clearwater, Florida

Robert S. Zeiger, MD, PhD
Clinical Associate Professor
Division of Allergy/Immunology
Department of Pediatrics
University of California, San Diego
Chief of Allergy
Kaiser Permanente Medical Center
San Diego, California

Moshe E. Zilberstein, MD
Assistant Professor
Department of Physiology and Biophysics
University of Illinois at Chicago
Chicago, Illinois

Preface

To be asked to produce a second edition of so large a textbook is not only a compliment to all participants of the first edition—authors and section editors alike—but it is also a tribute to the position this text has reached in a short time period as a reference resource for internists and obstetricians who treat pregnant women with medical problems.

The format of the book remains the same, though some chapters and sections have been rearranged. Obviously, *all* medical knowledge has been updated. While we believed that the first edition covered all medically relevant problems in pregnancy, correspondence with many readers taught us otherwise. Consequently, areas such as breast diseases and genetics were covered in more detail. The importance of AIDS as an obstetrical problem has grown—leading to a more in-depth review of this disease in this edition. Similarly, the knowledge about immunologically induced pregnancy loss has increased, resulting in coverage in two separate chapters. The updating and addition of new chapters resulted in approximately 1000 additional manuscript pages for the second edition and made a comprehensive book even more complete. Despite a reduction in size of type by a notch, this second edition still contains close to 100 more printed pages in 22 more chapters than its predecessor. We are pleased and thankful that the publisher was willing to support our effort to provide encyclopedic coverage of medical problems in pregnancy at an even lower book price than the first edition carried.

We are also indebted to a highly competent and dedicated editor in the person of Craig Percy. His support was crucial in establishing an unusually quick publication schedule, which guaranteed that the information provided in this book is as current as one can expect.

The editing process for the second edition also did not change. Authors were recruited by section editors, who also were responsible for the initial review. Only when the section editor was satisfied with a manuscript was it forwarded to the central editorial office, where yet another review and revision process took place. Each chapter thus underwent multiple reviews and revisions, and I am greatly indebted to all authors and section editors for their patience and effort in this rather tedious and repetitive process. Considering the magnitude of this project, one cannot but marvel at the speed with which authors and editors accomplished their respective tasks.

A final point of appreciation has to be made to all the secretaries and editorial assistants who carried the brunt of the pressure between authors and editors. The relentless pursuit of deadlines would not have been possible without their help. We hope that they all will accept this acknowledgment as a small token of our appreciation, first among them my own editorial assistant, Diana Turk, without whose help this book would not be in front of you now.

Norbert Gleicher, MD, Editor
Chicago, Illinois
March, 1991

PART I General Aspects of Medical Care in Pregnancy

Norbert Gleicher, Section Editor

Chapter One

Fertility Control in the Female Patient with Medical Disease

Norbert Gleicher and Uri Elkayam

1

The control of fertility in the female with medical disease has attracted only limited attention in the medical literature. Especially in conjunction with cardiac disease, the occurrence of a medically contraindicated pregnancy represents a failure of the medical community to appropriately counsel and treat.[1] However, the same also applies to other medical disorders affecting a woman during her reproductive years. While medical texts frequently address the possibility of termination in medically contraindicated pregnancies, only limited reference is made to the far more important aspects of *preconceptional counseling.* Correct family planning advice to the female with medical disease is important. It has to include discussions of contraindications of pregnancy and the particular choice of a contraceptive in the presence of a specific disease situation. Good medical care in very early gestation may be of particular importance in certain diseases because it may prevent injury to the fetus. Consequently, planned conception in patients with medical disease will often improve maternal, as well as fetal, outcome.

Preconceptional counseling comprises three major issues: First, medically contraindicated pregnancies have to be prevented because of maternal considerations. Second, pregnancies in patients with medical diseases have to be carefully planned to maximize fetal outcome. Third, a birth control method for the individual patient, which is compatible with her underlying medical problems, has to be chosen. All three issues require considerable expertise and experience because they usually require individualization. Individualization of the consulting effort represents the most important aspect of preconceptional counseling. The purpose of this chapter is to explain this process.

PRECONCEPTIONAL COUNSELING

The rationale for preconceptional counseling has been outlined above. The concept comes from the field of medical genetics, in which preconceptional counseling has been commonly practiced for years. Unfortunately, preconceptional counseling in females with disease during their reproductive years has not achieved the same level of prominence in medical literature or clinical practice.

As noted previously, the occurrence of a contraindicated pregnancy represents a failure of medical care. A medically indicated abortion becomes necessary only for maternal indications. The occurrence of a pregnancy in such a situation represents either a misjudgment of the woman's medical disease state before conception or failure of appropriate birth control. Evaluation of both of these aspects represents an integral part of the preconceptional counseling process. Because obstetricians rarely see patients before conception has occurred, close cooperation among different medical specialties is essential in this process.

Since medical diseases are generally affected by pregnancy and pregnancy is affected by diseases, an appropriate analysis will define these effects for a specific patient. This analysis serves as a cornerstone of the preconceptional counseling process (see also Chapter 2). The more severe the medical problem, the more likely it will influence pregnancy and the more likely it will be affected by pregnancy.

Available data for such a counseling process are limited. The more severe the predicted effects are on mother and fetus, the more important is the counseling process concerning appropriate birth control. Unfortunately, as the severity of the disease increases, the difficulty in choosing an appropriate birth control also often increases. Although very few absolute contraindications exist regarding the use of contraceptives in conjunction with specific diseases, relative contraindications are innumerable.

If the preconceptional counseling process succeeds, medically indicated abortions should become a rarity. Because this is not yet the case, a more detailed review of medically indicated abortions is warranted.

The Medically Indicated Abortion

The abortion issue has been the center of attention for decades. The ethical issue of *right to life* versus *the right to decide about one's own body* has made this an important issue on a political, social, and medical level. Because an individual's personal beliefs frequently enter into the decision-making process regarding any form of abortion, a clear definition of a medically indicated abortion is required.

A medically indicated abortion is based only on maternal indications and should therefore be recommended by a physician only when maternal well-being is endangered. Table 1–1 lists factors important in the decision-making process for a medically indicated termination of pregnancy. Objective factors are related to maternal well-being and include considerations such as maternal short-term morbidity and mortality, maternal long-term morbidity and mortality, evidence that improvement of short- and long-term maternal morbidity and mortality could be achieved by interrupting the pregnancy, and evidence that continuation of pregnancy would increase maternal risks. Unfortunately, only limited data are available in the medical literature to address these issues in conjunction with most medical disorders. The matter is further complicated by the fact that the definition of an *acceptable risk* to the mother or her family will vary, depending on cultural, religious, and personal considerations.

If maternal short-term morbidity and mortality are increased by continuation of the pregnancy, the decision will be simple. For many diseases, however, long-term effects of pregnancy are only poorly defined. Therefore, maternal long-term morbidity and mortality are much more difficult to assess. Furthermore, demonstrating an increase in short- or long-term maternal morbidity and mortality with continued pregnancy is not enough to recommend a medically indicated termination of pregnancy. It must also be proven that interruption of pregnancy will, in fact, void this increased risk. Systemic lupus erythematosus represents a good example. Interruption of pregnancy at any gestational age has been reported not to decrease the incidence of exacerbation of the disease. Interruption of pregnancy to prevent exacerbation of this disease is therefore almost never indicated.[2] An exception is the occurrence of progressive renal or cardiac involvement, which may lead to increasing damage. If this progression of damage can be prevented by pregnancy termination, then such a termination is indicated.[3] Progressive diabetic retinopathy is another indication for termination.[4] As part of this risk–benefit assessment, it also has to be established that the maternal risk from termination (from the technical procedure itself) does not exceed the risks of continued pregnancy.

TABLE 1–1. IMPORTANT FACTORS IN THE DECISION-MAKING PROCESS OF A MEDICALLY INDICATED TERMINATION OF PREGNANCY[a]

Objective Factors
Maternal short-term morbidity and mortality
Maternal long-term morbidity and mortality
Improvement of short- or long-term maternal morbidity and mortality by interruption of pregnancy
Increasing maternal risk with continuation of gestation
Subjective Factors
Quality of medical care
Patient compliance
Financial considerations
Social considerations

[a] No fetal considerations should enter into the decision-making process.
Modified from Gleicher and Elkayam.[1]

Subjective factors in the decision-making process for a medically indicated abortion are more difficult to assess. These include quality of medical care in a particular location, patient compliance, financial considerations, and related social considerations. Although it is possible to carry patients with elevated maternal risks safely in major medical centers, the same patients in smaller community hospitals with no tertiary-care capacity may have to undergo termination.

Differences in care based on the availability of resources are not only restricted to the termination issue. For example, a consensus development conference on cesarean section deliveries recommended that information about availability of care be given to affected patients so that they can make an informed choice about their site of delivery.[5] Care to the pregnant patient with a medical problem should follow similar guidelines. As an example, the cardiac patient in functional Class III (*New York Heart Association Classification*) may be strongly advised against delivering in a small community hospital setting but often can deliver with an acceptable safety margin in a larger medical center. In a situation with no available tertiary care, this pregnant patient may undergo medically indicated abortion; whereas with available tertiary care, the patient may be allowed to carry.[1] The establishment of *perinatal networks* has already greatly improved the referral situation in the United States. Unfortunately, in most established networks maternal referrals still lag behind neonatal referrals.

Even though the physician's decision for or against a medically indicated termination should be based only on maternal criteria, the patient, in her decision-making process, may take into account fetal considerations. For example, prematurity is associated with severe maternal cardiac disease, particularly if the patient is cyanotic.[6] A patient receiving medical care in an area without a tertiary-care nursery capable of caring for premature infants may therefore decide against the risk of pregnancy. In a situation in which tertiary care is available, the maternal decision may be different. A patient's subjective considerations will probably always contain fetal considerations.

The physician should serve only as the source of data. The decision for or against a medically indicated termination must be made by the patient and her family.

Major medical centers have the expertise to handle most medical problems during pregnancy. Exceptions are rare and are restricted to conditions such as primary pulmonary hypertension, Eisenmenger's syndrome, active systemic lupus erythematosus with cardiac or renal involvement, and rapidly progressing diabetic retinopathy. This should be considered before pregnancy termination is recommended.

An additional aspect warrants consideration. Only rarely will a medical disorder improve clinically with time. Most disease processes, particularly if chronic, will increase in severity with time. Therefore, an existing pregnancy may, in fact, represent the patient's last opportunity to conceive and carry a pregnancy. This also should be considered in the counseling process. Exceptions to this consideration of deterioration exist however. For example, a patient with severe valvular heart disease may functionally greatly improve after cardiac surgery. In such a patient, it may be advisable to terminate an existing pregnancy so that she may undergo corrective cardiac surgery. The risks to this patient with a subsequent pregnancy will then be decreased.[7] Unfortunately, such corrective interventions are rarely possible. In the majority of cases, the performance of a medically indicated abortion will abort the last chance for the patient to ever carry a pregnancy to viability.

The Prevention of Adverse Effects on the Fetus

The counselor has a responsibility to inform a patient and her family about fetal effects of the maternal disease. Not only have clear associations between maternal disease and subsequent fetal effects been recognized, but in some clinical situations, it has become possible to prevent fetal effects of maternal disease by appropriately timed intervention.

Short-term effects will be recognizable either during pregnancy or in the immediate postpartum period. Intrauterine growth retardation and prematurity represent excellent examples of nonspecific effects that occur in association with many maternal disease entities. Although these effects of medical diseases on the fetus must be recognized, it also must be recognized that even state-of-the-art medical treatment can affect these occurrences only to a limited extent. Prematurity may be treated more easily than growth retardation.[8] Undoubtedly, the more severe the maternal disease, the more difficult the prevention of nonspecific side effects will be.

Specific effects refer to a particular disease entity and its effects on the fetus. Some diseases, such as diabetes mellitus, systemic lupus erythematosus, congenital heart disease, and viral diseases have been found to be statistically associated with major congenital abnormalities of offspring.[6,9–11] Other diseases, particularly those of infectious etiology, may affect the fetus in different ways. Although congenital abnormalities can be associated with viral infections such as rubella, cytomegalovirus,[11–13] and possibly influenza, statistically, fetal infections will be a more frequent concern.[14] Individual disease entities are discussed in detail elsewhere, but preconceptional counseling can be of utmost importance with viral diseases, such as herpes virus, cytomegalovirus, viral hepatitis, and, more recently, acquired immune deficiency syndrome (AIDS), and with bacterial diseases, such as streptococcus B and Listeria monocytogenes. Some infectious agents can have a devastating effect on conception, ranging from miscarriage to prematurity to severe and sometimes fetal neonatal disease.

While infectious effects on the fetus often can be circumvented with appropriate prenatal and intrapartum management, some morphologic effects caused by maternal disease states have only recently become amenable to medical therapy. Diabetes mellitus is an excellent example. It has been suggested that the increased incidence of congenital abnormalities observed in the offspring of diabetic mothers can be reduced if maternal glucose levels are tightly controlled during early pregnancy stages.[9] This observation is important to the diabetic patient and represents a classic example of the value of preconceptional counseling in conjunction with maternal disease. Because obstetricians usually do not see pregnant patients before 6 to 12 weeks of gestation, the critical gestational period for the prevention of congenital abnormalities is frequently passed by the time the patient seeks medical care. The responsibility for prevention of congenital abnormalities in the offspring of the diabetic patient consequently must lie with the health care provider who assumes the responsibility for that patient before she is transferred to obstetric care. Preconceptional counseling has to be given to the patient at an early enough stage to allow timed conception under tight blood sugar control (see also Chapter 2).

As another example, for more than a decade, maternal systemic lupus erythematosus has been associated with congenital heart block in offspring. Only recently, however, has the presence of particular antibodies, Ro(SS-A) antibodies, in the mother been associated with the occurrence of complete block in the fetus[15] (see also Chapters 50 and 51). Therapeutic trials attempting to suppress these antibodies in affected mothers are underway.

Long-term effects of maternal diseases on the fetus must also be considered in the counseling process. They are frequently less recognizable and are often more difficult to counsel about. Long-term effects are largely restricted to growth defects, effects on intelligence, fetal carrier state of the maternal disease (such as in the cases of hepatitis), and recurrence of the maternal disease in her offspring. To continue with the example of diabetes, it is well recognized that diabetes mellitus is a familial disease. Most authorities consider it appropriate to discuss the increased chance of each offspring developing diabetes mellitus during preconceptional counseling. A similar familial occurrence must be considered with other medical conditions, such as hypertension, cardiovascular disease, and a variety of autoimmune disorders.

The counseling process concerning fetal effects of maternal disease should thus be concerned with two major aspects: First, the affected patient should be given appropriate information to make her own choice about the pregnancy. Second, whenever applicable, the counseling process should facilitate the prevention of preventable effects of maternal disease on the fetus.

THE CHOICE OF CONTRACEPTIVE

The choice of contraceptive for the patient with a medical disorder is often difficult. The more severe the medical disorder, the more difficult the choice of contraceptive is. With the exception of male sterilization and condom use, contraceptive responsibility, unfortunately, is solely the woman's. When sterilization is considered because of medical problems in the woman, the possibility of male rather than female sterilization should always be an alternative. Table 1–2 represents a listing of available and applicable contraceptive methods. It exceeds the framework of this chapter to give a detailed description of each of these methods; therefore, this chapter provides a general discussion of various means of birth control and their specific relevance to medical problems.

Epidemiologic Considerations

Contraceptive trends are constantly changing. It is remarkable, however, that approximately one third of the US population has remained steady in their refusal to use any means of birth control. This is of considerable interest because no data suggest a different trend in female patients with medical disorders. It thus seems reasonable to assume that approximately one third of women in their reproductive years, suffering from a medical disorder, do not use any

TABLE 1–2. CONTRACEPTIVE METHODS

Devices
- Diaphragms
- Intrauterine devices
  - Special devices: Progestasert (releases 65 μg/d progesterone for 1 year), Alza Corporation
  - Copper containing: ParaGuard, GynoPharma
- Contraceptive sponge
- Cervical cap

Oral Contraceptives
- Estrogen–progestin contraceptives at different dose levels
- Progestins only ("minipill")

Injectable Contraceptives
- Medroxyprogesterone acetate (Depo-Provera)

Implants
- Capsules
- Rods

Postcoital Contraceptives
- Estrogens: stilbestrol 25 mg B.I.D. for 5 days within 3 days of intercourse, conjugated equine estrogen (Premarin) 10 mg T.I.D. for 5 days following intercourse

Topical Contraceptives
- Foams
- Creams
- Jellies
- Suppositories

Rhythmic Abstinence

Sterilization
- Female sterilization (tubal interruption)
- Male sterilization (vasectomy)

contraception. Also, a considerable number of couples practice natural family planning or use contraceptive methods with relatively high failure rates; therefore, the problem of inadequate birth control for the female patient with medical problems is a major one.

Effectiveness of Individual Contraceptives

Effectiveness of contraceptive use is especially important in the patient for whom pregnancy is contraindicated. The definition of purpose of contraception is also important, as shown in Table 1–3. Failure rates of individual contraceptive methods vary depending on whether the original intention was to delay birth or to prevent birth. A variation between these two purposes is observed with every contraceptive method except oral contraceptives. A detailed evaluation of individual means of birth control is presented in Table 1–4.

TABLE 1–3. USE EFFECTIVENESS BY METHOD IN UNITED STATES[a]

Method	Intention: Delay Birth	Intention: Prevent Birth	Standardized
Pill	2.0	2.0	2.0
IUD	5.6	2.9	4.2
Condom	13.7	6.6	10.1
Diaphragm	15.9	10.3	13.1
Spermicides only	16.7	13.1	14.9
Natural family planning	28.8	9.5	19.1

[a] Failure rates are per 100 married women, aged 15 to 44, in the first year of use (1970–1973).

Adapted from Troen et al.[16]

Adverse Effects of Contraceptive Methods

Unwanted pregnancy is only one of many possible complications of contraceptive use. Although an unwanted pregnancy and a necessary termination represent a significant risk to the patient with a medical disorder, nonpregnancy-related risks of contraceptives also must be considered. They range from minor risks to mortality. Contraceptive failure rates and method-associated risk rates must be known to establish the individual risk-to-benefit ratio for a particular patient.

Diaphragms. First year failure rates for the diaphragm have been reported to range from 2.1 to 18.6 pregnancies per 100 women.[17]

It is recommended that diaphragms be used in conjunction with spermicidal vaginal creams. Diaphragms serve two purposes: to stop the sperm from entering the cervical canal and to hold the spermicide. Various diaphragms and spermicidal creams are available. Most diaphragms are made of pure elastic latex rubber, fitted over a coil spring, which usually is tension adjusted.

Possible complications of diaphragm use are relatively minor. They include vaginal aberrations caused by improper fitting of the diaphragm, difficulty of removal of the diaphragm, and allergic reactions to the spermidical agents. Although no direct association has been made, individual cases of toxic shock syndrome have been reported with use of the diaphragm. If true, this represents the most potentially dangerous complication. However, despite the low number of complications, even the diaphragm may be associated with death, as shown in Table 1–5, which summarizes estimated annual deaths associated with birth control. The risk of death includes those caused by pregnancy. Table 1–5 shows that the risk of death associated

TABLE 1–4. NUMBER OF PREGNANCIES PER 100 WOMAN-YEARS OF CONTRACEPTIVE PRACTICE[a]

Contraceptive Practice	Number of Pregnancies
No contraceptives	60–80
Oral contraceptives[b]	1
IUD	1–6
Diaphragm with spermicidal product	2–20
Condom	3–36
Aerosol foams	2–29
Jellies and creams	4–36
Periodic abstinence (rhythm)	
All types	1–47
Calendar method	14–47
Temperature method	1–20
Temperature method and intercourse in postovulatory phase only	1–7
Mucus method	1–25

[a] The efficacy of these means of contraception (except the IUD) depends on the degree of adherence to the method.

[b] Containing 35 μg of ethynyl estradiol or 50 μg of mestranol.

Modified from the Physician's Desk Reference.[21]

TABLE 1–5. ESTIMATED ANNUAL DEATHS ASSOCIATED WITH VARYING METHODS OF BIRTH CONTROL PER 100,000 NONSTERILE WOMEN ACCORDING TO METHOD AND PATIENT AGE

	Age of Study Groups (years)					
	15–19	**20–24**	**25–29**	**30–34**	**35–39**	**40–44**
No contraception	5–6	6–7	7	13–14	21	22–23
Abortion	1–2	2	2	2	2	2
Oral contraceptives (nonsmokers)	1–2	1–2	1–2	3	5	7–8
Oral contraceptives (smokers)	2	2	2	10–11	13–14	59–60
IUD	1	1	1	2	2	2
Diaphragm and condom	1–2	1–2	2	3	5–6	4–5
Diaphragm, condom, and abortion	1	1	1	1	1	1

Modified from Physician's Desk Reference.[21]

with contraceptive methods such as the diaphragm and condom is higher if pregnancy is allowed to continue than if the pregnancy is terminated. This applies to large populations who are overwhelmingly healthy and not affected by any medical disorder. The correlation in patients with a specific medical disorder should be determined, but such associations can probably be expected. As discussed earlier in this chapter, an abortion is only medically indicated if the maternal risk with continued pregnancy is higher than the maternal risk of abortion.

Problems that may occur with diaphragm use are occurrence of the toxic shock syndrome, recurrent urinary tract infections, allergic reactions to the latex or spermicide, foul smelling vaginal discharge (especially associated with prolonged use of the diaphragm), and pelvic discomfort caused by pressure on the bladder and rectum. Vaginal trauma and ulcerations from excessive rim pressure can also occur. The most common problem, however, appears to be spermicide sensitivity.[17]

Diaphragm use is also associated with clear benefits that are separate from its contraceptive action. They include protection against sexually transmitted infection, pelvic inflammatory disease, and cervical intraepithelial neoplasia (CIN), which is probably an antiviral effect.[17]

Intrauterine Devices. Many standard intrauterine devices (IUDs) are made of polyethylene and have a fine, usually double-thread "tail" made of polyethylene suture monofilament attached to the lower end. The monofilamentous thread represents a standard feature of IUDs used today because of past experience with polyfilamentous tails, which led to the removal of the Dalkon shield from the market.

The exact mechanism by which standard IUDs exert their contraceptive action is still unknown; however, it is believed that they interfere with nidation of an already existing embryo in the endometrium. The IUDs are contraindicated if pregnancy exists or is suspected, if the uterine cavity is distorted as a result of abnormalities of the uterus, during an acute episode of pelvic inflammatory disease or if a history of repeated bouts of pelvic inflammatory disease exists, during postpartum endometritis or with a history of an infected abortion in the past 3 months, with known or suspected uterine cervical malignancy (including an unresolved history of abnormal pap smear), with genital bleeding of unknown etiology, and with an apparent cervicitis until the infection is controlled.

Intrauterine devices have been associated with an increased incidence of septic abortions, at times associated with septicemia, septic shock, and death, in patients becoming pregnant with an IUD in place. It is therefore generally recommended that the IUD be removed if pregnancy occurs. If the string is not visible or if removal is difficult, termination of pregnancy should be considered and must be offered to the patient as an option. If the patient decides to continue the pregnancy, she must be informed about an increased risk of spontaneous abortion and sepsis. Removal of the IUD when pregnancy is detected decreases the later spontaneous abortion rate from 50% to 25%.[18] If the patient decides to continue her pregnancy, she must be observed closely even for nonspecific symptoms because initial symptoms of septicemia frequently may be insidious and difficult to notice.

Statistics suggest that pregnancies that occur with an IUD in place are more likely to be extrauterine than intrauterine. Consequently, any pregnancy occurring in a patient using an IUD should be carefully evaluated to rule out the presence of an ectopic pregnancy.

The most frequently associated risk with the IUD is that of pelvic infection.[19] Considerable evidence suggests that the IUD string serves as a conduit for bacteria entering the vagina into the endometrial cavity and beyond. An increased incidence of unilateral and bilateral tubo-ovarian abscesses have been reported in addition to an increased incidence of minor forms of pelvic inflammatory disease. Although the bacteriology of IUD-associated pelvic inflammatory disease seems to vary greatly, a clear association with rare actinomycosis infection has been reported.[20] It is therefore recommended that all pap smears in IUD wearers be specifically evaluated for the presence of actinomycosis. The American College of Obstetricians and Gynecologists suggests that patients with susceptibility to infection receive appropriate antibiotic coverage for 1 month after insertion of an IUD. Patients at risk include those on chronic steroid therapy and those with leukopenia or leukemia. It also suggests that IUD use in anticoagulated patients or those suffering from a coagulopathy may be contraindicated.[18]

Other complications reported with the use of IUDs are embedment of the IUD in the endometrium, which may cause difficult removal of the IUD and perforation of the uterus.

Only limited recommendations have been made regarding IUD use in patients with medical problems. It is recommended that IUDs be used only with caution in patients who have anemia or a history of menorrhagia or hypermenorrhea. Patients experiencing menorrhagia or metrorrhagia following IUD insertion may be at risk for the development of hyperchromic microcytic anemia. It also is recommended that IUDs be used with caution in patients receiving anticoagulation therapy and in patients who suffer from microangiopathy. Syncope, bradycardia, and other neurovascular episodes may occur during insertion or removal of an IUD. These episodes may be especially frequent in patients with previous dispositions to these conditions.[21]

The use of IUDs in patients with valvular or congenital heart disease is not contraindicated. It should be noted, however, that patients with valvular or congenital heart disease are more prone to develop subacute bacterial endocarditis. The use of an IUD in such a patient may consequently represent a potential source of septic emboli.[21] An IUD will therefore be relatively contraindicated in patients with cardiac disease; however, this relative contraindication must be balanced against the risks of unwanted pregnancy and competing contraceptive methods. Reports of endocarditis in IUD users are sparce. Sparks recently found two reports in the literature, one a fatality.[22] The problem thus does not represent a major one.

Medical diathermy, either short wave or microwave, may be indicated in patients with certain medical disorders. In patients with metal-containing IUDs, such therapy may cause heat injury to the surrounding tissue.[21]

No other recommendations are currently made concerning the use of unmedicated IUDs in conjunction with any other medical disorder. It is particularly noteworthy that no mention is made in the Physician's Desk Reference (PDR) about the use of the IUD in diabetic patients. Erroneously, diabetes mellitus is frequently considered a relative or absolute contraindication to the use of IUDs.

The intrauterine progesterone contraceptive system, *Progestasert*, is different from unmedicated IUDs in that its contraceptive effectiveness is allegedly increased by the continuous release of progesterone at an average rate of 65 μg/d for 1 year. It is believed that the progesterone effect resulting from this release is only local and not systemic. Investigations of luteinizing hormone, estradiol, and progesterone indicate a regular cycle pattern suggestive of ovulation. Blood chemistry studies relating to liver, kidney, and ovarian function also have revealed no systemic effects.[21] All of these investigations suggest that no systemic considerations concerning progesterone need be taken into account in the patient with medical problems.

Contraindication for the Progestasert are the same as listed for unmedicated IUDs. In addition, a history of previous ectopic pregnancies; of one or more episodes of venereal disease, including gonorrhea, syphilis, or Chlamydia infection; and of previous pelvic surgery are contraindications for the use of this device.[21]

It also has been suggested that the incidence of ectopic pregnancies in users of progesterone-containing IUDs may be higher than that shown with other IUDs.

Systemically administered sex steroids, which include some progestational agents, have been associated with an increased risk for congenital abnormalities in offspring. It is unknown whether progesterone-releasing IUDs affect congenital abnormality rates in pregnancies occurring with IUDs in place.

Copper-containing intrauterine contraceptive devices, such as the *ParaGuard*, the only copper-containing IUD on the US market, have been developed based on the observation that the minute amount of copper released by these devices increases contraceptive effectiveness. The exact mechanism by which this effect is achieved is unknown.

Contraindications to the use of copper-containing intrauterine devices are the same as those listed for nonmedicated IUDs. Additionally, some specific contraindications exist based on the copper content. Copper-containing IUDs are contraindicated in patients with diagnosed Wilson's disease and in patients with proven or suspected allergy to copper. Leukemia or the use of chronic corticosteroid therapy is also considered a contraindication for the use of these IUDs, because these conditions are considered more susceptible to infections that may be introduced during IUD insertion (see also previously noted ACOG recommendations). Copper from copper-containing IUDs is systemically absorbed and may precipitate symptoms in women with undiagnosed Wilson's disease.[21]

Most IUDs have been removed from the US market because of excessive (and often unwarranted) legal claims against their manufacturers. It is estimated that approximately 85 million people use IUDs worldwide, with 70% of users residing in China.[17]

Contraceptive Sponge. Only limited information is available concerning this over-the-counter product. Individual reports have associated the use of the contraceptive sponge with the occurrence of toxic shock syndrome; however, this association has remained controversial.[17]

The sponge is moistened with tap water before use. Its protective effects last approximately 24 hours and are based on the release of spermicide from the sponge and its barrier function.

First-year failure rates have been reported to be 17 to 24.5 pregnancies per 100 women. However, these data have been questioned because they may not reflect the differences between nulliparous and parous women.[17]

Cervical Cap. Cervical caps presently are *not* approved for use in the United States. Caps that are produced in Great Britain are available only under research protocols.

Condom. Except for male sterilization and withdrawal, the condom represents the only contraceptive method that is male determined. Because female contraception may be contraindicated at times because of female medical disease, condom use by the male may represent an attractive alternative. This alternative is too often overlooked during the counseling process.

The use of condoms has greatly increased in recent years. This is largely due to the AIDS crisis, for which condom use has become the battle cry. Among perfect users, the failure rate during an initial year of use has been estimated at approximately 2%.[17]

Condoms are now regulated by the Food and Drug Administration (FDA) and have been assigned a Class II designation. All manufacturers of latex condoms are authorized by the FDA to list the prevention of sexually transmitted diseases, including AIDS, as a medical purpose in addition to its contraceptive action.

Oral Contraceptives. Oral contraceptives are divided into those containing an estrogen and progestogen (*combination pill*) and those containing only progestins (*minipill*). Combination oral contraceptives are distributed in prepackaged form containing either 21 or 28 tablets. Packages of 28 tablets contain 21 progestogen–estrogen pills, followed by seven inert tablets usually representing a sugar.

The 1989 *Physician's Desk Reference* (*PDR*) lists many different oral contraceptives. Outside the United States, the number of available contraceptives is even higher. In many places, sequential oral contraceptive pills are still on the market; however, in the United States, sequential pills were removed from the market because of alleged carcinogenicity.

In contrast to sequential oral contraceptives, which

were designed to provide an estrogen compound alone for the first 2 weeks and the combination of estrogen and a progestational agent for the third week, combination pills contain both estrogen and progesterone in each pill throughout the 3-week cycle. The estrogenic component of birth control pills is usually ethynyl estradiol or mestranol, which is the 3-methyl ether of estradiol. The progestational components of each pill may vary but may contain such compounds as norgestrel, ethynodiol diacetate, or norethindrone.

Oral contraceptives are contraindicated in association with the following conditions[21]: thrombophlebitis or thromboembolic disorders, a past history of deep vein thrombophlebitis or thromboembolic disorders, cerebral vascular disease, myocardial infarction or coronary artery disease or any past history of any of these conditions, known or suspected carcinoma of the breast, known or suspected estrogen-dependent neoplasia of any kind, undiagnosed abnormal genital bleeding, known or suspected pregnancy, and past or present benign or malignant liver tumors among women who develop these tumors while using oral contraceptives or other estrogen-containing products.

It should be noted that neither cardiac disease, hypertension, nor diabetes mellitus are among absolutely contraindicated medical conditions unless associated with any of the previously listed absolute contraindications.

It has been suggested that cigarette smoking increases the risk of serious cardiovascular side effects from oral contraceptives. This risk further increases with age and with heavy smoking (50 or more cigarettes per day). The increased risk becomes particularly marked above the age of 35. It is generally recommended that women who use oral contraceptives should not smoke. Estimated annual death rates in association with oral contraceptive use in both smokers and nonsmokers are presented in Table 1–5.

The use of oral contraceptives has been associated with an increased risk for a variety of serious conditions including venous and arterial thromboembolism, thrombotic and hemorrhagic stroke, myocardial infarction, visual disorders, hepatic tumors, gallbladder disease, hypertension, and fetal abnormalities if used during pregnancy. Furthermore, oral contraceptive use has been associated with changes in lipid metabolism, glucose metabolism, and bile salt metabolism.[23,24] More recently, in two contraversial studies, the use of oral contraceptives was associated with an increased risk for breast cancer and cervical carcinoma.[25,26]

Many of the various risks associated with the use of oral contraceptives have been found to be dose related. Studies have shown a positive correlation between the dose of estrogen in oral contraceptives and the risk for thromboembolism. Similar reports have indicated an association between progestogen dose and lipid abnormalities. Consequently, the oral contraceptive product prescribed for any patient should be the product that contains the smallest amount of hormonal compound that is compatible with an acceptable pregnancy rate and patient acceptance. It is particularly recommended that new users of oral contraceptives be started on preparations containing 50 μg or less of estrogen.[21]

More recent reports also suggest that side effects may vary with progestational agent. This observation particularly refers to changes in lipid metabolism. Final conclusions can not be made, however, and the reader is referred to package inserts of individual oral contraceptives, which are constantly updated in conjunction with new developments.

It was noted previously that sequential oral contraceptives were considered carcinogenic. This suggestion, although unproven, refers only to the development of endometrial adenocarcinoma. Sequential pills were therefore removed from the US market. Presently no convincing evidence exists of carcinogenic effects of combination or progesterone-only oral contraceptives on any other organ system. Some associations with malignancies are highly controversial. The majority of published studies refute any carcinogenic effects of birth control pills. Some studies even indicate a protective effect, particularly on ovarian carcinoma. Two recent studies of questionable quality indicate an association with cervix carcinoma and breast carcinoma.[25,26] The literature concerning carcinogenic effects of oral contraceptives is too complicated to be reviewed here in detail; the interested reader is referred to detailed reviews in the *PDR*.[23,27]

A decrease in glucose tolerance has been observed in a significant percentage of patients taking oral contraceptives. It is therefore recommended that prediabetic and diabetic patients be observed carefully while receiving oral contraceptives. It should be noted, however, that neither the prediabetic nor the diabetic state represent a contraindication to the use of oral contraceptives. The clinical significance of observed changes in lipid metabolism remains to be determined. As noted previously, recent investigations suggest a correlation with progestational agents.

A clear association has been shown between the use of oral contraceptives and an increase in blood pressure. It has been suggested that the degree of developing hypertension may correlate with progesterone dosage. Although the incidence of hypertension in first-year users may be normal, the prevalence of hypertension increases with exposure, and in the first few years, it reaches 2.5 to 3 times that of control groups. It is also important to note that the incidence of hypertension in oral contraceptive users increases with age.[21]

It has been suggested that women with a history of hypertension, preexisting renal disease, a history of preeclampsia–eclampsia or any other form of hypertensive disease of pregnancy, a family history of hypertension or its consequences, a history of excessive weight gain, or fluid retention during the menstrual cycle are more likely to develop hypertension while using oral contraceptives. Consequently, it is recommended that women falling into any of these risk groups be monitored closely for the development of hypertension while on oral contraceptives. However, none of these conditions should be considered absolute contraindications for the prescription of oral contraceptives. An individual risk–benefit ratio has to be established with every patient.

Hypertension that develops in association with the use of oral contraceptives may or may not recede after discontinuation of the medication.

An increased incidence of headaches has been reported in association with the use of oral contraceptives. If migraines begin or are exacerbated or if any form of headache that is recurrent, persistent, or severe develops, oral contraceptives should be discontinued and the cause evaluated.

Oral contraceptives obviously affect the endocrine status of a woman. It is generally accepted that oral contraceptives exert their contraceptive effect by inhibiting ovulation through gonadotropin suppression. Undoubtedly, additional effects of oral contraceptives occur by way of changes in the genital tract, such as changes in the cervical mucus and endometrium, preventing sperm penetration and implantation.

Although the effects on the female endocrine system

are profound, they are quickly reversible. *Past-user anovulation* in women with normal menstrual patterns before using oral contraceptives is rare but can occur. The use of oral contraceptives has been associated with a high incidence of galactorrhea and pituitary prolactinomas. Although generally not listed as a contraindication, the use of oral contraceptives may be contraindicated in a patient with a prolactin-producing pituitary tumor.[21]

In contrast to intrauterine devices, oral contraceptives protect women from extrauterine pregnancies. In patients with a history of previous ectopic pregnancies, oral contraceptives would thus be the birth control of choice.

The risk for many of the major adverse side effects of oral contraceptives persists after discontinuation. Such a persistence of risk has been reported for circulatory disease in general, for coronary heart disease, and for cerebral vascular disease including cerebral hemorrhage, cerebral thrombosis, and ischemic attacks.

Oral contraceptive use has also been associated with less severe side effects. For example, preexisting uterine leiomyomata may increase with oral contraceptive use. Oral contraceptive use seems to be associated with an increased incidence of mental depression. A patient with a tendency toward depression or patients who develop depression while using oral contraceptives should be evaluated carefully. Oral contraceptives may increase fluid retention. They should consequently be used only with caution in association with conditions aggravated by fluid retention, such as convulsive disorders, migraine syndrome, asthma, cardiac conditions, or renal insufficiency. A patient with a history of jaundice during pregnancy will have an increased risk of jaundice while using birth control pills; if jaundice develops, oral birth control pills must be discontinued. Also, various steroids may be incompletely metabolized in patients with impaired liver function. Oral contraceptives should therefore be administered with caution in such patients. The use of oral contraceptives may result in a relative pyridoxine and folate deficiency. The influence of prolonged oral contraceptive therapy on pituitary, ovarian, adrenal, hepatic, and uterine function has not been established. Although steroid hormones are known to affect various immune parameters, the influence of prolonged oral contraceptive use on the immune system has also not been established.[17]

A large variety of laboratory results may be affected by the use of oral contraceptives. This particularly applies to endocrine and liver function tests. Table 1–6 lists observed alterations. Because of this, it is recommended that every abnormal test be repeated after the specific oral contraceptive has been discontinued for 2 months.

Drug interactions between oral contraceptives and a large variety of other drugs have been reported. These interactions may result in a decreased effectiveness of oral contraceptives or of other drugs. Because patients with medical problems frequently use many of these drugs concomitantly with oral contraceptives, their interaction represents an important point of consideration (Table 1–7).

Table 1–8 summarizes adverse reactions in association with the use of oral contraceptives.

The failure rate of oral contraceptives is generally considered the lowest amongst the different means of birth control. However, first-year failure rates are often surprisingly high, especially in women younger than age 22. A large part of this failure rate is the consequence of attrition. Only 50 to 75% of first-time users are still using the pill after one year.[17]

TABLE 1–6. OBSERVED ALTERATION IN LABORATORY RESULTS WITH USE OF ORAL CONTRACEPTIVES

Hepatic function: Increased sulfobromophthalein retention and other abnormalities in tests of liver function
Coagulation tests: Increased prothrombin and coagulation factors VII, VIII, IX, and X; decreased antithrombin III; increased platelet aggregability
Thyroid function: Increased thyroid-binding globulin (TBG) leading to increased circulating total thyroid hormone as measured by protein-bound iodine (PBI) or T_4 by column or radioimmunoassay; free T_3 resin uptake is decreased, reflecting the elevated TBG; free T_4 concentration is unaltered
Decreased pregnanediol excretion
Reduced response to metyrapone test
Increased blood transcortin and corticosteroid levels
Increased blood triglyceride and phospholipid concentrations
Impaired glucose tolerance
Altered plasma levels of trace minerals (increased ceruloplasmin)

Modified from Physician's Desk Reference.[21]

Injectable Contraceptives. Medroxyprogesterone acetate (Depo-Provera) is widely used in many countries, particularly in the underdeveloped world. Its use for contraceptive purposes in the United States is not approved. The advantage of this progestational compound is its prolonged contraceptive effectiveness, which is comparable to that of combined oral contraceptives. In contrast to oral contraceptive pills, its long action requires injections; however, they are needed only two to four times a year.

Postcoital Contraceptives. Postcoital contraceptives are generally called the "morning after pill." Two standard regimens are recommended. Both are listed in Table 1–2.

Topical Contraceptives. These include most of the over-the-counter contraceptives. Their efficiency varies from compound to compound and in the majority of cases, is poorly investigated. In most female medical diseases in

TABLE 1–7. DRUG INTERACTIONS WITH ORAL CONTRACEPTIVES

Drugs that decrease effectiveness of oral contraceptives	
Rifampin	Sulfonamides
Isoniazid	Nitrofurantoin
Ampicillin	Barbiturates
Neomycin	Phenytoin
Penicillin V	Primidone
Tetracycline	Phenylbutazone
Chloramphenicol	Analgesics
Tranquilizers	Antimigraine preparations
Drugs that may be affected by oral contraceptives	
Oral Anticoagulants	Vitamins
Anticonvulsants	Hypoglycemic agents
Tranquilizers (eg, diazepam)	Acetaminophen
Tricyclic antidepressants	Antihypertensive agents (eg, guanethidine)

Modified from Physician's Desk Reference.[21]

TABLE 1–8. ADVERSE REACTIONS IN ASSOCIATION WITH THE USE OF ORAL CONTRACEPTIVES

An increased risk of the following serious adverse reactions has been associated with the use of oral contraceptives:

- Thrombophlebitis and thrombosis
- Pulmonary embolism
- Arterial thromboembolism
- Raynaud's disease
- Myocardial infarction and coronary thrombosis
- Cerebral thrombosis
- Cerebral hemorrhage
- Hypertension
- Gallbladder disease
- Benign adenomas and other hepatic lesions with or without intra-abdominal bleeding
- Congenital anomalies

There is evidence of an association between the following conditions and the use of oral contraceptives, although confirmatory studies have not been executed:

- Mesenteric thrombosis
- Budd–Chiari syndrome
- Neuro-ocular lesions (eg, retinal thrombosis and optic neuritis)

The following adverse reactions have been reported in patients receiving oral contraceptives and are believed to be drug related:

- Nausea and vomiting (usually the most common adverse reactions, occurring in approximately 10% or fewer patients during the first cycle; other reactions, as a general rule, are seen much less frequently)
- Gastrointestinal symptoms (eg, abdominal cramps and bloating)
- Breakthrough bleeding
- Spotting
- Change in menstrual flow
- Dysmenorrhea
- Amenorrhea during and after use
- Infertility after discontinuation
- Edema
- Chloasma or melasma (may persist when the drug is discontinued)
- Breast changes: tenderness, enlargement, and secretion
- Change in weight (increase or decrease)
- Change in cervical erosion and secretion
- Endocervical hyperplasia
- Possible diminution in lactation when given immediately postpartum
- Cholestatic jaundice
- Migraine
- Increase in size of uterine leiomyomata
- Rash (allergic)
- Mental depression
- Reduced tolerance to carbohydrates
- Vaginal candidiasis
- Change in corneal curvature (steepening)
- Intolerance to contact lenses

The following adverse reactions or conditions have been reported in users of oral contraceptives, and the association has been neither confirmed nor refuted:

- Premenstrual-like syndrome
- Cataracts
- Changes in libido
- Chorea
- Changes in appetite
- Cystitis-like syndrome
- Headache
- Paresthesia
- Nervousness
- Dizziness
- Auditory disturbances
- Rhinitis
- Fatigue
- Backache
- Hirsutism
- Loss of scalp hair
- Erythema multiforme
- Erythema nodosum
- Hemorrhagic eruption
- Hemolytic uremic syndrome
- Itching
- Vaginitis
- Porphyria
- Impaired renal function
- Anemia
- Pancreatitis
- Hepatitis
- Colitis
- Gingivitis
- Dry socket
- Lupus erythematosus
- Rheumatoid arthritis
- Pituitary tumors (eg, adenoma) with amenorrhea or galactorrhea after oral contraceptive use
- Malignant melanoma
- Endometrial, cervical, and breast carcinoma

Modified from Physician's Desk Reference.[21]

which effective birth control is important, these contraceptive methods cannot be recommended.

Rhythm Abstinence. As noted, large segments of the population of the United States do not use any birth control. It may be assumed that rhythm abstinence is practiced by a considerable percentage of these couples. All available studies suggest that rhythm abstinence is an unreliable method of birth control. It therefore cannot be recommended to a patient with medical complications in whom prevention of pregnancy is important.

Considerable efforts have been made in recent years to develop LH-surge detector kits that would allow women to determine their ovulation 24 to 28 hours in advance.

Sterilization. Sterilization represents the ultimate means of birth control. The adverse effects of most other contraceptive methods make it understandable that sterilization has become one of the most popular methods of birth control. Figure 1–1 demonstrates male and female sterilization rates in the United States between 1971 and 1981. Various forms of tubal interruption represent the main methods of sterilization in the female. Hysterectomy is generally not an acceptable sterilization procedure unless associated with distinctive pelvic pathology. Vasectomy is the standard male sterilization procedure. As may be seen from Figure 1–1, vasectomies have decreased since 1971. This may be partially because of reports, which have since been refuted, indicating an increased risk for coronary artery disease and

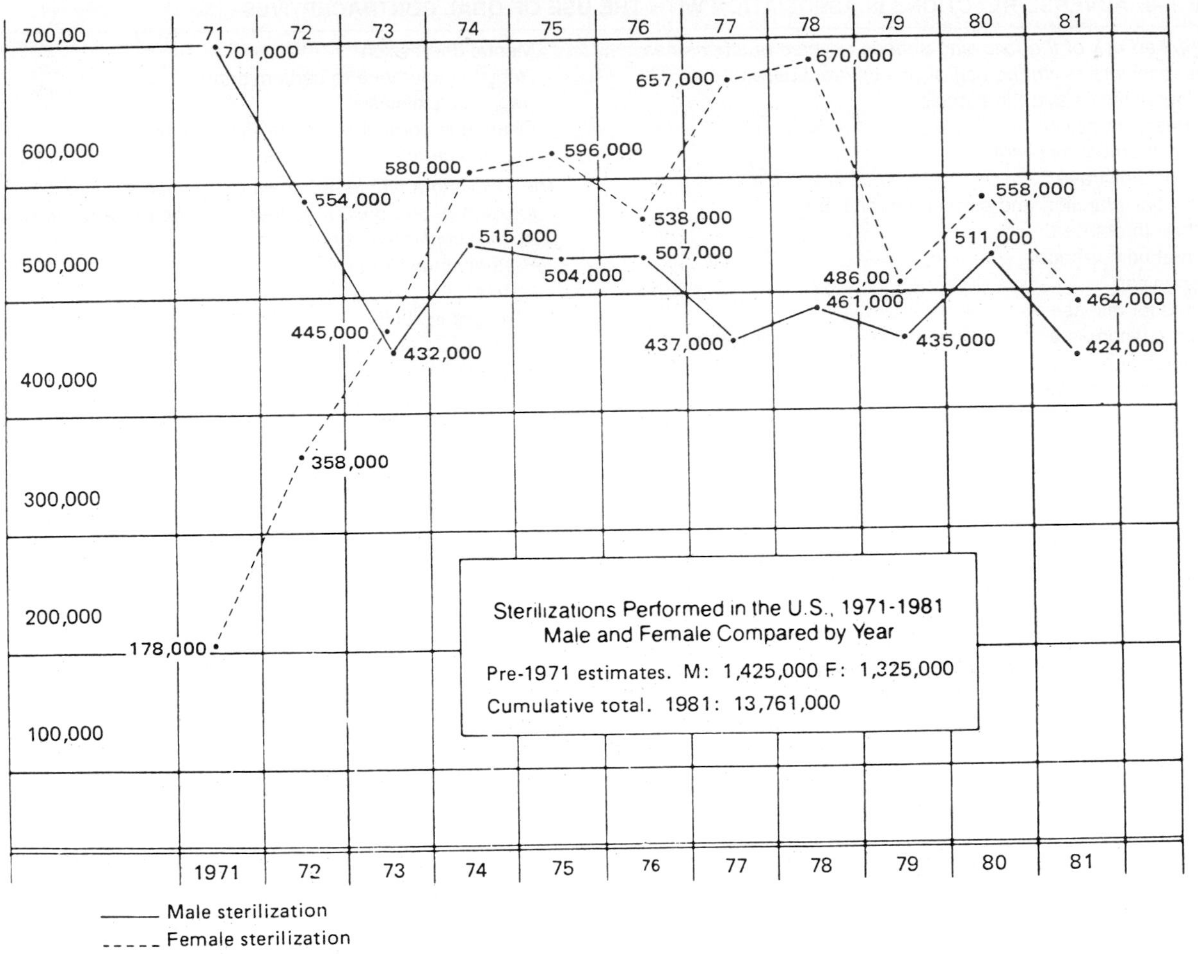

Figure 1–1. Sterilization in the United States, 1971–1981. (*From Association for Voluntary Sterilization, Inc., 1982; reprinted with permission.*)

possibly autoimmunity in males undergoing vasectomy.

The principal dangers associated with female sterilization are those associated with any form of surgery. Although tubal interruption can be performed under local anesthesia, these risk factors do not apply to male sterilization. Except for an overall failure rate of approximately 1% for tubal interruption procedures, additional complications of female sterilization include bleeding, infection, technical failures, and even death.[24] In the 1979 American Association of Gynecologic Laparoscopists' membership survey,[25] two deaths were reported out of 88,986 procedures, representing a death rate of two per 100,000. The Centers for Disease Control (CDC) identified 29 deaths attributable to tubal sterilization.[26] It also should be noted that in addition to intrauterine pregnancy, ectopic pregnancy is a risk after tubal sterilization: 4.5–7.4% of all ectopic pregnancies are preceded by an earlier tubal sterilization.[24]

The reversal of tubal sterilization and vasectomy is becoming increasingly popular. Both procedures should still, however, be considered permanent. Success rates of reversals are not ideal. The choice of sterilization as a means of birth control should therefore be only made if permanence is desired or required. In the patient with serious medical problems, the benefits of such permanent birth control must be considered against the dangers of the surgical procedure. Medical disease will rarely be severe enough to prohibit minor surgery but allow sexual intercourse. Such a situation may, however, exist; for example, Eisenmenger's syndrome is a condition associated with high surgical mortality during or close to pregnancy.[28] The possibility of male sterilization should always be considered a respectable alternative. In some situations, male sterilization may, in fact, represent the only acceptable alternative.

REFERENCES

1. Gleicher N, Elkayam U. Birth control and abortion in the cardiac patient. In: Elkayam U, Gleicher N, eds. *Cardiac Problems in Pregnancy*. New York, NY: Alan R Liss; 1989.
2. Friedman EA, Rutherford TW. Pregnancy and lupus erythematosus. *Obstet Gynecol*. 1956;8:601.
3. DeVoe LD, Taylor R. Systemic lupus erythematosus in pregnancy. *Am J Obstet Gynecol*. 1979;135:473.
4. Dibble CM, Kochenour NK, Wosley RT, et al. Effect of pregnancy on diabetic retinopathy. *Obstet Gynecol*. 1982;59:699.
5. Gleicher N. Cesarean section rate in the US: the short-term failure of the Consensus Development Conference in 1982. *JAMA*. 1984;252:3273.
6. Cobb T, Gleicher N, Elkayam U. Congenital heart disease and pregnancy. In: Elkayam U, Gleicher N, eds. *Cardiac Problems in Pregnancy*. New York, NY: Alan R Liss; 1982:61.
7. Noller KL. Pregnancy after cardiac surgery. In: Elkayam U, Gleicher N, eds. *Cardiac Problems in Pregnancy*. New York: Alan R Liss; 1982:207.
8. Herron MA, Katz M, Creasy RK. Evaluation of preterm birth prevention program: preliminary report. *Obstet Gynecol*. 1982;59:452.
9. Miller E, Hare JW, Cloherty TP, et al. Elevated maternal hemoglobin A_{Ic} in early pregnancy and major congential anomalies in infants of diabetic mothers. *N Engl J Med*. 1981;304:1331.

10. Scott JS. Corrective tissue antibodies and pregnancy. *Am J Reprod Immunol.* 1984;6:19.
11. Gregg NM. Congenital cataract following German measles in the mother. *Trans Ophthalmol Soc Aust.* 1942;3:35.
12. Brown EG, Ainbender E. Infectious causes of congenital abnormalities. In: Elkayam U, Gleicher N, eds. *Cardiac Problems in Pregnancy.* New York, NY: Alan R Liss; 1982:419.
13. Pritchard TA, MacDonald PC. *Williams Obstetrics.* 16th ed. New York: Appleton-Century-Crofts; 1980:766.
14. Wong VCW, Ip H, Reesink HW, et al. Prevention of HBsAg carrier state in newborn infants of mothers who are chronic carriers of HBsAg and HBeAg by administration of hepatitis-B vaccine and hepatitis-B immunoglobulin. *Lancet.* 1984;1:921.
15. Scott JS, Maddison PT, Taylor PV, et al. Connective-tissue disease, antibodies to microneucleoprotein, and congenital heart block. *N Engl J Med.* 1983;309:209.
16. Troen P, Bialy G, Catt K. *Contraceptive Development.* Washington, DC: Government Printing Office; 1981. US Department of Health, Education, and Welfare publication NIH 82–2304.
17. Hatcher RA, Guest F, Stewart F, et al. *Contraceptive Technology 1988–1989.* 14th ed. New York, NY: Irvington Publishers, Inc.
18. American College of Obstetrics and Gynecology. *ACOG Technical Bulletin.* June 1976.
19. Mishell DR Jr, Mayer DL. Association of pelvic inflammatory disease with the intrauterine device. *Clin Obstet Gynecol.* 1969;12:179.
20. Keebler C, Chatwaui A, Schwartz R. Antinomycosis infection associated with intrauterine contraceptive devices. *Am J Obstet Gynecol.* 1983;145:596.
21. *Physician's Desk Reference.* 38th ed. Oradell, NJ: Medical Economics; 1989.
22. Sparks RA. Endocarditis and the intrauterine contraceptive device. *Lancet.* 1984;1:957.
23. Vessey MP, Lawless M, McPherson K, et al. Neoplasia of cervix uteri and contraception—a possible adverse effect of the pill. *Lancet.* 1983;2:930.
24. Huggins GR, Sandheimer SJ. Complications of female sterilization: Immediate and delayed. *Fertil Steril.* 1984;41:337.
25. Phillips TM, Hulha TF, Hulha B, et al. 1979 AAGL membership survey. *J Reprod Med.* 1981;26:529.
26. Peterson HB, DeStefano F, Rubin GL, et al. Deaths attributable to tubal sterilization in the United States, 1977 to 1981. *Am J Obstet Gynecol.* 1983;146:135.
27. Pike MC, Henderson BE, Krailo MD, et al. Breast cancer in young women and use of oral contraceptives: Possible modifying effect of formulation and age at use. *Lancet.* 1983;2:926.
28. Gleicher N, Midwall T, Hochberger D, et al. Eisenmenger's syndrome and pregnancy. *Obstet Gynecol Surv.* 1979;34:721.

Chapter Two

Principles of Medical Care

Norbert Gleicher and Uri Elkayam

2

The considerations of management of medical problems during pregnancy are different than in the nonpregnant state. The major difference is that medical practice has to take into account two patients, the mother and the fetus. This makes the management of medical problems during pregnancy an area of special expertise, requiring not only knowledge about the specific medical condition, but also about pregnancy in general and maternal–fetal medicine in particular. Four principles of clinical management summarize the approach to the pregnant patient afflicted by a medical problem.

FOUR PRINCIPLES OF MEDICAL CARE IN PREGNANCY

Principle I: Pregnancy Affects Disease

While the pathophysiologic mechanism by which pregnancy affects medical diseases may vary between medical entities, the principle that pregnancy affects a disease is almost universal. For example, hemodynamic changes of pregnancy will be responsible for effects on patients with hypertension or cardiac disease.[1,2] The so-called diabetogenic state of pregnancy is responsible for the occurrence of gestational diabetes and for increasing insulin requirements of insulin-dependent diabetic patients.[3] Immunologic diseases, on the other hand, are affected by other mechanisms, often poorly understood.[4] Systemic lupus erythematosus and other collagen vascular diseases may exacerbate with pregnancy. Medical diseases in pregnancy exhibit an exacerbative pattern. However, some entities, such as rheumatoid arthritis, seem to improve, while others have shown a one-third distribution between improvement, no change, and exacerbation. Progression of disease does not occur only during pregnancy but may carry over into the immediate postpartum period, a time particularly affected by autoimmune diseases and cardiovascular diseases associated with pulmonary hypertension.[4,5]

Unfortunately, the available data on the effect of pregnancy on various diseases have remained scarce. Most information is anecdotal and poorly controlled. This is worrisome because management decisions are frequently made on the basis of inadequate data. The lack of well-controlled information also prevents the use of the pregnancy model to research the pathophysiology of individual disease entities and to predict future disease activity. Pregnancy could serve as a "model of nature" for the investigation of various diseases. The recent association by Scott et al[6] of maternal Ro(SS-A) antibodies (antibodies to a soluble tissue ribonucleoprotein antigen) with congenital heart block in offspring is only one example of the contribution of pregnancy to the understanding of disease states. Similarly, Chesley's work on the long-term follow up of hypertensive toxemic patients clearly established the validity of pregnancy as a predictor of later disease occurrence.[7] Patients who develop gestational diabetes during pregnancy have an increased incidence of later-occurring type II diabetes mellitus. Pregnancy as a window into the medical future of female patients has nevertheless remained largely underused.

Principle II: Disease Affects Pregnancy

The mechanisms by which diseases affect pregnancy also may vary. However, the universal principle applies and if appropriately recognized, will result in the correct association between disease effects and resultant management. For example, diabetes mellitus affects pregnancy, but the effect on the products of conception may vary with the severity of maternal disease. The use of this principle can result in appropriate association of a potential danger for macrosomia with milder forms of diabetes mellitus and fetal growth retardation with the most severe forms of this disease. Similarly, chronic hypertension in the mother is associated with fetal intrauterine growth retardation (IUGR). Again, the mere association will lead to a search for the associated condition and will therefore allow for the appropriate diagnosis. Examples of associations can be given *ad infinitum*. Asymptomatic bacterial and urinary tract infections are associated with amnionitis and premature labor. Cardiac disease, particularly if it produces cyanosis, is highly associated with prematurity and sometimes with IUGR. A sample listing of such associations between individual disease entities and associated fetal conditions is presented in Table 2–1.

Although the mechanisms by which these associations occur may be important to understand individual disease processes, the recognition of the association alone is sufficient to allow an improved rate of diagnosis for the fetus.

Principle III: Pregnancy Affects Diagnosis

Pregnancy predisposes the patient to the false diagnosis of medical diseases. This is caused by a variety of factors. First, even a normal pregnancy will cause a large number of signs and symptoms that in the nonpregnant state would be considered abnormal. Table 2–2 presents a sample list of symptoms and complaints frequently heard during pregnancy. Although these signs and symptoms may appear in a normal pregnancy, they may also represent the clinical picture of a disease state. Consequently, the differentiation may be difficult.

Nausea and vomiting, particularly during the early stages of pregnancy, are frequently observed clinical complaints and will most often represent morning sickness. Nevertheless, the same symptoms may represent gastric malignancy. Often such abnormal situations will be overlooked because signs and symptoms are automatically attributed to pregnancy.

As an example of the other extreme, maternal cardiac disease may easily be overdiagnosed. Seemingly abnormal heart tones, heart murmurs, and heart configuration during physical examination and routine chest x-ray, all normal findings for pregnancy, may be misleading.[8] Although modern noninvasive cardiac diagnostic tools, such as echocardiography, may have made a correct diagnosis during pregnancy more readily available, the diagnosis of medical disorders during pregnancy is still more difficult than in the nonpregnant state. Consequently, it is recommended that any medical condition originally diagnosed during pregnancy be reevaluated 6 to 8 weeks postpartum.

TABLE 2–1. FETOPLACENTAL CONSEQUENCES OF MATERNAL DISEASE[a]

Maternal Disease	Fetoplacental Effect
Diabetes mellitus	Macrosomia, hyperplacentosis, IUGR, congenital abnormalities
Hypertensive disease	IUGR, placental abruption
Cardiac disease	Prematurity, IUGR, congenital heart disease
Hepatitis	Hepatitis or carrier state
Other viral diseases	Fetal infection, congenital abnormalities
Bacterial diseases	Prematurity, fetal infection
Urinary tract infections	Prematurity, amnionitis
Immunologic diseases	Neonatal immunologic diseases, congenital heart block, fetal wastage
Thyroid disease	Fetal thyroid disease, fetal wastage

[a] This table represents selected examples in an attempt to demonstrate the necessity to associate fetal sequelae with maternal diseases.

TABLE 2–2. SIGNS, SYMPTOMS, AND LABORATORY DATA THAT ARE NORMAL IN PREGNANCY BUT ABNORMAL IN THE NONPREGNANT STATE[a]

Signs and Symptoms
- Nausea and vomiting
- Weight gain
- Increase in abdominal girth
- Changes in bowel habits
- Change in urinary habits (frequency)
- Palpitations
- Shortness of breath
- Prominent apex beat
- Sternal upheave
- Split heart sounds
- Heart murmurs
- Peripheral edema
- Tachycardia

Laboratory Findings
- Leukocytosis
- Elevated sedimentation rate
- Elevated alkaline phosphatase
- False positive
  - Rheumatoid factor
  - VDRL
  - LE-prep

[a] This list represents selected examples. For more detail, the reader is referred to chapters on individual diseases and their respective differential diagnoses.

More than signs and symptoms may be misleading during pregnancy. The laboratory evaluation of the pregnant patient is also more difficult. Many laboratory tests that would be considered abnormal in the nonpregnant state represent normal situations in the pregnant state. Furthermore, some of even the most basic laboratory parameters are only poorly defined during pregnancy. For example, basic laboratory tests, such as white blood cell differentials and erythrocyte sedimentation rate, are incompletely defined for normal pregnancy. Large variations in individual parameters represent a major problem for the clinician and for the investigator trying to establish abnormal values for disease entities in comparison to normal values in normal pregnancy. Finally, basic laboratory tests, such as tests for syphilis, rheumatoid factor, and lupus erythematosus cells have been reported as false positive in varying percentages of pregnancies. The occurrence of such a false-positive test rate makes diagnosis of disease states more complicated and points to the need for reevaluation of every patient after cessation of pregnancy.

Principle IV: Pregnancy Affects Treatment

Pregnancy represents a unique therapeutic problem because two patients exist, the mother and the fetus. At times, the mutual benefits of a particular therapy do not concur. A maternal condition may benefit from a particular drug therapy, which could adversely affect fetal well-being. It is in these situations that the treating physician, either the internist or perinatalogist, must make difficult decisions. Although most physicians will agree that the benefit to the mother is the first consideration, there is an obvious desire to prevent any major iatrogenic impact on the fetus. Drug therapy in the pregnant state will therefore frequently be different from that in the nonpregnant state. This principle applies not only to choices of medications, but also to amounts. As discussed in Chapter 7, the maternal volume expansion will require different dosages to achieve equal results. Therefore, as a principle, both quality and quantity of medication given to the pregnant patient usually will be different from those in the nonpregnant state.

The four principles that have been outlined should not be considered a comprehensive review of medical management principles during pregnancy. Such a review is given in the chapters referring to specific disease entities. These four principles may, however, be considered for each patient exhibiting a medical problem during pregnancy. The consideration of these four principles will allow a systematic approach to the diagnosis and therapy of the medical problem, taking into account the uniqueness of the two-patient situation during pregnancy.

GENERAL CONSIDERATIONS

Medical problems may afflict a woman during her pregnancy as they may through any other period of her life. In our society, the average age of menarche has decreased, the age of conception has increased, and improved medical care has led to longer survival and better disease control in women affected with a variety of medical problems. Because of these developments, the incidence and range of associations between medical conditions and pregnancy has grown. Only 20–25 years ago, patients with severe heart disease, diabetes, and many other medical disorders either never survived into childbearing years or experienced such a high rate of fetal wastage that the management of pregnancy hardly ever became a reality. In modern-day practice, this situation has changed. Not only do improved survival and better control of medical disorders allow women to conceive, but improved medical management almost guarantees maternal as well as fetal survival.

Maternal mortality in association with pregnancy has decreased drastically in all developed countries. The decrease in maternal mortality in the United States between 1920 and 1979 is shown in Table 2–3.[9] Although it is impossible to separate and define the percentage of maternal mortality caused solely by maternal medical problems, it is obvious that the total decline in mortality could not have been achieved without a corresponding decline in mortality from medical complications. Medical advances have also resulted in more sick patients conceiving because of better disease control. Diabetes mellitus represents a classic example. Early in this century, before the availability of insulin, most diabetic women never conceived. Williams reported in 1915 that he encountered only one pregnant diabetic in 13 years as chief of the Obstetrical Service of the Johns Hopkins Hospital.[10] Of the few women who did conceive during that time period, about 25% died during pregnancy. Perinatal mortality, reported at 50%, was even worse.[11]

The advent of insulin and increasingly sophisticated care of the diabetic patient have restored normal fertility rates in all but the most severe diabetics. Diabetic patients and those with any other significant medical illness will, however, require more medical care to achieve normal outcomes during pregnancy, and a satisfying perinatal outcome can not always be guaranteed. In some more severe diseases, the only result of such an extensive effort may be the conversion of a previously nonviable pregnancy into

TABLE 2–3. MATERNAL MORTALITY IN THE UNITED STATES FROM 1920 TO 1979

Year	Number of Maternal Deaths	Maternal Mortality Rate (Deaths per 100,000 Live Births)
1920	N.A.	799.0
1930	14,833	673.0
1940	8874	376.0
1945	5668	207.2
1950	2950	83.3
1955	1901	47.0
1960	1575	37.1
1965	1189	31.6
1970	803	21.5
1977	390	11.2
1978	321	9.6
1979	270 (provisional)	7.8

Compiled from National Institutes of Health statistics data.[9]

a delivery requiring prolonged subsequent intensive care. The resulting costs for society are not restricted to intensive care but also to acceptance of major handicaps in a certain portion of these offspring. In view of the socioeconomic impact of these developments, total perinatal morbidity and mortality may, in fact, exceed many other medical developments in importance. Any other improvement in medical care will at best result in the prolongation of a shortened life span. The successful provision of perinatal care, however, provides a full life span.

As society looks more and more consciously and critically at socioeconomic issues relating to medical developments, it will have to consider this fact. On the other hand, despite major advances in perinatal care, major problems remain to be resolved.

Medical advances affect society in a variety of complex ways. Although the general trend is toward improvement of outcome, the complexity of the issue must be recognized. No rules should be made either by physician or legislative representatives that would restrict reproduction for a sick individual. The final decision about pregnancy, whether in a healthy woman or in a woman with a medical problem, is her decision. However, the medical community has the responsibility of providing the data base for societal discussion, which, in turn, will allow the final decision to be made by the individual.

Pregnancy as a Research Model

Reproduction has always been at the forefront of societal developments. Undoubtedly it will remain there as our understanding of biologic processes and our capability to influence them will place us into constantly evolving areas of ethical responsibility.

One such area is the recognition that pregnancy, associated with diagnosed or undiagnosed medical disorders, represents an excellent research tool.

Pregnancy as a Tool in Preventive Medicine. Although it is widely recognized that pregnancy will exacerbate a wide variety of medical conditions, the importance of this principle for the practice of preventive medicine is slowly emerging. Patients with gestational diabetes have a higher probability of developing diabetes later in life.[12] Similarly, multiparous pregnant patients with pregnancy-induced hypertension show an increased incidence of hypertension with advancing age. Although these and many other examples of the predictive value of pregnancy have been known for many years, the importance of pregnancy for the practice of preventive medicine has not been adequately used. No long-term study has attempted to determine whether any form of behavior modification, based on the appearance of certain medical complications during pregnancy, could change long-term predicted disease occurrences. Nor has the exact predictive value of disease entities during pregnancy been established. As an example, it would be reasonable to assume that the functional capacity of the cardiac patient during pregnancy, the available or nonavailable reserve, could correlate to the patient's future cardiac performance. In other words, pregnancy could be used as a "stress test" for a variety of medical conditions. This has not been done despite the fact that the theoretical concept for such an approach has been available for quite some time.

Pregnancy as a Natural Research Model. The placenta has been called the "forgotten laboratory animal." In view of the magnitude of active processes in the placenta, this statement is appropriate. J. S. Scott, from the University of Leeds, once stated that the investigation of systemic lupus erythematosus could be greatly enhanced if only a small proportion of the effort directed toward this disease syndrome was redirected toward its association with pregnancy.[13] He correctly felt that the transplacental passage of humoral factors, producing transient neonatal systemic lupus erythematosus in the fetus, would represent an ideal model for the principal investigation of this disease. Although only recently was he again able to prove this concept to be correct[6], the placenta has unfortunately remained the forgotten laboratory animal. This oversight cannot be ignored, considering, for example, the drastic histopathologic changes that chronic hypertensive disease inflicts upon the placenta in the short period of gestation.

Great strides have been made in the understanding, diagnosis, and management of medical disorders complicating pregnancy. Undoubtedly, progress will continue and lead to further improvement in maternal and perinatal outcome. It is important, however, to recognize that the association of medical disease and pregnancy requires more than a one-sided look at the outcome. An understanding of the socioeconomic consequences of the improvements of care is required. Furthermore, pregnancy can serve as an almost unlimited research tool for our understanding of disease in general, not just in the pregnant state. Finally, pregnancy may provide an excellent way to practice preventive medicine for at least one half of our population, the female population.

REFERENCES

1. Elkayam U, Gleicher N. Cardiovascular physiology in pregnancy. In: Elkayam U, Gleicher N, eds. *Cardiac Problems in Pregnancy.* New York, NY: Alan R Liss; 1982:5.
2. Benedetti TJ. Hypertensive pregnancy. In: Elkayam U, Gleicher N, eds. *Cardiac Problems in Pregnancy.* New York, NY: Alan R Liss; 1982:179.
3. Kalkhoff RK, Kissebah AH, Kim A-J. Carbohydrate and lipid metabolism during normal pregnancy: relationship to gestational hormone action. In: Merkatiz IR, Adam RAJ, eds. *The Diabetic Pregnancy.* New York, NY: Grune & Stratton; 1979:3.
4. Smolen JS, Steinberg AD. Systemic lupus erythematosus and pregnancy: Clinical, immunological and theoretical aspects. In: Gleicher N, ed. *Reproductive Immunology.* New York, NY: Alan R Liss; 1981:283.
5. Gleicher N, Midwall J, Hochberger D, et al. Eisenmenger's syndrome and pregnancy. *Obstet Gynecol Surv.* 1979;34:721.
6. Scott JS, Maddison PJ, Taylor PV, et al. Connective tissue disease, antibodies to ribonucleoprotein, and congenital heart block. *N Engl J Med.* 1983;309:209.
7. Chesley LC. Remote prognosis after eclampsia. In: Lindheimer MD, Katz AL, Zuspan FP, eds. *Hypertension in Pregnancy.* New York, NY: John Wiley & Sons; 1976:31.
8. Gleicher N, Knutzen V, Eklayam U, et al. Rheumatic heart disease diagnosed during pregnancy: A 30 year follow-up. *Int J Gynaecol Obstet.* 1979;17:51.
9. Quilligan EJ. *Pregnancy, Birth and the Infant.* Washington, DC: Child Health and Human Development; 1983. US Dept of Health and Human Services, NIH publication 82–2304.
10. Williams JW. The limitations and possibilities of prenatal care. *JAMA.* 1915;64:95.
11. Pritchard JA, MacDonald PC. Diabetes mellitus. In: Pritchard JA, McDonald PC, eds. *Williams' Obstetrics.* 16th ed. New York, NY: Appleton-Century-Crofts; 1980:740.
12. Simpson JL. Genetics of diabetes mellitus and anomalies in offspring of diabetic mothers. In: Merkatz IR, Adam PAJ, eds. *The Diabetic Pregnancy.* New York, NY: Grune & Stratton; 1979:235.
13. Scott JS. Systemic lupus in the newborn. *Lancet.* 1979;1:983.

Chapter Three

Medical Records and Statistics

Stephen A. Myers and Norbert Gleicher

3

Medical records are an absolute necessity in patient care. They serve as documentation of medical events and as a means of communication between members of the health care team. In order for the records to fulfill this role, they have to be well organized, clear, and legible. They should reflect the identity and problems of the patient, the plan of management, and the outcome. In a structured record, information is clear and can be retrieved easily. Many problems can arise as a result of improper documentation of discussions with patients, of clinical decisions, and of medical procedures.

The problem-oriented record can serve the purposes mentioned previously and has four essential components: (1) a *data base* that includes history, physical examination, and initially necessary laboratory tests; (2) a *list of diagnoses* or *problems;* (3) a *plan of management* for each of the problems listed; and (4) a *documentation of progress* or *outcome.*

One difficulty frequently encountered is that patients

may receive medical care by different providers and, at times, at different institutions. This can hamper good medical care and may necessitate undue repeated routine testing (eg, pap smear, blood types, sickle cell screening). The solution to these problems is difficult.

Recently, many elements of medical care have become computerized, including the medical record. As further development enables this area to become more standardized, many difficulties related to patient records will be overcome. Moreover, as quality assurance and risk management functions become more widespread, the need for accurate information regarding patient care activities, procedures, and outcome will become essential. In many ways, an automated data base can fulfill not only the traditional medical record function of the chart, but emerging quality assurance and risk management requirements as well.

THE PRENATAL RECORD

The importance of a good prenatal record cannot be overemphasized. It serves as a means of communication among the members of the obstetric and neonatal teams. Consequently, all information should be obtainable with a quick review of the record. It is used during prenatal care by the nursing and medical staff, the nutritionist, the social worker, and the genetic counselor. Involvement of additional members of the health care team is important with high-risk patients. During the intrapartum period, the record should be available to the obstetric staff, to pediatricians, and to other team members of the labor floor. It is a common practice at most institutions to make a copy of the complete prenatal record available on the labor floor as the patient approaches 36 weeks' gestational age. This information is essential whenever a pregnant woman presents to the labor floor. When emergencies occur or when antepartum admissions are required, it is also helpful to have access to the prenatal record prior to 36 weeks of gestational age, even when outpatient facilities or private doctors' offices are closed.

The prenatal record is a problem-oriented record. Various prenatal chart models are used by different providers and prenatal clinics. The OB/GYN department at Mount Sinai Hospital Medical Center, Chicago, uses a self-designed prenatal chart (Appendix 3–1). In December of 1989, the American College of Obstetricians and Gynecologists (ACOG) released a new four-page prenatal record, developed over a 2-year period. Both are formatted to be similar to a routine history and physical examination. Family history and past medical problems are listed to prevent omissions. Screening for high-risk pregnancies is part of history and physical examination and is discussed later in this chapter. Evaluations and recommendations for social workers and nutritionists also are frequently included.

The third page contains the list of problems, plan of management, and a tabulation of weekly visits. Furthermore, planning for childbirth and delivery must be reviewed with the patient and must be recorded. Finally, it is of utmost importance that all medication used during the pregnancy be recorded.

Unlike the bi-fold form designed by ACOG, the Mount Sinai prenatal form is in triplicate using carbonless paper. One copy goes to the hospital's medical records department with the maternal record, another remains with the newborn chart, and the third copy becomes part of the woman's outpatient record either in the hospital's ambulatory facility or the physician's office. In this way, multiple photocopies are not needed. It is extremely important that all physicians practicing in a department use the same record system. Use of identical records also has been strongly suggested within perinatal networks.

The common problem, particularly in urban areas, is that patients present in labor after having received prenatal care at another institution. The absence of medical information about previously obtained laboratory results and prenatal visits precludes provisions for good intrapartum care. This is especially true regarding evaluation of size and data discrepancies, previous treatments, and assessment of longitudinal changes in any maternal, physical, or chemical parameter. Again, patients close to term should carry with them a copy of their prenatal records or at least minimally pertinent information. Obstetric patients can then be given a card, which is updated frequently. This practice follows the trend toward medical identification cards given to special patient groups, such as diabetics and cardiac patients, in nonpregnant states.

Obstetric History

A detailed medical, social, and reproductive history is essential for good prenatal management. Many details that seem trivial in the nonpregnant state are important factors in the screening process of high-risk pregnancies. Marital status, occupation, ethnic group, and parity represent examples. Emotional problems in pregnancy related to the acceptance of pregnancy may relate to subsequent patient compliance. Therefore, questions such as "was the pregnancy planned or unplanned?" and if unplanned, "is it wanted or unwanted?" have to be asked.

Past medical history should be investigated with direct and actively leading questions. Important medical information may be forgotten by patients but can be recorded using a check list of the most common disorders.

Personal and family histories of genetic disorders, including congenital malformation, mental retardation, and of other hereditary diseases are important for the management and prognosis of pregnancy (see also Chapters 13 and 17). Many authorities suggest that a genetic questionnaire be completed during the first prenatal visit or preferably during preconception counseling. Patients should be evaluated for risk of certain genetic diseases and certain congenital anomalies. The ACOG has a genetic questionnaire available to identify patients in these groups (Appendix 3–2).

Medical disorders and their complications in pregnancy have a significant impact on management and prognosis. In addition to the fetal and neonatal risks, maternal mortality and morbidity are increased when underlying cardiovascular or severe metabolic disease exists. Hypertension is a major complicating factor during pregnancy, and screening for this disease is primarily historic. The family history, patient's age, ethnic group, and body build are important factors. Past medical history can help identify the patient who is predisposed to essential hypertension and who may demonstrate overt disease in pregnancy. An earlier adverse response to the use of estrogen–progestogen combination oral contraceptives or to previous pregnancy may represent a clue to this diagnosis. This is especially important for the nullipara who presents in late pregnancy for prenatal care and has increased blood pressure. Historic data can help to differentiate between preeclampsia and chronic hypertension. Previous history of fetal growth retardation, fetal death, or abruption of the placenta may indicate underlying chronic hypertension or renal disease.

Diabetes is yet another medical disorder that interphases very strongly with pregnancy. Even cases of gestational diabetes that are not identified or not managed properly have a significantly increased risk for perinatal morbidity. Patients with repetitive abortions, fetal deaths, and previous deliveries of infants with congenital heart block require screening for systemic lupus erythematosus (SLE) or other autoimmune phenomena. Previous delivery of a mentally retarded child requires evaluation of the recurrence risk.

Uncertainty about gestational age is a common problem in obstetric practice, especially in a "clinic population." Clarification of the last menstrual period (LMP) and the previous menstrual period (PMP) is important. Direct questioning is necessary to determine whether the LMP was normal and whether the patient is misrepresenting the date of her first missed menses.

The reproductive history should be as detailed as possible. The outcome of each pregnancy, including prenatal, intrapartum, and neonatal complications, must be recorded. The early development of each child should be ascertained if possible. Time intervals between successive pregnancies are important because optimal spacing of pregnancies improves outcome. A complete and detailed review of complicated or unsuccessful pregnancies (eg, miscarriages, premature labor, fetal or neonatal death) is important for management and prognosis of future pregnancies. Previous medical records should be requested and reviewed in order to corroborate the medical history.

SCREENING FOR HIGH-RISK PREGNANCY

Screening and identification of disease states and early intervention are important preventive measures in medicine. The screening methods used should be as sensitive and specific as possible and should be performed at a time amenable to intervention and therapy.

After a substantial decrease in maternal mortality in the fifth and sixth decades of this century, attention turned to perinatal outcome. The United States Collaborative Project and the British Perinatal Mortality Study[1] helped identify some risk factors with the recognition that only 20–30% of the obstetrical population contributes 70–80% of the perinatal morbidity and mortality. This led to the idea of screening patients to determine who might be susceptible to "high-risk pregnancies." The assumption was that if high-risk patients can be recognized early in pregnancy or even before conception, special preventive and interventional measures would substantially reduce the perinatal mortality and morbidity.

The identification of high-risk pregnancies has become more practical during the last 20 years since fetal surveillance has become clinically available. It was logical that the most cost-effective and rewarding approach would be to apply various surveillance techniques to the high-risk group, which contributes so extensively to the perinatal mortality. The natural evolution of this concept led to the development of high-risk clinics, to perinatal centers and networks, and to maternal–fetal medicine as a subspecialty in obstetrics and gynecology in the United States. A similar counterpart within internal medicine exists in some medical centers within the British system.

Many methods of screening for high-risk pregnancies have been suggested. The unfortunate implication is that no superior approach has been found. The variables used by different authors, however, are the same. Most authors assume that risk factors are additive; therefore, a pregnancy with a few minor risk factors scores high in the total evaluation. The cut-off lines for low, moderate, and high risks are also arbitrary. A list of the most frequently used risk factors is presented in Appendix 3–3. They can be divided into four groups: (1) demographic, social, and personal risk factors; (2) medical complications; (3) previous reproductive history; (4) current pregnancy and intrapartum risk factors.

Demographic, Social, and Personal Risk Factors

Many of these risk factors are known to be related to obstetric outcome. However, an exact quantification of the risk that each of the factors implies is not available. The list presented in Appendix 3–3 is not inclusive, and other variables may also be important.

Medical Complications

Many medical diseases occurring during pregnancy are associated with an increase in adverse maternal and perinatal outcome. Hypertensive diseases of pregnancy, which include preexisting silent or overt chronic hypertension, are the leading causes of maternal deaths. The perinatal mortality and morbidity in this group of patients are also increased if fetal death, fetal growth retardation, placental infarctions and separation, and the frequently indicated premature delivery occur. Screening and proper management will improve the perinatal outcome and decrease maternal risks. This concept has been well demonstrated in diabetic pregnancies. Identification and improved control of diabetes during pregnancy has decreased perinatal mortality to a range approaching that of the general population. The screening for gestational diabetes and the regulation of diet and insulin in women who have overt diabetes before or immediately after the pregnancy have had a major impact on the decrease of perinatal mortality.

The importance of screening for medical complications is not in the identification of those who have a clear history of disease. Recognition of individuals who are predisposed, who have latent disease, or who suffer from a condition that can become overt and affect pregnancy represents the main purpose of screening.

Previous Reproductive History

Factors in the previous reproductive history can contribute to fetal wastage in the present pregnancy and are therefore important risk factors. They are heavily weighed in most scoring systems.

Current Pregnancy and Intrapartum Risk Factors

Pregnancy is a dynamic process; therefore, the screening process should be continuous. Complications in the present pregnancy or labor have a major impact on neonatal outcome. Some authors have suggested screening the neonates for risk factors or morbidity. These can be correlated with prenatal and intrapartum scoring. No long-term follow up of infants is available for correlation with high-risk pregnancy scoring systems.

HIGH-RISK SCREENING SYSTEMS

Goodwin et al established a very rigid scoring system.[2] In their population, only 20% were screened as high risk. The score predicted 87% of perinatal mortality and 60% of cases with apgar scores of less than 4 (Table 3–1). Yeh et al reported a good correlation between Goodwin's scores and neonatal outcome as judged by fetal scalp pH and Apgar scores.[3]

TABLE 3–1. COMPARISON OF DIFFERENT METHODS FOR SCREENING HIGH-RISK PREGNANCIES

Author	Number of Variables	Study Group	Screened as High Risk (%)	Contribution to Perinatal Mortality and Morbidity (%)	False-Positive (%)	False-Negative (%)
Goodwin et al[2]	31	936	20	71.7	28.3	3.8
Nesbitt and Aubrey[4]						
Antepartum high risk	33	1001	30	47.0	53.0	8.3
Hobel et al[5]						
High-risk pregnancy	51	738	34	55.0	45.0	13.0
High-risk and labor	91	738	16	41.0	59.0	6.7
Edwards et al[7]	67	2085	47	76.0	24.0	13.2

Nesbitt and Aubrey established a high-risk scoring index by arbitrarily using 33 variables.[4] The risk scoring was evaluated in 1000 pregnant patients but was not used in their care; 30% were judged to be high risk. The incidence of miscarriage, preterm delivery, low birth weight, and fetal death was high in the high-risk group (Table 3–2). However, with antepartum screening, only 47% of cases of perinatal mortality and morbidity were detected. The addition of a labor index increased the yield to 75%.

Hobel et al screened pregnant women in the first visit and then again at 30, 35, and 39 weeks' gestation for prenatal factors and on admission to labor for intrapartum factors.[5] Using an arbitrary scoring system for 126 variables, they screened patients for high-risk pregnancy and for high-risk labor (see Table 3–1). They also developed a list of neonatal risk factors. Neonatal scoring correlated well with both the prenatal and the intrapartum scoring indexes. The perinatal mortality and morbidity were found to be increased in high-risk pregnancy. However, high-risk labor contributed more to poor outcome than high-risk pregnancy (Table 3–3). The sensitivity of the antepartum and intrapartum screening was good; 96% of prenatal mortality cases and 80% of neonatal complications were predicted. This scoring system is also known as the *Problem-Oriented Perinatal Risk Assessment* (POPRAS).

Sokol et al using Hobel's system, screened 1275 patients and found that 25% were at high risk both antepartum and intrapartum.[6] They contributed 80% of perinatal deaths. This correlation to the neonatal outcome was based only on Apgar score and neonatal mortality. Prematurity and birth weight were not correlated with the risk scores.

Edwards et al suggested a simplified scoring system using 67 variables.[7] He screened 2085 pregnant women at their initial visit, at 36 weeks' gestation, and on admission for delivery. They reported an excellent correlation between risk assessment and perinatal outcome—78% of fetal deaths, all neonatal deaths, and 75% of neonatal morbidity came from the high-risk group (Table 3–4).

Table 3–1 summarizes some of the screening systems. The Goodwin method shows the lowest false-negative rate, even though only 20% of patients present as high-risk pregnancies. The antepartum screening system of Hobel has high false-positive and -negative rates, with 34% of pregnancies screened as high risk. The Edwards scoring system has attained a low false-positive rate at the expense of a high false-negative rate. Unfortunately, the general rules of evaluating a screening method by calculation of specificity and sensitivity are impossible to implement accurately in the screening for high-risk pregnancy. A clear definition of high-risk pregnancy is thus lacking. Does a high-risk pregnancy necessarily mean a bad outcome? If a screened high-risk pregnancy results in a good outcome, does this represent a false-positive assignment?

Because the universal purpose of screening for high risk pregnancy is prevention of perinatal death and morbidity, overdiagnosis is acceptable, but the false-negative rate should be as low as possible. The suggested definition of high-risk screening by Sokol, "to recognize, document and accumulate factors to predict complications in mother, fetus, and neonate," is therefore incomplete, Many authors suggest using "screening to channel patients to appropriate clinics and management protocols." Morrison et al have used an intrapartum screening system to decide who should be referred to tertiary perinatal centers.[8] Antepartum screening methods can also be used to direct patients to different levels of perinatal care.

If the screening for high-risk pregnancies is so important, why has its use not spread to practicing obstetricians and to community hospitals? The guidelines for perinatal care, published by the American Association of Pediatricians and the ACOG, do not include quantitative scoring for high-risk pregnancy but instead give a list of high-risk factors.[9] One of the most widely used screening methods, the Hollister record, is not quantitative.

The future of high-risk screening, as more comprehensive care for all pregnancies becomes commonplace, has become uncertain. Emphasis will be placed on antepartum screening of all patients for the most frequent problems.

TABLE 3–2. ANTEPARTUM HIGH-RISK SCREENING AND PERINATAL OUTCOME (%)

	Miscarriages <20 Weeks	Premature Births <35 Weeks	Low Birth Weight <2500 g	Fetal Distress	Fetal Death	Neonatal Death
Low Risk	0	4.6	10.0	6.4	1.3	1.3
Moderate risk	0.8	4.4	11.3	8.2	1.0	1.3
High risk	2.4	7.8	19.6	10.0	3.1	1.4

Adapted from Nesbitt and Aubrey.[4]

TABLE 3–3. RISK SCORING AND PERINATAL OUTCOME

Risk		Percent of Patients	Perinatal Mortality	Neonatal Morbidity
Prenatal	Intrapartum			
Low	Low	46	3/1000	6.5%
High	Low	18	22/1000	11.8%
Low	High	20	35/1000	24.5%
High	High	16	145/1000	35.0%

(n = 738)
Adapted from Hobel et al.[5]

This should be part of the prenatal record because most risk factors are historic. Consequently, routine testing for Hepatitis B, human immunodeficiency virus, group B beta streptococcus, renal function, and platelets are part of the initial data base on every patient. Additionally, a 1- or a 3-hour glucose challenge test (GTT) is performed on every patient. Serial fetal evaluation by ultrasound and antepartum testing is tabulated on the prenatal record. Serial recording of the gestational age by LMP, ultrasounds, fundal height (FHT), recordings of fetal heart (by Doppler or fetoscope), are designed to pinpoint gestational age accurately or identify altered fetal growth.

Prematurity remains the most significant factor causing perinatal mortality. Therefore, if patients who are at risk for premature labor could be accurately identified, significant benefit could be derived. In fact, quantitative screening methods for premature labor are available.[10–17] A variety of special protocols for such patients have been proposed to decrease the incidence of preterm labor and resultant perinatal mortality. Unfortunately, little or no improvement has been reported. Recently, experience with home contraction monitors has been reported. Although initially promising, difficulty in distinguishing the effect of the "care" from the effect of the monitor information has made it impossible to establish certain benefit. Moreover, until more effective therapy can be provided for premature delivery, even early diagnosis should not be equated with less prematurity. The true use of prospective programs for prematurity prevention has yet to be identified.

Intrauterine growth retardation is an important factor in perinatal mortality and short- and long-term morbidity. Patients at risk for this complication should be identified, grouped, and managed with ultrasound follow-up of fetal growth and antepartum surveillance.

As the obstetric practice changes, some factors that are more amenable to therapy will lose their influence on perinatal outcome, and others will become more prominent or more frequent. Prevention of Rh hemolytic disease by the use of anti-D-globulin and the improved control of diabetes in pregnancy have decreased the perinatal complications of these entities. On the other hand, the contribution of genetic diseases and of congenital malformations to perinatal mortality has increased during the last decade. An ongoing evaluation of current screening systems is necessary. Indeed, Hobel has found that many of his risk factors are no longer important in predicting neonatal morbidity, and consequently, he suggests that changes in perinatal care affect the impact of risk factors on outcome.[12]

TABLE 3–4. RISK SCORING AND PERINATAL OUTCOME

	High Risk (n = 979)		Low Risk (n =1106)	
	Rate (%)	Contribution (%)	Rate (%)	Contribution (%)
Percent of total group (n = 2085)		47.0		53.0
Fetal death	2.96	77.8	7.2	22.2
Neonatal death	3.47	100.0	0.0	0.0
Perinatal death	6.33	88.6	7.2	11.4
Neonatal morbidity	42.1	75.0	12.5	25.0

Adapted from Edwards et al.[7]

Present screening methods are imperfect. However, they serve a useful purpose by identifying a large group of potentially complicated pregnancies.

MATERNAL AND PERINATAL MORTALITY STATISTICS

Maternal Mortality

Maternal death is defined as death during pregnancy or in the 6 weeks of puerperium, irrespective of cause. It is divided into *direct maternal death,* caused by obstetric complications, *indirect maternal death,* caused by preexisting or recent medical or surgical disease, and *nonobstetric death,* caused by accidents (eg, car accident) that are not related to pregnancy or disease entities.

Maternal death rate is reported per 100,000 live births and is still high in some areas of the world. In the United States, the maternal mortality rate has decreased from 582.1 in 1935 to 7.8 in 1985. Most of the changes occurred between 1940 and 1960.[13] The major risk factors for maternal deaths are race, age, and parity. The maternal mortality in black populations is still three to four times that of whites. Age and parity independently increase the maternal risk.

Approximately 60–70% of maternal mortality cases are related to pregnancy complications, but the contribution of direct causes is decreasing. The major causes of direct maternal death, the triad of hemorrhage, infection, and toxemia, are decreasing but still contribute 50% of maternal mortality.[14–16] Maternal deaths from other nonobstetric causes, such as vascular accidents, anesthesia, and pulmonary embolism are increasing. This suggests that since an absolute and relative decrease of total direct maternal mortality has occurred, a review of indirect, nonmaternal causes may be warranted. Among indirect causes, the main increase is related to cardiac diseases. Among nonmaternal causes, a significant increase in accidents and homicides has been observed. A recent report of the maternal mortality collaborative summarizes the results in the United States from 1980–1985.[16]

Another way to analyze maternal mortality is to divide it into gestational time periods. In the US statistics for 1968–1975, the maternal mortality rate was 18.9 per 100,000 deliveries, but 23% of the deaths occurred in the first half of pregnancy. This included terminations, miscarriages, and ectopic pregnancies. By 1985, although the overall mortality rate declined, 20% of maternal deaths still occurred in the first half of pregnancy.[16] Pregnancy complications were responsible for 27% of maternal deaths, toxemia being the most common cause. Complications during delivery were responsible for 25% of cases, hemorrhage being the most common cause. The remaining 25% of cases were caused by puerperal complications, most commonly pulmonary embolism.

When a mother has a medical complication such as hypertension, renal disease, or heart disease, the risk for maternal death is increased significantly. These patients should be regarded as high risk not just for fetal, but for maternal outcome as well. Control of the underlying disease will help to decrease maternal mortality and morbidity.

Perinatal Mortality

Fetal death rate is the number of stillborns weighing more than 500 g per 1000 deliveries. *Neonatal mortality rate* (NMR) is the number of neonatal deaths of infants weighing 500 g or more at birth, occurring in the first 28 days of life per 1000 live births. *Perinatal mortality rate* (PNMR) is the sum of fetal and neonatal death rates. This is also called *PNM period II,* in contrast to *PNM period I* used in some countries in Europe. This term refers to fetal death weighing more than 1000 g and neonatal deaths during the first 7 days.

Fetal death is sometimes divided into antepartum (occurring before labor) and intrapartum (occurring during labor) death. The latter is rare because of the increased use of fetal heart rate monitoring during labor.

Neonatal death is sometimes divided into early neonatal death, which occurs in the first 7 days, and late neonatal death, which occurs between days 8 and 27. Neonatal deaths are the first component in infant mortality, which covers death from the time of birth to the age of 1 year. The second component of infant mortality is postneonatal mortality, which includes death between day 28 and 1 year of age. With the increasing intensity of neonatal care, postneonatal deaths are sometimes still related to obstetric and neonatal events.

The perinatal mortality rate has decreased drastically over the last 3 decades (Table 3–5). Statistical analysis of various mortality rates is helpful if the results from different hospitals, communities, states, and countries can be compared. This is why it is important to have clear definitions of what is to be described within each entity. Moreover, it is apparent that crude PNM rates cannot be compared because differences in birth weight distribution in large populations are common. Birth-weight–specific mortality rates have become a reasonable way to compare qualities of health care systems. Standardization of weight distribution between Massachusetts and Swedish NMR has yielded close neonatal rates[17] (Table 3–6). The high PNM rate in the United States results from the high incidence of prematurity, which is almost twice that of Sweden. This, in turn, is the result of the special characteristics of the obstetric population, including teenage pregnancies and heterogeneous socioeconomic groups with a higher birth rate. Improvement in neonatal outcome has been observed across all weight groups as represented by lower mortality in specific weight groups.[18]

The second important consideration when evaluating PNM rates is the analysis of causes of death in weight-specific groups. The corrected PNM rate is then given after lethal congenital malformations are excluded. The contributions of anomalies to the neonatal death (NND) rate increase as the neonatal weight rises[19] (Table 3–7).

Major causes of fetal death include growth retardation, infection (especially syphillis), placental abruption, and infarctions. Prematurity is the main cause of neonatal mortality; the causes of death are respiratory distress syndrome, central nervous system hemorrhages, and infections. There are no national data available on the contribution of these causes to total perinatal mortality.

Every department of obstetrics and neonatology should have a monthly perinatal mortality review for its own use. This should include total perinatal mortality with a breakdown of fetal and neonatal rates. Birth-weight–specific mortality, including a breakdown in 100 g groups below 1000 g, should be obtained. These numbers are important in judging the quality of the individual perinatal and neonatal service and in making prospective decisions concerning future cases.

A detailed list of all fetal and neonatal deaths should be included in the monthly perinatal mortality review. The gestational age, prenatal complications, weight, Apgar scores, and cause of death should be evaluated. These monthly statistics can be used for educational purposes and improvement in perinatal care.

The data base should also include the incidence of maternal complications during pregnancy. Maternal risk

TABLE 3–5. PERINATAL MORTALITY IN THE UNITED STATES, 1950 THROUGH 1985

Year	Perinatal Rate[a,d]	Fetal Rate[b]	Neonatal Rate[c,e]
1950	39.0	18.8	20.5
1960	34.3	15.8	18.7
1970	28.9	10.6	15.1
1975	22.1	10.6	11.6
1980	17.5	9.1	8.5
1983	15.6	8.4	7.3
1985	14.7	7.8	7.0

[a] Perinatal definition II is used, which includes fetal deaths of 20 weeks' gestation or greater and infant deaths of less than 28 days.
[b] Fetal deaths of 20 weeks' gestation or more.
[c] Infanta/neonatal deaths of less than 29 days.
[d] Rate per 1000 live births and fetal deaths.
[e] Rate per 1000 live births.

TABLE 3–6. NEONATAL MORTALITY[a]

	Crude Rate, Massachusetts	Standardized Rates	
		Massachusetts	Sweden
1977	8.49	5.41	5.83
1978	7.94	5.06	5.28
1979	7.86	4.84	4.99

[a] Rate per 1000 live births.
Adapted from Guyer et al.[17]

TABLE 3–7. NEONATAL MORTALITY RATES, ALABAMA 1978–1980[a]

Birth Weight (g)	Neonatal Mortality Rate	Lethal Congenital Anomalies (%)
500–999	594.6	2
1000–1499	100.6	14
1500–1999	48.4	27
2000–2499	13.5	38
2500–3999	2.9	43
>3999	3.5	41
Total	7.8	23

[a]Rate per 1000 live births.
Adapted from Goldenberg et al.[19]

factors influence perinatal outcome; therefore, the incidence of high-risk pregnancies must be known when evaluating the quality of obstetrics and neonatology on the basis of perinatal outcome.

The rate of obstetric interventions should also be monitored, especially the cesarean birth rates. The individual indications for primary cesarean births should be followed. Maternal morbidity and mortality must be individually reviewed. Many states require a detailed review of every maternal death.

At Mount Sinai Hospital Medical Center in Chicago, this data collection and reporting are accomplished by means of an automated perinatal data base (BPM, Inc., Wilshire Blvd., Los Angeles, CA). Detailed information is collected as part of the maternal and newborn medical records (Appendix 3–4). These data are then used to generate reports of obstetrics and newborn outcome (Appendix 3–5). This system has the additional flexibility to examine outcome not only for departmental analysis, but for individual physicians or individual clinical situations. The obstetric report details information about route of delivery, cesarean section indications, and breech delivery, and it lists patients with previous cesareans. On the second page, other complications are tabulated, along with Apgar score data.

The newborn report is structured as a birth-weight–specific morbidity report. Because these large birth-weight groups significantly influence the occurrence of certain morbidities, the ability to separate the effect of birth weight is crucial when analyzing simple occurrence rates.

The birth-weight distribution is reported on the fourth page of the report and includes stillbirths and neonatal deaths, as well as the distribution of births in each birth-weight group.

All of these reports are generated regularly for the department as well as annually for individuals. Longitudinal comparisons to previous time periods, to other individuals, or within the department allow for trend analysis or the identification of certain "outliers." Such information is crucial if reasonable quality assurance activities are to be performed, as recommended by the ACOG.

REFERENCES

1. Butler NR, Alberman ED. *Perinatal Problems: The Second Report of the 1958 British Perinatal Mortality Survey*. Edinburgh, London: E & S Livingstone; 1969.
2. Goodwin JW, Dunne JT, Thomas BW. Antepartum identification of the fetus at risk. *Can Med Assoc J*. 1969;101:458.
3. Yeh SY, Forsythe A, Lowensohn RI, et al. A study of the relationship between Goodwin's high-risk score and fetal outcome. *Am J Obstet Gynecol*. 1977;127:50.
4. Nesbitt REL, Aubrey RH. High risk obstetrics. II. Value of semiobjective grading system in identifying the vulnerable group. *Am J Obstet Gynecol*. 1969;103:372.
5. Hobel CH, Hyvarinen MA, Okada DM, et al. Prenatal and intrapartum high-risk screening. I. Prediction of the highrisk neonate. *Am J Obstet Gynecol*. 1973;117:1.
6. Sokol RH, Rosen MG, Stojkov J, et al. Clinical application of high-risk scoring on an obstetric service. *Am J Obstet Gynecol*. 1977;128:652.
7. Edwards LE, Barrada I, Tatreau RE, et al. A simplified antepartum risk scoring system. *Obstet Gynecol*. 1979;54:237.
8. Morrison I, Carter L, McNamara S, et al. A simplified intrapartum numerical scoring system. The prediction of high risk in labor. *Am J Obstet Gynecol*. 1980;138:175.
9. Brann AW, Cefalo RC, Frigoletto FD, et al, eds. *Guidelines for Perinatal Care*. Evanston, Washington: American Academy of Pediatricians and American College of Obstetricians and Gynecologists; 1983:53.
10. Creasy RK, Grummer BA, Liggins GC. System for predicting spontaneous preterm birth. *Obstet Gynecol*. 1980;55:692.
11. Herron MA, Katz M, Creasy RK. Evaluation of a preterm birth prevention program: preliminary report. *Obstet Gynecol*. 1982;59:452.
12. Hobel CJ, Youkeles L, Forsythe A. Prenatal and intrapartum high-risk screening II. Risk factors reassessed. *Am J Obstet Gynecol*. 1979;135:1051.
13. Pritchard JA, MacDonald PC. Williams Obstetrics. 18th ed. New York, NY: Appleton-Century-Crofts; 1989:3.
14. Hardy WE, Freeman MG, Thompson JD. A ten-year review of maternal mortality. *Obstet Gynecol*. 1974;43:65.
15. Hughes EC, Cochrane NE, Czyz PL. Maternal mortality study, 1970–1975. *Ny State J Med*. 1976;76:2208.
16. Rochat RW, Koonin LM, Atrash HK, Jewett JF. Maternal mortality in the United States: report from the maternal mortality collaborative. *Obstet Gynecol*. 1988;72:91.
17. Guyer B, Wallach LA, Rosen SL. Birth-weight–standardized neonatal mortality rates and the prevention of low birth weight: how does Massachusetts compare with Sweden? *New Engl J Med*. 1982;306:1230.
18. Lee KS, Paneth N, Gartner LM, et al. Neonatal mortality: an analysis of the recent improvements in the United States. *Am J Pub Health*. 1980;70:15.
19. Goldenberg RL, Humphrey JL, Hale CB. Lethal congenital anomalies as a cause of birth-weight–specific neonatal mortality. *JAMA*. 1983;250:513.

Appendix 3–1
Prenatal Chart Model

Mount Sinai Hospital
Medical Center
California Avenue at 15th St.
Chicago, Illinois 60608

Department of Obstetrics and Gynecology
Prenatal Record — 1 · History

Name:_______________ Attending:_______________

Age____Race ____ Religion _____ Marital Status _____Years Married ____Education _______Occupation _______

Home Address _______________Home tel. __________Work tel. __________

Nearest Relative _______________Relative's Employer _______________Work tel.

Pregnancy History	Gr	T	P	A	L	FDLMP	PMP	EDC

No.	Month/ Year	Sex	Weight At Birth	Wks. Gest.	Hrs in Labor	Type of Delivery	MAT. Compl.	NEO. Compl.	Hosp.	Comments
1										
2										
3										
4										
5										
6										
7										
8										

Medical History	Patient	Family
1. Congenital anomalies		
2. Genetic diseases		
3. Multiple births		
4. Diabetes mellitus		
5. Malignancies		
6. Hypertension		
7. Heart disease		
8. Rheumatic fever		
9. Pulmonary disease		
10. GI problems		
11. Renal disease		
12. Other urinary tract problems		
13. Genitourinary anomalies		
14. Abnormal uterine bleeding		
15. Infertility		
16. Veneral disease		
17. Phlebitis, varicosities		
18. Nervous/mental disorders		
19. Convulsive disorders		
20. Metabol./endocrine disorders		
21. Anemia/hemoglobinopathy		
22. Blood dyscrasias		
23. Drug addiction		
24. Smoking/alcohol		
25. Infectious diseases		
26. Operations/accidents		
27. Blood transfusions		
28. Other hospitalizations		

Check and detail positive findings including date and place of treatment. Precede findings by reference number.

Sensitivities (detail positive findings)

- ☐ Antibiotics
- ☐ Analgesics
- ☐ Sedatives
- ☐ Anesthesia
- ☐ Other

_______________ M.D.

F1-705-1 6/89 OUTPATIENT RECORD

Appendix 3–1 (*Continued*)

Mount Sinai Hospital
Medical Center
California Avenue at 15th St.
Chicago, Illinois 60608

Department of Obstetrics and Gynecology
Prenatal Record — 2 · Exam/Lab

INITIAL PHYSICAL EXAM: Date ______________ Gest. Age ______________

Check if Normal: Detail Abnormal Physical Findings

	NORM.	ABNORMAL		NORM.	ABNORMAL	CLINICAL PELVIMETRY:
Thyroid			Pelvic			D.C. ______
Heent			Ext. Genit.			Sacaram ______
Heart			Perineum			Sidewalls ______
Lungs			Vagina			Spines ______
Extrem			Cervix			Post. Sag M.P. ______
Neuro			Uterus			Bitub. ______
Breasts			Adnexa			Arch. ______
Abdomen			Rectal			BORDERLINE ☐ ADEQUATE ☐

LABORATORY

ALL PATIENTS	INITIAL									
	Date	Results	Date	Results	Date	Results	Date	Results	Date	Results
Pap Smear										
Blood Type										
Antibodies										
Tine Test										
Rubella Titer										
H.I.V.										
MSAFP										
HBS										
VDRL										
GC										
GBBS V / R										
HB / HCT										
WBC / PLTS										
PT / PTT										
BUN / CR										
3 Hr GTT		FBS	1 Hr.		2 Hr.		3 Hr.			
UA										
UR C & S										
24 Hr CCL										
24 Hr TOT PROT.										
Ultrasound		EGA-US / EFW		EGA-US / EFW		EGA-US / EFW		EGA-US / EFW		EGA-US / EFW
NST / OCT										

PROGNOSIS:

Normal ☐ Trial of Labor ☐

Guarded ☐ Planned C/S ☐

Examiner ______________________ M.D.
RESIDENT

Examiner ______________________ M.D.
ATTENDING

F1-705-1 6/89

OUTPATIENT RECORD

Appendix 3–1 (*Continued*)

Mount Sinai Hospital
Medical Center
California Avenue at 15th St.
Chicago, Illinois 60608

Department of Obstetrics and Gynecology
Prenatal Record — 3 · Problem List/Visits

LIST OF PROBLEMS:

1.
2.
3.
4.
5.
6.
7.

MANAGEMENT PLAN:

1.
2.
3.
4.
5.
6. Genetic DX indicated: Yes / No Done: Yes / No
7. Breast/Bottle
8. Tubal Ligation Yes / No

Prepregnancy Wt.:

Date	Wt.	B/P	Edema	URINE			LMP GA	U/S GA	Fundus (cm)	FHT Doppl	FHT Fetos	FM	Remarks	Initials
				Prot.	Glu.	Acet.								
1.														
2.														
3.														
4.														
5.														
6.														
7.														
8.														
9.														
10.														
11.														
12.														
13.														
14.														
15.														
16.														
17.														
18.														
19.														
20.														
21.														
22.														
23.														

MEDICATIONS	Dose	Date Started	Date Stopped	MEDICATIONS	Dose	Date Started	Date Stopped
RHOGAM							

F1-705-1 6/89

OUTPATIENT RECORD

Mount Sinai Hospital
Medical Center
California Avenue at 15th St.
Chicago, Illinois 60608

Department of Obstetrics and Gynecology
Prenatal Record — 4 · Progress Notes

Date	GA	

F1-705-1 6/89 OUTPATIENT RECORD

Mount Sinai Hospital
Medical Center
California Avenue at 15th St.
Chicago, Illinois 60608

Department of Obstetrics and Gynecology

Prenatal Record — 5 · Post-Partum

PROGRESS NOTES:

Date	GA	

POST PARTUM CHECK-UP

Breastfeeding: YES NO

Pelvic Exam ______________________

Physical Exam ______________________

Pap Smear ______________________

Birth Control ______________________

Recommendation for P.P. Work-up ______________________

Disposition of Patient: ______________________

PREGNANCY OUTCOME:

Delivery Date ______________________

Method-Delivery ______________________

GA ______________________

Weight ______________________

APGAR ______________________

Complications: ______________________

____

______________________ M.D.

F1-705-1 6/89

OUTPATIENT RECORD

Appendix 3–2
Sample Prenatal Genetic Screen*

Name__________ Patient#__________ Date__________

1. Will you be 35 years or older when the baby is due? Yes_____ No_____
2. Have you, the baby's father, or anyone in either of your families ever had any of the following disorders? Yes_____ No_____
   - Down syndrome (mongolism) Yes_____ No_____
   - Other chromosomal abnormality Yes_____ No_____
   - Neural tube defect, ie, spina bifida (meningomyelocele or open spine), anencephaly Yes_____ No_____
   - Hemophilia Yes_____ No_____
   - Muscular dystrophy Yes_____ No_____
   - Cystic fibrosis Yes_____ No_____

   If yes, indicate the relationship of the affected person to you or to the baby's father: __________
3. Do you or the baby's father have a birth defect? Yes_____ No_____
   If yes, who has the defect and what is it?__________
4. In any previous marriages, have you or the baby's father had a child, born dead or alive, with a birth defect not listed in question 2 above? Yes_____ No_____
   If yes, what was the defect and who had it? __________
5. Do you or the baby's father have any close relatives with mental retardation? Yes_____ No_____
   If yes, indicate the relationship of the affected person to you or to the baby's father: __________
   Indicate the cause, if known: __________
6. Do you, the baby's father, or a close relative in either of your families have a birth defect, any familial disorder, or a chromosomal abnormality not listed above? Yes_____ No_____
   If yes, indicate the condition and the relationship of the affected person to you or to the baby's father: __________
7. In any previous marriages, have you or the baby's father had a stillborn child or three or more first-trimester spontaneous pregnancy losses? Yes_____ No_____
   Have either of you had a chromosomal study? Yes_____ No_____
   If yes, indicate who and the results: __________
8. If you or the baby's father are of Jewish ancestry, have either of you been screened for Tay–Sachs disease? Yes_____ No_____
   If yes, indicate who and the results: __________
9. If you or the baby's father are black, have either of you been screened for sickle cell trait? Yes_____ No_____
   If yes, indicate who and the results: __________
10. If you or the baby's father are of Italian, Greek, or Mediterranean background, have either of you been tested for β-thalassemia? Yes_____ No_____
    If yes, indicate who and the results: __________
11. If you or the baby's father are of Philippine or Southeast Asian ancestry, have either of you been tested for α-thalassemia? Yes_____ No_____
    If yes, indicate who and the results: __________
12. Excluding iron and vitamins, have you taken any medications or recreational drugs since being pregnant or since your last menstrual period? (include nonprescription drugs.) Yes_____ No_____
    If yes, give name of medication and time taken during pregnancy:__________

*Any patient replying "YES" to questions should be offered appropriate counseling. If the patient declines further counseling or testing, this should be noted in the chart. Given that genetics is a field in a state of flux, alterations or updates to this form will be required periodically.

Appendix 3–3
Antepartum Risk Factors

Demographic, Social, and Personal	Medical Complications	Previous Reproductive History	Current Pregnancy and Intrapartum
Age	Diabetes[a]	Infertility	Multiple pregnancy
Ethnic group	Hypertension[a]	Miscarriages	Polyhydramnios
Marital status	Heart disease	Uterine anomaly	Macrosomia
Parity	Urinary tract infection	Cervical incompetence	Vaginal bleeding
Planned or unplanned	Renal disease	Uterine fibroid	Inadequate weight gain
Unwanted pregnancies	Thyroid disorders	Rh sensitization	Preeclampsia
Spacing of pregnancies	Epilepsy	Previous cesarean section	Premature rupture of membranes
Education	Sickle cell trait or disease	Premature deliveries	Threatened premature labor
Income	Lung disease	Low birth-weight babies (<2500 g)	Postdate pregnancy
Housing		Fetal or neonatal death	Previous cesarean section
Nutrition		Congenital anomalies	Abnormal presentation
Underweight or overweight		Mental retardation	Meconium-stained fluid
Anemia		Cerebral palsy	Prolonged labor
When started			Placenta previa
Number of visits			Abruptio placentae
Psychoemotional problems			Fetal distress
Alcohol use			Indicated induction of labor
Smoking			
Sexually transmitted disease			

[a] In the patient or in first-degree relatives.

Appendix 3–4

Perinatal Mortality Review Committee Maternal Data for the Period of Jan. 1, 1989 through June 30, 1989

	TOTAL	%	1988		1987	
A. Mothers delivered	1320		2430		2301	
Babies delivered	1341		2472		2345	
1. Single pregnancy	1300	98.4	2390	98.3	2257	98.0
2. Multiple pregnancy	20	1.5	40	1.6	44	1.9
3. Nulliparas	369	27.9	761	31.3	666	28.9
4. Multiparas	951	72.0	1669	68.6	1635	71.0
5. Private	671	50.8	1471	60.5	1410	61.2
6. Faculty	649	49.1	959	39.4	891	38.7
7. Walk-ins	39	2.9	104	4.2	69	2.9
8. Home births	23	1.7	40	1.6	35	1.5
B. Vaginal deliveries	1175	89.0	2132	87.7	2035	88.4
1. NSVD	1107	83.8	1997	82.1	1895	82.3
2. Outlet forceps	28	2.1	63	2.5	70	3.0
3. Breech	34	2.5	55	2.2	43	1.8
4. Midpelvic delivery	5	0.3	15	0.6	27	1.1
A. Low or mid forceps	3	0.2	2	0.0		0.0
B. Mid forceps	2	0.1	10	0.4	13	0.5
C. Vacuum Extractions		0.0	3	0.1	14	0.6
C. Abdominal Deliveries	145	10.9	298	12.2	265	11.5
1. Private	76	5.7	193	7.9	168	7.3
2. Faculty	69	5.2	105	4.3	97	4.2
3. Low transverse	131	9.9	293	12.0	265	11.5
4. Low vertical	11	0.8	4	0.1		0.0
5. Classical	3	0.2	1	0.0		0.0
6. Second opinion	24	20.1	18	7.5		0.0
7. Primary	99	7.5	191	7.8	160	6.9
A. Dystocia	44	44.4	76	39.7	54	33.7
B. Breech	13	13.1	20	10.4	29	18.1
C. Fetal distress	23	23.2	51	26.7	46	28.7
D. Other	19	19.1	44	23.0	31	19.3
8. Repeat	46	3.4	107	4.4	105	4.5
9. Hysterectomy	1	0.0		0.0		0.0
D. Previous cesarean section	125	9.4	275	11.3	265	11.5
1. Elective	12	9.6	32	11.6	37	13.9
2. Trival of labor	113	90.4	243	88.3	228	86.0
A. Vaginal	79	69.9	167	68.7	160	70.1
B. Failed trial	34	30.0	76	31.2	68	29.8
E. Breech deliveries	54	4.0	109	4.4	113	4.8
1. Spontaneous breech	3	5.5	16	14.6	18	15.9
2. Assisted breech	27	50.0	40	36.6	23	20.3
3. Breech extraction	3	5.5	3	2.7	7	6.1
4. Cesarean section	21	38.8	49	44.9	65	57.5
A. Breech primary	15	71.4	29	59.1	38	58.4
B. Breech repeat	6	28.5	20	40.8	27	41.5
F. Multigestational deliveries						
1. Mothers	20	1.5	40	1.6	44	1.9
2. Babies	41	3.0	82	3.3	88	3.7
3. Babies vaginal	25	1.8	52	2.1	53	2.2
4. Babies cesarean section	16	1.1	30	1.2	35	1.4
A. Primaries	16	1.1	20	0.8	27	1.1
B. Repeats		0.0	10	0.4	8	0.3

Appendix 3–4 (*Continued*)

	TOTAL	%	1988		1987	
G. Gestational hypertension	59	4.4	155	6.3	174	7.5
1. Mild preeclampsia	30	2.2	88	3.6	97	4.2
2. Severe preeclampsia	11	0.8	14	0.5	10	0.4
3. Eclampsia	1	0.0	3	0.1	2	0.0
4. Chronic hypertension	17	1.2	46	1.8	58	2.5
5. Mild preeclamp and hypertension		0.0	2	0.0	5	0.2
6. Severe preeclamp and hypertension		0.0	2	0.0	2	0.0
7. Eclampsia hypertension		0.0		0.0		0.0
H. Episiotomy						
1. No episiotomy	565	48.0	1240	58.0	1163	56.9
A. No episiotomy or laceration	550	97.3	1211	97.6	1147	98.6
B. No episiotomy–third degree	12	2.1	17	1.3	12	1.0
C. No episiotomy–fourth degree	3	0.5	12	0.9	4	0.3
2. Episiotomy	611	51.9	897	41.9	879	43.0
A. Midline	256	41.8	441	49.1	506	57.5
1. Midline no laceration	237	92.5	374	84.8	439	86.7
2. Midline third degree	14	5.4	42	9.5	35	6.9
3. Midline fourth degree	5	1.9	25	5.6	32	6.3
B. Mediolateral	355	58.1	456	50.8	373	42.4
1. Mediolateral laceration	346	97.4	433	94.9	362	97.0
2. Mediolateral third degree	7	1.9	23	5.0	7	1.8
3. Mediolateral fourth degree	2	0.5		0.0	4	1.0
3. Cervical laceration	10	0.8	7	0.3		0.0
4. Vaginal laceration	8	0.6	4	0.1		0.0
I. Miscellaneous Complications						
1. Premature labor	268	20.3	474	19.5	464	20.1
2. Induced labor	113	8.5	325	13.3	333	14.4
3. Previa abruption	15	1.1	27	1.1	22	0.9
4. Srom before labor	210	15.9	480	19.7	412	17.9
5. Drug abuse total	96	7.2	123	5.0	120	5.2
A. Suspected	15	1.1	11	0.4	12	0.5
B. Admitted	81	6.1	112	4.6	108	4.6
6. 1 min apgar <7	99	7.3	257	10.3	253	10.7
7. 1 min apgar <3	7	0.5	44	1.7	41	1.7
8. 1 min apgar <7	16	1.1	70	2.8	76	3.2
9. 1 min apgar <3	2	0.1	12	0.4	6	0.2
10. Stillbirths >500 g	26	1.9	35	1.4	21	0.8

Appendix 3–4 (*Continued*)

Birthweight-Specific Neonatal Outcome for the Period of Jan. 1, 1987 through Dec. 31, 1987

Birthweight	> 2500 g		1500–2499 g		1500–1499 g	
	TOTAL	%	TOTAL	%	TOTAL	%
A. Babies delivered	2001	86.0	245	10.9	71	3.1
1. 1 min apgar < 7	171	8.5	42	16.5	40	56.
2. 1 min apgar < 3	18	0.8	9	3.5	14	19.
3. 5 min apgar < 7	41	2.0	16	6.2	19	26.
4. 5 min apgar < 3	3	0.1	1	0.3	2	2.
Babies and Morbidity Data	1808	90.3	210	82.6	35	4.9
B. Cardiorespiratory						
1. Endotracheal tube	22	1.2	22	10.4	21	60.
2. Chest tube	7	0.3	7	3.3	10	28.
3. Ventilator	14	0.7	22	10.4	19	54.
4. Maximum F102 > 60% 02	10	0.5	7	3.3	11	31.
5. Acidosis pH < 7.2	14	0.7	10	4.7	10	28.
6. Pneumo th/med	2	0.1		0.0		0.
7. Meconium aspiration	14	0.7		0.0		0.
8. Pneumonia	1	0.0		0.0		0.
C. Hematologic						
1. Bilirubin > 10mg/dL	71	3.9	47	22.3	15	42.
2. Phototherapy	73	4.0	51	24.2	22	62.
3. EXC. transfusion		0.0		0.0	1	2.
4. RBC transfusion	5	0.2	5	2.3	13	37.
D. Neurologic						
1. Seizures	3	0.1		0.0		0.
2. Paralysis		0.0		0.0		0.
3. CNS hemorrhage	2	0.1	2	0.9	3	8.
4. Hydrocephalus	2	0.1		0.0		0.
5. Other	14	0.7	2	0.9		0.
E. Infection						
1. Sepsis	7	0.3	3	1.4	2	5.
2. Scalp		0.0	2	0.9		0.
3. Lung	2	0.1	1	0.4	3	8.
4. Other	12	0.6	3	1.4	2	5.
F. Miscellaneous						
1. Genetic abnormality	6	0.3	1	0.4		0.
2. GI Abnormality	35	1.9	15	7.1	7	20.
3. Fracture	1	0.0		0.0	1	2.
4. Peripheral IV	111	6.1	49	23.3	10	28.
5. Central IV	113	6.2	50	23.8	13	37.

Appendix 3–4 (*Continued*)

Perinatal Mortality Review Committee Data Sheet

Birthweight (g)	December, 1988 Total	%	Live	Still-births	Neonatal Deaths	Out	Ndo	Year-to-Date Total	%	Live	Still-births	Neonatal Deaths	Out	Ndo
All	217		216	1	1	1	0	2472		2424	48	26	37	2
> 2500	181	83.4	181	0	0	0	0	2091	84.5	2083	8	2	12	0
2250–2499	17	7.8	17	0	0	0	0	130	5.2	126	4	1	2	0
2000–2249	3	1.3	3	0	0	0	0	74	2.9	72	2	0	3	0
1750–1999	6	2.7	6	0	0	0	0	43	1.7	41	2	0	0	0
1500–1749	4	1.8	3	1	0	1	0	33	1.3	30	3	0	4	0
1250–1499	4	1.8	4	0	0	0	0	28	1.1	23	5	2	4	0
1000–1249	1	0.4	1	0	0	0	0	14	0.5	12	2	1	3	0
900–999	0	0.0	0	0	0	0	0	7	0.2	6	1	1	1	0
800–899	0	0.0	0	0	0	0	0	8	0.3	6	2	3	5	0
750–799	0	0.0	0	0	0	0	0	2	0.05	2	0	0	1	0
700–749	1	0.4	1	0	1	0	0	5	0.2	5	0	1	0	0
600–699	0	0.0	0	0	0	0	0	6	0.2	4	2	2	1	1
500–599	0	0.0	0	0	0	0	0	10	0.4	6	4	5	0	0
<500	0	0.0	0	0	0	0	0	21	0.8	8	13	8	1	1

December, 1988: PRM 9.2; NMR 4.6; FMR 4.6.
Rates per 1000 and exclude any stillborn under 500 g.

Year-to-Date: PRM 24.8; NRM 10.7; FMR 14.1.
Rates per 1000 and exclude any stillborn under 500 g.

Appendix 3–5
Perinatal Chart Model

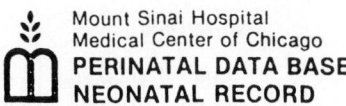

Mount Sinai Hospital
Medical Center of Chicago
PERINATAL DATA BASE
NEONATAL RECORD

MATERNAL ID

ID
_ _ _ _ _ _

LAST NAME
_ _ _ _ _ _ _ _ _ _ _ _ _ _ _

FIRST NAME
_ _ _ _ _ _ _ _ _ _

DELIVERY DATE
_____/_____/_____

NEONATAL ID

AGE ON ADMISSION (Hrs)
_ _ _

INFANT'S PHYSICIAN
_ _ _

REFERRING HOSPITAL
_ _ _

INFANT'S ID NUMBER
_ _ _ _ _ _ _ _

HOSPITAL CARE

SURGERY — _ _
0. None
1. Circumcision
2. Cardiac
3. GI
4. CNS
5. Renal
6. Multiple of above
8. Other

LINES — _
0. None
1. Intermittent sampling - no IV
2. Peripheral IV
3. Umbilical artery
4. Umbilical vein
5. Umbilical vein and artery
8. Other

TUBES — _
0. None
1. Endotracheal
2. Chest
3. Nasogastric
4. Multiple of above
8. Other

VENTILATOR SUPPORT — _
0. None
1. Ventilator
2. CPAP
3. Other

MAX F10$_2$ — _
0. Room air
1. ◄40% O$_2$
2. 40-60% O$_2$
3. 61-80% O$_2$
4. ►80% O$_2$

CARDIOVASCULAR PROCEDURES — _
0. None
1. ECG
2. Echocardiogram
3. Cardiac catheterization
8. Other

TRANSFUSION — _ _
0. None
1. Packed cells
2. Albumin/plasma
3. Platelets
4. Multiple of above
5. Exchange transfusion
8. Other

THERAPY OF JAUNDICE — _
0. None
1. Phototherapy
2. Exchange transfusion
3. Phototherapy and exchange

MISCELLANEOUS PROCEDURES — _ _
0. None
1. CT scan
2. Ultrasound (non-cardiac)
3. Lumbar puncture
4. Paracentesis
5. Suprapubic tap
6. Multiple of above
8. Other

FEEDING — _
0. None
1. Bottle/breast
2. Gavage
3. Nasal/jejunal-duodenal
4. Hyperalimentation
8. Other

MEDICATIONS (Table C)
_ _,_ _,_ _

CLINICAL COURSE

GROWTH — _
0. AGA
1. SGA
2. LGA

NEUROPHYSICAL EXAM (WKS)
_ _

GENETIC — _
0. None
1. Downs syndrome - trisomy 21
2. Trisomy 13
3. Trisomy 18
4. Other chromosomal syndrome
5. Karotype normal
6. Multiple malformations -no syndrome
7. Inborn error of metabolism
8. Other

COGENITAL ANOMALY (Table E) — _ _
1. Anen/Spina Bifida
2. Hydrocephalus
3. Other NS Anomaly
4. Eyes
5. Cleft Lip/Palate
6. Heart
7. Respiratory System
8. G-U System
9. Down's Syndrome

TEMPERATURE — _
0. Euthermia
1. Hypothermia - ◄97°F
2. Fever - ►100°F
3. Hypo/hyperthermia

RESPIRATORY — _ _
0. None
1. TTN/wet lung
2. Pneumothorax/mediastinum
3. Interstitial emphysema
4. Pneumopericardium
5. Broncho-pulmonary dysplasia
6. Pulomnary hemorrhage
7. Meconium aspiration
8. Formula
A. Pneumonia
B. RDS
C. Apnea
D. Other

PERINATAL ACIDOSIS — _
0. None
1. Mild pH◄7.2
2. Moderate pH◄7.1
3. Severe pH◄7.0

Appendix 3–5 (*Continued*)

Mount Sinai Hospital
Medical Center of Chicago

PERINATAL DATA BASE
MATERNAL RECORD AND
LABOR AND DELIVERY SUMMARY
Page 1 of 2

MATERNAL ID

REFERRING HOSPITAL — — — —

ID — — — — — — — —

LAST NAME — — — — — — — — — — — — — — — —

FIRST NAME — — — — — — — — — —

PHYSICIAN — — —

MATERNAL DEMOGRAPHICS

AGE — —   GR/T/P/A/L — — — — —

HEIGHT (INS) — —   WEIGHT (LBS) — — —

RACE —
1. White
2. Black
3. Asian
4. American Indian
5. Refused to State
6. Hispanic

WEEK OF 1ST VISIT/ RESPON. PHYS. — —/—
A. None
B. PVT MD (Non-GF)
C. BOH
D. PVT GF, Kling
E. PVT GF, River North
F. PVT GF, 55th
G. PVT GF, Cicero
H. PVT GF, TJ/AS, Nr. North
I. PVT GF, TJ/AS, Madison
J. PVT GF, TJ/AS, Warren
K. PVT GF, JK/MG, Komed

PREVIOUS MEDICAL HISTORY

MED/SURG HISTORY (Table A) — —,— —,— —,— —,— —

MEDICATIONS — —,— —,— —

PREVIOUS PREGNANCIES

MAT. COMPLICATIONS (Table D) — —,— —,— —

FETAL COMPLICATIONS — —
0. No previous pregnancy
1. Normal outcome
2. Stillbirth
3. Neonatal death
4. Anomaly
5. Handicap
6. Premature
7. Macrosomia
8. Fetal distress
9. Non-vertex presentation
A. Trauma
B. SIDS

FETAL COMPLICATIONS Cont.
C. Jaundice
D. Multiple
E. Spont. Ab. (s)
F. Induced Ab.(s)
G. IUGR

OBSTETRICAL COMPLICATIONS — —
0. No previous delivery
1. Uneventful
2. C/S labor abnormality
3. C/S other
4. Midforceps
5. Breech
6. Multiple births
7. Shoulder dystocia
8. Placenta previa-abruption
9. Incompetent cervix
A. Difficult delivery
B. Previous C/S x 2
C. Previous C/S 3- or more

PRESENT PREGNANCY

LAST MENSTRUAL PERIOD ______ / ______ / ______

ANTEPARTUM TESTING —
0. None
1. NST
2. NST/CST
3. NST/BPP
4. CST
5. BPP
6. CST/BPP

ULTRASOUND —
0. None
1. First trimester
2. Second trimester
3. Third trimester
4. Serial

AMNIOCENTESIS —
0. None
1. Genetic
2. Rh
3. Maturity
4. Multiple
5. Complication
8. Other

GESTATIONAL HYPERTENSION (P.I.H.) —
0. None
1. Mild pre-eclampsia
2. Severe pre-eclampsia
3. Eclampsia
4. Chronic hypertension
5. (4 + 1)
6. (4 + 2)
7. (4 + 3)

DIABETES —
0. None
N. GTT Negative
A. Class A
B. Class B
C. Class C
D. Class D
F. Class F
H. Class H
X. Class F/R

HEMORRHAGE —
0. None
1. First trimester
2. Second trimester
3. Third trimester

INFECTION — —
0. None
1. Uterine
2. Urinary
3. Respiratory
4. Undetermined origin
5. Hepatitis
6. Herpes HX
7. Herpes Confirmed
8. Other
9. GC
A. HIV
B. Syphlis

RH FACTOR/ANTIBODIES TYPE/RH/AB(±) — —/—/—

OTHER COMPLICATIONS/PROCEDURES — — —
0. None
1. Rhogam
2. Excessive weight gain
3. Inadequate weight gain
4. Premature labor
5. Previous hospitalization-other cause
6. Incompetent cervix/cerclage
7. IUGR
8. Breech version attempt
9. Pelvic surgery
A. Other surgery
B. Pelvimetry
C. Fetoscopy
D. Cone biopsy
E. Multiple
F. Tocolysis

DRUG ABUSE —
0. None
1. Smoking
2. Alcohol
3. Smoking/alcohol
4. Drugs suspected
5. Drug abuse (list type)

MEDICATIONS — —,— —,— —

ADMISSION

STATUS —
1. In labor
2. Not in labor
3. Post partum

EGA — —

BASIS-EGA —
1. Exam-HX
2. Amnio/LS
3. U/S

EFW (100 g) — — — —

ADMISSION TIME (0001-2400 Hrs) — — — —

ADMISSION DATE ______ / ______ / ______

LABOR

LABOR ONSET —
0. None
1. Spontaneous
2. Induced-elective
3. Induced-fetal test result
4. Induced-maternal
5. Induced-others
6. No trial of labor/No labor
7. No trial/spont. labor

MEMBRANES —
0. Non ruptured (C/S)
1. Spontaneous-before labor
2. Spontaneous-during labor
3. Artificial-induction
4. Artificial-in labor

PRESENTATION —
1. Frank
2. Complete
3. Footling
0. Oblique
T. Transverse
V. Vertex

POSITION — — —

MECONIUM —
0. Absent
1. Before labor
2. During labor
3. At delivery

OXYTOCIN —
0. Not used
1. Induction
2. Augmentation
3. Both

DYSFUNCTIONAL LABOR — —
0. No labor
1. Normal
2. Prolonged latent phase
3. Failed descent
4. Protracted dilatation/descent
5. Arrest of dilatation/descent
6. Combined (protraction and arrest)
7. Precipitous birth

FETAL MONITORING (EFM) —
0. None
1. External only
2. Internal only
3. Both
4. EFM and SS

ANALGESIA FOR LABOR — —
0. None
1. Narcotic
2. Local/pudendal
3. Narcotic and tranquilizer
4. Epidural
5. PCB

ANESTHESIA FOR DELIVERY —
0. None
1. Local/pudendal
2. Epidural
3. Spinal
4. General

MEDICATIONS — —,— —,— —

DELIVERY

METHOD OF DELIVERY —
0. Spontaneous vaginal
1. Low forceps
2. Mid forceps (list)
3. Vaccum extraction
4. CS (Low transverse)
5. Breech forceps
6. Breech assisted
7. Breech extraction
8. Low Mid forceps
9. CS (Low vertical)
A. CS (Classical)

WHITE — CHART COPY   YELLOW — NEWBORN RECORD   PINK — FILE RECORD   GOLDEN ROD — DATA BASE   F1-16 9/86   Revised 9/88

Mount Sinai Hospital
Medical Center of Chicago

PERINATAL DATA BASE MATERNAL RECORD AND LABOR AND DELIVERY SUMMARY
Page 2 of 2

INDICATION FOR OPERATIVE DELIVERY —
0. Not applicable
1. Dysfunctional labor
2. Breech, malpresentation
3. Previa, abruption
4. Fetal distress
5. Cord prolapse
6. Maternal (list)
7. Elective Repeat C/S
8. Elective 1° C/S
A. Multigest
B. Premature
C. Postmature
D. CPD
E. Failed TOL

ESPISOTOMY/LACERATION — —
0. No episiotomy, no lacerations
1. No Episiotomy 3rd degree
2. No Episiotomy 4th degree
3. Midline
4. Midline 3rd degree
5. Midline 4th degree
6. Med/lat
7. Med/lat 3rd degree
8. Med/lat 4th degree
9. Cervical
A. 1° Perineal
B. 2° Perineal
C. Vaginal

ESTIMATED BLOOD LOSS —
0. <500 cc
1. 500-750 cc
2. 750-1000 cc
3. 1000-1500 cc
4. 1500-2000 cc
5. >2000 cc

Onset of Labor ____________ ____________

DURATION OF LABOR (HRS) — —

Membranes Ruptured ____________ ____________

DURATION OR ROM (HRS) — — —

COMPLETE DILATION
Date ____________ ____________

DELIVERY TIME (0001-2400 Hrs) — — —

DELIVERY DATE
______ / ______ / ______

DELIVERY OF PLACENTA
Date ____________ ____________

LOCATION —
1. Delivery
2. Labor room
3. Birthing center
4. Home delivery
5. E.R.

RESPONSIBLE PHYSICIAN
Attending — — —
Primary Resident — — —
Secondary Resident — — —

COMPLICATIONS

MATERNAL COMPLICATION(S) LABOR/DELIVERY (Table D)
— —,— —,— —

FETAL COMPLICATIONS — — —
0. None
1. Fetal distress
2. Hemorrhage
3. Prolapsed extremity
4. Prolapsed cord
5. Arrhythmia
6. Hydrops
7. Tachycardia
8. Bradycardia
A. Decels
B. Decreased Var
C. IUFD ante.
D. IUFD intra.

OBSTETRIC COMPLICATION(S) — —
0. None
1. Malpresentation
2. Transverse lie
3. Placenta previa
4. Placenta abruptio
5. Contraction ring/tetany
6. Inversion of uterus
7. Trail/failed forceps/vacuum
8. Pelvic disproportion
9. Hemorrhage
A. Shoulder dystocia
B. Uterine Dehiscene (occult)
C. Uterine Rupture

ANESTHESIA COMPLICATION(S) — —
0. None
1. Convulsions
2. Hypertension
3. Hypotension
4. Total spinal
9. Unknown

INTRAPARTUM PROCEDURES — —
0. None
1. Tubal ligation
2. Hysterectomy
3. Appendectomy
4. Salpingo-oophorectomy/cystectomy
5. D and C
6. Hypogastric artery ligation
7. Breech version
8. Blood transfusion
9. Hysterectomy & A.Lig
A. Manual removal of placenta

POSTPARTUM PROCEDURES —
0. None
1. Transfusion
2. D and C
3. Surgery - tubal
4. Surgery - elective
5. Hysterectomy

CORD/PLACENTAL PATHOLOGY — —
0. None
1. Nuchal cord
2. Vasa previa
3. Succenturiate lobe
4. Placenta (per) accreta
5. Placental infarct

MEDICATION POSTPARTUM (Table C)
— —,— —,— —

MAT. OUTCOME —

MAT. HOSP. DAYS — —

NEONATAL DELIVERY ROOM

SEX —
0. Male
1. Female

BIRTH ORDER —
1. First or singleton
2. Second
3. Third
4. Fourth
5. Fifth

MULTIPLE GESTATION —
1. Singleton
2. Twins
3. Triplets
4. Quads
5. Quints

APGAR

	Heart rate	Respiration	Tone	Reflex	Color	Totals
1 min.						
5 min.						

PEDIATRICIAN
☐ Yes ☐ No
Name:

RESUSCITATION — —
0. None
1. Stimulation/suction
2. Supplemental O_2
3. Positive pressure (mask)
4. Intubation/suction
5. Intubation - positive pressure
6. Cardiac massage
7. Umbilical catheter/meds
8. Other
9. Unknown
A. Delee Suction
B. Laryngoscopy/cord vis.

BIRTH WEIGHT (GRAMS) — — — —

BIRTH TRAUMA/ANOMALY — —
0. None
1. Moulding/caput-marked
2. Cephalhematoma
3. Scleral hemorrhage
4. Bruising
5. Palsy
6. Fracture
7. Multiple trauma
8. Other
9. Unknown
A. Anomaly

I.D. Bracelet No. ____________

PREP ☐YES ☐NO ☐ABDOMINAL ☐PERINEAL

BABY TRANS TO —
1. Normal new born
2. Intermediate nursery
3. IICU

BREAST ☐ BOTTLE ☐

FETAL BLOOD DATA
☐No samples obtained

	pH	pCO_2	pO_2	HCO_3	BE
Fetal 1					
Fetal 2					
Fetal 3					
Maternal					

CORD BLOOD GASSES

	pH	pCO_2	pO_2	HCO_3	BE
UMB_A					
UMB_V					
MATERNAL					

MOTHER TRANSFERRED TO:
T P R BP

NOTES: ____________

Attending Physician ____________

Resident ____________

Midwife ____________

Med Student ____________

2° OPINION ☐ YES ☐ NO
If Yes — — —

Nurse

WHITE — CHART COPY YELLOW — NEWBORN RECORD PINK — FILE RECORD GOLDEN ROD — DATA BASE F1-16 9/86 Revised 9/88

Chapter Four
Physiologic Changes in Normal Pregnancy

Stephen A. Myers and Norbert Gleicher

4

Pregnancy induces a multitude of anatomic, physiologic, biochemical, and psychological changes. It is imperative that a physician caring for pregnant patients be familiar with normal changes, lest they be interpreted as abnormal. Sinus tachycardia, systolic heart murmur, apparent cardiac enlargement, and dependent edema, which are common changes in pregnancy, can easily be interpreted erroneously as signs of heart disease. Thyroid enlargement, sinus tachycardia, and the finding of high protein-bound iodine can lead to the false diagnosis of hyperthyroidism if a physician is not aware that these findings are normal changes of pregnancy.

Most physiologic changes in pregnancy have a teleological basis; that is, they serve to protect the mother from the risks of pregnancy and delivery and facilitate fetal growth and development. The increase in blood volume and red blood cell (RBC) mass protects the mother from blood loss during delivery. The deposition of fat in the first half of pregnancy provides a supply of substrate during late pregnancy and the breast-feeding period.

Appreciation of changes in blood volume, total body water, and renal clearance also is important for prescribing drugs during pregnancy. Serum drug levels may decrease in pregnancy because of significant hemodilution or increased renal clearance. Unless an adjustment of dose is made, a therapeutic level may not be maintained. This often occurs with hydantoin and aminophylline levels in patients with epilepsy and asthma, respectively. Principles of drug therapy in pregnancy are discussed in more detail in Chapter 7.

One of the principal goals of the subspecialty of *maternal–fetal medicine* (*perinatology*) is to provide expertise in areas that overlap those of internists and obstetricians who care for the patient with medical complications during pregnancy. A medical counterpart (internist) to such an obstetric subspecialist has been established primarily in the British medical system but also could be beneficial within the American system.

WEIGHT GAIN

Weight gain represents one of the most obvious physiologic changes in pregnancy. The average normal weight gain is 12.5 kg or 27.5 lbs, but a wide range of weight gain from 7–20 kg (15–45 pounds) is compatible with a normal outcome.[1] Younger patients tend to gain more weight, and parity has little effect on weight gain. Also, no clear correlation exists between prepregnancy weight and weight gain during pregnancy.[2]

Weight gain during pregnancy seems to be linear after the first trimester and amounts to 0.45 kg or 1 lb per week. In the first trimester, a minimal gain of 1–1.5 kg (2–4 lb) occurs. Hytten and Chamberlain[1] divided pregnancy into quarters. They suggest that the expected weight gained at 10 weeks should be 0.65 kg (1.5 lbs), at 20 weeks 4 kg (9 lbs), at 30 weeks 8.3 kg (15 lbs), and at term 12.5 kg (27.5 lbs).

Fetal growth and gestational-age-adjusted birth weights were found to correlate well with prepregnancy weight and weight gain during pregnancy.[3]

One of the most important components in maternal weight gain is expansion of total body water.[4] This reflects intracellular expansion in growing organs, including the uterus, placenta, and fetus, and extracellular expansion, including the expansion of plasma volume, fluid in the different organs, and amniotic fluid. An excess of 5 kg (11 lbs) is unaccountable after all components are taken into account but probably represents fluid accumulated in connective tissues and subcutaneous fat. Under the hormonal influences of pregnancy, more mucopolysaccharides are synthesized in the ground substance, which increases water retention in these tissues. This is the cause of the observed relaxation of joints and ligaments during pregnancy. The collagen of skin and subcutaneous tissues can accumulate water, causing clinical edema. Thomson et al[5] have found that patients with generalized edema without hypertension and proteinuria have larger babies than patients without edema. Such edema thus represents a normal and probably reassuring finding.

In view of societal concerns about the net weight gain after completion of pregnancy, it is of utmost importance that patients and physicians understand the components of weight gain. A detailed explanation of the distribution of added weight will help pregnant women to understand the nutritional guidelines that will result in adequate weight gain. Table 4–1 summarizes individual components contributing to overall weight gain in pregnancy.

Table 4–2 summarizes the distribution of the individual components of weight gain at different gestational ages. From this table, it is apparent that significant expansion in maternal components occurs during the first half of pregnancy, before the significant physiologic demands of the uterus in later gestation. The largest growth of the fetal–placental unit occurs in the second half of pregnancy. The main growth of the placenta and fetus occurs between

TABLE 4–1. INDIVIDUAL COMPONENTS CONTRIBUTING TO WEIGHT GAIN IN PREGNANCY

	Pounds	Kilograms
Fetus	7.5	3.4
Placenta	1.5	0.6
Amniotic fluid	2.0	0.8
Uterus	2.5	1.0
Blood volume increment	0.25	1.5
Fat deposits	0.25	3.3
Interstitial fluid	0.25	1.5
Breast tissue	1.0	0.5
Total	27.5	12.5

Adapted from Hytten and Chamberlain.[1]

TABLE 4–2. DISTRIBUTION OF WEIGHT (G) AT DIFFERENT GESTATIONAL AGES

	Uterus and Conceptus			
	10 Weeks	20 Weeks	30 Weeks	40 Weeks
Uterine				
Fetus	5	300	1500	3400
Placenta	20	170	430	600
Placental to fetal weight ratio	4	0.5	0.25	0.20
Amniotic fluid	40	320	600	1000
Uterus	140	320	600	1000
Maternal				
Breast	50	100	400	500
Fat storage[a]	328	2050	3480	3345
Blood volume	100	600	1300	1500
Extravascular fluid[b]	—	30	80	1680
Total body water	—	1740	4300	7500

[a] Includes deposit in breasts and other organs.
[b] In pregnancy with no edema.
Adapted from Hytten and Chamberlain.[1]

TABLE 4–3. RECOMMENDED DIETARY ALLOWANCES IN PREGNANT AND NONPREGNANT FEMALES OF REPRODUCTIVE AGE (15–35)

	Nonpregnant Females	Additional Requirements	
		Pregnancy	Lactation
Calories (kcal)	2000	300	500
Protein (g)	45	30	20
Vitamin A (mg)	800	200	400
Vitamin B (mg)	7.5	5	5
Vitamin C (mg)	60	20	40
Folic acid (mg)	400	400	100
Niacin (mg)	13	2	5
Riboflavin (mg)	1.2	0.3	0.5
Thiamin (mg)	1.0	0.4	0.5
B_6 (mg)	2.0	0.6	0.5
B_{12} (μg)	3.0	1.0	1.0
Calcium (mg)	800	400	400
Phosphorus (mg)	800	400	400

Adapted from Pitkin.[6]

weeks 20 to 30, when each increases three to five times in weight. The placental–fetal ratio decreases with gestational age, however, which may help to explain the decreased fetal growth rate at term and post-term. The consequence is a relative decrease in placental capacity thus lowering the margin of safety ordinarily available.

Maternal fat storage is used for milk production and as a source of calories in the last trimester and during the breast-feeding period. The patient who nurses will continue to lose weight after delivery and will return more rapidly to her prepregnancy weight. Large maternal weight gain in the first half of pregnancy usually represents excessive fat deposition. Women who have this tendency may increase their nonpregnant weight with parity unless weight loss can be accomplished between pregnancies.

Rapid weight gain in pregnancy increases nutritional requirements. It is estimated that the total caloric cost of pregnancy is about 75,000 kcal.[6] There are variations with respect to age, activity, height, and prepregnancy weight. It is normal for the weight gain in the first trimester to be small compared to that in the last two trimesters, and this should be reflected in food intake. The recommended dietary allowance (RDA) in pregnancy contains 300 kcal/d more than nonpregnant intake. The World Health Organization recommends an addition of only 150 kcal/d in the first trimester and 350 kcal/d later in pregnancy.[6] The total caloric intake for pregnancy should amount to 2300–2400 kcal/d (Table 4–3).

Amino acids are used by the mother and fetus for growth and for plasma volume expansion. The recommended daily protein intake is 1.2 g/kg. In teenage pregnancy, this should be increased to 1.5 g/kg.[6] A large part of the protein should be from animal sources (milk, eggs, meat, fish, and poultry). The efficient use of protein depends on adequate caloric intake. A balanced diet should contain about 100 g of fat and 200 g of carbohydrates.

Iron requirements increase in pregnancy and usually cannot be met by diet alone. Supplemental elemental iron is recommended in the amount of 60 mg per day or more if iron stores are chronically depleted. A detailed discussion of this topic is presented under Hematologic Changes in this chapter.

Folic acid and other vitamins are required in increased amounts in pregnancy (see Table 4–3). The routine use of prenatal vitamins is controversial.[6] They are used to ensure that patients with an inadequate diet receive the recommended daily allowance of folic acid and other vitamins.

The caloric and metabolic requirements of pregnancy often are used as justification for temporary nutritional support, usually in the form of *maternal hyperalimentation.* However, although clinically feasible, this is rarely a physiologic necessity. It has been estimated, based on extensive physiologic studies,[7,8] that daily fetoplacental caloric requirements are less than 100 kcal/kg. Table 4–1 shows that such requirements are less than 200 kcal before the last few weeks of pregnancy, and is negligible before 20 weeks gestation. Therefore, this "fetal indication" can easily be met with means other than hyperalimentation. There are few conditions in which prolonged nutritional support should be considered; these are primarily severe inflammatory bowel disease and burn injuries. In most instances, hyperemesis and postoperative recovery do not cause sufficiently prolonged periods of poor nutrition to warrant nutritional support for fetal indication. Good prenatal care should obviously include nutritional evaluation and counseling if either diet or weight gain is inappropriate.

CARDIOVASCULAR CHANGES

The increase in maternal blood volume represents one of the most important changes of pregnancy and results in an increase in cardiac output and in renal and uterine blood flow.

Blood Volume

Blood volume significantly increases in early pregnancy, reaching a peak at 32 weeks and a plateau thereafter.[9] This observation was made from measurements taken in the left lateral position. When subjects were tested in a supine position, an alleged decrease in blood volume was noted during the last few weeks of pregnancy. This discrepancy between earlier reports in the literature, suggesting a decrease in volume after 36 weeks' gestational age, and more recent reports can be explained by the aortocaval compression caused by the uterus in the supine position. The result of this compression is a decrease in venous return to the heart.[9]

Blood volume increases during normal singleton pregnancy an average of 1600 mL, but the normal range is wide. This represents a 40–50% increase above prepregnancy levels, reaching values of 73–96 mL/kg. Multigravidas and women carrying multiple fetuses demonstrate a larger increase in blood volume than primigravidas.[10] Most of the increased blood volume is plasma, increasing by an average of 1300 mL. The increase in RBC mass is only 400 mL.[9] The net effect of this discrepancy is a reduction of the maternal hemoglobin concentration, the *dilutional anemia* or *physiologic anemia* of pregnancy.

Along with the increase in blood volume, a decrease in vascular resistance occurs. The cause-and-effect relationship between these parameters is not fully understood. Many investigators believe that the decrease in vascular resistance is the primary event, which is followed by the increase in blood volume to fill the created space.[11] The observed decrease in vascular resistance is caused by two components: First, systemic vasodilation occurs, caused by vascular resistance to circulating vasoactive compounds. Second, blood flow in the placenta functions as a large volume, low-resistance arteriovenous fistula. A good correlation among placental mass, birth weight, and blood volume increase in pregnancy has been observed. Patients whose blood volume fails to expand adequately are reported to have smaller babies.[12]

Arterial Blood Pressure

Arterial blood pressure during pregnancy reflects the decreased vascular resistance and, indirectly, the blood volume. A small decrease in systolic blood pressure (10–15 mm Hg) is accompanied by a significant decrease in diastolic blood pressure (20–25 mm Hg), resulting in a wider pulse pressure.[13] This change is maximal during midpregnancy and returns to nonpregnant values around term. It is not unusual to observe pressures in the range of 80/50 to 90/60 in a normal gravida during midpregnancy. Mean arterial pressure (MAP) (diastolic pressure + ⅓ pulse pressure) in the second trimester (MAP II) has been used to predict pregnancy outcome in chronic hypertensive patients.

Many factors affect blood pressure; for example, increasing age and parity correlate with an increase in blood pressure.[13] Position of the patient at the time of measurement also clearly has an effect on arterial blood pressure values. In comparison to the sitting position, which is the standard position for blood pressure measurement in the office, the left lateral position is associated with lower blood pressure values. In most pregnant patients, the supine blood pressure will be lower than the left lateral blood pressure because of varying degrees of caval compression.[14] A paradoxical increase of the diastolic pressure of more than 20 mm Hg after a change from the lateral to the supine position was suggested to predict preeclampsia (positive *roll-over test*).[15] About 0.5–11.2% of pregnant women will show a significant increase in blood pressure in the supine position.[14] This is called the *supine hypotension syndrome* and is the result of aortocaval pressure exerted by the uterus on the large vessels.[16] Caval compression decreases the venous return, the cardiac output, and consequently the arterial pressure. Aortic compression will increase the brachial arterial pressure and decrease the femoral arterial pressure.[17]

Brachial artery pressure may not represent the uterine artery pressure in the supine position. This is clinically important in patients receiving epidural anesthesia during labor because in some cases, the brachial blood pressure will be normal, while signs of fetal distress are seen related to the anesthesia. The net effect of the supine posture on the arterial blood pressure depends on the degree of caval versus aortic compression, the existence of paravertebral collateral venous circulation, the vascular sensitivity to angiotensin, and the patient's tendency toward a vasovagal reflex or baroreceptor sensitivity. The bradycardia that is frequently part of the supine hypotension syndrome is a vasovagal baroreceptor response to the aortic compression.[16]

Renin, Angiotensin, and Prostaglandins

The renin–angiotensin system is important in the regulation of blood volume and systemic blood pressure. The renin concentration is the limiting factor in determining the concentration of angiotensin II (A-II), which is the active pressor substance. Renin is synthesized in small amounts in the arterial tree but mainly in the afferent artery of the glomerulus. Hypovolemia resulting in a decrease of perfusion pressure will stimulate renin secretion and A-II production, thus increasing systemic blood pressure. Hyponatremia will stimulate the macula densa in the distal tubule, resulting in increased renin, A-II, and aldosterone concentrations.[18] Angiotensin II has multiple effects: It increases the synthesis of aldosterone, thus compensating for the hypovolemia or hyponatremia. At the same time, A-II stimulates prostaglandin (PG) production, which is important in the intrinsic autoregulation of the renal blood flow.[19] Prostaglandin E_2 and PGI_2 are vasodilators synthesized in the kidney and uterus. Prostaglandin E_2 is active locally and is inactivated rapidly by the pulmonary capillaries. Prostaglandin I_2 is a systemic vasodilator synthesized in blood vessel walls. Both prostaglandins prevent vasoconstriction by A-II and keep a constant blood flow in the kidney. This mechanism prevents ischemia of vital organs and counteracts the increase in pressor substances (A-II, catecholamines) in case of hypovolemia (see also Chapter 142).

A similar system of prostanoid autoregulation of flow is in operation in the uteroplacental unit. Both renin and PG can be synthesized by the uteroplacental unit[19,20]; however, their effect on uteroplacental flow during normal pregnancy is uncertain. Estrogen increases the synthesis of renin substrate. The relative hyponatremia caused by the natriuretic effect of progesterone also stimulates the renin–angiotensin system. The result is an increase in renin, A-II, and aldosterone during pregnancy. In the normal nonpregnant state, this situation will exist to compensate for hypovolemia. With expansion of blood volume, the renin–aldosterone concentration will decrease. It is paradoxical that pregnancy is characterized by high renin–angiotensin and aldosterone, expansion of blood volume, and increased renal blood flow. Moreover, the arterial blood pressure is not increased in response to the high A-II levels, but rather the vascular resistance and the diastolic blood pressure are decreased.

The explanation for this hemodynamic situation is decreased sensitivity to pressor substances, such as A-II and catecholamines. A decrease of angiotensin sensitivity has been documented in pregnancy and is probably a result of the synthesis of prostaglandins by the uteroplacental unit.[15] Prostaglandin I_2 production has been found to increase during pregnancy.[21] The actions of PGI_2 and PGE_2 are mediated by the changes in the arteriolar wall's sodium concentrations that occur in pregnancy. In the nonpregnant state, infusion of PGE_2 will not modify the pressor response to A-II.[22] The high renin, angiotensin, and aldosterone in conjunction with expanded blood volume and lower blood pressure are specific to pregnancy and resemble secondary aldosteronism and *Bartter's* syndrome. This is a rare syndrome of angiotensin insensitivity and includes high renin, low to normal blood pressure, and elevated PGE_2.[23] Loss of angiotensin resistance in pregnancy has been related to development of preeclampsia[14] (see Chapter 138) and is likely mediated by decreased prostaglandin production.[19,20]

The Heart

In the third trimester, the increase in intra-abdominal pressure displaces the heart upward and rotates it forward. On chest x-rays, the left border is straightened, simulating left atrial hypertrophy seen in mitral stenosis.[24] The anteroposterior diameter and cardiothoracic ratio are increased, reflecting the more horizontal position of the heart. Diastolic heart volume is increased with progression of pregnancy, resulting in an increased stroke volume. There is, however, no significant increase in left ventricular wall thickness.[25]

In auscultation of the heart, the first sound is louder and split as a result of the hyperkinetic circulation and the earlier mitral valve closing.[26] The second sound is more intense and sometimes loses its physiologic splitting. A third heart sound is rarely detected by auscultation but can be detected by phonocardiography in approximately 16% of pregnancies.[26]

Systolic ejection murmurs are common in pregnancy and result from the hyperkinetic circulation. Diastolic murmurs are less frequent and might either represent a tricuspid flow murmur or an extracardiac murmur.[26] Continuous murmurs are occasionally heard over the base of the heart, are frequently caused by mammary vessel flow, and can be modified by changes in position or by compression of the stethoscope.[27]

The observed electrocardiogram (ECG) changes are caused by positional changes of the heart in the thoracic cavity. Left-axis deviation of the QRS complex during pregnancy has been reported by many authors.[28] Recently, Schwartz and Schamroth found a normal distribution of the frontal QRS in late pregnancy.[29] Transient ST and T changes are common in pregnancy, as are Q waves and inverted T waves in lead III.

Cardiac Output

The increase in intravascular volume in pregnancy leads to a rise in cardiac output. Cardiac output in the lateral recumbent position increases 30–50% over the prepregnancy values (from 4–4.5 to 6 L/min). Most of this increase occurs in the first trimester, with a peak at 20–24 weeks' gestation.[25,30]

A decrease in cardiac output in the supine postion in the last 8–10 weeks of pregnancy has been reported. In the left lateral position, this decrease is small and not statistically significant.[25] The aortocaval compression in the supine position increases with gestational age and may be responsible for the decreased cardiac output reported during the last trimester.[30]

Increased cardiac output is attributed to an increased stroke volume and a slightly increased maternal heart rate. In late pregnancy, the stroke volume declines to a prepregnant range, and a substantial increase in heart rate becomes the predominant factor for the increased cardiac output[30] (Fig. 4–1). In multiple pregnancies, the increase in cardiac output is larger than that in singleton pregnancies.[10]

Although most of the increase in cardiac output occurs in the first half of the pregnancy, oxygen consumption increases mainly in the second half, reaching 20–30% above the nonpregnant state at term.[31] The asynchrony between the increased hemodynamics and oxygen requirements decreases the oxygen arteriovenous differences in the first half of pregnancy and increases it to nonpregnant levels at term.[31] This fact may represent a preparatory step for the growing oxygen needs in late pregnancy and may compensate for the "dilutional anemia." The rise in total hemoglobin (not hemoglobin concentration) and the increased cardiac output thus meet the additional oxygen requirement of pregnancy.

The Distribution of Cardiac Output. The uterus receives the largest noncarcass portion of the increased cardiac output. Uterine blood flow increases from less than 50 mL/min in early pregnancy to 500 mL/min at term, approximately 15–18% of the cardiac output.[32] Renal blood flow increases about 30% above the nonpregnant state by midpregnancy.[33] As pregnancy progresses, the renal blood flow, measured in the lateral recumbent position, remains unchanged.[34] An increased blood flow to skin, extremities, and breasts also occurs. Clinically, pregnant patients frequently complain of heat and may have warm skin and hands. For these reasons, there is improvement in cases with Raynaud's phenomenon. Other signs of peripheral vasodilation commonly seen in pregnancy are palmar erythema and spider angiomata. Blood flow through the liver and brain are unchanged in pregnancy.

Venous Pressure and Edema

Venous pressure in the upper extremities does not change in pregnancy, but the femoral venous pressure increases from 9 cm H_2O at 10 weeks to 20 cm H_2O at term.[35] Between the inferior vena cava and the femoral vein there are no venous valves. In the nonpregnant state, the femoral venous pressure is similar to the central venous pressure in the horizontal position. Because central venous pressure is nor-

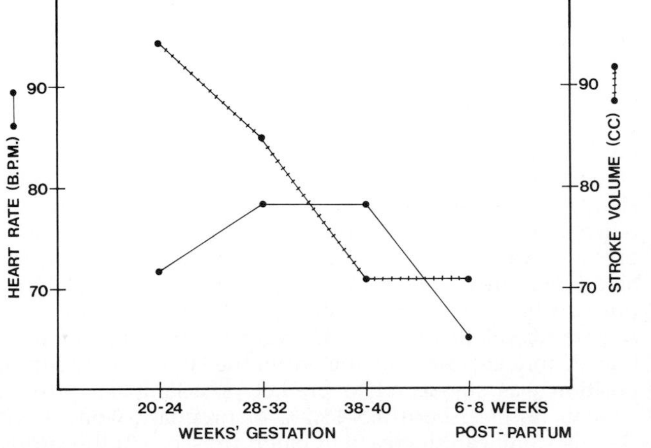

Figure 4–1. Stroke volume (mL) and heart rate (beats per minute) at different gestational ages and postpartum in the left lateral position. (*Adapted from Ueland et al.*[30])

mal in pregnancy, the increased femoral pressure in pregnancy is explained by mechanical pressure of the uterus and fetal head on the iliac vein and inferior vena cava and by retrograde flow from the uterine vein. Consequently, the blood flow rate is decreased in the veins of the lower extremities. The resulting increased pressure and the progesterone-induced changes in the venous system result in an increased incidence of leg and vulvar varicosities and of hemorrhoids.

Dependent leg edema is common in normal pregnancy. Various factors may be involved, including the previously-noted venous pressure in the lower extremities and a normally occurring decrease in colloid osmotic pressure. Lying horizontally decreases the venous pressure and changes the Starling's equation. As a result, the edema diminishes, contributing to the clinical nocturia of late pregnancy.

Cardiovascular Changes in the Intrapartum and Postpartum Periods

During labor, an increase in cardiac output occurs with every contraction and a cumulative increase occurs as labor progresses[36,37] (Fig. 4–2). During contractions, blood vessels are compressed, and blood is diverted out of the uterus and into the systemic circulation. Venous return, cardiac output, and blood pressure are increased. Aortocaval compression, more commonly seen in the supine position, is relieved during contractions. This explains why the hemodynamic changes of the contraction are more significant in the supine than in the lateral position. In fact, in the lateral position, only a minimal change during contractions occurs.[37] Other factors affecting the cardiovascular system are existence of pain and anxiety, type of anesthesia, and stage and duration of labor. The multiple factors involved explain some of the disagreement among investigators about the effects of contractions on maternal heart rate.

After delivery, because of the relief of caval compression, uterine transfusion of blood, infusions of large volumes of crystaloid, and reduced venous pooling in the uterus, cardiac output is increased significantly; This increase may reach 20–30%. A relative sinus bradycardia also occurs. Therefore, most of the increased cardiac output is a result of increased stroke volume.[38] Blood volume decreases about 10% during the first day postpartum and keeps declining over the next few days.[9]

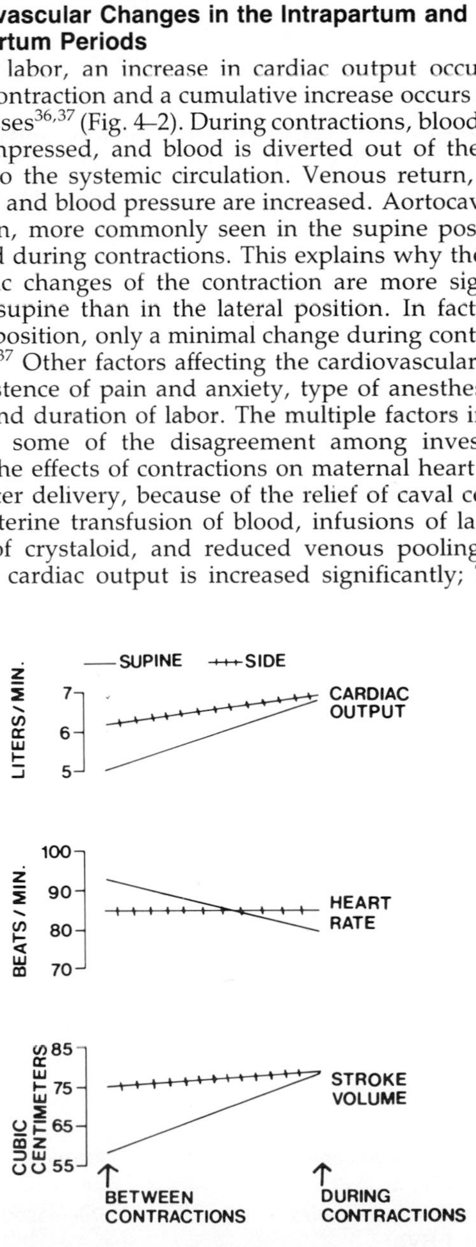

Figure 4–2. Changes in maternal cardiac output, heart rate, and stroke volume during and between uterine contractions in the supine and lateral positions. (*From Metcalfe and Ueland*[37] *with permission.*)

Exercise in Pregnancy

With an increasing number of women in the work force and with increasing emphasis on physical fitness, it is relevant to review the effect of exercise and work on mother and fetus. In general, exercise increases cardiac output to meet the increased oxygen requirements and the resultant heat dissipation. Cardiac output is redistributed. Blood flow to the skeletal muscles and skin is increased, and conversely the flow to the splanchnic and renal systems is decreased. Exercise tolerance and physical fitness mean good cardiac output reserve. Well-conditioned people have the capacity to increase stroke volume and therefore cardiac output without excessive tachycardia.

As pregnancy progresses, partly because of the weight gain, a subjective difficulty exists when performing hard physical work. When body weight is not a factor, as in static exercise (e.g., bicycle ergometer), there is no difference in the energy cost of exertion between pregnant and nonpregnant women.[39] With moderate exercise, the increased cardiac output that occurs during pregnancy is larger than in the nonpregnant state. Because the base-line cardiac output is already increased in pregnancy, exercise will bring the cardiac output to higher absolute values as compared to the nonpregnant state.[30,40] In advanced pregnancy, the resting cardiac output increases, and therefore the cardiac reserve and the subsequent rise in cardiac output after exercise become small as pregnancy progresses.[30,40]

The effect of exercise on pregnancy is controversial. Because strenuous exercise results in a redistribution of the cardiac output, and blood flow is diverted from the splanchnic area, which includes the uterine vasculature, decreased uterine blood flow may occur. This decreased flow can decrease oxygen transfer to the fetus and the dissipation of heat from the fetus to the mother. Increased fetal temperature will compromise umbilical circulation and decrease fetal cardiac function.[41,42] Animal studies have shown that exercise reduces uterine blood flow and fetal oxygen levels.[41] Other studies have found this decrease only in already compromised pregnancies or when the animals were exhausted.[42] Human studies have shown a 95% decrease in uterine clearance of radioactive sodium after exercise.[43] Exercise in pregnancy was used by Hon and Wholgemuth[44] and Pomerance et al[45] to detect fetal distress in already compromised human pregnancies.

It seems that the fetal response to exercise depends on maternal fitness and cardiac reserve and on the fetoplacental reserve. Erkkola suggests that athletic pregnant patients who routinely exercised demonstrated an improved reproductive outcome.[39] In a retrospective study, Jarrett and Spellacy found that jogging in pregnancy had no deleterious effect on the mother or the fetus if the woman had been accustomed to jogging before her pregnancy.[46]

Recently, the American College of Obstetricians and Gynecologists has reported recommendations for exercise in pregnancy.[47] From their recommendations, one can conclude that extended periods of exercise that result in heart rates above 120 beats per minute for extended periods should be avoided. Similarly, high impact or potentially traumatic exercise should be avoided. The avoidance of overheating is equally important when counseling patients about exercise in pregnancy.

During counseling, emphasis should be placed on individual response. The desire to stay fit has to be balanced with potential effects on the mother and fetus. Women who are well conditioned before pregnancy may continue their activity at reduced levels. For a majority of women who have had no exposure to cardiovascular conditioning, the initiation of such a program during pregnancy should be avoided.

PULMONARY PHYSIOLOGY

The main function of the respiratory system is oxygen–carbon dioxide exchange (see also Chapter 118). The respiratory center, controlled by PO_2, PCO_2, and pH, determines the rate and amplitude of the respiratory effort. Mechanical and hormonal alterations in pregnancy cause many changes in the respiratory system.

Anatomic Changes

The increased intra-abdominal pressure during pregnancy causes changes in the thoracic cavity. The transverse diameter increases by about 2 cm. A flaring of the lower ribs occurs, and the costal angle increases from 68.5 to 103 degrees.[48] These changes are reversible and disappear a few weeks after delivery. The diaphragmatic motion is increased, and breathing in pregnancy is more diaphragmatic than costal.[49]

Hormonal Factors

The tidal volume and minute ventilation are increased during pregnancy, leading to arterial blood gas changes similar to a compensated respiratory alkalosis.[50] Although the increased oxygen consumption and the decreased PCO_2 can be explained teleologically, the exact mechanism for the increased ventilation is not clear. Prowse and Gaensler reported a fourfold increase in ventilation after a PCO_2 increase of 1 mm Hg in a pregnant woman compared to a nonpregnant woman.[50] Progesterone administration was found to increase the respiratory center sensitivity to CO_2.[51] Some investigators believe that progesterone can directly stimulate the respiratory center.[52]

Prostaglandins have an effect on the bronchial tree. Most of the prostaglandins produced in pregnancy (E series) have a bronchodilating effect.[53] However, their clinical significance for pulmonary function in pregnancy is unclear. From a teleologic perspective, it is conceivable that the decreased resistance of the large airways and the general bronchodilation during pregnancy can be explained by the prostaglandins produced in pregnancy. However, it is doubtful that uteroplacental prostinoids reach the pulmonary vasculature in appreciable quantities.

Lung Volumes and Capacities

All lung volumes can be measured by spirometry except the residual volume (RV), which is the remaining volume after forced expiration. The total lung capacity can be divided into four basic volumes: (1) the *RV*, which is mentioned above; (2) the *expiratory reserve volume*, which is the exhaled volume in forced expiration (after normal expiration); (3) the *tidal volume*, which is the volume inspired and expired in normal respiration; and (4) the *inspiratory reserve volume*, which is the volume inhaled in deep maximum inspiration above the tidal volume (Fig. 4–3).

Combinations of volumes will give different capacities: *Total lung capacity* includes all volumes; *inspiratory capacity* is the sum of the tidal volume and inspiratory reserve volume; *vital capacity* includes the tidal, expiratory, and inspiratory reserve volumes; and *functional residual capacity* is the residual volume combined with the expiratory reserve volume (see Fig. 4–3).

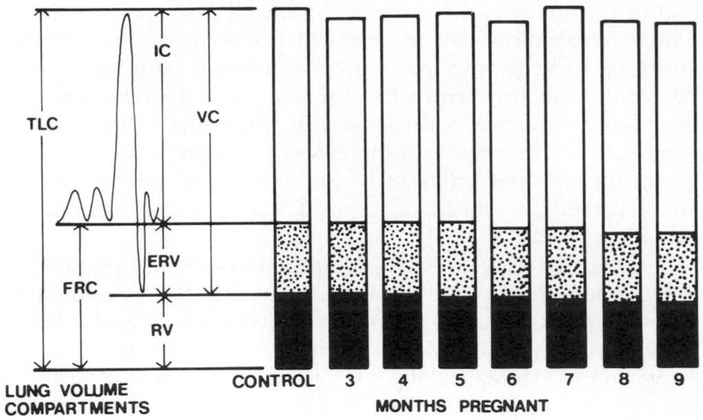

Figure 4–3. Serial measurements of lung volume compartments during pregnancy. (TLC, total lung capacity; FRC, functional residual capacity; IC, inspiratory capacity; ERV, expiratory reserve volume; RV, residual volume; VC, vital capacity.) (*From Prowse and Gaensler,[50] with permission.*)

Lung volumes are not changed in the first half of pregnancy. In the second half of pregnancy, the main change is gradual reduction of the residual volume[54,55] (Table 4–4 and Figure 4–4). The change results mainly from the elevation of the diaphragm and the changes in the chest configuration. Another factor that is important in the determination of the residual volume includes chest wall stiffness, which is decreased in pregnancy, allowing for more inward movement and reduction in the residual trapped volume.[56] The airway closure volume, which is increased in pregnancy because of congestion of the small airways is also reduced.[57] This increase is overcome by the elevation of the diaphragm and the decreased stiffness of the thoracic wall, creating a net decrease of the residual volume. The residual volume is decreased from 1500 to 1200 mL, and the expiratory reserve volume is decreased by 200 mL, bringing the decrease of the functional residual capacity to 500 mL.[55] The vital capacity shows a slight increase. An increase in tidal volume from 500 to 700 mL occurs.[54] Total lung capacity does not change, but the volumes are rearranged with an increase in the tidal respiratory volume and a decrease in the residual and expiratory volumes (see Fig. 4–4).

TABLE 4–4. CHANGES IN VOLUMES AND CAPACITIES IN THE SECOND HALF OF PREGNANCY

Volumes	
Inspiratory reserve volume (IRV)	Increased 300 mL
Tidal volume (TV)	Increased 200 mL
Expiratory reserve volume (ERV)	Decreased 200 mL
Residual volume (RV)	Decreased 300 mL
Capacities	
Inspiratory reserve capacity (TV + IRV)	Increased 500 mL
Functional residual capacity (RV + ERV)	Decreased 500 mL
Vital capacity (TV + IRV + ERV)	Increased 300 mL
Total lung capacity	Unchanged

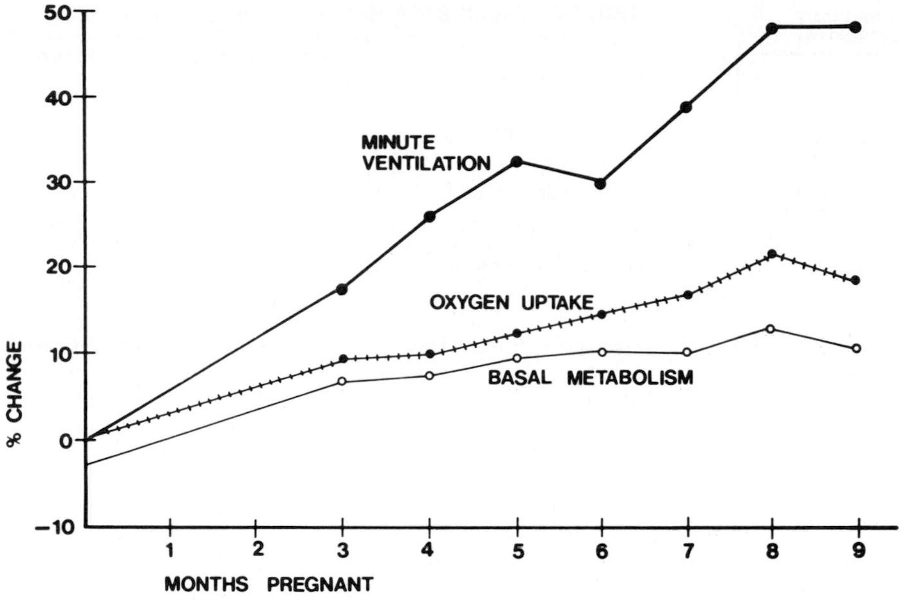

Figure 4–4. Time course of percent changes in minute ventilation, oxygen uptake, and basal metabolism during pregnancy. (*From Prowse and Gaensler[50] with permission.*)

Airway Function

Lung function can be measured by three main parameters: air flow, ventilation, and diffusing capacity (Table 4–5). The air flow depends on the resistance at the different levels of the respiratory tract. The two most important factors in the resistance to air flow are the bronchial smooth muscle tone and the degree of congestion of bronchial wall capillaries. Pregnancy is characterized by decreased resistance and increased flow in the large airways, in which blood vessel congestion plays a minor role. Bronchodilation may be caused by the increase in prostaglandin production during pregnancy.[53] In the small airways, vascular congestion plays a more significant role than bronchial relaxation, and, consequently, air flow will be decreased. According to various authors, the total airway resistance in pregnancy is either minimally decreased or unchanged.[57]

Large airway function is measured using the *forced expiration volume* in one section after maximal inspiration (FEV_1). About 80–85% of the *forced vital capacity* (FVC) is expired in the first second in healthy pregnant and nonpregnant women.[58] This useful clinical measurement can be used to differentiate patients with respiratory insufficiency secondary to asthma from other causes. Because of the bronchoconstriction, the FEV_1/FVC is sharply diminished in pregnant and nonpregnant patients.

The small airway diameter can be assessed by measuring the closing volume. As noted above, vascular congestion in the bronchial wall in pregnancy causes the increase in this volume.[57] If the closing capacity exceeds the functional residual capacity, then the airway closure occurs during tidal breathing.[59] This could decrease the ventilation–perfusion ratio in lung bases where most of the closing volume exists, and can consequently decrease the PO_2. However, studies during pregnancy did not confirm such an increase in the closing volume; they attribute the reduced differences between closing capacity and functional residual capacity to a decreased expiratory reserve volume and functional capacity, which occurs during pregnancy.[60,61] Other small airway tests, such as the maximal expiratory flow-volume curve, are not changed in pregnancy, supporting the theory that there is no alteration in small airway function.[60]

TABLE 4–5. PULMONARY FUNCTIONS IN PREGNANCY

Forced expiratory volume (FEV_1)	Unchanged
Closing volume	Small increase or unchanged
Minute volume	40–50% increase
Alveolar ventilation	40–50% increase
Respiratory rate	No change
Oxygen consumption at rest	15−20% increase

Ventilation

The *minute volume* (tidal volume × respiratory rate) is increased in pregnancy by 40% from 7.5 to 10.5 L/min (see Table 4–4).[50,51] An increase in both respiratory rate and tidal volume occurs.[58] The *alveolar ventilation* in pregnancy ([tidal volume − dead space] × respiratory rate) is increased by 50% despite a 60-mL increase in the dead space caused by bronchodilation.[58] These changes easily explain the common clinical observation by pregnant patients early in their pregnancy that they feel short of breath. Later in pregnancy, the sensation is augmented by increased pressure on the diaphragm.

The increase in minute volume in pregnancy occurs not only before any significant physiologic demand, but also exceeds the additional oxygen consumption (Figure 4–5).[50] This hyperventilation is explained by the direct effect of progesterone on the respiratory center or on its sensitivity to CO_2.[51,52]

Pregnancy imposes less stress on the respiratory system than on the cardiovascular system. Although both systems increase their functional capacity by 30–40% in pregnancy, their reserve capacities are different. The minute ventilation can increase tenfold to 80 L/min during exercise compared to a cardiac output reserve that is only threefold of the pregnancy resting value.[62] Because respiratory reserve is far greater than cardiac reserve, exacerbations of respiratory diseases during pregnancy often are better tolerated than those of cardiac disease.[62]

Exercise in pregnancy is not limited by the respiratory reserve. The response to exercise represents a greater in-

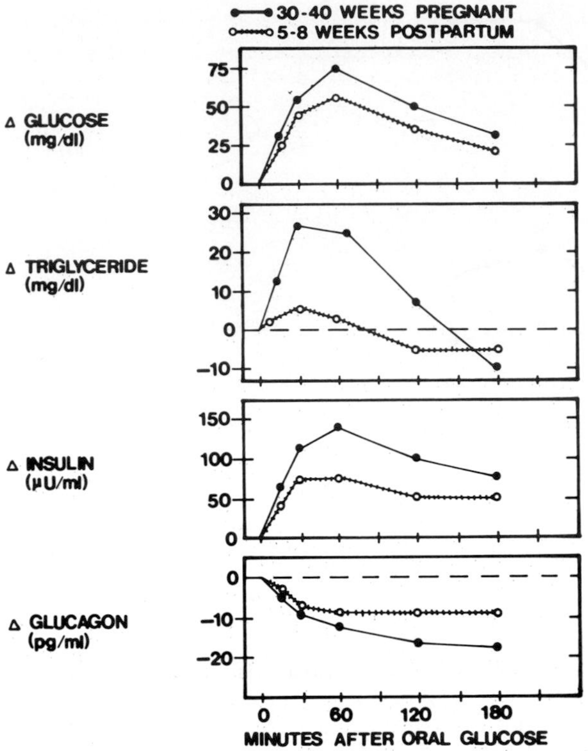

Figure 4–5. The effect of oral glucose administration on maternal plasma glucose, triglyceride, insulin, and glucagon concentrations. The data are expressed as changes from the basal concentrations. (*From Freinkel*[129] *with permission.*)

crease in oxygen consumption and ventilation compared to the nonpregnant state. Moreover, the increase in ventilation is disproportionately greater than the increase in oxygen consumption.

Oxygen consumption at rest increases by 15–20% (30–40 mL/min) in late pregnancy (Figure 4–4 and Table 4–5).[50] The ventilatory equivalent, which is the minute volume divided by the oxygen consumption, is therefore also increased.

Diffusing Capacity

The diffusing capacity of oxygen from the alveolus to the pulmonary capillary depends on the thickness of the intervening membranes and on the pulmonary blood flow. Milne and coworkers,[63] using carbon monoxide to evaluate the diffusing capacity, found an increase in early pregnancy followed by a decrease until 24 to 27 weeks. The values remain constant in the last trimester and increase again in the postpartum period. The increase in early pregnancy can be explained by increased pulmonary blood flow. In the second trimester, the hemodilution decreases the hemoglobin concentration and the oxygen diffusion. The decrease in the diffusing capacity is compensated by an increase in alveolar ventilation, improved gas mixing, and higher PO_2 in the alveoli.

Acid-Base Balance and Blood Gases

Arterial PCO_2 is decreased in pregnancy, reflecting the increased ventilation.[64] It is approximately 30 mm Hg compared to 35–40 mm Hg in the nonpregnant state (Table 4–5 and Table 4–6). This decrease in PCO_2 facilitates CO_2 transfer from the fetal to the maternal circulation and thus is teleologically advantageous. To compensate, bicarbonate is secreted through the kidney to maintain the pH in the normal range of 7.4–7.45.[64] Some authors have found the pH to be in the mildly alkaline range of 7.41–7.47.[65] Serum bicarbonate and sodium decrease, resulting in a slight fall in osmolality. An increase in base deficit to 3.4 mEq/L is the consequence.[65]

TABLE 4–6. ACID-BASE BALANCE AND BLOOD GASES

	Nonpregnant	Pregnant
PO_2 (mm Hg)	98–100	101–104
PCO_2 (mm Hg)	35–40	25–30
Arterial pH	7.38–7.44	7.40–7.45
Bicarbonate (mEq/L)	24–30	18–21
Base deficit (mEq/L)	0.07	3–4

Adapted from references 63-65.

Arterial PO_2 increases in pregnancy compared to the nonpregnant state.[66] The increase in PO_2 is explained by the relative increase in alveolar ventilation compared to the additional requirement of pregnancy. This increase occurs despite a decrease in diffusing capacity[63] and an increase in alveolar–arterial gradients.[66] The increase in PO_2 has a minor effect on oxygen saturation in healthy subjects at sea level. However, at high altitudes, the effect of pregnancy on oxygen saturation can be significant. In two studies of pregnant women at high altitudes, the arterial PO_2 was approximately 60 mm Hg compared to 50 mm Hg in the nonpregnant state.[67,68] This compensatory increase in ventilation and PO_2 has a significant effect on oxygen saturation because it affects the oxyhemoglobin saturation curve in the area of its maximal slope. Moreover, at high altitudes, the hyperventilation of pregnancy seems to be accentuated.[69] This mechanism of compensation helps pregnant women under hypoxic conditions to maintain higher PO_2 relative to nonpregnant subjects.[67,68]

In summary, the major changes in the respiratory function in pregnancy are decreased residual volume, increased sensitivity of the respiratory center to PCO_2, increased ventilation, increased PO_2, decreased PO_2, and blood gases resembling a compensated respiratory alkalosis.

THE URINARY SYSTEM

The urinary tract undergoes many changes during pregnancy. The main factors affecting these changes are the mechanical pressure by the growing uterus, the hormonal milieu, and the increase in cardiac output and renal blood flow. The practitioner caring for pregnant patients must be familiar with the pregnancy-related changes of kidney function, which affect serum values of electrolytes and other solutes (see also Chapter 142).

Anatomic Changes

The kidney undergoes slight enlargement in pregnancy. Reviews of pyelographies performed in the immediate postpartum period and compared to those performed 6 months later indicate an increased kidney length of 1 cm in late pregnancy.[70] The kidney in pregnancy weighs about 50 g more than in the nonpregnant state.[71] Most of this increase probably represents increased blood or water content.[72] The histology of the kidney is similar in the pregnant and nonpregnant states.[73]

Changes in the collecting system (renal pelvis, calyces, and ureters) are more significant. A dilatation of the entire system that begins early in pregnancy and is more pronounced on the right side has been reported.[70] One mechanism responsible for ureteral dilatation is partial ureteral obstruction at the pelvic brim by the growing uterus. This obstruction is more pronounced on the right side because of the normal uterine dextrorotation caused by the rectosigmoid. The general smooth muscle relaxation of pregnancy, which is hormonally mediated, also affects the ureter.[70,74] It persists up to 3 months after delivery. Another possible factor in the dilatation of the collecting system is the increased urine volume of pregnancy.[75] This suggestion is based on experience with diabetes insipidus, in which urine volume is also increased.[76]

Renal Hemodynamics

Renal plasma flow and glomerular filtration rate (GFR) increase in the first trimester. They peak in the second trimester to values 30–50% above those in the nonpregnant state.[77] Although most authors have documented the increase in renal hemodynamics, differences exist in the amplitude of the reported change and pattern late in pregnancy. Many factors can affect the various measurements of renal function, especially in the pregnant state. As an example, the increased dead space created by the dilatation of the collecting system may interfere with timed urine collection. Intravenous fluid increases renal hemodynamics, and as a result the patient should be maintained on oral fluids during 24-hour urine collection. Sodium restriction tends to decrease the renal plasma flow and glomerular filtration rate; therefore, sodium intake should be standardized.[78]

Most authors have found that late in pregnancy, supine or sitting positions decrease the renal plasma flow, glomerular filtration rate, sodium excretion, and urine flow.[79] Measurements of renal function in the lateral recumbent position result in stable values after the peak of the second trimester.[80] Renal plasma flow, as estimated by para-aminohippuric acid clearance, increases from about 500 mL/min in the nonpregnant state to 700 mL/min. Glomerular filtration, as estimated by 24-hour creatinine clearance, increases from about 100 mL/min to 140–150 mL/min in the second trimester and shows some decline toward the end of pregnancy.[81] Measurement of the glomerular filtration rate by intravenous insulin or creatinine clearance reveals higher maximal values (160–170 mL/min) without a decrease in the last trimester.[81] This is explained by the temporary increase in intravascular volume and renal plasma flow.

Filtration Fraction

The proportion of renal plasma flow that is filtered through the glomerulus is the filtration fraction. In the nonpregnant state, it is 20%. In the first 30 weeks of pregnancy, it decreases to 10% because of a fall in the postglomerular afferent arterial resistance. In the last 10 weeks of pregnancy, the filtration fraction rises to 22%.[77] This rise is explained by the fall in plasma oncotic pressure and the efferent vasoconstriction.

Mechanisms of the Increased Renal Hemodynamics

The distribution of the increased cardiac output favors the uteroplacental unit and kidneys. Renal blood flow is increased by 40%.[77,79] The preferential increase in flow to the kidneys and uterus may be explained by local production of prostaglandins, causing vasodilation and decreased vascular resistance. This concept of autoregulation, suggesting that an organ controls its own blood flow, has been demonstrated in the kidney[82,83] and is discussed in more detail under Cardiovascular Changes.

Glucose Filtration and Reabsorption

Glucose is filtered by the glomerulus and reabsorbed by the renal tubule. The old concept of *maximal tubular reabsorption capacity for glucose* (TMG) has been challenged. The tubular reabsorption of glucose has been shown to continue to rise as the GFR increases.[84] Most of the glucose reabsorption occurs in the proximal tubule, and many factors are involved. Increased GFR and decreased sodium and bicarbonate reabsorption affect glucose reabsorption. Some of the glucose reabsorption occurs in the distal tubule. In the nonpregnant patient, the TMG will be determined by the GFR–reabsorption ratio.

In pregnancy, glucose reabsorption is less effective, causing an increase in the GFR–tubular reabsorption ratio.[84] This causes a decrease in TMG. Welsh and Sims[84] report that the TMG in the nonpregnant state is 366 mg/min. In two groups of pregnant women with the same GFR, 13 patients with glucosuria had a TMG of 310 mg/min compared to 378 mg/min in 16 nonglucosuric pregnant women. As a result of these changes, glucosuria can occur in normal pregnancy because of the increased GFR coupled with a diminished capacity for reabsorption. The decrease in sodium and bicarbonate reabsorption, caused by the volume expansion in pregnancy, leads to a decrease in glucose reabsorption. A decreased glucose reabsorption also occurs in the distal tubule.[84] Women with a lower capacity for glucose reabsorption (TMG) in the nonpregnant state will have glucosuria in pregnancy once the GFR starts to increase.[85] The incidence of glucosuria in pregnancy may be as high as 50%.[86] It can start early in pregnancy and peak between 8 and 11 weeks. In some patients, marked glucosuria also can be manifested in late pregnancy. The blood glucose threshold for glucosuria is 155 ± 17 mg/dL in the pregnant state compared to 194 ± 6 mg/dL in the nonpregnant state.[87] Nonpregnant patients with normal carbohydrate metabolism loose less than 100 mg of glucose daily. In pregnancy, 90% of women excrete daily more than 100 mg of glucose, many of them more than 1 g, and some up to 10 g.[86]

Amino Acids and Protein

As a result of the increase in GFR and the decrease in tubular reabsorption, increased urinary excretion of most amino acids occurs in pregnancy. Coupled with the increased uterine uptake, the plasma levels of most amino acids are reduced. Hytten and Cheyne studied the excretion of 19 amino acids during pregnancy and found different patterns of excretion for different amino acids.[88] The urinary loss of amino acids can reach 2 g/d, which might be important in the nutritional counseling of malnourished populations.

In the nonpregnant state, the upper limit for "physiological proteinuria" is 150 mg/24 hours.[89] In pregnancy, most consider the upper limit to be 300 mg/24 hours. This is a result of the increased glomerular filtration. Orthostatic proteinuria is more common in pregnancy but does not increase the risks of these individuals; however, it is important to rule out other causes of proteinuria.

Uric Acid

Uric acid is filtered in the glomerulus, reabsorbed in the proximal tubule, and actively excreted in the distal tubule. In pregnancy, the amount of uric acid excreted daily does not change. Urate clearance is increased from 6–12 mL/min in the nonpregnant state to 12–20 mL/min in the pregnant state. The serum level decreases from 4.2 ± 1.2 mg/dL to 3 ± 0.17 mg/dL, respectively.[90] Most of the increase in clearance is caused by an increase in proximal tubular excretion as a result of increased renal plasma flow (RPF). The net tubular reabsorption is decreased.[90] In late pregnancy, urate clearance decreases, and serum volumes approach those of nonpregnant women. This is mainly a result of a decrease in distal tubular secretion and a net increase in tubular reabsorption.[90] Urate clearance is sensitive to changes in renal plasma flow. The decrease in renal plasma flow and in renal clearance of urate accounts for the hyperuricemia often observed in patients with preeclampsia. In patients known to have normal serum urate levels, acute elevations may be one of the earliest signs of preeclampsia. A laboratory test, therefore, can be useful in distinguishing preeclampsia from other clinical problems.

Sodium Balance

The kidneys regulate sodium. In pregnancy, a retention of about 1000 mEq of sodium has been reported, which is used for the expansion of the intravascular and extravascular fluid compartment.[91] The increase in GFR is accomplished by increased tubular absorption of sodium to prevent sodium depletion. This represents one of the major renal adaptations during pregnancy. In spite of the hypervolemia and the increase in filtered sodium, pregnant women have a similar response to changes in sodium intake as nonpregnant women. On a low-sodium diet, however, a more significant increase in aldosterone occurs in the pregnant, rather than nonpregnant, state.[81] On a high-sodium diet, the decrease in aldosterone is less than expected from nonpregnant women. In pregnancy, plasma sodium decreased by 3–4 mEq/L, and 24-hour urine sodium excretion increased by 20–30 mEq compared to the nonpregnant state.[91]

Potassium Balance

Pregnant patients tend to form alkaline urine because of the increased excretion of bicarbonate. As a result of the bicarbonate excretion, increased aldosterone levels, and other mineralocorticoids, potassium loss should be expected. However, pregnant patients are resistant to potassium loss, and about 350 mEq are retained during pregnancy. The antagonistic action of progesterone to the mineralocorticoids is responsible for the potassium conservation.[92] In fact, the hypokalemia of primary aldosteronism is improved in pregnancy.

Acid-Base Balance

Because of the increased ventilation in pregnancy, there is a decrease in PCO_2. To compensate for this, bicarbonate excretion increases, creating serum values in pregnancy of 17–22 mEq/L compared to 24–28 mEq/L in the nonpregnant state.[64] The arterial pH increases from 7.40 to 7.44, a state sometimes referred to as *compensated respiratory alkalosis* (see Table 4–4). This results in a decreased buffering capacity leaving the pregnant patient more susceptible to ketoacidosis or lactoacidosis.

Water Excretion and Osmolality

In pregnancy, a decrease in plasma osmolality of 10 mOsm/kg occurs compared to the nonpregnant state.[91] However, antidiuretic hormone (ADH) level does not decrease as expected, suggesting the osmoreceptor system is set on a lower plasma osmolality. As a result, water loading or deprivation will lead to urine dilution or concentration, respectively, as in the nonpregnant situation.[78,83] Urine volume is increased about 25% in pregnancy, and daily sodium excretion also is increased.[91] Consequently, urine osmolality is not significantly different. However, in pregnant patients assuming the lateral recumbent position, urine osmolality decreases. Renal concentration tests are therefore less reliable in this position compared to sitting or supine positions, in which the urine flow is decreased.[93] Urinary dilution, on the other hand, is better tested in the lateral recumbent position.

Clinical Application

The anatomic changes of pregnancy in the collecting system are reversed 8–12 weeks postpartum. Hence, the interpretation of intravenous pyelography before this period should include considerations of pregnancy's effects.

Because of the increased GFR, an increased amount of glucose and amino acids enters the urine. This, coupled with the increased urinary dead space caused by ureteral dilatation, may predispose patients to an increased incidence of urinary tract infections. Similarly, acute pyelitis in pregnant women with asymptomatic bacteriuria may occur more often than in nonpregnant women.

As a result of the increase in GFR, decreased blood levels of blood urea nitrogen, creatinine, and uric acid occur. More proteinuria exists, up to 300 mg/24 hours, compared to 150 mg/24 hours, in the nonpregnant state. The clearance of water-soluble vitamins is increased in pregnancy. Glucosuria is more common in pregnancy; it may be intermittent, and day-to-day variations are frequent. Glucosuria is not always related to blood levels of glucose; therefore, blood levels of glucose and not those of urine should be used for control of diabetes.

Because the supine position decreases the GFR and consequently urine output and natriuresis[93], lateral recumbency is the preferred position for pregnant women.

THE DIGESTIVE TRACT

Gastrointestinal complaints are common in pregnancy. Nausea and vomiting are frequent in early pregnancy, and heartburn primarily occurs in late pregnancy. Gastrointestinal symptoms can mimic disease states such as cholecystitis, pancreatitis, and appendicitis; sometimes a delay in diagnosis or operative intervention may occur in patients with significant disease because symptoms may be attributed to pregnancy. To allow for a proper differential diagnosis, it is essential to be familiar with the anatomic and physiologic changes of the gastrointestinal tract during pregnancy.

Mouth

The amount of saliva is not increased in pregnancy.[94] Ptyalism, excessive secretion of saliva, is common in women with nausea who might have difficulties in swallowing their saliva. This should not be confused with emesis. The gums become hyperemic and edematous during pregnancy and may tend to bleed. The edema is partly caused by chemical changes in the connective tissue with an increase in mucopolysaccharides, which are hydrophilic.[95]

Esophagus

Lower esophageal sphincter (LES) pressure is decreased in pregnancy. The decrease correlates positively with gestational age and returns to normal 1 to 7 weeks postpartum.[96] This decrease in pressure is the main cause of heartburn during pregnancy. The decrease in sphincter pressure is attributed to the smooth-muscle-relaxing activity of progesterone, as is also demonstrated in patients using oral contraceptives.[97] Heartburn is the result of reflux of hydrochloric and bile acids into the esophagus. The reflux results not only from low LES pressure, but also from the increased intra-abdominal pressure of pregnancy as term approaches. An additional factor in the subsequent development of reflux esophagitis is the decreased motility of the distal esophagus, which prevents appropriate drainage of the refluxed acid back into the stomach.[98]

Stomach

The effect of pregnancy on gastric acid secretion is not clear. Van Thiel et al have found no change in basal or postprandial secretion of gastric acid.[96] Murray, et al report a decrease in the basal and histamine-stimulated gastric acid secretion in the second trimester.[99] The secretion of pepsin parallels the changes in the output of gastric acid.[100] The reduced gastric secretion could account for the improvement of peptic ulcers sometimes observed in pregnancy.

The stomach is both hypomotile and hypotonic in pregnancy. This effect is also caused by the systemic relaxation of smooth muscles by progesterone. Davison et al report that the gastric emptying time is prolonged in pregnancy and even more so after ingestion of solid foods.[101] This observation can be explained by slower digestion, which is a result of decreased gastric acid and pepsin secretion. The delayed gastric emptying also is responsible for the delayed absorption after a glucose meal.[102] This explains why aspiration of gastric contents at the time of anesthesia for cesarean section results in high maternal mortality.

Small Intestine

Absorption of iron and calcium is improved in pregnancy.[103] This may be caused by a combination of decreased intestinal motility and better absorption, or it may represent a response to an increasing need. Parry et al have documented decreased motility of the small bowel during pregnancy.[104] The compensatory increase in small-bowel efficiency in pregnancy has been demonstrated in patients after resection of large segments of the small bowel.[105]

Large Intestine

Constipation, which is a frequent complaint during pregnancy, is attributed to decreased motility of the colon and increased water absorption during pregnancy.[106] More water and sodium are absorbed in pregnancy than in the nonpregnant state. Angiotensin and aldosterone, both increased in pregnancy, have been implicated in this phenomenon.[107] Iron supplementation also may contribute to constipation.

Liver

Pregnancy has a significant effect on liver function (see also Chapter 15). Estrogen and progesterone modify the metabolism and excretion of bilirubin. During pregnancy and in women using oral contraceptives, an increased incidence of cholestatic jaundice has been reported.[108] Some pregnant patients may have only pruritus related to biliary stasis. Spider angiomata, pruritus, and elevated levels of alkaline phosphatase (of placental origin) and lipids, all common observations in normal pregnancy, can mimic liver disease.

In a review of autopsy records of pregnant patients, Combes and Adams did not find an increase in liver size compared to nonpregnant controls.[108] Also, there was no evidence suggesting an increase in hepatic blood flow. The histologic picture of the liver during normal pregnancy demonstrates only minor, nonspecific changes, such as increased fat and glycogen storage and variations in the size of individual cells.[109] In pregnant monkeys and after estrogen stimulation, enhanced phagocytosis and proliferation of the reticuloendothelial cells (Kupffer's cells) have been reported.[110,111]

Both pregnant women and those using birth control pills who have cholestatic jaundice show on histology dilated canaliculi and increased bile viscosity.[110,112]

Pregnancy and exogenous estrogens modify the synthesis of proteins in the liver. Fibrinogen synthesis increases significantly during pregnancy.[113] Estrogens and pregnancy increase the synthesis of binding proteins, which explains the increase in protein-bound iodine, corticosteroids, and testosterone. Total serum protein decreases in pregnancy, mainly because of the decrease in serum albumin concentration.[114] The decrease in serum albumin is attributed to the hemodilution of pregnancy and to decreased synthesis. Globulins show a small increase, resulting in a net albumin–globulin ratio of close to 1.[114]

The liver is capable of conjugating and excreting toxic waste substances in pregnancy. Sulfobromophthalein (BSP) clearance, once commonly used to assess this function, is reduced for a number of reasons,[115] including increased protein binding and storage in the liver and decreased biliary excretion. With the standard BSP test, the pregnant patient retains 10% of the BSP after 45 min compared to 5% in the nonpregnant state.[116] Tindall reports that, when using a modified BSP test (serial sampling of BSP for 60 min after intravenous injection), the excretory efficiency decreased from 85–95% in the nonpregnant state to 55–66% with singleton pregnancy. In twin gestation, the values were even lower, approaching 40–50%.[117] Estrogen administration was found to decrease excretory function of the liver, and estrogens are probably responsible for these changes in pregnancy.[118]

Bilirubin is handled as BSP by conjugation and excretion. However, there is disagreement in the literature about normal bilirubin levels in pregnancy. Some authors report increased levels in pregnancy, while others find no changes.[119,120] It is possible that these different results represent the fact that some patients are more prone to bilirubin retention. Steroid hormones can act as inhibitors of glucoronyl transferase. Pruritus and cholestatic jaundice of pregnancy are extreme manifestations of the previously mentioned changes and may represent increased sensitivity of the liver to estrogen.[121] Women in Scandinavia and Chile are genetically predisposed to cholestatic jaundice of pregnancy.[119]

The serum transminases, aspartate aminotransferase (formerly SGOT) and alanine aminotransferase (formerly SGPT), are not increased in pregnancy. Alkaline phosphatase is increased twofold to fourfold. Most of the increase results from synthesis by the placenta. Placental alkaline phosphatase is heat stable, and its measurement was once used as a placental function test and test of fetal well-being. Other fetal surveillance techniques have replaced this.

Gallbladder

Pregnancy increases the size and decreases the motility of the gallbladder.[122] The residual gallbladder volume after emptying is twice as large as in the nonpregnant state. The increase in gallbladder volume dilutes the bile and decreases its solubility of cholesterol. The cholesterol then precipitates to form crystals and stones. Pregnancy and estrogen–progesterone compounds decrease the concentration of chenodeoxycholic acid and increase the cholesterol concentration.[123] The decrease in motility and increase in volume, combined with changes in the bile and its composition, explain the correlation between the incidence of cholelithiasis and parity. Cholelithiasis should be considered when pregnant women have upper abdominal complaints, especially because diagnostic ultrasound of the gallbladder is easily accomplished. The clinical presentation of this disease often occurs toward the end of the woman's reproductive period.

METABOLIC CHANGES

The need of the growing fetus for substrates to satisfy the caloric requirements for growth and metabolism necessitate major changes in the metabolism of the three main nutrients—protein, fat, and carbohydrates—during pregnancy (see also Chapter 29). Hormonal changes, particularly the increase in steroid hormones and insulin with insulin antagonists, are the basis for these metabolic changes. Human placental lactogen (HPL), also called human chorionic somatotropin, probably represents the most important hormone responsible for the increased use of lipids for maternal caloric needs. Its purpose is presumably to spare the available glucose and amino acids for fetal use.

The fasting blood glucose is physiologically important because it represents the actual glucose level during most hours of the day.[124] The basal glucose level depends on the production and consumption of glucose. The production, which occurs mostly by glycogenolysis and gluconeogenesis in the liver, depends on low circulating levels of insulin, allowing increased release of glucagon.[125]

With an intake of carbohydrates or proteins, a release of insulin occurs, which facilitates the uptake of glucose and amino acids by the tissues. Glucagon release is suppressed by glucose but stimulated by protein intake. Glucagon prevents the hypoglycemia that will follow the release of insulin by the protein meal.[125] Insulin levels increase twofold to tenfold, but with intermittent feedings of mixed meals, blood glucose excursions generally stay within a range of 30–40 mg/dL over basal values.[126] After an oral glucose load of 50 g, the glucose peaks at 30 minutes, and the fasting value is achieved at 60 minutes. The peak increase in glucose values should be no more than 30–35 mg/dL.[127] The plasma insulin curve is similar to that of glucose, but the peak is reached after 45 minutes, and the basal level is reached 2 hours after the glucose load. Insulin levels increase from 6–40 μU/mL (Fig. 4–5).[127]

The Fasting State in Pregnancy

Fasting plasma glucose is reduced as soon as 10–15 weeks of pregnancy by 5–10 mg/dL compared to the nonpregnant state.[127,128] It is not clear whether a further decrease occurs as pregnancy progresses.[127] The duration of fasting might be critical in the determination of fasting values. Felig and Lynch report that 12–14 hours of fasting are required to produce a significant difference in glucose levels between pregnant and nonpregnant women.[128] As the fasting time is prolonged, the discrepancy between fasting glucose values in pregnant and nonpregnant women increases. After 35 hours of fasting, pregnant women drop their plasma glucose to a hypoglycemic range of approximately 50 mg/dL compared to 70 mg/dL in the nonpregnant state.[128] Plasma glucose levels during sleep in late pregnancy are lower than in nonpregnant women. Freinkel characterizes this change as accelerated starvation.[129]

The mechanism for the decreased fasting glucose levels is not completely understood. Many factors are involved. Glucose and amino acid uptake by the uteroplacental fetal unit occurs. Renal clearance of glucose and amino acids increases, and the low levels of amino acids, caused by hemodilution, make amino acids less available for gluconeogenesis. Hepatic glucose production is therefore subnormal in pregnancy. Glycogenolysis, normally stimulated by a low insulin–glucagon ratio, is decreased in pregnancy because of the increase of this ratio.[128] Estrogen and progesterone also favor glycogenesis and decrease the glucagon-induced glycogenolysis. The increase in glucose consumption by the fetus and placenta in the second half of pregnancy and the concomitant decrease in hepatic production result in accelerated starvation, lower fasting glucose values, and the use of fatty acids stored in early pregnancy to satisfy maternal caloric requirements.

Lipolysis in the fasting state is increased during the second half of pregnancy. The levels of free fatty acids are increased compared to the nonpregnant state, as are metabolites of its β-oxidation, ketone bodies, which are also found in higher levels after fasting.[128] After an overnight fast, blood levels of ketone bodies are elevated in pregnancy twofold to fourfold compared to the nonpregnant state. As a result, fasting ketonuria should not automatically be interpreted as pathologic. Lipolytic hormones include steroids, ACTH, growth hormones, and glucagon. The insulin–glucagon ratio is increased, indicating that glucagon is not responsible for the enhanced lipolysis. The level of growth hormone decreases in the second half of the pregnancy. The main lipolytic factor in pregnancy is human placental lactogen. This hormone also is hyperglycemic, contributes to insulin resistance and the diabetogenicity of pregnancy, and is discussed later in more detail.

The Fed State in Pregnancy

After a 50-g glucose load, the plasma glucose peak is delayed compared to the nonpregnant state, and the delay becomes longer as pregnancy progresses[129] (Fig. 4–6). At 20 weeks it is 37 min, compared to 55 min at term. The plasma glucose peak concentration is increased over that in the nonpregnant state.[127,129] A concomitant increase in insulin secretion after a glucose load occurs in the last 10 weeks of pregnancy (Fig. 4–6). The insulin peak occurs at 60 min, and levels are still elevated from the baseline at 180 minutes.[129] The glucagon decrease in response to a glucose load is more pronounced in the pregnant woman (Fig. 4–5).

The characteristics of the fed state in late pregnancy as compared with the nonpregnant state include increased hyperglycemic and hyperinsulinemic responses and a diminished peripheral sensitivity to insulin.[129] Pregnancy is a state of decreased tolerance to carbohydrates and has therefore been referred to as a *diabetogenic state.* Indeed, patients, who before pregnancy had normal tolerance to glucose or only latent chemical diabetes, can progress during pregnancy to abnormal tolerance or overt diabetes (see also Chapter 43).

Factors involved in decreased glucose tolerance during pregnancy are multiple. Freinkel has shown that insulin response to the same glucose levels is higher for the pregnant than for the nonpregnant state.[129] On the other hand, glucose uptake after a given dose of insulin is lower in the pregnant than in the nonpregnant state.[130] Tissue sensitivity to insulin has reportedly decreased as much as 80% in pregnancy.[131] This increased resistance does not occur at the insulin receptor level because insulin binding to red blood cells was found to rise during pregnancy.[132] To compensate for the increased insulin resistance, pancreatic β cells hypertrophy, resulting in increased insulin production and serum levels. The high circulating insulin levels cannot

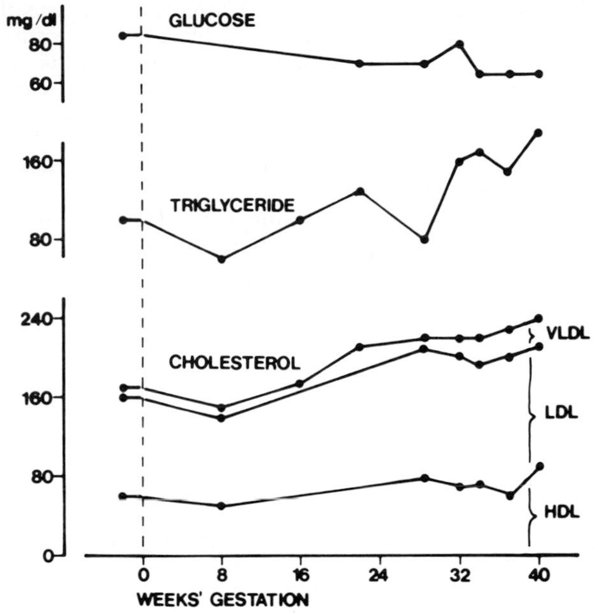

Figure 4–6. Serial changes in concentrations of glucose and lipids during normal pregnancy. (VLDL, very-low density lipoproteins; LDL, low-density lipoproteins; HDL, high-density lipoproteins.) (*From Knopp*[136], *with permission.*)

be explained by either an increase in the inactive proinsulin, which stays at the normal 5–15% range of total insulin, or the total immunoreactive insulin. Insulin destruction by placental or liver insulinase is not increased in pregnancy as had been thought previously. Also, the half-life of insulin is the same in the pregnant as in the nonpregnant state.[132] Carbohydrate metabolism is significantly altered by human placental lactogen. This hormone reduces the sensitivity of peripheral tissues and of the liver to the effect of insulin.[54]

Many hormones are thought to be insulin antagonists. Synthetic estrogen administered to healthy individuals decreases the tolerance to carbohydrates, and resulting insulin levels are increased.[133] Naturally occurring estrogens and progesterones contribute to hyperinsulinemia, but glucose tolerance is improved.[134] Glucagon suppression after glucose load is more pronounced in pregnancy than in the nonpregnant state; therefore, it cannot play a role in the insulin resistance of pregnancy.[129] The same is true for pituitary growth hormone, which decreases as pregnancy progresses.

The main hyperglycemic factor of pregnancy is human placental lactogen (HPL). This polypeptide hormone, which has a metabolic action similar to that of pituitary growth hormone, is synthesized in large amounts by the syncytiotrophoblast of the placenta. The HPL levels increase as pregnancy progresses and plateau after 30 weeks. This coincides with the findings that decreased carbohydrate tolerance is maximal at approximately 30 weeks' gestation. The HPL levels correlate with functional placental mass, and HPL levels are high in twin pregnancy and macrosomia. As a result, the incidence of abnormal glucose tolerance in these conditions is increased. Prolonged infusion of HPL into nonpregnant subjects decreases glucose use and increases insulin levels.[135]

The metabolic actions of HPL include lipolysis, increased free fatty acid blood levels, and decreased sensitivity to exogenous or endogenous insulin. As a result, a net decrease of glucose and amino acid use occurs because these compounds are spared for the fetus. The exact action of HPL on glucose metabolism is not entirely clear. It may induce cellular or metabolic actions that increase the tissue resistance to insulin. Adipose tissues retain normal sensitivity to insulin in early pregnancy when fat deposition occurs. In late pregnancy, HPL increases, and lipolysis is enhanced (see also Chapter 37).

Lipid Metabolism

The accelerated starvation of the second half of pregnancy increases the use of lipids for the energy requirements of pregnancy. Triglycerides and cholesterol increase as pregnancy progresses, and this increase is most marked at term.[136] The increase in triglyceride levels after an oral glucose load is much more significant in late pregnancy (Fig. 4–6). Triglycerides rise progressively throughout pregnancy, and their level is more than tripled at term.[136] The increase occurs proportionately in all lipoprotein fractions. Most of the cholesterol increase during pregnancy occurs in the last trimester and in the low- and very-low-density lipoprotein fraction.[136] The high-density lipoprotein fraction shows little change compared with the nonpregnant state. The increase in triglycerides results mainly from increased synthesis stimulated by estrogen.[137] The mechanism for the rise of cholesterol is, however, unclear. Free fatty acid (FFA) levels are hard to measure and are influenced by many factors. Nevertheless, the pattern shows a decrease in midpregnancy and an increase in the last trimester.[138] The first half of the pregnancy is characterized by fat storage. Insulin is still effective and converts glucose to triglycerides, diminishing the FFA release. In the last trimester, HPL, by its lypolytic action and antagonism to insulin, increases the levels of FFA. This is the time in pregnancy when most of the lipid increase occurs. The FFAs are used by the maternal tissues for the generation of energy; however, some also may be transferred to the fetus, especially the essential fatty acids.[139] In the last trimester, the availability of FFA decreases the use of glucose and amino acids for increased maternal energy requirements and spares them for the fetus. The major hormone affecting this change is HPL.

Fetal Metabolic Considerations

Glucose is used by the fetus and the placenta for caloric requirements and glycogen and fat synthesis. The uptake of glucose each minute by the third trimester fetus is 6 mg/kg compared to 4.2 in the neonate and 2–2.5 in the adult.[7,8] Glucose is transferred from the mother to the fetus by a carrier system (facilitated diffusion). The levels in the fetus are 10–20 mg below maternal values. Amino acids are actively transferred by the placenta and serve as substrates for protein, gluconeogenesis, and oxidative metabolism. Essential fatty acids are transferred to the fetus for anabolic needs. Ketone bodies can be used by the fetal brain and liver and are readily transferred to the fetus.[8]

Insulin, glucagon, and other polypeptides such as HPL are not transferred from the maternal to the fetal circulation. Fetal insulin is secreted in response to fetal glucose and amino acid levels.[140] Persistent fetal hyperglycemia, as a result of maternal hyperglycemia, will result in fetal hyperinsulinemia, and β-cell hyperplasia, causing macrosomia and neonatal hypoglycemia in the offspring of diabetic mothers.

Clinical Fetal Metabolic Considerations

The acceleration of starvation makes the pregnant patient more susceptible to ketosis. Pregnant diabetic patients who are already susceptible to acidosis because of lower bicarbonate value may develop ketoacidosis with only moderate hyperglycemia. The metabolic changes during the fasting and fed states are much more profound in late pregnancy compared to the nonpregnant state. Ideally, pregnant patients should never fast for more than 6–8 hours.

Increased hyperglycemia and hyperinsulinemia after a carbohydrate load necessitate screening for diabetes. Current recommendations include screening all pregnant patients for carbohydrate intolerance at 26–28 weeks' gestation when the maximal diabetogenic effect of HPL occurs. This is performed by measuring serum glucose after a 30-g oral carbohydrate food. Blood sugar >135 mg/dL should be considered abnormal, necessitating standard 3-hour glucose tolerance testing. Clinical screening should, however, be instituted as early as possible when a diabetic state in the mother is suspected (see also Chapter 43).

In summary, the metabolism of carbohydrates, protein, and fat changes with pregnancy. The change serves two purposes: (1) to spare glucose and amino acids for the fetus, which is growing rapidly in the second half of the pregnancy; and (2) to increase fat deposition in the first half of pregnancy, which will be available for maternal use in late pregnancy and during lactation.

The increased insulin resistance in all tissues except fat enhances the conversion of glucose to fat in early pregnancy. In late pregnancy, HPL increases lipolysis and the maternal use of lipids. Fasting blood glucose is lower in pregnancy than in the nonpregnant state, and the tolerance to glucose load is decreased. The paradox of high glucose and high insulin is explained by insulin antagonists, mainly HPL, but is still not completely understood.

HEMATOLOGIC CHANGES

The major changes of the hematologic system during pregnancy include the increase in blood volume and the change in the coagulation system. The increase in blood volume is important for the perfusion of the uteroplacental bed. The increased red blood cell (RBC) mass is important in the protection of the mother against blood loss.

Blood Volume and Red Blood Cell Mass

Blood volume increases 40–50% during pregnancy, about 1600 mL more than the nonpregnant state.[7] The rise starts early in pregnancy, reaches its peak around 30–34 weeks, and plateaus thereafter. Changes in blood volume and related physiologic mechanisms are discussed in detail earlier in this chapter.

Seventy-five percent of the increase in blood volume represents plasma expansion. Only 25% is an increase in RBC mass, which increases by 450 mL (from 1350 mL to 1800 mL).[7] The rise in RBC mass starts later than the rise of plasma volume and continues until delivery.[141] The differences in timing and magnitude of the changes between plasma volume and RBC mass explain the changes in hematocrit observed during pregnancy. As plasma volume increases in the first trimester, hematocrit decreases and reaches its lowest values at 32–34 weeks. In the last 8–10 weeks, the plasma volume reaches a plateau, while RBC mass still increases, resulting in a slight rise in hematocrit. The decrease in hemoglobulin concentration, also called *physiological anemia of pregnancy,* is caused by hemodilution. The total RBC mass is increased.

Red Blood Cell Production

Red blood cell production is increased in pregnancy. Reticulocyte count is higher in the last trimester of pregnancy, and the increased proportion of young cells increases the mean corpuscular volume (MCV).[142] Injected iron is incorporated into the RBC faster in pregnancy than in the nonpregnant state.[143] The RBC half-life is unchanged.[7] The bone marrow is hyperplastic, and the main stimulus is increased levels of erythropoietin,[144] although other hormones, such as HPL and progesterone, may play a role in that change. A slight increase in the synthesis of fetal hemoglobin occurs, reflected as an increased number of fetal cells in the circulation.[145] The physiologic significance of this change is not clear. The compensated respiratory alkalosis of pregnancy tends to shift the oxyhemoglobin saturation curve to the left. However, the increase in 2,3-diphosphoglycerate in maternal RBCs facilitates oxygen release to the fetus. The fetal hemoglobin on the other side of the placental barrier has a higher affinity for oxygen, facilitating an easy exchange.

Iron Metabolism

The increase in RBC mass and fetal requirements modifies the maternal iron metabolism during pregnancy. In the normal adult, total body iron is 3–4 g. In the female, it can be as low as 2 g.[146] Red blood cells contain 60–70% of this iron, and the rest is stored in liver, spleen, and bone marrow. A small fraction (3–4%) is found in myoglobin and other enzyme systems. Obligatory loss by way of the gastrointestinal tract and skin desquamation is about 1 mg/d. Estimated blood loss in the normal menstruating female is 40–60 mL per cycle, which is equal to 20–30 mg iron[147] (1 mL of blood contains 0.5 mg iron). Consequently, the iron requirement in the nonpregnant state is about 2 mg/d. Most American diets contain 10–12 mg iron, and about 10% of this is absorbed.[148] Heme iron, derived from animals (meat and liver), is more readily absorbed than inorganic iron found in vegetables. In pregnancy, the iron requirement is increased to 4 mg/d or about 800 mg for the entire pregnancy.[149] Most of this iron is needed in the second half of pregnancy, when RBC mass and fetus are growing rapidly. The total iron requirement in pregnancy is about 1 g per 450-mg increase in RBC mass. Of that, 350 mg are transferred to the fetus and placenta. A 200-mg obligatory loss through the gut and a 200-mg blood loss during normal singleton delivery occur as well.

Serum iron decreases in pregnancy, whereas the total iron-binding capacity increases as a result of enhanced synthesis of transferrin. The percentage of iron saturation decreases in nonpregnant patients. Serum ferritin levels are a sensitive index of iron stores; normal values are about 35 ng/mL.[150] During pregnancy, however, seemingly normal serum ferritin levels can accompany significant iron deficiency. As a result, calculation of transferrin saturation (from iron binding capacity) may be more predictive. Values less than 16% saturation are considered diagnostic. Ferritin levels, serum iron, and transferrin saturation decrease in the last trimester of pregnancy if iron prophylaxis is not administered.[151] The decreased ferritin levels are not clearly associated with decreased hemoglobin or mean corpuscular volume (MCV).[151] However, some authors have reported such a decrease in unsupplemented patients,[152] while others have documented a larger increase in RBC mass after iron supplementation.[153]

Pregnancy increases the iron requirement beyond the intake from a regular diet. Iron absorption is improved during pregnancy, but maximal absorption from a normal diet is only up to 2.6 mg.

The question of routine iron prophylaxis during pregnancy is still not completely settled. In the well-nourished woman, the iron stores will be partially depleted during pregnancy and replenished afterward. Red blood cell production will not be affected even if iron is not supplemented. On the other hand, in women who are prone to iron deficiency because of multiparity, inadequate spacing of pregnancies, and suboptimal nutrition, iron stores already may be depleted, and RBC production will thus be affected if iron supplements are not used. This is why in low socioeconomic groups, iron prophylaxis is indicated during pregnancy.

In normal pregnancy, a patient can lose as much as 25% of her total blood volume during delivery without any need for compensatory increase in volume after the loss.[145] The blood loss in such a case will be approximately equal to the increase in blood volume during gestation, and the resulting hematocrit will be the same as in the last trimester. If the blood loss is less than 500 mL, as in a normal singleton delivery, the plasma volume will decrease in the first few days postpartum as a result of diuresis. The hematocrit will stablize to the prepregnancy levels as a result of decreased RBC production and destruction of the additional RBC mass formed in pregnancy.

White Blood Cells

Total leukocyte count and, more specifically, the neutrophil count increase during the estrogen peak of the menstrual cycle. If conception occurs, the total white blood cell (WBC) count further increases with a peak at 30 weeks and a plateau thereafter.[154] The mean WBC count in pregnancy is 9000/mm^3, but 30% of normal pregnant women have counts over 10,000/mm^3.[3,155] With the onset of labor, the WBC count can increase up to 25,000–40,000/mm^3, most of the increase reflecting neutrophilia.[156] Normal values are then achieved within the first postpartum week.

There is a major change in the differential count of WBC. The absolute number and percentage of sequential neutrophils increase. Lymphocytes, on the other hand, decrease in absolute number and percentage. Monocytes increase in number but do not change in percentage of total WBC. This leads to a change in the lymphocyte–monocyte ratio, which may affect the immune response.[157] Changes occur in subsets of lymphocytes in pregnancy: B lymphocytes do not change, while T lymphocytes decrease in absolute number.[158] This decline is probably more pronounced in helper T cells because the suppressor T-cell subsets are found to increase.[159] Greatly varying data, however, are reported in the literature.

Platelets

The results of platelet studies are not consistent.[160,161] Most authors report a slight decrease in platelet count in the last trimester, but rarely to below 150,000/mm^2.[161] The mechanism for the decrease is not fully understood. Some authors ascribe the change to hemodilution alone.[161] There is, however, ample evidence that increased use of platelets in pregnancy may be related to chronic localized intravascular clotting in the placenta.[162] The number of platelets further decreases after delivery, but from the third to fifth day postpartum, a sharp increase is noted. As the platelet count decreases during pregnancy, platelet diameter and volume increase. This is a result of the increased platelet formation and decreased life span, resulting in more young platelets in the circulation.[161]

Coagulation Factors

A significant change in coagulation factors occurs in pregnancy (see also Chapter 167). The fibrinogen is increased from the nonpregnant level of 250–400 mg/dL to as high as 600 mg/dL.[163] The high fibrinogen is the main reason for the increased sedimentation rate in pregnancy. The changes in other blood levels are seen in Table 4–7. All levels increased significantly except for factor XI and factor XIII (fibrin stabilizing factor).

The degree of blood coagulability is determined by a dynamic equilibrium between coagulation and fibrinolysis. This has been reviewed in detail elsewhere.[164] The traditional interpretation has been that pregnancy results in a hypercoagulable state as a result of increased coagulation and inhibited fibrinolysis. Ample evidence exists for the activation of the coagulation cascade; fibrinopeptide A, which results from the action of thrombin on fibrinogen, is increased.[165] An increase in fibrin monomers and a decrease in antithrombin III activity, which is a natural anticoagulant, occur.[166]

Whether serum fibrinolytic activity *in vivo* is decreased during pregnancy, however, is less certain. Fletcher et al have suggested that an appropriate fibrinolytic response exists but levels of plasminogen activation are depressed because of sequestration at sites of fibrin deposition.[166] Adequate fibrinolysis also may be inferred from the observation that significant numbers of normal pregnancies at term have detectable fibrin split products in their blood.[167]

At delivery, although a significant amount of fibrinogen is used to cover the placental site, uterine contraction repre-

TABLE 4–7. PLASMA COAGULATION FACTORS AND INHIBITORS IN PREGNANCY

Roman Numeral	Coagulation Factor	Inhibitor	Change in Pregnancy
I	Fibrinogen	Fibrinogen	4.0–6.5 g/l
II	Prothrombin	Factor II	100–125%
IV	Ionic calcium		
V	Proaccelerin	Factor V	100–150%
VII	Proconvertin	Factor VII	150–250%
VIII	Antihemophilic factor A (AHF)	Factor VIII	200–500%
IX	Antihemophilic factor B (Christmas factor)	Factor IX	100–150%
X	Stuart Prower factor	Factor X	150–250%
XI	Antihemophilic factor C	Factor XI	50–100%
XII	Hageman factor	Factor XII	100–200%
XIII	Fibrin-stabilizing factor	Factor XIII	35–75%
		Antihemophilic III	75–100%
		Antifactor Xa	75–100%

Modified from Romero.[164]

sents the primary factor in postpartum hemostasis. Platelets and fibrinogen are consumed after placental separation, and their level decreases. Those levels start to rise again on the third to fifth day postpartum. Fibrinolysis, however, returns to normal within a few hours after delivery of the placenta.[168]

REFERENCES

1. Hytten FE, Chamberlain G. *Clinical Physiology in Obstetrics*. Oxford, England: Blackwell Scientific; 1980;193.
2. Brown JE, Jacobson HN, Askue LH, et al. Influence of pregnancy weight gain on the size of infants born to underweight women. *Obstet Gynecol*. 1981;57:13.
3. Niswander K, Jackson EC. Physical characteristics of the gravida and their association with birth weight and perinatal death. *Am J Obstet Gynecol*. 1974;119:306.
4. Lindheimer M, Katz AI. Sodium and diuretics in pregnancy. *N Engl J Med*. 1973;288:891.
5. Thomson AM, Hytten FE, Billewicz WZ. The epidemiology of edema during pregnancy. *Obstet Gynaecol Br Commonw*. 1967;74:1.
6. Pitkin RM. Nutritional support in obstetrics and gynecology. *Clin Obstet Gynecol*. 1976;19:489.
7. Sparks JW, Girard JR, Battaglia FC. An estimate of the calorie requirements of the human fetus. *Biol Neonate* 1980;38:113.
8. Battaglia FC. The comparative physiology of fetal nutrition. *Am J Obstet Gynecol*. 1984;148:850.
9. Pritchard JA. Changes in the blood volume during pregnancy and delivery. *Anesthesiology*. 1965;26:393.
10. Rovinsky JJ, Jaffin H. Cardiovascular hemodynamics in pregnancy. I. Blood and plasma volumes in multiple pregnancy. *Am J Obstet Gynecol*. 1965;93:1.
11. Assali NS, Vaughn DL. Blood volume in pre-eclampsia: Fantasy and reality. *Am J Obstet Gynecol*. 1977;129:355.
12. Arias F. Expansion of intravascular volume and fetal outcome in patients with chronic hypertension and pregnancy. *Am J Obstet Gynecol*. 1975; 123:610.
13. Christianson RE. Studies on blood pressure during pregnancy. I. Influence of parity and age. *Am J Obstet Gynecol*. 1976;125:509.
14. Quilligan EJ, Tyler C. Postural effects on the cardiovascular status in pregnancy: A comparison on the lateral and supine postures. *Am J Obstet Gynecol*. 1978;130:194.
15. Gant NF, Chand S, Worley RF, et al. A clinical test useful for predicting the development of acute hypertension in pregnancy. *Am J Obstet Gynecol*. 1974;120:1.
16. Kerr MG, Scott DB, Samuel E. Studies of the inferior vena cava in late pregnancy. *Br Med J*. 1964;1:532.
17. Marx GF, Husain FJ, Shiau HF. Brachial and femoral blood pressures during prenatal period. *Am J Obstet Gynecol*. 1980;136:11.
18. Ferris TF. Toxemia and hypertension. In: Burrow GN, Ferris TF, eds. *Medical Complications During Pregnancy*. Philadelphia, PA: WB Saunders; 1982:1.
19. Speroff L. An autoregulatory role for prostaglandins in placental hemodynamics: Their possible influence on blood pressure in pregnancy. *J Reprod Med*. 1975;15:181.
20. Franklin GO, Dowd AJ, Caldwell BV, et al. The effect of angiotensin-II intravenous infusion on plasma renin activity and prostaglandins A, E, and F levels in the uterine vein of the pregnant monkey. *Prostaglandins*. 1974;6:271.
21. Goodman RP, Killam AP, Brash AR, et al. Prostacyclin production during pregnancy and pregnancy complicated by hypertension. *Am J Obstet Gynecol*. 1982;142:817.
22. Pipkin FB, Hunter JC, Turner SR, et al. Prostaglandin E_2 attenuates the pressor response to angiotensin II in pregnant subjects but not in nonpregnant subjects. *Am J Obstet Gynecol*. 1982;142:168.
23. Gullner HG, Barter FC, Cerlett C, et al. Prostacyclin overproduction in Barter's syndrome. *Lancet*. 1979;2:767.
24. Turner AF. The chest radiograph in pregnancy. *Clin Obstet Gynecol*. 1975;18:65.
25. Rubler S, Prabodhkumar MD, Pinto ER. Cardiac size and performance during pregnancy estimated with echocardiography. *Clin Obstet Gynecol*. 1977;40:534.
26. Cutforth R, MacDonald MB. Heart sounds and murmurs in pregnancy. *Am Heart J*. 1966;71:741.
27. Tabatznik B, Randall TW, Hersch C. The mammary souffle of pregnancy and lactation. *Circulation*. 1960;22:1069.
28. Perloff JK. Pregnancy and cardiovascular disease. In: Braunwald E, ed. *Heart Disease*. Philadelphia, PA: WB Saunders; 1980:1871.
29. Schwartz DB, Schamroth L. The effect of pregnancy on the frontal plane QRS axis. *J Electrocardiol*. 1979;12:279.
30. Ueland K, Novy MJ, Peterson EN, et al. Maternal cardiovascular dynamics. IV. The influence of gestational age on the maternal cardiovascular response to posture and exercise. *Am J Obstet Gynecol*. 1969;104:856.
31. Bader RA, Bader ME, Rose DJ, et al. Hemodynamics at rest and during exercise in normal pregnancy as studied by cardiac catherization. *J Clin Invest*. 1955;34:1524.
32. Assali NS, Rauramo L, Peltonen T. Measurement of uterine blood flow and uterine metabolism. VII. Uterine and fetal blood flow and oxygen consumption in early human pregnancy. *Am J Obstet Gynecol*. 1960;19:86.
33. Chesley LC. Renal functional changes in normal pregnancy. *Clin Obstet Gynecol*. 1960;3:349.
34. Chesley LC, Sloan DM. The effect of posture on renal function in late pregnancy. *Am J Obstet Gynecol*. 1964;89:754.
35. McLennan CE. Antecubital and femoral venous pressure in normal and toxemic pregnancy. *Am J Obstet Gynecol*. 1943;45:568.
36. Winner W, Romney SL. Cardiovascular responses to labor and delivery. *Am J Obstet Gynecol*. 1966;95:1104.
37. Metcalfe J, Ueland K. Maternal cardiovascular adjustments to pregnancy. *Prog Cardiovasc Dis*. 1974;16:363.
38. Kjeldsen J. Hemodynamic investigations during labor and delivery. *Acta Obstet Gynecol Scand*. 1979;89(suppl):1.
39. Erkkola R. The influence of physical training during pregnancy on physical work capacity and circulatory parameters. *Scan J Clin Lab Invest*. 1976;36:747.
40. Ueland K, Novy MJ, Metcalfe J. Cardiorespiratory responses to pregnancy and exercise in normal women and patients with heart disease. *Am J Obstet Gynecol*. 1973;115:4.
41. Longo LD, Hewitt CW, Lorijn RHW, et al. To what extent does maternal exercise affect fetal oxygenation and uterine blood flow? In: *Proceedings of the 25th Annual Meeting of the Society for Gynecologic Investigations*. 1978:10. Abstract.
42. Emmanouilides GC, Hobel CH, Yashiro K, et al. Fetal responses to maternal exercises in sheep. *Am J Obstet Gynecol*. 1972;112:130.
43. Morris N, Osbor SB, Wright HP, et al. Effective uterine blood flow during exercise in normal and preeclamptic pregnancies. *Lancet*. 1956; 2:481.
44. Hon EH, Wholgemuth R. The electronic evaluation of fetal heart rate. IV. The effect of maternal exercise. *Am J Obstet Gynecol*. 1961;81:361.
45. Pomerance JJ, Gluck L, Lynch VA. Physical fitness in pregnancy: Its effects on pregnancy outcome. *Am J Obstet Gynecol*. 1974;119:867.
46. Jarrett II JC, Spellacy WN. Jogging during pregnancy: An improved outcome? *Obstet Gynecol*. 1983;61:705.
47. American College of Obstetricians and Gynecologists. *ACOG Technical Bulletin 87*.
48. Thomson KJ, Cohen ME. Studies on the circulation in pregnancy II. Vital capacity observations in normal pregnant women. *Surg Gynecol Obstet*. 1938;66:591.
49. McGinty AP. Comparative effects of pregnancy and phrenic nerve interruption on the diaphragm and their relation to pulmonary tuberculosis. *Am J Obstet Gynecol*. 1938;36:237.
50. Prowse CM, Gaensler EA. Respiratory and acid-base changes during pregnancy. *Anesthesiology*. 1965;26:381.
51. Lyons HA, Antonio R. The sensitivity of the respiratory center in pregnancy and after the administration of progesterone. *Trans Assoc Am Physicians*. 1959;72:173.
52. Skatrud JB, Dempsey JA, Kaiser DG. Ventilatory response to medroxyprogesterone acetate in normal subjects: Time course and mechanism. *J Appl Physiol Respir Environ Exercise Physiol*. 1978;44:939.
53. Hyman AL, Spannhake EW, Kadowitz PF. Prostaglandins and the lung: State of the art. *Am Rev Respir Dis*. 1978;117:111.
54. Cruikshank DP, Hays PM. Physiology of Pregnancy. In: Gabbe SG, Niebyl JR, Simpson JL, eds. *Obstetrics: Normal and Problem Pregnancies*. Edinburgh, Scotland: Churchhill, Livingstone; 1986.
55. Alaily AB, Carrol KB. Pulmonary ventilation in pregnancy. *Br J Obstet Gynaecol*. 1978;85:518.
56. Leith DB, Mead J. Mechanisms determining residual volume. *J Appl Physiol*. 1967;23:221.
57. Gerrard BS, Littler WA, Redman CWG. Closing volume during pregnancy. *Thorax*. 1978;33:488.
58. Niederman MS, Matthar RA. Asthma and other severe respiratory disease during pregnancy. In: Berkowitz R, ed. *Critical Care of the Obstetric Patient*. Edinburgh: Churchhill, Livingstone; 1983: Ch. 12.
59. Bevan DR, Holdcroft A, Loh L, et al. Closing volume and pregnancy. *Br Med J*. 1974;1:13.
60. Baldwin GR, Moorthi DS, Whelton AJ, et al. New lung functions and pregnancy. *Am J Obstet Gynecol*. 1977;127:235.
61. Holdcroft A, Bevan DR, O'Sullivan JC, et al. Airway closure and pregnancy. *Anaesthesia*. 1977;32:517.
62. Comroe JJ, Forster RE, Dubois AB, et al. *The Lung, Clinical Physiology and Pulmonary Function Tests*. Chicago, IL: Year Book Medical Publishers; 1962.

63. Milne JA, Mills RJ, Coutts JRT, et al. The effect of human pregnancy on the pulmonary transfer factor for carbon monoxide as measured by the single breath method. *Clin Sci Mol Med*. 1977;53:271.
64. Lim VS, Katz AL, Lindheimer MD. Acid-base metabolism in pregnancy. *Am J Physiol*. 1976;231:1764.
65. Lucius H, Gahlenbeck H, Klein HO, et al. Respiratory functions, buffer system, and electrolyte concentrations of blood during human pregnancy. *Respir Physiol*. 1970;9:3111.
66. Templeton A, Kelan GR. Maternal blood gases, (P_AO_2-P_aO_2), physiological shunt and V_D/V_T in normal pregnancy. *Br J Anaesth*. 1976; 48:1001.
67. Hellegers A, Metcalfe J, Huckabee W, et al. The alveolar PCO_2 & PO_2 in pregnant and nonpregnant women at high altitude. *Am J Obstet Gynecol*. 1961;82:241.
68. Sobrevilla LA, Cassinelli MT, Carcelen A, et al. Human fetal and maternal oxygen tension and acid-base status during delivery at high altitude. *Am J Obstet Gynecol*. 1971;111:1111.
69. Moore LG, Jahnigen D, Rounds SS, et al. Maternal hyperventilation helps preserve arterial oxygenation during high-altitude pregnancy. *J Appl Physiol*. 1982;52:690.
70. Bailey RR, Rolleston GL. Kidney length and ureteric dilatation in the puerperium. *J Obstet Gynaecol Br Commonw*. 1971;78:55.
71. Sheehan HL, Lynch JB. *Pathology of Toxaemia of Pregnancy*. Edinburgh, Scotland: Churchill, Livingstone; 1973:177.
72. Davison JM, Lindheimer MD. Changes in renal haemodynamics and kidney weight during pregnancy in the unanesthetised rat. *J Physiol*. (London) 1980;301:129.
73. Pollak VE, Nettles JB. The kidney in toxaemia of pregnancy, a clinical and pathological study based on renal biopsies. *Medicine*. 1960;39:469.
74. Guyer PB, Delany D. Urinary tract dilation and oral contraceptives. *Br Med J*. 1970;4:548.
75. Fitzsimons JT. The physiological basis of thirst. *Kidney Int*. 1976;10:3.
76. Marchant DJ. Alterations in anatomy and function of the urinary tract during pregnancy. *Clin Obstet Gynecol*. 1978;21:855.
77. Davison JM. Changes in renal function and other aspects of homeostasis in early pregnancy. *J Obstet Gynaecol Br Commonw*. 1974;81:1000.
78. Lindheimer MD, Weston PV. Effects of hypotonic expansion of sodium, water and urea excretion in late pregnancy: the influence of posture on these results. *J Clin Invest*. 1969;48:947.
79. Chesley LC, Sloan DM. The effect of posture on renal function in late pregnancy. *Am J Obstet Gynecol*. 1964;89:754.
80. Davison JM, Hyteen FE. Glomerular filtration during and after pregnancy. *J Obstet Gynaecol Br Commonw*. 1975;81:588.
81. Davison JM, Dunlop W, Ezimokhai M. 24-Hour creatinine clearance during the third trimester of normal pregnancy. *Br J Obstet Gynaecol*. 1980;87:106.
82. Bay WH, Ferris TF. Factors controlling plasma renin and aldosterone during pregnancy. *Hypertension*. 1979;1:410.
83. Lewis PJ, Boylan P, Friedman LA, et al. Prostacyclin in pregnancy. *Br Med J*. 1980;280:1581.
84. Welsh GW, Sims EAH. The mechanisms of renal glucosuria in pregnancy. *Diabetes*. 1960;9:363.
85. Davison JM, Hytten FE. The effect of pregnancy on the renal handling of glucose. *J Obstet Gynaecol Br Commonw*. 1975;82:374.
86. Lind T, Hytten FE. The excretion of glucose during normal pregnancy. *J Obstet Gynaecol Br Commonw*. 1972;79:961.
87. Christensen PJ. Tubular reabsorption of glucose during pregnancy. *Scand J Clin Lab Invest*. 1958;10:364.
88. Hytten FE, Cheyne GA. The aminoaciduria of pregnancy. *J Obstet Gynaecol Br Commonw*. 1972;79:424.
89. Vejlsgaard R. Bacteriuria in patients with diabetes mellitus. In: Kass EH, eds. *Progress in Pyelonephritis*. Philadelphia, PA: FA Davis; 1965:475.
90. Dunlop W, Davison JM. The effect of normal pregnancy upon the renal handling of uric acid. *Br J Obstet Gynaecol*. 1977;84:13.
91. Davison JM, Vallotton MB, Lindheimer MD. Plasma osmolality and urinary concentration and dilution during and after pregnancy: Evidence that lateral recumbency inhibits maximal urinary concentrating ability. *Br J Obstet Gynaecol*. 1981;88:472.
92. Ehrlich EN, Lindheimer MD. Effect of administered mineralocorticoids or ACTH in pregnant women: attenuation of kaliuretic influence of mineralocorticoids during pregnancy. *J Clin Invest*. 1972;51:1301.
93. Lindheimer MD, Ehrlich EN. Postural effects on renal function and volume homeostasis during pregnancy. *J Rep Med*. 1979;23:135.
94. Marder MZ, Wotman S, Mandel ID. Salivary electrolyte changes during pregnancy. I. Normal pregnancy. *Am J Obstet Gynecol*. 1972;112:233.
95. Gersh I, Catchpole HR. The nature of ground substance of connective tissue. *Perspect Biol Med*. 1960;3:282.
96. Van Thiel DH, Galvaler JS, Joshi SN, et al. Heartburn of pregnancy. *Gastroenterology*. 1977;72:666.
97. Van Thiel DH, Gavaler JS, Stremple J. Lower esophageal sphincter pressure in women using sequential oral contraceptives. *Gastroenterology*. 1976;71:232.
98. Ulmsten U, Sundstrom G. Esophageal manometry in pregnant and nonpregnant women. *Am J Obstet Gynecol*. 1978;132:260.
99. Murray FA, Erskine JP, Fielding J. Gastric secretion in pregnancy. *J Obstet Gynaecol Br Emp*. 1957;64:373.
100. Gryboski WA, Spiro HM. The effect of pregnancy on gastric secretion. *N Engl J Med*. 1956;255:1131.
101. Davison JS, Davis MC, Hay DM. Gastric emptying time in late pregnancy and labour. *J Obstet Gynaecol Br Commonw*. 1970;77:37.
102. Lind T, Hytten FE. Blood glucose following oral loads of glucose, maltose and starch during pregnancy. *Proc Nutr Soc*. 1969;28:64A.
103. Svanberg B. Iron absorption in early pregnancy. A study of the absorption of non-haeme iron and ferrous iron in early pregnancy. *Acta Obstet Gynecol Scan*. 1975;48(suppl):69.
104. Parry E, Shields R, Turnbull AC. Transit time in the small intestine in pregnancy. *J Obstet Gynaecol Br Commonw*. 1970;77:900.
105. Montgomery TL, Pincus IG. A nutritional problem in pregnancy resulting from extensive resection of the small bowel. *Am J Obstet Gynecol*. 1955;69:865.
106. Parry E, Shields R, Turnbull AC. The effect of pregnancy on the colonic absorption of sodium, potassium and water. *J Obstet Gynaecol Br Commonw*. 1970;77:616.
107. Munday KA, Parsons BJ, Shaikh DM. The control of colon fluid transport by aldosterone and angiotensin. *J Physiol*. (London) 1970;206:39.
108. Combes B, Adams RH. Pathophysiology of the liver in pregnancy. In: Assali NS, ed. *Pathophysiology of Gestation*. New York, NY: Academic; 1971:vol I.
109. Ingerslev M, Teilum G. Biopsy studies on the liver in pregnancy. II. Liver biopsy on normal pregnant women. *Acta Obstet Gynecol Scand*. 1945;25:352.
110. Song CS, Rifkind AB, Gillette PH, et al. Hormones and the liver. The effect of estrogens, prosetins and pregnancy on hepatic function. *Am J Obstet Gynecol*. 1969;105:813.
111. Wexler WM, Kantor FS. Reticuloendothelial function in pregnancy. *Yale J Biol Med*. 1966;38:315.
112. Adlercreutz H, Svanborg A, Anberg A. Recurrent jaundice in pregnancy. I. A clinical and ultrastructural study. *Am J Med*. 1967;42:335.
113. Regoeczi E, Hobbs KR. Fibrinogen turnover in pregnancy. *Scand J Haematol*. 1969;6:175.
114. Studd J. The plasma proteins in pregnancy. *Clin Obstet Gynaecol*. 1975; 2:285.
115. Combes B, Shibata H, Adams R, et al. Alterations in sulfobromophtalein sodium-removal mechanisms from blood during normal pregnancy. *J Clin Invest*. 1963;42:1431.
116. Brewer DW, Aubry RH. The physiology of pregnancy. Clinical pathologic correlations: Part 2. *Postgrad Med*. 1973;52:221.
117. Tindall VR. The liver in pregnancy. *Clin Obstet Gynaecol*. 1965;2:441.
118. Mueller MN, Kappas A. Estrogen pharmacology. I. The influence of estradiol and estriol on hepatic disposal of sulphobromophthalein (BSP) in man. *J Clin Invest*. 1964;43:1905.
119. Ikonen E. Jaundice in late pregnancy. *Acta Obstet Gynaecol Scand*. 1964; 43(suppl):1.
120. Haemmerli UP. Jaundice during pregnancy with special emphasis on recurrent jaundice during pregnancy and its differential diagnosis. *Acta Med Scand*. 1967;444(suppl):1.
121. Tikkanen MJ, Adlercreutz H. Recurrent jaundice in pregnancy. III. Quantitative determination of urinary estriol conjugates, including studies in pruritus gravidarum. *Am J Med*. 1973;54:600.
122. Braverman DZ, Johnson ML, Kern F. Effects of pregnancy and contraceptive steroids on gallbladder function. *N Engl J Med*. 1980;302:362.
123. Bennion IJ, Grundy SM. Risk factors for the development of cholelithiasis in man. *N Engl J Med*. 1978;299:1161.
124. Gillmer MDG, Beard RW, Brooke FM, et al. Carbohydrate metabolism in pregnancy Part 1. Diurnal plasma glucose profiles in normal and diabetic women. *Br Med J*. 1975;3:399.
125. Alford FP, Bloom SR, Hall R, et al. Glucagon control of fasting glucose in men. *Lancet*. 1974;2:974.
126. Cousins L, Rigg L, Hollingsworth D, et al. The 24-hour excursion and diurnal rhythm of glucose, insulin and C-peptide in normal pregnancy. *Am J Obstet Gynecol*. 1980;136:483.
127. Lind T, Billewicz WZ, Brown G. A serial study of changes occurring in the oral glucose tolerance test during pregnancy. *J Obstet Gynaecol Br Commonw*. 1973;90:1003.
128. Felig P, Lynch V. Starvation in human pregnancy: Hypoglycemia, hypoinsulinemia, and hyperketonemia. *Science*. 1970;170:990.
129. Freinkel N. Banting Lecture 1980. Of pregnancy and progeny. *Diabetes*. 1980;29:1023.
130. Lind T, Bell S, Gilmore E, et al. Insulin disappearance rate in pregnant and nonpregnant women, and in nonpregnant women given GHRIH. *Eur J Clin Invest*. 1977;7:47.
131. Fisher PM, Sutherland HW, Bewsher PD. Insulin response to glucose infusion in normal human pregnancy. *Diabetologia*. 1980;19:15.
132. Moore P, Kolterman O, Weyant J, et al. Insulin binding in human pregnancy: Comparisons to the postpartum, luteal and follicular states. *J Clin Endocrinol Metab*. 1981;52:937.
133. Javier Z, Gershberg H, Hulse M. Ovulatory suppressants, estrogens, and carbohydrate metabolism. *Metabolism*. 1968;17:443.

134. Costrini NV, Kalkhoff RK. Relative effects of pregnancy, estradiol, and progesterone on plasma insulin and pancreatic islet secretion. *J Clin Invest*. 1971;50:992.
135. Kalkhoff RK, Richardson BL, Beck P. Relative effects of pregnancy, human placental lactogen and prednisone on carbohydrate tolerance in normal and subclinical diabetic subjects. *Diabetes*. 1969;18:153.
136. Knopp RH. Fuel metabolism in pregnancy. *Contemp Ob/Gyn*. 1978;12:83.
137. Humphrey JL, Childs MT, Montes A, et al. Lipid metabolism in pregnancy, VII. Kinetics of chylomicron triglyceride removal in fed pregnant rats. *Am J Physiol*. 1980;239:E81.
138. McDonald-Gibson RG, Young M, Hytten FE. Changes in plasma nonesterified fatty acids and serum glycerol in pregnancy. *Br J Obstet Gynaecol*. 1975;82:460.
139. Samsioe G, Johnson P, Gustafson A. Studies in normal pregnancy. I. Serum lipids and fatty acid composition of serum phosphoglycerides. *Acta Obstet Gynecol Scand*. 1975;54:265.
140. Obsenshain SS, Adam PAJ, King KC, et al. Human fetal insulin response to sustained maternal hyperglycemia. *N Engl J Med*. 1970;283:566.
141. Lund CJ, Donovan JC. Blood volume during pregnancy: Significance of plasma and red cell volumes. *Am J Obstet Gynecol*. 1967;98:393.
142. Traill LM. Reticulocytes in healthy pregnancy. *Med J Aust*. 1975;1:205.
143. Pritchard JA, Adams RH. Erythrocyte production and destruction during pregnancy. *Am J Obstet Gynecol*. 1960;79:750.
144. Manasc B, Jepson J. Erthropoietin in plasma and urine during human pregnancy. *Can Med Assoc J*. 1969;100:687.
145. Chesley LC. Plasma and red cell volumes during pregnancy. *Am J Obstet Gynecol*. 1972;112:440.
146. Pitkin RM. Nutritional influences during pregnancy. *Med Clin North Am*. 1977;61:3.
147. Hallberg L, Hogdahl AM, Milsson L, et al. Menstrual blood loss: A population study. *Acta Obstet Gynaecol Scand*. 1966;45:320.
148. Greger JL, Higgins MM, Abernathy RP, et al. Nutritional status of adolescent girls in regard to zinc, copper and iron. *Am J Clin Nutr*. 1978;31:269.
149. Deleeuw NKM, Lowenstein L, Hsieh YS. Iron deficiency and hydremia of normal pregnancy. *Medicine*. 1966;45:291.
150. Jacobs A, Miller F, Worwood M, et al. Ferritin in the serum of normal subjects and patients with iron deficiency and iron overload. *Br Med J*. 1972;4:206.
151. Fenton V, Cavill I, Fisher J. Iron stores in pregnancy. *Br J Haematol*. 1977;37:145.
152. Deleeuw NKM, Brunton L. Maternal hematologic changes, iron metabolism and anemias of pregnancy. In: Goodwin JW, Godden JO, Chance GW, eds. *Perinatal Medicine*. Baltimore, MD: Williams & Wilkins; 1976:425.
153. Jepson JH. Endocrin control of maternal and fetal erythropoiesis. *Can Med Assoc J*. 1968;98:844.
154. Efrati P, Presenty B, Margalith M, et al. Leukocytes of normal pregnant women. *Obstet Gynecol*. 1964;12:429.
155. Kuvin SF, Brecher G. Differential neutrophil counts in pregnancy. *N Engl J Med*. 1962;266:877.
156. Gibson A. On leucocyte changes during labour and puerperium. *J Obstet Gynaecol Br Emp*. 1937;44:500.
157. Siegel I, Gleicher N. Peripheral white blood cell alterations in early labor. *Diagn Gynecol Obstet*. 1981;3:123.
158. Scott JR, Feldbush TL. T- and B-cell distribution in pregnancy. *JAMA*. 1978;239:2769.
159. Sumiyoshi J, Gorai I, Hirahara F, et al. Cellular immunity in normal pregnancy and absorption: Subpopulations of T lymphocytes bearing Fc receptors for IgG and IgM. *Am J Reprod Immunol*. 1981;1:145.
160. Sejeny SA, Eastman RD, Baker SR. Platelet counts during pregnancy. *J Clin Pathol*. 1975;28:812.
161. Fay RA, Hughes AO, Farron NT. Platelets in pregnancy: Hyperdestruction in pregnancy. *Obstet Gynecol*. 1983;61:238.
162. McKay DG. Chronic intravascular coagulation in normal pregnancy and preeclampsia. *Clin Nephrol*. 1981;15:108.
163. Bonnar J, McNicol GP, Douglas AS. Coagulation and fibrinolytic mechanisms during and after normal childbirth. *Br Med J*. 1970;2:200.
164. Romero R. The management of acquired hemophilic failure in pregnancy. In: Berhowitz RL, ed. *Critical Care of the Obstetric Patient*. Churchill, Livingstone; 1983:Chapter 9.
165. Hathaway WE, Bonnar J. *Perinatal Coagulation*. New York, NY: Grune & Stratton; 1978:17.
166. Fletcher AP, Alkjaersig NK, Burstein R. The influence of pregnancy upon blood coagulation and plasma fibrinolytic enzyme function. *Am J Obstet Gynecol*. 1979;134:743.
167. Trofatter KF, Howell ML, Greenberg CS, Hage ML. Use of the fibrin D-dimer in screening for coagulation abnormalities in preeclampsia. *Obstet Gynecol*. 1989;73:435.
168. Bonnar J, McNicol GP, Douglas AS. Fibrinolytic enzyme system and pregnancy. *Br Med J*. 1969;3:387.

Chapter Five
Diagnostic Procedures

Howard T. Strassner

5

Frequently during pregnancy, medical, surgical, or obstetric problems may arise that pose a threat to the health of the mother, the fetus, or both. Almost invariably some diagnostic modality is required to delineate the nature or magnitude of the problem and aid in formulating a therapeutic plan. Because common physiologic complaints of pregnancy may suggest pathology, cautious judgment must be exercised when selecting the complaints that require diagnostic intervention. Further, because of the maternal adaptations to pregnancy, benign anatomic and physiologic alterations may mimic pathologic changes. These occurrences may complicate diagnostic interpretations; misdiagnosis and the performance of unneeded procedures may place the mother and fetus at risk.

Diagnostic procedures alone are rarely a substantial risk to the mother. However, there is concern as to whether a diagnostic procedure may impart significant risk to the fetus. Where there is known risk, the clinician must weigh the expected benefit of the procedure to the mother against the risk to the fetus. From another perspective it must be appreciated that the fetus is viewed as a distinct patient in modern obstetric practice. Specific diagnostic modalities and even therapies are now available for the fetal patient. In circumstances in which procedures may be performed specifically for fetal diagnosis or treatment, the benefit must be balanced by an acceptable maternal and fetal risk.

ETIOLOGY OF DISEASE

A woman may enter pregnancy with any preexisting disorder or disease encountered in medical and surgical practice. These conditions may require new or continued diagnostic investigation during pregnancy. Similarly, a disorder may arise or first be detected during pregnancy and require extensive evaluation to establish a diagnosis. Further, any number of maternal complaints may arouse sufficient concern about the potential for organ system pathology that investigation during pregnancy may be warranted. The patient's presenting complaints, her diagnostic workup, and the therapeutic plans evolved are described in detail in the chapters covering the pathology of specific organ systems and disease states.

EFFECT OF PREGNANCY ON DIAGNOSTIC PROCEDURES

The diagnostic procedures may involve the areas of radiology, ultrasound, endoscopy, biopsy, or miscellaneous tests. Among the most widely used procedures and those of most concern are the radiologic studies. The concerns, however, are related to potential fetal risk. Clearly, no radiologic examination should be performed in pregnancy without medical necessity. It should be just as clear, however, that if diagnostic procedures are considered necessary for patient care, they should not be withheld. The well-being and survival of the mother should never be jeopardized because of a fear of using indicated radiologic diagnostic tools. Indeed, delay in diagnosis or treatment of maternal disease may pose a significant risk to the fetus. When radiologic procedures must be performed, special efforts should be made whenever possible to minimize the dose received by the fetus.

Maternal Diagnostic Procedures

Radiology. The radiologic examinations used for evaluating maternal disorders are external ionizing radiation and nuclear medicine studies, which use administered radioisotopes. The detrimental effects of very high-dose radiation (> 1 Gy) are well known and feared (eg, radiation sickness, tissue destruction, death). Fortunately, such radiation levels are never required or attained in diagnostic studies. The scientific data on the gestational effects of irradiation are mainly derived from animal studies. Exposure of the developing embryo to high-dose radiation (as in therapeutic irradiation) may lead to malformation, growth retardation, or death. Before implantation, and perhaps for 3 to 7 days after implantation (in humans), a sufficient dose of radiation may cause embryonic death. However, a surviving embryo will generally develop normally after implantation.

Throughout the subsequent period of organogenesis, the fetus is at risk for major malformation from teratogenic agents, including radiation. The developing central nervous system is particularly sensitive to the teratogenic effects of radiation. Microcephaly, mental retardation, and eye malformations are prominent adverse effects. In fact, no well-documented radiation-induced morphologic malformation has occurred in a child without the association of central nervous system abnormalities or growth retardation.[1] The severity of radiation-induced abnormalities is related to the dose received. However, the dose level of radiation that will not produce a teratogenic effect is difficult to determine. It appears that no major congenital malformation results from radiation dosage below .25 Gy from 14 days' gestation until term.[2] However, it is possible that more subtle deleterious changes may result from smaller doses. Consequently, the recommended maximum radiation dose is well below the known teratogenic dose.

Intrauterine growth retardation can result from irradiation received at any time after implantation to term. Embryos irradiated during organogenesis exhibit the most marked growth retardation at term, but irradiation of the fetus later in pregnancy produces the largest degree of permanent growth retardation. However, eventual growth retardation as an adult is not known to occur with less than .25 Gy irradiation administered at any time during pregnancy (Table 5–1).

An additional concern regarding prenatal irradiation is subsequent childhood malignancies, particularly childhood leukemia. Although 0.01–0.02 Gy of in utero irradiation is considered to increase the possibility of subsequent leukemia by 1.5–2, the etiologic relationship is unclear, and the epidemiologic data supporting the conclusion have been subject to criticism.[3] For example, subjects studied who were exposed to diagnostic x-rays were selected on the basis of medical indication; therefore, the observed results might have been influenced by the selection bias. In either event, the actual risk of malignancy after diagnostic radiation is low (Table 5–2). Termination of pregnancy would not be advised solely on the basis of this potential risk.

For practical purposes, .10 Gy has been suggested as the level of exposure above which fetal damage may occur.[4] Though clearly an arbitrary threshold, the proposed level is reasonable in attempting to ensure safety. In fact, patients exposed to standard diagnostic x-ray procedures will receive considerably less than this amount of exposure (Table 5–3). Even with abdominal and pelvic diagnostic x-ray procedures, the dose of radiation is generally less than 0.01 Gy. Deleterious fetal effects from less than 0.05 Gy have not been demonstrated. However, absolute assurance of safety

TABLE 5–1. ESTIMATION OF THE ACUTE-DOSE LD_{50} AND MINIMAL MALFORMING DOSES OF RADIATION FOR THE HUMAN EMBRYO BASED ON COMPILATION OF MOUSE, RAT, AND HUMAN DATA

Age	Approximate Minimal Lethal Dose	Approximate LD_{50}	Minimum Dose for Nonrecuperable Growth Retardation in Adult	Minimum Dose for Recognizable Gross Malformations	Minimum Dose for Induction of Genetic, Carcinogenic, and Minimal Cell-Depletion Phenomena
Day 1	10 R	70–100 R	[a]	[b]	Unknown
Day 14	25 R	140 R	>25 R	25 R	Unknown
Day 18	50 R	150 R	50–100 R	25–50 R	Unknown
Day 28	>50 R	220 R	>50 R	50 R	Unknown
Day 50	>100 R	260 R	>50 R	>50 R	Unknown
Late fetus to term		300–400 R	>50 R		Unknown

[a] Surviving embryos do not exhibit growth retardation even after high radiation exposure.
[b] Malformation incidence is low even after high doses of radiation.
From Brent [2] with permission.

TABLE 5–2 RISK OF LEUKEMIA IN VARIOUS GROUPS WITH SPECIFIED EPIDEMIOLOGIC AND PATHOLOGIC CHARACTERISTICS

Group	Approximate Risk	Increased Risk Over Control Population	Occurrence
Identical twin of leukemic twin	1:3	1000	Weeks to months
Radiation-treated polycythemia vera	1:6	500	10–15 years
Bloom syndrome	1:8	375	<30 years of age
Hiroshima survivors who were within 1000 meters of the hypocenter	1:60	50	Average 12 years
Down's syndrome	1:95	30	<10 years of age
Radiation-treated patients with ankylosing spondylitis	1:270	10	15 years
Siblings of leukemic children	1:720	4	To 10 years
Children exposed to pelvimetry in utero (gestational exposure)	1:2000	1.5	<10 years
White children <15 years of age in the United States	1:2880	1	To 10 years

From Brent[2] with permission.

can never be given; more subtle effects, as yet undetectable or unverifiable statistically, may exist. Consequently, it is important to emphasize that well-documented medical need should be present before performing any radiologic study during pregnancy, particularly during organogenesis. Alternative means of obtaining the needed information should be considered. If radiologic studies are required, the fetus should be shielded if possible without compromising the value of the study. However, examination of parts of the body distant from the fetus will result in little or no radiation to the fetus. Finally, the possibility of pregnancy must always be considered in any fertile woman undergoing radiologic studies so that inadvertent irradiation of a fetus may be avoided.

TABLE 5–3. ESTIMATED AVERAGE EMBRYONIC OR FETAL DOSE PER DIAGNOSTIC ROENTGENOGRAPHIC EXAMINATION

Examination	Dose to Embryo (mR)	Percent of All Examinations
Skull	4	7
Cervical spine	2	
Upper extremity	1	8
Lower extremity	1	8
Shoulder	1	
Chest		
Radiography	8	50
Photofluorography		8
Fluoroscopy	70	
Thoracic spine	9	
Upper gastrointestinal series		
Radiography	360	
Fluoroscopy	200	
Total	560	
Barium enema		27
Radiography	440	
Fluoroscopy	360	
Total	800	
Cholecystography	200	
Intravenous or retrograde pyelography	400	
Abdomen	290	
Lumbar spine	275	
Pelvis	40	
Hip	300	

From Brent[2] with permission.

Nuclear Medicine. Nuclear medicine studies using radioisotopes are infrequently used in pregnancy, and their gestational effects are less studied than the effects of external irradiation. Radioisotopes may vary in chemical form and in the type and energy of the emitted radiation; therefore, generalizations are difficult. A specific agent may or may not cross the placenta; it may concentrate in specific target organs; its distribution of radiation may not be random; metabolism of its radioactive elements may vary between persons or with disease states; and its change in dose rate with time may be difficult to evaluate.[5] Estimation of potential hazards produced by a radioisotope requires determining the dose to the fetus or to a fetal organ, the dose rate and its variability with time, and the stage of gestation when the radiation is received. Radioactive isotopes of iodine, ^{125}I and ^{131}I, are commonly used in nuclear medicine for such studies as thyroid and lung scans. The isotope may be administered as the inorganic ion or attached to proteins or hormones. Inorganic iodides readily cross the placenta and enter the fetal circulation. From the 10th week of gestation, the fetal thyroid avidly binds iodides. For example, administration of a therapeutic dose of ^{131}I during pregnancy may result in total fetal thyroid destruction, even though the fetal whole-body dose may be low. Protein-bound radioactive iodine compounds may not directly cross the placenta; however, with time, radioactive iodine may be released from the compound and reach the fetal circulation. Estimates of fetal exposure from such diagnostic studies have been made.[2] Even when tracer doses of ^{131}I are used, at least a theoretical concern remains for the possibility of inducing thyroid cancer by the exposure of the fetal thyroid to radioactive iodine. Consequently, for fetal considerations, all administration of radioactive iodine should be avoided during pregnancy unless overwhelming maternal indications require its use.

Technetium (^{99m}Tc) is a frequently used radioisotope for diagnostic imaging including brain, lung, thyroid, renal, and (rarely) placental scans. Advantages of ^{99m}Tc include short half-life, rapid excretion, and lack of B emissions.[5] Total-body radiation dose is lower, and there is little concern for radiation injury to a specific fetal organ. However, actual studies of the effects of this isotope on intrauterine development are lacking. It is uncommon for other radioactive elements, such as potassium, sodium, phosphorus, cesium, or strontium, to be used in diagnostic nuclear medicine studies. Consequently, it is rare for a pregnant patient to be exposed to these agents. Animal experiments have indicated that embryonic pathology and death may result if a large enough dose of radioactive phosphorus or strontium is given.

If nuclear medicine studies are necessary during pregnancy, the attending physician should seek active consultation with the radiologist. It may be possible to undertake measures to reduce the radiation exposure to the fetus. For example, a reduction in the dose of an administered isotope may be possible. Maternal hydration may be recommended to speed excretion of the isotope. In some cases, catheterization and continuous drainage of the bladder may help to decrease fetal exposure to radioactive agents that are excreted in the urine, which might otherwise remain for a longer time in close proximity to the fetus.

Endoscopy. Diagnostic endoscopy includes such procedures as gastroscopy, sigmoidoscopy, colonoscopy, anoscopy, and panendoscopy for diagnosis of gastrointestinal disorders; urethroscopy and cystoscopy for urologic evaluation; laparoscopy for intra-abdominal and pelvic evaluation; and hysteroscopy and colposcopy for other gynecologic evaluation. Endoscopies are performed for maternal indications to aid the physician in diagnosing conditions that may jeopardize the health of the pregnant patient. Any effect of these procedures on the fetus is strictly incidental. For the fetus, the major concern is generally not from the procedure but from the drugs that are administered to sedate, relax, or anesthetize the pregnant patient. Some procedures, however, can be performed without this risk. For example, with the new flexible endoscopes, particularly the pediatric size, panendoscopy can be carried out without premedication because the procedure is relatively comfortable for the patient.

Biopsy and Diagnostic Surgical Procedures. As with endoscopies, the major risk to the fetus of maternal biopsies and other diagnostic surgical procedures comes from anesthetics or medications used to relieve pain and anxiety. Local anesthetics, if clinically acceptable, are preferred to general or regional anesthetics, because no adverse effects on human embryos from local anesthetics have yet been reported. The risks for human embryos and fetuses to acute maternal exposure of anesthetics are not fully known. Studies of pregnant animals exposed to clinical concentrations of anesthetic gases have shown that fetal death rates and the number of offspring born with congenital defects increased. These increases were greatest after exposure during critical periods, such as the first trimester, and with prolonged exposure. In humans, however, there are no definitive studies proving that the clinical administration of anesthetics is harmful to the fetus. One reviewer notes that several epidemiologic studies have shown increases in spontaneous abortions after surgery and short-term acute exposure to anesthetics.[6] However, data regarding the type of anesthetic used, the nature of the procedure performed, and possible maternal exposure to other drugs or fetal toxins have often been lacking. Studies have not demonstrated a significant difference in the rate of congenital anomalies among pregnant patients having surgery and anesthesia compared to pregnant controls.[7] In addition, the impact of the underlying disease state that prompted the need for the anesthetic and diagnostic or therapeutic procedure is likely the most important consideration; therefore, this should not be overlooked when assessing the effect of a procedure.

The surgical condition, not the anesthesia or surgery itself, appears to be most important in determining perinatal wastage. Intraoperative or postoperative complications, such as hypoxia or shock also seem to have an adverse effect on pregnancy outcome. The occurrence of premature labor in the immediate postoperative period often has been blamed on anesthesia and surgery, especially intra-abdominal procedures. The risk of postoperative premature labor is greatest, however, only if the uterus is affected by the disease process or has been manipulated during the operation. There has been no association between nonabdominal surgery and an increased incidence of postoperative premature labor.

For reasons not totally defined, there appears to be an increased incidence of fetal loss after surgery or after exposure to anesthesia during the first and second trimesters of pregnancy.[7] Because of this, it is recommended that all but urgent surgery be deferred during these time periods.[6] However, it is likely that the surgical condition is a more important factor than the anesthesia or the operation. For example, one procedure that commonly must be performed in early pregnancy is the placement of a cervical cerclage for treatment of an incompetent cervix, a condition that is associated with increased fetal loss. In this instance, the surgical procedure and the accompanying anesthesia are often essential for a successful pregnancy. Therefore, in such cases, the risk must be taken.

If a surgical procedure must be performed during late pregnancy and uterine manipulation is anticipated, it has been recommended that inhalation agents such as halothane and enflurane be used for anesthesia. These agents may decrease uterine tone and inhibit uterine contractions, thus protecting against possible intraoperative and immediate postoperative premature labor. It also is prudent in late pregnancy to consider fetal heart rate monitoring when feasible during the surgical procedure. The value of this assessment in maintaining fetal well-being during surgery has been described.[8]

If emergency surgery is necessary for diagnosis or therapy during the first trimester (e.g., diagnostic laparoscopy), the anesthesiologist and surgeon should use whatever best-suited anesthetic for the patient and procedure to be performed. No commonly used anesthetic agent or technique is safer than another as long as the anesthetic is administered competently and to the appropriate patient. Also, no anesthetic drug has been definitively proven to be teratogenic in humans. As long as maternal blood pressure and oxygenation are satisfactorily maintained, there is probably little support of the use of one anesthetic technique (regional anesthesia) over another (general anesthesia) (see also Chapter 201).

Fetal Diagnostic Procedures

The practice in obstetrics of viewing the developing fetus as a distinct patient is possible because of the development and use of techniques to evaluate fetal condition. For much of the history of obstetrics, prenatal assessment of the fetus was limited to what the hand could feel or the stethoscope could hear. The advent of techniques allowing the obstetrician to view and sample the fetal environment has introduced an era of true fetal diagnostics and therapeutics. Among the major fetal diagnostic procedures in use are amniocentesis, ultrasound, and electronic fetal heart rate monitoring.

Amniocentesis. Amniocentesis provided the first window into the world of the fetus. Though first described in the 1880s, the procedure did not become a fetal diagnostic tool until the 1950s. In 1956, Bevis[80] reported on the significance of increased blood pigments in the amniotic fluid of Rh-sensitized pregnancies. Spectrophotometric analysis of the amniotic fluid provided the first useful means of assessing the severity of the effect of Rh disease on the fetus. During the subsequent years, use of the procedure increased dramatically, as more tests were developed to allow diagnosis of fetal disorders based on analysis of the amniotic fluid (see also Chapters 16 and 17).

Amniocentesis is the procedure of withdrawing amniotic fluid from the intrauterine amniotic sac. The procedure allows the study of the fluid or its cellular contents in order to diagnose fetal abnormalities. The route is virtually always transabdominal. The technical goal is to obtain amniotic fluid under sterile conditions while avoiding traumatic injury to the fetus or placenta. The procedure is generally performed for diagnostic purposes, although therapeutic amniocentesis occasionally is required for treatment of symptomatic polyhydramnios. The procedure is performed only during the second or third trimester. In the second trimester, the indication for the procedure primarily is to determine whether the fetus has, or is at high risk for, a genetic or developmental disorder. In the third trimester, assessment of fetal maturity and surveillance of the effect of Rh sensitization are the primary reasons for performing the procedure.

Amniocentesis is performed by an obstetrician with special training in the procedure, particularly in the case of genetic amniocentesis. The procedure is always immediately preceded by an ultrasound examination. Ultrasonography before amniocentesis allows confirmation of fetal life and age and selection of the best site for the procedure based on the relative location of the fetus, placenta, and pockets of amniotic fluid. After ultrasound site selection, the site is cleansed with an antiseptic solution, and a sterile field is established with sterile drapes. Local anesthesia may be used if desired, although the discomfort of the local infiltration often exceeds that of an amniocentesis alone. A 22-gauge needle with an appropriate length for the size of the patient (usually 3.5 inches) is then inserted with stylet in place through the maternal abdominal wall into the amniotic sac. The stylet is removed, a syringe is attached to the needle, and the volume of amniotic fluid required for the specific test is withdrawn and placed into sterile vials. If blood-tinged amniotic fluid is obtained initially, it frequently will clear. If blood persists, the location of the needle should be reassessed. Continuous ultrasound monitoring of the procedure will provide additional assurance of a safe, atraumatic procedure (Fig. 5–1). The amount of amniotic fluid required for testing is usually small relative to the total volume, even in the second trimester, and is rapidly replaced.

Amniocentesis is not without risks, but the overall complication rate is low. Maternal complications are uncommon, but risks include bleeding or hematoma formation in the abdominal wall, uterus, or pelvic vessels; infection (chorioamnionitis); vaginal bleeding; amniotic fluid leakage; pain at the site of needle insertion; and sensitization of the Rh-negative mother. An avoidable maternal complication is Rh sensitization. The blood group and Rh should be known for all patients undergoing amniocentesis, and Rh immunoglobulin prophylaxis is provided for all Rh-negative women who have the procedure.

The greatest concerns relate to the fetal risks of the procedure. Fetal risks ultimately relate to the complication of fetal loss after amniocentesis. This may occur as a result of fetal or placental bleeding, other fetal traumatic injury, or chorioamnionitis. A prospective controlled study to evaluate the risk of midtrimester (genetic) amniocentesis was initiated in 1971 by the National Institute of Child Health and Human Development. The study involved 1040 subjects and 992 controls. The results of the study showed no statistically significant difference in the rate of fetal loss between women undergoing midtrimester amniocentesis and their matched controls (3.5% for subjects, 3.2% for controls).[9] Furthermore, there were no significant differences in complications of pregnancy or in newborn evaluations through the first year of life. The study also found the diagnostic accuracy of genetic amniocentesis to be 99.4%. A comparable study of safety and accuracy performed in Canada yielded similar results. Results of a study addressing the same question performed in the United Kingdom suggested a higher rate of fetal loss with amniocentesis. However, an analysis of the design of this study casts doubt on the validity of the conflicting findings.[10] Overall, the data support the conclusion that midtrimester amniocentesis is highly accurate and safe and does not significantly increase the rate of fetal loss or injury.

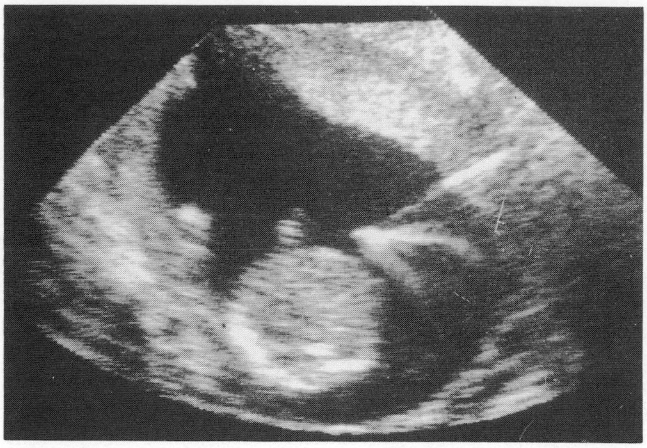

Figure 5–1. Continuous ultrasound monitoring of amniocentesis showing needle in amniotic fluid. (*Courtesy of Jason C. Birnholz, M.D., Rush-Presbyterian-St. Luke's Medical Center, Chicago.*)

Currently the majority of amniocenteses performed may be categorized as genetic amniocenteses (Chapter 16). A genetic amniocentesis diagnoses cytogenetic, neural tube, or certain metabolic abnormalities in the fetuses of women at high risk for delivering infants with these abnormalities. If a fetus without these abnormalities is detected, this may allay much of the concern and anxiety of high-risk parents. If an affected fetus is diagnosed, the mother can elect to terminate the pregnancy. On the other hand, the knowledge also may allow the couple to prepare themselves, their families, and their resources for the special needs of the child if they decide to continue the pregnancy. A genetic amniocentesis is usually performed during the 16th week of gestation, although there is increasing interest in performing early amniocentesis at 12–15 weeks' gestation. By 15–16 weeks' gestation enough amniotic fluid exists to obtain safely an adequate volume of fluid sample; cell growth in the laboratory is usually successful; the fetus is small enough to minimize the chance of injuring it; and the results of the cytogenetic and biochemical tests are available in time for a midtrimester termination of pregnancy if an abnormal fetus is detected. Early amniocentesis (before 15 weeks) has the advantage of earlier results at the expense of increased technical difficulty and less laboratory experience with biochemical tests such as alphafetoprotein. This is being investigated.

The most common indication for genetic amniocentesis today is advanced maternal age. It is recommended that pregnant women who will be 35 years of age or more at the time of delivery should receive counseling and be offered genetic amniocentesis. Down's syndrome is the most common cytogenetic abnormality and is usually the one about which the patient has heard the most and is most concerned. It is, however, only one of the potential cytogenetic abnormalities. At age 35, the chance of a mother giving birth to an infant with Down's syndrome is 1 in 365. However, other cytogenetic abnormalities also are associated with advanced maternal age, including trisomy 13 and 18 and sex chromosomal trisomies such as 47,XXY and 47,XXX. Overall, at a maternal age of 35, the likelihood of diagnosing a significant cytogenetic abnormality is 1 in 180.[11]

Genetic amniocentesis for fetal karyotype is also indicated if a couple has had a child with a chromosomal abnormality. After the birth of a child with trisomy 21 or with a sex chromosome trisomy, the risk of recurrence is approximately 1% regardless of parental age. Other cytogenetic indications for genetic amniocentesis include a history of Down's syndrome or other chromosomal abnormality in a close family member or a maternal history of multiple (three or more) spontaneous abortions. If either parent has a known chromosomal abnormality, a genetic amniocentesis also is indicated. For example, approximately 3% of all cases of Down's syndrome occur as a result of unbalanced chromosome translocation, most commonly a 14/21 (D/G) translocation. In nearly half of such cases, one parent will be a carrier of a balanced translocation. Because there is neither an absence nor an excess of genetic information in the balanced carrier, he or she is phenotypically normal. However, the balanced carrier is at high risk for producing genetically "unbalanced" offspring. The empiric risk of this occurring depends on which parent is the translocation carrier and the type of translocation involved. If a maternal chromosome number 21 is translocated onto a chromosome of the D group (eg, a 14/21 translocation), the child has a 10% chance of having Down's syndrome. If, however, a similar translocation is present in the father, there would be approximately a 2% chance of the child having a Down's syndrome. If either parent has a translocation between chromosomes of the same number (eg, a 21/21 translocation), only a monosomic or trisomic fetus is possible. Such a translocation carries a 100% risk of abnormality for all children delivered.

A less frequent indication for genetic amniocentesis is for fetal sex determination. This information may be important in pregnancies at risk for X-linked hereditary disorders. Such disorders include Duchenne muscular dystrophy, hemophilia, X-linked mental retardation, and X-linked hydrocephalus. For most X-linked disorders, only the potential for the disease can be determined by identifying that the fetus is male. This can present the parents with a difficult decision regarding pregnancy termination because a male fetus carries only a 50% chance of being affected.

Certain metabolic abnormalities also can be detected prenatally by cellular enzyme analysis of cultured amniotic fluid cells. In addition to several X-linked disorders, more than 100 autosomal recessive biochemical genetic disorders can be diagnosed by cellular-enzyme analysis for abnormalities of lipid, carbohydrate, macopolysaccharide, or amino acid metabolism. If a couple has had a child with an autosomal recessive biochemical genetic disorder that is detectable prenatally, they are candidates for genetic amniocentesis because these conditions have a 25% recurrence risk.

A history of delivering an infant with a neural tube defect is another indication for genetic amniocentesis. The recurrence risk for this defect is approximately 2–5%. Prenatal diagnosis also should be offered to siblings and children of an affected person and to the nieces, nephews, and maternal cousins. An assay of the amniotic fluid for alphafetoprotein is the diagnostic test for open neural tube defects. A thorough ultrasound examination of the fetal spine also is indicated. A fetal karyotype is not necessary in these cases; however, chromosome analysis of amniotic fluid cells also is performed to detect any "incidental" chromosomal abnormalities.

Although many conditions can now be diagnosed by prenatal genetic amniocentesis, prenatal genetic testing is not available for many birth defects. Examples of these include cleft lip and palate, congenital heart defects, congenital liver defects, club feet, blindness, deafness, and mental retardation from causes other than chromosomal and certain metabolic abnormalities. Thus, it is important that parents understand that a normal result from a prenatal karyotype, alphafetoprotein determination, or selected biochemical enzyme analysis does not guarantee a healthy baby.

The most frequent third-trimester indication for amniocentesis is for assessment of fetal maturity. A major clinical problem in obstetrics has been the accurate determination of fetal maturity. Before the availability and widespread use of amniotic fluid maturity tests, clinical estimates of fetal maturity resulted in significant occurrences of premature delivery, neonatal respiratory distress syndrome (RDS), and neonatal death because of ill-timed delivery. Discovery of the biochemical basis of RDS and the relationship of amniotic fluid phospholipids to the process led to specific tests to evaluate fetal pulmonary maturation. Consequently, the inadvertent delivery of a premature infant should no longer occur.

Chorionic Villus Sampling. Chorionic villus sampling is a new and promising technique for prenatal genetic diagnosis (Chapter 16). Virtually all genetic diagnoses that can be made by amniocentesis can be made by chorionic villus sampling. Its main advantage is that the technique can be used in the first trimester (approximately 10 weeks' gestation), allowing results to be obtained earlier than with midtrimester amniocentesis. It is an ultrasound-guided procedure, and both transcervical and transabdominal approaches have been used. Worldwide experience with the procedure is increasing, and in general, results have been encouraging.[12] Fetal loss rates appear to be higher than with traditional amniocentesis, but, when balanced against earlier availability of diagnosis, this is acceptable for many high-risk patients. With more providers gaining experience with this procedure, chorionic villus sampling will likely become a routine method offered for prenatal diagnosis.

Ultrasound. The applications of ultrasound in medicine have expanded rapidly; in fact, nearly half of all ultrasound examinations are performed in the field of obstetrics. In many instances, ultrasound is an acceptable or even preferred modality for evaluating maternal symptomatology and thereby avoiding the use of radiologic procedures during pregnancy (Chapter 6). However, the majority of ultrasound examinations in pregnancy are performed only to evaluate the fetus.

Ultrasound is mechanical wave energy with sound frequencies above the audible range in humans (i.e., greater than 20,000 Hz). Diagnostic ultrasound equipment operates in the 1–10 million-Hz range, with 3–5 million Hz most commonly used in obstetrics. Since its introduction in obstetrics by Donald in the late 1950s, ultrasonography has expanded from an investigational tool to a routine procedure, often performed in the obstetrician's office. This expansion has been aided primarily by major technological advances in ultrasound imaging and by the introduction of compact portable real-time ultrasound equipment. Experience in the performance and interpretation of obstetric ultrasound is now considered an integral part of obstetric training.

Common indications for obstetric ultrasound include determination of gestational age, placental localization, evaluation of bleeding in pregnancy, evaluation of discrepancy between uterine size and gestational dating, evaluation of fetal growth, diagnosis of multiple gestation, direction of amniocentesis and other intrauterine procedures, detection of congenital anomalies, estimation of fetal weight, determination of fetal sex, and determination of fetal well-being. Standard information that should be obtained from an obstetric ultrasound examination includes fetal number, fetal cardiac activity, fetal lie or presentation, gestational age by multiple parameters, placental localization, amount of amniotic fluid, major fetal landmarks, evaluation of uterus and adnexa, and presence of fetal abnormalities.[13] Sequential ultrasound examinations allow assessment of the adequacy of fetal growth and confirm or rule out suspected intrauterine fetal growth retardation. With continued improvement in image quality, an even greater ability to diagnose congenital abnormalities will exist.

Recently, the application of ultrasound has been extended to the assessment of fetal well-being. Most estimates of fetal well-being have been based on biochemical testing (eg, estriol levels) or fetal heart rate monitoring. The availability of ultrasound has allowed additional fetal characteristics to be observed. In particular, the presence of fetal breathing movements has been shown to predict good fetal condition.[14] Other observed biophysical parameters, such as the presence of fetal tone and fetal body movements, have been similarly suggestive of good fetal condition. Without these signs of fetal health, it has been demonstrated that the fetus is at increased risk for perinatal morbidity and mortality.[15,16] Doppler ultrasound evaluation of fetal umbilical blood flow is the most recent advance in ultrasound assessment of fetal well-being. As a predictor of placental insufficiency, fetal growth retardation, and fetal compromise, Doppler flow studies appear to be among the most promising tools for fetal assessment.[17]

The safety of diagnostic ultrasound is generally accepted. Studies and experience have not disclosed any adverse effects of diagnostic ultrasound on the human adult or fetus. Certainly there is sufficient experience and assurance to warrant use of ultrasound whenever it is indicated in pregnancy. However, an unresolved debate concerns the question of whether all fetuses should be evaluated with at least one ultrasound examination in pregnancy.

Electronic Fetal Monitoring. Electronic fetal monitoring is the major fetal diagnostic procedure used in obstetrics. As an intrapartum procedure, it is applied to most patients in labor. In the antepartum period, it is frequently used to assess fetal well-being in high-risk pregnancies. The fetal monitor is capable of providing continuous instantaneous information on fetal heart rate and on uterine contractions. The information is displayed on a continuous paper tracing, which may become a permanent addition to the maternal record. Monitoring of these parameters may be indirect (external) or direct (internal). External monitoring is most frequently used, although internal methods provide the most complete data. The data may be obtained externally in several ways. Generally, the fetal heart rate is obtained from a Doppler ultrasound applied to the maternal abdomen and held in place by a belt. Heart rate is measured by application of the Doppler principle, which calculates the difference in frequency of the ultrasound signal transmitted to and reflected from the fetal heart. Uncommonly, phonocardiography or abdominal wall electrocardiography may be used for antepartum assessment. Indirect uterine activity is monitored with a tocodynamometer applied to the maternal abdomen over the uterine fundus and held in place by a belt. As the uterine shape changes with contractions, pressure against the transducer is recorded. Advantages of external techniques are that they are noninvasive, can be applied for antepartum assessment, do not require rupture of membranes, and are easily applied. Recently, self-administration of external uterine activity monitoring has been used at home by selected patients at risk for preterm labor. As an aid to early diagnosis of preterm labor, home uterine activity monitoring is undergoing extensive investigation.

The most informative and reliable techniques of fetal monitoring measure the fetal ECG signal and the intrauterine pressure. The internal modes require rupture of membranes, the presence of cervical dilatation, and expertise in application. The fetal heart rate is measured by way of an electrode attached directly to the fetal presenting part. The fetal ECG is obtained from the electrode, and the heart rate is calculated from the signals received. The most important information regarding fetal heart rate variability and patterns can be obtained only from fetal ECG data. Direct uterine activity is measured by placement of a fluid-filled catheter into the uterine cavity. The catheter is attached to a strain gauge, and intrauterine pressure is thereby transmitted to the monitor. The baseline uterine tone, strength and duration of contractions, and contraction frequency can be measured. Information regarding the time relationship between the beginning and end of uterine contractions and the beginning and end of fetal heart rate decelerations can be accurately determined with the aid of intrauterine pressure monitoring. This information may be extremely valuable in evaluating certain fetal heart patterns suggestive of fetal distress.

Electronic fetal monitoring is used to assess the well-being of the fetus and its risk of death from perinatal asphyxia. The occurrence of perinatal death and neonatal morbidity related to intrapartum asphyxia provided the impetus for the development and widespread use of these improved methods of fetal assessment. Before the availability of continuous electronic fetal monitoring, auscultation of the fetal heart beat, inspection of the amniotic fluid for meconium, and palpation of the uterus were the only means of estimating the occurrence of fetal distress and the quality of uterine activity. Obvious clinical problems with simple auscultation of the fetal heart rate include the intermittent nature of the assessment, the inability to appreciate fetal heart rate patterns, and intrinsic errors of the method. With the use of the fetal monitor, observation of normal fetal heart rate patterns provides reassurance of good fetal condition and adequate fetal oxygenation. Observation of non-reassuring fetal heart rate characteristics (eg, tachycardia, bradycardia, decreased variability) or ominous fetal heart rate patterns (eg, late decelerations, severe variable decelerations) allows early and prompt reassessment of overall clinical status and prompt intervention, including intrauterine resuscitation or delivery.

Complications of fetal monitoring are uncommon. With external monitoring, essentially the only complications are supine hypotension and its sequelae, which might occur if the mother is made to remain on her back to obtain a satisfactory tracing. Perhaps the most important complication of internal or external monitoring is unwarranted operative intervention (eg, cesarean section or forceps delivery) or failure to intervene because of misinterpretation of fetal heart rate data. Internal monitoring carries the possible risk of increased maternal infection if cesarean delivery is required, although this is more likely to be a complication of the labor and patient risk factors than of fetal monitoring itself. For the neonate, scalp abscess is the most frequent complication of internal monitoring, occurring in approximately 0.5% of cases. They are generally self-limited and respond to local measures and antibiotics. However, isolated cases of serious sequelae of scalp infection associated with scalp electrodes have been reported, including bacterial sepsis, osteomyelitis, and disseminated herpes simplex. Other rare complications for the neonate include scalp bleeding, scalp hematoma, scalp laceration, and cerebrospinal fluid leakage.

Other Fetal Diagnostic Procedures. Fetal scalp blood sampling is performed to obtain blood for pH measurement. The purpose is to better assess fetal condition and to confirm or deny the diagnosis of fetal distress in labor. The diagnosis of fetal distress based on interpretation of fetal heart rate patterns can be difficult, and false predictions occur. The aim of fetal blood sampling is to decrease the occurrence of false predictions. The procedure will be influenced by the experience and skill of the clinician in interpreting fetal heart rate tracings and in performing scalp blood sampling. The pH of fetal blood represents an indirect indication of fetal oxygenation. A normal fetal scalp blood pH ($\geq$7.25) indicates the absence of fetal distress, whereas a distinctly abnormal result ($<$7.20) supports the diagnosis. The procedure of obtaining the fetal blood requires ruptured membranes and sufficient cervical dilatation to admit a conical endoscope. The patient must be in a lithotomy or, preferably, a lateral Sims' position. After introducing the endoscope through the cervix and onto the fetal scalp, the scalp is dried with swabs, silicone gel is applied, and scalp puncture is performed using a 2-mm blade designed for this purpose. The fetal scalp blood is collected in heparinized capillary tubes and analyzed immediately. Firm pressure must be applied to the puncture site for several minutes (through two uterine contractions) after the procedure, and then the site is reinspected to ensure that all bleeding has stopped. Potential complications include maternal discomfort from the performance of the procedure, fetal scalp laceration, persistent bleeding from the puncture site, scalp infection, and cerebrospinal fluid leakage.

Because of the value of fetal pH assessment and the limitations of intermittent techniques, work has been directed toward the development of methods to continuously monitor fetal tissue pH. Methods of assessing continuous pH through electrodes applied to the fetal scalp have been developed and tested with promising results.[18] However, this technology is not yet used for general clinical management of patients. In addition, similar research has been applied to the development of PO_2 electrodes for continuous monitoring of fetal oxygenation. This technique also is under investigation and is not yet available for general use.

Another method of obtaining fetal blood for diagnostic purposes is percutaneous umbilical blood sampling or cordocentesis. This procedure involves direct puncture of the umbilical cord.[19,20] It is done under ultrasound guidance and is applicable in a wide variety of clinical disorders including suspected genetic anomalies, assessment of fetal status in isoimmunization, suspected fetal thrombocytopenia or anemia, and fetal acid-base assessment. The approach also may be used for fetal therapy such as fetal intravascular transfusion. The continuing experience with this invasive procedure remains encouraging and the potential uses for this method are enormous. The considerable enthusiasm regarding its potential in fetal diagnostics appears justified.

Fetoscopy has been performed to obtain direct visualization of the fetus in order to diagnose external malformations. The transabdominal placement of an endoscope into the amniotic sac is a high-risk procedure and is currently performed clinically in only a few centers throughout the world. The procedure carries a substantial risk of fetal loss and allows a limited view of the fetus. In the future, the major indications for using fetoscopy likely will be to allow performance of associated procedures such as fetal skin biopsy, fetal internal organ biopsy, or fetal blood sampling for the midtrimester prenatal diagnosis of specific inherited diseases. Even some of these procedures may be adequately directed by ultrasound. When visualization of the fetus is all that is required, it is likely that fetoscopy will be supplanted entirely through improvements in ultrasound imaging.

REFERENCES

1. Brent RL. Teratogenic and carcinogenic effects of in utero irradiation. In: Bolognese RJ, Schwarz RH, Schneider J, eds. *Perinatal Medicine*. 2nd ed. Baltimore, London: Williams & Wilkins, 1982:85.
2. Brent RL. Irradiation in pregnancy. In: Gerbie AB, Sciarra JJ, eds. *Gynecology and Obstetrics*. Philadelphia, PA: Harper & Row; 1981;2:1.
3. Oppenheim BE, Griem ML, Meir P. The effects of diagnostic X-ray exposure on the human fetus: An examination of the evidence. *Radiology*. 1975;114:529.
4. National Council on Radiation Protection and Measurements. Medical Radiation Exposure of Pregnant and Potentially Pregnant Women. Washington, DC; NCRP report No. 54, 1977.
5. Russell LB. Irradiation damage to the embryo, fetus, and neonate. In: Fullerton GD, Koop DT, Waggener RG, et al, eds. *Biological Risks of Medical Irradiations*. New York, NY: American Association of Physicists in Medicine; 1980:33.
6. Brodsky JB. Anesthesia and surgery during early pregnancy and fetal outcome. *Clin Obstet Gynecol*. 1983;26:440.
7. Duncan PG, Pope B, Cohen MM, Greer N. Fetal risk of anesthesia and surgery during pregnancy. *Anesthesiology*. 1986;64:790.
8. Katz JD, Hook R, Barash PG: Fetal heart rate monitoring in pregnant patients undergoing surgery. *Am J Obstet Gynecol*. 1976;125:267.

8a. Bevis, DCA. Blood pigments in hemolytic disease of the newborn. *J Obstet Gynaecol Br Commonw*. 1956;63:68.

9. NICHD. National Registry for Amniocentesis Study Group. Midtrimester amniocentesis for prenatal diagnosis: Safety and accuracy. *JAMA*. 1976;236:1471.
10. Antenatal Diagnosis. Report of Consensus Development Conference. Bethesda, MD: US Dept. of Health, Education, and Welfare. NIH Publication 79–1973.
11. Hook E. Rates of chromosome abnormalities at different maternal ages. *Obstet Gynecol*. 1981;58:282.
12. Rhoads GG, Jackson LG, Schlesselman SE, et al. The safety and efficacy of chorionic villus sampling for early prenatal diagnosis of cytogenetic abnormalities. *N Engl J Med*. 1989;320:609.
13. ACOG. *Ultrasound in Pregnancy*. Technical Bulletin. Number 16, May 1988.
14. Platt LD, Manning FA, Lemay M, et al. Human fetal breathing: Relationship to condition. *Am J Obstet Gynecol*. 1978;132:514.

15. Manning FA, Platt LD, Sipos L. Antepartum fetal evaluation: development of a fetal biophysical profile. *Am J Obstet Gynecol.* 1980;136:787.
16. Manning FA, Morrison I, Lange IR, et al. Fetal assessment based on fetal biophysical profile scoring: experience in 12,620 referred high-risk pregnancies. *Am J Obstet Gynecol.* 1985;151:343.
17. Divon MY, Guidetti D, Braverman JI, et al. Intrauterine growth retardation—a prospective study of the diagnostic value of real-time sonography combined with umbilical artery flow velocimetry. *Obstet Gynecol.* 1988;72:611.
18. Lauersen NH, Hochberg HM. *Clinical Perinatal Biochemical Monitoring.* Baltimore, London: Williams & Wilkins, 1981.
19. Daffos F, Capello–Pavlowsky M, Forestier F. Fetal blood sampling during pregnancy with use of needle guided by ultrasound: a study of 606 consecutive cases. *Am J Obstet Gynecol.* 1985;153:655.
20. Weiner CP. Cordocentesis for diagnostic indications: two years experience. *Obstet Gynecol.* 1987;70:664.

Chapter Six

The Ultrasonic Obstetric Examination

Jason C. Birnholz

6

Ultrasound is a powerful physical examination technique. In its simplest obstetric form, it provides basic information about fetal number, position, viability, and stage. Another level of implementation achieves portrayal of fetal and uterine anatomy, and, in its most sophisticated form, combined observations disclose facets of fetal and fetomaternal physiology. The trends in obstetric ultrasound have increasing use (including routine screening and integration of ultrasound into community practice) and progressive clinical complexity of these studies. This chapter considers the nature and content of obstetric ultrasound studies as they apply to prospective patient evaluations, including extrauterine components relevant to maternal medical therapy.

The obstetric ultrasound examination is a hodgepodge of fetal and maternal features that continue to develop through individual experience and different forms of instrumentation. Both facets are necessary and inseparable for the obstetric goal of optimizing outcome for mother and child. First-trimester studies combine maternal issues of conception and implantation with fetal issues of early growth and development. Second-trimester studies fuse fetal anatomic features with maternal environmental issues, such as uteroplacental vascularity and structural integrity of the lower segment. In the third trimester, when infant survival is possible, central issues are recognition and prevention of hypoxic (fetal) brain injury, which involve evaluating supply line function and monitoring fetal condition. These issues influence the timing, urgency, and location of delivery. Other factors pertain to the route of delivery. Maternal scope of the study will be governed by clinical indications and can include any region that can be approached ultrasonically (ie, not shielded on all sides by gas or bone).

Obstetric applications of ultrasound have a relatively short history of three decades starting with the pioneering work of Donald and colleagues in Glasgow.[1] Many notions about ultrasound use were developed during the early academic proliferation of the method approximately 20 years ago. They have not been fully revised, even though that early experience bears little relevance to current practice. At that time, studies tended to be lengthy, and they focused on specific clinical questions rather than general diagnostic issues. Execution was often through the agency of a technologist, who would acquire a series of images for later interpretation. The study tended to be considered a "special procedure," performed according to specific indications late in the course of an evaluation when other forms of data indicated an abnormality. Two specific biases pertained specifically to obstetric studies. First, because physical measurements (such as cranial diameter) are part of data collection, the procedure might have been regarded as a type of laboratory procedure in which limited, typically "raw," data are relayed to the referring physician who interprets them in the context of other information before formulating a management plan. Second, the method was elected because of its safety, not because of its actual information content (i.e., ultrasound forms a triage for invasive or radiographic study rather than standing on its own as a final diagnostic entity). Additionally, a tendency has existed to subdivide ultrasound use by anatomic region or specialty, rather than pursuing a united developmental effort that encompasses mother, fetus, and newborn infant.

References on ultrasonic imaging tend to cite the theory and achievement of sonar in France at the start of the first World War as the origin of ultrasound. Sonar is an ancestor of ultrasound; however, the medical and conceptual origin can probably be traced to the 18th century and the descriptions of Auenbrugger on percussion as a physical examination method.[2] Ultrasound replaces the percussing finger with an electromechanical transducer. Instead of a few, relatively low-frequency shock waves, a stream of several thousand inaudible acoustic bursts per second are precisely formed by transducer design and excitation form. Instead of feeling a vibratory response (mediate percussion) or listening for an audible tone (immediate percussion), a pattern of echoes for each pulse is displayed visually on a screen, forming a map of structures deep to the skin.

This distinction in history is important because we believe strongly that the optimal use of ultrasound is as a physical examination technique, extending (and in the case of fetal studies, replacing) the traditional physical examination. While some specific components of the study can be identified for routine acquisition (ie, fetal measurements, Doppler waveforms), the examination should be performed primarily by a physician knowledgeable in the pathology pertaining to the case at hand. The physician also should be knowledgeable about instrument use and data acquisition and be capable of tailoring the study to clinical information (including material elicited during the study) and image findings. Furthermore, he or she should be capable of forming a professional, interactive relationship with the expectant couple (Figs. 6–1, 6–2). Every study is exploratory and includes many screening concerns pertinent to fetal anatomy, stage, condition, and premature labor risk (that cannot be anticipated by clinical history or conventional physical examination). Moreover, causes of abnormalities must be sought before management can be defined. For example, after diagnosing breech position at term, the physician must

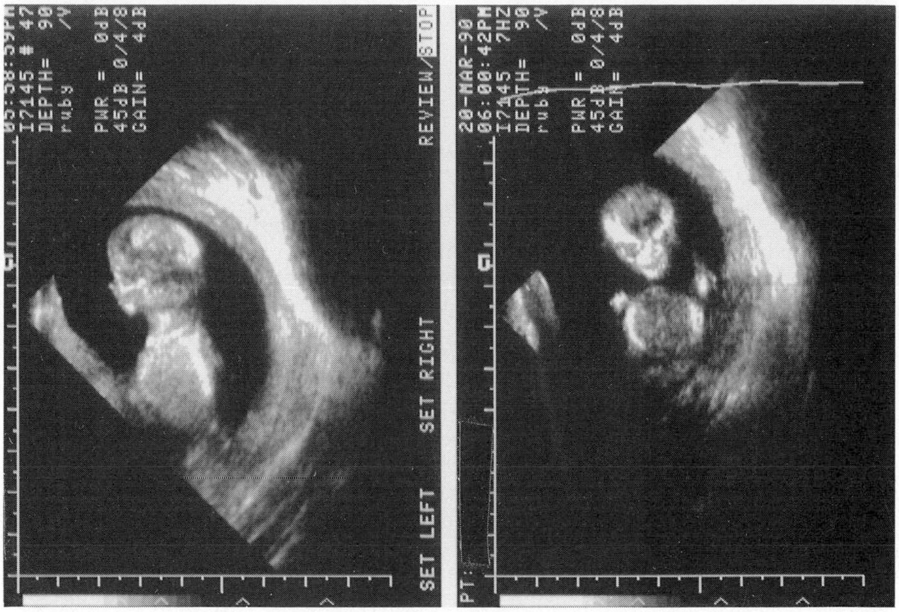

Figure 6–1. Fetal portraiture in an essential part of the interactive ultrasound examination, providing a reference point for the expectant couple. (Frontal and lateral pair, 9 weeks' gestation.)

exclude pathologic causes that will affect delivery. Other examples are estimating lung volume when oligohydramnios is present or distinguishing isolated anomalies from a multisystem complex of malformations.[3] Likewise, the examination should be extended to any extrauterine region when that information will enrich care, as in defining coincident renal or gastrointestinal disease, monitoring cardiovascular function, or indicating activity of collagen–vascular disease.

TECHNICAL FOUNDATIONS

The accuracy and extent of an ultrasound examination depends ultimately on the nature of acoustic pulse propagation in tissue, while it depends immediately on instrument performance. Individual images represent a composite of anatomic features and instrument factors; clinical results depend on the particular pathology that is occurring, the tissue it is occurring in, the depth of that tissue, the habitus of the subject, the particular instrument that is used, the way the instrument is operated, and the characteristics of the display medium. The goal of instrument development is to maximize anatomic display fidelity and decrease the instrument component (including noise and artifacts of various types); however, this goal is approached differently (and with different levels of success) by individual manufacturers. This section reviews instrument features that are pertinent to routine ultrasonic scanning.

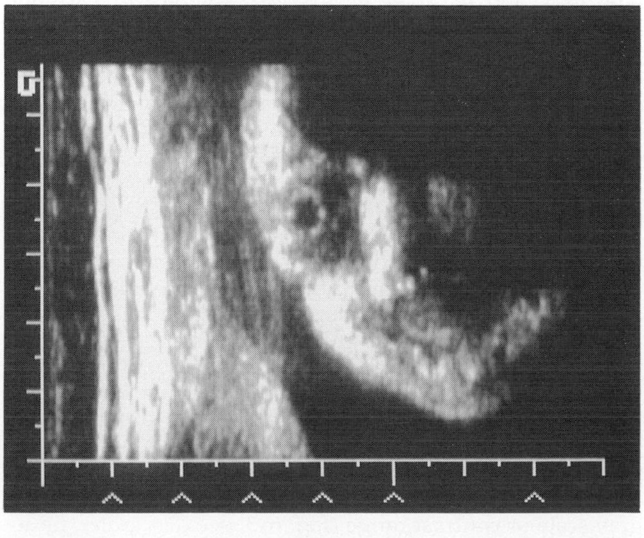

Figure 6–2. Frontal portrait (lateral coronal view) at 23 weeks' gestation. All images in this chapter were obtained with a large aperture, dynamically focused array instrument.

Without yet exploring the nature of the ultrasound image, detail, or spatial, resolution can be taken as primary instrument performance feature. A technical definition might focus on the smallest distance at which two reflectors with specific properties still appear separate in the final image, although a more practical measure is our ability to visualize fetal anatomic features at each gestational age. There is a fundamental limit to spatial resolution, which is about one wavelength in extent (wavelength = velocity/frequency). Early devices achieved about 25 wave lengths resolution, but new devices operate much closer to the Rayleigh limit.

The physical factor that controls detail resolution is the space occupied by the acoustic pulse as it travels through tissue. Pulses interact with tissues. There are scattering reactions (including the backscatter production of echoes forming the images), and there is attenuation with loss of energy to tissue. It is usual to refer to the dominant frequency of the transducer as *the* frequency of a pulse; however, this can be misleading when judging performance or selecting an instrument. Pulses contain a range of frequencies centered around the dominant frequency, called the *bandwidth.* The shorter the pulse duration, the broader the bandwidth, and the better the resolution capabilities. Shock excitation and damping of the transducer was the first means of producing short, spatially small pulses. Unfortunately, pulse size and shape and bandwidth change continuously as a pulse propagates and interacts with tissue. Higher frequency components are lost first. Resolution is better, for example, in the upper half of an image than in the lower portion. Phrased another way, the imaging close to one probe may be 5 MHz, but less than 2 MHz further on in the imaging field. Another consequence is that performance can be judged only from the image itself and not from transducer labeling alone. For example, one system operating at 3 MHz with a relatively broad band pulse could easily achieve better resolution performance than another labeled at 6 MHz, but having narrow band signal characteristics, when other signal processing features are the same.

The first instruments used single element transducers and formed images on a line-by-line basis. The larger the aperture (diameter in number of wavelengths), the smaller the size of the beam at its optimal focal depth and the better the resolution performance. Unfortunately, tight focus is associated with unfavorable focal characteristics elsewhere in the imaging field, resulting in compromised resolution to maintain a reasonable depth of field. Another feature of single-element transducers is that resolution is considerably better along the axis of the beam than at right angles to it (with specific consequences both for anatomic studies and for measurement precision). The first units used widely in the United States required manual scanning for a large field of view and took several seconds for image generation. Later, similar transducers were attached to motors for high-speed, mechanical scanning of a fixed, relatively small tissue region. All of these units produce images that are cross sectional with depth from the skin surface, and are referred to generically as B-mode imaging from international radar nomenclature.

Developments in the mid-1970s replaced the single-element transducer with an array of small adjacent elements, which were switched electronically for high-speed scanning. These devices were initially subdivided into simple linear arrays, which were inexpensive, durable, and reasonably small. However, they had limited performance features and a phased array (or electronic sector scanner) in which more elements were combined during pulse formation and data reception with exact time delay relations calculated and implemented for each data line by a dedicated, high-speed computer.

Rectilinear and phased linear arrays were improved greatly during the 1980s, resulting in several affordable types of equipment that have been marketed specifically for obstetric office practice. Mechanical scanning systems tend to be combined with separate linear array transducers or to use concentric ring arrays. Spatial resolution performance of all of these devices is similar and the choice depends on other performance features.

In theory, array transducers should outperform single-element devices by achieving dynamic focusing (ie, shifting a tight focus around the field as the image is formed); however, early experience was to the contrary. Critical factors in beam forming and receive focusing were found to depend on the number of data channels and on the active aperture (the number of elements used for each data line, not the length of the array itself). Large aperture, dynamically focused ultrasound imaging was released commercially in 1983 and continues to have the best performance features for diagnostic studies. This chapter is intended to reinforce the idea that all ultrasound instruments are not alike, and that the literature often may reflect minimal rather than maximal standards as ongoing instrument advances that extend diagnostic capabilities and improve diagnostic confidence and thoroughness.

Most instruments display images on a television (faster scan) monitor. Acoustic data are translated (or scan converted) to television format. This process usually is implemented in computer memory by alternately writing data into a three-dimensional matrix (with two values for position and one for signal intensity) and reading those values out to the display, possibly after intermediate steps of image processing or manipulation. The display can be regarded as consisting of individual units (ie, picture elements or pixels), each representing a volume element or voxel of tissue.

There are three practical concerns of the display matrix model. The first is that the number of pixels per tissue millimeter governs image resolution. If the matrix is too small, detail will be poor at any examination frequency. Likewise, a large field of view, or panorama, will have low detail resolution. Newer systems concentrate the area of scanning and allocate the entire display matrix to that tissue region (ie, image magnification) for optimal detail rendition. The second concern is temporal resolution or the ability to detect tissue movement during visually continuous imaging. Images consist of separate lines, each requiring a minimal time for acoustic pulse transmit from the deepest reflector and back. A predetermined number of lines create an image frame. Image cosmetics depend on line density with high-speed scanning (many frames per second) achieved at the expense of sparse data. The elements of temporal resolution are the rates of data acquisition and image updating, data registration (for successive frames), and display magnification. A reflector must appear in different pixels in subsequent frames before motion is observed. Electronic scanning units have exact registration, while mechanical scanning systems do not. Magnification imaging will reveal fetal cardiac motion from 5.4 weeks gestational age, while mechanical scanning systems may not demonstrate viability directly before 8 to 9 weeks.

Spatial resolution involves identifying image details by their location. Contrast resolution refers to identifying structures by their relative reflectivity, or gray scale properties, which is the third component of the display matrix. A matrix with a 6-bit depth will be able to display 2^6 or 64 gray shades. Ultrasound backscatter signal amplitudes depend on the local elastic moduli of the tissue under study, and consequently ultrasound images are maps of these elasticity features. In many instances, the collagenous histology of tissue can be displayed, as in the relative echodensity of decidua versus myometrium, reflectivity differences of fetal lung and liver, or progressive changes in placental reflectivity with age. Alternate examples relating to tissue macrostructure or material integrity (rather than collagen content) are appearances of simple serous cysts and effusions versus hemorrhagic, inflammatory, or neoplastic collections and the sonic differentiation of renal pyramids and cortex. Contrast features have not been explored thoroughly in fetal studies; however, they underlie the ability to discern anatomic features.

Endovaginal scanning is a great advance in obstetric and gynecologic ultrasound. Noise and beam distortion are introduced by sound transmission through layers of skin, fat, fascia, and muscle. Coupling the transducer to the vaginal wall or cervix greatly reduces these effects and yields "clean," sharply focused images. The improvement is most marked with small aperture imaging devices. As in conventional scanning, the larger the aperture, the larger the number of data channels, and the higher the center frequency, the better the image detail. Lower noise content with this form of imaging also results in a more realistic gray scale or contrast range (Fig. 6–3, see *color plate*). Endovaginal scanning has been used with increasing accuracy in first-trimester viewing of the uterus and its adnexa; how-

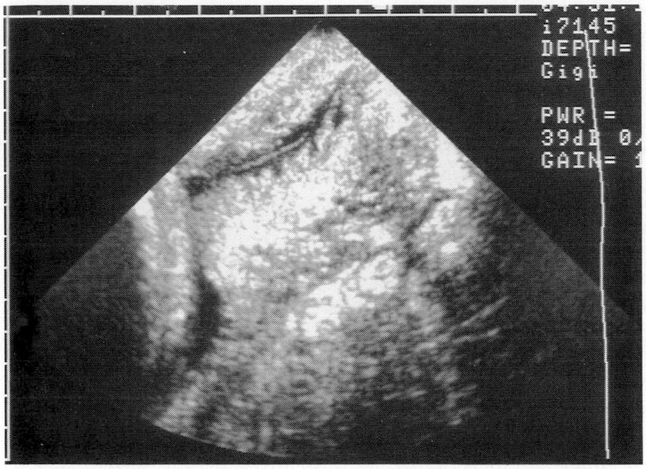

Figure 6–4. Arbor vitae form the rugose boundary of the endocervical canal. (7 MHz, endovaginal view.)

ever, it is the best way to visualize the endocervical canal at any age (Fig. 6–4), and it has specific advantages for detailed study of the temporal bone, eyes, and brain when the vertex presents. Other intracavitary probes have been developed for transrectal and transesophageal viewing, and microprobes are being studied for intravascular scanning.

The final technical topic pertinent to routine scanning is Doppler ultrasound. Motion (and attenuation) alters the frequency content of an ultrasound pulse or beam. The velocity of motion along the beam axis is directly proportional to the frequency shift. Blood flow within the fetal heart or larger arteries will induce Doppler shifts of a low-megahertz ultrasound pulse into an audible range. Conversely, the velocity of flow can then be determined by measuring the frequency shift between emitted and received pulses. Ultrasonic heart rate monitors use separate sending and receiving transducers, typically arranged as a V, focused at a predetermined depth below the skin. Ultrasound emission is continuous, and frequency shifts are induced by motion anywhere along the beam path.

Pulsed Doppler, like pulse echo imaging, uses acoustic pulses several microseconds in duration with most scanning time occupied by passive listening. Doppler shifts are determined for range compartments (or gates) a particular distance from the transducer surface. Originally, pulsed Doppler probes were combined with B-mode imaging for "duplex" scanning. The imaging portion was used for aiming, a picture frozen, and the Doppler activated for sampling. Two flaws in this arrangement are that the actual location of the Doppler gate does not correspond to image appearance at all times because beam refraction changes with angle of insonification and that target tracking is difficult for moving fields like the fetus, umbilical cord, or maternal kidney during breathing. These limitations are overcome with array imaging systems in which imaging and Doppler sampling incorporate the same elements: The gate and the target can be superimposed precisely, and imaging can be continuous by electronically alternating between two forms of data collection.

Conventional pulsed Doppler samples a single range gate. The display is a tracing of motion velocity toward or away from the probe. Motion along the beam axis is detected fully, while movement purely perpendicular to the beam is not detected at all; for motion in between, signal strength is related to the cosine of the angle of incidence. Geometry is a critical concern in Doppler sampling, particularly when flow velocity and channel size (cross-sectional area) are used to calculate volume flow, as in the umbilical or portal veins. Flow direction is indicated by the algebraic sign (+ or −) of the frequency shift.

Two-dimensional Doppler imaging[4] is achieved by using multiple range gates simultaneously. The frequency shift is portrayed as a color overlaying the B-mode image, hence the term *color flow* Doppler ultrasound (Fig. 6–5, see *color plate*). The range of velocities that can be detected and the size of vessels that can be portrayed with one- and two-dimensional Doppler depend on interrogating frequency and target depth. Just as imaging performance depends on particular instrument features, individual clinical applications of Doppler depend on available transducers and signal processing regimes.

MATERNAL EXAMINATION SCOPE

Scanning time is devoted primarily to the fetal examination in healthy, normotensive pregnant women; however, an upper abdominal survey can be completed in 1–2 minutes and can be implemented by protocol or clinical indication at any time. A phased array is used for surveying because of the large field of view and small probe contact area, which is especially important for intercostal viewing of the diaphragm, liver, gallbladder, spleen, adrenals, and heart. A larger aperture array is used for detail viewing when indicated by primary survey findings.

Gallbladder screening[5] is not established during pregnancy, although it is included in the examination protocol informally if the mother is obese. Just as a significant percentage of women with gestational diabetes will develop maturity-onset diabetes later, so too can women with intrabiliary particulates[6] during pregnancy be expected to have an increased risk of cholelithiasis. This screening may be helpful with the current advances in pharmacologic prevention of stones or their chemical dissolution.[7] Sonomammography is another potential screening examination for mammary dysplasia, ductal ectasia (Fig. 6–6), or a solid nodule.

Ultrasound permits definition of the incidence of hydronephrosis in pregnancy[8], although it is not clear that dilatation of the upper tracts has prognostic significance in the asymptomatic subject. Renal evaluation is enhanced by Doppler studies of intrarenal blood flow, and increasing arterial resistance at interlobar or arcuate artery level defines a cortical level functional abnormality. Likewise, color flow Doppler imaging of urine flow jets within the urinary bladder provides a noninvasive means to test split renal function (Fig. 6–7, see *color plate*). Renal imaging should be routine with hypertension. Unilateral renal disease can be identified, although this is an unlikely cause. Of practical significance, however, is the finding of perirenal fluid transudation, which heralds clinical decompensation in a patient with preeclampsia. Predictive studies of positional variations in renal blood flow may be developed as an ultrasonic form of rollover test.

Most maternal ultrasound studies in the second or third trimester are prompted by pelvic pain or by previous or concurrent systemic disease. Particular concerns of pelvic pain (assuming exclusion of extrauterine pregnancy) are renal calculus, appendicitis, red degeneration of a myoma,

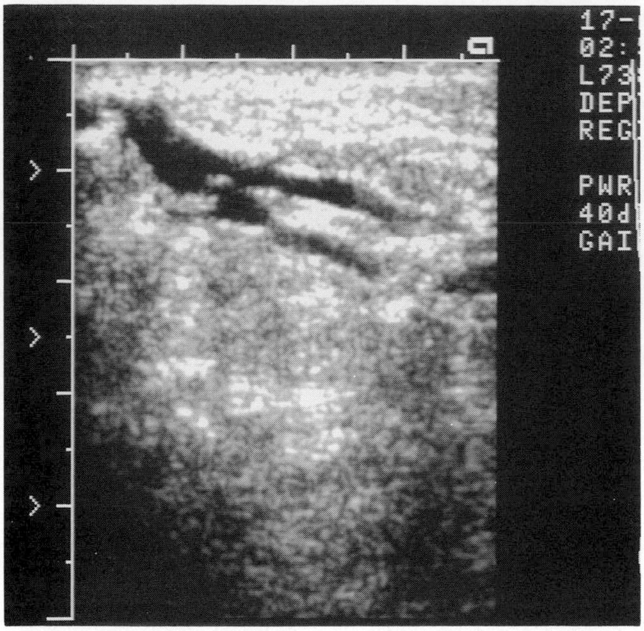

Figure 6–6. Ectatic ductal group at 2 o'clock in the left breast. Scale markers represent 5-mm tissue spacings.

hemorrhagic or infarcting ovarian cyst, or ruptured dermoid; each has a specific ultrasonic finding. Following are some basic maternal uses for ultrasound: for neoplastic disease—detection and staging of primary lesion, localization for biopsy, and diagnosis of metastatic foci, especially in liver or regional nodes; for collagen vascular disease—detection of effusions, especially of pleura or pericardium, evaluation of renal parenchyma and intrarenal blood flow, and detection of venous thromboses; for inflammatory disease—identification of abscesses or phlegmons and guidance for their drainage, and, in the case of inflammatory disease of the gastrointestinal tract, study of bowel wall features (Fig. 6–8).

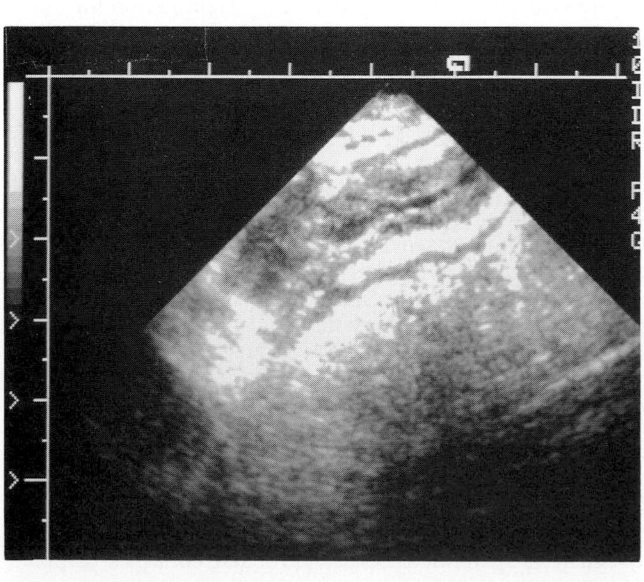

Figure 6–8. This segment of ileum has a reflective outer boundary, a very thick, rigid submucosal layer, and effaced mucosa (regional enteritis).

Ultrasonic study is usually not used for maternal neurologic conditions; however, the eyes are imaged easily with high-frequency probes, which may be helpful if chorioretinal components exist or when neuro-opthalmologic features are discernable from pupillary responses (Fig. 6–9). Vascular disease, particularly peripheral varicosities and thrombophlebitis, is amenable to ultrasonic evaluation through demonstration of thrombi directly[9] or inferred from altered flow patterns.

A well-developed segment of ultrasound is used for the cardiovascular system, but it tends to be limited in obstetric practice to conditions such as myocarditis during pregnancy or a gravid subject with congenital heart disease. Noninvasive physiologic vascular studies, however, may be useful for monitoring central venous volume flow or myocardial contractility with beta mimetic drug therapy. Lower segment movements can be monitored ultrasonically in these same patients to indicate a drug's effect and to contribute to drug dose titration.

Ultrasound images are synthesized on a line-by-line basis with each data line representing an acoustic pulse path. Any structure that is visualized ultrasonically can be entered physically by replacing a data line with a needle. Techniques are available that continually monitor ultrasonic needle passage.[10] This use of ultrasound is familiar from genetic amniocentesis (Fig. 6–10) and is identical conceptually to guided nephrostomy, biliary decompression, abscess drainage, aspiration of a simple cyst, thoracentesis, paracentesis, fetal transfusion, or biopsy of a solid mass, any of which might apply diagnostically or therapeutically during pregnancy.

The uterus can be considered during the maternal examination. One of the most important capabilities of high-frequency endovaginal and endorectal scanning is detailed visualization of the endocervical canal (see Fig. 6–4) and measurement of its length.[11] *Arbor vitae* are discerned cen-

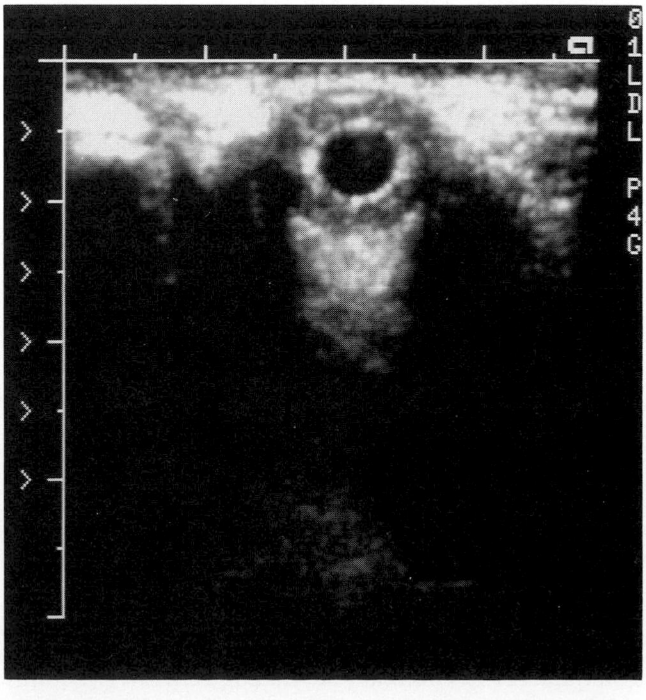

Figure 6–9. The iris and pupil are shown in coronal section. M-mode data lines permit quantitation of pupillary dynamics.

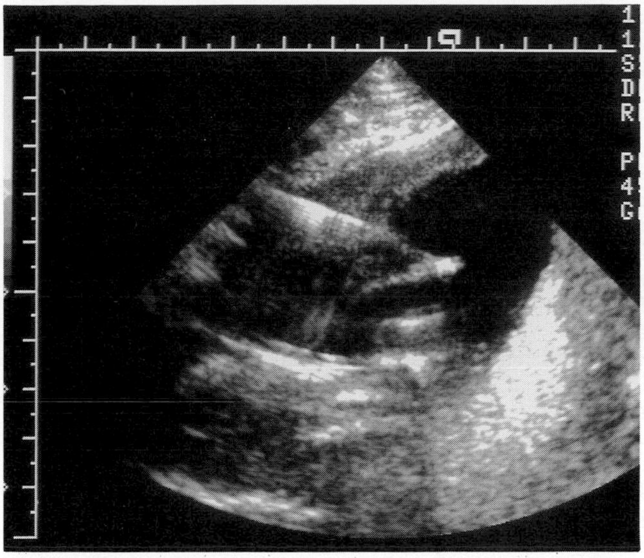

Figure 6–10. A #22 spinal needle enters from 10 o'clock. A sonic flare marks the needle tip within amniotic fluid.

trally, and full thickness wall features, vascularity, and contractility of the canal region are displayed. Examinations should distinguish mechanical failure of the canal (shortening, fluid distension, incompetent cervix) and organized contractions at the internal os. This same viewing portal facilitates definition of relations between a low-lying placenta and the internal os. Also, color flow Doppler imaging adds the dimension of detecting *vasa praevia* graphically.

ULTRASONIC MONITORING OF MATERNAL–FETAL INTERACTIONS

Maternal–fetal interactions include a broad range of potential adverse fetal effects of maternal disease or toxic exposures, a limited group of maternal conditions directly attributable to pregnancy, and a descriptively nebulous collection of dyadic, psychophysiologic interrelations between mother and fetus. Examples of these groups are fetal A-V block with maternal lupus (Fig. 6–11, see *color plate*), maternal liver infarcts with toxemia, fetal nephrolithiasis with maternal diuretic use,[12] and fetal tachycardia with maternal anxiety (presumably mediated by catecholamines).

Ultrasonic fetal studies may be divided into visualization of anatomy, observation of dynamics (principally neuromotor behavior and blood flow patterns), and inference of physiologic information from changing anatomic features, such as monitoring growth or staging a fetus from serial somatic measurements. The practical use of ultrasound for studying maternal–fetal interactions or for evaluating the fetus primarily depends on instrument performance and operational thoroughness in all three areas.

Ultrasound is an anatomic imaging process. The images describe tissue elasticity which, in many instances, translates to collagen distribution at a macroscopic level of organization. Contrast has been mentioned as a fundamental determinant of anatomic visualization. If there is no contrast between a structure and its surroundings, it will be "invisible." A glass stirring rod is visually invisible in water. Maximal spatial resolution is achieved when there is maximal contrast for the target, and as the contrast declines, details become blurred.

The chronology of visualization depends on contrast gradients. A minute but featureless gestational sac appears about 9 days after conception, the yolk sac appears approximately 6 days later, and finally a 1-mm fetus adjacent to a 3- to 4-mm yolk sac appears around day 20. These are fluid–soft tissue gradients. The first intrafetal features to be discerned are the spine at 7 weeks' gestation and the third vesicle posteriorly in the cranium. These represent hard versus soft tissue and fluid–solid (maximal contrast) gradients. Skeletal features, including cartilaginous portions of fingers and toes, are easily studied by 2½ months using higher frequency endovaginal scanning. The heart is recognized by its motion as early as 5½ weeks' gestation; however, a clear depiction of valves, septa, and myocardium is unusual with the same scanning regimen before 11 weeks because of the lower contrast gradients for these structures.

An early survey for anatomic defects is indicated by maternal drug use or toxic exposure around the time of conception (eg, oral contraceptives, lithium, dilantin, tetracycline, theophylline, fever, x-rays, lead, gases, or fumes) or by a family history of a malformation sequence. Typically, an all-or-nothing effect is expected from early exposures regarding the possibility of specific organ or system defects after the fifth week. Recent studies with endovaginal probes have indicated that true blighted ovum or anembryonic pregnancy is uncommon with sacs persistent beyond 6 weeks, and that "emptiness" in suprapubic views represents a technical limitation of that approach. Missed abortion usually appears as a small amniotic bubble containing a macerated fetal pole, typically without a well-formed adjacent yolk sac. Yolk sac failures have been noted with diabetes and with neural tube defects.[13] Fetal demise is defined (or excluded) explicitly by the absence of cardiac activity, which should always be visible with electronically scanned systems by 6 weeks' gestation. Occasionally, intracardiac gas will be seen in a first trimester fetus 4 days or more after demise. A heart rate below 80, even at 6 weeks, is a poor prognostic sign.[14]

The effects of the time course of organ development and the concept of vulnerable periods are illustrated by directed ultrasonic anatomic studies of the fetal brain. Cranial and spinal integrity are demonstrable around 7–8 weeks' gestation. Exencephaly in the middle of the first trimester is associated with proliferative fibrovascular material that reabsorbs, forming the typical appearance of anencephaly in the second trimester (Fig. 6–12, see *color plate*). A simianlike disproportion in arm length[15] and coarse facial features also are evident early. Division into hemispheres is defined by the appearance of paired choroid glomi by the eighth week, permitting early diagnosis of alobar holoprosencephaly. The first major phase of neuronal proliferation occurs around 14–16½ weeks, followed by the first phase of neuronal migration, followed then by glial proliferation. These phases are indicated ultrasonically by the time course of cortical thickness.[16] High-resolution imaging demonstrates cortical layering, which is established by 21 weeks (Fig. 6–13). The corpus callosum is fully formed by 22 weeks,[17] and its thickness and shape may provide a global marker of cortical development. Sulcation occurs in the third trimester. Consequently, abnormalities involving neuronal proliferation cannot be detected in the first trimester because that stage of development has not yet occurred. Likewise, migration disorders are not detectable before sulcation is established in the third trimester. Similarly, the first phase of neuronal migration is a time of particular

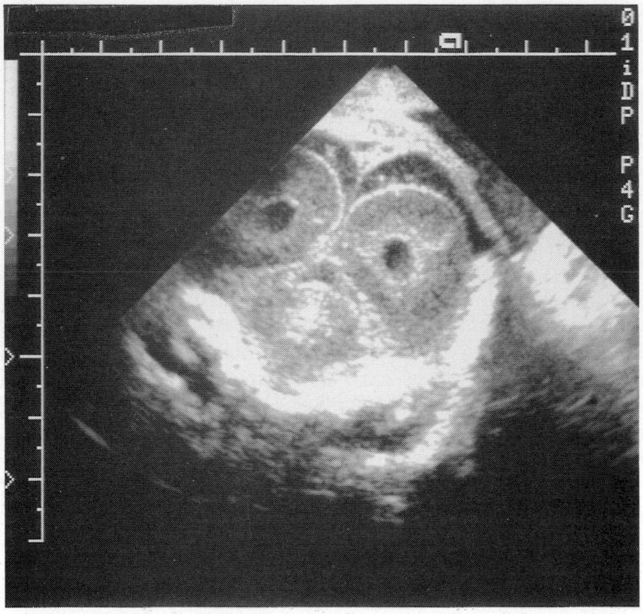

Figure 6–13. The germinal layer borders the ventricle and is echodense. Layers appear within the cortex later in the second trimester.

vulnerability to external insults, such as ionizing radiation[18] and alcohol.

Late effects are illustrated by maternal cocaine use; vasospastic injuries are associated with cerebral infarction, gastrointestinal atresias, or placental abruptions. Fetal distortions, such as clubbed feet or wrist contractures from oligohydramnios and immobility of a body part, are another source of deformity supervening on normal anatomic development. The most common form of acquired abnormality is hypoxic brain injury, which will be discussed later in this chapter.

Growth implies a progressive increase; therefore, clinical and physiologic studies of fetal growth require specific definitions. Somatic growth is monitored by serial changes in length, area, or volume of part or all of the body. Analysis includes calculation of a global measure, such as weight,[19] and of proportions between measured values. The acquisition of physiologic competence for extrauterine survival is referred to as maturation and is another aspect of growth. Somatic growth is depressed with chromosome abnormalities and with TORCH infections because of a primary decrease in cell division rates.[20] Severe growth deficits (as with triploidy) are associated with generalized soft-tissue hypoplasia and can be detected in the first trimester. Milder forms (eg, Down's syndrome) may be evident only through delayed neuronal proliferation (with transient, secondary ventriculomegaly at 16 weeks' gestation) or delayed lymphatic proliferation (with suboccipital skin thickening persisting after 13 weeks).

For the most part, clinical attention has been directed toward recognizing fetal growth retardation from placental–vascular insufficiency, paying particular attention to maternal hypertension, collagen vascular disease, insulin-dependent diabetes with eye or renal findings, or a history of maternal growth retardation. This emphasis on growth retardation is, however, clinically inappropriate. If the placenta begins to fall, the fetus can invoke several compensatory mechanisms.[21] On the circulatory side, the normally closed *ductus venosus* opens to increase venous return to the heart and alter blood flow streaming effects in the right atrium. Persistent portal steal through the ductus results in delayed growth of the right lobe of the liver, which accounts for the pattern of asymmetrical growth retardation. Also, blood flow is redistributed for preferential support of the brain, heart, and adrenals. Decreased renal blood flow[22] eventuates in diminished amniotic fluid volume. Energy is conserved by decreasing oxygen expenditure; heart rate decreases 10–16 beats per minute, all body movements are decreased (by way of central inhibition), and less time is spent in a rapid eye movement (REM) behavioral state. Finally, there is decreased growth factor secretion from the fetal gut, resulting in a global decrease in growth rate, which is perhaps associated directly with some acceleration of functional maturation of the lungs and brain. This type of growth retardation is part of the biologic compensation for deteriorating environmental conditions and represents cases in whom the compromise has been chronic and mild. In other words, a fetus may be normal in size but in serious jeopardy. A small fetus is at increased risk of hypoxic injury, but that injury may not occur.

There has been considerable technical interest in Doppler monitoring of fetal circulatory features. The most widely used technique evaluates the waveform of umbilical artery flow velocity to detect small vessel disease within the placenta from increased forward flow resistance (manifested through decreased or absent diastolic flow components).[23] The situation is similar to that of growth retardation because high resistance indicates a risk state but not that fetal injury has been sustained (or that growth has been affected). Conversely, normal flow may not be reassuring because there are other forms of placental pathology (e.g., biochemical transport capabilities) that can compromise the fetus greatly, but because they have no vascular components, there will be no direct Doppler sign.

The umbilical cord is an integral part of the maternal–fetal supply line, often regarded as a passive conduit; however, the potential for intrauterine or perinatal compromise in umbilical flow has been well documented since the classic review of Browne.[24] Nuchal coils are present in about one fourth of all deliveries.[25] Umbilical cords are easily seen with color flow Doppler (Fig. 6–14, see *color plate*), because of the flow velocities that occur normally. We have found that the incidence of nuchal coiling *in utero* is approximately 35% overall for the second and third trimesters, with a 40% transition probability of forming or losing a nuchal coil between random studies (Fig. 6–15, see *color plate*). Nuchal coils are more common with increased cord length and increased fetal motility, that is, with male sex, growth acceleration, and hydramnios. The incidence is also increased with depressed amniotic fluid volume and with decreased somatic growth. Nuchal cords, particularly those that are relatively straight (Fig. 6–16, see *color plate*), are easily compressed externally, and we have shown spontaneous decreases in umbilical vein volume flow with nuchal coiling. We interpret these findings as indicating that a nuchal cord can potentiate primary placental insufficiency or induce a supply line deficit by itself and observe that the perinatal etiology of cerebral palsy is not resolved.[26,27] Also noted is that the presence or absence of a nuchal coil at delivery does not indicate its prenatal occurrence at a critical developmental juncture. We have observed nuchal coils in three cases of middle second trimester hydrocephalus, although this may have been coincidental or related secondarily through an altered movement pattern.

There has been some attempt to predict the third-trimester occurrence of supply line deficiency from diminished

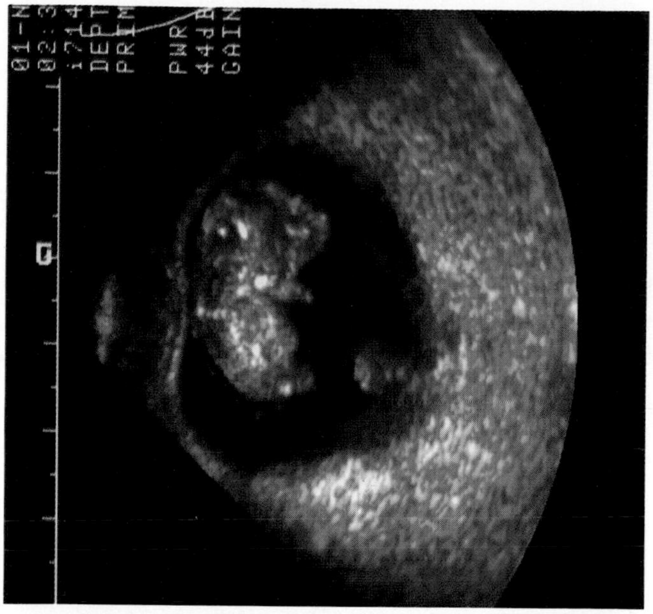

Figure 6–3. The gray scale of this 7 MHz endovaginal view of an early first trimester fetus has been translated (by computer) into color for perceptual enhancement.

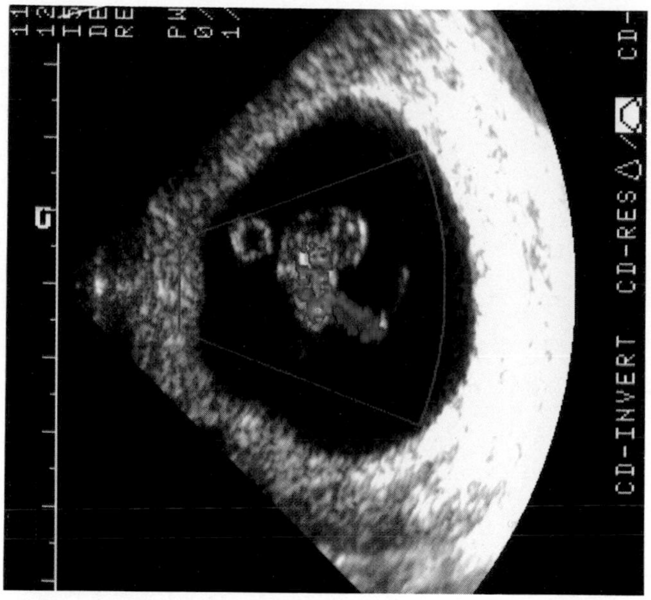

Figure 6–5. Blood flow in larger vessels and heart appear in color. This is a 15 mm fetus.

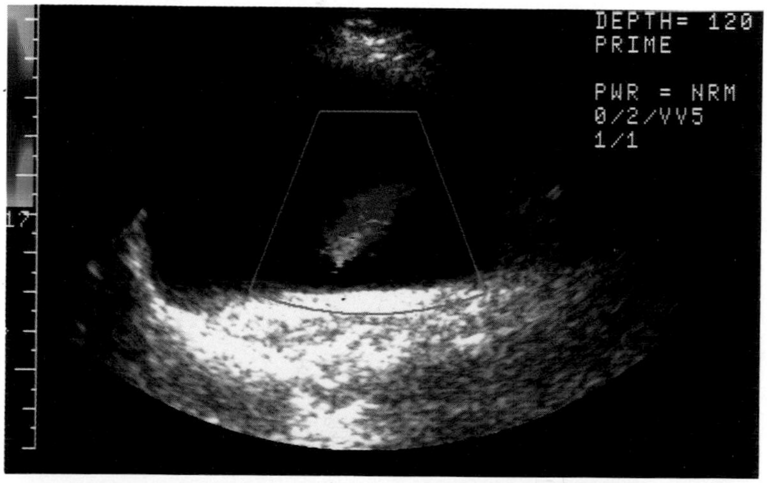

Figure 6–7. Color flow image of a pulse of urine injected into the bladder from the right uterovesicle junction (subject supine).

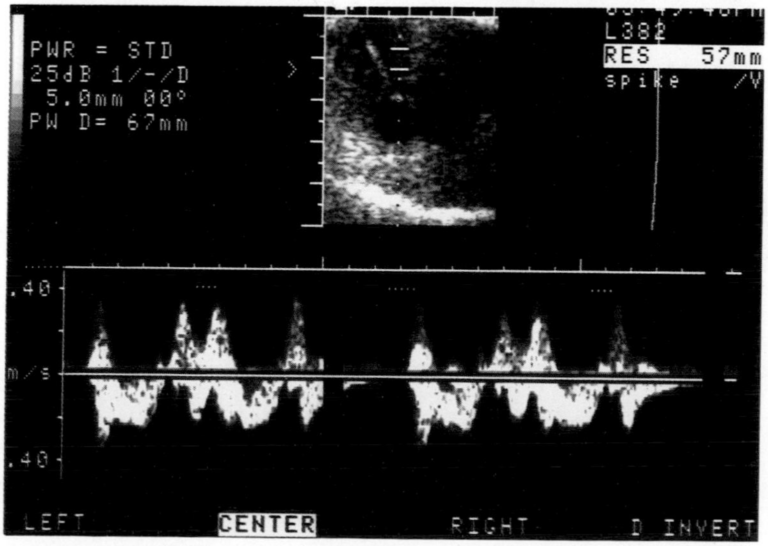

Figure 6–11. This fetal left ventricular cavity pulsed Doppler tracing shows a recurrent triplet complex of escape, normal, and aberrant atrial beats. Baseline heart rate was 125. These patterns may precede fixed heart block.

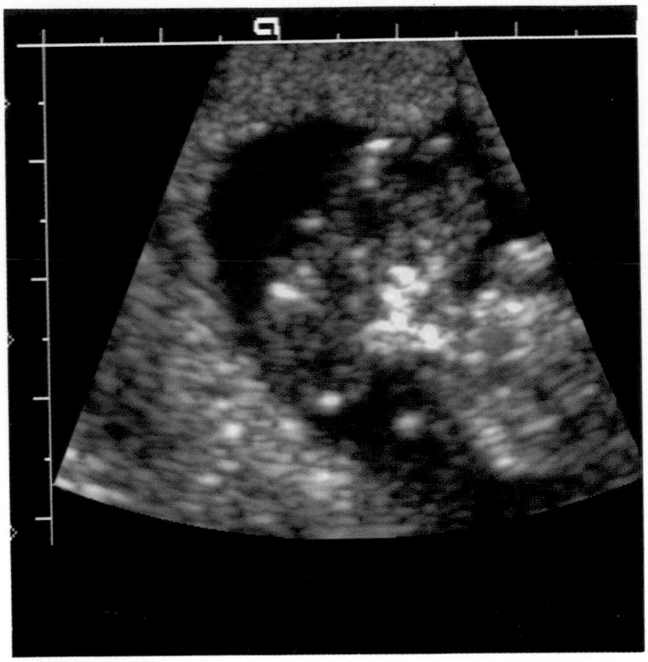

Figure 6–12. Exencephaly, first trimester. There is no cranium; facial bones are coarse, and fibrovascular material extends like a ram's horn.

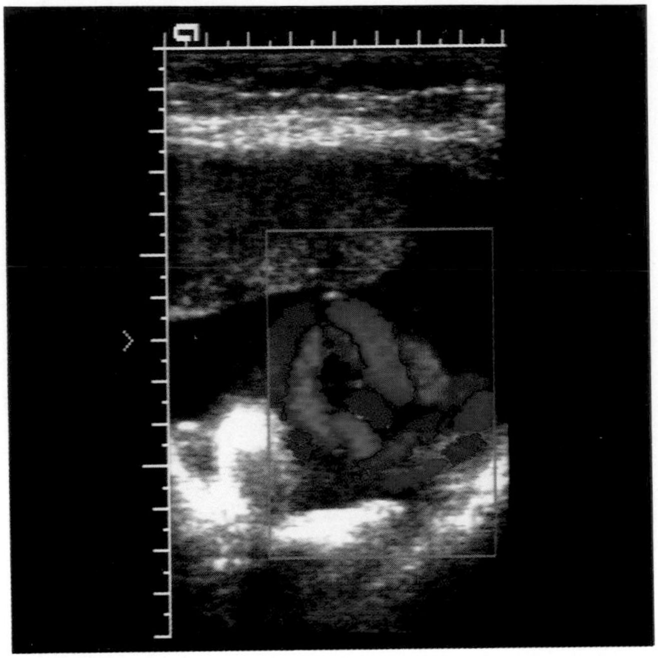

Figure 6–14. Umbilical cords are depicted graphically with color flow Doppler. Knots rarely tighten in utero.

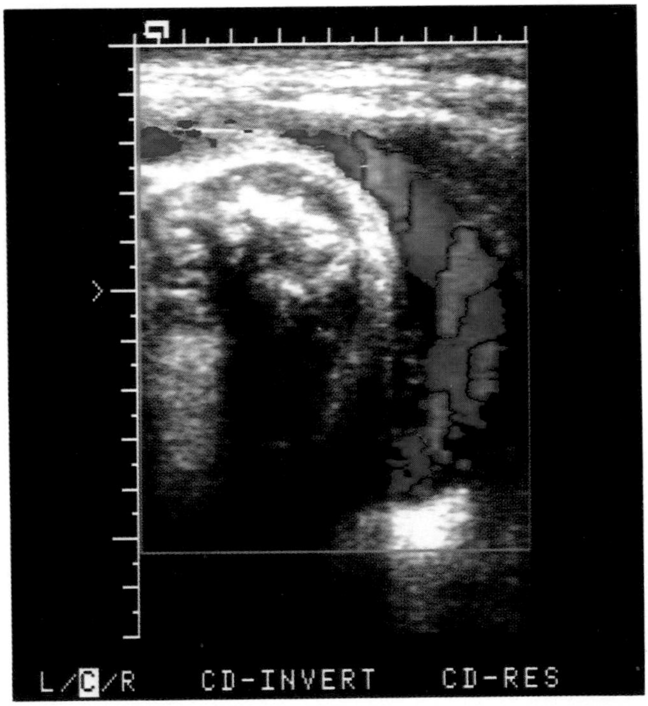

Figure 6–15. The neck is situated at the shallowest portion of the gravid uterus when the head presents. Nuchal cords can be compressed in utero.

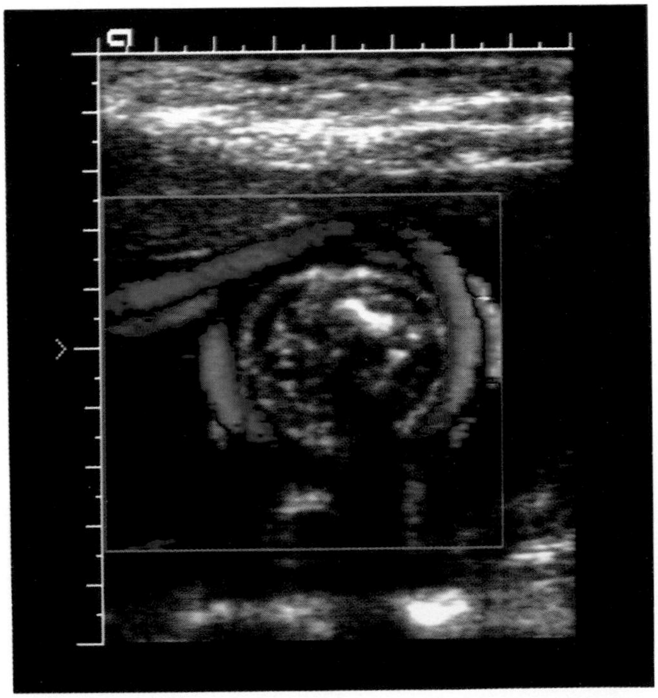

Figure 6–16. Straight nuchal cords appear to be particularly vulnerable to compression (compare with Figure 6–15).

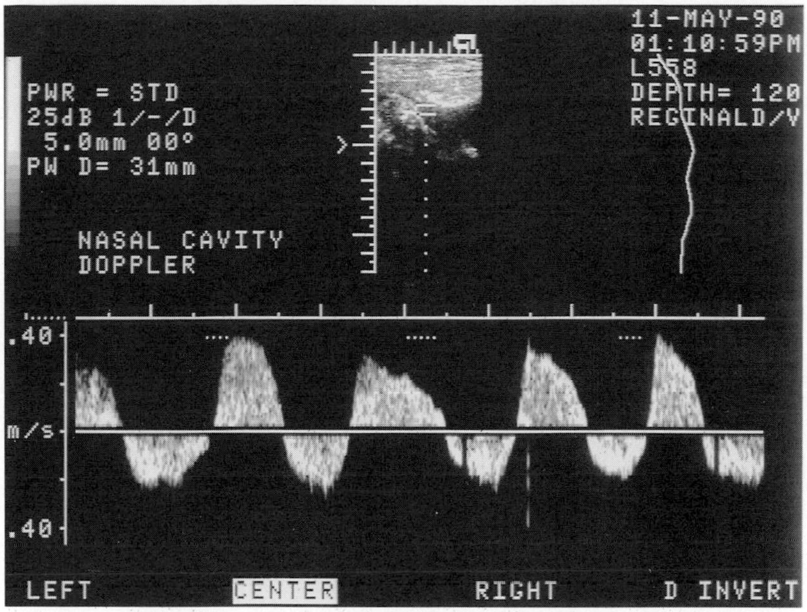

Figure 6–17. Pulsed and color flow Doppler permit approaches to fetal breathing studies. Patterns of fluid flow through the nose relate to behavioral state; breath-to-breath variations in waveform indicate baroreceptor and chemoreceptor effects.

uterine artery flow[28] and placental dimensions in the second trimester.[29] Maternal blood pressure may be elevated persistently or vary on a minute or hour time scale. Also, uterine blood flow may undergo short-term moderation, potentially representing an extraplacental pathway through which maternal stress may affect the fetal environment abruptly. Observations of changes in fetal movement patterns related to maternal emotional stress[30] preceded Doppler study capability.

A body of descriptive literature on fetal movements has evolved since the advent of high-speed ultrasonic imaging[31], which extends earlier works on maternal perception of movement or pressure transducer sensing through the maternal abdominal wall. Noninvasive studies of the human fetal sensorium have been limited primarily to hearing,[32] although anecdotal accounts and early invasive experience refer to taste and smell.[33] These modalities, unlike vision, function early in gestation and appear to require prenatal stimulation for their development. Maternal voice and gastrointestinal sounds are an integral part of the fetal acoustic environment.[34] Recent studies of newborn infants have demonstrated recognition and preference for maternal voice,[35] showing a fetal–maternal interaction with psychologic implications. This may be moderated prenatally through intention or when adverse environmental conditions depress presumptive fetal awareness (Fig. 6–17).

CONCLUSIONS

Progressive advances in ultrasound imaging technology have occurred during the past 20 years. While newer instrument types that permit structuring high-risk studies are diffusing into community practice, a trend toward distinguishing screening and detailed forms of study has occurred, chiefly by the expertise and thoroughness of the examiner.

Ultrasound is a form of physical examination that yields clinical information. It uses anatomic appearances and physiologic inference of dynamic observation, including blood flow volumes and patterns. The study technique requires a knowledge of instrument capabilities and performance. Ultrasound examinations provide a wealth of data about both maternal and fetal health. Examination emphasis and interpretation depend on all available information before the study and on material elicited during scanning. Findings must be reconciled with knowledge of potential pathology and pathophysiology.

When approached in the context of a problem-oriented physical examination, this detailed study, which uses low noise magnification techniques, is unique in the information retrieved. In this setting, reducing data to a manageable form can be difficult, particularly for purposes of forming a long-term prognosis or identifying new sources of maternal or fetal injury. Optimality scoring[36] may provide an interim solution as databases are developed.

REFERENCES

1. Donald I, Mac Vicar J, Brown TG. Investigation of abdominal masses by pulsed ultrasound. *Lancet*. 1958;I:1188.
2. Auenbrugger L. *Inventum Novum*. Vienna, Austria: Trattner, 1761.
3. Birnholz JC. Fetal syndromes. In: Hobbins JC, Benacerraf BR, eds. *Diagnosis and Therapy of Fetal Anomalies*. New York, NY: Churchill Livingstone, 1989:1.
4. Kasai C, Namekawa K, Koyano A, Omoto R. Real-time two dimensional blood flow imaging using an autocorrelation technique. *IEEE Trans Sonics Ultrasonics SU-32*. 1985;3:447.
5. Birnholz JC. Population survey ultrasonic cholecystography. *Gastroint Radiol*. 1982;7:165.
6. Filly RA, Allen B, Minton MJ, et al. *In vitro* investigation of the origin of echoes in thin biliary sludge. *J Clin Ultrasound*. 1980;8:193.
7. Broomfield PH, Chopra R, Sheinbaum RC, et al. Effects of ursodeoxycholic acid and aspirin on the formation of lithogenic bile and gallstones during loss of weight. *N Engl J Med*. 1988;319:1567.
8. Lindheimer MD, Katz AI. The kidney in pregnancy. *New Engl J Med*. 1970;283:1095.
9. Greer IA, Barry J, Mackon N, Allan PL. Diagnosis of deep venous thrombosis in pregnancy: A new role for diagnostic ultrasound. *Brit J Obstet Gynecol*. 1990;97:53.
10. Frigoletto FD, Birnholz JC, Rothchild SB, et al. Intrauterine transfusions with the use of phased array ultrasonography: a new technique. *Am J Obstet Gynecol*. 1978;131:273.
11. Ayers JWT, DeGrood RM, Compton AA, et al. Sonographic evaluation of cervical length in pregnancy: Diagnosis and management of preterm cervical effacement in patients at risk for premature delivery. *Obstet Gynecol*. 1988;71:939.

12. Fischer AF, Parker BR, Stevenson DK. Nephrolithiasis following *in utero* diuretic exposure: an unusual case. *Ped.* 1988;81:712.
13. Pinter E, Reece AE, Leranth CZ, et al. Yolk sac failure in embryopathy due to hyperglycemia. Ultrastructural analysis of yolk sac differentiation associated with embryopathy in rat conceptuses under hyperglycemic conditions. *Teratology* 1986;33:73.
14. Laboda L, Estroff J, Benacerraf BR. First trimester bradycardia. *J Ultrasound Med.* 1989;8:706.
15. Nañages JJC. A Comparison of the growth of the body dimensions of anencephalic human fetuses with normal fetal growth as determined by graphic analysis and empirical formulae. *Am J Anat.* 1925;35:455.
16. Birnholz JC. Ultrasonic studies of human fetal brain development. *Trends Neurosci.* 1986;9:329.
17. Rakic P, Yakovlev PE. Development of the corpus callosum and the *cavum sapti* in man. *J Comp Neurol.* 1968;132:45.
18. Gaulden ME, Murray RC. Medical radiation and possible adverse effects on the human embryo. In: Meyn RE, Winthers HR, eds. *Radiation Biology in Cancer Research.* New York, NY: Raven Press, 1980:277.
19. Birnholz JC. An algorithmic approach to accurate ultrasonic fetal weight estimation. *Invest Radiol.* 1986;21:571.
20. Paton GR, Silver MF, Allison AC. Comparison of cell cycle time in normal and trisomic cells. *Hum Genet.* 1974;23:173.
21. Birnholz JC. Ecologic physiology of the fetus. *Radiol Clin North Am.* 1990;28:179.
22. Mari G, Moise JJ Jr, Deter RL, et al. Doppler assessment of the renal blood flow velocity waveform during indomethacin therapy for preterm labor and polyhydramnios. *Obstet Gynecol.* 1990;75:199.
23. Trudinger BJ, Giles WB, Cook CM, et al. Fetal umbilical artery flow velocity waveforms and placental resistance: Clinical significance. *Br J Obstet Gynecol.* 1985;92:23.
24. Browne FJ. On the abnormalities of the umbilical cord which may cause antenatal death. *J Obstet Gynaecol Br Comm.* 1925;32:17.
25. Spellacy WN, Gravem H, Fisch RO. The umbilical cord complications of true knots, nuchal coils, and cords around the body. *Am J Obstet Gynecol.* 1966;94:1136.
26. Shields JR, Schifrin BS. Perinatal antecedants of cerebral palsy. *Obstet Gynecol.* 1988;71:899.
27. Mann LI. Pregnancy events and brain damage. *Am J Obstet Gynecol.* 1986;155:6.
28. Campbell S, Pearse JMF, Hackett G, et al. Qualitative assessment of uteroplacental blood flow: early screening test for high risk pregnancies. *Obstet Gynecol.* 1986;68:649.
29. Wolf H, Oosting H, Treffers PE. Second trimester placental volume measurement by ultrasound: prediction of fetal outcome. *Am J Obstet Gynecol.* 1989;160:121.
30. Ianniruberto A, Tajani E. Ultrasonic study of fetal movement. *Sem Perinatol.* 1981;5:175.
31. deVries JIP, Visser GHA, Prechtl HFR. The emergence of fetal behavior. I. Qualitative aspects. *Early Hum Dev.* 1982;7:301.
32. Birnholz JC, Benacerraf BR. The development of human fetal hearing. *Science.* 1983;222:516.
33. DeSnoo K. Das Trinkende Kind im Uterus. *Monat Geburt Gynaekol.* 1937;105:**88.**
34. Vince MA, Billing AE, Baldwin BA, et al. Maternal vocalizations and other sound in the fetal lamb's sound environment. *Inf Behav & Dev.* 1985;11:179.
35. DeCasper AJ, Fifer WP. Of human bonding: newborns prefer their mothers' voices. *Science.* 1980;208:1174.
36. Prechtl HFR. The optimality concept. *Early Hum Dev.* 1980;4:201.

Chapter Seven

Principles of Drug Therapy

Gary C. Cupit and Heschi H. Rotmensch

7

The past several decades have witnessed major advances in the practice of therapeutics. It is now recognized that the nature, duration, and intensity of drug action are dependent not only on the intrinsic properties of the drug, but also on the interaction with the host to whom the drug is being administered. Although research has been proceeding at a rapid rate in adult medicine, developments in drug therapy during pregnancy, the perinatal period, and the neonate are lagging far behind the other disciplines. This is because research in humans during pregnancy is limited by ethical and practical considerations. Therefore, present drug use in pregnancy is based on cautious empiricism, with therapeutic misadventures acting as warning signals.

This chapter deals with the concepts of drug therapy based on clinical pharmacologic principles and the alterations occurring during the course of pregnancy. Although information regarding the pharmacokinetics of drugs during pregnancy is limited, general principles in conjunction with good clinical judgment are helpful in guiding therapy. Furthermore, the mechanisms of placental and breast-milk transfer, as well as concepts of teratogenicity or potential effects on the fetus, are discussed.

CLINICAL PHARMACOLOGY CONCEPTS AND THE PREGNANT PATIENT

For a drug to be therapeutically effective, it must reach the site of its intended pharmacologic activity within the body at a sufficient rate and in sufficient amounts to yield an effective concentration. Most drugs act at specific receptor sites, thereby affecting biochemical or physiologic processes. Whether pregnancy, with its marked physiologic changes, influences the binding and affinity of drugs to receptors and thus modifies maternal responses has not been sufficiently evaluated. Pharmacokinetic differences among individuals account for variation in drug concentrations at receptor sites and in the time course of drug action. Factors that are important in drug concentrations attained in serum and eventually at receptor sites include absorption, distribution, biotransformation, elimination, genetic factors, and drug interactions (Fig. 7–1).

Absorption

Oral medications account for the majority of all drugs prescribed. Thus, absorption from the gastrointestinal tract becomes a critical factor for determining the concentration of a drug in the plasma and its subsequent therapeutic effect. Absorption of a drug from the gastrointestinal tract is a complex process. It is influenced by physicochemical properties of the drug (eg, pK_a, molecular weight, lipid solubility) and manufacturing techniques as well as physiologic factors in the patient, such as the rate of gastric emptying, gastrointestinal motility, and food intake.

An orally administered drug must first be released from its dosage form and dissolve in the gastrointestinal fluids before it can be absorbed. Decomposition may occur in the gastrointestinal lumen. Once an orally administered

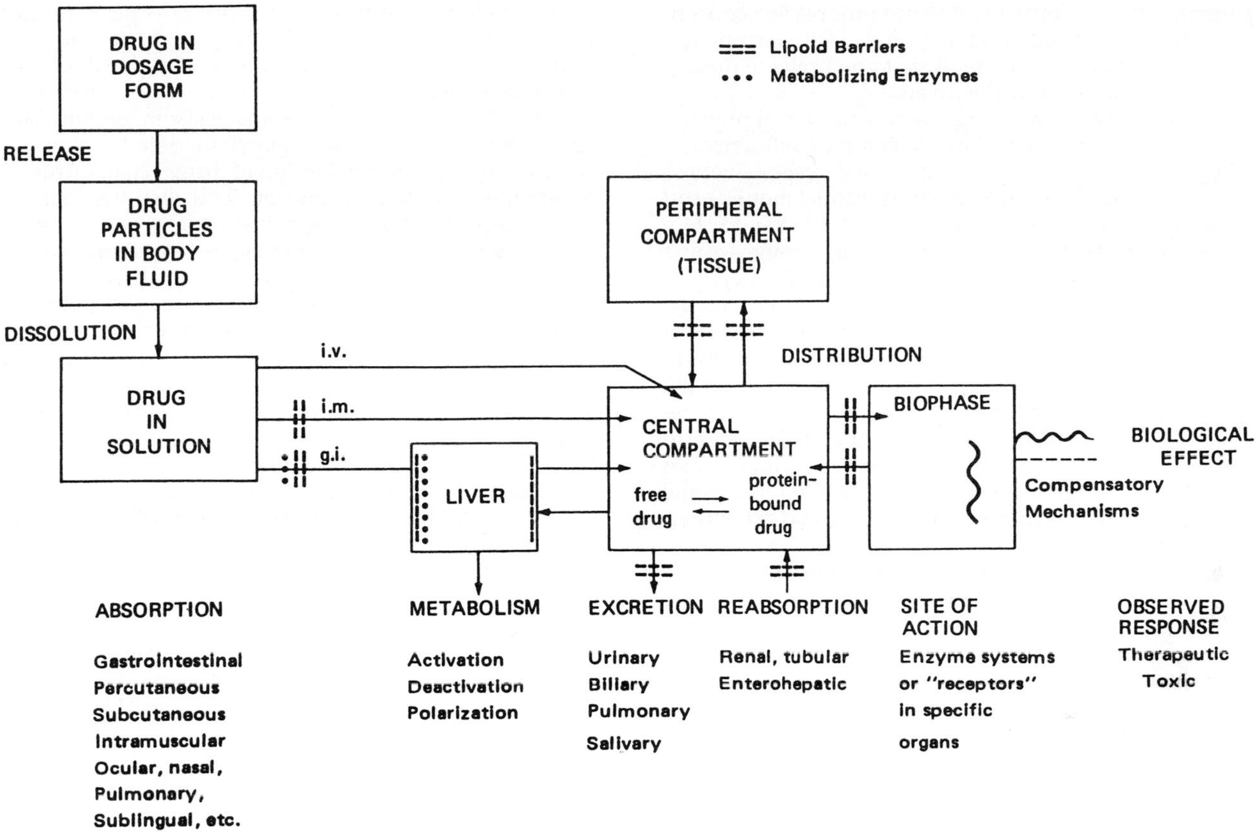

Figure 7–1. Diagram illustrating the factors that influence onset, duration, and intensity of drug effects. (*From Barr*[67] *with permission.*)

drug has been absorbed, it traverses the hepatic portal system and liver before reaching the systemic circulation. During this passage, drugs may be metabolized by enzymes in the liver (first-pass elimination). Thus, only a portion of a drug administered orally may reach the systemic circulation.

Drugs shown to undergo extensive first-past metabolism include propranolol[1], lidocaine[2], and nitroglycerin.[3] This partially explains the greater response to an intravenous dose of these drugs than to an equivalent oral dose.

Absorption does not only occur after oral administration of chemicals; it is equally applicable to events following the intramuscular, subcutaneous, topical, or inhalation route of drug administration. Incomplete or erratic absorption may occur following intramuscular and subcutaneous drug administration. With these routes of administration, blood flow to the injection site and drug solubility at pH 7.4 are the major determinants of bioavailability. For example, phenytoin has been shown to precipitate from its diluent at the pH of muscle tissue and is only slowly absorbed after intramuscular injection.[4] Shock reduces skeletal muscle blood flow and delays absorption of intramuscularly or subcutaneously injected drugs. (Table 7–1 summarizes drugs to avoid administering by the intramuscular route.) Monitoring the plasma concentration of a drug offers a useful means of assessing the entry of the drug into the body from any site of administration.

The term *bioavailability* describes the extent to which and the rate at which an administered drug dose reaches the systemic circulation unchanged. The bioavailability of a drug administered intravenously is equal to unity, whereas the bioavailability of the compound administered as an oral, intramuscular, or subcutaneous formulation is assessed in relation to an intravenous drug.

Although 100% bioavailability is ideal, predictable uniform bioavailability is satisfactory for therapeutic purposes. However, preparations of the same drug produced by different manufacturers may not be equivalent, and, thus, a change in brand may produce marked changes in serum concentrations as well as in the drug's therapeutic or toxic effects. In addition, switching from one route of administration to another may be associated with substantial serum concentration changes.[5] Significant differences in plasma drug concentrations after administration of different dosage forms and different brands of phenytoin, thyroid, prednisone, and digoxin have prompted many physicians to main-

TABLE 7–1. SELECTED AGENTS WITH ERRATIC ABSORPTION AFTER INTRAMUSCULAR ADMINISTRATION

Chlordiazepoxide
Diazepam
Digoxin
Haloperidol
Heparin
Insulin
Phenytoin
Phytonadione
Propranolol
Quinidine
Theophylline

tain patients on one product and to monitor plasma concentrations when switching dosage forms. This concept has become more critical as the use of sustained-release dosage forms is becoming more widespread.

The progressively changing maternal and fetal physiology during pregnancy may have a complex influence on drug disposition and, thus, on maternal responsiveness of therapy. During pregnancy; gastrointestinal motility and the composition of intestinal secretions may change. Elevated plasma progesterone concentrations, thought to be associated with the reduction in intestinal motility, decrease the gastric and intestinal emptying rate by 30–50% in the pregnant woman.[6] Furthermore, it has been shown that there is a reduction in gastric acid secretion, especially in the first and second trimesters, which may be up to 40% less than in the nonpregnant state.[7] Although there is reduced peptic activity, there is a considerable increase in mucus secretion. These alterations result in an increase in gastric pH and buffer capacity, which will influence the ionization of weakly acidic or basic drugs and alter their absorption characteristics.

The consequence of slower gastric emptying may be a reduction in the rate of drug absorption related to the delay in entering the small intestine. The slowed passage of drugs along the small intestine, however, may increase the absorption of some drugs.[8]

Although during pregnancy, circulatory plasma volume increases by 50%[9] and cardiac output by about 30%,[10] hepatic blood flow does not appear to be altered substantially.[11] Therefore, the magnitude of the first-pass metabolism, which is flow dependent, is not expected to differ from that in the nonpregnant woman.

For the majority of therapeutic agents, however, oral bioavailability in the pregnant patient has not been assessed.

Pulmonary absorption of therapeutic agents also may be altered during pregnancy. Absorption of drugs across the alveolar membrane is known to be influenced by both hemodynamic and ventilatory factors. Because cardiac output is increased in pregnancy, a higher pulmonary blood flow would favor alveolar drug uptake. Hyperventilation resulting from the increased tidal volume shown in pregnancy also results in a more rapid rate of transport across the alveolar membrane than in the nonpregnant woman.[12] These alterations should be considered in administration of drugs by inhalation to pregnant patients.

Distribution

Once absorption is complete, drugs distribute into tissues and other body fluids. The rate at which equilibrium between tissue and plasma concentrations is achieved depends on three major factors: blood perfusion rate to organs, drug lipid solubility, and drug binding to proteins or tissue.

Distribution of a drug is achieved at different rates within different compartments depending on the tissue vascularity. In a simple model, the body can be divided into two compartments: (1) the central compartment consisting of the plasma and extracellular fluid and highly vascular tissue (eg, red blood cells, lungs, liver, kidney), and (2) a compartment of poorly perfused tissues (eg, fat, muscle, skin). Drug distribution into poorly perfused tissues will require a longer time. If, for example, the site of action of a drug is located within a poorly perfused organ, the measurement of plasma concentration before equilibrium being attained may not reflect concentrations of the drug at the site of action.

Distribution of a drug also depends on its physicochemical properties including lipid solubility. The property of lipid solubility allows drugs to cross biologic barriers such as cell membranes, the blood–brain barrier, and the placenta, whereas highly water-soluble drugs will cross such membranes only if they are of small molecular size.

In addition, both tissue and plasma protein binding have been recognized as important determinants of the apparent volume of distribution of drugs. Acidic drugs commonly bind to albumin, and basic drugs often bind to α_1-acid glycoproteins and lipoproteins. Many endogenous substances, vitamins, and metal ions, are bound predominantly to globulins. Because only the nonprotein-bound (free) drug, which is pharmacologically active, is capable of distributing to tissues, drugs highly bound to serum proteins have a small volume of distribution. The presence of renal or hepatic disease affecting plasma protein concentrations may result in considerable changes in the percentage of drugs bound to protein, thus altering its volume of distribution as well as its biologic effects.

The apparent volume of distribution is defined as the volume of fluid into which a drug distributes, assuming a concentration equal to that measured in the blood. The concept of distribution volume is clinically useful because it defines the relationship between prescribed drug dose and expected plasma concentration. When a drug has a volume of distribution less than body weight, it usually is found preferentially in one compartment. This is the case with gentamicin, in which volume of distribution is 0.25 L/kg or 25% of total body weight.[13] Calculation of the apparent volume of distribution, however, may exceed body weight. This, for example, is the case with digoxin, in which volume of distribution is 7–9 L/kg,[14] indicating extensive accumulation in extravascular sites. (Selected volumes of distribution of compounds are listed in Table 7–2). The volumes of distribution of some drugs may be affected by intercurrent illnesses such as congestive heart failure or liver or kidney diseases.

The progressive expansion of maternal intravascular and extravascular fluid volumes as well as tissue volumes that accompany growth of the uterus, placenta, and fetus is likely to affect drug distribution. As mentioned previously, by the 30th to 34th week of gestation, the circulatory plasma volume has increased by about 50%, with cardiac output increasing by about 30%. Renal, uterine, and pulmonary blood flow increase in accordance with the increased cardiac output.

In addition to the hemodynamic changes, important alterations in body water compartments have been demonstrated.[15] The total increase of body water at term in a normal primagravida amounts to about 8 L, of which approximately 60% is in the product of conception (fetus, placenta, uterus, amniotic fluid). These adaptive changes

TABLE 7–2. SELECTED VOLUMES OF DISTRIBUTION

Drug	V_d(L/kg)
Digoxin	7.3
Digitoxin	0.45
Gentamicin	0.25
Lidocaine	1.3
Phenobarbital	0.7
Phenytoin	0.7
Procainamide	2.0
Quinidine	3.0
Theophylline	0.5

in body water distribution may influence drug distribution and elimination. The distribution of drugs into a larger physiologic volume implies that acute administration of a single dose of a drug is likely to result in lower plasma concentrations in pregnant than in nonpregnant women. Therefore, in order to achieve a desired drug plasma concentration, higher loading doses may be needed in pregnant women. Steady-state plasma concentrations of the drug, resulting from chronic administration, would not be expected to change significantly unless factors associated with pregnancy alter drug clearance from the body.

As mentioned previously, another important factor determining the distribution volume as well as the biologic activity of a drug is plasma protein binding.[16] There is increasing evidence that during pregnancy, plasma protein binding capacity decreases. As a result of the major expansion of the extracellular volume during pregnancy, concentrations of plasma proteins such as albumin[17] tend to fall. However, in addition to the changes in protein concentration, it has been postulated that a gradual rise in endogenous inhibitors of drug binding in plasma may account for the observed reduction in binding capacity. Pregnancy is associated with important hormonal changes, with a rise in total plasma lipids and free fatty acids, and with alterations in the concentrations of a variety of endogenous substances. Preliminary studies indicate that at equal concentrations of serum albumin, the unbound (free) fraction of diazepam, a highly protein-bound compound, is higher in the plasma of pregnant women than in controls.[18] This suggests that the binding capacity of albumin is reduced. This could reflect either intrinsic alterations in the properties of the albumin molecule or interference by endogenous binding inhibitors. An inverse relationship between free drug fraction and the concentration of albumin in the serum of pregnant women has been demonstrated for a number of drugs, including diazepam[19], phenytoin[20], phenobarbital[20], valproic acid,[20] sulfisoxazole,[21] and salicylic acid.[21] In contrast, some endogenous compounds such as copper, iron, and thyroid hormones frequently increase during pregnancy.

The alterations in drug-binding capacity during pregnancy may have several therapeutic implications when drugs are administered that are extensively protein bound (>90%). Because only the unbound fraction of a drug is biologically active, the reduced binding capacity may alter the response. For example, when a drug is administered rapidly by an intravenous injection, a decrease in protein binding may result in a higher concentration of free drug reaching highly perfused tissues such as the heart, brain, and placenta. This could result in a transient enhancement of the pharmacologic response.

For example, when diazepam is administered intravenously during pregnancy, there may be a potentiation of its immediate central nervous system effects because of the higher unbound fraction.

With chronic dosing, the consequences of a change in the plasma-binding capacity depend on the pharmacokinetic properties of a particular agent. Drugs in which elimination is not blood-flow dependent will achieve lower steady-state plasma concentrations of total drug even though the concentration of free drug remains the same. In other words, total drug concentrations will underestimate the concentration of free, biologically active drug, so that the "therapeutic" concentration of total drug needed to elicit a given effect may be diminished.

For drugs that are subject to flow-dependent elimination, a reduction in plasma-binding capacity may actually decrease the clearance and raise the concentration of free drug, resulting in an enhancement of the pharmacologic response. These potential changes must be considered when one is interpreting plasma drug concentrations in clinical practice.

Elimination

Drugs are removed from the body by metabolic or renal excretory pathways. Water-soluble drugs are excreted mainly unchanged by the kidneys, whereas lipid-soluble drugs generally are metabolized to more polar compounds before they are excreted into the urine.

Some chemicals must be metabolized before they are active (eg, cyclophosphamide to phosphoramide mustard); some compounds have both the parent molecule and the metabolite as active substances (eg, both amitriptyline and its metabolite nortriptyline); and metabolites of some compounds may be toxic (eg, methanol to the toxic metabolite formic acid). Although most drugs primarily are metabolized by the liver, other organs, such as the lungs, kidneys, and intestine, also have metabolizing capacity.

There are two types of metabolic processes in the liver: one in which more polar groups are introduced into the drug molecule by oxidation, reduction, or hydrolysis, and the other, a synthetic reaction that involves conjugation of the drug with glucuronic acid, sulfate, glycerin, or other groups.

The elimination of most drugs is a first-order process; the rate of drug elimination is directly proportional to the drug concentration in plasma. Although the term elimination half-life (ie, the time required for a 50% fall in plasma drug concentration) is commonly used to characterize the elimination of drugs, it is preferable to use the concept of elimination clearance.

Total-body clearance is the sum of all clearances, hepatic and nonhepatic, serving to eliminate the drug from the body. The two principal physiological variables controlling hepatic clearance are hepatic blood flow and the intrinsic capacity of elimination mechanisms (intrinsic hepatic clearance).

If one assumes complete drug absorption, the mean steady-state plasma concentration of a drug obeying first-order kinetics is related to the drug dosing rate and elimination clearance by a simple equation: drug plasma concentration = dosing rate/clearance. Thus, a measured plasma concentration provides a guide to dose adjustment because a linear relationship exists between administered dose and steady-state plasma concentrations. Body clearance, therefore, offers a more precise measurement of elimination than half-life because it is independent of drug distribution processes.

The elimination of some drugs, however, does not follow first-order kinetics. The primary pathway of phenytoin, for example, consists of initial metabolism to form a *para*-hydroxylated metabolite followed by glucuronide conjugation. Because the enzyme system that forms this metabolite is partially saturated at therapeutic phenytoin concentrations, phenytoin plasma concentrations rise disproportionately as the dosage is increased (Fig. 7–2).

This nonlinear relationship between phenytoin dose and plasma concentration complicates patient management. When using drugs that are disproportionate in their plasma concentration in relation to dosage (e.g., aspirin, warfarin, alcohol), it is prudent to increase the dose in small amounts and to rely on careful monitoring of clinical response and actual measurements of plasma drug concentrations.

The influence of disease states (eg, renal and hepatic dysfunction) also must be considered in evaluating elimina-

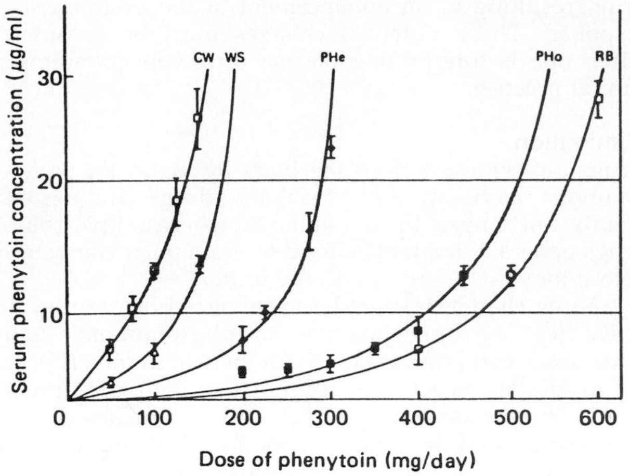

Figure 7–2. Relationship between serum phenytoin concentration and daily dose in five epileptic patients. (*From Richens and Dunlop*[68] *with permission.*)

tion capacity in a patient. Renal dysfunction is evaluated easily by determination of creatinine clearance. For those compounds that are renally eliminated, several equations and nomograms have been developed to account for their altered elimination in the face of renal impairment.

Unfortunately, a major impediment to estimating proper doses for drugs metabolized by the liver is that the hepatic clearance of drugs cannot be predicted accurately from standard tests of liver function. In these situations, it has been necessary to rely on therapeutic drug monitoring to assist in the evaluation of the liver's capacity to eliminate a compound.

Genetic control of drug metabolism is recognized as an important determinant in the elimination of compounds. For example, the ability to acetylate drugs in the liver by the *N*-acetyltransferase system is inherited as an autosomal recessive trait. On the basis of the activity of this enzyme, individuals may be categorized as fast or slow acetylators. Slow acetylators have higher concentrations of the parent compound, whereas rapid acetylators have increased concentrations of the metabolites. Agents such as procainamide, hydralazine, and isoniazid are all metabolized by this route. The clinical importance of this genetic predisposition has been realized in the last decade. Specifically, an agent such as procainamide has been determined to induce systemic lupus erythematosus in susceptible individuals. The metabolite *N*-acetylprocainamide (NAPA) is not thought to possess this side effect. In the face of renal failure, however, NAPA accumulates and possesses antiarrhythmic properties and toxicities similar to the parent compound, procainamide. For this reason, plasma concentrations of both procainamide and NAPA must always be monitored.

During pregnancy, clearances of drugs with a high hepatic extraction ratio, that is, those whose clearance is limited by blood flow, have been evaluated.[22] For example, clearance of lidocaine was found to be comparable in pregnant women and in nonpregnant controls. These data substantiate the observation that hepatic blood flow is not altered during pregnancy.[11]

The systemic clearance of drugs that are extensively metabolized by the liver (ie, hepatic intrinsic clearance) will, however, depend on the capacity of the liver to biotransform the drug. Because progesterone is known to enhance the activity of the hepatic microsomal oxidation system,[8] pregnancy might be expected to increase the rate of biotransformation of many drugs, resulting in a decrease in plasma drug concentration relative to dose. Recent studies with phenytoin, carbamazepine, and metoprolol suggest such an increase in metabolic clearance, but in neither study is the evidence conclusive. The situation may be complicated by the fact that the increased load of steroidal sex hormones might compete with some drugs for the biotransformation capacity of the induced enzyme systems.[23]

Renal physiology is substantially altered by pregnancy and may therefore influence drug elimination. Glomerular filtration rate (GFR) increases 30–50%, and effective renal plasma flow (ERPF) by about 25%.[24] Therefore, the drugs or their metabolites that are eliminated primarily by renal excretion are expected to be cleared more rapidly during pregnancy, leading to the possibility of subtherapeutic plasma concentrations with normal dosage regimens. For example, serum concentrations of digoxin, which is eliminated chiefly by renal excretion, have been found to be lower in maternal plasma during pregnancy than after delivery, probably because of enhanced renal elimination. Studies with gentamicin[25] and ampicillin[26], however, have not confirmed this observation; dosing requirements and elimination rates of these compounds during pregnancy were unchanged. As in the nonpregnant patient, significant variation in volumes of distribution and renal elimination of aminoglycosides occur, making an individual approach to aminoglycoside drug therapy mandatory.

The effects of absorption, distribution, and elimination of drugs can be represented in a two-compartment model by a semilogarithmic plot of drug plasma concentrations versus time (Fig. 7–3). After oral administration, serum concentrations initially rise, reflecting absorption of the drug from the gastrointestinal tract. Drug concentrations reach a peak level once the absorption rate of the drug is equal to its elimination rate. Subsequently, drug levels decline in a biphasic manner as a result of distribution of the drug from the systemic circulation to tissues and elimination of the drug. On intravenous administration, there is no absorption step, so peak serum concentrations are obtained instantaneously (see Fig. 7–3). The initial steeper decline of the curve reflects distribution of the drug, whereas the more gradual decline reflects the elimination of drug from the body.

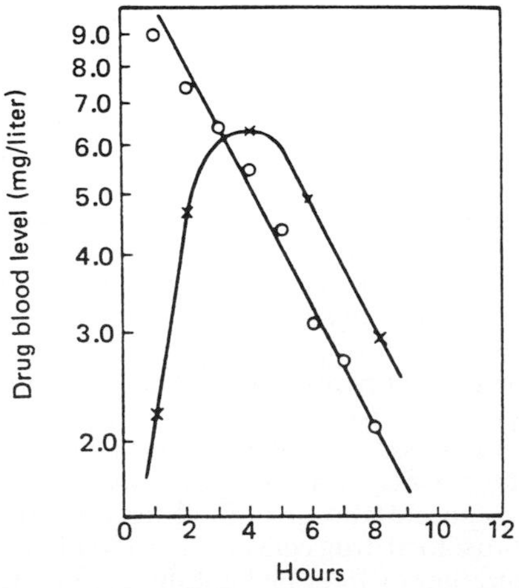

Figure 7–3. Average blood levels of theophylline in 11 subjects receiving 0.5 g of aminophylline by rapid intravenous injection (O) and one subject receiving 0.5 g of aminophylline orally (X). Note that after absorption is complete, blood levels of theophylline after oral administration decline parallel to those after intravenous administration (*From Swintosky*[69] *with permission.*)

Steady State

With repetitive dosing of a drug, serum drug concentrations gradually rise and eventually reach a plateau. When a state of equilibrium between the rate of drug administration and the rate of elimination is reached, a *steady state* is said to exist. This concept may be illustrated by considering what occurs during the intravenous infusion of a compound. Using theophylline as an example, it is apparent that when a constant infusion is started, the amount of drug in the body is zero. As the infusion continues, the amount of drug in the body rises and continues to do so until the rate of elimination matches the rate of infusion. When this state is reached, there will be a plateau or steady-state drug concentration of theophylline achieved (Fig. 7–4). A delay always exists between the initiation of drug therapy and the establishment of the steady-state concentration. The sole factor controlling the time to establish this steady state is the half-life or clearance of the drug. The amount of drug in the body, or plasma concentration, expressed as a percent of the plateau level may be calculated using the theoretical half-life of a compound. In one half-life, the level in the body is 50% of the plateau; in two half-lives, it is 75% of the plateau (Fig. 7–5). For practical purposes, however, the plateau may be considered to have been reached after three half-lives (87% of the plateau). Therefore, the shorter the half-life, the more rapidly the plateau is attained. For example, penicillin G (half-life of 30 minutes) reaches a plateau within minutes (three half-lives, 90 minutes), whereas it takes 2 to 3 weeks of constant phenobarbital administration (half-life 5 days) before the plateau is reached. The important concept is that the time required to achieve steady-state plasma concentrations depends solely on the half-life of the drug.

The same concept that applies to the accumulation of a drug during an infusion may also be applied to the elimination of a compound after the infusion has been discontinued. At this point, the plasma concentration falls by half each half-life of the drug. For practical purposes, it may be assumed that 87% of the compound is eliminated by three half-lives.

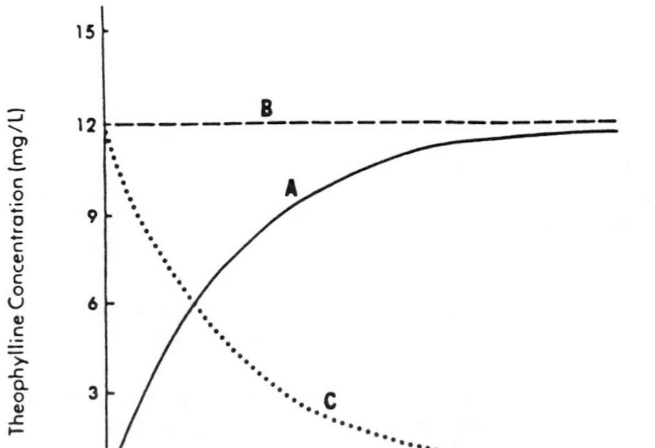

Figure 7–4. Time course of the plasma theophylline concentration following the constant-rate IV infusion of 42.5 mg/h of aminophylline without (— curve A) and with (--- curve B) the administration of an IV loading dose of 500 mg of aminophylline to patient A. Curve C (···) shows drug remaining from the loading dose. (*From Berkow*[70] *with permission.*)

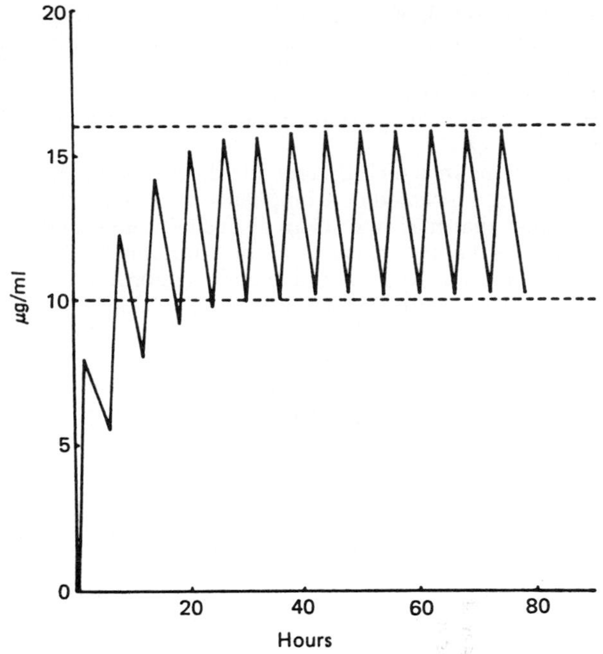

Figure 7–5. A graph illustrating the delay in achieving steady-state plasma concentration of orally administered theophylline.

Loading and Maintenance Doses

Initiation of drug therapy, in most instances, requires the administration of a loading dose followed by maintenance therapy.

The rationale for administering a loading dose is to establish rapidly therapeutic serum concentrations of a drug. This loading dose serves to occupy the volume of distribution and can be calculated by multiplying the volume of distribution by the desired serum drug concentration. If a loading dose is not administered, it would take approximately 20 hours of a constant infusion of theophylline, for example, before a desired plateau concentration is reached. It would take even longer for drugs that have half-lives greater than that of theophylline. In clinical practice, however, situations often demand that the therapeutic concentration be reached more rapidly. After therapy is started with a loading dose, it is usually continued with maintenance doses of the drug in order to maintain a desired serum concentration and, thus, a therapeutic effect. The daily maintenance dosage administered to replace the amount of drug that has been excreted or metabolized may be assessed by multiplying the clearance of a particular drug (available from pooled population data) with the desired steady-state plasma concentration.

THERAPEUTIC DRUG MONITORING

Determination of plasma drug concentrations may provide valuable information for rational drug therapy. For many compounds the intensity of the pharmacologic effect correlates better with the steady-state concentration of the drug in the plasma than with the daily dose; therefore, it is desirable to ensure a plasma drug concentration within the *therapeutic range*. This range is associated with optimal therapeutic effects and minimal adverse reactions. Some drugs at plasma concentrations above the upper limit of the therapeutic range are likely to cause adverse reactions, whereas concentrations below the lower limit most often are ineffective. Because of the marked interindividual variability in plasma drug concentrations attained after administration of the same dose, therapeutic drug monitoring is particularly important when drugs with a narrow therapeutic range are administered.

Situations in which therapeutic drug monitoring may be useful are suspected noncompliance or toxicity; intercurrent illness that may alter drug disposition; a dosage regimen that is being adjusted or the formulation is being changed; and an expected therapeutic response that is not achieved. Thus, drug therapy can be individualized to the requirements of a particular patient. It has to be emphasized, however, that interpretation of plasma drug concentrations must be performed in conjunction with a patient's clinical evaluation. In monitoring plasma drug concentrations, it is important that blood samples be obtained at appropriate time intervals. In general, blood samples should be taken in the elimination phase of drug disposition (ie, after both absorption and distribution of the drug have occurred). For many drugs, it is only at this time that serum concentrations correlate with pharmacologic effects.

Relatively little is known about monitoring drug concentrations in maternal plasma during pregnancy. Drug monitoring is usually performed in those women in whom it would be done ordinarily, based on the previously mentioned indications, regardless of the state of pregnancy.

Although the physiologic changes occurring during pregnancy may be expected to alter certain pharmacokinetic parameters of drug disposition, for most therapeutic agents, the magnitude of these changes and their clinical relevance remain to be established.

Despite the relative dearth of data on plasma drug level monitoring during pregnancy, there is reasonable evidence to suggest that the dosage of a few drugs may need to be adjusted during pregnancy in order to maintain satisfactory therapeutic responses.

In epileptic women, phenytoin plasma concentrations tend to fall during pregnancy despite the continued administration of an unchanged daily dosage. The underlying mechanisms of this effect are probably related to changes in protein binding capacity and to an increased plasma clearance because of enhanced hepatic metabolism.[27] In some pregnant women, phenytoin clearance may increase by more than 100%, and this may be accompanied by increased seizure activity. In this situation, dosage adjustment is required in order to maintain a desirable plasma phenytoin concentration, although serum albumin concentrations and a reduction in binding capacity need to be taken into account. For drugs that are highly protein bound, like phenytoin, determination of the unbound fraction of the drug may be a more reliable guide to dosage adjustment than the total concentration. Because phenytoin concentrations may fall early in pregnancy, it is prudent to measure drug levels every 4 weeks from the onset of pregnancy. The dosage requirement decreases to prepregnancy values during the puerperium. Similar changes have been reported to occur in plasma phenobarbital concentrations during pregnancy and the puerperium.[28]

Several reports have indicated that dosage requirements of digoxin and lithium also may increase during pregnancy, presumably because of enhanced elimination.[29]

PLACENTAL TRANSFER OF DRUGS

New developments in monitoring and assay techniques have produced major revisions in the understanding of the transfer of drugs across the placenta. The assumption, for example, that the maternal administration of respiratory depressants does not affect fetal respiration has been evaluated. Use of transcutaneous (Tc) Po_2 monitoring during labor indicated that 5 mg diazepam or 100 mg meperidine may decrease fetal Po_2 from 100 to a low of 30 mm Hg in some infants.[30] This degree of anoxia was sufficient to produce heart rate abnormalities. In contrast, phenoterol, a drug administered to suppress labor, produced a rise in Tc Po_2 that coincided with decreased uterine contractions. Without this new technique, neither drug effect could have been documented. It appears that advances in monitoring technology will be decisive factors in extending knowledge of fetal drug effects.

The advent of microassay techniques also has introduced the possibility of intrauterine sampling of compounds for a better understanding of placental drug transfer. Previous analytic techniques required large volumes of blood that were impractical to use prenatally or even neonatally. The movement of drug molecules through biologic membranes occurs through different processes, several of which are relevant to drug transfer across the placenta.

Passive Diffusion

Most drugs cross the placenta by simple diffusion, which is dependent on molecular weight, degree of ionization, and lipid solubility. The net movement is proportional to a maternal–fetal concentration gradient. Additional factors that influence this rate of diffusion across placental membranes include the surface area available for transfer and the thickness of the membrane.

Active Transport

Drugs that are transported across the placenta, that require an expenditure of metabolic energy, and that can move against a concentration gradient fulfill the basic criteria of an active transport process. Relatively few drugs are transported by this mechanism. Only vitamin B_{12}, creatinine, and certain amino acids are known to be actively transported from the mother to the fetus.

Facilitated Diffusion

Processes in which the rate of movement of a drug molecule across the placenta is greater than that obtainable by diffusion alone represent facilitated diffusion. Examples of facilitated diffusion include the transfer of glucose between the maternal and fetal circulations.

Properties Determining Placental Transfer of Drugs

The ability of compounds to cross the placenta is dependent on their molecular charge, molecular size, and lipid solubility. Drugs penetrate membranes more rapidly in their nonionized form. Substances such as thiopental and antipyrine that are nonionized at physiologic pH cross the placenta rapidly with minimal resistance to diffusion. In contrast, acidic drugs with a low pK_a, such as heparin and succinylocholine, which are ionized at physiologic pH, diffuse across membranes slowly. If a sufficiently high maternal-to-fetal concentration gradient exists, however, these compounds may cross the placenta and affect the fetus. For example, numerous reports have appeared of "floppy infants" after the administration of succinylocholine to the mother. A further influence on the ionization and partitioning of drugs is the respective differences in pH of the maternal and fetal blood. The maternal blood has a pH of 0.1 to 0.15 pH units greater than the mixed fetal blood in the umbilical vessels. This may lead to a net transfer of nonionized drugs from the mother to the fetus.

Therapeutic agents with low molecular weights diffuse more readily across membranes than do larger molecules. Because diffusion rates vary inversely with mass, compounds with molecular weights less than 600 invariably cross the placenta in significant quantities. Compounds with molecular weights above 1000 (such as heparin) or substances with molecular weights between 600 and 1000 (such as thyroxin) are variably transferred across the placenta.

As lipid solubility increases, the ability to penetrate the placenta increases. For example, a polar drug such as phenobarbital will obtain equal concentrations in the fetus and the mother.[27]

Another factor that works in concert with the previously mentioned factors is protein binding. Major differences exist between the binding affinities of fetal and maternal serum proteins for drugs. The binding of most drugs to plasma proteins in the fetus is considerably less than that observed in the mother. This has been reported for a variety of drugs including phenytoin, phenobarbital, and ampicillin.[16]

In summary, small, lipid-soluble, noncharged and non-protein-bound compounds diffuse most rapidly across the placenta.

FETAL DRUG METABOLISM

Until recently, it was thought that the fetus lacked the enzymes responsible for the biotransformation of drugs and other xenobiotics. Through improved analytic methodology it is now known that the fetal liver possesses some of the metabolic capabilities of the adult liver. Although the capacity of biotransformation of drugs by the mixed-function oxidases in the fetal liver is substantially less than that observed at later stages of postnatal development, generalizations regarding the enzymatic capabilities of the fetus cannot be made because sulfuration and glucuronidation, for example, may actually be increased in the fetus in comparison to the neonate or adult.

Initial studies conducted with liver homogenates prepared from neonatal guinea pigs, rats, and rabbits showed that these species were devoid of any drug-metabolizing activity in the early postnatal period. These observations are of significance because they reaffirm the distinction between experimental models and the human species regarding this aspect of drug disposition. It is interesting to note that the human fetus, when compared to the rodent fetus, has a higher capacity for oxidizing drugs, even during early gestation.

Factors complicating a critical comparison between human fetal and adult data are the wide variation in liver enzyme activity among individual fetuses and the fact that fetal tissues contain less protein per gram of tissue weight than adult tissues. Despite these shortcomings, oxidative metabolic processes in the fetus have been observed as early as the eighth week of gestation, increasing rapidly to reach levels that are constant for the remainder of gestation. The human fetal liver has a cytochrome P_{450} and NADPH-cytochrome *c* reductase activity equivalent to that of the adult when expressed in terms of activity per unit of weight. One must consider that the human fetal liver constitutes about 4% of total body weight compared to 2% in the adult. A variety of different drugs and substrates has been reported to undergo metabolism by homogenates of fetal liver (e.g., testosterone, ethylmorphine, desmethylimipramine, and bilirubin).[31]

It is generally assumed that unless fetal tissues are capable of metabolizing a drug more rapidly than the maternal tissues, fetal drug metabolism usually will not alter steady-state plasma concentrations of drugs or their metabolites in the mother. The size and activity of the maternal drug-biotransforming tissues, however, make it unlikely that fetal drug metabolism would occur at a more rapid rate than maternal metabolism. Total body clearances of drugs determined during pregnancy accounts for the metabolic processes contributed by fetal metabolism.

Of greatest concern regarding the fetal metabolism of drugs is the potential formation of reactive intermediary metabolites. These metabolites include epoxides, diolepoxides, hydroxylamines, carbonium ions, and other intermediates that have been implicated in the development of cancer, birth defects, immunosuppression, and cell death.[31] Although the data are far from conclusive at this time, they do suggest that humans may be more vulnerable than smaller experimental animals to the toxic effects of foreign organic chemicals during prenatal life (see below).

TERATOGENICITY

One of the greatest concerns of drug administration during pregnancy is the induction of a teratogenic side effect. Although historically, drugs with teratogenic potential were considered to have the capacity to produce major overt morphologic abnormalities, today the definition has been broadened to include minor and latent structural as well as functional and behavioral abnormalities.

In the United States, 200,000 birth defects are recorded each year, accounting for 7% of all live births.[32,33] More than 560,000 infant deaths, spontaneous abortions, stillbirths, and miscarriages are attributed to defective fetal development. It is estimated that 1–5% of these congenital defects may be drug- or chemical-related. Several epidemiologic surveys have confirmed that most women ingest drugs during pregnancy.[34] Women of childbearing age also are exposed occupationally to industrial chemicals. About 125,000 women in the United States work in environments containing potential teratogens, such as solvents and chemical reagents.[35] At present, the contribution of environmental and chemical contamination to the incidence of birth defects is unknown.

Manifestation of ill effects to the fetus can be recognized as including early death, abortion, and stillbirth; anatomic defects such as malformations, minor deviations, and fetal injuries; and growth disorders, postnatal developmental defects, and oncogenesis. It is well established that susceptibility to teratogenic agents varies with the developmental stage at the time of exposure. Factors that may determine a drug's effect include dosage, duration of exposure, mode of administration, concurrent use with other drugs, generation and accumulation of toxic metabolites, and genetic susceptibility. In the human, the critical period of embryonic development extends from the third week to the end of the third month of pregnancy. Compounds ingested before the first 3 weeks of gestation may have no effect or result in abortion before differentiation can occur.

The most well-known and tragic occurrence of a drug-induced teratogenic effect is that by thalidomide. This compound, a sedative hypnotic introduced in the late 1950s in Europe, was considered nontoxic at therapeutic doses. However, soon after the introduction of thalidomide, there was an increase in the number of infants born with phocomelia. Whereas not a single case of phocomelia was seen in the period between 1949–1959 at the University Pediatric Clinic in Hamburg, 30 cases in 1960 and 154 cases in 1961 were reported. In every case, thalidomide was ingested between the third and eighth weeks of pregnancy. Ultimately, 10,000 infants worldwide were deformed by thalidomide, and the drug was withdrawn from the market.[36]

Prompted by the thalidomide incident, regulatory agencies initiated requirements for animal testing of therapeutic drugs that could detect teratogenic potential before their widespread distribution. However, because of the great species variability regarding embryopathic susceptibility and fetal capacity to form reactive metabolites, it appears that teratogenic testing in animals has poor predictability of teratogenic potential in humans.

In recognition of the difficulty of obtaining information and performing testing on the teratogenicity of compounds, the Food and Drug Administration (FDA) has established five categories (A, B, C, D, X) to indicate a drug's potential for causing fetal defects. For each drug that is systemically absorbed and might be administered during pregnancy, the labeling describes the information appropriate to the category in which the drug has been placed.

Category A applies to drugs for which well-controlled studies in women failed to demonstrate a risk to the fetus. Although such studies can never entirely exclude a risk, the presumption can be made that when such drugs are used during pregnancy, the possibility of fetal harm is remote. However, as with other drugs, they should be used during pregnancy only when clearly needed.

Category B indicates either that animal studies have not demonstrated a fetal risk but that there are no adequate studies in women or that animal studies have uncovered some risks that have not been confirmed in controlled human studies.

Category C indicates that studies in animals have revealed adverse effects in the fetus and there are no adequate control studies in women or that studies in women and animals are not available.

Category D includes drugs that in human experiments have been shown to be associated with birth defects, but the potential benefits of the drug may be acceptable despite their known risk. A category D drug would be indicated for use only in a life-threatening situation or serious disease for which alternative drugs are not available. If a category D drug is given to a pregnant woman, or the patient becomes pregnant while taking it, she should be informed of the potential risk to the fetus.

Category X includes drugs for which fetal abnormalities have been demonstrated in animals or humans and the potential risk of which clearly outweighs the potential benefits. Such drugs are definitely contraindicated for use during pregnancy. Selected therapeutic agents and their teratogenic classification are listed in Table 7–3.

Under these guidelines, drugs also are labeled for their effect on reproduction when known and for any nonteratogenic adverse effects (eg, narcotic withdrawal symptoms, fetal hypoglycemia). The labeling must also include information for drugs with a recognized use in labor and delivery and detail the available information regarding their effect on the mother and child. This includes the effects of a drug on the duration of labor or delivery, the possibility that forceps or other intervention or resuscitation on the newborn may be necessary, and the effect of the drug on the later growth, development, and functional maturation of the child. If any of this information is not known, it is stated in the labeling. Also included in the labeling is information on drug excretion in human milk and the effects on the nursing infant.

It is anticipated that in the next decade this increased availability of information will greatly improve the safety and delivery of medications to pregnant patients.

TABLE 7–3. RISK FACTOR ASSIGNMENT OF SELECTED THERAPEUTIC AGENTS[a]

Acetaminophen	B	Hydrochlorothiazide	D
Amikacin	C_M	Ibuprofen	B
Amiloride	B_M	Insulin	B
Aminophylline	C	Isoniazid	C
Amitriptyline	C_M	Lincomycin	B
Amoxicillin	C	Lithium	D_M
Ampicillin	C	Magnesium sulfate	B
Aspirin	C	Meperidine	B
Betamethasone	C	Methicillin	B
Carbamazepine	C_M	Methyldopa	C
Carbenicillin	B	Morphine	B
Cefaclor	B	Nadolol	C_M
Cefazolin	B_M	Naproxen	B_M
Cefoxitin	B	Nitrofurantoin	B
Chloramphenicol	C	Nystatin	B
Chlordiazepoxide	C	Penicillin G	A_M
Chlorpromazine	C	Phenobarbital	B
Clindamycin	B	Phenacetin	B
Dexamethasone	C	Phenytoin	D
Diazepam	C	Prednisone	C
Digitalis	B	Propranolol	C
Ephedrine	C	Rifampin	C
Erythromycin	B_M	Sulfonamides	B
Ethambutol	C	Tetracycline	C_M
Ethacrynic acid	D	Theophylline	C
Furosemide	C	Tobramycin	D_M
Gentamicin	C	Trimethoprim–sulfamethoxazole	C_M
Heparin	D	Warfarin	X
Hydralazine	B		

[a] Since most drugs have not yet been given an FDA-approved letter rating, the risk factor assignments are tentative and made based on recommendations by Briggs et al.[66] Letters with subscript M are those assigned by the manufacturer.

INTRAUTERINE DRUG THERAPY

The development of prenatal diagnostic methods for the detection of diseases in the fetus has advanced rapidly in the last decade. Amniocentesis, ultrasonography, and intrauterine electrocardiography and echocardiography have facilitated the diagnosis of pathologic processes in the developing fetus that may require pharmacologic therapy.

Pharmacologic agents have been administered to the mother for entry into the fetal compartment. The most common examples of such an approach are the following:

1. Maternal antibiotic therapy for the treatment of intrauterine infections. Following premature rupture of the membranes, an ascending infection may lead to fetal or neonatal pneumonia or septicemia. Attempts to treat this condition, therefore, by maternal drug administration are dependent on the agents crossing into the amniotic fluid as well as the fetal compartment.
2. Antepartum maternal steroid therapy to prevent neonatal respiratory distress syndrome. Maternal parenteral administration of corticosteroids such as betamethasone,

dexamethasone, prednisolone, and intravenous cortisone have been used for this purpose. Presently, betamethasone appears to achieve the highest concentrations in the fetus and is more effective than the other corticosteroids.[37] The relative placental impermeability of other corticosteroids renders betamethasone the agent of choice.[38]

3. Treatment of intrauterine fetal arrhythmias has accumulated perhaps the greatest experience in maternal administration of drugs for the treatment of a fetal disorder. To date, agents such as digoxin[39-41], propranolol,[42] and procainamide[43] have all been used successfully in the management of paroxysmal supraventricular tachycardia. Concentrations of digoxin, propranolol, and procainamide at the time of delivery were found to be 90–100%, 20%, and 25% of the maternal concentrations, respectively. Of these agents, the safest has been digoxin. Risks are present for propranolol in inducing bradycardia, hypoglycemia, and small birth weight,[44,45] whereas procainamide may be associated with hypotension and endangering the fetal–placental unit.[43]

Because the fluids surrounding the fetus may provide more direct pharmacologic access to the fetal compartment, there has been increasing interest in amniotic fluid physiology in the last 15 years. It has been shown that many drugs administered to the mother are found in amniotic fluid. In humans, selected examples of these include antibiotics,[46,47] meperidine[48], diazepam[49], digoxin[41], cortisol[50], and betamethasone;[51] in animals, examples include digoxin[52], barbiturates[53], mannitol[54], and thyroxin.[55]

Amniotic fluid in the last trimester of pregnancy is a product of numerous active exchanges by the fetus.[56] Fetal swallowing, 200–450 mL/d at term, and fetal urine production, 600–800 mL/d at term, are the most visible sites of exchange. Significant reabsorption, however, of amniotic fluid could occur across respiratory tract epithelium. This concept evolved from measurements of large inflow and outflow, 600–800 mL/d at term, of amniotic fluid through fetal lungs in response to active fetal respiratory movements.[57] Additional exchanges of amniotic fluid are postulated across the chorionic plate on the posterior surface of the placenta and are possible across fetal skin. Although fetal skin keratinizes at 24 to 26 weeks' gestation and is rendered impermeable to most solutes, low molecular-weight, highly lipid-soluble compounds such as inert gases and carbon dioxide may cross in significant quantities.

Direct transfer of solute and water across the chorioamnion between maternal and amniotic compartments is very small because of the lack of vascularization and significant perfusion of this exchange surface. It is imperative that the understanding of amniotic fluid formation, reabsorption, and regulation be combined with experimental data to understand the concepts effecting maternal–fetal amniotic drug transfer. Compounds introduced into the maternal compartment do not cross in the amniotic fluid in significant quantities unless they are first readily transfered to the fetus. There is little or no direct transfer between the mother and amniotic fluid.

Water-soluble substances such as antibiotics may reach peak fetal concentrations within 30–60 minutes after maternal intravenous infusion and appear in amniotic fluid in highest concentrations between 4 to 24 hours.[46,47] The delay in appearance of these agents in the amniotic fluid indicates that the excretion of these solutes in fetal urine serves as a major pathway for amniotic fluid drug concentrations. The peak amniotic fluid levels far exceed simultaneous fetal or maternal levels, corresponding to high fetal urinary levels for these water-soluble substances. This indicates that equilibration of these compounds with the fetus is very slow.

Lipid-soluble compounds, however, such as phenobarbital or meperidine diffuse rapidly from the mother to the fetus, attaining peak concentrations within minutes and appearing in the amniotic fluid in large quantities within hours.[58] Concentrations of small, highly lipophilic substances such as carbon dioxide and nitrous oxide appear in amniotic fluid in equilibrium with fetal levels.[59] These small, lipid-soluble substances cross rapidly to the fetus and equilibrate rapidly in amniotic fluid, probably by diffusion across exchange sites such as fetal skin.

Another type of maternal–fetal amniotic fluid exchange is demonstrated by compounds such as phenytoin, which readily cross the placenta but are rapidly metabolized in the fetal liver, appearing in very small concentrations in amniotic fluid.[60]

The previously discussed equilibrium between fetal and amniotic fluid compartments has suggested the possibility that direct diffusion of drugs in the amniotic fluid may provide more immediate access to fetal circulation and successful *in utero* treatment. This route would bypass problems of placental permeability. The ultimate clinical use of infusions into the amniotic fluid will depend on the reliability and consistency of amniotic fluid transfer of these agents into the fetal circulation. This approach, however, is to be considered of experimental interest. With further development, this may prove to be a valuable route for drug treatment in pregnancy.

DRUGS IN BREAST MILK

The prevalence of breast feeding has increased substantially during the past decade. Therefore, knowledge concerning drug therapy and exposure to environmental pollutants during lactation is becoming more important. The long-term consequences to infants exposed to drugs by way of breast milk remain unknown. Weaning as a precaution during drug therapy can be evaluated only after accurate information is gathered about the drug's concentration in breast milk and its effects on the infant.

Adequate pharmacokinetic studies on drugs and chemicals ingested during lactation are limited, with most human data reporting only a small number of patients. Single determinations of concentrations of drugs in breast milk are of limited value. Animal studies may be misleading because of species variations in pH, milk composition, and differences in metabolic pathways. Many assay procedures in the past lacked sensitivity and specificity for reliable drug determination. An understanding of the pharmacokinetic properties of the drug and serum measurement of drug concentrations in maternal plasma, breast milk, and infant plasma are necessary. Drug therapy that is beneficial for the mother and not detrimental to the infant is the ultimate goal.

Plasma–Milk Transfer

Principles of drug transfer into breast milk and effect on the infant encompass absorption, distribution, metabolism, and elimination of a drug in both the mother and infant.

Drug transfer and concentration in breast milk are influenced by the drug's physical and chemical properties (molecular weight, ionization, solubility, and protein binding). The majority of clinically useful drugs have molecular weights between 250 and 500, and their passage into breast milk depends on their lipid solubility and degree of ionization. It is the un-ionized lipid-soluble form that passes through the cell membrane. The degree of ionization of weak acids and bases is related to the pH of the medium and to the drug dissociation constant (pK_a). The pH of breast milk ranges from 6.8–7.3, which is higher than that of plasma and interstitial fluid.[61] Weak bases are less ionized in the higher pH of the plasma and pass readily into more acidic milk where they become ionized and "trapped." This creates a higher concentration of a compound in breast milk than in plasma. Weak acids, however, have an equal or lower concentration in milk than in plasma. (Examples of these compounds would be barbiturates, organic acids, sulfonamides, diuretics, and benzylpenicillin.) Medications present in maternal blood must cross the capillary endothelium, extracellular spaces, and the hydrophobic barrier created by the alveolar cell membrane before entering breast milk. Most drug transfer occurs by passive diffusion, in which the concentration gradient governs solute movement. As maternal plasma concentrations decrease, the drug concentration in the milk decreases by back diffusion.[62]

Some ionized particles and small hydrophilic drugs with molecular weights less than 200 penetrate the membrane through aqueous channels or pores.[63] Facilitated diffusion explains the passage of water-soluble substances that are too large to pass through membrane pores. Substances that are actively transported across the membrane include glucose, amino acids, calcium, and magnesium.

Because only the unbound fraction of a drug exerts the pharmacologic action and can be metabolized and excreted, the extent and affinity of drug binding to both plasma and milk proteins affect drug concentration in milk. Displacement of a particular drug from albumin can occur by competitive binding with endogenous or exogenous substances and creates a higher concentration of free drug.

Though passage of drugs into breast milk is a cause for concern, the magnitude of breast milk production and the influence that drugs exert should also be considered. Mammary blood flow determines the rate of drug presentation to breast milk. Factors regulating mammary blood flow include metabolic activity, release of lactogenic hormones, a decrease of intramammary pressure after feeding, and the use of certain drugs. Mammary blood vessels are sensitive to vasoconstrictors and sympathomimetics, which can decrease blood flow and milk yield. Large amounts of nicotine in mothers who smoke heavily (more than two packs per day) can decrease milk supply.[63]

Breast milk secretion, which is under hormonal control, is also affected by drugs. Levodopa, ergocriptine, bromocriptine, pyridoxine, and monoamine oxidase inhibitors cause stimulation of dopamine receptors either directly or indirectly in the hypothalamus, which decreases the release of prolactin inhibitory factor. Conversely, drugs acting on the hypothalamus to suppress the secretion of prolactin inhibitory factor include phenothiazines, cimetidine, metoclopramide, methysergide, and certain antihypertensive agents, such as clonidine and methyldopa.[64] Metoclopramide, a potent stimulator of prolactin release, has been used to restore milk flow in women whose volume has decreased.[65]

Despite drug concentrations in breast milk that are equal to or even higher than those in the maternal blood, the daily amount of milk ingested by the infant may be relatively small, so that the total amount of drug ingested may not necessarily produce pharmacologic responses in the child.

REFERENCES

1. Wood AJJ, Carr K, Vestal RE, et al. Direct measurement of the propranolol bioavailability during accumulation to steady-state. *Br J Clin Pharmacol.* 1978;6:345.
2. Huet M, LeLorier J, Pomier G, et al. Bioavailability of lidocaine in normal volunteers and cirrhotics. *Gastroenterology.* 1978;75:968A.
3. Hill N, Antman EM, Green LH, et al. Intravenous nitroglycerin—a review of pharmacology, indications, therapeutic effects and complications. *Chest.* 1981;79:69.
4. Kostenbauder HB, Rapp RP, McGovern JP, et al. Bioavailability and single-dose pharmacokinetics of intramuscular phenytoin. *Clin Pharmacol Ther.* 1975;18:449.
5. Wilder BJ, Serrano EE, Ramsey E, et al. A method of shifting from oral to intramuscular diphenylhydantoin administration. *Clin Pharmacol Ther.* 1974;16:507.
6. Davison JS, Davison MC, Hay DM. Gastric emptying time in late pregnancy and labour. *J Obstet Gynaecol Br Commonw.* 1970;77:37.
7. Gryboski WA, Spiro HM. The effect of pregnancy on gastric secretion. *N Engl J Med.* 1956;255:1131.
8. Krauer B, Krauer F. Drug kinetics in pregnancy. *Clin Pharmacokinet.* 1977;2:167.
9. Pirani BKK, Campbell DM, MacGillivray I. Plasma volume in normal pregnancy. *J Obstet Gynaecol Br Commonw.* 1973;80:884.
10. Katz R, Karliner JS, Resnik R. Effects of a natural volume overload state (pregnancy) on left ventricular performance in normal human subjects. *Circulation* 1978;58:434.
11. Munnell EW, Taylor HC. Liver blood flow in pregnancy—hepatic vein catheterization. *J Clin Invest.* 1947;26:952.
12. Krauer B, Krauer F, Hytten FE. Drug disposition and pharmacokinetics in the maternal–placental–fetal unit. *Pharmacol Ther.* 1980;10:301.
13. Appel GB, Neu HC. Gentamicin in 1978. *Ann Intern Med.* 1978;89:528.
14. Aronson JK. Clinical pharmacokinetics of digoxin 1980. *Clin Pharmacokinet.* 1980;5:137.
15. Robertson EG. Physiologic adjustments in pregnancy: Water metabolism. *Clin Obstet Gynecol.* 1975;2:431.
16. Perucca E, Crema A. Plasma protein binding of drugs in pregnancy. *Clin Pharmacokinet.* 1982;7:336.
17. Reboud P, Groulade J, Groslambert P, et al. The influence of normal pregnancy and the postpartum state of plasma proteins and lipids. *Am J Obstet Gynecol.* 1963;86:820.
18. Wood M, Wood AJJ. Changes in plasma drug binding and α_1-acid glycoprotein in mother and newborn infant. *Clin Pharmacol Ther.* 1981;29:522.
19. Perucca E, Ruprah M, Richens A. Decreased serum protein binding of diazepam and valproic acid in pregnant women. *Br J Clin Pharmacol.* 1981;12:276P.
20. Chen SS, Perucca E, Lee JN, et al. Serum protein binding and free concentration of phenytoin and phenobarbitone in pregnancy. *Br J Clin Pharmacol.* 1982;13:547.
21. Dean M, Stock B, Patterson RJ, et al. Serum protein binding of drugs during and after pregnancy in humans. *Clin Pharmacol Ther.* 1980;28:253.
22. Dvorchik BH. Drug disposition during pregnancy. *Biol Res Preg.* 1982;3:129.
23. Davis M, Simmons GJ, Dordoni B, et al. Induction of hepatic enzymes during normal human pregnancy. *J Obstet Gynaecol Br Commonw.* 1973;81:690.
24. Davison JM, Hytten FE. Glomerular filtration during and after pregnancy. *J Obstet Gynaecol Br Commonw.* 1974;81:588.
25. Zaske DE, Cipolle RJ, Strate RG, et al. Rapid gentamicin elimination in obstetric patients. *Obstet Gynecol.* 1980;56:559.
26. Kubacka RT, Johnstone HE, Tan HSI, et al. Intravenous ampicillin pharmacokinetics in the third trimester of pregnancy. *Ther Drug Monit.* 1983;5:55.
27. Nau H, Kunz W, Egger HJ, et al. Anticonvulsants during pregnancy and lactation—transplacental, maternal and neonatal pharmacokinetics. *Clin Pharmacokinet.* 1982;7:508.
28. Lander CM, Edwards VE, Eadie MJ, et al. Plasma anticonvulsant concentrations during pregnancy. *Neurology (Minneap.)* 1977;27:128.
29. Eadie MJ, Lander CM, Tyrer JH. Plasma drug level monitoring in pregnancy. *Clin Pharmacokinet.* 1977;2:427.
30. Peabody JL. Transcutaneous oxygen measurement to evaluate drug effects. *Clin Perinatol.* 1979;6:109.
31. Juchau MR, Chao ST, Omiecinski CJ. Drug metabolism by the human fetus. *Clin Pharmacokinet.* 1980;5:320.
32. National Foundation—"March of Dimes." *Facts.* White Plains, New York; 1979.
33. Wilson JG. Embryotoxicity of drugs in man. In: Wilson JG, Fraser FC, eds. *Handbook of Teratology.* New York, NY: Plenum Press; 1977;1:309.
34. Bleyer WA, Au WYW, Lang WA, et al. Studies on the detection of adverse drug reactions in the newborn. I. Fetal exposure to maternal medication. *JAMA.* 1970;213:2046.
35. Yager JW. Congenital malformations and environmental influence: The

occupational environment of the laboratory worker. *J Occup Med.* 1973;15:724.
36. Stern L. *In vivo* assessment of the teratogenic potential of drugs in humans. *Obstet Gynecol.* 1981;58:3S.
37. Ballard PL, Ballard RA. Corticosteroids and respiratory distress syndrome: Status 1979. *Pediatrics.* 1979;63:163.
38. Petersen MC, Nation RL, Ashley JJ, et al. The placental transfer of betamethasone. *Eur J Clin Pharmacol.* 1980;18:245.
39. Harrigan JT, Kangos JJ, Sikka A, et al. Successful treatment of fetal congestive heart failure secondary to tachycardia. *N Engl J Med.* 1981;304:1527.
40. Newburger JW, Keane JF. Intrauterine supraventricular tachycardia. *J Pediatr.* 1979;95:780.
41. Kerenyi TD, Gleicher N, Meller J, et al. Transplacental cardioversion in intrauterine supraventricular tachycardia and digitalis. *Lancet.* 1980;2:393.
42. Klein AM, Holzman IA, Austin EM. Fetal tachycardia prior to the development of hydrops. Attempted pharmacologic cardioversion: case report. *Am J Obstet Gynecol.* 1979;134:347.
43. Dumesic DA, Silverman NH, Tobias S et al. Transplacental cardioversion of fetal supraventricular tachycardia with procainamide. *N Engl J Med.* 1982;307:1128.
44. Gladstone GR, Hordorf A, Gersony WM. Propranolol administration during pregnancy: effects on the fetus. *J Pediatr.* 1975;86:962.
45. Habib A, McCarthy JS. Effects on the neonate of propranolol administered during pregnancy. *J Pediatr.* 1977;91:808.
46. Bray RE, Boe RW, Johnson WL. Transfer of ampicillin into the fetus and amniotic fluid from maternal plasma in late pregnancy. *Am J Obstet Gynecol.* 1966;96:938.
47. Depp RC, Kind AC, Kirby WMM, et al. Transplacental passage of methicillin and dicloxacillin into the fetus and amniotic fluid. *Am J Obstet Gynecol.* 1970;107:1054.
48. Szeto HH, Mann LI, Ghaktharathsalan A, et al. Meperidine pharmacokinetics in the maternal–fetal unit. *J Pharmacol Exp Ther.* 1978;206:448.
49. Idanpaan-Heikkala JE, Jouppila JE, Poulakka, et al. Placental transfer and fetal metabolism of diazepam in early human pregnancy. *Am J Obstet Gynecol.* 1971;109:1011.
50. Abramovich DR, Wade DP. Transplacental passage of steroids: The presence of corticosteroids in amniotic fluid. *J Obstet Gynecol Br Commonw.* 1969;76:610.
51. Anderson ABM, Gennser G, Jeremy JY, et al. Placental transfer and metabolism of betamethasone in human pregnancy. *Obstet Gynecol.* 1977;49:471.
52. Fouron JC. Dynamics of the placental transfer of digoxin in the dog. *Biol Neonate.* 1973;23:116.
53. Carrier G, Hume AS, Douglas BH, et al. Disposition of barbiturates in the maternal blood, fetal blood and amniotic fluid. *Am J Obstet Gynecol.* 1969;105:1069.
54. Basso A, Fernandez A, Olthade O, et al. Passage of mannitol from mother to amniotic fluid to fetus. *Obstet Gynecol.* 1977;49:628.
55. Sack J, Fischer DA, Lam RW. Thyroid hormone metabolism in amniotic and allantoic fluids of the sheep. *Pediatr Res.* 1975;9:837.
56. Seeds AE. Current concepts of amniotic fluid dynamics. *Am J Obstet Gynecol.* 1980;138:575.
57. Duenhoeffer JH, Pritchard JA. Fetal respiration: quantitative measurements of amniotic fluid inspired near term by human and rhesus fetuses. *Am J Obstet Gynecol.* 1976;125:306.
58. Shier RW, Sprague AD, Dilts PV. Placental transfer of meperidine HCI. Part II. *Am J Obstet Gynecol.* 1973;115:556.
59. Seeds AE. Basic concepts of maternal–fetal amniotic fluid exchange—their relevance to fetal therapeutics. *Pediatr Clin North Am.* 1981;28:231.
60. Shoeman DW, Kaufman RE, Azarnoff DL, et al. Placental transfer of diphenylhydantoin in the goat. *Biochem Pharmacol.* 1972;21:1237.
61. Lien EJ, Kuwahara J, Koda RT. Diffusion of drugs into prostatic fluid and milk. *Drug Intell Clin Pharm.* 1974;8:470.
62. Catz CS, Giacoia GP. Drugs in breast milk. *Pediatr Clin North Am.* 1972;19:151.
63. Vorheer H. Drug excretion in breast milk. *Postgrad Med.* 1974;56:97.
64. Dickey RP. Drugs affecting lactation. *Semin Perinatol.* 1979;3:279.
65. Sousa PLR. Reestablishment of lactation with metoclopramide. *J Trop Pediatr.* 1975;21:214.
66. Briggs CG, Bodendorfer TW, Freeman RK, et al. *Drugs in Pregnancy and Lactation. A Reference Guide to Fetal and Neonatal Risk.* Baltimore, London; Williams & Wilkins: 1983.
67. Barr WH. Principles of biopharmaceutics. *Am J Pharm Educ.* 1968;52:958.
68. Richens AL, Dunlop A. Serum-phenytoin levels in the management of epilepsy. *Lancet.* 1975;2:247.
69. Swintosky JV. Illustrations and pharmaceutical interpretations of first order drug elimination rate from the bloodstream. *J Am Pharm Assoc Sci Ed.* 1956;45:395.
70. Berkow R, ed. *Merck Manual,* 14th ed. Rahway, NJ: Merck Sharp and Dohme Research Laboratories; 1982:2255.

Chapter Eight

Consequences of Alcohol Abuse

Ernest L. Abel and Robert J. Sokol

8

It has been more than 15 years since the first clinical descriptions of fetal alcohol syndrome (FAS).[1,2] Since then, alcohol's teratogenic potential has been firmly established; effects range from spontaneous abortion to a collective group of abnormalities called FAS, to subtle behavioral anomalies, such as attention deficits in the absence of observable physical abnormalities. More than 5000 relevant articles have been published on this topic.[3] Obviously, it is not possible to review all of this literature. Psychological concomitants of alcohol abuse in pregnancy, associated patterns of family stress, and treatment of alcohol intoxication and withdrawal syndromes have been detailed elsewhere.[4,5]

Recognition of alcohol's potential as a teratogen followed the appearance of two key articles in 1973 by Jones, Smith, and their colleagues[1,2] describing growth retardation, craniofacial and cardiac defects, and developmental delay in 11 children born to alcoholic women. The impact of these two publications was greater than might have been expected because they appeared during a period of increased public and professional interest and concern with maternal, fetal, and infant health. Perhaps, in retrospect, the most important contribution of these articles was the author's coining of the term fetal alcohol syndrome, which dramatically refocused interest on an important medical problem.

Approximately 550 cases of FAS have been described in the scientific literature.[6] These cases have been reported from all over the world (eg, Australia, Belgium, Brazil, Canada, Chile, Czechoslovakia, France, Germany, Hungary, Ireland, Italy, Japan, Réunion, South Africa, Spain, Sweden, Switzerland, and the United States).[7] As might be expected, no standardized criteria were used in making these diagnoses. In 1980, however, the Fetal Alcohol Study Group of the Research Society on Alcoholism proposed criteria.[8] A slight modification to this standard has recently been recommended.[9] It requires that at least one feature from each of the following three categories be present for a diagnosis of FAS:

1. Prenatal or postnatal growth retardation (weight, length, or height below the 10th percentile when corrected for gestational age).
2. A pattern of abnormal features of the face and head, such as microcephaly, microphthalmia, or midfacial hypoplasia, including a flattened bridge and short length of nose and absence or decreased prominence of the philtrum (the vertical groove between the nose and mouth).
3. Evidence of central nervous system abnormality, including, for example, attention deficit syndrome, mental retardation, or other evidence of abnormal neurobehavioral development.

None of these features is pathognomonic of fetal alcohol exposure. Other nonspecific abnormalities also seen in conjunction with FAS include ocular retinal tortuosity; cardiac abnormalities, particularly septal defects; renal anomalies, such as hydronephrosis; genital anomalies, such as hypospadias and undescended testes; hemangiomas; dermatoglyphic abnormalities; and other anomalies, such as hernias. Any of these abnormalities may be seen individually even when there is no maternal drinking. We prefer the term *alcohol-related birth defects* rather than *fetal alcohol effects* for these individual anomalies.

The reported prevalence of FAS is variable and no firm national data for the United States are available. Depending on the location and the population under study, the overall prevalance has varied from 0.4 per 1000 in Cleveland to 3.1 per 1000 in Boston. Estimates from Europe have ranged from 1.6 per 1000 in Sweden[10] to 2.9 per 1000 in France. The overall prevalence of FAS in the Western World appears to be 1.9 per 1000 births.[11] When only women identified as problem drinkers or alcohol abusers are considered, estimates of the frequency of FAS are more consistent and higher, with the overall average about 59 per 1000. Thus, although only relatively few children may be born with enough stigmata to be diagnosed as FAS, effects attributable to prenatal alcohol exposure occur relatively often among infants born to women who drink heavily during pregnancy and may be responsible for about 5% of all congenital anomalies.[12] Mental retardation is the most serious and damaging of all alcohol-related birth defects, and maternal alcohol abuse during pregnancy now seems to be the most common teratogenic cause of mental retardation in the Western world.[11]

Because experimental administration of alcohol to pregnant women is clearly unethical, studies of alcohol and pregnancy in humans are limited to clinical observation or nonexperimental, noninvasive designs. Clinical reports, however, can be of particular importance in unique cases. For instance, a case in which one fraternal twin was more severely affected with FAS than the other indicates that genetic factors are significant in determining fetal susceptibility to alcohol's damaging effects.[13] This may help explain why two women can consume the same amount of alcohol, yet one may give birth to a child with FAS and the other may not.

Observational studies involving large numbers of patients rather than single cases can be more difficult to interpret. Detailed critical reviews of such studies have recently been published and have identified two general problem areas.[14,15] The first involves the issue of bias. In many published case reports and studies, the diagnosis of alcohol-related birth defects has not been blind to the history of maternal alcohol abuse. This leads to the possibility that some of the observed associations may be artifactual (i.e., found purely because they were being studied).

A second major problem in human fetal alcohol studies is *confounding*. Alcohol is one of a multitude of possible pregnancy risks (cofactors), which include maternal characteristics, medical diseases, pregnancy complications, exposure to environmental pollutants, and lifestyle factors, such as abuse of substances other than alcohol.[16,17] In epidemiologic studies, complex statistical techniques can be used to try to control and adjust for as many factors as possible to support inferences linking observed effects to alcohol. Many pregnancy risks remain unknown, however, and there are limitations in these statistical techniques. Therefore, it is not possible to adjust completely for confounding. Although human studies can document associations between alcohol and adverse pregnancy outcome, they cannot *prove* causality.[18] Studies in animals, on the other hand, when rigorously designed and performed, allow greater control and greater certainty in inferring a causal role for alcohol as a teratogen.

Alcohol-related birth defects comparable to those occurring in humans have been observed in mice,[19] rats,[20] beagles[21], sheep[22], miniature swine[23], and monkeys.[24] These studies have documented direct dose-response effects of alcohol on perinatal mortality, infant weight, and soft-tissue malformation.

Additional compelling evidence for a direct effect of alcohol as a teratogen comes from *in vitro* models. In one study,[25] rat embryos exposed to 0.15 or 0.3 g of alcohol per 100 mL of culture medium (0.1 g per 100 mL blood is considered intoxicating) had decreased crown–rump and head lengths, decreased total cell counts, and retarded development compared to controls after only 24 hours of exposure. Because rat embryos at this stage cannot metabolize alcohol to their primary metabolite, acetaldehyde, this study strongly supports a causative role of alcohol as an agent directly toxic to the fetus. In another *in vitro* study,[26] a fraction of rat liver and a source of energy were added to the culture medium to make metabolism of alcohol to its metabolite, acetaldehyde, possible. Fetal malformations similar to those obtained with the direct action of acetaldehyde were observed, providing further support that alcohol or its metabolities has a direct toxic effect on the fetus.

ALCOHOL ABUSE

About 60% of American women drink alcoholic beverages, and about 3% can be classified as problem drinkers.[7] The proportion of women in reproductive years (age 18–34) who drink an average of at least two drinks per day (i.e., 14 drinks per week) is about 5.5%. During pregnancy, the proportion of women who drink this much decreases to about 2%.[7] Different populations of gravidas, however, appear to behave differently—in a study in California[27], 0.5%, and in a study in Buffalo[28], 16% of gravidas reportedly drank 14 or more drinks per week. These estimates pose two interesting issues: (1) Because alcohol crosses the placenta, most people in the United States probably have been exposed to some alcohol prenatally; and (2) a considerable number of fetuses probably have been exposed to a lot of alcohol. Despite such exposures, however, relatively few Americans have suffered adverse consequences. Statements to the effect that "social" or "moderate" drinking is inexorably damaging to the fetus are therefore of dubious wisdom. We feel that statements about the dangers of a single drink have no basis in fact.

Determining the amount and timing of alcohol consumption that puts the fetus at risk is an elusive problem because of difficulties in obtaining reliable drinking histories and in quantitating drinking, a complex human behavior. To complicate the problem further, drinking patterns often change during pregnancy.

Identification of drinking patterns during pregnancy generally depends on self-reports of patients and are usually imprecise. A drink, for instance, can vary from 1–8 oz depending on the respondent and the way questions are posed.[29] Using self-report data to estimate relations between numbers of drinks per day and a particular risk to the fetus also is problematic because of denial or inability to recall actual alcohol intake. In all likelihood, the greater the drinking, the more inaccurate the response, and, typically, the lower the estimate compared with actual intake.[30,31] Such underreporting will have the effect of exaggerating the risk to the fetus from an apparent two drinks per day. For example, Ernhart et al[32] found that drinking reports given four to five years after the pregnancy correlated with pregnancy reports, but for 41% of the women, the later reports were higher than those obtained during the pregnancy. Especially noteworthy was the fact that the retrospective report was a better predictor of alcohol-related birth defects than the pregnancy reports. This improved predictive validity suggests the higher reports were more accurate and, the higher the drinking, the greater the underreporting. The implication is that women most at risk for fetuses with alcohol-related birth defects are those most likely to grossly underestimate their drinking. The corollary is that the risk to the fetus of what might appear to be two drinks a day is likely to be the result of much more than two drinks.

A second stumbling block in estimating risk levels of drinking is the multitude of definitions of *problem drinking, abusive drinking, heavy drinking,* and *alcohol dependence.* For example, in the Boston prenatal study, heavy drinking was defined as the consumption of 45 drinks per month and at least five drinks on some occasions[33]; in a study from Loma Linda, California, it was defined as the consumption of at least 2 oz of absolute alcohol per day (about four drinks per day).[34] In Seattle, where much of the early work in this area was conducted, it was defined as daily consumption of 1 oz of absolute alcohol (about two drinks per day)[34]; however, in the Cleveland prospective study, the Michigan Alcoholism Screening Test (MAST), a well-validated, widely used instrument to identify individuals with drinking-related psychosocial disruption, was used.[36] Such differences in definition and approach make comparisons across studies and estimates of fetal risk from maternal drinking more difficult.

Assessing risk levels is further complicated by the well-documented spontaneous decrease in drinking as pregnancy progresses.[29,36,37] This is a salubrious occurrence inasmuch as decreases in drinking should improve pregnancy outcome. However, it underscores the problem of trying to summarize an individual's alcohol consumption throughout pregnancy by a single number (eg, two drinks per day, or as 2 oz of absolute alcohol per day), calculated to two-decimal-place precision. The variability and complexity of human drinking behavior must always be kept in mind when interpreting studies of drinking during pregnancy.

Paternal Drinking

Women who drink heavily tend to consort with men who drink heavily.[38] Conceivably, some alcohol-related birth defects could be caused by paternal drinking. Abnormalities in sperm morphology have been observed in male alcoholics[39], and, thus, fertilization with defective sperm could result in fetal anomalies. Only one study has reported such effects (decreased birth weight) in humans.[40] In animals, offspring sired by alcohol-consuming fathers have been found to result in decreased activity and increased susceptibility to infection.[41–44] Conceivably, some of the effects attributed to *in utero* alcohol exposure may be caused by mutagenic effects of alcohol on sperm.

EFFECTS OF ALCOHOL

Spontaneous Abortion and Stillbirths

Maternal consumption of intoxicating levels of alcohol over prolonged periods is clearly associated with a range of specific adverse fetal outcomes. The risk for *spontaneous abortion* may be increased twofold in pregnancies complicated by maternal drinking, although perhaps only among women who are heavy or frequent drinkers (about 3–5% of women).[17,27,45,46] Pregnant monkeys also tend to abort after alcohol exposure[47], as do rodents[48,49], as is indicated by an increased rate of resorption, the analogue of spontaneous abortion in humans.

Data concerning *stillbirth* rate are less clear. In some studies, an increase in stillbirth rate has been noted[50], but in other studies[17,51], no such effect was observed. Likewise, studies in animals are equivocal with respect to alcohol and stillbirths.[38]

Low Birth Weight

Lowered birth weight is the most reliably observed effect of prenatal alcohol exposure in humans and animals. In a recent review of more than 550 reported cases of FAS, the average birth weight of such children was 2100 g[6], compared to the median birth weight for all infants in the United States of more than 3300 g.[52] Decreased birth weight also has been noted in the absence of full FAS.[6] Alcohol-related decreases in birth weight could be attributable to intrauterine growth retardation (IUGR) or preterm delivery, both of which are associated with an increased risk for mortality and morbidity. In a study by Sokol et al[17] of more than 12,000 pregnancies, birth weight was decreased by about 190 g in 204 pregnancies complicated by alcohol abuse with no effect on pregnancy duration.[34] The frequency of small-for-gestational-age infants was significantly increased. These findings of alcohol-related IUGR in humans are confirmed in numerous animal studies.[7,21,22,49] The IUGR is dose dependent and is related to treatment period. Exposure during the third trimester has a more severe effect on birth weight than exposure earlier in gestation.[53,54] It has even been observed after a single administration of alcohol shortly before term.[54,55] These observations in animals are consistent with studies in humans that indicate that women who reduce drinking during the third trimester give birth to infants with greater birth weights than women who do not reduce drinking during this period.[56]

Studies in animals also have suggested mechanisms by which prenatal alcohol exposure might induce IUGR. In addition to the direct effects of alcohol and acetaldehyde on fetal growth noted above[25,26], chronic fetal hypoxia has been suggested from indirect evidence to have a contributing role.[57] More direct evidence recently has been provided by an experiment in which high doses of alcohol were administered intravenously to pregnant monkeys, producing blood alcohol levels of 0.25 g/100 ml. The alcohol caused a collapse of umbilical vasculature, resulting in severe fetal hypoxia.[58] Savoy-Moore et al[59] also have reported that as little as 1 mg% of alcohol can cause contraction of the umbilical cord. Other possible mechanisms responsible for alcohol's effects on fetal growth include alcohol-induced fetal hypoglycemia[60], interference with the passage of amino acids across the placenta,[61] and decreased incorporation of amino acids into protein in fetuses.[62] Although alcohol-related decreased maternal zinc levels also have been suggested to contribute to growth retardation[63], the evidence on this issue is contradictory.[64]

Whether the lower birth weight of infants prenatally exposed to alcohol also may be attributable to preterm delivery is controversial. Alcohol-related prematurity was not identified in a study of more than 12,000 pregnancies[17], but it was noted in a case-control study of 175 mothers of singleton preterm infants and 313 mothers of singleton term infants when eight other risks for prematurity were controlled.[65] In a more detailed analysis of the same data set, heavy alcohol consumption (an average of two or more drinks every day) during pregnancy was associated with approximately a threefold increase in risk for preterm delivery, but no such association was identified for lighter drinking.[66]

Neurobehavioral and Neural Abnormality

If the fetus survives, arguably the most severe alcohol-related birth defects are those involving the central nervous system. Abnormal behavior development and anatomic, electrophysiologic, and biochemical abnormalities in the brain, which may underlie the observed behavioral deficits, have been documented in conjunction with fetal alcohol exposure in humans and animals.

Behavioral Development

The adverse effects of alcohol on behavioral development can first be detected in the neonatal period. Neonates born to heavy drinkers are more restless during sleep and sleep less than other children.[67] Abnormal electroencephalographic (EEG) activity during sleep has been noted for as long as 6 weeks after birth in some children. In fact, the EEG during some stages of sleep was so unusual in these children that the investigators were able to identify 20 of 22 children whose mothers were alcoholics on the basis of the EEG records alone.[68]

Slower mental and motor development in 8-month-old infants prenatally exposed to alcohol who did not exhibit full FAS was reported.[69,70] Streissguth et al[71] also have reported that children born to mothers who had three or more drinks per day during pregnancy had IQ scores about five points below those whose mothers drank less. Children in this study were tested at 4 years of age, and the analysis was adjusted for variables, such as maternal and paternal education. Although the authors interpreted these results as evidence that maternal consumption of more than three drinks per day in early pregnancy may "triple the risk of subnormal IQ," a decrease of five points in IQ is not the same as subnormal IQ. In fact, IQ scores for these children are not stated except for stating that they are in the "normal range." The implication of this study is similar to those showing a decrease in birth weight for children born to women who consumed around two drinks per day during pregnancy[72]—the relationship may be statistically significant but clinically unimportant.

Amounts of alcohol consumption leading to FAS, on the other hand, are linked with considerably lower IQ scores in several studies.[7] About 50% of all individuals with FAS have IQs below 70.[3] Also noteworthy is a report from Sweden[10] indicating that cerebral palsy occurred in 8.3 of 1000 births of children born to alcoholic women compared with 0.2 per 1000 births for the country as a whole.

Hyperactivity in children with FAS has been noted in several clinical case studies[7] and in 15 children who did not exhibit physical abnormalities consistent with FAS.[73] In conjunction with the later study, IQ scores were within normal limits, but all children eventually were recommended for special education services because of restlessness, short attention spans, and distractibility.

As is the case of physical anomalies, studies in animals have been able to duplicate many of the behavioral abnormalities noted in association with fetal alcohol exposure in humans. For example, hyperactivity and learning difficulties have been noted in rats prenatally exposed to alcohol[74–76], which may be related to an underlying problem in response inhibition.[77]

Neural Development

Neuroanatomic and biochemical abnormalities undoubtedly underlie the abnormal behavioral development observed in conjunction with fetal alcohol exposure. Microcephaly, a frequent characteristic of FAS, reflects an overall decrease in brain growth. Specific anatomic abnormalities observed in brains of children born to alcoholic women as studied at autopsy, as well as in animals prenatally exposed to alcohol, include hydrocephalus, absence of the corpus callosum, and abnormal migration of nerve and supportive glial cells.[48,78–80]

More subtle changes in brain structure have been noted in animals prenatally exposed to alcohol, such as abnormally distributed nerve fibers in the hippocampus[81], decreased cell content in the hippocampus[82], and decreased dendritic structure of hippocampal nerve cells.[83] The latter also has been observed in the hippocampus of a child with FAS.[84] Because the hippocampus is known to be involved in learning and memory performance and in inhibitory control of behavior, these anatomic abnormalities may be the structural basis for some of the behavioral abnormalities observed in humans and animal studies.

RESEARCH FRONTIERS

Prevention of alcohol-related birth defects depends, in part, on obtaining answers to at least three major questions concerning alcohol and pregnancy:[85] How do timing of alcohol exposure, pattern of exposure, and beverage source affect pregnancy outcome?[53] Is there a threshold for alcohol exposure below which there is no danger to the conceptus?[86] Can women who are susceptible to alcohol-related birth defects be identified?

Timing, Pattern, and Beverage Source

There is no "safe" time during pregnancy for drinking. Different alcohol-related birth defects can result from drinking during different critical periods (eg, early or late in pregnancy). Knowing when exposure occurs is important in anticipating different kinds of alcohol-related abnormalities (eg, facial versus central nervous system). A large but brief exposure to alcohol (binging) does not necessarily cause significant biologic damage to the human conceptus.[87] For damage to occur, drinking must be heavy and sustained.[87,88]

Beverage source is not a major determinant of infant outcome. Animal studies have been few and inconclusive.[86,89] Beer has been found to produce a small but significant risk for alcohol-related birth defects in three epidemiologic studies.[34,51,66] Determining if beverage source, in conjunction with the more direct effects of alcohol itself, contributes to alcohol-related birth defects might be useful for improving prevention strategies.

Threshold

One of the most frequently asked questions about alcohol and pregnancy is whether there is a safe level of alcohol intake and, if so, what it is. In July of 1981, the Surgeon General advised "women who are pregnant or considering pregnancy not to drink alcoholic beverages. . . ."[90] This advice is reasonable and conservative, but simplistic. Recommending abstinence to an alcoholic has no more chance of eliminating alcohol-related birth defects than it has of preventing alcohol abuse in general. Alcohol-related birth defects are a generic problem within the framework of alcohol abuse and alcohol dependence. Failing abstinence, specifying a safe level of alcohol intake would be useful for direct patient care.

Recent data from ongoing epidemiologic studies[91] now places the threshold for FAS at six drinks per day. This threshold was determined by focusing on 25 cases of FAS out of 1290 prospectively studied pregnancies. Pregnancies were divided into five exposure groups consisting of zero, more than zero but less than two drinks per day, up to six or more drinks per day. There were no significant increments in risk up to six drinks per day. When projected to the total study population, less than 1% of the women were drinking at or above this amount, but in this group, the risk for FAS was substantial.

Studies in animals similarly suggest that low to moderate doses of alcohol, resulting in blood alcohol levels below 100 mg/100 mL, have no or minimal fetal effects in offspring.[7,85] Reports of limited alcohol intake producing lowered birth weight,[72] abnormal neurobehavioral development,[70,71] and spontaneous abortion[8,28] are dependent on reported intakes, the method of data analysis, and the population being sampled.[8,12,18,46] In the ongoing debate as to whether there is a safe level of alcohol, personal experience is the ultimate guide. In the United States, about 60% of all women drink to some extent. This means that most Americans were very likely exposed to some alcohol *in utero*, and most of our children also have been exposed. Either most of us and our children are less than we might be as a result of a drink or two during our gestations, or there is a "no effect" zone of exposure that appears to be about 1–2 drinks per day. Although statistically significant effects have been reported at this level, none of these are biologically significant. Even in pregnancies complicated by very heavy alcohol use, only 2–3% of the offspring demonstrate full FAS, and about one half of the infants in such pregnancies show no effects attributable to alcohol at all.[17]

The identification of thresholds for alcohol-related birth defects provides a rational basis for advice to women in clinical care. A threshold for the expression of anatomic alcohol-related defects is in the range of three drinks per day, or 21 drinks per week. A clear dose-response relationship was detected above that level but a "no effect" response below it.[92] Only about 2–3% of women drank above the threshold. We do not mean to imply that alcohol-abusing gravidas are not placing their fetuses at risk, but that we need to concentrate our efforts on such women, the *risk-drinkers*.

Susceptibility

Some people are affected more by the same amount of alcohol than others.[7] Different species and different strains within a species of animals also differ in susceptibility to alcohol's teratogenic effects.[7] In humans, fraternal twins may not be equally affected by alcohol exposure.[13] This evidence suggests that differential susceptibility based on genetic factors contributes to determining whether alcohol will adversely affect the developing fetus. This difference should not be interpreted to mean that relatively small amounts of alcohol can be damaging depending on genetic susceptibility. Twins in these studies are born to alcohol-abusing women, not "social" drinkers. Instead, the implication is that if drinking is great enough (ie abused enough) to produce damage, genetic factors will contribute to the severity of such damage. Susceptibility also might be affected by the presence or absence of other pregnancy risks, such as poor nutrition, use of other drugs, or medical illnesses. A profile of patients particularly at risk for the adverse effects of *in utero* alcohol exposure would be useful to clinicians who provide direct patient care. Indeed, we have reported in a carefully controlled study, adjusted for the amount of fetal alcohol exposure, that black infants are about sevenfold more likely to develop FAS than white infants. This was only seen above a high threshold for exposure.[91] Minorities, including blacks and native Americans, may constitute high-risk groups, for whom prevention efforts might be focused.

PREVENTION

The most conservative advice from a prevention standpoint is abstention from alcohol from the time of conception throughout the entire perinatal period.[93] Such advice has been disseminated through public and professional education efforts.[90] Broad media coverage has been obtained for public health advisories regarding the use of alcohol during pregnancy. In one survey, 90% of the respondents knew that drinking during pregnancy might be harmful, but three fourths of these respondents believed that an average of more than three drinks per day was safe[94], and more recent surveys suggest that an even lower proportion of women are aware of the perinatal risks of alcohol. This suggests that public education programs may not be as successful as desired in modifying attitudes toward drinking during pregnancy. Furthermore, a survey of drinking patterns over a 6-year period indicated that although the proportion of women drinking during pregnancy had decreased, the proportion of women drinking at least two drinks per day was relatively constant.[95] Because it is precisely this limited proportion of the population, probably less than 10%, that incurs the greatest risk for alcohol-related birth defects, these results suggest that mass media-based public education efforts may not modify attitudes or behavior sufficiently and therefore are not the answer to abusive drinking during pregnancy. Whether placing warning labels on alcoholic beverages in the United States will have any appreciable impact on the frequency of "risk-drinking" also remains an open question.

An alternative approach is to focus on prevention in the clinic or physician's office.[33,96] Considerable evidence exists that this approach may be effective in decreasing alcohol intake or attaining abstinence during pregnancy and in improving pregnancy outcome.[29,33,36,56,96] The major problem here is that obstetricians and gynecologists are not yet expert in identifying alcohol abuse in their patients.

Diagnosing Alcohol Abuse

The first step in managing alcohol abuse is detecting the problem. We have no valid biologic markers for detecting alcohol abuse. Obtaining an alcohol history as a routine part of an obstetric or gynecologic history and physical examination is a viable alternative, but these histories are subject to denial.[17] Detailed history-taking might reveal alcohol abuse, but the ability of this approach is limited by the time available to the physician to devote to such activity.

We have recently described a new validated questionnaire that takes little time and is more sensitive than other available questionnaires, such as the Michigan Alcohol Screening Test (MAST) and CAGE, for identifying pregnant alcohol abusers.[31] It is called T-ACE, and it is a variant of the CAGE. It asks four questions having to do with tolerance (T = tolerance), annoyance at being asked about drinking (A = annoyance), attempts to cut down (C = cut down), and drinking early in the morning (E = eye opener). The questionnaire identified 69% of a group of risk drinkers and is the first validated questionnaire for use in obstetric and gynecologic practice.[31]

CONCLUSIONS

Alcohol has been clearly established as a teratogen in humans. The effects of *in utero* exposure to alcohol include a characteristic collection of anomalies called fetal alcohol syndrome (FAS) and subtle behavioral disturbances in children who bear no physical stigmata of prenatal alcohol exposure.

Extensive public education efforts have alerted women to the dangers of drinking during pregnancy, and labeling alcoholic beverages may have some effect. However, women who are heavy or abusive drinkers may have difficulty in decreasing their drinking, whether they are pregnant or not. These women (about 5–10%) may be subjecting their unborn children to a significant risk for well-documented embryotoxic and teratogenic effects. If women are able to cut their drinking down to occasional drinks, the evidence from animal and human studies suggests that their babies will be healthier.

Effective prevention strategies for FAS and alcohol-related birth defects probably relate to prevention of alcohol abuse in general. More information is needed about alcohol abuse and dependence in young women, so that more focused approaches to prevention can be developed. Professional education and involvement of physicians, nurses, and other health care providers may offer a rational and cost-effective approach to prevention of alcohol-related birth defects. If these individuals take an active role in influencing the drinking habits of their patients, it may be possible to decrease the occurrence of alcohol-related birth defects and improve pregnancy outcome.

REFERENCES

1. Jones KL, Smith DW, Ulleland CN, et al. Pattern of malformation in offspring of chronic alcoholic mothers. *Lancet*. 1973;1:1267.
2. Jones KL, Smith DW. Recognition of the fetal alcohol syndrome in early infancy. *Lancet*. 1973;2:999.
3. Abel EL. *New Literature on Fetal Alcohol Exposure and Effects*. Westport, CT: Greenwood Press; 1990.
4. Bowen OR, Sammons JH. The alcohol-abusing patient: a challenge to the profession. *JAMA*. 1988;260:2267.
5. Jessup M, Green JR. Treatment of the pregnant alcohol-dependent woman. *J Psychoact Drugs*. 1987;19:193.
6. Abel EL. *Fetal Alcohol Syndrome: Historical, Epidemiological, Medical and Economic Aspects*. Medical Economics. In press, 1989.
7. Abel EL. *Marijuana, Tobacco, Alcohol and Reproduction*. Boca Raton, FL: CRC Press; 1983.
8. Rosett HL. A clinical perspective of the fetal alcohol syndrome. *Alcohol Clin Exp Res*. 1980;4:119.
9. Sokol RJ, Clarren SK. Guidelines for use of terminology describing the impact of prenatal alcohol on the offspring. *Alcohol Clin Exp Res*. 1989; 3:597.
10. Olegard R, Sabel KG, Aronsson M, et al. Effects on the child of alcohol abuse during pregnancy. Retrospective and prospective studies. *Acta Paediat Scand Suppl*. 1979;275:112.
11. Abel EL, Sokol RJ. Incidence of fetal alcohol syndrome and economic impact of FAS-related anomalies. *Drug Alc Depend*. 1987;19:51.
12. Sokol RJ. Alcohol and abnormal outcomes of pregnancy. *Can Med Assoc J*. 1981;125:143.
13. Chasnoff IJ. Fetal alcohol syndrome in twin pregnancy. *Acta Genet Med Gemellol* 1985;34:229.
14. Abel EL, Sokol RJ. Alcohol consumption during pregnancy: the dangers of moderate drinking. In: Goedde HW, Agarwal DP, eds. *Alcoholism: Biochemical and Genetic Aspects*. New York, NY: Pergamon Press; 1989: 228.
15. Neugut RH. Epidemiological appraisal of the literature on the fetal alcohol syndrome in humans. *Early Human Develop*. 1981;5:411.
16. Plant ML, Plant MA. Family alcohol problems among pregnant women. Links with maternal substance abuse and birth abnormalities. *Drug Alc Depend*. 1987;20:213.
17. Sokol RJ, Miller SI, Reed G. Alcohol abuse during pregnancy: An epidemiologic study. *Alcohol Clin Exp Res*. 1980;4:135.
18. Sokol RJ. Alcohol abuse during pregnancy: clinical research problems. Neurobehav Toxicol. 1980;2:157.
19. Boggan WO, Monroe B, Turner WR, et al. Effect of prenatal ethanol administration on the urogenital system of mice. *Alcohol Clin Exp Res*. 1989;13:206.
20. Blanchard BA, Riley EP. Effects of physostigmine on shuttle amardincin rats exposed prenatally to ethanol. *Alcohol*. 1988;5:27.
21. Switzer BR, Anderson JJB, Pick JR. Effects of dietary protein and ethanol intake on pregnant beagles fed purified diets. *J Nutri*. 1986;116:689.
22. Potter BJ, Belling GB, Mano MT, et al. Experimental production of growth retardation in the sheep fetus after exposure to alcohol. *Med J Journal of Aust*. 1980;2:191.
23. Dexter JD, Tumbleson ME, Decker JD, et al. Fetal alcohol syndrome in Sinclair (S-1) miniature swine. *Alcohol Clin Exp Res*. 1980;4:146.
24. Clarren SK, Astley SJ, Bowden DM. Physical anomalies and developmental delays in nonhuman primate infants exposed to weekly doses of ethanol during gestation. *Teratology*. 1988;37:561.
25. Brown NA, Goulding EH, Fabro S, et al. Ethanol embryotoxicity: direct effects on mammalian embryos *in vitro*. *Science*. 1979;206:573.
26. Popov VB, Vaisman BL, Puchkov VF, et al. Embryotoxic effect of ethanol and products of its biotransformation in postimplanted rat embryo cultures. *Bull Exper Biol Med*. 1981;92:725.
27. Harlap S, Shiono PH. Alcohol, smoking and incidence of spontaneous abortions in the first and second trimester. *Lancet*. 1980;2:173.
28. Russell M, Bigler LR. Screening for alcohol-related problems in an outpatient obstetric–gynecologic clinic. *Am J Obstet Gynecol*. 1979;34:4.
29. Weiner L, Rosett HL, Edelin KC, et al. Alcohol consumption by pregnant women. *Obstet Gynecol*. 1983;61:6.
30. Morrow-Tlucak M, Ernhart C, Sokol RJ, et al. Underreporting of alcohol use in pregnancy: relationship to alcohol problem history. *Alcohol: Clin Exper Res*. 1989;13:399.
31. Sokol RJ, Martier SS, Ager JW. The T-ACE questions: Practical prenatal detection of risk-drinking. *Am J Obstet Gynecol*. 1989;160:863.
32. Ernhart CB, Morrow-Tlucak M, Sokol RJ, Martier S. Underreporting of alcohol use in pregnancy. *Alcohol: Clin Exper Res*. 1988;12:506.
33. Rosett HL, Weiner L. Identifying and treating pregnant patients at risk from alcohol. *Can Med Assoc J*. 1981;125:149.
34. Kuzma JW, Sokol RJ. Maternal drinking behavior and decreased intrauterine growth. *Alcohol Clin Exp Res*. 1983;6:396.
35. Hanson JW, Streissguth AP, Smith DW. The effects of moderate alcohol consumption during pregnancy on fetal growth and morphogenesis. *J Pediat*. 1978;92:457.
36. Sokol RJ, Miller SI, Debanne S, et al. The Cleveland NIAAA prospective alcohol-in-pregnancy study: The first year. *Neurobehav Toxicol Teratol*. 1981;3:203.
37. Little RE, Schultz FA, Mandell W, et al. Drinking during pregnancy. *J Stud Alc*. 1976;37:375.
38. Abel EL. *Fetal Alcohol Syndrome/Fetal Alcohol Effects*. New York, NY: Plenum Press; 1984.
39. Lester R, VanThiel DH. Gonadal function in chronic alcoholic men. *Adv Exper Med Biol*. 1977;85a:399.
40. Little R, Sing C. Father's drinking and infant birth weight: report of an association. *Teratology*. 1987;36:59.

41. Abel EL, Lee JA. Paternal alcohol exposure affects offspring behavior but not body or organ weights in mice. *Alcohol Clin Exp Res.* 1988;12:349.
42. Abel EL, Tan SE. Effects of paternal alcohol consumption on pregnancy outcome in rats. *Neurotoxicol Teratol.* 1988;10:187.
43. Berk RS, Nowicki-Montgomery I, Hazlett LD, Abel EL. Paternal alcohol consumption: Effects on ocular response and serum antibody response to *Pseudomonas aeruginosa* infection in offspring. In submission.
44. Hazlett LD, Barrett RP, Berk RS, Abel EL. Maternal and paternal alcohol consumption increase offspring susceptibility to *P. aeruginosa* ocular infection. *Ophthal Res.* In press.
45. Kline J, Shrout P, Stein Z, et al. Drinking during pregnancy and spontaneous abortion. *Lancet.* 1980;2:176.
46. Sokol RJ. Alcohol and spontaneous abortion. *Lancet.* 1980;2:1079.
47. Altshuler HL, Shippenberg TS. A subhuman primate model for fetal alcohol syndrome research. *Neurobehav Toxicol Teratol.* 1981;3:121.
48. Chernoff GF. The fetal alcohol syndrome in mice: An animal model. *Teratology.* 1977;15:223.
49. Randall CL, Lochry EA, Hughes SS, et al. Dose response effect of prenatal alcohol exposure on fetal growth and development in mice. *Subst Alc Actions/Misuse.* 1981;2:349.
50. Kaminski M, Rumeau-Rouquette C, Schwartz D, et al. Alcohol consumption in pregnant women and the outcome of pregnancy. *Alcohol Clin Exp Res.* 1981;2:155.
51. Kaminski M, Franc M, Lebouvier M, et al. Moderate alcohol use and pregnancy outcome. *Neurobehav Toxicol Teratol.* 1978; 3:173.
52. *Monthly Vital Statistics Report: Annual Summary for the United States, 1979.* Hyattsville, MD; National Center for Health Statistics; 1980.
53. Abel EL. Effects of ethanol exposure during different gestation weeks of pregnancy on maternal weight gain and intrauterine growth retardation in the rat. *Neurobehav Toxicol.* 1979;1:145.
54. Lochry EA, Randall CL, Goldsmith AA, et al. Effects of acute alcohol exposure during selected days of gestation in C3H mice. *Neurobehav Toxicol Teratol.* 1982;4:15.
55. Greizerstein HB, Abel EL. Acute effects of ethanol on fetal body composition and electrolyte content in the rat. *Bull Psycho Soc* 1979;14:355.
56. Rosett HL, Ouellette EM, Weiner L, et al. Therapy of heavy drinking during pregnancy. *Am J Obstet Gynecol.* 1978;51:41.
57. Abel EL. Consumption of alcohol during pregnancy: Effects on growth and development of offspring. *Human Biol.* 1982;4:421.
58. Mukherjee AB, Hodgen GD. Maternal ethanol exposure induces transient impairment of umbilical circulation and fetal hypoxia in monkeys. *Science.* 1982;218:700.
59. Savoy-Moore RT, Dombrowski MP, Cheng A, et al. Low dose alcohol contracts the human umbilical artery *in vitro*. *Alcohol Clin Exp Res.* 1989; 13(1):40.
60. Tanaka H, Suzuki N, Arima M, et al. Hypoglycemia in the fetal alcohol syndrome in the rat. *Brain Develop.* 1982;4:97.
61. Henderson GI, Turner D, Patwardhan RV, et al. Inhibition of placental valine uptake after acute and chronic maternal ethanol consumption. *J Pharmacol Exper Ther.* 1981;216:465.
62. Henderson GI, Hoyumpa AM Jr, Rothschild MA, et al. Effect of ethanol and ethanol-induced hypothermia on protein synthesis in pregnant and fetal rats. *Alcohol Clin Exp Res.* 1980;4:165.
63. Flynn A, Miller SI, Martier SS, et al. Zinc status of pregnant alcoholic women: A determinant of fetal outcome. *Lancet.* 1981;1:572.
64. Fisher SE, Alcock NW, Amirian J, Altshuler HL. Neonatal and maternal hair zinc levels in a nonhuman primate model of the fetal alcohol syndrome. *Alcohol Clin Exp Res.* 1988;12:417.
65. Berkowitz GS. An epidemiologic study of preterm delivery. *Am J Epidemiol.* 1981;110:355.
66. Berkowitz GS, Holford TR, Berkowitz RL, et al. Effects of cigarette smoking, alcohol, coffee and tea consumption on preterm delivery. *J Early Human Develop.* 1982;7:239.
67. Rosett HL, Synder P, Sander LW, et al. Effects of maternal drinking on neonatal state regulation. *Develop Med Child Neurol.* 1979;21:464.
68. Havlicek V, Childiaeva R, Chernick V, et al. EEG frequency spectrum characteristics of sleep rates in infants of alcoholic mothers. *Neuropaediat.* 1977;8:360.
69. Golden NL, Sokol RJ, Kuhnert BR, et al. Maternal alcohol use and infant development. *Pediatrics.* 1982;70:931.
70. Streissguth AP, Barr HM, Martin DC, et al. Effects of maternal alcohol, nicotine and caffeine use during pregnancy on infant mental and motor developments at eight months. *Alcohol Clin Exp Res.* 1980;4:152.
71. Streissguth AP, Barr HM, Sampson PD, et al. IQ at age 4 in relation to maternal alcohol use and smoking during pregnancy. *Develop Psychol.* 1989;25:3.
72. Little RE. Moderate alcohol use during pregnancy and decreased infant birth weight. *Am J Publ Hlth.* 1977;67:1154.
73. Shaywitz SE, Cohen DJ, Shaywitz BA, et al. Behavior and learning deficits in children of normal intelligence born to alcoholic mothers. *J Pediat.* 1980;96:978.
74. Abel EL, Dintcheff BA. Effects of prenatal alcohol exposure in nose poking in year-old rats. *Alcohol.* 1986;3:201.
75. Becker HC, Randall CL. Effects of prenatal ethanol exposure in C57 BL mice in locomotor activity and passive avoidance behavior. *Psychopharmacol.* 1989;97:40.
76. Bond NW. Prenatal alcohol exposure and offspring hyperactivity. *Neurobehav Toxicol Teratol.* 1986;8:287.
77. Meyer LS, Riley EP. Behavioral teratology of alcohol. In: Riley EP, Vorhees CL, eds. *Handbook of Behavioral Teratology.* New York, NY: Plenum Press; 1986;101.
78. Clarren SK, Bowden DM, Astley S. The brain in the fetal alcohol syndrome: Observations in human and nonhuman primates. *Alcohol Hlth Res Wld.* 1985;10:20.
79. Pfeiffer J, Majewski F, Fischbach H, et al. Alcohol embryo and fetopathy: Neuropathology of three children and three fetuses. *J Neurol Sci.* 1979; 41:125.
80. Rasmussen BB, Christensen N. Teratogenic effect of maternal alcohol consumption on the mouse fetus. A histo-pathological study. *Act Pathol Microbiol Scand.* 1980;88:285.
81. West JR, Hodges CA, Black AC, et al. Prenatal exposure to ethanol alters the organization of hippocampal mossy fibers in rats. *Science.* 1981;211:957.
82. Barnes DE, Walker DW. Prenatal ethanol exposure permanently reduces the number of pyramidal neurons in rat hippocampus. *Development Brain Res.* 1981;1:3.
83. Abel EL, Jacobson S, Sherwin BT. *In utero* alcohol exposure: Functional and structural brain damage. *Neurobehav Toxicol Teratol.* 1983;5:363.
84. Ferrer I, Galofre E. Dendritic spine anomalies in fetal alcohol syndrome. *Neuropediatrics.* 1987;18:161.
85. Abel EL. Effects of ethanol on pregnant rats and their offspring. *Psychopharmacol (Berlin).* 1978;57:5.
86. Abel EL. Prenatal effects of beverage alcohol on fetal growth. In: Messiha FS, Tyner GS, eds. *Endocrinology Aspects of Alcoholism. Progress in Biochemical Pharmacology 18.* Basel, Switzerland: S. Karger; 1981:111.
87. Jones KL, Chernoff FG, Kelley CD. Outcome of pregnancy in women who "binge" drink during the first trimester of pregnancy. *Clin Res.* 1984;32:114A.
88. Majewski F. Alcohol embryopathy: Some facts and speculations about pathogenesis. *Neurobehav Toxicol Teratol.* 1981;3:129.
89. Abel EL, Dintcheff BA, Bush R, et al. Behavioral teratology of alcoholic beverages compared to ethanol. *Neurobehav Toxicol Teratol.* 1981;3:339.
90. US Department of Health and Human Services. Surgeon General's Advisory on Alcohol and Pregnancy. *FDA Drug Bull.* 1981;11:9.
91. Sokol RJ, Ager J, Martier S, et al. Significant determinants of susceptibility to alcohol teratogenicity. *Ann New York Acad Sci.* 1986;477:87.
92. Fraser, Sauve, Parboosingh, et al. A randomized controlled trial of the effect of early amniotomy: II, Effect on fetal and early neonatal status. *Am J Obstet Gynecol.* In press.
93. Rosett HL, Weiner L. Prevention of fetal alcohol effects. *Pediatrics.* 1982; 69:813.
94. Little RE, Grathwohl HL, Streissguth AP, et al. Public awareness and knowledge about the risks of drinking during pregnancy in Mulnomah County, Oregon. *Am J Publ Hlth.* 1981;71:312.
95. Streissguth AP, Darby BD, Barr HM, et al. Comparison of drinking and smoking patterns during pregnancy over a six-year period. *Alcohol Clin Exp Res.* 1982;6:154.
96. Rosett HL, Weiner L, Edelin KC, et al. Strategies for prevention of fetal alcohol effects. *Obstet Gynecol.* 1981;57:1.

Chapter Nine
Tobacco Smoking

Siegfried T. Rotmensch, José A. Nores, and John C. Hobbins

9

The association between tobacco smoking and adverse effects on reproductive biology has been extensively documented. Despite its declining prevalence in Western society, smoking remains an important preventable cause of perinatal morbidity and mortality. Over the last two decades, the gender gap among smokers has narrowed substantially, and if trends continue, women will outsmoke men by the mid-1990s. About one third of women in reproductive age smoke, and more than 80% of those continue to do so during pregnancy.[1] Rates of smoking are higher among less educated, lower income, and minority groups, which are already disproportionately burdened with illness. Smoking in pregnancy is a fetal and maternal risk factor that should be identified and addressed by counseling and a higher index of suspicion for a variety of obstetric complications.

This chapter will focus on the effects of smoking on the pregnant mother and her offspring with particular emphasis on pathophysiologic data which should be helpful in perinatal counseling and management. A description of the adverse effects of chronic smoking on general health is beyond the scope of this chapter but readily available in the medical literature (see also Chapter 10).

MATERNAL ASPECTS

Tobacco smoke consists of more than 3800 identified components in the form of particulate matter, vaporphase, compounds, and gases. So far, biologic effects were demonstrated for many of these, including nicotine, cyanate, cadmium, and carbon monoxide.[2] There is evidence that many of these compounds are absorbed into the maternal circulation, resulting in elevated serum, saliva, and tissue levels.[3,4] A multitude of metabolic effects of tobacco smoke has been described; however, their mechanism of action has not been elucidated in all cases.

Prepregnancy weight of smokers is significantly lower than in nonsmokers.[5] According to cross-sectional studies, smokers weigh 5–10 lb less than nonsmokers of comparable age and height.[6] Animal studies suggest that nicotine is the agent responsible for this effect. Even though smokers appear to have a similar or higher caloric intake, remarkable differences in diet composition and energy expenditure for comparable physical activity seem to be present. Whether maternal weight gain during pregnancy is affected by smoking is still controversial[5], and, unfortunately, many studies fail to control for confounding factors such as socioeconomic status and concurrent substance abuse.

The maternal endocrine milieu appears to be affected by smoking from early in gestation. First trimester levels of estradiol, sex hormone-binding globulin, and human chorionic gonadotropin were shown to be significantly lower in smokers in a dose-response correlation.[7] These findings are consistent with multiple studies demonstrating an inhibitory effect of nicotine on steroidogenesis *in vivo* and *in vitro*[8] because of aromatase and 20,22-desmolase inhibition. Similarly, urinary estriol levels and serum human placental lactogen levels in advanced pregnancy were reported to be significantly lowered.[9] It is unclear whether the latter findings reflect placental dysfunction or changes in metabolism.

Hematologic alterations with maternal smoking consist mainly of an increase in hemoglobin concentration. This is largely a response to carbon monoxide-related impairment of oxygen transport and utilization. In contrast to the nonpregnant state, pregnant smokers do not demonstrate a compensatory change in 2,3-diphosphoglycerate and the oxyhemoglobin P_{50}.[10] The reason for the lack of this adaptive response in pregnancy is unclear; however, the physiologic implication is that oxygen delivery is mildly decreased to maternal tissues and to the uteroplacental–fetal unit. This mechanism could have an added detrimental effect in pregnant diabetics who already have an altered hemoglobin oxygenation curve because of elevated levels of hemoglobin A_{1c}. Other hematologic effects of smoking in pregnancy relate to increased platelet reactivity[11] and an apparently lowered prostacyclin production by the vascular endothelium.[12] Some investigators suggest that the latter finding could explain decreased uteroplacental perfusion in pregnant smokers due to vasoconstriction. This vasoactive effect, however, does not appear to be generalized because the only physiologically "beneficial" effect of smoking in pregnancy is a decreased incidence of hypertension.[13] It appears, therefore, that smoking has a more complex effect on prostaglandin metabolism in pregnancy than previously suggested.

Acute effects of smoking in pregnancy consist of an increase in maternal heart rate and mean arterial pressure within minutes after inhaling tobacco smoke.[14] These cardiovascular responses are consistent with rapid elevations in maternal plasma norepinephrine and epinephrine levels during smoking, probably initiated by nicotine activation of adrenergic discharge.[15] In the short run, none of these effects appears to be of major consequence to the gravid mother, but it is conceivable that a detrimental impact on the fetus occurs.

Finally, expectant mothers with preexisting pulmonary disease are more vulnerable to acute effects of tobacco smoking. Irritation of the bronchial tree and reactive mucus production can precipitate bronchoconstriction in asthmatics and predispose to respiratory infections.

Obstetric Complications

Multiple epidemiologic studies have linked maternal smoking to a higher incidence of spontaneous abortions, intrauterine growth retardation, premature labor, preterm premature rupture of membranes, *abruptio placentae,* and *placenta previa.* Based on currently limited pathophysiologic understanding of these complications, it can be theorized that the common denominator is hypoxic or toxic trophoblast damage. This theory is supported by the demonstration of decreased levels of placental hormones throughout pregnancy[7-9] and is consistent with findings of structural changes observed in trophoblastic tissue.[16] Pathologic placental changes observed in smokers include large and small infarcts, fibrinoid changes in arteries, avascular stem villi, thickened basement membranes of trophoblast, smaller vessels in terminal villi, and necrosis at the margin of the placenta.

Smoking during pregnancy is associated with a significantly increased rate of loss of chromosomally normal abortuses in a dose-response fashion.[17-19] This association persists after adjusting for confounding factors, such as maternal age, parity, history of previous abortions, socioeconomic background, and alcohol use.

The risk of premature labor and delivery appears to be substantially increased in smoking mothers. In a large epidemiologic study in England, the risk was found to be 2.3 times higher when the mother smoked 20 cigarettes or more per day.[20] Part of the increased incidence can be attributed to preterm premature rupture of membranes.[21] The mechanism of this smoking-related phenomenon is obscure, as is true for premature labor in general but is conceivably associated with minor degrees of placental separation.[22] *Abruptio placentae* is indeed a well-documented risk associated with maternal smoking.[23,24] Light smoking increases the risk by 24%, and smoking more than 20 cigarettes per day increases the risk by 68%. The pathophysiology of placental abruption in this setting appears to be related to degenerative changes in the arterial lining of decidual vessels. Such changes have been demonstrated with long-term exposure to low oxygen, carbon monoxide, and maternal smoking. Furthermore, the increased platelet reactivity[11] and thromboxane production[25] in smokers could result in thrombotic events in the placental circulation, leading to infarcts and abruptions. Another important bleeding complication associated with maternal smoking is *placenta previa*. The incidence increased from 25% with less than one pack of cigarettes smoked per day to up to 92% in heavier smokers.[23,24] Even though placental weight in smokers is not increased, it is conceivable that the total surface area is enlarged, similar to placentas of pregnancies at high altitudes. Cytotrophoblastic hyperplasia can be reproduced *in vitro* with low oxygen tension.[26]

FETAL ASPECTS

Most of the biologically active compounds in tobacco smoke cross the placenta freely and can be detected in fetal tissues. The fetal compartment is dependent on the maternal compartment for the excretion of various metabolic products and the physiologic environments differ remarkably. It is not surprising, therefore, that some tobacco smoke-derived compounds accumulate in the fetal circulation to a disproportionately higher degree. The concentration of carboxyhemoglobin in umbilical cord blood, for example, is 2.5 times higher than in maternal blood.[10] Adverse effects on the fetus are therefore the most consistently reported consequence of maternal smoking.

Abundant evidence exists that the fetus experiences the effects of maternal smoking within minutes. An increase in the frequency of fetal breathing movements has been demonstrated by ultrasonographic techniques.[27] Fetal activity decreases and heart rate increases acutely in response to maternal cigarette smoke inhalation.[14] During prolonged observation, however, there is a higher incidence of nonreactive nonstress tests[28] and decreased baseline variability[14] among fetuses of women who smoke.

Intrauterine growth retardation (IUGR) is the most consistently observed chronic effect of maternal tobacco consumption. Smoking 10–20 cigarettes per day throughout pregnancy reduces birth weight by approximately 200 g.[23] Anthropometric studies indicate that weight reduction is mainly caused by a targeted effect on lean, not fat, tissue growth.[29] It is unclear to what degree IUGR contributes to excess in perinatal mortality associated with smoking. Multiple hypotheses have been proposed to explain decreased fetal growth. Placental blood flow studies using the dehydroepiandrosterone sulfate conversion method,[30] radionuclides,[31] and Doppler technique[32] demonstrated decreased perfusion of the uteroplacental unit. It has been proposed that this is caused by the vasoconstrictive properties of nicotine[33] or the decreased prostacyclin production by the umbilical artery endothelium.[12] Other authors suggest that the disproportionate increase in fetal carboxyhemoglobin levels, relative hypoxia, or direct toxicity of nicotine and thiocyanate account for the growth impairment.[34] An interesting observation is the lowered zinc level in erythrocytes of fetuses exposed to maternal smoking.[35] Zinc deficiency has been linked with IUGR in many studies.[36] Tobacco-derived cadmium decreases zinc levels by inducing production of a low molecular weight protein, metallothionein, that binds both cadmium and zinc. There is preliminary evidence that both cadmium and zinc are sequestered in the placentas of smoking mothers.[35] Caloric intake does not appear to be an important factor in causing IUGR in this setting.

A wide range of congenital malformations, including neural tube defects, orofacial clefts, congenital heart disease, and limb reduction defects, have been reported in relation to tobacco smoking.[34] Virtually all of the studies neglect to control for important confounding variables and contradictory results, which makes it difficult to determine whether tobacco smoke contains important teratogens.

Considering the previously mentioned obstetric complications and the described direct effects, the fetus of a smoking mother is at significantly higher risk for perinatal morbidity and mortality. Most of the excess risk is contributed by complications of prematurity in spite of an overall lower incidence of respiratory distress syndrome in premature infants of smoking mothers.[37] Multiple logistic regression analysis of data on 369,000 singleton births in Missouri revealed a 36% greater risk of intrauterine fetal death and a 14% greater risk of neonatal death for primiparas who smoke less than 1 pack of cigarettes per day.[38] Those who smoked one or more packs per day had a 62% greater risk of intrauterine fetal death and a 42% greater risk of neonatal death. The offspring of multiparous mothers were at a somewhat lower perinatal death risk but significantly higher infant mortality risk.The authors estimated that if all pregnant women stopped smoking, the number of fetal and infant deaths would be reduced by approximately 10%. Similar results were obtained in a Swedish study with a relatively large study population.[39] Smoking mothers older than 35 years in this study had the highest perinatal mortality of all age groups. This might suggest that the detrimental effect of maternal smoking is modified by age-specific parameters. It is evident from the previously mentioned data, that tobacco smoking is a major preventable cause of fetal, neonatal, and infant mortality.

DEVELOPMENTAL AND LONG-TERM EFFECTS

The literature provides increasing evidence that fetal effects of maternal smoking during pregnancy are not limited to immediate complications of gestation. Large epidemiologic studies and animal research have linked maternal smoking to the sudden infant death syndrome (SIDS), delay in neurologic, intellectual and physical development, lower respiratory tract disease, and childhood malignancies.

In a prospective evaluation of more than 19,000 live births, SIDS occurred twice as often among babies of smoking mothers compared to babies of nonsmokers.[40] It is unclear whether this effect has its onset after birth or *in utero*. Animal research, however, demonstrates evidence of histologic brain-stem damage in rat fetuses exposed to maternal smoking during pregnancy.[41] This finding is consistent with reports on brain stem gliosis in human victims of SIDS.[42] Furthermore, considering the ultrasonographic evidence of changes in fetal respiratory movements during maternal smoking, a long-term effect on respiratory centers in the brain stem is conceivable.

Infants of mothers who smoked during pregnancy were reported to have less satisfactory neurologic and intellectual development to the age of 6.5 years.[43] Children aged 5–15 years with hyperactivity syndrome were more likely to be born to mothers who smoked in pregnancy. A thorough follow-up of 1,800 children in Finland to age 14 found that offspring of smoking mothers were shorter, and their mean school performance in theoretical subjects was poorer compared to nonsmoking mothers.[44] These differences remained significant after adjusting for maternal height, age, social class, number of older and younger children, and sex of the child. Animal research seems to support the notion that some of the developmental effects associated with maternal smoking occurs *in utero*. Studies on the ontogenetic pattern of the development of cholinergic binding sites in the rat brain revealed marked disruption of receptor acquisition in fetuses exposed to maternal smoking.[45] Since nicotine is an acetylcholine receptor agonist, it might be the mediator of this effect. Failure of animals to habituate to repeated stimuli also has been reported after prenatal exposure to maternal smoking. A normal habituation pattern reflects intact central nervous system function.

Lower respiratory tract illness in childhood seems to be significantly more frequent among children whose mothers smoked in pregnancy and discontinued the habit after delivery. These data were gathered from a large epidemiologic study in England in which 12,700 children were followed up to age 5.[46] Interestingly, prenatal exposure to tobacco smoke was a more significant risk factor for bronchitis and hospital admissions than postnatal passive smoking. This finding suggests that smoking during pregnancy may cause congenital damage to the developing respiratory system. It also has been proposed that prenatal exposure to tobacco smoke could interfere with the developing immune system and thereby predispose the fetus to respiratory infections.

Another concerning aspect of maternal smoking during pregnancy is the presumably increased incidence of a variety of childhood cancers.[47] The highest risk was seen for acute lymphoblastic leukemia and non-Hodgkin's lymphoma, followed by an excess of cases of Wilms' tumor. A postnatal effect of continued passive smoking exposure could not be controlled for in this study. It can be concluded from animal data, however, that a variety of tumors, including leukemia, can be induced by transplacental carcinogens.[48] Many of these carcinogens are known components of tobacco smoke.

COUNSELING

Pregnancy offers a unique opportunity to quit smoking. The growing awareness of impending motherhood and the concern for the fetus can be extremely motivating. In fact, it has been demonstrated that pregnant smokers are more likely to quit smoking after seeing their fetuses on an ultrasound scan (Stuart Campbell, personal communication). Under these circumstances it is the obligation of the health care provider to elicit a history about smoking habits at the first prenatal visit, and counsel the patient accordingly. Counseling should be based on facts and encouragement rather than on judgmental attitude. Most smokers say they want to quit, and many have tried unsuccessfully. Continuation of smoking is not only a choice, but also an addictive habit. The widespread availability of cigarettes, their social acceptability in large parts of our society, the fear of gaining weight, and the occurrence of withdrawal symptoms present major barriers to smoking cessation. Educational pamphlets, smoking cessation groups, and cigarette substitutes can be helpful in this process. Women should be encouraged that if cessation of smoking occurs before 20 weeks' gestation, the vast majority of perinatal complications can be prevented. Inclusion of the patient's partner can be equally important in coping with the stresses of smoking cessation. If he is a smoker, it should be emphasized that recent evidence links passive smoking to increased perinatal mortality and intrauterine growth retardation.[49]

CONCLUSIONS

Smoking in pregnancy is associated with a variety of adverse effects that mainly affect the fetus. It is a major preventable cause of perinatal morbidity and mortality. Recent evidence suggests the presence of behavioral teratologic effects that potentially affect the early development of children born to smoking mothers. The efforts invested in proper counseling are frequently rewarding and should be an integral part of modern prenatal care.

REFERENCES

1. Prager K, Malin H, Speigler D, et al. Smoking and drinking behaviour before and during pregnancy of married mothers of liveborn infants and stillborn infants. *Public Health Rep*. 1984;99:117.
2. World Health Organization, International Agency for Research on Cancer. Evaluation of the carcinogenic risk of chemicals to humans: Tobacco smoking. *IARC Monographs*. 1985;38.
3. Nowicki P, Sexton M, Hebel JR. Salivary thiocyanate in pregnant smokers: A comparison of two collection methods. *Addict Behav*. 1984;9:33.
4. Visnejevac V, Mikov M. Smoking and carboxyhemoglobin concentrations in mothers and their newborn infants. *Hum Toxicol*. 1986;5:175.
5. Garn SM. Smoking and human biology. *Hum Biol*. 1985;57:505.
6. Rigotti NA. Cigarette smoking and body weight. *N Engl J Med*. 1989;320:931.
7. Bernstein L, Pike MC, Lobo RA, et al. Cigarette smoking in pregnancy results in marked decrease in maternal hCG and oestradiol levels. *Br J Obstet Gynecol*. 1989;96:92.
8. Gunasegaram R, Loganath A, Peh KL, et al. Cigarette smoke induced cholesterol C-20,22 desmolase inhibition in pregnancy. *Ann Acad Med Singapore*. 1982;11:580.
9. Andersen AN, Rnn B, Tjenneland A, et al. Low maternal but normal fetal prolactin levels in cigarette smoking pregnant women. *Acta Obstet Gynecol Scand*. 1984;63:237.
10. Bureau MA, Shapcott D, Berthiaume Y, et al. Maternal cigarette smoking and fetal oxygen transport; A study of P50, 2,3-diphosphoglycerate, total hemoglobin, hematocrit and type F hemoglobin in fetal blood. *Pediatrics*. 1983;72:22.
11. Leuschen MP, Davis RB, Boyd D, et al. Comparative evaluation of antepartum and postpartum platelet function in smokers and nonsmokers. *Am J Obstet Gynecol*. 1986;155:1276.
12. Ahlsten G, Ewald U, Tuvemo T. Maternal smoking reduces prostacyclin formation in human umbilical arteries. *Acta Obstet Gynecol Scand*. 1986;65:645.
13. Duffus GM, MacGillivray I. The incidence of preeclamptic toxemia in smokers and nonsmokers. *Lancet*. 1968;1:994.

14. Kelly J, Mathews KA, O'Conor M. Smoking in pregnancy: Effects on mother and fetus. *Br J Obstet Gynecol.* 1984;91:111.
15. Quigley ME, Sheehan KL, Wilkes MM, et al. Effects of maternal smoking on circulating catecholamine levels and fetal heart rates. *Am J Obstet Gynecol.* 1979;33:685.
16. Rush D, Kristal A, Blanc W, et al. The effects of maternal cigarette smoking on placental morphology, histomorphometry and biochemistry. *Am J Perinatol.* 1986;3:263.
17. Himmelberger D, Brown B, Cohen E. Cigarette smoking during pregnancy and the occurrence of spontaneous abortion and congenital abnormality. *Am J Epidemiol.* 1978;108:470.
18. Kline J, Stein Z, Susser M, et al. Smoking: A risk factor for spontaneous abortion. *N Engl J Med.* 1977;297:793.
19. Kline J, Levin B, Shrout P, et al. Maternal smoking and trisomy among spontaneously aborted conceptions. *Am J Hum Genet.* 1983;35:421.
20. Fedrick J, Anderson ABM. Factors associated with spontaneous preterm birth. *Br J Obstet Gynecol.* 1976;83:342.
21. Meyer MB, Tonascia JA. Maternal smoking, pregnancy complications and perinatal mortality. *Am J Obstet Gynecol.* 1977;128:494.
22. Harris BA, Gore H, Flowers CE. Peripheral placental separation: A possible relationship to premature labor. *Obstet Gynecol.* 1985;66:774.
23. Meyer MB, Jonas BS, Tonascia JA. Perinatal events associated with maternal smoking during pregnancy. *Am J Epidemiol.* 1976;103:464.
24. Fielding JE. Smoking and pregnancy. *N Engl J Med.* 1978;298:337.
25. Wennmalm A. Interaction of nicotine and prostaglandins in the cardiovascular system. *Prostaglandins.* 1982;23:139.
26. Fox H. Effect of hypoxia on trophoblast in organ culture. *Am J Obstet Gynecol.* 1970;107:1058.
27. Thaler I, Goodman, JDS, Dawes GS. The effect of maternal smoking on fetal breathing rate and activity patterns. *Am J Obstet Gynecol.* 1980;138:282.
28. Phelan JP. Diminished fetal reactivity with smoking. *Am J Obstet Gynecol.* 1980;136:230.
29. Harrison GG, Branson KS, Vaucher YE. Association of maternal smoking with body composition of the newborn. *Am J Clin Nutr.* 1983;38:757.
30. Mochizuki M, Maruo T, Masuko K, et al. Effects of smoking on the fetoplacental–maternal system during pregnancy. *Am J Obstet Gynecol.* 1984;149:413.
31. Philipp K, Pateisky N, Endler M. Effects of smoking on uteroplacental blood flow. *Gynecol Obstet Invest.* 1984;17:179.
32. Morrow RJ, Ritchie JWK, Bull SB. Maternal cigarette smoking: The effects on umbilical and uterine blood flow velocity. *Am J Obstet Gynecol.* 1988;159:1069.
33. Trease GE, Evans WC. The pharmacological action of plant drugs. In: *Pharmacognosy.* 12th edition. London: Bailliere Tindall; 1983.
34. Werler MM, Pober BR, Holmes LB. Smoking and pregnancy. *Teratolosy.* 1985;32:473.
35. Kuhnert PM, Kuhnert PR, Erhard B, et al. The effect of smoking on placental and fetal zinc status. *Am J Obstet Gynecol.* 1987;157:1241.
36. Cunnane SC. *Zinc: Clinical and Biochemical Significance.* Boca Raton, FL: 1988.
37. Curet LB, Rao AV, Zachman RD, et al. Maternal smoking and respiratory distress syndrome. *Am J Obstet Gynecol.* 1983;147:446.
38. Kleinman JC, Pierre Jr MB, Madans JH, et al. The effects of maternal smoking on fetal and infant mortality. *Am J Epidemiol.* 1988; 127:274.
39. Cnattingius S, Haglund B, Meirik O. Cigarette smoking as risk factor for late fetal and early neonatal death. *Br Med J.* 1988;297:258.
40. Lewak N, van den Berg BJ, Beckwith JB. Sudden infant death syndrome risk factors. *Clin Pedriatr.* 1979;18:404.
41. Krous HF, Campbell GA, Fowler MW, et al. Maternal nicotine administration and fetal brain stem damage: a rat model with implications for sudden infant death syndrome. *Am J Obstet Gynecol.* 1981; 140:743.
42. Takashima S, Armstrong D, Becker L, et al. Cerebral hypoperfusion and the sudden infant death syndrome: brain stem gliosis and vasculature. *Ann Neurol.* 1978;4:257.
43. Dunn HG, McBurney AK, Ingram S, et al. Maternal cigarette smoking during pregnancy and the child's subsequent development. II. Neurological and intellectual maturation to the age of 6½ years. *Can J Publ Health.* 1977;68:43.
44. Rantakallio P. A follow-up study to the age of 14 of children whose mothers smoked during pregnancy. *Acta Pediatr Scand.* 1983;72:747.
45. Slotkin TA, Orband-Miller L, Queen KL. Development of (3H) nicotine binding sites in brain regions of rats exposed to nicotine prenatally via maternal injections or infusions. *J Pharmacol Exp Ther.* 1987;242:232.
46. Taylor B, Wadsworth J. Maternal smoking during pregnancy and lower respiratory tract illness in early life. *Arch Dis Chil.* 1987;62:786.
47. Stjernfeldt M, Berglund K, Lindsten J, et al. Maternal smoking during pregnancy and risk of childhood cancer. *Lancet.* 1986;1:1350.
48. Napalkov NP. Some general considerations on the problem of transplacental carcinogenesis. In: Tomatis L, Mohr U, eds. *Transplacental Carcinogenesis.* International Agency for Research on Cancer. Sci Publ No. 4. Lyon:IARC, 1973.
49. Martin TR, Bracken MB. Association of low birth weight with passive smoke exposure in pregnancy. *Am J Epidemiol.* 1986;124:633.

Chapter Ten

Environment and Pregnancy

Howard T. Strassner and Carolyn Weller Arnolds

10

Any deleterious potential of the environment deserves particularly acute attention in pregnancy, with its biologic, emotional, and societal concerns. Not only must the safety of a woman with a distinctly altered physiology continue to be a concern, but also the safety and relative risk imposed on her fetus. While the general appreciation of environmental hazards has increased, pregnant women also have increased their presence in many areas, including the industrial workplace. This has occurred as a result of changes in the social and economic structure of our society. Consequently, the exposure of women to potentially hazardous environmental conditions has increased. The potential for environmental alterations to deleteriously impact on pregnancy is therefore also increased.

The environment is considered the entire range of external physical and biologic influences that encompass and act on people. It is an extremely complex and dynamic system that continues to change as a result of nature's forces and, increasingly, human contributions. Human contribution to the quality of the environment dates as far back as the discovery of fire, the domestication of animals, and the pursuit of agriculture. Since the Industrial Revolution, however, the environmental alterations have become increasingly complex, occurring purposefully and inadvertently as a byproduct of achieving technologic and social progress. The soil, water, air, and food cycle and our levels of radiation exposure all have been affected. Indeed, human contributions have become nearly inseparable from the concept of the modern environment.

Over the last decade, society has become increasingly aware that this progress represents a double-edged sword, providing the comforts of an advanced industrial society and at the same time creating hazardous products and wastes from the industries. The general public and the medical community are becoming aware and concerned about the actual and potential health hazards from exposure to the agents. In general, a pregnant woman will be affected the same as any other adult by most environmental agents.

However, she is physiologically different from nonpregnant women, and consequently the mother might respond to certain environmental challenges differently.

The environment can have an effect on reproduction at any stage of the reproductive cycle. Although congenital defects often are singled out as the adverse pregnancy outcome of greatest concern, the human reproductive system is susceptible to environmental factors at many stages. Table 10–1 illustrates this range of possibilities. The production and release of adequate numbers of viable sperm and ova are primary prerequisites for successful human reproduction. If an environmental factor interferes with this, fertilization may not take place. For example, reduced sperm production secondary to occupational exposure could occur in the male. In the female, certain halogenated polycyclic hydrocarbons may block oogenesis or destory oocytes, leaving the ovary devoid of follicles.[1] Ovarian toxicity and oocyte destruction are produced by reactive electrophilic metabolites generated by the metabolism of the parent compound. Another example is ionizing radiation, which can destroy growing and preovulatory follicles. An environmental factor also could alter the DNA of the sperm or ova before fertilization. Early fetal wastage, stillbirth, or congenital defects could result if the insult occurs at this stage of susceptibility.[2] An environmental factor could interfere with fertilization itself. For example, smoking affects sperm motility, and altered sperm morphology or motility may prevent fertilization. After fertilization, but before implantation, damage to the developing organism has been viewed as an "all-or-none" phenomenon.[3] Because so few cells exist at this time, irreparable damage to some of them may be lethal to the entire organism. If the organism remains viable, however, it appears that organ-specific anomalies need not be a concern; repair or replacement of damaged cells at this stage should allow normal development. However, experimental research on preimplantation chemical insults challenges this concept.[4]

Once implantation has occurred, the embryo is then susceptible to environmental factors that could alter organogenesis, fetal and placental growth, and maturation. Similar incidents, which earlier were benign or lethal, now have the capability to produce organ-specific defects because replacement mechanisms are no longer operative. The first month of development is especially critical because during this time, the maternal–fetal circulation is established, the rudiments of the major systems—nervous, muscular, digestive, skeletal, and cardiovascular—are differentiated, and developmental refinements are programmed. An insult to any of these processes at this time can be lethal, leading to spontaneous abortion, or disruptive of many systems.[5] Regarding congenital anomalies, the second month also is a critically susceptible stage. Major organ systems are sequentially involved in developmental steps. Because all major organ systems are developing simultaneously and rapidly, a disruptive environmental toxin acting at this stage could have severe consequences. As an example, maternal infection with rubella early in pregnancy can be associated with spontaneous abortions; stillbirths; a variety of congenital malformations, such as ocular, cardiovascular, auditory, and mental retardation; and early-onset diabetes mellitus.[6] Organogenesis is completed by the end of the third month except for the brain, eyes, and gonads. Embryonic development thereafter is characterized primarily by increasing organ size and growth. Thus, an insult at this stage of development usually will not produce a visible malformation (brain and gonads excepted), but overall growth or size of a particular organ may be affected.[3]

Finally, the infant can be exposed even after birth to chemicals or toxins in maternal breast milk. For example, polycholorinated biphenyls (PCBs), methylmercury, and caffeine all are excreted in breast milk.

As can be seen, a successful reproductive outcome depends on a complex interdependent series of events. Human birth defects are not easy to attribute to specific causes. For example, malformations can be caused by complicated interactions between genetic and environmental factors.[7,8] Some malformations are determined by genes and some by environmental factors, and both groups of factors are involved in a large proportion of congenital malformations.

An example of the way in which many factors can interact and affect reproductive outcome is illustrated by the study of Hemminki et al[9] of an industrialized community in Finland. They studied the contribution of both parents to spontaneous abortion and reported a significant increase in risk of spontaneous abortions for women who worked in the textile industry and whose husbands worked in a large metallurgic factory. Their data suggested that two separate environmental factors, each acting singly on the mother and the father, acted synergistically in reproduction to increase the risk of spontaneous abortion.

THE AIR

Air is a mixture of gases, including nitrogen (78%), oxygen (21%), carbon dioxide, and others, as well as varying amounts of natural and artificial pollutants. Natural sources of air pollution include fog, airborne dust and soil, smoke, and pollens. Artificial pollutants arise from a variety of man-made activities.

Pollens are perhaps the most important and most abundant natural pollutant affecting humans. They are products of weeds, grasses, plants, and trees that require air currents for their release and distribution. This pollination process releases large amounts of airborn pollens to be widely distributed by wind.

Artificial pollution of the air also arises from multiple sources, including combustion of fuels in furnaces and automobiles, refineries, mills, chemical industries, and incineration. The common pollutants include nitrogen oxides (nitric oxide and nitrogen dioxide), sulfur dioxide (from sulfur impurities in fuels), carbon (soot), carbon monoxide, ozone, and lead.

Effect of Air Pollutants on Pregnancy and the Fetus

The principle adverse effects of natural environmental pollutants will be among people with allergic rhinitis, "hayfever," and asthma. During pregnancy, the course of these disorders is considered to be either unaltered or unpredictably affected. For example, pregnant women with asthma will show improved, worsened, and stable symptoms in similar proportions. However, a change in environmental exposure to allergenic agents may change the course of symptomatology in both pregnant and nonpregnant women. Most asthmatic patients will become increasingly symptomatic with increased concentrations of airborne environmental pollutants and antigens. Such environmental alterations may recur regularly with seasonal dispersion of pollens, or they may occur episodically, as in heavily industrialized urban areas where air quality is considered poor because of artificial pollutants. A variety of agents, plants, and animals found in the household as well as compounds used in the industrial workplace may contribute to airborne indoor pollution and allergic symptoms in susceptible people. Consequently, whenever an unusual worsening (or improvement) in allergic disorders occurs, a history of changes in environmental exposure should be sought. A rigorous

TABLE 10–1. MECHANISMS OF ADVERSE REPRODUCTIVE OUTCOMES

Stage of Susceptibility	Occurrence	Result	Effects
Stage 1	Inadequate number of viable sperm or ova	Infertility	Men and women
Stage 2	Mutations in the DNA of sperm or ova before fertilization not sufficient to preclude fertilization	Early fetal wastage, stillbirth, congenital defects (teratogenesis)	Men and women
Stage 3	Effect on sperm's fertilization capacity (conception)	Infertility	Men
Stage 4	Fertilized ovum unable to implant in uterus	Infertility	Women
Stage 5	Abnormal growth and development of fetus	Stillbirth, fetal wastage, congenital defects	Women, possibly men
Stage 6	Toxins in breast milk	Developmental abnormalities	Women

Modified from Pries.[2]

search for an etiologic change may be particularly necessary in pregnancy when many activities change, such as time spent outdoors, occupational exposures, and even household activities, such as cleaning and redecorating.

As with the natural pollutants, common environmental exposure to artificial air pollutants will have the greatest effects on people with respiratory disorders, particularly with increased concentrations. The combination of air pollution and pregnancy should not disproportionately affect the pregnant women. However, disagreeable odors that may accompany certain types of pollution frequently are a cause of concern to pregnant women in particular. Odors may warn of a harmful substance, and in such cases, identification of the source and substance is necessary to assess potential maternal and fetal effects. Commonly, however, odors are only a nuisance. For some susceptible pregnant women, noxious odors may, in fact, aggravate the nausea and vomiting of early pregnancy and thereby adversely affect maternal well-being.

The fetus generally will not be affected by natural sources of air pollution, such as dust and pollen, unless maternal health is seriously jeopardized, for example, in a severe asthmatic attack secondary to pollen exposure. Artificial pollution arising from the various man-made sources is the major focus of concern.

Of the common artificial air pollutants, carbon monoxide is probably the agent of greatest concern. Carbon monoxide is a colorless, ordorless gas produced by incomplete combustion of fuel. Although it is generated in many industrial processes, the automobile's internal combustion engine is the major source of carbon monoxide in the contemporary urban environment. In the home, unvented gas stoves used for cooking or supplemental heating may be a significant and dangerous source of carbon monoxide. On an individual basis, the greatest routine environmental exposure to carbon monoxide for the mother and fetus may result from maternal smoking. The concentration in cigarette smoke may approximate that found in automobile exhaust. Table 10–2 compares some environmental sources of carbon monoxide.

After inhalation, carbon monoxide is avidly bound to hemoglobin with an affinity more than 200 times that of oxygen and thereby decreases the oxygen capacity of blood. Fetal carboxyhemoglobin concentrations reflect those of the mother. Under steady-state conditions, the fetal carboxyhemoglobin concentration is 10 to 15% greater than that of the mother.[10] Carbon monoxide decreases the capacity of the blood to transport oxygen to the mother and fetus and shifts the blood-oxygen dissociation curves to the left. The combined effect is lowered fetal tissue oxygenation. The reduced neonatal birth weight that results from maternal smoking may be caused by the relative hypoxia of carbon monoxide. Although inconclusive, animal data and experience in humans suggest that overall effects of carbon monoxide on fetal development are hypoxic (mortality, neurologic damage) and not teratogenic. However, numerous other chemical agents also are present in cigarettes and smoke, and they also are likely to play a role in the adverse outcome. Pregnant women should be warned of the hazards of cigarettes and strongly advised not to smoke. Passive exposure to cigarette smoke also should be avoided.[11,12]

The known risks of cigarette smoking has led to concern regarding general environmental exposure to carbon monoxide in air pollution. A case-controlled study from Denver has investigated the relationship between low birth weight and the ambient levels of carbon monoxide in the mother's neighborhood. Within the limits of that study, an association between higher neighborhood carbon monoxide levels and higher odds of low birth weight could not be demonstrated. Further investigation of this subject is warranted.[13]

ALTITUDE

Life at high altitudes requires compensatory hematologic, respiratory, and cardiovascular adaptations to meet the demands of the environment. The primary environmental

TABLE 10–2. CARBON MONOXIDE CONCENTRATIONS IN AIR FROM VARIOUS SOURCES

Source	CO Concentration (ppm)[a]
Fresh sea air	0.06–0.5
Urban air	1–30
Street corner	5–50
Major interchange	50–100
Automobile exhaust	30,000–80,000
Cigarette smoke	20,000–60,000
Alveolar concentration in smoker	300–400
Smoke-filled room	25–100

[a] Parts per million by volume.
From Longo[10] *with permission.*

stress is the lowered partial pressure of oxygen and decreased oxygen availability as a result of decreased atmospheric pressure. Pregnancy at a high altitude will superimpose its additional physiologic demands on this. Physiologic adaptation to pregnancy is associated with increased ventilation, increased arterial pO_2, a slightly increased or unchanged alveolar–arterial oxygen gradient, and often a subjective sensation of dyspnea. In addition, hemoglobin concentration falls, and cardiac output and blood volume increase. A woman who is acclimated to a high altitude environment should handle pregnancy well. The normal pregnant woman who travels from sea level to high altitude may experience increased dyspnea, tachycardia, fatigue, headache, and difficulty with recent memory due to the decreased availability of oxygen in the air. Consequently, reduced activity should be maintained until acclimation occurs, particularly during pregnancy. On the other hand, individuals who have a marginally compensated cardiovascular or respiratory disease may not tolerate this environmental stress as well. For these women, the combination of pregnancy and ascent to high altitude could result in frank decompensation because of increased cardiorespiratory demands. The risk will depend on the degree of preexisting compromise and level of exertion. Also, cigarette smoking, which should always be avoided in pregnancy, may particularly aggravate or lead to symptomatology during acclimation, because the hypoxic effects of the carbon monoxide are similar to those of high altitude. The mother as well as the fetus may be particularly sensitive to this combination of hazards.

Related to the subject of altitude is the question of air travel during pregnancy for pregnant passengers and pregnant flight attendants.[14] Modern jet aircraft, although cruising at 20,000 to 40,000 feet, maintain a self-contained controlled environment pressurized to the equivalent of 5000–7000 feet. Exposure to this environment is relatively short-lived, intermittent, and accompanied by little physical exertion. Under these conditions, there is no evidence that flying is harmful to the pregnant patient or her fetus. Therefore, travel in commercial pressurized aircraft need not be restricted. Similarly, pregnant airline personnel need not be restricted until other attributes of pregnancy (eg, uterine size, difficulty with balance, nausea) make continued flight duties unwise.

The opposite extreme of atmospheric pressure exists in the increasingly popular recreational activity of scuba diving. Barometric pressure increases approximately one atmosphere per 33 feet of water depth. It must be appreciated that scuba diving involves inherent dangers whether one is pregnant or not[15], and proper training is essential. A general recommendation might be to avoid initiating this activity during pregnancy. However, with increasing numbers of trained divers, diving during pregnancy will occur. In addition to the inherent risks of the sport, some of the physiologic changes of pregnancy may increase the risk for the pregnant woman. Nausea and vomiting, fatigue, abdominal girth, and mucous membrane congestion are among the factors that may limit successful diving during pregnancy. When air breathing occurs at increased barometric pressure, inert gas, primarily nitrogen, is absorbed by body tissues. With rapid ascent (decreasing pressurc) after a dive, decompression sickness can result as gas bubbles are released from body tissues and fluids. Pain, infarction, and embolism are potential sequelae. Increased deposition of adipose tissue may increase the risk of decompression sickness; therefore, this risk also may be increased by the physiologic change that accompanies pregnancy.

Effect of Altitude on Pregnancy and the Fetus

Recent studies have suggested that pregnancy at high altitude may be associated with some added risk. Moore and associates[16] found a higher incidence of pregnancy-induced hypertension, proteinuria, and edema at a high altitude (3,100 m) than among pregnant women at a lower altitude. They also found that the degree of hypertension in pregnant women was inversely related to the level of maternal arterial oxygen saturation. The suggestion was raised that maternal hypoxia may play a role in the etiology of pregnancy-induced hypertension.

The fetus may be placed at increased risk of relative hypoxia by the decreased content of oxygen available at a high altitude. The degree of maternal acclimation, level of exertion, and state of maternal health play an important role. Infant birth weight is decreased at high altitude, though not all babies born at high elevations are growth retarded. Studies by Moore and associates[17] indicate that normal maternal arterial oxygenation is attained at high altitudes by compensatory hyperventilation. Mothers delivering low birth weight infants were distinguished by relative hypoventilation, falling hemoglobin concentration, and resultant reduction in arterial oxygenation.[18] Thus, the relative hypoxia of high altitude may be viewed as a factor limiting fetal growth potential in certain women. Importantly, maternal smoking at high altitudes was associated with a twofold to threefold greater reduction in birth weight than at sea level. The combination of these hypoxic events appears to have additive effects on birth weight reduction.

Fetal risks associated with the increased pressure encountered in scuba diving have been studied in animal models and surveyed in humans. Speculations exist that intravascular bubbles may form and obstruct fetal and placental blood flow even without signs of decompression sickness in the mother. Animal studies support the formation of bubbles after maternal decompression, but fetal malformation or death was not produced. There is minimal reported human experience with decompression sickness or hyperbaric oxygen therapy of decompression sickness.[15]

A survey of female divers was conducted by Bolton[19] to determine the extent of diving and the obstetric and fetal outcome after diving while pregnant. Although the group of 109 divers reported a significantly greater number of anomalies (5.5%) compared to women who refrained from diving during pregnancy (0.0%), the percentage was probably within the normal range for the general population. A recommendation is to discourage scuba diving during pregnancy. However, for women who choose to continue diving, Bolton recommends that they be informed of potential risks, encouraged to limit the depth of dives to 60 ft and the duration to one half the limits of the US Navy tables and to avoid strenuous dives, hypoventilation, and chilling.

TEMPERATURE

Environmental alterations in temperature may produce distressing symptoms to pregnant women. A pregnant woman's metabolic rate increases as a result of increased maternal and fetal metabolism. The fetus' temperature is approximately 1° above the mother's, and maternal thermoregulatory mechanisms must eliminate this additional excess heat. Consequently, pregnant women may be less tolerant of high environmental temperatures, whether naturally occurring or man-made (eg, saunas, hot tubs, occlusive garments). Symptoms, such as dizziness, fatigue, and fainting, may occur in pregnant women after such exposure. Again, patients with marginal cardiac reserve may be intolerant of the cardiovascular demand associated with elimination of excess heat. Therefore, these patients particularly should avoid such exposure during pregnancy.

Effect of Temperature on Pregnancy and the Fetus

Fetal concerns regarding temperature alterations are related to the potential of hyperthermia to produce fetal anomalies. Hyperthermia in the pregnant woman may be produced by high environmental temperatures, exertion in occlusive clothing, fever, or saunas and hot tubs. If maternal temperature rises, heat transfer from the fetus to the mother is reduced; therefore, fetal temperature also rises and continues to exceed that of the mother.

Hyperthermia has been shown to be teratogenic in animals under experimental conditions. Central nervous system abnormalities have been the most significant problems both in animal studies and in human case reports.[20] A threshold maternal temperature of 38.9°C appears to exist, and below this temperature, abnormalities are not seen. Although retrospective studies and case reports suggest a teratogenic role of hyperthermia at critical periods of development, no confirmatory prospective studies exist. Despite the lack of definitive proof, it is recommended that maternal hyperthermia be avoided by administering antipyretics for febrile illnesses and limiting exposure to environmental heat.

The association of hot tubs and saunas with central nervous system abnormalities is largely theoretical, but it is supported by isolated case reports. Most retrospective studies of hyperthermia actually have focused on maternal fever. However, on the basis of theoretical risks, Harvey and associates[21] studied the time in a sauna or hot tub required to raise body temperature to 38.9°C. They found that in all 20 pregnant study patients, maternal discomfort prevented them from remaining in a sauna at 81.4°C long enough for them to reach a core temperature of 38.9°C. In a hot tub, maternal temperatures of 38.9°C could be achieved, but not sooner than 10 minutes with a water temperature of 41.1°C, nor sooner than 15 minutes at a water temperature of 39°C. The data suggest that the normal use of hot tubs and saunas is unlikely to raise maternal temperatures to teratogenic levels. Therefore, 10- to 15-minute exposures should be reasonably safe.

NOISE

One of society's less tangible but increasing contributions to the environment is noise. Described as an "unwanted by-product of our mechanized society,"[22] noise is a form of pollution that has dramatically increased during the past few decades. Sources of noise include loud music, lawnmowers and chainsaws, household labor saving devices, street traffic, airplanes and airports, and industrial plants such as textile mills. Thus, in the workplace, community, and home, the pregnant woman in today's world may be exposing herself and her fetus to varying amounts of "noise." Though less publicized than other environmental contaminants, the potential hazards of noise should not be overlooked.

Because noise can be defined as "audible sound that may be harmful to health,"[23] its potential effect on the pregnant woman deserves consideration. Noise between 60 and 80 dB is stress producing and noise above 80 dB is harmful to hearing. A sudden loud noise can evoke a generalized stress reaction in a person, which is characterized by increased heart rate, respiration, blood pressure, gastrointestinal activity, size of pupils, and adrenal hormone secretion. The most thoroughly documented pathologic effect of excessive noise exposure is hearing loss.[22] Noise levels that can cause hearing impairment may be found in the industrial workplace. It has been estimated that 16 million American workers are exposed to occupational noise levels that endanger their hearing. Noise also may adversely affect work performance and efficiency.

Although the effects of overall environmental noise pollution generally are not as well defined as those associated with occupational noise exposure, environmental noise certainly can be a stressor. Reactions to the environmental effects of noise may include sleep disturbances, inability to relax, feelings of tension and edginess, and headaches.[22] A pregnant woman would be as vulnerable to these usual effects of noise as a nonpregnant woman. However, it is apparent that some of the reactions to noise are similar to complaints often expressed at various stages of gestation by women with normal pregnancies. Thus, noise may further exacerbate the usual complaints of pregnancy.

Effect of Noise on Pregnancy and the Fetus

Animal studies have examined the effects of noise on fertility and on maternal health. In the area of fertility, it was found that in rats, an auditory stimulus—the sound of an electric bell of about 110 dB—had an inhibitory effect on fertility.[24] The fertility rate decreased from 80% in a control group to 5.7% in a group that was exposed to the auditory stimulus for 14 to 26 days. Also, the number of offspring in the exposed group was 5.9% less than in the control group. When the sound stimulation time was reduced to 4 days, the fertility was reduced from 70% in a control group to 7.1% in the sound-exposed group, and the number of offspring was 3.3% less than the control rate. Furthermore, when the rats were exposed to audiogenic stimuli during the fourth to sixth days, seventh to ninth days, or eighth to tenth days of gestation, the fertility rates declined to 25%, 15%, and 5% respectively, as compared to the 80% control rate. Other investigators have found that pregnant mice who were exposed to high noise levels responded by gaining significantly less weight and reabsorbing significantly more fetuses than control mice.[25] The noise exposure was 100 dB of sound delivered at regular intervals for the first 6 minutes of each half hour on days 4 to 6, 7 to 10, or 11 to 14 of gestation. Though the animal studies show clear effects of noise under experimental conditions, the implications for human reproduction are not well defined.

Of the environmental elements that may adversely effect the developing fetus, one of the least frequently considered is noise. The concern, however, is twofold. First, the question arises whether acoustical stimulation can interfere with normal embryologic development and be a causative factor in congenital malformations. Second, the question as to whether the inner ear of the fetus is vulnerable to acoustic trauma arises. The question of risk of hearing impairment in children from mothers exposed to noise during pregnancy must be addressed.

Various animal studies have linked intrauterine noise exposure with malformations such as cleft palate, inhibition or retardation of osteogenesis,[26,27] polydactyly, encephalocele, cleft face,[28] and abnormal development of teeth.[29] These findings have not been universal, however. Other animal studies have indicated that noise is not a teratogenic agent.[25]

A human study, which suggests that noise deserves further study as a possible teratogen, examined the reportable birth defect rate of people living wholly or partially within the 90 dB loudness range under the landing patterns of Los Angeles International Airport.[30] The birth defect rate was higher in those areas under study than in the rest of the county. The authors point out that the results are not definitely conclusive in implicating noise because other aircraft or airport-related pollutants could be responsible; however, other investigators have come to similar conclusions regarding possible detrimental effects of noise on pregnancy.[31]

Acoustic stimuli can reach the inner ear of the fetus in women exposed to noise during pregnancy.[26,32] It is unclear whether there is an adverse effect on the fetus. It has been shown that acoustic stimuli of about 100 dB reaching the inner ear of the fetus are strong enough to excite the fetus. The resulting heart rate accelerations and movements provide evidence of the fetus' stimulation. It is not known, however, how vulnerable the inner ear of the fetus is to this acoustic trauma.

One study[26] compared hearing acuity, histologic preparations of Corti's organ and spiral ganglion, and histochemical preparations of cochlear structures of guinea pigs whose mothers were exposed to noise of 95 to 100 dB throughout their pregnancy with similar examinations of controls. The results did not show an impairing effect of noise on the structures of the inner ear of the fetus. However, conflicting findings exist that have shown hearing impairment in guinea pigs resulting from acoustic trauma suffered during intrauterine life. Although such studies certainly have not proven any specific effect of noise harmful to the developing human fetus, noise should nevertheless not be discounted as a potential danger.

THE WORKPLACE

In the past decade, the environment of the workplace is an increasing concern in regards to pregnancy. During this time, an increasing number of women have entered the labor force. In 1977, the number of new female workers increased by about 2 million, which was twice the number of new male workers.[33] In 1980, for the first time more than 50% of all women aged 16 to 64 were employed outside the home. These working women have not necessarily completed or decided to forego childbearing. The National Center for Health Statistics estimated in 1973 that about 42% of pregnancies occurred in working women[34], and this proportion probably has increased since then. Other statistics show that nearly 60% of women bearing their first child were employed during at least 6 months of their pregnancy and that 25% of women bearing second, third, and subsequent children were employed.[2] At the same time, concern about occupational hazards has grown dramatically, though the recognition that the workplace may pose a threat to those who work there certainly is not new. As early as the first century, the hazard of working with sulphur and zinc was described, and protective masks were worn by workers.[35]

Potential workplace hazards include chemical (eg, liquids, dust, fumes, mists, vapors, solvents, gases), physical (eg, ionizing radiation, nonionizing radiation, noise, vibrations, extremes of temperature or pressure), biologic, (eg, insects, rodents, fur animals, bacteria, viruses, mold, yeast, fungi), and ergonomic (eg, unusual body position, repetitive motion, fatigue, monotony, boredom).[35] Because of these potential hazards, many women have asked their physicians about the advisability of working during pregnancy. It is only by performing a thorough assessment that the physician will be able to address the patient's concerns. The assessment should begin with the usual evaluation of the patient's medical and obstetric status. It should then proceed to an evaluation of the patient's work activity and work environment.

The assessment of work exposures should be initiated during the patient's first prenatal visit and should be continually evaluated at subsequent visits. The questionnaire shown in Table 10–3 can be used as a guide. Initial data can be obtained by interviewing the patient. Additional data may need to be supplied by the physician, nurse, industrial hygienist in the company's employee health unit, plant safety director, or union representative. In some instances, it may be helpful to have the patient keep an hourly diary for several days, noting activities performed, subjective responses such as fatigue, and materials to which the patient is exposed or which she handles. To assist in determining the patient's risk, the physician may want to contact occupational health professionals in the company, designated state agencies, or one of the regional offices of the National Institute for Occupational Safety and Health (NIOSH).[36]

Analysis of these medical, obstetric, and work environment data may then enable the physician to make recommendations to the patient regarding the advisability of her working during pregnancy and ways to minimize potential hazards if necessary. These recommendations may be requested by the patient or by her employer to certify that she may safely remain on the job with or without modifications or that she is eligible for certain disability benefits. Disabilities of pregnancy fall into three basic categories: (1) disability of the pregnancy itself, as occurs at the time of labor, delivery, and postpartum; (2) disability related to complications, such as preeclampsia, premature labor, or cardiac disease; (3) disability related to job exposures, such as exposure to excessive levels of toxic substances.[33] The physician should consider these categories when making recommendations.

In the majority of cases, the patient will be able to continue work during pregnancy. In 1977, NIOSH funded a study that developed guidelines on pregnancy and work. They concluded that a woman with an uncomplicated pregnancy and a normal fetus in a job that presents no greater potential hazards than those encountered in normal daily life in the community may continue to work without interruption until the onset of labor and may resume working several weeks after an uncomplicated delivery.[36] Other than the recommendation that a woman may continue to work without change, the physician could recommend one of the following: (1) The woman may continue to work but with certain modifications of environment or activity. These modifications may be desirable (ie, the available evidence suggests that a modification of the work activity or environment will contribute to the worker's safety or comfort) or essential (ie, the seriousness of the potential effect or the probability that it will occur is such that a modification of occupational environment, activity, or location is necessary). (2) The woman should not work.[36] The flowchart in Figure 10–1 may assist in developing recommendations for the pregnant worker.

Although the potential work environment hazards will act on the pregnant woman (irrespective of the gametes, embryo, or fetus) as on any other individual, certain hazards will be intensified for the pregnant worker because of her altered physiology.

Among the chemical hazards to which the pregnant worker may be more vulnerable are asphyxiant agents, irritant gases, and airborne substances of particulate matter.

TABLE 10–3. QUESTIONS FOR OCCUPATIONAL HISTORY[a]

1. Type and Place of Work **Patient** / **Male partner** Job title Employer Union Supervisor Occupational health staff	This identifies the patient and persons to contact for further information. It is intended to augment the usual identifying and demographic data with information about the job setting. Information about the male partner is important if he is a potential carrier of toxic substances or infection.
2. Work Schedule Inquire about days worked, hours worked, schedule changes, frequency and amount of overtime, rest periods and breaks, frequency and regulation of work flow	This establishes the duration of work and the regularity of the work schedule. If rest periods are taken, ask whether these are on schedule or taken as needed. Adverse effects often can be obviated by altering the work schedule or changing the work–rest ratio. The flexibility of work flow is often important: Can the woman set her pace, or is it dictated by a process such as assembly-line work? Are there busy and slack times or is the pace steady?
3. Amenities Inquire about lavatory, rest areas, food and drink, access to emergency care.	This establishes the availability and accessibility of amenities that may be of special importance to pregnant workers. Can she go to the lavatory as needed? Is there a place to rest? To dine? Can arrangements be made for additional meals or rest periods as advised?
4. Physical Work Inquire about the nature of the activity, particularly sitting, standing, and other activities (such as walking, bending, climbing).	This establishes duration of continuous activity in hours and minutes, and the frequency per period in which these activities are performed. Continuous sitting may affect lower spine and venous return. Type of chair and availability of footstool are important. Bar-type chairs may be used to relieve the standing worker.
Inquire about the nature of the load handled by the worker.	This establishes the force (weight) required, size and shape, and type of handling such as lifting or pulling.
Inquire about task characteristics, including the balance and coordination required, risks of falling, task complexity, agility required by moving machinery or objects, sudden starts and stops, belts and harnesses.	This establishes information about any possible hazards related to the possibility of falling, either as a result of impaired balance or dizziness in pregnancy, or because of use of ladders or precarious positions. The risk of being struck or of the abdomen being impinged between spine and an external object is important.
5. Environmental Characteristics Inquire about exposure to important environmental factors such as: Climate, temperature Barometric pressure Noise, vibration Radiation Biologic agents Airborne dust, fumes, vapors Chemicals Special job characteristics	This establishes exposure to toxic factors in the environment. Each of these is discussed in more detail with respect to specific reproductive and systemic effects elsewhere in this document. Note the intensity—if possible in actual measurements—and the duration of the exposure. Also note any special job characteristics that may reduce or increase exposures: occlusive garments, ventilation, close quarters, isolation, available emergency equipment or transportation, emotional stress.

[a] This format may be used for assembling data about the employed patient and her partner to supplement the usual obstetric history and home information.
From American College of Obstetricians and Gynecologists[36] with permission.

Pregnancy is accompanied by increased respiration and oxygen demands, which are estimated to be 20–30% above the nonpregnant need. Because of these factors, asphyxiant agents that reduce the number of circulating red blood cells or interfere with oxygen uptake by hemoglobin may adversely affect the pregnant worker more than when she is not pregnant. Likewise, the respiratory demands of pregnancy may reduce the worker's usual tolerance for irritant gases, such as acid fumes and smoke. Also, the pregnant patient may inhale greater amounts of airborne substances than when she is not pregnant because of pregnancy-induced hyperventilation. The normal pregnant woman's ventilation rate increases from a nonpregnant average of 7 L/min to an average of 10 L/min by term. Other airborne particulate matter, such as flour, epoxy, or sawdust, may be more irritating to the pregnant worker because she has a hyperemic bronchopulmonary system.[36]

High temperatures and humidity in the work environment are among the physical hazards to which the pregnant worker may be more sensitive. As more women enter jobs requiring heavy manual labor or work in a hot environment, these stressors are becoming more important concerns. In addition, as noted earlier, the work environment is only one source of these stressors. The pregnant worker's response to extreme heat and humidity may require that she limit strenuous activity in such environments.

Biologic hazards may be a special concern to pregnant women employed in areas such as bacteriology and virology laboratories, pediatric clinics, or hospital contagious disease units. Although the pregnant patient does not seem to be more susceptible to infections during pregnancy, certain viral infections are likely to be more virulent.[37] In addition, fetal considerations may restrict the options for vaccination or drug therapy for an infection.

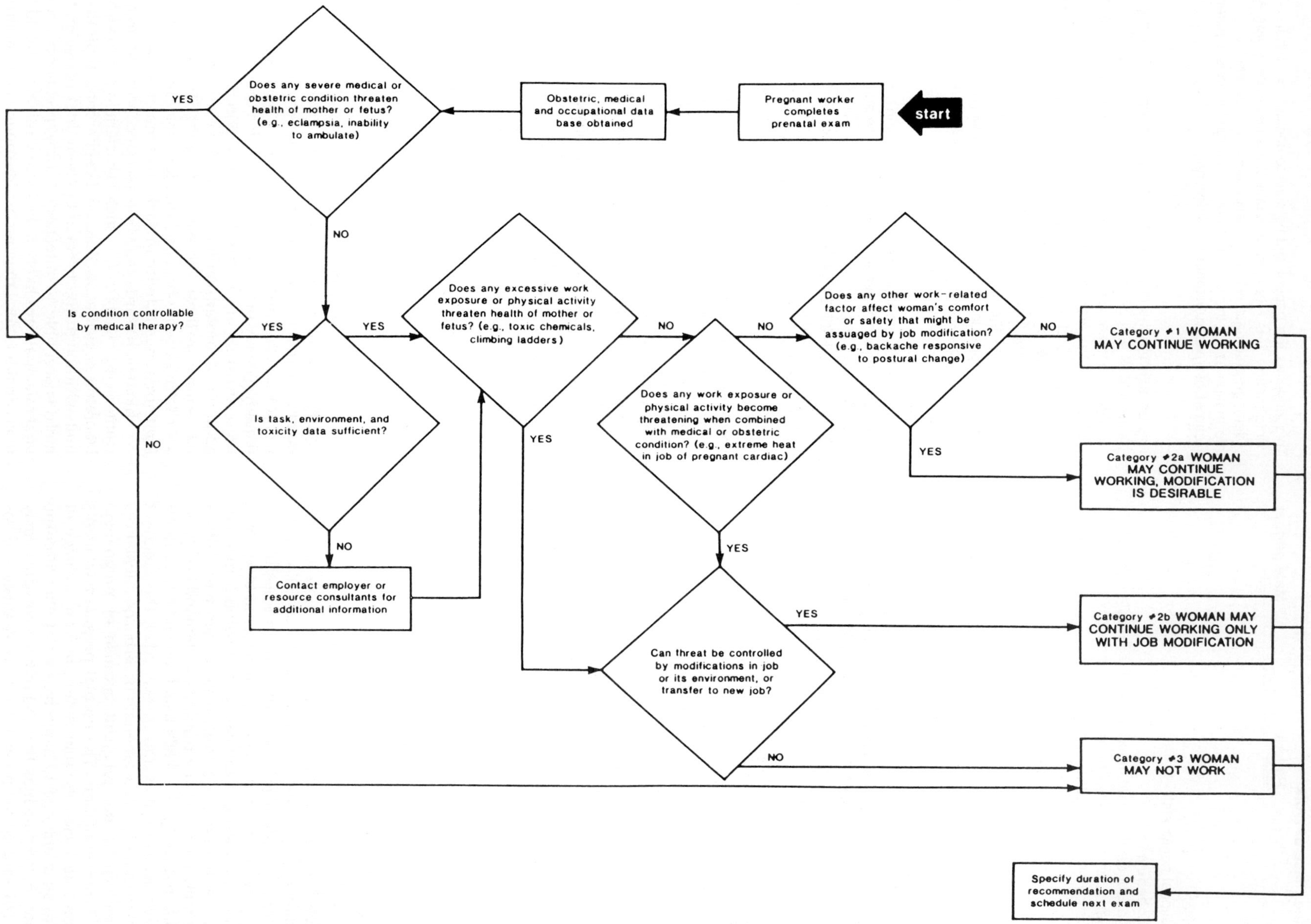

FIGURE 10–1 Steps for developing recommendations for the pregnant worker. *(From American College of Obstetricians and Gynecologists.[36])*

As with other types of hazards, the physical demands and erogonomic stresses to which the pregnant worker is exposed will vary widely depending on the specific job. The vulnerability of the pregnant worker to these demands and stresses will be determined by many factors. The worker's previous physical conditioning is of paramount importance. Generally speaking, pregnant women can continue to perform physical activities to which they have been accustomed.[36] Certain modifications, however, such as varying the rhythm of the work and rest cycles may be necessary. In addition, certain precautions need to be taken because of some normal musculoskeletal changes during pregnancy. The rising gravid uterus and the increasing weight of the breasts move the patient's center of gravity backward in the lumbar region and forward in the neck region. This altered balance and equilibrium can put the pregnant worker at greater risk for falling, especially when lifting or carrying loads or climbing a ladder. In addition, the act of lifting loads may be more difficult in the last trimester because of the protruding abdomen. Another consideration is the posture changes necessary to lift a load in front. This may further stress a pregnancy-stressed lumbar spine. The capability of a woman to lift a given load safely will vary with the individual. If a woman can handle a load easily when not pregnant, she will probably not be under stress when pregnant. However, if the load lifted before pregnancy required near maximum effort, it most likely will exceed the woman's capabilities in late pregnancy. Therefore, the load would need to be reduced. A load that was maximum before pregnancy should be reduced 20–25% during late pregnancy.[36]

Prolonged standing can cause dizziness and/or syncope in some pregnant women. These reactions are attributed to decreased cardiac output resulting from lowered venous return from the legs and the dilatation of peripheral vessels to dissipate body heat. Therefore, pregnant workers may need to avoid prolonged standing. Altered venous return from the legs also necessitates that the pregnant worker be allowed to change her posture frequently, and when seated, she should avoid pressure in the suprapopliteal region. A small foot stool can be useful to the seated pregnant worker.

Effect of the Workplace on Pregnancy and the Fetus

It is estimated that more than 1 million infants will be born each year to women who were employed at some time during their pregnancy.[33] As embryos and fetuses, these infants were thus potentially exposed to the chemical, physical, biologic, and ergonomic hazards that may have existed in the mother's work environment. The effect of these hazards on a pregnant woman, as noted earlier, will be about the same as for any other individual. The embryo-fetus, however, may be far more sensitive to these hazards.

The act of the mother working, all other related potential environmental factors aside, might be considered a risk for the growing fetus.[38] Analysis of selected data collected for the Collaborative Perinatal Project of the National Institute of Neurological and Communicative Disorders and Stroke showed that newborns of women who worked in the third trimester weighed 150 to 400 g less than newborns of mothers who remained at home. The only normally grown newborns of working mothers were the offspring of mothers who had sit-down work and no children at home. Growth retardation was greatest when mothers were underweight before pregnancy and had low pregnancy weight gain, when they were hypertensive, or when their work required standing. Shorter gestations were not the cause of the lower birth weights associated with maternal work outside the home, as there was no difference in the length of gestation among women who were at home throughout pregnancy or who worked at either sit-down or stand-up jobs after midpregnancy. Similarly, the lower birth weights associated with maternal work were not caused by lower maternal pregnancy weight gains, lower pregravid body weights, or differences in maternal blood pressures during pregnancy.

In addition to the differences in birth weight, the frequency of large (greater than 3 cm in diameter) placental infarcts progressively increased when women continued stand-up work into late gestation. For women who continued stand-up work after the 37th week, the frequency of large infarcts at term was 250 of 1000 births compared to 53 of 1000 when mothers remained at home and 47 of 1000 for stand-up workers who quit work before the 33rd week of gestation. The likely mechanism for diminished birth weight and large placental infarcts is low uteroplacental blood flow.

The association between work in various occupations and the occurrence of low birth weight, preterm birth,[39] spontaneous abortion, and fetal death[40] has been investigated. Increased adverse outcomes were observed in occupations in which work requirements exposed women to high levels of physical stress, such as heavy lifting, standing, long hours of work, noise, and vibration.

The embryo is particularly susceptible to hazards during the early weeks of pregnancy.[3] At that time it contains few cells, a higher proportion of undifferentiated cells, and rapid rates of proliferation. Embryonic cells have immature repair and detoxification mechanisms and possibly immature immunosurveillance mechanisms. Also, normal development during this period requires precise temporospatial sequencing, which may be affected by toxins.[2] In the early weeks, the placental barrier is immature, increasing the vulnerability further. Development of the placenta, however, does not guarantee safety for the fetus. Thus, the fetus is exposed despite its apparent sequestered location within the uterus. The placenta is not the complete protective barrier that it was once thought to be. The placenta is permeable to many substances taken into the pregnant woman and the fetus may even concentrate certain toxins.

Not only is the embryo–fetus possibly more sensitive to workplace hazards, but unfortunately defined occupational safety standards and exposure limits have not been developed with the embryo–fetus as the primary concern. Most hygienic standards and norms have been established to protect workers from acute toxicity of industrial exposures.[41] The teratogenicity of industrial compounds or properties, such as their potential to cause childhood cancer after maternal exposure, has not been an important factor influencing the setting of these standards. Thus, although the pregnant worker can limit her exposure to comply with the accepted standards and supposedly limit her own vulnerability, the embryo–fetus is not necessarily protected. Acceptable standards for adult workers may not be stringent enough to protect the embryo or fetus and the subsequent infant.

Even acceptable standards, however, do not take into account the effects that "mixtures" of hazards may pose, and the workplace offers a plethora of potential mixtures. The fetus may be exposed to a given chemical in a hot and noisy environment in which the mother stands most of the day. Under such conditions of mixtures, even stimuli of lesser intensity, which normally would cause no harmful effects, may produce an impairment.[26]

Chemical Hazards. Looking at potential chemical hazards alone, the magnitude of the threat to the embryo–fetus is staggering. The computer register of the American Chemical Society Abstracts Service contained more than 4 million distinct entries in 1977, with an average growth rate of approximately 6000 per week.[42] Roughly 63,000 chemicals are in use, and about 1000 new compounds are introduced onto the market each year. Only a fraction of these substances has been tested for toxicity, carcinogenicity, mutagenicity, and teratogenicity. The importance of these numbers to the potential hazards of the mother's work environment is recognized by considering that wherever environmental chemicals end up, they usually originate from industrial facilities where they are produced or first used. The occupational environment where the hazardous chemicals are manufactured is thus the first and possibly the most significant site of exposure to pollutants. Certain retrospective epidemiologic surveys and animal studies have shown that contaminated working environments are associated with spontaneous abortions, stillbirth, decreased birth weight, and increased frequency of birth defects.[40,43] The results do not unequivocally prove a cause and effect relationship, however.

Heavy Metals. Occupational exposure to heavy metals, such as lead, mercury, cadmium, nickel, and others, occurs in a variety of industries. In addition, industrialization has increased the general environmental level of certain heavy metals, such as lead and mercury. Occupational exposure added to a heavy environmental load may place the fetus at increased risk. Placental transfer of heavy metals does occur, and correlations between maternal blood, cord blood, placenta, and umbilical cord levels have been made.[44] Significant adverse perinatal effects from heavy metal contamination resulting from both fetal and neonatal (by way of breast milk) exposure have been documented (see also Chapter 28). Because general environmental levels cannot be easily controlled, minimizing maternal exposure in the workplace is crucial.

Waste Anesthetic Gases. Many embryo–fetuses are exposed daily to trace amounts of waste anesthetic gases if their mothers breathe the air while working in operating rooms and dental offices. Although the total amount of anesthetic agents present in the air of operating rooms or dental offices is small at any given time and measurable only in parts per million, the occupational exposure for physicians, nurses, technicians, and dental personnel is chronic. The effect of this exposure on the developing fetus is not fully known.

The data now available strongly suggest an association between women who work in anesthetic-contaminated rooms and increased rates of abnormal pregnancies. However, as Brodsky emphasizes in his review of the subject, for humans "there is no direct proof of a unique link between exposure to anesthetic and undesirable reproductive outcome."[45]

Exposing pregnant animals to clinical concentrations of anesthetic gases has persistently, though not uniformly, resulted in poor reproductive outcomes.[45] The results of exposing pregnant animals to trace concentrations of different anesthetic gases, however, have not been as consistent.[46] Several studies have shown repeated exposure to very low concentrations of inhalation anesthetics is associated with teratogenecity,[47,48] while other have not.[49,50]

An Ad Hoc Committee on the Effect of Trace Anesthetics on the Health of Operating Room Personnel studied the problem in humans.[51] They reported the following: (1) Statistically significant evidence exists that the risk of spontaneous abortion is increased for women exposed to the operating room environment during the first trimester of pregnancy and during the preceding year. The risk is estimated to be 1.3–2 times that of unexposed women. (2) There appears to be no increased risk of spontaneous abortion for the wives of exposed male personnel compared with the wives of unexposed male personnel. (3) Evidence exists for an increased risk of congenital abnormalities among the live babies of exposed female workers. (4) There was an increase in the incidence of congenital abnormalities for the wives of exposed male physician anesthetists. This national epidemiologic study was conducted by mailing questionnaires to exposed operating room personnel in four professional societies and to unexposed individuals in two professional societies serving as a comparison group.

Two early surveys in the United States examined spontaneous miscarriage rates between exposed female operating room nurses and unexposed female general duty nurses and between female anesthesiologists and female physicians in specialties other than anesthesia.[52] In both studies, the anesthesia-exposed group had approximately a three times greater spontaneous miscarriage rate. It also was reported that the miscarriages occurred earlier in both anesthesia-exposed groups compared with their control groups (8th versus 10th weeks), suggesting fetal lethality.

Corbett et al[53] looked at the incidence of birth defects among children of female nurse anesthetists. They found that 16.4% of children whose mothers worked during pregnancy had birth defects versus 5.7% of children whose mothers did not work during pregnancy. The difference was significant ($P < 0.005$). Waste anesthetic gases, however, were not necessarily blamed for this increased incidence of birth defects. As the authors note, their study was not designed to determine which of several factors (ie, low concentration of anesthetic gases, transmissible viruses, or radiation) was responsible for the increased incidence of birth defects among female anesthetists.

Another study[54] compared the incidence of congenital abnormalities, spontaneous abortions, and involuntary infertility between married women anesthetists and women doctor controls. The anesthetists group was then further broken down into those who worked during pregnancy and those who did not work. Anesthetists who worked during pregnancy were found to have a significantly higher frequency of children with congenital abnormalities (6.5%) than those who did not work (2.5%), but not significantly more than the control group (4.9%). Anesthetists who worked during pregnancy also had a significantly increased frequency of spontaneous abortions (18.2%) compared to the control group, but not compared to anesthetists who did not work. There was no difference regarding the type of congenital abnormality and no significant difference between the anesthetists and controls in the frequency of stillbirths or neonatal deaths. One variable not studied in some of the other studies was involuntary infertility. The frequency of this condition was twice as high among the anesthetists when compared to the controls, but no level of significance was noted.

A large-scale survey of dentists and female chairside assistants added more data on the effects of chronic exposure to trace anesthetic gases.[55] Dental personnel are exposed to twofold to threefold higher concentrations of anesthetic gases than hospital operating room personnel. In addition, many dentists who use inhalation anesthetics exclusively use nitrous oxide. This study therefore allowed for specific analysis of the reproductive effects of exposure to this drug alone. Paternal or maternal exposure to waste anesthetic gases was associated with an increased rate of spontaneous abortion. Wives of male dentists who had heavy exposure in the year before conception had a 50% higher rate of spontaneous abortions. Although this finding varies with the data reported in the large-scale survey of operating room personnel, which showed that wives of exposed male personnel were not at an increased risk for having a spontaneous abortion, this difference could possibly be attributed to the fact that the concentration of waste gases is higher in the dental operatory than in the hospital operating room. Among female chairside assistants, the risk of spontaneous abortion was 1.7 to 2.3 times higher, and appears to be dose-related, and a difference was noted between light and heavy exposure. In addition, women exposed solely to nitrous oxide showed twice the rate of spontaneous abortions compared to women not exposed to nitrous oxide.

Paternal exposure did not seem to affect the risk of congenital abnormalities in offspring, although maternal exposure did significantly increase this risk. There was a 1.4 to 1.6 times increase in congenital abnormalities among children of female chairside assistants exposed to all anesthetic gases. Maternal exposure to nitrous oxide alone resulted in a statistically significant 1.5 times increase in the incidence of congenital abnormalities in their offspring. Further dividing congenital abnormalities by type, it was found that the rate of musculoskeletal abnormalities doubled among children of exposed chairside assistants when compared to unexposed controls.

Although the majority of studies have noted an adverse reproductive outcome among women working in anesthetic-contaminated environments, not all have noted major problems. Ericson and Kallen[56] found that the delivery outcome of women known to have worked in operating rooms during pregnancy does not differ from that of women working in other medical occupations. No differences in the incidence of threatened abortions, low birthweight, perinatal death rate, or congenital malformations were found. The only suggested difference was a possibly increased incidence of pregnancies lasting less than 37 weeks. These results were based on data gathered from a government medical registry. The authors make a fairly strong case for their "unbiased" registry data collection method over the "biased" retrospective questionnaire-type of data collection used in most other studies.

Plastic Monomers and Additives. Plastic monomers, especially ethene and vinyl chloride, are among the major organic compounds produced today. The plastic monomers are reactive because of their chemical application in forming large polymers. Several of the plastic monomers have been tested for teratogenicity in experimental animals.[41] Acrylonitrile, methylacrylate esters (used in industry and for prosthetic devices and artificial eyes), phthalate esters (common additives in plastic products), urethane, and vinyl chloride have been found to be teratogenic in various laboratory animals. Styrene, used in the reinforced plastic industry, has been found to be fetotoxic as well as teratogenic in certain experimental animals. In addition, there have been increased rates of spontaneous abortion in wives of men exposed to vinyl chloride, and neighborhood exposures have been associated with increased rates of malformations.[57]

Solvents. Embryo–fetuses of mothers working in many types of industries are exposed to solvents such as benzene and carbon disulfide. Benzene has been associated with minor skeletal malformations in mice after inhalation exposure to 500 parts per million.[41] Carbon disulfide, used extensively in the viscose rayon industry, was teratogenic in the rat at relatively low doses. In humans, a survey[58] of female spinners in rayon factories exposed to carbon disulfide in the air at a level of 37–56 $\mu g/m^3$ showed higher incidences of pregnancy toxemia in exposed spinners than in a control group of nonexposed finishers. In addition, cord blood levels provided evidence that carbon disulfide transfers to the fetus through the placenta. Breast milk from exposed spinners also was found to contain carbon disulfide even after 23–56 days off the job. And 5 out of 10 breast-fed babies whose mothers were exposed to carbon disulfide had carbon disulfide present in their urine. Other industrial solvents, such as dimethyl formamide, dimethylsulfoxide, and propylene glycol, also have been found to cause malformations in various laboratory animals.[41]

Certain chlorinated hydrocarbons, such as methylene chloride, 1,1,1-trichloroethane, 1,1,2-trichloroethane, trichloroethylene, and tetrachloroethylene, also have been noted to cause malformations in chick embryos. Furthermore, minor skeletal malformations were seen in rats or mice after exposure to methylene chloride, trichloroethylene, and tetrachloroethylene.[41]

Toulene and xylene are among the most widely used industrial solvents today. Exposures in printing and painting are especially high. Minor skeletal defects in rats have been noted after exposure to these chemicals.

In humans, a 2-year study of mothers of children with congenital central nervous sytem (CNS) defects and their matched controls looked at maternal exposure to noxious influences during pregancy.[59] Significantly more case mothers than control mothers had been exposed to organic solvents during the first trimester of pregnancy ($P < 0.01$). The solvents included styrene, acetone, denatured alcohol, ethylene oxide, alkylphenol, dyes, benzene, dichlormethane, methanol, ether, white spirit (mixture of C7-9 aliphatic hydrocarbons), toulene, xylene, methylethylketone, petrol, and mixed aromatic or aliphatic solvents. Exposure occurred in plastics manufacturing, the leather industry, the textile industry, a community services laboratory, cultural services (museum), printing and publishing, rubber products manufacturing, metal products manufacturing, building, and handicrafts at home. This association between early pregnancy exposure to organic solvents and CNS defects in the offspring of exposed women has, however, not been confirmed.[60]

An incident of infant illness secondary to breast milk contamination with tetrachloroethylene also has been reported.[61] Tetrachloroethylene, a chlorinated hydrocarbon, is widely used as a solvent in the dry-cleaning industry. In the reported case, a 6-week-old breast-fed infant presented with obstructive jaundice. After other causes of the jaundice were ruled out, analysis of the mother's breast milk showed tetrachloroethylene to be present. The mother had been repeatedly exposed to tetrachloroethylene fumes at the family dry-cleaning plant during daily lunch-hour visits with her husband at the plant. The infant was never directly exposed to the father's working environment or to freshly dry-cleaned clothes. Although there have not been extensive studies on the transfer of occupational chemicals through breast milk and their effect on the suckling infant, this incident shows the potential for such transmission of at least one of the chlorinated hydrocarbons.

Hexachlorophene (HCP) has been reported to be teratogenic in humans.[62] Washing with HCP-containing soaps was associated with an increased incidence of birth defects among hospital nurses who washed their hands up to 60 times per day. HCP, although applied topically, is a drug with known systemic toxicity that can penetrate the placental barrier. Its teratogenicity in experimental animals has been known for more than a decade.

Chlorinated Dioxin Derivatives and Phenols. The chlorinated dibenzo-*p*-dioxins are among the most toxic substances known. They occur as contaminants in many substances, such as chlorinated pesticides (e.g., 2,4,5-T) and commercial polychlorinated phenols (e.g., the wood preservative, pentachlorophenol).[41,63] 2,3,7,8-tetrachlorodibenzo-*p*-dioxin (TCDD), a representative of this group, is an extremely potent teratogen in experimental animals, producing malformations at a dose of 0.006 mg/kg.[41] Data in humans are less extensive and conclusive. However, one Environmental Protection Agency study, completed early in 1979, examined the effects of 2,4,5-T in Oregon, which was sprayed to increase the productivity of commercial forests.[64] This study demonstrated an increased abortion rate throughout the spraying area. It also noted that most of the miscarriages had occurred in June and July, just after the peak spraying period in March and April. The route of transmission and the mechanism of action were not determined. Table 10–4 summarizes data on other industrial compounds.

Much of the data on occupational chemicals and their potential for causing harm to the developing human embryo–fetus are based on laboratory animal tests. Severe limitations should be placed on the extrapolation of these data to humans, and caution in interpretation also is required. However, the limited data available suggest that humans are at least as sensitive, if not more so, to the teratogenic effect of some chemicals as compared to experimental animals.[41] In addition, chronic exposure of the pregnant worker on the job may lead to the accumulation of the compound and chronic level effects, which the short-term animal experiment cannot predict. Thus, ignoring the results of such animal research also does not seem to be warranted. Occupational limits of exposure to certain industrial compounds, where they exist, definitely need to be heeded and continually re-evaluated. Until more data are gathered, it is not known whether current standards will ensure the safety of the developing human fetus. In fact, some standards already have been questioned. One reviewer[41] notes that the present standards of acrylonitrile, methacrylate esters, styrene, carbon disulfide, chloroform, methylene chloride, and possibly toulene and xylene may not provide an adequate margin of safety for the human embryo–fetus as extrapolated from the results of animal experiments.

Biologic Hazards. Pregnant women whose work frequently exposes them to certain infectious organisms may be putting their embryo–fetus at risk because some infectious organisms can cross the placenta and harm the fetus. In addition, certain maternal manifestations of the disease process, such as hyperthermia, may adversely affect the fetus. Hospital workers, elementary school teachers, and workers in infectious laboratories may comprise an "at risk" group. A maternal viral infection, depending on its nature and timing relative to fetal organogenesis, may lead to abortion, fetal death, fetal infection, or fetal abnormality. The more common viral diseases are rubella, measles, mumps, herpes zoster, herpes simplex, influenza, lymphocytic choriomeningitis, cytomegalovirus, hepatitis A, hepatitis B, coxsackievirus, and chickenpox. Human immunodeficiency virus is of increasing concern. Bacterial pneumonia can have a variable impact on the developing fetus, depending on the presence and degree of hypoxia, hypoglycemia, metabolic acidosis, and hyperthermia. Certain acquired protozoan agents, such as *Toxoplasma gondii,* plasmodia (malaria), and trypanosomes, also may cross the placenta and cause congenital disease or persistent postnatal infections.

THE HOME

For the health and safety of both the pregnant woman and her growing embryo–fetus, an assessment of the home environment must not be forgotten. Activities and exposures at home often are overlooked as the physician determines dangers in the work environment. Women who work spend a portion of each day at home, and women who do not work may spend even more time within the home environment. The home is not without its risks. Sometimes greater levels of physical activity and more hazardous environmental exposures can be found at home than on the

TABLE 10–4. OTHER INDUSTRIAL ORGANIC COMPOUNDS

Compound	Use of Representative Chemical Group	Observed Effect
Aminoazobenzene		Malformation in mice
Azo dyes, trypan blue		Malformation in rats
Detergents, such as alkylbenzene sulfonate, alcohol sulfate, olefin sulfonate, Triton	Washing powder, industrial emulsifiers	Malformations or minor defects in high doses in mice and rabbits
7,12-Dimethylbenzanthracene	Polycyclic aromatic hydrocarbons	Malformations in rats
Ethylenethiourea	Rubber industry and degradation product of a group of fungicides	Malformations in rats
Hydrazine	Oxygen-trapping agent in water	Malformations in chicks
Pentachlorobenzene	Fire retardant and fungicide	Skeletal malformations in rats
Thiram	Rubber industry and pesticides	Malformations in hamsters, rats, and mice
Disulfiram	Rubber industry	Malformation in hamsters

From Hemminiki[41] with permission.

job. The same careful detail regarding the workplace history should be applied to the home history.

The location of the house can reveal potential hazards. Proximity to a chemical manufacturing plant or commercial disposal site could put a pregnant woman at risk for inhaling or ingesting harmful chemicals.[43] For example, the lead consumed by animals and humans is affected by the proximity to major highways or smelters.[65] Also, the lead content of plants correlates with surface depositions more than the soil content of lead. Polychlorinated biphenyl has been detected in house dust from residences of occupationally exposed populations in southwestern Michigan.[66] Home well water from sources close to drainage fields of chemical plants or agricultural areas also could be potentially hazardous.[43]

Effect of the Home on Pregnancy and the Fetus

The activities that a pregnant woman engages in at home and the products she uses should be assessed. Lifting heavy groceries or laundry poses the same risks to the pregnant woman that heavy lifting on the job does.[36] Household cleaning can expose a pregnant woman and her fetus to a variety of potentially toxic chemicals. Home improvement products such as oil-based paints and lacquer thinner contain the organic solvents methyl alcohol, benzene trichloroethylene, toulene, and xylene, among others.[60] Also, 90% of tested commercial oxidative-type hair dye formulations were found to be mutagenic and hair dye compounds absorb through the skin.[7]

Biologic hazards in the home also can pose a threat to the pregnant woman and her fetus. If she has young school-aged children or children in a preschool play group, the pregnant woman could be exposed to a multitude of infections, such as chickenpox, rubella, or measles. Thus, for a complete assessment of the environment of the pregnant woman and her growing fetus, assessment of the home must be included.

FOOD

When considering food pollution and its possible effect on pregnancy, man-made contaminants, such as insecticides, or industrial pollutants such as methylmercury, usually come to mind. Although these man-made contaminants are extremely important, there also are many naturally occurring pollutants that deserve consideration. An explanation of this phenomenon was thoroughly reviewed by Ames.[67] Some examples, selected from this review, are discussed below.

Plants in nature, including those that are part of the human diet, synthesize toxic chemicals in large amounts. These toxic chemicals apparently serve as a primary defense against bacterial, fungal, and insect or other animal predator attacks. Although toxicologic studies have been completed for only small percentages of these chemicals, some naturally occurring mutagens, teratogens, and carcinogens have been identified in the human diet.

In addition to nature's contaminants, many man-made chemical contaminants, including industrial wastes, have unfortunately found their way into the human diet. In some cases, the results have been acute and catastrophic, others chronic and indolent, and for many, the final effects are unknown. Examples of these phenomena are mercury, pesticides, polychlorinated biphenyl (PCB), and polybrominated biphenyl (PBB).

Effect of Food on Pregnancy and the Fetus

Caffeine. Caffeine is a known, and in many cases desired, component of various beverages and foods. Caffeine crosses the placenta and reaches the developing fetus. Maternal ingestion of coffee, tea, cola drinks, chocolate, and other caffeine-containing foods therefore can cause the fetus to be exposed to caffeine. Concern that caffeine may be teratogenic led the Food and Drug Administration in 1980 to advise pregnant women that caffeine-containing food and drugs should be avoided or used sparingly. Animal studies indicating growth retardation and malformations in offspring of caffeine-exposed rats raised concern about the possible harmful effects of caffeine.[68] Data regarding the human teratogenicity of caffeine are sparse.

Two recent studies suggest that if there is a risk from caffeine use during pregnancy it is less than the 2–3% major malformation risk that women face in any pregnancy.[60] Rosenberg et al[69] in a case-control study of 2030 malformed infants, evaluated six selected birth defects—inguinal hernia, cleft lip with or without cleft palate, cardiac defects, pyloric stenosis, isolated cleft palate, and neural tube fusion defects—in relation to maternal ingestion during pregnancy of tea, coffee, and cola. For the levels of caffeine intake studied, the results indicated that such intake is not associated with large increases in the rates of the abnormalities selected. Because only 11% of the mothers ingested as much caffeine per day as is contained in four cups of coffee, it was not possible to evaluate birth defects in relation to very high levels of caffeine consumption.

A cohort study[68] assessed the effects of coffee consumption in more than 12,000 women interviewed at the time of hospitalization for delivery. After controlling for smoking and other habits Linn et al[68] found no relation between low birth weight or short gestation and heavy coffee consumption (defined as drinking four or more cups of coffee per day). Also, there were no excess malformations among coffee drinkers. High levels of coffee consumption could not be evaluated because less than 1% of the women in their population reported drinking seven or more cups of coffee daily. In addition, data about the consumption of soft drinks, cocoa, or chocolate, all of which contain caffeine, although in considerably smaller amounts than coffee, were not collected in this study. Although both of these studies appear to be reassuring regarding the safety of caffeine in pregnancy, as one author[69] warns, ". . . much larger samples are required to rule out smaller increases (in the rates of some common birth defects among women who drink caffeine-containing beverages), as well as to permit adequate evaluation of less common malformations." Specifically, much larger numbers of pregnant women need to be studied to exclude an increased risk of less common, though major, malformations such as limb reduction defects.

Caffeine also is excreted in breast milk, and can accumulate in the infant. If a nursing mother drank more than six to eight cups of any caffeine-containing beverage in a day, her infant could accumulate enough caffeine to be symptomatic (ie, wakeful, hyperactive).[70]

"Natural" Contaminants. Among nature's contaminants[67], the potato glycoalkaloids, solanine, and chaconine have been identified as possible teratogens. They are strong cholinesterase inhibitors and present at about 15 mg/200 g of potato. Potato disease, bruising, or exposure to light can cause glycoalkaloids to reach levels that can be lethal to humans. Theobromine, present in tea and cocoa powder, has been shown to be genotoxic, to potentiate DNA damage

by various carcinogens in human cells, and to cause testicular atrophy and spermatogenic cell abnormalities in rats. Pyrolizidine alkaloids are present in thousands of plant species (often greater than 1% by weight) and may be ingested by humans in certain herbs and herbal teas and occasionally in honey. These alkaloids have been found to be carcinogenic, mutagenic, and teratogenic. Human consumption of gossypol, found in cottonseed and cottonseed oil, may be significant in countries such as Egypt where fairly crude cottonseed oils (containing 100–750 mg/100 mL gossypol) are commonly used in cooking. Gossypol causes pathologic changes in rat and human testes, abnormal sperm, and male sterility. In fact, it has been investigated and used as a male contraceptive in China. Gossypol-treated male rats who were taken off gossypol and then allowed to mate produced embryos with dominant lethal mutations.

Leguminous plants, such as lupine, also have been found to contain teratogens. Offspring born to cows and goats who forage on these plants may have severe teratogenic abnormalities. The "crooked calf" abnormality, caused by maternal ingestion of anagyrine from lupine, is one such abnormality. Because these teratogens also can be transferred to the animal's milk, drinking the milk from the animal during pregnancy can pose a teratogenic hazard. One report noted that a baby boy, a litter of puppies, and goat kids all had the "crooked" bone birth-defect; the pregnant mother and pregnant dog had been drinking milk from the family goats, which had been foraging on lupine.

The human dietary intake of "nature's pesticides" is likely to be several grams per day—probably 10,000 times higher than the dietary intake of man-made pesticides.[67] However, the significance to the pregnant woman and her fetus is not clear. Not eating certainly is not an alternative, and no human diet can be entirely free of mutagens or carcinogens. The foods discussed above are only representative examples. Clearly, more research is needed in this area so that the pregnant woman can be counseled as to how to most safety meet the nutritional requirements for herself and her growing fetus.

Pesticides. Pesticides have turned out to be another double-edged sword. They protect crops from attack by certain insects, but they also contaminate the environment with a multitude of chemicals, many with long-term and reproductive effects that are not fully known. The Environmental Protection Agency has estimated there may be as many as 1500 different active ingredients in pesticides.[42]

Chlorinated pesticides such as toxaphene, Kepone, and mirex are accumulating in the food chain.[7] Organic chemicals containing chlorine are not used in natural mammalian biochemical processes and may not have been present in the human diet until the advent of the chemical age.[7] Once in the food chain, chlorinated pesticides are not easily eliminated. For example, toxaphene, one of the most widely used chlorinated pesticides, persists for at least several years in soils and lake sediments.[71] In addition, as with other fat-soluble chlorinated hydrocarbons, it contaminates fish. Because toxaphene is such a complex chemical mixture, it is difficult to analyze for it, and little else is known about toxaphene residues in humans and the environment. Some pesticides that have been banned in the United States are still being detected as residue on fruits and vegetables imported from other countries. For example, a 1978 survey by the Food and Drug Administration (FDA) found residues of dichlorodiphenyltrichloroethane (DDT), benzohexachlorophane (BHC), lindane, dieldrin, and heptachlor on coffee beans.[72]

Malathion, parathion, and mipafox are insecticides of the organophosphate class. Their toxic properties are most likely caused by their ability to act as esterase inhibitors in the central and peripheral nervous systems. A study by Duffy et al[73] confirmed the ability of organophosphate compounds to induce persistent abnormalities in the electric activity of the human brain.

The fetus is exposed to insecticides. It has been shown that DDT and other insecticides are transmitted from the mother to the fetus through the placenta.[74] Pesticides also can be excreted in human breast milk.[75] DDT and less widespread pesticides such as dieldrin, heptachlor epoxide (a metabolite of heptachlor), and oxychlordane (a metabolite of chlordane) have been found in breast milk. Regarding DDT, Rogan et al[75] reported that, "It seems reasonable to conclude that such contamination results from ambient rather than specific occupational exposure and that there are no obvious clinical or dietary predictors."

What is the hazard to the embryo–fetus and infant from these pesticides? As is the case with many environmental contaminants, the answer is not known. Some laboratory studies have been conducted. Toxaphene, for example, has been found to be highly mutagenic in the *Salmonella* test.[71] But long-term clinical studies on reproductive capacity have not been carried out, and newborns, who may be more susceptible than adults to toxic effects, have not been studied at all.[75]

Polychlorinated Biphenyls. Polychlorinated biphenyls are a group of chlorinated organic compounds with many industrial applications. They have been most widely used in the electrical industries to produce electric capacitators and transformers, but also have been used in heat exchange systems, hydraulic fluids and lubricants, plasticizers and adhesives, and sealants and printing inks.[76,77]

Past uncontrolled use of PCBs has led to environmental contamination, including contamination of the human food chain. Disposal and leakage of industrial fluids into rivers and coastal waters have been the principle mechanisms of this contamination, although leaks from sealed transformers and heat exchangers, leaks of PCB-containing fluids from hydraulic systems that are only partially sealed, and vaporization from PCB-containing formulates are other possible ways that PCBs get into the environment.[78] The total rate of loss of PCBs into the environment is estimated to have been $1.5–2 \times 10^3$ tons per year into the atmosphere, $4–5 \times 10^3$ tons per year into fresh and coastal waters, and 1.8×10^4 tons per year into dumps and landfills.[78] A significant portion of the population has been exposed. Polychlorinated biphenyl residues were found in approximately 30–40% of tissues analyzed in the early 1970s in one study,[79] and 41–45% of the general population had levels of 1.0 or more parts per million in another study.[66]

Pregnant women can be exposed to residues of PCBs in food in many forms; the original industrial product may be introduced accidently into the food, or the PCBs may have been subjected to other reactions in the food chain.[80] Human ingestion of various forms of PCB can occur as a result of PCB introduction directly to food, as in rice oil; PCB in paperboard may transfer to food; PCB in animal food, then humans eat the animal tissue; PCB contamination of fish, then humans eat the fish; PCB contamination of fish, which is a component of animal food, then humans eat the animal tissue.

In Japan, a direct contamination of rice cooking oil with a commercial brand of PCB resulted in an epidemic of a peculiar skin disease similar to chloracne, later labeled Yusho (oil disease). As described by Kuratsune and associates[81], the concentration of PCB in the oil was 2000–3000 parts per million. On an average, each of the patients consumed about 800 mL of the oil, resulting in an average ingestion of 2 g of PCB. The outcome of maternal ingestion of this contaminated oil during pregnancy was noted in 13 women. Two stillbirths resulted, and most of the live infants had greyish, dark-brown stained skin, while half had similar pigmentations of the gingiva and nails. A number of the fetuses were smaller than the national standards, and four of them were small-for-gestational-age babies. PCBs also were found in the breast milk of mothers with Yusho, and children who were breast fed had higher serum levels than controls.[75] Slight but clinically important neurologic and developmental impairments were noted in some of these children in follow-up studies approximately 9 years later.[75] A number of authors[75,76], however, have warned that findings from the Yusho patients should be interpreted cautiously because the rice oil was contaminated by a PCB mixture that contained other highly toxic impurities. In addition, the kind of exposure Yusho patients had was very different from that usually experienced by the general population.

Because PCBs are highly soluble in fat and tend to collect in the fatty tissues of animals, including humans, they may be bioconcentrated in the food chain. Aquatic invertebrates and fish can accumulate PCB levels between 3×10^3 and 7×10^4 higher than those in ambient water. Thus in the long food chain characteristic of marine systems, the levels in the top predators may be 10^7 times higher than those in the ambient water.[78]

An FDA study in the early 1970s found that PCB migration from cardboard containers and dividers could be another source of PCB contamination in the human diet.[77] Crackers, breadcrumbs, dry infant cereals, macaroni and noodle products, prepared mixes, ready-to-eat breakfast cereals, pretzels, and chips were all found to be a source of PCB because of their packaging. The use of reclaimed or recycled paper in the manufacture of the cardboard packaging material used for these foods was apparently the cause of the PCB contamination.

Contamination of PCB in animal food also may be responsible for human PCB contamination. Apparent misuse of PCB-containing transformer fluid for defoliant spraying operations adjacent to dairy pastures has been responsible for milk contamination.[77] In addition, PCB-contaminated fish meal, a component of poultry and fish food, was responsible for PCB residues in poultry, eggs, and commercially raised catfish.[77]

Fish are the primary dietary source of PCB. The highest concentrations of PCB residues in fresh water fish occur in rivers that are associated with industrialized areas (eg, in the United States the Hudson, Ohio, and Allegheny rivers.[82]

Polychlorinated biphenyls also have been found in human breast milk[75], and transfer of PCBs to the newborn by way of breast milk may be more important than placental transfer. For certain fat-soluble chemicals such as PCB, nursing infants are regarded as living at the top of the food chain. They are exposed to much more than background levels of the chemical. In Michigan, a major industrial state, environmental contamination by PCBs has been widely reported. Of 1057 breast-milk samples tested in Michigan during 1977 and 1978, PCB residues were detected in all, varying from trace amounts to 5.100 parts per million (fat weight basis).[76] The mean PCB level was 1.496 parts per million (standard deviation 0.796 parts per million); the median PCB level was 1.354 parts per million. Of these, 49.5% had PCB residues of 1 to 2 parts per million, 17.4% had 2–3 parts per million, and 6.14% had more than 3 parts per million. The PCB residues in four samples exceeded 4 parts per million. The FDA's present tolerance limit of PCBs in dairy products is 1.50 parts per million (fat weight basis); therefore, half of the breast milk samples in this study contained only slightly less than the FDA's present tolerance limit.[76]

On the basis of the data from the Michigan study, a theoretical infant weighing 8.97 kilograms at 8 months (50th percentile of weight for age growth), whose mother had a breast milk concentration of PCBs equal to the mean value of 1.496 parts per million would have an estimated body burden of PCBs of 0.89 parts per million. For the entire group of infants born to women in the study population, approximately 35% would have a body burden of 1 or more parts per million of PCBs at age 9 months.[76] Although no illnesses occurring in breast-fed children have been attributed to population levels of PCBs[83], the long-term health implications on infantile growth and development are currently unknown.

The benefits of breast-feeding, whether nutritional, immunologic, or emotional, are well recognized; however, in light of reports of breast-milk contamination, some physicians and patients may question the advisability of breast feeding. Although testing unselected mothers has not been proposed in the United States as a whole, the state of Wisconsin and the Canadian Ministry of Health have considered testing the milk of mothers who have a potentially high exposure to PCBs or whose breast-fed infants are ill. Canada has adopted an advisory level of 0.050 parts per million on a whole-milk basis, and Wisconsin has adopted an advisory level of 2.5 parts per million on a fat basis. However, the clinical usefulness of such testing seems minimal because laboratory analysis can take up to 6 weeks. In addition, the clinical importance of the advisory level is only conjectural because there are no directly applicable human studies.[75]

Until more is known about the risks of PCB-contaminated human breast milk, some[76,84] feel that it is premature to recommend any major changes in breast-feeding practices. A policy statement from the American Academy of Pediatrics recommends breast-feeding and mentions testing for PCBs only in women who have eaten large amounts of sport fish or who have been occupationally exposed. As a precaution, however, it is recommended that pregnant women and nursing mothers reduce or eliminate consumption of fish from PCB-contaminated waters.[75,84] In addition, they should be advised to avoid excessive weight reduction, because this may mobilize chemicals stored in their fat tissue.

For mothers who have potentially high exposure to PCBs and still choose to breast-feed, a determination of fat content and of the level of PCBs in their breast milk may help them decide the length of time they will breast-feed their infant. PCB body burden accumulates over time, and estimates of PCB body burden accumulating in the infant suggest that reducing the duration of breast-feeding from 12 months to 6 months could reduce the accumulation of infant PCB body burden by as much as 30%.[76] This would provide the infant with the benefits of breast-feeding and still reduce the potential risk of PCBs being transmitted to the infant through the breast milk.

Polybrominated Biphenyls. Polybrominated biphenyls (PBBs) are bromine analogues of PCBs. In 1973 and 1974, several thousand Michigan dairy farms were contaminated with PBBs when they were packed in bags mistakenly identified as a component of cattle feed.[85] Adverse effects on human pregnancy were not reported, although contamination of meat, milk, and eggs was demonstrated[86] along with an increased incidence of stillbirth among cattle that had consumed the contaminated feed.[85] As could be expected from the fact that PBBs are fat soluble organohalides like PCB and DDT, a 1976 survey of nursing mothers in the lower peninsula of Michigan showed that PBB residues were present in 96% of breast milk.[85] In the dose range demonstrated in the Michigan incident, no short-term toxicity to the breast-fed infant was detected.[82] Long-term implications are unknown.

It should also be noted that although routes of PBB contamination to humans have virtually been cut off except for a few designated farm areas where the soil is contaminated, the contaminated mothers are still a source to the fetus and newborns through the placenta and lactation. The only significant route of excretion of PBBs from the body is in the accompaniment of fat. Thus for practical purposes, PBBs only escape through the milk or through the placenta to the fetus. Consequently, a mother whose contamination level of PBB was rather high after the initial incidence and who chose not to breast feed her infant for that reason can pose the same potential risk to subsequent infants if her depot fats are mobilized.

REFERENCES

1. Mattison DR, Nightingale MS, Shironmizu K. Effects of toxic substances on female reproduction. *Environ Health Perspect.* 1983;48:43.
2. Pries C. Reproductive effects of occupational exposures. *Am Family Physician.* 1981;24:161.
3. Simpson JL, Golbus MS, Martin AO, et al. Principles of human embryology and teratogenesis. In: *Genetics in Obstetrics and Gynecology.* New York, NY: Grune & Stratton; 1982;202.
4. Iannaccone PM, Bossert NL, Connelly CS. Disruption of embryonic and fetal development due to preimplantation chemical insults: A critical review. *Am J Obstet Gynecol.* 1987;157:476.
5. Pernoll ML. Abortion induced by chemicals encountered in the environment. *Clin Obstet Gynecol.* 1986;29:953.
6. Simpson JL, Golbus MS, Martin AO, et al. Viruses and infectious agents. In *Genetics in Obstetrics and Gynecology.* New York, NY: Grune & Stratton; 1982;228.
7. Ames BN. Identifying environmental chemicals causing mutations and cancer. *Science.* 1979;204:589.
8. Fanghanel J, Schumacher GH. Environmental effects on normogenesis and teratogenesis, with special regard to noise and vibration. In: Persaud TVN, ed. *Advances in the Study of Birth Defects, Teratological Testing.* Baltimore, MD: University Park Press; 1979;2:325.
9. Hemminki K, Kyyronen P, Niemi ML, et al. Spontaneous abortion in an industrialized community in Finland. *Am J Publ Health.* 1983;73:32.
10. Longo DL. The biological effects of carbon monoxide on the pregnant woman, fetus, and newborn. *Am J Obstet Gynecol.* 1977;129:69.
11. Remmer H. Passively inhaled tobacco smoke: A challenge to toxicology and preventive medicine. *Arch Toxicol.* 1987;61:89.
12. Haddow JE, Knight GJ, et al. Second-trimester serum cotinine levels in nonsmokers in relation to birth weight. *Am J Obstet Gynecol.* 1988;159:481.
13. Alderman BW, Baron AE, Savitz DA. Maternal exposure to neighborhood carbon monoxide and risk of low infant birth weight. *Publ Health Reports.* 1987;102:410.
14. Cameron RG. Should air hostesses continue flight duty during the first trimester of pregnancy? *Aerospace Med.* 1973;44:552.
15. Jennings RT. Women and the hazardous environment: When the pregnant patient requires hyperbaric oxygen therapy. *Aviat Space Environ.* 1987;58:370.
16. Moore LG, Hershey DW, Jahnigen D, et al. The incidence of pregnancy-induced hypertension is increased among Colorado residents at high altitude. *Am J Obstet Gynecol.* 1982;144:423.
17. Moore LG, Jahnigen D, Rounds SS, et al. Maternal hyperventilation helps preserve arterial oxygenation during high-altitude pregnancy. *J Appl Physiol Respir Environ Exercise Physiol.* 1982;52:690.
18. Moore LG, Rounds SS, Jahnigen D, et al. Infant birth weight is related to maternal arterial oxygenation at high altitude. *J Appl Physiol Respir Environ Exercise Physiol.* 1982;52:695.
19. Bolton ME. Scuba diving and fetal well-being. A survey of 208 women. *Undersea Biomed Res.* 1980;7:183.
20. Fisher NL, Smith DW. Occipital encephalocele and early gestational hyperthermia. *Pediatrics.* 1981;68:480.
21. Harvey MAS, McRorie MM, Smith DW. Suggested limits to the use of the hot tub and sauna by pregnant women. *Can Med Assoc J.* 1981;125:50.
22. Dickman DM. Noise and its effect on human health and welfare. *Ear Nose Throat J.* 1977;56:61.
23. Welch BL. Physiological effects of noise: An overview. *Fed Proc.* 1973;32:2091.
24. Zondek B, Tamari I. Effect of audiogenic stimulation on genital function and reproduction. *Am J Obstet Gynecol.* 1960;80:1041.
25. Kimmel CA, Cook RO, Staples RE. Teratogenic potential of noise in mice and rats. *Toxicol Appl Pharmacol.* 1976;36:239.
26. Szmeja Z, Slomko Z, Sikorski K, et al. The risk of hearing impairment in children from mothers exposed to noise during pregnancy. *Int J Pediatr Otorhinolaryngol.* 1979;1:221.
27. Geber WF. Inhibition of fetal osteogenesis by maternal noise stress. *Fed Proc.* 1973;32:2101.
28. Ishii H, Yokobori K. Experimental studies on teratogenic activity of noise stimulation. *Gunma J Med Sci.* 1960;9:153.
29. Siegel MI, Smookler HH. Fluctuating dental asymmetry and audiogenic stress. *Growth.* 1973;37:35.
30. Jones FN, Tauscher J. Residence under an airport landing pattern as a factor in teratism. *Arch Environ Health.* 1978;33:10.
31. Ando Y, Hattori H. Statistical studies on the effects of intense noise during human life. *J Sound Vibration.* 1973;27:101.
32. Dwornicka B, Jasineske A, Smolarz W, et al. Attempt of determining the fetal reaction to acoustic stimulation. *Acta Otolaryngol.* 1964;57:571.
33. *Pregnancy, Work, and Disability.* Chicago, IL: American College of Obstetricians and Gynecologists; Tech Bull. No 58: 1980.
34. Brix K. Environmental and occupational hazards to the fetus. *J Reprod.* 1982;7:557.
35. Koren H. Occupational environment. In: *Handbook of Environmental Health and Safety.* New York, NY: Pergamon Press; 1980:263.
36. The American College of Obstetricians and Gynecologists. *Guidelines on Pregnancy and Work.* Chicago, IL: United States Department of Health, Education, and Welfare; 1977.
37. Horstmann DM. Viral infections. In: Burrow GN, Ferris TF, eds. *Medical Complications During Pregnancy.* 2nd ed. Philadelphia, PA: W.B. Saunders; 1982:333.
38. Naeye RL, Peters EC. Working during pregnancy: Effects on the fetus. *Pediatrics.* 1982;69:724.
39. McDonald AD, McDonald JC, et al. Prematurity and work in pregnancy, *Br J Indust Med.* 1988;45:56.
40. McDonald AD, McDonald JC, et al. Fetal death and work in pregnancy. *Br J Indust Med.* 1988;45:148.
41. Hemminki K. Occupational chemicals tested for teratogenicity. *Arch Occup Environ Health.* 1980;47:191.
42. Haugh T. Chemicals: How many are there? *Science.* 1978;199:162.
43. Heinrichs WL. Reproductive hazards of the workplace and the home. *Clin Obstet Gynecol.* 1983;26:429.
44. Tsuchiya H, Mitani K, Kodama K, et al. Placental transfer of heavy metals in normal pregnant Japanese women. *Arch Environ Health.* 1984;39:11.
45. Brodsky JB. Anesthesia and surgery during early pregnancy and fetal outcome. *Clin Obstet Gynecol.* 1983;26:449.
46. Brodsky JB, Cohen EN. Occupational exposure to anesthetic gases and pregnancy. *Dent Assist.* 1981;50:20.
47. Corbett TH, Cornell RG, Endres JL, et al. Effects of low concentrations of nitrous oxide on rat pregnancy. *Anesthesiology.* 1973;39:299.
48. Vieira E, Cleaton-Jones P, Austin JC, et al. Effects of low concentrations of nitrous oxide on rat fetuses. *Anesth Analg (Cleve).* 1980;59:175.
49. Bruce DL. Murine fertility unaffected by traces of halothane. *Anesthesiology.* 1973;38:473.
50. Coate WB, Kapp RW, Lewis TR. Chronic exposure to low concentrations of halothane-nitrous oxide. *Anesthesiology.* 1979;50:310.
51. Ad Hoc Committee on the Effect of Trace Anesthetics on the Health of Operating Room Personnel, American Society of Anesthesiologists. Occupational disease among operating room personnel: A national study. *Anesthesiology.* 1974;41:321.
52. Cohen EN, Bellville JW, Brown BW. Anesthesia, pregnancy, and miscarriage: A study of operating room nurses and anesthetists. *Anesthesiology.* 1971;35:343.
53. Corbett TH, Cornell RG, Endres JL, et al. Birth defects among children of nurse-anesthetists. *Anesthesiology.* 1974;41:341.
54. Knill-Jones RP, Moir DD, Rodriques LV, et al. Anesthetic practice and pregnancy: Controlled survey of women anaesthetists in the United Kingdom. *Lancet.* 1972;1:1326.
55. Cohen EN, Brown BW, Wu ML, et al. Occupational disease in dentistry and chronic exposure to trace anesthetic gases. *J Am Dent Assoc.* 1980;101:21.
56. Ericson A, Kallen B. Survey of infants born in 1973 or 1975 to Swedish women working in operating rooms during their pregnancy. *Anesth Analg (Cleve).* 1979;58:302.

57. Infante PF, McMichael AJ, Wagoner JK, et al. Genetic risks of vinyl chloride. *Lancet*. 1976;1:734.
58. Cai SX, Bao YS. Placental transfer, secretion into mother's milk of carbon disulphide and the effects on maternal function of female ciscose rayon workers. *Indust Health*. 1981;19:15.
59. Holmberg PC. Central-nervous-system defects in children born to mothers exposed to organic solvents during pregnancy. *Lancet*. 1979;2:177.
60. Cordero JF, Oakley GP Jr. Drug exposure during pregnancy: Some epidemiologic considerations. *Clin Obstet Gynecol*. 1983;26:418.
61. Bagnell P, Ellenberger H. Obstructive jaundice due to a chlorinated hydrocarbon in breast milk. *Can Med Assoc J*. 1977;117:1047.
62. Check W. New study shows hexachlorophene is teratogenic in humans. *JAMA*. 1978;240:513.
63. Longo LD. Environmental pollution and pregnancy: Risks and uncertainties for the fetus and infant. *Am J Obstet Gynecol*. 1980;137:162.
64. Smith J. EPA halts most use of herbicide 2,4,5-T. *Science*. 1979;203:1090.
65. Browder AA, Joselow M, Lauria D. The problem of lead poisoning. *Medicine*. 1973;52:121.
66. Price HA, Welch RL. Occurrence of PCBs in humans. *Environ Health Perspect*. 1972;1:73.
67. Ames BN. Dietary carcinogens and anticarcinogen. *Science*. 1983; 221:1256.
68. Linn S, Schoenbaum SC, Monson RR, et al. No association between coffee consumption and adverse outcomes of pregnancy. *N Engl J Med*. 1982;306:141.
69. Rosenberg L, Mitchell AA, Shapiro S, et al. Selected birth defects in relation to caffeine-containing beverages. JAMA. 1982;247:1429.
70. Lawrence R. *Breast-Feeding, A Guide for the Medicial Profession*. St. Louis, MO: CV Mosby; 1980:167.
71. Hooper NK, Ames BN, Saleh MA, et al. Toxaphene, a complex mixture of polychloroterpenes and a major insecticide, is mutagenic. *Science*. 1979;205:591.
72. Smith RJ. U.S. beginning to act on banned pesticides. *Science*. 1979;204:1391.
73. Duffy FH, Burchfield JL, Bartels PH, et al. Long-term effects of an organophosphate upon the human electroencephalogram. *Toxicol Appl Pharmacol*. 1979;47:161.
74. Bakken A, Seip M. Insecticides in human breast milk. *Acta Paediatr Scand*. 1976;65:535.
75. Rogan WJ, Bagniewska A, Damstra T. Pollutants in breast milk. *N Engl J Med*. 1980;302:1450.
76. Wickizer TM, Brilliant LB, Copeland R, et al. Polychlorinated biphenyl contamination of nursing mothers' milk in Michigan. *Am J Publ Health*. 1981;71:132.
77. Kolbye AC Jr. Food exposures to polychlorinated biphenyl. *Environ Health Perspect*. 1972;1:85.
78. Nisbet ICT, Sarofim AF. Rates and routes of transport of PCBs in the environment. *Environ Health Perspect*. 1972;1:21.
79. Yobs AR. Levels of polychlorinated biphenyls in adipose tissue of the general population of the nation. *Environ Health Perspect*. 1972;1:79.
80. Cook JW. Some chemical aspects of polychlorinated biphenyls (PCBs). *Environ Health Perspect*. 1972;1:3.
81. Kuratsune M, Yoshimura T, Matsuzaka J, et al. Epidemiologic study on yusho, a poisoning caused by ingestion of rice oil contaminated with commercial brand of polychlorinated biphenyls. *Environ Health Perspect*. 1972;1:119.
82. Stelling DL, Mayer FL. Toxicities of PCBs on fish and environmental residues. *Environ Health Perspect*. 1972;1:1159.
83. Rogan W, Gladen B. Monitoring breast milk contamination to detect hazards from waste disposal. *Environ Health Perspect*. 1983;48:87.
84. Miller R. PCBs and cola-colored babies. *J Pediatr*. 1977;90:510.
85. Brilliant LB, Van Amburg G, Isbister J, et al. Breast milk monitoring to measure Michigan's contamination with polybrominated biphenyls. *Lancet*. 1978;2:643.
86. Finberg L. PBBs: The ladies' milk is not for burning. *J Pediatr*. 1977;90:511.

Chapter Eleven

Effects of Pregnancy on Work Performance[a]

American Medical Association Council on Scientific Affairs[b]

11

Amended Resolution 126 (A-80) of the House of Delegates, "Professional Awareness of Reproductive Hazards to Pregnant Workers," urged the American Medical Association to heighten awareness of physicians about circumstances associated with the reproductive health of workers and to familiarize them with the *Guidelines on Pregnancy and Work*, published by the American College of Obstetricians and Gynecologists (ACOG). The adopted resolution was referred through the Board of Trustees to the AMA Council on Scientific Affairs.

The Council appointed an Advisory Panel on Reproductive Hazards in the Workplace to prepare a report. The panel recommended, with Council concurrence, that the report should consider all phases of the reproductive cycle including male and female fertility, mutagenicity, teratogenicity, fetotoxicity, and postnatal effects. The task was divided into three projects, namely: (1) Effects of Physical Forces on the Reproductive Cycle; (2) Effects of Toxic Chemicals on the Reproductive Cycle; and (3) Effects of Pregnancy on Work Performance.

The following report on the "Effects of Pregnancy on Work Performance" should be a useful guide to physicians. Suggestions are offered regarding safe and healthful job placement for the patient and her conceptus during the various stages of pregnancy.

WHAT WE KNOW VERSUS WHAT WE THINK WE KNOW

The impact of pregnancy on a worker's ability to perform her job has only recently become an area considered suitable for scientific inquiry. The advice given by generations of physicians regarding work during normal pregnancy has historically been more the result of social and cultural beliefs

[a] Reprinted from *Journal of the American Medical Association* 1984;251:1995, with permission.

[b] Members of the Council on Scientific Affairs include the following: John R. Beljan, M.D., Dayton, OH; George M. Bohigian, M.D., St. Louis; Theodore Cooper, M.D., Kalamazoo, MI; William D. Dolan, M.D., Arlington, VA, Past Chairman; Ira R. Friedlander, M.D., Chicago, Resident Physician; Ray W. Gifford, Jr., M.D., Cleveland, Chairman; Michael B. Kastan, St. Louis, Medical Student; John H. Moxley III, M.D., Beverly Hills, CA, Vice Chairman; Joseph H. Skom, M.D., Chicago; Rogers J. Smith, M.D., Portland, OR; James B. Snow, Jr., M.D., Philadelphia; C. John Tupper, M.D., CA; and Richard J. Jones, M.D., Chicago, Secretary; with the assistance of Jermyn F. McCahan, M.D. The Advisory Panel includes the following: Marcus B. Bond, M.D., Ernest M. Dixon, M.D.; Palmer C. Evans, M.D.; Bruce W. Karrh, M.D.; Martin L. Pernoll, M.D., Chairman; Richard T. F. Schmidt, M.D., Council Liaison Member; James H. Spraul, M.D.; John R. Venable, M.D.; and Jermyn F. McCahan, M.D., Secretary.

about the nature of pregnancy (and of pregnant women) than the result of any documented medical experience with pregnancy and work.[1] In attempting to review the available literature on the effect of gestation on ability to work, it is impressive to realize how few of our standard medical beliefs about the physical and emotional characteristics of pregnancy have any scientific basis.

Progress is being made, however. Researchers are now presenting results of work examining the emotional and physical impact of pregnancy on women.[2] To our knowledge, no specific studies have been reported applying these fledgling data to women in the work force. In assessing the relationship between pregnancy and work, therefore, it is essential to guard against accepting the traditional standard assumptions about pregnancy as fact. Culturally influenced beliefs about pregnancy, even though they may be supported empirically by physician experience, must be identified as the "softest" of data when one is formulating a protocol of medical advice.

THE STAGES OF PREGNANCY AND THEIR IMPACT ON ABILITY TO WORK

In our culture, certain symptoms are accepted as characteristic of early pregnancy—including nausea and emotional lability—and physicians expect women to exhibit such symptoms.[1,2] There are very little scientific data, however, to validate the frequency of such symptoms, or even their occurrence.

In reviewing literature, Lips[2] found that some early research seemed to document a generalized lack of psychological well-being among pregnant women, but researchers failed to distinguish between complaints attributable to the physical changes of pregnancy and psychosomatic symptoms suggestive of emotional disturbance. Other studies sought enumeration of negative aspects of the effects of pregnancy on well-being while failing to consider positive effects. Some research yields little conclusive information because of the lack of comparison with nonpregnant controls.

The way in which normative data from a comparison group can place a finding about pregnant women in proper perspective is illustrated by responses in their study to a question asking women whether they felt they were going to have a nervous breakdown. Twenty-four percent of the pregnant sample gave positive responses—a proportion that, the authors note, seems "alarming until one notes that 57% of the nonpregnant sample in the current study expressed the identical concern."[3]

It is important to realize that interpretation of day-to-day empirical experience with pregnancy symptoms may be similarly skewed—would we see equal amounts of fatigue, emotional lability, or digestive complaints in nonpregnant women if we looked for them?

In fact, the study by Lips that compared pregnant women with controls and enabled the enumeration of positive as well as negative effects of pregnancy on perceptions of well-being showed that the responses of women in the first 5 months of pregnancy differ very little from those of men and nonpregnant women. The two areas of response substantially altered by pregnancy were fairly predictable: pregnant women scored higher in indices of "feeling ill" and "feeling overweight." In spite of their more frequent reporting of "feeling ill," however, expectant women reported the least impact of their physical condition on their performance of any of the four groups studied (expectant women, prospective fathers, and nonexpectant women and men). Both partners of expecting couples expressed fewer "negative emotional state" responses than did nonexpectant couples. If conclusions are to be drawn from this work, then we would have to say that pregnancy has very little effect on perceived well-being.

It is through research such as this that we will begin to amass a scientific basis for our advice on pregnancy and working. In addition to subjective work such as that by Lips, it will be important to evaluate objectively the alteration of physical capabilities (if any) in early pregnancy by means of ergonomic testing and oxygen consumption testing along with other tests. Compilation by industry of figures on the actual frequency of absences and the need for altered working conditions because of symptoms would be most helpful. (At least two large industries are beginning to compile such data.)

It must be specified that in any discussion of the effect of pregnancy on women and working, generalizations are made for "normal" and uncomplicated pregnancies only. Complications that impinge on the health and well-being of the mother and/or fetus would, of course, require substantially different management than for healthy pregnant women.

Late Normal Pregnancy (from Six Months to Delivery)

Our culture also provides, for physicians and laymen alike, expectations of the physical and emotional condition of women in later pregnancy. The woman with swollen ankles who is exhausted and having trouble sleeping embodies our stereotype of the norm for this phase of gestation. Again, however, we have no data to measure how many women experience late pregnancy symptoms such as these and how many of the women who do experience them find their work substantially affected. (Lips's work is ongoing and should yield some useful data in the future.)

Certainly, some credence may be given to the reliability of data informally amassed by physicians in years of clinical practice. Few obstetricians would dispute the assertion that women in the final trimester of pregnancy seem to tire more easily than their nonpregnant co-workers. Nor would many deny that a shift in posture to counterbalance a growing abdomen may predispose a woman to backache. The crucial point, however, is that the extent to which such symptoms necessitate alteration in work activity is variable at best and presently completely unquantified. At this time, we are probably wise to undergeneralize by adapting the recommendations of the National Institute for Occupational Safety and Health (NIOSH) and the ACOG *Guidelines on Pregnancy and Work* to each woman based on individual demands and capabilities.[4] Only when we have satisfactory data on the physical capabilities of women in this phase of pregnancy will we be able to speak authoritatively about the capabilities of pregnant women as a group.

The Postpartum Period

As with pregnancy itself, our ability to speak knowledgeably about postpartum ability to work is badly hampered by lack of scientific data. Research—physical and psychological, laboratory and clinical, prospective and retrospective—is badly needed. The "magic" 6 weeks currently designated as the postpartum period may be no more reasonable when rationally evaluated than would 10 weeks or two.

Work During Pregnancy

The determination that a pregnant employee can or cannot perform a particular job should be made on a case-by-case basis. The determination is dependent on the types of activities and tasks the job requires, the general physical condition of the employee, and the length of gestation. For most industrial jobs that require lifting, standing, walking, or climbing, physical problems associated with balance secondary to posture and alteration of the center of gravity are important in determining suitable job placement.[5-7]

The pregnant employee should be able, in most cases, to continue productive work until the onset of labor.[8] Substantial complications of pregnancy, such as preeclampsia, premature rupture of the membranes, vaginal bleeding, or threatened abortion, require consideration on an individual basis and may be disabling for further work until after delivery.

Some medical conditions are severely compromised by pregnancy. Others predispose the pregnant patient to an increased likelihood of complications of the pregnancy. These medical conditions are not totally disabling by themselves, nor is a pregnant patient disabled because she has one or more of these conditions. However, patients with the following conditions must be carefully evaluated to determine if they should continue to work during the pregnancy or if it may be best to leave the job until after the delivery.[9]

1. Those who have been delivered of two premature infants weighing less than 2000 g.
2. Those with incompetent cervices and histories of previous fetal losses or cervical cerclage.
3. Those with uterine anomalies who have lost a fetus.
4. Those with cardiac status greater than Class II, which affects the ability to tolerate the massive increase in cardiac output and blood volume imposed by pregnancy.
5. Those with Marfan's syndrome.
6. Those with hemoglobinopathies, including thalassemia.
7. Those with pulmonary hypertension or arterial hypertension.
8. Those with retinopathy greater than Stage I, renal changes with abnormal creatinine clearance, preeclampsia, or polyhydramnios.
9. Those with herpes gestationis if discomfort is great.
10. Those with severe anemia—8 g/dL of hemoglobin or less.

Table 11–1 shows the period of time that healthy employees with normal uncomplicated pregnancies should be able to perform specific tasks without undue difficulty or risk to the pregnancy. It should not be interpreted to mean that all pregnant employees need stop these activities at the exact time of gestation noted but should be used as a guide to evaluate each case. An employee's job may require strenuous activity, such as lifting, and the anatomic changes of pregnancy make performing these tasks difficult. If the employee is not disabled for another type of work, placement on an alternative lighter job assignment until the employee becomes unable to work may be appropriate.

TABLE 11–1. GUIDELINES FOR THE TERMINATION OF VARIOUS LEVELS OF WORK DURING A NORMAL, UNCOMPLICATED PREGNANCY[a]

Job Function	Week of Gestation
Secretarial and light clerical	40
Professional and managerial	40
Sitting with light tasks	
Prolonged (>4 h)	40
Intermittent	40
Standing	
Prolonged (>4 h)	24
Intermittent	
(>30 min/h)	32
(<30 min/h)	40
Stooping and bending below knee level	
Repetitive	
(>10 times/h)	20
(<2 times/h)	40
Climbing	
Vertical ladders and poles	
Repetitive	
(≥4 times/8-h shift)	20
Intermittent	
(<4 times/8-h shift)	28
Stairs	
Repetitive	
(≥4 times/8-h shift)	28
Intermittent	
(<4 times/8-h shift)	40
Lifting	
Repetitive	
>23 kg	20
<23, >11 kg	24
<11 kg	40
Intermittent	
>23 kg	30
<14, >11 kg	40
>11 kg	40

[a] The report contained in the booklet is not intended to be construed or to serve as a standard of medical care. Standards of medical care are determined on the basis of all of the facts and circumstances involved in an individual case and are subject to change as scientific knowledge and technology advance and patterns of practice evolve. This report reflects the views of scientific literature as of September 1988.

Modified from Informational Report of the Council on Scientific Affairs, December, 1988 (1–88) Book II. Presented by George M. Bohigian, M.D., Chairman.

RECOMMENDATIONS

The Council on Scientific Affairs recommends that the American Medical Association:

1. Continue to endorse the *Guidelines on Pregnancy and Work* from ACOG and NIOSH, recognizing that they were prepared prior to The Pregnancy Discrimination Act (Pub L No. 95-555).
2. Continue to encourage, sponsor, and participate in research to document the physical and emotional impact of pregnancy on women and their ability to work. An interdisciplinary study group composed of occupational medicine, obstetrician/gynecologist, and pediatric physicians, representatives of industry and the various sciences—psychology, toxicology, or epidemiology—working together, could vastly expand our ability to understand pregnancy as it affects ability to work.
3. Encourage physicians to remain aware of the potential discrepancies between cultural beliefs, myths, and taboos about pregnancy and scientific data.
4. Remind physicians of the ever-present need to adapt recommendations on pregnancy, like all general guidelines, to each pregnant woman individually.

REFERENCES

1. Gries MR. Overcoming male myths and taboos. *Occup Health Safety.* 1981;50:58.
2. Lips HM. Somatic and emotional aspects of the normal pregnancy experience: The first five months. *Am J Obstet Gynecol.* 1982;142:524.
3. Barclay RI, Barclay ML. Aspects of the normal psychology of pregnancy: The mid-trimester. *Am J Obstet Gynecol.* 1976;125:207.
4. American College of Obstetricians and Gynecologists, National Institute for Occupational Safety and Health. *Guidelines on Pregnancy and Work.* Washington, Department of Health, Education, and Welfare, 1978.
5. Kuntz WD. Pregnant working women: What advice should you give them? *Contemp Obstet Gynecol.* 1980;15:69.
6. American College of Obstetricians and Gynecologists. *Pregnancy, Work and Disability, Technical Bulletin 58.* Chicago, American College of Obstetricians and Gynecologists Publications, 1980.
7. Lerner S. As quoted in Is she or isn't she? *Occup Health Safety.* 1976;May, June:27.
8. Jimenez MH, Newton N. Activity and work during pregnancy and the postpartum period: A cross-cultural study of 202 societies. *Am J. Obstet Gynecol.* 1979;135:171.
9. Carney P (moderator). Working in pregnancy: How long? How hard? What's your role? *Contemp Obstet Gynecol.* 1980;16:154.

Chapter Twelve

Medicolegal Aspects of Obstetric Care

Stephen A. Myers

12

The moral, ethical, and legal dilemmas that have emerged during the later half of this century concerning the topic of fetal rights could occupy volumes. These issues are as complex as they are numerous. Moreover, as continued technology and scientific advances turn medical science fiction into medical fact, that ability of society to adjust is often overwhelmed. Adding to this difficult situation is burgeoning medical liability. The physician caring for a pregnant patient and her fetus not only has the well-being of two patients to keep in mind, but also must continually balance concerns for the needs of each. The physician is always aware that a wrong step may not only result in an undesirable medical outcome, but in an adverse legal one as well. Detailed descriptions of the law and its relationship to the mother–fetus dyad are beyond the scope of this chapter. Several texts are available; an excellent text is *Obstetrics/Gynecology and the Law,* by Keith Feenberg (Health Administration President, 1984). This chapter will instead concentrate on some of the more important legal issues related to the care of the pregnant patient and her fetus. Other related issues are discussed in Chapter 18.

TORT LAW AND MEDICAL MALPRACTICE

Prenatal Injury

Although a fetus is not defined as a person by the US Constitution, as a result of the Supreme Court's decision in *Roe v Wade*[1], a fetus may be considered a person for the purposes of state law, particularly the law of torts. Tort law involves a civil wrong for which courts will provide a remedy in the form of an action for damages. Historically, the law of torts did not consider or recognize the fetus as an independently protectable being and therefore did not award compensation for prenatal injuries. Gradually, however, courts explicitly held that a child could recover damages for injuries inflicted before birth or during delivery.

Today, if a child is born alive, every state allows an action for the consequences of prenatal injuries.[2] Thus, if a physician negligently prescribes a drug to a pregnant woman carrying a viable fetus and the child is consequently born with serious defects, all jurisdictions permit the child to bring a lawsuit against the physician. Negligence on the part of the physician during delivery, which result in injury to the child, is another familiar example of tort liability for prenatal harm.

A growing number of courts now recognize tort liability suits on behalf of the child injured by harm that occurred before conception.[3,4] Such notable cases involve negligence that causes rhesus isoimmunization when the "damaged" individual did not even exist at the time of the negligent act. A case has even been brought against seven liquor companies, alleging that children were born with fetal alcohol syndrome as a result of failure by the companies to warn against the dangers of drinking during pregnancy.[5]

Such recognition of a tort duty to unborn children does not necessarily establish that, for all legal purposes, any and every fetus is a person under the law. Courts and legal commentators often characterize the tort law with respect to prenatal injuries as a reflection of a child's right to be born with sound mind and body rather than as a broad validation of fetal personhood.[6-8]

Wrongful Death

Under the tort law, if a person negligently or intentionally causes the death of another person, the estate or beneficiaries of the deceased person may sue the tortfeasor, the wrongdoer who caused the death, for damages under wrongful death statutes. In the case of the death of a child, most states permit the beneficiaries in a wrongful death lawsuit to recover economic damages as well as nonpecuniary damages for loss of the child's society (the loss of the comfort and companionship of children). All jurisdictions permit wrongful death damage suits when a child born alive subsequently dies as a result of negligently inflicted injuries received *in utero.* In the case of a stillborn fetus, resulting from injuries received *in utero,* states differ over whether a stillborn fetus is a person within the meaning of the state's wrongful death statutes. Unlike the case of a liveborn child injured before birth, cases of stillbirth directly raise the question of legal status of the fetus as a person under state tort law. Consequently, it is a contradiction that a tortfeasor may be awarded for killing, rather than maiming, a fetus. This, arguably, could create incentive to withhold maximal efforts to save the life of a fetus.

Wrongful Life and Wrongful Birth Suits

If a child is born in a defective condition as result of negligent action of a physician or genetic counselor, some courts have recognized the concept of *wrongful life* by granting suits on behalf of the infant. Also, many courts allow a *wrongful birth* suit on behalf of the infant's parents.

Tort liability may pertain if a physician negligently fails to diagnose prenatal defects in a timely manner or fails to warn about the effects of maternal disease or exposure to toxins on the developing fetus. Because of the advances in the ability to screen for and detect genetic and birth defects and potentially harmful conditions in the fetus through genetic counseling, ultrasonography, maternal alpha fetoprotein screening, amniocentesis, and chorionic villus sampling,[8] the expansion of wrongful birth liability related to prenatal diagnosis of defects, is troublesome. Until now, most wrongful birth actions related to the actual birth process or associated care.

The theory behind wrongful birth claims assumes that, had the mother been warned of the risks to her fetus sooner, she would have terminated the pregnancy. Many states have, however, refused to allow damages for the missed opportunity to abort a fetus. While a wrongful birth claim may be brought by parents in a majority of jurisdictions, only a few states permit a wrongful life claim on behalf of the child. In a wrongful life suit, the parent or guardian brings suit on behalf of the handicapped child and asserts that the child's condition is so bad that he or she should never have been born. For the most part, courts have reasoned that human existence is preferable to nonexistence.[9]

Maternal and Parental Conflicts with the Fetus

An emerging question in law and medicine concerns the extent to which the law will protect or compensate a fetus whose life or health is harmed by the mothers prenatal conduct. For example, a mother who must undergo a cesarean delivery to prevent the death or grave injury of a viable fetus refuses surgery on religious grounds. In another situation, a mother with phenylketonuria refuses the special diet that is vitally necessary during pregnancy to prevent brain damage to the fetus. In a final example, physicians detect a blocked urinary tract in a 23-week-old fetus and inform the mother that surgery to the fetus is necessary to improve the survival of the fetus, but the mother denies consent. As new techniques increase the ability to treat and prevent abnormalities of the fetus,[10] physicians and lawyers must confront situations in which pregnant women, who intend to deliver, refuse necessary treatment. In a 1987 study, based on a national survey of heads of maternal–fetal medicine fellowship programs, we conclude that sharp division in the obstetric community over court-ordered procedures exists.

The issues of maternal–fetal conflicts are complex and involve a number of areas of law. Detailed legal reviews on the emerging rights of the fetus are available from Lenow[11] and Shaw.[12] Although no definitive direction in the law has yet arisen, more courts and legislatures are willing to recognize a specific interest of the fetus, particularly of the viable fetus. This interest needs to be balanced with the health and privacy interests of the mother and family. For example, the Court of Appeals for the District of Columbia has noted that in cases involving unborn children, the state's interest in preserving the fetus's health may directly oppose the woman's interest of bodily integrity. In that case, the court concluded that a cesarean section would not significantly affect the woman's condition and that the child had a chance of surviving delivery.[13]

Similarly, in another case, an appellate court in Washington, DC, vacated and remanded a lower court decision ordering cesarean delivery in a woman with terminal cancer at 27 weeks' gestation. The woman died within days of surgery and the premature infant succumbed to the effects of extreme prematurity. Although decided years after the event, the court went out of its way to say that its decision was valid. This decision should not be seen as the court's interpretation that maternal right of privacy should prevail; instead, the decision should be viewed as an attempt to establish more rigid guidelines for such court-ordered interventions.[14]

Other courts have reached similar conclusions in cases in which a woman refused to consent to medical treatment deemed necessary to the health of the fetus. According to one study, court-ordered cesareans have been obtained in 11 states, hospital detentions in two states, and intrauterine transfusions in one state.[13] In a California case that drew widespread publicity, the district attorney's office brought child abuse charges against a woman whose son was born brain dead, allegedly as a result of maternal drug abuse. The charges were ultimately dropped, but the use of child abuse statutes may receive more attention in the future.[15]

The emergence of duties to protect the fetus from harm and abuse raises a number of ethical and legal issues, including a woman's right to have an abortion. Nearly all of the cases justifying forced medical treatment or tort liability of the mother have involved a viable fetus. The judicial readiness to impose a duty to refrain from harming a viable fetus appears consistent with the Supreme Court's holding in *Roe v. Wade* that the state has an interest in the potential life of the fetus.

If the fetus is not viable, however, it may be argued that because a woman has the right to abort her fetus, she may not be compelled to consent to any medical treatment aimed at benefiting her unborn child. This presumes that viability is an important and controlling aspect. Such a theory can in large measure only be proposed because the Supreme Court in *Roe v Wade* chose to place such importance on the viability standard. Recognizing the right to terminate a pregnancy does not, however, automatically require the recognition that pregnant women have a right to inflict physical damage on the fetus and bear children with devastating handicaps.

A common clinical dilemma often arises for women who are close to delivering severely premature infants for whom survival may not be certain. The patient's expectation for such a premature infant clearly will affect her decision about intensity of prenatal care given to her pregnancy. Issues related to documentation of the patient's decision about consent for operative intervention, the role of fetal monitoring, and obligations relating to resuscitation recently have been reviewed.[16] Fetuses with a chance for intermediate viability require yet other considerations and may allow some latitude in the decision-making process. These concepts are summarized in Table 12–1.

Probably the most complex medicolegal problem relates to the balance between a mother's rights to autonomy and privacy (as well as the father's and family's rights) and the interests of the fetus to be born and to be born without handicaps. This issue may, in part, have arisen from an overly broad interpretation of abortion rights and the presumed interests of the state.[17] Chervenak and McCullough have characterized these conflicts into four groups:[18] (1) conflicts between maternal autonomy-based obligations of physician and maternal beneficence-based obligations of physician; (2) conflicts between fetal beneficence-based obligations of mother and fetal beneficence-based obligations of physician; (3) conflicts between maternal autonomy-based obligations of physician and fetal beneficence-based obligations of physician; and (4) conflicts between maternal

TABLE 12–1. HOSPITAL GUIDELINES FOR FETAL VIABILITY ASSESSMENT AND POSTDECISION RESPONSIBILITIES BEFORE, DURING, AND AFTER DELIVERY

	Best Obstetric Estimate of Gestational Age		
	Less than 22 Wks (under 500 g)	**22 1/7 to 23 6/7 Wks (500–700 g)**	**24 Wks and Older (over 700 g)**
Viability assessment	Previable (<10% survival)	Intermediate viability (borderline 20–40% survive)	Viable (>50% survival)
Chart documentation of all data with specific numbers	Yes	Yes	Yes
Patient's acknowledgment of receiving above information	Yes	Yes	Yes
If patient declines operative intervention for fetal distress	Declining is appropriate	Declining may be appropriate	Consider contacting clergy, hospital administration, family, legal
Fetal monitoring	Unnecessary	Optional	Necessary
Nonsurgical Rx for fetal distress	Unnecessary	Recommended	Necessary
Result: Resuscitation			
Stillborn	N/A	Pediatric staff in attendance/appropriate resuscitation	N/A
Liveborn	Pediatric staff in attendance/appropriate resuscitation	N/A	Pediatric staff in attendance

Modified from Myers.[16]

beneficence-based obligations of physician and fetal beneficence-based obligations of physician. Even with clear identification of all issues in an individual case, however, there is often no clear resolution. Competing obligations appear to have equal weight.

Categorical opposition to the recognition of fetal rights and a refusal to balance maternal-parental interests with fetal–state interests minimizes the importance of the growing legal recognition of fetal interests and rights of children to avoid prenatal harm. Consequently, a physician or hospital who acquiesces to a mother's decision, which results in harm to her fetus, may face a legal liability situation if the child is born injured. In a recent survey of heads of fellowship programs in maternal–fetal medicine, 26 of 57 (46%) believed that mothers who refused medical advice and thereby endangered the life of the fetus should be detained in hospitals or other facilities so that compliance could be ensured.[19] This study may have implications for the generally applicable standard of care. Some authorities have suggested that maternal liberty is primary. A similar opinion recently was expressed by the court. One must remember, however, that liberties are not absolute. For example, people may be drafted into war or may have to undergo vaccination against diseases even though the vaccination may have obvious risks.

From the physician's perspective, the issues are principally medical: How significant is the risk to the fetus of a mother's action or inaction? Will treatment to assist the fetus pose material risk to the mother? When the potential for serious harm to the fetus is significant and treatment or therapy does not involve undue burdens on the mother's health or freedom, health care providers must consider whether court intervention is warranted. Bowes and Selgestad[20] suggest that institutions should develop a plan on how to face such situations *before* they occur. In 1983, federal legislation, initiated by the *"Baby Doe"* case, mandated the formation of hospital ethics committees to deal with these issues. The committees were to be composed of a mixture of lay and professional personnel from a variety of disciplines. Currently, however, such committees function at different levels at different institutions, without uniform approach or guidelines. Moreover, the interests of the patient or the patient's family seem disproportionately small when confronted by a large number of diverse interests. Many of these complex issues have been addressed by the American College of Obstetricians and Gynecologists.[21] Table 12–2 outlines an approach that provides organization while remaining flexible. It emphasizes that clear solutions are rarely achieved, while reiterating that the interests of the fetus should only rarely override a patient's own autonomy.[22] Each case must be evaluated and handled on a individual basis.

In view of new reproductive technologies, potential rights of human embryos pose additional legal, moral, and ethical challenges. Noncoital reproductive techniques, such as *in vitro* fertilization, artificial insemination by donor, embryo transfer, surrogate motherhood, and frozen embryo technology raise a wide array of related, but distinct, legal and ethical questions regarding fetal rights. Similarly, fetal experimentation and the use of fetal tissue for organ donation have been controversial issues, subject to strict federal and state regulations.

TABLE 12–2. GUIDELINES FOR ETHICAL DECISION MAKING

Identify decision makers
Collect data, establish facts
Identify options
Evaluate options according to values and principles involved
Identify conflicts and set priorities
Select options that can *best* be justified
Re-evaluate the decision after it is acted on

From ACOG.[21]

A person's feelings about the legal rights of a fetus depend to a large degree on nonmedical issues, such as personal moral beliefs and religious considerations. To create a more objective approach, given the legal recognition of brain death as the end of human existence, Gertler has suggested that human "personhood" should be equated with brain birth.[23] Such an approach focuses on points at which the fetus exhibits the capacity to feel pain or, later, possesses the capacity for conscious thought. This would represent a developmental continuum of rights and would move from viability as the principal reference point. For now, however, the issue remains unsettled.

REFERENCES

1. *Roe v Wade,* 410 vs 113, (1973).
2. Collins EF. An overview and analysis: Prenatal torts, preconception torts, wrongful life, wrongful death, and wrongful birth: Time for a new framework. *J Fam L.* 1984;22:68.
3. *Curlender v Bio-Science Laboratories,* 106 Cal. App. 3d 811, 165 Cal Rptr. 477 (1980).
4. *Renslow v Mennonite Hosp,* 67 Ill. 2d 348, 367 N.E. 2d 1250 (1977).
5. Moss DC. Parents sue liquor companies, cite lack of warnings about fetal alcohol syndrome. *ABAJ.* 1988;17.
6. *Grodin v Grodin,* 102 Mich. App. 396, 301 N.W. 2d 869 (1981).
7. *Smith v Brennan,* 31 N.J. 353, 157 A.2d 497 (1960).
8. Elias S, Annas G. *Reproductive Genetics and the Law.* Chicago, IL: Yearbook Publishers; 1987;253.
9. *Berman v Allen,* 80 N.J. 421, 404 A. 2d 8 (1979).
10. Callahan P. How technology is framing the abortion debate. *Hastings Cent Rep.* 1986;33.
11. Lenow JL. The fetus as a patient: emerging rights as a person? *Am J Law Medicine.* 1983;9:1.
12. Shaw MW. Conditional prospective rights of the fetus. *J Legal Med.* 1984;5:63.
13. In re A.C., 533 A. 2d 611 (D.C. 1987).
14. In re, A.C., 87-609 (App. D.C., April 26, 1990) (Lex15116).
15. Fetal abuse isn't a crime; court dismisses charges against a mother who ignored doctor's orders. *ABAJ.* 1987;37:150.
16. Myers SA. Hospital guidelines for fetal viability assessment and post-decision responsibilities. *Mt. Sinai J Med.* 1987;54:191.
17. Fletcher JC. The fetus as a patient: ethical issues. *JAMA.* 1981;772.
18. Chervenak FA, McCullough LB. Perinatal ethics: A practical method of analysis of obligations to mother and fetus. *Obstet Gynecol.* 1985;66:442.
19. Kolder E, Gallagher J, Parsons MT. Court-ordered obstetrical interventions. *N Engl J Med.* 1987;1192:316.
20. Bowes WA Jr, Selgestad D. Fetal versus maternal rights: medical and legal prospectives. *Obstet Gynecol.* 1982;58:209.
21. American College of Obstetricians and Gynecologistis. *Ethical Decision Making in Obstetrics and Gynecology.* Washington, DC: ACOG Technical Bulletin 136;1989.
22. American College of Obstetricians and Gynecologists. *Patient Choice: Maternal–Fetal Conflicts.* Washington, DC: ACOG Committee Opinion 55; 1989.
23. Gertler GB. Brain Birth: A proposal for defining when a fetus is entitled to human life status. *S Cal L Rev.* 1986;59:1061.

PART II Genetic Considerations Before and During Pregnancy

Gloria E. Sarto, Section Editor

Chapter Thirteen

General Genetics Principles: Chromosomal, Mendelian, and Principles of Teratology

Renata Laxova and Paula F. Feldman

13

When an attempt is made, before conception to determine whether a future pregnancy is at risk for an unfavorable outcome, many factors must be considered by family and physician. The potential for an unfavorable outcome may not be suspected until suddenly, during the course of the pregnancy, abnormalities are detected.

Pregnancies at known risk for an unfavorable outcome before conception include those associated with a risk for *cytogenetic abnormality,* those associated with a disorder caused by a *single gene* or a combination of genes and environmental factors (*multifactorially determined disorders*), and those at risk associated with *environmental exposure* to potentially hazardous agents.

PRINCIPLES OF CYTOGENETICS

According to Hsu[1], human cytogenetics has undergone four evolutionary stages: the *dark ages* before 1952, the *hypotonic period* from 1952–58 (the battle for clearer preparations), the *trisomy period* from 1959–69, and the *chromosome banding era* that started in 1970. A fifth stage should now be added, the *molecular period.*

Chromosomes, within a cell's nucleus, are the package that carries genetic information. One chromosome is a long molecule of deoxyribonucleic acid (DNA) and specific proteins associated with it, condensed into the nucleus. It is estimated that DNA within a cell is 2 m long. The nucleus can be as small as one hundred thousandth of a meter. Hence, unless prepared with specific techniques, the chromosomes are not usually visible within the nucleus.

The cell also contains a *nucleolus,* composed of ribonucleic acid (RNA) and protein. It is the site of ribosome production and is found in a specific region of the short arms of the five pairs of acrocentric (see below) chromosomes. It is called the nucleolar organizer region (NOR) and has been suspected of being associated with the incidence of nondisjunctional events.

Each nucleated human cell contains 46 chromosomes, divided into 23 pairs, 22 of which are called autosomes (each member of a pair is *like* the other). Each pair is numbered from 1 through 22, from longest to shortest. The 23rd pair is the hetero (different) or sex chromosomes, containing two X chromosomes in females and one X and one Y chromosome in males (Fig. 13–1). One of each pair of chromosomes is transmitted to the zygote through the sperm and one through the egg. Hence, exactly one half of our genetic information is inherited from each parent.

The presence of an X and Y or two X chromosomes (ie, the indication of sex) is the only characteristic that distinguishes one human karyotype from another. Our chromosomes appear similar even with sophisticated banding techniques. The genetic information, however, is identical only in identical twins. Because there are two chromosomes in each of 23 pairs and only one of these is transmitted from each of two parents, the number of possible combinations for any individual person is $2^{23} \times 2^{23}$. Furthermore, crossing over (recombination) can occur during pairing of homologous chromosomes in meiosis and adds to the amount of variation.

Chromosomes are most frequently analyzed in blood from short-term (72 hours) lymphocyte cultures, in bone marrow (immediate or 24-hour preparation) from skin fibroblasts in long-term (3–4 weeks) tissue cultures, and from

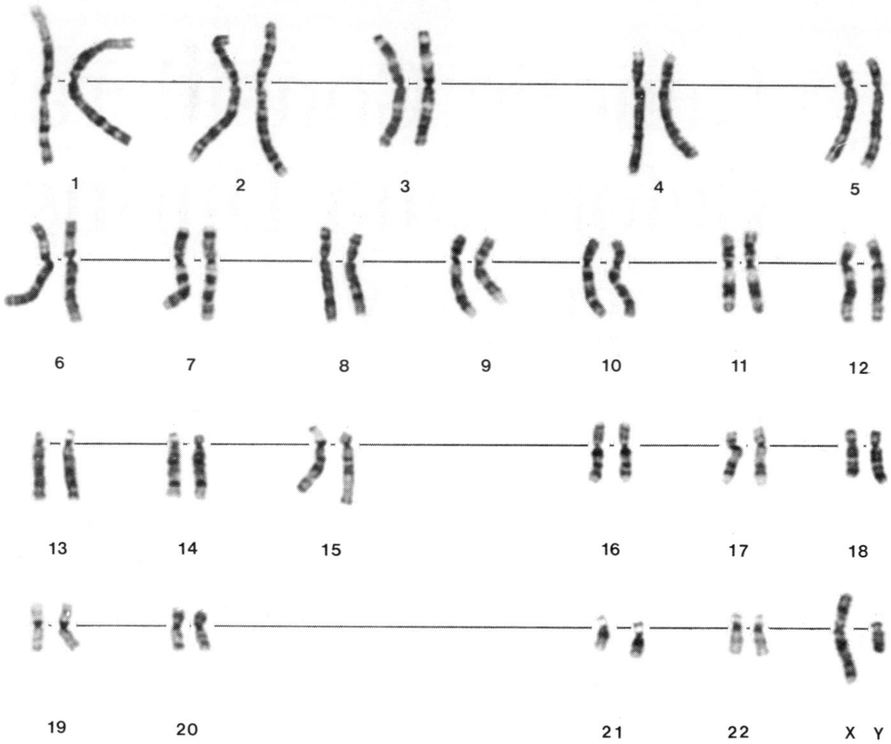

Figure 13–1. Normal male karyotype in metaphase.

amniotic fluid cells or chorionic villi. Cytogenetic analysis also can be performed theoretically on any nucleated cell, including tumors and gonads. The most frequent indication for chromosome analysis is for diagnostic purposes in a patient (or relative of a patient) or for prenatal diagnosis in a fetus; hence, in practice, peripheral lymphocyte and amniocyte or chorionic villus cultures exceed other analyses.

Karyotype

A *karyotype* is a carefully analyzed, photographic document of the paired chromosomes in one typical cell. While most cells of a referred patient are analyzed under the microscope, one to two karyotypes per patient are usually prepared in most laboratories (see Fig. 13–1 and Fig. 13–2). Standard banding techniques using G (Giemsa) or Q (quinacrine mustard, which highlights similar regions but uses fluorescence), R (reverse—the light and dark bands are a mirror image of those in G or Q banding), C (centromere), or T (telomere) banding reveal about 420 bands on chromosomes analyzed in mitotic metaphase. If mitosis is stopped in prometaphase when the chromosomes are less condensed, as many as 1200 or 2000 bands can be seen (Fig. 13–3). It is interesting to note that G/Q and R bands are not only visual opposites (a dark G band stains lightly with R banding and vice versa), but also appear to have opposite molecular functions (Table 13–1). It has recently been observed[2] that the enzyme family Alu, which recognizes short interspersed repeated DNA sequences on the chromosome, predominates in R bands. Long interspersed repeated DNA sequences, on the other hand, which are recognized by the enzyme family LI, predominate in G/Q bands. This is a first attempt to explain chromosome banding on a molecular basis and has far reaching implications.

Mitosis

The *transmission* of genetic information occurs through two types of cell division, *mitosis* and *meiosis*. Mitosis or somatic cell division applies to the fertilized ovum and to all other cells to which it gives rise during development and during the life of the organism. The principle of mitosis is simple: It consists of one replication of each of the 46 chromosomes and one cell division. Two daughter cells are formed with 46 chromosomes (23 pairs) containing identical genetic information to that in the parent cell. The process begins in interphase, continues through actual mitosis (in four phases), and ends by division of the cytoplasm, called cytokinesis.

The *interphase* cycle of cell division consists of the G1 (first gap), S (synthesis), and G2 (second gap) phases. Before division, during the S phase, the DNA double helix of each chromosome replicates to form two identical chromatids, each containing a double DNA strand and thus identical genetic information; they are linked to each other at a point called the centromere. Actual mitosis takes place in four stages. In *prophase*, the two sister chromatids are very close to each other, and they are long. As the chromatids begin to contract, a bipolar spindle is formed and the nuclear membrane begins to fragment. This occurs before metaphase, in *prometaphase*. Because the chromatids are not yet condensed, both prophase and prometaphase are useful for "high resolution analysis." Greater detail (see Fig. 13–3) is seen than in *metaphase* when the chromatids are exactly halfway through division. They align halfway between the poles of the cell and are easily visible by light microscopy, each as two distinct chromatids. Homologous chromosomes do not associate in any specific way during mitosis. As the sister chromatids separate at the centromere, one of each pair of chromatids moves to opposite poles of the cell. This is called *anaphase*. If, by chance both chroma-

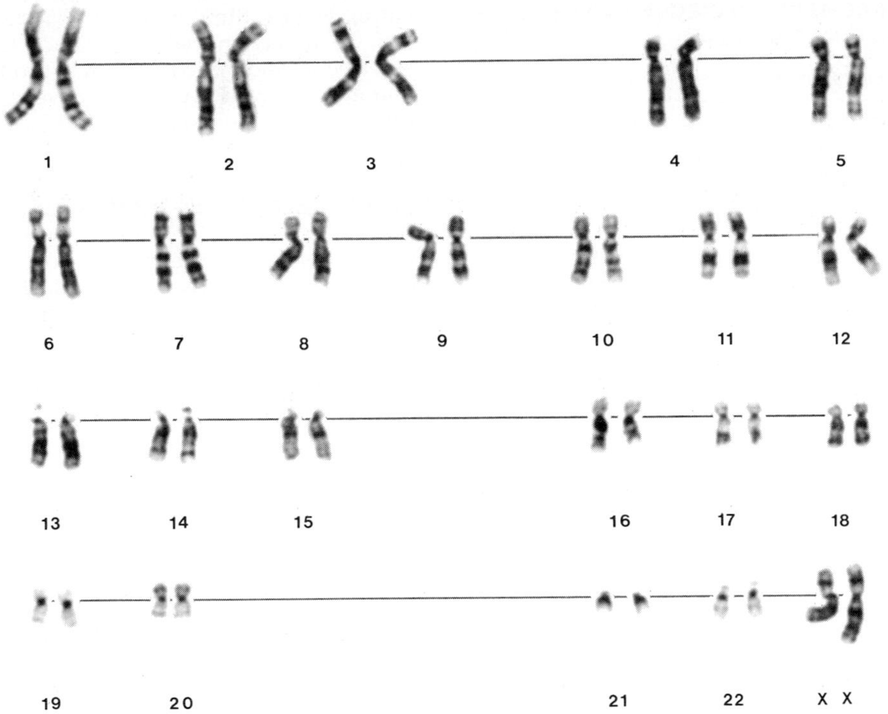

Figure 13–2. Normal female karyotype in metaphase.

tids of a pair move to the same pole of the cell, then the subsequent daughter cell will have one too many chromosomes. This is a very important phenomenon called *mitotic nondisjunction* (nonseparation) and provides the explanation for some types of chromosomal abnormalities and for *mosaicism*. If, on the other hand, a chromatid is left behind during anaphase, the daughter cell will have one missing chromosome, known as *anaphase lag*. During the final phase of mitosis proper, *telophase*, the chromatids stretch out again or decondense, and the nucleus begins to surround them. The whole process is completed by the division of the cytoplasm called *cytokinesis*, and two new daughter cells with identical genetic information to that in the parent cell are formed. Each has 23 pairs of chromosomes (46 chromosomes), and for that reason, these cells are called *diploid*.

Meiosis

The gametes are the only cells in the organism that contain only 23 chromosomes, one of each pair. They are called *haploid*. If the zygote were to receive a whole set, namely 46 chromosomes for each gamete, the next generation would have 92 chromosomes. In understanding the concept of *meiosis*, or *reductive cell division*, it is helpful to remember that our ancestors and our descendants all had, and will have, 46 chromosomes. Meiosis enables the reduction of the number of chromosomes to the haploid number of 23

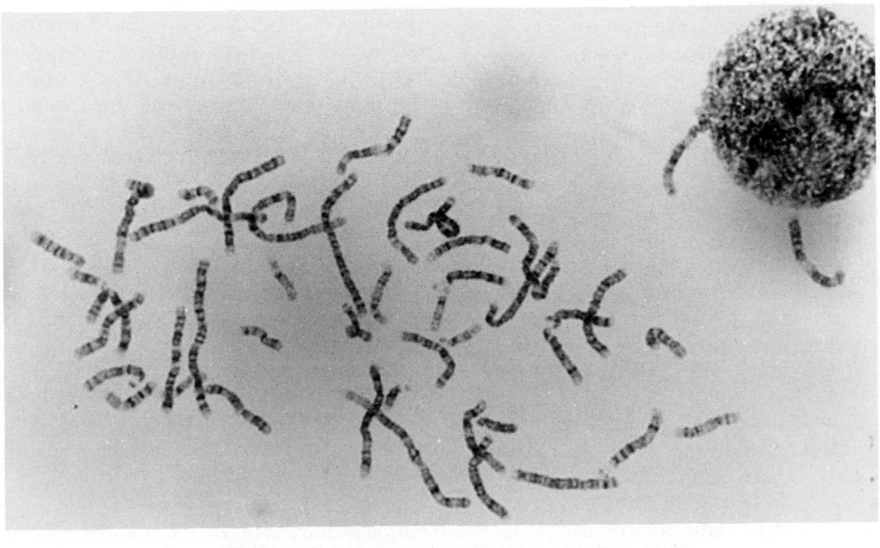

Figure 13–3. Normal karyotype in prometaphase.

TABLE 13–1. DIFFERENCE BETWEEN GIEMSA AND REVERSE BANDING AT THE MOLECULAR LEVEL

	G/Q Bands	R Bands
Rich in	Adenine thymine (AT)	Guanine cytosine (GC)
Replicate	Late in DNA synthesis	Early
Condense	Early during mitosis	Late
Reflect	Meiotic chromomere pattern	—
Gene expression	Poor in expressed genes	Rich in active genes

Adapted from Korenberg.[2]

and enables the recombination of genes through a phenomenon called *crossing over* between homologous chromosomes. Meiosis results in the transmission of exactly one half of our genetic information from each parent. There are two main reduction divisions, called *meiosis I* and *meiosis II.* Each is characterized by the same four phases as those that take place in mitosis, prophase I (subdivided into five stages), metaphase I, anaphase I, telophase I, cytokinesis, prophase II, metaphase II, and so forth.

Meiosis also begins in S phase when each chromosome replicates to form two identical chromatids that are very close together and appear as one during prophase. The first stage of *prophase I* is called *leptotene,* during which the chromosomes have condensed to such an extent that they are visible. In *zygotene,* homologous chromosomes pair up and align precisely, probably according to homology of the DNA nucleotide sequences, and are linked by a protein structure attached to the nuclear envelope called the synaptonemal complex. Once this is complete, the process continues through *pachytene,* the stage during which crossing over of genetic material from one chromatid to another of a homologous pair of chromosomes occurs. As the chromosome pair moves apart, in *diplotene,* it also begins to decondense. In the last stage of prophase I, the chromosomes recondense, and each of the four chromatids in each pair is visible. This is called *diakinesis.* The locations at which chromatids from homologous chromosomes (not sister chromatids) have crossed over, are called *chiasmata,* and these are visible as prophase I proceeds into *metaphase I.* The chromosomes pair up exactly and as they move apart, and chiasmata become apparent; they are the points of overlap chromatids and are important for the exchange of genetic material, called crossing over or recombination. They are, in a slightly hyperbolic sense, responsible for evolution. In *anaphase I* sister chromatids remain attached at the centromere. *Telophase I,* followed by *cytokinesis* or cytoplasmic division, is characterized by only one set of chromosomes, the haploid number of 23 in each of the two new resulting cells. *Meiosis II* resembles mitosis but is applied to 23 instead of 46 chromosomes. However, after telophase II and cytokinesis II, the result is four cells (meiosis II begins with two cells), each with a single set of chromosomes, one of each pair, corresponding to one of the four chromatids that were aligned so closely in the zygotene stage of prophase I.

The difference in oogenesis and spermatogenesis, which results in the respective gametes, is discussed elsewhere. Important differences, however, include the following. In females, only one of the four meiotic division products develops into a mature oocyte. The oocyte transmits inherited characteristics outside the nucleus called mitochondria or mRNA (see section on mitochondrial inheritance). Hence, the possibility of additional, nonchromosomal, or mitochondrial inheritance (mitochondropathies), must be considered. In the male, on the other hand, all four meiotic division products develop into mature spermocytes.

CHROMOSOME ABNORMALITIES

Chromosome abnormalities are not uncommon. They occur in about 30% of early spontaneously aborted pregnancies (trisomy 16, monosomy X, and triploidy are the most common) and in 5.6% to 6% of stillborn infants (20 weeks or older);[3] this is confirmed by findings among 800 infants evaluated by the Wisconsin Stillbirth Service Project in 1990. Even among the 0.6% liveborn infants with chromosome abnormalities, those with trisomy 13 and 18 rarely survive beyond the first weeks or months of life.

Chromosome abnormalities can be divided into those that affect the number and those that affect the structure of chromosomes.

Numeric Abnormalities

Numeric abnormalities result in a change in the total number of chromosomes per cell. They account for a little more than one half of the 0.6% of chromosome abnormalities in live births.

Trisomy. The most frequent numeric abnormality is trisomy, in which three copies of a given chromosome exist instead of two, resulting in a total of 47 chromosomes per cell. For example, trisomy 21 means that there are three #21 chromosomes in the cells. It is written as 47,XX or XY, +21.

The most frequent cause of trisomy is a phenomenon known as *nondisjunction;* instead of the separation of a pair of chromatids to opposite poles of the cell during anaphase, they migrate to the same pole. This occurs in maternal meiosis I and II and paternal meiosis I and II, in decreasing order of frequency. Approximately 20% of additional chromosomes resulting from nondisjunctional events are of paternal origin.[4] They are usually present in offspring of younger parents, as opposed to maternal nondisjunction, which tends to occur more frequently (but not always) during gametogenesis of women older than 35 years (the maternal age effect). The most frequent complete (i.e., involving a whole additional chromosome) autosomal trisomies in liveborn infants are trisomy 21, 18, and 13, respectively. Trisomy 16 and other rarer autosomal trisomies are infrequently seen in spontaneous abortions but never in liveborns. The most frequent sex chromosomal trisomies are 47,XXY, 47,XXX, and 47,XYY, respectively, all occurring in about 1 in 1000 live births.

Monosomy. Monosomy means that only one of a given chromosome pair is present instead of two. The only monosomy known in humans that is compatible with life is monosomy X, or Turner's syndrome. It is written as 45,X. Even in this unique situation, the majority of conceptions with a missing X chromosome are aborted spontaneously, under rather specific circumstances, while 2% to 4% are liveborn with the characteristic clinical picture and life expectancy of Turner's syndrome.

Partial Monosomy or Trisomy. Partial monosomy and partial trisomy are more common. They usually involve loss or gain of a short "p," or less frequently a long "q," arm of a chromosome. For example, a male patient with additional material from the short arms of chromosome 9 may have a characteristic phenotype, and his chromosome complement would be written 46,XY, 9p+. (*Note:* If a whole additional chromosome is present or missing the + or − sign is written *before* the number of the chromosome in question; eg, 47,XX +13). If a partial abnormality is present, the sign is written *after* the chromosome number and arm designation (eg, 46,XY, 5p−; missing portion of short arm of 5). The nomenclature that describes a specific abnormality of a portion of the chromosome uses the banding patterns. Prominent bands, called regions, are numbered consecutively starting from the centromere up on the short arm (p) down on the long arm (q). Smaller bands within the larger ones are numbered similarly. Thus, if the terminal band of the long arm of chromosome #14 is missing, the designation would be 46,XX or XY, 14q32.3− (Fig. 13–4).

Triploidy (Tetraploidy). Triploidy and tetraploidy (69 or 92 chromosomes per cell) rarely exist in viable humans, and they exist in mosaic form only. Triploidy, however, is one of the three most common findings in spontaneous abortions (along with trisomy 16 and monosomy X), and the fetus (like that with monosomy X) is relatively easy to recognize clinically (Fig. 13–5). Triploidy is sometimes associated with a hydatidiform mole or molar pregnancy. It may arise as the result of one of four phenomena, which include a tetraploid spermatogonium or oogonium, an error in first or second meiotic division, or a result of dispermy (fertilization with two spermatozoa). Recently, uniparental disomy also has been implicated in the origin of triploidy.

Mosaicism. Nondisjunction also can occur postmitotically and result in *mosaicism*. This means that at least two cell lines are present: the original one, derived from the zygote, and the second, derived after the nondisjunctional event. The degree of mosaicism depends on the percentage of cells and the number of tissues in which it is present. It may be written as follows: 46,XY (50%)/47,XY +21 (50%). If less than 20–25% of cells in all tissues available for karyo-

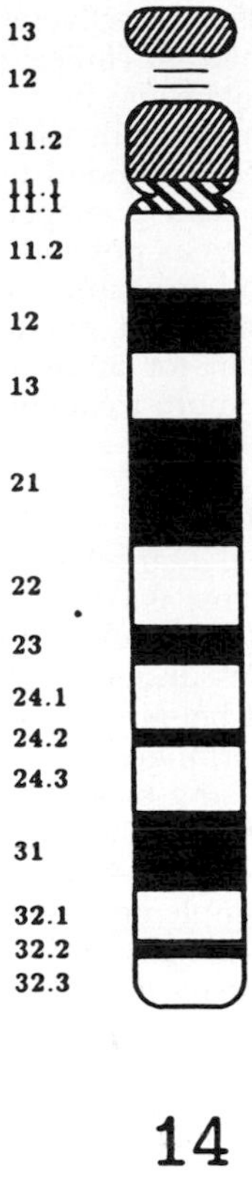

Figure 13–4. Diagram of Giemsa-banded chromosome #14.

typing have the abnormal cell line, mosaicism probably will be insignificant for the phenotype. For example, in a newborn male infant, an amniocentesis culture revealed 85% of cells with a karyotype of 46,XY, and the remaining 15% were 47,XY +21. His blood was tested, and a chromosome complement of 46,XY and 47,XY +21 was found in

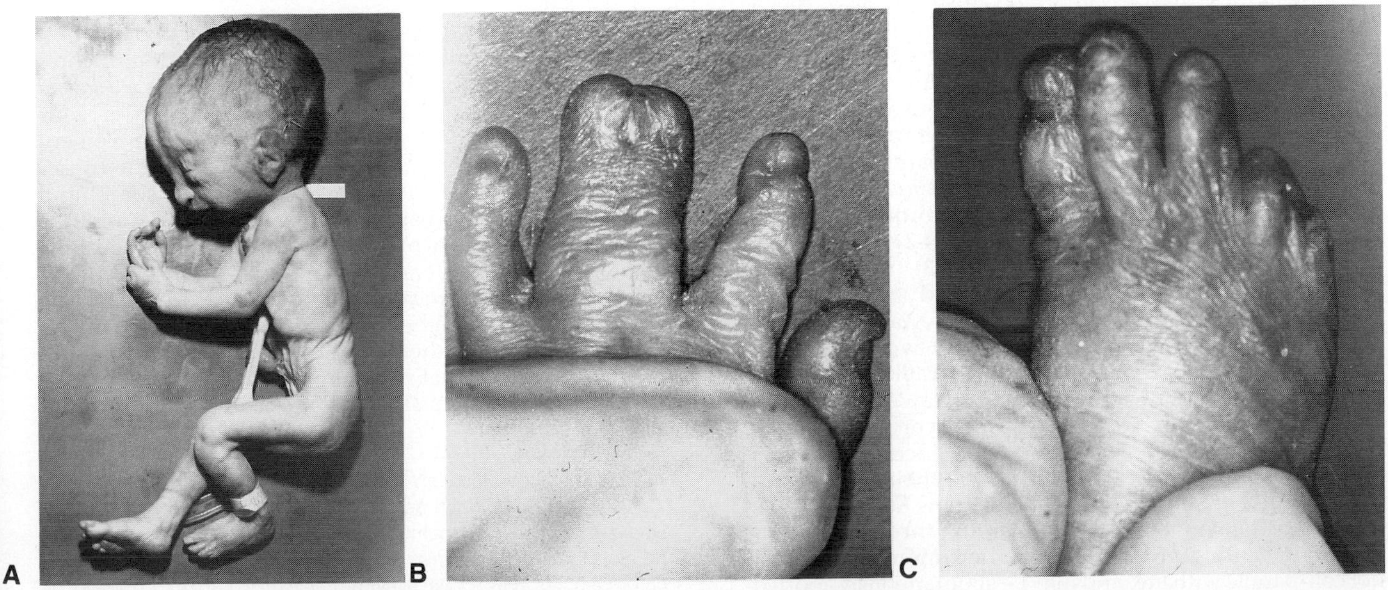

Figure 13–5. Twenty-one week fetus with 69,XXY. (*A*) Abnormal profile, mandibular micrognathia, microphthalmia. (*B*) Hand—hypoplastic nails, 3,4 syndactyly. (*C*) Foot—hypoplastic nails, short syndactylous fourth and fifth toes.

95 and 5% of his cells, respectively. At 4 years, he was developing well and had no clinical signs of Down's syndrome. It is possible that he may be at risk, during reproduction, for having an infant with trisomy 21, and prenatal diagnosis would be recommended for him and his future wife. Whenever mosaicism is suspected, it is essential to evaluate as many tissues as possible because it is the predominant cell line, and probably the tissues in which it occurs that are clinically and phenotypically significant. Chromosome mosaicism for autosomal trisomies is relatively rare; it is much more frequent in sex chromosomal abnormalities.

Structural Abnormalities

Structural chromosomal rearrangements, which occur in about 1 in 500 live births, is one of the most challenging situations facing genetic counselors attempting to help families and their physicians understand what has happened. The concept that must be stressed is that no matter what the arrangement or rearrangement of chromosomal material, none must be missing or additionally present for an individual to be *un*affected. There must be a complete set of the material of 46 chromosomes within the cells; that is, the chromosomal complement must be *balanced.* If material is missing or additionally present, the chromosomal complement will be *unbalanced,* and will result in phenotypic effects. The second difficult issue is that the opposite does not apply. While an individual with abnormal amounts of chromosomal material will almost always be affected, someone with completely normal chromosomes will not necessarily be genetically perfectly healthy and normal. The latter will not have the abnormality caused by an imbalance in chromosomal material, but by no means will all (in fact very few) pathologic processes be detectable through a structural abnormality of the chromosomes.

There are two basic types of translocations: robertsonian and reciprocal. Each can be either inherited (familial) or occur *de novo* for the first time in an individual.

Robertsonian Translocations. Robertsonian translocations result in the centric fusion (with usually one centromere or two, with one inactivated) of two whole, most frequently acrocentric, #13, 14, 15, 21, or 22 chromosomes. The most common of these are 13/14 and 14/21, respectively. A robertsonian translocation may be *balanced,* with no phenotypic or clinical effects except risks associated with the birth of an infant during reproduction with an unbalanced karyotype. It also may be *unbalanced,* in which case trisomy or monosomy of one of the fused chromosomes usually results. It can be seen from Figure 13–6 that if a parent is a healthy (eg, 14/21) translocation carrier, then *theoretically* six possible types of gametes and zygotes can be formed. They are normal (see Fig. 13–6, #1), balanced 14/21 translocation carrier (like parent) (#2), trisomy 21 (#3), monosomy 21 (#4), trisomy 14 (#5), and monosomy 14 (#6). Of these, the first three instances can result in a viable infant, of which two will be normal, and one will have Down's syndrome from an unbalanced 14/21) translocation. (*Note:* phenotypically, patients with this type of Down's syndrome, while microscopically different, are like every other patient with Down's syndrome caused by the effects of an additional chromosome #21. In other words, their disorder also is caused by trisomy 21, which happens to have arisen through a translocation). The remaining three gametes resulting in monosomy 21, trisomy, and monosomy 14 are not compatible with life, and may be spontaneously aborted. Hence, the risk for a parent who is a balanced 14/21 translocation carrier[a] is theoretically 50% for a viable infant (one third of which, about 16%, could result in Down's syndrome) and 50% spontaneous miscarriage. The couple's risk for having a Down's syndrome child (since that is the only viable possibility for an affected child) is theoretically 33% that if the child goes to term, he or she will have Down's syndrome.

The practical situation is, fortunately, very different from what would be expected from segregation analysis. Statistical studies have shown more favorable empirical risks. If the parental carrier is the mother, her risk for translocation Down's syndrome in her offspring is about 11%; if the carrier is the father, his risk is around 2.4%.[5]

Similar situations apply to other robertsonian translocations (eg, 13/14), in which the chance of normal (or balanced carrier) offspring is usually greater than would be expected theoretically. However, if a balanced translocation carrier is identified within a family, usually through the birth of a malformed infant with an unbalanced karyotype, it is imperative that other family members be evaluated, their chromosomes analyzed, information and supportive genetic counseling be provided, and prenatal diagnosis be offered as applicable. One of the few situations in medical genetics in which there is a 100% risk for an abnormal outcome is in the presence of a homologous robertsonian translocation, such as that in a balanced 21/21 translocation carrier. Unless such a carrier is mosaic for the translocation and has some cells (gonadal or other) with the normal chromosomal complement, the resulting zygotes will be either trisomic or monosomic for chromosome #21 and will result in an abnormal pregnancy outcome. It also is important to remember that this type of translocation *cannot be inherited;* if it could be, the carrier would be trisomic for chromosome #21. Therefore, no one else in the family is at risk for carrying or transmitting such a translocation. If balanced, it is always a *de novo* event. Prenatal diagnosis in this situation will reveal either a monosomic or trisomic fetus. On the other hand, recurrence risks for a couple who has had an infant with aneuploidy resulting from a spontaneous, noninherited or *de novo* robertsonian translocation are empirically comparable to the recurrence risks for a nondisjunctional event, about 1–2% or less. Prenatal diagnosis is indicated in all such situations during a subsequent pregnancy.

Reciprocal Translocations. If chromosomes of two different pairs exchange segments without loss or addition of chromosomal material, the phenomenon is known as a *balanced reciprocal translocation.* During gametogenesis, there are four possibilities (Fig. 13–7): a normal chromosome complement (#1); a balanced rearrangement, as in the parent carrier (#2); too much of one chromosome (partial trisomy) and too little of the other (partial monosomy) (#3); or too little of one and too much of the other (#4). Once a couple has had an infant with an unbalanced karyotype resulting from a parental reciprocal translocation, theoretically they have a 50% risk for another pregnancy resulting in an unbalanced (one or the other) karyotype. Practically, little is known about the actual risks for specific translocations because they are individually rare and involve so many differ-

[a] A balanced translocation carrier father's karyotype (see Fig. 13–6B) would be written as follows: 45,XY, −14, −21, t(14q/21q) where 45 is the total number of chromosomes (including XY) a normal 14 and 21 is missing and replaced by the translocated chromosomes. His Down's syndrome son's karyotype would be written as follows: 46,XY, −14, t(14q/21q).

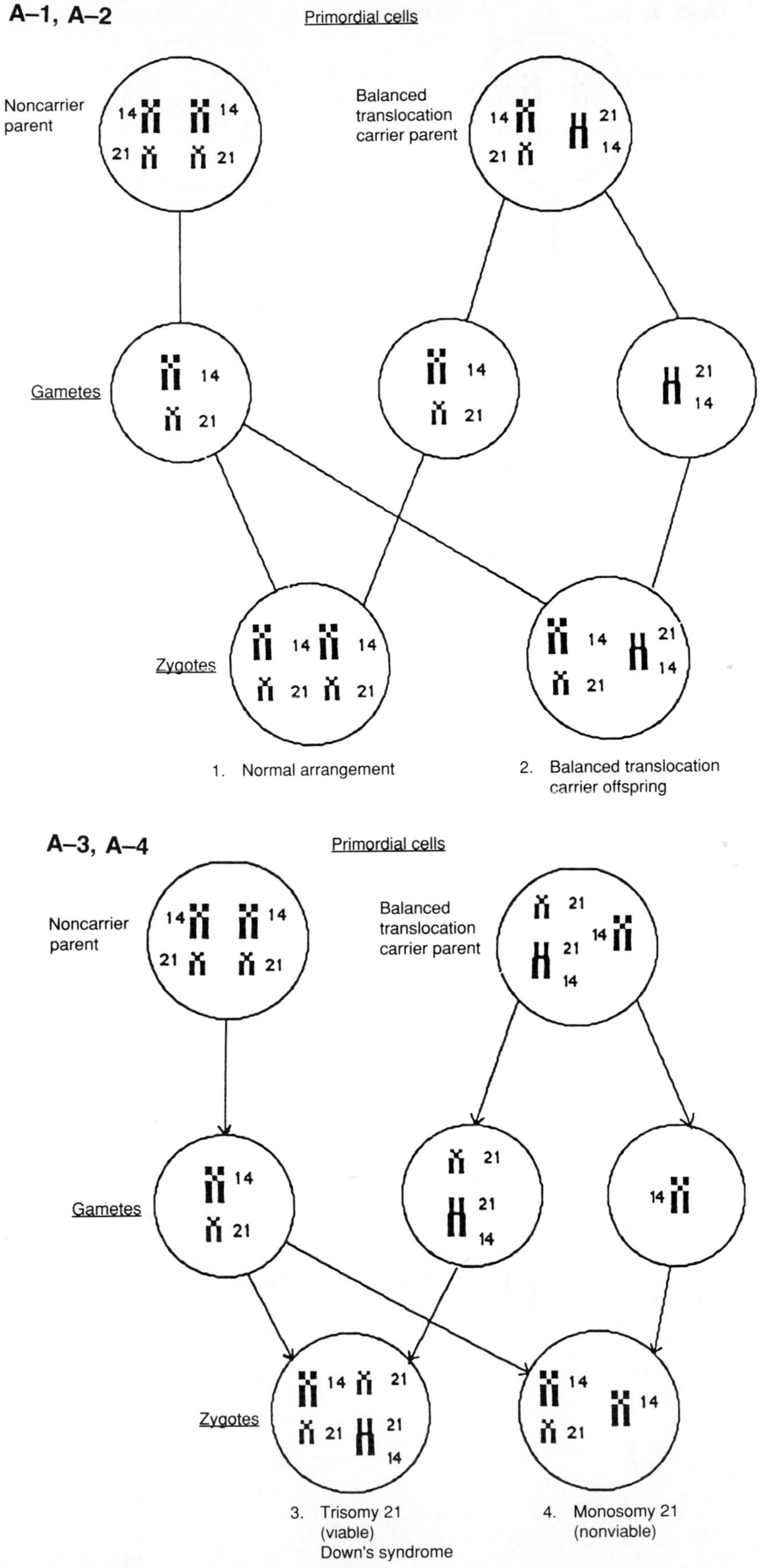

Figure 13–6. (*A*) Diagrammatic transmission of a 14/21 translocation (*continued*).

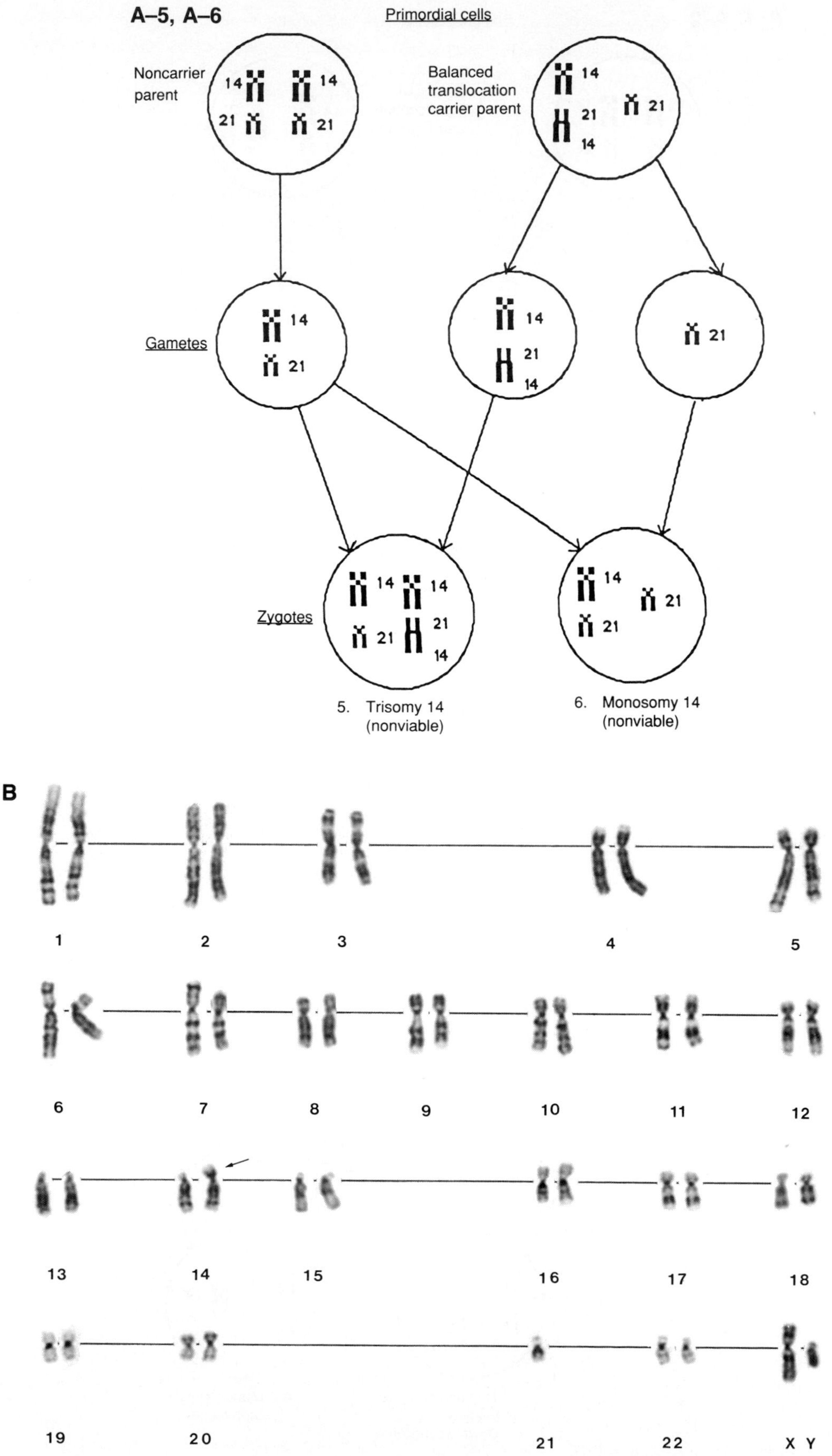

Figure 13–6. (*A*) *continued.* (*B*) Karyotype of a male with a balanced 14/21 translocation.

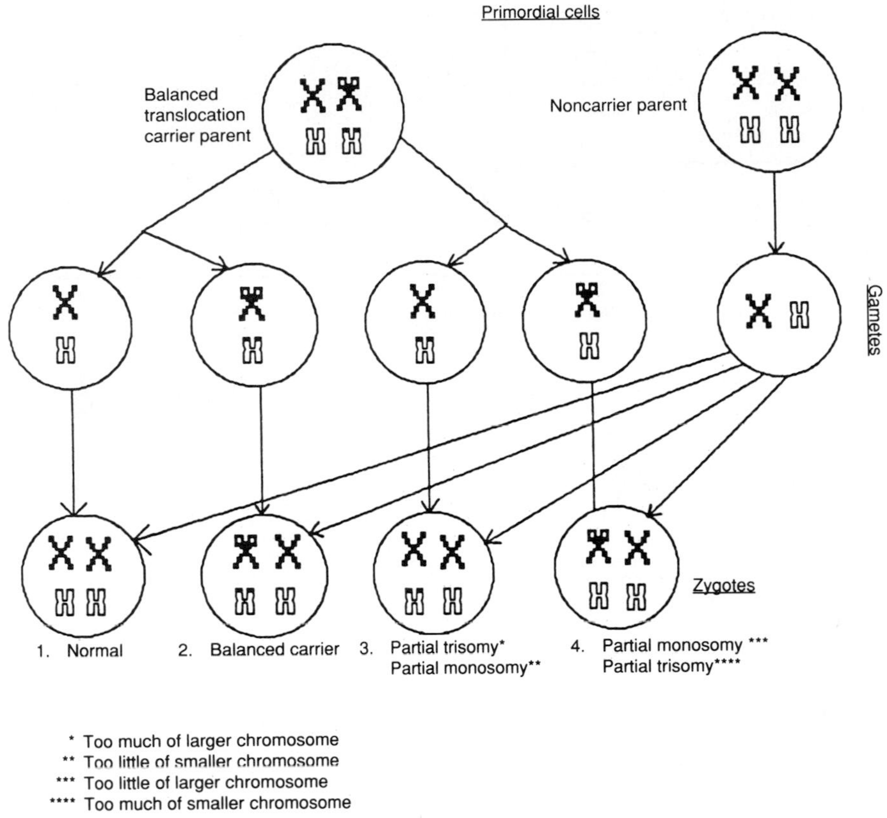

Figure 13–7. Diagrammatic transmission of a reciprocal translocation.

ent segments of different chromosomes. It is recommended in counseling a couple in which one partner is a known carrier of a reciprocal translocation that general principles be explained to them but that current information be sought on the specific translocation in question. Prenatal diagnosis is strongly indicated in all instances of translocation, and family studies are recommended. Figure 13–8 shows a pedigree of a family with a reciprocal translocation, which had affected three generations of infants and children before the cause of this "family curse," as the proposita (indicated by an arrow) put it, was identified. Figure 13–8A shows an actual karyotype of a reciprocal translocation involving chromosomes 2q and 18q.

Chromosome Breaks. Chromosome breaks, resulting in deletions and therefore in the loss of genetic material, are usually associated with phenotypic manifestations. Deletions, the phenotypic effects of which are known and recognizable, include 46,XX or XY 5p− or cri du chat syndrome, 46,XX or XY4p− or Wolf-Hirschhorn syndrome, and 46,XX or XY18p−, 18q−. Unless caused by a parental reciprocal translocation, deletions in a previous infant usually are not associated with an increased risk for recurrence, although prenatal diagnosis usually is offered for reassurance. Inversions and duplications of chromosomal material also may be encountered. The former, if complete, usually are without phenotypic effect, although this depends on whether the inversion takes place outside the centromere (*paracentric*) or whether it includes the centromere (*pericentric*). Duplications, on the other hand, almost always are associated with deleterious phenotypic effects, although they depend on the specific segment in question.

PREGNANCIES AT KNOWN RISK FOR CYTOGENETIC ABNORMALITIES

Families at risk of having an infant with a chromosomal abnormality can be divided into the following groups: those associated with increased parental age; those who have had a previous child with a *de novo* or inherited chromosomal abnormality; and those in which one of the parents is a carrier of a balanced translocation.

Parental Age

Mothers, 35 years or older, are at increased risk for having an infant with an additional chromosome as a result of a nondisjunctional event. The risks for such an event are given in Table 13–2 and are compared to the proportion of Down's syndrome births. It may be helpful to realize that, despite the validity of the maternal age effect,[6] most infants with additional chromosomes are born to women younger than 35 years. The reason for this is that only about 5% of all pregnancies are in women aged 35 or older; approximately 4% are between ages 35 and 39, and 1% are 40 or older. This proportion of pregnancies (5%) results in about 28%, 30%, and 32% of all infants with Down's syndrome, trisomy 18, and Klinefelter's syndrome, respectively. The remaining 95% of women younger than age 35, give birth, respectively, to 72%, 70%, and 68% of infants with the above syndromes.[7] It should be emphasized also that one half of the specific age related risk is for trisomy 21, the remaining half is for any other nondisjunctional event (see Table 13–2). The effect of increased paternal age is more controversial. Nondisjunction may occur slightly more frequently in conceptions fathered by males aged 55

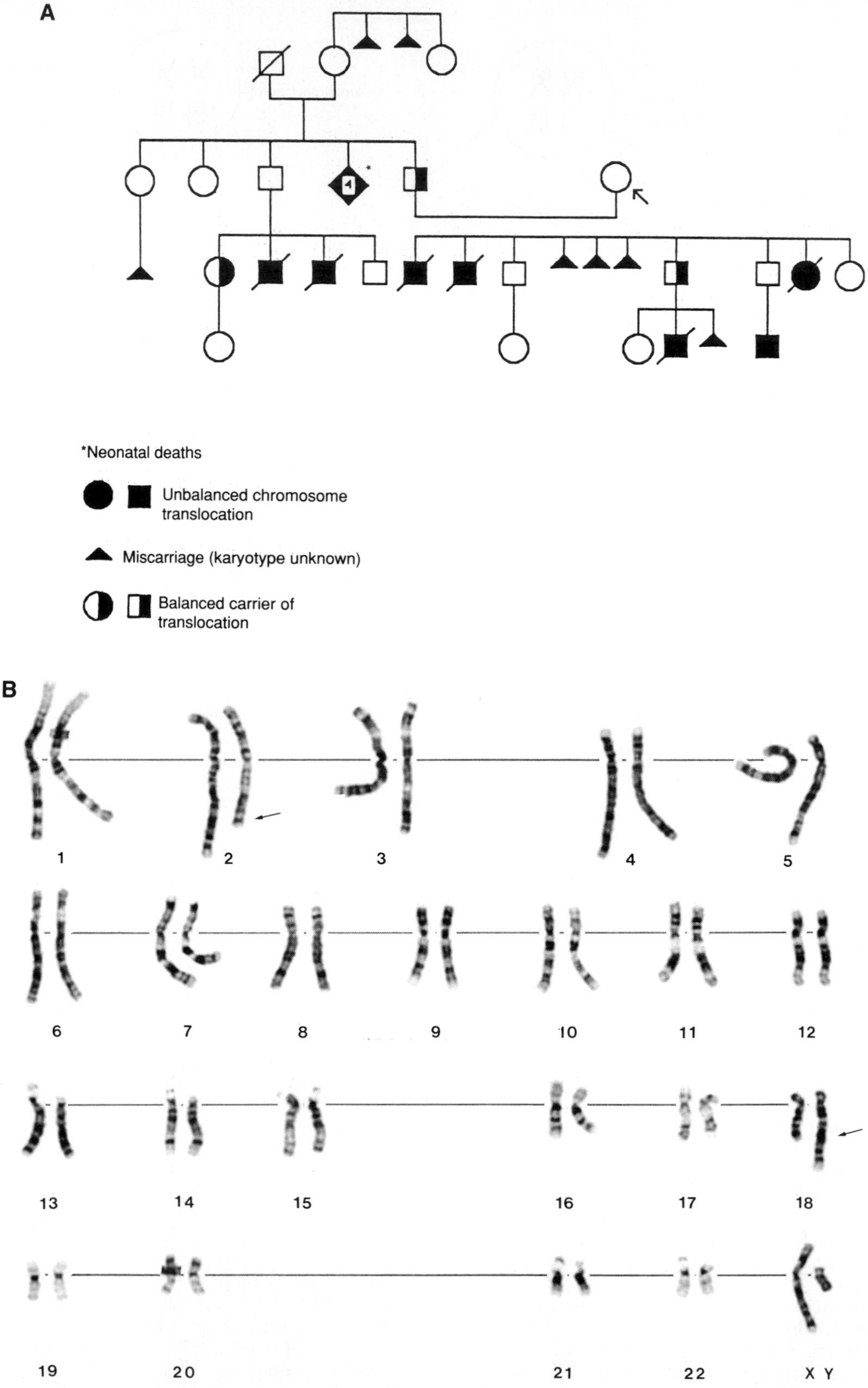

Figure 13–8. (*A*) Pedigree of a family with a 3q/7q reciprocal translocation. (*B*) Karyotype of a male with 2q/18q reciprocal translocation.

or over, and prenatal diagnosis may be indicated in such situations. The risk for dominant mutations in offspring of older fathers is higher than that in the general population[8], and, although it should be mentioned during prenatal counseling to a couple at risk, there is no technique that can prenatally detect an otherwise undefined dominant mutation in the fetus, unless it is a severe structural abnormality that might be detected on routine ultrasound.

TABLE 13–2. CHROMOSOME ABNORMALITIES DETECTED DURING SECOND-TRIMESTER AMNIOCENTESIS IN 17,859 WOMEN, AGED 35 OR OLDER

17,859 Women ≥35 y	All Chromosome Abnormalities Detected		Trisomy 21 Only	
	Number	Percent	Number	Percent
35–39	148	1.54	76	0.79
40	305	3.99	185	2.42
Total	453	~2.5	261	~1.5

Adapted from Milunsky A, ed. Genetics Disorders and the Fetus. *New York, NY: Plenum Press; 1979.*

At the other end of the spectrum, it is well known that pregnancies in young teenagers are at higher risk for prematurity and low-birth-weight infants. There is weak evidence that age alone predisposes teenaged mothers to a higher risk than the general population for infants with nondisjunctional events.[9]

Previous Child With Chromosome Abnormality

Families who have had an infant with a chromosome abnormality can be divided into two groups: those with an infant with a nondisjunctional event or a noninherited *de novo* chromosomal rearrangement, and those with an inherited chromosomal rearrangement.

Not Inherited. A spontaneous nondisjunctional event resulting in trisomy 21, 18, 13, sex chromosomal aneuploidy, and trisomies associated with a *de novo* robertsonian translocation, all have an empiric recurrence risk of approximately 1%. It is possible that this overall, statistically derived figure encompasses some situations in which the risk for recurrence is higher, for example, if one member of a couple has gonadal mosaicism, or if there is a tendency toward nondisjunction within a family (Figure 13–9). It should be noted that one half of the 1–2% risk for recurrence of a nondisjunctional event, like that associated with increased maternal age, is for trisomy 21, and the remaining half for other trisomies.

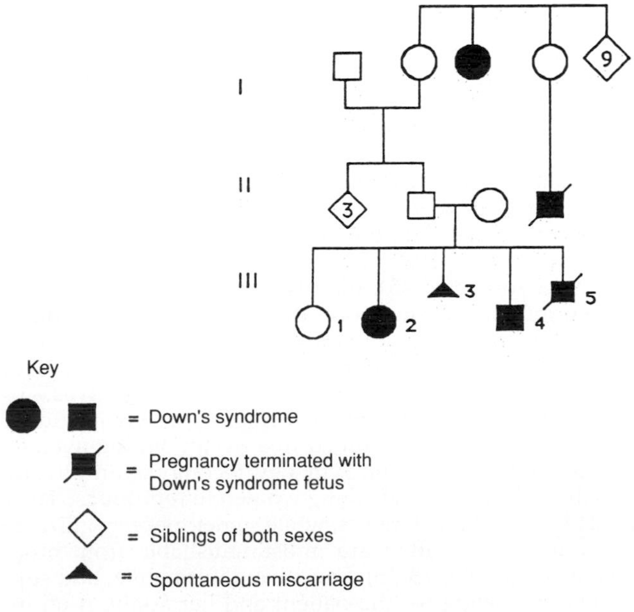

Figure 13–9. Pedigree of a family with an increased incidence of nondisjunction.

Noninherited reciprocal translocations are not known to be associated with an increased recurrence risk; they result from breaks rather than from nondisjunctional events and are not likely to recur. Similarly, *de novo* interstitial deletions would not be expected to recur in subsequent pregnancies. Thus, fetal karyotyping, although usually offered, is not strongly indicated during subsequent pregnancies because the outlook is no less favorable than that in the general population. It must be emphasized, however, that immediate counseling of couples in whose pregnancies *de novo* rearrangements or deletions have occurred unexpectedly can be extremely difficult and filled with anguish and uncertainty. The question of whether a seemingly balanced *de novo* reciprocal translocation is truly balanced and without phenotypic effect can never be answered with certainty. Even more difficult is the question of the nature of the phenotypic effects, if any, because the rearrangements seen in most reciprocal translocations are individually rare, sometimes unique, and have little precedent in the literature. Information as to an identical occurrence and its outcome is rarely available, and again, empiric risks are used, which are nonspecific and unsatisfactory. A detailed anomaly scan with ultrasound can rule out severe abnormalities of anatomy or growth but is not completely reassuring as to the absence of mental retardation or other future problems. Empirically, according to Warburton[10], the risk of abnormality in a *de novo* reciprocal, seemingly balanced translocation is 6–10%.

The finding of an unexpected deletion or duplication in the chromosomes of a fetus whose karyotype was evaluated for different reasons (eg, maternal age) can be a painful and difficult situation for the parents and the geneticist. The parents' question as to the significance of the finding can rarely be answered with accuracy. If the deletion (duplication) is on a chromosome site that is not associated with a known clinical picture, it is probably rare (even unique) and unlikely that it was clearly and unequivocally delineated in the literature in association with specific clinical manifestations. Also, if it has been reported, the chromosomal segments involved, while similar, usually differ in size. Even a series of reported patients with a duplication of 3p[11] will have different clinical manifestations, sometimes correlated to the size of the segment. Hence, information provided to parents is vague and can never be concrete.

A potential solution to these situations may come from the close collaboration between cytogeneticist, molecular geneticist, and clinician, regarding the concept of *contiguous genes,* coined by Schmickel.[12] Some previously well-defined clinical entities, such as Prader-Willi, Langer-Giedion, Miller-Dieker, DiGeorge syndromes, retinoblastoma, and Wilm's tumor aniridia complex, are characterized by small cytogenetic duplications or deletions, namely 15q11, 8q24, 17p13, 22q11, 13q14, and 11p13 respectively, in some patients. Recent evidence from the laboratory of van Tuinen et al[63], has demonstrated that patients with Miller-Dieker syndrome (MDS) who did not have a cytogenetically visible deletion of 17p13 did have a molecular deletion, thought to be less than 3 megabases long with one or more expressed genes mapping to it. Hence, while genetic material in these patients was not deleted microscopically, it is deleted at the molecular level and clearly associated with the severe clinical picture seen in MDS. Similar submicroscopic molecular deletions exist in the syndromes mentioned previously, which are known to have "chromosomal" and "nonchromosomal" forms. Ideally, once the human genome is saturated with probes, it will be possible to evaluate unexpected, apparently balanced *de novo* translocations, deletions, and duplications at the molecular level and, if the genetic material is altered, understand at least whether the rearrangements are likely to cause a phenotypic effect.

Inherited. If an infant is born with an unanticipated chromosomal rearrangement, parental chromosomal analysis is imperative so that inherited abnormalities and risks for other relatives can be identified. If one parent is a balanced translocation carrier, evaluation of the relevant grandparents and (if positive) other relatives is indicated. If grandparents are not available, the translocation carrier's siblings all must be evaluated. Recurrence risks for subsequent pregnancies would be the same as for those in the following group.

Parental Translocation

For families at risk because one parent is a balanced translocation carrier (see Fig. 13–8A), theoretical and practical recurrence risks are given in the section that discusses robertsonian and reciprocal translocations. It should be re-emphasized that the literature should be consulted for each individual rearrangement encountered because, apart from the situation associated with the most common translocations (eg, 14/21 and 13/14), many are unique for the family in question and recurrence risks differ within each family (Fig. 13–8).

DISORDERS ASSOCIATED WITH CHROMOSOMAL ABNORMALITIES

Only some of the more general, pregnancy related issues will be discussed here. The reader is referred to texts that describe these disorders in greater detail.[13–16]

Down's Syndrome

Down's syndrome occurs in about 1 in 700 births, although recently the incidence has decreased to about 1 in 1000. It is always caused by the presence of an additional #21 chromosome. Of liveborns with Down's syndrome, 94% have standard nondisjunctional trisomy 21; 4% have a robertsonian translocation (14/21, 21/22), one half of which (2% of the total) is inherited, the other half occurs *de novo;* and 2% have mosaicism. It is unclear whether their outlook for learning is better than those without recognizable mosaicism—it depends on the cells involved, the degree of mosaicism, and probably the individual in question. Ninety-eight percent of all patients with Down's syndrome have a noninherited type. Table 13–3 provides an overview of some medical concerns and their management, which may enhance the well-being of a person with Down's syndrome. Table 13–4 represents an algorithm for the cytogenetic evaluation of a family in which a relative is known or reported to have Down's syndrome. When facing new parents of an infant with unanticipated Down's syndrome, it is important that the informing physician acknowledges the baby's birth by congratulating them. At the same time, however, the parents' feelings of devastation, disappointment, and isolation also should be recognized. During the family conference, the many positive, delightful attributes of a child with Down's syndrome also should be stressed, and siblings and grandparents should be involved in family conferences.

Trisomy 18 and 13

Trisomy 18 and 13 are the second most frequent autosomal chromosome abnormalities caused by nondisjunction, occurring in about 1 in 2000 and 1 in 5000 live births, respectively. The phenotype is easily recognized at birth (Fig. 13–10 and 13–11) and, when present, is a medical genetics emergency. An accurate diagnosis, even before chromosome evaluation, can prevent distress, pain, and prolonged anguish if it is known that an infant has trisomy 18 or 13 before intubation. Parents and families should be encouraged to spend as much time as possible with their dying infant; it is a myth that distance alleviates grieving. Parents are already attached—they have imagined and anticipated the birth of their child, and they planned and wanted him or her. Time spent with their infant will provide precious memories, which, in the long run, will help them and their families cope with their loss. It is unclear why the majority (~97%) of infants with trisomy 13 or 18 die within the first days, weeks, or months of life. Many die of complex, inoperable congenital heart disease. It is usually inoperable because, even if anatomically reparable, the infant's general status is so debilitated that they rarely survive anesthesia or major surgical procedures. Some die of general "failure to live"; they deteriorate in spite of good medical care. Occasionally, if they survive long enough, they succumb to liver complications, biliary atresia, and other complications. Figure 13–12 is that of a 2½-year-old boy who survived with nonmosaic trisomy 13 until age 3 when he died, unexpectedly, of aspiration. He was a delightful, interactive, and cherished member of his family.

Monosomy X, Turner's Syndrome. The majority of conceptions with monosomy X attributed to anaphase lag rather than a nondisjunctional event are aborted spontaneously. Its incidence is not thought to be related to maternal age. With the advent of ultrasound, these fetuses are increasingly being recognized. The presenting symptom often is a large posterior cystic hygroma of the neck, seen on ultrasound performed for other reasons (Fig. 13–13). Monosomy X, and less frequently trisomy 21, are at the top of the list of differential diagnoses. Amniocentesis for chromosome analysis is always indicated in these instances, and parents and physicians are faced with a difficult dilemma. While it is highly probable that a fetus with the degree of severity as seen in Figure 13–13 will develop generalized hydrops and die *in utero,* it is still unclear whether this or a slightly smaller cystic neck mass could be partially resorbed and result in one of the few conceptions with monosomy X who are born alive, such as girls with Turner's syndrome (Fig. 13–14). The cause of posterior cystic neck hygroma is usually obstruction (eg, stricture, atresia) at the connection between the lymphatic sac and jugular junction; in many fetuses with monosomy X, it is associated with a very small heart and frequent coarctation of the aorta. It is interesting to note that in our own series of stillborn and miscarried fetuses, the majority were females (45X *and* 46XX); those who survived were males. It seems that not only a karyotype of 45X but also of 46XX is a risk factor of such infants. Furthermore, the presence on ultrasound of other malformations and intrauterine growth retardation is associated with risk for unfavorable outcome. Girls with Turner's syndrome can lead normal, meaningful lives. Although combined replacement therapy, possibly including growth hormone, has resulted in a disappointing average increase in stature of about 3 cm, new techniques are already available to enable these young women to reproduce. Their facial physical characteristics, while sometimes recognizable to a trained eye, often are indistinguishable from other girls their age (Fig. 13–15). Sensitive, informative, and supportive counseling for the patient and her family is an inseparable component of her medical care.

TABLE 13–3. PROTOCOL FOR MANAGEMENT OF PATIENTS WITH DOWN'S SYNDROME

	Birth	Early Infancy	Pre-school	Child-hood	Puberty	Adoles-cence	Adult-hood	Aging
Confirm diagnosis, test relatives (as needed)	Chromosomes	Keep records for family members						
Congenital Malformations: Cardiac (40%) Gastrointestinal (20%) Other	Echocardiogram evaluate rule out	GE Reflux?	Follow				Follow	Follow annually for acq. heart disease
General Physical Evaluation + Dental	–	+	At least	Annually	Annually	Annually	Annually	2/y
Sensory: Hearing	structural malformation	BEAR	Behavioral audiology	Annually	Biennial	Same	Same	Annually
Vision	dilated peds. eval.	+	Evaluate annually	Same	Same	Same	Same	Same
Smell			Evaluate					
Thyroid function tests	+ screen	at 12 months	Annual	Biennially > 5 years age			Annually	Annually
Cervical subluxation		X-ray at 18–24 months						
Hematology		Anemia?	CBC 2/y	Annual	p.r.n.			
Plastic surgery			Tongue reduction?		Patient should participate in decision			
Development: gross motor, fine motor, speech and lang., social/emotion.	*Bonding* Hypotonia	*EIS* hypo. PT	*ECP* PT PT S&L	*SEP* PT OT S&L	*SEP*	*Vocational training* Encourage independence	*Work*	
Sexuality:				Build self esteem—remember guardianship Educate	Educate Evaluate fertility Ovulation? Sperm count?	Educate		

GE = gastroesophageal; BEAR = brain evoked auditory response; acq. = acquired; PT = physical therapy; OT = occupational therapy; S&L = speech and language; EIS = early infant stimulation, 0–3; ECP = early childhood program, 3–5; SEP = special education program, 5–21.

TABLE 13–4. PROCEDURE IN SITUATIONS IN WHICH FAMILY MEMBER HAS (HAD) DOWN'S SYNDROME

A. Affected Family Member is *Alive* and Available for Testing

1. Arrange for chromosome analysis in affected person
2. If analysis is already available, obtain written report

Results

a) Noninherited, nondisjunctional event (trisomy 21)—96% of cases. Risks for all family members (other than parents of affected person) are equal to those in general population of comparable age. Offer prenatal diagnosis to *parents* only.

b) Translocation (4%). 1) Investigate parents of affected person; if normal chromosomes (2%), risks as for a. 2) If carrier detected (2%), or parents not available, investigate chromosomes of siblings and of other relatives of affected person for translocation carrier status. Offer prenatal diagnosis to *all carriers*.

c) Chromosomes of affected person normal. Affected individual does not have Down's syndrome. Recurrence risks for Down's syndrome for all family members equal to those in general population at comparable age. Attempt *must* be made to investigate affected person and establish diagnosis.

B. Affected Family Member *Not Alive* or Not Available for Testing

1. Confirm diagnosis with report of chromosome analysis; if available, proceed as for A2 a), b), or c).
2. If *not* available, request *photographs* of affected person
   - If photographs indicate Down's syndrome, investigate parents' chromosomes, if available, and proceed as for A 2b).
   - If photographs definitely do not indicate Down's syndrome, proceed as for A 2c).
3. No photographs available, but sufficient suspicion exists of Down's syndrome—proceed as for A 2b).

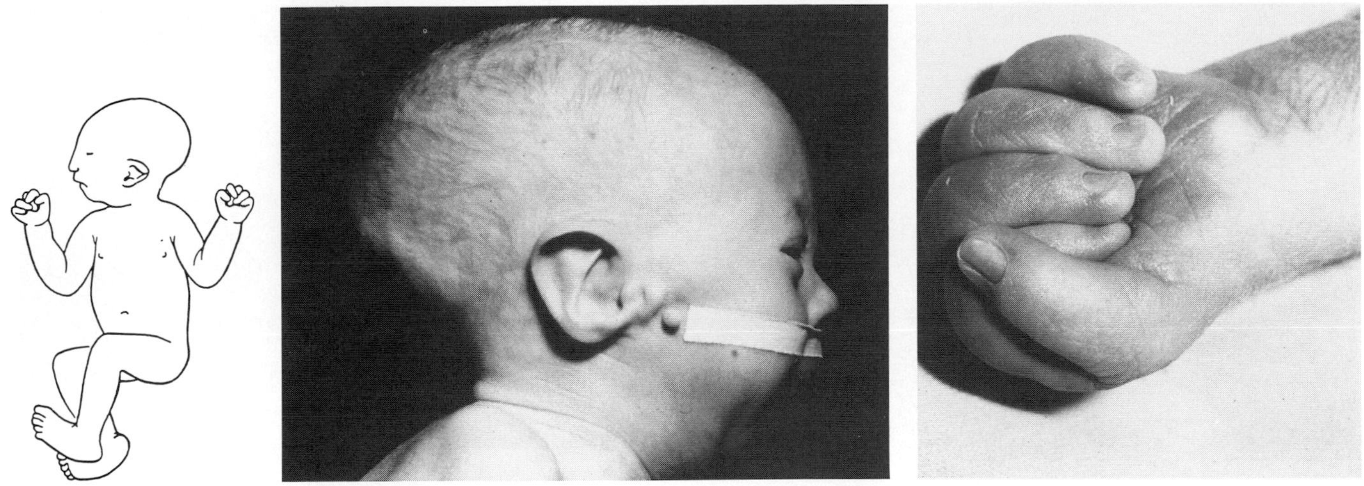

Figure 13–10. Infant with trisomy 18. This is a general diagram showing prominent occiput; large, abnormally configurated ears with pits; and preauricular ear tag, marked mandibular micrognathia. Characteristic hand with hypoplastic nails and overlapping digits.

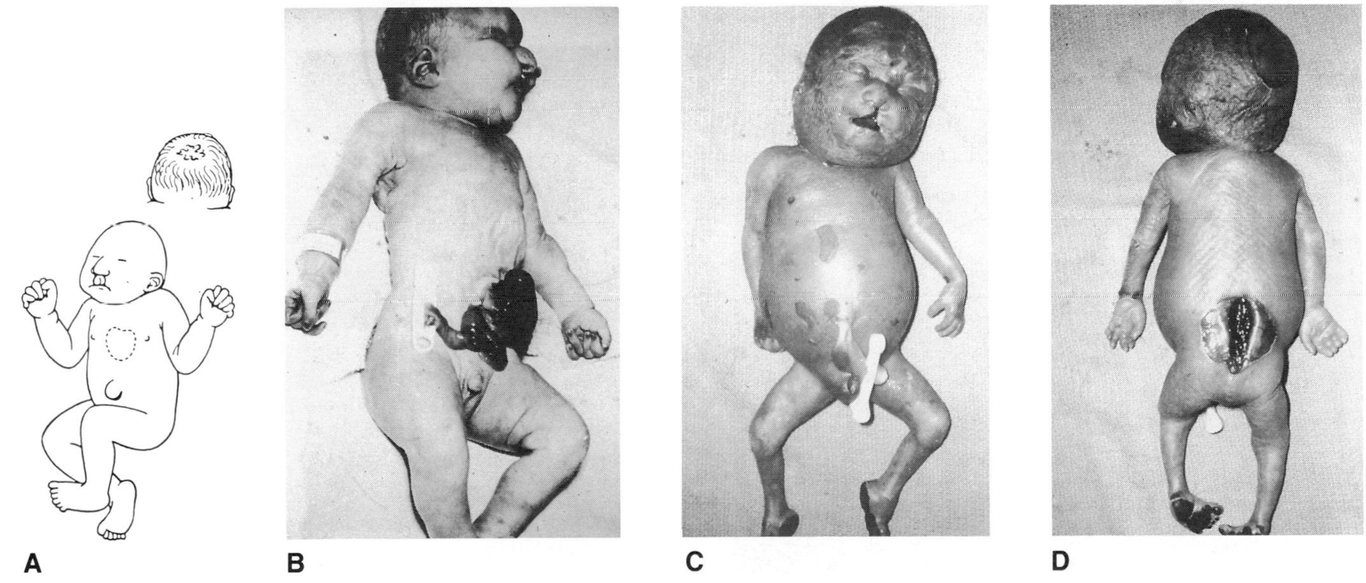

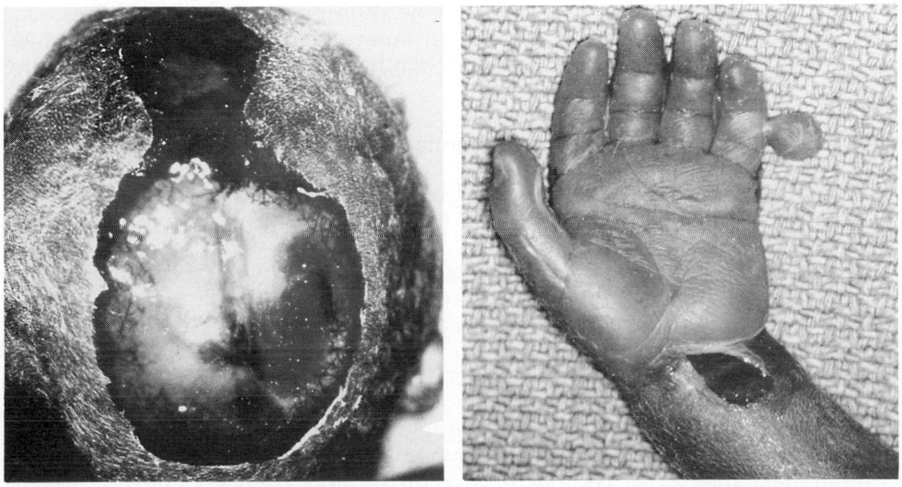

Figure 13–11. Infant with trisomy 13. (*A*) General diagram. (*B*) General view with midline clefting malformation, microphthalmia, polydactyly, omphalocele. (*C*) Front and (*D*) back views with lumbosacral meningomyelocele, (*E*) scalp defect, and (*F*) polydactyly.

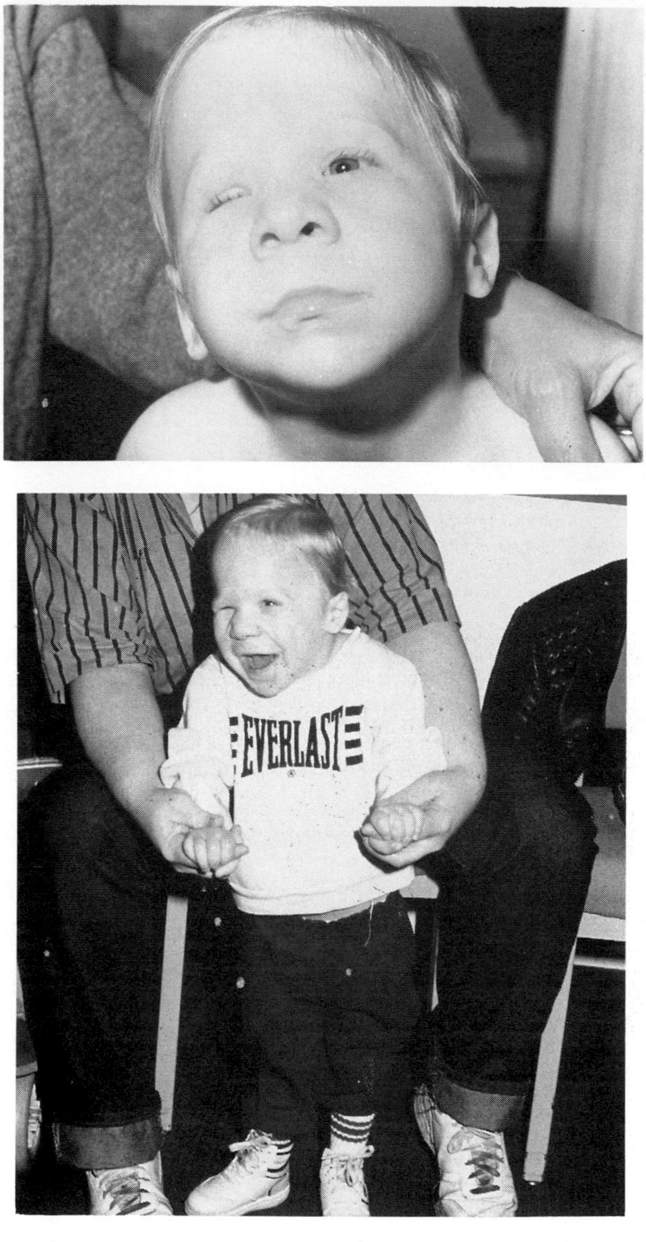

Figure 13–12. 2½-year-old boy with nonmosaic trisomy 13.

Klinefelter's and 47,XYY Syndromes. While the dilemma of a fetus with monosomy X is sometimes resolved by nature, the dilemma of a fetus with 47,XXX, 47,XXY, or XYY detected *in utero* is even greater. As with intrauterine Down's syndrome, there are no clues to the degree of severity of these disorders. It is known that the more sex chromosomes that are present, the greater the probability of mental retardation in the child. The best information available to these parents comes from the prospective studies of newborn populations.[17] Tables 13–5 and 13–6 show correlations of IQ, school performance, and behavior in children with sex chromosomal abnormalities within the family setting. Such information, along with a description of the physical, emotional, and medical problems involved, is sometimes helpful to parents who are desperately trying to make the right decision for them, their lives, and their family.

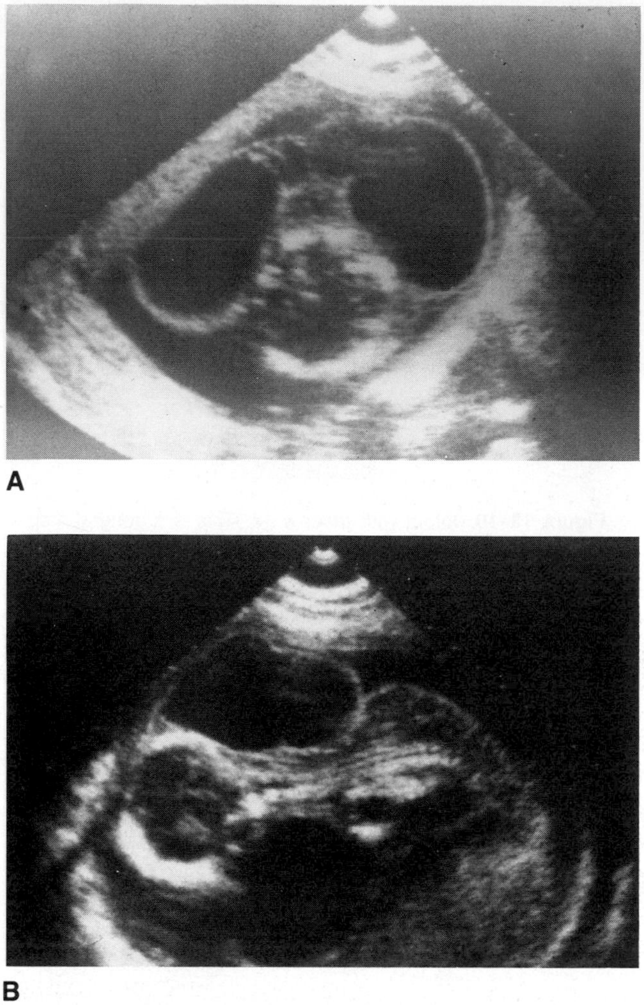

Figure 13–13. Ultrasound at 17 weeks' gestation with bilateral posterior bilocular cystic hygroma of the neck. (*A*) Transverse, and (*B*) longitudinal section.

CONCLUSIONS

In summary, the following issues or factors should alert the physician to the need for pregnancy-related cytogenetic analysis. In some instances, the indications will be known before conception; in others, they will be identified during pregnancy.

Indications Potentially Known Before Conception

1. Previous child with a known chromosomal abnormality
2. Previous child with a suspected chromosomal abnormality (child died or is otherwise unavailable for testing), who was thought to have multiple congenital malformations, mental retardation, or short stature
3. Parent who is a known carrier of a chromosomal rearrangement
4. Parent of advanced age (mother ≥35 years or father ≥55 years)
5. History of multiple miscarriages (chromosomes in parents' blood can be evaluated directly, but even if normal, the risk of a recurring nondisjunctional event may be increased)

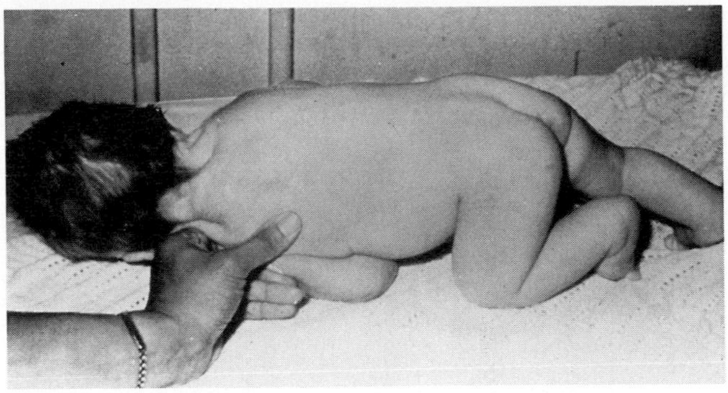

Figure 13–14. Healthy liveborn infant with Turner's syndrome with excess skin in neck area.

6. Instances in which fetal sex determination is indicated (eg, sex-linked disease, Fragile X syndrome)
7. Previous child with known syndrome associated with chromosome breakage (eg, Fanconi's syndrome, Bloom's syndrome, ataxia telangiectasia)

Chromosomes are usually analyzed even if the primary reason for prenatal testing is not cytogenetic (eg, DNA or AFP evaluations).

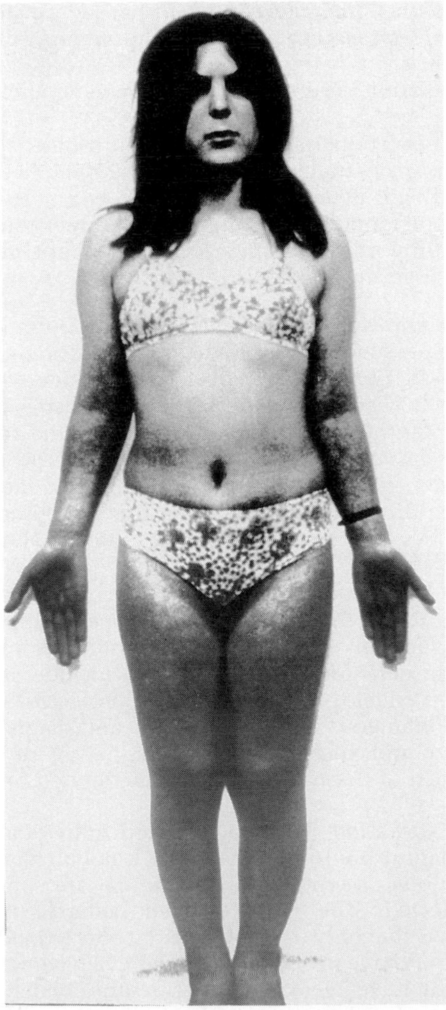

Figure 13–15. Seventeen-year-old girl with nonmosaic untreated Turner's syndrome. Note bilateral cubitus valgus.

TABLE 13–5. DEVELOPMENTAL AND PSYCHOMETRIC FACTORS IN CHILDREN WITH SEX CHROMOSOMAL ABNORMALITIES

	FULL SCALE IQ		
	N	X	SD
XXY	73	97.74	15.7
Control	60	103.60	12.9
XXY	28	105.00	15.2
Control	8	104.60	12.3
XXX	32	90.00	14.8
Control	25	108.40	13.3

Factors Identified During Pregnancy

1. Any one of the above eight indications that was not known/identified before conception
2. Unexpected abnormal findings on ultrasound that could potentially be associated with a chromosome abnormality (eg, malformations, fetal hydrops, cystic hygroma, or intrauterine growth retardation)
3. Significantly low levels of maternal serum alpha fetoprotein (AFP), which are known to be associated with an increased risk of chromosomal abnormalities and include trisomies and chromosomal rearrangements (see section on prenatal diagnosis and AFP)

PRINCIPLES OF MENDELIAN GENETICS

It is fortunate that a financially struggling teacher, Gregor Mendel, "realized that it was impossible for him to endure such exertions* any longer . . ." and that he . . . "therefore felt compelled to step into a position which would free him from the bitter struggle for existence" (from Mendel's application for admission to the Augustinian monastery in Brno, now Czechoslovakia). His laws of heredity and his basic concept of particles as the units of heredity, published in 1865, became the foundation for the modern science of genetics. His name has become permanently associated with the branch of genetics that studies the transmission of single genes. Ignored for 40 years, Mendel's discoveries surfaced at the beginning of the 20th century, around the time one of the first examples of an inherited metabolic disease, alkaptonuria, was observed by Archibald Garrod.

At the same time, the concept of mathematical and population genetics emerged, largely because of the contributions of R. A. Fisher and J. B. S. Haldane in Britain and Sewell Wright, H. K. Muller, and James F. Crow in the United States. After a period of bitter controversy, abuse, and misinterpretation of Mendel's laws before and during World War II, genetics resurfaced.

McKusick's catalog of Mendelian Inheritance in Man was first published in 1966 listed 1487 disorders. The ninth edition, published in 1990[18], is now computerized and continuously updated. It contains 4937 entries, of which 3047 are (or may be) autosomal dominant, 1554 are (or may be) autosomal recessive, and 336 are (or may be) X-linked.

Like cytogenetics 30 years ago, molecular genetics today has revolutionized the ability to help humans with

* refers to financial

TABLE 13–6. EFFECTS OF FAMILY FUNCTIONING ON IQ AND BEHAVIOR OF CHILDREN WITH SEX CHROMOSOMAL ABNORMALITIES

	Family Problems: Present/Absent			
	Verbal IQ	Performance IQ	Educational Difficulties	Behavioral Difficulties
XXY PRESENT	81	96	22/23	16/23
ABSENT	92	104	22/42	3/42
XYY PRESENT	96	108	6/7	5/6
ABSENT	100	106	9/21	5/21
XXX PRESENT	76	84	10/10	8/10
ABSENT	90	98	15/25	3/25
CONTROLS:				
MALE				
PRESENT	99	102	13/28	16/27
ABSENT	108	106	6/44	2/44
FEMALE				
PRESENT	98	113	7/11	6/11
ABSENT	109	103	2/18	5/18

genetic diseases. The search for genes causing devastating human diseases, such as Huntington's, cystic fibrosis, and muscular dystrophies, is now a routine activity in many laboratories around the world, and in the case of cystic fibrosis, it has become a spectacular success. The debate concerning the construction of a map of the whole human genome occupied scientific and popular media for many months. Truly causative treatment of genetic diseases through gene manipulation is no longer a dream of the distant future. Medical geneticists will now be able to do something they have never done before: They will treat and cure their patients.

The principles of mendelian genetics are simple. Their applications are far reaching and complex, with many problems and pitfalls. An understanding is imperative if appropriate information is to be provided to couples contemplating pregnancy. Mendel introduced the two mechanisms of inheritance, *dominance* and *recessivity*. Each of these depends on whether the gene(s) in question is (are) located on the autosomes or on the sex chromosomes. Dominance is a situation in which the presence of one allele is sufficient to result in phenotypic effects.

An allele is the DNA sequence occupying the same locus on each of two homologous chromosomes. It is another (allelus (-a), (-um) = the other) version of the gene. Some genes have several versions or alleles (eg, the ABO blood type has three, and all are normal). If a change occurs in an allele (in the DNA sequence), the result may be dysfunction or abnormality. If different (heterogeneous) alleles are present on each member of a pair of chromosomes, that individual is said to be heterozygous for that characteristic (eg, a person with blood type AO). If the same allele is present on both chromosomes, the person is homozygous (eg, AA).

Autosomal Dominant Inheritance

General Principles

1. In dominantly inherited disorders, affected individuals (ie, those who manifest the disorder) are always (or almost always) heterozygous for the allele causing their disorder.
2. Because it is located only on one of a pair of autosomes, every affected person has a 50% chance of transmitting the dysfunctional allele to offspring. Hence, there is a 1 in 2 or 50/50 segregation ratio in the offspring of affected parents.
3. Transmission occurs vertically, from generation to generation.
4. The dysfunctional allele is on an autosome; therefore, male to male transmission exists, and both sexes are affected with equal frequency.
5. When one member of a couple has a known autosomally dominantly inherited disorder, the risk of similarly affected offspring is 50%.

For example, in the pedigree in Figure 13–16, four generations of people of both sexes have *Waardenburg's syndrome type 1* (WS I). Complete manifestations include wide nasal bridge, or telecanthus, caused by lateral displacement of the inner canthi; pigmentary dysplasia in the form of a white (or darker) forelock of hair and heterochromia of the irides; cochlear deafness; and aganglionic megacolon, or Hirschsprung's disease. WS I in this family and many other families is inherited in a classic, autosomal dominant way.

Many additional complicating issues must be considered when attempting to provide accurate and helpful information to families with classically inherited disorders who are seeking genetics counseling. They include such phenomena as variable phenotypic expression, decreased penetrance, spontaneous mutation, genetic and diagnostic heterogeneity, and the availability and nature of prenatal testing. Each of these issues will be mentioned briefly.

Variable Expression. While all affected individuals in the family in Figure 13–16 truly have WS I, not all have similar manifestations of symptoms, and not all are similarly severely affected. The more detailed pedigree in Figure 13–17 shows that only three of the eight affected individuals are deaf, four have iris heterochromia, five have white forelocks, eight have increased inner canthic distances, and no one in this family has megacolon congenitum. The abnormal gene is expressed variably in different individuals, and there is no doubt that there is a 50% chance that the now

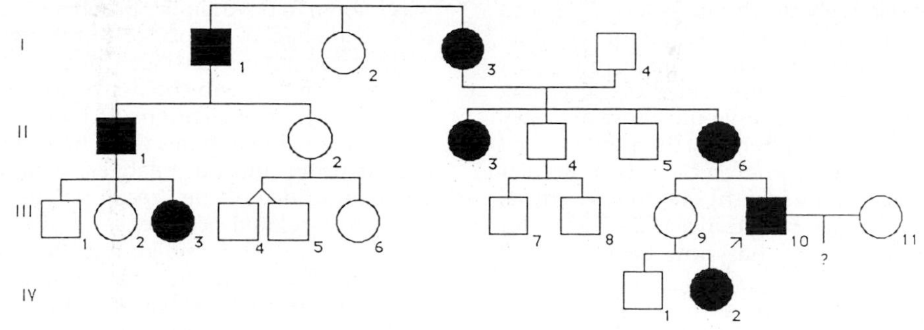

Figure 13–16. Pedigree of family with Waardenburg's syndrome type I.

conceived IV/III fetus will have WS I and a 50% chance that it will not. However, the reason that the couple III/10 and III/11 sought help was not for recurrence of WS I. Neither they nor their relatives were aware of the existence of WS I in their family. Their anxiety was for risks of severe hearing impairment, as present in III/10's niece and maternal aunt. They were hoping that deafness was "too distant" to affect their infant but sought reassurance. They were shocked to hear that their family history, review of medical records, and family photo album (all important components of a genetics evaluation) had resulted in the establishment of a diagnosis of WS I in the family and in the father of the infant. The chance was 1 in 2 that their infant would inherit it; the risk for deafness, while less than 50%, was unknown and unpredictable. Neither severity nor the extent of phenotypic manifestation can be predicted in dominantly inherited disorders. WS I cannot be diagnosed *in utero;* hence, the couple's options were limited to facing the risk or terminating the pregnancy.

Marfan's syndrome is another common, well-known, dominantly inherited disorder, affecting connective tissues (see also Chapters 36 and 134). It results in dolichostenomelia, arachnodactyly, tall (for the family) stature, dislocated lenses, midfacial hypoplasia, hyperextensible and easily dislocated joints, *pectus excavatum,* and (of greatest concern) a risk for dissecting aortic aneurysms. It is impossible to predict whether a child with a grandparent and great uncle who died at age 33 of dissecting aortic aneurysms will be equally, less, or more severely affected. It is important to stress two factors, however. (1) If the diagnosis in the grandparent or great uncle, was not established by the genetics "detectives" (as they were in the WS I family), no accurate information would be available to the families at all. (2) For Marfan's syndrome, prophylactic management with beta blockers is available and is thought to have beneficial effects.

Penetrance. Penetrance is the frequency with which a genotype is expressed as the expected phenotype within a family. For example in Figure 13–17, the sister of the propositus, III/9, who was the mother of a severely affected daughter, was evaluated and had no phenotypically demonstrable or measurable (eg, increased outer canthic distances) signs of WS I. This is known as *reduced penetrance.* In my opinion, it replaces the term *unknown factors* or *inability to delineate phenotype.* If, for example, it were not yet known that telecanthus was a component of WS I, female III/3 in Figure 13–17 would not have been classified as affected. We may be unaware of many inapparent physical, biochemical, and organic manifestations. This failure forces the use

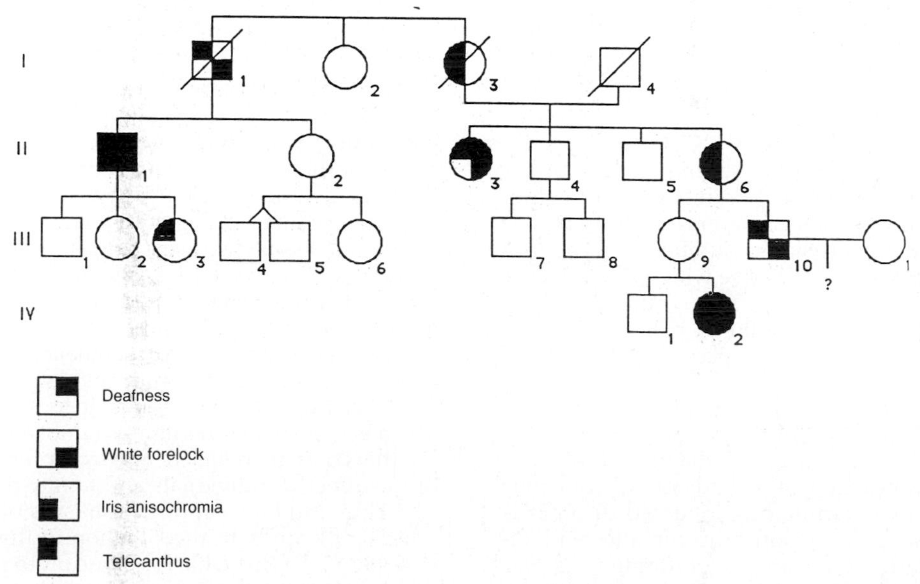

Figure 13–17. Pedigree of same family demonstrating variable expression of Waardenburg's syndrome type I.

of the mathematic but relatively meaningless term, reduced penetrance. On the other hand, the existence of this phenomenon, even if it is caused by lack of knowledge, must not be ignored. Had female III/9 sought genetics counseling before the birth of her children, she would most probably have been told she was at no higher risk than the general population. In the near future, analysis at the molecular level may provide more accurate insight into the superficial phenomenon now known as penetrance. The locus for Waardenburg's syndrome type I has now been mapped to chromosome 2q35−37.3.

Spontaneous Mutation. Spontaneous mutation is a permanent change in the genetic information; it is heritable (future generations can, but need not, be affected), but it is not inherited. It has occurred as a change, for the first time, in the person in question. The decision, whether the disorder is caused by spontaneous mutation or inherited from an affected parent in whom the phenotypic expression is so mild that it is inapparent, is a geneticist's nightmare. It is the difference between negligible (general population) risks and a 50% chance of further affected offspring. It also is the difference between managing, evaluating, and following one patient as opposed to many family members in whom signs of the disease have not yet developed.

Dominant disorders, particularly neurocutaneous disorders, present many such dilemmas for families and professionals. *Neurofibromatosis* is a common (occurring in about 1 in 3000) group of dominantly inherited disorders that affects growth of cells of neural crest origin. There are at least two types. Neurofibromatosis (NF) 1, or peripheral NF (located on chromosome 17q), is characterized by 1) multiple hyperpigmented, *café au lait* macules (CLM); 2) peripheral neurofibromata; 3) axillary freckling; 4) iris Lisch nodules; 5) optic gliomata; 6) osseous lesions, or scoliosis; 7) seizures; and 8) learning disabilities. Neurofibromatosis 1 is sometimes progressive and may be associated with considerable morbidity or even mortality. The second type, NF2, (located on chromosome 22q), is much rarer (estimated incidence is 1 in 50,000) and is characterized by acoustic neuromata and other CNS tumors including meningioma and intraspinal tumors. As for other autosomally dominantly inherited disorders, expression varies intrafamilially and interfamilially, and although the National Institutes of Health Consensus Conference developed minimal diagnostic criteria[19], they are not always helpful in the provision of information to families. For example, the mother of a child with an established diagnosis of NF1 has three large CLM on her skin. Her husband has two CLM and a history of childhood seizures of unknown origin. The remainder of both family histories is negative. Minimal diagnostic criteria according to the Consensus conference include two or more of the following seven signs: numbers 1 through 6 under NF1, and a known direct relative with NF1. However the criterion for CLM is six or more. This mother had three large CLM (2 × 3 cm). Is this child at risk for similarly affected siblings, or did his disorder occur as the result of a new mutation?

In another instance, a young woman was concerned about risks to her future offspring of familial adenomatous polyposis coli (FAPC). The FAPC was diagnosed in her at the early age of 9 years when thousands of adenomatous polyps were found. This dominantly inherited disorder is associated with 100% risk for colon cancer in affected individuals unless an early colectomy is performed, as was the case with this patient. She was one of seven siblings (including one miscarriage) and aside from a sister, no one was known to have similar problems in her extended family. Her sister had a history of rectal bleeding for 2–3 years, with visualization and subsequent disappearance of two polyps on proctoscopy on two occasions. Careful colonoscopies and other evaluations of both parents (in their early 60s) were negative. If this was a new mutation in the patient, her offspring, but not relatives, would be at risk. What is the significance of the "rectal polyps" in her sister? Were they an unrelated occurrence? It was suggested that their transience and the ambiguity of her rectal bleeding could have been an attention-seeking behavior in this sibling of a very sick patient. However, if this was not the situation, could this be an example of genetic heterogeneity (ie, could FAPC in this family be caused by an autosomal recessive gene)? If so, the patient's offspring were at no increased risk.

The geneticist is obliged to evaluate apparently healthy family members with expensive tests if they lead to preventive measures (eg, echocardiograms in family members of Marfan's patients to detect dilated aortic roots and to identify affected family members). When testing is purely for genetic counseling and diagnostic reasons, it may encounter strong opposition of third-party carriers. The molecular geneticist will provide answers to many of these questions. DNA analysis is already underway in the FAPC family because the FAPC gene was assigned to 5q.[20]

Gonadal Mosaicism. The presence of a mutated gene in some gonadal cells of a parent is another factor that contributes to the complexity of genetic analysis in some families. Two or more offspring with a known well-defined autosomal dominant disorder from parents who are clearly unaffected cannot be explained by a single spontaneous mutation. For example, increasing evidence exists that one of the congenitally severe forms of osteogenesis imperfecta, previously thought to be autosomal recessive, is dominant, and, in the absence of phenotypically affected parents, it is thought to be caused by a mutated gene present in some cells of one of the parental gonads. Strong suspicion also exists for gonadal mosaicism in healthy parents of some siblings with an unequivocal diagnosis of tuberous sclerosis (a neurocutaneous disorder characterized by skin changes, fibroadenomata, and other cutaneous abnormalities; visceral hamartomata; seizures; slow progression; and frequently concomitant mental retardation).

Genetic Heterogeneity. Genetic heterogeneity, which is the existence of the same phenotype in association with different genotypes and therefore different mechanisms of heredity, is another extremely frustrating and confusing situation for families and geneticists. For example, a young male, the only member of his family known to be affected with a heterogeneous disorder such as *cerebellar ataxia* or nightblindness, is concerned about potential manifestations in future offspring. This situation represents a major medical, economical, and socioemotional undertaking of enormous complexity. Many types of cerebellar ataxia or nightblindness exist, each inherited in several different ways. On a superficial level, all types result in similar manifestation. The mechanism of inheritance cannot always be determined on the basis of detailed and comprehensive evaluations of the affected individuals and family members.

Thus the types and mechanisms of inheritance, all of which may apply to the situation in this family, are given in Table 13–7. This table is not meant to provide a simplistic review of mendelian inheritance; it is meant to emphasize the complexity of a family counseling situation in which,

TABLE 13–7. RECURRENCE RISKS FOR OFFSPRING OR SIBLINGS OF MALE WHO IS THE ONLY AFFECTED INDIVIDUAL WITH POTENTIALLY GENETIC DISORDER OF UNKNOWN MECHANISM OF INHERITANCE

Patient (Male)		Offspring	Siblings
IF AD:	Parent affected	50%	50%
	New mutation	50%	Ø
	Parental gonadal mosaicism	50%	? but >0
IF AR:	Both parents carriers	0[a]	25%
IF XLR:	Mother carrier	0[b]	50% for males
	New mutation	0[b]	0

[a] Unless he marries a heterozygous carrier for the disorder (unlikely).
[b] All daughters will be carriers.

because of genetic heterogeneity, it is impossible to provide accurate genetics information. All eventualities must be explained, discussed, and understood by the family.

When the biochemical basis and, more importantly, the molecular genetics is understood in each of these disorders, they probably will be distinguishable on the basis of DNA analysis. The problems associated with genetics heterogeneity will then diminish.

Diagnostic Heterogeneity. The importance of an accurate diagnosis was emphasized in the discussion of the family with *Waardenburg's syndrome.* Another example stresses this even more dramatically. A young man was referred "for reassurance" because his father had died of metastatic disease resulting from renal cell carcinoma. The young man was interested in the risk of this disease to him and his future offspring. Review of the father's records revealed that renal disease had originated from a hypernephroma and that in his youth several "eye tumors" had been treated. The geneticist's suspicion of Hippel-Lindau disease was confirmed when an ophthalmologic evaluation of the young man detected several retinal angiomata, and an MRI showed multiple cerebellar and spinal hemangioblastomas. The presence of this devastating autosomal dominant disease represents significant (50%) risks to future generations, and because of its variable age of onset, it also must be evaluated in all presymptomatic relatives at risk. Because some of its extremely severe complications can be prevented by early detection, complicated and expensive protocols exist for all family members at risk. We have no choice but to offer and follow such protocols, until the localization of the gene or other molecular testing enables the presymptomatic differentiation of affected individuals.

Counseling Dilemmas, Huntington's Disease. A discussion of autosomal dominant disorders would be inappropriate without mention of *Huntington's disease,* a well-known, progressive neurodegenerative basal ganglia disorder with predominantly adult onset of symptoms. Mutations are rare; the majority of families in the United States are thought to be descendants of the original family of Simon Huntington, who came to this country in 1633 bringing the gene from Norwich in the county of Norfolk in East Anglia.[21] The disease is usually characterized by involuntary movements, personality change, memory loss, and dementia, and a diagnosis of schizophrenia precedes the recognition of the true diagnosis in many families. It is relentlessly progressive and leads to death within 5–15 years from onset of symptoms, before which the majority of patients at risk are unaware that they are affected. This means that many have transmitted the dominant gene to children and grandchildren before the disease is recognized in them. Life with an affected parent or sibling or with the knowledge of risk may be a devastating experience. Huntington's disease families have one of the highest known rates of suicide, 4%, compared to that in the general population, which is about 1%.[22] Until about 6 years ago, a person at risk (child, grandchild, niece, or nephew of an affected patient) who was aware of the magnitude of the risk, had no option than to observe with anguish the symptoms if they appeared. In the past, the diagnosis and its implications were rarely discussed within families. This was sometimes in the hope that once the affected member(s) died, the disease would be eliminated and perhaps more frequently, because relatives were unaware and uninformed about the genetic aspects involved. The gene for Huntington's disease is on chromosome 4p,[23] and molecular markers in its close vicinity have enabled the differentiation between affected and unaffected individuals. Although this is a major scientific breakthrough, it has done little to alleviate the suffering of those at risk. Many who are aware of the available information choose not to be tested. They elect to continue to live with the hope that they have escaped the disease, rather than live with the knowledge that they have not. Extensive counseling and support must be available to families seeking information and testing for Huntington's disease. Confirmation of the diagnosis (a crucial step in the evaluation process) should be followed by several informative and explanatory sessions with the family and individuals at risk. If the family is available for testing and found to be informative, more support, counseling, and discussions are needed before the collection of blood from individuals at risk. It must be clear that they may reconsider whether they wish to know the results at any time during the process—even after testing is complete. The above also applies, of course, to couples contemplating pregnancy. Prenatal diagnosis of Huntington's disease is available if desired, as is testing of the member of the couple at risk. The magnitude of the decision whether to terminate the pregnancy of an affected fetus is immeasurable. There are centers in this country where prenatal diagnosis of Huntington's disease will not be offered unless the couple agrees to terminate the pregnancy of an affected fetus. In my opinion, that is a paternalistic attitude because Huntington's disease is not different from other prenatally detectable late-onset diseases. The parents, prepared by counselors for the decision-making process, are helped to make the one that is right for them, their family, and their lives. However, as for all other genetic diseases, preparation for prenatal diagnosis in the form of confirmation, discussions, and identification of relevant family members for testing must be made before or as soon after conception as possible.

A list of some autosomal-dominant inherited disorders for which prenatal testing may be contemplated is provided in Table 13–8.

Autosomal Recessive Inheritance

General Principles. The difference between autosomal dominant and recessive inheritance is simple. In the former, the *abnormal* (or dysfunctional) gene dominates, and therefore the trait or disease is manifested in heterozygotes. In the latter, the *normal* gene dominates, and therefore the trait or disease usually is not manifested in heterozygotes. It is apparent only in individuals who are homozygous for the abnormal or dysfunctional gene, which must be present on both chromosomes of a homologous pair. Thus, heterozygote carriers of an abnormal recessive gene are healthy and have no overt signs of disease; the gene is carried silently, with no implications for health, development, or reproduction. It is well known that about eight to ten deleterious recessive genes exist in heterozygous

TABLE 13–8. COMMON AUTOSOMAL-DOMINANT DISORDERS FOR WHICH PRENATAL TESTING MAY BE CONTEMPLATED

Diagnosis	Characteristics	Prenatal Testing	Comment
Acrocephalosyndactyly group	Unusual head shape; digital anomalies with or without MR; with or without additional malformations	Serial ultrasound—limbs, head shape	Variable expression
Bone Dysplasias			
Achondroplasia	Short-limbed rhizomelic dwarfism	Ultrasound but very difficult to distinguish from normal measurement <20 weeks	Accurate diagnosis in newborn period important
Heterozygous	Nonlethal, characteristic phenotype and radiology		
Homozygous	Lethal—in early infancy or childhood	Ultrasound (serial measurement rhizomelic shortening)	Both parents affected
Osteogenesis imperfecta multiple types	Blue sclerae; increased number of fractures; otosclerosis	Ultrasound (serial scans and measurement)—bowing, fractures, thinning	Accurate diagnosis before testing
Connective Tissue Dysplasias			
Marfan syndrome	Tall stature (for family); dolichostenomelia; arachnodactyly; joint hyperextensibility; *pectus excavatum;* scoliosis; dislocation of lens; aortic root dilatation	Ultrasound, limb measurement (not reliable)	Management of mother during pregnancy
Stickler syndrome	Cleft palate; mandibular micrognathia; Pierre Robin sequence; myopia; deafness; hypotonia; loose joints	Ultrasound (oral clefting); no other reliable yet chromosome 12q in some families	Feeding difficulty in newborn
Huntington's Disease	Involuntary movements; progressive personality change; dementia; degeneration; loss of all functions	Gene on 4pter—p16.2 DNA analysis (CVS, amniocentesis) preceded by comprehensive counseling and information	Counseling support for patient and family
Multiple Malformation Syndromes	Depends on type	Serial ultrasound	
Opitz-Frias	Ocular hypertelorism; oral clefting; laryngotracheoesophageal clefting; congenital heart disease; umbilical hernia; hypospadias; bifid scrotum; imperforate anus	Serial ultrasound (polyhydramnios, clefting)	LTE complications may lead to sudden death
Neurocutaneous Disorders			
Neurofibromatosis type I	Cutaneous *cafe-au-lait* macules; neurofibromata; osseous changes; learning and developmental delays; seizures; optic glioma	Gene on 17q11.2 DNA analysis (CVS or amnio)	Variable expression
Neurofibromatosis type II	"Central" form; meningiomata, central and spinal; acoustic neuroma	Gene on 22q11-q13 DNA analysis (CVS or amnio)	Frequent recurrence of tumors
Tuberous sclerosis	Cutaneous pigmented and depigmented patches; fibroadenomas; hamartomas; CNS; mental retardation progression; seizures	Gene on chromosome 9q DNA analysis (CVS or amnio); ultrasound (fetal rhabdomyoma)	Very variable expression
Waardenburg's Syndrome	See text	Gene on chromosome 2q35 − 37.3	

form in the genome of every human being. They are transmitted silently and inapparently from generation to generation, and their existence remains unknown. If a union takes place of two related individuals (consanguinity), two individuals of common ethnic origin, or two unrelated individuals who both are heterozygous carriers of the same dysfunctional, deleterious gene, then their offspring have an increased risk of inheriting the unfavorable gene from each parent. This results in homozygosity and therefore in the expression of the disease.

Characteristics of autosomal recessive inheritance include (1) manifestations are present in one sibship only; (2) parents are unaffected, healthy heterozygous carriers of the gene; (3) Both sexes are affected equally; (4) Only two healthy heterozygous parent carriers can transmit the disease—they have a 1 in 4 or 25% risk of having affected offspring; (5) the degree of severity usually is not as variable as in dominantly inherited disorders.

Clinical manifestations of autosomally recessively inherited disorders are, in general, caused by the effects of the absence of a normal gene product or enzyme (eg, the alpha subunit of hexosaminidase A [hex A] in Tay-Sachs disease or α-1-iduronidase in Hurler's syndrome) or by the presence of an abnormal gene product (eg, Hemoglobin S in sickle cell disease). In single (heterozygous) form, the effects of abnormal genes are masked by the presence of the normal allele. For example, although a person heterozygous for Tay-Sachs Disease has less total activity of hex A than someone who is homozygous for both normal alleles, the remaining hex A activity ensures normal metabolism. Similarly, a heterozygote for Hurler Syndrome is no different from the general population, and, in fact, enzyme levels of heterozygotes frequently overlap with those of healthy homozygotes. Because the absence of the normal gene product is needed for manifestation of a recessive disorder, it is more probable that a consanguineous couple with genes in common will have a child with an autosomal recessive disorder than a couple who is unrelated. However, the risk for any recessive disorder in the offspring of a first cousin union is not greater than 2%. It is this risk on which the ruling of the Catholic Church is based, forbidding first cousin marriages in many states of this country. It is probable, however, that the true reason was unclear to the original authors of the ban.

In considering pregnancy in association with autosomal recessive disorders, several issues are raised. They include the type of the disorder, whether it is a parent who is affected or a fetus who is at risk, and whether and by what method the disorder is prenatally detectable.

Types of Disorders. For the purposes of this discussion, autosomal recessive disorders can be divided into three groups: those detectable in heterozygotes before the birth of an affected child, those detectable only after the birth of an affected child, and those that cannot be detected in heterozygotes at all.

DETECTABLE IN HETEROZYGOTES. Many inborn errors of metabolism are inherited in an autosomal recessive way. In some, the enzyme deficiency is known and detectable in heterozygotes before the birth of a first affected infant. As mentioned previously, carriers of Tay-Sachs disease, occurring more frequently in persons of Ashkenazi Jewish origin, can be detected by determining hex A levels in the population at risk. If two carriers are contemplating pregnancy, there is a 25% or 1 in 4 risk for an affected child, and prenatal diagnosis can be offered. Preparation for pregnancy is important in this situation also because serum hex A levels are decreased during early pregnancy, and testing during that time may lead to false positive results.

Accepted protocol for prenatal diagnosis of Tay-Sachs disease consists of carrier testing of the population at risk before conception. If a woman is pregnant, only the father should be tested; if he is not heterozygous, there is no risk to the pregnancy. If he is found to be a carrier, the mother's leucocyte hex A level must be tested (a much more accurate test than that in the serum). If the mother is found to be at carrier level, only then should fetal hex A be tested, either in chorionic villus sampling (CVS) (before 11 weeks) or in amniocytes.

Detectable After the Birth of an Affected Child. Risks for other inborn errors of metabolism (eg, lysosomal or other storage disorders) either cannot be detected in heterozygotes before the birth of a first affected child or are so rare and not known to occur more in any particular population group, that, even if detectable in heterozygotes, it is currently not feasible to screen the general population to identify carriers. After the birth of an affected child and the establishment of the accurate biochemical diagnosis of an autosomal recessive disorder, however, it is important to obtain specific information about the type of prenatal testing available and the nationally centralized laboratories or centers performing it. Most enzymes are detectable on samples from chorionic villi and from amniocytes, and early and systematically planned prenatal testing is most beneficial. The Catalog of Prenatally Diagnosed Conditions[24] is a helpful resource.

NOT DETECTABLE IN HETEROZYGOTES. The causes of many autosomally recessively inherited disorders have eluded us. For example, Smith-Lemli-Opitz syndrome or ectodactyly and ectodermal dysplasia clefting (EEC) syndrome at least are characterized by structural malformations. If clearly defined as part of the syndrome, they are potentially detectable on ultrasound (Fig. 13–18) and therefore also are prenatally detectable. Other disorders which are not associated with a known biochemical or molecular defect or with structural malformations cannot be diagnosed prenatally, and currently, the only information available to families about recurrence is in the form of statistical risks.

Parents Affected with Autosomal Recessive Disorders. If a parent is known to have an autosomal recessive disorder, there is no risk that offspring will be similarly affected, unless the other parent also is affected or heterozygous for the gene in question. This is unlikely because while cumulatively common, individual recessive genes are usually rare. Therefore, the hazards for the fetus of a mother with an autosomal recessive metabolic disorder originate not from risks for recurrence of the disease, but from the unfavorable intrauterine environment created by the affected mother's impaired metabolism. For example, a young woman diagnosed at birth with *phenylketonuria* (PKU) and treated by the appropriate low phenylalanine diet, has successfully avoided the mental retardation and other complications associated with untreated PKU. She has led a normal life and conceived. Phenylketonuria is caused by a deficiency of the enzyme phenylalanine hydroxylase (see also Chapters 30–31); this leads to secondary accumulation of the amino acid phenylalanine and results in mental retardation and other toxic effects. Treatment consists of a diet that avoids phenylalanine throughout childhood. It has been well documented that young women with treated

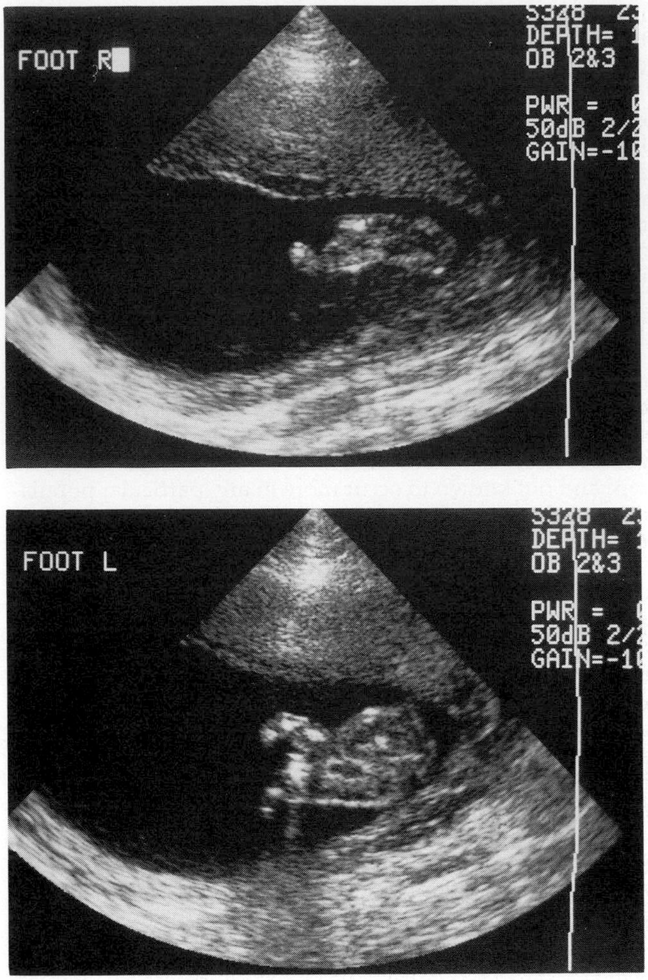

Figure 13–18. Ultrasound of feet of 20-week-old fetus with ectodactyly.

PKU have offspring who are mentally retarded, microcephalic, and otherwise malformed.[25] The reasons are unclear. All offspring are heterozygous; they do not have PKU, yet they are all mentally retarded. It is possible that if the mother follows the phenylalanine-free diet from before conception throughout pregnancy, fetal complications could be prevented, but insufficient experience exists. It is hoped that the national collaborative study on maternal PKU will provide answers to some of these questions. Similar risks apply to offspring of young women with other appropriately treated metabolic disorders.

In summary, it is essential that a young woman with a known autosomal recessive metabolic disorder seek counseling from an informed geneticist long before she considers conception so that all available management and options can be discussed.

Methods of Detection of Autosomal Recessive Disorders. Until recently, only statistical risks for disease recurrence or carrier status were available to families with autosomal recessive disorders of unknown etiology. For example, the recurrence risk for a couple with a child with *cystic fibrosis* (CF), as for any autosomally recessively inherited disorder, is 1 in 4 or 25%. The risk that the sibling of a patient with CF would have similarly affected offspring is the product of the probability that he or she is a carrier ($\frac{2}{3}$); the probability that the partner, if unrelated, is a carrier ($\frac{1}{20}$, the carrier rate for CF in the general population); and the probability that they would have an affected child ($\frac{1}{4}$). The risk, then, to a sibling of an affected patient for offspring with CF is $\frac{2}{3} \times \frac{1}{20} \times \frac{1}{4} = \frac{1}{120}$. Before molecular diagnosis of CF, its prenatal diagnosis was unreliable. Even though it was known that alkaline phosphatase activity was decreased or absent in the amniotic fluid of most fetuses with CF,[26] the test had a relatively high error rate, 2% to 5%, and it was not possible to confirm the presence or absence of disease in terminated pregnancies.

It is now known that the gene for CF is located on chromosome 7q31–32.[27] With the help of markers in its vicinity and with the recent recognition of specific molecular haplotypes that occur more frequently in individuals with the CF gene than in those without, it is possible to diagnose the disease prenatally by comparing markers of parents and affected patients with those of the fetus and to identify carriers by evaluating their haplotypes (see also Chapter 14).

Although still valid, this method was obsolete the day it was written. On August 23, 1989, a press release was issued that the CF gene had been isolated as a result of collaboration between scientists at the Hospital for Sick Children in Toronto (Lap-Chee Tsui and John Riordan and colleagues) and Francis Collins and colleagues at the Howard Hughes Medical Institute at the University of Michigan, Ann Arbor. The protein produced by the gene is called the *CF transmembrane regulator* (CFTR)[30]. In about 70% of people who have the gene, there is a three-base pair deletion which results in mutation and malfunction of the CFTR. This is called the ΔF508 mutation. The remaining 30% of CF patients do not have this mutation; it is estimated that they have about 40 additional mutations, many of which are as yet undectectable.

There are enormous problems and confusion. For example, the absence of the ΔF508 mutation in an individual (or fetus) does not preclude carrier or disease status. Does the presence of ΔF508 mutation in one parent but not the other of a CF-affected child indicate nonpaternity? Does it indicate the presence of one of the other undetectable gene mutations? Does the presence of the ΔF508 mutation in one but not the other member of a childless couple indicate that they are not at risk for having an affected child or does it just decrease their risk? By how much? Will the presence or absence of the ΔF508 mutation in a patient with CF be correlated with the severity, prophylaxis and types of treatment of the disease? How should this be explained to families, to their physicians, their insurance companies? How can they be helped to make informed decisions with this overwhelming amount of confusing information?

Couples desiring information about CF carrier status or risks for offspring are referred to a genetics center where up-to-date testing can be indicated, initiated, and applied to the family. The situation in 1991 is not yet favorable for mass screening of the general population for carrier status.

A list of some autosomally recessively inherited disorders for which prenatal diagnosis can be contemplated is given in Table 13–9.

Sex-Linked Inheritance

Y-Linked Inheritance. If a mutant gene is located on the X chromosome, its effects are said to be X-linked. If it is on the Y chromosome, it would be Y-linked. For practical pur-

TABLE 13–9. COMMON AUTOSOMAL-RECESSIVE DISORDERS FOR WHICH PRENATAL DIAGNOSIS MAY BE CONTEMPLATED

Diagnosis	Characteristics	Prenatal Testing	Comment
Bone Dysplasia Osteogenesis imperfecta type II	Depends on type; severe multiple fractures; lethal	Ultrasound; fractures, bowing, thinning	Accurate diagnosis before conception
Cystic Fibrosis	Viscous secretions of exocrine glands; digestive, respiratory symptoms; meconium ileus neonatally; respiratory failure later; growth failure; early death	Gene on 7q31-32; In families at increased risk DNA analysis before conception, before death of affected patient; fetal DNA analysis (CVS, amnio)	[a]
Metabolic Disorder[b]			
Hurler syndrome	Progressive mucopolysaccharidosis type I; coarse features; deterioration; dysostosis; hepatosplenomegaly; childhood death	Gene not localized; evaluate deficiency of enzyme α iduronidase in CVS or amnio.	Carrier detection not reliable
Others	Depends on metabolic defect in question	If enzyme deficiency known	See references 24 and 41
Hemoglobinopathies Sickle cell disease	Depends on type; sickling crises; pain; infections; strokes	β gene on 16p15.5 direct detection (CVS, amnio) of mutated gene	
Malformation Syndromes Smith-Lemli-Opitz	IUGR; microcephaly; GI, GU malformations; polydactyly; hypotonia; developmental delays	Ultrasound; serial scans	Spectrum varies from mild to severe; physical and developmental abnormalities not always correlated

[a] Information about the isolation of the CF gene was released on August 23, 1989. Therefore, prenatal diagnosis will probably be base analysis (CVS, amnio) in the majority of families, and carrier testing will be available for the general population.

[b] The reader is referred to references 24 and 41 for lists of prenatally diagnosable disorders and detailed metabolic disorders, respectively.

poses, the important genes on the Y chromosome are those that determine maleness. They include the testis differentiating factor and others that control the Y histocompatibility (H–Y) antigen. That is why individuals who have at least one Y chromosome, irrespective of the number of Xs (eg, 49,XXXXY) are always male. No diseases are known to be transmitted through the Y chromosome, and only one trait, hairy ears, is questionably and controversially thought to be. It is more probable that hairy ears are Y limited rather than Y linked. There is some evidence that tooth size also could be Y determined.[28] In situations of phenotypic sexual ambiguity, however, it may be helpful to use Y-linked DNA probes to detect the presence of Y chromosomal material in individuals in whom it would be undetectable.[29]

X-Linked Dominant Inheritance. Genes on the X chromosome may be dominantly or recessively inherited. Characteristics of X-linked dominant inheritance include the following:

1. Absence of male-to-male transmission
2. Prevalence of affected females
3. Because affected males are hemizygous and heterozygous females have the benefit of a "normal" allele on their other X chromosome, expression of an X-linked dominant disorder is expected to be so much more severe in males that it is frequently lethal.
4. Statistical risks indicate that 50% of the daughters of an affected mother will be affected and 50% of the sons of an affected mother will be affected. The latter can, in many instances result in prenatal or perinatal loss.
5. All daughters of affected males would be affected.

Examples of disorders inherited in this manner include the Xg blood group, Aarskog syndrome, *incontinentia pigmenti,* vitamin D resistant hypophosphatemic rickets, and ornithine transcarbamylase deficiency.

The problems and pitfalls mentioned in the discussion of autosomal dominant inheritance, such as the existence of new mutations, variable expression, and diagnostic accuracy, apply here also. For example, a couple was referred for genetics evaluation because they had lost two pregnancies and had a mentally retarded daughter (the oldest of two). The older daughter's medical history revealed a characteristic picture of *incontinentia pigmenti* with typical transitory skin changes documented in infancy (erythema, blisters, pigmentation). This X-linked dominant disorder is variably associated with mental retardation. On evaluation at age 5 years, the child was developmentally delayed with typical dysplastic pigmentary skin changes (the acute pemphiginous morphs had disappeared). The parents' concern was mental retardation in future offspring. Careful evaluation of the younger daughter revealed milder but characteristic pigmentary changes. She had had no other rashes and was intellectually advanced for her age. This was obviously not a new mutation in the older daughter. The mother was unaware of any abnormalities in her own skin until detailed questioning of the maternal grandmother revealed that in early childhood the mother had had rashes which "had disappeared," similar to those in her older daughter. She had remnants of mild pigmentary dysplasia. The risk, therefore, was 50% that another daughter would be affected and that a son could be lost prenatally or perinatally. The risk for mental retardation was less than 50%, but unknown.

Methods and techniques for prenatal diagnosis in situations of X-linked dominant inheritance depend, as always, on the specific disorder. If it is a metabolic disorder, such as *ornithine transcarbamylase* (OTC) *deficiency,* evaluation will be predominantly biochemical; if it is a structural disorder, ultrasound can be informative. If, as in *incontinentia pigmenti,* there are no prenatally detectable signs of the disease, the only option available to the family (aside from adoption or refraining from pregnancy) is sex determination and the provision of as much information as possible about the clinical course and spectrum of the disease. In addition, if the location of the gene on the X chromosome is known, it may be possible to determine whether or not the fetus inherited the X with or without the abnormal gene. Sex selection before implantation and possibly even selection of the "normal" X chromosome is a new, not completely reliable, rapidly developing technique. Thus, molecular diagnosis is already changing the outlook for the prenatal diagnosis of many of these diseases, and specific up-to-date information should be sought for each individual couple before or as early during the pregnancy as possible[24] (see also Chapter 14).

X-Linked Recessive Inheritance

Disorders inherited in an X-linked recessive manner are more common than those caused by dominant genes on the X-chromosome. Characteristics include the following:

1. Absence of male-to-male transmission
2. Affected males are prevalent. Although hemizygous, the mutant recessive gene is expressed in males in a single dose because there is no "normal" allele to mitigate the dysfunction of the mutant one (genes on the Y chromosome are different and not allelic to those on the X).
3. The classic pattern of inheritance in pedigrees is from unaffected females to affected males. Unaffected males cannot transmit the disorder. All daughters of affected males are carriers, half the daughters of female carriers are carriers, and half their sons are affected.
4. Truly affected females must be homozygous; that is, they must be the daughters of a carrier female–affected male union.
5. Heterozygous females should be, theoretically, unaffected as are heterozygotes for autosomal recessive traits. The X chromosome, however, is different from the autosomes because *only one* of all X chromosomes per cell (two in normal females, three in 47,XXX females, four in 49,XXXXY males) is active and functional.

In a female with normal chromosomes (46,XX), one X chromosome becomes inactivated at an early (possibly the 16 cell) stage of embryonic development. This was first suggested in 1961 by Mary Lyon and is known as the *Lyon hypothesis*.[31] Inactivation of one of the X chromosomes in female cells is random. That is, either the paternal or the maternal X may be inactivated or remain active. On average, inactivation of the maternal and paternal X occurs equally. However, if by chance the X containing the normal allele is inactivated in more than 50% of the cells and more than 50% of the cells have an active X with the mutant allele, then the effects of the mutant allele will be manifested in a female who is truly heterozygous. Before the stage of inactivation in normal females, both X chromosomes are active. The lack of function of both X chromosomes before inactivation is thought to be one of the causes of the phenotypic abnormalities in females with Turner's syndrome, who are lacking one of their chromosomes from the zygous state.

Examples of common disorders inherited in an X-linked recessive way include red–green color blindness, hemophilia A and B, Duchenne muscular dystrophy (DMD), and X-linked mental retardation (Table 13–10).

Counseling for families with X-linked disorders has become easier with therapeutic and technologic advances. Ten years ago if a woman with a son who had Hemophilia A or DMD became pregnant, she had no choice other than fetal sex determination and, if male, to risk the birth of an affected son or the termination of a healthy one. Our experience shows that most couples in this situation chose the former option. It was impossible to distinguish between an affected and unaffected male fetus. Advances in treatment of hemophilia have improved the outlook for the life of affected boys, and earlier prenatal testing (chorionic

TABLE 13–10. COMMON X-LINKED RECESSIVE DISORDERS FOR WHICH PRENATAL TESTING MAY BE CONTEMPLATED

Diagnosis	Characteristics	Prenatal Testing	Comment
Duchenne muscular dystrophy	Progressive clumsiness; weakness; inability to walk; respiratory failure	Gene: Xp21; family DNA analysis; fetal sex (CVS, amnio); fetal DNA analysis	Carrier detection of females by DNA analysis before conception
Fragile X syndrome	Macro-orchidism; characteristic long face, ears; connective tissue dysplasia; characteristic personality; mental retardation	Gene: Xq27.3; fetal sex (CVS, amnio); fragile X testing; DNA analysis	Carrier detection of females by fragile X and DNA analysis
Hemophilia A	Bleeding diathesis affects large joints	Gene: Xq28; family DNA analysis; fetal sex (CVS, amnio) fetal DNA analysis	Carrier detection of females; treatment of patients
Hemophilia B	Less severe than A	Gene: Xq26.3–27.2; as above	As above
Hunter syndrome	Progressive storage disorder; Mucopolysaccharidosis type II; coarsening of features; dysostosis; hepatosplenomegaly lethal	Gene: Xq27–28; fetal sex (CVS, amnio, deficient iduronate sulfatase activity in CV or amniotic cells)	Carrier detection not reliable
X-Linked hydrocephalus	Congenital hydrocephalus; aqueductal stenosis; hypoplastic thumbs; mental retardation	Gene not located; ultrasound (CNS and thumb abnormalities)	No known carrier detection
X-Linked mental retardation (several types)	Depends on type (spastic diplegia) macrocephaly, seizures	Some genes located; fetal sex determination, DNA analysis if applicable	Carrier detection not possible (unless gene location known)

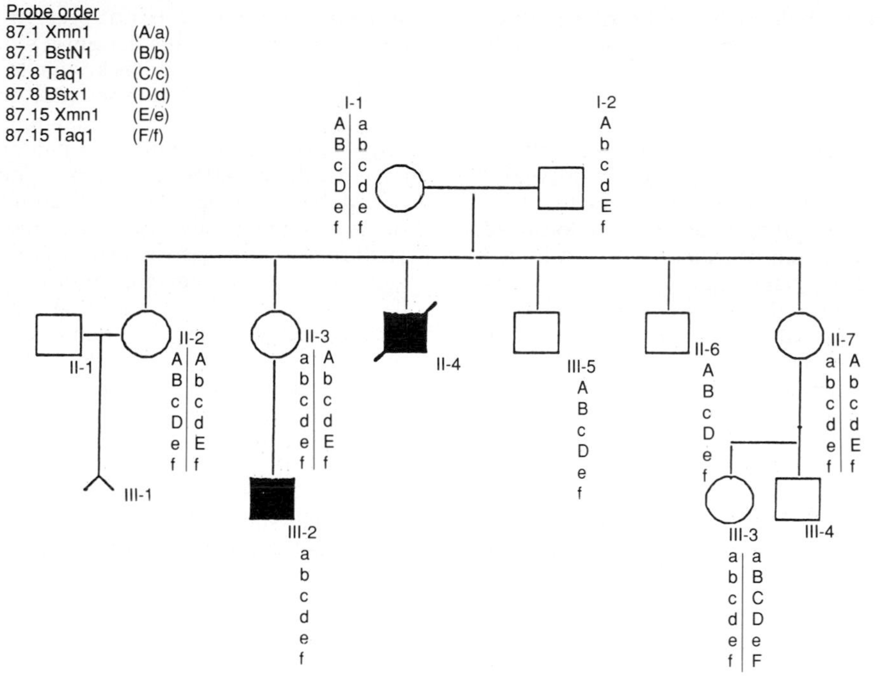

Figure 13–19. Pedigree of family with Duchenne muscular dystrophy showing origin of X chromosome in at-risk females. Note: grandmother I–1, daughters II–3 and II–7, grandson III–2 and granddaughter III–3 all have X chromosome with DMD gene.

villus sampling at 9–11 weeks) and molecular analysis have contributed to the greater specificity of information available to families in these tragic situations (Fig. 13–19).

Fragile X Mental Retardation. Fragile X mental retardation is the only disorder inherited in mendelian fashion that has an identifiable cytogenetic marker. It is estimated that mental retardation associated with the cytogenetic phenomenon known as fragile X (Fig. 13–20) occurs in about 1 in 1000 births. Its incidence therefore equals that of Down's syndrome, and since it is inherited, it is the most common recognizable inherited disorder that results in mental retardation.

The history of this complex type of familial mental retardation is characterized by the confluence of what were originally thought to be two artifacts. The first was the explanation of the predominance of males in the mentally retarded population, recognized as early as the 1930s. Because most retarded populations surveyed were residents of institutions,[32] the larger population of males within them was attributable to social, rather than mathematical, phenomena. Retarded males were more likely to be institutionalized, while females were more likely to be kept at home to help with simple chores.

The second artifact was the observation by Lubs[33] that the X chromosome of each of two retarded brothers, analyzed by chance in folate-deficient medium, had what he thought were satellites on the distal portion of the long arms. The medium was no longer in routine use, and the phenomenon, although reported, was not considered significant, particularly because other investigators using more current media were unable to reproduce it.

It was not until 1971 that Turner and colleagues[34] and Davison[35] found that the excess of males among the mentally retarded population was a real phenomenon, attributable to a gene or genes on the X chromosome. In 1973, Sutherland[36] confirmed that in some retarded males, a real marker, now known as the fragile X site (Fig. 13–20), occurred in chromosomes cultured in folic acid or thymidine-deficient medium. It is now known that the marker site is located on Xq27.3. Another recently recognized common fragile site, Xq27.1, is present in many individuals and is not associated with retardation or other known pathology. This has been the cause of some confusion and should be carefully differentiated from the true marker. Further confusion in the diagnosis, particularly prenatal diagnosis (see below), is caused by the presence of the fragile site in only a proportion of the cells of affected individuals, ranging from 3–40%, and in an even more variable number of cells in carrier females.

The clinical manifestations in individuals with fragile X mental retardation are characterized by a triad of symptoms frequently associated with signs of overgrowth. They include a characteristic facial appearance (long face with a large, prominent mandible); long, anteriorly cupped ears; and macro-orchidism demonstrable even in childhood. Testicular volume in adults is frequently twice or three times above that in the general population, which is about 25 cm^3. It is thought to be caused by histologic hypocellularity associated with an abundance of hydrophillic glycoprotein granules. This finding has been observed in the testicular tissue of fetuses. The personality of individuals with fragile X mental retardation also is characteristic. Perseverative behaviors and speech are common, as are some autistic features and mannerisms. Children frequently are hyperactive and difficult to control. Aversion of glance during con-

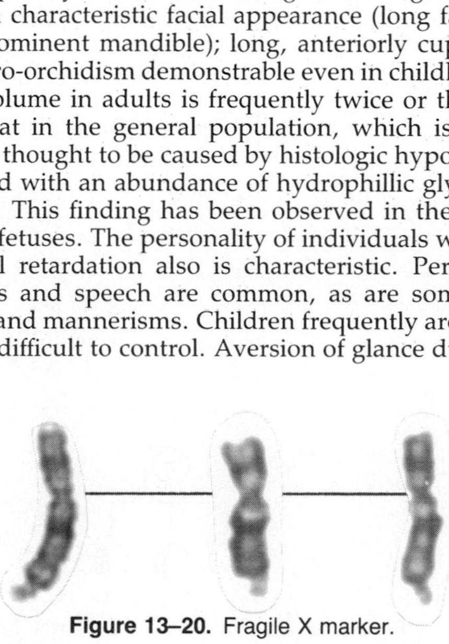

Figure 13–20. Fragile X marker.

versation may characterize both males and carrier females, and sudden emotional outbursts may cease as unexpectedly as they begin.

GENETICS. Fragile X mental retardation is one of the most complicated stories in medical genetics. In most families it is associated with the presence of the fragile site on Xq27.3, and, although it is probable that the gene causing the disorder is also on the X chromosome, it has not been localized. The most probable mechanism of inheritance is X-linked, but there are several factors that complicate this hypothesis and that are different from the situation in most other X-linked recessive or dominant disorders. For example, in families with fragile X mental retardation, 30% of females who have the gene in single dose (carriers) have some degree of involvement ranging from mild to severe mental retardation. Secondly, 50% of obligate carriers (with affected sons and brothers) do not express the fragile site. Thirdly, it was found[37] that pedigree analysis resulted in 20% fewer affected males than would be expected if this disorder were inherited in a classic X-linked recessive way. The number of affected males was not decreased, but although males in these families had the mutation (they expressed or transmitted the cytogenetic phenomenon of the fragile X site), some of them were neither mentally retarded nor differed in any recognizable way from the general population. For example, it can be seen from Figure 13–21 that III, the grandfather of the propositus V, was unaffected (he was a university professor), but each of his three daughters, his sister, and his maternal female cousin are known carriers.

The theory that provides the best explanation for these unusual phenomena was suggested by Laird[38], who postulates that two phenomena are needed to account for the unusual segregation ratios in fragile X families. The first is called imprinting of the X chromosome; the second is the presence of the fragile site at Xq27.3 (the fragile X mutation). Imprinting occurs in preoogonial cells in which half of the randomly inactivated X chromosomes are reactivated. If the fragile site at Xq27.3 is present on that chromosome, the reactivation process is blocked at that site. Hence, the gene product(s) from that site will be absent, deleted, or will malfunction and will lead to the clinical picture of fragile X syndrome, even in females if there is a disproportionately large number of imprinted (reactivated) X chromosomes with the Xq27.3 mutation. Furthermore, imprinting occurs only in preoogonial cells; therefore, if the mutation occurs in a male, imprinting is not present until the mutation is transmitted through his daughter's oogonia.

No specific treatment is known to ameliorate the behavioral symptoms or developmental delays present in boys and girls with fragile X mental retardation. Psychogenic drugs have been used in some patients, and folic acid may have a calming effect on others. The hope that the latter would have therapeutic implications because the fragile site is cytogenetically expressed only in folic acid deficient medium has not been realized. Patients are not folic-acid deficient, and the metabolism of folic acid is not impaired. Behavioral and educational programming directed specifically at patients' individual needs has been most beneficial.

GENETIC COUNSELING. Chromosome analysis with a specific request for fragile X testing is indicated in any retarded male whose symptoms, appearance, or behaviors are suggestive of the fragile X syndrome. Once established, the diagnosis affects the whole family, and as many relatives as possible should be informed, evaluated, and provided with sensitive and supportive counseling. Options available to males and females of reproductive age must be discussed and offered.

PRENATAL DIAGNOSIS. It is important that the couple at risk be referred to a genetics center with experience in all aspects of diagnosis, and counseling for fragile X syndrome evaluation. In addition, the referring physician should ensure that the laboratories in which cytogenetic or molecular testing will be performed are equally familiar with the problems and pitfalls of this complex situation. At least two false negative results currently have been reported from chorionic villus sampling for fragile X. Hence, it seems that amniocentesis is the most reliable method to detect the presence of fragile X in fetal cells and to avoid false positive and false negative results. Even amniocytes, however, should be evaluated by two or more culture techniques to avoid error. Because female offspring also can be retarded, early sex determination is unhelpful in this case. Analysis of DNA to identify the X chromosome of the fetus for comparison with that of the parents and other family members (who ideally should have been evaluated before pregnancy), together with evaluation of fragile X in amniocytes using several methods followed by periumbilical blood sampling (PUBS) if appropriate, is probably the most reliable combination of tests for fragile X syndrome. If the fetus has the same X chromosome as the carrier mother or other affected

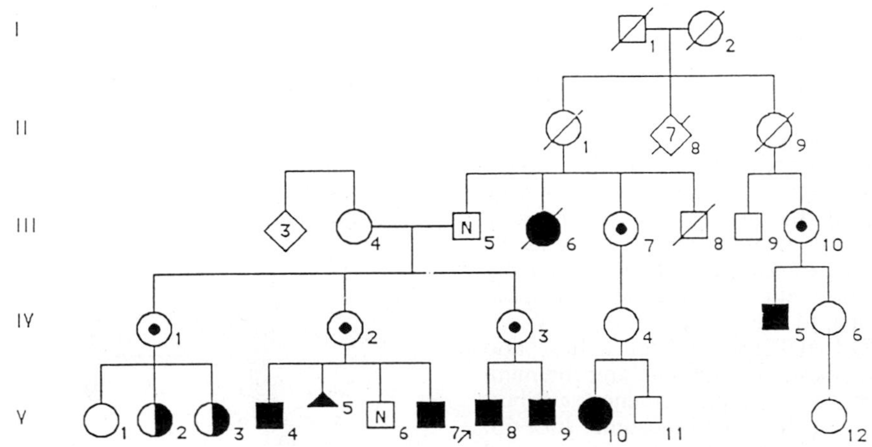

Figure 13–21. Pedigree of family with fragile X mental retardation, showing healthy, transmitting male, III/5.

individuals, the probability of recombination (crossing over) also must be considered and factored into the probability whether or not the fetus is affected. The newborn infant (or fetus if applicable) should be evaluated clinically and cytogenetically, and if affected, ongoing support and help for the family should be offered. See also Chapter 16.

MITOCHONDRIAL INHERITANCE

General Principles

Both chromosomal and mendelian inheritance discussed in the previous sections are characterized by the transmission of chromosomes to successive generations and with them, genes within the cell's nucleus. Hence, chromosomal and mendelian inheritance represent *nuclear inheritance* of DNA. DNA also exists outside the nucleus within the *cytoplasmic mitochondria.* Every human cell contains thousands of molecules of mitochondrial DNA (mtDNA), which is circular and consists of about 17,000 base pairs. Mitochondria contain separate types of RNA and ribosomes, which divide. They code for several of the subunits of the enzymes of adenosine triphosphate (ATP) generating oxidative phosphorylation. Because mitochondria are maternally derived, it is fascinating to speculate about the validity of recent findings published by the news media[39] attesting to the common origins of mitochondrial DNA of 147 females from five different geographic regions.

It is not the purpose of this chapter to provide a detailed review of mitochondrial inheritance; however, its existence cannot be ignored if accurate information is to be provided to couples in whom, or in whose family, there is suspicion of a mitochondrially transmitted disorder.

The genetic features of mitochondrial inheritance include the following:

1. It is inherited from the mother to the offspring of both sexes. Daughters then transmit it to their offspring. There is no male-to-male or male-to-female transmission; males do not transmit mitochondrial DNA.
2. If the mitochondrial genotype consists of both normal and mutant mtDNA, it is known as *heteroplasmic;* if it consists of only one type, it is *homoplasmic.* During cytokinesis (see Mitosis and Meiosis), mitochondria are partitioned randomly into daughter cells; therefore, the mtDNA genotype of a cell can shift from predominantly heteroplasmic to homoplasmic (mutant or normal) and vice versa.
3. The mtDNA cell phenotype depends on the proportion of mutant mtDNA and on the needs of the cell in question for intact mitochondrial function. Different tissues rely differently on energy derived through the mitochondrial oxidative phosphorylation process. Potential targets include the central nervous system, skeletal muscle, kidney, and liver in decreasing order of dependency.
4. It is thought that the frequency of deleterious mutations in a mtDNA oxidative phosphorylation gene is higher than that in its nuclear counterpart.

Disorders Thought to Be Transmitted by Mitochondrial Inheritance

The spectrum of diseases associated with changes in mtDNA is characterized by the following broad categories, depending on the nature of the mutation, the severity of the effects of the enzyme defect, and the presence or absence of heteroplasmy: *Leber's hereditary optic neuropathy* (LHON) consists of rapid, adolescent onset central vision loss through optic nerve death and inconsistent cardiac dysrhythmia. Affected individuals are always related through females; no paternal transmission has ever been documented. Expression can vary. Molecularly, this disease is thought to be the result of a conversion of arginine to histidine in a region that is important for electron transport. This results in reduced optic nerve cell ATP production and cell death. *Myoclonic epilepsy and ragged red muscle fiber disease* (MERRF) is probably caused by a point mutation in mtDNA through maternal lineage. It is characterized by signs such as subclinical changes in EEG, visual evoked response, myopathy (ragged red muscle fibers by Gomori stain), sensorineural hearing loss, myoclonic epilepsy, and cerebellar symptomatology. Ophthalmoplegia, retinopathy, dementia, seizures, strokes, and mitochondrial myopathy are characteristics of *Kearns-Sayre syndrome,* which is associated with a heteroplasmic mtDNA deletion at the molecular level. This is usually a sporadic event, and with one reported exception of an affected mother–daughter pair, a patient with Kearns-Sayre syndrome is usually the only affected member of the family.

If a family or medical history arouses suspicion of a mitochondropathy, it is recommended that a genetics center with experience in molecular diagnosis be contacted before or as early during the pregnancy as possible.

The principal differences between pedigrees indicative of mitochondrial and X-linked dominant inheritance are the absence of paternal transmission in the former and a significant predominance of affected females in the latter. Unfortunately, neither of these phenomena may be immediately apparent during the evaluation of a single family. For this reason, it is important to be aware of the existence of mitochondrial inheritance.

MULTIFACTORIAL INHERITANCE

General Principles

Individuals who have disorders inherited through mechanisms described in the previous sections are usually easily distinguishable from the general population because they have or have not inherited the abnormal gene or chromosomal rearrangement in question. Therefore, they are genotypically clearly discontinuous from the general population, and the incidence of the disorder follows a binomial or trinomial curve. For example, if the gene for cystic fibrosis is considered, one in 1600 individuals in the population at risk will be affected homozygotes; one in 20 will be heterozygotes; and the remaining, about 95%, will be unaffected homozygotes. However, not all inherited disorders are caused by microscopically visible changes in the chromosomes, by abnormalities in single genes, or even by isolated changes in mitochondrial DNA. Some normal physiologic characteristics are determined by a combination of genetic and nongenetic or environmental factors. Many of these characteristics account for variations within families and populations such as height; weight; head circumference; intelligence; blood pressure; birth defects, such as neural tube or congenital heart defects; cleft lip with or without cleft palate; commonly occurring diseases such as mental illness; some types of diabetes mellitus, and coronary heart disease. They are said to be *multifactorially inherited.*

If an attempt is made to determine the mechanism whereby the genetic component of these traits is transmitted, it becomes clear that there is no dominance and *many* genes are involved. When it is possible to express such a trait mathematically as a function of incidence in the population, it usually follows a unimodal continuous distribution in the form of a normal or Gaussian curve. However, it is well known that even the curve depicting IQ in the population is not perfectly bellshaped: there are more individuals at the lower end (IQs below 70) than at the upper end (IQs above 130). This phenomenon can be explained by the partition within the mentally retarded population of some disorders with an unknown, but definitive, genetic component. A similar concept applies to the presence within the population of a combination of additive *polygenic* and environmental factors. If present in a "favorable" constellation, this combination may lead to the occurrence of a birth defect, such as cleft lip with or without cleft palate or a neural tube defect.

It is not possible to construct a mathematically accurate function of the combination of genetic and environmental factors contributing to the occurrence, within a population, of a given birth defect. It is possible, however, to assume that for some birth defects or commonly occurring diseases, there is a graded continuum of causal parameters. The parameters are several genes plus the necessary environmental factors which, in a specific combination, give rise to the disease or birth defect. This continuum is called *liability*, and, in the general population, it forms a bell-shaped curve. Once the combination of liability factors results in a birth defect, it has exceeded beyond the threshold of liability and entered the sphere of increased risk. Because relatives have genes in common (offspring and siblings have one half, grandchildren one quarter, first cousins one eighth, and identical twins all their genes in common), there is always a greater probability that the risk of recurrence within a family of a multifactorially determined birth defect or disease will be greater than its incidence in the general population. The bell-shaped curve will shift to the right, and the probability of exceeding the threshold is greater the closer the relationship between the affected and at-risk individual (Fig. 13–22). The incidence and recurrence risks for some commonly occurring birth defects and diseases given in Table 13–10 serve as a useful guide for the practicing physician. The multifactorial model of inheritance of some birth defects is one of many suggested, but never completely applicable, mathematic theories for their incidence and recurrence risks.[39a] A recent new development using molecular techniques deserves mention. Ardinger and colleagues[39b] have suggested that a major-locus model best

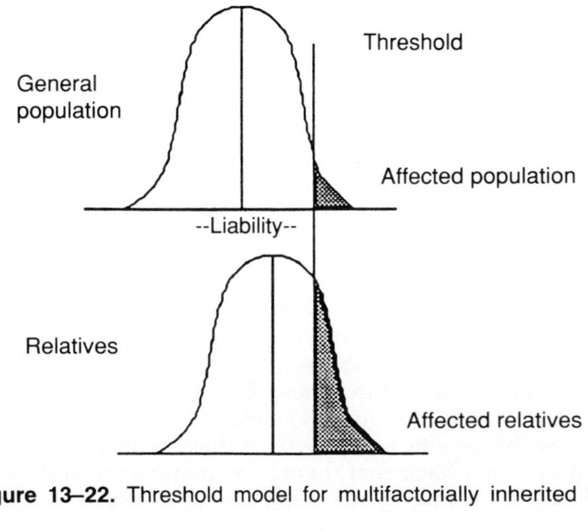

Figure 13–22. Threshold model for multifactorially inherited trait.

explains the recurrence of cleft lip and palate in Caucasian families. They found a significant association between two restriction fragment length polymorphisms at the locus, called transforming growth factor alpha on chromosome 2p13, in some individuals with nonsyndromic cleft lip and palate. This is one of the first attempts to explore molecularly the events underlying the occurrence of clefting malformations in humans.

Five practical considerations must be kept in mind before genetic counseling is offered for the disorders mentioned in Table 13–11.

1. As always in medical genetics, an accurate diagnosis is of utmost importance. For example, in a series of stillbirths[40-42], the diagnosis of anencephaly (part of the spectrum of neural tube defects) was reported on four of the fetal death forms. In reality, only two had true anencephaly, and the others were examples of the limb body wall disruption sequence.
2. Multifactorially determined birth defects are frequently single, isolated birth defects. Before the provision of information about recurrence, it is important to ensure that the condition in question is truly an isolated, single malformation of the type under consideration. If it is not, recurrence risks may differ dramatically. For example, a midline facial clefting malformation can be part of a *developmental field defect*, which affects the midline structures of the brain and may result in a clinical picture known as alobar holoprosencephaly. This can be inherited as a single gene disorder and may manifest genetic heterogeneity. Minor signs in a parent can indicate dominance, while similarly affected siblings from unaffected parents are characteristic of autosomal recessive inheritance; both have been reported, as have instances of new dominant mutations. All of these are different from the approximate 4% recurrence risk for the sibling of one child affected with an isolated cleft lip and palate.
3. Although multifactorially determined birth defects tend to have generally applicable recurrence risks within families, some, such as certain rare congenital heart defects, specifically have a lower recurrence risk than would be generally expected.
4. The incidence of specific birth defects may vary in different populations. For example, it is well known that neural tube defects (NTD) occur in as many as 8 per 1000 newborns in Ireland and only in 1–2 per 1000 in Wisconsin. Recurrence risks are correlated with incidence and although the risk for recurrence after the birth of an infant with a NTD in the former population is 5%, that in the latter is only 3%.
5. Prenatal diagnosis in the form of alpha fetoprotein (AFP) screening, ultrasound, fetal echocardiogram, and amniocentesis, must be considered and offered. Although the prevention of neural tube defects by the addition of folic acid to the mother's diet before and during pregnancy has not been documented definitively, it is an option that can be considered.

PRINCIPLES OF APPLIED TERATOLOGY

General Principles

It is estimated that 9–10% of birth defects are the result of maternal exposure to exogenous agents.[43] It is, therefore, impossible to address the causes of human malformations without also considering the role of the environment. Many of the questions asked by pregnant women concern the

TABLE 13–11. EMPIRIC RECURRENCE RISKS FOR COMMON MULTIFACTORIALLY DETERMINED DISORDERS FOR WHICH PRENATAL DIAGNOSIS MAY BE CONTEMPLATED

	Approximate Recurrence Risk (%) If Affected Relative(s)					
	None	One sibling or parent	Two siblings or one sibling one parent	2°[a]	Prenatal Testing	Comment
Cleft lip with or without palate	0.1	4	10–11	<1	↑ AFP (unreliable) U/S	Beware of single gene syndromes—e.g.
Cleft palate only	0.04	2–7	15	<1	↑ AFP (Unreliable) U/S polyhydramnios	Stickler syndrome; evaluate
Open neural tube defects						
Anenecephaly	0.1	3	8	1	↑ AFP and U/S and amniotic fluid acetylcholinesterase	Recurrence risk applies to any NTD
Meningomyelocele	0.1	3	8	1		
Congenital heart disease						
Any type	0.3	4–5	10–11	1	Fetal echocardiogram	Beware of concomitant malformation or syndromes; evaluate
Ventricular septal defect		3–4	10	<1	Fetal echocardiogram	
Patent ductus arteriosus		3–4	10	<1	Fetal echocardiogram	
Atrial septal defect		2–3	8	<1	Fetal echocardiogram	
Tetralogy of fallot		2–3	8		Fetal echocardiogram	
Pulmonary stenosis		2–3	6		Fetal echocardiogram	
Aortic stenosis		2–3	6		Fetal echocardiogram	
Hypoplastic left heart		2	6		Fetal echocardiogram	Can be autosomal dominant
VACTERL syndrome–association	*Characteristics:* Vertebral, anal, cardiac, tracheoesophageal, renal, limb (radial) malformations				AFP and ultrasound and fetal echocardiogram	Occurs more frequently in infants of diabetic mothers

[a] 2° = second degree relatives.
[b] *From Nova JJ, Fraser, FC.* Medical Genetics: Principles and Practice. *3rd ed. Philadelphia, PA: Lea & Febiger; 1989.*

effects of environmental factors, such as medication, maternal disease, alcohol, and drugs, on the developing fetus. In the past, their questions were addressed by obstetricians, primary care physicians, nurses, poison control centers, toxicologists, and others to whom the patient may have had access. Fortunately, in recent years, teratogen information services have been established around the country, and attempts are being made to address these issues more accurately.

Many teratogen information services are affiliated with genetics clinics because medical geneticists, trained in dysmorphology, are able to consider prenatal exposure to environmental agents as part of the differential diagnosis during the evaluation of patients with birth defects. Thalidomide, rubella infection, and alcohol are examples of known exogenous agents that can result in recognizable malformation syndromes. Future parents are concerned about many more situations, although it is generally surprising how few environmental agents have been clearly documented as teratogenic. It is usually difficult to establish a causal relationship between a congenital anomaly and prenatal exposure to an environmental agent. Of all the chemicals, pharmaceutical agents, and exogenous agents to which we are potentially exposed, less than 50 are proven teratogens.

In the literal context, a *teratogen* is a producer of monsters. A more recent and acceptable definition is any exogenous agent, chemical or physical, that can produce a permanent abnormality of structure or function in an organism that is exposed during embryonic or fetal life. Teratogenic effects, therefore, include structural malformations and functional deficits, such as mental retardation and behavioral abnormalities, which are not necessarily associated with gross malformations of the brain. A *mutagen,* on the other hand, is any agent that can alter the genetic material in somatic or germ cells. For example, ethylene oxide (a chemical frequently used to sterilize surgical instruments) has been associated with gross chromosome aberrations in the lymphocyte preparations of exposed workers.[44] It is therefore mutagenic, but there is no evidence that intrauterine exposure to ethylene oxide is associated with an increased incidence of structural malformations or functional abnormalities. Mutagenic effects are very different from teratogenic effects. Many mutagens also are teratogens, but not vice versa. It is not the purpose of this section to discuss mutagens, but the difference between a teratogen and a mutagen should be understood.

Not every pregnant woman who is exposed even to a proven teratogen faces an increased risk for an adverse pregnancy outcome. In order to accurately determine the significance of maternal exposure to an exogenous agent, many factors must be considered. They include the type of exposure, timing, route of administration, dosage, and duration of exposure. In addition, because many congenital defects are caused by a combination of several genes and environmental agents (see Multifactorial Inheritance), a family history must be taken into account as well. A discussion of these factors as well as general comments that apply to counseling patients at risk for unfavorable outcome of pregnancy as a result of potential exposure to hazardous agents follow.

Types of Exposure

This section is not inclusive, and it is not the only system of classifying potentially hazardous agents. However, its practical nature makes it convenient. A list of agents proven or virtually proven to be teratogenic and their potential effects is included at the end.

Drugs. A variety of pharmacologic agents has been demonstrated to be teratogenic in humans. Some of these (eg, lithium, tetracycline, streptomycin, progestins, and testosterone) are associated with well-documented isolated abnormalities. Maternal exposure to lithium is associated with an increased incidence of congenital heart disease, with particular affinity for the right heart.[45] Maternal exposure to tetracycline after the deciduous teeth begin to calcify (at around 5 or 6 months' gestation) results in dentine staining.[46] Intrauterine exposure to the aminoglycoside antibiotic, streptomycin, may result in eighth cranial nerve damage,[47] and maternal exposure to *synthetic progestins* and *testosterone* may result in transient masculinization of the external genitalia.[48] See also Chapter 7.

Other pharmacologic agents (eg, Dilantin, valproic acid, isotretinoin, Coumadin, and alcohol) have been associated with malformation syndromes. Prenatal exposure to several anticonvulsants has been associated with characteristic craniofacial features and other birth defects. Because polydrug therapy is common in patients with seizure disorders, it is difficult to indict any one drug of the several in use. However, it has been fairly well documented that children born to mothers treated with hydantoin anticonvulsants (Dilantin) are at increased risk for craniofacial anomalies, nail and digital hypoplasia, growth retardation, and possibly congenital heart disease and oral clefting.[49] Valproic acid also has been associated with craniofacial anomalies and approximately a 1–2% increased incidence of neural tube defects.[50]

Isotretinoin (Accutane), a vitamin A isomer used for treatment of cystic acne, has recently been found to be one of the most potent human teratogens. Maternal exposure to isotretinoin has been associated with a syndrome that may consist of all or part of the following: central nervous system damage, craniofacial abnormalities, and congenital heart disease.[51]

Coumarin derivatives such as warfarin are associated with an embryopathy consisting of a characteristic facial appearance, including nasal underdevelopment and abnormal calcification of epiphyseal regions of bones. Other adverse effects may include central nervous system and eye abnormalities.[52] The timing of exposure to warfarin, and all other drugs, is crucial when assessing the potential risks.

No recognizable pattern of malformations has been associated with most illicit durgs (including marijuana, methadone, and lysergic acid diethylamide). The teratogenic potential of cocaine is under investigation, but its vasoconstrictive effects are thought to be associated with risks for early spontaneous pregnancy loss, placental abruption and prematurity, genitourinary abnormalities, and even sudden infant death syndrome. Adverse fetal effects associated with maternal exposure to alcohol have been well publicized. The majority of information available on alcohol use during pregnancy is based on data obtained from chronic and heavy use (ie, 10–12 drinks per day throughout pregnancy). This level of maternal alcohol exposure results in about a 30% risk of true fetal alcohol syndrome (growth retardation, mental retardation, and characteristic facial anomalies). Such children also are at increased risk for speech and language delays, limb defects, heart disease, spina bifida, and other structural and functional abnormalities. Acute and more moderate alcohol consumption also may lead to adverse pregnancy outcome and to behavioral and learning disabilities (called fetal alcohol effects).[53] An absolutely safe amount of alcohol consumption during pregnancy is not known.

There is no conclusive evidence that maternal cigarette smoking causes congenital malformations. However, it is known to be associated with an increased incidence of pregnancy loss (spontaneous abortion and stillbirth), intrauterine growth retardation, and prematurity. It has been postulated that nicotine, a vasoconstrictor, compromises uteroplacental blood flow and results in intrauterine growth retardation.[54] Recent investigations have suggested that women who stop smoking during the first half of their pregnancy may not be at increased risk for low-birthweight infants.[55]

Physical Agents. Radiation, one of the first human teratogens described, can result in growthretardation and central nervous system damage after intrauterine exposure (see also chapters 5 and 26). Most data on radiation-related abnormalities are derived from Hiroshima and Nagasaki studies. Diagnostic x-rays, which result in far lower levels of radiation exposure than the atomic bomb, are less likely to be associated with adverse pregnancy outcome. Fetal risk assessment associated with maternal radiation exposure is based on the stage of gestation at which exposure occurred and fetal dosimetry. These factors will be discussed below.

Experimentally induced maternal hyperthermia is teratogenic in laboratory animals and frequently affects the central nervous system. The potential teratogenicity of high fever in humans has been more difficult to evaluate because fever most often accompanies infection, which could be the causative factor of adverse pregnancy outcome. Data are currently inconclusive, and the possible teratogenicity of hyperthermia must be assessed with regard to timing, degree, and duration of exposure. However, maternal hyperthermia cannot be completely excluded as a potential factor in the development of some congenital malformations. Recent studies have suggested that maternal hyperthermia may be associated with an increased risk for neural tube defects, although a causal connection has not been established.[56]

Chemical Agents. Few environmental chemicals are confirmed teratogens. Controversial evidence exists about many occupational agents, including organic solvents and anesthetic gases. More studies are needed before a causal relationship between maternal exposure and adverse pregnancy outcome can be established.

Maternal Factors. Several maternal factors are known to be associated with an increased incidence of malformations and other adverse effects. They include infections (rubella, toxoplasmosis, human parvovirus B19, cytomegalovirus), metabolic diseases (maternal phenylketonuria), and other maternal diseases (diabetes mellitus, myotonic dystrophy). Other maternal factors are mechanical in nature and include amnion disruption, compression, and constraint.

Paternal Factors. Paternal exposure to hazardous agents rarely results in fetal structural or functional defects. However, there are several situations in which paternal exposure can result in adverse pregnancy outcome. If the agent is a mutagen and affects the germ cell or sperm, a clastogenic or mutagenic event could occur. Also, paternal exposure to certain chemotherapeutic agents, such as methotrexate, may decrease fertility through oligospermia.[57]

Most teratogen information services receive frequent inquiries about paternal exposure to Agent Orange, alcohol, cocaine, marijuana, and lysergic acid diethylamide. No scientific evidence suggests that any of these is mutagenic, and paternal exposure has not been associated with structural or functional abnormalities. However, some studies suggest that paternal exposure to some (eg, alcohol and marijuana) could be associated with decreased testosterone levels and decreased fertility.[58,59] Social effects of paternal exposure and an increased probability of concomitant maternal exposure also must be kept in mind.

Timing

Teratogenic effects can be divided into three categories. (1) If exposure occurs before about 21 days after conception, it will most likely result in one of two events: either the embryonic tissue will not be harmed or the effects will be so devastating that they result in embryonic death and subsequent abortion. This is referred to as an "all or none response." (2) In general, the most sensitive periods (resulting in viable infants with malformations) occur between the third and ninth weeks after conception. During the time of organogenesis, each organ has its own periods of vulnerability or *critical periods.* If maternal exposure to a specific environmental agent has the potential to interfere with the development of a particular structure or organ, then exposure to that agent during that organ's critical periods of development may result in malformative damage, such as congenital heart disease, oral clefting, or facial dysmorphology. (3) If exposure to a teratogen occurs after 9 weeks' gestation (when organogenesis for all systems except the central nervous system is complete), more subtle effects on organ function may be expected. Fetal effects resulting from exposure in the second or third trimester can include growth and central nervous system abnormalities (the central nervous system develops throughout prenatal and early postnatal life). In addition to the timing of exposure in assessing potential reproductive risk, it is important to consider the half-life of the specific substance in question. If an agent remains in the human system after maternal exposure has ceased, the potential for embryonic fetal exposure and therefore damage remains.

Route of Exposure

The extent of fetal exposure depends on the route through which it occurs, and the method of maternal administration (inhalation, ingestion, dermal contact, intravenous, subcutaneous, intramuscular) may determine whether or not fetal exposure will occur. For example, an agent taken orally may not enter the maternal systemic circulation if it cannot be absorbed through the intestinal mucosa. On the other hand, intravenous administration of the same agent can potentially interfere with fetal development.

Dosage and Duration of Exposure

Teratogens often show threshold and dose-response effects. For example, there may be no demonstrable effects below a certain level. Once the level of exposure is above the threshold, the effects observed may be proportional to the dosage. The atomic bombing of Hiroshima and Nagasaki provided some information about this principle. No other group of pregnant women exposed to radiation has been studied so completely as Japanese survivors of the atomic bomb. Average exposure was about 2 Gy. It was clear from the investigations that maternal exposure to very high levels of radiation was associated with increased fetal risks, including pregnancy loss, growth retardation, and central nervous system abnormalities. A recent report on the prevalence of mental retardation in children exposed *in utero* to the atomic bomb suggested that the increased risk for severe mental retardation was 0.4% per .01 Gy of radiation.[60] However, potential risks associated with lower levels of exposure (ie, less than a total of .50 Gy) are less clear. Limited, direct empiric data on lower level radiation exposures indicate that there may be no significant association between risks for mental retardation and exposures below about .25–.50 Gy; however, there is evidence for increasing risks for fetal growth retardation at exposure levels of .10 Gy or more. Because most diagnostic x-rays are associated with less than .10 Gy of fetal exposure, the majority of pregnant women concerned about diagnostic x-rays can be reassured. Unfortunately, because the range of dose used for pharmacologic agents is usually very narrow, dose-response relationships for most medications are difficult to verify.

The duration of exposure also influences the magnitude of fetal risk. If, for example, a woman is exposed to methylene chloride (an organic solvent metabolized into carbon monoxide) throughout the second and third trimesters, her fetus may be at increased risk for growth retardation. If, on the other hand, her exposure is discontinued after several weeks, there may be no increased risk.

Family History

In the presence of a positive family history for a specific birth defect, an environmental agent known to be associated with that abnormality could further increase fetal risk.

Review and Interpretation of Available Literature

After the previously discussed factors (type, timing, route, dosage, duration of exposure, and family history) are considered, a thorough search of the literature should be undertaken, and an attempt should be made to interpret it in a way that is relevant and applicable to specific concerns.

Interpretation of the literature is sometimes difficult. Most studies about exposures to various agents during pregnancy have been conducted on animals, for obvious ethical and practical reasons. Occasionally, human population "studies" exist, usually when many pregnant women have been exposed to a particular agent and a higher than expected incidence of birth defects is detected. Less frequently, single case reports of adverse pregnancy outcomes may be reported after exposure to a particular agent. Many factors must be considered before conclusions can be drawn from animal studies, population studies, and case reports of this kind. They include the following:

1. Different species of animals have different levels of sensitivity after exposure to the same agent, caused by differences in physiology, metabolism, and embryonic development.
2. Experimental animals often receive doses many times higher than those given to humans, and the route of administration may be different.
3. Case reports are usually less than helpful because it is not possible to draw cause-and-effect conclusions as to whether the agent in question actually caused the adverse outcome.
4. Retrospective human studies usually fail to report the total number of women exposed to the agent in question who had normal pregnancy outcomes.
5. Few, if any, of the studies in the literature have taken into account the individuality of human response to an agent (ie, genetic predisposition or susceptibility).

6. Most studies do not follow pregnancy outcome past birth or 6 months, so there is little information about long-term effects or risks.
7. Almost no information is available on the potential synergistic effects of exposure to more than one agent.

Known Human Teratogens

A list of drugs and other agents that are certain or virtually certain human teratogens follows in Appendix 13–1. The reader should bear in mind how few agents have been clearly demonstrated to be teratogenic, and how the study of environmental causes of birth defects remains incomplete. In addition, all the factors mentioned above must be considered in detail, before any conclusions about specific effects of an exposure can be reached and before information is provided to a patient.

REFERENCES

1. Hsu TC. Human and mammalian cytogenetics: An historical perspective. In: Therman E: *Human Chromosomes: Structure, Behavior, Effects*. 2nd ed. Heidelberg: Springer; 1985:1.
2. Korenberg J, Rykowski MC. Human genome organization, Alu, Lines, and the molecular structure of metaphase chromosome bands. *Cell*. 1988;53:391.
3. Machin GA. Chromosome abnormality and perinatal death. *Lancet*. 1974;1:549.
4. Langenbeck U, Hausmann I, Hinney B, Hönig V. On the origin of the supernumerary chromosome in autosomal trisomies—with special reference to Down's Syndrome. *Hum Genet*. 1976;33:89.
5. Hamerton JL. Robertsonian translocations. In: Jacobs PA, Price WH, Law P, eds. *Human Population Genetics*. Baltimore, MD: Williams & Wilkins; 1970:63.
6. Penrose LS. The relative effects of paternal and maternal age in mongolism. *J Genet*. 1933;27:219.
7. Vogel F, Motulsky AG. Genome and chromosome mutations in man. In: *Human Genetics, Problems and Approaches*. 2nd ed. Heidelberg: Springer Verlag; 1986:339.
8. Vogel F, Motulsky AG. Gene mutation: Analysis at the phenotype level. In: *Human Genetics, Problems, and Approaches*. 2nd ed. Heidelberg: Springer Verlag; 1986:359.
9. MacDonald K. Incidence of major malformations in infants born to teenaged mothers. Madison, WI: University of Wisconsin—Madison; 1981. Thesis.
10. Warburton D. Outcome of cases of *de novo* structural rearrangements diagnosed at amniocentesis. *Prenatal Diagnosis*. 1984;4:69.
11. Martin NJ, Steinberg BG. The dup(3)(p25-->pter) Syndrome: A case with holoprosencephaly. *Am J Med Genet*. 1983;14:767.
12. Schmickel RD. Contiguous gene syndromes—A component of recognizable syndromes. *J Peds*. 1986;109:231.
13. Schinzel A. *Catalogue of unbalanced chromosome aberrations in man*. Berlin, Germany: W. de Gruyter; 1984.
14. Pueschel S, Tingey C, Rynders JE, et al, eds. *New Perspective on Down Syndrome*. Baltimore, MD: Paul H. Brookes; 1987.
15. Emery AEH, Rimoin DL, eds. *Principles and Practice of Medical Genetics*. Churchill Livingstone: 1983.
16. Jones KL. *Smith's Recognizable Patterns of Human Malformation*. 4th ed. Philadelphia: WB Saunders; 1988.
17. Ratcliffe SG, Paul N, eds. Prospective studies on children with sex chromosome aneuploidy. *M.O.D.B.D.O.A.S.* 23(3). New York, NY: Alan Liss; 1986.
18. McKusick VA. *Mendelian Inheritance in Man; Catalogs of Automsomal Dominant, Autosomal Recessive and X-linked Phenotypes*. 9th ed. Baltimore, MD: Johns Hopkins University Press; 1990.
19. Neurofibromatosis Conference. NIH Consensus development conference. *Arch Neurol*. 1988;45:575.
20. Nakamura Y, Lathrop M, Leppert M, et al. Localization of the genetic defect in familial adenomatous polyposis within a small region of chromosome 5. *Am J Hum Genet*. 1988;43:638.
21. Critchley M. Great Britain and the early history of Huntington's chorea. In: *Advances in Neurology, 1: Huntington's Chorea, 1872–1972*. New York, NY: Raven Press; 1973:13.
22. Kessler S. The dilemma of suicide and Huntington's disease. *Am J Med Genet*. 1987;26:315.
23. Gusella JF, Wexler NS, Conneally PM, et al. A polymorphic DNA marker genetically linked to Huntington's disease. *Nature*. 1983;306:234.
24. Weaver DD. *Catalog of Prenatally Diagnosed Conditions*. Baltimore, MD: Johns Hopkins University Press: 1989.
25. Levy HL, Waisbern SE. Effects of untreated maternal phenylketonuria and hyperphenylalanine on the fetus. *N Engl J Med*. 1983;309:1269.
26. Brock DJH. Amniotic fluid alkaline phosphatase isoenzymes in the early prenatal diagnosis of cystic fibrosis. *J Med Genet*. 1984;21:140.
27. Tsui LC, Buchwald M, Barker D, et al. Cystic fibrosis locus defined by a genetically linked polymorphic DNA marker. *Science*. 1985;230:1054.
28. Alvesalo L, Chappelle A. Tooth sizes in two males with deletions of the long arm of the Y chromosome. *Ann Hum Genet*. 1981;45:49.
29. Stalvez JRD, Erickson RP, Dasouki M, et al. Clarification of chromosomal abnormalities associated with sexual ambiguity by studies with Y-chromosomal DNA sequences. *Cytogenet Cell Genetics*. 1988;47:140.
30. Rommens JM, Iannuzzi MC, Kerem B, et al. *Science*. Chromosome walking and jumping. 1989;245,4922:1059.
31. Lyon MF. Gene action in the X chromosome of the mouse (*Mus musculus L*). *Nature*. 1961;190:372.
32. Penrose LS. A clinical and genetic study of 1,280 cases of mental defect. *Special Report Series, #229*. London, England: MRC: 1938.
33. Lubs HA. A marker X chromosome. *Am J Hum Genet*. 1969;21:231.
34. Turner G, Collins E, Turner D. Recurrence risk of mental retardation in sibs. *Med J Austr*. 1971;1:1165.
35. Davison CBC. Genetic studies in mental subnormality. *Br J Psychiatr*. 1973; Special Publ. 8.
36. Sutherland JR. Fragile sites on human chromosomes: Demonstration of their dependence on the type of tissue culture medium. *Science*. 1977;197:265.
37. Sherman S, Jacobs P, Morton N, et al. Further segregation analysis of the fragile X syndrome with special reference to transmitting males. *Hum Genet*. 1985;69:289.
38. Laird CD. Proposed mechanism of inheritance and expression of the human fragile X syndrome of mental retardation. *Genetics*. 1987;117:587.
39. Tierney J, Wright L, Springen K. The Search for Adam and Eve. *Newsweek*. 1988; Jan. 11:46.

39a. Fraser FC. Mapping the cleft lip genes: The first fix? *Am J Hum Genet*. 1989;45:345. Editorial.

39b. Ardinger HH, Buetow KH, Bell IG, et al. Association of genetic variation of the transforming growth factor alpha gene with cleft lip and palate. *Am J Hum Genet*. 1989;45:348.

40. Greb AE, Pauli RM, Kirby RS. Accuracy of fetal death reports: Comparison with data from an independent stillbirth assessment program. *Am J Publ Health*. 1987;77:1202.
41. Stanbury JB, Wyngaarden JB, Fredrickson DS, et al, eds. *The Metabolic Basis of Inherited Disease*. 6th ed. New York, NY: McGraw-Hill; 1989.
42. Brent RL. The complexities of solving the problem of human malformations. In: Sever JL, Brent RL, eds. *Teratogen Update: Environmentally Induced Birth Defect Risks*. New York, NY: Alan R. Liss; 1986:189.
43. Barlow SM, Sullivan FS. *Reproductive Hazards of Industrial Chemicals*. London, England: Academic Press; 1982.
44. Weinstein MR. Recent advances in clinical pharmacology. I. Lithium update. *Hosp Formul*. 1977;12:759.
45. Cohlan SQ. Tetracycline staining of the teeth. *Teratology*. 1977;15:127.
46. Donald PR, Sellers SL. Streptomycin ototoxicity on the unborn child. *S Afr Med J*. 1981;60:316.
47. Wilson JG, Brent RL. Are female sex hormones teratogenic? *Am J Obstet Gynecol*. 1981;141:567.
48. Hanson JW. Teratogen update: Fetal hydantoin effects. *Teratology*. 1986;33:349.
49. Lammer EG, Sever LS, Oakley GP. Teratogen update. Valproic acid. *Teratology*. 1987;35:465.
50. Lammer EJ, Chen DT, Hoar RM, et al. Retinoic acid embryopathy. *N Engl J Med*. 1985;313:837.
51. Hall JG, Pauli RM, Wilson KM. Maternal and fetal sequelae of anticoagulation during pregnancy. *Am J Med Genet*. 1980;68:122.
52. Abel EJ. Prenatal effects of alcohol. *Drug Alcohol Depend*. 1984;14:1.
53. Phillip K, Pateisky N, Endler M. Effects of smoking on uterine blood flow. *Gynecol Obstet Invest*. 1984;17:179.
54. Butler N, Goldstein H, Ross E. Cigarette smoking in pregnancy: Its influence on birth weight and perinatal mortality. *Br Med J Clin Res*. 1972;2:127.
55. Warkeny J. Teratogen update: Hyperthermia. *Teratology*. 1986;33:365.
56. Sussman A, Leonard JM. Psoriasis, methotrexate, and oligospermia. *Arch Dermatol*. 1980;116:215.
57. Joffe JM, Soyka LF. Paternal drug exposure: Effects on reproduction and progeny. *Sem Perinatol*. 1982;6:116.
58. Jones RT. Cannabis and health. *Ann Rev Med*. 1983;34:247.
59. Otake M, Schull WJ. *In utero* exposure to A-bomb radiation and mental retardation: A reassessment. *Br J Radiol*. 1984;57:409.

Appendix 13–1.

Agents Proved or Virtually Certain to be Human Teratogens

Agent	Effect(s)
Drugs	
Alcohol	Fetal alcohol syndrome or effects
Aminopterin (and other antifolates)	Aminopterine syndrome
Cigarettes	Intrauterine growth retardation
Cocaine	
Curare (chronic use only)	Arthrogryposis
Diazepam (Valium)	Oral clefting
Diethylstilbesterol	Vaginal clear cell carcinoma
Hydantoins (Dilantin)	Fetal hydantoin effects
Iodine	Thyroid abnormalities
Isotretinoin (Accutane)	Isotretinoin embryopathy
Lithium	Cardiac malformations
Propylthiouracil	Thyroid abnormalities
Progestins (synthetic)	Masculinization
Streptomycin	Hearing loss
Testosterone	Masculinization
Tetracycline	Tooth enamel abnormalities
Thalidomide	Thalidomide syndrome
Trimethadione	Trimethodione syndrome
Valproic acid	Fetal valproate syndrome
Warfarin (Coumadin)	Warfarin embryopathy
Physical Agents	
Radiation	CNS, eye, pregnancy loss, intrauterine growth retardation
Chemical Agents	
Lead	CNS
Mercury	Fetal minimata disease
Polychlorinated biphenyls (PCB)	Skin discoloration, growth retardation

Causes	Effect(s)
Maternal Factors	
Mechanical	
Amnion disruption	Fetal deformities
Compression	Abnormalities associated with craniofacial pressure and ischemia
Constraint	Clubfoot, scoliosis, and other postural deformities
Disease	
Diabetes Mellitus	CNS, others, caudal regression, other malformations included among those comprising the VACTERL association
Hyperphenylalanemia (including PKU)	Mental retardation, others
Myotonic dystrophy	Congenital myotonic dystrophy
Infections:	
Cytomegalovirus	CNS, others
Parvovirus	Hydrops, fetal death
Rubella	Congenital rubella syndrome
Syphilis	Congenital Syphilis
Toxoplasmosis	CNS, eye, others
Varicella (chicken pox)	Limb, skin, cataracts

Chapter Fourteen

Molecular Genetics: DNA Technology and Recent Developments

Carole Ober and David H. Lynch

14

The field of medical genetics has undergone striking changes in recent years, primarily as a result of the application of recombinant deoxyribonucleic acid (DNA) technology to clinical genetics. The potential for identifying and isolating human genes already has been realized; more than 3500 genes and other markers have been mapped to human chromosomes.[1] Furthermore, the number of single gene disorders potentially amenable to prenatal diagnosis is now virtually unlimited. In no other area of clinical medicine has this technology had such an immediate and dramatic impact as in reproductive genetics. This chapter reviews the principles of molecular genetics and DNA technology and describes some recent developments in this field as they are applied to prenatal diagnosis of human disease.

ADVANTAGES OF DNA-BASED DIAGNOSES

Before the application of recombinant DNA technology, prenatal diagnosis of mendelian genetic disorders was limited to those for which the biochemical defects were known and expressed by fetal tissues (eg, amniotic fluid cells, chorionic villi, blood, skin, liver). For example, hemophilia A and sickle cell anemia were diagnosable only through fetal blood sampling, and phenylketonuria (PKU) required fetal liver biopsies. These procedures confer considerable risk to the fetus. Other disorders, such as cystic fibrosis (CF), were not detectable prenatally because the biochemical basis for the disease was not known. Indeed, of the more than 2000 known Mendelian disorders[2], less than 100 are amenable to prenatal diagnosis using biochemical or morphologic markers in fetal tissues.[3] However, through the use of recombinant DNA technology all Mendelian disorders are, at least in theory, amenable to prenatal diagnosis. In the following sections, the basic molecular techniques that are now being used for prenatally diagnosing mendelian disorders, as well as some their advantages and disadvantages, are discussed.

THE BASIC TECHNIQUES OF PRENATAL DIAGNOSIS USING RECOMBINANT DNA TECHNOLOGY

Virtually every cell in the body contains a complete chromosomal complement. Therefore, each cell contains the full complement of DNA, and even if a gene is not expressed by a particular cell, the DNA coding for that gene product is present. For example, although the genes encoding hemoglobin are expressed only by reticulocytes, the DNA coding for hemoglobin is present in all cells, including amniotic fluid cells and chorionic villi. Furthermore, even if the biochemical or molecular defect is unknown, such as in CF, the DNA coding for the mutant gene is present in each cell.

Using DNA-based genetic analysis, there are virtually unlimited numbers of nucleotide sequence differences in the DNA of different individuals that can be detected by direct sequencing of the mutated DNA or by restriction fragment length polymorphism (RFLP, discussed below) analysis. Restriction fragment length polymorphism (RFLPs) serves as a marker for mutant genes that cause disease and allow diagnosis of affected individuals in families, even if the exact genetic defect (ie, mutation) is unknown. For example, this approach is now widely applied to the prenatal diagnosis of CF, even though the molecular and biochemical defects causing CF are still unknown. Thus, recombinant DNA technology provides a potentially powerful tool for the diagnosis of genetic disorders.

The DNA-based analysis of genetic disease involves three basic technologies: (1) the use of *restriction endonucleases* (restriction enzymes), (2) *southern blotting and hybridization,* and (3) the *polymerase chain reaction* (PCR). (Other techniques, such as DNA sequencing and gene cloning, will not be discussed here because their application to prenatal diagnosis is limited.[4,5]) Restriction endonucleases are bacterial enzymes that recognize and cut double-stranded DNA at specific nucleotide sequences. There are currently more than 400 known restriction enzymes that recognize and cut unique DNA sequences. Examples of restriction enzymes are listed in Table 14–1. The sequences of DNA recognized by specific restriction enzymes are called *restriction sites.* Several different restriction sites may be found within or surrounding any gene and are randomly distributed throughout the genome. However, because more than 95% of human DNA does not code for gene products, most restriction sites are, by chance, located within the noncoding portion of genes. The DNA between two restriction sites is called a *restriction fragment.* The size of a given restriction fragment is determined by the distance between two restriction sites and can vary from a few hundred to several thousand base pairs in length. Thus, when DNA is digested with a restriction enzyme, it is cut into many fragments of varying lengths.

One of the remarkable features of the human genome is that nucleotide sequences vary considerably from person

TABLE 14–1. EXAMPLES OF RESTRICTION ENZYMES AND NUCLEOTIDE RECOGNITION SITES

Enzyme	Recognition Sequence
*Pvu*II	CAG^CTG
*Eco*RI	G^AATTC
*Mst*II	CC^TNAGG
*Cvn*I	CC^TNAGG
*Msp*I	C^CGG
*Taq*I	T^CGA

^ = cutting site.
N = any nucleotide.

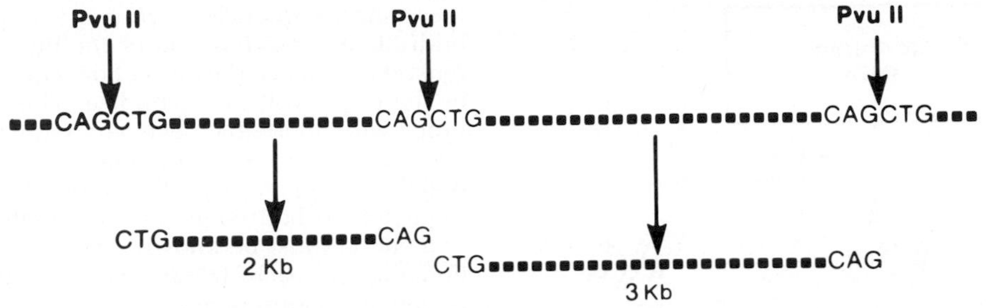

Figure 14–1. This simplified scheme shows the way in which restriction endonucleases cut specific DNA sequences to generate RFLPs. DNA nucleotide sequence is shown as single stranded. *PvuII* recognizes the sequence CAGCTG and cuts between the G-C. The length of the restriction fragments generated by *PvuII* is determined by the distance between the two sites. In this case, 2-kbp and 3-kbp fragments are generated. In: individuals lacking the middle *PvuII* site, only a 5-kbp fragment would result from digestion with this enzyme. (*From Ober C, Lynch DH. Molecular genetics. In Sciarra JJ, ed.* Gynecology and Obstetrics. *Philadelphia, PA: JB Lippincott, 1989.*)

to person, particularly within noncoding regions of DNA. In fact, if two chromosomes of any pair are compared, a single base change is found in approximately every 100–200 base pairs. As a result, individuals will vary with respect to the number of restriction sites that any one particular enzyme will recognize. Because the presence or absence of a restriction site will affect the length of the restriction fragment between two sites, individuals also will vary with respect to restriction fragment lengths. For example, in the theoretical case depicted in Figure 14–1, individuals lacking the second *Pvu*II restriction site will have one restriction fragment 5000 base pairs (or 5 kilobase pairs [kbp]) long, whereas individuals with the second restriction site will have two fragments of 3 kbp and 2 kbp in length. These variations in fragment lengths among individuals are called *restriction fragment length polymorphisms* (RFLPs). A polymorphism refers to the occurrence of two or more forms of a gene in a population, the least common having a frequency of at least 1%. Classic examples of human genetic polymorphisms are the ABO blood groups, serum transferrin, or the red cell enzyme G6PD. However, unlike RFLPs, the number of antigen, serum, or red cell polymorphisms are limited in the human genome to less than 50 loci. RFLPs, on the other hand, provide geneticists with a virtually unlimited source of genetic markers through which diseases can be traced in families.

When genomic DNA is digested with a particular restriction enzyme, fragments of many sizes result. The various size fragments can be made single stranded and physically separated on the basis of size by agarose gel electrophoresis because larger restriction fragments migrate through the gel more slowly than smaller fragments. After electrophoresis, digested DNA stained with ethidium bromide is visualized under ultraviolet light as a continuous smear (Fig. 14–2). To localize a gene of interest within the many different fragments on a gel, the fragments are transferred to a membrane (such as nitrocellulose or charged nylon) using a method called *southern blotting*.[6] During the transfer, the spatial orientation of the restriction fragments are maintained, resulting in band patterns on the membrane that are identical to those in the gel. The DNA is then *hybridized* to a specific radioactively (or enzymatically) labelled probe that contains DNA from the gene of interest or from DNA sequences that are located very close to (ie, linked to) the gene of interest. The probe will hybridize (ie, pair) to DNA that is complementary to the probe's DNA because both are single stranded. After hybridization, the excess unhybridized probe is washed away, and only the restriction fragments that contain DNA sequences complementary to the probe (and to which the probe hybridized) will be radioactively labeled. The southern blot is then exposed to photographic film for an appropriate period of time. After the film is developed, the restriction fragments containing the DNA that hybridized to the radioactive probe can be seen as dark bands. These steps are illustrated in Figure 14–3.

The *polymerase chain reaction* (PCR) is an *in vitro* method for amplifying, or making multiple copies of, specific DNA sequences.[7] This powerful technique is capable of synthesizing more than 1 million copies of specific DNA sequences that are up to 2.5 kbp long in just a few hours. The PCR

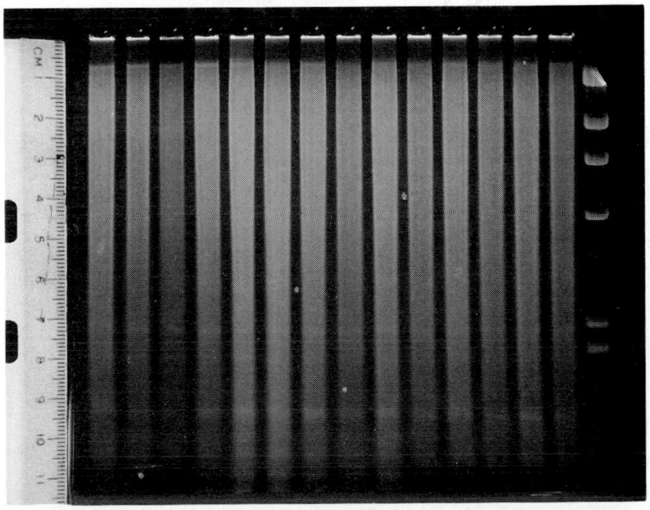

Figure 14–2. DNA digested with restriction enzyme *XbaI* after electrophoresis in an agarose gel. After electrophoresis, DNA was stained with ethidium bromide and visualized under an ultraviolet light. Each lane represents DNA from a different individual. The largest bands are on the top and the smallest on the bottom. Bands in the lane on the right are lambda size markers corresponding to (from top to bottom) 23,130, 9,416, 6,557, 4,361, 2,322, and 2,027 base pairs. (*From Ober C, Lynch DH. Molecular genetics. In: Sciarra JJ, ed.* Gynecology and Obstetrics. *Philadelphia, PA: J.B. Lippincott, 1989.*)

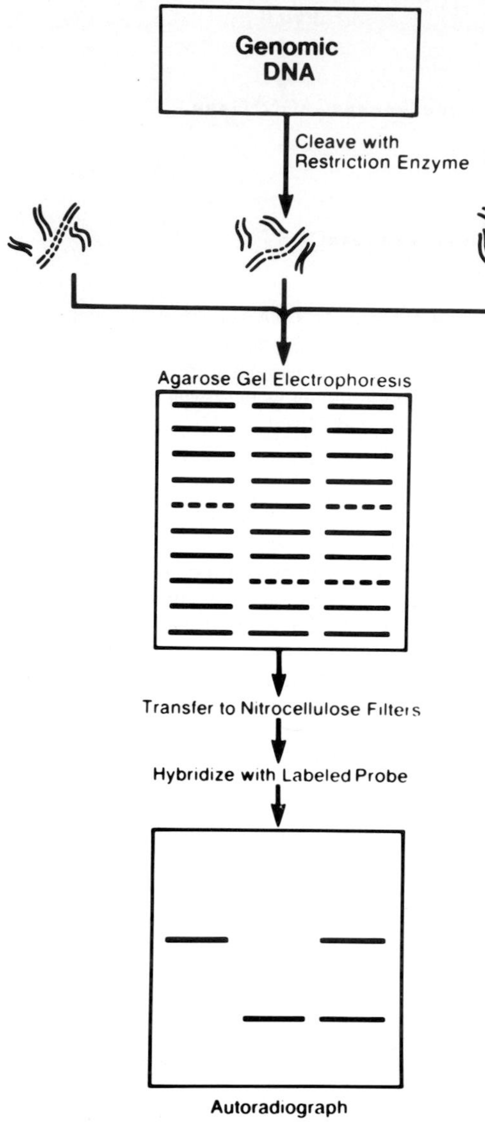

Figure 14–3. Visualizing RFLPs. DNA is cleaved with restriction enzyme, and the digested DNA is separated by size using agarose gel electrophoresis. The DNA is then transferred to a membrane, such as nitrocellulose, by southern blotting. The orientation of the bands on the membrane is identical to the orientation of the bands in the gel. The membrane is hybridized to a radioactively labeled probe. DNA fragments that hybridize to the probe are visualized after autoradiography. (From Ober C, Lynch DH. Molecular genetics. In: Sciarra JJ, ed. *Gynecology and Obstetrics.* Philadelphia, PA: J.B. Lippincott; 1989.)

not only allows diagnoses to be made from small amounts of DNA (ie, eliminating the need to culture cells to obtain larger amounts of DNA), but also makes possible the potential for eliminating several steps in the procedure and reducing the time required to make a diagnosis by up to 2 weeks. Diagnoses can be made on amplified DNA either by direct visualization of the amplified product under ultraviolet light (see the section on diagnosis of cystic fibrosis below) or after hybridization to *oligonucleotide probes* (see section on diagnosis of sickle cell anemia below). An oligonucleotide probe is a sequence of approximately 20 or less nucleotides that is synthesized in the laboratory. The usefulness of these short sequences as probes is that, under certain hybridization conditions, all of the nucleotides in the probe must *exactly* match the nucleotide sequence in genomic DNA or the probe will not hybridize. Thus, an oligonucleotide probe will differentiate between sequences that differ with respect to one base pair only (eg, sickle versus normal β-globin gene). A major limitation of PCR is that the DNA sequence on both sides of the mutation (ie, the flanking sequences) must be known. However, despite this limitation, this approach already has been applied to the diagnosis of genetic disorders and promises to become the method of choice for all diagnoses.

APPLICATIONS TO PRENATAL DIAGNOSIS

There are two general approaches to prenatal diagnosis through DNA analysis. The first, called the *direct method,* is the preferred method for prenatal diagnosis. With this approach, DNA from the at-risk fetus is directly tested for the presence or absence of the abnormal gene. There are few potential sources of error with this method, provided the clinical diagnosis of the disease is correct. However, if more than one mutation results in a similar clinical phenotype (such as in families with Duchenne's muscular dystrophy), a direct test would not be appropriate unless the specific mutation in that family is first identified. This potential genetic heterogeneity must always be excluded before direct DNA analysis can be considered. Therefore, the direct method is limited to genetic diseases in which the precise molecular defect is known. Although this is considered the ultimate goal for diagnosis of genetic disorders, few genetic diseases can be diagnosed using the direct method of DNA analysis.

The *indirect method,* based on linkage analysis, is generally applicable to all Mendelian (or single gene) disorders. This approach requires identifying RFLPs that are linked (lie within approximately 1000 kbp) to the disease gene. As discussed previously, RFLPs are randomly distributed through the genome. Thus, it is possible to identify RFLPs that demonstrate linkage to a disease in family studies, even if the abnormal gene has not been isolated or characterized. The RFLP can then be used to trace the abnormal gene in families.

Despite the potential power of this approach, there are several limitations and sources of error because the indirect method does not directly diagnose the defective gene. One requisite of the indirect method is that it requires studying family members, including, in many cases, at least one living relative affected with the disease. Another limitation of the indirect method is that it may not be diagnostic in all at-risk fetuses. Determining whether linkage studies are feasible requires studying the linkage relationship between the RFLP and the disease in each family requesting prenatal diagnosis, a costly and time consuming process. A third limitation of this approach is the possibility of genetic recombination between the genes that produce disease and the linked marker in one of the parents' gametes. Because this possibility always introduces a potential source of error in the diagnosis, the accuracy of the diagnosis using linked RFLPs is *always* less than 100%. The probability of recombination is proportional to the chromosomal distance between the mutant gene and the RFLP. Thus, restriction sites that lie within the gene are the most accurate for diagnosis, and the greater the distance between the site and the disease gene, the less accurate the test. Whenever possible, several different RFLPs that map to either side of the defective gene should be used so that if recombination occurs between the gene of interest and one RFLP, recombination also will occur between the two RFLPs and can be detected. The last potential source of error is false paternity. Obviously, if the biologic father is not included in the family studies, erroneous diagnoses may result.

PRENATAL DIAGNOSIS USING THE DIRECT METHOD

As discussed previously, the direct method of DNA analysis is feasible only when the molecular defect causing the disease is known. Direct detection of affected fetuses has been successful for genetic defects caused by gene deletions and single nucleotide substitutions. Examples of these follow.

Gene Deletions

The first genetic disorder to be diagnosed prenatally using direct DNA techniques was α-thalassemia,[8] a relatively common disease among Asian and African populations. This disorder, which causes anemia of varying severity, results from a deletion of chromosomal material that includes the alpha-globin genes. Because normal individuals have four α-globin genes (two on each chromosome), a spectrum of clinical symptoms results from the deletion of one, two, three, or four α-globin genes. The clinical picture associated with each of these defects is called α-thalassemia-1, heterozygous α-thalassemia, hemoglobin H disease, and homozygous α-thalassemia, respectively. The clinical spectrum ranges from no symptoms (α-thalassemia-1) to anemia of lethal severity (homozygous α-thalassemia).

When genomic DNA is digested with the restriction endonuclease *Eco*RI, the alpha-globin gene is contained within a 13.7 kbp fragment of DNA that can be separated and identified using electrophoresis, southern blotting, and hybridization to an alpha-globin gene probe. DNA from normal fetuses will reveal one dark band (13.7 kbp) after autoradiography. However, DNA from fetuses with homozygous α-thalassemia will not hybridize with the α-globin probe and no bands will appear after autoradiography. Fetuses with only two or three α-globin genes will show a 13.7 kbp band of intermediate intensity, which can be quantitated for diagnosis.

This general approach can be applied for diagnosis of any defect caused by a gene deletion, provided a probe for the gene is available. A possible error in interpretation of results could arise if the probe is not specific for the precise deletion. Thus, a fetus with a gene deletion may go undetected if the probe hybridizes to DNA around the deleted portion of the chromosome. This may be a particular concern if a defect involves a partial gene deletion. Therefore, this approach is applicable only if the probe does *not* hybridize to the gene outside of the deleted area. Furthermore, because diagnosis is based on the absence of a band, an error could result if fetal DNA is accidentally left out of the gel. In this case, a normal fetus may be diagnosed as affected. To avoid this potential error, a second probe specific for another gene should always be used to confirm the presence of DNA in the gel.

Mutations that Coincide with a Restriction Site

Sickle cell anemia is an autosomal recessive disorder affecting one out of 200 black children in the United States. The clinical manifestations include anemia, jaundice, and "sickle cell crises" marked by impaction of sickled cells, vascular obstruction, and painful infarcts in tissues, such as the bone, spleen, and lungs. The defect results from a single nucleotide substitution (A to T) in the sixth codon (GAG to GTG) of the β-globin gene. This mutation leads to the translation of valine instead of glutamic acid at position 6 of the β-globin polypeptide. The abnormal β-globin chains cause the red cells to assume a characteristic sickle shape if the oxygen tension or pH is reduced.

The mutation causing sickle cell anemia coincidentally resides within the recognition sites of restriction enzymes *Mst* II and *Cvn*I. Both of these enzymes recognize the nucleotide sequence CC^TNAGG, and thus an RFLP is created by the sickle cell mutation. Individuals with the sickle cell mutation lack the restriction site that is present in individuals with normal β-globin genes. The procedure for diagnosing fetuses affected with sickle cell anemia using RFLP analysis is illustrated in Figure 14–4. The only potential source of error with this procedure is if the disease is caused by a different mutation in a particular family (ie, genetic heterogeneity). Although the hemoglobinopathies are generally characterized by many different mutations causing similar clinical phenotypes, this is less common with sickle cell anemia. To avoid this possibility, family studies also can be performed to confirm the presence of the suspected mutation. This simple direct method has been applied only to sickle cell anemia; however, it should be applicable whenever a restriction site coincides with a mutation causing a disease.

Other Methods of Direct Diagnosis

New technologies that allow a more rapid diagnosis of genetic diseases are becoming increasingly available. How-

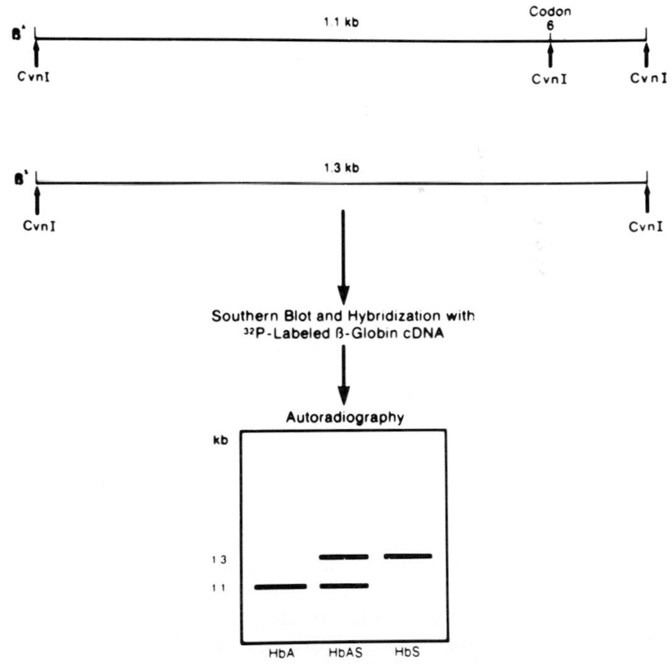

Figure 14–4. Use of a radioactively labeled β-globin probe to diagnose sickle cell anemia. The mutation causing the disease coincides with a *CvnI* site. Chromosomes with the sickle mutation lack the site that chromosomes with normal β-globin genes have. After digestion with *CvnI* and hybridization to a β-globin probe, DNA from individuals with sickle cell anemia yields a 1.3-kbp fragment, DNA from individuals with two normal β-globin genes yields a 1.1-kbp fragment, and carriers have 1.1- and 1.3-kbp fragments. (*From Ober C, Lynch DH. Molecular genetics. In: Sciarra JJ, ed.* Gynecology and Obstetrics. *Philadelphia, PA: J.B. Lippincott; 1989.*)

ever, these are only applicable when the DNA sequences flanking the specific mutation are known. One application, using PCR and allele-specific oligonucleotide (ASO) probes, is now the preferred method for diagnosis of sickle cell anemia.[9] This method quickly determines whether an individual carries zero, one, or two copies of the sickle cell gene. First, the β-globin gene DNA containing the point mutation that causes sickle cell anemia (ie, codon 6) is amplified. After 30 PCR cycles (2.5 hours), approximately 10^7 copies of the targeted β-globin sequence (a 536-base-pair fragment containing codon 6) are synthesized. The amplified segments are made single stranded and blotted in duplicate directly onto a membrane as "dot blots." Each filter is then hybridized to one of two 15-base-pair ASO. One ASO anneals with normal β-globin sequences but has a single nucleotide mismatch with abnormal (sickle cell) gene sequences. The second ASO anneals with sickle β-globin sequences but has a single nucleotide mismatch with normal gene sequences. The β-globin genotype of each sample of amplified DNA is determined by direct observation of the presence or absence of a colorimetric reaction with each probe. DNA that reacted to both ASO would be genotyped as HbAS (HbS carrier); DNA that reacted to the normal ASO only would be genotyped as HbAA (normal, noncarrier); and DNA that reacted to the sickle ASO only would be genotyped as HbSS (sickle cell anemia). The procedure requires one to two days to complete and can be performed on as little as 20 ng of DNA. (Standard RFLP or southern blot analysis requires 1–5 μg of DNA, and 1–2 weeks to complete). In addition to testing for sickle cell anemia, this approach also has been used to test for certain β-thalassemias.[9]

Unfortunately, few genetic disorders are as well characterized at the molecular level as the hemoglobinopathies or as genetically homogeneous as sickle cell anemia. Therefore, for most genetic disorders linkage-based family studies may be the more appropriate method for prenatal diagnosis and carrier detection.

PRENATAL DIAGNOSIS USING THE INDIRECT METHOD

The indirect method of DNA analysis through linkage-based family studies is, at least in theory, applicable to all genetic disorders. This strategy relies on finding an RFLP that is linked to the disease of interest. The RFLPs are used as codominant Mendelian markers to follow the inheritance pattern of the disease through families. It has been estimated that if RFLPs are identified an average of every 20,000 kbp throughout the genome, linkage studies will be possible for any genetic trait. Although this concept of a linkage map of the human genome was only first proposed in 1980[10], the rapid progress in this area has already made possible the prenatal diagnosis of many important genetic diseases, such as Duchenne's muscular dystrophy, polycystic kidney disease, neurofibromatosis, Huntington's disease, hemophilia A and B, and cystic fibrosis.

The basic principles and limitations of RFLP linkage analyses are illustrated in the following examples of family studies and prenatal diagnosis of CF and congenital adrenal hyperplasia (CAH).

Indirect DNA Diagnosis When the Biochemical Defect Is Unknown

Cystic fibrosis (CF) is the most common autosomal recessive genetic disorder among northern Europeans; approximately 4% are carriers (heterozygotes) and one child in 2500 births is affected with CF. Affected individuals rarely live past their twenties and suffer from debilitating pulmonary and digestive disorders. Linkage between CF and RFLPs on chromosome 7 was shown by mapping the CF gene to this chromosome in 1985.[10–14] The CF gene itself was identified recently.[15–17] A three-base pair deletion, resulting in loss of a phenylalanine residue at position 508 (ΔF508), was found in 75% of CF chromosomes[17]; the remainder each carry one of many (70+) less common mutations.

Direct detection of ΔF508 does not require studying an affected relative and could be used to screen the population for CF carrier status.[17] Because approximately 75% of CF carriers have ΔF508, 25% of carriers would go undetected. Thus, 25% of true carriers (approximately 1% of screened individuals) will have a negative test but are CF carriers. In addition, the frequency of the ΔF508 mutation is lower in ethnic groups other than northern European, non-Ashkenazi Caucasians. Among blacks, Ashnekazi Jews, and southern and eastern Europeans, it occurs in 30–60%. Thus, screening for CF mutations is recommended only for relatives with CF and for spouses of known CF carriers. Screening for CF carrier status in the general population is not recommended until more mutations can be tested for, thereby reducing the false-positive rate and increasing the sensitivity of the screen.[18,19] Direct testing for ΔF508 or other mutations is useful in families with a CF child. However, not all CF carriers have detectable mutations, and linkage analysis using RFLPs is still required in some families. Direct testing for ΔF508 is described elsewhere[20]; the indirect method of diagnosis is presented below.

Figures 14–5A and B illustrate the relationship between the CF gene and a closely linked RFLP in a family with three affected and two unaffected children, after southern blotting and hybridization analyses. The probe used is called *MetH*, which is cloned DNA from a gene on chromosome 7.[14] This probe hybridizes to DNA containing a polymorphic *Msp* I restriction site. DNA digested with *Msp* I and hybridized to the *Met*H probe yields DNA fragments of 5.5, 2.3, or 1.8 kbp or a combination of any two fragment lengths (each individual has two copies of each gene). The banding patterns after autoradiography for *Msp* I-digested DNA hybridized to the *Met*H probe are shown in Figure 14–5A, and the pedigree of the family with CF is shown in Figure 14–5B. The parents (I.1 and I.2) are presumed to be heterozygous carriers of the CF gene because they have three affected children. The affected children are assumed to be homozygous for the CF gene. The unaffected children can be either heterozygous carriers of the CF gene or can inherit normal genes from both parents and be homozygous normal. After DNA analysis (see Figure 14–5A), it is determined that the parents also are heterozygous at the *Msp* I site; the father has 5.5 and 2.3 kbp bands, and the mother has 2.3 and 1.8 kbp bands. RFLP analysis of DNA from the three affected children demonstrates 5.5 and 1.8 kbp bands. Thus, we can deduce that each affected child inherited a chromosome containing the 5.5 kbp *Msp* I fragment from their father and the 1.8 kbp *Msp* I fragment from their mother; and therefore, the CF gene must be on these parental chromosomes. Both parental chromosomes with the 2.3 kbp fragment must therefore carry the normal gene. We can further deduce that the sister with genotype 2.3/2.3 inherited the normal gene from each parent and is not a carrier for CF. The brother with genotype 5.5/2.3, on the other hand, inherited the chromosome with the normal gene from his mother

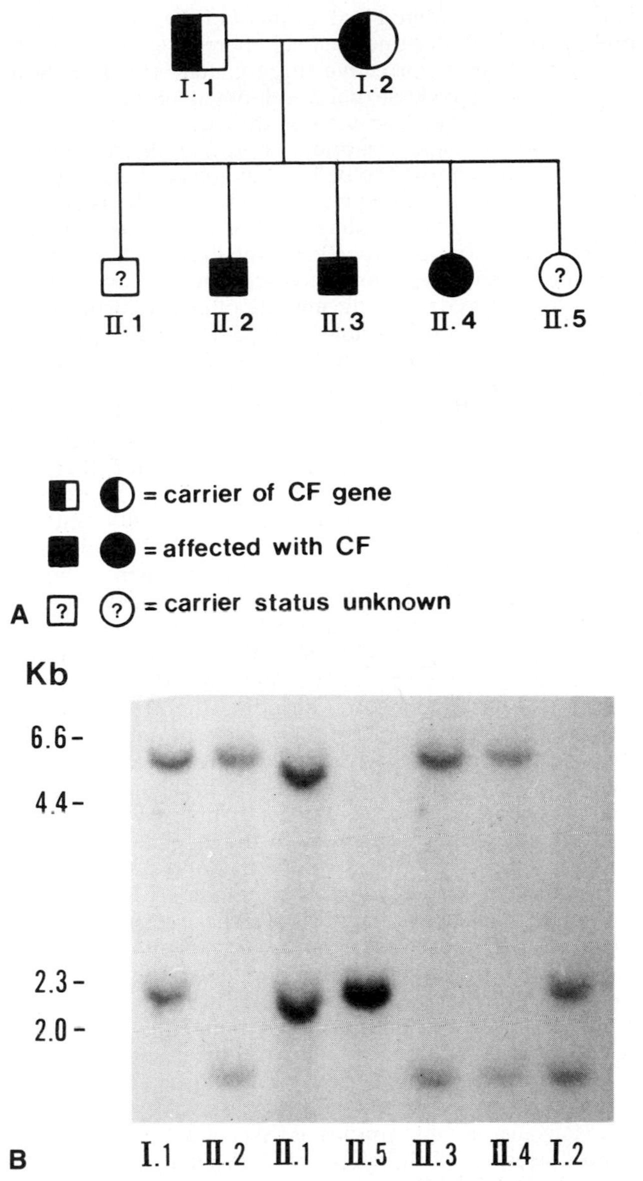

Figure 14–5. (*A*) DNA studies of family with cystic fibrosis. DNA digested with restriction enzyme *Msp*I and hybridized with probe *Met-H*. Resulting band sizes are 5.5 kbp, 2.3 kbp, or 1.8 kbp. (*From Ober C, Lynch DH. Molecular genetics. In: Sciarra JJ, ed.* Gynecology and Obstetrics. *Philadelphia, PA: J.B. Lippincott; 1989.*) (*B*) A family with cystic fibrosis. Children II.2, II.3, and II.4 are affected with CF. Parents are assumed to be carriers of the CF gene because they have affected children. After DNA studies of this family (*A*), it is determined that son II.1 is a carrier of the CF gene and daughter II.5 is homozygous healthy. See text for details. (*From Ober C, Lynch DH. Molecular genetics. In: Sciarra JJ, ed.* Gynecology and Obstetrics. *Philadelphia: J.B. Lippincott; 1989.*)

(2.3 kbp fragment) and the chromosome with the CF gene from his father (5.5 kbp fragment) and is presumed to be a carrier for CF.

Prenatal diagnosis of CF in subsequent pregnancies in this family also is possible. Fetal DNA derived from chorionic villi at 9–11 weeks' gestation or from amniotic fluid cells at 14–18 weeks' gestation could be genotyped for the *Msp* I polymorphism site using the methods described above. Thus, the CF status of the fetus could be deduced, and reproductive decisions could be made based on this information. As discussed previously, the major potential source of error in linkage studies is the probability of recombination between the restriction site and the abnormal gene in the parents' gametes. For example, if there was a meiotic cross-over in one of the father's gametes between the *Msp* I site and the CF gene, the CF gene may be on the chromosome with the paternal 2.3 kbp fragment in an offspring conceived from that gamete. If DNA from the fetus was determined to contain both the 2.3 and 1.8 *Msp* I fragments (genotype 1.8/2.3), a diagnosis of carrier would be made, but the fetus may be affected with CF. Thus, results from prenatal testing must always be given as a probability, considering the probability of recombination. For example, the recombination frequency between the *Msp* I site and the CF gene, determined from family studies, is less than 2%.[21] Thus, if prenatal testing of a subsequent pregnancy in the couple in Figure 14–5B revealed a 2.3/2.3 genotype, they should be counseled that the probability that the fetus does not have CF is equal to the probability that recombination has occurred between the CF gene and the RFLP in the maternal or paternal chromosome.

Recently, more rapid diagnoses of CF using PCR have been reported.[22,23] These methods still rely on family linkage studies, but they allow a diagnosis to be made in more than 70% of families at risk in 1–2 days after DNA is extracted from fetal tissue, instead of the 1–2 weeks required for standard RFLP analysis. In one method,[22] DNA that contains a polymorphic locus (*KM.19*) that is identified by the restriction enzyme, *Pst* I, is amplified. *KM.19* is within 100 kpb of the CF gene. Amplified DNA is digested with the restriction enzyme *Pst* I, and restriction fragments are electrophoresed. Banding patterns can be directly visualized under ultraviolet light, eliminating the need for southern blotting and hybridization. An example of this is depicted in Figure 14–6.

As illustrated in the previous examples, the indirect method of DNA analysis has already proven to be an invaluable tool for prenatal diagnosis of mendelian disorders. This general application is being applied to many genetic disorders in which the biochemical and molecular defects are unknown. Progress in this area is rapid, so it should not be long before prenatal diagnosis of any Mendelian disorder is feasible.

Indirect DNA Diagnosis When the Biochemical Defect Is Known

Congenital adrenal hyperplasia is an autosomal recessive disorder of cortisol biosynthesis, which is caused in 95% of cases by a deficiency in the enzyme steroid 21-hydroxylase.[24] This enzyme is required for the conversion of progesterone and 17-hydroxyprogesterone to 11-deoxycorticosterone and 11-deoxycorticosterol, which are intermediate products in mineralocorticoid and glucocorticoid biosynthesis, respectively.[25] Because of a lack of feedback suppression of this pathway in CAH, there is a compensatory increase in ACTH, leading to adrenal hyperplasia and excessive secretion of precursor steroids. The increased secretion of adrenal androgens (such as DHEA and DHEAS) leads to increased conversion of these products to testosterone and dihydrotestosterone.

Congenital adrenal hyperplasia occurs in a number of forms, ranging from mild to severe. The milder forms often

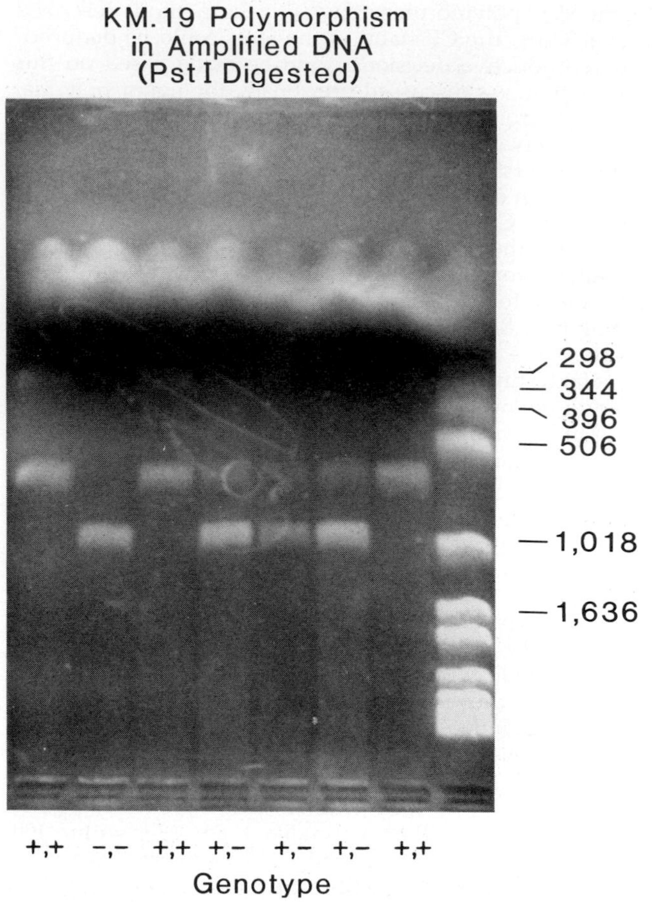

Figure 14–6. Diagnosis of cystic fibrosis in amplified DNA. DNA was amplified using PCR. Amplified DNA was digested with restriction enzyme *Pst* I and electrophoresed. DNA is labeled with ethidium bromide and visualized under ultraviolet light. Chromosomes that lack the *Pst* I cutting site ("−") appear as a single 950 base pair band (the size of the amplified DNA fragments). Chromosomes that have the cutting site ("+") appear as 650 and 300 base pair bands. The smallest 300 base pair band can not always be seen in the heterozygote.

present during childhood. More attenuated forms present at puberty (or even after puberty), with menstrual irregularities and infertility in women. The severe form is characterized by early virilization of female fetuses *in utero,* leading to marked masculinization of the external genitalia. Affected females may, in fact, be mistaken for males at birth, with bilateral cryptorchidism and hypospadias. The diagnosis may not be as obvious in males because the external genitalia are normal. Unless there is a recognized family history or indications of salt wastage (from a deficiency in the mineralocorticoids, which leads to hyperkalemia and sodium depletion, dehydration, and hypertension and compensatory hyper-reninemia), the disease process often is not diagnosed until later in infancy. Indeed, unrecognized salt wasting in CAH is often fatal because the inadequacy of glucocorticoids can lead to vascular collapse, shock, and death. The severe form of CAH occurs in 1 in 5000–10,000 births, and the milder (or attenuated) forms occur in approximately 1 in 1000 births.[26,27]

The virilization process *in utero* begins early in pregnancy because the genital ridge forms at 9–10 weeks' gestation. Fortunately, the virilization process of female fetuses *in utero* can be inhibited by treatment of the mother during pregnancy with dexamethasone, thereby eliminating the need for extensive corrective surgery after birth and allowing for normal psychosexual development and sexual function. However, because steroid treatment of the mother is not totally benign, treatment should be discontinued if the fetus is determined to be homozygous or heterozygous for the normal 21-hydroxylase genes or if the fetus is male. Thus, early and correct diagnosis of this genetic disease is of great importance. However, prenatal detection of CAH using biochemical tests for increased concentrations of amniotic fluid 17-hydroxyprogesterone often are inconclusive and usually are only feasible after 13–14 weeks' gestation.

The gene encoding the enzyme 21-hydroxylase has been mapped to the short arm of chromosome 6, closely linked to the HLA-B locus.[27–29] Gene probes for the 21-hydroxylase gene have been developed, and molecular genetic studies of this region have demonstrated that two copies of the 21-hydroxylase gene (called A and B) are present in this region.[27,30] These two genes can be differentiated by hybridizing 21-hydroxylase gene probes to *Taq* I-digested DNA; the A gene is detected on a 3.2 kbp fragment, whereas the B gene resides on a 3.7 kbp fragment. Detailed sequence analysis of the two genes has revealed that they are more than 90% homologous. However, three deleterious mutations in the A gene render it nonfunctional, whereas the B gene is a functional gene, encoding the 21-hydroxylase enzyme.[31,32] Analysis of southern blots of genomic DNA obtained from patients with salt wasting syndrome, using the cloned 21-hydroxylase gene as the probe, has revealed that in about 25% of patients, the 21-hydroxylase B gene is either deleted or converted to the A gene.[33] In these families, a direct diagnosis can be made to determine the presence or absence of the 3.7-kbp fragment. This application is analagous to the diagnosis of α-thalassemia discussed previously. In most cases, however, patients with CAH have the 3.7-kbp *Taq* I fragment (B gene) in their genomes; therefore, prenatal diagnosis of CAH in most families depends on the indirect method, even though the biochemical defects for this disorder are known. Probes specific for the 3′ untranslated region of the HLA-B locus have proven particularly useful for linkage studies in CAH families.

Molecular genetic studies of CAH families suggest that in most cases, small alterations of DNA (such as point mutations or small deletions or insertions) may inactivate the 21-hydroxylase B gene. These findings also underscore the fact that most genetic diseases are genetically heterogeneous. Thus, family studies using RFLP analysis with a number of probes closely linked to the abnormal gene will, in general, prove to be more accurate and useful in the molecular genetic diagnosis of congenital diseases, even for diseases in which the biochemical defects are known.

CONCLUSIONS

There is no doubt that DNA diagnosis has made striking contributions to the diagnosis of many genetic disorders, including the hemoglobinopathies, hemophilia A, Duchenne muscular dystrophy, cystic fibrosis, and congenital adrenal hyperplasia. The development of DNA probes linked to numerous other disorders (such as neurofibromatosis, Huntington's disease, and polycystic kidney disease) are becoming available at an almost dizzying rate, and their transfer into the clinical environment is already leading to simpler, faster, and more accurate diagnoses. This is clearly a field "whose time has come," and recombinant DNA techniques will play an important role in the diagnosis of disease now and in the future.

REFERENCES

1. Human Gene Mapping 9. Ninth international workshop on human gene mapping. *Cytog Cell Genet.* 1987;46:1.
2. McKusick VA. *Mendelian Inheritance in Man.* 8th ed. Baltimore, MD: Johns Hopkins Press; 1988.
3. Crawfurd M d'A. Prenatal diagnosis of common genetic disorders. *Brit Med J.* 1989;297:502.
4. Maniatis T, Fritsch EF, Sambrook J. *Molecular Cloning: A Laboratory Manual.* Cold Spring Harbor, NY: Cold Spring Harbor Laboratory; 1982.
5. Davis LG, Dibner MD, Battey JF. *Basic Methods in Molecular Biology.* New York, NY: Elsevier; 1986.
6. Southern EM. Detection of specific sequences among DNA fragments separated by gel electrophoresis. *J Molec Biol.* 1975;98:503.
7. Erlich HA, Gelfand DH, Saiki RK. Specific DNA amplification. *Nature.* 1988;331:461.
8. Kan YW, Golbus MS, Dozy AM. Prenatal diagnosis of alpha-thalassemia. Clinical application of molecular hybridization. *N Engl J Med.* 1976;295:1165.
9. Saiki RK, Chu-An C, Lenenson CH, et al. Diagnosis of sickle cell anemia and β-thalassemia with enzymatically amplified DNA and nonradioactive allele-specific oligonucleotide probes. *N Engl J Med.* 1988;319:537.
10. Botstein D, White RL, Skolnick M, Davis RW. Construction of a genetic linkage map using restriction fragment length polymorphisms. *Am J Hum Gen.* 1980;32:314.
11. Knowlton RG, Cohen-Haguenauer O, Van Cong N, et al. A polymorphic DNA marker linked to cystic fibrosis is located on chromosome 7. *Nature.* 1985;318:380.
12. Tsui L-C, Buchwald M, Barker D, et al. Cystic fibrosis locus defined by a genetically linked polymorphic DNA marker. *Science.* 1985;230:1054.
13. Wainwright BJ, Scambler PJ, Schmidtke J, et al. Localization of cystic fibrosis locus to human chromosome 7cen-q22. *Nature.* 1985;318:384.
14. White R, Woodward S, Leppert M, et al. A closely linked genetic marker for cystic fibrosis. *Nature.* 1985;318:382.
15. Rommens JM, Iannuzi MC, Kerem B, et al. Identification of the cystic fibrosis gene: chromosome walking and jumping. *Science.* 1989;245:1059.
16. Riordan JR, Rommens JM, Kerem B-S, et al. Identification of the cystic fibrosis gene: cloning and characterization of complementary DNA. *Science.* 1989;245:1066.
17. Kerem B-S, Rommens JM, Buchanan JA, et al. Identification of the cystic fibrosis gene: genetic analysis. *Science.* 1989;245:1073.
18. Wilfond BS, Fost N. The cystic fibrosis gene: medical and social implications for heterozygote detection. *JAMA.* 1990;263:2777.
19. Roberts L. CF screening delayed for awhile, perhaps forever. *Science.* 1990;247:1296.
20. Lemna WK, Feldman GL, Kerem B-S, et al. Mutation analysis for heterozygote detection and the prenatal diagnosis of cystic fibrosis. *New Eng J Med.* 1990;322:291.
21. Beaudet A, Bowcock A, Buchwald M, et al. Linkage of cystic fibrosis to two tightly linked DNA markers: Joint report from a collaborative study. *Amer J Hum Gen.* 1986;39:681.
22. Feldman GL, Williamson R, Beaudet AL, O'Brien WE. Prenatal diagnosis of cystic fibrosis by DNA amplification for detection of KM-19 polymorphism. *Lancet.* 1988;2:102.
23. Williams C, Williamson R, Coutelle C, et al. Same day, first-trimester antenatal diagnosis for cystic fibrosis by gene amplification. *Lancet.* 1988;2:102.
24. Childs BM, Grumbach MM, Van Wyk JJ. Virilizing adrenal hyperplasia, a genetic and hormonal study. *J Clin Invest.* 1962;35:213.
25. New MI, Levine LS. Recent advances in 21-hydroxylase deficiency. *Ann Rev Med.* 1984;35:649.
26. Speiser PW, Dupont B, Rubinstein P, et al. High frequency of nonclassical steroid 21-hydroxylase deficiency. *Am J Hum Genet.* 1985;37:650.
27. Carroll MC, Campbell RC, Porter RR. Mapping of steroid 21-hydroxylase genes adjacent to complement component C4 genes in HLA, the major histocompatibility complex in man. *Proc Nat Acad Sci, USA.* 1985;82:521.
28. Dupont B, Oberfield SE, Smithwick EM, et al. Close genetic linkage between HLA and congenital adrenal hyperplasia (21-hydroxylase deficiency). *Lancet.* 1977;2:1309.
29. Dupont B, Virdis R, Lerner AJ, et al. Distinct HLA-B antigen association for the salt-wasting and simple virilizing forms of congenital adrenal hyperplasia due to 21-hydroxylase deficiency. In: Terasaki PI, ed. *Histocompatibility Testing.* Heidelberg: Springer; 1984:660.
30. White PC, Grossberger D, Onufer BJ, et al: Two genes encoding steroid 21-hydroxylase are located near the gene encoding the fourth component of complement in man. *Proc Nat Acad Sci, USA.* 1985;82:1089.
31. White PC, New MI, Dupont B. Structure of human steroid 21-hydroxylase genes. *Proc Nat Acad Sci, USA.* 1986;83:5111.
32. Higashi Y, Yoshioka H, Yamani M, et al. Complete nucleotide sequences of two steroid 21-hydroxylase genes tandemly arranged in the human genome. *Proc Nat Acad Sci, USA.* 1986;83:2841.
33. Werkmeister JW, New MI, Dupont B, White PC. Frequent deletion and duplication of the steroid 21-hydroxylase genes. *Am J Hum Genet.* 1986;39:461.

Chapter Fifteen

Genetics of Spontaneous Abortion and Fetal Loss

Kathryn D. McGowan and Karin J. Blakemore

15

The understanding of genetic factors responsible for spontaneous abortion and fetal loss evolved with advances in modern cytogenetics. Before the development of karyotyping techniques, postulations regarding embryonic or fetal factors in pregnancy loss were limited to causes that could be visualized with the naked eye or with a microscope. Recognizable gross alterations in fetal structure were described in terms of growth retardation, major and minor malformations, or empty sacs. Increasing knowledge of human genetic endowment, starting with the role of chromosomal abnormalities in congenital malformation and disease, allowed for the emergence of a far more complex picture of fetal loss.

Chromosomal analysis of affected liveborns showed the full range of severity in cases of known syndromes, such as *Down's (trisomy 21), Patau's (trisomy 13),* or *Edwards' (trisomy 18)* syndromes. In general, the liveborn data preceded our knowledge of abnormalities during fetal life. Soon chromosomal etiologies became apparent in abortuses who resembled affected liveborns, and in abortuses displaying cytogenetic aberrancies that were never seen in liveborns. Large series elucidated the incidence of chromosomal aberrations in liveborns, abortuses, and pregnancies undergoing prenatal diagnosis, confirming the significant number of chromosomally abnormal pregnancies that never go to term. Innate nonviability, diagnosed by karyotype, joined the differential diagnosis for pregnancy loss, along with preterm labor, cervical incompetence, other abnormalities of maternal anatomy, hormonal or placental insufficiency, infections, maternal diseases (such as systemic lupus erythematosus), and exposure to environmental agents or teratogens.

Coincident with the advances in cytogenetics were developments in the more accurate diagnosis of early pregnancy by measuring the serum beta subunit of human chorionic gonadotropin and by performing prenatal ultrasound.

The role of chromosomal aberrations in the loss of early pregnancies was then apparent. Expanding fertility technology will hasten the use of prenatal diagnosis of genetic disorders at the preimplantation stage, to optimize an infertile couple's chance of carrying to term an infant who will survive and be healthy.[1,2]

INCIDENCE

Approximately 15% to 20% of clinically recognized pregnancies result in spontaneous loss. It has been well established that the rate of chromosomal abnormalities in first trimester abortions is approximately 50%.[3,8] As data from preimplantation conceptuses become available, this percentage is expected to increase.[1]

Landmark data were provided by Boué, Boué, and Lazar[9], who studied 1500 abortuses collected between 1966 and 1972, limited to pregnancies less than 14 weeks from the last menstrual period or 12 weeks' gestation on pathologic examination. They estimated that this duration of pregnancy includes at least 80% of the spontaneous abortions in recognized pregnancies because the frequency of loss declines with advancing gestational age. Their study is notable for the large number of early specimens obtained. Women seeking medical advice for symptoms of threatened abortion were provided with containers in which to collect the tissue at home if the pregnancy were lost. An average of 61% of the abortuses studied showed chromosomal abnormalities, with the range from 47–65%. When the first 2 years of study were excluded, the range narrowed to 62–65%. They compared this with an incidence of 0.5% for chromosomal abnormalities in newborns. The categories and incidence of abnormalities described have been confirmed in other studies.[3–5,7,10] These include *monosomy* (usually of the X chromosome), autosomal trisomies, *polyploidy* or duplications of the entire complement of chromosomes (most frequently *triploidy*), *mosaics,* and structural abnormalities of chromosomes (such as *translocations*).

The most frequent single chromosomal abnormality encountered in the first trimester is monosomy X, the cause of *Turner's syndrome.* This represented approximately 18% of the chromosomal anomalies recorded by Boué et al[9,11], and as many as 29% in other studies extending further in gestation.[7,10,12,13] At least 95% of 45,X conceptuses are lost prenatally, most commonly following arrest of development at approximately 6 weeks' gestation.

The largest category of chromosomal abnormalities found in spontaneous abortions is the *autosomal trisomies.* These comprise about one half of the chromosomal abnormalities seen in abortuses through the first 16 weeks of pregnancy. Unlike the trisomies seen in liveborn individuals, primarily affecting chromosomes 21, 13, 18, and the sex chromosomes, abortuses from the first trimester involve every autosome except 1 and only rarely involve the sex chromosomes. The most common autosomal trisomy among these abortuses involves chromosome 16, accounting for about 15% of the total samples collected.[9–11] Trisomy 16 is not seen in liveborn infants and can sometimes result in partial molar pregnancies similar to those seen in triploidy.[14]

Errors in chromosome number result from *nondisjunction* (improper division) during meiosis. Resulting conceptuses, which are either monosomic or trisomic, are generally so severely developmentally disrupted that they are eliminated before pregnancies are recognized, even using modern serum tests or ultrasound. Only a few of the autosomal trisomies survive past the first trimester, and these are generally the same disorders encountered in living individuals.

Unlike the case with 45,X conceptuses, there is a maternal age effect on the incidence of autosomal trisomies. This effect is most apparent on the acrocentric chromosomes of the D(13–15) and G(21–22) groups. This undoubtedly contributes to the increased incidence of spontaneous loss among older women.

Polyploidy contributes 20% to 25% of spontaneous abortions, most commonly in the form of *triploidy.* These conceptions usually result in empty sacs or simply very early losses, but some triploid conceptions result in *partial molar* pregnancies,[14] which show some recognizable evidence of fetal development.[15,16] Few triploid conceptions will reach viability, and these fetuses have a host of characteristic congenital anomalies.

Mosaicism comprises less than 5% of the cytogenetic abnormalities seen in spontaneous abortions. Mosaicism implies the presence of two or more chromosomal complements or populations of cells. There may be a normal (46,XX or 46,XY) cell line and an abnormal cell line. In assessing the incidence of mosaicism among abortuses, it is important to consider the presence of maternal (46,XX) tissue that may have contaminated the specimen. In addition, there may have been only placental tissue and not fetal or embryonic tissue available for culture after a spontaneous abortion. Although the villi of the early placenta generally reflect the genotype of the fetus, a propensity exists for placental tissue to exhibit mosaicism not actually present in the fetus itself. An abnormal cell line in the placenta does not appear to have as great an impact on the ability of a pregnancy to continue as does an abnormal cell line in the embryo or fetus itself. Sufficient numbers of cells within the placenta with a normal chromosomal complement may allow a pregnancy to continue to term, despite the presence of placental mosaicism.

Structural abnormalities of chromosomes, including translocations, inversions, and deletions, appear to contribute to less than 5% of chromosomally abnormal abortuses. Improved cytogenetic and recent DNA analysis techniques have allowed the identification of subtle forms of these errors, sometimes involving the loss or malfunction of single genes. In general, however, structural abnormalities refer to those visible to the cytogeneticist under the microscope. In the presence of these findings, examination of the parental karyotypes is necessary before speculating on the role of such an abnormality in future pregnancy loss for the couple. Structural abnormalities may occur *de novo;* that is, neither member of the couple shows any abnormality in his or her chromosomes, and the abortus' structural rearrangement represents an accident in the original germ cell. Occasionally, however, when couples are screened because of repeated pregnancy losses, one member is carrying a balanced rearrangement of chromosomal material. While that individual is phenotypically normal, his or her gametes can receive an abnormal complement of chromosomal material during oogenesis or spermatogenesis. This, in turn, can lead to miscarriage.

The incidence of chromosomal abnormalities among pregnancies lost at later gestational ages declines to approximately 20% to 30% in the second trimester and 5% to 10% in the third trimester.[5,7,9,17,18] These abnormalities of later gestation more closely reflect the types of abnormalities described in newborns. Because stillbirths may exhibit varying degrees of maceration, tissue growth in the cytogenetics laboratory may be precluded. This failure in tissue culture can result in underestimates of the true incidences of cytogenetic abnormalities.

Nonchromosomal embryonic or fetal abnormalities also may play a significant role in spontaneous pregnancy loss.[4,8] Embryos with multiple major malformations, which may be caused by a multifactorial, teratogenic, or unknown etiology, also may be unable to accomplish development beyond the early weeks of pregnancy.

RECURRENCE RISKS AND RECURRENT PREGNANCY LOSS

Despite the fact that at least one half of all early losses and possibly one third of all second-trimester losses are chromosomally abnormal, recurrence risks have been difficult to determine. In Lauritsen's group of 288 women whose spontaneous abortuses were karyotyped, the risk of subsequent abortion showed a positive correlation with the number of previous abortions; the karyotype of the index fetus also was relevant. If the karyotype was normal and this was the woman's first pregnancy loss, 85% of patients subsequently sustained a pregnancy to term; twenty-six percent had at least one subsequent abortion. For women in this group (ie, with a normal karyotype for the index abortus) who had had previous pregnancy losses, 45% would have a subsequent spontaneous abortion. If the karyotype of the index fetus was abnormal and this was the woman's first loss, only about 14% had subsequent abortions. With a history of repetitive losses, the incidence of subsequent abortions rose to 20% in this group.[7]

Warburton et al[18] performed a similar study on women with two consecutive abortions. Their data indicate that if a woman has a chromosomally abnormal index abortus, the incidence of an abnormal karyotype in the subsequent abortus was no higher than the 50–60% risk for the general population. If the index abortus was karyotypically normal, the odds for the subsequent abortus to likewise be chromosomally normal were higher (72–83%) than expected for the general population (40–50%). In other words, fewer than the "background risk" of 50–60% had an abnormal karyotype on the products of conception. This may reflect the likelihood that the causes for the miscarriages in the latter group of women include nongenetic etiologies, such as uterine anomalies, infections, or medical conditions such as systemic lupus erythematosus.

According to Alberman et al,[19] there may be an increased risk of trisomy 21 in offspring of women whose abortuses are chromosomally abnormal. This finding was not confirmed by Warburton et al.[18] Until further information is available on the significance of various chromosomal abnormalities in early abortuses, the subsequent risk for trisomic conceptuses surviving past the first or second trimester is unknown.

Individuals experiencing recurrent pregnancy loss are candidates for a detailed evaluation that includes a chromosomal analysis of both members of the couple. A heparinized blood sample is drawn using the usual aseptic technique. A culture of the lymphocytes is then obtained from this specimen. The incidence of chromosomal abnormalities in one member of the couple varies with the definitions of recurrent loss and abnormality. FitzSimmons et al[20] examined three of the most commonly used definitions of recurrent loss in their study of 740 individuals referred to a university genetics center for the evaluation of recurrent loss. Patients were grouped according to the pregnancy history recorded at the time of referral, between 1972 and 1979. Of 340 men and women (165 couples and 10 single women) with a history of two consecutive spontaneous losses, six chromosomal abnormalities were detected, representing approximately 2% of the men and women. This percentage was not significantly different from the number of abnormalities found in 305 individuals (144 couples and 17 single women) with three or more consecutive losses. A smaller, third group included men and women with a fetal loss rate greater than 50% who had conceived at least two pregnancies; these losses were not necessarily consecutive and did not include neonatal deaths. This third group comprised 26 couples and three single women, including only one person with a chromosomal abnormality, also equalling 2%. The incidences and abnormalities detected (primarily translocations, pericentric inversions, and sex chromosome abnormalities) in the three groups studied were not dissimilar to those found in other studies.[21–25] The actual percentage of such couples showing an abnormal karyotype ranges from 0%[24] to 31%.[26] An average taken from published data provides an incidence of 6–9%.[24,27] Even the 2% figure is, nevertheless, relatively large when compared to the incidence of such abnormalities in the general population, which is well under 1%.[22,26] Even a subtle structural abnormality in a parent can predispose to abnormal pairing or separation of chromosomes during gametogenesis and can lead to pregnancy loss.

In addition to performing blood lymphocyte karyotypes on both members of the couple, karyotyping any subsequent abortus may be beneficial if a future miscarriage occurs. If the abortus is chromosomally abnormal, the couple can be reassured as to the etiology and proceed directly to conceiving again. If the abortus' karyotype is normal, further investigation into other nongenetic causes of habitual abortion may be warranted.

EVALUATION AND RECOMMENDATIONS

The importance of eliciting a careful obstetric and family history of all patients of reproductive age cannot be overemphasized. The history should include the outcomes of pregnancies with prior partners, neonatal deaths, and spontaneous losses in the present and previous two generations. Any individuals born with congenital anomalies or who developed inherited diseases should be ascertained. The sex of any abnormal offspring should be noted whenever possible because this may allow the elucidation of sex-linked disorders within the family. Ethnic origins and the presence of consanguineous unions also are important. By carefully constructing the pedigree, genetic etiologies for spontaneous loss may become apparent.

The work-up for habitual losses in the first trimester includes karyotypes on both members of the couple. In addition, the products of future conceptions, if there are any subsequent miscarriages, generally should be submitted for cytogenetic study. For example, a couple undergoes a thorough evaluation, including normal blood (lymphocyte) karyotypes, and the woman is diagnosed with hypothyroidism, for which she is treated. She conceives and again suffers a first-trimester loss. Her obstetrician–gynecologist sends fetal tissue and chorionic villi for cytogenetic analysis, and the results show trisomy 16. This couple can be reassured that this last miscarriage was almost certainly caused by the trisomy 16, and any further work-up is not indicated for the history of reproductive losses.

Any couple experiencing repeated miscarriages may benefit from a chromosomal study on the products of conception, not just on the couple themselves. The tissue should be handled in as sterile a manner as possible and placed into sterile tissue culture media. This is usually available in microbiology and cytogenetic laboratories. If no media is available, the tissue should be covered with a saline-moistened gauze in a capped sterile container, or the serum spun from a blood specimen can be used to transport the sample to the laboratory. It is best *not* to immerse the tissue in saline.

It is important to submit tissue that is representative of the products of conception to the cytogenetics laboratory. The laboratory personnel must then recognize maternal decidua and discard it. A sample of chorionic villi may be the only viable, and perhaps the only recognizable tissue available for submission at the time of an early miscarriage. Although fetal tissue samples may grow exceptionally well in culture, maceration after fetal demise may preclude any growth at all. If maceration or the procedure of suction curettage prohibits accurately identifying tissue as fetal in origin, it is probably better to submit chorionic villi, which are easily recognizable under a dissecting or inverted microscope or by gross examination. Villi are useful to submit at all gestational ages when a fetal karyotype is desired because they may represent the most viable tissue. For term stillbirths, a small wedge of placenta can be submitted, along with any fetal tissue samples.

Autopsy and chromosomal analyses should be encouraged on all stillborn and congenitally malformed offspring. A higher culture success rate may be expected by performing an amniocentesis or chorionic villus sampling antenatally as soon as a malformation or intrauterine demise is diagnosed instead of postponing the recovery of samples for cytogenetic study to after delivery. Bacterial or fungal contamination contributes to culture failure when specimens are not collected until after delivery. Likewise, the importance of a fetal autopsy cannot be overemphasized. Although it is a difficult time for the parents emotionally, patients whose fetuses have died *in utero* should be encouraged sensitively that such information may be of great importance. Subsequent review of all studies, with both members of the couple present, should be offered as a routine part of follow-up care in the months after the loss and before any future pregnancies. Consultation with subspecialists in genetics, perinatology, neonatology, or pathology may result in a differential diagnosis for the loss, which can indicate further studies on the couple or prenatal diagnostic studies in future pregnancies.

A subsequent pregnancy is commonly conceived before counseling and a proper work-up have been accomplished. However, pregnant women should not receive less comprehensive evaluations of their past history simply because they are already pregnant. The evaluation should proceed as quickly as possible. Many evaluations can be undertaken in pregnancy, even though certain tests (such as a hysterosalpingogram) cannot. Studies begun even late in pregnancy may influence a couple's choice of site and mode of delivery and allow for consultation with specialists familiar with prognosis and treatment after birth, if a fetal abnormality is detected.

Couples who have experienced the loss of a wanted pregnancy undergo a grief reaction similar to the experience of losing a loved one they may have known all their lives. The question of *why* is invariably raised. An understanding of the underlying causes and pursuit of the proper evaluations are of great value in these circumstances. This can contribute to the couple's peace of mind and emotional healing and afford them a sound management plan for future pregnancies.

REFERENCES

1. Wramsby H, Fredga K, Liedholm P. Chromosome analysis of human oocytes recovered from preovulatory follicles in stimulated cycles. *N Engl J Med*. 1987;316:121.
2. Warburton D. Reproductive loss: How much is preventable? *N Engl J Med*. 1987;316:158.
3. Alberman ED, Creasy MR. Frequency of chromosomal abnormalities in miscarriages and perinatal deaths. *J Med Genet*. 1977;14:313.
4. Byrne J, Warburton D, Kline J, et al. Morphology of early fetal deaths and their chromosomal characteristics. *Teratology*. 1985;32:297.
5. Creasy MR, Crolla JA, Alberman ED. A cytogenetic study of human spontaneous abortions using banding techniques. *Hum Genet*. 1976;31:177.
6. Hassold T, Chen N, Funkhouser J, et al. A cytogenetic study of 1000 spontaneous abortions. *Ann Hum Genet*. 1980;44:151.
7. Lauritsen JG. Aetiology of spontaneous abortion. *Acta Obstetricia et Gynecologica Scandinavica*. 1976;52(suppl):1.
8. Poland BJ, Miller JR, Harris M, et al. Spontaneous abortion: A study of 1,961 women and their conceptuses. *Acta Obstetricia et Gynecologica Scandinavica*. 1981;102(suppl):1.
9. Boué J, Boué A, Lazar P.: The epidemiology of human spontaneous abortions with chromosomal anomalies. In: Blandau RJ, Witschi E, eds. *International Symposium on Aging Gametes*. New York, NY: S. Karger; 1975:330.
10. Carr DH, Gedeon M. Population cytogenetics of human abortuses. In: Hook EB, Porter IH, eds. *Symposium on Human Population Cytogenetics*. New York, NY: Academic Press; 1977:1.
11. Boué J, Boué A. Chromosomal abnormalities and abortion. In: Coutinho EM, Fuchs F, eds. *Physiology and Genetics of Reproduction, Part B*. New York, NY: Plenum Press; 1975:317.
12. Martin AO. Cytogenetics. In: Sciarra JJ, ed. *Gynecology and Obstetrics, Volume Five: Reproductive Endocrinology, Infertility and Genetics*. Philadelphia, PA: J.B. Lippincott; 1988:1.
13. Martin AO. Genetics of spontaneous abortion. In: Sciarra JJ, ed. *Gynecology and Obstetrics, Volume Five: Reproductive Endocrinology, Infertility and Genetics*. Philadelphia, PA: J.B. Lippincott; 1988:1.
14. Vassilakas P, Riotton G, Kajii T. Hydatidiform mole, two entities: A morphological and cytogenetic study with some clinical considerations. *Am J Obstet Gynecol*. 1977:127:167.
15. Szulman AE, Surti U. The syndromes of hydatidiform mole, I: Cytogenetic and morphologic correlations. *Am J Obstet Gynecol*. 1978;131:665.
16. Szulman AE, Surti U. The syndrome of hydatidiform mole, II: Morphologic evolution of the complete and partial mole. *Am J Obstet Gynecol*. 1978;132:20.
17. Kajii T, Ferrier, A, Nikawa N, et al. Anatomic and chromosomal anomalies in 639 spontaneous abortuses. *Hum Genet*. 1980;55:87.
18. Warburton D, Kline J, Stine F, et al. Does the karyotype of a spontaneous abortion predict the karyotype of a subsequent abortion?—Evidence from 273 women with two karyotyped spontaneous abortions. *Am J Hum Genet*. 1987;41:465.
19. Alberman E, Elliott M, Creasy M, et al. Previous reproductive history in mothers presenting with spontaneous abortions. *Br J Obst Gynecol*. 1975;82:366.
20. FitzSimmons J, Wapner RJ, Jackson LG. Repeated pregnancy loss. *Am J Med Genet*. 1983;16:7.
21. Portnoi MF, Joye N, Van Den Akker J, et al. Karyotypes of 1142 couples with recurrent abortion. *Obstet Gynecol*. 1988;72:31.
22. Pantzar JT, Allanson JE, Kalousek SK, et al. Cytogenetic findings in 318 couples with repeated spontaneous abortion: A review of experience in British Columbia. *Am J Med Genet*. 1984;17:615.
23. Lyberatou-Moraitou E, Grigori-Kostaraki P, Retzepopoulou Z, et al. Cytogenetics of recurrent abortions. *Clin Genet*. 1983;23:294.
24. Ward BE, Henry GP, Robison A. Cytogenetic studies in 100 couples with recurrent spontaneous abortions. *Am J Hum Genet*. 1980;32:549.
25. Michaels VV, Medrano C, Venne VL, et al. Chromosome translocations in couples with multiple spontaneous abortions. *Am J Hum Genet*. 1982;34:507.
26. Stenchever MA, Parks KJ, Daines TL, et al. Cytogenetics of habitual abortion and other reproductive wastage. *Am J Obstet Gynecol*. 1977;127:143.
27. Schwartz S, Palmer CG. Chromosomal findings in 164 couples with repeated spontaneous abortions with special consideration to prior reproductive history. *Hum Genet*. 1983;63:28.

Chapter Sixteen
Prenatal Diagnosis of Genetic Disorders

Marion S. Verp

16

Prenatal diagnosis was first performed in the mid 1950s when Fuchs and Riis[1] and several other groups demonstrated that fetal sex could be determined by X-chromatin analysis of amniotic fluid cells. In 1966, Steele and Breg[2] cultured and karyotyped amniotic fluid cells, leading to the first antenatal diagnosis of a chromosome abnormality. Simultaneously, Nadler[3] reported *in utero* detection of an enyzme abnormality—galactosemia—using amniotic fluid cells. Antenatal diagnosis is now an accepted component of prenatal care for women at increased risk for a child with a genetic or chromosomal abnormality. This chapter, which reflects my previous communications,[4,5] reviews currently accepted indications and techniques for antenatal genetic diagnosis, considers additional indications that may prove valid, and discusses the development of less invasive approaches to early detection of fetal disorders.

For most genetic disorders, fetal cells are required for diagnosis. Several techniques are available to obtain fetal cells with a reasonable degree of safety.

AMNIOCENTESIS

In early gestation, solutes are present in amniotic fluid in concentrations similar to those found in maternal serum. Amniotic fluid also contains fetal proteins (e.g., alpha-fetoprotein) and cells desquamated from amnion, fetal skin, gastrointestinal, genitourinary, and respiratory tracts. The diagnosis of chromosomal disorders and many enzyme deficiencies require amniotic fluid cells to be cultured before analysis, accounting for the 2–4-week interval from procedure to results. Less commonly, biochemical or DNA studies can be performed on the amniotic fluid or on uncultured cells, shortening the time of diagnosis substantially.

Technique

Amniocentesis, the aspiration of amniotic fluid, is traditionally performed at 15–17 weeks' gestation (menstrual weeks) because at this stage of gestation, sufficient amniotic fluid is present, the uterus is accessible to a transabdominal approach, the ratio of viable to nonviable cells is greatest, and adequate time is available to complete the diagnosis before fetal viability. Some investigators have been exploring the possibility of performing amniocentesis earlier in gestation (ie, at 12 to 14 weeks). Whether performed at the traditional time or earlier, the technique is similar. An ultrasound examination (preferably dynamic imaging) is performed immediately before amniocentesis to determine fetal biparietal diameter and femur length (to confirm gestational age), position of the placenta, location of amniotic fluid, presence of fetal cardiac activity or fetal movement, and number of fetuses (see also Chapter 6). Lidocaine may be infiltrated in the subcutaneous tissue, followed by transabdominal passage of a 20- or 22-gauge spinal needle into the uterus. Ultrasound monitoring can be continued during needle insertion. The initial drops of amniotic fluid are discarded to minimize the possibility of maternal cell contamination. Fifteen to thirty cubic centimeters of amniotic fluid are aspirated into two or three syringes, the amount withdrawn varying with individual laboratory requirements and gestational age (less amniotic fluid is removed from earlier gestations, see below). Grossly blood-stained amniotic fluid is aspirated occasionally; fortunately, blood usually does not adversely affect amniotic cell growth. In experienced hands, failure to aspirate fluid during an amniocentesis occurs only rarely (approximately 1%).

Amniocentesis can be reliably performed on twin gestations by the injection of dilute indigo carmine into the first sac after aspiration of fluid. A second amniocentesis is then performed in the ultrasonographically determined location of the second sac.[6,7] Aspiration of clear amniotic fluid confirms that the second sac has been entered.

Safety

Amniocentesis involves risk to both mother and fetus; however, maternal risks are low. For example, minor maternal complications (eg, transient vaginal spotting, minimal amniotic fluid leakage) occurred in 2–3% of cases, but serious complications (amnionitis) occurred in only one of 1040 patients in a study conducted by the United States National Institute for Child Health and Human Development (NICHD).[8] Anti–Rh (D) immune globulin is administered to Rh-negative women in most centers to avoid the possibility of Rh-immunization.[9,10]

Potential fetal risks include needle puncture, umbilical cord hematoma and occlusion, placental separation, chorioamnionitis, and premature labor. Reported major injuries have been extremely rare. The question of increased fetal loss after amniocentesis has been addressed by several large collaborative studies[8,11–13] and reviewed elsewhere[5,10] (Table 16–1). Briefly, in the US study[8], 3.5% of pregnant women who underwent amniocentesis experienced fetal loss between the time of the procedure and delivery, compared to 3.2% of controls; the small difference was not statistically significant and disappeared completely when corrected for maternal age. In a Canadian study,[11] matched controls were not recruited; however, the fetal loss rate in the amniocentesis group was 3.3%, not different from that of the US controls.

A third major collaborative study, undertaken by the United Kingdom Medical Research Council[12], reached different conclusions. This study found that the rate of fetal loss after amniocentesis was increased by 1.0–1.5%. However, subjects were significantly older than controls and of significantly greater parity, differences that might account

TABLE 16–1. FETAL LOSS RATES AFTER AMNIOCENTESIS[a]

	Study Patients	Controls
NICHD[8]	2.8%	2.4%
U.K.[12]	2.6%	1.1%
Tabor et al[13]	1.7%	0.7%

[a] To 28 weeks' gestation.

for the increase in fetal loss and antepartum hemorrhage. In fact, when the data were reanalyzed to control for age and parity, the difference in fetal loss rates were only borderline in significance.

Criticisms have been directed toward the selection of controls in the UK study, which initially was biased by the elimination of a small number who aborted soon after enlistment in the study, and selection of controls whose gestation was more advanced at the time of entry. However, these concerns were recognized and dealt with in a supplementary study.[12] The supplementary study included 1026 subjects and 1026 controls matched to exclude the foregoing oversights. The subjects still were found to have increased fetal losses compared to controls (2.6% versus 1.1%).

Recently, a randomized controlled study of amniocentesis was performed in Denmark[13] on 4606 women aged 25–34 years who were without known risk factors for fetal genetic abnormalities. Women with a number of risk factors for pregnancy loss were excluded. Maternal age, previous pregnancy history, social group, and smoking history were comparable in the study and control groups, as was gestational age at time of entry into the study. The spontaneous abortion rate after 16 weeks was 1.7% in amniocentesis patients compared to 0.7% in controls ($p < 0.01$). The authors also noted a 2.6 times higher relative risk of spontaneously aborting if the placenta was traversed.[13,14] In contrast, Crane and Kopta,[15] and Hanson et al[16] showed no difference in loss rates between groups in which the placenta was or was not perforated.

The Danish study,[13] the British study,[12] and animal studies[17] suggest that respiratory problems may occur more often in children born after amniocentesis. However, respiratory problems have not been consistently observed by other investigators.[18] Moreover, long-term follow-up (ie, 5–7 years) of 62 children whose mothers had undergone amniocentesis indicated no increase in physical or neurodevelopmental problems.[19]

To summarize, the risk of fetal loss associated with amniocentesis is relatively low. In counseling patients, a 0.5% risk of abortion secondary to amniocentesis may be cited. Patients also should be told that serious maternal complications and fetal injuries are reported but are very rare.

Early Amniocentesis

The studies cited above have assessed the risk of amniocentesis performed between 15–20 weeks' gestation. Recently, with the development of higher resolution ultrasound equipment and experienced sonologists, some centers have begun offering amniocentesis before 15 weeks' gestation. The majority of early amniocenteses have been performed at 13–14 weeks; only a few centers have sampled amniotic fluid before 13 weeks in pregnancies intended to continue. The technique is similar to that of routine amniocentesis, except that a smaller volume of fluid is removed because total amniotic fluid volume averages only 30–40 cc at 10–11 weeks and 50–100 cc at 12 to 14 weeks' gestation. Ultrasound guidance is particularly important because of the relatively small target area and the need to avoid the maternal bladder and bowel, which may obstruct the most desirable path to the uterus.

Because the number of such procedures reported to date is small, the efficacy and safety of early amniocentesis is still unknown. Initial reports of total pregnancy loss rates following early amniocentesis range from 0.9% to 6.5%.[5] These figures represent total fetal losses; that is, they include background losses and procedure-related losses. The number of amniocenteses performed at each gestational week is so small that it is difficult to evaluate whether procedure-related losses are increased over that of amniocentesis at 15 weeks or later. Fetal injuries and pulmonary and orthopedic disorders following early amniocentesis have not been assessed. A prospective randomized study will be necessary to determine whether the complication rate for early amniocentesis is greater than that of routine amniocentesis or chorionic villus sampling. If not, experienced clinicians probably will choose to offer amniocentesis for chromosome diagnosis somewhat earlier in gestation than is now the case. Early amniocentesis, however, may prove less reliable for measuring acetylcholinesterase than amniocentesis at 16 weeks[20]; therefore, it may prove disadvantageous for the patient at increased risk for a fetal neural tube defect (see below).

CHORIONIC VILLUS SAMPLING

Technique

Because amniocentesis results are not usually available before the middle of the second trimester, couples frequently experience great anxiety awaiting results. If an abnormality is diagnosed and pregnancy termination is chosen, maternal risk, expense, and psychologic stress are considerably greater than they would have been for a first-trimester pregnancy termination.

These concerns have led to the development of a diagnostic procedure that can be performed in the first trimester, chorionic villus sampling (CVS). Chorionic tissue is derived from the same fertilized cell as the fetus; therefore, fetal genetic abnormalities should be reflected in the chorion. Chorionic villus sampling is usually performed at 9–12 weeks' gestation by way of the cervix or abdomen. In transcervical CVS, a narrow-gauge catheter is introduced through the cervix into the uterus and a small amount of chorionic villus (placental) tissue is aspirated with a syringe. Ultrasound is used to monitor and direct the movement of the catheter (Fig. 16–1). The transabdominal approach to CVS requires insertion of an 18- to 20-gauge needle under ultrasound guidance through the maternal abdominal wall into the placenta, with aspiration of villus tissue. With either approach, the sample is examined immediately to assure

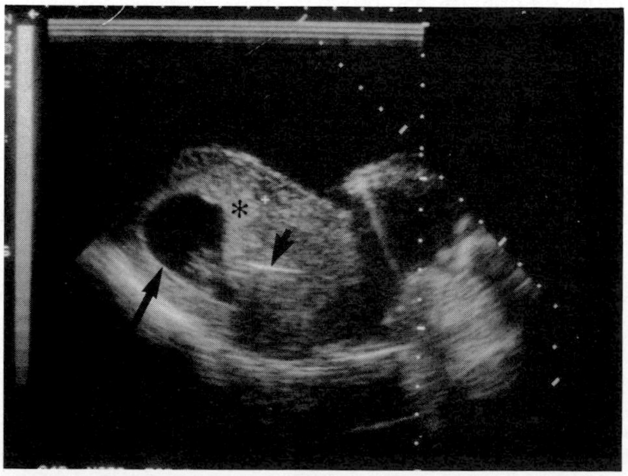

Figure 16–1. Ultrasound visualization of transcervical CVS. (* = anterior placenta; short arrow = indicates sampling catheter; long arrow = posterior surface of amniotic cavity.)

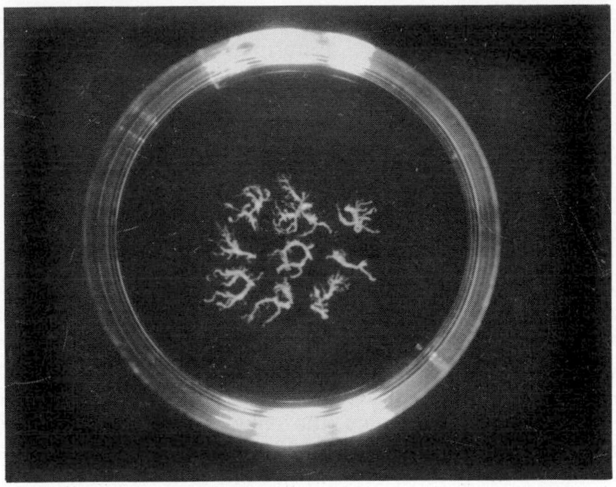

Figure 16–2. A 15–20 mg sample of chorionic villi. The characteristic villus structure can be seen.

that adequate villus material has been obtained. (Villus tissue is identified by characteristic morphologic features. See Fig. 16–2.) If the sample is insufficient or contains only maternal decidua rather than chorionic villi, a new sterile catheter or needle can be placed for a second attempt.

With each sampling, ten to 25 mg of villi are obtained. Many diagnoses (chromosomal, biochemical, DNA) can be performed directly on the villus tissue without culturing the cells first. In the case of chromosome analysis, this possibility exists because, in contrast to amniotic fluid cells, early trophoblastic tissue contains many spontaneously dividing (mitotic) cells. In addition to direct chromosome analysis, most laboratories also culture a portion of villus tissue for confirmatory diagnosis. Direct analysis can usually be completed within 2 days for chormosome or biochemical diagnosis; results from cultured cells are available in 1–2 weeks.

Only rarely is a CVS not technically appropriate or feasible by the transcervical or transabdominal route. Active cervvcal infection, presence of an intrauterine device, cervical stenosis, or fibroids may dictate one approach or the other. However, choice of method is usually made based on position of the placenta and uterus (eg, the transabdominal procedure for an anterior or fundal position in an anteverted uterus and the transcervical for a posterior placenta in the same uterus). Transabdominal CVS is also possible in the second and third trimesters and is useful when a high-risk patient has registered late for prenatal care or when ultrasound examination has detected anomalies consistent with a chromosome abnormality.

Rh immune globulin usually is given to Rh-negative women after CVS, just as in amniocentesis.

Safety

Both maternal and fetal risks exist with CVS. Following transcervical CVS, maternal spotting and bleeding are common (30%)[21,22]; these events are rarer after transabdominal CVS. Two cases of serious maternal infection have been reported, but a recent series of 4268 women undergoing transcervical CVS showed no serious maternal infections.[21]

Theoretical fetal risks include induction of deformation secondary to disruption of the amniotic sac and intrauterine growth retardation from placental loss or injury. Although at least one report of a fetus with amniotic band syndrome after CVS has been published, the overall frequency of congenital defects and low birth weight does not appear increased in CVS patients.[21–23]

The question of the fetal loss rate associated with CVS has been addressed by two large collaborative studies. In a Canadian study, 2787 women aged 35 years or older were randomized to either CVS or amniocentesis.[22] Total losses (spontaneous abortions, induced abortions, stillbirths) were 7.6% in the CVS group and 7.0% in the amniocentesis group. The difference was not statistically significant. These investigators also noted a shift to late pregnancy losses in the CVS group, but again this trend did not reach statistical significance.

The second study, performed at seven US centers, compared pregnancy outcome in 2278 women who had CVS and 671 women who underwent amniocentesis.[21] The patients were not randomized, but all procedures were performed at the same seven centers. Losses from spontaneous abortions, induced abortions, stillbirths, and neonatal deaths were 7.2% in the CVS patients, and 5.7% in the amniocentesis group. Adjustment for differences in gestational and maternal age yielded an excess loss rate in the CVS group of 0.8%, (80% CI −0.6% to 2.2%), not a statistically significant difference. In contrast to the Canadian data, excess losses occurred before 16 weeks gestation only.

In summary, although more data are needed to produce a precise risk estimate, the risk of loss associated with CVS is probably between 0.5% and 1.0% when performed by experienced individuals.

FETAL TISSUE SAMPLING

It is possible to perform chromosome, biochemical, or DNA studies on fetal lymphocytes aspirated from umbilical vessels under fetoscopic or ultrasound guidance (cordocentesis). For certain genetic disorders, fetal serum is used for diagnosis. Results frequently can be obtained from fetal blood in less than 1 week. Fetal blood sampling is performed in the second and third trimesters for a variety of indications, including pregnancy at high risk for a genetic disorder with late presentation for care or ultrasound diagnosis of a fetal anomaly. Details regarding technique and risks are given in Chapter 212.

Fetal skin biopsy for detection of severe dermatologic disorders is possible, but the associated fetal loss rate is about 5%.[24] Finally, fetal liver biopsy has been performed in a limited number of cases for detection of metabolic disorders not expressed in other more accessible tissues. Fetal loss rate is similar to that following skin biopsy.

INTERPRETIVE PROBLEMS IN CYTOGENETIC DIAGNOSIS

Variation naturally exists as a function of the experience and techniques of a given laboratory; however, in most well-established laboratories, the success rate for amniotic fluid and chorionic villus cultures is high. Nonetheless, there are several potential sources of error or confusion. First, in a particular case, poor growth may provide insufficient cells for proper analysis. Direct preparation of spontaneously dividng CVS cells usually yields metaphases of poorer quality than those obtained from cultures.

A second potential problem is that maternal, rather than fetal, cells may cultured. This phenomenon occurs in 0.3% of amniocentesis[25] and 2% of cultured CVS specimens.[26] Almost all cases of 46.XX/46.XY mosaicism in amniotic fluid or CVS cultures are caused by maternal cell contamination (MCC) of a sample from a normal male fetus. In addition to creating some difficulties in cytogenetic interpretation, MCC may be devastating if undetected in a sample destined for biochemical or DNA diagnosis. The incidence of MCC in amniotic fluid is minimized by not using the first few drops of aspirated fluid for cell culture. In CVS, careful separation of villus from decidual tissue is mandatory. Using a direct CVS preparation minimizes the chance of misinterpretation caused by maternal contamination because spontaneous mitoses from maternal decidua are very rare.

A third potential source of error is *in vitro* origin of aberrations. *In vitro* aberrations arise in all culture systems and should be suspected if many different aberrations are detected in the same specimen or if an abnormality is detected in only one of several cultures initiated from the same specimen. The problem of *in vitro* aberrations is considered in more detail elsewhere,[27] but, briefly, cells containing an extra chromosome (N = 47) occur in about 3% of amniotic fluid and CVS specimens. If the aberrant cell(s) are confined to a single clone (*in situ* technique) or culture (flask technique) and multiple other clones or cultures do not contain cells with the identical aberration, the finding is termed *pseudomosaicism* and is without clinical significance in almost all cases. Tetraploidy occurs normally in human amnion and villi and should not cause concern.

In contrast to pseudomosaicism, *true fetal mosaicism* may be present if cells with the same abnormal complement are detected in more than one flask of clone. True fetal mosaicism occurred in only 0.25% of a large collaborative study of amniotic fluid cells. When consistent abnormalities were present, the neonate was subsequently confirmed to be a mosaic in 70% of cases. Autosomal mosaicism was much more frequently associated with phenotypic anomalies at birth or abortion (35%) than was sex chromosome mosaicism (8%).[28] More common than in amniotic fluid cultures, the finding of true mosaicism in chorionic villi occurs in about 1% of cases.[26] Because in most cases the abnormality has proved to be limited to villi and is not present in the fetus, amniocentesis is usually recommended for clarification of fetal status.

Finally, true mosaicism may not be detected prenatally if the minority cell line is limited to tissues not sampled or if the line is of low frequency. Despite potential for error, however, accuracy in cytogenetic diagnosis is greater than 99%.

Apart from errors, dilemmas in interpretation may arise. For example, difficulty in predicting the phenotype arises when an apparently balanced translocation, inversion, or small supernumerary chromosome is detected. In such cases, parental chromosomes should be analyzed immediately. If a phenotypically normal parent has the identical translocation, inversion, or supernumerary chromosome, the fetus also can be expected to be phenotypically normal. On the other hand, if the translocation, inversion, or supernumerary chromosome has arisen *de novo* in the fetus, pooled data indicate that 10% to 20% of these fetuses will be phenotypically abnormal.[29] The finding of a sex chromosome abnormality also creates a quandary. Although abnormal phenotype and slow development are associated with 45,X, 47,XXX, 47,XXY, and 47,XYY, most individuals with these complements are neither severely retarded nor grossly malformed. Parents may have great difficulty in deciding whether or not to terminate such a pregnancy. In a study at Northwestern University, only 41% of pregnancies with sex chromosome abnormalities diagnosed at amniocentesis were terminated, in contrast to 88% of those with autosomal trisomies, and none with *de novo* balanced structural abnormalities.[30]

ACCEPTED INDICATIONS FOR ANTENATAL CYTOGENETIC STUDIES

Cytogenetic studies can be performed readily from amniotic fluid cells, chorionic villus cells, or fetal lymphocytes. Thus, chromosomal disorders are potentially detectable in all pregnancies. Although technically feasible, however, it is not appropriate to determine the complement of every fetus because for many couples, the risks of prenatal diagnosis outweigh the potential benefits. In this section, unequivocal indications for cytogenetic studies are considered.

Advanced Maternal Age

Eighty-five to ninety percent of all prenatal diagnosis is performed solely for advanced maternal age. There is still no widely accepted explanation for the relationship between aneuploidy and advanced maternal age. One hypothesis is that chiasmata between homologous chromosomes decrease in aging oocytes, leading to nondisjunction and chromosomally abnormal ova. A second theory is that cumulative risk for exposure to an unknown environmental toxin increases with age, again leading to nondisjunction. In contrast to the overall incidence of trisomy 21 (one per 800 live births in the United States),[31] the likelihood of a 35-year-old mother having a child with trisomy 21 is one in 385; at age 39, the risk is one in 137, and at age 45 the risk is one in 30 (Table 16–2).[32]

Trisomy 21 is not the only chromosomal abnormality that increases with maternal age. Trisomy 13, trisomy 18, 47,XXX, and 47,XXY also occur more frequently with increased maternal age.[32] Based on these data, most American authorities believe prenatal diagnosis should be offered to all women who will be 35 years old or older when their infant is born. However, the choice of a particular age is largely arbitrary because the risk for a chromosomally abnormal child increases steadily each year, even among younger women. Therefore, flexibility is desirable when confronted by an inquiry from a woman younger than 35 years. Some women younger than age 35 may be relatively less concerned about the risk of miscarriage than the risk of a chromosomally abnormal liveborn, and they may wish to have a diagnostic procedure despite the ostensibly unfavorable risk to benefit ratio.

The risk figures cited previously are based on detection in liveborns. In fact, the prevalence of abnormalities in antenatal studies at 16–18 weeks' gestation is about 50% higher than that in liveborn infants,[32] and the prevalence in first trimester CVS studies is even higher.[33] Discrepancies between the frequencies in liveborns and in first- and second-trimester fetuses are accounted for by the disproportionate number of chromosomally abnormal fetuses that abort spontaneously before livebirth.[32,33]

Previous Child With Chromosome Abnormality

After the birth of one child with an autosomal trisomy or a sex chromosome abnormality, the likelihood that subsequent progeny will have a chromosome abnormality traditionally has been considered increased, even if parental chromosome complements are normal. Actually, the risk for a second offspring with Down's syndrome or another

TABLE 16–2. CHROMOSOME ABNORMALITIES AT BIRTH AND AT AMNIOCENTESIS[a]

Maternal Age	Risk of Down's Syndrome at Birth	Risk of a Chromosome Abnormality at Birth	Risk of a Chromosome Abnormality at 16–20 Weeks' Gestation
20	1/1667	1/526[b]	
21	1/1667	1/526[b]	
22	1/1429	1/500[b]	
23	1/1429	1/500[b]	
24	1/1250	1/476[b]	
25	1/1250	1/476[b]	
26	1/1176	1/476[b]	
27	1/1111	1/455[b]	
28	1/1053	1/435[b]	
29	1/1000	1/417[b]	
30	1/952	1/384[b]	
31	1/909	1/384[b]	
32	1/769	1/322[b]	
33	1/625	1/317	1/185
34	1/500	1/260	1/154
35	1/385	1/204	1/125
36	1/294	1/164	1/101
37	1/227	1/130	1/82
38	1/175	1/103	1/66
39	1/137	1/82	1/53
40	1/106	1/65	1/42
41	1/82	1/51	1/33
42	1/64	1/40	1/27
43	1/50	1/32	1/21
44	1/38	1/25	1/17
45	1/30	1/20	1/13
46	1/23	1/15	1/10
47	1/18	1/12	1/8
48	1/14	1/10	1/6
49	1/11	1/7	1/5

[a] Because sample size for some intervals is relatively small, 95% confidence limits are sometimes relatively large. Nonetheless, these figures are suitable for genetic counseling.
[b] 47,XXX excluded for ages 20–32 (data not given).
From Hook[39] and Hook et al.[32]

chromosome abnormality appears to be increased only for mothers age 29 or younger at the time of the birth of the proband with Down's syndrome. Nonetheless, parental anxiety dictates that antenatal chromosomal studies at least be offered to all couples who have previously had a Down's syndrome child.

Information concerning recurrence risk after the birth of a child with a chromosomal abnormality other than trisomy 21 is limited, but data from four collaborative studies indicate that the risk is 1–2% for the same or a different chromosomal abnormality.[34–37] Thus, antenatal studies also should be offered to these couples.

Parental Translocation, Inversion, or Aneuploidy

Translocation. A third, less common, cytogenetic indication for antenatal diagnosis is the presence of a balanced translocation, inversion, or numerical chromosomal abnormality (aneuploidy) in a parent. For example, 5% of children who have Down's syndrome do not have three free chromosome 21s, but rather an unbalanced translocation between a chromosome 21 and another acrocentric chromosome. (Translocations between two acrocentric chromosomes [13, 14, 15, 21, 22] are called *robertsonian translocations* (see also Chapter 13). Of children who have Down's syndrome as a result of a translocation (eg, 46,XX,-14,+t[14q;21q]), one parent has the same translocation chromosome in a balanced state (eg, 45,XX-14,−21,+t[14q;21q]) in 25–50% of cases. Empiric risks are less than theoretic risks that a parent carrying a t(14q;21q) chromosome will have a child with Down's syndrome. If the father carries the translocation, the risk is at most 2%; whereas, if the mother carries the translocation, the risk is about 10–15%. This sex-specific difference has been found in cases ascertained through chromosomally abnormal liveborns and in collaborative reports of amniotic fluid[38] and CVS studies[37] (Table 16–3). Risks are similar

TABLE 16–3. RISK OF AN UNBALANCED REARRANGEMENT IN A FETUS WHOSE PARENT HAS A BALANCED REARRANGEMENT (CARRIER)

		Fetus		
Rearrangement	Sex of Carrier	Normal	Carrier	Unbalanced
t(14q;21q)[a]	Female	58	87	25 (14.7%)
	Male	24	34	0
t(13q;14q)	Female	69	88	0
	Male	27	46	0
Reciprocal translocations (pooled)	Female	168	166	44 (11.6%)
	Male	97	107	27 (11.7%)
Inversions (pooled)	Female	32	30	5 (7.5%)
	Male	14	35	2 (4%)

[a] Also includes CVS data from reference 37.
From Boué and Gallano.[38]

for other robertsonian translocations involving chromosome 21 (eg, t[13q;21q], t[15q;21q], t[21q;22q]), but robertsonian translocations that do not include chomosome 21 apparently carry much lower risks for unbalanced offspring. In fact, t(13q;14q), the most common robertsonian translocation found in normal individuals, apparently carries less than a 1% risk (see Table 16–3).

Reciprocal translocations do not involve centromeric fusion and, hence, usually do not involve acrocentric chromosomes. Unfortunately, because of their rarity, specific empiric data for most translocations are not available, and generalizations must be made based on pooled data derived from many different translocations. Again, theoretic risks for abnormal (unbalanced) offspring are greater than empiric risks, which are approximately 12% for maternal or paternal carriers[38] (see Table 16–3).

Inversions. In a chromosomal inversion, the normal sequence of genes on the chromosome is altered. Like those with balanced translocations, subjects with such inversions are phenotypically normal; however, they may produce unbalanced gametes if during meiosis I, crossing over (recombination) occurs within the inverted sequence. Thus, certain genes would be duplicated and others would be deficient in the unbalanced gamete[40] (Fig. 16–3). Pericentric inversions and inversions involving long segments are more likely to be associated with anomalous offspring than paracentric or short-inversion segments.[40] Empiric data are not available for specific inversions, but pooled data for all inversions indicate about a 5% risk for abnormal progeny, with maternal carriers at greater risk than paternal carriers[38] (see Table 16–3). An exception is inv(9), which is a common variant and is thought to be without clinical significance.

Aneuploidy. If a parent has a numerical chromosomal abnormality (aneuploidy), the risk to offspring is increased. For example, approximately 35% (but less than the theoretical 50%) of offspring of women with 47,XX,+21 (Down's syndrome) are aneuploid[41]; Therefore, antenatal chromosomal studies are indicated in a pregnant woman with Down's syndrome. Men with Down's syndrome are sterile. If a parent is mosaic for trisomy 21, antenatal diagnosis is in order. Although risk figures are plainly biased by the method of ascertainment, approximately 20% of offspring of fertile 45,X, 45,X/46,XX, and 45,X/46,XX/47,XXX subjects are said to show chromosome abnormalities.[41] Women with 47,XXX or 46,XX/47,XXX also have produced children with chromosome abnormalities. Theoretically, 47,XYY men are at increased risk for chromosomally abnormal offspring, but only a few abnormal offspring have been reported. Men with 47,XXY (Klinefelter's syndrome) are sterile, but those with mosaicism (46,XY/47,XXY) may be fertile. Antenatal diagnosis should be offered to all aneuploid individuals.

Relationship of Ascertainment to Empiric Risk. Mode of ascertainment is a significant determinant of empiric risk for an unbalanced liveborn. That is, when a family with a trans-

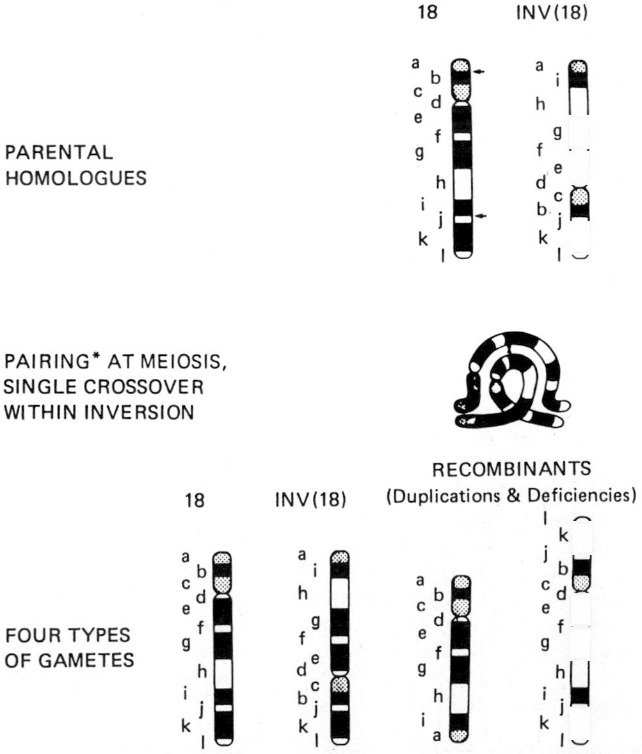

Figure 16–3. The effects of a single crossover within a pericentric inversion loop. Both normal and abnormal gametes result. Only two of the four strands are shown. (*From Simpson*[40] *with permission.*)

location is ascertained through a balanced proband, the risk for an unbalanced liveborn is lower than when ascertainment is through an unbalanced individual. Presumably, with some translocations, unbalanced gametes do not arise during meiosis, or, alternatively, unbalanced products are not selected at the gametic or early embryonic level. For example, if a rearrangement has been ascertained during an evaluation for repetitive abortions, the risk for an unbalanced liveborn is lower than the risk expected following ascertainment through an anomalous liveborn.[38]

Mendelian Disorders Associated With Chromosome Breakage

Several inherited disorders are characterized by chromosome breakage *in vivo* and *in vitro*. Individuals with these disorders often show increased propensity for neoplasia, growth retardation, and various somatic anomalies. Bloom syndrome, ataxia telangiectasia, and Fanconi's anemia are examples of these disorders. In some, the precise molecular defect is not known, but in each, distinctive cytogenetic features may permit antenatal diagnosis. For example, Voss and coworkers diagnosed Fanconi's anemia in a second-trimester fetus on the basis of high frequencies of spontaneous and clastogen-induced chromosome breakage in amniotic fluid cells.[42] More recently, similar studies have been performed with chorionic villus tissue and fetal blood. The disorders discussed in this section are inherited in autosomal recessive fashion; therefore, couples who have had an affected child have a 25% recurrence risk in each pregnancy. Antenatal diagnosis should be offered to these families.

Fragile X Syndrome and Other X-Linked Recessive Disorders

The fragile X syndrome is an X-linked disorder characterized in males by moderate mental retardation, macro-orchidism, a long face, and a prominent jaw. About one third of female carriers (heterozygotes) are mildly retarded, and two thirds have a normal phenotype. This syndrome accounts for a significant proportion of cases of familial X-linked mental retardation. The gene responsible for the condition is linked to a "fragile site" on the long arm of the X chromosome, visible as a break or gap in the chromosome structure. The fragile site is seen only when cells are grown in a special medium deficient in folic acid and thymidine or when an antimetabolite, such as 5-fluorodoxyuridine or methotrexate, is added to the culture medium.

Each male or female offspring of a female heterozygote has a 50% chance of inheriting the fragile X chromosome. Prenatal diagnosis has been accomplished by visualization of the fragile site in amniotic fluid cells, chorionic villus tissue, and fetal blood.[43] Unfortunately, both false-negative and false-positive results have occurred in amniotic fluid and CVS samples. Fetal blood cultures may prove more reliable. Molecular (DNA) methods also have been used to diagnose fragile X syndrome. However, genetic heterogeneity exists because in some families, the fragile X site is only loosely linked to the available probes. Therefore, DNA studies are not applicable to all families.

In other X-linked recessive or male-limited autosomal dominant traits, ordinarily only males are affected. It is possible to distinguish affected male fetuses in some sex-limited disorders. In others, affected infants can be consistently avoided only by terminating all pregnancies in which the fetus is male. In these cases, antenatal chromosomal studies to determine fetal sex may be indicated.

POTENTIAL INDICATIONS FOR CYTOGENETIC STUDIES

Even if use of antenatal cytogenetic studies increases greatly, the incidence of liveborns with chromosomal abnormalities would not be greatly decreased so long as the studies are performed only for the indications cited previously. Offering antenatal diagnosis only to women aged 35 and older decreases the frequency of trisomy 21 by less than 20%. Monitoring on the basis of the other cytogenetic indications contributes even less to decreasing the overall frequency of liveborns with chromosomal abnormalities. On the other hand, offering antenatal diagnosis to all women does not seem justified because of the small, yet finite, risk of invasive procedures. Therefore, optimally younger women whose risk of having a chromosomally abnormal fetus justifies the risk of prenatal diagnosis would be identified. That is, these women would constitute a high-risk group based on factors such as previous reproductive or medical history or fetal characteristics. A discussion of potential indications for antenatal studies follows.

Low Maternal Serum Alpha-Fetoprotein

Maternal serum alpha-fetoprotein (MSAFP) screening was initially developed for detection of fetal neural tube defects that are associated with elevated values of MSAFP (see below). However, more recently, investigators have shown that women with low MSAFP are at increased risk for a fetus with an autosomal trisomy, particularly trisomy 21.[44] Why MSAFP is decreased in such pregnancies is still uncertain, but it probably relates to decreased fetal production of alpha-fetoprotein. A number of pilot programs are now prospectively investigating the efficiency and feasibility of detection of trisomy 21 with MSAFP screening. In one study, an algorithm based on maternal age and MSAFP level was used to identify women younger than 35 years whose estimated risk for a fetus with Down's syndrome was ≥ one in 270 (2.1% of the total group of 51,141).[45] Of the patients selected, one in 81 had a fetus with trisomy 21, and one in 58 had a fetus with trisomy 21 or trisomy 18. Likewise, DiMaio et al[46] using a similar protocol, screened 34,354 women younger than age 35 and offered amniocentesis to 4.3%. One in 161 women had a Down's syndrome fetus, and one in 112 had Down's syndrome or another autosomal trisomy. DiMaio et al[46] calculated that MSAFP screening had detected 26% of the Down's syndrome cases expected in this group of pregnant women, as compared with the 10–20% that are detected by performing amniocentesis only on women age 35 or greater. Use of MSAFP to screen for chromosomal abnormalities is investigational. However, if further data support the sensitivity and specificity already reported, it is likely that low MSAFP will become an accepted indication for fetal chromosome analysis. Also of interest is a preliminary report that suggests that fetal trisomies may be detectable in the first trimester using a sensitive immunoradiometric assay for MSAFP.[47] Further research in this area can be expected.

In addition to alpha-fetoprotein, the usefulness of two other fetal–placental products in prenatal screening for Down's syndrome are under investigation. Bogart et al[48] have shown that human chorionic gonadotropin (hCG) is elevated in many pregnancies with chromosomally abnormal fetuses, and Canick et al[49] have reported depressed levels of unconjugated estriol in the same circumstances. This work has led to the suggestion that screening based on the aggregate values of maternal age, MSAFP, estriol, and hCG will be more efficient than maternal age and

MSAFP alone.[50] If additional work verifies this model and the cost to benefit analysis shows it to be feasible, the Down's syndrome detection rate should be increased without unduly increasing the number of amniocenteses performed.

Advanced Paternal Age

Although the relationship between aneuploidy and increased maternal age is better recognized and more established, in some studies, Down's syndrome also has been associated with advanced paternal age. Stene and coworkers[51] and others found that the risk of siring offspring with trisomy 21 increased by paternal age 55 and possibly earlier. Other investigators, however, have found a much smaller or no effect.[52–54] Therefore, advanced paternal age alone is probably not a sufficient indication for prenatal studies.

Previous Stillborn or Spontaneous Abortions

Couples experiencing *repetitive abortions* should undergo cytogenetic studies to exclude the presence of a parental translocation or inversion, either of which clearly justifies antenatal chromosomal studies. In the absence of a parental chromosome rearrangement, it is uncertain whether the risk for a trisomic liveborn is increased in couples with recurrent spontaneous abortions, even if their abortus is known to have been trisomic.[5] Because of this uncertainty, we generally offer prenatal diagnosis in the latter situation but not when the abortuses are known to have had normal chromosomes or when chromosome studies were not performed on the abortus.

Exposure to Irradiation or Chemotherapeutic Agents

Retrospective case-control studies have shown that women whose pregnancies produced liveborn offspring with Down's syndrome received significantly more X-irradiation before conception than controls. Irradiation occurred 2 to 10 years before conception, and doses as small as .02 Gy appeared to predispose to aneuploidy.[55] These studies are highly suggestive, and other studies revealed no such correlation.[56] Therefore, antenatal diagnosis does not seem warranted after diagnostic radiation before pregnancy and certainly not if exposure occurred during pregnancy.

Evaluation of risk following therapeutic radiation therapy is more complex. Radiation can cause gametic chromosomal and genetic damage, and men treated with testicular radiation doses of 0.4–5.0 Gy have shown an increased number of chromosome abnormalities in sperm.[57] However, empirically, no increase in congenital anomalies has been found in the offspring of individuals treated with X-irradiation for Hodgkin's disease or other cancers.[58,59] Japanese women exposed to X-irradiation through proximity to the atomic bomb explosions also did not show an increased prevalence of Down's syndrome offspring.[60] Therefore, antenatal cytogenetic studies might be discussed, but not encouraged, for women (or men) who have undergone radiation therapy. Couples electing to undergo antenatal diagnostic studies must realize that only numeric and structural chromosome abnormalities can be assessed. There is no possibility of monitoring for gene mutations, which also would be predicted to increase following irradiation.

Similar reasoning might also apply to men and women who have received chemotherapeutic agents because many agents used to treat neoplasia produce *in vitro* chromosomal damage and induce mutations. A person who had previously received such agents would thus theoretically be at increased risk for chromosomally abnormal progeny. Analogous to irradiation data, no increase in the actual rate of anomalies has been observed in liveborn infants of such couples.[58,59,61] Thus, antenatal cytogenetic studies are not necessarily indicated in this situation, although the issue may be worthy of discussion.

Fetuses Manifesting Anomalies on Ultrasound Examination

Gross anomalies frequently can be visualized in fetuses with chromosome abnormalities (see also Chapters 6 and 213). Antenatal chromosomal studies using amniocentesis, transabdominal CVS, or fetal blood sampling are appropriate if an abnormal fetus is detected on ultrasound examination. Even if chromosomal studies cannot be obtained soon enough to permit pregnancy termination, cesarean section for fetal distress in a fetus with a lethal abnormality might be avoided.

Recently, Lockwood et al[62] and Benacerraf et al[63] have reported sonographic screening methods for detecting Down's syndrome based on an elevated biparietal diameter to femur length ratio and the presence of a thickened nuchal skin fold. Although their results appear promising, other groups have not been able to satisfactorily discriminate between Down's syndrome and normal fetuses. Whether ultrasound detection of Down's syndrome will be applicable generally remains to be established.

Future Directions

It would be ideal if fetal chromosomal abnormalities could be detected without invasive procedures. If noninvasive techniques were available, all pregnant patients could be screened irrespective of history or age.

One approach being investigated involves recovery of fetal lymphocytes from maternal blood. Fetal lymphocytes are present in the maternal circulation during pregnancy, and analysis of many metaphases from blood samples of pregnant women usually shows a few nucleated fetal cells. To enrich the sample, it is necessary to separate fetal from maternal cells. Iverson and colleagues have attempted to do so by the presence of a paternal cell surface antigen (HLA) and Y-chromatin in fetal cells.[64] However, fetal lymphocytes isolated in this fashion are not transformed. Without transformation, the mitotic cells required for cytogenetic analysis cannot be obtained. One alternative to transformation might involve the use of quantitative hybridization with chromosome-specific DNA probes. For example, Julien and colleagues incubated a probe for chromosome 21 with amniotic fluid cells and counted the number of hybridized loci per cell.[65] The presence of three "spots" indicated trisomy 21, and the finding was confirmed with fetal blood studies. Similar studies might be possible on fetal cells extracted from the maternal circulation. A second possibility is measurement of relative DNA content of fetal cells with flow cytometry,[66] increased DNA content implying the presenne of an additional chromosome. Because DNA studies can be performed on interphase cells, the need for inducing mitosis is obviated, and the time from sampling to diagnosis could be a matter of days.

The approaches described previously are still potentially unreliable because fetal cells sometimes persist from previous pregnancies. However, if a reliable method of isolating fetal cells from maternal blood were available, a screening approach similar to that used for neural tube defects could be initiated. Blood could be obtained from all pregnant patients who desired testing. Those women whose blood samples revealed fetal chromosomal abnormalities would then be offered CVS, amniocentesis, or fetal blood sampling for confirmation. If universal screening were implemented, however, the demands for cytogenetic evaluation would be so great that automated methods for chromosomal analysis would likely be required. Automated systems for metaphase location and karyotyping already are available, and development or automated specimen-preparation systems is under investigation.

MENDELIAN DISORDERS

Mendelian disorders result from single mutant genes transmitted in dominant or recessive fashion, on an autosome or an X chromosome. Most Mendelian disorders individually are rare, although collectively, Mendelian disorders cause abnormalities in approximately 1% of liveborn infants. Typically, a couple will be identified to be at risk for a child with a Mendelian disorder because previously they had an affected child. In other cases, screening programs will identify heterozygotes for recessive disorders (eg, sickle cell anemia, Tay–Sachs disease) before the birth of an affected child.

The diagnosis of a Mendelian disorder is a more difficult undertaking than that of cytogenetic diagnosis. First, the correct diagnosis of a previously affected child must be confirmed so that the appropriate antenatal test can be performed. Second, detection of abnormalities requires that an aberrant or deficient gene product be expressed in amniotic fluid cells, chorionic villi, or fetal blood or that a DNA diagnosis is possible. Because some proteins are produced only in certain tissues (eg, ornithine carbamyl transferase in liver), fetal blood, amniotic fluid, and chorionic villus cells may not necessarily be used interchangeably for diagnosis. Third, one must be aware of the developmental pattern of normal fetal metabolism and not perform sampling before the age when discrimination between affected and healthy individuals is possible. Gestational-age matched controls are necessary. Fourth, diagnosis of rare mendelian disorders may be performed only in one or two referral laboratories. Physicians who are not geneticists cannot be expected to be fully informed about this complex area, and most patients at risk for a Mendelian disorder should be referred to a geneticist for consultation (see also Chapter 17).

Inborn Errors of Metabolism

Several compendia of metabolic disorders detectable *in utero* have been published.[67,68] Although almost immediately out-of-date because of rapid advances in the field, they are useful resources. Only a few examples of disorders that can be diagnosed prenatally will be discussed.

Tay–Sachs Disease. Tay–Sachs disease (G_{M2}-gangliosidosis type I) is an example of a recessive inborn error of metabolism for which screening programs have been developed and antenatal diagnosis is possible. In this disorder, hexosaminidase A, the enzyme necessary for metabolism of G_{M2}-ganglioside, a sphingolipid, is virtually absent. Sphingolipids accumulate, interfere with neurologic development, and result in death by 3 to 4 years of age. Heterozygotes for Tay–Sachs disease are rare in the non-Jewish population (one in 300) but are much more common among Ashkenazi Jews (one in 27). Intensive education programs aimed at the latter population have resulted in widespread screening for heterozygote detection. At-risk pregnancies can be monitored by assay of the hexosaminidase A level in amniotic fluid fibroblasts or chorionic villi. Affected fetuses can thus be recognized and pregnancy termination offered.

Serum hexosaminidase A activity decreases relative to total hexosamidase during pregnancy. Therefore, pregnant women mistakenly may be diagnosed as heterozygotes (false-positives). Thus, leukocyte assays should be available when a pregnant woman is tested.

Cystic Fibrosis. Cystic fibrosis is the most common serious Mendelian disorder in the Caucasian population. Life expectancy averages only 20–30 years, with death usually caused by respiratory failure or meconium ileus.

Cystic fibrosis is transmitted in an autosomal recessive pattern. Heterozygote detection is not yet routinely available; therefore, at-risk couples are usually identified after the birth of an affected child. DNA analysis is now possible for many at-risk families (see also Chapter 14). For others for whom DNA diagnosis may not prove informative, measurement of amniotic fluid microvillar intestinal enzymes (ie, alkaline phosphatase, gamma-glutamyl transpeptidase, leucine amniopeptidase) may be useful, albeit not 100% sensitive or specific.[69]

Hemoglobinopathies

In sickle cell anemia, α-thalassemia, β-thalassemia, and other disorders of hemoglobin biosynthesis, the metabolic derangment is limited to erythrocytes. Fetal blood may be obtained by aspiration from the umbilical vessels under fetoscopic of ultrasonic guidance (cordocentesis). If necessary, fetal cells can be separated from maternal cells by selective hemolysis. The final (pure) fetal sample is then incubated with radioactive leucine. The relative rates of synthesis of new globin chains (β:α ratio) can be measured to determine the presence or absence of β-thalassemia. The types of globin synthesized (eg, B^A or B^s) can be determined for diagnosis of sickle cell anemia. Hemoglobin assays have been more than 99% accurate.[70]

Fetal blood sampling for diagnosis of hemoglobinopathies has become almost obsolete, however, because recent developments in molecular genetics permit diagnosis of hemoglobinopathies by analysis of DNA from amniotic fluid fibroblasts or chorionic villi (see also Chapter 14). CVS and amniocentesis can be performed earlier in pregnancy than fetal blood sampling, and are probably safer.

Hemophilia and Other Disorders Detectable by Fetal Serum Assays

Many fetal disorders are potentially diagnosable by analysis of sera, rather than erythrocytes. Hemophilia A is reliably detectable based on the ratio between factor VIII-related antigen and factor VIII-coagulant antigen; the latter is decreased in hemophiliac fetuses.[71] Hemophilia B (factor IX deficiency) can be detected by similar methodology[71], as can homozygous von Willebrand disease. However, recent advances in DNA technology have obviated the need for fetal serum sampling for most disorders.

Dermatologic Disorders Detectable by Fetal Skin Sampling

Mutant genes may produce life-threatening dermatologic disorders. Examples include several different forms of epidermolysis bullosa and ichthyosis. Although autosomal dominant and X-linked recessive forms of each also exist, it is usually the autosomal recessive forms that are severe enough to justify antenatal diagnosis. Because neither the metabolic basis nor the gene defect responsible for these disorders is known, the only available method of antenatal diagnosis is histologic examination of fetal skin biopsy. Either fetoscopy or ultrasonography is used to direct the biopsy. The risk of subsequent abortion is about 5%. Diagnoses have been made for harlequin ichthyosis, epidermolytic hyperkeratosis, epidermolysis bullosa letalis, and others.[24]

Structural Defects

Certain mendelian and polygenic disorders characterized by structural anomalies are amenable to diagnosis by visualization using ultrasound, roentgenography, or fetoscopy. This topic is reviewed in Chapter 213.

ALPHA-FETOPROTEIN ANALYSIS

Failure of embryonic neural tube closure leads to anencephaly or *spina bifida* (myelomeningocele or meningocele). *Anencephaly* is incompatible with life, but spina bifida is not. Spina bifida may lead to hemiparesis, urinary incontinence, hydrocephalus, and mental retardation. Anencephaly and spina bifida represent different manifestations of the same pathogenic process—failure of neural tube closure. Other neural tube defects include encephalocele, exencephaly, and iniencephaly; however, hydrocephalus without spina bifida is etiologically distinct.

In the United States, if the proband has anencephaly, the likelihood that a first-degree relative will have either anencephaly or spina bifida is 2%; if the proband has spina bifida, the total risks also are 2% for either anencephaly or spina bifida. Families with more than one member affected have higher recurrence risks. Risks for second-degree relatives (nieces, nephews, grandchildren) and third-degree relatives (first cousins) of probands also appear to be increased.[72] It is important to establish a definitive diagnosis before offering recurrence risks because, although most neural tube defects result from polygenic or multifactorial inheritance with the previously mentioned recurrence risks, a minority are caused by single mutant genes (eg, Meckel's syndrome), chromosome abnormalities (eg, trisomy 13), or teratogens (eg, valproic acid). Recurrence risks would, of course, differ in these situations.

Antenatal diagnosis of neural tube defects can be accomplished by ultrasonography or assay of amniotic fluid alpha-fetoprotein (AFP). Ultrasonography by experienced investigators can exclude reliably anencephaly before 20 weeks' gestation, and spina bifida frequently can be visualized through serial views of the vertebral column. However, relatively few centers possess the technical sophistication to reliably detect spina bifida. By contrast, analysis of amniotic fluid AFP levels is more readily available. (AFP is the major serum protein in fetuses. It also is present in amniotic fluid and maternal serum. AFP enters amniotic fluid by fetal renal excretion and by transudation across fetal skin. If an open fetal defect exists, excess amounts of AFP are found in amniotic fluid.)

Amniotic fluid AFP determination is accurate but not without pitfalls. For example, AFP may be falsely elevated if the amniotic fluid is contaminated with fetal blood. This source of error can be eliminated if the presence of fetal hemoglobin and acetylcholinesterase are sought in the amniotic fluid. Elevated AFP and presence of acetylcholinesterase in amniotic fluid indicates that a neural tube defect,[73] or other fetal defect is present. In contrast, a false-positive amniotic fluid AFP caused by fetal blood contamination would be identified by the presence of fetal hemoglobin and the absence of acetylcholinesterase.

Elevated AFP is sometimes associated with anomalies other than neural tube defects (eg, omphalocele, gastroschisis, cystic hygroma, and congenital nephrosis). Acetylcholinesterase may be present or absent. Thus, detailed ultrasonographic studies should be performed when amniotic fluid AFP is elevated to determine the exact nature of the defect.

Alpha-fetoprotein Screening

Of the 1500 children born each year in the United States with spina bifida, only 5-10% occur in families with previously affected offspring. The other 90-95% are born to families with no known risk factors; therefore, a method to screen all pregnant women is desirable. The basis for screening is the finding that MSAFP levels usually are elevated in pregnancies with fetal neural tube defects. However, there is substantial overlap between MSAFP values in normal pregnancies and in pregnancies with a fetal neural tube defect or other abnormality.[74] Because MSAFP values increase with gestational age, the pregnancy must be dated accurately to interpret correctly the MSAFP level. In addition, because MSAFP varies inversely with maternal weight[75] and because insulin-requiring diabetics may have lower values than nondiabetics[76], laboratories must be given sufficient clinical information to interpret their results correctly.

An appropriate protocol for MSAFP screening is to draw a blood sample at 16–18 weeks' gestation, following a discussion with the patient and the consent (not necessarily written) for screening. If the MSAFP level is elevated, ultrasound examination should be performed. Previously,

TABLE 16–4. DEFECTS DETECTED IN PREGNANCIES WITH ELEVATED MSAFP

	Macri and Weiss[77]	Burton et al[78]	Milunsky et al[79]
Patients screened	17,703	12,084	35,500
Elevated MSAFP	692 (3.9%)	255 (2.1%)	387 (1.1%)
Neural tube defect detected with ultrasound, amniocentesis not done	0	3	23
Amniocentesis performed	365 (2.1%)	117 (1.0%)	107 (0.3%)
Neural tube defect detected with amniocentesis	20 (1:18 amniocenteses)	11 (1:10 amniocenteses)	8 (1:13 amniocenteses)
Other defects detected (↑ AFAFP)	5	1	11
Neural tube defect missed (normal MSAFP)	2	4 (2[a])	5[a]

[a] Because of screening at incorrect gestational age, closed NTD, or twins.

a second sample was recommended to confirm an elevated MSAFP. However, because of gestational time constraints and the likelihood that a second value will remain elevated, many large screening programs no longer require a second specimen. Ultrasound will allow correction of gestational dates and detection of multiple gestation or fetal demise, either of which may account for an elevated level. If no explanation is found, the patient should be counseled and offered amniocentesis for measurement of amniotic fluid AFP. For every 15 women requiring amniocentesis because of elevated MSAFP, one or two will have fetuses with a neural tube defect or other open fetal defect[77–79] (Table 16–4). Ninety percent of cases of anencephaly and 80% of those with spina bifida will be identified.[79] Women with elevated MSAFP but normal amniotic fluid AFP and a normal fetus are at increased risk for obstetric complications, such as late pregnancy loss, intrauterine growth retardation, and premature delivery.[77–79]

For a review of low MSAFP values, see discussion above.

CONCLUSIONS

Prenatal diagnosis is now a standard component of obstetric care. Techniques include amniocentesis, chorionic villus sampling, fetal blood or tissue sampling, and ultrasonography. Antenatal diagnosis should be offered to all couples at increased risk for a genetic disorder or structural anomaly.

REFERENCES

1. Fuchs F, Riis P. Antenatal sex determinants. *Nature.* 1966;177:330.
2. Steele MW, Breg WR Jr. Chromosome analysis of human amniotic fluid cells. *Lancet.* 1966;1:383.
3. Nadler HL. Antenatal detection of hereditary disorders. *Pediatr.* 1968;42.912.
4. Verp MS. Antenatal diagnosis of chromosome abnormalities. In: Sciarra JJ, ed. *Gynecology and Obstetrics.* Philadelphia, PA: Harper & Row; 1989:3; Chap. 102.
5. Verp MS, Simpson JL. Amniocentesis for prenatal genetic diagnosis. In: Filkins K, Russo JF, eds. *Human Prenatal Diagnosis.* 2nd ed. New York, NY; Marcel Dekker; 1990:305.
6. Elias S, Gerbie AB, Simpson JL, et al. Genetic amniocentesis in twin gestations. *Am J Obstet Gynecol.* 1980;138:169.
7. Verp MS, Elias S, Simpson JL. Further comments on amniocentesis in twin gestations. *Am J Med Genet.* 1983;14:397.
8. NICHD National Registry for Amniocentesis Study Group. Midtrimester amniocentesis for prenatal diagnosis. Safety and accuracy. *JAMA.* 1976;236:1471.
9. American College of Obstetricians and Gynecologists. *The selective use of* Rh_0 *(D)* Immune globulin (*RhIG*). ACOG Technical Bulletin No. 61, 1981.
10. Verp MS, Gerbie AB. Amniocentesis for prenatal diagnosis. *Clin Obstet Gynecol.* 1981;24:1007.
11. Simpson NE, Dallaire L, Miller JR, et al. Prenatal diagnosis of genetic disease in Canada: Report of a collaborative study. *Can Med Assoc J.* 1976;115:739.
12. United Kingdom Medical Research Council. Working party on amniocentesis. An assessment of the hazards of amniocentesis. *Br J Obstet Gynaecol.* 1978;85(suppl 2):1.
13. Tabor A, Philip J, Madsen M, et al. Randomized controlled trial of genetic amniocentesis in 4606 low-risk women. *Lancet.* 1986;1:1287.
14. Tabor A, Philip J, Bang J, et al. Safety of amniocentesis. *Prenat Diagn.* 1988;8:167.
15. Crane JP, Kopta MM. Genetic amniocentesis: Impact of placental position upon the risk of pregnancy loss. *Am J Obstet Gynecol.* 1984;150:813.
16. Hanson FW, Tennant FR, Zorn EM, Samuels S. Analysis of 2136 genetic amniocenteses: Experience of a single physician. *Am J Obstet Gynecol.* 1985;152:436.
17. Hislop A, Fairweather DVI. Amniocentesis and lung growth: An animal experiment with clinical implications. *Lancet.* 1982;2:1271.
18. Hunter AG. Neonatal lung function following mid-trimester amniocentesis. *Prenatal Diagn.* 1987;7:433.
19. Gillberg C, Rasmussen P, Wahlstrom J. Long-term following up of children born after amniocentesis. *Clin Genet.* 1982;21:69.
20. Drugan A, Syner FN, Greb A, Evans MI. Amniotic fluid alpha-fetoprotein acetylcholinesterase in early genetic amniocentesis. *Obstet Gynecol.* 1988;72:35.
21. Rhoads GG, Jackson LG, Schlesselman SE, et al. The safety and efficacy of chorionic villus sampling for early prenatal diagnosis. *N Engl J Med.* 1989;320:609.
22. Canadian Collaborative CVS-Amniocentesis Clinical Trial Group. Multicentre randomized clinical trial of chorion villus sampling and amniocentesis. First report. *Lancet.* 1989;1:1.
23. WHO Consultation on First Trimester Fetal Diagnosis. Risk evaluation in chorion villus sampling. *Prenat Diagn.* 1986;6:451.
24. Elias S, Esterly N. Prenatal diagnosis of hereditary skin disorders. *Clin Obstet Gynecol.* 1981;24:1069.
25. Benn PA, Hsu LYF. Maternal cell contamination of amniotic fluid cell cultures: Results of a U.S. nationwide survey. *Am J Med Genet.* 1983;15:297.
26. Ledbetter DH, Martin AO, Verlinsky Y, et al. Cytogenetic results of chorionic villus sampling. *Am J Obstet Gynecol.* 1990;162:495.
27. Simpson JL, Martin AO, Verp MS, et al. Hypermodal cells in amniotic fluid cultures: Frequency, interpretation, and clinical significance. *Am J Obstet Gynecol.* 1982;143:250.
28. Hsu LYF. Prenatal diagnosis of chromosome abnormalities. In: Milunsky A, ed. *Genetic Disorders and the Fetus.* 2nd ed. New York, NY: Plenum Press; 1986:115.
29. Warburton D. Outcome of cases of *de novo* structural rearrangements diagnosed at amniocentesis. *Prenat Diagn.* 1984;4:69.
30. Verp MS, Bombard AT, Simpson JL, Elias S. Parental decision following prenatal diagnosis of fetal chromosome abnormality. *Am J Med Genet.* 1988;29:613.
31. Hook EB, Hamerton JL. The frequency of chromosome abnormalities detected in consecutive newborn studies: differences between studies; results by sex and by severity of phenotypic involvement. In: Hook EB, Porter IH, eds. *Population Cytogenetics.* New York: Academic Press; 1978;63.
32. Hook EB, Cross PK, Schreinemachers DM. Chromosomal abnormality rates at amniocentesis and in live-born infants. *JAMA.* 1983;249:2034.
33. Hook EB, Cross PK, Jackson LG, et al. Maternal age-specific rates of 47, +21 and other cytogenetic abnormalities diagnosed in the first trimester of pregnancy in chorionic villus biopsy samples: Comparison with rates expected from observations at amniocentesis. *Am J Hum Genet.* 1988;42:797.
34. Mikkelsen M, Stene J: Previous child with Down's syndrome and other chromosome aberrations. In: Murken JD, Stengel-Rutkowski S, Schwinger E, eds. *Prenatal Diagnosis: Proceedings of the Third European Conference on Prenatal Diagnosis of Genetic Disorders.* Stuttgart: F Enke; 1979:22.
35. Simoni G, Fraccaro M, Arslanian A, et al. Cytogenetic finding in 4952 prenatal diagnoses: An Italian collaborative study. *Hum Genet.* 1982;60:63.
36. Stene J, Stene E, Mikkelsen M. Risk for chromosome abnormality at amniocentesis following a child with a non-inherited chromosome aberration. *Prenat diagn.* 1984;4(special issue):81.
37. Mikkelsen M. *CVS Newsletter.* (ed), 1986;19:7.
38. Boué A, Gallano P. A collaborative study of the segregation of inherited chromosome structural rearrangements in 1356 prenatal diagnoses. *Prenat Diag.* 1984;4(special issue):45.
39. Hook EB. Rates of chromosome abnormalities at different maternal ages. *Obstet Gynecol.* 1981;58:282.
40. Simpson JL. Pregnancies in women with chromosomal abnormalities. In: Schulman JD, Simpson JL, eds. *Genetic Diseases in Pregnancy.* New York, NY: Academic Press; 1981:440.
41. Verp MS. Chromosomal disorders in pregnancy. In: Gleicher N, ed. *Principles of Medical Therapy in Pregnancy.* 1st ed. New York, NY: Plenum Medical Book Co; 1985:1223.
42. Voss R, Kohn G, Shaham M, et al. Prenatal diagnosis of Fanconi anemia. *Clin Genet.* 1981;20:185.
43. Jenkins EC, Brown WT. The prenatal diagnosis of the fragile X syndrome. In: Milunsky A, ed. *Genetic Disorders and the Fetus.* 2nd ed. New York, NY: Plenum Press; 1986:185.
44. Merkatz IR, Nitowsky HM, Macri JM, Johnson WE. An association between low maternal serum alpha-fetoprotein and fetal chromosome abnormalities. *Am J Obstet Gynecol.* 1984;148:886.
45. Palomaki GE. Collaborative study of Down syndrome screening using maternal serum alpha-fetoprotein and maternal age. *Lancet.* 1986;2:1460.
46. DiMaio MS, Baumgarten A, Greenstein RM, et al. Screening for fetal Down's syndrome in pregnancy by measuring maternal serum alpha-fetoprotein levels. *N Engl J Med.* 1987;317:342.
47. Brambati B, Simoni G, Bonacchi I, Piceni L. Fetal chromosomal aneuploidies and maternal serum alpha-fetoprotein levels in first trimester. *Lancet.* 1986;2:165.
48. Bogart MH, Pandian MR, Jones OW. Abnormal maternal serum chorionic

gonadotropin levels in pregnancies with fetal chromosome abnormalities. *Prenatal Diagn.* 1987;7:623.
49. Canick JA, Knight GJ, Palomaki GE, et al. Low second trimester maternal serum unconjugated oestriol in pregnancies with Down's syndrome. *Br J Obstet Gynaecol.* 1988;95:330.
50. Wald NJ, Cuckle HS, Densem JW, et al. Maternal serum screening for Down's syndrome in early pregnancy. *Br Med J.* 1988;297:883.
51. Stene J, Fischer G, Stene E, et al. Paternal age effect in Down syndrome. *Ann Hum Genet.* 1977;40:299.
52. Hook EB, Cross PK. Paternal age and Down's syndrome genotypes diagnosed prenatally: No association in New York data. *Hum Genet.* 1982;62:167.
53. Roth M-P, Feingold J, Baumgarten A, et al. Re-examination of paternal age effect in Down's syndrome. *Hum Genet.* 1983;63:149.
54. Ferguson-Smith MA, Yates JRW. Maternal age specific rates for chromosome aberrations and factors influencing them: Report of a collaborative European study on 52,965 amniocenteses. *Prenat Diagn.* 1984;4:5.
55. Uchida IA, Holunga R, Lawler C. Maternal radiation and chromosome aberrations. *Lancet.* 1968;2:1045.
56. Cohen BH, Lilienfeld AM, Kramer S, et al. Parental factors in Down's syndrome—results of the second Baltimore case-control study. In: Hook EB, Porter IH, eds. *Population Cytogenetics.* New York, NY: Academic Press. 1977:301.
57. Martin RH. Chromosomal abnormalities in human sperm. In: Dellarco VL, Voytek PE, Hollaender A, eds. *Aneuploidy: Etiology and Mechanisms.* New York, NY: Plenum Press; 1985:91.
58. Horning SJ, Hoppe RT, Kaplan HS, Rosenberg SA. Female reproductive potential after treatment for Hodgkin's disease. *N Engl J Med.* 1981;304:1377.
59. Mulvihill JJ, McKeen EA, Rosner F, Zarrabi MH. Pregnancy outcome in cancer patients. Experience in a large cooperative group. *Cancer.* 1987;60:1143.
60. Schull WJ, Otake M, Neel JV. Genetic effects of the atomic bombs: A reappraisal. *Science.* 213:1220.
61. Walden PAM, Bagshawe KD. Pregnancies after chemotherapy for gestational trophoblastic tumors. *Lancet.* 1979;2:1241.
62. Lockwood C, Benacerraf B, Krinsky A, et al. A sonographic screening method for Down' syndrome. *Am J Obstet Gynecol.* 1987;157:803.
63. Benacerraf BR, Gelman R, Frigoletto FD Jr. Sonographic identification of second-trimester fetuses with Down's syndrome. *N Engl J Med.* 1987;317:1371.
64. Iverson GM, Bianchi DW, Cann HM, Herzenberg LA. Detection and isolation of fetal cells from maternal blood using the fluoroscence activated cell sorter (FACS). *Prenat diagn.* 1981;1:61.
65. Julien C, Bazin A, Guyot B, et al. Rapid prenatal diagnosis of Down's syndrome with *in situ* hybridization of fluorescent DNA probes. *Lancet.* 1986;2:863.
66. Elias S, Chandler RW, Wachtel S. Relative DNA content of interphase leukocytes by flow cytometry: A method for indirect diagnosis of chromosomal abnormalities with potential for prenatal diagnosis. *Am J Obstet Gynecol.* 1988;158:808.
67. Desnick RJ, Grabowski GA, Hirschhorn K. Prenatal metabolic diagnosis. In: Filkins K, Russo JF, eds. *Human Prenatal Diagnosis.* New York, NY: Marcel Dekker; 1985:59.
68. Weaver DD. A survey of prenatally diagnosed disorders. *Clin Obstet Gynecol.* 1988;31:253.
69. Brock DJH, Clarke HAK, Barron L. Prenatal diagnosis of cystic fibrosis by microvillar enzyme assay on a sequence of 258 pregnancies. *Hum Genet.* 1988;78:271.
70. Alter BP. Prenatal diagnosis of haemoglobinopathies: A status report. *Lancet.* 1981;2:1152.
71. Mibashan RS, Rodeck CH, Thumpston JK, et al. Plasma assay of fetal factors VIII C and IX for prenatal diagnosis of haemophilia. *Lancet.* 1979;1:1309.
72. Toriello HV, Higgins JV. Occurrence of neural tube defects among first-, second-, and third-degree relatives of probands: Results of a United States study. *Am J Med Genet.* 1983;15:601.
73. Collaborative Acetylcholinesterase Study. Amniotic fluid acetylcholinesterase electrophoresis as a secondary test in the diagnosis of anencephaly and open spina bifida in early pregnancy. *Lancet.* 1981;2:321.
74. Macri JN, Haddow JE, Weiss RR. Screening for neural tube defects in the United States. *Am J Obstet Gynecol.* 1979;133:119.
75. Wald N, Cuckle H, Boreham J, et al. The effect of maternal weight on maternal serum alpha-fetoprotein levels. *Br J Obstet Gynaecol.* 1981;88:1094.
76. Wald NJ, Cuckle HS, Boreham J, et al. Maternal serum alpha-fetoprotein and diabetes mellitus. Br J Obstet Gynaecol. 1979;86:101.
77. Macri JN, Weiss RR. Prenatal serum α-fetoprotein screening for neural tube defects. *Obstet Gynecol.* 1982; 59:633.
78. Burton BK, Sowers SG, Nelson LH. Maternal serum α-fetoprotein screening in North Carolina: Experience with more than twelve thousand pregnancies. *Am J Obstet Gynecol.* 1983;146:439.
79. Milunsky A. The prenatal diagnosis of neural tube and other congenital defects. In: Milunsky A, ed. *Genetic Disorders and the Fetus.* 2nd ed. New York, NY: Plenum Press; 1986:453.

Chapter Seventeen

Genetic Counseling and Screening

Patricia N. Olney, Teresa Castellano, and Gloria E. Sarto

17

The need to counsel people regarding inherited disorders exists in many disciplines of medicine: In obstetrics, it entails advising pregnant women with a family history of dominant genetic conditions; in psychiatry, it involves caring for a woman with a bipolar mental illness; and in internal medicine, it means attending to a woman with a dominant connective tissue disorder. All of these patients have the concern of the risk of passing their condition on to their offspring. An assessment of the patient's needs or desires for genetic counseling should be made at an initial interview, preferably before pregnancy.

The most common indications for genetic counseling in obstetrics and gynecology are listed in Table 17–1. *Advanced maternal age* is generally considered to be 35 years or older at time of delivery. A genetic *condition of ethnic origin* includes conditions in which the carrier state of a recessive trait, such as Tay-Sachs in Jewish individuals of eastern European background or sickle cell anemia in the black population, exists.

A comprehensive genetic counseling service consists of a team of geneticists, genetic counselors, cytogeneticists, and frequently perinatologists. Most major medical centers have these individuals on staff and thus provide the interdisciplinary team approach that may be needed for diagnosis and counseling of severe disorders.

Genetic counselors provide informative and supportive services to help patients reach decisions, but they do not make decisions for the patient. Table 17–2 outlines the format for a genetic counseling session. It is important to define a couple's education, social background, and religious attitudes to facilitate the presentation of information in an effective way at the level of the individual's understanding. Genetic counseling sessions require approximately 1 hour. A second session may be indicated if test results or further diagnostic information needs to be presented.

FAMILY HISTORY

Counseling should always include a detailed three-generation family history. Consequently a pedigree should be

TABLE 17–1. MOST COMMON INDICATIONS FOR GENETIC COUNSELING

Advanced maternal age
Previous child with genetic abnormality
Family history of genetic abnormality
Ethnic history of recessive trait
History of X-linked trait
Abnormal alpha-fetoprotein screen
Exposure to teratogens

drawn, including siblings of the proband (or couple), their children, their parents, and the parents' siblings. Age, sex, and health status of each individual should be addressed as well as the occurrence of stillbirths, neonatal deaths, and multiple spontaneous abortions. The cause and age of death should be investigated for every deceased. With a chronic illness, the age of onset should be determined. Detailed information about the site and nature of congenital malformations, the basis of acquired disease, and the primary site of malignancies also should be recorded.

If the pedigree is obtained because of a history of a birth defect or genetic disease, the information sought should be pertinent to the diagnosis in question. Particular attention should be given to assess the presence of milder forms of the disorder in family members. This may require physical or specific laboratory examinations. The question of consanguinity should be addressed. If there is common ancestry, one should ask about common relatives, common last names, or a common geographic origin. If consanguinity exists, the background risk for genetic disease in offspring is higher than usual, depending on the degree of the consanguinity.

The ethnic background can be important because some genetic diseases are more common among certain ethnic groups. Ideally, carrier testing should always take place before conception. This maximizes the couple's reproductive choices. If the couple is at risk of having a child with a specific genetic disease, the option of prenatal diagnosis should be presented. For example, a couple with Eastern European Jewish ancestry should be offered testing for the carrier status of Tay–Sachs disease. Though the mutant gene for Tay–Sachs is more common among Jews of eastern European ancestry, the gene frequency in nonJews may be as high as 1 in 150. Therefore, carrier testing should be considered even within mixed marriages. If the husband and wife are carriers, prenatal diagnosis should be offered by chorionic villi sampling or amniocentesis. Table 17–3 presents the most frequently occurring ethnically distributed inherited diseases.

TABLE 17–2. FORMAT OF A GENETIC COUNSELING SESSION

Obtain family and pregnancy history.
Establish exact diagnosis of genetic disease or birth defect.
Determine type of inheritance.
Calculate risk of recurrence.
Present risk to individual or couple.
Present prognosis associated with disorder to individual or couple.
Assess subjective interpretation of risk and evaluate family goals.
Present reproductive options and facilitate decision making.
Offer appropriate prenatal diagnostic testing.

TABLE 17–3. ETHNIC DISTRIBUTION OF SOME INHERITED DISEASES

Ashkenazi Jews	Tay–Sachs disease Niemann–Pick disease
Africans	Hemoglobinopathies: sickle cell anemia, hemoglobin C disease, thalassemia, G6PD
Mediterranean people (Italians, Greeks, Sephardic Jews)	β-Thalassemia
Chinese or Southeast Asians	α-Thalassemia

PREGNANCY HISTORY

All previous pregnancies, including abortions, stillbirths, and neonatal deaths, should be recorded. If a stillbirth or neonatal death has occurred, an attempt should be made to ascertain the cause.

If the patient is already pregnant, the gestational age should be assessed and a history of bleeding, cramping, or illness during the pregnancy should be determined. Any exposure to possible teratogens, including alcohol, cigarettes, recreational drugs, radiation or chemical agents, and prescription and nonprescription drugs also has to be recorded. In addition, the obstetric history of the patient should be noted, including birth dates and sex of the offspring, birth weights, estimated gestational ages and mode of delivery, complications of pregnancy, and all birth defects.

CONFIRMATION OF DIAGNOSIS

The accurate diagnosis of any genetic disorder is the most basic prerequisite of genetic counseling. If a couple had a previous child with a birth defect, a confirmed diagnosis of that child must be made before further genetic counseling can be provided. If the child is alive and a diagnosis has not been established, referral to a geneticist or dysmorphologist may be necessary. Other family members also often need to be examined to rule out the presence of milder forms of the same genetic defect. If the child is deceased, x-rays, laboratory data, and medical records should be reviewed. Photographs also may be helpful in this process.

PATTERNS OF INHERITANCE

Once an accurate diagnosis is established and the pattern of inheritance for the disorder is determined, a risk of recurrence can be provided. A commonly used source of reference that delineates the pattern of inheritance for over 4344 disorders is McKusick's *Mendelian Inheritance in Man*.[1] This catalog of inherited disorders is updated on a regular basis. Depending on whether the inheritance pattern is multifactorial, autosomal recessive, autosomal dominant, or X-linked recessive, the recurrence risk may range from 2–4% to up to 50% (see Tables 17–4 and 17–5). Some clinical disorders are inherited in more than one inheritance pattern. This is termed *genetic heterogeneity* and is an important consideration in genetic counseling.

Polygenic Multifactorial Inheritance

Isolated structural defects or malformations, such as cleft lip with or without cleft palate, cardiac defects, and neural

TABLE 17–4. APPROXIMATE RECURRENCE RISKS FOR VARIOUS GENETIC ABNORMALITIES

Abnormality	Risk of Recurrence (%)
Mendelian Mutations	
Autosomal-Recessive	25
Autosomal-Dominant	50 (unless new mutation or unless penetrance is reduced)
X-linked Recessive	
For Carrier Females	25 overall, 50 sons
For Affected Males	100 carrier daughters, 100 normal sons
X-linked Dominant	
For Affected Females	50 overall
For Affected Males	100 affected daughters, 100 normal sons
Common Multifactorial Conditions	2 to 5 (increases with each affected child)
Chromosome Abnormalities	
Trisomy syndrome, parents chromosomally normal	1 to 2
Balanced translocation, carrier parent	2 to 100

tube defects, have a multifactorial or polygenic inheritance pattern (see also Chapters 13 and 16).

Based on empiric data, for most isolated structural defects, the risk of recurrence in a subsequent pregnancy is approximately 2–5%. Recurrence risks for some isolated structural defects are listed in Table 17–5. Some risks are greater in one sex than the other. If more than one offspring is affected, the risk can be twofold to threefold. In some of these conditions, prenatal diagnosis is feasible.

Autosomal Recessive Inheritance

Autosomal recessive disorders are manifested only in individuals homozygous for the mutant gene. Because carriers for the mutant gene are phenotypically normal (in some conditions, the carrier status of parents can be determined biochemically), the carrier status of the parents is confirmed only when a child is born with a recessive condition. Thus, counseling is usually sought only after a couple has had an affected child. Affected individuals tend to be limited to siblings. Males and females are equally affected and the risk for subsequent affected individuals is one in four. For most recessive disorders, the mutant gene in the population is rare, and the probability that any two individuals who carry the same mutant allele would mate consequently also is low.

TABLE 17–5. RECURRENCE RISKS FOR MULTIFACTORIAL CONDITIONS

Cleft lip with or without cleft palate	4 to 5%
Cleft palate alone	2 to 6%
Cardiac defect (common types)	3 to 4%
Pyloric stenosis	3%
Hirschsprung's anomaly	3 to 5%
Neural tube defects	3 to 5%
Clubfoot	2 to 8%
Dislocation of hip	3 to 4%

From Jones K[3] with permission.

Frequently, unaffected siblings of individuals with autosomal recessive disorders will seek counseling to assess their risks of having an affected child. In order to calculate that risk, the chance that the unaffected offspring is a carrier ($\frac{2}{3}$) is multiplied by the risk of carrier status for the mate (the population frequency for the respective gene), and by the chance that each parent would pass the mutant gene to an offspring ($\frac{1}{4}$). For example, the carrier frequency for *cystic fibrosis* is one in 20.[2] Therefore, the chance that an unaffected sibling of an affected individual would have a child with cystic fibrosis is $(\frac{2}{3})(\frac{1}{20})(\frac{1}{4}) = \frac{1}{120}$.

Related individuals have an increased chance of carrying the same altered gene inherited from a common relative, and are therefore more likely to have children with rare recessive disorders. In consanguineous relationships, the risk depends on the closeness of the relation; for example, first cousins have one eighth of their genes in common. Many metabolic disorders, such as cystic fibrosis, Tay-Sachs, and phenylketonuria, are inherited in an autosomal recessive fashion.

Autosomal Dominant Inheritance

An autosomal dominant disorder is caused by a single mutant gene on an autosome. The transmission from an affected parent is independent of sex, and each offspring has a 50% chance of receiving the mutant gene assuming complete penetrance. Vertical transmission is evident on pedigree analysis. Consequently, affected individuals usually have an affected parent.

Exceptions to this rule occur, however. For example, with *incomplete penetrance,* an individual may inherit the mutant gene, pass it on to an offspring, and be found phenotypically normal. The gene is present, but it is not manifested in the parent. When it is passed on to a child, however, the trait is expressed. Whenever the gene is expressed, the expression is an all-or-none phenomenon. In order to determine the degree of penetrance of a disorder, a large number of pedigrees have to be studied. Penetrance is thus a statistical concept; for example, if eight of 10 obligate heterozygotes express the disorder, the gene shows 80% penetrance. On an individual basis, it means that an individual carrying that mutant gene has an 80% chance of expressing the disorder. Both the risk of receiving the gene and the degree of penetrance should be presented in genetic counseling for dominant disorders.

Variable expressivity, sometimes confused with penetrance, is another characteristic of autosomal dominant traits. Whereas penetrance is an all-or-none phenomenon, varying expressivity refers to the degree of severity of expression. For example, neurofibromatosis is an autosomal dominant condition with high penetrance and a wide variability in expression. The clinical features range in severity from *cafe au lait* spots as one of the only manifestations, to more serious subcutaneous tumors and associated seizures. Approximately 50% of the affected individuals are new mutations.[3]

Occasionally, a dominantly inherited disorder will appear as a *sporadic* case in a family with no other affected individuals. This most likely represents a new mutation occurring in one individual. Parents of a child with a new mutation have a neglible risk of recurrence in subsequent pregnancies. Approximately 90% of cases of *achondroplastic dwarfism* are new mutations.[3] There is evidence that increased paternal age may increase the risk for such spontaneous mutations.

Some autosomal dominant inherited disorders are not manifested until later in life (eg, *Huntington's disease*). The average age of onset for Huntington's disease is about 35 years. With such disorders, it is possible that an affected individual who has children dies from an unrelated cause before demonstrating the disease. When the child manifests the disorder, it erroneously appears to represent a new mutation of an affected offspring with an unaffected parent. Another possibility that may lead to the erroneous diagnosis of a sporadic case of autosomal dominant inheritance is the situation in which the perceived father is not the biologic father of the child.

In most dominantly inherited disorders, prenatal diagnosis still is not possible. Advances in molecular genetics, however, have allowed the prenatal diagnosis of some of the dominant conditions, which are linked to certain restriction fragment length polymorphisms (see also Chapter 14). For example, markers have been found close to the gene for Huntington's disease, making it possible to determine the presence of the mutant gene in an at-risk individual with 99% certainty. Other dominant disorders that now lend themselves to prenatal diagnosis include neurofibromatosis, osteogenesis imperfecta, and polycystic kidney disease.[4]

X-linked Recessive Inheritance

X-linked recessive genetic disorders are carried on the X chromosome and are passed from carrier females to male offspring. Carrier females are generally unaffected. Each son has a 50% chance of inheriting the mutant gene and of being affected. Daughters have the same 50% chance of inheriting the mutant gene and of being carriers. Because of a normal second X chromosome from the father, daughters are clinically unaffected. Unaffected sons cannot transmit the condition, and affected sons will have normal sons who cannot transmit the condition. Rarely, females will express an X-linked disorder. This may occur, for example, when the mutant gene is sufficiently common and the female is homozygous. Differences in the degree of lyonization of the X chromosome also may allow for expression of an X-linked recessive disorder in a heterozygous female. Random inactivation of the paternal or maternal X occurs very early in development. If, by chance, a higher percent of paternal X chromosomes are inactivated, the maternal mutant X chromosome may be expressed. Consequently, the individual would manifest the X-linked recessive disorder.

X-linked Dominant Inheritance

X-linked dominant inheritance also is characterized by the absence of male-to-male transmission because the mutant gene is on the X-chromosome. Because it is a dominant gene mutation, however, females also are affected. All daughters of an affected male will be affected, and 50% of all sons and daughters of an affected female will be affected. In contrast, all sons of an affected male will be normal. Vitamin D-resistant (hypophosphatemic) rickets is an example of a disorder inherited in this fashion.[1]

Once an inheritance pattern has been established as X-linked, the carrier status of the mother should be assessed. In some X-linked disorders, as noted above, the female may have mild expression and can thus be detected. In other conditions, such as hemophilia, her status may be confirmed biochemically or by DNA technology.

CHROMOSOME ABNORMALITIES

Aneuploidy and unbalanced rearrangements as a cause of congenital malformations occur in approximately 5 out of 1000 newborns. Among these, the most common is trisomy 21 or *Down's syndrome.*

The risk of having a child with Down's syndrome increases with maternal but not paternal age.[2] Consequently,

TABLE 17–6. ESTIMATED RATES OF CYTOGENETIC ABNORMALITIES PER 1000 LIVEBIRTHS IN ABSENCE OF SELECTIVE ABORTION

Maternal Age[a]	47,+21	47,+18	47,+13	47,XXX	47,XXY	Other Clinically Significant Abnormalities	All Abnormalities
33	1.6	0.2	0.2	0.4	0.4	0.7	2.9–3.4
34	2.0	0.2	0.2	0.5	0.4	0.7	3.6–4.1
35	2.6	0.3	0.3	0.5	0.6	0.8	4.7–5.1
36	3.4	0.4	0.3	0.6	0.7	0.9	5.9–6.3
37	4.4	0.5	0.4	0.8	0.9	0.9	7.6–7.8
38	5.7	0.6	0.4	0.9	1.1	1.0	9.7–9.7
39	7.3	0.8	0.5	1.1	1.4	1.1	12.4–12.1
40	9.4	1.0	0.5	1.3	1.7	1.2	15.8–15.2
41	12.2	1.2	0.6	1.6	2.2	1.3	20.2–19.1
42	15.7	1.6	0.7	1.9	2.7	1.4	25.7–24.0
43	20.2	2.0	0.8	2.2	3.4	1.5	32.9–30.2
44	26.1	2.5	1.0	2.7	4.3	1.6	41.9–38.2
45	33.7	3.2	1.1	3.2	5.4	1.7	53.5–48.3
46	43.4	4.0	1.3	3.8	6.8	1.8	68.4–61.2
47	56.0	5.1	1.5	4.6	8.5	2.0	87.3–77.7
48	72.3	6.4	1.8	5.5	10.7	2.1	111.4–98.7
49	93.3	8.1	2.0	6.5	13.4	2.3	142.2–125.6

[a] Maternal age is at time of expected livebirth.

the most common reason for genetic counseling is the risk of Down's syndrome associated with advanced maternal age (Table 17–6). The risk for women in the 15 to 19 year age group is about 1 in 2300, while the risk for women older than 45 years is 1 in 46.

Ninety-five percent of individuals with Down's syndrome have trisomy 21. Five percent are the result of a translocation between chromosomes 21 and 14, but a translocation between chromosomes 21 and 13 or 15 may occur as well. If the mother is a carrier of a 14/21 translocation, the risk of a Down's syndrome child is approximately 8–10%. If the father carries the translocation, the risk of an affected child is less than 5%. A carrier for a translocation between two 21 chromosomes provides gametes that are either trisomic or nullisomic for this chromosome; therefore, all liveborns from such a mating would have Down's syndrome. Established risk figures from one type of translocation cannot be transferred to another. Consequently, risk figures vary between 14 out of 21 and 15 out of 21. For each translocation, empiric risk figures must be established from pedigrees reported in the literature or from the proband's pedigree if it is sufficiently large (see Table 17–4).

PRENATAL DIAGNOSIS COUNSELING

Genetic counseling for advanced maternal age is based on balancing the risk of having a child with a chromosomal abnormality against the risks of either amniocentesis or chorionic villi sampling (CVS) (see also Chapter 16).

A maternal age of 35 at term has generally been selected as the age to offer prenatal diagnosis, although practices in different locales may vary and be as low as 33 years of age (personal communication). The risk of the procedure at that age has been shown to be equal to or lower than the risk of a chromosomal abnormality. A genetic counseling session should occur before the procedure to discuss the risks and benefits along with details of the diagnostic procedure. Additionally, a full pedigree should be obtained to determine any additional risks that may be relevant to the pregnancy or medical health of the individual(s).

Pregnancy termination, adoption, or the possibility of raising an abnormal child are issues that may be discussed if an abnormality is found. Couples also always should be told of the limitations of prenatal diagnosis. A normal result with prenatal testing does not guarantee a normal child.

Another common indication for prenatal genetic counseling is an abnormally elevated or low maternal serum alpha-fetoprotein (MSAFP). This is only a screening test. Though the risk for open neural tube and other birth defects is increased if the MSAFP is elevated, most women with elevated results do not carry an abnormal fetus. An elevated MSAFP may be caused by a twin gestation or a fetal demise. Even in an accurately dated pregnanacy, an elevated result is associated with an overall risk of approximately 1 in 30 for having an affected fetus.[6]

A detailed ultrasound scan and an amniocentesis are usually offered in follow-up whenever the MSAFP is elevated. A pregnancy with elevated MSAFP but normal amniotic fluid AFP should be followed and monitored for such complications as premature rupture of membranes or small-for-gestational age fetal development. A low MSAFP has been associated with an increased risk of Down's syndrome. The MSAFP value is combined with the woman's age to give a statistical risk for Down's syndrome.[5] (The formula for the calculation is based on information from the company providing the RIA assay or the Foundation for Blood Research.)

EFFECTIVENESS OF GENETIC COUNSELING

Historically, genetic counseling has shifted from the concept of preventive medicine, primarily aimed at the prevention of birth defects, to a person-oriented counseling process including psychosocial ramifications of genetic disease.

In 1975, the Ad Hoc Committee on Genetics Counseling defined the generally accepted counseling goals as follows:

> Genetic counseling is a communication process which deals with the human problems associated with the occurrence, or the risk of occurrence, of a genetic disorder in a family. This process involves the following goals:
>
> 1. Comprehend the medical facts, including the diagnosis, the probable course of the disorder, and the available management.
> 2. Appreciate . . . the risk of recurrence in specified relatives.
> 3. Understand the options for dealing with the risk of recurrence.
> 4. Choose the course of action which seems appropriate in view of their risk and their family goals, and act in accordance with that decision.
> 5. Make the best possible adjustment to the disorder . . . and to the risk of recurrence of that disorder.[7]

Information is provided to the patient, parent, and guardian about the transmission of a genetic condition, the prognosis, and the potential preventive measures. One might assume that reproductive decisions are made based on the available risk information. However, it has been shown in several studies that only about one half of all individuals affirm that counseling has influenced their reproductive decisions.[8] More important considerations appear to be a desire to have more children, the potential burden of the disease, and the degree of uncertainty the couple faces.[9]

To be effective, the timing of a genetic counseling session is important. After the birth of an abnormal infant, most couples are in a state of shock or disbelief. At that point, it is most appropriate to offer emotional support and to establish a rapport with the family. Counseling regarding recurrence risks for future offspring and availability of prenatal testing are appropriate at a later time when the couple is psychologically ready to hear this information. A nondirective approach should be maintained while exploring all the issues.

REFERENCES

1. McKusick V. *Mendelian Inheritance in Man*. 8th ed. Baltimore, MD: Johns Hopkins University Press; 1988.

2. Harper PS. *Practical Genetic Counseling*. 3rd ed. Bristol, England: Butterworth and Co. Ltd.; 1988.
3. Jones KL. *Smith's Recognizable Patterns of Human Malformation*. 4th ed. Philadelphia, PA: WB Saunders; 1988.
4. King CR. Prenatal diagnosis of genetic disease with molecular genetic technology. *Obstet Gynecol Surv*. 1988;43:493.
5. Cuckle HS, Wald NJ, and Thompson SG. Estimating a woman's risk of having a pregnancy associated with Down syndrome using her age and serum alpha-fetoprotein level. *Br J Obstet Gynecol*. 1987;94:387.
6. Burton BK. Elevated maternal serum alphafetoprotein (MSAFP): Interpretation and follow-up. *Clin Obstet Gynecol*. 1988;31:293.
7. Ad Hoc Committee on Genetic Counseling. *Am J Hum Genet*. 1975;27: 240.
8. Evers-Kieboom G, van den Berghe H. Impact of genetic counseling: A review of published follow-up studies. *Clin Genet*. 1979;15:465.
9. Wertz D, Sorenson J, Heeren T. Genetic counseling and reproductive uncertainty. *Am J Med Genet*. 1984;18:79.

Chapter Eighteen

Ethical and Legal Issues in Obstetrics

George J. Annas and Sherman Elias

18

The 1989 Annual Clinical Meeting of the American College of Obstetricians and Gynecologists (ACOG) clearly showed that legal and ethical issues have become major concerns in the clinical practice and research of obstetrics. In fact, the president of the ACOG, Dr. Robert C. Park, chose the topic, "Applied Ethics for the Obstetrician–Gynecologist," for the president's program at the first scientific session. Other topics on the program at the meeting included the following:

- Perinatal Asphyxia: Diagnosis, Etiology, Neurologic Sequelae, and Legal Ramifications
- New Responsibilities: Genetic Counseling, When to Offer New Technologies, and the Liability for Not
- Ethics and Ethical Decision-Making
- Medical–Legal Considerations of Cesarean Birth
- Your Best Witness in Malpractice
- The Development of "No Fault" Obstetric Malpractice Insurance
- AIDS & Women: What are the Odds, Options, Laws, and Ethics?
- Medical–Legal Considerations of Antepartum Fetal Surveillance

It is impossible in a single chapter to provide an in-depth discussion of each of these topics or others of equal importance. This chapter focuses instead on selected issues that are particularly timely. This chapter is adapted from previous works by the authors.[1-3]

GENETICS

Genetic Screening

Genetic screening is the ". . . search in a population for persons possessing certain genotypes that (1) are already associated with disease or predisposed to disease, (2) may lead to disease in their descendants, or (3) may produce other variations not known to be associated with disease."[4] Persons in the first category are identified for treatment. The second group is identified so that individuals in it can receive counseling about their reproductive options and risks. Both of these categories also are counted for epidemiologic studies establishing incidence or prevalence figures. The third group is identified for research purposes, specifically to help determine the genetic constitutions of populations. Thus, genetic screening has different meanings and contexts and may be almost any size, ranging from selected individuals to all individuals regardless of age or clinical state.

Whereas traditional medicine responds to illness and injury presented to physicians, screening is a public health endeavor that actively seeks out asymptomatic people, many of whom are not otherwise receiving medical care. Screening tests have become pervasive and accepted in our society, even though they raise serious questions of autonomy, stigmatization, confidentiality, informed consent, and efficacy. In the field of genetics particularly, the past two decades have witnessed three waves of newborn genetic screening laws that have covered most of the states in the country. Phenylketonuria (PKU) screening programs were mandated by 43 states between 1963 and 1968; from 1971 to 1974, 17 states passed laws to promote screening for sickle cell anemia; and by 1986, 48 states and the District of Columbia had statutes (usually based on their original PKU enactment) governing newborn screening.[5-7]

From a clinical standpoint, *carrier screening* in obstetric practice generally refers to identification of heterozygotes (ie, carriers) for an autosomal or X-linked recessive disorder. The most common indication for carrier screening is to provide prospective parents with reproductive alternatives, such as possible termination of affected fetuses, artificial insemination, or deferral of childbearing. Screening all individuals for carrier status, regardless of family history or ethnic background, is impossible. The decision of who should be screened is generally based on several criteria, including the availability of a simple, accurate, inexpensive test for the identification of carriers; an ethnic, racial, or geographic heritage associated with an increased risk for that specific genetic disorder; and treatment or reproductive options for identified individuals.

In the United States, three disorders meet the above criteria for routine genetic screening in obstetric practice: Tay–Sachs disease, sickle cell anemia, and the thalassemias. For other diseases not routinely screened, carrier detection sometimes can be performed if the family history indicates an increased risk. An example would be a pregnant woman with a brother affected with Duchenne muscular dystrophy. Molecular techniques usually can alter substantially her empiric risk (50% risk of carrying the Duchenne's gene), sometimes obviating the need for invasive prenatal diagnostic procedures. Carrier testing for a growing number of diseases, including cystic fibrosis and Huntington's disease, is available when indicated by a positive family history. Participation of multiple family members, including affected individuals, usually is required for the most accurate risk assessment.

Increased demand and limited resources for genetic screening are forcing decisions about who should be screened and how the choice of diseases to be screened should be made. Important factors include frequency and severity of the condition; availability of a proven therapy; extent to which detection by screening improves the outcome; validity and safety of the screening tests; adequacy of resources to assure effective screening and follow-up; cost; and acceptance of the screening program by the community, including consumers and practicing physicians.[8] The optimal genetic program would be initiated only after adequate public education and only with community support and involvement in the program. Those screened would be informed of the purpose of the screening and would give consent, and confidentiality would be maintained. Results would be conveyed through nondirective counseling, and screening tests would be inexpensive, simple, and accurate. Finally, there would be sufficient qualified personnel and laboratory facilities for required follow-up, and the program would provide a means of self-assessment.

A major legal issue in all types of genetic screening is whether the program should be voluntary or mandatory. In 1975, the National Academy of Sciences recommended that "participation in a genetic screening program should not be mandatory by law, but should be left to the discretion of the person tested or, if a minor, of the parents or legal guardian."[4] In 1983, the President's Bioethics Commission endorsed voluntary screening, but noted that mandatory programs "requiring the performance of low-risk, minimally intrusive procedures may be justified if voluntary testing would fail to prevent an avoidable, serious injury to people—such as children—who are unable to protect themselves."[9] However, the vast majority of newborn genetic screening programs remain mandatory.

Confidentiality of genetic screening results is a second major legal issue. In 1983, the President's Bioethics Commission[9] underlined the importance of confidentiality by recommending the following:

- Genetic information should not be given to unrelated third parties, such as insurers or employers, without the explicit and informed consent of the person screened or a surrogate for that person.
- Private and governmental agencies that use data banks for genetic-related information should require that sorted information be coded whenever that is compatible with the purpose of the data bank.

In view of the history of genetics screening and the possible stigmatization that can result from possession of even a recessive gene, these recommendations seem minimal and should be followed. In addition, the President's Bioethics Commission[9] recommended that screening programs should not be undertaken at all unless the results that are produced were consistently valid, and a full range of prescreening and follow-up services for the population in question should be available before a screening program is introduced. We believe these recommendations are reasonable and that they should be followed.[2]

Prenatal Diagnosis

The standard of care that obstetricians are expected to provide with respect to genetic counseling and prenatal diagnosis has been clearly defined in the 1989 edition of Standards for Obstetric–Gynecologic Services, developed by the Committee on Professional Standards of the American College of Obstetricians and Gynecologists.[10]

> *The gynecologist should be alert to any indication of genetic disorders or conditions in a patient that might lead to birth defects in her offspring. Screening for genetic disorders begins with a careful evaluation of family medical history, drug use, and environmental factors. The physician should inquire about the outcome of previous pregnancies, mental retardation in family members, and known or suspected inherited or metabolic disease. Whenever possible, disorders should be diagnosed prior to pregnancy.*
>
> *When a genetic disorder is suspected, the gynecologist should discuss with the patient the ways in which the genetic disorder may affect her health, her reproductive capabilities, or the development of her offspring. A couple with a suspected genetic abnormality should receive the information necessary for them to decide based on the potential social, emotional, and economic consequences whether to proceed with further investigation. The gynecologist may wish to refer patients with potential genetic disorders to qualified genetic counseling and evaluation centers. . . .*
>
> *Antenatal screening for genetic disorders is an integral part of obstetric care. In some instances, identification of possible risks and appropriate diagnostic measures can be undertaken prior to pregnancy.*
>
> *The history obtained during the initial evaluation should be reviewed to detect signs that suggest a risk of genetic disorders:*
>
> - *Advanced parental age (mother 35 years of age or older at the expected time of delivery)*
> - *Previous offspring with a chromosomal aberration, particularly autosomal trisomy*
> - *Chromosomal abnormality in either parent, particularly a translocation*
> - *Family history of a sex-linked condition*
> - *Inborn errors of metabolism*
> - *Neural tube defects*
> - *Hemoglobinopathies*
> - *Ancestry indicating risk for Tay-Sachs, beta-thalassemia, or alpha-thalassemia*
>
> *Couples who have increased risks for producing abnormal offspring may undergo antenatal diagnostic studies after appropriate counseling.*

We have proposed the following guidelines concerning the legal and ethical obligations of the obstetrician in relation to genetic counseling and prenatal diagnosis[1]: First, genetic counseling should be nondirective; the counselor should remain impartial and objective in giving information that will allow patients to make their own rational decision. The Judicial Council of the American Medical Association has given the following opinion[11]:

> *Physicians, whether they oppose or do not oppose contraception, sterilization, or abortion, may decide that they can engage in genetic counseling and screening, but should avoid the imposition of their personal moral values and the substitution of their own moral judgment for that of the prospective parents. The ethical and moral decisions have to be made by the family and should not be imposed by the physician.*

Second, an obstetrician cannot be required to perform a genetic amniocentesis, chorionic villus sampling, or any other prenatal diagnostic procedure. Indeed, many are not qualified to perform such procedures and for them to do so may be malpractice. In such circumstances, referral to a specialist is usually the proper course. As stated by the Judicial Council of the American Medical Association,[11]

> *Physicians who consider the legal and ethical requirements applicable to genetic counseling to be in conflict with their moral values and conscience may choose to limit such service to preconception diagnosis and advice or not provide any genetic services. However, there are circumstances in which the physician who is so disposed is nevertheless obligated to alert prospective parents that a potential genetic problem does exist, that the physician does not offer genetic services, and that the patient should seek medical genetic counseling from another qualified specialist.*

Third, the law requires physicians to give accurate information to the parents and forbids the withholding of vital information from them. These principles are consistent with the doctrine of *informed consent* and the reasonable expectations of pregnant women under a physician's care.[12] The physician does not guarantee a healthy child, but the patient expects to be apprised of any information that the child might be defective and of the alternative ways to proceed so that she can determine the action to take.[13]

Finally, strict nondisclosure policies to nonfamily members should be maintained unless and until specific legislation is enacted that would clearly delineate the circumstances in which confidentiality must be breached, analogous to certain contagious diseases, gunshot wounds, and child abuse. To ensure the patient's interest in both autonomy and privacy, no information obtained in genetic counseling or screening should be disclosed to any third party, including insurers and employers, without the patient's informed consent.[9,12] On the other hand, counselors should be permitted to attempt to persuade patients to make disclosures of important information to potentially affected relatives. We recommend that the genetic counselor make clear, both verbally and in writing, the policy that he or she follows so that the patient can refuse to be screened or counseled if he or she is not in agreement with the policy. Such agreements will encourage people to participate voluntarily in screening and counseling and will serve to heighten the public's confidence in genetic counseling.

MATERNAL–FETAL CONFLICT: FORCED CESAREAN SECTION

The clinical application of new technologies, including ultrasonography, amniotic fluid studies, and electronic fetal monitoring, has enabled obstetricians to diagnose fetal disorders and recommend interventions for the sake of the fetus, as in cesarean section. Such obstetric "rescue efforts" reflect the concept that the viable fetus is a patient whose well-being should be promoted. The pregnant woman receiving the obstetrician's care is, of course, a patient as well.[14] A difficult ethical problem, and an important one in obstetrics, concerns how to balance the rights of fetus and mother when they conflict. As psychiatrist Jay Katz has noted, although these are called "maternal–fetal conflicts," the real conflict is usually between the obstetrician and the pregnant woman. There are two situations in which such conflict can occur. The first is if a pregnant woman engages in behavior that may endanger her fetus, such as abusing drugs or alcohol or working or living in an environment that is hazardous to the fetus. The second is a situation in which the pregnant woman refuses medical intervention that is required in the best interest of her fetus. Not all of these cases involve women who refuse treatment on religious grounds; some are motivated by different reasons, such as fear of surgery, distrust of the advice given by the obstetrician, or a feeling that a cesarean section somehow represents a failure (see also Chapter 12).

Disagreements between obstetricians and their pregnant patients can be emotionally devastating to physicians because of their feelings of helplessness and vulnerability in the face of potential catastrophy, but such disagreements inevitably occur. The question is how they should be resolved. Traditionally, physicians have not been eager to involve judges in medical treatment decisions, often arguing that this would interfere with the doctor–patient relationship. Thus, it is ironic that some obstetricians—the specialty that sees itself as most besieged by malpractice litigation—seek judicial intervention at the bedside. We must ask, is this a trend that should be encouraged?[15]

In a US survey in 1987, Kolder et al[16] found that court orders have been obtained for cesarean sections in 11 states, for hospital detentions in two states, and for intrauterine transfusions in one state. Among the 21 cases in which court orders were sought, the orders were obtained in 18 cases; in 15 of those cases, the orders were obtained within 6 hours. The majority of the women involved were black, Asian, or Hispanic. Nearly one half were unmarried, and one fourth did not speak English as their primary language. We must recognize that women from various ethnic backgrounds may have widely differing religious and personal beliefs—beliefs that often are misunderstood or even discounted by some physicians. Kolder and colleagues[16] make the point that the handful of court-ordered obstetric treatment cases rest on dubious legal grounds. In almost all of these cases, judges were called on an emergency basis and ordered intervention within hours. The judge usually went to the hospital. Physicians should remember what most lawyers and almost all judges know: When a judge arrives at the hospital and responds to an emergency call, he or she is acting much more like a lay person than a jurist. Without the time to analyze the issues, hear from the pregnant woman, reflect on the situation, or review the relevant law and in an unfamiliar setting with a calm physician and a woman who easily could be labelled "hysterical," the judge will almost always order whatever the doctor recommends.[15]

In addition to concern about maternal and fetal well-being, physicians invariably also fear liability when a woman refuses advice. If the child is injured, the physician may fear liability for malpractice. However, if the pregnant woman has made an informed refusal, this fear is unwarranted. The rights to bodily integrity and self determination are firmly grounded in common-law principles, and these rights are most explicitly articulated in the doctrine of informed consent. As Judge Benjamin Cardoza stated in 1914 in the case of *Schloendorff v Society of New York Hospital*,[17] medical treatment given without consent constitutes battery. If a competent adult refuses treatment, the exceptions to the informed consent rule for emergencies specifically are not applicable. Thus, in such cases, obtaining a court order may appear to be in the doctor's best interest. But the legitimacy is deceptive; the judge has acted injudiciously, and there is no opportunity for meaningful appeal. Also, the medical situation has not changed, except that more time has been lost that should have been devoted to discussion directly with the woman. Finally, the physician has now helped transform herself or himself into an agent of the state's authority.[15]

An established principle of ethics and law is that competent adults have a right to refuse treatment for themselves, even life-saving procedures. On the other hand, the right of parents to refuse treatment for their children has limits when refusal of treatment is likely to cause serious harm to the child. We do not think that child abuse and neglect laws should be extended to fetuses. Unlike a child, the fetus is absolutely dependent on its mother and cannot be treated without invading the mother in some way. In other words, the mother and fetus are not two separate individuals with separate rights. Treating them separately before birth can be done only by favoring one over the other in disputes. Nothing in *Roe v. Wade* or any other legal precedent gives judges or physicians the right to favor the life or health of the fetus over that of the pregnant woman. Even in the case of children, no mother can be legally required to donate a kidney or provide bone marrow or blood to save the life of her dying child. Therefore, there is no legal precedent to force a woman to submit to more invasive surgical procedures for the sake of her *fetus*.[15,18]

Those who support intervention to protect fetuses are not clear about the central important questions: What degree of risk would justify intervention by the legal system? What degree of certainty about that risk would be required? Physicians often disagree about the appropriateness of obstetric interventions, and they can be mistaken. This frequently has been the case when court-ordered cesarean sections have been sought. But even assuming 100% accuracy, we believe that pregnant women should still be permitted to refuse surgery to protect their liberty and human dignity. Practical considerations also support the rights of the woman over those of the fetus. Women may take matters into their own hands and not deliver in hospitals. Other interventions to which they might consent will be unavailable at home, and an opportunity to change their minds will be lost. The question of how to handle a woman who refuses treatment in the face of a court order remains. Do we really want to restrain, forcibly medicate, and operate on a competent refusing adult? Such a procedure may be legal, especially when viewed from a judicial perspective that the woman is irrational, hysterical, or evil-minded, but it is brutish and not what is generally associated with medical care.[2] It also encourages an adversarial relationship between the obstetrician and the patient, rather than the traditional positive relationship of the obstetrician working with the woman to achieve the goal of a healthy child born to a healthy mother.

Child neglect statutes cannot be applied to fetuses even when the mother appears to be acting irresponsibly and possibly is endangering her fetus. We may all agree that mothers should take care of themselves and their fetuses, but it is unlikely that the prospect of a damaged child suing its mother will be an effective deterrent or a useful means of compensating the child. It is not helpful to use the law to convert a woman's moral responsibility to her fetus into the woman's legal responsibility alone. The best chance we have to protect fetuses is to enhance the status of all women with programs of education, maternal and child health programs, and medical research to prevent complications of pregnancy.[2,15]

The Committee on Ethics of the ACOG published a Committee Opinion on Patient Choice: Maternal–Fetal Conflicts, which we support.[19] The following conclusions were set forth to provide guidance to the obstetrician:

1. With advances in medical technology, the fetus has become more accessible to diagnostic and treatment modalities. The maternal–fetal relationship remains a unique one, requiring a balance of maternal health, autonomy, and fetal needs. Every reasonable effort should be made to protect the fetus, but the pregnant woman's autonomy should be respected.
2. The vast majority of pregnant women are willing to assume significant risk for the welfare of the fetus. Problems arise only when this potentially beneficial advice is rejected. The role of the obstetrician should be one of an informed educator and counselor, weighing the risks and benefits to both patients as well as realizing that tests, judgments, and decisions are fallible. Consultation with others, including an institutional ethics committee, should be sought when appropriate to aid the pregnant woman and obstetrician in making decisions. The use of the courts to resolve these conflicts is almost never warranted.
3. Obstetricians should refrain from performing procedures that are unwanted by a pregnant woman. The use of judicial authority to implement treatment regimens in order to protect the fetus violates the pregnant woman's autonomy. Furthermore, inappropriate reliance on judicial authority may lead to undesirable societal consequences, such as the criminalization of noncompliance with medical recommendations.

(See also Chapter 12.)

FETAL RESEARCH

Fetal research is one of the most controversial and complex areas in the field of human experimentation. The National Commission for the Protection of Human Subjects of Biomedical and Behavioral Research spent the first year of its existence (1974–1975) working under a congressional mandate to make recommendations regarding fetal research before working on any other topic. This mandate was most influenced by *Roe v. Wade,* the 1973 decision of the US Supreme Court, which provided that the government could not interfere with the decision of a woman and her physician regarding abortion before fetal viability.[20] This decision invalidated criminal laws against abortion, increasing the number of fetuses aborted, and therefore, the number of fetuses potentially available for research.

As adopted by the US Department of Health and Human Services, federal regulations require that, before experimentation involving human fetuses, appropriate animal studies be done and that researchers have no role in any decision to terminate a pregnancy. The purpose of an *in utero* experiment must be to meet the health needs of the fetus, and the fetus can be placed at risk only to the minimum extent necessary to meet such needs. In the case of nontherapeutic research, the risk to the fetus must be minimal, and the knowledge to be gained must be important and not obtainable by other means. The consent of both the mother and the father is required unless the father's identity is not known, he is not reasonably available, or the pregnancy resulted from rape.

The research protocol must be reviewed by an institutional review board (IRB), which, in addition to its normal duties, must take special care to review the subject selection process and the methods by which informed consent is obtained. The consent process itself should probably be audited by a representative of the IRB as well. It also has been recommended that a special advocate for the fetus be appointed to help caution the parents against consenting to an experimental procedure on their fetus that they may not understand or that they incorrectly may see as therapeutic. It appears, however, that by the time parents reach the major medical centers involved in this research, they already have made up their minds to do what they consider the last hope their fetus may have. Thus, the advocate notion may be too little too late if its purpose is to beneficially influence the consent process.

These federal human experimentation regulations technically apply only to those researchers who receive federal funds or who are affiliated with institutions that have signed an agreement with HHS that all research in their institutions (and by their faculty and staff in other institutions) will be reviewed by their IRB. Nonetheless, these regulations are so fundamental to the protection of the integrity of the fetus, the potential parents, and the research enterprise, that they should be followed voluntarily in all institutions doing fetal research.

TRANSPLANTATION OF HUMAN FETAL TISSUE

Current federal regulations permit the use of tissue from dead fetuses in experimental transplantation when it is conducted in accordance with state law.[21] All but eight states (Arizona, Arkansas, Illinois, Indiana, Louisiana, New Mexico, Ohio, and Oklahoma) permit such experiments. Nonetheless, ethical concerns remain, and there has been contined political resistance to funding such research with public money.

The most recent series of disputes began in October 1987, when the National Institutes of Health (NIH) submitted a request to the Assistant Secretary for Health to fund the transplantation of human fetal tissue into the brain of a patient with Parkinson's disease. In March, 1988, Assistant Secretary Robert Windom asked that the NIH establish a special advisory panel to study 10 questions about fetal–tissue research. In May, a moratorium was announced on the use of fetuses from elective abortions in federally funded research.

The 21-member human tissue fetal transplant research panel subsequently created by the NIH invited more than 50 people, including the representatives of 16 groups, to present their views in public sessions. On December 5, the panel finalized its report, and on December 14, the advisory committee to the NIH director adopted it unanimously. The panel began by deciding to separate questions concerning abortion from the use of fetal tissue. Although legally and ethically appropriate, this separation may prove a politically untenable one. The panel also decided to limit discussion to the use of tissue from dead fetuses and to reject any payment for fetal tissue or intrafamilial donations—rulings consistent with an October 1988, amendment to the National Organ Transplant Act. The panel concluded that although it was of "moral relevance" that the fetal tissue be obtained from an induced abortion (rather than a spontaneous abortion or an interrupted ectopic pregnancy), the use of the tissue in research was "acceptable public policy" because "abortion is legal and . . . the research in question is intended to achieve significant medical goals."[22] This conclusion was accepted on a vote of 15 to 2, and included recommendations that the decision to abort be kept independent of the decision to retrieve and use fetal tissue, that recipients be informed of the tissue's fetal origins, and that fetal tissue be accorded the same respect given other cadaveric human tissue.[22] In answer to the remaining questions, the panel adopted the following recommendations: the decision to abort must be made before the use of the tissue is discussed; anonymity should be maintained between donor and recipient; the timing and method of the abortion should not be influenced by the potential use of the fetal tissues; and the consent of the pregnant woman is necessary and sufficient for the use of tissue unless the father objects.[22] The panel also concluded that "there is sufficient evidence from animal experimentation to justify proceeding with human clinical trials in Parkinson's disease and juvenile diabetes."[22] Many of these recommendations were adopted unanimously, and no more than two panel members dissented from any of them.

A second independent group, the Stanford University Medical Center Committee on Ethics,[23] was in fundamental agreement with the NIH panel. However, one important difference between the two reports was that the Stanford committee attempted to sidestep the question of elective abortion by recommending that "if tissue from spontaneous abortions can satisfy the medical demands for both quantity and quality of tissue, it would be preferable to avoid the ethical problems of using induced abortions."[23] The use of tissues from fetuses aborted spontaneously is particularly problematic. It is now well recognized that at least one half of spontaneously aborted first-trimester fetuses are chromosomally abnormal. Moreover, spontaneous abortions have been associated with a variety of infectious microorganisms (eg, Ureaplasma, urealyticum, cytomegalovirus, toxoplasma). It would be indefensible to transplant abnormal or infected fetal tissue that could increase the risk of a transplant failure and infection in the recipient. Tissue from spontaneously aborted fetuses should not be used for transplantation into a human subject.[3] Despite this difference between the NIH panel and Stanford committee, these two reports show strong agreement in the medical community on the major issues involved in the use of human fetal tissue for transplantation.

The primary objection to the use of fetal tissues from elective abortions appears to be a political one: If it were therapeutically successful, such use would create a new constituency—sick people who would benefit from such transplants and their families—who would be opposed to the prohibition of elective abortion. Of course, from a scientific and ethical standpoint, the central issue is whether it is reasonable to perform transplant experiments with fetal tissue at this time, a question neither panel attempted to examine in any depth. The politics of abortion have thus led us to focus on the tangential question of the tissue's source rather than the central question of its benefits to sick people. The subjects of the proposed transplant research are not the fetuses (which are dead), but the tissue recipients.[3]

There is no method of regulating the clinical trials of new surgical procedures (as there is of trials of new drugs) and no effective way to regulate experiments financed privately. We believe that such regulation should exist. It would be most beneficial to science and the public if such experimentation could be confined to a few centers of established excellence, where careful research could be pursued until the safety and efficacy of such transplantations are demonstrated. Additional scientific data are needed to better understand a variety of issues, such as graft-versus-host reactions, transplant function, and cellular growth patterns.

We have made the following recommendations for the transplantation of human fetal tissue[3]:

- The woman should be asked about the use of her fetus as a source of tissue after she has decided to have an abortion, but before the abortion has taken place. Afterward, she should be given an opportunity to withdraw her consent.
- When the physician has performed the standard inspection of the tissue to make sure that the abortion is complete, the tissue should be taken from the operating room and given to the researcher. The dissection of the tissues should be performed in a restricted facility designed to optimize the success of the procedure (eg, a sterile environment and proper dissecting instruments).
- To avoid conflict of interest, there should be no academic incentive (such as coauthorship of publications or grant support) or other incentive for the physician performing the abortion or anyone else involved in the woman's care, to obtain her agreement for the use of fetal tissue.

Society has generally been highly supportive of transplantation when it serves the purpose of saving a life that otherwise would have been lost. But transplantation involving fetal tissue is much more problematic, and the public may be less forgiving of ethical shortcuts. Saving a life usually is not at issue, and the source of the tissue, although not illicit, is troublesome to many. It is a general rule that whatever is technically possible will be attempted. Use of human fetal tissue for therapy and research must be soundly grounded in science, ethics, and compassionate patient care.

CONCLUSIONS

The development of ethical principles in the practice of obstetrics and genetics is no easy task. We believe, however, that a few general principles can be formulated to protect the autonomy and human dignity of obstetric patients. First, because of their interests in dignity and bodily integrity, competent patients should have the right to refuse *any* medical intervention that has risks to them. Second, obstetric patients have the right to full knowledge about the availability of genetic tests and screening procedures that can lessen the risk of giving birth to a handicapped child. Third, decisions in obstetric care should be *joint* decisions between the patient and physician to protect the dignity and autonomy of the patient and to foster a mutually respectful doctor–patient relationship that will enhance the likelihood of appropriate medical care for the pregnant woman and her fetus.

REFERENCES

1. Annas GJ, Elias S. Legal and ethical issues in perinatology. In: Gabbe SG, Niebyl JR, Simpson JL, eds. *Obstetrics: Normal and Problem Pregnancies.* New York, NY: Churchill Livingston: 1986;1079.
2. Elias S, Annas GJ. *Reproductive Genetics and the Law.* Chicago, IL: Year Book Medical Publishers; 1987.
3. Annas GJ, Elias S. The politics of transplantation of human fetal tissue. *N Engl J Med.* 1989;320:1079.
4. *Genetic Screening: Programs, Principles and Research.* Washington, DC: National Academy of Sciences; 1975.
5. Reilly P. *Genetics, Law and Social Policy.* Cambridge, MA: Harvard University Press; 1977.
6. Andrews LB. *State Laws and Regulations Governing Newborn Screening.* Chicago, IL: American Bar Association; 1985.
7. Andrews LB. *Legal Liability and Quality Assurance in Newborn Screening.* Chicago, IL: American Bar Association; 1985.
8. Holtzman NA. *Newborn Screening for Genetic–Metabolic Diseases: Progress, Principles and Recommendation.* Washington, DC: 1977. US Dept of Health, Education, and Welfare publication NIH 78-5207.
9. President's Commission for the Study of Ethical Problems in Medicine and Biomedical and Behavioral Research. *Screening and Counseling for Genetic Conditions.* Washington, DC: US Government Printing Office; Feb. 1983.
10. *Standards for Obstetric–Gynecologic Services.* 7th ed. The American College of Obstetricians and Gynecologists, 1989.
11. Recent opinions of the Judicial Council of the American Medical Association. *JAMA.* 1984;251:2078.
12. Annas GJ. Problems of informed consent and confidentiality in genetic counseling. In: Milunsky A, Annas GJ, eds. *Genetics and the Law.* New York, NY: Plenum Press; 1976;111.
13. Annas GJ, Coyne B. "Fitness" for birth and reproduction: Legal implications of genetic screening. *Family Law Q.* 1975;9:463.
14. Strong C. Ethical conflicts between mother and fetus in Obstetrics. *Clin Perinatol.* 1987;14:313.
15. Annas GJ. Protecting the liberty of pregnant patients. *N Engl J Med.* 1987;316:1213.
16. Kolder UEB, Gallagher J, Parsons MT. Court-ordered obstetrical interventions. *N Engl J Med.* 1987;316:1192.
17. *Schloendorff v. Society of New York Hospital,* 211 N.Y. 125, 105 N.E. 92 (1914).
18. Annas GJ. Forced cesareans: The most unkind cut of all. *Hastings Cent Rep.* 1982;12:16.
19. ACOG Committee Opinion No. 55, Committee on Ethics. *Patient Choice: Maternal–fetal Conflict.* Washington, DC: 1987.
20. *Roe v Wade,* 410 U.S. 113 (1973).
21. Robertson JA. Fetal tissue transplants. *Washington Univ Law Q.* 1988;66:443.
22. Consultants of the Advisory Committee to the Director of the National Institutes of Health. *Report of the Human Fetal Tissue Transplant Panel.* Washington, DC: National Institutes of Health; 1988.
23. Greely HT, Hamm T, Johnson R, et al. The ethical use of human fetal tissue in medicine. *N Engl J Med.* 1989;320:1093.

PART III Nutritional Requirements and Disturbances

Baha M. Sibai, Section Editor

Chapter Nineteen

Vitamins and Minerals

George M. Kazzi, Thomas L. Gross, and Mary Helen Quigg

19

The prescribing of vitamins and mineral supplements during pregnancy has become standard in obstetric practice. The recommendations, which suggest that these supplements improve maternal and fetal outcome, however, often are based on studies with serious deficiencies. Moreover, the increase in vitamin requirements during pregnancy usually can be more than adequately provided by dietary sources, assuming appropriate caloric intake and the consumption of animal protein. Much knowledge regarding transport of vitamins across the placenta is derived from animal studies and simple case reports. The animal data are generally obtained using study designs in which vitamins are totally excluded or administered to excess. This type of study design has little potential application to the human experience, even in a severely malnourished mother or a mother who is taking "megadose" vitamins. Human studies of pregnancy complications associated with vitamin deficiencies are generally uncontrolled; frequently they are performed in populations of patients with generally poor nutrition and multiple vitamin and mineral deficiencies. For this reason, it is difficult to extrapolate from these data to populations of pregnant women with well-balanced and nutritionally complete diets. Finally, there is no agreement on what constitutes normal serum levels of vitamins during pregnancy. Normal values for the nonpregnant state do not correspond to values in the pregnant state. This is because of the normal physiologic changes of pregnancy, which result in a decrease in many binding globulins and an increase in plasma volume. Both of these physiologic changes result in a decreased serum level of vitamins, in many cases to levels which would be considered deficient in the nonpregnant state.

While it is generally agreed that the scientific evidence for universal vitamin and mineral supplementation during pregnancy is ambiguous, when undertaken with reason, it represents a benign therapy with potential for improved outcome. Newer data support more conclusively the therapeutic benefit of some vitamin supplementation to prevent specific diseases. Examples are vitamin use for the prevention of neural tube defects, and calcium use for pregnancy-induced hypertension. On the other hand, frequently uncontrolled vitamin use, especially of megavitamins, may cause increased risks to pregnancies.

PLACENTAL TRANSPORT

In general, lipid-soluble vitamins cross the placenta more readily than water-soluble vitamins. The transport of vitamins and minerals across the placenta, like all nutritional substrates, uses several mechanisms, depending on the physical and chemical properties of the vitamin or mineral to be transported. These mechanisms are summarized below.[1]

Simple Diffusion

Diffusion occurs across the placenta because of a concentration gradient. The amount of maternal substance crossing into the fetal compartment is directly proportional to the concentration of this substance in the maternal compartment and the electrochemical properties of the substance in question. The fetal concentration is usually lower than the maternal concentration. Factors that play a role in simple diffusion include lipid solubility, molecular weight of the substance, thickness of membranes and surface area of placental membranes, and the membranes' chemical composition. Substances crossing by this mechanism include lipid-soluble vitamins.

Active Transport

This process involves energy expenditure because substances are pumped against a gradient. It usually results in the transfer of substances from the mother to the fetus, concentrating this substance in the fetal compartment at greater levels than would be expected with simple diffusion alone. Consequently, the resulting maternal level is often lower at delivery than the fetal level. Vitamins and minerals crossing the placenta by active transport include water-soluble vitamins and some ions, such as calcium, magnesium, and iron.

The changes that occur in the placenta as gestation advances have a direct influence on the transport mechanism, whether it is active or passive. Histologic studies have shown that the intervillous surface area increases significantly from 20–40 weeks' gestation. At the same time, the cellular number increases only minimally. The thickness of the placental membrane thus decreases, which results in more optimal conditions for passive diffusion. Hence, all vitamins that cross the placenta by simple diffusion, such as lipid-soluble vitamins, cross more readily at term than at an earlier gestational age. Although the active transport mechanism is not as well understood with respect to the developing placenta, studies have shown that placental oxygen consumption and ATP production decrease as pregnancy advances. This suggests that active transport may decrease late in pregnancy compared to earlier in gestation. The transport of the water-soluble vitamins may thus be decreased during later parts of gestation.

The *Recommended Dietary Allowances (RDA's)* for vitamins and minerals in the pregnant patient are listed in Table 19–1. Dietary sources for these vitamins and minerals are shown in Table 19–2.

TABLE 19–1. RECOMMENDED DIETARY ALLOWANCES FOR WOMEN AGES 19–50[a]

Nutrient	Nonpregnant	Pregnant	Lactating
Energy (kcal)[b]	1700–2500	+300	+500
Lipid-soluble vitamins			
Vitamin A (mg)	800	+200	+400
Vitamin D (μg)	5–7.5	+5	+5
Vitamin E (mg)	8	+2	+3
Vitamin K (μg)[c]	70–140	—	—
Water-soluble vitamins[c]			
Vitamin C (mg)	60	+20	+40
Thiamine (mg)	1.0–1.1	+0.4	+0.5
Riboflavin (mg)	1.2–1.3	+0.3	+0.5
Niacin (mg)	13–14	+2	+5
Vitamin B_6 (mg)	2.0	+0.6	+0.5
Folic acid (μg)	400	+400	+100
Vitamin B_{12} (μg)	3.0	+1.0	+1.0
Biotin (μg)[c]	100–200	—	—
Pantothenic acid (mg)[c]	4–7	—	—
Minerals			
Calcium (mg)	800	+400	+400
Phosphorus (mg)	800	+400	+400
Magnesium (mg)	300	+150	+150
Iron (mg)	18	+30–60	+30–60
Zinc (mg)	15	+5	+10
Iodine (μg)	150	+25	+50
Chromium (mg)[c]	0.05–0.2	—	—
Copper (mg)[c]	2–3	—	—
Manganese (mg)[c]	2.5–5.0	—	—

[a] *The National Research Council, Committee on Dietary Allowances, Food and Nutrition Board. Recommended Dietary Allowances. 9th ed. Washington, DC: National Academy of Science. 1980.*
[b] *The National Research Council Committee on Dietary Allowances, Food and Nutrition Board. Recommended Dietary Allowances. 9th ed. Washington, DC: National Academy of Science. 1980:23.*
[c] *The National Research Council Committee on Dietary Allowances, Food and Nutrition Board. Recommended Dietary Allowances. 9th ed. Washington, DC: National Academy of Science. 1980:178.*

WATER-SOLUBLE VITAMINS

Vitamin B1—Thiamine

Thiamine requirements during pregnancy may increase as much as threefold. The level of thiamine in maternal serum is lower in the pregnant than in the nonpregnant patient. Also, the thiamine level in cord blood is twice that of maternal serum, possibly because of an active transport mechanism in the placenta.[2] Thiamine deficiency in the American pregnant population is very rare because of the thiamine rich US diet. However, in third–world countries, such as Korea, the Philippines, and Vietnam where the diet consists of nonenriched wheat and rice or large amounts of raw fish contaminated by thiaminases from bacterial sources, *Beriberi* is still affecting significant numbers of women.[3] Earlier studies reported severe cardiac decompensation in mothers with severe thiamine deficiency and maternal *Beriberi.*[4] Infants born to mothers with thiamine deficiency may be normal at birth. If the condition is not promptly detected and treated with thiamine replacement, the infants deteriorate suddenly in the neonatal period and gradually experience cyanotic congestive heart failure. The outcome is death, unless the condition is diagnosed and treated quickly. In one study, Heller and associates[2] measured serum thiamine levels in 600 mothers and concluded that, based on concentrations in serum, one third were deficient in thiamine. This study is supported by a European study that concluded that 30% of clinically well-nourished pregnant women were thiamine-deficient.[5] No differences in either neonatal or maternal outcome between the deficient pregnancies and those with adequate thiamine levels were reported, however. These studies suggest that genuine thiamine deficiency can result in serious maternal and fetal sequelae. Maternal serum levels are of only poorly diagnostic quality to diagnose deficiency. There is no evidence that thiamine supplementation is needed during pregnancy in the United States. However, in countries with more unbalanced diets, supplementing with additional thiamine can be beneficial.

Excessive intake of thiamine at many times therapeutic doses can result in nausea, vomiting, anorexia, and lethargy.[3] The doses required to produce this syndrome are much greater than the typical megadose levels.

Vitamin B_2—Riboflavin

Riboflavin is a coenzyme in tissue oxidation–reduction reactions and in energy production through respiration. As such, it is involved in protein and energy metabolism and in erythropoiesis. The exact mechanism of riboflavin transport across the placenta is not well studied. One hypothesis is that flavin–adenine dinveleotied (FAD) enters the placenta from maternal blood and is there cleaved to riboflavin, which is released into the fetal circulation. The fetus then presumably synthesizes its own FAD from riboflavin.

Several national nutritional surveys have reported that up to 11% of US schools children have subclinical evidence

TABLE 19–2. DIETARY SOURCES OF VITAMINS AND ESSENTIAL MINERALS

Vitamin or Mineral	Dietary Source
Water-Soluble Vitamins	
Thiamine	Pork, organ meats, whole grains, legumes
Riboflavin	Widely distributed in foods
Niacin	Liver, lean meats, grains, legumes
Pyridoxine	Meats, vegetables, whole-grain cereals
Pantothenic acid	Widely distributed in foods
Folic acid	Legumes, green vegetables, whole-wheat products
Vitamin B_{12}	Muscle meats, eggs, dairy products (not present in plant foods)
Biotin	Legumes, vegetables, meats
Choline	Egg yolk, liver, grains, legumes
Vitamin C	Citrus fruits, tomatoes, green peppers, salad greens
Lipid-Soluble Vitamins	
Vitamin A	Provitamin A, beta carotene is widely distributed in green vegetables. Retinol is present in milk, butter, cheese, fortified margarine.
Vitamin D	Cod-liver oil, eggs, dairy products, fortified milk, and margarine
Vitamin E	Seeds, green leafy vegetables, margarine, shortenings
Vitamin D	Green leafy vegetables, small amount in cereals, fruits, and meats
Minerals	
Calcium	Mild cheese, dark green vegetables, dried legumes
Phosphorus	Milk, cheese, meat, poultry, grains
Magnesium	Whole grains, green leafy vegetables
Iron	Eggs, lean meats, legumes, whole grains, green leafy vegetables
Zinc	Widely distributed in foods
Copper	Meats, drinking water
Manganese	Widely distributed in foods
Iodine	Marine fish and shellfish, dairy products, many vegetables
Chromium	Fats, vegetable oils, meats

Adapted from Scrimshaw NS, Young, VR. The requirements of human nutrition. Sci Am. *1976;235:50.*

of riboflavin deficiency.[6] Recently, Heller and coworkers reported that deficiency is present in 25% of pregnant patients in the first trimester and in 40% by the third trimester, as measured by the glutathione reductase assay.[7] There is very little evidence to suggest that the reported riboflavin deficiency has any clinical significance in the United States. One study has suggested that there is an association between riboflavin deficiency, anemia, prematurity, and intrauterine fetal death; but a more recent study found no deleterious effects of maternal riboflavin deficiency on fetal or neonatal outcome.[7] Although some investigators[8] have noted an increased incidence of congenital malformations in the offspring of rats deficient in riboflavin, this has never been documented in humans. In these animal studies, a total deprivation of riboflavin, folic acid, and vitamin B_{12} is needed for such a syndrome to be produced. This clinical situation is unlikely to occur in humans except under conditions of extreme starvation. Riboflavin supplementation in pregnancy has been recommended, but support for this view is inconclusive. Riboflavin in high doses has not been reported to cause toxic effects in animal or human studies. This is in part because of the gastrointestinal tract's inability to absorb large amounts at a given treatment.[10]

Vitamin B_3—Pantothenic Acid

The exact requirements for pantothenic acid in nonpregnant and pregnant patients have not been established. It has been suggested that pantothenic acid decreases in pregnancy and returns to normal in the first week postpartum.[1] Although pantothenic acid deficiency was associated with cerebral abnormalities in rats[8], there is no evidence in humans that it causes congenital malformations.

Vitamin B_5—Nicotinic Acid or Niacin

Niacin is a component of two important enzymes that are needed in glycolysis and tissue respiration. Hundreds of enzyme reactions require the nicotinamide component found within nucleotide adenine diphosphate (NAD or NADP). The maternal serum level of niacin decreases during pregnancy and the urinary excretion of niacin metabolites increases.[8] It is doubtful that this is evidence of deficiency because the decrease in concentration may be a result of the increase in blood volume and glomerular filtration rate in pregnancy. The American diet is rich in niacin and clinically significant deficiency is rare. There is no evidence that a deficiency or an excess of niacin causes any adverse effect on prenancy outcome.

Vitamin B_6—Pyridoxine

Pyridoxine is an essential vitamin required in multiple enzymatic reactions involving the metabolism of lipids, proteins, and carbohydrates. The maternal serum level of pyridoxine is decreased during pregnancy compared to the nonpregnant state.[9] Urinary xanthurenic acid excretion after a test dose of tryptophan, which is the classic laboratory test to assess pyridoxine deficiency, has been found to increase progressively throughout gestation and reach about 15 times the nonpregnant level around term. Supplementation with daily doses of pyridoxine of 6–10 mg has been shown to normalize the blood levels of pyridoxine and to increase the xanthurenic acid excretion level.[9] Pitkin suggested that these biochemical changes in the blood level and in urinary excretion of xanthurenic acid represent physiologic adjustments, perhaps caused by the increase in blood volume, rather than a general vitamin B_6 deficiency.[9] The cord blood level of pyridoxine is twice the maternal blood level and may be evidence of an active transport mechanism.

The significance of pyridoxine deficiency in pregnancy is not clear. Several pregnancy complications have been associated with this deficiency, including pregnancy-induced hypertension, glucose intolerance, and hyperemesis gravidarum. Neurologic and arthrosclerotic changes have been reported in the offspring of reportedly deficient pregnancies.[8,11] The causal relationship between pyridoxine and any of these clinical complications is far from established. However, based on the limited data available, pyridoxine supplementation during pregnancy is recommended.

Very high doses of pyridoxine are required to produce toxic effects in adults, in the range of 2 to 6 g/d. This toxicity was discovered when megadoses of pyridoxine were used to treat carpal tunnel syndrome and preeclampsia. A peripheral neuropathy develops when using these tremendously high doses.[13] No adverse effects to the fetus from excess pyridoxine have been reported.

Vitamin B_{12}—Cobalamin

Vitamin B_{12} is a coenzyme required for erythropoiesis and for the metabolism of lipids, carbohydrates, and proteins. It is produced in the liver and was originally named *extrinsic factor*. It functions in all cells but has a major role in the cells of the bone marrow, gastrointestinal tract, and nervous system. In the bone marrow, it serves as a cofactor required for the synthesis of deoxyribonucleic acid (DNA). If it is not present, there is inadequate DNA synthesis, and the erthroblasts do not divide and are released into the circulation as megaloblasts, producing megaloblastic anemia. It is unclear whether this is the sole function of vitamin B_{12} or if it occurs in conjunction with folate.

Little is known concerning the requirements for vitamin B_{12} during pregnancy, yet several studies have shown that serum levels of vitamin B_{12} decrease progressively throughout pregnancy. When the urinary excretion of methylmalonic acid (MMA) was measured in a group of pregnant women who had low serum B_{12} levels, after a valine load most of the patients were found to have normal MMA urinary excretion. This suggests an adequate functional level of vitamin B_{12}. Attempts to reverse the decrease in serum levels in pregnancy using B_{12} supplementation have failed. This supports the theory that the decrease in serum vitamin B_{12} is independent of the dietary intake and does not necessarily reflect a depletion of the maternal B_{12} stores.[9] Animal studies have suggested that B_{12} deficiency in pregnancy may cause intrauterine growth retardation and hydrocephalus[12], but no such observations have been made in humans. The average American diet is more than sufficient to supply the required amount of vitamin B_{12} during pregnancy. The only patients of concern would be strict vegetarians, who may require oral supplementation. Patients who take excessive doses of vitamin C also may develop clinical B_{12} deficiency.

There is no evidence to suggest that megadoses of vitamin B_{12} are toxic either to pregnant women or to their fetuses. The amount of serum binding protein available limits the amount of vitamin retained in the body. Unbound vitamin B_{12} is excreted in the urine.

Folic Acid or Folicin

Folic acid or folicin is metabolized by the body to a coenzyme, tetrahydrofolate, which is required for the synthesis of purines and pyrimidines. Together with vitamin B_{12}, it is required for the synthesis of DNA. Folic acid appears to be concentrated in the bone marrow at levels greater than that found in the serum, which suggests an active transport mechanism.[14] As in vitamin B_{12} deficiency, a lack of folic acid also results in anemia. In the presence of folate deficiency, DNA is synthesized at a reduced rate, and the mitotic activity of the cells in the body is usually decreased. After iron deficiency, folate is the most common deficiency found in the pregnant patient.[15] The etiology of folate deficiency in pregnancy could be decreased intestinal absorption, impaired use, or increased demand.[16] The impaired use process is thought to be related to the increased level of estrogen during pregnancy. This is supported by the finding that folic acid deficiency also has been described in women on birth control pills. However, another important factor responsible for folate deficiency is the increase in the metabolic demands of pregnancy.

In addition to megaloblastic anemia, several reports have found that folic acid deficiency may cause several pregnancy complications, including antepartum hemorrhage, *abruptio placentae*, spontaneous abortions, preeclampsia, limited fetal growth, and congenital malformations.[17]

The last decade has seen multiple reports in animals and humans illustrating an alleged relationship between folic acid deficiency and the production of neural tube defects. Folate supplementation apparently can reduce the incidence of these defects.[18–22] Unfortunately, these studies are not conclusive. The majority of studies have been retrospective. This is in part because of a feeling that the available epidemiologic evidence is strong enough to support supplementation and that withholding folic acid would be unethical. Wild et al[19] analyzed two cohorts of women at high risk for producing a child with a neural tube defect. These women were divided into two groups: one that received vitamin supplementation (Pregvite Forte F beginning at least 28 days before conception; and one that did not receive supplementation. The groups were self-selecting. In addition, confounding factors were assessed including number of children with neural tube defects; social class; place of residence; and reproductive history, including spontaneous abortions, number of therapeutic abortions, and time between pregnancies. None of these factors altered the incidence of neural tube defects. The conclusion from the study was that the only significant factor was the presence or absence of vitamin supplementation with folic acid.

The majority of data concerning the beneficial effects of preconceptional vitamin supplementation have been derived from United Kingdom sources. The background risk of a neural tube defect is significantly higher in the United Kingdom than it is in the United States. Two recent studies with conflicting conclusions have been published using American data. The first used data from the *Atlanta Birth Defects Case Study* and retrospectively looked at 347 infants born with neural tube defects who were compared to 2829 randomly selected normal infants from the same population. All mothers were then questioned concerning vitamin usage before and during pregnancy. Periconceptional vitamin use was defined as taking vitamins three months before pregnancy and for the first 3 months of pregnancy. Nonusers where those women who did not take vitamins in this 6-month period. Only 14% of mothers reported periconceptional vitamin usage. This included 7% of study mothers and 14% of control mothers. Significant variations in the demographics of user and nonuser women were noted. The study concluded that periconceptual vitamins do have a protective effect against neural tube defects.[20]

The second major American study, from the *National Institute of Child Health and Human Development Neural Tube Study Group*, retrospectively examined whether periconceptional vitamin or folate supplementation decreased the risk of neural tube defects. The study population included 571 women who had produced a fetus with a neural tube defect. The control populations included 546 women who had had a malformed infant or stillbirth and 573 women with normal infants. They found that women who had infants with neural tube defects did not have a significantly lower rate of folate use when compared to either of the control groups.[21]

The authors noted that the differences between the two studies may be caused by the difference in time-lapse for interviews after delivery. The Atlanta study had a very long time-lapse, which may have increased recall bias. Moreover, the geographic variation in the incidence of neural tube defects also may have contributed to the differing results. Finally, as noted previously, the incidence of neural tube defects is small in the United States, requiring a large sample population to see small variations in results.[21] Based on published results, it is unlikely that a prospective study could be done in the litigious American atmosphere. The medical research council in Great Britain is completing a 5-year randomized prospective study of this issue.[22]

Vitamin C—Ascorbic Acid

Vitamin C is an essential vitamin for tissue collagen, absorption of iron, and the metabolism of folic acid. The serum level of ascorbic acid decreases in pregnancy, with serum levels at 40 weeks' gestation approximately one half the levels seen at midpregnancy. The umbilical cord serum levels of ascorbic acid have been reported to be 50% higher than maternal values.[8] Ascorbic acid deficiency is very rare in developed countries, and the clinical importance of vitamin C deficiency in pregnancy is not well known. There are unsubstantiated reports of an association of low vitamin C levels with premature rupture of the membranes, preeclampsia, and congenital abnormalities. The potential toxicity to the fetus from excessive doses of vitamin C, such as the 5 g/d dose suggested to prevent the common cold, has not been evaluated. However, the majority of the excess vitamin ingested is excreted rather than retained. Pregnant women should be cautioned against the use of large doses of vitamin C, particularly in the first trimester. The current recommended requirement during pregnancy is provided by the normal daily diet, and there is no additional benefit found by supplementation.

LIPID-SOLUBLE VITAMINS

The lipid-soluble vitamins, A, D, E, and K, are usually stored in the liver and are available when the need arises. In clinical situations, the deficiency of fat-soluble vitamins is rare. However, contrary to water-soluble vitamins, urinary excretion of lipid-soluble vitamins is usually limited. Because of this, megadose therapy with lipid-soluble vitamins can result in toxicity.

Vitamin A—Retinol

Vitamin A is needed for vision, development of epithelial tissue, bone growth, spermatogenesis, and fetal development of several organ systems. The maternal levels of vitamin A and its precursor, carotene, are variable during pregnancy but generally decrease progressively until term. Vitamin A is thought to cross the placenta by simple diffusion. Fetal levels of both carotene and vitamin A are usually slightly lower than the maternal level. The maternal serum level of vitamin A may be influenced by socioeconomic class, fetal sex, and vitamin supplementation. Deficiency of vitamin A has been associated with congenital malformation in animals[23], but this has not been confirmed in humans. Hypervitaminosis A also is reported to be associated with teratogenesis in animal experiments. There are reports of renal congenital malformations and central nervous system anomalies in human neonates whose mothers took excessive doses of vitamin A during gestation.[23] Most pregnant women are able to obtain the needed amount of vitamin A from their daily diet without resorting to additional supplementation.

Vitamin A analogues, such as isotretinoic acid (Accutane) and etretinate are presently on the market for the treatment of several dermatologic conditions, specifically cystic acne and psoriasis. Unfortunately although these drugs give dramatic relief from those conditions, they result in a 25% major congenital malformation rate and a 40% spontaneous pregnancy loss rate if ingested in the first trimester of pregnancy. In children born after maternal dose, ingestion during pregnancy, a 40% mental impairment rate has been reported.[24] The described effects include central nervous system malformations, ear malformations, craniofacial malformations, congenital heart disease, and thymic malformations.[25]

Vitamin D

Vitamin D promotes calcium absorption and regulates bone mineralization. It is taken in the diet or synthesized from cholesterol by ultraviolet radiation exposure of the skin. Deficiencies are not common in adults unless exposure to sunlight is very restricted. Maternal and fetal metabolism of vitamin D are very complex. 25-hydroxycholecalciferol vitamin D decreases, while 1,25-dihydroxycholecalciferol vitamin D increases as pregnancy progresses until term.[26] Both changes are consistent with the increased secretion of parathyroid hormone, which occurs during pregnancy in response to the decrease in free calcium.[8] Although a deficiency state of vitamin D is usually rare, neonatal tetany, abnormal development of the teeth, fetal rickets, and postnatal ricketic bone changes have been described in association with vitamin D deficiency in human pregnancy.[27] As with all other lipid-soluble vitamins, an excess of vitamin D causes more problems than a deficiency. Administration of very high quantities of vitamin D to pregnant laboratory animals causes defects in teeth formation and aortic lesions in offspring.[28] Similar lesions have been associated with excessive intake in humans, but without a reliable assay to determine the level of vitamin D, the evidence remains circumstantial. Vitamin D requirement is not increased in pregnancy and the required amount is present in a normal diet. Excessive doses of vitamin D can cause hypercalcemia. This toxicity is thought to be the result of excessive circulating levels of 25-hydroxycholecalciferol vitamin D, which substitutes for 1,25-dihydroxycholecalciferol vitamin D on the receptors. This results in a high rate of calcium transport and bone resorption.[29]

Vitamin E—Tocopherol

The main physiologic effect attributed to vitamin E is that of an antioxidant. The maternal level of vitamin E increases during gestation, reaching a peak at approximately 37 weeks' gestation and declining immediately after birth to the nonpregnant level.[30] The etiology of the increase in vitamin E during pregnancy could be related to an increased demand caused by fetal growth, but it probably reflects the normal hyperlipidemic state associated with pregnancy. The mechanism of vitamin E transport from the maternal to the fetal circulation is not clear, but the serum tocopherol level of cord blood is approximately one third of the maternal level. In animals, vitamin E deficiency is associated with gonadal atrophy, degeneration of the placenta, possible resorption of the embryo, and increased hemolysis of erythrocytes. Studies from Japan have linked vitamin E deficiency in human pregnancy to threatened abortion, premature labor, intrauterine growth retardation, and neonatal hemolytic anemia.[46] The dietary sources of vitamin E are abundant, and supplementation is unnecessary in pregnant women.

Vitamin K

Vitamin K functions as a cofactor in the liver for the production of prothrombin, factors VII, IX, and X. The only clinical implication related to vitamin K during the perinatal period is the fact that premature infants develop deficiency of vitamin K more frequently than term infants. This happens because of decreased tissue stores and impairment of intestinal absorption. Therefore, premature infants are more likely to manifest a coagulation deficit as a sign of vitamin K deficiency. Pregnant patients who are on coumadin therapy, a vitamin K antagonist, during pregnancy are exposed, as are their fetuses, to the hazard of intrauterine hemorrhage. The mechanism for transport of vitamin K across the placenta is not well understood. Studies in rats have suggested a facilitated diffusion pathway. Large doses of vitamin A and E may interfere with the absorption of vitamin K from the gut. The oral ingestion of sulfa drugs and of other oral antibiotics, such as neomycin, also may interfere with vitamin K absorption. Biliary obstruction, malabsorption syndrome, and liver disease all may result in vitamin K deficiency. As with all lipid-soluble vitamins, excessive doses of vitamin K will accumulate in the body and be toxic. The average American diet provides more than adequate amounts of vitamin K, and its routine supplementation in pregnancy is therefore not required. Recently, vitamin K has been experimentally used antenatally to determine if it will prevent intraventicular hemorrhage in the neonate.[44,45]

MINERALS IN PREGNANCY

Growth and development of the fetus *in utero* depends not only on the adequate supply of such nutrients as protein, carbohydrates, lipids, and vitamins, but also on adequate minerals. Essential minerals can be divided into *bulk minerals,* such as calcium, phosphorus, sodium, and potassium and *trace elements,* which are usually present in only very small amounts of living tissue. They can be essential, possibly essential, or nonessential[8] (see also Chapter 22).

Calcium

Calicum metabolism undergoes extensive changes during pregnancy in response to maternal changes and fetoplacental transfer. Many hormones, including human placental lactogen, estrogen, parathyroid hormone, and calcitonin, are involved in the changes in calcium metabolism. The net effect of this interrelated hormonal adjustment is to maintain the maternal calcium level. The total serum calcium level usually declines about 0.6–0.8 mg/100 mL over the course of pregnancy. The decline in calcium involves only the protein-bound fraction, while the free ionic calcium remains relatively constant, probably because of the increase in the parathyroid hormone. The decrease in serum calcium is most probably caused by hypoalbuminemia, with the pattern of change in total serum calcium similar to that of serum albumin.[9] There is an active transport of calcium across the placenta from the maternal to the fetal side, rendering the fetus hypercalcemic relative to the mother. Most of the fetal calcium is accumulated in the third trimester. The calcification of the skeletal system of the fetus starts around 9–10 weeks; at 26 weeks the fetal calcium content is 6 g and reaches 30 g by 40 weeks' gestation.[31] Calcium deficiency in pregnancy is rare. Most cases are caused by hypoparathyroidism. Cases of dietary inadequacy are uncommon. There is no evidence that maternal calcium deficiency or excess results in congenital anomalies. Milk and various dairy products represent the principal source of calcium in the diet. One quart of milk supplies the necessary recommended dietary allowance of 1200 mg/d in pregnancy. A high calcium intake will not cause hypercalcemia; however, megadose vitamin D therapy can result in hypercalcemia.

A series of epidemiologic studies have been published that link relative calcium deficiency to the development of pregnancy-induced hypertension (PIH). These epidemiologic studies demonstrate an inverse relationship between the ingestion of calcium and the incidence of eclampsia–preeclampsia.[32] Taufield et al[33] studied 40 women in the third trimester for an association between calcium and PIH. They found that the serum levels of calcium did not vary in their study population, but patients with PIH had hypocalciuria because of increased renal tubular reabsorption of calcium.[33] Another study, using a prospective double-blind clinical trial, looked at calcium supplementation after 26 weeks' gestation. This study analyzed 52 healthy pregnant women without evidence of either PIH or chronic hypertension. They received either 1.5 g of elemental clacium per day or a placebo. The calcium group had a PIH incidence of 4%, while the placebo group had an incidence of 11%. Because of the small sample size, these numbers were not statistically different, however, there was a significant reduction in diastolic blood pressure in the calcium group compared to the placebo group.[34] One theory to explain this preventive action of calcium is that it is mediated by a decrease in parathyroid hormone in association with high calcium levels. This is thought to cause a decrease in intracellular calcium with resultant vasodilation and decreased blood pressure.[32]

Iron

Iron is an essential component of hemoglobin, which is responsible for carrying oxygen to all organs in the body. Pregnancy is associated with significant physiologic changes that increase the demand for iron; these changes include an increase in blood volume of 40–50%, enhanced erythropoiesis with an increase in erythrocyte volume of 250–400 mL, and bone marrow hyperplasia. An average of 500 mg of elemental iron is needed to accommodate these pregnancy changes of erythropoiesis. The amount of iron present in the fetus and the placenta is additional 200–400 mg. If the amount of iron saved due to the amenorrhea of pregnancy, estimated at 120 mg, is then subtracted, the total iron requirement for pregnancy is about 800 mg.

The American diet supples 10–15 mg of elemental iron daily with only 10–15% of it absorbed. The amount of iron absorbed depends on the body's needs, iron stores, type of food consumed, and amount of iron ingested. Whenever iron deficiency exists, such as in anemia, hypoxia, and pregnancy, the rate of iron absorption increases. Despite the increase in the absorption rate of iron in pregnancy, the dietary source is still inadequate, especially in the presence of predisposing factors for iron deficiency, such as vaginal bleeding, twin gestation, poor dietary habits, and rapid successive pregnancies.

Iron deficiency anemia during pregnancy usually is preventable by furnishing every patient with iron supplements in addition to a well-balanced diet. In some countries, particularly Europe, only patients that are anemic or who are at high risk for iron deficiency are supplemented. All iron preparations are potentially toxic and the ingestion of large doses, especially by children, may lead to severe toxic symptoms and even death.[8,9,15]

Zinc

Zinc is one of the most widely studied trace elements in humans (see also Chapter 22). It has an essential role in protein and nucleic acid metabolism, and it constitutes the metal component of many enzymes that regulate various metabolic pathways. As pregnancy progresses, maternal blood levels of zinc decrease gradually from 80–100 μg/100 mL early in pregnancy, to a nadir of 45–50 μg/100 mL in the early third trimester.[35] This decrease in zinc with increasing gestation age probably does not represent a deficiency. Because this metal binds to albumin, the serum decrease may be caused by the hypoalbuminemia that occurs with gestation, redistribution of zinc between plasma and erythrocytes, or the dilutional effect of the normal increasein plasma volume of pregnancy. Zinc crosses the placenta readily, and by term, the fetal content is 50–60 mg.

In experimental animals, zinc deficiency during pregnancy was found to be associated with congenital anomalies of the skeletal system and soft tissue and with subsequent behavioral and learning disabilities of the surviving offspring.[36] In humans, unsubstantiated reports exist that associate zinc deficiency with several pregnancy complications, including dysmaturity, prolonged labor, atonic uteri, postpartum hemorrhage, premature labor, anemia, and congenital malformations.[37] Other studies have shown significant correlations between maternal zinc level and infant birth weight as well as the risk for fetal alcohol syndrome.[38] Studies on the bactericidal effect of amniotic fluid have shown that a zinc–protein complex may be involved in the inhibitory action of bacterial growth. The source of zinc in the diet is from animal protein, and a diet with normal protein has more than an adequate supply of zinc. Supplementation is not recommended except in the presence of severe malnutrition.

Copper

Copper is needed for hemoglobin synthesis and for other important enzymatic functions (see also Chapter 87). Blood copper levels in the mother increase as pregnancy progresses. About 95% of copper is bound by ceruloplasmin and 5% by albumin. The copper supply to the tissue is from the albumin-bound fraction.[39] The increase in copper level is caused by an increase in ceruloplasmin, which may be due to the endogenous estrogen increase because oral contraceptives are known to have similar effects.[40]

In animals, the offspring of copper-deficient rats were observed to have abnormal brain, hair, and skin development. In humans, low maternal copper levels have been associated with intrauterine fetal death. Water that is deficient in copper has been incriminated as a potential cause of neural tube defects in certain areas of the United Kingdom.[41] The clinical importance of these case reports is unknown. Because severe copper deficiency is rare, supplementation during pregnancy is not recommended.

Chromium

This trace element may have a role in the synthesis of fatty acids and cholesterol. Recently, it has been described to have an essential role in carbohydrate metabolism by increasing the affinity of insulin to cell membrane receptors. Chromium may form a complex with amino acids to form a *glucose tolerance factor*, the structure and function of which is unknown.[42] The lack of a maternal chromium response to glucose load indicates that it may play a role in gestational diabetes mellitus.[43] The average daily requirement of chromium in pregnancy is 10–60 μg. No evidence exists that supplementation in pregnancy is needed (see also Chapter 22).

Iodine

Iodine is the main component needed for the synthesis of thyroid hormone. Iodine deficiency during pregnancy may result in cretinism, especially if the deficiency is severe.[36] The fact that few pregnancies result in cretins, even in endemic areas, indicates that factors other than the severity of iodine deficiency also are important. In the United States, iodized salt is sufficient to provide the necessary amount of iodine.

Manganese

Manganese is the metal component of mitochondrial energy-producing enzyme systems. It also may be needed for the biosynethesis of mucopolysaccharides of the skeletal system. In animals, antenatal manganese deficiency has been associated with postnatal uncoordination, ataxia, and lack of equilibrium. The role of manganese in pregnancy is not well delineated. Manganese deficiency has not been demonstrated in human pregnancy.[8]

Magnesium

Magnesium is one of the most abundant trace elements on earth. Magnesium deficiency has been associated wtih neuromuscular symptoms, cardiac arrthymias, gastrointestinal disorders, alcoholism, and endocrinopathies.[8] No effects of magnesium deficiency on human pregnancy have been demonstrated.

CONCLUSIONS

Deficiencies of a number of different vitamins and trace elements have been associated with various pregnancy complications and abnormal fetal development. However, nearly all of these data are obtained from animal studies, in which the dosages are dissimilar to those used in human pregnancies, or from poorly controlled human studies. Prescribing vitamin and mineral preparations during pregnancy has become standard practice in the United States. This has occurred in spite of the fact that the increased requirements of pregnancy for nearly all of the vitamins and minerals are thought to be supplied by any diet adequate in calories and well balanced in protein, carbohydrates, and lipids. When this type of well-balanced diet is present, little evidence suggests that vitamin supplements are beneficial to maternal or fetal well-being. The *Committee on Maternal Nutrition of the National Research Council* states that prenatal vitamin and mineral preparations generally are not needed, with the major exception of iron supplementation. As noted previously, some evidence supports the supplementation with pyridoxine, folic acid, and calcium. The approach of the National Research Council is the most appropriate to follow until further research can document the need for other vitamin or mineral supplements.

REFERENCES

1. Malone JI. Vitamin passage across the placenta. *Clin Perinatol*. 1975;2:295.
2. Heller S, Salkfeld RM, Korner WF. Vitamin B_1 status in pregnancy. *Am J Clin Nutr*. 1974;27:1221.
3. McCormick DB. Thiamin. In: Shils M, Young V, eds. *Modern Nutrition in Health and Disease*. 7th ed. Philadelphia, PA: Lea and Febiger; 1988:355.
4. Blegen SD. Postpartum congestive heart failure. Beriberi heart disease. *Acta Med Scan*. 1965;178:515.
5. Hytten F, Chamberlain G, eds. *Clinical Physiology in Obstetrics*. 1980:163.
6. Lopez R, Cole HS, Montoya MF, Cooperman J. Riboflavin deficiency in a pediatric population of low socioeconomic status in New York City. *J Ped*. 1975;87:420.

7. Heller S, Salkfeld RM, Korner WF. Riboflavin status in pregnancy. *Am J Clin Nutr.* 1974;27:1225.
8. Moghissi KS. Risks and benefits of nutritional supplements during pregnancy. *Obstet Gynecol.* 1981;58:68S.
9. Pitkin RM. Vitamins and minerals in pregnancy. *Clin Perinatol.* 1975;2:221.
10. McCormick D. Riboflavin. In: Shils M, Young V, eds. *Modern Nutrition in Health and Disease.* 7th ed. Philadelphia, PA: Lea and Febiger; 1988;362.
11. Spellacy WN, Buhi SC, Birk SA. Vitamin B_6 treatment of gestational diabetes mellitus: studies of blood glucose and plasma insulin. *Am J Obstet Gynecol.* 1977;127:599.
12. Newberne PM, Young VR. Marginal vitamin B_{12} intake during gestation in the rat has long term effects on the offspring. *Nature.* 1973;242:263.
13. McCormick D. Vitamin B_6. In: Shils M, Young V, eds. *Modern Nutrition in Health Disease.* 7th ed. Philadelphia, PA: Lea and Febiger; 1988:376.
14. Herbert VD, Colman N. Folic acid and vitamin B_{12}. In: Shils M, Young V, eds. *Modern Nutrition in Health and Disease.* 7th ed. Philadelphia, PA: Lea and Febiger; 1988:400.
15. Pritchard J. Anemias of Pregnancy and Puerperium. In: *Maternal Nutrition and the Course of Pregnancy.* Washington DC: National Academy of Science; 1970:74.
16. Kitay DZ. Folic acid deficiency in pregnancy. *Am J Obstet Gynecol.* 1969;104:1067.
17. Mogan BLG, Winick N. The effects of folic acid supplementation during pregnancy in the rat. *Br J Nutrit.* 1978;40:529.
18. Smithells RW, Shephard S, Schorack CJ, et al. Possible prevention of neural tube defects by peri conceptual vitamin supplementation. *Lancet.* 1980;1:339.
19. Wild J, Read AP, Sheppard S, et al. Recurrent neural tube defects, risk factors and vitamins. *Arch Dis Child.* 1986;61:440.
20. Mulinare J, Cordero JF, Erickson JD, Berry RJ. Periconceptional use of multivitamins and the occurrence of neural tube defects. *JAMA.* 1988;260(21):3141.
21. Mills JL, Rhoads G, Simpson JL, et al. The absence of a relation between the periconceptional use of vitamins and neural tube defects. *N Engl J Med.* 1989;321(7):430.
22. Wald NJ, Plani PE. Neural-tube defects and vitamins: the need for a randomized clinical trial. *Br J Obstet Gynecol.* 1984;91:516.
23. Bernhardt JB, Dorsey DJ. Hypervitaminosis A and congenital renal anomalies in a human infant. *Obstet Gynecol.* 1974;43:750.
24. Lammer EJ. Retinoic Acid Teratogenicity, Human Teratogens. May 8–10, 1989.
25. Lammer EJ, Chen DT, Hoar RM, et al. Retinoic Acid Embryopathy. *N Engl J Med.* 1985;313:827.
26. Rosen JJ, Roginsky M, Natheson G, Finberg L. 25, hydroxyvitamin D plasma levels in mothers and their premature infants with neonatal hypocalcemia. *Am J Dis Child.* 1974;127:220.
27. Roberts SA, Cohen MD, Farfar JO. Antenatal factors associated with neonatal hypocalcemia convulsions. *Lancet.* 1973;2:809.
28. Friedman WF, Mills LF. The relationship between vitamin D and the craniofacial and dental anomalies of the supravalvular aortic stenosis syndrome. *Pediatrics.* 1969;43:12.
29. DeLuca HF. Vitamin D and its metabolites. In: Shils M, Young V, eds. *Modern Nutrition in Health and Disease.* 7th ed. Philadelphia, PA: Lea and Febiger; 1988:313.
30. Mino N, Nishimo H. Fetal and maternal relationship in serum vitamin E level. *J Nutr Sci Vitaminol.* 1973;19:475.
31. Widdowson EM. Changes in body proportions and composition during growth. In: David JA, Dobbings J, eds. *Scientific Foundation of Pediatrics.* Philadelphia, PA: WB Saunders; 1974:153.
32. Belizan JM, Villar J, Repke J. The relationship between calcium intake and pregnancy-inducted hypertension: up-to-date evidence. *Am J Obstet Gynecol.* 1988;158:898.
33. Taufield PA, Ales DL, Resnick LM, et al. Hypocalciuria in preeclampsia. *N Engl J Med.* 1987;316:715.
34. Villar J, Repke J, Belizan JM, Pareja G. Calicum supplementation reduced blood pressure during pregnancy: results of a randomized controlled clinical trial. *Obstet Gynecol.* 1987;70:317.
35. Metcoff J. Maternal nutrition and fetal growth. In: McLaren DS, Burnam D, eds. *Textbook of Pediatric Nutrition.* 2nd ed. London: Churchill Livingstone; 1982:18.
36. Hurley LS. Perinatal effects of trace element deficiencies. In: Prasad AS, ed. *Trace Elements in Human Health and Disease.* New York, NY: Academic Press; 1976;2:301.
37. Jameson S. Variations in maternal serum zinc during pregnancy and correlation to congenital malformation, dysmaturity and abnormal parturition. *Acta Med Scand.* 1976; (suppl) 21:593.
38. Flynn A, Miller SI, Martier SS, et al. Zinc status of pregnant alcoholic women: a determinant of fetal outcome. *Lancet.* 1981;1:572.
39. Fattah NMA, Ibrahim FK, Ramadan MA, Samnour MB. Ceruloplasmin and copper level in maternal cord blood and in the placenta in normal pregnancy and in pre-eclampsia. *Acta Obstet Gynecol Scand.* 1976;55:383.
40. Prasad AS, Oberleas D, Lei KY, et al. Effect of oral contraceptive agents on nutrients. I. Minerals. *Am J Clin Nutr.* 1975;28:377.
41. Morton MS, Elwood PC, Abernathy M. Trace elements in water and congenital malformation of central nervous system in South Wales. *Br J Prev Soc Med.* 1976;30:36.
42. Mertz W. Chromium and its relation to carbohydrate metabolism. *Med Clin North Am.* 1976;60:739.
43. Davison JM, Burt RL. Physiologic changes in plasma chromium of normal and pregnant women: effect on glucose load. *Am J Obstet Gynecol.* 1973;116:601.
44. Kazzi NJ, Ilagan NB, Liang K-C, et al. Maternal Administration of vitamin K does not improve coagulation profile of preterm infants. *Pediatrics.* (In press).
45. Kazzi NJ, Ilagan NB, Liang K-C, et al. Transfer of vitamin K-1 across the placental barrier in preterm pregnancies. *Am J Obstet Gynecol.* (In press).
46. Tateno M, Ohshima A. The relationship between serum vitamin and levels in the perinatal period and the birth weight of the neonate. *Acta Obstet Gynecol Jap.* 1972;20:177.

Chapter Twenty
Normal Fetal Growth

Thomas L. Gross and Honor M. Wolfe

20

Fetal growth involves the maternal–placental–fetal unit. Normal fetal growth is the result of a complex interaction of function among these three components. The maternal factor that is most frequently related to fetal growth and is of most interest to clinicians is the nutritional status of the mother. Before understanding how abnormal maternal nutrition can affect fetal growth, information regarding normal fetal growth and development is necessary. This includes the effects of maternal prepregnancy weight and pregnancy weight gain on birth weight; the components of maternal and fetal weight gain, including the prominent role that the storage of fat plays in both; and an understanding of how the recommended number of extra calories and protein needed during pregnancy was derived. Finally, a review of the relationship between carbohydrate, lipid, and protein metabolism and normal fetal growth is important before a discussion concerning abnormal maternal nutrition.

No mention of the average birth weight is recorded in early biblical, Greek, Roman, or Arabic writings; however, historically birth weight has been the only outcome variable used to assess fetal growth and development. The earliest known record of average birth weight was 14 to 15 lb in the textbook by Mauriceau. It is unknown what confusion led to this early estimate, but other early writers recorded similar high birth weights.

OUTCOME VARIABLES

Birth weight alone was the variable used to assess the adequacy of fetal growth in the past, and gestational age and birth weight percentile were not considered. Babies weighing less than 2500 g were defined as *premature*; those weighing more than 2500 g were *mature*. Many of the early studies of maternal nutrition, including all of the findings in the Collaborative Perinatal Project, used this definition. In order to more accurately describe fetal growth and maturity, newborns are now classified soon after birth according to their birth weight, gestational age, and birth-weight percentile.

Birth Weight

Babies weighing less than 2500 g at delivery are referred to as low birth weight. However, these babies are now divided into one of two groups—premature or small-for-gestational-age (SGA)—based on the definitions listed below. One other definition based on birth weight is that of *macrosomia*. The term macrosomic is used to describe neonates with a birth weight of more than 4000 g with some authors using greater than 4500 g.

Gestational Age

Obstetric. The obstetric estimate of gestational age is generally based on the mother's last menstrual period. The interval from the first day of the last period to the estimated date of confinement is 280 days. Often the date of the last menstrual period is inaccurate. Other factors also are used, including uterine size in the first trimester (most accurate at 6 to 10 weeks' gestation), maternal perception of fetal quickening (normally occurs at 16 to 18 weeks), and first unamplified fetal heart tones (usually heard at 18 to 20 weeks). The definitions used are preterm, less than 38 weeks; term, 38 to 42 weeks; and postterm, more than 42 weeks' gestation.

Pediatric. The estimate of gestational age can be determined accurately by assessing groups of physical and neurologic characteristics of the newborn. Many pediatricians have devised newborn examinations for this purpose, but the American Academy of Pediatrics has recommended using the Ballard modification of the Dubowitz examination.[2] Based on the numerical score achieved on the neuromuscular and physical examination, the neonate is assigned a gestational age. This can be of great value if obstetric dating is not available. However, the pediatric estimate has limitations in the very premature, the asphyxiated, and the heavily sedated neonate.

Birth-Weight Percentile

By comparing the pediatric estimate of gestational age to the birth weight, the rate of intrauterine growth can be approximated. This results in dividing the entire population into three groups: below the 10th percentile for gestational age, small for gestational age (SGA); between the 10th and 90th percentiles, appropriate for gestational age (AGA); and above the 90th percentile, large for gestational age (LGA). Each of the birth weight percentile groups can be further divided into preterm, term, and post-term, based on their gestational age.

All of the definitions are important for assessing neonatal outcome. The most significant factor contributing to neonatal morbidity and mortality is premature birth. However, both of the extremes in the gestational age category (preterm and post-term) and both extremes in the birth-weight percentile groups (SGA and LGA) have increased perinatal risk to varying degrees.

FETAL GROWTH CURVE AND COMPOSITION

Fetal Growth Curve

Singleton Gestation. Figure 20–1 from the monograph by Hytten and Leitch[1] contrasts the average curve of fetal and placental growth and change in amniotic fluid volume; in late gestation, growth in the fetus slows, placental growth nearly stops, and the volume of amniotic fluid declines. During the first half of pregnancy, there is strong agreement that the average fetal weight is about 5 g at 10 weeks and 300 g at 20 weeks. Intrauterine growth in the human follows a linear pattern between 28 and 38 weeks.[3] Beyond 38 weeks, there is probably a reduction in growth rate caused by a physiologic uteroplacental insufficiency. However, the neonatal growth then accelerates to the rapid growth rate seen *in utero* before 38 weeks. One explanation for this late slowing in growth is that there is a normal decline in the supply of nutrients shunted transplacentally in late pregnancy, resulting in an expected slowing of growth. This is supported by the fact that the curve for the average placental weight also plateaus late in pregnancy. However, whether this late slowing of fetal growth is a real finding in the individual pregnancy must be evaluated cautiously. It is well known that the fetus may continue rapid growth beyond term and that one of the strongest risks for a macrosomic neonate (more than 4000 g) is a pregnancy that extends beyond the estimated date of confinement. The findings in Figure 20–1 are not longitudinal studies in which fetal growth is followed serially throughout pregnancy; instead, the findings are based on a large number of pregnancies delivered at varying gestational ages and including high-risk mothers. Each pregnancy represents one point on the regression line. Stembera studied a country-wide population of patients and attempted to examine only those fetuses growing normally. The late slowing of the growth curve was not seen in this group of fetuses.[4] Longitudinal studies in which multiple ultrasound parameters are used

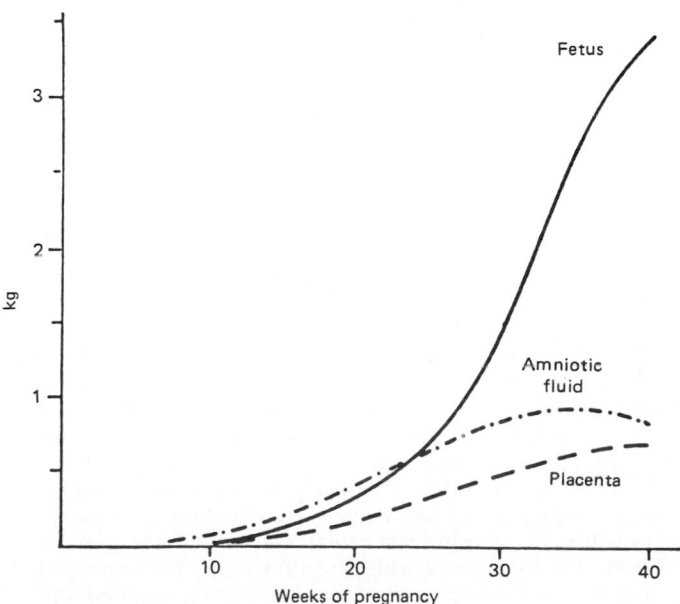

FIGURE 20–1. The growth curve of the human fetus with increasing gestational age compared to that of the placenta and the change in volume of amniotic fluid. (*From Hytten and Leitch*[1] *with permission.*)

to estimate serially fetal growth may be able to answer this question.

Multiple Gestation. Early studies have shown that as the number of fetuses increases there is increasing deviation from the usual singleton growth curve.[5] Birth weights in twins are similar to singleton pregnancies until approximately 30 weeks' gestation. Beyond this stage in pregnancy, the twins' mean birth weights are statistically less.[6] As the number of fetuses increases, including triplets and quadruplets, the increase in the growth curve slows earlier in gestation.[5]

Studies are now available that follow intrauterine growth of twins by ultrasound. Fetal measurements by ultrasound, which include individual measurements such as biparietal diameter, often correlate poorly with birth weight. Because of this, earlier fetal studies do not always agree with the birth weight studies.[7]

Recent ultrasound studies in which multiple fetal parameters (including fetal head, femur, and abdominal circumference) are measured suggest that twins without other complications grow at rates similar to singletons in the second trimester.[8] Studies of twin growth in the third trimester are more confusing. In cross-sectional studies, mean growth curves of a series of twins fall progressively below the lines of singletons.[9] However, in nearly half of the patients studied by individual growth curves and cross-sectional curves, both twins grew normally. This suggests that twins need to be assessed individually and that the cross-sectional studies may be misleading.[8,9]

Twins usually grow at similar rates, with the mean difference in birth weight approximately 11%.[10] The ultrasound assessment of fetal growth in multiple gestation is an important method of assessing fetal development and welfare. This is beyond the scope of this chapter, but it is addressed in detail elsewhere.[10]

Longitudinal studies of fetal growth using multiple anatomic parameters are now available.[11,12] Ultrasound can be used to diagnose intrauterine growth retardation, which is described in detail elsewhere.[13] For the future, growth models will likely be used to characterize prenatal growth with each fetus acting as its own control.[14]

Fetal Composition of Fat and Protein

The data in the literature regarding fetal composition of fat and protein have been summarized by Hytten and Leitch.[1] The data are a combination of normal abortus material and fetuses from abnormal pregnancies. Beyond 20 weeks' gestation, all of the newborns that were examined died either *in utero* or in the immediate neonatal period, so they can be considered only an approximation of fetal composition. However, data from macerated fetuses and severe congenital abnormalities were excluded.

Fat. The fetal fat and water content varies markedly with advancing gestation. Figure 20–2 shows the fetal water and fat content plotted against total fetal weight. The water content falls from a mean of 94% in the first-trimester fetus to approximately 70% at term. Up to 500 g fetal weight, the percent of body fat is relatively constant at approximately 0.5–1%. Beyond 500 g total fetal weight, the percent of body lipid increases with gestational age; the increased deposition of fat is extremely rapid as term is reached and even beyond. Below 500 g, the fetal lipid is presumed to be primarily structural, but late in pregnancy the rapid increase in lipid content is primarily deposited in the subcutaneous tissue. The amount of depot fat is highly variable; it is likely that some of this variability can be explained by maternal obesity, pregnancy duration, and dietary intake. Obese mothers deliver infants who have increased depot fat. On the other hand, the growth-retarded fetus loses subcutaneous fat first. The deposition of subcutaneous fat in the fetus is a normal phenomenon that occurs with increasing gestational age. Pregnancy prolonged beyond 40 weeks often is associated with increased fetal fat, and, again, one of the most common causes of fetal macrosomia is a post-term pregnancy.

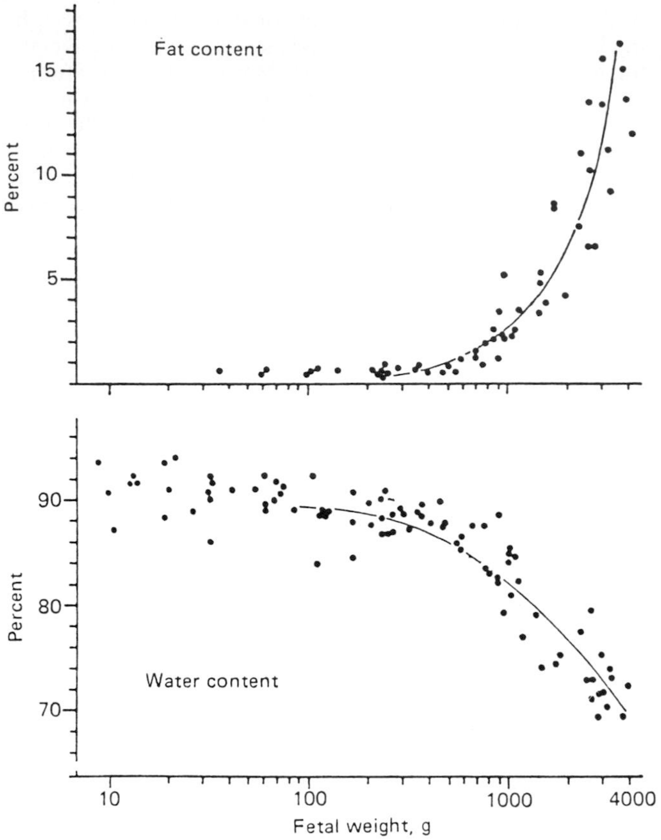

FIGURE 20–2. The fat and water content of the fetus plotted as percent of the total fetal weight, shown for range of total fetal weights from 10 to 4000 g. (*From Hytten and Leich[1] with permission.*)

Protein. The deposition of fetal protein increases rapidly as pregnancy progresses. Figure 20–3 shows the total mass of fetal nitrogen plotted against total fetal weight. In fetuses weighing more than 500 g, the regression line for protein has a sigmoid shape. The decrease in nitrogen content that occurs when a fetal weight of approximately 3000 g is reached is believed to be secondary to the rapidly increasing proportion of body fat. When the fetal nitrogen content is expressed as a percentage of total fetal fat-free weight, there is a slow increase throughout pregnancy from 1% in early pregnancy to 2.5% at term. Based on these studies, it appears that near term, the deposition of fetal body fat far exceeds the increase in nitrogen content.

DETERMINANTS OF FETAL GROWTH

Maternal Prepregnancy Weight and Pregnancy Weight Gain

Virtually all major studies have found that a positive association exists between prepregnancy maternal weight and ma-

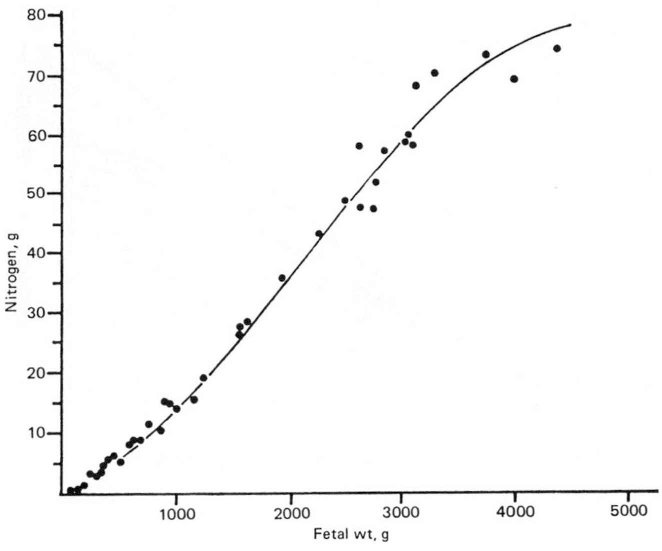

FIGURE 20–3. Nitrogen content of the fetus plotted in total grams and shown for range of total fetal weight from 10 to 4000 g. (*From Hytten and Leich[1] with permission.*)

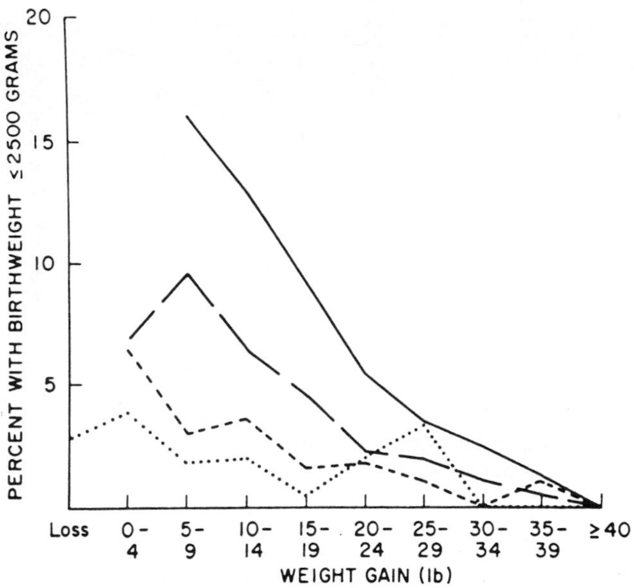

FIGURE 20–5. Association of both the prepregnancy weight of the mother and the maternal weight gain during pregnancy with the percent of low-birth-weight offspring (≤2500 g). (*From Niswander et al[15], with permission.*) Prepregnant weights are indicated by plotted lines. (——) ≤109, (— —) 110–129, (------) 130–149, (. . . .) ≥150.

ternal weight gain during pregnancy and birth weight of the offspring (Figs. 20–4, 20–5).[15] Both increasing prepregnancy weight of the mother and maternal weight gain during pregnancy are associated with higher mean birth weight (Fig. 20–4) and fewer low-birth-weight infants (see Fig. 20–5). Studies from the Collaborative Perinatal Project indicate that of 30 maternal variables examined, prepregnancy weight gain and maternal pregnancy weight were the strongest factors affecting birth weight.[2] Figures 20–4 and 20–5 show the influence of prepregnancy weight and weight gain during pregnancy on mean birth weight in term pregnancies. The data shown are for black patients only, although similar associations were seen when white patients were examined separately. Although weight gain during pregnancy is usually more important as a determinant of birth weight than maternal prepregnancy weight (as shown in Figs. 20–4 and 20–5), the association between pregnancy weight gain and birth weight changes as the maternal prepregnancy weight increases. The increasing maternal weight gain during pregnancy has the strongest effect on increasing birth weight in the lower weight mothers, but this effect is nearly lost in mothers weighing 190 lb or more. These findings are present even when diabetic mothers are excluded.

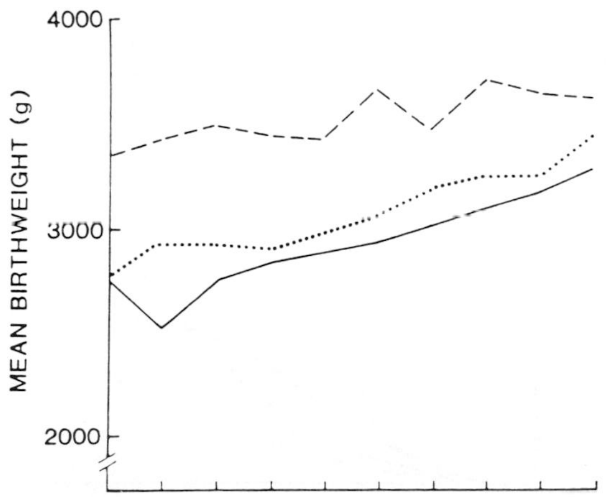

FIGURE 20–4. Association of both the prepregnancy weight of the mother and maternal weight gain during pregnancy with mean birth weight. (*From Niswander et al[15], with permission.*) Prepregnant weights are indicated by plotted lines. (———) ≤109 lb, (. . . .) 130–149 lb, and (------) ≥190 lb.

Other Variables Affecting Fetal Growth

Multiple variables influence fetal growth. By far, the strongest variable affecting growth of the fetus is increasing gestational age. The effect of maternal prepregnancy weight and weight gain during pregnancy has been described. Other important variables that have an impact on fetal growth are maternal medical and obstetric complications, parity, ethnic background, social class, and altitude. Many of the maternal variables may be interrelated. For example, it is known that when maternal prepregnancy weight is introduced into a multiple-regression model, it can replace both maternal age and parity as significantly affecting birth weight. This suggests that the increasing maternal age and parity may be associated significantly with increasing birth weight because older and more parous mothers tend to have progressively increasing body weight. Similar interactions have been suggested between maternal social class, ethnic background, height, and body weight.

OPTIMAL WEIGHT GAIN IN PREGNANCY

Maternal pregnancy weight gain associated with optimal fetal growth has been the subject of endless controversy. Early in the 19th century, maternal dietary restriction was used to retard fetal growth in an effort to reduce cephalopelvic disproportion. For much of the first half of the 20th

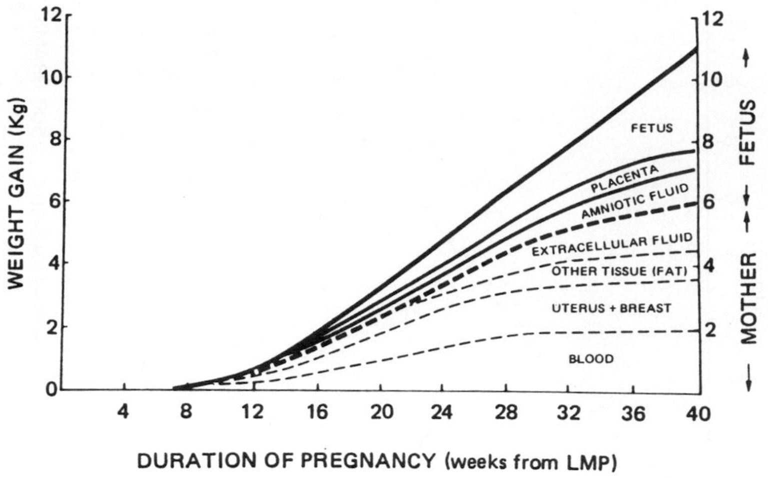

FIGURE 20–6. The pattern of growth and components of maternal weight gain with increasing gestational age. (*From Pitkin[16], with permission.*)

century, obstetricians restricted maternal weight gain in an attempt to prevent toxemia. Of course, this is no longer appropriate, and the emphasis has shifted to choosing maternal weight gain associated with the best fetal outcome. The optimal amount of maternal weight gain is still unclear in pregnancies complicated by obesity or malnutrition because of the lack of follow-up studies in these populations. However, guidelines can be followed in the normal patient.

Average Weight Gain in Normal Pregnancy

The healthy pregnant woman eating with no restrictions on her diet gains an average of 24–28 lb (11–12.5 kg) body weight during pregnancy. The pattern in which the weight is gained during pregnancy also is important. Minimal gain is expected in the first trimester, and an average gain of 0.4 kg (0.8 lb) per week throughout the second and third trimesters is the general rule. A maternal weight gain of 24–28 lb is not based on pregnancy outcome but is the average gain during pregnancy in a large group of normal women. There is a tremendously wide scatter of maternal weight gain that can be associated with normal fetal growth and outcome. In addition to the average maternal weight gain, there are some additional data, including the analysis of the individual components of weight gain and the theoretical calculations of increased caloric requirements of pregnancy, that can help to define the optimal weight gain or to approximate the number of additional calories needed throughout the pregnancy.

Individual Components of Weight Gain

At term, the weight of the individual components of mother and fetus that are absolutely necessary in a normal pregnancy comprise approximately 9 kg.[16] These include fetus (3.5 kg), placenta (0.5 kg), amniotic fluid (1 kg), extracellular fluid (1.5 kg), uterine and breast hypertrophy (1.5 kg), and increased blood volume (1.5 kg) (Fig. 20–6). The balance, approximately 2.5–3.5 kg, is likely maternal adipose tissue. The patterns in which these components are deposited are quite different between the fetal compartment (fetus, placenta, and amniotic fluid) and the maternal compartment (extracellular fluid and tissue, including fat, uterus, breast, and blood). The fetal components start to grow very slowly, comprising a small amount of pregnancy weight gain during the first 16 weeks of gestation. By late in the second trimester, fetal growth has reached its maximum and remains until late in pregnancy. Growth of maternal components vary; some tissue growth is maximum during the first two trimesters but slows dramatically by the beginning of the last trimester, but other maternal components continue to increase throughout gestation. The maternal intravascular volume reaches a maximum by early in the third trimester, but extravascular fluids continue to increase until the end of pregnancy. Maternal subcutaneous fat deposition is the component of weight gain that shows the most dramatic difference compared to fetal growth.

Changes in Maternal Fat Stores

The pattern of accumulation of maternal adipose tissue differs from that of other components—deposition of fat begins in early pregnancy, shows maximum gain in midpregnancy, and almost stops by early in the last trimester (Fig. 20–7).[1] This pattern, described by Hytten and Leitch[1], was based on autopsy data later confirmed by caliper measurements of skinfold thickness in the pregnant patient (Fig. 20–8). Measurement of skinfold thickness at multiple sites—thigh, suprailiac, subscapular, biceps, and triceps—can provide a useful index of total body fat. As shown in Figure 20–8, increased maternal fat during pregnancy is distributed primarily over the lower back, hips, and upper thighs. Be-

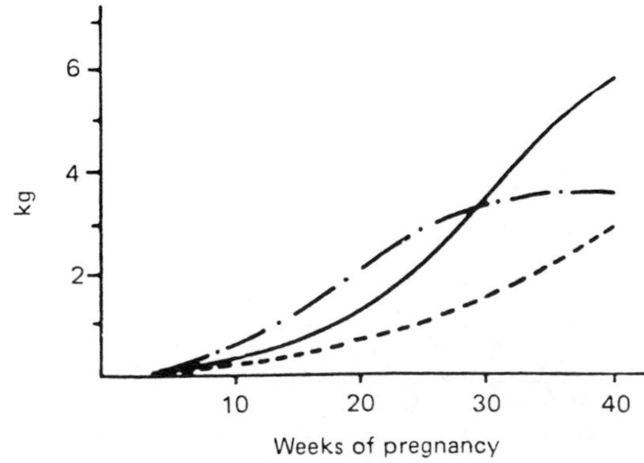

FIGURE 20–7. The pattern of increased growth with gestational age plotted in three categories—uterus and contents, (——), maternal body fluids (------), and maternal stores (adipose tissue) (–.–.–). Data from mothers with no edema or leg edema only. (*From Hytten and Leitch[1], with permission.*)

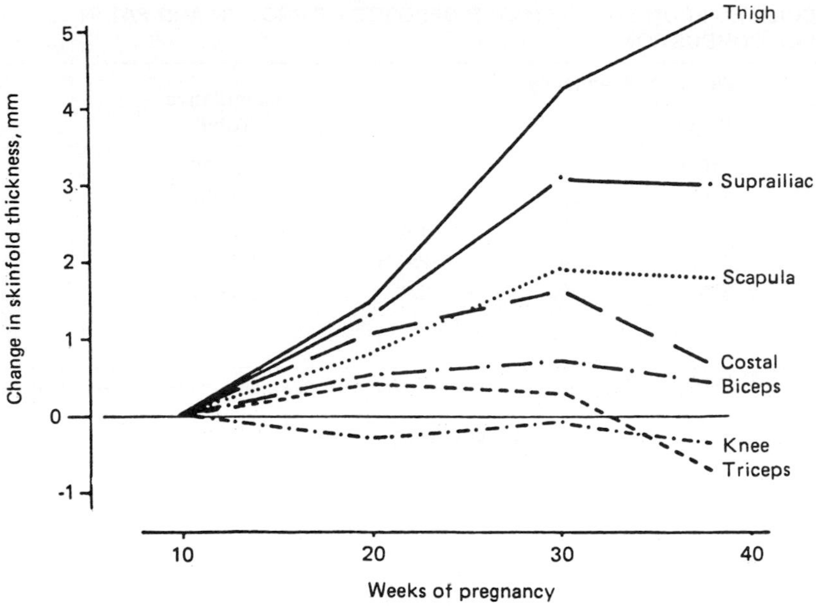

FIGURE 20–8. Increase in maternal skinfold thickness measured with calipers at seven sites during pregnancy. No increase occurred beyond 30 weeks except for small change in maternal thigh. *(From Hytten and Leitch[1] with permission.)*

cause of this accumulation of depot fat by midgestation, the normal patient enters the third trimester of pregnancy with significant energy stores, which may be used during the last months of pregnancy when nutritional needs of the fetus are at their maximum.

Caloric Requirement During Pregnancy

An additional 75,000 kcal are required during a normal human pregnancy. It is important to evaluate how this value was determined to understand how much of an estimate it represents. First, the theoretical estimates of protein and fat gained during pregnancy were calculated. Table 20–1, taken from Hytten and Leitch[1], shows the estimates of mean daily increments of protein and fat deposited in maternal and fetal tissue from the four quarters of pregnancy. This estimated increased tissue formation was converted to its net energy equivalent based on the heat of combustion, as shown in Table 20–2. The net energy cost of maintaining the fetus and extra maternal tissue was calculated from studies measuring the oxygen consumption of pregnancy patients. Because the efficiency for converting total net energy to metabolizable energy is not known, a figure of 10% was used as a reasonable estimate, and this was added to the total. Of the 75,000 kcal calculated to be required during pregnancy (cumulative energy cost of pregnancy), nearly 50% is accumulated as fat stores in the mother and fetus. If the increased need for calories was evenly divided over a 280-day gestation (which it is not), this would amount to an increased need of 270 kcal/d. This is then rounded off to 300 kcal/d, which is the usual clinical recommendation for increased kilocalories need during pregnancy.

Other investigators have used respiratory calorimetry to calculate the net energy cost of maintaining the fetus and additional maternal tissue and have estimated 27,000 kcal to be necessary for the entire pregnancy.[17] Because these more recent studies did not include estimates of kilocalories for stored fat and protein, the 27,000-kcal value is actually similar to that calculated by Hytten and Leitch.

In addition to the energy needs of pregnancy for adding maternal and fetal tissue and increased needs of maternal metabolism, the potential exists for an increased workload associated with a heavier body during pregnancy. It also has been hypothesized that the additional energy requirement during pregnancy may be compensated completely or in part by reduced physical activity in pregnant patients; however, there are no data to document this.

CARBOHYDRATE METABOLISM IN PREGNANCY

Pregnancy is associated with profound changes in carbohydrate metabolism. A detailed description of these changes is presented in Chapters 4 and 43. In this section, changes in carbohydrate metabolism that occur in the normal pregnancy and that have been directly related to fetal growth and development are highlighted:

TABLE 20–1. INCREMENTS OF PROTEIN AND FAT IN FETAL AND MATERNAL BODY AS MEAN DAILY INCREMENT FOR EACH QUARTER OF PREGNANCY AND THE CUMULATIVE TOTAL FOR THE ENTIRE PREGNANCY

	Weeks of Pregnancy				Cumulative Total
	0–10[a]	10–20	20–30	30–40	
Protein (g)	0.64	1.84	4.76	6.1	925
Fat (g)	5.85	24.80	21.85	3.3	3825

[a] For the first 10-week period, the total increment is divided by 56 since pregnancy is dated from the last menstrual period.

From Hytten and Leitch[1] with permission.

TABLE 20–2. ENERGY COST OF PREGNANCY CALCULATED FROM THE ESTIMATED DEPOSITS OF PROTEIN AND FAT IN MATERNAL AND FETAL TISSUE AND THEIR HEATS OF COMBUSTION[a]

	Weeks of Pregnancy				Cumulative
	0–10[b]	10–20	20–30	30–40	Total[c]
Protein	3.6	10.3	26.7	34.2	5,180
Fat	55.6	235.6	207.6	31.3	36,337
Oxygen consumption	19.9	62.0	110.9	186.1	26,244
Total net energy	79.1	307.9	345.2	251.6	67,761
Metabolizable energy (total net energy + 10%)	87	339	380	277	74,537

[a] Energy cost of maintaining the fetus and additional maternal tissue is derived from an RQ of 0.90, shown as mean daily equivalents of energy in kcal for each quarter of pregnancy and a cumulative total for the entire pregnancy.

[b] For the first 10-week period, total increment is divided by 56 since pregnancy is dated from the last menstrual period.

[c] Taken as 5.6 kcal/g for protein and 9.5 kcal/g for fat.

From Hytten and Leitch[1] with permission.

1. A combination of maternal fasting hypoglycemia and ketonuria occurs in the normal pregnancy.
2. Glucose is the major source of calories for energy for the fetus.
3. Fetal insulin plays a central role in fetal growth.
4. Both an excess and deficiency of glucose may have marked effects on fetal growth, so the changes in the maternal serum glucose and insulin response can be examined in the context of how they promote the supply of glucose for the placenta and fetus.

Maternal Changes in Pregnancy

During pregnancy, the combination of fasting hypoglycemia and glucose intolerance develop with advancing gestation. As early as the 15th week of gestation, maternal fasting levels of plasma glucose are 15–20 mg/100 mL lower than the prepregnancy levels.[18] This decrease in glucose after a fast results in lower levels of serum insulin. These changes can result in increased starvation ketosis, and blood levels of β-hydroxybutyric acid and acetoacetic acid are two to four times higher after an overnight fast in the pregnant patient. This combination of changes during pregnancy has been referred to as *accelerated starvation.*

The maternal metabolic response to feeding in pregnancy is characterized by hyperglycemia and hyperinsulinism. Figure 20–9 illustrates the effect of pregnancy on the response of plasma glucose and immunoreactive insulin to 100 g of glucose ingested orally after a 14-hour overnight fast.[18] The increased response of plasma glucose and insulin to orally administered glucose progressively increases throughout pregnancy and is most marked during the third trimester. A rise in glucagon also occurs. Accompanying the increased insulin levels is an associated hyperplasia of the β cells of the maternal pancreas. This hyperglycemia after an oral or intravenous carbohydrate load during pregnancy, accompanied by an increase in insulin that occurs in normal pregnancy, has resulted in pregnancy being referred to as a *diabetogenic state.*

The combination of a maternal tendency toward fasting hypoglycemia and elevated postprandial glucose can be explained only by referring to a combination of factors involving the maternal–placental–fetal unit. The maternal fasting hypoglycemia is the result of the continual drain of glucose from mother to fetus. Various maternal tissues (adipose, muscle, and liver) and less sensitive to insulin as pregnancy progresses, and the postprandial maternal hyperglycemia is presumed to be related to this insulin resistance. Recent studies in animals have attempted to quantify the insulin resistance by measuring the response of the plasma insulin to a fixed degree of hyperglycemia. These studies suggest that tissue sensitivity to insulin is reduced by as much as 80% in normal human pregnancy.[19]

Insulinases have been found in placental preparations, and in the past, these enzymes had been postulated as a cause of maternal hyperglycemia. However, this is no longer considered a mechanism for glucose changes in pregnancy because the rate of degradation of radiolabeled insulin *in vivo* does not appear to differ between pregnant and nonpregnant patients. The factors that are most often credited with the insulin resistance of pregnancy are placental hormones, mostly found in the protein hormone, human placental lactogen and the steroid hormones, progesterone and estrogen. All three hormones can be detected in the human trophoblast as early as the third to the seventh week of gestation, and placental production of each increases progressively throughout pregnancy.

Although evidence suggests that each of the three hormones—human placental lactogen, estrogen, and progesterone—can contribute to the insulin resistance of pregnancy, evidence does not support any of them individually causing the changes seen with advancing gestation. The mechanism by which insulin resistance occurs is unknown. An increase in insulin-binding by erythrocytes, hepatocytes, and adipocytes in human and animal pregnancies has been demonstrated in many studies. However, Jarrett has recently shown that in adipocytes from term human pregnancies, the prolactin hormone decreased insulin-binding and the hormone relaxin increased insulin binding.[20] This finding suggests that the hormone prolactin can interact with its own receptor to alter the affinity of another receptor for insulin. The increased insulin resistance in pregnancy could be the result of a combination of changes in several hormones, but research examining the interaction between hormones is just beginning.

Fetal Glucose Supply

Although other substrates cross the placenta (Fig. 20–10), glucose is considered the major source of calories for fetal energy and growth. Because the uteroplacental glucose transfer is greater than is accountable by diffusion alone, it is described as carrier mediated or facilitated; however,

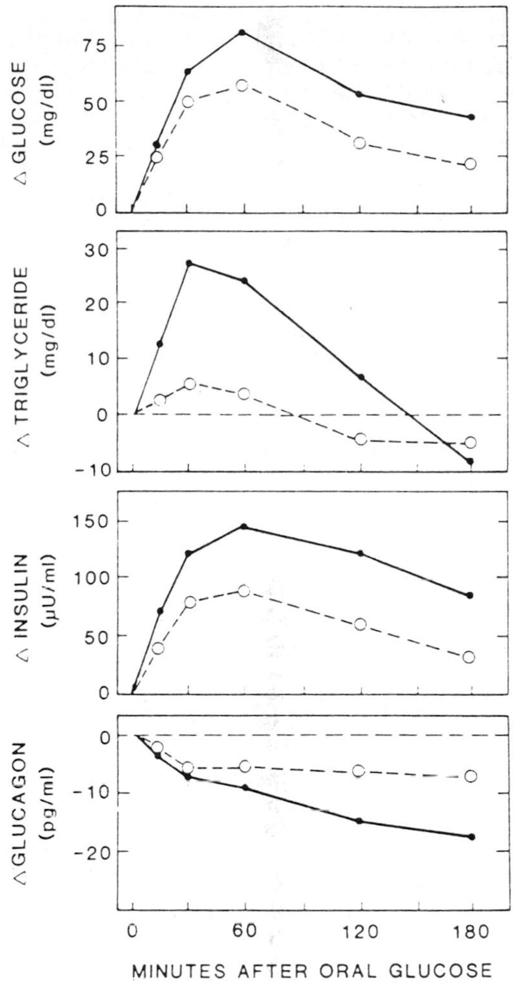

FIGURE 20–9. The effect of pregnancy on the response of plasma, glucose, triglyceride, immunoreactive insulin, and glucagon to a 100-g oral glucose load. Results are shown as the change from basal concentrations. (●) 20–40 weeks pregnant, (○) 5–8 weeks postpartum. In pregnancy, the administration of oral glucose results in increased levels of glucose, triglyceride, and insulin and a greater suppression of glucagon. (*From Freinkel*[18] *with permission.*)

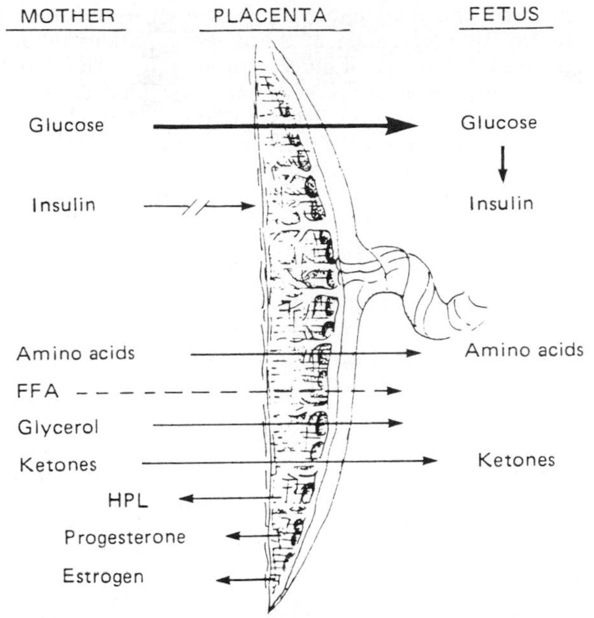

FIGURE 20–10. Maternal–fetal transfer of fuels and placental production of hormones. Glucose, amino acids, glycerol, and ketones are transferred from mother to fetus. Free fatty acids are transferred to a limited extent. Insulin is not transferred, and insulin present in the fetus is produced by the fetal pancreas. Placental hormones, including human placental lactogen, estrogen, and progesterone have known effects on maternal carbohydrate metabolism.

this is not an established fact. Oakley et al examined the maternal–fetal difference in plasma glucose levels in humans during normal and hyperglycemic states.[21] Fetal scalp capillary blood was obtained after rupture of membranes in normal patients. These studies showed that when the maternal plasma glucose was within the physiologic range, the maternal level is a mean of 20 mg/100 mL higher than the fetal level. When the maternal plasma glucose was raised well above the physiologic range, the fetal level rose significantly but plateaued at a level far below the maternal level; the usual 20 mg/100 mL difference between maternal and fetal plasma was not present. This suggests that there is an upper limit of maternal plasma glucose beyond which increased maternal hyperglycemia does not affect fetal glucose. This supports the hypothesis that a facilitated diffusion system is operating and that it is saturated at a particular level of maternal glucose.

The mechanisms regulating the placental transfer of glucose are not completely understood. The effect of insulin in stimulating placental transport of glucose has been studied in pregnant sheep. Marked elevations in maternal insulin are produced artificially, while maintaining glucose levels constant by a glucose clamp technique.[22] Glucose levels in the mother and fetus were not altered, suggesting that insulin plays little role in stimulating the uteroplacental uptake of glucose. Another factor that can affect placental transport of some substances directly is uterine blood flow. In animal studies, decreased uterine blood flow does not decrease placental transport of glucose until a blood flow less than 50% of normal is reached. Thus, in the usual range of uterine blood flow that could be anticipated clinically, even in pathologic conditions, other variables must be affecting the changes in placental glucose transfer.

The primary factor regulating the placental transfer of glucose appears to be the maternal plasma glucose concentration. Hay et al[23] studied glucose uptake in the three compartments—maternal–nonuterine, uteroplacental, and fetal—in a chronic preparation of pregnant sheep. The glucose uptake in each of these areas was directly related to the maternal plasma glucose level. In addition, the percentage of glucose distributed among the three compartments did not differ between normoglycemic and hypoglycemic sheep. Thus, in this animal model, maternal plasma glucose level was the primary factor that determined the delivery of glucose to the fetus, and there was no evidence that glucose was provided preferentially to the conceptus at low maternal glucose levels.

Fetal Insulin—A Growth Hormone

Insulin has been called the fetal growth hormone. This is based primarily on the observation that insulin levels are high in the umbilical cord of macrosomic infants of diabetic mothers. Insulin does not cross the placenta in any significant amount, so fetal insulin levels depend entirely on production by the fetal pancreas. It is well established that maternal hyperglycemia in the diabetic patient results in an increased delivery of glucose to the fetus. The resulting fetal hyperglycemia then stimulates the fetal pancreas to secrete increased insulin. The resulting fetal hyperglycemia and associated hyperinsulinemia are considered responsible for the excess growth seen in certain diabetic patients.

The importance of fetal hyperinsulinemia and hyperglycemia as a major mechanism in excessive fetal growth in diabetic pregnancies is well documented. Elevated umbilical cord insulin levels also have been reported in nondiabetic LGA infants and decreased insulin levels reported in SGA infants.[24] The questions of whether increased glucose supply to the fetus with subsequent hyperinsulinemia as associated with fetal macrosomia in nondiabetic patients and whether decreased fetal glucose or insulin levels are an important mechanism related to fetal growth retardation are not known.

LIPID METABOLISM DURING PREGNANCY

Maternal Changes in Pregnancy

Pregnancy is associated with major maternal changes in lipid metabolism (see also Chapters 4 and 35). There may be a slight decrease in total serum concentration of lipid in the first trimester, but starting at the end of the first trimester, serum levels rise; by term, maternal serum levels are nearly 50% above nonpregnant levels. The triglyceride and cholesterol fractions show the largest increase, but all serum lipids are increased. It is known that human placental lactogen produced by the placenta and released primarily into the maternal circulation can mobilize free fatty acids in normal pregnant patients, and this placental hormone may account for part of the increase in the maternal levels of free fatty acid seen in late pregnancy.

Fetal Lipid Metabolism

Although glucose appears to be the major metabolic fuel of the developing fetus, fatty acids also are probably required for normal fetal development. Free fatty acid transfer to the fetus provides essential fatty acids for synthesis of structural components of the fetus. The precise role of fatty acids in providing combustible fuel for fetal energy production is unclear. Very little data support either of these uses of fatty acids in the human fetus. It is obvious that fat plays a prominent role in the normal fetus for the storage of energy, resulting in large amounts of adipose tissue stores in the normal fetus. A shown in Figure 20–2, by late in gestation, the deposition of fetal subcutaneous fat rises rapidly. At 32 weeks' gestation, the fat content in the human fetus is about 3.5% of body weight; at full term, fat makes up 16% of body weight. In the normal fetus, more calories are stored as fat than any other storage fuel. Because complete oxidation of 1 mole of the 16-carbon palmitic acid results in 140 moles of ATP compared to 38 moles for complete oxidation of glucose, this makes the stored fat an efficient energy source.

The precursor of stored fetal fat is an interesting question. The large amount of glucose that is known to be shunted transplacentally could probably account for most, if not all, of the fat synthesis. The enzyme systems necessary to incorporate acetate, glucose, and amino acids into lipids are present in human fetal tissue as early as the first trimester.[25]

Placental transfer of lipids, including glycerol and free fatty acids, does occur. Maternal serum free fatty acids are increased in late pregnancy, but the extent of placental transport and their role in fetal growth are unclear. It has been hypothesized that the increased supply of maternal free fatty acids may be used to supply energy for maternal tissue and thus spare maternal glucose for placental delivery. The question of whether the increased maternal levels of free fatty acids results in an increased transport to the fetus is not known. In many animal species, the administration of essential and nonessential free fatty acids to the mother is accompanied by a rapid transfer of these fatty acids to the fetus and incorporation into tissue. The extent of placental transport of free fatty acids in the human fetus is not well known. Based on *in vitro* placental perfusion studies, it appears that active transfer of palmitic acid from mother to fetus occurs in the rhesus monkey.[26] Thus, it is likely that similar transfer also occurs in humans (see Fig. 20–10).

It is unknown what role the free fatty acids transported from mother to fetus play in fetal metabolism. Studies in nonhuman species have demonstrated that fatty acids are not a significant source of combustible fuel during fetal development in the normal pregnancy. In human pregnancy, the final answer awaits study. However, the large amount of maternal and fetal fat stores that are deposited as pregnancy progresses makes this an important research area.

PROTEIN METABOLISM DURING PREGNANCY

Protein is essential for the synthesis of new tissue (see also Chapter 4). Protein metabolism cannot be separated from metabolism of other nutrients because the lack of sufficient glucose and fat for energy will interfere with the deposition of new protein. There is an increased requirement for protein intake during pregnancy, but the actual amount of the increase varies.

Few quantitative estimates of protein deposition have been performed in human pregnancy. Hytten and Leitch based their estimates on direct chemical analysis of the products of conception and indirect estimates of the increased protein deposited in maternal tissue.[1] From this, they calculated a theoretical estimate that 925 g of new protein are deposited in the fetal and maternal tissue. The estimated mean daily increment of protein deposited increased with pregnancy as follows: 0 to 10 weeks, 0.64 g; 10 to 20 weeks, 1.84 g; 20 to 30 weeks, 4.76; and 30 to 40 weeks, 6.1 g. These estimates suggest a tenfold increase in the mean daily increment of protein deposited in mother and fetus as gestational age increases. However, these fetal and maternal composition studies are only theoretical estimates.

Protein balance studies in which the actual intake and output of protein are measured over 72 hours suggest that the actual protein retained in the pregnant patient is as high as 30 g/d.[27] The values in the balance studies reviewed by Hytten and Leitch, in which the theoretical estimate of protein deposited was calculated, are considerably higher than can be accounted for. In addition, the balance studies have shown no significant increase with gestational age in deposited protein. One explanation for the increased protein requirement found in the balance studies could be that some protein is deposited in maternal nonuterine tissue.

Maternal Protein Storage

In the past, much of the interest in maternal protein concerned maternal storage of protein during pregnancy. A study by King and associates suggests that maternal protein storage occurs during pregnancy. Total body potassium [^{40}K] was used to estimate maternal fat-free tissue.[27] This study showed that potassium accumulation was greater than the theoretical gain attributable to the fetus, placenta, and maternal pregnancy-related tissue, and the authors hypothesized that the additional potassium may indicate an increase in maternal storage of protein. There is very little direct evidence to prove or disprove the question of whether protein is stored in the maternal organism during pregnancy. However, based on indirect evidence, it is believed that most of the unexplained maternal weight gain during pregnancy represents stored fat instead of protein.

Maternal Protein Turnover

Animal Studies. Neither the nitrogen balance studies nor the studies using labeled potassium (described previously) could detect if a shift of protein from maternal tissue to fetal tissue occurs. Some data from animal studies suggest that nitrogen metabolism in the pregnant rat follows a biphasic course shown diagrammatically in Figure 20–11.[28] During the first 14 days of the normal 21-day gestational period, the protein content of maternal muscle increases by an amount roughly equivalent to one half the protein in the conceptus at term; this has been termed the anabolic phase. The final trimester of gestation, the time of rapid fetal growth when the maternal protein reserve is depleted, is referred to as the catabolic phase. It has been postulated that this catabolic phase occurs regardless of the protein intake of the mother. There are no studies confirming this finding of anabolic and catabolic phases of maternal protein metabolism during pregnancy, however. Some studies have attempted to confirm this theory by selectively instituting protein deprivation at specific times during gestation based on the hypothesis that maternal starvation should have different effects during the anabolic compared to the catabolic phase.[29] At present, these studies are inconclusive, and more exact animal studies are needed in which actual maternal protein stores are evaluated during the presumed anabolic and catabolic periods as well as isotope studies evaluating protein turnover.

Human Studies. Little is known regarding successive changes in protein turnover as pregnancy progresses in humans. Naismith has performed preliminary studies in human pregnancy by quantifying the rates of urinary excretion of 3-methylhistidine at monthly intervals throughout gestation.[30] 3-Methylhistidine is an amino acid exclusive to muscle proteins that is not metabolized; therefore, its rate of urinary excretion is a measure of muscle protein catabolism. Patients were studied at monthly intervals throughout pregnancy; the rates of urinary excretion of 3-methylhistidine were stable throughout the first two trimesters of pregnancy, but a pronounced rise was seen around 30 weeks' gestation. One explanation of this would be that an increase in maternal muscle protein catabolism occurred around 30 weeks' gestation. This supports the hypothesis that early in pregnancy, maternal stores of protein are increased, and then late in gestation, the mother redistributes amino acids from her protein stores to supply the fetus at the time of maximal fetal growth. However, these findings must be considered preliminary because other factors, including the amount of animal protein in the maternal diet, also can affect 3-methylhistidine excretion. There are no studies using stable isotopes of amino acids to measure protein turnover during pregnancy.

Fetal Protein Synthesis

Although the fetus can catabolize some amino acids for energy production if carbohydrates and fats are not consumed in sufficient amounts, the use of amino acids by the fetus in normal pregnancy is assumed to be mainly for anabolic purposes. Both *in vivo* and *in vitro* studies have shown that many amino acids are transported transplacentally from a lower concentration in the maternal circulation to a higher concentration in the fetus. This supports the possibility that active placental transport exists for many of the amino acids. Although placental transport is the predominant transfer mechanism of amino acids to the fetus, one study performed late in gestation in the rhesus

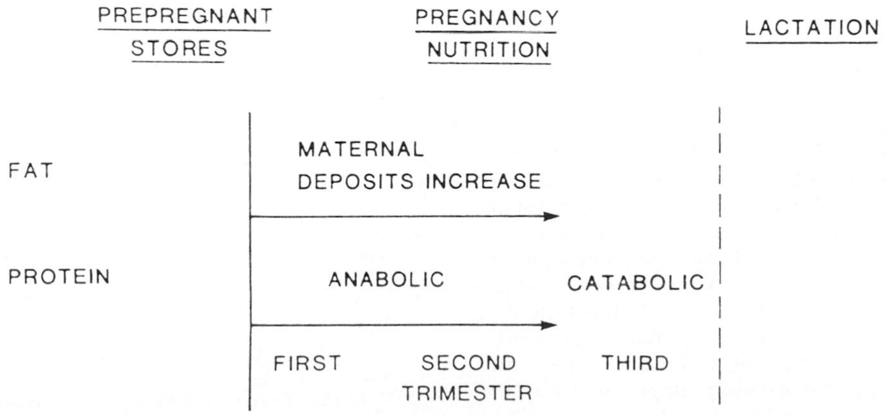

FIGURE 20–11. Diagram of the three stages of fat and protein nutrition important to pregnancy: prepregnant stores, pregnancy nutrition, and nutrition during lactation. Prepregnancy maternal stores as measured by maternal weight prior to pregnancy have a significant effect on birth weight. Maternal fat and protein may increase only through the first two trimesters of pregnancy to serve as a storage bank to supply rapid fetal growth in the third trimester or to supply lactation. This concept of a biphasic course during pergnancy (anabolic then catabolic) is well established for fat metabolism but only hypothesized for protein.

monkey found that up to 15% of fetal protein may be obtained by the fetus swallowing amniotic fluid.[31]

There is some indirect evidence that the maternal organism during normal pregnancy may have adaptations that allow more amino acids to be available to shunt transplacentally to the fetus. Naismith has demonstrated that enzymes regulating amino acid deamination and urea synthesis decline markedly during pregnancy in the rat.[28] This results in decreased amino acid catabolism followed by a lower plasma urea concentration. The result of the decreased maternal production of urea may be that more plasma amino acids are available to shunt to the fetus. There is some support for this concept from data of human pregnancies. Kalhan et al have measured urea synthesis and excretion in mothers during late pregnancy using a prime constant infusion of the stable isotope [$^{15}N_2$] urea.[32] These studies demonstrated a significant decrease in the rate of maternal urea synthesis, levels of blood urea nitrogen, and urinary excretion of urea in the pregnant patient.

Several important conclusions are suggested by these findings. First, the well-recognized decrease in maternal blood urea nitrogen that occurs with increasing gestation in human pregnancies was previously thought to result from an accelerated urinary excretion of urea secondary to the increased urinary output that occurs in pregnancy. The studies of Kalhan and associates suggest that the decreased blood urea may reflect a decreased maternal production of urea.[32] In addition, because urea production is an indirect measure of amino acid breakdown, this decrease in synthesis of urea during pregnancy could be a result of the decrease in the activity of urea cycle enzymes previously described in pregnant rats. Kalhan et al postulated that a more likely explanation is that the plasma levels of most amino acids decrease in nearly all previous studies of human pregnancies, and this decreased level results in decreased amino acids delivered to the liver for urea synthesis.[32] The decrease in maternal plasma levels of amino acids could be the result of redirecting amino acids to the fetus; however, another explanation could be the known hemodilution, which progressively increases throughout gestation, resulting in decreased plasma levels of many fuels.

Protein Requirement in Pregnancy

The additional daily protein requirement recommended because of pregnancy varies from 5 g/d in some countries to 30 g/d in the United States. Several lines of evidence played a key role in determining the estimate used in this country. First, the theoretical estimate of protein deposited in mother and fetus is as high as 6 g/d in late pregnancy. Second, the use of dietary nitrogen has been reported to be less efficient during pregnancy, with as little as 25–30% of dietary nitrogen used in the pregnant patient compared to the usual 75% in the nonpregnant patient.[27] Because of this, the theoretical estimate of protein deposited is multiplied by a factor of three to four. Finally, at each step, the recommended dietary requirement is overestimated because too little dietary protein could cause fetal damage, whereas an overestimate represents no risk. This latter assumption may not be accurate and is discussed in more depth in Chapter 21.

REFERENCES

1. Hytten FE, Leitch I. *The Physiology of Human Pregnancy*. London, England: Blackwell Scientific Publications; 1971.
2. Ballard JL, Novak K, Driver M. A simplified score for assessment of fetal maturation of newborn infants. *J Pediatr*. 1979;95:769.
3. Mendez H. Introduction to the study of pre- and postnatal growth in humans: a review. *Am J Med Genet*. 1985;20:63.
4. Stembera Z, Kovarik J, Jungmannova C. Frequency of fetal growth deviations diagnosed by ultrasonic measurement and analysis of their causes. *Acta Paediatr Scand*. 1985;319(suppl):48.
5. McKeown T, Record RG. Observations on fetal growth in multiple pregnancies in man. *J Endocrinol*. 1952;8:386.
6. Daw E, Walker J. Growth differences in twin pregnancy. *Br J Clin Pract*. 1975;29:150.
7. Sabbagha RE. Intrauterine growth retardation: antenatal diagnosis by ultrasound. *Obstet Gynecol*. 1978;52:252.
8. Stefos T, Deter RL, Hill RM, Simon N. Individual growth curve standards in twins: growth in the second trimester. *JCU*. 1989;17:641.
9. Simon NV, Deter RL, Hassinger KK, et al. Evaluation of fetal growth by ultrasonography in twin pregnancy: a comparison between individual and cross-sectional growth curve standards. *JCU*. 1989;17:633.
10. Bronsteen RA, Mariona FE, Sokol RJ. Intrauterine growth retardation in twins. In: Gross TL, Sokol RJ, eds. *Intrauterine Growth Retardation: A Practical Approach*. Chicago, IL: Year Book Medical Publishers; 1989:81.
11. Simon NV, Deter RL, Shearer DM, Levisky JS. Prediction of normal fetal growth by the Rossavik growth model using two scans before 27 weeks menstrual age. JCU. 1989;17:237.
12. Deter RL, Rossavik IK, Hill RM, et al. Longitudinal studies of femur growth in normal fetuses. *JCU*. 1987;15:299.
13. Horenstein J. Ultrasound assessment of fetal growth and fetal measurements. *Semin Perinatol*. 1988;12:23.
14. Deter RL, Hill RM, Tennyson LM. Predicting the birth characteristics of normal fetuses 14 weeks before delivery. *JCU*. 1989;17:89.
15. Niswander KR, Singer J, Westphal M, et al. Weight gain during pregnancy and pre-pregnancy weight, association with birth weight of term gestation. *Obstet Gynecol*. 1969;33:482.
16. Pitkin RM. Nutritional support in obstetrics and gynecology. *Clin Obstet Gynecol*. 1976;19:489.
17. Emerson K, Saxena B, Poindexter EL. Caloric cost of normal pregnancy. *Obstet Gynecol*. 1972;40:786.
18. Freinkel N. Of pregnancy and progeny. *Diabetes*. 1980;29:1023.
19. Fisher PM, Sutherland HW, Bewsher PD. Insulin response to glucose infusion in normal human pregnancy. *Diabetologia*. 1980;19:15.
20. Jarrett JC, Ballejo G, Saleen TH, et al. The effect of prolactin and relaxin on insulin binding by adipocytes from pregnant women. *Am J Obstet Gynecol*. 1984;149:250.
21. Oakley NW, Beard RW, Turner RC. Effect of sustained maternal hyperglycemia on the fetus in normal and diabetic pregnancies. *Br Med J*. 1972;1:466.
22. Hay WW, Sparks JW, Gilbert M, et al. Comparison of insulin effect in maternal hind limb, uterine and fetal glucose and oxygen extractions in conscious, pregnant sheep. *Fed Proc*. 1982;41:973.
23. Hay WW, Sparks JW, Wilkening RB, et al. Partition of maternal glucose production between conceptus and maternal tissues in sheep. *Am J Physiol*. 1983;245:E347.
24. Brinsmead MW, Liggins GC. Somatomedin-like activity, prolactin growth hormone and insulin in human cord blood. *Aust NZ J Obstet Gynaecol*. 1979;19:129.
25. Roux JF, Takeda Y, Grigorian A. Lipid concentration and composition in human fetal tissue during development. *Pediatrics*. 1971;48:540.
26. Portman OW, Behrman RE, Soltys P. Transfer of free fatty acids across the primate placenta. *Am J Physiol*. 1969;216:143.
27. King JC, Calloway DH, Margen S. Nitrogen retention, total body ^{40}K and weight gain in teenage pregnant girls. *J Nutr*. 1973;103:772.
28. Naismith DJ. The requirement for protein and the utilization of protein and calcium during pregnancy. *Metabolism*. 1966;15:582.
29. Anderson GD, Ahokas RA, Lipshitz J, et al. Effect of maternal dietary restriction during pregnancy on maternal weight gain and fetal birth weight in the rat. *J Nutr*. 1980;110:883.
30. Naismith DJ. Symposium on nutrition of the mother and child: maternal nutrition and outcome of pregnancy—a cultural appraisal. *Proc Nutr Soc*. 1980;39:1.
31. Pitkin RM, Reynolds WA. Fetal ingestion and metabolism of amniotic fluid protein. *Am J Obstet Gynecol*. 1975;123:356.
32. Kalhan SC, Tserng KY, Gilfillan C, et al. Metabolism of urea and glucose in normal and diabetic pregnancy. *Metabolism*. 1982;31:824.

Chapter Twenty-One

Effects of Maternal Malnutrition and Obesity

Honor M. Wolfe, Thomas L. Gross, and George M. Kazzi

21

Throughout history, the importance of nutrition during pregnancy has been marked by major change. Aristotle and Hippocrates both felt that improving maternal nutrition could decrease the incidence of spontaneous abortions and premature deliveries. During the 18th and 19th centuries, maternal nutritional advice generally was to devise various starvation diets in an attempt to reduce fetal size and prevent dystocia. The lack of regard for adequate maternal nutrition continued into the mid-20th century. Since then, the pendulum has swung back. The major emphasis now is improving the mother's diet, which in turn can improve fetal growth and long-term development of the neonate.

This chapter reviews the two aspects of abnormal nutrition, maternal malnutrition and maternal obesity, and their effects on pregnancy outcome.

MATERNAL MALNUTRITION

Several types of studies have, during the past 20 years, resulted in a change of the perspective on the importance of diet in pregnancy. These include starvation studies in animals; administration of food supplements to populations of chronically malnourished patients; natural disasters, including famines caused by wars; and other epidemiologic studies regarding maternal weight gain in pregnancy.

Numerous studies in animals have suggested that inadequate maternal nutrition during pregnancy, including protein- and energy-deficient diets, leads to adverse effects on birth weight and brain development and to an increased perinatal mortality rate. Caloric restriction of rats in the second half of pregnancy results in a significant decrease in fetal body weight, placental weight, brain weight, and cerebral deoxyribonucleic acid (DNA) in offspring. Other studies have found that the offspring of rats that were starved during pregnancy have lowered intelligence and more behavioral abnormalities later in life.[1]

However, it is unclear whether most of these studies apply to the clinical management of human pregnancy. First, the degree of starvation in these pregnant animals is more severe than would commonly occur in malnourished patients in a developed country. The restriction of protein or carbohydrates in the diet of a maternal animal commonly amounts to 50% or more of the normal intake. Consequently, the maternal animal often loses weight throughout the pregnancy. In addition, the placental structure and probably the transport of nutrients are different in animal pregnancy. Most importantly, however, there are marked differences in number of fetuses, fetal-to-maternal weight ratio, and the length of gestation between human and animal pregnancy. The pregnant rat, which is the animal model most frequently used in dietary control studies, has a large litter size with a total fetal weight of approximately 25% of maternal weight and a normal length of gestation of 21 days. This contrasts sharply with the human singleton pregnancy in which the fetal weight is only 5% or less of maternal weight, and the average gestational length is 280 days. Maternal dietary deficiency may have different fetal effects based on the ratio of fetal-to-maternal weight and length of gestation. Finally, one of the most frequent effects of starvation in the rodent is a decrease in litter size. This effect could actually mask the consequences of malnutrition by making more of the limited nutrients available to the remaining fetuses.

Thus, even though animal studies cannot directly be applied to the clinical management of human pregnancy, dietary manipulation studies in animals are nevertheless important for various research reports. For example, they allowed identification of the interaction of protein and carbohydrate deficiency[2], the possible biphasic nature (anabolic and catabolic) of protein metabolism[3], and the effect of malnutrition on placental transport.[4]

Natural experiments, such as famines caused by blockades during World Wars I and II, caused sudden and severe malnutrition. From the limited data available, it is clear that maternal starvation was quite severe. Fetuses developing during these times were smaller at the time of delivery than those born at other times.

The most thoroughly analyzed famines involve two countries invaded during World War II, the Soviet Union during the siege of Leningrad and the Netherlands during the Dutch hunger winter of 1944–1945. The siege of Leningrad lasted from August 1941 to August 1943. Severe famine conditions existed. Some pregnant women received rations as low as 450 kcal per person per day with average daily rations below 750 kcal for at least 6 months.[5] The mean birth weight of babies carried to term was decreased by more than 500 g during this period of starvation, compared to the period immediately preceding the siege. In addition, fetal mortality was reportedly doubled.

Similar data were recorded for pregnancies during the Dutch hunger winter of 1944–1945. The women in the blockaded cities were believed to be reasonably well nourished before the acute starvation. This study is important because the investigators found that a 300-g decrease in birth weight, caused by the famine, was manifested only when the starvation was present during the third trimester. An overall increase in perinatal mortality rate was not seen during the famine, even though these patients were believed to have daily rations as low as 800 kcal and only 40 g of protein. A group of women who were malnourished during the first trimester and then suddenly restored to a normal diet in the second trimester had slightly increased stillbirths.

The possibility that maternal starvation may have detrimental effects on the long-term neurologic development of the fetus represents an important concept. The military system in Holland requires all young men to undergo psychologic testing at age 18. Stein et al[6], have analyzed the results of the psychologic tests in the young men exposed to famine *in utero*. When compared to similar men in Dutch cities not exposed to famine, there were no differences in scores on intelligence tests or frequencies of severe or minor mental retardation (Fig. 21–1). This is described in more detail below.

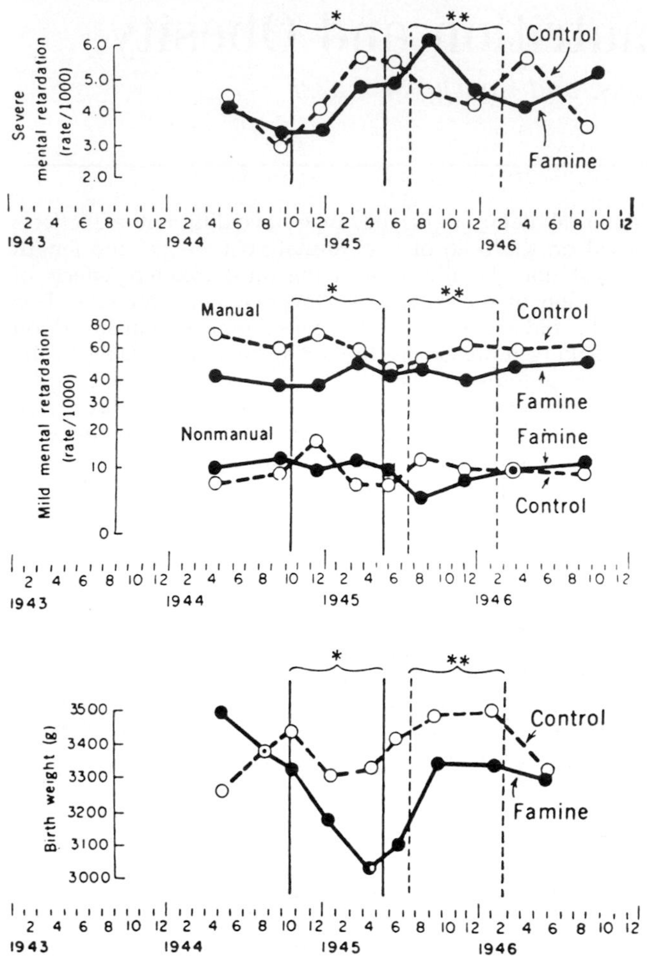

Figure 21–1. The outcome of mean birth weight in grams, frequencies of mild mental retardation, and severe mental retardation per 1000 men examined at age 19 from famine cities (*closed circles*) and control cities (*open circles*) from the Dutch hunger winter. Solid vertical lines bracket the period of famine, and broken vertical lines show the period when births occurred from pregnancies conceived during the famine. The data for mild mental retardation are stratified into manual and nonmanual workers. (*From Stein et al*[6] *with permission.*)

There can be no doubt that severe maternal starvation to the degree that occurred in the famines listed previously reduces birth weight. The starvation in Holland reduced birth weight by about 10%. Multiple aspects make these studies only poorly applicable to the clinical management of human pregnancies, however. The decrease in birth weight during the famine may underestimate the effects of maternal malnutrition for several reasons. Natural experiments, such as famines, represent a model of sudden acute starvation, occurring only during pregnancy in previously well-nourished women. This has only little relation to a clinical situation in which malnutrition is usually chronic and extends over a lifetime. Patients who are chronically malnourished before pregancy can be expected to have a poorer perinatal outcome than mothers from the famine studies who were starved only during pregnancy. In fact, one explanation for the more marked effect on birth weight after the siege of Leningrad, compared to the Dutch hunger winter is that the mothers in Holland were better nourished before the acute starvation.

One of the strongest variables that can lead to underestimation of the effect of maternal starvation on overall neonatal outcome is the selection process for determining who conceives during this type of social unrest. Failure to conceive has been consistently reported in nearly all of the famines in which reproductive outcome has been described. In addition to the many social factors involved, amenorrhea is common. Up to 50% of women were amenorrheic during the Dutch hunger winter.[7] This could mean that women who conceive are a select population, perhaps wealthier and better nourished.

Hytten also suggested other factors that could have resulted in an overestimation of the effects of maternal malnutrition on pregnancy outcome.[7] In addition to starvation, the women also were subjected to severe physical strain, reflected in long work hours throughout the winter with little rest and heat in their homes. Extreme physical exertion to the point of maternal exhaustion has been reported to have an adverse effect on pregnancy outcome.[7] There also were no exact records kept of the maternal-based rations. The possibility exists that pregnant women either were given preference in food distribution or women may have given their food rations to their living children and thus may have had a lower intake than has been estimated.

Studies in such underdeveloped countries as Guatemala[8] and in indigent populations in the United States[9] have shown that providing food supplements during pregnancy can increase maternal weight gain and neonatal birth weight. These studies usually deal with severely malnourished mothers and demonstrate a small increase in birth weight, varying from 40–100 g in newborns of mothers receiving food supplementation. This increase in birth weight probably directly relates to the actual number of kilocalories consumed by the supplemented patients. Lawrence et al[10] examined the effect of dietary supplementation on maternal fat deposition and birth weight in an area of rural Africa subject to annual preharvest food shortages. Supplementation, averaging 430 kcal/d, increased caloric intake from 1470–1900 kcal/d. Mean birth weight increased by 224 g among pregnancies supplemented during periods of food shortage. No such effect was observed during other seasons, however. The authors consequently hypothesized that the observed increase in maternal fat stores reduced the magnitude of change in seasonal energy use and was thus instrumental in increasing birth weight.

A unique approach to the study of maternal food supplementation during pregnancy is ongoing at the Royal Victoria Hospital in Montreal.[11] Unlike previous studies, this project begins with an assessment of caloric and protein nutritional needs for each patient. Patients are then supplemented to bring them to an optimal nutritional level based on their height and weight, with an additional supplement given if the patient was underweight before pregnancy. The average total daily requirement was calculated to be 3009 kcal and 107 g of protein per patient. Individual patient supplements ranged from an additional 784 kcal and 43 g of protein per day in those assessed to be of poor nutritional status, to 210 kcal and 16 g of protein per day in those patients assessed as well nourished. This method led to an increase in fetal birth weight in supplemented patients similar to those reported in previous studies. The Montreal study, however, also is cited to demonstrate that diet supplementation decreases the incidence of prematurity. Prematurity was defined as birth weight below 2500 g, which is an old definition no longer in use. Supplemented patients were also reported to have a lower perinatal mortality rate. Unfortunately, like nearly all other food supplementation studies, this one suffers from lack of an adequate control group because patients were not matched with properly selected controls.

One of the few randomized controlled trials examining the effect of food supplements during pregnancy was conducted in New York City.[9] Patients were recruited into the study only if they had known risk factors for poor maternal nutrition or a history of previous low birth weight infants. They were then randomly assigned to one of three study groups: the supplement group, which received an additional 40 g of protein and 470 kcal/d; the complement group, which received an additional 6 g of protein and 322 kcal/d; and the control group, which did not receive additional protein or kilocalories. Selected dietary histories were taken to estimate how much of the supplementation was being consumed. This study revealed no significant increase in mean birth weight for the supplement or complement group compared to the control group. Women given the high-protein supplement actually demonstrated an increased rate of prematurity and higher perinatal mortality than controls. This rather surprising finding caused the authors to conclude that high-protein dietary supplementation should be abandoned.[9]

Many studies reported a positive correlation between total maternal weight gain during pregnancy and neonatal birth weight. A second variable, acting independently in its influence on neonatal birth weight, is the mother's prepregnancy weight. Maternal prepregnancy weight is, however, usually less significant in its effect on birth weight than maternal weight gain during pregnancy. The interaction of maternal prepregnancy weight and weight gain during pregnancy is illustrated by data from the Collaborative Perinatal Project (see Fig. 20–5). This study was carried out by the National Institutes of Neurological and Communicative Disorders and Strokes, in which 53,518 pregnancies were prospectively followed in 12 US hospitals between 1959 and 1966.[12] This study demonstrated that increased maternal prepregnancy weight and increased weight gain during pregnancy are associated with fewer low birth weight newborns (<2500 g). The association with pregnancy weight gain is most marked in underweight mothers. In contrast, women weighing more than 190 lb demonstrated very little effect from increased pregnancy weight gain. At the time of this study, the concept of intrauterine fetal growth retardation was not recognized and the description of neonates as either small-for-gestational age or large-for-gestational age was not used. As a result, this study did not prospectively examine whether these low birth weight babies had signs of intrauterine fetal growth retardation. Because the data from the collaborative study (see Fig. 20–5) were restricted to mothers at 39–42 weeks' gestation, it appears retrospectively that the increased frequency of lower birth weight was, in fact, caused by fetal growth retardation.

One of the most important variables in the association of maternal nutrition and pregnancy outcome is infant growth and development in the first year of life. Follow-up data on 10,000 children in the Collaborative Study of Cerebral Palsy demonstrated that the percentage of infants with abnormal motor and mental test scores, growth, and neurologic findings decreased with increasing maternal weight gain.[13] This suggests that maternal nutrition, as recorded by weight gain during pregnancy, may affect long-term development of the infant.

In such epidemiologic studies, pregnancy weight gain is used to define the relationship between consumed kilocalories and maternal and fetal needs. A slow and steady maternal weight gain is usually a reassuring sign because it suggests that increased maternal metabolic requirements and fetal needs are satisfied by enough food stuff to supply maternal stores. However, maternal weight gain is a relatively inaccurate measure of maternal nutrition. Many questions regarding the actual relationship of maternal diet to neonatal outcome remain and will be answered only by carefully controlled longitudinal studies in which accurate maternal dietary histories and comprehensive neonatal outcome data are available.

Energy Deprivation Versus Protein Deprivation

It is established that maternal malnutrition can significantly alter fetal growth and development. Whether deprivation of maternal calories or lack of protein is more of a contributing factor, however, has remained controversial.

Animal models can play a major role in differentiating between the importance of energy deficiency and protein deficiency on fetal growth. However, even in animals, it is not simple to separate the effects of carbohydrates and proteins because protein-deprived rats often eat less carbohydrates as well. Most investigators have concluded that the energy in the diet plays the primary role in fetal growth.[3] A minority of studies suggested, however, that the availability of protein may be the primary limiting factor and that an energy-deficit diet may play only a secondary role in fetal growth.[14] Naismith examined this question in rats in which the maternal diet was patterned after previous dietary supplement studies in humans.[3] This study is important because it is one of the few in which dietary restrictions of the maternal animals were designed to simulate the moderate starvation of human malnutrition. Maternal rats were given different diets: high energy and high protein, low energy and low protein, high energy and low protein, and low energy and high protein. None of the dietary groups demonstrated a decrease in litter size. The animals on the low-energy and low-protein diet demonstrated a 14% decreased fetal weight compared to the high-energy and high-protein groups. Rats fed a carbohydrate supplement in their high-energy and low-protein diet showed considerable recovery in fetal weight, which had been decreased by 14% compared to the high-energy and high-protein group. Rats fed a carbohydrate supplement in their high-energy and low-protein diet showed considerable recovery in birth weight, while protein supplementation in the low-energy and high-protein diet demonstrated no such effect. This study supports the importance of energy supplementation for fetal growth.

The inclusion of protein in the usual food supplement of chronically malnourished women appears to have no effect on birth weight as described in the earlier study of chronically malnourished women in Guatemala.[8] The incidence of low birth weight infants was decreased by 50% in patients receiving an energy supplement during pregnancy, but the inclusion of protein in the supplement had no further effect.

Protein deprivation during pregnancy may affect fetal organ development, even though birth weight is not affected. Maternal rats deprived of protein early in pregnancy and then switched to an adequate diet in the final 20% of their gestation demonstrated no effect on fetal weight but did show a decrease in cell numbers of various organs, including the brain. Therefore, the effect was not reversed by providing an adequate diet in the final 20% of pregnancy.[15]

It appears that carbohydrate deprivation during pregnancy exerts a greater impact on fetal growth than protein deficiency. However, it should be noted that protein deprivation also may cause deficits in fetal, and possibly neonatal, development. Because a lack of maternal protein appears potentially more harmful than an excess, it is prudent to overestimate, rather than underestimate, protein requirement. Some caution is required, however, as noted below.

There is no general agreement as to how much extra protein is needed to supply normal maternal and fetal growth during pregnancy. The usual requirement suggested in the United States is 1.3 g/kg of lean body weight. This amounts to approximately an extra 20 to 30 g for the pregnant patient (see Appendix 21–1). The recommendations vary among countries from an additional 5 g of protein per day in the United Kingdom to approximately 30 g/d in the United States.[16]

Some studies in rhesus monkeys suggest that a high-protein diet may be harmful. Riopelle and associates divided diets of maternal animals into three groups and fed them 1, 2, or 4 g of protein per kilogram of maternal body weight per day throughout pregnancy.[17] Animals on the highest protein diet of 4 g/kg per day did not have bigger offspring. On closer evaluation, this was attributed to the fact that this group delivered significantly earlier in gestation than the mothers on the 1 or 2 g/kg per day protein diets. The application of the results of this study to human pregnancy is difficult because the level of Ug/bp/a protein associated with an apparent risk for prematurity is much higher than any dietary protein recommendation in humans.

However, there is some confirming evidence that high-protein dietary supplementation may increase the risk for prematurity in humans. As noted previously, the New York dietary supplement study found no significant difference in neonatal birth weights among three dietary controlled patient groups managed with either a low-protein supplement or a high-protein supplement compared to a control group.[9] On closer examination, it was found that the women given the high-protein supplement (an additional 40 g/d) experienced an increased premature delivery rate and an increased neonatal death rate.

Protein has commonly been thought to be deficient in diets of indigent populations. It also has been assumed that high-protein supplementation causes potential harm. Based on previously discussed studies, some detrimental effects of high-protein diets cannot be ruled out. Protein supplementation should therefore proceed with some caution.

Major Neonatal Morbidity

The concept that good maternal nutrition will decrease the frequency of major neonatal morbidity measures, such as prematurity, perinatal mortality, and long-term neurologic deficiencies, has remained controversial. Neonatal morbidity and mortality, related to prematurity and fetal growth retardation, are the most significant problems facing obstetricians and neonatologists today. Maternal malnutrition is commonly reported to be a major cause of premature delivery and retardation of fetal growth.

As noted previously, epidemiologic studies have supported an association between decreased prematurity rate and higher prepregnancy weight and increased weight gain during pregnancy.[12] Lower rates of prematurity also are reported in mothers receiving food supplements during pregnancy compared to those receiving no protein or caloric help.[11] A major problem with nearly all of these studies is that prematurity was almost universally defined as a birth weight of less than 2500 g. The assumption that all low birth weight infants are premature is obviously wrong and is based on old definitions of prematurity that have not been used for many years.

Low birth weight infants are now divided into those that are small because of *prematurity* and those that are small because of *intrauterine fetal growth retardation*. Prematurity is a gestational age estimate of less than 38 weeks. The definition of intrauterine growth retardation is based on a *birth weight percentile score* determined by a physical and neurologic examination of the newborn, which is compared to the remainder of the population at that hospital or to published values from other hospital populations. The lowest 10% of the newborn population, based on birth weight percentiles at any gestational age, are considered *small-for-gestational age*. This is the most frequently used criterion to define the population of newborns that are believed to be growth retarded *in utero*. Potential errors exist when calculating the pediatric estimate of gestational age and birth weight percentile. Even though these definitions are imperfect, they represent a great improvement over studies that assumed that all low birth weight infants were premature.

Only a few studies of maternal nutrition have attempted to divide low birth weight offspring into those that are premature and those that are growth retarded. As noted previously, an analysis of data from the Dutch famine suggested that a 300-g decrease in birth weight was present when maternal starvation was the worst.[7] This effect appeared because of intrauterine growth retardation, and length of gestation was not affected.

As discussed previously, data from the Collaborative Study of Cerebral Palsy examined the relationship of maternal weight gain with low birth weight and length of gestation. As shown in Table 21–1, the number of pregnancies attaining 37 weeks' gestation were fewer in mothers who experienced only a weight gain of 0–15 lb compared to those gaining 26–35 lb. However, this does not necessarily indicate a cause-and-effect relationship between improved

TABLE 21–1. PERCENTAGE OF PREGNANCIES DELIVERING AT PROGRESSIVELY INCREASING GESTATIONAL AGE SHOWN FOR FOUR CATEGORIES OF MATERNAL WEIGHT GAIN

	Length of Gestation (weeks)				
Pregnancy Weight Gain (lb)	28–30 (percent)	31–33 (percent)	34–36 (percent)	⩾37 (percent)	Total (percent)
0–15	1.3	4.3	12.5	81.7	100
16–25	0.7	2.5	8.8	87.8	100
26–35	0.4	1.4	7.9	90.1	100
⩾36	1.0	2.0	6.6	90.2	100

Adapted from Singer et al.[13]

maternal nutrition, as measured by increased maternal weight, and longer gestation. Maternal weight exponentially increases. Consequently, patients with longer pregnancy have more time to gain weight and reach the optimal level of weight. Conversely, patients may deliver prematurely regardless of their nutritional status. They simply have fewer weeks to reach the optimal level of pregnancy weight gain. A more meaningful analysis would examine the correlation of rate of weight gain in appropriate trimesters of pregnancy with premature delivery. This type of study has not yet been performed.

The increased rate of premature delivery in lower socioeconomic patient groups has frequently led to the assumption that malnutrition causes prematurity. This concept is based primarily on studies in which inaccurate definitions of prematurity were used. Patients in lower socioeconomic groups have many other potential causes for increased prematurity. From available data, it appears that the major benefit of improving maternal nutrition is increased fetal growth. There is, in fact, little to suggest that maternal malnutrition has a direct effect on stimulating premature labor. A recent study of 40 women documented an apparently adequate mean birth weight (2885 g) and a 10% incidence of low birth weight despite a calorie deficit of 700 kcal/d over the last two trimesters of pregnancy.[18] The authors concluded that pregnancy can be successful even in the presence of marginal energy intake.

Perinatal Mortality

Whether maternal malnutrition can be reflected in an increased perinatal mortality is controversial. Supportive evidence comes from studies of famines during the world wars. A paradoxical decrease in stillbirth rate from 38 in 1000 to 28 in 1000 occurred in Britain during World War II.[7] This improved fetal outcome could not be explained by an improvement in medical care, and in fact, prenatal care was actually felt to be worse because of the war. During this time, pregnant women received priority for food rations, and this has led some authors to ascribe the decreased rate of stillbirths to improved maternal nutrition. There are major weaknesses in this assumption. As noted previously, other investigators have suggested that during periods of famine and starvation, there is a selection process as to who conceives. Patients at highest risk for poor pregnancy outcome, such as lower socioeconomic groups, may be less likely to conceive. Pregnancy outcome during famines can therefore be expected to improve.

Some evidence from the Collaborative Perinatal Project suggests a correlation between maternal prepregnancy and pregnancy weight gain and perinatal mortality rate.[19] The pregnancy weight gain associated with the lowest perinatal mortality rate in normal-weight women was 20 lb. In underweight women, the weight gain associated with the lowest perinatal mortality rate was, however, 30 lb (Fig. 21–2). This suggests that the association of improved maternal nutrition with decreased perinatal mortality rate is most marked in underweight women.

Several studies in which food supplements were administered to pregnant women have attempted to examine the relationship of maternal intake of either kilocalories or protein with perinatal mortality rate. Most of these studies have been poorly controlled because patients chosen to receive food supplements were selected nonrandomly. Although a lower perinatal mortality rate often is seen in the supplemented patients, it should be emphasized that this could be entirely related to the selection process of

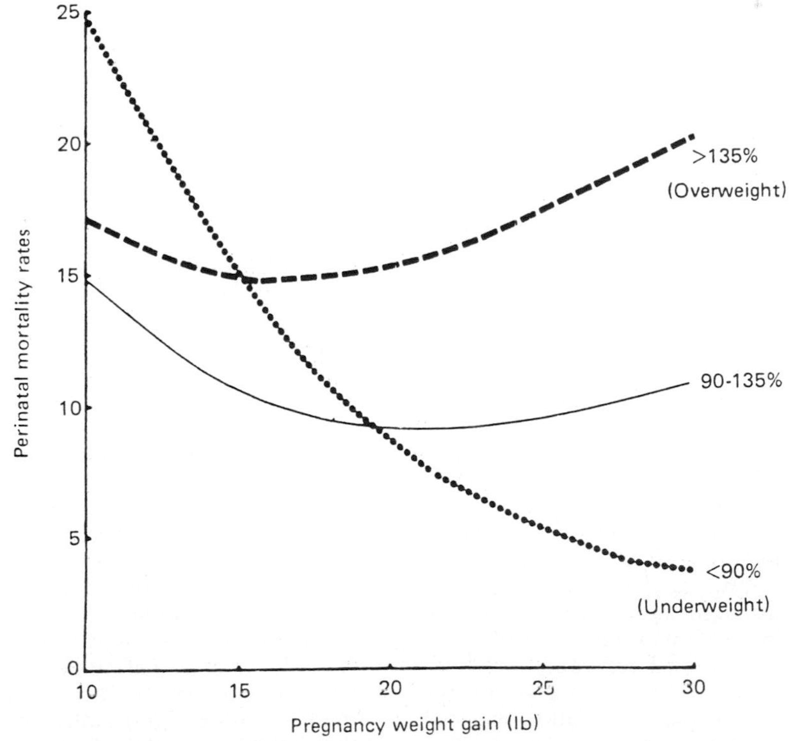

Figure 21–2. The relationship between weight gain in pregnancy and perinatal mortality rate shown for women divided into three categories of prepregnancy weight for height based on Metropolitan Life Insurance tables—underweight (<90%), normal weight (90–135%), and overweight (>135%). Curves are plotted as a percent of mean prepregnancy weight for height values (*Metropolitan*). (*From Naeye*[19] *with permission.*)

choosing the treated patients. In one prospective randomized trial in which women at nutritional risk were divided into groups either receiving or not receiving food supplements, the perinatal mortality rate was not improved in supplemented patients.[9]

The possible effect of maternal malnutrition on perinatal mortality may be too small to be detected by various research designs. The decrease in stillbirth rate ascribed to improved maternal nutrition during World War II went from 38 deaths per 1000 live births to 28 in 1000. To prove that such a change is significant in a controlled study of food supplementation would require approximately 10,000 study subjects.[20]

Long-Term Neurologic Development

The effect of malnutrition on the developing fetal brain and subsequent mental performance has attracted attention in the past 20 years. Low birth weight infants experience slower growth and development and demonstrate lower scores on follow-up intelligence tests when compared to the rest of the neonatal population. Because malnutrition during pregnancy increases the risk of a low birth weight infant, various investigators have attempted to correlate maternal malnutrition to retardation in mental development.

Animal studies have demonstrated that restricting maternal kilocalories during pregnancy reduces the total number of brain cells and the amount of DNA in the neonatal brain at delivery.[21] These studies suggest that the effect of the nutritional insult depends on duration and severity of the starvation and the stage of brain development at the time of insult. The degree of starvation in these animal studies is often too severe to extrapolate the results to humans even in a severely malnourished population. Based on these findings in animals, therefore, it is not reasonable to assume that malnutrition also may effect neurologic development in humans.

Data from the Collaborative Perinatal Project suggested that the effect of increasing maternal weight during pregnancy improves subsequent motor, mental, and neurologic outcome in infants and children.[13] In this study, approximately 10,000 infants were followed up to 1 year of age. An attempt was made to control for the confounding factors. Increasing maternal weight was associated with significant improvement in all examined areas except for the neurologic examination (Table 21–2).

TABLE 21–2. PERCENTAGE OF ABNORMAL INFANTS FOR EACH OF THREE GROWTH AND DEVELOPMENT MEASURES[a]

Pregnancy Weight Gain (lb)	Infant Measurements (% Abnormal)		
	Mental	Motor	Neurologic
0–15	12.5	11.3	8.8
16–25	9.3	8.0	7.5
26–35	8.3	6.8	7.9
≥36+	7.5	5.2	7.1

[a] Mental and motor scores were measured at 8 months, and neurologic tests were given at 12 months of age. Results are given for four categories of maternal weight gain during pregnancy. The decrease in percent abnormal outcome with increasing weight gain was statistically significant for mental and motor scores.

Adapted from Singer et al.[13]

Famines. Long-term follow-up studies of 20,000 adults demonstrated no significant impairment in mental performance of those that suffered acute exposure to famine *in utero.*[6] The records show that a mean of 450 kcal per person was available each day at the lowest point, and for 6 months, daily rations were below 750 kcal per person. The famine in Holland occurred suddenly in October of 1944 and was restricted to certain parts of the country. This allowed a detailed retroactive assessment of the famine. Figure 21–1 shows the results for the three outcome variables: birth weight, mild mental retardation, and severe retardation for males aged 18 years in the famine and control cities. Although a large effect of maternal starvation on birth weight during the months of the famine is apparent, the frequency of mild or severe mental retardation was not influenced by the famine. In fact, severe mental retardation increased slightly in both famine and control cities during the study period. There also was no correlation between maternal malnutrition at various stages of pregnancy and the intelligence quotient (IQ). Even though no effect on mental performance could be found in the offspring of mothers exposed to the famine, there was a significant association between the fathers' occupation and subsequent intelligence of the infant. Both mild mental retardation (Fig. 21–2) and decreased IQ were significantly more common in the offspring of manual laborers. This study shows convincingly that severe acute maternal starvation during pregnancy had no detectable effects on mental performance in 18-year-old male offspring; mental performance was not related to the decreased birth weight seen during the famine; and there was a strong association between the parents' social class and mental performance in the offspring.

As noted previously, a criticism of this study is that the majority of mothers were well nourished before the famine and became acutely malnourished only during the famine. This type of malnutrition does not usually occur in a clinical setting because malnourished mothers usually have chronically depleted nutritional reserves when they enter pregnancy and continue to be malnourished throughout the pregnancy.

Dietary intervention with food supplements has been reported from many different populations, but very few have included long-term follow-up. In the previously described controlled trial from New York City, patients receiving a high-protein supplementation (40 g of protein and 470 kcal) were compared to a group receiving a low-protein diet (6 g of protein and 322 kcal) and to a control group receiving no protein or caloric supplement.[9] The group receiving the high-protein supplementation demonstrated significant improvement in three psychologic measures at 1 year of age, but seven other psychologic measures were not different between the groups.

The observation that is most frequently used to associate maternal malnutrition with worsened long-term infant outcome is the association of maternal acetonuria with reduced intelligence of the newborn. Studies from the Collaborative Perinatal Project found IQ scores of 4-year-old children, whose nondiabetic mothers had acetonuria during pregnancy, to be significantly lower than those of matched controls.[22] Additional studies from the Collaborative Perinatal Project report that infants of acetone-positive diabetic mothers show significantly more developmental defects than infants of matched controls.[23] There are many problems with these studies, even though both the acetone-positive diabetic and nondiabetic patients were matched for maternal race, age, socioeconomic index, neonatal sex, and birth order to control for patients with no acetonuria.

While it is generally assumed that the presence of acetonuria serves as a marker of chronic malnutrition, a patient was considered acetone-positive if only one urine test was positive for "1+ or more ketones" during the 24 hours before delivery. The authors point out that a patient who is positive one day could be negative all other days. Unfortunately, these studies did not exclude maternal prepregnancy weight and pregnancy weight gain as contributing factors, and these weights were not given to permit estimation of whether these patients were chronically malnourished. Naeye and Chez relate acetonuria, weight loss, and low weight gain during pregnancy in both diabetic and nondiabetic patients to the infants' subsequent psychomotor development until 7 years of age.[24] No consistent evidence exists of motor or mental impairment in either black or white patients in whom acetonuria and low pregnancy weight gain or weight loss were present. Both of the previous studies are based on follow-up data from the same Collaborative Perinatal Project, but their results differ. Naeye and Chez suggest that the study failed to find an effect of maternal acetonuria and decreased pregnancy weight gain because they controlled for various non-nutritional factors that can influence psychomotor development.

Stehbens reported an association of maternal acetonuria and low intellectual status on a small group of diabetics.[25] The acetone-negative mothers had infants who, at 5 years of age, had significantly higher IQ scores than those in the acetone-positive group. However, this study did not evaluate normal control patients and did not control crucial factors affecting long-term development, such as delivery complications, social class, and gestational age.

The alleged association of maternal acetonuria with a subsequent deficit in an infant's neurologic development, reported for diabetic as well as nondiabetic patients, has probably influenced clinical care more than any other finding related to maternal malnutrition. This is the case even though the presented data are very weak. Even if the association between maternal ketonuria and decreased neonatal intelligence is confirmed, it remains to be established what is responsible for the toxic effect on fetal development. Serum acetone is increased during normal pregnancy, and it is unlikely that the presence of ketones alone alters fetal development. Other possibly contributing metabolic factors, including acidosis and hypoglycemia, were not evaluated in earlier studies. Basic cell culture and animal studies will be needed to investigate the potential toxicity of ketones and other metabolic factors. Ketoacids may simply serve as markers for other biochemical factors, which may affect development.

Is the Fetus a Parasite?

It is an old concept that the fetus can, even in the malnourished mother, grow well by parasitizing the maternal tissue. Even though this is now known to be a simplistic view, it is valuable to review some of the observations that led to this concept. This theory suggested that nutrients are distributed from the maternal blood into various tissues according to their metabolic needs. The fetus normally has a higher metabolic rate than the mother, and thus the fetal side of the placenta would receive more nutrients per kilogram of body weight than the mother. If nutrients become less available, the fetus could compete advantageously with the mother and receive a proportionately larger share. If severe protein or dietary restriction were imposed during pregnancy, the mother may even use a significant amount of her own tissue to support fetal growth. At some point, the dietary intake would reach a level so low that the mother could no longer supply fetal growth and the conceptus may then be affected.

Maternal malnutrition, even in severely malnourished patients, results in only relatively universal documented effects on neonatal outcome.[17] This observation has been used to support the concept that the fetus may receive preference for maternal nutrients.

Several animal studies failed to support the hypothesis that the mother preferentially supplies fetal growth, even to the point of breaking down her own tissue.[26,27] In most animal species, when maternal malnutrition is induced during pregnancy, the loss of maternal body weight is proportionally less than the loss of fetal body weight.

The primary maternal metabolic changes that have been studied in relation to fetal growth retardation have been the levels of blood glucose. Glucose is one of the major substrates of metabolism for the fetus. Numerous studies in animals and humans have documented the relationship between increased substrate delivery, such as in maternal diabetes mellitus, and the birth of infants who are large-for-gestational age. This has led to the possibility that the converse also may be true (ie, decreased maternal levels of glucose may be associated with limited fetal growth). Maternal hypoglycemia in animals, induced by insulin, results in lower body weight offspring. Whether a mechanism exists by which the fetus can parasitize maternal stores of glucose if the maternal serum level is decreased, also has been examined. Hay examined the distribution of glucose between fetal, uteroplacental, and maternal nonuterine compartments in chronic preparations of pregnant sheep (Fig. 21–3).[28] The sheep were not starved but were studied during periods of normoglycemia, after which hypoglycemia was induced. Radioactive tracers of glucose were used to measure the net glucose uptake by the fetal, uteroplacental, and nonuterine maternal tissues in pregnant sheep near term gestation. The study demonstrated that the uteropla-

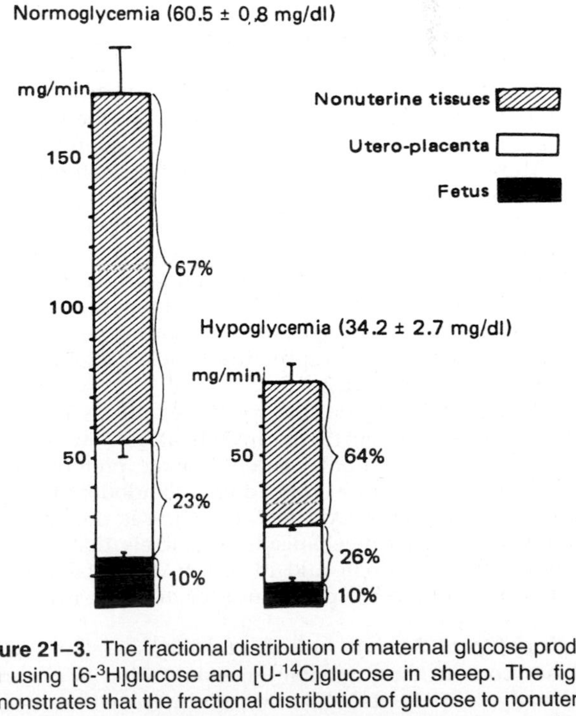

Figure 21–3. The fractional distribution of maternal glucose production using [6-^{3}H]glucose and [U-^{14}C]glucose in sheep. The figure demonstrates that the fractional distribution of glucose to nonuterine maternal tissue, uteroplacental tissue, and fetus was not altered by hypoglycemia. (*From Hay et al*[28], *with permission.*)

cental unit and the fetus respond to maternal hypoglycemia by decreasing uptake of maternal glucose. This suggests that glucose is not shunted preferentially to the fetus at low maternal glucose levels and argues against the concept of a parasitic fetus.

Although it appears convincing that altered maternal carbohydrate metabolism is associated with fetal growth retardation in animals, the clinical significance of this finding for humans is not known. Some preliminary observations in humans have supported the concept that hypoglycemia is associated with fetal growth retardation. A significant correlation between maternal hypoglycemia, occurring during glucose tolerance tests, and the birth of a small-for-gestational age infant has been observed.

Changes in lipid metabolism associated with malnutrition in pregnancy are poorly studied in animal and human pregnancy. Maternal starvation increases maternal levels of human placental lactogen (HPL). This could result in increased supply of fetal fuel by several mechanisms.[29] The increased supply of free fatty acids that are mobilized by HPL can be used by maternal tissue and therefore spare more glucose for placental transfer. The increased levels of fatty acids also could be shunted transplacentally. In the rabbit, evidence exists that maternal fasting is associated with increased placental transfer of fatty acids from mother to fetus. Although few studies examining lipid metabolism in malnourished patients are available, a model to examine the effect of altered maternal lipid metabolism has been established by Roux and associates.[30,31] Postmaturity, which is one cause of decreased placental transfer of substrates, is induced in pregnant rabbits by injecting chorionic gonadotropin. Radioactive tracers are then used to measure the transplacental mobilization of fatty acids. These studies suggest that in the postmature rabbit, there is a breakdown in placental transport, as documented by a slower rate of fetal uptake of maternally injected [1-14C] palmitate, followed by a dramatic mobilization of fetal liver glycogen and fetal lipid stores.

Rosso measured the placental transfer of a nonmetabolizable amino acid, [14C]-α-aminoisobutyric acid, in starved (6% casein diet) and control (27% casein diet) maternal rats.[4] In malnourished rats, the radioactively labeled amino acid had a slower rate of disappearance from the maternal plasma and was transported in reduced amounts to the fetus. These data suggest that during severe maternal starvation in rats, placental transfer of basic nutrients is reduced overall. However, not all animal models support this concept. Similar studies performed in guinea pigs, using a nonmetabolizable amino acid, amino isobutyric acid, in calorie- or protein-restricted animals, showed that the placental transfer of the nonmetabolizable amino acid per gram of fetus was increased in the protein-restricted pigs but was not affected by calorie restriction.[32]

This suggests that the concept of the fetus as a parasite is an oversimplification. Some investigators now support the concept that the mother receives some preference for available nutrients, while others do not. Undoubtedly, normal maternal placental and fetal nutrition is the result of a variety of complex mechanisms. It is likely that in some situations, the maternal, and in others, the fetal, side of the placenta will receive preference for different nutrients.

Relationship of Poverty and Malnutrition

A major confounding variable of malnutrition is poverty. Essentially, all patients who are chronically malnourished, except for an occasional food faddist, are living in poverty. Poverty, with many of its associated variables, clearly has a detrimental effect on pregnancy outcome. Because malnutrition so closely interacts with poverty, it is important to control these confounding variables in all studies of malnutrition.

Affluent mothers tend to have bigger babies than poor mothers. The fact that there are known differences in dietary intake between groups is often seen as proof that small changes in maternal diet can markedly affect birth weight. However, mothers in different socioeconomic groups usually also differ in other factors that can affect fetal growth, including race, age, parity, height, general health, increased frequency of infections, education, genetics, and living and working conditions.

Naeye et al reported on 469 pregnancies in which a fetal or neonatal death occurred and autopsy data were available.[33] Patients were stratified into poor and nonpoor on the basis of family income and family size. The mean body weight of infants from lower income families was 17% lower than that of higher income families. The organ weights were affected disproportionately, and thymus, liver, and adrenal glands were affected most. No differences were seen, however, in brain weights between income groups. These findings suggest that decreased birth weight in low income patients is caused not only by decreased subcutaneous adipose tissue, but also by altered weight in some fetal organs. The decreased organ weight in fetuses of poor mothers was still seen when maternal race, age, parity, and height were excluded as confounding factors.

In addition to malnutrition, many additional factors can worsen developmental outcome of an infant living in poverty. They include the opportunity for formal and informal education and the infant's genetic makeup.

PREGNANCY IN AN OBESE WOMAN

Obesity is one of the most common nutritional problems complicating pregnancy. However, no universally accepted definition of obesity exists. Consequently, there can be no consensus as to its prevalence. A body weight of greater than 20% above the normal weight for height is often used to define obesity in nonpregnant patients. Fat thickness evaluated by calipers measuring various skin folds is also used. These standard definitions of obesity are difficult to apply to obstetric patients because the prepregnant weight often is not known. However, normal weight gain during pregnancy can be dramatic.

Maternal obesity in pregnancy is consequently defined by varying parameters. Some authors use an actual body weight of greater than 80–114 kg (175–250 lb).[34,35] Others use a body weight based on height, and the definitions vary from greater than 50–300% above ideal prepregnant weight for height.[36,37] The most frequent definition of *morbid obesity* is a maternal weight of above 90 kg (200 lb).[38] However, this definition ignores the mother's height and does not consider mothers with a prepegnancy weight of greater than 90 kg in contrast to those who reach this weight based on massive gain during pregnancy. More recent studies have used weight for height to define relative maternal size.[39,40]

There is general agreement that maternal medical complications, including chronic hypertension and diabetes mellitus, are increased in obese mothers (Table 21–3). Many authors feel that overweight women also are at increased risk for albuminuria and preeclampsia, although there is no evidence of an increased risk for eclampsia.[41] In addition, a history of previous stillborn infants and inadequate mater-

TABLE 21–3. PREVALENCES OF COMPLICATIONS (PERCENT) DURING PREGNANCY IN OBESE WOMEN

Complications	Prevalences (%) All Study Groups (Median and Range)	Fraction of Publications With Significantly Increased Risks in Obese Women
Hypertension	17 (5–44)	11/13
Edema	35 (30–41)	5/5
Albuminuria	13 (5–39)	4/5
Preeclampsia	17 (9–36)	5/8
Eclampsia	1 (0–6)	0/2
Glycosuria	8 (2–10)	1/4
Diabetes[a]	7 (0–20)	5/8
Thrombophlebitis	2 (0–10)	1/3
Varicose veins	28 (22–33)	3/3
Urinary tract infection	9 (3–11)	2/7
Antepartum hemorrhage	9 (4–14)	0/2
Prolonged pregnancy	10 (3–23)	2/4
Inadequate weight gain	24 (10–67)	6/6

[a] Latent or manifest.
Modified from Ruge et al[41] with permission.

TABLE 21–4. PREVALENCES OF PUERPERAL COMPLICATIONS IN OBESE WOMEN

Complications	Prevalences (%) All Study Groups (Median and Range)	Fraction of Publications With Significantly Increased Risks in Obese Women
Endometritis	3 (3–17)	1/3
Urinary tract infection	8 (5–16)	1/4
Wound infection	5 (4–5)	1/2[a]
Thrombophlebitis	3 (0–9)	2/4
Subinvolution	22 (10–35)	1/2
Maternal mortality	0 (0–4)	0/4

[a] One publication demonstrated a decreased risk in obese women.
Adapted from Ruge et al[41] with permission.

nal weight gain also are observed more frequently in obese women. An increased frequency of fetal macrosomia and increased induction rate for medical complications have led some authors to suggest that obese women are at increased risk for cesarean delivery. Obese mothers also may be at increased risk for postpartum complications, such as endometritis, wound infection, thrombophlebitis, and urinary tract infection (Table 21–4). Although obesity is clearly an operative risk factor, a recent study suggests that varying degrees of maternal obesity and accompanying medical problems, such as hypertension and diabetes mellitus, may not be associated with greater operative morbidity.[42] Anemia is generally less frequent in obese than in nonobese patients. Obese mothers generally are also older and more parous than nonobese mothers. Increased age and parity may then represent confounding factors for a variety of medical complications. The fact that older, more parous mothers are likely to be overweight is thought to be one reason why birth weight tends to increase with advancing maternal age and parity. Past studies of obese mothers also report a significantly increased incidence of twin gestations. This observation probably also is related to the fact that twins are more common with increased maternal age and parity.

It is generally accepted that obese mothers deliver infants with larger mean birth weights. An increase in macrosomic (>4000 g) neonates and a decrease in low birth weight (<2500 g) neonates occur in obese mothers, even though maternal weight loss is common in these pregnancies. Whether these infants are larger because of increased deposition of subcutaneous fat or because of enhanced maturity is discussed in the following paragraphs.

In earlier studies of obese mothers, prematurity was defined as a neonatal birth weight below 2500 g. As in previously discussed malnutrition studies, no classification of pediatric age–weight relationships was performed.[12] These earlier studies suggest that obese mothers were three to five times less likely to deliver premature infants. In the Collaborative Perinatal Project, obese mothers were found to carry a threefold decrease in risk of delivering a low birth weight infant at term.[12] This study was, however, also performed before the classification of neonates as small-for-gestational age. As noted earlier, this newer classification representing low birth weight can be caused by either prematurity or poor intrauterine growth (small-for-gestational age).

In pregnant obese patients, the prepregnant maternal weight carries the most significant influence on birth weight. Weight gain during pregnancy is clearly less important. This is converse to what happens to nonobese mothers, in whom maternal weight gain during pregnancy has the overriding impact on birth weight. Consequently, it appears that obese women can mobilize large nutritional reserves that supply fuel for fetal growth. Kliegman et al examined the fetal growth of infants of obese mothers by comparing 12 neonates born to massively obese mothers to a group of neonates born to nonobese controls.[43] Diabetic patients were excluded. Comparison of the ponderal indices between the two groups indicated augmented body weight in infants of obese mothers but no increase in linear growth. Triceps and scapular skin fold thicknesses were significantly increased in neonates of obese mothers. This suggests that the increased birth weight of infants of overweight patients is contributed partly by an increased deposition of neonatal subcutaneous adipose tissue, without a concomitant increase in body length.

Gross et al compared a group of 279 women who weighed at least 90 kg during pregnancy (obese group) to a large number of normal weight women (nonobese group), extending on a previous study (Table 21–5).[38] Based on infant weight and pediatric estimate of infant maturity in the nursery, obese mothers were found to be only one half as likely to deliver a small-for-gestational age infant and 2.5 times more likely to deliver a large-for-gestational age infant than the nonobese mothers. Obese mothers also were found to be only about one half as likely to deliver preterm and 3.5 times more likely to deliver post-term than nonobese women. It is important that the shift toward higher infant birth weight percentiles in obese mothers was obvious, even in the presence of an increase in factors that might be expected to lower birth weight, such as inadequate maternal weight gain, chronic hypertension, and multiple

TABLE 21.5 COMPARISONS OF GESTATIONAL DURATION AND BIRTH WEIGHT OF INFANTS OF OBESE AND NONOBESE GRAVIDAS

	Obese (*N* = 284)	Nonobese (*N* = 2481)	*P*
Birth weight (g)			
Low birth weight (<2500 g)	5.6	12.2	<.001
Macrosomia (>4000 g)	15.1	4.2	<.0001
Gestational duration			
Preterm (<38 wk)			
Obstetric estimate	9.9	19.9	<.0001
Pediatric estimate	8.1	14.3	<.005
Post-term (>42 wk)			
Obstetric estimate	6.3	4.2	NS
Pediatric estimate	4.6	1.3	<.0001
Age–weight classification			
Small-for-gestational age	3.2	6.2	<.05
Large-for-gestational age	31.0	12.6	<.0001

[a] NS, not significant.
From Gross et al[38] with permission.

gestation (see Table 21–3). Because the obese mother also is at increased risk for glucose intolerance, this factor also could raise birth weight percentiles. Spellacy suggested a "high-risk triad" of obesity, diabetes, and postdates for the development of macrosomia.[44]

The higher fetal weight in infants of obese mothers is caused not only by increased adipose tissue mass, but also by increased maturity in these babies. The increased deposition of fat reported by some authors in infants of obese mothers and an increased level of maturity seen by others are not inconsistent. Both factors could, alone or in combination, be responsible for the increased size of these babies.

A low perinatal mortality rate has been observed in many studies of obese mothers. This is even more striking in view of major risk factors that are apparent in these patients. Obese mothers may experience an overriding metabolic effect that overcomes multiple risk factors that predispose to small-for-gestational-age infants. What this factor is and whether it is related to an altered maternal fetal flux of metabolites is unknown. One recent study in British literature questions the perinatal benefit of maternal obesity and suggests that premature infants born to obese women may be at increased risk for perinatal mortality.[45] After adjusting for major demographic and antenatal factors, maternal obesity was second in importance only to gestational age in predicting the death of preterm infants. Unlike term gestations, maternal obesity was associated with reduced birth weight and a nearly fourfold increase in the relative risk for death among preterm infants. Also, an increase in large-for-gestational age infants can be expected to increase the incidence of delivery trauma and of other neonatal morbidity.

Convincing evidence now exists that body size and relative obesity are the result of a strong genetic component[46], placing infants of obese women at long-term risk for obesity. Preliminary studies suggest that reduced energy expenditure, particularly on physical activity, may be an important factor in the rapid weight gain observed during the first year of life in infants born to overweight mothers.[47] The long-term significance of this finding is unknown. Among Pima Indians, maternal diabetes is more predictive of obesity in offspring at 5–19 years of age than birth weight or relative maternal body size.[48]

Weight gain in pregnancy is the consequence of the relationship between amount of energy in the diet and calories consumed for fuel. It is generally reassuring that the increased maternal metabolic requirements of pregnancy and fetal nutritional demands are met with varying amounts of food stuff apparently left over to serve as maternal storage requirements. Maternal fuel is stored during pregnancy primarily as adipose tissue. Consequently, fat can be accumulated rapidly during pregnancy. In an otherwise healthy, normal-weight pregnant patient, this is not a problem because extra fat stores can easily be lost postpartum. However, some patients become obese for the first time during pregnancy, and others become overweight later in life because of weight gained, and not lost, during successive pregnancies.[49] The obese patient that is encouraged to gain weight during pregnancy appears less likely to lose the weight postpartum.[50] These potential effects should be considered when the optimal weight gain during pregnancy is evaluated for an obese mother.

Recommendations for weight gain during pregnancy in an obese mother are variable. Early studies emphasized the importance of good maternal nutrition on fetal growth in nonobese mothers but recommended no weight gain in obese mothers. This was partially because of the belief that increased maternal weight gain caused toxemia. More recently, all mothers, irrespective of their prepregnancy weights, have been encouraged to gain approximately 12.5 kg through an entire pregnancy. Such practice is based on the following findings discussed previously in this chapter:

1. A decreasing perinatal mortality rate is seen with increasing pregnancy weight gain.
2. A positive correlation between severe maternal malnutrition and low birth weight infants has been described.
3. In nonobese patients, increasing pregnancy weight gain is associated with increasing birth weight.
4. Data from the Collaborative Perinatal Project have suggested that a maternal weight gain of greater than 18 kg during pregnancy was associated with the best neurologic outcome in infants at 1 year of age.[13]
5. Ketonuria during pregnancy, in studies of diabetic and malnourished mothers[22,23], possibly has been correlated with abnormal fetal development.

None of these findings has been examined in studies considering the role of maternal nutritional reserves on fetal growth, so the following findings are often overlooked when optimal weight gain in an obese patient is established.

1. The positive correlation between maternal weight gain and birth weight is lost when maternal obesity is considered[12] (see Figure 20–4).
2. The association of poor fetal growth with decreased maternal caloric intake has been observed primarily in severely malnourished nonobese patients.
3. There is an increased incidence of fetal macrosomia in obese pregnant patients, even when pregnancy weight gain is inadequate.[36]
4. Weight gain during pregnancy may increase the obese mother's risk of enhanced obesity in the future.

In the nonobese patient, poor maternal weight gain can have an important effect on fetal outcome. The unresolved relationship between inadequate maternal weight gain and fetal development in an obese mother can be addressed by asking whether decreased weight gain during pregnancy is associated with the following:

1. Higher perinatal mortality rate
2. Fetal growth retardation

3. Worsened long-term neurologic outcome
4. Adverse metabolic changes in obese pregnant patients
5. Tissue changes in animals

Data from the Collaborative Perinatal Project suggest that the maternal weight gain associated with the lowest perinatal mortality rate varied with the mothers' prepregnant stores.[19] Mothers were divided into three weight-for-height groups based on their prepregnancy weight, using Metropolitan Life Insurance tables (<90%, 90–135%, and >135% ideal body weight). Several variables that can affect outcome, such as maternal age, parity, race, and medical complications, were controlled for. An attempt to control for the multiple effects of socioeconomic status was made by stratifying the patients by family income. The relationship between weight gain during pregnancy and perinatal mortality rate is shown in Figure 21–2. The authors conclude that the pregnancy weight gain associated with the lowest perinatal mortality rate in underweight mothers was 30 lb; in normally proportioned mothers, 20 lbs; and in overweight mothers, 16 lb. This is one of the few studies that suggests that maternal nutritional stores, present before pregnancy, may be an important factor in determining the appropriate amount of maternal weight to be gained during pregnancy. However, even this study must be interpreted cautiously. The increasing perinatal mortality rate observed in the study with a maternal weight gain of above 16 lb in obese females may have been caused by massive edema from severe hypertension. Thus, the hypertensive disease could have been the cause of the increased perinatal mortaltiy rate, rather than factors related to nutrition. However, it was not noted whether the regression lines, shown in Figure 21–2, demonstrated statistically valid differences in the perinatal mortality rate between the three groups.

This study is nevertheless important because it suggests that the optimal weight gain during pregnancy varies with maternal prepregnancy weight. It appears that an increased pregnancy weight gain is important in the underweight mother while a decreased weight gain is preferred in the obese mother.

Early studies reported that obese patients who lost weight during pregnancy still had larger babies than nonobese patients who gained up to 20 lbs.[51] In the Collaborative Perinatal Project, there was little effect of increasing pregnancy weight gain on birth weight in patients weighing more than 190 lb (See Figs. 20–4 and 20–5). This finding was not related to the fact that diabetes mellitus is more common in obese patients because patients with diabetes were excluded from these earlier studies. However, it is likely that glucose intolerance was not diagnosed as reliably then as now. Edwards and associates[36] recently compared a group of nondiabetic massively obese patients (>150% above ideal body weight) to a nonobese group. Obese mothers with inadequate pregnancy weight gain (<12 lb during all of pregnancy) delivered infants with an average birth weight of 3300 g. This was 600 g more than the nonobese patients with inadequate weight gain. In fact, obese patients with inadequate weight gain had larger babies than nonobese patients with normal maternal weight gain.

Decreased maternal weight gain during pregnancy is related to an increased frequency of small-for-gestational age neonates in underweight and normal-weight mothers. It is unlikely that this relationship also is present in obese mothers. Too few studies have examined this concept in obese mothers to reach statistically valid conclusions at this time.[52,53]

The improvement of infant outcome on motor, mental, and neurologic tests has been associated with increased pregnancy weight gain in unselected obstetric populations. However, this has not been studied in the obese population. As noted in the previous section, increased adipose tissue stores in an obese mother may allow for more caloric reserves which the fetus can draw on for growth. Whether these caloric stores can lessen the effect on neurologic development is unknown.

There are numerous parallels between metabolic changes secondary to obesity and those related to pregnancy. Obesity in the nonpregnant patient is associated with increased circulating insulin concentrations and insulin resistance. Pregnancy also is characterized by hyperinsulinism and insulin resistance. Insulin requirements with obesity are decreased by weight reduction. Insulin requirements during pregnancy are reversed by delivery. Despite these similarities, few studies of the metabolic changes in the pregnant obese patient have been conducted. Borburg, et al[54] compared a group of patients who were 90–110% of their ideal weight with a group of mildly obese women above 120% of their ideal body weight. The obese patients were divided into two groups—those in whom carbohydrate intake was restricted to 150–180 g/d and those allowed to eat according to their appetite. The dieting group lost a mean of 2.3 kg, while the nondieting group gained a mean of 4.9 kg during the pregnancy. At 16 weeks' gestation, the basal- and glucose-stimulated insulin concentrations were higher in the two obese groups than in the nonobese group. The mean basal- and glucose-stimulated insulin concentrations doubled between 16 and 36 weeks in the obese and nonobese subjects. However, a much smaller increase in insulin concentration occurred between 16 and 36 weeks in the dieting obese compared to the nondieting obese patients. The urines of the nonobese, obese dieting, and obese nondieting patients were negative for ketones at every antenatal clinical visit, and no significant difference was seen in the mean fasting blood levels of β-hydroxybutyrate between the two obese groups. As previously discussed, ketonuria is always a concern in pregnant patients because it has been associated with impaired intellectual development in infants. This study was therefore important in demonstrating that carbohydrates could be restricted to a degree resulting in maternal weight loss without causing elevation of maternal serum or of urinary ketones. The only difference between the dieting and nondieting obese groups in this study was the lower insulin levels in patients who dieted to the point of weight loss. Because there is no known clinical importance of lower maternal insulin levels, this observation should not be used as a reason to restrict diets in obese pregnant patients to the point of weight loss.

Preliminary studies also have examined the effect of food restriction on maternal tissue changes in an animal model of obese rats.[55] Restriction of food intake by 60% in both obese and nonobese rats resulted in weight loss in all maternal animals. The weight loss in obese rats was entirely caused by loss of body fat, whereas nonobese rats lost lean tissue as well. Obese rats had the same carcass weight and composition as the *ad libitum* fed nonobese rats at the end of the food-restriction period. However, the fetal and placental weights were reduced 25% in the food-restricted obese and nonobese rats. This suggests that the rat fetus cannot parasitize increased maternal stores in the genetically obese rat.

Pregnancy After Jejunoileal Bypass

Surgical procedures to manage severe obesity have been used increasingly over the last 20 years. The most common procedure is the jejunoileal bypass. It can be associated with multiple maternal complications during pregnancy, including severe diarrhea, metabolic derangements, and liver failure. Pregnancy outcome in these patients has been reviewed in detail elsewhere.[56]

Metabolic changes can include reductions in serum potassium, sodium, calcium, magnesium, total protein, albumin, cholesterol, and triglycerides. There are no convincing data that pregnancy worsens the diarrhea or the metabolic changes associated with this surgery.

An adverse effect on fetal growth and delivery of a small-for-gestational age infant was initially considered a common complication of pregnancy after a jejunoileal bypass. Hey[57] reported on a group of 38 patients following jejunoileal bypass, and compared seven pregnancies that occurred before the bypass to 14 that occurred after the procedure. Birth weight, body length, and placental weight were all significantly reduced in pregnancies following surgery. Consequently, there can be no doubt that this type of gastrointestinal bypass surgery has a significant effect on fetal growth. Of 21 pregnancies after jejunoileal bypass reported by Ingardia, four (19%) of the neonates were diagnosed as small-for-gestational age.[58] Knudsen noted an increased rate of prematurity and growth retardation in 77 women after intestinal bypass surgery for obesity.[59] Interestingly, Deitel[60] reported not only a lower mean birth weight after intestinal bypass, but also a significant decline in maternal medical complications during these pregnancies.

A review of the literature[59] found six out of 179 (3.4%) pregnancies with serious malformations, including hydrocephalus and esophageal atresia. No specificity exists among these malformations. Too few pregnancies have been studied to determine whether the metabolic changes associated with bypass surgery confer an increased risk for fetal malformation.

Several recommendations can be made regarding pregnancies in patients after jejunoileal bypass. Fat-soluble vitamins and perhaps vitamin B_{12} are less readily absorbed in these patients. Consequently, supplementation is recommended during pregnancy. The risk to deliver a growth-retarded neonate appears the greatest during the period of most rapid weight loss. This time period varies from 6 months to 2 years after surgery. Because of this observation, the recommendation was initially made that pregnancy be deferred for at least 2 years after any jejunoileal bypass. However, no definite relation between the time elapsed from surgery and birth weight has been observed[59], suggesting that the effect on fetal growth persists longer than 2 years after bypass surgery. At present, it appears justified to make recommendations on an individualized basis, depending on the maternal condition until maternal diarrhea has decreased, body weight has stabilized, and liver failure has been ruled out. During pregnancy, these patients should then be followed carefully to document normal fetal growth.

NUTRITIONAL ASSESSMENT DURING PREGNANCY

The major nutritional assessment used to document the adequacy of diet in pregnancy is maternal weight gain based on total weight and the pattern of weight gain as pregnancy progresses. A major outcome variable used to retrospectively assess the maternal diet is neonatal birth weight. Weight gain during pregnancy is used by the obstetrician to measure the relationship between calories in maternal diet and maternal fetal needs. A slow, steady maternal weight gain is a reassuring sign.

Pregnancy weight gain and neonatal birth weight, however, are nonspecific and can be influenced by many factors other than nutrition. This limits their usefulness in research protocols.

Medical History

There are historic and clinical factors that may be important in predicting increased nutritional risk during pregnancy. These factors, as listed by the Task Force on Nutrition of the American College of Obstetricians and Gynecologists are shown in Table 21–6.[61] As noted previously, poor maternal nutrition has not been documented as a primary cause of specific pregnancy complications in some of the risk groups listed. However, there are valid theoretical reasons that patients in each of these groups may be at increased nutritional risk during pregnancy. This list is therefore useful as a clinical screening tool for pregnant patients. Patient groups at nutritional risk include the following: Women with short interpregnancy intervals or short time intervals between previous lactation and subsequent pregnancy are at risk. Pregnancy and lactation can deplete body stores and perhaps leave less fuel available to supply normal fetal growth in adolescent pregnancy. The expectant adolescent mother is at risk because the demands for growth of the maternal body in the pregnant teenager are added to the known nutritional demands of pregnancy. Patients in whom pregnancy follows immediately after therapy with oral contraceptives may be at increased risk because of the known deficiencies of folate and vitamin B_6 induced by birth control pills.

In the practical setting, the obstetrician rarely sets out to perform any laboratory assessment of maternal nutritional adequacy. Although laboratory tests routinely obtained during pregnancy, such as urinalysis, complete blood count, and 2-hour postprandial blood sugar, are all potentially related to nutrition, more direct tests of dietary adequacy are not included in the routine prenatal evaluation of the pregnant woman.

The urinary urea nitrogen to total nitrogen ratio and urinary urea nitrogen to creatinine ratio, measured in spot and 24-hour urine, have been suggested to assess maternal protein intake.[62] Although both have been correlated with maternal dietary intake and neonatal birth weight, neither test is used clinically. Other parameters, such as urinary acetone, serum folate, vitamin B_{12}, calcium, phosphorus, triglycerides, cholesterol, albumin, serum iron, and iron-binding capacity have some value in assessing nutrition

TABLE 21–6. WOMEN WITH POTENTIALLY INCREASED NUTRITIONAL RISK DURING PREGNANCY

Past Medical History
Poor reproductive history
Three or more pregnancies within 2 years
Short interval following lactation with previous pregnancy
Adolescent (younger than 16 years old)
Pregnancy within 6 months of taking oral contraceptives
Therapeutic diet for chronic disease
Food faddist
Heavy smoker or history of drug or alcohol abuse
Economic deprivation
Clinical Course—Present Pregnancy
Less than 9 lb weight gain first half of pregnancy
Weight gain less than 2 lb/mo during second and third trimesters
Weight gain greater than 2 lb/wk
Anemia (hemoglobin $<$11.0 g, hematocrit $<$33%)

Adapted from Task Force on Maternal Nutrition.[61]

in individual patients but are obviously not specifically related to pregnancy.

NUTRITIONAL COUNSELING DURING PREGNANCY

Nutritional counseling during pregnancy is primarily based on maternal prepregnancy weight, pregnancy weight gain, and dietary histories of actual protein and energy intake. Although abnormal maternal weight gain is a crude index of dietary intake, this is usually the first sign observed by the clinician.

The primary goal of managing maternal weight gain during pregnancy should be to advise a weight gain consistent with optimal fetal outcome. A second goal, often ignored, is to keep the mother from accumulating excess adipose tissue so that, after delivery, she can attain her prepregnancy weight.

The average weight gain during pregnancy in a healthy patient eating without restrictions is 24–28 lb (11–13 kg).[63] This represents an average not determined by neonatal outcome, which can vary greatly, even in normal pregnancy. In addition to absolute numbers, the time pattern of weight gain during pregnancy also is very important. A weight gain of 8 lb during the first twenty weeks of pregnancy, followed by a gain of 1 pound per week during the final 20 weeks represents the average. Patients gaining less than 8 lb in the first half of pregnancy or less than 2 lb/mo during the final 20 weeks should have detailed dietary histories taken by a person trained in nutritional counseling.

The pattern of maternal weight gain also is important in predicting patients who may have an increased risk of obesity after pregnancy. Patients gaining an average of 24–28 lb during pregnancy add only approximately 8 lb of fat stores, which can easily be lost postpartum. The patient who gains an excessive amount of weight during the first half of pregnancy is, however, at risk for permanent obesity. For example, a patient who gains up to 30 lb in the first 20 weeks of pregnancy has gained up to 25 lb of maternal fat stores. Because the majority of weight gained during the latter half of pregnancy represents supportive tissues to fetus or placenta, this patient must still be advised to gain 20 lb during the final 20 weeks. A recent retrospective study of 158 low risk mothers concluded that poor maternal weight gain between 28 and 32 weeks' gestation was predictive of small-for-gestational age births, even when corrected for other variables, including overall weight gain and weight at the first prenatal visit.[64]

Dietary counseling, given to the normal-weight patient, is relatively simple. The recommended daily requirements are shown in Appendix I. In the patient who is well nourished before pregnancy, the additional requirements due to pregnancy can be supplied in one quart of whole milk (30 g of protein and 600 kcal).[49] This recommendation of one quart of milk, in addition to a normally balanced diet, is all that is needed for energy and protein requirements of a normal pregnancy. The recommendations for iron and vitamin supplements vary between countries and are detailed in Chapter 19. In the United States, supplements of iron, Vitamin B_{12}, and folate are usually recommended in the amounts shown in Appendix I.

Underweight pregnant women are at higher risk than normal patients. The risk is primarily an increased frequency of spontaneous abortions and delivering more small-for-gestational age infants. Nutritional counseling is indicated at the first prenatal visit so that patients with inadequate diets can be detected and receive appropriate dietary counseling. This group of patients should be advised to gain the usual 24–28 lb, and nutritional counseling should outline the appropriate kilocalories and protein intake.

A more aggressive approach has been advised by others. It has been suggested that underweight females should receive additional calories and protein so that they gain up to 40–50 lb during the pregnancy. The intent is to replace body stores during the pregnancy in addition to gaining the usual 24–28 lb. There is no clear evidence that such additional supplementation improves pregnancy outcome. In fact, some data detailed earlier in this chapter suggest that a high protein supplement should be avoided. The most suitable approach to the undernourished patient is to recommend the protein and caloric intake and pregnancy weight gain that is optimal for normal patients.

Nutritional counseling in the obese pregnant patient should reflect several special considerations. The question arises as to whether the obese woman's adipose tissue reserves serve to supply some of the fuel needed for fetal growth, resulting in a lower requirement for maternal carbohydrate intake. The effect of diet control on the frequency of large-for-gestational-age infants is not known. An additional concern is whether the obese woman increases her risk of more severe obesity in the future by gaining extra weight during pregnancy.

While much is unknown, it appears that weight loss is not advised during pregnancy. While obese patients have likely been overnourished in caloric intake at some time during their lives, they may not necessarily be well nourished at the time of pregnancy. Therefore, a careful dietary history should be taken in all of these patients to determine the actual caloric and protein intake at that time. Some practical recommendations can be made for overweight patients. For patients who are 120–150% above ideal body weight, a routine recommendation for weight gain and dietary intake should be given. For massively obese patients (>150% above ideal body weight), some variation in weight gain is recommended. While some authors have recommended the usual 24-to-28 lb weight gain[65], others[66] suggest that weight gain during pregnancy should be based on the mother's prepregnancy weight for height, with a minimal weight gain of 7 kg for women with a prepregnancy weight over 120% of the "standard."

Experts in nutrition will continue the search for the maternal diet associated with optimal pregnancy outcome. Some practical guidelines, however, can be established: As discussed elsewhere[67], such a practical approach will result in an excellent outcome.

1. The healthy expectant mother should be advised to continue to eat a balanced diet. Food intake should be similar to that before pregnancy, with the addition of a quart of whole milk.
2. The patient should be questioned to ensure that there is an adequate food intake, particularly in patients of lower socioeconomic class.
3. Maternal weight gain should be recorded to be certain the patient is gaining weight at a rate equivalent to approximately 20 lb for the entire pregnancy. A wide range of weight gain is associated with normal outcome.
4. The patient should be questioned throughout the pregnancy to uncover any food fads or other bizarre diets.
5. For underweight mothers, the following is appropriate:
   a. The clinician should be more aggressive in obtaining a history of dietary intake and arranging for formal dietary counseling.
   b. The patient should receive formal dietary instruc-

tions, including the proper number of calories and amount of protein, using foods the patient is familiar with.

c. A nutritionally oriented follow-up should be provided throughout pregnancy.

d. There is no evidence that adding extra calories beyond the recommended amount for normal mothers improves pregnancy outcome.

6. For overweight mothers the following is appropriate:
   a. In mildly obese patients (>120% but <150% standard weight for height), the usual weight gain and dietary intake for normal pregnancy should be recommended.
   b. In massively obese patients (>150% standard weight for height), the mother should not lose weight during pregnancy. The optimal amount of maternal weight gain during pregnancy is not clear. Some clinicians recommend the usual 24 to 28 lb, but most feel that 10 to 15 lb is adequate.
   c. The patient should be encouraged to lose the excess weight postpartum.

Maternal nutrition is generally accepted as one of the most important maternal factors affecting pregnancy outcome. Proper nutrition is an important component of general health of mother and fetus. Poorly controlled studies of severe maternal starvation show that body stores of adipose tissue before pregnancy and maternal intake during pregnancy directly affect the birth weight of the offspring. However, the importance of less severe maternal malnutrition must be kept in perspective because there are many other factors that are related to poor pregnancy outcome. Osofsky has evaluated one of the previous maternal dietary surveys in which prematurity was defined as less than 2500 g birth weight.[68] Of the explained variance in birth weight in the study, 25% was accounted for by gestational age, 7% by maternal size, 7% by maternal weight gain during pregnancy, 1.5% by maternal caloric intake, and 0.8% by maternal protein intake. More than 50% of the variance in birth weight was unexplained and leaves many unanswered questions regarding maternal nutrition and neonatal outcome. Because of the many non-nutritional variables affecting neonatal outcome, careful prospective randomized trials are needed to answer many of the remaining questions.

REFERENCES

1. Latham MC, Cobos F. The effects of malnutrition on intellectual development and learning. *Am J Public Health.* 1971;61:1307.
2. Lederman SA, Rosso P. Effects of protein and carbohydrate supplements on fetal and maternal weight and on body composition in food-restricted rats. *Am J Clin Nutr.* 1980;33:1912.
3. Naismith DJ. The fetus as a parasite. *Proc Nutr Soc.* 1969;28:25.
4. Rosso P. Maternal–fetal exchange during protein malnutrition in the rat. Placental transfer of alpha amino isobutyric acid. *J Nutr.* 1977;107:2002.
5. Stein Z, Susser M, Rush D. Prenatal nutrition and birthweight. Experiments and quasi-experiments in the past decade. *J Reprod Med.* 1978;21:287.
6. Stein Z, Susser M, Saegner G, et al. Nutrition and mental performance. *Science.* 1972;178:708.
7. Hytten FE. Nutrition in pregnancy. *Postgrad Med J.* 1979;55:295.
8. Lechtig A, Habicht JP, Delgado H, et al. Effect of food supplementation during pregnancy on birthweight. *Pediatr.* 1975;56:508.
9. Rush D, Stein Z, Susser M. A randomized controlled trial of prenatal nutrition supplementation in New York City. *Pediatr.* 1980;65:683.
10. Lawrence M, Coward WA, Lawrence F, et al. Fat gain during pregnancy in rural African women: The effect of season and dietary status. *Am J Clin Nutr.* 1987;45:1442.
11. Higgins AC. Nutritional status and the outcome of pregnancy. *Can Diet Assoc.* 1976;37:17.
12. Niswander KR, Singer JE, Westphal M, et al. Weight gain during pregnancy and prepregnancy weight. Association with birthweight of term gestation. *Obstet Gynecol.* 1969;33:482.
13. Singer JE, Westphal M, Niswander K. Relationship of weight gain during pregnancy to birth weight and infant growth and development in the first year of life. A report from the Collaborative Study of Cerebral Palsy. *Obstet Gynecol.* 1968;31:417.
14. Hastings-Roberts MM, Zeman FJ. Effects of protein deficiency, pair-feeding, or diet supplementation on maternal, fetal and placental growth in rats. *J Nutr.* 1977;107:973.
15. Rosso P. Maternal nutrition, nutrient exchange, and fetal growth. *Curr Concepts Nutr.* 1977;5:3.
16. King JC. Protein metabolism during pregnancy. *Clin Perinatol.* 1975;2:243.
17. Riopelle AJ, Penelope AH. Nutritional and environmental factors affecting gestational length in rhesus monkeys. *Am J Clin Nutr.* 1975;28:1170.
18. Tuazon MA, VanRaaij JM, Hautvast JG, et al. Energy requirements of pregnancy in the Philippines. *Lancet.* 1987;2:1129.
19. Naeye RL. Weight gain and the outcome of pregnancy. *Am J Obstet Gynecol.* 1979;135:3.
20. Duncan EHL, Baird D, Thomson AM. The causes and prevention of stillbirths and first week deaths. I. The evidence of vital statistics. *Br J Obstet Gynaecol.* (London) 1952;59:183.
21. Winick M. Cellular growth in intrauterine malnutrition. *Pediatr Clin North Am.* 1970;17:69.
22. Churchill JA. FActors in intrauterine impoverishment. In: Moghissi KS, Evans TN, eds. *Nutritional Impacts on Women Throughout Life with Emphasis on Reproduction.* Hagerstown, PA: Harper and Row; 1977:72.
23. Churchill JA, Berendes HW, Nemore J. Neuropsychology deficits in children of diabetic mothers. *Am J Obstet Gynecol.* 1969;105:257.
24. Naeye RL, Chez RA. Effects of maternal acetonuria and low pregnancy weight gain on children's psychomotor development. *Am J Obstet Gynecol.* 1981;139:189.
25. Stehbens JA, Baker GH, Kitchell M. Outcome at ages 1, 3 and 5 years of children born to diabetic women. *Am J Obstet Gynecol.* 1977;127:408.
26. Thomson AM. Diet in pregnancy. 3. Diet in relation to the course and outcome of pregnancy. *Br J Nutr.* 1959;13:509.
27. McGanity WJ, Cannon RO, Bridgforth EB, et al. The Vanderbilt cooperative study of maternal and infant nutrition. Relationship of obstetric performance to nutrition. *Am J Obstet Gynecol.* 1954;67:501.
28. Hay WW, Sparks JW, Wilkening RB, et al. Partition of maternal glucose production between conceptus and maternal tissues in sheep. *Am J Physiol.* 1983;245:E347.
29. Warshaw JB. Fatty acid metabolism during development. *Semin Perinat.* 1979;3:131.
30. Roux JF, Yoshioka T. Lipid metabolism in the fetus during development. *Clin Obstet Gynecol.* 1970;13:595.
31. Mosse D, Roux JF, Harlow A, et al. *In vitro* palmitate and glucose metabolism in the postmature fetus. *Am J Obstet Gynecol.* 1980;136:505.
32. Young M, Widdowson EM, The influence of diets deficient in energy or in protein on conceptus weight and placental transfer of a nonmetabolizable amino acid in the guinea pig. *Biol Neonate.* 1975;27:184.
33. Naeye RL, Diener MM, Harcke HT, et al. Relation of poverty and race to birth weight and organ and cell structure in the newborn. *Ped Res.* 1971;5:17.
34. Roopnarinesingh SS, Pathak UN. Obesity in the Jamaican parturient. *J Obstet Gynaecol Br Commonw.* 1970;77:895.
35. Tracy TA, Miller GL. Obstetric problems of the massively obese. *Obstet Gynecol.* 1969;33:204.
36. Edwards LE, Dickes WF, Alton IR. Pregnancy in the massively obese: Course, outcome and obesity prognosis of the infant. *Am J Obstet Gynecol.* 1978;131:479.
37. Freedman MA, Wilds PL, George WM. Grotesque obesity: A serious complication of labor and delivery. *S Med J.* 1972;65:732.
38. Gross TL, Sokol RJ, King KC. Obesity in pregnancy: Risks and outcome. *Obstet Gynecol.* 1980;56:446.
39. Abrams BF, Laros RK. Prepregnancy weight, weight gain and birth weight. *Am J Obstet Gynecol.* 1986;154:503.
40. Garbaciak JA, Richter M, Miller S, et al. Maternal weight and pregnancy complications. *Am J Obstet Gynecol.* 1985;152:238.
41. Ruge S, Anderson T. Obstetric risk in obesity. An analysis of the literature. *Obstet Gynecol Survey.* 1985;40:57.
42. Wolfe HM, Gross TL, Sokol RJ, et al. Determinants of morbidity in women delivered by cesarean. *Obstet Gynecol.* 1988;71:691.
43. Kliegman R, Gross TL, Morton S, et al. Intrauterine growth and postnatal fasting metabolism in infants of obese mothers. *J Pediatr.* 1984;104:601.
44. Spellacy WN, Miller S, Winegar A, et al. Macrosomia: Maternal characteristics and infant complications. *Obstet Gynecol.* 1985;66:158.
45. Lucas A, Morley R, Cole TJ, et al. Maternal fatness and viability of preterm infants. *Br Med J.* 1988;296:1495.
46. Stunkard AJ, Sorenson TIA, Hanes C, et al. An adoption study of human obesity. *N Engl J Med.* 1986;314:193.

47. Roberts SE, Savage J, Coward WA, et al. Energy expenditures and intake in infants born to lean and overweight mothers. *N Engl J Med.* 188;318:461.
48. Pettitt DJ, Knowler WC, Bennett PH, et al. Obesity in offspring of diabetic Pima Indian women despite normal birthweight. *Diabetes Care.* 1987;10:76.
49. Pitkin RM. Nutritional support in obstetrics and gynecology. *Clin Obstet Gynecol.* 1976;19:489.
50. Greene GW, Smiciklas-Wright H, Schell TO, et al. Postpartum weight change: How much of the weight gained in pregnancy will be lost after delivery? *Obstet Gynecol.* 1988;71:701.
51. Eastman NJ, Jackson E. Weight relationships in pregnancy. *Obstet Gynecol Surv.* 1968;23:1003.
52. Harrison GG, Udall JN, Morrow G. Maternal obesity, weight gain in pregnancy and infant birth weight. *Am J Obstet Gynecol.* 1980;136:411.
53. Luke B, Dickenson C, Petrie RH. Intrauterine growth: Correlations of maternal nutritional status and rates of gestational weight gain. *Europ J Obstet Gynecol Reprod Biol.* 1981;12:113.
54. Borberg C, Gillmer MDG, Brunner EJ, et al. Obesity in pregnancy: The effect of dietary advice. *Diabetes Care.* 1980;3:476.
55. Lederman SA, Rosso P. Effects of obesity, food restriction and pregnancy on fetal and maternal weight and on body composition in rats. *J Nutr.* 1981;111:2162.
56. Woods JR, Brinkman CR. The jejunoileal bypass and pregnancy. *Obstet Gynecol Surv.* 1978;33:697.
57. Hey H, Niebuhr-Jorgensen U. Jejunoileal bypass surgery in obesity. Gynecological and obstetrical aspects. *Acta Obstet Gynecol Scand.* 1981;60:135.
58. Ingardia JC, Fisher RJ. Pregnancy after jejunoileal bypass surgery and the small-for-gestational-age infant. *Obstet Gynecol.* 1978;52:215.
59. Knudsen LB, Kallam B. Intestinal bypass operation and pregnancy outcome. *Acta Obstet Gynecol Scand.* 1986;65:831.
60. Deitel M, Stone E, Kassam HA. Gynecologic–obstetric changes after loss of massive excess weight following bariatic surgery. *J Am Coll Nutr.* 1988;7:142.
61. Task Force on Nutrition. *Assessment of Maternal Nutrition.* Washington, DC: American College of Obstetricians and Gynecologists and American Dietetic Association; 1978.
62. Luke B. *Maternal Nutrition.* Boston, MA: Little, Brown and Co; 1979:45.
63. Thomson AM, Billewicz WZ. Clinical significance of weight trends during pregnancy. *Br Med J.* 1957;1:243.
64. Lawton FG, Masson GC, Kelly KA, et al. Poor maternal weight gain between 28 and 32 weeks gestation may predict small-for-gestational age infants. *Br J Obstet Gynecol.* 1988;95:884.
65. Anonymous. Nutritional management of obese pregnant women. *Bulletin, Pan Am Health Organization.* 1979;13:201.
66. Rosso P. A new chart to monitor weight gain during pregnancy. *Am J Clin Nutr.* 1985;41:644.
67. Cunningham FG, MacDonald PC, Gant NF, eds. *Williams Obstetrics.* 18th ed. Norwalk, CT: Appleton & Lange; 1989:267.
68. Osofsky HJ. Relationships between nutrition during pregnancy and subsequent infant and child development. *Obstet Gynecol Surv.* 1975;30:227.
69. National Research Council. *Recommended Dietary Allowances.* 9th ed. Washington, DC: National Academy of Sciences; 1980.
70. National Center for Health Statistics. Maternal weight gain and the outcome of pregnancy, United States 1980. In: *Advance Data from Vital and Health Statistics.* Washington, DC: Government Printing Office; DHHS Publication No. (PHS) 86–1922, 1986.

Appendix 21–1

Daily Dietary Allowances for Calories, Proteins, Vitamins, and Minerals[a]

Dietary Allowance	Nonpregnant Females	Additions for Pregnancy	Additions for Lactation
Calories (kcal)	2100[b]	300	500
Protein (gm)	46[c]	30	20
Water-soluble vitamins			
Thiamine (mg)	1.1	0.4	0.5
Riboflavin (mg)	1.3	0.3	0.5
Niacin (mg equivalents)	14	2	5
Pyridoxine B_6 (mg)	2	0.6	0.5
Cobalamin B_{12} (μg)	3	1	1
Folacin (μg)	400	400	100
Ascorbic acid (mg)	60	20	40
Fat-soluble vitamins			
A (μg RE)[d]	800	200	400
D (μg)	10	5	5
E (mgα-TE)[e]	8	2	3
Minerals			
Calcium (mg)	800	400	400
Phosphorus (mg)	800	400	400
Iodine (μg)	150	25	50
Iron (mg of ferrous iron)	18	30–60	30–60
Magnesium (mg)	300	150	150

[a] Values are given for nonpregnant women with suggested additions for pregnancy and lactation.
[b] 2000 kcal if under 19 years of age.
[c] 44 g if under 19 years of age.
[d] 1 μg retinol = 1 retinol equivalent (RE).
[e] TE = tocopherol equivalent.
Adapted from Task Force on Nutrition[61], *National Research Council*[69], *and National Center for Health Statistics.*[70]

Chapter Twenty-Two

Nutritional Deficiencies as Causes of Obstetric Complications: Minerals and Trace Elements

John T. Repke and José Villar

22

For many years, it has been widely recognized that nutrition during pregnancy can have profound effects on perinatal outcome. In fact, for many years, it was believed that larger birth weights, seen among the upper socioeconomic classes, were caused by better nutrition. Since then, many advances in the understanding of nutritional needs during pregnancy have been made.

Although much data have been generated regarding nutritional intake of proteins, carbohydrates, and fats in relationship to birth outcome, it has only recently become clear that minerals and trace elements play an important role in pregnancy outcome.[1] Moreover, while caloric intake affects the incidence of low birth weight infants, the intake of certain minerals can have a similar effect.[2]

CALCIUM

Normal pregnancy places an increased calcium demand on the body (see also Chapter 19). By term, approximately 30 g of calcium have been deposited into the fetal skeleton, with more than 80% occurring in the third trimester.[3] Calcium transport during pregnancy also is enhanced, reaching a maximum level of maternal-to-fetal transfer at approximately 35 weeks' gestation.[4] In fact, several studies have demonstrated that at term, cord blood levels of ionized calcium exceed maternal levels by a considerable amount.[5,6] Additionally, it has been suggested that the placenta may possess mechanisms that facilitate calcium transport from mother to fetus.

To meet the increasing demand for calcium by the fetus, several maternal adjustments must take place. Alterations in maternal levels of parathyroid hormone and vitamin D are two of the changes that account for the alteration in calcium absorption and transport.

Maternal intestinal absorption of calcium is enhanced by hypocalcemia, vitamin D, parathyroid hormone, human growth hormone, dietary phosphate, lactose, reduced calcium intake, and intestinal acidity. Intestinal absorption of calcium may be inhibited by excessive intake of fat, phytate, fiber, cellulose, alcohol, and cortisol.[7] The change in calcium absorption during pregnancy begins in the first trimester and can increase to 50% by term.

Recent data have begun to clarify the role of vitamin D on calcium absorption. In a series of animal experiments, pregnant and vitamin D-deficient rats demonstrated no alteration in their ability to absorb calcium.[8] This observation suggests that perhaps during pregnancy, the role of vitamin D in calcium absorption is minor compared to the nonpregnant state. Calcium mobilization from bone and intestine, with an increase in placental calcium transfer, can be potentially regulated by prolactin.[9] Confirmation of this using human studies is not available, however.

Pregnancy also is a time of increased urinary calcium excretion. A number of metabolic studies have demonstrated a high urinary calcium output despite the obligatory positive calcium balance that occurs during normal pregnancy. This has led to the hypothesis that pregnancy is a time of obligatory physiologic hypercalciuria.[10]

Bone calcium reabsorption is affected by normal pregnancy. In a carefully controlled metabolic study[11], increased bone calcium accretion was found to be progressive throughout pregnancy. While calcium reabsorption from bone was initially depressed, there was a rise as pregnancy progressed. The authors of this study concluded that, despite the increase in absorption of calcium during normal pregnancy, pregnancy may cause a net loss of maternal bone calcium of approximately 10 g. The literature has, however, remained contradictory.[12] Women with multiple pregnancies do not appear to demonstrate radiologic evidence of bone loss.[13]

During normal pregnancy, serum calcium levels progressively decrease. Most of this decrease can be explained by reduced serum albumin secondary to intravascular volume expansion. Because of this net reduction in serum calcium, a compensatory increase in parathyroid hormone has been demonstrated during normal pregnancy.[14,15] The increase in parathyroid hormone has been suggested to be a physiologic hyperparathyroidism. This serves to maintain extracellular calcium ion concentration within the normal range in conjunction with increased renal excretion, large fetal requirements for calcium, and expanding maternal intravascular volume.[14]

Effects of Calcium on Obstetric Complications

Maternal hypertension, fetal prematurity, and low birth weight, major complications of pregnancy, recently have been suggested to have an association with calcium levels.[2] An association between calcium intake and blood pressure has been supported by numerous articles.[15-19] The blood pressure-lowering effect of calcium is thought to be mediated by alterations in plasma renin activity and parathyroid hormone.[17] Additionally, abnormalities in calcium metabolism resulting in reduced ionized calcium serum levels have been described in humans with untreated hypertension.[20,21] Data from the National Health and Nutrition Examination Survey I (HANES I) also demonstrated a significant negative association between calcium intake and blood pressure.[22]

Vascular sensitivity to angiotensin II is decreased in patients given calcium supplementation.[23] This reduction is presumably mediated by alterations in plasma renin activity and parathyroid hormone, resulting in direct smooth muscle relaxation.[17] Smooth muscle relaxation may, in turn, affect the uterus and account for the recently reported reduction in prematurity and low birth weight among a calcium-supplemented patient population at high risk for these two conditions.[2]

Maternal–Fetal Implications

Because pregnancy is a time of increased calcium demand, it is beneficial for pregnant women to receive at least the recommended dietary allowance (RDA) of calcium. Currently, this amount is 1200 mg of elemental calcium per day for adult pregnant women and for pregnant adolescents. Although evidence suggests that humans can adapt to very low calcium intake, the overall consequences of low dietary calcium intake remain to be established.

MAGNESIUM

Magnesium is another divalent cation that has profound effects on pregnancy (see also Chapter 19). While magnesium deficiency is rare among healthy individuals, it is common among chronic alcohol users and has been associated with a variety of physiologic alterations, including hypertension.[24] Obstetric interest in magnesium stems in part from the fact that magnesium sulfate has been a drug of choice in the treatment of pregnancy-induced hypertension and its seizure complications.[25] The drug also is used by some as a tocolytic agent.[26] The effect of magnesium on smooth muscle tone in the arteriolar bed and the uterus apparently relates to its interaction with calcium.[24,26] Myocyte contraction can be enhanced by placing prepared smooth muscle cells into magnesium-deficient media.[27] This type of experimental finding has led to the speculation that relative magnesium deficiency could result in elevated blood pressure on the basis of an increased smooth muscle tone.[27] It also has been speculated that magnesium supplementation may prevent the occurrence of preeclampsia.[28]

Serum magnesium in pregnancy is frequently lower than in the nonpregnant state. This is believed to be caused by the intravascular volume expansion of pregnancy. It also has been demonstrated that urinary excretion of magnesium and serum magnesium levels may be influenced by maternal calcium intake.[17] In normal pregnancy, total plasma magnesium and ultra-filterable plasma magnesium appear to decrease progressively as gestation progresses.[29] In contrast, urinary magnesium excretion, glomerular filtered load of the ultra-filterable portion of plasma magnesium, and the tubular reabsorption of magnesium remain unchanged.[29] This presumably occurs because of the physiologic increase in glomerular filtration during pregnancy.

Recently, there also has been interest in magnesium supplementation during pregnancy to prevent hypertension and reduce low birth weight.[28] Kovacs et al[30] reported a reduced incidence of prematurity and of low birth weight infants among women receiving magnesium. A reduced incidence of preeclampsia in supplemented patients has led to the recommendation that magnesium supplementation should represent a routine part of antenatal care.[30] Similar results have been reported in a retrospective study[31] but have not been corroborated by a more recent prospective randomized, double blind, clinical trial.[28]

Excessive magnesium administration may inhibit calcium absorption; however, the reverse is not true.[17] It also has been demonstrated that serum magnesium is elevated among individuals with low renin hypertension.[21] This observation is consistent with calcium, in which serum ionized calcium is lowest among low renin hypertensive patients.

The overall effect of magnesium has remained controversial because study results are contradictory. Magnesium depletion was not evident in a group of pregnant teenagers who developed pregnancy-induced hypertension.[32] In another investigation, magnesium supplementation was provided in a randomized prospective, double blind, clinical trial and was associated with reduced maternal hospitalization, a reduced preterm delivery rate, and fewer referrals of the newborn to the neonatal intensive care unit. These authors concluded that magnesium supplementation during pregnancy significantly influenced fetal and maternal outcomes before and after delivery.[33]

Maternal–Fetal Considerations

As the second most plentiful intracellular cation, magnesium appears to play an important role in pregnancy. Magnesium is a cofactor for all enzymatic reactions involving phosphate transfer and plays a vital role in binding messenger RNA to ribosomes. Hypomagnesemia may be seen in protein–calorie malnutrition and also may manifest itself as a neuromuscular dysfunction or as neuromuscular irritability.[34]

Hypermagnesemia may manifest itself as muscle weakness, hypotension, cardiac arrhythmias, and sedation.[34] One report suggests that long-term administration of magnesium sulfate for tocolysis may result in fetal parathyroid gland suppression, transient hypocalcemia, and other abnormalities resembling rickets.[35] It is now recommended that pregnant women receive the RDA of magnesium, and if documented magnesium deficiency exists, supplementation may be entertained. Its use in preeclampsia and as a tocolytic is well established but not without consequences. Magnesium supplementation above the RDA cannot be recommended. Clinical trials, which attempted to determine the potential effects of such supplementation, have remained inconclusive. The RDA for magnesium during pregnancy is 320 mg. Magnesium deficiency, occurring exclusively as a result of pregnancy, has not been reported.

ZINC

Zinc is a trace element that is essential for normal reproduction (see also Chapter 19). There are approximately 2 to 3 g of zinc in the body of the average adult. Its presence in human tissue is required as a catalyst of several steps in oxidative metabolism. Zinc also is an essential component of the enzyme systems of deoxyribonucleic acid (DNA) and ribonucleic acid (RNA) polymerases and plays a role in immune processes and membrane stabilization. The requirements for zinc increase when the body is undergoing repair or when rapid growth and development occur. Fetal requirements for zinc undergo a 50-fold increase during the second and third trimesters of pregnancy.[36]

The RDA for zinc during pregnancy is approximately 15 mg/d. This is about 3 mg/d more than the nonpregnant requirement. This requirement assumes that the woman is otherwise healthy and is excreting zinc at a predictable rate and absorbing it in an appropriate fashion. Zinc absorption depends on bioavailability. Animal experiments suggest that zinc absorption efficiency increases during gestation, but similar observations in humans have not confirmed this. It also has been suggested that preconceptional zinc deficiency may result in severe congenital malformations affecting all organ systems.[37] Also, prolonged labor and excessive bleeding at parturition have been observed in zinc-deficient animals.[38]

Several events of pregnancy will affect zinc metabolism. Volume expansion reduces serum zinc concentration. Estrogen and progesterone also have been found to reduce circulating zinc levels.[39] Because both of these steroid hormones are elevated during pregnancy, their effect on zinc concentration may be additive. Multiple studies have, however, failed to allow for a consistent nutritional interpretation of the observed decline in plasma zinc that occurs during normal pregnancy.

Congenital Malformations in Zinc Deficiency

Given zinc's role as a cofactor in reactions involving DNA and RNA polymerases, it is interesting to speculate on zinc's role in teratogenesis. The first study to demonstrate the teratogenic potential of zinc deficiency involved laboratory rats. The reported abnormalities affected the skeletal, nervous, pulmonary, and urogenital systems.[40] It also seems that the timing of zinc deficiency is crucial to the type of malformation observed.[41] It is impossible to duplicate in humans the level of zinc deficiency that can be achieved in an animal laboratory setting. In order to achieve similar levels of zinc deficiency in the human, the degree of nutritional deficiency would be so great that malnutrition and infertility would be a greater concern than zinc deficiency. With this in mind, the applicability of animal to the human condition remains questionable.

Clinical Presentations

Acrodermatitis enteropathica manifests itself clinically as a zinc-deficiency syndrome. Before the recognition that this syndrome was caused by zinc deficiency, this syndrome was usually fatal in childhood. However, occasionally a patient survived to childbearing age, and an increased teratogenesis in these pregnancies has been reported.[42] Once zinc supplementation is provided to these individuals, pregnancy outcome appears to normalize.[43]

Two other clinical entities associated with a disturbed zinc metabolism are the fetal alcohol syndrome and neural tube defects. A geographic association between diets low in zinc and the prevalence of neural tube defects has been reported.[44] Additional reports of anencephaly associated with low maternal serum zinc support this possible association.[45]

Relative zinc deficiency also is known to exist among alcoholics. The types of abnormalities seen in fetal alcohol syndrome have led at least one investigator to suggest that the fetal alcohol syndrome may be related to a relative zinc deficiency.[46] Animal data have confirmed a synergistic effect of ethanol exposure and zinc deficiency.[47]

It is difficult to establish a cause-and-effect relationship between intrauterine growth retardation and zinc deficiency because zinc deficiency is frequently related to malnutrition and poor protein intake. Significant correlations between birth weight and zinc concentration in the mother have been reported.[48,49] However, the strength of these associations is not overwhelming, and further study is needed before determining whether zinc availability to the fetus ultimately affects fetal growth in otherwise normal healthy pregnant women.

Zinc and Amniotic Fluid

Many investigators have studied zinc concentrations in amniotic fluid. Normal zinc levels in amniotic fluid are less than 2 μg/dL in the first trimester and rise to 25 μg/dL by 20 weeks' gestation.[50] It has been demonstrated that in chorioamnionitis, amniotic fluid zinc concentrations are reduced.[51] What remains to be resolved is whether this reduction in amniotic fluid zinc represents an acute phase response to infection or whether a preexisting low level of amniotic fluid zinc predispose to the development of infection.

Several studies have linked reduced amniotic fluid zinc levels to intrauterine growth retardation, pregnancy-induced hypertension, and post-term pregnancy. Other investigators have suggested that adverse pregnancy outcome is associated with increased levels of intra-amniotic zinc. A more recent prospective study failed to demonstrate any predictive value of amniotic fluid zinc level with regard to adverse pregnancy outcome.[52]

Maternal–Fetal Implications

There is no question that pregnancy is a time of altered zinc metabolism, but zinc deficiency appears to be a relatively rare occurrence, even in the most high-risk populations. The observations in human studies have varied, frequently with contradictory conclusions. A recent study suggested that zinc may be trapped in the placenta of cigarette smokers.[53] This may be related to cadmium concentrations in cigarette smoke, which may render the otherwise normal fetus marginally zinc deficient. Cigarette-smoking mothers may therefore potentially benefit from nutritional counseling concerning zinc supplementation. These same investigators also demonstrated that a depletion of zinc stores in older, multiparous women has been observed, and the older gravida who smokes may be at highest risk for relative zinc deficiency in her fetus.[54]

COPPER

Pregnancy is characterized by an increased copper concentration, probably caused by increased ceruloplasmin. While there is animal evidence to suggest that copper deficiency may result in fetal abnormality and fetal wastage, human studies do not confirm this.[55]

CHROMIUM

While it has been suggested that chromium deficiency may be associated with low birth weight[55], at least one study has demonstrated that premature and growth-retarded infants have lower than normal concentrations of chromium in hair samples.[56] It is probable that relative chromium deficiency is not uncommon in pregnancy and is of no major clinical consequence.

FLUORIDE

Fluoride is a trace element that has been recognized for years as effective in the prevention of dental caries. In one study, pregnant women were administered 1 mg of fluoride every day in the last two trimesters of their pregnancy. Their children were subsequently followed and found to have a reduction in the incidence of dental caries and a sixfold increase in the fluoride content of the tooth enamel compared to the nonsupplemented group.[57] The placenta provides some protection against fetal concentrations of fluoride. Normal supplementation, as is found in fluorinated drinking water or fluoride in vitamin and mineral tablets, has not been associated with adverse effects for mother or newborn. There has been a report of Down's syndrome associated with the fluoride content of drinking water, but more recent studies have not supported this observation.[58,59]

LEAD

Most lead exposure is environmental. In the United States, most lead exposure is caused by ingestion of paint chips, water transmitted through lead pipes or inhalation of industrial pollutants containing lead, most frequently automobile emissions. Of particular concern is the observation that past exposure to lead may correlate with umbilical cord blood levels because pregnancy is a time of relative lead mobilization.[60] A strong association between elevated lead levels and congenital anomalies has been reported[61], and one study demonstrated that even moderately elevated blood lead levels in the newborn may increase the risk for subsequent mental retardation.[62]

CONCLUSIONS

Pregnancy is a time of important nutritional needs. Investigations have now established the importance of normal intake of certain minerals, and benefits that may be associated with intakes above the RDA.[63] Calcium supplementation may reduce blood pressure and may improve pregnancy outcome with respect to birth weight and gestational age. Avoiding states of relative zinc deficiency also may be of maternal and fetal benefit. The role of magnesium in pregnancy for health and disease is less clear, although its effects are certainly important because it remains a mainstay in the treatment of premature labor and pregnancy-induced hypertension.

REFERENCES

1. Stein Z, Susser M, Saenger G, Marolla F. *Famine and Human Development: The Dutch Hunger Winter of 1944–1945.* New York, NY: Oxford University Press; 1975.
2. Villar J, Repke JT. Calcium supplementation during pregnancy may reduce preterm delivery in high-risk populations. *J Obstet Gynecol.* 1990;163:1124.
3. Pitkin RM. Calcium metabolism in pregnancy. A review. *Am J Obstet Gynecol.* 1975;121:724.
4. Forbes GB. Calcium accumulation by the human fetus. *Pediatr.* 1976;57:976.
5. Tan CM, Raman A, Sinnathray TA. Serum ionic calcium levels during pregnancy. *J Obstet Gynecol Br Commonw.* 1972;79:694.
6. Reitz RE, Daane TA, Woods JR, Weinstein RL. Calcium, magnesium, phosphorus and parathyroid hormone interrelationships in pregnancy and newborn infants. *Obstet Gynecol.* 1977;50:701.
7. Villar J, Belizan JM. Calcium during pregnancy. *Clin Nutr.* 1986;5:55.
8. Halloran BP, DeLuca HF. Calcium transport in small intestine during pregnancy and lactation. *Am J Physiol.* 1980;239:E64.
9. Prolactin and calcium metabolism in pregnancy and lactation. *Nutr Rev.* 1982;40:216. Editorial.
10. Gertner J, Corestan D, Klinger D. Pregnancy as a state of physiologic, absorptive, hypercalciuria. *Am J Med.* 1986;81:451.
11. Heaney RP, Skillman TG. Calcium metabolism in normal human pregnancy. *J Clin Endocrin.* 1971;33:661.
12. Christiansen C, Rodbro P, Heinild B. Unchanged total body calcium in normal human pregnancy. *Acta Obstet Gynecol Scand.* 1976;55:141.
13. Walker ARP, Richardson B, Walker F. The influence of numerous pregnancies and lactations on bone dimensions in South African Bantu and Caucasian mothers. *Clin Sci.* 1972;42:189.
14. Pitkin RM. Calcium metabolism in pregnancy and the perinatal period: a review. *Am J Obstet Gynecol.* 1985;151:99.
15. Villar J, Belizan JM, Repke J, Bryce GF. The effect of calcium intake on the blood pressure of young healthy individuals. *Ann NY Acad Sci.* 1985;435:509.
16. Villar J, Repke J, Belizan JM, Pareja G. Calcium supplementation reduces blood pressure during pregnancy: results of a randomized, controlled clinical trial. *Obstet Gynecol.* 1987;70:317.
17. Repke JT, Villar J, Anderson C, et al. Biochemical changes associated with blood pressure reduction induced by calcium supplementation during pregnancy. *Am J Obstet Gynecol.* 1989;160:684.
18. Villar J, Repke J, Belizan JM. Calcium and blood pressure. *Clin Nutr.* 1986;5:153.
19. Belizan JM, Villar J, Repke J. The relationship between calcium intake and pregnancy-induced hypertension: up-to-date evidence. *Am J Obstet Gynecol.* 1988;158:898.
20. McCarron DA. Low serum concentrations of ionized calcium in patients with hypertension. *N Engl J Med.* 1982;307:226.
21. Resnick LM, Laragh JH, Sealey JE, Alderman MH. Divalent cations in essential hypertension. *N Engl J Med.* 1983;309:888.
22. Ackley S, Barrett-Connor E, Suarez L. Dairy products, calcium and blood pressure. *Am J Clin Nutr.* 1983;38:457.
23. Kawasaki N, Matsui K, Nakamura T, et al. Effect of calcium supplementation on the vascular sensitivity to angiotensin II in pregnant women. *Am J Obstet Gynecol.* 1985;153:576.
24. Morris CD, Reusser ME, McCarron DA. Dietary calcium and blood pressure: Clinical studies and metabolic changes. *Clin Nutr.* 1989;8:164.
25. Hypertension in pregnancy. In: Cunningham FG, McDonald PC, Gant NF, eds. *Williams Obstetrics.* 18th ed. Norwalk, CT: Appleton & Lange; 1989:653.
26. Petrie RH. Tocolysis using magnesium sulfate. *Semin Perinatol.* 1981;5:266.
27. Altura BM, Altura BT, Carella A. Magnesium deficiency induced spasm of umbilical vessels: Relation to pre-eclampsia, hypertension, growth retardation. *Science.* 1983;221:376.
28. Sibai BM, Villar MA, Bray E. Magnesium supplementation during pregnancy: A double-blind, randomized, controlled clinical trial. *Am J Obstet Gynecol.* 1989;161:115.
29. Colussi G, Surian M, DeFerrari ME, et al. The changes in plasma diffusible levels and renal tubular handling of magnesium during pregnancy: a longitudinal study. *Bone Miner.* 1987;2:311.
30. Kovacs L, Molnar BG, Huhn E, Bodis L. Magnesium substitution in pregnancy. A prospective randomized double blind study. *Geburtshilfe Frauenheilkd.* 1988;48:595.
31. Conradt A, Weidinger H, Algayer H. On the role of magnesium in fetal hypotrophy, pregnancy-induced hypertension, and pre-eclampsia. *Mag Bull.* 1984;6:68.
32. Boston JL, Beauchene RE, Cruikshank DP. Erythrocyte and plasma magnesium during teenage pregnancy relationship with blood pressure and pregnancy-induced hypertension. *Obstet Gynecol.* 1989;73:169.
33. Spatling L, Spatling G. Magnesium supplementation in pregnancy. A double-blind study. *Br J Obstet Gynecol.* 1988;95:120.
34. Smith LH. Disorders of magnesium metabolism. In: Wyngaarden LH, Smith JB, eds. *Cecil Textbook of Medicine.* Philadelphia, PA: WB Saunders; 1982.
35. Lamm CI, Norton KI, Murphy RJ, et al. Congenital rickets associated with magnesium sulfate infusion for tocolysis. *J Pediatr.* 1988;113:1078.
36. Chaube S, Nishimura H, Swinyard CA. Zinc and calcium in normal human embryos and fetuses. *Arch Env Hlth.* 1973;26:237.
37. Hurley LS. Zinc deficiency in prenatal and neonatal development. In: Brewer GJ, Prasad AS, eds. *Zinc Metabolism: Current Aspects in Health and Disease.* New York, NY: Alan R. Liss; 1977:47.
38. Apgar J. Effect of zinc deprivation from day 12, 15, or 18 of gestation on parturition in the rat. *J Nutr.* 1972;102:343.
39. O'Leary JA, Spellacy WN. Zinc and copper levels in pregnant women and those taking oral contraceptives. *Am J Obstet Gynecol.* 1969;103:131.
40. Hurley LS, Swenerton H. Congenital malformations resulting from zinc deficiency in rats. *Proc Soc Exp Biol Med.* 1966;123:692.
41. Hurley LS, Govan J, Swenerton H. Teratogenic effects of short term and transitory zinc deficiency in rats. *Teratology.* 1971;4:199.
42. Verburg B, Burd L, Hoxtell E, Merrill L. Acrodermatitis enteropathica in pregnancy. *Obstet Gynecol.* 1974;44:233.
43. Brenton DP, Jackson MJ, Young A. Two pregnancies in a patient with acrodermatitis enteropathica treated with zinc sulphate. *Lancet.* 1981;2:500.
44. Sever LE, Emanuel I. Is there a connection between maternal zinc deficiency and congenital malformation of the central nervous system in men? *Teratology.* 1973;7:117.
45. Cadvar AO, Arcasoy A, Baycu T, Himmetoglu O. Zinc deficiency and anencephaly in Turkey. *Teratology.* 1980;22:141.
46. Flynn A, Miller SI, Martiet SS, et al. Zinc status of pregnant alcoholic women: A determinant of fetal outcome. *Lancet.* 1981;1:572.
47. Ruth RE, Goldsmith SK. Interaction between zinc deprivation and acute ethanol intoxication during pregnancy in rats. *J Nutr.* 1981;111:2034.
48. Jameson S. Effects of zinc deficiency in human reproduction. *Acta Med Scand.* 1976;593:5.
49. Crosby WM, Metcoff, Costilloe JP, et al. Fetal malnutrition: An appraisal of correlated factors. *Am J Obstet Gynecol.* 1977;128:22.
50. Chez RA, Henkin RI, Fox R. Amniotic fluid copper and zinc concentrations in human pregnancy. *Obstet Gynecol.* 1978;52:125.
51. Solomons NW, Helitzer-Allen DL, Villar J. Zinc needs during pregnancy. *Clin Nutr.* 1986;5:63.
52. Rosick U, Rosick E, Bratter P, Kynast G. Determination of zinc in amniotic fluid in normal and high risk pregnancies. *J Clin Chem Clin Biochem.* 1983;21:363.
53. Kuhnert BR, Kuhnert PM, Lazebnik N, Erhard P. The effect of maternal smoking on the relationship between maternal and fetal zinc status and infant birth weight. *J Am Coll Nutr.* 1988;7:309.
54. Kuhnert BR, Kuhnert PM, Zarlingo TJ. Associations between placental cadmium and zinc and age and parity in pregnant women who smoke. *Obstet Gynecol.* 1988;71:67.

55. Allen LH. Trace minerals and outcome of human pregnancy. *Clin Nutr.* 1986;5:72.
56. Hambidgh KM, Baum JD. Chromium nutrition in the mother and the growing child. In: Mertz W, Cornatzer W, eds. *Newer Trace Elements in Nutrition.* New York, NY: BC Decker; 1970:169.
57. Glenn FB, Glenn WD, Duncan RC. Fluoride tablet supplementation during pregnancy for caries immunity: A study of the offspring produced. *Am J Obstet Gynecol.* 1982;143:560.
58. Erickson JD, Oakley GP, Flynt JW, et al. Water fluoridation and congenital malformations: No association. *J Am Dent Assoc.* 1976;93:981.
59. Needleman HL, Pueschel SM, Rothman KJ. Fluoridation and the occurrence of Down's syndrome. *N Eng J Med.* 1974;291:821.
60. Buchet JP, Roels H, Hubermont G, Lauwerys R. Placental transfer of lead, mercury, cadmium, and carbon monoxide in women. II. Influence of some epidemiological factors on frequency distributions of the biological indices in maternal and umbilical cord blood. *Envir Res.* 1978;15:494.
61. Needleman HL, Rabinowitz M, Leviton A, et al. The relationship between prenatal exposure to lead and congenital anomalies. *JAMA.* 1984;251:2956.
62. Beattie AD, Moore MR, Goldberg A, et al. Role of chronic low level lead exposure in the etiology of mental retardation. *Lancet.* 1975;I:589.
63. National Research Council. *Recommended Dietary Allowances.* 10th ed. Washington, DC: National Academy Press; 1989.

PART IV Diseases Caused by Chemical and Physical Agents

Stanley A. Gall, Section Editor

Chapter Twenty-Three

Bites and Stings

Katharine D. Wenstrom

23

The average pregnant patient can maintain her usual social and recreational activities throughout pregnancy. While she is gardening, hiking, picnicking, and camping, she will be exposed to the same snakes, insects, and animals as the nongravid individual. The Obstetrician will therefore be required to treat injuries resulting from such exposure and should be cognizant of appropriate therapies and special considerations that should be applied to the gravida.

SNAKEBITES

Of the 3500 known species of snakes, less than 10% are venomous. Only two families of poisonous snakes (elapidae and crotalidae) are found in North America. Nevertheless, approximately 8000 snakebites are reported in the United States each year.[1] Although fewer than 20 result in death in nongravid individuals, several case reports suggest that morbidity and mortality after snakebite may be considerably higher in a pregnant patient. Little information on this subject exists in obstetric literature. The reader is referred to a thorough general review by Wallace[1], from which the following summary is derived.

Coral snakes (a variety of elapidae) are found throughout the South from Florida to Arizona. They can be identified by alternating bands of red and black separated by yellow rings, although black and albino varieties also exist. Generally nocturnal and reclusive, they will bite if provoked. Their short permanently erect fangs eject venom during a series of chewing movements, resulting in multiple fang marks on the victim. The venom is neurotoxic and usually causes little local pain or swelling. Within 10–15 minutes, however, neuromuscular transmission is impaired and local numbness and weakness are followed by central nervous system abnormalities. Ataxia, ptosis, pupillary dilatation, palatal and pharyngeal paralysis, salivation, nausea, and vomiting may be present before respiratory paralysis and seizures result in death, which occurs within 8–72 hours.

Pit vipers (crotalidae) have a small pit located between the eye and the nostril, and they have a triangular shaped head as a result of large venom glands located in the temporal region. When these aggressive snakes strike, their posteriorly folded fangs become instantly erect and eject venom as soon as contact is made. Pit viper venom contains several toxic proteins and enzymes that produce both local and systemic effects. Severe local burning and pain are followed by edema and ecchymosis and eventually by gangrene of skin and subcutaneous tissues. Systemic effects include fever, nausea and vomiting, bleeding secondary to disseminated intravascular coagulopathy, circulatory collapse, cramping, pupillary constriction, delirium and convulsions, and death within 6–48 hours.

Many factors influence the severity of snakebites, including the size of the victim and the snake, the general health and age of the victim, the location of the bite, the introduction of bacteria into the wound, and the subsequent activity of the victim. Although all snakebites should be evaluated in a hospital, first aid measures undertaken before transport may significantly improve outcome. The victim should rest immediately because activity increases the rate of absorption of toxin. The bitten extremity should be immobilized and a tourniquet placed above the bite mark to impede lymphatic (but not venous) flow. Linear incisions (1.0 cm long × 0.5 cm deep) should be made over each fang mark and suction applied to remove as much venom as possible. Suction must be continued until antivenin has been administered. The extremity should not be cooled because this may increase local tissue damage resulting from ischemia. Every attempt should be made to identify the snake to facilitate antivenin therapy.

In the emergency room, attention should be directed to maintaining an airway and providing circulatory support. A polyvalent antivenin effective against all North American pit vipers and a coral snake-specific antivenin are commercially available in the United States. As soon as sensitivity to horse serum, from which these antivenins are made, has been ruled out, a dose appropriate to the size of the patient and the estimated venom exposure must be given intravenously. After antivenin has been given, tetanus toxoid should be administered and pain relief provided. Both aerobic and anaerobic cultures of the wound should be performed because many snakes harbor gram-negative pathogens in their oral cavities. A broad-spectrum antibiotic may be given prophylactically. If local edema is significant, fasciotomy should be considered to prevent further compressive ischemic injury. The pregnant patient should be positioned on her side so that the gravid uterus is displaced off the great vessels, and the fetus should be monitored.

Laboratory evaluation should include a complete blood count, coagulation profile, and blood chemistries. The progression of anemia, thrombocytopenia, coagulopathy, and azotemia may herald the onset of shock and should be treated with volume replacement and component therapy. Treatment with steroids has not been shown to improve outcome of snakebite victims.[2]

In general, the pregnant patient should receive the same care as any other snakebite victim. Antivenin must be administered and tetanus toxoid given prophylactically. Tetanus toxoid has proven safe for use during pregnancy and may even provide transplacental immunization to the fetus.[3] Intravascular volume and blood pressure must be maintained because the supine hypotension commonly seen during pregnancy may predispose the gravid victim to circulatory compromise, which has been implicated in maternal death after snakebite.[4] Medications used to combat hypotension (ie, epinephrine) may contribute to placental insufficiency and possibly fetal death if the fetal response is not carefully evaluated during therapy.[5] Monitoring for uterine contractions should be instituted because several snake venoms have been shown to cause contractions in animals[6,7] and may contribute to the onset of labor or spontaneous abortion.[8] Laboratory parameters must be evaluated serially and coagulopathy treated aggressively. *Abruptio placentae* have been reported as the first sign of coagulation disorder in a gravid snakebite victim.[9]

Snakebite does not invariably lead to morbidity and mortality in the pregnant victim. Patients with minimal to moderate envenomation who receive prompt, appropriate care will recover well. One report documents the complete recovery of three such patients and their delivery at term of apparently unaffected infants.[8]

HYMENOPTERA STINGS

Bees, wasps, yellow jackets, hornets, and fire ants are all capable of inflicting painful stings or bites. The venoms of these hymenoptera contain vasoactive substances, such as histamine, kinins, hyaluronidase, and phospholipase, and they produce hemolytic, neurotoxic, and hypersensitizing effects.[1] The usual reaction to such stings is local pain and urticaria. Local erythema may develop but usually subsides within a few hours. After careful removal of the stinger, the affected area should be cooled and a topical antipruritic applied. An oral antihistamine also may help to relieve itching. Such a local injury should not affect the fetus in any way, and the gravida should receive the same care as any other patient.

Approximately 1% of the population, however, exhibits hypersensitivity to hymenoptera stings. Such reactions are mediated by immunoglobulin E (IgE). IgE bound to mast cells or basophils binds antigen, and as a result, histamine, eosinophilic chemotactic factor, and slow-reacting substances of anaphylaxis are released. Leukotrienes also may play a role in bronchial constriction. The clinical effect of these substances is devastating, and even a single sting in susceptible individuals can result in severe systemic manifestations of anaphylaxis. Massive edema of the face and glottis and bronchospasm produce dyspnea and cyanosis. Nausea, abdominal or uterine cramps, severe urticaria, hypotension, vascular collapse, and eventually coma ensue. Renal failure and convulsions have been associated with fatality.[10] Although IgE essentially does not cross the placenta and therefore poses no threat to the fetus, the maternal effects of IgE can severely compromise blood flow and oxygen delivery to the fetoplacental unit and have been associated with significant fetal morbidity and mortality. A case report of maternal anaphylaxis from shellfish ingestion[11] described fetal distress that was relieved with treatment of maternal hypotension and hypovolemia. Anaphylaxis after snakebite has been described, and severe maternal hypotension was thought to be related to the delivery of a brain damaged infant who subsequently expired.[5] A report of maternal bee sting anaphylaxis during the 30th week of pregnancy relates severe maternal hypotension to the occurrence of fetal hypoxia followed by fetal cerebral edema, hypoxic spinal cord damage, and patchy cerebral infarction. The severely depressed neonate died shortly after birth. Autopsy revealed cerebral atrophy, cavitation, and germinal hemorrhage described collectively as multicystic encephalomalacia.[12]

Every effort must be made to support maternal blood pressure and volume and to reverse the most severe symptoms associated with anaphylaxis. Immediate treatment should include placement of a tourniquet above the affected area and administration of 0.2–0.5 mL of 1:1000 epinephrine subcutaneously. Any theoretic teratogenic effects of epinephrine are outweighed by its beneficial effects in this situation.[13] If maternal condition warrants and cardiac status is carefully monitored, epinephrine boluses may be repeated every 3 minutes. The patient should be placed in a left lateral decubitus position with continuous fetal monitoring, and normal saline or Ringer's lactate solution given intravenously to maintain maternal intravascular volume. The maternal systolic blood pressure should not fall below 90 mm Hg. Vasopressive agents and volume expanders may be required to prevent this.

Respiratory distress must be treated expeditiously. Fetal hypoxemia is related to maternal oxygen levels and can be avoided if the maternal arterial PO_2 is kept above 60 mm Hg.[13] Supplemental oxygen should be administered by a face mask. Respiratory therapy with 0.5 mL of isoproterenol (diluted 1:200 with saline) or a small dose of aminophylline (0.25–0.5 g intravenously over 15–30 minutes) may relieve bronchospasm. Intubation may be required if laryngeal edema is significant and respiratory function fails to respond to these measures.

Prevention of hymenoptera bites is easier than their treatment. Susceptible patients should avoid such insects; should not wear bright clothing, perfumes, or flowers; and should not walk barefoot outdoors.[14] Nests and colonies of such insects near the home should be exterminated. Patients should obtain several insect bite kits and place them in accessible areas (ie, glove compartment of the car, vacation home, gardening shed). Family members should be instructed in the use of these kits so that they may render immediate assistance.

SPIDER AND SCORPION BITES

More than 100,000 species of spiders have been identified throughout the world, of which less than 1% are poisonous to humans.[15] The only two poisonous species found in North America are the *Loxosceles*, or recluse spiders, and the *Lactrodectus*, or widow spiders.

The brown *recluse* or *fiddler spider* is the most common *Loxosceles* in the United States and can be found throughout the Southeast. It is brown with short body hair and can be identified by the presence of a dark band in the shape of a violin on the cephalothorax. At least six other varieties of the recluse spider are found in California, Arizona, Utah, Nevada, New Mexico, and Texas. These shy, nocturnal spiders inhabit dark protected spaces (eg, barns, garages, sheds), and bite only if provoked. Their venom contains neurotoxins, hemotoxins, cytotoxins, levarterenol, hemolysins, and a spreading factor.[15] Reaction to the venom is local and systemic. Initial stinging and pruritis are followed by the appearance of marked erythema and edema. Local arterial spasm and hemolysis produce a bluish skin discoloration that changes to black as necrosis occurs. Systemic manifestations include fever and chills, nausea and vomiting, weakness, joint pain, and the development of a morbilliform rash. Rapid hemolysis may provoke a coagulopathy, and fibrinogen and platelets may be depleted. Eventual sloughing of the eschar over the bite leaves a depression that will gradually fill in with scar tissue.

Treatment should consist of pain relief, tetanus toxoid, and immobilization of the affected area. The patient with "systemic arachnidism," who is in danger of going into shock, will benefit from steroid administration and support of intravascular volume and electrolyte balance. No specific antivenin is available. The theory that early surgical excision of the bite might lessen symptoms and improve healing has been rejected in favor of allowing the necrotic margins of the wound to become apparent before attempting surgery.[14] Severe hemolytic anemia may be corrected by blood transfusion, and temporary renal failure may require dialysis. With proper care, recovery is complete and immunity results.

The *black widow spider* is found throughout the United States. It is black with a mark shaped like a red hourglass on its underside. It also nests in dry, dark spaces, and under rocks and logs. Its bite feels like a mild pin prick, but its venom contains a neurotoxin that rapidly produces systemic effects. Local erythema of the bitten area is followed by blanching. Severe muscle cramps in the chest, abdomen, and extremities begin within 1–3 hours because of depleted acetylcholine at neuromuscular junctions. Abdominal rigidity and muscle fibrillations quickly follow. Hypertension, bradycardia, electrocardiogram changes, fever, hyperglycemia, and neutrophilia may be manifest[14], as well as nausea, vomiting, respiratory difficulty, and oliguria. The patient is extremely anxious and in intense pain.

Treatment should begin with a hot bath and an intravenous injection of 10.0 mL of 10% calcium gluconate to temporarily relieve muscle spasms. Black widow antivenin is generally available and should be given to patients with severe symptoms, to small children, and to those with medical problems. Narcotics may be required to ensure pain relief. Appropriately treated patients should recover well, while untreated patients may have symptoms for 2–3 days and are at risk of death from respiratory or heart failure.

The two dangerous species of scorpion in the United States are *Centuroides sculpturatus* and *gertschi*. Both are found in Arizona and neighboring states. These eight-legged arthropods are nocturnal and usually sting humans by accident when they are discovered in shoes and other clothing. The neurotoxic venom contained in a stinger under the tail causes local pain, edema, and ecchymosis, followed by local paresthesia and numbness. These sensations spread, and eventually systemic symptoms, such as excessive salivation, respiratory stridor, nystagmus, nausea, vomiting, and incontinence, occur. The patient may be agitated and hyperactive but eventually lapses into coma. Convulsions may occur, and myocarditis with arrhythmias and heart failure may develop. If untreated, death occurs within 12–48 hours.

A tourniquet should be applied above the sting and the extremity kept cold to diminish spread of the venom. Antivenin is available in many areas, and should be administered while the patient is carefully observed for respiratory compromise or shock. If these or other severe symptoms develop, the patient should be monitored in an intensive care unit.

ANIMAL BITES

Between 1 and 2 million significant animal bites are reported each year, and they account for approximately 1% of all emergency room visits.[16] More men than women are bitten by dogs, but women are twice as likely to be bitten by cats.[17] Morbidity from such wounds results from infection, bleeding, and crush injury. Dogs may bite with a force of 150–450 lb/sq in, which results in devitalization of tissues and deep innoculation of microorganisms.[18]

Only a small proportion of appropriately treated animal bites become infected. In one large study[19], 88% of dog bites seen in the emergency room were clinically uninfected. Seventy percent of these wounds yielded no bacterial isolates or revealed *Staphylococcus epidermides* only. Of the remaining 30% that produced positive bacterial cultures, only 2.7% became infected. The oral flora of dogs usually includes multiple organisms, such as *Pasteurella multocida, Streptococcus species, Neisseria species*, several varieties of *Staphylococcus*, and numerous anaerobic bacteria. Of these, *P multocida* has been associated with the most rapid onset of infection and the most virulent course. All wounds may become infected if not properly treated. Immediate care should include copious irrigation with saline or iodine solution, cleansing, and careful debridement of devitalized tissue. Although most bites of the face are closed primarily for cosmetic reasons, bites on areas especially prone to infection (ie, the hand) should be left open. A plastic surgeon should be consulted if the bite is likely to be disfiguring. The use of prophylactic antibiotics for dog bite wounds is questionable, especially because no one agent successfully covers all potential pathogens. Penicillin is effective against *P multocida*, but the combination drug amoxicillin–clavulanate potassium may provide wider coverage. If antibiotics are prescribed, it is important to obtain cultures before treatment because complications, such as osteomyelitis, septic arthritis, cellulitis, and abscesses, may be avoided if antibiotic therapy is adjusted according to the identity of the invading organism and its sensitivities. It is important to minimize swelling, which could diminish blood supply and antibiotic delivery to the affected area. The affected part should be elevated, and injured hands should be immobilized. Rabies vaccine should be considered if the history makes rabies infection likely. Finally, although tetanus related to dog bite is uncommon, administration of a tetanus toxoid booster (if the previous booster was given more than 10 years before the bite) is prudent.

P multocida is the predominant pathologic organism in the oral flora of healthy cats, and the spectrum of bacteria commonly present is similar to that of dogs. Because cat bites seem more likely to become infected than dog bites, cleansing and irrigation of wounds should be especially vigorous and antibiotics given routinely. Monkey bites are occasionally reported but little is known about their microbiology. After appropriate cultures, they should be cared for in the same way as dog and cat bites.

HUMAN BITES

Human bites are reputed to cause more serious injury than animal bites. Most wounds involve the hand or the upper extremities. Women also are likely to be bitten on the breasts, although bites may occur anywhere on the body. When a hand injury occurs as a result of striking another person in the mouth, damage to the bones, tendons, and joint capsules of the hand may be extensive.

A major complication of a human bite wound is infection. In one large study[20], approximately 18% of such wounds become infected. Common pathogens of human bites include *S aureus, streptococci, Eikenella corrodens, Bacteroides species*, and other anaerobes.[18] *E corrodens* and alpha hemolytic streptococci frequently act synergistically in clenched fist injuries and may result in serious complications. Occasionally, an infectious disease may be transmitted by a human bite. Hepatitis B, syphilis, and actinomycoses have been transmitted in this manner. Theoretically, human immunodeficiency virus can be passed on by a human bite, but this has not yet been reported. Complications associated with human bites include osteomyelitis, septic arthritis, and tenosynovitis.[18] Such complications may lead to amputation.

Human bite wounds should receive the same initial treatment as animal bite wounds: copious irrigation, cleansing, and debridement of devitalized areas. A plastic surgeon or hand surgeon should be consulted for face or hand injuries as necessary, and tetanus booster administration should be considered. The patient may benefit from the use of prophylactic antibiotics. Pathogens in human bites are frequently resistant to penicillin, penicillinase, and betalactamase resistant penicillins, and first generation cephalosporins. A good antibiotic choice would therefore be amoxicillin–clavulanate potassium. Patients who are immunocompromised or who have complications such as osteomyelitis or cellulitis should be hospitalized for intravenous antibiotic therapy.

REFERENCES

1. Wallace JF. Disorders caused by venoms, bites, and stings. In: Braunwald E, Isselbacher KJ, Petersdorf RG, et al, eds. *Harrison's Principles of Internal Medicine*. New York, NY: McGraw-Hill; 1987:831.
2. Schottler WHA. Antihistamine, ACTH, cortisone, hydrocortisone, and anesthetics in snakebite. *Am J Trop Med*. 1954;3:1083.
3. Gill TJ, Repetti CF, Mettay LA, et al. Transplacental immunization of the human fetus to tetanus by immunization of the mother. *J Clin Invest*. 1983;72:987.
4. Sutherland SK, Duncan AW, Tibballs J. Death from a snakebite associated with the supine hypotension syndrome of pregnancy. *Med J Aust*. 1982;4:238.
5. Entman SS, Moise KJ. Anaphylaxis in pregnancy. *S Med J*. 1984;77:402.
6. Essex HE. The physiologic action of the venom of the water moccasin (*Agkistrodon piscivorus*). *Am J Physiol*. 1932;99:681.
7. Essex HE, Markowitz J. The physiologic action of rattlesnake venom (crotalin) II. The effect of crotalin on surviving organs. *Am J Physiol*. 1930;92:329.
8. Parrish HM, Khan MS. Snakebite during pregnancy. Report of 4 cases. *Obstet Gynecol*. 1966;27:468.
9. Zugalb M, deBarros ACSD, Bittar RE, et al. *Abruptio placentae* following snakebite. *Am J Obstet Gynecol*. 1985;151:754.
10. Staweski MA. Insect bites and stings. *Emerg Med Clin North Am*. 1985;3:785.
11. Klein VR, Harris AP, Abraham RA, et al. Fetal distress during a maternal systemic allergic reaction. *Obstet Gynecol*. 1984;64:15S.
12. Erasmus C, Blackwood W, Wilson J. Infantile multicystic encephalomalacia after maternal bee string anaphylaxis during pregnancy. *Arch Dis Child*. 1982;57:785.
13. Witter FR, Niebyl JR. Drug intoxication and anaphylactic shock in the obstetric patient. In: Berkowitz RL, ed. *Critical Care of the Obstetric Patient*. New York, NY: Churchill Livingstone; 1983:527.
14. Stawiski MA. Insect bites and stings. *Emerg Med Clin North Am*. 1985;3:785.
15. Williams RW. Necrotic arachnidism. In: Hoeprich PD, ed. *Infectious Disease*. 2nd ed. New York, NY: Harper & Row; 1977:874.
16. Underman AE. Bite wounds inflicted by dogs and cats. *Vet Clin North Am Small Anim Pract*. 1987;17:195.
17. Kizer KW, Town M. Epidemiologic and clinical aspects of animal bite injuries. *J Am Coll Emerg Phys*. 1979;8:134.
18. Goldstein EJC, Richwald GA. Human and animal bite wounds. *Am Fam Prac*. 1987;36:101.
19. Ordog GJ. The bacteriology of dog bite wounds on initial presentation. *Ann Emerg Med*. 1986;15:1324.
20. Lindsey D, Christopher M, Hollenbach J, et al. Natural course of the human bite wound. Incidence of infection and complications in 434 bites and 803 lacerations in the same group of patients. *J Trauma*. 1987;27:45.

Chapter Twenty-Four
Radiation Injury

Patricia M. Garcia

24

Radiation exposure in pregnancy is an anxiety-provoking and often misunderstood issue (see also Chapter 10). However, as Brent[1] has noted, more is known about radiation exposure than any other environmental teratogen. Although not complete, enough information is available to help patients and health care providers make appropriate use of important diagnostic and therapeutic radiation procedures and to help them make informed choices before planned exposures and after inadvertent ones. The goal of this chapter is to reduce the number of anxious patients and physicians who overestimate the risk from x-rays, which delays appropriate treatment and to guard against physicians who underestimate the risk and cavalierly overuse radiologic tests.

Radiation is characterized by the specific type of emission, the energy associated with the emission, and for radionuclides, the rate of disintegration. The biggest concern is high energy, *ionizing* radiation of which there are two main forms of emission: electromagnetic waves (x-rays, gamma waves) and particles (alpha and beta particles). Radiation of high enough energy, whether in the form of waves or particles, can pass through tissue and transfer energy. This transfer of energy to atoms results in the removal of electrons and the formation of ion pairs, hence the term ionizing radiation. It is this energy transfer and deposition that leads directly to molecular damage (usually cell death, disruption of function, or mutation) by breaking chemical bonds in essential biomolecules, such as DNA, proteins, and lipids. Ionizing radiation also can produce molecular damage indirectly by producing reactive chemical species from cellular water (free radicals), which also can alter chemical bonds. The linear energy transfer (LET) is the amount of energy transferred to tissue per unit length. Tissue damage depends not only on the amount of energy transferred, but also on the penetrating ability of the specific type of emission.

Particle and wave emissions have different energies and penetrating capabilities. Ionizing electromagnetic waves (x-rays and gamma waves) are characterized by a short wavelength, high frequency, and relatively high energy. They differ from other electromagnetic waves (radiowaves, microwaves, visible light waves), which are of longer wavelength and lower energy, because they are able to transfer energy and produce ionization while deeply penetrating tissues. In contrast to ionizing electromagnetic waves, high-energy particles, such as alpha particles, produce a greater quantity of ionizations but penetrate tissue poorly. The important clinical implication of this information is that radionuclides, which are particle emitters, may be relatively safe to the fetus when outside the mother. Once introduced into the body and concentrated near the fetus (eg, in the maternal bladder), they may represent a significant source of radiation exposure.

In order to estimate and quantify the risk of radiation exposure, the units by which it is measured and the dosimetry must be clearly understood. These units of measure differ according to the type of radiation, its energy, the medium through which it travels, and the qualities of the biologic matter that are absorbing the radiation. The basic unit that describes the amount or dose of radiation exposure is the roentgen (R). This applies only to x-rays or gamma rays ionizing air. In order to describe the tissue effects of radiation, the *absorbed* dose is used, which is defined as the quantity of energy absorbed per unit mass of a medium. The rad (radiation absorbed dose), which equals 0.01 joule/kg, was chosen because one R of exposure is approximately equivalent to 1 rad of absorbed dose in tissue. More recently, the International System of unit's term for absorbed dose, the gray (Gy), has gained wide acceptance and usage. One Gy is equivalent to 100 rads or 1 rad = 1 cGy.

Any type of ionizing radiation (x-rays, gamma rays, alpha, or beta particles) can be quantified in terms of grays or rads; however, to describe the biologic effectiveness of ionizing radiation; a special unit that takes into account the specific type of radiation, its energy, and the qualities of the tissue absorbing the radiation has been defined. This is called the dose-equivalent unit. The dose-equivalent unit is called rem (roentgen equivalents mammal) or the sievert (Sv) in the International System. The rem is equivalent to the rad multiplied by a quality factor. Fortunately, for ionizing radiation in mammalian tissue, the quality factor is 1; therefore, 1 rem = 1 rad and 1 Sv = 1 Gy. Radionuclides emit ionizing radiation in the form of x-rays, gamma rays, and alpha and beta particles. The unit of measure for radionuclide particulate radiation is the curie and is quantified in disintegrations per unit time where 1 Ci = 37×10^9 disintegrations per sec. Lastly, in defining radiation exposure and its potential harmful effects, the rate of exposure over time is an important factor. Acute exposures tend to produce a greater effect than the same amount chronically administered; therefore, the potential biologic damage of 1 Sv absorbed over 1 day is not equivalent to 1 Sv absorbed over an entire year.

Sources of exposure to ionizing radiation are natural (cosmic rays, decaying natural isotopes), man-made (medical diagnostic imaging x-rays, fission by-products of nuclear reactors), external (x-rays from a computed tomography [CT] scanner), and internal (radiopharmaceuticals inhaled for a V/Q scan). Natural background radiation from the combination of atmospheric sources (ionizing cosmic rays, 0.28 mSv), terrestrial sources (radionuclide decay from soil, rocks, and building materials, 0.39 mSv), and internal sources (decaying natural radionuclides inside the body, 0.26 mSv) totals about 0.8–1.2 mSv annual absorbed dose.[2] This can vary dramatically by geographic location and lifestyle considerations (eg, time spent in air travel, outdoors, at high altitudes, or near certain geographic formations with high concentrations of natural radionuclides). The contribution to background environmental radiation from man-made sources, such as nuclear power generation, has been estimated to be in the range of 0.1 mSv annually.[2]

By far, the largest man-made contributor to the total population exposure and the source of most concern for obstetricians is medical and dental diagnostic ionizing radiation[3] (standard x-ray imaging, single-photon emission computerized tomography [SPECT], positron emission tomography [PET], CT, and radionuclide imaging). Maternal and fetal radiation dose estimates (dose estimates are for the average skin entrance exposure in mrads) for common x-ray imaging studies are as follows: chest—P/A (maternal—12–25 mrads; fetal—0.1 mrads); abdomen—KUB (375–700 mrads; 105 mrads), IVP (475–850 mrads; 150 mrads), thoracic spine (300–500; 0.15 mrads), fluoroscopy (500–5000 mrads/min; depends on site and duration of exposure), lumbosacral spine (450–800 mrads; 55 mrads), xeromammogram (800–1700 mrads; 0) and head CT (2000–5000 mrads; 0).[3] The estimated fetal dose for standard x-ray pelvimetry ranges from 1–2 rads and can be reduced to 0.23 rads by using a low-exposure CT technique.[4] With judicious use of limited, shielded procedures, the radiologic diagnosis of deep venous thrombosis can be made with fetal radiation exposure of less than 0.50 rads, and pulmonary embolism can be diagnosed with less than 0.05 rads of fetal exposure.[5]

Radiopharmaceuticals represent an internal source of exposure for the developing embryo. Radiation doses from standard radionuclide studies are usually low and depend on the specific radionuclide. Its energy emission and half-life, the distribution in the maternal system (elements such as technetium, which accumulate in the maternal bladder, produce a greater fetal exposure), the dose used, and placental permeability. Bone scanning produces an estimated fetal dose of 17 mrad/mCi administered in an 8-week-old fetus.[6] A lung perfusion scan using ^{99m}Tc gives a fetal dose of 6–18 mrads, while the ventilation scan produces a similarly low dose of 4–19 mrads from ^{133}Xe. An ^{125}I-fibrinogen leg scan, however, produces a fetal dose of about 2.0 rads because it crosses the placenta and accumulates in the fetal thyroid starting at about 8 weeks' gestation.

PATHOPHYSIOLOGY

The sequence of events that leads from cellular damage and tissue interaction to the observed clinical effects of ionizing radiation is not completely understood. As previously described, energy transfer produces free ion pairs, which directly and indirectly cause the disruption of chemical bonds, most importantly in deoxyribonucleic acid (DNA). This produces breaks in both single- and double-stranded DNA along with base deletion and chemical cross-linking of strands. It is in the most rapidly proliferating cells that DNA damage is most apparent; therefore, rapidly dividing fetal central nervous system (CNS) cells are extremely sensitive to radiation damage. The most obvious consequence of DNA damage is cell death and depletion. This may result in populations of cells dying and account for the clinical effect of embryonic death, or it may result in permanent cell depletion, which yields organ hypoplasia (eg, growth retardation) or dysfunction (eg, mental retardation). Nonlethal cell damage also may occur and result in mitotic delay, mutation of the gene sequence, alterations in macromolecular or chromosomal structure, or disturbances of cell migration. The contribution of these mechanisms remains speculative. The progression from molecular and cellular radiation damage to the clinical effects of cell death, teratogenesis, mutagenesis, and carcinogenesis is unknown. These clinical outcomes are discussed later in this chapter.

An important concept related to the biologic effects of radiation is the notion of threshold. Radiation effects are classically described as a stochastic or nonstochastic phenomenon. Stochastic refers to effects induced by damage to a single cell that show no threshold of response so that the probability of occurrence, rather than the severity of effect, is a function of the dose. Carcinogenesis and mutagenesis are examples of this. Effects that are produced by damage to many cells and that exhibit a threshold dose below which no adverse effects are seen are labeled nonstochastic.[7] The severity of the effect is thought to be a function of the dose of exposure. Growth retardation and teratogenesis are examples of this. This is the rationale for making 5 rads of exposure the minimum safe dose for inadvertent x-ray exposure because no human teratogenic effect has been noted below this dose.[1] Recent data suggest this simple dichotomy may not be true for all radiation effects because mental retardation and diminution in IQ may be observed below what was previously thought to be the threshold level.[8]

It is not only the dose that determines the probability and extent of radiation damage. The timing of the exposure also is critical in accounting for the clinical effects of radiation injury. For the fetus, with respect to the lethal, teratogenic, and growth retarding effects, the timing of exposure directly influences the type and extent of damage.[9] The differential sensitivity of embryonic and fetal tissue reflects the progression of development. Before the blastocyst stage, the embryo is most sensitive to the lethal effects of irradiation.[10] If death does not result from the radiation exposure, the embryo usually develops normally without evidence of any growth retarding or teratogenic effect. This is the "all-or-none" effect. The period of greatest sensitivity for CNS damage is from 8–15 weeks after conception when the most rapid proliferation and migration of neurons is taking place.[11] During this period of early organogenesis, the embryo also is sensitive to the lethal and growth-retarding effects, although it can recover postnatally from the growth retardation to some extent.[1] Fifteen weeks after conception, the fetus is resistent to radiation-induced teratogenic effects. After 15 weeks, sensitivity remains for the development of growth retardation (which does not recover postnatally) and in the CNS for the potential development of mental retardation.[1] The last consideration relevant to timing is acuity versus chronicity of exposure. A dose of 50 rads delivered acutely is more likely to produce serious congenital malformations than fractionated doses totaling 50 rads delivered over many months. However, this may not be true for cancer risk. Finally, in addition to timing, host factors also may alter susceptibility to radiation effects. Various chemicals or physical factors may act as potentiators of radiation effect. Different hormones, immune status and nutritional status may modulate the clinical manifestations of radiation damage.

CLINICAL EFFECTS

Although the precise pathophysiologic mechanisms of radiation injury may not be known, the clinical effects on humans have been well delineated. A large body of information on fetal effects has accumulated since the early 1920s and 1930s. Doses of approximately 350 rads were used to induce abortion (unsuccessfully in a large percentage of cases). High doses of ionizing radiation to the pelvic area were used therapeutically to treat a variety of gynecologic (abnormal uterine bleeding, leiomyomata, malignancies) and nongynecologic (sacroiliac joint arthritis, tuberculous involvement of the bone) diseases. Examination of surviving fetuses revealed growth retardation, mental retardation, microcephaly, microphthalmus, and cataracts.[12] Since that time, follow up of adults and their offspring among atomic bomb survivors exposed in Hiroshima and Nagasaki in the 1940s has added to our information about early and late human radiation effects. Series of patients, such as children irradiated for "enlarged" thymuses and scalp ring-worm and women for postpartum mastitis, also have expanded the understanding of radiation-induced cancers.

Radiation effects can be classified as acute or late. Acute effects of ionizing radiation occur at doses of at least 0.2–0.5 Gy (20–50 rads) whole-body exposure. The lowest dose, 0.2 Gy, can cause transient hematologic changes (decreased lymphocyte and platelet counts), while higher doses cause more severe hematologic disturbances, such as skin burns, hair loss, bone marrow depletion, gastrointestinal tract mucosal destruction, organ failure, and even death.[3] These effects may take hours to weeks to manifest depending on the dose of exposure. Diagnostic radiation used in medical imaging does *not* cause acute radiation effects because the dosages are many orders of magnitude less (see previous section) than those causing signs of acute radiation sickness. Late effects of radiation can be caused by low and high levels of radiation exposure. Late effects have a long latent period, anywhere from months to years, before clinical manifestations become apparent. Late effects include mutagenesis, carcinogenesis, and teratogenesis.

Maternal Effects

Radiation can induce solid and hematopoietic tumors. With few exceptions, tumor induction has been observed in virtually all tissues. The carcinogenic risk of radiation exposure is associated with low to moderate doses of x-rays and with high-dose exposures. Studies have shown an increase in basal cell carcinoma of the skin after 300–600 rem to the scalp and 50–250 rem to the face and neck.[13] Latency periods range from 2 years for leukemias to 10–30 years for solid tumors, such as breast, thyroid, brain, and lung.[3]

Irradiation of germ cells in the female gonad poses a risk of inducing sterility from oocyte destruction and of inducing genetic effects from chromosomal aberrations and mutations, which can be transmitted to the next generation. Radiation-induced DNA breakage and chromosomal rearrangement resulting in reciprocal translocations are the most probable chromosomal abnormality but are not major contributors to radiation-caused genetic damage. A greater contributor is the mutagenic potential of ionizing radiation, although the magnitude of the effect is extremely small. The United Nations Scientific Committee on the Effects of Atomic Radiation (UNSCEAR) assessed the risk for induction of mutations leading to abnormal children in the next generation to be in the range of 0–20 per million live births per 0.01 Gy.[14]

Fetal Effects

Exposure of the embryo and fetus to ionizing radiation *in utero* can produce embryonic or fetal death, malformations, growth retardation, postnatal functional impairment and possibly an excess of childhood cancers. As noted previously, prenatal development is highly radiosensitive because of the rapid cell proliferation, migration, and differentiation taking place. This is true in particular for the fetal central nervous system, which retains its sensitivity to radiation for a long period during development. The radiation dose and timing of exposure with respect to the stage of development is critical in determining the specific clinical effects.

The main effect of irradiation on the preimplantation and early postimplantation embryo is embryonic death. During this period, the embryo is highly sensitive to the lethal effects and relatively resistent to the teratogenic and growth retarding effects of x-rays because of the enhanced proliferation of undifferentiated cells that survive.[10,15] No reliable human data exist, but animal data show the critical dose for embryonic death to be in the range of 1 Gy (100 rads) for the LD_{50}.[16] During organogenesis (days 15–50 after conception), the embryo is highly sensitive to the teratogenic effects of radiation and also can exhibit growth retarding effects, although postnatal catch-up growth is possible.[1] As gestation progresses, the risk of multiple organ system malformation diminishes and becomes nonexistent in the later fetal stages, but the CNS retains some susceptibility to radiation effects.[1] The fetus remains sensitive to growth retardation as gestation progresses and is less able to compensate postnatally. In later fetal stages, high doses of radiation can theoretically affect postnatal function by causing permanent cell depletion and producing conditions such as sterility.

The major human malformations that result from radiation exposure are primarily microcephaly, mental retardation, and eye malformations, although neural tube defects and skeletal defects have been described.[17] The greatest risk of microcephaly occurs during 6–11 weeks' gestation.[18] Eight to fifteen weeks after conception is the period of greatest sensitivity for the development of mental retardation. Most animal and human data support a threshold dose effect in the range of 10–50 cGy for these teratogenic effects of radiation.[3] Recently, some epidemiologic data from a reassessment of Japanese atomic bomb survivors suggest that exposures as low as 1–9 cGy can induce small head size and mental retardation.[11] This study showed no detectable threshold of response for severe mental retardation and estimated the probability of occurrence of mental retardation at 0.4% per gray.[11] This study contradicts most data, which fail to reveal any increase in malformation or growth retardation below 5 cGy (5 rads). A minimum dose range of 25–50 cGy to produce nonrecuperable growth retardation in the human embryo is estimated.[16] With regard to postnatal functional impairment, Hicks and D'Amato have demonstrated decreased behavioral performances in animals at doses of 25–50 cGy, and no studies have shown human effects at exposures below 25 cGy.[19]

Whether diagnostic radiation exposure *in utero* results in an increase in postnatal cancer is disputed. The original epidemiologic study that described an increase in childhood leukemia from prenatal x-ray exposure was conducted in England and reported an increased relative risk of about 5 in the first trimester and 1.5 in the second and third trimesters from 1–2 cGy exposures.[20] Despite other studies that support this inference, a dose response relationship has never been demonstrated; animal data does not support it, and Japanese atomic bomb data fail to show an increase in childhood cancer.[21] There is, however, an increased cancer rate in *adult* life for those exposed *in utero* to atomic bomb radiation.[22] The consensus from UNSCEAR in 1986 reveals an excess of cancer deaths of 2.0–2.5% per gray for fetal radiation.

PREVENTION AND COUNSELING

The most essential feature of counseling pregnant patients with regard to diagnostic radiation exposure is accurate knowledge of the risks of exposure as compared to the natural background rates of spontaneous abortion, congenital malformations, genetic diseases, and cancer. For each inadvertent or planned exposure, these risks must be weighed along with the potential benefit of the study. One cannot counsel pregnant patients without first placing the risks of radiation into the context of general risks of human reproduction. It must be remembered that approximately 30–50% of known conceptions spontaneously abort and that the background rate of major congenital malformations at birth is about 27.5 per 1000, which increases to approximately 100 per 1000 when all malformations and genetic diseases become manifest. As detailed previously, the usual dosages for medical imaging range from 20–5000 mrads (0.02–5.0 cGy). The teratogenic, growth-retarding, and mutagenic risks from such exposures are extremely small. As Brent has pointed out, no such effects have been noted at exposures less than 5 rads.[1] In each case, the spontaneous risks far outweigh the radiation-induced risks. The carcinogenic risk is more questionable. If the upper limit for increased risk in the first trimester using Stewart's data is assumed to be a relative risk of 5, the fetus may be subject to a 1:200 chance of childhood malignancy versus a normal incidence of 1:1000. Brent[1] considers the cancer induction risk of a 1 cGy exposure to be in the order of 1:2000 for leukemia instead of the natural background rate of 1:3000.

The approach to counseling must be uniform and thorough. Brent has delineated nine key steps in the counseling process to obtain the essential information for effective counseling:[1]

1. The exact stage of gestation at time exposure
2. Menstrual history
3. Previous pregnancy history
4. History of congenital malformations
5. Other potentially harmful environmental exposures
6. Maternal and paternal ages
7. Exact type, dates, and number of radiologic studies performed or proposed

8. Calculation of the embryonic or fetal exposure by a medical physicist, radiation biologist, or experienced radiologist
9. Status of the pregnancy (wanted or unwanted)

For planning diagnostic studies in pregnant patients, the radiation risks of the procedure must be weighed against the harm of avoiding the procedure (eg, failing to diagnose, failing to treat, assuming a diagnosis, and exposing a patient to unnecessary treatment). For example, with judicious technique, deep venous thrombosis can usually be diagnosed with less than a 0.5-rad exposure to the fetus. Thus, if the study is negative, it avoids unnecessary heparinization in the current and in future pregnancies and avoids denial of oral contraceptives for the rest of a patient's reproductive life. Suggestions for minimizing exposures include using shielding to minimize scatter, using Tc-sulphur colloid instead of Tc-DTPA for ventilation scans, using a brachial approach for pulmonary angiography, constantly draining the bladder and aggressively hydrating the mother during bone scanning, using CT pelvimetry instead of standard pelvimetry when needed, and reducing radionuclide dosages by increasing scanning times. Although most diagnostic imaging studies fall well below the dosage necessary to induce malformations and growth retardation, unnecessary, routine, and elective x-rays should be avoided in pregnancy. Medically necessary imaging studies should rarely, if ever, be avoided during pregnancy if other nonionizing imaging techniques are not appropriate.

REFERENCES

1. Brent RL. The effects of embryonic and fetal exposure to x-ray, microwaves and ultrasound. *Clin Perinatol*. 1986;13:615.
2. Radionuclides in pregnancy. Reproductive Toxicology Center. Washington, DC: *Reprod Toxicol*. 1986;5:17.
3. Edwards FM. Risks of medical imaging. In: Putman CE, Ravin CE, eds. *Textbook of Diagnostic Imaging*. Philadelphia, PA: WB Saunders; 1988:91.
4. Moore MM, Shearer DR. Fetal dose estimates for CT pelvimetry. *Radiology*. 1989;171:265.
5. Ginsburg JS, Hirsh J, Rainbow AJ, Cotes G. Risks to the fetus of radiologic procedures used in the diagnosis of maternal venous thromboembolic disease. *Thrombos. Hemost*. 1989;61:189.
6. Hedrick WR, DiSimone RN, Wolf BH, Langer A. Absorbed dose to the fetus during bone scintigraphy. *Radiology*. 1988;168:245.
7. International Commission on Radiologic Protection. *Recommendations of the ICRP*. Oxford: Pergamon Press; 1977.
8. Mays CW. Stochastic and nonstochastic concepts: Is revision needed? *Health Physics*. 1988;55:437.
9. Dekabon AS. Abnormalities in children exposed to x-radiation during various stages of gestation: Tentative timetable of radiation injury to the human fetus, Part I. *J Nucl Med*. 1968;9:471.
10. Brent RL, Bolden BT. The indirect effect of irradiation on embryonic development. III. The contribution of ovarian irradiation, uterine irradiation and zygote irradiation to fetal mortality and growth retardation in the rat. *Radiat Res*. 1967;30:759.
11. Otake M, Schull WJ. *In utero* exposure to A-bomb radiation and mental retardation: a reassessment. *Br J Radiol*. 1984;57:409.
12. Murphy DP. The outcome of 625 pregnancies in women subjected to pelvic radium or roentgen irradiation. *Am J Obstet Gynecol*. 1929;18:179.
13. Shore RE. Radiation epidemiology: Old and new challenges. *Environ Hth Perspect*. 1989;81:153.
14. Russell JGB. Diagnostic radiation, pregnancy and termination. *Br J Radiol*. 1989;62:92.
15. Russell LB, Russell WL. The effects of radiation on the preimplantation stages of the mouse embryo. *Anat Res*. 1950;108:521.
16. Michel C. Radiation embryology. *Experientia*. 1989;45:60.
17. Committee on the Biological Effects of Ionizing Radiation. The effects on populations of exposure to low levels of ionizing radiation. Washington, DC: National Academy Press; 1980.
18. International Commission on Radiological Protection. *Developmental Effects of Irradiation on the Brain of the Embryo and Fetus*. Oxford: Pergamon Press; 1986.
19. Hicks SP, D'Amato CJ. Effects of ionizing radiation on mammalian development. In: Woodlam. *Advances in Teratology*. London, England: Logos Press; 1966;1:196.
20. Stewart A, Webb J, Hewitt D. A survey of childhood malignancies. *Br Med J*. 1958;1:1495.
21. Jablon S, Kato H. Childhood cancer in relation to prenatal exposure to A-bomb radiation. *Lancet*. 1970;2:1000.
22. Yashimoto Y, Kato H, Schull W. Risk of cancer among children exposed *in utero* to A-bomb radiations, 1950–1984. *Lancet*. 1988;2:665.

Chapter Twenty-Five

Electrical Injury

Patricia M. Garcia

25

Electrical injury, although rare, can have a devastating effect on pregnancy, even when maternal injury is apparently minor. Pregnant women are potentially susceptible to electrical injury from two sources. The major source of exposure is *low voltage current* (110 V, 220 V) from appliances primarily in the household setting. However, as more women enter the work force, especially in nontraditional jobs, their exposure to industrial sources of electrical injury increases. Seventeen cases of low-voltage electrical injury to pregnant women have been reported (Table 25–1). Of these, one case resulted in maternal, but not fetal, death, and only five of the 17 fetuses survived.[1-8]

The second major source of electrical injury is *lightning*. Outdoor activities place women at risk of high-voltage electrical discharge from lightning strikes. Reports indicate that approximately 300 deaths occur annually from lightning.[9] In the obstetric literature, 12 cases of lightning injury, all nonfatal to the mother, have been reported since 1833 (Table 25–2). The fetuses survived in six of these cases.[1,10-14]

Lastly, health care workers must be aware of the potential hazards of electrical equipment for patients. Exposure to electrical current commonly occurs in the hospital setting, but reports of injury are rare. One case of fetal injury (scalp burn) was reported as a result of a fetal scalp electrode applied during intrapartum fetal heart rate monitoring.[15] A postpartum patient undergoing emergency laparotomy was electrocuted, suffered cardiac arrest, and subsequently died because of a faulty switch in an operating table with electrocardiogram leads completing the circuit.[16] The intentional application of electrical current, as with electroconvulsive therapy for depressed patients who are pregnant, has not been associated with adverse pregnancy outcomes.[17-20]

TABLE 25–1. LITERATURE REPORTS OF ELECTRICAL CURRENT INJURY TO PREGNANT WOMEN

Year	Author	Gestational Age at Time of Injury	Voltage/ Source	Maternal Effects	Fetal Effects and Pregnancy Outcome	Immediate Labor
1933	Cathala[a]	7 mo	110 V	None	Liveborn SUD at 8 mo, neonatal death at 3 d[b]	No
1936	Sosa y Sanchez[a]	3 mo	220 V	Superficial burns	Inevitable abortion; D&C	Yes
1957	Baldi[a]	8½ mo	220 V	None	Immediate intrauterine fetal demise, SVD 6 d later	No
1957	Dordelman[a]	8 mo	220 V	None	Immediate intrauterine fetal demise, SVD 5 d later	No
1963	Hrozek[2]	Third trimester	220 V light bulb	Paresthesia	Immediate intrauterine fetal demise	?
	Hrozek[2]	Third trimester	220 V lamp cord	Paresthesia	Immediate intrauterine fetal demise	?
1986	Lieberman et al[3]	26 wk	110 V	None	Immediate intrauterine fetal demise, 700 g	No
	Lieberman et al[3]	21 wk	110 V	None	Intrauterine growth retardation, stillbirth 12 wk, subsequently 1000 g	No
	Lieberman et al[3]	40 wk	110 V	None	Immediate intrauterine fetal demise, 2400 g	No
	Lieberman et al[3]	32 wk	110 V	None	Livebirth, oligohydramnios, 2830 g	No
	Lieberman et al[3]	20 wk	110 V	None	Livebirth, oligohydramnios, 3070 g	No
	Lieberman et al[3]	40 wk	110 V	None	Livebirth, 3400 g	No
1972	Peppler et al[4]	29–30 wk	110 V power line	Paresthesia	Immediate intrauterine fetal demise	No
1987	Mazor, Lieberman[5]	9 wk	220 V	None	Fetal death	No
1987	Strong et al[6c]	30 wk	110 V[c]	None	Abnormal fetal heart rate tracing precipitated cesarean delivery, liveborn, oligohydramnios	No
1972	Toongsuwan[7]	38 wk	220 V power cable	Maternal death	Perimortem cesarean delivery, severely depressed liveborn, 2530 g	No
1986	Jaffe et al[8]	13 wk	220 V appliance	None	Immediate intrauterine fetal demise	Yes

[a] As reported by Rees WD.[1]
[b] Infant reported to have burn marks on nose, ears, neck, temporomaxillary area, dorsal surfaces of hands and feet, knees, elbows, and extensor surfaces.
[c] Before severe electrical shock at 30 weeks, patient experienced several previous mild shocks since 18 weeks' gestation.

PATHOPHYSIOLOGY

Electricity produces its biologic effect on tissues through two mechanisms.[21] Direct physiologic changes (eg, cardiac conduction disturbances and arrest, intense muscular contractions, respiratory center depression and arrest, and seizures) result as a current passes through various organs. Aside from this direct physical effect, current flowing through tissues also can produce injury through the generation of heat. Joule's law relates heat production (measured in Joules) to the intensity of the current (measured in amps), the resistance of the tissue (measured in ohms), and the duration of contact ($J = IRT$). Kobernick translates this physical property of electricity into physiologic terms and states that thermal injury depends on the following factors: the type of current, its strength, the pathway through the body, and time of contact.[21] Lastly, the tissue itself and the inherent physical attributes that make it more or less resistant to current flow also influence the extent of injury.[21]

Current can be either direct or alternating. Alternating current (AC) is produced by electromagnetic generators at extremely high voltages. Transformers reduce it to smaller voltages and power lines distribute the current for residential and commercial use. A unique property of alternating current is its ability to produce tetanic muscle contractions that may prevent the victim from letting go of the source of contact. The direct current (DC) from lightning is produced by electrical discharge from the negatively charged cloud to the positively charged ground. Low-voltage AC is more dangerous than low-voltage DC.

TABLE 25–2. LITERATURE REPORTS OF LIGHTNING INJURY AMONG PREGNANT WOMEN

Year	Author	Gestational Age at Time of Injury	Location of Strike	Maternal Effects	Fetal Effects and Pregnancy Outcome	Immediate Labor
1883	Schieffer[a]	8 mo	Left shoulder	Fall, superficial burns	Livebirth at term	No
1844	Alexander[a]	7 mo	Left shoulder	Superficial burns	Livebirth	?
1891	Ebertz[a]	7 mo	Right shoulder	LOC, superficial burns	Livebirth at term	No
1906	Troggler[a]	7 mo	Left shoulder	None	Immediate intrauterine fetal demise, stillbirth 3–4 mo subsequent	No
1959	Samsoenarjo[a]	6 mo	Abdomen	LOC, severe burns ruptured uterus, mother survived	Immediate fetal death	—
1965	Rees[1]	10 wk	Back of neck	LOC, fall, superficial burns	Normal term, livebirth 2550 g	No
1972	Chan and Sivasamboo[10]	Term	Abdomen, chest	LOC, superficial burns	Livebirth, neonatal death at 15 h of life	Yes
	Chan and Sivasamboo[10]	Term	Right shoulder	Fall, superficial burns	Livebirth	Yes
1979	Guha-Ray[11]	Term	Right forehead, arm	LOC, superficial burns	Immediate intrauterine fetal demise, stillbirth 7 d later	No
1986	Pierce et al[12]	7 mo	Neck, sternum, abdomen	LOC, burns, cardiopulmonary arrest	Immediate intrauterine fetal demise	No
1979	Weinstein[13]	34 wk	Chest	LOC, respiratory arrest, burns	Immediate intrauterine fetal demise, stillbirth 48 h later	No
1982	Flannery and Wiles[14]	7 mo	Right arm	Fall, paresthesia	Term livebirth	No

[a] As reported by Rees.[1]

The strength of the current or voltage is the electromotive force of the system. Typical household current is 110–220 V. High-tension power lines that lead from generators to transformers carry more than 100,000 V, and power lines from transformers carry between 7000 and 8000 V before the reduction to the 110–220 V for individual users. In stark contrast, lightning produces an extremely high-voltage electrical discharge often containing millions of volts.[22] Although greater voltages are more likely to produce more extensive injuries, low voltages (110 V household current) can cause death usually by cardiac defibrillation.

The third factor that determines tissue damage is the pathway the current takes through the body. For a current to pass through a victim, it must have an entry or contact point and an exit point to complete the circuit. Most typical household accidents involve a hand-to-foot pathway, which allows the current to pass through the lungs, heart, and, in pregnant patients, the uterus and fetus. Current that passes from head to foot also can produce devastating central nervous system effects (arrest of respiratory center, seizures, coma, and amnesia). Contact with lightning may be in the form of a direct strike (the most dangerous), a side flash (discharges from the direct strike spray through the air to a nearby object), a stride potential (current flowing through the ground enters one leg and exits through the other) or a flash-over phenomenon (current is conducted around the outside of the body with less energy flowing through the victim).[22]

Tissue resistance helps to determine, but does not dictate, the current's pathway through the body. The highest resistance to current flow is from bone, fat, and tendon. Skin produces an intermediate resistance to flow that can be reduced by moisture and increased by thickness (ie, callouses). Muscle, blood, and nerve are the least resistant to current flow and resist flow in decreasing order. Although not proven, amniotic fluid probably provides very little resistance to current flow, thereby increasing the propensity for electrical injury to the fetus and contributing to the high incidence of poor pregnancy outcome in these cases.

CLINICAL MANIFESTATIONS

Electrical injury produces diverse, multisystem organ damage. As stated previously, injury results from the direct effect of current on certain tissues and from heat production that damages deep structures by tissue necrosis. Cutaneous burns are common. They may be thermal burns, flame burns, or "arc" burns, which occur from current traveling across flexed joints.[21] Lightning produces a characteristic surface burn described as feathery or arborescent. Aside from cutaneous burns, high-voltage electricity and lightning may produce extensive deep-tissue destruction that resembles crush injury more than burn injury. Both lightning and electrical current can produce ventricular fibrillation and respiratory arrest through direct effects on the heart and respiratory center. Central nervous system and peripheral nervous system changes also occur from electrical injury and range from motor deficits and paresis to quadriplegia, coma, and seizures. These changes may be acute, but delayed neurologic sequelae from lightning injury also have been noted. Orthopedic injuries also are common, especially in lightning strikes in which the victim is often thrown to the ground.

In terms of pregnancy outcome, lightning and electrical current injuries produce significant maternal and perinatal morbidity and mortality. Maternal effects are no different than those previously described for nonpregnant individuals. Fetuses appear to be at special risk of electrical injury because of the increased conductivity of the amniotic fluid compartment. Electrical current and lightning injuries in the mother and fetus are individually discussed.

Electrical Current

Electrical alternating current produces the same injuries in pregnant patients as in nonpregnant individuals. There are 17 reported cases of low-voltage (110 V, 220 V) injuries associated with home- or work-related electrical appliances (16 cases) and one power cable accident (see Table 25–1). In 16 of the cases, maternal injury was minor without any loss of consciousness, cutaneous burns, or tissue injury. In a few of the cases, transient paresthesias with cold extremities were noted. All cases involved a hand-to-foot pathway, and therefore theoretically the current passed through the uterus. In one case, maternal death resulted from a 220-V power cable accident.[7] Although it seems plausible that electrical current could precipitate labor, no case of labor immediately following an electrical accident was documented in any second- or third-trimester exposure. It would, however, be more likely in the case of severe electrical burn injury associated with extensive tissue damage and massive fluid shifts.

Pregnancy outcomes in cases of electrical injury are quite poor despite the lack of maternal morbidity. Of the 17 cases, fetuses survived in only five (see Table 25–1). No subsequent livebirths occurred from first-trimester electrical exposure because immediate fetal death was documented in all three of these instances.[1,5,9] One of three fetuses exposed in the second-trimester survived,[3] but most surviving fetuses (four of five) resulted from third trimester exposures.[3,6,7] In the cases of second- and third-trimester exposure in which an intrauterine death resulted, immediate cessation of fetal movement was noted by the mothers in all cases but one. No placental or fetal pathologic lesion detected in any of these cases. These observations lead to a speculation that the mechanism of fetal injury is direct, perhaps as a result of a cardiac conduction disturbance, and not from an induced change in the placental vasculature. However, in one case of intrauterine demise, 12 weeks after the electrical shock intrauterine growth retardation developed before the eventual demise.

Interesting observations have been made in the case of livebirths following electrical accidents. Cutaneous burns were noted over the prominent parts of a neonate delivered 1 month after an electrical accident suffered by the mother. This infant subsequently died after 3 days of life.[1] Of the five cases in which infants survived the neonatal period, no gross lesions of the infants or placentas were noted. However, in three of these cases, oligohydramnios developed.[3,6] It is especially noteworthy that decreased amniotic fluid developed in a case of repetitive mild electrical shocks. These occurred from 18 weeks' gestation before a severe shock at 30 weeks, which immediately preceded the infant's delivery.[6] One surviving infant was delivered by perimortem caesarean section and although severely depressed, responded to resuscitation.[1] A second surviving infant was delivered operatively for FHR abnormalities following a 110-V electrical shock in the mother.[6]

Lightning Injury

In contrast to electrical injury reports in pregnant women, maternal injuries are much more severe from lightning. They are the same as in nonpregnant individuals with a significant incidence of loss of consciousness, cardiorespiratory arrest, and burns. As opposed to electrical injury, lightning strikes have been associated with precipitating immediate labor in two of the 12 reported cases. One case of uterine rupture that resulted in fetal, but not maternal death also was reported.[1]

For the 12 reported cases of maternal lightning injury, a perinatal survival rate of 50% was noted (see Table 25–2). Exposures are reported in all trimesters with one of one first-trimester, zero of one second-trimester, and five of 10 third-trimester fetuses surviving. In all cases of intrauterine demise, death occurred immediately after the lightning strike. No placental or fetal pathologic lesions were documented. One liveborn infant died at 15½ hours of life, and autopsy findings were consistent with congestive heart failure, interstitial pulmonary hemorrhages, epicardial hemorrhages, and hemorrhagic meninges.[10] The worst prognostic factor appears not to be the trimester of exposure or extent of maternal injuries, but rather the location of the strike. In all instances in which the lightning strike was to the anterior chest or abdomen, the pregnancy resulted in fetal death, and in a high percentage of cases, immediate labor ensued.[1,10,12,13] In one case, the outcome was especially catastrophic because a ruptured uterus resulted.[1] Of the five liveborn infants who survived beyond the neonatal period, long-term follow-up in at least one child at 19 months of age revealed no abnormalities.[14]

Treatment and Prevention Considerations

The initial treatment of electrical injury is directed toward removing the victim from the current source and providing basic and advanced life support for cardiac and respiratory arrest. In electrical accidents, the victim represents a potential hazard to the rescuer if current continues to flow. The victim must be approached with extreme caution and removed from the electrical source with something that does not conduct electricity. Once removed from the source, immediate resuscitation can begin. Cardiorespiratory arrest from lightning strikes necessitates vigorous and prolonged resuscitation. Reports of good outcomes are common after prolonged periods of arrest if aggressive and persistent resuscitative efforts are maintained. The pregnant patient in the third trimester represents a potential problem. Cardiopulmonary resuscitation (CPR) may be ineffective in late pregnancy because of caval occlusion by the large, gravid uterus.[23,24] Consideration must be given to delivery as a maternal life-saving procedure in the third trimester if CPR is ineffective.

Most victims of serious injury should be cared for in trauma centers that are experienced in burn injuries. A search for orthopedic, muscle, and nervous system injury must be conducted. Fluid resuscitation and treatment of acidosis and myoglobinuria should be instituted in cases of high-voltage electrical injury associated with deep-tissue damage, burns, and massive fluid shifts. Cardiac arrhythmias must be diagnosed and treated.

When the maternal condition is stabilized, the fetal status should be assessed quickly by fetal heart rate monitoring and ultrasound. Continuous monitoring for fetal heart rate abnormalities and uterine activity should be conducted. In the long term, the pregnancy must be followed closely for the development of growth retardation and oligohydramnios.

Careful consideration should be given to preventing electrical accidents. The entire household should periodically undergo scrutiny for potential electrical hazards. Household appliances should be checked for proper functioning, insulation, and shock hazard. Proper precautions must be taken when outdoors during thunderstorms. Shelter in a building or car should be sought immediately. If no shelter is available, a stand of trees obviously shorter than the adjacent grove is preferable to open areas; however, isolated trees should be avoided. In an open area, seek out the lowest possible ground and lie down. Remove and discard any metal objects (jewelry, hairpins, umbrellas, golf clubs). Be mindful of the possibility of the side-flash phenomenon. Any pregnant woman who experiences an electrical shock or lightning strike in pregnancy should be followed carefully as cases of subsequent oligohydramnios and intrauterine growth retardation have been noted.

REFERENCES

1. Rees WD. Pregnant women struck by lightning. *Br Med J*. 1965;1:103.
2. Hrozek O. Intrauterine death of the fetus in a mother shocked by electric current. *Zbl Gynak*. 1963;85:203.
3. Leiberman JR, Mazor M, Molcho J, et al. Electrical accidents during pregnancy. *Obstet Gynecol*. 1986;67:861.
4. Peppler RD, La Granche FJ, Comeaux JJ. Intrauterine death of a fetus in a mother shocked by electrical current: A case report. *J Louisiana State Med Soc*. 1973;124:37.
5. Mazor M, Leiberman JR. Abortion caused by electrical current. *Arch Gynecol Obstet*. 1987;241:71.
6. Strong TH, Gocke SE, Levy AV, et al. Electrical shock in pregnancy: A case report. *J Emergency Med*. 1987;5:381.
7. Toongsuwan S. Postmortem cesarean section following death by electrocution. *Aust N Zeal J Obstet Gynaecol*. 1972;12:265.
8. Jaffe R, Fejgin M, Ben-Aderet N. Fetal death in early pregnancy due to electric current. *Acta Obstet Gynecol Scand*. 1986;65:283.
9. Apfelberg DB, Masters FW, Robinson DW. Pathophysiology and treatment of lightning injuries. *J Trauma*. 1974;14:453.
10. Chan Y-F, Sivasamboo R. Lightning accidents in pregnancy. *J Obstet Gynaecol Brit Commonw*. 1972;79:761.
11. Guha-Ray DK. Fetal death at term due to lightning. *Am J Obstet Gynecol*. 1979;134:103.
12. Pierce MR, Henderson RA, Mitchell JM. Cardiopulmonary arrest secondary to lightning injury in a pregnant woman. *Ann Intern Med*. 1986;15:597.
13. Weinstein L. Lightning: A rare cause of intrauterine death with maternal survival. *Southern Med J*. 1979;72:632.
14. Flannery DB, Wiles H. Follow-up of a survivor of intrauterine lightning exposure. *Am J Obstet Gynecol*. 1982;142:238.
15. Akhter MS. An unusual complication of intrapartum fetal monitoring. *Am J Obstet Gynecol*. 1976;124:657.
16. Chambers JJ, Saha AK. Electrocution during anesthesia. *Anesthesia*. 1979;34:173.
17. Repke JT, Berger NG. Electroconvulsive therapy in pregnancy. *Obstet Gynecol*. 1984;63:395.
18. Smith S. The use of electroplexy (ECT) in psychiatric syndromes complicating pregnancy. *J Ment Sci*. 1956;102:796.
19. Sobel DE. Fetal damage due to ECT, insulin coma, chlorpromazine or reserpine. *Arch General Psych*. 1960;2:606.
20. Levine R, Frost EAM. Arterial blood gas analysis during electroconvulsive therapy in a parturient. *Anesthesia Analg*. 1975;54:203.
21. Kobernick M. Electrical injuries: Pathophysiology and emergency management. *Ann Emergency Med*. 1982;11:633.
22. Cwinn AA, Cantrill SV. Lightning injuries. *J Emergency Med*. 1985;379.
23. Oates, S, Williams GL, Rees GA. Cardiopulmonary resuscitation in late pregnancy. *Brit Med J*. 1988;297:404.
24. Rees GA, Willis BA. Resuscitation in late pregnancy. *Anesthesia*. 1988;43:347.

Chapter Twenty-Six

Drowning and Near-Drowning

Laura DiGiovanni

26

Drowning is the fourth leading cause of accidental death in adults.[1] More than 8000 deaths occur each year in the United States as a result of drowning.[2] The actual incidence of near-drowning is more difficult to determine; however, it is estimated more than 80,000 near-drowning accidents occur annually in the United States.[2] The pregnant immersion victim is rarely encountered; however, with the increasing popularity of aquatic sports, it is important to have an understanding of the pathophysiology and management of immersion accidents.

A variety of terms are used when discussing immersion accidents. *Drowning* is acute death from asphyxiation by submersion in water. *Near-drowning* refers to survival, at least temporarily, after asphyxia from submersion in water.[3] Approximately 10–15% of drowning victims die from asphyxia without aspiration of water into their lungs. This is referred to as *dry-drowning* and is the result of prolonged laryngospasm precipitated by fluid contacting the larynx preventing aspiration.[3,4] These victims usually recover quickly after resuscitation because they do not suffer the pulmonary injury present in *wet drowning*, in which there is fluid filling of alveoli. The majority (80–90%) of submersion victims, however, do aspirate water into their lungs.[5] *Secondary drowning* refers to delayed death subsequent to near-drowning caused by pulmonary or cerebral insult. *Secondary drowning* may occur hours or days later and occurs in 10–25% of near-drowning victims.[6,7]

The most important and prognostically significant variable in a submersion episode is the duration of hypoxia. Unfortunately, this is usually unknown in near-drowning cases. A number of factors contribute to the magnitude of hypoxia and to the victim's ability to withstand it: salt water versus fresh water, alcohol or drug intoxication[8], immersion hypothermia[9], seizures, hypoglycemia, head or cervical spine trauma[4], and whether immediate resuscitation was given at the scene of the accident.[10] The critically important clinical assessment and management of the pregnant immersion victim depends on a clear understanding of the pathophysiology of near-drowning.

PATHOPHYSIOLOGY

The major pathophysiology of drowning is asphyxia, hypoxia, hypercarbia, and acidosis, which terminate in cardiopulmonary arrest regardless of the quantity of water aspirated. This process is directly related to the duration of submersion and produces a combined metabolic and respiratory acidosis. Submersion is a multisystem injury, with pulmonary injury and resultant hypoxemia as the foremost problems.

It was previously thought that the aspiration of fresh water versus salt water led to differences in electrolyte imbalances. Early literature on drowning suggested that aspiration of salt water, which has an osmolality three to four times higher than plasma, led to decreased blood volume secondary to osmotic forces pulling plasma into the alveoli and thus to more concentrated serum electrolytes.[11] Fresh water was believed to produce the opposite effect—aspiration of this hypotonic medium led to hypervolemia and a dilutional effect on serum electrolytes. However, studies by Modell and others confirmed that at least 22 mL/kg of fluid must be aspirated before significant electrolyte changes occur.[12-14] Only 15% of drowning victims aspirate that much fluid and most near-drowning victims aspirate less than 4 mL/kg.[12,15] It has been shown that in near-drowning patients no clinically significant difference exists in serum electrolytes and hemoconcentration following fresh water versus salt water aspiration.[7,16]

There are, however, differences in the pathophysiology and mortality of salt water versus fresh water near-drownings.[5,17] The mechanism of the pulmonary injury is different in fresh water and salt water aspiration.[5] Although the amount of fluid aspirated is rarely enough to cause significant electrolyte and blood volume changes, aspiration of as little as 1 mL/kg body weight results in profound impairment of gas exchange.[13,14] Fresh-water aspiration washes out surfactant, causing increased surface tension, alveolar collapse, and atelectasis.[5,18-20] Salt water, because of its hypertonicity, draws fluid into the alveoli and produces pulmonary edema. Although the surfactant may be diluted by salt water in the alveoli, its surface active properties are not significantly altered.[5] Direct damage to alveolar capillaries occurs in both salt-water and fresh-water aspiration, resulting in increased membrane permeability, exudation of fluid and plasma proteins into the alveoli, and pulmonary edema.[5,18,19] Whatever the mechanism, the result is ventilation–perfusion mismatch, hypoxemia, and intrapulmonary shunting. A combined respiratory and metabolic acidosis occurs because of the hypercapnia and anaerobic metabolism.

Aspiration of salt water or fresh water also involves the aspiration of contaminants. Seventy percent of victims aspirate foreign material such as mud, sand, algae, sewage, chlorine, bacteria, or vomitus.[4] Salt water is twice as lethal as fresh water per unit volume, not because of the osmolarity, but because it contains more contaminants.[21] Aspiration of large particulate matter may occlude bronchi and compound impaired gas exchange.

Regardless of the mechanism, the most important consequence of immersion accidents is hypoxemia and its effects on various organs. Hypoxia is the common denominator in all of the organ injuries following a submersion accident. Most seriously affected are the pulmonary and central nervous systems. Prolonged hypoxia causes profound disturbance of Central Nervous System (CNS) function. Significant CNS injury is present in 12–27% of near-drowning victims.[22] The pathogenesis of hypoxic encephalopathy is poorly understood. Several reports of full neurologic recovery following prolonged submersions of up to 40 minutes[23,24] make it impossible to reliably predict the outcome of resuscitation of a given individual victim, even those arriving in the emergency department without spontaneous cardiac activity. Therefore, all submersion victims must be aggressively resuscitated.[20,25] Adult respiratory distress syndrome (ARDS) may develop in the near-drowning victim as a result of CNS hypoxia. This is usually seen 12–24 hours after the acute insult; therefore, all submersion victims should be closely observed for 24 hours after the incident regardless of how benign the initial clinical presentation appears.[20,26]

Acidemia and hypoxemia may lead to the development of cardiac arrhythmias, which may greatly complicate resuscitation and survival after the initial rescue. Cardiac arrhythmias usually respond to treatment of the underlying acidosis and hypoxia. However, cardiogenic shock may result if hypoxic damage to the myocardium has occurred. Most patients with fresh water and salt water aspiration have low left ventricular filling pressure. This is caused by an excessive permeability of pulmonary and systemic capillaries resulting in hypovolemia. Central venous pressure (CVP) may be elevated despite hypovolemia because hypoxia and acidosis may lead to pulmonary arterial hypertension.[5]

Near-drowning also affects other organ systems. Renal failure may occur after 24–48 hours. Acute tubular necrosis secondary to hypoxia is the most common renal injury.[17] Renal failure also may be due to myoglobinuria or lactic acidosis.[21,27] Disseminated intravascular coagulation occasionally is seen and develops in up to 50% of cases complicated by ARDS.[24] Infection may be seen in the first few days, and unusual organisms should always be considered in these patients.

Immersion Hypothermia

Immersion in cold water may alter the pathophysiology of near-drowning because of the effects of hypothermia. Hypothermia is a core temperature below 35°C. Cold water may prolong survival in near-drowning. The record nonfatal submersion in cold fresh water is 40 minutes, in cold salt water is 17 minutes, and in warm fresh water is only 10 minutes.[23,27] Hypothermia causes a decrease in basal metabolic rate, which is reduced to 50% of normal at a core temperature of 28°C.[28] Hypothermia affects the cardiovascular system, causing a gradual decline in heart rate and cardiac output, conduction abnormalities such as brady cardia, inverted T wave, and atrial fibrillation may also occur. Spontaneous ventricular fibrillation may occur at core temperatures below 28°C and asystole can occur at 22°C.[5,28]

Blood gas measurements in a hypothermic patient may yield erroneous results. Arterial blood gas is usually performed at 37°C; therefore, the arterial blood gas results must be corrected for the patient's body temperature. Each 1°C decrease in core temperature will decrease pH by 0.015 and increase PCO_2 and PO_2 by 4.4% and 7.2%, respectively.[28,29] Uncorrected blood gas values in a hypothermic patient may therefore give a falsely high pH and falsely low $PaCO_2$ and PaO_2. However, it is controversial whether arterial blood gases need to be temperature corrected or make a difference in clinical management.[26]

Hypothermia also inhibits insulin release, makes tissues resistant to its action, and decreases glucose use by the body, resulting in hyperglycemia.[28]

Hypothermia may have profound effects on cerebral metabolism. Cerebral blood flow decreases 6–7% per 1°C temperature drop, resulting in significant depression of sensorium.[28] Unconsciousness, absence of deep tendon reflexes, and dilated pupils are seen at core temperatures below 30°C.[30] Hypothermia results in decreased cerebral metabolic requirements, thereby protecting the brain for some time. The patient may appear to be dead because of the cardiovascular and cerebral manifestations of hypothermia at a time when resuscitation and complete neurologic recovery is still possible. Resuscitation should never be stopped until the body temperature has been raised to 31°C.[17,28]

The same physiologic changes may occur in the fetus in response to hypothermia and may therefore provide some protection against prolonged hypoxia in the fetus; however, there is no literature to support this.

MANAGEMENT

Management on the Scene

The most important determinant of survival and maximal brain salvage in near-drowning is prompt correction of hypoxemia and acidosis. Immediate cardiopulmonary resuscitation (CPR) at the site of the accident is of paramount importance and is the single most important factor influencing the outcome.[5,31] Patients who are successfully resuscitated at the site of the accident and are conscious on hospital arrival have an excellent chance of complete recovery.[31] The duration of submersion should not be a consideration in the decision to initiate immediate resuscitation. All near-drowning victims should receive prompt CPR regardless of clinical appearance or estimated duration of submersion.[17,30]

Ensuring adequacy of the airway, breathing, and circulation (the ABCs) are the goals of basic life support. CPR must be started immediately after rescue if airway and cardiopulmonary status are inadequate. The fundamentals of basic life support are the same after near-drowning in the pregnant victim as for any other situation requiring CPR. Injury to the cervical spine and back must be considered and the head and spine properly immobilized. When available, 100% oxygen should be administered during resuscitation and transport to a medical facility. All near-drowning patients should be evaluated at a hospital and admitted for at least 24 hours, even if they appear clinically normal.[20,22,26,30]

Hospital Management

Correction of hypoxia and acidosis from the pulmonary injury is the main priority. The goal is to establish adequate ventilation and circulation before cerebral hypoxia occurs or worsens. Upon arrival in the emergency room, establishing an adequate airway, respiration, and peripheral perfusion are essential. The level of consciousness should be assessed. Supplemental 100% oxygen and an intravenous infusion of isotonic crystalloid (Ringer's lactate) should be initiated. Resuscitation should be guided by arterial blood gas results and the patient's neurologic status. Patients with respiratory acidosis, PaO_2 less than 60 mm Hg, or who are unconscious require endotracheal intubation and ventilation. In addition to arterial blood gases, immediate laboratory tests should include complete blood count, electrolytes, blood urea nitrogen, creatinine, glucose, coagulation profile, urinalysis, tracheal cultures, blood alcohol level, and urine toxicology screen.[20,30] Assessment of fetal heart tones and gestational age also should be done.

An initial blood gas and chest x-ray should be performed on all victims of submersion accidents regardless of condition. The initial pulmonary radiographic findings may be much less than expected on the basis of the arterial blood gases. However, initially normal or minimally abnormal chest x-rays may show severe pulmonary edema in 6–12 hours.[26] No matter what the first chest x-ray film shows, decisions regarding treatment should be based on the arterial blood gases, which are the most reliable indicators of the severity of pulmonary injury.

The goal of respiratory management is to maintain PaO_2 above 70 mm Hg. Seventy percent of near-drowning victims have a significant intrapulmonary shunt and require aggressive respiratory therapy[27], which should be guided by serial arterial blood gases. With adequate resuscitation, normocapnia or hypocapnia is usually achieved while hypoxemia persists, indicating a significant ventilation–perfusion mismatch and an intrapulmonary shunt. The addition of positive end-expiratory pressure (PEEP) will decrease the degree of intrapulmonary shunting, reduce the ventilation–perfusion mismatch, and increase functional residual capacity, all of which will result in an increased PaO_2.[20,27,32-36] If aspiration of particulate matter is suspected, fiberoptic bronchoscopy should be performed when the patient is stabilized.[20]

Victims of near-drowning have a combined respiratory and metabolic acidosis. Metabolic acidosis should be treated with sodium bicarbonate, and respiratory acidosis must be managed by improving ventilation. Seventy percent of near-drowning victims have severe metabolic acidosis requiring correction with sodium bicarbonate.[37]

Once the immediately life threatening hypoxia and acidosis have been controlled, attention should be turned to treatment of the cardiovascular system, hypothermia, and any associated injuries. The initial x-ray evaluation also should include views of the cervical spine, and head computed tomography should be considered if there is decreased level of consciousness and evidence of head injury. Near-drowning does not significantly lower hematocrit; therefore, a low hematocrit should raise the question of occult hemorrhage.

An electrocardiogram should be obtained, and the patient should have continuous cardiac monitoring. Cardiac arrhythmias, if present, usually will respond to correction of acidosis and hypoxemia. A CVP line or a flow-directed pulmonary artery catheter is extremely valuable for assessment of cardiovascular status and management of intravascular volume. A nasogastric tube and Foley catheter should be placed, and a chest x-ray should be repeated every 8 hours; arterial blood gases should be measured every hour until the patient's condition is stable.[26]

The prophylactic use of antibiotics and steroids is controversial; the data at this time do not support the use of prophylactic antibiotics for pneumonia. The use of steroids for cerebral and pulmonary resuscitation also remains controversial.[17,26]

Once resuscitated, the severity of CNS injury determines survival and long-term neurologic sequelae from near-drowning. The classification criterion of Modell and associates[38] and Conn and colleagues[39] are extremely useful in assessing the severity of cerebral dysfunction in the early postimmersion period. The neurologic status can be categorized as category A (awake), category B (blunted), or category C (comatose). Category C is subclassified into C1 (decorticate), C2 (decerebrate), and C3 (flaccid). Ninety to 100% of patients in categories A and B will survive and remain neurologically intact. This group will require only appropriate cardiopulmonary support for complete recovery.[5,17] It is difficult to manage patients in category C and to determine which of these patients are likely to survive, and which will die or sustain severe neurologic sequelae. Retrospective reports of category C patients have revealed that 55% will have complete recovery, 10% will have neurologic sequelae, and 34% will die.[32,37-39] Vigorous cerebral resuscitation is recommended for optimal survival of patients in category C.[37] This includes the managing cerebral edema, controlling intracranial hypertension, and decreasing cerebral metabolic requirements. Investigators have been unable to predict survival rates in the comatose patient using such variables as elevated intracranial pressure[40], cerebral perfusion pressure[41], or cardiac arrest.[42] Because accurate prediction of survival is not possible and the initial presentation of the patient is often deceptive, every near-drowning victim should receive full and aggressive resuscitation efforts.[17,43]

There is a lack of information on the pathophysiologic effects of near-drowning on the fetus. Initial resuscitation of the mother and correction of the hypoxia and acidosis should take top priority when confronted with the rare case of a pregnant near-drowning victim. There also is a lack of case reports or literature on fetal management in the pregnant drowning or near-drowning patient. Depending on gestational age and fetal viability, an emergency cesarean section should be considered in special circumstances when, despite maximal resuscitation measures, the maternal condition is deteriorating rapidly. In cases of gestation remote from term in a comatose woman with no neural activity on serial EEG, continuing mechanical support in the mother to achieve fetal viability should be considered on an individual basis. This requires careful multidisciplinary consideration of legal and moral issues.

PREVENTION

Prevention is the best therapy. It is much easier to prevent near-drowning than to treat it. Most immersion accidents are preventable. Increased public awareness, safety, and education programs, training in CPR, and resuscitation of drowning victims at the scene will reduce morbidity from drowning and near-drowning accidents.

REFERENCES

1. *Accident Facts.* Chicago, IL: National Safety Council; 1988.
2. Baker SP, O'Neill B, Karpf RD. *The Injury Fact Book.* Lexington, MA: DC Heath & Co; 1984:155.
3. Modell JH. Drown versus near-drown: A discussion of definitions. *Crit Care Med.* 1981;9:351.
4. Kizer KW. Resuscitation of submersion casualties. *Emerg Med Clin North Am.* 1983;1(3):643.
5. Sarnaik AP, Vohra MP. Near-drowning: fresh, salt, and cold water immersion. *Clin Sports Med.* 1986;5(1):33.
6. Frates RC Analysis of predictive factors in the assessment of warm water near drowning in children. *Am J Dis Child.* 1981;135:1006.
7. Modell JH, Graves SA, Ketover A. Clinical course of 91 consecutive near drowning victims. *Chest.* 1976;70:231.
8. Mackie I. Alcohol and aquatic disasters. *Practitioner.* 1979;222:662.
9. Conn AW, Barker GA, Edmonds JF, Bohn DJ. Submersion Hypothermia and near-drowning. In: Pozos RS, Wittmers LE, eds. *The Nature and Treatment of Hypothermia.* Minneapolis, MN: University of Minnesota Press; 1983:152.
10. Copley DP, Mantle JA, Rigers WJ, et al. Improved outcome for prehospital cardiopulmonary collapse with resuscitation by bystanders. *Circulation.* 1977;56:901.
11. Knopp R. Near drowning. *J Am Coll Emerg Phys.* 1978;7:249.
12. Modell JH, Davis JH. Electrolyte changes in human drowning victims. *Anesthesiology* 1969;30:414.
13. Modell JH, Moya F. Effects of volume of aspirated fluid during chlorinated fresh water drowning. *Anesthesiology.* 1966;27:662.
14. Modell JH, Moya F, Newby EJ, et al. The effects of fluid volume in sea water drowning. *Ann Intern Med.* 1967;67:68.
15. Harries MG. Drowning in man. *Crit Care Med.* 1981;9:407.
16. Yagil R, Etzion Z, Oren A. The physiology of drowning. *Comp Biochem Physiol.* 1983;74A:189.
17. Neal JM. Near-drowning. *J. Emerg Med.* 1985;3:41.
18. Giammona ST, Modell JH. Drowning by total immersion. Effects on pulmonary surfactant of distilled water, isotonic saline and sea water. *Am J Dis Child.* 1967;114:612.
19. Modell JH. The pathophysiology and treatment of drowning and near-drowning. Springfield, IL: Charles C. Thomas; 1971.
20. Kram JA, Kizer KW. Submersion injury. *Emerg Med Clin North Am.* 1984;2(3):545.
21. Modell JH, Moya F, Newby EJ, et al. The effects of fluid volume in seawater drowning. *Ann Intern Med.* 1967;67(1):68.
22. Knopp R. Near Drowning. In: Rosen P, ed. *Emergency Medicine: Concepts and Clinical Practice.* St. Louis, MO: CB Mosby Co; 1983:470.
23. Siebke H, Breivik H, Rod T, et al. Survival after forty minutes submersion without cerebral sequelae. *Lancet.* 1975;1:1275.
24. Sekar TS, MacDonnell KF, Namsirikul P, et al. Survival after prolonged submersion in cold water without neurologic sequelae. *Arch Intern Med.* 1980;140:775.
25. Oakes DD, Sherck JP, Maloney JR, et al. Prognosis and management of victims of near drowning. *J Trauma.* 1982;22:544.
26. Orlowski JP. Drowning, near-drowning, and ice-water submersions. *Ped Clin North Am.* 1987;34(1):75.
27. Modell J. Drowning and near drowning. *Soc Crit Care Med.* 1980;1:10.
28. Reuler JB. Hypothermia: Pathophysiology, clinical settings and management. *Ann Intern Med.* 1978;89:519.
29. Meyers RAM, Britten JS, Cowley RA. Hypothermia: Quantitative aspects of therapy. *J Am Coll Emerg Phys.* 1979;8:523.
30. Martin TG. Near drowning and cold water immersion. *Ann Emerg Med.* 1984;13(4):263.
31. Modell JH, Graves SA, Kuck EJ. Near-drowning: Correlation of level of consciousness and survival. *Can Anaesth Soc J.* 1980;27:211.
32. Gonzalez-Rothi RJ. Near-drowning: consensus and controversies in pulmonary and cerebral resuscitation. *Heart and Lung.* 1987;16(5):474.
33. Pruessner HT, Zenner GO, Hansel NK. Management of the near-drowning victim. *AFP.* 1988;37(5):251.
34. Orlowski JP. Prognostic factors in pediatric cases of drowning and near-drowning. *J Am Coll Emerg Phys.* 1979;8:176.
35. Modell JH. Biology of drowning. *Ann Rev Med.* 1978;29:1.
36. Hoff BH. Multisystem failure. A review with special reference to drowning. *Crit Care Med.* 1979;7:310.
37. Conn AW, Edmonds JF, Barker GA. Cerebral resuscitation in near-drowning. *Ped Clin North Am.* 1979;26:691.
38. Modell JH, Graves SA, Kuck EJ. Near-drowning: Correlation of level of consciousness and survival. *Can Anaesth Soc J.* 1980;27:211.
39. Conn AW, Montes JE, Barker GA, et al. Cerebral salvage in near-drowning following neurological classification by triage. *Can Anaesth Soc J.* 1980;27:201.
40. Dean JM, McComb JG. Intracranial pressure monitoring in severe pediatric near-drowning. *Neurosurgery.* 1981;9:627.
41. Nussbaum E, Galant SP. Intracranial pressure monitoring as a guide to prognosis in the nearly drowned, severely comatose child. *J Pediatr.* 1983;102:215.
42. Oakes DD, Sherck JP, Maloney JR, et al. Prognosis and management of victims of near-drowning. *J Trauma.* 1982;22:544.
43. Dean JM, Kaufman ND. Prognostic indicators in pediatric near-drowning: The Glasgow Coma Scale. *Crit Care Med.* 1981;9:536.

Chapter Twenty-Seven
Common Poisons

Thomas N. Balaskas

27

Poisoning in pregnancy is usually secondary to a suicide attempt. The frequency of successful suicide in pregnancy is low and is equal to that of nonpregnant women. As in nonpregnant women, suicide attempts greatly outnumber successful suicides. Suicide attempts may occur at any time during the pregnancy but occur mainly in the first two trimesters.[1] The suicide *gesture* involves a single method, usually the ingestion of an easily accessible prescription or over-the-counter medication. The most frequently ingested substances, in decreasing order of frequency, are analgesics, mainly acetaminophen; vitamin preparations; iron; sedatives; antibiotics; and antihistamines.[2] Poisoning in pregnancy also may be caused by the movement away from conventional medical care and the use of home remedies in the form of herbal preparations. Herbal substances may not be used for primary medical care, but may include termination of an unwanted pregnancy.[3]

Drugs ingested by pregnant women have the ability to produce acute toxicologic effects in the mother and fetus if taken in high enough doses, and they may result in long-term sequelae to the fetus depending on gestational age and duration of exposure. If exposure to a toxin occurs during fetal organogenesis, congenital anomalies may be produced. If exposure occurs just after implantation, the toxin may only be embryocidal, and if long-term low-dose exposure occurs, fetal growth and physiology may be altered, resulting in intrauterine growth retardation.

Fetal risks may be quite different than maternal risks because of the pharmacokinetics of drugs during pregnancy. Thus, drugs may be trapped on the fetal side of the placenta; the placenta may protect the fetus by preventing the passage of toxic substances or by metabolizing these compounds.

Diffusion is not the only means of transfer of toxins across the placenta. Transfer of substances into the fetal compartment depends on lipid solubility and molecular weight and on whether the substance is ionized, free, or protein-bound.[4]

Exposure to environmental toxins within the home, workplace, or outdoors also have been responsible for some poisonings of pregnant women (see also Chapter 10); yet the frequency of these poisonings is small. Unfortunately, very little literature addresses this subject.

Most poison control centers treat pregnant patients with few exceptions in the same manner as nonpregnant patients.

PHYSIOLOGIC CHANGES IN PREGNANCY

Many physiologic changes in pregnancy may affect the absorption, transfer, metabolism, and excretion of toxins in an exposed pregnant woman. They are discussed in more detail in Chapter 4. In short, *cardiovascular changes* include a 30–50% increase in cardiac output, which is secondary to increases in stroke volume and heart rate. These changes may predispose the pregnant woman to greater tissue concentrations of absorbed substances, especially in organs that receive a large portion of cardiac output, such as the uterus, placental bed, kidneys, and skin.

Pulmonary changes in general promote the absorption of inhaled soluble toxicants through the lung. This includes an increased diffusing capacity of the lungs in early pregnancy, which also predisposes the patient to an increased absorption of inhaled agents.[5]

Plasma volume increases in pregnancy result in an altered volume of distribution, producing a dilutional effect.

Plasma albumin decreases in early pregnancy by approximately 20%. This fall in plasma albumin along with increases in plasma volume results in decreased protein binding of drugs.[6] Decreased protein binding of drugs leads to increases in the free fraction of a drug in the plasma. Because the free fraction of the compound possesses the most activity, a larger portion of toxin is presented to maternal and fetal tissues.

Fat storage occurs primarily in the second trimester of pregnancy. The fat is centrally located and is mobilized in late pregnancy, depending on the nutritional demands of the fetus. The increased fat deposits may act as storage centers for lipid-soluble toxins, which when released in pregnancy, may expose the mother and fetus to high levels of previously ingested toxins. Mobilization of fat stores also may result in competition for albumin-binding sites by free fatty acids, further increasing the free fraction of a drug within the plasma.[4,7]

Renal function also undergoes major changes in pregnancy. The glomerular filtration rate (GFR) begins to increase early in pregnancy at about 6–8 weeks' gestation and peaks in the second trimester at about 50% above nonpregnant values. The GFR then plateaus or gradually rises in the third trimester until term. Variable changes have been reported in the GFR in the third trimester, which may be caused by changes in patient position. Renal plasma flow also increases in pregnancy, beginning early in the first trimester by rising to a level 40% greater than nonpregnant values. It may gradually rise in the third trimester until term. Because the major form of elimination of many toxins is by way of the renal system, increases in renal function may increase clearance of both free and conjugated drugs within the plasma.

Pregnancy also results in a prolonged gastric emptying time and in delayed transport through the small intestine, which may lead to increased absorption of ingested toxins.

Hepatic blood flow, size, and histology remain unchanged in pregnancy. Serum concentrations of many proteins produced by the liver are increased in pregnancy secondary to the increases in serum estrogen. Hepatic biotransformation of compounds is variable, depending on the nature of the ingested substrate. Unfortunately, very little information exists on the hepatic biotransformation of toxic substrates in pregnancy, which makes the coordination of treatment in an acutely poisoned pregnant patient much more difficult.[4,6,7]

MANAGEMENT OF THE ACUTELY POISONED PREGNANT PATIENT

Treatment of a pregnant patient who is acutely intoxicated with an ingested poison is not different from that of a non-pregnant patient. It involves stabilization, evaluation through history, physical examination and laboratory tests when the patient is stabilized, prevention of absorption, improvement of elimination, and specific antidote administration while assessing fetal well-being with electronic fetal heart rate monitoring.

Stabilization involves maintenance of airway, breathing, and circulation. Airway maintenance may involve the chin lift or jaw thrust to remove obstruction by the tongue. Removal of foreign bodies and secretions, along with nasopharyngeal or oropharyngeal intubation, may be necessary to maintain an airway and assist in ventilation of a comatose patient. Intubation also protects against aspiration. If ventilation is inadequate, supplemental oxygen and intubation are necessary. Vital signs should be obtained to assess circulatory status with continuous electrocardiographic monitoring.[8]

The patient should be placed in a left lateral recumbent position to improve maternal cardiac output, and the fetus should be continuously electronically monitored.

A large bore IV should be placed, and arterial blood gases, electrolytes, glucose, and necessary toxicologic screening tests should be obtained. If inadequate circulation is apparent, intravenous fluid challenge with crystalloid solution, combined with central monitoring using a Swan-Ganz catheter or central venous pressure line to assess intravascular volume and cardiac output may be necessary.

Neurologic status should be assessed after stabilizing ventilation and circulatory parameters. If the patient presents with a depressed mental status, 50 cm^3 of 50% dextrose in water (D50W) should be administered intravenously. A blood glucose level must be drawn before administration of D50W. Naloxone, 2 mg, should be given if narcotic intoxication is suspected or if the patient is comatose. Thiamine, 100 mg intravenously or intramuscularly, should be administered before glucose administration if alcoholism is suspected because glucose administration may deplete thiamine stores and worsen an existing Wernicke's encephalopathy.[9]

Poisoning victims may exhibit seizures, which should be treated with maintenance of oxygenation, followed by immediate treatment with diazepam, phenobarbital, or phenytoin.

If a metabolic etiology is identified (eg, hypocalcemia, hypoglycemia, electrolyte alterations or hypoxemia), attempts should be made to correct it immediately.

If anticonvulsant treatment is unsuccessful and the patient is in *status epilepticus,* general anesthesia may be required. Electronic fetal monitoring should be continued, with the addition of ultrasound to assess fetal well-being.

Prevention of absorption of ingested toxic substances involves induction of emesis, gastric lavage, administration of activated charcoal, and cathartics.

Emesis is useful for evacuating gastric contents and can be induced by using syrup of ipecac and apomorphine. Mechanical stimulation of the posterior pharynx with a smooth object, such as a spoon, finger, or tongue blade, is not as effective as syrup of ipecac and should be reserved for patients without medical supplies.

Syrup of ipecac is the emetic of choice because of its effectiveness, rapid onset of action, and few adverse effects. It is recommended for poisoned victims who are awake, alert, and have a gag reflex. Contraindications include ingestion of caustic or corrosive agents that may produce further destruction on emesis. It also is contraindicated in patients who have ingested petroleum distillate hydrocarbons, such as gasoline, kerosene, and mineral spirits, when the risk of aspiration is greater than the potential toxicity of the substance.[10]

Apomorphine may be used as an emetic agent and is equally effective, although it may produce sedation, respiratory depression, and prolonged vomiting. Syrup of ipecac is not specifically approved for use in pregnancy. Although there is a paucity of data on its effects in pregnancy and the risks of teratogenesis, it does not appear to place the fetus at increased risk. It is therefore important to individualize each case and weigh the benefits and risks of its use.

Gastric lavage is another means of preventing absorption of ingested poisons. It is as effective as syrup of ipecac and is ideal for patients with loss of consciousness, who are convulsing, or who have lost their gag reflex.

The patient should be placed in the left lateral position with the head down. Often intubation is required for airway protection, although lavage can be performed without intubation in a patient with an intact gag reflex. A large-bore orogastric tube is placed, and gastric contents are aspirated. Lavage is then performed with aliquots of 200–300 mL of warmed saline or water and allowed to drain. Gastric lavage should be continued until the aspirate is clear. Contraindications to this procedure include ingestion of caustic agents and sharp objects.

Complications include trauma to the esophagus, pulmonary aspiration, and the possibility of electrolyte imbalance if other lavage solutions are used.

Clinical toxicology has supported the administration of activated charcoal to prevent absorption of ingested toxins.

Activated charcoal is made by burning wood pulp, washing it, and activating it with acids or steam. The activation increases the absorption ability of the charcoal by removing absorbed substances and increasing the surface area. Activated charcoal can bind many drugs and substances and effectively prevents absorption within 1 hr after ingestion of the poison.

A study by Tenenbein and colleagues simulated an ampicillin overdose and demonstrated that activated charcoal without a gastric emptying procedure reduced ampicillin absorption by 57%, whereas gastric lavage reduced it by only 32%, and syrup of ipecac by 38%. Orogastric lavage appeared to be the least effective procedure.[11]

Activated charcoal is administered in a slurry form, in a dose of 60–100 g in an aqueous solution. It can be administered orally or through an orogastric tube. It is usually recommended in all poisonings after an initial treatment of emesis induction or lavage.

A contraindication to activated charcoal is ingestion of caustic agents because it does not absorb acids or alkali and may interfere with endoscopy. It should not be administered before an antidote administration because it may absorb the antidote and prevent its action. This has been seen with N-acetylcysteine, an antidote for acetaminophen poisoning.

Another method that may be helpful in preventing absorption is whole-bowel irrigation. This is a technique that has been used to cleanse the gastrointestinal tract before diagnostic procedures such as colonoscopy. Whole-bowel irrigation involves administration of a polyethylene glycol electrolyte solution orally or using a nasogastric tube until the rectal effluent is clear. Its use has been described in a pregnant woman with iron overdose in the third trimester of pregnancy. The patient was successfully treated without complications and delivered a normal term female infant 5 weeks later without perinatal complications.[12] This may prove to be an easy, effective, and safe way to prevent absorption of ingested toxins in pregnant and nonpregnant patients. More studies need to be performed, however, to assess its final value.

Cathartics may be used to reduce absorption of poisons. Common cathartics are magnesium sulfate, magnesium citrate, disodium phosphate, and sorbitol. Cathartics are thought to cause osmotic retention of water within the gastrointestinal tract and, at the same time, stimulate the release of cholycystokinin, which produces peristalsis.[13] These agents are taken orally and are contraindicated after the ingestion of caustic substances. Sodium-containing cathartics should be avoided in patients with severe hypertension, congestive heart failure, and renal disease, while magnesium cathartics should be avoided in patients with chronic renal disease or who have ingested nephrotoxins.

Enhancement of elimination includes the alteration of urine pH and the increase of urine flow by forced diuresis. Diuresis is achieved by the forced intravenous administration of fluids. In certain instances, mannitol or furosemide may be used to improve elimination of some toxins.

Alkaline diuresis involves the intravenous administration of sodium bicarbonate with dextrose and saline solutions every 3–4 hours until alkaline urine pH is achieved, usually in the range of a pH 7–8. Contraindications to this procedure involve renal or cardiac failure. *Acid diuresis* includes more intense patient monitoring and involves the intravenous administration of ammonium chloride or of a 0.1 M solution of hydrochloric acid until a urine pH of 5.5–6.0 is achieved. Contraindications to acid diuresis include renal failure, cardiac failure, and the presence of myoglobinuria.

Complications of forced diuresis with alteration of urine pH include fluid overload in the form of pulmonary edema, cerebral edema, electrolyte and acid-base imbalances.

It is important to maintain a pregnant patient in the left lateral recumbent position, which will improve diuresis. It is also essential to continue monitoring fetal well-being. Unfortunately, only few drugs fulfill the criteria for forced diuresis and alteration of pH, resulting in infrequent use of this method.

Forced diuresis and alteration of pH are useful in the primary and combination treatment of salicylate, phenobarbital, and 2,4 dichlorophenoxyacetic acid poisoning, using alkaline diuresis. The treatment of phencyclidine (PCP), amphetamine, quinidine, and strychnine poisoning may be successful through acid diuresis.[14]

Hemodialysis has benefits and risks. It has the ability to remove many types of toxins, yet it is limited by the physical properties of the toxin. The toxin must be water soluble, of low molecular weight (less than 500 d), poorly protein bound, and have a low volume of distribution.

The decision to perform dialysis depends on several factors, including prolonged coma, unstable vital signs, ingestion of a lethal dose of toxin, detection of a lethal blood level of toxin, and the presence of nonfunctional physiologic excretion routes.

Hemodialysis is useful in the removal of toxins, such as bromide, chloryl hydrate, ethanol, isopropyl alcohol, lithium, methanol, and salicylates.[15] Complications of this procedure include hypotension, electrolyte abnormalities, acute hemorrhage, hypoproteinemia, infection, air embolus, and acute hemorrhage.

There is limited information on hemodialysis for the use of toxin removal in pregnancy; however, there are reports of chronic hemodialysis in pregnant patients with chronic renal failure, resulting in preterm labor, preterm delivery, and intrauterine growth retardation.

Hemoperfusion is a method of removing a toxin from the blood by pumping it over an absorbent material, such as activated charcoal or an amberlite resin. Clinical features required to perform this procedure are similar to those for hemodialysis. The limitations of the two procedures differ, however, in that hemoperfusion is not limited by the molecular weight, protein binding, and water solubility of a substance.

Hemoperfusion can effectively remove phenytoin, chloramphenicol, theophylline, methotrexate, and phenobarbital. Complications consist of thrombocytopenia, leukopenia, hemorrhage, hypotension, and electrolyte imbalance.[16]

SPECIFIC POISONS

Although a paucity of information about the treatment of poisoning in pregnancy exists, it is important that regional poisoning centers be contacted when questions arise about the management of patients.

Acetaminophen

Acetaminophen is a widely prescribed, effective analgesic–antipyretic agent used in pregnant and nonpregnant individuals. It was developed in the 1950s and has become popular because it does not produce many of the potential adverse effects seen with salicylates, such as an increased risk of bleeding, sensitization in asthmatic patients, gastrointestinal irritation, development of Reye's syndrome in children, and premature closure of the fetal ductus arteriosus. Studies on drug use in pregnancy reveal that acetaminophen is the most commonly ingested drug in pregnancy second to iron and vitamins. It is taken four times more frequently than aspirin.[17]

Rayburn et al[2] reviewed suicide attempts in pregnancy and found that drug ingestion was the primary method of choice. Analgesics were the most common substances, with acetaminophen being the most frequently ingested analgesic.[2]

The liver metabolizes acetaminophen by the process of sulfation (52%) and glucuronidation (42%). Approximately 4% is metabolized by the cytochrome oxidase P-450 system, which results in the formation of a toxic metabolite.[18] This toxic metabolite is then conjugated with glutathione and excreted in the urine as mercaptopurate, which is nontoxic. Two percent of acetaminophen is excreted unchanged.

When patients ingest an overdose of acetaminophen, the glutathione is rapidly used, and the pathway is overwhelmed, causing an increase in unbound toxic metabolite. This can covalently bind to hepatocytes and produce necrosis with the possibility of fulminant liver failure. Ingestion of more than 7.5 g of acetaminophen is considered toxic and may cause acute liver damage. However, the severity of liver damage does not appear to be directly correlated to the amount of acetaminophen ingested. Other factors, such as age, nutritional status, and other ingested compounds, may affect the amount of cytochrome P-450 oxidase present. Drugs such as phenobarbital, which induce hepatic enzymes, actually may enhance acetaminophen toxicity. Renal failure, myocardial damage, and pancreatitis also have been seen in patients with acetaminophen overdoses.

Acetaminophen can cross the placenta and may pose a significant risk not only to the mother but to the fetus.[19] The actual amount of acetaminophen reaching the fetus in cases of maternal overdose is unknown. The human fetus possesses functioning liver enzymes that have the ability to metabolize drugs as early as 8 weeks' gestation.[20] Rollins et al, using *in vitro* preparations of fetal hepatocytes from 18–23 weeks' gestation, demonstrated that the fetal liver can detoxify acetaminophen by sulfation and can oxidize this compound to its toxic metabolite. This oxidation ability was measured as one tenth that of adult liver and appeared to increase with gestational age.[21] These findings suggest the possibility of increased risk of hepatic damage to the fetus if a large amount of acetaminophen crosses the placenta as in maternal overdose. Although only a small amount of literature exists on maternal and fetal outcomes after toxic ingestion of acetaminophen, varying outcomes have been seen. Toxic maternal exposure to acetaminophen at 16–36 weeks' gestation that required intensive treatment and resulted in good pregnancy outcomes at term have been reported.[22-27] Fetal distress, premature labor, premature delivery, and fetal demise also have been seen after maternal overdose.[28-30] Haibach described a case of fetal demise in which autopsy revealed significant lysis of fetal hepatocytes, consistent with acetaminophen toxicity, incriminating this drug as the primary cause of fetal death.[28] No studies have revealed an increase in fetal malformations caused by maternal toxic exposure to acetaminophen.

Diagnosis of acetaminophen overdose requires observance of clinical findings consistent with poisoning and a toxic plasma level of acetaminophen more than 4 hours after ingestion. Shortly after ingestion of a toxic dose, the patient may experience nausea, vomiting, diaphoresis, malaise, and pallor, which may last up to 24 hours.

If hepatic toxicity ensues, there is usually a latent period of 24–48 hours in which the patient may feel well. At some time during this period, the patient develops right upper quadrant pain and a rise in bilirubin, hepatic enzymes, and prolongation of prothrombin time. During days 3–5, if hepatic damage progresses, nausea, vomiting, jaundice, and hepatosplenomegaly begin, progressing to coagulopathy, hypoglycemia, and hepatic encephalopathy if hepatic injury is severe. If the patient survives and liver damage is reversible, the liver damage begins to resolve in 5 days, with total resolution by 3 months.

Plasma levels for acetaminophen should be obtained at least 4 hours after ingestion. Plasma levels greater than 120 mg/mL are usually considered toxic and require treatment. Those patients in which the time of ingestion is unknown also should be treated.

Treatment of acetaminophen poisoning in pregnant patients should not differ from that of nonpregnant patients. Management includes prevention of absorption, with syrup of ipecac or gastric lavage. The use of activated charcoal is controversial because *in vitro* studies have revealed binding of the antidote N-acetylcysteine (Mucomyst), which may prevent detoxification.[31] Activated charcoal followed by lavage before administration of N-acetylcysteine may be necessary. N-acetylcysteine is a safe and effective antidote that is specific for the treatment of acetaminophen poisoning. This compound is thought to be a precursor of glutathione, and can increase glutathione levels and thereby facilitate the metabolism of the toxic intermediate of acetaminophen. N-acetylcysteine should be administered immediately to patients with toxic plasma levels of greater than 120 mg/mL 4 hours after ingestion. If the patient has a documented history of ingestion of greater than 7.5 g of acetaminophen, the antidote also should be administered. N-acetylysteine may be administered orally or intravenously. When administered orally, a loading dose of 140 mg/kg should be administered, followed by 70 mg/kg every 4 hours for 17 doses.[32] Intravenous administration of N-acetylcysteine has been suggested at a dose of 300 mg/mL over 20 hours. Nausea and vomiting may limit the effectiveness of oral acetylcysteine.[33] Whatever route of administration is chosen, it is important to administer the antidote at least 10–12 hours after ingestion of the toxin for maximal effectiveness.

Other glutathione precursors, such as cysteamine and methionine, are less effective and less safe in the treatment of acetaminophen poisoning. Hemodialysis and hemoperfusion may be used selectively in patients with significantly high plasma acetaminophen levels.

Supportive therapy also should be carried out during the treatment period, accompanied by monitoring of fetal well-being in the form of electronic fetal heart rate monitoring or ultrasound evaluation. Delivery should be considered if fetal distress ensues.

Salicylates

Aspirin, or acetylsalicylic acid, is a commonly used analgesic. Its popularity and use in pregnancy has decreased because of some adverse effects of the drug and the advent of acetaminophen. Acetylsalicylic acid is a weak acid and is rapidly absorbed from the gastrointestinal tract. It is hydrolyzed in the gastrointestinal tract and in blood to form salicylic acid and acetic acid. Salicylic acid is the therapeutic component that produces the anti-inflammatory and toxic effects in overdosage. Acetylsalicylic acid prevents prostaglandin synthesis by acetylating and inactivating cyclooxygenase, which converts arachidonic acid to endoperoxide prostaglandin G_2. This prevents formation of other prostaglandins, including thromboxane A_2 and prostacyclin, exerting an antiplatelet aggregating effect (see also Chapter 15). Salicylic acid does not appear to possess this ability *in vitro*.[34] A majority of salicylic acid is bound to albumin, and at therapeutic doses, it is metabolized in the liver to form glycine and glucuronide conjugates before elimination. With overdose, the enzymatic pathways are saturated, and renal elimination occurs. Toxic levels of salicyclates will alter acid-base balance. Salicylates may stimulate directly the respiratory center, resulting in respiratory alkalosis, which is followed by excretion of bicarbonate, sodium, and potassium by the kidneys to compensate for this change. This alters the hydrogen ion concentrations, resulting in metabolic acidosis. Salicylates also uncouple oxidative phosphorylation, altering the Krebs cycle, which results in the formation of organic acids and metabolic acidosis. Uncoupling of oxidative phosphorylation results in a hypermetabolic state, which manifests as hyperthermia, hyperglycemia secondary to increased glycogenolysis, and possibly hypoglycemia secondary to increased glucose use. These pathophysiologic changes result in many of the clinical findings seen in acutely poisoned patients.

Salicylates have been shown to cause adverse effects in pregnancy even at therapeutic levels. Late in pregnancy, those may include an increased incidence of post-term pregnancy, postpartum hemorrhage, and prolonged labor. Because aspirin crosses the placenta, it may cause adverse fetal effects as well. Some studies have suggested that salicylates have teratogenic effects on the developing fetus if taken in the first trimester of pregnancy.[35] Other studies have refuted these claims.[36] Aspirin also may have adverse effects on fetal coagulation. Rumack et al found a significant increase in intraventricular hemorrhage in premature infants of mothers who had taken aspirin within 1 week of delivery, compared to infants of mothers who did not consume aspirin.[37] Inhibition of prostaglandin synthesis by aspirin also may cause premature closure of the ductus arterosus in the fetus. Reports of toxic ingestion of salicylates and of treatment in pregnancy are few and demonstrate varying outcomes.

Stillbirth has been reported after acute toxic ingestion of salicylates at 32–34 weeks' gestation. Detoxification therapy was instituted immediately, with apparent establishment of fetal well-being, followed by fetal death 20 hours after admission. Fetal autopsy revealed toxic levels of salicylates in the brain, liver, and blood.[38] It therefore appears that the fetus does not have the ability to effectively metabolize salicylates, as also demonstrated by reports of higher levels of salicylates in fetal serum.[39,40] This may be because of immature fetal glucuronidation and renal excretion capabilities.[7,39]

Patients with salicylate poisoning usually present with nausea, vomiting, and tinnitus. In moderate to severe cases, patients often develop hyperventilation, hyperthermia, hyperglycemia or hypoglycemia, lethargy, coma, and convulsions. As mentioned previously, acid-base disturbances, dehydration, and electrolyte abnormalities, such as hyponatremia, hypernatremia, hypokalemia, and hypocalcemia, may be seen. Hematologic changes caused by salicylate poisoning include decreases in factor VII, prothrombin, and platelet function. In severe toxicities, acute renal failure and noncardiogenic pulmonary edema also can occur. Serum salicylate levels are a valuable tool in assessing the severity of intoxication. The level should be obtained 6 hours after ingestion of salicylate, and serum levels greater than 30 mg/dL are considered toxic. Levels taken after a single ingestion are helpful, but not in patients with chronic ingestions who may display symptoms even if well below a serum level of 30 mg/dL.[41]

Treatment of patients with salicylate poisoning involves stabilization and supportive care. Intravenous fluids should be initiated immediately because most patients are dehydrated on presentation. Electrolyte levels, serum glucose, and blood pH must be assessed carefully. Acidosis should be treated immediately with intravenous sodium bicarbonate and potassium supplements if there is coexisting hypokalemia. If hyperthermia is present, a cooling blanket or ice can be used, along with careful monitoring of temperature.

Convulsions suggest severe intoxication and usually indicate the need for hemodialysis. Convulsions should be treated acutely with diazepam and a metabolic etiology must be investigated. If pulmonary edema ensues, the patient usually requires intubation, oxygen, and positive end–expiratory pressure PEEP ventilation. These patients usually require central monitoring to assess cardiac output, which may be decreased with PEEP.

Gastrointestinal decontamination involves induction of emesis and gastric lavage. Activated charcoal can be administered orally, followed by a cathartic such as magnesium sulfate. To enhance elimination, forced alkalinization of urine has proved helpful in patients with salicylate poisoning. This is accomplished by raising the urine pH to greater than 7.5 with intravenous administration of sodium bicarbonate. It is important to continually monitor electrolyte status and correct any abnormalities that exist during this period.

Hemodialysis or hemoperfusion usually is not required. However, strict criteria for instituting this therapy should be followed, including a serum salicylate level of greater than 120 mg/dL, renal failure, acidosis, unresponsiveness to therapy, pulmonary edema, or persistent central nervous system abnormalities (ie, convulsion, coma).[42]

The treatment of salicylate poisoning in pregnancy should not differ from conventional management, although continuous fetal monitoring should be maintained throughout treatment. Delivery should be considered for obstetric indications if the fetus has reached viability.

Iron

Iron is commonly used during pregnancy in the form of prenatal vitamins and iron supplements. It is the most frequently ingested drug in pregnancy and the second most commonly used drug in suicide attempts during pregnancy.[2,17]

Iron is absorbed in the gastrointestinal tract primarily within the duodenum. Approximately 15% of ingested iron actually is absorbed. The percentage absorbed may double in states of iron deficiency.

Iron is absorbed in its ferrous state by intestinal mucosal cells, where it is oxidized to the ferric state and binds to ferritin. Depending on the need for iron, it is actively transported to the plasma where it is bound to the beta-globulin, transferrin. Transferrin transfers the iron to areas of hematopoiesis and storage sites. It is usually 30% saturated with iron. Absorption of iron stimulates the production of both storage proteins, ferritin and hemosiderin.

During iron overdose, active transport, storage, and transfer systems are overwhelmed. This results in increased free serum iron and hemosiderin. Free serum iron is responsible for the toxic effects of overdose. It exerts a direct toxicologic effect on gastrointestinal mucosa by causing ulcerations and hemorrhage, on blood vessels by causing increased capillary permeability and decreased vascular tone, and on hepatocytes by causing fatty change and necrosis. Iron also may cause metabolic acidosis by altering oxidation and electron transport mechanisms within cells.

Iron appears to cross the placenta by the same protein active receptor transport mediated mechanism seen in other cell membranes. The few reports of maternal iron overdose in pregnancy suggest that the fetus may be protected against iron toxicity. These reports of maternal iron overdose in second and late third trimesters of pregnancy have revealed good neonatal outcomes despite two maternal deaths.[43-45] Fetal serum iron concentrations in cases studied revealed levels well within the normal range, and no evidence of increased iron deposition has been identified in placental studies.[43-45]

These findings suggest that despite toxic maternal levels of iron, even with poor maternal outcome, iron does not appear to cross the placenta that readily, thereby protecting the fetus from toxic insult.

Iron overdose patients initially present with nausea, vomiting, abdominal pain, hematemesis, and melena. Bleeding is secondary to irritation and ulceration of the gastrointestinal mucosa. Lethargy, restlessness, tachycardia, and hypotension also are seen. A latent period may occur in the first 24 hours in which signs of toxicity abate. Overdose patients during this period recover or progress to more severe toxicity. In the next 2 days, fever, shock, metabolic acidosis, and hyperglycemia are seen, progressing to hepatic necrosis, coagulation defects, cardiovascular collapse, pulmonary edema, and renal failure. Coma or convulsions also may be seen.

Serum iron levels and iron binding capacity obtained within 4 hours of ingestion can be helpful in the management of iron overdose patients. If serum iron levels exceed iron-binding capacity, patients are at significant risks of toxicity because free serum iron is present. Iron levels of 100–350 μg/dL are consistent with iron poisoning and require treatment. Levels of 1000 μg/dL or greater are associated with severe toxicity.[46]

Abdominal radiographs can aid in detecting radiopaque tablets within the stomach and help guide the removal of iron from the gastrointestinal tract. Other investigations, such as the detection of leukocytosis and hyperglycemia and radiographs and iron levels, may help predict severity of toxicity and guide management.

Treatment of patients with iron overdose involves induction of emesis or gastric lavage. It is suggested that gastric lavage be performed with sodium bicarbonate to form a less soluble form of iron, ferrous carbonate. Abdominal radiographs should be repeated after therapy, and if tablets remain, lavage should be repeated. If concretions are present or tablets remain despite repeated decontamination attempts, endoscopic removal may be necessary. Cathartics may be used unless diarrhea is present. Activated charcoal is not helpful because it does not bind iron well. Enhancement of elimination is not effective in removing iron. Hemodialysis will remove iron-deferoximine complexes but not iron.

Deferoxamine, a specific iron chelating agent, is the agent of choice in patients with significant iron toxicity. It has the ability to bind free iron, iron of ferritin, and iron of hemosiderin. Deferoxamine therapy should be instituted in patients with hypotension, coma, bleeding, serum iron levels greater than 350 μg/dL, or iron levels greater than the iron-binding capacity.

The use of deferoxamine in pregnancy is controversial because the manufacturer's listing suggests it may be teratogenic in rabbits and mice. Deferoxamine has been administered in the second and third trimesters of pregnancy in the treatment of maternal iron overdose with good perinatal outcomes.[43,45,47]

Throughout treatment, supportive care must be maintained by preventing hypovolemia with adequate volume replacement, monitoring the patient for gastrointestinal bleeding, correcting acidosis and hypoglycemia, and following renal and liver functions closely. Treatment of iron poisoning in pregnant women should not differ from that of nonpregnant patients. It is important that the fetal well-being be assessed throughout the treatment period.

Fluoride

Fluoride is a halogen that is found in numerous products and serves multiple uses in the home and industry. It is used in toothpaste and drinking water for the prevention of dental caries and also is found in vitamin preparations, manufacturing, and in some pesticides.

Drinking water contains approximately 0.1–4 ppm of fluoride. Fluoride concentrations of 0.7 ppm are considered adequate, not requiring supplementation. At levels greater than 2 ppm, dental fluorosis or discoloration and mottling of teeth may be seen in children.[48] Chronic exposure with concentrations exceeding 4 ppm may result in bone deformities. Overfluoridation of water is a potential problem that has resulted in mass toxic exposures.[49]

Fluoride ion crosses the placenta and has been found in fetal blood. Current data are conflicting, however, as to whether fluoride administration to pregnant women will reduce the incidence of dental caries in their children.[50,51]

Concern also has been raised regarding the use of the general anesthetics methoxyflurane and enflurane in pregnant women because they are metabolized to inorganic fluoride, exposing the fetus to potentially increased levels. This could result in fetal toxicity although no such toxic effects have been reported.[52-54] Biotransformation of these anesthetic agents in adults has been associated with high output renal failure.

Sodium fluoride in drinking water and vitamin supplements are rapidly absorbed from the stomach and small intestine. In its gaseous state, fluoride also is absorbed by the respiratory tract. Because of the rapid absorption, peak serum levels are seen 30 minutes to 1 hour after ingestion of an overdose. Fluoride exists in a free ionic state and is primarily deposited within teeth, bone, thyroid gland, and kidney. It is excreted primarily in the urine.

In acute fluoride poisoning, fluoride binds calcium ions, resulting in lowered calcium levels in serum and tissues. It exerts direct toxic effects on muscle, nervous tissue, and multiple enzyme systems. It forms hydrofluoric acid within the stomach, which results in significant irritation and ulceration of the gastrointestinal tract.

Patients with acute fluoride overdose usually present with nausea, vomiting, diarrhea, and hematemesis. Tetany, hyperreflexia, visual changes, and convulsions are neurologic findings that may be seen. Cardiovascular abnormalities consist of hypotension and cardiac arrhythmias. Pulmonary edema also may occur.

Hypocalcemia, hypomagnesemia, hypokalemia, or hyperkalemia, along with electrocardiographic changes revealing prolonged Q–T intervals, peaked T-waves and cardiac arrhythmias often are seen on evaluation of the patient.

Treatment involves stabilization and supportive care, with intense monitoring of electrolyte and electrocardiographic changes. Removal of fluoride is facilitated with induction of emesis and gastric lavage, using calcium hydroxide or calcium chloride solutions. In patients who have ingested more than 15 mg/kg body weight of fluoride or in patients demonstrating hypocalcemia, electrocardiographic changes or tetany, it is necessary to administer intravenous calcium gluconate or calcium chloride.

Hemodialysis or hemoperfusion usually is not recommended unless renal failure exists. The treatment of pregnant patients should not differ from that of nonpregnant individuals, and assessment of fetal well-being is mandatory throughout the treatment period.

Organophosphate Insecticides

Numerous chemical insecticides are used in agriculture to kill insects and improve production of crops. DDT, a chlorinated hydrocarbon insecticide introduced in the 1940s, was successful in reducing many insect-borne diseases, such as malaria and typhus. It was banned in the United States in the 1970s because of its accumulation in animal tissues, human tissues, and the environment. It also was found to have adverse effects on the reproduction of certain species of birds. Since the banning of DDT, organophosphate insecticides have become popular for insect control. Unlike DDT, they are broken down rapidly and are not concentrated in living tissues or within the environment.

Although organophosphate pesticides do not accumulate like the chlorinated hydrocarbon insecticides, they exhibit much more toxicity. Most acute poisonings with organophosphate insecticides are caused by occupational exposure and carelessness in use within the home.[55] Few cases of poisoning have been reported in pregnancy, but most exposures are suicide attempts.

These compounds are absorbed effectively by gastrointestinal, dermal, and respiratory routes and are metabolized in the liver primarily by cytochrome P–450 enzymes.

Organosphosphate compounds exert toxicity by covalently binding to acetylcholinesterase, thereby inactivating this enzyme. This is considered an irreversible binding. Because acetylcholine is normally metabolized by acetylcholinesterase, inhibition of the enzyme leads to an accumulation of acetylcholine in the synapse. This initially causes overstimulation and then paralyzes transmission in the cholinergic synapses of the central and peripheral nervous systems. The clinical effects of poisoning are caused by the stimulation of muscarinic, nicotinic, central nervous system receptors, and effector organs.

The signs and symptoms of acute organophosphate poisoning consist of muscarinic, nicotinic, and central nervous system effects. *Muscarinic effects* involve the respiratory tract, gastrointestinal tract, cardiovascular system, and other organs. Respiratory tract effects involve increased production of secretions, bronchospasm, and shortness of breath, while the effects on the gastrointestinal tract include nausea, vomiting, and diarrhea. The cardiovascular effect seen primarily is bradycardia, while other signs common to muscarinic stimulation include miosis, increased salivation, lacrimation, and urinary and fecal incontinence. *Nicotinic effects* include muscle twitching, muscle weakness, respiratory paralysis, hypertension, tachycardia, and pallor. *Central nervous system changes* include restlessness, confusion, seizures, and coma. If death ensues, it is usually caused by respiratory failure.

Diagnosis of acute organophosphate poisoning involves a history of exposure to the organophosphate insecticide and observance of the signs and symptoms mentioned. Diagnosis may be difficult if no evidence of exposure is present because signs and symptoms may be variable and are similar to many other drug intoxications. In addition, red blood cell true cholinesterase and serum pseudocholinesterase levels should be obtained because they can aid in diagnosis and monitoring of treatment. Cholinesterase levels of 50% below baseline indicate acute toxicity.[56]

From the small amount of existing literature on organophosphate insecticide poisoning in pregnancy, it appears that this compound crosses the placenta and exerts similar effects on the fetus.[57,58] No literature identifies any teratogenic effects of organophosphates in humans. Organophosphate poisoning has been reported in the second and third trimesters of pregnancy, with successful maternal treatment and good neonatal outcome at term.[57,59] In a case described by Weiss et al of maternal organophosphate poisoning at 35 weeks' gestation, the infant displayed significant signs of cholinesterase inhibition at delivery, which required mechanical ventilation and continued atropine administration. This suggests that organophosphates not only cross the placenta but may not be adequately treated *in utero* during maternal treatment.[57]

Treatment of acute organophosphate insecticide poisoning involves stabilization with adequate maintenance of airway and ventilation. This may involve intubation and mechanical ventilation with continuous suctioning to remove excess secretions. The patient should undergo removal of the poison, if ingested orally, by induction of emesis, gastric lavage, administration of activated charcoal, or cathartics, such as magnesium sulfate. It also is important to remove all the patient's clothing and thoroughly wash the skin with soap and water because organophosphates can be absorbed rapidly through the skin.

Antidotes for treatment of organophosphate poisoning include atropine and pralidoxime. Atropine blocks the muscarinic and central nervous system effects of organophosphates. It does not have any effect on nicotinic receptors, however, which are responsible for respiratory paralysis and muscle weakness. Two milligrams of atropine are administered intravenously. This is followed by 2–4 mg every 15–30 minutes until the secretions are dried, signifying adequate treatment. Pralidoxime (2-PAM, Protopam) is an antidote that actually breaks the phosphate bond between the organophosphate and acetylcholinesterase. Pralidoxime should be administered with atropine because it acts primarily at nicotinic sites to reverse muscle weakness and respiratory paralysis. It is administered intravenously in the dose of 1–2 g and is repeated every 8 hours if symptoms persist. To be effective, pralidoxime must be administered in the first 36 hours after ingestion.[56]

Treatment of pregnant patients should not differ from nonpregnant patients, although continuous fetal monitoring should be maintained throughout the treatment period. Because organophosphates cross the placenta and may have adverse effects on the fetus, immediate delivery may be required if fetal distress ensues and if the mother is stable. The patient must be delivered in a center where neonatologists and other personnel trained in resuscitation and detoxification can be present at delivery to administer immediate treatment if necessary.

Petroleum Distillates

Petroleum distillates are hydrocarbons made from crude oil. They are found in the industry and within the home. These petroleum distillates include gasoline, kerosene, motor oil, mineral seal oil (furniture polish), paint thinners, and petroleum jelly.

Ingested petroleum distillates affect the gastrointestinal tract, pulmonary system, and central nervous system. The greatest effect of the toxin is on the pulmonary system caused by aspiration of ingested substances. These hydrocarbons produce significant pulmonary damage in the form of a marked inflammatory response. Direct irritation of the gastrointestinal mucosa is seen in central nervous system depression and is thought to be caused by the hypoxia produced secondary to pulmonary aspiration.

The risk of aspiration is related to the viscosity of the agent, with lower-viscosity substances associated with a high rate of aspiration pneumonitis compared to high-viscosity substances.[60]

Patients with petroleum distillate poisoning may present with nausea, vomiting, abdominal pain, and burning of mouth and throat. If aspiration has occurred, the patient usually presents with coughing, gasping, chest pain, and cyanosis. Respiratory symptoms usually occur immediately after aspiration, but in some cases, they may not appear for 2 or more hours. Central nervous system findings include lethargy, dizziness, coma, and convulsions. Aromatic hydrocarbon poisoning appears to be commonly associated with central nervous system findings. Patients also commonly present with fever, which resolves in 24 to 48 hours and does not appear to be associated with an infectious etiology.

There is a paucity of literature on acute toxicity in pregnant women exposed to petroleum distillates. Maternal hypoxia secondary to chemical pneumonitis has direct effects on the fetus. Transplacental passage of hydrocarbons has been suggested in reports of pregnant women who ingested moth balls (napthalene). These women displayed signs of hemolytic anemia secondary to napthalene poisoning and delivered infants at term who also had significant hemolytic anemia. These findings suggest that napthalene or metabolites of napthalene may have crossed the placenta and produced a hemolytic anemia within the fetuses.[61,62]

Petroleum distillate poisoning is diagnosed by a history of ingestion and presentation of the signs and symptoms mentioned. Identification of the ingested compound is important because the viscosity of the compound will determine the type of decontamination procedure required. Chest radiographs may reveal abnormalities, such as bibasilar and perihilar infiltrates. They do not, however, correlate well with clinical findings and may lag behind clinical changes. Hypoxia may be identified on arterial blood gas determinations and leukocytosis also is frequently seen. Hydrocarbon blood levels are not helpful, although assays for other toxic substances added to the hydrocarbon, such as insecticides or metals, may be useful in the management of the patient.

Treatment primarily involves supportive care and stabilization of the patient because the major effects of toxicity involve aspiration and respiratory failure. Patients may require mechanical ventilation if severe hypoxia is evident.

Controversy exists regarding decontamination procedures that should be used in patients who have ingested hydrocarbons. The controversy is primarily because of concern over aspiration if emesis is induced. Generally, ingestion of agents that may produce systemic toxicity should require induction of emesis or gastric lavage. Low viscosity compounds that can produce severe chemical pneumonitis, such as mineral seal oil, furniture polish, and signal oil, are compounds for which emesis should not be induced. Compounds that can produce central nervous system toxicity, such as gasoline, kerosene, lighter fluid agents containing heavy metals, or insecticides, require induction of emesis. Compounds with high viscosity and low toxicity, such as mineral oil, fuel oil, and motor oil, do not require induction of emesis.[63] Gastric lavage may be performed in obtunded patients who require decontamination. Activated charcoal and cathartics also may be helpful.

Supportive care is the key to management, and respiratory status, acid-base changes, and fluid balance should be continually assessed. Pregnant patients should be managed in the same manner as nonpregnant patients, along with assessment of fetal well-being throughout the treatment period.

Carbon Monoxide

Carbon monoxide is a colorless and odorless gas found throughout the environment and is primarily produced by the incomplete combustion of fossil fuels. It is a product of cigarette smoking, automobile exhaust, faulty heating systems and fires; it also is endogenously produced by the catabolism of heme proteins within humans.

Carbon monoxide is rapidly absorbed through the respiratory tract and binds to hemoglobin with an affinity 250–300 times greater than oxygen. This reduces the oxygen-carrying capacity of hemoglobin and shifts the oxyhemoglobin dissociation curve to the left, which decreases the oxygen available to the tissues. It binds to cytochrome oxidases within the cells and to myoglobin within skeletal and cardiac muscles. All of these changes are responsible for tissue hypoxia and the clinical findings seen with carbon monoxide poisoning.

Carbon monoxide crosses the placenta and binds to fetal hemoglobin with high affinity. Fetal hemoglobin levels exceed maternal levels by approximately 10 to 15%. The oxyhemoglobin curve of the fetus normally lies to the left of the maternal curve, with the partial pressure of oxygen in fetal blood 20–30 mm Hg compared to normal maternal values of 100 mm Hg. Increase in maternal carboxyhemoglobin concentration lead to decreased oxygen-carrying capacity and a shift in the fetal oxyhemoglobin curve further to the left, resulting in tissue hypoxia.[64,65]

Acute maternal carbon monoxide poisoning in the first, second, and third trimesters of pregnancy has been reported with varying outcomes. Stillbirths and growth retardation were seen despite successful treatment of mothers.[66-68] Chronic low-level carbon monoxide exposure in pregnant smokers has been implicated as the cause of intrauterine growth retardation and increases in perinatal mortality.[69,70]

Carbon monoxide exerts major toxic effects on tissues with high metabolic rates, mainly the heart, central nervous system, and the skin. Angina, arrhythmias, and myocardial infarcts may occur secondary to tissue hypoxia. The central nervous system effects include cerebral edema, necrosis, and infarcts within various regions of the brain, while skin lesions involving necrosis of the epidermis with bullae formation appear.

Patients with acute carbon monoxide toxicity may present with a variety of symptoms and signs. These include central nervous system findings, such as headache, dizziness, lethargy, coma, and convulsions. Cardiovascular and pulmonary symptoms may include chest pain, shortness of breath, palpitations, hypotension, and respiratory failure.

Diagnosis of acute carbon monoxide toxicity is made by a history of exposure, signs, and symptoms described previously and by measurement of the carboxyhemoglobin level within the blood. Carboxyhemoglobin levels do not correlate exactly with clinical findings, but they help to identify the poison involved, the severity of toxicity, and the adequacy of treatment.

At carboxyhemoglobin concentrations of 10–20%, mild headache and fatigue usually are seen; at 20–30%, headache and dyspnea on exertion; at 30–40%, nausea, vomiting, and syncope; at 40–50%, convulsions and tachycardia; at 50–60%, coma and convulsions and depressed respiration, and at 60–70%, cardiorespiratory failure and death.[71] Carboxyhemoglobin concentrations in the normal range may not reflect the true status of the patient.

Arterial blood gases usually reflect a normal partial pressure of oxygen, decreased oxygen saturation and metabolic acidosis. The electrocardiogram helps to assess ischemic changes and arrhythmias of the heart, and chest radiographs may assist in the diagnosis of pulmonary edema. Other laboratory tests should include a complete blood count, urinalysis, and evaluation of cardiac enzymes.

Treatment involves stabilization of the patient and administration of 100% oxygen by tight mask or endotracheal tube. Hyperbaric oxygen also may be used for treatment and has the advantage of rapidly eliminating carboxyhemoglobin while increasing levels of dissolved oxygen within the plasma.

The half-life of carboxyhemoglobin in room air is 5 hours; in 100% oxygen 1.5 hours; and in hyperbaric oxygen at 2–3 atmospheres of pressure, 20–30 minutes. Hyperbaric oxygen is available only at a small number of centers. It is advocated as the primary treatment modality by many authors. Patients who are candidates for hyperbaric oxygen for treatment of carbon monoxide toxicity include those with severe poisoning, such as patients who are comatose or have significant neurologic findings; patients with carboxyhemoglobin concentrations greater than 40%; and pregnant patients with carboxyhemoglobin concentrations of 20% or with fetal distress.[72] Hyperbaric oxygen therapy carries potential risks of oxygen toxicity, barotrauma to tympanic membranes or sinuses, and exacerbation of tension pneumothorax. The risks of hyperbaric oxygen therapy to the fetus are unknown; however, a small number of cases of carbon monoxide poisoning in pregnancy treated with hyperbaric oxygen have reported good maternal and fetal outcomes.[73,74] Oxygen therapy is usually continued until carboxyhemoglobin concentrations are below 15%. The treatment of pregnant patients with carbon monoxide poisoning is similar to that of nonpregnant patients but may require more aggressive management because of the risks to fetus. It is imperative that fetal monitoring be continued throughout the treatment period.

REFERENCES

1. Whitlock FA, Edwards JE. Pregnancy and attempted suicide. *Comp Psychiatry*. 1968;9:1.
2. Rayburn W, Anonow R, DeLancey B, Hogan MJ. Drug overdose during pregnancy: An overview from a metropolitan poison control center. *Obstet Gynecol*. 1984;64:611.
3. Gold J, Cates W. Herbal abortifacients. *JAMA*. 1980;243:1365. Editorial.
4. Krauer B, Krauer F, Hytten FE. Drug disposition and pharmacokinetics in the maternal-placental-fetal unit. *Pharmacol Ther*. 1980;10:301.
5. Milne JA, Mills RJ, Howie AD, Pack AI. Large airways function during pregnancy. *Br J Obstet Gynecol*. 1977;84:448.
6. Perucca E, Crema A. Plasma protein binding of drugs in pregnancy. *Clin Pharmacokinet*. 1982;7:336.
7. Levy G. Pharmacokinetics of fetal and neonatal exposure to drugs. *Obstet Gynecol*. 1981;58:9S.
8. Ellenhorn MJ, Barceloux DG. Introduction and initial evaluation. In: Ellenhorn MJ, Barceloux DG, eds. *Medical Toxicology*. New York, NY: Elsevier; 1988:8.
9. Flomenbaum NE, Goldfrank LR, Kulberg AG, Weisman RS. General management of the poisoned or overdosed patient. In Goldfrank LR, Flomenbaum NE, Lewin NA, et al. eds. *Goldfrank's Toxicologic Emergencies*. Norwalk, CT: Appleton-Century-Crofts; 1986:3.
10. Wanke LA. Prevention of absorption: dilution, emesis, gastric lavage, absorption, catharsis. In: Bayer MJ, Rumack BH, Wanke LA, eds. *Toxicologic Emergencies*. Bowie, MD: Robert J. Brady; 1984:37.
11. Tenenbien M, Cohen S, Sitar DS. Efficacy of ipecac-induced emesis, orogastric lavage and activated charcoal for acute drug overdose. *Ann Emerg Med*. 1987;16:838.
12. Van Ameyde KJ, Tenenbein M. Whole bowel irrigation during pregnancy. *Am J Obstet Gynecol*. 1989;160:646.
13. Harvey RF, Read AE. Mode of action of saline purgatives. *Am Heart J*. 1975;89:810.
14. Ellenhorn MJ, Barceloux DG. Enhancement of elimination. In: Ellenhorn MJ, Barceloux DG, eds. *Medical Toxicology*. New York, NY: Elsevier; 1988:66.
15. Wanke LA, Bennett WM. Enhancement of elimination. In: Bayer MJ, Rumack BH, Wanke LA, eds. *Toxicologic Emergencies*. MD: Robert J. Brady; 1984:56
16. Pond SA. Renal principles; Diuresis, dialysis and hemoperfusion. In: Goldfrank LR, Flomenbaum NE, Lewin NA, et al, eds. *Goldfrank's Toxicologic Emergencies*. Norwalk, CT: Appleton-Century-Crofts; 1986:108.
17. Rayburn W, Wible-Kant J, Bledsoe P. Changing trends in drug use during pregnancy. *J Reprod Med*. 1982;27:569.
18. Rumack BH, Lovejoy FH Jr. Clinical toxicology. In: Klaasen CD, Ambur MO, Doull J, eds. *Casarett and Doull's Toxicology*. New York, NY: MacMillan; 1986:884.
19. Levy G, Garretson LK, Soda DM. Evidence of placental transfer of acetaminophen. *Pediatrics*. 1975;55:895.
20. Perucca E. Drug metabolism in pregnancy, infancy and childhood. *Pharmacol Ther*. 1987;34:129.
21. Rollins DE, Glauman H, Moldeus P, Rane A. Acetaminophen. Potentially toxic metabolite formed by human fetal and adult liver microsomes and isolated fetal liver cells. *Science*. 1979;205:1414.
22. Ludmir J, Main DM, Landon MB, Gabbe SG. Maternal acetaminophen overdose at 15 weeks gestation. *Obstet Gynecol*. 1986;67:750.
23. Byer AJ, Traylor TR, Semmer JR. Acetaminophen overdose in the third trimester of pregnancy. *JAMA*. 1982;247:3114.
24. Roberts I, Robinson MJ, Mughal MZ, et al. Paracetamol metabolites in the neonate following maternal overdose. *Br J Clin Pharmacol*. 1984;18:201.
25. Stokes IM. Paracetamol overdose in the second trimester of pregnancy. *Br J Obstet Gynecol*. 1984;91:286.
26. Robertson RG, Van Cleave BL, Collins JJ Jr. Acetaminophen overdose in the second trimester of pregnancy. *J Fam Pract*. 1986;23:267.
27. Ruthnum P, Goel KM. ABC of poisoning: Paracetamol. *Br Med J*. 1984:289;1538.
28. Haibach H, Akhter JE, Muscato MS, et al. Acetaminophen overdose with fetal demise. *Am J Clin Pathol*. 1984;82:240.
29. Rosevear SK, Hope PL. Favourable neonatal outcome following maternal paracetamol overdose and severe fetal distress. *Br J Obstet Gynecol*. 1989;96:491.
30. Lederman S, Fysh WJ, Tredger M, Gamsu HR. Neonatal paracetamol poisoning: treatment by exchange transfusion. *Arch Dis Child*. 1983;58:631.
31. Klein-Schwartz W, Oderda GM. Absorption of oral antidotes for acetaminophen poisoning (methionine and N-acetylcysteine) by activated charcoal. *Clin Toxicol*. 1981;18:283.
32. Ellenhorn MJ, Barceloux DG. Acetaminophen (Paracetamol). In: Ellenhorn MJ, Barceloux DG. eds. *Medical Toxicology*. New York, NY: Elsevier; 1988:156.
33. Prescott LF. Treatment of severe acetaminophen poisoning with intravenous acetylcysteine. *Arch Intern Med*. 1981;141:386.
34. Sibai BM, Amon EA. Aspirin safety during pregnancy. In: Petrie RH, ed. *Perinatal Pharmacology*. Oradell, NJ: Medical Economics; 1989:53.
35. McNiel JR. The possible teratogenic effect of salicylates on the developing fetus. *Clin Pediatr*. 1973;12:347.
36. Slone D, Heinonen OP, Kaufman DW, et al. Aspirin and congenital malformations. *Lancet*. 1976;1:1373.
37. Rumack CM, Guggenheim MA, Rumack BH, et al. Neonatal intracranial hemorrhage and maternal use of aspirin. *Obstet Gynecol*. 1981;58:52S
38. Rejent TA, Baik S. Fatal in utero salicylism. *J Forensic Sci*. 1985;30:942.
39. Garretson LK, Procknal JA, Levy G, Fetal acquisition and neonatal elimination of a large amount of salicylate, *Clin Pharmacol Ther*. 1975;17:98.
40. Levy G, Procknal JA, Garretson LK, Distribution of salicylate between neonatal and maternal serum at diffusion equilibrium, *Clin Pharmacol Ther*. 1975;18:210.
41. Ellenhorn MJ, Barceloux DG. Salicylates. In: Ellenhorn MJ, Barceloux DG eds. *Medical Toxicology*. New York, NY: Elsevier; 1988:562.
42. Goldfrank LR, Bresnitz EA, Hartnett L. Salicylates. In: Goldfrank LR, Flomenbaum NE, Lewin NA, et al, eds. *Goldfrank's Toxicologic Emergencies*, Norwalk, CT: Appleton-Century-Crofts; 1986:233.
43. Olenmark M, Biber B, Dottori O, Rybo G. Fatal iron intoxication in late pregnancy. *J Toxicol Clin Toxicol*. 1987;25:347.
44. Strom RL, Schiller P, Seeds AE, Bensel RT. Fatal iron poisoning in a pregnant female. Case report. *Minn Med*. 1976;59:483.
45. Rayburn WF, Donn SM, Wulf ME. Iron overdose during pregnancy: Successful therapy with deferoxamine. *Am J Obstet Gynecol*. 1983;147:717.
46. Moorhead JC. Iron poisoning. In: Bayer MJ, Rumck BH, Wanke LA, eds. *Toxicologic Emergencies*. Bowie, MD: Robert J. Brady; 1984:183.
47. Blanc P, Hryhorczuk D, Danel I. Deferoxamine treatment of acute iron intoxication in pregnancy. *Obstet Gynecol*. 1984;64:12S.
48. Ligh R. Fluoride therapy. *Hawaii Dent J*. 1985;16:8.
49. Waldbott GL. Accidental overfluoridation. *Kiln Wochenschr* 1982;60:813. Letter.
50. Horowitz HS, Heifetz SB. Effects of prenatal exposure to fluoridation on dental caries. *Public Health Rep*. 1967;82:297.
51. Glenn FB, Glenn WD, Duncan RC. Fluoride tablet supplementation during pregnancy for caries immunity: A study of offspring produced. *Am J Obstet Gynecol*. 1982;143:560.
52. Maduska AI, Ahokas RA, Anderson GD, et al. Placental transfer of intravenous fluoride in the pregnant ewe. *Am J Obstet Gynecol*. 1980;136:84.
53. Armstrong WD, Singer L, Markowski EL. Placental transfer of fluoride and calcium. *Am J Obstet Gynecol*. 1970;107:432.
54. Clark RB, Beard AG, Thompson DS. Renal function in newborns and mothers exposed to methoxyflurane analgesia for labor and delivery. *Anesthesiology*. 1979;51:464.
55. Murphy SD. Toxic effects of pesticides. In: Klaassen CD, Amdur MO, Doull J, eds. *Casarett and Doull's Toxicology*. New York, NY: MacMillan; 1986:519.
56. Tafuri J, Roberts J. Organophosphate poisoning. *Ann Emerg Med*. 1987;16:193.
57. Weiss OF, Muller FO, Lyell H, et al. Materno-fetal cholinesterase inhibitor poisoning. *Anesth Analg*. 1983;62:233.
58. Papadopoulou–Tsoukali H, Njau S. Mother–fetus post mortem toxicologic analysis in a fatal overdose with mecarban. *Forensic Sci Int*. 1987;35:249.
59. Karalliedde L, Senanayake N, Ariaratam A. Acute organophosphorus insecticide poisoning during pregnancy. *Human Toxicol*. 1988;7:363.
60. Kulig K, Rumack BH. Hydrocarbon ingestion. In: Bayer MJ. Rumack BH, Wanke LA, eds. *Toxicologic Emergencies*. Bowie, MD: Robert J. Brady; 1984:229.
61. Zinkham WH, Childs B. A defect of glutathione metabolism in erythro-

cytes from patients with napthalene included hemolytic anemia. *Pediatrics*. 1958;22:461.
62. Anziulewicz JA, Dick HJ, Chiarulli EE. Transplacental napthalene poisoning. *Am J Obstet Gynecol*. 1959;78:519.
63. Rumack BH, Lovejoy FH Jr. Clinical toxicology. In: Klaassen DC, Amdur MO, Doull J, eds. *Casarett and Doull's Toxicology*. New York, NY: MacMillan; 1986:890.
64. Longo LD. The biological effects of carbon monoxide on the pregnant woman, fetus and newborn infant. *Am J Obstet Gynecol*. 1977;129:69.
65. Fogh-Anderson N, Eriksen PS, Grinsted J, Siggaard-Anderson O. Gas-chromatographic measurement of carboxyhemoglobin in blood from mothers and newborns. *Clin Chem*. 1988;34:24.
66. Copel JA, Bowen F, Bolognese RJ. Carbon monoxide intoxication in early pregnancy. *Obstet Gynecol*. 1982;59:26S.
67. Margulies J. Acute carbon monoxide poisoning during pregnancy. *Am J Emerg Med*. 1986;4:516.
68. Caravati EM, Adams CJ, Joyce SM, Schafer NC. Fetal toxicity associated with maternal carbon monoxide poisoning. *Ann Emerg Med*. 1988;17:714.
69. Visnjevac V, Mikov M. Smoking and carboxyhaemoglobin concentrations in mothers and their newborn infants. *Human Toxicol*. 1986;5:175.
70. Harrison KL, Robinson AG. The effect of maternal smoking on carboxyhemoglobin levels and acid-base balance of the fetus. *Clin Toxicol*. 1981;18:165.
71. Winter PM, Miller JN. Carbon monoxide poisoning. *JAMA*. 1976;236:1502.
72. Ellenhorn MJ, Barceloux DG. Carbon monoxide. In: Ellenhorn MJ, Barceloux DG, eds. *Medical Toxicology*. New York, NY: Elsevier; 1988:826.
73. Van-Hoesen KB, Camporesi EM, Moon RE, Haga ML. Should hyperbaric oxygen be used to treat the pregnant patient for acute carbon monoxide poisoning? *JAMA*. 1989;261:1039.
74. Hollander DI, Nagey DA, Welch R, Pupkin M. Hyperbaric oxygen for the treatment of acute carbon monoxide poisoning in pregnancy. A case report. *J Reprod Med*. 1987;32:615.

Chapter Twenty-Eight
Heavy Metals

Howard T. Strassner

28

Many exogenous substances can cause disease when introduced into humans. Among these are heavy metals. Of the heavy metals, lead, cadmium, and mercury have demonstrated considerable potential for adverse fetal effects as a result of maternal exposure. Therefore, exposure to one or more of these elements in pregnancy causes concern for the production of disease and disability in the mother and for the safety and well-being of the fetus.

ETIOLOGY OF DISEASE

There is a common etiologic source of the disease and disorders resulting from heavy metal exposure. Generally, the most important source of heavy metal contamination is the industrial workplace. When human disease from heavy metal contamination occurs, from chronic exposure or acute poisoning, it often originates in the workplace. As a by-product of industrialization, however, these elements and other toxic compounds have been deposited in the atmosphere, on land, and in waters; they have produced some degree of contamination of the usual food chain (see also Chapter 10). Consequently, an increased toxic burden may result from activities of daily living.

Maternal exposure to heavy metals can be hazardous to the fetus. In animal studies, all heavy metals were capable of crossing the placental barrier and causing fetal malformations and death. For some of these elements, adverse outcomes similar to those produced in animal studies have been documented in human fetuses. The possibility exists that environmental levels of certain heavy metals may be an added hazard for fetuses who are exposed in maternal occupations. The burden of maternal occupational exposure to these metals may be further increased for the embryo–fetus. Thus, women who are exposed today in the workplace may be at greater risk for poor pregnancy outcome than in previous years. Acute maternal poisoning also could have decidedly detrimental effects on the developing fetus and on the mother.

LEAD

Lead is widely used in industry, and therefore workers in a large number of industries receive significant lead exposure. Such occupations include lead (and other metals) smelter work, mining, welding, storage battery work, pottery making, and manufacture painting. Work in the printing, painting, shipping, and automobile manufacturing industries may pose significant risk.

In the lead-contaminated work environment, the most important source of lead intake for exposed workers is inhalation. Ingestion of lead-contaminated dust on fingers, lips, or cigarettes also can account for significant occupational exposure. Although ingestion is a less frequent source of contamination in adults, it is the primary route of lead poisoning in children, usually from ingestion of old lead-based paint chips found in aging urban dwellings. Acutely, maternal poisoning can result from inhalation of fumes from burning storage batteries or spray painting or from ingestion of home-made whiskey contaminated by lead solder in the pipes of stills. Because the amount of lead in printing ink is significant, repeated burning of newspapers and magazines could lead to significant inhalation exposure.

Lead also may enter a pregnant woman from many other sources. For the general urban dweller with no unusual source of lead exposure, diet and ambient air are the main sources of lead. In urban areas, approximately one third of the lead absorbed by the adult body comes from inhalation of lead-contaminated air. The lead in air is primarily derived from motor vehicle emissions caused by combustion of leaded gasoline.[1] Consequently, living in high traffic areas may add to maternal contamination.

Manifestations of lead poisoning include severe abdominal pain (lead colic), anemia, and a variety of central and peripheral nervous system symptoms. Renal (interstitial nephritis), cardiac (arrhythmias, cardiomegaly), and liver function abnormalities also may occur. Lead absorption and excretion are slow. Poisoning results from chronic exposure, although the onset of symptoms may be sudden. Because most of the body lead burden accumulates in bone, reabsorption of bone may lead to further or continued signs of lead toxicity even after all sources of lead intake have been eliminated.

Effect of Pregnancy on Lead Poisoning

Women, particularly during periods such as pregnancy, may be particularly vulnerable to lead poisoning.[2] Pregnancy may increase the susceptibility of women to lead intoxication because it is a state in which the skeletal storage sites of lead may be mobilized. In addition, iron deficiency and calcium deficiency, for which women are at increased risk during pregnancy, increase the susceptibility to lead. Further, it has been found that maternal life-style habits may affect lead levels. Maternal alcohol use and cigarette smoking have been related to increased lead levels in maternal and cord blood.[3] This is an additional reason to emphasize avoidance of these agents in pregnancy.

Effect of Lead Poisoning on Pregnancy and the Fetus

Exposure to lead can pose a threat to the fetus. An one reviewer[4] notes, it has been shown that human placental transfer of lead begins as early as 12 weeks' gestation and the total content of lead in the fetus increases throughout pregnancy. The highest fetal concentrations have been found in bone and liver tissue, with significant amounts also in the blood, placenta, brain, heart, and kidney. Bridbord[1] and others have demonstrated that concentrations of lead in the mother's blood are comparable to concentrations of lead in umbilical cord blood at birth.

Increased levels of maternal and fetal blood lead have been associated with premature rupture of membranes and premature birth.[2] Furthermore, placental lead concentrations have been found to be higher in pregnancies with increased perinatal deaths.[5] Increased lead levels also have been associated with increased maternal blood pressure and increased occurrence of hypertension in pregnancy.

Lead has long been used as an abortifacient, and its toxic properties in this regard are well established. It is less clear, however, whether human lead exposure below that leading to abortion exerts any teratogenic effect.[4] The evidence in this area is conflicting. An increase in minor (but not major) malformations with increasing blood lead levels has been described in humans.[6] The suggestion also has been made that lead may be a behavioral teratogen, and lead exposure during pregnancy has been associated with decreased IQ scores at least up to 24 months of age.[6] Animal studies also have found lead to be teratogenic, with the incidence of malformations increasing with the dose of lead.[5]

Diagnosis of Lead Poisoning

Diagnosis of lead intoxication can be made by the finding of elevated levels of erythrocyte protoporphyrin and zinc protoporphyrin. Urinary delta-amniolevulinic acid and coproporphyrin levels also are increased. The finding of elevated levels indicates excessive exposure and, in the presence of related clinical symptoms, suggests toxicity from lead.

Excess exposure to lead has an early effect on the hematopoietic system through inhibition of the heme biosynthetic pathway. Damage to the nervous system emerges after greater exposure. One indicator of this early effect is interference with the enzyme aminolevulinic acid dehydrase (ALAD). Effects of lead on ALAD are first measurable at blood lead levels in the range of 10–20 μg/100 mL, and significant impairment to the maternal ALAD system occurs as blood lead levels rise above 30 μg/100 mL. In pregnancy, there is a correlation between ALAD activity in human mothers and their fetuses. Significantly, inhibition of erythrocyte ALAD activity related to lead has been observed in pregnant women and their fetuses.[1] Furthermore, a number of studies suggest adverse effects on the neurologic system in children at blood lead levels above 30–40 μg/100 mL. Because of the relationship between maternal and fetal blood lead level and between lead exposure and maternal and fetal ALAD activity, it has been recommended that maternal blood lead levels be kept under 30 μg/100 mL.[1]

Treatment of Lead Poisoning

As with all toxic exposures, the first step in the treatment of lead poisoning is eliminating the source of contamination. Supportive care and treatment of complications may be sufficient, but in severe cases, therapy with chelating agents may be required to remove the metal from the body. Dimercaprol (British antilewisite, BAL), calcium disodium edetate, and penicillamine are used for treatment of poisoning from many heavy metals. Successful treatment can be expected for the mother, except for a woman with encephalopathy, in which residual mentation deficit may remain. The chelating agents can have serious adverse side effects, and therefore they should not be used without urgent need. Furthermore, none of these agents have been adequately studied in pregnancy, and they cannot be presumed to be safe. Consequently, the chelating agents should be used in pregnancy only for treatment of life-threatening poisoning, in which the anticipated maternal benefit clearly justifies the maternal and fetal risks.

Preconceptional counseling plays an important role when potential excessive heavy metal exposure is anticipated. As noted previously, because of the relationship between maternal and fetal blood lead levels, it has been recommended as a first line of defense against fetal and newborn lead toxicity that maternal blood lead levels be kept below 30 μg/100 mL.[1] Translated to limits of exposure to airborne lead in the workplace, 40-hour weekly air lead exposure should be no higher than 50 $\mu g/cm^3$ for the female entering the work force with a pre-employment blood level that reflected no significant past exposure to lead.[1] Alteration of a patient's work environment may be necessary to achieve this objective.

The nonoccupationally exposed pregnant patient, by awareness and avoidance of potentially harmful lead sources, also may reduce her fetus' exposure to lead. A pregnant patient should avoid outdoor urban activities during hours when airborne lead pollution may be excessive. She also may choose to avoid such activities as spray painting in unventilated rooms. Of course, there may be even greater benefit for an occupationally exposed woman to avoid these exposures.

CADMIUM

Cadmium is a highly toxic element distributed widely in the earth's minerals. The major source of cadmium contamination is from industrial processes, such as smelting and refining of lead and zinc ores, combustion of coal and oil, waste disposal, and scrap metal recovery. For those not exposed in industry, food is the main source of the small amount of cadmium entering the body. Symptoms of cadmium toxicity are related to the pulmonary, gastrointestinal, and renal systems, and include dyspnea, cough, and wheezing. After years of exposure, symptoms include emphysema; nausea, vomiting, abdominal pain, and diarrhea, which develop rapidly with acute exposure; and nephropathy from damage to the proximal tubule, which occurs after chronic cadmium exposure and is heralded by the onset of proteinuria.

Effects of Cadmium on Pregnancy and the Fetus

Cadmium exposure may represent a hazard to the developing embryo–fetus. Exposure to cadmium can place an additional burden on fetuses of mothers who work in industries such as electroplating. Animal studies have shown fetal growth retardation and severe newborn anemia in the offspring of mothers who were exposed to cadmium throughout pregnancy.[7] Cadmium also has been associated with fetal malformations in hamsters, mice, and rats.[8] Impairment of iron metabolism or reduced intestinal iron absorption may be the primary effect of cadmium toxicity. Also, cadmium has an affinity for the placenta. Thus, another mechanism for cadmium's fetal toxicity may be that it interferes with nutrient transport in the placenta. If cadmium interferes with placental transport of nutrients such as iron, it is possible that very low exposure levels of cadmium could have little or no effect on the mother but could interfere with growth and blood formation in the fetus.

Diagnosis and Treatment of Cadmium Toxicity

Acute exposure to cadmium fumes can be diagnosed by the exposure history and the characteristic clinical manifestations. Cadmium can be measured in blood and urine. It also may be monitored by beta 2-microglobulin in urine, which occurs subsequent to renal tubular damages. With supportive care, the acute pulmonary and gastrointestinal symptoms generally resolve. However, in unusually severe cases, the pulmonary complications can be lethal.

MERCURY

Mercury exposure occurs in a large number of occupations. These include dental practice and the manufacture of mercury-containing lamps, lights, batteries, electrical equipment, jewelry, pesticides, and fungicides. Table 28–1 presents some guidelines for occupational exposure to mercury for women of childbearing age. Unfortunately, because of industrial contamination of lakes and rivers, mercury also has been introduced into the food chain through contaminated fish.

The primary nonoccupational source of mercury exposure is consumption of contaminated fish and fish products. The contamination occurs almost entirely in the form of methylmercury. An excellent critical review of the health effects of methylmercury in humans, including pregnant women and the fetus, has been provided by Inskip and Piotrowski.[9] Contamination of fish may result from mercury contamination in water from pollution from natural sources (eg, geothermal processes) and from man-made sources (eg, chlorine-alkali plants using mercury as an electrode and smelting and burning of fossil fuels). Microorganisms naturally present in water convert these inorganic and organic mercurial compounds into the most toxic mercury compound, methylmercury. Thus, all major forms of mercury entering the water are potential precursors to methylmercury. Methylmercury is taken into fish directly through the gills and indirectly through the ingestion of contaminated food. The fish effectively bioconcentrate the toxin

TABLE 28–1. EXPOSURE LIMITS FOR WOMEN OF CHILDBEARING AGE

	Previous Guidelines	Present Recommendations
Occupations		
Mercury vapor	Should not be exposed to elevated levels	<0.01 mg/M^{3}of air
Aerosols of inorganic mercury salts	Should not be exposed to elevated levels	<0.02 mg/M^{3}of air
Phenylmercury	Should not be exposed to elevated levels	<0.02 mg/M^{3}of air
Methylmercury	—	—

Modified from Koos BJ, Longo LD.[10]

TABLE 28–2. EXPOSURE LIMITS FOR WOMEN OF CHILDBEARING AGE

	Previous Guidelines	Present Recommendations
Fish		
Fish concentration	<0.25 μg of Hg/g	—
Total methylmercury ingestion	<0.025 μg of Hg/d (for 60 Kg woman)	—
Quantity of fish	—	350 g/wk[a]

[a] This value is based on a total methylmercury consumption of 0.025 μg/d and a fish concentration of 0.5 μg of Hg/g.
Modified from Koos BJ, Longo LD.[10]

because the methylmercury excretion half-life is up to several hundred days.[10] Because of the slow clearance time, the level of methylmercury can accumulate to concentrations thousands of times greater than in the surrounding water. When contaminated fish are ingested by humans, the methylmercury is readily absorbed from the gastrointestinal tract and widely throughout the body. Adverse effects of mercury exposure include pulmonary, renal, and central nervous system damage, including permanent brain damage. Gastrointestinal symptoms also may result.

Because methylmercury compounds are used as antifungal seed-dressing agents, it also is possible that methylmercury enters the human food chain through other foods such as flour or meat. Other than fish, however, most foods do not contain mercury in significant concentrations to be dangerous.[11] Even if contaminated meat were to reach the market, it is not likely that human illness would result because of the wide distribution in the various parts of the animal.[12] This ensures that a consumer would receive only a small fraction of the affected carcass. Unless the individual was receiving abnormal amounts of mercury from other sources (eg, industrial exposure), this would not cause abnormally high mercury levels. The only other significant source of mercury-contaminated food is game birds.[13]

Effect of Mercury on Pregnancy and the Fetus

Fetal mercury toxicity can result from maternal ingestion of mercury-contaminated food or maternal occupational exposure to mercury. This subject has been extensively reviewed by Koos and Long.[10] Mercury crosses the placenta and presents a special hazard to the fetus because it is concentrated in fetal blood and brain tissue. The greatest damage occurs to nervous tissues because mercury accumulates to the greatest extent there. Data of fetal effects of maternal mercury ingestion have been obtained from several epidemics of mercury poisoning resulting from environmental contamination.

The first epidemic of mercury poisoning occurred in Japan in the 1950s.[14] In the area around Minamata Bay, an outbreak of severe cases of neurologic disease occurred. Eventually it was discovered that the symptoms were caused by ingestion of methylmercury, an effluent into the bay from a nearby acetaldehyde plant. The methylmercury was transmitted through seafood taken from the contaminated bay; therefore, the disease was named Minamata disease. Subsequent epidemiologic, clinical, and pathologic studies in children born to mothers in the area confirmed the existence of methylmercury poisoning by way of the placenta (ie, congenital Minamata disease). The mothers of these infants appeared to be unaffected or only mildy affected by the ingestion of the contaminated fish. In addition, no conspicuous abnormalities or differences in birth weight or gestation were observed at birth. At 6 months, however, the following severe neurologic and mental symptoms were detected in the affected children: instability of the neck, convulsions, failure of the eyes to follow, intelligence disturbance, disruption of primitive reflex, cerebellar symptoms, disturbances of body growth and nutrition, dysarthria, deformity of limbs, hyperkinesia, hypersalivation, paroxysmal symptoms, strabismus, and pyramidal symptoms.

Grain contamination by organic mercurial pesticides has caused other epidemics with significant implications for the fetus. A severe episode of methylmercury poisoning occurred in Iraq in 1972 as a result of the ingestion of homemade bread prepared from wheat treated with methylmercury fungicide.[15] In this case, there also were reports of fetal poisoning secondary to maternal ingestion of the contaminated bread. In addition, mothers' breast milk was a continuing source of methylmercury for the infants. In all but one of the cases reported in a study from this population, the infants' blood mercury levels were higher than their mothers' during the first 4 months after birth. On the basis of the data from this study, it was not possible to tell which trimester of pregnancy is most hazardous to the fetus in terms of methylmercury exposure. Some of the affected infants were exposed only in the last 3 months of gestation, indicating that the fetus is sensitive to mercury poisoning during the last trimester. Another affected infant was maximally exposed during the first trimester, although exposure did occur throughout gestation.

An outbreak of alkyl mercury poisoning occurred in the United States after members of a family ingested mercury-contaminated pork.[12] The hogs had been fed a waste grain that had been treated with an alkyl mercury fungicide. A woman in the early stages of her pregnancy ate the contaminated pork and demonstrated no clinical symptoms of mercury poisoning other than slight slurring of speech. She subsequently delivered a male infant who had intermittent gross tremulous movements of the extremities in the first days of life and who later developed myoclonic convulsions. At 1 year of age, the child was blind and could not sit up.

Embryotoxic and teratogenic effects of methylmercury also have been reported in laboratory animals. For example, mice receiving methylmercury in food 30 days before gestation and up to 18 days after gestation had affected estrous cycles; decreased litter size accompanied by increased implantation sites, resorptions, dead embryos, and dead fetuses; increased incidence of cleft palate; and retarded fetal growth.[16] Other studies have shown altered neuronal migration in the cerebral cortex of methylmercury-exposed fetal mice, suggesting a morphologic basis for behavioral abnormalities secondary to fetal methylmercury exposure.[17]

DIAGNOSIS AND TREATMENT OF MERCURY TOXICITY

The diagnosis of mercury intoxication comes from a history of exposure and the presence of symptoms. Urinary and blood levels of mercury, blood levels of methylmercury, and hair and placenta mercury concentrations may aid in the diagnosis. Hair analysis for methylmercury is gaining importance.[9] Hair analysis has been applied to the study of fetal methylmercury exposure.[18]

With metallic and inorganic mercury intoxication, removal from the source of exposure is the first step. When necessary, treatment with chelating agents will improve maternal symptoms, but these should be used only with clear need and with great caution during pregnancy. With methylmercury intoxication, treatment is largely symptomatic because chelating agents are of limited value.

In pregnancy, the hallmark of treatment must be prevention because toxic effects on the fetus are irreversible. The placenta does not prevent fetal blood mercury accumulation during chronic maternal exposure. More importantly, because mercury is known to accumulate in fetal tissues, particularly in the brain, chronic exposure may result in tissue concentrations much higher than those predictable after an acute exposure. To help safeguard the fetus, pregnant women must limit their occupational exposure to mercury and their intake of mercury-contaminated fish. Table 28–2 provides some guidelines for mercury exposure from fish consumption in women of childbearing age. It has been suggested that pregnant women should not regularly consume fish with 0.5 ppm or more of methylmercury.[19] Further, it has been recommended they consume no more than 350 g of fish per week to allow for a margin of safety for the fetus.[10] Methylmercury consumption in the United States has been reviewed and related information provided regarding the US Food and Drug Administration (FDA) regulatory level of mercury in fish (1 ppm).[20] Though higher than the recommendations from the previous studies, the FDA believes this to provide adequate protection for the average consumer and young children.

For infants, breast milk also must be considered a major potential source of mercury contamination. Organic mercury is more readily transferrable across the placenta than inorganic mercury. Both forms of mercury are transferred through milk with approximately the same efficiency in the rat.[16] The mercury composition of human breast milk varies but is approximately 5% of the serum level.[20] It is prudent for mothers with significant histories of mercury exposure to avoid breastfeeding their babies.

REFERENCES

1. Bridbord K. Occupational lead exposure and women. *Prev Med.* 1978;7:311.
2. Rom WN. Effects of lead on the female and reproduction: a review. *Mt Sinai J Med.* 1976;43:542.
3. Ernhart CB, Wolf AW, Sokol RJ, et al. Fetal lead exposure: Antenatal factors. *Environ Research.* 1985;38:54.
4. Clayton BE: Lead: The relation of environment and experimental work. *Br Med Bull.* 1975;31:236.
5. Wibberley DG, Khera AK, Edwards JH, et al. Lead levels in human placentae from normal and malformed births. *J Med Genet.* 1977;14:339.
6. Needleman HL. The neurotoxic, teratogenic, and behavioral teratogenic effects of lead at low dose: A paradigm for transplacental toxicants. In: Scarpelli DG, Migaki G, eds. *Transplacental Effects on Fetal Health.* New York, NY: Alan R. Liss; 1988;281:279.
7. Webster WS. Cadmium-induced fetal growth retardation in the mouse. *Arch Environ Health.* 1978;33:36.
8. Hemminki K. Occupational chemicals tested for teratogenicity. *Int Arch Occup Environ Health.* 1980;47:191.
9. Inskip MJ, Piotrowski JK. Review of the health effects of methylmercury. *J Applied Toxicol.* 1985;5:113.
10. Koos BJ, Longo LD. Mercury toxicity in the pregnant woman, fetus, and newborn infant: A review. *Am J Obstet Gynecol.* 1976;126:390.
11. Tanner JT, Friedman M, Lincoln D. Mercury content of common foods determined by neutron activation analysis. *Science.* 1972;177:1102.
12. Pierce P, Thompson J, Likosky W, et al. Alkyl mercury poisonings in humans. *JAMA.* 1972;220:1439.
13. Eyl T. Alkylmercury contamination of foods. *JAMA.* 1971;215:287.
14. Harada M. Congenital minamata disease: intrauterine methylmercury poisoning. *Teratology.* 1978;18:285.
15. Amin-Zaki L, Elhassani S, Majeed MA, et al. Intrauterine methylmercury poisoning in Iraq. *Pediatrics.* 1974;54:587.
16. Nobunga T, Satch H, Suzuki T. Effect of sodium selenite and methylmercury embryotoxicity and teratogenicity in mice. *Toxicol Appl Pharmacol.* 1979;47:79.
17. Choi BH. Methylmercury poisoning of the developing nervous system: I. Pattern of neuronal migration in the cerebral cortex. *Neuro Toxicol.* 1986;7:591.
18. Marsh DO, Clarkson TW, Cox C, et al. Fetal methylmercury poisoning: Relationship between concentration in single strands of maternal hair and child effects. *Arch Neurol.* 1987;44:1017.
19. Kahn E. Perspective on tuna fish. *N Engl J Med.* 1971;285:49.
20. Tollefson L, Cordle F. Methylmercury in fish: A review of residue levels, fish consumption and regulatory action in the United States. *Environ Health Perspect.* 1986;68:203.

PART V | Metabolic Diseases

Norbert Gleicher, Section Editor

Chapter Twenty-Nine

Metabolism

Edmond Confino and Norbert Gleicher

29

Pregnancy represents a unique metabolic state. The rapidly growing fetus changes the maternal homeostasis and imposes increasing metabolic challenges to the mother. The hormonal fetomaternal feedback readjusts many enzymatic systems and metabolic pathways. The hormonally adjusted physiologic hyperthermia of pregnancy resets many enzymatic systems and elevates the basic metabolic rate.[1] Consequently, many laboratory values in the pregnant state may reach abnormal levels when compared to the nonpregnant state (see also Chapters 2 and 4).

Fetal nutritional requirements are the last to be affected, and maternal reserves are the first to be exhausted. Fetal and maternal metabolic changes of carbohydrates, amino acids, proteins, and lipids are described in detail in other chapters. Systems that are dominated by smooth muscle, such as the urinary and the gastrointestinal tracts, demonstrate slow peristalsis and ureteral reflux, resulting in constipation and an increased incidence of urinary tract infections. Therefore, the general statement that pregnancy is a hyperactive state must be restricted to systems that are directly involved in the production of energy.

ENERGY REQUIREMENTS IN PREGNANCY

Fuel requirements of the rapidly developing fetus are primarily met by glucose supply.[2] The small, readily available and quickly degradable glucose molecule is the perfect fuel for the rapidly growing fetal organism. The central nervous system remains exclusively dependent on glucose throughout life, while other systems depend on other energy sources in the adult organism, such as fatty acids.[3,4] Energy supply to the fetus is similar to that to the central nervous system. Only when rapid fetal cell division decreases and delivery occurs will the newborn rely on less readily available energy sources, such as lipids.[5,6]

Detailed studies of glucose metabolism in pregnancy demonstrate these principles. Transplacental transfer of glucose is more rapid than expected, based on a fetomaternal gradient of 10–20 mg/100 mL. This phenomenon is explained by carrier-mediated facilitated glucose diffusion. The process is not energy-dependent[5], and is thus more economical to the fetus than an enzyme-dependent active pump. Facilitated diffusion provides a wide margin of safety and a constant glucose supply, even when maternal serum glucose levels drop. Maternal insulin and glucagon fail to cross the placenta; therefore, fetal glucose homeostasis is not affected by maternal events. Fetal insulin, enhanced by glucose and aminogenic stimulation, plays a major role in the fetal growth process.[7,8]

Fetal birthweight depends on two additional variables that alter the metabolic demands during pregnancy: total fetal mass and length of gestation. Consequently, glucose metabolism in pregnancy is a major determinant of fetal growth. It is obvious that an excess supply of glucose to the fetus converts into fat deposits. These fat deposits are extremely important for thermoregulation and form most of the long-term energy storage. Fat accumulation is independent of the amount of maternal fat deposits; therefore, total fetal mass expressed as a percentage of maternal weight will vary. This phenomenon is probably species specific. The human fetus is exceptional because it contains as much as 16% fat at birth compared to only 10% in the guinea pig.[9] Moreover, in the human, this process occurs predominantly in the third trimester of pregnancy. Fat accounts for 80% of fetal caloric accumulation in the last few weeks of gestation.[9]

THE FETOPLACENTAL UNIT

Placental metabolism and physiology are discussed elsewhere. Some metabolic aspects, however, deserve additional emphasis. The placenta is unique because under dynamic steady-state conditions, high metabolic rates are obtained. Uteroplacental energy requirements are measured by subtracting the glucose–oxygen quotient entering the uterus from the fetal compartment. The differential represents placental and uterine energy use only, which is typically larger than fetal use.[10]

Unfortunately, fetomaternal gradients are difficult to evaluate. Preparation artifacts, acute changes, or dose-dependent metabolic changes may alter the results. The metabolism of lactate demonstrates this principle. An association between umbilical arteriovenous concentration gradient and fetal lactate levels can be observed. The well-

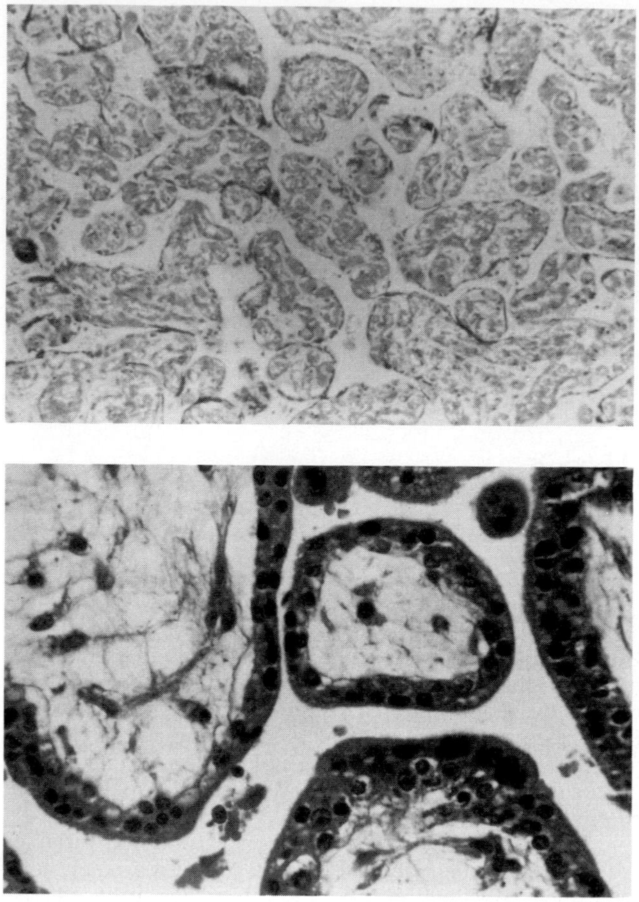

Figure 29–1. First trimester chorionic villi (*lower*) are thicker than third trimester chorionic villi (*upper*). This change allows improved transport of nutrients along the placental barrier with advancing placental age. (*Reproduced with permission from Vellios F. Pathology Learning Program in Obstetrics and Gynecology—Placenta. American Society of Clinical Pathologists, Chicago, IL, 1980.*)

oxygenated fetus demonstrates a low arterial concentration of lactate and an arteriovenous gradient. These circumstantial data suggest that lactate may represent an important nutrient for the human fetus. If oxygen supply to the fetus is interrupted, however, acute changes in lactate concentrations and placental metabolism will occur, resulting in difficulty in separating fetal from the placental relative contribution to the metabolic imbalance.[10]

The placenta supplies fetal metabolic precursors. Placental structural and biochemical adaptations throughout pregnancy maintain the increasing fetal demands. The placenta grows and hypertrophies as a compensatory mechanism. New villi are formed, increasing placental surface area from about 5 m^2 at 28 weeks' gestation to 10 m^2 at term.[11] In early pregnancy, the villi are plump with a central fetal blood vessel separated from the maternal intervillous blood by a thick layer of trophoblast. At term, the villi are smaller and the trophoblast is thinner. In some places, only a nuclear membranous layer separates fetal and maternal capillaries (Fig. 29–1).[12] These anatomic changes help to explain the compensatory mechanism that allows increased substrate transfer.

The fetus is equipped with mechanisms to help it survive even when maternal shortage of a substrate occurs. This principle is illustrated by transplacental iron transfer. Infants born to anemic mothers are rarely anemic. A diversion of iron to the fetus occurs even at the expense of the mother.[13] Only if maternal iron deficiency is significantly prolonged will fetal liver ferritin be reduced.[14] The fetus is more efficient than the mother in extracting iron from the maternal circulation because placental receptor sites to transferrin have a higher affinity at low iron levels than the maternal blood marrow. Consequently, radio-labeled iron, injected into the maternal circulation, reaches the fetus within 12 minutes.[13]

METABOLIC PROTECTIVE MECHANISMS

Many fetal metabolic pathways are superior compared to maternal pathways. Some organ systems demonstrate significant reserves that compensate sudden changes in the fetal or maternal environments. Fetal oxygen transport demonstrates this principle.

Fetal erythrocytes have a considerably greater affinity to oxygen than adult erythrocytes. Furthermore, maternal oxygen affinity is lower than in normal male adults.[15] This unique fetal capacity may be related to fetal hemogloblin. *In vitro* experiments, however, do not support this contention. Fetal hemoglobin in pure solution has similar dissociation curves to adult hemoglobin. Oxygen affinity may even be determined by 2,3 diphosphoglycerate, which competes for oxygen-binding sites on the hemoglobin molecule and thus regulates oxygen attachment to the molecule. Diphosphoglycerate is bound less effectively to fetal hemoglobin; therefore, fetal erythrocyte oxygen affinity may be increased.[16] High oxygen affinity may be advantageous for oxygen extraction from the maternal circulation. However, it also may be detrimental to fetal tissues because it results in impaired release of oxygen into the tissues. The fetal compensates with a steeper oxygen dissociation curve. A small decrease in fetal oxygen partial pressure will cause a relatively large oxygen release. Moreover, the fetus tolerates low oxygen levels of 25–30 mm Hg. Higher tissue oxygen tensions result in adjustments, such as closure of the ductus arteriosus. Such an occurrence *in utero* can be fatal. To prevent this, placental blood flow is reduced whenever oxygen partial pressure is high.[17]

The fetus is protected from maternal metabolic acidosis by the placenta, which readily disposes of carbon dioxide. Induced acidosis during cesarean section using infusion of ammonium chloride causes a rapid decrease in maternal plasma bicarbonate. A lower maternal plasma pH, however, does not immediately change the fetal metabolic acid-base balance.[18] Low placental permeability to bicarbonate and hydrogen ions explains this protective mechanism.

Oxygen supply to the fetus is of major importance. In chronic maternal oxygen depletion observed at high altitudes, fetal and maternal polycytemia are occasionally associated with placental hypertrophy.[19] Placental tissue cultures subjected to low oxygen levels demonstrate clustering of nuclei and protoplasm at the tip of the villi, with marked thinning of the syncytium.[20] This process may represent another fetal adaptation to effectively protect against compromised maternal metabolism.

REFERENCES

1. Quilligan EL. Maternal physiology. In: Danforth DN, ed. *Obstetrics and Gynecology*. 4th ed. Philadelphia, PA: Harper and Row; 1982:326.

2. Battaglia FC, Meshia G. Principle substrates of fetal metabolism. *Physiol Rev.* 1978;58:499.
3. Page EW. Human fetal nutrition and growth. *Am J Obstet Gynecol.* 1969; 104:378.
4. Kalhan SC, Savin SM, Adam PAJ. Attenuated glucose production rate in newborn infants of insulin-dependent diabetic mothers. *N Engl J Med.* 1977;296:375.
5. Felig P. Maternal and fetal fuel homeostasis in human pregnancy. *Am J Clin Nutr.* 1973;26:998.
6. Persson B, Gentz J. The pattern of blood lipids glycerol and ketone bodies during the neonatal period infancy and childhood. *Acta Paediatr Scan.* 1966;55:353.
7. Obenshain SS, Adam PAJ, King KC, et al. Human fetal insulin response to sustained maternal hyperglycemia. *N Engl J Med.* 1970;283:566.
8. Brinsmead MW, Liggins GC. Somato medin like activity, prolactin, growth hormone and insulin in human cord blood. *Aust NZ J Obstet Gynaecol.* 1979;19:129.
9. Battaglia F. The comparative physiology of fetal nutrition. *Am J Obstet Gynecol.* 1984;148:850.
10. Sparks JW, Hay WW, Meshia G, et al. Partition of maternal nutrients to the placenta and fetus in the sheep. *Eur J Obstet Gynaecol Reprod Biol.* 1983;14:331.
11. Hytten FE. Placental transfer. In: Hytten FE, Chamberlein G, eds. *Clinical Physiology in Obstetrics.* Oxford: Blackwell Scientific Publications; 1980:468.
12. Fox H. The correlation between placental structure and transfer function. In: Chamberlain G, et al, eds. *Placental Transfer.* Turnbridge Wells, England: Pitman Medical; 1979.
13. Fletcher J, Suter PEN. The transport of iron by the human placenta. *Clinic Science.* 1969;36:209.
14. Iyengar L, Apte SV. Nutrient stores in human fetal livers. *Br J Nutr.* 1972;27:313.
15. Bauer C, Ludwig M, Ludwig I, et al. Factors governing the oxygen affinity of human adult and fetal blood. *Resp Physiol.* 1969;7:271.
16. Tyuma I, Shimizu K. Effect of organic phosphates on the difference in oxygen affinity between fetal and adult human hemoglobin. *Fed Proc.* 1970;29:1112.
17. Tominaga T, Page EW. Accomodation of the human placenta to hypoxia. *Am J Obstet Gynecol.* 1966;94:679.
18. Blechner JN, Stenger VG, Eitzman DV, el al. Effects of maternal metabolic acidosis on the human fetus and newborn infant. *Am J Obstet Gynecol.* 1967;99:46.
19. Kruger H, Arias-Stella L. The placenta and the newborn infant at high altitudes. *Am J Obstet Gynecol.* 1970;106:586.
20. Josimovich JB, Kosor B, Bocella L, et al. Placental lactogen in maternal serum as an index of fetal death. *Obstet Gynecol.* 1970;36:244.

Chapter Thirty
Disorders of Amino Acid Metabolism

Michael Vermesh and Norbert Gleicher

30

The disorders of amino acid metabolism, although relatively uncommon, have become of interest to the clinician and are usually relatively easy to diagnose and treat. The accumulation of knowledge since Dent published his first papers[1,2] has been virtually exponential. Screening methods have been applied on a massive scale, particularly to the newborn infant, to recognize the biochemical imbalance during its latent early stages and thereby prevent its development into a clinical disease. These disorders are of particular interest to the medical specialist because an increasing number of women with these diseases now survive into the reproductive years. Many defects are modified in their expression by gestation. Furthermore, in some of the disorders, gestation may be altered by direct or indirect effects of the disease on mother or fetus, and therefore preconceptional counseling becomes important when pregnancy is contemplated. Some of the inborn errors of amino acid metabolism are now detectable *in utero* (Table 30–1). The obstetrician must be familiar with those diagnosable *in utero,* as he or she is required to perform the diagnostic tests and must act on the results.

PHYSIOLOGY OF AMINO ACID METABOLISM

Amino acids are the basic constituents of proteins. Although about 300 amino acids occur in nature, only 21 of these occur in proteins. The human body can biosynthesize only about one half of those. The remainder are termed *essential amino acids* because they must be supplied in the diet. Approximately 50% of digested protein is derived from ingested food; the rest comes from desquamated mucosal

TABLE 30–1. INBORN ERRORS OF AMINO ACID METABOLISM DETECTABLE *IN UTERO* BY STUDY OF AMNIOTIC FLUID CONTENTS

Disease	Enzyme Deficiency	Substance Accumulated
Argininosuccinic aciduria	Argininosuccinase	Argininosuccinic acid
Cystathioninuria	Cystathionase	
Cystinosis		Cystine
Histidinemia	Histidase	
Homocystinuria	Cystathionine synthetase	
Hypervalinemia	Valine transaminase	
Maple syrup urine disease	Branched-chain ketoacid decarboxylase	
Methylmalonic aciduria		
B_{12} unresponsive	Methylmalonyl-CoA mutase	Methylmalonate
B_{12} responsive	Vitamine B_{12} coenzyme	Methylmalonate
Ornithinemia	Ornithine α-ketoacid transaminase	
Propionic acidemia	Propionyl-CoA carboxylase	

cells and various secretions that are present within the digestive tract. Proteins that enter the digestive tract initially are cleaved in the stomach by pepsin enzymes into smaller units called peptides. Further digestion occurs in the duodenum and small intestine, where pancreatic proteolytic enzymes (trypsin, chymotrypsin, elastase) reduce the peptides into smaller units. Finally, the small peptides are split into amino acids by the action of pancreatic carboxypeptidases, intestinal aminopeptidases, and dipeptidases. Amino acids are rapidly absorbed from the intestine into the portal blood. The transport of most amino acids across the intestine is active and energy dependent. It has been suggested that neutral amino acids and basic amino acids have separate transport systems and that congenital defects in these systems in the intestine and renal tubules cause *Hartnup disease* and *cystinuria,* respectively.[3]

In infants, considerable quantities of undigested proteins can be absorbed by pinocytosis. This process is important because the absorption of protein antibodies derived from maternal colostrum contributes to passive immunity against infection. As the cells mature, they normally lose the ability to absorb by pinocytosis, and absorption of intact protein molecules in the adult is negligible. However, in some adults, the absorption of whole proteins may persist, as shown by the fact that some individuals develop allergic reactions after eating certain food proteins.[4]

The concentration of amino acids in blood is between 35 and 65 mg/dL. Following a meal, the concentration rises for a short period of time but returns to normal within minutes because a rapid active transport into cells takes place throughout the entire body. In the cells, amino acids are conjugated into proteins under the influence of intracellular enzymes. Under normal circumstances, the clearance of amino acids by the kidneys is low; most of the filtered pool of amino acids is actively reabsorbed by the proximal tubular epithelium. In a healthy person, the loss of amino acids in the urine is insignificant. However, in disorders of membrane transport of amino acids, amino aciduria may be present, as in *cystinuria* and *Fanconi syndrome.*

AMINO ACID METABOLISM IN PREGNANCY

In pregnancy, the plasma levels of amino acids tend to be lower than in the nonpregnant state. The mechanisms and role of this phenomenon are unknown. It has been suggested that a general lowering of amino acid levels in plasma produces a balance that favors transfer to the fetus rather than to the maternal compartment. The placenta is capable of actively transferring amino acids against a concentration gradient from maternal to fetal blood. It has been shown that the concentration of amino acids is higher in fetal blood than in maternal blood.[5] The concentration in the placenta exceeds both.[6,7] Studies in animals and humans have suggested that amino acids are major substrates for fetal energy production and growth. The total fetal uptake of amino acids exceeds their net accretion rate during fetal life, an observation that supports the role of amino acids as fuels during fetal life.[8,9]

A recent study compared umbilical plasma amino acid concentration differences in healthy and growth-retarded fetuses at term.[10] Small-for-gestational age fetuses had significantly lower concentrations of α-aminonitrogen, compared with those of appropriate-for-gestational age fetuses, in the umbilical artery and vein. Most of the difference was accounted for by the branched chain amino acids valine, leucine, and isoleucine. In contrast, hydroxyproline concentration was significantly higher in the umbilical artery and vein of small-for-gestational age fetuses. The increased excretion of amino acids by the kidneys during pregnancy may play a role in reducing their plasma concentration. The levels of most amino acids in urine during pregnancy increase in response to an increase in glomerular filtration rate coupled with reduced tubular reabsorption.[11] Pregnancy-induced *amino aciduria* is so common that an increase in urinary histidine has been used for years as a test for pregnancy. However, excretion of certain other amino acids (eg, aspartic acid, glutamic acid, methionine) does not increase at any time during pregnancy.

PATHOPHYSIOLOGY

Through the action of a variety of enzymes, amino acids are conjugated to form proteins or are converted into hormones, such as thyroxine, catecholamines, histamine, or serotonin. A defect or deficiency in any of these enzymes may lead to a deficiency in a compound or an excessive accumulation of toxic by-products. Disorders in enzymatic systems that facilitate amino acid transport through cell membrane may, in addition, cause excessive loss of amino acids in urine and stool, resulting in low plasma levels of certain amino acids.

More than 70 inherited aminoacidopathies are now known. Most are caused by defects in the intracellular metabolism. Only a selected group of diseases that are of special interest to the medical management of pregnancy are discussed in this chapter.

HOMOCYSTINURIA

This disease comprises a group of autosomal recessive disorders of sulfur amino acid metabolism. The most common type is related to a deficiency of *cystathionine synthase,* a pyridoxal-phosphate-dependent enzyme that catalyzes the reaction of serine with homocystine to form cystathionine. This enzyme defect results in raised blood and urine levels of homocystine, methionine, and other sulfur amino acids. The incidence of this error of metabolism is estimated at one in 160,000 births. Two forms of the disease are known: a vitamin-B_6 (pyridoxine)-responsive form and a vitamin-B_6-unresponsive form. Clinical manifestations include dislocation of the ocular lenses, osteoporosis, thromboembolic episodes, and mental retardation.

At least 50 pregnancies in 19 homocystinuric women have been reported.[12-20] Eighteen pregnancies resulted in fetal losses: six in the first trimester, one in the second trimester, four in the third trimester, and seven at an unspecified gestational age. All but one occurred in untreated patients. Three women underwent a therapeutic termination of pregnancy after amniocentesis and diagnosis of the disorder *in utero.* Ten women with pyridoxine-responsive homocystinuria who received pyridoxine therapy during pregnancy gave birth to 19 children, of which 17 were normal, one had brain damage, and one had trisomy 21. One patient with untreated homocystinuria had a therapeutic abortion at 18 weeks' gestation, and no obvious pathologic changes were present in the fetus.[15] Also, no pathologic abnormalities were found in fetal tissues recovered following a death *in utero* at the seventh month of gestation.[15]

These data suggest a very high risk of fetal loss in women with untreated homocystinuria. More data are needed to determine the long-term consequences to the infants born to such women. Administration of large doses of pyridoxine (250–500 mg daily) in combination with folic acid is expected to improve the outcome of pregnancy, particularly in women with the pyridoxine-responsive form. The effectiveness of a low-methionine diet is unclear. The risk of the fetus having the disease is very low (<1%) if the mother is affected and there is no parental consanguinity. Intrauterine diagnosis of the affected fetus is possible by demonstration of a decreased amniotic fluid level of the enzyme cystathionine synthetase (see Table 30–1).

HISTIDINEMIA

This autosomal recessive disease is characterized by the excessive accumulation of histidine in the plasma as a result of a deficiency in the enzyme *histidase,* which converts histidine to urocanic acid. The incidence of this disorder is about six cases per 100,000, and it is more common in Caucasians. The clinical manifestations of the disease are secondary to impaired development of the nervous system, and they include mental retardation and speech difficulty. It is, however, still difficult to know whether observed clinical features are related to the histidinemia or whether they represent coincidental features. Some studies indicate that histidinemia is not associated with any symptoms.[21]

A total of 50 pregnancies in 10 histidinemic patients have been reported. The incidence of miscarriages (14%) was not higher than expected, and the prenatal course was normal in all cases. The offspring of histidinemic mothers did not have mental retardation, and the speech defects that were encountered in some histidinemic children of one family also were present in nonhistidinemic members of the same family.[22]

There has been only limited experience with the treatment of histidinemia, and no claims can be made for clinical improvement of histidinemic patients treated by diet alone. On the other hand, it has been suggested that somatic growth of the fetus may be impaired if a histidine-restricted diet is maintained. It should be kept in mind that the fetal-maternal gradient for histidine is about 2.3.[23] It is thus possible for the fetus to be exposed to considerable amounts of histidine *in utero.*

HYDROXYPROLINEMIA

This is a benign biochemical trait that is characterized by elevated plasma levels of *4-hydroxyproline.* The exact nature of the enzymatic defect is not known. No correlation between the biochemical defect and clinical manifestations has been demonstrated. One pregnancy has been described in an affected individual[24], who had three normal children.

HARTNUP DISEASE

This is a rare autosomal recessive disorder of the renal and intestinal transport of neutral monoaminocarboxylic amino acids, which share a common reabsorption mechanism. These amino acids are alanine, serine, threonine, asparagine, glutamine, valine, leucine, isoleucine, phenylalanine, tryosine, tryptophan, histidine, and citrulline. The amino acids that are retained in the intestine are converted by intestinal bacteria into decomposition products that are toxic to the central nervous system. Patients with this disorder also may develop a pellagralike rash secondary to diminished synthesis of niacin from tryptophan. Only eight preg nancies of patients with Hartnup disease have been reported. Of these, seven resulted in healthy babies following uneventful pregnancies, and one offspring died of a nonrelated cause.

Treatment of pregnant women with Hartnup disease is not established. In general, patients have responded satisfactorily to prolonged oral administration of niacin.

PHENYLKETONURIA

Phenylketonuria is discussed in detail in Chapter 31.

REFERENCES

1. Dent CE. Detection of amino acids in urine and other fluids. *Lancet.* 1946;2:637.
2. Dent CE. A study of the behaviour of some sixty amino acids and other ninhydrin reacting substances on phenol- "collidine" filter paper chromatograms with notes as to the occurrence of some of them in biological fluids. *Biochem J.* 1948;43:169.
3. Navab F, Asatoor AM. Studies on intestinal absorption of amino acids and a dipeptide in a case of Hartnup disease. *Gut.* 1970;11:373.
4. Orten JM, Neuhaus OW. Metabolism of amino acids. In: Orten JM, Neuhaus OW, eds. *Human Biochemistry.* 10th ed. St Louis, MO: CV Mosby; 1982:320.
5. Young M. Foetus and placenta. In: Klopper A, Diczfalusy E, eds. *Fetus and Placenta.* Oxford: Blackwell Scientific; 1969.
6. Pearse WH, Sornson H. Free amino acids of normal and abnormal human placenta. *Am J Obstet Gynecol.* 1969;105:696.
7. Lemons JA. Fetal–placental nitrogen metabolism. *Semin Perinatol.* 1979; 3:177.
8. Battaglia FC. Umbilical uptake of substrates and their role in fetal metabolism. In: Visser HKA, ed. *Nutrition and Metablism of the Fetus and Infant.* Fifth Nutrician Symposium. The Hague: Martinus Nijhuff; 1979:83.
9. Van Veon LCP, Meschia G, Hay WW Jr., Battaglia FC. Léucine disposal and oxidation rates in the fetal lamb. *Metabolism.* 1987;36.48.
10. Cetin I, Marconi AM, Bozzetti, et al. Umbilical amino acid concentrations in appropriate and small for gestational age infants: A biochemical difference present *in utero. Am J Obstet Gynecol.* 1988;158:120.
11. Page EW, Glendening MB, Dignam W, et al. The causes of histidinuria in normal pregnancy. *Am J Obstet Gynecol.* 1954;68:110.
12. McKusick VA, Hall JG, Char F. The clinical and genetic characteristics of homocystinuria. In: Carson NAJ, Raine DN, eds. *Inherited Disorders of Sulfur Metabolism.* London, England: Churchill Livingstone; 1971:179.
13. Van-Sprang FJ. General discussion on the treatment of homocystinuria. In: Carson NAJ, Raine DN, eds. *Inherited Disorders of Sulfur Metabolism.* London, England: Churchill Livingstone; 1971:305.
14. Ritchie JWK, Carson NAJ. Pregnancy and homocystinuria. *J Obstet Gynecol.* 1973;80:664.
15. Hilden M, Brandt NJ, Nilsson IM, et al. Investigations of coagulation and fibrinolysis in homocystinuria. *Acta Med Scand.* 1974;195:533.
16. Brenton DP, Cusworth DC, Biddle SD, et al. Pregnancy and homocystinuria. *Ann Clin Biochem.* 1977;14:161.
17. Komrower GM. Pregnancy and inherited metabolic disease: An emerging medical problem. Presented at the Annual Meeting of the Canadian Paediatric Society, Edmonton, Alberta, June 23–27, 1979.
18. Kurcynski TW, Muir WA, Fleisher LD, et al. Maternal homocystinuria: Studies of an untreated mother and fetus. *Arch Dis Child.* 1980;55:721.
19. Drayer JIM, Cleophas AJM, Trijbels JMF, et al. Symptoms, diagnostic pitfalls and treatment of homocystinuria in seven adult patients. *Neth J Med.* 1980;23:89.
20. Fowler B, Borresen AL, Boman N. Prenatal diagnosis of homocystinuria. *Lancet.* 1982;2:875.
21. Levy HL, Shih VE, Madigan PM. Routine newborn screening for histidinemia. Clinical and biochemical results. *N Engl J Med.* 1974;291:1214.
22. Bruckman C, Berry HK, Dasenbrock RJ. Histidinemia in two successive generations. *Am J Dis Child.* 1970;119:221.
23. Butterfield LJ, O'Brian D. The effect of maternal toxemia and diabetes on transplacental gradients of free amino acids. *Arch Dis Child.* 1963; 38:326.
24. Pelkonen R, Kivirikko KI. Hydroxyprolinemia. An apparently harmless familial metabolic disorder. *N Engl J Med.* 1970;282:451.

Chapter Thirty-One

Maternal Hyperphenylalaninemia

Roger R. Lenke and Thaddeus W. Kurczynski

31

MATERNAL ASPECTS

Definition

The hyperphenylalaninemias result from the impaired conversion of phenylalanine to tyrosine. Classic phenylketonuria (PKU) is the most widely known and was originally identified in 1934 by Folling. If untreated, this disorder usually results in mental retardation and other manifestations of neurologic damage. In recent years, other forms of hyperphenylalaninemia have been described (Table 31-1).

Etiology and Pathogenesis

Phenylalanine is normally converted to tyrosine by phenylalanine hydroxylase. This enzyme is present only in the liver and kidney. In classic PKU, the converting enzyme is lacking in enzyme activity. In atypical and mild forms of the disease, some residual enzyme activity exists. Transient hyperphenylalaninemia is believed to result from a delay in the maturation of the enzyme system. Approximately 2% of cases of hyperphenylalaninemia are caused by a deficiency of various enzymes involved in biopterin metabolism, including *dihydropteridine reductase, guanosine triphosphate cyclohydrolase I,* and other pterin biosynthetic defects.[1] *Tetrahydrobiopterin* is an essential cofactor for phenylalanine hydroxylase and for tyrosine hydroxylase and tryptophan hydroxylase. The latter two enzymes are important in the synthesis of key neurotransmitters, including dopamine, epinephrine, norepinephrine, and serotonin. Pterin defects may lead to severe and progressive neurologic disease unresponsive to standard dietary therapy and associated with various neurotransmitter deficiencies.

The imparied hydroxylation results in reduced tyrosine formation and phenylalanine accumulation in the blood and urine. Alternate pathways of phenylalanine metabolism then lead to the accumulation of phenylpyruvate, phenylacetate, phenyllactate, and other derivatives that are cleared by the kidney and exreted in the urine. The resultant brain damage in affected individuals is believed to result from the elevated levels of phenylalanine and its breakdown products. The hypopigmentation of hair and skin is related to the reduced levels of tyrosine, a melanin precursor.

TABLE 31–1. DISORDERS SHOWING INCREASED SERUM PHENYLALANINE

Disorder	Blood Phenylalanine Level (mg/dL)	Treatment
"Classic" PKU	>20	Diet
"Atypical" PKU	12–20	? Diet
Persistent mild hyperphenylalaninemia	2–12	None necessary
Transient PKU	2–20	None necessary
Pterin deficiencies	12–20	L-Dopa 5-Hydroxytryptophan Tetrahydrobiopterin Folinic acid

Incidence

The hyperphenylalaninemias are inherited as autosomal recessive traits. They are widely distributed among caucasian and oriental people. The disease is rare in black people. Newborn screening programs detect hyperphenylalaninemia in approximately one in 10,000 births. Classic PKU accounts for approximately one half of these cases. Only about 2% of the hyperphenylalaninemias are the result of pterin deficiencies.

Manifestations

Newborns with PKU are indistinguishable from healthy infants. Before the use of screening programs and the institution of dietary therapy, classic PKU would invariably result in progressive brain damage with IQ scores usually less than 50. Seizure disorders and other neurologic sequelae also were common. Children with transient or persistent mild hyperphenylalaninemia are not at risk for these clinical consequences. Pterin deficiency may be transient or severe and may respond to treatment with tetrahydrobiopterin, L-dopa and 5-hydroxytryptophan, and folinic acid.

Diagnosis and Prevention

Each state has some newborn screening program for hyperphenylalaninemia, but the states differ considerably in their laws and practices for newborn screening. Only a few states have a mandatory program with no exclusions. Delaware has a voluntary program with no state law or public health regulation regarding newborn screening. Practitioners should become familiar with the procedures in their state. Prevention of the sequelae of the disease is based on the effectiveness of newborn screening programs.

Newborn blood samples are collected on filter paper before discharge and after protein feeding is established. Very early collection of samples could lead to false-negative results. All confirmed elevations of phenylalanine should be evaluated for PKU, and consideration should be given to dietary therapy in an experienced center or clinic. Pterin defects should be considered in cases not responsive to a low phenylalanine diet.

The structural gene for phenylalanine hydroxylase has been isolated and mapped to chromosome 12. Restriction fragment length polymorphisms at the phenylalanine hydroxylase locus have been used for prenatal diagnosis of PKU. They are applicable in about 90% of families for assessing carriers and affected individuals.[2] In order to apply this technique, a previously diagnosed relative from whom a blood sample can be obtained is necessary. Molecular deoxyribonucleic acid (DNA) analysis has further demonstrated that classic PKU and milk hyperphenylalaninemia are allelic within families. Such studies indicate that multiple and distinct mutations of the phenylalanine hydroxylase gene exist, which, in different combinations, result in varying degrees of hyperphenylalaninemia.

Treatment

Bickel was the first to treat classic PKU patients with a diet in which the bulk of the protein was replaced by an artificial amino acid mixture low in phenylalanine. He noticed a dramatic improvement in clinical status. Subsequently, this dietary therapy was instituted at birth in affected newborns. A number of studies in the United States and Europe studied children detected by newborn screening who were treated with dietary therapy from birth and found that the disastrous effects of the disease could be avoided. As noted previously, this dietary therapy is not effective for the pterin deficiencies.

When or whether dietary therapy should be discontinued has remained unresolved. It was common practice to terminate the diet in a young school-aged child. More recent data suggests, however, that some children are adversely affected by discontinuation, exhibiting lower IQs and attention-deficit disorders. The Collaborative Study of Children Treated for Phenylketonuria recommends continued dietary treatment after 8 years of age.[3]

Female PKU patients pose a special problem. Maternal PKU syndrome can result at any time after menses occurs. Many teenaged pregnancies are unplanned, and dietary management imposed after conception is of limited value. In addition, the introduction of a restricted diet after an early discontinuation is difficult and is often met with resistance. Thus, to prevent the possibility of adverse fetal effects, female children should continue dietary therapy during their reproductive years.

FETAL ASPECTS

Pathogenesis and Pathology

Dent first directed attention to the maternal PKU syndrome in 1957 when he reported on three nonphenylketonuric mentally retarded offspring of a PKU mother. Maternal PKU syndrome has come to include the offspring abnormalities of mental retardation, microcephaly, congenital heart disease, and low birth weight. The mothers also may have a slightly increased incidence of spontaneous abortions. In a review of 524 pregnancies from 155 women, it was found that 95% of mothers with blood phenylalanine concentrations of 20 mg/dL or greater had at least one mentally retarded child.[4] There also was an increased risk for women who had phenylalanine concentrations in the range of 16–19 mg/dL. Women with maternal phenylalanine levels between 3 and 15 mg/dL also may have a greater risk of fetal damage, but the available data are insufficient for definitive measurement of this risk. The fetal damage that occurs at lower levels of hyperphenylalaninemia may partially be explained by the increased concentration gradient of phenylalanine in the fetus. Fetal phenylalanine levels consistently run approximately 50% higher than those found in the maternal serum.

Incidence and Manifestations

Table 31–2 shows the observed incidence of damage in infants born to women with various degrees of hyperphenylalaninemia. As emphasized in the original report, even though these data are subject to ascertainment bias, they definitely point to an increased incidence of fetal abnormalities in pregnant women with PKU. Several factors from the original study should be emphasized. First, although there appears to be an increased frequency of spontaneous abortion in mothers with blood phenylalanine concentrations above 15 mg/dL, this increase could be explained by bias in ascertainment and inclusion of several families with exceptional fetal wastage. Second, although the occurrence of microcephaly and mental retardation appear to correlate with maternal phenylalanine levels above 15 mg/dL, the data on mothers with levels below 15 mg/dL should be taken with caution. Many of these families came to attention because of a clinical abnormality in the offspring. Future prospective studies are needed to better assess the risk of fetal damage at lower levels of hyperphenylalaninemia.

Although there was a definite increase in the incidence of congenital heart disease with maternal phenylalanine levels above 10 mg/dL, no pathognomonic lesion could be identified. Other structural defects were random, except esophageal atresia, which occurred more frequently than would be expected.

The study found a surprisingly increased incidence of offspring who had PKU or a lesser degree of hyperphenylalaninemia. The carrier frequency for the PKU gene is approximately one in 50; with random mating, only three of the 155 mothers would be expected to have had offspring with PKU or hyperphenylalaninemia. In fact, the study found 27 mothers who had offspring with elevated phenylalanine levels. These results possibly may be explained by bias in ascertainment, nonrandom mating, or other alleles at the hydroxylase locus, but further data are needed to clarify this matter.

TREATMENT

The successful dietary treatment of newborns with phenylketonuria has led many physicians to believe that dietary control of the biochemical abnormality during pregnancy would protect the fetus from damage. Table 31–3 shows the results of dietrary treatment instituted after conception.[5] It is obvious from these results that postconception dietary therapy did not prevent deleterious fetal effects. Of the

TABLE 31–2. OUTCOME OF UNTREATED PREGNANCIES OF WOMEN WITH PHENYLKETONURIA OR HYPERPHENYLALANINEMIA

Maternal Blood Phenylalanine Level (mg/dL)	IQ (DQ) >75	Normal Head Size	No Heart Disease	Birthweight >2500 g	Spontaneous Abortion
≥20	8%	27%	88%	60%	24%
16–19	27%	32%	85%	48%	30%
11–15	78%	65%	94%	44%	0%
3–10	79%	76%	100%	87%	8%
Controls	95%	95%	99%	90%	15–20%

TABLE 31–3. OUTCOME OF MATERNAL PKU PREGNANCIES WITH POSTCONCEPTION TREATMENT

Start of Treatment	Number of Offspring	IQ or DQ <90	Microcephaly	Congenital Heart Disease	Birth Weight <2500 g
First trimester	11	29% (2/7)	30% (3/10)	36% (4/11)	0% (0/4)
Second trimester	16	62% (4/13)	64% (4/14)	13% (2/16)	33% (4/12)
Third trimester	4	67% (2/3)	67% (2/3)	0 (0/4)	0 (0/2)

TABLE 31–4. OUTCOME OF MATERNAL PKU PREGNANCIES WITH PRECONCEPTUAL TREATMENT

Maternal Blood Phenylalanine (mg/dl)						
Pretreatment	Treatment	Birth Weight (g)	DQ	Microcephaly	Heart Disease	Age Last Observed
18	4–9	3500	—	No	No	1 mo
23	1–15	3300	100	No	No	2 y
20	?	3300	80	+/−	No	5 y
25	—	—	"Normal"	No	No	1 y
35	5–9	3314	—	No	No	6 mo
19	5–7	3120	—	No	No	6 mo
15	3–10	3500	"Normal"	No	No	10 mo
25	4–14	3300	"Normal"	No	No	6 mo

TABLE 31–5. MATERNAL PKU RECOMMENDATIONS FOR PREGNANCY MANAGEMENT

- Diet therapy (begin preconceptionally)
  - Phenylalanine (4–8 mg/dL)
  - Tyrosine (>1 g/dL)
- Weekly
  - Phenylalanine and tyrosine levels
- Every 4 weeks
  - Blood (3 mL)
  - Amino acids
  - Total protein and albumin
  - Hemoglobin, hematocrit
- Urine
  - Amino acids
  - Phenylketones
- Every 12 weeks
  - Blood (12 mL)
  - Folic acid
  - B_{12}
  - Zinc
  - Magnesium
  - Calcium
  - Phosphorus
  - Alkaline phosphatase
  - Iron
- Ultrasound examinations
- Assess:
  - Gestational age
  - Head development
  - Fetal growth
  - Obtain at 16, 20, 24, 30, and 36 weeks or as indicated.

31 pregnancies in mothers with PKU or hyperphenylalaninemia treated in this manner, outcomes varied from neonatal death with congenital heart disease to mental normality with no evidence of fetal effect.

Preconception treatment appears to give better results (Table 31–4). It should be noted, however, that almost all of these children are still less than 1 year of age, and their mental status cannot be fully evaluated. More preconceptionally treated cases must be studied before final recommendations are made.

If a women with PKU does contemplate pregnancy, she should be advised of the possibility of a poor fetal outcome, even with good dietary control. If she still elects to become pregnant, she should be placed on a low-phenylalanine diet before conception. Recommendations for dietary therapy include maintaining the phenylalanine level between 4 and 8 mg/dL. Tyrosine supplementation is given if the maternal serum tyrosine level falls below 1 mg/dL. Pregnancy and dietary therapy should be undertaken only in collaboration with a PKU center. The mother must receive a diet that has adequate calories, protein, calcium, minerals, and vitamins. Routine prenatal vitamins should not be given because many of these vitamins are already supplied in the dietary preparation. In addition to basic obstetric care, recommendations for follow-up during the pregnancy include obtaining the various blood and urine assays shown in Table 31–5. Ultrasound examinations also are valuable to assess gestational age, head development, cardiac development, and overall fetal growth. Several authors have implied that ultrasonography could detect fetal microcephaly before 24 weeks' gestation; however, a recent report shows that the diagnosis cannot be confirmed until well into the third trimester.[6] Thus, early ultrasonography should not be relied on to assure the mother that the fetus will have a normal head size later in the gestation or at birth.

PREVENTION

To evaluate the effects of PKU on pregnancy outcome, a Maternal PKU Collaborative Study (MPKUCS) was organized in 1984. This 7-year study involves all 50 states, the District of Columbia, and all of the provinces of Canada. Regional centers and a network of clinics have been established with funding from the National Institute of Child Health and Human Development. These centers are interested in providing hyperphenylalaninemic women (blood phenylalanine concentrations of >4 mg% while on a nonrestricted diet) of childbearing age with information and reproductive counseling. The goal of the project is to evaluate the effectiveness of a phenylalanine-restricted diet on pregnancy outcome. Because of the high incidence of teenage pregnancy, it is important that all clinics caring for young women with PKU discuss the possibility of pregnancy with their patients. Birth control and continuation of diet are strongly recommended in a young woman with PKU. If a pregnancy is contemplated, preconception dietary therapy is the goal. If a pregnancy occurs without preconception treatment, the patient should be counseled as to the possibility of poor pregnancy outcome, and termination should be considered.

Screening of all pregnant women for PKU would not be cost-effective compared with keeping contact with those patients identified by newborn screening. Most women consult their obstetricians after the pregnancy is established, and the available data indicate that the risk for fetal damage is high if dietary therapy is not instituted preconceptionally.

The identification of pregnancies at risk from maternal PKU lies with follow up of patients detected in newborn screening programs.[7] Whereas most patients with phenylalanine levels above 15 mg/dL have maintained contact with their PKU clinics, many patients with mild degrees of hyperphenylalaninemia have been lost to follow up. From the limited data available, these women may be at increased risk for fetal damage. The increased fetal risk at lower levels of hyperphenylalaninemia may be related to the fact that the fetus concentrates phenylalanine and maintains levels approximately 50% higher than in the maternal serum.

REFERENCES

1. Scriver CR, Kaufman S, Woo SLC. The Hyperphenylalaninemias. In: Scriver CR, Beaudet AL, Sly WS, Valle D, eds. *The Metabolic Basis of Inherited Disease*. New York, NY: McGraw-Hill; 1989:495.
2. Woo SLC, Lidsky AS, Suttler F, et al. Prenatal diagnosis of classical phenylketonuria by gene mapping. *JAMA*. 1984;251:1998.
3. Holtzman NA, Kronmal RA, Van Doorninck W, et al. Effect of age at loss of dietary control in intellectual performance and behavior of children with phenylketonuria. *N Engl J Med*. 1986;314:593.
4. Lenke RR, Levy HL. Maternal phenylketonuria and hyperphenylalaninemia. *N Engl J Med*. 1980;303:1202.
5. Lenke RR, Levy HL. Maternal phenylketonuria—results of dietary therapy. *Am J Obstet Gynecol*. 1982;142:548.
6. Lenke RR, Platt LD, Koch R. Ultrasonographic failure of early detection of fetal microcephaly in maternal phenylketonuria. *J Ultrasound Med*. 1983; 2:177.
7. Waisbren SE, Doherty LB, Bailey IV, et al. The New England Maternal PKU Project: Identification of at-risk women. *Am J Pub Health*. 1988;78:789.

Chapter Thirty-Two
Disorders of Nucleic Acid Metabolism

Pamela E. Smith

32

The indispensable contributions of nucleic acids to growth, development, differentiation, heredity, and the sustenance of life are self-evident. This chapter presents a basic review of relevant aspects of nucleic acid metabolism and clinical syndromes associated with abnormalities in metabolism, deoxyribonucleic acid (DNA) replication, and repair.

THE STRUCTURE AND REPLICATION OF DNA

Dietary nucleic acids are digested by pancreatic enzymes to mononucleotides, which are in turn converted to mononucleosides and free bases. The phosphates and sugars generated by this process can be reused, whereas most of the bases will be catabolized and subsequently excreted. An understanding of the principles of nucleic acid metabolic disease must therefore consider the biosynthesis of nucleic acid precursors.

Complete hydrolysis of a nucleic acid yields three major constituents: bases (purines and pyrimidines), sugars (ribose and deoxyribose), and phosphoric acid. Both DNA and ribonucleic acid (RNA) contain the purine bases adenine and guanine. DNA contains the pyrimidines, thymine and cytosine, and RNA contains cytosine and uracil. Partial hydrolysis by nucleases yields mononucleotides, which contain equimolar amounts of a nitrogenous base, sugars, and phosphoric acid. Further action by phosphatases yields inorganic phosphate and nucleosides. Representative structures of these compounds are illustrated in Figure 32–1.

Exonucleases are enzymes that cleave one mononucleotide at a time from the end of a polynucleotide chain. Endonucleases, in contrast, cleave polynucleotides at internal positions. Both enzymes are classified as phosphodiesterases because they cleave phosphodiester bonds, and both enzymes are extremely important in replication and repair of DNA.

The discovery that DNA is structured as a base-paired double helix and the observation that the molar concentraton of adenine equals that of thymine and that cytosine equals that of guanine laid the foundation for the *theory of semiconservative replication of DNA*. This theory proposed that the double-helical DNA strand "unwound" with the sequence of bases on one strand serving as a template for the synthesis of the other. Later experiments firmly

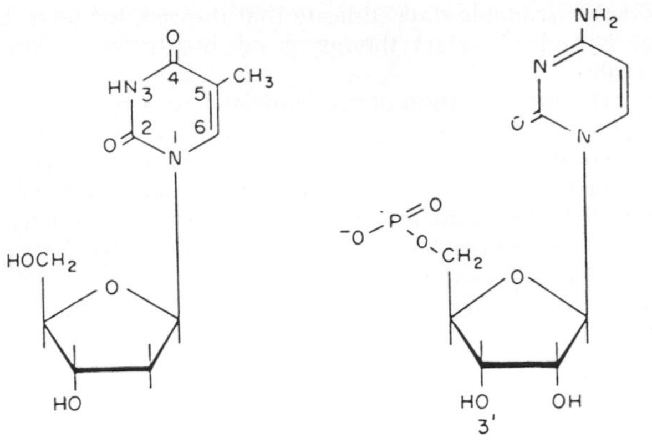

FIGURE 32–1. Structural examples of thymidine, a nucleoside (A) and thymidylic acid, a nucleotide (B).

established this hypothesis, but the mechanism responsible for the unwinding and subsequent transcription of nuclear material was still in question.

Experiments with mutant strains of E. coli provided invaluable insight into possible mechanisms of DNA replication and repair. As can be expected, the process of DNA synthesis is complex and involves multiple enzymes and cytoplasmic factors. Central to all these actions, however, is the function of an enzyme known as DNA polymerase. Three DNA polymerases have been isolated from E. coli and have been designated as I, II, and III. DNA polymerase I is most remarkable because it catalyzes three separate chemical reactions, a polymerizing reaction and two exonucleolytic activities. Consequently, the present hypothesis of DNA replication follows:

The DNA duplex opens slightly to allow the introduction of RNA polymerase, which catalyzes the synthesis of a short strand of RNA complementary to the exposed DNA strand. The free, single-stranded region of the DNA template becomes bound with a binding protein. The DNA binding protein and the polymerase interact with each other, while the protein holds the two DNA strands apart at the site of replication. The DNA polymerase then proceeds with the extension of the RNA primer. In a similar process, the opposite strand of the DNA template is copied. The result is newly synthesized DNA interspersed with segments of RNA. The exonucleases then remove the RNA segments, and DNA ligase joins the separated DNA fragments.[1]

Cooperation of endonucleases, exonucleases, and DNA ligase is again illustrated in mechanisms used to repair damaged DNA molecules. Three such mechanisms have been proposed: photoreactivation or reversal of UV light-induced thymidine dimers; excision repair, which serves to correct damage incured by UV light, x-ray, and chemical mutagens and involves the excision of the damaged segment and replication by the semiconservation model described previously[2]; and postreplication repair or replication of damaged DNA fragments.[2,3]

These mechanisms should be kept in mind because they are most important in the pathophysiology of the inherited disorder xeroderma pigmentosa.

PURINE BIOSYNTHESIS AND CATABOLISM

Figure 32–2 outlines purine biosynthesis and interconversions.[4] In consideration of the pathophysiology involved in the many purine metabolic disorders, the following factors should be kept in mind:

1. The formation of 5-phosphoribosyl-1-pyrophosphate (PRPP), an important intermediate in purine and pyrimidine synthesis, is catalized by PRPP synthetase (reaction #3) and involves the reactants ribose-5-phosphate and adenosine triphosphate (ATP).

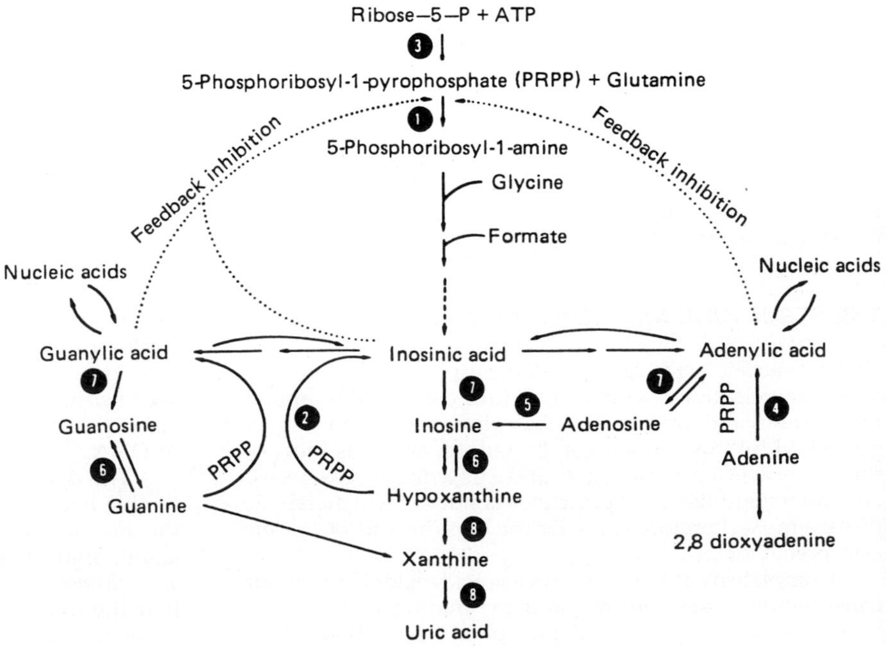

FIGURE 32–2. Purine synthesis and interconversions. Enzymes catalyzing the reactions are (1) amidophyosphoribosyltransferase, (2) hypoxanthine-guanine phosphoribosyltransferase, (3) PRPP synthetase, (4) adenine phosphoribosyltransferase, (5) adenosine deaminase, (6) purine nucleoside phosphorylase, (7) 5′-nucleotidase, and (8) xanthine oxidase. *(From Kelley[4] with permission.)*

2. The purine ring is synthesized entirely on the preexisting ribose molecule and involves the interaction of the amino acids glycine, glutamine, and aspartate, formic acid, and CO_2.
3. The first committed and rate-limiting step of purine biosynthesis involves PRPP and glutamine. A reaction catalyzed by glutamine PRPP aminotransferase (reaction #1).
4. The initial product of purine biosynthesis is inosinic acid, which can be converted to guanylic and adenylic acids.
5. A salvage pathway exists by which mononucleotides can be resynthesized from guanine, hypoxanthine, and PRPP. This reaction is catalized by hypoxanthine guanine phosphoribosyltranferase (HPRT) (reaction #2). Because PRPP is a substrate in this reaction, inactivity of HPRT may lead to increased production of xanthine and uric acid.
6. Feedback inhibition of aminotranferase (reaction #1) by nucleotides is an important control mechanism of purine biosynthesis.
7. Uric acid, the excretory product of purine metabolism in humans, is a poorly soluble substance and normally exists at near saturation concentrations in serum.

A thorough understanding of such disorders as gout, 2,8-dihydroxyadenine lithiosis, xanthinuria, and certain immunodeficiency disorders requires familiarity with the previously described metabolic reactions.

PYRIMIDINE BIOSYNTHESIS AND METABOLISM

Reactions involved in pyrimidine biosynthesis are outlined in Figure 32–3.[5] Important points to emphasize follow:

1. Unlike purine biosynthesis, the pyrimidine ring is formed before its attachment to ribose phosphate.
2. The first committed and rate-limiting reaction in pyrimidine biosynthesis involves aspartate and carbamyl phosphate and is catabolyzed by carbamyl phosphate synthetase.
3. The first pyrimidine nucleotide synthesized is uridine-5-monophosphate (UMP), which can serve as a precursor for the synthesis of thymidine and cytosine.
4. Pyrimidines are catabolized in the liver by reduction with NADPH. Unlike the excretory products of purine degradation, the products of pyrimidine metabolism are more soluble (ie, malonate and methylmalonate). Thus, there is no pyrimidine metabolic dysfunction analogous to gout.
5. Although, in general, dietary nucleosides are poorly absorbed, enough uridine can be absorbed to satisfy daily requirements.

Orotic aciduria represents the only reported defect in pyrimidine biosynthesis.

INTERCONNECTING PATHWAYS AND THE IMPORTANCE OF FOLATE

The biosynthesis of purines and pyrimidines are similar in many ways. In both pathways, for example, the initial reactions are irreversible, and therefore they determine the entire sequence of the reactions that follow. Aspartate transcarbamylase and PRPP aminotransferase, the rate-limiting enzymes for pyrimidine and purine synthesis, respectively, also are examples of enzymes controlled by the allosteric effects of their end products, namely, nucleotides.

Perhaps more important from an obstetric point of view is the pivotal position of folate coenzymes in nucleic acid metablism. Folate deficiency is one of the most common vitamin deficiencies in the world. Deficiences may be caused by infections, hemorrhage, pregnancy, or ingestion of certain drugs. Dietary folic acid is converted to tetrahydrofolate (THF), and it is this derivative that acts as the coenzyme acceptor of one-carbon units in the synthesis of precursors of nucleic acids. Table 32–1 lists the various reactions involved.

In light of such information, the genesis of most megaloblastic anemias in pregnancy can be understood. Likewise, theoretically, the administration of folic acid analogues should slow down growing cells. This would include cancer cells and cells of the developing fetus. Use of such drugs (eg, methotrexate, aminopterine) should therefore be avoided during pregnancy; however, there have been case reports of normal infants delivered who were exposed to these substances before birth (see Chapter 173).[1,3]

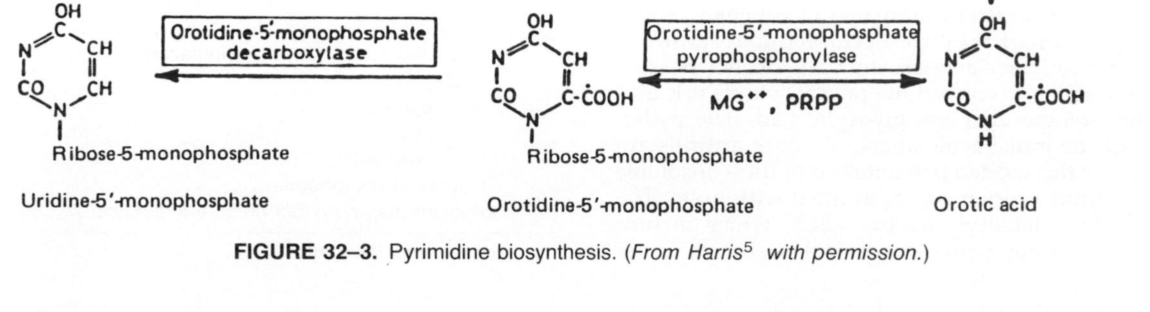

FIGURE 32–3. Pyrimidine biosynthesis. (*From Harris*[5] *with permission.*)

TABLE 32–1. ONE-CARBON TRANSFER REACTIONS UTILIZING TETRAHYDROFOLATE (THF) COFACTORS

Coenzyme	Reaction
5,10-Methylene-THF	dUMP→dTMP
5,10-Methenyl-THF	Glycine amide ribotide→formylglycine amide ribotide
10-Formyl-THF	Aminoimidazole carboxamide ribotide→formamidoimidazole carboxamide ribotide

CLINICAL SYNDROMES: ABNORMALITIES IN METABOLISM

Gout

Among the disorders of nucleic acid metablism, gout is most frequently recognized and described during pregnancy. The term gout refers to a derangement in purine metablism manifested by hyperuricemia, recurrent attacks of acute arthritis, and in some instances, the deposition of tophaceous collections of monosodium urate. It consists of two main forms: *primary gout*, a disease state that sometimes results from an inborn error of metabolism, and *secondary gout*, which refers to the occurrence of gout resulting from increased metabolism or decreased renal clearance of nucleic acid precursors. This occurs in response to another pathophysiologic process, such as rapid turnover of blood cells in leukemia.

According to Kelley[3,6], the clinical features of gout can be categorized as in the following sections (see also Chapter 52).

Asymptomatic Hyperuricemia. In this initial stage, the serum urate level is high, but arthritic symptoms, tophi, or stones are absent. It must be kept in mind, however, that a considerable number of people who are hyperuricemic never develop gout. All gouty subjects, in contrast, are hyperuricemic.

Acute Gouty Arthritis. As mentioned previously, serum concentrations of urate are normally near saturation levels in adults. Serum is saturated at a concentraton of 6.4 mg/100 mL, and normal men have serum values from 5–7 mg/100 mL; values in premenopausal females range from 4–5.7 mg/100 mL. With these values in mind, any increase in serum urate levels clearly leads to the danger of crystal precipitation, the situation in an acute gouty attack.

Interval Gout. After the initial acute attack, the patient enters an asymptomatic phase that may last from weeks to years. Seven percent of patients will not experience a recurrent attack for 10 years or more. This period of symptomatic relief is referred to as interval gout.

Chronic Gouty Arthritis. The presence of visible tophaceous involvement accompanied by permanent joint changes and chronic symptoms mark the onset of chronic gouty arthritis.

In contrast to lower animals, humans do not possess the enzymatic ability to convert the poorly soluble uric acid to the highly soluble urea and glyoxylic acid. The pathophysiology of the initial acute attack of gouty arthritis appears to involve the sudden precipitation of these insoluble microcrystals from a serum supersaturated with urate. The crystals are then phagocytosed by WBCs, which in turn enter lysosomes, resulting in subsequent lysosomal rupture and release of numerous enzymes that incite the intense inflammatory reaction. The presence of hyperuricemia antedates all of these reactions and can be produced by a variety of mechanisms.

In primary gout, increased availability of PRPP appears to be one of the mechanisms leading to an overabundance of uric acid. This can result from a deficiency of HPRT or from increased activity of the enzyme PRPP synthetase. The X-linked recessive *Lesch–Nyhan syndrome* is an example of the former mechanism but, because of its inheritance pattern, is a condition expressed only in the hemizygous male. Both mechanisms represent inborn errors of metabolism but account for less than 15% of all patients who have primary hyperuricemia associated with overproduction. The cause of the overproduction in the majority of these patients has yet to be defined.

The majority of patients with secondary hyperuricemia have this condition in response to an increased turnover of nucleic acids, for example, the rapid turnover of blood cells in leukemia or the production of hyperuricemia in patients with glucose-6-phosphatase deficiency. In the latter condition, called lactic acidosis, a direct consequence of the primary metabolic defect leads to decreased renal excretion of uric acid and enhanced nucleotide catabolism (see also Chapters 52 and 142).

Acute gouty arthritis is primarily a disease of the lower extremities. It presents initially as a monoarticular disorder predominantly affecting the great toe and is so painful that the patient may not be able to tolerate the weight of bed clothing. Recurrent attacks tend to be polyarticular and accompanied by fever. Specific events also may trigger the onset of an attack, such as trauma, alcohol ingestion, certain drugs (Table 32–2), dietary excess, or surgery.[6,7]

Acute attacks are managed by the administration of colchicine. Prophylaxis against recurrent attacks also can be managed by the daily use of colchicine or indomethacin, weight reduction, avoidance of precipitating factors, and in some cases, the use of uricosuric agents, such as probenecid or sulfinpyrazone, or the use of allopurinol, a drug that inhibits xanthine oxidase and decreases uric acid production.

Gout in Pregnancy. Lamon et al[8] reviewed the literature regarding the occurrence of gout in pregnancy. Originally, gout was thought to be primarily a disease that affected males and when it occurred in females, its onset

TABLE 32–2. DRUGS THAT AFFECT SERUM URIC ACID CONCENTRATION

Drugs that may increase serum uric acid concentrations
Small doses of salicylate (less than 2 g per 24 h)
Thiazide diuretics
Acetazolamide
Pyrizinamide
Ethambutal
Drugs that may decrease serum uric acid concentrations
Large doses of salicylates (4–6 g per 24 h)
Phenylbutazone, oxyphenylbutazone
Probenicid
Sulfinpyrazone
Allopurinol
Corticosteroids
Coumarin compounds
Colchicine has no effect on serum uric acid

Adapted from Newcombe.[7]

was most often during the postmenopausal period. This observation proved to be somewhat inaccurate because a number of case reports document the coexistence of gout with pregnancy. However, the biased nature of these reports does not allow for any general conclusions.

Until 1967, Talbott[9] reported at least 28 pregnancies complicated by gout. All produced normal, healthy term infants. The association of high-risk medical factors with gout must be considered when an attempt is made to gauge the impact of the disease on pregnancy. These factors include hypertension, obesity, and hyperlipidemia. There also is a questionable association between gout and diabetes mellitus. The presence of nephrolithiasis may be secondary to gout or a primary renal problem. There is some suggestion of an increased risk for those females who conceive and have gouty nephropathy.[8] In addition, reports of azotemia complicating gout in pregnancy and of postpartum gouty exacerbations have appeared.[10]

Probenecid, high fluid intake, and colchicine are recommended for the treatment of gout in pregnancy.[8]

Xanthinuria

Xanthinuria is a rare disorder of purine metabolism inherited as an autosomal recessive disease and associated with reduced activity of xanthine oxidase (see Fig. 32–2), an enzyme normally found in colostrum, liver, and intestinal mucosa. Its decreased activity results in low levels of serum urine acid and high levels of xanthine and hypoxanthine as metabolic end products of purine metabolism. Xanthine is less soluble at the urinary pH of 5–7 than uric acid. Therefore, in approximately 30% of patients, there is an increased tendency toward stone formation or patients may present asymptomatically with a skeletal myopathy caused by hypoxanthine and xanthine crystal deposits in muscle. Harkness et al[11] using retrospective and prospective data, report less than one case per 100,000 pregnant patients. From reports in the literature, xanthinuria does not adversely affect pregnancy outcome. Simmonds et al[12] report a dramatic increase in plasma uric acid concentrations in a pregnant xanthinuric female and attributes this to fetal uric acid production. Other investigators have confirmed this report.[11]

High fluid intake, reduction of dietary purines, alkalinization of urine, and administration of allopurinol were prophylactic measures suggested to decrease the risk of formation of urinary stones in these patients.

Orotic Aciduria

Orotic aciduria is inherited as an autosomal recessive disorder of the pyrimidine metabolism that manifests itself clinically by hypochromic anemia, vitamin B_{12}-unresponsive megaloblastic anemia, mental retardation, failure to thrive, and excessive urinary excretion of orotic acid (see Fig. 32–3). Two enzymatic defects have been discovered that produce an identical clinical syndrome. The first (*Type I*) one involves deficient activities of orotate phosphoribosyltransferase and orotidine-5′-phosphate decarboxylase. In the second, *hereditary orotic aciduria* (*Type II*), orotidine-5′-phosphate decarboxylase is deficient, although the activity of orotate phosphoribosyltransferase is increased.

Only nine patients with this disorder have been described in the literature, and of these, two were female children, ages 2 months and 6½ years, for whom follow-up reports of reproductive capacity were not available.[3]

As noted previously, use of dietary nucleotide bases is extremely poor, but effective treatment sometimes can be obtained with oral uridine.

MISCELLANEOUS DISORDERS OF PURINE METABOLISM

Congential disorders of purine metabolism resulting in immunodeficiency syndromes are primarily lethal autosomal recessive disorders of childhood and have not been reported in the homozygous state in pregnant women. Severe combined immunodeficiency disease (SCID) results from a lack of adenine deaminase activity (ADA, reaction #5). This is an enzyme whose production is controlled by a structural gene on chromosome 20. Pahwa[13], however, reports two children with ADA deficiency who were immunocompetent (one was a 10-year-old boy). Subsequent studies revealed a total lack of erythrocyte ADA with 25% lymphocytic ADA. Treatment for this disorder consists of bone marrow transplantation from a histocompatible sibling. There also is some evidence for a X-linked recessive inheritance pattern.[14]

Deficiency of purine nucleoside phosphorylase (reaction #6) results in severe lymphopenia and T-cell dysfunction, while humoral immunity remains intact. Production of this enzyme is controlled by a gene located on chromosome 14.

2,8-Dihydrozyadenine lithiasis is the clinical syndrome of renal stones secondary to a deficiency in the enzyme adenine phosphoribosyltransferease (reaction #4). Caused by structural similarities, it frequently has been misdiagnosed as gout.[3]

Myoadenylate deaminase deficiency is a disorder marked by easy fatigability, cramps, and myalgias following exercise. Evidence suggests that it follows an autosomal recessive inheritance pattern.

Clinical Syndromes: Disorders of DNA Replication and Repair

Apparently, females who are heterozygous for disorders of purine and pyrimidine metabolism have normal antenatal courses and remain clinically asymptomatic throughout life. In contrast, mounting evidence suggests that heterozygous carriers of DNA replication or repair disorders experience a higher incidence of malignant neoplasias[16,17] (compared to the general population, but lower than their homozygous counterparts), and thus these disorders can potentially impact on maternal and fetal health. Examples include xeroderma pigmentosum, Fanconi's (aplastic) anemia, Bloom's syndrome, and ataxia telangiectasia. All are inherited in an autosomal recessive pattern.

Bloom's Syndrome. This disorder is characterized clinically in the infant by intrauterine and postnatal growth retardation, sensitivity to sunlight, and telangiectatic erythema in the face and upper extremities. It is predominatly seen in men of consanguinous parents. There are immunologic deficiencies of IgA, IgG, or IgM as well as hypogonadism and various malignant neoplasms.[18,19] Cytogenetically, there is a tendency toward chromosomal breakage and rearrangement with frequent sister chromatid exchanges.

Fanconi's Anemia. Fanconi's anemia is characterized by chromosome breakage resulting in pancytopenia, congenital malformations, and a predisposition to malignancies.[20]

Ataxia Telangiectasia. Ataxia telangiectasia is presumed to be a disorder of DNA repair, although the specific defect has not been clearly defined. Clinically, there is progressive neural degeneration, immunodeficiency, cancer proneness, and extreme sensitivity to gamma radiation (x-rays). This is in contrast to xeroderma pigmentosum, in which a sensitivity to ultraviolet radiation exists. The symptomatic homozygous state is reported at an incidence of one in 40,000, while the asymptomatic carriers are estimated at one in 100.[16] The suspected predisposition of the heterozygous state to malignant transformation, coupled with its frequency, is of most concern regarding maternal health. Antenatal syndromes or complications associated with the heterozygous state have not been described.

Xeroderma Pigmentosum. Xeroderma pigmentosum is a disorder of DNA repair that manifests itself in a variety of neurologic disorders and sunlight-induced skin cancers. Its frequency in the homozygous state varies from one in 250,000 (United States and Europe) to one in 40,000 (Japan).[20] Complementation analysis has documented nine different groups, presumably representing nine different genetic mutations. Groups C, A, D, and variant are common in the United States and Europe, whereas group F is more common in Japan. The non-neurologic forms of xeroderma pigmentosum include groups C, E, F, and variant. The neurologic forms included groups A, B, D, and G.[3]

Normal cells use photoreactivation, excision repair, and postreplication repair to repair DNA damage. Patients with groups A through G are deficient in gene products required for the initial excision of damaged DNA. Patients with the variant variety are unable to complete semiconservative replication past damaged DNA sites.

Stages of skin changes associated with xeroderma pigmentosum include the following:

1. *Early inflammation*—this is secondary to extreme photosensitivity in those areas of the body exposed to light.
2. *Hyperpigmentation*—this is demonstrated by early freckling and lentigens that indicate areas of melanin collection.
3. *Atrophic and hypertrophic stages*—these are represented by atrophy, telangiectasias, and verrucous and malignant neoplasms.

Patients with the most common form of xeroderma pigmentosum (group C) frequently reach reproductive age. They are mentally and physically normal with the exception of the skin disease, which can be minimalized by surgical and environmental measures (eg, strict avoidance of sun light, wearing a sun barrier substance such as *p*-amino benzoic acid, which absorbs ultraviolet radiation). Apparently, specific allelic defects predispose to different types of skin cancers. Fischer et al[21] describe three sisters with the xeroderma pigmentosum-E defect who developed basal cell carcinomas between the ages of 16 and 20. Squamous cell carcinomas are more frequently found in groups A and C and lentigo maligna melanomas in group D.[20] Malignant melanoma, however, remains the most important skin malignancy concerning fetal–maternal health.

Melanomas represent 1% of the cancers diagnosed in the United States, with an overall incidence of 4.2 in 100,000.[22,23] With a peak incidence in the third and fourth decades of life, melanoma is concentrated among women in their reproductive years. There has been considerable concern over the possible exacerbating effects that pregnancy may have on the clinical course of malignant melanoma (see also Chapter 179).

Notwithstanding these observations, there is still considerable debate regarding the extent of the impact that pregnancy has on the prognosis of malignant melanoma. The consensus appears to be that the depth of invasion and location of the lesion are strong prognostic factors[23] (see also Chapter 179).

REFERENCES

1. Montgomery R, Dryper R, Conway T, et al. Nucleic acids and nucleotides and nucleic acid and protein biosynthesis. In: Montgomery R, Dryer R, Conway T, et al, eds. *Biochemistry: A Case Oriented Approach.* 2nd ed. St. Louis, MO: CV Mosby; 1977:519.
2. German J. Oncogenic implications of chromosomal instability. In: McKusick V, Claibourne R, eds. *Medical Genetics.* New York, NY: HP Publishing; 1974:39.
3. Wyngarden J, Kelley W, Simmonds H, et al. Disorders of purine and pyrimidine metabolism. In: Stanbury J, Wyngarden J, Fredrickson D, et al, eds. *The Metabolic Basis of Inherited Disease.* 5th ed. New York, NY: McGraw-Hill; 1983:1043.
4. Kelley W. Purine and deoxypurine metabolism. In: Kelley W, Harris E, Ruddy S, eds. *Textbook of Rheumatology.* 1st ed. Philadelphia, PA: WB Saunders; 1981:317.
5. Harris H. *The Principles of Human Biochemical Genetics.* 2nd ed. New York, NY: American Elsevier; 1975:385.
6. Kelley W, Mitchell B. Disorders of nucleic acid metabolism. In: Petersdorf R, Adams R, Braunwald E, eds. *Harrison's Principles of Internal Medicine.* New York, NY: McGraw-Hill; 1983:517.
7. Newcombe D. Gout and pseudogout. In: Harvey A, Johns R, McKusick V, et al, eds. *The Principles and Practice of Medicine.* New York, NY: Appleton-Century-Crofts; 1980:1153.
8. Lamon J, Lenke R, Levy H, et al. Selected metabolic diseases. In: Schulman J, Simpson J, eds. *Genetic Disease in Pregnancy.* New York, NY: Academic Press; 1981:15.
9. Talbott J. *Gout.* New York, NY: Grune & Stratton; 1967:146.
10. Meyers O, Monteagudo F. Gout in females: an analysis of 922 patients. *Clin Exp Rheum.* 1985;3:105.
11. Harkness R, et al. Pregnancy in and incidence of xanthine oxidase deficiency. *J Inher Metab Dis.* 1986;9:407.
12. Simmonds H, Spencer R, et al. Pregnancy in xanthinuria: demonstration of Fetal Uric Acid Production. *J Inher Metab Dis.* 1984;7:77.
13. Pahwa S. Defects of purine metabolism and immunodeficiency diseases. In: Wapnir R, ed. *Congenital Metabolic Diseases.* New York, NY: Marcel Dekker; 1985:385.
14. Bradford M, Krakoff I, Leeper R, et al. Study of purine metabolism in a xanthinuric female. *J Clin Invest.* 1968;47:1325.
15. Galjaard H. *Inborn Errors in Nucleic Acid Metabolism in Genetic Metabolic Diseases.* New York, NY: Elsevier; 1980:415.
16. McKinnon P. Ataxia-telangiectasia: An inherited disorder or ionizing-radiation sensitivity in man. *Hum Genet.* 1987;75:197.
17. Swift M, Morrell D, et al. The incidence and gene frequency of ataxia–telangiectasia in the United States. *Am J Hum Genet.* 1986;39:573.
18. Codeweyckx M, Fryns J, et al: Bloom's syndrome: Pitfalls in diagnosis. *AJDC.* 1984;138:812.
19. Kerckhove C, Ceuppens J, et al. Bloom's syndrome. *AJDC.* 1988; 142:1089.
20. Fujiwara Y, Matsumoto A, Ichihashi M, et al. Heritable disorders of DNA repair: Xeroderm pigmentosum and Fanconi's anemia. *Curr Prob Derm.* 1987;17:182.
21. Fischer E, et al: Report of three sisters with XP-E, a rare xeroderma pigmentosum complementation group. *Photoderm.* 1984;1:232.
22. Orr J, Shingleton H. *Cancer in Pregnancy.* Chicago, IL: Yearbook Medical Publisher; 1983.
23. Donegan W. Cancer and pregnancy. *Cancer.* 1983;33:194.

Chapter Thirty-Three
Disorders of Metals and Metalloproteins

Edward A. Zbella

33

WILSON'S DISEASE

Wilson's disease, or hepatolenticular degeneration, is a rare disease of metabolic dysfunction characterized by an excessive accumulation of copper in various organ systems of the body. The disease is transmitted by an autosomal recessive gene, and a high degree of consanguinity has been noted in the parents of affected individuals.[1] There is no racial or geographic predilection for the disease, and the prevalence is one in 10,000 people.

Copper appears to play a role in fertility[2-4], and women affected by Wilson's disease demonstrate a marked impairment in fertility. Primary amenorrhea and oligomenorrhea are common in untreated individuals. Pregnancy in affected women who remain untreated generally results in spontaneous abortions. Today, with an effective therapeutic agent for treatment, pregnancy in women with Wilson's disease is not uncommon and the obstetrician should be aware of its medical, obstetric, and neonatal aspects. Contraception has consequently become an issue. Copper-containing IUDs are considered contraindicated in these patients.

Pathogenesis

Copper is an essential element in certain proteins and enzymes in human tissue. These include cytochrome oxidase, tyrosinase, erythrocuprein, and ceruloplasmin. The average daily intake of copper is 2 g. Copper homeostasis is maintained by partial excretion of hepatic copper following its incorporation into ceruloplasmin and partially by way of bile excretion into the intestines. Copper is excreted mainly by the fecal route. The metabolic defect in Wilson's disease is an inability to maintain copper homeostasis. It is characterized by a deficient plasma ceruloplasmin, reduction of biliary copper excretion, elevation of plasma copper levels, and deposition of copper into various tissues of the body.

The primary genetic defect of the disease is unknown; however, different hypotheses have been proposed. Among these is the suggestion that the primary metabolic defect may be an abnormal intracellular protein that has an increased affinity for copper.[5] Another is that biliary copper may exist in a form that is more readily available for intestinal reabsorption.[6] Inadequate ceruloplasmin synthesis with subsequent low plasma copper levels and increased intestinal absorption of copper also have been suggested.[7-8]

Wilson's disease presents as one of two clinically distinct stages: an acute, hepatic form that presents in childhood and a subacute form, generally manifesting neurologic symptoms of late onset and presenting in adulthood. Most systems in the body are affected, and the liver appears to be the first organ affected. Up to 50% of patients present with signs and symptoms of liver disease. In untreated patients, the liver disease may progress to subacute hepatitis and cirrhosis, which may be irreversible even when therapy is instituted. Neurologic symptoms may include intention tremors, spasticity, dysphagia, chorea, and dementia. Although copper is frequently deposited in the kidney, renal dysfunction is rare. Deposition of copper in the inner surface of Descemet's membranes in the cornea occurs and produces the sign known as Kayser–Fleisher rings. These corneal deposits do not impair vision. Other reported effects include osteoporosis and hemolytic anemia.

Diagnosis

The diagnosis of Wilson's disease should be contemplated in the patient who presents with neurologic symptoms, liver disease, or Kayser–Fleisher rings. The diagnosis may be determined by measuring the serum ceruloplasmin level (less than 20 mg/dL), urinary copper excretion (greater than 100 μg/24 hours), or by liver biopsy demonstrating greater than 250 μg copper per gram dry weight of liver. However, hepatic copper elevations also have been reported in biliary cirrhosis, biliary atresia, and cholestatic syndromes.[9] When the diagnosis of Wilson's disease is definitive, further family evaluation for the disease should be undertaken.

Therapy

Treatment of Wilson's disease consists of removing excess tissue copper. D-Penicillamine (B,B-dimethylcysteine) is the drug of choice to promote copper excretion. It is administered in a dose of 1–2 g/d. Because D-penicillamine has an antipyridoxine effect, pyridoxine (25–50 mg/d) also must be given. A low-copper diet also is recommended. Toxic reactions to D-penicillamine have been reported and include fever, rash, lymphadenopathy, leukopenia, thrombocytopenia, and optic neuritis. The drug should be discontinued and slowly reinstituted when desensitization with steroids has been accomplished. An alternative drug for treatment is triethylene tetramine dihydrochloride. Once treatment has begun, it must be continued for life.

Pregnancy

There is an increase in the level of free copper and copper-bound ceruloplasmin during pregnancy. Ceruloplasmin levels may reach a level of 84 mg/dL at term, and mean serum copper levels have been noted to increase twofold at term (Table 33–1). Copper bound to ceruloplasmin does

TABLE 33–1. COPPER AND CERULOPLASMIN LEVELS AS AFFECTED BY PREGNANCY AND WILSON'S DISEASE

	Normal	Pregnant	Wilson's Disease
Total plasma copper	87–153 μg/dL	240–320 μg/dL	
Ceruloplasmin	20–30 mg/dL	48–84 mg/dL	0–20 mg/dL
Total body copper	100–150 mg		
Liver copper concentration	20–45 μg/g dry tissue		94–1800 μg/g dry tissue
Urinary copper excretion	5–25 μg/24 h		

not cross the placenta, whereas nonceruloplasmin copper appears to cross by diffusion. The elevated serum copper levels in pregnancy may provide a concentration gradient that allows the simple diffusion of copper across the placenta to the fetus.

Only a few cases of successful pregnancies in patients with Wilson's disease have been reported, and in most of these, the patient has been treated with D-penicillamine.[10-12] There also have been reports of women successfully managed with zinc[13] or trientine[14] during pregnancy. Some reports[15,16] have noted an improvement in the disease during pregnancy, attributed to an uptake of maternal copper by the fetus and the increased serum ceruloplasmin concentration noted during pregnancy. Continuation of D-penicillamine during pregnancy has had no adverse maternal effects. It therefore is recommended to continue during pregnancy, although the dose may be reduced safely. Pregnancy, however, is not advisable for patients with Wilson's disease who have hepatic insufficiency or evidence of portal hypertension.[17]

Some authors recommend reducing the dose of D-penicillamine 6 weeks before delivery if a cesarean section is planned.[18] The rationale is that this lower dose is less likely to interfere with wound healing while maintaining cupruresis. Because D-penicillamine crosses the placental barrier, some authors recommend its discontinuation during the sixth through the twelfth week of gestation, the period of organogenesis.[17,19] A single case of a minor congenital anomaly (cutis laxa and inguinal hernia) has been reported in an infant of a woman with Wilson's disease who was treated throughout her gestation with D-penicillamine. Mjolnerod et al[20] reports a case of a mother with cystinuria who was treated during pregnancy with D-penicillamine and delivered an infant with generalized connective tissue disease. Similarly, Solomon and associates[21] reports an infant with generalized connective tissue disease born to a mother who had received D-penicillamine therapy during pregnancy. Walshe[14] reports an infant whose mother was treated with trientine and was found to have the chromosomal defect, isochromex.[14]

All infants born to mothers with Wilson's disease and treated throughout pregnancy with D-penicillamine have demonstrated normal serum ceruloplasmin and copper concentrations. At birth, their serum ceruloplasmin levels are significantly lower than those in the adult, and the infants' tissue copper concentrations are more elevated. However, by the end of the first year of life, these levels approach those of a normal adult.

HEMOCHROMATOSIS

Hemochromatosis is a disorder of iron storage in which there is a generalized deposition of iron in the parenchymal cells of various organs in the body. This results in tissue damage, fibrosis, and dysfunction of the severely affected organs. The disease appears to be transmitted by an autosomal recessive gene and has been associated with the histocompatibility antigens HLA-A3, HLA-B7, and LLA-B14.[22] Hemochromatosis is observed more frequently in males than in females. The prevalence of the disease is one in 10,000 individuals.

The symptoms of this disease are generally not manifested until after the age of 40. However, with increasing awareness by physicians and screening of family members of individuals who have the disease, asymptomatic individuals are being recognized and treated at an early age.

Pathogenesis

The normal body content of iron is 4 g with the normal daily absorption and excretion 1 mg in males and 1.5 mg in menstruating females. The absorption of iron during the second half of pregnancy is 6–7 mg/d. An abnormality in absorption that can affect this homeostasis may lead to iron accumulation. Among the mechanisms proposed is that the intestinal mucosa absorbs amounts of iron in excess of the body's needs. Iron overload is observed with disorders of erythropoiesis, such as sideroblastic anemia, thalassemia, and porphyria cutanea tarda. Excess iron accumulation also may occur from excess iron ingestion. This has been documented in the Bantu tribe of South Africa in which excessive iron from fermented drinks is ingested because the liquid is brewed in iron containers.[23] Medicinal tonics and frequent red wine consumption are two additional sources of excessive dietary iron.

Parenteral administration of iron, by multiple blood transfusions or iron preparations, also may lead to an accumulation in the body. However, in these conditions, the accumulated iron is predominantly found in reticuloendothelial cells. Alcohol also enhances iron absorption and chronic alcoholism may lead to hemochromatosis. The exact metabolic defect leading to increased iron absorption in hemochromatosis still must be elucidated.

The iron accumulation in affected tissues is highest in the liver and pancreas, reaching levels of 50–100 times normal. Iron accumulation is 25 times normal in the thyroid, ten times normal in the heart and adrenals, and five times normal in the skin, spleen, kidney, and stomach.[24] The liver is usually the first organ involved and enlarges to an average weight of 2400 g. Splenomegaly occurs in 50% of cases. Hepatic function is usually unaltered, and the disease, in general, runs a benign course; however, episodes of hepatic failure may occur. Portal hypertension and esophageal varices may occur and hepatocellular carcinoma has been reported frequently.

A characteristic bronzing of the skin occurs in the majority of affected individuals as a result of an excess of melanin in the dermis. The face, neck, lower legs, genitals, and scars are particularly affected. Fibrosis of the pancreas with damage to the islets of Langerhans leads to symptoms of diabetes mellitus and is noted in most individuals with hemochromatosis. Cardiomyopathies are present in up to 15% of individuals, with congestive heart failure or cardiac arrhythmias the most common cardiac manifestations.

Arthropathies affect 25–75% of individuals and may be the initial symptom of the disease. The metacarpophalangeal joints initially are involved with a progressive arthropathy involving the knees, shoulders, and hips. Chondrocalcinosis may be present and is associated with episodes of acute synovitis. Erythropoiesis is normal and hematologic changes usually are not remarkable.

Diagnosis

The classic triad of cirrhosis, diabetes mellitus, and skin pigmentation should alert the physician to the diagnosis of hemochromatosis. Other frequently associated conditions include heart disease and arthritis.

Laboratory tests helpful in establishing a diagnosis of hemochromatosis include plasma iron concentration, percent saturation of transferrin, and serum ferritin concentration. The normal plasma iron concentration ranges from 50–100 μg/dL, and in affected individuals the levels are generally greater than 200 μg/dL. The saturation of transferrin is increased from a normal of 20–50 μg/dL to 50–100 μg/dL. Parenchymal iron can be estimated by measuring the serum ferritin concentration. The ferritin concentration normally is 50–200 ng/mL, whereas individuals with hemochromatosis usually have concentrations greater than 1000 ng/mL. Another method to estimate iron stores is to use the chelating agent desferrioxamine (Desferal). After injection of desferrioxamine, the urine iron level correlates well with the amount of iron stores. However, needle biopsy of the liver provides the definitive diagnosis, with histopathology demonstrating parenchymal localization of hemosiderin and varying degrees of fibrosis, depending on the severity of the disease.

Therapy

The specific treatment for hemochromatosis is to deplete the excess iron that has accumulated. The preferred method is by weekly or biweekly phlebotomy. One unit of blood contains 200–250 mg of iron. As the iron stores are decreased, there is a reflective decrease in the serum ferritin concentration. A noted decrease in plasma iron concentration marks the removal of iron stores. The process of depleting iron stores by phlebotomy usually takes 2–3 years. Following removal of iron stores, phlebotomy is required every 2–3 months. The chelating agent, desferrioxamine, parenterally given daily in a dose of 10–20 mg has been effective. Alternatively, a subcutaneous infusion pump of desferrioxamine also has been used to deplete iron stores. However, this drug is expensive and administration inconvenient.

The affected organs and the resulting pathophysiologic conditions must be treated. Diabetes mellitus should be treated with insulin. If cardiac arrhythmias or congestive heart failure occur, appropriate pharmaceutical treatment is mandatory.

When hemochromatosis is not treated, the disease is fatal with a 5-year survival rate of only 18%. Removal of the iron stores increases the survival rate to 66%.[25] However, of the individuals treated, one third eventually die from hepatocellular carcinoma. With treatment, the hepatomegaly and splenomegaly regress, and liver function becomes normal unless cirrhosis already has occurred, at which point the disease is not reversible. Pigmentary changes disappear, and cardiomyopathies regress. Insulin requirements also may diminish.

The physician should screen family members of affected individuals. If asymptomatic individuals are discovered, therapy should be instituted, and a better prognosis can then be expected.

Pregnancy

As noted previously, hemochromatosis generally becomes symptomatic after the age of 40. Consequently, there has been no report of a pregnant women with the disease. However, because the mode of inheritance and an association with certain histocompatibility antigens have been established, earlier recognition of the disease in relatives of affected individuals is anticipated.

Pregnancy requries only 1 g of additional iron to meet the requirements of the fetus, placenta, and expanded maternal red cell mass. Therefore, pregnancy will only slightly improve hemochromatosis. The use of desferrioxamine in pregnancy has not been established, and potential teratogenic affects are unknown. Phlebotomy should continue to be the mode of therapy in a pregnant woman. Iron supplementation should not be given to a pregnant woman with hemochromatosis.

THE PORPHYRIAS

The porphyrias are related disorders characterized by an excessive production and excretion of porphyrin, porphyrin precursors (aminolevulinic acid and porphobiligen), or both. There are six genetically recognized disorders in man and each type of porphyria represents a primary defect of heme biosynthsis, either in the liver or in the bone narrow (Table 33–2).

Clinical manifestations of the porphyrias usually involve cutaneous photosensitivity or neurologic abnormalities. Symptoms include abdominal pain, paralysis, psychosis, and coma. When excessive porphyrins are produced, cutaneous photosensitivity is noted, and when excessive porphyrin precursors are produced, neurologic symptoms are noted.

Pregnancy is not contraindicated in a woman with porphyria, and the obstetrician may even be the first physician to recognize and diagnose this disorder. Although pregnancy has been reported to have a deleterious effect on the course of acute porphyria, the maternal and perinatal risk is low. The obstetrician should be familiar with the primary symptoms or acute exacerbations of the disorder, avoid medication that may precipitate the disorder, and counsel the patient on the genetic aspects of the disease.

Congenital Erythropoietic Porphyria

Congenital erythropoietic porphyria (*Günther's disease*) is the least common form of the porphyrias and is characterized by a decrease in the enzyme uroporphyrinogen III cosynthetase with a subsequent increase in urinary uroporphyrin I. The mode of inheritance appears to be autosomal recessive. It affects males and females equally and has been reported in various racial and ethnic groups.

The most prominent and striking manifestation of congenital erythropoietic porphyria is the marked severity of cutaneous photosensitivity. Scarring, infections, and ulceration of the cutaneous lesions occur, with progressive disfigurement and mutilation reported. Hypertrichosis of affected areas is common. A mild hemolytic anemia may occur and splenomegaly is relatively common. Neurologic symptoms have not been reported.

Therapy involves the avoidance of sunlight and the prompt treatment of infected skin lesions. Splenectomy may improve the hemolytic anemia.

Few cases of pregnancy in women with congenital erythropoietic porphyria have been reported, and this reflects the rarity of this disorder. However, one maternal death during pregnancy has been reported.[26] Liver disease

TABLE 33–2. MODES OF INHERITANCE AND PRIMARY DEFECTS OF THE PORPHYRIAS

Porphyria	Heredity	Enzyme Abnormality
Congenital erythropoietic	Recessive	Uroporphyrinogen III cosynthetase
Protoporphyria	Dominant	Ferrochelatase
Cutanea tarda	Dominant	Uroporphyrinogen decarboxylase
Acute intermittent	Dominant	Uroporphyrinogen I synthetase
Variegate	Dominant	Protoporphyrinogen oxidase
Coproporphyria	Dominant	Coproporphyrinogen oxidase

and an increased risk of infection subsequent to splenectomy must be monitored. Although porphyrin has been noted to cross the placenta, no porphyrin elevation is detected in breast milk.

Brown-colored amniotic fluid has been reported at the 15th week of gestation in a fetus affected with congenital erythropoietic porphyria.[27] Nitowsky et al[28] demonstrates that reduced uroporphyrin III cosynthetase activity in cells cultured from amniotic fluid will establish a diagnosis of congenital erythropoietic porphyria.

Protoporphyria

Protoporphyria is a relatively common disorder characterized by a deficiency of ferrochelatase and a subsequent increase of protoporphyrin in erythrocytes, plasma, and feces. The mode of inheritance is autosomal dominant with variable penetrance, and it appears to occur more commonly in males than in females.

The disease usually presents in childhood and is characterized by mild to moderate cutaneous photosensitivity. Sunlight generally causes a burning or prickling sensation in exposed skin, which is followed by edema and erythema. The lesions usually disappear within a few hours; however, recurrent episodes may lead to skin thickening (solar eczema). Although protoporphyria generally is considered a benign disorder, associated abnormalities of the biliary tract and liver have been noted. There is an increased incidence of chololithiasis and progressive liver disease with subsequent fatal cirrhosis.[29] Therapy consists of avoidance of sunlight and administration of β-carotene in a dosage regimen of 120–180 mg/d, which increases the patient's tolerance to sunlight. Routine liver function tests should be performed regularly to screen for hepatic involvement.

A marked decrease and total disappearance of cutaneous lesions have been reported in pregnancy.[30] No reports of abnormal gestational or fetal effects have been associated with protoporphyria in pregnancy.

Porphyria Cutanea Tarda

Porphyria cutanea tarda is the most common form of porphyria and is characterized by a deficiency of the enzyme uroporphyrinogen decarboxylase. The enzyme deficiency usually occurs in the liver but also has been noted in erythrocytes, lymphocytes, and cultured skin fibroblasts. An increased urinary excretion of uroporphyrin I and 7-carboxylporphyrin is noted. The mode of inheritance is autosomal dominant with variable penetrance. Porphyria cutanea tarda usually presents in adulthood and, until recently, a preponderance of males affected by the disease has been reported. However, the disease now appears to be equally distributed among males and females, and this is thought to be related to the widespread use of estrogenic hormones by women.[31] Estrogens have been reported to be an etiologic factor in porphyria cutanea tarda. This disease also is precipitated by alcohol use and excessive iron ingestion. The disease is prevalent among the Bantu tribe of South Africa (see also section on hemochromatosis).

Skin lesions of porphyria cutanea tarda are characterized by mechanical fragility and vesicle formation. Milia are commonly noted on the hands and face. Hypertrichosis is common and especially frequent on the face. Hepatic siderosis is noted in most patients. No neurologic abnormalities are seen.

Therapy consists of the removal of precipitating factors. Abstinence from alcohol and the discontinuation of estrogen are important. Removal of hepatic iron by phlebotomy is frequently helpful. Avoidance of sunlight is recommended and sunscreens are helpful. The administration of small amounts of chloroquine apparently removes uroporphyrin from the liver but may cause hepatic necrosis and, therefore, is not advised.

Recent reports on porphyria cutanea tarda during pregnancy indicate that a symptomatic exacerbation may occur in the first trimester with a subsequent improvement in the latter half of pregnancy.[32-34] This is consistent with the increased levels of estrogen during the first trimester and the decreased levels of stored iron in the second and third trimesters. Increased estrogen may exacerbate symptoms, and lower levels of iron may improve symptoms. Iron supplementation in pregnancy should be avoided.

Amniotic fluid porphyrin levels have been reported to be three times those of the maternal serum level at 16 weeks' gestation.[32] No abnormal fetal effects have been reported in women with prophyria cutanea tarda.

Acute Intermittent Porphyria

Acute intermittent porphyria (pyrroloporphyria) is a disorder characterized by reduction activity of uroporphyrinogen I synthase and an excess production of the heme precursors aminolevulinic acid and porphobilinogen. The established mode of inheritance is autosomal dominant with variable expressivity. The estimated prevalence of the disorder is one to two per 100,000 individuals; however, the incidence in Sweden has been reported to be as high as 7.7 per 100,000 individuals.[35] Females have been noted to have clinically active disease more frequently than males, and symptoms generally occur at an earlier age in females than in males.

The disease occurs after puberty and is characterized by recurrent episodes of abdominal, neurologic, or psychiatric symptoms, with abdominal pain the most common complaint. The abdominal pain is usually crampy or colicky in nature and is often accompanied by constipation and vomiting. Neurologic manifestations are variable, with paresthesias, foot drop, and wrist drop frequently reported. Paraplegia, quadriplegia, and respiratory paralysis have been reported. Hyponatremia and tachycardia may occur during acute episodes. Mental symptoms include anxiety, confusion, hallucinations, and schizophreniclike behavior. Photosensitivity does not occur.

The characteristic abnormality of acute intermittent porphyria is excessive urinary excretion of aminolevulinic acid and porphobilinogen, which may be determined by the Watson–Schwartz or Hoesch tests. Aminolevulinic acid and porphobilinogen also are elevated in the serum and correlate with the severity of the symptoms during an acute episode. Liver functions are usually normal.

Acute attacks of porphyria may be precipitated by agents that induce hepatic cytochrome P-450, which, in turn, induces hepatic aminolevulinic acid synthase. These agents are listed in Table 33–3.

Treatment of acute intermittent porphyria includes avoidance or withdrawal of precipitating agents. Repression of aminolevulinic acid synthase may be accomplished by the administration of a large glucose load (at least 300 g/24 hours) orally or intravenously. The mechanism of action of glucose in repressing the enzyme is unknown. A second method involves the administration of hematin (hydroxyheme). Hematin is given intravenously in a dose of 4 mg/kg body weight at 12–24-hour intervals. A third approach is the administration of sodium benzoate, which diverts glycine, the direct precursor of aminolevulinic acid. Other measures include the correction of hyponatremia and the administration of phenothiazines to control pain and mental symptoms.

TABLE 33–3. AGENTS THAT MAY PRECIPITATE PORPHYRIA WITH NEUROLOGIC MANIFESTATIONS

Alcohol
Barbiturates
Chlordiazepoxide
Chloroquine
Diphenylhydantoin
Ergot derivatives
Estrogens
Griesofulvin
Imipramine
Meprobamate
Methaqualone
Methyldopa
Metoclopramide
Primidone
Progesterone
Sulfonamides

Acute intermittent porphyria is not a contraindication to pregnancy, and pregnancy appears to be well tolerated by women with this disorder. Brodie et al[36] demonstrated that pregnancy exacerbates acute intermittent porphyria in 54% of women and that only 24% have significant symptoms. Brodie et al also observed no difference in the attack rate during pregnancy for women known to have acute intermittent pophyria before pregnancy as opposed to women diagnosed during pregnancy. Only one maternal death, which occurred in 1954, has been associated with this disorder.

The physician must be aware of agents that may precipitate acute attacks of this disease and avoid their use.[37] Morphine and meperidine may be used safely for analgesia. Local anesthesia and epidural anesthesia are well tolerated.

A high incidence of prematurity has been reported in infants of women with acute intermittent porphyria.[36,38] The birth weights of infants born to mothers with this disorder who experience an acute attack during the pregnancy were significantly lower than the birth weights of infants born to affected women who were asymptomatic during gestation. The perinatal mortality is not increased in infants born to women with acute intermittent porphyria. However, Olund[39] reports a case of a woman with acute intermittent porphyria complicated by intrauterine growth retardation in two pregnancies that necessitated premature delivery. The neonate died of respiratory distress syndrome in the first pregnancy, while the second pregnancy resulted in a healthy child. The possible adverse effects of the therapeutic agent hematin on the fetus are unknown.

Uroporphyrinogen I synthase deficiency has been demonstrated in cultured amniotic fluid cells of a fetus from a mother with acute intermittent porphyria. The diagnosis was confirmed after delivery.[40]

Variegate Porphyria

Variegate porphyria is a rare disorder involving a deficiency of the enzyme protoporphyrinogen oxidase and characterized by excess excretion of all of the heme precursors. It is most common in the white population of South Africa and is inherited as an autosomal dominant trait.

The disorder usually presents in the second or third decade of life and has neurologic symptoms similar to those described for acute intermittent porphyria. Cutaneous lesions are characteristic in sun-exposed areas. During acute attacks, aminolevulinic acid and porphobilinogen are excreted in large amounts in the urine. However, the characteristic laboratory finding is large amounts of protoporphyria and coproporphyrin excreted in the feces.

Treatment is similar to that of acute intermittent porphyria, and precipitating agents should be avoided.

The reported maternal and fetal effects of this disease in pregnancy are similar to those of acute intermittent porphyria. No prenatal diagnosis of variegate porphyria has been reported.

Hereditary Coproporphyria

Hereditary coproporphyria is a rare disorder characterized by an overproduction of coproporphyrin III as a result of a deficiency of the enzyme coproporphyrinogen oxidase. The defect is inherited as an autosomal dominant trait.

Clinical symptoms are similar to those of acute intermittent porphyria, except that approximately 30% of individuals manifest cutaneous lesions. Treatment is similar to that outlined for acute intermittent porphyria and variegate porphyria; however, chlorpromazine has been reported to precipitate acute attacks in hereditary coproporphyria and should be avoided.

The reported maternal and fetal effects of this disorder are similar to those of acute intermittent porphyria. As with variegate porphyria, no prenatal diagnosis has been reported.

REFERENCES

1. Sass-Kortsak A, Bearn AG. Wilson's disease. In: Standbury JB, Wyngaarden JB, Fredrickson DS, eds. *The Metabolic Basis of Inherited Disease.* 4th ed. New York, NY: McGraw Hill; 1978,1098.
2. Suzuki M, Watanabe S, Hoshii M. Effect of estrogen on copper-induced ovulation in the rabbit. *Endocrinology.* 1965;76:1205.
3. Terajima T. Studies of the copper induced ovulation in the rabbit, with special reference to the action of D-penicillamine. *Acta Obstet Gynaecol Jpn.* 1971;18:59.
4. Underwood EJ. In: Bourne GH, Kidder GW, eds. *Biochemistry and Physiology of Nutrition.* London, England: Academic Books; 1953;2:426.
5. Uzaman LL. The intrahepatic distribution of copper in relation to the pathogenesis of hepatolenticular degeneration. *Arch Pathol.* 1957;64:464.
6. Gitlin D, Hughes WL, Janeway CA. Absorption and excretion of copper in mice. *Nature.* 1960;188:150.
7. Bearn AG. Wilson's disease: an inborn error of metabolism with multiple manifestations. *Am J Med.* 1957;22:747.
8. Scheinberg IH. *Wilson's Disease, Some Current Concepts.* Oxford: Blackwell Scientific; 1971;4.
9. Sternlieb I. Diagnosis of Wilson's disease. *Gastroenterology.* 1978;74:787.
10. Toaff R, Toaff ME, Pryser MR, et al. Hepatolenticular degeneration (Wilson's disease) and pregnancy. *Obstet Gynecol Surv.* 1977;32:497.
11. Biller J, Swiontoniowski M, Brazis PW. Successful pregnancy in Wilson's disease: a case report and review of the literature. *Eur Neurol.* 1985;24:306.
12. Morimoto I, Ninomiya H, Komatsu K, et al. Pregnancy and penicillamine treatment in a patient with Wilson's disease. *Jpn J Med.* 1986;25:59.
13. Lao TT, Chin RK, Cockram CS, et al. Pregnancy in a woman with Wilson's disease treated with zinc. *Asia Oceania J Obstet Gynaecol.* 1988;14:167.
14. Walshe JM. The management of pregnancy in Wilson's disease treated with trientine. *Q J Med.* 1986;58:81.
15. Dreifuss FE, McKinney WM. Wilson's disease (hepaticolenticular degeneration) and pregnancy. *JAMA.* 1966;195:960.
16. Albukerk JN. Wilson's disease and pregnancy, a case report. *Fertil Steril.* 1973;24:494.
17. Walsche JM. Pregnancy in Wilson's disease. *Q J Med.* 1977;46:73.
18. Schienberg IH, Sternlieb I. Pregnancy in penicillamine treated patients with Wilson's disease. *N Engl J Med.* 1975;293:1300.
19. Komrower GM, Sardharwalla IB, Coutts JMJ, et al. Management of phenylketonuria: An emerging clinical problem. *Br Med J.* 1977;1:1383.
20. Mjolnerod OK, Dommenud SA, Rasmussen K, et al. Congenital connective tissue defect probably due to D-penicillamine treatment in pregnancy. *Lancet.* 1971;1:637.
21. Solomon L, Abrams G, Pras M, et al. Neonatal abnormalities associated with D-penicillamine treatment during pregnancy. *N Engl J Med.* 1977;296:54.
22. Simon M, Bourel M, Genetet B, et al. Idiopathic hemochromatosis. Dem-

onstration of recessive transmission and early detection by family HLA typing. *N Engl J Med*. 1977;297:1017.
23. Bothwell TH, Settel H, Jacobs P, et al. Iron overload in Bantu subjects. Studies on the availability of iron in Bantu beer. *Am J Clin Nutr*. 1964;14:47.
24. Bothwell TH, Charlton RW, Motulsky AG. Idiopathic hemochromatosis. In: Stanbury JB, Wyngaarden JB, Fredrickson DS, et al, eds. *The Metabolic Basis of Inherited Disease*. 5th ed. New York, NY: McGraw-Hill; 1983;1127.
25. Bomford A, Williams R. Long term results of venesection therapy in idiopathic hemochromatosis. *J Med*. 1976;45:611.
26. Townes PL. Transplacentally acquired erythrodontia. *J Pediatr*. 1965;67:600.
27. Kaiser IH. Brown amniotic fluid in congenital erythropoietic porphyria. *Obstet Gynecol*. 1980;56:383.
28. Nitowsky HM, Sassa S, Nakagawa S, et al. Prenatal diagnosis of congenital erythropoietic porphyria. *Pediatr Res*. 1978;12:455.
29. Cripps DJ, Goldfarb SS. Erythropoietic protoporphyria: hepatic cirrhosis. *Br J Dermatol*. 1978;98:349.
30. Schmidt H, Smitker G, Thomsen K, et al. Erythropoietic porphyria: a clinical study based on 29 cases in 14 families. *Arch Dermatol*. 1974;110:58.
31. Stein KM, Rague CJ, Ziegerman JH, et al. Porphyria cutanea tarda induced by natural estrogens. *Obstet Gynecol*. 1971;38:755.
32. Baxi LV, Rubeo TJ, Katz B, et al. Porphyria cutanea tarda and pregnancy. *Am J Obstet Gynecol*. 1983;146:333.
33. Rajka G. Pregnancy and porphyria cutanea tarda. *Acta Derm Venereol*. 1984;64:444.
34. Lamon JM, Frykholm BC. Pregnancy and porphyria cutanea tarda. *Johns Hopkins Med J*. 1979;145:235.
35. Wetterberg L. *A Neuropsychiatric and General Investigation of Acute Intermittent Porphyria*. Stockholm; Svenska Bokforlaget; 1967.
36. Brodie MJ, Moore MR, Thompson GG, et al. Pregnancy and the acute porphyrias. *J Obstet Gynaecol Br Commonw*. 1977;84:726.
37. Milo R, Neuman M, Klein C, et al. Acute intermittent porphyria and pregnancy. *Obstet Gynecol*. 1989;73:450.
38. Zimmerman TS, McMillin JM, Watson CJ. Onset on manifestation of hepatic porphyria in relation to the influence of female sex hormones. *Arch Intern Med*. 1966;118:229.
39. Olund A. Acute intermittent porphyria complicated by pregnancy. *Clin Exp Obstet Gynecol*. 1988;15:168.
40. Sassa S, Solish G, Levere RD, et al. Studies in porphyria expression of the gene defect of acute intermittent porphyria in cultured human skin fibroblasts and amniotic cells. Prenatal diagnosis of the porphyric trait. *J Exp Med*. 1975;1442:722.

Chapter Thirty-Four

Disorders of Carbohydrate Metabolism

Leo R. Boler, Jr. and Norbert Gleicher

34

Fuel metabolism is a complicated and finely regulated process. This chapter concentrates on disorders of carbohydrate metabolism as they relate to the pregnant state, but does not review carbohydrate metabolism in pregnancy in detail. For this purpose, the reader is referred to Chapters 4 and 21 and standard references.[1,2] The main dietary carbohydrates are starch, sucrose, and lactose, which are degraded into free sugars, glucose, fructose, and galactose. After absorption from the intestinal tract, most of the fructose and galactose is immediately converted into glucose. Glucose thus becomes the final common pathway for transport of almost all carbohydrates to a tissue's cells. Fructose is rapidly used by the liver and is converted to glucose and lactate. When it is given intravenously, its conversion may be so intense that lactic acidosis may occur. Also, fructose-1-phosphate accumulates in the liver, causing depletion of phosphate and adenosine triphosphate, followed by conversion of nucleotides to uric acid, resulting in hyperuricemia.[3] Galactose is used by the liver. Its metabolism normally causes no problem. Only in congenital galactosemia does galactose accumulate in the blood.

Pregnancy is potentially diabetogenic. Clinical diabetes may appear in some women only during pregnancy. In others, existing diabetes may be aggravated. In the pregnant nondiabetic woman, circulating levels of glucose and amino acids are reduced; levels of free fatty acids, ketones, and triglycerides are increased; and the secretion of insulin in response to glucose is augmented. The metabolic state during pregnancy has been characterized as one of *accelerated starvation*. Diabetes is discussed in more detail in Chapter 43.

GALACTOSEMIAS

The term *galactosemia* describes two autosomal recessively inherited inborn errors of metabolism, in which blocks exist in the normal galactose-to-galactose metabolism pathway. Galactose levels thus become elevated in blood and urine.

Classic Galactosemia

This inborn error of metabolism results from a deficiency of *galactose-1-phosphate uridyltransferase* activity and represents the more widely recognized of these two metabolic disorders. Features of classic galactosemia are persistent galactose-1-phosphate uridyltransferase deficiency throughout life and a very toxic galactose-1-phosphate. A galactose-free diet is not harmful and is relatively simple to compose.

The incidence of galactosemia is one in 65,000.[4] In addition to galactose-1-phosphate, other metabolites accumulate in the body. Affected infants are clinically normal at birth, but often vomiting, hepatomegaly, and jaundice develop early in infancy. Weight gain frequently is retarded when using formulas containing milk. Some infants may die in the first weeks of life.

Galactokinase Deficiency

This is the second inborn error. It is much less common than transferase deficiency. Early onset of cataracts is the only known manifestation. Carriers of this trait have been found to have a higher incidence of cataracts than the general population.

Clinical Experience

Only five cases of maternal galactosemia have been reported.[5-8] Pregnancy, delivery, and offspring appear to be normal in all cases. Two of the five women were black. In one of these women, lactose deficiency, which is common in blacks, was established. No reports of pregnancies in untreated or partially treated maternal galactosemia have been published.

Only one case of maternal galactokinase deficiency has been reported.[9] This patient did not receive diet therapy. Although she had cataracts, they were not present in her four living offspring.

GLYCOGEN STORAGE DISEASES

The first description of a glycogen storage disease is attributed to Von Gierke in 1929. In all glycogen storage diseases, glycogen, which may be of an abnormal structure, is abnormally stored. Glycogen storage diseases have an overall frequency of approximately one in 60,000 live births. Almost all are autosomally recessively inherited. However, some exceptions to this pattern have been reported. Both autosomal recessive and sex-linked forms of type II (liver phosphorylase deficiency) have been described. Within the group of glycogen storage diseases, varying degrees of severity exist. For example, types II and IV are almost invariably lethal within the first 3–12 months of life, whereas type III is usually relatively mild. Varying degrees of severity also exist within the same enzyme defect. This is exemplified in type I (glucose-6-phosphate deficiency). Diagnoses of these disorders rely on direct enzyme analyses of suitable tissue. The most suitable tissues for enzymologic examination are usually muscle or liver, but in some disorders, leukocytes, erythrocytes, or fibroblasts can be used. The type of tissue preferred for each disease and the method of assay are shown in Table 34–1. Amniotic fluid cells have been useful in assessing fetuses at risk for the lethal types II and IV. An innovative method used in the diagnosis of type II involves the use of electron microscopy on uncultured amniotic fluid cells.[10] This method can give results in 3–6 days, whereas it takes 3–6 weeks to make the diagnosis by enzymatic analysis of cultured amniotic fluid cells. If an affected infant is diagnosed, abortion is usually offered to the mother.

Glycogen storage disease groups with relevancy to pregnancy are reviewed below.

TABLE 34–1. MAJOR GLYCOGEN STORAGE DISEASES

Type	Tissue Involved	Tissue Assayed	Glycogen Structure
I	Liver	Liver	Normal
	Intestine		Normal
II	Generalized	Leukocytes	Normal
	Liver	Amniotic fluid	
	Heart		
	Muscle		
	RBC		
	WBC		
	Amniotic cells		
III	Generalized	Leukocytes	Abnormal
	Liver		Abnormal
	RBC		Abnormal
	WBC		Abnormal
IV	Generalized	Liver	Abnormal
	Liver		Abnormal
	RBC		Abnormal
	WBC		Abnormal
V	Muscle	Skeletal muscle	
	RBC		Abnormal
	WBC		Abnormal
	Liver		
VI	Liver	Liver	Normal
	Kidney		Normal
	RBC		Normal
	WBC		Normal

Type I: Glucose-6-Phosphate Deficiency

This is an autosomal recessive disorder with clinical onset in infancy and characterized by hepatic enlargement, adiposity, flabby musculature, renal enlargement, hyperlipidemia, xanthomas, hyperuricemia, gout, and a bleeding diathesis related to impaired platelet function. Renal compromise and uremic death may occur.[11] The disease is compatible with survival into adult life and thus with both male and female reproduction. This disease has been reported to increase the risk of hepatocellular carcinoma and hepatoblastoma.[12] Pregnant patients with type I disease may be predisposed to a variety of complications. Renal disease may increase the risk of superimposed preeclampsia or eclampsia. Hypoglycemic convulsions, rare beyond childhood, also may affect fetal well-being.

Type II: Acid Maltase Deficiency

Deficient activity of the enzyme alpha-1,4 glucosidase leads to intralysosomal glycogen accumulation. This disease exists in at least three forms that may reflect different pathophysiologic mechanisms. *Type Ii,* the infantile form, is always fatal. Type *IIb,* the adult form, and a juvenile variant with marked hepatomegaly are compatible with life. The disease is inherited in an autosomal recessive mode. Parents with a type Ii child have a 25% chance of having another affected child with each subsequent pregnancy. Hypotonia and cardiac failure usually cause death before 1 year of age in type II. There are three reported cases of pregnancy in women with the adult variety[13-15], with no indications that labor or delivery were abnormal. The offspring were apparently healthy. Recent reports have shown the usefulness of chorionic villous sampling as a means of making first-trimester diagnosis of this disorder.[16]

Type V

This is a recessively inherited syndrome characterized by deficient activity of *muscle phosphorylase.* It presents clinically with muscle fatigue, cramps during exercise, and occasional myoglobinuria. There have been successful pregnancies reported in patients with this disease.[17] These pregnancies were uncomplicated, and spontaneous labor occurred at term. No muscle cramps were noted, and myoglobinuria was absent postpartum except in one case. The offspring were normal.

GLYCOLYTIC PATHWAY DEFECTS

The glycolytic pathway may exhibit enzymatic defects associated with hemolytic anemias and may range from mild to moderate. Of these defects, the only reported cases associated with pregnancy involve a *pyruvate kinase deficiency.*[18] This is the most common form of red cell glycolytic defect associated with chronic hemolysis. Hemolysis is moderate to severe and preventable by splenectomy. As with many of the inherited hemolytic anemias, a hemolytic crisis may be precipitated by biologic stress states, including pregnancy. The disorder is inherited as an autosomal recessive trait (see also Chapter 164).

HEXOSE-MONOPHOSPHATE-SHUNT DEFECTS

Glucose-6-phosphate dehydrogenase (G-6-PD) *deficiency* is the most common inherited form of hemolytic anemia and is found in more than 100 million people of all races throughout the world. More than 70 variants of the enzyme have been described, with at least 20 variants with chronic hemolysis. This enzyme is the first step in the hexose monophosphate shunt, which is involved in maintaining the level of reduced glutathione in the red cell by protecting it against oxidants. The severity of hemolysis is related to the specific enzyme variant, the severity of the deficiency, and the exposure to biologic stress or oxidizing agents. The major G-6-PD variant is found in the black population, and deficiency of this variant occurs in 10% of black American males and 3% of black American females. It is usually associated with episodic hemolysis but not a chronic hemolytic state. Hemolysis induced by fava beans (*favism*) is seen in caucasian and oriental individuals with certain G-6-PD variants but is most frequent in the black population.

Pregnancy in the patient with G-6-PD deficiency is associated with a number of specific complications.[19] Decreased G-6-PD activity has been reported in one third of normal patients in the third trimester. This may predispose these women to hemolytic episodes. The G-6-PD-affected fetus is at risk before and after delivery. Exposure to maternally ingested oxidants may produce hemolysis, hydrops, and death. The G-6-PD deficiency is inherited as an X-linked trait. A number of other enzymatic defects in the hexose monophosphate shunt have been associated with hemolytic anemias, but none has been reported in pregnancy (see also Chapter 164).

REFERENCES

1. Cunningham FG, Macdonald PC, Gant NF. *Williams Obstetrics*. 18th ed. East Norwalk, CN: Appleton & Lange, 1989;136.
2. Burrow GW, Ferris TF. *Medical Complications during Pregnancy*. 2nd ed. Philadelphia, WB Saunders; 1982;36.
3. Burman D, Holton JB, Pennock CA. *Inherited Disorders of Carbohydrate Metabolism*. Baltimore, MD: University Park Press; 1980;202.
4. Levy HL. Genetic screening. *Adv Hum Genet*. 1973;4:1.
5. Roe TF, Hallat JG, Donnell GN, et al. Childbearing by a galactosemic woman. *J Pediatr*. 1971;78:1026.
6. Tedesco TA, Morrow G, Mellman WJ. Normal pregnancy and childbirth in a galactosemic woman. *J Pediatr*. 1972;81:1159.
7. Samuels S, Sun SC, Verasestakul S. Normal infant birth in white galactosemic women. *J Med Soc NJ*. 1976;73:309.
8. Komrower GM. Pregnancy and inherited metabolic disease: an emerging medical problem. Presented at the Annual Meeting of the Canadian Paediatric Society. Edmonton; Alberta; June 23–27, 1979.
9. Gitzelmann R. Hereditary galactokinase deficiency, a newly recognized cause of juvenile cataracts. *Pediatr Res*. 1967;1:14.
10. Hug G, Soukup S, Ryan M, et al. Rapid prenatal diagnosis of glycogen storage disease type II by electron microscopy of uncultured amniotic fluid cells. *N Engl J Med*. 1984;310:1018.
11. Howell RR. The glycogen storage diseases. In: Stanbury JB, Wyngaarden JB, eds. *The Metabolic Basis of Inherited Disease*. 4th ed. New York, NY, McGraw-Hill; 1978;137.
12. Etsuro I, et al. Type Ia glycogen storage disease with hepatoblastoma in siblings. *Cancer*. 1987;59:1776.
13. Hudgson P, Gardener-Medwin DG, Worsfold M, et al. Adult myopathy from glycogen storage disease due to acid maltase deficiency. *Brain*. 1968;91:435.
14. Engel AG. Acid maltase deficiency in adults: studies in four cases of a syndrome which may mimic muscular dystrophy or other myopathies. *Brain*. 1970;93:599.
15. Hyam I, et al. Acid maltase deficiency: a case study and review of the pathophysiological changes and proposed therapeutic measures. *J Neurol Neurosurg Psych*. 1986;49:1011.
16. Grubisic A, Shin YS, Meyer W, et al. First trimester diagnosis of Pompe's disease (glycogenosis type 2) with normal outcome: assay of acid alpha-glucosidase chorionic villous biopsy using antibodies. *Clin Gen*. 1986;30:298.
17. Cochrane P, Alderman B. Normal pregnancy and successful delivery in myophosphorylase deficiency (McArdle's syndrome). *J Neurol Neurosurg Psychiatry*. 1973;36:225.
18. Collier HB, Ashford DR, Bell RE. Three cases of hemolytic anemia with erythrocyte pyruvate kinase deficiency in Alberta. *Can Med Assoc J*. 1966;95:1188.
19. Perkins RP. The significance of glucose-6-phosphate dehydrogenase deficiency in pregnancy. *Am J Obstet Gynecol*. 1976;125:215.

Chapter Thirty-Five

Disorders of Lipid Metabolism

Edmond Confino and Norbert Gleicher

35

Hyperlipoproteinemias are disturbances of lipid transport resulting from abnormalities in the synthesis or degradation of plasma lipoproteins, which may enhance atherosclerosis and induce pancreatitis.[1] Primary hyperlipoproteinemias are caused by an inherited aberration in the metabolism of lipoprotein particles. In secondary hyperlipoproteinemia, lipid levels are elevated because of alterations in related metabolic systems, such as hypothyroidism, hypoinsulinism, alcohol consumption, or oral contraceptives.[1]

Primary hyperlipoproteinemias can be divided into two groups according to their genetic transmission. The first category includes simple dominant or recessive single-gene hyperlipoproteinemias. In the second category, the cause is multifactorial. Interaction of several genes and environmental factors result in a familial disorder with a different severity of symptoms.[2,3]

PHYSIOLOGY OF LIPID METABOLISM

Nonpolar insoluble triglycerides and cholesterol esters are transported in the serum by globular particles, which have a nonpolar core and a polar surface coat. The hydrophobic core forms a lipid droplet and accounts for most of the particle's volume. The surface coat is composed of polar phospholipids that solubilize the particle. In the surface coat, small amounts of cholesterol and apoproteins bind the particle to enzymes, transport proteins, and cell membranes.

This microstructure of lipid droplets allows controlled emulsion formation, effective rapid transport of dietary fat, and efficient elimination by the liver (Figure 35–1).

The major lipoproteins in human plasma are classified according to their density, composition and electrophoretic mobility. Table 35–1 presents those particles and their characteristics. Although there are differences in their content, electrophoretic mobility, and apoproteins, they have arbitrarily been divided into several density groups. Various amounts of lipids are enzymatically removed in different sites changing each particle's size and characteristics. The large chylomicrons (800–5000 in number) are reduced in size in a stepwise fashion to high-density lipoproteins (HDL) particles (50–1200 in number). This changing scale of lipid particles allows differential transport and delivery

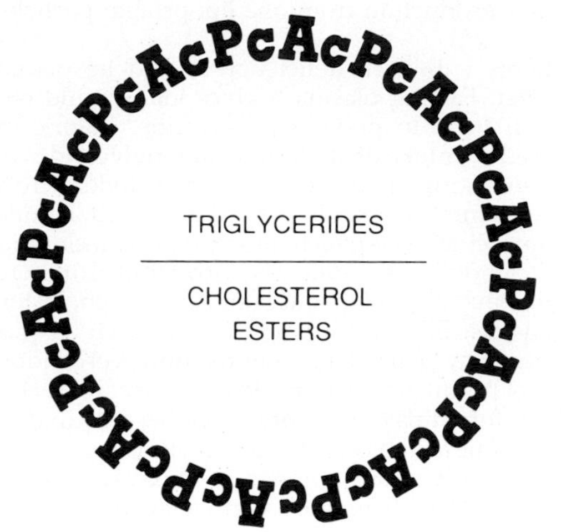

Figure 35–1. A lipoprotein particle. Different particles are separated during ultracentrifugation based on size and various ratios of the nonpolar lipids of the core and the polar soluble phospholipids of the surface coat. (A = apoprotein; P = phospholipid; C = nonesterified cholesterol)

of different proportions of cholesterol and triglycerides.

An average of 100 g of dietary triglycerides and 1 g of cholesterol are transported daily by the lipoproteins in the nonpregnant state. They are incorporated in the intestinal epithelial cells into large chylomicrons, and by way of the intestinal lymphatics are bloodborne to capillaries of various tissues, such as adipose tissue and skeletal muscle. *Lipoprotein lipase* (LPL) hydrolyses the triglycerides of the chylomicrons, releasing free fatty acids and monoglycerides. The fatty acids pass through the endothelial cells and are re-esterified to triglycerides or oxidized in the adipocytes and myocytes.[1]

Chylomicrons exchange some of the apoproteins with other plasma lipoproteins, lose most of the core triglycerides, and re-enter the circulation as remnant particles enriched in cholesteryl esters. These particles are transported to the liver and degraded, and some of the cholesterol contents are transformed into bile acids.

Endogenous triglycerides are synthetized in the liver and secreted into the blood stream in the large core of *very low density lipoproteins* (VLDL). The characteristics and apoprotein contents are similar to the chylomicrons. After triglyceride hydrolysis, VLDL remnants undergo an apoprotein transformation, and the triglycerides are replaced with cholesteryl esters. The new cholesterol enriched particle, *low density lipoprotein* (LDL), is the main source for cholesterol in various tissues, especially in the adrenal cortex. The LDL is hydrolysed by lysosomes of the target cells. Released cholesterol is used for steroidogenesis, membrane formation and in many other metabolic pathways. Whenever LDL reaches high blood levels, phagocytic cells in the reticuloendothelial system remove some of the particles. These scavenger cells eventually die, and the released cholesterol binds to serum HDL particles. The cholesterol is esterified with fatty acids by the plasma enzyme *lecithin-cholesterol acyl-transferase* (LCAT). Thereafter, the cholesterol esters are transferred to VLDL and later to LDL. This cycle delivers cholesterol to extrahepatic cells, and cholesterol is recycled by way of HDL.[4]

Lipid Metabolism in Pregnancy

Hyperlipidemia in pregnancy has been recognized for many years.[5,6] Hyperlipoproteinemias are divided into five types based on electrophoretic migration, and pregnancy is defined as type IV hyperlipoproteinemia.[7] The advent of ultracentrifugation improved the understanding of lipid transport in pregnancy and allowed quantitative determination of different lipoproteins.[8] Triglyceride content is increased in VLDL, LDL, and HDL with maximal concentration in LDL particles. Corresponding increases of cholesterol content are noted in VLDL and LDL and none in HDL.[9]

Most of the previously mentioned changes occurred in the second trimester and became maximal at 31–36 weeks' gestation. Lipoproteins remain high until delivery.[10] In midpregnancy, triglyceride contents of VLDL increase. This elevation is detected in pre-β-lipoprotein electrophoretic band, which corresponds to VLDL on ultracentrifugation.[11] Protein contents of VLDL simultaneously change with lipid changes. Apolipoprotein β, plasma apolipoprotein β, and plasma apolipoprotein α increase maximally in the third trimester.[12,13]

Plasma cholesterol and triglyceride concentrations fall rapidly within the first 24 hours after delivery. Plasma triglyceride levels decrease slowly compared to cholesterol. Plasma LDL cholesterol levels may rebound on the fifth day postpartum, probably because of rapid metabolism VLDL and conversion to LDL.[6] Elevation of all lipid plasma carriers during pregnancy correlates with the increase in fetal caloric demands.

The underlying control mechanism is probably hormonal. Some indirect data support hormonal regulation of lipoproteins. Distribution of lipoproteins, triglycerides, and cholesterol in women using oral contraceptives is comparable to third-trimester levels.[8] Furthermore, in young women with myocardial infarctions, one of the predisposing factors believed to contribute to the pathophysiology of coronary occlusion is elevated levels of LDL. Clinically,

TABLE 35–1. HUMAN PLASMA LIPOPROTEINS AND THEIR CHARACTERISTICS

Lipoproteins	Core Contents	Major Apoproteins	Electrophoretic Mobility
Chylomicrons	Dietary triglycerides	AI-II, B CI-III	nonmobile
Very low density lipoproteins	Endogenous triglycerides	B, CI-III, E	Prebeta
Remnants	Cholesteryl esters, triglycerides	B, CIII, E	Slow prebeta
Low density lipoproteins	Cholesterol esters	B	Beta
High density lipoproteins (HDL_2, HDL_3)	Cholesterol esters	A, I-II	Alpha

Adapted from Brown MS, Goldstein JL[1] and Upton V.[15]

they present with hypercholesterolemia and less often with hypertriglyceridemia.[13,14]

However, there is no unequivocal evidence for or against hormonally induced lipid changes and cardiovascular disease. Therefore, these rare cases may, in fact, represent genetic or other predisposing factors.[15] Even in the presence of clearly altered LDL–HDL ratios observed during danzol treatment of endometriosis, a cause-and-effect relationship with cardiovascular compromise is difficult to establish.[16]

DISORDERS OF LIPID METABOLISM

The Hyperlipoproteinemias

Hyperlipoproteinemia is considered to be present in any individual younger than age 20 whose total plasma cholesterol levels exceed 200 mg/100 mL or whose triglyceride levels exceed 140 mg/100 mL. In individuals older than age 20, the disease is defined as plasma cholesterol levels exceeding 240 mg/100 mL or triglyceride levels exceeding 200 mg/100 mL.[1] This definition is arbitrary because lipoprotein concentrations are influenced by many environmental and genetic factors. Table 35–2 summarizes six patterns of elevated lipoproteins.

Elevated lipoproteins in Table 35–2 illustrate the plasma pattern, not necessarily a specific disease. Various combinations of elevated lipoproteins may occur in one disease, while different diseases may display a similar lipoprotein pattern. Table 35–3 demonstrates this principle in detail. Numbers 1–5 in Table 35–3 are inherited disorders that affect some of the proteins involved in lipoprotein synthesis. In all, there are signs of lipid accumulation in the skin. With the milder forms, xanthelasmas will occur, while in the severe forms, eruptive xanthomas will appear. Except for LPL deficiency, all inherited conditions are associated with an increased incidence of premature atherosclerosis. Atherosclerosis in a young patient may result in myocardial infarction, cerebrovascular accidents, or acute pancreatitis. Table 35–3 depicts secondary hyperlipoproteinemias.[6-19] The underlying diseases cause increased secretion of one specific particle, frequently VLDL, and conversion into other particles such as LDL. Enzymatic inhibition of *lipoprotein lipase (LPL)*, increased hepatic lecithin secretion (see Table 35–3, acute hepatitis), lack of feedback inhibition of hepatic cholesterol synthesis by dietary cholesterol (see Table 35–3, hepatoma), immunoglobulin binding of remnants of VLDL (see Table 35–3, monoclonal gammopathy), decreased catabolism, and increased secretion of VLDL (see Table 35–3, stress), and insulin resistance result in decreased catabolism and use of the particles (see Table 35–3, diabetes mellitus, acromegaly, hypothyroidism). These may all result in shifts of production from one lipoprotein particle to another.

TABLE 35–2. ELEVATED PLASMA LIPOPROTEINS AND LIPIDS

Type	Elevated Lipoproteins	Elevated Lipids
1	Chylomicrons	TG
2a	LDL	CH
2b	LDL + VLDL	CH + TG
3	Remnants	CH + TG
4	VLDL	TG
5	VLDL + chylomicrons	CH + TG

TG = triglycerides; CH = cholesterol
Adapted from Brown MS, Goldstein JL.[1]

Patients with LPL deficiency should be placed on a low-fat diet. Fasting plasma triglycerides should be below 1000 mg/100 mL to prevent pancreatitis. Caloric input is maintained by intake of medium-chain triglycerides because they are not normally incorporated into chylomicrons. Fat-soluble vitamins also should be supplemented. Familial dysbetalipoproteinemia is effectively treated with clofibrate and reduced caloric intake. Patients with familial hypercholesterolemia have high LDL and should avoid cholesterol and saturated fats. Bile acid binding resins, such as cholestyramine, also may be used. Frequently, however, endogenous cholesterol production is induced because of bile acid depletion. Therefore, this treatment is effective only in the beginning. Nicotinic acid blocks endogenous cholesterol production and improves the potency of cholestyramine resin.[1] Familial hypertriglyceridemia with elevated VLDL levels also is treated with a low-fat diet and clofibrate. Secondary hyperlipoproteinemias are caused by diseases such as diabetes mellitus and hypothyroidism, alcohol consumption, and hormonal exposure, such as the contraceptive pill. Secondary hypolipoproteinemias are treated according to the underlying pathology; diabetes mellitus should be controlled and alcohol and oral contraceptives should be avoided.[1]

DISORDERS OF LIPID METABOLISM IN PREGNANCY

Diseases associated with hyperlipoproteinemia are described in Table 35–3. Some of these disorders, such as alcoholism and diabetes mellitus, can affect the mother and the fetus. For further information, the reader is referred to Chapters 8 and 43. Diagnostic effort and treatment should be directed to preventing immediate and long-term fetal and maternal sequelae of the underlying disease.

Familial hyperlipoproteinemias are usually long-standing diseases. Special efforts should be made to change dietary support in pregnancy as discussed previously in this chapter. Possible teratogenic effects of some of the drugs in use, such as clofibrate, should be weighed against the severity of the disease and possible benefits of treatment. The principles of medication selection and use in pregnancy are outlined in Chapter 7. Maternal age does not significantly affect plasma cholesterol levels[10], probably because some of the hyperlipoproteinemias appear only later in life. Therefore, the incidence of hyperlipoproteinemias in pregnancy is less frequent than the incidence of hyperlipoproteinemias in the general population.

Plasma cholesterol levels in preeclampsia are higher than in normal pregnancy, although the increase is not always significant.[5,18,19] An increase in the whole-plasma triglyceride concentration with elevated VLDL levels has been reported.[9] It is unclear whether the previously mentioned changes are specific to preeclampsia, or result from stress, hemoconcentration, and toxemia.

Pancreatitis in pregnancy is a rare complication associated with hyperlipoproteinemia.[19] Long-term nasogastric suction of pregnant women with pancreatitis may interfere with adequate caloric intake, may result in electrolite imbalance, and may result in fetal death.[20] Total parenteral nutrition may be safely and effectively administered to pregnant hyperlipidemic patients.[21] Most women with familial type I and IV hyperlipoproteinemias do not develop pancreatitis during pregnancy.[22] Only in severe hyperlipoproteinemias will the pancreatic vascular bed be obstructed with clumped lipid particles and result in full-blown pancreatitis.[23] Only anecdotal reports in the literature de-

TABLE 35–3. DISEASES ASSOCIATED WITH HYPERLIPOPROTEINEMIAS

Genetic Disorder	Biochemical Defect	Lipoprotein Pattern	Clinical Findings
Familial lipoprotein lipase deficiency	Lipoprotein lipase deficiency	I	Eruptive xanthomas, pancreatitis
Familial dysbetalipoproteinemia	Deficiency of apoprotein E III or VLDL	III	Xanthelasma, tuberous palmar creases, premature artherosclerosis
Familial hypercholesterolemia	LDL receptor deficiency	IIa	Xanthelasma, premature artherosclerosis
Familial hypertriglyceridemia	Unknown	IV	Eruptive, xanthoma, artherosclerosis
Familial combined hyperlipidemia	Unknown	IIa-b, IV, rarely V	Premature artherosclerosis
Diabetes mellitus	Reduced lipoprotein lipase activity, decreased VLDL catabolism, increased VLDL secretion	IV, rarely V	Overweight, lipodystrophies, hypertension, artherosclerosis, hypertension
Glycogenois type I (Von Gierke's disease)	Glucose-6 phosphatase deficiency	IV, rarely V	Accumulation of glycogen in liver, kidney, small bowel, decreased insulin secretion, hypoglycemia
Acromegaly	Insulin resistance	IV	Giantism, macrognatia hyperglycemia
Hypothyroidism	Insulin resistance	IIa, rarely III	Overweight, hypothermia, low BMR, decreased bowel activity
Anorexia nervosa	Psychogenic, reduced biliary excretion of cholesterol and bile acids	IIa	Cahexia, amenorrhea
Alcohol	Increased secretion of LDL in predisposed individuals	IV or V	Various degrees of alcohol intoxication, liver damage
Oral contraceptives	Increased secretion of VLDL in predisposed individuals	IV, rarely V	—
Glucocorticosteroids	Increased secretion of VLDL and conversion to LDL	IIa–b	Cushing's syndrome
Uremia	Increased secretion of VLDL, reduced lipoprotein lipase activity	IV	Yellow skin, odor, electrolite disturbances, anemia
Acute hepatitis	Decreased hepatic lecithin secretion	IV	Jaundice, liver function impairment
Hepatoma	Lack of feedback inhibition of hepatic cholesterol synthesis by dietary cholesterol	IIa	Abdominal mass biliary obstruction
Systemic lupus erythematosus	Decreased lipoprotein lipase activity	I	Skin lesions, cerebritis renal impairment, arthritis, anemia
Monoclonal gammopathy	Binding of remnants or VLDL, cholesterol, and bile acids	III, IV	Frequently asymptomatic
Stress	Decreased catobolism, increased secretion of VLDL	IV	Emotional, myocardial damage, burns, sepsis

Adapted from Brown MS, Goldstein JL.[1]

scribe severe complications of hyperlipoproteinemia in pregnancy, such as severe hemorrhagic pancreatitis of pregnancy and subsequent intrauterine fetal death.[24]

Whenever familial hyperlipoproteinemia is documented before pregnancy, a careful follow-up of plasma cholesterol and triglycerides should be carried out. Triglyceride levels above 100 mg/mL identify patients at risk and allow timely dietary intervention.[25] A cholesterol-free diet in pregnancy controls hypercholesterolemia, LDL levels, and pancreatitis.[26]

Familial hypercholesterolemia is usually asymptomatic, although cholesterol levels are elevated in the heterozygous female. Only homozygous individuals have accelerated atherosclerosis, and early death limits the opportunity for reproduction. Nevertheless, normal gestation, parturition, and lactation have been reported by several authors of homozygous hyperlipidemic women.[27]

Hyperlipoproteinemia may be diagnosed for the first time during pregnancy. Xanthomas, xanthelasmas, unexplained abdominal pain, or elevated cholesterol and triglyceride levels may be the presenting symptoms. Asymptomatic pregnant women with a family history suggestive of hyperlipoproteinemia should have a laboratory lipid work-up. Institution of an appropriate low-fat diet is necessary if a diagnosis of hyperlipoproteinemia is established. Diets high in cholesterol and saturated fats will result in lipid changes in pregnancy.[27-29] A cholesterol-free diet reduces LDL and total cholesterol levels in heterozygous type II patients by 19–33%.[23,30] Low-cholesterol diets in pregnancy should contain quality proteins, vitamins, minerals, and calories to meet the nutritional recommendations for pregnant women.[31]

Clofibrate lowers VLDL levels and triglyceride levels. It interrupts cholesterol biosynthesis before mevalonate formation.[32] It is indicated mainly for primary dysbetalipoproteinemia (type III), which does not adequately respond to diet. This drug also is effective in patients with very high triglyceride levels in type II and V hyperlipoproteinemia. Clofibrate should be avoided in pregnancy, although animal studies have failed to demonstrate any clear teratogenic potential. Clofibrate, however, accumulates in fetal serum in laboratory animals.[29]

Fetal Hyperlipoproteinemia

Fetal hyperlipoproteinemia is readily detected by umbilical cord blood sampling. Interpretation of cholesterol and triglyceride values, however, differ in the fetus compared to the adult. Although the passage of triglyceride molecules across the placenta has not been documented, a positive umbilical venous-arterial differential suggests possible transplacental transfer.[33] Maternal starvation results in elevated free fatty acids caused by triglyceride degradation.[34] These free fatty acids cross the placenta and can be incorporated into fetal triglycerides.[35] During short maternal starvation of less than 24 hours, umbilical lipid level changes are not detected.[36] This model suggests a mechanism of indirect increase in fetal lipids during inadequate maternal caloric intake.

Fetal asphyxia is frequently associated with free fatty acid release into the blood stream.[37,38] The free fatty acids are incorporated rapidly in the fetal liver and appear in experimental animals in serum lipoproteins within 10–20 minutes.[39] Only prolonged fetal anoxia results in cord hypertriglyceridemia in the human model.[34] A similar mechanism explains umbilical cord hyperlipoproteinemia in an intrauterine growth-retarded fetus.[35]

Newborns with hyperlipoproteinemia do not suffer necessarily from hyperlipoproteinemia.[40] Diseases such as preeclampsia and diabetes mellitus affect maternal, but not fetal, serum lipids.[17,41] An association between maternal obesity, increased placental flow of free fatty acids, and elevated cord triglycerides has been described.[36,42] Therefore, fetal and maternal measurements of lipid profiles on every newborn with a familial history of hyperlipoproteinemia is mandatory. Cord triglyceride levels alone as an indicator of fetal distress are therefore of limited value.[35] A careful family history of the mother will alert the physician to treat both fetus and mother in a timely fashion and reduces the complications associated with betalipoproteinemias.

REFERENCES

1. Brown MS, Goldstein JL. The hyperlipoproteinemias and other disorders of lipid metabolism. In: *Harrison's Principles of Internal Medicine.* 9th ed. New York, NY: McGraw-Hill; 1987;1650.
2. Motulsky AG. The genetic hyperlipidemias. *N Engl J Med.* 1976;294:823.
3. Frederickson DS, et al. The familial hyperlipoproteinemias. In: Stanbury JB, Wyngarden JB, eds. *The Metabolic Basis of Inherited Disease.* 4th ed. New York, NY: McGraw-Hill; 1978.
4. Brobeck JR. *Best and Taylor's Physiological Basis of Medical Practice.* 6th ed. Baltimore, MD: Williams and Wilkins; 1979;3:90.
5. Boyd EM. The lipemia of pregnancy. *J Clin Invest.* 1934;13:347.
6. Peters LP, Heinemann M, Man EB. The lipids of serum in pregnancy. *J Clin Invest.* 1951;30:388.
7. Fredrickson DS, Levy RI, Lees RS. Fat transport in lipoproteins—an integrated approach to mechanisms and disorders. *N Engl J Med.* 1967;276:34.
8. Knopp RH, Bergelin RO, Wahl PW, et al. Population based lipoprotein lipid reference values for pregnant women compared to non-pregnant women classified by sex hormone usage. *Am J Obstet Gynecol.* 1982;143:626.
9. Knopp RH, Warth MR, Carrol CJ. Lipid metabolism in pregnancy: in changes in lipoprotein triglyceride and cholesterol in normal pregnancy and the effects of diabetes mellitus. *J Reprod Med.* 1973;10:3.
10. Potter JM, Nestel PJ. The hyperlipidemia of pregnancy in normal and complicated pregnancies. *Am J Obstet Gynecol.* 1979;133:165.
11. Patelakis SN, Cameron AH, Davidson S, et al. The diabetic pregnancy. A study of serum lipids in maternal and umbilical cord blood and of the uterine and placental vasculature. *Arch Dis Child.* 1964;39:334.
12. Hillman L, Schonfeld G, Miller JP, et al. Apolipoproteins in human pregnancy. *Metabolism.* 1975;24:943.
13. Schonfeld G, Pfleger B. The structure of plasma high density lipoprotein and the levels of apolipoprotein in plasma as determined by radioimmunoassay. *Clin Invest.* 1974;54:236.
14. Stokes T, Wynn V. Serum–lipids in women on oral contraceptives. *Lancet.* 1971;2:677.
15. Upton GV. Lipids, cardiovascular disease, and oral contraceptives: a practical perspective. *Fertil Steril.* 1990;53:1.
16. Teichman AT, Cremer P, Wieland H, et al. Lipid metabolic changes during hormonal treatment of endometriosis. *Maturitas.* 1988;10:27.
17. Konttinen A, Pyorala T, Carpen E. Serum lipid pattern in normal pregnancy and preeclampsia. *Br J Obstet Gynaecol.* 1964;71:453.
18. DeAlvarez RR, Baratvold GE. Serum lipids in preeclampsia–eclampsia. *Am J Obstet Gynecol.* 1961;81:1140.
19. Corlett RL, Mishell DR. Pancreatitis in pregnancy. *Am J Obstet Gynecol.* 1972;113:281.
20. Jouppila P, Mokka R, Larmi TKI. Acute pancreatitis in pregnancy. *Surg Gynecol Obstet.* 1974;313:879.
21. Weinberg RB, Sitrin GM, et al. Treatment of hyperlipidemic pancreatitis in pregnancy with total parental nutrition. *Gastroenterology.* 1982;83: 1300.
22. Cameron JL, Capuzzi DM, Zuiodema GD, et al. Acute pancreatitis with hyperlipemia. The incidence of lipid abnormalities in acute pancreatitis. *Ann Surg.* 1973;177:483.
23. Klatskin G, Gorden M. Relationship between relapsing pancreatitis and essential hyperlipidemia. *Am J Med.* 1952;12:3.
24. Bremmer WF, Third JLHC. Type I lipoproteinemia and the pancreas. *Am J Med.* 1978;64:912.
25. Glueck CJ, Christopher C, Mishkel MA, et al. Pancreatitis, familial hypertriglyceridemia and pregnancy. *Am J Obstet Gynecol.* 1980;136:755.
26. Glueck CJ, Christopher C, Tsang RC, et al. Cholesterol free diet and the diet and the physiologic hyperlipidemia of pregnancy in familial hypercholesterolemia. *Metabolism.* 1980;29:10.
27. Stein EA, Meany C, Spitz L, et al. Portacaval shunt in four patients with homozygous hypercholesterolemia. *Lancet.* 1975;1:832.
28. Green JG. Serum cholesterol changes in pregnancy. *Am J Obstet Gynecol.* 1966;95:387.
29. De Alvarez RR, Gaiser DF, Simkins EK, et al. Serial studies of serum lipids in normal human pregnancy. *Am J Obstet Gynecol.* 1959;77:743.
30. Connor WE, Fry MM, Goplerud CP. The effects of dietary cholesterol upon the hypercholesterolemia and sterol balance in pregnancy. *Clin Res.* 1977;25:521A.
31. *Maternal nutrition and the course of pregnancy.* Washington, DC: National Academy of Sciences; 1970:1.
32. Angel JE. Clofibrate. In: *Physician's Desk Reference.* 3rd ed. Oradell, NJ: Medical Economic Company; 1984.
33. Sheath L, Grimwade L, Waldron K, et al. Arteriovenous nonesterified fatty acids and glycerol differences in the umbilical cord at term and their relationship to fetal metabolism. *Am J Obstet Gynecol.* 1972;113:358.
34. Kim YJ, Felig P. Maternal and amniotic fluid substrate levels during caloric deprivation in human pregnancy. *Metabolism.* 1972;21:507.
35. Elphich MC, Harrison AT, Lawlor JP. Cord blood hypertriglyceridemia as an index of fetal distress: use of simple screening test and results of further biochemical analysis. *Br J Obstet Gynaecol.* 1978;85:303.
36. Keele DK, Kay JL, Brown J, et al. Plasma free fatty acid and blood sugar levels in newborn infants and their mothers. *Pediatrics.* 1966;73:597.
37. Sabata V, Wolf M, Lansmann S. Glycerol levels in the maternal and umbilical cord blood under various conditions. *Biol Neonate.* 1970;15:123.
38. Anderson GE, Friis-Hansen B. Neonatal hypertriglyceridemia: a new index of antepartum–intrauterine fetal stress? *Acta Paediatr Scan.* 1976;165:369.
39. Van Duyne CM, Havel RJ, Felts JM. Placental transfer of palmitic acid 1G[14] in rabbits. *Am J Obstet Gynecol.* 1962;84:1069.
40. Goldstein JL, Albers JJ, Hazzard WR, et al. Genetic and medical significance of neonatal hyperlipidemia. *J Clin Invest.* 1973;52:35a. Abstract.
41. Chen CH, Adam PAJ, Laskowski DE, et al. The plasma free fatty acid composition and blood glucose of normal and diabetic pregnant women and of their newborns. *Pediatrics.* 1965;36:843.
42. Szabo AJ, Szabo O. Placental free fatty acid transfer acid fetal adipose tissue development: an explanation of adiposity in infants of diabetic mothers. *Lancet.* 1974;2:498.

Chapter Thirty-Six

Disorders of Connective Tissue

Ilan Tur-Kaspa and Norbert Gleicher

36

Connective tissue disorders are clinically, genetically, and biochemically a heterogeneous group of inherited diseases. Their primary defect resides in a component of the connective tissue matrix. They must be differentiated from collagen vascular disorders, which are primarily autoimmune conditions with impact on connective tissue. Clinical manifestations generally involve the eyes, skin, and skeletal and cardiovascular systems. Because normal pregnancy is associated with alterations in connective tissue, the potential problems for the mother and fetus with these disorders can easily be understood.

Because of the multisystem involvement of connective tissue disorders, a multidisciplinary team is essential for complete clinical management. In order to achieve this optimal management, obstetricians, internists, orthopedists, anesthesiologists, pediatricians, and geneticists should be familiar with these disorders and their complications during pregnancy, labor, and the postpartum period.

MARFAN'S SYNDROME

Marfan's syndrome (see also Chapter 134) is a genetic disorder of connective tissue. The main clinical manifestations are abnormalities of the eye, skeletal, and cardiovascular systems (Table 36–1).[1,2]

Marfan's syndrome is probably caused by mutations in the genes for collagen, elastin, or the enzymes that process these proteins.[3,4] It is estimated that one in 10,000 Americans has this syndrome.[2] There is no difference in prevalence between races and ethnic groups, and males and females are equally affected. Marfan's syndrome is inherited as an autosomal dominant trait with a high degree of penetrance. About 25–35% of new cases are sporadic and are most likely the result of a new mutation occurring in a germ cell of one of the parents. Such mutations occur more frequently with increasing paternal age.[2]

The diagnosis of Marfan's syndrome is established on the basis of characteristic abnormalities of the skeletal, cardiovascular, and ocular systems. When Marfan's syndrome is suspected, the two most important tests for diagnosis are echocardiography of the heart and aortic root and slit-lamp examination through a dilated pupil (see Table 36–1). A family history also can be important in establishing a diagnosis. Because most of the clinical symptoms of Marfan's syndrome are age-dependent, it is often easier to diagnose the syndrome in adolescents and adults than in infants and children.[2,5]

TABLE 36–1. CLINICAL FEATURES OF MARFAN'S SYNDROME

Cardiovascular
Aortic aneurism
Mitral regurgitation
Mitral valve prolapse
Aortic regurgitation
Skeletal
Tall stature
Disproportionate body
Dolichostenomelia
Arachrondactyly
Joint hyperextensibility
High-arched palate
Anterior chest deformity
Scoliosis
Ocular
Subluxation of the lens
Myopia
Retinal detachment
Flat cornea
Central Nervous System
Sacral meningocele
Dilated cisterna magna
Dural ectasia
Pulmonary
Spontaneous pneumonthorax

Genetic Counseling

Women affected by Marfan's syndrome have a 50% risk that any offspring (male or female) will inherit the syndrome. When a child is diagnosed with Marfan's syndrome, maternal and paternal families must be studied before assurances can be given that future risk to offspring approaches the lower mutation rate.[1]

Maternal Complications

Marfan patients without cardiovascular involvement and without ocular and skeletal manifestations face no contraindication to conception.

The natural history of Marfan's syndrome and the adverse effects of hemodynamic stresses of pregnancy on the aorta dictate an interdisciplinary approach to the pregnant woman with Marfan's syndrome. Because cardiovascular problems tend to progress during adulthood, women should be encouraged to conceive as early as possible.[3] *Dissecting aneurism* of the aorta is the most serious and life-threatening complication of this disease (see also Chapter 134).

The risk of death is low for pregnant women with Marfan's syndrome who have only minimal cardiovascular disease. Women with aortic dilatation of more than 40 mm, aortic regurgitation, or significant mitral valve dysfunction are, however, at high risk for death, during and shortly after pregnancy. Pregnancy in these females is therefore generally considered contraindicated and termination of inadvertently occurring pregnancy is recommended. Pregnant women with Marfan's syndrome should have serial echocardiography every 4–8 weeks in order to detect early changes in aortic root dilatation.[2,7,8]

Eighteen percent of all aortic dissections in women with Marfan's syndrome are associated with pregnancy.[9] Dissecting aneurism of the aorta may occur at any time during pregnancy, labor, and the early puerperium, but the majority of dissections have been reported during the third trimester. The earliest symptoms and signs of this potentially fatal complication are chest or back pain, hypotension, and fetal distress.[8,10,11] Computed tomography (CT), magnetic resonance imaging (MRI), and arteriography are effective modalities for making the diagnosis of aortic aneurism.[2] Modern diagnosis, preoperative antihypertensive drug therapy, and cardiovascular surgery (see also Chapter 136) have reduced the almost 50% mortality rate reported in 1944[12] for dissecting aortic aneurism during pregnancy.[8,13]

Cesarean section delivery should be reserved for patients with suspicion of impending aortic dissection or for obstetric indications. Otherwise, vaginal delivery is the preferred route. Epidural anesthesia and hemodynamic monitoring (including Swan–Ganz catheter) is recommended for all cesarean sections and for potentially complicated pregnancies.[8] Cardiac output and stroke volume increases similarly with epidural and general anesthesia.[14] However, with epidural anesthesia, afterload reduction prevents the sharp rise in blood pressure during intubation, which can be hazardous to patients with Marfan's syndrome.

Fetal Complications

The rate of spontaneous abortion and of low birth-weight infants appears to be higher in Marfan patients. However, both of these rates do not grossly exceed expectation.[7] One intrapartum death of an infant with recognizable cardiac defects of Marfan's syndrome has been reported.[15] Fetal distress may be caused by the hypotension resulting from dissection of an aortic aneurism.

OSTEOGENESIS IMPERFECTA

Osteogenesis imperfecta is an inherited heterogenous disorder of connective tissue. Susceptibility of affected individuals to bone fractures is the most significant clinical feature. Blue sclerae, dentinogenesis imperfecta, hearing loss, growth retardation, easy bruising, and cardiopulmonary and other skeletal abnormalities are other manifestations of this syndrome. Table 36–2 depicts the clinical and genetic classification of osteogenesis imperfecta.[16,17]

The incidence for osteogenesis imperfecta identifiable at birth is one in 20,000–30,000 individuals, and there is no preferential distribution by gender, race, or ethnic group.[17]

Molecular defects in the synthesis or structure of type I collagen or its precursor type I procollagen are the hallmark of this disease. Defective pro-α-chain of type I procollagen prevents the procollagen molecule from folding into a stable triple helix.[3] Deletion of some bases in the allele for the pro-α-chain 1 (I) gene or even a single-base mutation that substitutes cysteine or argenin for glycine[18], may disrupt the conformation of the protein and produce a lethal phenotype.

Genetic Counseling

The risk of any offspring from an individual with progressive deforming osteogenesis imperfecta (with an unaffected spouse) is 50% because of the dominant inheritance of the condition. Parents of a child with the lethal form of osteogenesis imperfecta generally have a recurrence risk of only 5%–7%, because most lethal osteogenesis imperfecta appears from new mutations. Parents of a child with progressive osteogenesis imperfecta and no family history of the disease should be counseled that the recurrence risk for them may be 5–25%.[17]

Prenatal Diagnosis

Prenatal diagnosis is based on molecular biology techniques. Prenatal diagnosis of osteogenesis imperfecta by Southern blot analysis of DNA extracted from chorionic villus sampling (CVS)[19] or by collagen studies using cultured cells from CVS[17], have been reported recently.

Prenatal ultrasonographic diagnosis depends on the type of osteogenesis imperfecta (see Table 36–2).[20,21] Types I and III have been diagnosed before 20 weeks' gestation. Shortened long bones of the lower extremities and fractures are ultrasonic findings compatible with these types of osteogenesis imperfecta. However, even several sonographic scans can fail to diagnose the syndrome with certainty.

The sonographic finding of type II osteogenesis imperfecta usually involves long bones, skull, ribs, and spine and also can be diagnosed before 20 weeks' gestation. Long bones, mainly the femur, may show fractures, shortening, and bowing. The skull may be thinner than usual, and the weight of the ultrasound probe may deform the head quite easily. Fetal movements often are decreased.[20]

Maternal Complications and Obstetric Management

Pregnancy has been reported in dwarfed and severely deformed women as a result of osteogenesis imperfecta.[22-24] Pregnancy has no adverse effects on the disease; however, pregnancy may decrease the degree of ambulatory mobility and cause bone pain and dental problems.

Delivery by cesarean section is the method of choice for most of these patients because of the increased risk of cephalopelvic disproportion, pelvic fractures, uterine rupture, and intrapartum or postpartum hemorrhage. Because of the associated kyphoscoliosis, there may be technical difficulties in inserting an epidural catheter. Nevertheless

TABLE 36–2. CLASSIFICATION OF OSTEOGENESIS IMPERFECTA

Type	Clinical Manifestations	Inheritance
I (Dominant with blue sclerae)	Bone fragility, blue sclerae, hearing impairment IA: Normal teeth IB: Dentinogenesis imperfecta	Autosomal dominant
II (Lethal perinatal)	Extreme bone fragility, blue sclerae, perinatal death	Autosomal recessive or new dominant mutation
III (Progessive deforming)	Bone fragility, growth retardation, progressive skeletal deformity, dentinogenesis imperfecta, normal sclerae	Autosomal recessive
IV (Dominant with normal sclerae)	Bone fragility, growth retardation, skeletal deformity, normal sclerae IVA: Normal teeth IVB: Dentinogenesis imperfecta	Autosomal dominant

epidural anesthesia is preferred, whenever possible, for cesarean section.[25] The skeletal deformities may cause difficulty with intubation and adversely affect pulmonary function. In addition, a mild hyperthermia, with features similar to those of patients with malignant hyperphyrexia, may occur with general anesthesia.

Fetal Complications

Type II osteogenesis imperfecta is lethal. Infants are stillborn or die shortly after birth. The option of pregnancy termination can be offered whenever a type II osteogenesis imperfecta is diagnosed.[20]

Types I and III are compatible with life, but affected individuals may suffer significant handicaps. Type IV has the best prognosis because fractures and deformities are uncommon. Early prenatal diagnosis permits couples to make a choice concerning termination of pregnancy. After viability, plans can be made for delivery by cesarean section to optimize the infant's chances of survival.[17] The risks of vaginal delivery include intracranial hemorrhage, evulsion of fragile body parts, and fractures of the thoracic cage and long bones.

EHLERS–DANLOS SYNDROME

Ehlers–Danlos syndrome is characterized by hyperextensibility of skin and joints, fragile tissue, and poor wound healing. Severe complications, such as spontaneous arterial or intestinal rupture, may occur rarely. At least 10 distinct variants can be recognized on the basis of clinical, genetic, and biochemical factors (Table 36–3).[3,26-34] Some forms are produced by mutations in genes for type I or type III procollagens, but others are produced by defects in enzymes required for the assembly or processing of the procollagens.[3] The estimated incidence of Ehlers–Danlos syndrome is one in 150,000 individuals. Males and females are equally affected, except for types V and IX, the X-linked forms, in which only males are affected.

Pregnancy in patients with Ehlers–Danlos syndrome carries risks for the mother and the child. Obstetric complications depend mainly on the type of Ehlers–Danlos syndrome, and patients with milder degrees of tissue laxity do not always have fewer complications.

Maternal Complications

Patients with Ehlers–Danlos syndrome who become pregnant can expect their symptoms to worsen during pregnancy. Complications in pregnancy include marked increase in joint laxity, back pain, abdominal hernias, increased bruising, varicose veins, symphysiolysis, antepartum and postpartum hemorrhage, tissue fragility making episiotomy repair and cesarean closure difficult, slow healing of perineal wounds, uterine prolapse, and maternal death from ruptures of the uterus, aorta, vena cava, and sigmoid colon.[26]

Recent reports of pregnancy with Ehlers–Danlos syndrome clearly correlate clinical course and prognosis with the type of Ehlers–Danlos syndrome.[27-33] Although many women with type I have no problems, the obstetrician should be prepared for major complications associated with tissue laxity and hemorrhage from extensive vaginal laceration. No maternal deaths have been reported with type I, and only patients with a severe form of this syndrome should be advised against pregnancy.[29]

Patients with Ehlers–Danlos syndrome type IV should be counseled against pregnancy because the risk of lethal complications appears to be augmented by pregnancy, and the maternal mortality rate for women with type IV is calculated to be 25% per pregnancy.[28] For women who become pregnant and decline termination of the pregnancy, extremely close observations for bowel and arterial rupture must be maintained. The periods of greatest risk appear to be during labor and the postpartum period.

Types II[32] and X[27] have minimal morbidity during pregnancy, and type III[33] may at times require early delivery by cesarean section to relieve symptoms.

The mode of delivery should be tailored to the individual patient. Except for type IV, vaginal delivery can be accomplished when appropriate. Common problems encountered during surgery on Ehlers–Danlos syndrome patients are hemorrhage, poor wound healing, and wound dehiscence. Using nonabsorbable or retention sutures and ligation of bleeding vessels with hemoclips may overcome some of these problems when performing cesarean sections.[30]

TABLE 36–3. CLASSIFICATION OF EHLERS–DANLOS SYNDROME

Type	Percent of Ehlers-Danlos Syndrome	Clinical Manifestations	Inheritance	Bichemical Defect
I (Gravis)	30–50	Varicose veins, musculoskeletal deformities, prematurity	Autosomal dominant	Unknown
II (Mitis)	30	Milder variation of the gravis type	Autosomal dominant	Unknown
III (Benign hypermobile)	10–30	Dislocations, arthritis, mitral valve prolapse	Autosomal dominant	Unknown
IV (Arterial)	<10	Easy bruisability, rupture of hollow viscera	Autosomal dominant or recessive	Type III procollagen defect
V (X-linked)	Rare	Joint hypermobility, hyperextensible skin	X-Linked recessive	Lysyl oxidase deficiency
VI (Ocular)	Rare	Glaucoma, retinal detachment, corneal and scleral fragility	Autosomal recessive	Lysyl hydroxylase deficiency
VII (Arthrochalasia multiplex congenita)	Rare	Joint hypermobility	Autosomal dominant or recessive	Procollagen peptidase deficiency
VIII (Periodontal)	Rare	Progressive periodontal disease	Autosomal dominant	Unknown
IX (X-linked skeletal)	Rare	Obstructive uropathy	X-linked recessive	Abnormal copper metabolism
X (Dysfibronectemic)	Rare	Hemostatic defect	Autosomal recessive	Fibronectin

Fetal Complications

Infants with Ehlers–Danlos syndrome have a high incidence (35–78%) of premature delivery and low birth weight. This has been attributed to a defect in the connective tissue of the fetal membranes.[26,34] Difficulties in ligature of the umbilical cord may be encountered because of its friability.[30]

PSEUDOXANTHOMA ELASTICUM

Pseudoxanthoma elasticum is a familial disorder characterized by degeneration of elastic tissue. Clinical expression of pseudoxanthoma elasticum is found mainly in the skin, the eye, and the cardiovascular system. The changes in the skin often are not clinically recognizable before the second decade of life. The skin in involved areas becomes lax, redundant, relatively inelastic, and may demonstrate yellowish plaques resembling xanthomata. Similar changes may affect the buccal, rectal, and vaginal mucosae. The characteristic changes in the eye consist of angioid streaking of the fundus, which are breaks in Bruch's internal elastic membrane beneath the retina, appearing as reddish-brown striae radiating from the optic disk. Cardiovascular manifestations include coronary insufficiency, hypertension, premature calcification of vessels, weakness or absence of pulses in the extremities, upper gastrointestinal tract hemorrhage, and severe uterine bleeding. The prevalance of pseudoxanthoma elasticum is one in 70,000 to one in 160,000 individuals. There are two autosomal dominant and two autosomal recessive types; the latter is more common.[35]

Maternal Complications

Eighty-three pregnancies in 31 women with pseudoxanthoma elasticum have been described.[35-38] Pregnancy may aggravate the vascular effect of pseudoxanthoma elasticum. Bleeding may be a chief complication during pregnancy, such as gastrointestinal bleeding with massive hematemesis (in nine of the pregnancies)[35,36], presenting with microscopic hematuria[37] or with epistaxis.[35]

In the largest single study of obstetric implications of pseudoxanthoma elasticum[38], hypertension occurred in seven of 20 pregnant women. Three women were treated only with bed rest and the other four with antihypertensive drugs.

The eyes and other organ systems involved in pseudoxanthoma elasticum usually are unaffected by pregnancy.[38] Abdominal striae developed in all patients, but the severity correlated primarily with weight gain and parity. Vaginal delivery is usually unremarkable.

Fetal Complications

Maternal vascular compromise may be the cause for the 26% first-trimester miscarriage rate reported with pseudoxanthoma elasticum.[38] Intrauterine growth retardation also may be associated with pseudoxanthoma elasticum.[37]

REFERENCES

1. Pyeritz RE, McKusick VA. The Marfan's Syndrome: diagnosis and management. *N Engl J Med.* 1979;300:772.
2. Pyeritz RE. The Marfan's Syndrome. *Am Family Physician.* 1986;34:83.
3. Prockop DJ, Kivirikko KI. Heritable diseases of collagen. *N Engl J Med.* 1984;311:376.
4. Pyeritz RE, McKusick VA. Basic defects in the Marfan's Syndrome. *N Engl J Med.* 1981;305:1011.
5. Sisk HE, Zahka KG, Pyeritz RE. The Marfan's Syndrome in early childhood: Analysis of 15 patients diagnosed at less than 4 years of age. *Am J Cardiol.* 1983;52:353.
6. Gott VL, Pyeritz RE, Magovern GJ, et al. Surgical treatment of aneurysms of the ascending aorta in the Marfan's Syndrome: Results of composite-graft repair in 50 patients. *N Engl J Med.* 1986;314:1070.
7. Pyeritz RE. Maternal and fetal complications of pregnancy in the Marfan's Syndrome. *Am J Med.* 1981;71:784.
8. Mor-Yosef S, Younis J, Granat M, et al. Marfan's Syndrome in pregnancy. *Obstet Gynecol Surv.* 1988;43:382.
9. Douglas PS. Rheumatic heart disease and other valvular disorders in women. In: Douglas PS, ed. *Heart Disease in Women.* Philadelphia, PA: FA Davis; 1989:259.
10. Ferguson JE, Ueland K, Stinson EB, Maly RP. Marfan's syndrome: Acute aortic dissection during labor, resulting in fetal distress and cesarean section, followed by successful surgical repair. *Am J Obstet Gynecol.* 1983;147:759.
11. Rosenblum NG, Grossman AR, Gabbe SG, et al. Failure of serial echocardiographic studies to predict aortic dissection in a pregnant patient with Marfan's syndrome. *Am J Obstet Gynecol.* 1983;146:470.
12. Schnitker MA, Bayer CA. Dissecting aneurysm of the aorta in young individuals, particularly in association with pregnancy. *Ann Intern Med.* 1944;20:486.
13. Cola LM, Lavin JP. Pregnancy complicated by Marfan's Syndrome with aortic arch dissection, subsequent aortic arch replacement and triple coronary artery bypass grafts. *J Reprod Med.* 1985;30:685.
14. James CF, Banner T, Caton D. Cardiac output in women undergoing cesarean section with epidural or general anesthesia. *Am J Obstet Gynecol.* 1989;160:1178.
15. Buchanan R, Wyatt GP. Marfan's syndrome presenting as an intrapartum death. *Arch Dis Child.* 1985;60:1074.
16. Sillence DO, Senn A, Danks DM. Genetic hetrogeneity in osteogenesis imperfecta. *J Med Genet.* 1979;16:101.
17. Marini JC. Osteogenesis imperfecta: comprehensive management. *Adv Pediatr.* 1988;35:391.
18. Constantinou CD, Nielsen KB, Prockop DJ. A lethal variant of osteogenesis imperfecta has a single base mutation that substitutes cysteine for glycine 904 of the α1(1) chain of type I procollagen. *J Clin Invest.* 1989;83:574.
19. Tsipouras P, Schwartz RC, Goldberg JD, et al. Prenatal prediction of osteogenesis imperfecta (OI type IV): exclusion of inheritance using a collagen gene probe. *J Med Genet.* 1987;24:406.
20. Romero R, Pilu G, Jeanty P, et al. Osteogenesis imperfecta. In: Romero R, et al, eds. *Prenatal Diagnosis of Congenital Anomalies.* East Norwalk, CT: Appleton & Lange; 1988;354.
21. Brons JTJ, van der Harten HJ, Wladimiroff JW, et al. Prenatal ultrasonographic diagnosis of osteogenesis imperfecta. *Am J Obstet Gynecol.* 1988;159:176.
22. Roberts JM, Solomons CC. Management of pregnancy in osteogenesis imperfecta: new perspectives. *Obstet Gynecol.* 1975;45:168.
23. Key TC, Horger ED. Osteogenesis imperfecta as a complication of pregnancy. *Obstet Gynecol.* 1978;51:67.
24. Young BK, Gorstein F. Maternal osteogenesis imperfecta. *Obstet Gynecol.* 1968;31:461.
25. Cunningham AJ, Donnelly M, Comerford J. Osteogenesis imperfecta: anesthetic management of a patient for cesarean section: A case report. *Anesthesiology.* 1984;61:91.
26. Taylor DJ, Wilcox I, Russell JK. Ehlers-Danlos Syndrome during pregnancy: A case report and review of the literature. *Obstet Gynecol Surv.* 1981;36:277.
27. Hammerschmidt DE, Arneson MA, Larson SL, et al. Maternal Ehlers-Danlos Syndrome Type X—Successful management of pregnancy and parturition. *JAMA.* 1982;248:2487.
28. Rudd NL, Holbrook KA, Nimrod C, Byers PH. Pregnancy complications in TYPE IV Ehlers-Danlos Syndrome. *Lancet.* 1983;i:50.
29. Snyder RR, Gilstrap LC, Hauth JC. Ehlers-Danlos Syndrome and pregnancy. *Obstet Gynecol.* 1983;61:649.
30. Rivera-Alsina ME, Kwan P, Zavisca FG, et al. Complications of the Ehlers-Danlos Syndrome in pregnancy. A case report. *J Reprod Med.* 1984;29:757.
31. Kiilholma P, Gronroos M, Nanto V, Paul R. Pregnancy and delivery in Ehlers-Danlos Syndrome, role of copper and zinc. *Acta Obstet Gynecol Scand.* 1984;63:437.
32. Peaceman AM, Cruikshank DP. Ehlers-Danlos Syndrome and pregnancy: association of type IV disease with maternal death. *Obstet Gynecol.* 1987;69:428.
33. Atalla A, Page I. Ehlers-Danlos Syndrome type III in pregnancy. *Obstet Gynecol.* 1988;71:508.
34. Barabas AP. Ehlers-Danlos Syndrome: Associated with prematurity and premature rupture of foetal membranes. Possible increase in incidence. *Br Med J.* 1968;2:682.
35. Berde C, Willis DC, Sandberg EC. Pregnancy in women with pseudoxanthoma elasticum. *Obstet Gynecol Surv.* 1983;38:339.
36. Lao TT, Walters BNJ, DeSwiet M. Pseudoxanthoma elasticum and pregnancy. Two case reports. *Br J Obstet Gynaecol.* 1984;91:1049.
37. Broekhuizen FF, Hamilton PR. Pseudoxanthoma elasticum and intrauterine growth retardation. *Am J Obstet Gynecol.* 1984;148:112.
38. Viljoen DL, Beatty S, Beighton P. The obstetric and gynaecological implications of pseudoxanthoma elasticum. *Br J Obstet Gynaecol.* 1987;94:884.

PART VI | Hormonal Diseases

Norbert Gleicher, Section Editor

Chapter Thirty-Seven

Endocrinology

Moshe E. Zilberstein and Norbert Gleicher

37

The primary function of the female reproductive system is achievement of conception and maintenance of pregnancy until delivery of the newborn. At the primordial steps, the communication between the developing embryo and the mother depends on direct physical contact, probably using autocrine and paracrine mechanisms. The system later develops into an intricate complexity of *local* communications between amniotic fluid, amnion, chorion laeve, decidua vera, myometrium, and *systemic* communications, which result in the placenta passively or actively interexchanging nutrients and biochemical signals between maternal and fetal circulations.[1] The initial codes for embryonal development reside within the genetic information and are conferred on the embryo by both parents.[2] The genetic embryonic apparatus must rely on the presupposition that the site of ideal conception is ready for its arrival. Rather than being an indifferent bystander of pregnancy, it has recently been revealed that the embryo–fetus is an important active driving force along gestation. The conceptus appears to influence significantly its own navigation through the tube and its intrauterine attachment, implantation, maintenance, immunoprotection, communication, nutrient and hormone transfer, initiation of labor, and parturition.

This chapter describes the endocrinologic processes involved in securing the reproductive steps, with special emphasis on the clinical and pathologic significance of aberrations in those processes. Because of the very broad topic, the chapter primarily concentrates on information that is pertinent to humans.

THE PLACENTA

This unique organ, which only evolves during pregnancy and whose life span is limited to pregnancy, deserves special attention. The placenta is the site of nutrient transfer and metabolite exchange between the mother and fetus. The human placenta elaborates an assortment of proteins, peptides, growth factors, cytokines, and steroidal hormones and is the largest endocrine gland in the human. Trophoblast cells are the origin of the copious synthetic activity. Because of this phenomenal output, the placenta is considered by many to be a separate compartment from that of the mother and her fetus.

Most of the hormones that are produced in the placenta are synthesized in the syncytiotrophoblast. These multinucleated syncytial formations are the products of fusion of mononucleated cytotrophoblast cells.[3,4] It has been proposed that cytotrophoblast cells produce releasing hormones, such as gonadotropin-releasing hormone (GnRH) and corticotropin-releasing factor (CRF), somatostatin, but also inhibin and activin. However, they synthesize only miniscule amounts of the classic trophoblast hormones. The fusion of cytotrophoblast cells demarcates the differentiation of the cells into the characteristic mature syncytiotrophoblasts. Cell division ceases, and the syncytial trophoblasts, which are equipped with a well-developed rough endoplasmic reticulum and golgi apparatus, exhibit a typically accelerated synthetic activity.[4,5] During pregnancy, the placenta produces striking amounts of steroids, human chorionic gonadotropin (hCG), human placental lactogen (hPL), adrenocorticotrophic hormone (ACTH), pro-opiomelanocortin, human chorionic thyrotropin (hCT), thyrotropin-releasing hormone (TRH), gonadotropin-releasing hormone (GnRH), corticotropin-releasing factor (CRF), somatostatin, inhibin, renin, angiotensinogen, angiotensin II, and placental proteins. Hence, two differentiation patterns can be recognized in the trophoblast: *morphologic* and *biochemical*. These two processes can be dissociated *in vitro*. HCG subunits and hPL can be detected by immunocytochemistry in mononucleated and syncytial cells.[6] It also appears that the formation of syncytium is not a prerequisite for hCG gene expression. For example, cyclic AMP has been shown to stimulate hCG and steroid production by cultured cytotrophoblast[7-10] (Fig. 37–1).

During the first trimester, the placenta undergoes rapid growth based on the multiplication of cytotrophoblast cells. Columns of cytotrophoblast cells invade the placentation site. The cytotrophoblast cells mature and terminally differentiate into syncytiotrophoblasts.

In the second and third trimesters, the relative portion of the syncytium in the placenta increases dramatically, and concomitantly, the growth of the placenta subsides. Only recently has it been possible to begin the elucidation of the mechanisms that control cytotrophoblast cell replication. Autocrine and paracrine agents have been implicated as regulators of cytotrophoblast replication. Several growth factors are produced in the placenta. Placental tissue also

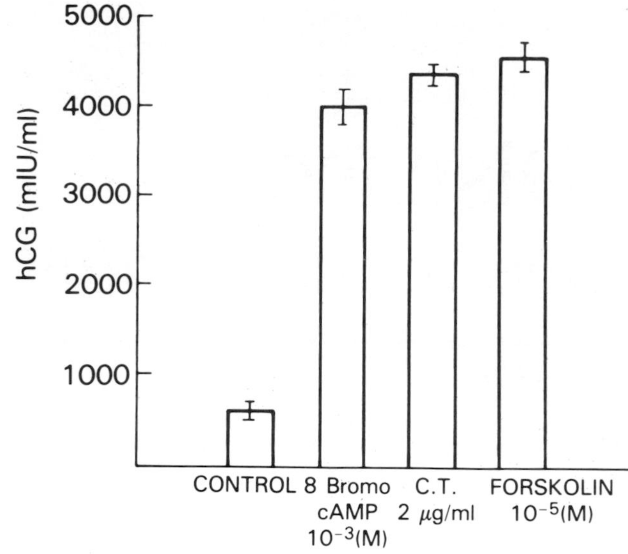

Figure 37–1. Stimulation of hCG production by 8-bromo-cAMP, cholera toxin (CT) and forskolin in human term placental cytotrophoblasts in culture. (*Zilberstein M, Das C, Catt KJ, unpublished data*).

is endowed with specific receptors for the growth factors, insulin, insulin-like growth factor (IGF), and epidermal growth factor (EGF). It also produces a host of oncogene products.[11] The IGFs, specifically IGF-II[12] act in an autocrine fashion. IGF-I also has a possible paracrine action.[13] It also has been suggested that platelet-derived growth factor (PDGF) induces DNA synthesis mediated by c-myc oncogen expression in cells of placental origin.[14,15]

Most of the proto-oncogen proteins that have been discovered also are present in the placenta. In fact, the placenta and placental c-DNA libraries are a plentiful source for the isolation of oncogenes, growth factor genes, hormones, and proteins. Several proto-oncogene protein products are highly expressed in the placenta and in the extra embryonic tissues. These include c-erb-B, c-erb-A, c-fms, c-fos, c-myc, c-sis, and c-ras. All have been suggested to have a role in placental growth and development. The proto-oncogen product of c-erb-B is similar to the EGF receptor, and c-fms is homologous to the CSF-1 receptor. Therefore, a potential role in placental cellular growth for these products can be envisioned. It has been demonstrated that trophoblast cells are capable of producing c-sis, which is a platelet-derived growth factor (PDGF)-like protein that can interact in an autocrine manner with the authentic PDGF receptors on the trophoblast cell membrane. None of the proto-oncogenes appear to be placental-specific, and extensive research is underway to elucidate their potential role in placental ontogeny and embryogenesis. This topic is extensively reviewed elsewhere.[11]

Although growth factors are primarily known for their mitogenic activities, they also appear to influence hormone formation, cellular division, and growth in the placenta. Hence, growth factors in the placenta demonstrate possible differentiating properties. In different systems, EGF was shown to increase hCG and hPL production or to have no effect on the secretion of these hormones. The receptors for EGF were shown to be expressed mainly in the syncytiotrophoblast. EGF was thus suggested to be mainly involved in trophoblast differentiation.[16,17] Among the IGFs, mRNA for IGF-I and IGF-II have been demonstrated in the trophoblast.[7,18-20] Moreover, IGF-II is preferentially expressed in relative abundance in trophoblast cells.[20,21]

EARLY MATERNAL–FETAL DIALOGUE

The corpus luteum develops subsequent to ovulation from the dominant follicle and secretes steroid hormones and, possibly, other peptide hormones. Progesterone is the steroid product that is intended for the maintenance of pregnancy during the periimplantation period.[22] In most mammals, a normal functioning corpus luteum requires the trophic support of luteinizing hormone (LH). In humans, the production of progesterone coincides with LH secretion during the luteal phase of the cycle.[23,24] Aberrations in corpus luteum function have been implicated in conception failures and early abortions.[25] A crucial event and a prerequisite for the resumption of a new cycle is luteolysis in a nonfertile cycle.[26] The mechanisms that bring about the regression of the corpus luteum in primates are widely unknown. When implantation occurs, the pivotal early requirement is the rescue of the corpus luteum.

The implanted embryo is responsible for signaling the mother and notifying its presence in the uterus. These embryonal messages lead to the extension of the life span and activity of the corpus luteum. In humans, it has been shown unequivocally that hCG, which is produced by the trophoblast and secreted into the maternal circulation at the time of expected corpus luteum demise, mediates the rescue of the corpus luteum.[27,28] Recently, it also has been suggested that two other ovarian peptides may be involved in the maintenance of early pregnancy; these peptides are relaxin and prorenin. Their role is discussed later in this chapter.

In order to achieve a successful pregnancy that will subsequently yield an adequately developed newborn, both mother and fetus collaborate and invest intensively in establishing a maternal-fetal communication system. For an effective maternal-fetal dialogue, the bidirectional signals should reach their targets in a timely fashion and at the exact magnitude. The receptive organ should be endowed with the capabilities to receive, decipher, and react to those messages. This precisely orchestrated system evolves and functions within a predetermined and relatively short timetable. The eventual success of the pregnancy attests to one of the most complex and amazing achievements of evolutionary processes. Growing evidence suggests that maternal-fetal communication is established shortly after fertilization in the fallopian tubes.[28,29] A flow of events directs the zygote to the optimal site of implantation in the uterus. However, little is known about the precise nature of that primordial communication system that seems to exist in the prenidatory period.

A possible paracrine influence was attributed to the corona radiate cells, which stay attached and may accompany the oocyte for up to 48 hours after ovulation. These cells are capable of hormone production (estrogen, progesterone, and prostaglandins)[30,31], which may transduce signals to the fertilized oocyte or to maternal organs (uterus and tubes). Moreover, recent information also suggests that polypeptide hormones (hCG-like)[32] and steroids[30,33,34] may be the products of the fertilized oocyte or the cleaving embryo. It is not clear whether the prenidatory embryo is capable of producing these chemicals, but these hormones and growth factors, if produced, might be responsible for the local events necessary for implantation. Peptide hormones, steroids, growth factors, and *pregnancy proteins* produced by the blastocysts can be envisioned as mediators of a maternal endometrial *acceptance reaction*. Maternal reaction involves vasodilation, angiogenesis, increased local blood flow, immunologic protection, enhanced metabolic and nutrient transfer, and rescue of the corpus luteum.

IMPLANTATION

The common site of fertilization is the fallopian tube. The zygote, which is the product of fertilization, undergoes cleavage into totipotential cells called *blastomers*. For 72 hours, the zygote resides in the tube, slowly dividing into a strawberry-shaped *morula*, which can be recovered from the uterine lumen at the 12–16 cell stage. Just before implantation, the morula hatches out of the zona pellucida and begins to organize into a *blastocyst*. Fluid accumulates within the conceptus. The inner cell mass at one pole is the progenitor of the embryo, and the outer cell mass will become the trophoblast. The blastocyst attaches to the endometrium in the uterus and erodes its way through the epithelium to become totally embedded within the endometrium. The mechanisms for this extraordinary tumorlike behavior of the conceptus are yet unclear. The trophoblast cells are the outermost areas of the conceptus, which actively invade the endometrium, are multinucleated syncytial formations called the *syncytiotrophoblast*. These unique cells do not divide and on immunohistochemical staining, it appears that they are the endocrinologically active compartment of the trophoblast by producing *in vivo* hCG, hPL, and steroid hormones. From *in vitro* and *in vivo* studies, there is evidence that the innermost cell layer of the trophoblast is composed of the *cytotrophoblast*. These are mononucleated and mitotically active cells that fuse to differentiate into the syncytiotrophoblast. This differentiation process depends on local regulation, probably mediated by growth factors and cAMP.[7,10] (See also Fig. 37–1.)

Implantation of the human blastocyst takes place 6 days after fertilization. Proper differentiation of trophoblast cells leads to the local production of facilitating factors, which are proteases that play a crucial role in the successful implantation. The later formation of the mature placenta in the human is referred to as *hemochorioendothelial* because the trophoblast is in direct contact with maternal blood but separated from fetal blood by the walls of capillaries. The early trophoblast is comprised of relatively large amounts of cytotrophoblast cells, but near term, the cytotrophoblast component of the trophoblast is neglgible.

Decidualization

Decidualization involves the proliferation and differentiation of endometrial stromal cells. The initial macroscopically identifiable signs of implantation involve demarcated areas adjacent to the implantation site of the blastocyst, where an increase in endometrial vascular permeability precedes cellular differentiation. This localized phenomenon suggests the local production of chemicals, which may be separated into vascular response and cellular decidual reaction. The fact that implantation also can occur in ectopic locations suggests that the role of the decidua is limited in comparison to aggressive and self-propelled events led by the zygote.

Histamine was first proposed as the prime inducer of decidualization by Shelesnyak.[35] It was suggested that mast cells produce histamine in response to a certain degree of tissue damage. Evidence for the existence of these mechanisms is derived mainly from studies in rodents and from pseudodecidualization models.[36] Indeed, the rodent blastocysts are capable of histamine production[33,34,37,38], and the administration of histidine decarboxylase inhibitor into the rabbit's uterine cavity interrupts implantation. Furthermore, rodent blastocysts and endometriums contain H_2 and H_1 receptors.[39] Conflicting data about H_1 and H_2 antagonist actions exist, however. Moreover, a third type of receptor, H_3, which has been linked to the control of blood circulation, also may have a role in implantation.[40]

Evidence suggests interaction between histamine and prostaglandins within the uterus that reverses the antiprostaglandin effect of drugs. The relevance of histamine for events taking place during human implantation, however, is not clear.

Prostaglandins and Leukotrienes

Prostaglandins (PG) are known to mediate vascular permeability and convincing evidence exists for a crucial role that they may play in affecting decidual changes in many species. Indomethacin, which is a well-characterized prostaglandin biosynthesis inhibitor, inhibits local vascular events and delays decidualization as well as implantation in rodents.[41,41] Endometrium and the blastocyst may be the source of prostaglandins. Areas of increased permeability contain higher levels of prostaglandins. In species in which decidualization can be induced artificially, augmentation of prostaglandin biosynthesis precedes these changes.[42,43] It is less obvious which prostaglandins are involved in the decidual, cellular, and vascular reactions. The biosynthesis of prostaglandins of the E, F, and I series was stimulated locally at the site of implantation. PGE_2 and $PGF_{2\alpha}$ have been shown to produce an adequate decidual manifestation in indomethacin-pretreated rats. The same effect can be achieved with 6-OXO-PGE_1 but not with PGI_2. In general, PGE_2 is equipotent to $PGF_{2\alpha}$ in producing decidualization in the rat.[44,45] However, in light of reported evidence that PGE_2, but not $PGF_{2\alpha}$, receptors exist in the endometrium, the physiologic role of $PGF_{2\alpha}$ is less clear.[46-48] It has been therefore suggested that $PGF_{2\alpha}$ can in the endometrium be converted to PGE_2.[44] Estrogens stimulate PG production in an unexplained mechanism, possibly after conversion into catechol estrogen in the uterus.[49]

Leukotrienes have well-documented vasoactive properties. LTC_4 was shown to be produced and have specific binding sites in the human endometrium throughout the cycle.[50,51] LTC_4 also induces decidualization, an effect further augmented in the rat in cooperation with PGE_2. The use of leukotriene inhibitors (NDGA) or of a LTC_4 antagonist (FPL 55712) inhibits a decidual reaction that can be restored by LTC_4 and PGE_2.[52,53] The relevance of these experiments is limited, however, because NDGA can inhibit both pathways of lypoxygenase and of cycloxygenase.

PLACENTAL HORMONES

Polypeptide Hormones

Human Chorionic Gonadotropin. HCG was discovered after LH-like activity was recognized in the urine of pregnant women.[54] This activity was used by Aschheim and Zondek to diagnose the existence of pregnancy. HCG is a glycoprotein of molecular weight (Mr 36,700 d)[55,57] with the highest carbohydrate content among human hormones. Human hCG is composed of two nonidentical single-chained subunits, alpha (α) and beta (β), which are linked noncovalently.[55,56] The *alpha subunit* is a 92 amino acid chain, while the *beta subunit* consists of 145 amino acids. Structurally, and to a lesser extent functionally, hCG is related to other glycoprotein hormones of pituitary origin, such as LH, FSH, and TSH, which also are dimers composed from similar alpha and beta subunits. The alpha subunits of all four hormones have a similar amino acid composition and differ only in the carbohydrate elements.[55] The beta subunits are responsible for the specific biologic activities of the various glycoproteins and show significant variation in both amino acid and carbohydrate composition.[58-60] For biologic activity and for the receptor binding properties[61], an intact hCG molecule is required. The β-hCG shows the highest (80%) sequence homology with β-LH, at the first 121 amino-terminal amino acids. However, β-hCG contains 24 more amino acids at the carboxy terminus.[62] The fact that both hLH and hCG bind to the same receptor, despite the fact that hCG contains amino acid extensions at the end of the molecule, suggests that this part is unimportant for receptor binding. HCG molecules contain carbohydrate moieties that are probably important for the coupling of the hormone-receptor complex to adenylate cyclase in an undetermined mechanism. Sialic acid residues located at the terminal sugars of the oligosaccharide chains of both hCG subunits seem to confer protection against the degradation of the hCG molecule.

The alpha subunits of all four glycoprotein hormones are encoded by one gene. Its location has remained controversial.[63,64] Eight genes code for the beta subunit of hCG and of hLH. All of these genes are linked and are localized to chromosome 19 (Fig. 37–2).[65,66] Each subunit of hCG is synthesized as a prepeptide from a specific mRNA and is later processed to a mature subunit by way of cleavage of the signal peptide. mRNA for the alpha-subunit was localized to cytotrophoblast, intermediate trophoblast, and syncytial cells. mRNA for the beta-subunit is localized to intermediate cells and syncytial cells.[67,68] The alpha-subunit is synthesized in more abundance than the beta-subunit because of differences in message levels and synthesis rates.[69] The alpha- and beta-subunit ratios increase from 1:2 to 2:3 in later pregnancy. The synthesized hCG is released immediately.[70] Trophoblast cells contain few secretory granules, and hCG in the syncytiotrophoblast is not associated with secretory granules.

Regulation of hCG Production. The rate of hCG production by the placenta determines the level of the hormone in the serum because all produced peptide is instantly secreted. Placental cells and tissue in the culture seem to produce hCG in a constitutive manner. HCG subunit genes are expressed and mRNA is produced in trophoblast cells before their terminal differentiation. The relative amount of cytotrophoblast cells and intermediate cells reaches a maximum at about 12 weeks of pregnancy and gradually declines thereafter, to be terminally replaced by increasing amounts of syncytiotrophoblast cells.[4]

The rate and magnitude of hCG synthesis thus determines the serum profile in pregnancy. The metabolic clearance rate is constant and independent of serum levels. The relative amounts of syncytiotrophoblast cells and cytotrophoblast cells determines the hCG profile in gestation.[14]

HCG has been localized mainly to the syncytiotrophoblast[67,71], but it also was demonstrated in intermediate and cytotrophoblast cells. Both mRNAs for alpha and beta subunits appear before the terminal differentiation into syncytiotrophoblast. Alpha-subunit hCG gene expression can be demonstrated earlier[68], than the appearance of mRNA for beta-subunit hCG in placental cells (see Fig. 37–2). The gene expression of both subunits can be induced by cAMP analogues to appear in cytotrophoblast.[10] It has been shown that early placental preparations secrete significantly more hCG than term preparations. The gene expression of both subunits is higher in early placenta compared to term.[69]

Although traditionally the production of hCG has been attributed primarily to the syncytiotrophoblast, levels of hCG in maternal plasma demonstrate a temporal correlation with the numbers of cytotrophoblasts in the placenta. In pregnancy disorders that involve *hyperplacentosis* and after increases in cytotrophoblast cell number, there also are increased concentrations of hCG. Shortly after implantation, the rapid increase in cell number is held accountable for the rapid hCG rise.

HCG concentrations in maternal blood fluctuate during pregnancy. There are, however, no rhythmic diurnal changes in hCG production.[72] During implantation, when the trophoblast comes into direct contact with the maternal blood (8–10 days after ovulation), the intact hCG can first be detected in maternal serum. Serum levels of hCG increase thereafter and reach their highest levels (between 10,000 mIU and 100,000 mIU/mL) between 8 weeks and 12 weeks of pregnancy (Fig. 37–3). The levels then decline until they reach a nadir at 18 weeks and stay constant at about 10,000 mIU/mL for the rest of pregnancy.[73,74]

The free alpha subunit of hCG appears in maternal blood at 6 weeks, and the concentration increases constantly until 36 weeks. Levels stay at less than 10% of intact hCG.[75] Free beta subunit concentrations are nondetected or very low throughout pregnancy.

The levels of hCG in fetal blood are 3% of maternal levels and are not influenced by fetal sex. Amniotic fluid levels follow a similar gestational pattern as do fetal and maternal serum concentrations. Absolute amniotic levels are similar to those of maternal serum at the beginning of the pregnancy and then decline to about 20% of those in maternal serum. To complicate the situation further, it has been suggested that the fetal kidney is responsible for amniotic fluid levels of hCG. Because hCG is secreted in the urine as an intact molecule, it can be derived partially from the fetus. One fourth of hCG is cleared in this way, while the rest is metabolized in the kidney and liver.

A large amount of data concerning second messengers in the regulation of hCG secretion has been reported. So far, however, the complete regulation of hCG production by the placenta has not been unequivocally established. The placenta is known to produce GnRH-like material[76], and the pattern of this GnRH production coincides with fluctuations of hCG secretion into maternal serum. It also has been demonstrated that the cytotrophoblast is the element of the trophoblast that secretes GnRH.[77] GnRH in physiologic concentrations is capable of inducing hCG secretion *in vitro* when incubated with placental explants from all stages of pregnancy. Moreover, GnRH antagonists inhibit hCG production.[78,79] The placenta possesses binding sites for GnRH.[80] Taken together, these data suggest that GnRH may be a local regulator of hCG in the placenta. It is, however, not clear whether GnRH is the physiologic secretagogue for hCG. *In vivo,* low doses of GnRH fail to stimulate hCG production.[81] Moreover, GnRH levels stay constant through 23 weeks' gestation, while hCG levels decline.[82]

Reports about the effect of progesterone on hCG production are conflicting. Progesterone at physiologic pregnancy concentrations, according to some authors, actually inhibits hCG secretion *in vitro,* while others suggest that progesterone has no effect.[83] Prolactin also was suggested as a regulator of hCG synthesis because its levels parallel those of hCG in maternal serum.[84] The actual effect of PRL

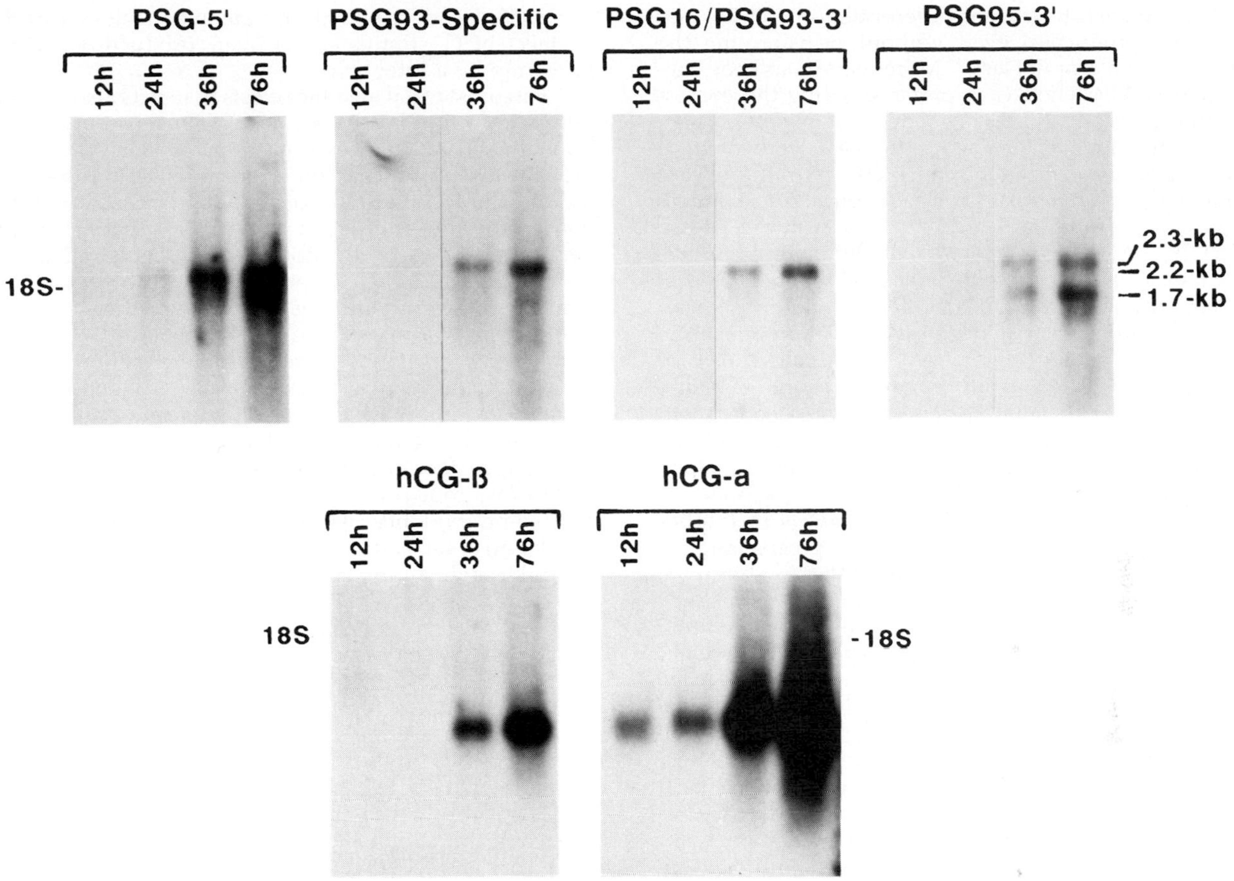

Figure 37–2. Expression of PsβG, hCGβ, and hCGα mRNAs during the differentiation of human cytotrophoblasts into syncytiotrophoblasts in culture. PSG-5′, PSG-93-Specific, PSG16/PSG93-3′, and PSG95-3′ are the probes used for PSβG. (*From Chou JY, Zilberstein M*[10] *with permission.*)

on hCG *in vivo* is still unknown. Somatostatin, androgen, and estrogen were reported to have no effect *in vitro,* while beta-adrenergic stimulation appears to augment hCG production.[85] As previously noted, EGF also has been examined as a possible regulator of hCG secretion; however, data regarding this growth factor have remained controversial. EGF stimulates hCG secretion in placental cell culture.[86,87]

From *in vitro* studies, it has been shown that under serum-supplemented conditions, mononucleated cytotrophoblast cells produce small amounts of hCG during the first 48 hours. By 72 hours, when most of the cells have formed a syncytium, a dramatic increase in this hCG production occurs.[71] While mRNA for alpha-subunit hCG is present in the cytotrophoblast, beta-subunit hCG gene expression appears only with the morphologic maturation into the syncytiotrophoblast (see Fig. 37–2).[30] Various factors can alter this pattern of hCG production. They include adenylate cyclase activators, such as cholera toxin and forskolin, beta-adrenergic drugs, and nondegradable cAMP analogues.[88,89] The action of cAMP in cytotrophoblast cells

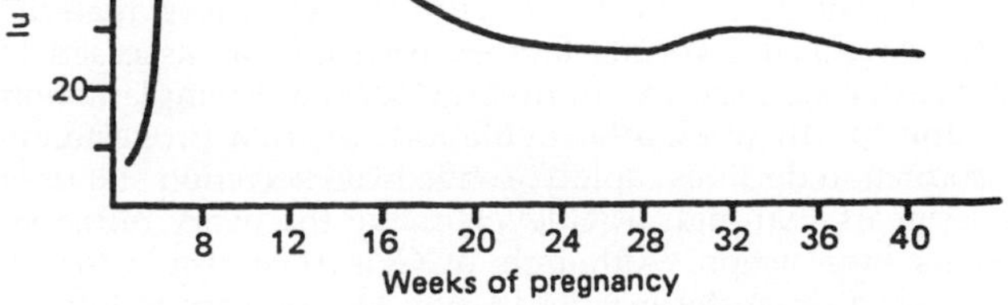

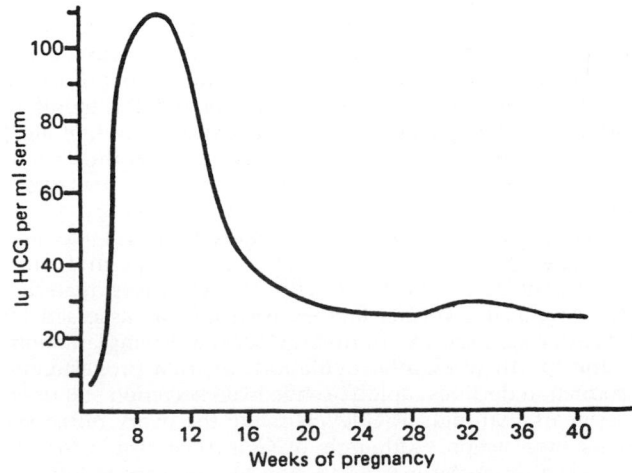

Figure 37–3. Serum hCG concentrations during the normal human pregnancy. (*From Mishell et al* [112] *with permission.*)

is to stimulate such functional differentiation as hCG and progesterone production even without transforming the cells into syncytial trophoblast.[89] Moreover, it has been suggested that cAMP action is in part regulating the expression of the subunits.[7,8,10] The level of adenylate cyclase activity is therefore a key factor in hCG production. It also has been shown that purified cytotrophoblasts are endowed with adenylate cyclase, coupled to stimulatory (Gs) and inhibitory (Gi) guanine nucleotides.[90] Presumably, cAMP acts through activation of a specific protein kinase A. The protein kinase inhibitor (H-7) prevents hCG induction by 8-bromo-cAMP and subsequent phosphorylation of several specific placental proteins. The addition of 8-bromo-cAMP to trophoblast cells causes *in vitro* an increased mRNA synthesis of alpha and beta subunit hCG.[9] The alpha-subunit gene also has been shown to contain cAMP-responsive elements (CRE), which may be involved in the induction of expression of the alpha CG gene.[8]

Several factors may regulate cAMP levels in trophoblast. They include β-adrenergic drugs, prostaglandins, high-density lipoproteins, corticotropin-releasing hormone (CRH), and hCG, as a stimulator of adenylate cyclase.[88] Other protein kinases that may be involved in the secretion of hCG include protein kinase C (PKC) and possibly calcium calmodulin kinases. However, their role in regulation awaits more investigation. Phorbol ester, which is a PKC activator, enhances hCG production in choriocarcinoma cells (JEG-3) and in normal cytotrophoblast.[87,91] Recently, a role for glucocorticoids has been suggested in the regulation of hCG production. Dexamethasone apparently stimulates the secretion of hCG production by inducing gene expression for the hCG subunits.[92] These effects can be inhibited by RU-486, which is a glucocorticoid antagonist. The dexamethazone effect probably occurs through an undetermined mechanism distinct from the cAMP pathway.[8,93] Because the alpha-subunit gene (but not the beta-subunit gene) of hCG contains a nucleotide sequence that resembles the glucocorticoid-responsive element (GRE), part of the glucocorticoid action may take place through the regulation of alpha-subunit gene expression.

Neither arachidonic acid nor diacylglycerol (DAG) affect the basal release of hCG. However, arachidonic acid potentiates EGF-stimulated hCG production in placental lines.[87]

Biologic Activity of hCG. The primary function of hCG is stimulation of steroidogenesis in responsive tissues. This effect of hCG has been best studied in reference to the regulation of steroidogenesis in the maternal ovaries. The luteotropic effect of hCG is well characterized. It is therefore widely accepted that hCG acts to rescue the corpus luteum.[94] An ovarian function in support of gestation is thus maintained until placental progesterone production is well established.

HCG directly stimulates the corpus luteum *in vivo*, and stimulates the secretion of progestins, androgens, and estrogens by the corpus luteum *in vitro*.[94-97] However, maternal hCG levels and corpus luteum function, as assessed by progesterone production, diverge soon after implantation. In the fourth week after ovulation, ovarian progesterone production declines rapidly, while hCG secretion still rises. It appears that high hCG levels make the ovary refractory to its own action. Although hCG is responsible for the excessive progesterone production by the corpus luteum, it is unlikely that it also directly prolongs the life span of the corpus luteum.

HCG is not a potent antiluteolytic factor in humans. In fact, hCG stimulates estrogen production, which is known to be a luteolytic agent.

Circumstantial evidence exists that hCG also modulates relaxin secretion by the ovaries.[98] The gestational production of both substances occurs in parallel. Thus, relaxin together with progesterone exert an effect on the maintenance of uterine quiescence. HCG also was shown to enhance prolactin production by decidua *in vitro*.[99] As in the ovary, hCG has been implicated in regulating placental steroidogenesis. These reports have, however, so far remained conflicting, and it is not clear whether hCG indeed has specific binding sites in the placenta.

During the period of sexual differentiation, hCG also regulates fetal testicular testosterone production.[100] Fetal peak testosterone levels coincide with maximum hCG levels. Through the activation of adenylate cyclase, hCG has been suggested to regulate fetal Leydig cell proliferation and testosterone production.[101,102] Although still controversial, some evidence also implicates hCG in the possible regulation of fetal adrenal steroidogenesis.[103] In the absence of ACTH, which appears after 16 weeks' gestation, dehydroepeandrosterone (DHEA-S) production commences in the fetal adrenal zone at about 10 weeks. This DHEA-S production coincides with peak hCG levels in fetal blood. HCG withdrawal after delivery may be the underlying cause for fetal adrenal zone regression (see also Chapter 42).

Fetal kidneys and liver also were shown to produce hCG[104], but the role of this hormone from these locations is unknown.

HCG also has been reported to have thyroid-stimulating activity and binding ability to thyroid tissue. HCG receptors, coupled to adenylate cyclase, exist on thyroid cell membranes.[105] Hyperthyroidism often accompanies the very high levels of hCG with trophoblastic diseases, such as hydatiform mole and choriocarcinoma. Although this thyrotropic effect of hCG is limited (1/4000 of TSH)[106], it is thought to be sufficient to contribute to the association of hyperthyroidism with gestational trophoblastic diseases.

HCG also has been described as immunosuppressive during pregnancy.[107,108] It is not clear, however, whether this is a direct effect of hCG or whether immunosuppression is mediated through other products, such as ovarian hormones.

Methods for hCG Quantitation. The first pregnancy test, developed by Aschheim and Zondek[54], was a bioassay measuring the effect of urinary hCG on the ovaries of immature female mice. This test was followed by many other bioassays, using a variety of animals. Because these types of assays were insensitive, allowing the diagnosis of pregnancy only 2 weeks after a missed menses, their clinical use was abandoned after the development of anti-hCG antibodies. Bioassays are, however, still used for research purposes, because the bioactivity of hCG may differ from its immunologically determined quantity.

Hemagglutination and latex agglutination inhibition tests require that hCG molecules be covalently linked to a carrier, either sheep red blood cells or latex particles. Addition of anti-hCG antibodies causes agglutination of the carrier. An antibody solution is therefore preincubated with the blood sample. Significant concentrations of hCG in the sample will bind to antibodies and thus reduce the amount of antibodies available to cause agglutination when subsequently incubated with the latex particles. Agglutination inhibition tests, based on antibodies against the β-subunit of hCG, increase the sensitivity of this assay and its accuracy by reducing cross-reactivity. Highly accurate results using such a method have been reported.[109]

Radioimmunoassays are accurate and sensitive. Antibodies can be directed to the intact molecule of hCG or to epitops of the β-subunit. Radiolabeled ligands and antibodies against the same ligands are used in this method. The unlabeled ligand in the sample is competing to displace the radiolabeled ligand from binding to the excess antibody. The counting is done for the "bound" radiolabeled ligand after the "free" radiolabeled ligand is separated and discarded. The level of bound radiolabeled ligand in the sample is then compared to a standard curve from which the amount of ligand in the sample can be extrapolated.

Enzyme-linked Immunoadsorbent assays (*ELISA*) provide the ability to detect small amounts of hCG without using radioactive materials. The counting is done by assessing the intensity of color produced by an enzyme that is linked to the second antibody or to the ligand, depending on the method used. The second antibody usually recognizes another epitope on the molecule rather than the first antibody and is added as a "sandwich." This second antibody is linked to an enzyme. The amount of enzyme that is attached to the sample hCG through its linkage with the second antibody can be estimated by a specific color reaction.

Radioreceptor assays are bioassays and use plasma membrane receptors of high affinity from tissues known to contain specific binding for hCG (ie, corpora lutea). The cross-reactivity with hLH is high because both hormones bind to the same receptor. Radiolabeled ligand binding curves are used to assess the competition of the hCG in the sample for receptor binding. The receptor is used for the same purpose as an antibody in a radioimmunoassay.

Clinical Application of hCG Measurements. The obvious primary use of hCG measurements in serum or in urine is the diagnosis of pregnancy. HCG is a specific marker for the existence of viable and active trophoblasts, except in rare cases of ectopic nontrophoblastic production of the hormone (see also Chapter 45). An exponential rise of hCG levels in the serum of pregnant women has been demonstrated in the 30–60 days from the last menstrual period, which can be correlated accurately to the date of pregnancy. In early pregnancy, hCG concentrations double about every 2 days.[110,111] Variations from this production profile of hCG may indicate pathology. Low concentrations suggest abnormal placentation, as in ectopic pregnancies, or reduction of the amount of viable trophoblast, as with impending abortion.[112] A low concentration of hCG also may indicate a relatively small amount of placental tissue because of a younger pregnancy than expected. In that case, levels should double every 2 days. In 80% of ectopic pregnancies, the hCG secretion pattern does not follow a normal doubling time.[113] Moreover, hCG levels over 2500 mIU/mL, in the absence of a demonstrable intrauterine pregnancy by competent vaginal ultrasonography, suggest an ectopic pregnancy.[114] Sensitive methods of measurement also have been used for infertility treatments, including *in vitro* fertilization management protocols for early detection of pregnancy. The ability to detect hCG levels before a menses is missed has demonstrated that many pregnancies occur as *"chemical pregnancies,"* characterized by pregnancy failure after a very brief period of hCG elevation.[115]

Inadequately high levels of hCG suggest an underestimation of gestation, age, a multiple pregnancy, or trophoblastic disease. While not all trophoblastic tumors produce excess hCG levels, levels exceeding 500,000 IU in 24 hours in urine or 200,000 mIU/mL in serum are highly suggestive of a molar pregnancy. Management and effectivity of treatment depend on accurate hCG measurements, as was first shown by Hertz et al in 1984.[116]

HUMAN PLACENTAL LACTOGEN (hPL)

HPL belongs to a group of three hormones that share similar structural and functional properties. The other two hormones that resemble hPL are prolactin (PRL) and human growth hormone (hGH). They are produced by the pituitary. The ability of placental tissue to stimulate mammary gland secretions indicates the presence of a lactogenic factor in the placenta.[117] Apart from prolactin-like activity, the placenta also demonstrates GH-like activity, which brought about the term *chorionic somatomammotropin* to designate this putative hormone.

HPL is a single-chain polypeptide of 191 amino acids and two disulfide bonds of molecular weight Mr 22,279. The amino acid sequence shows 96% homology to hGH. A similarily high level of homology (90%) also is shared between their respective genes. A lesser homology of 67% exists between the amino acid sequence of hPL and that of prolactin. This high level of homology between the three hormones led to the suggestion that their genes evolved from a common ancestral gene.

The lactogenic and immonologic characteristics of hPL are dictated by the amino terminus of the molecule. The carboxy-terminus is responsible for maintenance of conformation, while the disulfide bonds stabilize the molecule and are important for full immunogenic presentation.[118]

A higher molecular weight hPL appears in serum and placental extracts. It constantly represents 10% of all hPL in maternal serum.

The gene family consists of five linked genes positioned on chromosome 17. Two homologous (98%) genes, hCS-A and hCS-B, code for the hPL molecule.[119] A third gene, hCS-L, is not expressed. The respective hPL molecules, produced by these genes, differ in only one amino acid in the signal peptide; therefore, the end products are two identical hPL molecules. Syncytiotrophoblast, but not cytotrophoblast, contains mRNA for hPL, and it seems that hPL genes are expressed only after terminal differentiation of trophoblast cells.[67,68] The 25-amino acid signal peptide is cleaved cotranslationally in the syncytiotrophoblast. HPL cannot be found in secretory granules. However, some evidence suggests that two pools of hPL exist in cells. One is for immediate secretion, while the other is more stable.[119,120] The placenta hPL production reaches the amount of up to 1 g/day at term. The gene is thus highly expressed. Almost one fifth of the nonribosomal mRNA in term placenta is for hPL, attesting to the high level of secretion at this stage of gestation.

HPL can be detected 3 weeks after conception by radioimmunoassay in maternal serum, but it is present and can be localized in syncytiotrophoblast 1 week earlier. HPL levels constantly increase in the serum until 34 weeks' gestation and then plateau. The hormone is found in much lower amounts in fetal blood. Amniotic fluid levels are somewhat lower than maternal levels and rise toward term. The secretion of the hormone is episodic. Its half-life is 10–30 minutes, and the mechanisms for its disposal are unknown. Term placenta produces more hPL than early pregnancy placenta. This finding correlates with recent estimations that term placenta contains fourfold more specific hPL protein and mRNA. Furthermore, as the amount of syncytial cells increases toward term and more syncytial cells express the hPL gene, the level of production rises.[68,73,121]

Several factors have been examined to identify a short-term secretagauge. TRH, GnRH, somatostatin, acetylcholine, dopamine, and beta-adrenergic agonists and antagonists did not affect hPL secretion. The same is true for glucocorticosteroids, prolactin, glucagon, and thyroid hormone; conflicting results exist concerning the effects of progesterone and estrogen.[122-124] It is well established that fasting is followed by an increase of hPL levels in maternal blood.[125,126]

Unlike hCG, hPL secretion is probably not mediated by cAMP. On the other hand, incubation of placental tissue with phospholipase A_2 and arachidonic acid stimulates hPL production.[127,128] The activation of membranal phospholipase C, which stimulates phosphoinositide turnover, and the activation of the PKC and of the Ca^{2+} signaling systems cause increased production of hPL.[128,129]

Biologic Activity of hPL

While hPL is produced in the placenta in large quantities during pregnancy, its precise physiologic role is largely undetermined.[130] Structural similarity to GH and PRL led to the suggestion that hPL's metabolic actions also are similar. The somatotrophic effects of hPL are weaker than those described for GH.[131] Notwithstanding the possibility that the levels of hPL seen during pregnancy may influence placental or fetal growth, it has been suggested that the major metabolic effect of hPL is part of the mechanism ensuring constant glucose supply to the fetus during pregnancy. The *anti-insulinic* properties of hPL, together with estrogen and progesterone, inhibit glucose uptake and gluconeogenesis in the mother. Consequently, hPL induces an increase in maternal insulin levels.[132] Increased insulin levels, in turn, induce protein synthesis. HPL's diabetogenic effects on insulin economy also may be partially derived from a possible associated decrease in cellular response to insulin induced by the high levels of the hormone.[133] This type of effect also is responsible for the exaggerated insulin response to a glucose load observed during pregnancy.[134] Taken together, all these metabolic effects of hPL contribute to the *accelerated starvation state* observed in pregnancy. When prolonged starvation occurs in pregnancy, hPL levels increase.[126] Concomitantly, hPL increases the levels of free fatty acids (FFA) through increased lipolysis, thereby providing an abundant source of energy.[135,136]

The levels of hPL reach a maximum parallel with increased fetal metabolic requirements. Although the previously noted metabolic effects suggest an important role for hPL in the fetomaternal carbohydrate metabolism, successful and normal pregnancies have been described in the absence of any hPL production.[137]

STEROIDS

The placenta is responsible for an exceptionally large rate of steroidogenesis during pregnancy and hence for the elab-

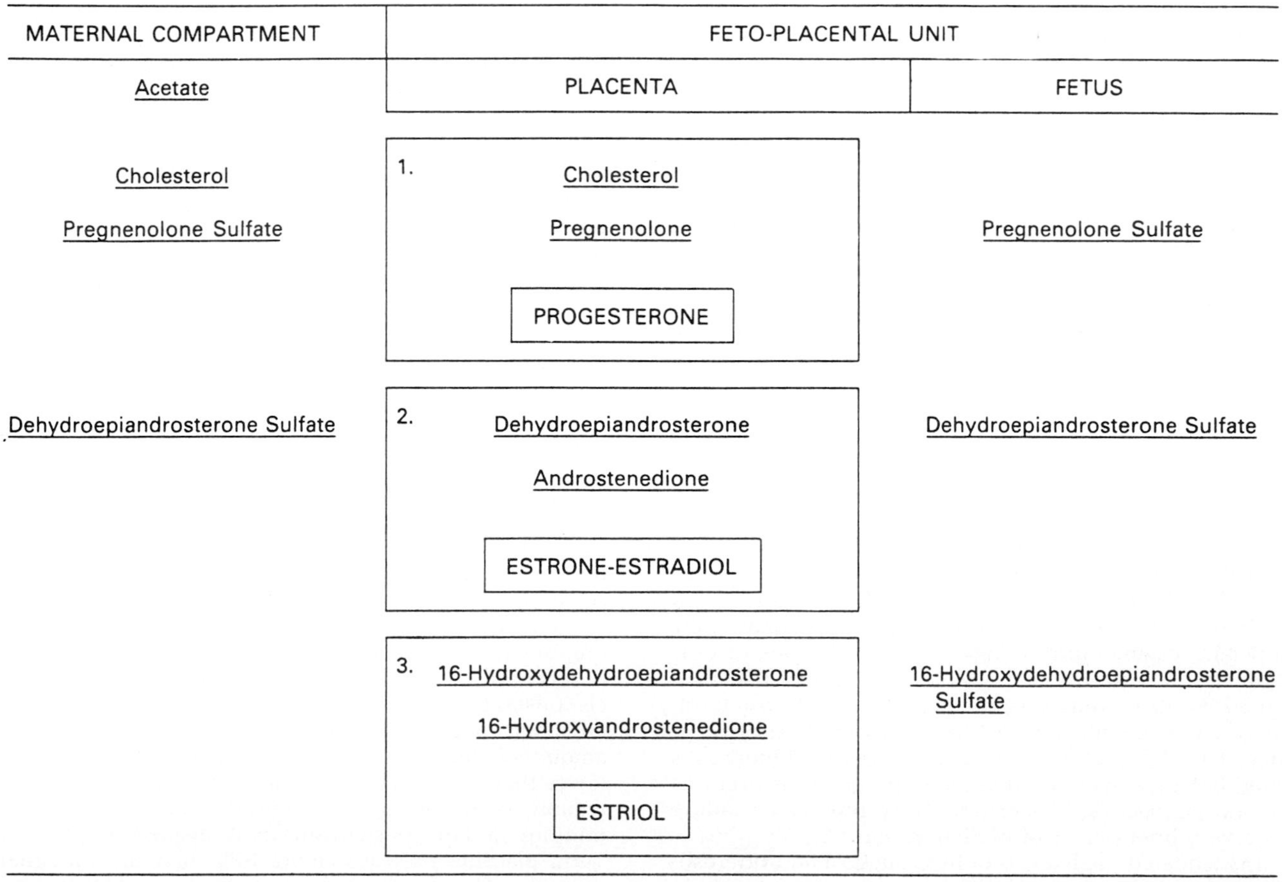

Figure 37–4. Major endocrine biosynthetic pathways in maternal and fetoplacental compartments. (*From Ryan KJ. Theoretical basis for endocrine control of gestation—a comparative approach. In Pecile A, Fenz; C, eds.* The Foetal Placental Unit. *Amsterdam: Excerpta Medica; 1964: 120 with permission.*)

oration of unprecedented amounts of estrogen and progesterone (Fig. 37–4). Steroids readily cross the placenta. Their production during pregnancy is the outcome of an unconventional collaboration between the fetoplacental unit and the mother. Curtailed enzymatic capabilities of involved tissues necessitate the critical cooperation between fetus, placenta, and mother. Early in pregnancy, the corpus luteum is a main source for steroid production. The corpus luteum produces progesterone until about 10 weeks' gestation. However, by the seventh week of pregnancy, the placenta assumes the responsibility of synthesizing adequate amounts of progesterone to maintain the pregnancy. Each day, 200 mg of progesterone are needed for the exogenous support of pregnancy during that time period.[138]

During nonconceptive cycles, the corpus luteum produces progesterone for 14 days before it regresses. However, in conception cycles, by virtue of hCG action on the ovary, the life span of the corpus luteum is extended; it becomes the corpus luteum of pregnancy. It appears that the pregnancy depends on the corpus lutuem for the first 4–6 weeks. During this period, ablation of the corpus luteum by ovariectomy will result in decreased steroidogenesis and abortion. After a transition period between weeks 7–12, the placenta takes over and produces rising levels of progesterone. These levels reach up to about 250–600 mg/day at term in singleton and multiple pregnancies, respectively. The levels of progesterone are in the range of 100–200 ng/mL. The corpus luteum maintains thereafter its steroidogenic capacity throughout pregnancy, but its function seems no longer vital for the maintenance of gestation.

PROGESTERONE

Because of limited 3-hydroxy-3-methylglutaryl coenzyme A (hMG-CoA) reductase activity in placental microsomes, hardly any *de novo* synthesis of cholesterol from acetate occurs in trophoblast. Only about 1–2% of total cholesterol is thus produced.[139] It also has been suggested that hMG-CoA reductase is further inhibited by cholesterol in placental cells. The placenta therefore depends on external sources for cholesterol. Convincing evidence exists that the fetus in the human is *not* the contributor of progesterone precursors because, even in the absence of a live fetus, the placental progesterone synthesis is uninterrupted.[138,140]

The placenta thus appears to use more than 90% of cholesterol principally derived from maternal plasma as the main precursor for progesterone biosynthesis. Low-density lipoprotein (LDL) cholesterol, and to a much lesser extent maternal high-density lipoproteins (HDL), provide an inexhaustible source for cholesterol.[141-143] LDL binds to specific high-affinity receptors on the trophoblast cell membrane and is endocytosed (internalized) into the cytoplasm.[144] The endocytotic vesicle, which contains the LDL-receptor complexes, then fuses with lysosomes, where LDL is hydrolyzed and the receptor can be recycled. Progesterone augments the amount of free cholesterol that is shuttled into steroidogenic pathways to meet the high placental need and increases the available free fatty acids.[143]

The first rate-limiting step in steroidogenesis is the generation of pregnenolone from cholesterol. This process is enzymatically and hormonally regulated and involves three consecutive reactions, a 20α-hydroxylation a 22-hydroxylation, and the cleavage of the cholesterol side chain between carbons 20 and 22. This cholesterol side-chain cleavage (CSCC) in the placenta is identical to the one in the adrenal. It was therefore suggested that three distinct enzymes comprise the CSCC complex to bring about the conversion of cholesterol to pregnenolone: a 20α-hydroxylase, a 22-hydroxylase, and a 20-, 22-lyase. Three moles of NADPH are consumed for conversion of 1 mol of cholesterol. However, recently it was shown that only a single enzyme P-450 scc on a single active site is responsible for all the chemical reactions in the CSCC. A single gene for P-450 scc has been cloned and sequenced in the bovine and human adrenal[146] and was localized on chromosome 15. The gene P-450 scc has been shown to be expressed in the human placenta from 10 weeks' gestation.[147]

In contrast to the placenta, the human decidua and fetal membranes also metabolize progesterone but prefer pregnenolone as the major substrate. Recently, dehydrogenase–isomerase was purified from the human placenta.[148] The enzyme is a monomer of about 41,000 d. Both enzymatic activities, isomerization and dehydrogenization for C_{19} and C_{21} steroids, are contained in a single protein.[149] Because 3 β-HSD in the human placenta is not a rate-limiting enzyme, pregnenolone conversion to progesterone occurs readily.[150] However, pregnenolone from the peripheral circulation contributes less than 3% to the rate of progesterone production at term. Interconversion of progesterone and 20 α-dihydroprogesterone occurs in the human placenta and 20 α-HSD catalizes the reaction in the mitochondria. The regulation of the enzyme and its activity is not clear, but it appears that in the human placenta, the reaction favors the production of progesterone during most of the pregnancy.

Regulation of Progesterone Production in the Placenta

In humans, the absence of a viable fetus, as in the case of intrauterine fetal death, has not been associated with immediate changes in the levels of progesterone or pregnandiol in serum. Some cases do, however, demonstrate a reduction in progesterone levels.[151] Data from subhuman primates suggest that the fetus may to some degree, be involved with maternal progesterone production.[152]

Numerous studies have shown no *in vitro* effect of hCG on progesterone synthesis in the placenta.[153] HCG has no effect on conversion of cholesterol to progesterone or on cholesterol side-chain cleavage activity.[154] In some reports, hCG has been shown to stimulate progesterone production in early pregnancy placentae *in vitro;* however, most data to date do not support such a role for hCG.

Placental GnRH, which is probably involved in the regulation of placental hCG, has been shown to inhibit progesterone production. Another trophic hormone, prolactin, has *in vitro* stimulatory effects on progesterone production.[155] However, *in vivo,* alterations of PRL levels do not affect progesterone levels in the maternal serum. Evidence from nonhuman primate experiments suggests a compensatory role for the corpus luteum in progesterone production when placental production is curtailed. The regulatory mechanism for such a compensation and whether it also exists in the human is unknown.

In vitro studies suggest a crucial role of cAMP in the regulation of progesterone production in normal and malignant placental tissue. The mechanism of cAMP action is similar to that described for regulation of hCG production. While it is difficult to assess the action of cAMP *in vivo,* it has been reported that adrenalin and vasopressin stimulation of progesterone production in early pregnancy was potentiated by theophylline and blocked by propranolol.[156] Thus it appears that, as in other tissues, beta-adrenergic receptor activation in the trophoblast increases the activation of adenylcyclase and of intrinsic cAMP generation, which in turn increases progesterone production. As with hCG, the production of progesterone in cytotrophoblast cells is stimulated by cAMP analogues, adenylcyclase stimulators, and phosphodiesterase inhibitors before terminal differentiation.[6,8]

Several investigators have demonstrated an inhibitory effect of androgens on progesterone synthesis.[157] These C_{19} steroids arise from the fetus and are suggested to affect the 3 β-HSD activity.[158]

The regulation of steroid synthesis in the placenta appears in part to use local autocrine and paracrine mechanisms. Recently, a role for various growth factors in placental function has been suggested. Reliable information is scarce and it appears that the in vitro role of these factors is to affect local modulation.

Progesterone appears in the amniotic fluid and reaches maximum concentrations in the second trimester. It later decreases gradually. The myometrium tends to concentrate progesterone in early pregnancy in comparison to maternal levels. At term, the levels become equal.

Progesterone Metabolites

During pregnancy a tenfold increase of 52-reduced metabolites occurs. The metabolite 5-pregnane-3, 20-dione is partially responsible for the uterine refractoriness to the pressor agent angiotensin II in pregnancy.[159] Deoxycorticosterone (DOC) at the end of pregnancy is 1200 times the nonpregnant level in the mother and fetus. Some of this is caused by the increase in cortisol-binding globulin (CBG) during pregnancy, but most of it occurs because of 21 α-hydroxylation of progesterone from the circulation. The physiologic role of DOC is unknown. Most DOC is produced extra-adrenally.[160,161]

The metabolic clearance rate of progesterone in pregnant women is the same as in nonpregnant women or men.

Biologic Action of Progesterone

Although an extraordinarily high rate of steroid synthesis denotes the state of pregnancy in humans, little is known about the specific functions for the various steroids produced during gestation. Progesterone has been implicated (even by nomenclature) as the prime hormone responsible for the maintenance of pregnancy.[162] Progesterone also is important for human implantation. Both estradiol and progesterone are massively produced by the corpus luteum early in pregnancy. However, it is generally agreed that successful implantation requires progesterone more than estradiol[163], whereas estrogens are needed for the endometrial priming effect. Progesterone also may play a role in the suppression of maternal immune responses to embryonal and trophoblast antigens. It has been proposed that progesterone together with hCG and decidual factors inhibits T-lymphocyte-mediated responses.[164]

Progesterone support for implantation and maintenance of pregnancy also can be achieved through its effect on smooth muscle. It is known as a potent relaxant of the uterotubal musculature and hence is capable of modulating tubal and uterine activity to create a favorable millieu for the conceptus.[165,166] Progesterone also affects maternal organs, causing gastrointestinal motility, constipation, heartburn, and regurgitation.

It is not clear to what extent progesterone and pregnenolone, produced by the placenta, are converted by the fetal adrenal to produce cortisol. The fetal adrenal is almost devoid of 3 β-HSD activity[167]; therefore, placental progesterone is used to overcome this enzyme deficiency. Hence, an important role for progesterone could be the supply of precursors for fetal adrenal production of glucocorticoids and mineralocorticoids. Relaxation of arteriolar smooth muscle by progesterone may be a cause of increased vascular capacitance, which results in a decrease in peripheral vascular resistance and thus lower blood pressure in early pregnancy. The same relaxing effect on the smooth muscle of the ureter partially may be the reason for the observed ureteral dilatation during pregnancy.

Progesterone also is implicated in well-recognized hyperventilation of pregnancy, probably by a central action on the respiratory center. Progesterone in nonhuman primates increases the plasma insulin response and probably also participates in the diabetogenic state of pregnancy.

Probably the most intriguing and controversial role of progesterone lies in the process of parturition. For many species, it has been established that progesterone withdrawal precedes the initiation of uterine contractions and subsequent labor. In many mammals, a decrease in maternal plasma progesterone is accompanied by a concomitant rise in estrogens. However, no evidence for such a temporal relationship exists in primates or humans.

ESTROGENS

Although ovarian steroidogenesis is constant throughout pregnancy, it is limited in comparison to the phenomenal production by the placenta. An increase of three estrogens is noted in maternal blood from 6–10 weeks' gestation. The three estrogens are estrone, estradiol, and estriol. Estrone and estradiol demonstrate an 100-fold and estriol an 1000-fold increase in pregnancy.[168,169] The metabolism of estrogens occurs in the maternal liver before their disposal in the urine.

In contrast to other mammalian species and other steroid-producing organs, the human placenta is devoid of 17 α-hydroxylase activity. The human placenta thus can not convert C_{21} to C_{19} steroids, with the latter being the precursors for estrogen production. The human placenta therefore cannot use either cholesterol or progesterone for the synthesis of estrogens. The human placenta is, however, equipped with a highly efficient mechanism of aromatization that converts C_{19} steroids into estrogens. The availability of C_{19} steroids thus becomes the limiting factor. In early pregnancy, most C_{19} steroids for placental use are maternal androgens. In the latter half of pregnancy, the fetus becomes the major supplier of androgen precursors for estrogen production.[170]

The placenta secretes large amounts of steroids into the maternal and fetal circulation. Steroids readily transverse between compartments. Those that appear in the fetal compartment are rapidly and efficiently conjugated with sulfate to generate inactive molecules. This conjugation and inactivation can be perceived as a protective mechanism against the overwhelming exposure of the fetus to highly potent steroids.

The placenta, on the other hand, is endowed with sulfatase activity that allows the prompt use of steroids derived from the embryo. For example, dehydroepiandrosterone sulfate (DHEA-S), provided by the fetal adrenal, is used by the placenta to produce estradiol and estrone. Maternal DHEA-S also can be used as an alternative precursor source for placental estrogen synthesis. As a third estrogen, estriol, which contains a 16-hydroxyl group, also is produced by the placenta. However, because the human placenta lacks 16-hydroxylation activity, most of the produced estriol is derived from the use of immediate fetal precursors and not by fetal conversion of estrone and estradiol.[171] Sixteen-hydroxydehydroepiandrosterone sulfate (16-OH-DHEA-S) is produced by the fetal liver from fetal adrenal-derived DHEA-S. The fetus does not have 3-β-HSD activity, and the 16-OH-DHEA-sulfate, which crosses into the placental compartment, is rapidly conjugated and converted into estriol. An alternative source for 16-OH-DHEA-S is the maternal liver. Ninety percent of estriol, which is produced during pregnancy, is thus obtained from the fetal compartment. This was the basis for estriol testing as a parameter of fetal well-being, a technique now largely abandoned.

Clinical Applications

Attempts to evaluate the quality of pregnancy by correlating its steroidogenic capacity were the result of recognizing that in pregnancy there is such a substantial increase in steroid production. Progesterone levels were found to be a poor indicator of fetal well-being, especially because, as previously noted, progesterone production is independent of the existence of a live fetus.

Estradiol and estrone are principally produced by the placenta with only a minor fetal contribution. Therefore, they do not mirror the condition of the fetus. Estriol, on the other hand, is a marker to which the fetus contributes 90% of precursors. The investigation of estriol has been suggested as valuable for the assessment of the fetoplacental unit and of fetal well-being.[172,173] Since the late 1970s, the monitoring of pregnancies with estriol has been replaced with antepartum testing because estriol evaluations were found to be less reliable. Estriol is a weak estrogen, 100 times less potent than estradiol. Unconjugated estriol rises during pregnancy from 0.05 mg/mL, at the onset of fetal adrenal function, to 15 mg/mL near term.

Estetrol is a 15-hydroxylation derivative of estriol. It is derived from estriol, which is the main source of its production. Hydroxylation occurs in positions 15 and 16 in the fetal liver. The 15-hydroxylation is an exclusive enzymatic property of the fetus, which is lost in adult life. Because its precursor, estriol, also depends on fetal metabolism, estetrol may represent the best potential biochemical monitor of fetal well-being.

PARTURITION

Normally, gestation is concluded at term, which is generally considered a gestational period of 38–42 weeks. Uterine contractions commence and labor progresses with the subsequent expelling of the fetus and placenta. Any deviation from this normal process, which usually maintains the conceptus in the uterus for at least 260 days, yields either parturition (abortion of premature delivery) or postmaturity. For the most part, neither maternal nor fetal factors involved in the sequence of events leading to parturition have been elucidated. Most of the existing data are derived from species other than humans. The sheep model has been investigated with the assumption that basic phenomena of parturition are similar. Substantial evidence has emerged, however, to suggest that the human parturition differs in many crucial aspects from most other mammalian species.

Several naturally occurring substances can elicit uterine contractions. Prostaglandins and oxytocin are used regularly for the induction of contractions and labor. Furthermore, angiotensin II, arginine vasopressin (AVP), and bradykinin also are potent stimulators of uterine contractions.[174] Many of these molecules are produced by the uterus or the conceptus and the uterus is endowed with their specific receptors.

Compounds that inhibit the formation of uterotonic agents or interfere with the binding to their specific receptors have been shown to induce different levels of uterine quiescence. Most hormones that are believed to be involved in the mediation of parturition also are very potent mediators of biologic events in other tissues and organs. When uterotonic activity peaks, there is no evidence for an extrauterine activation of related biologic mechanisms. Hence, the initiation of the biomolecular cascade most likely brings about uterine activity and labor and is, for the most part, locally regulated. Even less is known about the natural mechanisms that maintain uterine quiescence for most of the gestational period.

The Mechanisms of Uterine Activity

During muscle relaxation, Ca^{2+} ions are sequestered in intracellular sarcoplasmic storage vesicles. For the initiation of uterine muscle contractions, intracellular Ca^{2+} rises in the uterine muscle cells.[174,175] There also is evidence that during labor, gap junctions are formed between myometrial cells.[175,177] Gap junctions are means of communication between cells. Designated areas of the plasma membranes of adjacent cells fuse to form pores through which the cytoplasms of both cells are in direct contact. In myometrial cells, this type of communication facilitates the passage of current and metabolites between cells and allows the coordinated action of cells. A clear correlation exists between the appearance of gap junctions and subsequent labor. Almost no gap junctions are present in the quiescent uterus; they constantly increase during labor and rapidly disappear after delivery.[176,178] Prostaglandins PGE_2 and $PGF_{2\alpha}$, which are known to stimulate uterine activity, enhance the formation of gap junctions.[177] The number of gap junctions also seems to correlate with the number of estrogen and progesterone receptors. Progesterone inhibits, estrogen stimulates, and oxytocin has no effect on gap junction formation.[177,178]

A series of activations by phosphorylation occurs in the myometrial cell to bring about contractions. Any agent that increases intracellular ionic calcium concentration will induce myometrial activity. Calcium binds to its specific binding protein, calmodulin, which, in turn, causes the phosphorylation of myosin light chain kinase (MLCK). MLCK induces the phosphorylation of the light chain (20 kd) of myosin, thereby activating the ATPase of myosin. Hydrolysis of ATP by myosin ATPase supplies the energy for the cross-linking between myosin and actin filaments[179] and contractions. As mentioned previously, Ca^{2+} influx in order to raise its intracellular concentration is the primary signal for contraction. The flux of Ca^{2+} from sarcoplasmic storage by agonists that bind to muscle cell membrane receptors is probably transduced by activation of phospholipase C. This enzyme causes the hydrolysis of membranal phosphoinositides and the generation of IP_3 which, in turn, is capable of Ca^{2+} mobilization.[175,180,181] The concomitant generation of diacylglycerol (DAG) and protein kinase C (PKC) also activates MLCK.

Relaxation of smooth muscle is achieved by dephosphorylation of the myosin light chain or by reduction of intracellular Ca^{2+} levels. CAMP, for example, causes reduction of myosin light chain activity through two possible mechanisms: (1) by activation of protein kinase A and phosphorylation of MLCK at a site that, in turn, interferes with calmodulin activation; and (2) by indirectly reducing the intracellular Ca^{2+} concentration. Indeed, generation of intracellular cAMP by beta-adrenergic receptor or phosphodiesterase inhibitors causes smooth muscle relaxation.[182]

PROSTAGLANDINS

Prostaglandins in different species have been shown to be initiators and regulators of labor. They also seem to have an obligatory role in human parturition. Concentrations of PGE_2, $PGF_{2\alpha}$, and of their metabolites dramatically increase during labor in amniotic fluid, maternal blood and urine.[183-186] The administration of prostaglandins by any mode and at any stage of gestation has been shown to cause uterine contractions and expulsion of the conceptus. Administration of potent inhibitors of prostaglandin synthesis at any stage of pregnancy, in turn, suppresses uterine activity, prolongs labor, and inhibits premature labor. Furthermore, manipulations that are known to cause prostaglandin formation, such as cervical manipulation and rupture or stripping of membranes, also induce contractions.[174,187,188]

The principal precursor for prostaglandins is free arachidonic acid. It is commonly thought that the rate-limiting step in the generation of prostaglandins is the release of arachidonic acid. It is esterified into glycerophospholipids (ie, phosphatidylcholine), which is a constituent of every cell membrane. Arachidonic acid also is esterified into triglycerides and cholesterol esters.

It is the free arachidonic acid that can be used as substrate for the production of prostaglandins. Two pathways for the generation and release of arachidonic acid from membranal phospholipids exist: (1) phospholipase A_2 hydrolyses arachidonic acid at the Sn-2 position, preferentially from phosphatidylcholine, and phosphatidylethanolamine, and (2) phospholipase C cleaves 1,2 diacylglycerol (DAG) from phosphatidylinositol. In turn, diacylglycerol lipase (DG) and monoglyceride lipase (MG) liberate arachidonic acid from DAG.[184,187,189-191] Another route involves activation of phospholipase D-generated arachidonic acid.[181] Arachidonic acid will be recycled into phosphatidylinositol through the action of acyltransferases.[189,191] The latter might be inactivated by Ca^{2+} in the amnion and further increase the accumulation of arachidonic acid. Phospholipase A_2 and phospholipase C are regulated by Ca^{2+} and are thereby further stimulated to enhance the production of arachidonic acid.[192]

Cyclooxygenase is the microsomal enzyme that leads to the metabolism of arachidonic acid into prostaglandins. First, prostaglandin endoperoxide, PGG_2, is formed, which, in turn, is converted to endoperoxide PGH_2. This endoperoxide is the common percursor of biologically active prostaglandins. Specific synthetases form thromboxane and prostacyclin, respectively. Specific isomerases form prostaglandin E_2 and D_2, while $PGF_{2\alpha}$ is formed by reductase activity.[192-194] Nonsteroidal anti-inflammatory drugs, such as indomethacin and aspirin, specifically block cyclooxygenase activity. Therefore, they block the formation of PGG_2 and subsequently the formation of the aforementioned prostaglandins.

During the progression of labor, there is a constant increase in the concentration of arachidonic acid in amniotic fluid.[184] It also has been demonstrated that a local depletion exists in the phospholipid-arachidonic acid content of fetal membranes, which are in contact with amniotic fluid.[195] This observation suggests that, at least in part, the amniotic fluid arachidonic acid is liberated from adjacent fetal membrane glycerophospholipids. Another possible source for arachidonic acid is the decidua. This is suggested by the fact that fetal membrane arachidonic acid is replenished and levels in the amniotic fluid increase as labor progresses.[195]

There is no change in the characteristics of prostaglandin receptors during labor. Therefore the striking elevation in the amniotic fluid levels of PGE_2, $PGF_{2\alpha}$, and their circulating metabolites may have a crucial role in initiation and maintenance of uterine activity during labor. In contrast, prostacycline (PGI_2) production is hardly increased during induced labor. It therefore seems that there is preferential production of PGE_2 and $PGF_{2\alpha}$, which are stimulatory for the uterus, while PGI_2 may have inhibitory activities.[196]

In humans, all tissues participating in pregnancy are capable of producing prostaglandins. This includes fetal membranes, amnion, and chorion and maternal decidua and myometrium. While fetal membranes are producing PGE_2, the maternal decidua is producing the same amounts of PGE_2 and $PGF_{2\alpha}$.[197,198]

The produced PGE_2 is able to cross the fetal membrane.[199] It also was suggested that PGE_2, produced by the amnion, crosses toward the decidua, where it is metabolized into PGF_2.[200] The enzymatic activity that converts PGE_2 into $PGF_{2\alpha}$ has been demonstrated in the decidua.[200] This is one of the possible explanations for the observation that, in spite of PGE_2 formation in the amnion, the principal circulating metabolite is a $PGF_{2\alpha}$ metabolite.[185] It is also possible, however, that the accumulation of PGE_2 and its metabolites in amniotic fluid marks the primary role of prostaglandins produced by the decidua rather than that of fetal membrane-derived prostaglandins. The concomitant production in the decidua of such bioactive agents as arachidonic acid, prostaglandins (especially $PGF_{2\alpha}$ and its metabolite), platelet activating factor (PAF), and other cytokines, which are secreted into the amniotic fluid during labor, led Casey and MacDonald to imply a dominant role for the activated decidua in labor.[174,201] In such a context, the differentiated decidua has been compared to a macrophagelike body.

The myometrium also is capable of producing $PGF_{2\alpha}$.[202] This prostaglandin is, however, more likely to end up in the maternal circulation than to cross into amniotic fluid.

The mechanisms that regulate the enhanced prostaglandin production during labor are under intensive investigation. Progesterone withdrawal precedes the onset of parturition in most of the studied mammalian species. The decline in progesterone is a prerequisite for the initiation of labor in animals in which progesterone is produced to maintain pregnancy. A surge in estrogen production usually parallels the progesterone withdrawal in these species. This physiologic sequence also was observed in sheep, the most studied animal model.[203,204] In these animals, the withdrawal of progesterone is proceeded by increased prostaglandin synthesis. It is not clear whether progesterone withdrawal directly brings about the obligatory prostaglandin synthesis, which is required for initiation of labor. Instead, the rise in estrogen could be the key mechanism for releasing arachidonic acid and stimulating prostaglandins. Unfortunately, there is no human evidence to confirm that there is any significant change in the level of progesterone or estrogen.[205,206]

Progesterone withdrawal in humans can be recognized concomitantly with the expulsion of the conceptus in the third stage of labor. At that time, progesterone withdrawal serves a key role in the initiation of lactation.[207] The previous suggestion that, similar to other species, progesterone withdrawal occurs also in humans has not been confirmed. An overwhelming number of existing reports suggest the opposite.[206,208-210] Several recent reports have suggested the possibility of local regulation of progesterone concentrations at the sites that initiate labor.[211,212] This regulation could be through modulation of steroidogenesis enzymes or through regulation of the progesterone metabolism.

OXYTOCIN

Oxytocin is naturally and independently secreted by the fetus and mother and most probably does not cross the placenta. Oxytocin's effect on uterine activity is well investigated. It appears that late in pregnancy and close to term, oxytocin induces synchronous uterine contraction. Some level of uterine exitation and cervical readiness or "priming" is probably a prerequisite for oxytocin action in induction of labor.[213,214] Oxytocin has, however, limited effects on preterm myometrium, although it also is a potent agent in inducing contractions of the uterus after the expulsion of the conceptus. The decidua is endowed with specific binding sites for oxytocin that were shown to increase before labor.[203,215] Oxytocin also is a potent stimulator of prostaglandin $F_{2\alpha}$ and E_2 release in the endometrium and decidua.[203,215] It most probably does not have an effect on synchronization of contractions. This is the case because, as noted previously, it does not induce the formation of gap junctions. Oxytocin levels can be detected in the maternal circulation only very late in labor. Regulation of receptor characteristics by progesterone and estrogen may be the clue to its involvement in labor.

A rise in the levels of oxytocin during breast-feeing was reported by several investigators. Oxytocin is probably involved in the process of lactation (see also Chapter 188).

PREGNANCY PROTEINS

The primary function of the placenta is to secure the exchange of nutrients, gases, metabolites, and waste products between maternal and fetal compartments. A group of proteins that are transferred from the placenta to the maternal circulation were loosely termed *placenta-specific proteins*.[216-219] Much effort was invested in adjusting the measurements of these products to serve as indicators for placental–maternal transfer functions and hence as detectors of fetoplacental dysfunction.

SP_1 β_1-glycoprotein (PSβG)

Immunochemical studies of the protein composition of maternal serum during pregnancy have revealed the presence of this pregnancy-specific β_1-glycoprotein (PSβG). It is possible to detect PSβG during the first 2–3 weeks of pregnancy, and its level in maternal serum constantly rises with the progression of the gestation. The level of PSβG reaches 200–400 mg/mL at term. Very little is known about its function during pregnancy, although it is one of the major placental proteins. It was suggested that this protein may have some immunosuppressive activity. It also was suggested that PSβG may function in maintenance of placental cell growth.[10] PSβG is structurally similar to carcinoembryonic antigen (CEA), and it was therefore suggested that they belong to the same gene family.[220] Although PSβG was originally considered a placenta-specific protein, it is now known that skin fibroblasts and human fibroblasts in culture produce PSβG-like substances. PSβG-like activity also has been detected in the serum of nonpregnant women.[221] PSβG is, however, specific enough to be used as a pregnancy test. Patients who receive hCG for induction of ovulation can benefit from early pregnancy diagnosis using PSβG.

The trigger for the production of PSβG is unclear, but it appears in maternal serum concomitantly with implantation. Levels increase with placental size. PSβG production seems to be independent from the existence of a fetus. It also rises with ectopic gestation. The pace of increase in the levels of PSβG at the beginning of pregnancy is similar to that of hCG, doubling every 2–3 days.[217]

Immunohistochemical staining has localized PSβG to the syncytiotrophoblasts, and it also has been shown to be expressed in choriocarcinoma cells. PSβG also is found in the serum of untreated choriocarcinoma patients and in the serum of patients with malignant teratoma and other gonadal tumors.[222]

Placental Protein 5

Placental protein 5 (PP5) is a 36-kd glycoprotein that also was isolated from the placenta. It inhibits proteases, plasmin, and trypsin and antithrombin activities.[223,224] During pregnancy, PP5 can be detected at about 8 weeks' gestation, and it reaches peak levels in the last trimester of pregnancy. PP5 can be found in patients with hydatiform mole but cannot be detected in choriocarcinoma.[225]

Placental Protein 10

Placental protein 10 (PP10) is an alpha-glycoprotein with a molecular weight of 48 kd[226], and it is localized in the cytoplasm and nucleus of syncytiotrophoblast cells. It also appears in hydatiform mole but not in choriocarcinoma.[227]

Pregnancy-Associated Endometrial Alpha$_3$-globulin (α_2-*PEG*). This protein was first isolated from the decidua in the first-trimester and was named EP15. It also was found in amniotic fluid and term placenta, where it was known as PP14 and had a molecular weight of 25,000–28,000 d. It was then further characterized and found to be similar to progesterone-dependent endometrial protein PEP.[228,229] This protein has been shown to have sequence homology to β-lactoglobulins (milk proteins).[229,230] PP14 also was shown to have immunosuppressive qualities.[230,231]

Five to seven days after ovulation, the endometrium secretes PP14 in large amounts to become the major secretory product during the luteal phase. α_2-PEG is secreted by epithelial glands into the uterine lumen.[232] From early pregnancy, there appears to be a gradual decline in α_2-PEG secretion after a peak at 8–10 weeks. The amniotic fluid contains high levels of the protein, which are presumably derived from the decidua. Amniotic fluid levels decline after 15 weeks' gestation.[233] It seems therefore that α_2-PEG production follows the ontogeny of the endometrial glandular epithelium and declines with that tissue's regression.

PP12–α_3-PEG–EP14–Insulinlike Growth Factor Binding Protein. This protein demonstrates an interesting pattern of secretion by the human endometrium. During the menstrual cycle, it is one of the minor products of the endometrium. Its production is enhanced during luteal phase and decidual development, at which time it is detected around the blood vasculature. α_1-PEG was localized by immunohistochemical studies in pregnancy to decidual cells, where it represents a major product.[230,234] This protein appears to demonstrate IGF-binding properties. cDNA deduced sequencing and N-terminal amino acid sequence analysis demonstrated that α_1-PEG is identical to the low molecular-weight (34,000 d) IGF-binding protein (IGF-BP).

IGF-BP was isolated from amniotic protein (IGF-BP).[235,236] PP12, which originally was considered a placenta-specific protein but recently was demonstrated to be a decidual product, is immunochemically indistinguishable from α_1-PEG and demonstrates only minor amino acid sequence differences.[236] Many organs and tissues produce identical IGF-BP, and in different tissues, IGF-BP was shown to be stimulatory or inhibitory when bound to IGF. IGF-BP appears in amniotic fluid, where it reflects the synthetic activity of the endometrium. IGF-BP production is enhanced during pregnancy and can be detected in serum. Two peaks appear, one at mid pregnancy and one in the third trimester. The source of production is uncertain. Recently, it has been shown that in human serum, there is no change in levels of the binding proteins (IGFBP-1 25 kd; IGFBP-2 31kd; IGFBP-3 150kd complex) between secretory phase of the cycle and early pregnancy. However, IGFBP-3 declines during pregnancy after a 6-week gestation. IGFBP-2 decreases steadily during pregnancy. In contrast, IGFBP-I increases during pregnancy.[237]

IGF-BP of decidual origin appears concomitantly with peak levels of mRNA and production of IGF-I in the trophoblast. Hence, a paracrine interrelation can be envisioned. The placenta, and specifically the trophoblast, are the sources for IGF-II, which also can interact with IGF-BP. Both IGFs have been implicated in regulating placental growth and development.[7] This function can be regulated by IGF-BP.[234,238]

The nature of this paracrine action might be the local regulation and mediation of local stimulatory effects of IGF in light of unchanged circulatory levels of the growth factors. While the gene is not expressed in proliferative endometrium, mRNA for IGF-BP is found in secretory (predecidual) and decidual tissue, concomitantly with the progesterone-dominant period. This temporal relation might suggest progesterone regulation of gene expression.[234,239] Progesterone increases IGF-BP production in endometrial explants that were exposed to endogenous estradiol.[240] Other factors than progesterone might, however, be involved in the regulation of IGF-BP production and relaxin was implicated as one of these factors.[234] IGF-BP probably regulates IGF activity.

It has been reported that the human endometrium, during the late luteal phase, synthesizes a glycosilated form of prolactin. This makes the decidua the major source for extrapituitary prolactin during human pregnancy. Prolactin, which is a minor product of the endometrium during the luteal phase, becomes a major product of the differentiated decidua during pregnancy and is produced in parallel to IGF-BP.[234-241]

Pregnancy-Associated Plasma Protein-A

The molecular weight of pregnancy-associated plasma protein-A (PAPP-A) is 820,000 dd with a 20% carbohydrate content. It was shown to have various immunologic effects. Its other effects include anticomplimentory activity, inhibition of thrombin activity of plasmin, plasminogen activation, and activation of antithrombin II.[216,242]

PAPP-A was found in the serum of nonpregnant and pregnant women. It can be seen in trophoblast and decidua, in the female genital tracts, and in the male genital tract. It exists in the ovary at different stages of follicular development and also is localized in the cytoplasm of decidual cells.[216]

The clinical use for PAPP-A measurements has remained limited. With the *Cornelia de Lange's syndrome,* PAPP-A was absent in maternal blood.[243] It also was reported that dimished levels of PAPP-A were observed weeks before a spontaneous abortion. PAPP-A may be useful in predicting pregnancy outcome in imminent abortions. In cases of extrauterine pregnancy, it was shown that PAPP-A appears in lower than normal levels but only in one-half of the cases.[215]

Relaxin

Relaxin is produced by the corpus luteum in several species, including humans, during pregnancy and by the fetoplacental unit in other species. In primates, relaxin can be detected throughout pregnancy.[244] Relaxin has been known to be an effective myometrial relaxant. The effect probably involves cAMP generation, the lowering of intracellular Ca^{2+}, and the reduction of myosin light chain kinase activity by reducing its affinity to calmodulin and myosin. In the rat, relaxin is involved in the softening and priming of the cervix and in relaxing the symphysis pubis. As discussed previously, relaxin also has been demonstrated to induce IGF-BP by the endometrium. IGF-BP production appears to correlate with secreted relaxin. Relaxin also induces aromatase activity and prolactin production by endometrial cells in culture.[245,246]

Relaxin is a 63,000 d peptide and structurally resembles insulin. In lower primates, relaxin also is produced by the myometrium, decidua, and placenta and is localized to both cytotrophoblasts and syncytiotrophoblasts. Relaxin production can be stimulated by hCG in humans.[246,247]

In human pregnancies, relaxin can be detected within 3 weeks after conception. It reaches its maximal levels during the first trimester. After reduction to about 70% of maximal levels, it is maintained at a constant concentration until labor, in a pattern that resembles hCG. In rodents, relaxin levels increase before labor, but such a profile is absent in humans. HCG is probably the primary stimulator of relaxin production in the human. Administration of hCG to monkeys during the luteal phase induces the production and maintenance of relaxin levels. The time for relaxin production maintenance by hCG is days compared to the hours needed for hCG to stimulate progesterone production.[244,247] Hence, different mechanisms must be involved in these two pathways.

Prorenin

This is the high molecular-weight precursor of renin. Prorenin has been detected in the amniotic fluid and maternal circulation throughout pregnancy in the human. The fetoplacental unit is the source of this substance. About 10 days after conception, and within the first month of pregnancy, there is a significant rise in prorenin levels concomitantly with those of hCG.[249] Postpartum, hCG levels drop faster than prorenin levels, suggesting a source different than the placenta. The significant rise in prorenin originates in the maternal ovaries. While prorenin is considered inactive, its conversion results in the formation of active renin. The classic endocrinologic concept ties renin–angiotensin to the hormonal control of blood pressure. In that pathway, renin, a proteolytic enzyme is released primarily by the kidneys from its nonactive precursor, prorenin. The free circulating active renin converts angiotensinogen to angiotensin I, which, in turn, is the substrate for the pulmonary vasculature-converting enzymes. The converting enzymes catalize the formation of angiotensin II from the inactive angiotensin I. Angiotensin II is an effective vasoconstrictor and inducer of adrenal aldosterone production.

The reproductive system is a source of prorenin. During the menstrual cycle, prorenin levels increase during the luteal phase. Prorenin rises shortly after the LH surge and returns to baseline shortly after the LH peak is terminated. This temporal relationship suggests that prorenin levels are responsive to the LH surge.

The follicular fluid prorenin has been found by immunochemical and biochemical studies to be identical to the renal species. It appears therefore that the ovary begins to produce prorenin close to the LH surge. This production may be related to the normal profile of steroid production, with rising levels of gonadotropins augmenting prorenin production.[249]

The role of prorenins during the menstrual cycle and during early pregnancy is unclear. Renin has been found in follicular fluid and in amniotic fluid. However, it is still possible that prorenin exerts a direct action where it is produced.

INHIBIN

Inhibin is a glycoprotein hormone that is produced in the gonads and preferentially inhibits FSH production by the pituitary. In the ovaries, it is produced by granulosa cells. There are two forms of inhibin, inhibin A and inhibin B. Both have similar biologic effects. Two different subunits compose the intact heterodimers molecule (molecular weight 32,000 d). Each subunit is encoded by a specific mRNA. Both forms contain alpha-subunits, which are homologous to many species, including humans. The beta-subunits of the two forms, although highly homologous, are dissimilar. Inhibin A and B contain bA and bB, respectively.[250] Recently, it has been discovered that homodimers, which are composed of two bA or bA and bB chains occur naturally and can stimulate FSH secretion by the pituitary. These substances (28,000 d) have been called *activins* or FSH releasing peptides (FRP).[250,251] Inhibin and activin are related by the beta-subunit homology to a family of substances, which include transforming growth factor b (TGFb), Muellerian duct inhibiting factor (MIF), and others.[252]

The human placenta has been shown to be a source of bioactive and immunorecognizable inhibin[253,254], which inhibits FSH production in the pituitary with the same efficiency as the inhibition that was derived from follicular fluid. It appears therefore that the placental inhibin is undistinguishable from the follicular species. By immunocytochemical staining, the inhibin was localized to many of the cells in the cytotrophoblast layer.[255] In this also is the site on which other placental releasing and regulatory factors have been localized (ie, CRF, somatostatin and GnRH). CAMP analogues and cholera toxin cause release of inhibin from placental cell cultures. HCG also has been shown to stimulate inhibin production in placental cell cultures.[256] It has therefore been suggested that inhibin production in the placenta uses similar mechanisms as ovarian production. This entails gonadotropin (hCG) stimulation by way of cAMP. Vasoactive intestinal peptide (VIP) and neuropeptide Y (NPY) also are capable of inducing inhibin release, while somatostatin, substance P, and oxytocin are ineffective. Inhibin has recently been shown to affect hCG production. Hence, cytotrophoblast by way of inhibin production can theoretically regulate hCG production by the syncytiotrophoblast cells.[255] Placental inhibin may cause the low maternal FSH levels seen from the 10 weeks' gestation. Moreover, inhibin inhibition of hCG could occur through its inhibitory effect on placental GnRH, establishing a local paracrine axis. This implicated interaction in the placenta was suggested by experiments in which inhibin antibodies caused release of hCG and GnRH. Direct administration of purified inhibin, however, failed to show an increase in either GnRH or hCG.[255]

Activin is probably produced by the placenta where beta subunit inhibin mRNA also has been shown to be produced. Activin administration to cultured placental cells causes an increase in the measureable progesterone, GnRH, and GnRH-induced hCG.[255]

GONADOTROPIN-RELEASING HORMONE

The placenta has been shown to be a source for the production of GnRH-like substances. Human placental extracts were shown to have GnRH-like biologic activity in releasing LH in the rat pituitary.[257] Placental GnRH was purified, and it is identical to the hypothalamic hormone.[258,259] The placenta also can provide a target organ for GnRH action, as specific receptors have been shown to exist on placental membranes.[80] GnRH was localized by immunohistochemical staining to the cytotrophoblast component of the placenta. The intensity of staining declines with advancement of pregnancy and diminution of the cytotrophoblast elements. CAMP analogues and beta adrenergic receptor agonists, which are known to stimulate adenylate cyclase, cause the secretion of GnRH from placental cultures.[255] There is conflicting evidence probably because of the variation in methods of measurements, about the placental GnRH secretion profile. By RIA, the highest levels were measured between 12–23 weeks of pregnancy. An increase in secretion at the 8th week of pregnancy was measured by another method. As discussed previously, convincing evidence exists that suggests that GnRH might be involved in establishing an intraplacental axis for the regulation of hCG production. The administration of GnRH antagonists to pregnant baboons had a devastating effect on pregnancy outcome.[260]

The effect of GnRH on steroid production and prostaglandin generation in the placenta is less established.[261] Placental GnRH also might have an endocrine effect on the maternal pituitary by down-regulating pituitary function. It is probably released into the maternal circulation because plasma levels of GnRH are higher during gestation than in the nonpregnant state.

REFERENCES

1. Cunningham FG, Macdonald P, Gant NF. The placenta and fetal membranes. *Williams Obstetrics*, 18th ed. Norwalk, CT: Appleton and Lange; 1989:39.
2. McGrath J, Solter D. Completion of mouse embryogenesis requires both the maternal and paternal genomes. *Cell*. 1984;37:179.
3. Kliman HJ, Nestler JE, Sermasi E, et al. Purification, characterization and *in vitro* differentiation of cytotrophoblasts from human term placentae. *Endocrinology*. 1986;118:1567.

4. Hoshina M, Bothby M, Boime I. Cytological localization of chorionic gonadotropin alphs and placental lactogen mRNAs during development of human placenta. *J Cell Biol.* 1982;93:190.
5. Ender AC. A comparative study of the fine structure of the trophoblast in several Premochorial placentas. *Am J Anat.* 1965;116:29.
6. Feinman MA, Kliman HJ, Caltabiano S, Strauss JF III. 8 bromo-3', 5'-adenosin menophosphate stimulates the endocrine activity of human cytotrophoblasts in culture. *J Clin Endocrinol Metab.* 1986;63:1211.
7. Zilberstein M, Solan N, Das C, et al. Regulation of insulin like growth factor (IGF) gene expression in cultured cytotrophoblasts. *Biol Reprod.* 1989;40(supp):1.
8. Ringler GE, Kao L-C, Ulloa-Aguirre A, Strauss JF. Control of the endocrine function of the human placenta by cyclic AMP. In: Yoshinaga K, ed. *Blastocyst Implantation.* Boston, MA: Serone Symposia USA, Adams Publishing Group; 1989:209.
9. Ringler GE, Kao L-C, Miller WL, Strauss JF III. Effects of 8-bromo-cAMP on expression of endocrine functions by cultured human trophoblast cells. Regulation of specific mRNA. *Mol Cell Endocrinol.* 1989;61:13.
10. Chou JY, Zilberstein M. Expression of the pregnancy-specific beta, glycoprotein gene in cultured human trophoblasts. *Endocrinology.* 1990:127;2127.
11. Adamson ED. Expression of proto-oncogenes in the placenta. *Placenta.* 1987;8:449.
12. Ohlsson R, Holmgren L, Glaser A, et al. Insulin-like growth factor 2 and short-range stimulatory loops in control of human placental growth. *EMBO J.* 1989;8:1993.
13. Fant M, Munro H, Moses C. An autocrine/paracrine role for insulin-like growth factors in the regulation of human placental growth. *J Clin Endocrinol Metab.* 1986;63:499.
14. Goustin AS, Betsholtz C, Pfeifer-Ohlsson S, et al. Coexpression of the sis and myc proto-oncogenes in developing human placenta suggests autocrine control of trophoblast growth. *Cell.* 1985;41:301.
15. Taylor RN, Williams LT. Developmental expression of platelet-derived growth factor and its receptor in the human placenta. *Mol Endocrinol.* 1988;2:627.
16. Chen CF, Kurachi H, Fujita Y, et al. Changes in epidermal growth factor receptor and its messenger ribonucleic acid levels in human placenta and isolated trophoblast cells during pregnancy. *J Clin Endocrinol Metab.* 1988;67:1171.
17. Maruo T, Matsuo H, Oishi T, et al. Induction of differentiated trophoblast function by epidermal growth factor: relation of immunohistochemically detected cellular epidermal growth factor receptor levels. *J Clin Endocrinol Metab.* 1987;64:744.
18. Shen S-J, Wang C-Y, Nelson KK, et al. Expression of insulin-like growth factor II in human placentas from normal and diabetic pregnancies. *Proc Natl Acad Sci USA.* 1986;83:9179.
19. Wang C-Y, Daimon M, Shen S-J, et al. Insulin-like growth factor-I messenger ribonucleic acid in the developing human placenta and in term placenta of diabetics. *Mol Endo.* 1988;2:217.
20. Voutilainen R, Miller WL. Coordinate tropic hormone regulation of mRNAs for insulin-like growth factor II and the cholesterol side-chain cleavage enzyme P-450-ssc in human steroidogenic tissues. *Proc Natl Aca Sci USA.* 1987;84:1590.
21. Han VKM, Lund PK, Lee DC, D'Ercol AJ. Expression of somatomedian/insulin-like growth factor messenger ribonucleic acids in the human fetus: Identification, characterization and tissue distribution. *J Clin Endocrinol Metab.* 1988;66:422.
22. Tulchinsky D, Hobel CJ. Plasma human chorionic gonadotropin, estrone, estradiol, progesterone and 17-alpha hydroxyprogesterone in human pregnancy III. Early normal pregnancy. *Am J Obstet Gynecol.* 1973;117:884.
23. Filicori M, Butler JP, Crowley WF. Neuroendocrine regulation of the corpus luteum in the human evidence for pulsatile progesterone secretion. *J Clin Invest.* 1984;73:1638.
24. Mais V, Kazer RR, Cetel NS, et al. The dependency of folliculogenesis and corpus luteum function on pulsatile gonadotropin secretion in cycling women using a gonadotropin-releasing hormone antagonist as a probe. *J Clin Endocrinol Metab.* 1986;62:1250.
25. Soules MR, Wiebe RH, Aksel S, Hammond CB. The diagnosis and therapy of luteal phase deficiency. *Fertil Steril.* 1977;28:1033.
26. Goodman AL, Hodgen GD. The ovarian triad of the primate menstrual cycle. *Recent Prog Horm Res.* 1983;39:1.
27. Strott CA, Yoshimi T, Ross GT, Lipsett MB. Ovarian physiology: Relationship between plasma LH and steroidogenesis by the follicle and corpus luteum: effect of HCG. *J Clin Endocrinol Metab.* 1969;29:1157.
28. Ravindranath N, Moudgal NR. Hormonal requirement for the establishment of pregnancy in primates. In: Yoshinaga K, ed. *Blastocyst Implantation.* Serone Symposia USA; 1989:195.
29. Hearn JP. The embryo-maternal dialogue during early pregnancy in primates. *J Reprod Fertil.* 1986;76:809.
30. Shutt DA, Lopata A. The secretion of hormones during the culture of human preimplantation embryos with corona cells. *Fertil Steril.* 1981;35:413.
31. Shutt DA, Clark AH, Fraser IS, et al. Changes in concentration of prostaglandin F and steroids in human corpora lutea in relation to growth of the corpus luteum and luteolysis. *J Endocrinol.* 1976;71:453.
32. Levy C, Robel P, Gantray JP. Estradiol and progesterone receptors in human endometrium: Normal and abnormal menstrual cycles and early pregnancy. *Am J Obstet Gynecol.* 1980;136:646.
33. Ghosh D, Sengusta J. Patterns of estrogen and progesterone receptors in rhesus monkey endometrium during secretory phase of normal menstrual cycle and preimplantation stages of gestation. *J Steroid Biochem.* 1988;31(2):223.
34. Thomas K, DeHertogh R, Pizzaro M, et al. Plasma LH-hCG, 17-β estradiol, estrone and monitoring around ovulation and subsequent *nidation. Int J Fertil.* 1973;18:65.
35. Shelesnyak MC. Inhibition of decidual cell formation in the pseudopregnant rate by histamine antagonist. *Am J Physiol.* 1952;170:522.
36. Kraicer P, Shelesnyak MC. The induction of deciduomata in the pseudopregnant rat by systemic administration of histamine and histamine releasers. *J Endocrinol.* 1958;17:324.
37. Shelesnyak MC. Fall in uterine histamine associated with ovum implantation in pregnant rat. *Proc Soc Exp Biol Med.* 1959;100:380.
38. Dey SK, Johnson DC, Santos JG: Is histamine production by the blastocyst required for implantation in the rabbit? *Biol Reprod.* 1979;21:1169.
39. Dey SK, Villaneuva C, Abdou NI. Histamine receptors on rabbit blastocyst and endometrial cell membranes. *Nature.* 1979;278:648.
40. Ishikawa S, Sperelakis N. A novel class (H_3) of histamine receptors on perivascular nerve terminals. *Nature.* 1987;327:158.
41. Phillips CA, Poysner NL. Studies on the involvement of prostaglandins in implantation in the rat. *J Reprod Fertil.* 1981;62:73.
42. Kennedy TG. Evidence for a role for prostaglandin in the initiation of blastocyst implantation in the rat. *Biol Reprod.* 1977;16:286.
43. Kennedy TG. Prostaglandins and increased endometrial vascular permeability resulting from the application of an artificial stimulus to the uterus of the rat sensitized for the decidual cell reaction. *Biol Reprod.* 1979;20:560.
44. Kennedy TG, Lukash LA. Induction of decidualization in rat by the intrauterine infusion of prostaglandins. *Biol Reprod.* 1982;27:253.
45. Kennedy TG. Evidence for the involvement of prostaglandins throughout the decidual cell reaction in the rat. *Biol Reprod.* 1985;33:140.
46. Kennedy TG, Martel D, Psychoyos A. Endometrial prostaglandin E_2 binding: Characterization in rats sensitized for decidual cell reaction and changes during pseudopregnancy. *Biol Reprod.* 1983;29:556.
47. Martel D, Kennedy TG, Monier MN, Psychoyos A. Failure to detect specific binding sites for prostaglandin $F_{2\alpha}$ in membrane preparations from rat endometrium. *J Reprod Fertil.* 1985;75:265.
48. Hoffmann GE, Rao CV, DeLeon FD, et al. Human endometrial prostaglandin E_2 binding sites and their profiles during the menstrual cycle and in pathological states. *Am J Obstet Gynecol.* 1985;151:369.
49. Costracane VD, Jordan VC. Consideration into the mechanism of estrogen-stimulated uterine prostaglandin synthesis. *Prostaglandins.* 1976;12:243.
50. Rees MCP, DiMarzo V, Tippins JR, et al. Leukotriene release by endometrium and myometrium throughout the menstrual cycle in dysmenorrhoea and menorrhagia. *J Endocrinol.* 1987;113:291.
51. Chegini N, Rao CV. The presence of leukotriene C_4 and prostacyclin-binding sites in nonpregnant human uterine tissue. *J Clin Endocrinol Metab.* 1988;66:76.
52. Tawfik OW, Huet YM, Malothy PV, et al. Release of prostaglandins and leukotrienes from the rat uterus is an early estrogenic response. *Prostaglandins.* 1987;34:805.
53. Tawfik OW, Dey SK. Further evidence for role of leukotrienes as mediators of decidualization in the rat. *Prostaglandins.* 1988;35:379.
54. Aschheim S, Zondek B. Hypophysenvorderlappenhormon und ovarialhormon im harn von Schwangeren. *Klin Wochenschr.* 1927;6:1322.
55. Pierce JG. Gonadotropins: Chemistry and biosynthesis. In: Knobil E, Neil J, et al, eds. *The Physiology of Reproduction.* New York, NY: Raven Press; 1988:1335.
56. Hussa RO. Biosynthesis of human chorionic gonadotropin. *Endocrin Rev.* 1980;1:268.
57. Birken S. 1984 chemistry of human choriogonadotropin. *Ann Endocrinol (Paris).* 1984;45:297.
58. Bahl OP, Carlson RB, Bellisario R, Swaminathan N. Human chorionic gonadotropin amino acid sequence of the alpha and beta subunits. *Biochem Biophys Res Common.* 1972;48:416.
59. Morgan FJ, Birken S, Canfield RE. The amino acid sequence of human chorionic gonadotropin. The alpha subunit and beta subunit. *J Biol Chem.* 1975;250:5247.
60. Pierce JG, Parson TF. Glycoprotein hormones: Structures and Function Annu. *Rev Biochem.* 1981;50:465.
61. Strickland TW, Puett D. Contribution of subunits to the function of luteinizing hormone/human chorionic gonadotropin recombinants. *Endocrinology.* 1981;109:1933.
62. Fiddes JC, Talmagde K. Structure expression and evolution of the genes for the human glycoprotein hormones. *Recent Prog Horm Res.* 1984;40:43.
63. Fiddes JC, Goodman HM. The gene encoding the common α-subunit of the four human glycoprotein hormones. *J Mol Appl Genet.* 1981;1:3.

64. Boothby M, Ruddon RW, Anderson C, et al. A single gonadotropin α subunit gene in normal tissue and tumor-derived cell-lines. *J Biol Chem*. 1981;256:5121.
65. Naylor SL, Chin WW, Goodman HM, et al. Chromosome assignment of genes encoding the α and β subunit of glycoprotein hormones in man and in mouse somatic cell. *Mol Genet*. 1983;9:757.
66. Julier C, Weil D, Couillin P, et al. The beta chorionic gonadotropin beta luteinizing gene cluster maps to human chromosome 19. *Hum Genet*. 1984;67:174.
67. Hoshina M, Boothby M, Hussa R, et al. Linkage of human chorionic gonadotropin and placental lactogen biosynthesis to trophoblast differentiation and tumorogenesis. *Placenta*. 1985;6:163.
68. Boime I, Boothby M, Hoshina M, et al. Expression and structure of human placental hormone genes as a function of placental development. *Biol Reprod*. 1982;26:73.
69. Boothby M, Kukowska J, Boime I. Imbalanced synthesis of human choriogonadotropin α and β subunits reflects the steady state level of the corresponding mRNAs. *J Biol Chem*. 1983;258:9250.
70. Ruddon RW, Hartle RJ, Peters BP, et al. Biosynthesis and secretion of chorionic gonadotropin subunits by organ culture of first trimester human placenta. *J Biol Chem*. 1981;256:11389.
71. Kliman HJ, Nestler JE, Sermasi E, et al. Purification, characterization and in vitro differentiation of cytotrophoblasts from human term placentae. *Endocrinology*. 1986;118:1567.
72. Ayala AR, Bustos H, Aguilar RM. Daily rhythm of serum human chorionic gonadotropin and human chorionic somatomammotropin in normal pregnancy. *Int J Gynaecol Obstet*. 1984;22:173.
73. Braunstein GD, Rasor JL, Engrall E, Wade ME. Interrelationships of human chorionic gonadotropin human placental lactogen and pregnancy specific β_1-glycoprotein throughout normal human gestation. *Am J Obstet Gynecol*. 1980;138:1205.
74. Mishell DR, Wide L, Gemzell CA. Immunologic determination of human chorionic gonadotropin in serum. *J Clin Endocrinol Metab*. 1963;23:125.
75. Benveniste R, Scommegna A. Human chorionic gonadotropin α-subunit in pregnancy. *Am J Obstet Gynecol*. 1981;141:952.
76. Khodr GS, Siler-Khodr TM. Placental LRF and its synthesis. *Science*. 1980;207:315.
77. Khodr GS, Siler-Khodr TM. Localization of luteinizing hormone-releasing factor in the human placenta. *Fertil Steril*. 1978;29:523.
78. Siler-Khodr TM, Khodr GS, Valenzuela G, Rhode J. Gonadotropin-releasing hormone effects on placental hormones during gestation. I. Alpha-human chorionic gonadotropin, human chorionic gonadotropin and human chorionic somatomammotropin. *Biol Reprod*. 1986;34:245.
79. Siler-Khodr TM, Khodr GS, Vickery BH, Nestor JJ. Inhibition of hCG, α hCG and progesterone release from human placental tissue in vitro by a GnRH antagonist. *Life Sci*. 1983;32:2741.
80. Currie AJ, Fraser HM, Sharpe RM. Human placental receptors for luteinizing hormone releasing hormone. *Biochem Biophys Res Commun*. 1981;99:332.
81. Tamada T, Akabori A, Konuma S, Araki S. Lack of release of human chorionic gonadotropin by gonadotropin-releasing hormone. *Endocrinol Jpn*. 1976;23:531.
82. Siler-Khodr TM, Khodr GS. Content of luteinizing hormone-releasing factor in the human placenta. *Am J Obstet Gynecol*. 1978;130:216.
83. Wilson EA, Jawad MJ, Dickson LR. Suppression of human chorionic gonadotropin by progestational steroids. *Am J Obstet Gynecol*. 1980;138:708.
84. Kletzky OA, Rossman F, Bertolli SI, et al. Dynamics of human chorionic gonadotropin, prolactin, and growth hormone in serum and amniotic fluid throughout normal human pregnancy. *Am J Obstet Gynecol*. 1985;151:878.
85. Shu-rong Z, Bremme K, Eneroth P, Nordberg A. The regulation in vitro of placental release of human chorionic gonadotropin, placental lactogen, and prolactin. Effects of an adrenergic beta-receptor agonist and antagonist. *Am J Obstet Gynecol*. 1982;143:444.
86. Zilberstein M, Solan N, Chou JY, et al. Antibodies to EGF receptor inhibit basal and EGF stimulated hCG production in human term placental cells. *Endocrinology*. 1989;125:1037.
87. Ilekis J, Benveniste R. Effects of epidermal growth factor, phorbol myristate acetate and arachidonic acid on choriogonadotropin secretion by cultured choriocarcinoma cells. *Endocrinology*. 1985;116:2400.
88. Petraglia F, Lim AT, Vale W. Adenosine 3′,5′-monophosphate prostaglandins and epinephrine stimulate the secretion of immunoreactive gonadotropin releasing hormone from cultured human placenta cells. *J Clin Endocrinol Metab*. 1987;65:1020.
89. Feinman MA, Kliman JH, Caltabiano S, Strauss JF III. 8-bromo-3′,5′-adenosin monophosphate stimulates the endocrine activity of human cytotrophoblasts in culture. *J Clin Endocrinol Metab*. 1986;63:1211.
90. Nulsen JE, Woolbalis MJ, Kopf GS, Strauss JF III. Adenylate cyclase in human cytotrophoblasts: Characterization and its role in modulating hCG secretion. *J Clin Endocrinol Metab*. 1988;66:258.
91. Ritvos O, Bützow R, Jalkanen J, et al. Differential regulation of hCG and progesterone secretion by cholera toxin and phorbol ester in human cytotrophoblasts. *Mol Cell Endocrinol*. 1988;56:165.
92. Ringler GE, Kallen CB, Strauss JF III. Regulation of human trophoblast function by glucocorticoids: dexamethasone promotes increased secretion of chorionic gonadotropin. *Endocrinology*. 1989;124:1625.
93. Silvestr L, Dubois C, Renault M, et al. Voluntary interruption of pregnancy with mifepristone (RU 486) and prostaglandin analogue: a large scale French experience. *N Engl J Med*. 1990;322:645.
94. Bradbury JT, Brown WE, Gray LA. Maintenance of corpus luteum and physiologic actions of progesterone. *Recent Prog Horm Res*. 1950;5:51.
95. Rice BF, Hammerstein J, Savard K. Steroid hormone formation in the human ovary. II. Action of gonadotropins in vitro in the corpus luteum. *J Clin Endocrinol Metab*. 1964;24:606.
96. LeMaire WJ, Rice BF, Savard K. Steroid hormone formation in the human ovary: V Synthesis of progesterone in vitro in corpora lutea during the reproductive cycle. *J Clin Endocrinol Metab*. 1968;28:1249.
97. Savard K, Marsh JM, Rice BF. Gonadotropins and ovarian steroidogenesis. *Recent Prog Horm Res*. 1965;21:285.
98. Quagliarello J, Goldsmith L, Steinetz B, et al. Induction of relaxin secretion in nonpregnant women by chorionic gonadotropin. *J Clin Endocrinol Metab*. 1980;51:74.
99. Rosenberg SM, Bhatnagar AS. Sex steroids and human chorionic gonadotropin modulation of in vitro prolactin production by human term decidua. *Am J Obstet Gynecol*. 1984;148:461.
100. Albert A. Follicle-stimulating activity of human chorionic gonadotropin. *J Clin Endocrinol Metab*. 1969;29:1504.
101. Ahluwalia B, Williams J, Verma P. *In vitro* testosterone biosynthesis in the human fetal testis. II. Stimulation by cyclic cAMP and human chorionic gonadotropin (hCG). *Endocrinology*. 1974;95:1411.
102. Huhtaniemi IT, Korenbrot CC, Jaffe RB. HCG binding and stimulation of testosterone biosynthesis in the human fetal testis. *J Clin Endocrinol Metab*. 1977;44:963.
103. Reyes FI, Boroditsky RS, Winter JSD, Faiman C. Studies on human sexual development. II fetal and maternal serum gonadotropin and sex steroid concentrations. *J Clin Endocrinol Metab*. 1974;38:612.
104. Goldsmith PC, McGregor WG, Raymoure WJ, et al. Cellular localization of chorionic gonadotropin in human fetal kidney and liver. *J Clin Endocrinol Metab*. 1983;57:654.
105. Azukizaua M, Kurtzman G, Pekary AE, Hershman JM. Comparison of the binding characteristics of bovine thyrotropin and human chorionic gonadotropin to thyroid plasma membranes. *Endocrinology*. 1977;101:1880.
106. Nisula BC, Morgan FJ, Canfield RE. Evidence that chorionic gonadotropin has intrinisic thyrotropic activity. *Biochem Biophys Res Commun*. 1974;59:86.
107. Nisula B, Bartocci A. Choriogonadotropin and immunity: A reevaluation. *Ann Endocrinol (Paris)*. 1984;45:315.
108. Adock ED, Teasdale F, August CS. Human chorionic gonadotropin: Its possible role in maternal lymphocyte suppression. *Science*. 1973;181:845.
109. Hobson BM. Pregnancy diagnosis. *Lancet*. 1969;2:56.
110. Chartier M, Roger M, Barrat J, Michelon B. Measurement of plasma chorionic gonadotropin (hCG) and β-hCG activities in the late luteal phase: Evidence of the occurrence of spontaneous menstrual abortions in infertile women. *Fertil Steril*. 1979;31:134.
111. Batzer FR, Schlaff S, Goldfarb AF, Corson SL. Serial β-subunit human chorionic gonadotropin doubling time as a prognosticator of pregnancy outcome in an infertile population. *Fertil Steril*. 1981;35:307.
112. Mishell DR Jr, Davajan V. Quantitative immunologic assay of human chorionic gonadotropin in normal and abnormal pregnancies. *Am J Obstet Gynecol*. 1966;96:231.
113. Kadar N, Caldwell BV, Romero R. A method of screening for ectopic pregnancy and its indications. *Obstet Gynecol*. 1981;58:162.
114. Lavy G, DeCherney AH. The hormonal basis of ectopic pregnancy. *Clin Obs Gynecol*. 1987;30:217.
115. Edmonds DK, Lindsay KS, Miller JF, et al. Early embryonic mortality in women. *Fertil Steril*. 1982;38:447.
116. Hertz R, Ross GT, Lipsett MB. Primary chemotherapy of nonmetastatic trophoblastic disease in women. *Am J Obstet Gynecol*. 1963;86:808.
117. Talamantes F. *In vitro* demonstration of lactogenic activity in the mammalian placenta. *Am Zool*. 1975;15:279.
118. Handwerger S, Pang EC, Aloj SM, Sherwood LM. Correlation in the structure and function of human placental lactogen and human growth hormone. I. Nodification of the disulfide bonds. *Endocrinology*. 1972;91:721.
119. Selby MJ, Barta A, Baxter JD, et al. Analysis of a major human chorionic somatomammotropin gene. *J Biol Chem*. 1984;259:13131.
120. Suwa S, Friesen H. Biosynthesis of human placental proteins and human placental lactogen (HPL) *in vitro*. II. Dynamic studies of normal term placentas. *Endocrinology*. 1969;85:1037.
121. Ringler GE, Strauss JF Jr. *In vitro* systems for the study of human placental endocrine function. *Endocrin Review*. 1990;11:105.
122. Zeitler P, Markoff E, Handwerger S. Characterization of the synthesis and release of human placental lactogen and human chorionic gonado-

tropin by an enriched population of dispersed placental cells. *J Clin Endocrinol Metab.* 1983;57:812.
123. Bellevill F, Lasbennes A, Nabet P, Paysant P. HCS-HCS regulation in cultured placenta. *Acta Endocrinol (Copenh).* 1978;88:169.
124. Niven PAR, Buhi WC, Spellacy WN. The effect of intravenous estrogen injection on plasma human placental lactogen levels. *J Obstet Gynaecol Br Commonw.* 1974;81:466.
125. Felig P, Linch V. Starvation in human pregnancy: Hypoglycemia, hypoinsulinemia and hyperketonemia. *Science.* 1970;170:990.
126. Kim YJ, Felig P. Plasma chorionic somatomammotropin levels during starvation in mid-pregnancy. *J Clin Endocrinol Metab.* 1971;32:864.
127. Handwerger S, Barret J, Markoff BE, et al. Stimulation of human placental lactogen release by arachidonic acid. *Mol Pharmacol.* 1981;20:609.
128. Zeitler P, Murphy E, Handwerger S. Arachidonic acid stimulates ^{45}calcium efflux and hPL release in isolated trophoblast cells. *Life Sci.* 1986;38:99.
129. Zeitler P, Handwerger S. Arachidonic acid stimulates phosphoinositide hydrolysis and human placental lactogen release in an enriched praction of placental cells. *Mol Pharmacol.* 1985;28:549.
130. Letchworth AT. Human chorionic somatomammotropin. In: Klopper A, ed. *Plasma Hormone Assays in Evaluation of Fetal Well Being.* Edinburgh: Churchill Livingstone; 1976:147.
131. Grumbach MM, Kaplan SL, Vinek A. Human chorionic somatomammotropin (HCS). In: Berson SA, Yalow RS, eds. *Methods in Investigative and Diagnosis. Endocrinology.* Amsterdam: North Holland; 1973:797.
132. Josimovich JB, Atwood BL. Human placental lactogen (hPL), a trophoblastic hormone synergizing with chorionic gonadotropin and potentiating the anabolic effect of pituitary growth hormone. *Am J Obstet Gynecol.* 1964;88:867.
133. Lostroh AJ. Diabetogenic hormones (human choriosomatomammotropin and ovine growth hormone): Anti-insulin action in hypophysectomized rats. *Acta Endocrinol (Copenh).* 1974;77:96.
134. Tyson JE, Jones GS, Hutch J, et al. Pattens of insulin, growth hormone, and placental lactogen release after protein and glucose-protein ingestion in pregnancy. *Am J Obstet Gynecol.* 1971;110:934.
135. Grumbach MM, Kaplan SL, Abrams CL, et al. Plasma free fatty acid response to the administration of chorionic "growth hormone-prolactin." *J Clin Endocrinol Metabol.* 1966;26:478.
136. Desoye G, Shweditsch MO, Pfeiffer KP, et al. Correlation of hormones with lipids and lipoprotein levels during normal pregnancy and postpartum. *J Clin Endocrinol Metab.* 1987;64:704.
137. Nielsen PV, Pedersen H, Kampmann EM. Absence of human placental lactogen in an otherwise uneventful pregnancy. *Am J Obstet Gynecol.* 1979;135:322.
138. Speroff L, Glass RH, Kase NG. The endocrinology of pregnancy. In: *Clinical Gynecologic Endocrinology and Infertility.* 4th ed. Williams and Wilkins, 1989:317.
139. Simpson ER, Porter JC, Milewich L, et al. Regulation by plasma lipoproteins of progesterone biosynthesis and 3-hydroxy-3-methyl glutaryl coenzinae A reductase activity in cultured human choriocarcinoma cells. *J Clin Endocrinol Metab.* 1978;47:1099.
140. Lurie AO, Reid DE, Villee CA. The role of the fetus and placenta in maintenance of plasma progesterone. *Am J Obstet Gynecol.* 1966;96:670.
141. Simpson ER, Bilheimer DW, McDonald PC, Porter JC. Uptake and degradation of plasma lipoproteins by human choriocarcinoma cell in culture. *Endocrinology.* 1979;104:8.
142. Winkel CA, Snyder JM, MacDonald PC, Simpson ER. Regulation of cholesterol and progesterone synthesis in human placental cells in cultures by serum lipoproteins. *Endocrinology.* 1980;106:1054.
143. Winkel CA, Gilmore J, MacDonald PC, Simpson ER. Uptake and degradation of lipoproteins by human trophoblastic cells in primary culture. *Endocrinology.* 1980;107:1892.
144. Malassine A, Besse C, Roche A, et al. Ultrastructural localization visualization of the internalization of low density lipoproteins by human placental cells. *Histochemi.* 1987;87:457.
145. Simpson ER, Burkhart MF. Acyl CoA-cholesterol acyl transferase activity in human placental microsomes: inhibition by progesterone. *Arch Biochem Biophys.* 1980;200:79.
146. Miller WL. Molecular biology of steroid hormone synthesis. *Endocr Rev.* 1988;9:295.
147. Chung BC, Matteson KJ, Voutilainen R, et al. Human cholesterol side-chain cleavage enzyme P450scc: cDNA cloning, assignment of the gene to chromosome 15 and expression in the placenta. *Proc Natl Acad Sci USA.* 1986;83:8962.
148. Thomas JL, Myers RP, Strickler RC. Human placental 3β-hydroxy-5 ene-steroid dehydrogenase and steroid 5-4-ene-isomerase purification from mitochondria and kinetic profiles, biophysical characterization of the purified mitochondrial and microsomal enzymes. *J Steroid Biochem.* 1989;33:209.
149. Ishii-Ohba H, Saiki N, Inano H, Tamaoki B-I. Purification and Characterization of Rat Adrenal 3-5 Hydroxysteroid dehydrogenase with steroid 5-ene-4-ene-isomerase. *J Steroid Biochem.* 1988;24:753.
150. Henson MC, Pepe GJ, Albrecht ED. Transuterofetoplacental conversion of pregnenolone to progesterone in antiestrogen-treated baboons. *Endocrinology.* 1987;121:1265.
151. Dawood MY. Circulating maternal serum progesterone in high-risk pregnancies. *Am J Obstet Gynecol.* 1976;125:832.
152. Albrecht ED, Haskins AL, Pepe GJ. The influence of fetectomy at mid-gestation upon the serum concentration of progesterone, estrone and estradiol in baboons. *Endocrinology.* 1980;107:766.
153. Ryan KJ, Meigs R, Petro Z. The formation of progesterone by the human placenta. *Am J Obstet Gynecol.* 1966;96:676.
154. Macome JD, Bischoff K, Bai RU, Diczfalusy E. Factors influencing placental steroidogenesis invitro. *Steroids.* 1972;20:469.
155. Barnea ER, Fares F, Shahar K. Stimulatory effect of prolactin on human placental progesterone secretion at term *in vitro:* possible inhibitory effect on oestradiol secretion. *Placenta.* 1989;10:37.
156. Fylling P. Propanolol-blockade of vasopressin induced increase in plasma progesterone in early human pregnancy. *Acta Endocrinol. (Copenh).* 1971;66:283.
157. Siiteri PK, Seron-Ferre M. Some new thoughts on the fetoplacental unit and parturition in primates In: Novy MJ, Resko JA, eds. *Fetal Endocrinology.* New York, NY: Academic Press; 1981:1.
158. Grimshaw RN, Mitchell BF, Challis JRG. Steroid modulation of pregnenolone to progesterone conversion by human placental cells *in vitro.* *Am J Obstet Gynecol.* 1983;145:234.
159. Parker CR, Everett RB, Quirk JG, et al. Hormone production during pregnancy in the primigravid patient: I. Plasma levels of progesterone and 5α-pregnane-3, 20-dione throughout pregnancy of normal women and women who developed pregnancy induced hypertension. *Am J Obstet Gynecol.* 1979;135:778.
160. Parker CR, Everett RB, Whalley PJ, et al. Hormone production during pregnancy in the primigravid patient: II. Plasma levels of deoxycorticosterone throughout pregnancy of normal women and women who developed pregnancy-induced hypertension. *Am J Obstet Gynecol.* 1980;138:626.
161. Casey ML, MacDonald PC. Extraadrenal formation of a mineralocorticosteroid: deoxycorticosterone and deoxycorticosterone sulfate biosynthesis and metabolism. *Endocr Rev.* 1982;3:396.
162. Csapo AI, Pulkkinen MO, Ruttner B, et al. The significance of the human corpus luteum in pregnancy maintenance. I. Preliminary studies. *Am J Obstet Gynecol.* 1972;112:1061.
163. Rothchild I. Role of progesterone in initiating and maintaining pregnancy. In: Bardin CW, Milgrom E, Mauvais-Jarvis P, eds. *Progesterone and Progestins,* New York, NY: Raven Press; 1983:219.
164. Moriyama I, Sugawa T. Progesterone facilitates implantation of xenogenic cultured cells in hamster uterus. *Nature.* 1972;236:150.
165. Abraham GE, Samojlik E. Correlation between plasma unconjugated estriol and 16α-hydroxyprogesterone during human pregnancy. *Obstet Gynecol.* 1974;44:767.
166. Csapo AP, Wood C. The endocrine control of the initiation of labour in the human. In: James VHT, ed, *Recent Advances in Endocrinology.* London: Churchill; 1968:207.
167. Simonian MH, Capp MW. Characterization of steroidogenesis in cell cultures of the human fetal adrenal cortex: Comparison of definitive zone and fetal zone cells. *J Clin Endocrinol Metab.* 1984;59:643.
168. Buster JE, Abraham GE. The application of steroid hormone radioimmunoassays to clinical obstetrics. *Obstet Gynecol.* 1975;46:489.
169. Buster JE, Sakakini J Jr, Killam AP, et al. Serum conjugated estriol levels in the third trimester and their relationship to gestational age. *Am J Obstet Gynecol.* 1975;125:672.
170. Albrecht ED, Pepe GJ. Placental steroid hormone biosynthesis in primate pregnancy. *Endocr Rev.* 1990;11:124.
171. Madden JD, Gant NF, MacDonald PC. Study of the kinetics of conversion of maternal plasma dehydroisoandrosterone sulfate to 16α-hydroxydehydroisoandrosterone sulfate, estradiol, and estriol. *Am J Obstet Gynecol.* 1978;132:392.
172. Whittle MJ, Anderson D, Lowensohn RI, et al. Estriol in pregnancy. VI. Experience with unconjugated plasma estriol assays and antepartum fetal heart rate testing in diabetic pregnancy. *Am J Obstet Gynecol.* 1979;135:764.
173. Tulchinsky D. Placental secretion of unconjugated estrone estradiol and estriol into the maternal and fetal circulation. *J Clin Endocrinol Metab.* 1973;36:1079.
174. Cunningham FG, MacDonald PC, Gant NF. Parturition: biomolecular and physiological processes. In: *William Obstetrics,* 18th ed. Norwalk, CT: Appleton and Lange; 1989:187.
175. Roberts JM. Current understanding of pharmacologic mechanisms in the prevention of preterm birth. *Clin Obstet Gynecol.* 1984;27:592.
176. Garfield RE. Structural and functional studies of the control of myometrial contractility and labor. In: McNellis D, Challis JRG, MacDonald PC, et al, eds. *Cellular and Integrative Mechanisms in the Onset of Labor. An NICHD Workshop.* Ithaca, NY: Perinatology Press; 1988: 55.
177. Garfield RE. Control of myometrial function in preterm versus term labor. *Clin Obstet Gynecol.* 1984;27:572.

178. Garfield RE. Gap junctions: Their development, role, and regulation in the myometrium during parturition. In MacDonald PC, Porter JC, eds. *Initiation of Parturition: Prevention of Prematurity. Fourth Ross Conference on Obstetric Research, Ross Laboratories*. Columbus, OH: 1983;51.
179. Stull J, Taylor DA, MacKenzie LW, Casey ML. Biochemistry and physiology of smooth muscle contractility. In McNellis D, Challis JRG, MacDonald PC, et al, eds. *Cellular and Integrative Mechanisms in the Onset of Labor*. An NICHD Workshop. Ithaca, NY: Perinatology Press; 1988:17.
180. Nishizuka Y. The family of protein kinase c for signal transduction. *JAMA*. 1989;262:1826.
181. Naor Z. Signal transduction mechanisms: The case of gonadotropin releasing hormone. *Endocr Rev*. 1990;11:326.
182. Rasmussen H, Barret PQ. Calcium messenger system: An integrated view. *Physiol Rev*. 1984;64:938.
183. Challis JRG. Endocrinology of late pregnancy and parturition. *Int Rev Physiol*. 1980;22:277.
184. Bleasdale JE, Johnston JM. Prostaglandins and human parturition: regulation of arachidonic acid mobilization. *Rev Perinatal Med*. 1984;5:151.
185. Green K, Bygdeman M, Toppozada M, Wiquist N. The role of prostaglandin $F_{2\alpha}$ in human parturition. Endogenous plasma levels of 15-keto-13, 14-dihydro-prostaglandin $F_{2\alpha}$ during labor. *Am J Obstet Gynecol*. 1974;120:25.
186. Novy MJ, Liggins GC. Role of prostaglandin, prostacyclin, and thromboxanes in the physiologic control of the uterus and in parturition. *Semin Perinatol*. 1980;4:45.
187. Mitchell MD. Sources of eicosanoids within the uterus during pregnancy. In: McNellis D, Challis JRG, MacDonald PC, eds. *Cellular Integrative Mechanisms in the Onset of Labor. An NICHD Workshop*. Ithaca, NY: Perinatology Press; 1988:165.
188. Manabe Y, Okazaki T, Takahashi A. Prostaglandin E and F in amniotic fluid during stretched-induced cervical softening and labor at term. *Gynecol Obstet Invest*. 1981;15:343.
189. Irvine RF. How is the levels of free arachidonic acid controlled in mammalian cells. *Biochem J*. 1982;204:3.
190. Martin TW, Wysolmerski RB. CA^{2+} dependent and Ca^{2+} independent pathways for release of arachidonic acid from phosphatidylinositol in endothelial cells. *J Biol Chem*. 1987;262:13086.
191. Sammuelson B. Leukotrienes: Mediators of immediate hypersensitivity reactions and inflammation. *Science*. 1983;220:568.
192. Gerritsen ME. Eicosanoid production by the coronary microvascular endothelium. *Federation Proc*. 1987;46:47.
193. Mullane KM, Pinto A. Endothelium, arachidonic acid and coronary vascular tone. *Federation Proc*. 1987;46:54.
194. Ramwell PW, Foegh M, Loeb R, Leovey EMK. Synthesis and metabolism of prostaglandins, prostacyclin, and thromboxanes: the arachidonic acid cascade. *Seminars Perinatol*. 1980;4:3.
195. Okita JR, Johnston JM, MacDonald PC. Source of prostaglandin precursor in human fetal membranes: Arachidonic acid content of amnion and chorion laeve in diamniotic dichorionic twin placentas. *Am J Obstet Gynecol*. 1983;147:477.
196. Lye SJ, Challis JRG. Inhibition by PGI_2 of myometrial activity in vivo in non-pregnant ovariectomized sheep. *J Reprod Fert*. 1982;66:311.
197. Mitchell MD, Biddy J, Hicks BR, Turnbull AC. Specific production of prostaglandin E by human amnio *in vitro*. *Prostaglandins*. 1978;15:377.
198. Okazaki T, Casey ML, Okita JR, et al. Initiation of human parturition. XII. Biosynthesis and metabolism of prostaglandins in human fetal membranes and uterine decidua. *Am J Obstet Gynecol*. 1981;139:373.
199. Nakala S, Skimmer K, Mitchel BF, Challis JRG. Changes in prostaglandin transfer across human fetal membranes obtained after spontaneous labour. *Am J Obstet Gynecol*. 1986;155:1337.
200. Niesert S, Christopherson W, Korte K, et al. Prostaglandin E_2 9-ketreductase activity in human decidua vera tissue. *Am J Obstet Gynecol*. 1986;155:1348.
201. Casey ML, MacDonald PC. Biomolecular processes in the initiation of parturition decidual activation. *Clin Obstet Gynecol*. 1988;31:533.
202. Willman EA, Collins WP. Distribution of prostaglandin E_2 and $F_{2\alpha}$ within the fetoplacental unit throughout human pregnancy. J Endocrinol. 1976;69:413.
203. Liggins GC. Initiation of spontaneous labor. *Clin Obstet Gynecol*. 1983;26:47.
204. Liggins GC, Fairclough RJ, Grieves SA, et al. The mechanism of initiation of parturition in the ewe. *Recent Prog Horm Res*. 1973;29:111.
205. Smit DA, Essed GGM, Deltaan J. Predictive value of uterine contractility and the serum levels of progesterone and oestrogens with regard to preterm labour. *Gynecol Obstet Invest*. 1984;18:252.
206. Hanssens MCAJA, Selby C, Symonds EM. Sex steroid hormone concentrations in preterm labour and the outcome of treatment with ritodrin. *Br J Obstet Gynaecol*. 1985;92:698.
207. Topper Y. Multiple hormone interactions in the development of mammary gland *in vitro*. *Recet Prog Horm Res*. 1970;26:287.
208. Turnbull AC, Patten PT, Flint APF, et al. Significant fall in progesterone and rise in oestradiol levels in human peripheral plasma before onset of labour. *Lancet*. 1974;1:101.
209. Buster JE, Freeman AG, Tataryn IV, Hobel CJ. Time trend analysis of conjugated estriol concentrations in third trimester pregnancy. *Obstet Gynecol*. 1980;56:743.
210. Anderson PJB, Hancock KW, Oakey RE. Non-protein-bound oestradiol and progesterone in human peripheral plasma before labour and delivery. *J Endocrinol*. 1985;104:7.
211. Mitchell BF, Cruickshank B, Mclean D, Challis JRG. Local modulation of progesterone production in human fetal membranes. *J Clin Endocrinol Metab*. 1982;55:1237.
212. Gibb W, Lovoie JC, Roux JF. 3β-hydroxysteroid dehydrogenase activity in human fetal membranes. *Steroids*. 1978;32:365.
213. Turnbull AC. Influencing uterine contractility with oxytocin. In: Keirse MJNC, ed. *Human Parturition*. Martinus Nijhoff Publishers; 1979:143.
214. Calder AA. The management of the unripe cervix. In: Keirse MJNC, ed. *Human Parturition*. Martinus Nijhoff Publishers; 1979:201.
215. Fuchs AR, Fuchs F, Husslein P, et al. Oxytocin receptors and human parturition: A dual role for oxytocin in the initiation of labor. *Science*. 1982;215:1396.
216. Stabile I, Grudzinskas JG, Chard J. Clinical applications of pregnancy protein estimation with particular reference to pregnancy-associated plasma protein (PAPP-A). *Obstet Gynecol Survey*. 1988;43:73.
217. Grudzinskas JG, Westergaard JG, Teisner B. Biochemical assessment of placental function: early pregnancy clinics. *Obstet Gynecol*. 1986;13:553.
218. Westergaard JG, Teisner B, Grudzinskas JG. Biochemical assessment of placental function: late pregnancy clinics. *Obstet Gynecol*. 1986;13:571.
219. Chard T. Placental synthesis clinics. *Obstet Gynecol*. 1986;13:447.
220. Watanabe S, Chou JY. Human pregnancy-specific b-glycoprotein: A new member of the carcinoembryonic antigen gene family. *Biochem Res Commun*. 1988;152:762.
221. Mueller VW, Jones WR. Identification of an SP_1-like protein in non-pregnancy serum: Isolation using a monoclonal antibody. *J Reprod Immun*. 1985;8:111.
222. Seppala M, Iino K, Rutanen EM. Placental proteins in oncology clinics. *Obstet Gynecol*. 1986;13:593.
223. Bohn H, Winckler W. Isolierung und charaktesierung des plazenta-proteins PP5. *Arch Gynecol*. 1977;229:293.
224. Salem HT, Seppälä M, Chard T. The effect of thrombin on serum placental protein 5 (PP5): Is PP5 the naturally occurring antithrombin III of human placenta? *Placenta*. 1981;2:205.
225. Seppälä M, Wahlstrom T, Bohn H. Circulating levels and tissue localization of placental protein five (PP5) in pregnancy and trophoblastic disease. Absence of PP5 expression in malignant trophoblast. *Int J Cancer*. 1979;24:6.
226. Bohn H, Kraus W. Isolierung und charakterisierung eines neuen plazentaspezifischen protein (PP10). *Arch Gynecol*. 1980;227:125.
227. Wahlstrom T, Bohn H, Seppälä M. Immunohistochemical studies on pregnancy proteins. In: Grudzinskas JC, Seppala M, Teisner B, eds. *Pregnancy Proteins: Biology, Chemistry, and Clinical Application*. Sidney: Academic Press; 1982:415.
228. Joshi SG, Ebert KM, Swartz DP. Detection and synthesis of progesterone-dependent protein in the human endometrium. *J Reprod Fertil*. 1980;59:273.
229. Julkunen M, Raiker RS, Joshi SG, et al. Placental protein 14 and progesterone-dependent endometrial protein are immunologically indistinguishable. *Human Reprod*. 1986;1:7.
230. Bell SC, Fazleabas AT, Verhage HG. Comparative aspects of secretory proteins of the endometrium and decidua in human and non-human primates. In: Yoshinaga K, ed. *Blastocyst Implantation*. Boston, MA: Serono Symposia USA; 1989:151.
231. Fazleabas AT, Verhage HG, Bell SC. Steroid induced proteins of the primate oviduct and uterus: Potential regulators of reproductive function. In: Gulyas BJ, Lewis CK, eds. *Paracrine and Autocrine Interaction in Reproductive Endocrinology*. New York, NY: Plenum Press; 1989:115.
232. Bell SC, Patel SR, Kirwan PH, Drife JO. Protein synthesis and secretion by the human endometrium during the menstrual cycle and the effect of progesterone in vitro. *J Reprod Fert*. 1986;77:221.
233. Bell SC, Hales MW, Patel SR, et al. Amniotic fluid levels of secreted pregnancy-associated endometrial α 1- and α 2-globulins (α 1 and α 2-PEG). *Br J Obstet Gynaecol*. 1986;93:909.
234. Fazleabas AT, Verhage HG, Bell SC. Insulin-like growth factor binding protein and pregnancy: Regulation and function in the primate. In: Heyner S, Wiley L, eds. *Proceedings of the UCLA Symposium on Early Embryo Development and Paracrine Relationship*. New York, NY: Alan Liss; 1990. In Press.
235. Bell SC, Keyte JW. N-terminal amino acid sequence of human endometrial insulin-like growth factor binding protein-evidence for two forms of the small molecular weight IGF binding protein. *Endocrinology*. 1988;123:1202.
236. Bell SC, Bohn H. Immunochemical and biochemical relationship between human pregnancy-associated secreted endometrial α 1- and α

2-globulins (α 1- and α 2-PEG) and the soluble placental proteins 12 and 14 (PP12 and PP14). *Placenta*. 1986;7:283.
237. Giudice LC, Farrel EM, Pham H, et al. Insulin-like growth factor binding proteins in maternal serum throughout gestation and in the puerperium: Effects of a pregnancy associated serum protease activity. *J Clin Endocrinol Metab*. 1990;71:806.
238. Bell SC, Smith S. The endometrium as a paracrine organ. In: Chamberline GVP, ed. *Contemporary Obstetrics and Gynecology*. Butterworths Scientific; 1988:273.
239. Julkunen M, Koistinen R, Aalto-Setälä K, et al. Primary structure of human insulin-like growth factor-binding protein/placental protein 12 and tissue-specific expression of its mRNA. *FEBS Letters*. 1988;236:295.
240. Rutanen E-M, Koistinen R, Sjoberg J, et al. Synthesis of placental protein 12 by human endometrium. *Endocrinology*. 1986;118:1067.
241. Heffner LJ, Iddenden DA, Lyttle CR. Electrophoretic analysis of secreted human endometrial proteins: identification and characterization of luteal phase prolactin. *J Clin Endocrinol Metab*. 1986;62:1288.
242. Davey MW, Teisner B, Sinosich M, Grudzinskas JG. Interaction between heparin and human Pregnancy-Associated Plasma Protein-A (PAPP-A): A simple purification procedure. *Analyst Biochem*. 1983;131:18.
243. Westergaard JG, Chemnitz J, Teisner B, et al. Pregnancy-Associated Plasma Protein A: A possible marker in the classification and diagnosis of Cornelia de Lange Syndrome. *Prenat Diagn*. 1983;3:225.
244. Castracane VD, D'Eletto R, Weiss G. Relaxin secretion in the baboon (papio cynceplalus) In: Greenwald GS, Terranova PF, eds. *Factors Regulating Ovarian Functions*. New York, NY: Raven Press; 1983:415.
245. Sherwood OD, Downing SJ. The chemistry and physiology of relaxin. In: Greenwald GS, Terranova PF, eds. *Factors Regulating Ovarian Functions*. New York, NY: Raven Press; 1983:381.
246. Bryant-Greenwood GD. Relaxin is a new hormone. *Endocr Rev*. 1982;3:62.
247. Quagliarello J, Goldsmith L, Steinetz B, et al. Induction of relaxin secretion in nonpregnant women by human chorionic gonadotropin. *J Clin Endocrinol Metab*. 1980;51:74.
248. Schwabe C, Steinetz B, Weiss G, et al. Relaxin. *Recent Prog Horm Res*. 1978;34:123.
249. Hodgen GE, Itskovitz J. Recognition and maintenance of pregnancy In: Knobil E, Neil J, et al, eds. *The Physiology of Reproduction*. New York, NY: Raven Press; 1988:1995.
250. Mason AJ. Structure and recombinant expression of human inhibin and activin. In: Hodgen GD, Rosenwaks Z, Spieler JM, eds. *Nonsteroidal Gonadol Factors: Physiological Roles and Possibilities in Contraceptive Development*. Conrad Series, Jones Inst Press Va; 1988:19.
251. Ling N, Ying SY, Ueno N, et al. Pituitary FSH is released by an heterodimer of the b-subunits from the two forms of inhibin. *Nature*. 1986;321:779.
252. Massague J. The TGF-β family of growth and differentiation factors. *Cell*. 1987;49:437.
253. Vale W. Inhibin α-subunit cDNAs from porcine ovary and human placenta. *Proc Natl Acad Sci USA*. 1986;83:5849.
254. McLachlan RI, Healy DL, Robertson DM, et al. The human placenta: A novel source of inhibin. *Biochem Biophys Res Commun*. 1986;140:485.
255. Petraglia F, Vale W. Role of inhibin-related peptides in human placenta. In: Hodgen GD, Rosenwaks Z, Spieler JM, *Nonsteroidal Gonadal Factors: Physiological Roles and Possibilities in Contraceptive Development*. Conrad Series Jones Inst Press Va; 1988:181.
256. Mayo KE, Cerelli GM, Spiess J, et al. Localization, secretion and action of inhibin in human placenta. *Science*. 1987;237:187.
257. Gibbons JM, Mitnick M, Chieffo V. *In vitro* biosynthesis of TSH-, and LH-releasing factors by the human placenta. *Am J Obstet Gynecol*. 1975;121:127.
258. Tan L, Rousseau P. The chemical identity of the immunoreactive LHRH-like peptide biosynthesized in the human placenta. *Biochem Biophys Res Commun*. 1982;109:1061.
259. Khodr GS, Siler-Khodr TM. Placental luteinizing hormone releasing factor and its synthesis. *Science*. 1980;207:315.
260. Siler-Khodr TM, Khodr GS, Vickery BH, Nestor JJ. Inhibition of hCG alpha hCG and progesterone release from human placental tissue in vitro by a GnRH antagonist. *Life Sci*. 1983;32:2741.
261. Talamantes F, Ogren L. The placenta as an endocrine organ: Polypeptides. In: Knobil E, Neil J, et al, eds. *The Physiology of Reproduction*. New York: Raven Press; 1988:2093.

Chapter Thirty-Eight

Endorphins in Fetomaternal Physiology

Christina Gianoulakis and Michel Chrétien

38

Following the demonstration of specific opiate receptors in the nervous system of vertebrates and the isolation of a number of endogenous opioid ligands (β-endorphin, enkephalins, dynorphins, and neoendorphins) for these receptors, it was suggested that interactions of endogenous opioid peptides with opiate receptors may be involved in regulating some physiologic processes. Initially, the analgesic activity of the endogenous opioids was investigated. However, various types of stress stimulate the release of endogenous opioid peptides, suggesting that they may be important in the adaptation of the organism to various stressful situations. Endorphins also were found to modulate the release of prolactin (PRL) and of the gonadotropin hormones, luteinizing hormone (LH) and follicle-stimulating hormone (FSH), from the anterior pituitary in humans and experimental animals. They also influence the reproductive behavior in animals.

Furthermore, a number of publications indicate that during the latter stages of pregnancy and especially during labor, plasma β-endorphin levels are significantly increased in humans[1] and experimental animals.[2] It was suggested that these increased plasma β-endorphin levels were responsible for the increase of pain threshold observed in pregnant animals[3] and for some of the psychologic responses during pregnancy and parturition. Because endorphins are associated with feelings of euphoria and analgesia, it is possible that one of their functions during delivery is to enable the mother to cope with the severe pain of labor. This is very important for most animals because the mother must clean and feed the pups immediately after delivery. Undoubtedly, there was a time during the early evolution of humans when the mother herself had to clean and feed the human infant immediately after birth. Therefore, possibly a form of euphoria is produced by the increased release of β-endorphin during labor that acts as a positive reward and helps the mother to cope with the severe pain of labor. In this way, she is willing to care for her young infant and repeat the process of pregnancy and pain of labor.

Endorphins also may be important for the developing fetus because endorphinlike peptides have been detected in the fetal brain and pituitary gland very early in gestational life.[4,5] In this chapter, the various forms of endogenous opioid peptides, their origin, biosynthesis, distribution, and possible involvement in the processes of pregnancy and fetal development are discussed.

ENDOGENOUS OPIOID PEPTIDES

Shortly after the isolation of methionine–enkephalin (Met–Enk) and leucine–enkephalin (Leu–Enk) by Hughes and Kosterlitz, it was noticed that the pentapeptide sequence of Met–Enk (Tyr–Gly–Gly–Phe–Met) was identical to that of residues 61–65 of the hypophyseal hormone β-lipotropin (β-LPH). This observation led to the discovery, isolation, and characterization of β-endorphin (β-EP) by a number of investigators and in such varied species as camel, cow, pig, sheep, and human. β-Endorphin is the C-terminal fragment of β-LPH containing the β-LPH 61–91 amino acid residues and was shown to be a potent analgesic compound. The next endogenous opioids to be discovered were the dynorphins and neoendorphins. Both dynorphins and neoendorphins were isolated from posterior pituitary extracts.

CONCEPT OF PROHORMONES

The biosynthesis of enkephalins, endorphins, dynorphins, and neoendorphins involves the synthesis of larger proteins known as precursors or prohormones. The synthesis and maturation of these prohormones follow a sequence of events similar to those described for other secretory proteins. The first event is the initiation of protein synthesis on free ribosomes. This is followed by the attachment of the ribosomes to the membrane of the endoplasmic reticulum. This attachment is mediated by the presence of the signal peptides (the initial 15–30 amino acid residues of the prohormone), and the accompanying complex is called *signal peptide recognition particle* (SRP). The next step is the discharge of the peptide chain in the cisternal space of the rough endoplasmic reticulum with the simultaneous enzymatic cleavage of the signal peptide and glycosylation. The final step is the maturation of the prohormone into active molecules, which is completed during the transport through the Golgi complex and in the secretory granules. This maturation process involves different modifications such as N- and O-glycosylation; cleavage at sites characterized by the presence of pairs of basic amino acids, as was noted in 1967–1968 for the β-LPH and the proinsulin models; and chemical modifications of amino acid residues, such as acetylation, amidation, and phosphorylation.

To determine whether a protein is the precursor to a smaller peptide hormone, the following criteria must be satisfied:

1. Pulse-labeling and pulse-chase experiments must be carefully conducted to establish the precursor–product relationship between the high and low molecular weight forms of the proteins.
2. Immunoprecipitation experiments with well-characterized antibodies raised against the hormone must specifically precipitate the higher and the lower molecular weight forms of the hormones.
3. Peptide mapping of the precursor tryptic digestion fragments must demonstrate the existence, within the larger molecular weight form, of peptides characteristic of the active hormone together with additional fragments.
4. Sequence analysis of the putative precursor, the protein itself, or its cDNA counterpart, must reveal the existence of additional peptide(s) covalently linked to the active component(s).

Any of these findings alone constitutes suggestive evidence for the existence of a precursor for a given hormone, but conclusive proof can be obtained only through careful structural analysis of the putative precursor. Pulse-chase experiments and sequencing of the precursor to show an additional fragment covalently linked to the correct sequence for the active hormone constitute the final proof that the larger protein is the biosynthetic precursor of the smaller peptides.

Three distinct precursor proteins giving rise to opiate-active peptides have been characterized:

1. The precursor to β-EP, known as preproopiomelanocortin (POMC) because it also contains within its structure the sequence of adrenal corticotropic hormone (ACTH), of α-melanocyte-stimulating hormone (α-MSH) and of β-melanocyte-stimulating hormone (β-MSH)
2. The preproenkephalin, which contains within its sequence five molecules of Met–Enk and one molecule of Leu–Enk
3. The preprodynorphin, which is processed to dynorphins and neoendorphins

BIOSYNTHESIS AND POST-TRANSLATIONAL PROCESSING OF PREPROOPIOMELANOCORTIN

Cells able to synthesize POMC have been described in the anterior and intermediate lobes of the pituitary gland, the arcuate nucleus, and nucleus tractus solitarious of the brain and the placenta.[5,6] As previously shown for proinsulin, pairs of basic amino acids mark the major proteolytic cleavage sites of POMC (Fig. 38–1). Though similar precursor molecules are found in the anterior and intermediate lobes of the pituitary gland and in the arcuate nucleus and the placenta[5,6], the post-translational processing of the precursor molecules differs in the various tissues.[7] In the anterior lobe, POMC gives rise mainly to ACTH, β-LPH, γ-lipotropic hormone (γ-LPH), β-endorphin, the large N-terminal glycopeptide (HNT), and a joining peptide (HJP) separating it from the ACTH (see Fig. 38–1). In the human fetal intermediate lobe and in fetal and adult intermediate lobes in species such as the rat and in the brain arcuate nucleus, the final maturation products of POMC are α-MSH ($ACTH_{1-13}$) and the corticotropinlike intermediary peptide (CLIP) ($ACTH_{18-39}$) instead of ACTH and β-MSH (or γ-LPH in rat) and β-EP instead of β-LPH (Fig. 38–2).

Furthermore, studies have shown that $\beta\text{-EP}_{1-31}$ can be further processed to α-EP ($\beta\text{-EP}_{1-16}$), γ-EP ($\beta\text{-EP}_{1-17}$), and $\beta\text{-EP}_{1-27}$, $\beta\text{-EP}_{1-26}$, and their α-N-acetylated forms[7] (Fig. 38–3). The α-N-acetylation is very important because it alters the activity of the peptides; α-N-acetylation enhances the activity of α-MSH, whereas it decreases the steroidogenic potency of ACTH and abolishes the opiate activity of β-EP. Furthermore, it was found that different forms of β-EP fragments predominate in different regions of the pituitary and brain. In the anterior lobe and the hypothalamus, the opiate-active nonacetylated forms of β-EP predominate, whereas in the intermediate lobe, the opiate inactive α-N-acetylated forms of β-EP predominate (≈90%). The midbrain and amygdala contain $\beta\text{-EP}_{1-31}$ and $\beta\text{-EP}_{1-26}$ with negligible amounts of the acetylated fragments. However, the hippocampus, dorsal colliculi, and brainstem contain mainly the α-N-acetylated forms of $\beta\text{-EP}_{1-27}$ and $\beta\text{-EP}_{1-26}$. The fact that different forms of β-EP predominate in different regions of the pituitary and brain implies that there are region-

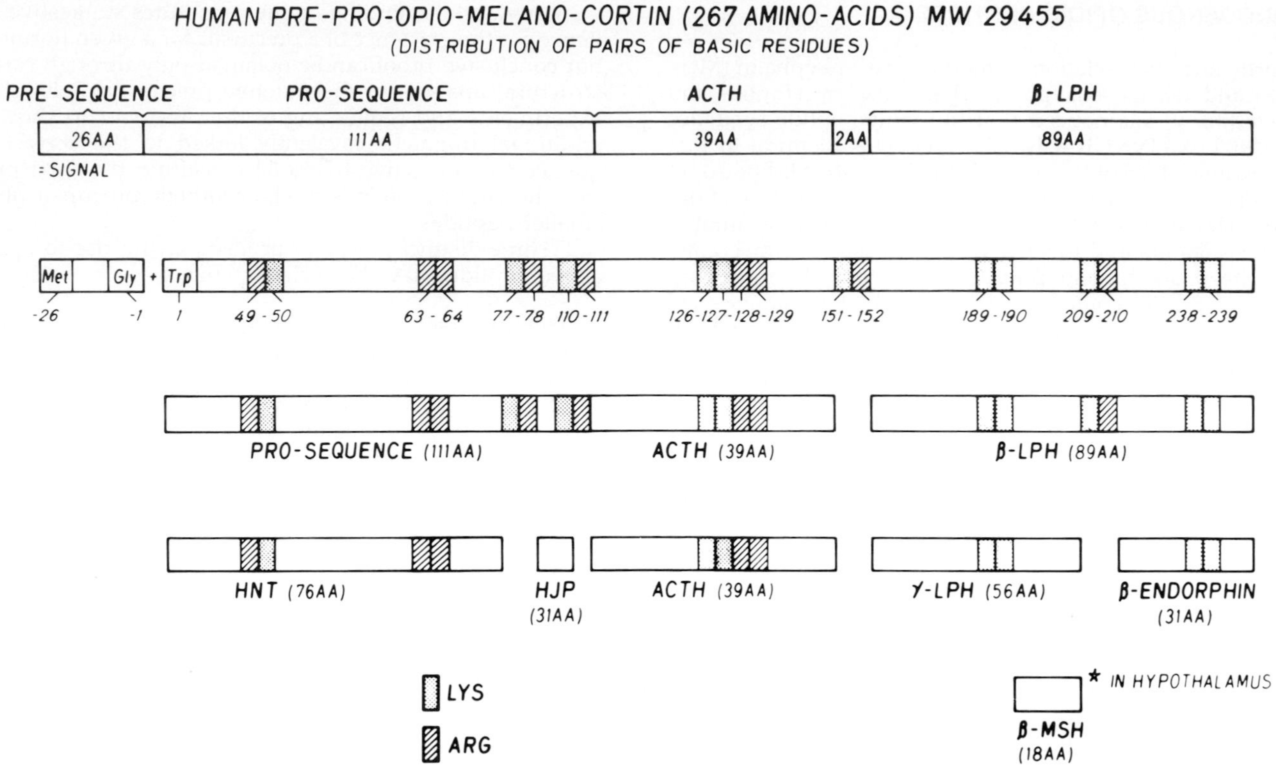

Figure 38–1. General model for maturation of human preproopiomelanocortin (POMC) molecule. (267 amino acids, molecular weight 29,455). The bottom part represents the isolated and completely characterized peptides from human pituitaries. The length of the human N-terminal (HNT) glycosylated peptide and the human joining peptide (HJP) isolated are given in parentheses as 76 and 31 amino acids, respectively. Exclusive cleavage at the pair of basic residues Lys–Arg is emphasized.

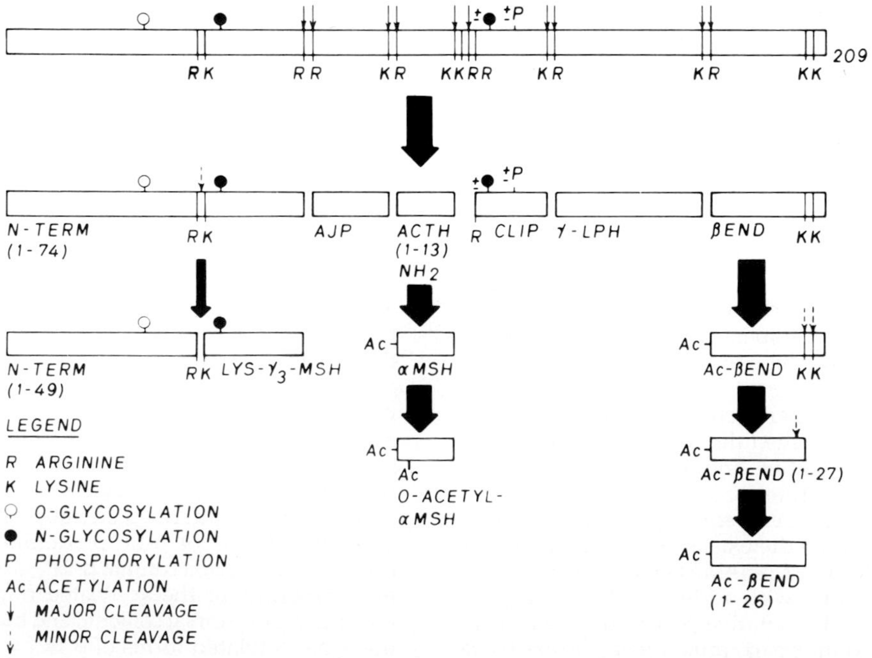

Figure 38–2. Model for the maturation of preproopiomelanocortin in rat pars intermedia and hypothalamus.

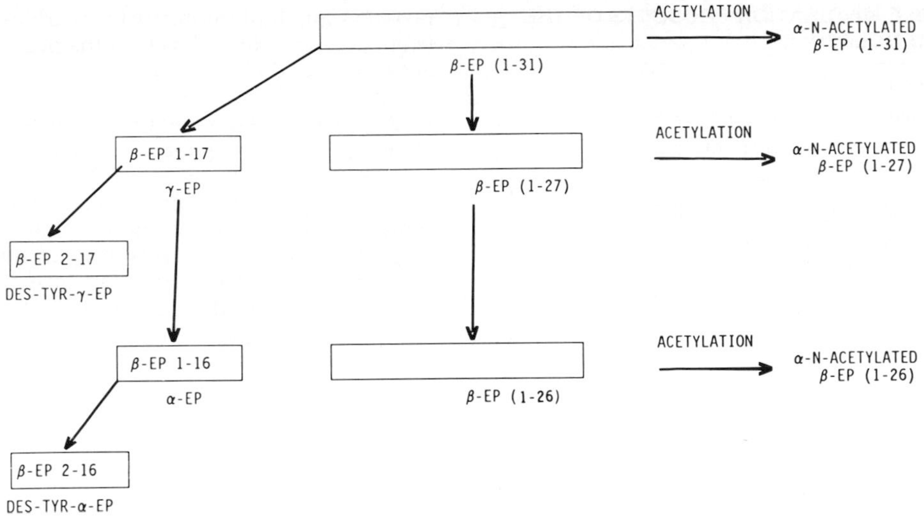

Figure 38–3. Secondary processing of β-endorphin 1–31 in pars intermedia or brain.

specific differences in the processing of POMC determined by the controlled action of specific enzymes located in those regions. It is uncertain whether the processing mechanisms of POMC are influenced by environmental stimuli and physiologic conditions, such as stress, pregnancy, age, sex, and drug treatments.

BIOSYNTHESIS AND POST-TRANSLATIONAL PROCESSING OF PROENKEPHALIN

Met–Enk and Leu–Enk were the first two endogenous opiate peptides to be isolated. The Met–Enk amino acid sequence is identical to the sequence of the first five amino acids of β-EP. However, Met–Enk and β-EP do not share the same precursor. Met–Enk is the maturation product of a distinctly different precursor protein known as preproenkephalin.[8] Preproenkephalin is synthesized in the brain, spinal cord, gut, and adrenal medulla.[9,10] The primary structure of the preproenkephalin has been demonstrated by use of the cDNA transcript of specific mRNA. If, as observed with POMC and other prohormones, the proteolytic cleavage on the preproenkephalin molecule occurs at the basic amino acids, then the preproenkephalin could give rise to one molecule of Met–Enk, one molecule of Leu–Enk, and five longer Met–Enk molecules ranging in length from seven to 48 amino acids (Fig. 38–4). These five long Met–Enk molecules could be cleaved further at pairs of basic amino acids and could give rise to three molecules of Met–Enk, one molecule of Met–Enk–Arg^6–Phe^7, and one molecule of Met–Enk–Arg^6–Gly^7–Leu^8 as well as a number of non-enkephalin-containing peptides (see Fig. 38–4 and Table 38–1). Because there are distinct neuronal systems expressing the preproenkephalin gene, the post-translational maturation processing of preproenkephalin may be different in each neuronal system, thus giving rise to different enkephalin molecules distinct for each system. Only pulse-chase experiments or purification studies of the maturation products will reveal the nature of the real secretory end products.

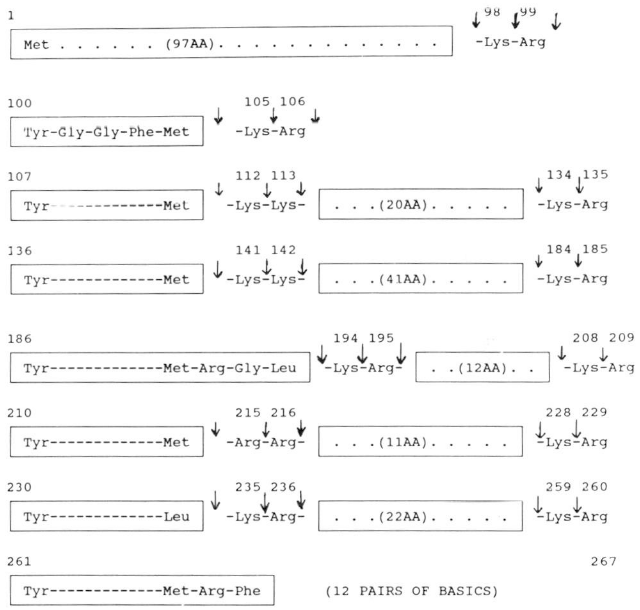

Figure 38–4. General model for the maturation of preproenkephalin. The sites of possible cleavages are indicated, and the end-products are described. If the Lys–Arg pair is the only cleavage site, the preproenkephalin molecule will give rise to one molecule each of Met–Enk (amino acids 100–104) and Leu–Enk (amino acids 230–234), one Met–Enk of 27 residues (amino acids 107–133), one Met–Enk of 48 residues (amino acids 136–183), one Met–Enk of eight residues (amino acids 186–193), one Met–Enk of 18 residues (amino acids 210–227), one Met–Enk of seven residues (amino acids 261–267), three nonenkephalin-related peptides, one of 97 residues (minus the signal peptide), one of 12 residues (amino acids 196–207), and one of 22 residues (amino acids 237–258). If the other pairs are cleaved, the secretory pattern becomes simpler. One gets one molecule of Leu–Enk and three types of Met–Enk: four molecules of regular Met–Enk and one each of seven and eight amino acids.

TABLE 38–1. POSSIBLE MATURATION PRODUCTS OF THE PREPROENKEPHALIN MOLECULE

One molecule of Met–Enk (5 AA)
One molecule of Met–Enk (5 or 27 AA)
One molecule of Met–Enk (5 or 48 AA)
One molecule of Met–Enk (8 AA)
One molecule of Met–Enk (5 or 18 AA)
One molecule of Leu–Enk (5 AA)
One molecule of Met–Enk (7 AA)

BIOSYNTHESIS AND POST-TRANSLATIONAL PROCESSING OF PRODYNORPHIN

Following the demonstration of the primary structures of POMC and preproenkephalin, it was noted that neither POMC nor preproenkephalin contained within its structure the sequences of α- and β-neoendorphin and dynorphin, suggesting a different precursor molecule for these peptides. The primary structure of a precursor protein containing both neoendorphins, dynorphin, and a third Leu–Enk sequence with a carboxyl extension was deduced from the cloned DNA sequence complementary to the porcine hypothalamic mRNA coding for dynorphin and neoendorphins.[11] This precursor protein, which is also called preproenkephalin B, gives rise to one molecule each of α- and β-neoendorphin, one molecule of dynorphin A, and one molecule of either dynorphin B or of an extended form of Leu–Enk (Fig. 38–5).

DISTRIBUTION OF ENDOGENOUS OPIATE PEPTIDES

Since the isolation of the endogenous opioid peptides, extensive studies have been performed using both radioimmunoassays and immunohistochemistry to investigate the distribution and relative levels of the opiate peptides in different tissues and brain areas.

β-Endorphinlike immunoreactivity has been demonstrated in the anterior and intermediate lobes of the pituitary gland, the brain, the pancreas, and the reproductive system. However, biosynthesis of β-EP has been seen only in the cells of the pituitary gland, brain arcuate nucleus, and placenta. Initially it was thought that brain β-EP was of pituitary origin because hypophysectomy did not alter the levels of brain β-EP, so an extrapituitary origin of the brain β-EP was strongly indicated. Most of the brain β-EP is synthesized in the cell bodies of hypothalamic neurons located in the arcuate nucleus. In addition, a small group of neurons in the nucleus tractus solitarious is synthesizing β-endorphinlike peptides. From the arcuate nucleus, endorphinergic neurons project to various areas of the brain.[12] From endorphinergic neurons of the nucleus tractus solitarious, fibers project to the spinal cord and to the hypothalamus.[12,13] Until recently, it was generally accepted that β-EP peptides are absent from the rat spinal cord except in early postnatal life.[14] However, the presence of fibers, but not cell bodies, containing POMC peptides has been demonstrated in the adult rat spinal cord.[15] The POMC, mRNA, and β-EPLPs also have been shown to exist in the gonads, pancreas, and placeba.[16] Highest concentrations of β-EP are found in the hypothalamus, central gray matter, amygdala, and nucleus accumbens. It is interesting that a similar pattern of distribution is found for ACTH (Table 38–2).

The enkephalins, Met–Enk and Leu–Enk, are widely distributed in the central and peripheral nervous systems. They also are found in the gut and in the adrenal medulla. Usually Met–Enk and Leu–Enk are found in the same areas, and Met–Enk is always present in higher concentration. In the brain, their distribution is uneven; some areas have higher amounts of enkephalins than others. Radioimmunoassay and immunohistochemical studies have been per-

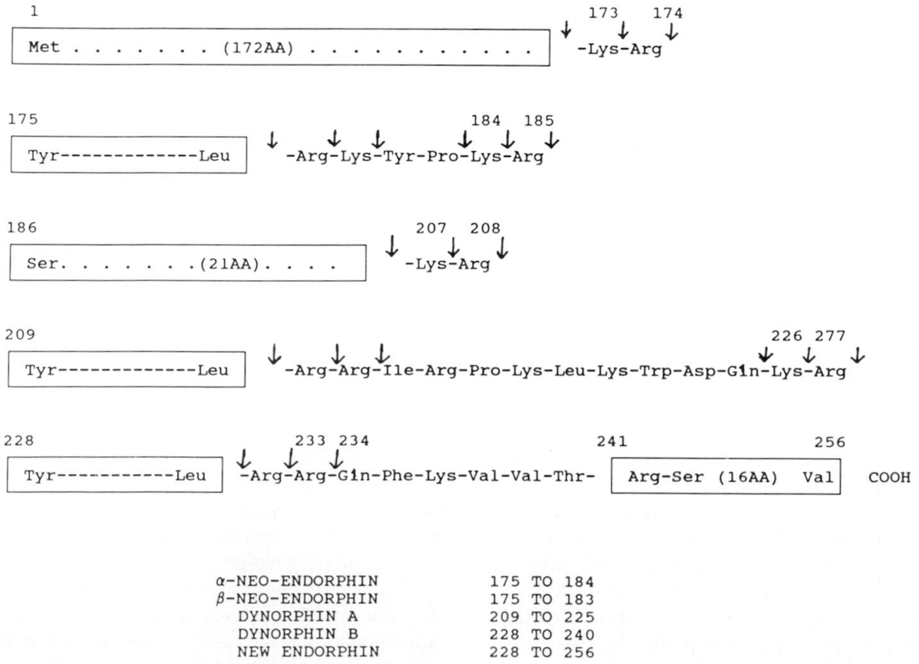

Figure 38–5. Model for the maturation of preprodynorphin and list of the final maturation products. Arrows indicate the possible sites of cleavage.

TABLE 38–2. COMPARATIVE DISTRIBUTION OF β-ENDORPHIN, ACTH, MET-ENK, AND DYNORPHIN IN THE RAT BRAIN

Brain Areas	β-Endorphin	ACTH	Met–Enk	Dynorphin
Hypothalamus	+++++	+++++	+++	+++++
Central gray matter	++++	++++	++++	Present
Midbrain	++++	++	+	++++
Amygdala	+++	+++	+++	Present
Nucleus accumbens	+++	++	++++	Present
Medulla	++	++++	+	++++
Pons	++	+++	+	++++
Cerebellum	++	++	+	+
Caudate–putamen	+	++	++++	+
Globus pallidus	+	+	+++++	++
Thalamus	+	++++	+	Absent
Hippocampus	+	++	+	+++

formed, and the results obtained are in agreement. Both types of studies show that the highest enkephalin levels are in the globus pallidus, followed by central gray matter of mesencephalon, nucleus accumbens, caudate–putamen, and amygdala (central amygdaloid nucleus). Cell bodies containing enkephalins are found in arcuate, retromedial, premamilary, paraventricular, and perifornical nuclei, nucleus raphe magnus, nucleus tractus spinalis of the fifth cranial nerve, and the dorsal horn of the spinal cord.[17,18] Leu–Enk and Met–Enk show the same pattern of distribution supporting their origin from the same precursor.[17,18] It is interesting that globus pallidus, an area rich in enkephalins is very poor in β-EP content (see Table 38–2). It also is noteworthy that there is a good correlation between the distributions of enkephalins and of opiate receptors.

The opioid peptide, dynorphin, which was originally extracted from porcine pituitaries, has been found in the neurohypophysis, hypothalamus, cortex, hippocampus, medulla–pons, spinal cord, and dorsal root ganglia of the rat as well as in the duodenum, the adrenal medulla, and the placenta. Immunohistochemical studies have demonstrated that the neoendorphins and dynorphins, peptides with the same precursor, coexist in the various areas of the brain. Cell bodies containing α-neoendorphin and dynorphin were seen in the supraoptic, retrochiasmatic supraoptic, paraventricular, and magnocellular accessory nuclei of the hypothalamus, and α-neoendorphin- and dynorphin-immunostainable fibers were found in the median forebrain bundle, the internal capsule, the substantia nigra, the hypothalamus, the nucleus accumbens, the hippocampus, and the medulla oblongata. Only a few fibers containing α-neoendorphin–dynorphin were seen in the cerebral cortex and striatum of rat brain.[19,20]

ENDOGENOUS OPIOIDS AND GONADOTROPINS

Although most of the research on opiates has centered on the effects of endogenous opioids on pain, stress, behavior, and psychiatric diseases, their presence in relatively high concentrations in the hypothalamus and pituitary suggests that they also may have endocrine functions. In fact, there is strong evidence indicating that the endogenous opioid peptides are involved in the regulation of pituitary hormone secretion. Administration of morphine, β-EP, and Met–Enk increased the serum concentration of PRL and growth hormone (GH) and decreased serum concentrations of LH and FSH.[21,22] These changes in the serum concentration of pituitary hormones after administration of either morphine or endogenous opioid peptides were prevented by the simultaneous administration of naloxone, a classic opiate antagonist. Furthermore, administration of naloxone alone to experimental animals decreased basal concentrations of GH and PRL and increased serum LH and FSH levels, indicating that endogenous opioid peptides influence basal secretion of anterior pituitary hormones. Further evidence that the endogenous opioid peptides may have a physiologic role in regulating PRL secretion was provided by the observation that the stress-induced PRL release could be inhibited by prior injection of naloxone or naltrexone. Stress is shown to increase the concentration of

TABLE 38–3. ENDORPHIN IN MATERNAL PLASMA AND CEREBROSPINAL FLUID

Physiologic Condition	Plasma β-EPLIA[a] (pg/mL)	CSF β-EPLIA (pg/mL)
Nonpregnant	63.5 ± 18.2[b1]	36.5 ± 15.8[b1]
	50.9 ± 6.2[b28]	
	232 ± 10[b29]	
	8.6 ± 1.5[c27]	
Pregnant	285 ± 19[b,d29]	60.1 ± 20.3[b,e1]
Elective cesarean	64.0 ± 12.2[b1]	57.5 ± 8.4[b1]
	85.8 ± 16.5[b28]	
	24.9 ± 3.7[c27]	
Active labor	110.8 ± 30.3[b1]	48.5 ± 8.3[b1]
	350 ± 19[b29]	
	29.9 ± 5.4[c28]	
Postpartum 24–48 h	7.8 ± 2.7[c28]	—

[a] β-EPLIA = β-endorphinlike immunoreactivity. Values are mean ± SEM β-Endorphin results published as femtomoles per milliliter have been multiplied by 3.4 to convert to picograms per milliliter. Direct comparison of all the results is difficult because of differences among antibodies, affinities, and specificities in the various studies.
[b] Values include β-endorphin and β-lipotropin.
[c] Values include β-endorphin only because the antiserum did not recognize β-lipotropin.
[d] Weeks 19–37 of pregnancy.
[e] Weeks 16–20 of pregnancy.

endogenous opioid peptides in the hypothalamus. This increased concentration of endogenous opioid peptides could mediate the increase in the PRL release after stress.

Administration of morphine during the critical period on the afternoon of proestrus in a rat prevented the normal LH surge and ovulation. In humans, a single injection of morphine was found to increase serum PRL. In addition, administration of methadone and pentazocine, two widely used analgesic opiates, increases serum PRL levels in women with breast cancer. Female narcotic addicts frequently exhibit amenorrhea, infertility, and spontaneous abortion. Injections of naloxone or naltrexone can inhibit the growth of PRL-dependent mammary tumors in rats, probably by decreasing the release of PRL.

It is clear that the endogenous opioids have an effect on the function of the pituitary gland. Many studies have been performed to elucidate the mechanism of action by which the opioid peptides influence the release of pituitary hormones. In general, opiates do not act directly on the pituitary gland because many of their effects cannot be demonstrated *in vitro*. However, there is convincing evidence that the action of opiates is mediated at least in part by their effects on the activity of hypothalamic neurons carrying biogenic amines or other neurotransmitters, which can influence the release of hypothalamic hypophysiotropic hormones into the portal vessels. It has been demonstrated that opiates decrease dopamine metabolism and increase serotonin metabolism in the hypothalamus. Furthermore, dopamine is known to decrease PRL and to increase GH release, whereas serotonin increases PRL and GH release and decreases LH and FSH release.[23] Thus, inhibition of dopamine by opiates would enhance PRL secretion, whereas stimulation of serotonin by opiates would induce an increased release of PRL and decreased release of LH and FSH.

As mentioned previously, neither morphine nor endogenous opioid peptides can alter PRL, FSH, and LH secretion by the pituitary gland *in vitro*. However, dopamine is known to have a direct *in vitro* inhibitory effect only on the PRL release by the pituitary gland. Recently, it was shown that although morphine and endogenous opioids have no effect on the basal release of prolactin *in vitro;* however, they could suppress the inhibitory effect of dopamine on PRL release, strongly suggesting a direct action of opioid peptides on the pituitary. Furthermore, this effect of opiates was dose dependent and naloxone reversible, indicating that it is mediated by specific opioid receptors on the anterior pituitary cells. In fact, opioid receptors have been identified in the pituitary gland in the anterior lobe and the neurohypophysis. High levels of β-endorphin have been demonstrated in the hypophyseal portal blood, suggesting that endogenous opioid peptides of hypothalamic origin are secreted into the portal blood and may directly influence the function of the anterior pituitary cell. Opiates bind to opiate receptors and interact with dopamine receptors to block the inhibitory effect of dopamine on PRL release.

ENDOGENOUS OPIOIDS IN PREGNANCY

Many studies have shown that plasma β-endorphin, β-LPH, and ACTH levels increase during pregnancy, reaching maximum levels during labor in women and in experimental animals.[23-28] Furthermore, β-EP was found in the placenta, and biosynthesis of β-EP by human placental trophoblastic cells in tissue culture has been demonstrated. Pulse-chase experiments suggested that the β-EP in the placenta is synthesized as part of a larger precursor protein similar to the proopiomelanocortin synthesized by the pituitary gland and brain arcuate nucleus.[6] The biosynthesis of POMC by the placental cells explains the observation that all the hormones originating from POMC (ACTH, β-LPH, β-EP, and β-MSH) are present in the human placenta. Recently, it was shown that the human placenta contains, in addition to β-EP, several forms of dynorphin peptides, which could account for about half of the total endogenous opiatelike peptides in the placenta. Because the placental concentration of dynorphin is 57.6 pmoles/g of tissue, comparable to the concentration in human brain and pituitary (3.0–120 pmoles/g of tissue), whereas the dynorphin in human plasma is less than 1 pmole/mL, it has been suggested that placental dynorphin is synthesized in the placenta itself. Not much placental opiate activity corresponding to enkephalins has been detected. However, the possibility that some enkephalins may be produced in some specialized placental cells cannot be excluded.

It is interesting that although in nonpregnant women the molar ratio of plasma β-LPH to β-EP is 6 to 1, in pregnant women, this ratio changes to 1 to 6. Thus, not only is the absolute amount of β-endorphinlike immunoreactivity (β-EPLIA) in the serum increased, but there also is a change in the molar ratio of β-LPH to β-EP.[27] It is not clear whether this change reflects changes in the usual biosynthetic pathways in the anterior pituitary or if a new source of β-EP is activated during pregnancy, such as the intermediate lobe, which is known to process POMC to β-EP rather than β-LPH. Although the fetal pituitary has an intermediate lobe, it involutes after parturition, and in the adult, no distinct intermediate lobe is found. However, it has been reported that pregnant women could develop a more distinct intermediate lobe, which could be responsible for the increased β-EP levels in circulation and the change in the relative molar ratio of β-LPH to β-EP.[27] The increased levels of α-MSH and β-MSH during pregnancy support this possibility. Because the intermediate lobe of the pituitary gland produces β-EP in the acetylated form, it would be interesting to investigate the proportion of nonacetylated β-EP to acetylated β-EP in the plasma of pregnant women.

Plasma levels of β-EP and β-LPH increase during pregnancy.[24-28] However, because of the blood–brain barrier, concentrations of β-EP and β-LPH in plasma may have no correlation with their levels in brain and cerebrospinal fluid (CSF), as shown by studies investigating the changes of β-EPLIA in CSF with pregnancy and labor.[1] These results, of course, do not exclude the possibility of changes in β-EP levels in such distinct brain areas as the hypothalamus and periaqueductal gray matter or changes of other such endogenous opioid peptides as enkephalins and dynorphins in both brain and CSF.

In view of the various known properties of opiates, it is possible to speculate on a number of physiologic effects of β-EP in pregnancy and in the process of parturition.

Analgesia and Mood Changes

β-Endorphin is a potent analgesic compound. It is possible that the increased plasma levels of β-EP during parturition help the mother to endure the severe pain of labor. In fact, it was shown that the pain threshold increases in the rat during pregnancy, reaching a maximum at the time of parturition, whereas during the postpartum period it shows a transient hyperalgesia before the pain threshold returns to baseline levels.[3] The plasma β-EP levels follow a similar pattern[27], increasing during pregnancy, reaching maximum levels during parturition, and decreasing postpartum (Table 38–3). The postpartum decrease of β-EP levels may be the cause of the observed hyperalgesia. Implantation of a naltrexone (opiate antagonist) pellet in pregnant rats prevented the increase in pain threshold, indicating the involvement of the opiate receptors. However, implantation of a naltrexone pellet in nonpregnant female rats has no effect on pain threshold.[3] It appears that during pregnancy in the rat, there is activation of an opioid system that is quiescent in nonpregnant female rats. Furthermore, because β-EP is associated with mood changes and is shown to suppress hostility, irritability, and anxiety, the increased β-EP levels during pregnancy may render the female psychologically better able to cope with the stress of pregnancy, whereas the decreased postpartum β-EP levels may be responsible for the postpartum depression often noticed in humans after parturition.

This hypothesis of the involvement of plasma β-EP in analgesia and mood disposition during pregnancy is very attractive; however, there is a great deal of evidence against it.

Plasma β-EP that is synthesized and secreted by the pituitary gland cannot easily penetrate the blood–brain barrier, so its concentration in the CSF does not change during the course of pregnancy and labor; therefore, plasma β-EP cannot reach the centers in the brain associated with analgesia and mood changes.

Following intravenous administration of β-EP, analgesic effects have been observed only when the β-EP concentration reaches levels that are much higher than the maximum plasma β-EP concentration observed in pregnant women during labor.

There is no correlation between plasma β-EP concentration and pain threshold or anxiety levels in pregnant women.[27] However, β-EP administered intrathecally to women during labor and delivery relieved the pain, suggesting a possible clinical use of β-EP or other endogenous opioid peptides.

Modulation of Hormone Release

In addition to the analgesic and behavioral effects of β-EP during pregnancy, another physiologic role of plasma β-EP could be to modulate the release of the reproductive hormones PRL, LH, and FSH and growth hormone by the anterior pituitary gland and of vasopressin by the neurohypophysis. The importance of PRL in the development of the mammary glands during pregnancy is well known, and β-EP increases the prolactin release. The opiate peptides of placental origin, β-EP and dynorphin, may be involved in controlling the release of the placental peptide hormones.

Peripheral Effects

A peripheral effect of plasma β-EP in gut motility is unlikely because a concentration range of 10^{-8} M is needed for such an effect, and the plasma β-EP levels during pregnancy reach a maximum concentration in the range of 10^{-10} M.

In summary, although a number of physiologic roles may be attributed to the increased plasma β-EP levels during pregnancy and parturition, these are speculative, and the exact role of plasma β-EP during pregnancy is not clear. It is possible that the changes in plasma β-EP observed during pregnancy are caused by a nonspecific response to stress. Also, they could be the result of changes in the concentration of sex steroid hormones during the course of pregnancy. Estrogen decreases the release of β-EP, whereas progesterone increases it.

ENDOGENOUS OPIOIDS IN THE FETUS

The importance of ACTH for fetal development has been well recognized; ACTH triggers the development and function of the fetal adrenal gland, and the ACTH–adrenal axis influences the development of adrenal medulla, liver, thyroid, thymus, lung, and gut and may even trigger the onset of parturition in some species. Since the discovery of a common precursor for ACTH and β-EP, the significance of the other peptides (α-MSH, CLIP, β-EP) sharing the same precursor with ACTH on fetal development has been under investigation.

Immediately after birth, the β-EPLIA in the unextracted plasma of neonates is significantly higher than the β-EPLIA in the plasma of control adults (300 pg/mL versus 230 pg/mL)[29] (Table 38–4). Furthermore, the plasma β-EP levels remain elevated for the first 4 days after birth and then decline, so that from the fifth day to the 24th day, the plasma β-EPLIA is similar to adult values.[29] The β-EP in the plasma of the neonate is considered to be produced by the neonate itself, and there is sufficient evidence supporting this hypothesis: 1. β-Endorphin is found in the fetal brain and pituitary gland early in development and at high concentrations. 2. If β-EP has been transferred from the mother's blood, it should have disappeared within several hours after birth because of its high turnover. However, β-EP remained high for 4 days after birth, indicating that biosynthesis of β-EP is taking place in the newborn itself. 3. If β-Ep had been transferred from the maternal blood, the umbilical vein should have a higher concentration of β-EPLIA than the umbilical artery. However, this is not the case (see Table 38–4).

Once the biosynthesis of β-EP by the fetus or newborn is accepted, the time of fetal development that the β-EP biosynthesis is initiated is unclear. In human, rat, and mouse fetuses, an early ontogenesis of the endogenous opioid system has been observed. Using *in situ* hybridization techniques, POMC mRNA was detected in the fetal mouse brain on 10–11 days' gestation in the area of the arcuate nucleus, on 12–13 days' gestation in the AL, and on 14–15 days' gestation in the NIL.[30] This early expression of the POMC gene was associated with an early establishment of dense fiber tracts, containing POMC-derived peptides

TABLE 38–4. β-ENDORPHINLIKE IMMUNOREACTIVITY (β-EPLIA) IN THE UMBILICAL ARTERY AND UMBILICAL VEIN IN INFANTS DELIVERED BY A CESAREAN SECTION WITHOUT LABOR OR VAGINALLY AND IN THE PLASMA OF NEWBORN INFANTS AT VARIOUS STAGES OF POSTNATAL DEVELOPMENT

	β-EPLIA (pg/mL)		
	Umbilical Artery	Umbilical Vein	Plasma
Elective cesarean	168.0 ± 46.5[1]	65.7 ± 13.7[1]	—
Active labor	89.6 ± 47.7[1]	58.8 ± 47.3[1]	—
(vaginal	264 ± 21[29]	299 ± 11[29]	—
delivery)	246.5[24]	263.5[24]	—
Neonatal			
Day 1	—	—	301 ± 2[29]
Day 4	—	—	294 ± 15[29]
Days 5–24	—	—	215 ± 15[29]
Adult	—	—	232 ± 10[29]

innervating specific regions of the brain.[30,31] Early development of the POMC system also was observed in the rat brain.[32] At birth, significant amounts of mRNA for POMC, proenkephalin and prodynorphin were detected in the rat brain.[33] During postnatal development, the levels of mRNA for each of the three opioid precursors presented changes that were tissue- and gene-specific.[33] In humans, POMC has been detected in brain cells on the 11th week of fetal development and in the pituitary on the 15th week. The β-EP content in the pituitary gland increased with the gestational age of the fetus. Though the adult human pituitary does not have a distinct intermediate lobe, the human fetal pituitary does have an intermediate lobe that involutes after birth.[34] Because the intermediate lobe processes POMC to α-MSH and β-EP, these peptides may play an important role in fetal development. In both human and rat, α-MSH is needed for the intrauterine growth of the fetus observed around 20 weeks of pregnancy in humans and 19 days in rats. Furthermore, because the hypothalamic cells producing POMC appear in an early period of fetal development before the formation of the arcuate nucleus, it is possible that the neurons containing POMC arise separately from the main mass of the arcuate nucleus cells and later become partly embedded inside and partly embedded outside the arcuate nucleus. Because the blood-brain barrier is immature in the fetus, neurons containing ACTH and related peptides may function as endocrine cells at the early stages of ontogenesis, particularly before the functional development of the pituitary gland. In the rat, the adrenal tissue first appears at 12 days' gestation, and the production of corticosterone can be demonstrated at 13 days' gestation.[35] Probably, hypothalamic ACTH is responsible for triggering the early adrenal function in the rat. Fetal hormones may be involved in processes that are different from the adult situation, and a study of the differences between fetal and adult endocrine systems might provide interesting results. The prenatal and postnatal ontogeny and post-translational processing of POMC have been studied using the rat as an experimental animal. Results indicate that the content of POMC-related peptides increased fivefold from birth to 28 days of life and another threefold by adulthood. In contrast, in the neurointermediate lobe, the content of POMC-related peptides increased 15-fold from birth to 4 weeks of life and another 10-fold by adulthood. At birth, the content of β-endorphinlike peptides (β-EPLPs) in the NIL was very low and significantly lower than in the AL. The post-translational processing of POMC by the AL was different in the early stages of postnatal life than in adulthood. In contrast, in the intermediate lobe of the pituitary gland, the processing of POMC is similar in the early postnatal life as in adulthood. In both ages, neonatal and adult β-endorphin and α-MSH sized peptides account for more than 90% of the content of the NIL immunoreactivity. Furthermore, α-MSH was mainly in the diacetyl form, and β-endorphin was mainly in the acetylated form. In addition, when the content of β-EPLIA was expressed per milligram of protein, it was noted that in both AL and the hypothalamus, there was a smaller increase in the concentration of β-EP peptides during days 4–14 (Fig. 38–6).[36] This is the period coinciding with the stress hyporesponsive period of the hypothalamic-

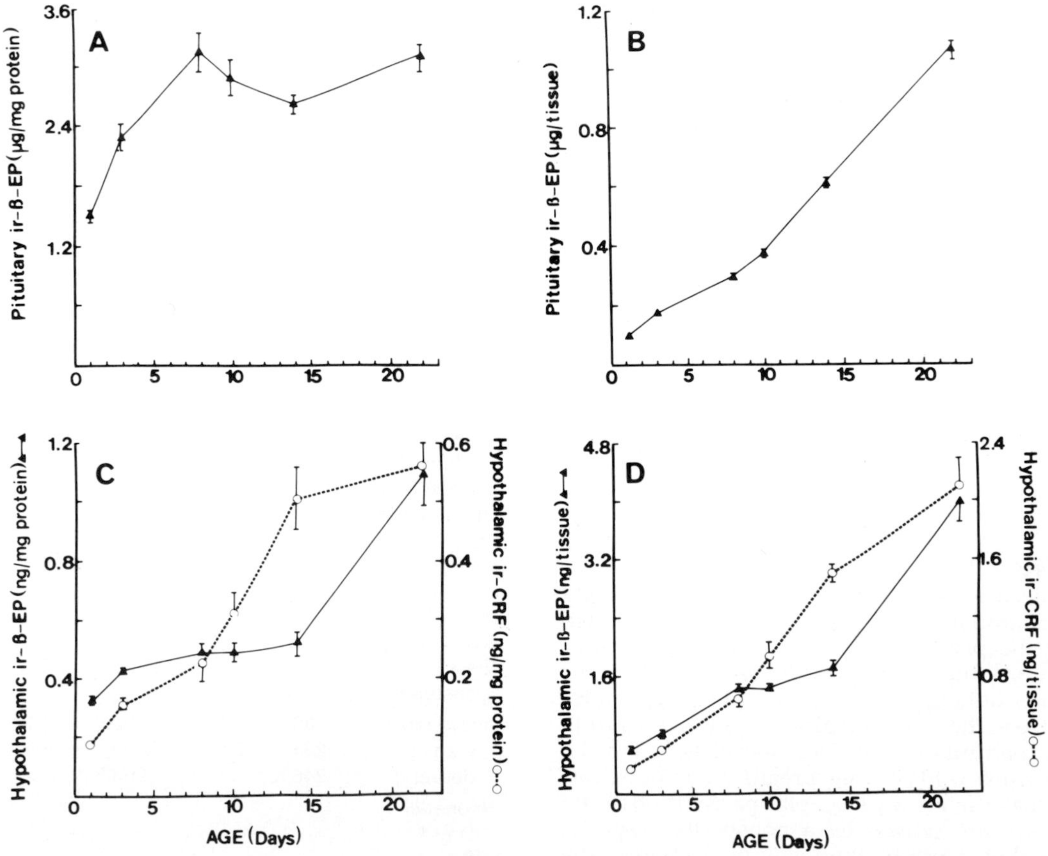

Figure 38–6. Pituitary concentration (*A*) and content (*B*) of immunoreactive β-endorphin (ir-β-EP) and hypothalamic concentration (*C*) and content (*D*) of ir-β-EP (▲—▲) and ir-CRF (○···○) at various ages of postnatal development in the rat. (*From Angelogianni and Gianoulakis,*[36] *with permission*).

pituitary-adrenal axis in the rat. Thus, during the stress hyporesponsive period, there is a small change or no change in the rate of synthesis and post-translational processing of POMC by the rat pituitary gland, which leads to a smaller increase in the content of ACTH and β-endorphin in the pituitary. Because a similar pattern is observed in the rate of increase of β-EPLIPs with age in the hypothalamus, a similar stress hyporesponsive period may exist in the hypothalamic POMC system.[36] This low rate of increase of POMC-related peptides is not associated with a low rate of increase of hypothalamic CRF content (See Fig. 38–6). However, during the stress hyporesponsive period, the serum β-EP and corticosterone contents are decreased (Fig. 38–7), reflecting the changes in the pituitary content of POMC peptides. Opiates have been shown to inhibit neural growth; thus, a decreased activity of the hypothalmic β-endorphin system during critical periods of brain development may be very important in allowing proper neural growth. A similar significance in the decrease of ACTH and cortisol production and their response to stress during this period has been shown.[37]

In addition to β-EP, the presence of other endogenous opioid peptides, such as enkephalins, dynorphins, and neoendorphins in the fetus and newborn, has been investigated. Enkephalinlike immunoreactivity was either undetectable or barely detectable on day 13 of fetal development in the rat. The enkephalin content in the brain increased slowly between days 13 and 16 and then increased at a faster rate between days 16 and 20 prenatally and postnatally to reach adult levels by day 25. Enkephalins also were found in the fetal gut on day 17. In the rat, there is a distinct difference between the ontogenesis of β-EP and enkephalins: By day 16, the regional distribution of β-EP is similar to the adult pattern. In contrast, the regional distribution of enkephalins in the fetal brain is different from their distribution in the adult brain. Dynorphins and neoendorphins are present at birth in the rat, and their concentrations in the neurohypophysis of the newborn rat increase in parallel.

The early ontogenesis of opioid peptides is associated with an early ontogenesis of opioid receptors. In the human fetus, μ and κ sites are present at 20 weeks' gestation in significant quantities, while δ sites are either absent or exist in lower amounts. Recent studies have demonstrated that endogenous opioid peptides and opioid receptors play an important role in the regulation of neural development by exerting an inhibitory effect on cell proliferation and differentiation.[38-40] The crucial role of the endogenous opioids on neural development has been demonstrated by the use of opioid antagonists such as naltrexone. Administration of opiates (morphine) inhibit neuronal growth, while administration of naltrexone (or naloxone) at high concentrations to produce a constant blockage of opioid receptors enhances neural growth.[38] On the other hand, administration of low doses of naltrexone, sufficient to produce only an intermittent daily blockage of opioid receptors, inhibits neural growth.[38] This inhibitory effect of intermittent naltrexone is attributed to up-regulation of opioid receptors by naltrexone, which could interact with the endogenous opioids during the interval when naltrexone is not available and the blockage is not occurring.[41] Furthermore, it appears that endogenous opioids control the pace of brain development by influencing cell replication without causing morphologic changes.[38-41] Thus, alterations on the endogenous opioid peptides–opioid receptor interactions from treatment with exogenous opiate agonists and antagonists may produce a number of defects on the development and function of various neuronal systems.

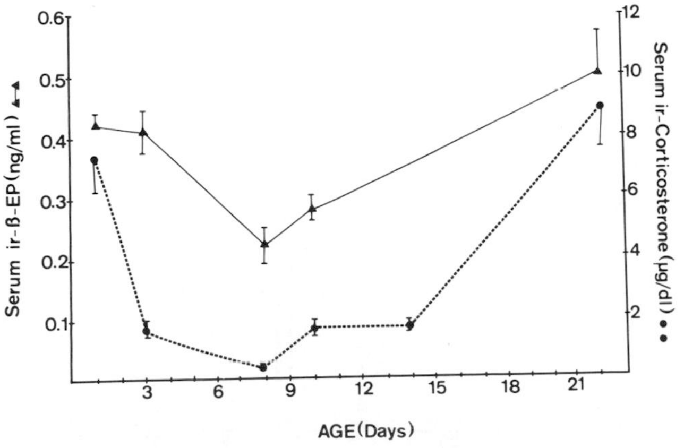

Figure 38–7. Serum levels of immunoreactive β-EP (ir-β-EP) (▲—▲) and ir-corticosterone (●···●) at various ages of postnatal development in the rat. (*From Angelogianni and Gianoulakis*[36], *with permission*).

POSSIBLE FUNCTIONS OF THE POMC-DERIVED PEPTIDES IN FETAL DEVELOPMENT

Although the role of ACTH on fetal development has been investigated extensively, the importance of the other POMC-derived peptides such as α-MSH, CLIP, and β-EP is not clear.

Adrenal Function and POMC-Derived Peptides

ACTH is the hormone responsible for the initiation of steroidogenesis by the adrenal cortex. Because hypothalamic ACTH is present earlier than pituitary ACTH, it is quite possible that the ACTH from the hypothalamus triggers the initiation of adrenal function. In humans, ACTH is the main initiator of steroidogenesis by the adrenal cortex and induces the synthesis of both dehydroisoandrosterone sulfate and cortisol. In contrast, α-MSH has little steroidogenic effect on undifferentiated cells of the adrenal cortex, but once the cells are differentiated by the action of ACTH, α-MSH could stimulate steroidogenesis. Thus, α-MSH is a secondary stimulating hormone.

Functions of the POMC-Derived Peptides Not Related to the Adrenal Glands

An important function of α-MSH on fetal development is its effect on the intrauterine growth of the fetus. In humans and rats, α-MSH was required for the intrauterine growth of the fetus observed around 20 weeks' gestation in humans and 19 days' gestation in rats. This fetal "growth spurt" is absent in anencephalic human fetuses[42] and in brain-aspirated rat fetuses.[43] Injections of a series of pituitary hormones could not induce growth in these fetuses. The only compound that could stimulate the intrauterine growth was α-MSH.

Recently, the $ACTH_{22\text{-}39}$ fragment, which is derived from proteolytic cleavage of CLIP ($ACTH_{18\text{-}39}$), was reported to stimulate insulin release by the pancreas. This fragment was named β-cell tropin.[44] The structure essential for the biologic activity of this peptide is the $ACTH_{22\text{-}24}$ sequence (Val–Tyr–Pro). $ACTH_{22\text{-}39}$ has been isolated by tryptic digestion of CLIP ($ACTH_{18\text{-}39}$), but its presence in extracts of the pituitary gland or brain has not been demonstrated.

However, a compound similar to $ACTH_{22\text{-}39}$ has been found in the serum of OB/OB strain of mice.

The importance of β-EP for fetal development is not clear. The early ontogenesis of β-EP in the brain and pituitary gland and the high levels of β-EP in the fetal plasma at the time of birth suggest a specific function of β-EP in fetal development. Because β-EP is a potent analgesic agent, one of its probable functions during delivery is to render the fetus better able to cope with the stress of delivery and the stress of the change of environment from the smooth, soft, and warm womb of the mother to the atmosphere. The high β-EP levels for the first 4 days after birth may help the newborn infant to adjust to environmental changes by controlling physiologic functions, such as thermoregulation and respiration. β-Endorphin and enkephalins cause respiratory depression, and hyperactivity of the endorphin system has been implicated in sudden infant death syndrome.[45] Infants of drug-dependent mothers show a higher incidence of sudden infant death syndrome[46], providing further support to the hypothesis of an abnormality of the endogenous opioid system involved in the pathogenesis of sudden infant death syndrome.

The sharp rise of β-EP immediately before birth may be significant in the process of parturition. Endorphins and enkephalins stimulate the release of arginine vasopressin by the neurohypophysis. In the rat fetal neurohypophysis, arginine vasopressin is not present. Instead, a similar compound, arginine vasotocin, is present. Arginine vasotocin also is found in the neurohypophysis of human fetuses at about 20 weeks' gestation. Furthermore, arginine vasotocin has been implicated in the process of parturition. If β-EP increases the release of arginine vasotocin, then β-EP is indirectly involved in the process of parturition. Endorphins also may be important in controlling the release of gonadotropins and thus the development of the reproductive system. The influence of various physiologic conditions and drug treatments on the ontogeny of the POMC system and its response to stress has been investigated. Thus, neonatal handling and prenatal exposure to two popular drugs of abuse, morphine and alcohol, have been shown to alter the development of the stress response of the HPA-axis and β-endorphin system in early postnatal and adult life.[37,47,48]

Daily administration of morphine in the drinking water from 4 days' gestation to parturition resulted in increased concentrations of pituitary and hypothalamic β-Endorphin in the offspring tested at 14 and 21 days' gestation and on the first day of life.[49] Similar changes may occur in the pituitary and hypothalamus of human infants of opiate-addicted mothers. Thus endogenous opioids may be involved in the pathogenesis of the behavioral changes observed in newborns of heroine-addicted mothers.[49] It was shown that the derangement of the sleep pattern of newborns of addicted mothers correlated well with the increased levels in plasma opioid peptides.[49] However, in other studies when morphine was administered by subcutaneous implantation of a 75-mg morphine base pellet on 9 and 13 days' gestation, the hypothalamic content of β-EPLP was lower than the controls on 19 and 20 days' gestation and on the first day of life. No significant difference was observed at later stages of development[48] (Fig. 38–8). When animals treated with morphine prenatally were challenged with stressful stimuli, such as the hot plate test, the stress-induced analgesia was significantly lower than in control

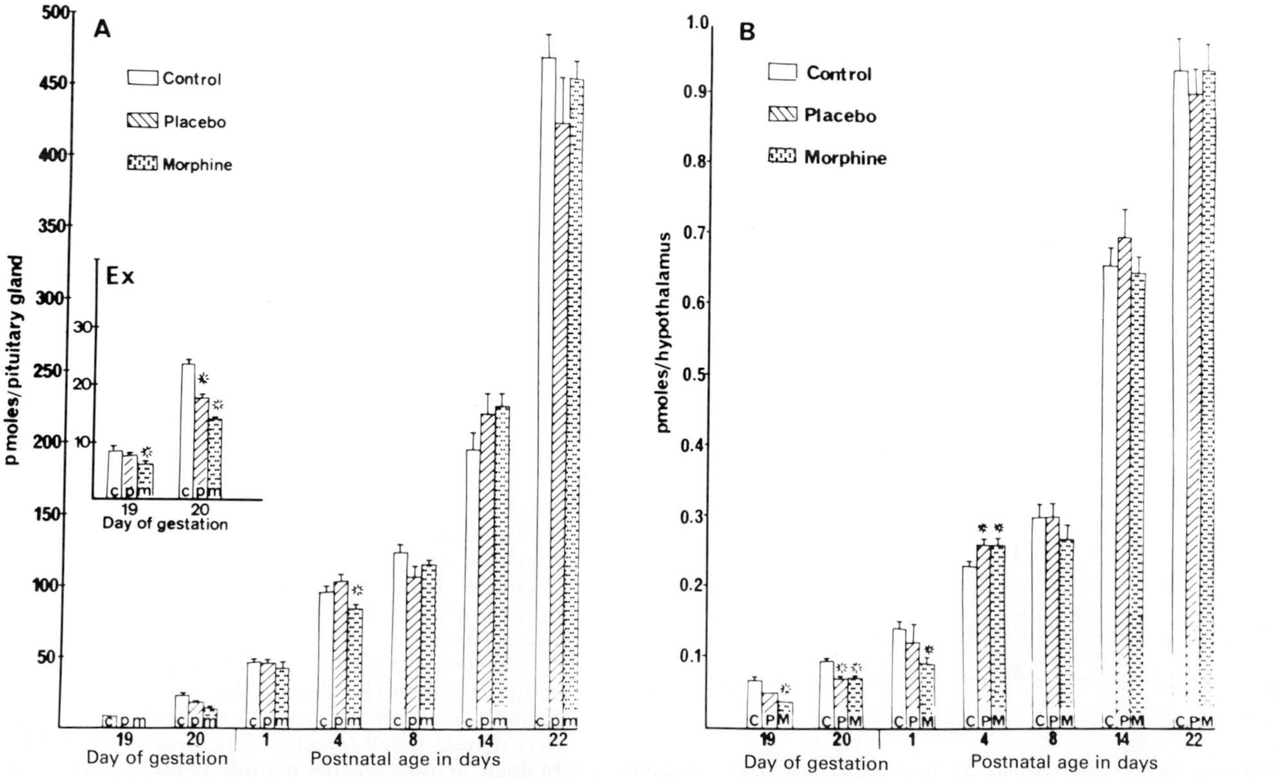

Figure 38–8. Effect of morphine treatment during gestation on the content of β-endorphinlike immunoreactivity in the pituitary gland (*A*) and hypothalamus (*B*) at various stages of prenatal and postnatal development. (Ex = expanded scale.) *Significantly different from controls $p \leq 0.05$)

animals[50], indicating a decreased release of endogenous opioid peptides or the presence of tolerance to endogenous opioids. Ethanol, another popular drug of abuse, has been shown to have a significant effect on the activity of the endogenous opioid system of offspring exposed to ethanol *in utero*. Thus, a lower content of β-endorphinlike peptides was found in the pituitary gland of offspring exposed to ethanol prenatally but not in the total hypothalamic content of either β-endorphin or CRF (Fig. 38–9). Both ethanol-treated and sucrose pair-fed offspring presented an increase in the concentration (ng β-EPLIA/mg protein) of hypothalamic β-EPLPs, indicating the influence of a nutritional factor and an ethanol associated factor on the observed changes of the activity of the POMC system. On the other hand, the content of β-EPLIA in the serum of rat offspring exposed to ethanol *in utero* was significantly higher than in control offspring on the first day of life but not at later stages of development (Fig. 38–10). Prenatal exposure to ethanol suppressed the β-endorphin and hypothalamic pituitary adrenal axis response to stress at an early postnatal age, while it enhanced the stress response at later stages of development (Fig. 38–11). This indicates that even though the content of POMC-related peptides has not been altered by prenatal ethanol exposure, the neural connections needed for normal response to stressful situations are not developed properly, allowing a more pronounced release of POMC peptides after stress. Also, animals exposed to ethanol *in utero* had difficulties in performing a number of learning and memory tasks. The difficulties presented by the offspring exposed to ethanol prenatally are similar to the problems that children of alcoholic mothers have such as difficulty in adjusting to various novel and stressful situations and deficits in learning and memory processes. Ethanol may exert its effects on the CNS by acting directly

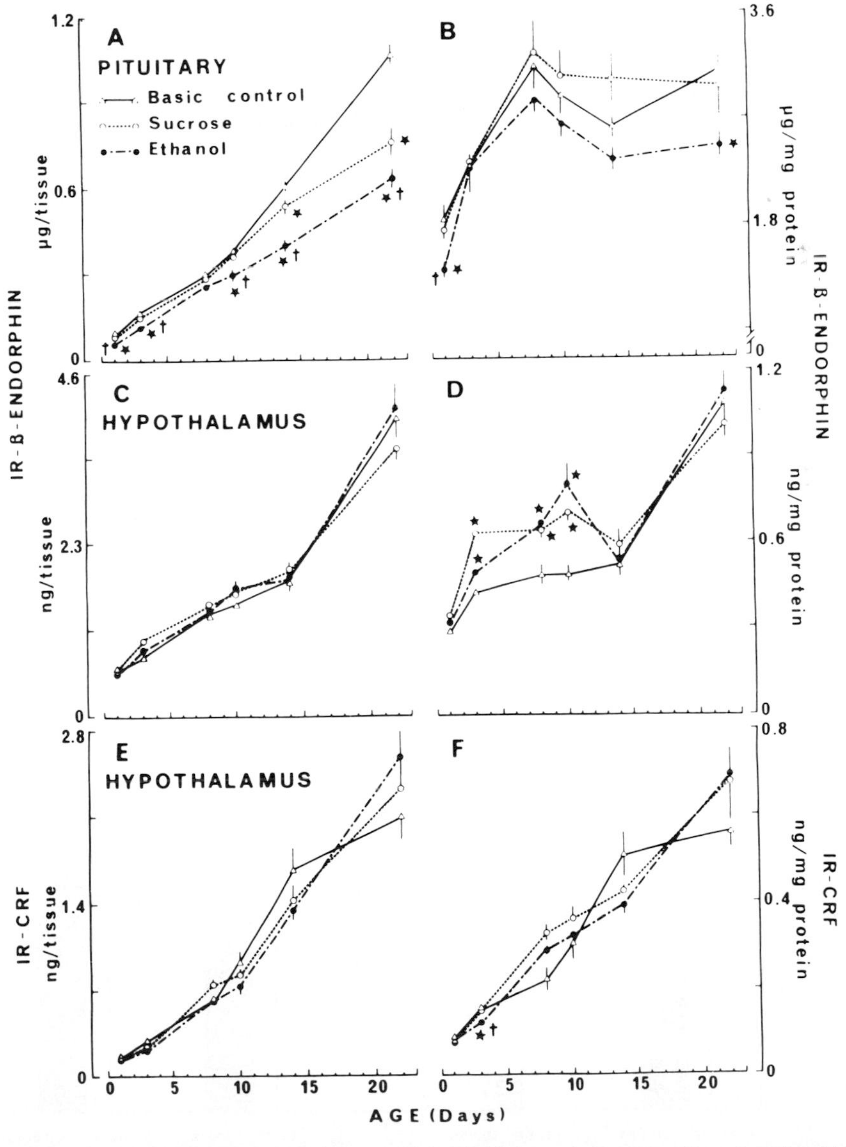

Figure 38–9. Mean total contents (*left*) and concentrations (*right*) of pituitary immunoreactive β-endorphin (ir-β-EP) (*A, B*), hypothalamic ir-β-EP (*C, D*), and ir-CRF (*E, F*) in offspring of ethanol-fed (●—●), pair-fed (○···○), and basic control dams (△—△) at various ages of development. *Significant difference from basic control group of same age ($p < 0.05$); †significant difference between ethanol and pair-fed group of same age ($p < 0.05$). (*From Angelogianni and Gianoulakis* [47] *with permission*).

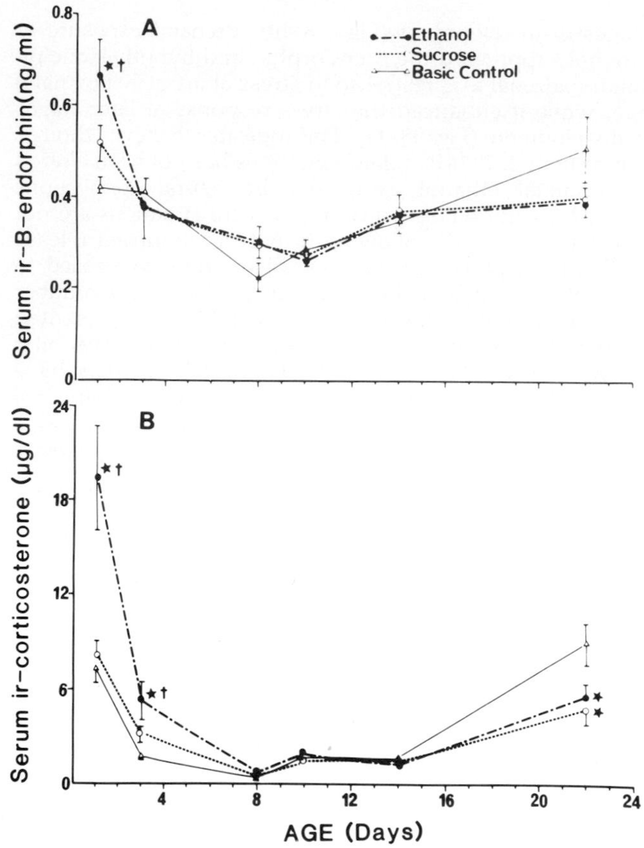

Figure 38–10. Serum levels of ir-β-EP (*A*) and ir-corticosterone (*B*) in offspring of ethanol-fed (●—●), pair-fed (○···○), and basic control dams (△—△) at various ages of development. *Significant difference from basic control group of same age ($p < 0.05$); †significant difference between ethanol and pair-fed groups of same age ($p < 0.05$). (*From Angelogianni and Gianoulakis.*[47] *with permission*).

on the various neuronal structures or by its effects on various neuroendocrine systems, which in turn may influence the development of the CNS. For example, offspring exposed to ethanol prenatally exhibit high levels of glucocorticoids in the first 3 days of life (see Fig. 38–10), and an enhanced response to stress by the pituitary–adrenal axis (leading to high levels of serum glucocorticoids) in early juvenile and adult life.[47] Similar to glucocorticoids, the content of β-endorphin is high on the first day of birth (see Fig. 38–10), and the response of the β-endorphin system to stress is more pronounced in young juvenile and adult rats exposed to ethanol *in utero*.[47] An excess of glucocorticoids has been shown to induce loss of hippocampal neurons and to induce deficits in hippocampal functions,[37] while an excess of opioids has been shown to decrease the neural development. Thus, this excessive glucocorticoid and β-endorphin activity at a young age (days 1–3 of life) and following stressful situations in juvenile and adult life by offspring exposed to ethanol prenatally may induce a decrease in neural development and hippocampal neurons and thus may be partially responsible for the problems of children born to alcoholic mothers.

CONCLUSIONS

In summary, although more information is available on the function of ACTH, the other POMC-derived peptides, α-MSH, CLIP, and β-EP, may be involved in important functions and control of normal fetal development. Thus a number of specific β-EP effects on fetal development can be postulated, including analgesic effect, adaptation to environmental changes, development of distinct behavioral patterns, and induction of the various types of opiate binding sites and neural growth. The end-products of the β-EP gene (POMC) have mostly been investigated, but the maturation end-products of the two other endogenous opioid genes, proenkephalin and prodynorphin, also need to be

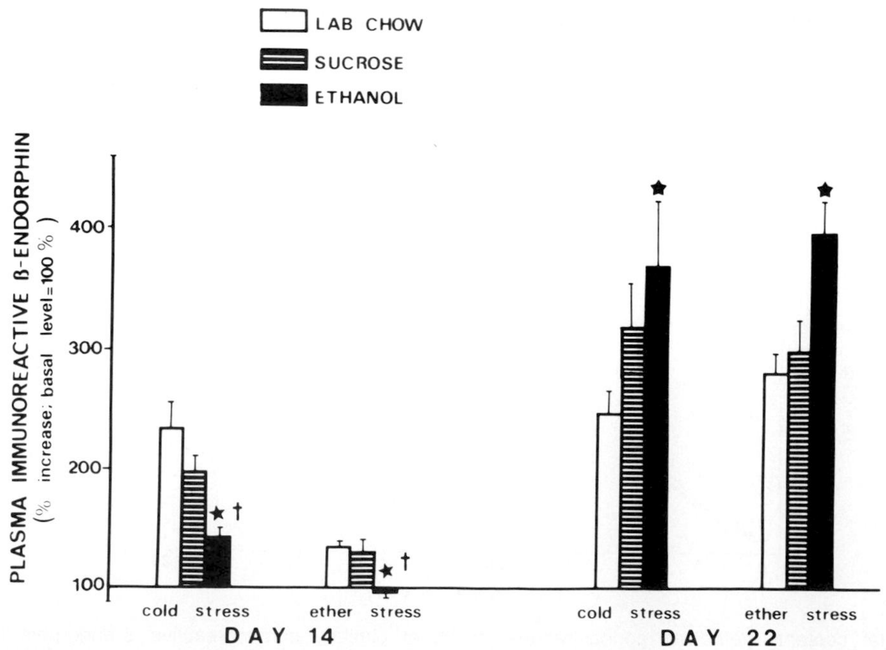

Figure 38–11. Effect of cold and ether stress on serum ir-β-EP concentrations expressed as percentages of unstressed levels in 14- and 22-day old offspring of ethanol-fed (■), pair-fed (□), and basic control (□) dams. *Significant difference between ethanol and basic control group of same age ($p < 0.05$); †significant difference between ethanol and sucrose pair-fed groups of same age ($p < 0.05$).

fully investigated. It is quite possible that these three distinct systems of endogenous opioid peptides might have regulatory roles in different important functions of fetal life and neurogenesis.

REFERENCES

1. Steinbrook AR, Carr DB, Datta S, et al. Dissociation of plasma and cerebrospinal fluid β-endorphin-like immunoreactivity levels during pregnancy and parturition. *Anesth Analg (Cleve)*. 1982;61:893.
2. Akil H, Watson SJ, Barchas JD, et al. β-Endorphin immunoreactivity in rat and human blood: Radioimmunoassay, comparative levels, and physiologic alterations. *Life Sci.* 1979;24:1659.
3. Gintzler AR. Endorphin-mediated increases in pain threshold during pregnancy. *Science.* 1980;210:193.
4. Silman RE, Chard T, Lowry PJ, et al. Human fetal pituitary peptides and parturition. *Nature.* 1976;260:716.
5. Bun NG T, Ho WKK, Tam PPL. Brain and pituitary β-endorphin levels at different developmental stages of the rat. *Int J Pept Prot Res.* 1984;24:141.
6. Liotta AS, Houghten R, Krieger DT. Identification of a β-endorphin-like peptide in cultured human placental cells. *Nature.* 1982;295:593.
7. Zakarian S, Smyth DG. Distribution of β-endorphin-related peptides in rat pituitary brain. *Biochem J.* 1982;202:561.
8. Comb M, Seeburg PH, Adelman J, et al. Primary structure of the human Met–and Leu–enkephalin precursor and its mRNA. *Nature.* 1982;295:663.
9. Fallon JH, Leslie FM. Distribution of dynorphin and enkephalin peptides in the rat brain. *J Comp Neurol.* 1986;249:293.
10. Schultzberg M, Hokfelt T, Lundberg JM, et al. Enkephalin-like immunoreactivity in nerve terminals in sympathetic ganglia and adrenal medulla and in adrenal medullary plant cells. *Acta Physiologica Scandinavia.* 1978;103:**475.**
11. Kakidani H, Furutani Y, Takahashi H, et al. Cloning and sequence analysis of cDNA for porcine β-neo-endorphin/dynorphin precursor. *Nature.* 1982;298:145.
12. Khachaturian H, Lewis ME, Schafer MKH, et al. Anatomy of the CNS opioid systems. *Trends Neurosci.* 1985;8:111.
13. Kohler C, Haglund L, Swanson LW. A diffuse α-MSH-immunoreactive projection to the hippocampus and spinal cord from individual neurons in the lateral hypothalamic area and zona incerta. *J Comp Neurol.* 1984;223:501.
14. Haynes LW, Smyth DG, Zakarian S. Immunocytochemical localization of β-endorphin (β-lipotropin C-fragment) in the developing rat spinal cord and hypothalamus. *Brain Res.* 1982;232:115.
15. Tsou K, Khachaturian H, Akil H, et al. Immunocytochemical localization of pro-opiomelanocortin-derived peptides in the adult rat spinal cord. *Brain Res.* 1986;378:28.
16. De Bold CR, Menefee JK, Nicholson WE, et al. Pro-opiomelanocortin gene is expressed in many normal human tissues and in tumors not associated with ectopic adrenocorticotropin syndrome. *Molec Endocrin.* 1988;2:862.
17. Schultzberg M, Dreyfus CF, Gerson MD, et al. VIP-, enkephalin-, substance P-, and somatostatin-like immunoreactivity in neurons intrinsic to the intestine: Immunohistochemical evidence from organotypic tissue cultures. *Brain Res.* 1978;155:239.
18. Pittius CW, Seizinger BR, Pasi A, et al. Distribution and characterization of opioid peptides derived from proenkephalin A in human and rat central nervous system. *Brain Res.* 1984;304:127.
19. Watson SJ, Akil H, Ghazarossian VE, et al. Dynorphin immunocytochemical localization in brain and peripheral nervous system: Preliminary studies. *Proc Natl Acad Sci USA.* 1981;78:1260.
20. McGinty JF, Van Der Kooy D, Bloom FE. The distribution and morphology of opioid peptides immunoreactive neurons in the cerebral cortex of rats. *J Neurosci.* 1984;4:1104.
21. Meites J, Bruni JF, Van Vugt DA, et al. Relation of endogenous opioid peptides and morphine to neuroendocrine functions. *Life Sci.* 1979;24:1325.
22. Olson Ga, Olson RD, Kastin AJ. Endogenous Opiates: 1987. *Peptides.* 1989; 10:205. Review.
23. Ieiri I, Chen HT, Meites J. Naloxone stimulation of luteinizing hormone release in pre-pubertal female rats; role of serotonergic system. *Life Sci.* 1980;26:1269.
24. Csontos K, Rust M, Hollt V, et al. Elevated plasma β-endorphin levels in pregnant women and their neonates. *Life Sci.* 1979;25:835.
25. Goland RS, Wardlaw SL, Stark RI, et al. Human plasma β-endorphin during pregnancy, labor and delivery. *J Clin Endocrinol Metab.* 1981;52:74.
26. Genazzani AR, Facchinetti F, Parrini D. β-Lipotropin and β-endorphin plasma levels during pregnancy. *Clin Endocrinol.* 1981;14:409.
27. Cahill C, Akil H. Plasma β-endorphin-like immunoreactivity, self-reported pain perception, and anxiety levels in women during pregnancy and labor. *Life Sci.* 1982;31:1871.
28. Kimball CD, Chang CM, Huang SM, et al. Immunoreactive endorphin peptides and prolactin in umbilical vein and maternal blood. *Am J Obstet Gynecol.* 1981;140:157.
29. Moss IM, Conner H, Yee WFH, et al. Human β-endorphin-like immunoreactivity in the perinatal/neonatal period. *J Pediatr.* 1982;101:443.
30. Elkabes S, Loh YP, Nieburg A, et al. Prenatal ontogenesis of proopiomelanocortin in the mouse central nervous system and pituitary gland: An *in situ* hybridization and immunocytochemical study. *Dev Brain Res.* 1989;46:85.
31. Nemeskeri A, Setalo G, Halasz B. Ontogenesis of the three parts of the fetal rat adenohypophysis. *Neuroendocrinology.* 1988;48:534.
32. Schwartzburg DG, Nakane PK. Ontogenesis of adrenocorticotropin-related peptide determinants in the hypothalamus and pituitary gland of the rat. *Endocrinology.* 1982;110:855.
33. Rosen H, Polakiewicz R. Postnatal expression of opioid genes in rat brain. *Dev Brain Res.* 1989;46:123.
34. Silman RE, Holland D, Chard T, et al. The ACTH "family tree" of the rhesus monkey with development. *Nature.* 1978;276:526.
35. Roos TB. Steroid synthesis in embryonic and fetal rat adrenal tissue. *Endocrinology.* 1967;81:716.
36. Angelogianni P, Gianoulakis C. Ontogeny of the β-endorphin response to stress in the rat: Role of the pituitary and hypothalamus. *Neuroendocrinology.* 1989;50:372.
37. Meaney MJ, Aitken DH, Van Berkel C, et al. Effect of neonatal handling on age-related impairments associated with the hippocampus. *Science.* 1988;239:766.
38. Hauser KF, McLaughlin PJ, Zagon IS. Endogenous opioids regulate dendritic growth and spine formation in developing rat brain. *Brain Res.* 1987;416:157.
39. Zagon IS, McLaughlin PJ. Opioid antagonist (naltrexone) modulation of cerebellar development: histological and morphometric studies. *J Neurosci.* 1986;6:1424.
40. Hess GD, Zagon IS. Endogenous opioid systems and neural development: Ultrastructural studies in the cerebellar cortex of infant and weanling rats. *Brain Res Bulletin.* 1988;20:473.
41. Zagon IS, McLaughlin PJ. Naltrexone modulates growth in infant rats. *Life Sci.* 1983;33:2449.
42. Honnebier WJ, Swaab DF. The influence of anencephaly upon intrauterine growth of fetus and placenta and upon gestation length. *J Obstet Gynaecol Br Commonw.* 1973;80:577.
43. Swaab DF, Honnebier WJ. The influence of removal of the fetal rat brain upon intrauterine growth of the fetus and the placenta and on gestation length. *J Obstet Gynaecol Br Commonw.* 1973;80:589.
44. Beloff-Chain A, Morton J, Dunmore S, et al. Evidence that the insulin secretagogue β-cell-tropin is ACTH 22–39. *Nature.* 1983;301:255.
45. Kuich TE, Zimmerman D. Could endorphins be implicated in sudden-infant-death syndrome? *N Engl J Med.* 1981;304:973.
46. Chavez DJ, Ostrea EM, Stryker JC, et al. Sudden infant death syndrome among infants of drug-dependent mothers. *J Pediatr.* 1979;93:407.
47. Angelogianni P, Gianoulakis C. Prenatal exposure to ethanol alters the ontogeny of the β-endorphin response to stress. *Alcoh Clin Exptl Res.* 1989;13:564.
48. Gianoulakis C. Effect of maternally administered opiates on the development of the β-endorphin system in the offspring. National Institute on Drug Abuse Research Monograph Series. *No. 75.* 1986:595.
49. Bianchi M, Marini A, Sacerdote P, et al. Effect of chronic morphine on plasma and brain beta-endorphin and methionine enkephalin in pregnant rats and in their fetuses or newborn. *Neuroendocrinology.* 1988; 47:89.
50. Lichtblau L, Messing RB, Sparber SB. Neonatal opiate withdrawal alters the reactivity of adult rats to the hot-plate. *Life Sci.* 1984;34:1725.

Chapter Thirty-Nine

Disorders of the Hypothalamus and Pituitary

Ilan Tur-Kaspa and Norbert Gleicher

39

Disorders of the hypothalamus and pituitary in pregnancy are not common. This is primarily because most of these disorders also are associated with infertility. Their diagnosis in pregnancy and the appropriate management before, during, and after pregnancy represent a unique challenge for a multispecialty team, often composed of gynecologists, endocrinologists, neurologists, neurosurgeons, ophthalmologists, and radiologists. The potential risks to mother or fetus from the disease or its treatment often complicate the management of these patients.

Disorders of the pituitary and hypothalamus result in decreased or increased secretion of pituitary hormones. It is not always easy to differentiate between excess hormone production that occurs because of *de novo* hyperplasia, an adenoma of the pituitary, or an excess secretion of a hypothalamic releasing factor. The same difficulty may arise in a hypofunction state. The placenta as an endocrine organ and the effect of pregnancy on the hypothalàmic–pituitary system further complicate diagnosis and management of these patients.

The pituitary gland consists of an anterior lobe (*adenohypophysis*) and a posterior lobe (*neurohypophysis*). Although three cell types have been classically recognized in the pars distalis of the anterior lobe (acidophils, basophils, and chromophobes), recent immunocytochemical staining and ultrastructural features of their secretory granules have identified at least five cell types.[1]

The *somatotroph* accounts for 50% of the pituitary cell population and secretes growth hormone (GH) and human placental lactogen (HPL). The *lactotroph* secretes prolactin (PRL) and vasoactive intestinal polypeptide (VIP). Adrenocorticotropic hormone (ACTH), β-lipotropin hormone (β-LPH), and γ-melanocyte-stimulating hormone (γ-MSH) are secreted from the *corticotroph* cell. The lactotroph and corticotroph consist of approximately 15% of the pituitary cells each. The *gonadotroph* produces mainly luteinizing hormone (LH) and follicle-stimulating hormone (FSH) and also dynorphin and atrial natriuretic peptide. Like the *thyrotroph*, which secretes the thyroid-stimulating hormone (TSH), each of these cell types accounts for 10% of the pituitary cell population.

The brain controls the secretion of each anterior pituitary hormone by vascular connections between the hypothalamus and the anterior lobe. However, the posterior lobe of the pituitary is an anatomic extension of the central nervous system (CNS), and consists primarily of the *pars nervosa* and the *pituitary stalk* or *infundibulum*. Two nuclear cell groups of the hypothalamus, the supraoptic and the paraventricular, project directly to the neurohypophysis and use neurophysin I and II as carrier proteins for the products of these cells, vasopressin and oxytocin.

PITUITARY GLAND GROWTH IN PREGNANCY

Autopsy studies have shown that pregnancy results in physiologic pituitary enlargement. The volume of the normal pituitary gland increases by approximately 70% during normal pregnancy.[2] An increase of 30–100% in the weight of the pituitary reportedly results mainly from hypertrophy and hyperplasia of the lactotroph cells.[3,4] Recently, Gonzalez et al[4] studied *in vivo* changes in the pituitary gland during pregnancy using magnetic resonance imaging (MRI). The MRI measurements in the first, second, and third trimesters showed a significant gradual increase in pituitary volume during pregnancy. At the end of the pregnancy, the hypophysis had increased 2.6 mm in vertical, anteroposterior, and transversal dimensions, with an overall increase of 136% when compared with the control group. Pituitary enlargement in the three dimensions did not produce any chiasmatic or cavernous sinus compression, and the pituitary stalk remained in the midline. These characteristics of normal pituitary growth in pregnancy may be used as a baseline for comparable measurements in pregnant women with hypothalamic or pituitary disorders.

PITUITARY TUMORS

Despite great advances in knowledge and understanding of pituitary hormone regulation, the pathogenesis of pituitary adenomas remains unknown.[1-1] There is evidence for and against the hypothesis that GH-, PRL-, and ACTH-secreting tumors arise as a result of hypothalamic dysregulation.[5] While 80–90% of these tumors appear to arise *de novo* within the pituitary; the remaining 10–20% may arise as a result of excess releasing hormones or decreased inhibiting hormones because of hypothalamic dysfunction. For example, it is not always clear whether hyperprolactinemia occurs because the tumor is a prolactinoma (a PRL-secreting adenoma) or because compression of the pituitary stalk by a nonsecreting tumor prevents access of the hypothalamic PRL inhibitor, dopamine.[9]

Pituitary tumors with no clinical evidence of hormone hypersecretion account for 25% to 30% of patients who present with a pituitary adenoma.[10] Most of the nonfunctioning adenomas produce gonadotropin hormones and subunits, but these nonsecreting tumors lack a characteristic hormone syndrome, and they usually present as large macroadenomas with neuro-ophthalmologic abnormalities secondary to their supracellar or extracellar extension. The close anatomic relationship of the pituitary to the optic nerve and chiasm renders these structures vulnerable to enlarging tumors of the gland. Visual loss, characteristically *bitemporal hemianopia*, is therefore an early and frequently the sole symptom of a pituitary tumor (see also Chapter 194).[11]

Magnetic resonance imaging and computerized tomography (CT) of the brain and pituitary have diminished the role of the ophthalmologist in making the diagnosis of a pituitary tumor.[11-13] Nevertheless, detailed neuro-ophthalmologic examination remains an essential part of the clinical evaluation. This has been recently reviewed by Melan.[11]

A pituitary adenoma of less than 10 mm in diameter, measured by radiologic[13] or pathologic[14] diagnosis, defines a *microadenoma*. A tumor larger than 10 mm is a *macroadenoma*. Microadenomas exist silently with the incidence in the general population varying between 2.7–27%. Forty to 50 percent of the tumors are prolactinomas.[2,7,13-16]

HYPERPROLACTINEMIA OR PROLACTINOMAS

Hyperprolactinemia is the most common hypothalamic–pituitary disorder. Prolactin-secreting adenomas are the most common type of secreting pituitary tumors.[2,16] The incidence of asymptomatic hyperprolactinemia in the general population is less than 1%.[17]

Pathologic hyperprolactinemia is defined in most laboratories as a consistant basal morning serum PRL level of greater than 20 ng/mL in the absence of pregnancy or postpartum lactation. Unfortunately, there is no clear consensus on the upper limit of normal. It can vary between 20–50 ng/mL.[16-18] A woman with a serum PRL of 20–50 ng/mL may be told in one center that she is healthy, while elsewhere she might be told that she has a microprolactinoma that requires further evaluation.[9]

The major concern in patients with prolactinomas is the known stimulatory effect of estrogen and progesterone on size and number of lactotrophs, the PRL-secreting pituitary cells, with a parallel increase in serum PRL levels.[19-21] Estrogens stimulate DNA synthesis, PRL mRNA levels, PRL synthesis, and lactotrophic mitotic activity. Progesterone also stimulates PRL secretion. Women with hyperprolactinemia, once pregnancy is confirmed, should therefore be followed closely for symptoms and signs of tumor expansion, such as headaches or visual disturbances.

However, only a small percentage (1.6%) of women with hyperprolactinemia and microprolactinomas will develop symptoms or signs of tumor growth during pregnancy.[22,23] The radiologic diagnosis of tumor enlargement was observed in 4.5% of asymptomatic women. The risk is higher with macroprolactinomas. Approximately 15% of such patients are symptomatic, and 9% demonstrate an asymptomatic enlargement of the prolactinoma.[22]

Headaches usually precede visual disturbance, and both may occur in any trimester.[24] There is no characteristic headache. Although bitemporal hemianopsia is the classic abnormal visual field finding, other defects also can occur. Except for tumor size, there are no prognostic indicators that can identify which patient is at risk for tumor expansion during pregnancy.

If a woman develops significant pituitary enlargement, management choices include observation, medical treatment with a dopamine agonist (bromocriptine), or surgery if the former choices have failed. Bromocriptine is the treatment of choice, and it has been shown to significantly decrease tumor size and improve headaches and visual defects during pregnancy.[2,22-26] The spontaneous regression of a PRL-producing pituitary adenoma during pregnancy also has been recently reported.[27]

Treatment

Regardless of the cause of secretory dysfunction, approximately 80% of hyperprolactinemic women achieve pregnancy after therapy.[23,24] Therapies of choice are bromocriptine or other dopamine agonists rather than pituitary surgery or irradiation, whether the diagnosis is idiopathic hyperprolactinemia, microprolactinoma, or macroprolactinoma.[2,16,22-46] Nevertheless, surgical or radiotherapy management in selected patients may be an acceptable, safe, and effective alternative (see also Chapter 181).[47-50]

Dopamine has been shown to be the primary physiologic inhibitor of PRL secretion in the hypothalamic-hypophyseal axis.[51] Bromocriptine, the active ingredient of Parlodel, a lysergic acid derivative, was the first dopaminergic agonist available for the clinical treatment of hyperprolactinemia.[33,34] Other ergoline derivatives, such as Metergoline[42], Hydergine[43], pergolide[52], and CU 32-085[53], also have been shown to treat hyperprolactinemia effectively. In pregnancy, only bromocriptine has been established as a probable safe drug.[22,23,33] The usual dosage is 2.5 mg orally twice a day, starting with an initial dose of 2.5 mg at bedtime. Its use during pregnancy has, however, remained controversial.

Bromocriptine has recently been shown to alter follicular fluid concentrations of PRL and estradiol. It also has a positive effect on human embryonic development *in vitro*. Oocyte fertilization and pregnancy rates were, however, unaffected.[54] Bromocriptine treatment during pregnancy lowers maternal and fetal blood levels of PRL. Nevertheless, no adverse effects on pregnancy or the newborn have been noted.[22-26,33] The drug does not affect amniotic fluid levels of PRL because this PRL derives from decidual tissue, and its secretion is controlled by estrogen and progesterone, not by dopamine.[24] Although no adverse effects of bromocriptine on offspring have been reported prenatally or postnatally, it is still recommended that bromocriptine therapy be stopped as soon as pregnancy is confirmed, unless a definite indication for its use has been established.[33] This is confirmed by a review of the literature involving more than 2000 reported pregnancies in hyperprolactinemic women.[16,17,22-46] Whether the drug increases the incidence of multiple pregnancies is controversial when correcting for concomitant therapy with other agents, especially ovulation-inducing drugs.[33]

Lactation

Hyperprolactinemia is not a reason to avoid breastfeeding.[22,24] Prolactin is crucial in the initiation of lactation.[55] Then, within 1–2 weeks after delivery, milk production primarily becomes a function of the amount withdrawn from the duct system, and the endocrine control of the process decreases in importance. This is why lactation does not affect hyperprolactinemic women, and hyperprolactinemia fails to improve lactation in the late peurperium.[56] The exact role of prolactin in establishing and maintaining milk production beyond the stage of initiation is still unclear. Prolactin is secreted in maternal milk. The effect of this PRL on the newborn also is not yet established. Prolactin secretion in milk continues for up to 40 weeks after delivery.[57]

The pharmacologic inhibition of lactation may be indicated in non-nursing hyperprolactinemic mothers. Bromocriptine for 14 days, starting on the day of delivery, has been the treatment of choice.[23]

Postpartum Follow-up

Prolactin levels can return to normal after pregnancy. This may occur spontaneously or after long-term bromocriptine treatment.[23,27,58-63] If bromocriptine therapy is initiated after a delivery, appropriate contraception should begin 14–21 days postpartum because ovulation can return in these women rapidly. When a new pregnancy is desired, there is no reason to advise against it, unless the patient is unstable because of tumor enlargement. There is also no contraindication to pharmacologic ovulation induction.[64]

CUSHING'S DISEASE IN PREGNANCY

Cushing's disease is caused by pituitary ACTH hypersecretion (see also Chapter 42). Pituitary adenomas are present in more than 80% of affected patients.[65] Although this is primarily a disorder that occurs in childbearing years, pregnancy is rare because amenorrhea, oligomenorrhea, and infertility characterize the disease, and because excess glucocorticoids suppress gonadotropin secretion.[66,67] A detailed description of the diagnosis and management of Cushing's syndrome in pregnancy has been presented.[66,67]

Diagnosis of Cushing's disease in pregnancy may be difficult. Delays occur frequently because nonaffected pregnant women also develop hypertension, edema, glucose intolerance, and striae. But diagnosis of Cushing's syndrome should be considered in any pregnant woman who develops hypertension, hyperglycemia, hypokalemia, and shows evidence of androgen excess, not only just when classic signs are present.[67]

Hypercortisolism during pregnancy can be diagnosed by the traditional dexamethasone suppression tests. ACTH measurement after corticotropin-releasing hormone (CRH) stimulation will distinguish pituitary causes of Cushing's disease from adrenal causes of Cushing's syndrome (see also Chapter 42). Computed tomography and MRI also can be used for this diagnosis.[68] An 80–90% remission rate after selective trans-sphenoidal resection of ACTH-secreting pituitary adenomas makes this surgical procedure the initial treatment of choice in Cushing's disease.[65]

Pickard et al[66] in a recent review of the literature summarized the management of 23 cases of Cushing's disease during pregnancy. Sixteen women required no treatment for their disease during pregnancy. One patient underwent a trans-sphenoidal hypophysectomy at 16 weeks' gestation, and another woman underwent trans-sphenoidal pituitary adenectomy at 22 weeks' gestation. One woman received pituitary irradiation during the second trimester, and bilateral adrenalectomy was performed during pregnancy in four patients between 12 to 22 weeks' gestation.[69] The maternal outcome in all women was successful. Two women were successfully treated with cyproheptadine before and during pregnancy. Cyproheptadine is a drug with antiserotoninergic, antihistaminic, anticholinergic, and antidopaminergic actions that inhibit ACTH secretion.[66] This drug is now not recommended because of its side effects.[64] Twelve of 23 pregnancies resulted in normal term deliveries; eight women (35%) gave birth to premature infants. One spontaneous abortion and two stillbirths also occurred in this series.[66] Steroid excess during pregnancy does not appear to increase the risk for congenital malformation, nor does it cause a significant risk of fetal adrenal insufficiency.[66,67,70]

ACROMEGALY

Acromegaly is a disease of GH overproduction. In more than 80% of cases, it results from a GH-secreting pituitary tumor.[71,72] Acromegaly is characterized by cosmetic disfiguration and metabolic abnormalities, such as glucose intolerance, hyperphosphatemia, and hypercalcemia. It also is frequently associated with systemic organ involvement, such as cardiomyopathy, neuropathy, arthropathy, and hypertension. The clinical course of patients with acromegaly may take the form of several syndromes: *excess of GH and GH-dependent tissue growth factors,* mainly insulinlike growth factor-I (IGF-I); *neuro-ophthalmic symptoms* and signs from the mass effects of the pituitary tumor; *pituitary hormone deficiency; associated hormonal hypersecretion,* mainly hyperprolactinemia.[71]

Forty percent of women of reproductive age with acromegaly have amenorrhea or oligomenorrhea resulting from low gonadotropin levels, with or without hyperprolactinemia. Thus, pregnancy in women with active disease is rare.[73,74] Pregnancy may induce worsening of acromegaly, and consequently, women with a GH-secreting tumor should be treated before pregnancy is attempted. Alternatively, if required, hypophysectomy can be performed in early pregnancy.[74] Treatment with bromocriptine has been effective in the treatment of acromegaly and in hyperprolactinemia. The dosage required to control the tumor may, however, be higher than for the treatment of PRL-secreting tumors.

DIABETES INSIPIDUS

The hypothalamus influences water homeostasis by controlling the pituitary secretion of arginine vasopressin in response to changes in osmolality and volume. Vasopressin enhances reabsorption of water by the distal renal tubules. *Central diabetes insipidus* occurs when the hypothalamic–pituitary system fails to secrete sufficient arginine vasopressin. Such a defect may be partial or complete.[75] It occurs in idiopathic fashion, or secondarily to a brain or a pituitary tumor, histiocytosis X, surgery, or rupture of an intracranial aneurism.

In the absence of vasopressin or if renal insensitivity to vasopressin develops (*nephrogenic diabetes insipidus*), the kidneys lose the ability to concentrate urine, and polyuria and compensatory polydipsia (increased water intake) develop. A third category of diabetes insipidus is seen only in pregnancy and is transient in nature.[75,76] This *transient diabetes insipidus in pregnancy* may be caused by the unmasking of a partial central diabetes insipidus by the diuretic effects of pregnancy or by excessive degradation of vasopressin by vasopressinase.[77]

Osmoregulation

Vasopressinase, an enzyme that rapidly inactivates vasopressin and oxytocin, increases steadily throughout pregnancy, with a 1000-fold increase until labor and delivery and a decrease thereafter, becoming undetectable by 4 weeks postpartum.[76] Vasopressinase is presumed to be of placental origin. Its activity *in vivo* and its role in osmoregulation in pregnancy are unknown.

During pregnancy, serum osmolality decreases by approximately 10 mOsm/kg. Thus, normal pregnancy is characterized by a resetting of the "osmostat" to a lower plasma osmolality (see also Chapters 4 and 142).[78,79] Pregnant women thus secrete vasopressin and experience thirst when their plasma sodium and osmolality rise to within the normal range for nonpregnant women. Conversely, an acute water load is rapidly excreted, and the urine quickly becomes maximally diluted. This pregnancy-induced state of physiologic superhydration presents a challenging diagnostic and therapeutic problem when diabetes insipidus and pregnancy coexist.

Diagnosis of Diabetes Insipidus

Pregnant women who present with polyuria and polydipsia should be evaluated for diabetes mellitus, preeclampsia, and liver and renal diseases. Psychogenic polydipsia also should be considered. The diagnosis of diabetes insipidus is made by using a water deprivation test.[75] Women with diabetes insipidus will not concentrate urine. A patient must lose up to 5% body weight before her dehydration is adequate to challenge the antidiuretic hormone (ADH) system.

Such dehydration is problematic in pregnancy because the resulting decrease in plasma volume may lead to uteroplacental insufficiency. Therefore, this test should be performed only on a labor floor with continuous fetal monitoring.[75]

In pregnant women, a threshold of 285 mOsm/kg is suggested for plasma levels that ensure dehydration, and not 295 mOsm/kg, as in a nonpregnant individual. If the patient has demonstrated rising serum osmolality with a urine osmolarity of less than 300 mOsm/kg, the diagnosis of diabetes insipidus is established. Antidiuretic hormone, such as 5 units of aqueous vasopressin, may be administered subcutaneously. The urine should concentrate within 1 hour. If after 2 hours the urine still does not concentrate, the vasopressinase-resistant dDAVP (1-desamino-8-D-arginine-vasopressin) may be given at 1 microgram of desmopressin by subcutaneous injection or as 10 micrograms by nasal spray. This will differentiate central diabetes insipidus from the transient vasopressin-resistant type of pregnancy.[75]

Central Diabetes Insipidus

The incidence of diabetes insipidus in pregnancy appears to be similar to the prevalence in the nonpregnant population (2–4 in 100,000).[76] Women with preexisting central diabetes insipidus usually experience increased thirst and require additional hormone replacement during pregnancy.[75,76,80-84] Whether this is caused by resistance of the kidneys to vasopressin or increased clearance of the administered vasopressin is unclear. Using the vasopressinase-resistant preparation, dDAVP, a synthetic analog of arginine vasopressin, may allow a distinction between these two possible explanations.[76] No complication to mother or fetus has been reported from the use of dDAVP.[75,76,85] Furthermore, dDAVP is poorly secreted in breast milk.[83]

Preeclampsia has been described in patients with diabetes insipidus[83,84], and the pressor and antidiuretic effects of vasopressin have been theorized to be involved in the pathogenesis of preeclampsia.[86] The fact that preeclampsia can occur in patients with complete central diabetes insipidus suggests, however, that vasopressin is not directly involved in the pathogenesis of pregnancy-induced hypertension.

Labor usually progresses normally in these patients. Dystocia and postpartum uterine atony and hemorrhage are infrequent.[76] Lactation may represent a potent nonosmotic stimulus for vasopressin release and often is associated with an improvement of the diabetes insipidus.[84] Thus, although increased requirement for fluid intake during lactation is anticipated, lactating mothers with diabetes insipidus experience decreased thirst and may reduce or, at times, discontinue exogenous antidiuretic hormone therapy while nursing.[76] If the mother does not nurse, a rapid return to the prepregnancy therapeutic regimen usually occurs.[76,81]

Transient Diabetes Insipidus of Pregnancy

Transient diabetes insipidus of pregnancy (*diabetes insipidus gravidarum*[87]) is a disease of late pregnancy and most often resolves spontaneously after delivery. Vasopressin-responsive (central) and vasopressin-resistant (initially thought to be nephrogenic) forms can be distinguished.

The transient vasopressin-responsive form of diabetes insipidus has a gradual onset and appears either idiopathic as an hereditary familial central diabetes insipidus, or in asymptomatic patients who have recovered from vasopressin-dependent central diabetes insipidus.[76] Whatever the etiology, it has a tendency to reoccur and occasionally to worsen in subsequent pregnancies.[87-89] Polyuria and polydipsia appear in the latter half of gestation and usually respond to hormone replacement. In the past, patients usually were treated with intramuscular injections of vasopressin tannate in oil (2.5 or 5 units), which has an antidiuretic effect for 24–72 hours. Desmopressin, a synthetic analogue of vasopressin (dDAVP), has prolonged antidiuretic activity with almost no pressor activity and is currently the drug of choice for treatment of diabetes insipidus. It has an antidiuretic effect for 12–24 hours in most patients when used intranasally in the amount of 10–20 μg (0.1–0.2 mL) or by subcutaneous injection (1–4 μg).

The transient vasopressin-resistant type of diabetes insipidus usually represents sporadic cases. With one exception[90], it has not recurred in subsequent pregnancies. A review of the literature[75,76] suggests that this form of diabetes insipidus is associated in most patients with preeclampsia, nausea, vomiting, and with laboratory abnormalities that indicate altered liver and renal functions. In general, only dDAVP is successful in treating these patients because vasopressinase does not break down dDAVP. Fluid restriction should be avoided because it will lead to dehydration and hemoconcentration.

Postpartum Diabetes Insipidus in Sheehan's Syndrome

It is highly unusual for isolated diabetes insipidus to occur after a normal delivery.[76,83] If Sheehan's syndrome is suspected, the anterior pituitary functions are usually extensively involved. However, only provocative tests of neurohypophyseal function will unmask subclinical diabetes insipidus.[76] When glucocorticoid deficiency is recognized and treated, urine volume increases and urine osmolality decreases. This observation suggests that the treatment of glucocorticoid deficiency may unmask subclinical diabetes insipidus.[91-94] Progress in reproductive endocrinology has allowed patients with Sheehan's syndrome to conceive.[94] Gynecologists and endocrinologists consequently must be aware of the very high incidence of latent central diabetes insipidus in patients with Sheehan's syndrome.

PITUITARY APOPLEXY AND SHEEHAN'S SYNDROME

Pituitary apoplexy may be highly variable in its clinical appearance. Sheehan and collegues established obstetric hemorrhage as a major cause of infarction of the nontumorous pituitary.[95,96] Tumor is the second most common predisposing condition to pituitary apoplexy.[97,98]

Reid et al[97] recently reviewed pituitary apoplexy. The clinical neurologic manifestations of pituitary apoplexy may be dramatic. The condition of some patients may deteriorate rapidly, leading to death within hours or days. In patients remaining conscious, conservative management with careful evaluation of hormonal status and appropriate replacement therapy are the only interventions necessary. Corticosteroid therapy should be initiated immediately when acute pituitary apoplexy is suspected. The progression of symptoms, with complete loss of vision, loss of consciousness, and evidence of hypothalamic damage, indicates that surgical decompression may be required.

In the absence of a tumor, the destruction of pituitary tissue leading to hypopituitarism initially causes few symptoms other than headache. Consequently, it frequently passes unnoticed until endocrine deficiencies become manifest or until autopsy.[97]

More than 1000 cases with Sheehan's syndrome have been reported since the original description of the disease.[99] In its classic form, patients have panhypopituitarism secondary to destruction of more than 95% of the anterior pituitary. The disease is characterized by failure of lactation, amenorrhea, loss of axillary and pubic hair, genital and breast atrophy, infertility, and symptoms and signs of hypothyroidism and adrenocortical insufficiency. Less extensive pituitary destruction (50–95%), is associated with mild or moderate hypopituitarism, which may be asymptomatic or present as an atypical form of the disease with loss of one or more tropic hormones.

Forty pregnancies in 20 patients with Sheehan's syndrome have been reported in the literature.[94,99] If hormonal replacement is adequate during pregnancy, a favorable outcome for the mother and baby can be expected. However, in 24 pregnancies in which hormonal replacement therapy was not provided, 42% ended in abortions, 1% were stillbirths, and only 54% were live births. Moreover, three of 11 patients (27%) who did not receive hormone replacement in the immediate postpartum period died. Early diagnosis and adequate therapy of hypopituitarism are vital to the mother and fetus.[99]

As noted previously, subclinical diabetes insipidus may appear in a Sheehan's patient during hormonal replacement therapy or during pregnancy.

EMPTY-SELLA SYNDROME

The empty-sella syndrome is either a radiologic or an autopsy diagnosis. In this syndrome, the sella turcica is found to be partially filled with cerebrospinal fluid. Incompetence of the diaphragma sellae is a prerequisite for the evolution of this syndrome. The diaphragma may be congenitally incompetent or thinned by tumor, surgery, or radiation. The syndrome also may develop as a result of infarction of a normal pituitary gland or of a pituitary tumor.[13,100] Empty-sella is found in approximately 5% of autopsies.[24]

The syndrome is more common in obese, parous, middle-aged females who frequently have headaches (50–80% of patients).[100,101] Although clinical hypopituitarism is not common, varying degrees of hypopituitarism are revealed in 30–40% of patients on detailed testing. Visual field defects are uncommon and are caused by herniation of the optic nerves into the sella.[100] Pituitary adenomas that may coexist with empty sellae have been described to secrete GH, ACTH, and prolactin.[101,102] Thus, in patients with endocrine indications of a secreting pituitary adenoma, a partially empty-sella should not preclude the correct diagnosis.

NELSON'S SYNDROME

Nelson and colleagues[103] described in 1958 the clinical appearance of an ACTH-secreting pituitary adenoma and of progressive hyperpigmentation following bilateral adrenalectomy in patients with Cushing's disease. Bilateral total adrenalectomy before the introduction of pituitary microsurgery was the preferred treatment for Cushing's disease. Currently, adrenalectomy is employed only in patients in whom other therapies are unsuccessful or unavailable.[65]

Rare cases of pregnancy in women with Nelson's syndrome have been reported.[104-106] Appropriate hormonal replacement therapy with glucocorticoids and mineralocorticoids is mandatory. In one patient, the pregnancy also was complicated by transient diabetes insipidus.[106]

THYROTROPIN-SECRETING PITUITARY TUMORS

Thyrotropin-secreting (TSH) pituitary tumors may be seen in two clinical situations.[107] Primary hypothyroidism may lead to compensatory pituitary enlargement, mostly a thyrotroph hyperplastic response, and rarely to an adenoma. Complete resolution of these "tumors" and reduction in sella's size are expected to occur after 1 month to 1 year of treatment with thyroxine. Conversely, thyrotroph adenomas may arise *de novo*, producing clinical thyrotoxicosis. Medical treatment can be directed at the thyroid or the pituitary gland (see also Chapter 40). However, pituitary surgery is the treatment of choice.

KALLMANN'S SYNDROME

The incidence of Kallmann's syndrome in women is one in 50,000 or about one fifth of the male incidence.[108] The pathologic findings include absence of the olfactory bulbs and tracts and a variable extent of hypothalamic hypoplasia with the clinical association of anosmia and hypogonadism.[109-111]

Aharoni and colleagues[108] recently reviewed seven reported pregnancies in women with Kallmann's syndrome. Pregnancies were achieved by induction of ovulation with either human menopausal gonadotropins and human chorionic gonadotropin (hMG–hCG) or by a gonadotropin-releasing hormone (GnRH) pump. Hormonal luteal phase support with hCG or progesterone may be considered in these patients because there is no endogenous luteinizing hormone to support the corpus luteum of pregnancy. Pregnancy proceeds essentially normally in such women, and labor can initiate spontaneously.

LYMPHOCYTIC ADENOHYPOPHYSITIS OF PREGNANCY

Lymphocytic adenohypophysitis is an autoimmune inflammatory disorder of the pituitary gland, characterized by the diffuse infiltration of the anterior pituitary with lymphocytes and plasma cells. Since first described in 1962 by Goudie and Pinkerton[112], nine cases of lymphocytic adenohypophysitis have been identified at autopsy[112-120] and eleven were proven by surgical biopsy.[121-130] With one exception[131], all were women, and most of them developed the symptoms toward the end of a normal pregnancy or during the postpartum period.

All women demonstrated clinical manifestations related to hypopituitarism or characteristic of a space-occupying lesion. Signs of the latter included headaches, visual loss, and blurring of vision. These patients seem to have a better prognosis, probably because the diagnosis was made earlier in the course of the disease and treatment with partial or total hypophysectomy and replacement therapy was initiated in a timely fashion.[120] Patients with hypoglycemic episodes or an acute illness (such as appendicitis, pneumonia, herpes labialis, or flu-like syndrome) that preceded the appearance of adrenocortical insufficiency and circulatory failure had a grave prognosis. Five patients died of the disease.[116-120]

The cause of lymphocytic adenohypophysitis remains poorly understood. Lymphocytes infiltrating the anterior pituitary were recently identified as a mixture of B and T cells, with a helper to suppressor ratio of 2 to 1.[130] The timing of occurrence suggests that this condition may be one of many recently reported peripartal autoimmune syndromes (see also Chapter 50). The relatively frequent association of other diseases considered to have an autoimmune etiology, such as lymphocytic thyroiditis, Hashimoto's disease, parathyroiditis, pernicious anemia, and retroperitoneal fibrosis[112,113,115,118-120], support an autoimmune etiology for lymphocytic adenohypophysitis.

Differentiation of a pituitary adenoma from lymphocytic adenohypophysitis by CT scan or MRI is practically impossible.[128] Surgical intervention is necessary to establish a diagnosis and may be necessary to reduce the size of the inflammatory lesion. This mass can compress surrounding structures, causing neuro-ophthalmic symptoms. In such a situation, radical surgery to remove all "tumor" tissue should be avoided.[128] The inflammatory tissue remaining after a subtotal resection can be treated with glucocorticoid therapy.

REFERENCES

1. Lechan RM. Neuroendocrinology of pituitary hormone regulation. *Endocrinol Metab Clin North Am.* 1987;16:475.
2. Vance ML, Thorner MO. Prolactinomas. *Endocrinol Metab Clin North Am.* 1987;16:731.
3. Bergland RM, Ray BS, Torack RM. Anatomical variations in the pituitary gland and adjacent structures in 225 human autopsy cases.*J Neurosurg.* 1968;28:93.
4. Gonzalez JG, Elizondo G, Saldivar D, et al. Pituitary gland growth during normal pregnancy: An *in vivo* study using magnetic resonance imaging. *Am J Med.* 1988;85:217.
5. Molitch ME. Pathogenesis of pituitary tumors. *Endocrinol Metab Clin North Am.* 1987;16:503.
6. Horvatch E, Kovacs K, Smyth HS. A novel type of pituitary adenoma: morphological features and clinical correlations. *J Clin Endocrinol Metab.* 1988;66:1111.
7. Abd El-Hamid MW, Joplin GF, Lewis PD. Incidentally found small pituitary ademonas may have no effect on fertility. *Acta Endocrinol* (*Copenh*). 1988;117:361.
8. Randall RV, Scheithauer BW, Laws ER, et al. Pituitary adenomas associated with hyperprolactinemia: a clinical and immunohistochemical study of 97 patients operated on transsphenoidally. *Mayo Clin Proc.* 1985;60:753.
9. Hyperprolactinaemia: When is a prolactinoma not a prolactinoma? *Lancet.* 1987;2:1002. Editorial.
10. Klibanski A. Nonsecreting pituitary tumors. *Endocrinol Metab Clin North Am.* 1987;16:703.
11. Melan O. Neuro-ophthalmologic features of pituitary tumors. *Endocrinol Metab Clin North Am.* 1987;16:585.
12. Colombo N, Berry I, Kucharczyk J, et al. Posterior pituitary gland: Appearance on MR images in normal and pathologic states. *Radiology.* 1987;165:481.
13. Wolpert SM. The radiology of pituitary adenomas. *Endocrinol Metab Clin North Am.* 1987;16:553.
14. Kovacs K, Horvath E. Pathology of pituitary tumors. *Endocrinol Metab Clin North Am.* 1987;16:529.
15. Burrow GN, Wortzman G, Rewcastle NB, et al. Microadenomas of the pituitary and abnormal sellar tomograms in an unselected autopsy series. *N. Engl J Med.* 1981;304:156.
16. Blackwell RE. Diagnosis and management of prolactinomas. *Fertil Steril.* 1985;43:5.
17. Dalkin AC, Marshall JC. Medical therapy of hyperprolactinemia. *Endocrinol Metab Clin North Am.* 1989;18:259.
18. Jeffcoate SL, Bacon RRA, Beastall GH, et al. Assay for prolactin: guidelines for the provision of a clinical biochemistry service. Ann Clin Biochem. 1986;23:638.
19. Rjosk HK, Fahlbusch R, von Werder K. Influence of pregnancies on prolactinomas. *Acta Endocrinol.* 1982;100:337.
20. Maurer RA. Relationship between estradiol, ergocryptine, and thyroid hormone: effects of prolactin synthesis and prolactin messenger ribonucleic acid levels. *Endocrinology.* 1982;110:1515.
21. Tyson JE, Hwang P, Guyda H, Friesen H. Studies of prolactin secretion in human pregnancy. *Am J Obstet Gynecol.* 1972;113:14.
22. Molitch ME. Pregnancy and the hyperprolactinemic woman. *N Engl J Med.* 1985;312:1364.
23. Velasco VR, Tolis G. Pregnancy in hyperprolactinemic women. *Fertil Steril.* 1984;41:793.
24. Speroff L, Glass RH, Kase NG. Amenorrhea. In: *Clinical Gynecologic Endocrinology and Infertility.* Baltimore, MD: William & Wilkins; 1989: 165.
25. Maeda T, Ushiroyama T, Okuda K, et al. Effective bromocriptine treatment of a pituitary macroadenoma during pregnancy. *Obstet Gynecol.* 1983;61:117.
26. Konopka P, Raymond JP, Merceron RE, Seneze J. Continuous administration of bromocriptine in the prevention of neurological complications in pregnant women with prolactinomas. *Am J Obstet Gynecol.* 1983;146:935.
27. Comtois R, Bertrand S, Beairegard H, et al. Spontaneous regression of a prolactin-producing pituitary adenoma during pregnancy. *Am J Med.* 1987;83:1105. Letter.
28. Jewelewicz R, Vande Wiele RL. Clinical course and outcome of pregnancy in twenty-five patients with pituitary microadenomas.*Am J Obstet Gynecol.* 1980;136:339.
29. vanRoon E, van der Vijver JCM, Gerretsen G. Rapid regression of a suprasellar extending prolactinoma after bromocriptine treatment during pregnancy. *Fertil Steril.* 1981;36:173.
30. Canales ES, Garcia IC, Ruiz JE, Zarate A. Bromocriptine as prophylactic therapy in prolactinoma during pregnancy. *Fertil Steril.* 1981;36:524.
31. Crosignani PG, Ferrari C, Scarduelli C, et al. Spontaneous and induced pregnancies in hyperprolactinemic women. *Obstet Gynecol.* 1981;58:708.
32. Landolt AM. Surgical treatment of pituitary prolactinomas: Postoperative prolactin and fertility in seventy patients. *Fertil Steril.* 1981;35:620.
33. Turkalj I, Braun P, Krupp P. Surveillance of bromocriptine in pregnancy. *JAMA.* 1982;247:1589.
34. Barbieri RL, Ryan KJ. Bromocriptin: endocrın pharmacology and therapeutic applications. *Fertil Steril.* 1983;39:727.
35. Bergh T, Nillius SJ, Wide L. Clinical course and outcome of pregnancies in amenorrhoeic women with hyperprolactinaemia and pituitary tumours. *Br Med J.* 1978;1:875.
36. Serri O, Rasio E, Beauregard H, et al. Recurrence of hyperprolactinemia after selective transsphenoidal adenomectomy in women with prolactinoma. *N Engl J Med.* 1983;309:208.
37. Hammond CB, Haney AF, Land MR, et al. The outcome of pregnancy in patients with treated and untreated prolactin-secreting pituitary tumors. *Am J Obstet Gynecol.* 1983;147:148.
38. Magyar DM, Marshall JR. Pituitary tumors and pregnancy. *Am J Obstet Gynecol.* 1978;132:739.
39. Samaan NA, Leavens ME, Sacca R, et al. The effects of pregnancy on patients with hyperprolactinemia. *Am J Obstet Gynecol.* 1984;148:466.
40. Molitch ME, Elton RL, Blackwell RE, et al. Bromocriptine as primary therapy for prolactin-secreting macroadenomas: Results of a prospective multicenter study. *J Clin Endocrinol Metab.* 1985;60:698.
41. Mornex R, Orgiazzi J, Hugues B, et al. Normal pregnancies after treatment of hyperprolactinemia with bromoergocryptine, despite suspected pituitary tumors. *J Clin Endocrinol Metab.* 1978;47:290.
42. Bohnet HG, Kato K, Wolf AS. Treatment of hyperprolactinemic amenorrhea with Metergolin. *Obstet Gynecol.* 1986;67:249.
43. Tamura T, Satoh T, Minakami H, Tamada T. Effect of hydergine in hyperprolactinemia. *J Clin Endocrinol Metab.* 1989;69:470.
44. Corenblum B. Successful outcome of ergocryptine-induced pregnancies in twenty-one women with prolactin-secreting pituitary adenomas. *Fertil Steril.* 1979;32:183.
45. Gemzell C, Wang CF. Outcome of pregnancy in women with pituitary adenoma. *Fertil Steril.* 1979;32:363.
46. Lamerts SWJ, Klign JGM, deLange SA, et al. The incidence of complications during pregnancy after treatment of hyperprolactinemia with bromocriptine in patients with radiologically evident pituitary tumors. *Fertil Steril.* 1979;31:614.
47. Halberg FE, Sheline GE. Radiotherapy of pituitary tumors. *Endocrinol Metab Clin North Am.* 1987;16:667.
48. Laws ER. Pituitary surgery. *Endocrinol Metab Clin North Am.* 1987;16:647.
49. Scanlon MF, Peters JR, Thomas JP, et al. Management of selected patients with hyperprolactinaemia by partial hypophysectomy. *Br Med J.* 1985;291:1547.
50. Thomson JA, Teasdale GM, Gordon D, et al. Treatment of presumed prolactinoma by transsphenoidal operation: early and late results. *Br Med J.* 1985;291:1550.
51. Jonathan NB. Dopamine: a prolactin-inhibiting hormone. *Endoc Rev.* 1985;6:564.
52. Kletzky OA, Borenstein R, Mileikowsky GN. Pergolide and bromocriptine for treatment of patients with hyperprolactinemia. *Am J Obstet Gynecol.* 1986;154:431.
53. Hesla JS, Rodman EF, Molitch ME, et al. The effect of the ergoline derivative, CU 32-085, on prolactin secretion in hyperprolactinemic women. *Fertil Steril.* 1987;48:555.
54. Sopelak VM, Whitworth NS, Norman PF, Cowan BD. Bromocriptine inhibition of anesthesia-induced hyperprolactinemia: Effect on serum and follicular fluid hormones, oocyte fertilization, and embryo cleavage rates during in vitro fertilization. *Fertil Steril.* 1989;52:627.
55. Speroff L, Glass RH, Kase NG. The breast. In: *Clinical Gynecologic Endocrinology and Infertility.* Baltimore, MD: Williams & Wilkins; 1989;283.
56. Barguno JM, de Pozo E, Cruz M, Figueras J. Failure of maintained hyperprolactinemia to improve lactational performance in late puerperium. *J Clin Endocrinol Metab.* 1988;66:876.

57. Yuen BH. Prolactin in human milk: the influence of nursing and the duration of postpartum lactation. *Am J Obstet Gynecol.* 1988;158:583.
58. Vaughn TC, Haney AF, Wiebe RH, et al. Spontaneous regression of prolactin-producing pituitary adenomas. *Am J Obstet Gynecol.* 1980;136:980.
59. Martin TL, Kim M, Malarkey WB. The natural history of idiopathic hyperprolactinemia. *J Clin Endocrinol Metab.* 1985;60:855.
60. Rasmussen C, Bergh T, Wide L. Prolactin secretion and menstrual function after long-term bromocriptine treatment. *Fertil Steril.* 1987;48:550.
61. Pereira MC, Sobrinho LG, Afonso AM, et al. Is idiopathic hyperprolactinemia a transitional stage toward prolactinoma? *Obstet Gynecol.* 1987;70:305.
62. Archer DF. Current concepts and treatment of hyperprolactinemia. *Obstet Gynecol Clin North Am.* 1987;14:979.
63. Malarkey WB, Jackson R, Wortsman J. Long-term assessment of patients with macroprolactinemia. *Fertil Steril.* 1988;50:413.
64. Blankstein J, Mashiach S. Lunenfeld B. Prolactin-inhibiting agents. In: *Ovulation Induction and In Vitro Fertilization.* Chicago, IL: Year Book Medical Publishers; 1986;77.
65. Aron DC, Findling JW, Tyrrell JB. Cushing's disease. *Endocrinol Metab Clin North Am.* 1987;16:705.
66. Pickard J, Jochen AL, Sadur CN, Hofeldt FD. Cushing's syndrome in pregnancy. *Obstet Gynecol Surv.* 1990;45:87.
67. Aron DC, Schnall AM, Sheeler LR. Cushing's syndrome and pregnancy. *Am J Obstet Gynecol.* 1990;162:244.
68. Dwyer AJ, Frank JA, Doppman JL, et al. Pituitary adenomas in patients with Cushing disease: Initial experience with Gd-DTPA-enhanced MR imaging. *Radiology.* 1987;163:421.
69. Casson IF, Davis JC, Jeffreys RV, et al. Successful management of Cushing's disease during pregnancy by transsphenoidal adenectomy. *Clin Endocrinol.* 1987;27:423.
70. Semple CG, McEwan H, Teasdale GM, et al. Recurrence of Cushing's disease in pregnancy. *Br J Obstet Gynecol.* 1985;92:295.
71. Barkan AL. Acromegaly. *Endocrinol Metab Clin North Am.* 1989;18:277.
72. Baumann G. Acromegaly. *Endocrinol Metab Clin North Am.* 1987;16:685.
73. Luboshitzky R, Dickstein G, Bazilai D. Bromocriptine-induced pregnancy in an acromegalic patient. *JAMA.* 1980;244:584.
74. Bigazzi M, Ronga R, Lancranjan I, et al. A pregnancy in a acromegalic woman during bromocriptine treatment: Effects on growth hormone and prolactin in the maternal, fetal and amniotic compartments. *J Clin Endocrinol Metab.* 1979;48:9.
75. Krege J, Katz FL, Bowes WA. Transient diabetes insipidus of pregnancy. *Obstet Gynecol Surv.* 1989;44:789.
76. Durr JA. Diabetes insipidus in pregnancy. *Am J Kidney Dis.* 1987;9:276.
77. Durr JA, Hoggard JG, Hunt JM, Schrier RW. Diabetes insipidus in pregnancy associated with abnormally high circulating vasopressinase activity. *N Engl J Med.* 1987;316:1070.
78. Lindheimer MD, Barron WM, Durr JA, et al. Water homeostasis and vasopressin secretion during gestation. *Adv Nephrol.* 1986;15:1.
79. Lindheimer MD, Barron WM, Durr JA, Davison JM. Water homeostasis and vasopressin release during rodent and human gestation. *Am J Kidney Dis.* 1987;9:270.
80. Carfagno SC, Durant TM, Shuman CR. Diabetes insipidus in pregnancy. *Arch Intern Med.* 1953;92:542.
81. Feldberg D, Samuel N, Dicker D, et al. Diabetes insipidus in pregnancy. *Israel J Med Sci.* 1985;21:695.
82. Amico JA. Diabetes insipidus and pregnancy. *Front Horm Res.* 1985;13:266.
83. Campbell JW. Diabetes insipidus and complicated pregnancy. *JAMA.* 1980;243:1744.
84. Hime MC, Richardson JA. Diabetes insipidus and pregnancy. Case report, incidence and review of literature. *Obstet Gynecol Surv.* 1978;33:375.
85. Shah S, Thakur V. Vasopressinase and diabetes insipidus of pregnancy. *Ann Intern Med.* 1988;109:435. Letter.
86. Burt RK. A hypothesis on the role of antidiuretic hormone in preeclampsia. *Med Hypoth.* 1983;12:61.
87. Frossman H. On the hereditary diabetes insipidus. *Acta Med Scan.* 1945;159 (Suppl): l.
88. Blotner H, Kunkel P. Diabetes insipidus and pregnancy. Report of two cases. *N Engl J Med.* 1942;227:287.
89. Baylis PH, Thompson C, Burd J, et al. Recurrent pregnancy-induced polyuria due to hypothalamic diabetes insipidus: an invitation into possible mechanisms responsible for polyuria. *Clin Endocrinol.* 1986;24:459.
90. Goodman H, Sachs BP, Phillippe M, et al. Transient, recurrent nephrogenic diabetes insipidus. *Am J Obstet Gynecol.* 1984;149:910.
91. Weiner P, Ben Israel J, Palvnick L. Sheehan's syndrome with diabetes insipidus. *Israel J Med Sci.* 1979;15:431.
92. Bakiri F, Benmiloud M. Antidiuretic function in Sheehan's syndrome. *Br Med J.* 1984;289:579.
93. Bakiri F, Benmiloud M, Vallotton MB. Argininepressin in postpartum panhypopituitarism: Urinary excretion and kidney response to osmolar load. *J Clin Endocrinol Metab.* 1984;55:511.
94. Barbieri RL, Randall RW, Saltzman DH. Diabetes insipidus occurring in a patient with Sheehan's syndrome during gonadotropin-induced pregnancy. *Fertil Steril.* 1985;44:529.
95. Sheehan HL, Murdock R. Postpartum necrosis of the anterior pituitary: Pathological and clinical aspects. *J Obstet Gynaecol Br Emp.* 1938;45:456.
96. Sheehan HL, Stanfield JP. The pathogenesis of postpartum necrosis of the anterior lobe of the pituitary gland. *Acta Endocrinol.* 1961;37:479.
97. Reid RL, Quigley ME, Yen SSC. Pituitary apoplexy. A review. *Arch Neurol.* 1985;42:712.
98. O'Donovan PA, O'Donovan PJ, Ritchie EH, et al. Apoplexy into a prolactin secreting macroadenoma during early pregnancy with successful outcome. Case report. *Br J Obstet Gynecol.* 1986;93:389.
99. Grimes HG, Brooks MH. Pregnancy in Sheehan's syndrome. Report of a case and review. *Obstet Gynecol Surv.* 1980;35:481.
100. Post KD, McCormick PC, Bello JA. Differential diagnosis of pituitary tumors. *Endocrinol Metab Clin North Am.* 1987;16:609.
101. Haney AF, Kramer RS, Wiebe RH, et al. Hypothalamic–pituitary function and radiographic evaluation of women with hyperprolactinemia and a "empty"sella turcica. *Am J Obstet Gynecol.* 1979;134:917.
102. Domingue JN, Wing SD, Wilson CB. Coexisting pituitary adenomas and partially empty sellas. *J Neurosurg.* 1978;48:23.
103. Nelson DH, Meakin JW, Dealy JB, et al. ACTH-producing tumor of the pituitary gland. *N Engl J Med.* 1958;259:161.
104. Leiba S, Kaufman H, Winkelsberg G. Pregnancy in a case of Nelson's syndrome. *Acta Obstet Gynecol Scand.* 1970;57:373.
105. Feeney JG, Craig GA, Hancoch KW. Pregnancy and Nelson's syndrome. Two case reports. *Br J Obstet Gynaecol.* 1978;85:715.
106. Reubens R, Thiery M, Vermeulen A. Pregnancy in Nelson's syndrome. *Z Geburtshilfe Perinatol.* 1979;183:303.
107. Smallridge RC. Thyrotropin-secreting pituitary tumors. *Endocrinol Metab Clin North Am.* 1987;16:765.
108. Aharoni A, Tal J, Paltieli Y, et al. Kallmann syndrome: a case of twin pregnancy and review of the literature. *Obstet Gynecol Surv.* 1989;44:491.
109. Tagatz G, Fialkow PJ, Smith D, Spandoni L. Hypogonadotropic hypogonadism associated with anosmia in the female. *N Engl J Med.* 1970;283:1326.
110. Spitz IM, Diamant Y, Rosen E, et al. Isolated gonadotropin deficiency: a heterogenous syndrome. *N Engl J Med.* 1974;290:10.
111. Soules MR, Hammond CB. Female Kallmann's syndrome: evidence for a hypothalamic luteinizing hormone-releasing hormone deficiency. *Fertil Steril.* 1980;33:82.
112. Goudie RB, Pinkerton PH. Anterior hypophysitis and Hashimoto's disease in young women. *J Pathol Bacteriol.* 1962;83:584.
113. Hume R, Roberts GH. Hypophysitis and hypopituitarism: report of a case. *Br Med J.* 1967;2:548.
114. Ceblin MS, Velasco ME, De Las Mulas JM, Druet RL. Galactorrhea associated with lymphocytic adenohypophysitis. *Br J Obstet Gynecol.* 1981;88:675.
115. Lack EE. Lymphoid hypophysitis with end organ insufficiency. *Arch Pathol.* 1975;99:215.
116. Engloff B, Fischbacker W, Von Goumoens E. Lymphomatose hypophysitis mit Hypophyseninsuffizienz. *Schweiz Med Wochenschr.* 1969;99:1499.
117. Richtsmeier AJ, Henry RA, Bloodworth JMB, Ehrlich EN. Lymphoid hypophysitis with selective adrenocorticotropic hormone deficiency. *Arch Intern Med.* 1980;140:1243.
118. Gleason TH, Stebbins PL, Shanahan MF. Lymphoid hypophysitis in a patient with hypoglycemic episodes. *Arch Pathol Lab Med.* 1978;102:46.
119. Sobrino-Simoes M, Brandao A, Pavia ME, et al. Lymphoid hypophysitis in a patient with lymphoid thyroiditis, lymphoid adrenalitis, and idiopathic retroperitoneal fibrosis. *Arch Pathol Lab Med.* 1985;109:230.
120. Gal R, Schwartz A, Gukovsky-Oren S, et al. Lymphoid hypophysitis associated with sudden maternal death: report of a case and review of the literature. *Obstet Gynecol Surv.* 1986;41:619.
121. Asa SL, Bilboa JM, Kovacs, et al. Lymphocytic hypophysitis of pregnancy resulting in hypopituitarism: a distinct clinicopathologic entity. *Ann Intern Med.* 1981;95:166.
122. Baskin DS, Townsend JJ, Wilson CB. Lymphocytic adenohypophysitis of pregnancy simulating a pituitary adenoma: a distinct pathological entity. *J Neurosurg.* 1982;56:148.
123. Hungerford GD, Biggs PJ, Levine JH, et al. Lymphoid adenohypophysitis with radiologic and clinical findings resembling a pituitary tumor. *AJNR.* 1982;3:444.
124. Mayfield RK, Levine JH, Gordon L, et al. Lymphoid adenohypophysitis presenting as a pituitary tumor. *Am J Med.* 1980;69:619.
125. Mazzone T, Kelly W, Ensick J. Lymphocytic hypophysitis associated with antiparietal cell antibodies and vitamin B12 deficiency. *Arch Intern Med.* 1983;143:1794.
126. Portocarrero CJ, Robinson AG, Taylor AL, Klein I. Lymphoid hypophysitis: an unusual cause of hyperprolactinemia and enlarged sella turcica. *JAMA.* 1981;246:1811.
127. Quencer RM. Lymphocytic adenohypophysitis: autoimmune disorder of the pituitary gland. *AJNR.* 1980;1:343.

128. Levine SN, Benzel EC, Fowler MR, et al. Lymphocytic adenohypophysitis: clinical, radiological and magnetic resonance imaging characterization. *Neurosurgery.* 1988;22:937.
129. McGrail KM, Beyerl BD, Black PM, et al. Lymphocytic adenohypophysitis of pregnancy with complete recovery. *Neurosurgery.* 1987;20:791.
130. Jensen MD, Handwerger BS, Scheithauer BW, et al. Lymphocytic hypophysitis with isolated corticotropin deficiency. *Ann Intern Med.* 1986;105:200.
131. Guay AT, Agnello V, Tronic BC, et al. Lymphocytic hypophysitis in a man. *J Clin Endocrinol Metab.* 1987;64:631.

Chapter Forty

Thyroid Diseases

Michael M. Kaplan

40

Thyroid diseases are commonly encountered during pregnancy because both hyperthyroidism and hypothyroidism are five to ten times more common in women than in men and because these diseases are readily treatable but rarely cured. Thus, a young woman who develops a thyroid disease will usually require treatment during all of her subsequent pregnancies. Estimates of prevalence rates for hyperthyroidism and hypothyroidism in women are 1–2% based on surveys of several largely Caucasian community populations. Pregnancy can alter the course of thyroid diseases; conversely, the manifestations of thyroid hormone excess or deficiency and the treatment of these conditions can have adverse effects on a pregnancy unless appropriate treatment is administered. There also is a tendency for some thyroid diseases to appear or to worsen in the first few months postpartum.

Many organs are targets for thyroid hormones. Almost any part of the body can exhibit the manifestations of thyroid hormone excess, called *hyperthyroidism,* when the thyroid gland is the source of the excess and more generally termed *thyrotoxicosis,* or of thyroid hormone deficiency, called *hypothyroidism.* When severe, hypothyroidism is called *myxedema,* although some reserve this term for the skin changes of hypothyroidism.

NORMAL THYROID HORMONE PHYSIOLOGY

Figure 40–1 illustrates the normal thyroid hormone economy. Thyroxine (T_4) is the main secretory product of the thyroid gland and the main form of thyroid hormone circulating in the blood. Within cells, however, 3,5,3′-triiodothyronine (T_3) is the main active form of thyroid hormone. All the T_4 in the body is secreted by the thyroid gland, but only about 20% of the T_3 is secreted by the thyroid. The majority of the circulating T_3 is made from T_4 outside of the thyroid by a process termed 5′-deiodination.

Biosynthesis of T_4 and T_3 in the thyroid gland involves several steps: (1) trapping of iodide from the plasma by active transport; (2) organification (ie, incorporation of the

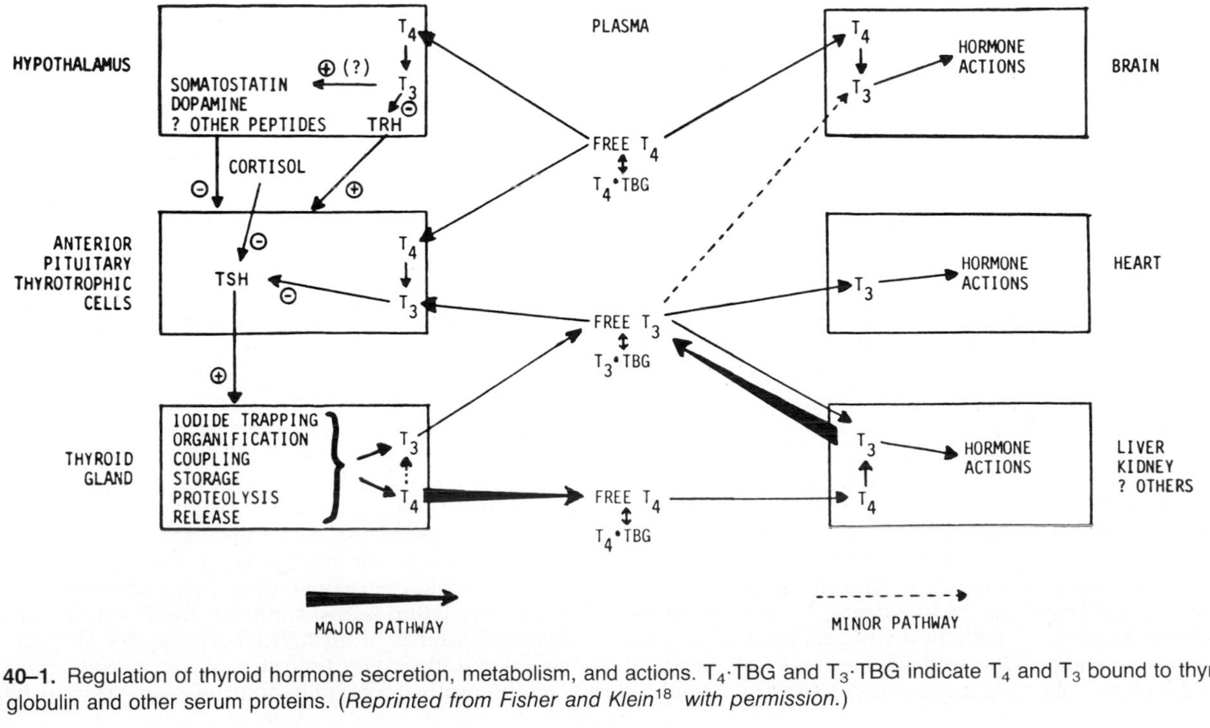

Figure 40–1. Regulation of thyroid hormone secretion, metabolism, and actions. T_4·TBG and T_3·TBG indicate T_4 and T_3 bound to thyroxine-binding globulin and other serum proteins. (*Reprinted from Fisher and Klein[18] with permission.*)

iodide into tyrosine residues on thyroglobulin, the colloid protein of the thyroid gland); (3) coupling of monoiodinated and diiodinated tyrosine residues to form thyronines, still part of the thyroglobulin molecule; (4) storage of thyroglobulin as colloid within the follicular lumen; (5) proteolysis and liberation of T_4 and T_3 from the thyroglobulin; and (6) release of T_4 and T_3 into the circulation. Some T_4 may be converted to T_3 within the thyroid gland before secretion.

Secretion of thyroid hormones is regulated by thyrotropin (thyroid-stimulating hormones, or TSH) secreted by the anterior pituitary gland. TSH accelerates all of the steps of thyroid hormone biosynthesis. Release of TSH is regulated by negative feedback of the thyroid hormones on the pituitary thyrotrophic cells and by stimulatory and inhibitory influences from the hypothalamus, as indicated in Figure 40–1. Stimulation by thyrotropin-releasing hormone (TRH) is by far the most important hypothalamic influence on TSH secretion. The feedback of serum T_4 and T_3 on TSH release is very finely tuned and includes a "long loop" feedback of serum T_4 and T_3 on TRH production. Even minimal degrees of hyperthyroidism or hypothyroidism cause marked suppression or stimulation, respectively, of basal TSH secretion and TRH-stimulated TSH release.

Most thyroid hormone actions are initiated by binding of intracellular T_3 to a specific nuclear receptor. The T_3-receptor binds to regulatory elements of certain genes, thereby directing production of specific messenger ribonucleic acids (mRNAs) and subsequent synthesis of their protein products. Some tissues, including the anterior pituitary and brain, produce a large fraction of their intracellular T_3 from T_4, whereas other tissues derive almost all their intracellular T_3 from plasma T_3 (see Fig. 40–1). The phenomenon of intracellular T_3 production from T_4 in the pituitary gland resolves the apparent paradox that serum TSH concentrations are often more closely correlated with serum T_4 than serum T_3 levels, even though T_3 is the main active form of thyroid hormone within cells.

CHANGES IN MATERNAL THYROID FUNCTION IN PREGNANCY

Almost all of the T_4 and T_3 in the plasma are bound strongly to plasma proteins, principally thyroxine-binding globulin (TBG). However, it is the concentrations of the free, or nonprotein bound, plasma T_4 and T_3 that determine the content of T_4 and T_3 in the tissues at the site(s) of action. It is common to have abnormalities of the serum TBG concentration in the absence of any thyroid disease; TBG production by the liver is stimulated by estrogens, and therefore serum TBG levels are high during pregnancy or during oral contraceptive treatment. In the case of a primary alteration in TBG, the total serum T_4 and T_3 concentrations will change in parallel with that of TBG, but the free T_4 and T_3 concentrations will change in parallel with that of TBG, but the free T_4 and T_3 concentrations remain normal. Thus, in pregnancy, there is a marked increase in the total serum T_4 and T_3 concentrations.

The great majority of pregnant women have values within the nonpregnant normal range for free T_4 and T_3 concentrations.[1] Measurements of the T_4 secretion rate from the thyroid gland during pregnancy also have been normal.[2] There are reports of unchanged, slightly increased, and slightly decreased mean serum free T_4 and T_3 concentrations in pregnant women[1,3,4], with an occasional individual who has a value outside of the nonpregnant normal range in either direction. There is no accepted "gold standard" method for the determination of the free hormone concentrations, and these minor discrepancies are probably due to methodologic variables.

Suppressibility of thyroid hormone secretion by exogenous T_3 is normal during pregnancy.[5] The basal serum TSH concentration and the normal range for the increase in serum TSH after stimulation by TRH are not substantially changed during pregnancy[6], although there is a slight decrease in the mean serum TSH concentration in the first trimester, a time when serum human chorionic gonadotropin (hCG) concentration are highest.[1] This decrease in TSH is probably a compensation for the weak thyrotropic effect of the high levels of hCG. The mean increment in TSH after TRH may be slightly increased in some pregnant women.[7]

In areas of the world with iodine deficiency or minimum degrees of iodine sufficiency, the thyroid gland may enlarge during pregnancy, creating a "goiter of pregnancy." The minimum dietary requirement for iodine is increased during pregnancy because of the increased renal excretion of iodide.[8] In North America where there is a superabundance of dietary iodine, thyroid enlargement in pregnant patients is almost always caused by clear-cut thyroid disease. This clinical impression is confirmed by recent systematic studies, which found no clinically important change in thyroid size during pregnancy in American women with no known thyroid disease.[9,10]

Laboratory Evaluation of Maternal Thyroid Function

Measurements of serum T_4, T_3, and TSH are readily available. Because of the major alterations in serum protein binding of T_4 and T_3 during pregnancy[11], the serum thyroid hormone levels always must be interpreted in the context of protein binding; that is, the free serum hormone concentrations must be estimated. Several techniques for measuring free T_4 and free T_3 are available commercially. The most accurate technique during pregnancy is the kinetic immunoextraction radioimmunoassay. Analog radioimmunoassays are adequate if they are formulated so that the reduction in serum albumin during pregnancy does not give artifactually low results. Less accurate in pregnancy is the method used most often: the free thyroxine index (FT_4I) obtained by multiplying the T_3 uptake test result by the serum T_4 concentration. The T_3 uptake value is proportional to the percent of free T_4 and percent of free T_3; however, the relationship becomes nonlinear at extremes of high or low percent of free hormone. Thus, the product of the serum T_4 (or T_3) and the T_3 uptake is proportional to the absolute free T_4 (or free T_3) concentration in most cases. However, in some normal pregnant women with very high TBG and total T_4 levels, the T_3 uptake underestimates the extent of T_4 binding to TBG and yields an erroneously high FT_4I. The T_3 uptake is not an independent test of thyroid function and does not measure the serum T_3 concentration.

Although measurement of the serum T_4 concentration or a free T_4 estimate have been the traditional first-line tests for evaluating thyroid function, a superior alternative, high-sensitivity serum TSH assays, has become available. These assays, which use monoclonal antibodies and chemiluminescent, enzymatic, or radiometric detection techniques (abbreviated ICMA, EIA, and IRMA, respectively), have increased the sensitivity of TSH measurements by 20- to 100-fold over conventional radioimmunoassays and, unlike the latter, can distinguish the low values found in hyperthyroidism from normal. The upper limit of normal also is slightly lower than that of many conventional TSH radioimmunoassays, allowing detection of mild hypothyroidism more readily. Serum total and free T_4 levels may be normal in cases of mild hypothyroidism and, less commonly, in mild hyperthyroidism. By contrast, results from high-sensitivity serum TSH assays are misleading only in the rare cases of TSH deficiency caused by pituitary or hypothalamic disease and the rarer cases of hyperthyroidism caused by TSH hypersecretion.

When a high-sensitivity TSH assay is used as a screening test for thyroid disease and the result is normal, the evaluation can stop. If a high-sensitivity TSH result is undetectably low, hyperthyroidism should be suggested, and estimates of serum free T_4 and free T_3 concentrations are needed to confirm the diagnosis and assess the severity of the disorder. In hyperthyroidism, the free T_3 and free T_3 index values are virtually always elevated, and the degree of elevation tends to be greater than that of the free T_4. Suppressed serum TSH concentrations also can be seen occasionally in women with severe morning sickness and no thyroid disease.[12] If the serum TSH result is high, hypothyroidism is probable. An estimate of the free T_4 level is indicated to help evaluate the severity of the thyroid hormone deficiency. The serum T_3 test is of little value in evaluating a patient for hypothyroidism because it remains within the normal range, usually in the lower part, in mild to moderate disease and falls below normal only in severe hypothyroidism.

More sensitive yet is the TRH stimulation test, performed by injecting 400–500 μg of synthetic TRH (protirelin) intravenously and measuring the serum TSH concentration before and 20 minutes afterward. If pituitary or hypothalamic abnormalities are being considered, additional 60- and 90-minute serum TSH measurements are useful. Patients should be told in advance that it is normal for TRH to induce transient (2–5 minutes) feelings of nausea, flushing, or an urge to urinate. When there is minimal thyrotoxicosis, or even when there, is largely autonomous but not excessive thyroid hormone secretion, the response to TRH is abolished (an increase of less than 2 μU TSH/mL at 30 minutes). A normal response to TRH provides assurance that borderline–high levels of free T_4 and T_3 are not pathologic. In even minimal hypothyroidism, the response to TRH is exaggerated, typically with an increase of more than 35 μU TSH/mL at 30 minutes. The TRH stimulation test is needed much less often when a high-sensitivity TSH assay is used for basal (unstimulated) TSH measurements than when a conventional TSH radioimmunoassay is used.

The normal ranges for the standard tests of thyroid function and the expected changes in different stages of pregnancy[1,11] are shown in Table 40–1. The interactions of the changes caused by thyroid diseases with the changes caused by pregnancy are shown in Table 40–2. Adjunctive tests, such as measurements of antithyroid antibodies and of thyroid-stimulating antibodies, may have some use in establishing the cause of a patient's thyroid disease or, as discussed below, assessing the risk of congenital hyperthyroidism, but they do not define the patient's thyroid status.

THYROID HORMONE ABNORMALITIES IN NONTHYROID ILLNESSES

In nonthyroidal illnesses, several patterns of alterations in thyroid hormone economy and thyroid function tests may occur. These do not represent thyroid disease and therefore must be recognized to avoid erroneous diagnoses of hyperthyroidism or hypothyroidism. The range of illnesses that can induce these abnormalities is vast, from simple fasting to infections, surgical stress, diabetes, and heart, kidney, and liver disease to shock. The most common changes in thyroid function are decreases in serum concentrations of total and free T_3 and the free T_3 index, with other tests remaining normal. In more severe illness, the serum total and free T_4 concentrations can be subnormal or elevated. In either setting, estimates of the serum free T_4 concentration by equilibrium dialysis, the free T_4 index, and other free T_4 methods often give different results, with the free T_4 index more often subnormal and the serum free T_4 by dialysis more often elevated. It is not clearly established whether one of these free T_4 estimates correlates better with tissue effects of thyroid hormone. Even when the estimated free T_4 concentration is elevated because of a nonthyroid illness, the total and free T_3 concentrations are low–normal or low.

TABLE 40–1. NORMAL VALUES FOR SERUM MEASUREMENTS USED TO EVALUATE THYROID FUNCTION

Measurement	Normal Range for Women Not Pregnant or Taking Estrogen	Changes in Mean Values in Pregnancy: First Trimester	Changes in Mean Values in Pregnancy: Second and Third Trimesters
Total T_4 concentration, μg/dL	5–11	Increased 30–40%	Increased 65%
TBG concentration, mg/L	15–30	Increased 90%	Increased 100–150%
Percent free T_4	0.018–0.030	Decreased 30%	Decreased 30–50%
T_3 uptake or equivalent[a]	Depends on method	Decreased 30%	Decreased 40%
Free T_4 concentration, ng/dL	0.7–2.2	Unchanged	Unchanged
Total T_3 concentration, ng/dL	70–200	Increased 30%	Increased 50–70%
Percent free T_3	0.18–0.45	Decreased 30%	Decreased 50–70%
Free T_3 concentration, pg/mL	200–500	Unchanged	Unchanged
TSH concentration, μU/mL	0.3–5.0	Unchanged	Unchanged
TSH response to exogenous TRH (400–500 μg IV), μU/mL	Increase of 5–25 above basal value	Unchanged	Unchanged

(The mean normal values for these tests and the limits of normal can vary as much as twofold among different methods and laboratories. The values in this table are typical.)

[a] Other terms are sometimes used for this test, including thyroid hormone binding ratio, TBG index, and thyroxine binding index.

TABLE 40–2. CHANGES IN SERUM HORMONE MEASUREMENTS CAUSED BY THYROID DISEASE IN PREGNANCY

	Hyperthyroidism		Hypothyroidism	
	Nonpregnant Patient	Pregnant Patient	Nonpregnant Patient	Pregnant Patient
Total T_4	↑	↑ ↑	↓	Normal or ↓
Free T_4 concentration	↑	↑	↓	↓
Free T_4 index	↑	↑	↓	↓
T_3 uptake	↑	Normal, slightly ↑, or slightly ↓	↓	↓ ↓
TBG concentration	Normal or slightly ↓	↑	Normal or slightly ↑	↑
T_4 to TBG ratio	↑	↑	↓	↓
Total T_3	↑	↑ ↑	Normal or ↓ [a]	Normal [a]
Free T_3 concentration	↑	↑	Normal or ↓ [a]	Normal[a]
TSH	↓	↓	↑	↑
TSH response to TRH	Absent	Absent	↑	↑

[a] The serum T_3 concentration does not fall below normal until hypothyroidism becomes severe. Even in severe hypothyroidism, the increase in serum T_3 concentration in pregnancy caused by increased binding to TBG may keep the total serum T_3 concentration normal.

When nonthyroidal illnesses of these types are present during pregnancy, alterations in thyroid function tests appear to be superimposed on the changes of pregnancy. Thus, some women with toxemia have total and free serum T_3 levels that are subnormal for pregnancy, and the mean total serum T_3 is significantly lower in preeclampsia than in uncomplicated pregnancy.[4] Also, with toxemia, there is a trend toward higher total and free serum T_4 levels than in an uncomplicated pregnancy.[4] Although the decrease in plasma volume in toxemia could cause an elevated total serum T_4, it would not alter the free T_4 and could not cause opposite changes in T_4 and T_3 concentrations. The changes in free T_4 and T_3 levels in hyperemesis gravidarum are more suggestive of hyperthyroidism, and are discussed in more detail below. During chronic therapy with the anticonvulsant drug phenytoin (diphenylhydantoin), the serum T_4 falls by a mean of 20–30%, occasionally more in some individuals. Partly because of a laboratory artifact and partly because of a true, mild fall in the free T_4, most techniques for measuring free T_4, including dialysis, frequently give subnormal readings in patients taking phenytoin, but these patients are not hypothyroid. Epileptic women often need to continue phenytoin during pregnancy, and they would be expected to show the effects of phenytoin on serum thyroxine levels superimposed on those of pregnancy.

THE PLACENTA AND THYROID HORMONE ECONOMY

The functions of the placenta that have an impact on thyroid hormones and thyroid disease are summarized in Table 40–3. Human chorionic gonadotropin has an intrinsic capacity to interact with the TSH receptor on thyroid cells but is only a weak thyroid stimulator.[12] The hCG and pituitary TSH are similar glycoprotein hormones, with virtually identical alpha subunits and with highly homologous beta subunits amino acid sequences. The serum hCG levels attained in normal pregnancy probably do not contribute to the overall thyroid hormone economy, except perhaps to a minor degree at the peak serum hCG levels present at 8–10 week's gestation. The higher serum hCG levels in trophoblastic diseases may cause hyperthyroidism, as discussed later. There is no compelling evidence for the existence of a human chorionic thyrotropin separate from chorionic gonadotropin. Human placenta contains material that resembles TRH by immunoassay and bioassay; its physiologic significance is unknown.

The placenta serves as a barrier between the hypothalamic–pituitary–thyroid axis of the mother and that of the fetus.[13,14] T_4, T_3, and TSH cross the placenta very poorly. When exogenous T_4 or T_3 was administered to pregnant women, doses equal to four to 10 times the normal daily production rates were required to deliver biologically signifi-

TABLE 40–3. FUNCTIONS OF THE PLACENTA IN THYROID HORMONE ECONOMY

1. HCG has intrinsic thyroid-stimulating activity. There is probably no other biologically significant placental thyroid stimulator. Alterations in the glycosylation of hCG can increase its thyrotrophic activity. This may occur in trophoblastic disease and probably contributes to the hyperthyroidism that is seen in some cases of hydatidiform mole and choriocarcinoma.
2. The placenta contains TRHlike material of uncertain biologic significance.
3. The placenta is poorly permeable to maternal T_4, T_3, and TSH. This property helps to maintain the fetal hypothalamic–pituitary–thyroid axis as a separate system from the mother's. Congenitally hypothyroid babies receive some thyroid hormone from the maternal circulation, partly protecting them from the effects of their own thyroid hormone deficiency.
4. The placenta has an enzyme that inactivates thyroid hormones by deiodination, converting T_4 to reverse-T_3 and converting T_3 to diiodothyronine. This enzyme appears to be a major component of the barrier separating the maternal and fetal thyroid hormone economies.
5. In maternal autoimmune thyroid disease, IgGs that can stimulate or inhibit thyroid function occasionally to cross the placenta in sufficient amounts to cause intrauterine and neonatal hyperthyroidism (congenital Graves' disease) or hypothyroidism.
6. Several drugs can affect the fetal thyroid to cross the placenta readily: thionamides, exogenous TRH, inorganic iodide (radioactive or nonradioactive), and beta-adrenergic blockers.

cant amounts to the fetus.[15,16] In completely athyreotic infants, the amount of maternal T_4 that crosses the placenta at term is only enough to maintain the average cord serum T_4 concentration at about half of the normal mean value.[17]

Recently it has been found that the placenta contains an enzyme, iodothyronine deiodinase type III, that deiodinates T_4 to an inactive metabolite, reverse-T_3, and also inactivates T_3 by conversion to diiodothyronine. This enzyme is probably the major factor that limits entry of maternal T_4 and T_3 into the fetal circulation[13], but physical barriers to the transport of iodothyronines across the placenta also may exist. There are two clinical implications of the independence of thyroid hormone levels in the maternal and fetal circulation. First, excess or deficient amount of thyroid hormones in the mother have no significant effect on the thyroid status of the fetus. Second, in the case of suspected intrauterine hypothyroidism, it is not possible to correct the fetal hormone deficiency by administration of thyroid hormone agonists to the mother without inducing maternal thyrotoxicosis.

Like many maternal immunoglobulins, the maternal thyroid-stimulating immunoglobulins of Graves' disease may cross the placenta in sufficient amounts to cause stimulation of the fetal thyroid. Similarly, the antithyroid antibodies of maternal autoimmune thyroiditis may cross the placenta and cause intrauterine hypothyroidism. Drugs used in the evaluation or treatment of maternal thyroid diseases cross the placenta in quantities sufficient to have biologic effects on the fetus. These include the thionamides (propylthiouracil, methimazole, and carbimazole), exogenous TRH, beta-adrenergic antagonists, and radioactive and nonradioactive iodide.[13]

THYROID FUNCTION IN THE FETUS

The human fetal thyroid gland can concentrate iodine by 12 weeks' gestation[18], at which time TSH can be detected in the fetal pituitary and TRH in the fetal hypothalamus. Between 16 and 30 weeks' gestation, there is a considerable increase in fetal pituitary TSH content and serum TSH concentrations, with a subsequent decrease in the serum level. The fetal serum T_4 level rises steadily between 10 and 30 weeks' gestation, probably because of a progressive rise in serum TBG concentration. The slower increase in serum T_4 after 30 weeks is not accompanied by an increase in TBG; thus, the serum free T_4 rises after 30 weeks. The reciprocal relationship of serum free T_4 and TSH in the normal fetus after 30 weeks suggests that the hypothalamic–pituitary-thyroid axis is fully operational by then. Further evidence is derived from the occurrence of elevated serum TSH concentrations in hypothyroid preterm infants as early as 28 weeks' gestation (Anast CS, Makowiak S, Kaplan MM, unpublished data). Amniotic fluid contains low concentrations of TSH[19], presumably of fetal origin.

Total and free serum T_3 levels are very low before 28–30 weeks' gestation. They rise somewhere thereafter but remain substantially below the adult values through labor and delivery. Reverse-T_3 is present in high concentrations in fetal serum after 28 weeks' gestation, in amniotic fluid, and in cord serum. Because much of the extrathyroidal conversion of T_4 to T_3 and the degradation of reverse-T_3 are carried out by the same enzyme, iodothyronine deiodinase type I, a low activity of this enzyme in fetal life, as found in animals, could account for the decreased serum T_3 and the increased serum reverse-T_3 in the fetus compared to the adult. However, studies in the rat suggest that maternal thyroid function may be more important than fetal thyroid function in determining amniotic fluid reverse-T_3 concentration.[13]

The physiologic significance of the low serum T_3 levels in fetal life is conjectural. It is possible that the effects of T_3 on the liver, brain, kidney, heart, and other organs are not needed in fetal life, and T_3 is accordingly not produced. It is even possible that exposure of some tissues to T_3 too early in development would lead to abnormal maturation. However, the relationship between serum T_4 and T_3 concentrations and intracellular T_3 concentrations are complex and vary from organ to organ (see Fig. 40–1). We have no clear idea of how tissue T_3 levels in the human fetus compare to levels later in life.

Dramatic changes in the serum thyroid hormone and TSH concentrations take place immediately after an infant is born (Fig. 40–2).[18] There is a marked surge in serum TSH, which peaks 30 minutes after birth; the trigger for this TSH surge is unknown. There follows a surge in serum T_3 and a more modest increase in serum T_4, both of which attain their maximum concentrations at 24 hours. The T_3 surge is largely caused by an increase in thyroidal secretion, but there also may be a rapid activation of the processes that convert T_4 to T_3 outside of the thyroid gland.

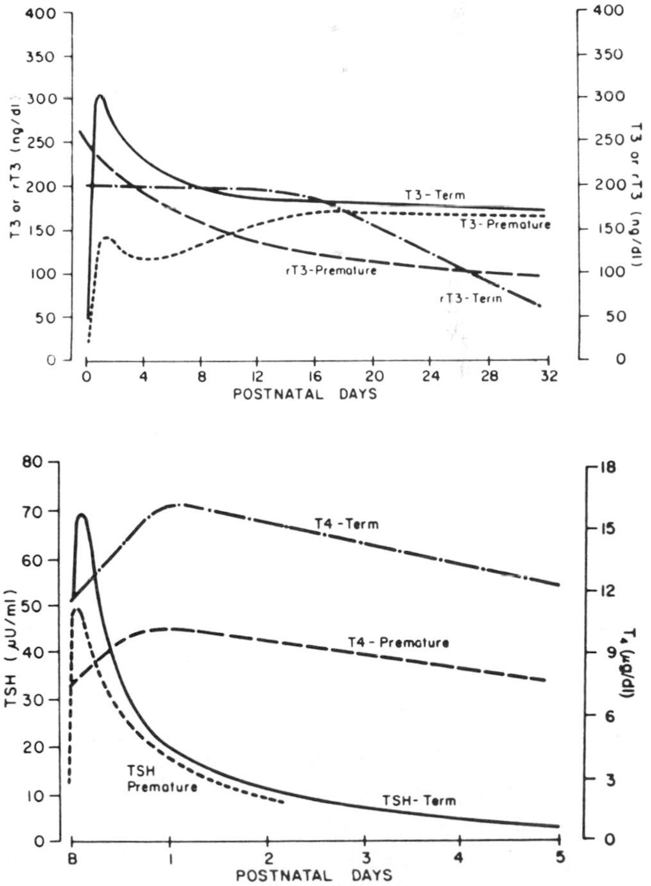

Figure 40–2. Changes in thyroid hormone and TSH blood levels in infants during the immediate postpartum period. rT_3 indicates the biologically inactive T_3 isomer reverse-T_3. (*Reprinted from Fisher and Klein*[18] *with permission.*)

HYPERTHYROIDISM

Causes

The various causes of thyrotoxicosis are listed in Table 40–4. *Graves' disease* is the most common, especially during pregnancy. Toxic multinodular goiter, the next most common cause, has a much higher incidence after age 50. Toxic autonomous thyroid nodules can occur at any age but are relatively uncommon. In a large series of women who carried pregnancies for 20 weeks or more, the frequency of recognized, concomitant hyperthyroidism was about two per 1000.[20] Another study reported a similar prevalence.[21] This is a minimum estimate and excludes women who had early abortions and those not diagnosed.

Graves' disease is an autoimmune process. The hypersecretion of thyroid hormones is caused by circulating immunoglobulins (IgGs) that bind to the TSH receptor on the thyroid follicular cells and stimulate thyroid hormone biosynthesis and secretion, just as TSH does. The antigen that triggers production of thyroid-stimulating IgGs is unknown. Although a body of literature suggests that emotional stress can precipitate Graves' disease, the reports are anecdotal, circumstantial, and inconsistent.

Graves' IgGs, because of their behavior in the original bioassays, were originally referred to as *long-acting thyroid stimulators* (*LATS*). Current assays measure displacement of radioactive TSH from thyroid membranes or measure adenylate cyclase stimulation in thyroid cells or thyroid cell membranes; therefore, the term LATS is outmoded, and the terms *thyroid-stimulating IgGs, anti-TSH receptor antibodies,* or *Graves' IgGs* are preferable. Graves' disease is associated with an increased frequency of other autoimmune diseases affecting the same patients: pernicious anemia, idiopathic thrombocytopenic purpura, systemic lupus erythematosus, and myasthenia gravis. There also is a genetic component to Graves' disease because many affected patients have a family history of autoimmune thyroid disease (Graves' or Hashimoto's diseases), and a higher risk of Graves' disease exists in individuals who possess histocompatability antigens HLA-B8, DR5, and DR3.

Clinical Features

The major clinical manifestations of thyrotoxicosis are listed in Table 40–5. The division of these features into the three categories, although somewhat arbitrary, has diagnostic and therapeutic implications. The sympatheticlike effects, along with Graves' ophthalmopathy, are responsible for the classic hyperthyroid appearance, and give the clinical impression of excessive beta-adrenergic discharge. These effects are not caused by increased catecholamine secretion or serum levels, which are normal to low. Instead, these signs and symptoms represent an increased sensitivity to circulating catecholamines. In some tissues, this may be caused by an increased number of beta-adrenergic receptors. The adrenergiclike signs and symptoms are the most responsive to treatment with beta-adrenergic blockers.

In some thyrotoxic patients, the predominant manifestations are designated intrinsic hormone effects (see Table 40–5). Especially in older individuals, the sympatheticlike features may be largely absent. In these cases, thyrotoxicosis can present primarily as a wasting disease, termed *apathetic thyrotoxicosis.* Some signs and symptoms are included in both categories in Table 40–5 because patients' pulse rates and oxygen consumption rates may remain elevated when complete beta-adrenergic blockade is achieved pharmacologically. The intrinsic hormone effects often are quite prominent in younger patients as well.

Graves' ophthalmopathy is clinically evident in about one third of patients with Graves' disease, but careful evaluation by orbital ultrasound, orbital-computed tomography, or intraocular pressure measurements in several eye positions reveal abnormalities in a majority of patients. The hyperthyroid state can cause stare and lid lag because of retraction of the upper eyelids. However, thyroid hormone excess alone does not cause the unique aspects of Graves' eye disease: infiltration of the retro-orbital tissues with lymphocytes and deposition of glycosaminoglycans in the extraocular muscles, retro-orbital tissues, and periorbital tissues. Abnormalities of both cellular and humoral immunity appear to be involved in the development of infiltrative ophthalmopathy, but the complete pathophysiologic picture has not been elucidated.

The clinical results of Graves' ophthalmopathy are eye irritation and photophobia, exophthalmos that can lead to corneal exposure and ulceration, extraocular muscle palsy causing double vision, and a rubbery swelling of the periorbital tissues. Deterioration of visual acuity is the most serious complication of Graves' ophthalmopathy, probably resulting from compression or stretching of the optic nerve by the swollen muscles and soft tissues constrained by the bony orbit. The mildest symptoms, irritation and photophobia, can sometimes be relieved by eyedrops, such as artificial tears. However, every patient with Graves' disease and symptoms or signs of ophthalmopathy should have a thorough ophthalmopathic evaluation, and manifestations that are more serious than irritation and periorbital swelling will best be managed by, or in close consultation with, an ophthalmologist.

The most severe form of hyperthyroidism is *thyroid storm* or *crisis,* which consists of extreme worsening of the abnormalities of thyrotoxicosis, especially the cardiovascular manifestations, along with delirium and hyperpyrexia. Circulatory collapse and death may occur. Usually there is a precipitating cause, such as sepsis or surgical stress. Fortunately, thyroid storm is much less common than in the past.

TABLE 40–4. CAUSES OF HYPERTHYROIDISM

Graves' disease (toxic diffuse goiter)
Toxic multinodular goiter
Subacute thyroiditis
Toxic autonomously functioning adenoma
Exogenous T_4 or T_3
Trophoblastic disease
Hyperemesis gravidarum
Iodide-induced thyrotoxicosis
Hashimoto's thyroiditis (rare)
Thyroid cancer (widespread disease)
Hypersecretion of TSH (rare)
Struma ovarii (very rare)

Special Considerations in Pregnancy

Women with marked hyperthyroidism have decreased fertility; thyrotoxicosis can cause loss of the midcycle gonadotropin surge, with anovulatory cycles and a tendency toward oligomenorrhea or amenorrhea (menometrorrhagia occurs less often). Women with treated Graves' disease or Graves' disease in remission probably will have normal

TABLE 40–5. CLINICAL FEATURES OF HYPERTHYROIDISM

Intrinsic Hormone Effects	Sympatheticlike Effects	Unique to Graves' Disease
	Symptoms	
FATIGUE	PALPITATION	Irritated, gritty, or sandy feeling in eyes
INCREASED APPETITE	HEAT INTOLERANCE	Diplopia
Weight loss (rarely weight gain)	EXCESSIVE SWEATING	Localized swelling of legs
Muscle weakness	SHORTNESS OF BREATH	
Fine, brittle hair	INCREASED URINARY FREQUENCY	
Itching of skin	NERVOUSNESS	
Brittle fingernails	EMOTIONAL LABILITY	
Oligomenorrhea or AMENORRHEA	INSOMNIA	
Increased bowel frequency	Tremor	
VOMITING	Brisk reflexes	
	Signs	
TACHYCARDIA	TACHYCARDIA	Diffuse goiter
Atrial fibrillation	CARDIAC FLOW MURMUR	Exophthalmos
Proximal myopathy	Increased pulse pressure	Periorbital swelling
Fine, warm, moist skin	Systolic hypertension	Extraocular muscle palsy
Onycholysis	Stare, lid lag	Infiltrative dermopathy (pretibial myxedema)
		Lymphadenopathy
		Splenomegaly
		Clubbing of fingers (thyroid acropachy)
	Laboratory Findings	
INCREASED OXYGEN CONSUMPTION	INCREASED OXYGEN CONSUMPTION	Thyroid-stimulating IgG
Hypercalcemia		Lymphocytosis
Elevated alkaline phosphatase		Neutropenia
Elevated transaminases		

(Findings that can occur due to pregnancy alone are capitalized. Thyroid enlargement (goiter), either diffuse or localized, is almost always present in young, hyperthyroid patients, regardless of the cause of hyperthyroidism.)

fertility. Sexually active hyperthyroid women who do not use contraception or are casual in its use should be advised that restoration of normal thyroid hormone blood levels will increase their chances of becoming pregnant.

Many of the clinical features of thyrotoxicosis also can occur in normal pregnancy (see Table 40–5), particularly from the second trimester on, when the hypermetabolism of pregnancy becomes more pronounced. This overlap of signs and symptoms can cause difficulty in making the clinical diagnosis of coexisting mild thyrotoxicosis. For example, in young patients with thyrotoxicosis, a resting pulse rate greater than 90 beats per minute is the rule, but because of the normal increase in pulse rate of about 10 beats per minute during pregnancy, a resting pulse of 90–100 becomes a less reliable indicator of thyroid hormone excess. In addition, the normal weight gain of pregnancy may overshadow the tendency toward weight loss in thyrotoxicosis. In this setting, therefore, the features of hyperthyroidism that are not also typical of pregnancy become especially important when suspecting hyperthyroidism: thyroid enlargement, eye signs, weight loss, increased bowel frequency, and myopathy.

Hyperthyroidism adversely affects the outcome of pregnancy. The incidence of first-trimester spontaneous abortion is increased, rates of stillbirth and neonatal deaths may be increased, and the frequency of low birthweight is increased twofold to threefold.[20,21] Heart failure is common in untreated maternal hyperthyroidism (five of eight cases in one series), usually in the setting of another stress, such as preeclampsia, infection, or anemia.[21] The frequency of these maternal and fetal complications is greatly reduced by treatment of the hyperthyroidism.[21] Thyroid storm occurs in approximately 2% of pregnant hyperthyroid patients whose thyroid disease is diagnosed during pregnancy and who receive treatment and in as many as 20% of untreated hyperthyroid pregnant women.[21]

There is a tendency for preexisting Graves' disease to worsen in the first trimester of pregnancy.[22] Conversely, Graves' disease tends to become less active in the second and third trimesters[23]; in this setting, maternal serum levels of thyroid-stimulating immunoglobulins fall in parallel with the activity of the Graves' disease. Women who require an antithyroid drug before they conceive or in the first trimester often need substantially lower doses and sometimes can discontinue the drug entirely in middle to late pregnancy.[24] This ameliorating trend, unfortunately, is not dependable and is frequently followed by a marked increase in the activity of the disease in the first weeks and months postpartum.[22] It is likely that the changes in the function of the immune system during and after pregnancy are responsible for the changes in the natural course of Graves' disease. There are no data suggesting that pregnancy alters the course of Graves' ophthalmopathy.

Two types of hyperthyroidism are unique to pregnancy: one occurring in the setting of hyperemesis gravidarum and one associated with trophoblastic disease.

A large fraction of women suffering from *hyperemesis gravidarum* have derangements of thyroid function tests suggesting hyperthyroidism. About 50% have elevated serum free T_4 or free T_4 index values compared to normal pregnant controls.[25-27] About 20% of the women who have had estimates of serum free T_3 levels during episodes of hyperemesis have had elevated values, and this fraction rises to about 50% in women with hyperemesis and elevated serum free T_4 values.[25-27] Eight of 10 such patients with high serum free T_4 levels had suppressed basal serum TSH concentrations as detected by a highly sensitive TSH assay.[26] Thirteen of 15 women with hyperemesis and high serum free T_4 values had blunted TSH responses to TRH stimulation, but none of the patients with hyperemesis and normal serum free T_4 values had such blunting.[27] Thus, all the biochemical criteria for a true hyperthyroid state are present, although not in every patient and generally to a mild degree.

Patients with hyperemesis gravidarum are not reported to exhibit specific clinical manifestations of thyrotoxicosis, although rarely, patients with thyrotoxicosis have nausea and vomiting as prominent symptoms. The abnormal laboratory tests of thyroid function resolve without antithyroid treatment within 1 month of the alleviation of the hyperemesis. The general absence of maternal symptomatology is probably caused by the short duration of serum thyroid hormone elevation and perhaps to the absence of marked elevations of serum T_3. There is a trend toward low birthweight in children of the women with hyperemesis and elevated free T_4 indexes compared to offspring of those with hyperemesis and normal free T_4 indexes. There is one report of a possible case of thyrotoxic crisis in this setting, but it is not entirely convincing.[28]

The hyperthyroidism in patients with hyperemesis gravidarum is most likely caused by thyroid stimulation by high serum concentrations of hCG. A positive correlation has been found between serum hCG and free T_4 concentrations in women with hyperemesis.[27] Pregnant women with nausea alone, or nausea and vomiting not severe enough to be termed hyperemesis, occasionally have elevated serum free T_4 concentrations, and this phenomenon is associated with increased serum hCG concentrations compared to those of pregnant women with no nausea.[12] It is not known whether there is a direct causal relationship between high levels of hCG or high serum free T_4 concentration and the nausea and vomiting.

Hyperthyroidism is common in *gestational trophoblastic diseases*, both choriocarcinoma and hydatidiform mole.[29,30] The hyperthyroidism is of the classic type, with elevated T_4 secretion rates, elevated total and free serum T_4 and T_3 levels, and in some cases, clinical features of hypermetabolism.[29-33] In a large series, about 50% of women with gestational trophoblastic disease had at least biochemical evidence of hyperthyroidism. It seems fairly clear that hCG produced by the abnormal trophoblastic tissue is they thyroid stimulator in gestational trophoblastic disease. Serum TSH concentrations are suppressed below 0.1 μU/mL.[34] Although there are discrepancies among patients between the serum levels of hCG and thyroid status, there is a high correlation between serum hCG levels and bioassayable thyroid-stimulating activity. The discrepancies between hCG measurements and thyroid status can be explained by molecular alterations in the hCG, such as desialation, which increase the ratio of thyrotrophic to immunologic activities[35], and by species' differences that render the bioassay of thyrotrophic activity only semiquantitative in predicting patients' responses.

It is consistently observed in the hyperthyroidism of gestational trophoblastic disease that the clinical manifestations of thyrotoxicosis are often subtle or absent.[29,30,33] Goiter hardly ever occurs. Weight loss and fatigue are fairly common, but it is difficult to know whether these are caused by the hyperthyroidism or the trophoblastic disease. Some patients do have the classic manifestations of thyrotoxicosis, and some with elevated serum thyroid hormone levels and no symptoms have been observed to develop thyrotoxic symptoms and signs over a period of weeks. Most likely, these findings result from the short duration of the hyperthyroid state, providing insufficient time for hyperplasia of the thyroid gland to develop. The elevated thyroid hormone levels and the signs and symptoms of thyrotoxicosis return to normal very quickly after removal of the molar tissue or effective treatment of the choriocarcinoma.[29,30,33] Therefore, specific treatment directed toward the thyroid gland probably needs to be considered only when a metastatic choriocarcinoma is unresponsive to therapy.

Diagnosis

Severe thyrotoxicosis is difficult to mistake for any other condition, especially when accompanied by a goiter or Graves' ophthalmopathy. Anxiety and agitated psychiatric states can mimic mild thyrotoxicosis. Pheochromocytoma can cause some of the same hypermetabolic abnormalities.

The laboratory diagnosis of thyrotoxicosis centers on establishing elevated serum levels of free T_4 and free T_3. The different techniques used for the estimation of these levels are discussed in detail above. When measurements of the serum thyroid hormone levels are inconclusive, determination of the serum TSH concentration by a high sensitivity TSH assay will establish or exclude the diagnosis of hyperthyroidism. In the presence of mild thyroid hormone excess, the serum TSH concentration is suppressed below normal, and with the best of these assays, it is reliably suppressed below 0.1 μU/mL or less. Conversely, a normal serum TSH concentration determined by such an assay excludes thyrotoxicosis with near certainty.

The changes in the total T_4, T_3 uptake, and free T_4 index tests resulting from hyperthyroidism and resulting from pregnancy are additive when the two conditions coexist (see Table 40–2). Thus, in the pregnant thyrotoxic woman, the total serum T_4 concentration may be very high with only mild to moderate thyrotoxicosis. The T_3 uptake is usually normal, slightly decreased, or slightly increased, instead of very low as in normal pregnancy or high as is typical for hyperthyroidism in the nonpregnant state. The upper limit of normal for the free T_4 index is often uncertain during the second and third trimesters because of imprecision in the serum T_4 measurement at high levels and because of the nonlinear relationship between the T_3 uptake value and the percent of free T_4 at high serum TBG concentrations. When the serum free T_4 level is measured by immunoextraction radioimmunoassay or equilibrium dialysis, the upper limit of normal is the same as for nonpregnant women. The behavior of analog free T_4 radioimmunoassays is variable during pregnancy.

If the suspicion of thyrotoxicosis is low, a first-line screening test can be a measurement of either the serum free T_4 concentration with consideration for any changes during pregnancy in the normal range for the method used or the serum TSH concentration by high-sensitivity assay. Analysis of the relative cost-effectiveness and comparative sensitivity and specificity for these two screening strategies is difficult because of the rapid evolution of the methods for both tests. I prefer the high sensitivity TSH assay. If the screening test is abnormal or suspicion is high, assessment of the patient's thyroid function is best made with a combination of tests to estimate the serum free T_4, free T_3, and TSH concentrations. Occasional hyperthyroid patients have isolated T_3 excess, which occurs in 3–5% of cases in iodine-sufficient areas. Typically, the rise in T_3 is proportionately greater than that of T_4 when the thyroid is stimulated. However, in hyperthyroidism caused by gestational trophoblastic disease or by hyperemesis gravidarum, the rise in T_3 is proportionately equal to or less than that of T_4.[25,30]

If the estimates of free T_4 and T_3 are equivocal and a high-sensitivity TSH assay is not available, a TRH stimulation test may be useful to establish or exclude autonomous thyroid secretion. Even though TRH crosses the placenta and can cause stimulation of the fetal thyroid by increasing fetal TSH, its short duration of action (a few hours) makes it unlikely that a TRH test would have any adverse effects on the fetus of a pregnant woman. Therefore, when establishment of thyrotoxicosis would alter a woman's management, pregnancy does not preclude a TRH test, although a basal serum TSH measurement using a high-sensitivity assay is preferable.

Even in the nonpregnant state, isotopic tests of thyroid function, including the thyroidal radioiodine uptake and thyroid scanning, are not necessary for establishing thyrotoxicosis. Rather, they establish the etiology of the thyrotoxic state and plan therapy. In pregnancy, these tests should not be performed; the same information often can be obtained in other ways, or the tests can be deferred. Graves' disease can usually be distinguished from a single toxic adenoma by palpation and from toxic multinodular goiter by palpation, by the presence of ophthalmopathy, or by elevated titers of antithyroid microsomal and antithyroglobulin antibodies. Elevated titers of these antibodies usually are present in the serum of patients with Graves' disease and absent with a multinodular goiter.

Treatment

All of the modalities available to treat hyperthyroidism are directed at the thyroid gland and serum thyroid hormone levels; none are directed at the production of thyroid-stimulating immunoglobulins. Antithyroid drugs, surgery, and radioiodine (sodium ^{131}I) are the three mainstays of therapy. Unfortunately, each has disadvantages during pregnancy. Still, the majority of women who have hyperthyroidism and want to bear children and who develop hyperthyroidism during pregnancy can have a successful pregnancy if diagnosis and treatment are prompt. It is almost never necessary to interrupt a pregnancy because of coexisting hyperthyroidism.

General supportive measures should be instituted. The patient should maintain adequate caloric intake, considering the increased caloric expenditure induced by pregnancy and thyrotoxicosis; she also should receive multiple vitamins because thyrotoxicosis may be accompanied by vitamin deficiency. Bed rest and protection of the patient from physical and psychologic stresses may cause a notable improvement in symptoms.

Thionamides. The thionamides are the drugs of choice for treating hyperthyroidism during pregnancy. In the United States, the two available agents are propylthiouracil (PTU) and methimazole (Tapazole). In other countries, a commonly used drug is carbimazole, which is rapidly converted to methimazole in the body and is equivalent to methimazole. Thionamides inhibit thyroid hormone biosynthesis at the steps of organification of iodide and coupling of iodotyrosines on the thyroglobulin molecule to form T_4 and T_3. PTU, but not methimazole, has the additional use of inhibiting extrathyroidal conversion of T_4 to T_3, and in the initial phase of treatment, PTU lowers the serum T_3 faster than methimazole. Methimazole is about 15 times more potent on a weight basis than PTU. Maternal serum drug concentrations after a given PTU dose appear to be lower in late pregnancy than postpartum.[36]

Sufficiently large doses of either drug (80–100 mg daily of methimazole or 800–1200 mg daily of PTU) will completely block thyroid hormone biosynthesis, but 300–450 mg of PTU daily divided into three doses is usually sufficient to achieve initial control of hyperthyroidism. Once the serum thyroid hormone levels in a hyperthyroid patient are restored to near-normal, the doses needed to control hyperthyroidism usually range from 50–300 mg daily for PTU and from 5–20 mg daily for methimazole. Many patients can be managed with a single daily oral dose of either drug, although some patients taking methimazole require two doses a day, and some taking PTU require as many as three doses a day. No parenteral formulations of PTU or methimazole are available. If a patient cannot take oral medications, methimazole can be administered rectally using suppositories.

Adverse reactions to PTU and methimazole are the same in nature and in frequency. The most common is a usually erythematous, maculopapular, and often pruritic skin rash, occurring in 2–8% of patients. Laryngospasm or bronchospasm, drug fever, oral ulcerations, dose-related neutropenia, and a lupuslike syndrome with arthralgias and vasculitis occur less commonly. The rarest but most dangerous complications are agranulocytosis and fulminant hepatitis. Agranulocytosis is an idiosyncratic reaction, different from the dose-related neutropenia; it occurs with a frequency of about one in 250 patients for both PTU and methimazole. It is most frequent in the first 3 months of treatment, is more common in older patients, and appears to be less common in patients taking less than 30 mg daily of methimazole than in those taking higher doses or those taking PTU. Thionamide-induced agranulocytosis is reversible when the drug is discontinued, unless a fatal infection supervenes, but that is a considerable danger.

Both PTU and methimazole cross the placenta, are taken up by the fetal thyroid gland early in the second trimester, and can inhibit function of the fetal thyroid gland.[13] Propylthiouracil crosses the placenta less efficiently than methimazole. When doses to the mother of more than 300 mg daily of PTU or 30 mg daily of methimazole are administered chronically, fetal goiter and hypothyroidism may occur, but they are unpredictable. On the other hand, when those doses or lower are used, even throughout the entire course of pregnancy, goiter and fetal hypothyroidism are much less common, and the clinical outcome both for the mother and the baby is usually satisfactory.[37] Cord serum PTU concentrations are higher than paired maternal serum levels.[36] The effect of PTU on fetal thyroid function at term is related to maternal serum concentrations but not to the PTU dose.[36]

A congenital skin lesion, *aplasia cutis,* consisting of circumscribed, usually small areas of undeveloped skin has been described in about 12 infants exposed to methimazole *in utero.*[38] The incidence of this lesion is low, and the precise relative risk of its occurrence in the setting of methimazole therapy is not known, but it has not been described in the setting of PTU treatment. Although it is theoretically possible that the fetus could have one of the hypersensitivity reactions to PTU or methimazole, no such case has been described.

The combined results from several published series totaling 362 women treated with thionamides during pregnancy show a total fetal mortality rate from all causes of

12.8% and a perinatal loss rate from all causes of 5.8%. These series include women treated with other drugs in addition to the thionamides, such as thyroid hormones, inorganic iodide, and beta-adrenergic blockers. These data were collected over more than 30 years, during which there have been many advances in obstetric and neonatal care. Current practice should therefore achieve complication rates no worse than these and probably better. In one study, even when PTU doses were kept at 200 mg/d or less, detailed examination of the infant's serum hormone levels showed a modest decrease in the mean cord serum free T_4 index, although only one of 11 infants had a value below normal, and the drug effect dissipated in about 24 hours.[37] In longer term follow-up studies of children exposed to these drugs *in utero,* there is no evidence of an abnormal incidence of developmental abnormalities; however, neither the number of children studied nor the number of years of follow-up are large enough to be completely definitive.

Use of PTU in pregnancy is preferable to use of methimazole for three reasons: the theoretical advantages of inhibition of extrathyroid conversion of T_4 to T_3, its lower efficiency of transplacental passage, and the apparent association of methimazole therapy with *aplasia cutis.* Nevertheless, if a patient has a mild allergic reaction to PTU, I would advise methimazole treatment rather than surgery, although a careful explanation to the patient of the advantages and disadvantages of each and her informed consent are essential.

It is exceedingly important to keep the thionamide dose as low as possible when treating a pregnant hyperthyroid patient. This will minimize the risk to the fetus of adverse effects. Clinical evaluation of the patient and estimates of serum free T_4 and free T_3 should be performed approximately every 3–4 weeks during the pregnancy. The dose of the drug should be adjusted to keep the thyroid hormone levels at or just above the upper limit of normal. Sometimes the free T_3 will remain substantially elevated after the free T_4 falls to normal; in this case, the drug dose may need to be increased, especially if the serum TSH level is still suppressed below detectability. The decision of exactly how far above normal to allow the serum hormone levels to remain depends on the clinical assessment of the degree of thyrotoxicosis. Whenever a patient's thyroid hormone blood levels are normal, the thionamide dose should be decreased. Because of the trend toward decreased activity of Graves' disease in middle to late pregnancy[22], sometimes the drug can be discontinued entirely without the reappearance of thyrotoxicosis. There appear to be no beneficial effects of adding oral thyroid hormone treatment to thionamide therapy. Because exogenous thyroid hormone treatment will not suppress thyroid secretion in Graves' disease, it will raise the serum thyroid hormone levels higher than they would otherwise be and increase the dose of thionamide required to achieve the therapeutic goal.

It is advisable to obtain a baseline white blood cell count and differential and liver function tests before initiating PTU treatment. There may be mild neutropenia from the Graves' disease alone, and only a significant decrease below the baseline level would necessitate discontinuation of the thionamide. Patients should be instructed to inform the physician immediately if there is a drug reaction, at which time the thionamide is stopped and a complete blood count is repeated. Inasmuch as idiosyncratic drug reactions can have an abrupt onset, regular complete blood counts and liver function tests cannot always predict problems; however, they may do so, particularly for liver damage, and therefore are advisable. About one third of patients who have allergic reactions to one of the thionamides also will be allergic to the other. Therefore, if a pregnant patient develops mild PTU hypersensitivity, an equivalent dose of methimazole sometimes can be substituted after the symptoms resolve.

During lactation, both methimazole and PTU are transported from maternal serum into the breast milk; methimazole is transported more efficiently. For PTU, the amount of drug in the milk is low enough that interference with the baby's thyroid function is unlikely.[39] The American Academy of Pediatrics Committee on Drugs includes PTU in a list of maternal medication "usually compatible with breast-feeding."[40] However, if a woman taking PTU does breast-feed, she should be advised of the possibility of effects on the baby's thyroid function and the baby's thyroid function should be monitored.

Other Drugs. Two other classes of drugs, iodide (nonradioactive) and beta-adrenergic blockers, occasionally are useful adjuncts in the treatment of thyrotoxicosis. Again, their use during pregnancy entails special considerations.

Iodide acutely inhibits the release of thyroid hormones already synthesized and stored in the thyroid gland. Most hyperthyroid patients will escape from this action of iodide in 10–14 days. In Graves' disease, iodide also decreases the vascularity of the thyroid gland and makes it firmer. Both of these changes make surgical thyroidectomy technically easier. Again, 10–14 days is sufficient to achieve this effect. Finally, iodide inhibits its own organification (the Wolff-Chaikoff effect). The effects of iodide and those of thionamides are additive.

Iodide crosses the placenta easily, and the fetal thyroid gland is uniquely sensitive to the several inhibitory actions of iodide.[13] Also, the fetal thyroid lacks the capability of the adult thyroid gland to adapt to or escape from these actions. For these reasons, chronic iodide administration to any pregnant woman, including one who is hyperthyroid, runs the risk of inducing a large fetal goiter, with or without hypothyroidism. Such a goiter can cause malpositioning of the fetal head at delivery and cause suffocation of the neonate. Inorganic iodide is cleared from the body within a few days, and the inhibitory effects on the thyroid do not persist after the iodide is excreted. Moreover, the induction of fetal goiter probably takes weeks. Therefore, although chronic treatment with inorganic iodide is absolutely contraindicated in pregnancy, its use for 7–10 days appears to be safe and is sometimes advisable in pregnant hyperthyroid women who have severe thyrotoxicosis or who are to be treated with thyroidectomy. Available preparations are intravenous sodium iodide, given in a dose of 1 g/d in a slow infusion, and Lugol's strong iodine solution and saturated solution of potassium iodide (SSKI) for oral use. Lugol's solution, which has a higher iodine concentration than SSKI, is effective in a dose of 3 drops in a glass of water taken once a day.

Beta-adrenergic blockers also have an adjunctive role in the treatment of thyrotoxicosis. They are particularly useful for ameliorating some of the sympatheticlike manifestations, such as tremor, tachycardia, and palpitations. Of the beta blockers available in the United States, only propranolol and atenolol have any effect on thyroid hormone blood levels because of their mild inhibitory effect on extrathyroidal conversion of T_4 to T_3, which is similar to the additive action of PTU. Because no other beta-blocker has any clear advantages over propranolol in the treatment of thyrotoxicosis and it is the least expensive beta-blocker, propranolol is the preferred beta-blocker.

In my opinion, beta-adrenergic blockade has a role in providing symptomatic relief in moderate to severe thyrotoxicosis in the days to weeks before other treatment can normalize the serum hormone levels, and it has a role in preparing a patient for thyroid or other surgery. It is not, by itself, adequate for long-term treatment. Even those signs and symptoms of thyrotoxicosis that tend to respond to beta-blockade show a more complete response to normalization of thyroid hormone blood levels.

The usual contraindictions to the use of beta-blockers, obstructive lung disease, heart block, heart failure, and insulin-dependent diabetes apply to the pregnant thyrotoxic woman. There also is some questionable evidence concerning occasional adverse effects of long-term maternal therapy during pregnancy with beta-adrenergic blockers, including intrauterine growth retardation and fetal cardiac distress and neonatal bradycardia and hypoglycemia.[41] The frequency of these adverse effects is probably not very high (see also Chapter 125). In the pregnant thyrotoxic woman in whom tremor, palpitation, and tachycardia are debilitating, it seems reasonable to treat with beta-blockers but to use the lowest effective dose for the shortest possible duration and to discontinue the drug when thyroid hormone levels fall to near-normal. The usual doses of propranolol needed to relieve symptoms and achieve a resting pulse rate of 100 or less are 40–80 mg orally, in three or four divided doses or as a single dose of a long-acting preparation.

Oral cholecystographic agents, such as iopanoate and sodium ipodate, have been used experimentally to treat hyperthyroidism. They are potent inhibitors of extrathyroidal conversion of T_4 to T_3, and iodide released from them inhibits thyroid hormone synthesis and release. The use of such agents during pregnancy is inadvisable because they are excreted slowly, and sustained exposure of the fetal thyroid to iodide is unavoidable.

Thyroidectomy. Subtotal thyroidectomy is an effective and generally safe treatment for hyperthyroidism. When thyroidectomy is performed by a surgeon expert in the technique, few patients will remain hyperthyroid, although there may be later recurrences. The incidence of immediate postsurgical hypothyroidism varies widely in reported series; its prevalence becomes considerable when patients are evaluated many years postoperatively. This, in part, probably reflects the natural history of Graves' disease, which includes late hypothyroidism in many cases. In skilled hands, the frequency of hypoparathyroidism and recurrent laryngeal nerve damage should be less than 1%. In addition to the specific complication of thyroidectomy, the complications of surgery in general and the impact of surgery on the outcome of pregnancy need to be considered. When weighing several factors (ie, short- and long-term effects on maternal thyroid status, complication of surgical and medical treatments, and outcome of the pregnancy), most thyroidologists consider medical treatment to be preferable. Surgical treatment is preferred when the mother is allergic to PTU and methimazole or when the hyperthyroidism cannot be controlled with daily doses of 300 mg of PTU or 30 mg of methimazole because higher doses substantially increase the risk of fetal hypothyroidism. To decrease the risks of surgery, the thyrotoxic state needs to be medically controlled as well as possible before operation. This may necessitate a short course of a beta-adrenergic blocker, with inorganic iodide (Lugol's solution) added 7–10 days before the surgery.

Radioactive Iodine

Radioactive iodine should never be used for diagnostic or therapeutic purposes during pregnancy. However, a discussion of its effects is pertinent because increasing numbers of women in childbearing years are being treated with radioiodine, and occasionally a woman who is treated discovers later that she had been pregnant at the time of the treatment.

The radioactive iodine isotopes in clinical use in the United States are ^{123}I and ^{131}I. In addition, ^{99m}Tc-pertechnetate is used for thyroid imaging. ^{131}I delivers much more radiation per administered microcurie than either ^{123}I or pertechnetate; therefore, the latter two agents are preferable for routine thyroid imaging. ^{131}I is used to treat hyperthyroidism. Estimates of whole-body radiation exposure to a first-trimester fetus inadvertently exposed to thyroid-related radiation are 0.00005–0.0002 Gy for a pertechnetate or sodium ^{123}I thyroid scan, and 0.015 Gy for treatment of hyperthyroidism with 10 mCi of sodium ^{131}I.[42,43] Children born after intrauterine exposure to ^{131}I given to treat maternal hyperthyroidism may suffer chromosomal breaks[44], but the incidence of this is unknown. The fetal thyroid concentrates ^{131}I avidly, and inadvertent exposure can cause congenital hypothyroidism; this occurred in six of 182 cases collected in a nationwide survey.[45] These children possibly may be at increased risk for leukemia, but no information is available on this. There is one report of combined congenital hypothyroidism and hypoparathyroidism after intrauterine ^{131}I exposure.[46] Although the number of reported cases is small, the risk of fetal or neonatal death or teratogenic effects after intrauterine ^{131}I exposure does not appear to be greatly increased.

For a woman inadvertently treated with radioactive iodine during pregnancy, a conservative approach would be to explain the potential risks carefully and thoroughly, but to leave the ultimate decision about termination of pregnancy to the woman and her family. Because the fetal thyroid does not begin to concentrate iodine until about 10–12 weeks' gestation the risk of congenital hypothyroidism is small if the exposure is earlier than that. If the exposure is in the 12th week or later and the pregnancy is discovered within a few days of the treatment, theoretically it would be beneficial to administer PTU until about 10 days after the ^{131}I treatment to try to reduce the exposure of the fetal thyroid to the radiation.[47] If fetal hypothyroidism eventually can be diagnosed, consideration could then be given to intra-amniotic thyroid hormone. Because treatment of congenital hypothyroidism diagnosed at birth is generally successful in preventing adverse effects, intra-amniotic thyroid hormone administration to fetuses exposed to radioactive iodine is not indicated.

Treatment of Thyroid Storm

When thyroid storm is present, maximally aggressive treatment is needed. If a thyrotoxic patient begins to decompensate, it is wise to treat as if thyroid storm is present because there are no definite diagnostic criteria. Moreover, because the mother's life may be at stake and the aggressive phase of treatment usually lasts only 1–2 weeks, the potentially adverse effects of high-dose PTU and iodide on the fetal thyroid are not considered. Precipitating causes must be evaluated thoroughly, and any that are identified must be treated vigorously.

The therapeutic regimen directed at the thyroid should include the following: (1) PTU should be given at 400 mg orally every 8 hours. If the patient cannot take medication orally, methimazole can be given rectally as a suppository in a dose of 30–40 mg every 8 hours. (2) sodium iodide, 1 g, should be given intravenously once daily. (3) Propranolol (if there is no heart failure) should be given initially 40 mg orally every 6 hours, with subsequent doses adjusted according to the cardiac response. If intravenous propranolol is necessary, 1 mg/min for 2–10 minutes can be given, during which pulse, blood pressure, and electrocardiogram must be carefully monitored. (4) Dexamethasone should be given 1 mg orally or intramuscularly every 6 hours to further inhibit extrathyroidal T_4 to T_3 conversion. (5) Oxygen, digitalis, fluid replacement, and antipyretics are indicated according to the clinical picture. Aspirin can acutely increase the percent of free T_4, so acetaminophen is preferred as an antipyretic.

CONGENITAL HYPERTHYROIDISM

Graves' disease occurs in the neonate, and a handful of cases have even been diagnosed *in utero*.[48-50] This phenomenon occurs almost exclusively in the offspring of women who have Graves' disease, but the congenital disease is independent of the mother's thyroid status. It can occur in women who have had treatment for their thyrotoxicosis and are euthyroid, who are hypothyroid and taking thyroid hormone replacement, or who are hyperthyroid. Autopsy of two fatal cases showed slim habitus, massive thyroid enlargement, hypertrophic cardiomyopathy, congestive visceromegaly, and signs of pulmonary hypertension.[51] When thyroid stimulating IgGs have been measured, maternal and cord serum levels in affected infants generally have been very high.[48,52] Neonatal Graves' disease occurs equally in both sexes as opposed to the great female predominance in other age groups. The incidence is probably in the range of 1–2% in infants of mothers with Graves' disease. The risk is substantially increased when the mother has previously delivered an affected child. The condition is usually transient, typically lasting 3–12 weeks. Based on these observations, it is probable that most, but not all,[49] cases of congenital hyperthyroidism are caused by transplacental passage of maternal thyroid-stimulating immunoglobulins.

Congenital hyperthyroidism is associated with considerable morbidity and 15–25% mortality in severe cases. In the fetus, tachycardia is the most common manifestation. The presence of a goiter may cause problems at delivery because of interference with respiration in the neonate. There is an increased incidence of low birth weight, but bone age may be accelerated. The infant often is very irritable and grows poorly or loses weight. Tachycardia exists, and heart failure may occur and is the most common cause of death in the fatal cases. Premature craniosynostosis is an uncommon but potentially devastating feature. Jaundice, hepatosplenomegaly, and thrombocytopenia also have been reported. If the mother is receiving thionamide treatment during pregnancy, the disorder may not appear until 8–9 days after birth, presumably because the drug effects have dissipated. Long-term follow-up of affected children indicates that minimal brain dysfunction is fairly common.[49]

A presumptive diagnosis of congenital hyperthyroidism can sometimes be made *in utero* if the pregnant woman has a history of Graves' disease and there is otherwise unexplained fetal tachycardia.[53,54] An elevated titer of maternal thyroid-stimulating IgG activity is a confirmatory finding, although the waiting time needed to obtain this test result may be too long to inititate therapy. Ultrasound could conceivably be helpful if it showed fetal goiter and cardiac hypertrophy. If this diagnosis is made, the woman should receive PTU in an initial dose of 200–300 mg daily, even if she does not require it, to treat the fetal hyperthyroidism. The fetal heart rate should be used to monitor the adequacy of the dose. Maternal serum thyroid hormone measurements should be followed to determine if levothyroxine treatment also is needed.

Even if there is no evidence of congenital hyperthyroidism during the pregnancy, every infant born to a mother with Graves' disease should be evaluated at birth for possible congenital hyperthyroidism, and especially if PTU has been administered, the infant should have follow-up evaluations over the first 2 weeks postpartum. Cord serum T_4, T_3, and free hormone estimations are readily and rapidly available and should be obtained for infants at high risk. Neonatal screening for hypothyroidism entails a T_4 measurement performed on a heel-stick blood sample at 2–3 days of age. However, many screening programs look only for low T_4 values, so screening is not reliable for the diagnosis of congenital Graves' disease.

If the severity of the clinical manifestations of congenital hyperthyroidism warrants treatment, PTU should be given in a dose of 5–10 mg/kg daily in three divided doses, and iodide should be given in the form of Lugol's solution, one drop orally every 8 hours.[48] If there are signs of heart failure, digitalis is indicated. Propranolol is sometimes given in a dose of 2 mg/kg daily in divided doses.[48]

PRECONCEPTION PLANNING

Because of the adverse effects of maternal hyperthyroidism on the outcome of pregnancy, it is desirable for a hyperthyroid woman to be rendered euthyroid before she tries to become pregnant. In my opinion, radioactive iodine (^{131}I) is the best therapeutic choice. Its use makes it easier to maintain a euthyroid maternal state in subsequent pregnancies, and spares the fetus exposure to antithyroid drugs. There is no way of administering antithyroid drugs during pregnancy to maintain maternal euthyroid status without risk of inhibition of fetal thyroid function.[55]

Radioactive iodine therapy has been used for almost 50 years. There is no evidence that hyperthyroid patients treated with it are at increased risk for subsequent development of thyroid cancer, leukemia, other malignancies, or excess mortality from any cause. The radiation dose to the adult ovary from a typical ^{131}I treatment dose for hyperthyroidism is 0.02–0.03 Gy[56]; this is the same range as the dose received during hysterosalpingography. In a published series of children treated for hyperthyroidism with radioactive iodine, none showed any resulting abnormality of their subsequent reproductive history.[57] Similarly, the reproductive history of a small number of young women treated with about 10-fold to 20-fold higher doses of ^{131}I for thyroid cancer appears to be normal.[58] As more accumulated experience fails to document the actual occurrence of theoretical, long-term, radiation-related side effects of radioactive iodine treatment for hyperthyroidism, its use in young patients has become routine in many centers. To guard against inadvertent administration of ^{131}I to a woman who is unknowingly pregnant, a pregnancy test should be done before such treatment if there is even the slightest chance of pregnancy.

After treatment of hyperthyroidism with ^{131}I, it is advisable for a woman to wait before trying to conceive until her thyroid function stabilizes and she becomes euthyroid. Most patients need oral levothyroxine therapy starting 1–3 months after the ^{131}I treatment. Waiting until a euthyroid state is achieved minimizes the occurrence of hyperthyroidism and hypothyroidism during the pregnancy. Usually 4–6 months are required for a stable euthyroid state to be achieved. The procedures for monitoring and adjusting the levothyroxine dosage are discussed in the section on hypothyroidism.

During pregnancy, it is helpful to determine the maternal serum level of thyroid-stimulating IgGs to assess the risk of congenital hyperthyroidism in the baby. This is accomplished best during the second trimester. The laboratory performing the test should be able to provide information about the level of thyroid-stimulating activity above which risk of congenital hyperthyroidism rises. With most assays, this threshold is approximately five times the upper limit of normal. Even when maternal serum thyroid-stimulating IgG activity is high, congenital hyperthyroidism is uncommon, but elevated levels should alert the obstetrician and the pediatrician to monitor the fetus and neonate very carefully for this possibility.

HYPOTHYROIDISM

Prevalence and Causes

In American women, the prevalence of hypothyroidism in pregnancies carried for at least 20 weeks is about six per 1000.[20] Like the frequency figure for hyperthyroidism, this is a minimum estimate. The prevalence of hypothyroidism during pregnancy may be considerably higher in women who have diabetes mellitus.

The causes of hypothyroidism are listed in Table 40–6. *Hashimoto's thyroiditis* and ablative treatment for hyperthyroidism account for the vast majority of cases. Hashimoto's thyroiditis is an autoimmune disease of unknown etiology. Characteristically it causes a rubbery, diffuse goiter and in most cases, hypothyroidism, although development of the latter may take years. A number of autoantibodies with several types of biologic effects are found in the serum of patients with Hashimoto's thyroiditis. Almost all patients with this disease have antithyroid microsomal antibodies (the antigen recognized by this antibody is the thyroid hormone biosynthetic enzyme thyroperoxidase), antithyroglobulin antibodies, or both. There also may be TSH-blocking antibodies, growth-promoting antibodies, growth-inhibiting antibodies, and cytotoxic antibodies. Differences between individuals exist in the balance of these activities. The probability that these antibodies can vary independently in their activity over time explains the wide range in size of the affected thyroid gland, the wide variability in the rate of development of hypothyroidism, and the rare spontaneous remission seen in this disease. In idiopathic myxedema, there is no goiter and antithyroid antibodies are not measurable, but this condition may be a variant of Hashimoto's thyroiditis, perhaps representing a disappearence of the autoimmune activity after the thyroid gland has been irreversibly destroyed. In subacute thyroiditis, both the painful and painless varieties, there often is a phase of hypothyroidism, usually lasting not more than 3–4 months.

Patients who have had external x-ray therapy to the neck region for cancer treatment have a high incidence of mild hypothyroidism. Young women who have been cured of metastatic Wilm's tumor or Hodgkin's disease may be fertile and should therefore be checked for hypothyroidism before and during pregnancy.

Iodine deficiency, though exceedingly rare in the United States, tragically continues to be a major public health problem and a major cause of hypothyroidism in many areas of the world. In pregnancy complicated by iodine deficiency, the fetus may be somewhat better protected than the mother against the deleterious effects, but there is a good correlation in this circumstance between maternal and fetal–neonatal thyroid status. This is not true in other causes of hypothyroidism because of the independence of the fetal pituitary-thyroid axis from that of the mother. Epidemiologic and physiologic studies clearly show that iodization improves the outcome of pregnancy in iodine-deficient areas.

Clinical Features

The common clinical manifestations of hypothyroidism are summarized in Table 40–7. Many of the features of mild hypothyroidism also are common in normal pregnancy, and most also are quite common in the general population. Also, most are symptoms, not signs. Therefore, the diagnosis of mild hypothyroidism cannot be established or excluded unequivocally without laboratory confirmation. When the thyroid hormone deficiency becomes moderate to severe, more readily observable physical signs appear, and the clinical diagnosis becomes more reliable. When examined carefully, the majority of hypothyroid patients have thyroid enlargement. It should be noted that weight gain of more than 5–8 kg is not a feature of hypothyroidism, despite the popular conception to the contrary. The reason is that hypothyroidism tends to decrease appetite, and food consumption falls in proportion to the decreased caloric expenditure. Moreover, most of the weight gain that occurs in hypothyroidism represents fluid retention. The most extreme form of hypothyroidism is myxedema coma, a condition with a high mortality; it is unlikely that a woman with such a severe degree of hypothyroidism would become pregnant.

Special Considerations in Pregnancy

Hypothyroid women have decreased fertility. In prolonged moderate to severe disease, hyperprolactinemia may occur, with resultant anovulation and amenorrhea with or without galactorrhea, sometimes accompanied by pituitary enlargement. The syndrome resolves entirely after restoration of the euthyroid state with exogenous thyroid hormone and therefore is unlikely to represent true pituitary adenoma formation. On the other hand, women with only mild hypothyroidism and hyperprolactinemia often have two separate diseases, and thyroid hormone replacement does not always normalize their serum prolactin. In severe hypothyroidism,

TABLE 40–6. CAUSES OF HYPOTHYROIDISM

Hashimoto's (chronic lymphocytic) thyroiditis
Idiopathic myxedema (probably a variant of Hashimoto's thyroiditis)
^{131}I therapy or thyroid surgery for hyperthyroidism; also may occur late (10–20 years) in the natural history of Graves' disease treated only with drugs
Subacute granulomatous (Quervain's) thyroiditis; usually self-limited
Subacute painless (lymphocytic) thyroiditis; usually self-limited
Radiation therapy for head, neck, or upper chest malignancies
Hypopituitarism (TSH deficiency)
Hypothalamic disease (thyrotropin-releasing hormone deficiency)
Antithyroid drugs: propylthiouracil or methimazole in overly high doses
Goitrogenic drugs: lithium, inorganic iodide, sulfonylureas (underlying thyroid disease exists in most cases); amiodarone can cause either hypothyroidism or hyperthyroidism
Infiltrative diseases: cystinosis, amyloidosis, leukemia (rare)
Iodine deficiency (virtually nonexistent in North America)
Congenital hypothyroidism; usually thyroid dysgenesis or agenesis, less often goitrous cretinism (intrathyroidal enzyme deficiency), rarely autoimmune
Syndromes of tissue resistance to thyroid hormone (very rare)

gonadotropin secretion also can be abnormal without a derangement of prolactin secretion. In the absence of laboratory evidence of hypothyroidism, there is no evidence for any beneficial effect of the administration of thyroid hormone to infertile women or to women who habitually abort.

Occasionally, a woman with moderate to severe hypothyroidism becomes pregnant. Maternal hypothyroidism during pregnancy can have adverse effects on the outcome of pregnancy. A large scale survey found that in pregnancies complicated by hypothyroidism, there is a twofold increase in stillbirths.[20] A recent series reported high frequencies of preeclampsia, *abruptio placentae,* anemia, postpartum hemorrhage caused by uterine atony, and low birth-weight infants in women with moderate to severe hypothyroidism.[59] In the same study, women with mild hypothyroidism had far fewer complications, and none clearly related to their hypothyroidism. Increased risks of perinatal mortality, congenital anomalies, and developmental abnormalities in offspring of hypothyroid women have been suggested but not proven. The studies that suggested these problems used questionable criteria for hypothyroidism. It is reasonable to conclude that most pregnant hypothyroid women will have a successful outcome of the pregnancy[60], but treatment of the hypothyroidism probably improves the chances of success and therefore always should be given.

There are occasional reports of spontaneous remission of chronic hypothyroidism during pregnancy.[61] It is not clear how often this happens because most chronically hypothyroid women take thyroid hormone, and it seems unwise to stop this therapy during pregnancy. It is common to see women who have taken thyroid hormone for years for unclear reasons; in some cases, they are hypothyroid but cannot recall the details of their previous symptoms or diagnostic evaluations, but in other cases, thyroid hormone has been administered for unnecessary reasons. When such an uncertain situation is encountered during pregnancy, it is advisable to continue treatment throughout pregnancy and lactation because there is no harm in taking replacement (not excessive) doses of thyroid hormone. Treatment can be withdrawn later to determine if the patient is actually hypothyroid.

Diagnosis

The most important laboratory test for establishing or excluding the diagnosis of hypothyroidism in pregnancy is the serum TSH concentration. This measurement is elevated above normal even in mild hypothyroidism, especially when a highly sensitive TSH assay is used, in which the upper limit of normal is approximately 5 μU/mL. Many patients with mild to moderate hypothyroidism have serum T_4 and free T_4 concentrations in the low normal range. If the serum TSH concentration is normal, primary hypothyroidism is excluded, except in patients taking high doses of glucocorticoids or receiving intravenous dopamine. Hypopituitarism and hypothalamic disease causing hypothyroidism are overlooked if serum TSH is used as the primary screening test. However, these are rare causes of hypothyroidism in the general population and are presumably even less common in pregnant women who needed normal gonadotropin function to become pregnant.

When there is a clear abnormality on examination of the thyroid gland in a woman suspected to be hypothyroid, or if the suspicion of hypothyroidism is high on clinical grounds, it is most efficient to determine the serum free T_4 concentration and antithyroid microsomal and antithyroglobulin antibody levels at the same time as the serum TSH level. Similarly, if the serum TSH level is used as a screening test and is abnormal, these other tests should be obtained.

The combination of the serum free T_4 and TSH concentrations define the severity of hypothyroidism. It is important to understand the relationship of total serum T_4 and serum TBG levels to the serum free T_4 concentration in making the laboratory diagnosis of hypothyroidism during pregnancy. Thus, in the hypothyroid pregnant woman, the total serum T_4 may be well within the nonpregnant normal range, while at the same time, the free T_4 concentration may be significantly subnormal. The presence of elevated titers of thyroglobulin antibodies or thyroid microsomal antibodies confirms that hypothyroidism is caused by autoimmune thyroiditis. If the antibody titers are not elevated, the other causes of hypothyroidism, listed in Table 40–6, must be considered; however, about 5% of patients with Hashimoto's thyroiditis have negative or borderline antibody test results. The serum T_3 concentration remains in the normal range until hypothyroidism becomes severe; therefore, this measurement is not diagnostically useful.

Treatment

Oral levothyroxine is the optimal treatment for hypothyroidism because adequate doses normalize all the clinical manifestations of thyroid hormone deficiency and restore serum T_4 and T_3, free T_4 and T_3, and TSH concentrations to normal. There is no advantage to combinations of T_4 and T_3, either as thyroid USP or in synthetic form. On the contrary, therapy with such preparations results in unphysiologic hour-to-hour excursions in the serum T_3 concentration, in serum T_4 and free T_4 levels that are sometimes difficult to interpret; and in a nullification of the body's ability to regulate circulating and intracellular T_3 concentrations in nonthyroid disease states. The average levothyroxine dose required to render hypothyroid patients euthyroid is about 125 μg as a single oral daily dose; the majority of patients require 50–200 μg daily, depending on age and body weight. It is safest to prescribe one levothyroxine brand that has been proven reliable instead of switching brands. There have been variations from the stated value of T_4 content in some generic levothyroxine preparations, and there may be variations in absorption of the T_4 from tablets of different manufacturers in some patients. Synthroid and Levothroid are the most commonly used brand name levothyroxine products in the United States.

TABLE 40–7. CLINICAL FEATURES OF HYPOTHYROIDISM

Mild Disease	Moderate to Severe Disease	Most Severe Disease
FATIGUE	Dry, thick skin	Hypothermia
CONSTIPATION	Thick, brittle hair	Hypoventilation
MUSCLE CRAMPS	Hoarse voice, thick tongue	Bradycardia
FLUID RETENTION	Hypertension	Depressed sensorium
Menometrorrhagia	Serous effusions	
Dry skin	Slow thinking and speech	
Cold intolerance	Decreased appetite	
	Delayed reflexes	
	CARPAL TUNNEL SYNDROME	

(Findings that can be caused by pregnancy alone are capitalized.)

Pregnancy imposes special considerations on the initiation of levothyroxine treatment in the newly diagnosed patient and on the dose needed for maintenance therapy. In the nonpregnant hypothyroid patient, it is advisable to begin levothyroxine therapy gradually if the hypothyroidism is long-standing, the patient has heart disease, or the patient is older than 50 and is at risk for occult heart disease. The rationale is that overly rapid restoration of the euthyroid state can precipitate myocardial ischemia. In the absence of known heart disease, these risks are remote in pregnancy, and the complications of hypothyroidism should be minimized, which makes it reasonable to start therapy in a pregnant hypothyroid woman with a full replacement dose of levothyroxine. Because this dose requires about 5 weeks to achieve a steady serum free T_4 concentration, consideration may be given to a loading dose, achieved by giving twice the estimated daily levothyroxine replacement dose for the first week. Treatment is monitored primarily by the serum TSH concentration; the levothyroxine dose should be adjusted every 4 weeks until the initially elevated serum TSH is restored to normal and not overly suppressed as judged by a highly sensitive TSH assay. When this is achieved, the serum free T_4 and free T_3 concentrations are virtually always satisfactory.

Some women who have hypothyroidism and are taking a satisfactory replacement levothyroxine dose and become pregnant need higher doses during the pregnancy. This need for an increased levothyroxine dose during pregnancy is reported to occur in about 20% of hypothyroid women taking replacement levothyroxine.[62] The reasons for the change in dose requirement are unclear. Measured T_4 production rates, corrected for body weight, are virtually identical in pregnant and nonpregnant women. Theoretically, there could be a decrease in the serum free T_4 concentration because of the rapid rise in TBG in early pregnancy if the T_4 "production rate" (ie, the T_4 dose) were constant. If a woman gained a large amount of weight during the pregnancy (other than retained water), her T_4 requirement might increase on that basis. There conceivably could be a decrease in the efficiency of gastrointestinal absorption of T_4 from the tablets.

In eight such patients in my practice, the elevation of the serum TSH concentration occurred as early as 8 weeks' gestation, and most of the women had gained less than 5 kg at the time of the first TSH elevation. The increase in serum TSH concentration was accompanied by a fall in the serum free T_4 concentration, suggestion no abnormality in the set point of the pituitary-thyroid axis. Most of the affected women had very little residual thyroid function, having had radioactive iodine treatment for hyperthyroidism, total thyroidectomy for cancer, or severe Hashimoto's thyroiditis. The average increase in the levothyroxine dose needed to restore a normal serum TSH level was about 65 μg daily, and the range of necessary increases was 25–125 μg daily.

After delivery, treatment with levothyroxine should not affect the mother's decision about whether to nurse her baby. T_4 is normally present in breast milk but in concentrations less than 4 ng/mL. Even if maternal serum T_4 concentrations were slightly supranormal (eg, in the setting of suppressive therapy with levothyroxine after removal of thyroid cancer), the amount of T_4 in the breast milk would be too small to make a significant impact on the infant.

There is a report that the relative risk of having a baby with cerebral palsy is associated with treatment with thyroid hormone, sometimes with concomitant estrogens, during pregnancy.[63] The relevance of this report to the treatment of hypothyroid women is dubious. No information was available about the thyroid hormone preparations used, the doses used, how the dose was monitored, or how well hypothyroidism was documented. One third of the mothers taking thyroid hormone had it prescribed for conditions other than thyroid disease, and for which thyroid hormone is not indicated according to present standards. Finally, the absolute risk of cerebral palsy in offspring of women taking thyroid hormone without estrogen was only 0.9%, and thyroid hormone administration without estrogens was not a significant predictor of cerebral palsy by multivariate analysis.[64]

Congenital Hypothyroidism

Congenital hypothyroidism is a relatively common disease, occurring in about one in 3500 liveborn infants.[65] Screening programs to detect this disease in operation throughout the United States, Canada, Europe, and Japan have been a tremendous medical and public health success. Even at examination after this diagnosis is established by screening studies, many of the affected infants have no stigmata by which the disease can be suspected clinically in the neonatal period[65], but if congenital hypothyroidism is not diagnosed and treated before 3 months of age, irreversible mental retardation commonly occurs. On the other hand, when treatment is instituted earlier than 3 months, this terrible complication can largely or entirely be avoided. Most cases are sporadic and are caused by an ectopic thyroid gland or thyroid agenesis. Inborn defects in thyroid hormone biosynthesis are rare, about one in 30,000 births, but these defects are often familial, with subsequent children of these families at risk. Cases of apparent transplacental passage of autoimmune thyroiditis causing transient neonatal hypothyroidism have been reported.[66] Maternal ingestion of goitrogens, particularly iodide and PTU, can cause fetal goiter and hypothyroidism.[13] This also has been reported with iodide exposure caused by release of iodide from radiocontrast agents used in amniofetography.[67]

The full-blown clinical syndrome of congenital hypothyroidism at birth includes lethargy, depressed nasal bridge, enlarged protuberant tongue, umbilical hernia, dry skin, muscle hypotonia, hyporeflexia, delayed neurologic development, delayed bone age, and epiphyseal dysgenesis. It must be emphasized that this is the exception even in clear-cut cases. The laboratory tests of thyroid function show a subnormal serum T_4 for age and an elevated serum TSH. Interpretation of the serum T_4 must be made carefully because the normal range changes almost daily in the first few days of life, and in preterm infants, the normal range depends on both age and birth weight (see Fig. 40–2).[13] The serum TSH is elevated, usually greatly so, except when the thyroid deficiency is secondary to congenital pituitary or hypothalamic disease. The combined incidence of the latter two conditions is less than 6% of primary thyroid disease. A thyroid scan is useful to determine whether the thyroid gland is absent, ectopic, or in the normal location but enlarged. It would be useful to be able to diagnose congenital hypothyroidism *in utero* in fetuses at risk, such as those in families with defects in hormone biosynthesis and those exposed to PTU, chronic, nonradioactive iodide, or radioiodine. Ultrasound examination can sometimes disclose a fetal goiter[68], and that may help in the planning of the delivery. However, amniotic fluid hormone measurements of T_4, reverse-T_3, or TSH do not predict fetal thyroid status in such high-risk pregnancies.

The initial treatment of congenital hypothyroidism consists of oral levothyroxine, 10 μg/kg daily as a single daily dose. The dose per kilogram decreases as the baby becomes older. Recommendations are available for levothyroxine dosages and comprehensive follow-up evaluations at different ages.[69] T_4 is absorbed from the amniotic fluid by the fetus and could theoretically be given in this way to treat congenital hypothyroidism in the fetus. However, besides our current inability to make this diagnosis reliably *in utero,* there is no information as to the appropriate levothyroxine dose or schedule of administration.

Intra-amniotic T_4 has been administered experimentally in the setting of a high risk for neonatal respiratory distress syndrome in the absence of hypothyroidism.[70] Although some infants with this respiratory disease have lower serum thyroid hormone levels than healthy infants, when gestational age and birth-weight are controlled for, there is no evidence that infants who develop respiratory distress syndrome have any abnormality of the thyroid gland. Rather, they show the abnormalities of thyroid function tests common to severe illness at any age. However, thyroid hormone promotes lung maturation, and it may prove that intra-amniotic thyroid hormone could decrease the risk of the respiratory distress syndrome on a pharmacologic basis, independent of the presence of thyroid disease. More studies are required to clarify this matter.

POSTPARTUM HYPERTHYROIDISM AND HYPOTHYROIDISM (SUBACUTE LYMPHOCYTIC THYROIDITIS)

Transient thyroid dysfunction is fairly common in the first several months postpartum[71,72], with an incidence of about 5% in Caucasian and oriental women, and 1–2% in black American women. The cause is a variety of autoimmune thyroiditis termed *silent* (or painless) *subacute thyroiditis, subacute lymphocytic thyroiditis,* or *lymphocytic thyroiditis with spontaneously resolving hyperthyroidism.* The thyroid gland shows lymphocytic infiltration and epithelial damage. The histology of this condition differs from that of classic, painful, subacute granulomatous (Quervain's) thyroiditis, and the exquisite thyroid tenderness, systemic symptoms, and elevated sedimentation rate characteristic of Quervain's thyroiditis are absent. Thyroid histology also differs from that of Hashimoto's thyroiditis. The cause of postpartum painless subacute thyroiditis and its relationship to other forms of autoimmune thyroiditis are not clear. Presenting features may be asymptomatic goiter, signs and symptoms of mild thyrotoxicosis (without the features unique to Graves' disease), or mild hypothyroidism. Patients often have a history of preexisting goiter, and transient thyroid dysfunction may occur in the same woman after successive pregnancies.[72]

When there is a hyperthyroid phase to this disease, it usually appears in the first 3 months postpartum and persists for several weeks to 3 months. The mechanism of the hyperthyroidism in this form of thyroiditis is release of previously synthesized and stored thyroid hormone because of widespread damage to the thyroid gland. In the hyperthyroid phase of postpartum subacute thyroiditis, the serum free T_4 and free T_3 are elevated, but the T_3 to T_4 ratio is not elevated, in contrast to the high ratio in Graves' disease. Because there is no external thyroid stimulation and because the excessive thyroid hormone concentrations suppress TSH secretion from the pituitary gland, the thyroidal radioiodine uptake is 1–2% or less at 24 hours. This is the most characteristic laboratory finding in postpartum subacute thyroiditis, which distinguishes it from Graves' disease, in which the radioiodine uptake is usually elevated (greater than 30% in the United States), and rarely below 20%. If a woman is nursing, it is best to defer isotopic testing, which is almost always possible. When a radioiodine uptake test is absolutely necessary, a very low dose of ^{131}I (0.1 μci) should be used for the uptake test, and the patient should stop breast feeding for 5 days after the test, during which time she should pump and discard breast milk; she may then resume nursing. ^{123}I is not suitable as a tracer in this situation because it may contain enough of the longer-lived isotope ^{124}I to deliver to the baby an undesirably high radiation exposure. Thyroid microsomal antibody titers often are elevated in subacute thyroiditis, but this is also true in other autoimmune thyroid diseases. Because of the mechanism of the hyperthyroidism and because of the self-limited nature of this phase of the disease, thionamide therapy is not indicated, but symptomatic treatment, perhaps including beta-adrenergic blockers, and reassurance are usually sufficient. After the hyperthyroidism resolves, a phase of hypothyroidism may occur, as detailed below. A goiter may persist for months or years.

In postpartum hypothyroidism caused by subacute thyroiditis, often there is no preceding phase of hyperthyroidism. There is nothing characteristic about the thyroid hormone and TSH serum levels. The radioiodine uptake is often low, but this occasionally may occur in Hashimoto's thyroiditis as well. On the other hand, hypothyroidism with a normal or high 24-hour thyroidal radioiodine uptake does not exclude subacute thyroiditis.

The hypothyroidism usually resolves by 9 months postpartum but may persist.[72] The decision to treat with levothyroxine or merely to follow the patient to make sure that recovery occurs must be individualized. I prefer to treat patients for 3–4 months with levothyroxine, 100 μg as a single daily oral dose, then to withdraw the levothyroxine and retest thyroid function. The rationale for treatment is that postpartum hypothyroidism is associated with an increased prevalence of depression, memory impairment, poor mental concentration, and increased carelessness.[73] Up to 30% of women who develop postpartum hypothyroidism because of subacute lymphocytic thyroiditis remain hypothyroid permanently.[74] This contrasts with the incidence of permanent hypothyroidism of less than 10% in patients whose subacute thyroiditis develops at other times. Thus, patients with this disease in the postpartum period must be followed carefully, with repeated assessment of thyroid function until the outcome is clear.

Preconception Planning

Hypothyroid women who are planning a pregnancy should have an evaluation of their thyroid function and adjustment of their levothyroxine dose as needed to achieve the euthyroid state as judged primarily by the serum TSH concentration. Thyroid function should be reassessed at about 8–10 weeks' gestation and again at about 6 months' gestation, with the necessary adjustments of the levothyroxine dose to maintain a normal serum TSH level. This approach will minimize the chances of complications caused by hypothyroidism during pregnancy. Subsequent testing of thyroid function should be carried out approximately 6 weeks postpartum. Women who need an increased levothyroxine dose during pregnancy usually need a decrease back to the preconception dose by that time. Also, at this time, the first signs of postpartum subacute lymphocytic thyroiditis may appear. Women who have goiters or have been found to have positive antithyroid antibody tests, regardless of their thyroid function before and during pregnancy, should be tested about 3 months postpartum because postpartum hypothyroidism is usually evident then.

THYROID NODULES AND THYROID CANCER

Thyroid nodules are present in 1–2% of young women, and may be discovered during pregnancy. The important question in this situation is whether there is significant risk that the nodule is a thyroid cancer. When multiple nodules are present, the cause is usually euthyroid multinodular goiter or Hashimoto's thyroiditis, and in either case, the incidence of cancer is low, unless there is a history of past therapeutic radiation exposure to the head or neck. A nodule presenting clinically as a single lesion usually proves to be a nodular goiter or a follicular adenoma, but may be a cyst, carcinoma, or dominant nodule in what is really a diffusely abnormal thyroid gland, again usually representing Hashimoto's disease or multinodular goiter. The overall prevalence of thyroid carcinoma in single thyroid nodules is 10–15%, but a given patient's cancer risk varies considerably according to age, size of the nodule, and other specifics of the clinical presentation.

Clinical evaluation of the patient with a single thyroid nodule should begin with an assessment of risk factors for thyroid cancer: history of previous head or neck x-ray therapy for benign or malignant disease, family history suggestive of multiple endocrine neoplasia types II or III, history of rapid growth of the nodule, or evidence of lymph node involvement or fixation of the nodule to surrounding structures. Laboratory evaluation includes estimates of serum free T_4 and free T_3 concentrations to assess the possibility of a toxic adenoma, which is almost never malignant but may necessitate treatment for thyrotoxicosis, and measurement of thyroglobulin antibodies and thyroid microsomal antibodies, which, when present in moderate to high titers, indicate Hashimoto's thyroiditis as a likely cause of the nodule. Ordinarily, a radionuclide thyroid scan is part of the evaluation, but this should not be performed in a pregnant patient. A thyroid ultrasound examination may show a purely cystic lesion, which decreases the likelihood of cancer but does not entirely exclude malignancy. Ultrasound imaging is not necessary if a needle biopsy is performed.

A fine-needle aspiration biopsy with cytologic examination of the aspirates is the most important part of the evaluation of a thyroid nodule. If the aspirates are adequate for cytologic diagnosis and cytology suggests a benign lesion, the patient can be observed. If cytologic or histologic findings are highly suspicious or definitely show malignancy, surgical removal of the nodule is indicated. If cytology is equivocal or the specimens are inadequate for diagnosis, all of the risk factors and laboratory results must be combined into an overall assessment of the patient's risk for cancer to decide between the options of observation or thyroid surgery. Surgical removal of a thyroid nodule, benign or malignant, does not carry an inordinate risk to the mother or fetus, although extensive neck exploration may increase the risk of spontaneous abortion.[75] If the patient proves to have a thyroid carcinoma, levothyroxine should be administered after surgery to suppress TSH secretion and decrease the risk of cancer recurrence. Most thyroidologists also advise treatment with levothyroxine after lobectomy for a benign nodule in the hope of preventing future nodule formation and avoiding the possibility of transient (or, rarely, permanent) mild hypothyroidism.

The great majority of thyroid cancers in young women are well-differentiated lesions of thyroid follicular cell origin, most having papillary or mixed papillary-follicular histology. Moreover, one half of all cases of these types of thyroid cancers in women are first detected during the childbearing years.[76] The majority of these lesions are cured surgically, and even when a cure is not achieved, it is typical for residual disease to be indolent for years. For all types of thyroid cancer, including the more aggressive, but less common, medullary and anaplastic varieties, the overall mortality rate from the thyroid lesions is about 10%, and the mortality from papillary and papillary-follicular cancers first diagnosed in women younger than age 50 is about 1%. Thus, the presence of a newly discovered or preexisting thyroid carcinoma in a pregnant women does not necessitate interruption of a pregnancy, except if there is evidence of progressive or widespread metastatic disease. In some cases, treatment after surgery with ^{131}I is desirable to improve the prognosis even further, but this can almost always be postponed until after the pregnancy, and if necessary, until breast-feeding is finished.

Preconception Planning

Evidence indicates that pregnancy does not alter the natural course of preexisting, well-differentiated thyroid carcinoma in patients with no evident residual disease and in those with known disease.[77,78] Therefore, patients in either category need not be proscribed from becoming pregnant unless it seems likely that ^{131}I therapy will be required in the near future. Previous ^{131}I therapy for thyroid cancer is accompanied by little or no increased risk for birth defects in patients' offspring. The dose of levothyroxine needed during pregnancy may rise, as discussed in the section on hypothyroidism.

REFERENCES

1. Harada A, Hershman JM, Reed AW, et al. Comparison of thyroid stimulators and thyroid hormone concentrations in sera of pregnant women. *J Clin Endocrinol Metab.* 1979;48:793.
2. Dowling JT, Appleton WG, Nicoloff JT. Thyroxine turnover during human pregnancy. *J Clin Endocrinol Metab.* 1967;27:1749.
3. Avruskin TW, Mitsuma T, Shenkman L, et al. Measurement of free and total serum T_3 and T_4 in pregnant subjects and neonates. *Am J Med Sci.* 1976;271:309.
4. Osathanondh R, Tulchinsky D, Chopra IJ. Total and free thyroxine and triiodothyronine in normal and complicated pregnancy. *J Clin Endocrinol Metab.* 1976;42:98.
5. Werner SC. The effect of triiodothyronine administration on the elevated protein bound iodine level in human pregnancy. *Am J Obstet Gynecol.* 1958;75:1193.
6. Ylikorkala O, Kivinen S, Reinila M. Serial prolactin and thyrotropin responses to thyrotropin-releasing hormone throughout normal human pregnancy. *J Clin Endocrinol Metab.* 1979;48:288.
7. Burrow GN, Polackwich R, Donabedian R. The hypothalamic–pituitary–thyroid axis in normal pregnancy. In: Fisher DA, Burrow, eds. *Perinatal Thyroid Physiology and Disease.* New York, NY: Raven Press; 1975:1.
8. Aboul-Khair SA, Crooks J, Turnbull AC, et al. The physiological changes in thyroid function during pregnancy. *Clin Sci.* 1964;27:195.
9. Levy RP, Newman DM, Rejali LS, et al. The myth of goiter in pregnancy. *Am J Obstet Gynecol.* 1980;137:701.
10. Nelson M, Wickus GG, Caplan RH, et al. Thyroid gland size in pregnancy: an ultrasound and clinical study. *J Reprod Med.* 1987;32:888.
11. Mulaisho C, Utiger RD. Serum thyroxine binding globulin: determination by competitive ligand-binding assay in thyroid disease and pregnancy. *Acta Endocrinol.* 1977;85:314.
12. Mori M, Amino N, Tamaki H, et al. Morning sickness and thyroid function in normal pregnancy. *Obstet Gynecol.* 1988;72:355.
13. Roti E, Gnudi A, Braverman LE. The placental transport, synthesis and metabolism of hormones and drugs which affect thyroid function. *Endocrine Rev.* 1983;4:131.
14. Grumbach MM, Werner SC. Transfer of thyroid hormone across the human placenta at term. *J Clin Endocrinol Metab.* 1956;16:1392.

15. Fisher DA, Lehman H, Lackey C. Placental transfer of thyroxine. *J Clin Endocrinol Metab.* 1964;24:393.
16. Raiti S, Holsman GB, Scott RL, et al. Evidence for the placental transfer of triiodothyronine in human beings. *N Engl J Med.* 1967;277:456.
17. Vulsma T, Gons MH, deVijlder JJM. Maternal–fetal transfer of thyroxine in congenital hypothyroidism due to a total organification defect or thyroid agenesis. *N Engl J Med.* 1989;321:13.
18. Fisher DA, Klein AH. Thyroid development and disorders of thyroid function in the newborn. *N Engl J Med.* 1981;304:702.
19. Hollingsworth DR, Alexander NM. Amniotic fluid concentrations of iodothyronines and thyrotropin do not reliably predict fetal thyroid status in pregnancies complicated by maternal thyroid disorders or anencephaly. *J Clin Endocrinol Metab.* 1983;57:349.
20. Thyroid dysfunction. In: Niswander KR, Gordon M, eds. *The Collaborative Perinatal Study of the National Institute of Neurological Disease and Stroke: The Women and Their Pregnancies.* US Department of Health, Education and Welfare; 1972:246.
21. Davis LE, Lucas MJ, Hankins GDV, et al. Thyrotoxicosis complicating pregnancy. *Am J Obstet Gynecol.* 1989;160:63.
22. Amino N, Tanizawa O, Mori H, et al. Aggravation of thyrotoxicosis in early pregnancy and after delivery in Graves' disease. *J Clin Endocrinol Metab.* 1982;55:108.
23. Hardisty CA, Munro DS. Serum long acting thyroid stimulator protector in pregnancy complicated by Graves' disease. *Br Med J.* 1983;1:934.
24. Montoro M, Mestman JH. Graves' disease and pregnancy. *N Engl J Med.* 1981;305:48.
25. Bouillon R, Naesens M, Van Assche FA, et al. Thyroid function in patients with hyperemesis gravidarum. *Am J Obstet Gynecol.* 1982;143:922.
26. Bober SA, McGill AC, Tunbridge WMG. Thyroid function in hyperemesis gravidarum. *Acta Endocrinol.* 1986;111:404.
27. Swaminathan R, Chin RK, Lao TTH, et al. Thyroid function in hyperemesis gravidarum. *Acta Endocrinol.* 1989;120:155.
28. Valentine BH, Jones C, Tyack AJ. Hyperemesis gravidarum due to thyrotoxicosis. *Postgrad Med J.* 1980;56:746.
29. Nagataki S, Mizune M, Sakamoto S, et al. Thyroid function in molar pregnancy. *J Clin Endocrinol Metab.* 1977;44:254.
30. Norman RJ, Green-Thompson RJ, Jialal I, et al. Hyperthyroidism in gestational trophoblastic neoplasia. *Clin Endocrinol.* 1981;15:395.
31. Cave WT, Dunn JT. Choriocarcinoma with hyperthyroidism: probable identity of the thyrotropin with human chorionic gonadotropin. *Ann Int Med.* 1976;85:60.
32. Cohen JD, Utiger RD. Metastatic choriocarcinoma associated with hyperthyroidism. *J Clin Endocrinol Metab.* 1970;30:423.
33. Higgins HP, Hershman JM, Kenimer JG, et al. The thyrotoxicosis of hydatidiform mole. *Ann Intern Med.* 1975;83:307.
34. Berghout A, Endert E, Wiersinga WM, et al. The application of an immunoradiometric assay of plasma thyrotropin (TSH-IRMA) in molar pregnancy. *J Endocrinol Invest.* 1988;11:15.
35. Amir S, Sullivan R, Ingbar SH. The effect of desialylation on the *in vitro* interaction of human chorionic gonadotropin with human thyroid plasma membranes. *Endocrinology.* 1981;109:1203.
36. Gardner DF, Cruikshank DP, Hays, PM, et al. Pharmacology of propylthiouracil (PTU) in pregnant hyperthyroid women: correlation of maternal PTU concentrations with cord serum thyroid function tests. *J Clin Endocrinol Metab.* 1986;62:217.
37. Cheron RG, Kaplan MM, Larsen PR, et al. Neonatal thyroid function after propylthiouracil therapy for maternal Graves' disease. *N Engl J Med.* 1981;304:525.
38. Van Dijke CP, Heydendael RJ, De Kleine MJ. Methimazole, carbimazole and congenital skin defects. *Ann Intern Med.* 1987;106:60.
39. Kampmann JP, Hansen JM, Johansen K, et al. Propythiouracil in human milk. *Lancet.* 1980;1:736.
40. American Academy of Pediatrics Committee on Drugs: The transfer of drugs and other chemicals into breast milk. *Pediatrics.* 1983;72:375.
41. Rubin PC. Beta-blockers in pregnancy. *N Engl J Med.* 1981;305:1323.
42. Smith EM, Warner CG. Estimates of radiation doses to the embryo from nuclear medicine procedures. *J Nucl Med.* 1976;17:146.
43. Husak V, Wiedermann M. Radiation absorbed dose estimates to the embryo from some nuclear medicine procedures. *Eur J Nucl Med.* 1980;5:202.
44. Goh G. Radioiodine treatment during pregnancy: chromosomal aberrations and cretinism associated with maternal iodine-131 treatment. *J Am Wom Med Assoc.* 1981;36:262.
45. Stoffer SS, Hamburger JI. Inadvertent ^{131}I therapy for hyperthyroidism in the first trimester of pregnancy. *J Nucl Med.* 1976;17:146.
46. Richards GE, Brewer ED, Conley SB, et al. Combined hypothyroidism and hypoparathyroidism after maternal ^{131}I administration. *J Pediatr.* 1981;99:141.
47. Burrow GN, Thyroid disease. In: Burrow GN, Ferris TF, eds. *Medical Complications During Pregnancy.* 2nd ed. Philadelphia, PA: WB Saunders; 1982:187.
48. Fisher DA. Pathogenesis and therapy of neonatal Graves' disease. *Am J Dis Child.* 1976;130:133.
49. Hollingsworth DR, Mabry CC. Congenital Graves' disease. Four familial cases with long-term follow-up and perspective. *Am J Dis Child.* 1976;130:148.
50. Check JH, Rezvani I, Goodner D, et al. Prenatal treatment of thyrotoxicosis to prevent intrauterine growth retardation. *Obstet Gynecol.* 1982;60:122.
51. Page DV, Brady K, Mitchell J, et al. The pathology of intrauterine thyrotoxicosis: two case reports. *Obstet Gynecol.* 1988;72:479.
52. Matsuura N, Konishi J, Fujieda K, et al. TSH-receptor antibodies in mothers with Graves' disease and outcome in their offspring. *Lancet.* 1988;2:14.
53. Robinson PL, O'Mullane NM, Alderman B. Prenatal treatment of fetal thyrotoxicosis. *Br Med J.* 1979;1:383.
54. Ramsay I. Attempted prevention of neonatal thyrotoxicosis. *Br Med J.* 1976;2:1110.
55. Momotani N, Noh J, Oyanagi H, et al. Antithyroid drug therapy for Graves' disease during pregnancy. *N Engl J Med.* 1986;315:24.
56. Robertson JS, Gorman CA. Gonadal radiation dose and its genetic significance in radioiodine therapy of hyperthyroidism. *J Nucl Med.* 1976;17:826.
57. Becker DV, Hurley JR. Current status of radioiodine (131I) treatment of hyperthyroidism. In: Freeman JM, Weissman HS, eds. *Nuclear Medicine Annual 1982.* New York, NY: Raven Press; 1982:265.
58. Sarker SD, Beierwaltes WH, Gill SP, et al. Subsequent fertility and birth histories of children and adolescents treated with ^{131}I for thyroid cancer. *J Nucl Med.* 1976;17:460.
59. Davis LE, Leveno KJ, Cunningham FG. Hypothyroidism complicating pregnancy. *Obstet Gynecol.* 1988;72:108.
60. Montoro M, Collea JV, Frasier SD, et al. Successful outcome of pregnancy in women with hypothyroidism. *Ann Int Med.* 1981;94:31.
61. Nelson JC, Palmer FJ. A remission of goitrous hypothyroidism during pregnancy. *J Clin Endocrinol Metab.* 1975;40:383.
62. Pekonen F, Teramo K, Ikonen E, et al. Women on thyroid hormone therapy: pregnancy course, fetal outcome, and amniotic fluid thyroid hormone level. *Obstet Gynecol.* 1984;63:635.
63. Nelson KB, Ellenberg JH. Antecedents of cerebral palsy. 1. Univariate analysis of risks. *Am J Dis Child.* 1985;139:1031.
64. Nelson KB, Ellenberg JH. Antecedents of cerebral palsy. Multivariate analysis of risk. *N Engl J Med.* 1986;315:81.
65. New England Congenital Hypothyroidism Collaborative. Characteristics of infantile hypothyroidism discovered on neonatal screening. *J Pediatr.* 1984;104:539.
66. Matsuura N, Yamada Y, Nohara Y, et al. Familial neonatal transient hypothyroidism due to maternal TSH binding inhibitor immunoglobulins. *N Engl J Med.* 1980;303:738.
67. Rodesch F, Camus M, Ermans AM, et al. Adverse effects of amniofetography on fetal thyroid function. *Am J Obstet Gynecol.* 1976;126:723.
68. Weiner S, Scharf JI, Bolognese RJ, et al. Antenatal diagnosis and treatment of a fetal goiter. *J Reprod Med.* 1980;24:39.
69. Fisher DA, Foley BL. Early treatment of congenital hypothyroidism. *Pediatrics.* 1989;83:785.
70. Mashiach S, Barkai G, Sack J, et al. Enhancement of fetal lung maturity by intraamniotic administration of thyroid hormone. *Am J Obstet Gynecol.* 1978;130:289.
71. Ginsberg J, Walfish PG. Post-partum transient thyrotoxicosis with painless thyroiditis. *Lancet.* 1977;1:1125.
72. Amino N, Mori H, Iwatani Y, et al. High prevalence of transient postpartum thyrotoxicosis and hypothyroidism. *N Engl J Med.* 1982;306:849.
73. Hayslip CC, Fein HG, O'Donnell VM. The value of serum antimicrosomal antibody testing in screening for symptomatic postpartum thyroid dysfunction. *Am J Obstet Gynecol.* 1988;159:203.
74. Nikolai TF, Turney SL, Roberts RC. Postpartum lymphocytic thyroiditis. Prevalence, clinical course. *Arch Intern Med.* 1987;147:221.
75. Cunningham MP, Slaughter DP. Surgical treatment of disease of the thyroid gland in pregnancy. *Surg Gynecol Obstet.* 1970;131:486.
76. Donegan WL. Cancer and pregnancy. *CA.* 1983;33:194.
77. Rosvoll RV, Winship T. Thyroid carcinoma and pregnancy. *Surg Gynecol Obstet.* 1965;121:1039.
78. Hill CS, Clark RL, Wolf M. The effect of subsequent pregnancy on patients with thyroid carcinoma. *Surg Gynecol Obstet.* 1966;122:1219.

Chapter Forty-One

Disorders of the Parathyroid Glands and Vitamin D

Michael M. Kaplan

41

CALCIUM HOMEOSTASIS IN PREGNANCY

Pregnancy presents a great challenge to a woman's calcium homeostasis because of the demands of fetal bone formation. Marked changes occur in virtually all aspects of her calcium economy. Moreover, because the fetus is more sensitive than its mother to disturbed calcium metabolism, it may suffer the brunt of parathyroid hormone or vitamin D disorders. In fact, neonatal skeletal or serum calcium abnormalities are sometimes the first clue to a maternal calcium disorder.

Calcium

Calcium exists in three forms in plasma: 40–45% is bound to albumin, and 5–10% is complexed with various anions. The rest is ionized, but only the ionized calcium exerts physiologic effects on cells. Direct measurement of ionized calcium is available in some laboratories, but the reproducibility of available methods is not optimal and care must be taken in drawing and processing the blood samples according to the requirements of the method for reliable results. When the serum albumin concentration decreases, the total serum calcium concentration also will fall. To determine whether a low serum calcium level is appropriate for the serum albumin, 0.8 mg/dL are added to the measured total calcium for every 1 g/dL below 4.6 in the serum albumin concentration. This corrected calcium value should fall within the normal range for total serum calcium.

During pregnancy, the maternal serum calcium and the maternal serum albumin concentrations fall progressively, the calcium by about 10% (Table 41–1)[1] and the albumin by about 20% at term. Maternal serum ionized calcium concentrations are unchanged in pregnancy (see Table 41–1).[1] Fetal serum ionized calcium concentrations are higher than maternal levels in the second and third trimesters and at term.[2,3] The total calcium is 1–2 mg/dL higher in cord serum than in paired maternal serum.[3] This calcium gradient is maintained by active transport of maternal calcium to the fetal circulation by the placenta. The term fetus has total body calcium stores of about 30 g, of which 20 g are supplied in the third trimester. This calcium requirement is met in part by considerably increased intestinal absorption of dietary calcium by the pregnant woman, rising from about 150 mg in the nonpregnant state to 400 mg daily by the second trimester.[4] This increased absorption is probably mediated by an increased serum level or the active form of vitamin D, calcitriol (see below). There is, however, a corresponding increase in daily maternal urinary calcium excretion from 90–300 mg[5], which must limit the positive gestational calcium balance.

Parathyroid Hormone

Parathyroid hormone (PTH) is a peptide hormone that regulates the serum-ionized calcium concentration by stimulating bone resorption, renal tubular calcium reabsorption, and synthesis of calcitriol by the kidney. Calcitriol, in turn, stimulates absorption of dietary calcium from the gut. The most important regulatory influence on PTH secretion is negative feedback by plasma-ionized calcium. Calcitriol also inhibits PTH secretion. Other factors that may regulate PTH secretion include catecholamines, histamine, and secretin.

The intact 84 amino acid PTH molecule is thought to be the biologically active circulating form, although inactive fragments also circulate in the blood. During pregnancy, the average serum concentration of the active form of PTH falls by about 50%. The reduction is seen in the first trimester, with no further change in the second and third trimesters (see Table 41–1).[1] Older studies, using assays that measured both intact PTH and inactive fragments, tended to show increased levels in pregnancy, but the lack of specificity of these assays makes their results unreliable. A reduced level of the active form of PTH in maternal serum during pregnancy is supported by a trend toward low levels of PTH biologic activity by two bioassays, an *in vitro* cytochemical assay and measurement of urinary excretion of cyclic-AMP generated in the kidney in normal pregnant women.[1,5]

The placenta has receptors for PTH, and incubation with placental tissue with PTH *in vitro* causes an increase in cyclic-AMP accumulation in the tissue. However, the precise role of PTH in placental calcium handling is not known. PTH does not cross the placenta. In sheep studies, fetal thyroparathyroidectomy reduced fetal serum calcium concentrations, but infusion of PTH did not restore the fetal serum calcium to normal.[6] Thus, the role of fetal PTH secretion also is uncertain.

Vitamin D

The vitamin D hormone system[4] includes several compounds: endogenous vitamin D_3 (cholecalciferol), which is produced in the skin under the influence of sunlight, and exogenous vitamin D_2 (ergocalciferol), which is obtained from plant sources. Both are relatively inactive and are hydroxylated in the liver to produce the most abundant form of vitamin D in circulation, 25-hydroxy-vitamin D (25-OHD), which also has only weak biologic potency. The principal active form of vitamin D is 1,25-dihydroxy-vitamin D, or calcitriol, produced from 25-OHD in the kidney. Renal synthesis of calcitriol is stimulated by PTH and by a decrease in the serum inorganic phosphate concentration. The main actions of calcitriol are stimulation of absorption of dietary calcium by the intestine and stimulation of bone resorption.

Maternal serum calcitriol concentrations rise early in pregnancy and remain elevated throughout gestation (see Table 41–1), although maternal serum 25-OHD levels do not change.[7] Part of this rise in calcitriol is caused by increased serum protein binding, but concentrations of unbound, or free, calcitriol also are significantly elevated. Total calcitriol concentrations in cord serum are slightly lower than those in paired maternal serum at term, but free calcitriol concentrations in the fetal circulation and cord blood are similar to maternal levels.[8] The fetal kidney can synthesize calcitriol, as can the placenta. The factors that regulate placental conversion of 25-OHD to calcitriol are not known. Both 25-OHD and calcitriol are transported across the placenta. Evidence suggests that placental production of calcitriol may be able to maintain normal maternal serum calcitriol concentrations when renal calcitriol production is deficient.[9] It seems likely that placental calcitriol synthesis

TABLE 41–1. AVERAGE SERUM CALCIUM, PTH, AND VITAMIN D CONCENTRATIONS DURING NORMAL PREGNANCY

Measurement	Nonpregnant	First Trimester	Second Trimester	Third Trimester
Total calcium, mg/dL	10.3	9.2	9.5	9.6
Ionized calcium, mg/dL	5.2	4.9	5.1	5.3
Intact parathyroid hormone, ng/L	25.0	13.0	16.0	14.0
25-hydroxy vitamin D, ng/mL	14.0	16.0	18.0	16.0
1,25-dihydroxy vitamin D (calcitriol), pg/mL	51.0	94.0	118.0	117.0

The normal range for serum PTH varies between assays. The normal range for 25-hydroxy-vitamin D varies according to geographic location and season of the year because both affect sunlight exposure.
From references 1, 5, and 7.

contributes to the rise in maternal serum free calcitriol levels.

The increased levels of calcitriol in pregnancy are probably responsible for the increased efficiency of maternal absorption of dietary calcium. The placenta has vitamin D receptors of the same type as in classic target tissues, and there is a placental vitamin D-dependent intracellular calcium binding protein similar to that in the intestine that mediates calcium absorption. Nonetheless, the precise effects of vitamin D on placental cells are not yet known. Also unclear is the role of the calcitriol synthesized by the fetal kidney.

Calcitonin

Calcitonin is a peptide hormone produced by the parafollicular cells, or C cells, of the thyroid gland. Calcitonin inhibits bone resorption, and by this mechanism, lowers serum calcium when administered acutely. However, chronic elevations in serum calcitonin leave the serum ionized calcium unaffected. It is postulated that calcitonin aids in accumulation of bone mineral because the main stimulus for calcitonin secretion is a rise in serum-ionized calcium, which may occur after eating. Fetal serum calcitonin levels are higher than those in maternal serum, presumably because of the higher ionized calcium concentrations in fetal serum.[3,6] There is a further rise in the serum calcitonin in infants in the first 48 hours after birth.[3]

Calcitonin does not cross the placenta, but the placenta has calcitonin receptors. As with PTH and vitamin D, the precise function of calcitonin in placental calcium metabolism is not known.

HYPERPARATHYROIDISM

Hyperparathyroidism is the syndrome caused by excessive secretion of the parathyroid hormone. Primary hyperparathyroidism results in raised serum ionized calcium concentrations, with potential adverse effects on many organs. Secondary hyperparathyroidism is the response of the parathyroid glands to chronically low serum ionized calcium concentrations (eg, in renal failure). Elevated serum PTH levels caused by primary or secondary hyperparathyroidism have direct effects on bone; therefore, both diseases can cause similar skeletal problems. Secondary hyperparathyroidism will not be discussed further in this chapter.

Incidence and Causes

Hyperparathyroidism is two to three times more common in women than in men and is much less common before the age of 40. The annual incidence rate rises progressively with age; in women younger than 40, there are an estimated eight new cases per year per 100,000 individuals.[10] Less than 100 cases of hyperparathyroidism during pregnancy have been reported in the medical literature.[11-15] This paucity of reports almost certainly underestimates the prevalence of the disease during pregnancy. A combination of factors probably accounts for the few reported cases: the absence of systematic surveys of unselected pregnancies; the possibility that mild disease is often asymptomatic as in the nonpregnant population; the unavailability until recently of reliable assays for serum levels of intact, biologically active PTH; the fact that mild elevation of serum total calcium and PTH concentrations during pregnancy will give values within the normal range for the nonpregnant population; and the likelihood that many cases are unreported[13] because they are diagnosed and treated successfully and uneventfully. Also, the pregnant woman might be partially protected against mild hyperparathyroidism because estrogens can antagonize the effects of PTH on bone resorption, and serum estrogen levels rise dramatically during pregnancy.

Primary hyperparathyroidism is caused by a single parathyroid adenoma in 80–90% of cases, multiglandular hyperplasia in 10–20% of cases, and parathyroid carcinoma in 1% or less. Ectopic secretion of parathyroid hormone by malignancies used to be considered common, but it is now evident that virtually all such cases are caused by secretion of other peptides with hypercalcemic effects. The set point for PTH secretion is generally changed in adenomatous and hyperplastic parathyroid glands; PTH secretion still can be stimulated and inhibited by changes in ionized calcium, but a higher serum-ionized calcium level than normal is required to inhibit PTH secretion.

Many cases of multiglandular parathyroid hyperplasia occur in the context of familial syndromes: multiple endocrine neoplasia types 1 and 2a, familial hyperparathyroidism, and familial hypocalciuric hypercalcemia (also called benign familial hypercalcemia).[4] Thus, the finding of multiple abnormal parathyroid glands at surgery should prompt family screening. Familial hypocalciuric hypercalcemia is usually an asymptomatic condition not requiring treatment, resulting from inheritance of one abnormal allele. However, homozygous neonates may have severe biochemical and skeletal abnormalities[16], which should be watched by the obstetrician and pediatrician because the infant may need immediate respiratory support after delivery. The other familial conditions cause the same spectrum of abnormalities as hyperparathyroidism caused by a single adenoma.

Clinical Features

The most common presentation of hyperparathyroidism is asymptomatic hypercalcemia, accounting for about one half of the cases reported since the advent of automated multiphasic serum chemistry panels.[10] Conversely, because malignancies are relatively uncommon in women in their childbearing years, hyperparathyroidism is probably the most common cause of asymptomatic hypercalcemia in this population.

When hyperparathyroidism is symptomatic, the most common manifestations are fatigue, weakness, renal stones, altered mentation, gastrointestinal symptoms, hypertension, headache, weight loss, and bone disease. Clearly, most of these conditions are nonspecific; even in patients presenting with renal stones, only a small fraction prove to have hyperparathyroidism. Hyperparathyroid bone disease has occurred in less than 10% of patients diagnosed in recent years. The most common finding is subperiosteal bone resorption, particularly in the phalanges of the fingers. The serum alkaline phosphatase activity usually is elevated when bone disease is present. Full-blown hyperparathyroid bone disease, called osteitis fibrosa cystica, includes bone pain, pathologic fractures, and localized bone swellings, which appear radiologically as lucent cystic lesions, the "brown tumors" of bone.

Sometimes a patient with hyperparathyroidism develops a hypercalcemic crisis—extreme hypercalcemia causing severe weakness, mental obtundation or even coma, and renal insufficiency.[4,17] The risk of this dangerous condition may be increased in the immediate postpartum period because of relative immobilization and dehydration.

Because hyperparathyroidism during pregnancy has been reported so infrequently, the literature may be biased toward the more severely involved end of the clinical spectrum. Nevertheless, the disease appears to cause substantial morbidity, with the fetus and neonate suffering most of the problems. In early series describing mostly untreated cases, fetal death or neonatal tetany occurred in 50–80% of cases. About 6% of cases of hyperparathyroidism reported in pregnant patients have been complicated by pancreatitis.[12,13,18] This is a much higher frequency than that of pancreatitis in nonpregnant hyperparathyroid patients and argues for aggressive therapy. However, some of these patients had additional predisposing risk factors for pancreatitis, and there may be a reporting bias.

The fetus and neonate suffer major adverse effects of maternal hyperparathyroidism. In untreated disease, spontaneous abortion or fetal death occur about 15% of the time, and neonatal hypocalcemic tetany, usually transient and sometimes fatal, occurs about 30% of the time. The etiology of neonatal tetany is thought to have two mechanisms: (1) sustained fetal hypercalcemia secondary to maternal hypercalcemia, resulting in more complete and prolonged suppression of neonatal PTH secretion than usual, and (2) neonatal hypomagnesemia, perhaps caused by maternal hypomagnesemia or by factors in the infant.[3]

Infants born to mothers with familial hypocalciuric hypercalcemia often manifest the hypercalcemia at birth. Some affected babies do well and do not require treatment. Others, who probably have a homozygous form of the disease, present with severe neonatal hyperparathyroidism, with exceedingly elevated serum calcium concentrations, severe bone disease, and muscle weakness, to the point that the chest wall is incapable of supporting respiration.[16] A history of familial hypocalciuric hypercalcemia in the father is as significant as that in the mother because the disease is inherited as an autosomal dominant condition, and affected infants have been born to healthy mothers.

Diagnosis

The characteristic laboratory findings of hyperparathyroidism include hypercalcemia; an elevated serum PTH concentration; hypophosphatemia caused by the phosphaturic effect of PTH on the renal tubule; a mild hyperchloremic metabolic acidosis, again caused by PTH effects on the kidney; elevated serum alkaline phosphatase activity, often absent in mild disease but the rule in hyperparathyroid bone disease; normal or only mildly elevated urinary calcium because PTH increases the efficiency of renal tubular calcium reabsorption from the glomerular filtrate; and high-normal or elevated serum calcitriol concentrations.

In the last few years, the technology of serum PTH measurement has advanced greatly, based on monoclonal antibody technology. PTH immunoradiometric assays are now available from commercial laboratories, and in kit form for use by any clinical laboratory, that can specifically measure the serum concentration of intact PTH (the molecule that is thought to be the main active form of the hormone), detect serum PTH levels below the lower limit of normal, and minimize the frequency of misleadingly normal or high readings in hypercalcemia of malignancy.[1] Determinations of serum 25-OHD and calcitriol concentrations also are readily available from commercial reference laboratories.

The work-up is initiated when hypercalcemia is discovered because this finding is rarely absent in hyperparathyroidism. The patient's medical history should be reviewed carefully for evidence of other causes of hypercalcemia, with special attention to calcium and vitamin D intake and thiazide therapy. Thiazides can cause mild hypercalcemia. In interpreting blood test results, the progressive decrease during pregnancy in the normal range for total serum calcium must be kept in mind when a gravida is being evaluated for possible hyperparathyroidism.

A reproducible elevation in serum calcium combined with an inappropriately high serum PTH concentration establishes the diagnosis of hyperparathyroidism, although a normal decrease in serum PTH concentrations occurs during pregnancy. It is important to verify the elevations in both the serum calcium and PTH levels on a second blood sample, particularly if a decision about surgical exploration hinges on the result. In doubtful cases, it is possible to use a bioassay for PTH by measuring urinary excretion of nephrogenous cyclic-AMP; however, this requires very careful processing of blood and urine samples.[4] The advent of the newer PTH assays should make this test rarely necessary. It is probably better in ambiguous cases to obtain PTH measurements by several different assays that use different antibodies. Consultation with the clinical laboratory can aid in the decision of which to use and how to interpret the results.

When hyperparathyroidism is diagnosed, the family history should be reviewed, and the ratio of urinary calcium clearance to creatinine clearance should be determined to exclude familial hypocalciuric hypercalcemia. The creatinine clearance obtained in the course of this evaluation also will indicate whether there has been any compromise of renal function caused by the hypercalcemia. Measurements of serum electrolytes, inorganic phosphate, and alkaline phosphatase are conventionally performed and often are confirmatory but frequently are normal. Serum alkaline phosphatase activity normally rises in the third trimester of pregnancy. This is because of an increase in the bone isoenzyme and the appearance of placental alkaline phosphatase in the blood.[19] The author's practice is to obtain a serum 25-OHD level to exclude hypervitaminosis D. Given the availability of vitamin D in any pharmacy, a patient may be ingesting inadvertently large amounts, and concomitant vitamin D excess could conceivably convert subclinical hyperparathyroidism to overt disease (the same is true for thiazide treatment).

The differential diagnosis of hyperparathyroidism includes sarcoidosis and other granulomatous diseases, hypercalcemia of malignancy, vitamin D or A intoxication, the milk-alkali syndrome, thiazide therapy, and the various causes of renal stones.

Treatment

In nonpregnant patients, the options that must be weighed in treating hyperparathyroidism are observation, medical treatment, and surgery. Because of the high frequency of fetal morbidity and mortality and the moderate frequency of maternal morbidity in reported cases of this disease in pregnant women, simple observation seems inadvisable. The medical therapy that has been used is oral phosphate, amounting to 1.5–2.5 g of elemental phosphorous per day.[14] This treatment may lower or normalize the serum calcium but can cause diarrhea, sometimes severe, and has the theoretical, albeit rarely observed, risk of nephrocalcinosis and renal damage. A few cases of hyperparathyroidism in pregnancy have been successfully managed with oral phosphate alone, but such an extremely small number of patients makes it impossible to define appropriate selection criteria for this therapy.

Surgical treatment appears to improve the outcome of pregnancies complicated by hyperparathyroidism.[12,13] Parathyroidectomy during pregnancy has been described in approximately 25 cases. Two operations were unsuccessful, leaving persistent hypercalcemia. In three other cases, spontaneous abortion or premature labor occurred within hours of surgery. In the other cases, three infants had neonatal tetany and the rest were healthy.[13] By contrast, in 50 hyperparathyroid pregnant women treated nonsurgically, fetal or maternal complications occurred in 41 of 79 pregnancies; the most common was neonatal tetany. In the absence of surgery, neonatal tetany remains common, occurring in infants of 11 out of 15 hyperparathyroid women reported in the last 20 years, including six out of eight pregnancies in which the mothers were asymptomatic.[12] Even though the neonatal tetany may be mild, transient, and without evident sequelae, there is no way of predicting which infants are at risk or what the severity will be.

Thus, parathyroidectomy must be considered the standard treatment for hyperparathyroidism during pregnancy, against which other options must be weighed in each patient. It is generally recommended that parathyroidectomy be performed in the second trimester to minimize the risks of the teratogenic effects of anesthetic agents and early spontaneous abortion in the first trimester and of premature labor in the third trimester.[13] High resolution neck ultrasound may be considered a possible means of localizing an adenoma preoperatively, thereby minimizing operative time. However, the accuracy of this imaging technique varies with the skill of the operator, and is suboptimal in sensitivity, especially for small adenomas and lesions located in the mediastinum or behind the trachea or esophagus, and specifically, because thyroid cysts and other thyroid lesions can have a similar ultrasound appearance to enlarged parathyroid glands. If the surgeon finds one parathyroid adenoma and evidence of at least one other normal parathyroid gland by frozen section, removal of only the adenoma usually cures the hyperparathyroidism. If multiple parathyroid glands are abnormal, removal of all but about 50 mg of the least abnormal appearing gland is recommended. In the case of multiglandular hyperplasia, some surgeons autotransplant the remaining tissue into the forearm. This makes reoperation easier; patients with hyperplasia are more likely to have late recurrences of hyperparathyroidism than patients with single adenomas.

Management of hypercalcemic crisis includes vigorous saline diuresis and administration of furosemide, both of which promote calciuresis. The intravenous saline also reverses the dehydration that is often present. During this treatment, potassium losses must be carefully monitored and replaced. Calcitonin may help control the hypercalcemia, at least transiently; injectable preparations of synthetic salmon and human calcitonin are available. Plicamycin (mithramycin) is sometimes used for hypercalcemic crises in the nonpregnant patient, but it may have adverse effects on the fetus, and should not be used in pregnancy. Inorganic phosphate is sometimes used, orally or intravenously, but should be a last resort because of the danger of deposition of calcium phosphate in soft tissues, including the kidneys, with resultant renal failure. After the patient is stabilized, parathyroidectomy should be performed as soon as possible to avoid a repeat crisis.

Preconception Planning

For a woman who is planning a pregnancy but has not yet conceived and who has asymptomatic or mild familial or sporadic hyperparathyroidism, surgical treatment is recommended. This approach will avoid the possible necessity for neck exploration during the pregnancy, even if nonsurgical management would otherwise be acceptable. There should at least be a full discussion with the patient concerning the possible problems attendant to hyperparathyroidism during pregnancy. In addition, if either member of a couple planning to have a child has a family member who is affected by a heritable syndrome including hyperparathyroidism, the couple should have counseling about the genetics of the disease; available screening techniques for adults, children, and fetuses; and the risks of potential clinical problems.

HYPOPARATHYROIDISM

Causes

Hypoparathyroidism is an uncommon disorder in which there is insufficient secretion of PTH to maintain a normal serum-ionized calcium concentration. It is most frequently a consequence of neck surgery, caused by inadvertent removal of all parathyroid tissue or irreversible damage to the parathyroid glands without actual removal.[20] Most often the surgery is for thyroid or parathyroid disease. The frequency of hypoparathyroidism after thyroidectomy depends on the extent of surgery, a history of prior neck surgery in the same patient, and the skill of the surgeon. It should happen less than 1% of the time when a less-than-total thyroidectomy is performed as a first neck operation. Hypoparathyroidism after ^{131}I treatment for hyperthyroidism is exceedingly rare—so rare that no causal relationship is clearly established.

Spontaneous hypoparathyroidism occurs sporadically and in the familial syndrome of multiple endocrine organ failure, sometimes accompanied by mucocutaneous candidiasis. Some of the clinical features of hypoparathyroidism, including hypocalcemia, also are seen in pseudohypoparathyroidism. This disease is an uncommon familial condition characterized by resistance to PTH at the level of the kidney, caused by a defect in the guanine nucleotide binding subunit of the PTH receptor-adenylate cyclase complex.[4] The patients also have resistance to other hormones that exert effects through adenylate cyclase. A secondary form of hypoparathyroidism is found in patients with severe hypomagnesemia, caused by a deficiency of PTH secretion and target organ resistance to PTH. This syndrome can be corrected completely by magnesium repletion.[20]

Clinical Features

The hallmark of hypoparathyroidism is hypocalcemia, leading to neuromuscular irritability manifested by paresthesias, carpopedal spasm, and occasionally seizures. Chvostek and Trousseau signs often are present. In addition, patients may have mental changes, ocular cataracts, increased intracranial pressure, and calcifications of the basal ganglia and cerebral falx. The basal ganglion calcifications are sometimes accompanied by extrapyramidal symptoms and signs.

Untreated maternal hypoparathyroidism during pregnancy can cause major fetal and neonatal morbidity. Birth weight less than 2500 g is frequent, and the infants have generalized skeletal demineralization and subperiosteal bone resorption.[3] Their serum calcium concentrations are low to normal, serum phosphate levels are normal to high, and the serum PTH concentration is elevated.[3] It is thought that maternal hypocalcemia causes fetal calcium deficiency, resulting in fetal parathyroid hyperplasia.[21] The excessive amounts of PTH in the fetal circulation cause hyperparathyroid bone disease, and possibly a state of vitamin D deficiency that worsens the bone disease. In affected infants who survive, the abnormalities resolve spontaneously over several months.[3] Although pseudohypoparathyroidism may present with hypocalcemia early in life,[4] the offspring of women with untreated pseudohypoparathyroidism also are at risk for neonatal hypoparathyroidism.[22]

Diagnosis

In hypoparathyroidism, the total and serum ionized calcium concentrations are low, and the serum PTH concentration is not appropriately elevated. There may be a measurable amount of PTH in the blood, but especially with the new, highly sensitive assays for intact PTH, PTH levels are in the low part of the normal range or subnormal and are clearly inappropriate for the hypocalcemia state. The serum inorganic phosphate level is elevated because of increased renal tubular phosphate resorption.

When hypocalcemia, not caused by hypoalbuminemia or renal failure, is discovered, a history of neck surgery, a family or personal history of other autoimmune endocrine deficiency diseases, or the presence of hyperphosphatemia strongly suggest hypoparathyroidism. Serum ionized calcium and PTH concentrations should be measured. The serum magnesium level also should be determined. Although it is relatively common for the serum magnesium concentration to fall during pregnancy, only severe hypomagnesemia causes secondary hypoparathyroidism. Serum 25-OHD and calcitriol measurements also are helpful in excluding vitamin D deficiency.

In pseudohypoparathyroidism, the serum PTH concentration is usually normal and sometimes elevated. Establishing this diagnosis requires the demonstration of a deficient renal response to exogenous PTH, with urinary phosphate and cyclic-AMP failing to rise. The presence of the characteristic phenotypic abnormalities—short stature, obesity, round face, thick neck, and short metacarpal bones, especially in the fourth and fifth fingers—together with hypocalcemia are strongly suggestive of pseudohypoparathyroidism.[4]

The differential diagnosis of hypocalcemia includes renal failure, hypomagnesemia, severe vitamin D deficiency or hereditary vitamin D resistance, severe acute hyperphosphatemia caused by tumor lysis or rhabdomyolysis, and "hungry bones." The latter is a transient syndrome that occurs occasionally after surgical correction of hyperparathyroidism or hyperthyroidism, in which the mineral deficit from the primary disease is severe, and abrupt correction of the primary disease permits such a rapid influx of calcium into the bones that hypocalcemia results.

Treatment

The goal of therapy is to keep the patient's serum ionized calcium, or the total calcium corrected for the serum albumin, close to the low end of normal. This is achieved with a combination of vitamin D and oral calcium supplementation. There are two potential problems when the serum calcium is kept in the middle or upper part of the normal range. In the absence of PTH, fractional excretion of calcium into the urine is increased. This can result in hypercalciuria and an increased risk of renal stones if the filtered calcium load is too high. Also, patient's dose requirements for vitamin D sometimes change for uncertain reasons and at unpredictable times. Hypercalcemia sometimes occurs as a result. If the baseline level of serum calcium is high normal, there may be an increased risk of this problem. For these reasons, a serum calcium concentration slightly below normal is acceptable in the asymptomatic nonpregnant patient. In the pregnant patient, it seems safer for the fetus if the maternal serum calcium level is in the low part of the normal range for pregnancy.

Parathyroid hormone is not available for therapeutic use. A synthetic fragment is available for diagnostic purposes, but it has a very short duration of action, and its use for treatment involves several injections daily. Therefore, the treatment of hypoparathyroidism consists of vitamin D, with or without oral calcium. Typical dose requirements are 50,000–100,000 units of vitamin D_2 daily (1 μg of vitamin D_2 or D_3 equals 40 USP units), although some patients require more. In one series, the average dose required to maintain a normal serum calcium in pregnant hypoparathyroid patients was slightly greater than 100,000 U daily.[23] Because of extensive storage of vitamin D in body fat, it takes several weeks for a patient to equilibrate when the dose is changed; therefore, increases should not be made more often than every 2–3 weeks.

Some physicians prefer to treat hypoparathyroid patients with dihydrotachysterol, a vitamin D analog that does not require the PTH-dependent step of 1-hydroxylation, or with calcitriol. Typical dose requirements are 0.5–1.0 mg daily of dihydrotachysterol and 0.25–1.0 μg daily of calcitriol. Both of these agents are much less extensively stored in fat than vitamin D, and both may therefore have a more rapid onset and offset of action. Calcitriol therapy may give a less stable serum calcium level in some patients than longer-acting preparations and a higher frequency of hypercalcemia.

When calcitriol has been used to treat pregnant hypoparathyroid women, the dose needed to maintain the desired serum calcium concentration sometimes increases progressively over a several-fold range, with a rapid decrease in the dose after parturition.[24-26] The doses of vitamin D and calcitriol needed to treat hypoparathyroidism in pregnancy do not appear to have adverse effects on the fetus.[23,27]

The reason for the increase in the calcitriol requirement during pregnancy is not known. Perhaps the high concentrations of estrogens or progestins antagonize the actions of vitamin D. During lactation, the calcitriol dose may fall dramatically.[26] The lactating breast makes a peptide, structurally related to PTH and having PTHlike actions on bone and kidney. It is conceivable that some of this peptide appears in the maternal circulation and serves as a PTH surrogate. It also has been speculated that prolactin may promote endogenous calcitriol synthesis. Although the mechanisms of the fluctuations in vitamin D dose requirements are not yet understood, it is clear that the pregnant hypoparathyroid patient needs careful and frequent monitoring of her serum calcium during and after the pregnancy.

Although calcium supplementation is not always needed in the management of hypoparathyroidism, it is prudent to recommend it during pregnancy because of the necessity to provide minerals for fetal bone development. The hypoparathyroid patient may need 2000–3000 mg daily. Calcium is available as calcium carbonate, lactate, and other salts; the percentage of elemental calcium in the salt must be taken into account when deciding the dosage, though most preparations specifically state their calcium content on the package. Prices of over the counter oral calcium preparations vary from a few pennies to more than 1 dollar per gram of calcium. There are no known advantages of the more expensive ones, so patients can be advised to choose an inexpensive product.

There have been reports of successful breast-feeding by hypoparathyroid women. Human milk contains about 400 mg of calcium per liter. This would seem to represent a considerable stress in a hypoparathyroid woman. Her milk also may have a higher than normal concentration of vitamin D, depending on therapy. However, with careful clinical monitoring of the mother and infant, breast-feeding can be permitted.

Preconception Planning

A woman with hypoparathyroidism should be informed that she will require frequent monitoring during the pregnancy to keep her calcium level in the suitable range. She should therefore consult her physician as soon as she thinks she may be pregnant. For a couple in which either member has pseudohypoparathyroidism or multiple autoimmune endocrine deficiency syndrome, genetic counseling is appropriate. They should be informed of the chances of an affected child and of symptoms in their children that may indicate the onset of the disease.

VITAMIN D DEFICIENCY

Vitamin D deficiency occurs in individuals with malabsorption, especially with biliary obstruction, in some patients treated chronically with anticonvulsants, and in individuals whose diets are deficient in vitamin D and who have insufficient exposure to sunlight to stimulate normal vitamin D synthesis in the skin. The latter combination is rare in the United States because of milk fortified with vitamin D, but it is seen in pregnancy in Asian immigrants in Great Britain.[28,29] There also are several rare syndromes of vitamin D resistance.[4]

In adults, mild vitamin D deficiency is often asymptomatic. When clinical manifestations occur, the most common are bone pain, especially during weight bearing, increased frequency of fractures, and x-ray evidence of bone demineralization. A characteristic radiologic finding is that of pseudofractures, or Looser's lines. Serum calcium and inorganic phosphate concentrations are normal to low, serum PTH levels are elevated, and the serum alkaline phosphatase often is elevated.

During pregnancy, asymptomatic or mild maternal vitamin D deficiency can cause serious problems for the fetus or neonate. The fetal parathyroid glands become hyperplastic and hypersecretory, presumably because of a subnormal fetal serum-ionized calcium concentration. The combination of fetal calcium deficiency, which impedes bone formation, and PTH excess, which stimulates bone resorption, can result in severely deficient bone mineralization, intrauterine growth retardation, and all of the other clinical features of rickets.

The diagnosis of vitamin D deficiency in a pregnant woman will more likely be suspect because of her medical and dietary history or socioeconomic circumstance than because of symptomatic disease. Laboratory verification can be obtained most directly by measurement or the serum 25-OHD concentration. This value must be interpreted in the context of normal values for the specific geographic area and time of year, although normal values do not change during pregnancy (unlike those of calcitriol). Interpretation of the serum alkaline phosphatase activity also must consider the normal rise in the third trimester, caused by an increase in the bone-derived fraction and the appearance of the placental isoenzyme.

Treatment consists of oral vitamin D supplementation. To counteract dietary deficiency, the initial dose is usually 50,000 U of vitamin D_2 twice a week. After several weeks, the body's stores are repleted, and thereafter administration of 400 U of vitamin D_2 daily should be an adequate maintenance dose.[30] For pregnant women taking the anticonvulsants phenytoin and carbamazepine, 400 U daily of oral vitamin D_2 maintain normal maternal serum concentrations of 25-OHD and calcitriol, although many values are in the lower part of the normal range.[31] In pregnant women taking anticonvulsants, maternal intake of 600 U of vitamin D plus 1 g of elemental calcium daily was sufficient to achieve normal bone mineral content and serum calcium concentrations in the women and their offspring.[32,33]

In vitamin D-resistant states, the treatment depends on the nature of the defect; some patients require high doses of vitamin D, while others respond to physiologic doses of calcitriol. In hypoparathyroid women, pregnancy appears to induce a vitamin D-deficiency state, which can be treated by maternal administration of oral calcitriol in doses that are somewhat higher than those appropriate for the prepregnant and postpregnant states. In contrast, one woman with pseudohypoparathyroidism exhibited a normal rise in serum calcitriol and an amelioration of her hypocalcemia during pregnancy.[9]

VITAMIN D EXCESS

Excessive vitamin D intake can cause hypercalcemia in adults and infants. There was an increased incidence of neonatal hypercalcemia in England during and after World War II because of inappropriately high levels of vitamin D supplementation in milk. Vitamin D intoxication is uncommon because it usually requires intake of several thousand units of vitamin D daily, and nonprescription vitamin preparations contain no more than 400 U per tablet or capsule. The diagnosis is established by the finding of an elevated maternal serum concentration of 25-OHD in a hypercalemic patient. Treatment consists of discontinuing the excessive intake, and during the weeks necessary for body stores of vitamin D to fall to normal, a low calcium diet and hydration.

Vitamin D-related hypercalcemia also occurs in sarcoidosis and other granulomatous diseases and in some lymphomas because of excessive synthesis of calcitriol by the granulomatous or malignant tissue. These patients have normal serum 25-OHD levels and no elevation of the serum PTH.

Neonatal hypercalcemia also is seen in association with a typical facial dysmorphism termed elfin facies, mental retardation, and supravalvular aortic stenosis in Williams' syndrome. A variety of abnormalities of vitamin D metabolism have been reported in studies of these rare patients; no coherent picture has emerged, but some effect of excessive vitamin D in these patients seems likely.[34]

REFERENCES

1. Davis OK, Hawkins DS, Rubin LP, et al. Serum parathyroid hormone (PTH) in pregnant women determined by an immunoradiometric assay for intact PTH. *J Clin Endocrinol Metab.* 1988;67:850.
2. Moniz CF, Nicolaides KH, Tzannatos C, et al. Calcium homeostasis in second trimester fetuses. *J Clin Pathol.* 1986;39:838.
3. Anast C. Disorders of mineral and bone metabolism. In: Avery ME, Taeusch HW, eds. *Schaffer's Diseases of the Newborn.* 5th ed. Philadelphia, PA: WB Saunders; 1984:464.
4. Aurbach GD, Marx SJ, Spiegel AM. Parathyroid hormone, calcitonin and the calciferols. In: Wilson JD, Foster DW, eds. *Williams' Textbook of Endocrinology.* 7th ed. Philadelphia, PA: WB Saunders; 1985:1137.
5. Gertner JM, Coustan DR, Kliger AS, et al. Pregnancy as a state of physiologic absorptive hypercalciuria. *Am J Med.* 1986;81:451.
6. Fisher DA. The unique endocrine milieu of the fetus. *J Clin Invest.* 1986;78:603.
7. Reddy GS, Normal AW, Willis DM, et al. Regulation of vitamin D metabolism in normal human pregnancy. *J Clin Endocrinol Metab.* 1983;56:363.
8. Bikle DD, Gee E, Halloran B, et al. Free 1,25-dihydroxyvitamin D levels in serum from normal subjects, pregnant subjects, and subjects with liver disease. *J Clin Invest.* 1984;74:1966.
9. Breslau N, Zerwekh JE. Relationship of estrogen and pregnancy to calcium homeostasis in pseudohypoparathyroidism. *J Clin Endocrinol Metab.* 1986;62:45.
10. Heath H III, Hodgson SF, Kennedy MA. Primary hyperparathyroidism. Incidence, morbidity and potential economical impact in a community. *N Engl J Med.* 1980;302:189.
11. Shangold MM, Dor N, Welt SI, et al. Hyperparathyroidism and pregnancy: a review. *Obstet Gynecol Survey.* 1982;37:217.
12. Kristoffersson A, Dahlgren S, Litnner F, et al. Primary hyperparathyroidism in pregnancy. *Surgery.* 1985;97:326.
13. Croom RD III, Thomas CG Jr. Primary hyperparathyroidism during pregnancy. *Surgery.* 1984;96:1109.
14. Montoro MN, Collea JV, Mestman JH. Management of hyperparathyroidism in pregnancy with oral phosphate therapy. *Obstet Gynecol.* 1980;55:431.
15. Lowe DK, Orwoll ES, McClung MR, et al. Hyperparathyroidism and pregnancy. *Am J Surg.* 1983;145:611.
16. Marx SJ, Fraser D, Rapoport A. Familial hypocalciuric hypercalcemia. Mild expression of the gene in heterozygotes and severe expression in homozygotes. *Am J Med.* 1985;78:15.
17. Fischinger W, Haufe S. Hyperkalzamische Krise bei primarem Hyperparathyreoidismus in der Schwangerschaft mit medullarer Nephrokalzinose. *Med Klin.* 1988;83:195.
18. Rajala B, Abbasi RA, Hutchinson HT, et al. Acute pancreatitis and primary hyperparathyroidism in pregnancy: treatment of hypercalcemia with magnesium sulfate. *Obstet Gynecol.* 1987;70:460.
19. Rodin A, Duncan A, Quartero WP, et al. Serum concentrations of alkaline phosphatase isoenzymes and osteocalcin in normal pregnancy. *J Clin Endocrinol Metab.* 1989;68:1123.
20. Nusynowitz M, Frame B, Kolb FO. The spectrum of hypoparathyroid states: a classification based on physiologic principles. *Medicine.* 1976;55:105.
21. Stuart C, Aceto T Jr, Kuhn JP, et al. Intrauterine hyperparathyroidism. Postmortem findings in two cases. *Am J Dis Child.* 1979;133:67.
22. Glass EJ, Barr DG. Transient neonatal hyperparathyroidism secondary to maternal pseudohypoparathyroidism. *Arch Dis Child.* 1981;56:565.
23. Goodenday LS, Gordan GS. No risk from vitamin D in pregnancy. *Ann Intern Med.* 1971;75:807.
24. Salle BL, Barthezene F, Glorieux FH, et al. Hypoparathyroidism during pregnancy: treatment with calcitriol. *J Clin Endocrinol Metab.* 1981;52:810.
25. Sadeghi-Nejad A, Wolfsdorf, Senior B. Hypoparathyroidism and pregnancy. Treatment with calcitriol. *JAMA.* 1980;243:254.
26. Bouillon R. Vitamin D metabolites in human pregnancy. In: Holick MF, Gray TK, Anast CS, eds. *Perinatal Calcium and Phosphorus Metabolism.* New York, NY: Elsevier Science Publishers; 1983:291.
27. Marx SJ, Swart EG Jr, Hamstra AJ, et al. Normal intrauterine development of the fetus of a woman receiving extraordinarily high doses of 1,25-dihydroxyvitamin D_3. *J Clin Endocrinol Metab.* 1980;51:1138.
28. Bashir T, MacDonald HN, Peacock M. Biochemical evidence of vitamin D deficiency in pregnant Asian women. *J Hum Nutr.* 1981;35:49.
29. Brooke DG, Brown IR, Bone CD, et al. Vitamin D supplements in pregnant Asian women: effects on calcium status and fetal growth. *Br Med J.* 1980;280:751.
30. Delvin EE, Salle BL, Glorieux FH, et al. Vitamin D supplementation during pregnancy: effect on neonatal calcium homeostasis. *J Pediatr.* 1986;109:328.
31. Markestad T, Ulstein M, Strandjord RE, et al. Anticonvulsant drug therapy in human pregnancy: effects on serum concentrations of vitamin D metabolites in maternal and cord blood. *Am J Obstet Gynecol.* 1984;150:254.
32. Christiansen C, Brandt NJ, Ebbesen F, et al. Bone mineral content during pregnancy in epileptics on anticonvulsant drugs and in their newborns. *Acta Obstet Gynecol Scand.* 1981;60:510.
33. Christiansen C, Brandt NJ, Ebbesen F, et al. Do newborns of epileptics on anticonvulsants develop biochemical signs of osteomalacia? *Acta Neurol Scand.* 1980;62:158.
34. Chesney RW, DeLuca HF, Gertner JM. Increased plasma 1,25-dihydroxyvitamin D in infants with hypercalcemia and elfin facies. *N Engl J Med.* 1985;313:889.

Chapter Forty-Two
Adrenal Disorders

Moshe E. Zilberstein, Michael Feingold, and Norbert Gleicher

42

In recent years, astounding advances have been made in the elucidation of endocrine, biochemical, and genetic mechanisms that control growth and function of the adrenals. During the pregnancies of most mammalian species, products that originate in the adrenals play an important role in the maturation of such fetal organs as the brain, retina, pancreas, gastrointestinal tract, and lungs. They also play a role in the maintenance of pregnancy after stress and possibly in the initiation of labor.[1]

Maternal adrenal dysfunction may have deleterious effects on fetal development and on maternal health. Pregnancies complicated by maternal adrenal dysfunction often may present a diagnostic challenge to the physician because these diseases are relatively rare in association with pregnancy. Furthermore, many baseline criteria for laboratory tests are not clearly defined for the pregnant state. Some diagnostic tools used in the routine evaluation of adrenal function may have undesired effects on the pregnancy. Because only limited data are available on their use in pregnancy, assessment of risk-benefit ratios for these procedures is extremely difficult.

The adrenals are pyramid-shaped organs that are

mounted on the upper poles of the kidneys. The adult adrenal weighs 5–6 g. Two distinct areas can be recognized: the outer yellowish ⅘ portion, which is the cortex, and the pearly-gray colored inner portion, the medulla. The cortex is comprised of three zones with distinctive ultrastructured cells: the outer zona glomerulosa, the middle zona fasciculata, and the inner zona reticularis. The zona glomerulosa is exclusively responsible for the production of aldosterone and responds to angiotensin and potassium. The zonae fasciculata and reticularis produce steroids, mainly of the C_{19} lineage. However, the zona reticularis produces more dehydroepiandrosterone sulfate (DHEA-S) than the zona fasciculata. Adrenocorticotropic hormone (ACTH) action increases steroid production and swelling of the adrenal cells and thus increases adrenal size.[2] During pregnancy, the maternal zona fasciculata increases in volume without significant impact on the total adrenal mass.

PITUITARY RELEVANCE TO ADRENAL FUNCTION

Classically, histologists have identified three cell types in the anterior pituitary by hematoxylin and eosin staining: acidophil, basophil, and chromophobe cells.[3] The association of acromegaly with acidophil cell tumors and of Cushing's disease with basophils elucidated the putative cellular source of growth hormone (GH) and ACTH, respectively. Immunohistochemical staining of electromicrographs and serially sectioned anterior pituitaries confirmed that the basophils are the ACTH-producing cells.[4] Through immunohistochemical staining studies of cellular granules, five cell types have been recognized: mammotrophs, somatotrophs, corticotrophs, thyrotrophs, and gonadotrophs.[4,5] ACTH is produced as part of a larger precursor that includes several other peptides, causing difficulties for the proper localization of ACTH in the corticotrophs.[6]

The corticotrophs are large, oval, and angular basophils, appearing alone or in clumps, and comprise 10–15% of the cells in the anterior pituitary. The secretory granules in the corticotrophs vary in density and size, with an average diameter of 350 μm. They contain a well-developed rough endoplasmic reticulum and Golgi apparatus and sparse mitochondria. The glycosylated precursor protein is produced in rough endoplasmic reticulum and is transferred into granules in the Golgi apparatus for post-translational processing. Pro-opiomelanocorticotropin (POMC) is cleaved predominately into an N-terminal glycosylated part, ACTH, and the C-terminal β-lipotrophin. In some of the corticotrophs, ACTH is further cleaved into melanocyte-stimulating hormone (MSH) and corticotropinlike intermediate lobe peptide (CLIP).[7]

Pregnancy represents an intriguing context for investigation of the classic release and feedback axis of the adrenals. Because most of the trophic and releasing hormones that occur in the hypothalamopituitary axis also are represented in the placenta, alternative pathways to the classic fetal hypothalamopituitary-adrenal axis that involve trophic hormones of placental origin in the regulation of the maternal adrenals can be envisioned.

ADRENAL STEROIDOGENESIS

Steroids are well recognized for their potent biological function and importance in regulating physiologic processes. They readily cross the cell membrane to interact with specific receptors. Steroid-receptor complexes bind to specific domains of many genes, where they exert their biological effect through the regulation of transcription.[8] With the progress of protein chemistry and molecular and cellular biology techniques, the long list of enzymes previously thought to be active in steroidogenesis pathways has been shortened. The realization that several of the known enzymatic activities occur through the action of distinct single enzymes, encoded by their respective identified genes, has revolutionized the understanding of these processes and opened new areas of clinical application. The principal pathways of human adrenal steroids are depicted in Figure 42–1.

Although steroids in different tissues arise from common pathways and demonstrate a basic structural similarity, their effects differ and extend into a broad array of paramount physiologic processes. The glucocorticoids mobilize carbohydrates and have numerous other effects related to stress tolerance. Mineralocorticoids are involved in sodium economy by regulating renal sodium retention. Progestins are essential for the maintenance of pregnancy and have a role in the menstrual cycle (see also Chapter 37). Androgens induce secondary male sex characteristics and support the male phenotype during the life of the adult. Estrogens, which are derived from androgens, are similar inducers and are vital in the maintenance of a female's secondary sex characteristics.

The basic steroid structure is a perhydrocyclopentanephenanthrene, which is a composition of three six-carbon rings and one five-carbon ring (Fig. 42–2). The rings of the molecule are considered to be in the same plane and constituents above and below that plane are designated β and α, respectively. Not all of the possible isomers exist in nature or are active steroids. The biosynthetic precursor for all steroids is cholesterol, and its conversion to pregnenolone in the mitchondria is the first rate-limiting and hormone-regulating step in steroidogenesis. Human steroidogenic tissues may synthesize cholesterol from acetate *de novo;* however, they preferably obtain cholesterol from low-density lipoproteins (LDL).[9] The rate-limiting enzyme in cholesterol synthesis in the human adrenal is 3-hydroxy-3-methylglutaryl coenzyme A (HMGCoA) reductase.[10] This enzyme and LDL uptake by receptors are stimulated by tropic hormones. However, LDL suppresses HMGCoA reductase, providing a regulatory function for cholesterol formation and availability. Cholesterol availability also is regulated by its storage levels in lipid droplets. ACTH has been shown to stimulate cholesterol esterase (cholesterol ester hydrolase) to inhibit cholesterol ester synthetase, thus increasing free cholesterol. Free cholesterol in turn is transported to the mitochondria by the sterol carrier protein 2 (SCP_2).[11] Most of the enzymes that are involved in steroidogenesis are oxidases of the cytochrome P-450 group.

Different metabolic and biosynthetic reactions are catalyzed by P-450 type enzymes in various tissues. The P-450 enzymes of the steroidogenic pathways are biochemically similar to all the other enzymes in the generic group.[12] The reactions that are catalyzed by the steroidogenic P-450 enzymes are either specific hydroxylation at a specific position on the molecule or consecutive reactions that will lead to aromatization of the A ring or cleavage of carbon bonds. The active site of the enzymes is associated with the heme part that binds the substrate and O_2.[12] The hydroxylation catalyzed by P-450 enzymes requires two electrons, H^+ and O_2. Specific electron carrier proteins are involved in transferring electrons from NADPH. In the mitochondrial P-450 systems, the flavoprotein adrenodoxin reductase receives the electron from NADPH and in turn transfers it to a ferredoxin adrenodoxin, thus establishing the means of electron transport. In the microsomal P-450 systems,

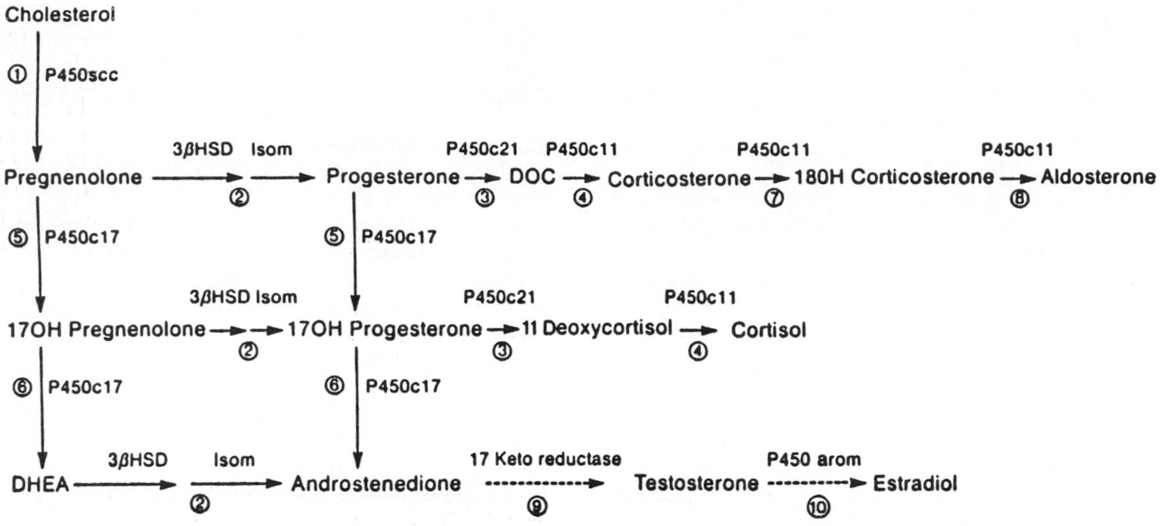

Figure 42–1. Principal pathways of human adrenal steroid hormone synthesis. Other quantitatively and physiologically minor steroids also are produced. The chemical identities of the enzymes are shown by each reaction, and the traditional names of the enzymatic activities correspond to the *circled numbers.* Reaction 1: Mitochondrial cytochrome P-450scc mediates 20α-hydroxylation, 22-hydroxylation, and scission of the C20–22 carbon bond, a set of reactions traditionally termed "20,22 desmolase." Reaction 2: A non-P-450 enzyme (or enzymes) bound to the endoplasmic reticulum mediates 3β-hydroxysteroid dehydrogenase and isomerase (Isom) activities. Reaction 3: P-450c21 in the endoplasmic reticulum mediates 21-hydroxylation. Reactions 4, 7, and 8: Mitochondrial P-450c11 exerts three clearly distinguishable activities: 11β-hydroxylation (4), 18-hydroxylation (7), and 18-methyl oxidase activity (8). Reactions 5 and 6: P-450c17 in the endoplasmic reticulum mediates both 17α-hydroxylase (5) and 17,20-lyase (6) activities. Reactions 9 and 10 are found principally in the testes and ovaries: 17-ketosteroid reductase, a non-P-450 enzyme of the endoplasmic reticulum, produces testosterone (9), which may then be converted to estradiol by P-450aro (10), another P-450 enzyme of the endoplasmic reticulum mediating the aromatization of the A ring of the steroid nucleus. (*Reprinted from Miller*[12], *with permission from* Endocrine Reviews.)

however, different flavoproteins, P-450 reductase and flavin mononucleotide, play a similar role.

In recent years, cDNAs have been isolated for most steroidogenic P-450 enzymes and for the electron transfer proteins. Most major steroidogenic P-450 enzymes are encoded by one or two functional genes. Hence, tissue-specific expression of steroidogenic enzymes in the various tissues is locally regulated.

The human adrenal mainly uses LDL-derived cholesterol. Cholesterol conversion into adrenocortical steroids requires a series of several enzyme-mediated steps, which include the removal of the cholesterol side chain, the introduction of hydroxyl groups, and the rearrangement of ring A. The first rate-limiting step is the conversion of cholesterol

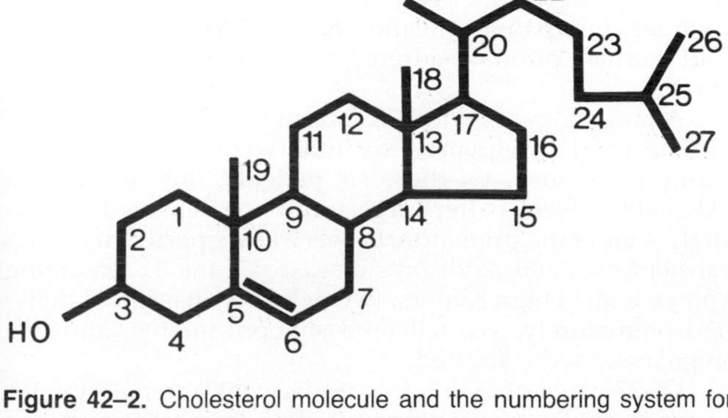

Figure 42–2. Cholesterol molecule and the numbering system for steroids. (*Reprinted from Speroff L, Glass RH, Kase NG. Hirsutism. In: Speroff L, Glass RH, Kase NG, eds.* Clinical Gynecologic Endocrinology and Infertility. *3rd ed. Baltimore: Williams & Wilkins; 1983; 201, with permission.*)

to pregnenolone. All enzymatic steps that produce pregnenolone from cholesterol (ie, 20 α-hydroxylation, 22-hydroxylation, and the cleavage of the bond between carbon 20 and 22) are catalyzed by a single enzyme on a single active site.[13] In the past, it was believed that three separate enzymes were responsible for this reaction. It also was shown that 3 mol of NADPH are required for the conversion of 1 mol of cholesterol to pregnenolone.

The purified protein has been characterized by immunostudies to be a single protein species. It is located in the inner mitochondrial membrane and is a 850-kd multimer, composed of 16 subunits.[14,15] Human data also prove that there exists a single P-450 scc gene located on *chromosome 15.*[16-18] The human adrenal and testicular P-450 scc cDNA clones are almost identical. Also loosely associated with the inner mitochrondrial membrane is adrenodoxin reductase; however, adrenodoxin resides in the solution content of the mitochondria.

Multiple genes for adrenodoxin exist in humans. One gene is functional and is located on chromosome 11q13→qter.[19] Two additional pseudogenes are on 20 cen→q 13.1. The adrenodoxin molecule forms a complex with one molecule of adrenodoxin reductase, then it dissociates and forms a complex with one molecule of the respective P-450 enzyme, transferring the electron to the enzyme. A P-450 enzyme, which is associated with its substrate, binds adrenodoxin more readily, directing the reaction toward the processing of the substrate.[20]

The single gene for adrenodoxin reductase is located on chromosome 17 cen→q25, and it is widely expressed in human tissues.[21] Alternate splicing of its mRNA brings about the formation of two forms of enzyme.

Pregnenolone is converted to either 17-hydroxypregnenolone or into progesterone. The enzymes that catalyze these reactions are P-450c17 and 3β-hydroxysteroid dehydrogenase/Δ5–Δ4 isomerase, respectively. P-450c17 also mediates the 17α-hydroxypregnenolone of progesterone, 17α-hydroxyprogesterone. Both 17α-hydroxypregnenolone and 17α-hydroxyprogesterone may then undergo conversion into dehydroepiandrosterone (DHEA) and androstendione, respectively. The 17,20 lyase activity resides in a single P-450c17, which is encoded by a single gene localized on the human chromosome 10.[22] This gene also is identical for the adrenal and testis.

The P-450c17 gene demonstrates sequences that resemble the consensus sequence for the glucocorticoids regulatory element (GRE), and also contains sequences that resemble regulatory elements of cAMP (CRE). It appears that P-450c17 prefers Δ5 substrates for its 17,20 lyase activity, and the adrenals of the fetus and adult produce mainly DHEA. The enzymes that are involved in the Δ5–Δ4 (3βHSD) conversion are not fully identified. A single enzyme probably exists and several isozymes were suggested to be involved in the different pathways. This is mainly supported by the fact that isolated 3βHSD deficiencies exist for the different pathways.[23] Both isomerase and 3βHSD activities reside in a single 45,000-d protein. Except for the conversion of pregnenolone to progesterone, it also catalyzes the conversion of 17-hydroxypregnenolone to 17-hydroxyprogesterone and of DHEA to androstendione. In the adrenal, progesterone and 17OHP are converted into deoxycorticosterone and 11-deoxycortisol, respectively. This hydroxylation at the 21 position is mediated by P-450c21, which resides in the smooth endoplasmic reticulum. Two genes for P-450c21 exist but only one of them is functional.[24]

It is now clear that one enzyme is responsible for the final steps in the production of mineralocorticoids and glucocorticoids. Both the 11β-hydroxylation of 11-deoxycortisol to cortisol and the conversion of deoxycorticosterone to aldosterone are mediated by a large protein enzyme (P-450c11). This enzyme has 11β-hydroxylase, 18-hydroxylase, and 18-oxidase activities. Two tandemly duplicated genes were localized on the long arm of chromosome 8.[25]

One step in the steroidogenic pathways is readily reversible and is mediated by 17-ketosteroid reductase. Interconversion of androstendione, DHEA, and estrone into testosterone, androstenediol, and estradiol, respectively, is mediated by this 35,000 d enzyme in the endoplasmic reticulum.

ADRENAL DISEASES

Adrenal Function in Pregnancy

During pregnancy, plasma cortisol concentration is increased twofold to threefold, and a similar increase has been described for plasma and urinary free cortisol.[26] This is partially caused by the increased levels of corticosteroid-binding globulin (CBG), which is similarly elevated because of the effect of high estrogen levels on hepatic production of CBG. Higher baseline levels and a wider diurnal variation in ACTH are observed during pregnancy because of high concentrations of unbound cortisol. Thus, it is possible that pregnancy, perhaps by way of high progesterone levels, induces some type of resistance against the suppression of ACTH by feedback control mechanisms. It also is possible that ACTH is generated by the placenta and is regulated differently. However, several pregnancy-induced features, such as abdominal striae, plethora, edema, rounded face, and glucose intolerance, can be explained as the product of exposure to higher levels of glucocorticoids. Both aldosterone production and plasma renin activity (PRA) are increased during pregnancy. Aldosterone production of maternal origin may be greater than 1 mg/d. However, an adequate response to sodium fluctuation is preserved.

Cushing's Syndrome

Cushing's syndrome (CS) is defined as the presence of chronic elevation of plasma cortisol or hypercortisolism. This can be the result of inappropriate secretion of ACTH from the pituitary gland or from an ACTH-producing tumor, leading to bilateral adrenal hyperplasia (*Cushing's disease*), adrenal adenoma, or adrenocorticol carcinoma. The chronic administration of synthetic corticosteroids for the treatment of medical problems also can lead to physical characteristics of Cushing's syndrome.

Two recent publications reviewed all reported cases of CS associated with pregnancy.[27,28] Pickard reviewed 53 cases and added one of his own. Aron's publication comprises 63 published cases and four cases from his own experience. Among the 63 case reports with known etiology, 27 (43%) had bilateral adrenal hyperplasia (BAH), 27 (43%) adrenal adenoma (AA), 7 (11%) adrenal carcinoma (AC), 1 (1.5%) nodular adrenal hyperplasia (NAH), and 1 (1.5%) ectopic ACTH syndrome (EAS).

The treatment of CS in a nonpregnant patient depends on whether hypercorticolism originates from pituitary, adrenal etiology, or from ectopic ACTH production.[29,30] Treatment in the nonpregnant state can be surgical, the removal of an adrenal or pituitary tumor; medical, the suppression or destruction of cortisol or ACTH-secreting tissue; or radiation treatment. When an adrenal tumor is the source of excessive cortisol production, a surgical approach generally is recommended.[30] The differentiation of an adenoma from a carcinoma may be difficult. Clinically, a rapid course, the production of abnormally high quantities of adrenal hormones or virilizing signs and symptoms, might suggest the presence of an adrenal carcinoma. A final diagnosis should, however, always rely on a histologic evaluation of the adrenal tumor, which can be difficult. In nonpregnant patients with adrenal cortical carcinoma, only 28% are biologically nonfunctional.

Most adrenal tumors are unilateral, and therefore unilateral adrenalectomy is usually sufficient. One should take into consideration that the long-lasting autonomous cortisol production by the adrenal tumor suppresses ACTH production and thus leads to an atrophic state of the remaining adrenal tissue of affected and contralateral glands. Therefore, presurgery and postsurgery replacement therapy with corticosteroids must be given in the same manner as given to patients on long-term corticosteroid treatment (ie, 100 mg of hydrocortisone every 6 hours beginning at the time of surgery for up to several months), with a gradual decrease until normal pituitary-adrenal function has been established.

Among 27 cases with CS caused by adrenocorticol benign tumors in pregnancy, six underwent adrenalectomies during pregnancy. Of these six patients, one delivered a 500-g fetus 3 weeks after surgery and one delivered prematurely. One of the premature babies was suspected of having transient neonatal Addison's disease. Of the 21 remaining women with benign tumors, two delivered at term, 11 delivered prematurely, six delivered stillborn infants, and two pregnancies were aborted.

Of 27 cases of BAH, five underwent adrenalectomies during pregnancy, which resulted in four term and one preterm infant. One received pituitary irradiation at 24 weeks' gestation and delivered at term and one had a transsphenoidol adenectomy at 22 weeks. Of the remaining 20 cases with BAH, one was treated with cyproheptadine, a serotonin antagonist, and delivered at 33 weeks. The rest were not treated during pregnancy and delivered nine preterm and eight term babies. Two pregnancies resulted in stillbirths at term and two in spontaneous abortions. None of the six reported cases of adenocortical carcinoma during pregnancy with CS had surgery during pregnancy. One had undergone an adrenalectomy before pregnancy and suffered from metastases to the liver. Of these six, three delivered at term, one delivered prematurely, one had an elective cesarean section, and one had a spontaneous abortion.

Cushing's Disease. The basophil cells in the anterior pituitary produce ACTH. They may undergo hyperplasia, result in microadenomas (less than 10 mm) or macroadenomas, and lead to bilateral adrenal hyperplasia.

The two approaches for treating Cushing's disease (CD) are trans-sphenoidal hypophectomy and pituitary irradiation. The former is associated with an approximate 70% success rate, while the latter can vary between 20% in adult disease to 80% in juvenile patients. Of the 23 reported cases of CD in pregnancy, 16 received no treatment during their pregnancy. One woman had trans-sphenoidal hypophysectomy and another underwent pituitary irradiation. Both treatments were given during the second trimester. In both cases, the women delivered normal babies at term.

Two patients were treated with cyproheptadine, the serotonin antagonist; one became pregnant while taking it and continued the treatment throughout pregnancy. She delivered an apparently normal boy at term, who died at 4 months of gastroenteritis. The second woman was treated with cyproheptadine before becoming pregnant and continued for 3 months into the pregnancy. She delivered a normal and healthy infant at 36 weeks. Two of the three women who had bilateral adrenalectomies during their pregnancies did well and delivered at term, while one had a preterm delivery. A total of 12 of the 23 reported cases of CD in pregnancy resulted in term delivery, eight in preterm delivery, two in stillborn deliveries, and one in spontaneous abortion. There are reported cases of complete remission of Cushing's syndrome following delivery or therapeutic abortion. Based on the latest review of the literature[27], this condition results in distinct maternal and fetal complications. Only 37% of the pregnancies ended in term deliveries. Forty-six percent were premature deliveries, and 17% were stillbirths or abortions.

Early diagnosis can lead to appropriate treatment at early stages of pregnancy. With close maternal and fetal follow-up and adequate supplementation of corticosteroids, a reasonable outcome for pregnant women with Cushing's syndrome can then be expected.

Clinical Manifestation. A nonpregnant patient with CS has distinct clinical manifestations. As a result of the high cortisol level, these patients are obese with mainly truncal distribution (centripetal obesity), a prominent cervicodorsal fat pad ("buffalo hump"), thin skin with striae, progressive weakness as a result of muscular wasting, hypertension, glucose intolerance leading to overt diabetes, and osteoporosis associated with hypercalcuria and renal stones. Many of these patients also demonstrate emotional or psychiatric problems.

The hyperandrogenic state that many manifest leads to hirsutism, acne, clitoromegaly, deepening of the voice, and male-type temporal hair loss. Most patients with CS have menstrual irregularities and 30–77% of them are amenorrheic. This explains the high rate of infertility among these patients.

These manifestations overlap with many normal changes of pregnancy, such as weight gain, striae, pigmentation, hypertension, and relative glucose intolerance. Table 42–1 summarizes the clinical manifestations in 67 reported cases of CS in pregnancy.

Laboratory Findings. The laboratory diagnosis of Cushing's syndrome in pregnancy relies on the same principles of diagnosis as in nonpregnant patients. However, the hormonal changes of pregnancy must be taken into consideration.

ACTH is produced in the anterior pituitary gland. Its production is controlled mainly by a positive feedback from the hypothalamus and a negative feedback from the adrenals. Stress, pain, emotion, and diurnal rhythms cause the central nervous system to act on the hypothalamus, which in turn produces corticotropin-releasing factor (CRF) that increases the ACTH production by the pituitary gland.[31] The ACTH acts in a negative-feedback mechanism to lower the CRF, while the glucocorticoids act at the level of the pituitary and hypothalamus.

The changes in ACTH levels during pregnancy are not clear. Some investigators show an increase[32,33], some show a decrease, and some show an increase with a decrease near term.[34,35] Normal ACTH levels range from 20–100 pg/mL and have a diurnal variation, with maximum levels in the morning.[36-38]

In patients with adrenal adenomas or carcinoma, the high cortisol levels cause a decrease in ACTH to undetectable levels; however, in Cushing's disease with a pituitary adenoma, the values are at a high-normal to slightly elevated range.

The diurnal variation of ACTH is responsible for the cortisol diurnal variation, with the highest levels in the morning (10–25 μg/dL) and the lowest at midnight (2 μg/dL).[39] In the evening, ACTH levels are usually less than 12 μg/dL, less than half of morning levels. This diurnal variation is maintained during pregnancy, although it decreases in amplitude.

Like all hormones, most cortisol is bound to plasma proteins: to corticosteroid-binding globulin (CBG-transcortin) in 70% and to plasma albumin.[40] The normally active part is free cortisol. Under the influence of the increased

TABLE 42–1. CLINICAL SYMPTOMS IN 67 WOMEN WITH REPORTED CUSHING'S SYNDROME IN PREGNANCY

Complication	Number of Patients (Out of 67)
Hirsutism	38
Hypertension	35
Diabetes mellitus	14
Electrolyte abnormalities	7
Congenital heart failure	5
Osteoporosis	5
Preeclampsia	4
Muscle weakness	4
Bone fracture	3
Infection	1
Psychosis	1

estrogen in pregnancy, CBG, albumin, and bound and free cortisol increase as pregnancy progresses. The combination of increased cortisol production and delayed plasma clearance can explain the reported increase in free cortisol in pregnancy. This free cortisol, which acts by binding to nuclear receptors, competes with the elevated progesterone concentrations of pregnancy for intracellular binding sites. Therefore, it is not clear whether the adrenal function at the cellular level is actually increased. The morning cortisol level in late pregnancy reaches three to four times the level in the nonpregnant state.

Urinary free cortisol levels of a third-trimester pregnant woman are between 200–500 μg per 24 hours compared to 150 μg per 24 hours, the upper limit of a healthy nonpregnant woman.[26,41]

In Cushing's syndrome, levels were found to be in a range of 600–900 μg per 24 hours and higher[26,42,43], but levels may overlap with pregnancy. 17-ketosteroid levels are, however, seldom used for diagnostic purposes. Dehydroepiandrosterone sulfate (DHEA-S) may be more valuable for this purpose. DHEA-S, which is primarily adrenal in origin, decreases progressively during pregnancy because of the increase in its metabolic clearance rate.[44-46]

Sex hormone-binding globulin (SHBG) is elevated in pregnancy as a result of the increased estrogen. This leads to elevated total testosterone levels but decreased free testosterone levels in pregnancy.[43,45,47,48]

Diagnosis. Using the previous information on hormonal levels in pregnancy, Cushing's syndrome in pregnancy can be diagnosed in stepwise fashion. First, a 24-hour urine collection for free cortisol should be obtained. If the value is not elevated, the diagnosis is excluded.[39,49-53] If the diagnosis is strongly suspected based on the clinical manifestations mentioned previously, a second collection should be obtained. Women with elevated values should be investigated further.

A plasma ACTH determination will then demonstrate undetectable or suppressed levels secondary to an adrenal tumor, or elevated or high-normal levels suggesting abnormal production by the pituitary gland. A selective ACTH sampling of the inferior petrosal sinuses can confirm these findings. Computed tomography (CT) of the sella turcica can reveal a microadenoma or macroadenoma of the pituitary gland. If neither the selective blood sampling nor the CT scan indicates the pituitary as the source of the elevated ACTH, an ectopic ACTH-producing tumor, like an oat-cell carcinoma, must be suspected (see also Chapter 45).

The use of dynamic tests, such as the CRF test or the dexamethasone suppression test can further clarify the etiology and distinguish between a pituitary etiology or adrenal tumor. There is, however, only limited experience with these tests in pregnancy. The single-dose dexamethasone test causes a marked decline in cortisol in the third trimester, from a mean of 30 to 4.6 μg/dL[54], but the complete suppression of nonpregnant healthy patients may not occur. Almost no data are available on low- and high-dose dexamethasone tests in pregnancy. Few case reports indicate suppression with a low dose of 17-OHCS in a patient with adrenal adenoma and partial suppression with a pituitary adenoma.[49,55] High-dose tests resulted in suppressed plasma cortisol with pituitary adenomas and no suppression in adrenal adenomas or carcinomas.[49,56-63]

The use of the metyrapone test in pregnancy is even more limited, and only minimal data are available on its effect on the fetus.[49] It therefore should be avoided during pregnancy.

An ultrasound evaluation might reveal an adrenal tumor or bilateral adrenal enlargement. Failure to visualize either does not exclude these possibilities, however, and an abdominal CT scan may be necessary if the uterus can be shielded.

It is almost impossible to distinguish between an adrenal adenoma or carcinoma without a thorough histologic evaluation. Malignant tumors are frequently larger than 7 cm and are accompanied by elevated DHEA-S levels. Both conditions will not respond to the dexamethasone suppression test.

Fetal Aspects. The effects of CS on the developing fetus are unclear. Theoretically, fetuses exposed to elevated levels of glucocorticosteroids and androgens should manifest the same symptoms as fetuses exposed to corticosteroid therapy. Experimental data show a possible correlation between hypercorticolism in mice and the formation of cleft palate[64], which also was reported in two women receiving pharmacologic doses of glucocorticoids during pregnancy. There is, however, only one case report of a preterm delivery at 36 weeks' gestation and a small-for-gestational age infant with cleft palate. Prematurity is common (61%) and contributes to the increased morbidity and mortality among babies delivered to women with CS. Although maternal cortisol and cortisone cross the placenta, neonatal adrenal insufficiency occurred in only one case, and fetal adrenal atrophy was found on autopsy in two cases. Thus, although neonatal adrenal insufficiency is rare, the appearance of hypoglycemia, seizures, circulatory collapse, fever, failure to thrive, hyperkalemia, or hyponathemia should alert the physician to this possibility.

ADDISON'S DISEASE

The inadequate production of adrenal corticosteroids—adrenal insufficiency—can be acute or chronic. It can result from a primary adrenocorticol deficiency, the inability of the adrenals to produce hormones, or as a result of insufficient ACTH production by the pituitary caused by a lack of stimulators. Hypoadrenalism also may occur when long-term administration of steroid medication is discontinued. The etiology of Addison's disease has changed over the years: In the past, the primary cause of Addison's disease was tuberculosis, while today, it is adrenal atrophy.[30,65,66] An autoimmune etiology has been suggested, and this same mechanism may be responsible for the polyendocrine disorders that are commonly associated with it (ie, ovarian failure, hypothyroidism, diabetes mellitus, and hypoparathyroid).[67-70]

Previous pituitary or adrenal surgery or irradiation may lead to iatrogenic Addison's disease. Other causes are the adrenogenital syndrome and inadequate replacement therapy. Rare etiologies for adrenocorticol deficiency are histoplasmosis, metastatic carcinoma of the adrenals, and treatment with 2,2-dis(chlorophenyl-4-chloropheny)-1-1-dichlorothane (OPDDD), which destroys cortisol-secreting cells.

The systemic effects of insufficient glucocorticoids include a tendency toward gastrointestinal disturbances, such as nausea, vomiting, abdominal pain, and weight loss; difficulty in maintaining fasting blood glucose levels; and spontaneous hypoglycemia.[70] Because of the low cortisol levels, there is a loss in the negative feedback, and ACTH is produced in excess along with melanocyte-stimulating hormone (MSH). This MSH is responsible for the typically increased pigmentation.

The elevated ACTH–MSH levels are not seen exclusively in Addison's disease. They also might be elevated in Cushing's disease and ectopic ACTH production. To distinguish between these conditions, the serum cortisol levels should be determined. The insufficiency in mineralocorticoids leads to a reduced ability to retain sodium and excrete potassium and decreased renal perfusion, cardiac output, intravascular volume, hypotension, and possibly shock.

Symptoms

The diagnosis of Addison's disease in pregnancy can be difficult because many of its symptoms normally occur during gestation. Weakness, lassitude, fatigue, increased pigmentation, weight loss, abdominal pain, anorexia, nervousness and personality changes, and postural hypotension with systolic blood pressure of less than 100 mm Hg occur in both states. When weight loss, nausea, vomiting, and weakness persist after the first trimester, the physician should be alerted to the possibility of Addison's disease.[70] As a result of increased diuresis and dehydration that may follow the delivery, women might develop adrenal crisis postpartum after an uneventful pregnancy.[71]

Laboratory Findings

The laboratory diagnosis of this condition consists of a serum electrolite assessment. A normal to low Na, elevated K, BUN, creatinine, elevated ACTH in most cases, 24-hour urinary free cortisol, or plasma cortisol below pregnancy levels and 17-OHCS are expected. Dynamic tests may follow the basal cortisol and 17-OHCS level determinations. The ACTH test by Cortrosyn infusion was used in pregnancy in some studies to demonstrate the existence or absence of adrenal reserves. If adrenal function is intact, 17-OHCS should increase after Cortrosyn. A more useful approach is the dexamethasone test, which can be diagnostic and therapeutic at the same time. This test should be performed immediately after basal cortisol and 17-OHCS are determined. Dexamethasone is superior to hydrocortisone because it has no effect on serum cortisol and 17-OHCS levels.

Fertility and Maintenance of the Pregnant Woman With Addison's Disease

Unlike women with Cushing's syndrome, most patients with Addison's disease have no menstrual irregularities. Irvine and Barres[66] report that 25% of women with idiopathic Addison's disease were amenorrheic. The steroid replacement therapy that a woman is on before gestation should be continued unchanged. Most replacement therapy consists of oral cortisol acetate, 25 mg each morning and 12.5 mg each evening.[72] In patients with no adrenal function, a salt-retaining hormone, 9-fluorohydrocortisone (Florinef) might be added. If prednisone is used, Florinef is usually added because it has no mineralocorticoid activity. Prednisone is less expensive but because of the decrease in its mineralocorticoid activity, Florinef must be added. If during pregnancy, hypertension or edema develop, the Florinef should be reduced. Any deviation from the normal course of pregnancy, such as infection or stress, requires upward adjustments in the steroid dosage. To avoid sudden adrenal insufficiency, these patients should carry with them 4 mg of dexamethazone in 1 mL H_2O in a sterile syringe at all times. During the delivery, the woman should maintain good hydration and should get cortisol hemisuccinate every 6 hours with 100 mg of cortisol in case of a prolonged delivery. This combination of intravenous fluids and steroids should be continued for several days after the delivery to avoid postpartum adrenal crisis.

Such a crisis was observed in 12 out of 22 patients who delivered at term. Burrow and Ferris[73] hypothesized that this tendency to develop an adrenal crisis postpartum is probably related to the diuresis and dehydration that may follow delivery. An interesting observation by Walsh et al[74] was that in cases of adrenal insufficiency in rhesus monkeys, the fetal adrenal can maintain both fetal and maternal levels of plasma cortisol.

Fetal Aspect. Because cortisol crosses the placenta, excessive steroid replacement therapy may lead to a transient decrease in fetal adrenal function. This may lead to an acute Addisonian reaction when the exogenous glucocorticoids are metabolized and the fetal adrenals are too suppressed to produce it. Symptoms will be similar to those described for fetal aspects of Cushing's disease. An immediate treatment consists of 2 mg/kg of cortisol every 8 hours and 10% glucose intravenously. This replacement therapy should be weaned off gradually.[72]

CONGENITAL ADRENAL HYPERPLASIA

Congenital adrenal hyperplasia (CAH) is an inherited disorder in which disruption of enzymatic pathways of steroidogenesis leads to chronic adrenal overactivity and histologic alterations.

The histologic changes in the adrenal and the clinical manifestations of CAH arise from the absence or the reduction of enzymatic activity in various steps of adrenal steroidogenesis. Each aberration of enzymatic function leads to alterations in the production patterns of a specific steroid and subsequent changes in the steroid's precursor levels. The wide range of metabolic clinical disturbances and genital abnormalities are the manifestations of varying degrees of steroid hormone imbalances. Nonclassic forms of the disease arise from partial defects in the enzymatic pathways that render themselves to diagnosis only with recently improved methods. The classic forms are the result of full expression of enzymatic failure and result in genital ambiguity and salt-retention disturbances in 75% of cases.

Pathology and Pathogenesis of CAH

The clinical manifestations of CAH are the result of the underlying enzyme deficiency. The levels of steroids that are produced beyond the points of the enzymatic blockage are decreased, while the steroid precursor preceding that step accumulate and appear in high levels. The identification of the nature of the steroid profile can lead to recognition of the specific enzymatic defect. ACTH production in the pituitary is stimulated in response to reduced plasma cortisol levels. Increased ACTH levels, in turn, further stimulate the adrenal cortical function, resulting in glandular overactivity and hyperplasia.[75] The adrenal changes in CAH can be explained on the basis of overproduction of ACTH in an attempt to compensate for the reduced glucocorticoid output. The weight of each adrenal in untreated neonates and children is 15 g (normal 1.5–3 g); in adults, it is 30–35 g.[76]

A diffusely convoluted brown surface is associated with typical microscopic findings of compact cells that dominate the cortex and extend from the medulla to the zona glomerulosa. Occasionally, a zone of lipid-rich cells separates the compact and glomerulosa cells. When a salt-losing syndrome exists and aldosterone production is not spared, compensatory hyperplasia of the zona glomerulosa is found.

The enzymatic blockage associated with CAH includes steroid 21-hydroxylase deficiency, which is the most frequent abnormality[35]; 11β-hydroxylase deficiency; 3β-HSD deficiency; steroid 17α-hydroxylase deficiency; cholesterol desmolase deficiency, which is extremely rare; and 18-hydroxylase or 18-hydroxysteroid dehydrogenase deficiencies.

Maternal manifestations of CAH depend on the level and type of steroids to which the affected individual is exposed. The timing of the exposure and the aberrant levels of the specific steroids also contribute to the characteristics of the disease. The disease may be diagnosed at different periods during life, depending on presenting symptoms; fetal ambiguous genitalia usually lead to diagnosis in the neonatal period. Metabolic disorders, such as skeletal growth abnormalities, usually lead to diagnosis during childhood. During the prepubertal period (*late onset*), the appearance of excess male characteristics and virilism leads to the diagnosis. All types of CAH are transmitted as autosomal recessive traits.[29] In one group of CAH disorders, overproduction from androgens of an adrenal source results in striking abnormalities of the fetal female phenotype, causing prenatal masculinization. The genitalia of male fetuses are not affected prenatally. A second group of CAH disorders, apart from cortisol production, affects the production of sex steroids in the gonads of female and male fetuses. Because adrenal steroids are essential for life, delayed forms of CAH that involve metabolic steroids must be incomplete.

Steroid 21-Hydroxylase Deficiency. This enzyme is essential for the conversion of 17α-hydroxyprogesterone to 11-deoxycortisol (cortisol pathway) and also for the conversion of progesterone to deoxycorticosterone (aldosterone pathway). This is the most commonly occurring type of CAH. Ninety-five percent of cases involve the steroid 21-hydroxylase. The accumulating precursors are shuttled to the sex hormone pathway (C_{19}/C_{18}), and androgens are overproduced. This type of enzymatic deficiency also may affect aldosterone production causing salt losses. It therefore presents as progressive simple virilization that is accompanied in 75% of cases by salt-wasting symptoms caused by abnormalities in sodium resorption. In one fourth of the cases, aldosterone production is spared and appears to reach normal or elevated levels.[77] Male fetal intrauterine development depends on fetal testicular androgen production. Testosterone supports the development of the Wolffian ducts to produce the epididymis, vas deferens, and seminal vesicles. The male external genitalia are affected primarily by the dihydrotestosterone-differentiating effect. Sertoli cells in the fetal testis also produce Müllerian inhibitory factor (MIF). MIF induces the degeneration and demise of the Müllerian structures, which are the fallopian tubes, uterus, and upper portion of the vagina, thus ensuring the development of the proper male phenotype. Fetuses that are not exposed *in utero* to MIF or androgens (normally all 46XX female) will develop an internal and external female phenotype.[78] In CAH females, the exposure to high androgens *in utero* will cause a virile differentiation of external genitalia, concomitant with the presence of normal female internal genitalia because MIF is not produced in these normal genetic 46XX females. The masculinization of a female can vary and genital ambiguity can range from labioscrotal fusion to the rare formation of a phallic urethra to mild clitoromegaly.[79] *Pseudohermaphroditism* in severe cases may cause a wrong-sex assignment after birth. Neonatally detected undescended testes should always raise the possibility of this type of CAH. At birth, the male fetus is normal, although genital hypopigmentation may be present. 21-Hydroxylase deficiency is the most common cause of ambiguous genitalia in the newborn.

The disorder also can be detected later in life during childhood. It is then characterized by progressive virilism with advanced somatic development. Early diagnosis is important because in females, the internal genitalia are intact, and the reproductive function can be preserved. In males, an enlarged penis in the presence of small testicles is caused by the suppression of hypothalamic-pituitary-gonadal axis by adrenal androgens. Both sexes demonstrate rapid growth and precocious closure of the epiphyses that eventually results in short stature. The symptoms vary later in childhood. They may include premature development of axillary or pubic hair, mild clitoromegaly or hirsutism, acne, and disorders of the menstrual cycle in pubertal girls. Both sexes may present different degrees of infertility. There are many cases that are asymptomatic and are revealed only by genetic HLA genotyping of 21-hydroxylase deficiency.

This type of disorder is the most common autosomal recessive disorder known in humans.[80,81] One in every 7000 persons has a genetic lesion of this enzyme. Approximately 60–80% of patients with CAH also present with salt loss.[82] It is difficult to explain the preserved aldosterone production in about 25% of the cases. A two-zone hypothesis has been presented, suggesting an intact enzyme activity in the zona glomerulosa of nonsalt-losers.[83] A compensatory effect of the kidney by high progesterone levels also has been proposed.

Severe salt wasting complicates many cases. Urinary salt loss is caused by impaired aldosterone secretion, as the mineralocorticoid pathway is affected. Often, sodium depletion leads to hyperkalemia, acidosis, dehydration, and vascular collapse. This necessitates rapid diagnosis and adequate treatment because it can rapidly become life-threatening. Such crises usually coincide with the maturation of the hepatic aldosterone pathways and can be aggravated by vomiting.

The newborn presents with decreased levels of plasma and urinary cortisol as well as aldosterone. Hypoglycemia, vasomotor collapse, hyperpigmentation, apneic spells, and seizures are the result of cortisol deficiency. Vomiting, hyponatremia, urinary salt wasting, hyperkalemia, dehydration hypotension, cyanosis, and shock result from reduced aldosterone levels. This presentation is typical of adrenal failure.[81,84]

The characterization of the P-450c21 protein and gene reveals that there is only one 21-hydroxylase and one functional gene in men. Cloning of P-450c21 cDNA[85] enables the localization of the gene for P-450c21 to the Class III region of the HLA supergene on the short arm of chromosome 6. Two P-450c21 genes are located immediately 3′ to one of two C_4 genes in the human genome.[86] However, it appears that only one P-450c21 gene is active.[87] It has been suggested that some cases with severe 21-hydroxylase deficiency experience deletions in the functional P-450c21 B gene, while deletions in the P-450c21 A have no clinical manifestations. That deletion also was shown by other groups but at a lower occurrence rate. Other nondeletional aberrations are under investigation.

Because of the high incidence of 21-hydroxylase CAH, screening for 21-hydroxylase deficiency was suggested.[88] In the face of the possible fatal outcome of a salt-losing crisis and to avoid the possible erroneous sex assignment of virilized females, prompt and early diagnosis is crucial. The later complications of virilization and growth aberrations and precocious development of secondary sex characteristics also command a diagnosis as early as possible. The suggested screening is by measuring 17-hydroxyprogesterone (17-OHP) in neonates. All babies with ambiguous genitalia or undescended testes should be evaluated. The initial evaluation includes a buccal smear, serum electrolites, serum 17-OHP, and urinary 17-KS. Also, parents of a child with CAH are carriers and have a 25% chance of giving birth to another affected fetus in a subsequent pregnancy.

Antenatal diagnosis[89] has been achieved by the detection of elevated 17-ketosteroids and pregnanetriol in the amniotic fluid. The most specific diagnostic tool for 21-hydroxylase deficiency is amniotic fluid evaluation of 17-OHP and the adjunctive measurements of Δ4-androstenedione. HLA genotyping of amniotic fluid cells based on the linkage between HLA and 21-hydroxylase genes, as described previously, is another method. A fetus sharing both HLA haplotypes with the affected proband (who is HLA-identical with the affected sibling) is predicted to have the disease, while carriers share one haplotype with the proband. With the introduction of chorionic villus sampling, HLA typing now can be achieved earlier. It should be recognized that late detection of the disease after the formation of the urogenital sinus voids any possibility of treatment. HLA genotyping is cumbersome and interpretation is difficult. The advance of molecular techniques, including the previously described isolation and elucidation of the P-450c21 gene structure, will enable the direct use of specific probes for the identification of genetic disorder in the future.

11-β-Hydroxylase Deficiency. This is the second most common type of CAH with an incidence of probably less than 5%. There is no linkage to HLA, as has been shown for 21-hydroxylase deficiency. It is not clear, however, whether in mild cases of biochemical 11-hydroxylase deficiency, the patients are actually heterozygotes. 11β-OH is the enzyme that catalyzes the conversion of 11-deoxycortisol (compound S) to cortisol and the conversion of deoxycorticosterone (DOC) to corticosterone (see Fig. 42–1). Therefore, it is the final enzyme in the synthesis of adrenal mineralocorticoids and glucocorticoids. It also mediates the final steps in the synthesis of aldosterone. A block at those steps causes an accumulation of 11-deoxycorticosterone and 11-deoxycortisol.

The circulating levels of cortisol and aldosterone, as measured in plasma and urine, are depressed. The metabolites of DOC and compound S in urine, tetrahydro-11-deoxycortisol (THS), and tetrahydrodeoxycorticosterone, are elevated. Another metabolite, 6α-THS, might be more specific for identifying the defect in newborns. Urinary 17OHCS is also elevated, as are androgens in the plasma and 17-ketosteroids in the urine. The notable characteristic of 11β-hydroxylase deficiency is hypertension, which appears frequently and is of malignant nature.[90] Virilism is similar to that described for 21-hydroxylase deficiency. The hypertension and hypokalemia are attributed to the mineralocorticoid activity of DOC.[91] The elevated fetal adrenal androgen *in utero* causes the virilization of external genitalia of female fetuses with preserved internal organs. Progressive masculinization and growth aberrations are seen in childhood and around puberty. Plasma renin activity is depressed in these cases. The presence of weak mineralocorticoid activity is probably the reason for the lack of the salt-wasting symptoms that occur with 21-hydroxylase deficiency.

The two disorders can be distinguished by the accumulation of DOC and compound S seen in 11β-hydroxylase deficiency. This is stimulated by ACTH administration, elevated urinary 17-ketosteroids, and suppressed plasma renin activity.[92] In 21-hydroxylase deficiency, serum levels of 17α-hydroxyprogesterone are elevated and urinary pregnanetriol also rises. Mild late-onset and asymptomatic cases of 11β-hydroxylase deficiency have been described.[90] Some of the obligated heterozygote parents show chemical evidence of the disease. In mild forms and with late onset, hirsutism and oligomenorrhea occurring after puberty are the principal features of the disease. Some patients with CAH have biochemical findings that suggest a combination of defects in 21α-hydroxylase and 11β-hydroxylase.[93] The gene for P-450c11 has been located on the long arm of chromsome 8.[25]

3β-Hydroxysteroid Dehydrogenase Deficiency. 3β-Hydroxysteroid dehydrogenase deficiency (3β-HSD) is the enzyme required for the conversion of 3β-Δ5 steroids to 3-keto-Δ4 configuration. It catalyzes 3β-hydroxysteroid dehydrogenation and isomerization of the double bond from the B ring to the A ring. A wide range of steroid production is affected in this enzymatic deficiency. Reduced production of aldosterone, cortisol, and testosterone are characteristic, but estrogen also is reduced, which is the product of 4 androgen aromatization. This rare form of CAH originally was described in male infants with pseudohermaphroditism and incomplete masculinization.[94] Cases of CAH in female infants were identified later, and they demonstrated mild clitoral enlargement. This presentation in the female is allegedly the consequence of very high levels of the weak androgen DHEA, which is elevated in this disorder. Also elevated are pregnenolone and 17-hydroxy pregnenolone in serum. The high ratio of Δ5/Δ4 steroids is typical for this disorder. This allows its distinction from a 21-hydroxylase deficiency where Δ4 steroids are equally high.

Because of low aldosterone and cortisol, cases of crises in infancy have been reported, with salt-losing combined with cortisol deficiency. Some patients survive. Clinically, it seems that 3β-HSD deficiency can be confined to a single steroidogenic pathway, implicating the possible existence of isozymes.[23,95] The exact characteristics of the involved enzymes are not clear and variable forms of 3β-HSD deficiency have been reported with various levels of penetration of symptoms. They may include mild developmental abnormalities with peripubertal onset. Appearance of gynecomastia and some spontaneous virilization also has been described. Late-onset forms present with hirsutism and menstrual irregularity in females. ACTH stimulation, administration of 0.25 mg IV Cortrosyn and 60-minute sampling will identify 3β-HSD defects with Δ5-hydroxyprogesterone, DHEA, and the Δ5–Δ4 ratios are high. The gene for 3β-HSD has not been cloned, and it is not an HLA-linked enzyme.

17α-Hydroxylase 17,20-Lyase Deficiency. This is a very rare disorder; approximately 50 cases are reported in the literature. A single enzyme is involved in the 17α-hydroxylation of pregnenolone and progesterone to 17α-hyeroxypregnenolone and 17α-hydroxyprogesterone, respectively. These latter products can further undergo scission of the C-17,20 carbon by the same enzyme to yield dehydroepiandrosterone (DHEA) and androstenedione, respectively. Enzymatic blockage of P-450c17 activity results in decreased steroid production by way of the glucocorticoid and sex steroid pathways. In turn, the augmented positive feedback on the pituitary gonadal axis causes an increase in ACTH production. Most adrenal steroid products are compromised by this defect. These include cortisol, sex steroids, and occasionally aldosterone. Aldosterone levels and plasma renin activity in some of the reported cases also have been compromised.[25] The consequence is excessive production of progesterone, pregnenolone, DOC, and corticosterone, while the corresponding products are depressed. 17α-hydroxyprogesterone, 17α-hydroxypregnenolone, urinary 17-OHCS, and 17-KS are low.

Most affected male infants have a female phenotype and may receive an erroneous sex assignment. After being raised as females, at puberty, amenorrhea, hypertension, and hypokalemia reveal the disorder. Low androgens in the male affect sexual differentiation. A large range of disorders can result from complete female appearance without the development of Müllerian-derived organs because MIF production is intact, to ambiguous genitalia, partial prenatal virilization, perineal hypospadias, small penis, and cryptorchism. In the female, the disease presents in sexual infantilism.[96] Serum concentrations of 17-deoxysteroids, DOC, and corticosterone are elevated and constitute enough glucocorticoid support for survival. The excess of DOC, however, is the supposed culprit in causing hypertension and hypokalemia while suppressing the renin–aldosterone system. Elevated 18-OH corticosterone also has been implicated in the hypertension.

No HLA association has been demonstrated for this defect. The gene for P-450c17 has been located recently on chromsome 10.[22] However, no clear association has been shown between disease and gross deletion or rearrangement in the gene. Also, the area of the gene has not been mapped for identification linkages.

Cholesterol Desmolase Deficiency. This is a very rare disorder; only about 40 cases are known. It is notable for a total enzyme block at the rate-limiting steroidogenesis step, the conversion of cholesterol to progesterone. This also is usually a fatal syndrome (*Prader-Willi Syndrome*). The result of such a defect so high in the steroidogenic pathway, when complete, is the failure to produce any adrenal steroids whatsoever. Of course, this type of disorder is devastating and incompatible with life. Cardiovascular collapse and death are caused by lack of mineralocorticoids. However, the survival of several patients[97] (11 out of 32 known), suggests the existence of partial blocks and milder forms that allow those patients to reach adulthood. Histologically, cholesterol accumulates in the enlarged adrenal cortex, producing a yellow foamy appearance, leading to the alternate name of the disease, *congenital lipid adrenal hyperplasia.*

Treatment consists of glucocorticoid and mineralocorticoid replacement. The levels of all steroids are low in serum. However, identification of the precise defect is compromised by the early death of the fetuses affected by the full-blown disorder. The total absence of steroids leads to the inability to produce androgen. Consequently, all patients are female, regardless of the genetic sex. None of the survivors that have been examined showed gross deletions in their genes. However, minor and point mutations are possible.[16] The possibility that adrenodoxin or adrenodoxin-reductase errors underlie this syndrome cannot be excluded. They may lead to the more fatal cases. Theoretically, early detection by molecular techniques allows early replacement therapy.

18-Hydroxylase–18-Hydroxysteroid Dehydrogenase Deficiency. This is a rare enzyme deficiency that affects the final steps in the synthesis of adrenal mineralocorticoids.[97] In this disorder, the adrenal is unable to synthesize aldosterone, which in turn leads to salt loss. Cortisol and androgen levels are unimpaired, and there is no sexual differentiation defect. In one type of the deficiency, corticosterone is not hydroxylated and both 18-hydroxycorticosterone and aldosterone are not produced. In the second type, 18-hydroxycorticosterone levels are increased because of an error in the dehydrogenation of the later precursor, and thus aldosterone is not produced.[98] In all cases, the levels of renin are elevated. Recently, it has been shown that a single enzyme P-450c11 has 11β-hydroxylase, 18-hydroxylase, and 18-oxydase activity.[99] The appearance of specific clinical deficiencies for each of these enzymatic activities can be explained by the existence of different sensitivities for each activity to deleterious effects and to confirmational changes. It also is possible to envision single-point mutations that affect one activity while sparing another.

Diagnosis of CAH

The differential diagnosis of nonpregnant young women with symptoms of androgen excess, such as hirutism, virilization, menstrual disorders, or amenorrhea, and with irregularities in glucocorticoids or mineralocorticoids must include the possibility of CAH. This notion is especially valid because at least 21-hydroxylase deficiency is a common genetic disorder with, at times, mild and cryptic presentation. Cushing's syndrome, polycystic ovarian disease, androgen-secreting tumors, and exogenous androgen therapy should be excluded. Gonadotropins, free and total testosterone, androstenedione and DHEA-S also can be detected by RIA, as can free cortisol in 24-hour urine. The type of CAH is diagnosed according to the detection of the levels of precursors and products of the inflicted enzyme.

Treatment

Recently, dexamethasone therapy has been proposed for pregnancies at risk for 21-hydroxylase deficiency.[100] The treatment is prescribed early in gestation (6–7 weeks) in order to suppress adrenal androgen secretion before the external genitalia are malformed. Oral 0.5-mg dexamethasone, twice daily, suppresses amniotic fluid androgens. However, the ability to suppress fetal adrenal function through the administration of replacement therapy to the mother is controversial, and its possible complications are under debate. The results are equivocal. However, it is logical that early treatment, later monitoring of the sex of the fetus (therapy in male fetuses should be stopped), and genetic assessment can establish a comprehensive management modality. In the immediate neonatal period, careful assignment of sex in a child with ambiguous genitalia can lead to the subsequent surgical repair of external genitalia. This, in turn, will allow for a normally functional vagina and preservation of the female reproductive capabilities. CAH is treated depending on the specific type of enzyme disorder. The primary treatment is the replacement of the adequate glucocorticoid. In cases complicated by the lack of salt, mineralocorticoids are replaced, and sodium cloride, supported by estrogen and testosterone therapy, may be indicated in specific cases. Cortisol is replaced directly with hydrocortisone or with dexamethasone (synthetic analogue). Correction of the cortisol deficiency suppresses ACTH overproduction. Dexamethasone, 0.25–0.5 mg before bed, or prednisone, 5 mg at night and 2.5 mg in the morning, are some of the possible maintenance protocols. Cortisone acetate, 50–100 mg, or prednisone or equivalents, 5–20 mg, are recommended. Dexamethasone readily crosses the placenta to the fetus. The levels of plasma 17-OHP and androgen are measured to follow the efficiency of treatment. Proper adjustment of glucocorticoid replacement prevents excessive androgen accumulation and protects the fetus from growth abnormalities and aberration in sexual development. Proper glucocorticoid replacement therapy also will conserve future fertility. A normal 17-hydroxyprogesterone level is less than 3 mg/mL. Controlled levels in the plasma range from 5–20 mg/mL. Monitoring the reduced levels of 17-hydroxyprogesterone assists in the achievement of close to normal levels of androgens. 17-hydroxyprogesterone levels and urinary levels of pregnenetriol are elevated in pregnancy and rise with advancing pregnancy. Pregnant women with CAH who are on replacement therapy may need an increase in glucocorticoid administration to adjust to the stress imposed by pregnancy. Any dose must be reduced to the minimum effective dose because of the controversial link to possible adverse effects on the fetus of steroid administration.[101] When the pregnant CAH patient needs mineralocorticoid replacement, 9α-fluorohydrocortisone (fluorocortisone) may be continued during pregnancy. The patient should be monitored carefully with weight measurements, blood pressure changes, and Cushinglike features recorded.

Recently, the importance of the renin–angiotensin system in CAH, exerting a primary influence on the adrenal secretion of aldosterone, was recognized. Even in cases of 21-hydroxylase deficiency, in which aldosterone production appears to be intact, plasma renin activity (PRA) is elevated. Similar findings occur in salt-wasting forms. It has been shown that even these simple cases may gain from the addition of mineralocorticoids to their management.[26,102] This addition usually allows the tapering of glucocorticoid therapy. When PRA levels were normal, additional improvement in skeletal growth was observed. PRA levels are elevated in salt-wasting forms and suppressed in mineralocorticoid-excess forms. If treatment is conducted adequately during the life of the CAH patient, she may conceive and undergo a relatively uneventful pregnancy. A vaginal delivery may be attempted, but many patients are eventually delivered operatively because of a contracted pelvis. A CAH patient may need additional steroids during the stressful period of delivery.

REFERENCES

1. Pepe GJ, Albrecht ED. Regulation of the primate fetal adrenal cortex. *Endocrine Reviews.* 1990;11:151.
2. Kahri AI, Huhtaniemi I, Salmenperä M. Steroid formation and differentiation of corticol cells in tissue culture of human fetal adrenals in the presence and absence of ACTH. *Endocrinology.* 1976;98:33.
3. Schonemann A. Hypophysis und thyroidea. *Virchows Arch* (*Pathol Anat*). 1892;129:310.
4. Pelletier G, Robert F, Hardy J. Identification of human anterior pituitary cells by immunoelectronmicroscopy. *J Clin Endocrinol Metab.* 1978;46:534.
5. Holmes RL, Ball JN. *The Pituitary Gland—A Comparative Account.* Cambridge, MA: Cambridge University Press; 1974:1.
6. Halmi NS, Krieger D. Immunocytochemistry of ACTH related peptides in the hypophysis. In: Bhatnagar AS, ed. *The Anterior Pituitary Gland.* New York, NY: Raven Press; 1983:1.
7. Krieger DT. The multiple faces of pro-opiomelanocortin, a prototype precursor molecule. *Clin Res.* 1983;31:342.
8. Catt KJ. Molecular mechanisms of hormone action: control of target cell function by peptide, steroid, and thyroid hormones. In: Felig P, Baxter JD, Broadus AE, Frohman LA, eds. *Endocrinology and Metabolism.* 2nd ed. New York, NY: McGraw Hill; 1988:82.
9. Brown MS, Kovanen PT, Goldstein JL. Receptor-mediated uptake of lipoprotein-cholesterol and its utilization for steroid synthesis in the adrenal cortex. *Recent Prog Horm Res.* 1979;35:215.
10. Mason JI, Rainey WE. Steroidogenesis in the human fetal adrenal: a role for cholesterol synthesized de-novo. *J Clin Endocrinol Metab.* 1987;64:140.
11. Chanderbhan R, Noland BJ, Scallen TJ, Vahouny GV. Sterol carrier protein 2: delivery of cholesterol from adrenal lipid droplets to mitochondria for pregnenolone synthesis. *J Biol Chem.* 1982;257:8928.
12. Miller WL. Molecular biology of steroid hormone synthesis. *Endocrine Reviews.* 1988;9:295.
13. Duque C, Morisaki M, Ikekawa N, Shikita M. The enzyme activity in bovine adrenocortical cytochrome P-450 producing pregnenolone from cholesterol: kinetic and electrophoretic studies on the reactivity of hydroxycholesterol intermediates. *Biochem Biophys Res Commun.* 1978;82:179.
14. Shikita M, Hall PF. Cytochrome P-450 from bovine adrenocortical mitochondria: an enzyme for the side chain cleavage of cholesterol. I. Purification and properties. *J Biol Chem.* 1973;248:5596.
15. Shikita M, Hall PF. Cytochrome P-450 from bovine adrenocortical mitochondria: an enzyme for the side chain cleavage of cholesterol. II. subunit structure. *J Biol Chem.* 1973;248:5605.
16. Matteson KJ, Chung BC, Urdea MS, Miller WL. Study of cholesterol side chain cleavage (20,22 desmolase) deficiency causing congenital lipoid adrenal hyperplasia using bovine-sequence P-450 scc oligodeoxyribonucleotide probes. *Endocrinology.* 1986;118:1296.
17. Nebert DW, Adesnik M, Coon MJ, et al. The P-450 gene superfamily: recommended nomenclature *DNA.* 1987;6:1.
18. Chung B, Matteson KJ, Voutilainen R, et al. Human cholesterol side-chain cleavage enzyme, P-450 scc: cDNA cloning, assignment of the gene to chromosome 15 and expression in the placenta. *Proc Natl Acad Sci USA.* 1986;83:8962.
19. Morel Y, Picado-Leonard J, Wu DA, et al. Assignment of the functional gene for human adrenodoxin to chromosome 11q13→qter and of adrenodoxin pseudogenes to chromosome 20cen→q13.1. *Am J Hum Genet.* 1988;43:52.
20. Lambeth JD, Pember SO. Cytochrome P-450-adrenodoxin complex: reduction properties of the substrate-associated cytochrome and relation of the reduction states of heme and iron sulfur centers to association of the proteins. *J Biol Chem.* 1983;258:5596.
21. Solish SB, Picardo-Leonard J, Morel Y, et al. Human adrenodoxin reductase: two mRNAs encoded by a single gene on chromosome 17cen→q25 are expressed in steroidogenic tissue. *Proc Natl Acad Sci USA.* 1988;85:7104.
22. Matteson KJ, Picado-Leonard J, Chung B-C, et al. Assignment of the gene for adrenal P-450c17 (steroid 17-hydroxylase/17, 20-lyase) to human chromosome 10. *J Clin Endocrinol Metab.* 1986;63:789.
23. Craviolo MDC, Vlloa-Aquirre A, Bermudez JA, et al. A new variant of the 3β-hydroxysteroid dehydrogenase-isomerase deficiency syndrome: evidence for the existence of two isozymes. *J Clin Endocrinol Metab.* 1986;63:360.
24. Higashi Y, Yoshioka H, Yamane M, et al. Complete nucleotide sequence of two steroid 21-hydroxylase genes tandemly arranged in human chromosomes: a pseudogene and a geniune gene. *Proc Natl Acad Sci USA.* 1986;83:2841.
25. Chua SC, Szabo P, Vitek A, et al. Cloning of cDNA encoding steroid 11β-hydroxylase (P-450c11). *Proc Natl Acad Sci USA.* 1987;84:7193.
26. Gibson M, Tulchinsky D. The maternal adrenal. In: Tulchinsky D, Ryan KI, eds. *Maternal–Fetal Endocrinology.* Philadelphia, PA: WB Saunders; 1980:129.
27. Pickard J, Jochem AL, Sadur CN, Hofeldt FD. Cushing's syndrome in pregnancy. *Obstet Gynecol Surv.* 1990;48:87.
28. Aron DC, Schvall AM, Sheeler CR. Cushing's syndrome and pregnancy. *Am J Obstet Gynecol.* 1990;162:244.
29. Rabin D, McKenna TJ. *Clinical Endocrinology and Metabolism. Principles and Practice of Clinical Medicine.* New York, NY: Grune Stratton; 1982;9:430.
30. Liddle GW. The adrenals. In: Williams RH, ed. *Textbook of Endocrinology.* 6th ed. Philadelphia, PA: WB Saunders; 1981:249.
31. Vale W, Spiess J, Rivier C, et al. Characterization of a residue ovine hypothalamic peptide that stimulates secretion of corticotropin and β-endorphin. *Science.* 1981;213:1396.
32. Genazzani AR, Fraioli F, Hurlimann J, et al. Immunoreactive ACTH and cortisol plasma levels during pregnancy. Detection and partial purification of corticotropin-like placental hormone: the human chorionic corticotropin (HCC). *Clin Endocrinol.* 1975;4:1.
33. Doknmov SI, Milanov SC, Trepetshov SP. Andrenocorticotrophic hormone in plasma of mother and newborn. *J Obstet Gynaecol Br Commonw.* 1984;81:220.
34. Mukherjee K, Swyer GIM. Plasma cortisol and adrenocorticotropin hormone in normal men and non-pregnant women, normal pregnant women and women with pre-eclampsia. *J Obstet Gynaecol Br Commonw.* 1972;79:504.
35. Genazzani AR, Felber JP, Fiovetti P. Immunoreactive ACTH, immunoreactive human chorionic somatomammotropin (HCS) and 11-OH steroids plasma levels in normal and pathological pregnancies. *Acta Endocrinol (Kbh).* 1976:83:800.
36. Winters AJ, Oliver C, Colston C, et al. Plasma ACTH levels in the human fetus and neonate as related to age and parturition. *J Clin Endocrinol Metab.* 1979;39:269.

37. Allen JP, Cook DM, Kendall JW, et al. Maternal fetal ACTH relationship in man. *J Clin Endocrinol Metab.* 1973;37:230.
38. Jubiz W. *Endocrinology: A Logical Approach for Clinicians.* New York, NY: McGraw-Hill; 1979:362.
39. Eddy RL, Jones AL, Gilliland PF, et al. Cushing's syndrome: a prospective study of diagnostic methods. *Am J Med.* 1973;55:621.
40. Rosenthal HE, Slaunwhite WR Jr, Sandberg AA. Transcortin: a corticosteroid-binding protein of plasma X cortisol and progesterone interplay and unbound levels of these steroids in pregnancy. *J Clin Endocrinol Metab.* 1969;29:352.
41. Oxley DK, Fischer CL. Ligand assays (immunoassay): principles and applications. In: Race GJ, ed. *Laboratory Medicine.* Philadelphia, PA: Harper & Row; 1982;1:1.
42. Murphy BEP. Clinical evaluation of urinary cortisol determinations by competitive protein-binding radioassay. *J Clin Endocrinol Metab.* 1968;28:343.
43. Mizuno M, Lobotsky J, Lloyd CW, et al. Plasma androstenedione and testosterone during pregnancy and in the newborn. *J Clin Endocrinol Metab.* 1968;28:1133.
44. Lobo RA, Paul WL, Goebelsman G. Dehydroepiandrosterone sulfate as an indicator of adrenal androgen function. *Obstet Gynecol.* 1989;57:69.
45. Gandy HM. Androgensin. In: Fuchs F, Klopper A, eds. *Endocrinology of Pregnancy.* 2nd ed. New York, NY: Harper & Row; 1977:123.
46. Belishe S, Osathanondh R, Tulchinsky D. The effect of constant infusion of unlabeled dehydroepiandrosterone sulfate on maternal plasma androgens and estrogens. *J Clin Endocrinol Metab.* 1979;5:544.
47. Demisch K, Grant JK, Black W. Plasma testosterone in women in late pregnancy and after delivery. *J Endocrinol.* 1968;42:477.
48. Forest MG, Ances IG, Tapper AJ, et al. Percentage binding of testosterone, androstenedione and dehydroisoandrosterone in plasma at the time of delivery. *J Clin Endocrinol Metab.* 1981;32:417.
49. Gormley MJJ, Hadden DR, Kennedy TL, et al. Cushing's syndrome in pregnancy-treatment with metyrapone. *Clin Endocrinol.* 1982;16:283.
50. Lin L, Jaffe R, Borowski GD, et al. Exacerbation of Cushing's disease during pregnancy. *Am J Obstet Gynecol.* 1983;145:110.
51. Check JH, Caro JF, Kendall B, et al. Cushing's syndrome in pregnancy: effect of associated diabetes on fetal and neonatal complications. *Am J Obstet Gynecol.* 1979;133:846.
52. Ross EJ, Marshal-Jones P, Friedmen M. Cushing's syndrome: diagnostic criteria. *Q J Med.* 1966;35:149.
53. Lope CL, Black EG. The reliability of some adrenal function tests. *Br Med J.* 1959;2:1117.
54. Nolten WE, Lindheimer MD, Oparil S, et al. Desoxycorticosterone in normal pregnancy. 1. Sequential studies of the secretory patterns of desoxycorticosterone, aldosterone and cortisol. *Am J Obstet Gynecol.* 1978;132:414.
55. Kreines K, Perin E, Salzer R. Pregnancy in Cushing's syndrome. *J Clin Endocrinol Metab.* 1964;24:75.
56. Liddle GW. The adrenals. In: Williams RH, ed. *Textbook of Endocrinology.* 6th ed. Philadelphia, PA: WB Saunders; 1981:249.
57. Eisenstein AB, Karsh R, Gall I. Occurrence of pregnancy in Cushing's syndrome. *J Clin Endocrinol Metab.* 1963;23:971.
58. Grimes EM, Fayez JA, Miller GL. Cushing's syndrome and pregnancy. *Obstet Gynecol.* 1973;42:550.
59. Wieland R, Schaffer M, Glove R. Cushing's syndrome complicating pregnancy. A case report. *Obstet Gynecol.* 1971;38:841.
60. MacDonald PC, Siitri PK. Origin of estrogen in women pregnant with an anencephalic fetus. *J Clin Invest.* 1965;44:465.
61. Bank H, Beer R, Lunenfeld B, et al. Recurrence of adrenal carcinoma during pregnancy with delivery of a normal child. *J Clin Endocrinol Metab.* 1965;25:359.
62. Beck P, Eaton CJ, Youn IS, et al. Metyrapone response in pregnancy. *Am J Obstet Gynecol.* 1968;100;327.
63. Brownie AL, Sprunt JG. Metopirone in the assessment of pituitary–adrenal function. *Lancet.* 1962;1:772.
64. Bongiovanni AM, McPadden AJ. Steroids during pregnancy and possible fetal consequences. *Fertil Steril.* 1960;11:181.
65. Robin D, McKenna TJ. Clinical endocrinology and metabolism. Principles and practice. In: Robin D, McKenna TJ, eds. *The Science and Practice of Clinical Medicine.* New York, NY: Grune & Stratton; 1982;9:430.
66. Irvine WJ, Barnes EW. Addison's disease, ovarian failure and hypoparathyroidism. *Clin Endocrinol Metab.* 1975;4:379.
67. Blizzard RN, Kyle M. Studies of the adrenal antigens and antibodies in Addison's disease. *J Clin Invest.* 1963;42:1653.
68. Neufeld M, MacLaren NK, Blizzard RM. Two types of autoimmune Addison's disease associated with different polyglandular autoimmune (PGA) syndrome. *Medicine.* 1981;60:355.
69. Brent F. Addison's disease and pregnancy. *Am J Surg.* 1950;79:645.
70. Drucker D, Shumak S, Angel A. Schmidt's syndrome presenting with intrauterine growth retardation and postpartum addisonian crises. *Am J Obstet Gynecol.* 1984;149:229.
71. Yanagibashi K, Haniu M, Shively JE, et al. The synthesis of aldosterone by the adrenal cortex: two zones (fasciculata and gomerulosa) possess one enzyme for 11β-18-hydroxylation, and aldehyde synthesis. *J Biol Chem.* 1986;261:3556.
72. Speiser PW, Laforgia N, Kato K, et al. First trimester treatment and molecular genetic diagnosis of congenital adrenal hyperplasia (21-hydroxylase deficiency). *J Clin Endocrinol Metab.* 1990;70:838.
73. Burrow GN, Ferris TF. *Medical Complications During Pregnancy.* Philadelphia, PA: WB Saunders; 1988:260.
74. Walsh SW, Norman RL, Novy MJ. *In utero* regulation of rhesus monkey fetal adrenals: effects of dexamethasone, adrenocorticotropin thyrotropin-releasing hormone, prolactin, human chorionic gonadotropin and α melanocyte-stimulating hormone on fetal and maternal plasma steroids. *Endocrinology.* 1979;104:1805.
75. Finkelstein M, Shaefer JM. Inborn errors of steroid biosynthesis. *Physiol Rev.* 1979;59:353.
76. Neville AM, O'Hare MJ. Histopathology of the human adrenal cortex. *Clin Endocrinol Metab.* 1985;14:791.
77. Kater CE, Biglieri EG. Distinctive plasma aldosterone, 18-hydroxycorticosterone and 18-hydroxydeoxycorticosterone profile in the 21- 17α and 11β-hydroxylase deficiency types of congenital adrenal hyperplasia. *Am J Med.* 1983;75:43.
78. Jost A, Vigier B, Prepin J, Perchellet JP. Studies on sex differentiation in mammals. *Recent Prg Horm Res.* 1973;29:1.
79. Savage MO. Ambiguous genitalia, small genitalia and undescended testes. *Clin Endocrinol Metab.* 1982;11:127.
80. Speiser PW, DuPont B, Rubinstein P, et al. High frequency of nonclassical steroid 21-hydroxylase deficiency. *Am J Hum Genet.* 1985;37:650.
81. Miller WL, Levine LS. Molecular and clinical advances in congenital adrenal hyperplasia. *J Pediatr.* 1987;111:1.
82. Fife D, Rappaport EB. Prevalence of salt-losing among congenital adrenal hyperplasia patients. *Clin Endocrinol.* 1983;18:259.
83. Kuhnle U, Chow D, Rappaport R, et al. The 21-hydroxylase activity in the glomerulosa and fasciculata of the adrenal cortex in congenital adrenal hyperplasia. *J Clin Endocrinol.* 1981;52:534.
84. Sperling MA. Newborn adaptation: adrenocorticol hormones and ACTH. In: Tulchinsky D, Ryan KJ, eds. *Maternal–Fetal Endocrinology.* Philadelphia, PA: WB Saunders; 1980:387.
85. White PC, New MI, DuPont B. Cloning and expression of cDNA encoding a bovine adrenal cytochrome P-450 specific for steroid 21-hydroxylation. *Proc Natl Acad Sci USA.* 1984;81:1986.
86. White PC, Grossberger D, Onufer BJ, et al. Two genes encoding steroid 21-hydroxylase are located near the genes encoding the fourth component of complement in man. *Proc Natl Acad Sci USA.* 1985;82:1089.
87. White PC, New MI, DuPont B. HLA-linked congenital adrenal hyperplasia results from a defective gene encoding a cytochrome P-450 specific for steroid 21-hydroxylation. *Proc Natl Acad Sci USA.* 1984;81:7505.
88. New MI, Josso N. Disorders of gonadal differentiation and congenital adrenal hyperplasia. *Endocrin Metab Clin North Am.* 1988;17:339.
89. Jeffcoate TNA, Fleigner JRH, Russel SH, et al. Diagnosis of the adrenogenital syndrome before birth. *Lancet.* 1965;2:553.
90. Rosler A, Leiberman E. Enzymatic defects of steroidogenesis: 11β-hydroxylase deficiency congenital adrenal hyperplasia. In: New MI, Levine LS, eds. *Adrenal Diseases in Childhood (Pediatric Adolescent Endocrinology).* Basel: S Karger; 1984;13:47.
91. Rosler A, Leiberman E, Sack J, et al. Clinical variability of congenital adrenal hyperplasia due to 11β-hydroxylase deficiency. *Horm Res.* 1982;16:133.
92. New MI, DuPont B, Pang S, et al. Metabolic errors of adrenal steroidogenesis. In: Martin L, James BHT, eds. *Current Topics in Experimental Endocrinology.* New York, NY: Academic Press; 1983;5:309.
93. Hurwitz A, Brautbar C, Milwidsky A, et al. Combined 21- and 11β-hydroxylase deficiency in familial congenital adrenal hyperplasia. *J Clin Endo Metab.* 1985;60:631.
94. Bongiovanini AM. The adrenogenital syndrome with deficiency of 3β-hydroxysteroid dehydrogenase. *J Clin Invest.* 1962;41:2080.
95. Pang S, Levine LS, Stoner E, et al. Non-salt-losing congenital adrenal hyperplasia due to 3β-hydroxysteroid dehydrogenase deficiency with normal glomerulosa function. *J Clin Endocrinol Metab.* 1983;56:808.
96. Biglieri EG, Herron MA, Brust N. 17-Hydroxylation deficiency in man. *J Clin Invest.* 1966;45:1946.
97. Hauffa BP, Miller WL, Grumbach MM, et al. Congenital adrenal hyperplasia due to deficient cholesterol side-chain cleavage activity (20,22-desmolase) in a patient treated for 18 years. *Clin Endocrinol.* 1985;23:481.
98. Buster JE. Fetal adrenal cortex. *Clin Obstet Gynecol.* 1980;23:803.
99. Ulick S. Diagnosis and nomenclature of the disorders of the terminal portion of the aldosterone biosynthetic pathway. *J Clin Endocrinol Metab.* 1976;43:92.
100. Evans MI, Chrousos GP, Mann DW, et al. Pharmacologic suppression of the fetal adrenal gland in utero. *JAMA.* 1985;253:1015.
101. Rosler A, Levine LS, Schneider B, et al. The interrelationship of sodium balance, plasma renin activity and ACTH in congenital adrenal hyperplasia. *J Clin Endocrinol Metab.* 1977;45:500.
102. Winter JSD. Current approach to the treatment of congenital adrenal hyperplasia. *J Pediatr.* 1980;97:81.

Chapter Forty-Three
Diabetes and Pregnancy

Mary J. O'Sullivan, Jay S. Skyler, Karen A. Raimer, and Alfred Abu-Hamad

43

During the past 15 years, there has been a dramatic change in the management and outcome of pregnancies complicated by diabetes mellitus—both insulin-dependent diabetes mellitus (*pregestational* diabetes) and diabetes developing during pregnancy (*gestational* diabetes).

Before the mid-1970s, most textbooks portrayed a relatively bleak picture of maternal survival and progression of diabetic complications and of substantial fetal morbidity and mortality, including the likelihood of unexplained intrauterine demise. Attention was focused on the occurrence and timing of early delivery. Caesarean sections were common either due to the planned early timing of delivery (to avoid intrauterine demise) or the need to avoid traumatic vaginal deliveries of macrosomic infants. Early deliveries often resulted in premature infants who developed respiratory distress syndrome, which led to high neonatal mortality. Infants of diabetic mothers (IDMs) were described as macrosomic with rampant neonatal hypoglycemia, hypocalcemia, hypomagnesemia, polycythemia, hyperviscosity, and hyperbilirubinemia. In addition, the rate of congenital malformations was more than threefold that of the general neonatal population.

Today, the picture is much different. The discovery of insulin has improved maternal mortality and has initiated an improvement in perinatal mortality (Fig. 43–1).[1] Modern obstetric and neonatal management has further decreased perinatal mortality and morbidity.

Over the past decade, radical changes have occurred in the management of diabetes in pregnancy and in the management of pregnancy itself. The introduction of self-monitoring of blood glucose (SMBG) launched the era of meticulous glycemic control during pregnancy without prolonged hospitalization. The attainment of excellent glycemic control has allowed diabetic women to continue their gestation to term and have spontaneous vaginal deliveries. The earlier problem of intrauterine demise during late gestation has nearly vanished. Overall perinatal survival rates are approaching those of healthy women. Today, the classic cherubic IDM baby is rare in the nurseries of major centers. Neonatal complications are dwindling markedly. Optimism prevails, and young women with diabetes no longer need to fear pregnancy.

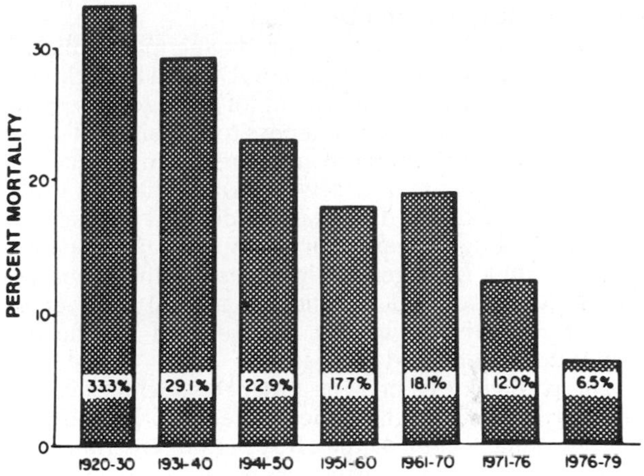

Figure 43–1. Perinatal mortality in pregnancies complicated by insulin-dependent diabetes (White Classes B–R), published in the *American Journal of Obstetrics and Gynecology* from 1920 through 1979. (*From Gabbe,[1] with permission.*)

OVERVIEW OF DIABETES MELLITUS

Recognized by elevated plasma glucose (hyperglycemia), diabetes mellitus is monitored by measuring the variation in glycemia. In *Type I* or *insulin-dependent diabetes mellitus* (IDDM), there is an absolute insulin deficiency requiring insulin therapy for the preservation of life. In *Type II*, or *noninsulin-dependent diabetes mellitus* (NIDDM), exogenous insulin is not generally required for the maintenance of life, but it may be required to control symptoms or correct a disordered metabolism.[2]

Diabetes management requires attention to be directed toward food intake, energy expenditure (activity), and medication. The patient should be involved in the treatment program on a daily basis. Patient behavior and motivation are critical to a successful therapeutic plan.

With time, many diabetics develop chronic vascular, neurologic, and organ-specific (particularly retinal and renal) complications.[3] The frequency, severity, and progression of these complications may be related to hyperglycemia, associated metabolic derangements, and the duration of the diabetes.[4,5]

Classification of Diabetes Mellitus

The classification of diabetes developed by the National Diabetes Data Group (NDDG) of the National Institutes of Health[6] is similar to that of the World Health Organization (WHO).[7] Insulin-dependent diabetes mellitus was previously called juvenile-onset or ketosis-prone diabetes, and noninsulin-dependent diabetes mellitus was called maturity-onset or ketosis-resistant diabetes. These major patterns of the diabetic syndrome are distinct in terms of etiology, pathogenesis, clinical presentation, and treatment strategies. Other subtypes include *tropical malnutrition diabetes* (Type III)[8], *Maturity-onset diabetes of the young* (MODY)[9], and a relatively newly defined entity occurring in young black people with features of both IDDM and NIDDM.[10]

Hyperglycemia may be secondary to or caused by primary pancreatic disease (pancreatic surgery, chronic pancreatitis, or cystic fibrosis), medication (eg, chronic steroid therapy), or other diseases (Cushing's syndrome, acromegaly, or pheochromocytoma) and is called secondary diabetes mellitus. It also is associated with some relatively uncommon genetic disorders.

Gestational diabetes mellitus (GDM) is first recognized during pregnancy. It is no longer required that glucose metabolism return to normal after pregnancy. Thus, GDM includes diabetes not recognized before pregnancy, either Type I or Type II, first diagnosed in pregnancy. The vast majority of GDM does remit postpartum and at that time is still classified as *previous abnormality* of carbohydrate metabolism by the NDDG classification.

Women with diabetes diagnosed before pregnancy are referred to as *pregestational diabetics* during pregnancy.

Characteristics of Type I Diabetes

A marked decrease of insulin-producing pancreatic islet beta cells is characteristic of Type I or IDDM. This is clinically reflected in an absolute deficiency of endogenous insulin secretion (insulinopenia), proneness to ketosis, and dependency on daily exogenous insulin for the maintenance of life.[11] This is the more rare, severe form of diabetes usually occurring in childhood. The peak incidence is between ages 10 and 13, although it may occur at any age, and the patients are usually thin. Management involves insulin two or more times daily and careful attention to a meal plan, energy expenditure (activity), insulin dosage, and routine daily self-monitoring of blood glucose.

The pathogenesis of Type I diabetes includes genetic, identified by the diabetic gene located on the short arm of chromosome 6 close to the HLA region; environmental, such as viral infections, noxious chemicals, or other unidentified environmental factors that in genetically susceptible individuals, appear to initiate damage to pancreatic islet beta cells; and an immune mechanism that lead to slow, progressive, pancreatic islet beta-cell damage and eventual destruction, often reflected by circulating islet cell antibodies (ICA), particularly at the onset of Type I diabetes.[12]

Characteristics of Type II Diabetes

In Type II or NIDDM, there is endogenous pancreatic insulin secretion with altered insulin secretory dynamics. Ketosis is absent, and insulin resistance is caused by diminished target cell response to insulin.[13,14] These patients usually are not dependent on insulin for prevention of ketosis or maintenance of life. They may require insulin for correction of symptomatic or persistent fasting hyperglycemia if control is not achieved by diet or medication. This is the milder, more common form of diabetes. Onset is generally after age 40, although it can occur as early as adolescence. The majority (80–90% in the United States) are obese. There are probably several subtypes of NIDDM. Effective weight reduction may help normalize the glycemia. Management includes weight reduction, increased physical activity, balanced nutrition, and medication. In the nonpregnant patient, medication may be either insulin or oral sulfonylureas. However, in pregnancy, sulfonylureas are not used.

Genetic and environmental factors also appear to be involved in the etiopathogenesis.[15] The specific genetics of NIDDM remain to be established. The environmental role in the pathogenesis of NIDDM became evident from studies of primitive societies undergoing "Westernization."[16] A sedentary lifestyle, especially coupled with obesity, leads to a marked rise in prevalence of NIDDM. Other diabetogenic factors are aging and multiparity.

Impaired islet beta-cell function and insulin action are the major pathogenic mechanisms in NIDDM.[13,17] Abnormal beta-cell function (impaired insulin secretion) is manifested in at least three ways:[18] (1) blunted or absent first phase insulin response to glucose; (2) decreased sensitivity of insulin response to glucose (ie, relative blindness to hyperglycemia); and (3) decreased insulin secretory capacity, particularly in more severe Type II diabetes. Although insulin secretory response is impaired, it is not static but dynamic. Chronic hyperglycemia may aggravate the impaired insulin secretion. Thus, with deterioration of NIDDM, there is a concomitant effect on insulin secretory response. Moreover, when hyperglycemia is corrected, endogenous insulin response to a meal challenge improves somewhat.

Insulin resistance is caused by an impaired insulin action at the target cell level.[19] Such abnormalities include receptor-binding defects caused by reduced numbers of receptors and postbinding (postreceptor) defects decreasing insulin action in the effector system beyond the cellular receptors, including a decreased glucose transport capacity. Additional defects cannot be excluded. Insulin binding can be altered. Insulin receptors are highly regulated and influenced by factors such as diet, activity, hormones, pharmacologic agents, and circulating concentrations of insulin. Postreceptor defects also can be reversed by vigorous insulin therapy. These too are subject to a complex regulatory scheme.

CLASSIFICATION OF DIABETES IN PREGNANCY

To classify diabetes in pregnancy, the clinician must consider two perspectives: (1) diabetes complicated by pregnancy (pregestational diabetes) and (2) pregnancy complicated by diabetes (gestational diabetes). This seems straightforward, yet the literature is confusing, primarily because most authors have not clearly distinguished between these two groups.

In 1949, Pricilla White published a classification scheme designed to assess perinatal risk in women with pregestational diabetes.[20] This scheme, subsequently updated[21] and reproduced in Table 43–1, assessed the patient's condition (duration of diabetes and the presence of diabetic complications) and its influence on pregnancy outcome. Obviously, duration of diabetes and the presence of complications cannot apply to gestational-onset diabetes. Therefore, in the original description[20] and as recently reemphasized by Hare and White[22] and others[23,24], only women with pregestational diabetes were included in the White classification scheme.

White's scheme has been used with many modifications, which has caused much confusion. Among these are Class A, which includes both gestational and pregestational diabetes treated without insulin and Class B when insulin is used (gestational Class B); Class A, which denotes gestational diabetes treated without insulin and Class B1 gestational diabetes when insulin is used; and Class B2, which is pregestational diabetes of short duration. Another scheme has used Class A to denote gestational diabetes treated without insulin and Class AB, Class B, gestational Class B, or Class Bg to denote gestational diabetes treated with insulin. Others have classified gestational diabetes using Class A1 for a fasting plasma glucose $<$ 105 mg/dL (5.8 mmol/L), Class A2 for a fasting glucose 105–130 mg/dL (5.8–7.2 mmol/L), and Class B1 for a fasting glucose $>$ 130 mg/dL (7.2 mmol/L).

This has been very confusing, and ironically, the White classification is becoming obsolete even in pregestational diabetes. From a therapeutic standpoint, it is of limited practical value. Moreover, duration of disease has become less important in determining pregnancy risk. Retinopathy may be treated with laser photocoagulation during pregnancy if indicated. The classification does retain some value, however, because fetal morbidity and mortality are increased in the presence of nephropathy (Classes F and RF). In addition, pregnancy threatens maternal survival in

TABLE 43–1. WHITE'S CLASSIFICATION OF DIABETES IN PREGNANCY[a]

Gestational Diabetes	Abnormal glucose tolerance test, but euglycemia maintained by diet alone. Diet alone insufficient; insulin required.
Pregestational Diabetes	
Class	
A	Euglycemia maintained by diet alone; diabetes may be of any duration and onset may have occurred at any age.
B	Onset at age 20 years or older and duration of less than 10 years
C	Onset during age range 10–19 or duration of 10–19 years
D	Onset younger than 10 years, duration of more than 20 years, background retinopathy, or hypertension (not preeclampsia)
R	Proliferative retinopathy or vitreous hemorrhage
F	Nephropathy with proteinuria exceeding 500 mg/dL
RF	Criteria for classes R and F coexist
H	Arteriosclerotic heart disease clinically evident
T	Prior renal transplantation

[a] All classes below A require insulin therapy. Classes R, F, RF, H, and T have no onset–duration criteria but usually occur in long-term diabetes. The development of a complication moves the patient to the lower class.
Adapted from Hare and White.[22]

Class H patients[25], and thus should possibly be avoided.

Many authors have tried to improve the classification system. Gabbe divides patients into three groups:[26] group I, gestational diabetes; group II, pregestational diabetes without complications; and group III, pregestational diabetes with complications (retinopathy, nephropathy, or vascular disease). Perinatal and maternal mortality increases with each group. Pyke's classification is similar to Gabbe's, but it incorporates glucose control as a prognostic indicator by dividing each of the aforementioned groups into (A) good control or (B) less than optimal control.[27] Pederson related poor prognosis to readily identifiable maternal characteristics, the prognostic bad signs of pregnancy (PBSP).[28-30] These are pyelonephritis, pre-coma or severe acidosis, preeclampsia (pregnancy-induced hypertension), and women who neglect prenatal care. When one or more of these are present, risk of poor pregnancy outcome is increased fourfold.[29]

SCREENING AND DIAGNOSIS OF GESTATIONAL DIABETES

Women with unrecognized, untreated gestational diabetes are at increased risk for poor pregnancy outcome.[31,32] To institute therapy, pregnant women need to be screened and diagnosed. Determining who should be screened, at what stage in gestation screening should occur, how screening should be accomplished, and how the diagnosis should be established are the center of debate.

Screening

For years, historic clinical risk factors were used to select women for a screening oral glucose challenge. These factors include family history of diabetes; maternal age greater than 30; obesity (body mass index [kg/(m)^2] ≥ 30); previous pregnancy with gestational diabetes, macrosomia, prematurity, unexplained fetal demise, stillbirth, or congenital malformations; parity of five or more; and glycosuria in the current pregnancy. When these criteria were used, they were found to have a sensitivity of 63% and a specificity of 56%.[33] Thus, 37% of women with gestational diabetes were missed. On the other hand, in an unselected indigent population, almost 40% of women had at least one of these risk factors.

Using random blood glucose determinations for screening a large pregnant population with 116 mg/dL [6.4 mmol/L] as a cutoff, 11.6% of women had elevated values.[34] In this series, using an oral glucose tolerance test (OGTT) to confirm the diagnosis, the frequency of gestational diabetes was only 0.9%, in contrast to 2–3% in other studies using universal screening.

The Second Workshop Conference on Gestational Diabetes sponsored by the American Diabetes Association (ADA) recommends that all pregnant women be screened for glucose intolerance; those not identified before the 24th week of gestation should have a 50-g oral glucose screening test between weeks 24 and 28, disregarding time of last meal or time of day; and a venous plasma glucose of 140 mg/dL [7.8 mmol/L] or more 1 hour after such a load signifies a need for a full 3-hour diagnostic oral glucose tolerance test.[32] The screening test may be repeated at 32 weeks' gestation in women at high risk for developing gestational diabetes (using the criteria outlined above) and in women who had previous positive screening results but negative OGTT results.

The American College of Obstetricians and Gynecologists (ACOG) recommends the same screening test but limits its application to women aged 30 and older and those who have the previously described risk factors.[35] Demographic and historic data on 6214 pregnant women universally screened showed that 56% with gestational diabetes were younger than 30 years. Forty-four percent of gestational diabetics had no risk factors. Thus, using the ACOG recommendation, 35% of gestational diabetes would go undiagnosed[36]; therefore, we endorse the ADA recommendation of universal screening.

Gabbe and Landon report that approximately 90% of perinatal specialists in the United States follow the ADA consensus in their practices. However, in a survey in the Los Angeles area, only a minority of general obstetricians had implemented universal screening.[37] Thus, in the United States, there seems to be a wide discrepancy between specialists and generalists concerning screening practices.

When originally described, the 50-g glucose screening test used a cutoff glucose of 130 mg/dL (7.2 mmol/L) in whole blood, with glucose measured by the Somogyi–Nelson technique. Today, most laboratories measure glucose in plasma rather than in whole blood and use the more specific glucose oxidase technique. The previous threshold of 130 mg/dL (7.2 mmol/L) in whole blood is equivalent to 143 mg/dL (7.9 mmol/L) in plasma with the glucose oxidase technique. This has been rounded off to 140 mg/dL (7.8 mmol/L) in the current recommendations.

When originally tested, this screening method yielded a sensitivity of 79% and a specificity of 87%. To increase sensitivity, a lower cutoff of 135 mg/dL (7.5 mmol/L) has been suggested.[38] This would detect an additional 15% of gestational diabetes, at the expense of performing an OGTT in 25% of the screened population versus 17% at 143 mg/dL (7.9 mmol/L).

The patient need not fast for the screening test. However, when the test was administered to women with known gestational diabetes, the result was significantly higher in patients who had fasted than those given a standard 600 kcal meal 1 hour before the test. Therefore, it has been suggested that the threshold for this challenge test be 130 mg/dL (7.2 mmol/L) when the test is administered in the fed state.[39]

Side effects of a glucose load include nausea, vomiting, abdominal bloating, and headache.[40] Vomiting will render interpretation difficult. Nausea and vomiting seem to be related to the high osmotic pressure and delayed absorption of glucose.[41] Using a more dilute solution may avoid this problem. A glucose polymer (polycose) with a smaller osmotic load than glucose is generally better tolerated and shows comparable results.[40]

Another screening tool, a 600-kcal breakfast tolerance test, uses 100 mg/dL (5.6 mmol/L) as a plasma glucose threshold. When compared to the 50-g glucose test, the sensitivity is 96%, and specificity is 74%.[42] Some have proposed that such a meal tolerance test could be used immediately for screening and diagnosis.

It would be ideal to screen on the basis of a single venous sample without any loading. The hope was that *glycosylated (glycated) hemoglobin levels* would serve this purpose. Glycation is the slow, nonenzymatic, irreversible binding of glucose or a phosphorylated sugar to hemoglobin. The glycosylated hemoglobin level reflects many weeks of glycemia. It is too insensitive for screening because of the inclusion in the window of observation of the period of normoglycemia that precedes development of gestational diabetes. In one series, glycosylated hemoglobin A1 (HbA1) was measured in 90 pregnant patients. All were screened with a 50-g glucose test, using a 140 mg/dL (7.8 mmol/L) threshold. Only four patients had an elevated HbA1, yet 18 had confirmed gestational diabetes.[43] A similar study of 806 prenatal patients, using a higher threshold of 150 mg/dL (8.3 mmol/L) on the challenge test, showed that the 1-hour glucose screening test had greater specificity, sensitivity, and predictive value for a positive diagnosis.[44]

Theoretically, glycosylated albumin, glycosylated serum protein, or fructosamine may prove to be better screening tools because these parameters reflect glycemia over several days, rather than several weeks as reflected by glycosylated hemoglobin.[45-48] However, these assessments have met with mixed reviews, and they generally lack the high sensitivity and specificity of the 50-g oral glucose load. Thus, this must remain the standard until sufficient data emerge to warrant a different consensus. What is needed, however, is a simple, convenient, inexpensive screening tool, requiring only one blood sample without glucose loading, and sufficiently high sensitivity and specificity to be used in all pregnant women.

Diagnosis

The classic criteria to establish the diagnosis of gestational diabetes are those of O'Sullivan and Mahan (Table 43–2).[49] These were initially proposed in 1963 and are still useful today. The authors performed OGTTs on 752 unselected pregnant women and analyzed the results statistically. The tests were performed with a 100-g oral glucose load, and four glucose determinations were performed: fasting and 1-, 2-, and 3-hours after consumption of glucose. An abnormal value was defined as two standard deviations above the mean for each of the four glucose values. By these criteria, gestational diabetes is defined as at least two abnormal glucose values. Two or more values were chosen to

TABLE 43–2. NORMAL LEVELS FOR ORAL GLUCOSE TOLERANCE TEST IN PREGNANCY

	Glucose mg/dL				
		Hour(s)			
OGTT[a]	Fasting	1	2	3	Specimen
NDDG[6b]	105	190	165	145	Plasma
Carpenter[38]	95	180	156	140	Plasma
O'Sullivan[49]	90	165	145	125	Whole Blood

[a] Oral glucose tolerance test.
[b] National Diabetes Data Group.

minimize laboratory error or occasional single high peaks resulting from unusually rapid absorption of glucose. In a subsequent study, a fourfold increase in perinatal mortality was demonstrated among 187 pregnancies in women with gestational diabetes diagnosed by these criteria, as compared to 259 pregnancies with normal OGTT values[50], which validated the criteria. The unique feature of the O'Sullivan data is that the women he studied have now been followed for 22–28 years.[51] Not only did the criteria predict pregnancy outcome, but they also predicted the future health of the mother, particularly the development of diabetes and of cardiovascular disease. Approximately 70% developed permanent diabetes[51,52] (Fig. 43–2). Other long-term risks include increased hypertension, hyperlipidemia, proteinuria, abnormal electrocardiograms, and cardiovascular disease.[51]

Performance of the OGTT. Preparation involves 2–3 days of unrestricted physical activity and an unrestricted diet containing at least 150 g of carbohydrates per day. Dietary priming avoids falsely high glucose values caused by carbohydrate depletion. The test is performed after an overnight fast of 8–12 hours. Patients should refrain from smoking, drinking, or eating during the test. The glucose solution should be ingested over 5 minutes, and if chilled, nausea and vomiting are less likely.

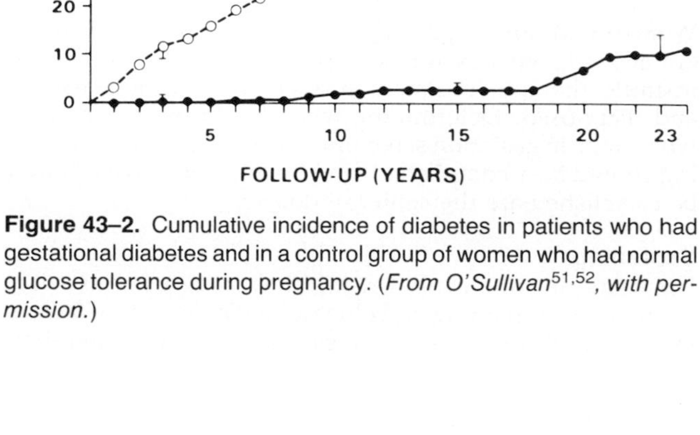

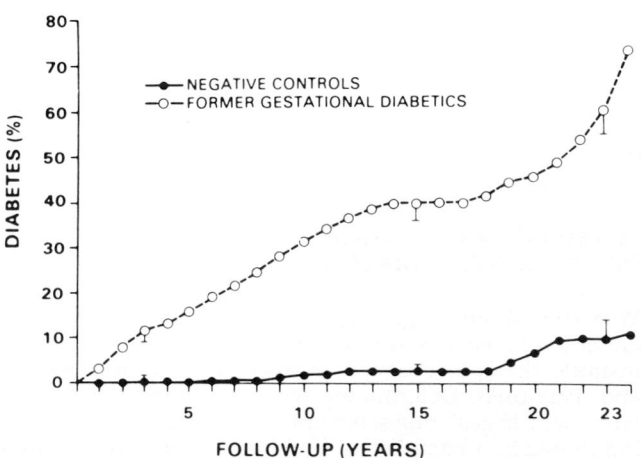

Figure 43–2. Cumulative incidence of diabetes in patients who had gestational diabetes and in a control group of women who had normal glucose tolerance during pregnancy. (*From O'Sullivan[51,52], with permission.*)

Diagnositc Criteria. O'Sullivan and Mahan measured glucose in whole blood, while today most laboratories perform glucose measurements in plasma. The latter is 14% higher than whole blood from the same sample using the same assay. As a consequence, the National Diabetes Data Group (NDDG) adjusted the O'Sullivan criteria for plasma by a 14% increase.[6] However, O'Sullivan and Mahan used the Somogyi–Nelson method to measure glucose. This method identifies other nonglucose-reducing substances (saccharides) in addition to glucose, whereas the glucose oxidase method, now commonly used, is specific for glucose. Thus, glucose values measured by the Somogyi–Nelson method are about 5 mg/dL higher than those by the glucose oxidase method. To correct for the reducing substances, Carpenter and Coustan subtracted 5 mg/dL from the original whole-blood values before adding 14% to correct for plasma.[38] Table 43–2 summarizes the original criteria and the corrections made by the NDDG and by Carpenter and Coustan.

To add to the confusion, the World Health Organization (WHO) recommends different criteria for gestational diabetes.[2] Women diagnosed with gestational diabetes by the O'Sullivan and Mahan criteria would not meet the WHO criteria, and vice versa.

Pragmatic issues also must be considered. The WHO uses a 75-g glucose load, which is more easily tolerated than the 100-g load. The WHO test spans 2 hours; the O'Sullivan takes 3 hours. The recently championed meal test is simpler, more palatable, and better tolerated than either glucose load, and it appears to be more reproducible.[53] The test meal, consisting of 453 kcal divided as 61% carbohydrate, 18% fat, and 16% protein, is more physiologic than a glucose load and thus perhaps more relevant to glucose control in pregnancy. More work is needed to establish its use as a potential replacement for an oral glucose load.

All diagnostic criteria are somewhat arbitrary. The basic question is whether the proportion of a given population is likely to develop gestational diabetes. This cannot be statistically defined or limited to a particular frequency in a specific population. Rather, the problem should be defined by outcome based on the level of glycemia that confers added risk to mother or fetus. For example, some authors have supported an increased risk with mild hyperglycemia not even fulfilling the O'Sullivan criteria. In one study, 139 pregnancies with one abnormal value on OGTT were compared to 725 randomly selected patients with a normal screen. Both macrosomia (18% frequency) and preeclampsia–eclampsia (7.9% frequency) were significantly increased in women with one abnormal OGTT value over that seen in the normal group (6.6% for macrosomia, 3.3% for preeclampsia–eclampsia).[54]

The selection of diagnostic criteria necessitates more sensitive outcome measures than used today. It requires consideration of confounding variables, such as ethnic background, maternal obesity, and nutrition. It also implies that intervention can influence outcome. We recently have used the O'Sullivan–Mahan criteria, as adapted by the NDDG (see Table 43–2). In the interim, these appear to be most appropriate.

Intravenous Glucose Tolerance Test. When a patient is intolerant of an oral glucose load, an intravenous glucose tolerance test may be used to identify gestational diabetes. The test involves an intravenous glucose load followed by measuring the disappearance curve of glucose. It is not a popular evaluation method because it is more complicated and less physiologic than the OGTT, which allows for gastrointestinal factors involved in insulin secretion.

FUEL METABOLISM IN PREGNANCY

Circulating insulin is the primary regulator of fuel metabolism. It coordinates the mobilization of fuel into and out of the various fuel storage depots to meet the needs of the organism, depending on the availability or lack of fuel in the environment. In response to nutrient input (ie, the fed state), insulin secretion is stimulated, which, in turn, stimulates the use and assimilation of substrates into their storage forms. Thus, relatively high levels of insulin herald the fed state. In contrast, in the interval between feedings (the fasted state), fuel is efficiently mobilized from storage depots to meet energy demands. Low circulating basal levels of insulin characterize the fasted state and facilitate fuel mobilization.

The availability and distribution of fuels in pregnancy change to meet the nutritional requirements of the growing fetus.[54-63] An organized sequence of hormonal adaptations ensure that glucose, the primary fuel of the fetus, is readily available. Glucose use by the fetus is substantial (as much as 6 mg/kg per minute) and is two to three times that of adults. During pregnancy, metabolic adjustments facilitate continuous delivery of glucose to the fetus in the fed and fasting states.

Glucose is transported across the placenta by facilitated diffusion.[64,65] The constant fetal use of glucose contributes to a reduced maternal plasma glucose concentration. Amino acids undergo active placental transport.[66] Alanine, the gluconeogenic amino acid, is of particular significance to blood glucose regulation. Its efflux from the maternal to the fetal compartment may contribute to decreased maternal alanine and other amino acids characteristic of pregnancy.[63]

The Fasted State

In the interval between feedings and the fasted or postabsorptive state (6–14 hours after a meal), plasma glucose levels are maintained in a narrow range because of a balance between hepatic glucose production and peripheral glucose use. These processes are regulated by insulin. Plasma insulin concentration decreases, thus permitting use of stored nutrients. Energy requirements are met by mobilizing fuel from a number of depots. In nonpregnant women, glucose is used as substrate by obligate glycolytic tissues, principally the brain. Other tissues that use glucose are blood cells, peripheral nerves, renal medulla, and to a lesser extent, skeletal muscle. However, in these, most glucose is metabolized by anaerobic glycolysis to lactate (or pyruvate), with the carbon skeleton recycled for gluconeogenesis (Cori cycle). Glucose consumption is virtually nonexistent in the rest of the body; most tissues use free fatty acids and ketoacids as substrates. Therefore, hepatic glucose output in the basal fasted state in the nonpregnant individual is principally determined by the need to provide glucose for the brain and obligate glycolytic tissue.

During pregnancy, the need for glucose is dramatically increased. Thus, there is greater activation of hepatic gluconeogenesis. Amino acids serve as a major gluconeogenic substrate, principally in the form of alanine derived from transamination of amino acids to pyruvate in muscle. They also serve as a source of delivery of amino acids to the liver (alanine cycle). The liver uses amino acids as substrate for gluconeogenesis but not for its own energy requirements. Lactate and glycerol also serve as major substrates for gluconeogenesis.

The metabolic fuel used by most tissue, apart from glucose, is derived from adipose tissue triglycerides as fatty acids or as ketones (beta-hydroxybutyrate and acetoacetate). With prolonged fasting, the brain diminishes its glucose consumption and uses ketoacids as its major substrate, requiring only a minimal amount of glucose. During pregnancy, there is a more rapid and profound mobilization of fat, with an exaggerated increase in use of fatty acids and ketones by maternal tissues.

Collectively, the modifications of fuel homeostasis during the fasted state in late pregnancy have been referred to as *accelerated starvation*.[56,57,63,67]

The Fed State

In response to nutrient input (ie, the fed state), insulin secretion is stimulated. In turn, insulin stimulates the use and assimilation of substrates into their storage forms. Thus, relatively high levels of insulin herald the fed state. These high levels are central to the control of carbohydrate metabolism; they stimulate glucose uptake and use and inhibit hepatic glucose production. In addition, some of the glucose retained in the liver is used for triglyceride formation, also stimulated by insulin. In terms of protein metabolism in the fed state, insulin enhances amino acid uptake and protein synthesis in skeletal muscle while inhibiting amino acid release and proteolysis. Regarding fat metabolism in the fed state, insulin stimulates hepatic triglyceride synthesis and very low density lipoprotein (VLDL) synthesis. Glucose use and fat deposition in adipose tissue is stimulated by insulin. Insulin promotes adipose tissue triglyceride accumulation by stimulating its synthesis and inhibiting triglyceride hydrolysis and liberation of free fatty acids. Insulin also inhibits ketogenesis.

During the fed state in pregnancy (particularly late pregnancy), there may be a greater rise in plasma glucose after ingestion of free carbohydrates[68,69], which facilitate access of ingested glucose to the fetus. The postprandial rise in triglycerides and VLDLs serve as maternal fuels.[68] This *facilitated anabolism* describes the fed state in pregnancy.[56,63,68] Thus, pregnancy magnifies the difference between the fasted and fed states.

Impact on the Mother

The effect of this redistribution of glucose and gluconeogenic substrate is a progressive decline in maternal fasting plasma glucose concentrations, from a mean of 73 ± 9 mg/dL (4.1 ± 0.5 mmol/L) in early pregnancy to a mean of 65 ± 9 mg/dL (3.6 ± 0.5 mmol/L) near term.[70] Plasma glucose levels in nondiabetic pregnant women rarely exceed 100 mg/dL (5.6 mmol/L), except in the first hour after a meal. The normal mean plasma glucose level is 82 ± 5 mg/dL (4.6 ± 0.3 mmol/L) in early pregnancy and 85 ± 5 mg/dL (4.7 ± 0.3 mmol/L) in late pregnancy (Fig. 43–3). The maximum level in nondiabetic early pregnancy is 107 ± 10 mg/dL (5.9 ± 0.6 mmol/L), and in late pregnancy, it is 114 ± 8 mg/dL (6.3 ± 0.4 mmol/L). The range of glucose excursions normally is 37 ± 8 mg/dL (2.1 ± 0.4 mmol/L) in early pregnancy and 47 ± 7 mg/dL (2.6 ± 0.4 mmol/L) in late pregnancy.[71]

Most maternal weight gain in early gestation is the result of expanded maternal fat stores.[72] Sensitivity to insulin is normal. There is only a modest increase in insulin secretion.[69,73]

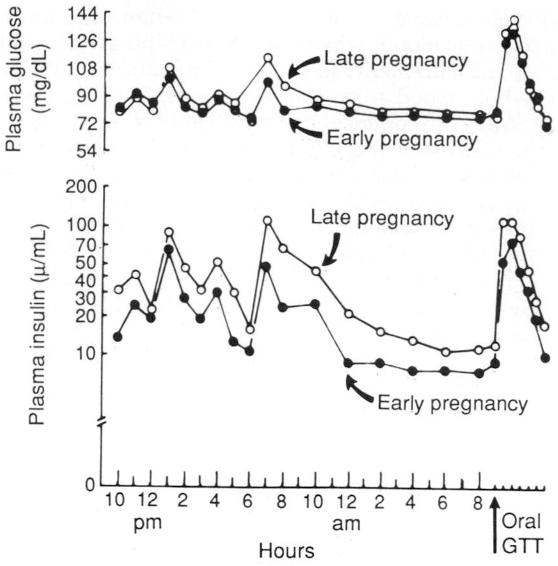

Figure 43–3. Plasma glucose and insulin concentrations during a diurnal profile and oral glucose tolerance test (OGTT) in nine nondiabetic women studied in the second and third trimesters of pregnancy. (*From Gillmer, et al*[71] *with permission.*)

Effects of Placental Hormones

As gestation progresses, the placenta produces increasing estrogen, progesterone, and human placental lactogen (human chorionic somatomammotropin) (Fig. 43–4).[74-78] These all have contrainsulin effects and are possibly responsible for the postreceptor resistance to insulin action during pregnancy (see also Chapter 37).

Placental hormone secretion is not influenced by plasma glucose excursions.[79-81] Contrainsulin effects are more obvious during the fasted state (low insulin levels) and somewhat offset by increased insulin secretion characteristic of the fed state. This all leads to availability of glucose to the fetus, a passive recipient of glucose from the mother. The primate fetal pancreas is relatively nonresponsive as long as glucose is within the physiologic range.[82-84] Sustained hyperglycemia may lead to fetal beta-cell hyperplasia and hyperinsulinemia. Thus, in the nondiabetic woman, fetal glucose parallels and is a direct function of maternal levels. Because insulin does not cross the placenta, maternal insulin is the principal arbiter of maternal (directly) and fetal (indirectly) fuel metabolism.[56]

Insulin Action in Pregnancy

In nondiabetic women, there is a progressive increase in insulin secretory response to glucose and a variety of other stimuli.[85-89] As pregnancy progresses, normoglycemia is associated with increasing circulating insulin levels.[63,85-89] Thus, pregnancy is characterized by hyperinsulinemia and euglycemia, fulfilling Berson and Yalow's definition of insulin resistance: "a state in which greater than normal amounts of insulin are required to elicit a quantitatively normal response."[90] Postpartum, the hyperinsulinemic state resolves.[85]

In a healthy human pregnancy, the blunted response to intravenous insulin further supports insulin resistance.[91,92] Progressive resistance is supported by the appearance of gestational diabetes in late pregnancy.[93] Such

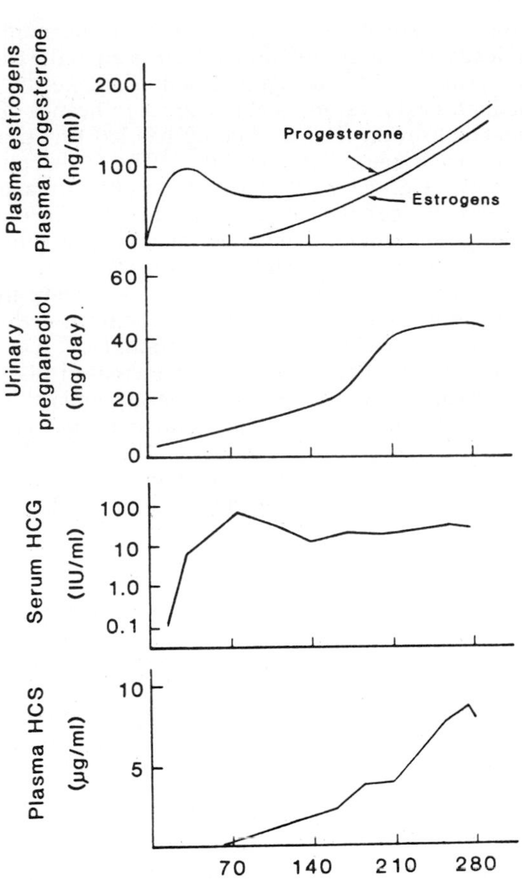

Figure 43–4. Plasma concentrations of estrogens, progesterone, human chorionic gonadotropin, human chorionic somatomammotropin, and daily urinary pregnanediol excretion during pregnancy. (*From Thau and Lanman*[78] *with permission.*)

patients often require large amounts of insulin to attain glycemic control[94], yet their condition is often cured after delivery.[49] Likewise, during pregnancy, women with IDDM require progressively increasing insulin to maintain glycemic control.[95]

The blunted response to exogenous insulin suggests a target-cell resistance to insulin action. This resistance may be caused by diminished target-cell receptors or defects beyond the initial binding of insulin, postreceptor (or postbinding) defects in insulin action. There is no decrease in insulin binding to receptors in pregnancy.[96-98] Thus, decreased binding to cellular receptors does not appear to be the cause of the insulin resistance characteristic of diabetes in pregnancy.

We have performed studies designed to characterize and quantify this resistance[99] and have confirmed that healthy human pregnancy is characterized by hyperinsulinemia and normal insulin binding to cellular receptors. Our data suggest insulin resistance is a consequence of a postreceptor defect in insulin action that resolves postpartum. Women with gestational-onset diabetes have a greater insulin resistance and a more severe defect in insulin action.

Maternal Carbohydrate Tolerance

Normal pregnancy-related alterations of insulin, glucose, and fuel dynamics impact on carbohydrate tolerance. There is blunted insulin action and increased insulin secretion in normal pregnancy. The latter parallels the fetal growth pattern.[99] Increased insulin secretion requires adequate beta-cell functional reserve. When this is exceeded, gestational diabetes mellitus emerges. Gestational diabetes should parallel the progression of pregnancy-related insulin resistance; therefore, it usually is diagnosed in the second half of pregnancy. Pregestational diabetics have a tendency to hypoglycemia and may experience ease of control in early pregnancy because of glucose use. Later, insulin requirements progressively increase, paralleling placental growth and progressive insulin resistance.[99]

MATERNAL GLYCEMIA AND FETAL MORBIDITY AND MORTALITY

Pregnancy complicated by diabetes is associated with increased perinatal morbidity and mortality. Fetal glucose is a direct function of maternal levels. When maternal diabetes is not controlled and hyperglycemia occurs, the fetus is exposed to this sustained or intermittent hyperglycemia related to meal intake. As a result, and by unresolved mechanisms, the fetal pancreatic beta cell adapts by induction of glucose-mediated insulin secretion and beta-cell hyperplasia[100,101], resulting in fetal hyperinsulinemia that parallels the prevailing maternal blood glucose.[83]

The fetal hyperinsulinemia and hyperglycemia contribute to many of the physical and morbid complications experienced by the IDMs (Fig. 43–5).[102]

Although glucose control can be related to pregnancy outcome, the view that hyperglycemia and fetal hyperinsulinemia account for all abnormalities is probably simplistic. In uncontrolled diabetes, there are abnormalities in all maternal fuels and therefore in fetal nutrient load.[56,102,103] Maternal glycemia may be only an index of overall control of diabetes, rather than the responsible mechanism. Nevertheless, maternal glycemia control is crucial for the best possible outcome of pregnancy.

Macrosomia

Fetal insulin production usually occurs after 12 weeks' gestation and is increased in uncontrolled diabetic pregnancies. Animal studies, which induce hyperinsulinemia by infusing insulin into the fetus, demonstrate that hyperinsulinemia results in increased use of transplacental nutrients and consequently increased body weight.[83,100,101] Comparing the

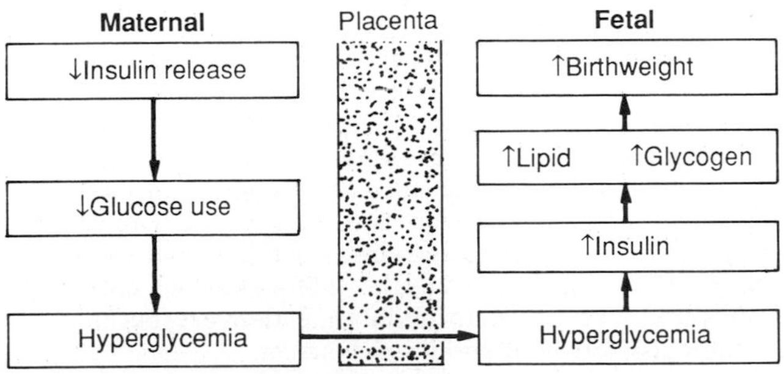

Figure 43–5. Fetal development in pregnant diabetic women. The classic hyperglycemic hyperinsulinemia hypothesis of Pedersen. Maternal hyperglycemia begets fetal hyperglycemia, which promotes fetal hyperinsulinemia. The combination of fetal hyperglycemia and hyperinsulinemia accounts for many of the morbid features of infants of diabetic mothers. (*From Freinkel and Metzger*[102] *with permission.*)

birth weight of rhesus monkey controls to those infused with low- and high-dose insulin, increasing insulin is associated with increased birth weight.[104] Several studies in human infants of diabetic mothers suggest hyperinsulinemia and increased use of nutrients are responsible for the increased body size.[102]

The mechanism whereby insulin stimulates fetal growth is not clear, but appears to be a result of the abnormal metabolic milieu to which the fetus is exposed. The Pedersen hypothesis of increased nutrient supply from the mother causing fetal hyperinsulinemia resulting in increased fetal growth appears true.[105] Fetal insulin may alter substrate entry into cells, enhancing lipogenesis, glycogen synthesis, and protein synthesis. Insulin may also act by way of receptors for insulinlike growth factors (IGF) to stimulate fetal growth (see also Chapter 37). This mechanism has been termed *receptor spillover*. Thus, fetal hyperinsulinemia can result in macrosomia, which accounts for the cherubic appearance of these infants at birth and possibly causes dystocia, complicating vaginal delivery.

Perinatal mortality of macrosomic infants is two to five times higher than in average-sized children.[106] Maternal mortality also is increased more than 10-fold in the presence of a macrosomic fetus.[105]

Control of maternal hyperglycemia is not the only factor involved in the prevention of macrosomia. Mean maternal glucose values in strictly controlled diabetic pregnancies do not correlate directly with the risk of macrosomia.[107] The fact that tight control has decreased, but not eliminated, macrosomia suggests a need for better answers. In our own institution, despite attempts at tight control, macrosomia and large-for-gestational-age (LGA) infants occur in 17% of our total diabetic group as compared to a 6–7% incidence in the total patient population. Among diabetic women with vascular disease, all tightly controlled, 25% of infants were LGA using the Lubchenko curve.[108]

This raises the issue of the definition of macrosomia. Some authors define macrosomia as babies weighing more than 4000 g. Most authors use weight related to gestational age (eg, the Lubchenko curve).[108] Others have used the macrosomia index, measured at ultrasonography by subtracting the biparietal diameter (BPD) from the average of the anteroposterior and transverse diameters of the chest. In one series, 87% of infants weighing more than 4000 g had a macrosomia index of 1.4 cm or greater; conversely, 92% of those weighing less than 4000 g had a macrosomia index of 1.3 cm or less.[109] It is clear that standarized reporting is necessary for series to be compared.

The complications of vaginal delivery of macrosomic infants can be prevented if recognized early by adequate sonographic evaluation of fetal size. A previous history of uneventful vaginal delivery of large infants, early recognition of fetal stress and distress in the presence of meconium, and careful monitoring for adequate progress of labor are helpful when vaginal delivery is contemplated. Vaginal delivery should be avoided if there is concern that the fetus is large. When an infant weighs 4500 g, serious consideration should be given to abdominal delivery because of the high risk (50%) of shoulder dystocia.[110]

Stillbirths

Unstable maternal glucose levels can lead to intrauterine deaths, previously characteristic of pregnancy in diabetic women. In the 1930s and 1940s, approximately 20% of pregnancies in diabetic women resulted in stillbirth.[111] Fetuses exposed to a hyperglycemic environment are more prone to asphyxia and acidosis. Ketoacidosis has been associated with intrauterine death. In hyperglycemic rhesus monkeys, hypoxia leads to an accumulation of lactic acid in the central nervous system and to subsequent brain damage.[112]

The increased awareness about the significance of maternal metabolism on fetal well-being has led to a proportional decrease in perinatal mortality.[113] The lowest perinatal mortality (Fig. 43–6) is associated with an average maternal blood sugar of 84 mg/dL (4.7 mmol/L). The perinatal mortality rate among diabetic women is approximately twice that of the general obstetric population.

Sonographically demonstrated fetal movement in the human is significantly decreased when maternal glucose levels are raised to 120 mg/dL (6.6 mmol/L).[114] Doppler wave form analysis has demonstrated increased placental vascular resistance with maternal hyperglycemia.[115] Oxygen delivery to the fetus is related to maternal glucose control, at least in diabetic pregnancies. Therefore, diabetic pregnancies should receive intensive fetal surveillance, especially if maternal glucose control is not optimal.

Respiratory Distress Syndrome

Because of the risk of intrauterine fetal demise and stillbirth, it was common obstetric practice in the 1940s through the 1970s to deliver IDMs at 35–37 weeks' gestation. Premature delivery was commonly associated with the presence of respiratory distress syndrome (RDS), often a consequence of hyaline membrane disease. Hyaline membrane disease in IDMs results not only from early delivery and prematurity, but also from delayed lung maturation secondary to fetal hyperinsulinemia, which inhibits pulmonary surfactant production.[116] It also may interfere with glucocorticoid enhancement of lung maturation by affecting lung production of fibroblast pneumocyte factor, which stimulates epithelial cell surfactant production.[117,118] Other factors affecting lung maturity include male sex (androgens may be inhibitory)[119-121] and asphyxia, either by direct cellular damage or by indirect effects of surfactant synthesis.[122-123] Yet only a small number of neonates with RDS have evidence of asphyxia.[124-127]

Markers of pulmonary maturation are based on measurement of phospholipids in the amniotic fluid. The lecithin–sphingomyelin (L–S) ratio was introduced in the 1970s. Measurement of other amniotic fluid phospholipids (eg, phosphatidyl glycerol) are more specific. With careful fetal surveillance and meticulous glycemic control, the risk of

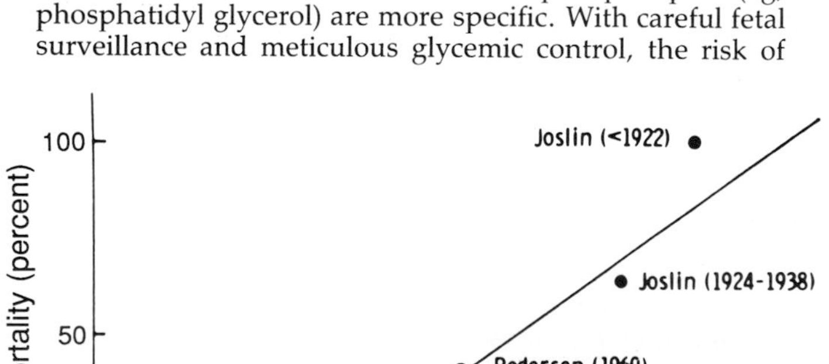

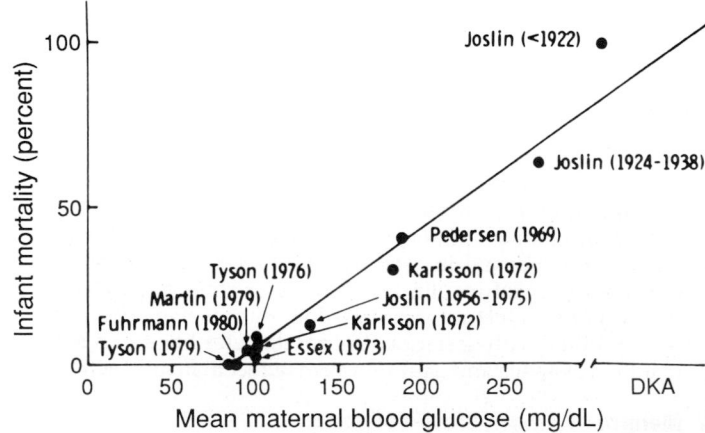

Figure 43–6. Mean maternal glucose levels versus infant mortality (1922–1980 selected series). (*From Jovanovic and Peterson[113] with permission.*)

intrauterine fetal demise and stillbirth has dramatically decreased and is almost obviated. Therefore, pregnancies are continued longer, usually to term, and RDS is almost nonexistent.

Prevention of RDS includes careful metabolic control of diabetes, expectation of spontaneous onset of labor at term, vaginal delivery, and close fetal monitoring throughout pregnancy and labor. Some factors necessitate early delivery. In some of these situations (intrauterine growth retardation, chronic fetal distress), lung maturation may be accelerated. If time permits and lungs are not mature by amniotic fluid testing, corticosteroids, thyroid-releasing hormone (TRH), or intra-amniotic thyroxin to enhance surfactant production (personal communication of K. Adamsons, University of Puerto Rico) may be considered. Corticosteroid therapy requires close monitoring of maternal glucose and increased insulin coverage.[128] An alternative treatment is TRH, which crosses the placenta to stimulate fetal TSH and subsequent thyroxine production by the fetal thyroid.[129] Thyroid hormone enhances lung maturation in the fetal rat but does not cross the placenta.[130] Umbilical cord T3 is decreased in the IDM. Whether TRH will be successful in diabetic pregnancies remains to be seen[131], but early clinical work is supportive.[132] A thyroid analogue DIMIT (3, 5-dimethyl-3′-isopropyl-L-thyronine) has been used in pregnant alloxan-induced diabetic rabbits with successful acceleration of lung maturation.[133]

Neonatal Metabolic Abnormalities

Persistence into neonatal life of the enhanced responsiveness of the fetal beta cell contributes to the infant's propensity to develop hypoglycemia after removal from the constant maternal source of glucose. The hyperinsulinemic state results in suppression of hepatic gluconeogenesis and glycogenolysis by the infant.[134] Neonatal glucose levels in term infants should be above 30–35 mg/dL and preterm infants above 20–25 mg/dL. Glucose decreases reaching a low level 1–1.5 hours after birth. Therefore, the monitoring of neonatal sugars is important. Early feeding helps prevent hypoglycemia, and glucose infusion may be necessary to treat the infant.

Hypocalcemia usually occurs on day 2–3 of life. It is generally asymptomatic and remains to be explained. Contributing factors may be immaturity of the neonatal parathyroid gland, resolving acidosis, or hypoglucagonemia.

Polycythemia, which usually is accompanied by hyperviscosity, is thought to be secondary to hypoxia with stimulation of erythropoietin and ultimate erythropoiesis.

Hyperbilirubinemia is increased in the IDM, when compared to gestational age-matched normal infants. The reason is unknown. However, polycythemia with increased red cell breakdown and turnover may contribute.

Neurobehavioral Deficits

Maternal ketonuria may be associated with significant lowering of the intelligence quotient and occurrence of neuropsychiatric deficits in offspring, particularly if the ketonuria is manifested during the third trimester.[135-139] Although these findings have been disputed by some[140], there is reason for concern. It should be noted that these often are subtle defects, which may not be appreciated until age 4 or 5 years and usually only by careful testing.

Congenital Malformations

Whether malformations are increased in the offspring of women with gestational diabetes is also controversial. However, in the progeny of women with IDDM, the rate of malformations is twofold to sixfold that of the general population.[141] They are multivaried, the most common being cardiac and neural tube defects, followed by skeletal, gastrointestinal, and urinary tract abnormalities.[142] Malformations occur during organogenesis, often before pregnancy is recognized. Factors influencing teratogenesis must be operative at the time.

The exact mechanisms by which malformations occur are unclear. Hyperglycemia before conception or during early pregnancy has been suggested.[143] Embryo cultures show disorganization of neural crest development in 100% of cases at high d-glucose levels; improvement is noted with decreased levels of glucose or with arachidonic acid.[144-150] Yolk sac developmental abnormalities also occur and may contribute to abnormal organogenesis.

Worldwide evidence supports the concepts that in early gestation, hyperglycemia is a critical determinant of the risk of congenital malformations and that meticulous glycemic control early in gestation, or preconceptionally, lessens that risk. Women who achieve good glycemic control preconceptionally or in early pregnancy have a lower malformation rate (0–3.3%) than those who enter for care later in pregnancy (6.6–10.5%).[151-155] Moreover, other studies have found a relationship between increased malformation rates and glycohemoglobin in the first trimester.[156-158] At least two centers that practice aggressive glycemic control reduced their malformation rates in IDMs to close to those of the general population. In a study from Copenhagen, the rate was 2.8%, compared to 1.7% in the general Danish population.[158] Likewise, a center in Aberdeen achieved a rate of 2.9%, compared with a 2% background malformation rate.[158]

In the American multicenter, Diabetes in Early Pregnancy Study (DIEPS), a malformation rate of 4.9% among 347 diabetic women enrolled within 21 days of conception was compared to a 9.0% rate among 279 diabetic women enrolled later. This represented a highly significant difference, supporting the concept of early enrollment and preconceptional counseling (see also Chapter 1).[141] This study was the first prospectively controlled trial to include a nondiabetic control group, in which both groups were followed concomitantly, with malformations ascertained in an identical manner. The control group (389 women) demonstrated a malformation rate of 2.1%, which was still significantly less than even that of the early enrolled diabetic group. It was therefore concluded that if glycemia contributes to malformations, there is a higher rate in late-entry than early-entry diabetic women, and the rate in both groups is higher than in nondiabetic control women.

At this point, data from five series, comparing early and late enrollment, clearly support the desirability of *planned* pregnancies and of early enrollment before conception (Table 43–3). Therefore, meticulous early pregnancy glucose control seems desirable. However, exactly how tight that control should be is still unclear.

The presence of maternal vascular disease may increase the malformation rate combined with poor glycemic control.[159] In our total pregestational diabetic population, the frequency of congenital malformations is 12.7%. The rate is, however, only 4.7% in our pregestational Class B group. This suggests an increased frequency of malformations with an increased severity of diabetes. A comparison with the general population is not available because IDMs are more carefully scrutinized. However, the malformation rate is only 3.4% in offspring of our diet-controlled gestational diabetic women.

TABLE 43–3. CONGENITAL MALFORMATION RATES IN OFFSPRING OF DIABETIC WOMEN IN FIVE SERIES COMPARING EARLY[a] AND LATE ENROLLMENT

Study	Early Enrollment Number of Malformations	Percent	Late Enrollment Number of Malformations	Percent
DIEPS[141b]	17/347	4.9	25/279	9.0
Fuhrmann[151]	2/185	1.1	31/473	6.6
Steel[152]	2/114	1.8	9/86	10.5
Goldman[153]	0 /52	0	3/31	9.6
Tamas[154]	3/92	3.3	34/479	7.1
Total	24/790	3.0	102/1348	7.6

[a] Often preconceptional.
[b] Diabetic in Early Pregnancy Study.

GLYCEMIC TARGETS

The establishment of glycemic targets for women with diabetes during pregnancy is based on several considerations. These include glucose levels that are normal in nondiabetic pregnant women, associated with the best neonatal outcome in diabetic women, associated with the lowest malformation rate among offspring of diabetic women, and achievable safely without undue risk of maternal (and also fetal) hypoglycemia. Each of these is considered below.

Normal Values in Pregnancy

As previously noted, in nondiabetic women, a progressive decline in maternal glycemia occurs during pregnancy. The fasting plasma glucose levels average 73 ± 9 mg/dL (4.1 ± 0.5 mmol/L) in early pregnancy and 65 ± 9 mg/dL (3.6 ± 0.5 mmol/L) near term.[70] Except in the first hour after a meal, plasma glucose rarely exceeds 100 mg/dL (5.6 mmol/L).

Neonatal Outcome

There has been a progressive improvement in perinatal mortality with increased awareness of, and attention to, the significance of maternal metabolism upon fetal wellbeing. In the classic study by Karlsson and Kjellmar[160], a mean maternal glucose level of more than 175 mg/dL (9.7 mmol/L) was associated with a perinatal mortality rate of 25%, while with a mean level of 115–175 mg/dL (6.4–9.7 mmol/L), the perinatal mortality rate declined to 15%. The rate was even lower (4%) when the glucose level was less than 115 mg/dL (6.4 mmol/L).[160] In a regression analysis of several series, Jovanovic estimated that the lowest perinatal mortality should be associated with a mean maternal glucose of 84 mg/dL (4.7 mmol/L) (see Fig. 43–6).[113]

Neonatal morbidity in IDMs is the concern today. An infant morbidity of 33% has been associated with a mean blood glucose of less than 110 mg/dL (6.1 mmol/L), which increased to 53% when the mean glucose was greater than 110 mg/dL (6.1 mmol/L). Significant differences also were observed for the frequency of neonatal hypoglycemia, macrosomia, and RDS. This study suggests a figure of 110 mg/dL (6.1 mmol/L) as an upper limit for mean maternal blood glucose.[161]

Malformation Rate

As discussed previously, it is unsettled what degree of glycemic control will minimize the risk of malformations. There is little information on this issue. In Furhmann's series, the 50th percentile mean blood glucose was approximately 90 mg/dL (5.0 mmol/L) in the prepregnancy group, compared to 130 mg/dL (7.2 mmol/L) in the late group.[151] In an Israeli series, first trimester mean blood glucose was 110 ± 6.9 (SD) mg/dL (6.1 ± 0.4 mmol/L) in the preconceptionally enrolled group and 163 ± 10.2 mg/dL (9.0 ± 0.6 mmol/L) in the late-entry group.[153] These two series had the lowest malformation rates among the five series summarized in Table 43–3, which suggests that malformations might be minimized with a mean maternal glucose of 110 mg/dL (6.1 mmol/L) or less.

Risk of Hypoglycemia

Although there are no direct data to that effect, maternal hypoglycemia may have an adverse influence on fetal outcome in humans. Freinkel et al found that maternal hypoglycemia has embryotoxic effects in the rat during a critical window of exposure corresponding to 16–26 days of human gestation.[162] Several authors advocate very low blood glucose targets without apparent concern about hypoglycemia.[159]

Although there are no direct data on neurologic deficits, hypoglycemia should not be disregarded. Thus both stringent glycemic targets and aversion of hypoglycemia should be the goal.

Definition of Glycemic Targets

It would seem that the standard for assessment of diabetic control in pregnancy should be the plasma glucose levels of nondiabetic pregnant women. Most recent studies used these goals, or values close to them. Whether diabetes precedes pregnancy or is diagnosed during pregnancy, the glycemic targets should be as close to normal as possible.

The attempted targets (Table 43–4) apply either to venous plasma or capillary whole blood. These are fasting glucose levels between 60 and 80 mg/dL (3.3–4.4 mmol/L) but preferably not above 90 mg/dL (5.0 mmol/L). Premeal (before lunch and dinner) glucose levels of 60–105 mg/dL (3.3–5.8 mmol/L) make it easier to keep the 2 hour postprandial value below 120 mg/dL (6.7 mmol/L). The 10:00 PM and 3:00 AM levels are targeted at 60–120 mg/dL (3.3–6.7 mmol/L). If attained, these targets should yield a 24-hour mean maternal glucose of less than 110 mg/dL (6.1 mmol/L).

MATERNAL EFFECTS OF DIABETES IN PREGNANCY

Well-controlled data, comparing obstetric complications in diabetic and nondiabetic pregnancies, are almost nonexis-

TABLE 43–4. TARGET BLOOD GLUCOSE LEVELS IN PREGNANCY

	mg/dL	mmol/L
Fasting	60–90	3.3–5.0
Preprandial	60–105	3.3–5.8
1-Hour postprandial	70–140	3.9–7.8
2-Hour postprandial	60–120	3.3–6.7
2:00 to 4:00 A.M.	Above 60	Above 3.3

tent. The following discussion reviews the literature regarding various obstetric complications in diabetic pregnancies.

Maternal Mortality

In 1882, the first published series on diabetes in pregnancy included 22 pregnancies in 15 women, most of whom apparently had gestational diabetes, and reported a 26.7% maternal mortality rate.[163] This decreased in the first major review since the discovery of insulin in 1933 to 9.3%.[164] A recent report quoted a maternal mortality rate of 0.11% from a review of 2614 diabetic pregnant patients during the past 2 decades[165], which is more than ten times the overall maternal mortality rate reported in the United States between 1970 and 1980.[166]

Hypertensive Diseases of Pregnancy

Because of inconsistencies in the definition of *Preeclampsia,* differences in the criteria for diagnosis and differences in patients reported by White's classification, it is difficult to assess the frequency of preeclampsia in diabetic pregnancies. At least two authors report that preeclampsia is not significantly increased in gestational diabetes.[167,168] In a prospective population-based study of women with gestational diabetes, the frequency of pregnancy-induced hypertension was no different than nondiabetic controls (3.8% versus 3.7%).[169] In contrast, at the University of Miami Jackson Memorial Hospital, the frequency of preeclampsia was 16.7%, which represents a twofold to threefold increase over the total patient population.[170] A thorough review of the literature by Cousins revealed a frequency of 11.7% for preeclampsia in 2968 diabetic pregnancies.[165]

There are fewer data on the frequency of preeclampsia in pregestational diabetes. Kitzmiller et al report frequency of 5% in 147 diabetic women, which was slightly higher than in his nondiabetic population (3.8%).[171] The only study with matched controls reported a twofold increase of preeclampsia.[172]

The frequency of *chronic hypertension* is increased in White Classes F, R, and RF (see also Chapters 138–141).

Preterm Labor

The spectre of sudden intrauterine fetal death prompted many obstetricians to deliver patients prematurely, especially before fetal surveillance testing was available. Therefore, data from the literature should be interpreted cautiously. Most early reports do not distinguish between iatrogenic and spontaneous preterm labor. Recent information suggests no significant increase in the incidence of preterm labor in diabetic pregnancies as compared to controls (6.2% and 7.1%, respectively).[169]

Cesarean Sections

The rate of cesarean sections is increased in gestational and pregestational diabetes. There appears to be a stepwise increase in cesarean section rates from Class A to Classes F and RF. Primary rates range from 26–47%, and total cesarean section rates range from 42–72%.[167,171] Fetal macrosomia, fetal distress, and induction of labor with an unripe cervix undoubtedly contribute to this increase.

At a New York Medical College, when allowing spontaneous labor in women with pregestational diabetes, a decrease in the cesarean section rate occurred from 40% in 1972–1973 with delivery 21 days before the calculated due date to 23% in 1974–1975 (with spontaneous labor) (Gugliucci C, O'Sullivan M, unpublished data). This was achieved without any increase in perinatal morbidity or mortality. Coustan summarized several publications and showed a wide range in cesarean section rates. At least two centers reported rates of 19% using management leading toward spontaneous labor whenever possible.[173,174] Such reduction in cesarean section rates requires careful attention to maternal glycemic control, fetal assessment, and avoidance of preterm induction unless fetal jeopardy is evident. This should be coupled with evaluation of fetal size and progress of labor to avoid the occurrence of shoulder dystocia.

Polyhydramanios

Defined as amniotic fluid volume exceeding 2000 mL, the frequency of polyhydramnios varies widely from 2.1% to more than 30%. This is probably caused by the lack of universally applicable criteria for the diagnosis. In the only report with matched controls, the frequency of polyhydramnios was higher in diabetic (29.4%) than nondiabetic women (0.99%), with no apparent etiology in 43.3% of cases.[172] The pathogenesis of polyhydramnios in diabetic pregnancies is unclear. There is no increase in fetal urine production[175] and no direct correlation between amniotic fluid glucose concentration and amniotic fluid volume.[176] Polyhydramnios is more common in poorly controlled diabetes. Pregnancies complicated by excess fluid pose a greater danger to the mother and baby. Preterm delivery is almost doubled.[171] There also is an increase in the congenital anomaly rate and a possible increase in perinatal mortality rate.[172] The frequency of polyhydramnios among diabetic women seems to be decreasing[177], perhaps reflecting the increased attention now paid to maternal glycemic control.

Pyelonephritis

Pyelonephritis is associated with a significantly increased perinatal mortality.[28] The frequency is approximately 1.0%, only slightly increased over that of the general population (0.3%).[169] Some have suggested higher rates among women with more severe diabetes (ie, White Classes C through F).[178] The expanded availability of prenatal care, with early and more frequent urine testing, may explain the decreased frequency of this infection (see also Chapter 143).

EFFECT OF PREGNANCY ON DIABETES

There is a paucity of information in the literature concerning the progression of diabetic complications in pregnancy. This is most likely because many factors influence the development of diabetic complications. It is extremely difficult to match patients with different stages of complications.

In one study, pregnant diabetic women were matched with childless controls for age, duration of disease, endogenous insulin secretion capacity, quality of blood glucose control, insulin requirements, hospitalization, and social status. Although the sample size was small (22 pairs of women), no differences could be demonstrated between the groups. Pregnancy did not result in development of retinopathy, nephropathy, or neuropathy in patients without these complications at the time of pregnancy.[179]

Diabetic Retinopathy

The effect of pregnancy on retinopathy generally depends on status before the pregnancy. A recent carefully controlled study found that pregnancy is associated with progression of retinopathy.[180] Apparent progression of retinopathy (usually transient) may occur with the introduction of meticulous glycemic control, independent of pregnancy status. Aggressive treatment of proliferative retinopathy is desirable. Patients treated with laser photocoagulation before pregnancy and who are well-controlled during pregnancy, generally do well.[181] In our population, among 26 patients who had proliferative retinopathy, three evidenced progression of disease (one received no treatment, two required laser photocoagulation and, one subsequently required vitrectomy). Most patients with nephropathy have background unproliferative retinopathy, which seldom progresses. However, macular edema and visual changes may occur when hypertension and proteinuria are present.[182]

Diabetic Nephropathy

Diabetic nephropathy is rarely seen before 10–15 years of diabetes. It is diagnosed by the presence of 300–500 mg protein per 24-hour urine in early pregnancy without infection or other causes of renal disease. Factors that significantly impact on pregnancy outcome are hypertension, especially if poorly controlled; severe proteinuria (>5 g/24h); renal failure (creatinine clearance ≤30 mL/min); serum creatinine (≥5 mg/dL); and associated arteriosclerotic heart disease.[183]

Most pregnant patients with diabetic nephropathy have increasing proteinuria, which usually returns to near prepregnancy levels postpartum. In our population with nephropathy but with no proliferative retinopathy, 50% had increasing proteinuria to 5–16 g/24 h. Some developed significant hypoalbuminemia and severe edema, which resolved very slowly postpartum and can be incapacitating. In the presence of diabetic nephropathy, creatinine clearance, which should be followed serially after establishment of baseline function in early pregnancy, may decline in one third of the patients. In our group, this occurred in 10%. The expected normal physiologic increase in creatinine clearance in pregnancy occurs in only one third of patients.[183,184] Meticulous glycemic control may decrease the degree of proteinuria or abnormality in creatinine clearance.

It is unclear what effect, if any, pregnancy has on long-term renal outcome. Progression of nephropathy does not appear to be affected by pregnancy because values return to pregestational levels in the majority of cases. Renal function returns to pregestational levels with the same progression seen in women, irrespective of pregnancy, as in men.[183,185] It is essential to control hypertension to prevent or decrease the rate of decline of renal function. The development of superimposed preeclampsia is often difficult to diagnose because of the frequently associated hypertension and proteinuria. Abnormal liver enzymes, decreasing platelets or clinical signs of either scotomata or epigastric pain are useful hints. Among 24 patients with Class F and FR disease at our institution, 50% were delivered because of a deterioration in renal status caused by severe preeclampsia.

Women with diabetic nephropathy are challenging to manage and should be cared for in a tertiary care facility. They are at risk for hypertension, nephrotic syndrome, anemia, intrauterine growth retardation, preterm delivery, and increased perinatal morbidity and mortality. Some may require renal dialysis during pregnancy.

The number of diabetic patients with renal transplants who have subsequently carried a pregnancy is small. Yet, there appears to be an increased incidence of superimposed preeclampsia (65%) over other renal transplant patients.[186] These women also are at risk for neurotropic bone and joint disease, as are all renal transplant recipients.

Coronary Artery Disease

Women with long-standing diabetes are at increased risk of coronary vascular disease.[187] These women, if pregnant, are labeled White Class H. Though the numbers are small, pregnancy has been associated with an increased maternal mortality.[188] Older pregnant women or those with long-standing diabetes should have an electrocardiogram and other indicated cardiovascular assessments early in gestation. Future developments in the management of coronary vascular disease may improve outcome. Such women may need counseling to avoid pregnancy. Moreover, the threat to maternal survival may justify termination of pregnancy (see also Chapter 133).

MANAGEMENT OF DIABETES IN PREGNANCY

Whether diabetes precedes pregnancy or is diagnosed during pregnancy, the main goal of management is the same: establish and maintain as normal an environment as possible. It is essential to achieve and maintain euglycemia. Targets are achieved by a combination of meal plan, insulin, glucose monitoring, and, when appropriate, exercise. The latter, however, varies from patient to patient, day to day, and trimester to trimester and requires patient education to manipulate calories, exercise, and insulin.

Diet

Recommended weight gain during pregnancy is 10–12 kg (22–26.5 lb), distributed as 1–2 kg during the first trimester and a progressive gain of approximately 350–400 g/wk throughout the second and third trimesters (Fig. 43–7).[189]

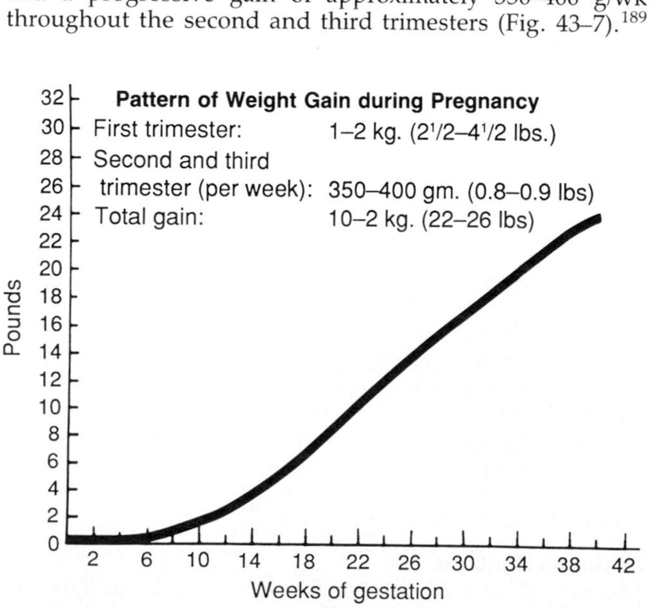

Figure 43–7. Pattern of recommended weight gain during pregnancy. (*From the National Research Council*[189] *with permission.*)

This ensures the adequacy of nutrition in both mother and fetus. Diabetes, therefore, should not influence projected weight gain.

Conventional wisdom suggests that obese women should gain weight during pregnancy. Two recent series discouraged weight gain in obese pregnant women, without apparent adverse effects.[190,191] In our experience, many obese women have such poor eating habits, that when placed on a meal plan, they tend to hold or lose weight without ketonuria when evaluated twice daily.

Caloric requirement depends on maternal age, activity, height, pregnancy weight, and stage of pregnancy. An increment of about 300 kcal/d above basal requirements should provide enough calories to meet the nutritional needs of pregnancy.[192-196] Forty-five to sixty percent of the calories (no less than 200 g, 50 g per day above nonpregnancy needs), should be in the form of carbohydrates.

The special needs of pregnancy require an additional 30 g of protein per day. Approximately 1.3 g of protein per kilogram of body weight will meet the protein needs during pregnancy; higher intakes (1.5–1.7 g/kg) are recommended for pregnant adolescents. In the meal plan, 20–30% of the kilocalories should be protein. The remainder of the calories are provided as fat.

Kilocalories are calculated as 25 kcal/kg of ideal body weight plus 100 additional kilocalories for each trimester, or 30 kcal/kg of actual body weight (not to exceed 2400 kcal), divided into three meals and two to four snacks per day (most commonly three). The heavier meals are lunch and dinner. A bedtime snack should include 25 g of carbohydrates and some protein to avert overnight hypoglycemia and starvation ketosis. Some women need two evening snacks if there is a long interval between dinner and bedtime. If urinary ketones (without glucose) occur consistently, 100 kcal are added to the preceding meal. If, despite a bedtime snack, morning ketonuria develops, an additional snack at 3:00 AM may be required.

The aim of meal planning is to limit hyperglycemia and minimize hypoglycemia and provide nutrients throughout the day that will meet the fuel requirements of the fetus. The importance of regular meals and snacks should be emphasized. The meal plan must fulfill the patient's routine (ie, night versus day work, weekends versus weekdays) and cultural food preferences. Patients should participate actively in their meal selection. Simple sugars and juices should be avoided and high fiber content foods should be encouraged. If patients keep a food diary combined with glucose levels, it will become apparent that some foods elicit different responses in different patients. They are eliminated if the response is hyperglycemia, and insulin adjustments are made as necessary.

INSULIN THERAPY

Insulin Regimens

All physiologic insulin regimens have multiple components of insulin availability, designed to coincide with each major meal and provide sustained insulin availability during the basal state overnight. Schematically depicted in Figure 43–8, these include (A) a split-mixed regimen with twice daily injections of regular- and intermediate-acting (NPH or lente)

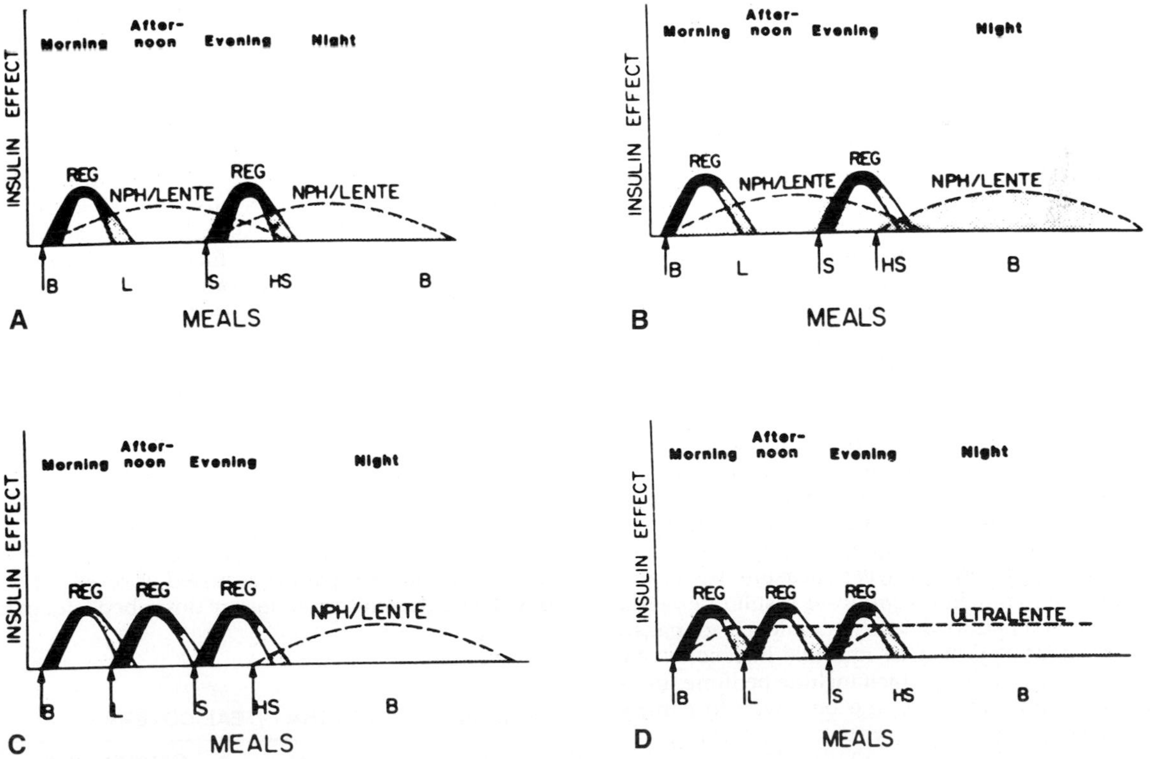

Figure 43–8. Effect of subcutaneous insulin regimens using regular (REG) insulin, intermediate-acting (NPH or LENTE) insulin, or long-acting ultralente insulin. (A) Split-mixed: Two daily doses each of regular and intermediate acting insulin. (B) Split-mixed: Evening intermediate insulin is delayed until bedtime, peak action coincides with prebreakfast glucose measurement. (C) Multiple dose: Three daily injections of regular before meals, and one of intermediate acting insulin at bedtime. (D) Multiple dose: Regular insulin before meals, and long-acting relatively peakless ultralente insulin for basal insulinemia. (B, breakfast; L, lunch; S, supper; HS, bedtime snack. Arrows indicate time of insulin injection, 30 minutes before meals.)

insulin; (B) a split-mixed regimen with a morning combination of regular- and intermediate-acting insulin, predinner regular insulin, and bedtime intermediate-acting insulin; (C) regular insulin before each meal and bedtime intermediate-acting insulin (often a small amount of intermediate-acting is included before breakfast to prevent depletion of daytime insulin); (D) regular insulin before each meal, coupled with a single daily peakless ultralente insulin to provide basal insulinemia.

Portable infusion pumps to deliver continuous subcutaneous insulin (CSII) at a basal rate in microliters of regular insulin, coupled with meal-related insulin boluses, are also used.

Pitfalls are associated with each of these regimens. In the common twice daily split-mixed regimen A, the evening intermediate-acting insulin peaks during the night, 8–10 hours after its administration. Therefore, attempts to normalize prebreakfast glucose values may result in nocturnal hypoglycemia. This risk is increased in pregnancy, when continuous glucose consumption by the fetus results in a nocturnal hypoglycemic tendency even in nondiabetic women. We rarely use this regimen during pregnancy.

With either of the split-mixed regimens, patients must eat on time, particularly lunch and dinner. A delay may result in hypoglycemia from the intermediate-acting insulin. Some patients treated with morning intermediate-acting insulin fail to attain the target glucose levels during the afternoon and may require the addition of regular insulin before lunch. With regimen C, meal delays may result in hyperglycemia from the waning effects of the previous regular insulin, unless prebreakfast intermediate-acting insulin is added. For regimen D, only beef ultralente preparations are truly peakless, but they are highly immunogenic and relatively contraindicated in pregnancy. Human ultralente often peaks about 14 hours after injection and may not last a full 24 hours. If used, some ultralente must be given in the evening (either before dinner or at bedtime) to prevent depletion of insulin overnight.

Continuous subcutaneous insulin infusion during pregnancy is controversial. Some physicians and insulin-pump manufacturers believe that glycemic control in pregnancy is best achieved with an infusion device. However, supportive evidence is lacking. In randomized studies comparing CSII and intensified conventional therapy, there was no difference in glycemic control or pregnancy outcome.[197,198] No advantages have been demonstrated with CSII during pregnancy. On the other hand, there is a unique risk of potential catheter occlusion and pump failure and consequent interruption of insulin delivery. Because there is no subcutaneous depot of insulin during CSII, this interruption imposes the risk of diabetic ketoacidosis. For this reason, CSII should be used during pregnancy only in conjunction with frequent blood glucose monitoring (no more than 4 hours between measurements) and careful attention to avoid interruption of insulin delivery.

In our opinion, insulin delivery should be managed by the more prudent approach of multiple injections. We favor regimen B or C, both of which include bedtime intermediate-acting insulin, which is the best way to control fasting glycemia.

Insulin Dose Calculation

The average insulin dose in women with pregestational diabetes in the first trimester is a total of 0.6–0.8 U/kg body weight, 0.7–0.9 U/kg and 0.8–1.2 U/kg in the second and third trimesters, respectively. Decreasing requirements in the third trimester may indicate fetal compromise and require careful fetal assessment. Only rarely will this result in early delivery.

Commonly, if using regimen B, insulin is divided as two thirds of the total dose in the morning and one third in the evening. The morning dose is subdivided into one-third regular and two-thirds intermediate-acting insulin, given 30–45 minutes before breakfast. The evening dose is divided as one-half regular insulin 30–45 minutes before dinner, and one-half intermediate-acting insulin subcutaneously between 10:00 PM and midnight, based on meal timing and daily pattern of activity. The morning regular insulin peaks approximately 2 hours after injection and provides insulinemia for breakfast and midmorning snack. It also may contribute to control of glycemia at lunch. The morning intermediate-acting insulin peaks about 8 hours after injection and provides insulinemia for part of lunch, midafternoon snack, and dinner. If its action is too late to satisfactorily control postlunch glycemia, it may be necessary to add prelunch regular insulin and reduce the morning dose of intermediate-acting insulin. The evening regular insulin provides insulinemia for dinner, while the bedtime intermediate-acting insulin provides overnight basal insulinemia and controls fasting glycemia.

Using regimen C, the total insulin dose is divided as 20–35% regular insulin, 30–45 minutes before breakfast; 18–25% regular 30–45 minutes before lunch; 18–30% regular, 30–45 minutes before dinner; and 20–25% intermediate-acting, between 10:00 PM and midnight, based on meal timing and daily pattern of activity. Each premeal dose provides insulinemia for that meal. The bedtime intermediate-acting insulin provides overnight basal insulinemia and controls fasting glycemia.

Algorithms are used to cover premeal glucose levels above the target value (Table 43–5). For each 25 mg/dL of glucose above 90 mg/dL fasting, an additional unit of regular insulin above basal is given. Following that concept, if the fasting blood sugar is 165 mg/dL, in addition to the calculated basal morning regular, the patient adds 4 U of regular insulin. The same system occurs for each 25 mg/dL above 105 mg/dL prelunch and predinner. At 3:00 AM, we cover with regular insulin if the glucose is above 150 mg/dL, following the same mg/dL, but generally to a maximum of 3 U of regular insulin. Based on additional coverage, basal insulin is increased by 10–20% until euglycemia is achieved. Once the patient's sensitivity to insulin is known, this algorithm may need minor or significant adjustment, as well as basal adjustments.

As part of the initial attempts to achieve control, if postmeal glucose is 150 mg/dL or greater, the snack is held. The blood test is repeated in 1 hour, and if glucose is below 150 mg/dL, at least half of the snack is consumed. However, if the glucose remains ≥150 mg/dL, the snack is held and the insulin or meal plan is adjusted appropriately the next day. Hypoglycemic episodes are described later in the chapter.

TABLE 43–5. ALGORITHM—MEAL COVERAGE

Units of Regular Insulin	Glucose mg/dL	
	Fasting	Prelunch, Predinner
1	91–105	106–125
2	106–125	126–150
3	126–150	157–175

The progressive increase in insulin requirements as gestation advances should be anticipated and doses should be adjusted accordingly (Fig. 43–9).[95]

Insulin in Gestational Diabetes

When to initiate insulin therapy is an area of considerable controversy. The extremes range from prophylactic insulin therapy in all women with gestational diabetes, to withholding insulin unless the fasting plasma glucose exceeds 140 mg/dL (7.8 mmol/L). Our approach operates on the assumption that the same degree of glycemic control should be attempted in these women as in those with pregestational diabetes.

There is generally less day-to-day glucose variability than in labile, pregestational diabetic women. Endogenous insulin secretion after meals may be sufficient to normalize meal-related glucose excursions. Thus, insulin regimens may be different, with less need for blood glucose monitoring several times per day.

Obese women with gestational diabetes, while following an appropriate meal plan, often have predominately fasting hyperglycemia. Therefore, when initiating insulin therapy in pregnancy in patients with only minimal elevation of the fasting plasma glucose levels (ie, less than 120 mg/dL [6.7 mmol/L] and postprandial excursions that are not high, we have successfully used intermediate-acting insulin at bedtime to normalize fasting glycemia. An initial dose might approximate 0.3–0.4 U/kg ideal body weight in lean patients and 0.5–0.7 U/kg ideal body weight in obese patients.

When fasting plasma glucose is less than 90 mg/dL (5.0 mmol/L), diurnal glycemic excursions should be examined to determine if additional insulin is required, and if it is, it is added as necessary. If initial fasting plasma glucose exceeds 120 mg/dL (6.7 mmol/L) or postprandial excursions are high (greater than 200 mg/dL [11.1 mmol/L]), the patient is started on a multiple component insulin regimen as in pregestational diabetes.

As pregnancy progresses, with increases in placental hormone production and peripheral insulin resistance, insulin requirements increase. Some obese women with gestational diabetes require as much as 2–3 U of insulin per kilogram of body weight in the third trimester.

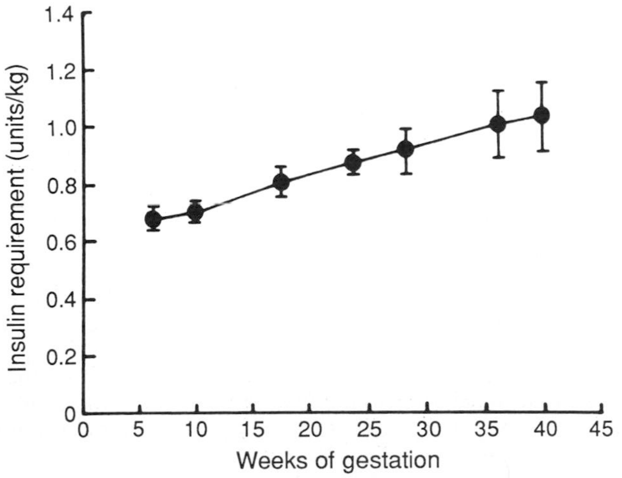

Figure 43–9. Insulin requirements during pregnancy in a group of insulin-dependent women in whom glucose was meticulously controlled. Solid dots represent the mean insulin requirement in units per kilogram per day. *(From Jovanovic, Druzin, and Peterson,[95] with permission.)*

Species of Insulin

Although free insulin does not cross the placenta[199,200], maternal anti-insulin antibodies do.[201-203] The transfer across the placenta of insulin specifically bound to maternal antibody has been described.[204] Potential adverse effects of anti-insulin antibodies in the fetus have not been proven. Nevertheless, it would seem desirable to minimize maternal anti-insulin antibody formation by using only human insulin during pregnancy. For two reasons this would seem particularly desirable in gestational diabetes: (1) There are no preexisting antibodies; and (2) adverse immunologic responses to insulin (ie, allergy or immunologic insulin resistance) are more likely to occur on rechallenge of patients with interrupted insulin therapy.[205]

Sulfonylureas. Most authorities do not use oral hypoglycemic agents during pregnancy because they stimulate fetal insulin production. They have, however, been used in some centers, especially outside the United States, without apparent adverse effects.

MONITORING OF DIABETIC CONTROL

Self-Monitoring of Blood Glucose

Because target glucose values are lower during pregnancy and exquisite glucose control is the aim, frequent monitoring of glycemia during pregnancy is necessary. In pregnant women with IDDM, we use four or more samples (preprandial and bedtime) daily as a minimum, with more complete profiles (eight or more samples, including postprandial values and a 2:00–4:00 A.M. value) at least once or twice weekly. Pregnant women are so highly motivated that they usually obtain more blood samples than requested. Because of the greater day-to-day stability of glycemia in women with NIDDM and in women with gestational diabetes, blood glucose monitoring can be less frequent in those patients.

For physiologic glucose control and because of the predictable progressive increases in insulin requirements (see Fig. 43–9), our algorithms for insulin dose regulation permit increases at a more rapid pace during pregnancy.

Urine Ketone Monitoring

Ketonuria, especially in the fasting state, may indicate starvation ketosis or nocturnal hypoglycemia. Nocturnal blood glucose monitoring and appropriate treatment, such as increasing the size of meals or snacks, are warranted.

Glycosylated Hemoglobin

Glycosylated hemoglobin (HbAlC) is used to monitor glycemic control over several weeks.[206,207] Measurement during pregnancy serves only to document that adequate glucose control is being attained. Values should fall into the normal range, although their correction may lag behind glucose by a few weeks[207] (Fig. 43–10).

A baseline HbAlC reflects previous glucose control. In the first 12–14 weeks of pregnancy, it is helpful for counseling patients because of the potential association between high HbAlC and congenital anomalies. Serially, it may serve as a cross check on home glucose-monitored patients and obviates the need for laboratory glucose measurements.

Glycosylated albumin or serum fructosamine levels reflect glycemia over a 2–3 week interval. Although used to

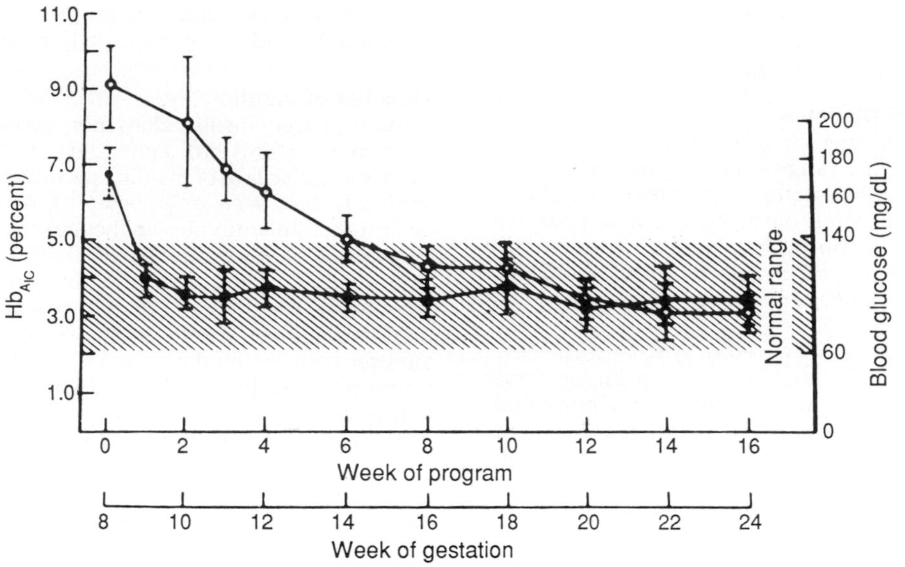

Figure 43–10. Time course for normalization of HbAIC and blood glucose for 10 insulin-dependent pregnant women treated in a program of meticulous glucose control. (*From Jovanovic and Peterson*[207] *with permission.*)

assess glycemic trends, they have not received the popularity of HbAIC.

HYPOGLYCEMIA

Because pregnant women are more prone to prolonged hypoglycemia than nonpregnant women, several groups have suggested that the episodes be treated with milk (skim or whole), rather than a simple carbohydrate.[190,208] One glass of milk provides carbohydrates, (12 g) for immediate correction of hypoglycemia, and protein, providing a more sustained source of calories and decreasing the likelihood that hypoglycemia will recur. The target is to raise the glucose above 60 mg/dL (3.3 mmol/L).

It also is possible to correct hypoglycemia with simple carbohydrates, such as cola beverages, gingerale, or honey. In more severe hypoglycemia, subcutaneous or intramuscular glucagon may be required. In the uncooperative or poorly responsive patient, honey in the buccal cavity usually raises the glucose.

EDUCATION

Most patients, regardless of socioeconomic status, who were insulin-dependent before pregnancy can be managed as outpatients to achieve reasonable control within 1 week, with fine tuning during the following week. In our setting, the patients receive individual or class teaching as outpatients and are seen in several sessions over 1–2 weeks, with contact daily or every other day. This requires dedicated personnel on-call 24 hours for patient and family support.

Even with initiation of insulin in pregnancy, patients rarely need admission for teaching and attainment of metabolic control. The patient who needs to be admitted is usually unwilling to learn or will require daily one-on-one education in all aspects of monitoring, diet, and insulin, or she is so out of control that admission for 1–3 days is desirable.

Prepregnancy Clinics

Education and attainment of glycemic control is optimally carried out before conception. Therefore, the concept of prepregnancy counseling has evolved (see also Chapter 1).

Preconceptional counseling is important for patient education, medical evaluation, and the attaining of good glycemic control. Several centers have prepregnancy clinics for diabetic patients to assess fitness for pregnancy by diagnosing retinopathy, nephropathy, hypertension, and ischemic heart disease; to ensure a planned pregnancy; to identify and treat infertility; to educate patients and their partners on good diabetes care; to obtain optimium diabetic control before conception; to identify the time of conception; to identify any gynecologic abnormality; to check immune status against rubella; and to encourage good general principles of health and hygiene.

Unfortunately, it is difficult to persuade some patients to attent a prepregnancy clinic.

SPECIAL CONSIDERATIONS IN OBSTETRIC MANAGEMENT

Fetal Evaluation

Ultrasound. Baseline sonography confirms or establishes gestational age best in the first trimester (see also Chapter 6). In the early second trimester, it is useful for detecting some major malformations. Pregestational diabetics, especially those with poor control or a history of cardiac anomalies, should have a four-chamber cardiac study and a fetal echocardiogram (16–20 weeks) when possible to determine cardiac anomalies.

Alpha-Fetoprotein. Maternal serum alpha-fetoprotein (MSAFP) should be offered as a screen for neural tube defects (NTD), which are increased 20-fold over nondiabetics.[209] Ideally performed at 15–16 (or as late as 20–21) weeks' gestation, corrections must be made for weight, race, and diabetes because values may be lower than in nondiabetics. With good control, the MSAFP may not be different from nondiabetics.[210,211] In 70–90% of cases, an elevated MSAFP suggests an open NTD (see also Chapter 16). False positive results occur in 3–4% if a cutoff of 2.5 multiples of the median (MOM) is used. If elevated, at least a high-resolution targeted ultrasound is indicated predominately to look for an NTD, although other malformations also should be sought. An amniocentesis to measure AFP and acetylcholinesterase (ACE) to confirm an NTD (false negative 0.5%) is suggested, especially when the sonogram does *not* confirm a defect.[212] Other conditions associated with an elevated ACE are omphalocoele, teratomas, Turner's syndrome and trisomy 21.[209] Counseling must consider an individual patient's wishes; some patients will not consider termination under any circumstances but still want to know, whereas others have no desire to pursue diagnostic studies because they will not abort an abnormal pregnancy. A majority of patients with a major abnormality will terminate. State laws concerning the timing of termination also must be considered.

Fetal Monitoring. In the absence of renal-vascular disease in diabetes, institution of fetal surveillance studies (eg, fetal movement counts, nonstress or stress testing, evaluation of biophysical profile, and Doppler velocimetry) should be performed based on history, glucose control, and associated medical or obstetric complications by 30–34 weeks in patients on insulin. The most important goal is to maintain fetal homeostasis by maternal metabolic control. All forms of biophysical monitoring should be used, keeping in mind that intervention is unnecessary for a healthy fetus. Serial sonography is important to assess adequacy of growth, rule out previously missed or later developed anomalies (eg, hydrocephalus), and determine amniotic fluid volume. Generally, fetuses decrease their activity as they become "ill" *in utero.* Therefore, fetal movement counts may be useful and are the least expensive of fetal status tests. A guide is a decrease to less than 10 movements in 12 hours or a 50% reduction.[213] Both nonstress testing (NST) and contraction stress testing (CST), on a serial basis, are more commonly used biophysical methods. The advantage of the NST is its noninvasiveness, ease, lack of contraindications, expense, and time required compared to a CST. The latter requires endogenous or exogenous oxytocin, is less physiologic, more expensive and time-consuming, may stimulate labor, and is relatively contraindicated in such conditions as preterm labor, premature rupture of membranes, and placenta previa. Yet, the CST is a better measure of placental reserve than the NST.[214-216]

Each can give false positive results. A nonreactive NST (less than two to four fetal movements associated with fetal heart accelerations of 15 beats per minute, lasting 15 seconds for 10–20 minutes, monitored for 40 minutes with or without stimulation or calories) occurs in approximately 10% of patients. A false positive CST (late decelerations with more than 50% of contractions) occurs at a rate of 30–50%. When comparing these two tests in relation to corrected antenatal death rates in a large survey of complicated pregnancies, the rate was 3.2 out of 1000 in the NST group, which was eightfold greater than the 0.4 out of 1000 in the CST group.[216] When selecting tests, it is important to keep in mind institutional abilities and cost. Additional testing possibilities, especially when there is an abnormal result, include acoustic stimulation, which is not widely used[217] and the biophysical profile. The latter is a good backup for the NST or the CST and evaluates fetal tone, body movement, respiratory movement, and amniotic fluid volume. It has been reported as the most reliable method of fetal assessment.[218] A score of 8 or greater (adding the NST) implies excellent fetal status, 4 or less suggests a need for delivery, and 6 is interpreted as a borderline result, requiring further exploration. Frequency of testing will depend on the test used, gestational age, and results of the last test. Generally, an NST is performed once or twice per week, CST once per week, and biophysical profiles once per week, occasionally interspersed with an NST.

Delivery. Timing of delivery should depend on maternal status, fetal status, and gestational age. With current technology for fetal surveillance and proper maternal metabolic control, spontaneous labor at term is ideal and safe for the fetus showing no evidence of jeopardy for the mother who is well controlled, with no other maternal indications requiring delivery.

In contrast, in advanced diabetes with nephropathy (F), only one third of our patients reach 37 weeks' gestation, predominantly because of complications requiring early delivery. Of those with significant retinopathy without nephropathy (R), two thirds carried for 37 weeks or more. Birth weight and gestational age at delivery for Classes F–R (1980–1987) are shown in Table 43–6. The cesarean section rate, however, was 100% in the last 10 years, as shown in Table 43–7. The perinatal mortality rate was 5.2%, with one death neonatally caused by a cardiac anomaly, and another fetal demise with severe IUGR at 27–28 weeks. Class D diabetics during the same period 74% went to ≥37 weeks but only 48% went into spontaneous labor, and only 29% delivered vaginally. The primary cesarean section rate was 57% (Table 43–8). The perinatal mortality rate (6.8%) included three fetal deaths at 28, 31, and 36 weeks and one neonatal death (cardiac anomaly with congenital herpes). In this group of advanced diabetics, despite home glucose monitoring, intensive fetal-maternal surveillance, and a concerted effort to allow as normal a pregnancy as possible, superimposed complications clearly dictated timing and method of delivery.

The majority of diabetics (gestational or pregestational), however, should be allowed to go into spontaneous labor. The mode of delivery should be dictated by the usual obstet-

TABLE 43–6. CLASSES F–R DIABETIC PREGNANCIES[a]

Class	F	FR	R
WEEKS:			
30–32	5	3	1
33–36	4	5	4
37+	3	3	9
Birth Weight (grams)			
1000–1250	—	1	—
1251–1500	2	3	—
1501–2000	5	2	—
2001–2500	2	1	2
2501–4000	3	2	10
>4000	—	2	2
Average-for-Gestational-Age	11	8	8
Small-for-Gestational-Age	—	1[b]	—
Large-for-Gestational-Age	1	2	6

[a] Jackson Memorial Hospital, 1980–1987.
[b] Stillborn—intrauterine fetal death, 27 wk, 575 g.

TABLE 43–7. CLASSES F–R DIABETIC PREGNANCIES[a]

	Method of Delivery			
Class	F	FR	R	Total
Cesarean section repeat	3	3	5	11
Primary	9	8	9	26
Total c-sections	12	11	14	37 = 100%
Indication				
Unknown		1	1	2
Failed induction (FI)	1	1		2
FI/severe PIH/renal[b]	7	5	3	15
Breech	1	2	1	4
Eyes—deterioration			2	2
Chronic fetal distress	1	1	1	3
Arrested progress	1		1	2
Previous myomectomy	1			1
Elective repeat		1	5	6

[a] Jackson Memorial Hospital, 1980–1987.
[b] Failed induction for pregnancy-induced hypertension or deteriorating renal function.

ric criteria and not necessarily by the diabetes. Excessive macrosomia usually dictates cesarean section. Therefore, careful assessment of fetal size, clinically and by sonography, should be performed in labor or just before. A previous low-segment transverse cesarean section is not a contraindication for trial of labor.

Labor and Delivery

Because most patients who go into spontaneous labor have eaten shortly before and have insulin with them, they often do not require further insulin in labor to keep the maternal glucose between 80–100 mg/dL (4.4–5.6 mmol/L).[219,220] If the level exceeds 120 mg/dL (6.7 mmol/L), an independent insulin drip (1 U regular insulin per cc of saline) may be used to titrate the glucose to the desired level using a pump, or 1 U of regular insulin per 100 cc may be added to the 5% dextrose intravenous solution. In the latter case, the amount of insulin in the solution may need adjustment up or down. For those who have not eaten or are being induced, 7.5–15 g of glucose will provide enough calories and prevent ketonuria in labor (150–300 cc of a 5% dextrose solution parenterally). Hourly capillary glucose levels should be obtained in all insulin-dependent diabetics and every 2–4 hours in those who are diet controlled. Labor should be managed actively and should be normoprogressive, with careful assessment for any evidence of fetal distress.

Insulin-dependent patients undergoing elective cesarean section should receive their usual bedtime or evening insulin the night preceding surgery. A fasting glucose should be obtained before starting the intravenous saline. If this is greater than 100–120 mg/dL (5.6–6.7 mmol/L), a glucose–insulin drip should be initiated to keep the maternal glucose between 80–100. Maternal hyperglycemia in normal and diabetic pregnancies in labor is associated with neonatal hypoglycemia, which is preventable.[134]

Whether delivery is abdominal or vaginal, if an insulin drip is used, it should be discontinued at delivery because requirements for insulin decrease rapidly after placental delivery, and the need for tight control can be relaxed.

TABLE 43–8. CLASS D DIABETIC PREGNANCIES[a]

	Number	Percent %
Labor and delivery	56	
Spontaneous labor	27	48
Inductions	14	25
Hypertensive disorders	8	
Premature rupture of membranes	3	
Unknown	3	
Vaginal delivery	16	29
Cesarean section	40	71
Primary cesarean section	32	57
Disproportion or arrested progress	11	
Fetal distress	7	
Failed induction	6	
Other	8	
Repeat	8	14

[a] Jackson Memorial Hospital, 1980–1987.

Postpartum

Postpartum management of diabetes is dictated by the maternal blood sugars, the method of delivery, and food intake. The gestational insulin-dependent diabetic almost never requires insulin postpartum. The pregestational insulin-dependent patient may not require insulin coverage for the first 24–48 hours. Initial coverage should be based on premeal sugars with the fasting starting at 120–140 mg/dL and prelunch or predinner at 140–160 mg/dL (2.8–2.9 mmol/L). A simple algorithm is 1 U regular per 25 mg/dL (7.4 mmol) above these targets. By day 2–3, split-mixed insulin is generally required. Most patients are still insulin sensitive. To prevent hypoglycemia, the initial insulin dose can be calculated as 0.25 U/kg of ideal body weight of split-mixed plus regular insulin coverage as required to maintain target levels. A meal plan with calories dictated by breast-feeding (ie, 25 kcal/kg ideal body weight [nonbreast feeding]) plus 500 kcal/day if breast-feeding is a good starting point. Thereafter, management should be dictated by the patient's need at the diabetologist's discretion.

Contraception

For the patient who is agreeable and who has completed her family, sterilization is the favored contraceptive method. Sterilization procedures can be performed for the diabetic female or her partner (see also (Chapter 1). An ideal birth control method is not available. The least likely method to produce metabolic abnormalities or infections is the barrier method, using a diaphragm or condoms and spermicidals for those desiring nonpermanent methods. The intrauterine device carries increased risk of pelvic infections, ectopic gestations, and perhaps a higher failure rate in diabetics. In addition, it is very expensive.[221-223] Among oral contraceptives available today, ie, combined low-dose triphasics or progestagen-only pills may have minimal metabolic effects on lipid metabolism and possibly carry a low risk of vascular complications in diabetics.[224-226] If oral contraceptives are prescribed, however, consideration should be given to limiting their use whenever possible to patients without vascular disease. Natural family planning, using cervical mucus to determine the fertile phase, requires a high degree of motivation of both partners but can be quite effective.

CONCLUSIONS

Although successful pregnancies in diabetic women have become a reality, management poses a continuous challenge, requiring both patient and caretaker vigilance, in a manner exemplifying shared responsibility. The short-term outcome is a healthy infant. In the long-term, the potential for enduring attitudinal and behavioral approaches to future diabetes care exist. The emphasis today is on outpatient management. The challenge for the future is to eliminate diabetes-related congenital malformations and significantly improve on neonatal morbidity.

REFERENCES

1. Gabbe SG. *Medical Complications of Pregnancy-Management of Diabetes in Pregnancy: Six Decades of Experience. Year Book of Obstetrics and Gynecology.* Chicago, IL: Year Book; 1980:37.
2. World Health Organization Expert Committee on Diabetes Mellitus. *Second Report.* Technical Report Series 646. Geneva: WHO; 1980.
3. Stowers JM, Beard RW. Special features of diabetic pregnancies and their progeny. In Keen H, Jarrett J, eds. *Complications of Diabetes.* 2nd ed. London, England: Arnold; 1982:215.
4. Skyler JS. Complications of diabetes mellitus: Relationship to metabolic dysfunction. *Diabetes Care.* 1979;2:499.
5. Skyler JS. Why control blood glucose? *Ped Ann.* 1987;16:713.
6. National Diabetes Data Group. Classification diagnosis of diabetes mellitus and other categories of glucose intolerance. *Diabetes.* 1979;28:1039.
7. World Health Organization Study Group on Diabetes Mellitus. *Technical report series 727.* Geneva: World Health Organization, 1985.
8. McMillan DE, Geevarghese PJ. Dietary cyanide and tropical malnutrition diabetes. *Diabetes Care.* 1979;2:202.
9. Tattersal RB, Fajans SS. A difference between the inheritance of classical juvenile-onset and maturity-onset type diabetes of young people. *Diabetes.* 1975;24:44.
10. Kappy MS, Spillar RP. Maturity-onset diabetes of youth in black Americans. *N Engl J Med.* 1987;316:282.
11. Skyler JS. Insulin-dependent diabetes mellitus. In: Kohler PO, ed. *Clinical Endocrinology.* New York, NY: John Wiley & Sons; 1986:491.
12. Skyler JS, Rabinovitch A. Etiology and pathogenesis of insulin-dependent diabetes mellitus. *Ped Ann.* 1987;16:682.
13. Lebovitz HE, Feinglos MN. Noninsulin-dependent diabetes mellitus. In: Kohler PO, ed. *Clinical endocrinology.* New York, NY: John Wiley & Sons, 1986:574.
14. Skyler JS. Non-insulin dependent diabetes mellitus—A clinical strategy. *Diabetes Care.* 1984;7(suppl):118.
15. Zimmet P. Type 2 (noninsulin-dependent) diabetes—An epidemiological overview. *Diabetologia.* 1982;22:**399.**
16. Zimmet P. Epidemiology of diabetes and its macrovascular manifestations in Pacific populations: The medical effects of social progress. *Diabetes Care.* 1979;2:144.
17. Porte D, Halter JB. The endocrine pancreas and diabetes mellitus. In: Williams RH, ed. *Textbook of Endocrinology.* Philadelphia, PA: WB Saunders; 1982:716.
18. Porte D, Pfeifer MA, Halter JB. Impaired B-cell function in noninsulin-dependent diabetes mellitus: The essential lesion? In: Skyler JS, ed. *Insulin Update.* Princeton, NJ: Excerpta Medica; 1982:1.
19. Olefsky JM. Insulin resistance and insulin action: An *in vitro* and *in vivo* perspective. *Diabetes.* 1981;30:148.
20. White P. Pregnancy-complicating diabetes. *Am J Med.* 1949;7:609.
21. White P. Pregnancy-complicating diabetes. *Am J Obstet Gynecol.* 1978; 130:228.
22. Hare J, White P. Gestational diabetes and the White classification. *Diabetes Care.* 1980;3:394.
23. Schwartz M, Brenner W. The need for adequate and consistent diagnostic classification for diabetes mellitus diagnosed during pregnancy. *Am J Obstet Gynecol.* 1982;143:119.
24. Leveno K, Whalley P. Dilemmas in the management of pregnancy complicated by diabetes. *Med Clin North Am.* 1982;66:1325.
25. Hare J, White P. Pregnancy in diabetes complicated by vascular disease. *Diabetes.* 1977;26:953.
26. Gabbe SG. Diabetes mellitus and pregnancy: Have all the problems been solved? *Am J Med.* 1981;70:613.
27. Essex NL, Pyke DA, Watkins PJ, et al. Diabetic pregnancy. *Br Med J.* 1973;4:89.
28. Pedersen J, Pedersen L. Prognosis of the outcome of pregnancies in diabetics: A new classification. *Acta Endocrinol.* 1965;50:70.
29. Pedersen J, Molsted-Pedersen L, Andersen B. Assessors of fetal perinatal mortality in diabetic pregnancy. *Diabetes.* 1974;23:302.
30. Pedersen J. *The Pregnant Diabetic and Her Newborn,* 2nd ed. Baltimore, MD: Williams & Wilkins; 1977:98.
31. American Diabetes Association. Workshop-Conference on Gestational Diabetes. Diabetes Care. 1980;3:399.
32. American Diabetes Association. Second Workshop-Conference on Gestational Diabetes. *Diabetes.* 1985;34(suppl):1.
33. O'Sullivan JB, Mahan CM, Charles D, Dandrow RV. Screening criteria for high-risk gestational diabetic patients. *Am J Obstet Gynecol.* 1973; 116:895.
34. Strangenberg M, Persson B, Nordlanden E. Random capillary blood glucose and conventional selection criteria for glucose tolerance testing during pregnancy. *Diabetes Research.* 1985;2:29.
35. American College of Obstetricians and Gynecologists. Management of diabetes mellitus in pregnancy. *ACOG Tech Bull.* 1986;92:1.
36. Coustan DR, Nelson C, Carpenter MW, et al. Maternal age and screening for gestational diabetes: a population-based study. *Obstet Gynecol.* 1989;73:557.
37. Gabbe SG, Landon MB. Management of diabetes mellitus in pregnancy: Survey of maternal-fetal medicine subspecialists in the United States. In: Sutherland HW, Stowers JM, Pearson DWM, eds. *Carbohydrate Metabolism in Pregnancy and the Newborn IV.* London, England: Springer-Verlag; 1989:309.
38. Carpenter MW, Coustan DR. Criteria for screening tests for gestational diabetes. *Am J Obstet Gynecol.* 1982;144:768.
39. Coustan DR, Widness JA, Carpenter MW, et al. Should the fifty-gram, one-hour plasma glucose screening test for gestational diabetes be administered in the fasting or fed state? *Am J Obstet Gynecol.* 1986;154:1031.
40. Reece EA, Holford T, Tuck S, et al. Screening for gestational diabetes: One-hour carbohydrate tolerance test performed by a virtually tasteless polymer of glucose. *Am J Obstet Gynecol.* 1987;156:132.
41. Court DJ, Stone PR, Killip M. Comparison of glucose and a glucose polymer for testing oral carbohydrate tolerance in pregnancy. *Obstet Gynecol.* 1984;64:251.
42. Coustan DR, Widness JA, Carpenter MW, et al. The "breakfast tolerance test": Screening for gestational diabetes with a standard mixed meal. *Am J Obstet Gynecol.* 1987;157:1113.
43. Shah BD, Cohen AW, May C, Gabbe SG. Comparison of glycohemoglobin determination and the one-hour oral glucose screen in the identification of gestational diabetes. *Am J Obstet Gynecol.* 1982;144:774.
44. Cousins L, Dattel BJ, Hollingsworth DR, Zettner A. Glycosylated hemoglobin as a screening test for carbohydrate intolerance in pregnancy. *Am J Obstet Gynecol.* 1984;150:445.
45. Bourgeois FJ, Harbert GM, Paulsen EP, Thiagarajah S. Glycosylated serum protein level as a screening and diagnostic test for gestational diabetes mellitus. *Am J Obstet Gynecol.* 1986;155:493.
46. Pollak A, Lischka A, Bartl W, et al. Glycated plasma proteins in normal and diabetic mothers and their offsprings. *Acta Endocrinol.* 1986; 227(suppl):141.
47. Roberts AB, Court DJ, Henley P, et al. Fructosamine in diabetic pregnancy. *Lancet.* 1983;2:998.
48. Paltieli Y, David M, Panski S, et al. Clinical usefulness of serum fructosamine levels as a screening test for gestational diabetes. *Society of Perinatal Obstetricians.* 1989. Abstract.
49. O'Sullivan JB, Mahan C. Criteria for the oral glucose tolerance test in pregnancy. *Diabetes.* 1964;13:278.
50. O'Sullivan JB, Charles D, Mahan CM, Dandrow RV. Gestational diabetes and perinatal mortality rate. *Am J Obstet Gynecol.* 1973;116:901.
51. O'Sullivan JB. Subsequent morbidity among gestational diabetic women. In: Sutherland HW, Stowers JM, eds. *Carbohydrate Metabolism in Pregnancy and the Newborn.* Edinburgh: Churchill Livingstone; 1984:181.
52. O'Sullivan JB, Mahan CM. Insulin treatment and high risk groups. *Diabetes Care.* 1980;3:482.
53. Sutherland HW, Pearson DWM, Lean MEJ, Campbell DM. Breakfast tolerance test in pregnancy. In: Sutherland HW, Stowers JM, Pearson DWM, eds. *Carbohydrate Metabolism in Pregnancy and the Newborn IV.* London, England: Springer-Verlag; 1989:267.
54. Lindsay MK, Graves W, Klein L. The relationship of one abnormal glucose tolerance test value and pregnancy complications. *Obstet Gynecol.* 1989;73:103.
55. Mintz D, Skyler J, Chez R. Diabetes mellitus and pregnancy. *Diabetes Care.* 1978;1:49.
56. Freinkel N. Of pregnancy and progeny. *Diabetes.* 1980;29;1023.
57. Freinkel N, Metzger B, Nitzan M, et al. "Accelerated starvation" and mechanisms for the conservation of maternal nitrogen during pregnancy. *Isr J Med Sci.* 1972;8:426.
58. Freinkel N, Metzer B. Some considerations of fuel economy in the fed state during late human pregnancy. In: Camerini-Davalos R, Cole H, eds. *Early Diabetes in Early Life.* New York, NY: Academic; 1975:289.
59. Metzger B, Freinkel N. Regulation of maternal protein metabolism and

gluconeogenesis in the fasted state. In: Camerini-Davalos R, Cole H, eds. *Early Diabetes in Early Life*. New York, NY: Academic; 1975:303.
60. Felig P, Lynch V. Starvation in human pregnancy: Hypoglycemia, hypoinsulinemia and hyperketonemia. *Science*. 1970;170:990.
61. Felig P, Kim Y, Lynch V, Hendler R. Amino acid metabolism during starvation in human pregnancy. *J Clin Invest*. 1972; 51:1195.
62. Felig P. Body fuel metabolism and diabetes mellitus in pregnancy. *Med Clin North Am*. 1977;61:43.
63. Freinkel N, Phelps R, Metzger B. Intermediary metabolism during normal pregnancy. In: Sutherland H, Stowers J, eds. *Carbohydrate Metabolism in Pregnancy and the Newborn*. New York, NY: Springer-Verlag; 1979:1.
64. Chinard F, Danesino V, Hartmann W, et al. The transmission of hexoses across the placenta in the human and the rhesus monkey (Macaca mulatta). *J Physiol*. 1956;132:289.
65. Simmons M, Battaglia F, Meschia G. Placental transfer of glucose. *J Dev Physiol*. 1979;1:227.
66. Young M. Placental transport of free amino acids. In Jonxis J, Visser H, Troelstra J, eds. *Nutricia Symposium: Metabolic Processes in the Fetus and Newborn Infant*. Baltimore, MD: Williams & Wilkins; 1971:97.
67. Freinkel N. Effects of the conceptus on maternal metabolism during pregnancy. In: Leibel B, Wrenshall G, eds. *On the Nature and Treatment of Diabetes*. Amsterdam: Excerpta Medica; 1965:679.
68. Freinkel N, Metzger B, Nitzan M, et al. Facilitated anabolism in late pregnancy: Some novel maternal compensations for accelerated starvation. In: Malaise W, Pirart J, eds. *Diabetes: Proceedings of the Eighth Congress of the International Diabetes Federation, International Congress Series No. 312*. Amsterdam: Excerpta Medica; 1974:474.
69. Kalkhoff R, Kissebah A, Kim H. Carbohydrate and lipid metabolism during normal pregnancy: Relationship to gestational hormone action. *Semin Perinatol*. 1978;2:291.
70. Victor A. Normal blood sugar variation during pregnancy. *Acta Obstet Gynecol Scand*. 1974;53:37.
71. Gillmer M, Beard R, Brooke F, Oakley N. Carbohydrate metabolism in pregnancy. I. Diurnal plasma glucose profile in normal and diabetic women. *Br Med J*. 1975;3:399.
72. Hytten F, Leitch I. *The Physiology of Human Pregnancy*. 2nd ed. Oxford: Blackwell Scientific; 1971.
73. Johannsson E. Plasma levels of progesterone in pregnancy measured by a rapid competitive protein binding technique. *Acta Endocrinol*. 1969; 61:607.
74. Spellacy W, Goetz F, Greenberg B, Ells J. Plasma insulin in normal "early" pregnancy. *Obstet Gynecol*. 1965;25:862.
75. De Hertogh R, Thomas K, Bietlot Y, et al. Plasma levels of unconjugated estrone, estradiol, and estriol and of HCS throughout pregnancy in normal women. *J Clin Endocrinol Metab*. 1975;40;93.
76. Josimovitch J, Kosor B, Bocella L, et al. Placental lactogen in maternal serum as an index of fetal health. *Obstet Gynecol*. 1970;36:244.
77. Pitkin R, Spellacy W. Physiologic adjustments in general, in Laboratory Indices of Nutritional Status in Pregnancy. Washington, DC: National Academy of Sciences; 1978:1.
78. Thau R, Lanman J. Endocrinological aspect of placental function. In: Gruenwald P, ed. *The Placenta and Its Maternal Supply Line: Effects of insufficiency of the fetus*. Baltimore, MD: University Books;1975:125.
79. Spellacy W, Buhi W, Schram J, et al. Control of human chorionic somatomammotropin levels during pregnancy. *Obstet Gynecol*. 1971;37:567.
80. Surmaczynska B, Nitzan M, Metzger B, Freinkel M. Carbohydrate metabolism in pregnancy. XII. The effect of oral glucose on plasma concentrations of human placental lactogen and chorionic gonadotropin during late pregnancy in normal subjects and gestational diabetics. *Isr J Med Sci*. 1974;10:1481.
81. Kuhl C, Gaede P, Klebe J, Pedersen J. Human placental lactogen concentration during physiological fluctuations of serum glucose in normal pregnant and gestational diabetic women. *Acta Endocrinol*. 1975;80:365.
82. Chez R, Mintz D, Reynolds W, Hutchinson D. Maternal–fetal plasma glucose relationships in late monkey pregnancy. *Am J Obstet Gynecol*. 1975;121:938.
83. Mintz D, Chez R, Hutchinson D. Subhuman primate pregnancy complicated by streptozotocin-induced diabetes mellitus. *J Clin Invest*. 1972; 51:837.
84. Chez R, Mintz D, Horger E III, Hutchinson D. Factors affecting the response to insulin in the normal subhuman pregnant primate. *J Clin Invest*. 1970;49:1517.
85. Spellacy WN, Goetz FC. Plasma insulin in normal late pregnancy. *N Engl J Med*. 1963;268:988.
86. Kalkhoff R, Schalch DS, Walker JL, et al. Diabetogenic factors associated with pregnancy. *Trans Assoc Am Phys*. 1964;77:270.
87. Bleicher SJ, O'Sullivan JB, Freinkel N. Carbohydrate metabolism in pregnancy. *N Engl J Med*. 1964;271:866.
88. Lind T, Billewicz WZ, Brown G. A serial study of changes occurring in the oral glucose tolerance test during pregnancy. *J Obstet Gynaecol Br Commonw*. 1973;80:1033.
89. Knopp RH, Montes A, Warth MR. Carbohydrate and lipid metabolism, in Laboratory Indices of Nutritional Status in Pregnancy. Washington, DC: National Academy of Sciences; 1978:35.
90. Berson SA, Yalow RS. Insulin "antagonists" and insulin resistance. In: Ellenberg M, Rifkin H, eds. *Diabetes Mellitus: Theory and Practice*. New York, NY: McGraw-Hill; 1970:388.
91. Burt RL. Peripheral utilization of glucose in pregnancy, III. Insulin tolerance. *Obstet Gynecol*. 1956;7:658.
92. Burt RL, Davidson IWF. Insulin half-life and utilization in normal pregnancy. *Obstet Gynecol*. 1974;43:161.
93. Mestman JH. Outcome of diabetes screening in pregnancy and perinatal morbidity in infants of mothers with mild impairment of glucose tolerance. *Diabetes Care*. 1980;3:447.
94. Roversi GD, Gargiulo M, Niolini U, et al. Maximal tolerated insulin therapy in gestational diabetes. Diabetes Care. 1980;3:489.
95. Jovanovic L, Druzin M, Peterson C. Effect of euglycemia on the outcome of pregnancy in insulin-dependent diabetic women as compared with normal control subjects. *Am J Med*. 1981;71:921.
96. Tsibris JCM, Raynor LO, Buhi WC, et al. Insulin receptors in circulating erythrocytes and monocytes from women on oral contraceptives or pregnant women near term. *J Clin Endocrinol Metab*. 1980;51:711.
97. Moore P, Lolterman O, Weyant J, Olefsky JM. Insulin binding in human pregnancy: Comparisons to the postpartum, luteal and follicular states. *J Clin Endocrinol Metab*. 1981;52:937.
98. Puavilai G, Drobny EC, Domont LA, Baumann G. Insulin receptors and insulin resistance in human pregnancy: Evidence for a postreceptor defect in insulin action. *J Clin Endocrinol Metab*. 1982;54:247.
99. Ryan EA, O'Sullivan MJ, Skyler JS. Insulin action during pregnancy: Studies with the euglycemic clamp technique. *Diabetes*. 1985;34:380.
100. Chez R, Mintz D, Hutchinson D. Carbohydrate metabolism in primate pregnancy. In: Scow R, ed. *Endocrinology: Proceedings, Fourth International Congress of Endocrinology, International Congress Series No. 273*. Amsterdam: Excerpta Medica; 1973:1057.
101. Chez R, Mintz D, Hutchinson D. The effect of theophylline on glucagon and glucose-mediated plasma insulin responses in the subhuman primate fetus and neonate. *Metal Clin Exp*. 1971;20;805.
102. Freinkel N, Metzger B. Pregnancy as a tissue culture experience: The critical implications of maternal metabolism for fetal development. In: *Pregnancy Metabolism, Diabetes and the Fetus: Ciba Foundation Symposium No. 63 (new series)*. Amsterdam: Excerpta Medica; 1979:3.
103. Metzger B, Phelps R, Freinkel N, Navickas I: Effects of gestational diabetes on diurnal profiles of plasma glucose, lipids and individual amino acids. *Diabetes Care*. 1980;3:402.
104. Susa JB, Gruppuso PA, Widness JA, et al. Chronic hyperinsulinemia in the rhesus monkey: Effects of physiologic hyperinsulinemia of fetal substrate hormones and hepatic enzymes. *Am J Obstet Gynecol*. 1984; 150:415.
105. Pedersen J. *The Pregnant Diabetic and Her Newborn*. 2nd ed. Baltimore, MD: Williams & Wilkins; 1977:56.
106. Koff AK, Potter EL. Complications associated with excessive development of the human fetus. *Am J Obstet Gynecol*. 1939;38:412.
107. Coustan DR, Berkowitz RL, Hobbins JC. Tight metabolic control of overt diabetes in pregnancy. *Am J Med*. 1980;68:845.
108. Lubchenco LO, Hansman C, Dressler M, Boyd E. Intrauterine growth as estimated from liveborn birth-weight data at 24 to 42 weeks of gestation. *Pediatrics*. 1963:793.
109. Elliott JP, Garite TJ, Freeman RK, et al. Ultrasonic prediction of fetal macrosomia in diabetic patients. *Obstet Gynecol*. 1982;60:159.
110. Acker DB, Sachs BP, Freidman RA. Risk factors for shoulder dystocia. *Obstet Gynecol*. 1985;66:762.
111. Miller HC, Hurwitz D, Kuder K. Fetal and neonatal mortality in pregnancies complicated by diabetes mellitus. *JAMA*. 1944;124:271.
112. Myers RE. Brain damage due to asphyxia: Mechanism of causation. *J Perinat Med*. 1981;9(suppl):78.
113. Jovanovic L, Peterson CM. Management of the pregnant, insulin-dependent diabetic woman. *Diabetes Care*. 1980;3:63.
114. Edelberg ST, Dierker LR, Kalhan S, et al. Decreased fetal movements with sustained maternal hyperglycemia using the glucose clamp technique. *Am J Obstet Gynecol*. 1987;156:1101.
115. Bracero L, Schulman H, Fleischer A, et al. Umbilical artery velocimetry in diabetes and pregnancy. *Obstet Gynecol*. 1986;68:654.
116. Quirk JG, Bleasdale JE. Fetal lung maturation in the pregnancy complicated by diabetes mellitus. In: DiRenzo GC, Hawkins PF, eds. *Perinatal Medicine: Updates and Controversies*. London, England: John Wiley & Sons; 1984.
117. Post M, Foros J, Smith BT. Inhibition of lung maturation by monoclonal antibodies against fibroblast-pneumocyte factor. *Nature*. 1984;308: 284.
118. Murphy BEP. Cortisol and cortisone levels in the cord blood at delivery of infants with and without the respiratory distress syndrome. *Am J Obstet Gynecol*. 1975;119:1112.
119. Torday J, Nielsen H, Fencl M, et al. Sex differences in fetal lung maturation. *Am Rev Respir Dis*. 1981;123:205.
120. Naeye R, Burt L, Wright D, et al. Neonatal mortality: The male disadvantage. *Pediatrics*. 1971;48:902.
121. Nielsòn H, Zinman H, Torday J. Dihydrotestosterone inhibits fetal rabbit pulmonary surfactant production. *J Clin Invest*. 1982;69:611.

122. Cassady G. The pathophysiologic picture of the postasphyxiated infant. In: Peckman G, Heymann M, eds. *Cardiovascular Sequelae of Asphyxia in the Newborn. 83rd Ross Conference in Pediatric Research, Columbus Ohio.* Columbus, OH: Ross Laboratories; 1982.
123. Cruz A, Buhi W, Birk S, et al. Respiratory distress syndrome with mature lecithin/sphingomyelin ratios: Diabetes mellitus and low Apgar scores. *Am J Obstet Gynecol.* 1976;126:78.
124. Duhring J, Thompson S. Amniotic fluid phospholipid analysis in normal and complicated pregnancies. *Am J Obstet Gynecol.* 1975;121:218.
125. Haukkamaa M, Nilsson C, Luukkaines T. Screening, management, and outcome of pregnancy in diabetic mothers. *Obstet Gynecol.* 1980; 55:596.
126. Gabbe S, Lowensohn R, Mestman J, et al. Lecithin/sphingomyelin ratio in pregnancies complicated by diabetes mellitus. *Am J Obstet Gynecol.* 1977;128:757.
127. Tabsh K, Brinkman C, Bashore R. Lecithin/sphingomyelin ratio in pregnancies complicated by insulin-dependent diabetes mellitus. *Obstet Gynecol.* 1982;59:353.
128. Berk J, Johnson J, Metzer W, et al. Glucocorticoids, hyperinsulinemia and fetal lung maturation. *Am J Obstet Gynecol.* 1981;139:465.
129. Rooney S, Marino P, Gobran, et al. Thyrotropin releasing hormone increases the amount of surfactant in lung lavage from fetal rabbit. *Pediatr Res.* 1979;13:623.
130. Gross I, Dynia D, Wilson C, et al. Glucocorticoid thyroid interactions in fetal rat lung. *Pediatr Res.* 1984;18:191.
131. Moya F, Mena P, Praiva E, et al. Thyrotropin releasing hormone (TRH) administration to pregnant women increases fetal T3 production. *Pediatr Res.* 1986;20:982.
132. Morales WJ, O'Brien WF, Angel JL, et al. Fetal lung maturation: the combined use of corticosteroids and thyrotropin-releasing hormone. *Obstet Gynecol.* 1989;73:111.
133. Newfield N, Melmed S. 3, 5 dimethyl-3'-isopropyl-L-thyronine therapy in diabetic pregnancy. *J Clin Invest.* 1981;68:1605.
134. Anderson O, Hertel J, Scholmolker L, et al. Influence of maternal plasma glucose concentration at delivery on the risk of hypoglycemia in infants of insulin dependent diabetic mothers. *Acta Pediatr Scan.* 1985;74:268.
135. Churchill J, Berendes H, Nemore J. Neuropsychological deficits in children of diabetic mothers: a report from the Collaborative Study of Cerebral Palsy. *Am J Obstet Gynecol.* 1969;105:257.
136. Berendes H. Effect of maternal acetonuria on I.Q. of offspring. In: Camerini-Davalos R, Cole H, eds. *Early Diabetes in Early Life.* New York, NY: Academic; 1975:135.
137. Stehbens J, Baker G, Kitchell M. Outcome at ages 1, 3, and 5 years of children born to diabetic women. *Am J Obstet Gynecol.* 1977;127:408.
138. Yssing M. Long-term prognosis of children born to mothers diabetic when pregnant. In: Camerini-Davalos R, Cole H, eds. *Early Diabetes in Early Life.* New York, NY: Academic; 1975:575.
139 Beibergeil H, Godel E, Amendt P. Diabetes and pregnancy: Early and late prognosis of children of diabetic mothers. In: Camerini-Davalos R, Cole H, eds. *Early Diabetes in Early Life.* New York, NY: Academic; 1975:427.
140. Naeye RL, Chez RA. Effects of maternal acetonuria and low pregnancy weight gain on children's psychomotor development. *Am J Obstet Gynecol.* 1981;139:189.
141. Mills JT, Knopp RH, Simpson JT, et al. Lack of relation of increased malformation rates in infants of diabetic mothers to glycemic control during organogenesis. *N Engl J Med.* 1988;318:11.
142. McCarter RJ, Keisler II, Comstock GW. Is diabetes mellitus a teratogen or a coteratogen? *Am J Epidemiol.* 1987;125:195.
143. Mills JT, Baker T, Goldman AS. Malformation in infants of diabetic mothers occur before the seventh gestational week: implications for treatment. *Diabetes.* 1979;28:292.
144. Reece EA, Pinter E, Lesanth CZ, et al. Malformations of the neural tube induced by *in vitro* hyperglycemia: an ultrastructural analysis. *Teratology.* 1985;32:363.
145. Penter E, Reece EA, Ogburn. Fetal arachidonic acid prevents hyperglycemia induced embryopathy: modifications on polyunsaturated fatty acids provide clues to pathogenesis. *Prac Soc Gyncol Invest.* 1986. Abstract.
146. Penter E, Reece EA, Teranth CZ, et al. Surface alterations of the embryogenic blood cells and the endodermal yolk sac layer under hyperglycemic conditions revealed by scanning electron microscopy. *Prac Soc Perinatal Obstet.* 1986. Abstract.
147. Penter E, Reece EA, Teranth CZ, et al. Yolk sac failure in embryopathy due to hyperglycemia: ultrastructural analysis of yolk sac differentiation associated with embryopathy in sac conceptuses under hyperglycemic conditions. *Teratology.* 1986;33:73.
148. Penter E, Reece EA, Teranth CZ, et al. Arachidonic acid prevents hyperglycemia associated yolk sac damage and embryopathy. *Am J Obstet Gynecol.* 1986;155:691.
149. Pettaway ZY, Moley KH, Vaughn WK, et al. Dose response impairment of mouse pre-embryo development in response of hyperglycemia. *Proc Soc Gynecol Invest.* 1989. Abstract.
150. Moley KH, de Cherney A, Vaughn WK, et al. Impaired development of pre-embryos from a spontaneous diabetic animal, the now obese diabetic (NOD) mouse: resolution by maternal in vivo insulin. *Proc Soc Gynecol Invest.* 1989. Abstract.
151. Fuhrmann K, Reiter H, Semmler H, et al. Prevention of congenital malformations in infants of insulin-dependent diabetic mothers. *Diabetes Care.* 1983;6:219.
152. Steel JM. Prepregnancy counselling and contraception in the insulin-dependent diabetic patient. *Clin Obstet Gynecol.* 1985;28:553.
153. Goldman JA, Dicker D, Feldberg D, et al. Pregnancy outcome in patients with insulin-dependent diabetes mellitus with preconceptional diabetic control: A comparative study. *Am J Obstet Gynecol.* 1986;155:293.
154. Tamas G, Demeter J, Baranyi E, et al. Use of NovoPen in pregnant diabetic women: First clinical experiences. Presented at the Third International Hvidore Symposium, Copenhagen, Denmark: May 28–29, 1985.
155. Lowy C, Beard RW, Goldschmidt JU. The confidential United Kingdom enquiry in the outcome of babies of diabetic mothers (1979–1980). *Diabetologia.* 1983;25:177.
156. Miller E, Hare JW, Cloherty, et al. Elevated maternal hemoglobin A_1C in early pregnancy and major congenital anomalies in infants of diabetic mothers. *N Engl J Med.* 1981;304:1331.
157. Ylinen K, Aula P, Stenman UH, et al. Risk of minor and major fetal malformations in diabetics with high haemoglobin A_1C values in early pregnancy. *Br Med J.* 1984;289:345.
158. Hare JW, Green MF, Cloherty JP, et al. First trimester glycemic risk for major malformations and spontaneous abortions. Aberdeen Colloquium, Poster Abstracts, 1988:7.
159. Pedersen LM, Tygstryes I, Pedersen J. Congenital malformations in newborn infants of diabetic women: correlations with maternal diabetes vascular complications. *Lancet.* 1964;1:1124.
160. Karlsson J, Kjellmer I. The outcome of diabetic pregnancies in relation to the mother's blood sugar level. *Am J Obstet Gynecol.* 1972;112: 213.
161. Landon MB, Gabbe SG, Piana R, et al. Neonatal morbidity in pregnancy complicated by diabetes mellitus: predictive value of maternal glycemic profiles. *Am J Obstet Gynecol.* 1987;156:1089.
162. Freinkel N, Lewis NJ, Akayawa S. The honeybee syndrome-implications of the teratogenicity of mannose in rat embryo culture. *N Engl J Med.* 1984;310:223.
163. Duncan JM. On puerperal diabetes. *Trans Obstet Soc Lond.* 1982;24:256.
164. Skipper E. Diabetes mellitus and pregnancy: a clinical and analytical study. *Quart J Med.* 1933; 2:353.
165. Causins L. Obstetric complications. In: Reece EA, Caustan D, eds. *Diabetes Mellitus in Pregnancy Principles and Practice.* Edinburgh: Churchill Livingstone; 1988:455.
166. Buehler J, Kaunitz A, Hogue C, et al. Maternal mortality in women aged 35 years or older: United States. *JAMA.* 1986;255:53.
167. Gabbe S, Mestman J, Freeman R, et al. Management and outcome of class A diabetes mellitus. *Am J Obstet Gynecol.* 1977;127:465.
168. Lavin J, Lovelace D, Miodovnik M, et al. Clinical experience with 107 diabetic pregnancies. *Am J Obstet Gynecol.* 1983;147:742.
169. Jacobson JD, Cousins L. A population-based study of maternal and perinatal outcome in patients with gestational diabetes. *Am J Obstet Gynecol.* 1989;161:981.
170. Beydoun SN. Avoidance of obstetric complications. In: Nywabid BS, Brinkman CR III, Lieb SM, eds. *Management of the Diabetic Pregnancy.* New York, NY: Elsevier; 1987:91.
171. Kitzmiller J, Cloherty J, Younger M, et al. Diabetic pregnancy and perinatal morbidity. *Am J Obstet Gynecol.* 1978;131:560.
172. Lufkin G, Nelson R, Hill L, et al. An analysis of diabetic pregnancies at Mayo Clinic, 1950–79. *Diabetes Care.* 1984;7:539.
173. Drury M, Stronge J, Foley M, et al. Pregnancy in the diabetic patient. Timing and mode of delivery. *Obstet Gynecol.* 1983;62:279.
174. Roversi G, Gargiulo M, Nicolini U, et al. A new approach to the treatment of diabetic pregnant women: report 479 cases seen from 1963–1975. *Am J Obstet Gynecol.* 1979;135:567.
175. VanOtterlo LC, Wladimiroff JW, Wallenburg HCS. Relationship between fetal urine production and amniotic fluid volume in normal pregnancy and pregnancy complicated by diabetes. *Br J Obstet Gynaecol.* 1977;84:205.
176. Spellacy WN, Buhi WC, Bradley B, et al. Maternal fetal and amniotic fluid levels of glucose, insulin and growth hormone. *Obstet Gynecol.* 41:323.
177. Ballard J, Holroyde J, Tsang R, et al. High malformation rates and decreased mortality in infants of diabetic mothers managed after the first trimester of pregnancy (1956–1978). *Am J Obstet Gynecol.* 1984; 148:1111.
178. Diamond M, Vaughn W, Salyer S. Efficacy of outpatient management of insulin-dependent diabetic pregnancies. *J Perinatol.* 1985;5:2.
179. Carstenser LL, Frast-Tarsen K, Fugleberg S, et al. Does pregnancy influence the prognosis of uncomplicated insulin-dependent diabetes mellitus? *Diabetes Care.* 1982;5:1.

180. Klein BEK, Moss SE, Klein R. Effect of pregnancy on progression of diabetic retinopathy. *Diabetes Care*. 1990;13:34.
181. Klein BEK, Klein R. Gravidity and diabetic retinopathy. *Am J Epidemicol*. 1984;119:564.
182. Sinclair S, Nelser C, Forman B, et al. Macular edema and pregnancy insulin-dependent diabetics. *Am J Ophthamol*. 1984;91:154.
183. Kitzmiller JC, Brown ER, Phillippe M, et al. Diabetic nephropathy and perinatal outcome. *Am J Obstet Gynecol*. 1981;141:741.
184. Jovanovic R, Jovanovic L. Obstetric management when normoglycemia is maintained in diabetic pregnant women with vascular compromise. *Am J Obstet Gynecol*. 1984;149:617.
185. Mogensen CE. Longterm antihypertensive treatment inhibiting progression of diabetic nephropathy. *Br Med J*. 1982;285:685.
186. Ogburn PL, Kitzmiller JL, Hare JW, et al. Pregnancy following renal transplantation in diabetes mellitus (Class T). *JAMA*. 1986;255:911.
187. Leland OS, Maki PC. Heart disease and diabetes mellitus. In: Marble A, Krall LP, Bradley RF, et al, eds. *Joslin's Diabetes Mellitus*. 12th ed. Philadelphia, PA: Lea & Febiger; 1985:553.
188. Olofsson P, Liedholm H, Sartor G, et al. Diabetes and pregnancy: a 21-year Swedish material. *Acta Obstet Gynecol Scand Suppl*. 1984; 122:3.
189. National Research Council. National Academy of Sciences, Committee on Maternal Nutrition, Food and Nutrition Board. *Clin. Obstet*. 1953.
190. Borberg C, Gillmer MDG, Brunner EJ, et al. Obesity in pregnancy: the effect of dietary advice. *Diabetes Care*. 1980;3:376.
191. Coetzee EJ, Jackson WPU. Pregnancy in established noninsulin dependent diabetics. *S Afr Med J*. 1981;60:795.
192. American College of Obstetricians and Gynecologists, Committee on Nutrition. Nutrition in Maternal Health Care, Chicago, IL: 1974.
193. Miller N, O'Sullivan M, Skyler J. Diabetes in pregnancy: nutritional management. *Perinatol/Neonatol*. 1983; 7:37.
194. Pitkin R. Nutritional influences during pregnancy. *Med Clin North Am*. 1977;61:3.
195. Jacobson H. Weight and weight gain in pregnancy. *Clin Perinatol*. 1975; 2:233.
196. National Research Council. National Academy of Sciences, Committee on Maternal Nutrition. *Maternal Nutrition and the Course of Pregnancy*. (NAS-NRC Publ 1961.) Washington DC: US Government Printing Office; 1970.
197. Coustan DR, Reece EA, Sherwin RS, et al. A randomized clinical trial of the insulin pump vs intensive conventional therapy in diabetic pregnancies. *JAMA*. 1986;255:631.
198. Kuhl C, Moller-Jensen B. Intensified insulin treatment in diabetic pregnancy. In: Sutherland HW, Stowers JM, Pearson DWM, eds. *Carbohydrate Metabolism in Pregnancy and the Newborn IV*. London, England: Springer-Verlag: 1989:161.
199. Adam P, Teramo K, Raiha H, et al. Human fetal insulin metabolism early in gestation: response to acute elevation of the fetal glucose concentration and placental transfer of human insulin-I-131. *Diabetes*. 1969;18:409.
200. Buse M, Roberts W, Buse J. The role of the human placenta in the transfer and metabolism of insulin. *J Clin Invest*. 1962;41:29.
201. Freinkel N, Goodner C. The metabolism of insulin by human placental tissue. *J Clin Invest*. 1958;37:895.
202. Spellacy W, Goetz F. Insulin antibodies in pregnancy. *Lancet*. 1963; 2:222.
203. Isles T, Farquhar J. The effect of endogenous antibody on insulin assay in the newborn infants of diabetic mothers. *Pediatr Res*. 1967;1:110.
204. Bauman W, Yalow R. Transplacental passage of insulin complexed to antibody. *Proc Natl Acad Sci USA*. 1981;78:4588.
205. Kahn C, Rosenthal A. Immunologic reactions to insulin: insulin allergy, insulin resistance, and the autoimmune insulin syndrome. *Diabetes Care*. 1979;2:283.
206. Bunn HF. Evaluation of glycosylated hemoglobin in diabetic patients. *Diabetes*. 1981;30:613.
207. Jovanovic L, Peterson CM. Clinical utility of glycosylated hemoglobin. *Am J Med*. 1981;70:331.
208. Jovanovic J, Peterson C. Optimal insulin delivery for the pregnant diabetic patient. *Diabetes Care*. 1982;5(suppl):24.
209. Wald NJ, Cuckle HS. Open NTD. In: Wald NJ, ed. *Antenatal and Neonatal Screening*. Oxford, England: Oxford University Press; 1984:25.
210. Milunsky A, Alpert E, Kitzmiller J, et al. Prenatal diagnosis of neural tube defects VIII. The importance of serum alpha fetoprotein screening in diabetic pregnant women. *Am J Obstet Gynecol* 1982;142:1030.
211. Reece RA, Davis W, Mahoney HH, et al. MSAFP in diabetic pregnancy, correlation with glycemic control. *Lancet*. 1987;1:275. Letter.
212. Report of the collaborative acetyl-cholinesterase study. Amniotic fluid acetyl-cholinesterase electrophoresis as a secondary test in the diagnosis of anencephaly and open spina bifida in early pregnancy. *Lancet*. 1981; 2:321.
213. Sadovsky E. Fetal movements and fetal health. *Semin Perinatol*. 1981; 5:131.
214. Freeman RR, Goebelsman U, Nochimson D, et al. An evaluation of the significance of a positive oxytocin challenge test. *Obstet Gynecol*. 1976;47:8.
215. Freeman RK. Contraction stress testing for primary fetal surveillance on patients at high risk for uteroplacental insufficiency. *Clin Perinatol*. 1982;9:265.
216. Freeman RK, Anderson G, Duchester W. A prospective multi-institutional study of antepartum fetal heart rate monitoring II. Contraction stress test vs nonstress test for primary surveillance. *Am J Obstet Gynecol*. 1982;143:778.
217. Smith CV, Phelan JP, Platt LD, et al. Fetal acoustic stimulation testing (The "FAS-TEST") II. A randomized clinical comparison with the nonstress test. *Am J Obstet Gynecol*. 1986;155:131.
218. Manning FA, Lange IR, Morrison I, et al. Fetal biophysical profile score and the nonstress test. A comparative trial. *Obstet Gynecol*. 1984; 64:326.
219. Goede SH, Good-Anderson B, Montoro M, et al. Insulin requirements during labor, a reappraisal. *Am J Obstet Gynecol*. 1982;144:556.
220. Jovanovic L, Peterson CM. Insulin and glucose requirements during the first stage of labor in insulin dependent diabetic women. *Am J Med*. 1983;75:607.
221. Skowby SO, Molsted-Pederson L. Intrauterine contraceptive devices for diabetics. *Lancet*. 1982;1:968.
222. Wiese J. Contraception in diabetic patients. *Acta Endocrin*. 1974; 182(suppl):87.
223. Thiery M, Van Kets H, Kierz K, et al. Intrauterine contraceptive devices used by diabetic women. *Br J Fam Plan*. 1982;8:55.
224. Skowby SO, Anderson O, Saurbrey M, et al. Oral contraception and insulin sensitivity: *In vivo* assessment in normal women and women with previous gestational diabetes. *J Clin Endocrin Metab*. 1987;64:519.
225. Radberg T, Gustafson A, Skryten A, et al. Oral contraception in diabetic women: diabetes control, serum and high density serum lipoprotein lipids during low dose progestogen, combined estrogen progestogen and non hormonal contraception. *Acta Endocrinol*. 1981;98:246.
226. Radberg T, Gustafson A, Skryten A, et al. Metabolic studies in women with previous gestational diabetes during contraceptive treatment: effects in serum lipids and high density lipoproteins. *Acta Endocrinol*. 1982;101:134.

Chapter Forty-Four
The Pineal Gland

Edward A. Zbella

44

Since the first description of the pineal gland over 2000 years ago by the anatomist Herophilus, the function and reputation of this tiny organ have been associated more with philosophic conjecture than with scientific foundation. Early anatomists regarded the pineal gland as "the valve that controlled the flow of memories, stored in the rear brain ventricle, forward to the consciousness serving part of the brain."[1] The 17th century philosopher Descartes regarded the human body as "an earthly machine presided over by the rational soul which occupied the pineal gland (seat of the soul), the little gland in the substance of the brain."[2] Another metaphysical epithet applied to the pineal gland because of its reputed ability to influence reproduction was the *chastity gland*.[3] Until the middle of the 20th century, debate about the function of the pineal gland varied between the extreme opinions that the gland was either a functionless vestige or a multipotent endocrine organ. During the last 25 years, research has confirmed that the pineal gland is a true secretory structure capable of producing a variety of biologically active substances and that pathologic tumors may arise within its structure. The precise role of the pineal gland in humans is still to be elucidated and its function in pregnancy is inferential.

ANATOMY

Embryologically, the pineal gland appears at 36 days of gestation as a small local evagination of the ependymal lining in the posterior part of the roof of the diencephalon. Later, the walls become thickened and the lumen obliterated. Shortly after birth, the gland loses all direct afferent and efferent neural connections with the brain. However, the gland continues to increase in size until 7 years of age, and it remains connected to the region by the pineal stalk.

The pineal gland derives its name from the pine cone, which it resembles in shape. It measures 5–9 mm in length, 3–6 mm in width, and 3–5 mm in thickness. The adult pineal gland weighs 100–180 mg. The gland is located beneath the posterior border of the corpus collosum, embedded between the superior colliculi.

Primary innervation and regulation of the mammalian pineal gland are derived from postganglionic sympathetic neurons consisting of noradrenergic nerve fibers that terminate in the interstitial space of the gland or on the plasma membrane of the pinealocyte. Preganglionic fibers in the superior cervical ganglion arise in the lateral column of the spinal cord. The sympathetic nerve cells are regulated by supraspinal impulses, some of which arise from a paired nucleus located in the hypothalamus just above the optic chiasm, termed the suprachiasmatic nucleus. The suprachiasmatic nucleus has an intrinsic oscillation that determines pineal and other circadian rhythms. The suprachiasmatic nucleus also receives a direct nerve input from the retina by way of the retinohypothalamic tract, which conveys information about light and dark independent of conscious perception. It is by way of this neural pathway that the retina serves to entrain the intrinsic rhythm to extrinsic rhythms.[4-6]

PHYSIOLOGY

The pineal gland contains many biologically active compounds. These include biogenic amines (norepinephrine, serotonin, histamine, melatonin, other related indoleamines, dopamine, and octopamine), peptides (gonadotropin-releasing hormone and thyrotropin-releasing hormone), and inhibitory neurotransmitters (GABA and epiphysin).[6] Melatonin was the first biologically active substance identified in the pineal gland and, hence, has been the most intensively studied. Melatonin is synthesized within the pineal parachymal cells from tryptophan. The pineal gland appears to mediate melatonin metabolism in response to light and darkness. Melatonin secretion is activated after exposure to darkness and is terminated on exposure to light.

In humans, melatonin administration causes a lowering of luteinizing hormone plasma levels, suppresses growth hormone secretion, induces drowsiness, changes the alpha-*wave pattern* on the electroencephalogram, and increases rapid-eye-movement sleep.[7-8]

With the exception of norepinephrine and dopamine, the physiologic function of other biologically active pineal substances is unclear. However, experimental evidence indicates that the pineal gland, by way of its indoleamines and polypeptides, may be affecting the synthesis and release of reproductive hormones either through a central action at the hypothalamic level or through direct action on the gonads.

The pineal gland has been implicated in the control of timing of a number of events in the reproductive cycle, including ovulation, puberty, and the onset of breeding. Not until 20 years ago was information available on whether the pineal gland affected parturition or whether pregnancy influenced pineal metabolism and function. The first observation of such a relationship was of decreased pineal weight in late pregnancy in rats bearing 10 or more embryos, and this was thought to indicate depressed pineal activity.[9] Other investigators noted increased pineal metabolic activity in guinea pigs during the latter half of pregnancy.[10] Nir and Hirschmann[11] noted that neither the basic pineal metabolism as reflected in nucleic acid and protein contents nor the hormonal indoleamines appeared to change during pregnancy.

There were, however, other indications associating the pineal gland with fertility and gestation. Rodents exposed to continuous darkness, to short daily photoperiods, or to decreased light intensity throughout pregnancy demonstrated significantly shorter lengths of gestation than controls in normal lighting.[12-13] Long daily photoperiods were reported to delay parturition. Pinealectomy did not abolish the effects of short photoperiods on the duration of gestation, which implies that the effect of darkness on gestation may not be mediated by the pineal gland. Neither exposure to low-intensity light, blinding, injection of melatonin, nor pinealectomy before fertilization had any subsequent effect on the number of offspring or length of gestation.[14-16] Significantly fewer living fetuses were found in animals pinealectomized during pregnancy than in controls.[17]

There are data on sheep to suggest that the pineal is functional in fetal life and that its activity may increase in the last 5 days of gestation, as indicated by the development of the capacity to both synthesize and to store melatonin at this time.[18] Melatonin also has been shown to cross into the fetus from the maternal circulation. It has been postulated that increased fetal pineal activity may affect the fetal hypothalamic-pituitary-adrenal axis involved in the timing of parturition.

Evidence implicating increased pineal activity in the human during pregnancy has included observations of increasing levels of melatonin in amniotic fluid before term and of high levels of melatonin excreted in maternal urine in the immediate delivery and postnatal period.[19-20] Women at 35–39 weeks' gestation were found to have significantly higher plasma melatonin levels than nonpregnant women or pregnant women at an earlier gestational age.[21]

There also is evidence that the rat pineal gland mediates an inhibitory visual reflex operating on milk ejection, probably by effecting the release of oxytocin induced by suckling.[22]

PATHOLOGY

Calcification of the pineal gland is a natural process that begins in childhood and apparently increases with age.

The calcified gland generally becomes visible on skull roentgenograms at puberty. This feature provides a pineal landmark to identify abnormal positional shifts of the pineal gland associated with an intracranial mass. The reported incidence of pineal calcifications is quite variable. Black people appear to have a lower incidence of pineal calcification.[23] It has been reported in the gerbil that exposure to constant light reduces calcium deposits, whereas blinding results in an increased number of concretions.[24]

In the past, calcification was taken as a sign of degeneration and involution of the pineal gland. However, studies of pineal enzyme activity have not shown any difference between calcified aged glands and glands without calcifications in young subjects.[24] Some reports even postulate that the formation of acervuli may reflect elaboration and secretion of pineal hormones, involving mechanisms similar to those linking calcium with secretion of posterior pituitary hormones.[25-26]

Pineal tumors are rare, composing 0.2–10% of brain neoplasms in caucasians and 2.7–4.5% in Japanese.[27-28] The histologic distribution of cell type is as follows: the parenchymal tumors, pinealcytoma and pinealblastoma, 30%; atypical teratomas, 23%; and nonparenchymal tumors, such as teratomas, 12%, gliomas, 23%, and cysts; and miscellaneous, 12%.[27,29,30]

Tumors occur most often in young men and only rarely in women. Consequently, the problem is rare in pregnancy. The earlier symptoms are those associated with increased intracranial pressure, such as headaches, nausea, and altered sensorium. Symptoms related to the cerebellum or to the motor system imply rapid spread of the tumor or a late stage of the disease process. The most common physical findings are associated with Parinaud's syndrome, which consists of upward gaze, pupillary areflexia arc to light, paralysis of convergence, and a wide-based gait. Rarely, pineal tumors cause hypothalamic dysfunction, which may be manifested by diabetes insipidus and consequent hypernatremia.

Precocious puberty was first associated with pineal tumors at the end of the 19th century. It has been noted that 10–15% of precocious men have a pineal tumor. However, pineal tumors associated with precocious puberty in women are extremely rare. Interestingly, hypogonadism or delayed puberty also is associated with pineal tumors.

A few case reports have noted choriocarcinoma of the pineal gland associated with high hCG secretion.[6,31]

Radiation therapy has been the standard mode of treatment for pineal tumors. Treatment protocols for pinealomas include entire brain irradiation of up to 40 Gy delivered over 4–5 weeks with a boosting dose of up to 55 Gy in 5.5–6 weeks. Surgical excision of these tumors is associated with a high mortality and, therefore, is not routinely used. Chemotherapeutic agents have been used infrequently.[6,29]

In pregnancy, there has been no report of a pineal tumor. However, choriocarcinoma of the pineal gland has been reported.[32]

REFERENCES

1. Altschule MD, ed. *Frontiers of Pineal Physiology*. Cambridge, MA: MIT Press; 1975:1.
2. Rolleston HD. The endocrine organs in health disease with a historical review. Oxford: Oxford University Press; 1936:452.
3. Reiter RJ, Fraschini F. Endocrine aspects of the mammalian pineal gland: a review. *Neuroendocrinology*. 1969;5:219.
4. Reiter RJ. Pineal regulation of hypothalamicopituitary axis gonadotropins. In: Knoble E, Sawyer WH, eds. *Handbook of Physiology, Endocrinology*. Part 2. Washington, DC: American Physiological Society; 1974:519.
5. Kappers JA, Smith AR, DeVries RAC. The mammalian pineal gland and its control of hypothalamic activity. In: Swaab DF, Schade JP, eds. *Progress in Brain Research*. Amsterdam: Elsevier; 1974:149.
6. Wurtman RJ, Cardinal DP. The pineal organ. In: Williams RH, ed. *Textbook of Endocrinology*. Philadelphia, PA: WB Saunders; 1981:625.
7. Wetterberg L. Melatonin in humans: physiological and clinical studies. *J Neural Transm*. 1978;13(suppl):289.
8. Watson SJ, Maden J. Melatonin and other pineal substances: psychiatric and other neurological implications. In: Usdin E, Hamburg DA, Barchas JD, eds. *Neuroregulators and Psychiatric Disorders*. New York, NY: Oxford University Press; 1977:193.
9. Huang CY, Everitt AV. The effect of pregnancy on pineal weight in the rat. *J Endocrinol*. 1965;32:261.
10. Vollrath L, Schmidt DS. Enzyme histochemical studies on the pineal gland of normal and pregnant guinea pigs. *Histochemie*. 1969;20:328.
11. Nir I, Hirschmann N. A possible role of the pineal gland in pregnancy and fertility. In: Matthews CD, Seamark RF, eds. *Pineal Function*. New York, NY: Elsevier/North-Holland Biomedical Press; 1981:421.
12. Ellendort F, Smidt D. Der Einfluss unterschiedlicher Belevchtung auf die neurosekretorische Akitvitat, Pubertat und Sexualfunktion von Mausen. *J Neurovisc Rel*. 1971;10(suppl):220.
13. Mitchell JA, Yochim JM. Influence of environmental lighting on duration of pregnancy of the rat. *Endocrinology*. 1971;87:472.
14. Tigchelaar PV, Nalbandov AV. The effect of pineal gland on ovulation and pregnancy in the rat. *Biol Reprod*. 1975;13:461.
15. Reiter RJ, Rudeen PK, Vaughn MK. Restoration of fertility in light-deprived female hamsters by chronic melatonin treatment. *J Comp Physiol*. 1976;111:7.
16. Misono H, Sensol N. Lack of effects of melatonin administration and pinealectomy on the milk ejection response in the rat. *Endocrinol Jpn*. 1970;17:417.
17. Guerra MO, Silva NOF, Gruimaraes CS, et al. Pinealectomy and blindness during pregnancy in the rat. *Am J Obstet Gynecol*. 1973;115:582.
18. Kennaway DJ, Matthews CD, Seamark RF, et al. On the presence of the melatonin in pineal glands and plasma of foetal sheep. *J Steroid Biochem*. 1977;8:559.
19. Mitchel MD, Sayers L, Keirse MJWC, et al. Melatonin in amniotic fluid during human parturition. *Br J Obstet Gynaecol*. 1978;85:684.
20. Grishenko VF, Demidenko DI, Koyada LD. Melatonin excretion at the end of pregnancy during normal labour and in postpartum women. *Akush Ginelol (Mosk)*. 1976;5:27.
21. Kennaway DJ, Matthews CSD, Seamark RF. Pineal function in pregnancy: studies in sheep and man. In: Matthews CD, Seamark RF, eds. *Pineal Function*. New York, NY: Elsevier/North-Holland Biomedical Press; 1981:123.
22. Prilvsky J, Deis RP. Inhibition of milk ejection by a visual stimulus in lactating rats: implication of the pineal gland. *Brain Res*. 1982;251:313.
23. Adeloye A, Felson B. Incidence of normal pineal gland calcification in skull roentagenograms of black and white Americans. *Am J Roentgenol*. 1974;122:503.
24. Welsh ML. Effects of superior cervical ganglionectomy, constant light, and blinding on the gerbil pineal gland: an ultrastructural analysis. *Anat Rec*. 1977;187:746.
25. Wurtman RJ, Axelrod J, Barchas JD. Age and enzyme activity in the human pineal. *J Clin Endocrinol Metab*. 1964;244:299.
26. Otani T, Gyorkey F, Farrell G. Enzymes of the human pineal body. *J Clin Endocrinol Metab*. 1968;28:349.
27. Obrador S, Soto M, Guttierrez-Diaz JA. Surgical management of tumors of the pineal gland. *Acta Neurochir*. 1976;34:159.
28. Arki C, Matsumoto SL. Statistical reevaluation of pinealoma and related tumors in Japan. *J Neurosurg*. 1979;30:146.
29. DeGrolami V. In: Shcmidek HH, ed. *Pineal Tumors*. New York, NY: Masson USA; 1977:1.
30. Greitz T. Tumors of the quadrigeminal plate and adjacent structures. *Acta Raadiol*. 1972;12:513.
31. Tod PA, Porter AJ, Jamieson KG. Pineal tumors. *Am J Roentgenol*. 1974;120:19.
32. Wass JA, Jones AE, Rees LH, et al. HCG beta producing pineal choriocarcinoma. *Clin Endocrinol*. 1982;17:423.

Chapter Forty-Five

Abnormal Hormone Production

Ilan Tur-Kaspa and Alan M. Neuman

45

Pregnancy is a dynamic state with complex normal metabolic and physiologic changes. The magnitude of these changes can mask and complicate the diagnosis of ectopic and abnormal hormone production. Nevertheless, early detection of abnormal hormone production in pregnancy is crucial because it may be associated with tumors and may affect the mother, the fetus, or both.

DEFINITION

Abnormal (eutropic) production of hormone refers to abnormal secretion of a hormone by the gland, or by a tumor of the gland, that normally secretes that hormone.[1] Hormone produced by tissue other than the endocrine gland that normally secretes it, represents *ectopic* hormone production. Table 45–1 depicts the criteria for the diagnosis of ectopic hormone production.[1,2] A spectrum of endocrine syndromes are associated with tumors derived from nonendocrine tissues. Increased awareness of the existence of such syndromes and the development of more sensitive and sophisticated techniques for detection and analysis of biologically active hormones make it possible to distinguish between *ectopic* and *abnormal* hormone production. For example, excessive androgen production by ovarian stroma in response to an invasion by a tumor represents abnormal (not ectopic) hormone production. Both ectopic and abnormal production of hormones in pregnancy may thus result in virilization of the mother or masculization of the fetus.[3,4] Hyperthyroidism, associated with high human chorionic gonadotropin (hCG) secreted by a trophoblastic tumor, also is an example of abnormal hormone production with possible maternal complications. Cervical carcinoma, secreting adrenocorticotropic hormone (ACTH)[5] or parathyroid hormone[6], and leiomyosarcoma of the small intestine, producing beta-hCG[7], are true ectopic hormone production syndromes.

INCIDENCE

The actual incidence of abnormal or ectopic hormone production during pregnancy is not known. It is estimated that less than 10% of patients with malignant tumors may have ectopic hormone production.[1] However, cancer is not common during the reproductive age, and thus it is rare in pregnancy.[8] The diagnosis of abnormal hormone production in pregnancy is less frequent than in the nonpregnant general population. True ectopic hormone production in pregnancy has not yet been reported.

PATHOGENESIS

The pathogenesis of ectopic hormone production is not clear. A variety of mechanisms have been postulated to explain this unique phenomenon. All somatic cells in the body contain the same genetic information. However, during the course of embryonic growth and development, these totopotential cells are programmed to express only certain segments of their respective genome. This results in the formation of specialized tissues and organ systems with well-defined hormonal products and functions. The theories of *dedifferentiation*[1] and *derepression*[9] refer to the return, partial or complete, to a totopotential state. Under these circumstances, genetic material that is not normally transcribed or translated becomes expressed by the affected cell. The hormone product may be identical to one produced elsewhere or may be slightly different, but it retains biologic or immunologic properties.

Warner's theory of cell hybridization refers to the fusing of malignant cells with normal neuroectodermal cells, resulting in a mixed hormone secreting phenotype.[10]

The ability of different tissues to secrete the same peptide hormone may occur because many cells are embryologically related to the precursors of normal endocrine tissues. This is the *APUD hypothesis* (amine precursor uptake and decarboxylation).[1] Neurosecretory granules, found in these cells, possess the biosynthetic pathways to produce peptide hormone. ACTH production, associated with cancer of the cervix[5,11], is an example of such a mechanism.

Oncogenes have been suggested as a trigger mechanism for the development of cancer in normal cells. This hypothesis also may explain the development of ectopic hormone production in humans. Growth factors, chromosomal translocations, and point mutations also have been implicated in the production of ectopic hormones.[12,13] It has been suggested that the immunologic mechanisms that are beneficial to the survival of the fetal allograft within the maternal immune system also may add to the "survival" of cancer.[14] Therefore, pregnancy also may influence the natural course of tumors associated with hormone production.[15]

VIRILIZATION IN PREGNANCY

Maternal virilization and masculinization of female fetuses may occur because of excess production of androgens by ovarian tumors. Because the tumor may be stimulated by hCG, this abnormal androgen production usually develops during or after the third month of pregnancy. Various degrees of maternal virilization may be caused by different durations of exposure to excess androgen. The clinical course may be one of rapid onset of generalized hirsutism, deepening and cracking of a woman's voice, acne, and enlargement of the clitoris.[16-20] When a virilization syndrome, or even excessive hirsutism develops during pregnancy, extraovarian causes must be excluded. These can include Cushing's syndrome or adrenal carcinoma. The possibility that drugs, such as androgens or progestins, cause virilization also should be considered.

The twofold to threefold increase in maternal serum testosterone and androsterone levels during normal pregnancy complicates the diagnosis of abnormal androgen production. Sex hormone-binding globulin, which binds testosterone, also is markedly elevated in the maternal circulation. An increased urinary excretion of 17-ketosteroids in pregnancy often is associated with abnormal androgen produc-

TABLE 45–1. CRITERIA FOR DIAGNOSIS OF ECTOPIC HORMONE PRODUCTION IN PREGNANCY

1. Presence of an endocrine syndrome in a pregnant woman with malignancy
2. Disappearance of the syndrome when the tumor is removed
3. Immunologic or histochemical localization of higher concentration of hormone in tumor cells than in adjacent normal tissue
4. Increased venous concentration of the hormone across the tumor vascular bed
5. Demonstration of hormone production by tumor cells *in vitro*
6. Recurrence of the syndrome with tumor regrowth or metastasis

tion.[21] Ultrasound is helpful for the diagnosis of ovarian or adrenal tumors. Recently, magnetic resonance imaging (MRI) also was used for the diagnosis of adrenal tumors in pregnancy.[22]

In utero exposure to excess androgens may masculinize the female fetus. Maternal tumors secreting androgens should be considered in the differential diagnosis of female newborns with *pseudohermaphroditism.* Because the external female phenotype is not completed until 140 days of fetal age, early androgen excess (7–12 weeks) may fully masculinize, whereas late exposure to androgen (18–29 weeks) may create limited ambiguity in the appearance of the female urogenital sinus and genital folds. The size of the clitoris depends on the quantity, rather than the timing, of androgen excess.[23]

Malignancy occurs in up to 5.7% of pregnancy-associated ovarian tumors.[24] With virilization, the malignancy rate increases dramatically to 50%. Reported tumors are arrhenoblastomas, granulosa–theca cell tumors, Krukenberg tumors, and ovarian mucinous cystoadenocarcinomas.[16] Benign dermoid tumors, luteomas of pregnancy, and Brenner tumors also may be associated with virilization in pregnancy. Because the possibility of malignancy is high, surgical exploration and histologic examination of the excised tissue are mandatory.

Following resection of the tumor, the virilization syndrome, including abnormal urinary and blood androgen levels, usually regresses, with the exception of hoarseness.[16] At least some of the virilizing tumors are stimulated by hCG. This is why virilizing features may start with pregnancy. Because the period of virilization is short, the prognosis is relatively good when the androgenic source is removed.[20]

ECTOPIC PRODUCTION OF CHORIONIC GONADOTROPIN COMPLICATING THE DIAGNOSIS OF PREGNANCY

Human chorionic gonadotropin is a placental hormone that maintains corpus luteum function during the early stages of gestation. Human chorionic gonadotropin also is a well-known tumor marker for malignant trophoblastic diseases and germ cell tumors. However, ectopic hormone production of alpha- or beta-subunits of hCG also has been associated with a variety of other tumors, including carcinoma of the lung or the breast, adenocarcinoma of the gastrointestinal tract, hepatoma, and melanoma.[1,25]

Beta-hCG and hCG are widely used for early diagnosis of pregnancy. Dynamics of hCG also are used for the diagnosis and monitoring of ectopic pregnancies and miscarriages.[26,27] Ectopic or abnormal hCG production may cause a false-positive pregnancy test.[7,28,29]

Ectopic hCG production may be mainly of the beta[28] or the alpha subunit.[29] Meredith et al[7] described a 22-year-old patient with primary leiomyosarcoma of the small bowel who presented with symptoms of nausea and vomiting, similar to hyperemesis gravidarum in a pregnant woman. She was found to have elevated levels of serum beta-hCG, which were localized later to the leiomyosarcoma cells. Morimoto et al[29] reported the discordance or quantitative discrepancy of hCG titrations among different types of immunologic pregnancy tests. These differences could be used to recognize the biologically inactive free subunit of hCG produced by a tumor. False-positive pregnancy tests also may be caused by heterophilic antibodies in the patient's serum that interfere with the immunoassays.[30] All these false-positive pregnancy tests may result in unnecessary diagnostic procedures.

Choriocarcinoma associated with a viable pregnancy is rare. The difficulty in establishing a diagnosis of this tumor, when associated with pregnancy, is considerable.[31]

CLINICAL SYNDROMES OF ECTOPIC HORMONE PRODUCTION

The clinical presentation of ectopic hormone production is frequently not as specific as in primary endocrinopathies.

Ectopic ACTH production has been described for a variety of tumors including oat-cell carcinoma of the lung, carcinoids, thymomas, pheochromocytomas, and cervical cancer.[1,5] Muscle weakness, hypokalemia, hyperpigmentation, and muscle wasting are commonly observed. Other classic symptoms of Cushing's syndrome, such as truncal obesity, hypertension, amenorrhea, purple abdominal striae, glucosuria, edema, and osteoporosis, however, are frequently absent. The ACTH secreted by these tumors differs from endogenous ACTH in some amino acids. The difference in the clinical course also may be caused by the rapidity of the development of the syndrome.[1]

Hypoglycemia can be induced by neoplastic states through the *production of ectopic insulin.* Symptoms include cold sweats, hypotension, confusion, weakness, apathy, and coma. Tumors associated with this occurrence include fibrosarcoma, mesothelioma, leiomyosarcoma, adrenal tumor, hepatocellular carcinoma, and cervical cancer.[1,32]

The development of nonpituitary *hyperthyroidism* is associated primarily with trophoblastic tumors but also may result from ectopically produced thyroid hormone by a *stroma ovarii* tumor. The thyrotropic activity seen in trophoblastic states probably is the result of elevated hCG rather than aberrant TSH synthesis. Patients clinically present with smooth skin, increased pulse pressure, tachycardia, tremor, and possibly a small goiter.[1]

Hyponatremic syndromes from ectopically produced antidiuretic hormone (*ADH*) have been observed in association with small-cell carcinoma of the lung, tumors of the pancreas and duodenum, thymomas, and lymphomas. Presenting symptoms include nausea, vomiting, headaches, anorexia, confusion, and coma.

Differentiating primary hyperparathyroidism from a *hypercalcemic syndrome,* secondary to malignancy, can be extremely difficult. Manifestations of this syndrome principally present in the central nervous system, kidneys, and gastrointestinal tract and include nausea, vomiting, anorexia, constipation, and polyuria. Breast carcinoma is the most common neoplasia associated with hypercalcemia, but it also has been observed with bronchogenic and renal-cell carcinomas and cancers of the vulva, cervix, and ovary.[1,2]

Carcinoid syndrome may manifest clinically by a complex of cutaneous flushing, disturbances of intestinal motility resulting in outbursts of diarrhea, bronchoconstriction, and cardiac symptoms related to tricuspid valvular insufficiency. It primarily occurs in conjunction with malignant cancers of the small intestine but also can be seen in bronchial and ovarian carcinomas.[10,33]

Rare ectopic *prolactin* or *oxytocin* production also has been reported in a few nonpregnant patients.[34-36] While hyperprolactinemia may cause infertility, increased serum bioactive oxytocin may cause premature contractions in pregnancy.

Treatment of these syndromes is primarily surgical and directed toward the underlying malignant disease.

CONCLUSIONS

Abnormal hormone production syndromes are infrequent in pregnancy. However, they frequently confound malignant disease, and the diagnosis of such a condition is difficult. The nature of presenting signs and symptoms often delays the recognition of abnormal hormone production in pregnancy. Nausea, vomiting, swelling, and fatigue are common and nonspecific complaints of pregnant women. Progression or persistence of these symptoms, however, needs to be noted and investigated, especially if they occur in an untimely fashion.

During the last decade, the rapidly advancing field of molecular biology has provided several new techniques that have enhanced the understanding of abnormal and ectopic hormone production.[37] They may lead, in the near future, to the discovery of the exact mechanisms by which these phenomena arise.

REFERENCES

1. Orth DN. Ectopic hormone production. In: Felig P, Baxter JD, Broadus AE, Frohman LA, eds. *Endocrinology and Metabolism*. New York, NY: McGraw-Hill Book Company; 1987:1692.
2. Shane JM, Naftolin F. Aberrant hormone activity by tumors of gynecologic importance. *Am J Obstet Gynecol*. 1975;121:133.
3. Novak ER, Lambrou CD, Woodruff JD. Ovarian tumors in pregnancy—an ovarian tumor registry review. *Obstet Gynecol*. 1975;46:401.
4. Fonseca JJS, Quesada GZ. Luteoma of pregnancy: report of a case and review of the literature. *J Reprod Med*. 1975;14:76.
5. Lojek MA, Fer MF, Kasselberg AG, et al. Cushing's syndrome with small cell carcinoma of the uterine cervix. *Am J Med*. 1980;69:140.
6. Hoeg JM, Saltopolsky E. Cervical carcinoma and ectopic hyperparathyroidism. *Arch Intern Med*. 1980;140:569.
7. Meredith RF, Wagman LD, Piper JA, et al. Beta-chain human chorionic gonadotropin-producing leiomyosarcoma of the small intestine. *Cancer*. 1986;58:131.
8. Hacker NF, Berek JS, Lagasse LD, et al. Carcinoma of the cervix associated with pregnancy. *Obstet Gynecol*. 1982;59:735.
9. Shields R. Gene derepression in tumors. *Nature*. 1977;269:752.
10. Shrider B, Manalo A. *Paraneoplastic Syndromes: Unusual Manifestations of Malignant Disease*. Chicago, IL: Year Book Medical Publishers; 1979:32.
11. Jones HW, Plymate S, Gluck FB, et al. Small cell nonkeratinizing carcinoma of the cervix associated with ACTH production. *Cancer*. 1976; 38:1629.
12. Buick RN, Pollak MN. Perspective on clonogenic tumor cells, stem cells, and ocogenes. *Cancer Res*. 1984;44:4909.
13. Person H, Hinnighausen L, Taub R, et al. Antibodies to human c-myc oncogene product: evidence of an evolutionarily conserved protein induced during cell proliferation. *Science*. 1984;225:687.
14. Tur-Kaspa I, Gleicher N. Immunology of the uterus. In: Altcheck A, Deligdisch L, eds. *The Uterus*. New York, NY: Springer-Verlag Publishers; 1990: in press.
15. Gleicher N, Siegel I, Francus K. Common denominators of pregnancy and malignancy. *Mt. Sinai J Med*. 1980;47:511.
16. Verhoeven ATM, Mastboom JL, Van Leusden HAIM, Van Der Velden WHM. Virilization in pregnancy coexisting with an (ovarian) mucinous cystadenoma: a case report and review of virilizing ovarian tumors in pregnancy. *Obstet Gynecol Surv*. 1973;28:597.
17. Chan LKC, Prathap K. Virilization in pregnancy associated with an ovarian mucinous cystadenoma. *Am J Obstet Gynecol*. 1970;108:946.
18. Fayez JA, Bunch TR, Miller GL. Virilization in pregnancy associated with an ovarian cystadenoma. *Am J Obstet Gynecol*. 1974;120:341.
19. Hamwi GJ, Byron RC, Besch PK, et al. Testosterone synthesis by a Brenner Tumor, Part 1. Clinical evidence of masculinization during pregnancy. *Am J Obstet Gynecol*. 1963;86:1015.
20. Novak DJ, Lauchlan SC, McCawley JC, Faiman C. Virilization during pregnancy. *Am J Med*. 1970;49:281.
21. Yen SSC. Endocrine physiology of pregnancy. In: Danforth DN, Scott JR, eds. *Obstetrics and Gynecology*. Philadelphia, PA: J.B. Lippincott Company; 1986:340.
22. Marks F, Young BK, Raghavendra BN, et al. Diagnosis of adrenal ganglioneuroma in pregnancy with magnetic resonance imaging and ultrasonography. A case report. *J Reprod Med*. 1989;34:59.
23. Speroff L, Glass RH, Kase NG. Normal and Abnormal Sexual Development. In: *Clinical Gynecologic Endocrinology and Infertility*. Baltimore, MD: Williams & Wilkins; 1989:379.
24. Tawa K. Ovarian tumors in pregnancy. *Am J Obstet Gynecol*. 1964;90:511.
25. Vaitukaitis JL. Ectopic hormonal syndromes. In: Yen SSC, Jaffe RB, eds. *Reproductive Endocrinology*. Philadelphia, PA: WB Saunders Company; 1986:631.
26. Kadar N, Romero R. Further observations on serial human chorionic gonadotropin patterns in ectopic pregnancies and spontaneous abortions. *Fertil Steril*. 1988;50:367.
27. Tur-Kaspa I, Confino E, Friberg J, et al. Ovarian stimulation protocol for *in vitro* fertilization with gonadotropins releasing hormone agonist widened the implantation window. *Fertil Steril*. 1990;53:859.
28. Nagelberg SB, Marmorstein B, Khazaeli MB, Rosen SW. Isolated ectopic production of the free beta subunit of chorionic gonadotropin by an epidermoid carcinoma of unknown primary site. *Cancer*. 1985;55:1924.
29. Morimoto N, Ozawa M, Nishimura R, et al. Discordant pregnancy tests in detection of alpha-subunit-producing tumors. *Obstet Gynecol*. 1983; 61:379.
30. Vladutiu AO, Sulewski JM, Pudlak KA, Stull CG. Heterophilic antibodies interfering with radioimmunoassay: a false-positive pregnancy test. *JAMA*. 1982;248:2489.
31. Cunanan RG, Lippes J, Tancinco PA. Choriocarcinoma of the ovary with coexisting normal pregnancy. *Obstet Gynecol*. 1980;55:669.
32. Shetty MR, Boghossian HM, Duffell D, et al. Tumor induced hypoglycemia: a result of ectopic insulin production. *Cancer*. 1982;49:1920.
33. Brown H, Lane M. Cushing's and malignant carcinoid syndromes from ovarian neoplasia. *Arch Intern Med*. 1965;115:490.
34. Wilson N, Ngser J. Large oxytocin and antidiuretic hormone from bronchogenic carcinoma in man. *Horm Metab Res*. 1980;12:708.
35. Turkinton RW. Ectopic production of prolactin. *N Engl J Med*. 1971;285:1455.
36. Hoffman WH, Gala RR, Kovacs K, Subramanian MG. Ectopic prolactin secretion from a gonadoblastoma. *Cancer*. 1987;60:2690.
37. Clark AJL. Ectopic hormone production. *Baillière's Clin Endocrinol Metab*. 1988;2:967.

PART VII The Immune System

Robert M. Galbraith, Section Editor

Chapter Forty-Six

Acquired Immune Deficiency Syndrome

Kwong-Yok Tsang

46

Acquired immune deficiency syndrome (AIDS) was conclusively shown to be caused by human immunodeficiency virus (HIV) in 1984. In March 31, 1989, the number of cases of AIDS reported to the Centers for Disease Control (CDC) reached 89,501. This number of cases did not include the 1.5–2.0 million HIV-infected asymptomatic individuals.

HIV is classified as a retrovirus. It is assigned to a subfamily of viruses known as the *Lentiviruses*. This classification is based on the observed similarities of HIV to "slow" viruses of sheep including the pulmonary disease virus maedi and the neurotropic virus visna.[1] HIV contains an RNA-dependent DNA polymerase (*reverse transcriptase*), that has a relatively low rate of transcriptional fidelity. The genetic variation in HIV is high. It has been reported that viral isolates may differ by as much as 20% of their amino acids.

HIV is transmitted by three primary routes: (1) exposure to infected blood or blood products, (2) sexual contact with infected individuals, and (3) perinatally from an infected mother to her baby. Table 46–1 shows the classification system developed by CDC for AIDS.[2]

Acute infection with HIV usually appears within 2–6 weeks of HIV infection, and the symptoms may include myalgia, arthralgia, headache, fever, photophobia, diarrhea, sore throat, lymphadenopathy, and maculopapular rash. Various neurologic manifestations also have been reported. Persistent antibodies to HIV usually develop within 3–6 months of HIV infection.

HIV INFECTION AND IMMUNOLOGIC MECHANISMS

The primary immunologic defect in HIV-infected individuals is a reduction in the level of CD_4-positive T cells. This reduction is usually rapid in the first year after infection for the seroconverted group, and the number plateaus at 200–1000/mm^3.[3] Studies of HIV-infected individuals in an effort to determine the relationship levels of CD_4-positive T cells to prognosis have shown a less favorable outcome for individuals with a low absolute count or a low CD_4 to CD_8 T cell ratio.[4] Many immunologic changes occur in individuals after HIV infection.

The following parameters are depressed: skin test reactivity; CD_4-positive T cells; CD_4 to CD_8 ratio; T cell proliferation response to mitogen and antigens; Interleukin-2 (IL-2) receptor expression; lymphokine production (eg, IL-2, γInterferon [γIFN]); natural killer (NK) cell activity; monocyte function; and chemotaxis and antigen presentation.

The following parameters are enhanced: lymphadenopathy; CD_8-positive T lymphocytes; immunoglobulins; Ig-secreting B cells; soluble IL-2 receptors; β_2-microglobulin; neopterin; and IL-6 and IL-production.

Several mechanisms have been reported to reduce the number of CD_4-positive cells in HIV infected cells *in vitro*. However, the exact mechanism of the cause of reduction of CD_4-positive T cells *in vivo* is still unclear.

The tropism of HIV for CD_4-positive T cells has been shown to reflect high-affinity interactions of the HIV envelope glycoprotein (gp)120 with the CD_4 molecule.[5] This binding is thought to be the primary event in the sequence of CD_4-positive cell depletion and as a consequence, leads to profound immune incompetence. A number of explanations have been offered for polyclonal loss of CD_4-positive cells. They include a direct cytopathic effect on antigen-driven CD_4-positive lymphocytes; cytotoxic T cell-mediated lysis of HIV infected cells; direct cytopathic effect on differentiating CD_4-bearing lymphocytes; antibody-triggered lysis of lymphocytes by way of CD_4–HIV complexes.

The interaction of gp120 and CD_4 uncovers another envelope protein called gp41. One end of the gp41 molecule embeds itself in the cell membranes, leading to the fusion of the viral and cell membranes. After HIV enters the cells, the viral genome may cause a persistent infection in which new virus particles are produced. In addition, infection may lead to the creation of syncytia, which die soon after formation. Syncytia are dominant effects of HIV infection in cell culture.

Immune mechanisms respond to HIV infection by induction of antibodies to proteins of HIV (gp160, gp120, gp41, p55, p24, p17). Whether or not cell-mediated immunity to the specific cytotoxic HIV-infected cells occurs is not clear because it is difficult to distinguish between specific cytotoxic reactions and antibody-dependent cell-mediated cytotoxicity (ADCC).

TABLE 46–1. CENTERS FOR DISEASE CONTROL CLASSIFICATION SYSTEM FOR HIV

Group I:	Acute infection
Group II:	Asymptomatic infection
Group III:	Persistent generalization lymphadenopathy
Group IV:	Other disease
Subgroup A:	Constitutional disease
Subgroup B:	Neurologic disease
Subgroup C:	Secondary infectious diseases
Category C-1:	Specified secondary infectious diseases listed in CDC surveillance definition for AIDS
Category C-2:	Other specified secondary infectious diseases
Subgroup D:	Secondary cancers
Subgroup E:	Other conditions

Many studies have suggested that antibody reactivity with p24 correlates with a higher level of ADCC than reactivity with gp160/120. The development of AIDS is preceded by a decline in antibody titer to the p24 antibody.[6] It also has been reported that progression to AIDS also is associated with a high red blood cell sedimentation rate, a low red blood cell count, and high β_2-microglobulin level. β_2-Microglobulin is a protein present on the membrane of all mediated cells. Other parameters associated with progression to AIDS are increased antibody to p17 (the other core protein of HIV), increased urinary and serum neopterin, higher titers of cytomegalovirus antibody, thrombocytopenia, the presence of α-interferon, and increased level of serum soluble IL-2 receptors.

Other cofactors may be necessary for the acquisition of HIV infection and for the development of specific manifestations of AIDS, progression to AIDS, or AIDS-related complex (ARC), among HIV-infected individuals.[7] The inducers are infectious agents, such as other viruses (eg, CMV and herpes simplex virus); behavioral cofactors, including the use of certain drugs (eg, hallucinogen); and age. However, the role of age as a cofactor among HIV-infected adults is not clear; genetic factors in the HIV infected individual (eg, HLA type) may be associated with the progression to AIDS. Whether pregnancy enhances the progression to AIDS in HIV-infected women is uncertain.

There are four major high-risk groups for AIDS: (1) homosexual and bisexual men; (2) hemophiliacs and transfusion recipients; (3) intravenous (IV) drug abusers; and (4) children born to HIV-infected mothers. Although the majority of AIDS cases in the next few years are expected to be confined to homosexual and bisexual men, IV drug users, and hemophiliacs, it has been predicted by the CDC that the number of children with AIDS acquired through perinatal transmission will increase. The CDC reported 583 children younger than 13 years of age with AIDS during 1988. The rate of perinatal transmission is about 40–50%.[8]

EFFECT OF PREGNANCY ON HIV INFECTION

Women account for about 7% of the reported cases of AIDS in the United States.[9] The majority of women with AIDS (78%) are in childbearing years. The primary risk factors for AIDS in women is heterosexual transmission (28%), IV drug use (49%), and transfusion (11%).[10] It was estimated that more than 2000 HIV-infected women gave birth in 1988.[9,11,12] Pregnancy may accelerate the disease progression in HIV-infected women.[13]

Scott et al[14] and Minkoff et al[15] reported that 45–75% of asymptomatic pregnant women develop symptoms 28–30 months postpartum. This rate of progression appears faster than the rate for other risk groups (homosexual men, IV drug users, and hemophiliacs) in which 13–34% of the asymptomatic carriers developed AIDS in a 6-year study.[16]

EFFECT OF HIV ON PREGNANCY

Johnstone et al[17] compared the effects of HIV on the outcome of pregnancy in 50 seropositive pregnant women (46 IV drug users, four with a seropositive partner) and 64 seronegative women (45 IV drug users, 19 with a seropositive partner) in Edinburgh. All these women were asymptomatic. Compared to the control group, the rate of prematurity and intrauterine growth retardation was increased almost twofold over those found in control subjects and the rate of low-birthweight babies was increased nearly fourfold. In this study, there was no evidence that HIV affects the outcome of pregnancy in asymptomatic women.

Fifty pregnant patients with HIV infection were investigated by Gloeb et al[18] with respect to the effects of HIV on pregnancy. The majority of the patients in the study group remained asymptomatic during their pregnancies. Three pregnant patients developed AIDS, and two others developed symptoms associated with the AIDS-related complex. Four patients were antenatally diagnosed with oral candidiasis. The patients followed in this study experienced several complications of pregnancy. More than one third of the pregnancies (34.6%) were complicated by preterm labor. Premature rupture of the membranes occurred in 15.4% of the patients. Approximately 33% of the patients experienced various kinds of infections, including urinary tract infection, syphilis, or gonorrhea. Urinary tract infections and sexually transmitted diseases are possible risk factors for perinatal HIV transmission. The mean (±SD) birthweight for the study was 2796±845 g with a range of 1000–5110 g. No neonates had congenital abnormalities. Ten of the patients are known to have had children with HIV infection. Nine neonates born in the study period are known to be infected with HIV.

Seventy-one infants born to mothers seropositive for HIV were studied as part of a project within the European community's research activities on AIDS.[19] Five developed symptoms of AIDS and AIDS-related complex, and three died. Eighteen of 71 infants had lost maternal antibodies by 10 months. It is estimated that 75% will lose antibody by 1 year of age. However, 2 of the 18 who lost antibodies were virus-positive. Thus, loss of antibodies does not necessarily indicate freedeom from infection. At present, insufficient data are available to draw a conclusion in regard to the association between mode of delivery or breast-feeding and the risk of AIDS and AIDS-related complex. It was suggested that the risk of AIDS and AIDS-related complex in infants is substantially greater if the mother has symptoms of HIV infection in pregnancy. However, it is not clear that the presence of maternal symptoms is a risk factor for infection or for early development of AIDS in the infant. The risk of intrapartum or congenital transmission of HIV from an infected woman to her fetus or newborn depends on many poorly defined factors. The estimates of risk for intrapartum congenital transmission from infected women ranges from 30–50%.[20] Cesarean section has not been proven to be protective. It is difficult to distinguish true infection in the newborn from passively acquired maternal HIV antibody. However, several studies have reported that

TABLE 46–2. TREATMENT OF HIV-RELATED INFECTIONS AND THE PERINATAL EFFECTS

Infections	Regimen	Reported Risks in Pregnancy
Candidiasis	Ketoconazole, 400 mg each day for 14 days, then each day for 5 d/mo for 6 months	No known risks[a]
Herpes simplex	Acyclovir sodium, 200 mg, five times daily	Safety in pregnancy is not known[a]
Pneumonia (*Pneumocystis carinii*)	Pentamidine 4 mg/kg/d IV Sulfamethoxazole, 100 mg/kg/d and trimethoprim, 20 mg/kg/d	Unknown[a] *Sulfonamides* cross the placenta and theoretically compete with bilirubin, potentially leading to kericterus caused by hyperbilirubinemia *Trimethoprin*, which crosses the placenta. Although it is a folate antagonist, no increase in fetal abnormality by this drug has been demonstrated.
Toxoplasmosis	Sulfadiazine sodium, 1 g orally 4 times each day and pyrimethamine isethionate, 25–50 mg/d	Most reports indicate no effects, but one case of gastroschisis, kernicterus.[a]

[a] Animal experiments have indicated adverse effects on the fetus (teratogenic, embryocidal) or no controlled experiments have been performed in women. Drugs should be administered only if the potential benefit justifies the potential risk to the fetus.

perinatally acquired HIV infection is associated with substantial morbidity and mortality. For example, in a study of 479 children born to HIV-infected mothers in Zaire[21], 81 (17%) died within the first year as compared to 18 (3%) of 574 children born to uninfected mothers.

Diagnosis of HIV infection in newborns is difficult because of the transplacental passage of maternal antibody to HIV in all infants. Both enzyme-linked immunosorbent assay (ELISA) and Western blot assay can be expected to be positive in infected and uninfected infants born to seropositive mothers. Passive-acquired HIV antibody decreases to undetectable levels in 50% of infants by 10 months and in 75% of infants by 12 months. As indicated previously, some infected infants who fail to develop HIV antibody give positive results in viral culture and antigen-detection assays. Additional tests for early detection of HIV infection in newborns include assay for HIV-specific IgM, HIV antigen, viral nucleic acids, and viral cultures. Furthermore, the polymerase chain reaction technique for amplification of the HIV genome has proven to be a very sensitive assay for early detection of HIV infection.

HIV can be transmitted sexually and perinatally. HIV-infected humans should therefore be screened for other diseases, such as gonorrhea and syphilis. Patients also should be screened for chlamydia infection and hepatitis B viral markers if they develop HIV-related infection.

TREATMENT OF HIV INFECTION

Social modifications of standard treatment regimens may be required during pregnancy. Table 46–2[22] describes some of the drugs used in patients with HIV-related infections and their perinatal effects.

Zidovudine is now being offered for treatment of symptomatic HIV infections. The safety of zidovudine in pregnancy has not been tested; however, the mode of action of zidovudine is inhibition of reverse transcriptase, which does not appear to pose a substantial risk to the fetus. In addition, *in vivo* and animal studies[23] have demonstrated that zidovudine does not cause mutagenicity and malformation.

There are no known instances of HIV infection acquired by exposure of infants to HIV-infected mothers at delivery. However, care must be focused on prevention of the nosocomial spread of HIV for those health care workers exposed to large amounts of maternal blood, amniotic fluid, and vaginal secretion. It is important that the infection control guidelines not be limited to patients known to be HIV antibody-positive but also are applied to patients known to be infected.

The risks of infection through mother's milk is not defined; however, it is recommended that HIV-infected mothers not breast-feed their children. Information in regard to the postpartum clinical course of HIV-infected women is scant. However, longer follow-up studies by Scott et al[14] and Minkoff et al[15] have revealed a high frequency of subsequent clinical illness in mothers whose children develop the disease.

REFERENCES

1. Narayan O, Wolinsky JS, Clements JE, et al. Slow virus replication: the role of macrophages in persistence of and expression of Visna viruses of sheep and goats. *J Gen Virol.* 1982;59:345.
2. Centers for Disease Control. Classification system for human T-lymphotropic virus type III/lymphadenopathy associated virus infection. *MMWR.* 1986;35:334.
3. Fahey JL, Giorgi J, Martinez-Maza, et al. Immune pathogenesis of AIDS and related syndrome. *Ann Inst Pasteur/Immunol.* 1987;138:245.
4. Taylor J, Afrasiabi R, Tahey JL, et al. Prognostically significant classification of immune change in AIDS with kaposi's sarcoma. *Blood.* 1986;67:666.
5. Dalgleish AG, Bevenley PCL, Claphan PR, et al. The CD4 (T4) antigen is an essential component of the receptor for the AIDS retrovirus. *Nature.* 1984;312:763.
6. Rozk AH, Lane HC, Folks T, et al. Sera from HTLV-III/LAV antibody positive individuals mediate antibody-dependent cellular cytotoxicity against HTLV-III/LAV injected T cell. *J Immunol.* 1987;138:1064.
7. Lifson AR, Rutherford GW, Jaffe HW. The national history of human immunodeficiency virus infection. *J Infect Dis.* 1988;156:1360.
8. Friedland GH, Klein RS. Transmission of immunodeficiency virus. *N Engl J Med.* 1987;317:1125.
9. Minkoff HL. Care of pregnant women infected with human immunodeficiency virus. *JAMA.* 1988;258:2714.
10. *AIDS Weekly Surveillance Report United States.* AIDS Program, Centers for Disease Control. February 29, 1987.
11. Minkoff, H. Confronting AIDS: what every woman's physician should know. Female Patient 1987;12:49.
12. Health Studies Task Force. HTLV-III/LAV antibody prevalence in US military recruit applicants. *MMUR.* 1986;35:421.
13. Dodson MG, Kerman RH, Lange CF, et al. T and B cells in pregnancy. *Obstet Gynecol.* 1977;49:299.
14. Scott GB, Fischl MA, Klimas N, et al. Mothers of infants with the acquired

immunodeficiency syndrome: evidence for both symptomatic and asymptomatic carries. *JAMA*. 1985;253:363.
15. Minkoff HL, Nanda D, Menez R, et al. Follow up to mothers of children with AIDS. *Obstet Gynecol*. 1987;87:288.
16. Goedert JJ, Riggar RJ, Weiss SH, et al. Three years incidence of AIDS in five cohorts of HTLV-III infected risk group members. *Science*. 1986;231:992.
17. Johnstone FD. Does infection with HIV affect the outcome of pregnancy? *Br Med J*. 1988;296:467.
18. Gloeb DJ, O'Sullivan MJ, Efantis J. Human immunodeficiency virus infection in women. I. The effects of human immunodeficiency virus on pregnancy. *Am J Obstet Gynecol*. 1988;159:756.
19. Mok, JQ, Rossi AD, Ades AE, et al. Infants born to mothers seropositive for human immunodeficiency virus. *Lancet*. 1987;1:1164.
20. Semprini A, Vucetich A, Pardi G, et al. HIV infection and AIDS and newborn babies of mothers positive for HIV antibody. *Br Med J*. 1987;294:610.
21. Ryder RW, Nsa W, Behets F, et al. Perinatal HIV transmission in two African hospitals: one year follow-up. Stockholm: Fourth International Conference on AIDS; 1988.
22. Fujisaki S, Mori N, Sasaki T, et al. Cell-mediated immunity in human pregnancy. *Microbiol*. 1979;23:899.
23. *Retrovirus Production Information*. Research Triangle Park, NC: Burroughs Wellcome Co; 1987.

Chapter Forty-Seven
Immunologic Disorders

Yacov Levy and Steven D. Douglas

47

During the childbearing age, women are often at peak risk of developing immunologic disorders, such as immunodeficiency or autoimmunity. Although these diseases may at times alter fertility or outcome of pregnancy, a considerable number of women who suffer from these disorders, especially with progressively improving care, give birth to live children.

Pregnancy is associated with important immunologic phenomena. The fetus, which can be considered as an allogeneic graft, grows in conditions that contradict the usual laws of transplantation immunogenetics. The failure of fetal rejection has been explained by a sequence of immunologic alterations that include anatomic changes in the uterus that render it a privileged site for implantation and survival[1], absence or ineffective expression of transplantation antigens on the trophoblast[2-4], changes in maternal lymphocyte subsets during pregnancy[4,5] with diminished cellular immune responses[6,7], and separation of maternal and fetal circulations.[1,8]

The maternal immune system is selectively depressed in part of its cellular repertoire during pregnancy. This suppression has been attributed to immunosuppressive factors present in the mother's serum, such as α_2-glucoproteins[9] and various hormones[10,11], rather than to intrinsic defects in lymphocytes.[12] For example, granulocyte chemotaxis was reported to be depressed when tested in the presence of pregnant women's serum.[13]

Pathologic events that occur in pregnant women take place in the mother and fetus as one whole system. The placenta facilitates the transport of immunoglobulin (class IgG) fractions from mother to fetus while blocking the transport of other immunoglobulin classes and subclasses. On the other hand, there is a passage of cells from mother to fetus, and vice versa, throughout pregnancy and labor.[14]

The pregnant woman also is susceptible to radical changes in her nutritional milieu (see also Chapter 21). Nutritional deficiencies in pregnancy include caloric malnutrition, iron and zinc deficiencies, hypocalcemia, hypovitaminosis, and changes in lipid metabolism[15,16], all of which can affect the immune system.

Immunologic diseases in the mother that involve IgG antibodies can be expected to be manifested in the fetus because of the passage of some IgG subclasses transplacentally. However, a protective fetal mechanism prevents some of this expression. Once a child is born, some maternal IgG antibodies can be found in the neonate but disappear within 3–6 months, based on the half-life of maternal IgG. Some drugs (eg, steroids and immunosuppressive agents) have variable capacities to cross the placental barrier. The appearance of neonatal symptoms caused by maternal antibodies may be delayed after birth because of the protective effect of such drugs given to the mother. These drugs usually have only a short duration of action. Their effect is therefore limited to a few days. Following this short interval, and on termination of the protective effect, the pathologic manifestations of antibodies may once again become evident.

IMMUNOLOGIC DISORDERS OCCURRING IN PREGNANT WOMEN

Hypogammaglobulinemias

The hypogammaglobulinemic disorders comprise a large and diverse group of B-cell immunodeficiencies with the common result a deficiency of immunoglobulins of some or all classes. Female patients with *common variable immunodeficiency* and *selective IgA deficiency* reach childbearing age.

Common Variable Immunodeficiency. Common variable immunodeficiency represents a heterogeneous group of patients who present after infancy, usually in the second or third decade, with a tendency for recurrent bacterial infections, markedly decreased serum immunoglobulins, and impaired antibody responses.[17] Cellular immunity is usually normal, but occasionally it is abnormal in patients or family members.[18,19] The presenting picture in most patients is of recurrent sinopulmonary infections that lead to bronchiectasis and chronic, persistent sinusitis. The organisms most frequently found in these patients are *Haemophilus influenzae, Streptococcus pneumoniae, Staphylococcus,* and *Mycoplasma*. On physical examination, there is usually a paucity of lymphoid tissue, although some patients may have hepatosplenomegaly and lymphadenopathy. Involvement of the gastrointestinal system is common. Many patients have a spruelike syndrome with steatorrhea, malabsorption of folate and vitamin B_{12}, lactose intolerance, protein-losing enteropathy, and abnormalities of the villous structure.[20] *Giar-*

dia lamblia is frequently found in the patient's small bowel and may be of pathophysiologic significance.[21] Enteric infections are common and tend to be protracted. Chronic *Campylobacter enteritis* has been reported in a hypogammaglobulinemic pregnant woman in association with recurrent abortions.[22] Although nodular lymphoid hyperplasia of the small bowel is associated with common variable immunodeficiency, these lymphocytic accumulations lack plasma cells.[23]

Autoimmune disorders and autoantibodies often are found in these patients and their families.[18,24] Disorders resembling rheumatoid arthritis, dermatomyositis, scleroderma, and systemic lupus erythematosus occur; autoimmune hemolytic anemia, pernicious anemia and immune thrombocytopenia also occur.[25,26]

Serum immunoglobulin levels are reduced, with IgG usually below 500 mg/dL (but seldom below 100 mg/dL). The IgM and IgA levels are undetectable in most patients, although normal levels are found in some. Isohemagglutinin titers are usually depressed, and the *Schick test* is positive. In most patients, the peripheral B cell number is normal, although a few patients lack them altogether. Immunization with new antigens usually invokes an antibody response. Despite immunologic memory, most patients cannot switch the antibody production from IgM to IgG after repeated immunizations.

T-lymphocyte function is normal in most patients with common variable immunodeficiency. However, some patients may present with negative delayed hypersensitivity skin tests, a low number of T cells, and depressed lymphocyte proliferation *in vitro* with mitogens, antigens, or alloantigens.[18,19,28]

A few cases have been described in which women with this syndrome gave birth to normal children.[27,29-31] The outcome of pregnancy in these women is related to the nature and severity of the infections occurring during the gestational period. The fetus is well protected against most bacterial infections. However, if the mother has severe septicemia or an acute exacerbation of her pulmonary disease, causing respiratory failure, the outcome may be grave, and the pregnancy may result in an abortion or a stillbirth.

Most important in the management of these patients is the administration of IgG, which was previously given as an intramuscular injection of γ-globulin 0.4–0.6 mL/kg (60–100 mg/kg), but is now often administered as an intravenous infusion of 8 mL/kg (400 mg/kg). This treatment usually is given every 21–28 days. Anaphylactic reactions to the intravenous infusion have been reported, and as a consequence, the infusion should not exceed a rate of 25 mL/h, with epinephrine and diphenhydramine available.[32] Patients who receive adequate doses of γ-globulin usually do not require prophylactic antibiotics; such therapy is used only for treatment of specific infections, which usually respond satisfactorily.

During the third trimester of pregnancy, there is an increased active passage of IgG transplacentally to the fetus.[33] This involves all four subclasses of IgG, but with somewhat less efficiency in the transport of IgG_2 and IgG_4.[34,35] As a consequence, the maternal IgG half-life is markedly reduced, and IgG levels may drop below the protective values.[36] During this period, immunoglobulin treatment should be given more frequently to keep maternal IgG levels above 200 mg/dL. Other alternatives are to use fresh frozen plasma (10 mL/kg) or to administer immunoglobulin subcutaneously.[31] In addition to concern for the mother's well-being, special attention should be given to the fetus. Fetal loss caused by intrauterine infections or fetal infections has been reported in hypogammaglobulinemic mothers who had inadequate IgG levels.[37,38] Intravenous gammaglobulin infusions given to the mother significantly increase the fetal IgG subgroups IgG_1, IgG_2, and IgG_3.[39]

If a patient becomes thrombocytopenic as part of an autoimmune disorder, this is a strong indication to administer immunoglobulin intravenously. Commercial γ-globulin preparations available for clinical use contain only traces of IgA and IgM. On the rare occasion when administration of these isotypes is desirable, fresh frozen plasma should be used.

Newborn infants born to hypogammaglobulinemic mothers have not been reported to have manifestations of the maternal disease.[28-31] However, levels of IgG in the serum of newborns of hypogammaglobulinemic mothers are slow to achieve normal values for age, and the antibody response to various antigens is delayed. These findings suggest that transplacental maternal antibodies play only a minor role, if any, in modulating total IgG production in the neonate. Maternal immunoglobulins may normally play a suppressive role in the neonate's immunoglobulin levels. Lack of this suppression from a hypogammaglobulinemic mother should result in a brisk elevation of the neonate's IgG. Failure of this elevation to occur suggests immaturity of B and T cells in the neonate rather than a lack of maternal suppressive effect.[30,40]

Selective IgA Deficiency. Selective IgA deficiency is the most common immunodeficiency disorder, with a prevalence of 1 in 400 to 1 in 800.[41,42] The low level of IgA in the serum (usually below 5 mg/dL) is the major immunologic finding. The basic defect in IgA deficiency has not been delineated. The presence of normal IgA-bearing B cells suggests that the defect is in the synthesis or release of IgA rather than in the quantity of IgA-producing cells. Deficiency of secretory IgA, the major immunoglobulin protecting the body's cavities (ie, respiratory tract, gastrointestinal lumen, mammary gland, urinary tract, middle ear, lacrimal tract), is responsible for the clinical abnormalities in these patients. Recurrent respiratory infections and chronic diarrhea may occur. Autoimmune disorders are common, especially systemic lupus erythematosus[41-43] and rheumatoid arthritis.[44] Although the pathogenesis of autoimmune manifestations in selective IgA deficiency is unclear, certain explanations have been proposed to account for this coincidence. The increased incidence of antibodies found in these patients directed against cow's milk and cow, sheep, and goat serum[45] may be secondary to a loss of selective absorption of proteins by the respiratory and gastrointestinal mucosa. Thus, antigens may enter the circulation and provoke the development of antibodies that react with human tissue or initiate immunopathologic mechanisms that culminate in autoimmunity. The absence of the secretory IgA may cause local disease because of the lack of local protection and the influence of normally restricted pathogens.

There is marked variability in the onset and severity of the disease, and several series report a high incidence of selective IgA deficiency among healthy populations.[46-48] There may be specific compensatory mechanisms in the IgA-deficient patient. Monomeric IgM has been found to be increased in the serum and in the secretions of these patients.[42] The intestinal biopsies of IgA-deficient patients contain many cells that stain for IgM.[49] The regulatory mechanisms for serum and secretory IgA are probably distinct, and in fact, a few patients have been described with normal secretory IgA despite the absence of serum IgA.[42,50]

The basic defect in these patients is not in the differentiation from earlier IgM precursors to mature IgA-producing cells, but rather in the terminal differentiation of IgA-secreting plasma cells, a process that is under thymic control.[51] A deficiency in production of IgA may imply a thymic abnormality[52], and lack or deficiency of T-suppressor cells could predispose to autoimmunity.

These patients show a large spectrum of associated clinical disorders. Most of the patients demonstrate allergic problems, primarily asthma.[42] The course of the asthma tends to be chronic and resistant to treatment. The greater incidence of gastrointestinal problems and pulmonary infections probably disrupts the fine equilibrium achieved by the treatment of asthma. These allergic or IgA-deficient patients have normal IgE-mediated responses.[42,53] The ability to synthesize IgG is also intact, and B cells are capable of responding briskly to any antigenic stimulation. If patients who completely lack IgA receive IgA from any source, it is treated as a foreign antigen, and an anti-IgA response and anaphylaxis may occur.[54] Thus, particular precautions should be taken when substances such as γ-globulin, fresh frozen plasma, or whole blood are given.

Selective IgA-deficient patients tend to have mild recurrent upper respiratory tract infections, which are more frequent during childhood and less frequent during adolescence. These infections, however, may result in chronic lung disease. Pulmonary hemosiderosis has been associated with selective IgA deficiency.[42,55]

These patients may present with celiac disease[56], intestinal nodular lymphoid hyperplasia[57], ulcerative colitis[41], regional ileitis[41], and pernicious anemia.[41,58] An association has been found between selective IgA deficiency and such chromosomal abnormalities as partial deletion of the short or long arm of chromosome 18 or a ring chromosome 18.[59,60] Familial expression of selective IgA has been described by various authors[61,62], but there is no consistent pattern of inheritance in these patients.

Infants may have low serum IgA levels, but the diagnosis cannot be made immediately because serum IgA achieves normal adult levels at age 10–12 years.

Selective IgA-deficient women who become pregnant do not manifest particular abnormalities other than those described previously. Most of these women are asymptomatic and do not require special therapy other than close follow-up. IgA-deficient pregnant women with allergic, gastrointestinal, or autoimmune disorders[63] should be treated accordingly.

Chronic Mucocutaneous Candidiasis

Chronic mucocutaneous candidiasis (CMC) is a cellular immunodeficiency characterized by chronic and prolonged infection of the mucous membranes, skin, scalp, and nails with *Candida* and other fungi. It is a relatively mild and restricted immunodeficiency limited to a selective inability to deal effectively with *Candida albicans* and antigenically related fungi. Immunity to viruses, bacteria, and other fungi is usually intact, and life-threatening infections do not usually occur. The onset of chronic *Candida* infection usually occurs in infancy but has been reported to begin at any time in the first 3 decades. The disorder usually presents as thrush, followed by involvement of the skin and nails. The illness may be very mild, involving only a single nail, or it may develop into generalized disease of almost the entire integument and intestinal tract. Most patients have a nearly normal life-span. Stiehm[64] has classified CMC patients into four clinical variants: (1) early onset, (2) late onset, (3) familial form, and (4) juvenile familial polyendocrinopathy with candidiasis.

The most severe and most typical is the early-onset form. *Candida granuloma* may occur in this form, and 50% of patients have an endocrinopathy, usually hypothyroidism. Late-onset candidiasis is the mildest form and may be limited to paronychia or to buccal mucosa involvement. In the familial form, endocrinopathy is uncommon; this form is inherited in an autosomal recessive pattern. The autosomal recessive juvenile familial polyendocrinopathy with candidiasis is associated with hypoparathyroidism or Addison's disease, which can precede the onset of the *Candida* infections.

The endocrine abnormalities usually develop several years after the candidiasis and include hypoparathyroidism, Addison's disease, diabetes, and hypothyroidism.[65] Autoantibodies to the affected endocrine glands often are found.[65] Other associated disorders include ovarian insufficiency, chronic active hepatitis[66], pernicious anemia[65], keratoconjunctivitis, alopecia, and iron-deficiency anemia.

The immunologic defects are heterogeneous, ranging from individuals with an apparently normal immune function to individuals with several different immunologic defects.[67] Most patients manifest skin anergy to *Candida* antigens; impaired *in vitro* lymphocyte proliferation responses to *Candida* antigen; and impaired synthesis of the lymphokine, migration inhibition factor (MIF), in response to *Candida* antigen.[68] The number of circulating B and T lymphocytes is usually normal. The immunoglobulin levels are normal or elevated, and antibody responses to *Candida* are also normal. Occasionally, allergies to different antigens in addition to *Candida* are found, and some patients have impaired lymphocyte proliferative response to phytohemagglutinin (PHA) and other mitogens in addition to the defective lymphocyte response to *Candida in vitro*. Defective monocyte cytotoxicity was shown in a few patients.[69] A monocyte chemotactic defect toward C_{5a} has been reported.[69] The serum complement levels and activity are normal. In a few patients, skin biopsies have shown deposits of C_3 and properdin in the basement membrane of the skin lesions. It has been proposed that the alternative complement pathway is activated by the candidal invasion and that a strong local inflammatory reaction may limit the spread of that pathogen.[70]

A *Candida*-specific T-cell defect is postulated as the defect in CMC. Specific failure of the T cells to respond to *Candida* could be related to a genetic restriction in responsiveness, to tolerance to the antigen, or to a cross-reactive antigen shared by *Candida* and an unknown tissue antigen. This tolerance may be a consequence of an active suppressor mechanism. The high incidence of autoimmune phenomena also suggests the possibility of disturbed suppressor mechanisms.

Women with CMC may experience a normal pregnancy, if the accompanying endocrinopathy is not severe. The most serious endocrine disorders are hypothyroidism and Addison's syndrome.

The two main therapeutic goals are to suppress the fungal infection and to potentiate immune responsiveness. Continuous antifungal therapy is usually necessary. During pregnancy, the local application of antifungal agents, such as mycostatin, clotrimazole, haloprogin, miconazole, amphotericin, and gentian violet is indicated. When applied to the skin or mucous membranes, such treatment will rarely lead to improvement but may prevent progression. Intravenous amphotericin B will result in improvement or complete clearing in most patients, but it is not a desirable treatment in pregnancy. Moreover, when treatment is stopped, relapse will usually occur. Nails are resistant to all forms of therapy except to surgical removal. Oral clotrimazole[71], fluorocytosine[72], ketoconazole, and intravenous miconazole[73] have been used successfully in some patients. The use of these agents during pregnancy is, however, not desirable and treatment should be postponed until after its termination. Because antimycotic agents cannot provide long-term remission, a variety of immunotherapy techniques have been used. The most commonly used is transfer factor, which is usually combined with intravenous amphotericin B.[74,75] Other treatments are transfusion of lymphocytes from *Candida* skin-test positive donors[76] and bone marrow transplantation.[77] All of these therapeutic approaches are experimental and are not routinely indicated in the treatment of the pregnant patient with chronic mucocutaneous candidiasis.

Hereditary Angioedema

The clinical syndrome of *C1-inhibitor deficiency* is inherited as an autosomal dominant trait. A critical plasma level of C1 inhibitor, about one third of normal, is required for normal inhibitor function.[78] During attacks of the disease, patients show sigificantly lower levels of the inhibitor than this critical concentration.

Hereditary angioedema is clinically manifested by recurrent attacks of nonpruritic, nonurticarial swelling of the extremities, face, trunk, abdominal viscera, and most importantly, the airway.[79] Swelling may occur spontaneously or in response to trauma, particularly dental manipulation. The biochemical mediator of this swelling has not been elucidated clearly. The patients show a depletion of early classic complement components (C4 and C2), while the alternative pathway components and terminal complement components remain intact. The patients are not at increased risk for infections, but usually are at increased risk for developing such autoimmune disorders as systemic lupus erythematosus, Sjörgren's syndrome, Crohn's disease, and scleroderma.

Approximately 85% of patients with hereditary angioedema have one normal and one silent C1-inhibitor gene. The remaining 15% are heterozygous for one of several antigenically normal but functionally deficient inhibitors. Thus, in about 15% of patients, symptoms occur in the presence of normal levels of C1 inhibitor but with low levels of C4.[78]

Menstruation and pregnancy have a major effect on disease activity. Women with angioedema reported an increased attack rate during the menstrual period.[79] During pregnancy and labor, the attack rate seems to decrease significantly. In one series of 10 women with a total of 25 pregnancies, none had an attack of angioedema at delivery, despite the obvious trauma to the birth canal. In 23 of 25 pregnancies, the women had markedly fewer or no attacks in the last two trimesters.[79] A recent report describes a pregnant woman with hereditary angioedema caused by decreased levels of C1 inhibitor associated with deficiency of IgA.[63] This patient had angioedema attacks before pregnancy and an increased rate of infections, which was attributed to the IgA deficiency.

Prophylactic treatment is given to patients with hereditary angioedema with life-threatening airway involvement or to patients who have very frequent attacks. Danazol, an androgenic steroid[80], or tranexamic acid[81] are usually used with positive results. Because the attack rate frequently increases during pregnancy, there is little indication for prophylactic treatment during pregnancy. Fibrinolytic therapy, using agents such as epsilon-amino caproic acid or tranexamic acid, is indicated for treatment of acute episodes[79]; interference with fibrinolytic activity is triggered by that complement activation in HAE. This treatment may induce thromboembolic processes as well as myalgias in the treated women.

Chronic Granulomatous Disease

Chronic granulomatous disease is a rare inherited disorder with phenotypic expression in 1 in 1,000,000 persons.[82] Patients with this disorder develop serious infections early in life, usually within the first year, that affect the skin, lungs, and liver. They usually present with abscesses and septicemia. Suppurative lymphadenitis, osteomyelitis, and meningitis are common. *Staphylococcus aureus* is the most common pathogen, but infections caused by gram-negative bacilli, *Serratia marcescens,* and fungi, such as *Candida* and *Aspergillus,* have been reported.[83] Granuloma may be found in the urinary tract, causing hydronephrosis or in the gastrointestinal tract, causing gastric outlet obstruction with intractable vomiting.

The main immunologic abnormality is the inability of intracellular killing by phagocytes, while chemotaxis and phagocytosis are generally intact. The killing defect involves the oxidative system. Consequently, the patient's phagocytes are unable to mount a respiratory burst or to generate hydrogen peroxide and oxygen radicals when stimulated.[84]

Chronic granulomatous disease is inherited predominantly in an X-linked fashion, although approximately 10–20% of the cases are transmitted by an autosomal recessive mode.[85] This observation suggests that the disease is a collection of disorders with a common clinical manifestation. The genetic heterogeneity of the disease probably reflects point mutations in the series of events that control the neutrophil oxidative metabolism. They include deficiency of leukocyte glucose-6-phosphate dehydrogenase, glutathione peroxidase[86], abnormal nincotinamide dinucleotide-phosphate-H (NADPH) oxidase affinity[87], and enzyme activation.[88] Dysfunction of an electron transport system involving flavoprotein[89], cytochrome b[90], and quionnes[91] also have been reported in a number of patients. A classification system has been created in which each of the defects is listed based on the mode of inheritance.[92]

Chronic granulomatous disease can be diagnosed by demonstrating the neutrophils' inability to kill bacteria. This defect is most pronounced when catalase-positive organisms, such as staphylococci, are tested. However a much more sensitive diagnostic assay system is to measure respiratory burst activity by evaluating oxygen consumption, hydrogen peroxide production, or superoxide generation.[91] Chemiluminescence is another indirect method that estimates the amount of respiratory burst that is usually defective in this disease. The most convenient assay for evaluation of the respiratory burst is the nitroblue tetrazolium (NBT) test. Here, the dye changes color from yellow to a purple formazan when the intracellular NADPH is reduced.

Various modes of therapy are effective in patients with chronic granulomatous disease. The most successful is the institution of prophylactic trimethoprim sulfamethoxazole, which significantly prolongs disease-free intervals to more than 2 months. During a severe, life-threatening infection, treatment with leukocyte transfusions can be considered. Bone marrow transplantation has been used with partial success.[93a,b,c] A possible additional treatment is the administration of γ-interferon to attempt to augment the phagocyte superoxide production.[94] A clinical trial of γ-interferon is underway.

Because of frequent severe infections during childhood, some patients with chronic granulomatous disease become debilitated and die in their early teens. Many patients, however, survive into adulthood. These patients probably have a milder variant of the disease. A 22-year-old woman with a mild case of chronic granulomatous disease had an uncomplicated pregnancy and gave birth to a normal male baby.[95] This patient did not require any treatment during pregnancy.

Hyperimmunoglobulinemia E Syndrome

The hyperimmunoglobulinemia E syndrome is a complex disease characterized by markedly elevated serum IgE levels, chronic dermatitis, and serious recurrent infections. Davis et al[96] reported the first two patients with this syndrome and noted an abnormal inflammatory response, resulting in the formation of "cold" staphylococcal abscesses. The syndrome was named *Job's syndrome* because "Job was afflicted with sore boils from the sole of his feet unto his crown." The major clinical features of the hyperimmunoglobulinemia E syndrome are recurrent severe pneumonias with pneumatoceles, furunculosis, pruritic eczematoid dermatitis with atypical distribution, and coarse facial features, usually with broad nasal bridge, prominent nose and irregularly proportioned cheeks and jaws.[97] Growth retardation, not explained by hormonal defects, also is found in a minority of the patients.[98]

The tendency to recurrent infections is usually well established at the age of 6 weeks. Deep-seated bacterial infections, however, usually become evident at the age of 6 months.[98] The manifestations of infections are skin abscesses, chronic otitis media, sinusitis, pneumonia with bronchiectasis, septic arthritis, and osteomyelitis. The major pathogen is *Staphylococcus aureus*. Other bacteria reported include *Haemophilus influenzae*, group A streptococcus, *Escherichia coli*, and *Pseudomonas*. Chronic candidal infection, affecting the mouth, nails, and skin, is very common. Cases have been reported with monilial infection of the gastrointestinal tract, meninges, and lungs.[98]

The mode of inheritance is not clear. Most of the reported cases are sporadic, although a family history of allergy and dermatitis is common. There are several reports, however, of familial occurrence of the syndrome, and in these cases, inheritance may conform to an autosomal dominant pattern with incomplete penetrance.

Hyperimmunoglobulinemia E patients have mild to moderate eosinophilia and elevated erythrocyte sedimentation rate. By definition, the patients have elevated serum IgE levels (greater than 2000 IU/mL).[99,100] The patients manifest a mild lymphocytic cellular defect with a cutaneous delayed hypersensitivity abnormality.[97] Using a radioimmunoassay, high levels of serum IgE antibodies directed to *Staphylococcus aureus* were found in all patients[101,102], and binding of more than 10% suggests this syndrome. IgE antibodies directed against other pathogens also were found in the sera of hyper-IgE syndrome patients. These pathogens include *Candida albicans*, *Streptococcus pneumoniae*, and *Haemophilus influenzae*.[98,102] The excessive production of specific IgE antibodies probably reflects underlying immunoregulatory abnormalities in this syndrome.

Clinical studies of hyper-IgE patients have demonstrated an impaired *in vitro* chemotactic response in some patients.[97,99] When present, the chemotactic defect may contribute to the increased susceptibility of the hyper-IgE patients to infections. A 61,000 d chemotactic inhibitor has been found in the supernatants of mononuclear cells of hyper-IgE patients[103], with a significant correlation between its level and the chemotactic defect.

Patients with the hyper-IgE syndrome have a low anamnestic response to immunization with DPT or DT[99] and to immunization with the capsular polysaccharide of *Haemophilus influenzae* type B (Hib-CP) and teichoic acid.[104] A deficiency of serum IgA against whole *Staphylococcus aureus*, as compared with healthy controls or patients with chronic granulomatous disease, also was found in hyper-IgE patients.[105]

Therapy in the hyperimmunoglobulinemia E-recurrent infections syndrome is directed at control of infections. Some clinicians use prophylactic, daily treatment with dicloxacillin, but the hazard of colonization with methicillin-resistant *S. aureus* is obvious. Others use daily trimethoprim-sulfamethoxazole similarly to patients with chronic granulomatous disease with favorable results. Surgical intervention and antistaphylococcal or anticandidal systemic treatment are required in cases of abscesses. The eczematoid dermatitis can be controlled with topical corticosteroids and oral antihistamines. The use of intravenous γ-globulin was suggested by Leung et al[98], to control particularly severe systemic infections. Plasmapheresis was used in a few severe cases that failed to respond to more conservative therapies and had a positive effect on eczematoid dermatitis and chemotactic defect.[106,107]

Recently, one of our patients with the hyper-IgE syndrome gave birth to a baby girl that was later diagnosed with the same syndrome.[108] During pregnancy, the mother had frequent sinobronchial infections that were promptly treated with antibiotics. She also had giardiasis and gingival abscesses that were treated by furazolidone and surgical drainage, respectively. The baby was born at 40 weeks' gestation and weighed 6 lb. 7 oz. At birth, she looked perfectly healthy, although she subsequently developed the syndrome. Adequate control of infections is essential for the favorable outcome of pregnancy in hyper-IgE-syndrome patients.

Acrodermatitis Enteropathica

Acrodermatitis enteropathica is a rare autosomal disease characterized by failure to thrive, skin lesions, alopecia, diarrhea, malabsorption, impaired immunity, intercurrent infections, and behavioral disturbances. This disorder is thought to be the consequence of zinc deficiency[109] (see also Chapter 19) and is more common in girls. Onset is insidious, usually during the first year of life. Initial symptoms often follow weaning from breast milk to cow's milk. The cutaneous eruptions consist of vesiculobullous and eczematous skin lesions in the perioral, acral, and perineal areas and on the cheeks, knees, and elbows. Initially, the lesions are intensely erythematous, but subsequently they become dry, hyperkeratotic, and psoriasiform. The hair becomes reddish, and alopecia is characteristic. Ocular manifestations include photophobia, conjunctivitis, blepharitis, and corneal dystrophy. Associated disorders are chronic diarrhea, stomatitis, glossitis, paronychia, nail dystrophy, growth retardation, personality changes, intermittent bacterial infections, and *Candida* infections. The course without treatment is chronic and intermittent but often progressive, terminating in severe marasmus and death. With less severe disease, only growth retardation and delayed development are evident.

Deficiencies of IgG and IgA[110], IgM and IgA[111], and

IgA alone[112] have been described in this disorder. Most patients, however, have normal or near normal immunoglobulins. One report describes two children, one of whom had absence of the thymus[113], and the other had a hypoplastic thymus and absent Peyer's patches. The T-cell immunodeficiency of protein calorie malnutrition has been associated with zinc deficiency.[114] Zinc treatment may enhance delayed skin reactions and reverse thymic atrophy.[115] Zinc-responsive neutrophil and monocyte chemotactic defects have been reported in three patients.[116] The other phagocytic and bactericidal functions of monocytes and neutrophils are normal in these patients.

A sustained remission was produced in the past by halogenated 8-hydroxyquinoline drugs, such as diodoquin.[117] The discovery that oral zinc therapy could produce complete remissions made this mode of therapy accepted.[109] Before initiation of diodoquin therapy, patients did not live beyond childhood. The first female survivors in their child-bearing years have appeared in the last decade. Hambidge et al[118] report that in three of seven diodoquin-treated or untreated cases, there was one spontaneous abortion and two major congenital malformations—an anencephalic baby and an achondroplastic dwarf.

During pregnancy, zinc sulfate should be given prophylactically at a dose of 300 mg/d (68 mg of elemental zinc).[119] This dose should be increased to 400 mg in the last month because transplacental passage increases at that period. The goal is to maintain a maternal plasma zinc level of 72–137 mg/dL.[120] None of the pregnant patients treated appropriately with zinc had babies with malformations, and zinc therapy significantly improves maternal immune function.

Pure Red Cell Aplasia

Pure red cell aplasia is a rare condition in which production of red cell precursors in the bone marrow is depressed. Associated disorders are dysgammaglobulinemia[121], leukopenia, and thymoma.[122] Alterations in the levels of immunoglobulins may lead to an immunodeficiency with bacterial infections of the sinobronchial tract. In one series of seven adult patients with acquired pure red cell aplasia, cytotoxicity for erythroblasts was identified in four.[123] Approximately one half of the patients had thymomas and manifested laboratory evidence of autoimmunity, including antinuclear factors[124], lupus erythematosus (LE) cells[124], paraproteins[124], and Coombs-positive hemolytic anemia.[122-124] Because 25–30% of patients undergo remission of the anemia when the thymomas are removed[125], it has been suggested that the disease is caused by an immunologic abnormality. In addition, some patients have responded to corticosteroids, and a few have responded to splenectomy.[125,126]

There are few published cases of pure red cell aplasia during pregnancy. Two women were reported[127] with well-documented red cell aplasia when not pregnant, and remission occurred with treatment. Subsequently, the women became anemic while pregnant; unfortunately, these cases were not substantiated by bone marrow studies. One 15-year-old primigravida developed pure red cell aplasia during pregnancy.[128] This worsened despite repeated transfusions, and the patient had a cesarean section at 30 weeks' gestation. The infant died of respiratory failure 24 hours after birth. There was no evidence of a thymoma, and the child's hematology values were normal for age. Immediately after the birth of the child, the mother experienced a rapid increase in hemoglobin, and 2 years later, she had an uneventful pregnancy during which the hemoglobin stayed above 11.5 g/dL. Another case was reported of a woman whose pregnancy was terminated artificially at 12 weeks' gestation, after which pure red cell aplasia was discovered.[129] After treatment with corticosteroids, the hemoglobin returned to normal values. No thymic enlargement was noted. Another 21-year-old woman had a second pregnancy and delivery; bone marrow aspiration documented pure red cell aplasia[130] developing during the second postpartum week and completely resolving 1 week later. When this patient's plasma was added to normal erythropoietic cell cultures, a significant depression of normal erythropoiesis was found.

By noninvasive studies, none of these patients with pure red cell aplasia during pregnancy had thymic enlargement. The relatively rapid remission in all of these cases after evacuation of the uterine contents indicates an association with pregnancy. The possible causes include alteration of the usual hormonal effect on erythropoiesis during pregnancy, an autoimmune mechanism, or an immune complex involving a cytotoxic factor.[131] The newborns of the affected mothers were always normal, which suggests that the causative agent does not cross the placenta. The management in this disorder involves two possible approaches. One approach is to treat the anemia with blood transfusions. In a second approach, the autoimmune phenomena can be treated with corticosteroids.

Thyroid Diseases

Graves' Disease. Thyrotoxicosis occurs in 1 in 2000 pregnancies (see also Chapter 40).[132] Neonatal thyrotoxicosis occurs in about 1% of mothers with Graves' disease.[133] In infants born to mothers with Graves' disease, hyperthyroidism may occur as a transitory phenomenon or as classic Graves' disease during the neonatal period. It is the most common endocrine disorder in pregnancy, with the exception of diabetes mellitus. Because thyroid-stimulating hormone does not cross the placenta, the fetal thyroid must function independently. The drugs used for treatment of maternal hyperthyroidism, especially those in the carbimazole group, easily cross the placental barrier.[134] These drugs act by blocking iodination of tyrosine of T_3 and T_4. The trophoblast produces and secretes a TSH-like substance.[135] Mothers with hyperthyroidism are known to produce a TSH-like substance, called long-acting thyroid stimulator (LATS). As an IgG-type immunoglobulin, it readily crosses the placental barrier. This substance and other immunoglobulins are elevated in mothers with Graves' disease.

The hyperthyroidism of Graves' disease is considered to be a consequence of stimulation of the thyroid by LATS and other related immunoglobulins. Many patients with Graves' disease do not demonstrate detectable LATS activity in the mouse bioassay.[136] At the same time, IgG from 90% of the patients protects LATS-positive serum from being adsorbed by human thyroid extracts. This activity of the patient's IgG is called the *LATS-protector.*[135] Thus, most LATS-negative sera contain LATS-protector immunoglobulins, which do not bind to and stimulate mouse thyroid gland, but are able to bind to human thyroid and compete with the binding of other thyroid-stimulating immunoglobulins.[135] Because TSH stimulates the thyroid by binding to its specific receptor on the plasma membrane of the thyroid cells, stimulating immunoglobulins that are present in the sera of patients with Graves' disease also interact with this membrane receptor.

An assay based on the ability of sera or immunoglobulins to compete with $[^{125}]$TSH for binding to its receptor on human thyroid membranes has been developed.[134]

Based on this assay, 60–100% of patients with Graves' disease have evidence of circulating anti-TSH receptor antibodies, called *human thyroid-stimulating immunoglobulin* (TSI), as opposed to the sera of patients with toxic nodular goiter or nontoxic goiter and normal controls.[136,137] This assay, however, lacks sensitivity, and many patients with Graves' disease are negative. On the other hand, there are a significant number of false-positive tests caused by nonspecific binding of normal human immunoglobulin to the thyroid receptor.

In general, most of the patients demonstrate a correlation between the inhibition test and thyroid activity. There are cases that fail to show this correlation and a few that show a negative correlation. This finding raises the question of whether some populations of antibodies might be primarily antagonists of TSH.[138] This potential existence of heterogeneous antibody populations suggests that assays based on the capacity to stimulate the thyroid would be better indicators of the presence of stimulatory factors. These assays use colloid droplet formation or cyclic AMP production as indicators of activity.[139] In these stimulation tests, the activity of the immunoglobulin lies in the Fab fragment and in the heavy chain. Consequently, it has been suggested that Graves' disease, Hashimoto's disease, and idiopathic myxedema may be manifestations of a similar underlying immunologic process.[140]

According to Volpe et al[138] interaction of T and B lymphocytes may produce the different immunologic pictures. In Graves' disease, TSI is the active factor, whereas in Hashimoto's disease, thyroid antibodies (antithyroglobulin and antimicrosomal fraction) of a nonstimulatory nature are present in greater quantity. These nonstimulatory antibodies may cooperate with T cells to produce cytotoxicity. Because the incidence of cretinism is not increased in babies born to mothers with Hashimoto's disease, the cytotoxic factor does not cross the placenta and thus does not affect the fetus.

Cellular and humoral immunity are thought to be involved in Graves' disease. Migration inhibitory factor (MIF) was shown to be produced in response to thyroid antibody by lymphocytes of patients with Graves' disease.[141] The percentage of T-lymphocytes is elevated in these patients, and the thymus is frequently enlarged. Lymphocyte subpopulations and functions are apparently normal in Graves' disease except for increased cytotonic cell activity, which may be present early in the course of the disease.[142]

Mothers with Graves' disease who have had surgical removal of the thyroid and who may be clinically asymptomatic or even myxedematous may still give birth to babies with the neonatal manifestations of hyperthyroidism because the end organ, rather than the basic immunologic process, was eliminated by the procedure. Thus, measurement of the maternal thyroid-stimulating immunoglobulin effect may be valuable in predicting the likelihood of neonatal disease. Another indicator is measurement of fetal heart rate or of excessive fetal movements.[132] The importance of antenatal diagnosis is stressed by the finding that intrauterine and neonatal thyrotoxicosis causes significant increases in the child's mortality rate.

Metabolic status at delivery correlates directly with pregnancy outcome, and women treated earlier in pregnancy with propylthiouracil are more likely to be euthyroid at delivery and have good outcomes.[132] Early diagnosis, preferably before pregnancy, increases the possibility of early treatment and good prognosis. Preterm delivery, perinatal mortality, and maternal heart failure are more common in women who remain thyrotoxic despite treatment and in those who are not treated.[132]

Hashimoto's Thyroiditis. Women with a history of goiter may develop transient hypothyroidism in the postpartum period (see also Chapter 40). The thyroid enlarges, and hypothyroidism occurs 3–5 months postpartum. This situation ends in a spontaneous remission after 5–10 months with a decrease in thyroid size but with persistent goiter. High titers of antithyroid microsomal antibodies are found.[143] This clinical behavior, with remission during pregnancy and a relapse after delivery, occurs in other autoimmune disorders as well, such as rheumatoid arthritis, systemic lupus erythematosus, and idiopathic thrombocytopenic purpura.[144,145]

Antibodies to thyroglobulin, detected by hemagglutination or radioimmunoassay, are found in the sera of almost all patients with thyroiditis.[146] Antibodies to a thyroid cell microsomal antigen, a precursor of thyroglobulin, are equally common.[143-146] Virtually all patients with Hashimoto's thyroiditis have antibodies to one of these antigens. Antimicrosomal antibodies usually are assayed by passive hemagglutination or by immunofluorescence.[143] Radioimmunoassay and complement fixation assay also are performed. Antibody to a surface antigen, unfixed monkey, or human thyroid cells can be detected by membrane immunofluorescence. This antibody can support complement-dependent and lymphocyte-dependent cytotoxicity against these cells.[146] Circulating immune complexes involving thyroid antigens have been detected[147] and reported to cause glomerulonephritis.[148]

Normal cellular immunity in this disorder is suggested by the presence of a significant mononuclear cell infiltration of the thyroid gland and by failure to induce thyroiditis in thymus-deficient animals. Peripheral blood lymphocytes of patients with thyroiditis can proliferate and release lymphokines in the presence of thyroglobulin. These cells show cytotoxicity for thyroglobulin-coated target cells.[149] The lymphocytes that infiltrate the thyroid gland in this disease also have been isolated and tested in the leukocyte inhibition factor assay. The cells did not respond better than control cells.[149] A possible explanation of this phenomenon may be inactivation of the lymphocytes by the excessive amount of the antigen present in the gland. K cells and other Fc-receptor-bearing lymphoid cells are present in the gland, but their activity has not been demonstrated clearly *in vivo*.[150] Except for thyroid autoimmunity, the immune system is normal in patients with Hashimoto's disease. Lymphocyte subpopulations are normal except for a slight excess of K cells.[142]

FETAL AND NEONATAL THYROID DISEASE. The newborns of hyperthyroid mothers may manifest signs of transient thyrotoxicosis in the perinatal period. Fetal and neonatal tachycardia are common.[151] These babies show intrauterine and postnatal failure to gain weight[152] as well as jitteriness, tachypnea, exophthalmos, goiter, and diarrhea. This condition can be diagnosed antenatally by recording the fetal heart rate and by the presence of TSI thyroid-stimulating immunoglobulin in the mother's blood. If this diagnosis is made, the mother should be treated with antithyroid drugs while the fetal heart rate is monitored.[153] The dose is administered to achieve maternal thyroid activity slightly above normal to prevent fetal cretinism. Antithyroid drugs cannot completely prevent the occurrence of postnatal hyperthyroidism because they have a much shorter half-life than that of TSI. If signs of hyperthyroidism appear in the newborn, the baby should be treated with antithyroid drugs for the first 3 months. TSI is responsible for this disorder and the long-acting thyroid-stimulating protector (LATS-P) is the main component involved.[153]

Infants of mothers with Hashimoto's disease do not manifest an increased evidence of cretinism.[140] Thus, the nonstimulatory antithyroid antibodies, which are believed to cause the maternal disease, either do not cross the placental barrier or do not influence the fetal thyroid gland.

Thrombocytopenic Purpura

Thrombocytopenia is a platelet deficiency that is commonly associated with purpuric and other hemorrhagic phenomena. It is evident that thrombocytopenic purpura is potentially hazardous during pregnancy. When antibodies to platelets of an IgG class are present in the mother's circulation and the fetus carries the relative antigen, it probably will experience transient thrombocytopenia, which will be spontaneously corrected in the first weeks of life. This is frequently seen in the most common type of autoimmune thrombocytopenic purpura, the *idiopathic* form (ITP). Neonatal thrombocytopenia may be caused by a direct antibody effect and may be associated with maternal ITP of the autoimmune type, maternal immunization against platelet antigens from the fetus, or rarely, drug-induced immunologic thrombocytopenia. It also may be caused by intravascular coagulation, intrauterine infection, septicemia with bone marrow depression, or failure of platelet production because of abnormalities of megakaryocytes (see also Chapter 165).

The most common form—ITP—is caused by increased destruction of circulating platelets, which have been damaged by an autoimmune antibody produced in response to an unknown stimulus. This IgG antibody is found in serum and bound to platelets of patients with ITP. Levels correlate with response to treatment with prednisone, splenectomy, or immunoglobulin therapy. The antibody is produced mainly in the spleen, where it is associated with platelet phagocytosis by splenic leukocytes. Some patients with ITP have lymphocytes that are stimulated *in vitro* by autologous platelets. This indicates a participation of cellular immunity in this process. The platelet antibodies may be agglutinating, complement fixing, or blockers of complement fixation.

The serum of mothers strongly suspected of having the disorder frequently shows incomplete or blocking antibodies, which can inhibit complement fixing by other antibodies. Incomplete antibodies are as effective as the complete type in causing thrombocytopenia; this coincides with clinical experience. Similar antibodies may induce thrombocytopenia in the common autoimmune form of the disease (ITP). The ITP factor may act similarly to the blocking type of antiplatelet isoantibodies, which probably accounts for the difficulty encountered in its identification. Splenic sequestration is the major mechanism by which the antibody-coated platelets are destroyed. Highly sensitized platelets are sequestered in the liver. This alternative pathway is probably a major cause of thrombocytopenia in the splenectomized patient. Steroids are believed to inhibit splenic sequestration of platelets with low-avidity antibody. The platelet antibodies may form complexes with antigen, and this can cause a delayed form of platelet aggregation, either directly or by way of complement activation. Some platelet antibodies were shown to inhibit clot retraction in reactive patients.[154]

The antigen involved in ITP has not been defined precisely, but it seems to have a low degree of polymorphism. Evidence for this comes from the fact that at least 70% of babies are affected by the mother's disease. More sensitive tests that correspond to the radioactive Coombs' test for erythrocytes should further elucidate the exact antigen(s) involved.

Mothers who have undergone splenectomy may still transfer the disease to the fetus, even if they are asymptomatic. The fetus has an active spleen that can sequester the sensitized platelets.

It is difficult to demonstrate the presence of the autoantibodies in ITP.[155] The diagnosis usually is made by ruling out other causes of thrombocytopenia. The best evidence for this disorder is the transplacental transfer of the disease to the fetus.

Isoimmune thrombocytopenia is similar to Rh isoimmunization. Sensitization may follow a delivery, abortion, or transfusion. The sensitization may be caused by platelets or cross-reactivity with leukocytes carrying the same antigen. The antibodies are found in patients who have had previous exposure to histocompatibility (HLA) antigens shared by platelets or specific platelet antigens of the HLA system that are not their own. The antibodies are measured by platelet radioactive serotonin release[156] or complement fixation.[157]

Platelet antibodies may exist in patients who demonstrate hypersensitivity to a drug or a chemical substance. The drug is a hapten that is bound to platelets or serum proteins and provokes the production of antibodies.[158] Complement is involved, and direct damage to the platelet may be caused by the drug–antibody complex adsorbed to the platelet surface nonspecifically and fixed complement.[158] Another proposed mechanism is that platelets are more adherent to red blood cells because of the action of drugs. The red blood cells are coated with complement, and as a result, platelet destruction is enhanced.[158]

Maternal Autoimmune Hemolytic Disease

Immune hemolysis is defined as destruction of red blood cells by immunologic mechanisms that involve antibody and complement, functioning together or alone. There are two types of this disorder, autoimmune and isoimmune. Maternal anemia caused by autoantibodies of the idiopathic type may occur in women of childbearing age. This disorder, unlike most autoimmune disorders, worsens during pregnancy and remits after delivery.[159] The degree of maternal anemia is of prognostic value to the outcome of the pregnancy. In one series, 20% of the pregnancies resulted in stillbirth, which was associated with a severe degree of maternal anemia (see also Chapter 164).[159]

Newborns seem to be unaffected by the maternal disease. They do not show signs of anemia or hydrops. It is postulated that the newborn displays a weak antigen on the membrane of erythrocytes or that the immunoglobulin responsible for the disease is of the IgG_4 subclass, which crosses the placenta only to a limited extent.

The treatment for autoimmune hemolytic anemia in pregnant women should include the usual treatment for nonpregnant patients with hemolytic anemia. Blood transfusions, corticosteroids, immunosuppressive drugs (azathioprine), and splenectomy are indicated in this disorder. Usually the treatment does not go beyond blood transfusions because of the benign course of this disorder in pregnant women.

Pernicious Anemia

Pernicious anemia is an organ-specific type of autoimmune disease with the gastric mucosa as the target. In this disease, there is an inability to secrete *gastric intrinsic factor,* a glycoprotein produced by the parietal cells of the gastric fundus. Intrinsic factor combines with the dietary vitamin B_{12} in a complex that is absorbed in the terminal ileum. The disease is more prevalent after the age of 40 years and therefore is rare in pregnancy. The antibodies found in pernicious anemia may be directed at the parietal cells or at the intrinsic factor itself. The intrinsic factor antibodies may prevent binding of the vitamin B_{12} complex or bind to an intrinsic factor—vitamin B_{12} complex. Antibodies occur in the gastric juice, which are probably synthesized by plasma cells in the stomach.

In one case, intrinsic factor antibodies were demonstrated in the cord blood, and at the age of 11 days, the baby's gastric juice did not contain intrinsic factor.[160] At the age of 12 weeks, the baby was clinically well, although vitamin B_{12} levels were low. Babies may show parietal cell antibodies transiently in the postnatal period.[161] However, these IgG-type antibodies are probably of no great immunopathologic importance.

Myasthenia Gravis

Myasthenia gravis is characterized by weakness of voluntary muscles following repetitive activity and a marked tendency to recover motor power after rest. Lymphocyte infiltration of skeletal muscle occurs in 50% of patients with myasthenia.[162] These changes resemble those found in many autoimmune disorders.[163] The thymus is frequently involved in myasthenia in the form of tumor or lymphoid hyperplasia. Often, clinical remission occurs after surgical thymectomy (see also Chapter 199).

The autoimmune characterization of this disease is now well accepted since the discovery that α-bungarotoxin, which is a venom of the krait *Bungarus multicinctus,* can be shown following ^{125}I labeling to bind specifically to acetylcholine receptors at the myoneural junction in humans.[164] Myasthenics carry a γ-globulin factor directed against acetylcholine (ACh) receptors, and studies have shown a reduction of 70% in the quantity of ACh receptors in myasthenics using competition techniques with α-bungarotoxin.[165] High titers of anti-ACh receptor immunoglobulin were identified in serum and thymic tissue of myasthenia gravis patients.[166] T-cell-mediated immunity involvement in this disorder was confirmed by a proliferative response of patients' lymphocytes to purified ACh receptor antigen.[167]

Circulating immunoglobulins that bind to skeletal muscle ACh receptor proteins reduce the number of motor end plates available to bind ACh. Failure to bind ACh inhibits the contractile ability of skeletal muscles but not those of smooth muscles; uterine contraction is thus unimpaired. This disorder is prevalent in women of childbearing age. If the disease is manifested during pregnancy, relapse is more frequent, and the medication requirement is higher.[168]

ANTENATAL DIAGNOSIS OF PRIMARY IMMUNODEFICIENCY DISORDERS

Primary immunodeficiency disorders usually are associated with debilitating morbidity and a high mortality rate. Unfortunately, treatment of patients with primary immunodeficiency is far from adequate and standard modes of treatment, such as bone marrow or fetal tissue transplantation, are associated with severe side effects and high mortality. Prevention should be considered when possible with a particular focus on antenatal diagnosis.

Most of the immunodeficiency syndromes have a known genetic inheritance pattern, usually X-linked or autosomal recessive.[169] In families who have already had a severely affected child, genetic counseling for carrier detection and prenatal diagnosis is an essential step in management. With the ongoing progress in the understanding of genetic and pathophysiologic mechanisms of immunodeficiency syndromes, it is now possible to advance treatment with the aid of prenatal diagnosis and interruption of pregnancy.

Several methods exist for prenatal diagnosis and carrier detection. Analysis of gene-point mutations that are responsible for the appearance of immunodeficiency syndromes is possible with the aid of DNA direct analysis by Southern blotting. This method has been termed *gene tracking.*[170] It requires a gene-specific or closely linked DNA probe that detects a restriction fragment length polymorphism, which is used to distinguish each chromosome of the pair in key family members. The method uses the close linkage between the disease and a DNA probe, even when the exact underlying defect is not known. Gene tracking is now possible for detection of X-linked agammaglobulinemia[171-173], X-linked severe combined immunodeficiency[174], X-linked hypogammaglobulinemia with high IgM[175], Wiskott–Aldrich syndrome[176], and X-linked lymphoproliferative disease.[177] For all these disorders, the gene map is established and can be used for detection by the gene tracking technique.[178]

Some immunodeficiency syndromes are associated with prominent biochemical or cellular defects. At least five such defects are known, and most of them are directly related to the pathophysiology of the immunodeficiency disorder. The disorders are (1) *inherited absence of adenosine deaminase* (ADA), which usually results in a clinical syndrome of severe combined immunodeficiency; (2) *genetic absence of purine nucleoside phosphorylase* (PNP), which results in a cellular immunodeficiency syndrome; (3) *absence of transcobalamin II,* which results in agammaglobulinemia, defects in hematopoietic stem cells, and a severe phagocytic deficiency; (4) *defective synthesis of a DNA-binding protein* (RF-X), which regulates the HLA class II gene promoter region, resulting in a defective expression of HLA class II molecules on the lymphocyte's membrane, and in the appearance of the *bare lymphocyte syndrome,* associated with severe combined immunodeficiency; and (5) *absence or residual expression of the β-chain common to all forms of leukocyte adhesion molecule families* (LFA-1, CR3, and gp 150,95), resulting in delayed separation of the umbilical cord and a phagocytic adhesion deficiency. Direct biochemical methods can measure the enzymatic activity of the purine pathway enzymes ADA and PNP[179] and the transcobalamin II isoprotein.[180] Monoclonal antibodies for class I and II HLA molecules[181], α and β chains of LFA-1[182], and run-off transcription and gel retardation assays for detection of RF-X[183] enable the diagnosis of defects in these systems.

The diagnosis of some of the immunodeficiency disorders can be established by measuring cellular function. An important example is the *nitroblue tetrazolium test* (NBT) and *superoxide generation* that have been studied in granulocytes of a 16-week-old fetus.[184] Absence of the superoxide generation on stimulation of the granulocytes with phorbol myristate acetate (PMA) and absence of NBT reduction with or without stimulation enables the diagnosis of chronic granulomatous disease.[185] In most instances, a maternal carrier state of linked chronic granulomatous disease can be shown by a phagocytic intracellular killing test where the mother's neutrophils show a bactericidal activity for *Staphylococcus aureus*, which is an intermediate between the maximal killing of a healthy control and the minimal or absent killing of an affected patient.

Chromosomal breakage syndromes frequently are associated with primary immunodeficiency. Among the syndromes are *ataxia-telangiectasia* with cellular immunodeficiency, absence of both IgA and IgE, increased spontaneous chromosomal breakage, and a presence of an abnormal clone with a 14/5 translocation. If spontaneous breakage is not significant, it may be induced *in vitro* by application of small doses of radiation or methotrexate.[186] Other syndromes of spontaneous chromosomal breakage associated with partial immunodeficiency are *Bloom's syndrome, Fanconi's anemia,* and *Down's syndrome.*

Using monoclonal antibodies, it is possible to diagnose defects in the ontogeny of various types of lymphocytes. This method is particularly effective when the possibility of severe combined immunodeficiency, X-linked agammaglobulinemia, and several ontogenic defects in the T-cell lineage are sought.[187,188] The monoclonal antibodies can be detected by fluorescent activated cell sorting analysis or by an immune-peroxidase staining.[178] *Chédiak–Higashi syndrome* is characterized by a partial oculocutaneous albinism; by phagocytic immunodeficiency that stems from an inability of the phagocytes to perform chemotaxis, phagocytosis, or nonoxidative intracellular killing; and by the presence of giant lysosomal inclusion bodies in the phagocyte's cytoplasm. The inclusion bodies have been visualized in the neutrophils at 18 weeks' gestation.[188]

An additional method has been proposed for detection of mothers who are carriers for X-linked disorders of the immune system. According to Lyon hypothesis, a permanent inactivation of one of the two X chromosomes randomly occurs in every somatic cell in the mother.[189] All progeny cells, therefore, inherit a stable pattern of chromosomes from the mother following this inactivation. Consequently, a female carrier of an X-linked immunodeficiency disorder has two distinct populations of lymphocyte precursors, if the gene is not essential for the development of that cell type (in that case only one set of healthy chromosomes will prevail). However, the ratio may vary from the expected 50–50 to as much as 90–10 in approximately 5% of normal women.[190] The finding of a ratio that violates this rule would thus indicate a selective usage of one chromosome. Allelic forms of the linked enzyme glucose-6-phosphate dehydrogenase (G-6-PD) can be used as markers.[191] However, because the method is only informative in certain families, Puck et al[192] have used a method based on the production of somatic cell hybrids between human and hamster cells. The hybrids tend to lose human chromosomes and because of the cultivation in a selective medium, only hybrids that retain the active human chromosome will survive. Based on this technique, carriers of linked *severe combined immunodeficiency*[193] and *X-linked agammaglobulinemia*[194] have been identified. A deviation from a stable and random X chromosome inactivation that is indicative for a state of maternal carriage was identified also in *Wiskott-Aldrich syndrome.*[195]

The management of immunodeficiency disorders should include the previously described strategies for detection of a carrier state in the mother or a disease state in the fetus. Biochemical or functional analysis that enables a precise diagnosis of the defect is the preferred technique when possible. In cases in which the exact pathogenetic mechanism is unknown, mapping of the gene by linkage studies using restriction fragment length polymorphisms can be used. Although more conditions are becoming amenable to diagnosis in the first trimester by analysis of chorionic villus biopsy specimens, at present most can only be diagnosed by analyzing fetal blood or amniotic fluid taken at 12–20 weeks' gestation. The number of cells recovered by these techniques is obviously the limiting factor for diagnosis, and laboratory micromethods for cellular, biochemical and genetic analysis are being devised to enable a precise diagnosis with a very small number of cells.[196]

REFERENCES

1. Stites DP, Pavia CS, Clemens LE, et al. Immunologic regulation in pregnancy. *Arthritis Rheum.* 1979;22:1300.
2. Faulk WP, Temple A, Lovins RE, et al. Antigens of human trophoblast: a working hypothesis for their role in normal and abnormal pregnancies. *Proc Natl Acad Sci USA.* 1978;75:1947.
3. Chatterjee-Hasrouni S, Lala P. Localization of H-2 antigens on mouse trophoblast cells. *J Exp Med.* 1979;149:1238.
4. Clements PJ, Yu DTY, Levy J, et al. Human lymphocyte subpopulations: the effect of pregnancy. *Proc Soc Exp Biol Med.* 1976;152:664.
5. Sridama V, Pacini F, Yang SL, et al. Decreased level of helper T-cells: a possible cause of immunodeficiency in pregnancy. *N Engl J Med.* 1982;307:352.
6. Brunham RC, Martin DH, Hubbard TW, et al. Depression of the lymphocyte transformation response to microbial antigens and to phytohemagglutinin during pregnancy. *J Clin Invest.* 1983;72:1629.
7. Goodfellow CF. Maternal lymphocyte responses during normal and abnormal pregnancies, measured *in vitro* using composite trophoblast antigens and phytohemagglutinin. *Immunol Rev.* 1983;75:61.
8. Rocklin RE, Kitzmiller JL, Kaye MD, et al. Immunobiology of the maternal-fetal relationship. *Annu Rev Med.* 1979;30:375.
9. Gangas JM. Glycoproteins in pregnancy serum which interact with concanavalin A and may suppress lymphocyte transformation. *Transplantation.* 1974;18:538.
10. Clemens LE, Siiteri PK, Stites DP. Mechanisms of immunosuppression of progesterone on lymphocyte activation during pregnancy. *J Immunol.* 1979;122:1978.
11. Mendelsohn J, Multer MM, Bernheim JL. Inhibition of human lymphocyte stimulation by steroid hormones: cytokinetic mechanisms. *Clin Exp Immunol.* 1977;27:127.
12. Poskitt PK, Kurt ET, Paul BB, et al. Responses to mitogen during pregnancy and the post partum period. *Obstet Gynecol.*1977;50:319.
13. Takeuchi A, Persellin RH. The inhibitory effect of pregnancy serum on polymorphonuclear leukocyte chemotaxis. *J Clin Lab Immunol.* 1980;3:121.
14. Parkman R, Mosier D, Umansky I, et al. GVH-disease after intrauterine exchange transfusions for hemolytic disease of the newborn. *N Engl J Med.* 1974;290:359.
15. Hytten FE. Nutrition in pregnancy. *Postgrad Med J.* 1979;55:295.
16. Jameson S. Zinc and pregnancy. In: Nriagu JO, ed. *Zinc in the Environment. Part II: Health Effects.* New York, NY: Wiley Co; 1980:183.
17. Hermans PE, Diaz-Buxo JA, Stobo JD. Idiopathic late-onset immunoglobulin deficiency: clinical observations in 50 patients. *Am J Med.* 1976;61:221.
18. Douglas SD, Goldberg LS, Fudenberg HH. Clinical, serologic and leukocyte function studies on patients with idiopathic "acquired agammaglobulinemia" and their families. *Am J Med.* 1970;48:48.
19. Waldmann TA, Durm M, Broder S, et al. Role of suppressor T cells in pathogenesis of common variable hypogammaglobulinemia. *Lancet.* 1974;2:609.
20. Ochs HD, Ament ME. Gastrointestinal tract and immunodeficiency. In: Ferguson A, McSween RNM, eds. *Immunological Aspects of the Liver and Gastrointestinal Tract.* Lancaster, PA: MTP Press; 1976:83.
21. Ament ME, Ochs HD, Davis SD. Structure and function of the gastrointestinal tract in primary immunodeficiency syndromes. A study of 39 patients. *Medicine.* 1973;52:227.
22. Pines A, Goldhammer E, Bregman J, et al. Campylobacter enteritis associated with recurrent abortions in agammaglobulinemia. *Acta Obstet Gynecol Scand.* 1980;62:279.
23. Hermans PE, Huizenga KA, Hoffman HN, et al. Dysgammaglobulinemia associated with nodular lymphoid hyperplasia of the small intestine. *Am J Med.* 1966;40:78.
24. Fudenberg HH, German JL III, Kunkel HG. The occurrence of rheumatoid factor and other abnormalities in families of patients with agammaglobulinemia. *Arthritis Rheum.* 1962;5:565.
25. Good RA, Yunis E. Association of autoimmunity, immunodeficiency and aging in man, rabbits and mice. *Fed Proc.* 1974;33:2040.
26. Schaller JG. Immunodeficiency and autoimmunity. In: Bergsma D, ed.

Immunodeficiency in Man and Animals. Birth Defects. March of Dimes; 1975;11:173.
27. Holland NH, Holland P. Immunological maturation in an infant of an agammaglobulinemic mother. *Lancet.* 1966;2:1152.
28. Preud'homme JL, Griscelli C, Seligmann M. Immunoglobulins on the surface of lymphocytes in fifty patients with primary immunodeficiency diseases. *Clin Immunol Immunopathol.* 1973;1:241.
29. Laursen HB, Christensen MF. Immunoglobulins in normal infant born of severe hypogammaglobulinemic mother. *Arch Dis Chil.* 1973;48:646.
30. Kobayashi RH, Hyman CJ, Stiehm ER. Immunologic maturation in an infant born to a mother with agammaglobulinemia. *Am J Dis Child.* 1980;1334:942.
31. Berger M, Cupps TR, Fauci AS. High-dose immunoglobulin replacement by slow subcutaneous infusion during pregnancy. *JAMA.* 1982;247:2824.
32. Day NK, Good RA, Wahn V. Adverse reaction in selected patients following intravenous infusions of gammaglobulin. *Am J Med.* 1984;76:25.
33. Gitlin D. Development and metabolism of the immune globulins. In: Kagan BM, Stiehm ER, eds. *Immunologic Incompetence.* Chicago, IL: Yearbook Medical Publishers; 1971:3.
34. Pitcher-Wilmott RW, Hindocha P, Wood CBS. The placental transfer of IgG subclasses in human pregnancy. *Clin Exp Immunol.* 1980;41:303.
35. Virella G, Amelia SNM, Tamagnini G. Placental transfer of human IgG subclasses. *Clin Exp Immunol.* 1972;10:475.
36. Sorensen RU, Tomford W, Gyves MT, et al. The use of intravenous immunoglobulin in pregnant women with common variable hypogammaglobulinemia. *Am J Med.* 1984;76:73.
37. Hausser C, Buriot D. Gammaglobulin therapy during pregnancy in mothers with hypogammaglobulinemia. *Am J Obstet Gynecol.* 1982;144:112.
38. Madsen DL, Catanzarite VA, Varela Gittling F. Common variable hypogammaglobulinemia in pregnancy: treatment with high dose immunoglobulin infusions. *Am J Hematol.* 1986;21:327.
39. Smith EC, Hammarstrom L. Intravenous immunoglobulin in pregnancy. *Obstet Gynecol.* 1985;66:395.
40. Hayward AR, Lawton AR. Induction of plasma cell differentiation of human fetal lymphocytes: evidence of functional immaturity of T and B cells. *J Immunol.* 1977;119:1213.
41. Claman HN, Merrill DA, Peakman D. Isolated severe gamma A deficiency: immunoglobulin levels, clinical disorders and chromosome studies. *J Lab Clin Med.* 1970;75:307.
42. Ammann AJ, Hong R. Selective IgA deficiency: presentation of 30 cases and a review of the literature. *Medicine.* 1971;50:223.
43. Cassidy JT, Petty R, Burt A, et al. Anti-IgA antibodies in patients with selective IgA deficiency and connective tissue diseases. *Clin Res.* 1969;17:351.
44. Bluestone R, Goldberg LS, Katz RM, et al. Juvenile rheumatoid arthritis: a serologic survey of 200 consecutive patients. *J Pediatr.* 1970;77:98.
45. Lopez M, Hyslop E. Precipitating antibody to bovidae serum proteins in dysgammaglobulinemic sera. *Fed Proc.* 1968;27:684.
46. Bachmann R. Studies on the serum γ-A-globulin level. III. The frequency of a-γ-A-globulinemia. *Scand J Clin Lab Invest.* 1965;17:316.
47. Hobbs JR. Immune imbalance in dysgammaglobulinemia type IV. *Lancet.* 1968;1:110.
48. Berg T, Johansson SGO. Immunoglobulin levels during childhood with special regard to IgE. *Acta Pediatr Scand.* 1969;58:513.
49. Crabbe PA, Heremans JF. Lack of gamma-A-immunoglobulin in serum of patients with steatorrhea. *Gut.* 1968;7:119.
50. Swanson V, Dyce B, Citron P, et al. Absence of IgA in serum with presence of IgA containing cells in the intestinal tract. *Clin Res.* 1968;16:119.
51. Lawton AF, Cooper MD. Modification of B lymphocyte differentiation by anti-immunoglobulin. In: Cooper MD, Warner NL, eds. *Contemporary Topics in Immunobiology.* New York, NY: Plenum Press; 1974;193.
52. Clough JD, Mims LH, Strober W. Deficient IgA antibody responses to arsanilic acid bovine serum albumin (BSA) in neonatally thymectomised rabbits. *J Immunol.* 1971;106:1624.
53. Ammann AJ, Hong R. Selective IgA deficiency and autoimmunity. *Clin Exp Immunol.* 1970;7:833.
54. Vyas GN, Perkins HA, Fudenberg HH. Anaphylactoid transfusion reactions associated with anti-IgA. *Lancet.* 1968;2:312.
55. Krieger I, Brough JA. Gamma-A-deficiency and hypochromic anemia due to defective iron mobilization. *N Engl J Med.* 1967;269:886.
56. Crabbe PA, Heremans JF. Selective IgA deficiency with steatorrhea. A new syndrome. *Am J Med.* 1967;42:319.
57. Gryboski JD, Self TW, Clemett A, et al. Selective IgA deficiency and intestinal nodular lymphoid hyperplasia: correction of diarrhea with antibiotics and plasma. *Pediatrics.* 1968;421:833.
58. Douglas SD, Goldberg LS, Fudenberg HH, et al. Agammaglobulinemia and co-existent pernicious anemia. *Clin Exp Immunol.* 1970;6:181.
59. Finley SC, Finley WH, Noto RA, et al. IgA absence associated with a ring-18 chromosome. *Lancet.* 1968;1:1095.
60. Stewart J, Go S, Ellis E, et al. Absent IgA and deletions of chromosome 18. *J Med Genet.* 1970;7:11.
61. Douglas SD, Goldberg LS, Fudenberg HH. Familial selective deficiency of IgA. *J Pediatr.* 1971;78:873.
62. Stocker F, Amman P, Rossie E. Selective γ-A-globulin deficiency with dominant autosomal inheritance in a Swiss family. *Arch Dis Child.* 1968;43:585.
63. Peters M, Riley D, Lockwood C. Hereditary angioedema and immunoglobulin A deficiency in pregnancy. *Obstet Gynecol.* 1988;72:454.
64. Stiehm ER. Chronic mucocutaneous candidiasis: clinical aspects. *Ann Intern Med.* 1978;89:91.
65. Blizzard RM, Gibbs JH. Candidiasis: Studies pertaining to its association with endocrinopathies and pernicious anemia. *Pediatrics.* 1968;42:231.
66. Wuepper KD, Fudenberg HH. Moniliasis, autoimmune polyendocrinopathy and immunologic family study. *Clin Exp Immunol.* 1968;2:71.
67. Valdimarsson H, Riches HRC, Holt L, et al. Lymphocyte abnormality in chronic mucocutaneous candidiasis. *Lancet.* 1970;1:1259.
68. Rocklin RE. Inhibition of cell migration as a correlate of cell-mediated immunity. In: Vyas GN, Stites DP, Brecher G, eds. *Laboratory Diagnosis of Immunologic Disorders.* New York, NY: Grune & Stratton; 1975:111.
69. Snyderman R, Altman LC, Frankel A, et al. Defective mononuclear leukocyte chemotaxis: a previously unrecognized immune dysfunction. Studies in patients with chronic mucocutaneous candidiasis. *Ann Intern Med.* 1973;78:509.
70. Sohnle PG, Frank MM, Kirkpatrick CH. Deposition of complement components in the cutaneous lesions of chronic mucocutaneous candidiasis. *Clin Immunol Immunopathol.* 1976;5:340.
71. Leikin S, Parrott R, Randolph J. Clotrimazole: treatment of chronic mucocutaneous candidiasis. *J Pediatr.* 1976;88:864.
72. Bennett JE. Drugs five years later. Fluorocytosine. *Ann Intern Med.* 1977;86:319.
73. Fischer TJ, Klein RB, Kershnar HE, et al. Miconazole in the treatment of chronic mucocutaneous candidiasis: a preliminary report. *J Pediatr.* 1977;91:815.
74. Kirkpatrick CH, Smith TK. Chronic mucocutaneous candidiasis: immunologic and antibiotic therapy. *Ann Intern Med.* 1974;80:310.
75. Validmarsson H, Wood CBS, Hobbs JR, et al. Immunological features in a case of chronic granulomatous candidiasis and its treatment with transfer factor. *Clin Exp Immunol.* 1972;11:151.
76. Validmarsson H, Moss PD, Holt PJL, et al. Treatment of chronic mucocutaneous candidiasis with leukocytes from HL-A compatible sibling. *Lancet.* 1972;1:469.
77. Buckley RH, Lucas ZJ, Hattler BG, et al. Defective cellular immunity associated with chronic mucocutaneous moniliasis and recurrent staphylococcal biotrymycosis: immunologic reconstitution by allogeneic bone marrow. *Clin Exp Immunol.* 1968;3:153.
78. Quastel M, Harrison R, Cicardi M, et al. Behavior in vivo of normal and dysfunctional C1—inhibitor in normal subjects and patients with hereditary angioneurotic edema. *J Clin Invest.* 1983;71:1041.
79. Frank MM, Gelfand JA, Atkinson JP. Hereditary angioedema: the clinical syndrome and its management. *Ann Int Med.* 1984;84:580.
80. Gelfand JA, Sherins RJ, Alling DW, et al. Treatment of hereditary angioedema with danazol: reversal of clinical and biochemical abnormalities. *N Engl J Med.* 1976;295:1444.
81. Sheffer AL, Fearon DT, Austen KF, et al. Tranexamic acid: preoperative prophylactic therapy for patients with hereditary angioneurotic edema. *J Aller Clin Immunol.* 1977;60:38.
82. Robertson D, Gallin JI. Disorders of phagocyte function. *Ann Rev Immunol.* 1987;5:127.
83. Tauber AI, Borregaard N, Simons E, et al. Chronic granulomatous disease: a syndrome of phagocyte oxidase deficiencies. *Medicine.* 1983;62:286.
84. Curnutte JT, Babior BM. Chronic granulomatous disease. *Adv Hum Genet.* 1987;16:229.
85. Forehand JR, Nauseef WH, Johnston RB Jr. Inherited disorders of phagocyte killing. In: Scriver CR, Beaudet A, Sly WS, Valle D, eds. *The Metabolic Basis of Inherited Disease.* New York, NY: McGraw-Hill; 1989;(2):2779.
86. Curnutte JT, Kipnes RS, Babior BM. Defect in pyridine nucleotide dependent superoxide production by a particulate fraction from the granulocytes of patients with chronic granulomatous disease. *N Engl J Med.* 1975;293:628.
87. Seager RA, Tiefenauer L, Matsunaga T, et al. Chronic granulomatous disease due to granulocytes with abnormal NADPH oxidase activity and deficient cytochrome-b. *Blood.* 1983;61:423.
88. Curnutte JT, Scott PJ, Kuver R, et al. NADPH oxidase activation cofactor: partial purification and absent activity in a patient with chronic granulomatous disease. *Clin Res.* 1986;34:445a.
89. Weening RS, Corbeel L, deBoer M, et al. Cytochrome b deficiency in an autosomal form of chronic granulomatous disease. *J Clin Invest.* 1985;75:915.
90. Segal AW. Cytochrome b-245 and its involvement in the molecular pathology of chronic granulomatous disease. *Hematol Oncol Clin North Am.* 1988;2:213.

91. Hassan NF, Campbell DE, Douglas SD. Clinical evaluation of defects in neutrophil oxidative metabolism. *Clin Immunol Newsletter*. 1988;9:37.
92. Curnutte JT. Classification of chronic granulomatous disease. *Hematol Oncol Clin North Am*. 1988;2:241.
93a. Kamani NR, August CS, Douglas SD, et al. Bone marrow transplantation in chronic granulomatous disease. *J Pediatr*. 1984;105:42.
93b. Kamani N, August CS, Campbell DE, et al. Marrow transplantation in chronic granulomatous disease: an update, with 6 year follow-up. *J Pediatr*. 1988;113:697.
93c. Kamani N, Douglas SD. Natural history of chronic granulomatous disease. *Diagn Clin Immunol*. 1988;5:314.
94. Ezekowitz RAB, Orkin SH, Newburger PE. Recombinant interferon gamma augments superoxide production and X-chronic granulomatous disease gene expression X-linked variant chronic granulomatous disease. *J Clin Invest*. 1987;80:1009.
95. Veille JC, Bigley R. Chronic granulomatous disease in pregnancy. *Obstet Gynecol*. 1985;66:85.
96. Davis SD, Schaller J, Wedgwood RJ. Job's syndrome: recurrent "colc" staphylococcal abscesses. *Lancet*. 1966;1:1013.
97. Donabedian HJ, Gallin JI. The hyperimmunoglobulin E-recurrent infection (Job's) syndrome. A review of the NIH experience and literature. *Medicine*. 1983;62:195.
98. Leung DYM, Guha RS. Clinical and immunological aspects of the hyperimmunoglobulin E syndrome. *Hematol Oncol Clin North Am*. 1988;2:81.
99. Buckley RH, Becker WG. Abnormalities in the regulation of human IgE synthesis. *Immunol Rev*. 1978;41:288.
100. Douglas SD, Lillie MA. Chemotaxis and hyper IgE. *Am Soc Clin Pathol*. 1981;5:1.
101. Schopfer K, Baerlocker K, Price P, et al. Staphylococcal IgE antibodies, hyperimmunoglobulinemia E and *Staphylococcus aureus* infections. *N Engl J Med*. 1979;300:835.
102. Berger M, Kirkpatrick CH, Goldsmith PK, et al. IgE antibodies to *Staphylococcus aureus* and *Candida albicans* in patients with the syndrome of hyperimmunoglobulinemia E and recurrent infections. *J Immunol*. 1980;125:2437.
103. Donabedian HJ, Gallin JI. Mononuclear cells from patients with the hyperimmunoglobulin E-recurrent infection syndrome produce an inhibitor of leukocyte chemotaxis. *J Clin Invest*. 1982;69:1155.
104. Leung DYM, Ambrosino DM, Arbeit RD, et al. Impaired antibody response in the hyperimmunoglobulin E syndrome. *J Allerg Clin Immunol*. 1988;81:1082.
105. Dreskin SC, Goldsmith PK, Gallin JI. Immunoglobulins in the hyperimmunoglobulin E and recurrent infection (Job's) syndrome. Deficiency of antistaphylococcus aureus immunoglobulin A. *J Clin Invest*. 1985;75:26.
106. Diprisco-Fuenmayor MC, Lynch NR, Lopez RI, et al. An unusual case of hyperproduction of IgE, treated by plasmapheresis. *Allergol Immunopathol*. 1986;14:1.
107. Chikazawa S, Nunoi H, Endo F, et al. Hyperimmunoglobulin E-associated recurrent infection syndrome accompanied by chemotactic inhibition of polymorphonuclear leukocytes and monocytes. *Ped Res*. 1984;18:365.
108. Lavoie A, Grodofsky M, Douglas SD. Hyperimmunoglobulinemia E-recurrent infection syndrome in infancy. *Am J Dis Child*. In press.
109. Moynahan EJ, Barnes PM. Zinc deficiency and a synthetic diet for lactose intolerance. *Lancet*. 1973;1:676.
110. Julius R, Schulkind M, Sprinkle T, et al. Acrodermatitis enteropathica with immunodeficiency. *J Pediatr*. 1973;83:1007.
111. Pass RF, Johnston RB, Cooper MD. Agammaglobulinemia with B lymphocytes in a neonate with acrodermatitis enteropathica. *Am J Dis Child*. 1974;128:251.
112. Beyer P, Wasmer A, Peter M, et al. Acrodermatitis enteropathica. *Pediatrie*. 1966;21:677.
113. Rodin AE, Goldman AS. Autopsy findings in acrodermatitis enteropathica. *Am J Clin Pathol*. 1969;51:315.
114. Golden MH, Jackson AA, Golden BE. Effect of zinc on the thymus of recently malnourished children. *Lancet*. 1977;2:1057.
115. Golden MH, Harland PS, Golden BE. Zinc and immunocompetence in protein-energy malnutrition. *Lancet*. 1978;1:1226.
116. Weston WL, Huff JC, Humber JR, et al. Zinc correction of defective chemotaxis in acrodermatitis enteropathica. *Arch Dermatol*. 1977;113:422.
117. Dillaha CJ, Lorinez AL, Aavik OR. Acrodermatitis enteropathica: a review of the literature and report of a case successfully treated with diodoquin. *JAMA*. 1953;152:509.
118. Hambidge KM, Nelden KH, Walraven PA. Zinc acrodermatitis enteropathica and congenital malformations. *Lancet*. 1973;1:577.
119. Brenton DP, Jackson MJ, Young A. Two pregnancies in a patient with acrodermatitis enteropathica treated with zinc sulfate. *Lancet*. 1981;2:500.
120. Successful outcome of two pregnancies in a patient with congenital acrodermatitis enteropathica. *Nutr Rev*. 1982;40:78.
121. DiGiacomo J, Furst SW, Nixon DD. Primary acquired red cell aplasia in the adult. *J Mt Sinai Hosp. NY*. 1966;33:382.
122. Schmid JR, Kiely JM, Harrison EG Jr, et al. Thymoma associated with pure red-cell agenesis: review of the literature and report of 4 cases. *Cancer*. 1965;18:216.
123. Zaentz SD, Krantz SB. Studies on pure red cell aplasia. VI. Development of two stage erythroblast cytotoxicity method and role of complement. *J Lab Clin Med*. 1973;82:31.
124. Barnes RD. Thymic neoplasms associated with refractory anemia. *Guys Hosp Rep*. 1965;114:73.
125. Roland AS. The syndrome of benign thymoma and primary aregenerative anemia: an analysis of 43 cases. *Am J Med Sci*. 1964;247:719.
126. Krantz SB. Pure red cell aplasia. *N Engl J Med*. 1974;291:345.
127. Skikne BS, Lynch RS, Bexwoda WR, et al. Pure red cell aplasia. *S Afr Med J*. 1976;50:1353.
128. Aggio MC, Zunini C. Reversible pure red cell aplasia in pregnancy. *N Engl J Med*. 1977;297:221.
129. Miyoshi I, Hikita T, Koi B, et al. Reversible pure red cell aplasia in pregnancy. *N Engl J Med*. 1978;299:777.
130. Seidenfeld AM, Owen J, Prchal JF. Pure red cell aplasia with an inhibitor to erythropoiesis. *Can Med Assoc J*. 1979;121:188.
131. Lehman G, Alcoff J. Reversible pure red cell hypoplasia in pregnancy. *JAMA*. 1982;247:1170.
132. Hodges RE, Evans TC, Bradbury JT, et al. The accumulation of radioactive iodine by human fetal thyroids. *J Clin Endocrinol Metab*. 1955;15:661.
133. Davis LE, Lucas MJ, Hankins GDV, et al. Thyrotoxicosis complicating pregnancy. *Am J Obstet Gynecol*. 1989;160:63.
134. Burrow GN. The management of thyrotoxicosis in pregnancy. *N Engl J Med*. 1985;313:562.
135. Adams DD, Kennedy TH. Evidence to suggest that LATS protector stimulates the human thyroid gland. *J Clin Endocrinol Metab*. 1971;33:47.
136. Smith BR, Hall R. Thyroid stimulating immunoglobulins in Graves' disease. *Lancet*. 1974;2:427.
137. Mukhtar ED, Smith BR, Pyle GA, et al. Relation of thyroid stimulating immunoglobulins to thyroid function and effect of surgery, radioiodine and antithyroid drugs. *Lancet*. 1975;1:713.
138. Endo K, Kasagi K, Konishi J, et al. Detection and properties of TSH binding inhibitor immunoglobulins in patients with Graves' disease and Hashimoto's thyroiditis. *J Clin Endocrinol*. 1978;46:734.
139. Onaya T, Kotani M, Yamada D, et al. New in vitro tests to detect the thyroid stimulator in sera from hyperthyroid patients by measuring colloid droplet formation and cyclic AMP in human thyroid slices. *J Clin Endocrinol*. 1973;36:859.
140. Volpe R, Farid NR, von Westarp C, et al. The pathogenesis of Graves' disease and Hashimoto's thyroiditis. *Clin Endocrinol*. 1974;3:239.
141. Mahieu P, Winand R. Demonstration of delayed hypersensitivity in retrobulbar and thyroid tissues in human exophtalmos. *J Clin Endocrinol Metab*. 1972;34:1090.
142. Calder EA, Irvine WJ, Davidson NM, et al. T, B and K cells in autoimmune thyroid disease. *Clin Exp Immunol*. 1976;24:17.
143. Amino N, Miyai K, Kuro R, et al. Transient post partum hypothyroidism. Fourteen cases with autoimmune thyroiditis. *Ann Intern Med*. 1977;87:155.
144. Scott JS. Immunological diseases in pregnancy. *Prog Allergy*. 1977;23:321.
145. Talal N. Disordered immunologic regulation and autoimmunity. *Transplant Rev*. 1977;31:516.
146. Doniach D. Humoral and genetic aspects of thyroid autoimmunity. *J Clin Endocrinol*. 1975;4:267.
147. Takeda Y, Kris JP. Radiometric measurements of thyroglobulin-antithyroglobulin immune complex in human sera. *J Clin Endocrinol Metab*. 1977;44:46.
148. O'Regan S, Fong JSC, Kaplan BS, et al. Thyroid antigen-antibody hepatitis. *Clin Immunol Immunopathol*. 1976;6:341.
149. Totterman TH, Hayry P, Andersson LC, et al. Blood and thyroid-infiltrating lymphocyte subclasses and functions in thyroid autoimmune disease. *Scand J Immunol*. 1977;6:1197.
150. Neville ME, Lischner HW. Lymphokine production by K cells upon interaction with antigen-antibody complexes. *J Reticuloendothel Soc*. 1977;22:45a.
151. Mahoney CP, Pyne GE, Stamm SJ, et al. Neonatal Graves' disease. *Am J Dis Child*. 1964;107:516.
152. Scott JS. Immunological disease and pregnancy. *Br Med J*. 1966;1:1559.
153. Ramsay I. Attempted prevention of neonatal thyrotoxicosis. *Br Med J*. 1976;2:1110.
154. Shulman NR, Aster RH, Leitner A, et al. Immune reactions involving platelets: V. Post transfusion purpura due to a complement-fixing antibody against a genetically controlled platelet antigen. *J Clin Invest*. 1961;40:1597.
155. Pitney WR. The purpuras. In: Haridsty and Weatherall DJ, eds. *Blood and Its Disorders*. Oxford: Blackwell; 1974:995.
156. Gockerman JP, Bowman RP, Connad ME. Detection of platelet isoantibodies by [^{3}H]serotonin platelet release and its clinical application to the problem of platelet matching. *J Clin Invest*. 1975;55:75.
157. Gockerman JP, Shulman NR. Isoantibody specificity in post transfusion purpura. *Blood*. 1973;41:817.

158. Karpatkin S. Drug induced thrombocytopenia. *Am J Med Sci.* 1971;262:69.
159. Chaplin H, Cohen R, Bloomberg G, et al. Pregnancy and idiopathic hemolytic anemia: a prospective study during 6 months gestation and 3 months post partum. *Br J Haematol.* 1973;24:219.
160. Barshany S, Herbert V. Transplacentally acquired antibody to intrinsic factor with vitamin B_{12} deficiency. *Blood.* 1967;30:777.
161. Fisher JM, Taylor KB. Placental transfer of gastric antibodies. *Lancet.* 1967;1:695.
162. Mendelow H. Pathology. In: Osserman K, ed. *Myasthenia Gravis.* New York, NY: Grune & Stratton; 1958:10.
163. Simpson JA. Myasthenia gravis: a new hypothesis. *Scot Med J.* 1960;5:419.
164. Lee CY. Chemistry and pharmacology of polypeptide toxins in snake venoms. *Annu Rev Pharmacol.* 1972;12:265.
165. Fambrough BM, Drachman DB, Satymurti S. Neuromuscular junctions in myasthenia gravis: decreased acetylcholine receptors. *Science.* 1972;182:293.
166. Appel SH, Almon RR, Levy N. Acetylcholine receptor antibodies in myasthenia gravis. *N Engl J Med.* 1975;293:760.
167. Abramsky O, Aharonov A, Webb C, et al. Cellular immune responses to acetylcholine receptor rich fraction in patients with myasthenia gravis. *Clin Exp Immunol.* 1975;19:11.
168. Giwa-Osagie OF, Newton JR, Larchner V. Obstetric performance of patients with myasthenia gravis. *Int J Gynecol Obstet.* 1981;19:267.
169. Report of World Health Organization Scientific Group. Primary immunodeficiency diseases. *Clin Immunol Immunopathol.* 1986;40:166.
170. Pembrey ME. Applications and limitations of direct DNA analysis in genetic prediction. *J Inher Metabol Dis.* 1986;9(suppl.):38.
171. Kwan SP, Kunkel L, Bruns GP, et al. Mapping of the X-linked agammaglobulinemia locus by use of restriction fragment-length polymorphism. *J Clin Invest.* 1986;77:649.
172. Mensink EJBM, Thompson A, Schot JDL, et al. Mapping of a gene for X-linked agammaglobulinemia and evidence for genetic heterogeneity. *Hum Genet.* 1986;73:327.
173. Malcolm S, de Saint Basile G, Arveiler B, et al. Close linkage of random DNA fragments from x q 21.3—22 to X-linked agammaglobulinemia. *Hum Genet.* 1987;77:172.
174. de Saint Basile G, Arveiler B, Oberle I, et al. Close linkage of the locus for X chromosome-linked severe combined immunodeficiency to polymorphic DNA markers in x q 11—q 13. *Proc Natl Acad Sci USA.* 1987;84:7576.
175. Mensink EJBM, Thompson A, Sandkuyl LA, et al. X-linked immunodeficiency with hyperimmunoglobulinemia M appears to be linked to the DXS 42 restriction fragment polymorphism locus. *Hum Genet.* 1987;76:96.
176. Peacocke M, Siminovitch KA. Linkage of the Wiskott-Aldrich syndrome with polymorphic DNA sequences from the human X chromosome. *Proc Natl Acad Sci USA.* 1987;84:3430.
177. Skare JC, Milunski A, Byron KS, et al. Mapping the x-linked lymphoproliferative syndrome. *Proc Natl Acad Sci USA.* 1987;84:2015.
178. Lau YL, Levinsky RJ. Prenatal diagnosis and carrier detection in primary immunodeficiency disorders. *Arch Dis Child.* 1988;63:758.
179. Hirschhorn R. Genetic deficiencies of adenosine deaminase and purine nucleoside phosphorilase: overview, genetic heterogeneity and therapy. *Birth defects.* 1983;19:73.
180. Frater-Schroder M, Hitzig WH, Butler R. Studies on transcobalamine. Detection of TC II isoproteins in human serum. *Blood.* 1979;53:193.
181. Touraine JL, Betuel H. The bare lymphocyte syndrome: immunodeficiency resulting from the lack of expression of HLA antigens. *Birth defects.* 1983;19:83.
182. Lisowska-Grospierre B, Bohler MC, Fischer A, et al. Defective membrane expression of the LFA-1 complex may be secondary to the absence of the beta-chain in a child with recurrent bacterial infections. *Eur J Immunol.* 1986;16:205.
183. Reith W, Satola C, Herrero Sanchez I, et al. Congenital immunodeficiency with a regulatory defect in MHC class II gene expression lacks a specific HLA-DR promoter binding promoter, RF-X. *Cell.* 1988;53:897.
184. Newburger PE, Cohen HJ, Rothchild SB, et al. Prenatal diagnosis of chronic granulomatous disease. *N Engl J Med.* 1979;300:178.
185. Levinsky RJ, Harvey BAM, Rodeck CH, et al. Phorbol myristate acetate stimulated NBT test: a simple method suitable for antenatal diagnosis of chronic granulomatous disease. *Clin Exp Immunol.* 1983;54:595.
186. Shaham M, Voss R, Becker Y, et al. Prenatal diagnosis of ataxia telangiectasia. *J Pediat.* 1982;100:134.
187. Linch DC, Levinsky RJ, Rodeck CH, et al. Prenatal diagnosis of three cases of severe combined immunodeficiency: severe T-cell deficiency during the first half of gestation in fetuses with adenosine deaminase deficiency. *Clin Exp Immunol.* 1984;56:223.
188. Durandy A, Dumex Y, Griscelli C. Prenatal diagnosis of severe inherited immunodeficiencies: a five year experience. In: Vossen J, Griscelli C, eds. *Progress in Immunodeficiency Research and Therapy II.* Amsterdam: Elsevier; 1986:323.
189. Lyon MF. X chromosome inactivation and developmental patterns in mammals. *Biol Rev.* 1972;47:1.
190. Fialkow PJ. Primordial cell pool size and lineage relationship of five human cell types. *Ann Hum Genet.* 1973;37:39.
191. Conley ME, Brown P, Pickard AR, et al. Expression of the gene defect in X-linked agammaglobulinemia. *N Engl J Med.* 1986;315:564.
192. Puck JM, Nussbaum RL, Conley ME. Carrier detection in X-linked severe combined immunodeficiency based on patterns of chromosome inactivation. *J Clin Invest.* 1987;79:1395.
193. Conley ME, Lavoie A, Briggs C, et al. Non random X chromosome inactivation in B cells from carriers of X chromosome-linked severe combined immunodeficiency. *Proc Natl Acad Sci USA.* 1988;85:3090.
194. Conley ME, Puck JM. Carrier detection in typical and atypical X-linked agammaglobulinemia. *J Pediat.* 1988;112:688.
195. Kohn DB, Fearon ER, Winkelstein JA, et al. Wiskott Aldrich syndrome carrier detection by X-chromosome inactivation analysis. *Ped Res.* 1987;21:313.
196. Linch DC, Rodeck CH, Simmonds NA, et al. Prenatal diagnosis for severe combined immunodeficiency. *Birth defects.* 1983;19:121.

Chapter Forty-Eight
The MHC Complex

Carole Ober

48

The human leukocyte antigens (HLA) are a group of genes located on human chromosome 6 that control cell-to-cell interactions and regulate immune responses. The HLA are cell surface glycoproteins that are antigenic. When exposed to cells from HLA-incompatible individuals of the same species, responding individuals form antibodies (alloantibodies) or cytotoxic T cells against foreign antigens. Thus, differences between individuals with respect to HLA types will result in rapid rejection of tissue grafts or organ transplants. Because of this important role in tissue and graft rejection, the HLA region is the major histocompatibility complex (MHC) in humans.

It was in the context of graft rejection that the role of HLA genes in pregnancy was first considered. The "riddle of the fetal allograft," or how the fetoplacental unit evades rejection by the maternal immune system was first proposed by Medawar in 1953 but remains unsolved today. The major transplantation antigens (HLA-A, B, C, DR, DQ) are not expressed on syncytiotrophoblast cell population in human pregnancy[1,2], which may help explain the success of the fetal allograft. However, maternal HLA cytotoxic antibody production, presumably elicited by fetal lymphocytes that cross the placenta, is not associated with spontaneous abortions, stillbirths, or developmental abnormalities. Furthermore, many other trophoblast proteins encoded by fetal genes are exposed to the maternal immune system[1-3] throughout pregnancy yet fail to elicit maternal rejection responses in normal pregnancy. Such proteins include novel

HLA antigens (ie, non–HLA-A, B, C, DR, DQ, DP), growth factors, and receptors for immunoglobulin and serum transferrin.

This chapter presents an overview of the biologic and genetic characteristics of the human MHC. A review of the studies investigating the role of HLA genes in recurrent spontaneous abortion and normal pregnancy follows. Finally, a discussion of the rationale for and status of immunotherapy for the prevention of spontaneous abortion is considered.

THE MAJOR HISTOCOMPATIBILITY COMPLEX

The MHC in humans and other mammals contains three subregions of genes, each coding for distinct gene products. These subregions are known as Class I, Class II, and Class III (Fig. 48–1). MHC genes on a single chromosome are generally inherited as a single unit, called a *haplotype.*

Structure and Function

Class I molecules are composed of a transmembrane glycoprotein (heavy chain) encoded by MHC genes and an associated β_2-microglobulin, encoded by a gene on chromosome 15. Class I genes include the serologically defined HLA-A, HLA-B, and HLA-C. These antigens have a ubiquitous tissue distribution; they are expressed on nearly all nucleated cells. A noteworthy exception is syncytiotrophoblast cells, which lack expression of HLA-A, HLA-B, and HLA-C, although novel class I antigens are present on early invasive cytotrophoblast.[4-6] Class I genes restrict antigen recognition predominantly by cytotoxic T lymphocytes. Recently, molecular genetic and biochemical studies have revealed at least 20 additional Class I genes in humans (eg, HLA-E, 6.0, 5.4 in Fig. 48–1).[7-11] The function, timing, and distribution of these genes are not known; however, they may be considered candidates for the unusual class I gene expressed in certain trophoblast cell populations.

Class II, or HLA-D region, molecules consist of two transmembrane glycoproteins (alpha and beta chains), both encoded by MHC genes. Class II genes include HLA-DR and HLA-DQ, which are serologically defined, and HLA-DP, which is defined by primed lymphocyte testing. Class II genes restrict antigen recognition by regulatory T cells. A cellular assay, the *mixed lymphocyte culture* (MLC), was used initially to identify what was thought to be a B cell-specific antigen. This antigen was called HLA-D. However, no single gene product has been identified that corresponds to HLA-D types, and HLA-D is now used to refer to a segment of the chromosome containing genes that determine reactivity of cells in MLC (ie, HLA-DR, HLA-DQ). Additional class II genes have been identified (eg, HLA-DO, HLA-DZ, HLA-DX in Fig. 48–1) by molecular genetic techniques, but it is not known whether these genes are expressed on the cell surface.[12] Class II antigens have more limited tissue distributions and are restricted to certain cell types. HLA-DR, HLA-DQ, and HLA-DP are primarily expressed on B lymphocytes, macrophages, endothelial cells, and activated T cells. Class II antigens are not expressed on any trophoblast cell population.

The Class III region contains genes that encode complement components, the alpha and beta chains of the tumor necrosis factor, and the enzyme 21, hydroxylase. Because little is known about the role of class III genes in pregnancy, these genes are not discussed further in this chapter.

Genetic Characteristics of HLA

MHC genes are unique not only because of their important biologic functions, but also because of their genetic characteristics. HLA are the most polymorphic loci in the human genome. For example, the 1987 International Histocompatibility Workshop identified at least 24 HLA-A, 50 HLA-B, 11 HLA-C, 18 HLA-DR, nine HLA-DQ, and five HLA-DP types. Rarely does the frequency of any one antigen exceed 30% in any population. This allows for more than 300 million genetically different individuals, which makes the probability that two unrelated individuals are HLA identical very unlikely.[13]

A second striking feature of the MHC is *linkage disequilibrium,* the nonrandom association of alleles at different loci. Some of the best examples of linkage disequilibrium in humans are the HLA antigens, such as the HLA-A1-B8 and HLA-B8-DR3 haplotypes among northern Europeans. These antigens occur together on a single haplotype (or chromosome) more than would be expected by chance. At least 5% of all possible paired combinations of HLA-antigens are in linkage disequilibrium in any given population.[13] Thus, disease associations with an antigen at one MHC locus could be produced by linkage disequilibrium with an antigen at another MHC locus. For example, associations with most autoimmune diseases can be attributed to HLA-DR locus antigens. Because of linkage disequilibrium between alleles at the HLA-DR and HLA-B loci, weaker associations with autoimmune disease and HLA-B antigens can be demonstrated. This explains why earlier studies showed associations between HLA-B8 and insulin-dependent diabetes mellitus, while the true association is now known to be with HLA-DR3. Linkage disequilibrium also will increase the probability that individuals with similar antigens at one MHC locus also will be similar with respect to antigens at a second MHC locus.

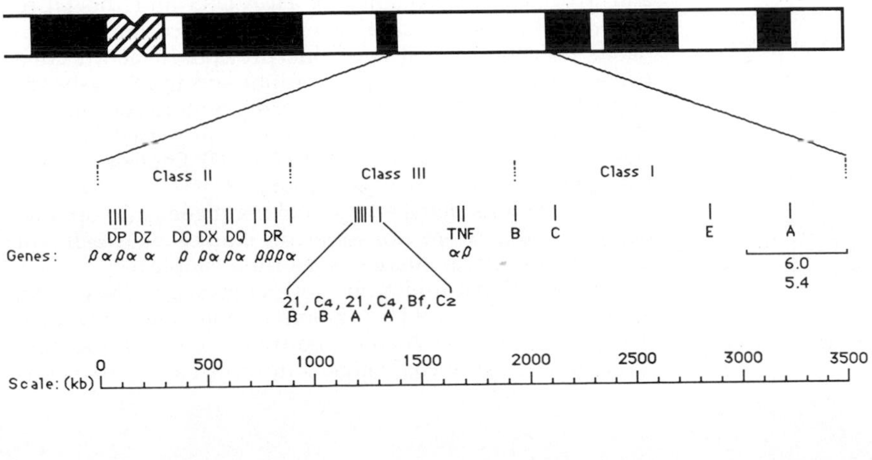

Figure 48–1. Molecular map of the human major histocompatibility complex. *(From Ober[62], with permission.)*

THE ROLE OF HLA GENES IN PREGNANCY

Shortly after the role of MHC genes in tumor and graft rejection was realized, Medawar[14] proposed that the mammalian embryo also should be at risk for maternal immunologic rejection because paternal and maternal MHC genes are expressed by fetal tissues. However, it became apparent that maternal recognition of paternally-derived HLA not only occurs in normal pregnancy, but may be beneficial.[15,16] Sensitization to paternal HLA occurs commonly in multiparous pregnancies without any ostensible deleterious effects but rarely occurs in women with recurrent spontaneous abortion.[15,17] It has been proposed that normal pregnancy requires maternal recognition of, and response to, paternally derived fetal antigens. Thus, pregnancy failure could result from inadequate or inappropriate maternal immune response to fetal antigens, or failure of the maternal immune system to recognize fetal antigens. The former may be related to maternal MHC haplotypes carrying particular immune response genes, while the latter may result from maternal-fetal histocompatibility (ie, fetuses whose paternally derived MHC antigens do not differ from maternal antigens).

Associations With Particular MHC Haplotypes

The hypothesis that specific MHC haplotypes or antigens are associated with spontaneous abortion is consistent with the following observations: (1) maternal autoimmune diseases may be associated with fetal losses[18-20]; and (2) many autoimmune diseases show population associations with specific HLA antigens.[21] Thus, it is likely that autoimmune-associated spontaneous abortion is also associated with particular MHC antigens or haplotypes. Autoimmune diseases that are associated with specific HLA antigens in Caucasians and for which information is available on fetal loss rates are shown in Table 48–1. It is curious that seven of eight autoimmune diseases associated with increased fetal wastage also are associated with HLA-B8 or HLA-DR3 antigens.

TABLE 48–1. FETAL LOSS IN HLA-ASSOCIATED AUTOIMMUNE DISEASES[a]

Autoimmune Disease	Associated with Fetal Losses[b]	HLA Antigen Association[c]
Systemic lupus erythematosus	+	B8,DR3[d]
Myasthenia gravis	+	B8[d],DR3
Polymyositis	+	B8,DR3[d]
Graves' disease	+	B8,DR3[d]
Insulin-dependent diabetes mellitus	+	B8,DR3[d] and B15,DR4[d]
Chronic active hepatitis	+	A1,B8[d],DR3
Herpes gestationis	+	B8,DR3[d]
Pemphigus vulgaris	+	DR4
Rheumatoid arthritis	–	DR4
Autoimmune thrombocytopenic purpura	–	DR2
Mutliple sclerosis	–	B7,DR2[d]

[a] Includes only autoimmune diseases for which HLA associations are demonstrated.
[b] Summarized from references 18–20.
[c] Summarized from reference 21, includes associations in Caucasians only.
[d] Primary association.

Autoimmune diseases associated with other antigens are not associated with fetal wastage, and this raises the possibility that the underlying pathogenesis of autoimmune-associated fetal wastage may be mediated by genes in linkage disequilibrium with HLA-B8 and HLA-DR3. Thus, the HLA-B8,DR3 haplotype may be a marker for autoimmune-associated spontaneous abortion.

Among couples with idiopathic recurrent spontaneous abortion, specific MHC haplotypes or antigens may be markers for a lack of maternal immunologic responsiveness. It is well accepted that MHC-linked genes influence immune responsiveness significantly. For example, associations between HLA antigens and responsiveness to specific pathogens[21], to nonspecific PHA stimulation[22], and to alloantigens in mixed lymphocyte culture[22] have been reported. Thus, it is possible that lack of maternal responsiveness to fetal alloantigens or to intrauterine pathogens could underlie spontaneous abortions in some couples. Indeed, associations between recurrent spontaneous abortions and HLA antigens have been reported by several investigators, but the mechanisms accounting for these associations are unclear.

Gerencer and colleagues reported an increased frequency of HLA-A9[23] and HLA-Dw5[24] in Yugoslavian women with recurrent gestational disorders of unknown etiology. They also report a greater proportion of women with recurrent spontaneous abortion who responded low to their husbands' lymphocytes (in mixed lymphocyte culture) compared to control women. Unfortunately, the HLA types of the women who were low responders were not reported. They suggest, however, that this may reflect their earlier finding of increased frequencies of HLA-Dw5 in spontaneous abortion[24] and the association between HLA-DR5 and low responsiveness to alloantigens in mixed lymphocyte culture.[22]

Reznikoff-Etievant and associates also reported increased frequencies of HLA-DR5 in 20 French wives and husbands with idiopathic recurrent spontaneous abortion compared to 100 control subjects but did not observe any differences in HLA-A or HLA-B antigen frequencies.[25] Jeannet et al[26], studying HLA-A, HLA-B, HLA-C, and HLA-DR antigens, report increased frequencies of HLA-A10 in 29 Swiss couples with recurrent spontaneous abortion compared to control couples.

Bolis and colleagues studied HLA-A, HLA-B, and HLA-C antigens in 20 Italian couples with recurrent spontaneous abortion.[27] They reported an increased frequency of HLA-B35 in women with recurrent spontaneous abortions compared to control subjects. Among Australian couples, Cauchi et al[28] report a decreased frequency of HLA-B35 in 31 women with recurrent spontaneous abortion and no previous liveborn children (ie, primary spontaneous abortion) and a decreased frequency of HLA-DR3 and the HLA-A1,B8,DR3 haplotype in 31 women with recurrent spontaneous abortion and at least one previous liveborn child (ie, secondary spontaneous abortion) and in 38 husbands of primary spontaneous abortion compared to control subjects. Johnson and colleagues[29] reported increased frequencies of the haplotype HLA-A,B12 in 80 English women with primary spontaneous abortion.

Associations between particular antigens and spontaneous abortion were not found in studies of Israeli[30] or US[31,32] recurrent spontaneous abortion couples.

An additional finding by several investigators was an increased frequency of HLA-B homozygotes among women with recurrent spontaneous abortion. Increased homozygosity for HLA-B locus antigens in recurrent spontaneous abortion couples has been reported in British[29], Australian[27], and US[33] studies. Homozygosity for HLA-B locus antigens may identify a subgroup of recurrent spontaneous abortion with a common immunologic defect involving low responsiveness to foreign antigens. Johnson and colleagues suggest that homozygosity for antigens at the HLA-B locus may be a marker for lack of responsiveness to cytomegalovirus (CMV) and to cell-surface alloantigens. This hypothesis is consistent with observations of selectively impaired antibody response to CMV in spontaneous abortions[34] and a low prevalence of serum anti-CMV antibodies in women with recurrent spontaneous abortion compared to age-matched controls.[35]

In aggregate, these studies suggest that in selected couples, MHC genes, haplotypes, or genotypes may be markers for spontaneous abortion. HLA associations may be found in women with autoimmune disease or in women who are low responders to foreign antigens (eg., viruses or fetal alloantigens). The fact that specific antigens associated with spontaneous abortion differ among studies and that spontaneous abortion in many couples does not appear to be associated with MHC genes suggests that these genes are probably not the cause of a significant proportion of recurrent spontaneous abortions.

Maternal-fetal Histocompatibility and Spontaneous Abortion

Initial data suggesting a role for MHC genes in human pregnancy were derived from retrospective studies of HLA sharing in couples with repetitive spontaneous abortion. These studies tested the hypothesis that maternal-fetal histocompatibility is associated with repetitive abortion by comparing the frequency of HLA sharing among recurrent spontaneous abortion and fertile control couples. Because only couples sharing HLA could produce compatible fetuses, increased HLA sharing among couples with recurrent spontaneous abortion would be consistent with the hypothesis that histocompatible fetuses are at a selective disadvantage during early pregnancy. Furthermore, linkage disequilibrium between alleles at MHC loci would increase the likelihood that couples sharing serologically determined MHC antigens (ie, HLA-A, HLA-B, HLA-C, HLA-DR) also share alleles at other MHC loci. Thus, the effects of histocompatibility for MHC genes other than HLA could be assessed indirectly by evaluating the degree of HLA sharing among couples with various reproductive histories.

Evidence for increased HLA sharing among couples with recurrent spontaneous abortion was first reported by Komlos and colleagues in 1979.[36] They compared the frequency of HLA-A and HLA-B sharing between 18 control couples with at lease two or more liveborn children and no history of abortion and three groups of experimental couples, including 13 couples with only one abortion, 23 with repeated abortions, and 25 with hydatidiform moles. The proportion of couples sharing HLA-A or HLA-B antigens was increased in all groups of experimental compared to control subjects, but the differences reached statistical significance in repetitive aborters only.

Since this initial investigation, many studies of HLA sharing in spontaneous abortion have been reported (Table 48–2), resulting in confusion in the literature. In general, a majority of the studies have reported increased sharing of HLA antigens in recurrent spontaneous abortion compared to control couples. However, among studies supporting a role for HLA sharing, there is little agreement with regard to the MHC gene or region associated with spontaneous abortion. Increased antigen sharing at the HLA-B and HLA-DR loci is often cited as the most obvious trend among these studies.[37,38] However, many studies demonstrate noticeable associations with HLA-A antigen sharing or with the total number of antigens shared (see Table 48–2).

The role of HLA sharing in primary versus secondary spontaneous abortion couples also is unclear. For example, McIntyre and colleagues report increased sharing of HLA-A, HLA-B, and HLA-DR antigens among primary but not secondary aborters[39], Komlos et al show data where there is more HLA-A sharing among primary aborters and more HLA-B sharing among secondary aborters (they did not study HLA-DR)[36], Schacter et al report increased HLA-A sharing among secondary aborters and increased HLA-B sharing among primary aborters.[40]

The discrepancy in the results between studies are difficult to reconcile. The conflicting data may be partly caused by differences between centers with regard to tissue typing methodology, the numbers of antigens tested for, the number of antigens present in a particular population, the choice and number of control couples, and the selection and stratification of recurrent spontaneous abortion couples. In addition, genetic heterogeneity could account for some of the results. That is, different MHC genes or regions may have distinct effects on fertility, which could explain some of the conflicting results regarding the role of HLA sharing in primary versus secondary spontaneous abortion.

To address the methodologic limitations discussed previously and to elucidate the reproductive effects of parental HLA sharing in a population not selected on the basis of reproductive outcome, Ober and colleagues initiated prospective, population-based studies in the Hutterites. These studies have provided data on the role of MHC genes in normal pregnancy.[41-43]

HLA Sharing in Normal Pregnancy: Studies in Hutterite Couples

The Hutterites are Anabaptists who originated in the Moravian Alps in the 1500s. In the 1870s, approximately 400 Hutterites migrated to the United States and established three communal farms, or colonies, in what is now South Dakota. Additional details of Hutterite history and population structure are discussed by Steinberg et al.[44]

Several features make the Hutterites a unique population to study the effects of genetic factors on fertility. First, the extant population of more than 30,000 Hutterites is derived from less than 100 founders who settled in South Dakota in the 1870s.[45] This small number of founding haplotypes increases the likelihood that many Hutterite couples share HLA antigens and that couples sharing antigens also will share alleles at nearby loci. The effects of sharing antigens at undefined MHC loci may be more easily studied in this population than in outbred couples. Second, Hutterites prohibit contraception. As a result, the length of the interval from marriage to last birth commonly exceeds 15 years and median completed family size is approximately nine. Only 2.3% of Hutterite couples are childless compared with 10% in the general population, and overall fertility rates are among the highest ever recorded. Third, the Hutterite communal lifestyle minimizes the effects of nongenetic factors that may affect fertility. For example, smoking is prohibited, alcohol consumption is moderate, and diet is relatively uniform among Hutterite colonies.

Studies of HLA in Hutterites reveal that the intervals from marriage to each birth are consistently longer among couples sharing one or more HLA-A, HLA-B, or HLA-DR antigens compared to couples sharing no antigens (Table

TABLE 48–2. HLA-SHARING IN COUPLES WITH UNEXPLAINED RECURRENT SPONTANEOUS ABORTION

Reference	Number of Couples	Increased Sharing by Locus[a] HLA-A	HLA-B	HLA-DR	Increased Antigen Sharing[a]	Hypo-responsive MLR[a,b]	Comments[c]
Beer[51]	237	+/−	+	+	+	+	1° versus 2° RSA not specified
Bolis[27]	20	+	+/−	NA	+	NA	1° versus 2° RSA not specified
Cauchi[28]	46	−	−	+/−	−	NA	1° RSA
Cauchi[28]	37	−	−	−	−	NA	2° RSA
Caudle[58]	12	−	−	−	−	NA	1° and 2° RSA
Coulam[33]	32	NA	NA	+	+	NA	1° RSA
Coulam[33]	27	NA	NA	+/−	+/−	NA	2° RSA
Gerencer[23]	105	−	+	+	+/−	+	1° and 2° RSA
Jeannet[26,d]	29	NA	NA	NA	+/−	NA	1° versus 2° RSA not specified
Johnson[29]	80	−	+	−	NA	NA	1° RSA
Johnson[29]	33	+/−	+/−	+/−	NA	NA	2° RSA
Komlos[36]	23	+	+	NA	+	NA	1° and 2° RSA
McIntyre[39]	35	+	+	+	+	NA	1° RSA compared to 2° RSA
Oksenberg[30,59]	60	−	−	−	−	+	1° RSA only
Reznikoff-Etievant[25]	20	−	+	+	−	NA	1° versus 2° not specified
Schacter[40]	16	−	+	−	NA	NA	1° RSA
Schacter[40]	36	+	−	−	NA	NA	2° RSA
Smith[53]	115	NA	NA	NA	−	NA	1° and 2° RSA; couples with explained RSA used as controls
Thomas[32,d]	21	−	−	−	NA	NA	1° and 2° RSA
Unander[60,d]	8	+/−	+/−	+	+	−	1° RSA
Vanoli[61]	47	+/−	−	+/−	NA	NA	1° versus 2° RSA not specified

[a] Recurrent spontaneous abortion compared to fertile controls unless otherwise noted. (+/− = increased sharing among recurrent spontaneous abortion but not statistically significant, NA = data not available.)
[b] + = Depressed mixed lymphocyte response.
[c] 1° RSA = primary recurrent spontaneous abortion, 2° RSA = secondary recurrent spontaneous abortion.
[d] Compared to theoretically derived population-based frequencies.

48–3). The differences in the distribution of the intervals (not shown) reach statistical significance by the second birth and remain significant through the sixth birth. There are no apparent differences between couples sharing one or more antigen. When effects of individual loci on interval lengths were examined, a significant HLA-DR sharing effect was revealed ($p = 0.025$); however, HLA-DR sharing alone does not account for all the differences in reproductive performance between couples sharing and not sharing antigens. For example, median completed family size is smaller among couples sharing HLA-DR compared to couples not sharing HLA-DR (median sizes equal 6.5 and 9.0, respectively, two-tailed $p = 0.082$), but nine of 26 Hutterite couples who shared HLA-DR had 10 or more children. Furthermore, there does not seem to be an association between any particular HLA antigen or haplotype and family size in Hutterite couples, but the sample size is too small to evaluate the relationship statistically.

Fetal loss rates after 4 weeks' gestation are 15% in Hutterite couples.[46] Approximately 4% of women have reported three or more losses, but all women reporting fetal losses also have had several liveborn. In fact, no primary aborters have been identified from more than 200 Hutterite women who were interviewed; therefore, all Hutterite couples with recurrent spontaneous abortion would be classified as *secondary aborters.* Increased HLA sharing was observed among couples experiencing fetal losses compared to couples who delivered at term, but differences did not reach statistical significance. Interestingly, loss rates were increased among Hutterite couples sharing Class I antigens, particularly at the HLA-B locus. Loss rates were 0.12 and 0.24 among couples sharing 0 or ≥1 HLA-B antigen, respectively (2-tailed $p = 0.057$). However, the number of fetal losses in this study is still small (N = 19) and the power of the analysis is correspondingly low.

Nevertheless, Hutterite couples sharing HLA-DR antigens take significantly longer to achieve pregnancy than couples not sharing HLA-DR. The median times to pregnancy (determined by home urine testing 30 days after the last period) were 4.66 (standard error [s.e.] = 0.35)

TABLE 48–3. INTERVALS (MONTHS) FROM MARRIAGE TO SUCCESSIVE BIRTHS IN HUTTERITE COUPLES[a]

	Shared HLA-A, HLA-B, Or HLA-DR Antigens			
Parity	0(N = 37)	1(N = 43)	>1(N = 31)	*p* value
1	12.00	15.08	14.00	.110
2	31.57	37.15	34.59	.007
3	50.62	59.25	52.69	.006
4	72.62	82.89	80.10	.030
5	91.51	105.51	104.33	.040
6	114.51	141.51	129.74	.019

[a] Upper quartile.
Upper quartiles (shown above) represent the upper 25th percentile of interval lengths (ie, 75% of couples who completed the interval from marriage to this birth within the number of months shown). Upper quartiles are estimated from time-to-birth curves generated from survival analysis; *p* values (two-tailed) are based on the log-rank test and compare the full time-to-birth curves for each parity.
From reference 43.

and 1.9 (s.e. = 0.44) months among couples sharing and not sharing HLA-DR ($p = 0.009$). After 10 months of unprotected intercourse, pregnancy rates were 85% for couples sharing HLA-DR compared to 100% among couples sharing HLA-A or HLA-B antigens.

Overall, these data demonstrate that although HLA sharing does not preclude normal fertility, it is associated with reduced fertility, even in a healthy, fertile population. Furthermore, studies of HLA in Hutterites suggest that there may be more than one MHC gene or region influencing reproductive outcome in humans. Maternal–fetal compatibility for HLA-DR or genes in linkage disequilibrium with HLA-DR may result in unrecognized losses, while compatibility for HLA-A or HLA-B region genes may result in clinically recognizable losses. These results suggest that in Hutterites, compatibility for genes linked to HLA-A or HLA-B may be associated with secondary spontaneous abortion. Associations between HLA-A or HLA-B sharing and secondary spontaneous abortion also has been observed in outbred couples[40] (see Table 48–2).

No primary aborters were identified among Hutterite couples, which makes it impossible to speculate which, if any, MHC region is likely to be associated with primary spontaneous abortion in outbred couples. However, pooled data from retrospective studies of primary spontaneous abortion (see Table 48–2) and results of immunotherapy in these couples support a role for MHC genes in primary recurrent abortion.

IMMUNOTHERAPY FOR RECURRENT SPONTANEOUS ABORTION

The scientific rationale behind immunotherapy for spontaneous abortion is based on the hypothesis that normal pregnancy requires maternal recognition of and appropriate response to fetal antigens. Idiopathic spontaneous abortion results from lack of recognition and response to fetal antigens. This statement is supported by the following observations: Couples with idiopathic spontaneous abortion tend to share more HLA antigens than fertile couples; serum factors that block cellular proliferation are associated with normal pregnancy but usually are not detectable in sera from women with recurrent spontaneous abortion; recurrent spontaneous abortion is rarely associated with maternal production of antipaternal lymphocytotoxic antibodies that are found in sera of women with normal pregnancies. Thus, the purpose of immunotherapy is to stimulate artificially normal immunologic responses that protect the fetoplacental unit in women who do not, on their own, recognize or respond to fetal antigens. Such responses include maternal production of lymphocytotoxic alloantibodies and serum blocking factors. This reasoning is analogous to the rationale for transfusing patients before kidney transplants, which significantly increases graft survival.[47]

Three approaches to immunotherapy have been described (see also Chapter 49). In the first, individual or pooled third-party (nonhusband) leukocytes are transfused before or throughout pregnancy. The rationale for using third-party cells is that the husband's cells are not sufficiently different with respect to histocompatibility antigens to stimulate the maternal immune system. Third-party leukocyte transfusions as a treatment for recurrent spontaneous abortions were first reported by Faulk and colleagues.[39,48,49] They report a success rate of approximately 82–89% for a term delivery of a healthy baby. Unander, using a similar protocol, reported a 72% success rate among 28 primary aborters and a 48% success rate among secondary aborters.[50] Unfortunately, these studies did not include control groups to evaluate the effects of placebo. Thus, the pregnancy successes can not be attributed conclusively to the treatment.

The second immunotherapeutic approach uses a husband's, instead of third-party, leukocytes. This method minimizes potential risks related to transfusing third-party cells but relies on the assumption that the route of transmission or concentration of paternal cells will provide the immunologic stimulation that the fetoplacental unit does not supply. Using husbands' leukocytes injected intradermally before conception, Beer and colleagues report a 79% success rate in 96 immunized couples.[17,51,52] Women who abort after immunization are reimmunized using third-party (nonpaternal) cells; in this group, the successful delivery rate is 72%. Among couples who decline immunotherapy after immunologic evaluation, the delivery rate was 25%.[51] Smith and Cowchock report an overall success rate of 66% among women immunized intravenously, intradermally, and subcutaneously with paternal cells.[53] In a smaller sample of 58 couples who underwent extensive immunologic evaluation before and after immunization, success rates were greater in primary aborters than in secondary aborters (54% versus 25%, respectively).[53]

A third approach has been described.[54] Johnson et al immunized recurrent spontaneous abortion women with a single intravenous infusion of isolated placental trophoblast plasma membrane vesicle preparations. The rationale for this approach is to mimic fetal antigen presentation that occurs in normal pregnancy. The success rate among the first 21 pregnancies in immunized women was 76%. The success rate was higher in secondary compared to primary spontaneous abortion (90% versus 55%, respectively).

Clinical trials evaluating the efficacy and safety of immunotherapy are underway.[19,54] Only one randomized, controlled trial has been completed.[55] Mowbray and colleagues reported significantly better outcomes in women immunized with a husband's compared to a wife's (placebo) cells. Women with recurrent spontaneous abortion were eligible to participate in the study if they met the following criteria: (1) negative for the known infective, metabolic, anatomic, or genetic causes of spontaneous abortion; (2) no detectable lymphocytotoxic antipaternal antibodies; and (3) no more than one previous liveborn. One hundred and seven couples met the study criteria and agreed to participate. Husbands and wives each donated blood for lymphocyte preparations; women were injected intravenously, intradermally, and subcutaneously with either their husband's or their own cell preparations. The choice of donor cells was determined by computer-generated random numbers; neither the couples nor the obstetricians knew which cells were used. At the end of the trial, 53 women had become pregnant. Pregnancy rates in the two groups were similar; however, immunization with paternal cells resulted in significantly more deliveries and fewer abortions than immunization with maternal cells. Spontaneous abortion rates were 0.22 and 0.63 in women immunized with paternal and maternal cells, respectively ($p = 0.01$). The overall success rate among women immunized with paternal cells was 0.78; this rate was slightly higher among secondary compared to primary aborters (0.82 versus 0.75, respectively). The dizygotic twinning rate was 4.5% and sex ratios did not differ from expected ratios.[56]

The safety of immunotherapy is still a primary concern, even though preliminary results suggest that risks to the mother and fetus may be small. No serious maternal complications following immunotherapy have been reported. Mowbray reported four major malformations among 109 infants delivered from immunized mothers.[55,56] Malformations included a small ventricular septal defect requiring surgery, a chromosomal defect (trisomy 15), an absent bladder associated with polycystic kidneys, and a Fallot's tetralogy that was surgically repaired. Johnson reported no abnormal outcomes in 21 infants of immunized mothers.[54] Smith and Cowchock observed one out of 29 infants delivered after immunization with neonatal alloimmune thrombocytopenia.[53] The authors speculated that this finding could be related to anti-P1^{A1} antibodies boosted in titer by platelets in the paternal cell innoculum. In addition, they reported one chromosomal abnormality (trisomy 22) in a pregnancy that was spontaneously aborted, and one chromosomal abnormality (trisomy 21) and one genetic defect (spina bifida) in pregnancies that were electively aborted.[53]

The distribution of birth weight did not differ from control populations among 20 infants delivered of mothers immunized with third-party cells[39], 92 infants delivered by mothers immunized with paternal cells[56], and 21 infants delivered by mothers immunized with trophoblast membrane preparations.[54] However, Beer et al described three severely growth-retarded infants among the first 26 infants born to immunized mothers.[51,52] They raise the possibility that intrauterine growth retardation may be a later manifestation of the same processes causing spontaneous abortion in these couples. The latter interpretation is consistent with reports of increased frequencies (as high as 30%) of low-birthweight babies born to mothers with three or more previous spontaneous abortions.[57] Intrauterine growth retardation or low birthweight among infants delivered of immunized mothers has not been observed by other investigators,[39,48,49,54-56] which suggests that there may be significant differences among centers with regard to patient selection criteria or referral patterns.

Although still experimental, immunization thus appears to be a promising therapy for couples with idiopathic recurrent spontaneous abortion. Differences between centers with respect to patient selection criteria, cells used for immunization, and route and timing of immunization make it difficult to draw inferences about the biologic processes underlying the success and failure of the various treatments. Notwithstanding these differences, the risks of immunotherapy to mother and fetus appear to be small. Conclusions regarding the safety and efficacy of immunotherapy await completion of additional clinical trials in the United States and abroad.

CONCLUSIONS

Although the mechanisms by which the fetal allograft escapes rejection are still poorly understood, the evidence for MHC genes mediating certain immunologic processes that enhance pregnancy outcome is compelling. Specific MHC genes, haplotypes, or genotypes may be associated with autoimmune-associated abortion or pregnancy loss resulting from low maternal responsiveness to fetal alloantigens or intrauterine pathogens. In addition, retrospective studies of recurrent spontaneous abortions and prospective studies in a fertile population suggest that maternal–fetal compatibility for Class I or Class II MHC antigens is associated with reduced fertility. Finally, the apparent successes of a variety of immunotherapeutic approaches suggest that augmentation of maternal immune responses does enhance pregnancy outcome. If these initial findings are confirmed by ongoing trials, immunotherapy may become a viable option for carefully selected couples with unexplained recurrent spontaneous abortions.

REFERENCES

1. Faulk WP, Hsi BL, McIntyre JA, et al. Antigens of the human extraembryonic membranes. *J Reprod Fertil*. 1982;31:181.
2. Johnson PM, Stern PL. Antigen expression at human materno-fetal interfaces. *Prog Immunol*. 1986;6:1056.
3. Galbraith RM, Werner P, Kantor RR, Galbraith GM. Studies of the interaction between human transferrin and specific receptors on the trophoblast membrane. *Placenta*. 1981;3:49.
4. Bulmer JN, Johnson PM. Antigen expression by trophoblast populations in the human placenta and their possible immunobiological relevance. *Placenta*. 1985;6:127.
5. Johnson PM, Risk JM, Bulmer JN, et al. Antigen expression at human materno-fetal interface. In: Gill TJ, Wegmann TG, eds. *Immunoregulation and Fetal Survival*. New York, NY: Oxford University Press; 1986:181.
6. Sunderland CA, Naiem M, Mason DY, et al. The expression of major histocompatibility antigens by human chorionic villi. *J Reprod Immunol*. 1981;3:356.
7. Geraghty DE, Koller BH, Orr HT. A human major histocompatibility complex class I gene that encodes a protein with a shortened cytoplasmic segment. *Proc Natl Acad Sci USA*. 1987;84:9145.
8. Lévi-Straus M, Carroll MC, Steinmetz M, Meo T. A previously undetected MHC gene with an unusual periodic structure. *Science*. 1988; 240:201.
9. Carroll MC, Katzman P, Alicot P, et al. Linkage map of the human histocompatibility complex including the tumor necrosis factor. *Proc Natl Acad Sci USA*. 1987;84:8535.
10. Koller BH, Geraghty DE, Shimizu Y, et al. HLA-E: a novel HLA class I gene expressed in resting T lymphocytes. *J Immunol*. 1988;141:897.
11. Fauchet R, Boscher M, Bouhallier O, et al. New class I in man: serological and molecular characterization. *Hum Immunol*. 1986;17:3.
12. Trowsdale J, Young JAT, Kelly AP, et al. Structure, sequence, and polymorphism in the HLA-D region. *Immunolog Rev*. 1985;85:5.
13. Bodmer W, Thomas G. Population genetics and evolution of the HLA system. In: Davsset J, Svejgaard A, eds. *HLA and Disease*. Copenhagen: Williams & Wilkins; 1977:280.
14. Medawar PB. Some immunological and endocrinological problems raised by the evolution of viviparity in vertebrates. *Symp Soc Exp Biol*. 1953;7:320.
15. Amos DB. HL-A, fertility, and natural selection. Karolinska Symposia on Research Methods in Reproductive Endocrinology, 7th Symposium. 1974;318.
16. Beer AE, Billingham RE. *The Immunobiology of Reproduction*. Englewood Cliffs, NJ: Prentice Hall; 1976.
17. Beer AE, Quebbeman JF, Ayers JWT, Haines RF. Major histocompatibility complex antigens, maternal and paternal immune responses, and chronic habitual abortions in human. *Am J Obstet Gynecol*. 1981;141:987.
18. Gleicher N, Siegel I. Pregnancy and the immune state. In: Davis T, ed. *Autoimmune Endocrine Disease*. New York, NY: John Wiley; 1983:225.

19. Scott JR, Rote NS, Branch DW. Immunologic aspects of recurrent abortion and fetal death. *Obstet Gynecol.* 1987;70:645.
20. Cowchock S, Dehoratius RD, Wapner RJ, et al. Subclinical autoimmune disease and unexplained abortion. *Am J Obstet Gynecol.* 1984;150:367.
21. Tiwari JL, Terasaki PI. *HLA and Disease Association.* New York, NY: Springer-Verlag; 1985.
22. Onody C, Buc M, Gerencer M, et al. Association between T lymphocyte reactivity and HLA. Joint report from HLA-DR intertransplant workshop 1979. *Tissue Antigens.* 1980;16:10.
23. Gerencer M, Singer Z, Pfeifer S, et al. HLA and red blood group antigens in pregnancy disorders. *Tissue Antigens.* 1988;32:130.
24. Gerencer M, Kastelan A. The role of HLA-D region in feto–maternal interactions. *Transplant Proc.* 1983;15:893.
25. Reznikoff-Etievant MF, Edelman P, Muller JY, et al. HLA-DR locus and maternal–foetal relation. *Tissue Antigens.* 1984;24:30.
26. Jeannet M, Bischof P, Bourrit B, Vaugnat P. Sharing of HLA antigens in fertile, subfertile, and infertile couples. *Transplant Proc.* 1985;17:903.
27. Bolis PF, Bianchi MM, Soro V, Belvedere M. HLA typing in couples with repetitive abortion. *Biol Res Pregnancy.* 1984;5:135.
28. Cauchi MN, Tait B, Wilshire MI, et al. Histocompatibility and habitual abortion. *Am J Reprod Immunol Microbol.* 1988;18:28.
29. Johnson PM, Chia KV, Risk JM, et al. Immunological and immunogenetic investigation of recurrent spontaneous abortion. *Disease Markers.* 1988;6:163.
30. Oksenberg JR, Persitz E, Amar A, Brautbar C. Maternal–paternal histocompatibility: lack of association with habitual abortions. *Fertil Steril.* 1984;42:389.
31. Schacter B, Muir A, Gyves M, Tasin M. HLA-A,B compatibility in parents of offspring with neural-tube defects or couples experiencing involuntary fetal wastage. *Lancet.* 1979;i:796.
32. Thomas ML, Harger JH, Wagener DK, et al. HLA sharing and spontaneous abortion in humans. *Am J Obstet Gynecol.* 1985;151:1053.
33. Coulam CB, Moore SB, O'Fallon WM. Association between major histocompatibility antigen and reproductive performance. *Am J Reprod Immunol Microbiol.* 1987;14:54.
34. Radcliffe JJ, Hart CA, Francis WJA, Johnson PM. Immunity to cytomegalovirus in women with unexplained recurrent spontaneous abortion. *Am J Reprod Immunol Microbiol.* 1986;12:103.
35. Johnson PM, Barnes RMR, Hart CA, Francis WJA. Determinants of immunological unresponsiveness in recurrent spontaneous abortion. *Transplantation.* 1984;38:280.
36. Komlos L, Zamir R, Joshua H, Halbrecht I. Common HLA antigens in couples with repeated abortions. *Clin Immunol Immunopath.* 1977;7:330.
37. Gill TJ III. Immunogenetics of spontaneous abortions in humans. *Transplantation.* 1983;35:1.
38. Risk JM, Johnson PM. Genetic studies of the MHC region in human recurrent spontaneous abortion. In: Gill TJ, Wegmann TG, eds. *Molecular and Cellular Nature of Maternal–Fetal Signalling.* New York, NY: Oxford University Press; 1989.
39. McIntyre JA, Faulk P, Nichols–Johnson VR, Taylor CG. Immunologic testing and immunotherapy in recurrent spontaneous abortion. *Obstet Gynecol.* 1986;67:169.
40. Schacter B, Weitkamp LR, Johnson WE. Parental HLA compatibility in parents of offspring with neural–tube defects: evidence for a T/t–like locus in humans. *Am J Hum Gen.* 1984;36:1082.
41. Ober C, Martin AO, Simpson JL, et al. Shared HLA antigens and reproductive performance in the Hutterites. *Am J Hum Gen.* 1983;35:994.
42. Ober C, Hauck WW, Kostyu DD, et al. Adverse effects of HLA-DR sharing on fertility: a cohort study in a human isolate. *Fert Steril.* 1985;44:227.
43. Ober C, Elias S, O'Brien E, et al. HLA sharing and fertility in Hutterite couples: evidence for prenatal selection against compatible fetuses. *Am J Reprod Immunol Microbiol.* 1988;18:111.
44. Steinberg AG, Bleibtreu HK, Kurczynski TW, et al. Genetic studies in an inbred human isolate. In: Crow JF, Neel JV, eds. *Proceedings of the Third International Congress of Human Genetics.* Baltimore, MD: Johns Hopkins University Press; 1967:267.
45. Martin AO. The founder effect in a human isolate: evolutionary implications. *Am J Phys Anthropol.* 1970;32:351.
46. Ober C, Elias S, Hauck WW, Kostyu D. Evidence for more than one MHC region influencing fertility in Hutterite couples. *Am J Hum Genet.* 1988;43:A219.
47. Norman DJ, Barry JM, Fischer S. The beneficial effect of pretransplant third-party blood transfusions on allograft rejection in HLA identical sibling kidney transplants. *Transplantation.* 1986;41:125.
48. Taylor C, Faulk WP. Prevention of abortion with leukocyte transfusion. *Lancet.* 1981;ii:68.
49. Taylor CG, Faulk WP, McIntyre JA. Prevention of recurrent spontaneous abortions by leukocyte transfusions. *J Roy Soc Med.* 1985;78:623.
50. Unander AM, Lindholm A. Transfusions of leukocyte-rich erythrocyte concentrates: a successful treatment in selected cases of habitual abortion. *Am J Obstet Gynecol.* 1986;154:516.
51. Beer AE, Semprini AE, Xiaoyu Z, Quebbeman JF. Pregnancy outcome in human couples with recurrent spontaneous abortions: HLA antigen profiles; female serum MLR blocking factors, and paternal leukocyte immunization. *Expl Clin Immunogenet.* 1985;2:137.
52. Beer AE, Quebbeman JF, Zhu X. Nonpaternal leukocyte immunization in women previously immunized with paternal leukocytes: immune responses and subsequent pregnancy outcome. In: Clark DA, Croy BA, eds. *Reproductive Immunology 1988.* New York, NY: Elsevier Science Publishers; 1986:261.
53. Smith JB, Cowchock FS. Immunological studies in recurrent spontaneous abortion: effects of immunization of women with paternal mononuclear cells on lymphocytotoxic and mixed lymphocyte reaction blocking antibodies and correlation with sharing of HLA and pregnancy outcome. *J Reprod Immunol.* 1988;14:99.
54. Johnson PM, Chia KV, Hart CA, et al. Trophoblast membrane infusion for unexplained recurrent miscarriage. *Br J Obstet Gynecol.* 1988;95:342.
55. Mowbray JF, Liddell H, Underwood JL, et al. Controlled trial of treatment of recurrent spontaneous abortion by immunisation with paternal cells. *Lancet.* 1985;i:941.
56. Mowbry JF. Immunology of early pregnancy. *Hum Reprod.* 1988;3:79.
57. Reginald PW, Beard RW, Chapple J, et al. Outcome in pregnancies progressing beyond 28 weeks gestation in women with a history of recurrent miscarriage. *Br J Obstet Gynecol.* 1987;94:643.
58. Caudle MR, Rote NS, Scott JR, et al. Histocompatibility in couples with recurrent spontaneous abortion and normal fertility. *Fertil Steril.* 1983;39:793.
59. Oksenberg JR, Persitz E, Amar A, et al. Mixed lymphocyte reactivity nonresponsiveness in couples with multiple spontaneous abortions. *Fertil Steril.* 1983;39:525.
60. Unander AM, Olding LB. Habitual abortion: parental sharing of HLA antigens, absence of maternal blocking antibody, and suppression of maternal lymphocytes. *Am J Reprod Immunol.* 1983;4:171.
61. Vanoli M, Fabio G, Bonara P, et al. Histocompatibility in Italian couples with recurrent spontaneous abortions of unknown origin and with normal fertility. *Tissue Antigens.* 1985;26:227.
62. Ober C, Weitkamp L. Immunogenetics. In: Coulam CB, Faulk WP, McIntyre JA, eds. *Immunologic Obstetrics.* New York, NY: W.W. Norton & Company; 1991. In press.

Chapter Forty-Nine

Alloimmunity

Salim Daya and David A. Clark

49

Spontaneous abortion is the most common complication of pregnancy. In North America, it is defined as the loss of a pregnancy before 20 weeks' gestation. Some women may have *recurrent* (ie, two or more consecutive spontaneous abortions) or *habitual* abortion (ie, three or more consecutive spontaneous abortions). The latter group may be further divided into a *primary* or *secondary* group, depending on whether there has been a previous live birth or stillbirth delivered after 20 weeks' gestation.

Spontaneous abortion usually occurs as an isolated

event, and in the vast majority of cases, the cause remains unknown. Chromosomal abnormalities were noted in 50–60% of first-trimester spontaneous abortions as determined by cytogenetic studies of the products of conception.[1-3] Hence, it is generally assumed that the cause of most early spontaneous abortions is a chromosomal abnormality in the conceptus. However, this figure represents only those products of conception successfully grown in culture, and because only a small proportion can be karyotyped successfully, the true incidence of chromosomal abnormalities is unknown. In contrast, women with habitual abortion are more likely to have losses of chromosomally *normal* conceptions.[4] Also, the risk of a second abortion following the abortion of a fetus with an abnormal karyotype is less than the risk for women who have had karyotypically normal abortuses.[1,2,5] Thus, causes other than genetic abnormality are likely in the pathogenesis of habitual abortion.

FREQUENCY OF ABORTION AND RISK OF RECURRENCE

The frequency of clinically recognized spontaneous abortion in the general population has been estimated to be about 15%.[4,6,7] The actual rate may be higher because patients may undergo complete abortions at home and may never reach treatment. Additionally, significant early fetal loss can occur soon after implantation and may be unrecognized.[8,9] Many attempts have been made to calculate the risk of abortion after a previous abortion. The initial estimates, based on mathematical calculations, indicate a substantially increased risk with each abortion.[10,11] More recently, data obtained from epidemiologic surveys confirm this increased risk, although the magnitude of the risk is much smaller.[4] For example, using data from more than 14,000 reproductive histories and taking into consideration the number of previous abortions and the sequence of abortions and live births, the risk after one, two, and three previous spontaneous abortions has been determined to be 23%, 29%, and 33%, respectively.[12] Similarly, pregnancy outcome data from patients recruited prospectively and preconceptually gave respective rates of 12%, 29%, and 36%.[13] There are few data on those patients with more than four consecutive abortions, but it is believed that the risk may increase even further. In contrast, a previous live birth seems to improve the prognosis for subsequent successful pregnancies.

Universally accepted information on the incidence of habitual abortion is not available. The current estimates are derived from antenatal clinics in which the frequency varies from 0.1–0.5%.[14,15]

Many etiological factors have been suggested in association with habitual abortion.[16] However, in many patients, a cause for the pregnancy loss cannot be established. In many of these patients with *unexplained* habitual abortion, the cause is believed to be an impairment in maternal *alloimmune* recognition, resulting in failure to produce a protective response toward the fetus.[17,18]

ANTIGENIC STATUS OF THE CONCEPTUS

The conceptus bears antigens that may render it foreign to the mother. During pregnancy, the conceptus undergoes several phases of development, each accompanied by changes in antigen expression and in susceptibility to particular effector mechanisms.[19] Some of these antigens represent paternally derived major and minor histocompatibility antigens and others represent organ-specific and embryonal antigens. There is increasing evidence that a pregnant female may recognize and mount immune responses against at least some of these antigens.

Mammalian fertilization involves the fusion of sperm and egg surface membranes, following which, sperm surface antigens continue to move freely over the zygote membrane.[20,21] Antisperm antibodies have been shown to interfere with fertility, causing an inhibition of fertilization.[22,23] Postfertilization fertility also may be affected as indicated by the increased spontaneous abortion rate in women with antisperm antibodies, although this association has remained controversial.[24-26]

The developing blastocyst at implantation consists of an inner cell mass, which will become the fetus, and an outer trophoblast layer, which will become the placenta, at the fetomaternal interface. Extensive studies on trophoblasts have confirmed that *syncytiotrophoblast* fails to express class I major histocompatibility complex (MHC) antigens.[27-29] However, trophoblast-specific TA_1 and TA_2 antigens have been detected on trophoblast cells.[30,31] In contrast to syncytiotrophoblast, early invasive *cytotrophoblast* (nonvillous trophoblast), which anchors the placenta to and is in direct contact with the maternal decidua, expresses readily detectable Class I MHC determinants.[27-29] Nonvillous trophoblast also produces physiologic modifications in the maternal spiral arteries of the placental bed in a way that invades and replaces the normal vascular endothelium.[32] Therefore, although syncytiotrophoblast does not express transplantation antigens, cytotrophoblast, which is in contact with maternal decidua and maternal blood, expresses strong transplantation antigens.

Several observations suggest that maternal immunologic reactions against the trophoblast can occur. A significant number of normal term plancentae are affected by a nonspecific *lymphocytic vilitis,* which is associated in severe cases with small infants and stillbirths.[33] In *pemphigoid gestationis,* there is increased expression of class II MHC antigens on villi, and inflammatory infiltrate can be observed at the site of trophoblast attachment.[34] In animal experiments, the trophoblast was found to be susceptible to specific lysis with antipaternal antibody, but damage required an exogenous source of complement *in vivo.*[35] The trophoblast was not susceptible to lysis by cytotoxic T lymphocytes (CTL) or antibody-dependent cell-mediated cytotoxicity. These data suggest that "natural" (ie, nonantigen-specific effector mechanisms (that can be boosted by cytokines released by specifically immune cells) deserve consideration. Fresh murine trophoblast cells were readily killed by lymphokine-activated killer cells.[36] Human trophoblast cells were weakly susceptible to lysis by allogeneic natural killer (NK) cells, and this killing activity could be enhanced by interferon.[37] Finally, passive immunization of rodents with antisera raised in rabbits against trophoblast cells produced abortions in rats.[38]

Abortion also can be caused by a variety of antibodies, neuraminidase (because of its endotoxic content), or endotoxin. The linking feature is activation of cells such as macrophages that produce tumor necrosis factor, a toxic cytokine that causes thrombosis in the vascular supply.[39] Collectively, these observations indicate that pregnancy failure may result from maternal immune reaction against the trophoblast. However, it is also possible for immune reactions to be beneficial to the fetus.

The postimplantation phase involves development of

a distinct fetus whose cells also begin to express paternal MHC antigens.[40]

SPONTANEOUS ABORTION CAUSED BY FETAL ALLOGRAFT REJECTION

Several observations support the idea that spontaneous abortion is a form of rejection by the mother, albeit by the natural effector cell mechanisms (NK cells, lymphokine-activated killer cells, macrophages). The evidence for embryo rejection is suggested by the observation that human *in vitro* fertilized embryos undergoing abortion were infiltrated by maternal mononuclear cells—a finding similar to that in graft rejection by both specific and natural effector mechanisms.[41]

Animal models of spontaneous abortion provide further evidence for the participation of immune reactions in abortion. Some of these models involve interspecies pregnancies such as goat–sheep mating and transfer of donkey embryos into horses.[42,43] The abortion is associated with a mononuclear cell infiltration of the fetus. Similarly, pregnancy in laboratory mice created by the transfer of *Mus Caroli* blastocysts into the uterus of *Mus Musculus* recipients is associated with a maternal nonantigen-specific cytotoxic T-lineage lymphocyte infiltration of the fetus after implantation in association with fetal death.[44]

It is believed that maternal production of serum factors, which block the reactivity of their lymphocytes against placental or paternal leukocyte antigens, is necessary to prevent immune rejection of the conceptus, and a failure of this response may cause some cases of first-trimester abortion.[45,46] Immunization of these women with paternal leukocytes to stimulate the production of antipaternal blocking antibodies is associated with a reduced risk of subsequent abortions.[46,47] Murine allopregnancy models of spontaneous abortions provide further indication that protection against abortion might be immunologically mediated because immunization of the female before the first conception with Balb/c spleen cells, compatible with the MHC of the paternal strain, reversed the occurrence of spontaneous abortion.[48,49] Protection could be transferred to naive females by an MHC-specific serum antibody. The question of how such protection comes about remains.

MECHANISMS PROTECTING THE FETUS

Decidualization of the endometrium is important in the preparation for implantation and nutrition of the blastocyst. The decidua also appears to play an important role in impairing certain aspects of graft rejection. During normal successful allopregnancy, suppressor cells accumulate at the implantation site in the uterine decidua.[50,51] In mice, these cells prevent the generation of CTL *in vitro*, and in humans, they suppress mitogen-induced proliferation of lymphocytes. These cells appear to be predominantly small, granule-containing, non-T lymphocytes from which a soluble factor that blocks the response of maternal T and NK cells to interleukin 2 (IL-2) and other cytokines can be isolated.[52,53] Induction of decidualization also is associated with the presence of a large suppressor cell, which also is present in early pregnancy, and whose activity can be induced with hormones alone.[50,51] This cell appears to alter the afferent limb of the CTL immune response without preventing development of humoral immunity and may inhibit the generation of cytotoxic cellular immune responses against non-MHC antigens, expressed by cells of the early developing conceptus.

The mechanism of activation of small postimplantation suppressor cells appears to be dependent on recruiting signals from trophoblast.[54,55] Such activation appears to be restricted to the implantation site in the uterus because no small cell activation was observed when the pregnancy was located at a site remote from the uterus.[54] The localization and trophoblast dependence of the suppressor cell suggests that it might be associated with events at the choriodecidual junction that lead to blockage of graft rejection mechanisms.

There is good evidence from human and animal models of spontaneous abortion that trophoblast-dependent suppressor cells play a role in fetal survival. Spontaneous abortion in allogeneic pregnancy established in CBA/J mice by DBA/2 males was associated with reduced suppressor cell activity at the implantation site, and the fetus was infiltrated by maternal CTL.[49,56] In contrast, fetal death was not preceded by suppressor cell deficiency in mice aborting because of the action of lethal T/t locus genes.[57] These findings imply that a deficiency of suppressor cells at the implantation site does not nonspecifically occur concomitant with fetal death but probably allows successful maternal immunologic rejection of the fetus. This concept is also supported by the observation that alloimmunization, which reduces the incidence of abortion, is associated with an increase in local suppressor cell activity.[56,58]

In human studies, which are more difficult to perform because of the limited availability of tissue from the implantation site, similar findings have been observed. Suppressor cell activity was absent in decidua in women with missed abortion but was present in decidua of women undergoing a therapeutic abortion for normal pregnancy.[59] Also, a deficiency of granulated cells, similar to the murine small lymphocytic, decidua-associated suppressor cell, has been noted in the placental bed before a spontaneous abortion.[60] The supernatants obtained from such samples also had significantly less suppressor activity in the spontaneous abortion group when compared with the normal pregnancy group.[57] Thus, suppressor cells and their soluble factors (which block cytokines such as IL-2) appear to be crucial for fetal survival. Further, failure of the trophoblast for any reason could lead to a deficiency of suppressor cell activation in the decidua, allowing maternal cytotoxic cells to cross into the fetus and result in pregnancy failure.

IMMUNOLOGIC TESTING IN WOMEN WITH RECURRENT PREGNANCY LOSS

In a significant proportion of women with recurrent pregnancy loss, no etiology can be identified by routine gynecologic testing. It is thought that this group of patients may have an underlying immunologic allorecognition defect accounting for their losses. This is further emphasized by the fact that women who have abortions with one partner may have successful pregnancies with another. This group is usually identified by a process of exclusion after chromosomal, infectious, hormonal, uterine, and autoimmune causes have been excluded.[16] Clinicians now realize that an immunologic diagnostic work-up must be part of the evaluation of couples with recurrent abortion when all other etiologies have been ruled out. There is no concensus on the appropriate immunologic tests to identify this subgroup of patients. Consequently, several tests are performed, and

TABLE 49–1. IMMUNOLOGIC TESTING IN UNEXPLAINED HABITUAL ABORTION

HLA-A, HLA-B, HLA-C, and HLA-DR typing of couple
MLR blocking
Antipaternal cytotoxic antibody

immunotherapy is offered based on the results of some or all of these tests (Table 49–1).

Human Leukocyte Antigen Sharing

Maternal recognition of paternally derived fetal antigens is believed to be necessary for a successful pregnancy. In situations in which paternally derived human leukocyte antigen (HLA) of the fetus does not differ from its maternal antigens, such a protective alloresponse is not possible. Thus, histocompatible fetuses, resulting from couples who share HLA, are believed to be at a disadvantage in pregnancy. Sharing of HLA between male and female partners in excess of expectation by random selection has been reported in couples with recurrent pregnancy loss.[61,62] Sharing occurs primarily at class II MHC loci[63], although this is not universally observed.[64] In Hutterites, HLA sharing, particularly at class II loci, is not associated with clinical miscarriage but rather with occult losses.[65] Much of the existing controversy concerning these data may stem from the insufficient characterization of aborting populations. It has been suggested that primary aborters share HLA and secondary aborters do not.[66] If this is correct, HLA typing could be useful in distinguishing primary from secondary aborters. However, HLA sharing may not be important. Some data suggest that the sharing of *trophoblast–lymphocyte* cross-reactive (TLX) alloantigens, which also appear to be associated with HLA may, in fact, represent the important factor.[67] This hypothesis may explain why some abortion-prone couples present without HLA sharing and some fertile couples share HLA but do not have a poor reproductive performance.

Mixed Lymphocyte Reaction

In vitro coincubation of maternal lymphocytes with paternal lyphocytes in serum from an unrelated donor results in immune recognition by the maternal lymphocytes, as measured by cellular proliferation and the production of lymphokines. If the incubation is performed in the presence of maternal serum, immune recognition is prevented.[68,69] When the experiment is performed using cells and serum from a woman with a history of recurrent, unexplained abortions, there is no inhibition of immune recognition, suggesting that these patients lack serum factors that block maternal recognition of paternal antigens. The time at which these *blocking factors* occur in a normal pregnancy is not yet known; nor is it known at what period during gestation these circulating factors are essential for fetal survival. It is unknown whether the presence of a blocking factor is necessary for a successful pregnancy, or if it only indicates a pregnancy that is already destined to be successful.

Antipaternal Cytotoxic Antibody

The *in vitro* ability to mount a cytotoxic response against paternal lymphocytes in the presence of complement is believed to be an important marker in patients with unexplained recurrent pregnancy loss. There appears to be a significant difference between primary and secondary aborting patients in their ability to demonstrate these responses. The primary aborters do not manifest antipaternal immunity, and their pregnancies are lost early.[70] In contrast, secondary aborters manifest polyspecific antipaternal lymphocytotoxic antibodies that are thought to represent inappropriate responses to TLX antigen allotypes because the activity can be removed by the trophoblast membrane from some pregnancy sera.[71] Despite these observations, there are some reports questioning the use of this test. It has been suggested that the absence of this antibody in aborting patients is merely related to the fact that they had insufficiently long gestations to produce a response.[13] Nevertheless, this test is still widely used and will continue to be used until better tests can be developed.

IMMUNOTHERAPY IN PATIENTS WITH RECURRENT ABORTION

Attempts at reducing spontaneous abortions have been made by simulating appropriate maternal responses by immunization against paternal antigens. This has been possible in several spontaneous abortion models in animals.[49,58,72] In the CBA × DBA/2 system, protection against abortion is mediated by soluble antigen-specific factors

TABLE 49–2. OUTCOME OF IMMUNIZATION WITH PATERNAL CELLS IN UNEXPLAINED HABITUAL ABORTION

Author	Dose	Frequency	Route[a]	Successful Pregnancy Proportion (%)	Status of Offspring
Mowbray[76]	Cells from one unit of blood	1	IV, SC, ID	17/22 (77)	Normal
Beer[83]	5 × 10⁷ cells	2, every 6 wk (if no antibody)	ID	100/121 (83)	15% IUGR
Alexander[81]	5 × 10⁷ cells	monthly until positive antibody	IV	20/26 (77)	4% IUGR 7% cong. anomaly
Reznikoff-Etievant[84]	2–4 × 10⁸ cells	1–3 monthly	IV, SC, ID	29/34 (85)	Normal
Carp[88]	—	—	—	43/66 (65)	Not reported
Fujii[85]	4 × 10⁷ cells	4, every 2 wk	ID	7/9 (78)	Normal
Takakuwa[86]	5–8 × 10⁷ cells	1 (1 in 3 pregnancies)	ID	5/7 (71)	Not reported

[a] Route of administration of cells was intravenous (IV), intradermal (ID), or a combination of IV, ID, and subcutaneous (SC).

TABLE 49–3. OUTCOME OF IMMUNIZATION WITH DONOR LEUKOCYTES IN UNEXPLAINED HABITUAL ABORTION

Author	Dose	Frequency	Route[a]	Successful Pregnancy Proportion (%)	Status of Offspring
Taylor[87]	250 mL leukocyte-rich preparation	2 every 3 wk to 26 wk gestation	IV	16/21 (76)	Normal
Beer[83]	5×10^7 cells	2 every 6 wk to 24 wk gestation	ID	15/21[b] (72)	Normal
Unander[88]	One unit packed cells	3–5, every 2 mo	IV	100/120 (83)	1.6% IUGR

[a] Route of administration of cells was intravenous (IV) or intradermal (ID).
[b] All these patients had failed to achieve successful pregnancy with paternal leukocyte immunization.

that boost local suppressor cell activity at the implantation site.[73]

In women with unexplained recurrent abortions and with no anti-paternal cytotoxic antibodies, immunization with paternal or third-party donor leukocytes has reduced the probability of spontaneous abortion (Tables 49–2 and 49–3). However, the risks of viral transmission, especially that of the human immunodeficiency virus (HIV), maternal sensitization to HLA, erythrocytes or platelet antigens, and the possibility of host-versus-graft disease make the use of donor leukocytes or blood transfusions less appealing to patients and their physicians. Other methods, such as the use of frozen donor leukocytes and trophoblast membranes, are being investigated.[74,75] Preliminary reports of leukocyte immunization were uncontrolled.

Subsequently, a randomized trial suggested a significantly improved pregnancy success rate with paternal leukocyte immunization (77%) compared with a control group (37%).[76] Similarly high success rates have been reported by others (see Table 49–2). Several ongoing controlled trials are testing the efficacy of this treatment. The mechanism by which immunization confers its suggested beneficial effects is not clearly understood. It also is unclear if antibodies, detected *in vitro*, are the actual mediators of changes in the uterine decidua that lead to fetal protection. The stimulation of circulating antibodies (antipaternal cytotoxic and MLR blocking antibodies) appears to be correlated with the overall success rate of pregnancy.[76,77] Women who seroconverted after immunization continued to have protection after treatment. In contrast, women who remained negative for cytotoxic antibodies and conceived more than 80 days after treatment were likely to experience spontaneous abortions.[78]

The dose of cells used for immunization has an effect on the success rate. However, the optimal dose necessary to achieve a successful outcome has not been established. When using a single immunizing dose before pregnancy, the success rate fell when the amount of cells fell below 110 million cells.[79] In most centers, repeated doses are given at fixed intervals (which vary from center to center) before conception is attempted (see Tables 49–2 and 49–3). The frequency of injections often is determined by testing for the presence of circulating antibodies. In some centers, reimmunization, especially with donor leukocytes, is carried out as soon as a pregnancy has been confirmed, and treatment is continued at regular intervals until the end of the second trimester (see Table 49–3).

The number of leukocyte injections necessary to achieve seroconversion is unclear. Single-dose treatment has been shown to achieve a high rate (65%) of seroconversion.[78] Patients who do not demonstrate antibodies after a single immunization should be offered a repeat dose of cells to boost their immune response. Repeated injections increase the probability of seroconversion, although some patients required up to 20 doses to achieve this end point.[80,81] Women who show no seroconversion and who become pregnant more than 3 months after treatment are given 50 million cells at the start of their pregnancy. Allegedly, high success rates are being observed with this approach.[77,79]

The route of immunization also may be important in producing a response. Treatment is given by one or a combination of subcutaneous, intradermal, and intravenous routes. The intradermal route is very effective for inducing an immune response, especially to T-cell antigens. The intravenous route, however, is more likely to induce a classic type of immune response. The concern that intrauterine growth retardation (IUGR) of the fetus (see Table 49–2) is the result of immunotherapy may be related to the route of immunization. A combined approach (ie, intravenous and intradermal) may be the best way to avoid this possible complication. It is quite possible, however, that IUGR in

TABLE 49–4. SPONTANEOUS CURE RATE IN PATIENTS WITH UNEXPLAINED HABITUAL ABORTION

Author	Treatment[a]	Successful Pregnancy Proportion (%)	Status of Offspring
Mowbray[76]	Autologous cells	10/27 (37)	Normal
Beer[83]	None	13/51 (25)	Normal
Reznikoff-Etievant[84]	None	10/28 (36)	Normal
Carp[88]	None	5/16 (31)	Not reported
Takakuwa[86]	None	1/3 (33)	Not reported

[a] The female partner in the control group of Mowbray's[76] trial was given an injection of leukocytes from 20 mL of her own blood. In all other studies, the control group of patients received no treatment.

TABLE 49–5. SUMMARY OF SUCCESSFUL PREGNANCY RATES FOLLOWING IMMUNOTHERAPY COMPARED WITH PATIENTS NOT RECEIVING SUCH TREATMENT

Treatment	Successful Pregnancy[a] Proportion (%)
Paternal cell immunization	221/283 (78)
Donor cell immunization	131/164 (80)
Placebo/No treatment	39/125 (31)

[a] Successful pregnancy rates were calculated as crude overall proportions after combining the data presented in Tables 49–2 through 49–3.

these patients is not related to immunotherapy but is the result of obstetric factors, such as hypertension and smoking.

Immunotherapy is offered in several centers, each claiming high success rates (see Tables 49–2 and 49–3). The spontaneous cure rate in this group of patients with unexplained habitual abortions appears to be quite low, ranging from 25–37% with an average rate of 31% (Table 49–4). It appears, therefore, that immunotherapy is efficacious in only a selected group of patients, resulting in a 2.5-fold rate increase of successful pregnancy (Table 49–5). It is hoped that the control trials that are being conducted will confirm this observation and determine ways of identifying the subgroup of patients to whom such therapy should be offered. Many additional questions remain unanswered, including the appropriate route, dose, and frequency of immunization and whether treatment should be continued in pregnancy. Also, the appropriate marker for successful treatment needs to be identified. Finally, a registry of infants born after immunotherapy must be established, especially since cases of intrauterine growth retardation and congenital abnormality have been reported.[81,82] Long-term follow-up of these children is important to identify if there are any developmental abnormalities that can be attributed to the immunization treatment. Until such time, immunization programs must be considered experimental.

REFERENCES

1. Boue J, Boue A, Lazar P. Retrospective and prospective epidemiological studies of 1500 karyotyped spontaneous human abortions. *Teratology.* 1975;12:11.
2. Lauritsen JG. Aetiology of spontaneous abortion. A cytogenetic and epidemiologic study of 288 abortuses and their parents. *Acta Obstet Gynecol Scand.* 1976;52 (suppl):1.
3. Huisjes HJ. *Spontaneous Abortion.* New York, NY: Churchill Livingstone; 1984.
4. Warburton D, Strobino B. Recurrent spontaneous abortion. In: Bennett MJ, Edmonds DK, eds. *Spontaneous and Recurrent Abortion.* Oxford: Blackwell Scientific; 1987:193.
5. Geisler M, Kleinebrecht J. Cytogenetic and histologic analyses of spontaneous abortions. *Hum Genet.* 1978;45:239.
6. Roth DB. The frequency of spontaneous abortion. *Int J Fert.* 1963;8:431.
7. Poland BJ, Miller JR, Jones DC, Trimble BK. Reproductive counselling in patients who have had a spontaneous abortion. *Am J Obstet Gynecol.* 1977;127:685.
8. Miller JF, Williamson E, Gordon YG, et al. Fetal loss after implantation. *Lancet.* 1980;ii:554.
9. Edmonds DK, Lindsay KS, Miller JF, et al. Early embryonic mortality in women. *Fertil Steril.* 1982;38:447.
10. Malpas PJ. A study of abortion sequences. *J Obstet Gynaecol Br Empire.* 1938;45:932.
11. Eastman NJ. Habitual abortion. In: Mergs JV, Sturgis S, eds. *Progress in Gynaecology.* New York, NY: Grune & Stratton; 1946;1:262.
12. Naylor AF, Warburton D. Sequential analysis of spontaneous abortion. II. Collaborative study data shows that gravidity determines a very substantial rise in risk. *Fertil Steril.* 1979;31:282.
13. Regan L. Spontaneous and recurrent abortion: Epidemiological and immunological considerations. In: Chapman M, Grudzinskas G, Chard T, eds. *Implantation: Biological and Clinical Aspects.* London: Springer-Verlag; 1988:183.
14. Bishop PMF. Studies on clinical endocrinology. II. Habitual abortion; its incidence and treatment with progesterone or vitamin E. *Guy's Hosp Rep.* 1937;87:362.
15. Javert CT. Habitual abortion. *NY St J Med.* 1948;48:2595.
16. Daya S. Habitual abortion. *SOGC Bulletin.* 1988;10:15.
17. Mowbray JF, Underwood JL. Immunology of abortion. *Clin Exp Immunol.* 1985;60:1.
18. Faulk WP, McIntyre JA. Trophoblast survival. *Transplantation.* 1981;32:1.
19. Clark DA. Current concepts of immuno regulation of implantation. In: Chapman M, Grudzinskas G, Chard T, eds. *Implantation: Biological and Clinical Aspects.* London: Springer-Verlag; 1988:163.
20. Gunderson GG, Medill L, Shapiro BM. Sperm surface proteins are incorporated into the egg membrane and cytoplasm after fertilization. *Dev Biol.* 1986;113:207.
21. Johnson M, Edidin M. Lateral diffusion in plasma membrane of mouse egg is restricted after fertilization. *Nature.* 1978;272:448.
22. Menge AC. Clinical immunological infertility: Diagnostic measures, incidence of antisperm antibodies, fertility and mechanism. In: Dhindsa DS, Schumacher GB, eds. *Immunological Aspects of Infertility and Fertility.* Holland: Elsevier-North; 1980:205.
23. Naz RK. The fertilization antigen: Applications in immunocontraception and infertility in humans. *Am J Reprod Immunol Microbiol.* 1988;16:21.
24. Jones WR. Immunological aspects of infertility. In: Scott S, Jones WR, eds. *Immunology of Reproduction.* London: Academic Press; 1976:375.
25. Mathur S, Baker ER, Williamson HO, et al. Clinical significance of sperm antibodies in infertility. *Fertil Steril.* 1981;36:486.
26. Menge AC, Medley NE, Mangione CM, Deitrich JW. The incidence and influence of antisperm antibodies in infertile human couple on sperm–cervical mucus interactions and subsequent infertility. *Fertil Steril.* 1982;38:439.
27. Bulmer J, Johnson PM. Antigen expression by trophoblast populations in the human placenta and their possible immunobiological relevance. *Placenta.* 1985;6:127.
28. Johnson PM, Risk JM, Bulmer JN, et al. Antigen expression at human maternofetal interfaces. In: Gill TJ, Wegmann TG, eds. *Immunoregulation and Fetal Survival.* New York, NY: Oxford University Press; 1987;181.
29. Sunderland CA, Naiem M, Mason DY, et al. The expression of major histocompatibility antigens by the human chorionic villi. *J Reprod Immunol.* 1981;3:323.
30. Whyte A, Loke YW. Antigens of the human trophoblast plasma membrane. *Clin Exp Immunol.* 1979;37:359.
31. Faulk WP, Temple A, Lovins RE, Smith N. Antigens of human trophoblasts: A working hypothesis for their role in normal and abnormal pregnancies. *Proc Natl Acad Sci USA.* 1978;75:1947.
32. Brosens IA. Morphological changes in the uteroplacental bed in pregnancy hypertension. *Clin Obstet Gynecol.* 1977;4:573.
33. Labarrere C, Althabe O, Tetenta M. Chronic villitis of unknown aetiology in placentae of idiopathic small for gestational age infants. *Placenta.* 1982;2:309.
34. Borthwick GM, Sunderland CA, Holmes RC, et al. Abnormal expression of HLA-DR antigen in the placenta of a patient with pemphigoid gestationis. *J Reprod Immunol.* 1984;6:393.
35. Zuckerman F, Head JR. Susceptibility of mouse trophoblast to antibody and complement-mediated damage. *Transplant Proc.* 1985;17:925.
36. Drake BL, Head JR. Murine trophoblast cells are susceptible to lymphokine-activated killer (LAK) cell lysis. *Am J Reprod Immunol Microbiol.* 1988;16:114.
37. Pross H, Mitchell H, Werkmeister J. The sensitivity of placental trophoblast cells to intraplacental and allogeneic cytotoxic lymphocytes. *Am J Reprod Immunol Microbiol.* 1985;8:1.
38. Beer AE, Billingham RE, Yang SL. Further evidence concerning the autoantigenic status of the trophoblast. *J Exp Med.* 1972;135:1177.
39. Head JR, Beer AE, Gasic GJ. Analysis of the abortifacient action of neuraminidase in mice. *Transplant Proc.* 1975;7:403.
40. Ozato K, Wan Y-J, Orrison BM. Mouse major histocompatibility class I gene expression begins at midsomite stage and is inducible in earlier-stage embryos by interferon. *Proc Natl Acad Sci USA.* 1985;82:2427.
41. Nebel L, Fern A, Rudak E, et al. Structural aspects of embryo failure following in-vitro fertilization and embryo transfer; immune rejection or malimplantation? In: Clark DA, Croy BA, eds. *Reproductive Immunology 1986.* Amsterdam: Elsevier Science; 1986:227.
42. McGovern PT. The effect of maternal immunity in survival of goat X sheep hybrid embryos. *J Reprod Fertil.* 1973;24:215.
43. Allen WR. Immunologic aspects of the endometrial cup reaction and the effect of xenogeneic pregnancy in horses and donkeys. *J Reprod Fertil Suppl.* 1982;31:57.
44. Croy BA, Rossant J, Clark DA. Histological and immunological studies of post implantation death of *Mus caroli* embryos in the *Mus musculus* uterus. *J Reprod Immunol.* 1982;4:277.
45. Rocklin RE, Kitzmiller JL, Carpenter CB, et al. Maternal–fetal relation: absence of an immunologic blocking factor from the serum of women with chronic abortion. *New Engl J Med.* 1976;295:1209.

46. Beer AE, Quebbeman JF, Zhu X. Non-paternal leukocyte immunization in women previously immunized with paternal leukocytes. In: Clark DA, Croy BA, eds. *Reproductive Immunology 1986*. Amsterdam: Elsevier Science; 1986:261.
47. Mowbray JF. Effect of immunization with paternal cells on recurrent spontaneous abortion. In: Clark DA, Croy BA, eds. *Reproductive Immunology 1986*. Amsterdam: Elsevier Science; 1986:269.
48. Chaouat G, Kiger N, Wegmann TG. Vaccination against spontaneous abortion in mice. *J Reprod Immunol*. 1983;5:389.
49. Clark DA, Chaput A, Tutton D. Active suppression of host-versus-graft reaction in pregnant mice. VII. Spontaneous abortion of allogeneic DBA/2 and CBA/J fetuses in the uterus of CBA/J mice correlates with deficient non-T suppressor cell activity. *J Immunol*. 1986;136:1668.
50. Clark DA, Brierley J, Slapsys R, et al. Trophoblast-dependent and trophoblast-independent suppressor cells of maternal origin in murine and human decidua. In: Clark DA, Croy BA, eds. *Reproductive Immunology 1986*. Amsterdam: Elsevier Science; 1986:219.
51. Daya S, Clark DA. Immunoregulation at the materno–fetal interface: The role of suppressor cells in preventing fetal allocraft rejection. In: *Immunology and Allergy Clinics of North America*, 1990;10:1.
52. Clark DA, Slapsys RM, Chaput A, et al. Immunoregulatory molecules of trophoblast and decidual suppressor cell origin at the materno fetal interface. *Am J Reprod Immunol Microbiol*. 1986;10:100.
53. Daya S, Rosenthal KL, Clark DA. Immunosuppressor factor(s) produced by decidua-associated suppressor cells—a proposed mechanism for fetal allograft survival. *Am J Obstet Gynecol*. 1987;156:344.
54. Daya S, Johnson PM, Clark DA. Trophoblast induction of suppressor type cell activity in human endometrial tissue. *Am J Reprod Immunol Microbiol*. 1989;19:65.
55. Slapsys RM, YoungLai E, Clark DA. A novel supressor cell is recruited to decidua by fetal trophoblast-type cells. *Regional Immunol*. 1988;1:182.
56. Clark DA, Croy BA, Wegmann TG, Chaouat G. Immunological and para-immunological mechanisms in spontaneous abortion: recent insights and future directions. *J Reprod Immunol*. 1987;12:1.
57. Clark DA. Host-immunoregulator mechanisms and the success of the conceptus fertilized *in-vivo* and *in-vitro*. In: Beard RW, Sharp F, eds. *Early Pregnancy Loss: Mechanisms and Treatment*. London: Royal College of Obstetricians and Gynaecologists; 1988:215.
58. Chaouat G, Kolb JP, Kiger N, et al. Immunologic consequences of vaccination against abortion in mice. *J Immunol*. 1985;134:1594.
59. Daya S, Clark DA, Devlin C, Jarrell J. Preliminary characterization of two types of suppressor cells in the human uterus. *Fertil Steril*. 1985;44:778.
60. Clark DA, Mowbray J, Underwood J, Liddell H. Histopathologic alterations in the dicidua of human spontaneous abortion: Loss of cells with large cytoplasmic granules. *Am J Reprod Immunol Microbiol*. 1987;13:19.
61. McIntyre JA, Faulk WP. Histocompatibility and recurrent abortions. *Fertil Steril*. 1984;41:653.
62. Beer AE, Quebbeman JF, Ayres JW, Haimes RF. Major histocompatibility complex antigen, maternal and paternal immune responses and chronic habitual abortions in humans. *Am J Obstet Gynecol*. 1981;141:987.
63. Thomas ML, Harger JH, Wagener DK, et al. HLA sharing and spontaneous abortion in humans. *Am J Obstet Gynecol*. 1985;8:1053.
64. Balasch J, Pastor M, Martorell J, et al. Shared HLA antigens between parents and recurrent spontaneous abortion. *Int J Fertil*. 1986;31:213.
65. Ober C, Elias S, O'Brien E, et al. HLA sharing and fertility in Hutterite couples: Evidence for prenatal selection against compatible fetuses. *Am J Reprod Immunol Microbiol*. 1988;18:111.
66. McIntyre JA, McConnachie PR, Taylor CG, Faulk WP. Clinical, immunological and genetical definitions of primary and secondary recurrent spontaneous abortions. *Fertil Steril*. 1984;42:849.
67. McIntyre JA, Faulk WP, Nichols-Johnson VR, Taylor CG. Immunologic testing and immunotherapy in recurrent spontaneous abortion. *Obstet Gynecol*. 1986;67:169.
68. Lauritsen JA, Kristensen T, Grunnet N. Depressed mixed lymphocyte culture reactivity in mothers with recurrent spontaneous abortion. *Am J Obstet Gynecol*. 1976;125:35.
69. Oksenberg JR, Persitz P, Amar A, et al. Mixed lymphocyte reactivity nonresponsiveness in couples with multiple spontaneous abortions. *Fertil Steril*. 1983;39:525.
70. McConnachie PR, McIntyre JA. Maternal antipaternal immunity in couples predisposed to repeated pregnancy losses. *Am J Reprod Immunol*. 1984;5:145.
71. Faulk WP, McIntyre JA. Immunological studies of human trophoblast: Markers, subsets and functions. *Immunol Rev*. 1983;75:139.
72. Allen WR, Kydd JH, Antczak DF. Successful application of immunotherapy to a model of pregnancy failure in equids. In: Clark DA, Croy BA, eds. *Reproductive Immunology 1986*. Amsterdam: Elsevier Science; 1986:253.
73. Clark DA, Kiger N, Guenet JL, Chaouat G. Local active suppression and vaccination against spontaneous abortion in CBA/J mice. *J Reprod Immunol*. 1987;10:79.
74. Denegri JF, Muzaffer A, McConnachie P., et al. Immunotherapy of primary immunological aborters: rationale for the use of pooled cryopreserved purified normal peripheral blood mononuclear cells. *Am J Reprod Immunol Microbiol*. 1986;12:65.
75. Johnson PM, Chia KV, Hart CA, et al. Trophoblast membrane infusion for unexplained recurrent miscarriage. *Br J Obstet Gynaecol*. 1988;95:342.
76. Mowbray JF, Liddell H, Underwood JL, et al. Controlled trial of treatment of recurrent spontaneous abortion by immunization with paternal cells. *Lancet*. 1985;i:941.
77. Mowbray JF, Underwood JL, Michel M, et al. Immunisation with paternal lymphocytes in women with recurrent miscarriage. *Lancet*. 1987;ii:679.
78. Mowbray JF. Effect of immunisation with paternal cells on recurrent spontaneous abortion. In: Clark DA, Croy BA, eds. *Reproductive Immunology 1986*. Amsterdam: Elsevier Science; 1986:269.
79. Mowbray JF. Success and failures of immunisation for recurrent spontaneous abortion. In: Beard RW, Sharp F, eds. *Early Pregnancy Loss: Mechanisms and Treatment*. London: Royal College of Obstetricians and Gynaecologists; 1988:325.
80. Reznikoff-Etievant MF, Durieux I, Huchet J, et al. Human MHC antigens and paternal leucocyte injections in recurrent spontaneous abortions. In: Beard RW, Sharp F, eds. *Early Pregnancy Loss: Mechanisms and Treatment*. London: Royal College of Obstetricians and Gynaecologists; 1988:375.
81. Alexander SA, Latinne D, Debruyere M, et al. Belgian experience with repeat immunisation in recurrent spontaneous abortions. In: Beard RW, Sharp F, eds. *Early Pregnancy Loss: Mechanisms and Treatment*. London: Royal College of Obstetricians and Gynaecologists; 1988:355.
82. Beer AE, Semprini AE, Zhu X, Quebbeman JF. Pregnancy outcome in human couples with recurrent spontaneous abortions: (1) HLA antigen profiles; (2) HLA antigen sharing; (3) Female serum MLR blocking factors and (4) Paternal leukocyte immunization. *Exp Clin Immunogenet*. 1985;2:137.
83. Beer AE. Pregnancy outcome in couples with recurrent abortions following immunological evaluation and therapy. In: Beard RW, Sharp F, eds. *Early Pregnancy Loss: Mechanisms and Treatment*. London: Royal College of Obstetricians and Gynaecologists; 1988:337.
84. Reznikoff-Etievant MF, Durieux I, Huchet J, et al. Paternal leukocyte injections in recurrent spontaneous abortion. *Lancet*. 1989;i:436.
85. Fujii T, Mizuno M, Kwana T, et al. Outcome of pregnancy after injection with mononuclear cells. *Am J Obstet Gynecol*. 1988;158:1015.
86. Takakuwa K, Kanazawa K, Takeuchi S. Production of blocking antibodies by vaccination with husband's lymphocytes in unexplained recurrent aborters: the role in successful pregnancy. *Am J Reprod Immunol Microbiol*. 1986;10:1.
87. Taylor CG, Faulk WP, McIntyre JA. Prevention of recurrent spontaneous abortions by leukocyte transfusions. *J R Soc Med*. 1985;78:623.
88. Beard RW, Sharp F, eds. *Early Pregnancy Loss: Mechanisms and Treatment*. London: Royal College of Obstetricians and Gynaecologists; 1988.

Chapter Fifty
Autoimmunity

Norbert Gleicher

50

Autoimmunity is generally defined as a disturbance in the immunologic tolerance of self. While the concept of clonal deletion is widely accepted as the basis for the tolerance of *self*, it is now accepted that even in normal individuals, complete clonal deletion may not always take place. Rather, normal tolerance of *self* may be characterized by the successful elimination of most cellular clones against self, resulting in only the generation of low normal autoantibody levels with usual low affinity. It is likely therefore that adequately sensitive assay systems could detect autoantibody reactivity against many self components. For example, if standard autoantibody groupings, such as antiphospholipid antibodies (APA), antihistones (AH), and antipolynucleotides (APN) are investigated in normal female and male populations, reactivity can be routinely detected. Normal autoantibody levels in females and males are not identical. In fact, significant differences can be detected, with females in general exhibiting higher levels.[1]

This significant difference in *normal* female and male autoantibody levels must have physiologic significance to survive evolutionary selection, even though higher autoantibody levels may, in fact, be a predisposing contributor to the significantly increased predisposition of women towards autoimmune disease. Only a very powerful benefit from higher autoantibody levels could then outweigh their adverse effects on females. It has been suggested that such a powerful benefit exists and relates to the female's biologic function to bear children.[2]

PREGNANCY AS AN AUTOGRAFT

Pregnancy has been recognized as an immunologic paradox for decades. The interest of immunologic investigations has, however, exclusively concentrated on the fetoplacental unit as an allograft (see also Chapter 49). This approach overlooks the fact that the products of conception contain autoantigenic specificities in equal amounts to alloantigens. An immunologic understanding of pregnancy requires not only an explanation for the tolerance of alloantigens but also of the female's capability to handle unusually large amounts of *self* antigens, even though they are derived from the parasitic fetus.

We have previously proposed that it is exactly this need for *tolerance* of increased self antigen loads during pregnancy that has resulted in higher autoantibody reactivity in females than males.[2] This hypothesis has recently been supported by many investigations; Ober et al[3], in a study of socially and genetically accurately defined Hutterites, confirmed significant differences in autoantibody levels between the sexes. More importantly, for the first time they were able to demonstrate that autoantibody patterns change with onset of sexual intercourse or pregnancy. El-Roeiy et al[4] expanded on this observation by demonstrating that autoantibody production in pregnancy increases (Table 50–1), although autoantibody levels in normal pregnancies generally remain within the nonpregnant range. Autoantibody levels during normal gestation remain static despite an increase in production because of the dilutional effect of the vascular expansion of pregnancy (see also Chapters 4 and 124). The specificity of the autoantibody response in pregnancy is documented by the fact that, in contrast to autoantibody levels, total immunoglobulin levels decrease in pregnancy because of intravascular volume expansion. Autoantibody levels appear to correlate directly with the amount of fetomaternal cell traffic.

As the volume of fetomaternal cells entering the maternal circulation increases with advancing gestational age, autoantibody levels also increase. It is well established that cell traffic peaks during labor and delivery and that this is the time of highest autoantibody levels, often exceeding a normal range for the nonpregnant state (see Table 50–1).

TABLE 50–1. A LONGITUDINAL INVESTIGATION OF IGM AUTOANTIBODY LEVELS THROUGHOUT GESTATION

	Nonpregnant Controls	Week of Pregnancy					Delivery (wk 39 ± 1.9)
		16	20	24	28	32	
Total IgM (mg/dL)	180 ± 70	155 ± 40	151 ± 64	161 ± 66	153 ± 54	158 ± 62	151 ± 55
Phospholipids							
Cardiolipin	24 ± 19	23 ± 19	11 ± 8	15 ± 10	29 ± 36	22 ± 13	24 ± 14
Phosphatidylserine	29 ± 31	14 ± 13	8 ± 11	14 ± 11	14 ± 13	35 ± 22	39 ± 24[a]
Phosphatidylglycerol	32 ± 38	33 ± 26	34 ± 18	23 ± 22	16 ± 22	39 ± 45	42 ± 49[a,b]
Phosphatidylethanolamine	5 ± 8	2 ± 3	3 ± 3	3 ± 4	3 ± 5	4 ± 4	5 ± 4
Phosphatidylinositol	26 ± 26	38 ± 22[c]	13 ± 8	39 ± 22	41 ± 24[c]	20 ± 17	22 ± 18
Phosphatidic acid	20 ± 24	32 ± 27[c]	19 ± 13	14 ± 10	15 ± 11	20 ± 24	22 ± 27
Histones							
H 1	56 ± 38	44 ± 30	45 ± 25	22 ± 25	27 ± 20	54 ± 32	60 ± 35[b]
H 2A	46 ± 36	61 ± 31	37 ± 25	26 ± 23	38 ± 21	63 ± 39	70 ± 43[b]
H 2B	48 ± 35	12 ± 18	29 ± 20	36 ± 22	34 ± 21	59 ± 38	65 ± 41[a,b]
H 3	47 ± 33	39 ± 21	29 ± 20	25 ± 22	25 ± 19	50 ± 27	55 ± 30[a]
H 4	139 ± 79	80 ± 72	73 ± 56	29 ± 23	46 ± 34	96 ± 60	105 ± 66
Polynucleotides							
ssDNA	115 ± 76	12 ± 25	33 ± 18	36 ± 27	18 ± 20	45 ± 29	50 ± 32
dsDNA	169 ± 84	85 ± 75	69 ± 97	87 ± 91	75 ± 77	119 ± 71	100 ± 81
Poly(I)	143 ± 86	79 ± 41	106 ± 80	80 ± 80	89 ± 44	127 ± 59	140 ± 64[a,b]
Poly(dT)	171 ± 102	68 ± 46	78 ± 48	75 ± 95	95 ± 77	117 ± 60	128 ± 66[a,b]

Ig = immunoglobulin.
Data are presented as optical density × 10^3 at 405 nm.
[a] Statistically increased level compared with levels at 16 weeks (before normalization) ($P < .05$).
[b] Statistically increased level compared with levels at 16 weeks (after normalization) ($P < .05$).
[c] Statistically increased level compared with nonpregnant controls ($P < .05$).
Similar observations also were made for IgG and IgA autoantibodies throughout gestation.
From El-Roeiy et al[4] with permission of author and publisher.

As expected, the *abnormal* autoantibody levels noted at that time are of IgM isotype, suggesting recent antigen stimulation. Normal pregnancy should thus be understood as a time of increased *auto*-antigen exposure, increased autoantibody response, and possibly as a consequence of the two, it is a time predisposed to an increased incidence of clinical autoimmune phenomena.

AUTOANTIBODY ABNORMALITIES IN PREGNANCY

As noted previously, in normal pregnancy, autoantibody levels rarely exceed the normal range of nonpregnant females. Moreover, exceptions to this rule are usually restricted to IgM specificities and occur exclusively in the peripartal period. The detection of abnormal IgG autoantibody levels must therefore always be considered an abnormal finding; however, abnormal IgM autoantibody levels, especially at term, should be considered with caution and should not be overinterpreted.

The detection of abnormal autoantibody specificities also will depend on the extent of the performed B lymphocyte evaluation.

The Detection of Autoantibody Abnormalities

"Search and you will find" could be the motto for the investigation of B lymphocyte function. Abnormal B cell function is almost never monoclonal in nature. Consequently, the investigation of single autoantibody specificities will often be inadequate.

Figure 50–1 demonstrates classic B lymphocyte activation patterns. As the figure demonstrates, normal individuals demonstrate a broad background pattern of antibody production. Single antigen immunization with, for example, tetanus will result in a specific antitetanus response peak; however, it also should be noted that the background oscillation, reflective of nonspecific antibody responses, also is increased. In a classic autoimmune disease, such as systemic lupus erythematosus (SLE), selective autoantibody specificities are exceedingly high, probably in response to specific antigen stimulation. However, in addition, the background oscillation is again elevated. In fact, background oscillation is higher than after tetanus immunization. This suggests an even stronger activating impulse on B lymphocytes, possibly caused by multiple antigenic stimulations. Moreover, these observations point out that antigenic stimulation of B cells always activates nonspecific clones in addition to specific responses. This indicates that polyclonal B cell activation, as demonstrated in the fourth cell of Figure 50–1, is a feature of any B lymphocyte activation. Only the degree of polyclonal activation varies.[5]

As a consequence, we have recommended that the practice of single-autoantibody investigation in conjunction with B lymphocyte dysfunction in pregnancy be abandoned. However, this leaves the question of which antibody specificities should be investigated. We have established an autoantibody profile, involving such classic autoantibody groupings as antiphospholipids, antihistones, and antipolynucleotides (Fig. 50–2). The latter two groupings involve specificities that are frequently elevated with autoimmune diseases such as SLE, while antiphospholipid antibodies are characteristically associated with pregnancy loss and other features of the *reproductive autoimmune failure syndrome* (RAFS), discussed later in this chapter. As a complete profile also involving specific isotypes, this establishes a broadly based reflection of B lymphocyte activity, clearly superior to any single marker. Nevertheless, no profile can be all encompassing.

Autoantibody abnormalities can occur in pregnancy in the absence of clinical autoimmune diseases. In fact, a majority of autoantibody abnormalities will probably be detected in clinically asymptomatic patients because clinical autoimmune disease is rare. Moreover, preexisting autoimmune disease will not necessarily demonstrate abnormal autoantibody levels during pregnancy because the volume expansion of pregnancy may reduce previously elevated levels to a normal range.

Autoantibody positivity also requires definition. Different laboratories define autoantibody positivity in different ways. Most establish positivity at a specific standard deviation of mean of a varying number of control patients. This mean can be based on as few as a single digit number of controls. While such an analysis would obviously be of only limited value, it also has become apparent that autoantibody abnormalities should *not* be assessed in that way. Autoantibodies, especially antiphospholipid and antihis-

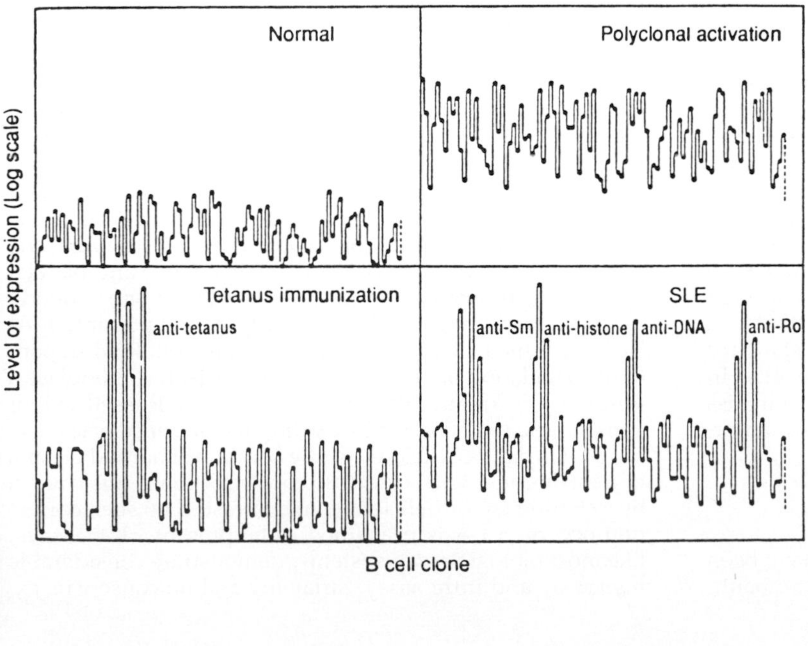

Figure 50–1. Various patterns of B cell activation. (*From Eisenberg and Cohen[5] with permission of authors and publishers.*)

AUTOANTIBODY SCREEN

Patient Name
Address

Phone
Date of Birth Account No.

Referring Physician DR. GLEICHER
Office Address 750 N ORLEANS
CHICAGO
Phone

DEPT PROV 210 BAT 255 CASE 14 REC 1167 REP 3308 SREP 3308 DOT 04/16/91
Patient Information
(by referring office) Diagnosis: 1. R/O RAFS
Gravida 0 2. PRE IVF
LMP 03/28/91 Para 0 3.
Premature 0 Medication: 1. ANANCIN 3 prn, VIT'S
Blood Drawn 04/12/91 Abortion 0 2. IRON SUPPLEMENT

IMMUNOGLOBULIN PANEL
o IgG 1376 (700-1700 mg/dl)
o IgM 435 * (70- 210 mg/dl)
o IgA 202 (70- 350 mg/dl)

o ANA 1: (20)
o Lupus Anticoagulant 1.29
(1.2-1.3 borderline; 1.30 abnormal)
o APTT 43 * (< 40)

AUTOANTIBODY SCREEN	IgG			IgM			IgA		
Phospholipids									
Cardiolipin	11.53 *	[100]	(5.00)	0.71	[ ]	(5.10)	4.00	[ ]	(9.00)
P. Serine	21.50 *	[100]	(8.20)	0.68	[ ]	(7.70)	2.71	[ ]	(23.00)
Phosphatidic A.	11.17 *	[99]	(10.60)	0.29	[ ]	(7.20)	2.67	[ ]	(10.30)
P. Ethanolamine	3.00	[ ]	(12.00)	4.33	[ ]	(12.00)	3.33	[ ]	(7.00)
P. Glycerol	8.73 *	[99]	(6.50)	0.47	[ ]	(5.30)	0.82	[ ]	(15.00)
P. Inositol	8.94 *	[100]	(5.00)	0.12	[ ]	(6.20)	2.00	[ ]	(6.70)
o Histones									
Total Histones	0.33	[ ]	(4.80)	0.43	[ ]	(3.30)	3.50	[ ]	(15.00)
H2A	0.89	[ ]	(6.00)	1.21	[ ]	(3.80)	8.50	[ ]	(14.00)
H2B	1.29	[ ]	(7.00)	0.70	[ ]	(3.30)	4.00	[ ]	(12.00)
H3	1.67	[ ]	(8.20)	2.15	[ ]	(3.80)	4.33	[ ]	(38.30)
H4	1.46	[ ]	(10.00)	0.41	[N/A]	(2.50)	1.25	[ ]	(4.30)
o Nucleotides									
ssDNA	2.95	[ ]	(4.00)	0.68	[ ]	(3.10)	1.42	[ ]	(8.00)
dsDNA	1.78	[ ]	(3.50)	0.97	[ ]	(4.10)	1.07	[ ]	(11.00)
PolyI	0.20	[ ]	(4.50)	0.36	[N/A]	(3.30)	0.52	[N/A]	(6.00)
Poly (dT)	0.56	[N/A]	(2.80)	0.77	[N/A]	(3.80)	0.48	[N/A]	(3.60)

OTHER TESTS:
SS-A (anti-Ro)
SS-B (anti-La)
Sm (anti-Smith)
COMMENTS: RAFS; To start babyaspirin ASAP; requires treatment.

Technician: GEORGE KABERLEIN M.D.: DR. GLEICHER
Laboratory Director: Alan Dudkiewicz, Ph.D.

* INDICATES ABNORMAL RESULT
NUMBERS IN [] INDICATE PERCENTILE OF MEDIAN OF 400 NORMAL CONTROL SERA > 94%
NUMBERS IN () INDICATE THE UPPER RANGE OF 99% OF 400 NORMAL CONTROL SERA.

Figure 50–2. Reproductive immunology consultation.

tone antibodies, are nonparametrically distributed in a normal population.[1,4] Such a distribution invalidates a statistical evaluation based on standard deviations and requires the establishment of confidence limits, which will vary for each antibody and each isotype. The reader is therefore encouraged to investigate their autoantibody assays before clinical decisions are made based on their results. These issues may be of minor importance with defined autoimmune diseases in which autoantibody levels can be exceedingly high, but they will be of crucial importance in clinically asymptomatic patients with B lymphocyte dysfunction, who may exhibit abnormal autoantibody levels, even though at a lower level than clinically symptomatic patients. A positive cutoff value based on a small number of standard deviations would result in many false-positive results. In contrast, a cutoff at too many standard deviations will miss a considerable number of affected patients with low abnormal autoantibody levels.

Autoantibody Abnormalities in the Absence of Autoimmune Diseases

Autoantibody abnormalities in early pregnancy have been associated primarily with pregnancy loss, while autoantibody abnormalities in late pregnancy have been linked with maternal hypertension and fetal intrauterine growth retardation.

Pregnancy Loss. In 1984, Lubbe et al were the first to associate abnormal B lymphocyte function with repeated pregnancy loss.[6] Their observation was the presence of the *lupus anticoagulant* (LA) in women with unexplained repeated pregnancy wastage. As Figure 50–3 demonstrates, LA is believed to interfere with the balance between thromboxane and prostacylin in favor of the vasoconstrictive and platelet aggregating thromboxane. LA is believed to be one antibody (or more than one) of either IgG or IgM (and possibly IgA) isotype, which, if present, prolongs phospholipid-dependent coagulation assays, such as the partial thromboplastin time (APTT), kaolin clotting time (KCT), and Russell's viper venom time (RVVT). While clotting factor deficiencies also can prolong any of these tests, the addition of normal plasma in a mixing test will correct the prolongation if it is caused by a clotting factor deficiency. In contrast, if no such correction occurs, a LA is presumed to be present.[7] LA assays, like most biologic assay systems, demonstrate considerable interassay and intra-assay variability and no consensus ex-

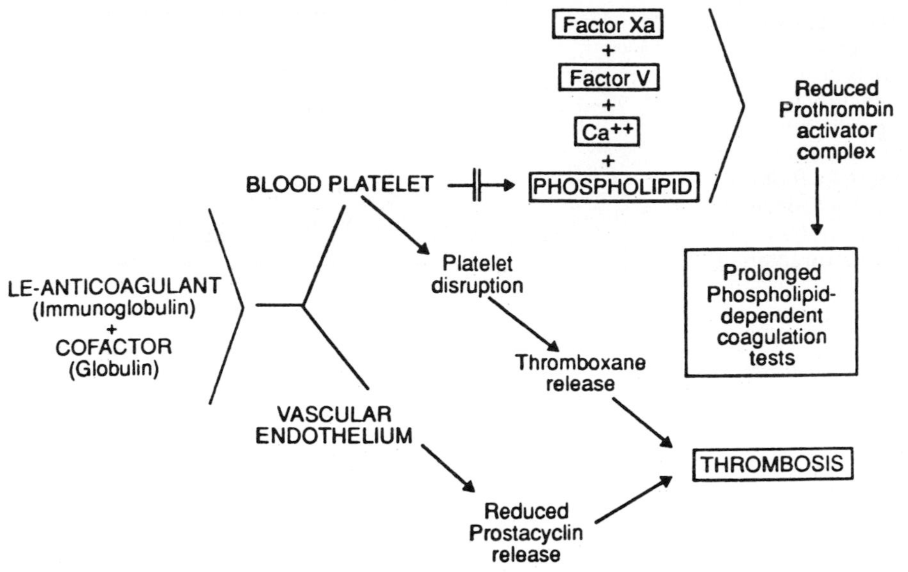

Figure 50–3. The proposed activity of lupus anticoagulant, affecting the thromboxane–prostacyclin balance. (*Modified from Lubbe and Liggins*[20], *with permission of authors and publishers.*)

ists as to which assay should be used to detect LA. In fact, consensus exists that no single assay is reliable enough, and that, therefore, at least two assays should be used before clinical decisions are made based on the detection of LA.

The presence of LA predisposes to the development of thromboembolic phenomena. In one study, the retroactive evaluation of women with repeated pregnancy loss and LA positivity revealed an exceedingly high incidence of previous thromboembolic phenomena.[8] Some authorities have suggested that pregnancy loss in these patients occurs as a consequence of thromboembolic events in the microcirculation of the placenta.

Lubbe's initial report on LA was rapidly followed by the recognition that LA was only one of many markers of abnormal B cell function in affected women.[9] Other abnormalities noted in these patients are listed in Table 50–2. In concurrence with the previously discussed activation patterns of B lymphocytes, B-cell activation in these patients is mostly polyclonal. Consequently, as noted previously, autoantibody investigations should not be restricted to single-antibody investigations. Some authorities have suggested otherwise, especially expanding the use of anticardiolipin antibodies as disease markers, either alone or in conjunction with LA.[10] We have opposed this approach as incomplete and have suggested the use of a more broadly based autoantibody profile (see Fig. 50–2) to identify affected patients.

Various terms have been coined by investigators to describe the association of autoantibody abnormalities with repeated pregnancy loss. They include the *cardiolipin antibody syndrome,* among those which have (wrongly) emphasized the predominance of anticardiolipin antibodies. The *phospholipid antibody syndrome* is preferred by proponents of a more correct view in that the whole family of antiphospholipid antibodies is closely associated with pregnancy loss (see also Chapter 51). Because antiphospholipid antibodies are not the only B cell abnormalities associated with pregnancy loss and because autoantibody abnormalities also are associated with other forms of reproductive failure, we coined the term *reproductive autoimmune failure syndrome-* (RAFS) to describe all forms of reproductive failure attributed to abnormal B lymphocyte function.

Whatever terminology is used, one has to recognize that the association between pregnancy loss and abnormal B cell function has, despite much research effort, remained an *association.* Causation has not been proven, even though experimental evidence is slowly being developed.

For example, some possible animal models have been reported, although none is satisfactory. The recent suggestion that antiphospholipid antibodies may affect signal transduction processes could provide a molecular explanation for the large variety of effects that antiphospholipid antibodies appear capable of exerting on reproductive processes.[11] Until effects of specific autoantibodies have been established, preferably in an animal model, causation of pregnancy loss by autoantibodies must remain unproven and be considered an association. This has to be considered before treatment regimens are instigated.

Diagnosis. Autoantibody abnormalities in women with pregnancy loss usually are detectable before conception. It has been our experience, however, that approximately 10% of patients exhibit no or too few abnormalities before conception to reach diagnosis. Their autoantibody profile deteriorates significantly as soon as pregnancy is achieved. Only a small minority of patients demonstrate autoantibody abnormalities for the first time at a later gestational age.

TABLE 50–2. FREQUENT FINDINGS IN HABITUAL ABORTERS WITHOUT AUTOIMMUNE DISEASE THAT SUGGEST ABNORMAL B LYMPHOCYTE FUNCTION

Laboratory
- Lupus anticoagulant
- Gammopathy (usually polyclonal, mostly IgM but also IgG and IgA)
- Antiphospholipid antibodies (mostly IgG but also IgM and IgA)
- Antihistone antibodies (mostly IgG but also IgM and IgA)
- Antipolynucleotide antibodies (mostly IgG but also IgM and IgA)
- Increased incidence of tissue specific autoantibodies
  - Antithyroid antibodies
  - Antismooth muscle antibodies

Clinical Findings
- Family history of autoimmune disease
- Patient history of autoimmune disease or compatible symptomatology that does *not* fully fulfill criteria for diagnosis of autoimmune disease
- Endometriosis

The diagnostic problem with autoantibody-associated pregnancy loss lies in the fact that the diagnosis depends on a history of previous pregnancy loss. There is no evidence that B-cell abnormalities in the absence of a history of pregnancy loss should be the basis of any therapeutic intervention. There are no data that would support treatment under such conditions, even though the withholding of therapy, especially with severe and multiple autoantibody abnormalities, can be a difficult decision. The decision can be especially difficult when the patient presents with a threatened abortion with vaginal bleeding.

The literature also is not clear as to how many miscarriages should qualify a patient for the diagnosis of autoantibody-associated pregnancy loss. While, for years, the general consensus in the investigation of repeated pregnancy loss has been that any diagnostic intervention was statistically not warranted before three miscarriages, most studies on autoantibody associated pregnancy loss contain patients with fewer losses. At what stage the diagnosis is attached to a patient has therefore been left to clinical judgment. The more autoantibody abnormalities a patient exhibits, the fewer miscarriages should be required before the diagnosis can be made. This suggestion represents another argument in favor of a more broadly based investigation of B lymphocyte function.

Some authorities suggest that the diagnosis can be exclusively based on the recognition of an LA. In our experience, LA positivity almost never exists in the absence of autoantibody positivity, although rare exceptions have been observed.[12] The use of LA testing as an exclusive screening test for affected females is inadequate. Such a diagnostic approach would miss a majority of affected patients. While an excellent correlation between LA positivity and a variety of phospholipid antibodies had initially been reported, it has since become apparent that this correlation is not as close as initially suggested.

Treatment. Whether there is any effective treatment for autoantibody-associated pregnancy loss is undetermined. A large number of studies has suggested such a benefit; however, none has been randomized prospectively. A beneficial effect from therapy was first suggested by Lubbe et al,[14] who recommended a regimen involving corticosteroid therapy and low-dose aspirin. The steroids suppress autoantibody production, while low-dose aspirin counteracts the thromboxane effect of platelet aggregation, instigated by phospholipid antibodies.

The most widely quoted study in the literature suggests that in patients, who, after retroactive case review, had close to 100% pregnancy wastage, close to 80% viability was achieved in the first treated pregnancy.[8] This study has also been cited as the reason that a prospective evaluation of treatment regimens compared to no treatment was ethically impossible. It also institutionalized the treatment of autoantibody-associated pregnancy loss with prednisone and aspirin. As noted previously, the concept of therapy was twofold; corticosteroid therapy was expected to suppress autoantibody production by B lymphocytes, while low dose ("baby") aspirin was thought to counteract the thromboxane effect of LA and antiphospholipid antibodies (see Fig. 50–3). Most therapeutic treatment regimens reported in the literature involve prednisone therapy of 30–60 mg and one "baby" aspirin daily. This therapy usually is carried through until delivery. Figure 50–4 demonstrates this treatment regimen in one of our earliest patients. Since then, we have learned that prescribing prednisone therapy until term is unnecessary. Most affected patients demonstrate a *critical period* during pregnancy, at which time autoantibody abnormalities peak. Once this critical period has been overcome, prednisone therapy can safely be tapered down to zero, as autoantibody abnormalities decrease in parallel. Autoantibody abnormalities usually resurge in the third trimester; however, at that point, our recommendation is to treat the patient obstetrically based on the clinical evaluation of the pregnancy, using ultrasound and antepartum testing.

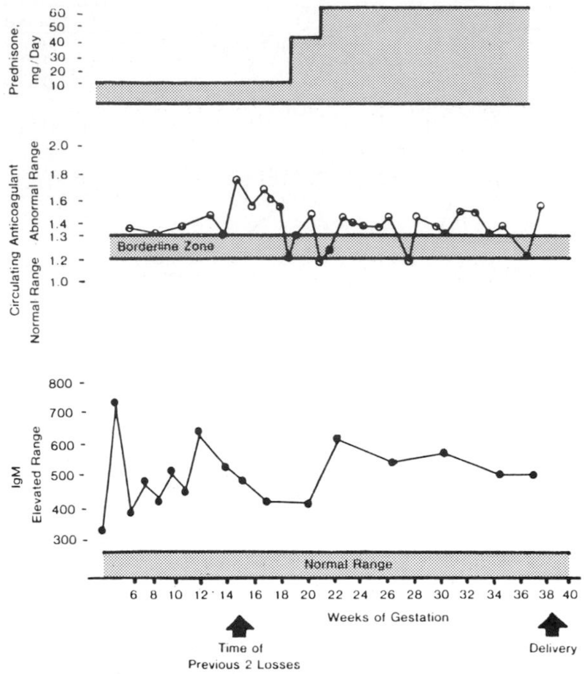

Figure 50–4 Antibody abnormalities and treatment protocol in habitual aborter. Treatment protocol of a very early patient with RAFS before the treatment period with prednisone was shortened (*From Gleicher and Friberg*[9] *with permission*).

Our protocol requires weekly autoantibody evaluation until the patient's critical period is passed by 2–3 weeks. The critical period is usually identical, or at least close, to maximal autoantibody abnormalities. However, it also usually corresponds to the times of previous pregnancy loss. Based on these weekly autoantibody assessments, the prednisone dose is adjusted weekly upward or downward.

Table 50–3 summarizes the treatment protocol that has been in place in our unit for more than 3 years. Treatment is usually instigated as soon as pregnancy is recognized or as soon as the patient presents. The decision as to when to instigate therapy also depends on the timing of previous pregnancy losses. While autoantibody-associated pregnancy wastage in most cases is *not* early pregnancy loss, it may be in a minority of patients. In these patients, early onset of therapy is especially important, and we often start treatment with 10 mg of prednisone *before* conception. As soon as pregnancy is recognized, prednisone therapy is increased to 30–40 mg daily, depending on body weight and severity of autoantibody abnormalities. As noted previously, prednisone is adjusted weekly according to autoantibody titers. The oral maximum dose is 60 mg daily. We recommend that this dose not be exceeded. In rare instances, where higher doses of corticosteroid therapy are required, we recommend that it be administered intravenously. Such treatment has only been necessary in our institution when patients break through at maximal oral dose and develop vaginal bleeding. These females are then

TABLE 50–3. TREATMENT PROTOCOL FOR HABITUAL ABORTERS WITH B-LYMPHOCYTE DYSFUNCTION

Miscarriages Before 4 Weeks Gestational Age

With pregnancy attempt, patient is started on:

Prednisone (0.17 mg/kg) and aspirin (81 mg daily): As soon as pregnancy is recognized (preferably before missed menses), Prednisone is increased to 0.5–1 mg/kg daily. The dose is adjusted weekly, dependent on the severity of autoantibody abnormalities noted (see Fig. 50–2).

Aspirin is maintained.

Miscarriages After 4 Weeks Gestational Age

Prednisone (0.5–1 mg/kg) as soon as pregnancy is diagnosed. Dose is adjusted weekly based on autoantibody profile (see Fig. 50–2).

Aspirin (81 mg daily)

Threatening Miscarriage Despite Maximal Oral Prednisone Dose (60 mg daily)

Patient admitted to hospital for intravenous therapy with corticosteroids until bleeding stops, then switched to maximal oral dose (60 mg daily). Heparin (10,000 u b.i.d.) may be added.

Length of Therapy

Prednisone is tapered off to zero, starting 2 weeks after the *latest* previous gestational week of pregnancy loss (*critical period*). Tapering takes place in 10 mg increments per week.

Aspirin continues to term.

Autoantibody abnormalities usually increase again toward term. At this point, we do not recommend pharmacologic suppression, but obstetric management. Patients who fail the standard protocol may receive experimental therapy with heparin or intravenous gammaglobulin.

admitted for intravenous steroid therapy, which is usually required for only 1–2 days.

Some authorities have suggested that the LA (or phospholipid antibodies) does not (or do not always) suppress on corticosteroid therapy. This is a correct observation, although only in a minority of cases. All reports on the inability to suppress autoantibodies were based on the evaluation of single or a small number of autoantibody specifities. Whether the inability to suppress, for example, anticardiolipin antibodies suggests that corticosteroid therapy is ineffective, remains to be established. Anticardiolipin antibodies, and for that matter, any other single autoantibody specificity, is only one among many disease *markers*. Neither has been directly implicated as a causative factor.

Consequently, we do not act on the fluctuation (or lack thereof) of any single autoantibody but attempt to get a broader impression of B lymphocyte activation, as previously described. If this assessment demonstrates that maximum corticosteroid therapy has been ineffective, alternative therapies are considered, although aspirin is always continued to term.

Alternative therapies are even less established than corticosteroid therapy. Treatment with subcutaneous heparin (2500–10,000 subcutaneously twice daily) has been recommended by some investigators. Some preliminary data suggest that this therapy may show similar effectiveness to corticosteroids. A prospective, randomized control study comparing heparin use with *no* treatment has not been performed. We substitute heparin therapy only in patients who are failing or have failed corticosteroid therapy in a previous pregnancy and are presently not using this treatment as a primary option. However, our approach is as anectodal as that of other investigators who may recommend a primary treatment protocol involving heparin.

A third treatment option that has been proposed in a limited number of case reports is the use of intravenous immunoglobulin preparations. Intravenous gammaglobulin preparations have been successfully used in a variety of autoimmune diseases to decrease autoantibody levels. Their mode of action is poorly understood, but they do not appear to interfere with the subsequent evaluation of autoantibody levels, even though they contain autoantibody specificities.[15]

In summary, while autoantibody-associated pregnancy loss appears to represent a factual entity, the best therapeutic approach to the problem remains to be established. Even the use of aspirin has not been assessed in controlled trials.

Effects on Pregnancy. It appears that any of the previously discussed treatment regimens will result in viable pregnancies. Affected pregnancies are still high risk because they are associated with a considerable complication rate. Reports suggest that the incidence of pregnancy-induced hypertension, diabetes mellitus, and intrauterine growth retardation (IUGR) is high.[8] While incidence numbers vary, it is clear that some of these complications are preventable while others are not.

For example, the incidence of diabetes mellitus appears to be directly related to the amount and length of corticosteroid therapy. We have experienced severely impaired glucose tolerance in more than half of all patients when corticosteroid therapy was continued to term. Since we have modified our treatment approach and have tapered off prednisone once the critical period is passed, the incidence of gestational diabetes has been reduced to normal background levels.

A similar observation was made in reference to pregnancy-induced hypertension. Early reports suggest a very high incidence of hypertensive disorders in affected patients. We believe that this incidence can be reduced if corticosteroid therapy is not continued to term. However, in contrast to diabetes, the incidence of pregnancy-associated hypertension remains high compared to control populations. In our experience, approximately one third of patients will develop hypertension, and often require early delivery.

This increased incidence of hypertension in affected females should not be a surprise because hypertensive disorders of pregnancy have been associated with abnormally increased autoantibody levels. The same association also was made with IUGR. Consequently, an increased incidence of IUGR also can be expected and, in fact, occurs.[16]

As noted previously, a second peak of autoantibody abnormalities can be observed in the third trimester. A theoretical discussion of the possible underlying pathophysiology also was presented previously. Autoantibody abnormalities in late pregnancy should not be treated medically. Because their signficance at that point primarily appears to lie in their effect on the fetus, we recommend exclusively obstetric management based on fetal condition. This will result in delivery before the 36th week of gestation in approximately one third of cases.

One issue requires further notice: A number of recent investigations have suggested that low-dose aspirin therapy can lower the incidence of pregnancy-induced hypertension.[17,18] These data are convincing because they were reported independently from different centers. As in patients with phospholipid antibodies, patients with pregnancy-induced hypertensive diseases have been suggested to suffer from a thromboxane–prostacyclin imbalance.[19] This observation, together with the recently reported high incidence of IgG phospholipid antibodies in hypertensive pregnant patients[16], creates a theoretical background for the successful use of aspirin. It is therefore tempting to speculate that low-dose aspirin therapy also could have a beneficial effect on patients with autoantibody-associated pregnancy loss. This theoretical concept influences us to prescribe low-dose aspirin until term, recognizing that confirmation of its benefits awaits prospective evaluation.

ABNORMALITIES IN THE PRESENCE OF AUTOIMMUNE DISEASES

The preceding parts of this chapter are largely dedicated to the discussion of autoantibody abnormalities in clinically normal pregnant individuals. This section reviews females with an autoimmune disease who conceive. Individual autoimmune diseases are discussed in their respective chapters. Consequently, this chapter only summarizes some principles.

The effects of pregnancy on autoimmune diseases vary. Many diseases appear unaffected or unaffected to a large extent. Others have been reported to exacerbate with pregnancy or, especially, in the puerperium. Lastly, some (eg, rheumatoid arthritis) may even improve.

Table 50–4 provides a list of medical conditions that have been associated with abnormal autoimmunity. A woman in her child-bearing years should always be advised on how pregnancy may affect her disease. Moreover, she should receive appropriate family planning counseling (see also Chapter 1) to assure that pregnancy occurs only when the patient is in the best possible physical condition for pregnancy. The concept of *preconceptional counseling* is discussed in detail in Chapter 1.

TABLE 50–4. MEDICAL CONDITIONS ASSOCIATED WITH ABNORMAL B-LYMPHOCYTE TO FUNCTION

Collagen vascular diseases
Rheumatoid arthritis
Systemic lupus erythematosus
Mixed connective tissue disease
Periateritis nodosa (necrotizing vasulitis)
Polymyositis
Systemic sclerosis
Ankylosing spondylitis
Felty's syndrome
Glomerulonephritis
Rheumatic fever
Cardiomyopathy
Dermatitis herpetiformis
Atopic diseases
Celiac disease
Herpes gestationis
Ulcerative colitis
Crohn's disease
Idiopathic interstitial pneumonia
Adult respiratory distress syndrome
Sarcoidosis
Multiple sclerosis
Amyotrophic lateral sclerosis
Myasthenia gravis
Uveitis
Tissue injury
Surgery
Transplantation
Behcet's syndrome
Chronic active hepatitis
Autoimmune hemolytic anemia
Immune thrombocytopenic purpura
Thyroid disease
Hyperthyroidism (Graves' disease)
Hypothyroidism (Hashimoto's thyroiditis)
Diabetes mellitus
Malignancy
AIDS
Endometriosis
Unconfirmed associations specific to pregnancy
"Laboratory only syndrome" with or without IgM-monoclonopathy, HELLP syndrome
Respiratory distress syndrome
Preeclampsia, eclampsia, and other hypertensive conditions of pregnancy

TABLE 50–5. MEDICAL CONDITIONS WITH DISTURBED B-LYMPHOCYTE FUNCTION THAT HISTORICALLY HAVE BEEN ASSOCIATED WITH INCREASED PREGNANCY LOSS

Collagen vascular diseases
Systemic lupus erythematosus
Mixed connective tissue disease
Systemic sclerosis
Dermatitis herpetiformis
Celiac disease
Herpes gestationis
Ulcerative colitis
Crohn's disease
Chronic active hepatitis
Thyroid disease
Diabetes mellitus
Endometriosis

Pregnancy Loss

It is surprising that the association between pregnancy loss and abnormal B lymphocyte function has only recently been recognized. Pregnancy loss as a feature of autoimmune diseases has been recognized for decades. The recent understanding of medical disorders, such as thyroid disease and diabetes mellitus, as autoimmune conditions suggests that all medical conditions that historically have been associated with increased pregnancy wastage are autoimmune in etiology (see Table 50–5). This observation strongly supports the concept of autoimmune-induced pregnancy loss. This concept also is supported by the observation of McHugh and Maddison[19] who report that the incidence of pregnancy loss with such autoimmune diseases as systemic lupus, systemic sclerosis, and rheumatoid arthritis is higher after than before the onset of disease.

REFERENCES

1. Gleicher N, El-Roeiy A. Autoantibody profile in normal females and males. Submitted for publication.
2. Gleicher N, El-Roeiy A. The reproductive autoimmune failure syndrome (RAFS). *Am J Obstet Gynecol*. 1988;195:223.
3. Ober C, Gleicher N, Elias S, Harlow L. Natural autoantibodies in Hutterites: 1. Sex differences in antibody levels. *Am J Reprod Immunol*. 1990;22:85. Abstract.
4. El-Roeiy A, Myers SA, Gleicher N. The prevalence of autoantibodies

and lupus anticoagulant in healthy pregnant women. *Obstet Gynecol.* 1990;75:390.
5. Eisenberg RA, Cohen PL. Mechanisms of autoantibody production in systemic lupus erythematosus. *Clin Aspects Autoimmun.* 1988;2:1.
6. Lubbe WF, Butler WS, Palmer SJ, Liggins GC. Lupus anticoagulant in pregnancy. *Br J Obstet Gynaecol.* 1984;91:359.
7. Lupus anticoagulant. *Lancet.* 1984;i:1117. Editorial.
8. Branch DW, Scott JR, Kochenour NK, Hershgold E. Obstetric complications associated with the lupus anticoagulant. *N Engl J Med.* 1986;313:1322.
9. Gleicher N, Friberg J. IgM gammopathy and the lupus anticoagulant syndrome in habitual aborters. *JAMA.* 1985;253:3278.
10. Harris EN, Chan JKH, Ashwerson RA, et al. Thrombosis, recurrent fetal loss and thrombocytopenia. Predictive value of anti-cardiolipin antibody test. *Arch Int Med.* 1986;146:2153.
11. Gleicher N, Harlow L, Silberstein M. The regulatory effect of antiphospholipid antibodies (APA) on signal transduction. A possible model for autoantibody induced reproductive failure. Submitted for publication.
12. Gleicher N, Harlow L, El-Roeiy A. The correlation between lupus anticoagulant and autoantibodies. *Mount Sinai J Med.* In press.
13. Rote NS, Dostal-Johnson D, Branch DW. Antiphospholipid antibodies and recurrent pregnancy loss: correlation between activated partial thromboplastin time and antibodies against phosphatidylserine and cardiolipin. *Am J Obstet Gynecol.* 1990;163:575.
14. Lubbe WF, Butler WS, Palmer SJ, Liggins GC. Fetal survival after prednisone suppression of maternal lupus anticoagulant. *Lancet.* 1983;i:1361.
15. Gleicher N, Harlow L. Commercial IgG immunoglobulin preparations exhibit IgG and IgA reactivity at pharmacological but not at physiological concentrations. *Mount Sinai J Med.* In press.
16. El-Roeiy A, Myers SA, Gleicher N. The relationship between autoantibodies and intrauterine growth retardation in hypertensive disorders of pregnancy. *Am J Obstet Gynecol.* In press.
17. Wallenburg HCS, Makovitz JW, Dekker GA, Rotmans P. Low-dose aspirin prevents pregnancy-induced hypertension and preeclampsia in angiotensin-sensitive primigravidae. *Lancet.* 1986;1:1.
18. Cunningham FG, Gant NF. Prevention of Preeclampsia—a reality? *N Engl J Med.* 1989;321:606.
19. McHugh NJ, Maddison PJ. Systemic lupus erythematosus: biological effects and management. In: Scott JS, Bird HA, eds. *Pregnancy, Autoimmunity and Connective Tissue Disorders.* Oxford, England: Oxford Press; 1990:81.
20. Lubbe LW, Liggins GC. Lupus anticoagulant and pregnancy. *Am J Obstet Gynecol.* 1985;153:322.

Chapter Fifty-One

Systemic Lupus Erythematosus, Connective Tissue Disorders, and the Vasculitides

Ann L. Parke

51

Systemic lupus erythematosus (SLE) and many of the other connective tissue diseases are more prevalent in women, especially women of childbearing age. In SLE, the male to female ratio is 1 to 15 during childbearing years and 1 to 9 overall. It is therefore not surprising that many women with SLE and other connective tissue diseases want to become pregnant. The following questions need to be addressed by physician and patient:

1. Is it safe for women with these connective tissue diseases to become pregnant? Can they safely tolerate the physiologic demands of pregnancy?
2. How will the disease affect the pregnancy with particular reference to fertility rates and fetal wastage rates? What are the factors that determine these rates?
3. How will the pregnancy affect the disease?
4. How should patients with connective tissue diseases be managed throughout pregnancy and in the postpartum period? Many of the drugs used to manage these connective tissue diseases are not recommended for use in pregnancy (Table 51–1).
5. Is breast-feeding advisable?
6. If it is determined that patients with these diseases should not get pregnant or that pregnancy should be delayed, what method of contraception would be the most desirable in such patients?

In addition to the well-defined connective tissue diseases, there are now two more recently described syndromes, the *phospholipid antibody syndrome* and the *neonatal lupus syndrome*. In these syndromes, the presence of certain maternal antibodies (phospholipid antibodies in the phospholipid antibody syndrome and antibodies to extractable nuclear antigen [ENA] ie, anti-Ro, anti-La, and RNP antibodies in the neonatal lupus syndrome) have been incriminated in the development of congenital abnormalities and even fetal death. Various therapies have been used during pregnancy in patients with these syndromes (Table 51–2) in an attempt to prevent adverse affects; however, the pathogenetic mechanisms and the precise relationship of these antibodies to fetal wastage and the development of congenital abnormalities have not been identified (see also Chapter 50). There also are numerous reports of women with these antibodies who have successfully completed pregnancy and have produced normal live infants. The use of aggressive therapies in these women must therefore be questioned.

SLE AND RELATED SYNDROMES

Systemic lupus erythematosus is a multisystem disease with the hallmarks of autoantibody production and vasculitis, usually small vessel vasculitis. The revised American Rheumatism Association (ARA) criteria for SLE established in 1982 define the disease[1] (Table 51–3); however, some patients with clinical complaints suggestive of SLE fail to meet four criteria and therefore cannot be labeled as having the disease. These patients clearly demonstrate the limitations of having criteria to establish a diagnosis, and recent developments have suggested that the concept of *subclinical* autoimmune disease is not as ridiculous as it may sound. Patients with subclinical autoimmune disease have no clinical complaints, but they have multiple laboratory markers of autoimmunity and clearly demonstrate pathology under certain circumstances, such as pregnancy when they only experience multiple fetal deaths or produce a child with neonatal lupus syndrome.

There is no difference between the rate of fertility in women with SLE and normal women.[2]

TABLE 51–1. DRUGS USED IN THE MANAGEMENT OF CONNECTIVE TISSUE DISEASES

Disease	Therapies Used to Treat Disease	Use in Pregnancy (Risk–Benefit Ratio)[a]
Systemic lupus erythematosis		
Systemic	Corticosteroids	D
	4-amino quinoline antimalarial drugs	C
	Azathioprine	D
	Cyclophosphamide	D
	Plasmapheresis	
Cutaneous	4-amino quinoline antimalarial drugs	C
	Dapsone	C[b]
	Accutane	X
	Oral gold	C[b]
Scleroderma	NSAIDs (excluding phenylbutazone)	B but becomes D if used in third trimester
	D-Penicillamine	D
	Nifedipine	Cm
	ACE (angiotensin-converting enzyme inhibitors ie, captopril)	Cm
Dermatomyositis	Corticosteroids	D
	Azathioprine	D
	Methotrexate	D
	Cyclophosphamide	D
Systemic vasculitides		
Wegener's granulomatosis	Corticosteroids	D
Polyarteritis nodosa	Cyclophosphamide	D
Behcet's syndrome	Azathioprine	D
Wegener's granulomatosis	Sulphonamide antibiotics	B

[a] Codes for risk–benefit ratio taken from Briggs GG, Freeman RK, Yaffe SJ, eds. *Drugs in Pregnancy and Lactation: A Reference Guide to Fetal and Neonatal Risk.* New York, NY: Williams & Wilkins; 1986.
[b] Codes for risk–benefit ratio taken from *Physician's Desk Reference* and definitions given in Chapter 7.

Fetal Wastage

Although fertility is not reduced in patients with SLE, fetal wastage is definitely increased.[2-7] A variety of factor are known to contribute to fetal wastage, including active disease at the time of conception and the presence of certain maternal antibodies.

Active disease at the time of conception is associated with increased fetal wastage[2,8,9], and it is our policy to advise patients to wait at least 6 months after their disease has been well controlled before attempting to become pregnant. We feel that disease control before conception is so important that we carefully review the risks of continuing a pregnancy and of continuing any medications with the lupus patient who becomes pregnant unexpectedly.

Another factor known to contribute to fetal wastage in patients with SLE is the presence of certain maternal antibodies. It has been suggested that lymphocytotoxic antibodies that react with trophoblast may contribute to fetal wastage[10], and more recently, Soloninka and Laskin et al have reported finding a noncytotoxic lymphocyte antibody in women with unexplained fetal wastage who do not fulfill criteria for SLE.[11]

Maternal antibodies are considered to be associated

TABLE 51–2. DRUG THERAPIES FOR CONNECTIVE TISSUE SYNDROMES

Syndrome	Therapies Used During Pregnancy
Phospholipid antibody syndrome	Corticosteroids
	Aspirin
	Subcutaneous heparin
	Dipyridamole
	Intravenous gammaglobulin
Neonatal lupus syndrome	Corticosteroids (including dexamethasone)
	Plasmapheresis

TABLE 51–3. THE 1982 AMERICAN RHEUMATISM ASSOCIATION REVISED CRITERIA FOR THE CLASSIFICATION OF SYSTEMIC LUPUS ERYTHEMATOSUS

1. Malar rash	Fixed erythema, nasolabial sparing
2. Discoid rash	Raised patches, scaling
3. Photosensitivity	Skin rash in sunlight
4. Oral ulcers	Usually painless
5. Arthritis	Nonerosive
6. Serositis	Pleurisy, pericarditis
7. Renal disorder	Proteinuria or cellular casts
8. Neurologic disorder	Seizures or psychosis
9. Hematologic disorder	Hemolytic anemia, leukopenia, lymphopenia, or thrombocytopenia
10. Immunologic disorder	Positive lupus erythematosus cell prep, anti-DNA, anti-Sm, or false-positive STS
11. Antinuclear antibody	Abnormal ANA titer

Classified as SLE if at least four of the 11 criteria are present.

with the development of two syndromes: the neonatal lupus syndrome and the phospholipid antibody syndrome. These syndromes are discussed in more detail at the end of the section on SLE; however, there is now considerable evidence that the presence of antibodies to negatively charged phospholipids predisposes both SLE mothers and normal women to an increased risk of fetal wastage (see Phospholipid Antibody Syndrome). The presence of maternal antibody to ribonuclear protein Ro (known to be associated with the predisposition to the development of neonatal lupus syndrome), does not appear to promote fetal wastage, although some children with this syndrome may die prematurely because of the cardiac complications associated with this syndrome (see Neonatal Lupus Syndrome).

Placental Pathology

Pathologic studies of placentae from SLE patients are few and far between. Abramowsky, reporting the histologic and immunofluorescent findings in 10 SLE placentae, found a necrotizing decidual vasculopathy in five of the 10 placentae studied.[12]

Hanly et al, studying 11 SLE patients, found that placentae from SLE patients were smaller and weighed less than placentae from normal controls and diabetic mothers. Reduced placental weight correlated with active SLE, the lupus anticoagulant, thrombocytopenia, and hypocomplementemia but did not necessarily correlate with reduced birth weight.[13] Placental infarction, as expected in patients with the phospholipid antibody syndrome, clearly compromises fetal growth and may contribute to fetal wastage, but prematurity and small-for-gestational-age babies are more common in lupus mothers in general.

Effect of Pregnancy on SLE

Pregnancy can exacerbate SLE. A review of the literature addressing the disease activity and maternal mortality in pregnant SLE patients concluded that there were exacerbations of disease activity in 50% of pregnancies, occurring during pregnancy or in the postpartum period.[14] The percentage of exacerbations remained constant during the three decades studied; however, the percentage of maternal deaths declined from 17% (1950–1959) to 1% (1970–1980), an encouraging trend that may be caused by better medical management of patients with active disease or a greater recognition of milder forms of the disease. After reviewing several reported series, Ramsey-Goldman concluded that 10–30% of pregnant SLE patients (in whom the disease was inactive at the time of conception) can anticipate an exacerbation of disease activity during pregnancy or in the postpartum period. This rate reportedly increased twofold to threefold in patients in whom the disease was active at the time of conception.[15]

One of the problems in evaluating the reports of flares of SLE activity during pregnancy has been the inability to ascertain the frequency of disease flares in the nonpregnant patient. This is because the triggers of disease activity are unknown and each patient's disease is different. In a case-controlled perspective study comparing pregnant SLE patients with age, race, organ system, and disease severity matched nonpregnant controls, Lockshin et al concluded that there was no greater frequency of flares in pregnant compared to nonpregnant patients.[16] Mintz et al also drew similar conclusions from their study where they compared 75 pregnant SLE patients with a group of SLE patients on contraceptives.[7]

We rarely advise the SLE patient against pregnancy except in those rare instances in which major organ damage would expose the mother to considerable risk. We feel that careful monitoring of the patient and fetus minimizes the risk to the mother and child.

Lupus nephritis is associated with significant mortality.[17] The patient with lupus nephropathy who wants to become pregnant therefore raises more questions. Not only must the eventual fetal outcome be considered, but the risk disease exacerbation with subsequent (possibly permanent) organ damage (which may contribute to maternal survival) must also be taken into account.

After studying 25 pregnancies in 23 women with moderate renal insufficiency (only one of whom had lupus nephritis), Hou et al concluded that pregnancy may contribute to a deterioration in renal function greater than that expected from the natural history of the disease in a nonpregnant individual. A significant deterioration in renal function was seen in seven of these 23 women with a more modest deterioration seen in an additional seven. Delivery did not reverse the decline in renal function, suggesting that precluding the onset of life-threatening hypertension, a significant deterioration in renal function is not an indication for termination of pregnancy.[18]

Earlier reports addressing the significance of lupus nephropathy in pregnancy suggested that lupus nephritis was a contraindication to pregnancy, being associated with frequent maternal deaths and postpartum exacerbations of nephritis.[3,4,5,19] Recent reports, however, are more encouraging.[20-22] Burkett summarized the results of six recent studies that reported 242 pregnancies in 156 women and concluded that there was a 7.1% chance of a permanent deterioration in renal function in pregnant women with lupus nephropathy and that in 57.2%, there was no change in renal function. Live births occurred in 69.2% of these pregnancies, but if the disease was well controlled throughout pregnancy, fetal survival was closer to 85%. Although a successful outcome of pregnancy was more likely in the women with more normal renal function, (ie, a serum creatinine of 1.5 mg/mL or less), a creatinine clearance of 50 cc/min or more and proteinuria of less than 3 g per 24 hours, the most important factor determining outcome was quiescent disease for at least 6 months before conception.[23] Tozman et al, studying 24 pregnancies in 18 lupus patients, concluded that even in patients with previous major organ involvement, if the disease was inactive at the time of conception, exacerbations of disease activity with increasing organ damage were not seen.[9] Most recently, Mintz et al studied 102 pregnancies in 75 women and reported an exacerbation of preexisting renal disease in six of 58 pregnancies and a new onset of renal disease in three of 44 pregnancies. This new onset of renal disease was not statistically different from the onset of renal disease in five of the same patients followed in the postpartum period or when compared to a group of lupus patients receiving contraceptives.[7]

The new onset of hypertension, proteinuria, and renal insufficiency in a pregnant lupus patient can herald the onset of active lupus nephritis or the development of *preeclampsia.* Differentiating between the onset of active SLE and *toxemia of pregnancy* can be difficult. Buyon et al recently studied four groups of patients: (1) normal nonpregnant women, (2) normal women in their third trimester of pregnancy with no complications, (3) normal women in their third trimester of pregnancy fulfilling criteria for preeclampsia, and (4) lupus mothers in their third trimester of pregnancy. They found that the levels of C_3 and C_4 were higher in the pregnant normal patients than in nonpregnant normal volunteers. The levels of C_4 were lower in the preeclamptic pregnancies compared to normal pregnancies, and SLE mothers had significantly lower levels of C_3 and C_4 compared to normal pregnant mothers. A decrease in the levels of C_3 and C_4 from prepregnancy levels in lupus patients heralded the onset of a flare of disease. One patient with SLE who developed preeclampsia had no change in complement levels. These findings suggest that the measurement of complement levels may be useful for differentiating between the onset of preeclampsia and a flare of disease in patients with SLE.[24] Other investigators question the value of complement evaluations.

The incidence of preeclampsia is increased in patients with SLE.[25] Patients with antiphospholipid antibodies, regardless of whether they fulfill the criteria for SLE, are also at risk for the development of toxemia and preeclampsia.[26]

Treatment

Numerous studies have shown that disease activity, either at the time of conception or throughout pregnancy, is detrimental to pregnancy and results in fetal distress or wastage or maternal morbidity. It is therefore absolutely essential to monitor the patient carefully throughout pregnancy for any signs of impending disease activity.

Complement levels rise during normal pregnancy, and even though pregnant SLE patients have lower complement levels than mothers without SLE, the serial measurement of complement levels throughout pregnancy is a vital part of the management of pregnant SLE patients.

We routinely see all pregnant lupus patients monthly or more frequently if there is evidence of possible disease activation. Complement levels, ANA, antibody to DNA (FARR test), and a CBC, platelet count, and urinalysis are ordered routinely. While we do not expect the titer of ANA to change, a change in pattern of the ANA (ie, to a peripheral pattern) may be the marker of potential problems. Any fall in complement levels should be treated promptly, but we do not routinely place patients on corticosteroids just because they are pregnant.

Routine assessments of fetal growth and development with regular ultrasound and fetal nonstress tests are indicated, especially in mothers who have experienced previous problems in completing pregnancy. Doppler measurements of umbilical blood flow may be useful in pregnancies in which placental insufficiency may be anticipated[27], although some feel that these measurements are no more useful than ultrasound.

Much of this chapter has been devoted to emphasizing the importance of controlling disease activity before and during pregnancy. This, of course, raises the question of which medications are comparatively safe to use during pregnancy and which must be avoided. Table 51–1 lists the drugs routinely used for the treatment of systemic features of SLE and therapies recommended for the cutaneous manifestations of this disease.

Corticosteroids, such as prednisone, which do not readily cross the placenta are comparatively safe to use during pregnancy, even at high dosages (60 mg daily). Although previous animal studies have suggested that there may be an increased incidence of cleft palate, premature placental aging, and severe growth retardation in fetuses exposed to corticosteroids, this has not been substantiated in humans, and our policy for managing disease activity during SLE pregnancies is to manage the patient with prednisone. We maintain this therapy at the same dosage for approximately 2 months postpartum. Even though recent studies have suggested that flares of disease may be less frequent during the postpartum period[16] than previously reported, we follow this protocol because the puerperium is an extremely stressful time for the new mother and stress can lead to disease exacerbation.

Antimalarial drugs containing the 4-aminoquinoline radicals are useful in the management of skin disease and arthritis in patients with SLE. There is no evidence that these drugs are valuable in the management of major organ involvement in SLE; however, previous reports have shown that the disease may flare in patients with SLE when antimalarial therapy is discontinued.[28] Chloroquine crosses the placenta and has been shown to accumulate in fetal tissues.[29] Many reports in the rheumatologic literature suggest that antimalarial drugs containing the 4-aminoquinoline radical cannot be used safely throughout pregnancy. Most of these reports quote a paper by Hart and Naunton, which described a mother of six with discoid lupus erythematosus who had taken chloroquine phosphate at some time throughout three of her six pregnancies with resulting congenital abnormalities seen only in the three children that were exposed to the drug.[30] Other authors addressing the question of malarial prophylaxis during pregnancy, however, state categorically that chloroquine is safe to use in pregnant patients requiring malarial prophylaxis[31], but the antimalarial dosage required for malarial prophylaxis is 500 mg chloroquine phosphate or 300 mg chloroquine weekly, a considerably smaller dose than recommended for use in patients with SLE.

We recently studied eight patients with SLE who had taken antimalarial drugs, either chloroquine phosphate (250–500 mg daily) or hydroxychloroquine sulfate (plaquenil, 200–400 mg daily) throughout the entire length of one pregnancy. These eight women had 14 pregnancies while taking antimalarial therapy. Although fetal wastage was high in these mothers, the resulting six full-term babies, having been exposed to antimalarial drugs throughout gestation, were all normal without any obvious congenital abnormalities. Long-term follow-up of one of these children has revealed no evidence of eye or ear damage when examined at the age of 13.[32]

Although we would prefer women not to take these antimalarial drugs throughout pregnancy (because of the concerns mentioned previously), we feel that these data indicate that it is safer for patients who require antimalarial therapy to control their disease to continue the therapy throughout pregnancy. The risk for producing a flare of disease activity is greater than that of producing an abnormal child if antimalarial therapy is continued throughout pregnancy. Our report confirms other reports that suggest that antimalarial drugs given at the dosage used in the management of rheumatic diseases may be given to pregnant mothers comparatively safely.[33] However, we would not knowingly start a pregnant patient on antimalarial therapy; instead, we use prednisone for the management of active disease during gestation. Any patient anticipating pregnancy is advised to ensure that the disease is well controlled on prednisone before conception, which may mean a wait of many months if antimalarial drugs have to be discontinued and the dosage of prednisone readjusted to control the disease.

The use of *azathioprine* during pregnancy is reasonably well documented because of its use in renal transplant patients. These patients also received corticosteroid therapy.

Although azathioprine and its metabolites cross the placenta, there are many reports of anatomically normal children born after exposure to azathioprine and its metabolites during pregnancy.[34,35] Immunosuppression appears to be more of a problem than teratogenicity for these infants, with reports of transient lymphopenia, low immunoglobulin levels, and persistent cytomegalovirus.[34-36] We would not knowingly initiate azathioprine in SLE patients known to be contemplating pregnancy, but patients requiring azathioprine to control their disease should not have this drug discontinued because of pregnancy. Azathioprine does not appear to affect fertility.

Cyclophosphamide is an alkalating agent that inhibits DNA synthesis. It is clearly teratogenic in animal studies, and no control studies have been performed in humans. There are several case reports documenting the use of cyclophosphamide in pregnancy with fetal abnormalities developing in some instances.[37,38] We feel that cyclophosphamide should be avoided early in pregnancy, and if at all possible, during late pregnancy, although the possible fetal effects are obviously less. Some reports have shown that women exposed to cyclophosphamide therapy before conception may successfully complete pregnancy; however, cyclophosphamide may induce ovarian failure, and the use of this drug in women who may subsequently wish to become pregnant must be discussed at length. Factors that appear to potentiate the onset of ovarian failure include more than 25 years of age at the time of administration, prolonged usage, and concurrent therapy, such as radiotherapy.[39]

Breast-feeding

We encourage our lupus mothers to breast-feed if possible because we feel the benefits to the mother and baby far outweigh possible detrimental effects. If the infant is underweight or premature and the mother is receiving large doses of corticosteroids, theoretically the amount of corticosteroid per kilogram of body weight to which the infant may be exposed in the breast milk may be worrisome; however, the amount of prednisolone secreted in breast milk is so small that we feel that the concern is mostly theoretical.[40] We usually manage these patients with prednisone once a day, knowing that almost all orally administered prednisone is removed from the circulation within 8 hours. By scheduling the time the prednisone is taken to follow a feeding, an infant requiring four hourly feedings will be exposed at only one feeding (4 hours after the prednisone is taken). If the mother is concerned about this, we suggest that this exposed feeding be given as formula.

Family Planning

Although the differences between drug-induced and idiopathic SLE have been emphasized, there are reports of drugs inducing flares of disease, even in patients with idiopathic disease.[41,42]

Jungers et al studied the effects of various oral contraceptives on the activity of SLE; they compared contraceptives containing ethinyl–estradiol at different dosages (30 mg or 50 mg with preparations containing progesterone alone). In 26 lupus nephropathy patients followed for up to 30 months after starting hormonal therapy, a flare of disease (with exacerbation of renal disease in four patients) was documented in 43% of the patients receiving estrogen-containing oral contraceptives, compared to no flares of disease in the patients receiving progesterone only.[42]

We routinely advise our patients not to take estrogen-containing oral contraceptives and similarly advise our postmenopausal patients, despite their steroid requirements and potential for osteoporosis.

Because fertility is not reduced in lupus patients and the timing of conception with relation to disease activity is vital, contraception is a major part of the management of lupus patients. We also are hesitant about the use of intrauterine devices in patients taking corticosteroids and immunosuppressive therapy who are at increased risk for infection. It seems that condoms or diaphragms are the safest methods for contraception in lupus patients, but they are the least effective. The potential for unwanted pregnancy must be considered when advising these patients about birth control.

The Phospholipid Antibody Syndrome

The most conclusive evidence demonstrating an association between the presence of certain maternal antibodies in fetal wastage is found in the literature addressing the significance of phospholipid antibodies. Phospholipid antibodies are routinely detected by three laboratory tests: the lupus anticoagulant, a biologically false-positive test for syphilis (VDRL), and cardiolipin antibodies. These antibodies are directed against negatively charged phospholipids and have been associated with a predisposition to arterial and venous thrombosis, thrombocytopenia, central nervous system disease, and fetal wastage. We routinely test for the presence of these antibodies in all pregnant lupus patients because it has suggested that presence of cardiolipin antibodies, especially IgG, is predictive of fetal distress or death in patients with SLE.[43,44] The fetal wastage associated with these antibodies has been attributed to the thrombotic diathesis associated with the presence of these antibodies that results in placental infarction and fetal death. Several reports have shown that a very high fetal wastage rate in women with lupus anticoagulants (some of whom fulfill criteria for SLE) could be lowered by treatment with corticosteroids and low-dose aspirin during pregnancy[26,45], although there are no well-controlled therapeutic trials addressing the management of these patients. Recent work by Lockshin et al suggest that prednisone does not prevent fetal death in women with phospholipid antibodies.[46] Our work concurs with the suggestion that steroidal suppression of antibodies is unnecessary[47], but we feel strongly that some sort of therapeutic intervention is useful. Recent reports have addressed the benefits of intravenous γ-globulin (IVIG)[47] or subcutaneous heparin (see Table 51–2); however, the optimum therapy for these phospholipid antibody patients is not known because randomized controlled studies have not been done (see also Chapter 50).

Neonatal Lupus Syndrome

The primary manifestations of the neonatal lupus syndrome are a transient photosensitive skin rash or the presence of permanent congenital complete heart block. The syndrome is associated with the presence of maternal antibody in the fetal circulation, although the pathogenesis and the relationship of the clinical complaints to the maternal antibody remains unknown.

Antibody to the ribonuclear protein Ro is most commonly associated with neonatal lupus syndrome, even in mothers who do not fulfill criteria for connective tissue disease.[48] However, McCune et al showed that during a 5-year follow-up period eight of 11 asymptomatic mothers of children with the neonatal lupus syndrome developed a connective tissue disease.[49] Other maternal antibodies associated with this syndrome are antibody to the ribonuclear protein La and antibody to RNP.

Depending on the assay used, antibody to Ro ribonuclear protein can be found in 20–80% or more of lupus patients. If antibodies to Ro and La nuclear proteins can be associated with the development of the neonatal lupus syndrome in mothers without lupus, what is the significance of Ro or La antibody in the pregnant lupus mother? Ramsey-Goldman reports that the risk for a lupus mother producing a child with congenital complete heart block was one in 60, but fell to one in 20 if the mother was anti-Ro positive.[50] The risk of producing a child with the neonatal lupus syndrome also was higher if the mother had had a previously affected child, although it is obvious that there are unidentified fetal determinants for the expression of the neonatal lupus syndrome. There have been case reports of one affected twin born to anti-Ro positive mothers.[51,52] Other determinants include the presence of HLA-DR3, which in white anti-Ro positive mothers, increases the risk of producing an infant with the neonatal lupus syndrome by 32 times.[53] Fetal HLA associations have not been shown.

Although there has been some suggestion that Ro antibody in the mother may predispose her to fetal wastage, there are several reports that suggest that this is not true.[50,54] However, the congenital complete heart block seen in the neonatal lupus syndrome is permanent, and some children require pacemakers. This heart block and some of the other cardiac abnormalities described as part of the neonatal lupus syndrome may contribute to neonatal deaths.[49,55] Attempts have been made to prevent cardiac damage by treating mothers with corticosteroids and plasmapheresis with the hope of lowering the levels of antibody[56,57] (see Table 51–2). This treatment presumes that these antibodies play a direct pathogenetic role, which has not been proven. Even in the cases in which healthy children have been delivered, it is impossible to conclude that the interventions played any part in the outcome. There is no way to predict a child at risk for developing neonatal lupus syndrome, even in mothers who have had children previously affected.

Discoid Lupus

Patients with discoid lupus may require management with topical steroid creams, antimalarial therapy, and even systemic corticosteroids. The use of antimalarial drugs and oral corticosteroids is discussed in the management of SLE. The steroid absorption of topical steroid creams is small, but steroids such as dexamethasone cross the placenta more readily than prednisone.

SYSTEMIC SCLEROSIS

Systemic sclerosis (scleroderma) is an uncommon disease with a female predominance of 8-10:1 (F:M) during the child-bearing years. The associated vasculopathy and the systemic uncontrolled proliferation of connective tissue with collagen deposition characteristic of this disease allows for unique problems in a pregnant patient with systemic sclerosis.

There are few reports of large series of pregnant patients with systemic sclerosis, which makes it difficult to evaluate the influence of systemic sclerosis on the outcome of pregnancy. Giordano et al compared 86 patients with systemic sclerosis to 86 healthy controls and found a significantly increased abortion rate in the patients compared to controls. The rate of fetal wastage was no different in the patients with limited disease compared to those with diffuse disease.[58] Silman and Black report similar findings with increased fetal wastage, but they also find an increased rate of fertility problems in systemic sclerosis patients, compared to healthy patients, that was present even before the onset of the disease.[59] Steen et al, however, were unable to show an increased rate of fetal wastage when comparing mothers with systemic sclerosis to two control groups of mothers. The groups were neighbors with the same social economic background and patients with rheumatoid arthritis. These authors found that there were significantly more small full-term babies born to mothers with systemic sclerosis; These small babies were born with equal frequency, before and after the onset of the clinical manifestations of systemic sclerosis.[60]

The paucity of reports in the literature makes it hard to draw any firm conclusions about the effect of pregnancy on systemic sclerosis. Case control studies, however, suggest better maternal outcomes than individual case reports, which frequently describe progression of maternal disease and even maternal death. Steen et al conclude that it is possible for women with systemic sclerosis to have uneventful, healthy, successful pregnancies, although they advise patients at risk for renal crisis to avoid pregnancy.[60]

Renal disease is the major cause of maternal death in patients with systemic sclerosis and may present during pregnancy with the onset of hypertension, which can be particularly difficult to treat. Black concludes from the data available that the presence of renal disease before conception is an indication for avoiding pregnancy and that the onset of renal disease during pregnancy should be an indication for termination of pregnancy.[61]

Involvement of other major organs also may dictate that pregnancy be avoided. Pulmonary hypertension and its consequent embarrassment of right heart function, as seen particularly in the patients with CREST syndrome (a limited form of scleroderma in which the patient presents with calcinosis, Raynaud's phenomenon, esophageal dysmotility, sclerodactyly, and telangectasia), gives rise to horrendous cardiovascular complications in pregnant patients. Similarly, bacterial overgrowth, malabsorption, and bowel stasis make it difficult to provide an adequate nutritional state conducive to pregnancy.

Treatment

Because there is no effective therapy for the management of systemic sclerosis, drug therapy during pregnancy is not a major problem. D-penicillamine, which is sometimes used to manage systemic sclerosis (especially the rapidly progressive cutaneous manifestations of systemic sclerosis), should be avoided during pregnancy.[62,63] Nifedipine may be given to manage Raynaud's phenomenon and can be administered during pregnancy; however, it is preferable to avoid all medications whenever possible.

Angiotensin-converting enzyme inhibitors have reduced the mortality of systemic sclerosis by reducing the complications of scleroderma renal crisis. The onset of severe hypertension during pregnancy must be treated, but it cannot be concluded that these drugs are safe for use during pregnancy. Fetal wastage has been described with both captopril and enalapril, although only scant reports address the use of these drugs in human pregnancy.[64-66]

Patients with systemic sclerosis must be monitored carefully throughout pregnancy. Frequent checks of renal function, including urinalysis, serum BUNs, and creatinines must be made. Cardiovascular status must be monitored frequently with any onset of hypertension promptly treated and signs of cardiac embarrassment monitored closely. Patients with gastrointestinal involvement are particularly at risk for a poor nutritional state.

DERMATOMYOSITIS

The majority of patients with dermatomyositis develop this disease after their child-bearing years. Mintz reviewed pregnancies in patients with previous childhood dermatomyositis and concluded that pregnancy may cause a previously quiescent disease to flare, although the outcome of pregnancy was good in seven of 10 pregnancies resulting in a live birth at term.[67] Addressing adult disease, Mintz divides patients with adult dermatomyositis into two groups: those with a preexisting diagnosis of dermatomyositis who become pregnant and those with the onset of disease during pregnancy. The numbers of patients reported in each group is small but those with new onset of the disease during pregnancy had a fetal wastage rate of 62.5% and showed the closest association between dermatomyositis and pregnancy. These patients experienced a dramatic improvement of the disease postpartum.[67]

Patients with active dermatomyositis should be managed with corticosteroids throughout pregnancy. Only in extremely resistant diseases should other therapies, such as azathioprine, be considered.

THE VASCULITIDES

The systemic vasculitides comprise a group of diseases that result in inflammation in blood vessels of different sizes and with different underlying pathologies. These diseases frequently are associated with a grave prognosis although the 5-year survival in Wegner's granulomatosis has dramatically improved with daily cyclophosphamide therapy.[68]

The literature addressing *Wegner's granulomatosis* and pregnancy is so scant that it is impossible to make generalized recommendations, especially because daily cyclophosphamide is indicated in the management of nonpregnant patients, but pregnancy makes the use of cyclophosphamide less desirable. Recent reports of the benefit of sulfonamides in treating this disease[69] may make the discussions of management of a pregnant patient with Wegners' granulomatosis easier in the future.

Patients in which *polyarteritis nodosa* has complicated pregnancy have been described and, in 11 reported cases, maternal deaths resulted in seven. Three of the four surviving patients had been diagnosed before conception, and in these cases, the disease was under good control at the time of conception. In contrast to the dreadful maternal outcome, fetal survival was surprisingly good with the successful delivery of eight infants.[70-72]

In one report, *cutaneous vasculitis* in both mother and infant was described.[73]

Behcet's syndrome is a systemic disease with the predominant features of oral and genital ulceration and inflammation in the eye. Other features include neurologic and gastrointestinal complaints as well as skin disease and thrombotic episodes. It has been suggested that there may be a hormonal influence over the expression of this disease and that oral contraceptives may be useful treatment.[74] The influence of pregnancy on clinical Behcet's syndrome, however, appears variable. Hamza et al reported 21 pregnancies in eight Behcet's patients and found that disease expression varied from patient to patient and from pregnancy to pregnancy. Three of the eight patients had a consistent response during pregnancy, two remitted and one exacerbated their disease. Four of the remaining patients had a variable response during pregnancy, and one patient had only one pregnancy, during which her disease went into remission.[75] Behcet's syndrome does not appear to affect pregnancy because all 21 pregnancies resulted in a live birth.[75]

Some patients with autoimmune disease defy classification because they manifest the features of more than one connective tissue disease. We prefer to label these patients as examples of an overlap syndrome. The management of these patients is dictated by their clinical complaints, and there are no good studies of the outcome of pregnancy because the definition of their disease is difficult, and the clinical expression of the disease is diverse.

Corticosteroids, such as prednisone, which do not readily cross the placenta, can be safely given during pregnancy, but the use of other drugs, such as cyclophosphamide or azathioprine, to manage aggressive vasculitis must be reviewed on an individual basis and used only when absolutely necessary. It appears from the limited reports available that pregnancy and polyarteritis nodosa are a particularly lethal combination which may be grounds for recommending a termination of pregnancy, whereas maternal and fetal outcome in a disease such as Behcet's syndrome appear to be much better.

REFERENCES

1. Tan EM, Cohen AS, Fries JF, et al. The 1982 revised criteria for the classification of systemic lupus erythematosus. *Arth Rheum.* 1982;25:127.
2. Fraga A, Mintz G, Orozco J, et al. Sterility and fertility rates, fetal wastage and maternal morbidity in systemic lupus erythematosus. *J Rheumatol.* 1974;1:293.
3. Donaldson LB, DeAlvarez RR. Further observations on lupus erythematosus associated with pregnancy. *Am J Obstet Gynecol.* 1962;83:1461.
4. Estes D, Larson DL. Systemic lupus erythematosus and pregnancy. *Clin Obstet Gynecol.* 1965;8:307.
5. Garsenstein M, Pollak VE, Kark RM. Systemic lupus erythematosus and pregnancy. *N Engl J Med.* 1962;267:165.
6. Zurier RB, Argyros TG, Urman JD, et al. SLE management during pregnancy. *Obstet Gyneceol.* 1977;51:178.
7. Mintz G, Niz J, Gutierrez G, et al. Prospective study of pregnancy in systemic lupus erythematosus. Results of a multidisciplinary approach. *J Rheum.* 1986;13:732.
8. Gimovsky ML, Montoro M, Paul RH. Pregnancy outcome in women with systemic lupus erythematosus. *Obstet Gynecol.* 1984;63:686.
9. Tozman ECS, Urowitz MB, Gladman DD. Systemic lupus erythematosus and pregnancy. *J Rheumatol.* 1980;7:624.
10. Bresnihan B, Grigor RR, Oliver M, et al. Immunological mechanisms for spontaneous abortion in systemic lupus erythematosus. *Lancet.* 1977;2:1205.
11. Soloninka CA, Laskin ZA, Chin W, et al. A noncytotoxic antilymphocyte antibody is highly specific in identifying women with unexplained recurrent fetal loss and subclinical autoimmunity. *Arth Rheum.* 1989;32:S123.
12. Abramowsky CR, Vegas ME, Swinehart G, et al. Decidual vasculopathy of the placenta in lupus erythematosus. *N Engl J Med.* 1980;303:668.
13. Hanly JG, Gladman DD, Rose TH, et al. Lupus pregnancy: a prospective study of placental changes. *Arth Rheum.* 1988;31:358.
14. Cecere FA, Persellin RH. The interaction of pregnancy and the rheumatic diseases. *Clin Rheum Dis.* 1981;7:747.
15. Ramsey-Goldman R. Pregnancy in systemic lupus erythematosus. *Rheum Dis Clinics North Am.* 1988;14:169.
16. Lockshin MD, Reinitz E, Druzin ML. Lupus pregnancy: case controlled prospective study demonstrating absence of lupus exacerbation during pregnancy. *Am J Med.* 1984;77:893.
17. Wallacy DJ, Podell TE, Weiner JM, et al. Systemic lupus erythematosus. Survival patterns. *JAMA.* 1981;245:934.
18. Hou SH, Grossman SD, Madias N. Pregnancy with renal disease and moderate renal insufficiency. *Am J Med.* 1985;78:185.
19. Bear R. Pregnancy and lupus nephritis. A detailed report of six cases with a review of the literature. *Obstet Gynecol.* 1976;47:715.
20. Hayslett JP, Lynn RI. Effect of pregnancy in patients with lupus nephropathy. *Kidney Int.* 1980;18:207.
21. Houser MT, Fish AJ, Tagatz GE, et al. Pregnancy and systemic lupus erythematosus. *Am J Obstet Gynecol.* 1980;138:409.
22. Jungers P, Dougados M, Pelissier C, et al. Lupus nephropathy and pregnancy. *Arch Intern Med.* 1982;142:771.
23. Burkett G. Lupus nephropathy in pregnancy. *Clin Obstet Gynecol.* 1985;28:310.

24. Buyon JP, Cronstein BN, Morris M, et al. Serum complement values (C_3 and C_4) to differentiate between systemic lupus activity and pre-eclampsia. *Am J Med.* 1986;81:194.
25. Zurier RB. Systemic lupus erythematosus and pregnancy. In: Lahita RG, ed. *Systemic Lupus Erythematosus.* New York, NY: John Wiley & Sons; 1987:545.
26. Branch WB, Scott JR, Kochenour NK, et al. Obstetric complications associated with the lupus anticoagulant. *New Engl J Med.* 1985;313:1321.
27. Rightmire DA. Clinical doppler ultrasonography: uterine and umbilical blood flow. *Clin Obstet and Gynecol* 1988;31:27.
28. Rudnicki RD, Gresham GE, Rothfield NF. The efficacy of antimalarials in systemic lupus erythematosus. *J Rheumatol.* 1975;2:323.
29. Ullberg S, Lindquist NJ, Sjostrand SE. Accumulation of chorioretinotoxic drugs in the fetal eye. *Nature.* 1970;227:1257.
30. Hart CN, Naunton RF. The ototoxicity of chloroquine phosphate. *Arch Otolaryngol Head Neck Surg.* 1964;80:407.
31. Bruce-Chwatt LJ. Malaria and pregnancy. *Br Med J.* 1983;286:1457.
32. Parke AL. Antimalarial drugs, systemic lupus erythematosus and pregnancy. *J Rheumatol.* 1988;15:607.
33. MacKenzie AH. Antimalarial drugs for rheumatoid arthritis. *Am J Med.* 1983;75:48.
34. Penn I, Makowski EL, Harris P. Parenthood following renal transplantation. *Kidney Int.* 1980;18:221.
35. Rudolph JE, Schweizer RT, Bartus SA. Pregnancy in renal transplant patients. *Transplantation.* 1979;27:26.
36. Hayes K, Symington G, Mackay IR. Maternal immunosuppression and cytomegalovirus infection of the fetus. *Aust NZJ Med.* 1979;9:430.
37. Greenberg LH, Tanaka KR. Congenital anomalies probably induced by cyclophosphamide. *JAMA.* 1964;188:423.
38. Toledo TM, Harper RC, Moser RH. Fetal effects during cyclophosphamide and irradiation therapy. *Ann Intern Med.* 1971;74:87.
39. Sanders JE, Buckner CD, Leonard JM, et al. Late effects on gonadal function of cyclophosphamide, total-body irradiation, and marrow transplantation. *Transplantation.* 1983;36:252.
40. Briggs GG, Bodendorfer TN, Freeman RK, et al. *Drugs in Pregnancy and Lactation.* Baltimore, MD: Williams and Wilkins; 1983:65.
41. Carr-Locke DL. Sulfasalazine-induced lupus syndrome in a patient with Crohn's disease. *Am J Gastroenterol.* 1982;77:614.
42. Jungers P, Dougados M, Pelissier C, et al. Influence of oral contraceptive therapy on the activity of systemic lupus erythematosus. *Arthritis Rhem.* 1982;25:618.
43. Lockshin MD, Druzin ML, Goci S, et al. Antibodies to cardiolipin as a predictor of fetal death in pregnant patients with systemic lupus erythematosus. *N Engl J Med.* 1985;313:152.
44. Derue GJ, Englert HJ, Harris EN, et al. Fetal loss in systemic lupus erythematosus: association with anticardiolipin antibodies. *J Obstet Gynecol.* 1985;5:207.
45. Lubbe WF, Palmer SJ, Butler WS, et al. Fetal survival after prednisone suppression of maternal lupus-anticoagulant. *Lancet.* 1983;1:1361.
46. Lockshin MD, Druzin ML, Qamar T. Prednisone does not prevent recurrent fetal death in woman with antiphospholipid antibody. *Am J Obstet Gynecol.* 1988;160:439.
47. Parke AL, Maier D, Wilson D, et al. Intravenous gamma globulin, antiphospholipid antibodies and pregnancy. *Ann Int Med.* 1989;110:495.
48. Scott JS, Maddison PJ, Taylor PV, et al. Connective tissue disease, antibodies to ribonucleoprotein, and congenital heart block. *N Engl J Med.* 1983;309:209.
49. McCune AB, Weston WL, Lee LA. Maternal and fetal outcome in neonatal lupus erythematosus. *Ann Int Med.* 1987;106:518.
50. Ramsey-Goldman R, Hom D, Deng JS, et al. Anti-SSA antibodies and fetal outcome in maternal systemic lupus erythematosus. *Arth Rheum.* 1986;29:1263.
51. Callen JP, Fowler JF, Kulick KB, et al. Neonatal lupus erythematosus occurring in one fraternal twin. *Arth Rheum.* 1985;28:271.
52. Harley JB, Kaine JL, Fox OF, et al. Ro (SS-A) antibody and antigen in a patient with congenital complete heart block. *Arth Rheum.* 1985;28:1321.
53. Lee LA, Weston WL. New findings in neonatal lupus syndrome. *Am J Dis Child.* 1984;138:233.
54. Watson RM, Braunstein BL, Watson AJ, et al. Fetal wastage in women with anti-Ro(SSA) antibody. *J Rheumatol.* 1986;13:90.
55. McCue CM, Mantakas ME, Tingelstad JB, et al. Congenital heart block in newborns of mothers with connective tissue disease. *Circulation.* 1977;56:82.
56. Buyon JP, Swersky SH, Fox HE, et al. Intrauterine therapy for presumptive fetal myocarditis with acquired heart block due to systemic lupus erythematosus. *Arth Rheum.* 1987;20:44.
57. Buyon J, Roubey R, Swersky S, et al. Complete congenital heart block: risks of occurrence and therapeutic applications to prevention. *J Rheumatol.* 1988;15:1104.
58. Giordano M, Valentini G, Lupoli S, et al. Pregnancy and systemic sclerosis. *Arth Rheum.* 1985;28:237.
59. Silman A, Black CM. Increased incidence of spontaneous abortion and infertility in women with scleroderma before disease onset: a controlled study. *Ann Rheum Dis.* 1988;47:441.
60. Steen VD, Conte C, Day N, et al. Pregnancy in women with systemic sclerosis. *Arth Rheum.* 1989;32:151.
61. Black CM, Stevens WM. Scleroderma. *Rheum Dis Clin North Am.* 1989;15:193.
62. Solomon L, Abrams G, Dinnesr M, et al. Neonatal abnormalities associated with D-penicillamine treatment during pregnancy. *N Engl J Med.* 1977;296:54.
63. Harpey JP, Jaudon MC, Clavel JP, et al. Cutis laxa and low serum zinc after antenatal exposure to penicillamine. *Lancet.* 1983;2:144.
64. Boutroy MJ, de Ligney BH, Miton A. Captopril administration in pregnancy impairs fetal angiotensin converting enzyme activity and neonatal adaptation. *Lancet.* 1984;935.
65. Duminy PC, Burger P du T. Fetal abnormality associated with the use of captopril during pregnancy. *South African Medical Journal.* 1981;60:805.
66. Lindheimer MD, Katz AI. Current Concepts. Hypertension in pregnancy. *N Engl J Med.* 1985;313:675.
67. Mintz G. Dermatomyositis. *Rheum Dis Clin North Am.* 1989;15:375.
68. Fauci AS, Hayns BF, Katz P, Wolff SM. Wegener's granulomatosis: prospective clinical and therapeutic experience with 85 patients for 21 years. *Ann Int Med.* 1983;98:76.
69. DeRemee RA, McDonald TJ, Weiland LH. Wegener's granulomatosis: observations on treatment with antimicrobial agents. *Mayo Clin Proc.* 1985;60:27.
70. Pitkin RM. Polyarteritis nodosa. *Clin Obstet Gyencol.* 1983;147:103.
71. Reed NR, Smith MR. Periarteritis nodosa in pregnancy. Report of a case and review of the literature. *Obstet Gynecol.* 1980;55:381.
72. Varriale P, Fusco JM, Acampora A, et al. Polyarteritis nodosa in pregnancy. *Obstet Gynecol.* 1965;25:866.
73. Boran RJ, Everett MA. Cutaneous vasculitis in mother and infant. *Arch Dermatol.* 1965;92:568.
74. Hewitt AB. Behcet's disease. Alleviation of buccal and genital ulceration by an oral contraceptive agent. *Br J Vener Dis.* 1971;47:52.
75. Hamza M, Elleuch M, Zribi A. Behcet's disease and pregnancy. *Ann Rheum Dis.* 1988;47:35

Chapter Fifty-Two

Rheumatic Diseases: The Arthropathies

W. Watson Buchanan, Christopher J. Needs, and Peter M. Brooks

52

Pregnancy holds an important place in the history of rheumatic diseases. The ameliorative effects of pregnancy in active rheumatoid arthritis led the late Dr. Philip S. Hench to the discovery of cortisone. This discovery is regarded as the most important scientific event in rheumatology, and as a result, Dr. Hench became rheumatology's first Nobel winner. Relatively little research has been performed on the reasons pregnancy has this effect, and it is only in the past decade that serious attention has been paid to the problem.

RHEUMATOID ARTHRITIS

In 1938, Hench[1] reported that 20 of 22 women had amelioration of their rheumatoid arthritis during 30 of 34 pregnancies. These observations have since been confirmed.[2-11] Overall 75% of patients experience improvement, while the remainder remain the same or worsen.[7,8] Approximately 50% of patients experience improvement during the first trimester, while maximum improvement occurs during the third trimester.[7,11] Regression of subcutaneous nodules has been described.[9] This improvement is even more impressive when one considers that many patients discontinue their second line medications, such as gold therapy, and many are even able to stop taking nonsteroidal anti-inflammatory analgesics.[10,12] However, even patients who improve during pregnancy may show fluctuations of disease activity.[8]

None of the clinical or laboratory features of pregnancy or rheumatoid arthritis predict which patient's arthritis will improve during gestation.[6,9,10,12,13,14] It seems reasonably well established, however, that women who improve can expect the same in subsequent pregnancies.[2,6,9,11,15,16-19] Ostensen and Husby[10,20] have suggested that elevation of immunoglobulin (IgG, IgM) and erthyrocyte sedimentation rate, but not rheumatoid factor, are associated with remission during pregnancy; however, this remains to be confirmed.

Pregnancy is not a cure for rheumatoid arthritis because relapse invariably occurs after delivery.[6-8,13,14] In two thirds of patients, relapse occurs within 2 months, and in all by 6 or 8 months.[2,4,5] Relapse does not appear to correlate with the onset of menses or with breast-feeding.[5] Usually the arthritis returns to the prepartum state[2,20], requiring reinstitution of medication.[9] Although many patients improve during pregnancy, a few deteriorate and develop fresh articular erosions.[9] A small number develop rheumatoid arthritis first during pregnancy[2,4,14,17], especially during the second and third trimesters[10] or in the postpartum period.[2,9] Patients who develop rheumatoid arthritis during pregnancy often show improvement, but then they relapse postpartum.[20] Therapeutic abortion for vasculitis or other serious complications is rarely required in patients with rheumatoid arthritis[3,11,21], but like spontaneous abortion, normal delivery frequently is followed by an exacerbation.[3]

Silman[22] has recently reviewed the evidence that nulliparity may be protective against seropositive rheumatoid arthritis and that increasing the number of pregnancies may increase the risk of developing the disease. Lawrence[23] found that the increased incidence of rheumatoid arthritis in women declined after menopause, so the incidence in both sexes was the same at age 70.[24] This, however, has not been confirmed by other investigators.[25] Moreover, although the US Health Examination Survey showed that rheumatoid arthritis occurred less frequently in nulliparous women and is highest in those with more than four children[26], other studies have failed to confirm this.[23,27-29] Kay and Bach[27] report reduced fertility among patients who subsequently developed rheumatoid arthritis. Clearly, further work is required to determine the role of pregnancy in the initiation of rheumatoid arthritis.[30] Such studies should include the HLA-DR4 status.

Why rheumatoid arthritis improves during pregnancy is still unknown. Hench[16] believed that it might be caused by excess production of adrenal hormones. Certainly, the free cortisol plasma concentration continues to rise steadily during pregnancy, almost doubling in the third trimester. However, there is a poor correlation between plasma concentration and remission of arthritis, and the level rapidly returns to normal after delivery, without necessarily causing an exacerbation of the disease. Moreover, the plasma cortisol elevation is insufficient to have a clinically significant effect on joint inflammation.[17] There has been much speculation on the role of sex hormones in the pathogenesis of autoimmune disease.[30,31] Sex hormones, especially estradiol, have been shown experimentally to have effects on lymphocytes and other cells, such as thymic epithelial and reticuloendothelial cells.[8] Prolactin receptors have been demonstrated on lymphocytes[32], and prolactin has been shown to increase immune responses.[33] These responses can be reduced by both chloroquine and cyclosporine A.[32] Experimental immune polyarthritis also can be modified by sex hormones, especially estrogens. Males with rheumatoid arthritis have a reduction in testosterone and dihydroepiandrosterone[34], and sporadic cases of rheumatoid arthritis have been reported in Klinefelter's syndrome, which may be the result of hyperestrogenism, although this is unconfirmed.

There has been much interest in the effects of oral contraceptive use. In a study of 50,000 women in general practice in the United Kingdom, these drugs were found to have a protective effect against developing rheumatoid arthritis.[35,36] Further studies using case-control designs have given conflicting results; some found benefit[25,36-40], while others did not.[41,42] The methodologic problems in these studies, which might account for their divergent results, have been the subject of considerable controversy.[42-45] Paradoxically, oral contraceptives have been reported to cause mild rheumatic symptoms, erythema nodosum, antinuclear antibodies, and changes in cell mediated immunity.[46] The effect of estrogen treatment (12.5 μg ethinyl estradiol) on the clinical and laboratory manifestations of rheumatiod arthritis has recently been studied in a 24-week prospective, double blind, crossover trial. The results, however, were not impressive.[47] Thus, the studies on oral contraceptives do not shed light on the cause of amelioration of rheumatoid arthritis during pregnancy.

Among the many changes in laboratory parameters during pregnancy[19], acute-phase reactants and the production of trophoblastic-decidual proteins, including pregnancy-associated plasma protein A, pregnancy-associated alpha-2 globulin, placental protein 14, pregnancy-specific beta-1 glycoprotein, and other pregnancy serum proteins[12,15,48], appear the most relevant in predicting and affecting the clinical outcome of rheumatoid arthritis during pregnancy. However, values of the acute-phase proteins, such as C-reactive protein, and the erythrocyte sedimentation rate appear to reflect disease activity of rheumatoid arthritis rather than its outcome. All of the placental proteins mentioned previously have been shown to have immunoregulatory or anti-inflammatory activity.[49] Of these, pregnancy-associated alpha-2 glycoprotein has been the most intensively studied.[12,49] This is a 36,400 d glycoprotein, which is synthesized, not as previously believed in the trophoblast, but by mononuclear leukocytes in the maternal decidua.[49] The normally low serum concentrations gradually rise during pregnancy,[48] although 25% of women do not develop an increase.[48] This protein has been shown to be effective *in vitro* in physiologic concentrations in many inflammatory and immune responses[12,49], including effects on polymorphonuclear leukocytes, inhibition of monocyte Fc receptor, and HLA-DR antigen expression. An inverse relationship between pregnancy-associated alpha-2-glycoprotein and disease activity has been reported by some workers[12], but was not confirmed by others.[48] Sany et al[49] have reported that approximately two thirds of patients with rheumatoid arthritis improved when treated with placenta-eluted gammaglobulins. Whether this effect is the result of masking HLA-DR antigens is not known. Further work is necessary concerning these pregnancy-associated proteins to further define their role in causing amelioration of rheumatoid arthritis during pregnancy.

Many hypotheses have been proposed to explain the amelioration of rheumatoid arthritis during pregnancy based on a mechanism of pregnancy-induced immunosuppression.[15] IgG concentrations have been noted to fall slightly during pregnancy, especially during the third trimester, although antibody levels to various vaccines are normal. Mannik and Nardella[50] and Pekelharing et al[51] have recently observed increased glycosylation of IgG during pregnancy. Conceivably, this could lead to reduction of formation of harmful IgG aggregates and amelioration of rheumatoid arthritis but requires further study.[52] There is evidence that the placenta may act as an immunoabsorbent sponge[15] and may be the reason that immune complexes have been reported to fall during pregnancy[53], leading to improvement of rheumatoid arthritis. Antigens from the placenta can result in maternal antibody production, and these may cross-react with leukocytes and have an immunosuppressive action. The fetus may produce a graft of suppressor T cells in the mother and alpha-fetoprotein, which might result in immunosuppression and cause gestational improvement in the arthritis.

Depression of cell-mediated immunity in pregnancy is supported by diminished reactions to tuberculin skin testing, prolongation of allogeneic skin grafts, and an increased incidence and severity of protozoal, fungal, and viral diseases. Circulating T cells decrease during pregnancy, especially helper–inducer T cells. Circulating T lymphocytes respond poorly to mitogens, such as phytohemagglutinin, and sera from pregnant women suppress lymphocytic proliferation. It has been suggested that the immunomodulating factors in pregnancy serum act by inhibiting interleukin 2.[54,55] A large number of suggestions have been made as to what these immunomodulating factors are, but all remain speculative.[15]

Pregnancy sera in experimental *in vivo* animal models have been shown to inhibit adjuvant arthritis and carrageenan-induced inflammation. Pregnant serum also has been shown to suppress polymorphonuclear leukocyte and macrophage function. However, it is not clear what role, if any, these changes have in improving arthritis.

Effect of Rheumatoid Arthritis on Pregnancy and the Fetus

Hargreaves[56] was the first to suggest that female patients with rheumatoid arthritis may have reduced fertility, and Kay and Bach[27] observed that this included patients who developed their disease after the menopause. However, a recent study by Kaplan[57] failed to confirm this observation. Rheumatoid factor of IgM type does not cross the placental barrier and no increased number of fetal abnormalities have been reported.[8,9,11,20,21] However, an increased incidence of stillbirths was reported in one study although not confirmed in two other studies.[58]

Sjögren's syndrome complicates seropositive erosive rheumatoid arthritis in 10–15% of patients. Sjögren's syndrome is associated with a plethora of serum autoantibodies, excepting autoantibodies to native ds DNA, unless coexisting systemic lupus erythematosus is present. Among the serum autoantibodies are *anti-Ro* (SSA) and *anti-La* (SSB).[59,60] which are present in nearly one half of the patients with rheumatoid arthritis and Sjögren's syndrome and in 5% of patients with rheumatoid arthritis.[61,62] Anti-Ro autoantibodies have been incriminated in the development of isolated congenital complete heart block.[61,63-69] Many of the cases described have been in newborns with the *neonatal lupus syndrome,* whose mothers have systemic lupus erythematosus. However, heart block also has occurred in children whose mothers do not express anti-Ro antibody.[61] Moreover, although the evidence linking anti-Ro antibody with congenital heart block is very strong, not all children born to mothers with the antibody are affected.

Labor and delivery pose no serious problems in patients with rheumatoid arthritis.[15,21] Mechanical interference with delivery may, however, occur with severe hip disease.[21] Vertebral subluxation of the cervical spine presents a potential hazard when endotracheal incubation is required, as may cricoarytenoid involvement.[11] Aspirin therapy may prolong gestation and labor and result in an increase in antepartum and postpartum hemorrhage.[70,71]

ANKYLOSING SPONDYLITIS

Ankylosing spondylitis was considered rare in women until the discovery of the association with HLA-B27. The disease occurs with approximately the same frequency in both sexes, but is less typical and milder in women, especially in terms of spinal ankylosis. Until recently, the effect of pregnancy on ankylosing spondylitis received little attention.[72] Although several authors have suggested that pregnancy may be an initiating factor in ankylosing spondylitis, the evidence is not particularly impressive[10], and the occurrence of the disease during pregnancy simply may be fortuitous.[72] Ostensen and Husby[72] have recently reviewed the results of pregnancy in ankylosing spondylitis in case reports and retrospective studies comprising 184 pregnancies. Only in 59 pregnancies did the activity of ankylosing spondylitis improve (32%), with the remainder showing either no change (40%) or worsening (28%). In one study, anterior uveitis occurred in 8% of patients.[72] Only two prospective studies have been performed involving altogether 27 pregnancies.[9,73] Eleven patients had an exacerbation of symptoms, 10 remained essentially no different from the prepregnancy state, and six improved. However, all six patients had ankylosing spondylitis associated with psoriatic arthritis or ulcerative colitis. Unlike rheumatoid arthritis, there does not appear to be any pattern to activity of disease during successive pregnancies.[9,73] All that can be concluded is that pregnancy does not improve the symptoms of ankylosing spondylitis. Postpartum flare is common within 6 months of delivery and may last for 2–4 months.[72]

Widespread peripheral joint disease, elevation of the erythrocyte sedimentation rate, and increased serum concentrations of IgA in the prepregnant state appeared in one study to predict best gestational amelioration of disease.[19]

Ankylosing spondylitis does not appear to adversely affect pregnancy, labor, or the fetus.[72,73] Total ankylosis of the sacroliac joints does not interfere with normal delivery, although fusion of the hip joint might.[72]

One of the major concerns of patients with ankylosing spondylitis is that they may pass it on to their children. This appears to occur in 10% of cases, especially in those carrying the HLA-B27 phenotype.

PSORIATRIC ARTHRITIS

The effect of pregnancy on the onset of psoriatic arthritis has recently been studied by McHugh and Laurent.[74] In this retrospective study, 18% of 33 patients had onset of arthritis within 3 months postpartum, which is similar to the occurrence of rheumatoid arthritis.[2] All of these patients had polyarthritis of the rheumatoid type. However, the beneficial effect of pregnancy appears to be less marked than with rheumatoid arthritis, although the numbers studied are small.[73,74] Pregnancy does not appear to affect the onset or the course of psoriasis.[74]

GOUT

Gout is relatively rare in premenopausal women who normally have a lower concentration of serum urate than men. During normal pregnancy, the serum urate concentration falls to extremely low concentrations during the first trimester but rises particularly in the third trimester because of the contribution of uric acid produced by the fetus. Hypouricemia can be considered an early diagnostic test for pregnancy. Only a few cases have been reported of pregnancy in patients with gouty arthritis and only one report of a patient having her first acute attack during pregnancy. Acute renal failure has been described, but the patients had preeclampsia, and there was no evidence that this complication arose as a result of gout. Talbott[75] suggests that patients with gouty arthritis might be subfertile. Five spontaneous abortions occurred out of 22 pregnancies, but a larger series would be required to determine whether this is higher than expected.

There is no information on the effect of gouty arthritis on pregnancy, labor, delivery, and the fetus (see also Chapter 32).

DRUG THERAPY OF ARTHROPATHIES

The physiologic changes that normally occur during pregnancy may affect the pharmacokinetic disposition of drugs. Thus, changes in gastric acid and mucus production and delay in gastric emptying time may affect absorption. The concurrent use of alkalis and iron preparations may affect the absorption of nonsteroidal anti-inflammatory analgesics and of D-penicillamine, respectively. An increase in blood volume may lead to an increase in the apparent volume of distribution. Reduction in serum albumin concentration has the potential of increasing the free fraction of a drug, although this appears to be only clinically relevant when hepatic biotransformation and excretory pathways are impaired. The protein binding of salicylates is slightly higher (84.4%) in neonatal plasma than in maternal plasma (77.9%).[76] Hepatic biotransformation is enhanced during pregnancy and may affect drugs that are largely metabolized by the liver. Serum cholinesterase activity is reduced during pregnancy, which may affect aspirin and methylprednisolone metabolism. Drugs that have a high enterohepatic circulation, such as indomethacin, piroxicam, salazopyrine, and sulindac may be affected by the cholestasis that occurs during pregnancy. Drugs that are primarily excreted by the kidney, such as azapropazone, might be expected to have a reduced plasma half-life, but this has not been confirmed.

Analgesics

Simple analgesics frequently are prescribed during pregnancy, and it is important to realize that they cross the placenta. Acetaminophen and codeine have not been found to cause fetal malformations. Several case reports have implicated dextropropoxyphene, but this was not confirmed in a large-scale study. Both codeine and dextropropoxyphene have been reported to cause a neonatal withdrawal syndrome. Acetaminophen may be the preferred drug for analgesia in the arthritic patient during pregnancy, but as Lee[77] has pointed out, the safety of this drug in pregnancy has not been studied directly.

Salicylates

Chronic aspirin ingestion by pregnant women has been implicated as a cause of stillbirths and low-birth weight infants[78], although the latter has not been confirmed[79] and may be related to concomitant use of simple analgesics.[80] Neonatal hemorrhage, especially in premature infants, is increased if aspirin has been taken up to 1 week before delivery.[81,82] Chronic aspirin use during pregnancy may prolong gestation and labor and may lead to increased blood loss at delivery[83] because of inhibition of prostaglandin production. Anemia during pregnancy also is significantly increased in mothers receiving aspirin compared with controls.[84]

Numerous animal studies, using doses of aspirin in excess of the therapeutic dose in humans, have shown a variety of fetal abnormalities, including learning difficulties. Retrospective studies in humans also have suggested that malformations in infants born to mothers taking therapeutic doses of aspirin during pregnancy may be increased, but this has not been confirmed by recent prospective studies.[85]

Nonsteroidal Anti-inflammatory Analgesics

Other nonsteroidal anti-inflammatory analgesics that inhibit prostaglandin synthesis also have the potential to prolong gestation and labor and lead to an increase in postpartum hemorrhage. In addition, in premature infants, respiratory distress has been reported in some[86] but not all reports[87] with the use of indomethacin, and severe hypoxia has been reported with naproxen in these infants.[88,89] Pulmonary hypertension has been reported in infants whose mothers have received indomethacin[90], and hyponatremia and fluid retention have occurred with naproxen.[91] The evidence that fetal malformations occur with the use of indomethacin is tenuous, and there is no evidence that any fetal malformations occur with any of the other nonsteroidal anti-inflammatory analgesics, such as diclofenac, diflunisal, and sulindac. Phenylbutazone is associated with chromosomal abnormalities in adults with rheumatic disease; its use in pregnancy is not recommended.

Chrysotherapy

Injectable gold complexes have been reported occasionally to cause fetal abnormalities in humans[92,93], but this has not been confirmed.[94,95] The number of patients studied, however, is too small to draw any definite conclusions. Because therapeutic concentrations of gold have been found in infants at time of delivery[95], it would seem prudent to avoid chrysotherapy during pregnancy. A small number of patients have been followed on auranofin therapy during pregnancy with no adverse effects to the mother or child.

However, because auranofin is a triethylphosphene compound, it seems prudent to eschew this medication during pregnancy.

D-Penicillamine

Despite the fact that D-penicillamine has been used in pregnancy in patients with Wilson's disease and rheumatoid arthritis without ill effects to the mother or child, there are disturbing reports of children being born with connective tissue defects similar to Ehlers–Danlos syndrome.[96-100] Its slow withdrawal during pregnancy or at least reduction in the dose is recommended.[97]

Antimalarials

Antimalarial drugs cross the placenta and can accumulate in the fetus, although the concentrations are much lower than in maternal tissue. Chromosomal damage has been reported *in vitro* with antimalarial drugs and fetal sensory-neural hearing loss has been reported after exposure to chloroquine phosphate prescribed during the first trimester.[101] Whether this occurs with hydrooxychloroquine, which is the preferred antimalarial drug in the treatment of rheumatoid arthritis, is unknown. Parke[102] concluded that fetal loss in systemic lupus erythematosus was not caused by antimalarial drug therapy but by the disease.

Sulphasalazine

This drug reduces the sperm count in males but does not appear to affect female fertility. Sulphasalazine and its metabolites, including sulphapyridine, cross the placenta, and case reports of children born with congenital malformations whose mothers received the drug during pregnancy have been reported.[103] However, no increased incidence of fetal malformations has been reported with the use of the drug in inflammatory bowel disease.

Corticosteroids

Despite the fact that cleft palate has been reported in a variety of animals from the use of corticosteroids during pregnancy, there is little evidence, despite an occasional case report, of ill effects in humans. It is debatable whether pregnancy outcome is affected by corticosteroid therapy. It seems that the primary disease for which corticosteroid therapy is prescribed is of greater importance than corticosteroid therapy, and in systemic lupus erythematosus, fetal immaturity may be reduced with corticosteroid treatment.[104]

Cytotoxic Drugs

Cytotoxic agents, such as chlorambucil, cyclophosphamide, azathoprine, and methotrexate, are teratogenic in humans, especially if used during the early months of pregnancy. Despite this, many healthy infants have been born to mothers who have received these drugs during pregnancy.[105] Bone marrow depression also may occur in the fetus as a result of these drugs.[105] The long-term effects of these drugs on the offspring of mothers requires study, especially concerning late carcinogenesis.

DRUG THERAPY

A number of factors determine the passage of drugs into breast milk. First, the mammary gland epithelium forms a lipid barrier with protein-lined pores. Second, milk is slightly more acidic (pH = 6.8) than blood (pH = 7.4). Third, acidic and basic drugs readily pass into milk, whereas highly protein-bound and large molecular size drugs do not.[77] Drugs with a long plasma half-life persist longer in breast milk than those with a short half-life. Back-diffusion into the systemic circulation is slow in general, so that the elimination of the drug in breast milk is much slower than in the blood. The nonsteroidal anti-inflammatory analgesics are highly protein bound, which reduces the amount of drug that passes into the milk. Glucuronide conjugates may be cleaved in the infant's gastrointestinal tract, but usually at a slower rate than in the adult.[106] It probably does not matter whether the mother takes medication before or after breast-feeding because the maximum concentration of most drugs will not be obtained in the 15 minutes it takes to breast-feed an infant. Of greater importance is the selection of a drug with a short plasma half-life.

Analgesics

Acetaminophen passes into breast milk in small amounts, less than 0.2% of a 500-mg dose, and the neonate excretes a greater proportion of unchanged acetaminophen than the mother. Acetaminophen is generally accepted as a safe analgesic for nursing mothers. The American Academy of Pediatrics[107] also considers codeine and propoxyphene acceptable for nursing mothers.

Salicylates

Single-dose studies, using relatively small doses of aspirin, 450–650 mg, have shown that up to 21% of a maternal dose enters the breast milk over a 24-hour period.[108,109] Peak concentrations in breast milk occur 2 hours later than in plasma.[108] The neonate may absorb free salicylate from cleavage of salicylphenolic glucuronide from the gastrointestinal tract[106], which may be important for mothers receiving high doses of salicylates. Further studies are required of the pharmacokinetic disposition of salicylates in breast milk and in neonates whose mothers are receiving full anti-inflammatory doses (ie, more than 3 g/d).

Nonsteroidal Anti-inflammatory Analgesics

Indomethacin and some other nonsteroidal anti-inflammatory analgesics demonstrate a high enterohepatic recycling of its metabolites. There is one case report of convulsions in a breast-fed infant whose mother was receiving indomethacin.[110] Indomethacin is therefore not recommended for mothers who are breast-feeding. Sulindac and diclofenac have long plasma half-lives and should probably be avoided. Despite its long plasma half-life, only very small amounts of piroxicam have been detected in breast milk[111], which makes it probably safe for nursing mothers. Likewise, only very small amounts of ibuprofen and naproxen have been detected in breast milk. Concentrations of other short half-life drugs, including diclofenac, fenbufen, and flurbiprofen, have not been estimated but probably are safe in nursing mothers. Fenoprofen and ketoprofen form glucuronides, but the concentrations in breast milk are sufficiently low to avoid problems in the infant.

Chrysotherapy

Trace amounts of gold have been detected in milk, but because it is not absorbed, it is unlikely to cause problems in the infant.[112] There are no data on the concentrations of auranofin in human breast milk, and until they become available, this drug should be avoided in nursing mothers.

Antimalarials

Both chloroquine and hydroxychloroquine can be found in small amounts in breast milk but in quantities inadequate to protect the infant from malaria. It has been estimated that a suckling infant receives 2% of the maternal dose of hydroxychloroquine.[113] The antimalarials have been used extensively as prophylactics against malaria without apparent injury to breast-fed infants. However, further studies are required to determine their safety in nursing mothers with rheumatoid arthritis before recommendations regarding their use can be made.

Sulphasalazine

Approximately 30% of sulphasalazine and 50% of sulphapyridine can be recovered in breast milk.[114] The amount is insufficient to displace bilirubin from its protein-binding sites. Nevertheless, this drug cannot be recommended to nursing mothers until further studies have been performed to determine its safety.

Corticosteroids

Corticosteroids exist at less than 0.3% of the maternal dose in human milk. Prednisolone binds to albumin and lactoferrin in the milk. In the dosage used for the treatment of rheumatoid arthritis or other inflammatory joint diseases, (ie, 10 mg or less by mouth per day of prednisone or prednisolone or equivalent), these drugs are probably safe to prescribe to nursing mothers.

Cytotoxic Drugs

Methotrexate and azathioprine are found in only very small amounts in human milk and are probably safe to prescribe during lactation. Cyclophosphamide, however, is contraindicated because it is present in very high concentrations.

REFERENCES

1. Hench PS. Amerliorating effect of pregnancy on chronic atrophic (infectious) rheumatoid arthritis, fibrositis and intermittent hydroarthrosis. *Proc Mayo Clin.* 1938;13:161.
2. Oka M. Effect of pregnancy on the onset and course of rheumatoid arthritis. *Ann Rheum Dis.* 1953;73:227.
3. Flebo M, Snorrason E. Pregnancy and the place of therapeutic abortion in rheumatoid arthritis. *Acta Obstet Gynecol Scand.* 1961;40:116.
4. Okam, Vainio U. Effect of pregnancy on the prognosis and serology of rheumatoid arthritis. *Acta Rheum Scand.* 1966:12:47.
5. Kaplan D, Diamond H. Rheumatoid arthritis and pregnancy. *Clin Obstet Gynecol.* 1965;8:286.
6. Neely NT, Persellin RH. Activity of rheumatoid arthritis during pregnancy. *Texas Med.* 1977;73:59.
7. Persellin RH. The effect of pregnancy on rheumatoid arthritis. *Bull Rheum Dis.* 1977;27:922.
8. Cecere FA, Persellin RH. The interaction of pregnancy and the rheumatic diseases. *Clin Rheum Dis.* 1981;7:747.
9. Ostensen M, Husby G. A prospective clinical study of the effect of pregnancy on rheumatoid arthritis and ankylosing spondylitis. *Arth Rheum.* 1983;26:1155.
10. Ostensen M, Husby G. Pregnancy and rheumatic disease. A review of recent studies in rheumatoid arthritis and ankylosing spondylitis. *Klin Wochenschr.* 1984;62:891.
11. Bulmash JM. Rheumatoid arthritis and pregnancy. *Obstet Gynecol.* 1985;8:223.
12. Unger A, Kay A, Griffin AJ, Panayi GS. Disease activity and pregnancy associated α2-glycoprotein in rheumatoid arthritis during pregnancy. *Br Med J* 1983;286:750.
13. Peckham CH, King RW. Study of intercurrent conditions observed during pregnancy. *Am J Obstet Gynecol.* 1963;87:609.
14. Betson JR Jr., Dorn RV. Forty cases of arthritis and pregnancy. *J Int Coll Surg* 1964;42:521.
15. Klipple GL, Cecere FA. Rheumatoid arthritis and pregnancy. *Rheum Dis Clinic North Am.* 1989;15:213.
16. Hench PA. The potential reversibility of rheumatoid arthritis. *Mayo Clin Proc.* 1949;7:167.
17. Persellin RH. Inhibitors of inflammatory and immune responses in pregnancy serum. *Clin Rheum Dis.* 1981;4:769.
18. Oka M. Activity of rheumatoid arthritis and plasm 17-hydroxycorticosteroids during pregnancy and following parturition. *Acta Rheum Scand.* 1958;4:243.
19. Ostensen M. The influence of pregnancy and blood parameters in patients with rheumatic disease. *Scand J Rheumatol.* 1984;13:203.
20. Ostensen M, Aune LB, Husby G. Effect of pregnancy and hormonal changes on the activity of rheumatoid arthritis. *Scand J Rheumatol.* 1983;12:69.
21. Thurnau GR. Rheumatoid arthritis. *Clin Obstet Gynecol.* 1983;26:558.
22. Silman AJ. Is pregnancy a risk factor in the causation of rheumatoid arthritis? *Ann Rheum Dis.* 1986;45:1031.
23. Lawrence JS. *Rheumatism in Populations.* London: Heinemann; 1977.
24. Wood PHN. Age and the rheumatic diseases. In: Bennett PH, Wood PHN, eds. *Population Studies of the Rheumatic Diseases.* Amsterdam: Excerpta Medica; 1968:26.
25. Linos A, Worthington JW, O'Fallon WM, Kurland LT. The epidemiology of rheumatoid arthritis in Rochester, Minnesota: A study of incidence, prevlance, and mortality. *Am J Epidemiol.* 1980;111:87.
26. Engel A. Rheumatoid arthritis in US adults 1960–62. In: Bennett PH, Wood PHN, eds. *Population Studies of the Rheumatic Diseases.* Amsterdam: Excerpta Medica; 1968.
27. Kay A, Bach F. Subfertility before and after the development of rheumatoid arthritis in women. *Ann Rheum Dis* 1965;24:169.
28. Hellgren L. Marital status in RA. *Acta Rheumatol Scand.* 1969;15:271.
29. Hochberg MC. Adult and juvenile rheumatoid arthritis. Current epidemiologic concepts. *Epidemiol Rev.* 1981;3:27.
30. Lahita RG. Sex steroids and the rheumatic diseases. *Arthr Rheum.* 1985;28:121.
31. Talal N, Ahmed SA. Immunomodulation by hormones—an area of growing importance. *J Rheumatol.* 1987;14:191.
32. Russell DH, Kibler, Matrision L, et al. Prolactin receptors on human T and B lymphocytes: Antagonism of prolactin bindings by cyclosporine. *J Immunol.* 1985;134:3027.
33. Lavalle, Layo, Paniagua R, et al. Correlation study between prolactin and androgens in male patients with systemic lupus erythematosus. *J Rheumatol.* 1987;14:268.
34. Catulo M, Balleari E, Accardo S, et al. Preliminary results of serum androgen level testing in men with rheumatoid arthritis. *Arthr Rheum.* 1984;27:958. Letter.
35. Royal College of General Practitioners. *Oral Contraceptives and Health: Interim Report.* London: Pitman; 1974.
36. Wingrove S, Kay CR. Reduction in incidence of rheumatoid arthritis associated with oral contraceptives. *Lancet.* 1978;1:569.
37. Vandenbroucke JP, Valkenburg HA, Boersma JW, et al. Oral contraceptives and rheumatoid arthritis: further evidence for a preventitive effect. *Lancet.* 1982;1:839.
38. Allebeck P, Ahlbom A, Ljungstrom K, Allander E. Do oral contraceptives reduce the incidence of rheumatoid arthritis? *Scand J Rheum.* 1984;13:140.
39. Vandenbroucke JP, Witteman JCM, Valkenburg HA, et al. Noncontraceptive hormones and rheumatoid arthritis in perimenopausal and postmenopausal women. *JAMA* 1986;255:1299.
40. Linos A, O'Fallon WM, Worthington JW, Kurland LT. Case control study of rheumatoid arthritis and prior use of oral contraceptives. *Lancet.* 1983;2:1299.
41. del Junco DJ, Annegers JF, Luthra HS, et al. Do oral contraceptives prevent rheumatoid arthritis. *J Am Med Assoc.* 1985;254:1938.
42. Kay CR, Wingrave SJ. Oral contraceptives and rheumatoid arthritis. *Lancet.* 1983;1:1437.
43. Vandenbroucke JP. Oral contraceptives and rheumatoid arthritis. *Lancet.* 1983;2:200.
44. Esdaile JM, Horwitz R. Resolving contradictory results in epidemiological studies of oral contraceptives and rheumatoid arthritis. *Clin Res.* 1984;32:462.
45. Silman AJ. Sex, hormones and rheumatoid arthritis. *Editorial Hospital Update.* 1988;14:1078.
46. Bole GG, Friedlaender MH, Smith CK. Rheumatic symptoms and serological abnormalities induced by oral contraceptives. *Lancet.* 1969;1:323.
47. Bijlsma WJ, Huber-Bruning O, Thijssen JHH. Effect of estrogen treatment on clinical and laboratory manifestations of rheumatoid arthritis. *Ann Rheum Dis.* 1987;46:777.
48. Ostensen M, von Schoultz B, Husby G. Comparison between serum α2 pregnancy-associated globulin and activity of rheumatoid arthritis and ankylosing spondylitis during pregnancy. *Scand J Rheumatol.* 1983;12:315.
49. Sany J, Clot J, Borneau M, Ardary M. Immunomodulating effect of human placenta–eluted gamma globulins in rheumatoid arthritis. *Arthr Rheum.* 1982;25:17.
50. Mannik M, Nardella FA. IgG rheumatoid factor and self-association of these antibodies. *Clin Rheum Dis.* 1985;11:551.
51. Pekelharing JM, Hepp, Kamerling JP, et al. Alterations in carbohydrate composition of serum IgG from patients with rheumatoid arthritis and from pregnant women. *Ann Rheum Dis.* 1988;47:91.
52. Stanworth DR. A possible immunochemical explanation for pregnancy

associated remissions in rheumatoid arthritis? *Ann Rheum Dis.* 1988;47:89.
53. Pope RM, Yoshinoya I, Rutstein JE, et al. Effect of pregnancy on immune complexes and rheumatoid factors in patients with rheumatoid arthritis. *Am J Med.* 1983;74:973.
54. Nicholas NS, Panayi GS, Nouri AME. Human Pregnancy serum inhibits interleukin-2 production. *Clin Exp Immunol.* 1984;58:587.
55. Nicholas NS, Panayi GS. Inhibition of interleukin-2 production by retroplacental sera. A possible mechanism for human fetal allograft survival. *Am J Reprod Immunol Microbiol.* 1985;9:6.
56. Hargreaves ER. A survey of rheumatoid arthritis in West Cornwall. A report to the Empire Rheumatism Council. *Ann Rheum Dis.* 1958;17:61.
57. Kaplan D. Fetal wastage in patients with rheumatoid arthritis. *J Rheumatol.* 1986;13:875.
58. Shapiro S, Monson RR, Kaufman DW, et al. Perinatal mortality and birth weight in relation to aspirin taken during pregnancy. *Lancet.* 1976;1:1375.
59. Alspaugh MA, Talal N, Tan, EM. Differentiation and characterization of autoantibodies and their antigens in Sjögren's syndrome. *Arth Rheum.* 1976;19:216.
60. Alexander EL, Hirsch TJ, Arnett FC, et al. Ro(SSA) and La(SSB) antibodies in the clinical spectrum of Sjögren's syndrome. *J Rheumatol.* 1982;9:239.
61. Maddison P, Mogavero H, Provost TT, et al. The clinical significance of autoantibodies to a soluble cytoplasmic antigen in systemic lupus erthyematosus and other connective tissue diseases. *J Rheumatol.* 1979;6:189.
62. Andonopoulos AP, Drosos AA, Skopouli FN, et al. Secondary Sjögren's syndrome in rheumatoid arthritis. *J Rheumatol.* 1987;14:1098.
63. Franco HL, Weston WL, Peebles C, et al. Autoantibodies directed against sicca syndrome antigens in the neonatal lupus syndrome. *J Am Acad Dermatol.* 1981;4:67.
64. Kephart DC, Hood AF, Provost TT. Neonatal lupus erythematosus: new serologic findings. *J Invest Dermatol.* 1981;77:331.
65. Lockshin DD, Gibofsky A, Carol L, et al. Neonatal lupus erythematosus with heart block: Family study of a patient with anti-SSA and anti-SSB antibodies. *Arth Rheum.* 1983;26:210.
66. Scott JS, Maddison PJ, Taylor PV. Connective tissue disease, antibodies to ribonucleoprotein, and congenital heart block. *N Engl J Med.* 1983;309:209.
67. Lockshin MD, Bonfa E, Elkon K, Druzin ML. Neonatal lupus risk to newborns of mothers with systemic lupus erythematosus. *Arth Rheum.* 1988;31:697.
68. Ramsey-Goldman R, Hom D, Deng J-S, et al. Anti-SSA antibodies and fetal outcome in maternal systemic lupus erythematosus. *Arth Rheum.* 1986;29:1269.
69. Petri M, Watson R, Hochberg MC. Anti-Ro antibodies and neonatal lupus. *Rheum Dis Clin North Am.* 1989;15:335.
70. Lewis RB, Schulman JD. Influence of acetysalicylic acid, and inhibitor of prostaglandin synthesis, on the duration of human gestation and labour. *Lancet.* 1973;2:1159.
71. Collins E, Turner G. Maternal effects of regular salicylate ingestion in pregnancy. *Lancet.* 1975;2:335.
72. Ostensen M, Husby G. Ankylosing spondylitis and pregnancy. *Rheum Dis North Am.* 1989;15:241.
73. Ostensen M. Pregnancy in psoriatic arthritis. *Scand J Rheumatol.* 1988;17:67.
74. McHugh NJ, Laurent MR. The effect of pregnancy on the onset of psoriatic arthritis. *Br J Rheumatol.* 1989;28:50.
75. Talbott JH. Remarks on gout and gouty arthritis. *Bull Hosp Joint Dis.* 1957;18:3.
76. Levy G. Salicylate pharmacokinetics in the human neonate. In: Morselli, Garatinni, and Serini, eds. *Basic and Therapeutic Apsects of Perinatal Pharmacology.* New York, NY: Raven Press; 1975;319.
77. Lee P. Anti-inflammatory therapy during pregnancy and lactation. *Clin Invest Med.* 1985;8:328.
78. Turner G, Collins E. Fetal effects of regular salicylate ingestion in pregnancy. *Lancet.* 1975;2:338.
79. Sloane D, Heinonen O, Kaufman DW, Shapiro S. Aspirin and congential malformations. *Lancet.* 1976;1:1373.
80. Corby DR. Aspirin in pregnancy: Maternal and fetal effects. *Pediatrics* 1978;62(suppl):930.
81. Bleyer WA, Breckenridge RT. Studies on the detection of adverse drug reactions in the newborn. II. The effects of prenatal aspirin on newborn hemostasis. *J Am Med Assoc.* 1970;213:2049.
82. Rumack CM, Guggenheim MA, Rumack BH. Neonatal intracranial haemorrhage and maternal use of aspirin. *Obstet Gynecol.* 1981;52(suppl):52.
83. Lewis RB, Shulman JD. Influence of acetylsalicylic acid, an inhibitor of prostaglandin synthesis, on the duration of human gestation and labour. *Lancet.* 1973;1:1159.
84. Collins E, Turner G. Maternal effects of regular salicylate ingestion during pregnancy. *Lancet.* 1975;2:335.
85. Needs CJ, Brooks PM. Anti-rheumatic medication in pregnancy. *Br J Rheum.* 1985;24:282.
86. Zuckerman H, Reiss V, Rubinstein I. Inhibition of human premature labour by indomethacin. *Obstet Gynecol* 1974;44:787.
87. Wiquist N, Lundstrom V, Green K. Premature labour and indomethacin. *Prostaglandin.* 1975;10:515.
88. Wilkinson AR, Aynsley-Green A, Mitchell MD. Persistent pulmonary hypertension and abnormal prostaglandin E. Levels in preterm infants after maternal treatment with naproxen. *Arch Dis Child.* 1979;54:942.
89. Wilkinson AR. Naproxen levels in preterm infants after maternal treatment. *Lancet.* 1980;2:591.
90. Manchester LD, Margolis HS, Sheldon RE. Possible association between maternal indomethacin therapy and primary pulmonary hypertension of the newborn. *Am J Obstet Gynecol.* 1976;126:467.
91. Alun-Jones E, Williams J. Hyponatremia and fluid retention in a neonate associated with maternal naproxen overdosage. *J Tox Clin Tox.* 1986;24:257.
92. Miyamato TS, Miyaji S, Horiuch, Y, et al. Gold therapy in bronchial asthma—special emphasis on blood levels of gold and its teratogenicity. *J Jap Soc Int Med.* 1974;63:1190.
93. Rogers JG, Anderson R McD, Chow CW et al. Possible teratogenic effect of gold. *Aust Paed J.* 1980;16:194.
94. Cohen DL, Orzel J, Taylor A. Infants of mothers receiving gold therapy. *Arth Rheum.* 1981:24:104.
95. Tarp U, Graudal H. A follow up study of children exposed to gold *in utero. Arth Rheum.* 1985;28:235.
96. Ostensen M, Husby G. Antirheumatic drug treatment during pregnancy and lactation. *Scand J Rheum.* 1985;14:1.
97. Lyle WH. Penicillamine in pregnancy. *Lancet.* 1978;1:606.
98. Soloman L, Abrams G, Dinner M, Berman L. Neonatal abnormalities associated with D-penicillamine treatment during pregnancy. *N Engl J Med.* 1977;296:54.
99. Endres W. D-penicillamine in pregnancy—to ban or not to ban. *Klinische Wochenschrift.* 1981;59:535.
100. Rosa FW. Teratogen update: Penicillamine. *Teratology.* 1986;33:127.
101. Hart CM, Naunton RF. The ototoxicity of chloroquine phosphate. *Arch Otolaryngol Head Neck Surg.* 1964;80:407.
102. Parke AL. Antimalarial drugs, systemic lupus erythematosus and pregnancy. *J Rheumatol.* 1988;15:607.
103. Newman NM, Correy JF. Possible teratogenicity of sulphasalazine. *Med J Austral.* 1983;1:528.
104. Hill RM, Stern L. Drugs in pregnancy: Effects on the fetus and the new born. *Drugs.* 1979;17:182.
105. Sokal JE, Lessman EM. Effects of cancer chemotherapeutic agents on the human fetus. *J Am Med Assoc.* 1966;172:1765.
106. Levy G. Clinical pharmacokinetics of aspirin. *Pediatrics.* 1978;62:867.
107. Committee on Drugs, American Academy of Pediatrics. The transfer of drugs and other chemicals into human breast milk. *Pediatrics.* 1983;72:375.
108. Berlin CM, Pascuzzie MJ, Yaffe SJ. Excretion of salicylate in human milk. *Clin Pharm Ther.* 1980;27:245.
109. Findlay JW, DeAngelis RL, Kearney MF, et al. Analgesic drugs in breast milk and plasma. *Clin Pharm Ther.* 1981;29:625.
110. Eeg-Olofsson O, Malmros I, Elwin CE, Steen B. Convulsion in a breast fed infant after maternal Indomethacin. *Lancet.* 1978;2:215.
111. Ostensen M. Piroxicam in human breast milk. *Eur J Clin Pharm.* 1983;25:829.
112. Ostensen M, Skavdal K, Myklebust G, et al. Excretion of gold in human breast milk. *Eur J Clin Pharm.* 1986;31:251.
113. Nation RL, Hackett LP, Dusci LJ, Ilett KF. Excretion of hydroxychloroquine in human milk. *Br J Clin Pharm.* 1984;17:368.
114. Kahn AKA, Truelove SC. Placental and mammary transfer of sulphasalazine. *Br Med J.* 1979;2:1553.

Chapter Fifty-Three
Allergic Diseases

Michael Schatz and Robert S. Zeiger

53

Forty to sixty million Americans suffer from allergic disorders that may involve the skin (atopic dermatitis or eczema, urticaria or angioedema), nose or eyes (allergic rhinitis or conjunctivitis), chest (asthma), or gastrointestinal tract (food allergy). Close to 20% of women of childbearing age suffer one or more of these allergic diseases, and up to 4% are affected by asthma during pregnancy. Combined with disorders that mimic allergies (ie, nonallergic rhinitis, sinusitis, and hereditary angioneurotic edema) and those entities in which definable allergies are uncommon (chronic urticaria and chronic dermatoses of pregnancy), these illnesses represent the most common group of medical conditions associated with or complicating pregnancy.

GENERAL CONSIDERATIONS

IgE-mediated Reactions

In the 1960s, conclusive studies demonstrated that IgE was the unrecognized class of immunoglobulins responsible for immediate hypersensitivity reactions. The mechanisms involved in IgE-mediated reactions are summarized in Figure 53–1.[1,2] Nonimmunologic events also may trigger mediator release from mast cells and basophils and thereby induce clinical symptoms and disorders similar to those caused by IgE. Examples include urticaria or angioedema and anaphylaxis activated by cold, heat, pressure, sunlight, strenuous exercise, emotion, contrast media, aspirin (ASA), and other nonsteroidal anti-inflammatory drugs (NSAIDs); asthma triggered by exercise, ASA, other NSAIDs, and viral infections; and rhinoconjunctivitis induced by ASA, other NSAIDs, and cold air.

Detection of IgE Sensitization

Specific IgE sensitization can be demonstrated most easily by the wheal and flare reaction that occurs within 15–20 minutes at the site of a prick or puncture or intradermal injection of allergen, a rather inexpensive, sensitive, and reliable procedure when performed by an experienced person.[3] Alternatively, somewhat less sensitive *in vitro* solid phase immunoassays may be used.[3,4] These tests, best exemplified by the radioallergosorbent test (RAST), determine by radioimmunoassay the titer of specific IgE antibody in sera. During pregnancy, selective RAST tests are preferred over skin testing when specific allergen sensitizations cannot be ascertained by a careful history alone because RAST testing circumvents the possibility of anaphylaxis (see Anaphylaxis). For allergens, such as the minor penicillin determinant, that are not available for testing by RAST or other *in vitro* solid-phase immunoassays, careful skin testing, starting at more dilute concentrations, is appropriate.

General Principles of Allergy Therapy

The three types of allergy treatment (in usual order of institution) include: (1) avoidance therapy, (2) pharmacotherapy to minimize or prevent allergen-induced symptoms (discussed in detail in subsequent sections), and (3) immunotherapy to lower or eliminate specific allergic sensitization.

Avoidance of allergic or nonspecific factors known to precipitate symptoms is especially important during pregnancy. Guidelines for environmental control measures effective in reducing exposure to mite, mold, and pollen are found elsewhere[5], but optimal, individualized environmental control measures are best provided to the allergic patient by an allergy specialist.

Immunotherapy, known alternatively as desensitization or hyposensitization, can be best understood in clinical and immunologic terms. Clinically, it is the administration of offending allergens in increasing concentrations in an attempt to prevent the symptoms associated with exposure to allergens. Immunologically, it is the manipulation of the body in an attempt to induce a state of relative tolerance to a specific allergen. The indications for determining candidates for immunotherapy are beyond the scope of this chapter[6,7], but in general terms, they include patients with documented IgE-induced diseases in whom environmental avoidance unsuccessfully affects exposure, pharmacotherapy does not ameliorate symptoms adequately, contraindicating conditions do not exist, and reliable allergens are available and effective.

Immunotherapy appears to be generally safe during pregnancy[8], although anaphylaxis caused by immunotherapy occasionally occurs and could be a threat to the fetus (see below). It is generally recommended that allergen immunotherapy be *continued* during pregnancy by women who are deriving benefit, are not prone to systemic reactions, and are at maintenance or at least receiving a substantial dosage. Dose reduction usually is appropriate to further decrease the risk of a systemic reaction, and for the same reason, patients early in the course of immunotherapy may be served best by discontinuing their immunotherapy during pregnancy. *Beginning* immunotherapy generally is not recommended during pregnancy because of the unknown potential in such a patient for benefit or systemic reactivity and because of the usual latency of several months before any substantial clinical benefit from immunotherapy is achieved. One possible exception to this may be immunotherapy for venom anaphylaxis in patients unable to avoid stinging insects (see Anaphylaxis).

ASTHMA

Definition

Clinical asthma manifests itself as a spectrum of illness ranging from infrequent, spontaneously remitting symptoms to acute, severe, fatal attacks, to a chronic unrelenting illness causing substantial disability (see also Chapter 122). From an operational standpoint, symptomatic asthma may be defined as fluctuating degrees of wheezing, dyspnea, chest tightness, or cough associated with reversible obstructive airway disease or demonstrable bronchial hyperreactivity. Each aspect of this definition of asthma may be scrutinized further.

Respiratory Symptoms and Signs. Most patients with asthma report the symptom of wheezing, which may be

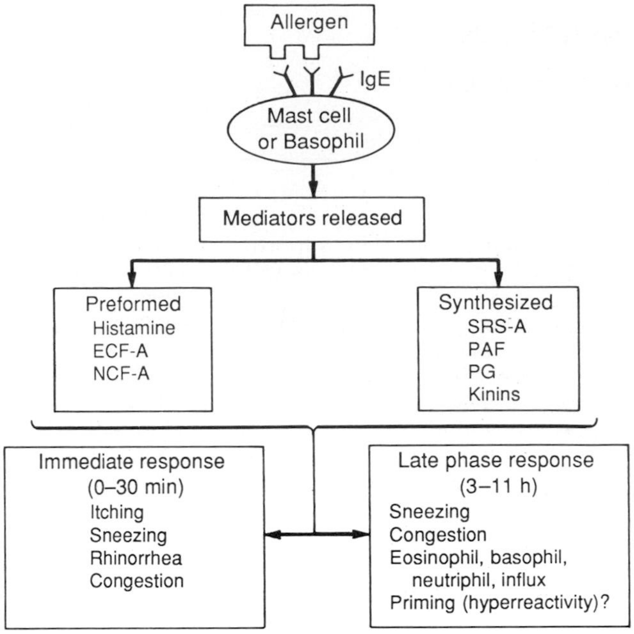

Figure 53–1. Nasal IgE-mediated allergic reaction initiated by allergen-bridging of two molecules of allergen-specific IgE bound to the surface of nasal mast cells or basophils. Similar reactions are documented in the skin and lungs. The mediators exert effects on target tissues, which include variable degrees of enhanced vasodilation, smooth muscle contraction, chemotaxis, vasopermeability, mucus secretion, platelet aggregation, and stimulation of pain receptors. In about 50% of patients exhibiting an immediate IgE-mediated reaction, a late phase reaction occurs. (ECF-A = Eosinophil chemotactic factors of anaphylaxis; NCF-A = Neutrophil chemotactic factors of anaphylaxis; SRS-A = Leukotrienes; PAF = Platelet activating factor; PG = Prostaglandins.

confirmed on chest auscultation during symptomatic episodes. Occasionally, cough[9] or dyspnea[10] without wheezing may represent the sole respiratory symptom in patients with asthma. Many patients with asthma report symptom-free periods of hours to months, spontaneously or in response to treatment, but some patients with more severe asthma or asthma that is inadequately treated may experience continuous symptoms.

Reversible Obstructive Airway Disease. The pulmonary function hallmark of asthma is airway obstruction with reversibility, although it is not clear what constitutes significant reversibility. Recent data[11] support the Intermountain Thoracic Society criteria for reversibility:[12] a 15% or more increase in the forced expiratory volume in 1 second (FEV_1) or a 25% or more improvement in maximum midexpiratory flow rate after an inhaled bronchodilator. It is increasingly evident that reversibility of airway obstruction may not be demonstrable after a single bronchodilator treatment but may require chronic therapy, sometimes with inhaled or oral corticosteroids, before the reversibility of the airway obstruction can be defined.

Bronchial Hyperreactivity. Airway hyper-responsiveness to a variety of stimuli is an almost universal feature of asthma, even when airway obstruction is not present. Such hyperreactivity may be reproducibly measured by the response to inhaled methacholine. Asthma is confirmed in subjects who experience a decrease in FEV_1 by 20% after provocative doses of methacholine of 225 breath units or less[13] or a concentration of 20 mg/mL or less.[14]

Etiology and Pathophysiology

The cause of asthma is unknown. However, certain pathophysiologic mechanisms are suspected to be important in the etiology of asthma, and a number of clinical triggering factors of asthma have been identified.

Pathophysiologic Mechanisms

GENETIC. Asthma occurs more frequently in patients with a family history of asthma. It is more common in allergic individuals, and the incidence of asymptomatic bronchial hyperreactivity is increased in allergic individuals without asthma and in asymptomatic family members of asthmatics.[15] These observations suggest that there is a genetic predisposition to asthma that is related to a genetic predisposition to allergy. However, the exact mode of inheritance and the specific inherited defect(s) remain to be defined.[15]

BRONCHOCONSTRICTION. The airway hyperreactivity of asthma confers an increased tendency to bronchoconstriction. Pathophysiologic factors potentially related to this increased bronchoconstriction in asthmatic subjects include abnormalities of smooth muscle, abnormalities of bronchoconstricting and bronchodilating neurogenic reflexes, beta-adrenergic hyporesponsiveness, and alpha-adrenergic hyperresponsiveness.[16]

AIRWAY INFLAMMATION. Airway mucosal inflammation is recognized as an important mechanism in the clinical manifestations and airway hyperreactivity of asthma. This inflammation may be triggered by IgE-mediated reactions to allergens, viral infections, and possibly other unidentified mechanisms. Frequently, it develops in response to the release of the chemotatic, vasoactive, and spasmogenic mediators from mast cells described previously.[17] Eosinophils appear to be the most important effector cells in the resulting mucosal inflammation of asthma, but neutrophils, lymphocytes, and monocytes also may play a role.[17]

ABNORMAL MUCOCILIARY FUNCTION. Abnormalities of mucus production and mucociliary function are documented in patients with asthma.[18] Whether these abnormalities are primary or secondary to the neurologic or inflammatory mechanisms previously alluded to, however, is unclear.

TRIGGERING FACTORS. A number of exposures trigger symptoms in patients with asthma.[19] *Allergies,* such as pollen, mite, mold spores, and animal dander, may be important triggers of symptoms. Intermittent allergen exposures may lead to intermittent symptoms. Chronic exposure may lead to chronic symptoms or chronic airway inflammation, which may lower the threshold to other triggers of asthmatic episodes. *Respiratory infections,* particularly viral infections and bacterial sinusitis, are probably the most important triggers of severe asthma and may lead to long-lasting bronchial hyperreactivity. *Emotional upset* may trigger episodes of asthma, but this is usually of minor importance in the overall symptomatology of most patients with asthma. *Exercise* will trigger asthma in the majority of patients if it is vigorous enough, and some patients experience wheezing only with exercise. *Aspirin* and other NSAIDs trigger wheezing in approximately 10% of adult patients, especially steroid-dependent patients and those with nasal polyps and sinusitis. The pathogenesis of aspirin-induced wheezing is undefined but does not appear to involve IgE-mediated mechanisms. *Irritants,* such as tobacco smoke, perfume, inorganic dusts, paint fumes, other chemical fumes, and aerosols may trigger symptoms in patients with asthma. *Aeropollutants,* such as sulfur dioxide, ozone, and oxides of nitrogen, may increase bronchial hyperreactivity or trigger overt bronchospasm in asthmatic patients. Changes in a number of *meteorologic* factors, such as ionization of the atmosphere, barometric pressure, temperature, wind velocity, and humidity, consistently trigger symptoms in some patients, although no single factor or combination of factors has been shown to have significant consistent effects on large populations of asthmatic subjects. Finally, approximately one third of women notice exacerbations of asthma in relation to their *menstrual cycle,* most commonly during the several days before the onset of menstruation.[20,21] Although these premenstrual exacerbations occur most commonly in women with more severe asthma, no relationship between the occurrence of premenstrual asthma exacerbations and the subsequent course of asthma during pregnancy has been clearly defined.

Effect of Pregnancy on Asthma

Asthma may improve, worsen, or remain unchanged during pregnancy. Although the change in the course of asthma during pregnancy in individual women is unpredictable, two studies have suggested that women with more severe asthma before pregnancy may be more likely to experience worsening of their asthma during pregnancy than women with milder disease.[22,23] In addition, experience during a previous pregnancy may be somewhat predictive because in approximately 60% of women, asthma course was similar in successive pregnancies.[22,24] The variable effect of pregnancy on the course of asthma appears to be more than just random fluctuation in the natural course of the disease because the changes in asthma that women attribute to pregnancy generally revert toward the prepregnancy course within 3 months postpartum.[24] The exact mechanisms involved in the change of asthma during pregnancy have not been defined, but a number of gestational physiologic changes have the potential to affect asthma[25] (Table 53–1).

Several observations have been made regarding the course of asthma and the stage of pregnancy. The peak incidence of flares during pregnancy appears to be between 24 and 26 weeks' gestation, especially in women whose asthma worsens during pregnancy.[23,24] In contrast, asthmatic women tend to experience fewer symptoms during the last 4 weeks of pregnancy than during any other 4-week gestational period, no matter what their gestational asthma course has been.[24] Finally, troublesome asthma during labor and delivery is extremely rare in prospectively managed asthmatic women.[24]

Effect of Asthma on Pregnancy

Retrospective data suggest that asthma complicates approximately 1% of pregnancies and is the most common potentially serious medical problem in pregnancy.[26] Available clinical data on the effect of asthma on pregnancy may be divided into studies in which maternal asthma was apparently not systematically managed by specialists (Table 53–2); and studies in which maternal asthma was actively managed by allergists or pulmonologists (see Table 53–2). These studies suggest that active asthma management may prevent the increased perinatal mortality that had been observed in infants of asthmatic mothers, but this management may not eliminate the increased risk of chronic hypertension, preeclampsia, and prematurity observed in the pregnancies of asthmatic women. Moreover, one recent study has suggested that the increased gestational hypertension in pregnant asthmatic women predisposes to the increased prematurity in their infants through necessitating preterm delivery intervention.[34]

Potential mechanisms that may explain the increased hypertension associated with increased prematurity in the pregnancies of asthmatic women include maternal smoking, uncontrolled asthma, inherent smooth muscles abnormalities, and asthma medications. The data supporting these various mechanisms are summarized in Table 53–3. Although an increased prevalence of maternal smoking in asthmatic women may contribute to the increased prematurity and perinatal mortality observed in studies that did not control for maternal smoking, recent observations suggest that the increased prematurity and chronic hypertension observed in the pregnancies of asthmatic women are beyond what could be attributed to maternal smoking.[34] Hospitalization for uncontrolled asthma has been associated with low birth weight in one study[31], but it is hard to differentiate the effects of uncontrolled asthma in this study from the effects of race, increased medication, and maternal smoking. Although prematurity, uterine hyperreactivity, and bronchial hyperreactivity were related in one study[45], the increased prematurity observed in asthmatic subjects in another study was not associated with increased preterm labor.[34] Another study of prematurely born infants could not confirm an increase in asthma or bronchial hyperreactivity in mothers.[49] Clearly, further studies are necessary to define the actual mechanisms of the increased perinatal

TABLE 53–1. PHYSIOLOGIC CHANGES DURING PREGNANCY THAT MAY AFFECT THE COURSE OF ASTHMA

Factors That May Improve Asthma
Progesterone-mediated bronchodilation
Estrogen or progesterone-mediated potentiation of beta-adrenergic stimulation
Decreased plasma histamine-mediated bronchoconstriction (caused by increased circulating histaminase)
Pulmonary effects of increased serum free cortisol
Increased glucocorticoid-mediated beta-adrenergic responsiveness
Increased prostaglandin E-mediated bronchodilation
Prostaglandin I_2-mediated bronchial stabilization
Increased half-life or decreased protein-binding of endogenous or exogenous bronchodilators
Factors That May Worsen Asthma
Pulmonary refractoriness to cortisol caused by competitive binding to glucocorticoid receptors by elevated progesterone, aldosterone, or deoxycorticosterone
Increased prostaglandin $F_{2}\alpha$-mediated bronchoconstriction
Decreased functional residual capacity with resultant airway closure during tidal breathing and altered ventilation-perfusion ratios
Increased major basic protein reaching the lung
Increased viral or bacterial respiratory infection-triggered asthma
Increased gastroesophageal reflux
Increased stress

Adapted from Schatz and Hoffman.[25]

TABLE 53–2. EFFECT OF ASTHMA ON PREGNANCY

Reference	Number of Pregnancies		Perinatal Outcomes in Asthmatic Versus Control Subjects		
	Asthmatics	Controls	Perinatal Mortality	Prematurity	Hypertension
		Studies in Which Asthma Was Not Systematically Managed			
26.	277	30,861	Increased	Not increased	Not reported
27.	381	125,423	Increased (neonatal)	Increased	Toxemia increased
28.	153	116	Not reported	Not reported	Chronic hypertension increased
		Studies In Which Asthma Was Actively Managed by Specialists			
29.	70	General population	Not increased	Increased	Not increased
30.	45	General population	Not increased	Increased	Not reported
31.	80	General population	Not increased	Increased	Not reported
32.	198	198	Not increased	Not reported	Preeclampsia increased
33.	290	Not reported	Not reported	Increased	Not reported
34.	360	295	Not increased	Increased	Chronic hypertension increased Preeclampsia increased in multiparas

morbidity in the pregnancies of asthmatic women. However, the previously discussed data suggest that optimal control of gestational asthma with carefully chosen medication reduces perinatal mortality and has the potential to reduce perinatal morbidity.

Diagnosis

General Diagnostic Criteria. Most patients who complain of wheezing associated with chest tightness, cough, or dyspnea have asthma. Although the demonstration of wheezing on chest auscultation is more objective than subjective wheezing, the objective diagnosis of asthma depends on the demonstration of reversible obstructive airway disease (as defined previously) on pulmonary function testing. Thus, a presumptive diagnosis of asthma during pregnancy usually can be made from the history and physical examination with the confirmation of diagnosis achieved by pulmonary function testing. Pulmonary function tests also represent an objective measurement of asthma severity, and

TABLE 53–3. FACTORS POTENTIALLY RELATED TO INCREASED PERINATAL MORTALITY AND MORBIDITY IN PREGNANCIES OF ASTHMATIC WOMEN

Factor	Observations
Maternal smoking	Increased incidence of smoking in asthmatic versus nonasthmatic pregnant women[28,34] Maternal smoking associated with increased perinatal mortality[35] Maternal smoking associated with increased prematurity[36]
Uncontrolled asthma	Acute asthma associated with hypertension,[37] which improves with amelioration of the asthma[38] Acute asthma may be associated with hypoxia, hypocapnia, and alkalosis[39] Maternal hypocapnia or alkalosis may impair fetal oxygenation[25] Relative maternal hypoxia associated with low birthweight in high-altitude pregnancies[40] Chronic maternal hypoxia associated with increased prematurity and intrauterine growth retardation in women with uncorrected congenital heart disease compared to women with corrected congenital heart disease[41] Lower birthweight in infants of mothers hospitalized for asthma during pregnancy (2920 g) versus infants of mothers not requiring emergency therapy for gestational asthma (3354 g)[31] Lower gestational pulmonary function associated with lower birthweight and asymmetric intrauterine growth retardation in infants of asthmatic mothers[42]
Inherent smooth muscle abnormalities	Relative vascular smooth muscle beta-adrenergic hyporesponsiveness to infused isoproterenol in asthmatic subjects[43]—may predispose to hypertension Vascular alpha-adrenergic hyperresponsiveness to intradermal phenylephrine in allergic asthmatic subjects[44]—may predispose to hypertension Increased bronchial hyperreactivity (to histamine) associated with uterine muscle hyperreactivity (preterm labor) in pregnancies producing premature infants[45]
Asthma medications	Beta-agonists may cause hypertension[46] Theophylline may cause vasoconstriction in certain vascular beds[47] Increased incidence of low birth weight infants and lower mean birthweight in infants of previously infertile mothers who received 10 mg of prednisone daily throughout pregnancy for pregnancy maintenance compared to control pregnancies[48] Chronic theophylline use associated with prematurity and maternal hypertension[34]

therefore some measurement of pulmonary function (FEV_1 or peak expiratory flow rate) should be performed on each clinic visit in an asthmatic patient.

It may be difficult to demonstrate airway obstruction in patients with infrequent asthma episodes or in those with cough variant asthma. In these circumstances, the diagnosis of asthma may be confirmed by methacholine testing (as described previously). However, methacholine testing is contraindicated during pregnancy.[46] Thus, pregnant patients with a history that is consistent with asthma but with pulmonary function confirmation lacking should be considered for therapeutic trials of bronchodilators or even corticosteroids after other causes of symptoms (see below) have been excluded. A positive clinical response to asthma therapy would then serve as the confirmation of asthma in these patients until methacholine testing can be performed postpartum.

Differential Diagnosis. Conditions to be considered in the differential diagnosis of asthma and important features distinguishing these conditions from asthma are shown in Table 53–4. Chronic bronchitis or emphysema should be considered in a smoker with irreversible obstructive airway disease, and α_1-antitrypsin deficiency should be considered in a nonsmoking pregnant woman with irreversible obstructive airway disease, especially if she has a family history of emphysema. Pulmonary edema may be associated with wheezing (*cardiac asthma*), and the diagnosis of pulmonary edema during pregnancy in a patient with known asthma requires particular vigilance. Further information on the diagnosis of cardiac disease during pregnancy can be found in Chapter 123, and the evaluation of possible pulmonary embolism during pregnancy is described in Chapter 119. Dyspnea of early or late pregnancy and hyperventilation can occur in asthmatic or nonasthmatic patients, but the absence of wheezing or airway obstruction during symptomatic episodes usually allows the patient and the physician to differentiate asthma from these dyspneas. Finally, the presentation of amniotic fluid embolism (see also Chapter 120) may occasionally include bronchospasm.

TABLE 53–4. DIFFERENTIAL DIAGNOSIS OF ASTHMA

	Distinguishing Features		
Condition	**History, Physical**	**Pulmonary Function**	**Laboratory**
Mechanical obstruction (larynx, trachea, main bronchi)	History of injury, aspiration, hemoptysis Wheezing over the trachea	Inspiratory and expiratory obstruction on flow volume loop No response to bronchodilators Normal maximum midexpiratory flow rate	Endoscopy diagnostic
Laryngeal dysfunction	Wheezing over the trachea	Same as above	Endoscopy reveals adduction of vocal cords during symptomatic episodes
Chronic bronchitis or emphysema	Smoking Daily productive cough Family history of emphysema	Irreversible airway obstruction	$Alpha_1$ antitrypsin deficiency
Pulmonary edema	Nocturnal dyspnea Wheezing may occur Cardiomegaly Gallop rhythm Valvular Disease Tocolytic therapy	Decreased forced vital capacity	Chest x-ray: cardiomegaly, pulmonary venous hypertension, interstitial edema Echocardiography: mitral or aortic valve disease, left ventricular dilatation, or hypertrophy, hypocontractile left ventricle in peripartum cardiomyopathy
Pulmonary embolism	*Sudden* onset of dyspnea or wheezing Chest pain Hemoptysis	—	Arterial hypoxemia Abnormal perfusion on ventilation perfusion scan Pulmonary angiography diagnostic
Carcinoid syndrome	Episodes of flushing, diarrhea, hypotension associated with wheezing	—	Urine 5-hydroxyindole acetic acid (5-HIAA) elevated
Dyspnea of pregnancy	No associated wheezing or cough Early or late pregnancy	Normal	—
Hyperventilation syndrome	Dyspnea without wheezing Perioral and peripheral paresthesias	Normal	Respiratory alkalosis (blood gases)
Amniotic fluid embolism	Acute respiratory distress during labor or delivery Cyanosis Shock Bleeding Wheezing may occur	—	Disseminated intravascular coagulation Demonstration of fetal elements in the maternal circulation

Data are adapted from reference 19.

Identification of Triggering Factors. The patient's history should help to identify the factors (discussed previously) that are likely to trigger each patient's asthma. Regarding allergens, patients may notice that animals, dust, freshly cut grass, or mildew trigger their wheezing, or the seasonal variation of their asthma may suggest triggering by pollen (spring or spring and fall), dust or dander (winter), or mold (spring and fall or fall through spring). Testing for specific IgE during pregnancy is discussed earlier in this chapter. Referral to an allergy specialist is the optimal means of evaluating historic and specific IgE data to determine the relative role of allergy-triggering factors in each woman's asthma.

Treatment

Nonpharmacologic Management. Avoidance of triggering factors is an obvious but often underused modality in the

TABLE 53–5. DATA ON THE SAFETY OF ASTHMA MEDICATIONS DURING PREGNANCY

Drug	FDA Pregnancy Classification	Human Data: Congenital Malformations (CM)	Human Data: Other[50]
Sympathomimetics			
Inhaled	—	No increase in CM or other perinatal complications in 259 asthmatic women using inhaled beta-agonist bronchodilators (IB) compared to 101 concurrently followed asthmatic women not using IB and 295 nonasthmatic controls[51]; 83% of subjects used metaproterenol, while 32% of subjects used more than one specific IB.	
Systemic–Specific			
Epinephrine	—	Increased CM ($p < .05$) in 189 subjects in collaborative perinatal project (CPP)[52]	May inhibit labor
Ephedrine	—	No increased CM in 373 subjects in CPP	—
Isoproterenol	—	No increased CM in 31 subjects in CPP	—
Isoetharine	—	—	—
Metaproterenol	C	—	May inhibit term labor
Terbutaline	B	—	May inhibit term labor; intravascular administration preserves or increases uteroplacental blood flow
Albuteral	C	—	May inhibit term labor
Bitolterol	C	—	—
Pirbuterol	C	—	—
Theophylline	C	No increased CM in 193 subjects in CPP	Neonatal symptoms of theophylline toxicity reported in eight infants whose asthmatic mothers received theophylline at term (cord blood levels 6–17 μg/mL); increased hypertension and prematurity in infants of women treated with chronic theophylline during pregnancy[34]; may inhibit uterine contractions.
Cromolyn	B	CM in 1.4% of 296 infants of asthmatics treated with cromolyn throughout their entire pregnancies[53]	No perinatal mortality or prematurity in 296 infants of asthmatics treated with cromolyn throughout their entire pregnancies[53]
Anticholinergics			
Atropine	—	No increased CM in 401 subjects in CPP	Fetal tachycardia and fall in breathing incidence reported after maternal intravenous atropine
Ipratropium	B	—	—
Corticosteroids			
Systemic	—	No increased CM in 154 subjects in CPP No increase in CM in 261 reported women receiving corticosteroids for asthma during pregnancy (compared to general population figures)[50]	No increase in perinatal mortality in 261 reported women receiving corticosteroids for asthma during pregnancy (compared to general population figures)
Inhaled			
Beclomethasone	C	No increase in CM in 45 pregnancies in 40 women (compared to general population figures)[30]	—
Flunisolide	C	—	—
Triamcinolone	D	—	—

decreased management of asthma. It is particularly beneficial during pregnancy when it may improve clinical well-being with a need for pharmacologic intervention. It is particularly important for the pregnant asthmatic woman to *discontinue smoking* during pregnancy because smoking may predispose to increased asthma, complicating bronchitis or sinusitis, and increase the need for medication; and the increased morbidity attributed to smoking may be additive to that conferred by maternal asthma.[34,42] Allergen immunotherapy during pregnancy has been previously discussed.

Pharmacologic Management. The pharmacologic management of asthma during pregnancy is not substantially different from such management in nonpregnant patients, and the usual goals of therapy (achieving symptomatic control, preventing acute episodes, and optimizing pulmonary function) appear to be beneficial for the fetus and for the mother (discussed previously). However, data on the use of asthma medications during pregnancy (Table 53–5) lead to certain specific recommendations for the pharmacologic management of asthma in pregnant women.

Medications recommended for the outpatient management of chronic asthma and the order of their use are shown in Table 53–6. The recent emphasis on the use of *inhaled* medications seems particularly appropriate for management of asthma during pregnancy, but the reliance on inhalational therapy requires that respiratory tract penetration of the drugs be optimized by appropriate inhaler technique and by spacer devices.[54] Medications generally should be added one by one until adequate control is achieved. Interpatient variability in asthma severity, compliance, and medication tolerance leads to a variety of dosages and combinations of these medications that are required to achieve acceptable asthma control in each patient. Monthly (or more often) visits to an allergist or pulmonologist who is assessing asthma severity and the response to treatment objectively (with pulmonary function tests) and subjectively appear to be the optimal way to achieve desired therapeutic goals in asthmatic patients who require regular medications during pregnancy.

The recommended management of subacute and acute asthma during pregnancy also are described in Table 53–6. It is essential that asthmatic patients are able to contact their physician so that subacute increases in symptoms can be treated appropriately and acute asthma prevented as much as possible. When approaching the patient with *acute* asthma during pregnancy, it must be rememberd that blood gas analysis in a healthy pregnant woman reveals a higher pO_2 (102–106 mm Hg) and a lower pCO_2 (28–30 mm Hg) than in nonpregnant patients. Thus, a $pCO_2 \geq 35$ mm Hg or a $pO_2 < 70$ mm Hg associated with acute asthma represents more severe respiratory compromise during pregnancy than similar blood gases in the nongravid state. Some authors recommend the use of subcutaneous epinephrine for the management of acute asthma during pregnancy because of its time-honored efficacy and apparent safety.[55] However, we prefer inhaled beta-agonists because inhaled beta-agonists are generally as effective as epinephrine with less systemic side effects[50] and available animal and human data are more reassuring for the gestational use of inhaled beta-agonists than for the use of epinephrine (see Table 53–4).

Pharmacokinetic studies have shown that theophylline's weight-corrected volume of distribution is unaffected by pregnancy, but its half-life is increased and clearance decreased, particularly during the third trimester.[50] Consequently, loading dose recommendations for theophylline are the same during pregnancy as in nonpregnant women, but initial maintenance dose guidelines are more conservative (see Table 53–6). Theophylline therapy must be individualized by means of serum theophylline determinations, generally aiming for levels of 5–15 μg/mL.

There are no analogous data on the pharmacokinetics of exogenous corticosteroids during pregnancy. However, the potential target organ corticosteroid-resistance conferred by the gestational increase in circulating competitive antagonists (progesterone, adolsterone, dexoycorticosterone)[25] suggests that higher doses of corticosteroids may be necessary during pregnancy than in nonpregnancy to achieve the same benefit.

In addition to medications, oxygen and intravenous hydration are important in the management of acute gestational asthma (see Table 53–6). The management of respiratory failure during pregnancy is described in Chapter 122.

The approach to asthma management during labor and delivery is shown in Table 53–6. Although only 10% of prospectively managed asthmatic women experience symptoms of asthma during labor or delivery[50], prophylactic medications should be continued. Of 366 asthmatic women enrolled in one prospective study of gestational asthma, 4.1% required inhaled bronchodilators, 0.5% required intravenous aminophylline, and none required intravenous corticosteroids for the treatment of asthma during labor and delivery.[50]

Obstetric Management. The obstetric management of asthmatic women during pregnancy is generally the same as for nonasthmatic women. However, in several circumstances, the presence of asthma may influence obstetric treatment decisions.[50] Because *prostaglandins* and *ergonavine* exacerbate asthma, substitutes should be used if possible. If there are no acceptable substitutes under the particular clinical circumstance, these drugs should be used with caution, monitoring clinical respiratory status and airway function closely and considering prophylactic therapy with intravenous corticosteroids. *Beta-adrenergic antagonists* also may exacerbate asthma[19]; they should be avoided in the management of gestational hypertension in asthmatic women if possible. When such drugs are essential for the management of recalcitrant hypertension during pregnancy in asthmatic women, metoprolol, a more selective beta-adrenergic antagonist, should be used.[50] However, because the cardioselectivity of metoprolol is relative rather than absolute, asthmatic women receiving metoprolol must be monitored carefully for possible deterioration of their respiratory status.

Obstetric management during labor and delivery of women with controlled asthma is identical to management in nonasthmatic women, including the preference for regional versus general anesthesia. When general anesthesia is required for cesarean section, the use of halogenated anesthetics to supplement balanced general anesthesia is not recommended because, although these agents possess bronchodilator qualities, their concomitant relaxing effect on uterine musculature has been associated with increased blood loss at cesarean section.[59]

RHINITIS

Incidence, Etiology, and Pathophysiology

Substantial symptoms of rhinitis have been reported in approximately 30% of pregnant women.[56] Essentially, any of the recognized forms of rhinitis may occur during preg-

TABLE 53–6. KAISER–PERMANENTE PROTOCOL FOR THE PHARMACOLOGIC MANAGEMENT OF ASTHMA DURING PREGNANCY[a]

A. Chronic outpatient[b]
  1. Inhaled terbutaline 1–2 puffs q4h p.r.n.
  2. Regular inhaled terbutaline (1–2 puffs q.i.d.)
  3. Regular inhaled cromolyn (2 puffs q.i.d.) following inhaled terbutaline (at least initially)
  4. Regular inhaled beclomethasone (2–4 puffs b.i.d.–q.i.d.) following inhaled terbutaline (at least initially)
  5. Regular oral theophylline[c]
  6. Oral prednisone
     course[d]
     alternate day
     daily

B. Subacute symptoms[e]
  1. Inhaled terbutaline (up to 3 puffs q3h)
  2. Oral theophylline[c]
  3. Oral corticosteroids[d] (may be added earlier with severe episode)
  4. Antibiotics for clinical findings of bacterial bronchitis, sinusitis, or pneumonia

C. Acute asthma (emergency room or hospital)
  1. Supplemental O_2
     Initially 3–4 L/min
     Then adjust to maintain $pO_2 \geq 70$ or O_2 saturation (pulse oximetry) ≥ 95
  2. Glucose-containing intravenous fluids[f]—at least 100 cc/h initially
  3. Nebulized terbutaline (2–4 mg + 2 cc saline)
     May be repeated every 20–30 min, monitoring pulse rate, until respiratory distress corrected, $pO_2 \geq 70$, $pCO_2 < 35$
     then taper to q4h maintenance (eg, q1h × 1–4, q2h × 1–4, q3h × 1–4, then q4h)
  4. Intravenous methylprednisolone[f] (should be given along with initial therapy to patients on regular corticosteroids, or those with poor response to initial terbutaline treatment)
     40–125 mg initially
     then 40–80 mg q4h until definite improvement
     then taper
  5. Consider intravenous aminophylline[g]
     For patients *not* receiving oral theophylline: 5 mg/kg over 20–30 min, then maintenance dose
     For patients receiving oral theophylline: stat theophylline level (<5 μg/mL: 2.5 mg/kg over 20–30 min, then maintenance dose; ≥5 μg/mL: proceed to maintenance dose)
     Maintenance dose (initially) 0.5 mg/kg/h, following response, side effects, and serum theophylline levels[h]
  6. Consider anticholinergics for patients responding poorly—nebulized atropine (.025–.050 mg/kg) or metered dose ipratropium (4 puffs with spacer device) q6h
  7. Subcutaneous terbutaline 0.25 mg if not responding to the above therapy
  8. Oral prednisone course after the acute symptoms are resolved unless:
     only one nebulized treatment is required to clear the episode, or
     normal pulmonary function tests are demonstrated after therapy (and the triggering event is not considered to be ongoing)

D. Management during labor and delivery
  1. Continue prelabor regimen of oral theophylline, inhaled cromolyn, or inhaled beclomethasone
  2. For asthma symptoms during labor
     Inhaled terbutaline (1–2 puffs or 2 mg nebulized as above q3–4h)
     Intravenous methylprednisolone (as above)
     Intravenous aminophylline (as above)
  3. For patients on regular corticosteroids or who have received frequent courses during pregnancy: 100 mg hydrocortisone intravenously at admission, followed by 100 mg intravenously q8h for 24 hours (or until absence of complications is established)

[a] Medications generally should be used sequentially as indicated.
[b] With no demonstrable evidence of a concurrent infection or a self-limited triggering factor
[c] Generally beginning with 200 mg sustained release preparations b.i.d.
[d] Generally beginning with 40–60 mg daily in divided doses and tapering over 10–14 d
[e] Increased symptoms without respiratory distress, usually associated with a specific precipitant, such as an upper respiratory infection
[f] Patient may be considered for oral therapy when respiratory distress corrected and patient receiving adequate oral fluids.
[g] The therapeutic index of IV aminophylline in patients receiving optimal inhaled beta-agonists and intravenous corticosteroids requires further study, but the benefits in general may not outweigh the risks.
[h] Obtained 3 hours after each new maintenance dose, then every morning while on IV aminophylline

nancy, but the most common types of rhinitis during pregnancy appear to be allergic rhinitis, bacterial rhinosinusitis, rhinitis medicamentosa, and vasomotor rhinitis.[57]

Allergic rhinitis is caused by an intranasal IgE-mediated reaction to inhaled allergens, such as pollen, mite, mold, or animal dander. It frequently preexists in women of childbearing age but may appear during pregnancy.

Bacterial rhinosinusitis may complicate another underlying cause of rhinitis or may follow a viral upper respiratory infection. The incidence of sinusitis in pregnancy has been reported to be 1.5%, an apparent sixfold increase over the nonpregnant population.[58]

Rhinitis Medicamentosa, the syndrome of rebound nasal congestion resulting from the overuse of topical vasoconstricting nose sprays, also may complicate another underlying cause of chronic rhinitis or a viral upper respiratory infection. Its frequency during pregnancy may be explained by the perceived desirability of using topical rather than systemic medications during pregnancy.

Many women notice some increase in nasal congestion associated with nasal dryness and epistaxis during pregnancy. These symptoms apparently are caused by nasal vascular pooling, which is secondary to the increased circulating blood volume and possibly enhanced by the vasodilating effect of progesterone.[57] In some women, this nasal congestion becomes very troublesome and requires treatment. Such *vasomotor rhinitis* usually improves postpartum, although a similar syndrome of noneosinophilic, noninfectious chronic nasal congestion may exist in young women independent of pregnancy.

Interrelationships Between Rhinitis and Pregnancy

Few data exist regarding the clinical effect of pregnancy on rhinitis or the effect of rhinitis on pregnancy. Estrogen and progesterone have been linked to nasal mucosal swelling, cyclic changes in female nasal mucus, and increased activity of nasal mucosal glands.[57] In addition, as described previously, nasal vascular pooling may occur during pregnancy. These changes may predispose to worsening of rhinitis during pregnancy. In contrast, the increased serum-free cortisol that occurs with advancing pregnancy may lead to improvement of eosinophilic rhinitis during pregnancy.[57] In one unpublished study, nasal symptoms worsened during pregnancy in 34% of women, improved in 15%, and remained unchanged in 45% of women surveyed.[57]

It seems unlikely that gestational rhinitis would have any direct adverse effect on the course of pregnancy, but severe rhinitis could indirectly affect pregnancy adversely by interfering with sleeping, eating, or emotional stability. In addition, uncontrolled rhinitis or sinusitis during pregnancy may exacerbate coexisting asthma.

Diagnosis

The etiology of rhinitis during pregnancy usually can be determined from the history, physical examination, and nasal cytology (Table 53–7). The use of skin or blood tests to confirm the presence of specific IgE has been discussed previously. Because the classic symptoms and signs of sinusitis were absent in nearly one half of the pregnant women with proven sinusitis in one study[58], clinical findings and a high index of suspicion may be supplemented by other diagnostic procedures. The use of A-mode ultrasonography is limited by the existence of false-negative and false-positive results.[57] Because the radiation exposure associated with sinus radiographs is small and is reduced by abdominal or pelvic shielding[50], sinus radiographs should be used during pregnancy when necessary to confirm or establish the diagnosis, especially if the patient is not responding adequately to treatment. Diagnostic sinus irrigations may be necessary during pregnancy in patients with abnormal sinus radiographs who are not responding to therapy.

Treatment

The treatment of specific rhinologic entities during pregnancy is summarized in Table 53–8. Medication choices are based on available data regarding the use of antihistamines and decongestants during pregnancy (Table 53–9), previously described data (see Table 53–5) on the gestational use of asthma medications (cromolyn, inhaled corticosteroids) that have been adapted for topical intranasal use, and the relative efficacy of the various medications for specific rhinitis syndromes. When possible, nonpharmacologic therapy should be used maximally to minimize the need for medications. The available data (see Table 53–9) do not allow absolute determination of the safest antihistamine during pregnancy. Based on the data, we generally use tripelennamine first, followed by chlorpheniramine or hydroxyzine if tripelennamine is not effective. Antihistamines are particularly helpful for sneezing, itching, and rhinorrhea, while decongestants are most helpful for nasal con-

TABLE 53–7. CLINICAL AND NASAL CYTOLOGIC FEATURES OF THE COMMON TYPES OF RHINITIS OCCURRING DURING PREGNANCY

Type	Major Symptoms	Exacerbating Factors[a]	Nasal Cytology
Allergic rhinitis	Sneezing, runny nose, nasal itching, eye itching	Seasonal Grass, house dust, animals Pregnancy in ⅓ of women	Eosinophils ± basophilic cells
Bacterial rhinosinusitis	Postnasal drainage Sinus distribution pain Purulent discharge	Following an upper respiratory infection Pregnancy (increased incidence)	Neutrophils ± bacteria (may be normal)
Rhinitis medicamentosa	Congestion	Vasoconstricting nose spray abuse	Normal
Nonspecific postnasal drainage	Postnasal drainage Clear or white mucus	Pregnancy	Normal
Vasomotor rhinitis	Congestion (particularly alternating nostril)	Pregnancy	Normal
Eosinophilic nonallergic rhinitis	Congestion, nose blowing, sneezing	None (nonseasonal)	Eosinophils ± basophilic cells
Nasal polyps	Obstruction, anosmia	None (nonseasonal)	Eosinophils ± basophilic cells

[a] Other than nonspecific precipitants, such as aerosols, alcohol, temperature changes, and smoke

Reprinted with permission from Schatz and Zeiger.[57]

TABLE 53–8. TREATMENT OF SPECIFIC RHINOLOGIC ENTITIES DURING PREGNANCY

Type of Rhinitis	Nonpharmacologic Therapy	Pharmacologic Therapy
Allergic rhinitis or conjunctivitis	Avoidance of antigens Immunotherapy (continuation, not initiation)	Intranasal cromolyn (1–2 sprays b.i.d.–t.i.d.) Ophthalmic cromolyn (1 gtt q4h) Tripelennamine[a] ± pseudoephedrine[b] Intranasal beclomethasone[c]
Bacterial rhinosinusitis	Sinus irrigation for recalcitrant disease	Topical oxymetazoline (2 b.i.d) ≤ 5 d Pseudoephedrine[b] Antibiotics for 3 w
Rhinitis medicamentosa	Discontinue vasoconstrictive nose spray	Intranasal beclomethasone[c] Pseudoephedrine[c] ± tripelennamine[a]
Nonspecific postnasal drip	Saline lavage	Tripelennamine[a]
Vasomotor rhinitis	Exercise (commensurate with pregnancy) Nasal saline spray	Pseudoephedrine[b]
Eosinophilic nonallergic rhinitis	—	Intranasal beclomethasone[c] Tripelennamine[a] ± pseudoephedrine[b] Treatment of complicating infection
Nasal polyps	Polypectomy under local anesthesia	Intranasal beclomethasone[c] Tripelennamine[a] ± pseudoephedrine[b] Treatment of complicating infections Prednisone for recalcitrant disease

[a] 25–50 mg q6h or 100 mg sustained-release b.i.d.
[b] 60 mg b.i.d.–q.i.d. or 120 mg sustained-release b.i.d.
[c] 2 sprays b.i.d. and taper to lowest effective dosage
Modified from Schatz and Zeiger[57]

gestion; combination therapy often is superior to the use of either type of medication alone. While oral medication may be most appropriate for intermittent symptoms of allergic rhinitis, intranasal cromolyn or (if not adequately effective) beclomethasone may be better for chronic symptoms. Some patients with severe eosinophilic rhinitis or rhinitis medicamentosa may require combinations of intranasal and regular oral therapy to achieve adequate control of their symptoms. The treatment of sinusitis is discussed in Chapter 195.

ANAPHYLAXIS

Definition

Anaphylaxis is an acute clinical episode characterized by dermatologic (urticaria or angioedema), respiratory (asthma, laryngeal edema), cardiovascular (hypotension, electrocardiographic alterations, and vascular collapse), and gastrointestinal (vomiting, spasmodic lower abdominal or flank pain, diarrhea, and incontinence) symptoms and signs, appearing alone or together.[62] Such a definition en-

TABLE 53–9. DATA ON THE SAFETY OF ANTIHISTAMINES AND DECONGESTANTS DURING PREGNANCY[a]

Drug	Teratogenic in Animals	Human Data
Brompheniramine	No data	Increased total congenital malformations (CM) in 65 subjects in Collaborative Perinatal Project (CPP)[52]
Chlorpheniramine	No	No increase in total CM in 1070 subjects in CPP, but increase in eye and ear malformations and inguinal hernia
Diphenhydramine	No	No increase in CM in 595 subjects in CPP Increased use by mothers of 549 infants with oral clefts in case-controlled study[60] Withdrawal syndrome reported in one infant after high dose regular maternal gestational use[57]
Hydroxyzine	Yes	No increase in CM in 50 subjects in CPP or 74 subjects in another study[61] Withdrawal syndrome reported in one infant after high-dose regular maternal gestational use[57]
Tripelennamine	No	No increase in CM in 100 subjects in CPP
Phenylephrine	Yes	No increase in total CM in 1249 subjects in CPP, but increase in eye and ear malformations and clubfoot
Phenylpropanolamine	No data	Increase in total and specific CM in 726 subjects in CPP
Pseudoephedrine	No	No increase in total CM in 39 subjects in CPP

[a] Includes only medications for which human data are available. Data from Group Health Cooperative Study[59] not included because of potential methodologic difficulties.

compasses the above clinical syndrome whether it is incited by an IgE- or non–IgE-mediated release of potent mast cell and basophil mediators. Anaphylaxis may range from mild to catastrophic, although an initially mild episode may progress to a severe one if not promptly recognized and treated.

Incidence, Etiology, and Pathophysiology

Precise incidence figures for the occurrence of anaphylaxis during pregnancy are unavailable, but the incidence is probably extremely low.[63] Potential etiologic agents that have triggered anaphylaxis in nonpregnant patients and have or could cause similar reactions during pregnancy are categorized by their proven or presumed mechanism of action in Table 53–10. In addition, some patients experience anaphylaxis during exercise, and other patients manifest anaphylaxis with no identifiable cause (idiopathic anaphylaxis).

Early reports implicated penicillin and procaine as the most common agents causing anaphylaxis during pregnancy[63], however, recently other agents have been implicated including intravenous iron[64], bee venom[65], snake antivenom[66], shellfish[67], oxytocins[68], human serum albumin[69], modified polygelatin solution[70], intravenous conjugated estrogens[71], endogenous progesterone[72], and exercise during labor and delivery.[73]

Effect of Anaphylaxis on Pregnancy

The fetus appears protected from anaphylaxis, possibly because of placental production and secretion of histaminase (discussed previously), which could catalyze the endogenous amines, including histamine, which are released during the reaction; and placental exclusion of maternal anaphylactic IgE.[74] However, maternal hypoxia and hypotension caused by anaphylaxis may be catastrophic to the mother and the fetus. Fetal distress manifested by repetitive late decelerations in fetal heart rate[67] and multicystic fetal[65] or infantile encephalomalacia[65,66] have been associated with maternal anaphylaxis. With prompt and aggressive therapy, fetal distress associated with maternal anaphylaxis may resolve totally without maternal or fetal compromise.[65] Alternatively, fetal or neonatal death may occur despite maternal survival, presumably because of diminished uteroplacental perfusion as a result of the rapidity and severity of the episode or inadequate antianaphylaxis treatment.[65,66]

TABLE 53–10. CAUSES OF ANAPHYLAXIS

IgE-mediated mechanisms
Antibiotics (particularly penicillins and cephalosporins)
Foreign proteins, including heterologous serum, ACTH, hormones, enzymes, venom, and protamine
Other therapeutic materials, such as allergen extracts, vaccines, muscle relaxants, ethylene oxide, and thiopental
Foods (especially egg, shellfish, nuts, seeds, fish, celery, milk, and legumes)
Immune complex or complement-mediated mechanisms
Whole blood
Cryoprecipitate
Immunoglobulin
Plasma
Methotrexate
Arachidonic acid metabolism modulating agents
Aspirin
Other nonsteroidal anti-inflammatory drugs
Direct mediator-releasing agents
Opiates
Curare
Radiocontrast media
Dextran
Mannitol
Pentamidine
Polymyxin B
Thiamine

Diagnosis

Clinical Findings. Patients with typical *severe anaphylaxis* present with the sudden and frightening onset of diffuse urticaria, wheezing, tachycardia, diaphoresis, disorientation, hypotension, shock, vascular collapse, and even sudden death within minutes. However, when anaphylaxis is *slowly evolving,* patients may present with a constellation of more subtle or mild symptoms and signs, frequently in combination with one another. Examples include cutaneous pruritus, burning, or flushing; urticaria or angioedema, which may be localized to the acral areas, such as the top of the head, palms, soles, or ears, or may be more generalized, involving the palate, throat, pharynx, and trunk; increased salivation, ocular and nasal symptoms, clearing of the throat, and swallowing difficulties; agitation, anxiousness, or foreboding feelings; abdominal discomfort or uterine cramps; coughing, chest tightness, and dyspnea; or persistent hypotension with bradycardia in patients taking beta-adrenergic blocking agents, which impede a homeostatic tachycardic response to shock.[75] Recognition of these milder or earlier symptoms and signs of anaphylaxis with concomitant aggressive therapy often prevents or aborts reactions that could be life-threatening. Anaphylaxis may reappear hours after apparent resolution of the early episode, analogous to the late-phase IgE-mediated reaction previously discussed.

Differential Diagnosis. Vasovagal reactions such as sudden fainting following injections, venipuncture, and other procedures, usually can be distinguished from anaphylaxis by the characteristic pallor, preceding nausea, diaphoresis, and bradycardia; absence of urticaria, pruritus, and respiratory symptoms; and generally rapid recovery with recumbency, elevation of extremities, inhalational ammonia, and atropine, if needed. In *hyperventilation,* breathlessness rarely progresses to collapse; symptoms generally appear more slowly; respiratory embarrassment and dermatologic signs are absent; lightheadedness, tingling, carpal pedal spasm, and stable pulse and blood pressure are characteristic; and treatment with breathing into a paper bag and reassurance are curative.[76]

Laryngeal stridor, a serious symptom of anaphylaxis, must be differentiated from the laryngeal edema reported during *preeclampsia*[77], and that associated with *laryngopathia gravidarum*[78] or *hereditary angioedema* (HANE)[79] (discussed below). Signs of preeclampsia, including hypertension, peripheral edema, and urinary abnormalities, as well as the prior diagnosis of preeclampsia, should prevent confusion. In laryngopathia gravidarum, laryngeal symptoms are usually less sudden and the acute form occurs just before parturition.[78] In HANE, the onset of laryngeal stridor is slower, abdominal pain is prominent, hypotension and urticaria are absent, and a family history of HANE can be obtained frequently.[79]

Disorders associated with acute collapse from *cardiac* (myocardial infarction, arrhythmia, major vessel rupture), *pulmonary* (embolism, aspiration), and *cranial* (seizure, hemorrhage) origin generally can be distinguished from anaphylaxis by careful history, absence of urticaria or angioedema, presence of localizing signs, results of therapy, and time.

Prevention and Treatment

Prevention. Probably nowhere in medicine is active prevention more mandatory and rewarding than in anaphylaxis. Guidelines that should reduce needless anaphylaxis include (1) care in history-taking to avoid using an agent or cross-reacting drug that previously induced anaphylaxis or allergy (ie, cephalosporin in penicillin-allergic patients and NSAID with aspirin sensitivity); (2) educate at-risk patients of their condition, the mechanisms of avoidance of exposure, and the need for them to carry an identification of their allergy (ie, Allergy Alert Bracelet); (3) prescribe an autoinjectable source of epinephrine (Epipen) to patients at risk for noniatrogenic anaphylaxis (sensitivity to foods, venom, exercise); (4) avoid parenteral administration of therapeutic agents whenever possible; (5) observe patients for at least 30 minutes after parenteral injections; (6) determine sensitivity (skin tests or RASTS) of all patients before receiving agents commonly associated with anaphylaxis (eg, heterologous antisera); and (7) refer patients suspected of sensitivity to any required drug or agent to an allergist for evaluation.

The prevention of hymenoptera sting anaphylaxis in venom-sensitive pregnant patients warrants specific comment. All pregnant women with a history of hymenoptera-sting anaphylaxis should receive renewed insect avoidance procedures and an up-to-date emergency kit containing injectable epinephrine, oral tripelennamine, and a tourniquet. Although only preliminary data are available supporting the safety of venom immunotherapy during pregnancy[80], benefit–risk considerations suggest that pregnant women receiving maintenance venom immunotherapy before pregnancy should continue treatment during pregnancy. Pregnant women with histories suggesting hymenoptera sting anaphylaxis should avoid skin testing until postpartum. If identification of venom-specific IgE is required, a venom RAST may be obtained. Finally, benefit–risk considerations do not appear to favor *beginning* venom immunotherapy during pregnancy in most women. However, venom immunotherapy can be initiated during pregnancy in the rare patient whose risk of a life-threatening hymenoptera sting reaction during pregnancy appears to be greater than the potential risk of anaphylaxis during immunotherapy.

Treatment. Management of anaphylaxis during pregnancy should be aggressive and expeditious, using similar medication as that routinely used in nonpregnant persons. Because of the altered circulatory and respiratory physiology during pregnancy, adequate intravascular volume repletion and oxygenation are particularly important in the management of anaphylaxis during pregnancy to prevent both maternal and fetal complications. Of the routine antianaphylactic medications, epinephrine and diphenhydramine have been possibly implicated in causing increased fetal malformations. However, the tentative nature of these data and the lack of equally effective substitutes suggest that these medications must be used during pregnancy for this life-threatening emergency.

All anaphylactic reactions should be considered potentially severe or life-threatening until resolved and therefore must be managed promptly. The extent of treatment depends on the severity of the reaction, which can only be determined during the course of therapy. Epinephrine (0.2–0.5 mL of 1:1000 injected intramuscularly) and oxygen (administered by nasal cannula or face mask) are the first agents to be used in treating anaphylaxis. Tourniquets placed proximal to injected material (drugs, allergenic extracts, insect stings), ice applied at the site, and epinephrine (0.2 mL of 1:1000) injected into the site are additional measures that have great efficacy and should not be neglected.

Anaphylactic reactions that rapidly resolve during

TABLE 53–11. KAISER–PERMANENTE SEVERE ANAPHYLAXIS PROTOCOL

Modify as desired, cross off nonapplicable orders.

1. Call a doctor STAT.
2. P,R, B/P q5min or q2min if B/P <90 mm Hg.
3. Patient wt ______ kg ______
4. O_2 at 6 L/min by nasal cannula.
5. If systolic B/P <90 mm Hg, use Trendelenburg position, place patient on left side and monitor EKG.
6. Continue ice and tourniquets if reaction secondary to injection, skin test, or sting.
7. Continue epinephrine (1:1000) 0.3 mL IM in deltoid, repeat q10min if reaction persists. In addition, give either half or equivalent dose into site of skin test injection or sting.
8. Start IV with 18- or 19-ga needle or intercath; infuse Ringer's lactate; start wide open then check with doctor for rate or volume (may require 3–10 L)

Consider:

9. Benadryl (50 mg/mL): 1 mL IV piggyback in 50 mL over 5 min.
10. Methylprednisolone (125 mg/2 mL) 2 mL in 50 mL IV piggyback over 5 min. Do not mix with benadryl.
11. If wheezing, use terbutaline (2 mg/mL) 2.0 mL added to 2 mL saline and nebulize.
12. If symptoms persist, ranitidine (50 mg/2 mL) 2 mL in 50 mL IV piggyback infused in 5 min.
13. If systolic BP less than 90 mm Hg and pulse less than 60 beats per min, give atropine (1 mg/10 mL) 5 mL IV push, may repeat 10 mL if necessary in 5–10 min.
14. If still hypotensive, or hypotension recurs, use maintenance epinephrine: 1 mL epinephrine (1:1000) to 10 mL saline and infuse over 10 min. Consider repeating if still hypotensive, perfusing immediately after previous dose.
15. If still hypotensive or if hypotension recurs, use maintenance epinephrine: 1 mL epinephrine (1:1000) in 250 mL D_5 W (4 µg/mL) and infuse at 15 mL/h (1 µg/min). Titrate q5min to maintain systolic B/P ≥90 mm Hg. Maximum dose 60 mL/h = 4 µg/min.
16. If still hypotensive, DC maintenance epinephrine and infuse dopamine (400 mg/5 mL): mix 5 mL with 250 mL IV solution (1.6 mg/mL) and start infusion at 0.15 × ___kg (4 µg/kg/min) = ___mL/h to maintain systolic B/P ≥90 mm Hg. Titrate q5min to maintain systolic B/P ≥90 mm Hg (usual maximum dose 5 × infusion rate = to 20 µg/kg/min).
17. If ventricular dysrhythmia occurs, use lidocaine (100 g/50 mL) acutely: 0.05 × ___kg = ___mL IV bolus, which may be repeated in 5 min. Consider twice the dose in 15 min if necessary.
18. If dysrhythmia persists, Lidocaine (2 g/50 mL) maintenance dosage: add 50 mL to 500 mL D_5 W, and start infusion at 30 mL/h (2 mg/min).
19. Consider glucagon if patient on beta-blocker and anaphylaxis persists. Add 1 mL glucagon diluting solution to glucagon vial and infuse 0.5 mL IV push. May repeat if necessary.
20. If wheezing persists and on no previous theophylline for past 24 hours, give bolus of Aminophylline (500 mg/20 mL) 0.2 × ___kg = ___mL IV in 50 mL IV solution over 20 min.

P, pulse; R, respiration; B/P, blood pressure; DC, discontinue.

treatment may have only required one dose of epinephrine, removal of a stinger, ice, tourniquets, oxygen, and possibly diphenhydramine (50 mg intramuscularly). More serious and prolonged anaphylactic reactions may require multiple doses of epinephrine, repeating intramuscular injections every 10–15 minutes or more frequently if necessary, while carefully monitoring maternal and fetal heart rates and cardiac rhythms. A complete protocol to treat anaphylaxis has been formulated (Table 53–11).

When treating hypotension during pregnancy, it has been recommended that a minimum maternal systolic blood pressure of 90 mm Hg be maintained to assure adequate placental perfusion.[81] The pregnant hypotensive patient should be placed on her left side to prevent added positional hypotension resulting from compression of the inferior vena cava by the gravid uterus.[81] Impending or existing hypotension must be reversed promptly with large volumes of intravenous fluids (up to 5–10 L are occasionally necessary), such as Ringer's lactate, normal saline, or preferably colloid. Intravenous epinephrine may be required, despite its potential to cause decreased uteroplacental blood flow.[66,67,82] If intravenous epinephrine becomes necessary, adverse affects can be reduced by infusing it slowly or continuously (see Table 53–11).[83] Some obstetricians and obstetric anesthesiologists prefer ephedrine (10–15 mg intravenous push) to treat hypotension during pregnancy because its predominant beta-adrenergic activity should cause less reduction in uterine blood flow compared to epinephrine.[66,67,82] However, several reports have demonstrated that epinephrine is more effective than ephedrine in reversing anaphylaxis-induced hypotension during pregnancy.[84,85] As such, epinephrine should be the drug of choice to treate anaphylaxis in the parous and nonparous states.

Though corticosteroids apparently do not reverse anaphylaxis acutely because of their delayed effects, they are helpful during prolonged, refractory, or recurrent anaphylaxis. Corticosteroids should therefore be administered early in the treatment of severe anaphylaxis to obtain its delayed effect sooner. Laryngeal spasm or edema unresponsive to medical management may require intubation and rarely tracheostomy. Though prompt and aggressive treatment to anaphylaxis should successfully resolve the insult and preserve maternal and fetal well-being, prevention of anaphylaxis (discussed previously) remains the best way to minimize maternal or fetal morbidity or mortality from this life-threatening emergency.

URTICARIA AND ANGIOEDEMA

Definition

Urticaria manifests as circumscribed, raised, pruritic, and erythematous lesions caused by edema involving the superficial dermis. Extension of the edema to deeper areas of the dermis, subcutaneous tissue, or submucosa generally leads to localized but more diffuse erythematous swelling, called *angioedema*. Symptoms that persist less than 6 weeks are termed *acute*, while those persisting longer are considered *chronic*.[86]

Incidence, Etiology, and Pathophysiology

While up to 20% of individuals may experience an episode of urticaria or angioedema at least once, probably less than 2% are afflicted chronically or recurrently.[86] In the latter chronic group, the causes for the urticaria or angioedema remain unknown in more than 90%, leading to the classification of idiopathic urticaria or angioedema. Urticaria or angioedema may occur during pregnancy from any of the causes, agents, and mechanisms noted in the nonpregnant state (Table 53–12), or may be limited to pregnancy, redeveloping in subsequent pregnancies. Champion et al[87] reported that three of 438 (0.5%) consecutive pregnant patients exhibited chronic pregnancy urticaria or angioedema syndrome. The etiology of this syndrome is uncertain, but some observations suggest possible allergic sensitization to endogenous hormones, particularly progesterone. For example, some nonpregnant women consistently manifest urticaria 7–10 days premenstrually[88], and intramuscular injections of progesterone reproduce symptoms within 1 hour in afflicted patients, while cyclically administered conjugated estrogens control the urticaria. In addition, endogenous progesterone has been implicated as a cause of recurrent anaphylaxis.[72]

HANE is an uncommon autosomal dominant disorder caused by a deficiency or malfunction of C1-esterase inhibitor, which, when normally present, functions to inhibit the first component of the complement cascade. Without normal C1-esterase inhibitor function to modulate an activated complement cascade, it is believed that kininlike fragments and other pharmacologically active mediators form that cause the clinical constellation of symptoms and signs of HANE: recurrent 1–4-day attacks of nonpruritic and nonurticarial angioedema of the extremities, abdomen, face, and, potentially most seriously, of the larynx.[79] Involvement of the bowel wall typically causes severe abdominal colic, vomiting, and guarding without fever, leucocytosis, elevated sedimentation rate, or rigidity. These HANE-induced abdominal attacks must be carefully differentiated from a surgical or obstetric abdominal emergency to avoid needless surgical exploration. Laryngeal edema leads to hoarseness, difficulty swallowing, and, when severe, life-threatening upper-airway obstruction. Episodes generally are sporadic but often are triggered by trauma (minor or major dental, surgical, and accidental), stress, infections, and extreme temperature fluctuations. A familial history of similar episodes frequently can be elicited with careful questioning.

Interrelationship Between HANE and Pregnancy

Frank et al[79] noted that 23 of 25 women experienced fewer or no HANE attacks during the last two trimesters of pregnancy and that 10 women with a total of 25 pregnancies did not experience angioedema during vaginal delivery, despite its traumatic potential. Although pregnancy generally appears to produce a profound calming effect on HANE, one woman experienced worsening of HANE during three pregnancies.[89] In addition, postpartum exacerbations have been reported[89], and one maternal death resulted after delivery from localized perineal swelling with secondary irreversible shock.[90]

Diagnosis

A thorough history and careful physical examination generally elicits the cause of urticaria or angioedema, if a cause exists. Laboratory evaluation generally is limited to screening with a complete blood count, urinalysis, and erythrocyte sedimentation rate (ESR). Specific diagnostic tests reserved for confirmation of diagnostic suspicions are noted in Table 53–12.

Gestational urticaria or angioedema must be differentiated from autoimmune progesterone dermatitis of pregnancy, polymorphic eruption of pregnancy (PEP), other pruritic dermatoses of pregnancy and laryngopathia gravidarum. *Autoimmune progesterone dermatitis of pregnancy* appears as a papulopustular eruption associated with transient

TABLE 53–12. DIAGNOSTIC TESTS FOR URTICARIA OR ANGIOEDEMA DURING PREGNANCY

Suspected Disorder	Procedure
Food[a], drug[a], or inhalant allergy	Diary and trial avoidance of causal agent; RAST
Physical	
Dermatographism	Stroke skin with tongue blade
Cold	Ice cube on forearm for 5 min Cryoglobulins, cyrofibrinogen
Cholinergic	Methacholine skin test (postpartum)
Solar	Expose skin to lightwave lengths Protoporphyrins or coproporphyrins
Vibratory	Vortex skin for 4 min
Pressure	Weights to extremity for 10 min
Aquagenic	Expose hand to tap-water at varying temperatures
Exercise	History
Infectious	Appropriate cultures or titers Stool for ova or parasites
Cutaneous or systemic vasculitis	Skin or tissue biopsy with immunofluorescence Immunoglobulin analysis Antinuclear antibody Thyroid antimicrosomal antibody Complement profile
Hereditary angioedema (HANE)	C4, C2, CH50 C1-esterase inhibitor by functional and protein analysis
Malignancy	CH50, C1, C1-esterase inhibitor
Idiopathic	History with negative tests

[a] Any of the causes of anaphylaxis listed in Table 53–10 may potentially cause urticaria or angioedema without other signs of anaphylaxis.

arthritis, peripheral and tissue eosinophilia, miscarriage, and delayed intradermal sensitivity to aqueous progesterone.[91] PEP is an urticarial, pruritic eruption that develops in and around the abdominal striae in about 0.5% of pregnancies.[92] Table 53–13 helps to distinguish PEP from several of the other pruritic dermatoses of pregnancy.

Laryngopathia gravidarum[78] has been described as an acute or chronic, noninfectious, mildly inflammatory process of the laryngeal tissues in multigravid patients. The acute form occurs just before parturition, while the chronic form occurs earlier in pregnancy and has recurred in subsequent pregnancies. Both forms spontaneously subside postpartum. Symptoms include progressive dypsnea (occasionally necessitating an artificial airway), hoarseness, sore throat, and odynophagia without fever, malaise, lymphadenopathy, or cough but with elevated white blood count and ESR (40–60 mm/h). The larynx and frequently the epiglottis demonstrate patchy localized edema and congestion, but the aryepiglotic folds, arytenoids, vestibular region, and true vocal cords are unaffected. Microscopically, the surface epithelium and mucus glands are normal, but the submucosa appears edematous and is infiltrated with lymphocytes and plasma cells. The pathogenesis of laryngopathia gravidarum remains speculative, but it may comprise several different entities. It has been attributed to an abnormal effect of pregnancy hormones on the laryngeal mucosa because of its rapid reduction after delivery.[78]

Prevention and Treatment

Ideally, identification and avoidance of offending agents or causes would prevent urticaria or angioedema symptoms and obviate pharmacologic treatment. When symptomatic therapy is required, tripelennamine (25–50 mg every 6 hours or 100 mg sustained release twice a day) is recommended as the initial H1-antihistamine of choice during pregnancy, based on the available data (see Table 53–9). Addition of ephedrine (25–50 mg every 6 hours) or substitution of hydroxyzine (10–25 mg every 6 hours) should be considered in refractory situations.[50] Rarely, systemic corticosteroids may be required for severe, recalcitrant urticaria or angioedema during pregnancy. Acute, severe urticaria or angioedema should be treated aggressively in a similar fashion to anaphylaxis (see Table 53–11).

During pregnancy, HANE does not generally require nor warrant attenuated androgen prophylaxis because of the potential for drug-related fetal damage[93], including female masculinization and pseudohermaphroditism, and the potential for spontaneous abortion.[94] Women of child-bearing years with HANE should maintain effective contraception while taking androgens to prevent these adverse fetal effects from occurring before confirmation of the pregnancy. Vaginal deliveries do not apparently trigger HANE attacks, thereby obviating the need for preventive measures[79]; however, cesarean sections do require preoperative transfusion of 2 U of fresh frozen plasma to prevent episodes.[93] Regional anesthesia should be instituted instead of general anesthesia to prevent laryngeal edema, which may be induced by endotracheal intubation. Life-threatening laryngeal edema caused by HANE during pregnancy requires rapid and aggressive therapy, including androgens (stanozolol 4 mg four times a day), standard emergency measures for reversing airway obstruction (endotracheal intubation and if necessary, tracheostomy), and intravenous fluid replacement for hypovolemia when present.[93] Although epinephrine, antihistamines, and corticosteroids may be attempted, they are generally effective only in a few patients during acute HANE attacks.[79] Though infrequent, postpartum HANE episodes must be identified quickly to permit aggressive therapy, including large-volume fluid replacement of third-space losses and reintroduction of appropriate prepregnancy treatment, most notably, androgenic therapy.[93]

ATOPIC DERMATITIS

Definition, Etiology, and Pathogenesis

Atopic dermatitis is an eczematous disorder occurring in about 1–2% of adults and is characterized by pruritus, chronicity, typical morphology and distribution, and association with a hereditary tendency to allergic rhinitis, asthma, and food allergy. Manifestations may be as severe as generalized exfoliative erythroderma or as mild as an isolated, small, circumscribed patch of chronic nummular dermatitis. Erythema, dermal edema, excoriations, and weeping characterize the acute condition, while scaling, thickening, hyperpigmentation, and fissuring denote the chronic state. Areas of predilection in adults include the antecubital and popliteal fossae, neck, upper trunk, perioral, and periorbital areas and hands.[95]

Individuals with atopic dermatitis, particularly those with concurrent allergic respiratory symptoms, evidence elevated serum IgE levels, peripheral eosinophilia and often

TABLE 53–13. COMPARATIVE CHARACTERISTICS OF THE PRURITIC DERMATOSES OF PREGNANCY

	Pemphigoid Gestationis[a]	Pruritic Folliculitis of Pregnancy	Prurigo of Pregnancy	Polymorphic Eruption of Pregnancy	Impetigo Herpetiformis[b]	Pruritus Gravidarum
Onset and incidence	Second trimester; rare	Fourth to ninth mo; rare	25th to 30th wk, 0.3–2%	Last trimester; 0.5%	Second half of pregnancy; rare	Last trimester; common (0.02–2.4%)
Gravidity preference	Multigravidas	None	None	Primigravidas	None	None
Distribution	Generalized; buttocks, abdomen, extremities, mucous membranes	Shoulders, back, buttocks, abdomen, thigh, "acne of pregnancy"	Trunk and extremities (extensor surfaces)	Abdomen with spread to extremities; striae involved; face spared	Intertriginous zones and thighs	Abdomen, trunk, extremities
Clinical lesions	Erythematous papules, vesicles, bullae Constitutional symptoms	Follicular erythematous papules	Excoriated erythematous papules	Erythematous papules and urticarial plaques; excoriations rare	Small, sometimes coalescent pustules; constitutional symptoms	No primary lesions; excoriations
Pruritus	Moderate–severe	Moderate	Moderate	Severe	Mild	Mild to severe
Histology	Subepidermal bullae often containing eosinophils	Acute sterile folliculitis, dermal edema, and perivascular infiltrates	Parakeratosis, acanthosis, with dermal perivesicular infiltration of lymphocytes	Spongiotic dermatitis with superficial mixed perivascular inflammation	Spongioform and intraepidermal pustules	Nonspecific cholestasis of liver; no skin biopsy data
Immunofluorescence	C_3 deposition at basement membranes in lesional skin	Negative	Negative	Negative	ND	ND
Laboratory abnormalities	Peripheral blood eosinophilia; ↑ HLA-B8 and DR3; circulating HG factor (autoantibody)	None	None, but associated with atopy	None	↓ Ca^{++}, ↑ ESR, ↑ WBC	↑ Bile acid; abnormal liver functions (variable)
Treatment	Systemic steroids as topical steroids usually inadequate	10% benzoyl peroxide and 1% hydrocortisone	Topical antipruritics, oral antihistamines	Topical steroids; systemic steroids if necessary	Ca^{++}, vitamin D, Systemic steroids	Topical antipruritics, cholestyramine
Complications	Maternal: increased infection; fetal: prematurity and stillbirth; blisters in neonate	None	None	None	Maternal: prostration, renal failure, cardiac failure, death; fetal: abortion, stillbirth, neonatal death	Maternal: none; fetal: prematurity
Prognosis	May flare postpartum Recurrences common in subsequent pregnancies	Clears postpartum Recurs in 1/3 of patients	Clears postpartum Recurrences uncommon	Clears postpartum Recurrence rare	Clears postpartum, recurs earlier in subsequent pregnancies	Clears postpartum Recurrences common in subsequent pregnancies

[a] Herpes gestationis (HG) older terminology.
[b] Possibly pustular psoriasis exacerbated by pregnancy.
ND, No data; ESR, erythrocyte sedimentation rate; WBC, white blood cell count.
Modified from Romero R, Olsen TG, Chervenak FA, Hobbins JC. J Reprod Med *1983;28:615. Using classification of Holmes RC, Black MM.* J Am Acad Dermatol. *1983;8:405. Reprinted with permission from Schatz, et al.*[50]

(up to 80%) specific IgE to foods and inhalants, which historically may be related to triggering cutaneous symptoms. The pathogenesis of atopic dermatitis, though uncertain, probably involves an abnormal immunologic mechanism that leads to the cutaneous release of mediators, such as histamine.[95,96]

Diagnosis

Hanifin and Lobitz[97] formulated diagnostic criteria to aid in the diagnosis of atopic dermatitis (Table 53–14). Classic atopic dermatitis should be easily differentiated from the following cutaneous disorders: (1) *seborrheic dermatitis* with its characteristic greasy, scaling areas on a yellow-red base over the scalp, forehead, and flexor areas; (2) *allergic contact dermatitis* with its acute, patchy, and streaky lesions and historic correlation to contactant exposure; (3) other immunologic disorders, including the *hyper-IgE syndrome* with its recurrent cold abscesses, severe local and systemic infections to candida and staphylococcus, coarse facies and skeletal abnormalities, and markedly elevated serum IgE levels; *dermatitis herpetiformis* with its severe, refractory pruritus, blistering, and excoriations frequently associated with sprue and wheat sensitivity; *Wiskott–Aldrich* syndrome with its purpura from thrombocytopenia and systemic infections from immunologic abnormalities; and *chronic granulomatous disease* with its recurrent skin abscesses, fistulas, pneumonia, hepatosplenomegaly, and abnormal NBT test; and (4) cutaneous lymphomas, such as mycosis fungoides, Sézary syndrome, and Hodgkin's disease, which may present early with pruritic, dermatitic lesions involving linear thickening of flexural surfaces, but typically progresses to more characteristic lesions.

TABLE 53–14. DIAGNOSTIC CRITERIA FOR ATOPIC DERMATITIS

Absolute features:
Pruritus
Flexural lichenification in adults
Chronic or recurrent tendency
Plus
Two or more of the following features:
Personal or family atopic history (asthma, allergic rhinitis, or atopic dermatitis)
Specific IgE (skin test or RAST)
White dermographism (a white line rather than a wheal in response to skin stroking) or delayed blanch to methacholine
Anterior subcapsular cataracts
Or
Four or more of the following features:
Xerosis, ichthyosis, or hyperlinear palms
Pityriasis alba
Keratosis pilaris
Facial pallor or infraorbital darkening
Dennie–Morgan infraorbital fold
Elevated serum IgE
Keratoconus
Tendency toward nonspecific hand dermatitis
Tendency toward recurrent dermal infections

From Hanifin and Lobitz [97] with permission.

Interrelationships Between Pregnancy and Atopic Dermatitis

Roth and Kierland[98] noted in 117 women with mild to severe atopic dermatitis that pregnancy was associated with clearing or definite improvement in 3% and definite exacerbation in 1%. Such observations suggest that pregnancy exerts no, or only minimal, effect on atopic dermatitis. We are aware of no published data regarding the outcome of pregnancy in women with atopic dermatitis.

Treatment

Therapy of atopic dermatitis during pregnancy must emphasize *avoidance* of triggering factors, including known food and inhalant allergens; irritating agents, such as wools and chemicals; excessive perspiration and heat; unwarranted stress; occlusive clothing; and any other known exacerbants. Efficacious topical care measures include moisturizers and lubricants to alleviate dryness (Neutrogena hand cream, Aveeno, Eucerin cream), cleansers, such as Cetophil lotion instead of soaps, and aluminum acetate (Burow's solution) or baking soda soaks to relieve inflammation, weeping, and pruritus. Oral antihistamines should be used at the lowest effective dosage if clinically indicated. Based on the available data (see Table 53–9), therapy with tripelennamine (25–50 mg every 6 hours or 100 mg sustained-release twice a day) is recommended initially, followed by hydroxyzine (10–50 mg at the hour of sleep) if tripelennamine proves inadequate. Topical corticosteroid therapy should be limited to more severe eruptions and initiated with the least potentially adrenal suppressive preparations, such as hydrocortisone (0.5–2.5%). More potent topical corticosteroid preparations should be reserved for more recalcitrant areas or patients. Intralesional or systemic corticosteroid injections should be avoided. Penicillinase-resistant synthetic penicillins or erythromycin (in penicillin-allergic patients) may be helpful for apparent infectious exacerbations generally caused by *Staphylococcus aureus*.[95]

DRUG ALLERGY

Etiology, Pathogenesis, and Incidence[99]

For the purposes of this discussion, such adverse drug-induced reactions as overdose, side effects, secondary effects, drug interactions, intolerances, and idiosyncrasies are omitted. Allergic drug reactions can be classified into four general immunologic mechanisms: (1) Type I reactions include anaphylaxis caused by the presence of IgE sensitivity to a drug (see Anaphylaxis) and those resembling anaphylaxis (anaphylactoid) in which IgE sensitivity cannot be demonstrated (eg, contrast media, polymyxin, NSAIDs, and opiates); (2) Type II reactions involve cytotoxic antibody-mediated responses, such as hemolytic anemia caused by penicillins or methyldopa; (3) Type III reactions consist of immune complex-mediated reactions, such as serum sicknesslike responses to dilantin, hydralazine, and heterologous sera; and (4) Type IV reactions are caused by delayed hypersensitivity mechanisms involving organs such as the skin (contact dermatitis to topical agents), the lung (to gold and nitrofurantoin) and the kidney (to NSAIDs). For this discussion, anaphylactic or anaphylactoid drug reactions are emphasized because of their acute and potentially life-threatening nature.

While no specific figures are available, the incidence of drug reactions during pregnancy must be considerably lower than in the nonpregnant state, probably because of the markedly reduced use of pharmacologic agents during this time. The decreased occurrence of anaphylaxis during pregnancy, noted previously, is consistent with this supposition.

Diagnosis

An exhaustive history generally identifies most agents that may be responsible for suspected drug-related reactions. The history should include the temporal relationship between exposure and symptoms; the route of administration, duration of therapy, and response to previous exposure; the presenting clinical manifestations; and the effect of drug discontinuation. Immediate skin testing should be considered when a drug becomes absolutely indicated for therapy and an IgE-mediated mechanism may exist (eg, penicillin, cephalosporin, insulin, toxoids, vaccines containing egg proteins, heterologous antisera, enzymes, hormones, and local anesthetics).

Prevention and Treatment

Prevention of reactions is the most effective way to minimize morbidity and mortality from drugs. Prevention entails avoidance of all drugs (and cross-reacting agents) suspected of causing previous reactions unless absolutely indicated for life-threatening illnesses. Documented cross-reactions occur between penicillins and cephalosporins, among the aminoglycosides (streptomycin, kanamycin, gentamycin, and neomycin), among the paraaminobenzene derivatives (sulfonamide antibiotics, sulfonylurea hypoglycemics, thiazide diuretics, acetazolamide, procaine, procainamide, and aminosalicylic acid), and between ASA and other NSAIDs.[99]

Treatment of drug reactions begins with the recognition of the association of symptoms and signs to the use of the drug, followed by its discontinuation and patient notification to avoid future exposure. If discontinuation fails to bring symptomatic relief, treatment of anaphylaxis, urticaria, asthma, or dermatitis should be instituted as described above. The approach to penicillin, insulin, and oxytocin allergy during pregnancy warrant additional comment.

Penicillin. Patients with histories of penicillin allergy who develop bacterial respiratory infections during pregnancy generally receive erythromycin because tetracyclines and sulfonamides are not recommended. For women who are intolerant to or unresponsive to erythromycin therapy, penicillin skin testing should be performed, preferably to penicillin G, penicilloyl polylysine (Prepen), and a minor determinant mixture. A negative skin test should be followed by oral administration of the penicillin or cephalosporin with physician observation for at least 30 minutes before parenteral or full-dose therapy begins. For pregnant patients with positive reactions to penicillin testing, antibiotics, such as clindamycin or chloramphenical, may be considered. Alternatively and depending on the specific clinical circumstances, penicillin desensitization may be indicated. On these rare occasions, an allergist or another physician skilled in desensitization should perform the procedure, preferably in an intensive care area equipped for anaphylaxis treatment and potential resuscitation.

Recently Wendel et al[100] described 15 pregnant women afflicted with serious infections (syphilis, listeriosis, and streptococcus viridins endocarditis) who had penicillin allergy documented by positive history (anaphylaxis, urticaria, asthma, or rash) and positive immediate skin tests (benzylpenicillin G, benxylpenicilloic acid, or penicilloyl polylysine). Using an oral desensitization protocol similar to one described recently[101], each patient was successfully desensitized over 4–6 hours permitting full-dose parenteral therapy with penicillin G or ampicillin immediately thereafter. During desensitization or early therapy, five of these 15 pregnant patients developed urticaria or pruritus. These reactions were mild, resolved spontaneously or after administration of diphenhydramine (25 mg intramuscularly) or intravenously and did not interfere with treatment. This study demonstrates that oral desensitization to penicillin in penicillin skin test-positive women permits relatively safe administration of penicillin to pregnant women with penicillin allergy and serious infections requiring penicillin.

Insulin. Diabetes may begin or be exacerbated during pregnancy (see also Chapter 43). Because oral hypoglycemic agents are contraindicated during pregnancy[102], certain women must therefore be started on insulin therapy during pregnancy. Some of these women may manifest local or systemic insulin allergy. Two recent cases of insulin allergy during pregnancy occurred in women with no history of insulin treatment. Gossain et al[103] described a four-month pregnant woman who developed generalized urticaria three weeks after initiation of therapy with mixed beef–pork insulin. Her reaction continued in spite of switching to purified pork and then to human insulin. She was subsequently successfully desensitized to human insulin. Yap[104] also described a 4-month pregnant patient who developed local reactions to pork insulin 11 days after initiation of therapy, associated with a strongly positive skin test to porcine insulin. Although she also was skin test-positive to human insulin, similar reactions did not occur when she was switched to human insulin.

Although these women manifested insulin allergy after institution of insulin for the first time, the majority of patients exhibiting allergic reactions to insulin have had interrupted insulin therapy. Because women with gestational diabetes may no longer need insulin therapy postpartum but may require it during a subsequent pregnancy, women with gestational diabetes mellitus may be at increased risk for intermittent insulin exposure and thus for development of insulin allergy. Because human insulin generally induces less specific IgE than nonhuman insulins[99], it would appear that human insulin should be used when insulin therapy is required for gestational diabetes. However, use of *human* insulin for gestational diabetes does not ensure that an immunologically mediated adverse reaction to insulin will not occur. Grammer et al[105] reported of a woman in whom the initiation of human insulin therapy for gestational diabetes caused large local reactions followed by insulin resistance associated with increased IgE and IgG against human insulin. In patients who manifest insulin allergy during pregnancy, skin testing and desensitization with human insulin is appropriate, as described in detail elsewhere.[99]

Oxytocin. Anaphylactoid reactions to oxytocin have been reported in several women. Most recently, oxytocin injection into several areas of the uterine myometrium and then systemically by infusion immediately after cesarean section caused severe anaphylaxis, manifested by facial and extremity numbness, chest tightness, urticaria or angioedema, and sustained hypotension, which required intravenous epinephrine for reversal.[84] Another woman experienced two separate cutaneous and hypotensive reactions within minutes following postpartum oxytocin administration[68], and a death attributed to oxytocin anaphylaxis has been described.[106] An anaphylactoid reaction during oxytocin infusion also occurred in another woman, but this episode could have been caused by thiopental.[106] Although the incidence of allergic reactions to oxytocin is undoubtedly small, obstetricians must recognize their presentation and intervene expeditiously.

PREVENTION OF ALLERGIC DISEASE IN THE INFANT

As mentioned in the beginning of this chapter, allergic disorders potentially cause morbidity in up to 20% of the population, and these illnesses appear to be increasing in prevalence and severity, as noted by increasing asthma deaths in the past decade. The phenotypic expression of allergic disease results from the interaction of the environment with an individual who is genotypically predisposed to react to minute amounts of allergen with a sustained allergen-specific IgE response. Efforts to prevent allergic disease must be directed toward modulating the environment to reduce the allergenic load and decrease nonspecific augmenting factors because genotypic manipulation remains unachievable. Even environmental preventive efforts remain formidable because they entail overcoming many risk factors (Table 53–15) that together act to induce IgE sensitization in at-risk infants.

Though not completely predictive of allergic disease, a family history of allergy and cord serum IgE levels appear to be important predictors of subsequent allergic disease. Infants born to parents with a uniparental or biparental history of allergic disease have a 30–60% chance, respectively, of developing allergies. Moreover, depending on the duration of follow-up, from 52–82% of infants with elevated cord IgE levels, compared with 5–30% of those with normal cord IgE levels, subsequently develop obvious or probable allergies during childhood (the higher percentages occurred with a follow-up of 8 years). Preventive efforts, if found rewarding, should be directed toward these high-risk infants.

The following recently documented findings have aided in delineating recommendations for allergic disease prevention. First, although the fetus possesses the immunologic capacity to produce nonspecific IgE as early as 11 weeks' gestation (which appears increased by maternal atopy, elevated IgE, and smoking), rarely does the infant evidence specific IgE to foods at birth.[107] Second, on *postnatal* ingestion of food, infants mount a brisk humoral immunologic response involving specific antibody of all the immunoglobulin classes. Specific food IgG, IgA, IgM, IgD, and a small transient IgE response represent the normal immunologic reaction of infants to foods. In contrast, infants with high atopic genotypes tend to show large and sustained IgE responses to these same foods that typically lead to food allergies.

Modulation of the infant's allergic response has been attempted prenatally and postnatally. Maternal avoidance of highly allergenic foods (milk and egg) *prenatally* during the third trimester *fails* to affect the incidence of allergic disease in high-risk infants.[108] Moreover, varying maternal diet *prenatally* with either a high or low content of egg or milk also fails to alter levels of cord blood IgE or IgG antibody against milk or egg.[107] Reductions in maternal weight gain during the third trimester also occur in mothers following these prenatal allergenic avoidance diets.[108, 109] Thus, maternal avoidance diets *must not* be instituted prenatally in an attempt to modify allergic disease in infancy[107] because they are ineffective and potentially malnutritious.

In contrast, recent studies suggest that delayed introduction of foods *postnatally* appears rewarding in reducing or delaying food allergy in infancy.[107,109-111] Maternal diets free of egg, milk, and fish during lactation for at least 3 months appear to reduce atopic dermatitis during the first 6 months of infancy.[110] Moreover, maternal avoidance diets during the entirety of lactation in infants supplemented or weaned with a casein hydrolysate formula (containing low molecular weight nonsensitizing peptides) instead of a cow's milk formula and avoiding solid foods for 6 months and all highly allergenic foods for 1 year appears to reduce food-induced allergic disorders (including atopic dermatitis, urticaria, and gastrointestinal disease) during the first year of life.[109] Because food allergy naturally wanes after the first year of life, differences were not observed by 2 years. Unfortunately, development of allergic rhinitis, asthma, and inhalant sensitization from infancy to 2 years of age are not affected by these food avoidance regimens.[109]

Much controversy still persists regarding whether breast-feeding prevents or reduces allergic disease because potentially allergenic food peptides pass through breast milk, which can sensitize susceptible infants. Specifically, exclusively breast-fed infants may develop anaphylaxis symptoms on their presumed first nonbreast exposure to egg, milk, or peanut.[119]

Nonfood environmental factors also affect the development of allergic disease. Maternal smoking during pregnancy increases geometric mean cord IgE levels and the incidence of elevated cord IgE levels.[112] Parental smoking postnatally increases infant serum IgE levels and increases incidences of specific IgE to pollen and foods, asthma, and allergic rhinitis.[112,113] Exposure to pollen and cat allergens in the first 6 months of life increases the risk of IgE sensitization and allergic disease.[114] Household dust mite antigen content above 2 μg/g in infancy increases the occurrence of dust mite sensitization by age 5.[115] Exposure to diesel exhaust fumes and other pollutants appears to increase greatly the risk of pollen allergy.[113] Finally, studies have indicated that viruses may function as cofactors to increase allergic disease in infants.[107]

Although it would be presumptuous to propose that allergic disease could be prevented entirely by implementation of specific environmental avoidance procedures, it may be possible to reduce, delay, or decrease the severity of certain types of infant allergy. It may be rewarding for those parents at high risk of producing an allergic infant to become knowledgeable about the factors influencing allergic sensitization and to implement preventive efforts with which they feel comfortable. An idealized strategy that could be implemented by interested and motivated parents

TABLE 53–15. RISK FACTORS IN DEVELOPMENT OF ATOPY

Hereditary (parental atopy)
Increased allergen exposure
Brief breast-feeding
Allergens in breast milk
Early solid food feeding
Increased household mite and pet exposure
Month or season of birth or weaning
Specific viral infections
Exposure to excessive cigarette smoke
Specific infant immunologic characteristics
Increased cord or serum IgE
Increased specific IgE (egg, mite)
Decreased T (T_8 subset) cells
Increased peripheral eosinophilia
Increased nasal eosinophilia or basophilia
Increased monocyte cyclic AMP phosphodieserase activity
Clinical signs
Recurrent wheezing in infancy
Recurrent croup

Reprinted with permission from Zeiger.[107]

TABLE 53–16. IDEALIZED STRATEGY AND METHODS FOR THE REDUCTION OF ALLERGIC DISEASE IN INFANTS

Strategy	Methods
1. Identify at-risk infant	Document biparental atopy Document elevated cord IgE
2. Prevent infant sensitization to	
a. Food allergens	
in breast milk	Maternal avoidance of major allergenic foods (egg, milk, peanut) during lactation (supplement with calcium 1500 mg daily)
in infant diet	Only breast milk or casein hydrolysate formula for at least 6 mo Delay introduction of solid foods until 6 mo Introduce allergenic foods as follows >1 year: cow's milk, soy, wheat, corn, citrus >2 years: egg, fish, peanut
b. Environmental allergens	Environmental control in home, especially child's room, for mite and mold No furry animals, carpeting, wool, or feathers. Air conditioner or purifier
3. Maximize immunologic competence	Breastfeed at least 6 mo
4. Minimize nonspecific enhancing factors	Discourage parental smoking; avoid viral illnesses (avoid daycare)

is summarized in Table 53–16. Such a strategy should not be prosletyzed but presented to those families requesting assistance.

REFERENCES

1. Ishizaka T. Mechanisms of IgE-mediated hypersensitivity. In: Middleton E Jr, Reed CE, Ellis EF, et al, eds. *Allergy: Principles and Practice.* 3rd ed. St. Louis, MO: CV Mosby Co; 1988:71.
2. Wasserman SI. Mediators of immediate hypersensitivity. *J All Clin Immunol.* 1983;72:101.
3. Saxon A. Immediate hypersensitivity: Approach to diagnosis. In: Lawlor GJ, Fischer TJ, eds. *Manual of Allergy and Immunology.* 2nd ed. Boston, MA: Little Brown & Co; 1988:15.
4. American Academy of Allergy. Position Statement. Skin testing and radio-allergosorbent testing (RAST) for diagnosis of specific allergens responsible for IgE-mediated diseases. *J All Clin Immunol.* 1983;72:515.
5. Haas F, Haas SS. *The Essential Asthma Book.* New York, NY: Ivy Books; 1987:158.
6. Zeiger RS, Schatz M. Immunotherapy of atopic disorders. Present state of the art and future perspectives. *Med Clin North Am.* 1981;65:987.
7. Van Metre TE, Adkinson MF. Immunotherapy for Aeroallergen Disease. In: Middleton E, Reed CE, Ellis EF, et al, eds. *Allergy: Principles and Practice.* 3rd ed. St. Louis, Mo: CV Mosby Co; 1988:1327.
8. Metzger WJ, Turner E, Patterson R. The safety of immunotherapy during pregnancy. *J All Clin Immunol.* 1978;61:268.
9. Corrao WH, Brenner SS, Irwin RS. Chronic cough as the sole presenting manifestation of bronchial asthma. *N Engl J Med.* 1979;300:633.
10. Lusk JA, Winterbauer DF, Dreis DF, et al. Dyspnea of unknown etiology: Prospective study of 92 consecutive cases. *Am Rev Respir Dis.* 1986;133:A56.
11. Pennock BE, Rogers RM, McCaffree DR. Changes in measured spirometric index. What is significant. *Chest.* 1981;80:97.
12. Kanner RE, Morris AH, eds. *Clinical Pulmonary Function Testing. A Manual of Uniform Laboratory Procedures for the Intermountain Area. Salt Lake City: Intermountain Thoracic Society; 1975:1.*
13. Chai H, Farr Rs, Froehlich LA, et al. Standardization of bronchial inhalation challenge procedures. *J All Clin Immunol.* 1975;56:323.
14. Hargreave FE, Ryan G, Thomson NC, et al. Bronchial responsiveness to histamine or methacholine in asthma: Management and clinical significance. *J All Clin Immunol.* 1981;68:347.
15. Gerrard JW. Genetic factors in the development of asthma. In: Weiss ER, Segal MS, Stein M, eds. *Bronchial Asthma: Mechanisms and Therapeutics.* 2nd ed. Boston, MA: Little, Brown and Co; 1985:24.
16. Nadel JL, Sheppard D. Mechanisms of bronchial hyperreactivity in asthma. In: Weiss ER, Segal MS, Stein M, eds. *Bronchial Asthma: Mechanisms and Therapeutics.* 2nd Ed. Boston, MA: Little, Brown and Co; 1985:30.
17. Busse WW, Reed CE. Asthma: Definition and pathogenesis. In: Middleton E, Reed CE, Ellis EF, et al, eds. *Allergy: Principles and Practices.* 3rd Ed. St. Louis, MO: CV Mosby Co; 1988:969.
18. Wanner A. Airway mucus and the mucociliary system. In: Middleton E, Reed CE, Ellis EF, et al, eds. *Allergy: Principles and Practice.* 3rd ed. St. Louis, MO: CV Mosby Co; 1988:541.
19. Mathison DA. Asthma in adults: Diagnosis and treatment. In: Middleton E, Reed CE, Ellis EF, et al, eds. *Allergy: Principles and Practices.* 3rd ed. St. Louis, MO: CV Mosby Co; 1988:1063.
20. Gibbs CJ, Coutts II, Lock R, et al. Premenstrual exacerbation of asthma. *Thorax.* 1984;39:833.
21. Eliasson O, Scherzer HH, DeGraff AC. Morbidity in asthma in relation to the menstrual cycle. *J All Clin Immunol.* 1986;77:87.
22. Williams DA. Asthma and pregnancy. *Acta Allergol (Kbh).* 1967;22:311.
23. Gluck JC, Gluck PA. The effects of pregnancy on asthma: A prospective study. *Ann All.* 1976;37:164.
24. Schatz M, Harden K, Forsythe A, et al. The course of asthma during pregnancy, postpartum and with successive pregnancies: A prospective analysis. *J All Clin Immunol.* 1988;81:509.
25. Schatz M, Hoffman C. Interrelationships between asthma and pregnancy: Clinical and mechanistic considerations. *Clin Rev All.* 1987;5:301.
26. Gordon M, Niswander KR, Berendes H, Kantor AG. Fetal morbidity following potentially anoxigenic obstetric conditions. VII. Bronchial asthma. *Am J Obstet Gynecol.* 1970;106:421.
27. Bhana SL, Bjerkedal T. The course and outcome of pregnancy in women with bronchial asthma. *Acta Allergol.* 1972;27:397.
28. Dombrowski MD, Bottoms SF, Boike GM, Wald J. Incidence of preeclampsia among asthmatic patients lower with theophylline. *Am J Obstet Gynecol.* 1986;155:265.
29. Schatz M, Patterson R, O'Rourke J, et al. Corticosteroid therapy for the pregnant asthmatic patient. *JAMA.* 1975;233:804.
30. Greenberger PA, Patterson R. Beclomethasone diproprionate for severe asthma during pregnancy. *Ann Intern Med.* 1983;98:478.
31. Greenberger PA, Patterson R. The outcome of pregnancy complicated by severe asthma. *Allergy Proc.* 1988;9:539.
32. Stenius-Aarniala R, Piirila P, Teramo K. Asthma and pregnancy: a prospective study of 198 pregnancies. *Thorax.* 1988;43:12.
33. Schaefer G, Silverman R. Pregnancy complicated by asthma. *Am J Obstet Gynecol.* 1961;82:182.
34. Schatz M, Zeiger RS, Hoffman CP. A prospective analysis of perinatal mortality and morbidity in 360 pregnancies complicated by maternal asthma. Submitted for publication.
35. Cnattingius S, Haglund B, Meirik O. Cigarette smoking as risk factors for late fetal and early neonatal death. *Br Med J.* 1988;297:258.
36. Shiono PH, Klebanoff MA, Rhoads GG. Smoking and drinking during pregnancy: Their effect on preterm birth. *JAMA.* 1986;255:82.
37. Fischl MA, Pitchenik A, Gardner LB. An index predicting relapse and need for hospitalization in patients with acute bronchial asthma. *N Engl J Med.* 1981;305:783.
38. Fanta CH, Rossing TH, McFadden ER Jr. Treatment of acute asthma. *Am J Med.* 1986;80:5.
39. Nowak RM, Tomlanovich MC, Sarkar DD, et al. Arterial blood gases and pulmonary function testing in acute bronchial asthma. *JAMA.* 1983;249:2043.
40. Moore LG, Rounds SS, Jahnigen D, et al. Infant birthweight is related to maternal arterial oxygenation at high altitude. *J Appl Physiol.* 1982;52:695.
41. Whittmore R, Hobbins JC, Engle MA. Pregnancy and its outcome in women with and without surgical treatment of congenital heart disease. *Am J Cardiol.* 1982;50:641.
42. Schatz M, Zeiger RS, Hoffman CP, et al. Intrauterine growth is related to gestational pulmonary function in pregnant asthmatic women. *Chest.* 1990; 98:389.
43. Larsson K. Studies of sympatho-adrenal reactivity and adrenoreceptor function in bronchial asthma. *Eur J Resp Dis.* 1985;66(suppl):1.
44. Kaliner M, Shelhamer JH, Davis PB, et al. Autonomic nervous system abnormalities and allergy. *Ann Intern Med.* 1982;96:349.
45. Bertrand JM, Riley SP, Papkin J, Coates AL. The long-term pulmonary sequelae of prematurity: The role of familial airway hyperreactivity and the respiratory distress syndrome. *N Engl J Med.* 1985;312:742.

46. Huff BB, ed. *Physicians' Desk Reference*. Oradell, New Jersey: Medical Economics Co; 1987:711.
47. Bowton DL, Alford PT, McLees BD, et al. The effect of aminophylline on cerebral blood flow in patients with chronic obstructive pulmonary disease. *Chest*. 1987;91:874.
48. Reinisch JM, Simon NG, Karow WG, Gandelman R. Prenatal exposure to prednisone in humans and animals retards intrauterine growth. *Science*. 1978;202:436.
49. Chan KN, Noble-Jamieson CM, Elliman A, et al. Airway responsiveness in low birthweight children and their mothers. *Arch Dis Child*. 1988;63:905.
50. Schatz M, Hoffman CP, Zeiger RS, et al. The course and management of asthma and allergic disease during pregnancy. In: Middleton E, Reed CE, Ellis EF, et al, eds. *Allergy: Principles and Practices*. 3rd Ed. St. Louis, MO: CV Mosby Co; 1988:1093.
51. Schatz M, Zeiger RS, Harden K, et al. The safety of inhaled beta-agonist bronchodilators during pregnancy. *J All Clin Immunol*. 1988;82:686.
52. Heinonen O, Slone D, Shapiro S. *Birth Defects and Drugs in Pregnancy*. Littleton, MA. PSG Publishing Co; 1977.
53. Wilson J. Utilization de cromoglycate de sodium a cours de la grossessa. *Acta Ther*. 1982;8(suppl):45.
54. Newhouse MT, Dolovich MG. Control of asthma by aerosols. *N Engl J Med*. 1986;315:870.
55. Greenberger PA, Paterson R. Management of asthma during pregnancy. *N Engl J Med*. 1985;312:897.
56. Mabry RL. Rhinitis of pregnancy. *South Med J*. 1986;79:965.
57. Schatz M, Zeiger RS. Diagnosis and management of rhinitis during pregnancy. *NER Allergy Proc*. 1988;9:545.
58. Sorri M, Hartikainen-Sorri AL, Karja J. Rhinitis during pregnancy. *Rhinology*. 1980;18:83.
59. Jick H, Holmes LB, Hunter JR, et al. First-trimester drug use and congenital disorders. *JAMA*. 1981;246:343.
60. Saxen I. Cleft palate and maternal diphenhydramine intake (letter). *Lancet*. 1974;1:407.
61. Erez S, Schifrin BS, Dirim O. Double-blind evaluation of hydroxyzine as an antiemetic in pregnancy. *J Reprod Med*. 1971;7:35.
62. Wasserman SI, Marquardt DL. Anaphylaxis. In: Middleton E, Reed CE, Ellis EF, et al, eds. *Allergy: Principles and Practice*. 3rd ed. St. Louis, MO: CV Mosby; 1988:1365.
63. Hayashi RH. Emergency care in pregnancy. In: Queenan JT, ed. *Management of High Risk Pregnancy*. Oradell, NJ: Medical Economics; 1985:447.
64. Sharpe O, Hall EG. Renal impairment, hypertension, and encephalomalacia in an infant surviving severe intrauterine anoxia. *Proc R Soc Med*. 1953;46:1063.
65. Erasmus C, Blackwood W, Wilson J. Infantile multicystic encephalomalacia after maternal anaphylaxis during pregnancy. *Arch Dis Child*. 1982;57:785.
66. Entman SS, Moise KJ. Anaphylaxis in pregnancy. *South Med J*. 1984;77:402.
67. Klein VR, Harris AP, Abraham RA, Neibyl JR. Fetal distress during a maternal systemic allergic reaction. *Obstet Gynecol*. 1984;64(suppl):158.
68. Slater RM, Bowles BJM, Pumphrey RSH. Anaphylactoid reactions to oxytocin in pregnancy. *Anaesthesia* 1985;40:655.
69. Stafford CT, Lobel SA, Fruge BC, et al. Anaphylaxis to human serum albumin. *Annals Allergy*. 1988;61:85.
70. Lund N. Anaphylactoid reaction to infusion of polygelatin (Haemacel), *Anaesthesia*. 1980;35:655.
71. Searcy CJ, Kushner M, Nell P, Beckmann CRB. Anaphylactic reaction to intravenous conjugated estrogens. *Clin Parm*. 1987;6:74
72. Meggs WJ, Pescouitz OH, Metcalfe D, et al. Progesterone sensitivity as a cause of recurrent anaphylaxis. *N Engl J Med*. 1984;311:1236.
73. Smith HS, Hare MJ, Hoggarth DE, Assen ESE. Delivery as a cause of exercise-induced anaphylactoid reaction: Case report. *Br J Obstet Gynaec*. 1985;92:1196.
74. Baraka A, Sfeir S. Anaphylactic cardiac arrest in a parturient: response of the newborn. *JAMA*. 1980;243:1745.
75. Lawlor GJ, Rosenblatt HM. Anaphylaxis. In: Lawlor GJ, Fischer TJ, eds. *Manual of Allergy and Immunology*. 2nd ed. Boston, MA: Little, Brown & Co; 1988:225.
76. Sheffer A. Anaphylaxis. *J All Clin Immunol*. 1985;75:227.
77. Seager SJ, MacDonald R. Laryngeal oedema and preeclampsia. *Anaesthesia*. 1980;35:360.
78. Bhatia PL, Singh MS, Jha BK. Laryngopathia gravidarum. *Ear Nose Throat J*. 1981;60:408.
79. Frank MM, Gelfand JA, Atkinson JP. Hereditary angioedema: The clinical syndrome and its management. *Ann Intern Med*. 1976;84:580.
80. Schartz HJ, Golden DBK, Lockey RF. Venom immunotherapy in the hymenoptera-allergic pregnant patient. *J All Clinc Immunol*. 1990;85:709.
81. Witter FR, Niebyl JR. Drug intoxication and anaphylactic shock in the obstetric patient. In: Berkowitz RL, ed. *Critical Care of the Obstetric Patient*. New York, NY: Churchill Livingstone; 1983:527.
82. Eng M, Berges PV, Voland K, et al. The effect of methoxamine and ephedrine in normotensive pregnant primates. *Anesth*. 1971;35:354.
83. Barach E, Nowak R, Tennyson G, Tomlanovich M. Epinephrine for treatment of anaphylactic shock. *JAMA*. 1984;251:2118.
84. Kawarabayashi T, Narisawa Y, Nakamura K, et al. Anaphylactoid reaction to oxytocin during cesarean section. *Gynecol Obstet Invest*. 1988;25:277.
85. Gallagher JS. Anaphylaxis in pregnancy. *Obst Gynecol*. 1988;71:491.
86. Soter NA, Wasserman SI. Clinical manifestations, pathogenesis and therapeutic approaches in urticaria/angioedema. *Dermatol. Dig*. 1979; 18:17.
87. Champion RH, Roberts SOB, Carpenter RG, Roger JH. Urticaria and angioedema. *Br J Dermatol*. 1969;81:588.
88. Farah F, Shtaklu A. Autoimmune progesterone urticaria. *J All Clin Immunol*. 1971;48:257.
89. Warin RD, Cunliffer WT, Greaves MW, Wallington TB. Recurrent angioedema: Familial and estrogen induced. *Br J Dermatol*. 1986;115:731.
90. Postnikoff IM, Pritzker KP. Hereditary angioneurotic edema: an unusual case of maternal mortality. *J Forensic Sci*. 1979;24:473.
91. Bierman SM. Autoimmune progesterone dermatitis of pregnancy. *Arch Dermatol*. 1973;107:896.
92. Holmes RC, Black MM. The specific dermatoses of pregnancy. *J Am Acad Dermatol*. 1983;8:405.
93. Stiller RJ, Kaplan BM, Andreoli JW. Hereditary angioedema and pregnancy. *Obstet Gynecol*. 1984;64:133.
94. Adverse effects of danazol in pregnancy. *Ann Intern Med*. 1982;96:672. Editorial.
95. Zeiger RS. Atopic dermatitis of childhood: Current concepts and management. *Immunol Allergy Practice*. 1981;3:198.
96. Hanifin JM. Atopic dermatitis. In: Middleton E, Reed EC, Ellis EF, et al, eds. *Allergy: Principles and Practice*. 3rd ed. St. Louis, MO: CV Mosby; 1988:1403.
97. Hanifin JM, Lobitz WC. Newer concepts of atopic dermatitis. *Arch Dermatol*. 1977;113:663.
98. Roth HL, Kierland RR. The natural history of atopic dermatitis. *Arch Dermatol*. 1964;89:209.
99. De Swarte RD, Schatz M, Grammer L, Greenberger PA. Drug allergy. In: Patterson R, ed. *Allergic Disease: Diagnosis and Management*. Philadelphia, PA: JB Lippincott; 1985:505.
100. Wendel GD, Stark BJ, Jamison RB, et al. Penicillin allergy and desensitization in serious infections during pregnancy. *N Engl J Med*. 1985;312:1229.
101. Sullivan TJ, Yecies LD, Shatz GS, et al. Desensitization of patients allergic to penicillin using orally administered beta-lactam antibiotics. *J All Clin Immunol*. 1982;69:275.
102. Adam PAJ, Schwartz R.: Diagnosis and treatment: Should oral hypoglycemic agents be used in pediatric and pregnant patients. *Pediatrics*. 1968;42:819.
103. Gossain VV, Rovner DR, Mohan K. Systemic allergy to human (recombinant DNA) insulin. *Ann Allegy*. 1985;55:116.
104. Yap PK. Primary allergy to monocomponent porcine insuline. *Postgrad Med J*. 1985;61:629.
105. Grammer LC, Metzger B, Fitzsimons R, et al. IgE and IgG against human (recombinant DNA) insulin in patients with local insulin allergy followed by immunologic insulin resistance (abstract). *J All Clin Immunol*. 1986;77:134.
106. Giuffrida JG, Singh S, Bizzarri DN. Anaphylaxis to thiopental or oxytocin. *Anesth Rev*. 1981;8:30.
107. Zeiger RS. Development and prevention of allergic disease in childhood. In: Middleton E, Reed EE, Ellis EF, et al, eds. *Allergy: Principles and Practice*. 3rd ed. St. Louis, MO: CV Mosby Co; 1988:930.
108. Falth-Magnusson K, Kjellman NIM. Development of atopic disease in babies whose mothers were receiving exclusion diet during pregnancy—A randomized study. *J All Clin Immunol*. 1987;80:868.
109. Zeiger RS, Heller S, Mellon MH, et al. Effect of combined maternal and infant food allergen avoidance on development of atopy in early infancy. A randomized study. *J All Clin Immunol*. 1989;84:72.
110. Hattevig G, Kjellman B, Sigurs N, et al. The effect of maternal avoidance of egg, cow's milk and fish during lactation upon allergic manifestations in infants. *Clin Exp Allergy*. 1989;19:27.
111. Chandra RK, Puri S, Suraiya C, Cheema PS. Influence of maternal food antigen avoidance during pregnancy and lactation on incidence of atopic eczema in infants. *Clinical Allergy*. 1986;16:563.
112. Magnusson CGM. Maternal smoking influences cord serum IgE and IgD levels and increases the risk for subsequent infant allergy. *J All Clin Immunol*. 1986;78:898.
113. Bjorksten B, Kjellman NIM. Perinatal factors influencing the development of allergy. *Clin Rev All*. 1987;5:339.
114. Kjellman NIM, Andrae S, Croner S, et al. Epidemiology and prevention of allergy. *Immunol Allergy Practice*. 1988;10:393.
115. Platts-Mills TAE, de Weck AL. Dust mite allergens in asthma. *J All Clin Immunol*. 1989;83:416.

PART VIII | Infectious Diseases

Stanley A. Gall, Section Editor

A

General Aspects of Infectious Diseases

Chapter Fifty-Four

The Approach to Infectious Diseases

Jay F. Dobkin

54

Several dramatic developments have remarkably altered the clinical approach to infectious diseases in recent years. New disease processes such as legionnaires' disease, Lyme disease, toxic shock syndrome, and acquired immune deficiency syndrome (AIDS) have appeared. Old diseases such as syphilis and tuberculosis have surged back into prominence. The techniques of modern biology have opened an era in which a recombinant hepatitis B vaccine and a growing roster of effective antiviral drugs have become realities. New classes of antibiotics, such as the advanced generation cephalosporins, and the quinolones, have been developed and promise to register a major impact on serious bacterial infections. The widening spectrum of infectious etiologies and the availability of more therapeutic modalities have made it even more important to adhere to the standard precepts of infectious disease practice in seeking, wherever possible, a specific etiology and using therapy as specifically tailored as possible to that etiology.

PATHOGENESIS OF INFECTION

The normal microbial flora of the body plays a critical role in both health and disease[1] (Table 54–1). Low virulence organisms, ordinarily found in areas such as the gastrointestinal tract, may, under such circumstances as aspiration of oral contents or penetration of the colon, cause infectious disease syndromes. Correspondingly, many pathogens must take up residence among the normal flora before they can invade and cause disease. The difficulty of implanting new organisms among the intact normal flora has been termed *colonization resistance.* Conditions or such iatrogenic interventions as antibiotics that disturb the normal flora appear to promote the proliferation of pathogens. Several disease processes appear to arise from disturbances of the normal flora balance without invasion by exogenous pathogens. One example is the syndrome of antibiotic-associated colitis, in which disturbance of the normal gut flora by antibiotics provokes *Clostridium difficile* to elaborate diarrhea-producing toxins.

The normal flora of the skin includes coagulase-negative staphylococci (*Staphylococcus epidermidis*) and a variety of anaerobic nonspore-forming gram-positive rods, especially *Propionibacterium acnes.* The oral cavity usually is colonized by facultative streptococci of the viridans group and a variety of microaerophilic and anaerobic organisms including *Fusobacterium* species and spirochetes. In the presence of gingival disease, the variety and density of anaerobic organisms increases dramatically and plays a major role in the pathogenesis of aspiration pneumonia. Oropharyngeal colonization with pathogens such as *Streptococcus pneumoniae, Hemophilus influenzae,* and *Neisseria meningitidis* may occur in 5–10% of adults without these infections. Short-term colonization with these organisms precedes actual infection.

Under normal conditions, the gastrointestinal tract has minimal bacterial flora between the stomach and the distal small intestine. In the large bowel, anaerobes predominate at a ratio of at least 100 to 1 over aerobes, with gram-positive nonspore-forming rods such as lactobacilli and *Eubacterium* species often the most common (Table 54–2).

The normal flora of the large intestine is the most com-

TABLE 54–1. PREDOMINANT MICROORGANISMS INHABITING VARIOUS SURFACES OF THE HEALTHY HUMAN BODY

Skin
Staphylococci
Corynebacteria
Propionibacteria
Candida species
Dermatophytic fungi
Oropharynx
Viridans (alpha hemolytic) streptococci
Staphylococci
Streptococcus pyogenes
Streptococcus pneumoniae
Branhamella catarrhalis
Neisseria species
Lactobacilli
Corynebacteria
Hemophilus species
Obligate anaerobes (not *Bacteroides fragilis*)
Candida albicans
Various protozoa
Nasopharynx
Staphylococci (including *Staphylococcus aureus*)
Streptococci (including *Streptococcus pneumoniae*)
Branhamella catarrhalis
Neisseria species
Hemophilus species
Conjunctiva
Staphylococci
Corynebacteria
Hemophilus species
Upper intestine
Streptococci
Lactobacilli
Candida species
Lower genitourinary tract (female)
See Table 54–3.
Large intestine and feces
See Table 54–2.

plex and probably the most significant in both health and disease. Most information on the colonic flora is derived from enumeration studies that are very laborious, semiquantitative at best, and difficult to reproduce. The normal human colon contains over 600 identifiable species of bacteria and many others that have never been taxonomically classified. With a density of 10^{12} organisms per gram of stool the complexity and magnitude of the normal human flora has made it difficult for investigators to define its precise physiologic role and the subtle disturbances that may contribute to or arise from disease processes.[2,3] More recent approaches using metabolic functions of the intact gut flora rather than the enumeration of bacterial species have demonstrated some striking properties. Metabolic functions such as the production of methane and the degradation of the cardiac glycoside digoxin are distinct and stable characteristics of the gut flora of a large fraction of healthy human subjects.[4-6] In contrast to the impression left by the enumeration studies, these recent investigations indicate that the metabolic activity of the gut flora undergoes a slow and progressive maturation during childhood and adolescence before the adult patterns are fully established.[7]

Clinical Microbiology of the Female Genital Tract

Although the fallopian tubes and endometrium are normally sterile, the cervix and vagina contain a complex microbial flora that changes with age, menstruation, and pregnancy (Table 54–3). In prepubertal girls, lactobacillus colonization of the vagina is less extensive than after menarche but *Bacteroides* are more common. Diphtheroids (gram-positive, nonspore-forming rods) are common in both groups. *S epidermidis*, yeasts, and *Gardnerella vaginalis* are present as well.[8,9] After menarche, an increase in colonization by lactobacilli occurs that is associated with and a possible cause of acidification of the vaginal contents that protects against colonization by pathogenic organisms. Lactobacilli are the predominant species in the adult female genital tract and are found in up to 95% of women studied.[10-13] Little change in the normal flora has been noted in pregnant women except for an increase in aerobic lactobacilli associated with an overall increase in total facultative organisms.[14] In the postpartum period, regardless of the method of delivery, substantial changes have been noted compared to late pregnancy, including a decrease in lactobacilli and increased *Bacteroides fragilis*, as well as other aerobic and anaerobic gram-negative rods.[10,13,15] Some variation has been noted during the menstrual cycle, with the number of detectable species increasing but the total quantity of bacteria decreasing during menstruation.[13] Among the gram-positive aerobic cocci group B streptococci are commonly found while group A streptococci are infrequent. Group B streptococci have become increasingly appreciated as important members of the vaginal flora and are found in up to 35% of healthy pregnant women. These organisms are important causes of postpartum sepsis in both the newborn and the mother. *S epidermidis* is another commonly isolated organism with minimal pathogenic potential in this setting, while *Staphylococcus aureus* is uncommonly found, although colonization may be promoted by tampon use and may lead to *toxic shock syndrome*.

The microflora of the female genital tract is probably influenced by its proximity to the rectum but differs in important ways from the fecal flora. Some colonic organisms, such as the enterococcus, are commonly found in the vaginal flora, but others, such as *Escherichia coli* and *B fragilis*, are uncommon. It appears that childbirth, surgery, or other forms of trauma promote vaginal colonization by these fecal strains, which are then positioned to establish urogenital infection.[10,13,16] Among the aerobic gram-negative bacilli, *E coli* is the most common organism isolated in vaginal specimens and is correspondingly the most common etiology for community-acquired urinary tract infections in women. Other coliform organisms such as *Klebsiella* species are found with a low frequency of less than 15% in normal vaginal contents. Other aerobic gram-negative rods resistant to commonly-used antibiotics, such as *Pseudomonas*, *Citrobacter*, and *Providencia*, are rarely isolated from the vaginal contents of normal healthy women but may be found in hospitalized patients, especially after treatment with antibiotics.

Anaerobic organisms account for a substantial portion of the normal vaginal flora. Anaerobic streptococci are commonly isolated and may be important pathogens, especially in mixed infections. Species of clostridia are found in less than 10% of asymptomatic women and are potential pathogens, but may be isolated from asymptomatic women also. Bacteroides species, including members of the *B fragilis* group and organisms such as *Bacteroides bivius* and *Bacteroides disiens*, are major pathogens in pelvic infectious processes and are usually resistant to penicillin drugs.

TABLE 54–2. NORMAL FLORA OF THE LARGE INTESTINE

Category or Species	Percent of Subjects Carrying Organism	Mean Count in Carriers (log 10)
Gram-negative bacilli (aerobic or facultative)		
Escherichia coli	86	6.5
Klebsiella pneumoniae	43	4.7
Enterobacter cloacae	28	3.9
Facultative streptococci		
Enterococcus faecalis	78	6.5
Other streptococci	100	8.0
Other facultative or aerobic organisms		
Bacillus species	86	4.2
Yeasts	50	4.5
Staphylococcus epidermidis	36	4.8
Lactobacillus species (all)	100	10.1
Anaerobic cocci (all)	78	9.6
Peptostreptococci	64	7.9
Bacteroides (all)	100	11.7
Bacteroides fragilis group	93	11.1
Eubacterium species (all)	93	10.4
Bifidobacterium (all)	64	7.8
Clostridium (all)	93	8.4

Modified from Finegold.[2]

Several other organisms recoverable from cervical and vaginal specimens are strongly associated with disease processes but may be recovered from asymptomatic individuals as well. The frequency of detecting such organisms as *Neisseria gonorrhoeae, Trichomonas vaginalis, Chlamydia trachomatis,* and herpes simplex reflects the degree of sexual exposure of the woman to these infectious agents.[17]

Microbial Virulence and the Pathogenesis of Infection

A rigid distinction is no longer made between virulent and nonvirulent microorganisms since it has become clear that any microbe capable of reproducing on or in human tissue is capable of producing infection under some circumstances. This is especially evident with debilitated and immunosuppressed hosts. The detailed examination of microbial viru-

TABLE 54–3. VAGINAL FLORA AT DIFFERENT STAGES OF LIFE

Frequency of Organism Isolated in Indicated Group	Prepubertal Girls	Normal Adult Women (Nonmenstruating)	Pregnant Women	Postmenopausal Women
More than 50%	Diphtheroids *Staphylococcus epidermidis* *Bacteroides melaninogenicus* Anaerobic gram-positive cocci	Diphtheroids *Staphylococcus epidermidis* Lactobacilli Anaerobic gram-positive cocci Group D streptococci	Diphtheroids Lactobacilli *Staphylococcus epidermidis* *Candida albicans* Group D streptococci	Diphtheroids Lactobacilli *Staphylococcus epidermidis*
20–50%	*Bacteroides fragilis* *Clostridium perfringens* *Escherichia coli* *Candida albicans* Lactobacilli Genital mycoplasmas *Streptococcus viridans*	*Bacteroides* species *Escherichia coli* *Streptococcus viridans* Anaerobic gram-positive cocci *Staphylococcus epidermidis*	*Escherichia coli* Anaerobic gram-positive cocci *Bacteroides* species	Gram-negative bacilli *Streptococcus viridans* *Bacteroides* species Group D streptococci
Fewer than 20%	*Corynebacterium vaginale* *Candida* species	Group B streptococci Group A streptococci *Staphylococcus aureus*	Group B streptococci Group A streptococci Anaerobic gram-positive cocci *Staphylococcus aureus*	

Adapted from references 8–17.

lence properties and host–microbe interactions has elucidated the means by which some microorganisms produce infection more readily than others. In clinical practice a distinction still needs to be made between infection, colonization, and contamination. In true infection, a reproducing microorganism causes signs and symptoms of disease or at least evidence of immunologic recognition by the host, usually reflected by production of a specific antibody. In colonization, the organism merely reproduces on the surface of the host. Contamination implies the false-positive identification of a microorganism that has entered a diagnostic specimen from the environment in the process of collection, transport, or laboratory processing.

The concept of microbial virulence is supported by the classic demonstration that the pneumococcal capsule is a major determinant of pathogenicity, since unencapsulated ("rough strain") mutants are noninfectious in animal models. Similar roles for bacterial encapsulation have been demonstrated for *H influenzae, Klebsiella,* and for the fungus *Cryptococcus neoformans.* Extracellular products of bacteria have long been recognized to be important pathogenic factors, as in the case of the DN-ase and hyaluronidase produced by group A streptococci, which promote connective tissue destruction, allowing organisms to spread and proliferate.

The concept of microbial virulence and interaction with host susceptibility has recently been substantially clarified with respect to urinary tract infections (UTIs). While *E coli* is known to be the most frequent pathogen, certain serotypes with distinct features cause UTIs with a disproportionately high frequency compared to their representation in the fecal flora. Ability to adhere to uroepithelial cells appears to be a key virulence factor.[18-20] Type 1 or *mannose-sensitive* fimbriae on many gram-negative rods mediate adherence to the lower tract epithelium, whereas the more restricted group of strains with *mannose-resistant P fimbriae* are much more likely to reach the renal pelvis and parenchyma.[21,22] It also appears that expression of this virulence factor can be modulated to the benefit of the bacterium and detriment of the host. Expression of the type 1 fimbriae, which facilitate adherence to urinary slime in the bladder[23] but also increase susceptibility to neutrophil phagocytosis, is decreased once the organism reaches the kidney.[18,24] Host variability may also play a role in pathogenesis since women with a high frequency of UTIs appear to have an increased density of uroepithelial receptors for bacterial fimbriae.[25]

Host Defenses

Susceptibility or resistance of the host to an infecting microbe is a function of specific as well as nonspecific defense mechanisms. Nonspecific defenses play a crucial role but are rarely appreciated, except when they fail. These include normal intact skin and mucous membranes, the unobstructed drainage of organs producing secretions, and such basic neuromuscular functions as the gag and pain reflexes. Even the ability to move and ambulate might be viewed as a host defense against skin breakdown and subsequent infection. Examples of defects in these systems that predispose to infection range from the obvious, such as a contaminated traumatic surgical wound, to the occult—a subclinical bronchogenic carcinoma, obstructing airway drainage and presenting as a postobstructive pneumonia.

The interrelation between microbial colonization, trauma, and instrumentation has been defined in the pathogenesis of postpartum endometritis.[26,27] Several factors contribute independently to the risk of amniotic fluid infection (labor, ruptured membranes), which, in turn, predispose to endometritis.[28-30] Iatrogenic factors contribute substantially to this risk, which is reflected in the strong association of endometritis with cesarean section.

Circulating polymorphonculear neutrophil leukocytes (PMNs) provide a nonspecific but vital first line of defense against invading bacteria and fungi. In granulocytopenia, which is most often a byproduct of cancer chemotherapy or other drug side effects, there is a quantitative inverse relationship between the number of PMNs and the risk of bacterial infection. When counts of circulating PMNs fall below 500 per milliliter, infection risk rises proportionally.[31] At counts below 100, the majority of patient days are complicated by infection, and the rapid development of sepsis with gram-negative rods such as *Pseudomonas aeruginosa* often occurs. Qualitative defects of certain granulocyte functions such as chemotaxis are established as the pathogenic mechanism in Job's syndrome[32] and may play an important role in the predisposition to infection in alcohol abusers.[33] Similarly, intracellular killing by PMNs is defective in chronic granulomatous disease and myeloperoxidase deficiency.[34]

Specific immunity to infecting pathogens traditionally has been divided between a humoral arm, in which antibodies are produced by B lymphocytes, and a cellular arm, in which T cells and other lymphocytes and macrophages interact to destroy tumor cells, cells infected with intracellular pathogens such as *Mycobacterium tuberculosis,* and viruses. Although the intricacy of the immunoregulatory pathways between the components of the immune system is becoming clearer[35], it is still useful to appreciate the clinical syndromes classically associated with a deficit in one, but not the other, of these arms.

The importance of antibody-mediated immunity, a major component of the humoral immune system, is well established, based on observations in patients with congenital absence of gamma globulin, in patients with chronic lymphocytic leukemia, and in patients with multiple myeloma who appear to lack quantitatively sufficient immunoglobulin.[36-38] Manifestations of immunoglobulin deficiency include susceptibility to encapsulated pyogenic bacterial infection, which reflects the importance of antibody in opsonizing these bacteria to facilitate phagocytosis. The development of intravenous gamma globulin maintenance therapy has proven to be very useful in congenital deficiency states. Its role appears minimal in conditions such as multiple myeloma, where increased catabolism rather than decreased production of IgG occurs.[39] Absence of certain complement components has been linked to increased susceptibility to infection with *Neisseria* species such as the gonococcus and meningococcus. Patients with recurrent infections with either of these organisms should be screened for the absence of the late complement components.[40] A combination of factors including antibody deficiency and hyposplenism is thought to be important in diseases such as sickle cell anemia, in which encapsulated bacteria are prominent pathogens.[41] A new and potentially sizeable source of adult patients with abnormal antibody production is HIV infection. Polyclonal hyperglobulinemia is a prominent manifestation of the syndrome, and inability to form antibody in response to polysaccharide antigens appears to be a relatively early manifestation of the immunoregulatory disorder of AIDS.[42] The role of HIV-associated humoral disorders in the pathogenesis of infectious complications is, however, not yet clear.

Deficient cell-mediated immunity has traditionally been defined by depression or loss of delayed hypersensitivity skin test reactivity. Clinical experience with disorders of the T lymphocyte-dependent arm of the immune system has expanded greatly with increased use of therapeutic immunosuppression for organ transplantation and with the appearance of the AIDS epidemic. The key role of the T lymphocyte in defense against viral, protozoan, and mycobacterial infection is well illustrated by the frequency of such diagnoses as cryptococcal meningitis, *Pneumocystis carinii* pneumonia, and disseminated cytomegalovirus infection in both organ transplant and AIDS patients.

Older literature suggests that pregnancy appears to be associated with diminished cell-mediated immunity, which could facilitate immune tolerance of the fetal allograft as well as a variety of other functional impairments of immunity.[43-51] Increased susceptibility to infection with *Listeria monocytogenes* in pregnancy, and especially the likelihood of severe fetoplacental infection, may be explained by the local inhibition of maternal cellular immune responsiveness, which has the benefit of preventing an antifetal response. In a murine model of fetoplacental listeriosis, the T lymphocytes and macrophages, which defended against listerial organisms in other tissues, were inhibited from entering the decidua basalis.[52]

CLINICAL ASSESSMENT

Fever is the cardinal sign of infectious diseases and is found nearly universally in seriously infected patients, even in those with profound immune deficiencies or severe granulocytopenia.[53] Defined as a rectal temperature of 100.5°F or more, fever may be absent in infected patients at the extremes of age or in patients with end stage cardiac or renal failure, and can be obscured by hypothermia due to environmental exposure or septic shock. The detection of fever plus any localizing signs and symptoms, along with a history of exposure to or particular susceptibility to infectious agents, is the initial basis on which the diagnostic evaluation rests.

The preservation of the febrile response, even in patients with profound granulocytopenia, reflects the basic mechanism in which a variety of stimuli, including microorganisms, their component parts or toxins, antigen–antibody complexes, physiologic conditions such as strenuous exercise or the period following ovulation, and a variety of chemical compounds (all of which can be designated *exogenous pyrogens*), induce the formation of interleukins-1 or -6, interferon alpha, or tumor necrosis factor (*endogenous pyrogens*) by reticuloendothelial system cells, particularly monocytes and macrophages.[53,54] The endogenous pyrogens then stimulate the hypothalamic febrile response, presumably by way of interaction with specific receptors on capillary endothelial cells, leading to elevated prostaglandin E2 levels.[55]

Increased PGE2 concentrations in the brain cause an upward resetting of the core temperature and neural responses, such as vasoconstriction and shivering, which raise body temperature to the new set point. Elevated temperature can also occur without elevation of the normal temperature set point and is then termed *hyperthermia* rather than fever. Heat stroke, in which defenses against environmental overheating such as sweating are ineffective or overwhelmed, is an extreme example. Hyperthyroidism also may produce mild hyperthermia. Some anesthetics or neuroleptic agents may result in severe hyperthermia.[56,57] It is important to distinguish fever from hyperthermia. Because when the temperature set point remains normal, antipyretics will not affect hyperthermia. Rather, the offending environmental or pharmacologic cause must be removed and, in severe cases, patients must be cooled by physical means such as ice water baths.

Antipyretic therapy, although widely employed in infections, remains controversial. In addition to the use of fever as a therapeutic modality, evidence has been reported of a beneficial effect of fever on various immune responses.[58,59] Widely accepted indications for use of antipyretic therapy do include advanced cardiac or pulmonary disease or seizure history in a child. The effectiveness of antipyretic drugs is a function of their inhibition of cyclooxygenase in the brain, reflecting the key role of prostaglandin E2 in producing fever. Agents with potent antipyretic activity include aspirin, acetaminophen, and nonsteroidal anti-inflammatory drugs. Corticosteroids are antipyretic at two levels: they block transcription of the messenger RNA for endogenous pyrogen and inhibit PGE2 synthesis.

Historical features may be crucial in the assessment and initial management of patients with infectious diseases. Host defense defects may be indicated by a history of diabetes, chronic cardiac, respiratory, or renal disease, or by a history of a malignant condition. Risk factors for AIDS should be routinely assessed. A history of prior infectious disease episodes may point directly to the etiology of the present illness. In particular, previous antibiotic treatment, whether prescribed by a physician or self-administered, may alter or obscure the pattern of an infection. In addition, recent antibiotic exposure substantially increases the likelihood that bacteria causing an acute infection will be resistant to some antibiotics, and it is therefore a critical historical feature in selecting empiric antibiotic therapy. For patients who are hospitalized or who have recently been discharged, a detailed review of their course as well as an understanding of the epidemiology of nosocomial infections is important. The two major determinants of frequency and type of hospital-acquired infections are the host defense status of the patient and the number and type of invasive diagnostic or therapeutic procedures. The most frequent hospital-acquired infections reflect the following procedures: urinary tract infections principally occur in patients who have had bladder catheterization; phlebitis and septicemia are increasingly a function of intravenous lines and other intravascular devices; wound infections are principally found in postoperative surgical patients; and pneumonia may complicate aspiration due to the alteration of the gag reflex by anesthesia or sedatives, or in neurology patients with defects of the gag reflex, or in consciousness.

Several other areas should be routinely addressed in history taking. Foreign travel or origin in a foreign country raise diagnostic possibilities such as malaria and typhoid fever which are not likely in nontravelers. Regional patterns of increased antimicrobial resistance—for example, high rates of drug-resistant tuberculosis in Southeast Asia—underscore the importance of geographic history taking. Even within the United States, the localization of certain pathogens, such as coccidioidomycosis in the Southwest and histoplasmosis in the Ohio River Valley and Puerto Rico, make geography a consideration, even in the absence of foreign travel.

Environmental history taking is vital in assessing patients with infectious diseases. Obviously, exposure to someone with active tuberculosis is a key question for any patient with this diagnostic possibility. Food exposure may be important to elicit in patients presenting with hepatitis or diarrhea syndromes. Outbreaks of listeriosis have in recent years been associated with consumption of milk in the Northeast and Mexican-style cheese in the Southwest.

Consumption of unusual foods such as unpasteurized milk or cheese may be important clues to the occurrence of unusual processes like brucellosis. Recreational and leisure activity history, including pets and exposure to outdoor areas, may raise diagnostic possibilities such as Lyme disease, Rocky Mountain spotted fever, and arboviral encephalitis.

DIAGNOSIS OF INFECTIOUS DISEASES

Diagnostic testing to confirm the presence and specific etiology of an infectious disease is virtually always desirable, especially in seriously ill patients. Even when historical findings and physical examination strongly indicate a specific site of infection, it is important to determine the microbial etiology and antibiotic sensitivity. The ordering of tests and their interpretation need to be tailored to the individual patient, even though the hallowed *fever workup* remains useful for a hospitalized febrile patient.

Direct Microscopy

The use of the microscope, especially in the physician's office or in the ward laboratory, is a potentially very rapid and efficient way to narrow down diagnostic possibilities. Assessment of body fluids and inflammatory exudates for both inflammatory cells and microorganisms can provide a high degree of diagnostic specificity within minutes. In patients with possible lower respiratory tract infection, aggressive attempts should be made to obtain sputum for Gram's stain and culture. The finding of 25 or more polymorphonuclear leukocytes (PMNs) and fewer than 10 epithelial cells per high power field indicates a low probability of specimen contamination and, hence, places greater significance on any microorganisms isolated on culture.[60] The presence of many PMNs, along with a predominant morphology of organisms such as gram-positive diplococci, is strongly suggestive of a specific etiology of pneumococcal pneumonia. Correspondingly, a sputum specimen with few PMNs or many epithelial cells probably represents oral contents, and organisms recovered from such cultures do not reflect the presence of lower respiratory tract infection. In the syndrome of aspiration pneumonia, which may be complicated by a putrid lung abscess, the characteristic sputum Gram's stain findings are numerous PMNs and mixed gram-negative and gram-positive rods and cocci reflecting the normal oral flora, which in this setting contribute synergistically to the pathogenesis of the infection.[61] Thus, the distinction between a truly significant sputum culture result and one that is falsely positive due to oral flora contamination rests primarily on the inflammatory and epithelial cell content of the sputum Gram's stain.

In the case of urinary tract infection, the urinalysis plays a similar role to the sputum Gram's stain in assessing the need for and significance of urine culture results. Although only semiquantitative, the standard urinalysis assay for PMNs can be very helpful since the overwhelming majority of patients with urinary tract infections will have an excess of inflammatory cells detectable in the urine. Thus, unless a patient is profoundly granulocytopenic, the absence of PMNs in the urine constitutes substantial evidence against the presence of a urinary tract infection. Quantitation of bacteriuria can also be done rapidly by microscopic examination of Gram's-stained urine, which correlates strongly with quantitative culture to establish the presence of a significant number of bacteria.[62]

In suspected meningitis the rapid and accurate evaluation of cerebrospinal fluid (CSF) is crucial to proper diagnosis and management. The number of cells present in CSF, as well as the morphologic differential between PMNs and mononuclear cells, provides one important means of distinguishing acute bacterial meningitis from viral and other forms of aseptic meningitis. Although Gram's stain identification of bacteria in CSF in acute bacterial meningitis occurs in less than 50% of cases, a positive result is obviously significant and can provide prompt, crucial help in treatment. A similar examination of all normally sterile body fluids that are aspirated in the course of a diagnostic work up should be performed with a cell count, differential, and Gram's stain, ideally done both by the physician and by the diagnostic laboratory.

Direct microscopic examination of vaginal secretions or of a penile discharge can be diagnostic for gonococcal disease. In females, the distinction between nonpathogenic neisseria and gonococci can be made by the finding of gram-negative diplococci within PMNs on cervical Gram's stain. In the case of a male discharge, the finding of gram-negative diplococci, not necessarily within PMNs, has the same significance, since the male urethra, unlike the female vagina, does not normally contain *Neisseria* species. Gram's stains of cervical or vaginal material will also accurately detect *Candida,* which appear as large oval budding gram-positive forms. Wet-mount examination may detect the characteristic motile flagellated morphology of *T vaginalis.*

In patients with diarrhea, microscopical stool examination may be useful for the detection of protozoon pathogens, although expert interpretation is often necessary for these diagnoses. The stool Gram's stain is worth performing on patients with significant diarrhea, since it may allow detection of fecal leukocytes that are associated with more invasive and destructive etiologies such as *Shigella, Campylobacter,* and antibiotic-associated colitis caused by *C difficile.*

SPECIMEN COLLECTION AND PROCESSING

The proper techniques of transport and processing are vital in the successful identification of microbial pathogens by the laboratory. Several important guidelines are worth emphasizing.[63] Materials submitted to the laboratory should be as representative as possible of the infected site. Therefore, biopsy or deeply aspirated material is preferred to a superficial swab of a wound or sinus tract. Reasonable quantities of material should be submitted whenever possible because division between several culture media may be necessary, and in the case of chronic infection or fastidious organisms the quantity of microorganisms may be small. Sterile technique must be practiced, especially in obtaining and handling specimens from normally sterile body fluids and sites. Prompt transport to the laboratory is important, since many organisms will deteriorate over time and fastidious ones may become completely unrecoverable. Perhaps of greatest significance is to obtain all possible specimens for culture before initiation of antimicrobial therapy, which may otherwise render cultures falsely negative. Cultures should often be obtained from more than just the presumed site of infection. In the case of female genital gonococcal infection, for instance, some patients have positive rectal cultures but negative cervical cultures. In patients with pneumonia or with evidence of sepsis arising from a local site, culture of blood is indicated and may often yield the diagnosis when cultures from the primary site, such as sputum, are negative or contaminated. In collecting speci-

TABLE 54–4. CLINICAL INFECTIOUS DISEASE SYNDROMES

Site of Infection	Probable Diagnosis	Status of Host	Community (C) or Hospital (H) Acquired?	Likely Pathogen(s)	Antimicrobial Resistance	Initial Therapy
Skin	Cellulitis	Normal	C	Group A Strep *Staphylococcus aureus*	Unlikely	Penicillin or oxacillin
Skin	Cellulitis	Leukemia + neutropenia	H	Staph/Strep, Pseudomonas, Candida	Likely	Ceftazidime or ticarcillin + aminoglycoside
Urine	Pyelonephritis	Pregnant; history UTIs	C	*Escherichia coli*	Possible	Trimethoprim/sulfa or cefotaxime
Urine	Pyelonephritis	ICU, catheter	H	Coliforms, *Pseudomonas*, *Serratia*, and others	Likely	Cefotaxime, aztreonam, imipenem
Lungs	Pneumonia—lobar	Elderly	C	*Pneumococcus*	Unlikely	Penicillin
Lungs	Pneumonia—diffuse	Elderly	C	*Legionella* (summer) Influenza A (winter)	—	Erythromycin Amantidine
Lungs	Pneumonia—diffuse	Drug abuser	C	*Pneumocystis* (AIDS)	—	Trimethoprim/sulfa or pentamidine
Heart	Endocarditis	Prior rheumatic fever	C	*Streptococcus viridans*	Unlikely	Penicillin
Heart	Endocarditis	Postoperative septic phlebitis	H	*Staph. aureus*, gram-negative rods	Likely	Oxacillin or vancomycin and/or cefotaxime

mens, use of preservative-containing irrigants should be avoided. Specimens from pelvic and intra-abdominal abscesses or other sites from which anaerobic organisms may be recovered should be handled with special precautions to maximize recovery. Anaerobic transport containers are widely available, but it is often best to cap and send the syringe used to aspirate liquid abscess material directly to the microbiology laboratory. Direct plating of certain specimens in the operating room or at the bedside may increase the yield of cultures, but care needs to be exercised to avoid contamination. In addition, proper selection of medium is important. For example, cervical or rectal culture for gonococcus should be inoculated onto Thayer–Martin medium, which contains antibiotics to inhibit normal flora. On the other hand, aspirates of joint fluid should be inoculated onto chocolate agar for maximum recovery of gonococci, some of which might be inhibited on Thayer–Martin medium.

CLINICAL SYNDROMES IN INFECTIOUS DISEASES

The fundamental practical questions in managing infectious diseases, such as what diagnostic studies to perform, whether to start antimicrobial agents, and which agents to choose, all derive from consideration of the patient's presenting syndrome and the setting in which it occurs. A healthy, sexually active young woman with dysuria, presenting in an outpatient office, and a postoperative patient with a Foley catheter, fever, and signs of impending sepsis, may both turn out to have urinary tract infections. The former will require minimal diagnostic efforts and may be successfully treated with a single oral dose of an antibiotic, while the latter will probably require substantial diagnostic efforts and will need broad-spectrum initial antibiotic coverage to deal with the possibility of a hospital-acquired resistant infection. Thus, the standard approach to evaluating infected patients begins by focusing on the probable site of infection and the range of potential pathogens. At the same time, it is necessary to define both the degree of host susceptibility and the probability that microorganisms causing the infection are resistant to antimicrobial agents. Although speed and accuracy of diagnostic microbiology labs have improved remarkably, immediate or even same-day identification and susceptibility testing of pathogens are not yet a reality. Therefore, almost all initial assessments of infected patients must answer the two questions of whether empiric antimicrobial therapy is needed, and, if so, which agents are appropriate. Table 54–4 provides several examples of this initial approach to the assessment of infected patients.

REFERENCES

1. Mackowiak PA. The normal microbial flora. *N Engl J Med.* 1982;307:83.
2. Finegold SM, Sutter VL. Fecal flora in different populations, with special reference to diet. *Am J Clin Nutr.* 1978;31:116.
3. Simon GL, Gorbach SL. Intestinal flora in health and disease. *Gastroenterology.* 1984;86:174.
4. Bond JH, Engel RR, Levitt MD. Factors influencing pulmonary methane excretion in man. *J Exp Med.* 1971;133:572.
5. Lindenbaum J, Rund DG, Butler VP Jr, et al. Inactivation of digoxin by the gut flora: reversal by antibiotic therapy. *New Engl J Med.* 1981; 305:789.
6. Dobkin JF, Saha JR, Butler VP Jr, et al. Digoxin-inactivating bacteria: identification in human gut flora. *Science.* 1983;220:325.
7. Linday L, Dobkin JF, Wang TC, et al. Digoxin inactivation by the gut flora in infancy and childhood. *Pediatrics.* 1987;79:544.
8. Hammerschlag MR, Alpert S, Rosner I, et al. Microbiology of the vagina in children: normal and potentially pathogenic organisms. *Pediatrics.* 1978;62:57.
9. Hammerschlag MR, Alpert S, Onderdonk AB, et al. Anaerobic microflora of the vagina in children. *J Obstet Gynecol.* 1978;131:853.
10. Larsen B, Galask RP. Vaginal microbial flora: composition and influences of host physiology. *Ann Int Med.* 1982;96:926.
11. Moberg P, Eneroth P, Harlin J, et al: Cervical bacterial flora in infertile and pregnant women. *Med Microbiol Immunol.* 1978;165:139.
12. Lindner JGEM, Plantena FHF, Hoogkamp-Korstanje JAA. Quantitative studies of the vaginal flora of healthy women and of obstetric and gynecology patients. *J Med Microbiol.* 1978;11:233.

13. Goperlud CP, Ohm MJ, Galask RP. Aerobic and anaerobic flora of the cervix during pregnancy and the puerperium. *Am J Obstet Gynecol.* 1976; 126:858.
14. Levison ME, Corman LC, Carrington, Kaye D. Quantitative microflora of the vagina. *Am J Obstet Gynecol.* 1977;127:80.
15. Thadepalli H, Chan WH, Maidman JE, Davidson EC Jr. Microflora of the cervix during normal labor and the puerperium. *J Inf Dis.* 1978; 137:568.
16. Larsen B, Galask R. Vaginal microbial flora: practical and theoretic relevance. *Obstet Gynecol.* 1980;55(Suppl):100S.
17. Shafer MA, Sweet RL, Ohm-Smith MJ, et al. Microbiology of the lower genital tract in postmenarchal adolescent girls: differences in sexual activity, contraception and presence of nonspecific vaginitis. *J Pediatr.* 1985; 107:974.
18. Svanborg-Eden C, Gotschlich EC, Korhonen TK, et al. Aspects of structure and function of uropathogenic *E coli. Prog Allergy.* 1983;33:189.
19. Iwahi T, Abe Y, Nakao M, et al. Role of type 1 fimbriae in the pathogenesis of ascending urinary tract infection induced by *Escherichia coli* in mice. *Infect Immun.* 1983;39:1307.
20. Svanborg-Eden C, Eriksson B, Hanson LA. Adhesion of *Escherichia coli* to human uroepithelial cells in vitro. *Infect Immun.* 1977;18:767.
21. Leffler H, Svanborg-Eden C. Glycolipid receptors for uropathogenic *Escherichia coli* binding to human erythrocytes and uroepithelial cells. *Infect Immun.* 1981;34:920.
22. O'Hanley P, Lark D, Falkow S, et al. Molecular basis of *Escherichia coli* colonization of the upper urinary tract in BALB/c mice: Gal-Gal pili immunization prevents *Escherichia coli* pyelonephritis in the BALB/c mouse model of human pyelonephritis. *J Clin Invest.* 1985;75:347.
23. Orskov I, Ferencz A, Orskov F. Tamm-Horsfall protein or uromucoid is the normal urinary slime that traps type I fimbriated *Escherichia coli. Lancet.* 1980;i:887.
24. Svanborg-Eden C, Bjursten LM, Hull R, et al. Influence of adhesions on the interaction of *Escherichia coli* with human phagocytes. *Infect Immun.* 1984;44:672.
25. Jacobson S, Carstensen A, Kallenius G, et al. Fluorescence-activated cell analysis of P-fimbriae receptor accessibility on uroepithelial cells of patients with renal scarring. *Eur J Clin Microbiol.* 1986;5:649.
26. Gibbs RS, Jones PM, Wilder CJY. Internal fetal monitoring and maternal infection following cesarean section: a prospective study. *Obstet Gynecol.* 1978;52:193.
27. Nielsen TF, Hokegard KH. Postoperative cesarean section morbidity: a prospective study. *Am J Obstet Gynecol.* 1983;146:911.
28. Awadalla SG, Perkins RP, Mercer LJ. Significance of endometrial cultures performed at cesarean section. *Obstet Gynecol.* 1986;68:220.
29. Rosene K, Eschenbach DA, Tompkins LS, et al. Polymicrobial early postpartum endometritis with facultative and anaerobic bacteria, genital mycoplasmas and *C. trachomatis:* treatment with piperacillin or cefoxitin. *J Infect Dis.* 1986;153:1028.
30. Williams CM, Okada DM, Marshall JR, et al. Clinical and microbiologic risk evaluation for post-cesarean section endometritis by multivariate discriminant analysis: role of intraoperative mycoplasma, aerobes, and anaerobes. *Am J Obstet Gynecol.* 1987;156:967.
31. Bodey GP, Buckley M, Sathe YS, et al. Quantitative relationships between circulating leukocytes and infection in patients with acute leukemia. *Ann Int Med.* 1966;64:328.
32. Donabedian H, Gallin JI. The hyperimmunoglobulin E recurrent-infection (Job's) syndrome. *Medicine* (Baltimore). 1983;62:195.
33. Gluckman SJ, Dvorak VC, MacGregor RR. Host defenses during prolonged alcohol consumption in a controlled environment. *Arch Intern Med.* 1977;137:1539.
34. Parry MF, Root RK, Metcalf JA, et al. Myeloperoxidase deficiency. Prevalence and clinical significance. *Ann Intern Med.* 1981;95:293.
35. Royer HD, Reinherz EL. T lymphocytes: ontogeny, function, and relevance to clinical disorders. *N Engl J Med.* 1987;317:1136.
36. Rosen FS, Cooper MD, Wedgwood RJP. Medical progress: the primary immunodeficiencies. *N Engl J Med.* 1984;311:235, 300.
37. Miller DG. Patterns of immunologic deficiency in lymphomas and leukemias. *Ann Intern Med.* 1972;57:703.
38. Savage DG, Lindenbaum J, Garrett TJ. Biphasic pattern of bacterial infection in multiple myeloma. *Ann Intern Med.* 1982;96:47.
39. Stiehm RE, Ashida E, Kim KS, et al. Intravenous immunoglobulins as therapeutic agents. *Ann Intern Med.* 1987;107:367.
40. Ross SC, Densen P. Complement deficiency states and infection: epidemiology, pathogenesis and consequences of neisserial and other infections in an immune deficiency. *Medicine,* (Baltimore). 1984;63:243.
41. Bjornson AB, Lobel JS. Direct evidence that decreased serum opsonization of *Streptococcus pneumoniae* via the alternative complement pathway in sickle cell disease is related to antibody deficiency. *J Clin Invest.* 1987; 79:388.
42. Lane HC, Masur H, Edgar LC, et al. Abnormalities of B-cell activation and immunoregulation in patients with the acquired immunodeficiency syndrome. *N Engl J Med.* 1983;309:453.
43. Gall SA. Maternal immune system during human gestation. *Semin Perinatol.* 1977;1:119.
44. Larsen B, Galask RP. Host–parasite interactions during pregnancy. *Obstet Gynecol Surv.* 1978;33:297.
45. Bjorksten B, Soderstrom T, Damber MG, et al. Polymorphonuclear leukocyte function during pregnancy. *Scand J Immunol.* 1978;8:257.
46. Noonan FP, Halliday WJ, Morton H, Clunie GJA. Early pregnancy factor is immunosuppressive. *Nature.* 1978;278:649.
47. Siiteri PK, Stites DP. Immunologic and endocrine interrelationships in pregnancy. *Biol Reprod.* 1982;26:1.
48. Sridama V, Pagini F, Yang S, et al. Decreased levels of helper T cells: a possible cause of immunodeficiency in pregnancy. *N Engl J Med.* 1982; 307:352.
49. Cotton DJ, Seligmann B, O'Brien WF, et al. Selective defect in human neutrophil superoxide anion generation elicited by the chemoattractant N-formylmethionylleucylphenylalanine in pregnancy. *J Infect Dis.* 1983; 148:194.
50. Lederman MM. Cell-mediated immunity and pregnancy. *Chest.* 1984; 86S:6.
51. Weinberg ED. Pregnancy-associated depression of cell-mediated immunity. *Rev Infect Dis.* 1984;6:814.
52. Redline RW, Lu CY. Specific defects in the anti-listerial immune response in discrete regions of the murine uterus and placenta account for susceptibility to infection. *J Immunol.* 1988;140:3947.
53. Dinarello CA, Cannon JG, Wolff SM. New concepts in the pathogenesis of fever. *Rev Infect Dis.* 1988;10:168.
54. Cannon JG, Dinarello CA. Increased plasma interleukin activity in women after ovulation. *Science.* 1985;227:1247.
55. Coceani F, Lees J, Bishai I. Further evidence implicating prostaglandin E2 in the genesis of pyrogen fever. *Am J Physiol.* 1988;254:R463.
56. Allsop P, Twigley AJ. The neuroleptic malignant syndrome. Case report with a review of the literature. *Anesthesia.* 1987;42:49.
57. Naylor AM, Ruwe WD, Veale WL. Antipyretic action of centrally administered arginine vasopressin but not oxytocin in the cat. *Brain Res.* 1986; 385:156.
58. Duff GW, Durum SK. Fever and immunoregulation: hyperthermia, interleukin-1 and 2, and T-cell proliferation. *Yale J Biol Med.* 1982;55:437.
59. Hanson DF, Murphy PA, Silicano R, et al. The effect of temperature on the activation of thymocytes by interleukin-1 and interleukin-2. *J Immunol.* 1983;130:216.
60. Murray PR, Washington JA II. Microscopic and bacteriologic analysis of sputum. *Mayo Clin Proc.* 1975;50:339.
61. Bartlett J, Gorbach S, Finegold S. The bacteriology of aspiration pneumonia. *Am J Med.* 1974;56:202.
62. Jenkins RD, Fenn JP, Matsen JM. Review of urine microscopy for bacteriuria. *JAMA.* 1986;255:3397.
63. Washington JA II: Bacteria, fungi and parasites. In: Mandell GL, Douglas RG Jr, Bennett JE, eds: *Principles and Practice of Infectious Diseases.* 3rd ed. New York: Churchill Livingstone; 1989:160.

Chapter Fifty-Five

Hospital-Acquired Infections

David L. Pitrak

55

NOSOCOMIAL INFECTIONS

Despite recent advances in our understanding of nosocomial infections and despite the institution of infection control programs in hospitals nationwide, these infections pose a major problem for clinicians and their patients. It is estimated that 5–6% of the approximately 40 million people hospitalized each year in the United States will develop nosocomial infections, and these infections are associated with significant morbidity and mortality.[1] Furthermore, the cost of prolonged hospitalization and treatment for these infections is staggering, an estimated $5–10 billion annually.[1] Obstetric patients are not excluded, although most obstetric patients do not have many of the risk factors associated with the development of nosocomial infections.

The increased morbidity and mortality associated with hospitals has long been recognized, and several authors have chronicled the evolution of our concept of nosocomial infections. It is of particular interest to obstetricians that early concerns about hospital-acquired infections often centered around puerperal sepsis. Oliver Wendell Holmes suggested in 1843 that puerperal sepsis was a hospital-acquired infection.[2] Soon afterward, Ignaz Semmelweis published his observations on the causes of puerperal fever or *childbed fever* over fifteen years of practice at the Vienna Medical School.[3] He demonstrated that maternal mortality as a result of puerperal sepsis was much greater when deliveries were performed by medical students in the First Division of the Vienna Lying-in Hospital, compared to that observed in the Second Division, where deliveries were performed by midwives. It was noted that the medical students frequently went from the autopsy suite to the delivery suite without washing their hands. Semmelweis proposed that the students were transferring an agent on their hands that resulted in puerperal sepsis. He also theorized that the offending agent may be transferred from patient to patient by way of contaminated examination beds, linen, and so on. He isolated infected patients and instituted a policy of washing hands with lime prior to deliveries and demonstrated that these simple maneuvers significantly decreased the incidence of puerperal sepsis. Many of these observations helped to build the foundation for the current approach to the control of nosocomial infections.

Definition

Nosocomial infections are defined as infections that develop during hospitalization and include infections with long incubation periods such as viral hepatitis, that may not become manifest clinically until well after the patient has been discharged. This definition excludes infections that are incubating at the time of admission. It is usually assumed for most bacterial infections that an infection occurring within the first 48 to 72 hours of hospitalization is a community-acquired infection, while those occurring after 72 hours should be considered nosocomial. Although this is not absolutely accurate, it is a good general rule. The first step in nosocomial infections is colonization with pathogenic bacteria associated with hospital-acquired infections. The risk of such colonization increases with the duration of hospitalization, but it may occur early. In one study of hospitalized patients, oropharyngeal colonization with enteric gram-negative rods occurred within 96 hours in 55% of patients classified as severely ill.[4] Patients in other altered environments, such as nursing homes and other chronic care facilities, are predisposed to the same types of infections with the same organisms as hospitalized patients, and infections in these patients should be managed as if they were hospital-acquired.

Documentation of fever alone is not sufficient to make a diagnosis of a hospital-acquired infection. In a prospective study of 2725 obstetric patients admitted to the hospital, fever occurred in 131 (5.8%), but an infectious etiology as evidenced by leukocytosis, clinical symptoms, radiographic abnormalities, and microbiologic data was established in only 63 patients (48%) of the patients with fever.[5] Other patients with fever generally had a low-grade fever that occurred a few hours after a surgical procedure and the administration of anesthesia and other drugs perioperatively. These patients generally felt well and the fever usually resolved by 48 hours. The concept of transient fever of a noninfectious etiology occurring in postoperative obstetric patients has been recognized by a number of investigators, and the term *one day fever* has been coined by Ledger.[6] It is important to recognize that not all fever is due to infection, in order to prevent unnecessary antibiotic therapy or inappropriate diagnostic testing.

Incidence

The problem of nosocomial infections has long been recognized, but the magnitude of the problem was not systematically studied until the 1960s. A 1965 a survey of all services over a six-month period at the Johns Hopkins Medical Center revealed a 4% incidence of nosocomial infections. Urinary tract infections accounted for 40%, followed by wound infections (30%), pneumonias (14.5%), and phlebitis (10.5%).[7] It was also in the 1960s that the Centers for Disease Control (CDC) developed the concept of hospital surveillance and infection control programs. The National Nosocomial Infections Study (NNIS) was established in 1969 as a surveillance system to provide the CDC with information on nosocomial infections from a variety of hospitals across the country, and since then the CDC has evaluated nosocomial infection rates yearly.[8] By 1970, it was recommended that all hospitals institute their own surveillance and infection control programs, and in 1976 this became a requirement for accreditation by the Joint Commission of Accreditation of Hospitals (JCAH). Overall, yearly nosocomial infection rates have varied from 3.12% to 3.58%. In general, rates have been higher for University-based hospitals, although this may reflect an increased risk of infection for high-risk populations. The rates reported from the NNIS are underestimations. Data from the Study on the Efficacy of Nosocomial Infection Control (SENIC) indicate that overall nosocomial infections rates are 5–6%.[9] The distribution of nosocomial infections has remained fairly constant, with urinary tract infections accounting for 35–40%, wound infections 25–30%, other soft tissue infections 5–10%, pneumonia 15–20%, bacteremia 5%, and other infections 5–10%. Ap-

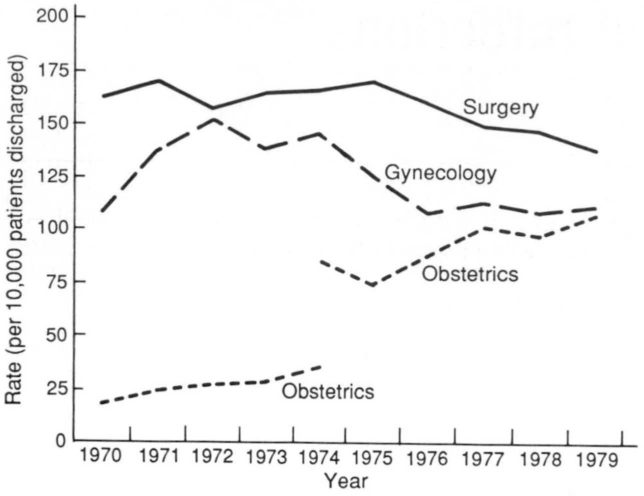

Figure 55–1. Frequency of surgical wound infections on obstetric services, National Nosocomial Infections Study (NNIS) hospitals, 1970–1979. (*From Allen et al*[12] *with permission.*)

TABLE 55–1. HOSPITAL-ASSOCIATED FEVER OF INFECTIOUS ORIGIN IN OBSTETRIC AND GYNECOLOGIC PATIENTS

Cause and Source of Fever	Total Cases No. (%)	Obstetric Patients No. (%)	Gynecologic Patients No. (%)
Wound	56(37)	37(59)	19(23)
Pelvic inflammatory	43(29)	—	43(50)
Urine	26(17)	11(16)	15(18)
Blood	7(5)	6(10)	1(1)
Pelvic abscess	4(3)	4(6)	—
Upper respiratory tract	3(2)	2(3)	1(1)
Gastrointestinal tract	3(2)	1(2)	2(2)
Lung	3(2)	1(2)	2(2)
Other	3(2)	1(2)	2(2)
Appendix	1(1)	—	1(1)
Total	149(100)	63(100)	86(100)

From Klimek, et al[5]*. with permission.*

proximately 95% of these infections are due to bacteria, and two thirds of these involve enteric gram-negative rods.[10]

Nosocomial infections may occur in epidemics, but this accounts for a relatively small proportion of nosocomial infections. These outbreaks have been important in studying the mode of nosocomial infections and the impact of infection control practices on nosocomial transmission. Such outbreaks are identified by an increased incidence of infections with unusual organisms or common organisms with unusual antibiotic susceptibility patterns. The distribution of sites of infection in epidemic nosocomial infection is also different from the distribution seen with endemic infections. The most frequent infections that occur in epidemics are gastroenteritis (21%), skin infections (12%), bacteremia (12%), meningitis (11%), and hepatitis (10%).[11]

Obstetric services have relatively low rates of nosocomial infections and the overall rate has varied little, but important changes have been noted for specific infections. From 1970 to 1979, while the rates of surgical wound infections on general surgery services were decreasing, the incidence of wound infections on obstetric services steadily increased, and this is likely to be due to the increased frequency of deliveries by cesarean section (Figure 55–1).[12] In obstetric patients, wound infections are the most common type of nosocomial infection, followed by urinary tract infections and gynecologic infections. In the study of hospital-acquired fever in obstetric patients by Klimek and coworkers, the overall infection rate for obstetric patients was 2.4%.[5] Sixty-three patients had infections, with skin and soft tissue infections (59%), urinary tract infections (16%), and bacteremias (10%) being most common (Table 55–1). Pelvic abscess, upper respiratory tract infection, pneumonia, gastroenteritis, and other infections were observed, but these were much less frequent. This same incidence and distribution of infections has been noted in other studies in developed countries. In developing countries, however, nosocomial infections are an even more common problem, with nosocomial infection rates in obstetric patients as high as 17% being reported.[13]

Morbidity and Mortality

Nosocomial infections are associated with significant morbidity and mortality. Nosocomial infections result in death in 0.5–1.1% of cases and contribute to death in another 2.8–3.9%.[14] Nosocomial infections may be directly responsible for 30,000 deaths annually in the United States.[15] Mortality is associated with severe underlying illness, and rates are highest for nosocomial pneumonias and bacteremias. Morbidity due to nosocomial infections results in prolonged hospital stays and increased hospitalization costs. In one study, postcesarean section endometritis extended the hospital stay by 3 days and increased the cost of the average hospitalization by $850 in 1980.[16]

Etiologic Agents

The microbial causes of nosocomial infections have changed little during the past decade, although some agents have only recently been recognized as nosocomial pathogens. Aerobic bacilli still account for 60% of cases, with *Escherichia coli* alone accounting for 20%. Other enteric gram-negative bacilli are also encountered, including *Klebsiella, Pseudomonas aeruginosa, Proteus, Serratia,* and others. *Staphylococcus aureus* and enterococci are also commonly involved, each accounting for 10% of cases. One change in these familiar organisms has been the emergence of antibiotic resistance by a variety of different mechanisms.[17]

A number of organisms have only recently been recognized to be nosocomial pathogens.[10,18-21] This group includes *Legionella* species (pneumonia and lung abscess), *Chlamydia trachomatis* (neonatal pneumonia), *Clostridium difficile* (antibiotic-associated colitis), and uncommon gram-negative bacilli, such as *Pseudomonas cepacia, Xanthomonas, Acinetobacter, Citrobacter, Enterobacter, Alcaligenes,* and *Flavobacterium.* The JK bacillus has become an important pathogen in prosthetic infections and septicemia in immunocompromised patients. Atypical mycobacteria (*Mycobacterium chelonei* and *Mycobacterium fortuitum*) have been implicated in wound infections, especially when foreign material is present.

The frequency of hospital-acquired infections with fungi is increasing.[21,22] *Candida albicans* and *Aspergillus fumigatus* remain important nosocomial pathogens, but other *Candida* species and *Aspergillus* species are also emerging as important nosocomial pathogens. Members of the class Zygomycetes, *Pseudallascheria,* and *Fusarium* may also be involved in hosptial-acquired infections. Other fungi newly recognized as significant pathogens include *Bipolaris, Curvularia, Alternaria, Exserohilum, Hansenula, Trichosporon, Microsporum,* and *Malassezia.* Many of these agents only cause infection in severely immunocompromised patients in association with cancer chemotherapy and immunosuppressive therapy for organ transplantation. Nosocomial fungal infections can be rapidly progressive and are often fatal.

Nosocomial viral infections also occur, and the incidence of these infections has been underestimated.[23] Infections with respiratory viruses are most frequent, with influenza and respiratory syncytial virus (RSV) being implicated most often. Other viruses that cause nosocomial infections are rhinovirus, parainfluenza virus, measles (rubeola), varicella zoster virus (VZV), enteroviruses, rotaviruses, and the Norwalklike agents. Nosocomial viral infections may occur in epidemic fashion (RSV, influenza, and measles).

The route of acquisition of nosocomial infections is of obvious concern with respect to infection control programs, and the route of infection differs with respect to the agents involved. Many nosocomial bacterial infections are the result of transmission on the hands of hospital personnel, but even some viral pathogens such as RSV are transmitted in this fashion. Person-to-person spread can also occur by way of airborne transmission in outbreaks of measles, varicella, influenza, and tuberculosis. The airborne route may not involve person-to-person spread, but rather transmission from an environmental source. This has been observed with *Legionella* species, *Aspergillus, P aeruginosa,* and atypical mycobacteria. Infection can also be acquired through contaminated blood products (non-A, non-B hepatitis, cytomegalovirus (CMV), Epstein–Barr virus (EBV), human immunodeficiency virus (HIV), and *Toxoplasma*). Other parasitic infections are rarely acquired through blood transfusions in the United States, but this is a significant problem in developing countries. Bacterial contamination with blood usually involves skin organisms, but this is rarely associated with clinical problems. Cold storage has helped eliminate the transmission of syphilis through blood transfusion. Some organisms, however, can survive cold storage, and this can result in sepsis related to blood transfusion (*Pseudomonas* and *Yersinia* species). Parenteral fluids may be contaminated, resulting in infusion-associated sepsis (*Enterobacter, Citrobacter,* and *Flavobacterium*). *Candida* and *Malassezia* have a propensity for contaminating hyperalimentation solutions. Other modes of transmission have recently been recognized, including contamination of drug delivery systems and pressure monitoring devices (*Pseudomonas* species and *Flavobacterium*).

Antibiotic Resistance

The emergence of antibiotic resistant organisms by a variety of mechanisms has become a major obstacle in treating patients with nosocomial infections, especially in referral centers.[17] One major problem has been the increasing incidence of methicillin resistance among gram-positive organisms. In many hospitals, methicillin-resistant strains of *S aureus* and coagulase-negative staphylococci are important causes of hospital-acquired infections. The usual mechanism of methicillin resistance is reduced affinity of penicillin-binding proteins for methicillin, although some methicillin-resistant strains may be hyperproducers of β-lactamase.[24] Vancomycin is the drug of choice for these infections, and the increased use of vancomycin has resulted in increased cost and drug toxicity associated with the treatment of these infections. Recently, vancomycin resistance has been observed in coagulase-negative staphylococci, and this may become a major problem in the future.[25] Strains of *S aureus* that are resistant to high levels of aminoglycosides have also been recovered.

Enterococci are another group of gram-positive organisms that are becoming increasingly drug resistant. These organisms, including the human pathogens *Enterococcus faecalis, Enterococcus faecium,* and *Enterococcus durans,* were previously classified as group D streptococci. These organisms are inhibited by penicillin G, ampicillin, and vancomycin, but are tolerant to the bactericidal activities of these drugs. Infections with these organisms often require the addition of an aminoglycoside for synergy with a β-lactam antibiotic or vancomycin. It has long been recognized that strains have become resistant to streptomycin, but currently up to 20% of enterococci are resistant to gentamicin and other aminoglycosides. In some instances, the aminoglycoside resistance is low-level and aminoglycosides may still be used for their synergistic effect, but in other cases there is very high level resistance (MIC $>$500 μg/mL) to aminoglycosides, including amikacin. The lack of a bactericidal combination makes treatment of serious enterococcal infections difficult, indeed. There are now reports of penicillin and ampicillin resistance due to β-lactamase production, and it appears that this property may have been acquired from staphylococci by conjugation.[26] There are also a few reports of plasmid-mediated vancomycin resistance due to these organisms.[27] Currently, vancomycin resistance is not a widespread problem, but the potential exists.

Enteric gram-negative rods associated with nosocomial infections are notorious for being resistant to multiple antibiotics. Strains resistant to β-lactam antibiotics and aminoglycosides are frequently recovered in patients with nosocomial infections, especially those strains associated with cross infections and epidemics in the hospital. Many of these bacteria possess plasmids, or R factors, that can transfer resistance from one bacterial strain to another. Bacteria may also acquire antibiotic resistance by spontaneous chromosomal mutations under selective pressure of antibiotic therapy. Resistance to β-lactam antibiotics may be due to decreased outer membrane permeability, alteration in the penicillin binding proteins, or production of enzymes that degrade the antibiotic. Production of β-lactamase is a very common mechanism of resistance. New β-lactamases are continuously being identified, and some enteric gram-negative rods now produce enzymes capable of destroying newer extended spectrum penicillins and cephalosporins that were previously considered β-lactamase-resistant. These newly recognized β-lactamases often are not inhibited by clavulanic acid or other β-lactamase inhibitors. Recently, it has been shown that β-lactamase production by some organisms can actually be induced by therapy with certain β-lactam antibiotics. This not only results in resistance to the inducing agent, but to other β-lactams as well. For example, it is well known that cefoxitin induces β-lactamase production by *Enterobacter.* Aminoglycoside resistance can be the result of decreased active transport into the cell, alteration of ribosomal binding sites, or enzymatic degradation. The wide array of mechanisms of antibiotic resistance exhibited by enteric gram-negative rods has made the treatment of nosocomial infections with these organisms a major challenge.

The solution to the problem of antibiotic resistance will not only rely on the development of newer agents, but also on the appropriate and judicious use of antibiotics. Antibiotic use clearly influences the development of resistance. Control of antibiotic usage, such as assuring proper dosing and reserving newer antibiotics for treatment of infections with resistant organisms, may help prevent or at least delay the development of resistance. Specific guidelines for improving antimicrobial usage have been proposed by the Infectious Diseases Society of America.[28]

Risk Factors

Obstetric patients lack many of the risk factors that predispose patients to nosocomial infections, and this accounts for the relatively low nosocomial infection rates observed on obstetric services.[29] The majority of these patients are well and do not have chronic underlying medical illnesses associated with an increased risk of acquiring nosocomial infections, although there are physiologic changes in pregnancy that predispose patients to certain infections. For example, there are a number of changes in the urinary tract of pregnant women that predispose them to the development of urinary tract infections. Furthermore, hospitalized obstetric patients are exposed to many of the same procedures as other hospitalized patients, such as urethral catheterization and intravenous cannulization, as well as invasive diagnostic and operative procedures unique to the obstetric patient, including cesarean section, amniocentesis, and intrauterine monitoring.

WOUND INFECTIONS

Clinical Manifestations

Surgical wound infections are characterized by purulent discharge from the incision site or other local evidence of infection such as erythema, warmth, induration, and tenderness. Wound infections usually occur a few days after delivery. The site of infection can be the episiotomy site following vaginal deliveries or the abdominal incision after cesarean section. Fever and leukocytosis are common, and these clinical features may precede local signs of infection. Fluctuance signals the formation of an abscess.

Serious complications of wound infections can occur, including bacteremia, necrotizing fasciitis, and myonecrosis. Necrotizing fasciitis is characterized by marked systemic toxicity, and blood cultures are often positive. Cutaneous anesthesia results from destruction of cutaneous nerves as they course through fascia. This may be an early sign of fasciitis preceding necrosis of the overlying skin. This infection can spread along fascial planes with resulting erythema and induration of the abdomen, thigh, or buttocks distant from the incision site. Crepitation or the presence of gas on x-rays is present in only half of the cases, and the presence and extent of fasciitis can only be determined by surgical exploration. Myonecrosis is another infrequent serious postoperative infection that is characterized by marked systemic toxicity. It may be a primary infection due to *Clostridium perfringens,* or it may occur as a late complication of necrotizing fasciitis. The diagnosis is made by demonstrating myonecrosis at surgery.

Incidence

Wound infections are the most common infections occurring on obstetric services. The incidence of wound infection following cesarean section varies from 6–11%. Episiotomy wound infections are less common, with rates of 0.09–0.3% being reported.[30] Data from the CDC shows that there has been a gradual decrease in wound infections on surgical services, but there has been an increase in the incidence of wound infections on obstetric services. Although data concerning the types of procedures associated with wound infections is unavailable through the NNIS, increased wound infection rates are most likely the result of the increased number of deliveries by cesarean section.

Pathogenesis

Tissues can become infected with skin flora or organisms that were colonizing the genital tract at the time of operation. A number of risk factors have been associated with wound infections.[31] Emergency surgery is associated with higher wound infection rates than elective surgery. Other factors include the duration of the operation, the use of electrocautery, and the placement of drains. Preexisting conditions, such as obesity and diabetes mellitus, also increase the incidence of wound infections. The rate of infection also correlates with the duration of hospitalization prior to surgery, although this may only reflect an increased risk for the high-risk patient. Preoperative shaving has also been associated with increased skin colonization and an increased incidence of wound infection.

Etiologic agents

Wound infections are due either to skin flora or organisms that have colonized the genital tract. In the study by Klimek and coworkers, wound and soft tissue infections accounted for 59% of infections, and cultures of wound drainage revealed *E coli* (21%), *bacteroides* species (14%), *S aureus* (11%), β-hemolytic streptococci (11%), *Staphylococcus epidermidis* (10%), enterococci (5%), *Klebsiella* (5%), and mixed flora (23%).[5] Other enteric aerobic gram-negative organisms may be recovered. Necrotizing fasciitis is often due to group A β-hemolytic streptococci, but mixed infection with anaerobes, facultative anaerobic streptococci, and enteric gram-negative rods also occurs. Clostridia rarely are involved, but can cause severe infections, and *C perfringens* is the agent classically associated with gas gangrene and myonecrosis. However, not all patients from whom clostridia are isolated have myonecrosis.

Treatment

Areas of fluctuance should be incised and drained. Patients with systemic toxicity should have the wound opened and explored. It is important to exclude necrotizing fasciitis and myonecrosis, as these infections require extensive debridement. The mortality rate for these infections is nearly 100% with antibiotic therapy alone, and even with surgery the mortality rate is high. Mortality is most dependent on the time from the onset of symptoms to diagnosis and surgical intervention. Empiric antibiotic therapy for wound infections should include coverage for staphylococci, streptococci, aerobic gram-negative bacilli, and anaerobes. Clindamycin plus an aminoglycoside is a good combination. This same combination should be given as adjunct to surgery in cases of necrotizing fasciitis. When the diagnosis of clostridial myonecrosis is made or suspected, penicillin G should be given. Therapy should be modified when results of blood or wound cultures are available.

Prevention

The importance of good surgical technique is obvious. A number of studies have shown that prophylactic antibiotics can reduce the incidence of wound infections that occur after cesarean section, as well as pelvic–peritoneal and urinary tract infections.[32] First generation cephalosporins have been shown to be effective. Broader spectrum second and third generation cephalosporins are at least as effective, but their cost may preclude their routine use for prophylaxis.[33] Recommendations as to which antibiotic is the agent of choice for prophylaxis will probably change as costs change and new agents become available. Irrigation and topical antibiotics have been evaluated, but the benefits of these interventions are less clear compared to systemic antibiotic therapy.

PELVIC INFECTIONS

Clinical Manifestations

Postpartum pelvic infections usually occur in the hospital setting and are therefore nosocomial. As with other nosocomial infections, cross infection or environmental contamination is possible. However, the vast majority of these infections are due to the patient's own colonizing flora. The diagnosis of postpartum pelvic infections may be difficult. Fever is common, but not invariable, and fever or leukocytosis are not specific for pelvic infection. Purulent lochia is a frequent manifestation of pelvic infections following vaginal delivery. Abdominal pain and tenderness are common features of pelvic infections complicating either vaginal deliveries or cesarean sections. In general, absence of uterine tenderness should suggest another site of infection. An adnexal mass suggests the development of a pelvic abscess. A complaint of hip pain may indicate a paracervical or paravaginal infection complicating a pudendal or paracervical anesthetic nerve block.[34] It is important to be aware of this sign, as early antibiotic therapy can prevent extensive subgluteal and retropsoas abscess formation. Blood cultures are often positive in postpartum endometritis, and this infection is the most common cause of nosocomial bacteremia in the obstetric population. Multiple or persistently positive blood cultures, septic pulmonary emboli, or persistent fever despite appropriate antibiotic therapy for a pelvic infection may indicate a diagnosis of septic pelvic thrombophlebitis occurring as a complication of a pelvic infection (see also Chapter 117).

Incidence

Along with wound infections, postpartum pelvic-peritoneal infections are the most common infections occurring in hospitalized obstetric patients. In one prospective study, 12% of all women delivering developed peripartum infections, and endometritis was the diagnosis in 3.8% of cases. The incidence was about 2.5% after vaginal delivery, but from 13–27% following delivery by cesarean section.[30] This had been shown repeatedly in other studies. The relative risk has been reported to be as high as 20 times, and delivering by cesarean section is the single most important risk factor for developing a postpartum uterine pelvic-peritoneal infection. Furthermore, these infections tend to be more severe in postoperative patients, and these women have a higher mortality. The incidence of infection is greater when surgery is performed in an emergency. The incidence of infection and maternal mortality seems to be greater for patients undergoing a classic cesarean section rather than a low transverse cesarean section. Labor prior to cesarean section may also increase the risk of postoperative endometritis, even with intact membranes. The role of contribution of general anesthesia to the development of this infection is unknown due to confounding variables present in most studies.

Premature rupture of membranes (PROM) occurs in 7–12% of labors and can result in amnionitis, puerperal infection, or both, and the risk is proportional to the length of time between rupture of membranes (ROM) and delivery. Some studies, however, indicate that the risk is actually due to the duration of labor and not the duration of ruptured membranes. Early studies suggested that there was an association between the use of internal fetal monitoring (IFM) and maternal infection, but other studies have not confirmed this association. If IFM does increase the risk of maternal infection, the risk is small compared to other risk factors. The number of pelvic exams prior to delivery has also been associated with an increased risk of infection, but, again, this may only reflect duration of labor. Other factors that may predispose patients to postpartum pelvic-peritoneal infections include anemia, low socioeconomic status, episiotomy, manual removal of the placenta, forceps delivery, or other trauma at the time of delivery (see also Chapter 113).[35]

Pathogenesis

Although the upper part of the endometrial cavity is sterile in most women after delivery, the vagina and cervix are heavily colonized with bacteria. These organisms enter the endometrial cavity during labor. While the organisms most often gain entry after ROM, labor can result in migration of bacteria across intact amniotic membranes into the amniotic cavity. *Listeria* was recognized as a pathogen that could cross intact membranes, but it is now known that many bacteria, including anaerobes, can do this. Infection can spread to vascular channels or fallopian tubes, resulting in parametritis or salpingitis, respectively. There are a number of explanations for the increased incidence of endometritis following cesarean section. Organisms may get into the myometrium by way of the incision, and surgically devitalized tissue may act as a nidus for infection. The uterine cavity and peritoneal cavity may also become contaminated with infected amniotic fluid during the procedure.

Etiologic agents

β-hemolytic streptococci (including groups A, B, D, and G) have been commonly implicated in cases, and in some instances outbreaks, of postpartum endometritis. *E coli* is frequently isolated, but other enteric gram-negative bacilli, such as *Klebsiella*, *Proteus*, *Pseudomonas*, and *Enterobacter*, are uncommon. Anaerobes are very commonly isolated, especially anaerobic streptococci and *Bacteroides* species (most often *Bacteroides bivius*, *Bacteroides disiens*, and *Bacteroides fragilis*). Clostridia may be isolated and have the potential to cause serious infection, but usually this is not the case. *S aureus* is infrequently involved in postpartum endometritis, and coagulase-negative staphylococci are probably only involved in mixed infections. *Gardnerella vaginalis*, *Mycoplasma hominis*, and *Ureaplasma urealyticum* have been isolated from blood in patients with postpartum endometritis. It is not known whether these organisms have a primary role in the infection or are only present as part of a mixed infection. The significance of isolating *Chlamydia trachomatis* from patients with endometritis is also unclear, although this infection occurs more often in women from whom *C trachomatis* was recovered prior to delivery or women whose children developed inclusion conjunctivitis.

Part of the difficulty in determining the probable pathogens in postpartum endometritis stems from interpreting endometrial cultures, and in individual patients interpretation of endometrial cultures can be extremely difficult. There is almost always a problem with contamination by the colonizing flora of the cervix. Collection of specimens with a double lumen tube with a brush inside has been evaluated, but this technique is costly and not of proven benefit. Transabdominal fundal aspiration has been attempted, and this technique does circumvent the problem of lower genital tract colonization. However, this technique is not very sensitive, and cultures may be negative in patients that clearly have endometritis by clinical criteria. Culdocentesis has also been used as an indirect method of identifying the bacteria involved in endometrial infections, but there is the possibility that the specimens obtained are contaminated by vaginal flora. Postpartum endometritis is a common cause of nosocomial bacteremia in obstetric patients, but blood cultures are insensitive. Even when blood cultures are positive, usually only one organism is isolated when the infection is most likely mixed. Nevertheless, the isolates are usually significant, and blood cultures should always be collected. Endocervical smears and cultures should also be done, despite their limitations. Therapy should be directed against predominant or unusual isolates, especially if the patient does not respond to empiric antibiotic therapy.

Treatment

Empiric therapy should include coverage against streptococci, gram-negative bacilli, and anaerobes, especially the *Bacteroides* species. Empiric coverage for staphylococci is unnecessary. Clindamycin plus an aminoglycoside is the standard combination regimen. Flagyl has good activity against anaerobes and is frequently used for intra-abdominal infections in combination with an aminoglycoside, but there is some concern about the lack of activity against certain species of streptococci that may be involved in these infections. Second or third generation cephalosporins with good anaerobic activity, including activity against *Bacteroides*, are an alternative, and studies have shown single agent therapy is just as effective as combination therapy, as well as less expensive.[36] Therapy should be modified to cover isolates from blood and predominant or unusual isolates from endocervical specimens, especially if there is a failure with the initial empiric regimen. Abscesses require surgical drainage. If septic pelvic thrombophlebitis is suspected, a trial of therapeutic heparin may be indicated. If there is a response within 48 hours, the heparin should be continued for a 10-day course.

Prevention

As with wound infections, the incidence of postpartum endometritis can be decreased with the use of perioperative antibiotics for delivery by cesarean section. Some authorities have suggested that prophylaxis only be given to patients considered to be at high risk for infection, but generally antibiotic prophylaxis is felt to be indicated for all patients undergoing cesarean section. First generation cephalosporins are effective prophylactic agents. Three perioperative doses are adequate for prophylaxis. There is no added benefit of using a third generation cephalosporin or an extended-spectrum penicillin, despite their broader spectrum of activity. Certainly, the cost of these agents makes them less attractive for prophylaxis. Even this short-term prophylaxis alters the patient's flora, but longer courses of prophylaxis compound this problem. When infections occur despite prophylaxis, resistant organisms are often responsible.[37] Therefore, it is prudent to give short-term prophylaxis with three perioperative doses of a first generation cephalosporin.

URINARY TRACT INFECTIONS

Clinical Manifestations

Urinary tract infections (UTIs) are common in hospitalized patients, including obstetric patients (see also Chapter 143). Recently, there has been a great deal of interest in pathogenesis, diagnosis, and therapy of urinary tract infections, and recent studies have resulted in many changes in the management of these infections.[38] In the past, the diagnosis of a UTI required the presence of significant bacteriuria, defined as $>10^5$ cfu bacteria/mL of urine in a clean catch urine sample. This level of bacteriuria identifies patients with UTI and excludes cases of contamination, but it is now known that many women with acute bacterial cystitis have infection with colony counts from 102–104 cfu/mL. The urinalysis is helpful in these patients, as the presence of pyuria indicates infection even when the quantitative urine culture does not demonstrate >105 cfu/mL. Recently, there has been an interest in other rapid tests to detect UTI, including dipstick tests for screening for pyuria and bacteriuria. Dipsticks that detect leukocyte esterase are fairly accurate in determining whether or not there is significant pyuria. A positive nitrite test on dipstick analysis of urine can be used to screen for bacteriuria. These tests may be more helpful than the time-honored quantitative urine culture in identifying patients with bacteriuria or UTI.

Patients with pyelonephritis should be distinguished from patients with cystitis, but this may not be easy on the basis of clinical signs and symptoms alone. Suprapubic tenderness suggests cystitis, and flank pain is characteristic of acute pyelonephritis, but it is well known that these clinical signs are not very accurate in identifying which patients have upper or lower tract infections. Fever, chills, nausea and vomiting, and other constitutional symptoms also suggest pyelonephritis, but patients without these symptoms may have upper UTI or occult pyelonephritis. A number of methods have been used to distinguish between upper and lower UTI, including ureteral catheterization, bladder washout techniques, and antibody-coated bacteria assays. Unfortunately, the antibody-coated bacteria test is less accurate than initially hoped, and the other techniques mentioned are not practical for the routine management of UTIs. Blood cultures may be positive in pyelonephritis, but the sensitivity of blood cultures is low. Currently, the best test for identifying patients with upper UTI, at least in certain populations such as young women with acute dysuria, is the response to single dose antibiotic therapy.[39] More than 90% of patients with uncomplicated cystitis will respond to single dose regimens. A failure or relapse with single-dose therapy may indicate an occult upper UTI.

Incidence

Overall, UTIs are the leading cause of nosocomial infections and account for 35% of these infections. In the obstetric population, UTIs are second only to wound and pelvic-peritoneal infections as a cause of nosocomial infection. In one study, UTIs were present in 4.4% of hospitalized obstetric patients. In hospitalized obstetric patients with fever, UTIs have been identified in 16% of cases.

Pathogenesis

Colonization of the periurethral epithelium is the first step in the development of a UTI in females. The reservoir for the colonizing organisms is the gastrointestinal tract. These organisms gain access to the bladder by retrograde migration along the urethra. In some cases, this seeding of the bladder is associated with sexual intercourse. Approximately 4% of pregnant women will develop asymptomatic bacteriuria with $>10^5$ cfu/mL early in the course of pregnancy.[40] Studies where suprapubic aspiration was performed indicate an even greater prevalence of bacteriuria by identifying bacteriuric women with $<10^5$ cfu/mL. It is these bacteriuric women who are at risk for developing symptomatic UTIs later in the course of pregnancy, usually the third trimester or postpartum period. These bacteriuric patients can be identified by screening in the first trimester and at the first antenatal visit. Women without bacteriuria are much less likely to develop symptomatic UTIs later on. A number of changes in the urinary tract, such as dilatation of the collecting system, decreased ureteral peristalsis, increased residual urine volume, and trauma during labor may account for the high incidence of UTIs in these bacteriuric women.

For nosocomial UTIs in general, the major risk factor is urethral catheterization.[41] Overall, 70–80% of nosocomial UTIs follow catheterization. Catheterization also is a risk factor for nosocomial UTI in the peripartum period. Intrapartum catheterization results in bacteriuria in 15% of patients, and this may be as high as 25% for women after a complicated delivery. The risk of infection increases by 5–10% per day of catheterization and by 14 days, as many as 50% of patients will be infected, even with closed urinary drainage systems. Bacteriuria from catheterization can result from introduction of bacteria at the time of catheter placement, by extraluminal migration of bacteria, or intraluminal migration. Although extraluminal migration is the most common route of infection, intraluminal migration is evidenced by the increased risk of UTIs when there is a break in the closed drainage system. Cross infection due to transfer of organisms from patient to patient by hospital staff occurs in 15% of cases.[42] Cross infection can be identified by recognizing clustering of cases. The organisms may be transferred on the hands of the staff or introduced by way of contaminated antiseptic or irrigation solutions, collection vessels, or urometers.

Etiologic Agents

Gram-negative rods are the most common organisms causing nosocomial UTIs. *E coli* accounts for ≥50% of cases, followed by *Klebsiella, Proteus* species, *P aeruginosa, Enterobacter, Serratia,* and *Citrobacter.* Enterococci are the most commonly isolated gram-positive organisms, followed by groups B streptococci and staphylococci. *Candida* may also cause infection in patients in association with urethral catheterization and prior antibiotic therapy. *E coli, Proteus,* and enterococci usually cause sporadic cases of UTI, while clusters of UTIs due to cross infection are caused by *Pseudomonas, Serratia,* and *Citrobacter.* These organisms involved in clusters of cases tend to be relatively more antibiotic-resistant.

Therapy

Patients with symptomatic UTI require treatment. Patients with fever, chills, other constitutional symptoms, or flank pain should receive empiric therapy with the combination of ampicillin plus an aminoglycoside. This combination will provide adequate coverage against most nosocomial pathogens, with the exception of staphylococci, *Candida,* and drug-resistant enteric gram-negative rods. Therapy can be directed when the results of cultures and susceptibilities are available. Parenteral therapy for presumed pyelonephritis should continue for 24 hours after fever resolves, and then oral therapy given until the patient has received a 10–14-day total course of antibiotics. One week after therapy a repeat urine culture should be performed, and patients with persistent bacteriuria given a 6-week course of antibiotics to eradicate the infection.

Patients with dysuria and pyuria indicating acute bacterial cystitis should be treated with oral antibiotics, even if there are $<10^5$ cfu/mL on quantitative urine culture. Short courses of therapy (1–3 days) are probably as effective as conventional 7–14-day courses in most women with cystitis.[38] Data on the effectivenesss of short course antibiotic therapy for nosocomial UTIs in pregnant or postpartum women is unavailable, and it may be prudent to give a conventional course of therapy in this situation. Again, therapy should be adjusted appropriately when culture results are available.

Patients with asymptomatic bacteriuria associated with urethral catheterization should not be treated if the catheter is to remain in place. Therapy in these patients will result in the emergence of resistant organisms. Symptomatic infection may be prevented by treatment of bacteriuria in patients when the catheter is removed or is to be removed within 96 hours.

Candiduria in association with urethral catheterization may resolve with removal of the catheter alone, but symptomatic infections may require antifungal therapy. Bladder irrigations with amphotericin B (continuous irrigation by way of a triple lumen catheter with 25–50 mg in one liter sterile water daily) is effective. Oral therapy with flucytosine is also effective in cases of fungal UTI. Ketoconazole has good tissue penetration, but it is not concentrated in the urine, and its role in the treatment of fungal UTIs has not been established. Intravenous amphotericin B is usually reserved for refractory cases because of its potential for toxicity, but there is evidence that a single dose of intravenous amphotericin B may be effective in eradicting *Candida* from the urinary tract.

Prevention

UTIs in the obstetric patient can be prevented by screening all pregnant women for bacteriuria at the time of the first antenatal visit. Therapy with a single dose of antibiotics is probably as effective as a conventional course of therapy, but some authorities still recommend a conventional 7–10-day course of therapy.[43] A follow-up culture should be performed one week after the completion of therapy and then every month until delivery. In cases of therapeutic failure or recurrence, a repeat course of therapy is given. Patients who have had symptomatic UTIs or recurrent episodes of asymptomatic bacteriuria should receive suppressive therapy until delivery.[40]

The incidence of UTI due to urethral catheterization can be reduced by paying attention to aseptic technique during insertion of the catheter. Closed drainage systems should be used. The system should remain closed if possible. If irrigation is necessary, this should also be performed by aseptic technique. Retrograde flow of urine from the collecting system should be avoided. Cross infection should be prevented by strict handwashing and avoidance of cross contamination with inanimate objects, such as collection vessels and urometers. Prevention of cross infection may be facilitated by isolating catheterized patients if feasible. The efficacy of daily care in preventing catheter infections has not been established. Finally, catheters should be removed as soon as possible.

INTRAVENOUS CATHETER SEPSIS

Clinical Manifestations

Nosocomial bacteremias may be primary or, more commonly, secondary to identifiable local infections.[44] In the hospital, bacteremias due to intravenous catheters or other intravascular devices are the leading cause of primary bacteremia and account for significant morbidity and mortality. Rarely, bacteremia may result from contamination of the infusate, and outbreaks have occurred. Improper handling of total parenteral nutrition (TPN) solutions has also resulted in outbreaks of infusion-related sepsis.

Local signs of infection around a catheter may be a clue to the diagnosis. This can include surrounding cellulitis or purulent discharge from the catheter site. A tunnel infection with a central venous catheter is characterized by erythema, warmth, and tenderness along the subcutaneous course of the catheter. However, the diagnosis of catheter sepsis is often difficult, and these local signs of inflammation are present in only 50% of catheter-associated infections. Blood cultures give important information, but the value of cultures drawn through the catheter is not clear. Culture of catheter tips in broth cultures are extremely sensitive, but a single contaminating organism can give a positive culture and result in an unacceptably high false positive rate. A semiquantitative technique has been developed where the tip of the catheter is rolled across an agar plate and the number of colonies counted. Most infections will result in confluent growth, but a colony count of 15 is considered significant.[45]

Suppurative thrombophlebitis is a distinct subset of catheter sepsis characterized by erythema, warmth, tenderness, and often a palpable cord due to an infected clot within the vein, as well as systemic toxicity. The infection can be documented by expressing or aspirating pus from the vein. In some cases, when the diagnosis is suspected it may be necessary to surgically explore the vein in order to make the diagnosis.

Incidence

Approximately 25,000 cases of nosocomial primary bacteremia due to intravascular devices occur each year in the United States.[44] The incidence of both secondary bacteremias and primary bacteremias due to catheter sepsis had increased from 1970–1979.[12] Reports from different studies range from 0% to as high as 27% in patients receiving long-term parenteral hyperalimentation. These rates are dependent on the duration and methods of intravenous cannulation, as well as the method of diagnosis. The morbidity, mortality, and economic cost of these infections is high.

Pathogenesis

The development of intravenous catheter sepsis is dependent on a number of factors, including the type of catheter, duration of placement, and host factors.[46] Infection usually begins with the formation of a fibrin clot on the surface of the catheter, which serves as a site of attachment for bacteria. Plastic and polyvinylchloride catheters are thrombogenic. Stainless steel needles are less thrombogenic and are associated with lower infection rates. Bacteria gain access to this attachment site by a number of routes. Hematogenous spread from a distant focus of infection is probably an uncommon route of infection, but it may be important, especially in patients with long-term central venous catheters. Migration of organisms from the skin site of insertion is of primary importance in infections of short intravenous catheters. There are a number of factors that alter the colonizing flora of the skin. The newer membrane dressings allow visualization of the catheter site, but are associated with a greater rate of skin colonization. Shaving the insertion site also results in increased skin colonization. Patient age (<1 yr, >60 yrs), preexisting skin conditions, granulocytopenia, abnormal granulocyte function, and other immunodeficiency states, including AIDS, are some of the host factors associated with an increased incidence of catheter sepsis. The most important risk factor for the development of catheter-related infections is the duration of catheterization. Rates of intravenous catheter colonization and sepsis markedly increase after the catheter has been in for >72 hours. The experience and skill of the person placing the catheter may also be important, and some studies have indicated that an I.V. team may reduce the incidence of catheter-associated infections. Cut down catheters have a greater risk of infection than catheters that are placed percutaneously.

Bacterial endocarditis may complicate catheter infection. This is especially true for patients with central venous catheters, which cross the tricuspid valve and can initially cause fibrin–platelet aggregates on the valve that serve as a focus of infection. Although right-sided endocarditis is more common, left-sided endocarditis can occur. Some patients may develop a localized metastatic focus of infection, such as septic arthritis, endophthalmitis, or osteomyelitis without endocarditis.

Pathogens

The most frequently isolated organisms in catheter sepsis include *S aureus*, coagulase-negative staphylococci, and enteric gram-negative rods, especially *Klebsiella*. Suppurative thrombophlebitis is most often due to *Klebsiella*, although *S aureus* is also involved in a significant number of these cases. Infections caused by contaminated infusates usually involve enteric gram-negative rods (*Enterobacter*, *Citrobacter*, non-aeruginosa *Pseudomonas*). *Candida* species can cause catheter sepsis, and the risk of this increases with previous broad-specturm antibiotic therapy and parenteral hyperalimentation.

Therapy

Catheters that may be infected should be removed and properly cultured. An exception may be long-term central venous catheters. Recent experience shows that these infections may be adequately treated with parenteral antibiotics without removal of the catheter, especially infections due to staphylococci and streptococci. Infections due to gram-negative bacilli and fungi are more difficult to cure, and catheter removal is often required. Exit site infection can be treated with the catheter in place, while tunnel infections usually require removal of the catheter, in addition to antibiotic therapy. Empiric antibiotic therapy with a penicillinase-resistant penicillin, a first generation cephalosporin, or vancomycin plus an aminoglycoside should be initiated pending the results of cultures.

Suppurative thrombophlebitis should be treated with aggressive surgical exploration and removal of the involved segment of vein. If a deep vein is involved, heparin therapy in addition to antibiotic therapy may be successful in clearing the infection. However, this condition is serious and associated with significant morbidity and mortality.

Prevention

Skill and attention to aseptic technique during catheter insertion are important. The use of antibiotic preparations at the site of insertion may be useful in preventing bacterial catheter infections. The most important infection control measure to prevent intravenous catheter infections is changing the catheter every 48–72 hours. The duration of central venous catheterization is a matter for discussion. Infection rates increase dramatically after seven days. Some authorities have recommended changing the catheters over guidewires every seven days, but this is controversial. Hickman indwelling catheters have low rates of infection, but this can be minimized by good aseptic technique and the avoidance of using the catheter for purposes other than parenteral hyperalimentation.

PNEUMONIAS

Clinical Manifestations

Nosocomial pneumonias are relatively uncommon in the obstetric population. These infections are characterized by new onset of fever and cough productive of purulent sputum in a patient without prior pulmonary infection, or by increased sputum production with fever in a patient admitted with pulmonary disease. The physical examination reveals rales, bronchial breath sounds, or signs of consolidation. Chest x-ray shows an infiltrate, although infiltrate occasionally can be absent early in the course (see also Chapter 121).

Incidence

Pneumonia is the third most common nosocomial infection accounting for 15% of cases, according to NNIS. However, this is not true, with obstetric services where the rate is 0.4% per 1000 discharges versus 6.5–7.5% per 1000 discharges on medical and surgical services.[14] In the study of Klimek and coworkers, pneumonia accounted for only 2% of cases of hospital-acquired fever in obstetric patients.[5] These infections, however, are associated with significant morbidity and mortality. Pneumonia is the most common cause of death among nosocomial infections, accounting for 60% of nosocomial-related deaths.[47]

Pathogenesis

The development of pneumonia usually indicates a defect in the host's respiratory tract defense mechanisms. Most organisms, with the exceptions of *pneumococcus* and *Legionella,* cannot cause pneumonia in a completely healthy host. Some patients may have a specific congenital condition predisposing them to respiratory tract infections, but this is rare and these patients usually can be identified by a history of recurrent infections. Other patients may have an acquired immune defect. These patients are predisposed to a pneumonia with a number of pathogens. Most patients, however, do not have a specific immune defect, but rather some type of chronic underlying medical illness that affects lung defense mechanisms. The conditions that predispose patients to pneumonia are many and the effects on the host may be varied, but in many cases these conditions predispose patients to pneumonia by altering the oral flora. Advanced age, diabetes, congestive heart failure, chronic obstructive pulmonary disease, alcoholism, acidosis, azotemia, and prior antibiotic therapy all increase the incidence of oropharyngeal colonization with pathogenic bacteria associated with hospital-acquired pneumonia.

The low incidence of nosocomial pneumonia in obstetric patients reflects the low incidence of chronic underlying medical illness in this patient population. However, obstetric patients do have some abnormalities that may put them at risk of developing pneumonia. General anesthesia predisposes patients to aspiration by altering consciousness and depressing cough reflexes and gag reflexes. Narcotic analgesics may do the same.

Etiologic Agents

Hospital-acquired pneumonias are most commonly caused by gram-negative bacilli. *P aeruginosa* is the single most common agent of pneumonia in the hospital, accounting for 15% of cases. Other gram-negative rods, such as *E coli, Klebsiella,* and *Enterobacter,* collectively account for another 45% of cases. *S aureus* is also more common in the hosptial setting, accounting for 10% of cases, and is the second most common single species. *Streptococcus pneumoniae* can also cause pneumonia in the hospitalized patient, but it accounts for less than 5% of hospital-acquired pneumonias, versus 60–90% of community-acquired pneumonias. *Legionella* may be a nosocomial pathogen and is associated with contaminated water sources. However, the incidence of *Legionella* pneumonia is quite variable, and this probably reflects geographic differences in the prevalence of *Legionella.* The importance of anaerobes in hospital-acquired pneumonia has been underestimated because techniques required for isolation of anaerobes have not been used in most studies of nosocomial pneumonia. Some studies indicate that anaerobes may be involved in up to 20% of cases of nosocomial pneumonia. Tuberculosis can also be a nosocomial pathogen. Viruses can cause outbreaks of nosocomial pneumonia, especially influenza, adenoviruses, and RSV.

Therapy

Therapy for pneumonia should be guided by the sputum Gram's stain. Cultures of expectorated sputum should be collected, but are of limited value. Oropharyngeal contamination can lead to false-positive sputum culture results. On the other hand, some pathogens are fastidious (*Pneumococcus, Hemophilus influenzae*) or require special culture techniques (*Legionella*), and this can result in false-negative cultures. Sputum cultures can be helpful in excluding pneumonia due to nonfastidious organisms such as *S aureus* and enteric gram-negative rods. Initial empiric therapy when the Gram's stain does not allow for an etiologic diagnosis should include a penicillinase-resistant penicillin or first generation cephalosporin in combination with an aminoglycoside to cover for *S aureus* and gram-negative rods. If there is a high incidence of methicillin-resistant *S aureus* infections in the hospital at the time, vancomycin plus aminoglycoside may be a reasonable alternative regimen. Patients who have developed pneumonia after aspirating oropharyngeal or gastric contents should be treated with penicillin G or clindamycin plus an aminoglycoside to cover for anaerobes and gram-negative rods. Obviously, the antibiotic regimen should be adjusted when results of smears and cultures are available, although interpretation of culture data may be difficult.

Prevention

There is great interest in developing approaches to the prevention of nosocomial pneumonia. Recently, it has been shown that antacids given to prevent stress ulcers in severely ill intensive care unit patients may result in colonization of the upper gastrointestinal tract and subsequent colonization of the oropharynx with enteric gram-negative rods. Colonization did not occur in patients receiving sucralfate, which does not cause an increase in gastric pH, and this may prevent the development of gram-negative rod pneumonia. Other approaches to the prevention of oropharyngeal colonization have included selective decontamination of the oropharynx using nonabsorbable antibiotic preparations in high risk patients. Other standard methods for prevention include sterilization of respiratory therapy equipment, attention to aseptic technique when suctioning patients, and strict handwashing to prevent cross infection. However, most of these interventions apply only to extremely high risk groups, specifically, intubated patients requiring mechanical ventilation.

BREAST INFECTIONS

Clinical Manifestations

Mastitis and breast abscesses are relatively common postpartum complications.[31] Mastitis is characterized by pain and tenderness, erythema, and swelling. A fluctuant area indicates that mastitis has progressed to abscess formation. Fever occurs, but systemic toxicity is rare. Mastitis and abscess usually occur in women who breast feed (see also Chapter 188).

Incidence

Approximately 1–5% of postpartum females will develop breast infections, but rates may be much higher when epidemics occur.

Pathogenesis

Breast-feeding is the major predisposing factor for the development of mastitis. There is considerable evidence that the initial event is contamination of the milk and ductal system with the oropharyngeal flora of the nursing infant. Most infants become colonized with *S aureus* during the first week of life, and the strains of staphylococci are usually hospital strains acquired from contaminated equipment or the hands of the staff.

Etiologic Agents

S aureus is recovered in 95% of the cases, and these organisms have the same susceptibility patterns as most hospital-acquired strains. Most are penicillin-resistant, and some may be methicillin-resistant. Other organisms may be recovered, including enterococci and coagulase-negative staphylococci. Enteric gram-negative rods are rarely recovered. Abscesses should be aspirated and specimens submitted for Gram's stain and culture and susceptibility testing. Breast milk can be cultured after properly prepping the nipple prior to expressing the sample.

Treatment and Prevention

Mastitis should be treated with a penicillinase-resistant penicillin or a first generation cephalosporin. Abscesses require surgical drainage. Prevention of this infection is difficult given the pathogenesis, but certainly epidemics can be controlled or perhaps prevented by careful handwashing and other infection control interventions. Mothers can continue to breast-feed while undergoing therapy for mastitis, but mothers with breast abscesses should refrain from nursing in order to prevent staphylococcal infection, pneumonia, or lung abscess in the neonate.

INFECTION CONTROL

It is estimated that as many as one third of nosocomial infections can be prevented.[1] Prevention in large part depends on effective hospital infection control programs. There must be ongoing surveillance to identify nosocomial infections and to institute infection control measures when a problem is identified. Data from SENIC show that hospitals without programs or with ineffective programs had a significant increase in nosocomial bacteremias, UTIs, wound infections, and pneumonia during the period from 1970–1976.[48] Hospitals with effective programs, however, had significant decreases in the rates of all these types of infections.

Proper control of nosocomial infections includes the appropriate isolation of patients with infections. While isolation is important in preventing the spread of infection, unnecessary precautions must be avoided. This is especially true of obstetric services where separation of the mother and infant is a major consideration. Guidelines for isolation have been published by a number of groups and government agencies. The CDC revised its recommendations for hospital isolation precautions in 1983.[49] The new guidelines allow hospitals to choose between category-specific or disease-specific isolation. Seven categories are recommended for category-specific isolation: strict isolation, contact isolation, respiratory isolation, tuberculosis isolation, enteric precautions, drainage–secretion precautions, and blood–body fluid precautions. The precautions for each category are applicable to a group of diseases with similar modes of transmission. In disease-specific isolation, only those precautions necessary for that particular disease are enforced. Each system has its advantages and disadvantages, and it is the responsibility of the infection control committee to decide which system will best suit the needs of the hospital. Hospital infection control committees also have the authority to devise their own isolation policies. The CDC has also proposed the concept of universal precautions for blood and body fluids to be applied to all hospitalized patients.[50] These recommendations have been developed to prevent the transmission of bloodborne infections to health care workers. Specific isolation guidelines for obstetric patients have been proposed by Weinstein, Boyer, and Linn.[51] These detailed guidelines can be very helpful to infection control committees in setting up their own policies for infection control on obstetric services.

REFERENCES

1. Wenzel RP. Nosocomial infections, diagnosis-related groups, and Study on the Efficacy of Nosocomial Infection Control. *Am J Med*. 1985;78(suppl 6B):3.
2. Holmes OW. On the contagiousness of puerperal fever. *Medical Classics*. 1936;1:211.
3. Semmelweis IP. The etiology, the concept, and the prophylaxis of childbed fever. *Medical Classics*. 1941;5:350.
4. Johanson WG, Pierce AK, Sanford JP. Changing pharyngeal flora of hospitalized patients. Emergence of gram-negative bacilli. *N Engl J Med*. 1969;281:1137.
5. Klimek JJ, Ajemian ER, Gracewski J, et al. A prospective analysis of hospital-acquired fever in obstetric and gynecologic patients. *JAMA*. 1982;247:3340.
6. Ledger WJ. *Infection in the Female*. 2nd ed. Philadelphia, PA: Lea & Febiger; 1986:268.
7. Thoburn R, Fekety FR, Cluff LE, Melvin VB. Infections acquired by hospitalized patients. *Arch Intern Med*. 1968;121:1.
8. Bennett JV, Scheckler WE, Maki DG, Brachman BS. Current national patterns—United States. In: Proceedings of the International Conference on Nosocomial Infections. Centers for Disease Control; August 3–6, 1970;42–9.
9. Haley RW, Culver DH, White JW, et al. The nationwide nosocomial infection rate. A new need for vital statistics. *Am J Epidemiol*. 1985; 121:159.
10. Harris AA, Levin S, Trenholme GM. Selected aspects of nosocomial infections in the 1980s. *Am J Med*. 1984;77(suppl 1B):3.
11. Stamm WE, Weinstein RA, Dixon RE. Comparison of endemic and epidemic nosomial infections. *Am J Med*. 1981;70:393.
12. Allen JR, Hightower AW, Martin SM, Dixon RE. Secular trends in nosocomial infections: 1970–9. *Am J Med*. 1981;70:389.
13. Gedebou M, Habte-Gabr E, Kronvall G, Yoseph S. Hospital-acquired infections among obstetric and gynecological patients at Tikur Anbessa Hospital, Addis Ababa. *J Hosp Infect*. 1988;11:50.
14. Centers for Disease Control. Nosocomial infections surveillance, 1984. (Reprinted from surveillance summaries). *MMWR*. 1986;35:17SS.
15. Wenzel RP. The mortality of hospital-acquired bloodstream infections: need for a new vital statistic. *Trans Amer Clin Climatol* 1986;98:43.
16. Donowitz LG, Wenzel RP. Endometritis following cesarean section. A controlled study of the increased duration of hospital stay and direct cost of hospitalization. *Am J Obstet Gynecol*. 1980;137:467.
17. Neu HC. Mechanisms of bacterial resistance. *Am J Med*. 1984;77(suppl 1B):11.
18. Fraser DW. Bacteria newly recognized as nosocomial pathogens. *Am J Med*. 1981;70:432.
19. Mayer KH, Zinner SH. Bacterial pathogens of increasing significance in hospital-acquired infections. *Rev Infect Dis*. 1985;7(suppl 3):S371.
20. Mayer KH, Opal SM. Unusual nosocomial pathogens. *Infect Dis Clin N Am*. 1989;3:883.
21. McGowan JE. Changing etiology of nosocomial bacteremia and fungemia and other hosptial-acquired infections. *Rev Infect Dis*. 1985;7(suppl 3):S357.
22. Anaissie E, Body GP. Nosocomial fungal infections. Old problems and new challenges. *Infect Dis Clin N Am*. 1989;3:867.

23. Valenti WM, Hall CB, Douglas RG, et al. Nosocomial viral infections: I. Epidemiology and significance. *Infect Control*. 1980;1:33.
24. Sabath LD. Mechanisms of resistance to beta-lactam antibiotics in strains of *Staphylococcus aureus*. *Ann Intern Med*. 1982;97:339.
25. Schwalbe RS, Stapleton JT, Gilligan PH. Emergence of vancomycin resistance in coagulase-negative staphylococci. *N Engl J Med*. 1987;316:927.
26. Murray BE, Mederski-Sanaroz B. Transferable B-lactamase: a new mechanism for *in vitro* penicillin resistance in *Streptococcus faecalis*. *J Clin Invest*. 1983;72:1168.
27. Leclercq R, Derlot E, Duval J, Courvalin P. Plasmid-mediated resistance to vancomycin and teichoplanin in *Enterococcus faecium*. *N Engl J Med*. 1988;319:157.
28. Marr JJ, Moffet HL, Kunin CM. Guidelines for improving the use of antimicrobial agents in hospitals: a statement by the Infectious Diseases Society of America. *J Infect Dis*. 1988;157:869.
29. Freeman J, McGowan JE. Risk factors for nosocomial infections. *J Infect Dis*. 1978;138:811.
30. Sweet RL, Ledger WJ. Puerperal infectious morbidity—a two-year review. *Am J Med*. 1973;117:1093.
31. Eschenbach DA, Wager GP. Puerperal infections. *Clin Obstet Gynecol*. 1980;23:1003.
32. Hirsch HA. Prophylactic antibiotics in obstetrics and gynecology. *Am J Med*. 1985;78(suppl 6B):170.
33. Herbst AL, Mercer LJ. Overview of therapeutic and prophylactic antibiotics in obstetrics and gynecology. *J Repro Med*. 1988;33(suppl):144.
34. Hibbard LT, Snyder EN, McVann RM. Subgluteal and retropsoal infection in obstetric practice. *Obstet Gynecol*. 1972;39:137.
35. Yonekura ML. Risk factors for postcesarean endometritis. *Am J Med*. 1985;78(suppl 6B):177.
36. Faro S, Sanders CV, Aldridge KE. Use of single-agent antimicrobial therapy in the treatment of polymicrobial female pelvic infections. *Obstet Gynecol*. 1982;60:232.
37. Gibbs RS, St Clair PJ, Castillo MS, Castenada YS. Bacteriologic effects of antibiotic prophylaxis in high-risk cesarean section. *Obstet Gynecol*. 1981;57:277.
38. Johnson JR, Stamm WE. Diagnosis and treatment of acute urinary tract infections. *Infect Dis Clin N Am*. 1987;1:773.
39. Ronald AR, Boutros P, Mourtada H. Bacteriuria localization and response to single-dose therapy in women. *JAMA*. 1976;256:1854.
40. Patterson TF, Andriole VT. Bacteriuria in pregnancy. *Infect Dis Clin N Am*. 1987;1:807.
41. Turck M, Stamm W. Nosocomial infection of the urinary tract. *Am J Med*. 1981;70:651.
42. Schaberg DR, Haley RW, Highsmith AK, et al. Nosocomial bacteriuria: a prospective study of case clustering and antimicrobial resistance. *Ann Intern Med*. 1980;93:420.
43. Masterton RG. Single-dose amoxicillin in the treatment of bacteriuria in pregnancy and the puerperium—a controlled clinical trial. *Br J Obstet Gynecol*. 1985;92:498.
44. Maki DG. Nosocomial bacteremia. An epidemiologic overview. *Am J Med*. 1981;70:719.
45. Maki DG, Weise C, Sarafin HW. A semiquantitative culture method for identifying intravenous-catheter-related infection. *N Engl J Med*. 1977; 296:1305.
46. Henderson DK. Bacteremia due to percutaneous intravascular devices. In: Mandell GL, Douglas FG, Bennett JE. 3rd ed. New York: John Wiley & Sons; 1989:2189.
47. LaForce FM. Hospital-acquired gram-negative rod pneumonias: an overview. *Am J Med*. 1981;70:664.
48. Haley RW, Culver DH, White JW, et al. The efficacy of infection surveillance and control programs in preventing nosocomial infections in US hospitals. *Am J Epidemiol*. 1985;121:182.
49. Garner JS, Simmons BP. CDC guidelines for isolation precautions in hospitals. *Infect Control*. 1983;12:103.
50. Centers for Disease Control. Update: Universal precautions for prevention of transmission of blood-borne pathogens in health-care settings. *MMWR*. 1988;37:377.
51. Weinstein RA, Boyer KM, Linn ES. Isolation guidelines for obstetric patients and newborns. *Am J Obstet Gynecol*. 1983;146:353.

Chapter Fifty-Six

Chemotherapy of Bacterial Infection

Jay F. Dobkin

56

The management of suspected bacterial infection in pregnancy is particularly challenging. Conditions such as cystitis and asymptomatic bacteriuria, which are benign in the nonpregnant woman, constitute a substantial threat to both mother and fetus if improperly managed. Correspondingly, however, unnecessary or improperly chosen antibiotics pose a threat to the patient and especially to the fetus. Thus, a judicious approach to determining the need for antibiotic therapy and to selection of the most effective and least toxic drug has special importance in this setting. This chapter focuses on the selection of antibacterial agents based on clinical diagnosis, laboratory identification of pathogens, and interpretation of *in vitro* sensitivity testing. Because many new antibacterial drugs have recently become available, particular attention is given to their potential use in pregnancy.

The association of particular organisms with certain infectious disease syndromes provides an important basis for the evaluation and initial therapy of the infected patient (Table 56–1). Individual assessment of each case is critical because the likelihood of unusual or "opportunistic" pathogens and particularly the probability of antibiotic resistance is largely predictable from historical factors, such as the presence of underlying diseases, recent instrumentation, hospitalization, or antibiotic therapy.

URINARY TRACT INFECTIONS

Because fully 5% of pregnant women have bacteriuria, and between 1% and 2.5% have acute cystitis or pyelonephritis, the importance of urinary tract infections (UTIs) in pregnancy is clear (see also Chapter 143).[1] The high rate of progression from *asymptomatic bacteriuria* to acute pyelonephritis in pregnancy (at least 30%) leads to the necessity for screening and treatment.[2,3] Once a prenatal patient is found to have asymptomatic bacteriuria, the physician faces several treatment choices. Single-dose therapy of cystitis in nonpregnant women and asymptomatic bacteriuria in pregnant women has been demonstrated to be usually effective with several agents other than first generation cephalosporins.[4,5] This approach remains controversial, however, due to the risk of complications from relapse or unsuspected upper tract disease, especially when follow-up culture cannot be assured after treatment. A seven- to 14-day course is, therefore, still advisable.[6,7] The appropriate choice of antibiotics is also problematic. Community-acquired UTIs are not as predictably caused by highly sensitive coliform organisms as in the past. If older, narrow-spectrum β-lactam drugs, such as ampicillin or cephalexin, are used, culture and sensitivity data and test-of-cure follow-up cultures become even more important.

TABLE 56–1. MICROORGANISMS CAUSING INFECTION IN WOMEN OF CHILDBEARING AGE

- Urinary Tract Infections
  - Community-acquired
    - Enterobacteriaceae (*Escherichia coli, Proteus mirabilis, Morganella morganii, Klebsiella pneumoniae*)
    - *Staphylococcus saprophyticus*
    - *Enterococcus faecalis*
  - Hospital-acquired or anatomic abnormality
    - Resistant Enterobacteriaceae (*Enterobacter* species, *Serratia, Providencia*)
    - *Acinetobacter* var. anitratus
    - *Pseudomonas aeruginosa*
    - *Pseudomonas* species (*Pseudomonas cepacia, Pseudomonas maltophilia*)
    - *Candida albicans*
  - Acute urethral syndrome
    - Enterobacteriaceae
    - *Neisseria gonorrhoeae*
    - *Chlamydia trachomatis*
    - *Staphylococcus saprophyticus*
    - Herpes simplex virus
- Pelvic Inflammatory Disease
  - First attacks, <24 years of Age
    - *Neisseria gonorrhoeae*
    - *Chlamydia trachomatis*
    - *Ureaplasma urealyticum*
    - *Mycoplasma hominis*
    - Vaginal anaerobes, aerobes
  - Subsequent attacks or first attack >24 years of age
    - Organisms above less common; organisms in vaginal flora more common
    - Anaerobes
      - *Bacteroides bivius, disiens* (common)
      - *Bacteroides fragilis* (less common)
      - Peptococcus, peptostreptococcus, *Veillonella*
      - *Clostridium* species
    - Aerobes
      - Enterobacteriaceae (*Escherichia coli, Proteus mirabilis*)
      - Streptococci (groups B,D)
      - *Staphylococcus epidermidis*
      - *Chlamydia trachomatis*
  - Chronic pelvic inflammatory disease
    - Vaginal aerobes and anaerobes
    - Actinomyces
    - *Chlamydia trachomatis*
    - *Mycoplasma hominis*
    - *Ureaplasma urealyticum*
    - *Mycobacterium tuberculosis* (rare)
  - Patients with intrauterine devices
    - Vaginal aerobes and anaerobes
    - Actinomyces
    - *Chlamydia trachomatis*
- Genital Lesions
  - Ulcers
    - *Treponema pallidum* (primary syphilis)
    - Herpes simplex virus
    - *Hemophilus ducreyi* (chancroid)
    - *Chlamydia trachomatis* (lymphogranuloma venerum)
    - *Candida albicans*
  - Papules
    - *Treponema pallidum* (secondary syphilis)
    - Human papillomavirus
    - Molluscum contagiosum
    - *Sarcoptes scabiei* (scabies)
    - *Candida albicans*
  - Inguinal adenopathy
    - Sexually Transmitted Diseases (STDs)
      - *Neisseria gonorrhoeae*
      - *Treponema pallidum* (primary syphilis)
      - Herpes simplex virus
      - *Hemophilus ducreyi* (chancroid)
      - *Chlamydia trachomatis* (lymphogranuloma venereum)
      - *Candida albicans*
    - Non-STD
      - *Staphylococcus aureus*
      - *Streptococcus pyogenes*
        - Rare: Cat-scratch disease bacillus
          - *Francisella tularensis* (tularemia)
          - *Mycobacterium tuberculosis*
          - Brucella species (Brucellosis)
- Postpartum Endometritis
  - Early infection (first 48 h)
    - Aerobic bacteria
      - *Escherichia coli*
      - *Klebsiella pneumoniae*
      - Streptococci (groups B and D)
      - *Staphylococcus epidermidis*
      - *Gardnerella vaginalis*
    - Anaerobic bacteria
      - *Bacteroides* (especially *Bacteroides bivius*)
      - Peptococci, peptostreptococci
    - Other
      - *Mycoplasma hominis*
      - *Ureaplasma urealyticum*
      - *Chlamydia trachomatis* (uncommon)
  - Late infection (2 days–6 weeks)
    - Not well established
    - *Chlamydia trachomatis* (30% of infections?)
- Amnionitis
  - Similar to bacteriology of early postpartum endometritis
  - Group B streptococci and alpha-hemolytic streptococci commonly involved
- Skin and soft-tissue infection
  - Cellulitis
    - *Staphylococcus aureus*
    - *Streptococcus pyogenes*
- Diabetic foot infections
  - Enterobacteriaceae (*Escherichia coli, Proteus*)
  - *Pseudomonas aeruginosa*
  - Anaerobic bacteria
- Pneumonia
  - Community-acquired
    - *Streptococcus pneumoniae*
    - *Mycoplasma pneumoniae*
    - *Chlamydia pneumoniae*
    - Viruses
      - Influenza A, B
      - Adenovirus
      - Varicella—zoster virus
    - *Hemophilus influenzae*
    - *Staphylococcus aureus*
    - *Legionella pneumophila*
    - *Neisseria meningitidis*
    - *Klebsiella pneumoniae*
    - Mixed oral anaerobes (aspiration pneumonia)
    - *Bacteroides melaninogenicus*
    - *Peptococcus* species
    - *Peptostreptococcus* species
    - *Fusobacterium* species
    - *Mycobacterium tuberculosis*
    - Unusual causes

TABLE 56–1 (*Continued*)

Fungi
- *Histoplasma capsulatum, Coccidioides immitis, Cryptococcus neoformans*
- *Chlamydia psittaci* (psittacosis)
- Actinomyces species (actinomycosis)
- *Branhamella catarrhalis*

Hospital-acquired
- *Streptococcus pneumoniae*
- *Staphylococcus aureus*
- Enterobacteriaceae (*Klebsiella pneumoniae, Enterobacter* species, *Escherichia coli, Proteus mirabilis, Serratia marcescens*)
- *Pseudomonas aeruginosa*
- *Acinetobacter* var. anitratus
- Oral anaerobes
- *Bacteroides fragilis*

Immunosuppressed Patients
- *Pneumocystis carinii*
- Fungi
  - *Aspergillus* species
  - *Candida* species
- *Legionella*
- Herpes simplex virus
- Cytomegalovirus
- *Strongyloides stercoralis*

Other drugs useful in this setting continue to be short-acting sulfa compounds, such as sulfisoxazole (not recommended in the third trimester), and perhaps trimethoprim-sulfamethoxazole, although this agent is, largely on theoretical grounds, regarded as potentially toxic to the fetus. Among the newer agents, the combination of amoxicillin with clavulanate, a penicillinase inhibitor, has activity comparable or superior to first-generation cephalosporins against penicillinase-producing strains of *Escherichia coli, Klebsiella, Enterobacter,* and *Proteus* and appears safe in pregnancy.[8] New oral second (cefuroxime axetil) or third (cefixime) generation cephalosporins, while expensive, offer the option of oral treatment for resistant organisms that previously would have required hospitalization and parenteral therapy. Unfortunately, ciprofloxacin and the other fluoroquinolones, which have exceptional utility in treating diarrheal diseases, bone infections, and sexually transmitted diseases (STDs), as well as UTIs, appear unsafe in pregnancy and childhood due to damage to developing cartilage.

Cystitis occurs in about 1% of pregnancies. Common symptoms include urinary frequency, dysuria, and urgency. Pyuria is nearly universal in cystitis, and urine cultures usually yield over 100,000 colonies of a single pathogen. It is now clear, however, that the same presentation may occur with low-count bacteriuria (100–1000 colonies per milliliter) or may be due to chlamydia or even herpes simplex when bacterial cultures are negative.[9] Cystitis most often develops during the second trimester, often in women with previously negative screening for asymptomatic bacteriuria.[10] Treatment options are the same as for asymptomatic bacteriuria.

Pyelonephritis is defined clinically by fever, chills, flank pain, and pyuria. Some cases present with mild symptoms suggesting cystitis and are inadvertently treated with single-dose therapy. The failure of single-dose therapy to clear a presumed lower tract infection has been shown to correlate strongly with tests that localize infection to the kidneys, such as the assay for antibody-coated bacteria or direct ureteral cultures by way of retrograde catheterization. Such upper-tract infection carries substantial risk of both maternal and fetal morbidity, so aggressive therapy is warranted. Bacteremia occurs in about 10% of cases and complications of sepsis, such as shock and disseminated intravascular coagulation, may ensue. Shock lung, also known as adult respiratory to distress syndrome (ARDS), may occur with a higher frequency in pregnant compared to nonpregnant women with pyelonephritis, even without confirmed bacteremia or other features of septicemia.[11] Hospitalization for pyelonephritis in pregnancy is necessary, and parenteral antibiotic treatment until the patient is afebrile for at least 48 hours is usually followed by oral treatment to complete a 14-day course. Therapeutic courses for pyelonephritis as short as five days or as long as three to six weeks have been investigated. Both appear undesirable due to high recurrence rates in the former case and more side effects as well as more chance of resistant reinfections in the latter.[12,13] Either continuous suppressive therapy or close monitoring for the duration of the pregnancy is warranted after an episode of pyelonephritis.[1,14-16]

Standard therapy for pyelonephritis has included a penicillin, such as ampicillin, or a first-generation cephalosporin, such as cefazolin, alone or with an aminoglycoside such as gentamicin. Such therapy is still likely to be effective in first episodes of community-acquired pyelonephritis, but the possibility of resistance must be strongly considered in patients who have had recent courses of antibiotics, hospitalization, or urinary tract instrumentation. The impact of new β-lactam drugs is substantial for pyelonephritis in pregnancy because all are concentrated in urine and appear safe in pregnancy. The third-generation cephalosporins provide excellent activity against the coliforms responsible for most UTIs, with ceftazidime also effective in severe infections due to *Pseudomonas aeruginosa.* The monobactam aztreonam covers the same broad gram-negative spectrum as the aminoglycosides, and imipenem offers exceptionally broad activity against these organisms, as well as against gram-positives and anaerobes.

PELVIC INFLAMMATORY DISEASE

The most common severe complication of STDs, pelvic inflammatory disease (PID), affects more than one million women in the United States annually (see also Chapter 116).[17] This entity involves several organs, a range of organisms, and various clinical patterns.[18] Risk factors for PID include prior episodes of gonorrhea, multiple sexual partners, the use of an intrauterine contraceptive device and not using other means of contraception. The general clinical pattern is one in which initial episodes in sexually active young women are produced by recognized STD pathogens, such as *Chlamydia trachomatis* and *Neisseria gonorrhoeae,* either alone or in a polymicrobial process.[19] With repeated or inadequately-treated infections, later episodes involve polymicrobial infection with the following organisms normally found in the vaginal or gut flora: aerobic gram-negative rods such as *E coli,* and anaerobes such as *Bacteroides, Peptococcus, Peptostreptococcus,* and *Veillonella* species. Although organisms such as *Mycoplasma hominis* and *Ureaplasma urealyticum* are detected frequently in cervical cultures of women with PID, direct culture of intraperitoneal or fallopian tube material in PID yields these organisms infrequently.[20] Current treatment regimens recognize the need for specific coverage of such organisms as *C trachomatis* and *Bacteroides* species.

POSTPARTUM ENDOMETRITIS

The pathogenesis of postpartum infection of the uterus and adjacent structures involves the complex and changing flora of the vagina and the effects of delivery (see also Chapters 113 and 117). The strong association of endometritis, especially the early form occurring within the first 48 hours after delivery, with cesarean section underscores the relative importance of these factors. The increase in vaginal anaerobes, especially *Bacteroides* species, in the first days after delivery appears significant, and such organisms are recovered in a majority of cases of endometritis. Aerobic gram-negative rods and gram-positive cocci, such as *Streptococcus faecalis,* group B streptococcus, and *Streptococcus viridans* are also common isolates.[21] When special selective media are used, *Gardnerella vaginalis* may be a very common isolate in endometritis.[22] *C trachomatis* and *M hominis* are occasionally implicated in these infections, but a more prominent role is not established.[23] *U urealyticum* has been isolated from the endometrium in a high percentage of cases when appropriate methods were employed, but its significance as a pathogen is unclear except in a few cases.[22]

In the past, standard therapy incorporated a β-lactam, such as ampicillin, or cefazolin with an aminoglycoside. Presently, either clindamycin or metronidazole is added for activity against resistant *Bacteroides* organisms. Such activity appears especially important in postcesarean infections.[24] Clindamycin plus gentamicin is a widely used initial regimen.[25] Alternatively, single-agent therapy with either cefoxitin or piperacillin may be used, both having good activity against the anaerobes and streptococci that are important in endometritis.[26,27] Among the newer agents, ampicillin/sulbactam alone or aztreonam plus clindamycin are potentially useful.[28,29]

AMNIONITIS

The bacteriology of amnionitis is similar to postpartum endometritis, that is, also reflecting the normal vaginal flora. Thus, *E coli* and *Bacteroides* species are prominently represented, as are group B and group D streptococci. *Mycoplasma, Ureaplasma,* and *Chlamydia* may play an important role as well but require special culture methods for detection, which are not widely available. Studies have conflicted on the importance of these organisms as causes of morbidity in pregnancy.[30-32]

SKIN AND SOFT TISSUE INFECTIONS

Skin and soft tissue infections that are community-acquired are most often caused by *Staphylococcus aureus* or group A streptococci (*Streptococcus pyogenes*). The latter organism remains universally susceptible to penicillin, and mild-to-moderate infections can be treated with an oral agent such as penicillin V. *S aureus* is now almost universally penicillin-resistant, and in many areas a high frequency of methicillin-resistant strains is encountered even among community-acquired infections. For methicillin-sensitive organisms, mild-to-moderate infections can be treated with oral agents such as dicloxacillin or cephalexin. Methicillin-resistant isolates, however, must be regarded as resistant to all β-lactam drugs, including the cephalosporins. In the case of serious infections with these organisms, intravenous vancomycin is required.

Would infections developing in the hospital, especially after surgical procedures involving nonsterile mucosal surfaces, have a more complex microbiology. Rapidly progressive soft tissue infections beginning within a day of delivery or surgery suggests *Clostridium perfringens* or *S pyogenes.* Clostridial soft tissue infections are often accompanied by profound toxicity and gas formation. Enteric gram-negative rods are an increasingly common cause of hospital-acquired soft tissue infections, which in diabetics may also form gas. Mixed processes in which aerobes such as *S aureus* and anaerobes such as *Bacteroides* act synergistically are relatively frequent after abdominal surgery.

Episiotomy infections often necessitate only local drainage, but more extensive infection, leading to fasciitis, may develop after vaginal delivery with third-or fourth-degree lacerations. The microbiology of this process reflects the polymicrobial vaginal and colonic flora. Because progressive soft tissue necrosis is the pathogenetic process, early detection and aggressive debridement are critical.[33-35] Antibiotic coverage should be broad and should include activity against coliforms and anaerobes. Because of its rapidly bactericidal action against *Bacteroides fragilis* and *C perfringens,* metronidazole may have an important place in the therapeutic regimen.

PHARMACOKINETIC CONSIDERATIONS

Although outweighed by concerns for potential toxicity to the fetus, several pharmacokinetic issues are important in the selection and use of antimicrobial agents in pregnancy.[36,37] The major increase in body water during pregnancy (50% increase by the eighth month) leads to a larger volume of distribution and, therefore, lower serum levels for a given drug dose compared to the nonpregnant state. The decline in albumin concentration early in pregnancy leads to a further decrease in intravascular drug levels for agents tightly bound to albumin. Increases in renal blood flow and glomerular filtration rate raise the clearance and lower the blood level for a given dose of any drug that is subject to substantial excretion by the kidneys, such as the β-lactams and aminoglycosides.[38-40] Drugs predominantly metabolized and excreted by the liver are also affected by pregnancy because progesterones may induce increased levels of hepatic metabolism.[41,42]

Orally administered ampicillin produces blood levels one third lower in pregnancy than in the same women after delivery, with the difference attributable to increased volume of distribution and rate of excretion.[40] The same variables appear to account for lower levels after intravenous ampicillin. Ceftriaxone, ceftazidime, and moxalactam levels also appear to be lower during pregnancy.[43,44] The serum levels of several other agents, including clindamycin and trimethoprim-sulfamethoxazole appear to be unchanged in pregnancy.[45]

The likely impact of these physiologic and consequent pharmacologic changes is underdosing and at possibly subtherapeutic blood levels of drugs in the β-lactam and aminoglycoside classes as well as erythromycin.[45] This result is more likely to be clinically significant with drugs such as the aminoglycosides, which are given in relatively low doses because of their potential toxicity, than with β-lactams such as ampicillin, which are inexpensive and have little dose-related toxicity, and therefore are administered in larger amounts. Another point of clinical significance may arise with infections such as osteomyelitis, meningitis, or endocarditis, where tissue barriers cause only a fraction of the serum level to penetrate to the infected site. A lower serum drug level in these situations might lead to therapeutic failure. Both monitoring of serum levels of drugs such as the aminoglycosides and dose increases may be necessary. For β-lactams, use of higher doses in severe infections may be needed without determining levels that are not widely available. Another variable affecting drug levels is decreased rate of gastric emptying and intestinal motility during pregnancy, which may lead to substantial variation in the absorption of orally administered agents.[46,47]

An additional consideration is the adequacy of antibiotic levels in the fetal circulation and amniotic fluid in cases where the fetus is involved in the infectious process. The adequacy of fetal blood and amniotic fluid levels depends on maternal drug levels and on characteristics of the drug, such as lipid solubility, protein binding, and ionization. The fetomaternal barrier produced by the placenta is also variable, becoming thinner as pregnancy advances and therefore allowing progressively more diffusion of drugs from maternal to fetal circulation.[48,49]

Actual measurements of maternal to fetal drug level ratios are difficult to carry out, and available data are not conclusive. With most agents studied, peak levels appear in cord blood about 30 to 60 minutes after a maternal dose. The fraction of the maternal peak level detected in cord blood is between 30% and 90% of ampicillin, clindamycin, cephalothin, carbenicillin, and the aminoglycosides.[37] For the penicillins, efficiency of transfer is proportional to serum protein binding, so ampicillin (20% bound) achieves high fetal and amniotic concentrations, while dicloxacillin (96% bound) does not. A substantial time lag occurs in achieving antibiotic levels in the amniotic fluid after an intravenous dose to the mother. This delay appears to be due to the fact that amniotic levels in the third trimester are dependent on fetal urinary excretion. Amniotic drug levels are therefore lower early in pregnancy and negligible with intrauterine fetal death.[45,50,51]

The therapeutics of amniotic and fetal infections may be complicated by these pharmacologic relationships. For instance, the aspiration of infected amniotic fluid can produce severe pneumonia, but antibiotic penetration to the amniotic fluid is delayed, and fetal circulation to the lungs is poor, so that prompt delivery at signs of fetal distress is needed in amnionitis.

Transfer of antibiotics to breast milk is determined by factors similar to those involved at the maternal-placental interface. Umbilical cord levels of drugs usually reflect maternal serum levels, so any of the drugs noted above that achieve lower levels in the pregnant woman will produce correspondingly lower fetal levels. Unionized, nonprotein-bound drugs enter the mammary alveolar cells. Since the pH of breast milk averages 6.8–7.0, weakly basic compounds are less ionized in maternal plasma and pass into the breast milk more readily than neutral compounds.[45,52,53] Most antimicrobial drugs can be detected in breast milk, but adverse effects on the neonate are uncommon, probably due to a combination of factors, including the low drug concentrations usually present, the presence of a fraction of the drug in metabolized form, and the further metabolism by the infant. In general, the potential for adverse effects is greater if the infant is premature or has hepatic or renal impairment.[37]

SUSCEPTIBILITY TESTING OF BACTERIAL PATHOGENS

Selection of antimicrobial therapy is a complex process requiring synthesis of several types of data. Intricate sequential probabilities are calculated (usually informally), such as the likelihood the patient is infected, the most probable organism, and its likely sensitivity pattern. Clinical and laboratory data may help to increase these odds in the physician's (and patient's) favor, but no single test or procedure provides an absolutely certain answer. Properly-obtained culture material that yields one or more pathogens whose antimicrobial susceptibility is then determined comes closest to a definitive guide to therapy.[54] The technicalities of *in vitro* susceptibility testing are of little consequence to the average clinician, but several facts and concepts are important. Some organisms such as *S pyogenes* have very predictable sensitivity patterns and may not need to be formally tested. Other organisms, such as *Streptococcus pneumoniae* (*Pneumococcus*), have developed uncommon exceptions to their reliable sensitivity patterns so that isolates from life-threatening blood stream or cerebrospinal fluid infections are screened for resistance by most laboratories. Other organisms, especially the gram-negative enteric rods, have widely variable sensitivity patterns that must be determined for each isolate. Some general trends in resistance may be clinically useful. Generally speaking, infections acquired in the hospital, following instrumentation, or while on antibiotics tend to be more antibiotic-resistant. Susceptibility patterns vary substantially over time, between different hospitals, and even among services or units in the same institution. Even so, several reliable patterns of sensitivity can be perceived, and these may form the basis for initial antimicrobial selection as outlined in Tables 56–2 through 56–6.

TOXICITY OF ANTIMICROBIAL AGENTS IN PREGNANCY

Penicillins and Cephalosporins

The β-lactam antibiotics in these two classes have proven to be the safest antimicrobial agents in pregnancy. Allergic reactions may occur as in the general population, but no specific maternal or fetal side effects have been determined.[50,51] In situations such as syphilis, where penicillin is superior to other agents, desensitization of pregnant patients with severe allergy is recommended over alternative drugs.[55]

Tetracyclines

Drugs of this class are contraindicated in pregnancy for several reasons.[56-60] Maternal renal and hepatic failure after intravenous administration appears to be increased in pregnancy, especially if complicated by renal insufficiency.[57,59] Fetal exposure during the first trimester may be teratogenic and may lead to bone and tooth damage during the second and third trimesters.[56,58,60]

Metronidazole

A valuable agent for anaerobic and certain parasitic infections, metronidazole is used with caution in pregnancy because of carcinogenic and mutagenic properties in laboratory tests[61] despite a long record of apparent safety in pregnant women.[62,63]

Erythromycins

Except for erythromycin estolate, erythromycins are safe agents in pregnancy and are important oral alternatives for penicillin-allergic patients with streptococcal infections. The estolate form may lead to subclinical hepatitis in 10–15% of women in late pregnancy by way of a hypersensitivity mechanism.[64] Other erythromycin preparations have also been associated with milder hepatic reactions.[65,66]

TABLE 56–2. FACULTATIVE GRAM-POSITIVE COCCI CAUSING INFECTION IN OBSTETRIC AND GYNECOLOGIC PATIENTS[a]

Organisms	Penicillin G	Ampicillin, Amoxicillin	Penicillinase-Resistant Anti-Staphylococcal Penicillins[b]	Carbenicillin, Ticarcillin, and Ureidopenicillins[c]	Cephalosporins First Generation[d]	Cephalosporins Second Generation[e]	Cephalosporins Third Generation[f]	Imipenem	Erythromycin	Vancomycin	Clindamycin
Staphylococcus aureus											
Penicillinase-negative	4+	4+	4+	4+	4+	3+	3+	4+	3+	3–4+	3+
Penicillinase-positive	0	0[k]	3+	0[l]	3–4+	3+	3+	4+	1+	3–4+	2+
Methicillin-resistant[g]	0	0	0	0	0	0	0	0	0	3–4+	2+
***Staphylococcus epidermidis*[h]**	0	0[k]	2+	0[l]	3+	0–1+	0–1+	3+	1+	3–4+[o]	1–2+
Streptococci											
Streptococcus viridans	4+	4+	3+	4+	3–4+	3–4+	3–4+	4+	3+	3–4+	3–4+
Streptococcus pneumoniae	4+	4+	3+	4+	3–4+	3–4+	3–4+	4+	3–4+	3–4+	3–4+
Groups A,B,G[i]	4+	4+	3+	4+	4+	4+[n]	3–4+	4+	3–4+	3+	3+
Enterococcus faecalis[j]	3+	3–4+	0	1–4+[m]	0	0	0	3+	1–2+	3–4+	0
Group D Streptococcus (non-*Enterococcus*)	3–4+	3–4+	2+	4+	3+	3+	3+	4+	2–3+	3–4+	3+

[a] Symbols: 0, universally resistant; 1+, majority resistant; 2+, at least 50% of isolates resistant; 3+, most susceptible; 4+, universally susceptible

[b] Oxacillin, dicloxacillin, nafcillin. Methicillin refers to entire class. Drugs of choice only for susceptible staphylococci

[c] Ureidopenicillins include piperacillin, mezlocillin, and azlocillin

[d] First-generation cephalosporins include cephalothin, cefazolin, cephalexin (oral), cefadroxil (oral), and cephradine (parenteral and oral)

[e] Second-generation cephalosporins include cefoxitin, cefamandole, cefotetan, cefaclor (oral), and cefuroxime axetil (oral)

[f] Third-generation cephalosporins include cefotaxime, ceftizoxime, moxalactam, cefoperzone, ceftazidime, ceftriaxone, and cefixime (oral). Susceptibility patterns may vary from agent to agent. These are not drugs of choice for infections caused by gram-positive cocci

[g] Methicillin-resistant *Staphylococcus aureus* may appear to be susceptible to cephalosporins *in vitro* but usually does not respond to these drugs clinically. Infections caused by these organisms should usually be treated by vancomycin. Potential oral alternatives: Trimethoprin-sulfamethoxazole, or if not pregnant, a quinolone (ciprofloxacin or norfloxacin)

[h] Penicillin-resistant, methicillin-sensitive. Many hospital-acquired strains are methicillin-resistant

[i] Penicillin or ampicillin are drugs of choice for infections caused by these organisms. Alternatives in the penicillin-allergic patient are erythromycin, clindamycin, or vancomycin; cephalosporins may also be considered if the allergy was not severe

[j] Formerly called *Streptococcus faecalis* or Enterococcus. Serious enterococcal infections, eg, endocarditis, should be treated with a combination of a penicillin (or, in the penicillin-allergic patient, vancomycin) and an aminoglycoside

[k] Combinations with β-lactamase inhibitors (amoxacillin/clavulanate (oral), ampicillin/sulbactam (parenteral) active against penicillinase positive staphylococci)

[l] Ticarcillin/clavulanate active against penicillinase-positive staphylococci

[m] Ureidopenicillins: very good activity; others: poor

[n] Cefoxitin not active against group B *Streptococcus*

[o] Active against methicillin-resistant strains also

TABLE 56–3. FACULTATIVE GRAM-NEGATIVE BACILLI CAUSING INFECTION IN OBSTETRIC AND GYNECOLOGIC PATIENTS

Organism	Ampicillin	Carbenicillin, Ticarcillin, and Ureidopenicillins[a]	Cephalosporins[b]			Imipenem	Aztreonam	Aminoglycosides[e]	TMP–SMX[f]
			First Generation	Second Generation[c]	Third Generation[d]				
Escherichia coli	3+	3+[h]	3–4+	3–4+	3–4+	4+	4+	3–4+	3–4+
Proteus mirabilis	3+	3+[h]	3–4+	3–4+	3–4+	4+	4+	3–4+	3–4+
Morganella morganii	0–1+	3+	3+	3–4+	3–4+	3–4+	3–4+	3–4+	3–4+
Klebsiella species	0–1+[g]	2–3+[i]	2–3+	3+	3–4+	4+	3–4+	3–4+	3+
Enterobacter species	0–1+	3+	1+	2+	3+	4+	2–3+	3–4+	3+
Pseudomonas aeruginosa	0	2–3+	0	0	2–3+	3–4+	3–4+	3–4+	0
Serratia marcescens	0	2–3+	0	2+	3+	3–4+	3–4+	3–4+	1+
Acinetobacter species	1–2+	2–3+	0	1–	1–2+	3–4+	0–1+	3+	2+
Providencia species	0–1+	3+	0	1–	3+	3–4+	3–4+	3+	3+
Citrobacter species	0–1+	3+	0	1–	3+	4+	2–3+	3+	3+

[a] Piperacillin and azlocillin are the most active penicillins against *Pseudomonas aeruginosa* but should be used in combination with an aminoglycoside for severe infections caused by this species
[b] See footnotes to Table 56–2 for members of the cephalosporin groups
[c] Cefoxitin, cefamandole, and cefuroxime differ in their activity; organisms should be tested for susceptibility
[d] Third-generation cephalosporins differ in their activity against individual isolates; organisms should be tested for susceptibility. Only ceftazidime has potent activity against *Pseudomonas aeruginosa* and might be used as single-drug treatment. In general, serious *Pseudomonas* infections should be treated with an aminoglycoside together with either broad-spectrum penicillin (see footnote *a*) or, possibly, a third-generation cephalosporin
[e] Aminoglycosides include gentamicin, tobramycin, netilmicin, and amikacin. Tobramycin is slightly more active than the others against *Pseudomonas aeruginosa*. Amikacin is the *congener* most likely to be active against strains that are resistant to the other aminoglycosides
[f] TMP–SMX = trimethoprim-sulfamethoxazole
[g] Combinations with β-lactamase inhibitors (amoxacillin/clavulanate, ampicillin/sulbactam) active against *Klebsiella*
[h] Ticarcillin/clavulanate active against β-lactamase-producing strains
[i] Combinations with β-lactamase inhibitors (amoxacillin/clavulanate, ampicillin/sulbactam, ticarcillin/clavulanate) active against *Klebsiella*

TABLE 56–4. OTHER FACULTATIVE BACTERIA CAUSING INFECTION IN OBSTETRIC AND GYNECOLOGIC PATIENTS[a]

Organism	Penicillin G	Ampicillin[b]	Carbenicillin, Ticarcillin[b], and Ureidopenicillins	Cephalosporins: First Generation	Cephalosporins: Second Generation	Cephalosporins: Third Generation	Imipenem	TMP–SMX	Chloramphenicol
Hemophilus influenzae	0	3+[e]	3+[f]	2+	3+[g]	3–4+	4+	3–4+	4+
Neisseria meningitidis	4+	4+	3+	3+	3+[g]	4+	4+	3–4+	3–4+
Neisseria gonorrhoeae[c]	3–4+	3–4+	3+	3+	3–4+	4+	3–4+	3–4+	3–4+
Listeria monocytogenes	3–4+[d]	3–4+[d]	3+	1+	1+	0	3–4+	3+	3+

[a] See Tables 56–2 and 56–3 for identification of antibiotics

[b] Amoxacillin/clavulanate, ticarcillin/clavulanate active against penicillinase–producing *Hemophilus influenzae, Neisseria gonorrhoeae*

[c] Because of the possibility of resistance, cultures should be obtained before treatment. Cefoxitin or a third-generation cephalosporin or spectinomycin is active against penicillinase-producing strains. Cefamandole is less effective than cefoxitin for gonorrhea

[d] Aminoglycosides show synergy *in vitro* with penicillin G or ampicillin. Some authors recommend the use of these combinations for severe or refractory infections caused by *Listeria monocytogenes*

[e] About 15–20% of strains are resistant to ampicillin because of β-lactamase production, or in a few instances, impermeability of the cell membrane

[f] Penicillinase-producing *Hemophilus influenzae*-resistant

[g] Only cefuroxime has adequate activity and central nervous system penetration for treatment of meningitis

TABLE 56–5. ANAEROBIC BACTERIA CAUSING INFECTION IN OBSTETRIC AND GYNECOLOGIC PATIENTS

Organism	Penicillin G, Ampicillin	Carbenicillin, Ticarcillin, and Ureidopenicillins	Cefoxitin	Cefotaxime	Cefoperazone	Moxalactam	Imipenem	Clindamycin	Metronidazole	Chloramphenicol	Tetracycline
Bacteroides											
B fragilis group	0–1+	3+[a]	3+	2–3+	2+	3+	3–4+	3–4+	4+	4+	1+
B bivius	0–1+	3+[a]	3+	2–3+	2+	3+	4+	3–4+	4+	4+	1+
B disiens	0–1+	3+[a]	3+	2–3+	2+	3+	4+	3–4+	4+	4+	1+
B melaninogenicus	3	3–4+	4+	2–3+	2+	3+	4+	4+	4+	4+	3–4+
Clostridium perfringens	3–4+	3–4+	3+	2–3+	2–3+	2–3+	3–4+	3+	3–4+	2–3+	1–2+
Peptococcus	3–4+	3–4+	4+	3+	3+	3–4+	4+	4+	3–4+	3–4+	2+
Peptostreptococcus	3–4+	3–4+	3–4+	3+	3+	3–4+	4+	4+	4+	3–4+	2+
Veillonella	3–4+	3–4+	4+	3+	3+	3–4+	3–4+	4+	3–4+	3–4+	2+

[a] Pipercillin is the most active of these drugs against *Bacteroides fragilis* group, *Bacteroides bivius,* and *Bacteroides disiens.* Ticarcillin/clavulanate is more active than ticarcillin.

TABLE 56–6. EMPIRIC ANTIBIOTIC TREATMENT OF COMMON INFECTIOUS SYNDROMES

Infection	Common Pathogens	Suggested Antimicrobial Regimen[a]
Skin and subcutaneous tissue		
Nondiabetic adults	*Staphylococcus aureus, Streptococcus pyogenes*	Mild infection (oral treatment): dicloxacillin, erythromycin, cephalexin or clindamycin. Severe infection (parenteral treatment): penicillin G and oxacillin[b] or cephalosporin I
Lower extremity in diabetic patient	Same as above plus Enterobacteriaceae, anaerobes	For mild infection: oxacillin (or dicloxacillin) or cephalosporin I. For more serious infection: oxacillin[b,c] and either an aminoglycoside or aztreonam, or ticarcillin/clavulanate or imipenem
Postsurgical wound infection (fulminant, first 24 h)	*Clostridium perfringens, Streptococcus pyogenes*	Penicillin G (additional coverage usually provided until gram-negative sepsis ruled out by blood culture)
Postsurgical wound infection (more than 24 h postoperative)	*Staphylococcus aureus*[c], Streptococci, Enterobacteriaceae anaerobes	One of the following plus an aminoglycoside or aztreonam: clindamycin, oxacillin (misses *Bacteroides* species) cefoxitin, cephalosporin III, piperacillin, or one of the following alone: ampicillin/sulbactam, ticarcillin/clavulanate, imipenem
Urinary tract infection		
Community-acquired cystitis or nonseptic pyelonephritis	*Escherichia coli, Proteus mirabilis, Klebsiella pneumoniae*	Ampicillin (misses *Klebsiella pneumoniae*), cephalexin, TMP–SMX
Hospital-acquired infection, septic patient, or anatomic abnormality	More resistant gram-negative bacilli, including *Pseudomonas aeruginosa, Enterococcus*	Ampicillin plus aminoglycoside or cephalosporin II or III (misses *Enterococcus*), or imipenem, ticarcillin/clavulanate, or aztreonam (gram-negatives only)
Pelvic inflammatory disease[d]	*Neisseria gonorrheae, Chlamydia trachomatis,* Enterobacteriaceae, streptococci, vaginal anaerobes, (genital mycoplasmas)	Cefoxitin (parenteral)[e] plus doxycyline[f] (oral), or clindamycin plus gentamicin (parenteral) plus doxycycline[g]
Postpartum endometritis[h] and amnionitis	Enterobacteriaceae, *Gardnerella vaginalis,* streptococci (including group B), vaginal anaerobes	One of the following agents plus an aminoglycoside: cefoxitin[e], clindamycin, ampicillin/sulbactam, or piperacillin
Breast (mastitis/abscess)		
Postpartum	*Staphylococcus aureus*	Dicloxacillin (ambulatory therapy) or oxacillin[b] (severe infection)
Nonpuerperal	*Staphylococcus aureus, Bacteroides* species, *Peptococcus* species	Clindamycin or ticarcillin/clavulante or oxacillin plus metronidazole
Diarrhea		
Dysentery[i]	*Shigella, Salmonella, Campylobacter,* Rotavirus, Enterotoxigenic *Escherichia coli*	Ampicillin (misses *Campylobacter* and some resistant strains of *Salmonella* or *Shigella*), TMP–SMX (misses *Campylobacter*), erythromycin (covers only *Campylobacter*)
Clostridium difficile colitis	*Clostridium difficile* (toxigenic)	Metronidazole (oral or IV), vancomycin (oral)
Peritonitis and intra-abdominal abscess		
"Spontaneous" bacterial peritonitis (cirrhotic or nephrotic patient)	*Streptococcus pneumoniae, Streptococcus pyogenes,* Enterobacteriaceae, *Staphylococcus aureus*	Ampicillin or cefoxitin or cephalosporin III
Community-acquired (secondary to bowel perforation or gynecologic infection)	Aerobes: Enterobacteriaceae, *Enterococcus faecalis, Neisseria gonorrhea* (gyn. source). Anaerobes: *Bacteroides* species, *Peptostreptococcus* species, *Fusobacterium* species, *Clostridium* species, *Eubacterium* species	Cefoxitin or a combination of: clindamycin or metronidazole plus an aminoglycoside or aztreonam
Hospital-acquired underlying illness, or recent antibiotics	Above plus resistant gram-negative bacilli (*Serratia marcescens, Pseudomonas aeruginosa, Acinetobacter* species)	One of the above combinations or imipenem or ticarcillin/clavulante
Cholangitis	Enterobacteriaceae, *Enterococcus faecalis, Bacteroides* species, *Clostridium* species	Same as for the community-acquired peritonitis, or ampicillin plus aminoglycoside
Pharyngitis[j]	*Streptococcus pyogenes, Mycoplasma pneumoniae*[k], *Chlamydia pneumoniae*[k], respiratory viruses, Epstein–Barr virus, (uncommon: *Neisseria gonorrhoeae*)	Penicillin (or benzathine penicillin I.M.), ampicillin (or amoxicillin), erythromycin (for penicillin allergy), cephalexin

TABLE 56–6 (*Continued*)

Infection	Common Pathogens	Suggested Antimicrobial Regimen[a]
Paranasal sinusitis or otitis media[j]	Respiratory viruses, *Streptococcus pneumoniae, Streptococcus pyogenes, Staphylococcus aureus, Hemophilus influenzae, Branhamella catarrhalis*	Ampicillin or amoxicillin (misses *Staphylococcus aureus,* resistant *Hemophilus influenzae*), TMP–SMX, cephalexin or cefaclor, cefuroxime axetil, amoxicillin/clavulanate (cover resistant *Hemophilus influenzae*)
Epiglottitis	*Hemophilus influenzae, Streptococcus pneumoniae, Staphylococcus aureus, Streptococcus pyogenes*	Cephalosporin III, cefuroxime, ampicillin/sulbactam, chloramphenicol
Pneumonia		
Community-acquired, previously healthy person	*Streptococcus pneumoniae, Mycoplasma pneumoniae,* viruses, *Legionella*	Penicillin G, ampicillin, or cefuroxime (miss *M pneumoniae* and *Legionella*), erythromycin
Community-acquired in alcoholic, diabetic, or COPD patient	Above plus *Hemophilus influenzae, Klebsiella pneumoniae, Staphylococcus aureus,* oral anaerobes	Cefuroxime or cephalosporin III, plus erythromycin for *Legionella*
Hospital-acquired	*Staphylococcus aureus,* Enterobacteriaceae, *Acinetobacter* species, *Pseudomonas aeruginosa,* oral anaerobes	Cephalosporin III (not highly active against *Pseudomonas*), ceftazidime (covers *Pseudomonas aeruginosa*), aztreonam, imipenem, ampicillin (or oxacillin or cephalosporin I) plus aminoglycoside (covers *Staphylococcus aureus*), broad-spectrum penicillin (ticarcillin or ureidopenicillin) plus aminoglycoside (potent combination against *Pseudomonas*), clindamycin plus aminoglycoside (if anaerobic or mixed infection suspected)
Empyema and putrid lung abscess	Oral anaerobes, *Staphylococcus aureus,* Enterobacteriaceae	Penicillin G or ampicillin (misses *Staphylococcus aureus,* Enterobacteriaceae), clindamycin (misses Enterobacteriaceae), cefoxitin
Bacterial endocarditis[l]		
Subacute	*Streptococcus viridans*	Penicillin G (or ampicillin)
Acute (parenteral drug abuser)	*Staphylococcus aureus*[b] (Rare: *Streptococcus faecalis, Pseudomonas,* Enterobacteriaceae, *Candida* species)	Oxacillin (or vancomycin) plus aminoglycoside pending culture results
Osteomyelitis	Staphylococci (Enterobacteriaceae, *Pseudomonas* species if contiguous source)	Depends on results of bone biopsy culture and sensitivity testing; may begin with oxacillin, cephalosporin II or III or ticarcillin/clavulanate (if gram-negatives suspected)
Arthritis	*Neisseria gonorrhoeae, Staphylococcus aureus, Streptococcus pyogenes,* Enterobacteriaceae	Depends on results of Gram's stains, cultures, and sensitivity testing. Penicillin or ampicillin (if sensitive GC likely), ceftriaxone (if resistant GC likely). If *Staphylococcus aureus* likely, add or substitute oxacillin[c]
Meningitis		
Adult or child	*Streptococcus pneumoniae, Neisseria meningitidis, Hemophilus influenzae*	Depends on results of cultures and sensitivity testing; may begin with ampicillin (misses resistant *Hemophilus influenzae*) or cephalosporin III
Neonate	Group B *Streptococcus,* Enterobacteriaceae, *Listeria monocytogenes*	Ampicillin (to cover streptococci and *Listeria*) plus either an aminoglycoside or cephalosporin III

[a] Initial therapy before culture data available
[b] May substitute nafcillin
[c] If methicillin-resistant isolate suspected or confirmed, vancomycin is required
[d] Regimens listed are for inpatient care. For ambulatory therapy, a single dose of cefoxitin or ceftriaxone (plus probenicid) and a tetracycline for 10–14 days is advised
[e] Cefotetan or a cephalosporin III may be substituted
[f] Erythromycin may be substituted if tetracycline is contraindicated
[g] Preferred regimen if Enterobacteriaceae are suspected as primary pathogens
[h] Most cases are presumed to be polymicrobial in etiology
[i] Ciprofloxacin or norfloxacin preferred initial therapy but contraindicated in pregnancy
[j] Oral treatment adequate in most cases
[k] Therapy requires a tetracycline or erythromycin. β-lactams inactive
[l] Treatment should be based on *in vitro* quantitative sensitivity testing (minimal inhibitory concentration, MIC) of blood culture isolate

Abbreviations and Terminology: Enterobacteriaceae, *Escherichia coli, Klebsiella* species, *Enterobacter* species, *Proteus* species, *Morganella morganii;* TMP–SMX, trimethoprim/sulfamethoxazole; aminoglycoside, gentamicin, tobramicin, amikacin; cephalosporin I, First generation cephalosporin: cefazolin, cephalothin, cephalexin (oral); cephalosporin III, Third generation cephalosporin without *Pseudomonas* activity: cefotaxime, ceftizoxime, ceftriaxone; ureidopenicillin, azlocillin, mezlocillin, piperacillin

Clindamycin

The widespread use of clindamycin for pelvic anaerobic infections and as a penicillin alternative for staphylococcal and streptococcal infections in pregnancy has established this agent as a particularly safe and useful one.[67] The concern for its one potentially severe side effect, pseudomembranous colitis, has been tempered by the availability of effective diagnostic and therapeutic measures to manage this complication.

Sulfonamides

As one of the earliest effective antimicrobial classes, sulfonamides have been widely used, particularly in UTIs, including those occurring in pregnant women. Concern for possible teratogenicity when these drugs are used in early pregnancy has been expressed, but actual fetal toxicity has not been documented.[37] Displacement of bilirubin from albumin in the newborn is a theoretical concern. Usage late in pregnancy is, therefore, contraindicated.[68,69]

Trimethoprim-sulfamethoxazole

This fixed-ratio combination is available in intravenous as well as oral preparations and has very broad use. Its sequential blockade of folate metabolism, however, raises the question of teratogenicity, and avoidance altogether or usage with caution is recommended.[37,70]

Aminoglycosides

Short-course treatment with the agents of this class appears safe in pregnancy. However, because of toxic potential, difficulty in administration, and the recent availability of new agents, such as third-generation cephalosporins and aztreonam with equivalent or superior efficacy, the need for these agents has diminished. Fetal toxicity manifested as sensorineural hearing loss and vestibular damage has been noted only in the instance of prolonged maternal treatment with streptomycin for tuberculosis.[71-73] Careful monitoring of serum levels and dose adjustment is needed when the aminoglycosides are used in pregnancy.

Vancomycin

This glycopeptide antibiotic is being used with increased frequency as infection with methicillin-resistant *S aureus* and *Staphylococcus epidermidis* become more common. Ototoxicity and nephrotoxicity are the major adverse effects in adults.[74] Since little data from humans is available on possible adverse effects to the fetus, vancomycin should be used with caution only for severe infections with the organisms noted above.

Chloramphenicol

Toxic accumulation of chloramphenicol given to premature infants can cause the *"gray baby syndrome,"* a multisystem process with high mortality.[75] This process theoretically might occur in neonates exposed to the drug *in utero* but has not been reported. The rare occurrence of fatal aplastic anemia and more common dose-related suppression of hematopoesis make chloramphenicol an infrequently needed back-up agent.

Nitrofurantoin

Concern about nitrofurantoin's potential for mutagenicity[76] and for precipitating hemolysis due to red-cell deficiency of glucose-6-phosphate dehydrogenase (G6PD) have limited its use in pregnancy.

Nalidixic Acid, Norfloxacin, and Ciprofloxacin

The DNA gyrase inhibitor 4-quinolones are an important new class of antimicrobial agents derived from the older drug, nalidixic acid. Nalidixic acid has been used extensively for UTIs in pregnancy but is best avoided now due to potential adverse effects on the fetal central nervous system. The new quinolone drugs are not approved for pregnant women or children due to their adverse effects on cartilage and bone growth.[77]

Antituberculous Agents

The standard agents for tuberculosis include isoniazid, rifampin, ethambutol, and pyrazinamide (see also Chapter 77). The first three have been widely used in pregnancy without adverse maternal or fetal consequences.[78,79] Active disease should be treated promptly, but the possibility of an increased risk of INH hepatotoxicity in pregnancy leads some experts to defer prophylaxis with this agent until after delivery.[80]

CHARACTERISTICS OF NEWER ANTIBACTERIAL AGENTS

Several new agents have become available since the last edition of this text, and these are reviewed below.

Oral Cephalosporins

Cefuroxime Axetil (Ceftin). This is an oral preparation of the second-generation parenteral cephalosporin cefuroxime. It is active against most strains of *N gonorrhoeae, Hemophilus influenzae,* and *Branhamella catarrhalis.* Many Enterobacteriaceae are susceptible, but *Serratia* species and *P aeruginosa* are not. This drug is less active than earlier-generation cephalosporins against *S aureus* and is not active against *B fragilis.* Cefuroxime axetil may be useful for respiratory tract infections involving *H influenzae* or *Branhamella.* It may also be useful in pregnancy for oral treatment of resistant gram-negative UTIs because alternative agents, such as trimethoprim-sulfamethoxazole or the quinolones, may be contraindicated.

Cefixime (Suprax). This new agent is considered an oral third-generation cephalosporin and is highly active against *N gonorrhoeae, H influenzae,* and *B catarrhalis.* It is more active than other oral cephalosporins against several gram-negative bacilli, such as *E coli, Klebsiella,* and *Serratia marcescens.* It has no activity against *S aureus* or *Pseudomonas,* and many strains of *Enterobacter* and *Acinetobacter* are also resistant. As with cefuroxime axetil, cefixime may be useful in otitis media or sinusitis, but several other agents appear equally effective. In addition, because of its extended gram-negative rod activity, it may be useful for oral treatment of resistant UTIs.

Monobactams

Aztreonam (Azactam). This is the first agent in the new monobactam class of β-lactam antibiotics and is highly active against most gram-negative bacilli, including *P aeruginosa,* but has no activity against gram-positive cocci or anaerobes. It may often be substituted where an aminoglycoside would ordinarily be used to treat severe gram-negative rod infection, often in combination with a β-lactam antibiotic to cover gram-positive cocci.

TABLE 56–7. ADVERSE REACTIONS TO ANTIMICROBIAL AGENTS IN PREGNANCY

Drug	Adverse Reactions Peculiar to Pregnancy	Fetal Toxicity or Teratogenicity	Recommended Usage in Pregnancy
Aminoglycosides	None reported	Ototoxicity (rarely) with streptomycin	Avoid or use cautiously[a]
Clindamycin	None reported	None reported	Probably safe
Chloramphenicol	None reported	"Gray baby" syndrome in neonates	Avoid near term[a]
Ciprofloxacin	None reported	Defective bone and cartilage growth	Contraindicated
Erythromycin	None except cholestatic hepatitis with estolate form	None reported	Probably safe (except estolate form)
Methenamine mandedate	None reported	None reported	Probably safe
Metronidazole	None reported	Teratatogenic in some animals	Avoid or use cautiously[a]
Nalidixic acid	None reported	Central nervous system damage in newborns	Contraindicated
Nitrofurantoin	None reported	Risk of hemolysis in fetus or neonate with G6PD deficiency	Contraindicated
Norfloxacin	None reported	Defective bone and cartilage growth	Contraindicated
Penicillins and other β-lactams[b]	None reported	None reported	Probably safe
Sulfonamides	None reported	Kernicterus in newborns exposed near term	Contraindicated at term; probably safe earlier in pregnancy
Tetracyclines	Renal and hepatic toxicity with IV use	Tooth discoloration and dysplasia; fetal bone growth inhibition	Contraindicated
Trimethoprim-sulfamethoxazole	None reported	Theoretical teratogenic antifolate effect; also kernicterus at term (see sulfonamides)	Contraindicated at term; avoid or use cautiously earlier in pregnancy[a]
Antituberculous drugs[c]			
Isoniazid	None reported	No human toxicity, but teratogenic in animals	Use cautiously
Ethambutol	None reported	No human toxicity, but teratogenic in animals	Use cautiously
Rifampin	None reported	No human toxicity, but teratogenic in animals	Use cautiously
Pyrazinamide	Unknown	Unknown	Avoid in pregnancy

[a] Alternate agents are available for most indications.
[b] Newer agents such as third-generation cephalosporins, Imipenem, and Aztreonam are expected to be equally safe as older pencillins and cephalosporins, but less data is available for these drugs.
[c] Active tuberculosis should be treated during pregnancy. Deferral of prophylactic isoniazid treatment is sometimes advised.

Quinolones

The new class of agents known as the 4-quinolones offers major advances compared to previous therapy for many conditions. Unfortunately, because of fetal toxicity these agents are contraindicated in pregnant and nursing women and in growing children (see Table 56–7). Two members of this class are currently available. *Norfloxacin (Noroxin)* is an oral agent that achieves therapeutic levels in the urine and is available for the treatment of UTIs due to gram-negative bacilli. The second agent to become available, *Ciprofloxacin (Cipro),* has a much broader spectrum of action and is a useful oral agent in a wide variety of conditions, including UTIs, STDs including resistant gonococcal infection, and infectious diarrheas due to *Salmonella, Shigella, Campylobacter jejuni, Aeromonas, Yersinia, E coli,* and *Vibrio.* It is also active against *P aeruginosa* and staphylococci and has been used in the treatment of conditions such as *Pseudomonas osteomyelitis*. These drugs are not active against anaerobes and should not be used for pneumococcal or streptococcal infections where other agents are more active.

β-Lactamase Inhibitor Combinations

Three agents are available that combine a β-lactam antibiotic with a β-lactamase inhibitor.

Amoxicillin/Clavulanate (Augmentin). The activity of amoxicillin is extended by the addition of the β-lactamase inhibitor clavulanate to include resistant strains of *staphylococci, gonococci* and *Hemophilus* as well as many strains of *E coli* and *Proteus mirabilis*. This combination is useful in treating sinusitis and otitis media as well as lower respiratory infections, such as bacterial bronchitis. Human bite wounds and diabetic foot infections are other settings where this agent may be useful.

Ticarcillin/Clavulanate (Timentin). In this combination, the spectrum of activity of ticarcillin is extended to include resistant β-lactamase-producing organisms such as *S aureus, H influenzae* and gram-negative anaerobes, such as *B fragilis.* It has been used to treat pneumonias such as aspiration pneumonia and intra-abdominal infections from intestinal or gynecologic sources, as well as cutaneous and bone infections.

Ampicillin/Sulbactam (Unasyn). The β-lactamase inhibitor sulbactam added to ampicillin in this parenteral preparation provides activity against organisms ordinarily resistant to ampicillin, including most staphylococci, *Klebsiella,* resistant *Hemophilus,* and *E coli* strains, and *Bacteroides* species. Sul-

Sulbactam itself is active against *Neisseria* species, *Bacteroides* species, and some *Acinetobacter*. This combination agent may be useful in treating mixed bacterial infections, such as intra-abdominal and pelvic abscesses as well as soft tissue and bone infections.

Carbapenems

Imipenem-cilastatin (Primaxin). This agent, often referred to as imipenem, offers the broadest antibacterial spectrum of any drug currently available. It has extensive activity against gram-positive cocci, including staphylococci and enterococci, is highly active against gram-negative rods, including *P aeruginosa, Serratia* and *Enterobacter* species, and is very active against most anaerobes, including the *B fragilis* group. Several uncommon organisms are predictably resistant and may produce superinfection in patients treated with imipenem. These include *Pseudomonas maltophilia* and *Pseudomonas cepacia*. This drug, which is available only in parenteral form, is extremely useful in severe infections due to resistant organisms. Ordinarily, use of imipenem is reserved for infections unresponsive and resistant to other available agents, such as third-generation cephalosporins and aminoglycosides.

REFERENCES

1. Klein EH. Urologic problems of pregnancy. *Obstet Gynecol Surv.* 1984;39:605.
2. Krieger JN. Complications and treatment of urinary tract infections during pregnancy. *Urol Clin North Am.* 1986;13:685.
3. Patterson TF, Andriole VT. Bacteriuria in pregnancy. *Infect Dis Clin North Am.* 1987;1:807.
4. Masterton RG, Evans DC, Strike PW. Single-dose amoxycillin in the treatment of bacteriuria in pregnancy and the puerperium—a controlled clinical trial. *Br J Obstet Gynecol.* 1985;92:498.
5. Jakobi P, Neiger R, Merzbach D, Paldi E. Single dose antimicrobial therapy in the treatment of asymptomatic bacteriuria in pregnancy. *Am J Obstet Gynecol.* 1987;156:1148.
6. McNeeley SG Jr. Treatment of urinary tract infections during pregnancy. *Clin Obstet Gynecol.* 1988;31:480.
7. Johnson JR, Stamm WE. Urinary tract infections in women: diagnosis and treatment. *Ann Intern Med.* 1989;111:906.
8. Pedler SJ, Bint AJ. Comparative study of amoxicillin-clavulanic acid and cephalexin in the treatment of bacteriuria during pregnancy. *Antimicrob Agents Chemother.* 1985;27:508.
9. Stamm WE, Wagner KF, Amsel R, et al. Causes of the acute urethral syndrome in women. *N Engl J Med.* 1980;303:409.
10. Harris, RE, Gilstrap LC. Cystitis during pregnancy: a distinct clinical entity. *Obstet Gynecol.* 1981;57:578.
11. Cunningham FG, Leveno KJ, Hankins GDV, Whalley PJ. Respiratory insufficiency associated with pyelonephritis during pregnancy. *Obstet Gynecol.* 1984;63:121.
12. Ronald AR. Optimal duration of treatment for kidney infection. *Ann Intern Med.* 1987;106:467.
13. Turck M, Anderson KN, Petersdorf RG. Relapse and reinfection in chronic bacteriuria. *N Engl J Med.* 1966;275:70.
14. Harris RE, Gilstrap LC. Prevention of recurrent pyelonephritis during pregnancy. *Obstet Gynecol.* 1974;44:637.
15. Lenke RR, VanDorsten JP, Schifrin BS. Pyelonephritis in pregnancy: a prospective randomized trial to prevent recurrent disease evaluating suppressive therapy with nitrofurantoin and close surveillance. *Am J Obstet Gynecol.* 1983;146:953.
16. Faro S, Pastorek JG, Plauche WC, et al. Short-course parenteral antibiotic therapy for pyelonephritis in pregnancy. *South Med J.* 1984;77:455.
17. Curran JW. Economic consequences of pelvic inflammatory disease in the United States. *Am J Obstet Gynecol.* 1980;138:848.
18. Sweet RL. Pelvic inflammatory disease. *Sex Trans Dis.* 1986;13:192.
19. Wasserheit JN, Bell TA, Kiviat MB, et al. Microbial causes of proven pelvic inflammatory disease and efficacy of clindamycin and tobramycin. *Ann Intern Med.* 1986;104:187.
20. Sweet RL, Draper DL, Schachter J, et al. Microbiology and pathogenesis of acute salpingitis as determined by laparoscopy: what is the appropriate site of sample? *Am J Obstet Gynecol.* 1980;138:985.
21. Gibbs RS. Infection after cesarean section. *Clin Obstet Gynecol.* 1985;28:697.
22. Rosene K. Eschenbach DA, Tompkins LS, et al. Polymicrobial early postpartum endometritis with facultative and anaerobic bacteria, genital mycoplasmas and *Chlamydia trachomatis. J Infect Dis.* 1986;153:1028.
23. Harrison HR, Alexander ER, Weinstein L, et al. Cervical *Chlamydia trachomatis* and mycoplasmal infections in pregnancy. Epidemiology and outcomes. *JAMA.* 1983;250:1721.
24. diZerega G, Yonekura L, Roy S, et al. A comparison of clindamycin and penicillin-gentamycin in the treatment of post cesarean section endomyometritis. *Am J Obstet Gynecol.* 1979;134:238.
25. Gibbs RS, Blanco JD, Castaneda YS, St Clair PJ. A double-blind, randomized comparison of clindamycin-gentamicin versus cefamandole for treatment of post-cesarean section endomyometritis. *Am J Obstet Gynecol.* 1982;144:261.
26. Gilstrap III LC, Maier RC, Gibbs RS, et al. Piperacillin versus clindamycin plus gentamicin for pelvic infections. *Obstet Gynecol.* 1984;64:762.
27. Sweet RL, Robbie MO, Ohm-Smith M, Hadley WK. Comparative study of piperacillin versus cefoxitin in the treatment of obstetric and gynecologic infections. *Am J Obstet Gynecol.* 1983;145:342.
28. Gibbs RS, Blanco JD, Lipscomb KA, et al. Aztreonam versus gentamicin, each with clindamycin, in the treatment of endometritis. *Obstet Gynecol.* 1985;65:825.
29. Pastorek JG, Cole C, Aldridge KE, Crapanzano JC. Aztreonam plus clindamycin as therapy for pelvic infections in women. *Am J Med.* 1985;78(2A):47.
30. Hillier SL, Martius J, Krohn M, et al. A case-control study of chorioamnionic infection and chorioamnionitis in prematurity. *N Engl J Med.* 1988;319:972.
31. Sweet RL, Landers DV, Walker C, Schachter J. *Chlamydia trachomatis* infection and pregnancy outcome. *Am J Obstet Gynecol.* 1987;156:824.
32. Lamont RF, Taylor-Robinson D, Wigglesworth JS, et al. The role of mycoplasmas, ureaplasmas, and chlamydiae in the genital tract of women presenting in spontaneous early preterm labour. *J Med Microbiol.* 1987;24:253.
33. Golde S, Ledger WJ. Necrotizing fasciitis in postpartum patients: a report of four cases. *Obstet Gynecol.* 1977;50:670.
34. Meltzer RM. Necrotizing fasciitis and progressive bacterial synergistic gangrene of the vulva. *Obstet Gynecol.* 1983;61:757.
35. Sutton GP, Smirz LR, Clark DH, Bennett JE. Group B streptococcal necrotizing fasciitis arising from an episiotomy. *Obstet Gynecol.* 1985;66:733.
36. Philipson A. Pharmacokinetics of antibiotics in pregnancy and labor. *Clin Pharmacokinet.* 1979;4:297.
37. Chow AW, Jewesson PJ. Pharmacokinetics and safety of antimicrobial agents during pregnancy. *Rev Infect Dis.* 1985;7:287.
38. Good RG, Johnson GN. The placental transfer of kanamycin during late pregnancy. *Obstet Gynecol.* 1971;38:60.
39. Weinstein AJ, Gibbs RS, Gailager M. Placental transfer of clindamycin and gentamicin in term pregnancy. *Am J Obstet Gynecol.* 1977;124:688.
40. Philipson A. Pharmacokinetics of ampicillin during pregnancy. *J Infect Dis.* 1977;136:370.
41. Krauer B, Krauer F. Drug kinetics in pregnancy. *Clin Pharmacokinet.* 1977;2:167.
42. Fever G. Action of pregnancy and various progesterones on hepatic microsomal activities. *Drug Metab Rev.* 1979;9:147.
43. Giamerellou H, Gazis J, Petrikkos G, et al. A study of cefoxitin, moxalactam, and ceftazidime kinetics in pregnancy. *Am J Obstet Gynecol.* 1983;147:914.
44. Kafetzis DA, Brater DC, Fanourgakis JE, et al. Ceftriaxone distribution between maternal blood and fetal blood and tissues at parturition and between blood and milk postpartum. *Antimicrob Agents Chemother.* 1983;23:870.
45. Landers DV, Green JR, Sweet RL. Antibiotic use during pregnancy and the postpartum period. *Clin Obstet Gynecol.* 1983;26:391.
46. Parry E, Shields R, Turnbull AC. Transit time in the small intestine in pregnancy. *Journal of Obstetrics and Gynaecology of the British Commonwealth.* 1970;77:900.
47. Eadie MJ, Lander CM, Tryer JH. Plasma drug level monitoring in pregnancy. *Clin Pharmacokinet.* 1977;2:427.
48. Mirkin BL. Perinatal pharmacology, placental transfer, fetal localization and neonatal distribution of drugs. *Anaesthesiology.* 1975;43:156.
49. Finster M, Pederson H. Placental transfer and fetal uptake of drugs. *Br J Anaesth.* 1979;51(suppl):25s.
50. Ledger WJ. Antibiotics in pregnancy. *Clin Obstet Gynecol.* 1977;20:411.
51. Schwarz RH. Considerations of antibiotic therapy during pregnancy. *Obstet Gynecol.* 1981;58(suppl):95S.
52. Vorherr H. Drug excretion in breast milk. *Postgrad Med.* 1974;56:97.
53. Beeley L. Drugs and breast feeding. *Clin Obstet Gynecol.* 1981;8:291.
54. Rosenblatt JE. Laboratory tests used to guide antimicrobial therapy. *Mayo Clin Proc.* 1987;62:799.
55. Wendel GD, Stark BJ, Jamison RB, et al: Penicillin allergy and desensitization in serious maternal/fetal infections. *New Engl J Med.* 1985;312:1229.
56. Wallman IS, Hilton HB. Teeth pigmented by tetracycline. *Lancet.* 1962;1:827.
57. Greene G. Tetracycline in pregnancy. *N Engl J Med.* 1976;295:512.

58. Beeley L. Adverse effects of drugs in later pregnancy. *Clin Obstet Gynecol.* 1981;8:275.
59. Whalley JP, Adams RH, Combes B. Tetracycline toxicity in pregnancy. *JAMA.* 1964;189:357.
60. Carter MP, Wilson F. Antibiotics and congenital malformations. *Lancet.* 1963;1:1267.
61. Sloan DA, Theiszer DM, Richards GN, et al. Increased incidence of experimental colon cancer associated with long-term metronidazole therapy. *Am J Surg.* 1983;145:66.
62. Peterson WF, Stauch JE, Ryder CD. Metronidazole in pregnancy. *Am J Obstet Gynecol.* 1966;94:343.
63. Robbie MO, Sweet RL. Metronidazole use in obstetrics and gynecology: a review. *Am J Obstet Gynecol.* 1983;145:865.
64. McCormack WM, George H, Donner A, et al. Hepatotoxicity of erythromycin estolate during pregnancy. *Antimicrob Agents Chemother.* 1977;12:630.
65. Viteri AL, Greene JR, Dyck WP. Erythromycin ethylsuccinate induced cholestasis. *Gastroenterol.* 1979;76:1007.
66. Sullivan D, Csuka ME, Blanchard B. Erythromycin ethylsuccinate hepatotoxicity. *JAMA.* 1980;243:1074.
67. Mickal A, Panzer JD. The safety of lincomycin in pregnancy. *Am J Obstet Gynecol.* 1975;121:1071.
68. Silverman WA, Anderssen DH, Blanc WS, et al. A difference in mortality rate and incidence of kernicterus among premature infants allotted to two prophylactic antibacterial regimens. *Pediatrics.* 1956;18:614.
69. Some hazards of sulphonamides. *Br Med J.* 1968;1:658. Leading Article.
70. Williams JD, Brumfitt W, Condie AP, et al. The treatment of bacteriuria in pregnant women with sulphamethoxazole and trimethoprim. A microbiological, clinical and toxicological study. *Postgrad Med J.* 1969; 45:S71.
71. Robinson GC, Combon KG. Hearing loss in infants of tuberculous mothers treated with streptomycin during pregnancy. *N Engl J Med.* 1964;271:949.
72. Conway N, Birt BD. Streptomycin in pregnancy: effect on fetal ear. *Br Med J.* 1965;2:260.
73. Assael BM, Parini R, Rusconi F. Ototoxicity of aminoglycoside antibiotics in infants and children. *Pediatr Infect Dis.* 1982;1:357.
74. Sorrell TC, PJ Collignon. A prospective study of adverse reactions associated with vancomycin therapy. *J Antimicrob Chemother.* 1985;16:235.
75. Burns LE, Hodgman JE, Cass B. Fatal circulatory collapse in premature infants receiving chloramphenicol. *N Engl J Med.* 1959;261:1318.
76. McCalla DR. Biological effects of nitrofurans. *J Antimicrob Chemother.* 1977;3:517.
77. Andriole VT. Quinolones. In: Mandell GL, Douglas RG Jr, Bennett JE, eds. *Principles and Practice of Infectious Diseases.* 3rd ed. New York; John Wiley & Sons; 1989.
78. Snider DE Jr, Layde PM, Johnson MW, Lyle MA. Treatment of tuberculosis during pregnancy. *Am Rev Respir Dis.* 1980;122:65.
79. Good JT, Iseman MD, Davidson PT. Tuberculosis in association with pregnancy. *Am J Obstet Gynecol.* 1981;140:492.
80. Moellering RC Jr. Special consideration of the use of antimicrobial agents during pregnancy, post partum, and in the newborn. *Clin Obstet Gynecol.* 1979;22:373.

Chapter Fifty-Seven

Prevention of Infection: Immunization and Antimicrobial Prophylaxis

Karen C. Cummiskey and Stanley A. Gall

57

Several methods exist to prevent infections. These methods may include: reducing the exposure to the offending microorganism, acquiring immunity either by active or passive regimens, and using antimicrobial agents to prevent colonization or enhance host resistance during possible exposure periods. For individuals, active immunization is the preferred method to obtain protection against infectious diseases. Unfortunately, vaccines are not available for many infectious diseases, and those that are available must be used with care during pregnancy. This chapter summarizes current recommendations for immunization, the impact on pregnancy, and current guidelines for using antimicrobial prophylaxis during pregnancy.

IMMUNIZATION

The objective of immunization schemes is to induce a state of immunity in the patient so that confrontation with the offending organism can be successful in protecting the host. The ultimate goal is to induce an immune state by vaccination equivalent to that found in the host following natural infection. The vaccines are prepared from inactivated, live-attenuated, modified, or mutant forms of the causative agents. It is of utmost importance that the vaccine contain the antigen that is important in the disease process, so that an antibody will be formed to react with the natural antigen.[1]

Immunization results in the production of antibodies directed against the infecting agent or its toxic products and may initiate cellular responses mediated by lymphocytes and macrophages. *Live vaccines* usually induce a prompt but transient production of specific IgM antibodies followed by a sustained production of specific IgG. *Inactivated vaccines* and *toxoids* usually produce a less complete response, and several doses of vaccine at appropriate intervals of time must be given to obtain an adequate and longlasting IgG response.

Active immunization with *live-attenuated vaccines* generally results in subclinical or mild clinical illness similar to the disease the vaccine was to prevent.[2] The protection provided is frequently long-lasting. Inactivated vaccines, such as influenza, rabies, typhoid, and cholera vaccines, do not cause infectivity but need several doses of antigen, larger doses of antigen, and a greater time period from vaccine administration to the presence of protective antibody.

The most important protective antibodies include those that inactivate soluble toxic protein products of bacteria (antitoxins), facilitate phagocytosis and intracellular ingestion of bacteria (opsonins), interact with complement component to damage the bacterial cell membranes (lysins), prevent proliferation of infectious virus (neutralizing antibodies), or interact with components of the bacterial surface to prevent adhesion to mucosal surfaces.

Induced or passive antibodies react with the offending antigen in the blood, extracellular fluid, and at mucosal surfaces. Antibodies cannot readily reach an intracellular site of infection.

TABLE 57–1. PASSIVE IMMUNIZATION

Disease	Product[a]	Dosage and Route	Comments
Black widow spider bite	Equine	1 vial (2.5 ml) IM or IV	If symptoms do not subside in 3 h, a second dose may be given.
Botulism	ABE polyvalent antitoxin, equine	1 vial IV and 1 vial IM; repeat after 2–4 h if symptoms worsen and after 24 h.	Available from CDC[b]. Type E antitoxin is active substance that can affect outcome; 20% incidence of serum reactions. Prophylaxis not recommended.
Diphtheria	Diphtheria antitoxin, equine	20,000–120,000 U IM or IV depending on severity and duration of symptoms	Nonimmune contacts are probably better treated with antibiotic prophylaxis. Contacts should be observed for illness and antitoxin administered if needed.
Hepatitis A	Immunoglobulin, human	0.02–0.06 mL/kg after exposure up to 6 wks; protective effect for 6 months	Infection is only modified, not prevented. Recommended for household and other contacts of similar intensity. Not to be used for school or office contacts unless epidemic. Recommended for travelers to epidemic areas.
Hepatitis B	Hepatitis B immunoglobulin, human	0.06 mg/kg IM as soon as possible after exposure; a second injection should be given 25–30 days after exposure.	To be used as prophylaxis for individuals following parenteral exposure or direct mucous membrane contact. Not to be given to individuals who are anti-HBsAG positive. Live vaccine should be delayed 2 months after concentrated immunoglobulin has been given. Infants born of mothers who are HBeAg positive at delivery should be given 0.5 mL at birth, 3, and 6 months to markedly decrease chronic carrier state.
Hypogammaglobulemia	Immunoglobulin,	0.6 mL/kg every 3–4 wks	Initial dose should be a double dose.
	Immunoglobulin IV, human	100–150 mg/kg IV	This product is chemically modified to be aggregate-free while retaining immunologic potency and ability to fix complement.
Measles	Immunoglobulin, human	0.25 mL/kg as soon as possible after exposure, up to 15 mL. This dose may be ineffective in immunoincompetent patients, who need 20–30 mL.	Live measles vaccine will prevent natural infection if given within 48 h following exposure. If immunoglobulin is given, delay live virus 3 months. Give to exposed susceptible pregnant females or immunodeficient persons.
Pertussis	Pertussis immunoglobulin, human	1.5 mL IM; repeat in 5–7 days.	Efficacy doubtful; may be given for treatment. No longer manufactured, but may be available.
Rabies	Rabies immunoglobulin, human	20 IU/kg: 50% is infiltrated locally, and 50% IM. If equine product used, dose is 40 IU/kg.	Give as soon as possible after exposure. To be used with both tissue culture and duck embryo rabies vaccine.
Rh isoimmunization	Rh(D) immunoglobulin, human	300 μg IM within 72 h of delivery, amniocentesis, ectopic pregnancy, or abortion in Rh(D)-negative female	May be effective at greater postexposure intervals. Give even if more than 72 h have elapsed. Can inhibit immune response to 12-mL fetomaternal bleed. May give multiple doses in mismatched Rh(D)-positive transfusions. Should be routinely administered at 28–30 weeks' gestation in an Rh(D)-negative, Coombs-negative woman.

TABLE 57–1 (Continued)

Disease	Product[a]	Dosage and Route	Comments
Snake bite	Antivenin coral snake, equine Antivenin rattlesnake, copperhead, and moccasin, equine	3–5 vials IV	Dose should be sufficient to reverse symptoms of venom. Consider antitetanus measures as well. For information on availability of nearest supply of antiserum, call Antivenin Index Center, Oklahoma City, OK, 73126, telephone (405) 271-5454.
Tetanus	Tetanus immunoglobulin, human (TIG); bovine and equine antitoxins not recommended	Prophylaxis: 250–500 units IM Therapy: 3000–6000 units IM	Give in separate syringes at separate site from simultaneously administered toxoid. Recommended only for major wounds in patients with fewer than 2 doses of toxoid at any time in the past.
Varicella	Varicella-zoster immunoglobulin human (VZIG)	1 vial/10 kg IM or fraction thereof, up to a maximum of 5 vials. Give within 96 h of exposure.	Available for prevention of varicella in immunosuppressed patients. For neonates whose mothers have developed varicella less than 5 days before or 48 h after delivery. May give to pregnant patient. VZIG modifies natural disease.

[a] Always question carefully, and test for hypersensitivity before administering animal sera. Immune antisera and globulin should always be given IM unless otherwise noted.
[b] Centers for Disease Control (CDC), telephone (404) 639-3311.
[c] Contact the regional blood center of the American Red Cross.

Contraindications to Vaccination

There are few indications to immunization with live or attenuated vaccines during pregnancy. Live vaccines have a variable ability to produce transplacental dissemination and fetal infections. Other contraindications to immunization would be the use of live-virus vaccines in immunosuppressed or immunodeficient patients. This would include patients receiving chemotherapy, radiation therapy, or corticosteroids. Patients with febrile disease should not be immunized until the acute illness has passed. Simultaneous administration of Rh immune globulin (IG) and rubella vaccine may decrease the antibody response to the live-attenuated rubella vaccine. Ideally, the rubella vaccine should not be given for at least six weeks and preferably three months after the Rh immune globulin administration. However, because of the concerns regarding adequate follow-up in these patients, the Centers for Disease Control (CDC) does recommend simultaneous administration at different sites and repeat testing in three months to assess rubella immunity.[3]

Passive Immunization

Immunization can be accomplished passively by administering either preformed cells or serum from a person or animal that has been adequately immunized. Antibody either as whole serum or concentrated immunoglobulin G obtained from persons who have recovered from the disease or professional donors who have been immunized may be administered. These antibodies provide immediate protection. Therefore, passive immunization is beneficial for patients who cannot form antibodies or for the normal host who might develop disease before the 7–10 days required for active immunization.

Antibodies may be obtained from humans or animals, but animal serum is always less desirable because these proteins give rise to immune reactions, rapid elimination, and serum sickness. No antiserum of nonhuman origin should be given without careful inquiry about prior exposure or allergic response to any product of that specific animal source. Patients with unrelated allergies should be tested also, as they are more prone to develop serum reactions. Table 57–1 presents a list of antisera generally available for passive immunization.[4]

Illness may occur following a single injection of foreign serum but is more common in patients who have previously been injected with proteins from the same species. Reactions range in severity from acute anaphylaxis with hives, back pain, dyspnea, and cardiovascular collapse, to even death from serum sickness, arising hours to weeks following treatment. The administration of human gamma globulin is rarely accompanied by similar allergic reactions.

It is very important to exercise care in avoiding intravenous injection with standard gamma globulin. The current preparations contain high-molecular-weight aggregated IgG, which can result in moderate to severe anaphylactic reactions. The standard immune globulin preparations must not be confused with recently-licensed immune globulin IV, which can be given safely intravenously.

Active Immunization

Primary active immunity develops more slowly than the incubation period of most infectious agents and must therefore be induced prior to exposure to the etiologic agent. The initial response by the host is a prompt but transient production of specific IgM followed by a sustained rise of IgG. Booster reimmunization provides a rapid secondary (*anamnestic*) increase in serum antibody, which outpaces development of infection. Oral vaccines may primarily cause development of IgA and IgG antibodies, whereas parenteral vaccines stimulate IgM and IgG antibody production.[5]

Recent studies in humans suggest that transplacental immunization of the human fetus to tetanus toxoid can be accomplished by immunizing the mother at 20 and 36 weeks' gestation. These infants who had IgM antibody in their blood showed a more rapid response to diphtheria, pertussis, tetanus (DPT) immunization than controls. This may be an excellent method of neonatal immunization if additional studies confirm these preliminary results.[6]

Active immunization may cause fever, malaise, and reaction at the injection site, whereas other reactions may be more specific for the particular vaccine, for example, arthralgia/arthritis following rubella vaccine. The reactions are much less frequent and less severe than those accompanying natural illness. Other conditions that usually contraindicate vaccination are these:

1. *Acute febrile illness.* It is feared that the vaccine antigen may accentuate the illness, or the preexisting viral illness may diminish the immune response through the role of interferon produced by the infecting virus. It is therefore recommended that the patient's febrile illness be resolved prior to vaccination.
2. *Immunodeficiency.* Immunodeficiency conditions resulting from most etiologies contraindicate the use of live viral vaccine because virus replication may occur following administration. This would apply to patients whose immune response has been depressed, as in leukemia, lymphoma, or systemic malignancy, and following therapy with corticosteroids, anticancer chemotherapy, and radiation therapy. Vaccination with inactivated vaccines usually produces an inadequate response, and additional booster injections may be needed for protection.

Pregnancy

The pregnant woman is immunologically competent and will react to immunization with live-virus vaccines, inactivated vaccines, and toxoids with unaltered response. However, because of the theoretical risk to the developing fetus, live-attenuated virus vaccines should not be given during pregnancy. If a patient demonstrates rubella susceptibility during pregnancy, immunization should be given during the postpartum period. The patient should be advised not to become pregnant for at least 3 months after administration of the vaccine.

Patients who have become pregnant within 3 months of receiving the *rubella vaccine* have been assessed for the risk of congenital rubella syndrome. In those patients who underwent interruption of pregnancy, the virus isolation rate from the embryo was 4%. In completed pregnancies, 2% of the neonates demonstrated serologic evidence of subclinical infection. None of the infants demonstrated the birth defects associated with congenital rubella syndrome (see also Chapter 89). Thus, the theoretical risk for congenital rubella syndrome after receiving the vaccine is 2–5%, with the observed risk being 0%. Termination of pregnancy is not recommended for pregnant patients receiving the rubella vaccine.[7]

Yellow fever vaccine and *oral polio vaccine* may be given to pregnant women who are at high risk of exposure to those natural infections. If international travel requirements constitute the only reason to vaccinate a pregnant woman, rather than an increased risk of infection, a waiver letter may be obtained from the patient's physician.

Pregnant women may be exposed to children or adults who have been immunized with live-virus vaccines. Persons who have been given measles, mumps, or rubella vaccines can shed but not transmit these viruses. These vaccines can be safely administered to children of pregnant women. Live polio virus is shed by recently-immunized persons (particularly after the first dose), but no fetal risk has been demonstrated.

Inactivated viral vaccines, bacterial vaccines, and toxoids have not been shown to be harmful to a pregnant woman or fetus. In general, waiting until the second or third trimester is a reasonable precaution to minimize concern over teratogenicity.[8]

The only vaccine virus isolated from breast milk is the rubella vaccine virus. There is no evidence that breast milk from women recently immunized against rubella is harmful to the infants.

Consultation on vaccination problems during pregnancy is available from the Center for Disease Control, Atlanta, Georgia, telephone (404) 639-1864. Recommendations regarding active immunization are listed in Table 57–2.

ANTIMICROBIAL PROPHYLAXIS IN OBSTETRICS

Antibiotics have been used prophylactically to prevent infection by an exogenous organism, prevent indigenous bacteria from infecting a normally sterile site, prevent an inactive pathologic organism from causing disease, and enhance host resistance during the period of surgery when a depression of innate host resistance occurs. In general, prophylaxis for medical diseases has been directed toward a single pathogen, with antibiotics administered over a moderate period of time. Examples of this approach are the prevention of recurrent episodes of rheumatic fever caused by group A streptococcal disease with benzathine penicillin, and the prevention of malaria with chloroquine.

Antibiotic prophylaxis in surgery has become extremely popular because it has been shown to be not only effective in reducing febrile morbidity but also in reducing serious infections. The principles of prophylaxis in surgery have been described by Burke and associates.[9] These include the observations that during the time of surgery and for a short time in the postoperative period, there is a state of abnormal physiology; during the period of abnormal physiology, there is a corresponding depression of host resistance; bacteria that enter the operative field do so when the initial incision is made, and subsequent infection results from contamination; and the presence of an antibiotic in the tissue when the incision is made provides the best opportunity to prevent infection, and administration of antibiotics even as soon as one hour after the operative incision may not provide any benefit.

Guidelines in the selection of operative procedures for use of prophylactic antibodies include: surgical procedures that have moderate to high rates of moderate to serious infections, surgical procedures with rare infections (but when infections occur the results are catastrophic), surgical procedures with a large bacterial contamination, surgical procedures in immunosuppressed patients, and surgical procedures that are very lengthy.

Guidelines for the administration of prophylactic antibodies are as follows: The antibiotic should be administered prior to the procedure in a time sequence that produces peak tissue concentrations when the surgical incision is made; the dose should be the maximum dose, especially the preoperative dose. Use of meager dosing schedules in cardiovascular surgery has led to severe *Staphylococcus epidermidis* infections. It is recommended that the appropriate dose of most β-lactam antibiotics in cesarean section be 2.0 g per dose; the elapsed time from the administration of the antibiotic until the surgical incision is made should be no more than two half-lives of the injected antibiotic; the prophylaxis should be done with one drug if possible; and the antibiotics should be continued for only a brief period postoperatively but never longer than 24 hours.

Adverse effects of prolonged prophylaxis can occur but rarely occur with short perioperative courses. These include development of a superinfection with an organism whose resistance has developed during therapy, increased side effects, such as allergic reactions, diarrhea, and vaginal overgrowth with *Candida albicans*, and increased cost.

Prophylactic antibiotics are commonly used during the perinatal period in several clinical situations. These include maternal vaginal carriers of group β-hemolytic *Streptococcus*, premature rupture of membranes, infective endocarditis prophylaxis in patients with valvular heart disease, and cesarean section.

Group B Streptococcal Infections

Group B streptococcus (GBS) is known to cause significant maternal and neonatal infections, including chorioamnionitis, postpartum endometritis, and early- and late-onset neonatal sepsis. It is also associated with an increased risk of premature labor and premature rupture of the membranes. Rates of maternal colonization vary from 5% to 30% depending on the site of the genital tract cultured, the number of times the patient is cultured, and the selectivity of the growth medium used.[10] The attack rate in infants of colonized mothers is 7% in preterm infants and 0.2% in term infants. In addition, GBS acts as a venereal disease during pregnancy and necessitates treatment of the partners.

Many different screening and treatment regimens have been implemented in the antenatal period to eradicate GBS colonization. Because of the high carrier rate with a relatively low attack rate, the intermittent nature of the carriage, and the rate of recurrence of GBS after antibiotic therapy, schemes requiring universal screening and prophylactic antibiotic treatment have been shown to be costly and ineffective. One such study demonstrated a significant reduction in colonization among mothers treated with ampicillin within three weeks of completion of therapy but found that this difference was not present at delivery.[11] In a more recent study, serial cultures were performed to evaluate the risk of perinatal complications in carriers and noncarriers. Neither inoculum size nor chronic carriage were predictive of morbidity. Because the majority (92%) of colonized women did not experience increased morbidity, the predictive value of a positive prenatal culture did not exceed 8% for any of the complications.[12]

GBS culture and intrapartum chemoprophylaxis in the subgroups at high risk for GBS complications have been offered as an alternative to universal screening and therapy.[13] These high-risk groups include those patients with preterm labor, preterm premature rupture of membranes, chorioamnionitis, and prolonged rupture of membranes at term. Antibiotic chemoprophylaxis with penicillin or ampicillin (erythromycin if penicillin allergy is present) should be initiated after obtaining the appropriate cultures.

Treatment of the newborn with single-dose penicillin prophylaxis against GBS infection has been evaluated as an alternative to maternal therapy. One such study did demonstrate a decrease in the GBS colonization rate of the treated newborns and a decreased incidence in all infections with penicillin-susceptible organisms. Of significance, there was an increased number of infections with penicillin-resistant organisms in the treated group.

Concerns for this approach include chemoprophylaxis of many newborns who would not require therapy and the unsuccessful treatment of newborns with symptomatic infection at birth.[14]

Numerous methods for rapid detection of GBS have been tested in an effort to identify carriers in the intrapartum period. Cervicovaginal Gram's stain performed at the time of sterile speculum exam has a low specificity and a high false-positive rate.[15,16] Rapid latex fixation tests allow GBS identification by 30 minutes to 5 hours (depending upon the test) after obtaining the specimen. These screens appear to be fairly sensitive and specific, although both false-positive and false-negative results have been demonstrated. No clinically significant perinatal infections were observed in the false-negative group, which had light colonization on culture. Initial studies appear to support a role for these rapid latex screening tests to identify those carriers who would benefit from chemoprophylaxis in labor, but more studies need to be performed[17-20]

Premature Rupture of Membranes

The rupture of membranes prior to labor is a common event, occurring in 10% of pregnancies. Many attempts have been made to overcome the greatest perceived problem, that is, development of maternal or fetal infection. Data could now support the concept that the development of chorioamnionitis in association with premature rupture of membranes (PROM) is directly related to the length of the latent period and inversely related to the length of gestation at the time PROM occurs. It appears that after 35 weeks' gestation, the incidence of infection is directly proportional to the length of the latent period, but before 35 weeks, incidence of chorioamnionitis is inversely proportional to the latent period. In the time period prior to 35 weeks, more neonates will die from respiratory distress syndrome than from infection. When chorioamnionitis occurs, it appears to significantly influence perinatal mortality in patients with PROM.

Although the use of prophylactic antibiotic therapy in PROM patients is still controversial, there are several recent studies that indicate beneficial effects. One such study randomized PROM patients less than 34 weeks' gestation with documented lecithin: sphingomyelin ratios of less than 2.0 to either controls or antibiotic therapy (ampicillin) at the time of admission. The group treated with ampicillin had a lower incidence of clinical chorioamnionitis and neonatal sepsis with no difference in latency period. This lower infection rate was specifically related to those patients colonized with GBS who received antibiotics.[21]

A second study looking at chemoprophylaxis with ampicillin in PROM patients showed a significant prolongation in the latency period in those patients receiving antibiotics. The median interval from randomization to delivery was 118 hours in the treated group compared with 49 hours in the untreated group. Also, the incidence of early neonatal sepsis was significantly lower in the treated group—2% versus 17%.[22]

In our institution, we routinely administer prophylactic antibiotics in PROM patients after obtaining the appropriate cervicovaginal cultures and continue therapy until the final culture results are available. If positive for *Neisseria gonorrhoeae*, *Chlamydia*, or group B streptococcus, the appropriate antibiotic therapy is given. All positive cultures are repeated after therapy.

Infective Endocarditis

Infective endocarditis is a disease in which microorganisms, usually bacteria, grow in patients with structural or flow

TABLE 57–2. ACTIVE IMMUNIZATION

Disease	Product (Source)	Type of Agent	Route	Primary Immunization	Duration of Effect
Cholera	Cholera vaccine	Killed bacteria	IM, subcutaneous, IO	Two doses 1 wk apart	6 months
Diphtheria, tetanus	—	Toxoid	IM	Primary, 3 doses at 1-month intervals; booster, 0.5 cc/10 yr	10 years
Hepatitis B	Hepatitis B vaccine (human carriers); recombinant hepatitis B vaccine (yeast)	Formalin-treated purified viral antigen; cultures of recombinant yeast strain	IM	Three doses at 0, 1, and 6 months	5 years (?)
Influenza	Influenza virus vaccine, monovalent or bivalent (chick embryo); composition depends on epidemiologic circumstances	Killed whole or split virus A or B	Im	Primary, 2 doses 6–8 wks apart in early fall; booster, single dose	1 year
Measles	Measles virus vaccine, live (chick embryo)	Live virus	Subcutaneous	One dose	Permanent
Meningococcus	Meningococcal polysaccharide vaccine group A or group C	Polysaccharide	Subcutaneous	One dose; antibody response requires at least 5 days	Permanent (?)
Mumps	Mump virus vaccine, live (chick embryo)	Live virus	Subcutaneous	One dose	Permanent
Plague	Plague vaccine	Killed bacteria	IM or subcutaneous	Three doses 4 wks apart	6 months
Pneumococcus	Pneumococcal polysaccharide vaccines, polyvalent	Polysaccharide	Subcutaneous, IM	0.5 mL once	Unknown; 5 years(?)
Poliomyelitis	Poliovirus vaccine, live oral trivalent (monkey kidney, human diploid)	Live virus types I, II, III	Oral	Two doses 6–8 wks apart	Permanent
Rabies	Rabies vaccine (human diploid); vaccine from infected duck embryo (DEV) is inferior and not recommended	Killed virus	IM	Preexposure, two doses 1 wk apart with third dose 2–3 wks later; postexposure, rabies immune globulin; see Table 57–1. If not immunized, give five doses on days 0, 3, 7, 14, and 28	2 years
Rubella	Rubella vaccine	Live virus	Subcutaneous	One dose	Permanent
Yellow fever	Yellow fever vaccine	Live virus	Subcutaneous	One dose	10 years

TABLE 57–2 (*Continued*)

Risk of Disease to Pregnancy	Risk of Disease to Fetus or Neonate	Risk of Vaccine to Fetus	Indication for Vaccination in Pregnancy	Comments
Significant morbidity, not altered by pregnancy	Not known	Probably none	Needed for international travel requirement or in epidemics	50% vaccine efficacy; need to repeat every 6 months
Severe morbidity, 10% mortality, not altered by pregnancy	Neonatal tetanus mortality 60%	Probably none	Lack of primary series or no booster in 10 years	Third dose should be given 6–12 months after second dose
Severe morbidity, small mortality; 10% develop chronic disease; disease more severe in pregnancy in underdeveloped countries	Significant Risk to fetus if HBeAg + Risk increased for carrier state with subsequent cirrhosis or hepatoma	Not determined but probably none	Household contacts of HB patients, selected medical and dental personnel, travel to third world	Length of time of protection may be longer than 5 years. Measure neonate for infection with HBsAg. See Table 57–1
Morbidity and mortality increased during epidemics of introduction of new strains	Increased abortion rate in epidemics; evidence of teratogenesis during epidemics	Probably none: prudent to avoid during first trimester: consult health authorities for current recommendations	Recommended for patients with severe underlying medical problems	Give immunization in early fall. Recommended especially for patients with cardiovascular diseases, diabetes, and other chronic diseases. Guillain-Barre syndrome may be rare complication.
Significant morbidity, rare mortality; more severe in pregnancy	Increased prematurity rate; no evidence of increased rates of abortion or congenital anomalies	Not known	Contraindicated	Administer immune serum globulin (ISG), 0.25 mL/kg, as soon as possible after exposure.
Significant mortality and morbidity; not altered by pregnancy	Small risk unless mother compromised	Probably none	Recommended in epidemic situations	Use antibiotic prophylaxis in preventing secondary cases in family contacts.
Moderate morbidity, rare mortality; not altered by pregnancy	No recent cases	Not known	Contraindicated	Virus particles have been recovered from placental tissue: therefore, do not use in pregnancy.
Significant morbidity and mortality; not altered by pregnancy	Not known	Probably none	Occupational exposure: exposed persons	Not for residents of endemic areas of S.W. United States.
Significant morbidity, low mortality; not altered by pregnancy	Not known	Probably none	Same population as influenza plus patients who are functionally or surgically asplenic	Effective against 23 pneumococcal types; booster doses should not be given because of the danger of adverse reactions.
Increased risk of severe disease	Anoxic fetal damage; 50% mortality in neonatal disease	None confirmed	Epidemics, travel to endemic areas	Individuals who have completed primary series may take a single booster dose if exposure risk is high; many adults already immune.
Nearly 100% fatal; not altered by pregnancy	Determined by maternal disease	Not known	Same as in nonpregnant patient	If previously immunized with diploid vaccine do not use serum therapy. Give two booster doses, one stat and one 3 days later. Check antibody titer after primary therapy. If not sufficient, 1:16, give booster and recheck titer 3 wks later. For animal bite, consider antitetanus measures as well.
Minimal morbidity; not altered by pregnancy	Significant risk of teratogenesis, especially in first trimester	Placental infection observed	Contraindicated	Give to women who are (HI) antibody-negative. Use contraception for 3 months after vaccine.
Significant mortality and morbidity; not altered by pregnancy	Not known	Unknown	Not indicated unless exposed	Postpone travel rather than have vaccination.

abnormalities of the heart or great vessels (see also Chapter 128). Since the bacteria must get to the heart by way of the blood, it has been recommended that antibiotic prophylaxis be used to prevent the occurrence. Therefore, patients with increased susceptibility to bacterial endocarditis should receive antibiotic prophylaxis during predictable periods of bacteremia. It is likely susceptible patients have valvular heart disease, prosthetic valve replacements, or a history of a previous episode of infective endocarditis. The American Heart Association (AHA) recommends routine prophylaxis for dental and urologic procedures, colon and rectal surgery, gastrointestinal tract procedures, and septic abortion. The AHA does not recommend prophylaxis routinely for proctoscopy, sigmoidoscopy, dilation and curettage (D&C), or pelvic examination. Patients undergoing cesarean section should receive prophylaxis.

The case for the routine use of prophylactic antibiotics in a patient with increased susceptibility for infective endocarditis during routine vaginal delivery is unproven. Most obstetricians will recommend the use of prophylaxis. A review by Fleming[23] presents data indicating the occurrence of infective endocarditis to be very rare in routine vaginal delivery. His recommendation was that no indication exists for routine prophylactic antibiotic during routine labor and vaginal delivery. The AHA has not recommended routine prophylaxis.

It has been widely advised, however, that antibiotic prophylaxis be used in susceptible patients. Ideally, prophylaxis requires the selection of antibiotics that are effective against the most likely pathogens to be encountered and the administration of doses sufficient to prevent infective endocarditis. The recommendations in Table 57–3 are directed against *Enterococcus, S epidermidis,* and gram-negative bacilli. It is important to note that these are empiric suggestions; no regimen has been proven effective, and prevention failures may occur with any regimen.

Cesarean Section

The highest risk factor for developing postpartum infection is cesarean section. Many studies have demonstrated significant reductions in postpartum febrile morbidity, endometritis, and wound infections with the administration of prophylactic antibiotics during cesarean section.[23-25] These studies have also shown prophylactic antibiotics to be cost effective, with healthier patients and shorter hospital stays.

It is important to identify the patient at risk for postpartum infection. Many different risk factors have been proposed, but the most consistently cited ones include duration of labor, length of rupture of membranes (term or preterm), and number of vaginal examinations prior to cesarean section. Patients undergoing primary cesarean section are at greater risk for infection than patients who have elective repeat cesarean sections. In Swartz's review of cesarean section prophylaxis, he found six studies that showed a reduction in febrile morbidity for both primary and repeat cesarean sections (primary, 50% in controls to 25% in treated; repeat, 35% in controls to 19% in treated).[26]

A short course of one to three doses of a single antibiotic is now the recommended regimen. The antibiotic should not be administered for greater than a 24-hour period. Multiple studies have shown equal efficacy with a single-dose regimen compared with a multiple-dose regimen.[27,28] In fact, one study demonstrated that a single dose of cefotetan was more effective than multiple doses of cefoxitin in reducing infectious morbidity.[29]

Many different antibiotics have been used, including ampicillin and first-, second-, and third-generation cephalosporins. All have been successful in decreasing the infectious morbidity associated with cesarean section. Individual variations in effectiveness have been noted. In Ford's study, he demonstrated differing rates of successful antibiotic prophylaxis: piperacillin, 98%; cefoxitin, 91%; cephalothin and ceftazidime, 82%; cefotaxime, 80%, and ampicillin, 77%. He recommended consideration of an antibiotic with a broader spectrum of coverage, such as piperacillin, which has an extremely low failure rate (2%). This minimizes the costs of treating the infections secondary to prophylactic failures.[30] In another recent study, Faro et al looked at 10 different regimens for prophylaxis in 1580 patients undergoing cesarean section. They demonstrated that a single dose of cefotetan was the most effective regimen. Piperacillin, cefazolin, and ampicillin were also useful as single-dose regimens.[31]

Controversy remains concerning the optimal timing of administration of prophylactic antibiotics. The work of Burke would suggest that the most scientifically sound concept is to have the antibiotic agent in the tissue when the incision is made.[9] Preoperative antibiotics with low levels in the umbilical cord at the time of delivery of the fetus have caused concern by pediatricians that this may mask an infection or obscure the cultures. This concept has not

TABLE 57–3. PROPHYLACTIC RECOMMENDATIONS AGAINST INFECTIVE ENDOCARDITIS

Condition	Recommendation
Labor, delivery	Ampicillin 2.0 g IV q 6 h plus aminoglycoside (gentamicin or tobramycin) 1.5 mg kg IV q 8 h. Continue at least 8 h postpartum.
Allergy to penicillin	Vancomycin 1.0 g IV slowly over 1 h plus aminoglycoside as outlined above
GI or GU procedures	Ampicillin 2.0 g IV and aminoglycoside (gentamicin or tobramycin) 1.5 mg/kg. To be given prior to procedure and 8 h later
Oral regimen for minor GI or GU tract procedures	Amoxicillin 3.0 g orally 1 h before and then 1.5 g 6 h later
Patient penicillin-sensitive	Erythromycin 1.0 g orally 1 h before and 0.5 g 6 h later

TABLE 57–4. CURRENT PROPHYLACTIC RECOMMENDATIONS IN CESAREAN SECTION

Condition	Recommendation
Primary cesarean section or elective cesarean section	Cefotetan, cefazolin, cefoxitin 2.0 g IV or piperacillin 4.0 g IV on call to OR or after cord is clamped. May continue for 1 or 2 doses postoperatively but single-dose regimen is effective.
Penicillin-allergic patients	Clindamycin 600 mg IV or gentamycin 1.5 mg/kg IV on call to OR or after cord is clamped. May continue for 1 or 2 doses postoperatively.

been proven but remains a potential concern. Most obstetricians opt for administering the antibiotics immediately after clamping of the umbilical cord, which appears to be equally efficacious to preoperative antibiotics. Interestingly, in a recent study by Rodriguez et al, it was shown that the timing of administration was critical to prophylaxis. If the patients received the antibiotic preoperatively or within three minutes after clamping of the umbilical cord, the antibiotic significantly decreased the infectious morbidity. If the patient received the antibiotic more than three minutes after cord clamping, the infection rate was significantly higher. There were no adverse effects seen in the neonates whose mothers received antibiotics preoperatively.[32] Current prophylactic recommendations in cesarean section are listed in Table 57–4.

REFERENCES

1. Harrison HR, Fulginiti VA. Bacterial immunization. *Am J Dis Child.* 1980;134:184.
2. Brunell PA, Weigle K, Murphy MD, et al. Antibody response following measles-mumps-rubella vaccine under conditions of customary use. *JAMA.* 1983;250:1409.
3. ACIP. General recommendations on immunization. *MMWR.* 1989; 38:205.
4. Immunization during pregnancy. ACOG Technical Bulletin. 1982;64:108.
5. Ogra PL, Fishaut M, Gallagher MR. Viral vaccination via mucosal routes. *Rev Infect Dis.* 1980;2:352.
6. Gill TJ, Repetti CF, Metlay LA, et al. Transplacental immunization of the human fetus to tetanus by immunization of the mother. *J Clin Invest.* 1983;72:987.
7. Centers for Disease Control. Rubella vaccination during pregnancy—United States 1971–1982 and congenital rubella syndrome. *Inf Dis Lett Ob Gyn.* 1984;6:21.
8. Centers for Disease Control. Health information for international travel 1988. U.S. Department of Health and Human Services, Public Health Service. 1988;73.
9. Burke JF. Preoperative antibiotics. *Surg Clin North Am.* 1963;43:665.
10. Anthony BF, Okada DM, Hobel CJ. Epidemiology of group B streptococcus: longitudinal observations during pregnancy. *J Inf Dis.* 1978;137:524.
11. Hall RT, Barnes W, Krishnan L, et al. Antibiotic treatment of parturient women colonized with group B streptococci. *Am J Obstet Gynecol.* 1976;124:630.
12. Bobitt JR, Damato JD, Sakarini J. Perinatal complications in group B streptococcal carriers: a longitudinal study of prenatal patients. *Am J Obstet Gynecol.* 1985;151:711.
13. Minkoff H, Mead P. An obstetric approach to the prevention of early-onset group B beta-hemolytic streptococcal sepsis. *Am J Obstet Gynecol.* 1986;154:973.
14. Siegal JD, McCracken GH, Threlkeld N, et al. Single-dose penicillin prophylaxis against group B beta-hemolytic streptococcal infections. *N Eng J Med.* 1980;303:769.
15. Holls WM, Thomas J, Troyer V. Cervical Gram stain for rapid detection of colonization with beta-streptococcus. *Obstet Gynecol.* 1987;69:354.
16. Sandy EA, Blumenfeld ML, Iams JD. Gram stain in the rapid determination of maternal colonization with group B beta-streptococcus. *Obstet Gynecol.* 1988;71:796.
17. Tuppurainen N, Hallman M. Prevention of neonatal group B streptococcal disease: intrapartum detection and chemoprophylaxis of heavily colonized parturients. *Obstet Gynecol.* 1989;73:583.
18. Isada NB, Grossman JH. A rapid screening test for the diagnosis of endocervical group B streptococci in pregnancy: microbiologic results and clinical outcome. *Obstet Gynecol.* 1987;70:139.
19. Brady K, Duff P, Schilhab JC, Herd M. Reliability of a rapid latex fixation test for detecting group B streptococci in the genital tract of parturients at term. *Obstet Gynecol.* 1989;73:678.
20. Morales WJ, Lim DV, Walsh AF. Prevention of neonatal group B streptococcal sepsis by the use of a rapid screening test and selective intrapartum chemoprophylaxis. *Am J Obstet Gynecol.* 1986;155:979.
21. Morales WJ, Angel JL, O'Brien WF, Knuppel RA. Use of ampicillin and corticosteroids in premature rupture of membranes: a randomized study. *Obstet Gynecol.* 1989;73:721.
22. Amon E, Lewis S, Sibai BM, Moretti M. Ampicillin prophylaxis in preterm premature rupture of membranes: a prospective randomized study. Presented at the Eighth Annual Meeting of the Society of Perinatal Obstetricians; February 1988; Las Vegas, NV.
23. Gilstrap LC. Prophylactic antibiotics for cesarean section and surgical procedures. *J Reprod Med.* 1988;33:588.
24. Rayburn WF. Prophylactic antibiotics during cesarean section: an overview of prior clinical investigations. *Clin Perinatol.* 1983;10:461.
25. Galask RP. Changing concepts in obstetric antibiotic prophylaxis. *Am J Obstet Gynecol.* 1987;157:491.
26. Swartz WH, Grolle K. The use of antibiotics in cesarean section. *J Reprod Med.* 1981;26:595.
27. Gall SA, Hill GB. Single-dose versus multiple-dose piperacillin prophylaxis in primary cesarean operation. *Am J Obstet Gynecol.* 1987;157:502.
28. Varner MW, Werner CP, Petzold R, Galask RP. Comparison of cefotetan and cefoxitin as prophylaxis in cesarean section. *Am J Obstet Gynecol.* 1986;154:951.
29. McGregor JA, Gordon SF, Krotec J, Poindexter AN. Results of a randomized, multicenter, comparative trial of a single dose of cefotetan versus multiple doses of cefoxitin as prophylaxis in cesarean section. *Am J Obstet Gynecol.* 1988;158:701.
30. Ford LC, Hammil HA, Lebherz TB. Cost-effective use of antibiotic prophylaxis for cesarean section. *Am J Obstet Gynecol.* 1987;157:506.
31. Faro S, Martens MG, Hammill HA, et al. Antibiotic prophylaxis: is there a difference? *Am J Obstet Gynecol.* 1990;162:900.
32. Rodriguez GC, Gall SA, Parsons MT. Timing of prophylactic antibiotic administration at cesarean section. Presented at the Tenth Annual Meeting of the Society of Perinatal Obstetricians; January, 1990; Houston, TX.

Chapter Fifty-Eight
Obstetric Bacteremia and Septic Shock

Ruth E. Tuomala

58

BACTEREMIA

Obstetric bacteremia is a frequent event. The exact incidence of bacteremia among hospitalized obstetric patients or among postpartum patients with or without fevers is not known. There have been no large-scale, prospective assessments of standardly obtained blood cultures in any group of obstetric patients.

Rates of bacteremia associated with postpartum febrile illness have been reported to be between 6% and 32.5%. The majority of such reports are from clinical trials of various antimicrobial regimens for the treatment of postpartum endometritis.[1-8] Three reviews of bacteremias from obstetric services, one review containing information from gynecologic patients, and only one review prospective, suggest overall rates of obstetric bacteremia between 9.7% and 12%.[9-11] In addition, the occurrence of positive blood cultures surrounding delivery in from 1–4.9% of cases has been reported.[12-14]

Bacteremia in obstetric patients is seen in association

with postpartum endometritis, septic events surrounding both spontaneous and induced abortions, pyelonephritis, wound infections, and various nonobstetric infections. The most common infection associated with postpartum bacteremia is endometritis. Patients who develop endometritis after cesarean section appear to have a greater risk for bacteremia than do those patients who develop endometritis after vaginal deliveries. Blanco et al have reported a rate of bacteremia after cesarean sections of 3% and a rate of bacteremia after vaginal deliveries of 0.1%.[9]

Risk factors for postpartum bacteremia in association with endometritis have been described.[5,9] In addition to cesarean section, these have included the occurrence of fever in labor, the presence of internal monitoring, duration of ruptured membranes, and questionably, duration of labor. The organisms isolated from blood cultures in cases of obstetric bacteremia are those that have been reported in various obstetric and gynecologic soft tissue infections. These include single organism isolation of both aerobic[15–17] and anaerobic organisms[18] as well as polymicrobial bacteremias.[19] Polymicrobial bacteremias have been reported in between 8% and 25% of bacteremias. Anaerobic bacteremias have been reported in between 15% and 86% of cases. β-hemolytic group B Streptococcus and aerobic gram-negative rods, chief among these being *Escherichia coli*, are major pathogens in many reported series of bacteremia. Aerobic gram-negative rods have been reported as isolates in cases of bacteremia between 7% and 50% of the time and group B Streptococcus between 16% and 40% of the time. There is scant data by which to assess any differences in clinical presentation for bacteremias associated with specific organisms. Blanco et al[9] have suggested that bacteremias due to different organisms have similar presentation in regard to time of onset, height of postpartum fever, the birth weight or gestational age of infants born to women with such postpartum fever, and also in the rates of response to therapy for associated complications. In a separate report, Gibbs and Blanco[16] suggested streptococcal obstetric bacteremia may be characterized by the occurrence of fever soon after delivery, 50% of the time without associated clinical findings of endometritis. They also reported a greater rate of group B streptococcal bacteremia in women who gave birth to premature infants. DiZerega et al[8] and Ledger et al[11] both suggested a more prolonged course of fever in association with anaerobic bacteremia and the need for more antibiotics. Additional antibiotics were associated both with treatment failures and with the occurrence of complicated infections such as abscesses.

Reports that have included clostridial bacteremias have noted the universally favorable outcome of postpartum clostridial bacteremia and the lack of severe manifestations of clostridial sepsis in these selected patient populations. Bacteremias due to *Staphylococcus aureus* and the enterococcus are included in multiple reports. Although there have been case reports of toxic shock syndrome in association with postpartum staphylococcal disease, the presentation of staphylococcal bacteremia as described is nondistinctive. Similarly, enterococcal bacteremia appears to have no distinctive presentation, and the specific role of enterococci as postpartum pathogens remains largely undefined.

There have been both case reports and small series of obstetric bacteremias associated with organisms that are common inhabitants of the lower genital tract, but which are typically thought not to be major pathogens in cases of invasive infections. Among these are lactobacilli, *Gardnerella vaginalis*, and mycoplasmas.[20-24] Series of both mycoplasma and *G vaginalis* bacteremias have suggested that these organisms may be isolated as sole pathogens but disproportionately in association with other bacterial species. Therapeutic response is uniformly good without regard to the use of antimicrobial therapy directed specifically against these organisms. In addition, blood culture media selected to enhance retrieval of these organisms has been used. Therefore, the exact role that these organisms may play in general postpartum bacteremia is unclear.

All authors who have reported on postpartum bacteremias have indicated the uniformly favorable outcome of patients with this complication. Antimicrobial therapy directed toward the underlying infection, most commonly endometritis, results in cure rates similar to patients without bacteremias, and with no differences in complication rates. Bryan et al[10] noted the much more favorable outcome in patients with bacteremia on the obstetric and gynecologic service compared to other patients, with mortality rates of 6.8% and 30.8%, respectively. Low rates of associated septic shock, from 0–12%, and of death, from 0–2.9%, have been noted in association with such bacteremias. However, over the last decade reports of bacteremias specifically from obstetric patients have almost universally included no reports of either septic shock or death. Current opinion is that cases of obstetric bacteremia in patients without compromising underlying medical conditions may be successfully treated with short courses of antimicrobial agents aimed toward routine therapy of underlying conditions, regardless of the organisms that are isolated from blood cultures.

SEPTIC SHOCK

Septic shock is a clinical condition of marked hemodynamic instability, metabolic acidosis, wide-spread tissue injury, and multi-organ failure. It is the most serious consequence of systemic sepsis. Reports of septic shock in the general population suggest rates of mortality ranging from 10–80%, and averaging in the 25–50% range.[25,26] Septic shock in obstetric patients is a relatively uncommon event. Therefore, there is a lack of reports of substantial series of obstetric patients suffering from septic shock. However, it is generally accepted that due to their underlying state of good health, obstetric patients have a much lower mortality rate due to septic shock than do other groups of patients. Obstetric patients with septic shock may present at any time during gestation, including the postpartum period. Since septic shock is relatively uncommon in obstetric patients, there have been no large case series by which to judge specific risk factors for its occurrence. Septic shock at any gestational age has been associated with infected abortions, both spontaneous and induced, and pyelonephritis. In addition, chorioamnionitis and prolonged ruptured membranes have both been associated with septic shock, as has endometritis and wound and episiotomy infections.[25-28] Despite its relatively uncommon occurrence in obstetrics, however, septic shock is always a life-threatening condition whose successful management requires aggressive diagnosis and therapy based on knowledge of the underlying pathophysiology.

Septic shock is most closely associated with gram-negative bacteremia but can also occur in association with gram-positive aerobic bacteremia and anaerobic bacteremia. The pathophysiologic mechanisms of septic shock are set into play by mediators released upon destruction of bacterial cell walls. The endotoxin that appears to be responsible for the major effects associated with gram-negative bacteremia appears to be the lipopolysaccharide portion of the cell wall, in particular the lipid A portion. Peptidoglycans of gram-positive cell walls also probably mediate septic shock.

Bacterial mediators are capable of both direct end organs effects and also of stimulating the production and release of various soluble mediators from target organs.[29] The major target organs and sources of endogenous mediators are the vascular endothelium, tissue macrophages, and circulating mononuclear cells. Some soluble mediators appear to be capable of inducing systemic effects that result in some of the major manifestations of septic shock, while others are probably responsible for more local, organ-specific effects.[30-32] Interactions among all of the various mediators probably influence their production, release, and individual target organ effects. The exact identification and actions of the soluble mediators involved in causing septic shock are not completely known. Attempts at defining the basic pathophysiology of septic shock have been complicated by inaccuracies in assays for suspected mediators in humans with septic shock, plus the incomparabilities inherent in studying animal models of experimentally-induced sepsis.

The actions of soluble mediators and endogenous enzymes in septic shock have been elucidated through measurements of levels of these substances in humans or animals with septic shock, observations of differential effects noted when blocking substances have been used as either pretreatment or during therapy, and by observation of direct effects of specific substances experimentally injected into animals. Major effects on cardiovascular physiology, volume regulation, respiratory function, and stimulation of both hematopoietic cells and the coagulation cascade seen in septic shock have been observed by investigation of various substances. Soluble mediators and enzymes that probably play a part in the pathophysiology of human septic shock include complement, interleukins, interferon, monokines, platelet activating factor, tissue plasminogen activator, histamine, serotonin, various kinins, and the major products of arachidonic acid metabolism, including prostaglandins, thromboxane, and leukotrienes. A partial listing of these factors and possible functions in septic shock is listed in Table 58–1.

While endotoxin itself is capable of causing direct end

TABLE 58–1. MEDIATORS OF SEPTIC SHOCK

Substance	Possible Role in Septic Shock
Complement	Promotes release of neutrophils; chemotaxis of neutrophils and monocytes Promotes degranulation of mast cells leading to release of histamine, leukotrienes, other mediators ? aggregates and promotes microembolization of white blood cells ? vasodilates
Endorphins (endogenous opioids)	Mediate hypotension Modify immunoregulatory effects
Histamine	? vasodilates
Interferon-γ	Increases phagocytic and cytotoxic activities of white cells Potentiates interleukin-1-induced alveolar macrophage secretion Enhances cachectin production Pyrogen

TABLE 58–1. MEDIATORS OF SEPTIC SHOCK (*Continued*)

Substance	Possible Role in Septic Shock
Interleukin-1	Acts synergistically with cachetin to stimulate the actions of platelet-activating factor and other mediators T and B lymphocyte activation Promotes endothelial cells' adhesiveness; induces release of procoagulants; inhibits tissue plasminogen activator Mediates acute phase liver protein synthesis Promotes alveolar macrophage secretion Pyrogen
Interleukin-2	Promotes induction of interferon-γ Lymphocyte proliferation and growth
Kinins	Mediate vasodilation and vascular permeability
Leukotrienes	Leukocyte chemotaxis; leukocyte aggregating agent Bronchoconstrict Vasoconstrict of renal, pulmonary, coronary vessels Decrease myocardial contractility ? mediate enhanced pulmonary vascular permeability
Monokines	Local paracrine function Mediate endocrine activity; promote initial protective metabolic effects (catabolism) Regulate the proliferation of bone-marrow-derived precursor cells Stimulate phagocytosis, cytolytic activity, secretion of proteases Promote prostaglandin synthesis
Platelet aggregating factor	Promotes platelet aggregation and secretion Promotes degranulation and margination of white blood cells Increases vascular permeability Smooth muscle contractor
Prostacyclin	? promotes hypotension ? vasodilation under hypoxic conditions
Prostaglandins	Induce interleukin-1 activity Inhibit platelet aggregation Promote tissue factor activity Promote macrophage phagocytosis Vasodilate; decrease peripheral vascular resistance ? regulate renal blood flow ? potentiate permeability changes
Serotonin	Increases pulmonary vasoconstriction and vascular resistance
Thromboxane	Vasoconstricts Promotes platelet release and aggregation ? acute pulmonary vasoconstriction ? promotes hypotension
Tissue factor activity	Induces extrinsic coagulation pathway Promotes microvascular thrombosis

organ effects, it is probable that many of the actions attributed to endotoxin are mediated through cachectin.[29,33,34] Cachectin is a substance that is released by tissue macrophages or monocytes under stimulation of endotoxin or other bacterial substances. Cachectin appears to be the same substance as tissue necrosis factor. It is directly toxic to vascular endothelial cells. Many of its effects on the cardiovascular and hematologic systems may be due both to this direct effect and to subsequent release of endogenous mediators. In addition, cachectin serves as a mediator of certain functions. It appears to possess specific endogenous pyrogeneic activity. Under the influence of cachectin, phagocytic and cytotoxic activity of polymorphonuclear leukocytes is stimulated, and their adhesion to endothelial surfaces is enhanced. Cachectin appears to induce coagulation changes through stimulation of endothelial tissue factor procoagulant activity. Cachectin activity appears to trigger the production or release of platelet activating factor, leukotrienes, and interleukin-1. It may also stimulate the cyclooxygenase pathway of arachidonic acid metabolism, leading to increased levels of prostaglandins and thromboxane. Its presence is associated with suppression or inhibition of the function of lipoprotein lipase.

As opposed to strictly categorizing the occurrence of changes of septic shock into defined stages, the multisystem changes associated with septic shock might better be viewed as occurring along a continuum of effects. Basic effects involve endothelial damage, altered vascular reactivity, fluctuations in sympathetic tone, decrease in tissue perfusion, local and generalized acidosis, and eventually, irreversible end organ hypoxia and death. Immediately prior to death, involvement of all organ systems is typical. However, the most prominent changes throughout this continuum of septic shock are typically manifested in the cardiovascular, respiratory, hematologic, and metabolic systems.

The cardiovascular changes of septic shock are somewhat dependent upon the baseline volume status and cardiovascular integrity of the host. Usually, initially there is a hyperdynamic appearance.[35-37] Typically early cardiovascular changes due to septic shock include a decrease in system vascular resistance and an increase in cardiac output and heart rate. Vascular dilatation may well be the earliest change, which then leads to a secondary increase in cardiac output because of adrenergic stimulation induced by the decrease in afterload. There may or may not be a slight decrease in blood pressure; however, hypotension is not usually a prominent initial manifestation of septic shock. Increased vascular permeability at the capillary level causes a shift of fluid from the intravascular space to the extravascular compartment, with the development of edema. Patterns of vascular dilatation and constriction lead to a central redistribution of blood flow. Metabolic demands of sepsis and hyperpyrexia also contribute to a decrease in intravascular volume. Eventually, further increases in cardiac output cannot compensate for decreases in intravascular volume, and hypotension ensues. Impaired myocardial performance is well described in septic shock. This may be due to a circulating myocardial depressant factor that some feel is elaborated by the ischemic pancreas. In particular, abnormal decreased left ventricular function is observed, including decreased ejection fraction and ventricular dilatation, and abnormal ventricular compliance with an abnormal left ventricular stroke work response to volume. This impaired myocardial function further results in decreased cardiac output and hypotension. Late in shock, perhaps in an attempt to compensate for profound hypovolemia, systemic vascular resistance may rise. The observation has been made that prior to death, nonsurvivors of septic shock may have a higher measurable systemic vascular resistance than those who eventually survive.

The initial respiratory changes of septic shock[37,38] include both tachypnea and hyperventilation, with a resultant respiratory alkalosis that may be quite marked, with measured P_{CO_2} levels of less than 30. This initial change may be due to a direct effect of endotoxin or other mediators, but also is probably contributed to by increases in sympathetic activity, hyperpyrexia, and eventually by changes in lung compliance plus metabolic acidosis. Decreased lung compliance, increased vascular resistance, and an increase in alveolar capillary permeability may be noted fairly early. Vascular congestion and an increase in capillary permeability lead to septal edema and alveolar collapse. The alveolar collapse leads to perfusion of unventilated tissue, and this mismatch leads to a decreased P_{O_2} level. Aggregation of platelets, red blood cells, and white blood cells, in addition to thrombi, further interfere with oxygen transfer. This type of right-to-left shunting refractory to administered oxygen therapy clearly occurs prior to, and may herald the onset of, adult respiratory distress syndrome (ARDS). ARDS is typified by increased capillary permeability with increased lung water, decreased pulmonary compliance, and diffuse infiltrates. The pulmonary capillary wedge pressure is normal. Hypoxia may be refractory due to the ventilation perfusion mismatch. A diagnosis of ARDS can be made on the basis of inability to achieve a P_{O_2} level of greater than 50 mm Hg with a FiO_2 of less than 50%. It is theorized that activated, sequestrated white blood cells along with mediators synthesized and metabolized in the lungs promote the inflammation and damage that leads to the acute pulmonary capillary leaks that eventuate in ARDS. Septic shock is the most common cause of ARDS, and when ARDS is present, the prognosis of septic shock is worse. Eventually, the increased work associated with the many respiratory changes of septic shock leads to failure of the respiratory muscles. A decrease in the respiratory rate with concomitant respiratory acidosis and an increase in the P_{CO_2} signifies end-state septic shock.

Disseminated intravascular coagulation, or DIC, is one of the primary events that occurs in septic shock.[36,37,39] DIC is probably precipitated by vascular endothelial damage that leads to collagen exposure and liberation of the various soluble factors that activate the intrinsic and extrinsic coagulation cascades. There is platelet adhesion, activation, and aggregation, and fibrin deposition. There is direct activation of the intrinsic clotting system by bacterial products and mediators and activation of the extrinsic coagulation system by the release of procoagulants and complement from macrophages and monocytes. Platelets, fibrinogen, and clotting factors are consumed. After fibrin deposition and clot formation occur, fibrinolytic mechanisms are activated. Tissue plasminogen activator activity increases. At various times, the manifestations of either intravascular coagulation or of inability of blood to clot may predominate. Platelet aggregation and fibrin deposition may contribute to a decrease in blood flow and local ischemia. Acidosis may serve to perpetuate the changes of DIC. Decreases in measurable clotting factors, an increase in fibrin degradation products, prolongation of clotting times, and thrombocytopenia are seen. Initially, there may be isolated thrombocytopenia.

Initial margination of white blood cells may result in a transient decrease in white blood cell count early in septic shock. Subsequently, the white blood count typically is markedly elevated with a left shift. There may be the release of less mature granulocyte forms from the marrow. Substances that facilitate the release of neutrophils and activate bone marrow stem cells probably include complement and other soluble factors. Functional changes in white blood cells are also facilitated, including increases in phagocytic and cytotoxic activity.

The changes in metabolic processes seen in septic shock are probably mediated both by soluble monokines and by both changes in circulating hormone levels and alterations in hormone receptor activity. Increases in insulin and glucagon levels have both been noted. In general, metabolic processes are diverted to catabolism and increased energy production.[31] Initial hyperglycemia reflects a decrease in glycogen synthesis and an increase in glycogenolysis. There is impaired hepatic gluconeogenesis. This may be due to hepatic dysfunction. As glycogen stores are depleted and gluconeogenesis fails, hypoglycemia results. Muscle protein is broken down. There is a decrease in adipose tissue of the lipoprotein lipase activity that prevents the uptake and storage of exogenous triglycerides, leading to an increase in circulating free fatty acids and hypertriglyceridemia. Hepatic ketogenesis is impaired.

Early in septic shock, lactic acid begins to accumulate, perhaps due to inadequate liver and renal metabolism. Peripheral hypoperfusion resulting in anaerobic metabolism leads to further accumulation of lactate. Cellular metabolism is further impaired. Even in the presence of adequate oxygen delivery to these tissues, there appears to be peripherally impaired oxygen utilization, perhaps due to a defect in mitochondrial function.[40]

Tissue hypoxia and damage to the liver may lead to hepatocellular dysfunction, with elevation of hepatocellular enzymes. Interference with the hepatic microcirculation may lead to a cholestatic picture. Pancreatic vasoconstriction may lead to hypoxia and elaboration of pancreatic enzymes, with attendant damage. Other gastrointestinal effects of septic shock may include stress-induced mucosal erosions and bleeding.

A variety of renal problems may be seen with septic shock, ranging from minimal proteinuria to acute renal failure. Decreased renal blood flow may lead to acute tubular necrosis (ATN). The development of ATN may be facilitated by an accumulation of cellular breakdown pigments as well as the renal toxic affects of various medications. Glomerulonephritis and interstitial nephritis may be seen. Fibrin deposition in renal blood vessels plus perivascular tubule inflammation may lead to focal necrosis. Acute cortical necrosis should be suspected in a normovolemic patient who is anuric.

Marked alteration in the sensorium is a bad prognostic sign in septic shock. Even in the absence of hypotension, severe hypoxia, or end-stage metabolic imbalance, however, central nervous system changes have been noted. The exact reason for this is unclear.

The outcome of septic shock is most associated with the underlying condition and state of health of the individual prior to the bacteremic insult. To some extent, the source of bacteremia also influences the prognosis, with intra-abdominal and respiratory infections more often being associated with death. Poor prognostic signs in septic shock include inability to maintain an effective circulating volume with a decreasing cardiac output and generalized signs of hypoperfusion, coma, steadily increasing acidosis and increasing blood lactate levels, and hypercarbia with a decrease in respiratory rate.

There is little evidence from human observational data that pregnant women have a worse prognosis from septic shock than do nonpregnant individuals of similar age groups and underlying good health. Data from experimental animals has suggested that pregnancy may predispose to more severe complications from septic shock.[41,42] Pregnant hamsters are more susceptible to the lethal effects of experimentally-induced septic shock. Pregnant minipigs were observed to die sooner and develop greater degrees of acidosis with experimentally-induced septic shock than their nonpregnant counterparts.

There is animal data to suggest that endotoxin may be associated with placental or fetal injury and pregnancy loss.[43-46] Injected endotoxin has resulted in placental injury with either embryo toxicity or fetal demise in mice, hamsters and rat species. There has been little evidence of any direct effects of endotoxin upon animal fetuses; however, one study suggested changes in the long bones and an increase in neuron necrosis in the brains of fetuses of mice injected with endotoxin. The exact mechanisms of tissue injury and pregnancy loss following endotoxin administration may be mediated by pathophysiologic mechanisms similar to those observed in the rest of the body. The presence of typical fibrin thrombi in the products of conception of endotoxin-treated mice plus the observation of placental injury in rats treated with specific interleukin-1 and tumor necrosis factor are interesting in this regard.

Experimentally induced hyperthermia in various animal species has suggested the possibility of neurological teratogenicity.[46-49] Congenital defects, such as arthrogryposis and microcephaly, as well as histologic and ultrastructural changes have been observed. It has been suggested that fever may have a synergistic teratogenetic effect with other environmental teratogens such as vitamin A and lead.[50,51] There have been case reports of hypotonia or dystonia, arthrogryposis, and other central nervous system manifestations in infants born to women with febrile illnesses between seven and 20 weeks of gestation. However, other observations of pregnant women with fevers and urinary tract infections and pregnant women exposed to hyperthermia in saunas have not supported any major teratogenic effect of fever in humans.[41,52]

Metabolic studies performed on cannulated fetuses of animals with induced sepsis have suggested that fetal compromise in sepsis is secondary to uterine hyperactivity and the eventual development of acidosis and metabolic instability in the pregnant animal. Currently, the major effects of septic shock on the human fetus are believed to be secondary to the effects of maternal metabolic and hemodynamic compromise.[53-56.]

Early management of septic shock is directed toward aggressively replacing intravascular volume and maximizing the cardiovascular dynamics and tissue oxygenation.[57] Although careful calculation of intake and output is important in volume restoration, adequate intravascular support may require massive volumes to correct for the marked third spacing of fluids caused by all of the pathophysiologic changes of septic shock. There is no consensus of opinion as to whether volume should be administered as crystalloid or colloid. The use of the Swan-Ganz catheter for measuring pulmonary capillary wedge pressure has not been documented to improve outcome in septic shock. However, its use may help to avoid errors of excessive volume replacement that can occur in association with alterations in left ventricular compliance and function.[26,35,36,57] In addition, the ability to determine cardiac output and oxygen consumption may provide an added advantage in the management of seriously ill patients. The goal should be to maintain a pulmonary capillary wedge pressure (PCWP) in the 10–14 range.

Adequate delivery of oxygen, including early intubation, is warranted to both improve tissue oxygenation and decrease the work of breathing. In particular, the earliest signs of increase in P_{CO_2} along with reversal in the respiratory alkalosis seen initially should prompt consideration of intubation.

Vasoactive medications are routinely administered in septic shock. Vasopressors should be begun only after aggressive attempts at volume replacement. Dopamine is the initial vasopressor of choice.[58] This drug, when used in low doses of less than 15 μg per kg per minute, improves myocardial contractility and cardiac output and, in addition, increases mesenteric and renal blood flow. Higher doses should not be employed, as the vasoconstrictive effects that then predominate may have an adverse affect. If hypotension persists, drugs with alpha-adrenergic effects, such as metaraminol, may be tried. All alpha-adrenergic vasoactive drugs, in particular isoproterenol, can cause an increase in cardiac work, and thus may be problematic. When there is evidence for myocardial dysfunction, digitalization is appropriate. Correction of acidosis with the administration of sodium bicarbonate to achieve a pH level between 7.2 and 7.3 can aid in stabilizing cardiovascular hemodynamics.

Intra-arterial catheters for the continual measurement of blood pressure and to aid in frequent assessments of arterial blood gases facilitate appropriate, aggressive management. Continuous ECG monitoring can be helpful in interpreting metabolic derangements and oxygen requirements. Echocardiograms can help in the early assessment of left ventricular function and may even highlight an indication for Swan-Ganz monitoring.

The efficacy of administration of high-dose steroids during septic shock has been controversial.[59] Animal models of steroid use have correlated improvements in survival with steroid administration prior to endotoxin or bacterial challenge. It has been apparent that delayed administration of steroids to patients with septic shock does not improve survival. Articles by Bone et al[60] and the Veterans Administration Systemic Sepsis Cooperative Study Group[61], published simultaneously in 1987, were the first large-scale, prospective, randomized, double-blind, placebo-controlled trials that included in their study designs the attempt to administer steroids early in the diagnosis of sepsis, even before the specific diagnosis of septic shock. Both studies were unable to show that the occurrence of septic shock or survival up to 14 days were affected by the administration of steroids. Bone et al suggested that higher rates of mortality with steroid use were observed in people with preexisting disease and in cases of secondary infection. Because there is no apparent benefit from the use of high-dose steroids in septic shock, and because their use may potentially be detrimental to some patient groups, their use is currently not justified.

Coincident with aggressive management, diagnostic modalities should be judiciously employed. All potentially infected sites should be aggressively cultured, and Gram's stains made of any potentially infected secretions. Culture sites should always include blood, urine, sputum, and wound sites including episiotomies. Considerations should be given to culturing the intrauterine contents in cases of both antepartum and postpartum septic shock. Frequent monitoring of arterial blood gases, electrolytes, and blood sugars can be helpful in judging metabolic changes in the success of therapeutic maneuvers. Periodic monitoring of both renal and hepatic function is necessary to guide the use of medications and fluids. All coagulation parameters should be closely monitored in order to assess the need for component replacement and reversal or coagulopathies.

Antibiotic management should be tailored to specific situations. Empiric therapy of most obstetric infections requires multidrug regimens to include a broad spectrum of antibacterial activity. Coverage for gram-negative organisms, in particular *E coli* and *Enterobacter* species, gram-positive organisms, including *S aureus,* all streptococcal species, including the *Enterococcus,* and anaerobes, including penicillin-resistant *Bacteroides* species, should be provided. Since many of the antimicrobial agents commonly selected are renal toxic, including aminoglycosides and vancomycin, their use should be carefully monitored and dosage schedules tailored to serum levels whenever possible.

Proper management of obstetric septic shock may include the aggressive use of surgical procedures to eliminate the source of sepsis. If the source of infection is thought to be the uterus, the uterus must be evacuated of all products of conception or retained tissue on an emergency basis. Speroff has reported that curettage has been followed by chills and an increase in temperature but not by deterioration in the clinical course.[62] The method chosen to evacuate the uterus should be guided by the clinical response to initial therapeutic maneuvers. When shock is profound, hysterotomy or immediate cesarean section may be necessary. Although surgery is usually avoided for maternal reasons in seriously ill parturients, the improvement of respiratory function and beginning reversal of shock have been reported upon evacuation of the near-term size uterus of patients in near end-stage shock. The need for hysterectomy in cases of septic shock is a matter of individual judgment. It has been suggested that hysterectomy is clearly indicated when microabscesses or tissue necrosis are present and when less invasive surgical procedures do not result in prompt stabilization of the clinical condition.[25,26,62,63] In cases of continued clinical deterioration, hysterectomy has been reported to be life-saving.

REFERENCES

1. Sorrell TC, Marshall JR, Yoshimori R, Chow AW. Antimicrobial therapy of postpartum endomyometritis II. Prospective, randomized trial of mezlocillin versus ampicillin. *Am J Obstet Gynecol.* 1981;141:246.
2. Gibbs RS, Blanco JD, Castaneda YS, St. Clair PJ. Therapy of obstetrical infections with moxalactam. *Antimicrob Ag Chemother.* 1980;17:1004.
3. Gibbs RS, Huff RW. Cefamandole therapy of endomyometritis following cesarean section. *Am J Obstet Gynecol.* 1980;136:32.
4. Cibbs RS, Blanco JD, Duff P, et al. A double-blind, randomized comparison of moxalactam versus clindamycin-gentamicin in treatment of endomyometritis after cesarean section delivery. *Am J Obstet Gynecol.* 1983;146:769.
5. Cunningham FG, Hauth JC, Strong JD, Kappus SS. Infectious morbidity following cesarean section: comparison of two treatment regimens. *Obstet Gynecol.* 1978;52:656.
6. Gibbs RS, Blanco JD, Casteneda YS, St. Clair PJ. A double-blind, randomized comparison of clindamycin-gentamicin versus cefamandole for treatment of post-cesarean section endomyometritis. *Am J Obstet Gynecol.* 1982;144:261.
7. Gibbs RS, Blanco JD, Lipscomb KA, St. Clair PJ. Aztreonam versus gentamicin, each with clindamycin in the treatment of endometritis. *Obstet Gynecol.* 1985;65:825.
8. DiZerega GS, Yonekura ML, Keegan K, et al. Bacteremia in post-cesarean section endomyometritis: differential response to therapy. *Obstet Gynecol.* 1980;55:587.
9. Blanco JD, Gibbs RS, Castaneda YS. Bacteremia in obstetrics: clinical course. *Obstet Gynecol.* 1981;58:621.
10. Bryan CS, Reynolds KL, Moore EE. Bacteremia in obstetrics and gynecology. *Obstet Gynecol.* 1984;64:155.
11. Ledger WJ, Norman M, Gee C, Lewis W. Bacteremia on an obstetric-gynecologic service. *Am J Obstet Gynecol.* 1975;121:205.
12. Redleaf PD, Fadell EJ. Bacteremia during parturition; prevention of subacute bacterial endocarditis. *JAMA.* 1959;169:1284.
13. Baker TH, Hubbell R. Reappraisal of asymptomatic puerperal bacteremia. *Am J Obstet Gynecol.* 1967;97:575.

14. Marraro RV, Harris RE, Hartwell S. Incidence of puerperal bacteremia. *South Med J*. 1979;72:1619.
15. Gibbs RS, Blanco JD, Bernstein S. Role of aerobic gram-negative bacilli in endometritis after cesarean section. *Rev Infect Dis*. 1985;7:S690.
16. Gibbs RS, Blanco JD. Streptococcal infections in pregnancy. A study of 48 bacteremias. *Am J Obstet Gynecol*. 1981;140:405.
17. Faro S. Group B beta-hemolytic streptococci and puerperal infections. *Am J Obstet Gynecol*. 1981;139:686.
18. Chow AW, Guze LB. Bacteriodaceae bacteremia: clinical experience with 112 patients. *Medicine*. 1974;53:93.
19. Monif GG, Baer H. Polymicrobial bacteremia in obstetric patients. *Obstet Gynecol*. 1976;48:167.
20. Cox SM, Phillips LE, Mercer LJ, et al. Lactobacillemia of amniotic fluid origin. *Obstet Gynecol*. 1986;68:134.
21. Lamey JR, Eschenbach DA, Mitchell SH, et al. Isolation of mycoplasmas and bacteria from the blood of postpartum women. *Am J. Obstet Gynecol*. 1982;143;104.
22. Kelly VN, Garland SM, Gilbert GL. Isolation of genital mycoplasmas from the blood of neonates and women with pelvic infection using conventional SPS-free blood culture media. *Pathology*. 1987;19:277.
23. Reimer LG, Reller LB. *Gardnerella vaginalis* bacteremia: a review of thirty cases. *Obstet Gynecol*. 1984;64:170.
24. Monif GRG, Baer H. *Haemophilus (Corynebacterium) vaginalis* septicemia. *Am J Obstet Gynecol*. 1974;120:1041.
25. Cavanagh D, Rao PS, Roberts WS. Septic shock in the gynecologic patient. *Clin Obstet Gynecol*. 1985;28:355.
26. Gonik B. Septic shock in obstetrics. *Clin Perinatol*. 1986;13:741.
27. Lee W, Clark SL, Cotton DB, et al. Septic shock during pregnancy. *Am J Obstet Gynecol*. 1988;159:410.
28. Cavanagh D. Shock and the pregnant patient. *Curr Surg*. 1986;43:91.
29. Morrison DC, Ryan JL. Endotoxins and disease mechanisms. *Ann Rev Med*. 1987;38:417.
30. Ball HA, Cook JA, Wise WC, Halushka PV. Role of thromboxane, prostaglandins and leukotrienes in endotoxic and septic shock. *Intensive Care Med*. 1986;12:116.
31. Filkins JP. Monokines and the metabolic pathophysiology of septic shock. *Fed Proc*. 1985;44:300.
32. Makaboli GL, Mandal AK, Morris JA. An assessment of the participatory role of prostaglandins and serotonin in the pathophysiology of endotoxic shock. *Am J Obstet Gynecol*. 1983;145:439.
33. Beutler B, Cerami A. Cachectin: more than a tumor necrosis factor. *New Engl J Med*. 1987;316;379.
34. Michie HR, Manogne KR, Spriggs DR. Detection of circulating tumor necrosis factor after endotoxin administration. *N Engl J Med*. 1988;318:1481.
35. Parillo JE. The cardiovascular pathophysiology of sepsis. *Ann Rev Med*. 1989;40:469.
36. Knuppell RA, Rao PS, Cavanagh D. Septic shock in obstetrics. *Clin Obstet Gynecol*. 1984;27:3.
37. Harris RL, Musher DM, Bloom K, et al. Manifestations of sepsis. *Arch Intern Med*. 1987;147:1895.
38. Newman JH. Sepsis and pulmonary edema. *Clin Chest Med*. 1985;6:371.
39. Beller FK. Sepsis and coagulation. *Clin Obstet Gynecol*. 1985;28:46.
40. Rackow EC, Astiz ME, Weil H. Cellular oxygen metabolism during sepsis and shock. *JAMA*. 1988;259:1989.
41. Ornoy A, Altshuler G. Maternal endotoxemia, fetal anomalies, and central nervous system damage: a rat model of a human problem. *Am J Obstet Gynecol*. 1976;124:196.
42. Beller FK, Schmidt EH, Holzgreve W, Hauss J. Septicemia during pregnancy: a study in different species of experimental animals. *Am J Obstet Gynecol*. 1985:151:967.
43. Haesaert B, Ornoy A. Transplacental effects of endotoxemia on fetal mouse brain, bone, and placental tissue. *Pediatr Pathol*. 1986;5:167.
44. Coid CR. Bacterial endotoxin and impaired fetal development. *Experientia*. 1976;32:735.
45. Silen ML, Firpo A, Morgello S, et al. Interleukin-1 alpha and tumor necrosis factor alpha cause placental injury in the rat. *Am J Pathol*. 1989;135:239.
46. Ivarsson SA, Henriksson P. Septic shock and hyperthermia as possible teratogenic factors. *Acta Paediatr Scand*. 1984;73:875.
47. Smith DW, Clarren SK, Harvey MAS. Hyperthermia as a possible teratogenic agent. *J Pediatr*. 1978;92:878.
48. Edwards MJ. The experimental production of arthrogryposis multiplex congenita in guinea-pigs by maternal hyperthermia during gestation. *J Pathol*. 1971;104:221.
49. Wanner RA, Edwards MJ, Wright RG. The effect of hyperthermia on the neuroepithelium of the 21-day guinea-pig foetus: histologic and ultrastructural study. *J Pathol*. 1976;118:235.
50. Ferm VH, Ferm RR. Teratogenic interaction of hyperthermia and vitamin A. *Biol Neonate*. 1979;36:168.
51. Edwards MJ, Beatson J. Effects of lead and hyperthermia on prenatal brain growth of guinea pigs. *Teratology*. 1984;30:413.
52. Sohar E, Schoenfeld Y, Shapiro Y, et al. Effects of exposure to Finnish sauna. *Isr J Med Sci*. 1976;12:1275.
53. Cefalo RC, Hellegers AE. The effects of maternal hyperthermia on maternal and fetal cardiovascular and respiratory function. *Am J Obstet Gynecol*. 1978;131:687.
54. O'Brien WF, Golden SM, Davis SE, Bibro MC. Endotoxemia in the neonatal lamb. *Am J Obstet Gynecol*. 1985;151:671.
55. O'Brien WF, Cefalo RC, Lewis FE, et al. The role of prostaglandins in endotoxemia and comparisons in response in the nonpregnant, maternal, and fetal models II. Alterations in prostaglandin physiology in the nonpregnant, pregnant, and fetal experimental animal. *Am J Obstet Gynecol*. 1981;139:535.
56. Morishima HO, Niemann WH, James LS. Effects of endotoxin on the pregnant baboon and fetus. *Am J Obstet Gynecol*. 1978;131:899.
57. Karakusis PH. Considerations in the therapy of septic shock. *Med Clin North Am*. 1986;70:933.
58. Rao PS, Cavanagh D. Endotoxic shock in the primate; some effects of dopamine administration. *Am J Obstet Gynecol*. 1982;144:61.
59. Sprung CL, Caralis PV, Marcial EH. The effects of high-dose corticosteroids in patients with septic shock. *N Engl J Med*. 1984;311:1137.
60. Bone RC, Fisher CJ Jr, Clemmer TP, et al. A controlled clinical trial of high-dose methylprednisolone in the treatment of severe sepsis and septic shock. *N Engl J Med*. 1987;317:653.
61. Veterans Administration Systemic Sepsis Cooperative Study Group. Effect of high-dose glucocorticoid therapy on mortality in patients with clinical signs of systemic sepsis. *New Engl J Med*. 1987;317:659.
62. Speroff L. Bacterial shock in obstetrics and gynecology; with emphasis on the surgical management of septic abortion. *Am J Obstet Gynecol*. 1966;95:139.
63. Lloyd T, Dougherty J, Karlen J. Infected intrauterine pregnancy presenting as septic shock. *Ann Emerg Med*. 1983;12:704.

Chapter Fifty-Nine
Abscesses and Local Infections

Stanley A. Gall, Jr.

59

Local bacterial infections manifest as a cellulitis or abscess in ducts and glands infected due to flow stasis or as a secondary infection in devitalized tissue. Surgical wounds are colonized and are also at risk for infection. These localized infections cause discomfort and have the potential for hematogenous seeding systemically or uncontrolled spread regionally. Treatment for the gravid or postpartum female may require modification to protect the fetus or breast-feeding infant. This applies most particularly to antibiotics (see also Chapter 56).

Abscesses and local infections occur when a combination of microbe and host factors coincide to provide favorable conditions for bacterial growth. Local factors predisposing to bacterial infection include stasis of glandular flow, endogenous flora, tissue compromise, and disruption of normally protective tissue planes. Systemic diseases, remote infections, and immunocompromise place the patient at further risk for infection.

Stasis of flow contributes to infectious morbidity in mastitis, hidradenitis, sinusitis, abscesses of the Bartholin's gland, and perirectal abscesses. Blockage of normal flow of secretions creates a static fluid collection that is a fertile culture medium. The bacterial inoculum, often endogenous flora, is normally kept at a dilute concentration by unobstructed flow. In the absence of flow, the bacteria propagate in a now-static fluid. The host response is frustrated by limited diffusion of immune elements into the fluid collection. Formed elements that do penetrate are relatively ineffective because of diminished phagocytosis in this progressively acidic compartment. A host inflammatory response that causes edema, swelling, or induration around the infection limits the extent of infection, brings host defenses into play, and contributes to abscess formation but may further reduce normal flow and ensure a continued lack of drainage. Once an adequate host response occurs, the infection is contained and becomes a recognizable fluctuant abscess. Reestablishing normal flow or draining this fluid collection is the cornerstone of treatment.

The profile of endogenous bacteria varies with the site. Hair follicles contain primarily *Staphylococcus,* while vaginal cultures demonstrate an average of 9.1 organisms per patient with a numeric predominance by anaerobes.[1] When the normal flora is altered by systemic disease such as diabetes or pregnancy or systemic broad-spectrum antibiotics, then potentially pathologic bacteria may be present. The mere presence of bacteria is not sufficient to cause an infection, however. Episiotomy wounds are clearly infested with vaginal and rectal flora but infrequently develop wound infection. Local factors outlined below increase the frequency of localized infections by lowering the minimum concentration of bacteria necessary to effect infection.

Tissue that has been traumatized, violated by surgical egress, or handled without care for Halsted's principles is damaged or devitalized. This tissue and excess foreign matter provide a nidus for bacterial growth, reducing the minimal inoculum needed to cause a wound infection. Devitalized tissue, hematomas, and fluid collections are also barriers to capillary ingrowth, limiting host response and slowing healing. Tissue planes opened during surgical procedures may violate natural boundaries to infection. Once inoculated, infection may spread easily in avascular planes and spaces.

Preexisting infection in remote sites heightens the risk of developing localized infections. Infections may be caused by direct spread or by hematogenous seeding—metastatic implantation. Bacteremic blood may inoculate hematomas or traumatized tissue, leading to infection. Pregnant women have an excess rate of urinary tract colonization. Twenty to forty percent of those colonized will progress to a symptomatic urinary tract infection.[2] Diabetes mellitus, malignancy, chemotherapy, corticosteroid use, and pregnancy all result in some level of immunocompromise. These patients have infections diagnosed at later stages and generally have the most severe complications. They are also at greater risk for uncontrolled local spread, such as necrotizing fasciitis.

Diabetes mellitus occurs in 2–4% of Americans and presents *de novo* in 1.5–6.0% of pregnancies.[3,4] This disease adversely affects host immunity while concomitantly providing an enriched culture medium favoring gram-positive cocci.[5] Although wound infection rates in the National Research Council Study[6] were not demonstrably different for diabetics after correction for age, other authors demonstrate a 25% increase in infectious complications in patients undergoing major vascular, abdominal, and femoral neck fracture surgery.[7] Cruse showed a five-fold increase in wound infection rates in diabetic patients.[8]

Elevated serum glucose levels inhibit bacterial phagocytosis by granulocytes and decrease granulocytic chemotaxis, killing of bacteria, and adherence.[5] Excess serum glucose adversely affects wound healing by decreasing synthesis of collagen and protocollagen, and impairing capillary ingrowth and fibroblast proliferation. These effects may be secondary to a decreased influx and activity of granulocytes responsible for orchestrating the inflammatory response requisite for wound healing. These defects are reversible with insulin administration.[9] Granulocyte function is normalized when serum glucose is maintained below 250 mg/dL.

Diabetics are also more obese than the normoglycemic population. The poorly vascularized fatty tissue of the obese patient presents particular problems during wound closure in avoiding tension, closing dead space, and ensuring an adequate tissue Po_2.[10] Fatty tissue tolerates contamination less well than better perfused tissues. Green and Sarubbi identified obesity as one of four factors significantly associated with febrile morbidity after cesarean delivery.[11] Nielsen and Hokegard's prospective study also identified obesity as a risk factor.[12] Their definition of obese (weight at delivery greater than desirable pregravid weight plus 30 pounds) was particularly severe. Despite an association with increased age and longer procedures, obesity is an independent factor in wound infection regardless of the degree of contamination.[11]

Patients using exogenous corticosteroids have an increased rate of wound infection and prolonged wound healing. These patients may not develop febrile morbidity or local symptoms from localized abscesses or infection, because corticosteroids inhibit all phases of the inflammatory response. Corticosteroids also decrease intracellular killing by monocytes but do not affect cell-mediated or humoral immunity. Host defenses are affected indirectly as corticosteroids severely reduce capillary dilatation, local edema, fibrin deposition, and local prostaglandin production, the vital components of the local inflammatory response to infection or incision. Additionally, inhibition of leukocyte migration and macrophage phagocytosis delay abscess formation and subsequent collagen production in the healing abscess or wound.

Alteration of immune responsiveness in the gravid female is inherent in a system that tolerates the fetal allograft.[13] While humoral and cellular immune responses may be blunted, natural killer activity and thymus-dependent leukocyte reactivity are reduced. Immunoglobulin G concentration declines continuously as gestation progresses, at least partially, due to increased catabolism. Immunity against gram-negative organisms is impaired, and the streptococcal colonization rate is higher.[14] Additionally, the pregnant female has an increased incidence of candidiasis and has greater susceptibility to *Hemophilus influenzae, Listeria monocytogenes,* and tuberculosis.[15] The pregnant female has not only an altered capability to defend against bacterial infection, but is at a higher risk for infectious morbidity due to a simultaneously increased colonization rate.

IMPETIGO AND ERYSIPELAS

Both impetigo and erysipelas, cutaneous manifestations of streptococcal infection and streptococcal pharyngitis, are important primarily for their risk of glomerulonephritis and rheumatic fever. These infections are treated with penicillin (see also Chapter 63). Cellulitis is the most frequent manifestation of cutaneous streptococcal infection. Like erysipelas, where lymphangitis and a sharply defined advancing border are present, cellulitis must be treated medically and is not amenable to surgical treatment. Cellulitis may arise *de novo* or secondary to trauma but occurs most frequently as a sign of wound infection, with redness, heat, and tenderness spreading from the incision.

SINUSITIS

Sinusitis is inflammation of the sinuses of the face and head[16] (see also Chapter 195). Suppurative sinusitis results from mucus stasis. Acute supporative sinusitis requires treatment to prevent the devastating complications of meningitis, epidural abscess, frontal lobe abscess, osteomyelitis, cavernous sinus thrombosis, or orbital involvement with cellulitis or abscess. The gravid female is predisposed to sinus disease, as the frequency of stuffiness of the nose is increased in pregnancy, apparently correlated with estrogen levels.[17]

The sinuses perform heat and moisture exchange and filtration of inspired air. The mucosal epithelium lining the sinuses clears secreted mucus with a mucociliary apparatus. Each sinus has an ostium communicating with the nasopharynx, which is at risk for blockage. Sinus stasis occurs when mucosal inflammation restricts the ostium, when ciliary function is diminished, after injection of infected water during swimming, or from hyperproduction of mucus that overwhelms the ciliary apparatus. Sinus stasis decreases sinus oxygenation, providing for an anaerobic and acidic environment ideal for bacterial growth.

The symptoms of sinusitis begin as a stuffy nose, with a slow increase in pressure over the affected sinus. Malaise and fever are present, and if stasis is not relieved, severe local pain and tenderness may result. Localization of symptoms is dependent on the involved sinus (Table 59–1).

The sinus discharge becomes purulent and may be blood-stained. The mucosa is hyperemic and edematous. Acute frontal and maxillary sinus involvement are most common because their draining ostia are not in a dependent position.

The microbiology of sinus infections reflects the normal flora of the nasopharynx. *Staphylococcus* is unusual, but *H influenzae, Pneumococcus,* and group A *Streptococcus* are more common. Anaerobic growth is more frequent in chronic cases, with *Bacteroides* species and *Peptostreptococcus* as the most frequent isolates.

Sinusitis is treated medically. Surgical intervention is reserved for chronic cases. Medical treatment is directed at pain relief, reducing swelling of the sinus and nasal mucosa, and control of infection. Pain control is accomplished with narcotics. Hot packs and the breathing of moisturized air can help with discomfort and reduce mucosal swelling. Topical vasoactive agents such as pseudoephedrine or phenylephrine may be required to reduce critical mucosal swelling. Intranasal saline lavage is beneficial in clearing mucus and opening sinus ostia. These maneuvers for relieving blockage are prerequisites for infection control. Antibiotics are also required, and an appropriate spectrum of activity is provided for by penicillin, ampicillin, amoxicillin, trimethoprim-sulfamethoxazole, and cefaclor.[18]

The pregnant female has increased sinus congestion, predisposing to more frequent sinus infections with the common symptoms and signs.[17] Penicillin and cephalosporins provide appropriate, safe antibiotic coverage. Vasoactive compounds should be used in limited fashion and only for the most severe symptoms. Cases that do not resolve with this medical routine should be referred to an otolaryngologist for evaluation.

TABLE 59–1. SYMPTOMATOLOGY OF ACUTE SINUSITIS

Involved Sinus	Distribution of Symptoms
Maxillary	Upper teeth, cheek
Ethmoid	Medial and deep to eye; Discomfort with eye movement
Frontal	Forehead over eyebrow
Sphenoid	Deep to eye, over occiput or radiating to the vertex

Adapted from Slavin.[16]

ABSCESSES AND INFECTIONS OF DRUG ABUSE

Abscess formation in the extremities is the most frequent infectious complication of drug abuse. Addicts are also afflicted by foreign body granulomas, sterile abscesses, thrombophlebitis, and necrotizing fasciitis, resulting from injection of impure substances or from using unsterile equipment. Although the injected material may be heated and initially sterile, it is often strained through nonsterile cotton and administered through hypodermic needles that have never been cleaned or that have merely been blown dry by mouth. The frequency of infections with oral flora is not surprising. Quinine, used as a base, induces a sterile abscess that then provides an acidic environment favorable to anaerobic and particularly clostridial organisms.[19] This population's high rate of anergy demonstrates their immunocompromised status.[20]

Parenteral access inoculates the circulatory system, resulting in thrombophlebitis or subacute bacterial endocarditis. Septic thrombophlebitis is treated by excising the infected vein. The approach to subacute bacterial endocarditis is covered in Chapter 128.

Repeated injection in the dorsum of the hand, where loose areolar tissue predisposes to extravasation, produces lymphedema.[21] This lymphatic obstruction causes the skin to become thick and fibrous. No treatment is possible for this condition, but it must be differentiated from a deep palmar space infection. A superimposed cellulitis may require antibiotic treatment.[22]

Treatment of abscesses consists of incision, drainage, curettage, and penicillinase-resistant antibiotics. An average of 2.4 organisms were isolated in such patients, with β-hemolytic *Streptococcus* and *Staphylococcus aureus* present in 68% of patients and accounting for 50% of isolates.[20] Oropharyngeal flora and gram-negative rods were also common. Definitive surgical drainage should not be delayed, as 23% of patients may have positive blood cultures indicating bacteremia. Pyogenic joints may result from direct inoculation or metastatic infection and require open drainage with continuous irrigation. These complications of drug abuse are treated identically in the gravid patient but following appropriate antibiotic guidelines. This population also has a notably higher incidence of acquired immune deficiency syndrome (AIDS), which will further contribute to their immunocompromise.

MASTITIS AND ABSCESSES OF THE BREAST

Mastitis occurs most frequently in the lactating breast, presenting as a spectrum of inflammation from milk stasis to frank abscess. Conversely, abscesses of the breast occur more frequently in the nonlactating, nonpregnant female (see also Chapter 188).

Inflammation of the nonlactating breast may be *Mondor's disease* or a developing abscess. Mondor's disease is a thrombophlebitis of subcutaneous veins over the breast, producing a cordlike swelling that is tender, usually oriented cranio-caudad, and occasionally erythematous.[23] This inflammation resolves spontaneously without surgical or medical treatment.

Abscesses of the breast may occur peripherally or subareolarly. Peripheral breast abscesses present as a tender mass with overlying erythema. Systemic symptoms include malaise and fever. Lymphangitis and adenopathy may occur. Peripheral abscesses of the breast occur most frequently as a result of trauma, representing fat necrosis with superimposed infection. Although the architecture of the breast, primarily the compartmentalizing Cooper's ligaments, prevents extension of the abscess throughout the breast, fluctuance characteristic of an abscess may not develop as the infection instead burrows deep into the breast. There should be no delay in drainage while waiting for a breast abscess to "ripen."

The incision should be made parallel to the areolar margin. This incision produces a less noticeable scar and better cosmetic results than the radially oriented incision. The abscess cavity is entered, and all loculations are broken down. Peripheral abscesses in the lactating or antepartum breast have the same etiology and are treated in a similar manner.[24] Simple incision and drainage with a course of oral antibiotics to cover *Staphylococcus* is usually adequate in these infections. Cephalosporins provide excellent, safe coverage.

Carcinoma may present as an abscess. Therefore, tissue for pathologic examination is always obtained at the time of incision and drainage. The patient must be seen in follow-up to ensure complete resolution of all masses. Residual masses may represent malignancy, but present as recurrent abscess. Excisional biopsy is then required to exclude carcinoma and to treat any residual abscess.

Subareolar abscesses of the breast occur secondary to stasis within the mammary ducts. In the nonpuerperal female, mammary duct ectasia, squamous metaplasia, or intraductal carcinoma result in stasis of ductal debris. In mammary duct ectasia, this collection of cellular debris imitates pus but may actually be sterile. Secondary infection produces an abscess. Hyperplasia of the normal squamous epithelium plugs the ducts. Chronic infection ensues with keratinized material acting as a foreign body. These abscesses are chronic and recur in 39% to 75% of cases.[25,26] In one study, 21% of patients went on to require formal excision of ducts by Hadfield's procedure.[27]

Subareolar abscesses were thought to be strictly staphylococcal before the advent of reliable anaerobic transport and culture techniques. Walker et al prospectively recovered an average of 3.6 different bacteria from culture-positive nonpuerperal breast abscesses, and although coagulase-negative *Staphylococcus* did indeed represent 60% of aerobic bacteria isolated, anaerobic isolates outnumbered aerobic species 2:1.[26] *Peptostreptococcus* represented 47% of these anaerobes, which were present in 70% of all specimens and 75% of patients with chronic abscesses. Brook studied 90 isolates in 41 women (2.2 isolates/specimen) that also contained a predominance of anaerobic species.[28] Anaerobes outnumbered aerobes 62 to 28, but here *Bacteroides* species (24 of 62) occurred with equivalent frequency to *Peptostreptococcus* (21 of 62). Aerobes were predominantly gram-positive cocci evenly divided between *streptococcus* and *staphylococcus*. This anaerobic predominance demonstrates the importance of fastidious anaerobic culture and transport techniques. Gram's stain specimens will frequently indicate the polymicrobial nature of infection but do not accurately identify organisms.

Medical management may be used to manage antepartum mastitis with good results.[24] Treatment with hospitalization and intravenous antibiotics to cover the anaerobic and aerobic components must be accompanied by frequent physical examination to ensure an appropriate course of recovery.

Mastitis in the puerperium is nearly always a function of milk stasis and presents with a spectrum of severity.[29] Thomsen et al used quantitative cultures and leukocyte counts of expressed milk to define this spectrum and guide therapy (Table 59–2).

Milk stasis is the focal breast engorgement resulting from inspissated secretions or a blocked mammary duct.[30] Symptoms include a swollen, firm, tender sector of the breast without fever or erythema.[29] Treatment is local massage, heat, and continued nursing. Manual expression may be helpful to completely empty the breast. Symptoms generally resolve in 2.1–2.3 days, with only 8% of patients having a prolonged course or recurrence.[29] Antibiotics are not indicated.

Noninfectious inflammation occurs in severe and persistent cases of milk stasis. This state is differentiated from milk stasis by increased tenderness and swelling, with an increase in breast milk leukocyte concentration but minimal or no bacterial involvement. Breast emptying is more critical here, reducing the duration of symptoms from a mean of 7.9 days to 3.2 days. Patients who did not undertake regular emptying of the breast achieved normal lactation in only 21% of cases.[29] Antibiotics were not employed for this process and probably are not indicated, as 90% of patients regained normal lactation with regular breast emptying alone.

Infectious mastitis occurs in 2.5% of nursing mothers.[31] Criteria for infectious mastitis (see Table 59–2) require bacterial growth. This infection may be either a cellulitis or mammary adenitis.[30] These patients present with a sector of erythema, tenderness, swelling, and breast soreness. They are febrile. Sporadic or endemic infection most likely results from fissured nipples and milk stasis, representing an infection by skin flora. *Endemic mastitis* presents at a mean of 5.5 weeks.[31] Nipple injury and increased breast engorgement are prominent during this period. A second peak of incidence occurs at the time of weaning, when the breast remains full during involution. Nipple fissuring

TABLE 59–2. QUANTITATIVE STRATIFICATION OF SEVERITY OF PUERPERAL MASTITIS

Diagnosis	Leukocyte Count	Bacteria Count
Milk stasis	$<1 \times 10E6/mL$	0
Noninfectious inflammation	$>1 \times 10E6/mL$	0
Infectious mastitis	$>1 \times 10E6/mL$	$>1 \times 10E3/mL$

Adapted from Thomsen et al.[29]

was present in only eight of 65 patients in one study, however.[31] Infections were preceded by milk stasis secondary to a missed feeding in nine of 65 patients.

In the absence of grossly purulent nipple discharge, it is safe and preferable to continue breast-feeding to effect maximal breast emptying. Treatment by regular breast emptying alone resulted in resolution of symptoms and resumption of lactation in 51% of patients. This compares to a good outcome in only 15% where no treatment was employed. The group with no treatment had a 10.9% rate of abscess formation and a 12.2% rate of recurrence.[29] In patients who weaned at the time of symptoms, 20% developed abscesses.[31] In contrast, treatment with oral antibiotics and regular breast emptying resulted in resumption of lactation in 96% and no abscess formation.

Staphylococcus is the most common isolate in mastitis, but β-hemolytic *Streptococcus, Enterococcus,* and *Escherichia coli* have been isolated as well.[29,31] A high percentage of these organisms demonstrated resistance to penicillin or ampicillin *in vitro.* No treatment failures occurred with these agents, though. A penicillinase-resistant antibiotic would be considered appropriate. The presence of enteric organisms, *E coli,* and *Enterococcus* in some infections represents lack of appropriate breast hygiene. Epidemic mastitis is caused by a particularly virulent staphylococcal infection acquired by the breast-feeding infant from nursery personnel. The infant's suckling inoculates the mammary ducts, and an adenitis results.[30] Discontinuing breast-feeding is encouraged until the infection resolves, but regular breast emptying must be continued. Continued breast-feeding may only serve to reinfect the breast from the infant.

Treatment of *puerperal abscess* begins with discontinuing breast-feeding. This prevents toxic inoculation of the infant with a high concentration of bacteria and spread to other family members.[2] Penicillinase-resistant antibiotics are employed, and may be substituted with erythromycin or a first-generation cephalosporin. Incision and drainage are mandatory at an early stage to limit parenchymal damage. The wound should be packed open and then periodic dressing changes should begin after 24 hours. One study treated puerperal abscess in six patients with repeated aspiration and antibiotics.[32] No prospective studies have confirmed the benefit of this technique. Benson et al employ traditional incision and drainage, then perform curettage and follow with primary closure.[33] Benson and Goodman compared this technique, originally proposed in the treatment of anorectal abscess, with standard incision, drainage, and packing, and showed more rapid wound healing rates (21 versus 27.9 days) with an identical recurrence rate (13%). This method requires strict attention to curettage to ensure that all the infected tissue that lines the abscess is removed.

Suppurative processes involving the perineum include Bartholin's gland abscess, hidradenitis suppurative, or pilonidal abscess. The *peri-rectal abscess* or *abscess-fistula in ano* is the most common local infection of the perineum.[34] In one study, eight of 49 women were pregnant or postpartum. These lesions arise as abscess of the anal glands in the acute stage and become a fistula in the chronic stage. The deep anal glands lie in the intermuscular space defined by the internal anal sphincter and conjoined longitudinal muscle of the rectum. They open into the crypts of Morgagni just above the dentate line. The glands coursing superiorly are simple, while those directed inferiorly exhibit more complex branching. Infection results from obstruction of the duct. These abscesses must be differentiated from Bartholins's gland abscesses, pilonidal cysts, or fistulae secondary to inflammatory disease. More infrequently, a perirectal abscess may arise from episiotomy, superinfected thrombosed hemorrhoid, or trauma.

Perianal abscess is an infection of the superficial perianal space and, as a tegumentary process, requires no more than simple incision and drainage. External perirectal abscess occurs in the ischiorectal space, and is not of anal glandular origin but instead the result of hematologic seeding, trauma, or foreign body. This abscess will point to the central portion of the ischiorectal fossa and is treated by incision and drainage.

Eisenhammer classifies the three main groups of cryptoglandular abscess as low (distal) intermuscular, high (proximal) intermuscular, and intermuscular transsphincteric or ischiorectal abscess-fistula *in ano.*[35] The low intermuscular abscess-fistula extends inferiorly from the dentate line, following the intermuscular space to the superficial anal space. These make up 85% of cryptoglandular abscesses. The greater proportion of glands lie posteriorly, accounting for the 90% frequency of posterior abscess. Posteriorly arising abscesses that spread in the posterolateral superficial anal space should not be confused with a laterally arising abscess.

The high intermuscular abscesses occur in only 3–5% of cases.[34] Infected liquid feces are less likely to infect these glands because they are superiorly directed, simple, unbranched, and short. This abscess dissects proximally in the intermuscular space and may be complicated by rupture at the supralevator level, inducing pelvic suppuration. The transsphincteric abscess-fistulae form 13% of cases. Again, the abscess has arisen from the anal glands, but dissects through the external anal sphincters to invade the fat of the ischiorectal space or posterior deep anal space.

Cryptoglandular abscesses are mixed infections with enteric bacteria and a high proportion of anaerobes. *E coli, Proteus mirabilis, Streptococcus,* and *Bacteroides* predominate. Clostridial species (welchii) produce a more fulminant toxic process.[34]

Systemic symptoms of perirectal abscess are malaise and pyrexia, while local inflammation produces steady pain that may progress to throbbing. Patients will generally be able to identify a point of maximum tenderness, but supralevator abscesses of abdominopelvic origin will be less well localized. Low abscesses will be associated with increased pain on defecation. The intramuscular abscesses induce spasm of the internal sphincter, appreciated only under anesthesia. Physical examination then must determine if the infection is indeed supralevator, a purely external ischiorectal fossa infection, superficial perianal abscess, or a true cryptoglandular abscess.

Physical examination begins externally, palpating the ischiorectal and perianal regions. Digital rectal exam is performed with bimanual palpation of the ischiorectal spaces. Ischiorectal fossa infections produce induration of the levator palpable on digital rectal exam and do not affect the internal anal sphincter. Low intramuscular fistula-abscess *in ano* are unilateral, localized to the distal intermuscular space, and most frequently posterior. The internal anal sphincter is in spasm below the dentate line, and the ischiorectal space is free of inflammation. These lesions may extend laterally. The high intramuscular abscess will be palpable only on digital rectal exam that reveals a fluctuant mass at or above the levator shelf. The high intramuscular abscesses occur almost exclusively posteriorly. The proximal internal anal sphincter is spastic. These infections warrant emergency treatment as extension to the supralevator space produces complicated rectovesical, retrorectal, or pelvic infection.[36]

The transsphincteric abscess-fistulae *in ano* are distinguished by deep postanal pain, but involvement with the deep ischiorectal fossa may be difficult to differentiate from a supralevator process. Transsphincteric infections, arising from a low intramuscular process, are more superficial and have readily palpable ischiorectal fossa induration.

Drainage is performed as soon as possible.[37] Delay only allows the abscess to become more complicated.[38] The procedure of choice is primary fistulectomy.[34] First, proctoscopy must be performed in all cases to identify the crypt of origin. A radial incision through this crypt lays open the fistula and is curative. If only simple incision and drainage are performed, the etiology of the cryptoglandular abscess has not been addressed, and the patient is likely to suffer a recurrence. More complex processes may require additional incisions.[35,38,39] Antibiotics are indicated for seven to 10 days; the cephalosporins provide excellent coverage and are acceptable in the gravid patient.

BARTHOLIN'S GLAND CYSTS AND ABSCESSES

The Bartholin's glands are paired structures with ducts opening into the introitus that provide vaginal lubrication. These are not palpable in the normal state but may develop cysts or abscesses.Cysts may occur in either the gland or the duct. They become noticeable only when their size interferes with daily activities.[39] These may become secondarily infected. The most common responsible organisms are Enterobacteriaceae, *Neisseria gonorrhoeae,* or a mixed infection of normal vaginal flora.[40] *Staphylococcus,* clostridia species, and streptococci have also been described.[41] Chlamydia is reported in a single case.[42]

Treatment prior to the 1960s most frequently consisted of excision of the gland. This procedure was complicated frequently by hemorrhage, hematoma, postoperative pain, and dyspareunia.[43] Methods of developing a cutaneous fistula were developed. Although the Word catheter was successful, with a low 13% recurrence rate, it never gained common use. Marsupialization was suggested by Davies in 1948.[43] This consisted of packing open the incised cyst/abscess until epithelialization occurred. True marsupialization, sewing the cyst wall to the labial skin, was introduced by Jacobson in 1960, but others could not duplicate his 2.5% rate of recurrence. Cheetham advocates a sterile aspiration of the mass to relieve the patient's discomfort and obtain material for Gram's stain, culture, and sensitivities.[41] He treated purulent aspirates with antibiotics, while those with no leukocytes on Gram's stain received no antibiotics. Normal function was not established in 15%, all of whom went on to marsupialization. Patients who are treated with incision and drainage or marsupialization require no antibiotics unless lymphangitis or cellulitis is present. Cheetham used metronidazole with either penicillin or erythromycin. Ampicillin would be the drug of choice if no gonococci are present on Gram's stain.

A severe complication of Bartholin's abscess is that of necrotizing fasciitis.[44] Roberts describes a group of six obese, diabetic patients who developed extensive necrotizing fasciitis with a 50% mortality. This process requires rapid, aggressive surgical debridement to limit the extent of infection (see below).

HIDRADENITIS SUPPURATIVA

The apocrine sweat glands form part of the pilosebaceous–apocrine apparatus limited to the skin of the axillae, groin, perianal region, sacrum, ear canal, areolae, eyelid, and umbilicus. In individuals prone to keratinous inspissation of these glands, inflammation, dilatation, and then rupture may proceed to hidradenitis suppurativa as other regional apocrine glands are affected.[45] First described in 1839 by Velpeau and specifically related to the apocrine apparatus by Schieflerdecker in 1912, this chronic inflammation progresses to suppuration with abscess and fistulous tract formation after ductal bacteria propagate in the rich milieu of apocrine secretions.[46] Prevalence is estimated at 1 in 3000. While no clear familiar inheritance is known, patients with hidradenitis do have a higher familial incidence of acneiform lesions.[47] Females are affected three times more frequently than males and have a predominance of axillary disease, while males have a tendency for perineal and perirectal disease.[48]

Apocrine glands become active during puberty under the influence of androgenic and estrogenic stimulation. While the condition may continue in patients late in life, presentation after the third decade is unusual. The disease is distributed in multiple regions in 65% of patients, affecting the axillae (61%), groin (48%), perineum (22%), and breast (13%).[49] The disease starts as small pustules formed when plugged glands rupture and become infected. These are accompanied by induration, swelling, and pain, then acute abscess. Apocrine lipids act as a foreign body and provide for chronic abscess and fistula formation, followed by cicatrization.

Differentiation must be made from tuberculosis, lymphogranuloma venerum, cat scratch fever, and tularemia. In perianal lesions, ulcerative colitis, pilonidal abscess, and perirectal abscess must be excluded. The early stages are sometimes adequately managed by improved hygiene. Avoiding irritating substances, clipping hair to avoid depilatory agents or shaving, wearing loose-fitting garments, losing weight if necessary, and washing several times daily with hexachlorophene or chlorhexidine are suggested. Hurley feels that topical and systemic antibiotics for a prolonged period are beneficial.[45] Dietary manipulation, ultraviolet or x-ray irradiation, vaccination, and steroids have no place in treatment. Reports of success with oral isotretinoin are not consistent.[51] While there are no reports of incidence in pregnancy, apocrine gland function is diminished in the hormone milieu of pregnancy.[50] Despite this, treatments that attempt to mimic pregnancy with exogenous estrogens or progesterone have failed.[48]

Acute abscesses in the gravid patient should be treated just as in the nongravid patient—with incision and drainage, oral antibiotics, hot packs, and frequent cleansing. Common isolates include *S aureus, E coli,* and alpha-hemolytic *Streptococcus.* While anaerobic organisms are occasionally involved, incision and drainage leads to resolution of the acute abscess.

When the disease has progressed to the point of abscesses and scarring, definitive treatment is effected only by excision of all apocrine gland-bearing skin in the affected areas. This therapy should be delayed until the postpartum period. Skin and subcutaneous tissue are excised to a depth such that all infected material is removed. Repair of the defect may be managed by primary closure, split thickness skin grafting, or skin flap.[52] In axillary hidradenitis, excision and skin grafting required reoperation in only 13% of patients, while primary closure required reoperation in 54%.[52] Reoperation was required for regions not adequately excised or from newly developed disease adjacent to the graft.[49] In perianal disease, colostomy formation may be avoided by allowing the wound to heal by secondary intention.[53]

This technique has approximately a 10% reoperation rate.[54] Treatment with isotretinoin is yet to be proved effective and is absolutely contraindicated in pregnancy because of its known teratogenic effects.

PUERPERAL INFECTIONS

The gravid female is at heightened risk for infections in the puerperium, whether the fetus is delivered vaginally or by cesarean section. Infections occurring after cesarean section include endometritis, wound infection, and intrapelvic infections. Vaginal delivery may be complicated by endometritis or episiotomy infection. Infection may also ensue as a complication of anesthesia, with epidural, retropsoas, or subgluteal infection. Puerperal sepsis is discussed in Chapter 117.

EPIDURAL AND SPINAL ABSCESSES

Epidural anesthesia is being employed with greater frequency in the management of labor and delivery. This procedure may inoculate the sterile epidural space directly or by introducing blood to the space. Although uncommon, spinal epidural abscess has devastating complications.[55] Without timely treatment, such infections may lead to hemiparesis or permanent neurologic deficit. Dawkins was unable to distinguish any case of epidural abscess in 32,000 cases of epidural anesthesia, while others[56] report no pyogenic complication in 65,677 to 78,746 cases. Male reported on the first puerperal spinal epidural abscess.[56] Baker et al report a rate of spinal epidural abscess of 0.2 to 1.2 per 10,000 hospital admissions annually.[57] North and Brophy reported on two cases felt to be secondary to direct contamination.[58] Patients who have remote infections often are bacteremic. Blood introduced during the procedure inoculates the epidural space. This space is poorly vascularized, offering little resistance to bacterial growth. The infection is not due to direct contamination, but rather made possible by the trauma of the procedure, exposing an otherwise sterile and protected space to infection. The source of infection is traceable to remote infections in 20–50%, and to direct extension by a vertebral osteomyelitis in 35–38%.[57,58]

The obstetric population is at higher risk of infection because of the frequency of epidural anesthesia and their propensity for excess colonization. In Baker's series, three patients were pregnant and two others had acute infection secondary to spread from wound infections. Symptoms include back pain, localized spinal tenderness, nerve root pain, weakness, urinary retention, or paralysis.[59] Back pain was present for an average of three days, followed by root symptoms for 4–5 days, and weakness for 24 hours when paralysis began.[57] The differential diagnosis includes meningitis, which usually presents with headache, a vascular lesion that usually occurs suddenly as a stroke, disk compression that may have a sudden or insidious onset of root pain, weakness, urinary retention, and vertebral osteomyelitis. The cerebrospinal fluid will be clear in disk compression or osteomyelitis. Myelography demonstrated root or cord compression or obstruction to flow of contrast in 27 of 27 cases.[57] *Staphylococcus* was the most frequently isolated organism, followed by *Streptococcus* and *E coli*. Treatment consists of laminectomy for drainage and intravenous antibiotics. Ten of 15 patients with acute abscess and 13 of 19 patients with chronic symptoms recovered.[57]

Prevention of epidural abscess requires avoiding this route of anesthesia in any patient with a remote infectious process; use of new, sterile equipment; meticulous sterile technique; and millipore filters for anesthetic injection. Any patient presenting with back pain after epidural anesthesia should prompt a neurosurgical consultation.

SUBGLUTEAL AND RETROPSOAS ABSCESSES

Hibbard et al first noted the complication of subgluteal and retropsoas infection.[60] Svancarek and colleagues added 11 further cases, while Wenger and Gitchell noted two others.[61,62] In Hibbard's study, three of five patients died of their infections, while in Svarancek's study, two of 11 died. These infections were traced to inoculations occurring with administration of paracervical or transvaginal pudendal anesthesia. The needle probably passed through the colon or rectum and carried colonic or vaginal organisms into the paracervical space. Infection spreads dorsally following the pudendal nerve, either leaving the pelvis through the lesser sciatic notch to infest the posterior hip capsule or to follow the sciatic nerve roots superiorly to inoculate the retropsoas space.[62] The retropsoas space may likewise be entered directly along the base of the broad ligament after paracervical injection.

Diagnosis of these infections is to be considered in any postpartum patient who had paracervical or pudendal block, has hip, flank, thigh, or buttock pain, or has a disturbed gait with any sign of systemic toxicity.[62] Physical exam is helpful especially if cellulitis or a psoas spasm is present. Psoas spasm was present in all cases of retropsoas abscess. Computed tomography is probably the diagnostic tool of choice to localize exactly the process and plan an operative or percutaneous drainage approach.

Treatment of these infections consists of early extensive debridement and antibiotics. Cultures of these infections demonstrated *Bacteroides, E coli, Streptococcus, Proteus, Pseudomonas, Klebsiella, Staphylococcus,* and *Enterococcus,* which are colonic or vaginal in origin. While adequate drainage may be established posteriorly, a perineal or anterior approach may also be required.

EPISIOTOMY

Episiotomy is performed during stage II of labor to enlarge the vaginal opening in hopes of preventing haphazard laceration to the vaginal mucosa and musculature by placing a more easily repaired surgical incision. The episiotomy may be made mediolateral—an approach of historical interest—or in the midline posteriorly. Vaginal laceration and episiotomy incisions are graded identically, from grade I, with only vaginal mucosal laceration, to grade IV, with all layers of vagina and rectum involved.

Infection at the episiotomy site ranges from a stitch abscess to wound infection with abscess formation. While cultures of episiotomy wounds are positive in 76% of cases, reflecting the proximity of the vagina and rectum, few clinical infections result. Clinical infections occur in 0.5–3.0% of cases.[63] When infection results, the wound must be opened and left packed open to heal by secondary intention. Antibiotics are indicated for any sign of cellulitis or vulvar edema. Degree of laceration makes no difference in rate of infection.

Rectovaginal fistula is a defined complication of episiotomy occurring in two of 9757 vaginal deliveries[64], while

Fleming reports one rectovaginal fistula requiring repair in every 3,055 episiotomies.[65] Episioproctotomy has a higher incidence of fistula (four in 225 cases).[66] Patients with inflammatory bowel disease may have an increased incidence and along with those patients using steroids have a prolonged course of healing.

Devastating complications of episiotomy are necrotizing fasciitis and clostridial myonecrosis. Clostridial myonecrosis occurs less frequently and is most commonly due to *Clostridium sordellii*.[67] As in necrotizing fasciitis, aggressive, timely surgery is the cornerstone of treatment. Necrotizing fasciitis originating in an episiotomy will behave similarly to necrotizing fasciitis arising from a Bartholin's abscess, with spread over the pubis into the groin, then superiorly along the abdominal wall and inferiorly along the fascia lata.

WOUND INFECTIONS AFTER CESAREAN SECTION

The incidence of febrile morbidity after cesarean section ranges from 53% with no prophylactic antibiotics[68], to 29.2% after primary cesarean section, and 13.7% after repeat cesarean section.[69] Wound infection rates for cesarean delivery are variable also, ranging from 4.7%[70] to 6.9%.[12] Farrell in 1980 surveyed several studies that had a range of 1.3% to 16.0% and reported an incidence of 4.1%.[71] In a retrospective matched case control review of 93 patients with no prophylactic antibiotics, 6% had wound infections.[68]

Cesarean delivery exposes the vaginal and uterine contents as microbial sources, transmitting their contaminants to the wound. A wound is universally considered to be infected when purulent material is discharged from it. Wounds that are inflamed but do not yet meet this description of drainage form a continuum from mild redness to cellulitis in the wound edges, are increasingly likely to be infected, and may be so considered if the skin edges are separated and a culture-positive exudate is present. These wounds must be opened and inspected for abscess, dehiscence, or necrotizing fasciitis. The flora isolated in the postcesarean delivery wound infection parallel amniotic flora and are similar to those in postpartum endometritis, with a mixed anaerobic and aerobic character. Gilstrap and Cunningham assessed amniotic contamination with transabdominal aspiration in patients with rupture of membranes greater than six hours.[72] They demonstrated bacterial growth in all specimens. A mixed polymicrobial spectrum was present in 63%, while 30% had anaerobes only. *Streptococcus* represented 72% of all isolates, while *Bacteroides* and *E coli* represented 23% and 21%, respectively. Some bacteria were normal vaginal flora; however, 61% were pathogenic species. *S aureus, E coli, P mirabilis, Bacteroides* species, β-hemolytic *Streptococcus,* and *Pseudomonas* are most common. Clostridial species are more rarely found.[73] This mixed infection creates a synergistic system between the aerobes and anaerobes that may follow a particularly fulminant course.

In examining risk factors for wound infection, Gibbs et al found that the use of internal fetal monitoring was relatively unimportant in relation to the duration of labor, presence of ruptured membranes, and vaginal examinations.[74] No studies have determined the independence of rupture of membranes, duration of labor, or number of vaginal exams, as these are probably interrelated in their contribution to alterations in the amniotic flora.

Abscesses in the pelvis or peritoneal cavity must be considered when patients are febrile for a prolonged period after cesarean section and when no wound, urinary, or pulmonary infection is present. Additional signs of abscess may be abdominal or pelvic tenderness. Pelvis exam may demonstrate a mass, fluctuance, or tenderness. A wound infection is also present in 40–50% of these patients.[75] Initial antibiotics may not provide an appropriate spectrum in 20% of these patients.[75] Ultrasound identifies the presence of masses or fluid collections in the pelvis but is nonspecific. Computed tomographic scanning has the advantages of distinguishing fluid collections from old blood (being particularly helpful in the large or obese patient who will not have an adequate ultrasound examination) and guiding aspiration of any fluid collections that are identified. Acholonu reported success with percutaneous catheter drainage in seven patients with bladder flap fluid collections.[76]

NECROTIZING FASCIITIS

Frank Meleney first described the infectious process now known as necrotizing fasciitis.[77] He noted it as a manifestation of streptococcal disease and so named it hemolytic streptococcal gangrene. He described 20 cases, primarily involving the extremities, each arising from a skin lesion. The extremity would develop swelling, redness, heat, and tenderness, with proximal and distal spread from the central lesion. Fevers and chills were followed by prostration. Beginning centrally, the skin was first red, then darker and necrotic, developing blisters and bullae. The surrounding skin became numb and then anesthetic. These cutaneous manifestations underestimated the true spread of the infection at the fascial and subcutaneous levels. This is classically described as undermining and represents metastasizing abscess of the subcutaneous space. No lymphagitis or adenopathy were present. Laboratory tests were significant for a striking leukocytosis, proteinuria, anemia, and bacteremia. He treated his cases with excision of demarcated dead skin and incisions extending to the boundaries of fascial necrosis. Amputation was performed only in cases where the osteomyelitis was present—always due to the inciting injury. Meleney clearly described the pathophysiology of the infection. The subcutaneous tissue would become gangrenous, interrupting and thrombosing the perforating vessels to the skin. First the veins are affected, leading to ecchymosis.[78] As the arteries are thrombosed, the nerves die, resulting in anesthesia.

Prior to Wilson's series, this infectious process was known by many other names, often incorrectly applied.[77,78] Necrotizing fasciitis has an indistinct cutaneous margin, undermining far in advance of skin changes, abscess of muscle or lymphatic involvement, and is rapidly progressive with systemic toxicity. Cellulitis affects the soft tissues only and has no undermining; the borders are sharp, lymphangitis is present, and antibiotics alone produce rapid relief. *Synergistic necrotizing cellulitis* is a slowly progressive mixed infection with anaerobes and gram-negative aerobes synergistically inducing necrosis of muscle and fascia. *Aerobic streptococcal myositis* is a muscle infection with gangrene.[79]

Necrotizing fasciitis occurs most frequently postoperatively or arising from an abscess. Less commonly, it may begin with a seemingly trivial wound, such as an insect bite or minor laceration. The majority of Meleney's cases involved the extremities. This process also occurs in the perineum and on the abdominal wall following vaginal delivery or cesarean section. Although most cases arise in older patients, necrotizing fasciitis following cesarean section, episiotomy, Bartholin's gland abscess, or pudendal anesthesia, is well documented in the younger and particularly in the diabetic population.[67,80-88] Golde and Ledger report an incidence of four cases in 109,531 deliveries.[83] Shy and Eschenbach report a rate of 0.5 maternal deaths per 100,000 live births from episiotomy related infections[85], while Ewing et al report three of four maternal deaths in 49,007 births secondary to postpartum vulvar edema.[82]

While Meleney described primarily streptococcal cultures in his patients, Wilson noted 80% of his gram-positive cocci to be *Staphylococcus*.[77,78] Giuliano et al investigated the bacteriology of necrotizing fasciitis in 16 patients.[89] This group included nine of 16 patients with extremity infections. These patients separated into two distinct groups of infecting organisms indistinguishable clinically or pathologically. The first group had synergistic infections of anaerobes in combination with facultative anaerobes such as Enterobacteriaceae or nongroup A *Streptococcus*. Giuliano emphasizes the important role of the facultative anaerobic component. Such synergism is understood to be based on the facultative organisms' capability to provide a more optimal environment for the anaerobes through oxygen usage to reduce the redox potential and catalase production.[89] The second group of patients had group A *Streptococcus* and *Staphylococcus* only. Other than microbiologic findings, there were no differences in the pathologic findings, signs, or symptoms that could differentiate these two groups.[81,89] Other studies report similar bacteriologic patterns in postpartum patients.[82-87] After *Streptococcus, Vibrio vulnificus* is the only other organism described to cause necrotizing fasciitis. *Vibrio* enters through lacerations from infected sea water, producing a particularly fulminant infection course that may result in death in only hours.[81]

Symptoms of infection in deep soft tissue, such as the perineum, are much more difficult to diagnose, are diagnosed late, and consequently have greater morbidity and mortality. In necrotizing fasciitis occurring from Bartholin's abscess, perirectal abscess, or episiotomy, the first symptoms are fever, malaise, and perineal pain and swelling. After episiotomy, these symptoms may involve one or both labia or the mons, and may extend to the thighs, abdomen, or buttocks. Occasionally, gait disturbance is present. This pain progresses as the infection spreads and signs of systemic toxicity appear.[90]

On physical examination, the involved areas are initially reddened with swelling that progresses to brawny edema radiating from the site of incision, laceration, or abscess. The site becomes progressively tense and turns dusky, then blue-black. These are late changes. Induration extends much further than the other skin changes. Addison et al also note crepitance on exam.[80] Fisher et al suggest roentgenographic evaluation of soft tissue gas in these patients to permit earlier diagnosis.[91]

Once this infection is suspected, operative treatment is mandatory. The incision is opened or the area of infection is incised. The necrotic, stringy fascia leaks serosanguinous dishwater-gray fluid. The subcutaneous tissue is necrotic centrally but may be viable centrifugally. The pathognomic sign of necrotizing fasciitis is ease of dissection of subcutaneous tissues off of the underlying muscle in the fascial plane. The infection extends to the limit of this blunt dissection.

The differential diagnosis is based on erythema, induration, characteristics of the margin of erythema, bullae, vesicles, ecchymosis, subcutaneous undermining, skin anesthesia, and systemic toxicity (Table 59–3).

Surgical intervention and adequate debridement are crucial to successful treatment of necrotizing fasciitis. Intervention must also be timely. Any postpartum vulvar edema or erythematous wound must be explored immediately. If the subcutaneous tissue does not separate from the underlying fascia easily, necrotizing fasciitis is probably not present but will be avoided by laying open the infected wound. If dissection in the fascial plane is without resistance, then dissection and excision must be carried to the full extent of fascial involvement. The wound is packed open and subjected to q 4–6 hour dressing changes. Antibiotics to cover anaerobes, gram-positive cocci, and Enterobacteriaceae should be administered intravenously. Empiric therapy should be started immediately and adjusted on the basis of intraoperative cultures. Hyperbaric oxygen therapy may be a useful, although not proven, adjunct but must *not* delay surgery.[92,93] These patients will require intensive care stays for wound care, invasive monitoring, nutrition, and treatment of third space losses, sepsis, and shock. They are at high risk for multiple organ system failure.

It may not be possible to complete excision of all infected tissue on the initial operation. Patients will benefit by daily return to the operating room for continued debridement until stable, healthy fascia is exposed on all wound margins.[94] After the infection is eradicated, dressing changes continue until granulation tissue adequate for split thickness skin grafting is present.

A combined mortality for multiple studies is 66 of 200 (33%) patients with necrotizing fasciitis of all sites. Patients with necrotizing fasciitis but following episiotomy or postpartum vulvar edema have a slightly higher mortality of 18 of 46 patients (39%). Achieving an adequate operation in a timely fashion to interrupt the infection is the single most important factor in improving mortality.[81,95]

TABLE 59–3. DIFFERENTIAL DIAGNOSIS OF SOFT TISSUE INFECTIONS

Infection	Systemic Toxicity	Erythema	Purulent Collection	Induration	Lymphatic Involvement	Borders	Muscle Involvement	Ecchymosis, Vesicles, Bullae	Emphysema	Undermining	Pace
Erysipelas	–	+	–	–	+	sharp	–	–	–	–	moderate
Necrotizing fasciitis	+	+	microabscesses	+	–	diffuse	–	late	±	+++	rapid
Cellulitis	–	+	–	+	+	sharp	–	–	–	–	slow
Myonecrosis	+	mild	+	+	+	sharp	+++	–	±	–	rapid
Synergistic necrotizing cellulitis	+	+	–	+	+	sharp	+	Eschar	–	–	slow

CONCLUSIONS

Abscesses and local infections result when local conditions combine with a bacterial inoculum to overcome the host's defenses. These most frequently occur in ducts and glands where flow is obstructed or in tissue that has been devitalized by either trauma or imprecise surgical technique. Static fluid collections are similar to devitalized tissue in that perfusion is absent and delivery and function of immune elements are compromised. The host inflammatory response may actually further impede normal ductal or glandular flow as the developing infection is cordoned off. Thus, the overriding principle of treatment is reestablishing normal flow or providing drainage. Most processes will require surgical therapy.

The infecting organisms are the endogenous flora of the region at the time of infection, but these may not be the normal flora. Systemic host diseases such as diabetes mellitus, immunocompromise, or exposure to broad-spectrum antibiotics substitute the normal flora with pathogenic species and at generally higher concentrations. Treatment of underlying medical conditions enhances the host's immune capability. Antibiotics are indicated for any process that shows signs of spread locally or systematically as evidenced by cellulitis, lymphangitis, or systemic toxicity. Antibiotic choice is important and is generally guided by culture and sensitivity testing.

The pregnant or lactating female is predisposed to a greater variety of infections exclusive of the febrile morbidity associated with delivery. These patients have an altered immune status and a concomitantly greater frequency of bacterial colonization. Most of these conditions are treated identically in the pregnant or lactating state, with major limitations attributable to the constraints of potential fetal or infant toxicities of antibiotic therapy and deferment of certain definitive procedures until the postpartum period.

REFERENCES

1. Gall SA. Infections in the female genital tract. *Comprehensive Therapy.* 1983;9:34.
2. Pritchard JA, MacDonald PC, Gant NF. *Williams Obstetrics.* Norwalk, CT: Appleton-Century-Crofts; 1985:581.
3. Amankwah KS, Prentice RL, Fleury FJ. The incidence of gestational diabetes. *Obstet Gynecol.* 1977;49:497.
4. Lavin JP, Barden TP, Miodovnik M. Clinical experience with a screening program for gestational diabetes. *Am J Obstet Gynecol.* 1981;141:491.
5. McMurry JF. Wound healing with diabetes mellitus. *Surg Clin N Am.* 1984;64:769.
6. National Academy of Sciences—National Research Council, Division of Medical Sciences, Ad Hoc Committee of the Committee on Trauma. Postoperative wound infections: the influence of ultraviolet irradiation of the operating room and of various other factors. *Ann Surg.* 1964;160:1.
7. Hjortrup A, Sorensen C, Dyremose E, et al. Influence of diabetes mellitus on operative risk. *Brit J Surg.* 1985;72:783.
8. Cruse P. Infection surveillance: identifying the problems and the high-risk patient. *Southern Med J.* 1977;70:4.
9. Goodson WH, Hunt TK. Wound healing and the diabetic patient. *Surg Gynecol & Obstet.* 1979;149:600.
10. Kuhn HH, Ullman U, Kuhn FW. New aspects on the pathophysiology of wound infection and wound healing—the problem of lowered oxygen pressure in the tissue. *Infection.* 1985;13:52.
11. Green SL, Sarubbi FA. Risk factors associated with post cesarean section febrile morbidity. *Obstet Gynecol.* 1977;49:686.
12. Nielsen TF, Hokegard KH. Postoperative cesarean section morbidity: a prospective study. *Am J Obstet Gynecol.* 1983;146:911.
13. Gall SA. Maternal adjustments in the immune system in normal pregnancy. *Clin Obstet Gynecol.* 1983;26:521.
14. Gall SA. Maternal immune system during human gestation. *Sem Perinat.* 1977;1:119.
15. Ho JL, Barza M. An approach to infectious disease. In: Gleicher N, ed. *Principles of Medical Therapy in Pregnancy.* New York, NY: Plenum Press, 1985:381.
16. Slavin RG. Sinusitis in adults. *J Allerg Clin Immunol.* 1988;81:1028.
17. Hill JH, Applebaum EL. Otolaryngology: head and neck problems in pregnancy. In: Gleicher N, ed. *Principles of Medical Therapy in Pregnancy.* New York, NY: Plenum Press; 1985:875.
18. Deweese DD, Saunders WH, Schuller DE, Schleuning AJ. *Otolaryngology—Head and Neck Surgery.* 7th ed. St. Louis, MO: CV Mosby; 1988.
19. Geelhoed GW, Joseph WL. Surgical sequelae of drug abuse. *Surg Gynecol & Obstet.* 1974;139:749.
20. Orangio GR, Pitlick SD, Latta PD, et al. Soft tissue infections in parenteral drug abusers. *Ann Surg.* 1984;199:97.
21. Clark DD. Surgical management of infections and other complications resulting from drug abuse. *Arch Surg.* 1970;101:619.
22. Ritland D, Butterfield W. Extremity complications of drug abuse. *Am J Surg.* 1973;126:639.
23. Schwartz GF. Benign neoplasms and "inflammations" of the breast. *Clin Obstet Gynecol.* 1982;25:373.
24. Wong MK, Smith CV, Phelan JP. Antepartum mastitis, a report of two cases. *J Reprod Med.* 1986;31:511.
25. Ekland DA, Zeigler MG. Abscess in the nonlactating breast. *Arch Surg.* 1973;107:398.
26. Walker AP, Edmiston CE, Krepel CJ, Condon RE. A prospective study of the microflora of nonpuerperal breast abscess. *Arch Surg.* 1988;123:908.
27. Scholefield JH, Duncan JL, Rogers K. Review of a hospital experience of breast abscesses. *Brit J Surg.* 1987;74:469.
28. Brook I. Microbiology of non-puerperal breast abscesses. *J Infect Dis.* 1988;157:377.
29. Thomsen AC, Esperson T, Maigaard S. Course and treatment of milk stasis, noninfectious inflammation of the breast, and infectious mastitis in nursing women. *Am J Obstet Gynecol.* 1984;149:492.
30. Niebyl JR, Spence MR, Parmley TH. Sporadic (nonepidemic) puerperal mastitis. *J Reprod Med.* 1978;20:97.
31. Marshall BR, Hepper JK, Zirbel CC. Sporadic puerperal mastitis. *JAMA.* 1975;233:1377.
32. Dixon JM. Repeated aspiration of breast abscesses in lactating women. *Brit Med J.* 1988;297:1517.
33. Benson EA, Goodman MA. Incision with primary suture in the treatment of acute puerperal breast abscess. *Brit J Surg.* 1970;57:55.
34. Kovalcik PJ, Peniston RL, Cross GH. Anorectal abscess. *Surg Gynecol & Obstet.* 1979;149:884.
35. Eisenhammer S. Emergency fistulectomy of the acute primary anorectal cryptoglandular intermuscular abscess-fistula *in ano. South Afr J Surg.* 1985;23:1.
36. Eisenhammer S. The final evaluation and classification of the surgical treatment of the primary anorectal cryptoglandular intermuscular (intersphincteric) fistulous abscess and fistula. *Dis Colon Rectum.* 1978;21:237.
37. McElwain JW, MacLean MD, Alexander RM, et al. Anorectal problems. *Dis Colon Rectum.* 1975;18:646.
38. Hanley PH. Anorectal problems. *Dis Colon Rectum.* 1975;18:657.
39. Azzan BB. Bartholin's cyst and abscess: a review of treatment of 53 cases. *Brit J Clin Prac.* 1978;32:101.
40. Lee YH, Rankin JS, Alpert S, et al. Microbiological investigation of Bartholin's gland abscesses and cysts. *Am J Obstet Gynecol.* 1977;129:150.
41. Cheetham DR. Bartholin's cyst: marsupialization or aspiration? *Am J Obstet Gynecol.* 1985;152:569.
42. Saul HM, Grossman MB. The role of *Chlamydia trachomatis* in Bartholin's gland abscess. *Am J Obstet Gynecol.* 1988;158:576.
43. Heah J. Methods of treatment for cysts and abscesses of Bartholin's gland. *Brit J Gynaecol Obstetric.* 1988;95:321.
44. Roberts DB, Hester LL. Progressive synergistic bacterial gangrene arising from abscess of the vulva and Bartholin's gland duct. *Am J Obstet Gynecol.* 1972;114:285.
45. Hurley HJD. Diseases of the apocrine and eccrine sweat glands. In Moschella SL, Hurley HJ, eds. *Dermatology.* 2nd ed. Philadelphia, PA: WB Saunders; 1985.
46. Thomas R, Barnhill D, Bibro M, Hoskins W. Hidradenitis suppurativa: a case presentation and review of the literature. *Obstet Gynecol.* 1985;66:592.
47. Fitzsimmons JS, Fitzsimmons EM, Gilbert G. Familial hidradenitis suppurativa: evidence in favour of single gene transmission. *J Med Genet.* 1984;21:281.
48. Jemec GBE. The symptomatology of hidradenitis suppurativa in women. *Brit J Dermatol.* 1988;119:345.
49. Broadwater JR, Bryant RL, Petrina RA, et al. Advanced hidradenitis suppurativa. *Am J Surgery.* 1982;144:668.
50. Cornbleet T. Pregnancy and apocrine gland diseases: hidradenitis, Fox–Fordyce disease. *Arch Dermatol Syphilology.* 1952;65:12.
51. Brown CF, Gallup DG, Brown VM. Hidradenitis suppurativa of the anogenital region: response to isotretinoin. *Am J Obstet Gynecol.* 1988;158:12.
52. Watson JD. Hidradenitis suppurativa—a clinical review. *Brit J Plast Surgery.* 1985;38:567.

53. Billet A, Stueber K, Vaughan L. Hidradenitis suppurativa of unusual severity. *Ann Plast Surg*. 1983;10:231.
54. Silverberg B, Smoot CE, Landa SJF, Parsons RW. Hidradenitis suppurativa: patient satisfaction with wound healing by secondary intention. *Plast Reconstr Surg*. 1987;79:555.
55. McDonough AJ, Cranney BS. Delayed presentation of an epidural abscess. *Anaesth Intens Care*. 1984;12:364.
56. Male CG, Martin R. Puerperal spinal epidural abscess. *Lancet*. 1973;1:608.
57. Baker AS, Ojemann RG, Swartz MN, Richardson EP. Spinal epidural abscess. *N Engl J Med*. 1975;293:463.
58. North JB, Brophy BP. Epidural abscess: a hazard of spinal epidural anaesthesia. Aust NZ J Surg. 1979;49:484.
59. Loarie DJ, Fairley HB. Epidural abscess following spinal anesthesia. *Anes Analg*. 1978;57:351.
60. Hibbard LT, Snyder EN, McVann RM. Subgluteal and retropsoal infection in obstetric practice. *Obstet Gynecol*. 1972;39:137.
61. Svancarek W, Chirino O, Schaefer G, Blythe JG. Retropsoas and subgluteal abscesses following paracervical and pudendal anesthesia. *JAMA*. 1977;237:892.
62. Wenger DR, Gitchell RH. Severe infections following pudendal block anesthesia: need for orthopaedic awareness. *J Bone Joint Surg*. 1973;55-A;202.
63. Thacker SB, Banta HD. Benefits and risks of episiotomy: an interpretative review of the English language literature, 1860–1980. *Obstet Gynecol Surv*. 1983;38:322.
64. Brantley JT, Burwell JC. A study of fourth degree perineal lacerations and their sequelae. *Am J Obstet Gynecol*. 1960;80:711.
65. Fleming AR. Complete perineotomy. *Obstet Gynecol*. 1960;16:172.
66. Norris F. Episioproctotomy. *Surg Clin N Am*. 1962;42:947.
67. Soper DE. Clostridial myonecrosis arising from an episiotomy. *Obstet Gynecol*. 1986;68:26S.
68. Blanco JD, Gibbs RS. Infections following classical cesarean section. *Obstet Gynecol*. 1980;55:167.
69. Hurry DJ, Larsen B, Charles D. Effects of postcesarean section febrile morbidity on subsequent fertility. *Obstet Gynecol*. 1984;64:256.
70. Hawrylyshyn PA, Bernstein P, Papsin FR. Risk factors associated with infection following cesarean section. *Am J Obstet Gynecol*. 1981;139:294.
71. Farrell SJ, Anderson HF, Work BA. Cesarean section: indications and postoperative morbidity. *Obstet Gynecol*. 1980;56:696.
72. Gilstrap LC, Cunningham FG. The bacterial pathogenesis of infection following cesarean section. *Obstet Gynecol*. 1979;53:545.
73. Sweet RL, Yonekura ML, Hill GB, et al. Appropriate use of antibiotics in serious obstetric and gynecologic infections. *Am J Obstet Gynecol*. 1983;146:719.
74. Gibbs RS, Jones PM, Wilder CJY. Internal fetal monitoring and maternal infection following cesarean section. *Obstet Gynecol*. 1978;52:193.
75. Gibbs RS. Severe infections in pregnancy. *Med Clin N Am*. 1989;73:713.
76. Acholonu F, Minkoff H, Delke I. Percutaneous drainage of fluid collections in the bladder flap of febrile post-cesarean-section patients. *J Reprod Med*. 1987;32:140.
77. Meleney FL. Hemolytic *Streptococcus* gangrene. *Arch Surg*. 1924.9:317.
78. Wilson B. Necrotizing fasciitis. *Am Surgeon*. 1982;18:416.
79. Janevicius RV, Hann SE, Batt MD. Necrotizing fasciitis. *Surg Gynecol Obstet*. 1982;154:97.
80. Addison WA, Livengood CH, Hill GB, et al. Necrotizing fasciitis of vulvar origin in diabetic patients. *Obstet Gynecol*. 1984;63:473.
81. Arenholz DH. Necrotizing soft-tissue infections. *Surg Clin N Am*. 1988;68:199.
82. Ewing TL, Smale LE, Elliott FA. Maternal deaths associated with postpartum vulvar edema. *Am J Obstet Gynecol*. 1979;134:173.
83. Golde S, Ledger WJ. Necrotizing fasciitis in postpartum patients. *Obstet Gynecol*. 1977;50:670.
84. Lowthian JT, Gillard LJ. Postpartum necrotizing fasciitis. *Obstet Gynecol*. 1980;56:661.
85. Shy KK, Eschenbach DA. Fatal perineal cellulitis from an episiotomy site. *Obstet Gynecol*. 1979;54:292.
86. Sutton GP, Smirz LR, Clark DH, Bennett JE. Group B streptococcal necrotizing fasciitis arising from an episiotomy. *Obstet Gynecol*. 1985;66:733.
87. Finkler NJ, Safon LE, Ryan KJ. Bilateral postpartun vulvar edema associated with maternal death. *Obstet Gynecol*. 1987;156:1188.
88. Cruikshank SH, McLauchlan L. A *de novo* case of vulvar synergistic necrotizing fasciitis. *Obstet Gynecol*. 1987;69:516.
89. Giuliano A, Lewis F, Hadley K, Blaisdell FW. Bacteriology of necrotizing fasciitis. *Am J Surg*. 1977;134:52.
90. Hammar H, Wanger L. Erysipelas and necrotizing fasciitis. *Brit J Dermatol*. 1977;96:409.
91. Fisher JR, Conway MJ, Takeshita RT, Sandoval MR. Necrotizing fasciitis: importance of roentgographic studies for soft-tissue gas. *JAMA*. 241:803.
92. Ledingham IM, Tehrani MA. Diagnosis, clinical course and treatment of acute dermal gangrene. *Brit J Surg*. 1975;62:364.
93. Gozal D, Ziser A, Shupak A, et al. Necrotizing fasciitis. *Arch Surg*. 1986;121:233.
94. Roberts DB. Necrotizing fasciitis of the vulva. *Am J Obstet Gynecol*. 1987;157:568.
95. Freischlag JA, Ajalat G, Busuttil RW. Treatment of necrotizing soft tissue infections. *Am J Surg*. 1985;149:751.

Chapter Sixty

Acute Bacterial Diarrhea and Bacterial Food Poisoning

Joseph G. Pastorek II and Joseph M. Miller, Jr.

60

Acute diarrheal disease caused by bacteria, along with food poisoning of bacterial etiology, is a major cause of morbidity throughout the world. Of particular interest in developing countries is the infant and child mortality associated with these gastrointestinal syndromes. However, even in the United States, acute diarrheal disease ranks second only to the common cold as a cause of absence from work. Roughly one third of all diarrheal diseases in this country appear to be food-related.[1] Therefore, the obstetrician should be familiar with some of the more common and more serious of these syndromes, because the pregnant patient will often present with such a malady.

Bacterial diarrhea and food poisoning are syndromes resulting from pathogenic bacteria or their products acting upon or through the gastrointestinal tract. Food poisoning may be defined as an acute illness involving the gastrointestinal tract or nervous system that affects two or more persons who have shared a meal within the past 72 hours. Diarrhea is present when there is an abnormally large amount of fluid present in the terminal stool, particularly when the content of the stool is abnormal (ie, the stool contains mucus or blood).

In spite of advances in medical microbiologic technology over the past few decades, the etiologic agents of perhaps half of the cases of diarrhea in this country remain obscure. This is due in part to improper handling of specimens, underequipped laboratories, and as yet unrecognized pathogens. In many cases of bacterial diarrhea and food poisoning, however, causative microorganisms may be found.

Organisms such as *Staphylococcus aureus, Bacillus cereus, Clostridium botulinum, Clostridium perfringens,* and enterotoxigenic *Escherichia coli* are known to produce various syndromes of food poisoning. Acute diarrheal syndromes may be produced by infection with *Vibrio cholerae, Salmonella* species, *Shigella* species, invasive *E coli, Vibrio parahaemolyticus, Yersinia enterocolitica,* and *Campylobacter jejuni* (previously considered a species of *Vibrio*).

PATHOPHYSIOLOGY

Diarrhea can occur from any one of, or a combination of several of, the following mechanisms: decreased fluid and electrolyte absorption; increased fluid and electrolyte secretion; abnormal permeability of the intestinal wall; osmotic effects of a large amount of nonabsorbable, osmotically active material within the intestinal lumen; and abnormally increased intestinal motility. In addition, extraintestinal effects of food poisoning and systemic effects of intestinal infection may be caused by absorption of bacterial toxin across the intestinal wall or by actual invasion by the responsible microorganisms. It is common to separate these acute intestinal disorders into two categories, toxigenic and invasive, based upon the mechanism by which the illness is caused (Table 60–1).

Toxigenic diarrheas, the category to which most food poisonings belong, result from the action of bacterial toxins, including cytotoxins and enterotoxins, which cause disorders in fluid and electrolyte metabolism in the intestinal wall. Cholera, due to *V cholerae,* is the prototypic toxigenic diarrhea. Strains of *E coli, S aureus, B cereus, C perfringens, C botulinum,* and *Campylobacter* also produce toxins. These may be preformed in food, leading to food poisoning, or may be produced directly within the bowel lumen. The toxins are thought to act by stimulation of mucosal adenyl cyclase, leading to the accumulation of intracellular cyclic AMP, which results in disorders in absorption and secretion of fluid and electrolytes across the bowel mucosa.

Cytotoxins cause their effects by directly killing the intestinal cells. Cell death causes abnormal absorption rather than disorders in secretion, of luminal fluid. The Shiga toxin, produced by *Shigella dysenteriae,* is the prototype of this class of substances. Shigalike toxins are also produced by some strains of *E coli* and *Clostridium difficile.*

Invasive diarrheas, typified by salmonellosis, are characterized by bacterial invasion of the intestinal mucosa leading to an acute inflammatory reaction, which disrupts bowel function, possibly through the same adenyl cyclase-cyclic AMP pathway, causing an increase in motility and fluid loss into the bowel lumen. Interestingly, invasive disease generally involves the colon, while toxigenic disease is usually of small bowel origin, sparing the large bowel. Bacteria causing invasive diarrheal syndromes are *Salmonella* species, *Shigella* species, and invasive strains of *E coli.* Some organisms, notably *V parahaemolyticus* and *Y enterocolitica,* may produce both toxic and invasive disease.[2]

TABLE 60–1. MECHANISMS OF BACTERIAL DISEASE

Mechanism	Pathogen
Enterotoxin production	*Vibrio cholera, Escherichia coli, Salmonella* species, *Campylobacter* species, *Bacillus cereus, Staphylococcus aureus, Yersinia enterocolitica*
Cytotoxin production	*Shigella* species, *Escherichia coli, Clostridium difficile, Salmonella* species, *Campylobacter jejuni*
Tissue invasion	*Shigella* species, *Salmonella* species, *Campylobacter* species, *Yersinia* species, *Escherichia coli*

The source of the organism causing a particular case of diarrhea or food poisoning often varies with the species of organism. Fecal-oral transmission of infection is common, particularly in underdeveloped or inner-city areas, and especially among the young. Bacteria commonly spread from person to person in this manner are *Shigella, Y enterocolitica* (occasionally), and perhaps the enteropathogenic types of *E coli,* which cause outbreaks of disease within the newborn nursery. Disease contracted from household pets such as puppies, kittens, and hamsters may be caused by *Campylobacter* and possibly *Yersinia.*

Waterborne diarrheal illness is characteristic of the *vibrios,* and to some extent, *C jejuni.* Salmonellosis is usually a disease derived from contaminated animal products, that is, meat, poultry, or milk, because the organism is essentially endemic in many populations of food animals.

Staphylococcal food poisoning is generally produced by the inoculation of prepared food by a food handler with an insignificantly-infected wound or with asymptomatic nasal carriage. The clostridial organisms are ever-present in soil and dust, and spores that settle on food products may germinate if given the proper conditions. *B cereus* is another ubiquitous bacterium disseminated in a manner similar to the clostridia.

When *S aureus* enterotoxin is ingested, the patient will experience increased sialorrhea, nausea, vomiting, some cramping, and watery diarrhea that may last for up to eight hours. Recovery in a day or two is expected. *C perfringens* produces a similar syndrome, though it is not so pronounced. The gastrointestinal disease caused by *C botulinum* toxin is even less severe, and it is usually overshadowed by the paralysis caused by the toxin's inhibition of acetylcholine release from nerve endings. *B cereus* can produce two types of gastrointestinal illness: a syndrome similar to staphylococcal poisoning with the same short (1 to 6 hours) incubation period is termed the *emetic form,* while a longer-incubating form, the *diarrheal form,* is similar to disease produced by *C perfringens* (incubation period of 8 to 16 hours).

Classic cholera, due to *V cholerae,* is a characteristically explosive small bowel disease with a one-to-three-day incubation period, resulting in abdominal cramping and profuse watery diarrhea. The stools may have some streaks of mucus in them, sometimes called "rice water" stools. There is rarely fever or vomiting with this disease. This same clinical syndrome may be produced by enterotoxigenic strains of *E coli, V parahaemolyticus,* and, occasionally, *Salmonella* and *Shigella.*

Shigellosis, caused by the four major types of *Shigella, S dysenteriae, Shigella flexneri, Shigella boydii,* and *Shigella sonnei,* is an illness that arises abruptly after a one- to two-day incubation period. Approximately one fourth of patients will exhibit high fever with little gastrointestinal symptomatology, whereas one fourth will have an illness characterized by abdominal cramping and watery diarrhea without fever. One half of infected individuals will present with a history of a short bout of fever followed by cramps and diarrhea for two to three days. This diarrhea may progress to dysentery, consisting of fever, abdominal cramping, bloody diarrhea, and tenesmus. In an otherwise healthy individual, the disease usually resolves within a week with only supportive treatment, though dehydration and resultant prostration may occur. There is rarely bacteremia, because the organism is generally localized to the superficial bowel mucosa. If untreated, an infected individual usually clears the stool of organisms spontaneously within four to six weeks.

Salmonellosis in the United States is usually caused by the organism *Salmonella enteritidis*, serotype *typhimurium*. An incubation period of up to two days is followed in two thirds of patients by a syndrome consisting of fever, chills, nausea, vomiting, and profuse, watery diarrhea. There may be a dysenterylike illness in the latter stages of the disease. A small percentage of patients, perhaps 3%, may develop bacteremia. This is especially true of neonates, the elderly, and persons with compromised immunity, including individuals with sickle cell disease. The higher incidence of bacteremia in salmonellosis compared to shigellosis may be due to the slightly more invasive nature of *Salmonella* species, as they tend to involve the lamina propria of the bowel wall and occasionally cause erosions and crypt abscesses of the large bowel. In the healthy patient, the illness usually spontaneously resolves in a week, with the bacterial shedding ending by two weeks, occasionally ending after a month or more. In less than 1% of persons, bacterial carriage will continue, asymptomatically, for more than a year. This carrier state is more common in elderly women, people with gallstones or other biliary tract disease, or patients with obstructive uropathy.

Toxigenic strains of *E coli* are thought to play a major role in the etiology of so-called traveler's diarrhea. These organisms are not thought to be a major cause of acute diarrhea in the United States, although a choleralike syndrome has been associated with them. A dysentery syndrome almost indistinguishable from shigella-induced dysentery has been ascribed to certain invasive strains of *E coli*, one outbreak in the early 1970s being blamed on imported French cheese. This particular illness is not common in the United States.

In the Scandinavian countries and on the European continent, *Y enterocolitica* has been shown to be the agent of food-borne and animal-carried outbreaks of an illness that may variously resemble salmonellosis, produce mesenteric adenitis, cause a necrotizing enteritis of the ileum and colon, and produce or mimic acute appendicitis. Septicemia and metastatic liver or splenic abscesses are not uncommon. Migratory polyarthritis, erythema nodosum, and Reiter's syndrome have also been associated with this organism. During the acute illness, the diarrheal feces are often filled with neutrophils and mononuclear cells.[3]

Because of an increased awareness and improved isolation techniques, the species of *Campylobacter* are increasingly recognized as human pathogens.[4] *Campylobacter fetus* is known to cause systemic disease. Enteritis is usually associated with *C jejuni* and begins after an incubation period of two to 11 days with diarrhea, abdominal pain, fever (rarely), and vomiting in up to one third of patients. The diarrheal stools may become profuse, watery, purulent, and foul-smelling. Blood and mucus may appear in the diarrhea after several days. The disease lasts for about a week, but the abdominal pain may remain even after normal stools have returned. Relapses may occur for up to nine months in some persons. The abdominal pain is sometimes mistaken for appendicitis or bowel perforation, and the histologic picture of chronic *Campylobacter* infection may be mistaken for ulcerative colitis or Crohn's disease.

PREGNANCY AND DIARRHEAL DISEASES

Because most of the syndromes described above do not entail a significant risk of maternal bacteremia, fetal risk from direct bacterial infection is low to nonexistent. Major hazard to the pregnancy comes from maternal dehydration and hypovolemia, which tends to reduce uterine artery flow and, thus, placental perfusion. Vigorous supportive care for the mother is often all the fetus needs for continued health and survival.

Toxins absorbed by the mother may theoretically pose a threat to the fetus. Information is scarce; however, a rabbit model of botulism poisoning would suggest that the botulism toxin will not cross the placenta. In addition, there is an anecdotal report of acute botulism during pregnancy with no obvious direct fetal poisoning, although the infant suffered hypoxia and possibly intracranial hemorrhage from a precipitous premature delivery during the acute maternal illness.[5]

The primary threat to the infant comes postnatally, when there is a risk of contracting various of the enteritides from the mother directly during handling, breast-feeding, and so on. Mothers with such diseases should be instructed, therefore, in strict handwashing techniques and care with toilet practices if they are to contact the infant directly. Breast-feeding should be encouraged as a mode of transmission of immunoglobulins to the infant's gut, which may help thwart the development of any such infection.

Since *Campylobacter* has been specifically implicated in abortion and perinatal sepsis[6,7], it is probably wise to treat any pregnant woman who is found to harbor the organism. Gravidas presenting with diarrheal illnesses should perhaps be appropriately evaluated for *Campylobacter*, even if the maternal disease appears to be spontaneously resolving, because recognition and treatment may improve fetal and neonatal outcome.

Diagnosis

The suspicion of food poisoning or infectious diarrhea may often be made on clinical grounds, taking into account the patient's symptoms and history of food ingestion or travel. If the agents considered in the above discussion are kept in mind by the physician, food products and stool may be properly cultured to yield the offending organism. In cases suspected of being caused by some of the more fastidious organisms, such as *Campylobacter*, the physician should alert laboratory personnel of any such suspicions so that adequate care may be taken to recover the organism by appropriate methods.

Gram's-stained stool specimens may be examined for evidence of invasiveness, such as polymorphonuclear leukocytes or mononuclear cells, to give the examiner some hint as to the general class of enteric pathogen involved in the illness. This may also serve to rule out other types of gastrointestinal disease, such as those caused by protozoans or helminths.

Recent advances in laboratory technology have provided a number of methods of rapid diagnosis, so that the physician may have at least a partial identity of the organism within hours, rather than the days necessary for culture diagnosis (Table 60–2). Of course, culture identification and especially antibiotic sensitivity determination are

TABLE 60–2. DIAGNOSTIC METHODOLOGIES IN BACTERIAL DIARRHEAS

Method	Specifics
Culture isolation	Stool specimens, rectal swabs, selective media
Serologic detection of antigen	Agglutination reactions (various species)
Toxin detection	Biologic assay, DNA hybridization, immunologic testing, serologic testing
DNA hybridization	Organisms, toxins, invasive plasmids, enteroadherence factors

still mandatory, both for public health reasons and for patient care considerations.

The physical examination is still all-important, for many of these illnesses resemble surgically correctable maladies, such as appendicitis or intussusception. Any extraintestinal manifestations may make the diagnosis much clearer, for example, paralysis in botulism poisoning or migratory polyarthritis in *Yersinia* infection.

Treatment

The majority of these illnesses are self-limiting and need no treatment in the healthy individual except for supportive care and attention to fluid and electrolyte balance. By the time the definitive culture reports are received, the patient is often recovering. However, some of the pathogens that cause significant systemic illness may need specific therapy.

Poisoning with botulism toxin carries the risk of respiratory arrest and should be treated with antitoxin and close observation. Should respiratory support be necessary, adequate facilities and personnel should be available. The patient poisoned with staphylococcal, *B cereus*, or *C perfringens* toxin need only to be supported, and the source of the contaminated food discovered.

Salmonellosis uncomplicated by severe systemic disease should not be treated other than with supportive care. It has been shown that antibiotic therapy does not shorten the course of the enteritis, and the emergence of antibiotic resistance is of concern. Similarly, *E coli* enteritis is basically a self-limiting disease and needs no special therapy, though traveler's diarrhea is said to be prevented by prophylactic use of antibiotics, notably doxycycline and trimethoprim-sulfamethoxazole. Similarly, since uncomplicated shigellosis is a self-limiting disease, antibiotics are often not used, in an effort to prevent the development of antibiotic resistance. It has been shown, however, that antibiotic therapy may shorten the length of the diarrheal episode in shigellosis.

Y enterocolitica is susceptible to trimethoprim-sulfamethoxazole, the quinolones, tetracycline, the third-generation cephalosporins, and the aminoglycosides, not all of which are safe for use in the pregnant patient. It is recommended that persons with severe or systemic disease, as well as those who are immunocompromised, be treated. However, there is evidence that uncomplicated enteritis need not be treated for the same reasons stated for salmonellosis. *Campylobacter* infections, on the other hand, are said to respond rapidly to treatment with erythromycin. However, highly erythromycin-resistant strains have been reported, and the therapeutic rationale for these infections is not clear.

Of course, the hallmark of therapy for food poisoning and bacterial diarrheas is prevention. Careful handling and proper storage of foodstuffs is generally recommended. Care in the preparation of food and avoidance of, or thorough screening of, raw food will likewise decrease the incidence of these illnesses. In less developed countries or urban areas, proper hygiene, handwashing, and general cleanliness should be the aim of educators and health care professionals.

Vaccination against cholera is required for travel in many areas of the world. For the agents of the rest of these enteritides, however, there is no vaccine in widespread use. In fact, enteritis caused by some of these organisms, notably salmonellosis, is not appreciably altered by the level of circulating humoral antibody.[8]

REFERENCES

1. Archer DL, Kvenberg JE. Incidence and cost of food-borne diseases in the United States. *J Food Protect.* 1985;48:887.
2. Ashkenazi S, Pickering LK. Pathogenesis and diagnosis of bacterial diarrhea. *Eur J Clin Microbiol Infect Dis.* 1989;8:203.
3. Cover TL, Aber RC. *Yersinia enterocolitica. N Engl J Med.* 1989;321:16.
4. Riley LW, Finch MJ. Results of the first year of national surveillance of *Campylobacter* infections in the United States. *J Infect Dis.* 1985;151:956.
5. St Clair EH, Dikiberti JH, O'Brien ML. Observations of an infant born to a mother with botulism (letter). *J Pediat.* 1975;87:658.
6. Tobak MA, Hart MD, Osborn LM. *Campylobacter* enteritis: prenatal and perinatal implications. *Am J Obstet Gynecol.* 1983;147:845.
7. Simor AE, Karmali MA, Jadavji T, et al. Abortion and perinatal sepsis associated with *Campylobacter* infection. *Rev Infect Dis.* 1986;8:397.
8. Guerrant RL. Principles and syndromes of enteric infection. In: Mandell GL, Douglas RG, Bennett JE, eds. *Principles and Practice of Infectious Diseases.* 3rd ed. New York, NY: Churchill Livingstone; 1989:837.

B

INFECTIONS CAUSED BY GRAM-POSITIVE COCCI

Chapter Sixty-One

Pneumococcal Infections

Patrick Duff

61

Streptococcus pneumoniae is responsible for a variety of infections in adults, children, and infants. From the perspective of the obstetrician, the most important maternal illnesses caused by this organism are pneumonia, meningitis, endocarditis, and genital tract infection. *S pneumoniae* also may be responsible for serious neonatal infections, such as pneumonia, meningitis, and septicemia.[1]

PATHOGENESIS

The organism usually enters the host through the upper respiratory tract. As many as 20% of adults harbor the organism in the oropharynx. In females, the genital tract is a second portal of entry, although only a small number of women have pneumococci in the vaginal flora. In the immunocompetent patient, there are various defense mechanisms that protect against invasive pneumococcal infection. In the respiratory tract, such mechanisms include the expulsive cough reflex, mucociliary transport, and phagocytosis by neutrophils and macrophages. In the genital tract, the intact chorioamniotic membrane normally protects the mother and fetus from ascending pneumococcal infection.

Humoral immunity is also important in protecting the host against infection. Although the polysaccharide capsule of *S pneumoniae* is not itself a toxin, it does retard engulfment of bacteria by white blood cells. Antibodies opsonize pneumococci and enhance phagocytosis even in the presence of the capsule. In the preantibiotic era, specific antiserum was used to treat patients with pneumococcal infection.

Certain disorders may disrupt these defense mechanisms and, thus, predispose the patient to invasive pneumococcal infection. General anesthesia, alcohol intoxication, convulsions, and oversedation may depress the cough reflex and result in aspiration of contaminated upper airway secretions. Inhalant gases, antecedent viral infection, debilitating systemic diseases such as lymphoproliferative disorders and acquired immune deficiency syndrome (AIDS), and immunosuppressive drugs also disturb normal mucociliary transport and polymorphonuclear leukocyte function. Rupture of the chorioamniotic membrane may expose the endometrial cavity to ascent of pathogenic bacteria from the vagina.

Patients with deficient levels of systemic antibodies, such as individuals with multiple myeloma, hypogammaglobulinemia, and asplenia, also are at high risk for developing disseminated pneumococcal infection. In addition, selected studies suggest that pregnant women may have greater difficulty than nonpregnant women in responding to pneumococcal infection.[2-4]

CLINICAL MANIFESTATIONS

Pneumonia

S pneumoniae is the most common cause of community-acquired bacterial pneumonia. Five hundred thousand cases of pneumonococcal pneumonia occur annually in the United States. The reported incidence of pneumonia in pregnancy ranges from 0.63% to 2.3%.[5] The pneumococcus is responsible for one third to one half of these cases. In the majority of instances, *S pneumoniae* is the sole pathogen. In some cases, pneumococci may be present in association with other pathogens, such as influenza virus and *Hemophilus influenzae*.

Pneumococcal pneumonia usually occurs as a primary pulmonic infection affecting the right lower, right middle, or left lower lobe. In some instances, it may develop as a complication of antecedent infection in the paranasal sinuses, mastoid bone, endocardium, or female genital tract.

Pneumococcal pneumonia typically begins abruptly with a single shaking chill. The chill is followed rapidly by high fever, headache, malaise, severe pleuritic pain, dyspnea, and cough productive of purulent, blood-tinged sputum.

On physical examination, the patient appears acutely ill. She usually has rapid, shallow respirations and mild cyanosis. Diaphragmatic excursion on the affected side is limited by splinting. When pulmonary consolidation is present, tactile fremitus is increased, and the affected lung is dull to percussion. Tubular breath sounds and fine crepitant rales also may be heard. Abdominal distention occurs frequently; at times, a profound adynamic ileus develops.

The chest radiograph usually shows a discrete area of consolidation occupying one or more lobes of the lung. A diffuse bronchopneumonia also may be present (Figure 61–1). Other x-ray findings may include loss of lung volume, pleural thickening, pleural effusion, and empyema. Complete resolution of chest x-ray abnormalities may require eight to 10 weeks, even in previously healthy women.

Patients with pneumococcal pneumonia are at risk for several major complications. Some disorders, such as lung abscess, subcutaneous abscess, empyema, and pericarditis, develop as a result of contiguous spread of infection from the primary focus within the lung. Others, such as arthritis, metastatic brain abscess, endocarditis, and peritonitis, may

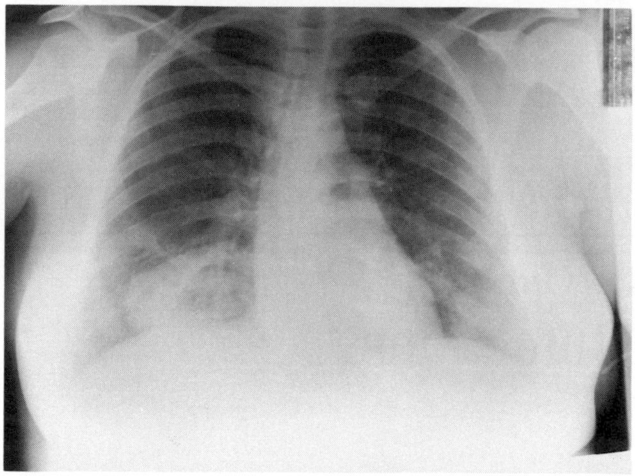

Figure 61–1. Chest x-ray of a 20-year-old woman demonstrates bilateral bronchopneumonia, with more severe changes noted in the right lower lobe. Gram's stain and culture of sputum were positive for pneumococci.

result from hematogenous or lymphatic dissemination of microorganisms. Bacteremia occurs in 25% to 30% of patients with pneumococcal pneumonia. Despite modern intensive care, the mortality in patients with pneumococcal bacteremia still ranges from 17% to 30%. It may be even higher in patients with advanced age, associated debilitating diseases, immunodeficiency disorders, and asplenia.[2–4]

In the preantibiotic era, 20% to 35% of pregnant women who had pneumococcal pneumonia died. Mortality was particularly high when infection occurred in the last trimester of pregnancy. Perinatal mortality in infected patients also was high, averaging 50% to 60% in most series. At the present time, pneumococcal pneumonia is unlikely to cause maternal death except in an immunocompromised host. Perinatal mortality appears to be increased slightly and is primarily the result of complications associated with preterm delivery.[4]

Meningitis

Next to *Neisseria meningitides, S pneumoniae* is the most common cause of bacterial meningitis in adults. Pneumococcal meningitis may present as a primary infection, but it occurs more frequently as a complication of infection in the lung, paranasal sinuses, mastoid bone, or endocardium. Pneumococcal meningitis also may develop as a result of skull fracture where an opening is created between the central nervous system and the nasopharynx.

The principal clinical manifestations of pneumococcal meningitis are chills, fever, headache, nuchal rigidity, and altered sensorium. Physical examination may demonstrate cranial nerve palsies and positive Kernig's and Brudzinski's signs. Cerebrospinal fluid analysis typically shows high protein, low glucose, many polymorphonuclear leukocytes, and gram-positive diplococci. In spite of improved medical therapy, approximately 30% of patients with pneumococcal meningitis die or suffer permanent neurologic sequelae.[2]

Endocarditis

In the preantibiotic era, *S pneumoniae* was responsible for approximately 15% of cases of endocarditis. At the present time, less than 2% of cases are due to this organism. Pneumonia and meningitis are the usual sites of primary infection in patients who subsequently develop pneumococcal endocarditis. This complication is particularly likely to occur in patients who have chronic illnesses, such as alcoholism and cirrhosis, immunodeficiency disorders, or preexisting valvular lesions.

After a brief period of apparent improvement in their primary infection, affected patients typically develop a high fever and intractable heart failure. Other serious complications include valve perforation, rupture of the chordae tendineae, annular abscess, and conduction disturbances. The case fatality rate varies from 30% to 70%. Age, timeliness of diagnosis, and severity of the patient's underlying disease process are the most important factors in determining the affected individual's ultimate prognosis.[6]

Genital Tract Infection

Peritonitis. Pneumococcal peritonitis may be primary or secondary. In primary peritonitis, peritoneal inflammation is the original manifestation of the disease process. This disorder is unique to females and occurs principally in girls less than 10 years of age. In secondary peritonitis, peritoneal inflammation develops as a result of pneumococcal infection in another organ system. Both disorders are rare.[7,8]

In primary peritonitis, *S pneumoniae* organisms ascend from the lower genital tract into the peritoneal cavity. Infection then begins as a localized pelvic peritonitis. If untreated, it may progress to generalized peritonitis and septicemia. In secondary peritonitis, dissemination of organisms occurs by way of the lymphatics or blood stream. Organisms also may enter the peritoneal cavity by contiguous spread from adjacent sites of infection, such as the lung, pericardium, or subcutaneous abscess.

Symptoms of pneumococcal peritonitis include pelvic and abdominal pain, nausea, vomiting, diarrhea, and urinary frequency. The principal physical findings are adynamic ileus, abdominal and pelvic tenderness, and peritoneal irritation. Some patients may have an associated pelvic abscess.

Intra-amniotic Infection. Intra-amniotic infection may occur as a result of dissemination of pneumococcal organisms from an extrapelvic site of infection or as a primary event. In the latter circumstance, organisms ascend from the vagina and cervix into the endometrial cavity following rupture of the chorioamniotic membrane. The clinical manifestations of intraamniotic infection are nonspecific and include maternal fever, uterine tenderness, foul amniotic fluid, and maternal and fetal tachycardia.[9]

Endomyometritis. In isolated cases, *S pneumoniae* may be one of the organisms responsible for postabortal or postpartum endomyometritis. In these instances, other pathogenic organisms usually are present at the site of infection. In addition, there may be evidence of extrapelvic pneumococcal infection. The usual clinical manifestations of endomyometritis are fever, tachycardia, uterine tenderness, and foul-smelling lochia.

Neonatal Infection. In rare instances, *S pneumoniae* may cause life-threatening infection in the neonate. The clinical presentation is similar to that of group B streptococcal infection. In early-onset disease, the infant demonstrates respiratory distress, cyanosis, temperature instability, and shock. The chest radiograph demonstrates rapidly progressive pneumonia, and blood cultures usually are positive for pneumococci. In late-onset disease, infants display fever, lethargy, and irritability and have bacteriologic evidence of central nervous system infection.

Overall, *S pneumoniae* is responsible for approximately 5% of cases of neonatal meningitis. Eighty percent of affected infants have positive blood cultures, and as many as 70% die as a result of their illness.[10]

DIAGNOSIS

The diagnosis of *S pneumoniae* infection may be confirmed by bacteriologic and immunologic techniques. In Gram's stain preparations, pneumococci typically appear in pairs or short chains of gram-positive, lancet-shaped cocci. In unusual circumstances, the organisms may stain gram-negative rather than gram-positive. In this case, they still preserve their characteristic morphology.

The optimal medium for isolating *S pneumoniae* is fresh beef-infusion broth containing 10% serum or blood. The bacteria can be grown satisfactorily, however, on regular blood agar plates that are incubated in 10% carbon dioxide. Pneumococci produce an incomplete zone of hemolysis on blood agar, and their colonial morphology resembles colonies of *Viridans streptococcus*. Tests for bile solubility and sensitivity to ethylhydrocupreine (Optochin) may be used to differentiate pneumococci from β-hemolytic streptococci.

S pneumoniae is enveloped by a capsule that is composed of complex polysaccharides. Differences in composition of the capsule have been used to classify pneumococci into more than 80 serotypes. Although all serotypes are pathogenic for humans, types 1, 3, 4, 7, 8, and 12 are the ones most commonly encountered in clinical practice. The polysaccharide capsules can be identified by suspending the bacteria in India ink or by treating them with type-specific anticapsular antibody [Neufeld's (quellung) reaction]. The quellung reaction may be a better rapid diagnostic test than the conventional Gram's stain because of the variable appearance of the organism in gram-stained preparations. Counterimmune electrophoresis also may be used to identify specific serotypes of *S pneumoniae*.

TREATMENT

The antibiotic of choice for treating confirmed pneumococcal infection is penicillin. Most serotypes of *S pneumoniae* are extremely sensitive to penicillin and have minimal inhibitory concentrations (less than or equal to 0.1 μg/mL. Approximately 2% of strains of *S pneumoniae* are resistant to penicillin. In addition, rare strains of pneumococci are resistant to multiple antibiotics, including chloramphenicol, tetracyclines, cephalosporins, erythromycin, clindamycin, and aminoglycosides.

For treatment of pneumococcal pneumonia, the appropriate dose of penicillin is 600,000 units every six hours. Patients who are seriously ill should be hospitalized and treated with intravenous antibiotics. Women who appear only mildly to moderately ill can be treated as outpatients with oral antibiotics.

Patients who have pneumococcal meningitis should be hospitalized and treated with high doses of intravenous aqueous penicillin G, five million units every four to six hours. Individuals with infectious endocarditis due to *S pneumoniae* also should be hospitalized and treated with this high dose of intravenous penicillin. In such patients, parenteral therapy should be continued for a minimum of four weeks.

Women with genital tract infections caused by *S pneumoniae* should receive similar doses of intravenous penicillin. They also should receive treatment with additional antibiotics that are effective against the mixed aerobic–anaerobic pelvic flora. One effective combination regimen is clindamycin (or metronidazole) plus penicillin plus gentamicin.

In patients who are allergic to penicillin, a first-generation cephalosporin is effective in treating pneumococcal pneumonia. For oral treatment, cephalexin, or cephradine, 250 mg every six hours, are appropriate selections. For intravenous therapy in more seriously ill patients, cefazolin, 1–2 g every eight hours, should be used. In patients who have pneumococcal meningitis, ceftriaxone[11], is the preferred cephalosporin.

Erythromycin, 250 to 500 mg every six hours, and clindamycin, 300 mg every six hours, also may be used to treat pneumococcal pneumonia. Vancomycin, 500 mg intravenously every six hours, should be used for treatment of disorders caused by pneumococci that are resistant to multiple antibiotics.

In addition to receiving antibiotic therapy, patients may require surgical intervention to eliminate foci of pneumococcal infection. Surgery may include procedures to drain a localized abscess or to replace a contaminated, dysfunctional heart valve.

Pregnant women with acute pneumococcal infection should be observed carefully for premature labor. External electronic fetal monitoring should be utilized to detect uterine contractions and to evaluate fetal heart rate. Pelvic examination should be performed to detect changes in cervical effacement and dilatation. Tocolytic therapy should be instituted if the diagnosis of premature labor is confirmed. Hyperthermia should be corrected by administration of an antipyretic, such as acetaminophen. Too-rapid decrease in body temperature by means of an ice bath or cooling blanket should be avoided, however. Additional supportive measures in the pregnant patient include correction of fluid and electrolyte imbalances and careful observation for onset of septic shock.

PREVENTION

At the present time, a polyvalent vaccine is available to immunize individuals who are at high risk for developing invasive pneumococcal infection. The current vaccine (Pneumovax 23, Merck Sharp & Dohme; and Pnu-Imune 23, Lederle Laboratories) is composed of purified capsular

TABLE 61–1. PRINCIPAL CONDITIONS THAT PREDISPOSE TO INVASIVE PNEUMOCOCCAL INFECTIONS IN ADULTS

Cardiovascular disease
Pulmonary disease
Diabetes mellitus
Cirrhosis
Splenic dysfunction or anatomic asplenia
Lymphoproliferative disorders
Multiple myeloma
Chronic renal failure
Organ transplantation associated with immunosuppression
Acquired immune deficiency syndrome (AIDS)

polysaccharide antigens of 23 types of *S pneumoniae*. These serotypes are responsible for approximately 90% of bacteremic pneumococcal disease in the United States. Each 0.5 mL dose of vaccine contains 25 μg of each polysaccharide antigen. The protective efficacy of the vaccine appears to range from 60% to 80%.[11] Vaccination is indicated for pregnant women who are at increased risk for acquiring invasive pneumococcal disease. Conditions that predispose to severe pneumococcal infection are summarized in Table 61–1.[11,12]

Following vaccination of healthy adults, protective levels of antibody persist for at least five years. Individuals with immunodeficiency disorders such as AIDS may have an impaired antibody response to the vaccine.

REFERENCES

1. Finland M, Dublin TD. Pneumococcic pneumonias complicating pregnancy and the puerperium. *JAMA*. 1939;112:1027.
2. Burman LA, Norrby R, Trollfors B. Invasive pneumococcal infections: incidence, predisposing factors and prognosis. *Rev Infect Dis*. 1985;7:133.
3. Bruyn GAW, van der Meer JWM, Hermans J, Knoppert W. Pneumococcal bacteremia in adults over a 10-year period at University Hospital, Leiden. *Rev Infect Dis*. 1988;10:446.
4. Gransden WR, Eykyn S, Phillips I. Pneumococcal bacteremia: 325 episodes diagnosed at St. Thomas's Hospital. *Br Med J*. 1985;290:505.
5. Benedetti TJ, Valle R, Ledger WJ. Antepartum pneumonia in pregnancy. *Am J Obstet Gynecol*. 1982;144:413.
6. Powderly WG, Stanley SL, Medoff G. Pneumococcal endocarditis: report of a series and review of the literature. *Rev Infect Dis*. 1986;8:786.
7. McCartney JE, Fraser J. Pneumococcal peritonitis. *Br J Surg*. 1922;9:479.
8. Nuchols HH, Hertig AT. *Pneumococcus* infection of the genital tract in women. *Am J Obstet Gynecol*. 1938;35:782.
9. Duff P, Gibbs RS. Acute intraamniotic infection due to *Streptococcus pneumoniae*. *Obstet Gynecol*. 1983;61:25S.
10. Fosson AF, Fine RN. Neonatal Meningitis. Presentation and discussion of 21 cases. *Clin Pediatr*. 1968;7:404.
11. Austrian R. The assessment of pneumococcal vaccine. *N Engl J Med*. 1980;303:578.
12. Pneumococcal polysaccharide vaccine. *MMWR*. 1989;38:64. Editorial.

Chapter Sixty-Two
Staphylococcal Infections

Patrick Duff

62

Staphylococci are responsible for a number of serious disorders in pregnant women, including toxic shock syndrome (TSS) and infections of the skin, subcutaneous tissue, genitourinary tract, cardiopulmonary system, and central nervous system. Staphylococcal organisms also may cause serious neonatal infections, such as scalded skin syndrome, osteomyelitis, bacteremia, and meningitis. The two species of staphylococci that are most likely to cause severe infections are *Staphylococcus aureus* and *Staphylococcus epidermidis*. *Staphylococcus saprophyticus* is of importance as a uropathogen.

PATHOGENESIS

Staphylococci are normal inhabitants of the skin and mucous membranes. *S aureus* may be present transiently in the nasopharynx of 70% to 90% of the population. Twenty to 30% of individuals are permanently colonized with this organism. Skin colonization usually correlates with nasopharyngeal colonization. Superficial and invasive staphylococcal infections develop when normal anatomic barriers are disrupted by lacerations, burns, animal bites, or chronic skin diseases. Invasive infections also occur with increased frequency in patients with debilitating conditions such as diabetes, cirrhosis, renal disease, disseminated malignancy, malnutrition, and immunodeficiency disorders, and in intravenous drug addicts. Pregnancy does not appear to increase the frequency or severity of staphylococcal infections.

Under ordinary circumstances, a large inoculum of staphylococci is required to produce overt clinical infection. The presence of a foreign body, however, reduces significantly the number of microorganisms necessary to establish infection. Therefore, patients with prosthetic implants also are at increased risk for developing invasive staphylococcal infection.

Cell-mediated host defenses are essential in containing staphylococcal infections. Antibody production also is necessary to opsonize bacteria and facilitate phagocytosis. Polymorphonuclear leukocytes rapidly enter infected tissue and ingest staphylococcal organisms. Thrombosis of surrounding capillaries occurs, fibrin is deposited around the periphery of the lesion, and an abscess cavity is formed. When host defenses are impaired or the bacterial inoculum is exceptionally large, staphylococci may invade the blood stream. Hematogenous dissemination results in metastatic foci of infection, principally in the long bones, lung, kidney, heart, liver, spleen, and brain.[1,2]

As noted in Table 62–1, staphylococci produce many substances that are important in the pathogenesis of infection. Toxin production is of particular interest in the pathogenesis of TSS. In patients affected by this disorder, elaboration of TSS toxin-I appears to be the result of acquisition of viral DNA (lysogeny) by particular strains of *S aureus*.[3]

CLINICAL MANIFESTATIONS

Skin Infection

Staphylococcal infection confined to a hair follicle is termed *folliculitis* and is manifested by a small erythematous nodule. When a more invasive infection of the hair follicle or sebaceous gland develops, the lesion is called a *furuncle* (*boil*). *Hidradenitis suppurativa* is a disorder characterized by extensive infection of sebaceous glands in the axilla and groin. A *carbuncle* is a more deeply invasive skin lesion with multiple discharging sinuses. It usually is present on the back of the neck or upper part of the thigh. Patients with carbun-

TABLE 62–1. PRODUCTS OF STAPHYLOCOCCAL ORGANISMS OF IMPORTANCE IN THE PATHOGENESIS OF INFECTION

Product	Pathophysiologic Effect
Lipolytic enzymes	Render bacteria resistant to bactericidal lipids of skin
Coagulase	Inhibits phagocytosis by host, promotes abscess formation, produces thrombotic effect on host's plasma proteins
Staphylokinase	Activates host's fibrinolytic system
Hyaluronidase	Degrades hyaluronic acid and facilitates penetration of connective tissue by bacterium
Hemolysin	Lyses host's red blood cells
Leukocidin	Causes degranulation and destruction of host's white blood cells
Enterotoxin	Causes nausea, vomiting, diarrhea
Exotoxins	Directly injure many organs, including myocardium, liver, peripheral vasculature, skin

cles often have fever and severe localized pain. Bacteremia occurs commonly in such individuals.

Bullous impetigo, an exfoliative pyoderma, also is caused by *S aureus.* In addition, although *Streptococcus pyogenes* is the more common cause of cellulitis, *S aureus* also may play an important role in the pathogenesis of this disorder.[4]

Pneumonia

S aureus is responsible for less than 1% of cases of community-acquired pneumonia but may be a more frequent pathogen among debilitated hospitalized patients. Staphylococcal pneumonia usually results from hematogenous dissemination of the organism from another site in the body. It is characterized by abrupt onset of high fever, chills, dyspnea, cyanosis, cough, and pleuritic pain. The sputum is purulent and often blood-tinged. Bacteremia occurs in 20% of patients. Chest radiograph usually shows irregular central infiltrates. Pneumatoceles, empyema, and lung abscess also may be present.[1,2]

Food Poisoning

If inoculated into food, *S aureus* multiplies rapidly when the food is maintained at ambient temperature. The organism produces a potent enterotoxin that causes severe nausea, vomiting, and diarrhea in the infected host. The incubation period of the illness is one to six hours, and the disorder usually resolves within 10 hours. Attack rates are very high among individuals exposed to the toxin. Foods that are particularly likely to be vehicles for propagation of staphylococcal infection are cream pastries, potato salad, and mayonnaise.[1,2]

Urinary Tract Infection

S saprophyticus is responsible for less than 5% of urinary tract infections in pregnant women. When these organisms are present in low colony counts in a single urine specimen obtained by clean void technique, they are likely to represent contamination of the urine by vaginal and perineal flora. When present in high colony counts in two consecutive clean void specimens or in a single specimen obtained by catheterization, however, the organisms should be considered uropathogens. Staphylococci typically cause only asymptomatic bacteriuria or cystitis. They rarely, if ever, cause acute pyelonephritis.[1,2]

Abdominal Wound Infection

The organisms most commonly responsible for wound infections after cesarean delivery are *S aureus, Escherichia coli,* aerobic streptococci, and anaerobes. *S aureus* can be isolated in pure or mixed culture from approximately 20% of women with postcesarean wound infection.

Affected patients usually have been treated initially for presumed endomyometritis. Despite appropriate antimicrobial therapy, they remain febrile. Their principal physical findings are erythema, induration, tenderness, and warmth at the margins of the incision. If the incision is opened, drainage of purulent material is evident. Wound infections predispose the patient to dehiscence and evisceration. If not treated properly, they may progress to necrotizing fasciitis or myonecrosis particularly in immunocompromised patients. When these sequelae develop, other pathogens such as *Clostridium* species and anaerobes become of predominant importance.

Puerperal Mastitis

S aureus and aerobic streptococci are the most common causes of puerperal mastitis. The usual clinical manifestations of this disorder are high fever, chills, and malaise. In addition, there is a discrete inflamed area in the breast that is extremely tender to touch. Milk from the affected breast may be purulent, and axillary lymph nodes typically are enlarged and tender. When delay in medical therapy occurs, a breast abscess may develop.

Genital Tract Infection

Chorioamnionitis and Endomyometritis. *S aureus* may be isolated from the amniotic fluid or endometrium in 1% to 5% of women with intrapartum or puerperal infection. Although the organism is considered to be of high virulence, it usually is present in association with other aerobic and anaerobic bacteria. *S epidermidis* may be isolated from 3% to 10% of patients with these infections and is usually considered to be an organism of low virulence.

The principal clinical manifestations of intra-amniotic infection are maternal fever, uterine tenderness, foul-smelling amniotic fluid, and maternal and fetal tachycardia. Corresponding signs of endomyometritis are fever, uterine tenderness, and foul-smelling lochia.

Toxic Shock Syndrome. A small number of cases of TSS have occurred in the immediate postpartum period. Some of these cases have occurred as a consequence of a localized skin or wound infection. The remainder have developed as a sequela of vaginal colonization with *S aureus.* Approximately 5% of women are colonized with this pathogen. Simultaneous development of TSS in mother and neonate also has been documented.

The three principal clinical manifestations of TSS are high fever, hypotension, and skin rash. The rash is a diffuse, nonpruritic, scarlatiniform eruption that is most prominent on the trunk and extremities. Subcutaneous edema may be present in association with the rash. One to two weeks after onset of the acute illness, desquamation of the skin occurs (Figure 62–1).

In addition to these findings, there is evidence of derangement in virtually every other organ system (Table 62–2). Gastrointestinal disturbances include nausea, vomiting, and diarrhea. Mucosal surfaces are intensely inflamed. Diffuse myalgias and myositis may be present. Renal abnormalities include oliguria, anuria, and pyuria. Hepatic dysfunction is indicated by bilirubin and transaminase enzyme elevation. The most prominent hematologic derangements

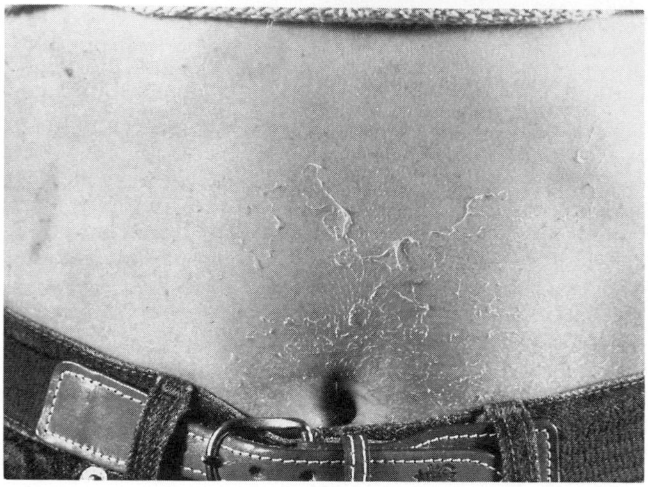

Figure 62–1. Photograph demonstrates the characteristic desquamation of the skin that occurs 1–2 weeks after the onset of toxic shock syndrome.

are thrombocytopenia and disseminated intravascular coagulation. Myocardial ischemia, left ventricular dysfunction, adult respiratory distress syndrome, and central nervous system abnormalities also may occur in the patient with TSS.[5-8]

Endocarditis

The incidence of bacteremia is approximately 7.5 per 1000 obstetric admissions. The three most common obstetric infections associated with bacteremia are endomyometritis, pyelonephritis, and intra-amniotic infection. *S aureus* is responsible for 4% to 5% of bacteremias in obstetric patients. *S epidermidis* is a less common isolate from blood cultures.[9]

In medical and general surgical patients who have *S aureus* bacteremia, the mortality is approximately 20%. Although fatalities from staphylococcal bacteremia are distinctly unusual in obstetric patients, serious complications of disseminated staphylococcal infection still occur. Such complications include lung abscess, osteomyelitis, renal and splenic abscess, brain abscess, and meningitis. The most ominous sequela of staphylococcal bacteremia is endocarditis. Fortunately, less than 10% of patients who have staphylococcal bacteremia develop this life-threatening complication.

TABLE 62–2. CASE DEFINITION OF TOXIC SHOCK SYNDROME

1. Fever ≧ 38.9°C, 102°F)
2. Characteristic skin rash—diffuse macular erythroderma
3. Desquamation of skin 1–2 weeks after onset of illness
4. Hypotension or orthostatic dizziness
5. Dysfunction of three or more of the following organ systems:
   a. Gastrointestinal (vomiting, diarrhea)
   b. Muscular (myalgia or CPK ≧ 2 × upper limit of normal)
   c. Mucous membrane (vaginal, oropharyngeal, conjunctival)
   d. Renal (BUN or creatinine ≧ 2 × upper limit of normal or ≧ 5 wbc/hpf on microscopic urinalysis)
   e. Hepatic (total bilirubin, SGOT, SGPT ≧ 2 × upper limit of normal)
   f. Hematologic (platelets ≧ 100,000 mm^3)
   g. CNS (altered sensorium)
6. Negative throat and cerebrospinal fluid culture (a positive blood culture for *Staphylococcus aureus* does not exclude a case from consideration)
7. Negative serologic tests for Rocky Mountain spotted fever, leptospirosis, measles

Adapted from multiple publications from the Centers for Disease Control.

The reported incidence of bacterial endocarditis in pregnancy ranges from 1 in 2000 to 1 in 5000 pregnancies. The disorder is most likely to occur in women with preexisting rheumatic or congenital heart disease, especially women with prosthetic heart valves. Drug addicts also are at increased risk for developing endocarditis.[10]

S epidermidis is responsible for infection primarily in patients with prosthetic heart valves. *S aureus*, however, may cause endocarditis even in women with normal cardiac anatomy. The organism produces fulminant, destructive lesions affecting primarily the aortic and mitral valves. The tricuspid valve also may be affected, particularly in drug addicts.

Frequent complications of staphylococcal endocarditis include valve perforation, rupture of the chordae tendineae, myocardial abscess, annular abscess, coronary artery embolization, suppurative pericarditis, and septic pulmonary embolization. Conduction disturbances, valvular incompetence, and myocardial dysfunction may develop as a result of these phenomena.

Metastatic brain abscess and meningitis also may occur as a consequence of septic embolization. Approximately 45% of patients with staphylococcal endocarditis have evidence of central nervous system infection. Because of these complications, the mortality in patients with staphylococcal endocarditis is exceptionally high, ranging from 40% to 80%.[1,2,11,12]

The patient with acute staphylococcal endocarditis typically has a high fever and appears severely ill. There usually is a localized staphylococcal lesion that is the source of bacteremia. There may be a new cardiac murmur or a change in a preexisting murmur. The most common auscultatory findings are aortic and mitral insufficiency. In peripheral areas of the body, there often is evidence of septic embolization and vasculitis. There also may be signs of central nervous system infection, manifested by major motor and cranial nerve dysfunction, meningeal irritation, and visual disturbances. Septic shock and disseminated intravascular coagulation also may be present.[1,2,11,12]

Chest x-ray usually demonstrates cardiomegaly and pulmonary edema. Conventional electrocardiography may show evidence of conduction disturbances and myocardial ischemia. Echocardiography is of great value in confirming the presence of endocardial vegetations.

The most comprehensive study of bacterial endocarditis in pregnancy was published in 1953. In that survey, Pedowitz and Hellman[13] observed a maternal mortality of 15% when acute bacterial endocarditis developed during pregnancy. In a more recent review, Seaworth and Durack[10] reported maternal and perinatal mortality rates of 29% and 23%, respectively. The majority of perinatal deaths are the direct result of complications associated with preterm delivery.

Neonatal Infections

Staphylococci may be inoculated onto the neonate's skin during passage through the maternal birth canal or during handling by nursery personnel. The most common manifestation of infection is the presence of isolated small pustules, usually found around the neck or in the axillae. Another common site of infection is the periumbilical area. In bullous impetigo (pemphigus neonatorum), large vesicles containing yellow fluid are distributed in the axillae, around the neck, and around the umbilicus. The most severe form of neonatal skin infection is the scalded skin syndrome. In certain respects, this disorder resembles TSS and usually presents as a diffuse, scarlatiniform eruption that progresses to extensive desquamation, exposing multiple raw areas of skin. Staphylococci also may cause localized scalp abscesses at the site of attachment of a monitoring electrode.

Most neonatal staphylococcal infections remain localized and respond promptly to antimicrobial therapy and local care of the lesions. In rare instances, dissemination of microorganisms results in metastatic foci of infection, usually affecting the central nervous system. Staphylococci are responsible for approximately 5% of cases of neonatal meningitis and bacteremia.[8]

DIAGNOSIS

The diagnosis of staphylococcal infection is confirmed by isolating the organism in culture. Staphylococci are nonmotile, nonspore-forming, gram-positive, spherical organisms. In Gram's stained smears of purulent material, they appear in small, grapelike clusters, often within the cytoplasm of polymorphonuclear leukocytes. In some smears, staphylococci appear as diploids or short chains. The length of the chain rarely exceeds four members.

Staphylococci are facultative anaerobes. They grow rapidly, however, on blood agar or Columbia colistin nalidixic acid agar incubated at 35–37°C under aerobic conditions. On solid agar media, *S aureus* and *S epidermidis* produce characteristic golden yellow and ivory white pigments, respectively.

Staphylococci are differentiated from streptococci on the basis of their positive catalase reaction. *S aureus* is distinguished from *S epidermidis* by its characteristic colonial morphology, ability to ferment mannitol, and production of coagulase. Individual strains of *S aureus* may be identified by phage typing.

The only serologic test for staphylococci that is of major clinical importance is the assay for antibodies to the teichoic acids, which are present in the cell wall of the organism. The antibodies are detected by counterimmunoelectrophoresis. The principal use of the assay is in determining the duration of parenteral antibiotic therapy in patients who have bacteremia (see below).[1,2]

TREATMENT

Selection of Antibiotic

The majority of strains of staphylococci that cause serious infections produce β-lactamase enzymes. Therefore, treatment should be initiated with a penicillinase-resistant antibiotic, such as methicillin (2 g every 4 h), oxacillin (1–2 g every 4 h), or nafcillin (1–2 g every 4 h). In recent reports, unfortunately, many strains of *S aureus* and *S epidermidis* also have been resistant to methicillin. In addition, such strains have a high degree of resistance to other antibiotics, including the aminoglycosides, erythromycin, clindamycin, tetracyclines, and quinolones.[14] As noted below, in institutions where such strains are endemic, vancomycin is the antibiotic of choice for treating invasive staphylococcal infections.

The first-generation cephalosporins, such as cephalothin (1–2 g every 4–6 h) or cefazolin (1–2 g every 8 h), also are of value for treatment of many staphylococcal infections. Most of the newer, extended-spectrum cephalosporins, however, do not provide acceptable coverage against this microorganism and, therefore, should not be used for treatment of invasive infections. In addition, cephalosporins must be administered with caution to patients who have a history of penicillin allergy. In individuals who have manifested an immediate hypersensitivity reaction to penicillin (laryngeal edema, bronchospasm, urticaria), cephalosporins are contraindicated.

Vancomycin has unique application in the treatment of staphylococcal infection, particularly in individuals who are allergic to penicillin. Vancomycin is effective against virtually all strains of coagulase-positive staphylococci. The appropriate intravenous dose of the drug is 1–1.5 g administered over a 30-to-40 minute period every 12 hours. Vancomycin should be considered the initial drug of choice for staphylococcal infection in hospitals with a high prevalence of both penicillin-resistant and methicillin-resistant staphylococci.

Other antibiotics, such as lincomycin, erythromycin, trimethoprim-sulfamethoxazole, clindamycin, and the aminoglycosides, also have activity against staphylococci. Although these drugs are not considered the treatment of choice for staphylococcal infection, they may be used in mild to moderately ill patients who are allergic to penicillins and cephalosporins. In more seriously ill patients, vancomycin remains the preferred agent.

In genital tract infections, staphylococci usually are present in association with other pathogens. In such instances, therapy must be broadened to include antimicrobials with efficacy against aerobic and anaerobic streptococci, aerobic gram-negative bacilli, and *Bacteroides* species.[1,2,12]

In patients with TSS, systemic antibiotics do not consistently hasten the resolution of the disorder but do appear to reduce the frequency of recurrences. Of more importance in these individuals is the prompt correction of fluid and electrolyte disturbances and support of the cardiopulmonary and renal systems.

Length of Antibiotic Therapy

Staphylococci are killed slowly by antibiotics. Relapses occur frequently, and duration of therapy often must be longer than in other bacterial infections. For most localized staphylococcal infections, antibiotic therapy should be continued for 48–72 hours beyond the time when the patient has become afebrile and asymptomatic and clinical evidence of infection has resolved.

There are two principal exceptions to this treatment guideline. Patients with osteomyelitis should be treated for a longer period of time, usually 28 days, because infections of the bone are exceptionally difficult to eradicate. Second, patients with documented staphylococcal endocarditis should receive extended therapy with parenteral antibiotics for 4–6 weeks. Shorter courses of therapy (10–14 days) appear to be acceptable in patients with bacteremia who have no evidence of endocarditis and who demonstrate prompt clinical improvement. Prior to discontinuing antibiotic therapy, such patients should be assessed for the presence of serum antibodies directed toward bacterial teichoic acids. A negative result is reassurance that metastatic dissemination of the infection has not occurred.[1,2,13,15]

Surgery

For well-localized, superficial staphylococcal infections, surgical debridement may be the only treatment necessary to effect a cure. In other situations, surgery may be the essential measure necessary to stabilize the critically ill patient. Skin, subcutaneous, and deep-seated abscesses must be opened and drained. Infected products of conception, devitalized bone, and contaminated intravascular catheters and prosthetic devices should be removed from the host.

Surgery appears to be particularly important in patients with endocarditis. The principal indication for valve replacement is worsening heart failure that is unresponsive to medical management. Valve replacement has been accomplished successfully in pregnant patients, and indicated surgery should not be delayed, regardless of the stage of gestation.[1,2,15]

Preventive Measures

At the present time, neither a staphylococcal vaccine nor an antitoxin is available for clinical use. Accordingly, preventive measures must be directed toward minimizing the risk of invasive staphylococcal infection, particularly bacteremia, in both the parturient and the neonate. Medical personnel who have overt staphylococcal lesions should be prohibited from working in the neonatal or obstetric units until their infections have resolved. Patients with large open staphylococcal lesions should be isolated from other patients. Medical and nursing personnel caring for these individuals must observe strict handwashing procedures and utilize protective gowns, caps, masks, and gloves as indicated.

In patients who have serious staphylococcal infections, it may be necessary to remove contaminated prosthetic devices and intravascular catheters. Women with artificial heart valves should receive prophylaxis for bacterial endocarditis during the intrapartum period. Prophylaxis should include antibiotics with coverage against staphylococci. Finally, patients with staphylococcal lesions should receive prompt medical and surgical therapy to prevent metastatic dissemination of these virulent microorganisms.

REFERENCES

1. Sheagren JN. *Staphylococcus aureus*. The persistent pathogen I. *N Engl J Med*. 1984;310:1368.
2. Sheagren JN. *Staphylococcus aureus*. The persistent pathogen II. *N Engl J Med*. 1984;310:1437.
3. Schlievert PM. Role of toxic shock syndrome toxin 1 in toxic shock syndrome: overview. *Rev Infect Dis*. 1989;11:S107.
4. Finch R. Skin and soft-tissue infections. *Lancet*. 1988;1:164.
5. Chesney PJ. Clinical aspects and spectrum of illness of toxic shock syndrome: overview. *Rev Infect Dis*. 1989;11:S1.
6. Broome CV. Epidemiology of toxic shock syndrome in the United States: overview. *Rev Infect Dis*. 1989;11:S14.
7. See RH, Chow AW. Microbiology of toxic shock syndrome: overview. *Rev Infect Dis*. 1989;11:S55.
8. Faden HS, Burke JP, Glasgow LA, et al. Nursery outbreak of scalded-skin syndrome. *Am J Dis Child*. 1976;130:265.
9. Blanco JD, Gibbs RS, Castaneda YS. Bacteremia in obstetrics: clinical course. *Obstet Gynecol*. 1981;58:621.
10. Seaworth BJ, Durack DT. Infective endocarditis in obstetric and gynecologic practice. *Am J Obstet Gynecol*. 1986;154:180.
11. Weinstein L, Schlesinger JJ. Pathoanatomic, pathophysiologic and clinical correlations in endocarditis. *N Engl J Med*. 1974;291:832.
12. Eykyn SQ. Staphylococcal sepsis. The changing pattern of disease and therapy. *Lancet*. 1988;1:100.
13. Pedowitz P, Hellman LM. Pregnancy and healed subacute bacterial endocarditis. *Am J Obstet Gynecol*. 1953;66:294.
14. Maple PAC, Hamilton-Miller JMT, Brumfitt W. World-wide antibiotic resistance in methicillin-resistant staphylococcus aureus. *Lancet*. 1989;1:537.
15. Richardson JV, Karp RB, Kirklin JW, et al. Treatment of infective endocarditis: a 10-year comparative analysis. *Circulation*. 1978;58:589.

Chapter Sixty-Three
Streptococcal Infections

Sebastian Faro

63

The streptococci are among the most frequent bacterial pathogens to cause infection in humans. This is an interesting group of bacteria because some, especially members of the groups A and B β-hemolytic streptococci, are considered primary pathogens, whereas others, such as the enterococci (now a separate genus *Enterococcus*), are considered secondary pathogens, and still others are considered not to be pathogens at all. The streptococci are responsible for a wide variety of infections, including erysipelas, pyoderma, cellulitis, lymphangitis, pharyngitis, pneumonia, scarlet fever, rheumatic fever, glomerulonephritis, endocarditis, cystitis, and puerperal sepsis.

The streptococci occupy a historic position in medicine and obstetrics. The cause of puerperal sepsis, group A β-hemolytic streptococcus, was first thought of as a contagion and was responsible for childbed fever. It was Dr. John Leak who, in 1772, first suggested that postpartum fever was contagious. This view was supported by Dr. Charles White, who in 1773 advised the isolation of affected women, that strict cleanliness be maintained, and that the patient be placed in a semirecumbent position to allow for adequate drainage of the lochia. Additional support for the management of septic women was obtained from Dr. Alexander Hamilton in 1781 and Dr. Alexander Gordon in 1795. Dr. Oliver Wendell Holmes, in 1843, showed that the infection could be traced to the lack of proper precautions on the part of all medical personnel attending affected patients. Dr. Ignaz Phillipp Semmelweis, in 1847, demonstrated that the disease was transmitted from an affected individual to a nonaffected individual by way of the carriage of contaminated material on the examining finger of the medical attendant.

CLASSIFICATION

The streptococci are gram-positive nonmotile bacteria, most of which are facultative anaerobes, although some are obligate anaerobes or microaerophilic, such as the peptococci or peptostreptococci. The streptococci are spherical or ovoid in shape and usually grow in pairs, chains, or tetrads. The family Streptococcaceae is made up of five genera: *Streptococ-*

cus, Leuconostoc, Pediococcus, Aerococcus, and *Gemella*. The genus *Streptococcus* is a heterogeneous group of bacteria consisting of approximately 21 species, and there is no single set of criteria available to differentiate one species from another. Species differentiation is based on growth characteristics, biochemical reactions, antigenic properties, and patterns of hemolysis when the bacteria are grown on blood agar. Lancefield differentiated the streptococci into serogroups by extracting cell wall antigens and identifying individual groups by precipitin reactions using specific antiserums.[1] She established groups A, B, C, D, E, F, G, H, and K to T. The majority of human pathogenic strains are β-hemolytic and belong to groups A, B, C, D, F, and G (Table 63–1).[1] However, the group D species, *Streptococcus faecalis*, commonly referred to as the enterococcus, does not cause hemolysis when grown on blood agar and is a human pathogen.

The hemolytic reaction caused by the streptococci when grown on blood agar not only serves as a taxonomic tool but also is useful in clinical situations. The streptococci produce three patterns of hemolysis: alpha, beta, and gamma. *Streptococcus pneumoniae*, an α-hemolytic strain, will cause partial hemolysis, which appears as an area of green discoloration around the colony when grown on blood agar. *Streptococcus pyogenes* and *Streptococcus agalactiae*, both important pathogens in causing infection in obstetric patients, are both β-hemolytic and cause complete hemolysis of red blood cells when grown on blood agar. β-hemolysis appears as a clear zone around the growing colony. The *enterococcus faecalis* does not have the ability to lyse red blood cells; therefore, no zone of hydrolysis appears when it is grown on blood agar.

Although there are many pathogenic species of streptococci, *S pneumoniae, S pyogenes, S agalactiae,* and *S faecalis* are the species most frequently involved in obstetric infections. *S pneumoniae* is still the predominant cause of pneumonia; *S agalactiae* has become a frequent cause of postpartum endometritis and neonatal pneumonia, sepsis, and meningitis.[2-4]; *E faecalis* is found in urinary tract infections and appears in patients with postpartum endometritis, especially in patients treated with antibiotics that lack coverage for the enterococcus; and *S pyogenes*, group A, β-hemolytic streptococci, at one time the predominant cause of puerperal sepsis, is found infrequently.

STREPTOCOCCUS PYOGENES

S pyogenes is a ubiquitous organism and is one of the most important bacterial pathogens. Pasteur isolated *S pyogenes* from the blood of a patient with puerperal sepsis in 1879. The role of streptococci as agents of disease was further advanced by Brown who, in 1919, demonstrated that these bacteria caused different degrees of hemolysis when grown on blood agar and introduced the terms alpha, beta, and gamma hemolysis. Lancefield found that most pathogenic strains of *S pyogenes* belonged to serogroup A.[1] Strains of *S pyogenes* could be further differentiated by antigenic determinants located in the cell wall, known as M-protein.

S pyogenes produces a number of clinically important somatic constituents and extracellular products. The cell wall is a complex structure containing clinically important antigens, known as the somatic constituents. The cell wall consists of three layers: the innermost layer is a peptidoglycan containing polymers of N-acetylglucosamine and N-acetylmuramic acid joined by amino acid side chains of alanine, glutamic acid, lysine, and glycine; the middle layer, known as the group-specific carbohydrate, is made up of rhamnose and N-acetylglucosamine in a ratio of 2:1; the outer layer of the cell wall contains protein and the clinically important M-protein and T protein. A capsule of hyaluronic acid surrounds the cell wall.

The M-protein is found on the surface of *S pyogenes* and only on virulent strains.[5] M-protein has been designated the major virulence factor. Strains possessing M-protein are resistant to phagocytosis. In addition, these strains multiply rapidly in human blood and are capable of initiating disease. Immunologic differences have been found in M-protein, and thus far 80 different serotypes have been identified. There have been many strains isolated, but their M-protein has not been serotyped because the typing sera is not available.[6] The complete amino acid sequence of M-6 protein has been determined, and a model has been constructed.[7] It is theorized that the protein originates in

TABLE 63–1. STREPTOCOCCI PATHOGENIC IN HUMANS

Species	Serogroup	Hemolysis	Diseases
1. *S pyogenes*	A	β	Pharyngitis, tonsillitis, erysipelas, impetigo, pneumonia, puerperal sepsis, scarlet fever, rheumatic fever, glomerulonephritis
2. *S agalactine*	B	β	Chorioamnionitis, puerperal sepsis, neonatal sepsis, pneumonia, meningitis
3. *S equi* *S zooepidemicis* *S equisimilis*	C	β	Erysipelas, wound infection, endocarditis
4. *S faecalis*	D	None	Bacteremia, endocarditis, genitourinary infection
5. *S minutus* *S anginosus*	F	β	Skin wound, brain abscess, bacteremia, endocarditis
6. *S canis*	G	β	Pharyngitis, skin wound, gynecologic infections
7. *S pneumoniae*	None	α	Pneumonia, empyrema, otitis media, mastoiditis, endocarditis, meningitis, peritonitis
8. *S milleri* *S mitior* *S mutans* *S salivarius* *S sanguis*	"Viridan"	α	Bacteremia, endocarditis in patients with congenital or acquired heart disease

the bacterial cell membrane, penetrates, and is intercalated within the cross-linked peptidoglycan of the wall. The alpha-helical coiled-coil rod segment extends beyond the surface of the cell wall.[8-10] Immunity to group A streptococcal infection occurs by way of the development of opsonic antibodies against the M-protein. Some strains produce undetectable amounts of M-protein and, therefore, cannot be serotyped, but strain differentiation can be accomplished by differences detected in T-protein. This antigen, T-protein, is not associated with virulence. The group A *Streptococcus* poses a second virulence factor, lipoteichoic acid (LTA), which has an affinity for cell membranes. The LTA enables the *Streptococcus* to adhere to human epithelial cells, thereby allowing the bacteria to colonize the host.[11]

The extracellular products produced by *S pyogenes* are responsible for various manifestations of streptococcal infection. A listing of some of the more important products is given in Table 63–2. Streptolysin O induces antibody formation. Titers of streptolysin O obtained by comparing acute and convalescent serum can be used to establish whether or not a patient has had a recent streptococcal infection. In addition to hemolysins, the organism produces DNases, hyaluronidase, and streptokinase, all of which function to cause liquefaction of pus and the advancement of the streptococci along tissue planes.[12]

Although *S pyogenes* is responsible for a variety of diseases, both suppurative and nonsuppurative infections (see Table 63–3), it is beyond the scope of this chapter to discuss all of these. The discussion is limited to those infections most likely to occur in the obstetric patient, namely, pharyngitis and puerperal sepsis. The nonsuppurative complications, acute rheumatic fever and acute glomerulonephritis, are usually preceded by streptococcal pharyngitis; therefore, patients who complain of sore throat should be properly evaluated for the possible existence of streptococcal pharyngitis.

Pharyngitis

Colonization and infection of the faucial areas by *S pyogenes* may produce peritonsillar cellulitis or abscess, or retropharyngeal abscess. The organism may extend up the eustachian tubes to produce otitis media or may advance up the pharyngeal epithelium to cause a cervical lymphadenitis, which may lead to penetration of the cribriform plate, producing brain abscesses, meningitis, or thrombosis of the intracranial venous sinuses. The organism may descend to the lower respiratory tract to cause pneumonia.

TABLE 63–2. EXTRACELLULAR PRODUCTS PRODUCED BY *STREPTOCOCCUS PYOGENES*

Substance	Manifestation
Erythrogenic toxin	Rash of scarlet fever
Streptolysin O	Hemolysis of RBCs Toxic to polymorphonuclear leukocytes, platelets
Streptolysin S	Damages membranes of polymorphonuclear leukocytes, platelets, and cellular organelles Hemolysis of RBCs
DNases A,B,C, and D	Degradation of deoxyribonucleic acid
Hyaluronidase	Degrades hyaluronic acid of connective tissue
Streptokinase	Dissolution of clots

TABLE 63–3. DISEASES CAUSED BY *STREPTOCOCCUS PYOGENES*

Pharyngitis	Scarlet fever
Erysipelas	Rheumatic fever
Pyoderma	Acute glomerulonephritis
Cellulitis	Puerperal sepsis
Lympharyngitis	

Streptococcal pharyngitis cannot be diagnosed by clinical examination; a throat culture is required in order to isolate and identify the organism. The most likely cause of pharyngitis is viral infection. Group A streptococci will be isolated from approximately one third of patients with pharyngitis. Among this group, only 50% will demonstrate a rise in antibody titer to one of the streptococcal antigens; the remainder will have fixed titers and represent the carrier state.[13] Therefore, it is extremely important that the specimen for culture be obtained appropriately. A sterile, cotton-tipped applicator should be passed over the tonsils or tonsillar fossae, oropharynx, and nasopharynx posterior to the uvula. The tongue, buccal mucosa, and gums should be avoided to reduce the possibility of retrieving normal oral flora. The swab should then be used to inoculate blood agar.

The diagnosis of *S pyogenes* is established by the isolation of gram-positive cocci that, when grown on blood agar, cause β-hemolysis. In addition, *S pyogenes* is very sensitive to bacitracin. Therefore, the ability to completely hemolyze red blood cells and extreme sensitivity to bacitracin are diagnostic of *S pyogenes*.

Therapy of streptococcal pharyngitis is designed to prevent the nonsuppurative complications of acute rheumatic fever and glomerulonephritis. *S pyogenes* remains sensitive to penicillin; therefore, penicillin is the drug of choice for the treatment of streptococcal pharyngitis. The prevention of acute poststreptococcal glomerulonephritis following the treatment of streptococcal pharyngitis with penicillin has not been established. Penicillin continues to be extremely efficacious in preventing acute rheumatic fever. The more expensive broad-spectrum semisynthetic penicillins and cephalosporins are not indicated for the treatment of streptococcal pharyngitis. A single intramuscular injection of the long-acting benzathine penicillin G, 1.2 million units, is sufficient for uncomplicated streptococcal pharyngitis. Oral treatment can be accomplished with penicillin G or V, 200,000 to 250,000 units, given four times daily for 10 days. Pregnant patients who are allergic to penicillin can be treated with erythromycin, 250 mg orally, four times daily for 10 days.

Tetracyclines are contraindicated in pregnancy and should not be used for the treatment of *S pyogenes* infection, because the organism is usually resistant to this antibiotic. Sulfonamides are not effective in eliminating streptococcal colonization of the pharynx or in the prevention of rheumatic fever. At the completion of therapy, the patient's throat should be recultured, and if the organism is still present, a second course of antibiotic should be instituted.

Puerperal Infection

S pyogenes has in the past been the causative agent for two serious obstetric infections, namely, postpartum endometritis (puerperal sepsis) and necrotizing fasciitis. These diseases may be caused solely by group A β-hemolytic streptococci; however, it is uncommon to find other bacteria growing in association with *S pyogenes*.

Puerperal sepsis secondary to *S pyogenes* infection consists of two phases. The initial phase may be an endometritis, endomyometritis, or endomyoparametritis. Spread to the parametrium occurs by way of the lymphatics. A peritonitis develops that may eventually lead to systemic infection. The disease usually becomes symptomatic within 48 hours after delivery. The patients develop an increase in oral body temperature, which may be as high as 105°F, leukocytosis, tachycardia, and a soft, tender uterus. If the patient has had a cesarean section, the uterine tenderness is out of proportion to the operative procedure. The lochia is serosanguineous and has no significant odor. The infection may be fulminating, and if not treated early, it progresses with extension beyond the pelvis. Patients develop diffuse peritonitis, marked abdominal distention secondary to an adynamic ileus, shaking chills, bacteremia with involvement of the cardiopulmonary system, and disseminated intravascular coagulopathy.[14]

If a Gram's stain of an endometrial specimen reveals the presence of gram-positive cocci, treatment should be instituted immediately. One of the new broad-spectrum semisynthetic penicillins should be administered intravenously, 4 g every 6 hours. These agents, that is, mezlocillin, piperacillin, and ticarcillin, will provide coverage against the streptococci and also are active against gram-negative aerobes and anaerobes. Patients allergic to penicillin may be treated with a cephamycin or erythromycin. The patient should be isolated, because this is a hospital-acquired organism and is easily transmitted from one patient to another by way of medical personnel.

Necrotizing Fasciitis

Meleny described in 1924 an infection of a surgical wound caused by group A β-hemolytic streptococci, known as hemolytic streptococcal gangrene. The condition was recognized during the Civil War and was referred to as hospital gangrene. Today, this disease is known as necrotizing fasciitis and is caused by the concomitant growth of *S pyogenes* and *Staphylococcus aureus*.[15]

The bacteria gain entrance through a surgical wound, thereby colonizing the subcutaneous tissue and fascia, causing a rapidly progressive infection that requires aggressive therapy. The patient becomes febrile, with a temperature of 103°F and a marked tachycardia. The wound edges at first appear erythematous and edematous; eventually the skin becomes dusky. Blisters form that contain a serosanguineous fluid. As the infection progresses, the original margins of the incision take on the characteristic gray-black color seen in gangrenous necrosis. The fascia liquefies and sloughs off. The patient often develops bacteremia, with distant foci of infection such as the lungs.

The diagnosis is established by the clinical findings and the isolation of *S pyogenes* and *S aureus*. This disease is distinctive from synergistic bacterial gangrene, which is caused by the growth of microaerophilic or anaerobic streptococci and *S aureus*. Synergistic bacterial gangrene usually presents as burrowing ulcers around retention sutures.

Therapy must be instituted immediately, as the bacteria spread rapidly by way of tissue planes by destruction of connective tissue through the elaboration of hyaluronidase. All necrotic tissue must be surgically excised. Secondary skin grafts are required when the disease has been eradicated. Antibiotic therapy should be immediately instituted with massive doses of intravenous penicillin G. However, the newer β-lactam antibiotics may prove to be as efficacious, if not more so.

Toxic Shock-like Syndrome

S pyogenes, prior to the late 1970s, had been associated with serious infection; however, during the period from 1980–1985, infections appeared to have decreased. In the past three years, there has been an increase in serious infections, for example, acute rheumatic fever and streptococcal pharyngitis.[16-18] The appearance of streptococcal toxic shock-like syndrome may herald a renewed virulence of the streptococcus.

S pyogenes produces a variety of toxins. The pyrogenic toxins, A, B, and C, are extracellular, or exotoxins, are produced by 90% of the group A isolates, and are capable of causing significant tissue injury.[19,20] These exotoxins are not associated with other strains of streptococci; therefore, they appear to be unique to the group A strains. The amino acid sequence of streptococcal pyogenic exotoxin A appears to be similar to staphylococcal enterotoxin B, which is associated with toxic shock syndrome (TSS) toxin-1 and with the nonmenstrual TSS.[21,22]

The toxic shock-like syndrome appears quite uncharacteristic for group A β-hemolytic streptococcal infections. The initial infection is atypical when it occurs in the immunocompromised or chronically debilitated patient. Earlier studies have shown that individuals who were elderly, diabetic, alcoholics, or drug abusers were at risk for group A streptococcal sepsis.[23,24] The initial infection usually presents as a cellulitis or necrotizing fasciitis or may present as endomyometritis, suppurative phlebitis, peritonitis, osteomyelitis, or endophthalmitis.[25] The infection is accompanied by a release of exotoxin A, which causes systemic toxicity. This results in septic shock or toxic shock-like syndrome, characterized by hypotension, renal dysfunction, respiratory failure, hypoalbuminemia, and hypocalcemia. The multisystem failure and clinical characteristics are similar to those seen in patients with staphylococcal TSS.[26-28] The similarity between the two syndromes, that is, streptococcal and staphylococcal TSS, may be due to the similarity in amino acid sequencing of the toxins. The two syndromes differ in that streptococcal toxic shock is typically associated with bacteremia, and a focus of infection is easily established. In a recent report, 20 patients were described, in whom a diagnosis of streptococcal TSS was made.[25] The median age was 36, with a range of 25 to 66 years of age. Thirteen of the patients had no underlying disease, whereas two were alcoholics, two were intravenous drug abusers, one had diabetes, and one had cerebellar ataxia. Eleven patients were male and nine were female. The most common initial infection was necrotizing fasciitis with or without myositis. The mortality rate in this group was 30%.

Treatment must be aggressive, utilizing a combination of surgical and medical intervention. The patients required fluid replacement, invasive monitoring, for example, a Swan–Ganz catheter, arterial line, antibiotic therapy, and surgical debridement. Surgical debridement must be performed early in the course of the disease and must be thorough. The surgical debridement must include the removal of all necrotic tissue, as well as tissue with a compromised vascular supply. Healthy tissue is characterized by the presence of brisk bleeding when the tissue is incised. Antibiotic therapy must be instituted immediately, without knowing the causative agent. A Gram's stain may be helpful; however, if it is not of particular benefit, it would be appropriate to begin Timentin, a combination of ticarcillin/clavulanic acid plus an aminoglycoside. After the specific bacterium has been identified as *S pyogenes,* intravenous crystalline penicillin G, 4 million units every 6 hours, should be administered until the patient's signs and symptoms have completely resolved.

STREPTOCOCCUS PNEUMONIAE

Pneumonia continues to be a major disease and is the result of infection by various microorganisms. However, *S pneumoniae,* formerly known as *Diplococcus pneumoniae,* continues to be the primary causative agent of pneumonia and occurs more frequently in the winter and early spring months. The frequency of pneumonia is estimated to be 2.1 cases in 1000 per year in the general population, with an overall mortality of 5–10%. Maternal mortality is estimated to be 2% to 3% in pregnant individuals with severe disease, and the fetal mortality may approach 30%.[2]

S pneumoniae is a gram-positive lancet-shaped bacteria found growing in pairs in clinical specimens, with their tapered ends in close approximation. This bacteria, when grown in the laboratory, may produce a capsule. It is then referred to as the *smooth form* and is virulent. The bacteria may grow without a capsule; it is then referred to as the *rough form,* and is avirulent. The smooth form produces mucoid colonies when grown on blood agar and produces α-hemolysis. However, when the bacteria are grown anaerobically, lysis results in release of pneumolysin O, which results in β-hemolysis. *S pneumoniae* can be rapidly identified in clinical specimens by Neufeld's reaction (quellung reaction). The quellung reaction is carried out by mixing the specimen with pneumococcal antiserum and methylene blue on a glass slide. The preparation is examined microscopically for the presence of bacteria surrounded by a large capsule. In addition to capsular polysaccharides, *S pneumoniae* and *S pyogenes* both possess M-protein and group-specific carbohydrates. The M-protein found in the *Pneumococcus* is not antiphagocytic and, therefore, is not a virulence factor. The capsular polysaccharides are antigenic and form the basis for distinguishing the various serotypes, of which 84 have been identified.

S pneumoniae is a member of the normal microflora of the upper respiratory tract in 5% to 70% of humans. Pneumococcal pneumonia occurs when the bacteria have been aspirated, thereby colonizing and multiplying within the alveolar spaces. The growth of bacteria causes an inflammatory response within the alveolar spaces, and this exudate favors multiplication and growth of bacteria. In the absence of antimicrobial therapy, the disease progresses through four phases. Initially, the lungs become congested secondary to hyperemia, edema, and migration of neutrophils. This is followed by red hepatization, in which the capillary network of the infected lung segment becomes congested, and the alveoli become laden with bacteria and red blood cells. Usually, by the fifth day of the infection, the affected segments become densely infiltrated with neutrophils, and there is a noticeable absence of bacteria; this stage is referred to as *gray hepatization.* This stage is followed by resolution of the disease, which is characterized by complete healing and the absence of tissue necrosis.

Symptoms of infection are usually abrupt in onset. The patient initially develops shaking chills and fever between 102°F and 105°F. Some patients develop a rusty sputum, chest pain, dyspnea, malaise, weakness, anorexia, tachycardia, and tachypnea. Auscultation of the lungs reveals signs of bronchopneumonia, such as consolidation. A complete blood count with white cell differential usually reveals an increase in both mature and immature neutrophils, as well as anemia. The indirect bilirubin may be elevated as a result of hemolysis of red blood cells. Arterial blood may reveal the presence of hypoxia. A sputum specimen should be obtained for culture, antibiotic sensitivities, quellung reaction, and Gram's stain. The presence of polynuclear leukocytes indicates that the specimen originated from a site of inflammation.

Antibiotic therapy should be started immediately with either intramuscular or intravenous penicillin. Intramuscular procaine penicillin, 300,000–600,000 units twice daily for 7–10 days, or procaine penicillin, 600,000 units intramuscularly, followed by phenoxymethylpenicillin, 250 mg orally four times daily, or intravenous aqueous penicillin, 5–10 million units daily as the recommended treatment regime. Patients who are allergic to penicillin should receive erythromycin. Penicillin remains the drug of choice in the treatment of pneumococcal pneumonia. *S pneumoniae* susceptibility to antimicrobial agents has not significantly changed in the United States and Canada in the past 15 years.

The patient with pneumococcal pneumonia receiving antibiotic therapy should show a definite response to antimicrobial therapy within 36 hours; in some instances, it may take up to 96 hours. The initial response is characterized by a decrease in the febrile response followed by a decrease in respiratory rate, cough, and chest pain. The radiologic changes do not show signs of resolution coincident with the physical findings, but are delayed two to three weeks. Patients who have persistent signs of infection, fever, tachycardia, and dyspnea should be evaluated for suppurative complications, such as extension to pleural or pericardial cavities, abscess formation, meningitis, endocarditis, or arthritis. Consideration should also be given to colonization by additional bacteria (see also Chapter 121).

STREPTOCOCCUS AGALACTIAE

The Lancefield group B β-hemolytic streptococci (GBBS), *S agalactiae,* are a major cause of maternal and neonatal infection.[3,4,29,30] Five serotypes have been identified, Ia, Ib, Ic, II, and III, based on a type-specific capsular polysaccharide and a single protein antigen. All serotypes possess sialic acid (N-acetylneuraminic acid) in the polysaccharide capsule in various concentrations, which may differ within a given serotype. Virulent strains appear to contain high concentrations of sialic acid and resist opsonization by the host serum.[31] These strains, which do not induce opsonic antibodies, would be resistant to phagocytosis. Individuals infected by GBBS appear to lack opsonic antibody.[32]

Reports in the literature implicating GBBS as a major cause of puerperal sepsis have been sporadic. Fry, in 1938, described seven cases of GBBS puerperal sepsis. Hood et al, in 1961, reported the isolation of GBBS in 8.4% of patients with antepartum fever and amnionitis.[33] Finn and Holden, in 1973, described six cases of postpartum endometritis caused by GBBS.[34] In 1980, Faro reported 40 cases of puerperal sepsis involving GBBS, of which 13 patients had bacteremia.[3,35] Ten of the 13 bacteremic patients had GBBS isolated from venous blood. The overall incidence of GBBS puerperal sepsis is not known; however, at Charity Hospital in New Orleans, approximately 10% of the cases of postpartum sepsis involve GBBS.

Puerperal sepsis secondary to GBBS infection is strongly reminiscent of the childbed fever described by Semmelweis. Patients who develop GBBS puerperal sepsis usually manifest signs and symptoms of infection early in the puerperium. Initially, within the first 24 hours after delivery, there is a rapid increase in oral body temperature, peaking at an average temperature of 38.5°C, with a concomitant rise in pulse rate. Abdominal distention secondary to an adynamic ileus occurs, which is a result of peritonitis of the pelvis and lower abdomen. The increase in abdominal girth causes an elevation of the diaphragm, with a resulting tachypnea. The uterus, adnexa, and parametrial areas are exquisitely tender on palpation and motion of the cervix. The patient may develop shaking chills. The lochia is usually serosanguineous, not purulent, nor is it malodorous. Patients in whom treatment is delayed may deteriorate rapidly because of the fulminant nature of this disease. Dissemination appears to occur rapidly by way of hematogenous and lymphatic routes. Bacteremia, urinary tract infection, and wound infections are frequently found in patients with puerperal sepsis secondary to GBBS infection.

Specimens obtained from the endometrial surface from patients in the immediate postpartum period must be regarded as highly suspicious because bacteria from the lower genital tract may contaminate the specimen. However, when only a single genus is reported, this should be considered a valid specimen. The most common cause of postpartum sepsis, endomyometritis, or endomyoparametritis, is thought to be both an aerobic and anaerobic infection. The polymicrobic nature of these infections, up until the last few years, dictated the use of antibiotic regimens that employed combinations of antibiotics, such as clindamycin and an aminoglycoside. However, the new broad-spectrum agents, such as ticarcillin, mezlocillin, piperacillin, cefoxitin, moxalactam, cefoperazone, and cefotetan, provide coverage for aerobic and anaerobic bacteria. Numerous studies have been reported that have demonstrated that these agents used alone are as efficacious as the combination of clindamycin plus an aminoglycoside in the treatment of postpartum sepsis.[36-38]

Colonization rates of the lower female genital tract by GBBS has been reported to range between 5% and 25% depending on the population and geographical location. Vogel et al studied sera from 200 pregnant women and found that 26% had antibody to GBBS serotype type Ia, 52% had antibody to type Ib, 82% had antibody to type II, and 45% had antibody to type III.[39] Although the colonization rates among newborns may reach as high as 33%, the attack rate ranges between 1 and 4 per 1000 births. However, the mortality rate in infants with early-onset disease (less than 10 days of age) ranges from 58% to 71%, whereas in infants with late-onset disease, the mortality rate is between 14% and 18%.[40] Early-onset neonatal GBBS disease has been most frequently associated with serotypes I and III and has high mortality. The mortality rate is higher for low-birth weight and premature infants. Infants who develop early-onset disease are usually delivered from women whose genital tracts are colonized with GBBS and frequently have had prolonged rupture of amniotic membranes (greater than 12 hours). The infection often mimics hyaline membrane disease or respiratory distress syndrome (RDS).[4] Infected infants develop respiratory distress shortly after birth, with severe apnea and signs of poor vascular perfusion. Bacteria can frequently be isolated from the infant's venous blood, cerebrospinal fluid, urine, pleural fluid, and tracheal aspirate. The chest x-ray is often consistent with that found in an infant with RDS.

Pregnant women who are admitted with premature labor or premature rupture of amniotic membranes should have a cervical specimen taken for the isolation of GBBS. If an amniocentesis is performed, amniotic fluid should be Gram's stained and cultured for aerobes and anaerobes. Several reports have been published documenting the presence of bacteria, GBBS in particular, in amniotic fluid in the presence of intact membranes.[29,41] If gram-positive cocci are seen on Gram's stain, or if GBBS are cultured, then the patient should be treated with penicillin and delivered. If no bacteria are seen on the Gram's stain and if the patient is not delivered, a WBC count should be followed daily. If the patient develops fever with or without a rising WBC and no focus of infection can be found, then chorioamnionitis should be suspected, and the patient should be delivered.

Pregnant women who have a history of fetal wastage should have cervical cultures done beginning at 30 weeks' gestation. Individuals who have positive cultures for GBBS should be treated, and their sexual partners should also be treated. It is difficult to develop criteria for the management of GBBS-colonized women; however, screening for GBBS colonization in a high-risk population is reasonable.

Antibiotic treatment of asymptomatic colonized women has been attempted but was found to be unsuccessful. Initially, the vagina and cervix can be cleared of GBBS following treatment with ampicillin, but they then may become recolonized. Two sources for recolonization exist: inoculation by way of sexual intercourse and fecal contamination of the genitalia. Treatment with ampicillin or penicillin does not rid the rectum of GBBS because of the large number of penicillinase-producing coliforms. Amstey[42] found 5.2% of women admitted to the hospital for pregnancy termination to be colonized with GBBS. None of these women were treated with antibiotics; however, none developed infection. Faro and colleagues (unpublished data) followed 50 women with serial cultures of cervix, throat, and rectum for the isolation of GBBS. Specimens were obtained every four weeks beginning in the first trimester. This group of women remained colonized, and none of the mothers or infants became infected. These findings are in agreement with other studies concerning maternal colonization and postpartum infection or neonatal infection.

Late-onset disease caused by GBBS begins insidiously and is frequently associated with meningitis. These infants usually have no manifestations of infection the first 10 to 12 days of life. Often, these infants are born to women who were not colonized with GBBS, and the obstetric history was unremarkable. Baker and Barrett[40] reported that the ratio of colonization to disease is 100 to 1 in neonates. Other investigators have observed that neonatal colonization increased from 23% at birth to 65% by discharge from the hospital. However, no change in maternal colonization was noted. No inanimate or human reservoir could be found to account for the increase in neonatal colonization. The mortality rate for late-onset GBBS neonatal infection is 25% to 40%, and those who survive often have neurologic sequelae.

REFERENCES

1. Lancefield RC. A serological differentiation of human and other groups of hemolytic streptococci. *J Exp Med.* 1933;57:571.
2. Benedetti TJ, Valle R, Ledger WJ. Antepartum pneumonia in pregnancy. *Am J Obstet Gynecol.* 1982;144:413.
3. Faro S. Group B, beta-hemolytic streptococci and puerperal infections. *Am J Obstet Gynecol.* 1980;139:686.
4. Albow RC, Driscoll SG, Effmann EL, et al. A comparison of early onset group B, streptococcal neonatal infection and the respiratory distress syndrome of the newborn. *N Engl J Med.* 1976;294:65.
5. Phillips GN, Flickes PF, Cohen C, et al. Streptococcal M protein: alpha-helical coiled structure and arrangement on the cell surface. *Proc Nat Acad Sci USA.* 1981;78:4689.

6. Quinn RW, VanderZwaag R, Lowry PN. Acquisition of a group of A streptococcal M protein antibodies. *Pediatr Infect Dis.* 1985;4:373.
7. Fischetti VA, Pany DAD, Trus BL, et al. Conformational characteristics of the complete sequence of Group A streptococcal M6 protein. *Proteins: Structure, Function and Genetics.* 1988;3:60.
8. Hollingshead SK, Fischetti VA, Scott JR. Complete nucleotide sequence of type 6 M protein of the group A streptococcus: repetitive structure and membrane anchor. *J Biol Chem.* 1986;261:1677.
9. Swanson J, Hsw KC, Gotschlich EC. Electron microscopic studies on streptococci. IM antigen. *J Exp Med.* 1969;130:1063.
10. Coligan JE, Kindt TJ, Krause RM. Structure of the streptococcal groups A, A-variant and C-carbohydrates. *Immunochemistry.* 1978;15:755.
11. Beachey EH, Ofek I. Epithelial cell binding of group A streptococci by lipoteichoic acid on fimbriae denuded of M protein. *J Exp Med.* 1976;143:759.
12. Duma RJ, Weinberg AN, Medrek TF, et al. Streptococcal infections. *Medicine.* 1969;48:87.
13. Widdowson JP, Maxted WR, Notley CM, et al. The antibody response in man to infection with different serotypes of group A streptococci. *J Med Microbiol.* 1974;7:483.
14. Gibberd GF. Puerperal sepsis. *J Obstet Gynaecol Br Commonw.* 1966;73:1.
15. Rea WJ, Wyrick WJ. Necrotizing fasciitis. *Ann Surg.* 1970;172:957.
16. Veasy LG, Wiedmeier SE, Orsmond GS, et al. Resurgence of acute rheumatic fever in the inter-mountain area of the United States. *N Engl J Med.* 1986;316:412.
17. Acute rheumatic fever at a Navy training center–San Diego, California. *MMWR.* 1988;37:101.
18. Gaworzewsku E, Coleman G. Changes in the patterns of infection caused by *Streptococcus pyogenes. Epidemiol Infect.* 1988;100:257.
19. Cone LA, Woodard DR, Schlievert PM, Tomory GS. Clinical and bacteriologic observations of a toxic shock-like syndrome due to *Streptococcus pyogenes. N Engl J Med.* 1987;317:146.
20. Schlievert PM, Bettin KM, Watson DW. Production of pyrogenic exotoxin by groups of streptococci: association with group A. *J Infect Dis.* 1979;140:676.
21. Johnson LP, L'Italien JJ, Schlievert PM. Streptococcal pyrogenic exotoxin type A (scarlet fever toxin) is related to *Staphylococcus aureus* enterotoxin B. *MGG.* 1986;203:354.
22. Schlievert PM. Staphylococcal enterotoxin B and toxic-shock syndrome toxin-1 are significantly associated with non-menstrual TSS. *Lancet.* 1986;1:149.
23. Bibler MR, Rowan GW. Cryptogenic group A streptococcal bacteremia: experience at an urban general hospital and review of the literature. *Rev Infect Dis.* 1986;8:941.
24. Ispahani P, Donald FE, Aveline AJ. *Streptococcus pyogenes* bacteremia: an old enemy subdued but not defeated. *J Infect.* 1988;16:37.
25. Stevens DL, Tanner MH, Winship J, et al. Severe group A streptococcal infections associated with a toxic shock-like syndrome and scarlet fever toxin A. *N Engl J Med.* 1989;321:1.
26. Todd J, Rishaut M. Toxic-shock syndrome associated with phage group 1 staphylococci. *Lancet.* 1978;2:1116.
27. Batter T, Dascal A, Canoli K, Curley FJ. "Toxic strep syndrome": manifestation of group A streptococcal infection. *Arch Intern Med.* 1988;148:1421.
28. Horibalova V. *Streptococcus pyogenes* and the toxic shock syndrome. *Ann Intern Med.* 1988;108:772.
29. Vigorita VJ, Pamley TH. Intramembranous localization of bacteria in beta-hemolytic Group B streptococcal chorioamnionitis. *Obstet Gynecol.* 1979;53(suppl):135.
30. Eickhoff TC, Klein JO, Daly AK, et al. Serious infections in adults due to group B streptococci. *Am J Med.* 1976;61:498.
31. Shigeoka AO, Rote NS, Santos JI, et al. Assessment of the virulence factors of group B streptococci: correlation with sialic acid content. *J Infect Dis.* 1983;147:857.
32. Baker CJ, Kasper DL. Correlation of maternal antibody deficiency with susceptibility to neonatal group B, streptococcal infection. *N Engl J Med.* 1976;294:753.
33. Hood M, Janney A, Dameron G. Beta-hemolytic streptococcus group B associated with problems of the perinatal period. *Am J Obstet Gynecol.* 1961;82:809.
34. Finn PD, Holden FA. Observations and comments concerning the isolation of group B beta-hemolytic streptococci from human sources. *Can Med Assoc J.* 1978;103:249.
35. Faro S. Group B streptococcus and puerperal sepsis. *Am J Obstet Gynecol.* 1980;138:1219.
36. Faro S, Sanders CV, Aldridge KE. Use of single agent therapy in the treatment of polymicrobial female pelvic infections. *Obstet Gynecol.* 1982;60:232.
37. Marier R, Faro S, Sander CV, et al. Moxalactam in the therapy of serious infections. *Antimicrob Agents Chemother.* 1982;21:650.
38. Sweet RL, Ledger WJ. Cefoxitin: single-agent treatment of mixed aerobic-anaerobic pelvic infections. *Obstet Gynecol.* 1979;54:193.
39. Vogel LC, Boyer KM, Gadzala GA, et al. Prevalence of type-specific group B streptococcal antibody in pregnant women. *J Pediatr.* 1980;96:1047.
40. Baker CJ, Barrett FF. Transmission of group B streptococci among parturient women and their mothers. *J Pediatr.* 1973;83:919.
41. Faro S, Walker C, Pierson RL. Amnionitis with intact amniotic membranes involving *Streptobacillus moniliformis. Obstet Gynecol.* 1980;55:9S.
42. Amstey MS. Low morbidity in the surgical patient with group B streptococci. *Obstet Gynecol.* 1977;50:428.

C

INFECTIONS CAUSED BY GRAM-NEGATIVE COCCI

Chapter Sixty-Four

Meningococcal Infections

Stefanie Schupp Christian and Patrick Duff

64

Neisseria meningitidis causes several rare but serious diseases in pregnancy. Infection occurs in both endemic and epidemic patterns. The major manifestations of meningococcal disease are acute meningococcemia and meningitis. Less frequent manifestations include pericarditis, endocarditis, septic arthritis, pneumonitis, sinusitis, conjunctivitis, and chronic meningococcemia.

N meningitidis is a fastidious aerobic gram-negative diplococcus. Meningococci can be divided into at least 13 serogroups on the basis of agglutination tests that detect capsular antigens. The major groups are A, B, C, D, X, Y, Z, W-135, and 29-E. These serologic groups can be subclassified into distinct serotypes on the basis of identification of subcapsular antigens.

The natural reservoirs for meningococcus are the nasopharynx and oropharynx. The principal means of transmission is through inhalation of droplets of infected nasopharyngeal secretions. The carrier rate among healthy adults during nonepidemic periods is 2–15% and may rise to 20–40% among close contacts of persons with sporadic cases of meningococcal disease. In closed populations or during epidemics, the carrier rate may increase to 75% or more. Although there are reported cases of individuals harboring *N meningitidis* for years, the carrier state usually is transient, lasting only weeks to months.

Since 1946 endemic rates of meningococcal disease in the United States have been stable at one to three cases per 1000 persons per year. Seasonal variations exist, and the peak incidence occurs in late winter and spring. Endemic disease also shows age-specific attack rates. Children between six months and one year have the highest attack rates, accounting for 46% of cases of meningococcal meningitis and 49% of cases of meningococcemia. However, more than 25% of cases of meningococcemia occur in adults over 20 years of age.[1]

In contrast to the stable rate of endemic disease, there is a cyclic variation in epidemic outbreaks of meningococcal disease. These outbreaks occur approximately every 8 to 12 years and last 4 to 6 years. From 1960 to 1980, meningococcal epidemics exhibited dramatic shifts in seroepidemiology. Recently in the United States, serogroup B has been the most common cause of meningococcal outbreaks, accounting for 50% of cases. Other important groups include serogroups C (20%), W-135 (15%), Y (10%), and A (1–2%). Elsewhere in the world, serogroup A is the most common cause of epidemics of meningococcal infections.[2]

Introduction of meningococcal infection into households is primarily by way of infected adults, and young children tend to be the last colonized. Overt infection, however, is predominantly a disease of infants and children, suggesting that natural immunity is age-dependent. Immunity correlates with the appearance of bactericidal antibodies in serum. Natural immunity results from asymptomatic meningococcal colonization of the nasopharynx. This carrier state leads to formation of antibodies to the infecting strain and the production of cross-reacting antibodies as well. As opposed to carrier state immunity, immunity resulting from meningococcal meningitis or meningococcemia is generally group-specific; thus, the patient remains at risk for infection caused by other serogroups.

The complement system is critical in the defense against both primary and recurrent infection. Deficiencies of C5, C6, C7, and C8 have been associated with recurrent meningococcal infection, even though the affected adults have serum antibody to meningococcus.

In most instances, infection with *N meningitidis* is asymptomatic or associated only with mild upper respiratory symptoms. Dissemination occurs through the bloodstream, and, in some patients, fulminant septicemia develops. In other cases, although the bacteremia is transient, it still leads to localized infections of one or more organ system, particularly the meninges. The tissue injury in meningococcal infection appears to result from the effects of an endotoxin similar to that of the enteric bacilli.[3]

The attack rate among close contacts of individuals with sporadic cases of meningococcal disease is 0.3% to 1.0%, a 300- to 1000-fold increase above that of the general population. In epidemic periods, the attack rate among close contacts may be nearly 100%. Persons at highest risk of contracting meningococcal infections are household contacts or health care personnel who have direct contact with a case and individuals in large groups who live under crowded conditions, such as in military camps and day care centers. Nearly one third of secondary cases occur in the first four days after the index patient is hospitalized.

With appropriate therapy, the survival rate for meningococcal infection is 85–95%. Survival is lower for children under two years of age, for adults over the age of 40, and for patients with meningococcemia. Early sequelae of meningococcal disease, including meningitis, are rare if the initial infection is treated appropriately. Seizures and focal neurologic deficits, which are often noted early in patients with meningitis, are transient and generally resolve. Cranial nerve damage, particularly of the auditory portion of CN VIII, occasionally persists. Late complications, such as communicating hydrocephalus, dural sinus thrombophlebitis, subdural effusions, and chronic adrenal insufficiency, are uncommon, but, of course, extremely serious.[4]

Pregnant women are not at increased risk for infection from *N meningitidis*. Conversely, there is no evidence that pregnancy worsens the prognosis for those who contract the infection.[5]

CLINICAL MANIFESTATIONS

Meningococcal infections may present in several ways. Each of the clinical manifestations will be discussed below. It is important to recognize that these infections are exceedingly rare in pregnancy, and that the literature on meningococcal diseases complicating pregnancy is surprisingly scant. In a review of standard obstetrics texts as well as several critical care texts that focus on care of the obstetric patient, we were unable to identify a single chapter devoted to this topic. Accordingly, we will make specific reference to infection in pregnancy only when specific data are available.

Meningococcemia

Thirty to fifty percent of patients who develop overt meningococcal disease present with meningococcemia without meningitis. Meningococcemia presents as a continuum ranging from a transient mild febrile illness to a fulminant, often fatal, disease. Common prodromal symptoms include cough, headache, and sore throat. In most patients, the prodrome is immediately followed by the onset of fever, chills, nausea, malaise, arthralgias, and myalgias. Infrequently, symptoms resolve spontaneously. More frequently, patients become increasingly ill and manifest high fever, tachycardia, tachypnea, hypotension, and prostration. Three fourths of patients with acute meningococcemia develop a characteristic rash composed of erythematous, nonpruritic blanching macular lesions, 2 to 15 mm in diameter, located primarily on the trunk and extremities. These lesions quickly are followed by a prominent petechial eruption in the same distribution. Rarely, the petechiae may develop into ulcerated purpuric nodules.

Acute Fulminant Meningococcemia

Acute fulminant meningococcal septicemia, or *Waterhouse–Friderichsen syndrome,* occurs in 10% to 20% of patients with meningococcemia and is associated with vasomotor collapse and shock. The onset usually is abrupt and is characterized by profound prostration. The purpuric eruptions enlarge rapidly, resulting in extensive intracutaneous hemorrhage. Early shock may be associated with generalized vasoconstriction and a functional high output cardiac state suggestive of endotoxemia. Subsequently, coma and biventricular failure develop. Disseminated intravascular coagulation also occurs commonly and is responsible for the bleeding diathesis, widespread arterial thrombosis, and adrenal hemorrhage characteristic of this disorder. It is the contention of most authors that massive adrenal hemorrhage contributes to the profound shock and sudden death of the patient with this syndrome.[5] There are very few cases of Waterhouse-Friderichsen syndrome reported in pregnancy. Of those that have been reported, most have resulted in maternal mortality.[5]

Chronic Meningococcemia

The least common of the meningococcemial infections is chronic meningococcemia. This disorder is characterized by fever, headache, rash, arthralgias, and arthritis. Fever and chills begin abruptly and follow an intermittent course in 60% of cases. During afebrile periods, patients look remarkably well. Ninety percent of affected patients have a characteristic rash composed of a generalized polymorphous eruption of maculopapular, erythematous lesions, 2 to 15 mm in diameter. Petechiae and tender erythematous nodules also may be present. Migratory arthralgias and occasional episodes of arthritis occur in two thirds of cases. Splenomegaly is detected in about 20% of cases.

Chronic meningococcemia is thought to result from a unique host–bacterium relationship that permits intermittent recurrent septicemia. If the diagnosis is not made and therapy is not initiated, localized infection such as meningitis, endocarditis, or arthritis ultimately can develop as a complication of the initial infection.

Meningitis

The most common form of localized meningococcal infection is meningitis. Next to *Streptococcus pneumoniae, N meningitidis* is the most common cause of bacterial meningitis in adults. Twenty to forty percent of patients with meningococcal disease have meningitis without clinical evidence of meningococcemia. The most common clinical manifestations are fever, vomiting, headache, confusion, lethargy, and meningismus. In patients with both meningitis and meningococcemia, the characteristic petechial rash is present, and the disease progression tends to be more rapid.

Other Localized Infections

Acute purulent pericarditis is present in 2% of patients with meningococcemia. It also can occur as a primary infection in patients who are not bacteremic. Purulent pericarditis is a serious complication because it frequently causes cardiac tamponade. The typical clinical picture includes a hectic febrile course and progressive cardiac decompensation.

Meningococcal pneumonia is acquired through inhalation of infected respiratory particles. The symptoms are primarily respiratory and progress in an indolent pattern. Pleuritic chest pain and small pleural effusions occur in 20% of affected patients; frank empyema is rare. Radiographically, 80% of cases present as patchy bronchoalveolar infiltrates, and the remaining 20% present as segmental or lobar consolidation. Bacteremia is uncommon in patients with meningococcal pneumonia.

N meningitidis has been isolated with increasing frequency from the genitourinary tract and anal canal of symptomatic and asymptomatic patients of both sexes. Actual symptomatic *urogenital tract infection,* however, is extremely uncommon. When it occurs, there may be a spectrum of illnesses similar to those produced by *Neisseria gonorrhoeae,* including cervicitis, salpingitis, urethritis, epididymitis, and proctitis.

Other rare, localized meningococcal infections include arthritis, conjunctivitis, sinusitis, endophthalmitis, and pleuritis. Joint involvement in meningococcal disease can present as either monoarticular or polyarticular arthritis. Aspirated synovial fluid is typically purulent.

Neonatal Infection

Meningococcal disease in neonates is rare because infants usually are protected from this infection by the transplacental transfer of maternal immunoglobulins. Relative immunity appears to persist up to the third month of life. Therefore, the neonate is likely to become infected only if its mother is immunocompromised.

There is one reported case of meningococcemia in a newborn infant whose mother had a lower genital tract infection due to meningococcus at the time of delivery.[6] Isolated cases of meningococcal conjunctivitis also have been reported. In our institution, we recently treated a case of neonatal meningococcal pneumonia associated with conjunctivitis. We believe this is the first such reported case of early neonatal respiratory infection (M. Tuggy, personal communication).

DIAGNOSIS

In the absence of prior antibiotic therapy, meningococci can be recovered readily from cultures of blood, cerebrospinal fluid, pericardial fluid, synovial fluid, and from fresh skin lesions. Meningococci grow well on solid or semisolid media containing blood, serum, or ascitic fluid, and thrive best at temperatures between 35°C and 37°C in an atmosphere of reduced oxygen tension and 5–10% carbon dioxide. In order to recover meningococci from specimens that contain large numbers of normal flora (for example, cervix, anus, or skin), specimens should be inoculated onto Thayer–Martin medium, which contains vancomycin, polymyxin, and nystatin. This medium is not necessary when culturing specimens that are normally sterile (for example, cerebrospinal, pericardial, or synovial fluid). In these instances, warmed chocolate agar is appropriate. Culture of secretions obtained by transtracheal aspiration is more likely to be diagnostic than is sputum culture.

Gram's stain is slightly less sensitive than culture in diagnosing meningococcal infection. On Gram's stain examination, the organism appears as a gram-negative diplococcus with flattened adjacent sides (Figure 64–1). The organism may be seen in stains from cerebrospinal fluid, pericardial and synovial fluids, aspirates of skin lesions, and the buffy coat of blood from patients with meningococcemia. In meningococcal meningitis, a smear of the spinal fluid is diagnostic in about 50–70% of patients. Diagnosis also can be made using countercurrent immunoelectrophoresis to detect specific meningococcal antigens in infected fluid or serum. The isolation of meningococci from the nasopharynx does not by itself indicate the presence of meningococcal disease.

Peripheral blood leukocyte counts usually are elevated in meningococcal meningitis, most commonly ranging from 12,000 to 40,000/mm.[3] However, in patients with meningococcemia, the leukocyte count may be normal or low. Examination of cerebrospinal fluid in meningococcal meningitis reveals abnormalities typical of pyogenic meningitis. Cerebrospinal fluid pressure and protein are increased. Glucose concentration is often depressed below 35 mg/100 ml. There usually is a pleocytosis ranging up to several thousand cells per mm^3, primarily polymorphonuclear leukocytes. Infected synovial and pericardial fluids are characteristically purulent; leukocyte counts may exceed 50,000/mm^3. Synovial fluid glucose typically is decreased, and the protein concentration is increased.[3]

Coagulation studies in meningococcal disease reflect varying degrees of disseminated intravascular coagulation. In mild coagulopathy, the platelet count is depressed and the prothrombin and partial thromboplastin times are elevated. As the coagulopathy becomes increasingly severe, hypofibrinogenemia, red blood cell fragmentation, increased thrombin time, and elevated levels of fibrin split products are seen.

The principal elements in the differential diagnosis of meningococcal infection are listed in Table 64–1. In differentiating these disorders, careful consideration must be given to the specific clinical features of the illness, laboratory data, travel history, and exposure to animal or insect vectors. In the absence of a clinical picture of meningococcemia, meningitis and other localized infections cannot be attributed to *Meningococcus* without supporting bacteriologic data. The diagnosis of meningococcal disease is unaffected by pregnancy.

MANAGEMENT

Antibiotic therapy should be initiated as soon as meningococcal disease is suspected and should be continued for five to seven days after the patient is afebrile and

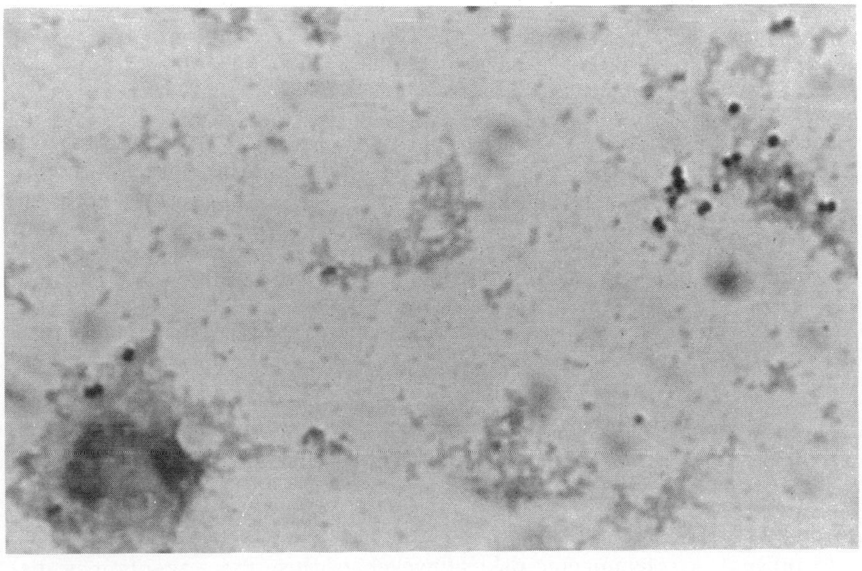

Figure 64–1. Gram's stain of cerebrospinal fluid demonstrates characteristic gram-negative diplococci with flattened adjacent sides. (1000 x). *(Photograph courtesy of Rodney A. Michael.)*

TABLE 64–1. DIFFERENTIAL DIAGNOSIS OF MENINGOCOCCAL INFECTIONS

Viral exanthems, such as echovirus type 9
Rickettsial diseases
Rocky Mountain spotted fever
Epidemic typhus
Brill–Zinsser disease
Infection due to *Streptobacillus moniliformis*
Infection due to *Streptobacillus minus*
Gonococcemia
Septicemia due to *Hemophilus influenzae* type b
Typhoid fever
Acute *Staphylococcus aureus* endocarditis
Vasculitis syndromes
Polyarteritis nodosa
Churg–Strauss syndrome
Anaphylactoid (Henoch–Schoenlein) purpura
Toxic shock syndrome

asymptomatic. The minimum course of therapy should be 10 days.[6] The antibiotic of choice for meningococcal infection is penicillin G. For adults with meningitis, the appropriate dose is 24 million units per day, administered intravenously, in divided doses every two hours. For patients who do not have meningitis, a total daily dose of 5–10 million units appears to be acceptable because it is not necessary to have high concentrations of antibiotic in the cerebrospinal fluid. Primary meningococcal pneumonia that is not associated with bacteremia can be treated with penicillin G in a dose of 600,000 units intramuscularly or intravenously every 8–12 hours.

Intravenous ampicillin in doses of 200–400 mg/kg/day is as effective as penicillin G and can be used if the diagnosis is uncertain and a broader-spectrum antibiotic is preferred. However, when bacteriologic evidence of meningococcal disease is available, antibiotic therapy should be changed to penicillin G because it is less expensive and is less likely to cause alterations in the flora of the bowel and vagina. Because of the high rate of sulfonamide resistance among meningococcal isolates, sulfonamides should not be used alone in the treatment of meningococcal disease unless the patient's isolate is susceptible to these drugs. Moreover, these agents are contraindicated in patients near term because of their association with hyperbilirubinemia of the newborn.

In cases of documented penicillin allergy, chloramphenicol, 100 mg/kg/day, given intravenously in divided doses every six hours may be used. However, chloramphenicol should not be used in term patients because of the theoretical risk of cardiovascular collapse and the gray baby syndrome in exposed infants.

First- and second-generation cephalosporins show incomplete cerebrospinal fluid penetration and thus are poor antibiotic choices for meningococcal infection. The third generation cephalosporins, such as cefotaxime, ceftizoxime, and ceftriaxone, however, are active against meningococci and yield cerebrospinal fluid levels that are adequate to treat meningitis. These antibiotics provide a suitable alternative to chloramphenicol for treating meningococcal meningitis in obstetric patients who are allergic to penicillin.

In addition to antimicrobial therapy, patients with meningococcal infection also require supportive therapy to maintain fluid and electrolyte balance and to prevent respiratory collapse. In patients with shock, visceral perfusion and acid–base status must be maintained. This may be accomplished by supporting intravascular fluid volume and treating cardiac failure. Management of shock is facilitated by Swan–Ganz catheter placement and the judicious use of vasoactive drugs such as dopamine or dobutamine. Digoxin may be necessary in the presence of myocarditis. Coma and respiratory failure require endotracheal intubation and mechanical ventilation.

As noted above, dehydration and hypovolemia are common complications of meningococcal infection. Intravenous fluid resuscitation is a particularly difficult problem in patients who have meningitis and cerebral edema. To prevent exacerbation of the edema, free water must be restricted to no more than 1500 cc/day. Deliberate hyperventilation combined with the administration of mannitol or dexamethasone may be necessary in severe cases in order to prevent brain stem herniation.

Hyperventilation can be accomplished in patients who have endotracheal tubes in place. The partial pressure of carbon dioxide should be maintained between 25 and 30 mm Hg in order to constrict the cerebral vascular beds, thus decreasing intracranial vascular volume. The peak effect is achieved in 2 to 30 minutes. A 20% solution of mannitol, made with 100 g mannitol in 500 ml, 5% dextrose and water, can be given in doses of 1–1.5 gm/kg as an intravenous infusion over 10 to 20 minutes. Therapeutic effects occur within minutes and reach a peak in 90 minutes. Doses can be repeated every four to six hours as needed. The principal risks of treatment with osmotic agents are the development of a marked osmotic diuresis, which can exacerbate dehydration and hyponatremia and, conversely, the development of increased intravascular volume, which can lead to pulmonary edema and congestive heart failure.

A final alternative in managing cerebral edema is the administration of dexamethasone 10 mg intravenously or intramuscularly, followed by 4 mg intravenously, intramuscularly, or orally every six hours. This regimen is less likely to cause the profound fluid shifts noted above.

Disseminated intravascular coagulation requires specific therapy with clotting factors and platelets only if active bleeding exists. Heparin should be given only as a last resort to patients who have persistent bleeding despite appropriate replacement of coagulation factors and platelets and correction of volume deficits.

Prevention of Infection

Prevention of spread of infection during epidemics is a major objective in the management of meningococcal disease. Therefore, prompt chemoprophylaxis is advised for all close contacts of an infected patient. The current recommendation for chemoprophylaxis is rifampin, unless the organism is known to be sensitive to sulfadiazine. Rifampin should be given orally, 600 mg twice a day for two days in adults. For use in pregnancy, rifampin is a category C drug; no controlled studies have linked the use of rifampin with congenital defects.

Sulfonamide resistance among meningococci has varied dramatically in recent years. In 1970, the overall prevalence of sulfonamide-resistant strains of *N meningitidis* was 67%. By 1980, the prevalence had declined to less than 15%. This apparent trend toward increasing sulfonamide susceptibility may be a result of the infrequent use of sulfonamides for prophylaxis against meningococcal disease.[7] The dosage for sulfadiazine in adults is 1 g twice a day for two days.[8] Sulfonamides do not appear to pose a significant teratogenic risk. However, because these agents may displace bilirubin from plasma protein binding sites, they have been associated with neonatal hyperbilirubinemia.

Minocycline also has been used as an alternative to either rifampin or sulfadiazine. However, the tetracyclines are category D drugs and should not be used in pregnancy. Possible adverse effects from use of tetracyclines during pregnancy include staining of fetal teeth and bones, maternal liver toxicity, and possible minor congenital defects including hypospadias, inguinal hernias, and limb hypoplasia.[9]

Systemic antimicrobial therapy of meningococcal disease does not reliably eradicate nasopharyngeal carriage of *N meningitidis.* Therefore, it is also important to give chemoprophylaxis to the index patient before discharge from the hospital.

A quadrivalent polysaccharide vaccine against disease caused by *N meningitidis* serogroups A, C, Y, and W-135 has been developed and is currently licensed in the United States. The vaccine has not been proven to be protective in children less than 18–24 months of age. However, it is effective for older children and adults and can be used to control epidemics. Specific monovalent vaccines against serogroups A and C have been studied and have been found to have an efficacy of 85–90%. Similar studies for the group Y and W-135 polysaccharides are not available.

Routine vaccination of the general population is not recommended. However, the vaccine has been shown to be useful during outbreaks caused by serogroups represented in the vaccine. In an outbreak, the serogroup should be determined and the population at risk should be defined and vaccinated. In addition, routine immunization is recommended for individuals at particularly high risk, such as those with terminal complement deficiencies and those with anatomic or functional asplenia. Vaccination also may benefit travelers to countries where meningococcal disease is endemic or where frequent epidemics occur, such as sub-Saharan Africa. Updated information on recent epidemics can be obtained from travelers' clinics, state health departments, and the Centers for Disease Control.

The vaccine is administered as a single 0.5 mL subcutaneous dose and can be given at the same time as other vaccines. Adequate antibody levels are achieved within 10 to 14 days after vaccination, but decline markedly during the first three years after administration. Revaccination may be indicated for individuals at high risk of infection, such as children who were first immunized at less than four years of age. The need for revaccination in older children and adults remains unclear.

On theoretical grounds, the use of meningococcal vaccine in pregnancy has been discouraged because of animal studies that showed that pneumococcal polysaccharide vaccine given to infant mice produced immune tolerance. Extensive vaccination with polysaccharide vaccine during a large epidemic of serogroups A and C meningococcal disease in Brazil during 1974–1975 allowed evaluation of the vaccine in pregnant women during an epidemic. Analysis of that data demonstrated that children born to mothers vaccinated during gestation, regardless of the trimester of vaccination, were not immunotolerant to groups A and C vaccine at six months of age.[10,11] Based on these data, vaccination with licensed meningococcal polysaccharide vaccines should not be withheld from pregnant women considered to be at high risk of contracting meningococcal infection.

REFERENCES

1. Surveillance Summary of CDC. Bacterial meningitis and meningococcemia—United States, 1978. *MMWR.* 28:276.
2. Recommendation of the Immunization Practices Advisory Committee (ACIP). Meningococcal vaccines 1985. *MMWR.* 34:255.
3. Beaty H. Meningococcal infections. In: Petersdorf R, Adams R, et al, eds. *Harrison's Principles of Internal Medicine.* 9th ed. New York, NY: McGraw-Hill, 1980:935.
4. Rubenstein E, Federman D, eds. *Scientific American Medicine.* New York, NY: Scientific American Inc; 1985:1.
5. Polayes SH, Ohlbaum C, Winston H. Meningococcus meningitis with massive hemorrhage of the adrenals (Waterhouse-Friderichsen syndrome) complicating pregnancy with pre-eclamptic toxemia. *Am J Obstet Gynecol.* 1953;65:192.
6. Sunderland WA, Harris HH, Spence DA, Lawson HW. Meningococcemia in a newborn infant whose mother had meningococcal vaginitis. *J Pediatr.* 1972;81:856.
7. Band JD, Chamberland ME, Platt T, et al. Trends in meningococcal disease in the United States, 1975–1980. *J Infect Dis.* 1983;148:754.
8. Meningococcal Disease Surveillance Group. Meningococcal disease: secondary attack rate and chemoprophylaxis in the United States, 1974. *JAMA.* 235:261.
9. Briggs G, Bodendorfer T, Freeman R, Yaffe S. *Drugs in Pregnancy and Lactation—A Reference Guide to Fetal and Neonatal Risk.* Baltimore, MD: Williams & Wilkins; 1983:322,339,344.
10. McCormick JB, Gusmao HH, Nakamura S, et al. Antibody response to serogroup A and C meningococcal polysaccharide vaccines in infants born of mothers vaccinated during pregnancy. *J Clin Invest.* 1980;65:1141.
11. Carvalho A, Giampaglia CM, Kimura H, Pereira OA. Maternal and infant antibody response to meningococcal vaccination in pregnancy. *Lancet.* 1977; 2:809.

Chapter Sixty-Five
Gonococcal Infections

Charles H. Livengood III

65

MATERNAL ASPECTS

Neisseria gonorrhoeae, the gonococcus, is one of the classic sexually transmissible organisms. As such, it is acquired by the intimacy of sexual activity or may be passed on to a fetus by an infected mother. Inoculation of mucosal surfaces with a columnar epithelium (endocervix, rectum, pharynx, urethral structures, conjunctiva) or the immature squamous epithelium of the premenarchal vagina results in primary infection of these sites. Such mucosal infection constitutes *gonorrhea,* a name conceived by Galen in 130 A.D., when male urethritis was thought to be the only manifestation of the disease. The word is derived from the Greek *gono* (seed) and the German *rhein* (to flow). Gonorrhea, not itself a benign disease, can be complicated by contiguous, hematogenous, or possible lymphatic spread of the organisms to generate upper genital tract infection in men and women, perihepatitis in women, fetal infection after rupture of membranes, and disseminated gonococcal infection with involvement of almost any organ. Despite the prolonged familiarity of medical science with this organism and predictions of its total eradication when penicillin became available, it continues to flourish today.

Etiology

N gonorrhoeae was first identified in male urethral exudate by Neisser in 1879; it was isolated by Leistikow in 1882. The currently utilized sugar fermentation profiles were identified by Elser and Huntoon in 1909. The organism occurs as a gram-negative oval or biscuit-shaped coccus 0.8 by 0.6 μm and is usually found in pairs. It is nonmotile, has no capsule, and produces an endotoxin lethal to laboratory animals. The gonococcus is an exceptionally fastidious organism *in vitro:* it will not tolerate drying or inoculation onto cold medium, it is killed by heat of 42°C in a few hours, and it requires a pH between 7.2 and 7.6. It is a delicate aerobe and facultative anaerobe, to the degree that room air is toxic and a CO_2 concentration of 2–10% is needed for cultivation. It is identified in the laboratory on the basis of its formation of grayish-white, smooth, convex colonies of 0.5–1 mm diameter, Gram's stain characteristics, synthesis of indophenol oxidase, and fermentation of glucose but not maltose, fructose, or sucrose. Gonococci can survive in urethral exudate outside the body on a towel for up to 24 hours and on a glass slide for up to 17 hours. Many of the other *Neisseria* species are oral, vaginal, and bowel commensals with limited pathogenic potential.

Although long neglected, the biology of the gonococcus is currently under intense investigation; available results portray a dynamic, adaptable organism, responsible for changes in the immediate host environment and in world antibiotic use. Kellogg and colleagues[1] identified four colony types of the organism. Types 1 and 2 grow in primary culture from infected specimens; their cells have fine appendages 85Å by 0.5–4.0 μm called *pili,* and they are more virulent than types 3 and 4, which arise during subculture and have no pili. All gonococci are capable of expressing all four types. Volunteers undergoing urethral inoculation with type 2, 3, or 4 organisms yielded type 1 colonies when their infections were recultured. Thus, pili are associated with virulence and have been shown to be involved in organism attachment to mammalian cells and in interference with cell-mediated killing of the organism. However, other properties important to virulence have been identified, including endotoxin and other toxin production and resistance to killing by serum. The latter property probably results from an antigenic structure that requires killing antibody to compete with blocking antibody for access to the organism and is an obligate property of strains causing hematogenous spread of infection.

James and Swanson[2] have demonstrated that gonococci isolated perimenstrually show enhanced trypsin resistance and a tendency to form transparent colonies, whereas those isolated at midcycle are trypsin-sensitive and form opaque colonies; also, trypsin-resistant colonies were more common in young women, and both of these cyclic variations were eliminated in oral contraceptive users. Other workers have evaluated patients with acute pelvic inflammatory disease (PID) and found transparent colonial phenotype among organisms from oviducts and peritoneal fluid and opaque forms in the endocervix. Both groups showed enhanced susceptibility to nonspecific killing by serum of the opaque colony type organisms. Thus, not only do gonococci respond to cervical physiologic changes, but these responses seem to result in enhanced virulence during the perimenstrual phase of the cycle. Variations in substrate requirements (auxotype) have been demonstrated among gonococci but do not seem to affect virulence.

Development of penicillin resistance among gonococci was identified during the 1970s. Two distinct strains of penicillin-resistant gonococci arose simultaneously, one in West Africa and one in the Far East; resistance in both of these strains is the result of plasmid-mediated β-lactamase production, but membrane resistance also exists among other strains. The rapidity of emergence of the Far East strain is remarkable: in 1976 only 0.1% of gonorrhea in Singapore was caused by these organisms, but in 1980 the figure was 30%. During this period the total number of gonorrhea cases doubled. Penicillinase-producing *N gonorrhoeae* (PPNG) arrived in the United States in the spring of 1976, apparently from the Far East. In addition to penicillinase production, gonococci with plasmid-mediated tetracycline resistance have appeared in sporadic US outbreaks. Most dangerous of all, however, are the chromosomally-mediated resistant *N gonorrhoeae* (CMRNG). While the β-lactam and tetracycline resistant strains have maintained susceptibility to other antibiotic agents, the CMRNG have a membrane-mediated mechanism of resistance that makes them impervious to multiple antibiotics. Strains with combinations of resistance mechanisms have been described. The annual US incidence of cases involving resistant gonococci increased from about 1000 in 1980 to 26,000 in 1987.[3] Thus, *N gonorrhoeae* must be respected as a survivor, a pathogen constantly adapting to its surroundings, and a pathogen unlikely to decline in clinical significance in the near future.

Pathogenesis and Pathology

When gonococci gain access to a columnar epithelium, either by direct inoculation or by spread from a primary focus, they attach avidly to the free surface of the epithelial cells, showing a preference for primary attachment to cilia and microvilli. These appendages of a single cell may become so densely laden with organisms that they resemble a "gonococcal tree;" such attachment is largely dependent on the presence of pili. It has been shown that attachment to urethral epithelium occurs within one hour after inoculation. Ward and coworkers[4] have elucidated subsequent pathogenetic events in elegant experiments with human oviduct organ cultures. They found that three hours after inoculation gonococci anchor to the host cell membrane with bundles of pili. Subsequently, there is pinocytosis of organisms, but only by nonciliated cells. Gonococci then spread to the subepithelial level both by traversing cells after inoculation and by passing through intercellular spaces. Within 24 hours after inoculation, dead and dying epithelial cells begin to slough off their basement membrane; ciliated cells containing no gonococci are lost as early as nonciliated cells with a large burden of intracellular organisms, suggesting effects of gonococcal toxin(s). *In vivo,* polymorphonuclear leukocytes accumulate rapidly at the subepithelial level and kill gonococci, but apparently host immune response does not contribute to endosalpingeal damage. Ciliary activity is lost within a few days after infection, but this is because of loss of ciliated cells rather than a direct effect on cilia themselves.

Harkness[5] has summarized early findings on the pathology of human gonococcal infection. He notes that gonococcal infection tends to be patchy, and that healing of affected areas consists of squamous metaplasia and eventually scarring with contraction and stricturing. The female urethra is lined by a stratified squamous epithelium, and especially after menarche this offers little opportunity for gonococcal invasion; the paraurethral glands (Skene's glands), on the other hand, contain columnar epithelium and drain poorly, and are thus fertile ground for gonococcal infection. Subsequent edema may obstruct the ducts, and a gonococcal paraurethral abscess ensues. Infection of the columnar epithelia of the Bartholin's ducts, endocervix, endometrium, endosalpinx, rectum, and pharynx all seem to follow the course described by Ward[4] in oviduct organ cultures. It is generally believed that canalicular routes are the mechanism of spread of gonococci in the female genital tract, and presently there is no reason to question this concept; nonetheless, gonococci have been observed invading lymphatic channels.

Infection of the premenarchal vagina seems to be a function of an alkaline environment in the absence of fermentable glycogen, widened intercellular spaces, and absence of a dense superficial horny layer of anuclear cells. In this setting, gonococci are found among the upper layers of squamous cells but do not penetrate to the basement membrane as in infection of columnar epithelium; a dense inflammatory cell infiltrate does develop at the basement membrane, however. Thus, the basement membrane is not exposed by loss of all overlying epithelial cells, and scarring does not occur.

It is generally accepted that gonococci cause upper genital tract infection in women by luminal migration. Why only 10–17%[6] of women with gonorrhea develop PID is not known, but a combination of host immune status, cervical physiology, and organism virulence is likely to be involved. It is known that gonococci are present in the oviducts only during the early days of PID, during which they are etiologic, and that these organisms are not found in a chronic state among post-PID pelvic adhesions. These findings spawned the currently accepted belief that gonococci pave the way for other pathogens found in PID and that the latter organisms, being more competitive for nutrients or more resistant to host immune mechanisms, subsequently eliminate gonococci from the site as the infection progresses. Sweet and coworkers[7] have shown that these other pathogens arrive in the oviducts very early in gonococcal PID. It should be noted that the term *gonococcal PID* is intended only as an etiologic descriptor, that is, that gonococci are present in the endocervix and thus probably initiated the episode, not that the PID itself is caused solely or even in part by gonococci at the time of diagnosis. The PID-associated perihepatitis has been assumed to result from carriage of organisms leaking from the abdominal ostea of the oviducts to the liver capsule by the general flow of peritoneal fluid toward the right hemidiaphragm. However, recent evidence raises the possibility of lymphatic dissemination of organisms from the pelvis to the liver surface, and failure to culture organisms from the liver surface in many cases leaves open the possibility of a chemical etiology.

The pathogenesis of gonococcal complications of pregnancy is not understood but presently is presumed to result from sequelae of contiguous inoculation of the gestational tissues. In pregnancy, PID is extremely rare, probably because of barrier-type phenomena inhibiting ascension of organisms. The cervical mucous plug of pregnancy, in addition to constituting a formidable physical barrier, contains a 100-fold higher concentration of lysozyme than that found in serum. Also, the uterine cavity is obliterated by the gestational sac by 16 weeks of gestation, further limiting upward migration of organisms.

Disseminated gonococcal infection (DGI) rarely coexists with PID and is reliably caused by gonococci with resistance to nonspecific killing by serum and marked sensitivity to penicillin (these properties vary independently), so that some organism specificity is prerequisite. However, the association of DGI with menses[8], pharyngeal gonorrhea[9], pregnancy[10], and terminal serum complement deficiencies suggests that host properties are involved in pathogenesis as well.

DGI is divided into two stages. The first stage is gonococcemia with skin lesions representing septic infarcts, polyarticular tenosynovitis, myalgias, and other constitutional signs. The skin lesions tend to occur in sites overlying involved distal joints. Histopathology of these skin lesions shows severe small vessel vasculitis and perivascular cuffing by polymorphonuclear leukocytes, intradermal neutrophilic pustules, involvement of deep as well as superficial vessels, pronounced hemorrhage, and microthrombi. Because isolation of gonococci from these lesions have proven elusive, a localized Shwartzman's phenomenon (reaction to endotoxin release from dying organisms) may be operative. Joint involvement in this stage is limited to periarticular inflammation. In the second stage, the process localizes to one or several joints with a frankly purulent synovial effusion, which progresses to irreversible destruction of cartilage if untreated. Increased pressure, acidification, decreased glucose concentration, and release of proteolytic enzymes from inflammatory cells within the joint space probably contribute to pathogenesis of gonococcal arthritis. Renal lesions, myocarditis, and meningitis with a fulminant Waterhouse-Friderichsen syndrome are rare complications of DGI and are not well understood.

Gonococcal infection is not chronic. Urethral infection in men resolves after about eight weeks, and their cultures become negative. Local secretary IgA, serum antibody, and cell-mediated mechanisms participate in eradicating the organism. Although solid immunity is not retained, partial resistance to reinfection does develop, but this may be strain-specific. The affinity of the gonococcus for young people, even when corrected for sexual behavior, suggests development of some degree of resistance.

Epidemiology

Gonorrhea is a major health problem in the United States. In recent years, nearly one million cases of gonorrhea have been reported annually, an incidence that has been stable since 1974 when the strategy of presumptive treatment of high risk persons was instituted; prior to that time, the incidence had been steadily increasing at 10–15% per year. It is probable that only one fourth of cases are reported. The annual national cost of gonorrhea is over $200 million, and if long-term sequelae of PID are considered, the figure is roughly $2 billion (assuming that 60–70% of PID is caused by the gonococcus). Taxpayers continue to bear the burden of these costs; it is, however, encouraging to note that without federally funded gonorrhea control efforts, that burden would have been greater by approximately $150 million annually.[11]

Risk factors for gonorrhea begin and rise with sexual activity; men with five or more sexual partners are at 20-fold greater risk than those with one partner. Nonwhites, the poor, and those from urban areas are at increased risk. The greatest age-specific incidence is in the 20- to 24-year-old group, followed by 15- to 19-year olds. A seasonal variation for gonorrhea exists, with peak incidence in the late summer.

Asymptomatic gonorrhea, presumably the major reservoir of infection, was evaluated by the study of nine million women during 1976; in private clinics, asymptomatic infection was found in 1.6%, and in venereal disease clinics, infection was found in 19%. Among all women with gonorrhea, an estimated 90% have no symptoms. It has been demonstrated that two thirds of men with urethral gonorrhea are inadequately impressed by their infection to seek medical care. Genital transmission of the gonococcus occurs equally from men to women and vice versa. Rates of transmission vary and have been reported from 5% to 20% to 50% to 75%.[12] It seems likely that the number of exposures to an infected person determines the rate of transmission, and it is possible that this may in turn be affected (dependently or independently) by female cervical physiology at the time(s) of exposure.[13] Pharyngeal gonorrhea is found in 20% of women or men practicing fellatio but in only about 4% of those practicing cunnilingus[14] and in fewer than 1% of those not practicing orogenital contact. Homosexual men now form the major source of cases of anorectal gonorrhea. Mouth-to-mouth and mouth-to-genital transmission are not known to occur.

In pregnancy, the prevalence of gonorrhea ranges from 2.5% to 7.5% in the United States. However, reinfection rates after treatment during the same pregnancy are as high as 30%.[15] In a large series, Waters and Roulston[16] reported that 71% of prenatal patients with cervical gonorrhea were asymptomatic, and over half of the remainder had vaginal discharge as their only symptom. Solola and coworkers[17] found anogenital gonorrhea in 11 of 117 gravidas presenting in labor; of those infected, four had had negative prenatal cultures, and seven had been positive, treated, and cure was confirmed. These authors implicate a history of PID as a risk factor for active gonorrhea at delivery and underscore the importance of obtaining repeat cultures near term in high-risk patients. It is of particular interest to note that Corman and coworkers[18] found pharyngeal gonorrhea in 12 of 31 (39%) pregnant women with gonorrhea at any site, and 11 of 12 were positive only from the pharynx. Although the reason for this is not clear, the relative resistance of pharyngeal infection to treatments effective against anogenital gonorrhea suggests that pregnant women at high risk or positive at another site should be evaluated for pharyngeal infection as well. As noted, PID complicating gonorrhea in pregnancy is rare. Acosta and coworkers[19] found 12 examples of gonococcal PID among 5124 consecutive pregnancy admissions, and all of these are not unquestionably documented. In reviewing the literature, Jafari and coworkers[20] found only 19 tubo-ovarian abscesses visually confirmed in pregnant women; all patients were asymptomatic, and none of the abscesses revealed *N gonorrhoeae* on culture.

DGI occurs in fewer than 0.5% of persons with gonorrhea; failure to report most cases of gonorrhea makes calculation of a more exact rate impossible. Although classically a disease of male predominance, the majority (up to 80%) of cases now occur in women. The age-specific incidence parallels that of gonorrhea, peaking in the teens and 20s, and the disease is rare in children. Pregnancy seems to increase the risk of dissemination of gonococci, accounting for 28–40% of patients in most series of DGI; late pregnancy seems to further enhance the risk. Persons with pharyngeal gonorrhea are at distinctly greater risk for dissemination than those with primary infections elsewhere. Other risk factors for DGI are the same as those for gonorrhea.

Manifestations

Male urethral gonorrhea has an incubation period of 3–4 (range 2–14) days. The majority of cases are symptomatic and present as a relatively profuse purulent penile discharge with dysuria. Prior to the advent of antibiotic therapy, 5–20% of these men went on to a unilateral epididymitis, but this complication is now rare. In women, gonorrhea is found in the endocervix, urethra, rectum, and pharynx, in that order of frequency, and the great majority are asymptomatic. Patients with evidence of infection may complain of bump dyspareunia and increased vaginal discharge; a purulent "dirty-yellow" endocervical discharge with or without friability and tenderness can be seen. Urethral infection (primarily the paraurethral glands) may manifest as dysuria, frequency, early-void pyuria, and intromission dyspareunia; on examination, the urethra is usually tender, a drop of pus may be milked from the length of the urethra to the meatus, and inflammatory masses in the periurethral tissue may be found. Hematuria is rare, and bladder mucosal infection is probably extremely rare. Anorectal infection is asymptomatic at diagnosis in two thirds of cases; when present, symptoms consist of burning anal pain, tenesmus, and mucopurulent or bloody discharge. Clinical features of pharyngitis do not correlate with pharyngeal gonorrhea; it is almost exclusively asymptomatic. Constitutional symptoms, signs, and laboratory findings are consistently absent in these primary mucosal gonococcal infections.

Gonococcal PID tends to be a fulminant, acute disease. Fever and leukocytosis are as likely to be found as not, and no reliable constellation of findings can be identified in this complication of endocervical gonorrhea. Perihepatitis (Fitz-Hugh–Curtis syndrome), consisting of inflammation of the liver capsule, is found in about one fourth of patients with PID, whether it is gonococcal or nongonococcal in etiology. The illness manifests as rapid onset of right upper quadrant abdominal pain, often with a pleuritic component and referral to the right shoulder. Transient elevation of liver enzymes in serum and nonvisualization of the gallbladder on oral cholecystogram are not uncommon, and fever, leukocytosis, and elevation of erythrocyte sedimentation rate are usually found. Most patients with perihepatitis, however, are asymptomatic.

Bartholin's gland duct may become infected by *N gonorrhoeae,* and this results in edematous occlusion with accumulation of secretions in the gland. Gonococci and potentially pathogenic vaginal and perineal commensal organisms sequestered within these secretions generate a bartholinitis, which usually presents as a unilateral, exquisitely tender cellulitis posterolateral to the fourchette. Within a week, an abscess evolves and drains spontaneously by way of the perineum, vagina, or rectum, in that order of frequency. Bartholinitis is usually associated with low-grade fever and leukocytosis. The tract heals in one to two weeks, and residual secretory epithelium of the gland may generate a chronic Bartholin's cyst, which may cause dyspareunia or may be asymptomatic. Recurrent bartholinitis is common and, like the primary infection, may or may not involve gonococci. Chronic rectoperineal and rectovaginal fistulas are rare complications.

Manifestations of *N gonorrhoeae* in pregnancy are not fully defined. On the basis of existing data, there is a clear association between endocervical gonorrhea and premature rupture of membranes (PROM). Handsfield and coworkers[21] found that of 14 neonates with gonococci in their orogastric aspirate, 11 resulted from pregnancy complicated by PROM. Of 23 gravidas with gonorrhea in the third trimester, Sarrel and Pruett[22] found eight patients with endocervical gonorrhea and PROM. Charles et al[23] studied pregnant gonorrhea patients and found PROM among 2.5% of those treated and 42% of those not treated. In this study, postpartum febrile morbidity occurred at a rate of 5.8% among those treated for gonorrhea and at 28% in the untreated, linking active gonorrhea to postpartum metritis. Amstey and Steadman[24] showed a significant correlation between both premature and prolonged rupture of membranes in pregnant patients with gonorrhea when compared to uninfected controls. Gonorrhea has also been weakly associated with septic abortion; its role in premature labor and other pregnancy complications awaits investigation.

DGI is associated with pregnancy in up to 40% of cases, and pregnancy with pharyngeal gonorrhea, which in turn carries a higher risk of DGI. There seems not to be any consistent temporal relationship between acquisition of gonorrhea and onset of DGI. DGI is characterized by the acute onset of symptoms, consisting of fever, chills, migratory arthralgias, myalgias, and polyarticular tenosynovitis-periarthritis (most commonly involving wrist or ankle) in the majority of patients. Some patients may display a frank arthritis early in the disease, and of these one third each are mono- , oligo- , and polyarticular.[25] One half of patients will present with a characteristic rash, most commonly found overlying affected distal joints, consisting of 5–20 petechial, papular, pustular, or hemorrhagic lesions, which are painful and evolve to central necrosis. This is the first stage of gonococcemia, and occurs in women within one week of the onset of menses in 50% of cases. Subsequently, and sometimes without history consistent with bacteremia stage, frank purulent arthritis develops, involving a mean of 2.6 joints. The upper limb joints are more commonly involved than the lower, and wrists, knees, and hands are the most frequent sites. These patients show evidence of systemic toxicity, with lassitude, fever, and leukocytosis; the picture of septic shock is uncommon. Five to 10% of patients will present in a "transition phase" with evidence of both gonococcemia and septic arthritis. The severity of illness correlates with the amount of joint leukocytosis. Failure of treatment of gonococcal arthritis results in irreversible joint damage in the majority of adult cases.

Diagnosis

The diagnosis of gonococcal infection rests almost entirely on isolation of the organism from properly procured and processed specimens on appropriate media. Serologic diagnosis of gonococcal infections is in its infancy but may evolve into an important modality.

The use of Gram's stain for diagnosis of infections caused by *N gonorrhoeae* was appropriate prior to the advent of selective media and our current understanding of factors important to the sensitive cultivation of the organism. The technique has only 50% sensitivity under the best of circumstances, with an experienced microbiologist investing 30 minutes in the examination of each slide. Specificity is confounded by the presence of other *Neisseria* species and gram-negative coccobacilli (*Moraxella* species, *Veillonella* species, excessively decolorized *Streptococcus* species, and so on) in the lower genital tract; additionally, in women being evaluated for acute pelvic pain, it must be remembered that PID complicates endocervical gonorrhea in only 10–17%, so that even the true positive finding of gonococci on Gram's stain of endocervical swabbings does not ensure that the abdominal process is PID. A presumptive diagnosis of gonorrhea based on the finding of gram-negative intracellular diplococci with a biscuit or kidney bean shape is probably justified only in male urethritis or at facilities with severely limited resources.

Endocervical swabbing for culture for *N gonorrhoeae* is the best single approach for screening and evaluating women suspected of upper genital infection and those with signs of cervicitis. Women with symptoms of dysuria, frequency, urgency, or expressible pus from the urethra should undergo intraurethral swabbing, as should men with these findings and men being screened. Anorectal symptoms require swabbings of that area, which requires that the columnar epithelium of the rectum be sampled. In bartholinitis, endocervical swabbings should be obtained if pus from the abscess is not available; if it is, both should be sampled. Because pharyngeal infection is usually asymptomatic, considerably less responsive to therapy than genital infection, common among pregnant women with gonorrhea, and associated with DGI more often than mucosal infection at other sites, physicians must consider obtaining pharyngeal swabbings for culture among high-risk patients who are pregnant, practicing fellatio, have any pharyngeal symptoms (sore throat) or signs, or have gonococcal infection at any other site.

Procuring a specimen for gonococcal culture requires vigorous swabbing of the affected epithelium because of the adherence property of the organism. Swabs should be immediately rolled in a Z pattern onto the surface of chocolate agar and Thayer–Martin or Martin–Lewis agar plates warmed to room temperature. Subsequently, drying, thermal shock, and atmosphere low in CO_2 must be avoided; this can be accomplished by placing the plates in a candle jar or one of the commercially available systems that provide for an atmosphere enriched in CO_2 and moisture within a few minutes after inoculation. Delivery to the laboratory for incubation under optimal conditions should be accomplished at least daily.

Several details of the diagnosis of gonorrhea by isolation of the organism, in addition to proper specimen handling, are of critical importance but not widely recognized. Important work by Johnson, Holmes, and their colleagues[26] showed that a single endocervical specimen missed one half the cases of gonorrhea and that the majority of this effect resulted from sampling near the time of ovulation (cycle days 16–20). The midcycle false-negative rate was offset by a disproportionately high number of positive cultures obtained during the menses. Physicians must be circumspect about ruling out the possibility of endocervical gonorrhea on the basis of a single negative culture, especially if that culture was obtained at midcycle. Next, cultures obtained after therapy to confirm cure must include a rectal specimen along with a specimen from the sites originally positive; 25% of treatment failures are positive only from the rectum. Finally, the concentrations of vancomycin and trimethoprim found in media selective for gonococci (Thayer–Martin and Martin–Lewis) are high enough to inhibit some strains of gonococci. Thus, a chocolate agar plate should always be inoculated as well, and the selective media are not recommended for specimens from sites where growth of commensal flora is not expected (that is, urethra, joint fluid).

The diagnosis of DGI is usually made by a suggestive clinical picture, especially the typical rash, in association with a positive culture for the gonococcus from the urethra, pharynx, rectum, or endocervix; all four of these sites must be sampled in women suspected of DGI. Blood cultures are usually positive in those few patients presenting within 48 hours of the onset of illness but are rarely so in the later septic joint stage. Culture of exudate from skin lesions is rarely positive, but fluorescent antigonococcal antibody staining of exudate and culture of lesion biopsies are positive in over one half of cases. Only one half of septic joint aspirates will be culture-positive in DGI. The differential diagnosis of DGI is formed primarily by acute rheumatic fever and Reiter's syndrome. In the former, temperature is usually higher (greater than 103°F) than in DGI, and skin lesions will differentiate the two when present; in the latter, conjunctivitis, gradual onset, less pronounced fever, and absence of tenosynovitis and migrating polyarthralgia are hallmarks in discriminating it from DGI. It has been proposed that 600,000 units of aqueous procaine penicillin G, given intramuscularly twice daily in the absence of antipyretic therapy, will result in marked improvement in patients with DGI within 48 hours but will change minimally if at all the course of patients with acute rheumatic fever or Reiter's syndrome. If aspirin is then added to the regimen of those unresponsive to penicillin, persons having acute rheumatic fever will become asymptomatic within hours, whereas patients with Reiter's syndrome will remain ill.

The diagnosis of PID complicating endocervical gonorrhea is a presumptive one unless the inflammatory process of the upper genital organ is viewed directly at laparoscopy or laparotomy. Such a diagnosis is justified if complaints of pelvic pain can be localized to the uterus or adnexae on bimanual pelvic examination in the absence of compelling evidence of another process. Vital signs, white blood count, erythrocyte sedimentation rate, and specific ancillary symptoms and signs are neither sensitive nor specific in the diagnosis of PID. The differential diagnosis is that of conditions causing pelvic pain in women and includes primarily ectopic gestation, chronic pelvic adhesive disease, endometriosis externa, ovarian tumors with or without torsion, uterine myomata, appendicitis, disease of the bowel and urinary tract, heavy metal intoxication, and porphyria. Fitz-Hugh–Curtis syndrome is usually diagnosed on the basis of pain and tenderness in the right upper quadrant of the abdomen in a patient thought to have PID. A friction rub may be heard over the liver in some patients. At laparoscopy, the diagnosis can be made by visualizing red and yellow mottling of the liver surface (unpublished data). Primary disease of the liver parenchyma, biliary system, and right lung must be considered in the differential diagnosis.

Treatment

The evolution of resistant strains of *N gonorrhoeae* during recent years has radically changed the therapy of gonococcal infections. A harbinger of our present situation is found in the 24-fold rise in the recommended penicillin dosage for genital gonorrhea during the period 1948–1985, from 200,000 to 4.8 million units. Now, for the first time, authorities[27] recommend that penicillins should be used only in uncomplicated gonorrhea and in areas routinely free of resistant strains of gonococcus, and when susceptibility testing and comprehensive test-of-cure evaluations are employed. In these circumstances, familiar regimens may be used: amoxicillin 3.0 g or ampicillin 3.5 g by mouth or aqueous procaine penicillin G, 4.8 million units intramuscularly, each preceded by probenecid 1 g orally.

For many situations now, ceftriaxone 250 mg intramuscularly as a single dose without probenecid is recommended for genital gonorrhea. Specifically, this regimen is clearly the treatment of choice in complicated gonorrhea (PID, DGI), primary treatment failures, gonorrhea in children, and for patients from areas experiencing episodes of resistant gonococcal strains. For patients intolerant of ceftriaxone, spectinomycin 2 g as a single intramuscular injection should be substituted; it is recommended that this substitution be made only when there is a history of specific cephalosporin allergy or history of anaphylactic response to penicillins, not when there is only a history of nonspecific reaction to penicillins.

For pharyngeal and anorectal gonorrhea, the same ceftriaxone regimen is clearly preferable. In pharyngeal gonorrhea, failure rates for other antibiotics are high; for example, the parenteral penicillin G dose will fail in about 10%, the ampicillin oral regimen in over 50%, and spectinomycin in over 25%. Anorectal gonorrhea also tends to be more resistant to treatment than genital infection. For gonococcal ophthalmitis, ceftriaxone 1 g daily for five days, either IM or IV, is recommended, along with buffered saline irrigation and consultation with an ophthalmologist. For DGI, ceftriaxone 1 g IV daily for seven days is recommended.

Pregnancy requires no deviation from the guidelines offered above, because no teratogenic effects of penicillin, procaine, probenecid, ceftriaxone, or spectinomycin are known.

The physician must bear in mind that administration of the appropriate antibiotic represents only partial treatment for gonorrhea, because there are four additional requirements for complete treatment. First, treatment for chlamydial infection must also be given because the coinfection rate approaches 50% in some populations; doxycycline 100 mg orally twice daily for at least seven days is suggested, and erythromycin base or stearate 1 g daily in divided doses for 14 days in pregnancy. Second, the patient must be made to understand that all sexual partners must be effectively treated, and that she will almost certainly be reinfected if they are not. Third, there has been an alarming rise in the rate of syphilis among women in recent years, and while the parenteral penicillin regimen used in the past was effective against incubating syphilis, spectinomycin is not and it is not known whether ceftriaxone is; a syphilis serology three months after treatment with either of the latter two regimens is suggested for the present. Fourth, a test-of-cure culture four to seven days after treatment remains necessary from all sites originally positive and from the rectum. Finally, it must be remembered that the ground we have gained with respect to gonorrhea control is largely a result of presumptive treatment strategies, which remain as important now as ever.

Prevention

Condoms provide reliable prophylaxis against the transmission of gonorrhea. Although the diaphragm will prevent acquisition and transmission of endocervical disease, spread of female urethral, anorectal, and pharyngeal infection will not be affected. The risk of PID complicating endocervical gonorrhea is diminished by 50% by oral contraceptive use, probably a reflection of chronic progestational influence on the cervical mucus. Intrauterine contraceptive devices should be avoided by those at high risk for, or with a history of, gonorrhea.

In vitro there is a profound inhibitory effect of nonoxynol 9 and other spermicides in topical contraceptives on gonococci. Additionally, the incidence of recurrent endocervical gonorrhea seems to be reduced by use of a topical contraceptive agent containing phenylmercuric acetate. The extent to which topical contraceptives protect against transmission of gonorrhea is not yet known with certainty. However, the presence of a 1% nonoxynol 9-containing gel in the vagina does not diminish the sensitivity of endocervical culture for the gonococcus or eradicate the organism over the short term (unpublished data).

Conscientious screening or presumptive treatment of high-risk individuals, administration of effective treatment to those infected, confirmation of cure, and treatment of all sexual partners of those infected are the basis of control of gonorrhea.

FETAL ASPECTS

Pathogenesis and Pathology

As noted, incomplete study has been devoted to the effects of the gonococcus on pregnancy or the fetus. Available data strongly support an association between endocervical gonorrhea and premature rupture of the membranes and premature delivery, although these may not be independent variables. There are no reports to suggest that transplacental or transamniotic infection of the fetus or amniotic fluid occurs; rather, the fetus acquires the organism by contiguous spread after rupture of the membranes, so that intrauterine as well as intrapartum fetal inoculation occurs. Portals of entry appear to be the fetal eye and possibly the bowel, but primary infection of the lung by aspiration has not been documented; the neonatal vagina is influenced by maternal estrogens and is thus not subject to infection. DGI in neonates has been shown to originate from conjunctival and rectal infections, but in most studies the site of primary infection is unclear. The skin lesions typical of DGI in the adult have not been described in neonatal infection, but it seems unlikely that this represents a difference in its pathogenesis. Funisitis and amnionitis are usually found in association with fetal infection but have no unique pathologic characteristics. The histopathogenesis of gonococcal ophthalmia neonatorum is as described for adult epithelial infection.

Epidemiology

The advent of silver nitrate topical prophylaxis against gonococcal ophthalmia neonatorum (GON) has dramatically reduced the incidence of clinical expression of neonatal gonococcal infection. In 1880, 10% of children born in Europe developed GON except among those in whose eyes Crede instilled a 2% solution of silver nitrate, where the rate of GON was only 1% and later fell to .03%. In the United States, 28% of children entering schools for the blind in 1908 had blindness resulting from GON, and the figure fell to 7% by 1941, when 46 states required 1% $AgNO_3$ prophylaxis. By 1959, the use of modern antibiotics had dropped the figure to less than 0.1%. Immediately prior to the institution of $AgNO_3$ prophylaxis in New York City in the 1950s, GON occurred in 183 in 100,000 live births, and thereafter fell 92% to 14 in 100,000. Although rates of GON have risen with the increase in frequency of maternal disease since then, it remains a relatiely rare disease. Male children are twice as likely to develop GON as females. Approximately 50% of mothers with genital gonorrhea will transmit the infection to their infants during the interval between rupture of membranes and delivery. Neonatal DGI is a very rare disease, with only a few cases reported in the antibiotic era.

Manifestations

Maternal gonorrhea during pregnancy, if treated and not reacquired, has no adverse effect on the fetus or newborn.

Gonococcal ophthalmia usually manifests at 2–5 days of age, although two thirds of cases begin after three days, when mother and infant have been discharged from the hospital if all else is well. Onset after eight days is rare, and onset after 12 days implies postpartum infection. The infant develops a tense bilateral blepharoedema with a profuse purulent ophthalmic discharge. Originally involving the eyelids, the infection rapidly spreads to the cornea as well. Once the cornea is involved, permanent damage to it is sustained in the form of ulceration with residual nebulae, perforation with infection and residual synechiae of the anterior chamber, and occasionally panophthalmitis requiring enucleation. Clearly, prompt diagnosis and treatment are critical in the management of this devastating infection. Interestingly, asymptomatic GON has been reported as well but apparently was not acquired intrapartum.

Neonatal DGI almost always presents as a septic arthritis. Holt[28] reported 26 cases of gonococcal arthritis in neonates in 1905, but only two had onset in the first month of life; 14 of these infants died from the infection. In Cooperman's review[29] of 53 nosocomial cases of gonococcal arthritis in 1927 (transmitted apparently by rectal thermometers), there were no deaths and a few infants with joint sequelae, all of which involved the hip. Although rash is described in these infants, the description is not that of the pustular, necrotic lesions seen in the gonococcemic stage of adult DGI. Mortality from neonatal DGI has not occurred since penicillin has been used for treatment. Kohen[30], in reviewing this disease in the postantibiotic era, notes that most infants present with nonspecific signs (irritability, poor feeding, and fever) for several days prior to the appearance of septic joint, and all are within the first month of life. He notes that most of these infants have a low-grade fever, and some are afebrile; there is leukocytosis from 10,200/mm^3 to 30,350/mm^3. Multiple joint involvement was seen in most of these babies, and knees and ankles were most commonly involved, although small joint involvement was seen as well.

Rhinitis, fetal death *in utero* 1 day after premature rupture of membranes (PROM), and meningitis have also been ascribed to gonococcal infections in neonates, and the organism has been implicated in sepsis and pneumonia.

Diagnosis

The diagnosis of GON must be entertained in any infant thought to have chemical conjunctivitis as a result of $AgNO_3$ instillation that appears more severe than usual during the first 24 hours of life or that begins, persists, or progresses at all beyond that time. Relative mean times of onset for the various causes of neonatal conjunctivitis are presented in Table 65–1. Although these temporal relationships are useful, their use must be tempered by the recollection that GON may occur at any time in the neonatal period and that its disastrous consequences can be avoided consistently but only by rapid institution of therapy. It is known that one in five infants with no evidence of conjunctivitis harbors potentially pathogenic bacteria in the eye during the first few days of life. Thus, when bacteria other than *N gonorrhoeae* are isolated from the conjunctiva of an infant with ophthalmia, these are not necessarily the etiology of the infection. Additionally, the high rate of maternal coinfec-

TABLE 65–1. ETIOLOGIES OF OPHTHALMIA NEONATORUM, LISTED IN DECREASING ORDER OF FREQUENCY

Etiology	Usual Time of Onset After Birth
Chemical conjunctivitis (silver nitrate)	6–24 h
Chlamydia trachomatis (TRIC agent)	>5 days
Neisseria gonorrhoeae	2–5 days
Staphylococcus aureus	4 days–3 weeks
Other bacteria	Variable
Herpes simplex	2 days–3 weeks

From Sandstrom et al,[33] with permission.

tions by *Chlamydia trachomatis* and *N gonorrhoeae* suggests that the finding of the former in neonatal conjunctivitis does not rule out, and in fact may enhance, the possibility of gonococcal infection as well. Although the identification of gram-negative intracellular diplococci on microscopic examination of conjunctival swabbings may make the physician more comfortable with the initiation of therapy directed against a gonococcal etiology, failure to initiate such treatment on the basis of absence of these organisms should be undertaken with extreme caution. It is wise to initiate therapy for GON in all infants with neonatal conjunctivitis because of the rapidly destructive potential of the disease. Conjunctival swabbings should be inoculated onto chocolate and Martin–Lewis or Thayer–Martin media for isolation of *N gonorrhoeae;* therapy may be amended later if cultures are negative.

The diagnosis of DGI of the neonate is suspected in any infant with septic arthritis and is confirmed by isolation of *N gonorrhoeae* from synovial fluid. Prior to therapy, cultures from blood, oropharynx, rectum, and conjunctivae should be obtained; in the event of synovial fluid Gram's stain suggestive of gonococci but negative by culture, isolation of *N gonorrhoeae* from one or more of these sites is adequate for diagnosis. All of these infants should undergo lumbar puncture on admission to provide cerebrospinal fluid for examination and culture for gonococci and other bacteria. The differential diagnosis includes traumatic and other bacterial causes.

Infants born to women with PROM or the development of intrapartum chorioamnionitis should have orogastric aspirate cultured for the gonococcus as well as other bacteria. The usefulness of cultures from other sites (rectum, vagina, external ear canal, conjunctiva, blood, umbilicus) is presently a matter of opinion.

Treatment

Gonococcal ophthalmia neonatorum is a highly infectious process until at least 24 hours of therapy have been given. Infants with this diagnosis should be admitted to the hospital and kept in isolation for the first day of therapy. Therapy should consist of ceftriaxone 25–50 mg/kg body weight IV or IM for 7 days. Affected eyes should be irrigated with saline or buffered ophthalmic solution hourly until the purulent exudate is resolved, and if only one eye is involved, the other should be covered with a patch during this interval to avoid cross infection, although this is unlikely after the initiation of therapy. Topical antibiotics are neither effective nor indicated when parenteral therapy is used. Both parents of the infant must be treated, and examination and conjunctival culture of siblings is indicated.

Neonatal gonococcal arthritis should be treated with hospitalization and administration of ceftriaxone 50 mg/kg body weight IV or IM daily for at least seven days. Affected joints should be repeatedly aspirated as long as effusion accumulates. Arthrotomy and antibiotic joint irrigation are not indicated. Although Cooperman[29] ascribed much of his success to joint immobilization, this technique is not currently recommended. Documentation of at least one negative culture from all sites originally positive is strongly recommended prior to termination of therapy.

Prevention

The effectiveness, in the prevention of GON, of 1% silver nitrate instilled into the eyes of every newborn in the delivery room is beyond question. In a comprehensive review, Rothenberg[31] notes a cumulative failure rate of 0.063% with this method. Holmes[32] suggests that most failures result from *in utero* establishment of GON after rupture of the membranes, irrigation of the eyes with saline (especially if this is done sooner than 15 seconds after application of $AgNO_3$), postpartum acquisition of the infections, or erroneous labeling of chlamydial conjunctivitis as gonococcal infection. Objections to the use of silver nitrate prophylaxis consist of the occurrence of failures, the almost inevitable chemical conjunctivitis it causes during the first day of life, and the serious corneal injury that results from mistaken use of solutions of higher concentration. Most important, however, is the failure of $AgNO_3$ to prevent neonatal conjunctivitis caused by *C trachomatis,* the most common etiologic agent in this infection in the United States today. Thus, currently recommended for prevention of GON is instillation of 0.5% erythromycin or 1% tetracycline ointment immediately after birth, without rinsing. These agents are highly effective against gonococcal and chlamydia conjunctivitis, do not cause chemical irritation, do not carry the risk of sensitization to the drug that topical administration of penicillin does, and have a smaller chance of technical error because rinsing is not performed. However, they are not effective against established infection or infection at other sites by either organism. Although other antimicrobials may prove equally effective, bacitracin has been shown to be little better than no prophylaxis against gonococcal infection.

Infants born to mothers having anogenital gonorrhea and those who are asymptomatic but have a positive screening culture (done for PROM, prematurity, or intrapartum chorioamnionitis) should be treated with a single intramuscular or intravenous dose of ceftriaxone 125 mg; for low-birth weight infants, 25–50 mg/kg body weight is sufficient. Topical ophthalmic prophylaxis does not protect these neonates from infection at other sites. These infants should be followed closely during the neonatal period, and prolonged therapy as described above instituted immediately if a clinical infection emerges.

REFERENCES

1. Kellogg DS Jr, Peacock WL Jr, Deacon WE, et al. *Neisseria* gonorrhoeae: I virulence genetically linked to colonal variations. *J Bacteriol.* 1963;85:1274.
2. James JF, Swanson J. Color/opacity colonial variants of *Neisseria gonorrhoeae* and their relationship to the menstrual cycle. In: Brooks GF, Gotschlich EC, Holmes KK, et al, eds. *Immunobiology of Neisseria Gonorrhoeae.* Washington, DC: American Society for Microbiology; 1978:338.
3. Centers for Disease Control. Antibiotic-resistant strains of *Neisseria gonorrhoeae.* MMWR. 1987;36(suppl 5):1.
4. Ward ME, Watt PJ, Robertson JN. The human fallopian tube: a laboratory model for gonococcal infection. *J Infect Dis.* 1974;129:650.
5. Harkness AH. The pathology of gonorrhoeae. *Br J Vener Dis.* 1948;24:137.
6. Rees E, Annels EH. Gonococcal salpingitis. *Br J Vener Dis.* 1969;45:205.
7. Sweet RL, Draper DL, Hadley WK. Etiology of acute salpingitis: influence or episode number and duration of symptoms. *Obstet Gynecol.* 1981;58:62.
8. Holmes KK, Counts GW, Beaty HN. Disseminated gonococcal infection. *Ann Intern Med.* 1971;74:979.
9. Handsfield HH. Disseminated gonococcal infection. *Clin Obstet Gynecol.* 1975;18:131.
10. Brown D. Gonococcal arthritis in pregnancy. *South Med J.* 1973;66:693.
11. Wiesner PJ, Paara WC. Sexually transmitted diseases: meeting the 1990 objectives—a challenge for the 1980s. *Public Health Rep.* 1982;97:409.
12. Holmes KK. Gonococcal infection: clinical, epidemiologic, and laboratory perspectives. *Adv Intern Med.* 1974;19:259.
13. Johnson DW, Holmes KK, Kvale PA, et al. An evaluation of gonorrhea case finding in the chronically infected female. *Am J Epidemiol.* 1969;90:438.
14. Bro-Jorgensen A, Jensen T. Gonococcal pharyngeal infections reported in 110 cases. *Br J Vener Dis.* 1973;49:491.
15. Jones DED, Brame RG, Jones CP. Gonorrhea in obstetric patients. *J Am Vener Dis Assoc.* 1976;2:30.

16. Waters JR, Roulston TM. Gonococcal infection in a prenatal clinic. *Am J Obstet Gynecol.* 1969;103:532.
17. Solola AS, Ryan GM, Ling FW. Gonorrhea during the intrapartum period. *Am J Obstet Gynecol.* 1982;144:351.
18. Corman LC, Levison ME, Knight R, et al. The high frequency of pharyngeal gonococcal infection in a prenatal clinic population. *JAMA.* 1974;230:568.
19. Acosta AA, Mabray CR, Kaufman RH. Intrauterine pregnancy and coexistent pelvic inflammatory disease. *Obstet Gynecol.* 1971;37:282.
20. Jafari K, Vilovic-Kos J, Webster A, et al. Tuboovarian abscesses in pregnancy. *Acta Obstet Gynecol Scand.* 1977;56:1.
21. Handsfield HH, Hodson WA, Holmes KK. Neonatal gonococcal infection I. Orogastric contamination with *Neisseria gonorrhoeae*. *JAMA.* 1973;225:697.
22. Sarrel PM, Pruett KA. Symptomatic gonorrhea during pregnancy. *Obstet Gynecol.* 1968;32:670.
23. Charles AG, Cohen S, Kass MB, et al. Asymptomatic gonorrhea in prenatal patients. *Am J Obstet Gynecol.* 1970;108:595.
24. Amstey MS, Steadman KT. Asymptomatic gonorrhea in pregnancy. *J Am Vener Dis Assoc.* 1976;3:14.
25. Garcia–Kutzbach A, Dismuke SE, Masi AT. Gonococcal arthritis: clinical features and results of penicillin therapy. *J Rheumatol.* 1974;1:210.
26. Johnson DW, Holmes KK, Kvale PA, et al. An evaluation of gonorrhea case finding in the chronically infected female. *Am J Epidemiol.* 1969;90:438.
27. Centers for Disease Control. 1985 STD Treatment Guidelines. *MMWR.* 1985;34(suppl 4):81S.
28. Holt LE. Gonococcus infections in children with special reference to their prevalence in institutions and means of prevention. *NY Med J.* 1905;81:521.
29. Cooperman MB. Gonococcus arthritis in infancy: a clinical study of forty-four cases. *Am J Dis Child.* 1927;33:932.
30. Kohen DP. Neonatal gonococcal arthritis: three cases and review of the literature. *Pediatrics.* 1974;53:436.
31. Rothenberg R. Ophthalmia neonatorum due to *Neisseria gonorrhoeae:* prevention and treatment. *Sex Trans Dis.* 1979;6(suppl):187.
32. Holmes KK. Gonococcal infection. In: Remington JS, Klein JO, eds. *Infectious Diseases of the Fetus and Newborn Infant.* Philadelphia, PA: WB Saunders; 1976:616.
33. Sandstrom KI, Bell TA, Chandler JW, et al. Diagnosis of neonatal purulent conjunctivitis caused by *Chlamydia trachomatis* and other organisms. In: Mardh PA, Holmes KK, Oriel JO, et al, eds. *Chlamydial Infections.* New York, NY: Elsevier; 1982:217.

D

AEROBIC BACTERIAL INFECTIONS

Chapter Sixty-Six

Gram-negative Bacillary Infections

Roger E. Bawdon and Larry C. Gilstrap III

66

The gram-negative aerobic bacilli, especially those belonging to the Enterobacteriaceae family, are commonly isolated from obstetric patients with infections. Moreover, the enteric gram-negative bacilli are indigenous to the female genital tract and account for a significant portion of the normal vaginal/cervical flora during pregnancy.[1,2]

ENTEROBACTERIACEAE

Etiology

This family of enteric aerobic organisms is a normal inhabitant of the gastrointestinal tract, living in a commensal relationship with its human host. The most common members of this group include *Escherichia, Klebsiella, Proteus,* and *Enterobacter.* The Enterobacteriaceae are nonspore-forming, gram-negative bacilli that ferment glucose. Moreover, the majority of these organisms will reduce nitrates to nitrites; this characteristic forms the basis for a useful clinical test that will be discussed later.

Pathogenesis

Because Enterobacteriaceae, especially *Escherichia coli,* are commonly found in the cervix and vagina in pregnant women, it is reasonable to assume that the majority of infections associated with these organisms arise either from direct contamination from these areas or by ascending infection, as would be the case in urinary infection. During labor, the lower uterine segment is usually inoculated with these organisms during digital examination to assess cervical dilatation.[2] Thus, if the fetal membranes are ruptured, these bacteria can readily enter the amniotic cavity, causing chorioamnionitis or postpartum endometritis (especially if the patient was delivered by operative delivery).

Enteric bacteria such as *E coli* or *Klebsiella* usually enter the lower urinary tract by way of urethral contamination. Moreover, during pregnancy there is increased urinary stasis secondary to both hormonal and mechanical factors, which in the presence of bacterial contamination may lead to symptomatic urinary tract infection, such as acute pyelonephritis (see Chapter 143). Once these organisms are associated with infection, they may spread to the other organs by way of the bloodstream (that is, septicemia).

E coli and other Enterobacteriaceae produce pili or p-fimbriae, which are important virulence factors for urinary tract infections in women.[3] Pili are flagellalike structures that originate in the plasma membrane of bacteria; they consist of a helical protein monomer, but are straighter, thinner, and shorter than flagella. They are important in attachment to epithelial cells, particularly in the urinary tract of humans. The strains of *E coli* bearing p-fimbriae correlate with pyelonephritis, whereas those patients with type I fimbriae had symptoms associated with acute cystitis, asymptomatic bacteriuria, and pyelonephritis. This p-fimbria appears to be important not only in acute lower urinary tract infections and asymptomatic bacteriuria, but also in ascending urinary tract infection.

Recently, it has also been reported that the Lewis blood group phenotype may be associated with recurrent urinary tract infections in women, the majority of which are caused by the gram-negative bacilli.[4] In this latter study, women with the nonsecretor (Le, a+b−) and recessive (Le, a−b−) phenotypes had a higher frequency of recurrent urinary infections.

Epidemiology

Of all enteric bacteria encountered in obstetric infections, *E Coli* is by far the most common, followed by *Klebsiella.* The majority of these organisms isolated are from pregnant women with urinary tract infections. Approximately 2–10% of pregnant women will have either an asymptomatic or symptomatic urinary tract infection, and *E coli* and *Klebsiella* account for the majority (75–80%) of these infections.[5-7]

As previously mentioned, the Enterobacteriaceae are among the most common aerobic organisms isolated from the lower genital tract in pregnant women and from postpartum endometrial infections.

Manifestations

The most common manifestations of enteric gram-negative bacillary infection during pregnancy are urinary tract infections, including asymptomatic bacteriuria, cystitis, and acute pyelonephritis. These organisms, especially *E coli,* are also commonly isolated from women with chorioamnionitis and postpartum endometritis.

Another more serious manifestation of the Enterobacteriaceae is bacteremia, which in turn may lead to septic shock. This is especially true for *E coli.* Because all members of the Enterobacteriaceae produce endotoxin, "gram-negative" shock is a potential manifestation of these infections. Enteric gram-negative bacteria can be associated with infections elsewhere in the body, such as the lungs, but these infections are uncommon during pregnancy unless preexisting pulmonary disease is present.

More recently, bacterial toxins in amniotic fluid have been shown to correlate with the onset of preterm labor.[8] The endotoxin or lipopolysaccharide portion of the cell wall of *E coli* has been found in amniotic fluid and correlates with the onset of preterm labor. The mechanism for the onset of labor includes involvement of macrophages, interleukin-1, acute phase reactions, and the eventual activation of the prostaglandin cascade. Because *E coli* is by far the most common gram-negative rod isolated from obstetric infections, this is a serious manifestation.

Diagnosis

The diagnosis of gram-negative bacillary infections is based primarily on culture results. Although Gram's stain is helpful in detecting gram-negative rods, it does not help to differentiate among specific organisms. The nitrate reduction test is also helpful in detecting gram-negative enteric organisms, but again does not identify the specific organisms. This latter test may be used as a screening test for the detection of bacteriuria during pregnancy, and because most cases of bacteriuria are secondary to *E coli* and *Klebsiella* infections, this particular test is especially useful clinically.

The gram-negative enteric bacilli are relatively easy to recover and to cultivate on various media and to identify by standard biochemical tests and specialized growth media.

There are few other useful laboratory tests that aid in the differential diagnosis of these infections. The white blood cell count is frequently elevated in gram-negative enteric infection, but is also elevated in the majority of other bacterial infections.

Treatment

The Enterobacteriaceae are sensitive to a variety of antimicrobials including the semisynthetic penicillins, ureidopenicillins, cephalosporins, penicillins and cephalosporins in combination with β-lactamase inhibitors, tetracyclines, sulfonamides, nitrofurantoins, quinolones, and aminoglycosides. Not all are approved for antimicrobial therapy in pregnancy. The penicillins and cephalosporins (including the newer ones) are Food and Drug Administration category B drugs and are relatively safe for use during pregnancy.[9] Nitrofurantoin and the sulfonamides are also category B drugs, although the former has been reported to cause hemolytic anemia in women with glucose-6-phosphate dehydrogenase deficiency[10] and the latter has been reported to be associated with hyperbilirubinemia in the newborn.[11] Fortunately, these complications are rare. The tetracyclines, including the newer ones, are category D drugs because of the potential to cause yellow-brown discoloration of the deciduous teeth in the newborn[12] and thus should be avoided during pregnancy except in unusual circumstances. Chloramphenicol and most of the aminoglycosides are category C drugs. According to their manufacturers, the quinolone antibiotics, norfloxacin and ciprofloxacin, may cause arthropathy in immature animals and are not generally recommended for use during pregnancy. They are listed as category C drugs.

Resistant strains are relatively common. The Enterobactericeae are especially sensitive to aminoglycosides and for the most part are resistant to macrolides such as erythromycin. Also, with the exception of *Proteus mirabilis,* most of these organisms are not sensitive to benzylpenicillin. Ideally, one should choose specific antimicrobial therapy based on sensitivity studies. However, this is often not practical from a clinical standpoint.

Prevention

Short of prophylactic antibiotics prior to surgical procedures or catheterization, there is little one can do to prevent actual infection secondary to gram-negative enteric organisms, because they constitute a significant portion of the normal gastrointestinal and genital tract flora. Urinary tract infections secondary to these organisms might be also reduced by limiting urethral catheterization and the length of time these catheters remain in place.

Fetal Aspects

The fetus may indirectly suffer from the effects of maternal urinary tract infections, especially acute pyelonephritis, arising from gram-negative enteric organisms. The neonate may also acquire a gram-negative bacillary infection secondary to maternal colonization or infection. These infections may be quite severe and life threatening to the neonate, resulting in bacteremia and meningitis. This is especially true for *E coli* infections.

OTHER GRAM-NEGATIVE BACILLI

Pseudomonas

Etiology and Epidemiology. The most common member of this species is *Pseudomonas aeruginosa,* which is a nonencapsulated gram-negative motile rod. It is commonly found on the skin in the axillary and genital areas. This particular microorganism is also a common hospital contaminant and is responsible for nosocomial infections, especially in older, debilitated patients. Moreover, it is a common source of infection in burns wards. *Pseudomonas* organisms are also commonly found in fresh water and are a frequent cause of ear infections.

Pathogenesis. These gram-negative organisms may enter the body in several different ways, although the most common ways are through contamination from the skin or from use of contaminated water and prepping solutions. They frequently enter the respiratory tract from contaminated equipment used in patients with chronic lung diseases. Chronic debilitating diseases and chronic antibiotic usage also predispose to *Pseudomonas* infections.

Manifestations. *P aeruginosa* may cause urinary tract infections, otitis externa, wound infections, and respiratory infection. It is frequently associated with skin infections in burn patients. It is an uncommon cause of bacteremia except in elderly and debilitated patients, patients with malignancies, and patients on protracted antibiotic therapy.

Treatment. *P aeruginosa* is usually sensitive to carbenicillin, ticarcillin, and piperacillin, as well as the aminoglycosides, especially amikacin. It is also very susceptible to polymyxin, but usually resistant to the cephalosporins.

Prevention. Nosocomial infections can be reduced by frequent surveillance and cleansing of commonly contaminated areas such as operating room scrub facilities and respiratory equipment.

Fetal Aspects. *Pseudomonas* infections are uncommon in the neonate. However, they are more common in the premature infant and may cause bacteremia and life-threatening illness. The same antibiotics can be used for these infections in the neonate as in the adult.

Salmonella

Etiology and Epidemiology. These gram-negative bacilli are motile rods that ferment glucose. The most common species that causes disease in man is *Salmonella typhi,* the etiologic agent of typhoid fever. The usual source of infection is contaminated food and water. Another source of infection is asymptomatic chronic carriers who excrete the organisms in the stool. The gallbladder is frequently a reservoir for these organisms.

Pathogenesis and Manifestations. *Salmonella* organisms enter the body through the gastrointestinal tract, where they multiply. Manifestations may include acute gastroenteritis and bacteremia. Clinically, the patient may manifest fever and chills, nausea and vomiting, abdominal pain, profuse watery diarrhea, and marked dehydration. Dehydration may be especially severe in the pregnant patient who is already experiencing hyperemesis from her pregnancy.

Diagnosis. Diagnosis can be confirmed by isolation of the causative organisms from the stool, bloodstream, or contaminated food. Included in the differential diagnosis are other causes of acute gastroenteritis, including viral and other bacterial agents. Shigellosis, which is caused by the nonmotile gram-negative bacillus *Shigella,* may produce identical symptomatology, such as fever, nausea and vomiting, pain, and watery diarrhea.

Treatment. In mild cases of *Salmonella* infections during pregnancy, supportive therapy with correction of electrolytes and fluid replacement may be the only therapy necessary. Ampicillin is usually effective against this organism. Pregnant patients who are allergic to penicillin and who are toxic may be treated with chloramphenicol. Pregnant patients with gastroenteritis without systemic symptoms who are allergic to penicillin should be treated with supportive therapy only.

Prevention. Detection and surveillance of chronic carriers, especially food handlers, will aid in reducing the number of acute infections.

Fetal Aspects. The main risk to the neonate is the acquisition of the infection from the mother. Newborn diarrheal illness from *Salmonella* can be life threatening. Obviously, infected mothers and their newborns should be isolated.

Shigella

The manifestations of the infection caused by this organism include fever and chills, nausea and vomiting, abdominal pain, and profuse diarrhea. Infection usually results from contact with chronic carriers. The disease is usually self-limited, and treatment is primarily supportive. The main risk to the pregnant woman and her fetus is dehydration. Ampicillin is usually the antibiotic of choice when drug therapy is deemed necessary.

Campylobacter (Vibrio)

Etiology and Epidemiology. These gram-negative rods are motile, slender, curved rods that are microaerophilic, requiring 3–15% CO_2 for growth, and do not ferment glucose. The most common species causing disease in man are *Campylobacter jejuni* and *Campylobacter fetus,* the etiologic agents of enteritis.[13] The usual source of infection is contaminated food and water, with poultry being high on the list.

Pathogenesis and Manifestations. *Campylobacter* probably causes as much enteritis as do *Salmonella* and *Shigella.* The organisms enter the body by penetrating the intact intestinal mucosa, then into the blood and reticuloendothelial system. Clinically, the patients may manifest fever and chills, nausea and vomiting, marked dehydration, and bloody diarrhea. *C fetus* may cause uterine infection with fever and respiratory involvement.

Diagnosis. Diagnosis can be confirmed by isolation of the causative agent from the stool, blood-stream, or the contaminated food. The selective media used is "Canpy" blood agar incubated in 5–15% CO_2. *Shigella* and *Salmonella* may produce similar clinical symptoms.

Treatment. Dehydration, as with *Salmonella* and *Shigella,* may be severe, and the patient should undergo fluid and electrolyte replacement.[14] This may be the only therapy necessary for the majority of patients. For those that need antimicrobial therapy, erythromycin is the drug of choice. However, in sepsis, treatment with gentamicin or chloramphenicol may be indicated.

Prevention. Avoid undercooked poultry, contaminated food, and raw milk.

Fetal Aspects. The main risk to the neonate is the acquisition of the infection from the mother. Newborn illnesses develop symptoms that may progress to meningitis and may be fatal.

Hemophilus

Etiology and Epidemiology. The most common organism of this genus causing infection in man is *Hemophilus influenzae,* a pleomorphic gram-negative bacillus. These organisms are commonly found in the upper respiratory tract, and infection may result from airborne spread.

Manifestations. The major clinical manifestations of infection secondary to this organism are pharyngitis, bronchitis, pneumonitis, and otitis media. This organism is also a common cause of meningitis in young children.

Diagnosis. The diagnosis of *H influenzae* is based on the recovery of the organism from suspected infected sites. It is relatively easy to cultivate on chocolate agar. Included in the differential diagnosis are infections caused by other bacteria such as streptococci and staphylococci.

Treatment. *H influenzae* organisms are sensitive to a variety of antibiotics including penicillin, ampicillin, chloramphenicol, tetracycline, and sulfonamides. For patients with meningitis, ampicillin or chloramphenicol are usually effective.

Fetal Aspects. Most neonates have passively acquired antibodies that are protective against *H influenzae* for the first two months of life. However, these organisms may be the etiologic agent in neonatal meningitis, pneumonia, and septicemia and may rarely be responsible for neonatal mortality.

Brucella

Brucellosis is an uncommon infection in humans in the United States and is a rare complication of pregnancy. It is caused by the gram-negative bacilli *Brucella abortus, Brucella suis,* and *Brucella melitensis.* Brucellosis is usually a self-limited disease. The major manifestations are low-grade fever, headache, and lethargy or a flulike syndrome. Diagnosis can be made by either isolating the organism using trypticase broth or, more practically, by serology using the tube-dilution agglutination test. The drug of choice is tetracycline in the nonpregnant patient. As a general rule, tetracycline should not be used in the pregnant patient. Alternatives for the pregnant patient include the aminoglycosides or chloramphenicol. The role of brucellosis in abortion in the human is not clear, although there have been reports of such an association.[15,16]

Tularemia

Tularemia is an uncommon infection caused by the gram-negative bacillus *Pasteurella tularensis* and usually occurs from contact with infected animals such as rabbits, squirrels, or rats. It may also be acquired from insects and ticks. The usual manifestations are a red ulcerative lesion and regional lymphadenopathy. Occasionally, the patient may have systemic involvement with pneumonitis. Clinically, the patient may experience fever, chills, lethargy, irritability, and myalgia. Diagnosis is usually based on serologic testing (agglutination). Plague must be considered in the differential diagnosis. There is little information regarding the association of tularemia in pregnancy and adverse fetal effects. The antibiotic of choice for tularemia is streptomycin. Chloramphenicol and tetracycline are also effective, although the latter should not be used during pregnancy.

Pasteurella

Pasteurella infections are uncommon in humans at the present time in the United States. The most famous *Pasteurella* infection is the plague caused by the gram-negative bacillus, *Yersinia pestis* (formerly called *Pasteurella pestis*). The main reservoir for this infection is the rodent, and the bacillus is usually transmitted to humans by fleas. The major manifestations of plague are high fever, chills, nausea and vomiting, headache, and extreme prostration. Bacteremia is relatively common, and pneumonitis may be present. Suppurations of the regional lymph nodes ("buboes") are common. The disease can run a fulminant course if not treated. Plague may be diagnosed both bacteriologically from cultures and serologically. Tularemia, typhoid, and lymphogranuloma venereum should be considered in the initial differential diagnosis.

Because plague is a rare disease in this country, there is little or no information regarding the association of this illness in pregnancy. Streptomycin and kanomycin, as well as tetracycline and chloramphenicol, are usually effective against the causative organism, *Y pestis*. Sulfonamides are also sometimes effective. Vaccines provide limited protection, and all personnel, including pregnant women, traveling to endemic areas should be vaccinated.

Another gram-negative bacillus, *Pasteurella multocida* (formerly called *Pasteurella septica*), can cause infection in humans. The main reservoirs are dogs and cats, and infection usually results from animal bites. The main manifestations are wound infection and cellulitis. Moreover, *P multocida* may be a causative agent of osteomyelitis.[17] Unlike *Y pestis*, this latter organism is highly susceptible to penicillin, which is the antibiotic of choice.

CONCLUSIONS

The aerobic gram-negative bacilli are frequently encountered in human infections. Many of these organisms make up a significant part of the normal genital tract flora in women and thus are a potential source of infection in obstetric patients. Members of the family Enterobacteriaceae, such as *E coli* and *Klebsiella*, are the most common encountered in obstetric infections.

REFERENCES

1. Wong R, Gee CL, Ledger WJ. Prophylactic use of cefazolin in monitored obstetric patients undergoing cesarean section. *Obstet Gynecol.* 1977;51:407.
2. Gilstrap LC, Cunningham FG. The bacterial pathogenesis of infection following cesarean section. *Obstet Gynecol.* 1979;53:545.
3. Latham RH, Stamm WE. Role of fimbriated *Escherichia coli* in urinary tract infections in adult women: correlation with localization studies. *J Infect Dis.* 1984;149:835.
4. Sheinfeld J, Schaeffer AJ, Cordon-Cardo C, et al. Association of the Lewis blood group phenotype with recurrent urinary tract infections in women. *N Engl J Med.* 1989;320:773.
5. Harris RE, Gilstrap LC. Cystitis during pregnancy: a distinct clinical entity. *Obstet Gynecol.* 1981;57:578.
6. Leveno KJ, Harris RE, Gilstrap LC, et al. Bladder versus renal bacteriuria during pregnancy: recurrence after treatment. *Am J Obstet Gynecol.* 1981;139:403.
7. Gilstrap LC, Cunningham FG, Whalley PJ. Acute pyelonephritis in pregnancy: an anterospective study. *Obstet Gynecol.* 1981;57:409.
8. Romero R, Roslonsky P, Ayarzum E, et al. Labor and infection. II. Bacterial endotoxin in amniotic fluid and its relationship to the onset of preterm labor. *Am J Obstet Gynecol.* 1989;158:1044.
9. Federal Drug Administration. Pregnancy and labeling: prescription drug categories. *FDA Drug Bull.* 1979;9:35.
10. Powell RD, DeGowin RL, Alving AS. Nitrofurantoin-induced hemolysis. *J Clin Med.* 1963;62:1002.
11. Lucey JF, Driscoll TJ. Hazard to newborn infants of administration of long-acting sulfonamides to pregnant women. *Pediatrics.* 1959;24:498.
12. Kutcher AH, Zegarelli EV, Tovell HM, Hochberg B. Discoloration of teeth induced by tetracycline. *JAMA.* 1963;184:586.
13. Blaser MJ. Campylobacter species. Infectious disease and their etiologic agents. In: Monde GL, Douglas RG, Bennett JE, eds. *Principles and Practice of Infectious Diseases.* 2nd ed. New York, NY: John Wiley & Sons; 1985;1221.
14. Marcy MS, Guernant RL. Microorganisms responsible for neonatal diarrhea. In: Remington JS, Klein JO, eds. *Infectious Diseases of the Fetus and Newborn Infant.* 2nd ed. Philadelphia, PA: WB Saunders Co; 1983:980.
15. Poole PM, Whitehouse DB, Gilchrist MM. A case of abortion consequent upon infection with *Brucella abortus*, biotype 2. *J Clin Pathol.* 1972;25:882.
16. Sarram M, Geiz J, Foruzandeh M, et al. Intrauterine fetal infections with *Brucella melitensis* as a possible cause of second-trimester abortion. *Am J Obstet Gynecol.* 1974;119:657.
17. Jarvis WR, Banko S, Snyder E, et al. *Pasteurella multocida.* Osteomyelitis following dog bites. *Am J Dis Child.* 1981;135:625.

Chapter Sixty-Seven
Chancroid

Charles H. Livengood III

67

MATERNAL ASPECTS

Definition

Chancroid is an acute ulcerative disease with remarkable specificity for genital tissues, involving the skin, mucosae, and lymphatics. It is usually a self-limited process with minimal sequelae, although destructive lesions may rarely occur.

Etiology

Chancroid results from infection by *Hemophilus ducreyi,* an extremely small, gram-negative bacillus 1.5 = 0.5 μm. The organism can be found singly or in clusters in pus from infected patients, and sometimes parallel chains form in strands of mucus to create the "school of fish" or "railroad tracks" appearance. It was first described by Ducrey in 1889[1], and Koch's postulates have been satisfied.

H ducreyi is a fastidious organism, a fact that has generated confusion in our understanding of chancroid, because accurate diagnosis requires isolation of the organism. Kraus et al[2] note that organisms described in some early studies were in fact not *H ducreyi,* so that the disease process characterized in these studies was not chancroid. Recent years have seen a great improvement in techniques for *H ducreyi* isolation based on selective media with vancomycin, enriched with serum and factor X (hemin), and incubation under more humid, capneic, and cool conditions.

Pathology

The lesion of chancroid begins as a tender macule or papule, develops into a vesicopustule, and ulcerates to form a soft, painful, sharply circumscribed chancre. The edges of the chancre are erythematous and undermined, and the base consists of friable granulation tissue, usually with a shaggy gray exudate covering it. Lesions vary in size from 1–25 mm.

The histopathology of the chancroid lesion has been described by Heyman et al[3], who ascribed to it a 90% diagnostic sensitivity. These workers identified three zones: most superficially, a thin layer of neutrophils, fibrin, erythrocytes, and necrosis (the exudate); next, a layer of vigorous neovascularization in which degenerative changes and thrombosis can be seen in some of the vessels (the granulating ulcer base); and finally, a deep zone consisting of an intense infiltrate of plasma cells and lymphocytes.

Epidemiology

Chancroid is transmitted by direct frictional contact with an active lesion, almost invariably during sexual activity, although rare accidental infections of medical personnel have been noted. Based on failure of examination of named sexual contacts to identify new cases[4,5], it seems likely that the transmission rate of chancroid is low.[6] Variations in the distribution of the disease between the sexes are found in the literature, with some sources reporting that 90–95% of cases are found in men, and other sources reporting only about 66% of cases found in men.[7] This apparent inequity may result from internal lesions in women that go unnoticed; more important, however, is the increasing evidence that an infectious carrier state in the absence of symptoms and lesions can exist in women, probably with the cervix as the reservoir.[8]

Although chancroid has traditionally been considered a tropical disease with only about 700 cases reported in the United States annually, recent dramatic increases in the incidence of chancroid believed to be associated with drug-related prostitution now result in thousands of cases each year. The prevalence of chancroid increased from 0.24 to 2.07 reported cases per 100,000 population during the interval from 1978 to 1987. The coexistence of other sexually transmitted diseases is discussed under Diagnosis.

Manifestations

The incubation period of chancroid is 1–14 days, with most cases occurring in the first week after exposure. The lesions are found almost exclusively on the genitalia, although extragenital chancroid of the mouth, fingers, and breasts is known, and autoinoculation to other body sites occurs. Generally, patients present within 1–2 weeks of onset of the lesions, which begin as a tender macule that forms into a pustule and ulcerates. This superficial genital ulcer is remarkable for its tenderness and lack of duration, both in contrast to the syphilis chancre. The edges are ragged, erythematous, and undermined, and the base consists of friable granulation tissue overlaid by a shaggy gray exudate (Figure 67–1). Single or multiple lesions may occur, and coalescence can be seen. Occasionally, deep ulcers are seen, complicated by bleeding, and mild induration may occur rarely. Chancroid ulcers heal with mild to moderate scarring.

Although inguinal adenitis is considered a hallmark of the disease, its appearance is variable, occurring in only 32–50% of patients. The adenitis is more often unilateral, beginning as tender, swollen, fixed nodes about one week after the primary lesion appears. In half of all cases, adenitis resolves spontaneously, and in the remainder, a fluctuant unilocular bubo develops (this occurs less frequently in women[9]), which may rupture and drain through a single ostium, as opposed to the multiple draining inguinal sinus tracts seen in lymphogranuloma venereum.

Systemic toxicity is rare in chancroid. Usually, the disease heals spontaneously over weeks. A bubo that is allowed to rupture spontaneously will drain for months and scar badly as it heals. Rarely, progressive extension of the disease occurs with genital destruction and fistula formation. This seems to occur with superinfection of the lesions, but some of these cases may actually represent granuloma inguinale or lymphogranuloma venereum.

The effects of chancroid on pregnancy have not been addressed in the literature, as revealed by an exhaustive search. However, because of the frequent coexistence of chancroid with other sexually transmissible diseases that are known to adversely affect pregnancy outcome, any pregnant patient found to have chancroid should have careful surveillance for syphilis, gonorrhea, and herpetic and chla-

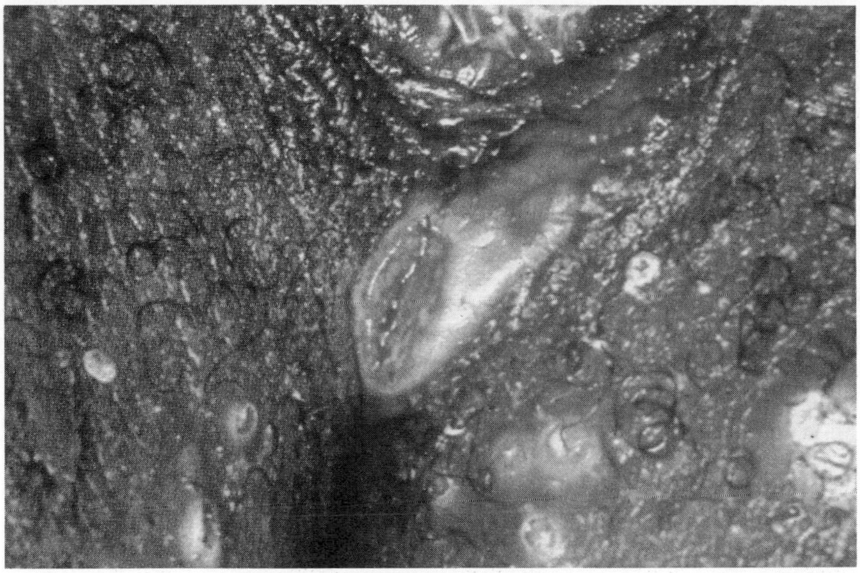

Figure 67–1. Large chancroid lesion of the perineum with multiple satellite lesions. Note the ragged, undermined edges. Unlike the primary chancre of syphilis, these chancroid ulcers are extremely tender and lack extensive underlying induration. (*From Meheus and Ursi*[22] *with permission.*)

mydial infections throughout gestation by the appropriate laboratory tests and genital examination.

Diagnosis

Exclusion of other genital ulcerative diseases in cases of suspected chancroid must be considered an integral aspect of diagnosis. First, even experienced venereologists correctly identify chancroid by history and examination in only 60% of cases[10]; the lesions can resemble those of herpes genitalis, lymphogranuloma venereum, hidradenitis suppurativa, syphilis, granuloma inguinale, and their variants too closely to be differentiated. Second, any of these diseases may coexist with chancroid. In the Sheffield epidemic of 1980, 59% of patients with chancroid had a history of previous sexually transmitted disease (STD), and 82% had other active coexistent STDs. Additionally, up to 19% have coexistent syphilis[11], usually in the primary stage, when serology may be negative.

The diagnosis of chancroid is based on isolation of the organism in the laboratory from vigorous ulcer swabbings. Bubo aspirates may also be cultured but are positive in only 50% of cases. As noted, previous difficulties in media and conditions for culture have been largely resolved, and isolation of *H ducreyi* can now be accomplished without undue expense or complexity. Most hospitals should offer this service, the details of which can be obtained from the literature.[12-15] and from the Centers for Disease Control.

Adjunctive diagnostic techniques include rolling a swabbing of the ulcer base on a slide for Gram's staining and identifying the "school of fish" pattern. Unfortunately, the false-negative rate of this test is 49%[16] or higher, and typical *H ducreyi* are rarely seen in bubo aspirates; the false-positive rate is also unacceptably high because of the similarity of the organism to other common commensals and pathogens. Biopsy of the lesion tends to yield nonspecific results, and skin testing is inaccurate and archaic. Culturing the organism in a tube of the patient's clotted blood has met with variable success, and there is no consensus on standardization of this technique.[17,18]

The evaluation of a patient suspected to have chancroid should consist of culture for *H ducreyi* and herpes simplex virus, dark-field microscopy to rule out *Treponema pallidum*, a crushed biopsy stained with Wright's or Giemsa stain to detect the Donovan bodies of granuloma inguinale, serology for syphilis and lymphogranuloma venereum, cytology or biopsy to rule out neoplasia and herpetic infection, and a knowledge of the appearance of hidradenitis suppurativa.

Treatment

H ducreyi antibiotic sensitivities have evolved significantly during the past decade. Whereas tetracyclines and sulfonamides have been the traditional drugs of choice in chancroid, their efficacy is now considered inadequate. Further, it has become clear that the antibiotic susceptibility pattern of the organism varies considerably from one locale to another, and physicians treating chancroid should avail themselves of information about sensitivities of recent isolates in their area. First-line therapy for chancroid is currently a single dose of ceftriaxone, 250 mg intramuscularly.[19] Cephalosporin-allergic patients should be treated with erythromycin base or stearate, 500 mg orally four times a day for seven days. Patients intolerant of both of these drugs should be treated after consultation with local or state health authorities. All sexual partners must be treated. Patients should be followed closely to confirm resolution of ulcerative lesions and adenitis, which should be evident within one week of initiation of therapy; if not, treatment failure should be suspected and the patient should be retreated using another drug.

An important aspect of treatment of chancroid is the management of inguinal adenitis. When a bubo is identified, both spontaneous rupture and incision for drainage must be avoided because delayed healing and a prolonged draining sinus tract and associated risk of superinfection usually result. Proper management of a bubo consists of aspiration of the contents with a needle placed through normal adjacent skin.

Prevention

Condoms and postcoital washing of the genitalia should diminish transmission rates of chancroid.

FETAL ASPECTS

As noted above, no information on chancroid during pregnancy can be identified, but fetuses of mothers with chancroid are clearly at high risk on epidemiologic grounds for exposure to other STDs and their attendant morbidities.

It is noted that chancroid is almost unknown in children[20], but a reference is made to rare cases of ophthalmia neonatorum caused by *H ducreyi,* with conjunctival ulcers typical of chancroid and ipsilateral preauricular lymphadenopathy.[21] Transmission to the neonate at delivery through infected genitalia is certainly feasible, and such infants should probably be treated with ceftriaxone.

REFERENCES

1. Ducrey A. Recherches experimentales sur la nature intime du principe contagieux du chancre mou. *Ann Dermatol Syph.* 1890;1:56.
2. Kraus SJ, Kaufman HW, Albritton WL, et al. Chancroid therapy: a review of cases confirmed by culture. *Rev Infect Dis.* 1982;4(suppl):848.
3. Heyman A, Beeson PB, Sheldon WH. Diagnosis of chancroid. *JAMA.* 1945;129:935.
4. Centers for Disease Control. Chancroid—California. *MMWR.* 1982;31:173.
5. Hafiz S, Kinghorn GR, McEntegart MG. Chancroid in Sheffield. A report of 22 cases diagnosed by isolating *Hemophilus ducreyi* in a modified medium. *Br J Vener Dis.* 1981;57:382.
6. Hand WL. *Hemophilus* species. Chancroid. In: Mandell GL, Douglas RG, Bennett JE, eds. *Principles and Practice of Infectious Diseases.* New York, NY: John Wiley & Sons; 1979:1770.
7. Gaison A, Heaton CL. Chancroid: alias the soft chancre. *Int J Dermatol.* 1975;14:188.
8. Hart G. Chancroid, donovanosis, lymphogranuloma venereum. *DHEW Publication No. (CDC) 75-8302;*1975.
9. Lykke-Olesen L, Pederson TG, Larsen L, et al. Epidemic of chancroid in Greenland 1977–78. *Lancet.* 1979;1:654.
10. Chapel TA, Brown WJ, Jeffries G, et al. How reliable is the morphological diagnosis of penile ulcerations? *Sex Transm Dis.* 1977;4:150.
11. Mauff AC, Ballard RC, Bilgeri YR, et al. Isolation of *Haemophilus ducreyi* from genital ulcerations in white men in Johannesburg. *S Afr Med J.* 1983;63:236.
12. California Department of Health Services. An outbreak of chancroid in Orange County. *Calif Morbid.* 1982;12:5.
13. Oberhofer TR, Back AE. Isolation and cultivation of *Haemophilus ducreyi. J Clin Microbiol.* 1983;15:625.
14. Sottnek FO, Biddle JW, Kraus SJ, et al. Isolation and identification of *Haemophilus ducreyi* in a clinical study. *J Clin Microbiol.* 1980;12:170.
15. Hammond GW, Lian CJ, Wilt JC, et al. Comparison of specimen collection and laboratory techniques for isolation of *Haemophilus ducreyi. J Clin Microbiol.* 1978;7:39.
16. Nsanze H, Fast MV, D'Costa LJ, et al. Genital ulcers in Kenya. Clinical and laboratory study. *Br J Vener Dis.* 1981;57:378.
17. Tan U, Rajan VS, Koe SL, et al. Chancroid: a study of 500 cases. *Asian J Infect Dis.* 1977;1:27.
18. Khoo R, Sng EH, Goh AJ. A study of sexually transmitted disease in 200 prostitutes in Singapore. *Asian J Infect Dis.* 1977;1:77.
19. Centers for Disease Control. 1989 STD treatment guidelines. *MMWR.* 1989;38(suppl 8):4.
20. Grossman M, Drutz DJ: Veneral disease in children. *Adv Pediatr.* 1974;21:97.
21. Ostler HB. Oculogenital disease. *Surv Ophthalmol.* 1976;20:233.
22. Meheus A, Ursi J-P. *Sexually Transmitted Diseases.* Kalamazoo, MI: The Upjohn Company; 1982:14.

Chapter Sixty-Eight

Anthrax

Sebastian Faro

68

Anthrax is a disease that dates back to 5000 BC. It occurred among farmers in Egypt and Mesopotamia. It was also considered to be the fifth plague of Egypt.[1,2] The disease was also recorded in ancient Greek and Hindu writings. Europe had not been exposed to significant infection by the anthrax bacillus until 1613, when an epidemic occurred in southern Europe. The first reported cases in the United States occurred in Louisiana in the 18th century. The first microscopic observation of the bacillus was reported by Delefond in 1838. In 1868, Devin demonstrated the infectivity of the bacillus, and in 1877, Koch, using his postulates for the first time, demonstrated that this bacillus was the agent responsible for anthrax. Pasteur subsequently developed a vaccine and inoculated animals to prevent and protect them from the anthrax bacillus. Penicillin was used successfully to treat humans in 1944.

Bacillus anthracis, the causative agent of anthrax, is a gram-positive rod that may assume an elliptical or cylindrical shape. The bacillus is encapsulated, nonmotile, and may possess a central spore. The spore forms are not found in living animals, but develop when environmental conditions are not favorable for vegetative reproduction. The spores are resistant to disinfectants and heat, but can be destroyed by boiling in water for 10 minutes or by dry heat of 104°C for three hours. The spores can survive dehydration for many years. Specimens obtained from blood or tissue when stained may reveal the presence of bacilli in chains or in pairs. Frequently, when the bacilli are arranged in chains, they resemble a reed of bamboo with a capsule surrounding the entire colony. The bacteria can be easily grown on blood agar. The colonies are nonhemolytic, raised, opaque, grayish-white and mucoid, often described as tenacious. Growth occurs best in a CO_2 rich environment.

B anthracis is found primarily in herbivores, for example, cattle, goats, horses, and sheep. Transmission to humans occurs by way of contact with infected animals or animal products containing spores. Anthrax is classified as being acquired usually in one of three settings; industrial, agricultural, or laboratory.[3] The number of cases occurring in the United States have steadily declined from 127 between 1916 and 1925 to 2.5 between 1970 and 1980. Coincident with a decrease in morbidity was a decline in mortality, with the majority of cases occurring prior to 1944, which preceded the introduction of penicillin. However, between 1955 and 1980, there was an increase in the number of cases—231 cases with 20 fatalities reported.[4,5] The greatest number of cases (80%) were related to industrial processes, for example, contact with goat's hair, wool, animal hides.[6] Individuals whose vocation is farming or ranching, butchering, or veterinary medicine are at greatest risk for acquiring the infection. The reservoir for anthrax spores is the soil, vegetation, and water. In the United States, the major endemic areas for spores are the Mississippi Delta, farming areas of California, Arkansas, Iowa, Nebraska, Louisiana, Oklahoma, Oregon, and Texas. The spores can be transported by way of various animal products. An important vehicle for transporting spores of the anthrax bacillus is bone meal used for fertilizer.

PATHOGENESIS

Anthrax may present in one of three primary forms or a combination of these forms: cutaneous, respiratory, or gastrointestinal. A complex presentation may be the initial presentation because the organism can be disseminated by way of the lymphatic or hematogenous routes. Meningitis may develop from the initial infection; although rare, it has been reported to occur in less than 5% of patients. In a review of 70 cases of anthrax meningitis, the most frequent primary infection was cutaneous (53%); initial respiratory infection occurred in 23%, and gastrointestinal occurred in 19%. No primary infection could be found in 12% of the patients.[6]

Cutaneous anthrax develops following inoculation through the skin, which most likely enters through small breaks in the dermis. The spores germinate below the epidermis, multiply, and produce toxin. The toxin causes necrosis of the surrounding tissue, thus producing a black eschar that heals with the formation of a scar. The bacilli may advance locally by way of regional lymphangitis or lymphadenopathy or become systemically transported by way of the lymphatic or hematogenous channels, resulting in bacteremia and systemic symptoms.

Respiratory anthrax results from inhalation of spores that are carried as contaminants on airborne particles. The spores are phagocytized and transported to regional lymph nodes, where germination, replication, and toxin production take place. This form of the disease may be the most severe because the organism can cause septicemia, general toxemia, and death. However, respiratory depression can occur by the enlarged necrotic and hemorrhagic mediastinal lymph nodes, which compress the respiratory passages. The toxin may also have a direct suppressant effect on the central nervous system. The development of anthrax pneumonia is uncommon, but secondary pneumonia may result. Death is usually the result of respiratory failure due to the formation of pulmonary capillary thrombosis.

Gastrointestinal disease results from the ingestion of spores. The spores migrate through the mucosa and germinate in the submucosal layers. Here they multiply and produce toxin, which results in necrosis of tissue and ulcers, most frequently found in the terminal ileum and cecum. The organism can cause hemorrhage and fistula formation and can migrate to regional lymph nodes.[7]

After entering the subepidermis, an incubation period of 1–7 days is necessary to allow the spores to germinate. At this time, a small papule develops and proceeds to a vesicle. Initially, a number of vesicles may be closely associated, which may coalesce to form a large vesicle. The tissue surrounding the vesicle becomes erythematous and edematous, which may also be associated with pruritus. The fluid in the vesicle is initially clear, but within a few days becomes blue-black. Eventually, the vesicle ruptures spontaneously, if not mechanically, and an ulcer with sharp walls results with the development of a black eschar in the center.

Systemic symptoms, such as a low-grade fever, malaise, regional lymphangitis, and lymphadenopathy, may develop. Rarely does the patient develop systemic toxicity. The eschar fully develops over a period of 10 days. Healing begins with the margins or border of the ulcer separating from the eschar, which eventually loosens and drops off. The center of the ulcer heals by the formation of granulation tissue, which leaves a scar behind. The lesions tend to form primarily on exposed parts of the body, the upper extremities being the most common site.

Occasionally, the cutaneous lesions may be quite severe and are associated with a significant degree of edema, induration, and systemic illness. This has been termed *malignant edema*.

Inhalation of anthrax spores is followed by an incubation period of 1–5 days, with the ensuring development of a flulike syndrome: malaise, myalgia, low-grade fever, fatigue, a nonproductive cough, and occasionally a sensation of heaviness overlying the precordium. This is considered to be the initial phase of infection, which is followed within 2–4 days by the second phase. Initially, the patient appears to improve, but suddenly develops severe respiratory distress, characterized by dyspnea, cyanosis, stridor, and diaphoresis. Edema of the subcutaneous tissues of the neck and chest may occur. The patient develops a pleural effusion, tachycardia, tachypnea, and fever. A chest x-ray usually shows widening of the mediastinum due to the expanding lymphadenopathy, hemorrhage, and necrosis of the mediastinal lymph nodes. The patient's condition progressively worsens, with the white blood cell count becoming moderately elevated, and may go on to develop shock. Death may occur within 24 hours of the development of the second phase of the infection.

Ingestion of contaminated foods, principally meats, is followed by the development of symptoms within 2–5 days. The patient notes anorexia and nausea, which are followed by vomiting and fever. Subsequently, the patient complains of abdominal pain and hematemesis, and may have bloody diarrhea. The patient's abdomen resembles that of an acute surgical abdomen. The disease may progress to a severe state with the development of shock and death.

Meningeal anthrax is rare and occurs in less than 5% of patients. Meningitis can be a complication of any of the forms of anthrax described, but is most commonly associated with cutaneous infection (53%), with gastrointestinal infection being the least likely to predispose the patient to central nervous system (CNS) infection.

PREGNANCY

The occurrence of anthrax in pregnant patients is rare. Three cases have been reported in the German literature. These cases occurred prior to 1900, at which time no treatment was available, and the patients all died of their disease. *B anthracis* was recovered from fetal tissues.[8,9] In 1964, a case was reported from Iran in which the patient developed a cutaneous lesion on her left eyelid, who within a 48-hour period went into labor, delivered an unaffected neonate. The mother subsequently expired.[10]

DIAGNOSIS

The appropriate diagnosis depends upon which form of the disease the patient has. Cutaneous anthrax is heralded by the presence of a painless vesicle which is accompanied by pruritus. The progression to the ulcerative stage that becomes necrotic and the formation of an eschar should raise the suspicion of anthrax. The lesion should be cultured in its early stage, avoiding the delay of waiting for spontaneous resolution.

Respiratory anthrax is more difficult to diagnosis because the early presentation resembles a flulike syndrome. The patient's history and association with animals, animal products, or employment in a laboratory that places the individual at risk would raise the physician's index of suspicion. It is important to remember that to contract respiratory disease, the spores must be inhaled, and therefore they must be aerosolized. Thus, a detailed history must be obtained to determine if the patient is at risk for contracting or being exposed to the organisms. The organisms can be isolated and identified from pleural fluid; however, a pleural effusion does not develop in the initial phase of respiratory anthrax. Additional evidence is the mediastinal widening that occurs in the second stage of the disease, which can be noted on chest x-ray. It is important to recall that the second stage often is associated with rapid deterioration of the patient leading to shock and death. Therefore, it is extremely important to consider anthrax when one is considering acute respiratory disease in the differential diagnosis if the history suggests there is possible exposure.

Gastrointestinal anthrax is probably the most difficult diagnosis to establish, because there are no unique features of this form of the infection. The best clue is the ingestion of poorly-cooked meat.

Isolation of the organism from the site of infection confirms the diagnosis. A Gram's stain showing chains of gram-positive rods or a bamboo-shaft resemblance is strongly indicative of the presence of *B anthracis*. The immunological diagnosis is based on a four-fold rise in titer directed against an antigen of the anthrax bacillus. The acute phase titer and convalescent titer should be tested in parallel.

TREATMENT

Specimens for cultures should be obtained prior to instituting antibiotic therapy. The treatment of choice for cutaneous anthrax is penicillin. In mild cases, oral penicillin is administered in a dose of 30 mg/kg of body weight, every six hours for seven days. More extensive disease should be treated with intravenously administered penicillin, two million units every six hours. Patients with malignant edema will require the addition of hydrocortisone, 100–200 mg/day.[11] Individuals allergic to penicillin can be treated with tetracycline, chloramphenicol, erythromycin, or streptomycin.

Respiratory anthrax requires high dose penicillin therapy, 18–24 million units/day. In addition, it is recommended that streptomycin, 1–2 g/day, be included because the two antibiotics may act synergistically. The difficulty with this form of anthrax is that the diagnosis is usually not made until the patient has entered the toxic phase and the prognosis is poor, even with the use of high doses of antibiotics. Meningitis secondary to *B anthracis* is also treated with high doses of penicillin, but treatment is prolonged, usually lasting 14 days.

The patient with untreated cutaneous anthrax has a 10–20% chance of having a fatal outcome. Treatment with penicillin will result in a 99% survival rate. During adequate antimicrobial therapy, the cutaneous lesion will follow the progressive changes to result in scarring. Antibiotic therapy will reduce the extent of local reaction, such as erythema and edema formation. The patient will typically develop antibodies, which offer protective immunity, although this does not guarantee total protection to future exposure.

Respiratory anthrax is almost always fatal. Gastrointestinal infection results in 25–50% mortality. Subclinical infections most likely occur, because antibody levels are detected in workers exposed to handling animal products but who have no history of ever having acute infection.

PREVENTION

The best approach to the prevention of anthrax in humans is to eliminate it at its source. However, because this is not entirely possible, several actions can be taken. Vaccination of domestic animals should be performed, especially in high endemic areas. Animals suspected of dying of anthrax should have the diagnosis confirmed. All animals suspected of or confirmed of dying from anthrax should be cremated. Individuals at high risk should be vaccinated. Employees who work in areas where dust and the possibility of aerosolized spores exist should be compelled to wear respirators. Better methods should be developed to reduce the production of aerosolized spores.

Individuals exposed to *B anthracis* should be quarantined for seven days; this is the maximum incubation period for the disease to manifest signs and symptoms. Antibiotics should be administered to those individuals suspected of ingesting contaminated meat or who have accidentally been inoculated with virulent bacilli through the skin. Penicillin should be administered as described earlier for seven days.

PERINATAL INFECTION

The bacillus can be transmitted by way of the hematogenous route transplacentally. This usually results in intrauterine fetal demise. Neonatal anthrax can be contracted if the infant comes into direct contact with a lesion. The possibility exists of acquiring the bacillus at the time of delivery if the mother is shedding the organism rectally.

REFERENCES

1. Brachman PS. Industrial inhalation of anthrax. *Bact Rev.* 1966;30:646.
2. Klemm DM, Klemm WR. History of anthrax. *J Vet Med Assoc.* 1959;135:458.
3. Brachman PA, Feeley JC, *Bacillus anthracis.* In: Blair JE, Lennett HE, Truant JP, eds. *Manual of Clinical Microbiology.* Bethesda, MD: American Society for Microbiology; 1970:106.
4. Centers for Disease Control. *MMWR.* 1976;25.
5. Glassman HN. World incidence of anthrax in man. *Public Health.* 1958;73:22.
6. Brachman PS, Fekety FR. Industrial anthrax. *Ann NY Acad Sci.* 1958;70:574.
7. Brachman PS. Anthrax. In: Hoeprich PD, ed. *Infectious Disease.* Philadelp hia, PA: Harper and Row Publishers; 1983:939.
8. Rostowzen MJ. Uber die Uehbergang von Milzbranbacillus bein menschen von die Mutter auf die Frucht bei Pustula maligna. *Gerburtshilfe Gynaekol.* 1897;37:542.
9. Ahfeld F, Marchand F. *Ahfelds' Lehrbuch der Gerburtshifle.* 1898;11:239.
10. Kohout E, Sehat A, Asharf M. Anthrax: a continuous problem in Southwest Iran. *Am J Med Sci.* 1964;247:565.
11. Poretz DM. *Bacillus anthracis* (anthrax). In: Mandell GL, Douglas RG, Bennett JE, eds. *Principles and Practice of Infectious Disease.* New York, NY: John Wiley and Sons; 1979:1634.

Chapter Sixty-Nine
Listeriosis

Joseph M. Miller, Jr. and Joseph G. Pastorek II

69

Listeria monocytogenes is a well recognized perinatal pathogen. Microbiologically, the organism is a gram-positive, nonspore-forming, aerobic rod that is motile at room temperature; weak β-hemolytic properties separate it from similar appearing diphtheroids. Gram's stains of clinical specimens may appear coccoid. It may occur in pairs and may be mistaken for the pneumococcus. The bacterium is catalase-positive and Voges–Proskauer-positive. There are at least 11 serotypes of *L monocytogenes*, but over 90% of human disease is caused by types Ia, Ib, and IVb.

L monocytogenes is ubiquitous. The organism has been isolated from soil, water, sewage, and nearly every type of animal, including asymptomatic humans. Fecal excretion is found in 1–5% of people without the disease. Carriage rates among poultry workers of 29% and among public health laboratory workers involved in Listeria isolation of 77% have been reported. Culture positivity among contacts of symptomatic patients is reported at 26%. These data support the idea of oral–fecal contamination. Vaginal and cervical carriage rates in women are only 1–2%.

Several recent reports support the role of transmission by food in epidemic disease.[1] In 1981 in Canada, manure-contaminated cabbage that had been cold stored was used to prepare coleslaw. Of 41 documented cases of listeriosis reported, 34 were in infants. In 1985, Jalisco brand Mexican-style cheese contaminated with *L monocytogenes* type IVb was linked to at least 103 cases. In 1987, another cheese-related outbreak occurred in Switzerland. In sporadic cases in adults, often neither the route of transmission nor the source of infection are evident. Venereal spread is known in animals and has been suggested in humans.

Listeriosis has a predilection for those under one year of age and those over 55. Patients who have chronic illness (for example, diabetes, tuberculosis) or are immunocompromised (for example, systemic lupus erythematosus or acquired immune deficiency syndrome [AIDS]) are also at higher risk. Pregnancy, independent of other risk factors, also appears to be associated with a greater risk of infection. Transplacental transmission may occur, giving rise to fetal involvement.

The neonate has unusual sensitivity to this pathogen. In part, this may be due to a selective defect in the immune system of the fetus. Animal work has shown that while *L monocytogenes* is phagocytosed normally, macrophage activation does not occur. This deficiency is associated with a lack of Ia antigen in the monocyte surface. Surface Ia antigen is required for effective macrophage helper T-cell interaction and lymphokine production. Without the presence of lymphokines, macrophage activation and killing of this intracellular pathogen do not happen. In the experimental animal, Ia antigen expression on the monocyte surface appears to be suppressed by alpha-fetoprotein.[2] The elevated alpha-fetoprotein level encountered in pregnancy and in the fetus may explain the predilection for the disease at this time.

Geographic and anatomic distribution of the various serotypes of *L monocytogenes* has been evaluated. There are no definite regional trends, and the most common serotypes vary from year to year. Types Ia and Ib are more common *in utero* and early-onset neonatal disease, while late onset is more often associated with type IVb.[3] Neither serotype nor phagotype is related to virulence. Virulence has been related to hemolysin production, however.

The pathogenesis of human listeriosis is poorly understood. The portal of entry is generally presumed to be the gastrointestinal tract, because this is the site most often colonized. Whether or not colonization gives rise to disease is dependent upon several factors: the state of the host (age, immunocompetence); the route of infection; the virulence of the strain; inoculum size; and pregnancy. Noninfectious diseases, primarily cirrhosis of the liver, diabetes mellitus, and various malignancies, often precede documented listeriosis. In some instances, the disease may follow contact with infected material. Certainly, foodborne transmisson is documented.[1] However, the incubation period is unknown, and the minimum infective dose is uncertain.

All virulent strains of *L monocytogenes* produce an extracellular SH-activated hemolysin, listeriolysis. This causes lysis of phagolysosomal membranes and ferritin vesicles, thereby freeing iron, a cation that stimulates growth of *L monocytogenes*. Bacterial hemolysin does not completely explain virulence.

L monocytogenes differs from other bacteria that cause more common foodborne disease in that this organism can act as an intracellular parasite within circulating lymphocytes. In such a setting, the bacterium may persist despite the action of host immune defenses and antibiotics. This resistance does not appear to be mediated by transformation to an L-form, but may help explain hematogenous spread. This facultative intracellular bacteria may also grow extracellularly. Host defenses require T lymphocyte interaction. Both helper and cytolytic cell lines contribute to acquired resistance.[4]

Macrophages are of key importance in this infection. The ability of these bacteria to grow within macrophages appears to be a prerequisite for proper antigen processing and presentation and for the generation of cell-mediated immunity to *L monocytogenes*. SH-activated hemolysis is correlated with the ability of the bacteria to survive and multiply within a macrophage.[5] Virulent bacteria may be actively involved in their own uptake. *L monocytogenes* is also able to penetrate fibroblasts.[5] It is quite likely that virulent bacteria are able to initiate their own entry into intestinal epithelial cells.

The basic pathologic lesion in listeriosis is miliary granulomatosis, with focal necrosis or suppuration in involved tissues. Such lesions may be visible in the liver, adrenals, and lungs. Meningeal localization is common, not appearing different from any other pyogenic meningitis.

EFFECTS OF PREGNANCY

L monocytogenes has a predilection for pregnancy; 50% of reported cases have been in pregnant women and fetuses. The presentation of listeriosis is different in pregnancy. While nonpregnant adults frequently have the symptoms of meningitis, gastrointestinal symptoms have been reported most often in pregnancy.[6] Maternal mortality is rare, likely reflecting the mild nature of the illness and the good health of the mother. Only two maternal deaths associated with listeriosis have been reported; one patient had AIDS[7], the other had systemic lupus erythematosus.[8]

Infection from *L monocytogenes* may occur anytime during pregnancy, but it is more common in the third trimester. During pregnancy, infected abortion and amnionitis may develop, although many patients have little clinical evidence of significant infection. Premature delivery is common. Patients often have only nonspecific signs and symptoms, such as fever, chills, myalgia, pharyngitis, or diarrhea.[6,7]

While genital listeriosis is rare, cervicovaginal carriage has been associated with miscarriage. Repeated abortion is not a clearly established sequela. Septic abortion may occur, however, even in the absence of genital carriage, presumably secondary to hematogenous spread from the gastrointestinal tract.

Preterm delivery may accompany listeriosis, although patients with bacteremia may occasionally experience no sequelae.[9] Fetal distress associated with listerial amnionitis has also been documented.[10] Direct fetal involvement is common, with premature birth of a dead infant. The term *granulomatosis infantiseptica* has been applied to this condition. Intrauterine infection may arise by either hematogenous or transcervical (ascending) routes. The former is more common, as many affected patients have negative cervicovaginal cultures.[9] The fetal membranes are nearly always intact.[6]

Neonatal listeriosis has both early- and late-onset clinical forms.[6] Early-onset disease is far more severe and is commonly associated with prematurity and congenital pneumonia. Disseminated abscesses or granulomas may be observed in multiple organs, including the liver, spleen, lungs, kidney, brain, and placenta. Conjunctivitis may also be present. Greenish discoloration or meconium staining of the amniotic fluid is common. Mortality is high (up to 40% of liveborns), but is improved if fully disseminated disease, granulomatosis infantiseptica, is absent.[6,9] Among survivors, pulmonary dysplasia may develop as a result of required ventilatory support.

Late-onset disease presents after the fifth day of life but generally within a month of delivery.[3] It is characterized by meningitis in a normal birth weight infant and an absence of obstetric complications. On occasion, listeria may be isolated in the mother. Nosocomial transmission may occur. When treated appropriately, mortality (4–10%) is far less than other bacterial meningitides.[3] Major sequelae may include hydrocephalus and mental retardation.

DIAGNOSIS

In pregnancy, the differential diagnosis of listeriosis in the absence of fetal distress or demise includes any febrile illness. Listeriosis is often not suspected because of the vague, nonspecific signs and flulike symptoms that include chills, myalgia, pharyngitis, diarrhea, and, occasionally, urinary tract symptoms. More advanced maternal disease may be present, such as endocarditis or meningitis. In adults, a positive blood culture is generally confirmatory. Amniotic fluid, Gram's stain, and culture may also prove beneficial. Carriage may also be sought in the stool, but cervicovaginal carriage, in the absence of ruptured membranes or delivery, is often absent.

If infection in the pregnant patient is unrecognized, stillbirth generally results. In early-onset disease, the newborn is often premature and may manifest signs of distress. Laboratory evaluation other than culture or Gram's stain is not always helpful. Chest x-ray will identify pulmonary involvement. Late-onset newborn disease can be confirmed by culture of cerebrospinal fluid. Blood cultures are occasionally positive.

TREATMENT

L monocytogenes is susceptible to many antibiotics, including penicillin, erythromycin, rifampin, trimethoprim, aminoglycosides, and tetracycline; sensitivities have changed little over the past 20 years. Ampicillin or penicillin plus tobramycin has maximal listericidal effects. Penicillin-allergic patients should receive erythromycin. Tetracycline or doxycycline should be avoided in the pregnant patient or neonate. Therapy should be continued for two to three weeks. Fetal survival rates of 80% have been reported when a prompt diagnosis has been made.[11] In the absence of fetal demise or evidence of fetal maturity, data support expectant medical management at any time during pregnancy even if the amniotic fluid is culture-positive.[11,12]

REFERENCES

1. Ryser ET, Marth EH. "New" food-borne pathogens of public health significance. *J Am Diet Assoc.* 1989;89:948.
2. Lu CY, Changelian PS, Unane ER. Alphafetoprotein inhibits macrophage expression of Ia antigen. *J Immunol.* 1984;132:1722.
3. Albritton WL, Wiggins GL, Feeley JC. Neonatal listeriosis: distribution of serotypes in relation to age at onset of disease. *J Pediat.* 1976;88:481.
4. Kaufmann SHE. Possible role of helper and cytolytic T lymphocytes in antibacterial defense: conclusions based on a murine model of listeriosis. *Rev Infec Dis.* 1987;9:S650.
5. Kuhn M, Kathariou S, Goebel W. Hemolysin supports survival but not entry of the intracellular bacterium *Listeria monocytogenes. Infect Immun.* 1988;56:79.
6. Halliday HL, Hirata T. Perinatal listerosis—a review of twelve patients. *Am J Obstet Gynecol.* 1979;133:405.
7. Wetli CV, Roldan EO, Fojaco RM. Listeriosis as a cause of maternal death: an obstetric complication of acquired immunodeficiency syndrome (AIDS). *Am J Obstet Gynecol.* 1983;147:7.
8. Fan Y-D, Pastorek JG, Janney FA, et al. Listeriosis as an obstetric complication in an immunocompromised patient. *S Med J.* 1989;82:1044.
9. Evans JR, Allen AC, Stirson DA, et al. Perinatal listeriosis: report of an outbreak. *Pediatr Inf Disease.* 1985;4:237.
10. Koh KS, Cole TL, Orkin AJ. Listeria amnionitis as a cause of fetal distress. *Am J Obstet Gynecol.* 1980;136:261.
11. Katz VL, Weinstein L. Antepartum treatment of *Listeria monocytogenes* septicemia. *S. Med J.* 1982;75:1353.
12. Cruikshank DP, Warenski JC. First-trimester maternal *listeria monocytogenes* sepsis and chorioamnionitis with normal neonatal outcome. *Obstet Gynecol.* 1989;73:469.

Chapter Seventy
Diphtheria

Sebastian Faro

70

Diphtheria, historically, is one of the most important infectious diseases because it encompasses many different aspects of microbiology and far reaching pathophysiology of infection. The understanding of the complex relationship between a bacterium, the pathophysiology, and the relationship to the resulting infection have made diphtheria one of the most well understood infections. The bacterium typically infects the pharynx, but cutaneous diphtheria also occurs. The systemic effect is due to an extracellular toxin produced by the bacterium.

An understanding of diphtheria began in 1883, when the bacillus was described by Klebs.[1] Loeffler, in 1884, described the morphological characteristics of the bacillus; in addition, he was able to culture and establish that the bacterium was the etiologic agent responsible for the infection.[2] The pathophysiology was further elucidated when Roux and Yersin, in 1888, demonstrated that cell-free filtrates of cultures of the bacillus killed guinea pigs.[3] This discovery led to the development of antiserum by von Behring and Kitasato in 1890.[4] Further research led von Behring to a program of active immunization using a toxin neutralized with antitoxin.[5] Glenny and Ramon developed toxoid[6,7], which is diphtheria toxin treated with 0.4% formaldehyde. Today, immunization with toxoid remains the primary means of preventing diphtheria; however, epidemics still occur.

Diphtheria occurs worldwide, usually in epidemics. The introduction of immunization programs has greatly reduced the incidence of diphtheria, but cases continue to be reported from Alaska, Arizona, New Mexico, South Dakota, and Washington.[8] These states have sizable American Indian populations, and the attack rate among this group is 10 to 100 times higher than that seen in other races. It also seems to attack the poorly-nourished and debilitated who are living in crowded conditions.[9]

There appears to be a bimodal distribution with respect to a predilection for particular age groups. Children ages 2 to 5 are a primary target for the bacillus and also have a high mortality rate. In addition to children, patients who are 50 years of age or older have become a primary target for infections.

The natural host for the bacillus is humans. The bacilli are transferred from one individual to another by way of one of two mechanisms. Respiratory transmission occurs by way of aerosolized droplets that are contaminated with the bacillus. A second mode of transmission is through contact with cutaneous lesions. Diphtheria is not seasonal, but there is a tendency to record an increased incidence in the colder months.

The bacillus *Corynebacterium diphtheriae* is a gram-positive, nonspore-forming pleomorphic bacterium. The organism is nonmotile, nonencapsulated, and aerobic. A septum can be seen between organisms that are attached or actively dividing, and, when stained, the transverse septum does not take up the stain, giving the bacilli a segmental appearance.

The bacterium can be cultured on media containing tissue extracts or agents that are toxic to other bacteria, thus allowing the diphtheria bacillus to grow. Typically, colonies of *C diphtheriae* are grayish-white when grown on Loeffler's medium. When the organism is grown on a medium containing tellurite, the diphtheria bacilli may be easily isolated. When a specimen is obtained from the pharynx, it is likely to be contaminated by other endogenous bacteria. Tellurite is an agent that inhibits the growth of other bacteria. Three morphological colonial forms can be differentiated on tellurite medium. *Mitis colonies* are black, smooth, and convex, and are capable of causing hemolysis, but do not ferment starch or glycogen. *Gravis colonies* are gray-to-black, semi-rough, flat, and are capable of fermenting starch, as well as glycogen, but are not hemolytic. *Intermedius colonies* have a black center with grayish borders, are small and smooth, do not ferment starch or glycogen, and are not hemolytic.[10,11]

A bacteriophage has been identified that infects the bacterium and carries a gene, tox^+, which enables the organism to produce diphtherial toxin.[12,13] Strains not infected with the bacteriophage carrying the tox^+ gene do not produce the toxin. The toxin interferes with protein synthesis by disrupting the association of ^{t}RNA and ribosomal RNA, thereby blocking protein synthesis.[14-16]

Other species of *Corynebacterium* can cause diphtheria-like illnesses. *Corynebacterium ulcerans* can be isolated from the nasopharynx of healthy patients, but can also be obtained from the throats of individuals with a diphtherialike illness. Another species that resembles *C diphtheriae* is *Corynebacterium pseudotuberculosis. Corynebacterium haemolyticum* causes pharyngitis that is associated with a scarlatiniform rash, but does not produce an exotoxin. It is haemolytic and does not grow on tellurite-containing medium. *Corynebacterium minutissimum* causes a chronic skin infection and is characterized by red to brownish patches on the medial aspect of the thighs, the scrotum, and the axilla. This condition is referred to as *erythrasma.*

PATHOGENESIS

Diphtheria can be asymptomatic or may manifest as nasal, tonsillar, pharyngeal, laryngeal, bronchial diphtheria, myocarditis, or infective endocarditis. The infection may be minimally symptomatic or may develop into a rapidly fulminant infection that results in death. The factors that determine whether or not the patient will be mildly, moderately, or severely infected depends upon the host's immunity toward the toxin, the virulence of the strain, and whether or not the strain possesses the bacteriophage that carries the tox^+ gene. The site of infection is also important, as is the age of the patient and any existing systemic disease.[17-19]

The incubation period is two to six days. Adults are more likely to complain of pharyngitis than children. The disease is somewhat insidious in that the patient may have mild symptoms but can be severely ill.

Nasal diphtheria is usually mild and is not commonly associated with systemic toxicity. The patient develops a thick mucopurulent nasal discharge. Examination of the internal nares may reveal the presence of a creamy yellowish membrane.

Tonsillar diphtheria is characterized by the development of a thick membrane covering the tonsils. The membrane becomes grayish-green and quite thick. The membrane adheres tenaciously to the tissue and may be difficult to dislodge. When the membrane is removed, there is often bleeding that results from denuding the surface epithelium of the tonsil. Patients frequently complain of a sore throat, pain with swallowing, headache, nausea, and vomiting.

The membrane in pharyngeal diphtheria covers the palatine tonsil, the uvula, and the soft palate and encompasses the pharyngeal wall. The tonsils tend to swell and become quite large, often preventing examination of the posterior aspect of the tonsils. Significant nasal bleeding may result if the nasal mucosa is involved. The patient frequently has significant halitosis, referred to as the *diphtheria fetor,* but this halitosis is also seen with mononucleosis and Vincent's angina (necrotizing ulcerative gingivitis). Edema of the neck may occur; upon resolution, prominent enlarged lymph nodes remain. The edema may be so marked that it obscures the angle of the mandible, the anterior border of the sternocleidomastoid muscle, the clavicle, as well as the superclavicular lymph nodes.

Patients with diphtheric myocarditis usually are toxic and have other systemic findings. Abnormalities of the electrocardiogram develop during the first week. Interestingly, nerve conduction defects in the peripheral nerves, for example, median, ulnar, and common peroneal nerves, is noted prior to the development of electroconduction defects in the myocardium.[19-21] Heart failure is rarely seen with nasal diphtheria, but may occur in up to 9% of the cases of pharyngeal–laryngeal diphtheria. This is due to the great likelihood of significant toxin production associated with pharyngeal and laryngeal infection. The patient develops pallor, hypotension, and collapsed peripheral pulses, and becomes diaphoretic. Individuals with diphtheria who develop ST-T changes have a 28% risk of death. Patients with myocarditis also have elevated aspirate aminotransferase (AST).

A rare complication of diphtheria is infective endocarditis. Blood cultures may reveal the presence of toxicogenic or nontoxicogenic *C diphtheriae,* which has a mortality rate of 70%. The bacterium may infect normal or abnormal valves.

Cutaneous diphtheria has assumed an important role in the evolution and perpetuation of the disease because it may serve as a reservoir of disease. The cutaneous form is commonly seen in the tropical climates and among indigent alcoholics in temperate areas. These individuals are more likely, as are respiratory carriers, to spread the disease. Cutaneous lesions persist longer than respiratory infections, and unlike the latter, cutaneous infection is not associated with systemic toxic manifestations. Therefore, complications such as myocarditis and endocarditis are rare.[22-24]

Diphtheria occurring in pregnancy is rare. Three cases have been reported.[25,26] One case occurred in a patient who was nine weeks pregnant and subsequently developed total paralysis, but delivered a normal infant. Two patients, delivered by cesarean section, experienced rapid deterioration during endotracheal intubation. One individual died of systemic toxicity and the other required a tracheotomy.

DIAGNOSIS

The disease is diagnosed by isolating the bacterium and identifying it by way of biochemical reactions to establish that it is *C diphtheriae.* The appropriate method is to obtain a specimen of membrane and transport it immediately to the laboratory in a moist, reducing, nonnutritious medium. This prevents the organism from drying, to which it is very sensitive, and inhibits the growth of other bacteria. The specimen should be plated out on Loeffler's medium as well as a medium containing tellurite. The presence of the bacteriophage carrying the tox^+ gene must be established, because these strains are associated with more severe illness.

The diagnosis is more difficult to establish if the patient has a mild case and if no membrane is present on the pharyngeal mucosa. The presence of an exudate on the pharyngeal mucosa may lead the physician to a diagnosis of viral or streptococcal infection, Vincent's angina, or mononucleosis.

TREATMENT

The treatment begins with the administration of antitoxin. In mild cases, 30,000 to 40,000 units are injected intramuscularly. Individuals with more severe disease should receive 40,000 to 80,000 units, administered intravenously over one hour. The antitoxin is developed from horse serum, and approximately 10% of patients develop an allergic reaction, a nonspecific fever, and serum sickness. Prior to administration of the antitoxin, the patient should be questioned as to possible allergy to horse serum; if not known, then conjunctival and intracutaneous skin tests for hypersensitivity should be performed. Epinephrine should be immediately available. If the patient tests positive, then she should be desensitized by administering increasing doses of antiserum.

Antibiotic therapy is essential to the successful treatment of acute diphtheria. This is necessary to eliminate the bacterium and thereby remove the source of toxin. In addition, the spread of the organism within the population is eliminated, and secondary infections can be effectively treated. In the absence of antibiotic therapy, approximately 1–15% of patients become carriers. Tonsillectomy and adenoidectomy may be required to eliminate the carrier state. The organism is susceptible to penicillin and procaine penicillin, 600,000 units, administered every 12 hours intramuscularly for two weeks. Erythromycin, 500 mg given four times daily for two weeks, is also effective. This regimen has been used to follow penicillin therapy in those individuals who have not had the bacterium eradicated with pencillin therapy.[27] Erythromycin may be used initially, especially in patients who are allergic to penicillin. Although erythromycin is considered the drug of choice, pregnant patients tend to have difficulty tolerating this antibiotic, and pencillin is a suitable alternative.

Following completion of antimicrobial therapy, specimens should be obtained from the nasopharynx and oropharynx to determine if the bacterium has been eradicated. The specimens should be obtained no sooner than one week after therapy has been concluded. This is imperative because it must be documented that the patient has not become a carrier.

PREVENTION

Diphtheria, although a communicable disease, is preventable. It is now routine to immunize all infants at two months of age, and documentation of immunization is required prior to entering school in many states. However, not everyone receives immunization. Booster doses should be administered every 10 years, although this is not routinely done. Analysis of antibodies in pregnant women reveal that approximately 50% have adequate antibody levels.[17] Individuals exposed to diphtheria who have been previously immunized should receive a booster of toxoid. If they have not been immunized, they should receive 3000 units of antitoxin and they should be cultured. If they subsequently develop symptoms, primary immunization and antimicrobial therapy should be started.

REFERENCES

1. Klebs E. Ueber Diptherie. *Verhandlungen des Congresses fur Innere Medicin*. 1883;1:139.
2. Loeffler F. Mitt Reichsgesundh Amt. 1884;2:421.
3. Roux E, Yersin A. Contribution a L'Etude de la Diptherie. *Ann Inst Pasteur*. 1888;2:40.
4. MacGregor RB, *Corynebacterium diphtheriae*. Mandell GL, Douglas RG, Bennett JE, eds. *Principles and Practice of Infectious Diseases*, 3rd ed. New York: Churchill Livingstone; 1990:1574.
5. Von Behring E, Unterschungun uber das Zustandkommen der Diptherie-Immunitat bei Thieren. *Dtsch Med Wochenschr*. 1890;16:1145.
6. Glenny AT, Pope CG. Diphtheria toxoid-antitoxin floccules. *J. Path Bact*. 1927;30:587.
7. Glenny AT, Ramon A, Pope CG, et al. Immunological notes: antigenic value of toxoid precipitated by potassium alum. *J. Path Bact*. 1926;27:38.
8. Naiditch MJ, Bower AG, Diphtheria: A study of 1433 cases observed during a ten-year period at the Los Angeles County Hospital. *Am J Med*. 1954;17:229.
9. Pedersen AHB, Spearman J, Tronca E, et al. Diphtheria on Skid Row, Seattle, Washington, 1972–75. *Public Health Rep*. 1977;92:336.
10. McCloskey RV. Corynebacteria Species (Including Diphtheria). In: Mandell GI, Douglas RG Jr, Bennett JE, eds. *Principals and Practice of Infectious Diseases*. New York, NY: John Wiley and Sons; 1979:1620.
11. Hoeprich PD. Diphtheria. In: Hoeprich PD, ed. *Infectious Diseases*. Philadelphia, PA: Harper and Row; 1983:300.
12. Pappenheimer AM Jr. Diphtheria toxin. *Ann Rev Biochem*. 1977;46:69.
13. Barksdale L, Arden SB. Persisting bacteriophage infections, lysogeny, and phage conversions. *Ann Rev Microbiol*. 1974;28:265.
14. Collier RJ. Diphtheria toxin: mode of action and structure. *Bact Rev*. 1975;39:54.
15. Bowman GC. Studies on the mode of action of diphtheria toxin III. Effect on subcellular components of protein synthesis from tissues of intoxicated guinea pigs and rats. *J Exp Med*. 1970;131:659.
16. Gill DM, Pappenheimer AM Jr, Uchida T. Diphtheria toxin protein synthesis and the cell. *Fed Proc*. 1973;32:1508.
17. Fisher AM, Cobb S. The clinical manifestations of the severe form of diphtheria. *Bulletin Johns Hopkins Hosp*. 1948;83:297.
18. Johnson WD, Kaye D. Serious infections caused by diphtheroids. *Ann NY Acad Sci*. 1970;174:568.
19. Boyer NH, Weinstein L. Diphtheric myocarditis. *New Engl J Med*. 1948; 239:301.
20. Altshuler SS, Hoffman KM, Fitzgerald PH. Electrocardiographic changes in diphtheria. *Am J Med*. 1948;29:294.
21. Burkhardt EA, Eggleston C, Smith LW. Electrocardiographic changes and peripheral nerve palsies in toxic diphtheria. *Am J Med Sci*. 1938; 195:301.
22. Belsey MA. *Corynebacterium diphtheriae* skin infections in Alabama and Louisiana. A factor in the epidemiology of diphtheria. *New Engl J Med*. 1969;280:135.
23. Koopman JS, Campbell J. The role of cutaneous diphtheria infections in a diphtheria epidemic. *J Infect Dis*. 1975;131:239.
24. Belsey MA, LeBlanc DR. Skin infections and the epidemiology of diphtheria. *Am J Epidemiol*. 1975;102:179.
25. Petchclai B, Cuwattika P. Diphtheria and tetanus antitoxin levels in the maternal and cord blood of Thai infants. *J Med Assoc Thai*. 1978; 61:672.
26. El Seed A, DaFalla AA, Aboud OI. Fetal immune response following maternal diphtheria during early pregnancy. *Ann Trop Paediatr*. 1981; 1:217.
27. McCloskey RV, Green M, Eller JJ, Smilack J. Treatment of diphtheria carriers; benzathine penicillin, erythromycin and clindamycin. *Ann Intern Med*. 1974;81:788.

Chapter Seventy-One

Cholera

Sebastian Faro

71

Cholera is an ancient disease, the signs and symptoms of which can be found in the writings of Hippocrates, Galen, and Wang-Shooho. The historic writings describe observations of ill individuals dying of severe dehydration due to diarrhea and vomiting. In the late fifteenth century, observations of this devastating illness were recorded from India and Asia. A devastating epidemic occurred in the Ganges River Delta in 1817. The disease then spread over Asia and the Middle East, finally arriving in Europe in 1829. It made its appearance in North America in 1832.[1] Cholera has spread across the world, causing significant epidemics and death on seven different occasions since 1817. Today, the disease remains primarily confined to southern Asia.

Humans are the natural hosts and victims of *Vibrio cholerae*, which is transmitted by the ingestion of contaminated water and food. However, during epidemics, food and water become contaminated with human excreta, which contains the organism, thus providing opportunity for the easy exposure of humans to the organism. Not everyone infected with the bacterium will develop significant symptoms and signs of infection. These individuals, who may be asymptomatic or may have a mild case, are considered carriers and play a significant role in transmission as well as dissemination of the disease. The ratio of asymptomatic carriers to symptomatic individuals ranges from 4 to 1 to 20 to 1, depending upon biotype of *V cholerae*. The gallbladder serves as a reservoir for the organism in approximately 3% of patients and is commonly found in the gallbladder of older convalescent patients. This condition is not found in the pediatric population and, therefore, does not appear to be the sole explanation for perpetuation of this disease. In endemic areas, the attack rates are greatest among children one to five years of age. When the organism invades geographic localities that have not become endemic areas, the organism does not seem to have a predilection for any particular age group.[2,3]

The bacterium *V cholerae* is a short, curved, gram-negative rod. The organism is easily isolated from infected water or excreta and readily grows on selected media. One medium that is particularly useful is thiosulfate-citrate-bile salt-sucrose agar (TCBS), because it does not require sterilization prior to use. It does not support the growth of a large variety of fecal organisms, thus facilitating isolation of *V cholerae.* Colonies of *V cholerae* can be easily selected from other enteric bacteria by their characteristic opaque, yellow colonies.

Vibrio is commonly found on the surface of waters around the world. There are two main pathogenic genera, *V cholerae* and *V parahaemolyticus*, both known to cause diarrhea. These bacteria differ in that *V parahaemolyticus* invades the mucosa of the colon, whereas *V cholerae* does not invade the mucosa and is found primarily in the small intestine.

The strains of *V cholerae* that cause epidemic disease can be identified by determining the presence of somatic antigens. The pathogenic strains have three somatic antigens; serotype Ogawa has both A and B antigens, Inaba has A and C, and Hikojima has antigens A, B, and C.[3,4] Gotschlich, in 1905, isolated six strains of *V cholerae* that produce hemolysins from dead patients who were quarantined at El Tor.[5] The fact that hemolytic strains of *V cholerae* could cause a significant disease was not generally accepted until 1961, when it was isolated frequently from infected patients in the Philippines.[5] The eltor biotype has since been isolated across Asia, the Middle East, Africa, and Europe. This strain has also been isolated from individual cases in North America and South America.

Certain characteristics of the eltor biotype make it a significant organism that will continue its journey around the world. This strain can produce the cholera toxin and can cause severe disease; however, the ratio of cases to carriers compared to the classic biotype is much less. For example, for the eltor biotype, the ratio is 1:30 to 1:100, whereas for the classic biotype, the ratio is 1:2 to 1:4.[6,7]

PATHOGENESIS

V cholerae enters the gastrointestinal tract by the ingestion of food. The organism does not invade any body tissues, but enters and colonizes the small intestine where, if appropriate conditions prevail, the organism replicates. The organism has the ability to penetrate the mucosa lining of the small intestine and colonize the epithelium, but does not enter the cells of the intestine. The intestine secretes an alkaline-rich bile solution that acts to enhance the growth of the bacterium. The organism secretes an enterotoxin that binds to the mucosal lining.[8,9] The enterotoxin produced by *V cholerae* is similar to the toxin produced by *Corynebacterium diphtheriae* and *Escherichia coli.*

The enterotoxin causes an increase in the secretion of chloride, which in turn stimulates and competes with agents that increase the production of cyclic AMP. Cholera enterotoxin has been demonstrated to activate adenylate cyclase in tissues that possess the enzyme.[10,11] The cells that are most affected by the toxin are the crypt cells of the small intestine. These cells are stimulated to secrete enormous amounts of fluid. The goblet cells are stimulated to secrete mucus and give the watery stool the appearance of containing rice, often referred to as "rice-water stools."

DIAGNOSIS

The clinical manifestations of the disease vary, ranging from the asymptomatic individual, to the individual with mild diarrhea, to the patient with the full-blown syndrome. It is important to point out that an individual who appears perfectly healthy and develops the full-blown disease may rapidly deteriorate and die within a few hours of the onset of symptoms. Typically, the patient develops liquid stools, and within 4 to 12 hours, the patient may progress to shock and may expire within 18 hours. Initially, the patient may develop lower abdominal cramping, a feeling of fullness, and gurgling in the abdomen. The initial stools are liquid but do not have the characteristic rice-water stools appearance which occurs later in the disease. The rice-water stools have a mild fishlike odor.

The patient becomes severely dehydrated because of the enormous amount of fluid loss due to diarrhea and vomiting. The patient quickly develops electrolyte imbalance due to shifts from the intravascular and extracellular compartments into the lumen of the bowel. Failure to institute aggressive fluid replacement results in severe dehydration and the development of hypovolemic shock. Some individuals may develop an ileus early in the course of the disease, and often do not have diarrhea, but also become severely dehydrated. These individuals also become hypovolemic because the fluid moves from the cellular and intravascular compartments to the lumen of the bowel. These patients also can develop shock because of severe hypovolemia or electrolyte imbalance. In this setting, it is often difficult to estimate the amount of fluid lost, because large quantities of fluid accumulate in the small and large intestine.[12] This presentation may be confusing because it may be mistaken for a bowel obstruction, because diarrhea is not present. These individuals also can experience a fulminant, rapidly deteriorating course.

The disease may also cause hypoglycemia, which is an extremely critical condition. The mechanism that produces hypoglycemia is not known. It does not seem to be directly related to the dehydration or to malnutrition.[13] These patients may develop seizures or may be unconscious.

In areas where the disease occurs in epidemics or is endemic, the diagnosis can be established on the clinical characteristics. The clinical presentation that is seen with infection caused by enterotoxin-producing strains of *E coli* is the same as that produced by *V cholerae.* Therefore, it is imperative that appropriate fluid and electrolyte replacement be instituted immediately and that no time is wasted attempting to determine appropriate antibiotic therapy.

Specimens of stool should be plated on TCBS medium. Within 18 hours, the characteristic opaque, yellow colonies will appear on the agar surface. Identification should be carried by agglutination with group- and type-specific antiserums. Biochemical characteristics must also be used to obtain appropriate identification.

TREATMENT

The hallmark of treatment is immediate and rapid replacement of fluids and electrolytes. Intravenous replacement should be instituted with sterile water containing 5 g sodium chloride, 4 g sodium bicarbonate, and 1 g potassium chloride, infused at a rate of 50–100 cc per minute. This can be alternated with lactated Ringer's solution. The infusion rate can be titrated according to the patient's pulse rate. Once the pulse rate returns to normal, the fluids should be infused at a rate that keeps pace with the total fluid losses. Adult patients can lose as much as one liter of isotonic liquid per hour during the first 24 hours.[14]

Inadequate fluid replacement results in severe dehydration, associated with electrolyte imbalance and renal insufficiency. Normal renal function usually returns with restoration of proper fluid and electrolyte balance. It is also important to monitor the fluid status of the patient closely, because the infusion of rapid and large amounts of fluid may result in pulmonary edema.

Hypoglycemia, and the accompanying hypokalemia, can be corrected by administering intravenous fluid containing 95 mEq/L of sodium, 65 mEq/L of chloride, 15 mEq/L of potassium, 45 mEq/L of bicarbonate, and 20 g/L of glucose. If this solution is alternated with lactated Ringer's solution, the patient should receive 5% glucose solution by mouth.

Antibiotic therapy will decrease the duration of diarrhea and facilitate fluid replacement. The antibiotic of choice is tetracycline[15,16]; however, this agent should not be used in the pregnant patient. Tetracycline has been found to shorten the duration of diarrhea by 60% and positive cultures by 80%. The pregnant patient who contracts cholera is very likely to undergo spontaneous abortion, and there is no evidence that antibiotics will reduce the risk of abortion.[17-19] Other antibiotics that have proven to be suitable alternatives to tetracycline are chloramphenicol, trimethoprim-sulfamethoxazole, and furazolidone.[20] The pregnant patient can adequately be treated with ampicillin, 250 mg every six hours.[15] It should be pointed out that the disease is self-limiting, and appropriate fluid replacement, avoidance, or prompt treatment of hypoglycemia often results in cure. Once an index case has been identified, antibiotics should be administered to all other household members. Approximately one fifth of the close contacts will be infected. Tetracyline, 1 g either administered as a single dose or in a divided dose, should be administered for five days.[21]

The severe effect on the fetus is not due to infection by *V cholerae*, but to the associated severe dehydration and shock. This undoubtedly results in poor placental perfusion with a decrease in fetal oxygenation. The mother becomes acidotic, which also is reflected in a fetal acidosis. Patients in the third trimester will frequently experience an intrauterine fetal demise. Vaccinating the mother can protect the mother and the fetus. An oral vaccine consisting of killed cholera whole cells with the B subunit component of toxin was found to immunize individuals against cholera in endemic areas successfully.[22]

REFERENCES

1. Baurua D, Burrows W. *Cholera*. Philadelphia, PA: WB Saunders; 1974:458.
2. Woodward WE, Mosley WH. The spectrum of cholera in rural Bangladesh II. Comparison of El Tor, Ogawa and classical Inaba infection. *Am J Epidemiol*. 1971;96:342.
3. Felsenfeld O. A review of recent trends in cholera research and control. *Bull WHO*. 1966;34:161.
4. Carpenter CCJ, Mitra PP, Sack RB. Clinical studies in Asiatic cholera, Parts I–VI. *Bull Hopkins Hosp*. 1966;118:165.
5. Dizon JJ. Studies on El Tor in the Philippines: (1) Characteristics of cholera El Tor in Negros Occidential Province, November 1961 to September 1962. *Bull WHO*. 1965;33:627.
6. Gerichter CB, Sechter I, Cohan J, et al. A serological survey for cholera antibodies in the population of Jerusalem and surroundings. *Israel J Med Sci*. 1973;9:980.
7. Bart KJ, Juq Z, Khan M, et al. Seroepidemiologic studies during simultaneous epidemic infection with El Tor, Ogawa and classical Inaba *Vibrio cholerae*. *J Infec Dis*. 1970;121:17.
8. Gill M. Mechanism of action of cholera toxin. *Adv Cyclic Nucleoride Res*. 1977;8:85.
9. Gangarosa EJ, Beisel WR, Benyajati C, et al. The nature of the gastrointestinal lesion in Asiatic cholera and its relation to pathogenesis: a biopsy study. *Am J Trop Med Hyg*. 1960;9:125.
10. Sharp GWG, Hynie S. Stimulation of intestinal adenylate cyclase by cholera toxin. *Nature*. 1971;229:266.
11. Kimberg DV, Field M, Johnson J, et al. Stimulation of intestinal mucosal adenylate cyclase by cholera enterotoxin and prostaglandins. *J Clin Invest*. 1971;50:1218.
12. Hirschhorn N, Kinzie JL, Sachar DB, et al. Decrease in net stool output in cholera during intestinal perfusion with glucose containing solutions. *N Engl J Med*. 1968;176:279.
13. Hirschhorn N, Lindebaum J, Greenough WB, Alam SM. Hypoglycemia in children with acute diarrhea. *Lancet*. 1966;2:128.
14. Carpenter CCJ. Cholera. In: Hoeprich PD, ed. *Infectious Diseases*. Philadelphia, PA: Harper and Row; 1983:669.
15. Carpenter CCJ, Sack RB, Mondal A, Mitra PP. Tetracycline therapy in cholera. *J Indian Med Assoc*. 1964;43:309.
16. Wallace CK, Anderson PN, Brown TC, et al. Optimal antibiotic therapy in cholera. *Bull WHO*. 1968;39:239.
17. Ayangade O. The significance of cholera outbreaks in the prognosis of pregnancy. *Int J Gynaecol Obstet*. 1981;19:403.
18. Khan PK. Asiatic cholera in pregnancy. *Int Surg*. 1969;51:138.
19. Hirschhorn N, Chowdhuury AKMA, Lindebaum J. Cholera in pregnant women. *Lancet*. 1969;1:1230.
20. Gharagogloo RA, Naficy K, Mouin M, et al. Comparative trial of tetracycline, chloramphenicol and trimethoprim-sulphamethoxazole in eradication of *Vibrio cholerae* El Tor. *Br Med J*. 1970;4:281.
21. McCormack WM, Chowdhuury AM, Jahanju N, et al. Tetracycline prophylaxis in families of cholera patients. *Bull WHO*. 1962;38:787.
22. Clemens JD, Sack DA, Harris JR, et al. Field trial of oral vaccines in Bangladesh. *Lancet*. 1986;2:124.

Chapter Seventy-Two

Campylobacter Infection

Sebastian Faro

72

The first human infections due to a suspected vibriolike organism were recorded in 1947.[1] Dysentery caused by *Vibrio fetus* was reported in 1963; however, the bacterium was not isolated from a stool specimen obtained from a symptomatic patient until 1972.[2,3] In 1978, *Campylobacter* was responsible for 2000 cases of enteritis that occurred in Vermont.[4]

Campylobacter fetus, formerly called *Vibrio fetus*, has been isolated from 3–8% of patients with diarrhea considered to have an infectious etiology. A large study was conducted in which 22,000 stool specimens, obtained over an 8-year period, were examined for the presence of *fetus subspecies jejuni*. Positive cultures were obtained from 5.9% of patients with diarrhea. Specimens obtained from asymptomatic, healthy individuals yielded an isolation rate of 1.3%, thus suggesting that there is a normal asymptomatic carrier state.[5]

Three subspecies of *C fetus* have been isolated from cattle and sheep, which acquire the bacterium from ingesting contaminated food and water. The organism can enter the vascular system and is hematogenously disseminated to various parts of the body, including the urogenital tract. The organism can be transmitted venerally and is a frequent cause of abortions in cattle and sheep.[6,7]

Human infection occurs mainly through the ingestion of contaminated food and water. Outbreaks of acute gastroenteritis from water have been reported from Vermont[4], and from California and Colorado, which were traced to ingestion of raw milk.[8] It has been hypothesized that *C fetus* may be sexually transmitted by humans, but the organism has never been isolated from the male genital tract. However, the bacterium has been recovered from human abortuses and has caused neonatal infection. The organism has been recovered from the vagina of pregnant women. There is a case report of the isolation of *C fetus* from the cervix of a patient who had aborted two months earlier.[7]

C fetus is a curved, nonspore-forming, gram-negative rod. The bacterium has a single, unipolar or bipolar flagella. The organism is classified under the family Spirillaceae, and there are three subspecies: *C fetus subspecies jejuni, C fetus subspecies intestinalis,* and *C fetus subspecies fetus.* All three subspecies have been isolated from cattle and sheep, but only *C fetus subspecies intestinalis* and *C fetus subspecies jejuni* have been isolated from humans. The organism grows readily on supplemented media and usually appears on the surface of the agar within 24–48 hours, although incubation time may require 72–96 hours or longer. Therefore, the culture plates should not be discarded until approximately two weeks have elapsed from the time of inoculation. The organism is microaerophilic.[9,10]

A second species has been identified, *Campylobacter pyloris.* This species appears to be implicated in the pathogenesis of human gastritis. The organism has been identified in the gastric mucus and at the intracellular junctions of gastric epithelial cells.[11]

DIAGNOSIS

The pathogenesis of the infection is not well understood. The organism does not appear to produce a toxin, nor does it seem to be invasive. The bacterium has a predilection for the small intestine and may cause inflammation of the mesenteric lymph nodes. Typically, the organism does not cause bacteremia in healthy individuals; however, persons with impaired immunity have been reported to develop *Campylobacter* bacteremia. This occurs in predominantly older men with alcoholic cirrhosis. In addition, individuals who are at risk for developing bacteremia are those with malignancies, hypoalbuminemia, and those with defects in cell-mediated immunity.[12]

The disease is usually preceded by the development of fever, malaise, headache, myalgias, and anorexia. Some individuals may develop significant pain, mimicking a surgical abdomen. Therefore, it is important that these individuals be carefully evaluated to rule out a bowel obstruction and to avoid unnecessary exploratory laparotomy. Soon after the onset of the clinical manifestations, usually within 24 hours, diarrhea occurs. The liquid stool initially is bile colored and then becomes watery or mucoid, turning to melena or frankly bloody.[13] The patient who will usually have diarrhea for 48–72 hours, which may resolve spontaneously, will not feel well for approximately two weeks. Examination of the stool reveals the presence of leukocytes in 80% of the cases and fresh blood in 66% of the cases. The disease may also be prolonged with exacerbations typified by the presence of fever, chills, and myalgias. Frequently, in such cases, a focus of infection cannot be established. Intermittent diarrhea or nonspecific abdominal pain will occur, without localizing signs. Antibiotic therapy will result in a cure; as a rule, however, fatalities may occur. In some instances, secondary seeding of organs may occur, leading to a more complicated infection such as endocarditis, pericarditis, septic arthritis, and meningitis.[14-16]

Secondary infection may frequently present as a vascular infection, for example, vascular necrosis, which is commonly associated with endocarditis.[17,18] There have been nine cases of thrombophlebitis reported in association with *C fetus* bacteremia.[18] Patients with bacteremia with no identifiable focus of infection should be considered to have septic thrombophlebitis.

Pregnant patients with *C fetus* infection usually present with an upper respiratory infection. These individuals usually have symptoms of pneumonitis, fever, and bacteremia. Typically, the mother will respond to antibiotic therapy. In a small series of five second trimester pregnancies, four mothers delivered dead fetuses and one individual treated with antibiotics delivered a healthy term infant.[19,20] There have not been enough cases for study and thus specific guidelines for pregnant patients with *Campylobacter* gastroenteritis are not available.

TREATMENT

Most patients with survive the acute episode of gastroenteritis; however, individuals with severe or systemic infection will require antibiotic therapy. *Campylobacter* is sensitive to erythromycin, clindamycin, tetracyclines, chloramphenicol, and aminoglycosides.[21] However, approximately 2–10% of the strains have been found to be resistant to erythromycin.[22] Furazolidone is active against 95% of isolates tested. Most strains are resistant to trimethoprim but are sensitive to sulfamethoxazole. Penicillins are typically ineffective against *Campylobacter,* as is cefoxitin and cephalosporins. Most strains of *Campylobacter* are capable of producing β-lactamase, thereby rendering β-lactam antibiotics useless.

The drug of choice is erythromycin for symptomatic infection with *Campylobacter.* The dose is 50 mg/kg/day, for five to seven days. It has been observed that treatment with erythromycin is associated with significant nausea in 10–20% of patients, and this may also be a significant problem with the pregnant patient. The pregnant patient should not be treated with doxycycline or tetracycline. Alternative treatment can be carried out with clindamycin or aminoglycosides. Patients with systemic illness should be treated with intravenously administered antibiotics.

In the absence of specific treatment guidelines for the pregnant patient, it would seem logical to institute replacement therapy of fluids and restore electrolyte balance. In addition, if erythromycin can be tolerated, then it should be administered. Obviously, individuals with more severe disease should receive intravenous antibiotic therapy.

REFERENCES

1. Vinzent R, Dumas J, Picard N. Septiceme grave au cours de la grossesse due a un vibrion: avortment consecutif. *Bull Acad Z Natl Med Paris.* 1947;131:90.
2. Mandel AD, Ellison RC. Acute dysentery syndrome caused by *Vibrio fetus:* report of a case. *JAMA.* 1963;185:36.

3. Deykeser P, Gossiun-Detrain M, Butzler JP, Sternon J. Acute enteritis due to related vibrio: first positive stool cultures. *J Infect Dis*. 1972;125:390.
4. Tiehan W, Vogt RL. Waterborne *Campylobacter* gastroenteritis—Vermont, *MMWR*. 1978;27:207.
5. Lauwers S, DeBock M, Butzler JP. *Campylobacter* enteritis in Brussels. *Lancet*. 1978;1:604. Letter.
6. Franklin B, Ulmer D. Human infection with *Vibrio fetus*. *West J Med*. 1967;120:200.
7. Hood M, Todd JM. *Vibrio fetus*—A cause of human abortion. *Am J Obstet Gynecol*. 1960;83:506.
8. Taylor PR, Weinstein WM, Bryner JH. *Campylobacter fetus* infections in human subjects; association with raw milk. *Am J Med*. 1979;66:779.
9. Holt JR, ed: *Bergey's Manual of Determinative Bacteriology*. 8th ed. Baltimore, MD: Williams and Wilkins; 1974:207.
10. Morris GK, Patton C. In: Lenette EH, Balows A, Hauser W, Shadomy HJ, eds. *Manual of Clinical Microbiology*. 4th Ed. Washington, DC: American Society of Microbiology; 1985:302.
11. Hazell SL, Lee A, Brady L, Hennessy W. *Campylobacter pyloris* and gastritis: association with intracellular spaces and adaptation to an environment of mucus as important factors in colonization of the gastric epithelium. *J Infect Dis*. 1986;153:658.
12. Park CH, McDonald F, Twohig AM, et al. Septicemia and gastroenteritis due to *Vibrio fetus*. *South Med J*. 1973;66:531.
13. Blaser MJ, Berkowitz ID, Laforce FM. *Campylobacter* enteritis: clinical and epidemiologic features. *Ann Intern Med*. 1979;91:179.
14. Collins HS, Blevins A, Baxter E. Protracted bacteremia and meningitis due to *Vibrio fetus*. *Arch Int Med*. 1964;113:361.
15. Lawrence R, Nibble AF, Levin S. Lung abscess secondary to *Vibrio fetus*, malabsorption syndrome and acquired agammaglobulinemia. *Chest*. 1971;60:191.
16. Loeb H, Bettag JL, Yantz NK, et al. *Vibrio fetus* endocarditis. *Am Heart J*. 1966;71:381.
17. Vesely D, MacIntyre S, Ratzan KR. Bilateral deep brachial vein thrombophlebitis due to *Vibrio fetus*. *Arch Int Med*. 1975;135:994.
18. Skirrow MB. Campylobacter enteritis: a new disease. *Br Med J*. 1977; 2:9.
19. Eden AN. Perinatal mortality caused by *Vibrio fetus*. Review and analysis. *J Ped*. 1966;68:297.
20. Gribble MJ, Salit IE, Isaac-Renton J, et al. *Campylobacter* infection in pregnancy. *Am J Obstet Gynecol*. 1981;140:423.
21. Butzler JP, Deykeser P, Lafontaine T. Susceptibility of related vibrios and *Vibrio fetus* to twelve antibiotics. *Antimicrob Agents Chemother*. 1974; 5:86.
22. Vanhoff R, Vanderlindon MP, Dierickx R, et al. Susceptibility of *Campylobacter fetus ss jejuni* to twenty-nine antimicrobial agents. *Antimicrob Agents Chemother*. 1978;14:553.

Chapter Seventy-Three
Bartonellosis

Joseph M. Miller, Jr. and Joseph G. Pastorek II

73

Cutaneous manifestations of bartonellosis, or benign *verruga peruana,* have been known in Peru for centuries. The acute form, *Oroya fever,* was recognized in the late 1800s. The common bacterial cause of both syndromes was established a century ago by Daniel Carrión while he was still a medical student.

Bartonella bacilliformis is a small, motile, aerobic, pleomorphic bacillus. It is gram-negative, but counterstains poorly; *B bacilliformis* stains best after growth on an enriched media. Colonies stain reddish-purple with Giemsa stain.

Bartonellosis is limited to areas of the Andes Mountains at altitudes of 2000–8000 feet where the sandfly vector *Phlebotomus verrucarum* resides. In these areas of Peru, Ecuador, and Colombia, the disease is endemic, with asymptomatic cases and long-term carriers serving as a reservoir of infection.

Among nonimmune persons, infection with *Bartonella* occurs through the bite of an infected sandfly. Large numbers of bacteria enter the blood stream, adhere to erythrocytes, and invade endothelial cells.[1] Anemia develops because of erythrocytic destruction and bone marrow suppression. Complicating infections, especially with *Salmonella,* occur commonly during the recovery phase. As immunity develops, organisms disappear from the blood. Most individuals go on to develop a chronic form of bartonellosis, verruga peruana. The incubation period is approximately three weeks, but marked variation occurs. Hemangiomatous nodules, which may contain *Bartonella,* develop in the skin and subcutaneous tissues over a period of three months to a year. Old cutaneous lesions may become quite fibrotic. On occasion, lesions recur in internal organs and tissues, including bone and central nervous system.

A variety of clinical manifestations are possible, but a patient may have as little as a positive blood culture to make the diagnosis. Usually when Oroya fever develops, the patient experiences chills, fever, headaches, diaphoresis, and changes in mentation. The sudden anemia and slight jaundice give the skin a peculiar color. The anemia is macrocytic, with polychromasia, poikilocytosis, Howell–Jolly bodies, and nucleated red blood cells present.[2] Erythrocyte counts may fall to as low as 500,000/mm^3. The characteristic feature is the presence of numerous organisms adherent to as many as 90% of erythrocytes. *B bacilliformis* is also found in phagocytic cells, such as the Kupffer's cells of the liver and spleen. In addition to anemia, thrombocytopenia with purpura may develop.[3] The leukocyte count is variable, but there is usually a shift to the left.

If the patient survives this preeruptive stage, a critical state ensues. The bacteria disappear from the erythrocytes. Fever diminishes and erythrocyte numbers increase. Intercurrent infection is common and accounts for more than half the mortality.[1] Salmonellosis, amebiasis, malaria, and tuberculosis are common complications.

After resolution of Oroya fever, myalgias and arthralgias may persist until the time of verruga development.[3] This cutaneous eruption may develop without prior symptoms. Nodules develop over one to two months, frequently on exposed parts of the body. Cutaneous lesions vary from red to purple and appear in crops. Lesions may be in various stages of growth and regression within the same patient.

The verrugas may be confluent, nodular, pedunculated, or miliary, with individual lesions of up to 2 mm in diameter. If secondarily infected, the verrugas may ulcerate or bleed. The organism may be cultured from cutaneous lesions and, occasionally, from blood and bone marrow.[3]

BARTONELLOSIS AND PREGNANCY

There is no information available on bartonellosis in pregnancy. Pregnancy would, however, not be expected to alter the course of the disease.

The high fever and bacteremia of bartonellosis could be expected to be associated with miscarriage, preterm delivery, or congenital infection. The absence of reported cases makes this conjectural. Maternal mortality would have the expected adverse outcome on the fetus.

Diagnosis

The diagnosis of bartonellosis can be made clinically where the disease is endemic. In the acute febrile form, the organisms are seen on peripheral blood smears and confirmed by blood culture. In the chronic benign form, bacteria can be cultured from the verrugas.

Treatment

Prevention of the disease requires control of the sandfly. Further individual protection can be afforded by use of insect repellents and bed netting. Community measures include the use of insecticide sprays, such as DDT.

Chloramphenicol and penicillin are useful in treating acute bartonellosis.[1] Streptomycin may also be effective. Although there is concern about use of chloramphenicol in later pregnancy, it should be considered the drug of choice, especially if *Salmonella* superinfection is present.[4] Choramphenicol, 2 gm or more daily for a minimum of 7 days, should be prescribed.[1] Supportive measures include blood transfusion. Cutaneous verrugal lesions have a variable response to antibiotic therapy. Larger or secondarily infected nodules may actually require excision.

REFERENCES

1. Urteaga BO, Payne EH. Treatment of the acute febrile phase of Carrión's disease with chloramphenicol. *Am J Trop Med.* 1955;4:507.
2. Reynafarje C, Ramos J. The hemolytic anemia of human bartonellosis. *Blood.* 1961;17:562.
3. Ricketts WE. Clinical manifestation of Carrión's disease. *Arch Intern Med.* 1949;84:751.
4. Cuadra M. Salmonellosis complications in human bartonellosis. *Tex Rep Biol Med.* 1956;14:97.

Chapter Seventy-Four
Granuloma Inguinale

Charles H. Livengood III

74

MATERNAL ASPECTS

Definition

Granuloma inguinale is a mildly contagious disease of chronic ulcerative granulomatous lesions affecting primarily the skin and subcutaneous tissues and found only in man. It has also been known as Donovanosis, granuloma contagiosa, granuloma pudendi tropicum, sclerosing granuloma, and other synonyms, which are now archaic. Granuloma inguinale was probably first described by McLeod[1] in 1882; the causative agent was identified by Donovan in 1905[2], and the first United States cases were reported by Grindon in 1913.[3]

Etiology

Granuloma inguinale results from infection by *Calymmatobacterium granulomatis,* a gram-negative bacterium measuring 1.5 × 0.7 μm that is very difficult to grow on artificial media and does not produce disease in animals. Anderson et al[4,5] were able to isolate and grow this organism in the chick embryo yolk sac after many previous failures and described its morphologic and immunologic features. These workers did adapt the organism to growth on artificial media, but only after considerable deviation in its properties. Felman and Nikitas[6] note that *C granulomatis* has a prominent capsule as well as seroreactivity, suggesting a relation to *Klebsiella* species, but the aforementioned complexity of laboratory cultivation has resulted in incomplete characterization of this organism, and its current taxonomy should be considered unconfirmed. Koch's postulates have not been fulfilled with *C granulomatis.*

Pathology

The gross pathology of the lesion is that of one or more indurated nodules, almost always initially occurring in the genital region, which erode the skin to form an ulcer of beefy, friable granulation tissue, although exophytic lesions may occur. Microscopically, enhanced vascularity and acanthosis are seen with dense dermal infiltrate of plasma cells and histiocytes, some foci of polymorphonuclear leukocytes, and rare lymphocytes.[7] The large "foamy" cytoplasmic inclusion, measuring 25–90 μm in diameter, of monocytes containing 20–30 deeply stained *C granulomatis* organisms within cystic spaces is the pathognomonic Donovan body of granuloma inguinale (Figure 74–1).

Epidemiology

Granuloma inguinale is a tropical disease particularly prevalent on the Coromandel coast of India, New Guinea, and the Caribbean, where as many as one fourth of the population is infected. Fewer than 100 cases are reported annually in the United States, and these tend to be from southern states. More commonly infected are those of lower socioeconomic status in the years of sexual activity and with other

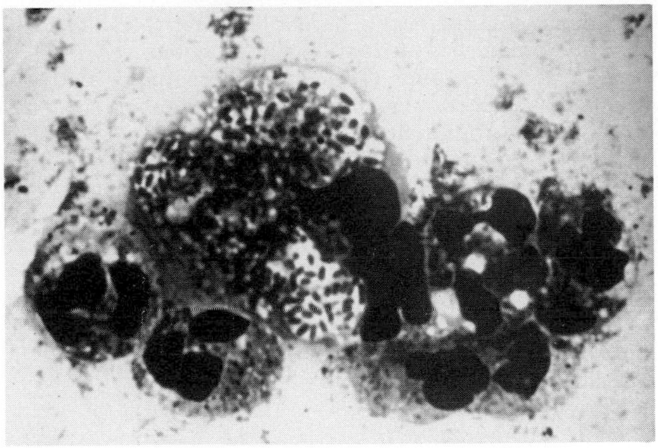

Figure 74–1. Donovan body, diagnostic of granuloma inguinale in crushed biopsy of ulcer base. Under light microscopy, these large, "foamy" cytoplasmic inclusions of monocytes contain numerous blue-black organisms with a "safety pin" appearance on Wright's stain.

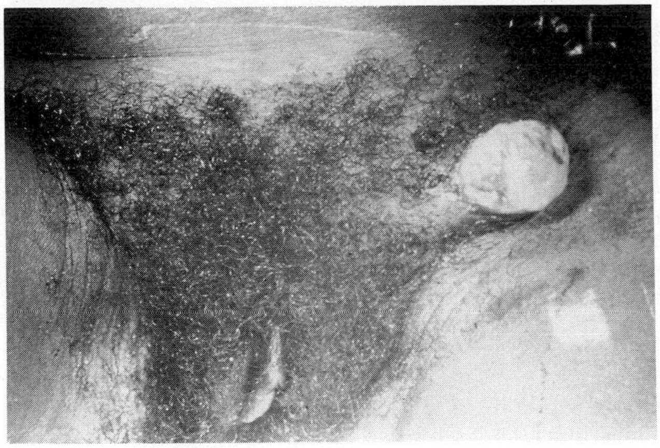

Figure 74–3. "Pseudobubo" of granuloma inguinale. Exophytic solid mass of granulation tissue occurring in the groin affects skin and subcutaneous tissue but actually spares the lymphatics.

sexually transmissible infections. Sexual distribution is essentially equal, although the lesions are more often apparent in men. Although nonsexual transmission and autoinoculation are quite common, this should be regarded as a mildly contagious sexually transmissible disease. Transmission to casual sexual contacts is rare, but 12–52% of steady sexual partners are infected.[8] There is good correlation between rectal disease in passive homosexuals and penile lesions in their active partners,[9] and the genitalia are involved in the vast majority of cases. An excess frequency of malignancy in old scars of granuloma inguinale has been suggested, but lacks documentation.

Manifestations

Although the incubation period may vary from 8 to 80 days, pus from infected persons injected into volunteers produced disease after about six weeks.[10,11] One or more small, nontender, pruritic, indurated nodules appear initially and may regress, only to reappear. Over weeks the nodules grow, forming the classic "pseudobubo" when they occur in the inguinal area, and the overlying skin becomes taut and glossy and eventually erodes away. The remaining painless ulcer has a soft, velvety, smooth base of granulation tissue coated with serosanguinous exudate and a well defined but irregular, rolled, indurated border (Figure 74–2). Some lesions are exophytic, so that a mass of granulation tissue seems to have erupted through the skin (Figure 74–3). Secondary infection may occur. These lesions grow slowly but inexorably and will not heal without therapy. Fibrosis, elephantiasislike change, and even complete genital destruction eventually ensue.

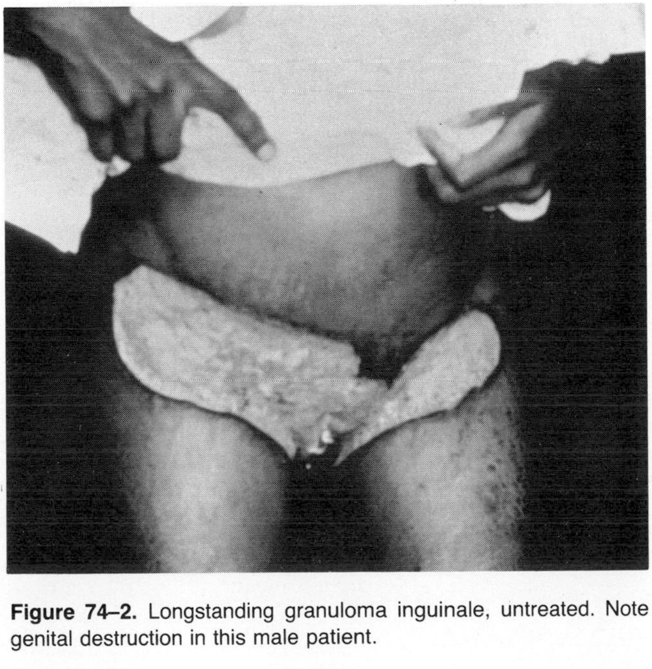

Figure 74–2. Longstanding granuloma inguinale, untreated. Note genital destruction in this male patient.

Genitalia are involved in 90% of cases, the inguinal region in 10%, the perianal region in 5–10%, and other sites in 5%.[12] Extragenital primary lesions of the oral mucosa and skin of the face and torso have been described.[13] A conspicuous absence of regional lymphadenopathy is characteristic; however, with vaginal and cervical lesions marked ipsilateral induration of the underlying tissues is the rule. Late manifestations may include systemic toxicity and infection of deep tissues such as cervix, adnexae, liver, and bone. Death, usually from cachexia, is rare.

Murugan et al[14] reported two cases of abnormal vaginal bleeding caused by granuloma inguinale of the vagina and cervix; one patient, at 24 weeks' gestation, was successfully treated, although the outcome of her pregnancy is not described. Several authors[15-17] in the preantibiotic era noted a "tendency toward progression and fatality" of the disease during pregnancy and the postpartum period, with several reports of deaths associated with involvement of the uterus and adnexae in the setting of isolated cervical lesions.

Diagnosis

Lesions of the disease are rather characteristic in appearance, duration, and lack of tenderness, although superinfection may obscure these features. Culture facilities for *C granulomatis* are rarely available. The diagnosis is based on clinical evaluation and confirmed by observation of Donovan bodies. The latter is performed by biopsy of clean granulation tissue, crushing the specimen between two glass slides, staining with Wright's, Giemsa, or Warthin–Starry stain, and identification of monocytes with large, foamy, cytoplasmic inclusions containing blue-black organisms with a "safety pin" appearance. This technique has good sensitivity and specificity in the diagnosis of granuloma inguinale. Donovan bodies are less readily identified by light microscopy in tissues that have been fixed, embedded, and sectioned, although electron microscopy can be used to identify the organisms.[18]

Diseases to be differentiated from granuloma inguinale include syphilis, chancroid, lymphogranuloma venereum, neoplasia, and herpes genitalis. These may be ruled out by dark-field microscopy and serology, culture for *Hemophilus ducreyi,* culture for *Chlamydia trachomatis* serotypes $L_{1\text{-}3}$, serology, biopsy, and culture for herpes simplex, and cytology, respectively.

Treatment

First-line therapy is tetracycline, 0.5 g every six hours orally. Ampicillin, 0.5 g every six hours orally, may be used but may require prolonged administration.[19] Failures may occur with both drugs and should be managed with gentamycin, 1 mg/kg twice daily intramuscularly, or chloramphenicol, 0.5 g every eight hours orally; these drugs will cure most lesions within three weeks. When successful therapy is begun, lesions will show evidence of regression within seven days. Treatment should be continued for a minimum of three weeks and until the lesions are healed.

There are no guidelines to govern treatment during pregnancy. Inpatient therapy should probably be undertaken to ensure compliance. Ampicillin, 2 g every six hours intravenously, is probably the best first choice. If this fails on the basis of no improvement in the appearance of lesions within seven days, then gentamycin in the doses above will be required. Wysoki et al[20] recently reported successful treatment of a woman in the third trimester of pregnancy using erythromycin.

Prevention

Yearly screening of males in an endemic area of New Guinea reduced the prevalence of disease to 1%.[21] Clearly, in the United States the low prevalence of disease makes this approach impractical. Sexual contacts, family, and intimate contacts of identified cases should be followed with examination for three months after resolution of the index case.

FETAL ASPECTS

Data addressing effects of granuloma inguinale on the fetus have not been identified since 1953; this attests to the extreme rarity of such an effect in modern times and probably to the efficacy of antibiotic therapy in pregnancy in avoiding fetal effects.

In 1953, Scott et al[22] reported a 5-month-old infant with lesions of granuloma inguinale involving the umbilicus, penis, middle ear, radius, and postauricular skin. His mother had granuloma inguinale of the vulva and delivered vaginally with a third-degree laceration. After a long delay in diagnosis, he was effectively treated with streptomycin but suffered permanent right facial paralysis. Wilson[16] described five intrauterine fetal deaths among 14 pregnancies complicated by this disease, and among 105 women with granuloma inguinale at Charity Hospital (New Orleans, LA), a "tendency toward stillbirth" is noted.[23] Arnell and Potekin described four cases during pregnancy with one spontaneous abortion at 10 weeks' gestation and cite a case of granuloma inguinale of the umbilicus in a 6-week-old infant born vaginally to a woman with vaginal disease.[17] One may conclude that vertical transmission at delivery does occur, that neonatal granuloma inguinale is a serious disease, and that intrauterine transmission with fetal death may occur. The histopathology, appearance, and diagnosis of the lesions in neonates are identical to those in adults.

Prevention of ill effects of the disease in pregnancy requires knowledge of granuloma inguinale during the physical examination.

REFERENCES

1. McLeod K. Precis of operations performed in the wards of the first surgeon, Medical College Hospital, during the year 1881. *Indian Med Gaz.* 1882;17:113.
2. Donovan C. Medical cases from Madras General Hospital. *Indian Med Gaz.* 1905;40:411.
3. Grindon J. Granuloma inguinale tropicum, report of three cases. *J Cutan Dis.* 1913;31:236.
4. Anderson K. The cultivation from granuloma inguinale of a microorganism having the characteristics of Donovan bodies in the yolk sac of chick embryos. *Science.* 1943;97:560.
5. Anderson K, DeMonbreum WA, Goodpasture EA. An experimental investigation of the etiology and immunology of granuloma inguinale. *Am J Syph Gonorr Vener Dis.* 1945;29:165.
6. Felman YM, Nikitas JA. Granuloma inguinale. *Cutis.* 1981;27:364.
7. Hart G. Donovanosis: granuloma inguinale. In: Mandell GL, Douglas RG, Bennett JE, eds. *Principles and Practices of Infectious Diseases.* New York, NY: John Wiley & Sons, 1979:1902.
8. Hart G. Chancroid, Donovanosis, lymphogranuloma venereum. *U.S. Department of Health, Education and Welfare Publication No. (CDC) 75-8302;* 1975.
9. Marmell M. Donovanosis of the anus in the male. An epidemiologic consideration. *Br J Vener Dis.* 1958;34:213.
10. Davis CM. Granuloma inguinale. *JAMA.* 1970;211:632.
11. Greenblatt RB. Management of chancroid, granuloma inguinale, lymphogranuloma venereum. *Public Health Service Publication No. 255.* United States Government Printing Office: 1958.
12. Zigas V. Medicine from the past-Donovanosis project in Goilala (1951–1954). *Papua New Guinea Med J.* 1971;14:148.
13. Rajam RV, Rangiah PN: Donovanosis. 1954;*WHO Monogr 24.*
14. Murugan S, Venkatram K, Renganathan PS. Vaginal bleeding in granuloma inguinale. Case reports. *Br J Vener Dis.* 1982;58:200.
15. Pund ER, McInnes GF. Granuloma venereum: a cause of death. Report of six fatal cases. *Clinics.* 1944;3:221.
16. Wilson LA. Pregnancy and labor complicated by granuloma inguinale. *JAMA.* 1930;95:1093.
17. Arnell RE, Potekin JS. Granuloma inguinale of the cervix. *Am J Obstet Gynecol.* 1940;39:626.
18. Dodson RF, Fritz GS, Hubler WR, et al. Donovanosis: a morphologic study. *J Invest Dermatol.* 1974;62:611.
19. Breschi LC, Goldman G, Shapiro SR. Granuloma inguinale in Vietnam: successful therapy with ampicillin and lincomycin. *J Am Vener Dis Assoc.* 1975;1:118.
20. Wysoki RS, Majmudar B, Willis D. Granuloma inguinale (donovanosis) in women. *J Reprod Med.* 1988;33:709.
21. Vogel LC. Een granuloma-venereum (Donovanosis)—epidemic in Suid New Guinea (1920). *Ned Tijdskr Geneeskd.* 1965;109:2425.
22. Scott CW, Harper D McC, Jason RS, et al. Neonatal granuloma inguinale. *Am J Dis Child.* 1953;85:308.
23. D'Aunoy R, von Hamm E. Granuloma inguinale. *Am J Trop Med.* 1937; 17:747.

Chapter Seventy-Five

Legionnaires' Disease

Joseph G. Pastorek II and Joseph M. Miller, Jr.

75

In Philadelphia in 1976, an outbreak of an acute, febrile, respiratory infection broke out among a group of persons attending an American Legion convention.[1] The causative agent was ultimately found to be a fastidious, pleomorphic, gram-negative bacillus that was later named *Legionella pneumophila*. It was subsequently discovered by a retrospective serologic study that *L pneumophila* was responsible not only for this outbreak of legionnaires' disease, but also for mysterious outbreaks of pulmonary illness in previous years. For example, a 1968 outbreak of an influenzalike pneumonitis syndrome in Michigan, termed *Pontiac fever*, was investigated through examination of frozen specimens and found to have been caused by *L pneumophila* as well.[2]

Finally, as more work was done in epidemiologic and bacteriologic study of new and past mini-epidemics of similar respiratory illnesses, a multitude of species of *Legionella* was discovered. Generally, these sporadic occurrences of disease were attributed either to *L pneumophila* or to similar organisms, termed *atypical legionellalike organisms*, or *ALLO*. Some identified species are listed in Table 75–1.

PATHOPHYSIOLOGY

Early reports of legionnaires' disease usually included many fatalities; therefore, autopsy material was readily available. Fulminant illness was thus easily characterized, and included acute bilateral pneumonia arising from bronchioles and spreading often to total lobar consolidation. Macroscopic, multiple, small abscesses are seen in perhaps a quarter of patients, while the histologic picture of alveolitis and hyaline membrane disease (that is, intra-alveolar collections of leukocytes and proteinaceous debris) is present microscopically. In addition, bacteria may be demonstrated in lung tissue with a variety of stains, though direct fluorescent antibody (DFA) stains must be used to specifically identify *Legionella*.

Extrapulmonary manifestations of legionnaires' disease are not commonly appreciated. Hyperplastic lymph nodes full of bacteria are present. Occasionally, congestive hepatosplenomegaly, myocarditis, and pericarditis are described. None of these findings is specific or even very common. And, although *Legionella* has been demonstrated in extrathoracic tissues, the bacteria are almost invariably found within cells of the reticuloendothelial system (RES), and not directly in the parenchyma of organs such as the heart and liver; as well, there is usually no associated inflammatory infiltrate in these areas, as there is within the lung.[3]

It is no coincidence that *Legionella* is found within the cells of the RES. These organisms are facultative, intracellular bacteria that grow both extracellularly and within certain cell types (for example, endothelial and exothelial cells). However, *Legionella* preferrentially replicates within mononuclear phagocytes. In a manner similar to *Mycobacterium tuberculosis*, *Legionella* inhibits the fusion of the lysosome with the phagosome, thus preventing digestion by host enzymes. Therefore, like bacteria such as *Listeria monocytogenes* and the mycobacteria, *Legionella* organisms elude the normal phagocytic immune system and incite, by a complicated mechanism, the helper and cytolytic T-cell functions of the patient. If an overly aggressive cytolytic response ensues, the immune system may actually cause damage to the infected host.[4]

Classic legionnaires' disease is a fulminant, pulmonary syndrome consisting of a number of characteristic signs and symptoms: fever, often as high as 40°C associated with shaking chills; a dry cough, which becomes productive of relatively nonpurulent sputum after 72–96 hours of illness; tachypnea, with rales heard on auscultation of the chest; intense headache early in the course of the disease, with some patients exhibiting confusion and hallucination; and watery stools, accompanying mild abdominal distention and tenderness, in up to one third or one half of patients. The onset of illness may be quite abrupt and dramatic, presenting as overt shock in some cases. Occasional patients have been reported with disseminated coagulopathy and thrombotic thrombocytopenia. As mentioned previously, pericarditis and myocarditis have been reported due to legionellosis, as have pyelonephritis, rhabdomyolysis, encephalitis, and skin rash. This typical presentation of *L pneumophila* infection may represent only the most virulent form of the disease.

Serologic studies of healthy persons indicate that up to one third of persons have had immunologic exposure to *Legionella*. One study of nearly two hundred mothers postpartally found a significant seropositive rate of 35.7%[5], indicating a high rate of subclinical infection. The syndrome of Pontiac fever, while manifest with similar symptoms (for example, high fever, chills, tachycardia, cough, and headache), is generally self-limiting. It would therefore be true to say that disease caused by *L pneumophila* (and the ALLO organisms as well) may clinically present as anything from asymptomatic, subclinical infection to fulminant, fatal legionnaires' disease.

TABLE 75–1. SOME SPECIES OF GENUS *LEGIONELLA*

Legionella pneumophila
L micdadei
L bozemanii
L dumoffii
L gormanii
L jordanis
L longbeachae
L wadsworthii
L oakridgensis

LEGIONELLA INFECTION AND PREGNANCY

Full-blown legionnaires' disease primarily attacks older people, and the male-to-female ratio approaches 3 in 1. Therefore, it is to be expected that women of childbearing age will rarely be seriously infected (though subclinical infection must be common, as mentioned above). Even so, case reports do exist of legionellosis in pregnancy.[6] However, many more patients will have to be treated to document what effect, if any, pregnancy has on legionnaires' disease and vice versa.

Theoretically, the increase in lung water and other alterations in pulmonary physiology attendant with pregnancy may make the gravida a bit more susceptible to severe disease. As well, immunologic changes of pregnancy may have unpredictable effects on the patient's handling of this pathogen, because cell-mediated, rather than humoral, mechanisms are primarily responsible for the immune response against it, as mentioned previously. In any event, the pregnant woman is also more sensitive to the hyperdynamic changes (for example, tachycardia, hypotension, hyperpyrexia) accompanying full-blown illness than is the nonpregnant woman.

Since *Legionella* bacteremia has been described, it is theoretically possible that fetal infection may occur. On the other hand, the organism has a distinct trophism for aerated lung, and so the infant *in utero* may enjoy a certain protection. What effect the organism may have on the placenta itself is unknown. It goes without saying that severe systemic disease in the mother may have adverse effects on her unborn child.

Diagnosis

Since the clinical presentation of legionnaires' disease is common to many different conditions (for example, pneumococcal pneumonia), it is not possible for the physician to make the diagnosis by examination alone. Certainly, if a patient presents with high fever, severe headache, and pulmonary symptomatology in a community where other cases of legionellosis have been reported, this diagnosis will be high on the practitioner's differential. However, without any epidemiologic hints, the identification of *Legionella* is made by ancillary testing.

Initially, there was thought to be a characteristic roentgenographic appearance of legionella pneumonia that served to differentiate it from other pulmonary infections. Though this is no longer thought to be true, there are certain common findings in the patient with pulmonary legionellosis that are at least suggestive, if not actually diagnostic. These include: progression of pulmonic infiltrates in spite of (appropriate) antibiotic therapy; pleural effusion, often anteceding or in the absence of infiltrates of the lung fields; pleuritic pain associated with periplural infiltrates (mimicking pulmonary embolism); slow resolution of the infiltrates, even with apparent clinical improvement; and circumscribed peripheral densities, even cavitation, occurring especially in the immunocompromised patient again progressing even in the face of clinical improvement).[7]

Serologic testing has been the mainstay of laboratory diagnosis of *Legionella* infection. A four-fold rise in antibody titer to greater than 1 in 28, or a single titer of 1 in 256 in a patient with appropriate signs and symptoms, is considered diagnostic. More specific is DFA staining of fresh or formalin-fixed tissue or fluids to directly demonstrate the organism. Likewise, culture techniques are now available that enable isolation of *L pneumophila* and the related ALLO in the laboratory.

Treatment

One important aspect of the therapy of legionellosis of any kind is prevention. It is appreciated now that these organisms are normal inhabitants of the aquatic environment of this planet. Certainly, the medical establishment cannot prevent patients from coming into contact with water in nature, but artificial sources of the bacteria, such as contaminated air conditioning condensors, should be cleaned, if detected. In fact, air conditioning equipment is especially important, because it is felt that the organism is spread by aerosolization and direct infection of the lungs. Institutional epidemics of the disease have been aborted by hyperchlorination of the suspected contaminated water supply.

The patient with acute legionellosis must initially receive intensive supportive care commensurate with the presenting condition and symptomatology. In full-blown legionnaires' disease, intubation and respiratory support are commonly needed. This is especially true in the pregnant patient, because even less severe systemic illnesses, such as pyelonephritis, may predispose her to cardiovascular and pulmonary compromise (that is, hypotension, adult respiratory distress syndrome). As well, maternal oxygenation is important for fetal well being.

Antibiotic therapy of *Legionella* infection consists of erythromycin, 2 g per day for two to three weeks. Treatment may be initiated intravenously and then followed with oral medication. Tetracycline is probably as efficacious as erythromycin, but tetracycline drugs are contraindicated in pregnancy due to hepatic toxicity in the mother and dental and bony effects in the fetus. Similarly, trimethoprin-sulfamethoxazole may be active against the organism, but trimethoprin is also contraindicated in pregnancy, especially in the first trimester, due to theoretic teratogenic effects.

In healthy patients, the fatality rate for appropriately treated legionnaires' disease is reported to be roughly 20%; many of these patients are older than the usual obstetric patient. In the immunocompromised subset of patients, fatality rates may be as high as 80%. The treated patient will usually respond clinically to erythromycin therapy within 24–48 hours, though the fever may persist for up to a week, and, as mentioned above, the chest roentgenographic findings may actually worsen in spite of obvious clinical improvement.

REFERENCES

1. Fraser DW, Tsai T, Orenstien W, et al. Legionnaires' disease: description of an epidemic of pneumonia. *N Engl J Med*. 1977;297:1183.
2. Glick TH, Gregg MB, Berman B, et al. Pontiac fever: epidemic of unknown etiology in a health department. I. Clinical and epidemiologic findings. *Am J Epidemiol*. 1978;107:149.
3. Evans CP, Winn WC. Extrathoracic localization of *Legionella pneumophila* in legionnaires' pneumonia. *Am J Clin Pathol*. 1981;76:813.
4. Kaufmann SHE. Possible role of helper and cytolytic T-lymphocytes in antibacterial defense: conclusions based upon a murine model of listeriosis. *Rev Infect Dis*. 1987;9:S650.
5. Silberg SL, Lawrence CH, Gutherie PJ. Transplacental transfer of *Legionella pneumophila* antibodies. *Pediatr Infect Dis J*. 1987;6:925.
6. Baker DA, Phillips CA. Association of legionnaires' disease and pregnancy. *Am J Obstet Gynecol*. 1979;134:227.
7. Muder RR, Yu VL, Parry MF. The radiologic manifestations of legionella pneumonia. *Semin Resp Infect*. 1987;2:242.

E

Anaerobic Bacterial Infections

Chapter Seventy-Six

Infections Caused by Anaerobic Organisms

Stephen J. Fortunato and Roger E. Bawdon

76

The existence and pathogenesis of anaerobic organisms have been recognized for many years. Although pure anaerobic infections due to toxins elaborated by the clostridia have been well characterized for decades, it was only in 1978 that the causative role of *Clostridium difficile* toxins in antibiotic-associated colitis (AAC) was discerned.[1,2] Recent advances in microbiology, permitting the recovery of the more fastidious anaerobes, have led to the finding that many genital tract infections are polymicrobial, with significant anaerobic involvement. This chapter will discuss several infections due purely to anaerobic organisms, as well as the mixed infections in which anaerobes play a large role.

DISEASES ASSOCIATED WITH CLOSTRIDIAL TOXINS

Pseudomembranous Colitis (Antibiotic-Associated)

Toxins elaborated by *C difficile* are causative of antibiotic-associated diarrhea and colitis.[1,2] Many mild cases of antibiotic-associated diarrhea without pseudomembranes in which *C difficile* toxins are present have now been reported.

Pseudomembranous colitis is caused by toxins elaborated by *C difficile*, a gram-positive spore-forming obligate anaerobe, which until recently was thought to be nonpathogenic in humans. The disease most commonly follows antibiotic administration. The incidence of this disease varies greatly from center to center, probably reflecting geographic differences in the carrier status of the populations studied.[3] The overall incidence of the disease in the United States has been estimated at less than one per 1000 treated patients. Nearly all antibiotics except vancomycin and systemic aminoglycosides can cause pseudomembranous colitis.[4] It is now second only to *Salmonella* as a bacterial cause of gastrointestinal disease in industrialized countries.

C difficile produces two toxins that have been implicated in AAC. In animal studies, hamsters immunized against both toxins were protected from the disease, while immunization, against one or the other gave no protection.[5,6] *Toxin A* induces fluid accumulation, an inflammatory exudate, and erythema, while *toxin B* is primarily cytotoxic. Despite these different pathologic effects, it would appear that both toxins are important in the disease process.

Ampicillin, amoxicillin, cephalosporins, and clindamycin are the antibiotics most frequently associated with AAC, presumably due to their frequency of use. It appears that suppression of inhibitory organisms is the most important effect allowing for overgrowth of *C difficile* in the gut. With stoppage of the causative antimicrobial or upon effective treatment, most patients spontaneously eliminate *C difficile* from the gut flora.

Pathologic changes in the colon of patients with *C difficile* toxin-positive AAC reflect a spectrum of severity. In the mildest cases, simple diarrhea without mucosal changes is seen. This contrasts with the classic picture of pseudomembranous colitis, consisting of elevated, beige-colored plaques on an erythematous, friable edematous base. The plaques are composed of fibrin, polymorphonuclear leukocytes, and cellular debris, but contain no bacteria. These are usually confined to the distal colon, but infrequently may involve the entirety of the colon. Polymorphonuclear infiltration of the lamina propria is common.

It has been suggested that the decreased intestinal motility accompanying pregnancy and a high carrier rate of *C difficle* in the female urogenital tract should predispose to a higher incidence of AAC in the pregnant population. The fact is, however, that the authors have been unable to locate any case reports of *C difficile*-related colitis in a continuing gestation. Many cases of AAC secondary to prophylactic antibiotics (primarily cephalosporins) at the time of cesarean section have, however, been reported. AAC has been documented after a single dose of cefazolin for prophylaxis in this setting.[7] The data are too sparse, however, to comment upon the incidence of this disease in pregnancy.

AAC is a disease produced by clostridial toxins. These toxins as a group are thought not to cross the placenta. In fact, *C difficile* toxins remain localized in the alimentary tract. The effects of the disease on the pregnancy, therefore, are primarily those associated with hypovolemia and infection.

The timely diagnosis of AAC requires a high index of suspicion. Any patient presenting with diarrhea within several weeks of antibiotic therapy should be suspect. The clinical presentation of AAC extends from several unformed stools per day to the classic picture of pseudomembranous colitis, consisting of severe abdominal pain with cramping, fever, chills, toxic megacolon, and collapse due to electrolyte imbalance and dehydration. The definitive diagnosis rests on demonstration of *C difficile* toxin in the stool. Culture of the organism is more difficult and time-consuming. Fecal leukocytes are present in only 50% of patients with AAC.

Occasionally, the stools may be bloody, but most commonly they are watery, large in volume, and without mucus or blood. The temperature is frequently elevated (38–39°C), and the white blood cell count is mildly to moderately increased ($<20,000/mm^3$).

Treatment. The treatment of AAC rests on four principles:

1. Discontinuation of the implicated antibiotic, if possible;
2. Enteric isolation of the patient to prevent the organism from spreading to other patients;
3. Administration of vancomycin or metronidazole, if indicated; and
4. Symptomatic support (that is, fluid and electrolyte replacement).

Many patients will show resolution of symptoms and clear the organism and toxin with simple cessation of the implicated antibiotic. In patients requiring continuation of the implicated antibiotic or of a substitute, or in those with persistent diarrhea after discontinuation of the antibiotic, specific therapy should be started. Additionally, patients who are systemically ill should be treated with vancomycin. The recommended dosage of vancomycin is 150–500 mg QID orally for 7–14 days. Systemic absorption after an oral dose is minimal, and maternal or fetal toxicity should be minimal. It is a category C drug in pregnancy.

Relapses after treatment are not uncommon (15–20%). The relapse rate is not related to the duration of treatment, dosage of drug used, or severity of illness. The organisms cultured from relapse patients remain sensitive to vancomycin. Patients who remain toxin-positive after a full course of therapy are at a greater risk of relapse. Retreatment of a relapsing patient with vancomycin will effect a good clinical response, although one third of the patients who suffer a relapse will have a second relapse.

Other drugs, such as metronidazole, tetracycline, and bacitracin, have proven effective in the treatment of *C difficile* colitis. Tetracycline should not be used in pregnancy. Metronidazole is much less expensive than vancomycin; however, its absorption from the intestine leads to unpredictable drug levels in the colon. Bacitracin, 25,000 U Q6h for a week, is not absorbed from the gut and should place the fetus at no risk.[8] It has been noted to be effective both in removing toxin from the gut and in producing a clinical response. For life threatening cases of pseudomembranous colitis, however, vancomycin remains the treatment of choice, as bacitracin seems to be less effective.

Tetanus

Tetanus is a disease caused by a neurotoxin elaborated by *Clostridium tetani,* a gram-positive, spore-forming anaerobic bacillus.

C tetani is ubiquitous in nature, with spores found primarily in soil and feces. Inoculation of the spores into tissue under suitably anaerobic conditions allows for conversion of the organism to the toxin-producing vegetative form. Minor puncture wounds are the most frequent source of infection.

The occurrence of clinical disease is directly related to the immunization status of the population. Because of this, tetanus remains a major health problem in the developing world.

The systemic symptomatology of tetanus is due to the neurotoxin. The bacillus itself remains localized at the site of infection. The negative redox potential, required for anaerobic infection and spore germination, is promoted by the presence of necrotic tissue and coexisting bacterial infection. The vegetative form of the bacteria releases a peptide neurotoxin that invades the central nervous system and skeletal muscles. The toxin travels by retrograde axonal transfer to the spinal cord, where it blocks inhibitory synapses, resulting in unopposed muscle contraction, loss of antagonistic muscle function, and generalized flexion contractures. Binding of the toxin to cerebral gangliosides leads to generalized seizures. Acetylcholine release from the motor end plate of the neuromuscular junction is inhibited, leading to dysfunction of polysynaptic reflexes, producing unopposed muscle spasms. The sympathetic nervous system may also be involved, producing diaphoresis, hypertension, vasoconstriction, fever, and tachycardia.

The clinical manifestations of tetanus begin after a variable incubation period of generally 7–21 days, although extremes are reported. The severity of disease and rapidity of onset is proportional to the amount of toxin available to neural tissue.

Approximately 75% of patients develop generalized tetanus, initially manifested by trismus with local spasm at the site of injury.[9] They may subsequently develop tonic contraction of voluntary muscles, nuchal rigidity, dysphagia, glottal and laryngeal spasm, lethargy, irritability, and sympathetic vaso-motor instability. There is a characteristic facial expression, *risus sardonicus,* a typically anxious facies with the eyebrows and corner of the mouth drawn up, the muscles of the neck and trunk rigid, and the back slightly arched. The sensorium remains clear. Minimal stimulation frequently produces a tetanic seizure.

Less commonly, the disease may remain localized with persistent rigidity of the site of injury on an extremity. Cephalic tetanus may develop, which is a variant form of local tetanus, following a head injury. The course of local tetanus is generally a benign one.

Pregnancy has little, if any, effect upon the disease process. If the patient requires critical life support systems, the physiologic differences in pregnancy must be kept in mind. A woman approaching term may prove difficult to ventilate artificially. The stimulation of fetal movement has been reported to cause tetanic seizures. Adequate sedation of both the mother and fetus should alleviate this problem.

The effects of tetanus on pregnancy are limited to its symptomatic consequences. The neurotoxin is not thought to cross the placenta. Obviously, the patient with trismus will suffer nutritional deprivation and this must be made up by enteral or parenteral nutrition with the caloric, vitamin, and mineral requirements of pregnancy in mind.

Neonatal tetanus is a disease of infants born without the benefit of aseptic technique to nonimmunized mothers. Inoculation usually occurs at birth, most commonly by way of an infected umbilical stump. As previously stated, transplacental passage of the toxin has not been demonstrated.

Although the diagnosis of tetanus is essentially clinical, Gram's stain of the wound site may reveal typical large gram-positive bacilli with terminal spores, and with careful anaerobic culture techniques the organism can be isolated. However, *C tetani* can be cultured from wounds in patients who never develop clinical tetanus. Consequently, isolation of the organisms does not indicate disease. Patients with tetanus usually have a leukocytosis and an elevated creatinine phosphokinase. The clinical differential diagnosis from disorders with similar neurologic findings is shown in Table 76–1.

Treatment. Treatment of tetanus is aggressive and multifactorial, yet mortality rates of 30–60% persist with generalized tetanus.[10] Parenteral antibiotic treatment with penicillin (aqueous penicillin G, 1 million units IV Q6h, or procaine

TABLE 76–1. DIFFERENTIAL DIAGNOSIS OF TETANUS IN ADULTS

Disorder	Similarity to Tetanus	Differentiating Features
Encephalitis	Trismus and muscular spasm may be present	Clouded sensorium
Purulent meningitis	Nuchal rigidity, seizures	Pleocytotic change of cerebrospinal fluid
Rabies	Muscular spasm, especially of muscles of respiration and deglutition	Trismus absent; cerebrospinal fluid may be pleocytotic
Strychnine	Trismus present, but a late symptom	Rapid progression of symptoms
Phenothiazine reaction	Dysphagia and trismus may be present	Also have athetoid movements, tremors, and torticollis; demonstrable serum and urine levels

penicillin G, 1,200,000 units IM qd) inhibits further growth of *C tetani* and indirectly stops further toxin production. Tetracycline and chloramphenicol may be used in the penicillin-allergic patient but have potentially adverse effects on the developing fetus. Erythromycin also has reported efficacy. Administration of human tetanus immune globulin, 3000–6000 units, provides pharmacologic antitoxin levels. Preliminary studies have recently shown encouraging results with direct intrathecal injection of immune globulin, given before the development of tetanic spasm. Subsequent progression to generalized spasm and death were markedly reduced when intrathecal administration was compared to immune globulin given intramuscularly in similar patients. No improvement was seen when immune globulin was given intrathecally after generalized spasms had begun. Heterologous antitoxin of bovine or equine serum has previously been used successfully, but its use was complicated by a high incidence of immunologic reactions to animal serum. It effectively binds circulating toxin but is entirely ineffective against toxin already bound to neurons or to the motor end plate of skeletal muscles. Because heterologous antitoxin does not cross the placenta, passive immunity in the fetus of an infected mother will not occur. The heterologous antitoxin should, therefore, be used only when human immune globulin is unavailable.

Surgical debridement of the local wound site after antitoxin has been administered is recommended to remove infected necrotic tissue. Uterine curettage in postabortal or postpartum cases is recommended to remove retained products of conception. The value of hysterectomy is unknown, and the potential benefit must be weighed against the operative mortality in these criticially ill patients.

Because stimulation may precipitate muscle spasms or seizures, patients with tetanus should be sedated and placed into a quiet environment. Sedation is usually instituted with barbiturates, benzodiazepines, or phenothiazines. If sedation fails, the patient may require paralysis and ventilatory assistance. If tetanus occurs during pregnancy and ventilatory assistance is required, it must be remembered that pregnant women normally maintain a mild respiratory alkalosis. When tetanus occurs late in pregnancy, the enlarged uterus may also cause mechanical difficulties with assisted ventilation.

Because patients with tetanus frequently lose weight from starvation, the disease has special significance during pregnancy, when caloric requirements are increased and where starvation ketosis can have potentially adverse effects on the fetus. Although many nonpregnant patients with moderate disease may be fed by a nasogastric tube, strong consideration should be given to either cuffed-tube endotracheal intubation or tracheostomy because of the increased risk of gastroesophageal reflux in pregnancy. Tracheostomy may also be indicated for uncontrolled laryngeal or generalized spasms, difficulty in managing oropharyngeal secretions, respiratory insufficiency, or prolonged intubation.

Tetanus is a preventable disease with proper immunization.[10] Adults who have not received full childhood immunization should be immunized with three monthly injections of tetanus toxoid followed by a booster immunization one year after the third injection. Additional booster injections are required every 7 to 10 years to maintain adequate serum antitoxin levels to prevent infection. When the immunization history is unknown and a clearly contaminated wound is present, 250 U of human tetanus immune globulin should be given to provide passive protection if full immunization as needed. Prophylactic immune globulin is not invariably protective, because approximately 5% of cases in the United States occur in patients given immune globulin at the time of injury. Although quantitative interference with active antibody formation has been demonstrated when immune globulin and toxoid are given at the same time, it has not been shown to be clinically significant. Injections should be given at separate sites and in different syringes, for instance, into opposite extremities. All persons surviving tetanus must receive full immunization, which should be initiated with other treatment, because a sublethal dose of tetanus toxin does not confer subsequent immunity. Recurrent tetanus has been reported. Toxoid administration with the occurrence of each injury in the face of adequately demonstrated previous immunization is to be avoided because excess antibody production has been demonstrated and may be responsible for the increased incidence of allergic reactions to tetanus toxoid.

Botulism

Botulism is a disease caused by ingestion of preformed neurotoxin produced by *Clostridium botulinum*.[11] Like other clostridial organisms, the offending bacterium, *C botulinum*, is an anaerobic spore-forming, gram-positive bacillus. The spores are endemic in distribution in the soil, allowing easy contamination of vegetables, meat, dairy products, and fish, from the soil and water. Germination of the spore in a favorable environment, with subsequent toxin formation, produces the characteristic disease by its action on cholinergic synapses of the nervous system and the motor end plates of skeletal muscle.

The toxin elaborated by *C botulinum* is a polypeptide and is one of the most lethal substances known. In contrast to the spore of *C botulinum*, which is heat-resistant, the toxin is heat labile and is destroyed by heating at 100°C for 20 minutes.[11]

The usual source of the toxin is contaminated food, although rarely the toxin may be introduced through a contaminated wound. When contaminated food is ingested, proteolysis does not occur in the gut, and the toxin is absorbed by both hematogenous and lymphatic routes. It then finds its way to cholinergic synapses, where it inhibits the release of acetylcholine, blocking synaptic transmission. Cranial nerve roots are characteristically affected first, followed by symmetric descending involvement manifest as skeletal muscle weakness or paralysis and autonomic dysfunction. The central nervous system is not affected.

Once the toxin is ingested there is a latent period of 12–48 hours before the patient becomes symptomatic, although a range of four hours to eight days has been reported. Initial symptoms are frequently gastrointestinal and include nausea, vomiting, and diarrhea. Visual blurring and diplopia are common because of impairment of extraocular muscle function. Dysarthria and dysphagia are also common. Neurologic progression is manifest as a symmetric muscular weakness or paralysis with a caudal progression. Respiratory failure is usually a later symptom but may occur abruptly. Characteristically absent are sensory abnormalities and mental status changes. There is no fever, unless additional infection is superimposed. Peripheral blood counts and electrolytes are normal, as are studies of the cerebrospinal fluid.

Obstetric association is coincidental, and pregnancy has no reported influence on the course of maternal disease. The effects of botulism on pregnancy are limited to the effects of the isolated disease process. Fetal and neonatal involvement have not been reported.[12]

The diagnosis is made on the basis of the clinical presentation and a history suspicious of contaminated food ingestion, or rarely, of a contaminated wound.[13] Confirmation of the diagnosis is through identification of the toxin in the serum or stool of the patient or in a sample of the suspected food. The differential diagnosis encompasses other causes of acute neurologic impairment, and common differentiating features are shown in Table 76–2.

Treatment. If botulism is suspected, early gastric lavage is completed to minimize toxin absorption. Evidence of neurologic involvement mandates intensive monitoring for the development of cardiorespiratory failure. Early respiratory support, maintaining a mild respiratory alkalosis in the pregnant patient, is advocated. Concern should be given to prevention of aspiration pneumonia, a complication that a pregnant patient is more likely to encounter. When the diagnosis is made clinically with reasonable certainty, trivalent antitoxin should be given. It is, however, derived from horse serum rather than human serum, and 10–15% of patients may have an anaphylactic reaction or develop serum sickness. Administration of antitoxin does not provide immediate symptomatic relief, and prolonged support may be necessary. In such cases, adequate nutrition for the patient and her fetus must be maintained.

TABLE 76–2. DIFFERENTIATING FEATURES OF OTHER NEUROLOGIC DISEASES FROM BOTULISM

Disorder	Differentiating Features
Myasthenia gravis	Accentuation of muscular fatigability during exercise Positive edrophonium (Tensilon) test Gastrointestinal symptoms uncommon except dysphagia
Guillain–Barré syndrome	History of preceding viral illness Presence of paresthesias Ascending motor paralysis Increased spinal fluid protein
Cerebrovascular disease	Presence of localizing signs Usually unilateral
Staphylococcal food poisoning	Absence of cranial nerve involvement
Chemical poisoning (methyl alcohol, organophosphates)	Rapid onset of symptoms (usually within 1 h)
Carbon monoxide poisoning	Rapid onset of symptoms Cranial nerves not affected

The use of antibiotics as part of the primary treatment is controversial. Proponents argue that it may help to prevent further toxin formation, whereas opponents feel that it has no proven benefit because the toxin is preformed and the disease is an intoxication rather than an ongoing infection.

Since 1950, the mortality from botulism has declined, and currently, only approximately one in four cases is fatal. A short incubation period and ingestion of large amounts of contaminated food typically predict a more severe course with a worse prognosis. When recovery occurs, it is usually complete. As for tetanus, subsequent protection is not conferred, and repeat episodes have been reported.

Prevention lies primarily with individuals in home food processing. Strict commercial food processing regulations have virtually eliminated public outbreaks.[14]

Gas Gangrene

Clostridial myonecrosis, or gas gangrene, is a disease caused both by infection and the toxins produced by several clostridial species. However, nearly 90% are a result of infection with *Clostridium perfringens* (*Clostridium welchii*).

C perfringens is a gram-positive, spore-forming, bacillus that exists primarily in a saprophytic spore form and is ubiquitously distributed in soil and feces. Vegetative conversion of the spore form may occur in the presence of low oxygen tension and traumatized or necrotic tissue. The development of clinical disease results from exotoxin production by the vegetative form of the organism.[15]

Clostridial infection is opportunistic, and only a small percentage of women who endogenously harbor or who are colonized with clostridia from an outside source develop a clinically significant infection.[16] Clostridial organisms are present in the intestine of 25–35% of humans and in the genital tract of 3–30% of women, with clostridials representing 2–9% of all anaerobic isolates. The largest study of obstetric clostridial sepsis was performed by Ramsey in 1949, and showed a 1.5% (23/1513) incidence of identifiable clostridia in postpartum sepsis.[17] However, only one of the 23 positive cultures could be definitely related to the clinical findings. Ramsey also reviewed postabortal sepsis and identified clostridia in 20% (190/965) of these patients. Twenty-eight, or 14%, had a positive blood culture. In 68% of these, the organism was considered a saprophyte, and only eight patients, or 4%, had true gas gangrene. Recent studies have not refuted these findings. As with other obstetric infections, women at increased risk include those with chronic vascular disease, premature rupture of membranes, prolonged labor, postpartum hemorrhage, retained products of conception, and prolonged fetal demise.

As with other anaerobic infections, a low redox potential in the infected tissue provides the most favorable conditions for the development of myonecrosis and its systemic manifestations. This is accomplished by tissue destruction, trauma, or infection. Clinical disease results from exotoxin production by the vegetative form of the organism. More than 10 toxins have been identified in association with C *perfringens* infection. Clinically, the α toxin is a lecithinase, which cleaves the lecithin of cell membranes, causing cellular lysis. Other toxins include a nonlecithinase necrotizing toxin, which digests the collagen of muscle and subcutaneous tissue. The organism may also produce a DNase, a bursting factor that enhances the activity of the other toxins, a fibrinolysin, a phagocyte-inhibiting toxin, and an enterotoxin that can cause profuse diarrhea. Damaged components provide substrate for bacterial metabolism with production of lactic acid, further lowering the redox potential. The infected tissue undergoes autolysis, putrefaction necrosis, and gas formation, which increase tissue tension and compromise blood flow, perpetuating the infectious process.

With severe infection, the patient becomes systemically ill with disseminated intravascular coagulation and renal failure. Renal failure is due to acute tubular necrosis (ATN). This tubular change is secondary to cast formation, toxic products of cellular necrosis, decreased renal perfusion with subsequent ischemia, and the vasopressor effects of free hemoglobin. This is analogous to the ATN seen in rhabdomyolysis.

The infected or traumatized pregnant uterus provides an excellent environment for proliferation of the vegetative form of *Clostridium*. The products of conception are excellent culture media for anaerobic growth when infected. The progression of infection and tissue destruction in chorioamnionitis, endometritis, and infectious intrauterine fetal demise allow for rapid clostridial growth when the organism is present.

The Effect of the Disease Upon Pregnancy. More than 95% of obstetric clostridial infections will remain localized to the uterus. The majority of these will be a mild endometritis, manifest by low-grade temperature, vaginal discharge, and uterine tenderness, with clostridial species identified on Gram's stain and culture. A mixed infection is the rule, however, with other anaerobes and gram-negative aerobic bacilli frequently identified as well.

Fetal emphysema may be seen with intrauterine fetal demise and prolonged retention of the dead fetus. It begins as a localized chorioamnionitis and generally runs a fairly benign course, although the clinical findings frequently suggest a more fulminant infection than is actually present. Typical findings include a gaseous vaginal discharge, crepitus of the uterine wall, and the radiologic finding of extensive fetal air. Characteristically, clostridia can only be isolated from fetal cultures and not from maternal cultures.[16]

Endomyometritis with necrosis, uterine perforation, and sepsis represent the fulminant obstetric clostridial infection. The incubation period is 1–4 days, after which the patient typically exhibits the sudden onset of marked restlessness and anxiety. There is uterine tenderness with a gaseous vaginal discharge that may have a putrid sweet odor. Tachycardia is out of proportion to temperature elevation, and marked diaphoresis and pallor are noted. As sepsis becomes apparent, the blood pressure falls, and rapidly advancing jaundice and evidence of disseminated coagulopathy are seen. With marked hemolysis and tissue destruction, portwine discoloration of the serum and urine is seen, reflecting the presence of free hemoglobin. Oliguria heralds the onset of renal failure. A rapidly falling hematocrit with rising free hemoglobin, rapidly rising bilirubin, and abnormal clotting studies mark advanced sepsis. Marked hyperkalemia develops as a result of cellular lysis, with release of intracellular potassium and the inability of the failing kidney to clear even a normal potassium load. Leukocytosis is present, and an abdominal radiograph may show a physometra. But this is a late finding and is not pathognomonic of clostridial sepsis. Clinically, the progression from a mild endometritis to fulminant myonecrosis is suggested by a slow response to antibiotic therapy, myalgias, and parametrial tenderness on pelvic examination. The presence of hemolysis portends a poor prognosis and in most instances heralds the onset of hypotension and oliguria, despite adequate hydration.

A "gas abscess" or "welch abscess" may also be seen as a localized wound infection at the site of abdominal incision or episiotomy. In these infections, clostridia are present as part of a mixed infection, and simple incision and drainage will ordinarily provide adequate treatment.

Neonatal clostridial sepsis, other than tetanus, attributed to transplacental or transvaginal colonization has rarely been reported. A review of the English literature shows only seven cases of neonatal clostridial sepsis (other than tetanus).[18]

The diagnosis of clostridial infection is largely clinical. A high index of suspicion in the appropriate clinical situation is mandatory, as microbiologic studies provide confirmation only after the diagnosis is grossly apparent in the moribund patient. Alternatively, the finding of clostridia on routine wound, endometrial, or even blood cultures does not invariably imply fulminant infection and must be evaluated in the context of the clinical presentation. A localized crepitant cellulitis may occasionally be associated with other nonclostridial endogenous pelvic pathogens. A mixed infection is usually present in these instances with a combination of aerobic coliforms, *Bacteroides*, and peptostreptococci. They are more commonly responsible for pelvic septic thrombophlebitis, in which clostridia are rarely reported.

Treatment. The treatment of clostridial infections depends on the site and extent of infection. Incidental culture without evidence of infection requires no therapy.[16] A mild endometritis generally responds to antibiotic therapy alone, with penicillin being the drug of choice in a pure clostridial infection. Curettage may occasionally be necessary and is advocated on a routine basis by some to remove the nidus of infection. Fetal emphysema is ordinarily adequately treated by high-dose penicillin and evacuation of the uterus. Localized cellulitis generally responds to local wound care and antibiotics, with coverage extended to include aerobic enteric pathogens and other anaerobes. Fulminant endomyometritis with systemic manifestations requires prompt and aggressive treatment. General measures include adequate hydration to maintain a brisk urine flow to prevent or minimize renal compromise and combat vascular collapse. Central venous pressure monitoring, although helpful, cannot reliably prevent pulmonary edema, as it may occur on a noncardiogenic basis, presumably secondary to direct pulmonary endothelial damage. Broad-spectrum antibiotics are needed. Chloramphenicol or clindamycin may also be used. Dosing should reflect the renal status of the individual patient. It should be noted that whereas *C perfringens* is uniformly sensitive to penicillin, other clostridial species, also capable of producing the same clinical picture, may be resistant to many of the antibiotics, including penicillin, the cephalosporins, and clindamycin. They are, however, sensitive thus far to chloramphenicol, metronidazole, and imipenam-cilastatin.

Early peritoneal dialysis or hemodialysis within 24–48 hours after the diagnosis of renal failure has been made facilitates removal of toxin and free hemoglobin as well as normalizing of the fluid and electrolyte balance. The use of heparin in the treatment of the coagulopathy has no proven benefit.

The role of hysterectomy in these patients remains controversial. Proponents argue that aggressive surgical intervention provides maximal chance for survival and that only a total abdominal hysterectomy with bilateral salpingo-oophorectomy (TAH-BSO) is adequate in the presence of sepsis and endomyometritis, because foci of infection are also frequently seen in the cervix, tubes, and ovaries. Opponents cite successful outcomes in the absence of surgery with its associated operative morbidity.

The use of antitoxin is disputed, but most feel that it is of no proven value either prophylactically or therapeutically.[19] The rationale for its use is the neutralization of any free toxin; however, the blood supply to the site of infection is poor, and the toxins are rapidly bound, rendering the antitoxin useless. Only an equine antitoxin is available. The development of serum sickness represents a possible complication under such treatment.

Hyperbaric oxygen therapy has been successfully used in cases of gas gangrene, although the benefit of its routine use is unproven and remains controversial.[19] Potential advantages lie in its provision of improved demarcation of necrotic and viable tissue, aiding surgical dissection, and possibly in reducing systemic toxicity. Its disadvantages are based on its bacteriostatic rather than bacteriocidal effect and some complications associated with its use. Once removed from high oxygen concentrations, the bacterium may again multiply and elaborate toxin. Additionally, any preformed toxin is unaffected by the oxygen. Pulmonary complications, including adult respiratory distress syndrome, and neurologic complications of mental confusion and convulsions at the time of peak oxygen pressure may cause additional morbidity.

If there is evidence of advancing infection at a wound site with muscular involvement, thorough debridement with excision of all devitalized and necrotic tissues becomes paramount to successful management. Antibiotic therapy and treatment of the systemic manifestations are the same as with fulminant endomyometritis.

Bacterial Anaerobic Vaginosis

Bacterial vaginosis (BV), previously known as nonspecific vaginitis, is a replacement of the normal vaginal flora (lactobacilli) by gram-negative coccobacilli consistent with *Gardnerella vaginalis,* together with other bacteria resembling anaerobic species, especially *Bacteroides* and *Mobiluncus* species.

BV is thought by some to be a sexually transmitted disease, although this is controversial. The nomenclature of this condition has recently been changed from nonspecific vaginitis as it is neither nonspecific nor an inflammation. Investigations into the microbiology of BV have demonstrated not only *G vaginalis,* but additionally an overgrowth of many species of anaerobic bacteria. It is now thought that the presence of *G vaginalis* may be but a marker of anaerobic overgrowth and that it is the colonization by anaerobic organisms that is responsible for symptoms associated with BV. The role of anaerobes in BV is supported by several findings. Most striking is the clinical responsiveness of this condition to metronidazole, which has excellent activity against anaerobic bacteria and limited activity against other organisms including *G vaginalis.* Additionally, the isolation of anaerobes in high concentrations and the detection of organic acids, produced by anaerobes from the vaginal discharge of BV patients, lend evidence to this theory.

There is a cyclic variability in anaerobic colonization of the vagina with respect to the menstrual cycle. Neary et al has found *Bacteroides* species in 17% of women in the follicular phase and 2.5% of women in the luteal phase of the menstrual cycle.[20] Correspondingly, 23% of women undergoing hysterectomy in the follicular phase and only 8% in luteal phase developed post operative infections. The bearing of these data on BV is uncertain.

BV does not appear to be an actual infection. There is no inflammation of the vaginal mucosa and the traditionally described vaginal discharge contains few inflammatory cells. The normally predominant lactobacilli are replaced by a high density of many types of anaerobic bacteria and the ecosystem accompanying them.[21] There is a characteristic pattern of organic acid secretion consisting of decreased lactate with increased succinate, butyrate, propionate, and other volatile fatty acids. The vaginal redox potential is low, and abnormally high amounts of putrescine, cadaverine, and other volatile amines are found.[22]

BV is not an uncommon finding in an otherwise normal pregnancy. It seems, however, that this condition should be more common in early gestation, as the vagina and cervix have been found to have a markedly different microflora in early versus late pregnancy (Figure 76–1).[23,24] Anaerobic bacteria are present in greater quantities in early gestation and decrease in colony count and number of species isolated as pregnancy progresses. These findings are suggestive that BV is a more pathologic condition in mid to late gestation than in early gestation.

There has been much interest lately in the association between vaginal, cervical, and amniochorionic microflora and the incidence of premature labor and preterm premature rupture of the fetal membranes. Many organisms have been implicated. Specifically, the presence of *G vaginalis* and of a higher concentration of anaerobic organisms have been associated with both preterm labor and preterm premature rupture of the fetal membranes. Additionally, using clinical criteria for diagnosis of BV, many authors have shown an association between BV and preterm birth.[25]

The diagnosis of BV is based on clinical parameters. Although cultures demonstrate a replacement of lactobacilli by *G vaginalis* and anaerobes, analysis by culture is not a practical means of diagnosis in the routine patient. The clinical triad of a fishy odor to vaginal secretions, clue cells on wet prep, and a vaginal pH >4.5 forms the basis for routine diagnosis in the office setting. Some investigators have recommended the use of the Gram's stain on vaginal discharge. This demonstrates lack of lactobacilli and the presence of clue cells (mixed and gram-negative to gram-variable coccobacilli adherent to vaginal epithelial cells).

Treatment. The treatment of choice for BV is metronidazole. Although very effective against the majority of anaerobic bacteria, metronidazole is not as effective against *G vaginalis.* The hydroxy metabolite of metronidazole, however, is more active against some species of *G vaginalis,* although not against all of them.[26] It has been proposed that the reestablishment of the normal vaginal flora (lactobacilli) is instrumental in establishing long-lasting cure. The use of ampicillin will inhibit lactobacilli as well as BV organisms, while metronidazole inhibits only the anaerobes and *G vaginalis* and not the lactobacilli. Theoretically, this gives the lactobacilli a chance to reestablish a more normal vaginal ecosystem, reducing the pH and increasing the redox potential to a level inhibitory to anaerobic organisms.

Although the use of metronidazole for the treatment of BV in pregnancy has remained somewhat controversial,

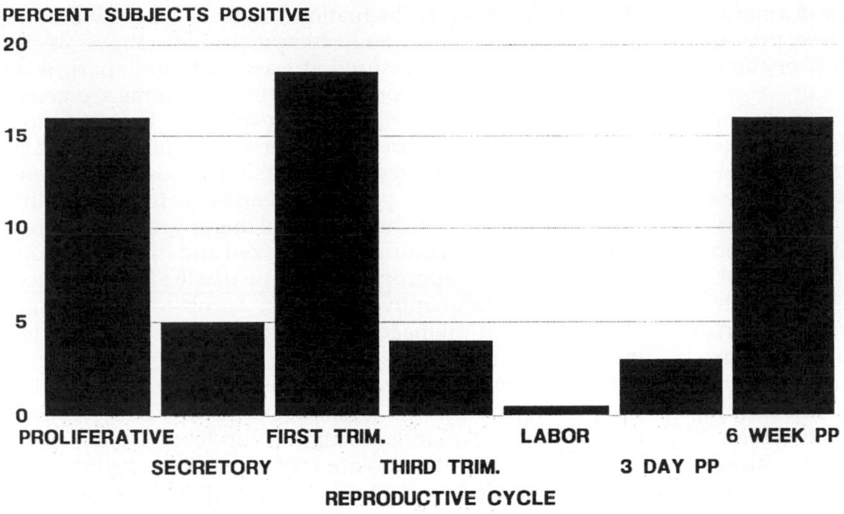

Figure 76–1 Percentage of women with positive cervical cultures for *Bacteroides fragilis* at various stages of the menstrual cycle and of pregnancy. (*Adapted from Thadepalli H*[24])

it is the opinion of the authors that the risk of BV-associated prematurity outweigh the theoretical risk of this drug in the last two trimesters of pregnancy (see also Chapter 115).

Mixed Aerobic-Anaerobic Infections in Obstetrics

Mixed aerobic-anaerobic infections are primarily caused by the endogenous saprophytic vaginal flora that are ever present in the female genital tract. In studies conducted at Parkland Memorial Hospital[27], flora isolated from these polymicrobial infections frequently include the bacteria shown in Table 76–3.

Microorganisms that are predominantly anaerobic exist in a commensal relationship with healthy women. They do not cause an infectious process unless the genital tract undergoes trauma, there are changes in the microbial flora due to inadequate treatment, or there is invasion by other potentially pathogenic bacteria. The oxidation reduction potential of the genital tract, plus the ability of some bacteria to produce superoxide dismutase and catalase, are important factors in the ability of anaerobic bacteria to produce an infection. There is a high correlation between anaerobic bacteria producing these enzymes and their ability to cause infection. There is also a correlation between normal anaerobic flora and their ability to produce these enzymes. Since the normal body oxidation reduction potential is about 150 millivolts, unless the anaerobes are oxygen-tolerant, the microbes will not survive.[28,29] Obstetric infections involving polymicrobic aerobic and anaerobic bacteria are listed in Table 76–4.

TABLE 76–3. BACTERIAL ISOLATES FROM PELVIC INFECTIONS AT PARKLAND MEMORIAL HOSPITAL

Aerobic	Anaerobic
Enterococcus	*Peptococcus* species
Group B *Streptococcus*	*Bacteroides fragilis* group
Escherichia coli	*Clostridium* species
Streptococcus viridans	*Fusobacterium* species
Other gram-negative rods	*Lactobacillus* species
Chlamydia trachomatis	*Bacteroides bivius*
Gardnerella vaginalis	*Bacteroides disiens*
Mycoplasma hominis	
Ureaplasma urealyticum	
Lactobacillus species	

Mixed aerobic-anaerobic infections are primarily a result of trauma to the genital tract in which aerobic bacteria, such as gram-negative rods, produce *endotoxins*, and gram-positive cocci produce *enterotoxins*. *Escherichia coli* and *Staphylococcus aureus* are examples of each, respectively. The anaerobic bacteria, normally implicated in obstetric infections, produce similar lipopolysaccharides and enzymes and combine with aerobic organisms to produce synergistic infections. In early studies by Gesner and Jenkins, it was found that septic thrombophlebitis was frequently caused by strains of bacteroides and fusobacteria.[30] This combination caused an increase in coagulation, although the exact mechanism could not be identified. Septic shock may be caused by either aerobic bacteria, anaerobic bacteria, or a mixed infection of both. Onderdonk et al found that neither aerobic nor anaerobic bacteria singularly would cause an abscess when injected intraperitoneally into rats, but when injected in combination, an abscess would form.[31]

Like most infectious processes, mixed infections are characterized by the presence of inflammatory cells in the discharge from the infection site. The isolation of both aerobic and anaerobic bacteria from the infection site may be the diagnostic criteria for pregnancy-related infections. Frequently, the microorganisms causing these infections consist of bacteria found in the normal vaginal flora. It is not uncommon to isolate three or more different species of anaerobic bacteria from an infection site.[32] As previously discussed, the bacterial flora is altered during pregnancy. Infection mainly occurs because there is a breach in the

TABLE 76–4. POLYMICROBIC OBSTETRIC INFECTIONS

Postpartum endometritis
Septic abortion
Cesarean section wounds
Septic thrombophlebitis
Chorioamnionitis
Episiotomy
Puerperal sepsis
Infected ectopic pregnancy

protective mechanisms (intact fetal membranes and a sterile amniotic cavity) that existed prior to delivery. These protective mechanisms are either complicated, reduced, or eliminated in the puerperium.

Labor contractions and frequent examinations during delivery allow movement of bacteria into the uterine cavity, with the resulting inoculum growing in a nutrient-rich environment, characterized by a reduced redox potential. The presence of bacteria in the uterus after delivery is common, but the development of clinical disease is contingent on the risk factors and the general well being of the patient. Infection rates at Parkland Memorial Hospital range up to 85% for high-risk indigent patients after cesarean section. Risk factors include ruptured membranes of more than six hours' duration cephalopelvic disproportion, internal fetal monitoring, and multiple vaginal exams.[33,34] Private hospitals frequently have much lower postpartum infection rates.

Many of the diseases caused by anaerobic or mixed anaerobic bacteria do not exist in the nonpregnant woman and are related directly to the postpartum period. Most of these infections, as mentioned earlier, are a result of manipulation of the genital tract or due to breaches in either skin or tissue, which allows these organisms to invade the genital tract. Amniotic fluid is bacteriostatic in most pregnancies; however, when infected, the products of conception provide an excellent medium for bacterial growth.

Any infection in pregnancy represents an inflammatory process, which causes activation of macrophages, the production of interleukin-1-β, and the stimulation of the prostaglandin cascade leading to the onset of labor.[35] Premature labor may thus result, with possible fetal or neonatal demise. It appears that preterm infections can result in premature delivery if not properly treated. Chorioamnionitis may be responsible for not only maternal sepsis, but infection of the fetus or neonate.

Properly collected cultures from the various anatomic sites are important in the laboratory diagnosis of polymicrobic infections during pregnancy. Special anaerobic culture collecting devices are available in most clinics. In most cases, specimens consisting of pus, wound discharge, and endometrial tissue and those obtained from sites remote from the cervicovaginal flora give good culture results. Specimens contaminated with bacteria from the vagina, cervix, and endocervix may be meaningless. The pipelle endometrial suction brush (Unimar Inc., Wilton, Connecticut) or the uterine sampling device (Medi-Tech Inc., Canton, Massachusetts) are excellent devices for collecting specimens that are not contaminated with vaginal flora. The submission of cervical cultures to the laboratory will frequently result in misleading data, as the report will frequently identify three or more aerobic and anaerobic microorganisms, which may or may not be related to the infectious process. Other tests that may be useful in the diagnosis of obstetric infections include a Gram's stain of the wound exudate and a leukocyte count ($>10,000/mm^2$). Recently, Mayberry and colleagues attempted to correlate C-reactive protein, leukocyte esterase activity, and fibronectin concentrations with the presence of chorioamnionitis. No correlation between chorioamnionitis and any of these tests, either singly or together, was noted.[36] Other tests that may be of value include three sets of blood cultures over a 24-hour period.

The clinical signs of an acute obstetric infection are not different following surgical procedures or a spontaneous event. Probably the most important clinical symptom, indicating the onset of an obstetric infection, is the presence of fever. Although there may be small changes in body temperature (36.5 to 37.8°C) from morning to evening, alteration in this normal fluctuation suggests a possible infection. The increase in body temperature to above 38.5°C on two occasions, measured at least six hours apart, is an indication of an infection. Postpartum infections are generally indicated by a febrile response after the first 24 hours. Once these temperatures are observed, cultures should be obtained from suspected infection sites if possible. Gram's stains of exudates may provide an early clue to the invading organism, and empiric antimicrobial therapy may be started. Once the bacterial cultures are analyzed and the antibiogram completed, more appropriate therapy may be implemented. Other signs, frequently present in an obstetric infection, include wound drainage, tachycardia, erythema, and uterine or pelvic tenderness.

Chorioamnionitis, or intra-amniotic infection (IAI), has been found in up to 1% of all pregnancies.[37] Despite histological evidence of inflammation in up to 40% of all membranes and placentas, isolation of an etiologic agent is frequently lacking. In fact, there is colonization of the amniotic fluid in 30% of pregnant women who deliver at term. About 8% of cultures contained organisms that were considered highly virulent.[38] Thus, the presence of bacteria in the amniotic fluid is not a clear indication of infection, and the clinical presentation is more important for the diagnosis. The microorganisms involved are generally from the cervical or vaginal flora and most likely include a mixture of anaerobic and aerobic bacteria. The clinical indicators of IAI are listed in Table 76–5 (see also Chapter 113).

Postpartum endometritis is defined by the United States Committee on Maternal Welfare as a temperature exceeding 38°C in the first 10 days postpartum, excluding the first 24 hours. The risk factors are defined in Table 76–6. The microbial population is mixed, and the most common isolates include *E coli* and *Bacteroides bivius* (see also Chapter 112).

Septic pelvic thrombophlebitis occurs at a frequency of about one case per 2000 deliveries. It most often follows obstetric surgery.[39] This infection is difficult to diagnose and is frequently a diagnosis of exclusion. In the event of persistent fever in spite of adequate antimicrobial therapy, the response to heparinization within two days generally confirms the diagnosis. Many species of bacteria may be isolated from the site, and a mixed infection is the rule. Recently, Brown et al developed criteria for diagnosis of septic pelvic thrombophlebitis on CT scan and MRI.[40]

Wound infections occur in about 5% of all cesarean sections and are the result of a number of factors, including the handling of the tissue during surgery, length of labor, bacterial contamination, the presence of hair on the surgical site, length of surgery, and the general health of the patient.[41-43] Wound infections may be categorized into early- and late-onset infections, which are defined as within two days and eight days, respectively. Early infections are generally characterized by one isolate, either an aerobe or an

TABLE 76–5. CLINICAL INDICATORS OF IAI

Maternal and fetal tachycardia
Ruptured membranes
Leukocytosis
Uterine tenderness
Foul smelling amniotic fluid
Maternal fever
Preterm labor

TABLE 76–6. RISK FACTORS FOR POSTPARTUM ENDOMETRITIS

Extended labor
Multiple vaginal exams
Cephalopelvic disproportion
Fetal scalp monitoring
Preexisting infections
Absence of prenatal care
Anemia
Poor socioeconomic status
Prolonged rupture of membranes

anaerobe, whereas late infections are characterized by a polymicrobic flora consisting of both aerobes and anaerobes. Therefore, the recommended treatment may be substantially different.

The incidence of *episiotomy infections* has been reported to be less than 3%.[44] There has been no reported relationship between lacerations caused by labor or episiotomy and infection, although the combination of both may enhance the possibility of infections. The incidence of maternal death from episiotomy infections is relatively low, but it does occur. There are several classifications of episiotomy infection: simple, superficial, fascial, and myonecrosis.[45] The latter is frequently caused by *C perfringens,* whereas the other infections are most likely caused by a combination of aerobic and anaerobic organisms. One of the problems associated with an episiotomy infection is that bacterial contamination of the surgical site is frequently observed without infection. In one study, 70 out of 76 cultures from episiotomy sites were positive for bacterial growth. As expected, the microorganisms isolated from these infections may include *E coli,* other gram-negative aerobic rods, bacteroides, and clostridia.

Septic abortion is a serious complication in obstetrics. Although the frequency of this infection has not been reported, it has diminished significantly with legalized abortion. The obvious cause of septic abortion is the contamination of the uterine cavity with vaginal or bowel flora. Bacteremia frequently follows this contamination, and blood cultures from these women indicate that *Peptococcus* and *E coli* are the most frequently isolated organisms.[46]

There exists only a little literature on *infected ectopic pregnancies.* Anaerobic and mixed infections probably do occur, but are most likely the complication of a previous sexually transmitted disease. The organisms isolated would be those seen in salpingo-oophoritis. There is little evidence that *spontaneous abortion* can be caused by anaerobic infections. It is possible, however, that bacteremia from an underlying disease may result in spontaneous abortion.

Treatment. Ideally, prior to antimicrobial treatment, cultures from the suspected infection site should be obtained. This is frequently difficult or impossible in obstetric infections, and therapy must often be started on an empiric basis. Antimicrobial treatment of bacteria from mixed infections should include coverage for both aerobic and anaerobic microbes, including the *Bacteroides* species. Antibiotic therapy should include an aminoglycoside and a penicillin, with or without a β-lactamase inhibitor such as sulbactam or a broad-spectrum cephalosporin such as cefoxitin, cefotetan, or ceftizoxime. Clindamycin or metronidazole may also be added for better anaerobic coverage. Eighty-five to 90% of infections will be successfully treated with single-agent broad-spectrum coverage. Cephalosporins will not effectively cover the *Enterococcus,* and the addition of ampicillin may be required. The incidence of enterococcal infection has been estimated at approximately 5% of obstetric infections. Although excellent single agent coverage is provided by a third-generation cephalosporin with good anaerobic coverage, ampicillin with a β-lactamase inhibitor, or the extended-spectrum penicillins, in cases of failure of these regimens, triple therapy (ampicillin, an aminoglycoside, or aztreonam and either metronidazole or clindamycin) may still be required.

REFERENCES

1. Chang TW. *Clostridium difficile* toxin and antimicrobial agent induced diarrhea. *J Infect Dis.* 1978;137:854.
2. Larson HE, Price AB, Honour P, Borriello SP. *Clostridium difficile* and the aetiology of pseudomembranous colitis. *Lancet.* 1978;1:1063.
3. Viscidi R, Willey S, Bartlett JG. Isolation rates and toxigenic potential of *Clostridium difficile* isolates from various patient populations. *Gastroenterology.* 1981;81:5.
4. Bartlett JG. Antimicrobial agents implicated in *Clostridium difficile* toxin-associated diarrhea or colitis. *Johns Hopkins Med J.* 1981;149:6.
5. Lyerly DM, Lockwood DE, Richardson SH, Wilkins TD. Biological activities of toxin A and B of *Clostridium difficile. Infect Immun.* 1982;35:1147.
6. Libby JM, Wilkins TD. Effects of two toxins of *Clostridium difficile* in antibiotic-associated cecitis in hamsters determined by active immunization and intracecal injection. Abstract No. 716. Presented at the 21st Interscience Conference on Antimicrobial Agents and Chemotherapy, Chicago, November 1981.
7. McNeeley SG Jr., Anderson GD, Sibai BM. *Clostridium difficile* colitis associated with single-dose cefazolin prophylaxis. *Obstet Gynecol.* 1985;66:737.
8. Chang TW, Gorbach SL, Bartlett JG, Saginur R. Bacitracin treatment of antibiotic-associated colitis and diarrhea caused by *Clostridium difficile* toxin. *Gastroenterology.* 1980;78:1584.
9. Januszkiewicz J, Galaska A, Adamczyk J, et al. Severe tetanus in late pregnancy. *Scand J Infect Dis.* 1973;5:233.
10. Rothstein RJ, Baker FJ. Tetanus prevention and treatment. *JAMA.* 1978;240:675.
11. Donadio JA, Gangarosa EJ, Faich GA. Diagnosis and treatment of botulism. *J Infect Dis.* 1971;124:108.
12. St. Clair EH, DiLiberti JH, O'Brien ML. Observations of an infant born to a mother with botulism. *J Pediatr.* 1975;56:658.
13. Merson MH, Dowell VR. Epidemiologic, clinical and laboratory aspects of wound botulism. *New Engl J Med.* 1973;289:1005.
14. Mersun MH, Hughes JM, Dowell VR, et al. Current trends in botulism in the United States. *JAMA.* 1974;229:1305.
15. Smith LP, McClean APH, Maughan GB. *Clostridium welchii* septicotoxemia. *Am J Obstet Gynecol.* 1974;110:135.
16. Ledger WJ, Hackett KA. Significance of clostridia in the female reproductive tract. *Obstet Gynecol.* 1973;41:525.
17. Ramsey AM. The significance of *Clostridium welchii* in the cervical swab and blood stream in postpartum and postabortum sepsis. *J Obstet Gynecol Brit Empire.* 1949;56/2:247.
18. Bogdan TC, Rapkin RC. *Clostridium* infection in the newborn. *Pediatrics* 1976;58:120.
19. Bornstein DL. Clostridial Myonecrosis. In: Braude A, Davis CE, Fierer J, eds. *Infectious Disease and Medical Microbiology.* Philadelphia, PA: WB Saunders; 1986:1490.
20. Neary MP, Allen J, Okubadejo OA, Payne DJH. Preoperative vaginal bacteria and post operative infections in gynecologic patients. *Lancet.* 1973;2:1291.
21. Holmes KK, Chen KCS, Lipinski CM, Eschenbach DA. Vaginal redox potential in bacterial vaginosis (nonspecific vaginosis). *J Infect Dis.* 1985;152:379.
22. Spiegel CA, Davick P, Totten PA, et al. *Gardnerella vaginalis* and anaerobic bacteria in the etiology of bacterial (nonspecific) vaginosis. *Scand J Infect Dis.* 1983;Suppl 40:41.
23. Goplerud CP, Ohm MJ, Galask RP. Aerobic and anaerobic flora of the cervix during pregnancy and the puerperium. *Am J Obstet Gynecol.* 1976;126:858.
24. Thadepalli H. Anaerobic infections of the female genital tract. *Scand J Infect Dis.* 1979;Suppl 19:80.
25. Martius J, Krohn MA, Hillier SL, et al. Relationship of vaginal lactobacillus species, cervical chlamydia trachomatis, and bacterial vaginosis to preterm birth. *Obstet Gynecol.* 1988;71:89.

26. Jones BM, Geary I, Alawattegama AB, et al. In vitro and in vivo activity of metronidazole against *Gardnerella vaginalis, bacteroides* spp. and *mobilluncus* spp. in bacterial vaginosis. *J Antimicrob Chemo.* 1985;16:189.
27. Bawdon, RE, Hemsell D. Personal communications.
28. Allen SD, Seder JA, Morier LM. Isolation and examination of anaerobic bacteria. In: Lennette EH, Ballows A, Hausler WJ Jr, Shadomy HJ., eds. Manual of *Clinical Microbiology.* 4th ed. Washington, DC: American Society for Microbiology; 1985.
29. Gorbach SL, Bartlett JG. Anaerobic infection (Third of three parts). *New Engl J Med.* 1974;290:1289.
30. Gesner BM, Jenkins CR. Production of heparinase by bacteroides. *J Bacteriol.* 1981;81:595.
31. Onderdonk AB, Bartlett JG, Louis T, et al. Microbial synergy for experimental intra-abdominal abscesses. *Infect and Immun.* 1976;12:22.
32. Platt LD, Yonekura ML, Ledger WJ. The role of anaerobic bacteria in postpartum endometritis. *Am J Obstet Gynecol.* 1979;135:814.
33. Cunningham FG, Hauth JC, Strong JD, et al. Infection morbidity following cesarean section—comparison of two treatment regimens. *Obstet Gynecol.* 1978;52:656.
34. Gilstrap LC, Cunningham FC. The bacterial pathogenesis of infection following cesarean section. *Obstet Gynecol.* 1979;53:545.
35. Romero R, Brody DT, Oyarum E, et al. Infection and labor, III. Interleukin-1: a signal for the onset of parturition. *Am J Obstet Gynecol.* 1989;160:1117.
36. Maberry M, Bawdon R, Little B, Gilstrap L. Biochemical markers in the amniotic fluid of pregnancies complicated by chorioamnionitis. Abstract #33. Presented at the Infectious Disease Society for Obstetrics and Gynecology, 1989.
37. Gonik. Intensive care monitoring of the critically ill pregnant patient. In: Creasy RK, Resnik R., eds. *Maternal/Fetal Medicine: Principles and Practice.* 2nd ed. Philadelphia, PA: WB Saunders and Company; 1989:
38. Gibbs RS, Blanco JD, St. Clair PJ, Castoneda YS. Quantitative bacteriology of amniotic fluid from women with clinical intraamnionitic infection at term. *J Infect Dis.* 1982;145:1.
39. Josey WE, Staggers SR. Heparin therapy in septic pelvic vein thrombophlebitis: a study of 46 cases. *Am J Obstet Gynecol.* 1974;120:228.
40. Brown CEL, Lowe TW, Cunningham FG, Weinreb JC. Puerperal pelvic thrombophlebitis: impact on diagnosis and treatment using x-ray computed tomography and magnetic resonance imaging. *Obstet Gynecol.* 1986;68:789.
41. Sweet RL, Ledger WJ. Puerperal infection, a two year review. *Am J Obstet Gynecol.* 1973;117:1093.
42. Howard JM, Baker WF, Culbertson WR, et al. Postoperating wound infections: the influence of ultraviolet irradiation of the operating room and various other factors. *Ann Surg.* 1960;160:1S.
43. Curse PJE, Loord RA. A five year prospective study of 23,649 surgical wounds. *Arch Surg.* 1973;107:206.
44. Thacker SB, Bonta HD. Benefit and risks of episiotomy: an interpretative review of the English language literature 1860–1980. *Obstet and Gynecol Sur.* 1983;38:322.
45. Sky KK, Eschenbach DA. Fatal perineal cellulitis from an episiotomy site. *Obstet Gynecol.* 1979;54:292.
46. Smith JW, Southern PM, Lehmann JD. Bacteremia in septic abortion: complications and treatment. *Obstet Gynecol.* 1970;35:704.

F

INFECTIONS CAUSED BY MYCOBACTERIA, ECTOPARASITES, AND SPIROCHETA

Chapter Seventy-Seven

Mycobacterial Infections

Constance A. Benson

77

From 1953 through 1984, the number of cases of disease due to *Mycobacterium tuberculosis* in the United States reported to the Centers for Disease Control (CDC) declined by 73.6%.[1] The annual risk of tuberculosis declined from 53.0 to 9.4 per 100,000 population; however, this decline was less among nonwhite than among white populations.[1] This downward trend leveled off in 1985 and reversed in 1986 when the reported number of cases actually rose. From 1985 to 1987, the largest national increase occurred in Hispanic and black populations in the 25- to 44-year age group, roughly coinciding with peak adult reproductive ages. The change in epidemiologic pattern and number of reported cases appears to be in part a consequence of the current epidemic spread of human immunodeficiency virus (HIV) infection, as the increases in the numbers of cases of tuberculosis have occurred most significantly in the demographic groups also affected by the acquired immune deficiency syndrome (AIDS).[1] While males are twofold more likely than females to have clinical tuberculosous disease, recognition and appropriate treatment of mycobacterial infections in women of reproductive age remains of continuing importance.

Disease due to nontuberculous atypical mycobacteria, while relatively uncommon in otherwise healthy adolescents and adults, may occur during pregnancy particularly when pregnancy is complicated by HIV infection. Atypical mycobacteria may produce disease similar to and often clinically indistinguishable from disease due to *M tuberculosis*. Microbiologic characteristics of some of the atypical mycobacteria are summarized in Table 77–1. Clinical manifestations and specific therapies depend on the isolate and on drug susceptibility testing and will not be further detailed here.

The focus of this chapter will be the etiology, pathogenesis, common clinical manifestations, diagnosis, treatment, and prevention of infections due to *M tuberculosis* and *Mycobacterium leprae* in women of reproductive age, with particular focus on the consequences of disease and its treatment during pregnancy and in the neonate.

HUMAN TUBERCULOSIS

Human tuberculosis is a bacterial infection caused by *M tuberculosis*. Rarely, the same clinical syndromes may result from infection due to *Mycobacterium bovis*, an organism normally causing disease in cows and rarely transmitted to humans through ingestion of contaminated milk products. *M tuberculosis* is a 0.2–0.5 × 2–4 micron aerobic, acid-fast, nonspore-forming, nonmotile bacillus.[2] Visible growth of the organism on agar takes from two to eight weeks at 37°C producing buff-colored, rough, friable colonies.[2] Differentiation from other mycobacterial species is based on growth pattern, colony appearance, and biochemical characteristics.

Infection due to *M tuberculosis* results from inhalation of droplet nuclei containing the organism.[3] The size of droplet nuclei enables their circumvention of normal mucociliary clearance, allowing penetration to distal airways, where they lodge and multiply locally. Prolonged exposure is usually required for infection to occur. Fomites are not significant vectors for disease transmission.

The most important factors associated with risk of transmission are the infectivity of the index case and the closeness of contacts. Those most highly infectious are individuals with cavitary pulmonary disease productive of sputum that is smear-positive for acid-fast bacilli (AFB). The risk is highest among household contacts, where transmission rates range from 27–50%, although crowded or closed environments such as nursing homes, the risk may be even higher in susceptible individuals.[4]

The risk of infection progressing to active disease is greatest in the first one to two years following infection and appears to vary with age. The risk is greatest in those under age three, in early adulthood, in elderly individuals, and in the immunosuppressed. In studies of large numbers of adolescents and young adults, the risk of progression to active disease following infection was 8–10%, with the majority of cases occurring within two years of known exposure or conversion to tuberculin-positive skin tests.[5] In elderly populations, the risk of disease progression may be as high as 30%.[4] The risk of progression to active disease is probably no greater during pregnancy than in the nonpregnant, otherwise healthy woman.[6]

Once mycobacteria reach terminal air spaces, local replication begins. The mid or lower lung fields are the initial foci of infection.[7] Bacteria are ingested by alveolar macrophages, in which they continue replicating. Infected alveolar macrophages may be ingested by and may recruit other phagocytic cells, with eventual spread to regional lymph

TABLE 77–1. CHARACTERISTICS OF ATYPICAL MYCOBACTERIA

Runyon Group	Colony Characteristics	Growth	Representative Organisms
I	Photochromogen: yellow/orange pigment after light exposure	Slow	*M kansasii* *M marinum* *M simiae*
II	Scotochromogen: orange/red pigment in the dark	Slow	*M scrofulaceum* *M xenopi* *M gordonae*
III	Cream-colored, smooth colonies	Slow	*M avium-intracellulare*
IV	Buff or cream-colored colonies	Rapid	*M fortuitum* *M chelonei*

nodes. Early after infection, when specific cell-mediated immunity and tissue hypersensitivity are absent, mycobacteria may spread by hematogenous routes to the lymphoreticular system, kidneys, epiphyseal areas of long bones, vertebral bodies, central nervous system, and the apical posterior portions of the lung. Ultimately, it is the apical posterior portions of the lung that most favor mycobacterial growth. Within six to eight weeks following initial infection, delayed cutaneous and tissue hypersensitivity develops coincident with development of cell-mediated immune responses to tuberculin antigen. This results in enhanced activation of tissue and circulating macrophages that continue to ingest mycobacteria, release high concentrations of lytic enzymes, and recruit and activate circulating lymphocytes capable of recognizing mycobacterial antigens.[7] The characteristic granulomatous tissue reaction that intervenes consists of activated macrophages, lymphocytes, fibroblasts, typical epithelioid cells (which are highly activated macrophages capable of stimulating fibroblast collagen production, allowing fibrous encapsulation of antigenic material), and Langhans' giant cells (which are fused, activated macrophages oriented around tuberculous antigen with multiple nuclei in a peripheral position).

The end result of this tissue hypersensitivity response is enhanced mycobactericidal activity. If the mycobacterial load is small and the degree of tissue hypersensitivity high, well-defined granulomata form, designed to contain infection. If the mycobacterial load is heavy and the tissue hypersensitivity response is poor, granulomata will be less organized and presumably less able to contain infection.

As the inflammatory reaction continues, tissue necrosis occurs due to release of lytic enzymes from degenerating macrophages, producing amorphous debris within the center of granulomata, referred to as *caseation necrosis*. The chemical environment and oxygen tension within caseous material are not favorable for continued mycobacterial metabolism and replication. Partial calcification may also arrest multiplication of mycobacteria. If liquefaction continues, granulomata may erode into adjacent parenchyma, air spaces, or bronchi producing a tuberculous cavity where conditions may be more optimal for mycobacterial multiplication.[7]

Further progression of infection depends on the continued interaction between local mycobacterial inoculum, cell-mediated immune response, and tissue hypersensitivity. In the majority of cases, these interactions result in bacterial destruction and infected persons show no evidence that infection has occurred other than a positive tuberculin skin test. When disease is progressive, the clinical manifestations will depend on the age and immune competence of the host. Extremes of age, general deterioration in health, poor nutritional status, and other immune-suppressing conditions favor progression of infection. While pregnancy was long regarded as a time of special risk, more recent studies suggest this risk is more likely to be related to underlying physical disease or malnutrition in the mother than to inherent immunocompromise during pregnancy.[6] Other specific factors that appear to be associated with increased risk of disease progression include therapy with corticosteroids or other immunosuppressive agents, hematologic malignancies, the postgastrectomy state, end-stage renal disease, and possibly certain viral illnesses such as influenza or measles.

Clinical Manifestations

The protean clinical manifestations of all disease entities produced by infection with *M tuberculosis* are beyond the scope of this chapter. Pulmonary disease, the most common manifestation for over 80% of all tuberculosis cases in the United States, will be detailed here, as will certain syndromes common to women and neonates. Fewer than 15% of cases present with extrapulmonary disease syndromes, some of which are outlined in Table 77–2. Early recognition and treatment of pulmonary disease in women of childbearing years may circumvent subsequent complications of pulmonary or extrapulmonary disease during pregnancy and in the neonate.

TABLE 77–2. OTHER ORGAN SYSTEM DISEASES ASSOCIATED WITH TUBERCULOSIS

Central nervous system tuberculosis
Tuberculous meningitis
Tuberculous pericarditis
Skeletal tuberculosis
Tuberculous spondylitis (Pott's disease)
Peripheral skeletal tuberculosis
Genitourinary tuberculosis
Male and female genital tuberculosis
Renal tuberculosis
Gastrointestinal tuberculosis
Tuberculous peritonitis
Tuberculous lymphadenitis
Cutaneous tuberculosis
Tuberculous laryngitis
Tuberculous otitis
Tuberculous mastitis
Uveal tuberculosis

The manifestations of *primary (initial) pulmonary disease* are age-dependent. Primary disease occurring in the neonate or infant as a consequence of perinatal transmission from an infected mother most often results in lymphohematogenous dissemination or primary progressive pulmonary disease. The initial focus begins in the lower and mid-lung fields. Extensive regional hilar or mediastinal lymphadenitis is common. Extension into bronchi may result in local progression of pneumonitis. For children over the age of three to five years, relative resistance to progressive disease develops, and the primary focus may involute, encapsulate, and calcify without overt disease progression.

Primary infection in the adolescent or young adult may have features similar to childhood primary progressive pneumonia, although the tendency to develop apical cavitation early after initial infection appears around the time of puberty and continues into young adulthood. First infections acquired in this age group are less likely to cause parenchymal and hilar calcification and are more likely to result in chronic upper lobe disease such as might be recognized in adulthood.[7]

Primary infection in the elderly, as with the infant, appears more likely to present with mid or lower lobe disease. Progressive consolidation with ill-defined cavitation may be seen. Involvement of mediastinal and hilar lymph nodes, however, is less likely than with primary progressive pulmonary disease of childhood.

Chronic pulmonary tuberculosis, characteristic of disease in adulthood and the most common disease manifestation in the pregnant woman, generally begins through activation of a bacterial colony in the subapical posterior portion of an upper lobe. A less common but also characteristic location is the apical portion of a lower lobe. Progression of the previously described granulomatous inflammatory response leads to an area of caseation necrosis surrounded by epithelioid cells and fibrosis. Caseous material may liquefy draining into the bronchial tree, which induces cough. Fibrous encapsulation prevents collapse resulting in cavitation and favoring continued mycobacterial replication. Aerosolization of material draining from such cavities results in bronchogenic spread to new foci. Regional lymphadenitis and hematogenous dissemination, while characteristic of primary infection in early childhood, is an uncommon feature of chronic pulmonary tuberculosis in adults.

Early pulmonary tuberculosis is generally an asymptomatic condition. As the mycobacterial inoculum reaches significant proportions, constitutional symptoms such as anorexia, fatigue, weight loss, chills, fever, and night sweats occur. These symptoms are late manifestations of disease gradual in onset but progressive. Cough and sputum production are the result of bronchial irritation from caseating material exuded from cavitary lesions. In late chronic disease, hemoptysis may occur as caseous material sloughs or endobronchial erosion of cavitary lesions into blood vessels occurs. Chest pain may result from extension of inflammation to the peripheral pleura, which may stimulate a serous pleural effusion.

Physical findings are nonspecific and depend on the extent of illness and the degree of change induced by constitutional symptoms. Signs of consolidation such as dullness to percussion or egophany occur with large cavitary lesions surrounded by large areas of pneumonitis.

Tuberculosis in the fetus (congenital tuberculosis) is thought to be transmitted by one of two means: (1) hematogenous spread from the infected placenta by way of the umbilical vein and (2) fetal aspiration of infected amniotic fluid *in utero* or at the time of birth.[8-10] The liver is the major site of involvement, followed by the lungs. Once the fetus has been infected, disseminated (miliary) disease is common with involvement of the central nervous system, bone marrow, gastrointestinal tract, lymphoreticular system, adrenal glands, kidney, and skin. Symptoms are usually present within the first few days up to the second or third week of life. They include respiratory distress, fever, poor weight gain, lethargy, and irritability. Physical findings include hepatosplenomegaly, peripheral lymphadenopathy, wasting, fever, and, occasionally, skin lesions. Approximately 50% of patients will have a miliary pattern on chest radiograph while the remainder will develop a pattern consistent with primary progressive pulmonary tuberculosis as previously described.[8,10]

Diagnosis

The chest roentgenogram is most often the study supporting the suspicion of pulmonary tuberculosis in the pregnant woman and should be performed with shielding of the fetus.[11,12] Primary or chronic pulmonary tuberculosis in the adolescent or adult woman most often presents with apical or subapical patchy infiltrates with cavitation that may be more readily appreciated on apical lordotic views. Occasionally, more ill-defined cavities may be seen in posterior lower lobes. Air fluid levels are seen in less than 10% of upper lobe cavities but may be more prevalent in lower lobe cavities. As the initial lesions heal, they form fibrotic scars that tend to contract with sharp margins, resulting in volume loss. Primary pulmonary infection occurring during childhood presents with middle or lower lobe infiltration with enlarged hilar and mediastinal lymph nodes.

Sputum smears will be positive for AFB in the majority of women presenting with pulmonary disease.[11,12] The yield will be highest if early morning sputum, collected on three consecutive days, is examined. In patients nonproductive of sputum, induction with aerosolized saline or aspiration of early morning gastric secretions may be useful ancillary studies. Bronchoscopy with endobronchial biopsy or bronchoalveolar lavage may be the most efficient and highest-yield alternative diagnostic procedure.[11] Culture and speciation of the organism provides the definitive diagnosis. Nonspecific laboratory abnormalities may accompany active disease. Normochromic normocytic anemia is common in later stages of tuberculosis but may be masked by the anemia of pregnancy. Decreased albumin and elevated globulin levels are generally present in patients with longer-term disease. The white blood cell count is usually normal but mild elevations in the range of 10,000/mm^3 to 15,000/mm^3 may be seen. A monocytosis, thought to be a classic finding in tuberculosis, is present in less than 10% of individuals.[7] Rarely, other hematologic abnormalities such as pancytopenia, leukomoid reactions, leukopenia, and thrombocytopenia may be present in the peripheral blood smear.

As previously discussed, neonatal disease may be congenital or perinatal in its transmission. The establishment of disease as congenital rests on the documentation of AFB in body fluids or tissue biopsy specimens or growth of *M tuberculosis* in culture from appropriate clinical material obtained at birth; demonstration of a primary disease complex in the liver; disease manifestations within the first days of life; and the exclusion of extrauterine/perinatal transmission.[8-10] However, whether or not disease is congenital or perinatal in origin matters little to the importance of immediate recognition and institution of antituberculous therapy. The tuberculin skin test is rarely positive in the infected neonate. Direct smears of middle ear fluid, bone marrow, tracheal aspirates, or biopsies of liver, skin lesions, peripheral lymph nodes, or lung may show AFB and are likely to yield positive cultures for *M tuberculosis*.[8] A high index of suspicion should be maintained, particularly when the mother is known to be infected.

Tuberculin skin testing with purified protein derivative (PPD) to detect delayed hypersensitivity responses to mycobacterial antigens is a reasonably effective ancillary diagnostic tool. Quantitative interpretation requires the use of the Mantoux test, which entails injection of PPD (five TU strength) intracutaneously to raise a blanched wheal. The reaction is measured in 48 to 72 hours. A positive test is defined as the presence of induration of greater than 10 mm in diameter.[7,13] Reactions of less than 5 mm induration are considered negative. Those between 5 and 10 mm are doubtful unless present in the context of immunosuppression, particularly HIV infection, when this may be considered a positive test.[1,7] Tuberculin skin tests may be negative in as many as 20% of cases of known tuberculosis when individuals are first tested, although repeat tests placed within two to three weeks will convert to positive. Skin testing of the neonate is not useful, as tests are rarely positive regardless of disease status.[8,10]

Factors associated with diminished or absent delayed hypersensitivity reactions to tuberculin antigen in the infected adult include malnutrition, intercurrent viral infection, reticuloendothelial malignancy, other immunosuppressive disorders or intercurrent therapy with corticosteroids or immunosuppressive agents. Pregnant women generally react to PPD skin testing to a similar degree and in a manner similar to the general population.[13] Tuberculin skin testing is safe during pregnancy.[13]

Uncommon Presentations of Tuberculosis

Miliary Tuberculosis (Disseminated). All primary tuberculous infections result in transient hematogenous dissemination that ceases with the development of cell-mediated immune responses and tissue hypersensitivity. In a small percentage of cases, progressive disseminated disease results; alternatively, in individuals with chronic organ tuberculosis that is quiescent, recurrent hematogenous seeding from chronic foci may occur in circumstances of advancing age, intercurrent illness, or immunosuppression resulting in widespread multiorgan system disease.

Miliary tuberculosis may be acute or subacute in onset associated with nonspecific symptoms of fever, malaise, weight loss, and more specific symptoms related to the organ systems involved. Table 77–3 outlines the most common disease manifestations and abnormalities associated with miliary tuberculosis.[14-16] The characteristic "millet seed" appearance or miliary infiltrate on the chest roentgenogram is often the first clue to the presence of dissemination, although chest radiographs may be normal early in disease. Up to 25% of individuals with miliary tuberculosis will have negative tuberculin skin tests.[16] The diagnosis generally is dependent upon the clinical setting and the demonstration of AFB in histopathologic specimens obtained from biopsy of involved organs. Sputum samples may be smear-negative although two thirds of patients will have positive sputum cultures in the presence of miliary spread. Urine cultures may be positive. Bronchoscopy with transbronchial biopsy or bronchoalveolar lavage sampling of endobronchial tissue may have a higher diagnostic yield than sputum culture and smear, particularly in those patients who are nonproductive of sputum. Other organs from which smear and culture are associated with a reasonably high diagnostic yield include lymph nodes, liver, and bone marrow.

TABLE 77–3. CLINICAL FINDINGS ASSOCIATED WITH MILIARY TUBERCULOSIS

Abnormality	Frequency
Miliary pattern on chest x-ray	93–97%
Positive tuberculin skin test	61–84%
Liver granulomata	66%
Positive sputum culture	63%
Positive sputum acid-fast bacilli (AFB)	31%
Anemia	29%
Other foci of tuberculosis	23–32%
Meningitis	17–19%
Bone marrow granulomata	16–33%
Splenomegaly	0.5–13%

Pooled from references 14, 15.

Serofibrinous Pleurisy With Effusion. This particular syndrome occurs most often in young adults usually within weeks following primary or initial infection and before the development of significant cell-mediated immune response to tuberculin antigen.[7] During this time, a subpleural focus of infection may develop with little or no tissue inflammatory reaction, resulting in pleural fluid accumulation at the time of onset of tissue hypersensitivity. Similarly, in patients with chronic pulmonary tuberculosis, visceral–parietal pleural fusion at a point of cavitation may allow antigenic material to drain into the pleural space, resulting in fluid and cell accumulation. In less than 10% of patients who present with this syndrome, the pathogenesis is hematogenous or miliary spread of mycobacteria.[7]

The onset of symptoms is usually abrupt, with high-grade fever, pleuritic chest pain, and cough. The chest radiograph generally shows a unilateral pleural effusion. Thoracentesis reveals pleural fluid containing between 500 and 2000 white cells with a lymphocytic predominance; the pH is usually less than 7.3, the AFB smear is usually negative, and culture of pleural fluid is positive in only 25% to 33%.[7] The tuberculin skin test is positive in greater than 90% of cases. The diagnosis may require pleural needle biopsy, which will demonstrate granulomata in 75% or open pleural biopsy, which will yield a diagnosis in nearly 100% of patients.[7]

Female Genital Tuberculosis. Of particular importance and more common in women of childbearing years in developing countries, female genital tuberculosis is a rare complication of disseminated disease in the United States. It is usually initiated by a hematogenous focus of spread in the endosalpinx; this is followed by subsequent spread to contiguous organs, with involvement of the ovaries, endometrium, and rarely the cervix. With cervical involvement, granulomatous masses resembling cervical carcinoma may be visualized by speculum examination. The symptoms associated with genital tuberculosis in the female are generally local. Lower abdominal pain, menstrual dysfunction, cervical motion tenderness, low-grade fever, and adnexal inflammatory masses palpable on exam may mimic pelvic inflammatory disease of other causes.[7] Persistence of symptoms unresponsive to antibacterial therapy may be a clue to the diagnosis. The diagnosis usually is dependent on demonstration of AFB and granulomata in tissue and culture of material obtained by way of laparoscopy, laparotomy, or dilatation and curettage.[17] Rarely, organisms may be cultured from menstrual blood or endocervical scrapings, although these tissues are usually AFB smear-negative.[7]

As with pelvic inflammatory disease of alternative etiologies, complications of genital tuberculosis include tubo-ovarian abscess, infertility, ectopic pregnancy, and chronic pelvic pain.[17] Another potential complication of pelvic tuberculosis is the occurrence of tuberculous peritonitis. Hysterosalpingography or tubal insufflation performed during the evaluation and treatment of sterility or the performance of other pelvic diagnostic or therapeutic procedures in the presence of untreated pelvic tuberculosis may result in the spread of tubercle bacilli to the peritoneum. When this occurs, signs of peritonitis result, including fever, abdominal pain, weight loss, anorexia, and rebound tenderness accompanied by the presence of ascites. Peritoneal fluid obtained in this setting is exudative with a lymphocytic pleocytosis of 500 to 2000 cells. The AFB smear is rarely positive, the culture is positive in only 25%, and the diagnosis most often requires peritoneal biopsy or biopsy of other tissue specimens.[7]

Treatment

The risk of untreated tuberculosis to the pregnant woman and the fetus far outweighs the risk of treatment. It is necessary that the diagnosis be made without delay and effective therapy be initiated as soon as possible thereafter. Isoniazid, ethambutol, and rifampin have all been used successfully during pregnancy and with relatively little risk of teratogenesis or maternal toxicity.[18-20] Snider et al., in an extensive review of the literature, concluded that 94% of all pregnancies treated with one or more of these agents resulted in delivery of healthy term infants.[18] The greatest range of experience is available for isoniazid and ethambutol. Women treated with these two agents delivered healthy term infants in greater than 95% of cases.[18] While rifampin has also been associated with a low congenital malformation rate, some fetuses born to women treated with rifampin demonstrated blood dyscrasias and limb malformation.[18] Studies have raised the theoretical caution that rifampin-induced inhibition of DNA-dependent RNA polymerases may cause fetal damage.[19] More recent studies suggest, however, that malformation rates associated with rifampin are no greater than background rates in otherwise normal women.[8,19] Streptomycin is associated with significant ototoxicity regardless of the trimester of exposure and is not recommended for treatment of tuberculosis during pregnancy.[18-20]

First-line agents recommended for treatment of pregnant women and neonates, including doses and common side effects, are outlined in Table 77–4. Ultimately, long-term treatment regimens should be based on antituberculous drug susceptibility testing. For patients not suspected of having drug-resistant disease, therapy with two drugs, isoniazid and rifampin, is recommended as initial treatment.[19] For patients with extensive or disseminated disease or for those suspected of being infected with isoniazid-resistant organisms, the addition of ethambutol as a third drug is advocated. Alternative antituberculous agents such as pyrazinamide, cycloserine, ethionamide, kanamycin, and capreomycin should be avoided, as little specific information about the effects of these agents on the fetus is available. Streptomycin, which has been shown to interfere with development of the ear and may cause congenital deafness, should not be used during pregnancy. Pyridoxine should be administered along with isoniazid to pregnant women to prevent the development of peripheral neuropathy. While minimal concentrations of antituberculous drugs do appear in breast milk, levels achieved are insufficient for effective treatment or prophylaxis for the nursing newborn. Alternatively, such levels have not been associated with significant toxicity in the neonate.[8]

Based on currently available data, six- and nine-month durations of therapy have been shown to be as effective as more extended durations.[21] There are, however, several exceptions that apply to pregnant women. When treating *nonpregnant* adults, regimens administered for less than nine months should include isoniazid, rifampin, and pyrazinamide administered daily for the first two months.[19,21] The second phase of treatment should consist of isoniazid and rifampin given daily or twice weekly for an additional four months. However, as pyrazinamide is not recommended for use during pregnancy, this six-month regimen should not be employed for the pregnant woman. Nine-month regimens using isoniazid and rifampin alone are

TABLE 77–4. INITIAL ANTITUBERCULOUS AGENTS RECOMMENDED FOR USE IN PREGNANT WOMEN AND NEONATES

Drug	Daily Dose	Maximum Daily Dose	Common Side Effects
Isoniazid[a]	10–20 mg/kg/d (p.o./IM)	300 mg/d	Elevated liver transaminases Hepatitis Peripheral neuropathy[a]
Rifampin	10–20 mg/kg/d (p.o.)	600 mg/d	Fever/myalgia syndrome Hepatitis Orange discoloration of secretions/urine Rarely, blood dyscrasia/thrombocytopenia
Ethambutol	15–25 mg/kg/d (p.o.)	2.5 gm	Optic neuritis Skin rash
Streptomycin[b]	20 mg/kg/d 5 days week (IM)	25–30 mg/kg	Ototoxicity (sensorineural hearing loss, vestibular abnormalities) Nephrotoxicity

[a] Pregnant women treated with isoniazid should receive concomitant therapy with pyridoxine, 25–50 mg orally daily, to prevent peripheral neuropathy.
[b] Should not be used during pregnancy; can be used for treatment of neonates.

probably equally effective to the six-month regimen.[19,21] If ethambutol is substituted for rifampin, the effectiveness of this regimen is probably decreased; therefore, treatment with isoniazid and ethambutol should be continued for a full twelve-month period.[19] Ethambutol should be added to the initial two or three drug regimen if drug resistance is suspected. Further management of drug-resistant cases must be individualized based on drug susceptibility testing.

The neonate born to a mother with active tuberculosis should be treated with isoniazid for the first two to three months of life or at least until the mother is known to be smear- and culture-negative and known to be in compliance with her treatment regimen.[8,19] After three months, if the mother has a negative sputum smear and culture and the infant is tuberculin-negative with a normal chest roentgenogram, isoniazid may be discontinued. If the infant has a substantial tuberculin skin reaction at three months or if the chest radiography or clinical signs or symptoms indicate the presence of disease, treatment with two drugs should be initiated. Rifampin should be the second drug of choice, although it has not been approved for use in neonates. Streptomycin may also be given to newborns. Ethambutol may be difficult to use in infants because of the inability to monitor visual acuity or color vision for evidence of toxicity.

Although widespread controlled clinical trials have not been conducted using six- and nine-month treatment regimens for extrapulmonary tuberculosis, these regimens are probably as effective as they are for pulmonary disease.[19,22] However, bone and joint disease, lymphadenitis, or disease in patients who are immunosuppressed will likely require longer-term therapy and should be managed on an individual basis.[19]

Monitoring the patient for adverse reactions and evaluation of response to therapy is necessary. Adults should have baseline measurements of liver enzymes, bilirubin, serum creatinine, complete blood count, and platelet count. In addition, a baseline ophthalmologic examination should be performed for patients who will be treated with ethambutol. These tests do not need to be routinely monitored during therapy unless patients develop symptoms suggesting an adverse reaction. However, patients should be evaluated clinically on at least a monthly basis and questioned concerning symptoms of drug toxicities. If such symptoms do occur, appropriate laboratory studies should be repeated. In addition, a sputum smear and culture should be obtained at monthly intervals until sputum conversion is documented.[19] Those patients who have not become smear- and culture-negative after three months of treatment with regimens containing isoniazid and rifampin should be reevaluated for drug resistance or poor compliance. If organisms are found to be resistant, the treatment regimen should be modified to include at least two drugs to which the organisms are susceptible.[19]

It may be more difficult to assess occurrence of adverse reactions or response to therapy in neonates; therefore, clinical, laboratory, and radiographic follow-up examinations are of greater necessity. As ophthalmologic abnormalities are difficult to assess in neonates and young infants, ethambutol should be avoided in therapeutic regimens employed for this age group.

Prevention

Those individuals with recent development of significant tuberculin skin test reactivity or significant exposure to infection require therapy to prevent disease. Preventive therapy with isoniazid given for a duration of six to twelve months is effective in decreasing the risk of future tuberculous disease.[19] This preventive protection is presumably effective for life.[23] Persons for whom preventive therapy is indicated include household members or other close contacts of infectious persons; recently infected individuals (within the past two years); persons with past untreated tuberculosis or with a significant tuberculin skin reaction and an abnormal chest radiograph for whom current active tuberculosis has been excluded; infected persons in special clinical situations, such as those with silicosis, diabetes, immunosuppression, hematologic and reticuloendothelial malignancies, end stage renal failure, or clinical conditions of rapid weight loss or chronic malnutrition; and tuberculin skin test reactors younger than 35 years of age.

The goal of preventive therapy with isoniazid is to balance the risk of adverse reactions to the drug with the risk of development of active tuberculosis. Hepatitis is the major adverse effect associated with isoniazid. In a study of 13,838 patients given isoniazid alone as preventive therapy, the rate of hepatitis increased in direct proportion to age; the risk was absent for those under 20, 0.3% for those 20 to 24 years of age, 1.2% for those 35 to 49 years of age, and 2.3% for those 50 to 64 years of age.[24] Although no harmful effects of isoniazid to the fetus have been observed, the general recommendation is that preventive therapy for the pregnant woman who otherwise meets criteria for prophylaxis should be delayed until after delivery.[6,8,19] Compared to others who may benefit from isoniazid prophylaxis, there does not appear to be a substantial increase in tuberculous risk for women during pregnancy, with the possible exception of pregnant women who have been recently infected.[6] This includes women who have had significant exposure to an infectious contact or tuberculin skin test conversion to positive within the past two years. For these women, isoniazid preventive therapy should begin when conversion is documented but after the first trimester.[6,8,19]

The perinatal management of the neonate born to an infectious mother has been previously detailed. Separation of the mother and infant is reasonable when the infant is continuously exposed to a highly infectious, untreated, or noncompliant caretaker.[19] If the newborn must be left in such a situation, isoniazid should be continued for the duration of the exposure.

For those who have been potentially infected with isoniazid-resistant organisms or exposed to close contacts who have isoniazid-resistant disease, preventive therapy for one year with rifampin and ethambutol is advocated.[19] The use of bacille Calmette–Guérin (BCG), a vaccine derived from an attenuated strain of *M bovis,* has been reported to result in protection rates that vary from 0–80% in areas where tuberculous disease is widespread.[7] BCG vaccination may be an alternative when isoniazid preventive therapy cannot be used. It may be considered for neonates who have no reaction to tuberculous skin testing and who have repeated exposure to infectious contact cases.[19] The presence of depressed host immunity or pregnancy are contraindications to BCG administration.[13,19]

LEPROSY

While leprosy remains a rare disease in women of childbearing age in developed countries, the number of reported cases in the United States is increasing as a consequence of importation from endemic areas. Between 1985 and 1987, there were 1139 reported cases; 75% of these were foreign-born individuals who were infected in endemic areas such as Mexico, the Philippines, India, and the Far East.[25] Recognition of cases and early treatment may not only improve the overall prognosis of mother and infant, but may interrupt the chain of transmission to other susceptible individuals.

Leprosy is caused by the organism *M leprae*. The organism cannot be cultivated in the laboratory on artificial media or in tissue culture. It is a small, acid-fast, curved bacillus, 0.5×4–7 microns, at times noted to have a metachromatic granule in the center or at one pole.[25] Differentiation of this organism from other acid-fast bacilli is based on growth and biochemical characteristics and its ability to preferentially infect peripheral nerves of humans or experimentally infected armadillos.

The distribution in nature of this organism and its transmission is poorly understood. Transmission is thought to result from skin-to-skin contact with an infected individual.[25] Individuals most infectious are those who have high bacillary loads. At highest risk of infection are household or close contacts of infectious individuals. Newer data support the hypothesis that the respiratory route may be of greater significance in transmission.[26] Large numbers of bacilli can be found in nasal secretions of infected patients, and organisms may maintain viability in dried secretions for several days.[26] Little is known about intrauterine transmission. Most neonates or infants are likely to be infected through contact with maternal skin lesions or respiratory secretions after birth. Other potential routes of transmission include infected breast milk and, possibly, biting insects.[27]

Diagnosis

Leprosy is characterized by a wide spectrum of disease ranging from limited (*tuberculoid*) to generalized (*lepromatous*). Disease is classified according to and progresses in the following manner: *Full tuberculoid* (TT) to *borderline tuberculoid* (BT) to *borderline* (BB) to *borderline lepromatous* (BL) to *full lepromatous* (LL).[25] Tuberculoid lesions are large, sharply demarcated, erythematous plaques, usually flat, dry, and hairless with notable cutaneous anesthesia. Damage to peripheral nerves is localized, and the surface area of skin involvement is limited. As disease progresses to borderline stages, lesions become more numerous and are associated with satellite lesions. They become more irregular in shape, poorly defined, with central hypopigmentation and less marked cutaneous anesthesia. The clinical characteristics of the lesions are closely paralleled by their histologic appearance. Tuberculoid lesions contain well-formed granulomata densely infiltrated with lymphocytes. Involved nerve bundles are swollen and infiltrated with mononuclear inflammatory cells. Acid-fast organisms may be few or absent. As skin disease progresses to borderline lesions, granulomata are progressively less well-demarcated and more often infiltrated with mononuclear cells. AFB are more extensively demonstrable throughout the lesions.

Lepromatous leprosy is notable for extensive skin involvement with a symmetric bilateral distribution of multiple erythematous, maculopapular nodules and plaques. The characteristic "leonine" facies are the result of thickening and infiltration of facial skin, with loss of eyebrows and eyelashes and widespread destruction of nasal and maxillary structures. Nerve involvement is diffuse, with patchy sensory loss typical of mononeuritis multiplex. Histologically, lepromatous disease demonstrates little or no granulomata formation and dense infiltration of skin with massive numbers of AFB.

Erythema nodosum leprosum (ENL) occurs in patients with disease at the lepromatous end of the spectrum.[25] Most patients develop this complication within the first year after initiation of therapy for their leprosy. ENL may be triggered by pregnancy.[28] ENL differs from other inflammatory causes of erythema nodosum by its widespread distribution and involvement of the face rather than localization to the anterior tibia or lower extremities. Histopathologically, a localized proliferative vasculitis is seen.[25] ENL may also be accompanied by polyarthralgia, neuritis resulting in sudden loss of peripheral nerve function, high fever, necrosis of the nodules, and leukemoid reactions. Untreated cases may result in death.

Reversal reactions are those in which skin lesions rapidly develop a raised indurated erythematous shiny character with or without ulceration, associated with neuritis and loss of motor function. These reactions are most common in patients with borderline or early forms of lepromatous leprosy and are thought to represent a localized host immune response to the organisms.[25]

Deformity of nasomaxillary facial structures is most often a consequence of primary infection with *M leprae*, while deformity of peripheral extremities is more often a consequence of peripheral neuritis, with loss of sensory and motor function. Repeated trauma and infection in areas of cutaneous anesthesia may result in chronic ulceration and resorption of bone.

Ophthalmic complications occur in 25–30% of patients with lepromatous leprosy.[25] The most frequent manifestations of these are conjunctivitis, keratitis, and leprotic iridocyclitis. Secondary damage to the cornea may occur as a result of corneal anesthesia resulting from involvement of the ophthalmic division of the fifth cranial nerve.

Diagnosis is generally made on clinical grounds and through biopsy of appropriate tissue. Skin testing may be helpful in some circumstances. Persons with tuberculoid stages of disease retain their capability of reacting to skin test antigens of *M leprae*. Those in lepromatous stages of disease are anergic. The most generally available antigen for skin testing is integral lepromin, made from nodules of lepromatous patients.[25] Patients tested with this preparation first manifest transient erythema and induration at 24 to 48 hours, followed by the development of a nodule at the site of the skin test. The reaction peaks at three to four weeks. A weak positive reaction is one in which nodule formation achieves a diameter of three to five millimeters; a strongly positive test is one with a diameter of greater than five millimeters with ulceration.

Treatment

There are only four major antibacterial drugs currently available for treatment of leprosy. Antibiotics are generally necessary for prolonged periods and in some cases for life. The four drugs currently in use include dapsone, rifampin, clofazimine, and ethionamide. Very little information about the use of any of these drugs is available for pregnant women. The most experience is available with the use of dapsone, a sulfone structural analog of para-aminobenzoic acid that interferes with folic acid metabolism. This drug has been used during pregnancy with no significant adverse effects on the fetus, with the possible exception of displacement of bilirubin from albumin in the neonate similar to the effect occurring with other sulfonamides. This requires careful attention to the newborn at the time of and shortly after birth. While clofazimine has been used during pregnancy in a small number of women without notable teratogenicity, experience is so limited that its use should not be recommended except in severe circumstances. Pigmentation of the skin has been observed in some infants, suggesting that placental transfer of this drug does occur. For pregnant women who require therapy, regimens of dapsone and rifampin will probably be the most reasonable.

Recommended treatment for high bacillary load forms of disease (BB, BL, and LL) includes multiple drug combinations. Dapsone in oral doses of 50–100 mg daily, clofazimine 50 mg daily, plus an extra 300 mg dose once per month, and oral rifampin 600 mg once monthly is the suggested regimen.[29] Ethionamide can be substituted for clofazimine when the latter is not tolerated. Combined therapy should be given for a minimum of two years and if possible until all skin scrapings and biopsies are negative for AFB. For treatment of low bacillary load forms (TT and BT), oral rifampin in a dose of 600 mg once per month for a six-month period plus oral dapsone 100 mg daily for six months are recommended.[29] Some experts recommend daily dapsone in doses of 50–100 mg plus daily rifampin in doses of 450–600 mg for a period of six months, followed by continual dapsone therapy for an additional period of two to five years.[29] Toxic effects of dapsone include hemolytic anemia in patients with glucose-6-phosphate dehydrogenase deficiency, agranulocytosis (rarely), hypoalbuminemia, and possibly an infectious mononucleosislike syndrome. Common side effects for rifampin are presented in Table 77–4.

Corticosteroids may be required for treatment of severe ENL or reversal reactions. For nonpregnant patients, thalidomide is also recommended and is effective in treating ENL. Oral doses of 300 mg per day will generally control even severe manifestations, and this dose can be tapered over weeks to months to lower doses of 100 mg once per day. Obviously, the teratogenic effects of thalidomide preclude its use during pregnancy.

Prophylaxis

Household contacts of patients with leprosy, especially neonates and children, should be examined and any suspicious lesions biopsied. Those with extensive household contact with highly infectious persons, such as those with lepromatous disease who are shedding organisms in nasal secretions or from open skin lesions, should be considered for dapsone prophylaxis. This has been demonstrated to be useful in infants and children under the age of 16 in previously recommended dosage schedules.[30] Adults appear to be less susceptible to leprosy, and the efficacy of dapsone prophylaxis has not been established in older age groups. Although specific data are lacking, infants born to mothers with highly infectious lesions may benefit from dapsone prophylaxis.

REFERENCES

1. Reider HL, Cauthen GM, Kelly GD, et al. Tuberculosis in the United States. *JAMA*. 1989;262:385.
2. Youmans AS. The morphology and metabolism of mycobacteria. In: Youmans GP, ed. *Tuberculosis*. Philadelphia, PA: WB Saunders; 1979:8.
3. Riley RL. Disease transmission and contagion control. *Am Rev Respir Dis*. 1982;125(No. 3, Pt. 2):16.
4. Comstock GW. Epidemiology of tuberculosis. *Am Rev Respir Dis*. 1982; 125(No. 3, Pt. 2):8.
5. Stead WW. Tuberculosis among elderly persons: an outbreak in a nursing home. *Ann Intern Med*. 1981;94:606.
6. Snider D. Pregnancy and tuberculosis. *Chest*. 1984;86(suppl):10S.
7. Des Pres RM, Heim CR. Mycobacterium tuberculosis. In: Mandell GL, Douglas RG Jr, Bennett JE, eds. *Principles and Practice of Infectious Disease*. New York, NY: Churchill Livingstone; 1990:1877.
8. Jacobs RF, Abernathy RS. Management of tuberculosis in pregnancy and the newborn. *Clin in Perinatol*. 1988;15:305.
9. Beitzke H. Uber die angeborene tuberkulose infeckion. *Ergb Ges Tuberk Forsch*. 1935;7:1.
10. Nemir RL, O'Hare D. Congenital tuberculosis. Review and diagnostic guidelines. *Am J Dis Child*. 1985;139:284.
11. Medchill MT, Gillum M. Diagnosis and management of tuberculosis during pregnancy. *Obstet Gynecol Survey*. 1989;44:81.
12. Good JT Jr, Iseman MD, Davidson PT, et al. Tuberculosis in association with pregnancy. *Am J Obstet Gynecol*. 1981;140:492.
13. Gillum MD, Maki DG. Brief report: tuberculin testing, BCG in pregnancy. *Infect Control Hosp Epidemiol*. 1988;9:119.
14. Biehl JP. Miliary tuberculosis. A review of sixty-eight adult patients admitted to a municipal general hospital. *Am Rev Tuberc*. 1958;77:605.
15. Munt PW. Miliary tuberculosis in the chemotherapy era: with a clinical review in 69 American adults. *Medicine (Balt)*. 1972;51:139.
16. Slavin RE, Walsh TJ, Pollack AD. Late generalized tuberculosis: a clinical pathologic analysis and comparison of 100 cases in the pre-antibiotic and antibiotic eras. *Medicine*. 1980;59:352.
17. Merchant R. Endoscopy in the diagnosis of genital tuberculosis. *J Reprod Med*. 1989;34:468.
18. Snider DE Jr, Layde PM, Johnson MW, Lyle MA. Treatment of tuberculosis during pregnancy. *Am Rev Respir Dis*. 1980;122:65.
19. American Thoracic Society, Centers for Disease Control. Treatment of tuberculosis and tuberculous infection in adults and children. *Am Rev Respir Dis*. 1986;134:355.
20. Holdiness MR. Teratology of the anti-tuberculous drugs. *Early Human Develop*. 1987;15:61.
21. Snider DE, Cohn DL, Davidson PT, et al. Standard therapy for tuberculosis. *Chest*. 1985;87(suppl):117S.
22. Dutt AK, Moers D, Stead WW. Short-course chemotherapy for extrapulmonary tuberculosis. *Ann Intern Med*. 1986;104:7.
23. Farer LS. Chemoprophylaxis. *Am Rev Respir Dis*. 1982;125:102.
24. Kopanoff DE, Snider DE, Caras GJ. Isoniazid related hepatitis. *Am Rev Respir Dis*. 1978;117:991.
25. Bullock WE. Mycobacterium leprae (leprosy). In: Mandell GL, Douglas RG Jr, Bennett JE, eds. *Principles and Practice of Infectious Disease*. New York, NY: Churchill Livingstone; 1990:1906.
26. Shepard CC. The nasal excretion of *Mycobacterium leprae* in leprosy. *Int J Lepr*. 1962;30:10.
27. Pedley JC. The presence of *M. leprae* in the nipple secretion and lumina of the hypertrophied mammary gland. In a case of gynecomastia associated with active and untreated lepromatous leprosy. *Lepr Rev*. 1968;39:67.
28. Rose P, McDougall D. Adverse reactions following pregnancy in patients with borderline (dimorphous) leprosy. *Lepr Rev*. 1975;46:109.
29. WHO Study Group. Chemotherapy of leprosy for control programmes. *WHO Tech Rep Ser*. 1982;675:7.
30. Filice GA, Fraser DW. Management of household contacts of leprosy patients. *Ann Intern Med*. 1978;88:538.

Chapter Seventy-Eight
Scabies, Lice, and Other Ectoparasites

Michael T. Parsons

78

An *ectoparasite* has been defined as an organism that attaches to the outside of the body of the host and derives sustenance from the host.[1,2] The definition has been extended to those parasites that temporarily burrow into the superficial tissues of the host's body, but continue communications with the environment.[1] An infestation, rather than an infection as seen with endoparasites, is the result.[2] Ectoparasites produce clinical problems both in the direct irritation they cause by tissue injury from the infestation and from the other diseases carried while acting as vectors. The primary problem with ectoparasitic infestations in pregnancy is the medication-related side effects that potentially could be harmful to the embryo or fetus.

SCABIES

Scabies is an immunologic response to the body mite *Sarcoptes scabiei* variety *hominis*, an obligate parasite to humans.[3,4] The discovery of the mite in 1687 by Bonomo made scabies the first human disease attributed to a known cause.[5] The disease is caused by a white, translucent, eyeless, oval mite with eight legs.[3] The male, which measures 200 × 150 μm, usually remains on the surface of the host's skin.[3] The female, 400 × 300 μm produces the primary lesion by burrowing in the stratum corneum to the boundary of stratum granulosum and remains for life, which is approximately 30 days.[4] The female produces an elevated, 0.5 mm × 10 mm tortuous tunnel in which she deposits eggs and feces. The eggs hatch in 3–4 days and the emerging larvae travel to the skin surface and mature to adults in 10–14 days.[5] Mating takes place on the skin surface; then they burrow back into the skin.[6] The usual number of mites in an infestation rarely exceeds fifty.

Scabies is spread through personal contact. The prevalence is estimated at 6–27%, the highest being among the young and the overcrowded.[3] Individuals sharing beds or having prolonged and intimate contact have an increased occurrence. Scabies is considered a sexually transmitted disease although its transmission is very often nonsexual, especially to children.[5] The mites can survive up to two days away from skin.

The clinical presentation is severe pruritus. Patients previously uninfested develop symptoms in a month, while patients previously infested may develop symptoms within 24 hours. Their degree of pruritus is similar. Areas most affected are finger webs, wrists, arms, legs, and tight clothing areas. The back, chest, and head are rarely involved in adults. The pruritus is most severe at night. Aggressive scratching can produce bleeding, spreading of infestation, and secondary infection including impetigo.[1,2,4,5]

In addition to the visible tunneling on the skin, an erythematous, papular rash may appear. A type IV immunologic reaction to the mite or its fecal pellets produces symptoms, with peripheral eosinophilia and lymphocytes and eosinophils around the tunnels.[3]

A less common condition, *Norwegian scabies*, occurs in patients with a defective immunologic response. In these cases, thousands of mites infest an individual, causing a condition that is only minimally pruritic, has extensive crusting, and is highly contagious.[3,6] Also uncommon is a presentation of clinical and pathologic vasculitis.[5]

Pregnancy has no effect on the prevalence or clinical presentation.[7] The major concern about scabies in pregnancy is the potential toxicity of therapeutic agents to the fetus.

In patients suspected of having scabies, a small, slightly elevated track may be identified on the skin. An opening to the tunnel and a small vesicle at the end of the tunnel can be seen with a magnifying glass.[6] The diagnosis of scabies can be made by using a scalpel to scrape a suspected area on the skin onto a microscope slide and identifying mites or eggs.[3] This may be best accomplished by identifying an unexcoriated burrow, unroofing the top of the burrow, and placing the contents with mineral oil on the slide. Even if scrapings are negative, a therapeutic trial of medication may be indicated.

The most common medication for treatment of scabies in nonpregnant patients is gamma benzene hexachloride (lindane, Kwell)[3], a miticide and pediculicide that is absorbed through the mite's exoskeleton and acts on its nervous system to produce convulsions and death.[8] A 1% lotion or cream is applied thinly over the entire body from the neck down, left on for 12 hours, then washed off.[9] Relief should occur within 48 hours, but all signs and symptoms may not clear for weeks. A repeat treatment in seven days may be necessary. Close household contacts and sexual partners should be treated. Toxic effects to the patient's central nervous system have been reported, but are mostly associated with misuse and in young patients.[10] Aplastic anemia has been reported after prolonged exposure.[8] Although it has not been shown to be teratogenic[11,12], the manufacturer of lindane (Kwell) recommends use with caution during pregnancy, and many investigators recommend refraining from use during pregnancy.[5] Even with the manufacturer's note of caution, lindane has been widely used in pregnancy with a shorter exposure time (<8 hours) with no reports of adverse fetal effects. In pregnancy, an alternate choice is 10% crotamiton cream or lotion (Eurax)[3,11], applied from the neck down every 24 hours for 2 or 3 applications. This also has an antipruritic effect, but needs more applications than lindane. The mechanisms of the scabicidal and antipruritic actions of crotamiton are unknown. A third choice is 5–6% sulfur precipitate in petrolatum nightly for three nights.[10,11] This is the oldest and probably the safest preparation, but it has the disadvantage of being foul-smelling and messy. The recommendations from the 1985 STD Treatment Guidelines from the Centers for Disease Control are that lindane not be used in pregnant and lactating women.[13] Their choice is crotamiton or sulphur (6%) in petrolatum. With all of the preparations, bed linens and clothes should be washed in hot water. The pruritis may remain until mite antigens slough off with skin.

LICE

Lice are wingless, parasitic, flat insects.[4,14,15] The adult measures 1–3 mm in diameter and has three pairs of legs with tarsal claws.[14] The three varieties of lice that affect humans are *Pediculus humanus corporis* (body louse), *Pediculus humanus capitis* (head louse) and *Phthirus pubis* (pubic crab louse).[4,14] The fertilized adult lays 0.5 mm oval, translucent eggs (nits) that are cemented to body hairs or clothing.[14] Small nymphs emerge from the eggs and molt three times before becoming an adult. The female produces 250 eggs over the next month before dying.[4] The adult louse anchors its mouth to the skin of the host and lives on the blood it sucks.[4] The life cycle is approximately 25 days.[5]

Infestation by lice causes problems in two ways. First, the adult lice release saliva upon entering the skin, which may produce an antigenic effect causing immunologic pruritus and dermatitis, called *pediculosis*.[4,14] The incubation period to pruritus is one month.[5] Symptoms vary from asymptomatic to severe itching with bluish papular or urticarial lesions, and secondary infection.[15] Second, body lice act as vectors for several severe epidemics, including epidemic typhus (by *Rickettsia prowazekii*) and epidemic relapsing fever (by *Borrelia recurrentis*).[14,15]

Head lice are spread by close personal contact and are most often seen in school-aged children.[4,15] The eggs are deposited on hairs of the head and neck.[14] Pruritus with subsequent scratching, infection, and lymphadenopathy may result.[4] The lice can survive for several days away from humans.

The body louse lives on clothing and bedding and feeds on the skin.[4] Very few are found on human hairs or on the body. Eggs are attached to fibers of clothing.[14,15] Infestation causes generalized itching and papular lesions. It is usually transmitted through infested clothing and is common in areas of poor hygiene, crowding, and heavy clothing.[14]

Pubic lice are most often found in the pubic hair, but other areas, including axillary, perianal, scalp, and trunk hair, can be infested. It is most frequently found in adults and is contracted through sexual partners, infested bedding, or clothing.[4,14] It also has been reported to spread in locker rooms and mats in gym class.[14] Other untreated sexually transmitted diseases are found in one third of patients with pediculosis pubis.[5]

Pregnancy does not appear to have any effect on the infestation of lice or its manifestations. As with scabies, the importance of lice associated with pregnancy is with the therapeutic agents used.

The diagnosis of lice infestation is made with history and physical examination of cutaneous lesions. Head lice may be seen on the scalp, but often it is the nit that is visible on the scalp hairs. With pubic lice, nits, bites, and the louse itself may be seen at the base of hairs.[15] The parasites are rust-colored after a blood meal. Microscopic examination of the parasite or its nit will confirm the diagnosis.

Treatment for head and pubic lice in nonpregnant patients is with lindane shampoo 1% for four minutes; the patient should rinse thoroughly, dry, then comb out remaining nits.[4,19] For pubic lice, sexual contacts should also be treated.[10] The same concerns with the use of lindane in pregnancy as discussed in the section on scabies apply here. Recommendations by the Centers for Disease Control (1985) include not using lindane shampoo for pregnant or lactating women.[11] Alternative treatment includes the over-the-counter combination preparation of 0.3% pyrethrins and 3% piperonyl butoxide (RID) applied to the affected area for 10 minutes, followed by bathing.[4,10] This should be repeated in 10 days. This combination acts synergistically to kill lice and eggs.[10] In addition to the medication, freshly laundered underwear and bed sheets should be used daily for one week.[10] Body lice usually do not require medication, but all clothes and bedding should be washed.[4,15] If any articles are hard to clean, storage for two weeks will completely rid them of living lice and eggs. If eyelashes are involved, 0.25% physostigmine opthalmic ointment or petrolatum can be used.[5] Patients with pubic lice should also be examined for other sexually transmitted diseases.

TICKS

Ticks are arcarid ectoparasites that suck blood from mammals. There are two families, the soft ticks (*Argasidae*) and hard ticks (*Ixodidae*).[16] They have an egg, larva, nymph, and eight-legged adult stage with a life cycle of up to two years.[16,17] Ticks have a large animal and human reservoir and are present in grasses along animal trails, and they attach to passing hosts.[17] Mating takes place either with the female attached to a host or off the host, and a single mating may result in thousands of eggs. After hatching, the tick gets blood from the host, then drops off.

Ticks attach to humans by inserting mouth parts into skin layers.[16] This initial bite and feeding of blood produces minimal if any discomfort to the host.[16,17] The adults engorge to 1 cm in size after feeding. The mouth parts in the host may provoke an inflammatory response, and salivary secretions inhibit coagulation of blood and cause histolysis at the site. Additional damage can result from attempting to remove the tick; the tick breaks off and leaves portions in the skin, and a tick bite granuloma may form.[4,16] After successful removal of the tick, a punctum surrounded by erythema is visible for over one week. A very rare but severe reaction to prolonged tick attachment is tick paralysis.[16,17] A neurotoxin has been isolated from the salivary gland that may produce cerebella ataxia, weakness, and reduced motor strength. The symptoms usually disappear after removal of the tick. A final problem is that ticks act as vectors for a variety of viruses, rickettsiae, bacteria, and protozoa, causing conditions such as Lyme disease, Rocky Mountain spotted fever, Q fever, relapsing fever, and encephalitis.[4,16]

No specific problems with simple infestation have been reported with pregnancy. Diagnosis is made by visualization of the tick or tick part attached to the skin. Ticks can be removed by applying ether, chloroform, acetone, or benzene to the head of the tick to relax its mouth parts. They can also be burned off or surgically removed.[4,16]

FLEAS

Fleas (*Siphonaptera*) are ectoparasites of mammals (humans, dogs, cats, rodents) and birds that attach to skin to suck their host's blood.[4,18] The female lays eggs after insemination on the host or surrounding area, which develop through larval stages into adults and can survive for a year. The adults are small (1–4 mm), wingless, brown insects with mouthparts for piercing the skin and sucking blood and long hind legs for jumping.[18] Flea bites on humans produce an irritating dermatitis on legs and other exposed parts of the body. The lesion is erythematous, papular, edematous, and pruritic, with occasional induration and secondary infections. Fleas also can act as vectors to rodents carrying plague (*Yersinia pestis*).[18]

There is no effect on the disease with pregnancy. Treatment of the dermatitis is with topical steroids and antihistamine for pruritus. Repellents such as benzyl benzoate may be useful. Dogs and cats can be treated with malathion, DDT powder, or flea collar (with dichlorvos). Frequent vacuuming for eggs, larvae, and adults will decrease the infestation.[4,18]

CHIGGERS

The common chigger (*Eutrombicula alfreddugési*) occasionally infests humans. The adult chigger has a fused head and thorax and six legs.[19] The adults feed on vegetable matter and deposit eggs in the soil or foodstuffs and hatch into small (1 mm), oval larvae. It is the larvae, not the adult, that attaches and feeds on humans and other hosts. Chiggers do not burrow into the skin, but bite and release a digestant.[19,20] The bite will become severely pruritic within 1–2 days, with the sometimes hemorrhagic papule lasting 5–6 days. Bites are common on the legs and other exposed skin areas. There are no special concerns with pregnancy. The process is self-limiting; the only treatment necessary is symptomatic, with application of topical or systemic antipruritics. Protective clothing and insect repellents may help prevent infestation.[19,20]

REFERENCES

1. Weary PE. Ectoparasites. Introduction. In: Mandell G, Douglas RG Jr, Bennett JE, eds. *Principles and Practice of Infectious Disease*. New York, NY: John Wiley and Sons, Inc; 1985:1589.
2. Beaver PC, Jung RC, Cupp EW. *Clinical Parasitology*. 9th ed. Philadelphia, PA: Lea and Febiger; 1984:4.
3. Burkhart CG. Scabies: an epidemiologic assessment. *Am J Intern Med*. 1983;98:498.
4. Pien FD, Grekin JL. Common ectoparasites. *West J Med*. 1983;139:382.
5. Orkin M, Mailbach HI. Current views of scabies and pediculosis pubis. *Cutis*. 1984;33:85.
6. Beaver PC, Jung RC, Cupp EW. *Clinical Parasitology*. 9th ed. Philadelphia, PA: Lea and Febiger; 1984:601.
7. Ross SM. Sexually transmitted diseases in pregnancy. *Clin Obstet Gynaecol*. 1982;9:365.
8. Berkowitz RL, Coustan DR, Mochizuki TK. *Handbook for Prescribing Medications During Pregnancy*. 2nd ed. Boston/Toronto. Little, Brown and Company; 1986:135.
9. Weary PE. Scabies. In: Mandell G, Douglas RG Jr, Bennett JE, eds. *Principles and Practice of Infectious Disease*. New York, NY: John Wiley and Sons, Inc; 1985:1591.
10. Crissey JT. Scabies and pediculosis pubis. *Urol Clin North Am*. 1984;11:171.
11. Gurevitch AW. Scabies and lice. *Pediat Clin North Am*. 1985;32:987.
12. Rasmussen JE. The problem of lindane. *J Am Acad Dermatol*. 1981;5:507.
13. Centers For Disease Control. *MMWR*. 1985;34.
14. Beaver PC, Jung RC, Cupp EW. *Clinical Parasitology*. 9th ed. Philadelphia, PA: Lea and Febiger; 1984:611.
15. Weary PE. Lice (Pediculosis). In: Mandell G, Douglas RG Jr, Bennett JE, eds. *Principles and Practice of Infectious Disease*. New York, NY: John Wiley and Sons, Inc; 1985:1590.
16. Beaver PC, Jung RC, Cupp EW. *Clinical Parasitology*. 9th ed. Philadelphia, PA: Lea and Febiger; 1984:581.
17. Weary PE. Ticks (Including Tick Paralysis). Mandell G, Douglas RG Jr, Bennett JE, eds. *Principles and Practice of Infectious Disease*. New York, NY: John Wiley and Sons, Inc; 1985:1594.
18. Beaver PC, Jung RC, Cupp EW. *Clinical Parasitology*. 9th ed. Philadelphia, PA: Lea and Febiger; 1984:696.
19. Weary PE. Chiggers (Mites). In: Mandell G, Douglas RG Jr, Bennett JE, eds. *Principles and Practice of Infectious Disease*. New York, NY: John Wiley and Sons, Inc; 1985:1593.
20. Braunwald E, Isselbacher KJ, Petersdorf RG, et al. *Harrison's Principles of Internal Medicine*. 11th ed. New York, NY: McGraw-Hill Book Company; 1987:829.

Chapter Seventy-Nine

Syphilis

George D. Wendel, Jr.

79

Syphilis is a complex, chronic, sexually transmissible disease caused by *Treponema pallidum* that can have profound effects on pregnancy. It is characterized by a three-week incubation period; a primary stage with a single cutaneous lesion and regional adenopathy; a secondary stage with diffuse mucocutaneous lesions, lymphadenopathy, and spirochetemia; a latent period of variable infectivity; and, finally, progression to late syphilis with a myriad of manifestations. It also causes one of the few transplacentally-acquired fetal bacterial infections that is preventable and treatable in humans.

After several years of declining rates of infectious syphilis in adults, the incidence of primary and secondary syphilis in the United States is rising. The declining incidence in the early 1980s, led by decreases in rates for homosexual males, has been replaced by marked increases in syphilis in heterosexuals, mostly in indigent, urban populations already plagued with drug abuse, prostitution, and human immunodeficiency virus (HIV) infection.[1-3] The most marked increases have occurred in areas of the United States already suffering the ravages of HIV infection, such as New York City, California, and Florida. Because most of the infectious syphilis is occurring in reproductive-age adults, it is not surprising that congenital syphilis also has reached the highest rates since the 1970s.[1,4] As the current urban epidemic of syphilis continues, it is imperative that obstetricians re-educate themselves about the effects of syphilis on the gravida, her sex partner(s), and her fetus.

The causative agent of syphilis, *T pallidum*, is a spirochete that is morphologically indistinguishable from the treponemes that cause nonvenereal infections such as pinta, yaws, and endemic syphilis (bejel).[5] It is 5 to 15 μm (average 10 μm) in length and generally slightly longer than the width of a red blood cell. The thin (0.15 μm), tightly coiled, helical organism has spiral waves 1.1 μm in length and 0.5 μm in width along its axis. *T pallidum* exhibits characteristic motility consisting of translation (slow forward or backward movement), rotation (slow or rapid corkscrewlike movement along the longitudinal axis), and flexion (elastic-like bending, twisting, or side-to-side undulation about the center of the organism).[6] The structure of the organism consists of an outer membrane that surrounds the endoflagella, cytoplasmic membrane, and protoplasmic cylinder of the organism. The outer membrane, a protein-deficient bilayer different from that of other gram-negative bacteria, is thought to possess the antigenic molecules important in the immunopathogenesis of syphilis. With new laboratory techniques, major immunogenic surface antigens have been identified and monoclonal antibodies developed that will allow further insight into the natural history of syphilitic infection.[7]

Unfortunately, *T pallidum* cannot be readily cultivated *in vitro*. Attempts have been made to maintain motile organisms in special enriched medium and in cell culture, but these techniques are still under investigation. The most widely used means to demonstrate or maintain virulent spirochetes is the rabbit infectivity test.[8] This involves inoculating clinical material into the animal host, usually into the testicle, intracutaneously or intravenously. Serial passage or transfer between rabbits by testicular inoculation allows maintenance of virulent organisms for investigation.

Syphilis can be acquired by intimate contact (kissing, touching, coitus, fellatio, cunnilingus) with an infected partner. It can be acquired by the fetus presumably by transplacental passage or by exposure to infectious maternal secretions, blood, or lesions at delivery. Direct inoculation by needle stick and by transfusion of infected blood products can occur, but rarely in the 1990s. Infection by *T pallidum* occurs probably through minute abrasions in skin or through mucous membranes. The sites of lesions in women are those that sustain microtrauma with coitus or intimate contact: the fourchette, the labia, the cervix, the anus, the lips, and the nipples. It is estimated from placebo-controlled studies of various regimens in preventing infection[9], that sexual partners of infected individuals in the previous 30 days have a 30% chance of acquiring syphilis.

After entry into the host, local replication of organisms occurs and dissemination begins by way of lymphatics. The replication time for treponemes is 30–33 hours, and clinical lesions develop when critical amounts of organisms (10^7 treponemes per gram of tissue) are reached. The incubation period after infection is usually three weeks (range 3–90 days), but varies inversely proportional to the infecting inoculum and poorly defined host factors.

PRIMARY SYPHILIS

The initial phase of infection is called the *primary stage* of syphilis. The characteristic lesion or chancre is a raised, red, nontender papule of 0.5–2.0 cm in size. With induration and ulceration, it acquires a characteristic rubbery or cartilaginous consistency. The central superficial erosion of the base gives rise to slightly raised borders. The lesion is usually round, but may be elongated when it occurs along tissue folds. Chancres are usually solitary, but multiple chancres are occasionally seen, particularly in HIV-coinfected adults. Atypical chancres are seen in patients with a prior history of syphilis, immunosuppression, or recent topical or systemic antimicrobial administration. Histopathologically, the chancre exhibits ulceration, plasma cellular infiltrate, and varying stages of obliterative endarteritis. The chancre is accompanied by a nontender, rubbery, regional lymphadenopathy in 80% of adults. Chancres uncommonly become secondarily infected, and the lymph nodes do no suppurate.

Chancres are not diagnosed in women as frequently as in men. Because chancres cause little discomfort, they may not result in gravida seeking medical attention. Cervical chancres are usually asymptomatic and undetected except by careful speculum examination.[10] Consequently, most women have secondary or latent syphilis at the time of diagnosis of syphilis. Untreated chancres resolve in 3–8 weeks, leaving minimal or no scarring. The adenopathy may take longer to resolve. It is common to see a persistent or healing chancre with early signs of secondary syphilis.

SECONDARY SYPHILIS

Despite local immunologic events that result in healing of the chancre, spirochetes systemically disseminate in the *secondary stage* of syphilis. Virtually all adults will progress to this stage of infection within 4 to 10 weeks (average, 6 weeks) of the appearance of their chancre. This is a stage of multiplication of *T pallidum* resulting in a large systemic organism load. Spirochetemia results in widespread dissemination and diffuse organ involvement. Typically, bilateral, symmetric skin lesions and systemic abnormalities occur. In the past, the protean clinical manifestations of this stage led to syphilis being called "the great imitator."

The dermatologic manifestations of secondary syphilis are the most commonly recognized. The lesions are always diffuse, bilateral, and symmetric. Initially, an evanescent macular rash occurs in the trunk and proximal extremities, which is often missed by the patient. This progresses in a variable fashion to a papular rash in several days to weeks. The typical lesions are round, red, or hyperpigmented and are 0.5–2 cm in size with discrete borders. Lesions involve the trunk, extremities, and face. Facial lesions called *annular syphilids* are readily diagnosed as are the palmar and plantar maculopapular targetlike lesions. Split papules can occur in nasolabial folds or at the corner of the mouth. Painless, erosive, mucosal lesions (mucous patches) can develop in the oral cavity, the genital area, or the anus.

The genital manifestations of secondary syphilis are also characteristically bilateral and symmetric. In intertriginous areas subject to friction, papules form moist, raised, white-grey plaques that often coalesce into large erosive painless lesions, called *condylomata lata*. Mucous patches also occur and may resemble genital herpes infection, but without the typical vesicles or tenderness. Bilateral painless inguinal lymphadenopathy is commonly noted with this stage of syphilis.

Systemic symptoms reflect the diffuse involvement of secondary syphilis. Many women will have constitutional symptoms such as transient fever, malaise, anorexia, headache, or pharyngitis. These symptoms are often misdiagnosed, delaying the diagnosis of syphilis. Generalized lymphadenopathy also occurs, particularly reflected by epitrochlear adenopathy. Patchy alopecia may appear. Syphilis may cause hepatitis or the nephrotic syndrome. Anterior uveitis and cranial nerve involvement occurs. Central nervous system (CNS) involvement is seen by meningeal signs or cerebrospinal fluid (CSF) abnormalities in protein and cell count in up to 40% of patients.[11-13] Virtually any organ system can be affected by this disseminated stage of syphilis.

LATENT SYPHILIS

Three to twelve weeks after the onset of secondary syphilis, the lesions heal and the patient enters an asymptomatic *latency period*. The diagnosis is made in this stage only by history, lack of signs of syphilis, and the presence of antitreponemal antibody. Unfortunately, this also may represent a heterogenous group of patients with misdiagnosed or inapparent lesions, those without a recollection of prior treatment, and those with partially treated syphilis.

Despite its name, this stage is characterized by infectivity and progression of infection. Latent syphilis can be complicated by relapses that resemble clinical secondary syphilis in up to 20–25% of adults. Ninety percent of these recurrences occur within the first year of infection.[13] Latent syphilis is called *early* if it is less than one year's duration and *late* if it is over one year's duration. Epidemiologically, the greatest infectivity for sexual or fetal transmission of syphilis coincides with the first year of infection. Many health care providers and organizations group primary, secondary, and the early latent stages together and call them early syphilis.[14] All three stages are infectious and can be treated with similar antimicrobial regimens.

LATE SYPHILIS

After a period of latency of over one year, and usually of many years, 20–30% of untreated adults will develop complications of *late* or *tertiary syphilis*. This stage is becoming less common in the 1990s in the United States as fewer patients escape detection and treatment.[15] Due to the slow development of this stage of infection, most of the clinical manifestations are not commonly seen in reproductive-age women or in pregnancy.

Benign late syphilis is characterized by destructive, granulomatous gummas of the skin, bone, or viscera; it develops in 15% of untreated adults.[13,16] *Cardiovascular syphilis* is manifest by syphilitic aortitis, and mediated by involvement of vasovasorum of the aorta, causing aortic medial necrosis.[17] It is seen in at least 10% of untreated adults, and possibly more when sought at autopsy.[13]

Neurosyphilis develops in 7% of untreated adults.[18] It is distinguished from CNS invasion by *T pallidum* and acute meningitis that can complicate secondary syphilis in up to 40% of immunocompetent adults. Neurosyphilis is divided into asymptomatic and symptomatic phases. Patients with normal neurologic examinations and CSF abnormalities (see Diagnosis) have asymptomatic neurosyphilis. Adults with symptomatic infection are divided into meningovascular and parenchymal neurosyphilis. The signs of meningovascular involvement represent the sequelae of an inflammatory endarteritis in the meninges, brain, and spinal cord causing hemiplegia, hemiparesis, aphasia, or seizures. The manifestations of parenchymal involvement are due to degeneration of nerve cells in the cerebral cortex causing general paresis or tabes dorsalis.

The pathogenesis of this stage of infection is beyond the scope of this chapter, but may be due to an exaggerated, delayed immune response to treponemal antigens rather than viable *T pallidum*. Several detailed reviews discuss the pathophysiology of the late complications of syphilis.[16-18]

EFFECT OF PREGNANCY ON SYPHILIS

Pregnancy probably has minimal effect on the natural history of syphilis. The immunosuppression of pregnancy that prevents the fetal allograft from being rejected is often cited in explaining decreases in cellular and humoral immunity in gravidas. Studies in the preantibiotic era observed less severe clinical manifestations of primary and secondary syphilis[19] and amelioration of the signs of neurosyphilis in pregnancy.[20] In the rabbit model, experimental syphilis is less evident in pregnant animals.[21] Recent investigators have not noted any differences in the spectrum or severity of clinical infection. In a small group of young women with latent syphilis, CSF antitreponemal antibody was detected in 19%[22], comparable to the incidence in adults with early syphilis.

The symptoms of early pregnancy may mimic the signs of secondary syphilis. Patchy alopecia may be erroneously attributed to pregnancy. Dermatologic manifestations of disseminated infection are sometimes misdiagnosed as pregnancy-induced palmar erythema, pruritus gravidarum, or livedo reticularis. Secondary syphilis may be diagnosed more commonly in gravidas due to prior, unrecognized cervical chancres. Cervical chancres are seen more commonly in pregnancy, presumably after inoculation of a hyperemic, friable, everted cervix, typically seen antepartum.[10]

The effect of pregnancy on maternal serologic tests for syphilis is unclear. Pregnancy is commonly listed as an etiology for false-positive serologies, but recent reports have not shown increased rates of such results in gravidas.[23,24] Anecdotal experience indicates that nontreponemal antibody titers may not drop as quickly in pregnancy after treatment. This makes it difficult to apply serologic criteria that indicate an adequate response to treatment to gravidas (see Treatment).

Despite some difficulties in diagnosing the clinical signs of syphilis in gravidas, pregnancy offers an opportunity to screen and treat a large group of sexually active, young women for syphilis. Although some areas of the United States do not have a high incidence of early syphilis, serologic testing for syphilis is cost-effective. In a cost–benefit analysis, first trimester serologic screening was cost-effective when the incidence of infectious syphilis was greater than five cases 100,000 gravidas.[25] Pregnancy is not known to alter the efficacy of therapy in treating maternal infection.[26-28] This is true despite increases in weight, blood volume, and glomerular filtration rate, which may alter antimicrobial levels in pregnancy.

EFFECT OF SYPHILIS ON PREGNANCY AND THE FETUS

Early syphilis profoundly can affect pregnancy outcome, causing preterm delivery, congenital syphilis, fetal demise, or neonatal death. Fetal risks for infection are directly proportional to the degree of maternal spirochetemia and duration of untreated maternal infection. Thus, the highest rates of congenital syphilis occur in women with secondary syphilis or latent syphilis with recently resolved signs of secondary syphilis. Fifty percent of the infants born to women with untreated primary or secondary syphilis will have congenital infection at birth.[29] The remainder will be inoculated at delivery and develop neonatal infection in several months. The maternal infectivity is less with latency. Forty percent of neonates born to women with early latent infection will have congenital syphilis, and 6–14% of infants will be affected with maternal late latent syphilis.[29] Infants with clinically evident congenital infection are more common with maternal infection that develops in first, second, and early third trimester. Asymptomatic infected infants are common with antepartum infection in the last weeks of pregnancy.

Although it is known that *T pallidum* can be found in fetal tissue at any stage of gestation[30], little is known about the pathophysiology of fetoplacental infection. Much of the current hypotheses about the natural history of fetal infection is inferred from indirect evidence. Recent studies have shown that *T pallidum* is able to traverse intact endothelial intercellular junctions *in vitro*.[31] This is a more plausible route to the placenta and fetus than after infarction and necrosis mediated by endarteritis in the placenta. Equally untenable is the role of the Langhans' layer in preventing transplacental passage of treponemes.[32] The fetal immune response to syphilis is understood poorly. Immature fetuses less than 18 weeks' gestation rarely have histologic evidence of syphilitic infection[32], presumably due to a relative immunoincompetence in the fetus until this time.[33] This may explain the nearly universal success of maternal therapy to prevent congenital syphilis when treatment occurs prior to 18 weeks.

Congenital syphilitic infants are usually of low birth weight, mostly due to preterm delivery[34,35] rather than growth retardation.[36] The mechanism for preterm labor in this *in utero* infection is unknown, but is currently being investigated. Severe fetoplacental infection can lead to fetal death, but the pathophysiology of this process is unknown.[37] Indirect evidence of fetal stress is present in the cord blood of syphilitic infants when the endocrine function of the fetoplacental unit is examined.[38] In most reports of congenital syphilis, 20–50% of infants are stillborn.[29,39] With the current association between crack cocaine drug abuse and syphilis[3], it will be important to determine the individual contribution and interaction between these factors in future fetal demises. At present, there is no information about the role of maternal HIV coinfection and risks of fetal infection with either pathogen.

Concurrent with fetal syphilis, placental infection occurs. The gross appearance is a thickened, heavy, pale, sometimes hydropic placenta. In stillborn infants with congenital syphilis, the umbilical cord also may exhibit severe involvement with a characteristic "barber pole" gross appearance and microscopic necrotizing funisitis.[40] Histologically, the placenta often does not have abnormalities unless the fetus is symptomatic or stillborn or unless the placenta is visibly abnormal. The typical histologic signs are a focal proliferative villitis, varying stages of endarteritis obliterans, and immature villi.[41] Spirochetes may be demonstrated by silver staining techniques[42], but may not be identified as frequently as in the fetus.

Although the precise mechanism of fetal infection is still unclear, the pathology of fetal infection is well described. Fetal infection is analogous to adult secondary syphilis, but there is an absence of genital lesions. Congenital syphilis is a truly disseminated infection, and histologic signs can be found in virtually every organ system.[37] The spirochete maybe detected by silver staining in many tissues. Small vessel vasculitis, lymphocytic and plasma cellular infiltrates, focal ischemia, necrosis, and fibrosis are seen.[43]

DIAGNOSIS

The absolute diagnosis of syphilis can be accomplished only by demonstration of *T pallidum* from material from a suspected host. Since *T pallidum* cannot be cultivated *in vitro,* the microbiologic diagnosis can be made by the previously mentioned rabbit infectivity test. Darkfield microscopy is widely available in hospital laboratories and sexually transmitted disease clinics, but the accuracy of this technique is dependent on a properly-obtained specimen and an experienced microscopist. Clinical material from moist genital lesions or regional lymph node aspirates is suitable, unless there is superinfection, prior antimicrobial treatment, or near healing. Special staining with silver impregnation techniques[42] or direct fluorescent antibody stains[44] on tissue can reveal treponemes and support histologic changes of syphilis.

Serologic tests for antibody production associated with syphilis allow the clinician to make a presumptive diagnosis of infection and define the latent stage.[6,45] There are two broad types of serologic tests for syphilis. The first is *nonspecific* or *nontreponemal* and measures antibodies to a mixture of lipids, including cardiolipin, presumed to be from tissue damage in the host. The rapid plasma reagin (RPR) and Venereal Disease Research Laboratory (VDRL) tests are commonly used nontreponemal tests that are utilized to screen and follow response to therapy. These tests are reported in titers that generally reflect the activity of infection, allowing serial testing to show declining titers after treatment. Pretreatment titers are consequently higher with secondary, primary, and latent syphilis, respectively. HIV coinfected adults may show extremely high titers or paradoxically seronegative titers with secondary syphilis.[46] RPR titers are generally higher than VDRL titers, creating potential confusion in interpretation of serial values if all are not of the same type of test. The second type of test detects antibody specifically directed against *T pallidum* and is called *treponemal* test. Commonly used tests are the microhemagglutination assay for antibodies to *T pallidum* (MHA-TP) or the fluorescent treponemal antibody-absorption (FTA-ABS) test. These tests are not given titers, but reported as positive or negative. They confirm true-positive nontreponemal tests, for nontreponemal antibody can be produced by nonsyphilitic states. False-positive testing (positive nontreponemal test but negative treponemal test) should rule out the diagnosis of syphilis. Treponemal tests remain reactive for life, excluding their use to assess response to therapy or reinfection. This permanent seropositivity proscribes their use in differentiating current from past infection.

The limitations of serologic testing for maternal syphilis mainly involve the nontreponemal tests. Nontreponemal antibody may not be detected in up to 20% of adults with chancres in the first week of primary syphilis.[6] Seronegative secondary syphilis has also been described in immunocompromised HIV coinfected adults.[46] Darkfield microscopy or biopsy of clinical lesions can make the diagnosis in either of these settings. In secondary syphilis, the nontreponemal tests are reactive in over 98% of patients, and as change to "j," the prozone phenomena (antibody excess leading to a false-negative test) are uncommon.[6] Transient false-positive tests occur in about 1% of patients tested and generally have low titers.[23] They are due to laboratory error, febrile infections, immunizations, and, doubtfully, pregnancy. Chronic (≥6 months) false-positive serologies can be due to autoimmune disease or drug abuse.

The examination of the CSF to diagnose *neurosyphilis* is plagued by the lack of a single diagnostic standard.[12,18,47] After a lumbar puncture, the CSF VDRL (not RPR) cell count and differential and protein should be performed. The CSF VDRL has a specificity of nearly 100% and is virtually diagnostic of neurosyphilis.[14] However, it is of variable sensitivity and should not be used to exclude neurosyphilis. The CSF FTA-ABS can be utilized in the latter setting due to its lower specificity and high sensitivity; thus, it has a low positive predictive valve and high negative predictive value for neurosyphilis.[14] The CSF protein is less useful than the CSF leukocyte count, which is usually elevated (>5 WBC/mm^3) in neurosyphilis. Serial CSF leukocyte counts have been advocated as a means to assess the response to treatment in neurosyphilis.[14]

Unfortunately, 40% of adults with untreated primary

TABLE 79–1. INDICATIONS FOR LUMBAR PUNCTURE IN LATENT SYPHILIS OF UNCERTAIN OR MORE THAN ONE YEAR'S DURATION

Neurologic signs or symptoms
Treatment failure
Serum RPR or VDRL titer of ≥1:32
Other evidence of active late syphilis:
Aortitis
Gumma
Iritis
Nonpenicillin treatment planned
Positive HIV antibody test

and secondary syphilis have evidence of CNS invasion by *T pallidum*.[17] The ultimate significance of this is uncertain, for most immunocompetent adults using currently recommended treatment guidelines do not develop neurosyphilis.[15,46] The Centers for Disease Control (CDC) does not recommend lumbar punctures for any adult with early syphilis, unless neurosyphilis is suspected by the presence of optic, auditory, cranial nerve, or meningeal symptoms or signs.[14] Ideally, all adults with latent syphilis of unknown or more than one year's duration should have pretreatment lumbar punctures, but the decision can be individualized. A CSF examination is indicated with late latent syphilis in certain settings (Table 79–1), but likely to be of limited value in older asymptomatic adults.[14]

Similar to problems with the diagnosis of neurosyphilis, there is no single standard for the diagnosis of *congenital syphilis*. In both cases, symptomatic infection does not present a diagnostic dilemma, but asymptomatic infection is difficult to detect. Several sets of clinical criteria have been used by clinicians to define congenital syphilis.[48–50] In general, they all use a combination of maternal and neonatal syphilis serology, neonatal examination, neonatal laboratory and radiologic evaluation, and neonatal lumbar puncture in determining the certainty of congenital infection. The current standard for diagnosis, outlined by the CDC in 1988, allows the rapid evaluation, treatment, reporting and follow-up of infants born to women with syphilis.[51] Cases are usually classified into practical categories based on the strength of evidence to support the diagnosis of congenital syphilis and to ensure that no infant at risk misses appropriate evaluation and treatment. The older terms of definite, probable, possible, and unlikely congenital syphilis have been combined into confirmed, compatible and unlikely categories.

Although congenital syphilis is divided into early (<1 year) and late (≥1 year) phases based on the age of the child at diagnosis, most attention is directed to detection and treatment in the immediate neonatal period before discharge from the hospital.[51] Unfortunately, most infected newborns have minimal or no clinical findings of congenital syphilis, but develop them in the first months of life. Those that are clinically affected exhibit a myriad of systemic signs of disseminated syphilis from their transplacental acquisition of infection. The clinical presentation of neonatal infection is distinct from that of older infants (Table 79–2).[48] Hepatosplenomegaly and skeletal involvement are nearly universal in both groups, but jaundice is more common in neonates, and skeletal symptoms, rash, anemia, and snuffles are more common in the older infant. Nonimmune hydrops, ascites, lymphadenopathy, pneumonitis, myocarditis, nephrosis, and pseudoparalysis can also be seen.[43]

TABLE 79–2. CLINICAL FEATURES OF EARLY CONGENITAL SYPHILIS

Feature	Age <4 Weeks (%)	Age >4 Weeks (%)
Hepatosplenomegaly	91	87
Joint swellings	3	34
Skin rash	31	55
Anemia	64	89
Jaundice	49	7
Snuffles	12	50
Metaphyseal dystrophy	95	91
Periostitis	34	80
Cerebrospinal fluid changes	44	37

Adapted from Hira SK, Bhat GJ, Patel JB, et al.[48]

Infants at risk for congenital syphilis are those born to women with syphilis in whom treatment was absent, recent (within a month of delivery), ineffective (nonpenicillin), a failure, uncertain, or undocumented. These infants should have a careful examination for signs of congenital syphilis, including an RPR or VDRL; a lumbar puncture for CSF VDRL, cell count, and protein; a long bone radiologic survey; and a hemotocrit, platelet count, and liver function tests.[14,51] A lumbar puncture is essential in the work-up, for 40% of infants have CSF abnormalities, including some that are otherwise asymptomatic.[35] If the lumbar puncture is unavailable, impractical, or unsuccessful, neurosyphilis cannot be excluded, and appropriate treatment should be instituted (Table 79–3).[14]

The cord blood or neonatal RPR or VDRL serology is difficult to evaluate due to transplacental transfer of maternal IgG antibody.[50] IgM antibody does not cross the placenta, so elevated levels in the neonate should reflect fetal production due to infection. Total IgM levels may be elevated from various nonsyphilitic etiologies, but specific antitreponemal IgM reflects fetal antibody production and correlates with congenital syphilis.[52–54] Unfortunately, such tests generally are not available yet in clinical laboratories. Several tests have been developed against major treponemal surface immunogens[55,56] and using a modified 19S-IgM FTA-ABS test.[54] These tests may be valuable in the future if they can accurately diagnose and exclude asymptomatic congenital infection. Currently, the initial serology is of value if it is fourfold higher or greater than the maternal titer, indicating a significant fetal IgG production, and as a baseline to follow after treatment.[51] A nonreactive RPR or VDRL from a neonate at risk does not exclude infection or the need to treat the infant for possible incubating syphilis.

Stillborn infants born to women with reactive serologies should undergo a thorough evaluation to determine the cause of death, including congenital syphilis. Postmortem

TABLE 79–3. RECOMMENDATIONS FOR TREATMENT OF SYMPTOMATIC OR ASYMPTOMATIC INFANTS

Aqueous crystalline penicillin G, 50,000 units/kg IM or IV daily, in two divided doses for at least 10 days

or

Aqueous procaine penicillin G, 50,000 units/kg IM daily, for at least 10 days gross and histologic examinations of the fetus[37] and placenta[41] often reveal signs suggestive of syphilis, unless there is autolysis from a long-standing demise. Silver or immunofluorescent staining techniques may detect spirochetes in fetal or placental tissue.[42,44] In the investigation of fetal death prior to labor in a gravida with syphilis, an amniocentesis may be indicated. Darkfield microscopic examination of amniotic fluid is often positive when the cause of fetal death is congenital syphilis.[57] Long bone survey by conventional radiography[58,59] or xeroradiography[60] can demonstrate osteochondritis and metaphyseal dystrophy, even in markedly macerated stillborns.

TREATMENT

Penicillin is the treatment of choice for adults and neonates with any stage of syphilis. *T pallidum* is extremely sensitive to penicillin at low concentrations (0.03 μg/mL) and has not developed resistance to penicillin[61], despite its capability to accept plasmid DNA.[62] Successful therapy of early syphilis is more dependent on consistent maintenance of treponemicidal penicillin levels for at least seven days than on the level of penicillin achievable by higher doses of penicillin.[63] Such levels are reached for three to four weeks in adults given 2.4 million units of benzathine penicillin intramuscularly. Increasing penicillin dosage beyond 0.6 mg/kg given every nine hours in humans[64], or increasing the level of penicillin above 0.1 μg/mL *in vitro*[65], does not improve the rate of elimination of *T pallidum* from lesions or immobilization of virulent treponemes, respectively. Thus, improvement in the efficacy of early syphilis therapy is, in immunocompetent women, likely to come from achieving prolonged, consistent, treponemicidal penicillin levels by increasing the duration of treatment rather than the dosage of penicillin.

The current CDC recommendations for treatment of syphilis were updated in 1989 (Table 79–4).[14] Controversy continues about the need for lumbar puncture prior to therapy and effective regimens in HIV coinfected individuals.[14,46] The recommendations should be viewed as minimum treatment guidelines that can be altered according to the individual patient. This is particularly true in the gravida who is coinfected with HIV and the gravida whose fetus is severely infected and hydropic *in utero*. There is little clinical experience in either of these settings to guide appropriate management. Close follow-up is essential in either case after treatment. In the case of severe fetal infection, the outcome may be preterm labor or a demise[66], so consideration should be given to delivery and neonatal treatment if pulmonary maturity is assured.

TABLE 79–4. RECOMMENDATIONS FOR TREATMENT OF SYPHILIS DURING PREGNANCY

Early Syphilis[a]
- Benzathine penicillin G 2.4 million units IM as a single injection

Syphilis of More Than 1 Year's Duration[b]
- Benzathine pencillin G 2.4 million units IM weekly for 3 doses

Neurosyphilis
- Aqueous crystalline penicillin G 2–4 million units IV every 4 hours for at least 10 days, followed by benzathine penicillin G 2.4 million units IM weekly for 3 doses
- Aqueous procaine penicillin G 2.4 million units IM daily, plus probenecid 500 mg orally 4 times daily, both for 10 days, followed by benzathine penicillin G 2.4 million units IM weekly for 3 doses

[a] Primary, secondary, and latent syphilis less than 1 year's duration.
[b] Latent syphilis of unknown or more than 1 year's duration, cardiovascular, or late benign syphilis.

TABLE 79–5. RECOMMENDATIONS FOR TREATMENT OF EARLY SYPHILIS IN PENICILLIN-ALLERGIC PATIENTS

Confirm Penicillin Allergy

Document penicillin, allergy history (pruritus, urticaria, dyspnea, bronchospasm, anaphylaxis)

Skin testing: major and minor determinant antigens

Recommended Regimen

Offer desensitization followed by appropriate penicillin dosage for stage of syphilis

Alternative Regimen

Erythromycin, 500 mg 4 times daily orally for 14 days

Tetracycline, 500 mg 4 times daily orally for 14 days

Doxycycline 100 mg 2 times daily orally for 14 days

Ceftriaxone 250 mg IM daily for 10 days or 500 mg IM every other day for 5 doses[a]

Nonpenicillin therapy for disease of greater than one year's duration *not* recommended

Asymptomatic infants born to women treated with nonpenicillin regimens should be treated with benzathine penicillin G, 50,000 units/kg intramuscularly in a single dose.

[a] Not tested in pregnancy.

The efficacy of the currently-recommended penicillin regimen for adult or antepartum early syphilis is 98%; most failures are really reinfections.[26,28,67] From 1983 to 1985, however, 19% of the congenital syphilis cases reported to the CDC were treatment failures.[4] The success of nonpenicillin regimens are lower[26,28] and probably unacceptable for use in pregnancy.[14] Documentation of penicillin allergy by history and skin testing is recommended to detect patients at risk for IgE antiody-mediated reactions, which can be life threatening.

The penicillin-allergic patient presents problems from a diagnostic and therapeutic approach (Table 79–5). She needs skin testing to the minor and major determinant antigens of penicillin.[68,69] If any are reactive, she is at risk for an IgE-mediated reaction that may be severe, if administered a therapeutic course of penicillin. The available regimens of erythromycin, tetracycline, or doxycycline for adults have not been tested in large studies in pregnancy.[27,28,70] Erythromycin is difficult to tolerate, crosses the placenta poorly[71,72], and is associated with treatment failures.[34,53,73-75] Tetracyclines can cause maternal liver dysfunction[76] and have untoward fetal effects.[77,78] These regimens require two weeks of compliance, which is difficult with the gastrointestinal upset common in early pregnancy. If nonpenicillin regimens are used, the neonate should be closely examined for congenital infection and treated prophylactically for asymptomatic infection.[14]

Penicillin desensitization followed by penicillin treatment is the best option for the penicillin-allergic gravida.[14] It can be accomplished during a short hospitalization by the oral[79] or parenteral route.[80] An oral regimen of gradually increasing doses of phenoxymethyl penicillin suspension over nearly four hours is widely used and results in a temporary tolerance to penicillin (Table 79–6).[79] This allows the

TABLE 79–6. ORAL PENICILLIN DESENSITIZATION PROTOCOL

Dose[a]	Phenoxymethyl Penicillin Suspension[b]	Cumulative Units	Cumulative Dose
1	1000 u/mL	100	100
2	"	200	300
3	"	400	700
4	"	800	1500
5	"	1600	3100
6	"	3200	6300
7	"	6400	12,700
8	10,000 u/mL	12,000	24,700
9	"	24,000	48,700
10	"	48,000	96,700
11	80,000 u/mL	80,000	176,700
12	"	160,000	336,700
13	"	320,000	656,700
14	"	640,000	1,296,700

Observe for 30 minutes prior to administration of penicillin

[a] Interval between doses—15 minutes.
[b] Phenoxymethyl penicillin suspension (penicillin V potassium) 250 mg/5 mL equals 80,000 units/mL.

administration of a therapeutic dose of parenteral penicillin, intravenously or intramuscularly. If multiple doses of benzathine penicillin are needed over several weeks, the procedure need not be repeated if the doses are administered weekly.[79]

Little is known about the efficacy of other drugs in the treatment of syphilis in pregnancy.[27,28,70] Various cephalosporins have efficacy in treating early syphilis in adults, but they may result in significant allergic reactions in penicillin-allergic women.[81] Limited experience indicates that ceftriaxone, 250 mg daily for 10 days, or 500 mg every other day for 5 doses, is effective in treating early syphilis.[82] Ceftriaxone given 2 g intravenously does cross the placenta, resulting in levels in the fetus and placenta that are treponemicidal for at least 12 hours.[83,84] However, there is no clinical or pharmacokinetic experience with lower dosages to safely predict efficacy in maternal-fetal infection.

PREGNANCY

In pregnancy, CDC guidelines should be followed in a setting of accessible prenatal care, with serologic screening at the first prenatal visit, at 28–32 weeks' gestation in high-risk groups, and at delivery.[51] Puerperal detection of maternal antibody is preferred over umbilical cord blood testing to improve the sensitivity of screening by detecting seronegative but exposed infants delivered by seropositive mothers with recent infection. Treatment prior to 20 weeks' gestation rarely results in failure to prevent congenital syphilis, barring maternal reinfection. No regimen will prevent or treat all cases of fetal syphilis, but treatment in pregnancy prevents congenital syphilis in 98% of gravidas.[26-28] Women with a history of recently resolved secondary syphilis or current secondary syphilis of over two weeks' duration may have well established fetal infection. Sonography is recommended to detect hydramnios, a thickened placenta, hepatomegaly, or ascites that might indicate severe fetal infection. Maternal treatment in this setting may precipitate preterm labor, fetal distress, or a demise.[66] The severely infected fetus may not be adequately treated by maternal therapy, so consideration should be given to an amniocentesis. Darkfield microscopy of the amniotic fluid can be performed and pulmonary maturity assessed. If pulmonary maturity is present, prompt delivery and neonatal treatment is a reasonable plan.

The Jarisch–Herxheimer reaction is common after the treatment of early syphilis and will complicate the treatment of most gravidas.[85] It is a systemic reaction of uncertain etiology that follows penicillin treatment of active syphilis, presumably related to the beginning of the killing of large numbers of spirochetes. It is not mediated by endotoxin, but probably through interleukins and prostaglandins.[86,87] Signs include fever, tachycardia, mild hypotension, vasodilation, malaise, headaches, and erythematous, painful lesions. It occurs several hours after treatment, is usually of little consequence in adults, and abates by 24 hours. In pregnant women, it may incite transient uterine contractions, premature labor, fetal tachycardia, decreased fetal movement, and late fetal heart rate decelerations.[66] As the changes may indicate a change in fetal status, women should report any decrease in fetal movement, increase in uterine activity, or fever in the first 24 hours after syphilis treatment.

Antipyretics may be administered with intravenous fluid and oxygen for preterm contractions and transient changes in fetal status. If preterm labor ensues soon after treatment, it is usually due to a severely syphilitic infant.[66] Tocolysis should be considered with this in mind, for it is usually unsuccessful in this setting. The value of prophylactic antipyretic, antiprostaglandin, or corticosteroid administration to gravidas to prevent the Jarisch–Herxheimer reaction and its possible sequelae warrants investigation.

After treatment, *epidemiologic investigation and contact tracing* should be performed. All adults with genital ulcer disease, including syphilis, should be offered counseling and testing for HIV antibody.[14] Routine visits for prenatal care are recommended with repeat titers of nontreponemal tests monthly until delivery.[51] Postpartum follow up should include serologies to meet the recommended 3-, 6-, and 12-month quantitative serologies for women with treated early syphilis. Those with latent infection of over one year's duration should have an additional serology at 24 months. HIV coinfected adults need serologies at 1, 2, and 3 months posttreatment and then every 3 months until a serologic response is noted.[14,46]

The expected serologic response in adults is a fourfold (2 tube dilution) decrease in the quantitative nontreponemal titer.[14] This occurs by three months for primary and secondary syphilis[88] and by six months for early latent infection.[89] Late latent stage titers are generally lower and tend to fall slowly. In patients with persistent high titers or a sustained increase in titer of fourfold or greater, treatment failure or reinfection is likely. Such women need a thorough physical examination and lumbar puncture for CSF examination. Unless reinfection is detected, retreatment, directed by the CSF findings, is indicated for late latent syphilis or neurosyphilis (see Table 79–4).[14]

The serologic response after treatment in pregnancy has not been studied. Anecdotally, clinicians have noted a slower decline in the quantitative RPR or VDRL titer in pregnancy than in adults. Often, delivery interrupts the follow up prior to an adequate time to document a serologic response. Regardless, the nonpregnant adult serologic response should be sought in gravidas, with the knowledge that more frequent retreatment may occur. It is important to use consistently the same nontreponemal test serially in pregnancy and in the neonate, if possible, to allow valid comparisons of antibody titers.

Women with persistently positive nontreponemal tests despite adequate prior treatment have serofast serologies. These are generally of low titer, but must be followed closely. The differentiation between a serofast syphilis serology and a reinfection in the early latent stage can tragically occur at the delivery of an unexpectedly infected infant. Consequently, it is prudent to consider gravidas with poor follow up after prior treatment to be infectious. An arbitrary VDRL titer of 1 in 4 or greater in any woman treated at least one year prior is an indication for antepartum therapy in one institution.[70]

HUMAN IMMUNODEFICIENCY VIRUS COINFECTION

Recent reports of adults with early syphilis who are HIV coinfected have questioned the effect of concurrent HIV infection on the natural course of syphilis.[47,90,91] HIV-infected individuals may present with unusual manifestations of syphilitic infection, sometimes with laboratory evidence of central nervous system involvement. Others have reported treatment failures or relapses in HIV coinfected adults with subsequent progression to neurosyphilis.[47,92] These reports suggest that the impaired cellular and hormonal immune response in HIV-infected adults may alter the presentation of syphilis and its response to therapy.[11,47,93] Seronegative secondary syphilis (biopsy confirmed) has also been reported.[94]

Currently, the CDC recommends no changes in the treatment of primary, secondary, or early latent syphilis in HIV-infected adults[14], but stresses the need for closer follow up in this group.[46] The CDC advises a CSF analysis prior to treatment of all HIV coinfected adults with latent syphilis of unknown or more than one year's duration. Benzathine penicillin G for treatment of asymptomatic neurosyphilis in HIV-infected adults should be avoided; parenteral aqueous penicillin G for at least 10 days is recommended (see Table 79–4).[46]

It is not known if the pregnant patient with HIV coinfection is at increased risk for treatment failure of maternal or fetal infection using currently recommended treatment guidelines.[14,46] Maternal therapy should be guided by the above-mentioned guidelines. Investigation of the influence of maternal HIV coinfection on the natural history of fetal and neonatal syphilis and on the efficacy of antepartum therapy to prevent congenital syphilis is anticipated. Given the principles of syphilotherapy[61], it is likely that longer therapy (that is, 2–3 weeks) for early syphilis with benzathine penicillin G may be a reasonable but untested guideline in this setting.

REFERENCES

1. Centers for Disease Control. Syphilis and congenital syphilis—United States, 1985–1988. *MMWR*. 1988;37:486.
2. Centers for Disease Control. Increases in primary and secondary syphilis, United States. *MMWR*. 1987;36:393.
3. Centers for Disease Control. Relationship of syphilis to drug use and prostitution—Connecticut and Philadelphia, Pennsylvania. *MMWR*. 1988;37:755.
4. Centers for Disease Control. Congenital syphilis, United States, 1983–1985. *MMWR*. 1986;35:625.
5. Musher DM. Biology of *Treponema pallidum*. In: Holmes KK, Mardh PA, Sparling PF, et al, eds. *Sexually Transmitted Diseases*. 2nd ed. New York, NY: McGraw-Hill; 1989:203.
6. Larsen SA, Hunter EF, McGrew BE. Syphilis. In: Wentworth BB, Judson FN, eds. *Laboratory Methods for the Diagnosis of Sexually Transmitted Diseases*. Washington, DC: American Public Health Association; 1984:1.
7. Norgard MV, Chamberlain NR, Swancutt MA, et al. Cloning and expression of the major 47-kilodalton surface immunogen of *Treponema pallidum* in *Escherichia coli*. *Infect Immun*. 1986;54:500.
8. Schell RF. Rabbit and hamster models of treponemal infection. In: Schell RF, Musher DM, eds. *Pathogenesis and Immunology of Treponemal Infection*. New York, NY: Marcel Dekker; 1983:121.
9. Schroeter AL, Turner RH, Lucas JB, Brown WJ. Therapy for incubating syphilis: effectiveness of gonorrhea treatment. *JAMA*. 1971;218:711.
10. Wendel GD. Syphilitic cervical chancres: an underdiagnosed entity. *Infectious Disease Society for Obstetrics and Gynecology*. 1987. Abstract.
11. Musher DM. How much penicillin cures early syphilis? *Ann Intern Med*. 1988;109:849. Editorial.
12. Weisel J, Rose DN, Silver AL, et al. Lumbar puncture in asymptomatic late syphilis. An analysis of the benefits and risks. *Arch Intern Med*. 1985;145:465.
13. Clark EG, Danbolt N. The Oslo study of the natural course of untreated syphilis: an epidemiologic based on re-study of the Boeck-Bruussgaard material. *Med Clin North Am*. 1964;48:613.
14. Centers for Disease Control. 1989 sexually transmitted disease treatment guidelines. *MMWR*. 1989;38(S-8):5.
15. Musher DM. Syphilis. *Infect Dis Clin*. 1987;1:83.
16. Kampmeier RH. Late benign syphilis. In: Holmes KK, Mardh PA, Sparling PF, et al, eds. *Sexually Transmitted Diseases*. 2nd ed. New York, NY: McGraw-Hill; 1989:251.
17. Healy BP. Cardiovascular syphilis. In: Holmes KK, Mardh PA, Sparling PF, et al, eds. *Sexually Transmitted Diseases*. 2nd ed. New York, NY: McGraw-Hill; 1984:247.
18. Swartz MN. Neurosyphilis. In: Holmes KK, Mardh PA, Sparling PF, et al, eds. *Sexually Transmitted Diseases*. 2nd ed. New York, NY: McGraw-Hill; 1984:231.
19. Moore JE. Studies on the influence of pregnancy. I. The course of syphilitic infection in pregnant women. *Johns Hopkins Med Bull*. 1923;34:89.
20. Moore JE. Studies in asymptomatic neurosyphilis. III. The apparent influence of pregnancy on the incidence of neurosyphilis in women. *Arch Int Med*. 1922;30:548.
21. Brown WH, Pearce L. On the reaction of pregnant and lactating females to inoculation with *Treponema pallidum*—a preliminary note. *Am J Syph*. 1920;4:593.
22. Jones JE, Harris RE. Diagnostic evaluation of syphilis during pregnancy. *Obstet Gynecol*. 1979;54:611.
23. Moore JE, Mohr CF. Biologically false positive serologic tests for syphilis. *JAMA*. 1952;150:467.
24. Manikowska-Lesinska W, Linda B, Zajac W. Specificity of the FTA-ABS and TPHA tests during pregnancy. *Br J Vener Dis*. 1978;54:295.
25. Stray-Pedersen B. Economic evaluation of maternal screening to prevent congenital syphilis. *Sex Transm Dis*. 1983;10:167.
26. Jackson FR, Vanderstoep EM, Knox JM, et al. Use of aqueous benzathine penicillin G in the treatment of syphilis in pregnant women. *Am J Obstet Gynecol*. 1962;83:1389.
27. Thompson SE. Treatment of syphilis in pregnancy. *J Amer Vener Dis Assoc*. 1976;3:159.
28. Brown S. Update on recommendations for the treatment of syphilis. *Rev Infect Dis*. 1982;4:837S.
29. Fiumara NJ, Fleming WL, Downing JG, et al. The incidence of prenatal syphilis at the Boston City Hospital. *New Engl J Med*. 1952;247:48.
30. Harter CA, Benirschke K. Fetal syphilis in the first trimester. *Am J Obstet Gynecol*. 1976;124:705.
31. Thomas DD, Navab J, Haake DA, et al. *Treponema pallidum* invades intercellular junctions of endothelial cell monolayers. *Proc Natl Acad Sci*. 1988;85:3608.
32. Dippel AL. The relationship of congenital syphilis to abortion and miscarriage, and the mechanism of intrauterine protection. *Am J Obstet Gynecol*. 1944;47:369.
33. Silverstein AM. Congenital syphilis and the timing of immunogenesis in the human fetus. *Nature*. 1962;194:196.
34. Mascola L, Pelosi R, Blount JH, et al. Congenital syphilis: why is it still occurring? *JAMA*. 1984;252:1719.
35. Mascola L, Pelosi R, Blount JH, et al. Congenital syphilis revisited. *Am J Dis Child*. 1985;139:575.
36. Naeye RL. Fetal growth with congenital syphilis. *Am J Clin Pathol*. 1971;55:228.
37. Oppenheimer EH, Hardy JB. Congenital syphilis in the newborn infant: clinical and pathological observations in recent cases. *Hopkins Med J*. 1971;129:63.
38. Parker CR, Wendel GD. The effects of syphilis on endocrine function of the fetoplacental unit. *Am J Obstet Gynecol*. 1988;159:1327.
39. Ingraham NR. The value of penicillin alone in the prevention and treatment of congenital syphilis. *Acta Derm Venereol*. 1951;31(S24):60.

40. Fojaco RM, Hensley GT, Moskowitz L. Congenital syphilis and necrotizing funisitis. *JAMA.* 1989;261:1788.
41. Russell P, Altshuler G. Placental abnormalities of congenital syphilis. *Am J Dis Child.* 1974;128:160.
42. Dorman HG, Sahyun PF. Identification and significance of spirochetes in the placenta. *Am J Obstet Gynecol.* 1937;33:954.
43. Schulz KF, Murphy FK, Patamasucon P, Meheus AZ. Congenital syphilis. In: Holmes KK, Mardh PA, Sparling PF, et al, eds. *Sexually Transmitted Diseases.* 2nd ed. New York, NY: McGraw-Hill; 1989:821.
44. Epstein H, King CR. Diagnosis of congenital syphilis by immunofluorescence following fetal death in utero. *Am J Obstet Gynecol.* 1985;152:689.
45. Hart G. Syphilis tests in diagnostic and therapeutic decision making. *Ann Intern Med.* 1986;104:368.
46. Centers for Disease Control. Recommendations for diagnosing and treating syphilis in HIV-infected patients. *MMWR.* 1988;37:600.
47. Lukehart SA, Hook EW, Baker-Zander SA, et al. Invasion of the central nervous system by *Treponema pallidum:* implications for diagnosis and treatment. Ann Intern Med. 1988;109:855.
48. Hira SK, Bhat GJ, Patel JB, et al. Early congenital syphilis: clinico-radiologic features in 202 patients. *Sex Transm Dis.* 1985;12:177.
49. Kaufman RE, Jones OG, Blount JH, et al. Questionnaire survey of reported early congenital syphilis: problems in diagnosis, prevention, and treatment. *Sex Transm Dis.* 1977;4:135.
50. Srinivasan G, Ramamurthy RS, Bharathi A, et al. Congenital syphilis: a diagnostic and therapeutic dilemma. *Ped Infect Dis.* 1983;2:436.
51. Centers for Disease Control. Guidelines for the prevention and control of congenital syphilis. *MMWR.* 1988;37(S-1):1.
52. Alford CA, Polt SS, Cassady JV, et al. Gamma M-fluorescent treponemal antibody in the diagnosis of congenital syphilis. *N Engl J Med.* 1969;280:1086.
53. Mamunes P, Cave UG, Budell JW, et al. Early diagnosis of neonatal syphilis: evaluation of a gamma M-fluorescent treponemal antibody test. *Am J Dis Child.* 1970;120:17.
54. Muller F. Specific immunoglobulin M and G antibodies in the rapid diagnosis of human treponemal infection. *Diagn Immunol.* 1986;4:1.
55. Norgard MV, Sanchez PJ, McCracken GH, et al. Molecular analysis of the fetal IgM response to *Treponema pallidum* antigens: implications for improved serodiagnosis of congenital syphilis. *J Infect Dis.* 1989;159:508.
56. Dobson SRM, Taber LH, Baughn RE. Recognition of *Treponema pallidum* antigens in IgM and IgG antibodies in congenitally infected newborns and their mothers. *J Infect Dis.* 1988;157:903.
57. Wendel GD, Maberry MC, Christmas JT, et al. Examination of amniotic fluid in diagnosing congenital syphilis with fetal death. *Obstet Gynecol.* In press.
58. Cremin BJ, Fisher RM. The lesions of congenital syphilis. *Br J Radiol.* 1970;43:333.
59. Cremin BJ, Draper R. The value of radiography in perinatal deaths. *Pediatr Radiol.* 1981;11:143.
60. Cox SM, Wendel GD. Xeroradiography and skeletal survey in the diagnosis of congenital syphilis following fetal death. *Society of Perinatal Obstetricians.* February, 1987. Abstract.
61. Rein MF. General principles of syphilotherapy. In: Holmes KK, Mardh PA, Sparling PF, et al, eds. *Sexually Transmitted Diseases.* New York, NY: McGraw-Hill; 1984:374.
62. Norgard MV, Miller JN. Plasmid DNA in *Treponema pallidum* (Nichols): potential for antibiotic resistance by syphilis bacteria. *Science.* 1981;213:553.
63. Idsoe O, Guthe T, Wilcox RR. Penicillin in the treatment of syphilis. The experience of three decades. *Bull WHO.* 1972;47(suppl):6.
64. Tucker HA, Robinson DCV. Disappearance time of *Treponema pallidum* from lesions of early syphilis following administration of crystalline penicillin G. *Bull Johns Hopkins.* 1947;80:169.
65. Nell EE. Comparative sensitivity of treponemes of syphilis, yaws and bejel to penicillin in vitro, with observations on factors affecting its treponemicidal action. *Am J Syph Gonor Vener Dis.* 1954;38:92.
66. Klein VR, Cox SM, Mitchell MD, Wendel GD. The Jarisch-Herxheimer reaction complicating syphilotherapy in pregnancy. *Obstet Gynecol.* 1990; 75:375.
67. Schroeter AL, Lucas JB, Price EV, et al. Treatment for early syphilis and reactivity of serologic tests. *JAMA.* 1972;221:471.
68. Sullivan TJ, Wedner HJ, Shatz GS, et al. Skin testing to detect penicillin allergy. *J Allergy Clin Immunol.* 1981;68:171.
69. Solley GO, Gleich GJ, VanDellen RG. Penicillin allergy. Clinical experience with a battery of skin test reagents. *J Allergy Clin Immunol.* 1982;69:238.
70. Wendel GD. Gestational and congenital syphilis. *Clin Perinatol.* 1988;15:287.
71. Kiefer L, Rubin A, McCoy JB, et al. The placental transfer of erythromycin. *Am J Obstet Gynecol.* 1955;69:174.
72. Philipson A, Sabath LD, Charles D. Transplacental passage of erythromycin and clindamycin. *N Engl J Med.* 1973;288:1219.
73. Fenton LJ, Irwin JL. Congenital syphilis after maternal treatment with erythromycin. *Obstet Gynecol.* 1976;47:492.
74. Hashisaki P, Wertzberger GG, Conrad CR, et al. Erythromycin failure in the treatment of syphilis in a pregnant woman. *Sex Trans Dis.* 1983;10:36.
75. South MA, Knox JM, Short DH. Failure of erythromycin estolate therapy in *in utero* syphilis. *JAMA.* 1964;190:182.
76. Whalley PJ, Adams RH, Combes B. Tetracycline toxicity in pregnancy. *JAMA.* 1984;189:357.
77. Cohlan SQ, Bevelander G, Tiamsic T. Growth inhibition of prematures receiving tetracycline. *Am J Dis Child.* 1963;105:453.
78. Genot MT, Golan HP, Porter PJ, et al. Effect of administration of tetracycline in pregnancy on the primary dentition of the offspring. *J Oral Med.* 1970;25:75.
79. Wendel GD, Stark BJ, Jamison RB, et al. Penicillin allergy and desensitization in serious maternal/fetal infections. *N Engl J Med.* 1985;312:1229.
80. Ziaya PR, Hankins GD, Gilstrap LC, et al. Intravenous penicillin desensitization and treatment during pregnancy. *JAMA.* 1986;256:2561.
81. Sullivan TJ. Pathogenesis and management of allergic reactions to penicillin and other beta-lactam antibiotics. *Pediatr Infect Dis.* 1982;1:344.
82. Hook EW, Roddy RE, Handsfield HH. Ceftriaxone therapy for incubating and early syphilis. *J Infect Dis.* 1988;158:881.
83. Kafetzis DA, Brater DC, Fanourgakis JE, et al. Ceftriaxone distribution between maternal blood and fetal blood and tissues at parturition and between blood and milk postpartum. *Antimicrob Agents Chemother.* 1983;23:870.
84. Johnson RC, Bey RF, Wolgamot SJ. Comparison of the activities of ceftriaxone and penicillin G against experimentally induced syphilis in rabbits. *Antimicrob Agents Chemother.* 1982;21:984.
85. Brown ST. Adverse reactions in syphilis therapy. *J Am Vener Dis Assoc.* 1976;3:172.
86. Young EJ, Weingerten NM, Baugh BE, et al. Studies on the pathogenesis of the Jarisch-Herxheimer reaction. *J Infect Dis.* 1982;146:606.
87. Shenep JL, Feldman S, Thornton D. Evaluation of endotoxemia in patients receiving penicillin therapy for secondary syphilis. *JAMA.* 1986;256:388.
88. Brown ST, Zaidi A, Larsen SA, et al. Serological response to syphilis treatment. *JAMA.* 1985;253:1296.
89. Fiumara NJ. Treatment of early latent syphilis of less than one year's duration. *Sex Transm Dis.* 1978;5:85.
90. Johns DR, Tierney M, Felsenstein D. Alteration in the natural history of neurosyphilis by concurrent infection with the human immunodeficiency virus. *N Engl J Med.* 1987;316:1569.
91. Radolf JD, Kaplan RP. Unusual manifestations of secondary syphilis and abnormal humoral immune response to *Treponema pallidum* antigens in a homosexual man with asymptomatic human immunodeficiency virus infection. *J Am Acad Dermatol.* 1988;18:423.
92. Berry CD, Hooton TM, Collier AC, et al. Neurologic relapse after benzathine penicillin therapy for secondary syphilis in a patient with HIV infection. *N Engl J Med.* 1987;316:1587.
93. Tramont EC. Treatment of syphilis in the AIDS era. *N Engl J Med.* 1988;316:1600.
94. Hicks CB, Benson PM, Lupton GP, et al. Seronegative secondary syphilis in a patient infected with the human immunodeficiency virus (HIV) with Kaposi sarcoma. *Ann Int Med.* 1987;107:492.

Chapter Eighty

Nonvenereal Treponematoses: Yaws, Pinta, and Endemic Syphilis

Joseph M. Miller, Jr. and Joseph G. Pastorek II

80

Pinta, yaws, and endemic syphilis constitute the nonvenereal treponematoses. These diseases are produced by morphologically indistinguishable treponemes and are found almost exclusively in underdeveloped populations of the tropical and semi-arid areas of the world. These illnesses are contact diseases that cause formation of indistinguishable antibodies. Yaws is caused by *Treponema pertenue*, pinta by *T carateum*, (sometimes also designated *T herrejani*), and endemic syphilis by *T pallidum*, (sometimes also designated *T endemicum*). Transmission is by skin or mucous membrane contact, generally occurring before adolescence. The causative treponemes differ only in the clinical response (serologic responses are identical), and not surprisingly, some degree of cross immunity develops.[1] It is unclear if the differences between the nonvenereal treponematoses and venereal syphilis are related to host and environmental factors or to as yet unidentified biologic differences.

While venereal syphilis is not unique to a particular social class or geographic area, the nonvenereal treponematoses are usually diseases of the underprivileged. Yaws is common in the tropical zones and endemic syphilis is common in the adjacent dry regions. Pinta occurs primarily among Indians in the central and the northern parts of South America.

Yaws and endemic syphilis are usually childhood diseases. Poor hygiene, close crowding, frequent skin trauma, and lack of protective clothing facilitate transmission of yaws by skin-to-skin contact, or perhaps by passive transfer of treponemes by insects. Endemic syphilis is transmitted through contaminated fomites, such as shared eating and drinking utensils. Pinta, a more benign disease, occurs only in the Western Hemisphere. The onset is typically later in life, usually between the ages of 10 and 20. It is also nonvenerally transmitted by skin-to-skin contact.[2]

The nonvenereal treponemes can be likened to syphilis, with its primary, secondary,and tertiary stages. After the treponemes invade the skin, the organisms proliferate. Spread may occur through the lymphatic and vascular systems during the incubation period. Spirochetes can be identified in the early lesions of these diseases, and serologic tests for syphilis all ultimately become positive.[3]

YAWS

The primary lesion is termed the *mother yaw*. Histologically, it is a papillary, inflammatory granuloma with hypertrophy and thickening of the epidermis. Chronic granulation tissue is present in the dermal and subcutaneous layers. Hyperkeratosis develops. In the nonulcerated phase, there is a mononuclear infiltrate accompanied by endothelial cell hypertrophy and proliferation. The lesions of secondary yaws are quite similar. Tertiary lesions involve gummata formation with necrosis and osteoperiostitis. Widespread involvement is common. Visceral, ocular, and neurologic involvement, although uncommon, may also occur.

This chronic childhood disease has many names, including framboesia, pian, and bouba. As with syphilis, a primary lesion appears at the site of initial invasion three to four weeks following introduction of the organism. The red-brown papule enlarges and becomes papillomatous. The surface sloughs and becomes secondarily infected. Spirochetes are present in the inflammatory focus. Regional lymphadenopathy occurs.

Two or three months later, generalized skin lesions mark the beginning of the secondary stage. The lesions vary from scaly macules to papules quite similar to the mother yaw. Less commonly, the secondary lesions involve the mucous membranes as a papillomatous condyloma, resembling the condyloma latum of syphilis.

Other manifestations of early yaws include nocturnal bone pain and polydactylitis due to periostitis. Infectious cutaneous relapses may occur at any time during the five years following inoculation.

Tertiary lesions usually appear five or more years after infection and involve gummas of the skin and bones, particularly of the legs. Other findings include hyperkeratoses of the soles and palms, osteitis, periostitis, juxta-articular nodes, and hydrarthrosis. Late lesions are extensive. Destruction of the nose, maxilla, palate, and pharynx, termed *gangosa*, or *rhinopharyngitis mutilans*, occurs. Hypertrophic osteoperiostitis of the nasal process of the maxilla gives rise to the distinctive facial appearance called *goundou*. Rarely, late disease has also been associated with aortic aneurysm or aortic valvular disease, myocardial lesions, and central nervous system abnormalities. One fourth of patients have cerebral spinal fluid abnormalities.[4]

The diagnosis is often evident upon examination. The age of the patient and endemic foci of prevalence aid the diagnosis. *T pertenue* can be identified by darkfield examination of scrapings of early cutaneous lesions, but should not be confused with other spirochetes found in tropical ulcers. Serologic tests for syphilis, including the rapid plasma reagin (RPR) and fluorescent treponemal antibody absorption (FTA-ABS), are positive.

PINTA

Pinta is an infectious disease of the skin caused by *T carateum*. There are three cutaneous stages marked by changes in skin color. Other organ systems are not involved. Disfigurement is the major disability.

The initial lesion is characterized by epidermal thickening and hyperkeratosis. There is a diffuse, scattered, mononuclear infiltrate, and the numbers of malanophores increase in the dermal connective tissues. Pigmentation increases in the basal cells of the stratum germinativum.

Treponemes are present. As the lesions age, vascularity diminishes and fibrous scarring occurs.

The secondary lesions are histologically similar. While a clear demarcation between secondary and tertiary pinta does not exist, the inflammatory components gradually subside, and pigmentation is lost. However, depigmented areas may be adjacent to hyperpigmented ones. Palmar and plantar hyperkeratosis may be present.

The primary papular lesion develops 2–3 weeks after inoculation. It enlarges and becomes irregular in shape, with a serpiginous, hyperpigmented border. Regional lymphadenopathy occurs.

A secondary eruption unassociated with lymphadenopathy appears 1–12 months later. The secondary lesions are termed *pintids* and vary greatly in color, from rose to brown-black. Color is lost as the lesions age.

White achromic lesions represent the late stage. *T carateum* can be found in the transudates from the initial, early, secondary, or dyschromic lesions. Serologic tests for syphilis are positive, but convert more slowly than in venereal syphilis.

ENDEMIC SYPHILIS

A primary lesion probably does not form in endemic syphilis. The earliest findings are highly infectious mucus patches of the oral cavity. Generalized infection occurs during the secondary stage, where multiple lesions develop in the mouth and on the lips, genitalia, and anal region. These lesions vary in type, but tend to be papular, squamous, annular, and erosive. Late lesions include cutaneous and osteoarticular gummata. Synonyms include *bejel, dichuchwa, njovera* and *balash.*

The first indication of the disease is usually a mucous patch in the mouth resembling condyloma latum. Treponemes are present in the early lesions, as well as in aspirates of regional lymph nodes. Serologic tests for syphilis are usually positive early in the disease.

Early lesions generally heal in about 12–18 months. After a variable latent period, late lesions appear, similar to those of late benign syphilis, including skin rashes, leaving discoloration, patchy loss of hair, bony osteoperiostitis, and periarticular nodules. Destructive gummata occur in the palate, nasal septum, and nasal bones, producing mutilation. Gummata occur on the nipple of mothers who have previously had endemic syphilis and who are breast-feeding infants with oral lesions. Over the last 30 years, endemic syphilis seems to have become clinically attenuated, with the majority of people having only latent disease.

PREGNANCY AND THE TREPONEMATOSES

Pregnancy neither improves nor worsens the nonvenereal treponematoses. Because of routine screening for syphilis, there is an increased likelihood of diagnosis while the patient is pregnant.

Transplacental passage of nonvenereal treponemes is strongly suspected. Certainly, confusion surrounding the diagnosis may exist as venereal syphilis may be acquired by a patient subsequent to yaws, endemic syphilis, or pinta. Nevertheless, congenital yaws very likely occurs, although less frequently than congenital syphilis. Fetal mortality appears to be only one fifth that of congenital syphilis. Positive cord blood serologies from newborns of mothers with active lesions of endemic syphilis have been reported, although IgM-specific studies were not performed.[5]

Diagnosis

Diagnosis of the nonvenereal treponematoses is not difficult because cases usually occur only in certain geographic locations. With yaws and endemic syphilis, clinical suspicions can easily be confirmed by demonstrating treponemes by darkfield examination. Serologic tests for syphilis, including the RPR and FTA-ABS, convert during the early stages of these three nonvenereal treponemal diseases.

In patients with early yaws or endemic syphilis, lesions caused by bromides or iodides should be considered. *Goundou* may be confused with acromegaly, syphilitic osteitis, and leontiasis ossea. *Gangosa* must be distinguished from syphilis, leprosy, and leishmaniasis. Juxta-articular nodules may require biopsy to distinguish between rheumatic, syphilitic, and onchocercal disease. The skin lesions of pinta are characteristic, but psoriasis, eczematous dermatitis, and leukodermia from other causes should be considered.

In Great Britain, the distinction between latent yaws and latent syphilis among immigrants from areas where yaws is endemic may be difficult. Often, histories may be nonspecific and serologic tests for syphilis may be positive. X-rays may reveal periostitis and serologic evaluation may reveal low titers, which are more common in yaws. The presence of aortitis or central nervous system involvement usually indicates syphilis. In many cases, an accurate distinction cannot be made.

Treatment

Intramuscular penicillin is the drug of choice for these treponematoses. Procaine penicillin with aluminum monostearate (PAM) or benzathine penicillin G (bicillin) have been used extensively. For yaws, 1.2 million units for adults and older children, or 600,000 units PAM for smaller children, is adequate. Pinta requires 1.2 million units of bicillin in adults and 300,000 to 600,000 units for children. Endemic syphilis is treated with 1.2 million units of bicillin with smaller doses for infants. The dose may be doubled if bony lesions are present. Contacts without overt signs of disease should receive preventive or "abortive" treatment with PAM whenever treponemal diseases constitute a public health threat.[6,7]

For patients who are allergic to penicillin, erythromycin or tetracycline (in children over eight years of age) are adequate drugs. Either may be given to older children or adults in doses of 500 mg by mouth four times a day for 15 days. A Jarisch–Herxheimer reaction may develop in response to effective treatment.

Pregnant patients with a positive serologic test for syphilis, even with documented treatment of a nonvenereal treponemal disease, should be treated with 600,000 units of procaine penicillin intramuscularly, daily for 10 days. Pregnant patients allergic to penicillin should receive 500 mg erythromycin four times daily for 15 days. At birth, the infant should then be treated with aqueous penicillin G, 500 units per kg parenterally, in two divided doses each day, or procaine penicillin G, 50,000 units per kg intramuscularly, daily for 10 days. Tetracycline should be avoided because bone growth may be impaired and deciduous teeth may be stained.

REFERENCES

1. Willcox RR. Changing pattern of treponemal disease. *Brit J Vener Dis.* 1974;50:169.
2. Cutler JC. Endemic syphilis, yaws and pinta. In: Johnson RC, ed. *The Biology of Parasitic Spirochetes.* New York, NY: Academic Press; 1976:365.
3. Taber LH, Feigin RE. Spirochetal infections. *Ped Clin NA.* 1979;26:392.
4. Roman GC, Roman LN. Occurrence of congenital, cardiovascular, visceral neurologic and neuro-opthalmologic complications of late yaws: a theme for future research. *Rev Infect Dis.* 1986;8:760.
5. Perine PL. Syphilis and endemic treponematosis. In: Strickland GE, ed. *Hunters Tropical Medicine.* 6th ed. Philadelphia, PA: WB Saunders; 1984:247.
6. Hopkins DR. Control of yaws and other endemic treponematoses; implementation of vertical and/or integrated programs. *Rev Infect Dis.* 1985;7:S339.
7. Willcox RR. Mass treatment campaigns against endemic treponematosis. *Rev Infect Dis.* 1985;7:S278.

Chapter Eighty-One

Leptospirosis

Joseph M. Miller, Jr. and Joseph G. Pastorek II

81

Leptospirosis is an acute febrile infectious disease caused by a single family of organisms of which there are multiple serogroups and serotypes. *Leptospira* contains only one pathogenic species, *Leptospira interrogans.* Nearly 180 serotypes have been arranged in over 20 serogroups. The serogroups *icterohaemorrhagiae, canicola, autumnalis, copenhageni* and *pomona* are the most well-known. Leptospires are slender, round, active, mobile spirochetes between 6 and 20 μm long. In liquid media, one or both ends are usually hooked.

Leptospirosis is a worldwide zoonotic disease with a wide range of animal reservoirs. Some serotypes, such as *icterohaemorrhagiae* and *canicola,* occur throughout the world, while others are more regional. Among mammals, rodents are the most important hosts, though virtually all mammals may be infected and can transmit the disease. In the United States, dogs are a prominent source of human infection. Although the leptospires have been assigned a variety of names related to geographic distribution and differ somewhat in their clinical manifestation, they should be considered a single clinical disease.

Transmission of leptospirosis to man follows contact with blood, urine, tissue of infected animals, or exposure to an environment contaminated by leptospires. Abraded skin often serves as the portal of entry. Occupation is a risk factor for infection; risk groups include rice farmers, gardeners, cane cutters, meat and fish processors, and sewage workers. In the United States, an increasing number of cases have resulted from recreational exposure, often from swimming or hunting.[1]

The leptospires probably invade the human through small breaks in the skin or intact mucosa. The initial site of multiplication is undetectable, and a local lesion does not develop. Leptospiremia occurs rapidly after inoculation. Organisms spread throughout the body to produce the protean manifestations of this disease. Pathogenicity may in part be the result of an enzyme or toxin elaborated by or released from lysed leptospires. Endotoxins have yet to be demonstrated convincingly.

A prominent feature of leptospirosis is the hemorrhagic diathesis. While serum prothrombin and platelet counts may be reduced, this is not a constant feature of the disease. The diathesis is thought to be the result of widespread capillary endothelial damage. Among patients most severely affected, hepatic, renal, and central nervous system involvement is common. Hemorrhage and bile staining are evident. Massive bleeding may also occur into the lungs and, on occasion, the adrenal medulla. Petechial hemorrhages are often found beneath the renal capsule, and the kidneys are swollen with a congested medulla. Skeletal muscle may also exhibit such petechial hemorrhage.

When striated muscle damage occurs, it is most evident in the soleus. Histologic changes consist of loss of striation with subsequent vacuolization and disintegration of the sarcoplasm. Leptospiral antigen demonstrated by fluorescent antibody staining is present. The damaged sarcoplasm is absorbed and the sarcolemma proliferates. Inflammation or fibrosis is limited. Similar changes in cardiac muscle have been described. A fibrinous pericarditis has also been described.

The major renal lesion is an interstitial nephritis associated with mesangial hyperplasia, glomerular swelling, and fusion of the foot processes of glomerular podocytes. Renal tubular involvment varies from dilatation of the distal convoluted tubules to degeneration, necrosis, and rupture of the basement membrane. Widespread edema and a mononuclear white cell infiltrate are evident in the interstitium. Numerous leptospira have been identified in the tubular lumen. Urinary excretion of leptospires is common for up to two months in humans.

Widespread hepatocytic intracellular and extracellular edema is evident. A mononuclear leukocytic infiltrate is most evident periportally. Kupffer's cells are often enlarged. Significant destruction does not occur, and bile duct proliferation or stasis is absent. Rarely, leptospires can be identified throughout the liver.

Leptospiral meningitis has been observed, but only late in the disease process after antibody has developed.

The severity of leptospirosis varies greatly, determined for the most part by the health of the host and by the infecting strain. Severe icteric disease, with a high fatality rate, is uncommon, but is more often associated with the serogroups *icterohaemorrhagiae* and *copenhageni.* Less severe and anicteric disease occurs far more often and is usually caused by serogroups *australis* and *pyrogenes.* Disease due to serogroups *tanicola, ballum* and *pomona* is usually mild.[2]

The incubation period averages 10 days, ranging from 2 to 21. The clinical illness is biphasic with an abrupt onset. During the leptospiremic phase, leptospires are present in the blood and cerebrospinal fluid. Symptoms include headache and myalgias, particularly in the thighs. Chills, fever, conjunctival suffusion, and gastrointestinal problems also occur. This phase lasts 4–7 days. Symptomatic improvement and defervescence coincide with the disappearance of leptospires from the blood and cerebrospinal fluid, but not the renal parenchyma. Antibody to leptospires, primarily IgM, develops quickly and marks the beginning of the second (immune) stage of this disorder, which lasts from 4–30 days. Leptospiruria is common and is generally not affected by antibiotic treatment. Hepatic or renal manifestations, when present, tend to occur toward the end of the first phase; meningitis begins during the second phase.

Most patients with leptospirosis are anicteric; these individuals may escape definitive diagnosis. Some patients experience only the leptospiremic phase and are asymptomatic after the first week. The principal manifestation of the immune stage is an aseptic meningitis, characterized by cerebrospinal fluid pleocytosis, often in the absence of signs or symptoms of meningeal irritation. Cell counts of the cerebrospinal fluid vary from normal up to 100 cells per cubic millimeter. Polymorphonuclear leukocytes predominate early, but mononuclear cells are noted later in the immune phase. Glucose concentrations are usually normal. Protein may reach 3000 mg per dL, even in the absence of pleocytosis.

Less common features of the immune stage include encephalitis, myelitis, and peripheral neuropathy. Iritis, iridocyclitis, and chorioretinitis may also be noted.

The most severe form of leptospirosis, often called Weil's disease, is characterized by jaundice and is usually accompanied by azotemia, hemorrhage, anemia, vascular collapse, and severe alterations in consciousness. Mortality rates, despite adequate care, are between 5 and 15%, predominantly in patients with hepatic and renal failure and generally from the latter. The distinctive features appear at the end of the leptospiremic stage and progress to the immune stage. Either renal or hepatic dysfunction may predominate. Hepatic manifestations include hepatomegaly and right upper quadrant tenderness. Transaminase values are minimally elevated. Hyperbilirubinemia, primarily direct, is observed, with maximal values of 80 mg/dL reported, resulting from the inability to excrete bilirubin after conjugation.

The most common renal abnormality is proteinuria, which is mild. Hyaline or granular casts and red and white cellular elements may be found in the urine. Acute tubular necrosis associated with oliguria may occur as early as the third day of clinical illness. Blood urea nitrogen levels peak on day five to seven and remain below 100 mg/dL. The long-term prognosis of the acute renal lesion is good, with glomerular filtration rates usually returning to normal; some patients exhibit a defect in concentrating ability, however.

Clinical hemorrhage may occur, as evidenced by epistaxis or by bleeding into the adrenal gland, subarachnoid space, lungs, or gastrointestinal tract. Hypoprothrombinemia and thrombocytopenia have been reported, but are not essential to this bleeding diathesis.

Leptospirosis may be found in up to 13% of cases of aseptic meningitis.[3] Numerous clinical manifestations may be present. Rarely, the disease presents as meningoencephalitis.

LEPTOSPIROSIS AND PREGNANCY

Pregnancy is not known to alter the basic disease process. Leptospirosis in the pregnant woman is clinically similar to infection in the nonpregnant patient. Leptospirosis during pregnancy is, however, associated with an increased risk of fetal loss.

Most fetal wastage is probably secondary to the effects of severe maternal disease and not direct fetal involvement. Intrauterine infection may occur, though, as the leptospires do cross the placenta.[4] Involvement of the fetal liver and kidney has been noted. Hepatocellular necrosis with relative sparing of periportal areas and renal tubular destruction have been described.

Diagnosis

The initial presentation of a patient with leptospirosis may bring to mind meningitis, viral hepatitis, nephritis, influenza, and miscellaneous other febrile illnesses. A diagnosis can be made by either culture of *Leptospira* or serologic proof of its presence. Direct demonstration of *Leptospira* by darkfield methods is unreliable because of artifacts and cellular debris. The organism may be isolated from blood or cerebrospinal fluid in the initial phase of the illness, or from urine in the second phase. A semisolid medium, such as Fletcher's medium, should be used. Animal inoculation or the use of a selective inhibitor such as 5-fluorouracil is helpful if the specimen is contaminated.[5]

Antibody appears a week after the onset of the disease and peaks 2–3 weeks later. The standard serologic test is microscopic agglutination, in which a fourfold or greater increase in titer of paired acute and convalescent sera is regarded as diagnostic. Infecting serotypes may be identified. The enzyme-linked immunosorbent assay (ELISA) distinguishes between old and current infection, but does not indicate the serotype. Macroscopic slide agglutination and complement fixation may also be performed.

Therapy

Penicillin, streptomycin, tetracycline, and erythromycin are effective *in vitro* and in experimental leptospiral infections. If initiated within two days of the onset of illness, antibiotic therapy is of benefit; it is of little use after the fourth day. Parenteral penicillin G, 600,000 units every four hours, is the preferred treatment. Tetracycline, 2 g/day in divided doses, or doxycycline, 100 mg orally twice daily for seven days, may be used in nonpregnant patients.[6] A Jarisch–Herxheimer reaction may occur and is regarded as a sign of effective treatment. In pregnancy, tetracycline should be avoided.

Early rest may minimize morbidity. Fluid and electrolyte therapy is important. Patients with acute renal failure may require hemodialysis. Exchange transfusion may be of benefit in patients with extremely high bilirubin levels. Analgesics, antipyretics, antiemetics, and sedatives are often required for symptomatic relief. In the pregnant woman, high fever should be avoided to prevent possible fetal damage and maternal cardiovascular compromise.

REFERENCES

1. Heath CW Jr, Alexander AD, Galton MM. Leptospirosis in the United States. *New Engl J Med*. 1973;273:857, 915.
2. Turner LH. Leptospirosis. *Br Med J*. 1973;1:537.
3. Sanford JP. Leptospirosis—time for a booster. *N Engl J Med*. 1984;310:524.
4. Lindsay S, Luke IW. Fatal leptospirosis (Weils's disease) in a newborn infant. *J Ped*. 1949;34:90.
5. Taber LH, Feigin RD. Spirochetal infections. *Ped Clin NA* 1979;26:400.
6. McClain JB. Doxyclycline therapy for leptospirosis. *Am Int Med*. 1984;100:696.

Chapter Eighty-Two
Relapsing Fever (Borreliosis)

Joseph M. Miller, Jr. and Joseph G. Pastorek II

82

Relapsing fever, an acute febrile infectious disease caused by spirochetes of the genus *Borrelia,* is clinically characterized by recurrent episodes of fever and apyrexia. The disease caused by these spirochetes may be divided into an epidemic form, which is louseborne, and an endemic form, which is tickborne.[1]

Borrelia are helical organisms 3 to 20 μm long and 0.2 to 0.5 μm wide. They have three to 30 uneven coils. Spirals are coarser and closer together than those of treponemes or leptospires. Unlike the other spirochetes, they stain with analine dyes.

Louseborne relapsing fever is caused by *Borrelia recurrentis.* Tickborne disease is caused by numerous strains of *Borrelia* including, in North America, *B. hermsii, B. parkeri,* and *B. turicatae.*

The vectors of tickborne borreliosis are ticks of the genus *Ornithodoros.* This species feeds exclusively on blood, often at night. The bite is painless and the tick usually feeds for less than one hour. When the tick bites a borrelemic host, the infecting *Borrelia* penetrates the tick's coelomic cavity. In subsequent feeding, the coxal or salivary fluid contaminates the bite. *Borrelia* may be passed transovarially to subsequent generation of ticks. Tickborne disease occurs throughout the world. In North America, it is more common in the western states.

The human head louse and body louse, *Pediculus humanus subspecies corporis* and *P humanus subspecies capitis,* are vectors of endemic relapsing fever. Spirochetes ingested during feeding penetrate the louse intestine and multiply in the body. Human infection occurs when the louse is crushed into a cut or abrasion. Animal reservoirs are unknown. The disease is more often seen in the Sudan, Ethiopia, South America, and Southeast Asia. Endemic relapsing fever often follows war or famine, when personal hygiene and general physical health may wane.

After inoculation, the *Borrelia* enters the blood stream and multiplies, producing spirochetemia and fever. There are no symptoms during the incubation period. Thrombocytopenia, which causes petechiae, results from platelet sequestration. With the appearance of antibodies several days later, spirochetemia and fever resolve. Approximately one week later, a new antigenic variant arises from the pool of sequestered *Borrelia.* Spirochetemia and fever recur. The process may be repeated. The symptoms and severity of relapsing fever depend upon the immune status of the host, geographic location, strain of *Borrelia,* and phase of the epidemic. The fatality rate is about 1 in 20, but intercurrent pneumonia or predisposing conditions such as famine may elevate this.

At autopsy, multiple small splenic and hepatic abscesses may be present. Congestion of both organs is common. Evidence of hepatocellular damage is found in most patients. Glomerular, meningeal, and cerebral congestion have also been described. An interstitial nephritis and myocarditis may also develop.

Following an incubation period of 2–18 days, the illness begins suddenly with fever, headache, muscle pain, weakness, and photophobia. Symptoms are usually mild on the first day and then progress in intensity. The initial attack lasts 3–7 days and is longer in louseborne than in tickborne disease. The fever, often as high as 40°C, is usually continuous.

Hepatomegaly, splenomegaly, and jaundice are common, more so in louseborne disease. Liver function tests indicate hepatocellular destruction. Bilirubin levels may be as high as 16 mg/dL and are primarily unconjugated. A consumptive thrombocytopenia, often with counts below 50,000/mm^3, is commonly seen, and both prothrombin and partial thromboplastin times may be prolonged. The white blood cell count is generally normal, but increased bands and decreased eosinophils may be demonstrated. Blood urea nitrogen levels are elevated in jaundiced patients.

A macular rash is more characteristic of the tickborne illness. Bronchitis, pneumonia, meningitis with or without encephalitis, and ocular disease are frequent. Myocarditis is less frequent and more often found in louseborne relapsing fever. Hemorrhagic manifestations include petechiae or purpura.

Spirochetes have been identified in cerebrospinal fluid; protein concentration may be increased and leukocytes may be present. A false-positive serologic test for syphilis may occur. Patients may develop agglutination antibodies to *Proteus* Ox-K antigens, part of the "febrile agglutinins" panel.

The initial attack ends in crisis, coincident with the immune response and lysis of the organisms. As the spirochetes disappear, the patient becomes flushed, diaphoretic, and hypotensive. Cardiovascular collapse occasionally occurs. The temperature then usually returns to normal, and the patient is asymptomatic until the next attack, 5–14 days later. Several relapses are characteristic of tickborne illness, but only one for louseborne illness.

THE EFFECT OF PREGNANCY

Pregnancy has not been associated with specific alterations in the disease process. As well, borreliosis does not uniquely affect the pregnant woman other than the fact that gravidas do not tolerate the hyperdynamic status associated with severe febrile illness as well as nonpregnant women. Relapsing fever may, however, adversely effect the fetus. Abortion is a well recognized complication of borreliosis, probably a result of the maternal hyperpyrexic and systemic illness. Maternal mortality would also be expected to be associated with poor fetal outcome.

Direct congenital infection may occur, since *Borrelia* crosses the placenta. Splenic and central nervous system dysfunction are prominent components of fetal disease. Hepatosplenomegaly, hyperbilirubinemia, and thrombocytopenia may be present in an infected newborn. Cerebrospinal fluid may contain spirochetes. Thickened meninges with a mononuclear cell infiltrate may be present. The enlarged spleen contains yellow miliary lesions of liquefaction.[2]

The diagnosis, if made, is fortuitous and depends upon the finding of *Borrelia* in a blood smear. Because of the rarity of relapsing fever, more common infectious processes, particularly viral, are generally considered first.

Diagnosis

The clinical presentation and demonstration of *Borrelia* in the blood (more likely to be seen early in the course of the illness) allow a definitive diagnosis. This may be accomplished by examining thick or thin blood films stained with Wright's or Giemsa stains. Serologic testing has been employed in endemic areas but is generally not commercially available.

Other acute febrile illnesses, including leptospirosis, typhus, dengue, rat bite fever, or malaria, may be confused with the initial febrile episode of relapsing fever. Viral illness due to adenovirus, influenza, and hepatitis, as well as *Mycoplasma pneumoniae* infections and Rocky Mountain spotted fever, should also be considered. The periodic nature of the fever in this illness clearly separates it from these other entities.[3]

Treatment

Oral or parenteral tetracycline, choramphenicol, and erythromycin are effective in eradicating *Borrelia*. Therapy with the penicillins has a somewhat higher relapse rate. Treatment is accompanied by a Jarisch–Herxheimer reaction resembling the spontaneous resolution of crisis.[4] Therefore, antibiotics should be given between relapses or at the beginning of the febrile episode and the patient followed carefully for the next two days. Attempts to block the severity of this reaction by using anti-inflammatory or antipyretic drugs have not been highly successful.

Tetracycline, the usual drug for treating relapsing fever, should be avoided in pregnancy and in newborns. Chloramphenicol may be used by the gravida not at term. Erythromycin may be used at any time during pregnancy.

While a single oral 500 mg dose of tetracycline will clear the blood of spirochetes, a 5- to 10-day course of 500 mg every 6 h is recommended to prevent relapse. In epidemics, 0.5 or 1.0 g oral chloramphenicol can be used.

REFERENCES

1. Southern PM, Sanford JP. Relapsing fever. A clinical and microbiological review. *Medicine*. 1969;48:129.
2. Fuchs PC, Oyama AA. Neonatal relapsing fever due to transplacental transmission of *Borrelia*. *JAMA*. 1969;208:609.
3. Sherts SR, Brown MS, Bobitt JR. Listerosis and borreliosis as causes of antepartum fever. *Obstet Gynecol*. 1983;62:256.
4. Butler T, Jones PK, Wallace CK. *Borrelia recurrentis* infection: single dose antibiotic regimen and management of the Jarisch-Herxheimer reaction. *J Infect Dis*. 1978;137:573.

Chapter Eighty-Three
Lyme Disease

Ruth E. Tuomala

83

Lyme disease is the most common arthropodborne disease in the United States.[1] Lyme disease, which is also called Lyme borreliosis, is caused by the spirochete *Borrelia burgdorferi*. This spirochete is transmitted by Ixodes ticks of the *Ixodes ricinus* genus. Lyme disease was first reported in 1977 from endemic areas in the northeastern and midwestern sections of the United States and eventually was associated with the tick *Ixodes dammini*. Spirochetal disease with similar presentations associated with other species of ixodes ticks had previously been reported from other continents. Currently, cases of *Lyme borreliosis* have been reported from at least 43 different states, as well as other continents. In addition to *I dammini*, the ticks associated with Lyme disease include *Ioxodes pacificus* in the western States, *I ricinus* in Europe, and *Ioxodes persulcatus* in Asia.

Both the complete life cycle of *I dammini* and infection of these ticks by *B burgdorferi* are dependent upon the proximity of preferred animal hosts. The life cycle of *I dammini* is two years, during which time there are three feeding cycles. In spring and early summer, nymphs feed on white-footed mice. If nymphs are infected with *B burgdorferi*, the spirochetes are injected into the mouse. The spirochetes breed inside of the mouse, which tolerates the presence of these organisms without signs of infection. In late summer, larval forms of the tick feed on the same mice and can in turn become infected with the spirochetes. The larval forms then mold into nymphs. The nymphs subsequently can infect other mice and also eventually become infected adults. The adults require white-tailed deer to complete their life cycle. New areas of endemic Lyme borreliosis are notable for the presence of these animal species and *I dammini*.[2] The vast majority of all cases of Lyme disease occur between May and November, with a primary peak of occurrence in June and July and a secondary peak between September and November. These time periods of disease correspond to the feeding cycles of the ixodes ticks.

Lyme disease is a multisystem illness with protean manifestations.[1,3] Similar to other spirochetal illnesses, there are typical stages of disease. *Early infection* may include both localized disease and also symptoms of disseminated infection. *Late* or *persistent infection* begins a year or more after the time of initial infection. In any stage of disease, multiple organ systems may be involved and any organ system may be involved with varying manifestations at different time periods during the disease. At any stage, symptoms may be intermittent or chronic.

The classical lesion of early Lyme disease is *erythema migrans* (formerly called *erythema chronicum migrans*). This skin lesion is the typical first presentation of disease. At least 80% of patients with Lyme disease present with erythema migrans; however, some patients never show evidence of this earliest stage of infection. Erythema migrans presents as a localized red macule or papule at the site of the tick bite. Within a week to a month (average nine days), the redness gradually expands. Typically, the outer area will be bright red and there will be partial central clearing of the erythema. Although usually single, these skin lesions can sometimes be multiple. Within a highly variable period of time, but average three to four weeks, these lesions fade. While erythema migrans is present, there may also be associated constitutional symptoms with fever, fatigue, myalgias, and regional lymphadenopathy.

Days to weeks after the initial tick bite and often (though not always) after resolution of erythema migrans, symptoms of disseminated infection may become apparent. Skin lesions of disseminated infection can include a malar rash, a secondary presentation of erythema migrans-like lesions, diffuse erythema, and urticaria. Various neurological manifestations may be prominent and may occur either in fleeting attacks or, particularly later on, for longer periods of time. These manifestations may include Bell's palsy, severe headaches, mild meningitis or encephalitis and radiculopathies. Migratory musculoskeletal pains are typical and may occur in areas of muscle, joints, bone, and tendons. Cardiac manifestations may include temporary atrioventricular block and myocarditis or pericarditis. Frequently, in association with other symptoms or by itself, there may be prolonged, severe malaise and fatigue. Less commonly, there may be signs of liver, respiratory, genitourinary, eye, and reticuloendothelial (RES) involvement. Symptoms of disseminated infection may evolve over weeks to months, may be chronic, or may spontaneously resolve. Patients who have intermittent episodes of migratory musculoskeletal pain may later begin to have discrete episodes of asymmetric arthritis, particularly of large joints. The knee is the most frequently involved site. Abnormal synovial fluid will be present and will display a leukocytosis.

Late infection is characterized either by recurrent episodes of discrete disease or chronic symptoms. The frequency of recurrences of symptomatic disease become less with time and, eventually, episodic disease ceases. In a small number of individuals, chronic symptoms or recurrent episodes may result in irreversible tissue damage and lifelong symptomatology. The most frequently described late manifestation of Lyme disease is large joint arthritis, again affecting most commonly the knee. Late neurological symptoms also occur and may include distal paresthesias, radicular pain, central manifestations such as dementia, and a progressive encephalomyelitis. A distinctive skin lesion of late Lyme disease has also been described. *Acrodermatitis chronica atrophicans* is described as a bluish-red discoloration first with swelling, then eventual atrophy. This lesion may last for years.

Lyme disease has been reported in all age groups. Males and females are affected approximately equally. There is no evidence that clinical disease is more severe or associated with any particular manifestations during pregnancy.

It is possible to demonstrate the spirochete, *B burgdorferi*, by stain or culture at various stages of illness. Spirochetes may be present in biopsy specimens taken from erythema migrans lesions. During dissemination of infection, spirochetes may be isolated from the blood stream. In later stage disease, spirochetes may occasionally be found in synovial or cerebral spinal fluid. However, spirochetes are often difficult to isolate by culture and are not always demonstrable by darkfield examination. Therefore, diagnosis of Lyme borreliosis is not ususally made by demonstration of the spirochete. Serologic tests are the most widely available and reliable tests for diagnosis of Lyme disease. Three to six weeks after exposure, antibody to *B burgdorferi* is measurable. Thus, when erythema migrans is first apparent, antibody testing may be negative. In most later stages of disease, antibody is usually present. The Enzyme-Linked Immunosorbent Assay (ELISA) test is currently the most sensitive and specific method of antibody assay. However, standards for interpretation and performance of this test are not uniform. In addition, often antibody testing is performed only in specialized laboratories and results may not be available for weeks. Positive antibody test results must be interpreted according to the presence of suggestive symptoms, and, often, proper management must be initiated based on the clinical diagnosis of symptoms suggestive of Lyme borreliosis.

The sequelae of Lyme disease during pregnancy are largely undefined.[4] Markowitz et al[5] reported five adverse outcomes among 19 pregnancies complicated by maternal Lyme disease. These five adverse outcomes were all different and included an intrauterine fetal demise, a small-for-gestational-age infant who delivered prematurely but subsequently had normal development, an infant with syndactyly, a full-term infant who later developed cortical blindness and developmental delay, and a term infant who developed a rash and hyperbilirubinemia in the neonatal period. None of these adverse outcomes were clearly associated with infection. Spirochetes were not isolated from products of conception, placentas, or any of the infants. In addition, there was no documentation of specific antibody to *B burgdorferi* in any of the infants. In addition, there was no association between occurrence of adverse pregnancy outcome and trimester of pregnancy during which maternal infection occurred or whether or not the pregnant woman received antibiotic therapy. Similarly, Nadal et al[6] reported on pregnancy outcome in 12 women who had possible Lyme disease during pregnancy based on the presence of antibodies. One woman, who also had clinically apparent Lyme disease during pregnancy, gave birth to an infant with a ventricular septal defect. Six other pregnancies resulted in adversely affected infants, including two infants with hyperbilirubinemia, one with muscular hypertonia, one with cardiac arrhythmias, one small-for-gestational-age infant, and one infant with macrocephaly. However, there was again no direct evidence of fetal or neonatal infection by *B burgdorferi*.

There is evidence that *B burgdorferi* can cross the placenta and infect the fetus. Schlesinger et al[7] reported a case of an infant born at 35 weeks' gestation who died at 39 hours of age. The mother had symptomatic Lyme disease in the first trimester of pregnancy, with recurrent arthralgias during the third trimester. Autopsy of the infant revealed complicated congenital cardiac defects and the presence of small numbers of spirochetes in the spleen, renal tubules, and bone marrow. There was no evidence of cardiac inflammation, and spirochetes were not isolated from cardiovascular tissue. Subsequently, MacDonald et al[8] reported the identification of spirochetes in fetal liver, myocardium, adrenal gland, and brain, as well as placenta of a stillborn fetus delivered from a woman who had symptoms of Lyme disease during the first trimester of pregnancy. In addition, a small atrioventricular canal ventricular septal defect was identified at autopsy. In neither of these two cases had the pregnant woman received antibiotic therapy for Lyme disease during pregnancy. In 1988, Weber et al[9] reported the identification of spirochetes from the brain and liver of an infant who died 23 hours after birth. The mother of this infant had erythema migrans diagnosed in the first trimester of pregnancy and had received antimicrobial therapy.

In summary, reported cases of adverse outcome associated with maternal Lyme disease during pregnancy have not consistently revealed a specific syndrome that can be associated with perinatal Lyme disease. The magnitude of any associated risk for adverse outcome of pregnancy is unknown. The *in utero* transmission of spirochetes from infected pregnant women to the fetus appears to have been documented. The magnitude of risk of such transmission is unknown, but probably small. The definition of any specific congenital anomalies caused by *in utero* fetal infection by *B burgdorferi* remains to be seen.

Antibiotic therapy of Lyme disease during its early stages appears to be effective in preventing major manifestations of late disease and ameliorating the presentation of disease at any stage.[10,11] However, minor symptoms of disease may recur or become persistent despite early antibiotic therapy. Joint or neurological involvement of late disease that occurs in patients who have not received prior antibiotic therapy or despite earlier antibiotic therapy may respond only partially or not at all to late-stage antimicrobial therapy. *B burgdorferi* is sensitive *in vitro* to tetracycline, ampicillin, ceftriaxone, and imipenem. It is moderately sensitive to penicillin, and not sensitive to aminoglycosides or rifampin. It is also sensitive to erythromycin. *In vivo* efficacy of tetracycline in preventing late disease manifestations appears to be greater than that of penicillin, and both appear to be more efficacious than erythromycin. Onset of therapy should depend on recognition of clinically obvious disease and should not be delayed by laboratory confirmation. The exact best length of therapy is unknown. Oral tetracycline, penicillin, or amoxycillin are given for 10–30 days depending on response for early Lyme disease. Late-stage disease, in particular neurological involvement, is typically treated with parenteral penicillin or ceftriaxone.

Current recommendations for the treatment of Lyme disease during pregnancy are for aggressive treatment with oral phenoxymethyl penicillin or amoxycillin in early-stage disease with a consideration for parenteral antibiotics in late-disease stages. The efficacy of maternal therapy in preventing intrauterine transmission, adverse pregnancy outcome, or fetal infection is absolutely unknown. Regardless, women who develop Lyme disease during pregnancy should receive antibiotic therapy for the clear-cut benefit of preventing or ameliorating maternal disease and preventing major manifestations of late disease.

REFERENCES

1. Steere AC. Lyme disease. *N Engl J Med*. 1989;321:586.
2. Lastavica CC, Wilson ML, Berardi VP, et al. Rapid emergence of a focal epidemic of Lyme disease in coastal Massachusetts. 1989;320:133.
3. Steere AC, Bartenhagen NH, Craft JE, et al. The early clinical manifestations of Lyme disease. *Ann Intern Med*. 1983;99:76.
4. Centers for Disease Control. Update: Lyme disease and cases occurring during pregnancy. *MMWR*. 1985;35:376,383.
5. Markowitz LE, Steere AC, Benach JL, et al. Lyme disease during pregnancy. *JAMA*. 1986;255:3394.
6. Nadal D, Hunziker UA, Bucher HU, et al. Infants born to mothers with antibodies against *Borrelia burgdorferi* at delivery. *Eur J Pediatr*. 1989;148:426.
7. Schlesinger PA, Duray PH, Burke BA, et al. Maternal-fetal transmission of the Lyme disease spirochete, *Borrelia burgdorferi*. *Ann Intern Med*. 1985;103:67.
8. MacDonald AB, Benach JL, Burgdorfer W. Stillbirth following maternal Lyme disease. *NY State J Med*. 1987;87:615.
9. Weber K, Bratzke HJ, Neubert U, et al. *Borrelia burgdorferi* in a newborn despite oral penicillin for Lyme borreliosis during pregnancy. *Pediatri Infect Dis J*. 1988;7:286.
10. Steere AC, Hutchinson GJ, Rahn DW, et al. Treatment of the early manifestations of Lyme disease. *Ann Intern Med*. 1983;99:22.
11. Duffy J. Lyme disease. *Infect Dis Clin North Am*. 1987;1:511.

G

Infections Caused by Actinomyces, Fungi, Rickettsia, Mycoplasma, and Chlamydia

Chapter Eighty-Four

Infections Caused by Fungi and Actinomyces

Elmer W. Koneman

84

Problems relevant to the diagnosis of fungal infections in pregnancy are exemplified by the following abstracted case study:[1]

> *On a prenatal check up, an obstetrician noticed two small pustules on the face of a 23-year-old black housewife. The diagnosis of impetigo was made and the patient was placed on a 10-day course of ampicillin. No note of the skin lesions was made at the time of the uneventful delivery of a seemingly healthy child. However, three weeks later, the infant died. At necropsy, diffuse pulmonary infiltrates due to* Blastomyces dermatitidis *were found.*
>
> *Two days before the infant's death, the mother again sought medical attention for her skin lesions. The diagnosis of impetigo was reconfirmed. Two weeks later, the lesions showed significant enlargement; specifically, a lesion on the right cheek measured 3 × 6 cm, and one on the forehead measured 3 × 7 cm. A 1 × 1-cm bulbous lesion of the left nostril, a 3 × 3-cm verrucous fungating lesion of the chin, and two 2-cm papular lesions on the right thigh were also present. These lesions were crusty and drained purulent material. Cultures of the facial lesions grew* B dermatitidis; *cultures of the sputum and urine were also positive for* B dermatitidis. *Roentgenograms of the chest revealed no signs of pulmonary blastomycosis.*

I experienced a similar case while in pathology practice in Denver, Colorado, a community not endemic for the agents causing disseminated fungal infections. A forester who had recently moved from Missouri consulted a local physician because of a draining ulcer on the mucosal surface of the lower lip. Culture revealed *Staphylococcus aureus*, and the patient was placed on a course of ampicillin. He had an allergic reaction, which was treated with corticosteroids. Two weeks later, multiple skin lesions clinically highly suggestive of impetigo erupted over the trunk and legs. One week later the patient died. At autopsy, disseminated blastomycosis was found; coincidentally, typical, large, broad-based budding yeast forms were demonstrated in the skin lesions.

Shweni et al[2] report a case of fatal mucormycosis in a 35-year-old diabetic woman that developed following long-term antibiotic and corticosteroid therapy administered for complications of a septic abortion. With candor, the authors concluded, "In general, gynecologists have no experience of mucormycosis . . . the delay in making the diagnosis was due to our ignorance as gynecologists about the condition."

The general uncommonness of deeply invasive and disseminated fungal infections in pregnancy and the rarity with which physicians working in nonendemic areas of the country encounter classic cases of fungal diseases in general lead to these disturbing case reports. The problem is compounded by the myriads of primary and secondary signs and symptoms occurring during pregnancy from much more common conditions that mask the possibility of a fungal infection as a differential diagnosis. However, being aware of a few basic concepts of the biology of fungal agents, their modes of infections, and common clinical manifestations can significantly reduce the frequency with which these unrecognized cases will occur.

THE SCOPE OF FUNGAL INFECTIONS

The general clinical classification of fungal infections as superficial, subcutaneous, and systemic, although simplistic and to some extent outdated, may still serve as a useful guide when considering the subpopulation of women who are pregnant. Of the several hundred fungal species that may be encountered in medical practice, only about two dozen account for greater than 98% of the clinically significant mycoses. These are listed in Table 84–1, which also serves as an outline for the discussion in this chapter.

When addressing the subject of fungal diseases in pregnancy, the basic issues are: (1) fungal infections in pregnancy are different from those in the general population, making recognition and diagnosis more difficult, (2) pregnancy alters the clinical course and prognosis of fungal infections in the mother, and (3) the developing fetus is in danger, either directly from the infective agent or secondarily from the antimicrobial therapy. The greatest concern is with the few mycotic agents that cause systemic and disseminated disease in pregnant women who have no other underlying conditions. Superficial, subcutaneous, and opportunistic fungal infections do not significantly dif-

TABLE 84–1. MOST COMMON FUNGAL AGENTS CAUSING HUMAN MYCOSES

Superficial Fungal Infections
Malassezia furfur (*Pityriasis versicolor*)
Dermatophytosis
Epidermophyton floccosum
Microsoporum canis
Microsporum gypseum
Trichophyton mentagrophytes
Trichophyton rubrum
Trichophyton tonsurans
Subcutaneous Fungal Infections
Sporothrix schenckii
Actinomycotic mycetoma
Actinomyces israelii
Nocardia asteroides
Streptomyces species (rare)
Eumycotic mycetoma
Petriellidium boydii
Exophiala jeanselmei
Opportunistic Fungal Infections
Aspergillosis
Aspergillus fumigatus
Aspergillus flavus
Aspergillus niger
Aspergillus terreus
Zygomycosis
Rhizopus species
Mucor species
Candidiasis
Candida albicans
Non-*albicans Candida* species
Torulopsis (*Candida*) *glabrata*
Cryptococcosis
Cryptococcus neoformans
Dimorphic Pathogenic Fungi
Blastomyces dermatitidis
Histoplasma capsulatum
Coccidioides immitis
Paracoccidioides brasiliensis
Sporothrix schenckii

fer in the infected pregnant and nonpregnant female, and the approaches to diagnosis and management are not substantially different.

Superficial Fungal Infections

The classical taenia or "ringworm" infections of the skin, hair, and nails, caused by three genera of dermatophytes, *Epidermophyton*, *Microsporum*, and *Trichophyton*, and the superficial skin condition, pityriasis versicolor, caused by the common endogenous cutaneous saprophyte, *Malassezia furfur*, present no differently and are no more frequent or severe during pregnancy.[3] The dermatophytoses present as several well-defined clinical syndromes referred to as *tinea capitis* (ringworm of the scalp), *tinea corporis* (smooth skin of the body), *tinea pedis* (feet), *tinea manus* (hands), *tinea cruris* (groin), *tinea unguium*, and *onychomycosis* (nails). Infections may present as transient scaling and itching or may progress to a superficial inflammatory cellulitis or vesicular and pustular eruptions if secondarily infected. The infections tend to recur, particularly during the more humid summer months, and are difficult to completely eradicate. For a detailed review of the various dermatophyte infections, see reference 4.

Pityriasis versicolor is characterized by macular hypopigmentation and fine scaling. The rash may be either asymptomatic or mildly pruritic and is primarily of cosmetic importance. Examination with a Wood's light reveals yellow fluorescence. The disease is most common in the 15- to 30-year-old age range and manifests most frequently in the summer months. Pregnancy may be a predisposing factor.[3]

The clinical diagnosis of a superficial dermatophyte infection is usually confirmed by placing superficial skin scales, plucked hairs (the use of an ultraviolet light Wood's lamp may be helpful in selecting the infected hairs, which often fluoresce), or material scraped from a nail bed in a drop of 10% potassium hydroxide on a glass slide and examining microscopically for the presence of typical hyphae.[5] The hyphae of the dermatophytes are 1–2 μm in diameter and have a tendency to break up into segments, called *arthroconidia*. In addition, spherical spores may be seen in cases of pityriasis, giving a so-called "spaghetti and meatball" effect.

This procedure requires some experience, as background debris and artifacts can make interpretation difficult. Gently heating the slide (short of boiling) and setting aside the mount for 30–60 minutes to allow clearing of background debris can increase the sensitivity of detection. Where a fluorescent microscope is available, the ease and rapidity of detecting fungal elements can be substantially increased by adding a drop of the fluorescent whitener, Calcofluor white (available from most laboratory supply companies), to the potassium hydroxide. The reagent firmly attaches to fungal cell walls and fluoresces brightly when excited with ultraviolet light. If hyphal elements are detected, most cases can be effectively treated locally.

Therapy of Superficial Infections. Mild cases of tinea corporis (and pityriasis) can often be managed by improving hygiene (frequent soapy baths or showers) or by using keratolytic agents such as Whitfield's ointment. The treatment of choice for pityriasis versicolor during pregnancy is selenium sulfide shampoo, used to soap the whole body for 10–15 minutes every other day for two weeks. Although a case of systemic *M furfur* infection has not been reported in pregnancy, positive blood cultures have been obtained from patients receiving hyperalimentation therapy.[6] In more severe cases of tinea pedis, tinea manus, and tinea cruris infections, topical antifungal creams or powders may be applied to the skin lesions. Several drugs are presently available, including tolnaftate (Tinactin), miconazole, clorimazole, bifanazole, naftinfine, ketoconazole, and econazole. Tinea capitis and onychomycosis are best managed by debriding infected hairs or nails.

Barkey[7] cautions against the use of combination corticosteroid and antifungal creams. I would caution that topical steroids may disguise cases of tinea corporis, may interfere with the therapeutic action of the antifungal agent when used in combination, and can result in unsightly striae in prolonged use during pregnancy. Systemic therapy with griseofulvin is not recommended during pregnancy[3], as its safety has not been determined. Various product inserts provided by the manufacturers of griseofulvin indicate that the drug has been found to be embryotoxic and teratogenic in studies performed in pregnant rats. Thus, present counsel advises to treat dermatophyte infections during pregnancy with topical agents and to reserve systemic therapy in severe cases until after delivery if at all possible.

Subcutaneous Fungal Infections

Clinicians must remain aware that deep-seated, disseminated mycoses may initially present as verrucous or pustular lesions of the skin, even in the absence of pulmonary disease. For example, the skin is involved in over 50% of cases of disseminated blastomycosis. The case history presented at the beginning of this chapter is cited as an example of how a systemic fungal disease can be missed if the importance of subcutaneous lesions is ignored. Any persistent subcutaneous lesion, particularly if it ulcerates to the surface and continues to exude serous or purulent material, must be thoroughly investigated for a fungal etiology. Direct potassium hydroxide mounts or smears of infected materials can be made; or, if the diagnosis is not confirmed, biopsies of such lesions may be necessary. Cultures should also always be ordered from any material obtained from these lesions, because organisms may be recovered in cases where fungal forms are not found in direct examination of excretions. We will return to a discussion of the cutaneous and mucous membrane manifestations of systemic mycoses later in this chapter.

Mycetoma. Mycetoma is a localized, indolent, often deforming deep infection of the skin and subcutaneous tissues, frequently of the feet (Madura foot) and hands, often extending into the underlying fascia or bone. The lesions are suppurative abscesses and draining sinuses, often containing soft or hard grains or granules (sulfur granules) within the purulent exudative material. These infections follow the traumatic implantation into the dermis and subcutaneous tissues of soil or vegetative matter that is infected with the spores or other forms of various species of fungi and bacteria. These infections are prevalent in the tropical regions of the world; they are rare in the United States. Pregnancy has no effect on the evolution, clinical manifestations, or prognosis of these disorders.

ACTINOMYCOTIC MYCETOMAS. Mycetomas can be divided into two broad categories, actinomycotic and eumycotic. The actinomycotic mycetomas are caused not by fungi but by filamentous, branching, gram-positive bacteria belonging to the genera *Actinomyces* and *Nocardia*. *Actinomyces israelii*, the species of *Actinomyces* causing most human infections, is a commensal of the human mouth and gastrointestinal tract, and subcutaneous or submucous infections may occur if there is a traumatic break in the squamous epithelium in an area where organisms are present. A common manifestation of actinomycosis is in the deep tissues of the pharynx and neck, causing a clinical syndrome known as "lumpy jaw." Pulmonary infections, caused by inhalation of spores, may lead to pleural infections with the production of suppurating sinus tracts that may extend through the intercostal spaces and penetrate the skin overlying the anterior or posterior thorax.

More than 25 cases of pelvic actinomycosis associated with long-term use of intrauterine contraceptive devices have also been reported.[3] Purulent material can be examined both visually and microscopically for the presence of granules. Microscopically, these granules are composed of tangled, filamentous, branching, gram-positive bacillary forms. *Actinomyces* species are obligate anaerobes; therefore, clinicians must alert microbiologists that actinomycosis is suspected so that appropriate culture medium and incubation conditions can be selected. Penicillin G continued for 2–12 months is the treatment of choice.[8]

The soil saprophytes, *Nocardia asteroides*, *N brasiliensis*, and *N caviae*, are the species most commonly causing nocardiosis in humans. Clinical syndromes include primary subcutaneous, primary pulmonary, and systemic forms. Most cases occur in immunocompromised patients, primarily as subacute or chronic pneumonia often simulating tuberculosis (in fact, *N asteroides* is most commonly recovered in the laboratory on tuberculosis or mycobacteria culture medium from pulmonary secretions submitted for acid-fast culture). Systemic nocardiosis has not been reported as a complication of pregnancy.[8]

Mycetomas caused by *Nocardia* species are relatively rare but clinically show the characteristic tumefaction, suppuration, and sinus formation characteristic of this lesion. Nocardia species generally do not form grains or granules. The bacterial filaments are partially acid-fast (a low concentration organic acid is used for decolorization in the acid-fast stain rather than the conventional more active acid–alcohol) and grow in culture aerobically on most primary isolation culture media. Sulfonamides or trimethoprim-sulfonamide combinations have been used to treat cases of nocardiosis in nonpregnant patients; I have not found a case in a literature search where a pregnant patient has been treated with these agents.

EUMYCOTIC MYCETOMAS. The term eumycotic mycetoma is used to describe classic lesions caused by a variety of true fungi. The etiologic agents include several species of dark or dematiaceous fungi, including pathogenic species belonging to the genera *Phialophora, Cladosporium, Exophiala,* and *Wangiella,* and saprophytic species in the genera *Alternaria, Curvularia,* and *Bipolaris.* Collectively, these mycetomatous infections are known as *phaeohyphomycosis,* to distinguish them from mycetomas caused by the light staining, hyaline group of fungi (hyalinohyphomycosis), of which *Pseudallescheria boydii* (formerly called *Petriellidium boydii* and *Allescheria boydii*) is worthy of mention.[9]

PSEUDALLESCHERIA BOYDII. *P boydii* is listed in the literature as *Monosporium* or *Scedosporium apiosperum,* which is the asexual phase of the organism and is a saprophytic fungus found in soil around the world. Subcutaneous infection is acquired by inoculation of the skin and subcutaneous tissue.[10] A small, painless papule develops into a progressive, granulomatous abscess forming sinus tracts draining pus that contain gray-white or gray-brown grains. Microscopically, these grains are composed of true, septate hyphae with a tendency to form clublike swellings at the periphery. Extracutaneous infections with *P boydii* include pneumonia secondary to inhalation of spores and "fungus ball" infections, both in preexistent cavities in the lungs or in the paranasal sinuses.

Only one infection due to *P boydii* during pregnancy has been reported.[3] This patient had Madura foot and was followed for 14 years; signs of inflammation and drainage frequently increased during menses. However, each of three pregnancies resulted in remissions, and supplemental estrogens appeared to suppress signs of activity. In the listing of several scores of cases of pseudallescheriasis culled from the medical literature, Rippon[4] found no cases occurring in pregnancy. A problem may arise should a rare case be encountered in the future, as most strains of *P boydii* are resistant to amphotericin B. Although miconozole in achievable blood concentrations has been found to inhibit *P boydii,* systemic use of this drug cannot be advocated.

EXOPHIALA JEANSELMEI. *Exophiala jeanselmei* is infrequently encountered and is mentioned here only for completeness. It is an agent of mycetoma and may occasionally be recovered from patients in the United States. It produces a slowly growing, black colony that initially may look like a yeast. In time, the colony will develop into a mold with a delicate, hairlike or suede surface. Microscopically, the hyphae are deep brown and septate and produce long conidiophores from the tips of which clusters of conidia can be seen. The differentiation of these etiologic agents of mycetomas must be left in the hands of competent mycologists. Mycetomas are often refractory to antibiotic therapy, and extensive debridement or amputation may be the only mode of therapy remaining in severe cases.

SPOROTRICHOSIS. The typical history of sporotrichosis of the skin is the appearance of a painless nodular or pustular lesion of the finger or hand (rarely the foot) that has been draining for several days to a few weeks without healing. The patient may remember that she stuck herself at that site with a rose thorn, splinter, or other piece of plant material or decaying vegetation. Careful examination may reveal nodular swellings along the lymphatic channels draining the hand or foot. In more severe cases, secondary ulcerating lesions may be seen along the course of the lymphatics where the organisms have infected underlying lymph nodes. Secondary spread from the subcutaneous tissue to underlying fascia, muscle, joints, and bone may occur. Rarely, systemic infections may occur in immunosuppressed people, and primary pulmonary infection has been reported, presumably from direct inhalation of spores. Farmhands, florists, and gardeners (thus the designation "rose gardener's disease") are the people at risk, although anyone handling packing material made from natural products can become infected.

Catanzaro[11] cites three cases of lymphocutaneous sporotrichosis that occurred during pregnancy. The first case cited was described by Plauche as an infection of the right leg incurred prior to conception and which persisted throughout pregnancy and the postpartum period with no effect on the delivery of a healthy infant. In the second cited case, reported by Romig in 1972, a lesion of the face developed during the first trimester and was successfully treated with local applications of heat. The patient gave birth to a healthy infant.

The third cited case, reported by Vanderveen et al[12], ended in delivery of a stillbirth. A 35-year-old mother was 22 weeks pregnant when lesions of the left wrist, right forearm, and right thigh were culture positive for *Sporothrix schenckii*. The authors felt this represented lesions from multiple inoculation sites rather than an expression of systemic disease. Treatment consisted of local application of heat to the skin lesions, as there was fear of fetal toxicity from amphotericin therapy. The lesions regressed in size and pregnancy progressed normally. However, a macerated fetus was delivered at full term. Tissue sections of fetal and placental tissue failed to reveal organisms; however, cultures at autopsy were not obtained. The authors concluded that placental transfer of the organism was unlikely in their case and that the fetal death was unrelated to the mother's disease, although proof was lacking.

The diagnosis of sporotrichosis rests upon isolation of *S schenckii* from exudates or from biopsy material. It is virtually impossible to demonstrate the organisms in tissue sections of suspected lesions even with special stains. No special culture medium is required for recovery of the organism. *S schenckii* is dimorphic; therefore, it will be recovered as a mold if the cultures are incubated at room temperature or at 30°C, usually within 3 to 5 days. However, the organism can grow on the sheep blood agar plates used routinely for the recovery of bacteria, and we recently had a case where recovery of the yeast form occurred after overnight incubation at 35°C. The laboratory identification is based strictly on recognizing in the mold form the typical daisyhead arrangement of single conidia connected by a thin hairlike attachment (thus, the genus name, *Sporothrix*) or demonstration of the elongated, cigar-shaped yeast cells in cultures incubated at 35°C.

THERAPY. As indicated by these case studies, cutaneous sporotrichosis can be cured by local application of heat. Application of hot packs (heated to greater than 40°C and applied for 30–60 minutes, 4–6 times daily for 6–9 months) and the use of battery-operated "pocket warmers" have been used.[4] Oral administration of a saturated solution of potassium iodide (3–5 drops of a saturated solution in milk, tid, up to 30–40 total drops) has been effective; however, Stamm and Dismukes[3] indicate that the use of SSKI during pregnancy has been associated with congenital hypothyroidism and nontoxic goiter. In nonpregnant patients, amphotericin B and 5-fluorocytosine have been used in the treatment of relapsed lymphocutaneous sporotrichosis and for pulmonary and disseminated disease. Dall and Salzman[13] have successfully used ketoconazole in the treatment of pulmonary sporotrichosis in nonpregnant patients, but use of this drug is currently not recommended in pregnant women. Vanderveen et al[12] report a case of lymphatic cutaneous sporotrichosis successfully treated in the mother with application of local heat, but terminating in a macerated fetus at term. They contemplated using amphotericin B during pregnancy; however, in retrospect, they expressed relief in the fact that drug toxicity was probably not implicated in the death of the fetus. Antibiotics may be necessary in cases where the cutaneous lesions have become secondarily infected with bacteria.

Opportunistic Fungal Infections

It may be somewhat artificial to segregate certain disseminated fungal infections as being opportunistic. However, the implication is that disseminated diseases, such as aspergillosis, zygomycosis (mucormycosis), candidiasis, and cryptococcosis occur only in patients who have preexistent diseases or conditions; that is, those who are immunosuppressed, have been receiving long-term antibiotic or corticosteroid therapy, are receiving chemotherapy, or have any one of a number of chronic, debilitating diseases (diabetes mellitus being prominent among these).[14]

The question also arises as to what effect pregnancy itself may have on host defenses. The following alterations have been found during pregnancy: (1) depression of first set skin graft rejection, (2) reduction in delayed-type hypersensitivity skin test response, (3) inhibition of most lymphocyte responses, including a reduction of migration inhibiting factor (MIF), and (4) decrease in lymphocyte transformation.[11] It is also well recognized that changes in hormonal concentrations during pregnancy predispose patients to candidal vaginitis[15], although the risk of systemic candidiasis is no greater during pregnancy than at other times. The above-cited alterations in host defenses, however, would not appear to be sufficiently profound to consider pregnancy as a predisposing condition for opportunistic fungal infections. However, the basic tenet here is that clinicians must consider the possibility of opportunistic fungal infection in any pregnant woman who also has an underlying predisposing condition. The case of mucormycosis lying predisposing condition. The case of mucormycosis in a pregnant diabetic mother cited at the beginning of this chapter is a classic example.

Aspergillosis. Although aspergillosis is one of the more commonly encountered opportunistic fungal infections in the general population, only one citation of this disease complicating pregnancy through 1983 had been reported, involving a mother with choriocarcinoma.[3] Schwartz et al[16] recently reported a fatal case of disseminated aspergillosis in a neonate. The low incidence of aspergillosis in pregnancy is somewhat surprising given the ubiquitous presence of conidia (spores) in soil, hay, grain, and other vegetative matter. Dissemination of conidia during hay fever season can also be heavy. *Aspergillus fumigatus* is the organism most commonly recovered from patients with systemic aspergillosis. *A flavus* can be associated with systemic disease; however, it is more frequently seen in cases of allergic bronchopulmonary disease. *A niger* is one of the more common causes of otitis externa (swimmer's ear) and has also been recovered from cases of fungal ball infections of the lung and of the paranasal sinuses. One danger of aspergillus infections in immunosuppressed people is the propensity for the organism to invade blood vessels. Thrombosis, infarction, and hematogenous dissemination to the brain, heart, liver, and other viscera are common findings at autopsy in fatal cases.

Zygomycosis (Mucormycosis). The key associations in making the diagnosis of zygomycosis are the sudden onset of facial or orbital edema or cellulitis, acute sinusitis (particularly if a dark brown-black hemorrhagic exudate from the nares is seen), and the presence of ketoacidosis from any cause (diabetes mellitus is the most common predisposing disease, but acidosis from uremia, dehydration, or other conditions may also predispose). If an exudate is seen from the eye or from the nares, it is not sufficient to obtain merely a swab culture. The hyphae of the zygomycetes invade deeply into the tissue; only rarely do they exfoliate into the secretions. I have witnessed cases in which treatment for a bacterial pathogen, such as *S aureus,* was initiated in cases of orbital zygomycosis based on the culture report on swab cultures obtained from conjunctival or nasal exudates. Delay in specific antifungal therapy can be deleterious, as orbital zygomycosis can become rapidly invasive, potentially causing cavernous sinus thrombosis, meningitis, and brain abscess, often with a fatal outcome. The hyphae of the zygomycetes, as with the aspergilli, also have a high propensity to invade blood vessels, causing thrombosis and infarction. This is the reason that debrided tissue from cases of sinusitis appear as if it has been scorched with a blow torch.

Three cases of mucormycosis during pregnancy have been reported, with symptoms and signs appearing in the sixth or seventh month.[3] One patient who presented with epigastric pain, intractable vomiting, and cough for one week was found to have pneumonia and empyema. *Mucor* species was recovered in culture. Glucosuria had been detected on one occasion prior to evaluation. As stated earlier, a second patient[2] ran a fatal course of mucormycosis following spontaneous delivery of a stillborn. The third patient[17] had a 10-year history of diabetes mellitus. Onset of rhino-orbital zygomycosis terminated in bilateral cavernous sinus thrombosis 25 days after the onset of illness.

Stamm and Dismukes[3] also cite two fatal cases of post-abortal zygomycosis in mothers who died within eight days after delivery and two cases in neonates. One baby became fussy on day five and developed fever and abdominal distension. Primary infection of the stomach was seen at autopsy, with extension into the liver, spleen, and pancreas. The second infant presented with vomiting, abdominal distension, and hematochezia on day nine. Perforation of the colon due to invasive zygomycosis was seen at autopsy.

LABORATORY ASPECTS. Several genera of the zygomycetes may be involved in human disease; however, *Rhizopus* species and *Mucor* species are by far the most common isolates. Although there is little difficulty in distinguishing these two genera from cultures (*Rhizopus* species possess rhizoids; *Mucor* species are devoid of rhizoids), there is little clinical reason to make the differentiation. The organisms are ubiquitous in nature, living as saprophytes in decaying vegetation and soil. They most commonly are recognized as dark molds on bread and fruit. The organisms sporulate heavily and can be easily inhaled or ingested. No special culture media are required. The organisms are among the most rapidly growing fungi, filling a culture dish with a gray-white mold within two days (growth is often so exuberant that the term "lid lifter" has been used when the lid of the Petri dish is literally lifted off). Because the hyphae of the zygomycetes are aseptate, care must be taken in processing specimens to ensure that they are not fractured. Specimens should not be ground in a tissue grinder; rather, the tissue should be cut into small pieces with a sterile, sharp scalpel and the bits and fragments buried beneath the agar surface. Even so, mycologists are often disappointed when cultures are negative from tissues received from patients presenting with classical clinical signs and symptoms and when biopsy material clearly shows the presence of ribbonlike, branching aseptate hyphae.

Candidiasis

VAGINAL CANDIDIASIS. *Candida* species are ubiquitous commensal microorganisms located in the oropharynx, gut, vagina, and on the skin. Vaginal cultures are positive in one third of pregnant women, twice the prevalence observed in nonpregnant females.[18] The increased frequency of candidal vaginitis is attributed to the high levels of reproductive hormones that provide a higher glycogen content in the vaginal environment.[15] The glycogen serves as a rich source of carbon to support growth and germination of the yeast forms. *Candida albicans* is the species recovered in about 80–95% of cases[18], presumably because the yeast cells adhere much more avidly to vaginal epithelial cells than other species. Non-*albicans Candida* species are capable of inducing vaginitis, and decisions must be made on an individual case whether definitive species identification is needed. (See also chapter 115.)

Because so many women carry *Candida* species in their vaginal tract, clinicians must decide whether the condition in any given patient warrants treatment, based on evaluation of the history, physical examination, and laboratory data. Before antifungal therapy is considered, a first step in managing clinically significant cases of vaginitis is to have the patient avoid the use of restricting and poorly-ventilated clothing and nylon underclothing. Such undergarments potentially can result in increased local and perineal moisture and temperature, conditions that are optimal for growth of the organism.

Antifungal therapy may be required in more severe cases of vulvovaginal candidiasis. Most commonly, local application of an antifungal agent is prescribed.[19] A variety of preparations are commercially available, most commonly either from the polyene group (candicidin and nystatin) or the imidazole groups (clotrimazole, miconazole, econazole). These preparations are safe to use during pregnancy without concern for systemic effects or fetal toxicity. Ainsworth[20] specifically notes that the use of topical miconazole (Monistat) is not harmful during pregnancy, despite the recommendation that this family of drugs not be used systemically during pregnancy.[21] Lindeque and van-Niekerk[22] report successful treatment of vaginal candidiasis by prescribing single 500 mg chlortrimazole vaginal pessaries.

SYSTEMIC CANDIDIASIS. Despite the increased overall prevalence of vaginal candidiasis, only 17 cases of disseminated infection in pregnant women had been reported through 1983.[3] A computer search of the current medical literature since 1983 reveals no additional reported cases. The risk factors for systemic candidiasis are identical for pregnant and nonpregnant individuals: disruption of mechanical barriers by intravenous therapy, burns, surgery, indwelling urinary catheters, or intrauterine contraceptive devices; alterations of normal bacterial flora by treatment with broad-spectrum antimicrobial agents; administration of glucocorticosteroids, resulting in impaired cell-mediated immunity and hyperglycemia; total parenteral nutrition requiring chronic intravenous catheterization and causing hyperglycemia; intravenous drug abuse; and uremia or advanced malignancy with adverse effects on the immune response. Although patients with acquired immune deficiency syndrome (AIDS) are particularly at risk, especially for mucocutaneous infections, which occur with almost 100% frequency, cases of disseminated candidiasis in pregnancy are rarely reported. Candidemia should be considered in patients who experience fever, chills, and hypotension. Blood cultures should be drawn, in conjunction with fever spikes if possible. The use of a lysis centrifuge system (Isolator System, DuPont Corp., Wilmington, DE) for obtaining blood cultures will increase the yield of positive cultures. Because metastatic disseminated disease may be present, with involvement of other organs, additional cultures of urine, sputum, and other sites where there may be evidence of disease should also be performed. In these cases, definitive identifications are necessary. If all cultures grow the same species, disseminated disease must be strongly considered.

The treatment of systemic candidiasis requires removal of any infected foreign bodies and drainage of abscesses. The chemotherapeutic agent of choice is amphotericin B, in a dose of 0.3–0.5 mg/kg/day. Patients with less serious disease may be effectively treated with doses as low as 20 mg/day continued for only 2–3 weeks. Patients with endocarditis and deeply invasive, suppurative disease may require 4–8 weeks of therapy. This treatment regimen with amphotericin B does not have ill effects on the fetus. Catanzaro[11] does mention, however, that anemia may occur in the course of treatment with amphotericin B and may exacerbate the anemia of pregnancy. Schonbeck and Segerbrand[5] report a case of *C albicans* septicemia occurring in the first half of pregnancy, successfully managed with 5-fluorocytocine. The report of a case of postpartum endophthalmitis by Cantrill et al[23] indicates that patients with fungal diseases during pregnancy must be followed after delivery for possible complications.

CHORIOAMNIONITIS AND NEWBORN CANDIDIASIS. Several cases of candidal chorioamnionitis have recently been reported. Morgan et al[24] present the case of a 23-year-old multiparous white woman who presented with a profuse yellowish-white vaginal discharge at 28.5 weeks' gestation. Pseudohyphae were seen in a Gram's stain of amniotic fluid obtained by amniocentesis. They cite eight additional cases in which the diagnosis of chorioamnionitis was diagnosed predelivery by amniocentesis. In their case, a 1470 g male neonate with Apgar scores of 6 and 7 at one and five minutes was delivered by cesarean section. The placenta showed severe acute chorioamnionitis and umbilical chord vasculitis. Cultures grew *C albicans*. The neonate had a generalized macular rash and a KOH preparation of skin scrapings revealed pseudohyphae. Skin cultures were positive for *C albicans*. The infant was given a 5-day course of amphotericin B. The respiratory distress resolved, and the neonate was discharged in good health.

Bider et al[25] report a case of intrauterine fetal death due to candidal chorioamnionitis. Spaun and Klunder[26] and Smith et al[27] report cases of candidal chorioamnionitis ending in fetal death in patients carrying intrauterine devices (IUDs), with seven additional cases cited from the literature. They theorize that the IUD string serves as a "ladder" for the vaginal *Candida* organisms to reach the placenta and fetus. Invasion from the vagina may also be facilitated by premature rupture of the membranes.[28]

Disease of the umbilical cord is characterized by multiple, barely visible, macular, white-yellow lesions. Superficial penetration of Wharton's jelly occurs with the formation of granulomas and foci of necrosis. Infection in the first trimester may result in spontaneous abortion. Fetal involvement may be manifest by macular, petechial, papular, vesicular, or pustular exanthems, exfoliative dermatitis, alveolitis, and petechial hemorrhages in the viscera.

LABORATORY ASPECTS. *Candida* species grow well on most primary isolation culture media, including sheep blood agar. The identification of an isolate as *C albicans* can be presumed if the two-hour germ tube test is positive. Laboratory personnel should be cautioned, however, that a negative germ tube test does not rule out the isolate as *C albicans*, and further observations must be made. The decision of whether to identify the species on non-*Candida* species must be evaluated on a case by case basis. In tissue sections utilizing special fungal stains, the diagnosis can be highly suspected if fungal elements are seen with characteristic pseudohyphae and budding yeast forms. *Candida* species are the only fungi presenting this picture. The case has been made that the presence of pseudohyphae indicates invasive disease. However, I have not seen a case where pseudohyphae have been absent, even in Gram's stained mounts of mucocutaneous disease. Although it has been demonstrated that pseudohyphae are necessary for invasion, their presence does not necessarily mean that one is dealing with systemic disease. There are no laboratory tests available to identify disseminated disease. High serum levels of Candida mannans may provide some clue; however, there is sufficient overlap of plasma levels in patients with disease confined to mucous membranes to make the sensitivity of this approach too low to be reliable.

Cryptococcosis. Whether one considers cryptococcosis as an opportunistic or an obligate mycosis is probably a moot point. Cryptococcosis is a rare complication of pregnancy, and congenital infections apparently do not occur, or are exceedingly rare. Animal experiments indicate that the organism does not cross the placenta.[29] Stamm and Dismukes[3] cited 22 reported cases of cryptococcosis complicating pregnancy through 1983. A computer search of the literature since then reveals no additional cases; however, many unreported cases in pregnant women with AIDS must have occurred. In the cases cited by Stamm and Dismukes[3], only two of the women had significant underlying disease or exposures. Almost all had meningoencephalitis with manifestations including fever, headache, nausea, and focal neurologic findings. Two patients had concomitant cryptococcal pneumonia, and one had progressive pneumonia and empyema without any signs of disseminated disease. Hemoptysis was the presenting complaint in two of these cases.[30]

The clinical features, course, and outcome of cryptococcal meningitis are seemingly not influenced by pregnancy, although symptoms worsened in the case reported by Stafford et al[29], leading us to believe that pregnancy may exacerbate the disease. About one half of the 22 patients were treated and cured with amphotericin B. The drug is usually given as an intravenous dose of 0.4–0.8 mg/kg/day, continued for 8–12 weeks. Fetal toxicity from the drug has not been reported, although Stafford et al[29] make the point that none of the patients previously reported was treated in the first trimester. Combination therapy with flucytosine is generally not recommended, due to its potential teratogenicity; however, Stafford et al report successful treatment of cryptococcal meningitis without evidence of fetal damage.

LABORATORY ASPECTS. *Cryptococcus neoformans* is the species causing virtually all human cryptococcal infections. Rapid diagnosis can be made by examining spinal fluid obtained from a fresh lumbar puncture for the presence of cryptococcal organisms in an India ink preparation. This procedure is performed by lightly centrifuging the spinal fluid to concentrate the organisms and examining the sediment. A drop of sediment is added to a drop of India ink or nigrosin on a microscope slide, a coverslip is overlaid, and the mount examined microscopically. The cryptococcal yeast cells range from 5 μ to 15 μ (with all sizes in between), are surrounded by a thick capsule, and characteristically show a single bud connected to the mother cell by a delicate, hairlike attachment. This form is diagnostic when seen in an India ink preparation.

In only about one third of confirmed light infections, organisms will be found in the India ink preparation. The latex agglutination test for the detection of capsular antigen in cerebrospinal fluid is considerably more sensitive, replacing the India ink test in some laboratories. In patients with AIDS, however, where infections tend to be heavy, the India ink test is of much greater value. Cerebrospinal fluid titers of >1:8 should be considered suspicious; we have seen titers approach 1:1 million in patients with AIDS. The organisms can also be readily visualized in tissue sections. The presence of the capsule and the irregularity in size of the yeast cells are the clues needed to make a presumptive tissue diagnosis. In cases of heavy infection, the aggregation of yeast cells may be so dense as to simulate a mucin-secreting carcinoma.

No special culture media is required to recover the organism. It grows in 2–5 days on Sabouraud's dextrose agar and other fungal recovery medium but will also grow on routine sheep blood agar plates. Colonies often have a mucoid appearance, and the presence of capsular material can be suspected. The identification of *C neoformans* can be made by demonstrating the production of caffeic acid by the isolate. This can be accomplished either by using niger seed (bird seed) agar and looking for the appearance of deep red-brown colonies after 48–72 hours' incubation at 35°C or by demonstrating the appearance of a dark brown color when a suspicious colony is streaked on filter paper impregnated with the caffeic acid reagent (commercially available). Carbohydrate assimilation studies may on occasion be necessary to identify atypical strains.

The Dimorphic Pathogenic Fungi

The five species of dimorphic fungi that cause human disease are *B dermatitidis, Coccidioides immitis, Histoplasma capsulatum, S schenckii,* and *Paracoccidioides brasiliensis.* Cutaneous *S schenckii* infection was discussed earlier; systemic disease in pregnancy due to this organism has not been reported. *P brasiliensis* is endemic in South America and only rarely encountered in the United States; therefore, it will not be discussed further here.

The term *dimorphic* refers to the property of these fungi to exist in two forms: (1) a mold form when exposed to ambient temperature, which is how the organism exists as a saprophyte in nature, representing the infective form for humans; and (2) the parasitic yeast (or spherule) form, found in human tissues or in the laboratory when cultures are incubated at 37°C. It is this property of thermal dimorphism, particularly the ability to convert to the parasitic yeast form, that allows this group of organisms to adapt to the unfavorable environment of the human host, to proliferate, and to cause invasive and disseminated disease.

A few salient characteristics of the mycoses caused by the dimorphic fungi are worth mentioning. These fungi are obligate pathogens and will cause disease even in healthy and immunocompetent humans when the inoculum is sufficiently heavy. However, in the vast majority of cases (over 90%), the infections are either asymptomatic or of short duration with complete resolution, conferring long-standing resistance to reinfection. Human-to-human transmission does not occur or is extremely rare, as the tissue forms are not infective at least by the usual routes of infection (an exception is in the transplant of infected organs, when, for example, histoplasmosis can be transferred to an immunosuppressed renal transplant recipient). Except for sporotrichosis, which has a wide distribution in nature, diseases caused by the dimorphic fungi are restricted geographically, and primary infections occur only when individuals live in or visit these endemic areas (blastomycosis is limited to the upper river valleys of the midwest United States, histoplasmosis is endemic in the more southern river valleys, and coccidioidomycosis is endemic in the desert regions of the southwest). These fungi are only infective within restricted time periods when the environmental conditions are ideal for sporulation. Therefore, it is important to obtain a careful history of travel itineraries and activities when assessing a patient with suspected fungal disease.

Modes of Infection and Clinical Presentations. Inhalation of airborne spores is the mode of infection, and in virtually all instances the initial infection is in the lungs. As mentioned above, the majority of infected patients remain asymptomatic, or the primary pulmonary disease manifests as grippe or an influenzalike syndrome—cough, fever, chills, headache, arthralgias, and dyspnea (called valley fever in the case of coccidioidomycosis). In most instances, the acute symptoms are short-lived and heal without sequelae. Only rarely does pulmonary disease progress into a chronic form where coin lesions, granulomas, fibrosis with cavitation, and other consolidative changes may be seen. Chest pain, severe shortness of breath, hemoptysis accompanied by weight loss, and easy fatigability are more prominent. It is unusual for the disease to become disseminated; this usually occurs in patients who are immunosuppressed or who have underlying debilitating disease.

As mentioned before, cutaneous and mucous membrane lesions in the form of pustules, nonhealing ulcers, verrucous growths, and the like may be the first manifestations of disseminated disease. For example, ulcerative lesions of the tongue, posterior pharynx, and buccal mucosa are only rarely caused by bacteria. When these ulcers become chronic, stained smears of scrapings and exudates or biopsy tissue sections must be examined for the presence of causative organisms and appropriate cultures must be obtained. The importance of making smears directly from suspected lesions and examining microscopically for the presence of characteristic yeast forms cannot be emphasized enough.

Culture Media. The dimorphic fungi require special culture media to maximize recovery from specimens. It is essential that clinicians are informed of the usual practices of the laboratory to which they submit specimens. If a deep-seated fungal disease is suspected, this should always be recorded on the request slip to alert laboratory personnel to select the appropriate culture medium. If Sabouraud's dextrose agar or equivalents such as Mycosel agar are used for the primary recovery of fungi, the ability to recover the dimorphic species will be severely compromised. An enriched medium, such as brain heart infusion agar or equivalents (such as inhibitory mold agar or SABHI agar), preferably with 10% blood, must be used. For specimens that are likely to be contaminated with bacteria or saprophytic fungi, one set of culture medium must also contain antimicrobial drugs. Chloramphenicol and cycloheximide (C & C) are commonly used. It is mandatory that fungus cultures be held for at least one month, even if a yeast or saprophytic mold is initially recovered. We have seen cases where a delayed growth of colonies of *H capsulatum* appears on top of more rapidly growing yeast or mold colonies. Close communication between clinicians and laboratory personnel is often essential if the diagnosis of fungal infections is to be made.

Occurrence in Pregnancy. Deep-seated mycoses are rare in pregnancy. Historically, fungal infections from the dimorphic pathogens in the general population have occurred more commonly in middle-aged males, particularly among those engaged in outdoor activities in rural areas. However, females are engaging in more and more outdoor activities such as camping, bicycling, and spelunking, and are more involved in outdoor occupations such as road construction. Even so, rates of infection are low. For example, Wack and associates[31], in a study of coccidioidomycosis in Tucson (AZ), found that the average annual incidence of symptomatic infection among susceptible young adults (skin test negative) was 0.4%. There were only 10 cases of coccidioidomycosis among 47,120 pregnancies (0.02%), making this association an extremely rare event.

Therapy for Infections With the Dimorphic Fungi. The antifungal drugs that are most commonly used in the treatment of human mycotic infections are the polyenes (amphotericin B and nystatin), the imidazoles (ketoconazole, miconazole, clotrimazole, econazole), the fluoridated pyrimidine, F-fluorocytosine (flucytosine), and the antidermatophyte drugs, griseofulvin and tonaftate. The action of amphotericin B requires that the drug combine with sterols, especially ergosterol in the cytoplasmic membrane of fungal cells.[32] This binding results in open pores in the fungus cell membranes, leading to dissolution and cell death. Although this action is primarily directed toward ergosterol, there is also some effect on the cholesterol in mammalian cells as well, thus explaining one underlying cause of toxicity in humans.

The primary action of the imidazoles is to inhibit the synthesis of ergosterol at the level of oxidative 14C-demethylation.[32] This results in a decreased uptake of ergosterol into the cytoplasmic membrane and the inability of the fungus to develop. Flucytosine works primarily to inhibit the synthesis of DNA by competitive inhibition of thymidine metabolism, again compromising the ability of the fungus to grow and replicate. The action of griseofulvin is not known.

Chow and Jewesson[21] have listed the human toxicities of several of the antifungal drugs commonly used:

- Amphotericin B: Nephrotoxicity, anemia, hypokalemia, idiosyncratic reactions
- Flucytosine: Hepatoxicity, teratogenicity in rats
- Griseofulvin: Allergic reactions, hepatotoxicity, teratogenicity in rats
- Ketoconazole: Hepatitis, adrenal suppression
- Miconazole: Hyperlipidemia, hyponatremia, thrombocytosis

In view of these potential complications, any physician treating a pregnant woman with any of these antifungal drugs is advised to monitor closely renal and hepatic function, determine serum sodium and potassium levels, and obtain peripheral blood counts using appropriate laboratory tests during the course of therapy. Physicians must also be alert for any physical signs or symptoms that may suggest untoward reactions.

Amphotericin B remains the treatment of choice for most systemic mycoses, particularly during pregnancy.[3] The drug is administered by slow intravenous infusion. An initial test dose of 1 mg in 100 mL of 5% dextrose in water (D5/W) is given over 30–60 minutes. In the absence of a serious adverse reaction, a therapeutic dose of 0.25 mg/kg in 500 mL of D5/W is delivered over 4–6 hours. Subsequent daily doses are determined in part by the patient's tolerance and susceptibility of the pathogen to the drug. Antipyretics, antiemetics, and hydrocortisone are often used concomitantly to combat adverse effects of fever, chills, nausea, vomiting, and phlebitis.

Ishmail and Lerner[33] reviewed 10 previously reported cases of disseminated fungal infections in pregnant women and added a case of disseminated blastomycosis. There were no adverse effects on the fetus reported. Following infusion of approximately 16 mg of amphotericin B in the 2 hours and 20 minutes prior to delivery, the concentration of amphotericin B in the maternal serum at delivery was 0.32 μg/mL, or about three times the concentration in the fetal cord serum (0.12 μg/mL). This 3:1 ratio is consistent with the experience of others.[11] Hager et al[34] reported simultaneous maternal to infant blood levels of amphotericin B at birth of 1.9 μg/mL and 1.3 μg/mL, with an amniotic fluid level of 0.3 μg/mL, following daily intravenous doses of 460 mg for 6 weeks. They also cite 21 previous cases of systemic mycoses in pregnancy, all ending in healthy neonates, except in two cases where there was evidence of transient "amphotericin nephrosis."

Newer antifungal agents cannot be recommended for use during pregnancy. McGregor and Pont[35] advise against the use of ketoconazole in pregnancy, citing the association with embryotoxicity and teratogenesis in experimental studies in rats and the blocking effect of ketoconazole on androgen and corticosteroid synthesis. They also indicate that other imidazoles may adversely influence cholesterol metabolism in mammalian cells, leading to other toxic effects.

Hager et al[34] cite animal studies in which administration of ketoconazole has resulted in syndactyly and oligodactyly. For more details, an excellent review of the mechanisms of action, spectrum of activity, and adverse reactions of ketoconazole in therapeutic use has been published by Van Tyle.[36]

Schonbeck and Segerbrand[5] report successful treatment of a case of candidal septicemia with flucytosine. However, the spectrum of antifungal activity is limited and rarely essential to therapy in most cases. There has been minimal experience during human pregnancy, and the drug is teratogenic in animals. Experience in griseofulvin in pregnancy is lacking, as this drug has also not received sanction for use due to its potential teratogenic effects.

Blastomycosis

Cohen[37] was able to find only four cases of blastomycosis in pregnancy reported in the medical literature prior to 1987. He added two more cases: a 34-year-old woman with twins diagnosed during her 22nd week of pregnancy and a 39-year-old woman admitted to the hospital in her 26th week of pregnancy. Each mother received a 10-week course of amphotericin B therapy (total dose 960 mg and 975 mg, respectively) leading to remission of symptoms. All three infants were healthy upon delivery and showed no observable effects from the amphotericin B therapy. The authors further commented from study of the previously reported case histories that amphotericin B does not seem to affect the neonates, even though the arterial cord levels reach about one third that in the maternal circulation. Daniel and Salit[38] also recommend that amphotericin B not be withheld from pregnant women after successful treatment of a patient with blastomycosis.

In a case reported both by Tuthill[39] and by Watts et al[1], the infected infant died at age three weeks with pulmonary blastomycosis. This case is remarkable in that the diagnosis was delayed because the appearance of pustules and bumps on the face were misdiagnosed as impetigo and treated with antibiotics. The authors concluded that intrauterine transmission was responsible for the infant's infection, although acquisition of infection during birth or postnatally could not be excluded.

B dermatitidis is a dimorphic fungus with reservoir in the soil. Infection occurs from inhalation of spores during very short and select periods when the fungus is sporulating in nature. The disease is endemic along the upper Mississippi, Missouri, and the Ohio river basins in the United States, and in Southern Manitoba and in regions north and east of Lake Superior in Canada. The diagnosis can be made by examining purulent material or biopsy specimens for the large, 8–15 μ, thick-walled yeast cells that form a single bud with a broad base. The diagnosis can be confirmed by culture, which usually is recovered in the mold form (30°C incubation of culture plates), usually within 1–2 weeks. Delicate septate, hyaline hyphae bearing single pyriform conidia supported by a short conidiophore (lollipops) is the diagnostic form. The final diagnosis can be confirmed by converting the mold form to the yeast form by incubating subcultures at 35°C, or by demonstrating exoantigens extracted from the fungal cell wall.

Histoplasmosis

Histoplasmosis in pregnancy is extremely rare. Stamm and Dismukes[3] cite only two reported cases through 1983. One was a woman with choriocarcinoma, and the other developed disseminated disease during the 1978–1979 outbreak in Indianapolis. Search of the medical literature since then reveals only one other reported case of histoplasmosis in pregnancy, manifesting clinically as meningoencephalitis.[40] The identification of *H capsulatum* as the causative agent was not made until the twelfth hospital day, when the mother's condition worsened. Cesarean section was mandated, and an 810-g, male, premature infant was delivered. The mother died of widespread meningoencephalitis shortly after delivery. The infant survived a hyaline membrane disease. The authors discuss the difficulty of treating central nervous system fungal infections because antifungal agents, cross the placenta poorly.

H capsulatum is a dimorphic fungus that is concentrated in bird manure and bat guano. Concentrations of organisms are highest in soil rich in lime (for example, in caves where bats thrive) or rich in nitrogen from bird droppings. Roosting starlings in particular are prone to carry *H capsulatum*, accounting for outbreaks when citizens attempt to clean up the debris in town squares and parks. Humans become infected by inhalation of dustborne spores. The majority of infections are asymptomatic, and over 95% of natives living in endemic areas show positive histoplasmin skin tests. Chronic cavitary pneumonia rarely occurs, and dissemination has been found in only 0.05% of infected patients, the majority of whom are immunocompromised.

In the tissues of infected persons, *H capsulatum* exists as yeast cells 2–4 μ in diameter surrounded by a halo originally thought to be a capsule (but subsequently shown to be a retraction artifact from the staining process), that grow within the cytoplasm of reticuloendothelial cells. Therefore, hepatomegaly, splenomegaly, and lymphadenopathy may be seen in varying degrees in disseminated cases. The bone marrow is an excellent site to demonstrate these intracellular yeast forms. We have observed *H capsulatum* yeast cells within circulating monocytes in patients with AIDS and histoplasmosis.

Laboratory Aspects. The organism grows relatively slowly in culture (2–3 weeks), although in recent cases in patients with AIDS, where the concentration of organisms may be extremely high, growth as soon as 5 days has been seen. In the tissue form, the organism exists as tiny yeast cells 2–3 μ in diameter within the cytoplasm of reticuloendothelial cells (macrophages) in the bone marrow, spleen, liver, and lymph nodes. These forms are only rarely seen in direct examination of expectorated sputum samples, and biopsies of infected organs or bone marrow aspirations are usually required to make the diagnosis. The mold form, as seen in culture incubated at 30°C, is characterized by the formation of delicate, septate hyphae that produce both pyriform microconidia resembling those produced by *B dermatitidis* and characteristic large macroconidia with a cell wall that becomes roughened and spiked (tuberculate). Serum serology studies may be of help in making the diagnosis in equivocal cases, particularly if both H and M precipitin bands are seen on double diffusion preparations.

Coccidioidomycosis

Of all the dimorphic mycoses, coccidioidomycosis is the one fungus that has caused major morbidity and mortality during pregnancy in endemic areas. Catanzaro[11] reviewed the medical literature up to 1984 and cited numerous studies where coccidioidomycosis in pregnancy led to fatal outcomes. An early 1951 study by Vaughan and Ramirez[8] is cited, where 33 cases of documented coccidioidomycosis during pregnancy in a survey of hospitals in Kern County, California, were reviewed (during the period 1942–1949). Of 12 women who had the diagnosis made during the first trimester, 11 had uneventful recoveries, in contrast to 11 patients who contracted the disease in the third trimester, all but four of whom died from disseminated disease. They cite a later survey by Smale and Waechter in Kern County and Tulare County, California, between 1950 and 1967, during which 15 cases of disseminated coccidioidomycosis during pregnancy were reported. Two of these cases had dissemination prior to pregnancy, one of whom died despite amphotericin B therapy. Of the 13 who had dissemination during pregnancy, only 4 survived, three of whom had received amphotericin B therapy. Eight patients died during pregnancy; four received amphotericin B and four did not.

Purtilo[14], on reviewing cases of fatal mycotic infection in 17 pregnant women from the files of the Armed Forces Institute of Pathology, found that coccidioidomycosis was the only fungal infection leading to the death of pregnant women who were not immunosuppressed. Pappagianis[41] reviewed the literature in 1980 and added an additional 16 cases, observing also that the risk of dissemination is highest during the third trimester of pregnancy. This may be related to the finding that 17-b-estradiol, in the concentrations found in the serum of pregnant women, causes a profound stimulation of the growth of *C immitis.*[42] Powell and Drutz[43] also conclude from their studies that the growth stimulatory effect of sex hormones on *C immitis,* even in nanomolar concentrations, may be mediated by a specific cytosol protein-binding system, which particularly in pregnancy induces pathogenicity and dissemination of the organism.

The placenta is directly involved in up to one quarter of cases of disseminated coccidioidomycosis. Many spherules may be seen in the placenta with extensive villous destruction; however, fetal infection is rare.[44] Pregnancy is not adversely affected in nondisseminated maternal coccidioidal disease, and healthy term babies are delivered in most instances. Even the high fetal mortality rates reported in the earlier literature in disseminated disease may be significantly improved today, as previously discussed. Following serologic tests in neonates may be helpful. The tests are initially positive due to the passive transfer of maternal antibodies. Titers fall to undetectable levels in the first months of life, and therapy is not advocated for healthy infants whose titers are decreasing.

The clinical features of coccidioidomycosis are similar in pregnant and nonpregnant persons. Chronic pulmonary disease may be manifest as persistent infiltrates, cavities, hilar adenopathy, or pleural effusions. This form of disease does not usually adversely affect the mother or fetus. Hematogenous dissemination most commonly affects the skin, subcutaneous tissues, lymph nodes, bones, joints, and meninges. The central nervous system is involved in about one third of cases. Because of poor permeability of the blood–brain barrier, intrathecal as well as intravenous dosing is required. Peterson et al[45] recommend the following combined intrathecal and intravenous treatment regimen: begin intrathecal therapy with a test dose of 0.05–0.1 mg, with 25 mg of hydrocortisone, and increase as tolerated to 0.25–0.50 mg every other day. Continue intrathecal treatment until at least three months have elapsed, checking that cerebrospinal *Coccidioides* complement fixation titers are negative. Raise intravenous doses incrementally 5–10 mg/day, after a 1-mg test dose, to a total dose of 0.5–1.5 mg/kg every other day. Current regimens administer approximately 2 g intravenously early in the course of treatment, usually along with antihistamines or hydrocortisone.

Two reviews since 1980 indicate that the rate of dissemination of coccidioidomycosis in pregnancy and mortality may be less than reported in the earlier literature.[11,30] In the first of these, Catanzaro[11] conducted an informal survey of obstetricians and infectious disease specialists in San Diego, Los Angeles, Bakersfield, Phoenix, and Tucson, who remembered very few cases of coccidioidomycosis in pregnancy.

The series of 10 cases among over 47,000 pregnancies as reported by Wack et al[31], from records culled from three health care facilities in Tucson, provide more definitive data on the lower rate of incidence and mortality. Of their 10 patients, 7 had the diagnosis made during the first trimester and all recovered from their infections. Two women developed fulminant disease in the postpartum period, and both had symptoms consistent with respiratory infection during the third trimester. Within 10 days after delivery, both developed disseminated coccidioidal infection with diffuse nodular infiltrates on the chest radiograph and meningitis. Intravenous and intrathecal amphotericin B was given, and both patients continued treatment more than four years later for chronic coccidioidal meningitis. The third patient developed pulmonary coccidioidomycosis one week postpartum and recovered with no complications.

The authors relate several factors that may account for the better prognostic findings in their study compared to previous surveys. Some cases may have escaped follow up due to restrictions of the research methods. The populations of people being studied during these two times may not be comparable; that is, the patients may have been a different age, of different racial background, and not at the same risk of exposure. In the earlier studies, maternal mortality may have been influenced by underlying conditions other than coccidioidomycosis. Yet, it is possible that improvements in medical care, particularly the introduction of antifungal therapy, may have played a role in reducing the mortality in the current study.

Coccidioidomycosis is endemic in the desert in the Southwest from San Joaquin Valley, California, to southwest Texas, and in much of Mexico and Central America. More than 90% of adults living in these areas have been infected, the majority with asymptomatic disease. Approximately one third of those infected develop a transient flulike illness; of these, only about 5% develop chronic pulmonary disease, and extrapulmonary dissemination occurs in only 0.2%. The risk of dissemination is much higher in blacks, American Indians, Mexicans, and Filipinos.

The diagnosis of coccidioidomycosis must be suspected in a pregnant woman who lives in or has traveled to an endemic area and then develops a flulike illness, particularly if pulmonary symptoms such as cough, fever, chest pain, headaches, and arthralgias persist. Chest x-rays should be obtained to determine if a pulmonary infiltrate is present or if there is evidence of hylar adenopathy. The skin and mucous membranes should be carefully examined for the presence of papules, ulcerations, or crusting. The tissue form of *C immitis* is the formation of spherules ranging from 10–200 μ in diameter. These are only rarely seen in direct examination of sputum or secretions; therefore, biopsy is usually required to confirm the diagnosis.

Laboratory Aspects. The organism grows in culture on most fungal isolation media, and rates of recovery as early as five days may be possible in heavy infections. Extreme care must be taken in the laboratory when working with any culture suspected of harboring *C immitis*. The tiny, barrel-shaped arthroconidia characteristic of the mold form of the organism are easily airborne and can cause laboratory-acquired infections. Examination of cultures must be done with great care only in a biologic safety hood. To minimize dangers in handling, an exoantigen test is available for confirming the identity of a suspicious culture.

A variety of serological tests are available to aid in making the diagnosis in equivocal cases. The complement fixation (CF) test is the time-honored method, and a titer of >1:16 is generally indicative of disseminated disease. The procedure, however, is time consuming and not available in many laboratories. Immunodiffusion (ID) and a latex particle agglutination test (LPA) are available and can be used for an initial diagnostic screen. If both reactions are negative, coccidioidomycosis can be ruled out; if the reactions are positive, a confirmatory CF test should be done to set a baseline for later serial examinations.

Treatment of all pregnant women with active disease is recommended, and Stamm and Dismukes[3] suggest the following treatment regimen: primary pulmonary infection—amphotericin B in a dose of 0.3–0.6 mg/kg/day or 0.6–1.0 mg/kg every other day, administered intravenously to a cumulative dose of 1 g, may be required. For disseminated disease, 0.5–0.75 mg/kg/day, and a cumulative dose of 2–4 g is usually necessary. Intrathecal therapy is required with central nervous system involvement. The regimen suggested by Peterson et al[45] was described earlier in this chapter.

REFERENCES

1. Watts EA, Gard PD Jr, Tuthill SW. First reported case of intrauterine transmission of blastomycosis. *Pediatr Infect Dis*. 1983;2:308.
2. Shweni PM, Moodley SC, Bishop BB. Septic abortion complicated by rhinocerebral phycomycosis (mucormycosis). A case report. *S Afr Med J*. 1986;69:515.
3. Stamm AM, Dismukes WE. Infections caused by fungi and higher bacteria. In: Gleicher N, ed. *Principles of Medical Therapy in Pregnancy*. Norwalk, CT: Appleton & Lange; 1985.
4. Rippon JW. *Medical Mycology: The pathogenic fungi and the pathogenic actinomycetes*. 3rd ed. Philadelphia, PA: WB Saunders; 1988:159.
5. Schonbeck J, Segerbrand E. *Candida albicans* septicemia during first half of pregnancy successfully treated with 5-fluorocytosine. *Br Med J*. 1973;4:337.
6. Marcon MJ, Posell DA. Epidemiology, diagnosis and management of *Malassezia furfur* systemic infection. *Diagn Microbiol Infect Dis*. 1987;7:161.
7. Barkey WF. Striae and persistent tinea corporis related to prolonged use of betamethazone dipropionate 0.05% cream/clotrimazole 1% cream. *J Am Acad Derm*. 1987;17:518.
8. Vaughan JE, Ramirez M. Coccidioidomycosis complicating pregnancy: report of 3 cases and review of the literature. *Obstet Gynecol*. 1951;28:401.
9. Travis LB, Roberts GD, Wilson WR. Clinical significance of *Pseudallescheria boydii*: a review of 10 years' experience. *Mayo Clin Proc*. 1985;60:531.
10. Mohr JA, Muchmore HG. Maduromycosis due to *Allescheria boydii*. *JAMA*. 1968;204:125.
11. Catanzaro A. Pulmonary mycosis in pregnant women. *Chest*. 1984;86(suppl):14.
12. Vanderveen EE, Messenger AL, Voorhees JJ. Sporotrichosis in pregnancy. *Cutis*. 1982;30:761.
13. Dall L, Salzman G. Treatment of pulmonary sporotrichosis with ketoconazole. *Rev Infect Dis*. 1987;9:795.
14. Purtilo DT. Opportunistic mycotic infections in pregnant women. *Am J Obstet Gynecol*. 1975;122:607.
15. Brabin BJ. Epidemiology of infection in pregnancy. *Rev Infect Dis*. 1985;7:579.
16. Schwartz DA, Jacquette M, Chawla HS. Disseminated neonatal aspergillosis: report of a fatal case and analysis of risk factors. *Ped Infect Dis J*. 1988;7:349.
17. Weisskopf A. Mucormycosis–a rhinologic disease. *Ann Otol Rhinol Laryngol*. 1964;73:16.
18. Sobel JD. Pathogenesis and epidemiology of vulvovaginal candidiasis. *Ann NY Acad Sci*. 1988;544:547.
19. Weisberg M. Treatment of vaginal candidiasis in pregnant women. *Clin Therap*. 1986;8:563.
20. Ainsworth RE. Use and safety of miconazole during pregnancy. *West J Med*. 1988;147:599. Letter.
21. Chow AW, Jewesson PJ. Use and safety of antimicrobial agents during pregnancy. *West J Med*. 1987;146:761.
22. Lindeque BG, van-Niekerk WA. Treatment of vaginal candidiasis in pregnancy with a single clortrimazole 500 mg vaginal pessary. *So Afr Med J*. 1984;65:123.
23. Cantrill HL, Rodman WP, Ramsey RC, et al. Postpartum *Candida* endophthalmitis. *JAMA*. 1980;243:1163.
24. Morgan MA, Pippitt CH, Thurnau GR. Antenatal diagnosis of *Candida* chorioamnionitis. *South Med J*. 1989;82:176. Letter.
25. Bider D, Ben-Rafael Z, Barkai G, Mashiach S. Intrauterine fetal death apparently due to *Candida* chorioamnionitis. *Arch Gynecol Obstet*. 1989;244:175.
26. Spaun E, Klunder K. *Candida* chorioamnionitis and intra-uterine contraceptive device. *Acta Obstet Gynecol Scand*. 1986;65:183.
27. Smith CV, Horenstein J, Platt LD. Intraamniotic infection with *Candida albicans* associated with a retained intrauterine contraceptive device: a case report. *Am J Obstet Gynecol*. 1988;159:123.
28. Schirar A, Rendu C, Vielh JP, et al. Congenital mycosis (*Candida albicans*). *Biol Neonate*. 1974;24:2173.
29. Stafford CR, Fisher JF, Fadel HE, et al. Cryptococcal meningitis in pregnancy. *Obstet Gynecol*. 1983;62(suppl):35S.
30. Silberfarb PM, Sarosi GA, Tosh FE. Cryptococcosis and pregnancy. *Am J Obstet Gynecol*. 1972;112:714.
31. Wack EE, Ampel NM, Galgiani JN, Bronnimann DA. Coccidioidomycosis during pregnancy. An analysis of ten cases among 47,120 pregnancies. *Chest*. 1988;94:376.
32. Walsh TJ. Recent advances in the treatment of systemic fungal infections: a brief review. *ASM News*. 1987;54:240.
33. Ismail MA, Lerner SA. Disseminated blastomycosis in a pregnant woman: review of amphotericin B usage during pregnancy. *Am Rev Respir Dis*. 1982;126:350.
34. Hager H, Welt SI, Cardasis JP, Alvarez S. Disseminated blastomycosis in a pregnant woman successfully treated with amphotericin-B. A case report. *J Reprod Med*. 1988;33:485.
35. McGregor JA, Pont A. Contraindication of ketoconazole in pregnancy. *Am J Obstet Gynecol*. 1984;150:793. Letter.
36. Van Tyle JH. Ketoconazole: mechanisms of action, spectrum of activity, pharmacokinetics, drug interactions, adverse reactions and therapeutic use. *Pharmacotherapy*. 1984;4:343.
37. Cohen I. Absence of congenital infection and teratogenesis in three children born to mothers with blastomycosis and treated with amphotericin B during pregnancy. *Pediatr Infect Dis*. 1987;6:76.
38. Daniel L, Salit IE. Blastomycosis during pregnancy. *Can Med Assoc J* 1984;131:759.
39. Tuthill SW. Disseminated blastomycosis with intrauterine transmission. *South Med J*. 1985;78:1526. Letter.
40. McGregor JA, et al. Meningoencephalitis caused by *Histoplasma capsulatum* complicating pregnancy. *Am J Obstet Gynecol*. 1986;154:925.
41. Pappagianis D. Epidemiology of coccidioidomycosis. In: Stevens D, ed. *Coccidioidomycosis*. New York, NY: Plenum; 1980:63.
42. Drutz DJ, Huppert M. Coccidioidomycosis: factors affecting the host–parasite interaction. *J Infect Dis*. 1983;147:372.
43. Powell BL, Drutz DJ. Confirmation of corticosterone and progesterone binding activity in *Candida albicans*. *J Infect Dis*. 1983;147:359.
44. McCaffree MA, Altschaler G, Benirschke K. Placental coccidioidomycosis without fetal disease. *Arch Pathol Lab Med*. 1978;102:512.
45. Peterson CM, Johnson SL, Kelly JV, Kelly PC. Coccidioidal meningitis and pregnancy: a case report. *Obstet Gynecol*. 1989;73:835.

Chapter Eighty-Five
Rickettsial Disease

John Segreti

85

The Rickettsiae are obligate intracellular parasites. These small, gram-negative coccobacilli are true bacteria specialized for intracellular growth. They multiply by binary fission and contain both RNA and DNA. Many of the *Rickettsiae* also contain endotoxin.[1] With the exception of *Coxiella burnetii* (the etiologic agent of Q fever), the Rickettsiae can survive only in a host. *C burnetii* is a relatively hardy organism that resists desiccation and is transmitted primarily by an airborne route. The other Rickettsiae are almost always transmitted by way of an insect vector. In the United States, the most common rickettsial diseases include Rocky Mountain spotted fever and Q fever. Other rickettsial diseases are summarized in Table 85–1.

ROCKY MOUNTAIN SPOTTED FEVER

Rocky Mountain spotted fever is caused by *Rickettsia rickettsii*. Despite its name, the incidence of Rocky Mountain spotted fever is highest in the south Atlantic states and in the west central region of the United States.[2] However, cases are reported from almost every state. The American dog tick, *Dermacentor variabilis*, is both the vector and the main reservoir of *R rickettsii*. However, other ticks have also been found to be able to harbor the organism. The organism is transmitted transovarially in ticks, thus maintaining the agent in nature.[2] The adult tick is the only form that feeds on humans, and the rickettsiae are transmitted during feeding.[2] The bite is painless and frequently goes unnoticed. After feeding, rickettsiae are released from the salivary glands. Although Rocky Mountain spotted fever is often considered a rural disease, the recent discovery of a focus in New York City emphasizes that Rocky Mountain spotted fever can be widely distributed.[3] The highest incidence of the disease is during this summer and early fall, primarily at times of greatest tick activity.[4]

Rickettsiae introduced into the skin spread to the regional lymphatics and small blood vessels, resulting in hematogenous dissemination. The rickettsiae attach to their target cells, the vascular endothelium, and proliferate intracellularly by binary fission.[5] This results in direct toxicity to the endothelial cells, which increases vascular permeability, which in turn results in edema, hypovolemia, hypotension, and hypoalbuminemia. Vascular injury and subsequent host response corresponds to the distribution of the rickettsiae and may include interstitial pneumonia, interstitial myocarditis, and vascular lesions in the skin, gastrointestinal tract, pancreas, liver, skeletal muscles, and kidneys.[2] Thrombocytopenia is observed in up to 50% of patients secondary to local consumption.[2] However, true disseminated intravascular coagulation rarely occurs.

The incubation period of Rocky Mountain spotted fever ranges from 2–14 days with a mean of 7 days.[2] The variation in incubation period depends on the initial inoculum of rickettsiae. The initial symptoms are fever, myalgia, and headache.[2] Nausea, vomiting, abdominal pain, diarrhea, and abdominal tenderness are also very common. The rash is the major diagnostic sign and usually occurs during the first five days of illness. Rash is found in over 90% of patients; however, Rocky Mountain "spotless" fever has also been described and seems to occur most commonly in older patients and in black patients.[2] The rash typically begins around the wrists and the ankles, but may start on the trunk or may even be diffuse at the onset. Involvement of the palms and soles is considered characteristic; however, the absence of this should not rule out the diagnosis.[4,6] The cerebrospinal fluid is usually unremarkable; however, leukocytes may be present in up to one third of patients.

The prognosis of Rocky Mountain spotted fever is largely related to the timeliness of appropriate therapy. In addition, cases with hepatomegaly, jaundice, stupor, and renal insufficiency are more likely to have a fatal outcome.[2]

The diagnosis of Rocky Mountain spotted fever is often based on clinical and epidemiologic factors. Rocky Mountain spotted fever may also be diagnosed by isolation of rickettsiae from the blood. However, few laboratories undertake this procedure, because this poses a significant biohazard.[7] Some hospital and reference laboratories are able to demonstrate rickettsiae in cutaneous biopsy specimens by direct immunofluorescence.[2] This is the only rapid diagnostic method during the acute phase of the infection. Serology is usually retrospective; however, it continues to be the

TABLE 85–1. FEATURES OF SELECTED RICKETTSIOSES

Disease	Organism	Insect Vector	Geographic Area
Rocky Mountain spotted fever	*Rickettsia rickettsii*	Tick	Western Hemisphere
Boutonneuse fever	*Riskettsia conorii*	Tick	Africa, the Mediterranean
Rickettsialpox	*Rickettsia akari*	Mite	US, USSR, Korea, Africa
Epidemic typhus	*Rickettsia prowazekii*	Body louse	Africa, Asia, South America
Murine typhus	*Rickettsia typhi*	Flea	Worldwide
Scrub typhus	*Rickettsia tsutsugamushi*	Mite	Asia, Australia
Q fever	*Coxiella burnetti*	—	Worldwide

usual method for confirmation of the diagnosis.[4] The Weil–Felix test, using *Proteus vulgaris* strains OX-19 and OX-2 agglutination, is not reliable. Indirect hemagglutination, indirect immunofluorescence, latex agglutination, and compliment fixation are more specific tests.

There are very few cases of Rocky Mountain spotted fever during pregnancy reported in the literature.[8,9] However, given the geographic distribution of potential cases of Rocky Mountain spotted fever, this diagnosis should be considered in pregnant women with fever and a characteristic rash. As in nonpregnant patients, early treatment is essential. The decision to treat a patient with a presumptive diagnosis of Rocky Mountain spotted fever should not await confirmatory laboratory testing. The tetracyclines and chloramphenicol appear to be equally effective in treating Rocky Mountain spotted fever.[2] However, tetracyclines are usually contraindicated in pregnancy. Serious hepatotoxicity and pancreatitis have been reported in pregnant women.[10] Tetracyclines cross the placenta and because of their affinity for calcium, are incorporated into calcifying teeth and bone, resulting in staining of the teeth and depression of skeletal growth.[10] Chloramphenicol appears to be safe during pregnancy for both the mother and the fetus. Use of chloramphenicol in the neonate, however, may result in gray syndrome.[10] This consists of abdominal distension, pallor, cyanosis, vasomotor collapse, and usually death. It appears to be related to immaturity of the hepatic enzyme system involved in conjugation and excretion of the drug. As in nonpregnant women, chloramphenicol may result in dose-related bone marrow suppression, which is reversible.[10] Irreversible aplastic anemia appears to be unrelated to dose and duration of treatment. This occurs in approximately 1:40,000 patients and is usually fatal.[10]

Prevention of Rocky Mountain spotted fever is of great importance. Pregnant women should be advised to avoid areas known to have heavy tick infestation. If such advice is impractical, women should be encouraged to wear protective clothing. Tick repellents containing DEET are rapidly absorbed through the skin. Adverse reactions to DEET have included serious neurologic reactions, including seizures and coma. Thus, the use of these products should not be advised in pregnancy. Pregnant women who are camping or walking through areas known to be endemic for Rocky Mountain spotted fever should carefully search their clothes, skin, and scalp for ticks. Ticks should be removed quickly, preferably with tweezers to try to avoid removing the body of the tick while leaving the head imbedded in the skin.

There is little information on the effects of Rocky Mountain spotted fever on the developing fetus. Because Rickettsiae cause vasculitis in various tissues, it is likely that the placenta will also be affected. This could conceivably result in decreased blood flow to the fetus and fetal damage. In the few reported cases of Rocky Mountain spotted fever in pregnant women, the fetus developed normally and was healthy on delivery.[8] In the French literature, there are scattered reports of abortion and premature delivery in women infected with Rickettsiae.[11,12] However, in a rat model of *C burnetii,* inapparent infection did not appear to have a detrimental effect on the pregnancy.[13] In other animal models, there was lack of transplacental infection with *Rickettsia tsutsugamushi* and *Rickettsia typhi.*[14,15]

Q FEVER

Q fever is due to infection with *C burnetii.* The animals most commonly infected with this organism are cattle, sheep, and goats. These animals can shed the organism in their urine, feces, milk, and especially the placenta.[16] Recently, exposure to parturient cats has been identified as a significant risk factor.[17] Humans are infected by inhalation of the contaminated aerosols. After an incubation period of approximately 20 days, the infected person becomes ill with headache, fever, chills, fatigue, and myalgias. Other manifestations can include pneumonia, endocarditis, and hepatitis.[16] There are a few reports of Q fever in pregnant women.[18,19] Some articles report an increased incidence of abortions and stillbirths.[18,19] One report described the infected placenta as showing large areas of necrosis.[18] Others have reported normal births of healthy babies even when the placenta was infected.[20] The diagnosis is usually made clinically and epidemiologically. Serology will confirm the diagnosis. Tetracycline is the treatment of choice, but chloramphenicol has also been used.[16] Quinolone antibiotics have good *in vitro* activity against *C burnetii,* but there is no clinical information on efficacy.[21] In addition, their use in pregnancies is not recommended.

HUMAN EHRLICHIOSIS

Ehrlichieae are intraleukocytic bacteria of the *Rickettsiaeae* family. *Ehrlichia sennetsu* is a human pathogen that was isolated in 1954 from a patient in Japan with an infectious mononucleosislike syndrome.[22] This illness has also been reported in Southeast Asia and the Philippines. There are no reported cases of *E sennetsu* in the United States or Europe. Most *Ehrlichia* organisms are pathogens of animals. The primary example of this is *Ehrlichia canis,* which is the cause of tropical canine pancytopenia.[23] The vector of *E canis* for dogs appears to be the brown dog tick *Rhipicephalus sanguineus.* In recent years, there have been reports of *E canis*-like organisms causing infection in humans.[24-27] Malaise was the most common prodrome; others included low back pain, nausea, and vomiting. Patients had sudden onset of high fever often accompanied by relative bradycardia. Headache is characteristic. The history of tick attachment and the clinical picture strongly suggests the diagnosis of Rocky Mountain spotted fever.[22] However, a rash is almost always absent in human ehrlichiosis.[22] Laboratory findings most commonly include an absolute lymphopenia, and thrombocytopenia is also reported. The illness is usually self-limited; however, there is a good response to tetracyclines. There is no evidence that chloramphenicol is helpful in these situations. Therefore, the potential treatment of pregnant women remains problematic.

REFERENCES

1. Saah AJ. Rickettsiosis. In: Mandell GL, Douglas RG, Bennett JE, eds. *Principles and Practice of Infectious Diseases.* New York, NY: Churchill Livingstone; 1989:1463.
2. Raoult D, Walker DH. *Rickettsia rickettsii and other spotted fever* Group Rickettsiae (Rocky Mountain spotted fever and other spotted fevers). In: Mandell GL, Douglas RG, Bennett JE, eds. *Principles and Practice of Infectious Disease* New York, NY: Churchill Livingstone; 1989:1465.
3. Salgo MP, Telzak EE, Currie B, et al. A focus of Rocky Mountain spotted fever within New York City. *N Engl J Med.* 1988;318:1345.
4. Taylor JP, Istre GR, McChesney TC. The epidemiology of Rocky Mountain spotted fever in Arkansas, Oklahoma, and Texas, 1981 through 1985. *Am J Epidemiol.* 1988;127:1295.
5. Walker TS. Rickettsial interactions with human endothelial cells in vitro: adherence and entry. *Infection and Immunity.* 1984;44:205.
6. Rocky Mountain spotted fever—United States, 1988. *MMWR.* 1989; 38:513.

7. Oster CN, Burke DS, Kenyon RH, et al. Laboratory-acquired Rocky Mountain spotted fever: the hazard of aerosol transmission. *N Engl J Med*. 1977;297:859.
8. Gallis HA, Agner RC, Painter CJ. Rocky Mountain spotted fever in pregnancy. *NC Med J*. 1984;45:187.
9. Herbert WP, Seeds JW, Koontz WL, Cefalo RC. Rocky Mountain spotted fever in pregnancy: differential diagnosis and treatment. *Southern Med J*. 1982;75:1063.
10. Segreti J, Trenholme GM. Beta-lactam antibiotics, the tetracyclines, chloramphenicol, erythromycin, clindamycin, metronidazole, and the quinolones. *Clin Chest Med*. 1986;7:393.
11. Gillet JY, Keller B, Muller P. Action of listeria, toxoplasmosis and rickettsia in the syndromes of interruption of pregnancy and neonatal deaths. Results of a presonal study. *Gynecologie et Obstetrique (Paris)*. 1968;67:51.
12. Museteanu C. Rickettsial endometritis, cause of spontaneous and recurrent abortion. *Revue Francaise de Gynecologie et d'Obstetrique*. 1969;64:425.
13. Giroud A, Giroud P, Martinet M, Deluchat C. Perturbations du Development Par Une Rickettsiose Inapparente (R. burneti). *Societe de Biologie*. 1957;11:553.
14. Shirai A, Chan TC, Gan E, Groves MG. Lack of transplacental infection with scrub typhus organisms in laboratory mice. *Am J Trop Med Hygiene*. 1984;33:285.
15. Arango-Jaramillo S, Wisseman CL, Azad AF. Newborn rats in the murine typhus enzootic infection cycle: studies on transplacental infection and passively acquired maternal antirickettsial antibodies. *Am J Trop Med and Hygiene*. 1988;39:391.
16. Marrie TJ. *Coxiella burnettii* (Q Fever). In: Mandell GL, Douglas RG, Bennett JE, eds. *Principles and Practice of Infectious Diseases*. New York, NY: Churchill Livingstone; 1989:1472.
17. Marrie TJ, Durant H, Williams JC, et al. Exposure to parturient cats: a risk factor for acquisition of Q fever in Maritime Canada. *J Infect Dis*. 1988;158:101.
18. Riechman N, Raz R, Keysary A, et al. Chronic Q fever and severe thrombocytopenia in a pregnant woman. *Am J Med*. 1988;85:253.
19. McGivern D, White R, Paul ID, et al. Concomitant zoonotic infections with ovine chlamydia and 'Q' fever in pregnancy: clinical features, diagnosis, management and public health implications. *Brit J Obstet Gynaecol*. 1988;95:294. Case Report.
20. Syrucek L, Sobeslavsky O, Gutvirth I. Isolation of *Coxiella burnettii* from human placentas. *J Hygiene, Epidemiol, Microbiol Immunol*. 1958;2:29.
21. Yeaman MR, Mitscher LA, Baca OG. In vitro susceptibility of *Coxiella burnettii* to antibiotics, including several quinolones. *Antimicrobial Agents Chemotherapy*. 1987;31:1079.
22. Saah AJ. *Ehrlichia* species (human ehrlichiosis). In: Mandell GL, Douglas RG, Bennett JE, eds. *Principles and Practice of Infectious Diseases*. New York, NY: Churchill Livingstone; 1989:1482.
23. Harvey JW, Simpson CF, Gaskin JM. Cyclic thrombocytopenia induced by a rickettsia-like agent in dogs. *J Infect Dis*. 1978;137:182.
24. Golden SE. Aseptic meningitis associated with *Ehrlichia canis* infection. *Ped Infect Dis J*. 1989;8:335.
25. Taylor JP, Betz TG, Fishbein DB, et al. Serologic evidence of possible human infection with *Ehrlichia* in Texas. *J Infect Dis*. 1988;158:217.
26. Maeda K, Markowitz N, Hawley RC, et al. Human infection with *Ehrlichia canis*, a leukocytic rickettsia. *N Engl J Med*. 1987;316:853.
27. Edwards MS, Jones JE, Leass DL, et al. Childhood infection caused by *Ehrlichia canis* or a closely related organism. *Ped Infect Dis J*. 1988;7:651.

Chapter Eighty-Six

Respiratory Infections With *Mycoplasma Pneumoniae*

Timothy W. Harstad and Larry C. Gilstrap III

86

Eaton et al in 1944 reported a filterable agent thought to be a cause of atypical pneumonia (Eaton agent).[1] This agent was felt to be a virus until 1961, when Marmion and Goodburn reported it to be a pleuropneumonia-like organism.[2] Mycoplasmas have been shown to consist of only three organelles: plasma membranes, ribosomes, and prokaryotic chromosomes. Similar to bacteria, they contain both RNA and DNA. The organisms are pleomorphic and lack a rigid cell wall. Pneumonia caused by *Mycoplasma pneumoniae* has been characterized by fever, cough, and pulmonary infiltrates that appear more extensive on x-ray than would be expected by physical exam. *M pneumoniae* may cause disease throughout the respiratory tract, including the nasopharynx, throat, trachea, bronchii, bronchioles, and alveoli, as well as the inner ear. The involvement of the upper respiratory tract may be either symptomatic or asymptomatic.

M pneumoniae has the following characteristics: (1) absence of a cell wall, (2) growth in cell-free media, (3) dependence on the availability of sterols for growth, (4) inhibition of growth by specific antibody, (5) susceptibility to antimicrobial agents that inhibit protein synthesis, and (6) resistance to agents that affect synthesis of cell walls.[3]

Mycoplasma can be divided on the basis of fermentation characteristics into two broad groups: fermenters and nonfermenters. *M pneumoniae, Mycoplasma fermentans,* and *Mycoplasma genitalium* ferment glucose. *M pneumoniae* may be distinguished from the others by rapid hemolysis of sheep or guinea pig erythrocytes. The organisms can also be detected serologically by fluorescent antibody, complement fixation, growth inhibition, indirect hemagglutinin, mycoplasmacidal tests, and by the Enzyme-Linked Immunosorbent assay (ELISA).[4,5]

M pneumoniae infections are the result of prolonged close contact with infected individuals and are probably spread by means of infected respiratory secretions.[6] Most *M pneumoniae* illnesses will affect people between the ages of 5 and 25 years, whereas bacteria-induced labor pneumonia tends to occur in the very young and elderly.[4] *M pneumoniae* infections can be detected throughout the year, but peaks are observed when close or crowded conditions are present. Populations of military groups or college students demonstrate 10–50% of the pneumonias due to this organism.[7] The recovery from *M pneumoniae* infections is based primarily on antibody development, as is subsequent resistance, which is related to the magnitude of antibody response. Subsequent infections are, therefore, reduced and attenuated due to the presence of antibodies.

Autopsy findings of eight patients with cold-hemagglutinin associated atypical pneumonia have been reported.[8] Essential changes included interstitial pneumonia and acute bronchiolitis. Findings such as thickening of the bronchiolar wall with edema, vascular congestion, and infiltrates of mononuclear and plasma cells were also described. Fatality due to this organism is quite rare. The pathogenesis of infection causing the symptoms clinically seen include attachment to respiratory mucosa at the cell membrane receptor (which consists of neuraminic acid), metabolic impairment of the cells, and interference with ciliary motion.

The organisms remain extracellular throughout the course of infection. There is some suggestion that pulmonary infiltrates may be due to an immunologic response to reinfection, based on the observation that pneumonia is rare in young children but increases in frequency and severity with age.[9]

The reports that have contained pregnant women with *M pneumoniae* infection, particularly pneumonia[10,11], have not documented any untoward effects of pregnancy upon this infection. The symptoms and duration of illness have been similar to that of the nonpregnant individual.

In 1982, Benedetti et al reported 39 patients with pneumonia during pregnancy. Two patients had serologic evidence for mycoplasma as the etiologic agent. One patient was lost to follow up and the other had a normal spontaneous vaginal delivery at term. The overall incidence of *M pneumoniae* in pregnancy is not clearly defined. Similarly, with the high rate of familial transmission, one might expect it to match that in the general population.[12] The diagnosis should be suspected in pregnant women presenting with persistent upper respiratory symptoms beyond two weeks or rales on auscultation. Appropriate serology and chest x-ray should be performed.

There are no reports suggesting transplacental transmission of this organism or fetal infection, and thus there is little data concerning the effect *M pneumoniae* infections may have on the fetus. In those few pregnancies reported with *M pneumoniae* infection, the neonatal outcome has been good.[10,13] Pneumonia from all causes has been shown to result in few preterm births. No effect was noted on the pregnancy or fetal development in thirteen women who had symptoms of lower respiratory tract infection and positive complement fixation test for *M pneumoniae*.[11]

Information regarding *M pneumoniae* infections in the newborn is sparse. Children less than five years of age generally do not become infected. However, two children under two years of age contracted *M pneumoniae* and developed pneumonia among 20 children up to age 10 in infrafamilial transmission studies.[12]

DIAGNOSIS

The incubation period of *M pneumoniae* is somewhat variable but generally is considered to be between two and three weeks.[4,6] Initial clinical manifestations include symptoms of upper respiratory infection, which may then progress to lower respiratory tract infection. Upper respiratory illness (25%), pharyngitis (6–59%), otitis (12%), tracheobronchitis (10%), and pneumonia (3–10%) are included in the clinical spectrum of this disease.[4,14] Ten percent will be asymptomatic. Involvement of the ear frequently occurs in children, whereas sinusitis is noted more commonly in adults. Physical examination may reveal myringitis, pharyngitis, cervical lymphadenopathy, and a temperature generally ranging from 38°C to 40°C. Pleural rubs and significant effusions are uncommon findings. Sputum Gram's stains reveal polymorphonuclear leukocytes and no predominant organisms.

The roentgenologic changes most often noted are confluent or patchy consolidations with involvement of only one lobe in 40% of patients. Lower lobes (77%) were involved more frequently than upper lobes (38%).[15] Complete resolution is generally the rule, with 40% clearing by four weeks and 96% by eight weeks.[15] Radiologic changes appear to resolve more quickly in treated patients.[16]

Nonrespiratory manifestations may include cold agglutinin hemolytic anemia, arthralgias and polyarthritis, skin rashes, Stevens–Johnson syndrome, meningoencephalitis, pericarditis, myocarditis, and intravascular coagulation.

The demonstration of complement fixing antibodies is probably the most useful serologic test. Acute and convalescent sera demonstrating a fourfold increase is usually diagnostic. A single convalescent titer of 1:64 or greater is suggestive of *M pneumoniae* infection.[8]

Cold agglutinins, which are IgM antibodies that bind to the erythrocyte I antigen, are present in over 50% of patients with *M pneumoniae*.[5] The titer of cold agglutinins correlate directly with the severity of pulmonary involvement, and they usually appear by the end of the first week of illness. They remain for approximately 2–6 weeks. The presence of cold agglutinins is not diagnostic of *M pneumoniae* and can be seen with viral infections, dysproteinemias, and infectious mononucleosis. Fluorescent antibody, indirect hemagglutination, and growth inhibition tests also yield specific diagnostic information. During acute illness, a leukocytosis of 10,000–15,000 cells/mm^3 occurs in about 25% of cases. Electrocardiogram, urinalysis, electrolyte, and liver function studies show no characteristic changes.

Pneumonia caused by *M pneumoniae* should be distinguished from pneumonia from other causes. It is usually less severe than pneumococcal and other bacterial-related pneumonias, occurs throughout the year, and x-ray changes are less dense. Tuberculosis may be present in asymptomatic individuals with a pulmonary infiltrate.

Influenza viral infections or their complications by pneumococcal, streptococcal, or staphylococcal species or *Haemophilus influenzae* should be considered. Q fever, psittacosis, and tularemia are less frequent causes of pneumonia but must be included in the differential diagnosis. Legionnaires' disease may resemble a severe case of *M pneumoniae* pneumonia. The diagnosis is generally made on the basis of history and physical examination with the aid of laboratory data (appropriate serology, WBC) and chest x-ray.

The respiratory manifestations of this infection in infants or young children is similar to that in the adult patient. In younger children, *M pneumoniae* infection may be asymptomatic or associated with upper respiratory symptoms including coryza and cough. The infection is infrequently associated with pneumonia. Diagnosis is based on the results of history, physical, serologic testing, and chest x-rays, when indicated.

TREATMENT

Erythromycin and tetracycline derivatives have been effective in the treatment of *M pneumoniae* infections. This treatment has shortened the duration of fever, rales, and cough, and has hastened the resolution of chest radiologic abnormalities. However, shedding of the organism may continue for several weeks after treatment. In pregnancy, erythromycin 500 mg orally 4 times daily for 14–21 days is the regimen of choice. Erythromycin is a category B drug (indicating relative safety) for usage during pregnancy[17], and very little erythromycin actually crosses the placenta because of significant protein binding.[18]

Although the tetracyclines as a group are very effective for the treatment of *M pneumoniae* infections, they are contraindicated during pregnancy. All of the tetracyclines, including the newer semisynthetic agents, are category D drugs. They may cause yellow-brown discoloration of the deciduous teeth if given in the second half of pregnancy.[19,20] Tetracyclines have also been reported to cause a syndrome of azotemia, jaundice, and pancreatitis in pregnant women with impaired renal function.[21]

There is no known method other than isolation to prevent *M pneumoniae* infections. Both killed and live attenuated agents have thus far been ineffective as vaccines. Transmission of infection is not altered by antimicrobials.[9]

Erythromycin administered at the appropriate dose for age and body weight should be used in the neonate or child. Infants may be passively protected by maternal IgG if the mother has previously been infected.

REFERENCES

1. Eaton MD, Meiklejohn G, van Herich W. Studies in etiology of primary atypical pneumonia. A filterable agent transmissable to Cotton rats, hamsters and chick embryos. *J Exp Med.* 1944; 79:649.
2. Marmion BP, Goodburn GM. Effect of an organic gold salt on Eaton's primary atypical pneumonia agent and other observations. *Nature (London).* 1961;189:247.
3. Freundt EA. Principles of mycoplasma classification. *Ann NY Acad Sci.* 1973;225:7.
4. Denny FW, Clyde WA Jr, Glezen WP. *Mycoplasma pneumoniae* disease. Clinical spectrum, pathophysiology, epidemiology and control. *J Infect Dis.* 1971;123:74.
5. Lin JL. Human mycoplasmal infections: serologic observations. *Rev Infect Dis.* 1985;7:216.
6. Foy HM, Grayston JT, Kenny GE, et al. Epidemiology of *Mycoplasma pneumoniae* infection in families. *JAMA.* 1966;197:859.
7. Mogabgab WJ. *Mycoplasma pneumoniae* and adenovirus respiratory illnesses in military and university personnel, 1959–1966. *Amer Rev Resp Dis.* 1968;97:345.
8. Parker F Jr, Jolliffe LS, Finland M. Primary atypical pneumonia: report of eight cases with autopsy. *Arch Path (Chicago).* 1947;44:581.
9. Snepar R. *Mycoplasma pneumoniae.* In: Levison ME, ed. *The Pneumonias.* Boston, MA: John Wright PSG Inc; 1984:419.
10. Benedetti TJ, Valle R, Ledger WJ. Antepartum pneumonia in pregnancy. *Am J Obstet Gynecol.* 1982;144:413.
11. Miller MJ, Enborn JA. Congenital *Mycoplasma pneumoniae* infection. In: Thalhammer O, ed. *Prenatal Infections. International Symposium of Vienna, Sept. 2–3, 1970.* New York, NY: Grune & Stratton Inc; 1970:22.
12. Balassanian N, Robbins FC. *Mycoplasma pneumoniae* infection in families. *N Engl J Med.* 1967;277:719.
13. Hopwood H. Pneumonia and pregnancy. *Obstet Gynecol.* 1965;25:875.
14. Cassell GH, Cole BC. Mycoplasmas as agents of human disease. *N Engl J Med.* 1981;304:80.
15. Finnegan OC, Fowles SJ, White RJ. Radiographic appearances of *Mycoplasma pneumoniae. Thorax.* 1981;36:469.
16. Mufson MA, Manko MA, Kingston JR, et al. Eaton agent pneumonia. Clinical features. *JAMA.* 1961;178:369.
17. Federal Drug Administration: Pregnancy categories for prescription drugs. *FDA Drug Bulletin.* Sept 1979.
18. Fenton LJ, Light LJ. Congenital syphilis after maternal treatment with erythromycin. *Obstet Gynecol.* 1976;47:492.
19. Rendle-Short TJ. Tetracycline and teeth and bone. *Lancet.* 1962;1:1188.
20. Kutcher AH, Zegarelli EV, Tovell HM, et al. Discoloration of deciduous teeth induced by administration of tetracycline antepartum. *Am J Obstet Gynecol.* 1966;96:291.
21. Whalley PJ, Adams RH, Combs B. Tetracycline toxicity in pregnancy. *JAMA.* 1964;189:357.

Chapter Eighty-Seven
Chlamydial Infections

Charles H. Livengood III

87

MATERNAL ASPECTS

The spectrum of diseases for which *Chlamydia trachomatis* is responsible is expanding rapidly. Until recently, the organism was felt to be involved in trachoma, still the leading cause of blindness in the world, lymphogranuloma venereum (LGV), a rare chronic sexually transmissible disease that can destroy the genitalia, and in occasional cases of ophthalmia neonatorum. Additional diseases in which *C trachomatis* is currently implicated as an etiologic agent include cervicitis, acute salpingitis, urethritis, postpartum fever, endometritis, cervical neoplasia, perihepatitis, Reiter's syndrome, intrauterine fetal death, most cases of ophthalmia neonatorum, infantile pneumonia, and otitis media. *Chlamydia psittaci* remains the cause of only the zoonosis psittacosis, a pneumonic process, and affects reproductive medicine only rarely.

Etiology

The nomenclature of chlamydiae has undergone many changes, which often makes comprehension of older literature difficult. Recent improvement in our knowledge of the biology of these organisms, which were previously classified under *Miyagawanella, Bedsonia,* and others, has resulted in establishment of the order Chlamydiales, with one family, Chlamydiaceae, one genus, *Chlamydia,* and two species, *C psittaci* and *C trachomatis.* Despite their biologic similarities, the two species show little DNA homology and are thus not genetically related. Whereas *C trachomatis* multiples within an iodine-staining matrix because of accumulation of glycogen, has a rigid inclusion membrane, and is susceptible to sulfonamides, *C psittaci* multiplies within widespread cytoplasmic vesicles that do not stain with iodine, and is sulfonamide-resistant. *C psittaci* causes diseases in over 100 species of animals, whereas *C trachomatis* infects only mice and man.

These organisms are prokaryotic obligate parasites of eukaryotic cells. However, they are bacteria (not viruses) on the basis of reproduction by binary fission, sensitivity to antibiotics, and presence of DNA, RNA, enzymes, and a cell wall[1] resembling that of the gram-negative bacteria in appearance and chemical composition. The metabolic machinery of *Chlamydia* lacks only the ability to generate energy, and it is for this commodity that they enter the host cell cytoplasm in order to reproduce.

The life cycle of the chlamydiae is unique and fascinating in its adaptation, as depicted in Figure 87–1. The infecting form is the elementary body, a metabolically dormant particle of 0.2–0.3 μm diameter containing both DNA and RNA, which binds to the host cell membrane by mechanisms involving both electrostatic forces and specific sialic acid residue receptors. The elementary body then induces its own phagocytosis even in typically nonphagocytic host

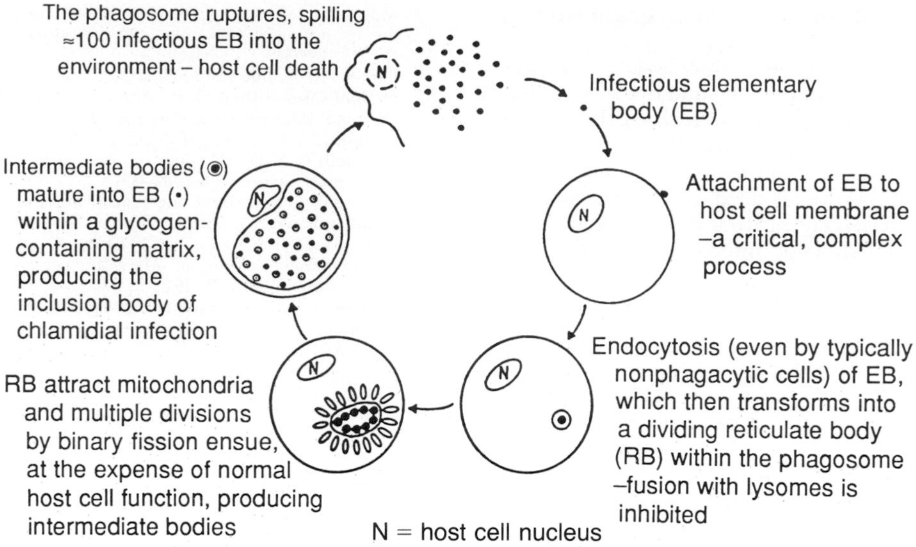

Figure 87–1. Life cycle of *Chlamydia trachomatis.*

cells and escapes killing by preventing fusion of the phagosome with lysosomes. It is known that prostaglandins play an important role in *Chlamydia* uptake by eukaryotic cells. The elementary body reorganizes during the first few hours in the phagosome into a reticulate body, the dividing form of chlamydiae. During the next 20–30 hours reticulate bodies divide rapidly, recruiting energy and metabolites and thus inhibiting normal function of the host cell, and the phagosome enlarges into the typical cytoplasmic inclusion body surrounded by energy-giving mitochondria. Reticulate bodies destined to mature rather than divide from intermediate bodies. At 48–72 hours after infection, presently undefined mechanisms result in inclusion lysis and host cell death with release of about 100 mature, infectious elementary bodies into the environment.

Chlamydiae have multiple antigens. There are group antigens shared by both species, and these react in the complement fixation and hemagglutination tests. Species-specific antigens exist but have proven difficult to purify. There are 15 type-specific antigens within the *C trachomatis* species, closely associated with the elementary body form, which also act as lethal toxins in mice; these react in the microimmunofluorescence (micro-IF) test.

Of the 15 serotypes of *C trachomatis,* three groups can be identified. Serotypes A, B, Ba, and C cause endemic trachoma. Serotypes D, E, F, G, H, I, J, and K are the oculogenital serotypes and are the group implicated in the current explosion of diseases that *C trachomatis* may cause. Serotypes L_1, L_2, and L_3 cause LGV. The first two groups are sometimes lumped under the term *TRIC agents,* for trachoma inclusion conjunctivitis agents.

Chlamydiae are highly temperature-sensitive. They have only limited survival rates at more than 37°C and less than 4°C unless frozen below −40°C. Survival of infectivity in media requires addition of stabilizing agents such as serum or milk.[2] *C psittaci* and the LGV strains show considerably more tolerance to *in vitro* conditions than the TRIC strains and are less delicate during isolation. *C trachomatis* is sensitive to tetracyclines, erythromycin, sulfonamides, rifampin, and chloramphenicol; penicillins have some inhibitory effect on multiplication *in vitro,* but after removal of drug, normal organism function resumes. *C psittaci* has the same antibiotic sensitivities with the exception of its resistance to sulfa drugs.

Cases of atypical pneumonia associated with exposure to wild birds were reported during the 19th century, but it was not until 1930 that the infectious origin of psittacosis was demonstrated by isolation of *C psittaci* from human and avian tissues. In 1909, cytoplasmic inclusions were found in Giemsa-stained conjunctival scrapings from infants with opththalmitis, and the similarity was noted for findings in like preparations from patients with trachoma. In 1910, cytoplasmic inclusions in conjunctival scrapings from a baby with conjunctivitis and the mother's cervix were described, and the agent was confirmed to be *C trachomatis* in a mother-infant pair in 1959. LGV has been described as a discrete disease entity since early in this century.

Pathogenesis and Pathology

Psittacosis results from inhalation of infected dried bird excreta, handling of contaminated feathers, and even brief exposure to infected birds, which usually appear healthy. Person-to-person transmission and infection by dressed poultry are extremely rare. After entering the bronchial tree, *C psittaci* reaches the reticuloendothelial cells of the liver and spleen, where it replicates. Subsequent hematogenous spread results in a systemic illness with most prominent involvement of the lung. Focal areas of edema, necrosis, and small hemorrhages occur particularly in the dependent lobes. Microscopically, the alveolar septa and air spaces are primarily involved, with a mononuclear infiltrate, serous exudate, and sometimes frank necrosis. The pleura and bronchial tree are generally spared, but hilar lymphadenitis is common. The hematogenous nature of the infection is expressed as focal inflammation and necrosis of the liver and spleen. Severe cases include involvement of the myocardium, pericardium, brain, meninges, and adrenals.[3]

Trachoma consists of a chronic follicular keratoconjunctivitis; after multiple infections, corneal scarring and vascularization (pannus formation) occur. Distortion of the eyelids may occur from scarring. Bacterial superinfection significantly augments these pathogenetic events. Some investigators conclude that trachoma is an immunopathogenic disease, noting that efforts at immunization with a lower titer of antigenic particles or with killed organisms predispose to more severe infection and more rapid evolution of blindness. Classically, trachoma is not a systemic disease, but it has been suggested that the increased incidence of pneumonia and diarrhea in these patients may reflect disseminated chlamydial infection.

LGV is a sexually transmitted disease occurring in three stages. First, an inconspicuous genital or anal papule or ulcer appears and heals quickly without scarring at the site of inoculation. Histologically, this lesion is a nonspecific ulceration with mononuclear infiltrate, edema, fibroblastic proliferation, endothelial hyperplasia, and vascular engorgement; sometimes inclusion bodies can be identified within phagocytes. In the second stage, the regional lymph nodes are the primary victims, although constitutional symptoms are common. These nodes initially enlarge with nonspecific hyperplasia and eventually mat together as perinodal tissue is involved. Histologically, small granulomas with necrotic centers develop, and these coalesce to form branching sinuses of suppurative necrosis with a granulomatous wall consisting of fibroblasts in a radial palisade arrangement, reticuloendothelial cells, and macrophages with an epithelioid appearance; plasma cells and lymphocytes surround this wall. Fibrosis and lymphedema are the hallmarks of the third stage, with strictures of the rectum, vagina, and urethra and elephantiasis of the genitalia common.

Our knowledge of the pathogenesis of female genital infection by the oculogenital serotypes of *C trachomatis* is in a phase of rapid evolution. It is currently believed that this organism behaves like *Neisseria gonorrhoeae* in many respects. That is, transmission is primarily by sexual contact with a male whose urethra harbors the organism, which may produce infection of the columnar epithelium of the endocervix, urethra, and rectum; upper genital infection and its sequelae may subsequently ensue in a certain fraction of these women as a result of canalicular ascent of the organism; and neonatal infection may occur as a result of intrapartum inoculation. Hare et al[4] and others have described the colposcopic and histologic features of chlamydial cervicitis. Generally, they report on colposcopy the finding of an exophytic follicular cervicitis with edematous ectopy and a follicular appearance to the transformation zone. Less uniformly, they report on histology the finding of subepithelial lymphoid follicles with otherwise nonspecific findings of an intense inflammatory cell infiltrate and intraepithelial microabscesses.

Mardh and coworkers[5] first suggested *C trachomatis* as an etiologic agent in acute pelvic inflammatory disease (PID), isolating the organism from the endocervix in 19 of 53 patients with PID and from the oviducts in 6 of 20 patients with PID. Subsequently, a large body of evidence from Scandinavia and Western Europe has accumulated to support their work. Studies in grivet monkeys have shown that *C trachomatis* instilled into the endocervix or endometrium produced an endosalpingitis identical to that caused by *N gonorrhoeae* in man, including the luminal route of ascent and associated perihepatitis (Fitz-Hugh–Curtis syndrome). Oviduct histology in two women with PID presumably caused by *Chlamydia* was found to be almost identical to that in gonococcal salpingitis. Curiously, Hutchinson and coworkers[6] were able to show replication of *C trachomatis* in human oviduct organ cultures in the absence of pathologic change; this finding is consistent with the immunopathogenic mechanism of damage suggested in trachoma.

The immunology of infection by the oculogenital strains of *C trachomatis* remains an unsettled issue. Both humoral and cell-mediated immunity are raised against these organisms, but neither seems to provide solid immunity to reinfection. Although some contend that chlamydial antibody titer and culture positivity are inversely related, others describe a direct relationship. Further difficulty in understanding humoral immune response to these agents arises as a result of the high positive background in most populations, variable antibody response to infection, difficulty in obtaining paired serum samples in the typically indolent diseases caused by *C trachomatis*, and blunting of antibody response by antibiotic administration. These same issues clearly have an impact on the use of serology in diagnosis of infection by these agents.

Epidemiology

Psittacosis is found all over the world, with about 50 cases annually in the United States. The disease occurs in sporadic outbreaks, and owners of pet birds account for half of all cases. Workers in pet stores, poultry workers, zoo workers, and veterinarians are at high risk as well. The incidence of psittacosis has declined markedly in the United States, probably because of the addition of tetracycline to poultry feed, the requirement for 30 days of medication prior to importation of psittacine (parrot-related) birds, and growth in the domestic breeding of parakeets. *C psittaci* may be acquired by women intimately exposed to aborting ewes and cows; septic abortion can in turn result for these women.

Trachoma is a disease prevalent in impoverished countries with limited public sanitation and absence of a tradition of personal hygiene. As human conditions improve in the world, the incidence of trachoma declines. Nonetheless, trachoma remains the single most common cause of blindness in the world, with an estimated 400 million people affected by the disease and resultant blindness in two million. North Africa, northern India, and the Middle East remain endemic areas.

Lymphogranuloma venereum is most prevalent in tropical countries, especially India, Indonesia, East Africa, Vietnam, and Central and South America. In the United States, the disease was most common after World War II but has declined since then to around 300 cases annually. As with the other sexually transmitted diseases, male homosexuals now comprise a significant portion of the reservoir of this disease; LGV is reported three times as often among men as it is among women. Additionally, persons of low socioeconomic status living in the Southeast and those returning from endemic areas are at increased risk[7], as are those with numerous sexual contacts.

The oculogenital serotypes of *C trachomatis* are presently estimated to be the most prevalent sexually transmitted disease agent in the developed world. Among PID patients in Western Europe, about 30% harbor this organism in the endocervix, as opposed to endocervical *N gonorrhoeae* in 10–20%. Among patients with clinically diagnosed mild PID in Vancouver, endocervical *Chlamydia* is found in one half and gonorrhea in one third. In the United States, one third of the cases of PID are presently caused by genital *Chlamydia* infection. *C trachomatis* has been isolated from the endocervix in 20% of women attending sexually transmitted disease clinics in the United States. Among asymptomatic patients in Vancouver and the United States[8], *C trachomatis* has been isolated from the endocervix two and ten times, respectively, more often than *N gonorrhoeae*. Among women with gornorrhea, *Chlamydia* is also found in the endocervix of 27–63%, and in Sweden the figure is as high as 79%. In addition to PID and gonorrhea, other factors increasing the likelihood of chlamydial endocervicitis are oral contraceptive use, younger age, absence of pelvic pain, and complaints of vaginal discharge. Sexual transmission rates from men to women of the oculogenital serotypes of *C trachomatis* have been reported at 45–74%, as opposed to about 80% for gonorrhea in the same study populations. Among women whose male partners have nongonococcal urethritis, 35–43% have been found to have chlamydial cervicitis.

Manifestations

Psittacosis exhibits a variable clinical course.[9] After an incubation period of one to two weeks (or longer), the patient experiences either sudden onset of a febrile illness or onset of malaise over several days. The pulse is often slow relative to the degree of fever, and malaise, myalgias, arthralgias, and anorexia are common. Headache is the most consistent complaint and is often severe. A persistent cough appears at onset of illness or a few days thereafter and is generally productive of only a small amount of sputum, sometimes streaked with blood. After a week of this illness, lassitude and confusion may occur and may progress to stupor and coma if hypoxia is severe. Gastrointestinal symptoms (nausea, vomiting, diarrhea) are less common, and jaundice occurs only in severely affected patients. On physical examination, fine rales in the lower lung fields, pleural and pericardial friction rubs, and hepatosplenomegaly may be found. X-ray findings vary from localized infiltrates to consolidation of a lung, but patchy infiltrates radiating out from the hilum are most common. The white blood count remains in or near the normal range, anemia is rare, and liver function tests and cerebrospinal fluid remain normal. Gram's stain of the sputum reveals only some leukocytes and no organisms.

Trachoma manifests after a 5- to 10-day incubation period as a sudden onset of conjunctivitis in a person in an area where the disease is endemic. Fingers, flies, and fomites transfer the disease from eye to eye. In such areas, 91% of children aged 5–9 years are infected. After several weeks, necrotic follicles of inflammatory cells develop beneath the conjunctival mucosa, usually at the edge of the upper eyelid. At this point, spontaneous healing occurs slowly unless there is reinfection. With multiple recurrent infections, especially when there is bacterial superinfection, corneal vascularization (pannus formation), usually beginning at the upper limbus, and conjunctival scarring with trichiasis and entropion eventually result in blindness.

LGV begins one to two weeks (range 3–30 days)[10] after infection as one (occasionally multiple) small vesiculopapule, which often degenerates into a superficial ulceration. This lesion is not tender, heals quickly, does not scar, and rarely causes the patient to see the physician. Only 25–35% of patients with LGV notice the primary lesion, which may occur within the vagina or rectum.[11] Several weeks later, unilateral (2/3 of cases) or bilateral (1/3 of cases) regional adenopathy develops, with firm, tender, discrete nodes at first. After a week, the nodes mat together and become fluctuant (*bubo formation*). In men, the inguinal and femoral nodes may be involved, with the inguinal ligament fixed between them, creating the "sign of the groove." This conformation is characteristic although not pathognomonic of LGV in men, but is rarely seen in women. The buboes eventually begin to drain through multiple cutaneous sinus tracts and tend to continue to do so for months prior to healing, which is accompanied by scarring. Among women with internal genital primary lesions, the internal pelvic nodes are affected, which is usually not identified on examination; thus, women are more likely than men to present in the last (tertiary) stage of the disease.

During the secondary stage, LGV commonly causes nonspecific constitutional symptoms of fever, chills, myalgia, and athralgia; erythema nodosum may be seen. Leukocytosis, an increase in the erythrocyte sedimentation rate, hypergammaglobulinemia, and elevated serum liver enzymes are common in this stage. In the years following the stage of adenopathy, chronic changes of lymphatic destruction occur and comprise the tertiary stage of disease. These changes consist of rectal, vaginal, and perineal fistula formation, fibrosis, stricturing of the urethra, vagina, and rectum, and lymphedema, which can progress to elephantiasis (Figure 87–2). Such scarring and deformity of the lower genitalia in parturients predispose to severe perineal laceration, and cesarean delivery should be considered for these patients. Extragenital LGV can occur, usually oropharyngeal in location, and is associated with cervical adenopathy and aseptic meningitis.

Manifestations of disease caused by the oculogenital *C trachomatis* are many and are not yet comfortably defined, but they generally follow a theme of prolonged, indolent, often subclinical disease. *C trachomatis* is now well-known to be a common cause of nongonococcal urethritis; it is the vector by which women contract chlamydial cervicitis during coitus. As noted above, chlamydial cervicitis manifests as an edematous, follicular, exophytic inflammation with a mucopurulent endocervical discharge; cervical tenderness is usually encountered. However, up to 50% of cases are asymptomatic, and Arya et al[12] report identification of only one third of cases of history and examination.

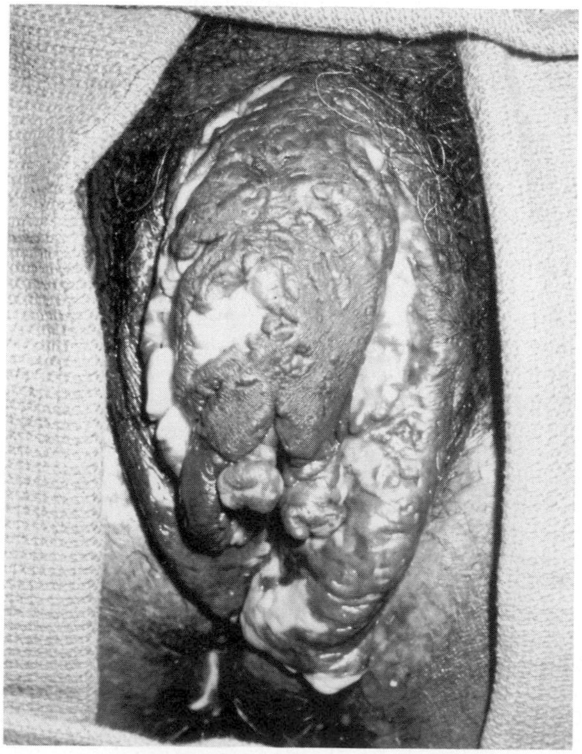

Figure 87–2. Chronic vulvar lymphedema in longstanding LGV. This mass was resected after three weeks of antibiotic therapy. Urethral, vaginal, and rectal strictures did not require therapy in this patient.

In the United States, McCormack et al[13] report that of seven untreated asymptomatic women with chlamydial cervicitis, four remained infected 15 or more months later. Thus, this infection frequently follows a protracted subclinical course. Preinvasive and invasive cervical neoplasia is reported in 8% and 18%, respectively, of women with positive *Chlamydia* cultures from the cervix, as opposed to 1% of controls without neoplasia. Antichlamydial cervical IgA has been found in 69% of women with neoplasia and in 12% of normal controls, and antichlamydial antibody in the serum is found twice as often among women with neoplasia as among controls matched carefully for other risk factors. Thus, *Chlamydia* and cervical neoplasia have a confirmed association, although a causative relationship is unproved. When the female urethral syndrome is defined as dysuria, pyuria, and fewer than 10^5 colonies/mL of a single organism on routine bacterial culture, over one half of such patients harbor *C trachomatis* in the urethra; unfortunately, relief of symptoms after treatment with antichlamydial drugs is variable.

Chlamydial endometritis has been reported in association with PID, providing further evidence for the luminal route of spread of this organism in PID. Wager et al[14] describe a fourfold rise in infectious morbidity after vaginal delivery among women with prenatal genital *Chlamydia* infections. Severe postcesarean pelvic infections requiring extirpation of the reproduction organs, apparently caused by *C trachomatis*, have been reported. Pelvic infection after therapeutic abortion appears to be another entity associated with chlamydial infection, increasing the incidence by three to ten times.[15] Treatment with antichlamydial antibiotics prior to the procedure appears to eliminate this excess morbidity. The well-founded belief that *C trachomatis* causes PID in a fashion similar to the gonococcus is described above. About 10% of women with chlamydial cervicitis will progress spontaneously to such upper genital infection, and these patients more commonly complain of abnormal vaginal bleeding and have a higher erythrocyte sedimentation rate at presentation than women with PID of other etiology. However, the most important aspect of PID associated with *C trachomatis* is the indolent, often subclinical nature of the disease despite major, ongoing tubal destruction. Among otherwise asymptomatic women undergoing laparoscopy prior to tuboplasty for infertility in Paris, Henry-Suchet and her colleagues identified *C trachomatis* in the upper genital tract in 20–25%.[16] Several groups of investigators have identified the presence of chlamydial antibodies in the serum as a powerful predictor of tubal disease in infertile women. *C trachomatis* also appears to be capable of inducing Fitz-Hugh–Curtis syndrome (PID-associated perihepatitis).

Adult conjunctivitis caused by oculogenital strains of *C trachomatis* is a great deal less common than the neonatal form. When it does occur, there is usually the acute onset of conjunctival irritation, mucopurulent discharge, and photophobia. The conjunctiva takes on an edematous, follicular appearance, but in the absence of reinfection and bacterial superinfection, healing without scarring occurs slowly over many months. Although these eye infections are less virulent than those caused by the trachoma strains, it should be noted that they differ little in most respects and that the potential for reinfection and serious sequelae by the oculogenital strains will probably be enhanced as sexual transmission increases their prevalence. Other adult diseases in which the oculogenital *C trachomatis* has been implicated include endocarditis, myocarditis, pneumonia, Reiter's syndrome, epididymitis, and meningoencephalitis.

Diagnosis

As a rule, the diagnosis of chlamydial diseases is difficult, time consuming, and often confirmed long after therapy. This is especially true for the oculogenital strains, and it continues to pose a major obstacle to our understanding of the diseases they cause.

Psittacosis is generally diagnosed by serology; isolation of *C psittaci* from sputum can also be used but poses considerable hazard to those in the laboratory, so that few hospitals offer this service. In the unusual instance in which isolation is required, physicians should contact the Virology Laboratories of the Centers for Disease Control for instructions as to submission of specimens. Confirmed serologic diagnosis requires a fourfold rise in titer of paired sera in the complement fixation assay. Antibody titers usually begin to rise by the end of the second week of illness, so the second specimen should not be drawn until this time; administration of antibiotics delays the appearance of antibody by several weeks. Presumptive diagnosis is often made by demonstration of a single titer of 1:16 or greater. Clinically, the presence of splenomegaly in a patient with pneumonia and a history of exposure to fowl or aborting pastoral animals is suggestive, especially when additional prominent features are headache, pulse–temperature disparity, high fever, and failure to improve with penicillin therapy. The differential diagnosis includes mycoplasmal pneumonia, tuberculosis, legionnaires' disease, fungal infection, and tularemia; brucellosis, hepatitis, and infectious mononucleosis must be considered when the pneumonic process is less pronounced.

Trachoma is suspected in patients with severe conjunctivitis involving primarily the upper palpebral and bulbar conjunctivae, a protracted course, and recent exposure to a trachoma-endemic area. Diagnosis is confirmed by scraping (swabbings are relatively useless, because inclusion bodies must be observed within host epithelial cells) the upper fornix with a sterile metal spatula, spreading this specimen on a clean glass microscopy slide, and looking for typical cytoplasmic chlamydial inclusions with Giemsa staining. Slides must be evaluated for 20 minutes by the clock prior to being declared negative.

LGV should always be considered in a patient with genital ulceration, although the benign nature of this disease rarely brings the patient to medical attention. Diagnosis at this stage is dependent on culture of the organism from scrapings of the lesion or procurement of an acute phase serum sample. The chancre of syphilis is usually more prominent and indurated and is associated with painless regional adenopathy, a positive darkfield evaluation, and sometimes a rash. Herpes genitalis usually presents with more painful crops of vesicles and ulcers, a positive viral culture or Tzanck preparation, and nonsuppurative adenopathy. In chancroid, the lesion or lesions are more tender and the adenopathy is more typical of a unilocular bubo. In granuloma inguinale, the lesion is chronic, progressive, and larger, and the regional adenopathy is not suppurative. The second stage of LGV presents with indurated, matted, tender inguinal or femoral adenopathy from which multiple draining sinuses may develop. Diagnosis at this stage is usually made by demonstration of complement-fixing antibodies at a titer of 1:64 or greater or by a fourfold rise in titer in the rare instance that an acute phase sample is available. Affected nodes should be aspirated for culture for *C trachomatis*; if pus cannot be aspirated, 1 cc of nonbacteriostatic saline should be injected and aspirated. Although some sources suggest that culture of bubo aspirates lacks sensitivity, their studies reflect older methods of isolating the organism, and the technique definitely should be included in evaluation of these patients. In the third stage of LGV, in which women commonly first present, cultures are rarely positive. Although LGV serology usually is positive, titers may have declined below the definitive level of 64 or greater, and the diagnosis is often made on clinical grounds. The female patient who presents with chronic vulvar lymphedematous change, stricturing of the vagina, urethra, or low rectum, inguinal cicatrix, and history compatible with LGV should be treated for LGV. It must be remembered that the other sexually transmitted diseases often accompany LGV, and they should be ruled out in these patients.

Diagnosis of infection by the oculogenital strains of *C trachomatis* should be made by isolation of the organism from infected tissue. This technique is demanding but not unreasonable; with the identification of these organisms as common pathogens, most hospitals should offer the service of *Chlamydia* culture. In 1991, a typical charge for *Chlamydia* culture is $50 to $75 per specimen. In specimen procurement, physicians must be aware that infected host cells are the only component of the specimen that will yield a positive culture; thus, vigorous swabbing, a biopsy, or scraping of the site must be employed, and pus should be excluded as much as possible. Also, Mardh and Zeeberg[17] and others have shown that swabs tipped with calcium alginate or charcoal granules, or those with wooden sticks are unsuitable for obtaining specimens for chlamydia culture; cotton- or rayon-tipped swabs on aluminum or plastic sticks yield the most sensitive results. Specimens are placed into transport medium and kept on ice until delivered to the laboratory within 24 hours. Culture technique subsequently involves inoculation of the specimens onto cell monolayers (tissue culture) treated with antimitotic agents, centrifugation, incubation, and staining with iodine, Giemsa stain, or fluorescein-labeled antibody to identify the typical cytoplasmic inclusions of *C trachomatis* infection.

Results are generally available three days after the specimen is inoculated, although some laboratories employ subculture, which requires twice as long to establish a final report. Such isolation can be considered to have essentially 100% specificity and 90–95% sensitivity when proper technique is employed, and it is the method of choice for confirmation of genital infection by these organisms. In women being evaluated for lower genital infection by oculogenital *C trachomatis*, endocervical specimens are taken, and an additional 15% of patients so infected will be identified by including a urethral specimen. In upper genital infection, endometrial aspirate, swabbings, or biopsy, and endosalpingeal swabbings or biopsy have been employed.

Direct examination of stained (Giemsa or immunofluorescent) scrapings from infected tissues is useful only in conjunctival infection by oculogenital *C trachomatis*. The technique is as described for trachoma, except that the lower eyelid conjunctiva is sampled rather than the upper. In such preparations, chlamydial inclusions are large, intracytoplasmic, granular, and often indent the nucleus, as shown in Figure 87–3. Under Giemsa stain, the DNA-predominant elementary bodies are red-purple. When a Giemsa-stained inclusion is viewed with darkfield microscopy, the elementary bodies show a golden-yellow autofluorescence. In genital infection, cytologic diagnosis by Papanicolaou's stain has been advocated, but its accuracy remains uncertain. Purola and Paavonen[18] convincingly warn against use of this modality for diagnosis.

Oculogenital *C trachomatis* is a much less effective antigen than the LGV strains or *C psittaci*. Thus, antibody response is variable, often weak, and adversely affected by curative or even suppressive antibiotic therapy; the prevalence of such antibodies is high in most populations. The micro-IF test must be used to detect such antibody and is exceptionally tedious, easily misinterpreted, and performed by very few laboratories. Although many studies have employed serology to evaluate the role of oculogenital *C trachomatis* in human infection, Schachter[19] and coworkers have shown that this modality is too inaccurate for individual diagnosis. An exception is in neonatal pneumonia, when a single titer of 1024 or greater is reliable. Evaluation of local antibody production may be proven in the future to be useful. An overview of diagnostic techniques is provided in Table 87–1.

Newer, rapid tests that are now available for diagnosis of oculogenital *C trachomatis* infection fall into two categories: enzyme immunoassay (Chlamydiazyme, Abbott Laboratories, and others) and direct fluorescent antibody staining (MicroTrak, Syva Company, and others). Enzyme immunoassay tests have the advantages of requiring no expertise

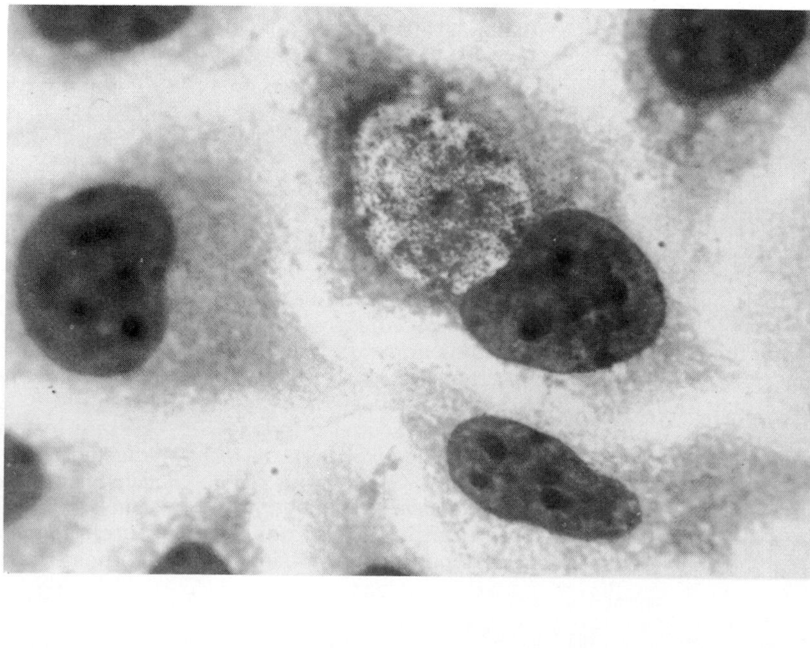

Figure 87–3. Giemsa stain of cytoplasmic inclusions of McCoy cell infected by *Chlamydia trachomatis*. Under light microscopy, these granular lesions contain blue-purple or red-purple organisms. Clear halo around perimeter of inclusion is characteristic. (*From Bird and Forrester*[2], with permission.)

TABLE 87–1. COMPARISON OF DIAGNOSTIC METHODS FOR *CHLAMYDIA TRACHOMATIS* INFECTION

	Direct Examination			Isolation			Serology	
Infection	IF	Giemsa	Iodine	Cell Culture (treated)	Eggs (yolk sac)	Mice	Micro-IF	CF
Eye								
Newborn	Excellent	Excellent	Good	Excellent	Excellent	—[a]	Good	—
Adult	Excellent	Good	—	Excellent	Good	—	Good	—
Genital								
Urethra	Good	Fair	—	Excellent	Good	—	Good	—
Cervix	Good	Good	—	Excellent	Good	—	Good	—
Bubo	—	—	—	Excellent	Excellent	Good	Good	Good
Fallopian tubes[b]				Excellent			Good	
Respiratory[b]				Excellent			Good	

[a] Not suitable
[b] Data limited
From Bird and Forester[2]

for interpretation, and they are inexpensive; their sensitivity varies in existing studies from 70–90% and their specificity varies from 75–99%. Direct fluorescent antibody stains are somewhat more accurate, with sensitivity reported at 80–99% and specificity at 96% or more in most studies; these tests are also rapid and inexpensive, but extensive interpreter experience and dedication are required for accurate results. In the absence of laboratory diagnostic technique with carefully documented accuracy, physicians are strongly encouraged to employ presumptive treatment strategies endorsed by the Centers for Disease Control in patients at risk as described in Table 87–2.

TABLE 87–2. WOMEN AT SUFFICIENT RISK FOR GENITAL *CHLAMYDIA* INFECTION TO JUSTIFY PRESUMPTIVE TREATMENT IN THE ABSENCE OF A HIGHLY RELIABLE LABORATORY DIAGNOSTIC TEST[a]

Male sexual partner with urethritis or epididymitis
Cervicitis, especially with mucopurulent discharge
Pelvic inflammatory disease
Infant with chlamydial infection
Any gonococcal infection
Any two: age <20 years, multiple sexual partners, oral contraceptive use, sexually active women of lower socioeconomic status
Late postpartum endometritis
Postabortal endometritis
Sterile pyuria
Any other newly acquired STD
Pelvic pain
Infertility
Ectopic pregnancy
Prepubertal vaginitis
Cervical neoplasia
Histologic severe endometritis
History of any of the above without intervening treatment for *Chlamydia trachomatis*

[a] Presented in approximate order of likelihood of infection

Treatment

Psittacosis in nonpregnant persons carries a low mortality, now less than 1%, when managed with appropriate supportive measures and antichlamydial chemotherapy. Recommended therapy is 2–3 g of tetracycline hydrochloride in divided doses daily; this should be continued for 2 weeks after a clear response, because relapses are common. Response usually is seen in 2–3 days after initiation of therapy, but may occur more slowly. Psittacosis in late pregnancy, based on the few case reports available, is a lethal disease. Beer and colleagues[20] report two cases of psittacosis contracted from sheep in the third trimester of gestation in which patients presented with fulminant sepsis, with resistant disseminated intravascular coagulation and hypoxemia the most conspicuous components. The authors felt that erythromycin therapy was ineffectual until delivery was effected, citing the placentophilic nature of *C psittaci* in animals and death in their patient whose delivery was delayed. When a patient with recent history of intimate avian or animal exposure presents in the third trimester with fulminant sepsis and other evidence of psittacosis, it would seem prudent to deliver promptly, include erythromycin or chloramphenicol in the choice of antibiotics, and obtain a serum sample for acute phase serology. Maternal complications of *C psittaci* infection in early pregnancy seem limited to spontaneous abortion, as described below.

Trachoma is localized to the eye, and thus the pregnant woman is at no increased risk. Treatment requires prolonged antimicrobial therapy with doxycycline, 2.5–4 mg/kg once daily, for 40 days. Data on therapy in pregnancy are outstanding, but an equally prolonged course of erythromycin (ethylsuccinate, base, or stearate), 500 mg by mouth four times daily, should be effective as well. Improved personal hygiene is an integral part of the treatment of trachoma.

Treatment of LGV should consist of at least two weeks of antichlamydial chemotherapy, treatment of all sexual partners, hot compresses to ulcerations, and needle aspiration of fluctuant lymph nodes through adjacent normal skin; incision and drainage of buboes are contraindicated, as chronic fistulae are thereby encouraged. Antibiotic choice in nonpregnant individuals may consist of tetracycline hydrochloride, 500 mg by mouth four times daily, or doxycycline, 100 mg by mouth twice daily; in pregnant patients use either erythromycin, 500 mg by mouth four times daily, or sulfamethoxazole 1 g by mouth four times daily.[21] In late LGV, chronically lymphedematous tissues will not resolve after medical therapy, and resection for cosmetic reasons is sometimes required; attempts to dilate symptomatic rectal strictures usually result in perforation, and a two-stage resection and reanastomosis are usually necessary.

Treatment of patients infected by the oculogenital strains of *C trachomatis* is not as prolonged as that for the other chlamydial diseases, but neither is it as straightforward as that for gonorrhea. At present, the suboptimal situation of relying on compliance of patients with a sexually transmitted disease exists in the treatment of these organisms, and this will undoubtedly contribute to their prevalence. For uncomplicated lower genital infection in women, therapy must be continued for at least seven days. First-line regimens are tetracycline hydrochloride, 500 mg by mouth four times daily, or doxycycline, 100 mg by mouth twice daily. In pregnancy, erythromycin, 500 mg by mouth four times daily, is recommended; gastrointestinal symptoms are frequently intractable with this dose, and erythromycin, 250 mg by mouth four times daily for 14 days, may be used. In pregnant women who cannot tolerate erythromycin, tetracycline, chloramphenicol, and rifampin are all contraindicated. The remaining drug from which efficacy might be expected is sulfamethoxazole or sulfisoxazole, and a dose of 1 g by mouth four times daily for a minimum of two weeks would seem reasonable. Scant data are available to support use of this regimen[22], and sulfa drugs should be avoided in the third trimester because of icterus induced by displacement of bilirubin from plasma proteins by these drugs. All male sexual partners must be treated as well.

Test-of-cure cultures from the site(s) originally positive are of great importance, but should not be undertaken until four weeks after treatment. Isolates resistant to one or more of the usually effective drugs have been described. Lack of efficacy against *C trachomatis* of the old and new penicillins and cephalosporins, aminoglycosides, aminocyclitols (spectinomycin), and imidazoles (metronidazole) has been demonstrated. Some early investigations suggest that macrolides other than erythromycin (clindamycin, rosarimicin) may be active against *Chlamydia*. New fluoroquinolones, particularly afloxacin and temafloxacin, show promise for treatment of genital chlamydial infection.

For upper genital and the deep soft tissue infections caused by oculogenital *C trachomatis*, a tetracycline or erythromycin in doses as for uncomplicated genital infection for a minimum of 10 or 14 days, respectively, is advised. In adult conjunctivitis caused by these agents, systemic, not topical, therapy with an effective antibiotic for at least two weeks is suggested.

Prevention

Prevention of psittacosis involves careful handwashing after intimate animal exposure, avoidance of imported psittacine birds without documentation of 30 days of antibiotic therapy, avoidance of avian excreta, and elimination of sick birds and chronically aborting animals from the environment. Pregnant women should not be exposed to persons with undiagnosed atypical pneumonia. Prevention of trachoma requires improved public sanitation and personal hygiene; these measures are actually more important in eradicating the disease and subsequent blindness than antibiotic therapy. LGV can be prevented by more selective sexual association, and transmission probably can be decreased by use of condoms. Further declines in LGV incidence may be achieved by more widespread use of empiric therapy for the oculogenital strains.

The first step in prevention of infections caused by oculogenital *C trachomatis* must be raising the index of suspicion of health care providers, especially obstetrician–gynecologists, urologists, and personnel in sexually transmitted disease clinics. Transmission is probably eliminated by use of condoms. Empiric therapy for those at high risk on epidemiologic grounds must become common. Finally, a rapid, simple, accurate method of diagnosing infection caused by these organisms is greatly needed, as are more data about the diseases they cause.

FETAL ASPECTS

Pathology

C psittaci is a known abortifacient in animals. This organism has been associated with human spontaneous abortion as well, but reported cases are limited to pastoral regions in Europe and Asia. Intrauterine fetal death is associated with maternal psittacosis in late pregnancy. Beer and colleagues[20] have suggested that *C psittaci* has an affinity for the placenta and that this is expressed as fetal wastage resulting from hematogenous dissemination of the organism during maternal infection. Fetal infection resulting from transplacental transmission occurs and is a cause of neonatal sepsis, although a healthy baby may be born to a woman with active *C psittaci* sepsis.

Although trachoma has no known effects on the fetus, acquisition of the disease early in life is the rule in endemic areas.

There are no reports of sequelae for the fetus arising from maternal LGV. Acquisition of the organism during passage through an infected birth canal has not been reported; if this were to occur, one would predict serious consequences for the neonate.

Whereas the oculogenital strains of *C trachomatis* carry distinct risks for the neonate, their effect on the fetus is unclear. Driscoll[23] in Boston has cultured placentas from equal numbers of three groups of infants: those with fetal or neonatal deaths, those requiring intensive care, and those who are healthy term infants. None of the 236 placentas tested has revealed the presence of *C trachomatis*. Martin et al[24] in Seattle demonstrated fetal or neonatal death ten times more often and a shorter mean pregnancy duration among women harboring *C trachomatis* in the endocervix than among uninfected controls. Heggie et al[25] in Cleveland found no increase in fetal or neonatal death, premature delivery, premature rupture of membranes, or spontaneous abortion associated with endocervical chlamydial infection. However, the great majority of recent literature clearly associates genital chlamydia infection in pregnancy with preterm premature rupture of membranes, preterm birth, preterm labor, and low birth weight.[26-29] At present, obstetricians should view maternal genital chlamydial infection as a major risk factor for adverse pregnancy outcome, and they should manage their patients accordingly.

Maternal-fetal transmission of oculogenital *C trachomatis* is thought to be a result of direct contact during the second stage of labor. It has been suggested that infants delivered from infected mothers by cesarean section with intact membranes can also acquire the organism, but this remains to be confirmed. The primary portal of entry for the fetus is believed to be the eye, with subsequent spread to the nasopharynx by way of the lacrimal ducts, and from there to the bronchial tree by aspiration or to the middle ear by the eustachian tubes. The fetus then becomes at risk for chlamydial infection at any of these sites. Neonatal chlamydial conjunctivitis (inclusion blennorrhea) is prevented by erythromycin (but not silver nitrate) drops[30] and pathologically is similar to the adult form of inclusion conjunctivitis with primarily lower lid involvement. However, lymphoid follicle formation is rare in neonates. The rapidity of onset correlates with the size of the inoculum, whereas the severity of illness does not. Asymptomatic cases have been reported. The infection heals slowly, with or without sequelae, over 1–2 months, but sometimes requires as long as 2 years. Nasopharyngeal infection alone seems to be an asymptomatic entity, but it presumably serves as the reservoir from which otitis media and pneumonia develop, and it is apparently not prevented even by topical erythromycin prophylaxis. These infants shed the organism from the respiratory tract for about one year.[31] There is strong evidence that neonatal vaginitis and proctitis can result from intrapartum acquisition of these organisms. Chlamydial pneumonia of the neonate is characterized pathologically by a nonspecific interstitial pneumonia, which may evolve into necrotizing bronchiolitis, pulmonary consolidation with mononuclear alveolar infiltrate, and pericarditis. Chlamydial inclusions are not detected in these lung sections, and it has been postulated that a hypersensitivity reaction may account for a significant portion of the pathogenesis of neonatal chlamydial pneumonia. Passive transfer of maternal antibody confers no protection to the exposed fetus.

Epidemiology

At present, maternal-fetal transmission of *C psittaci* must be considered an extremely rare event, especially in the United States. However, the organism should be considered in the setting of women with abortion or stillbirth with intimate exposure to animals or avians. Trachomas will be found almost exclusively in neonates with postnatal exposure to an endemic area. Neonatal LGV is extremely rare and apparently results only from postnatal exposure; clearly, it suggests sexual abuse of the infant.

The endocervix is colonized by oculogenital *C trachomatis* in 2–18% of pregnant women, and it has been suggested that these organisms are currently the most common sexually transmitted disease agents passed on to the fetus. Prospective mothers with multiple sexual partners are up to ten times more likely to have chlamydial cervicitis than those with one sexual partner; younger women and especially those whose sexual partners have nongonococcal urethritis are also at increased risk. About one half of the babies born to mothers with chlamydial cervicitis will develop conjunctivitis. This rate produces an estimated 42,000 cases annually in the United States, or 2–6% of all newborn infants.[32] Among infants less than six months of age with pneumonia, oculogenital *C trachomatis* is the cause in about half, comprising an estimated 24,000 United States cases annually. Fewer than 50% of infants with chlamydial pneumonia have a history of neonatal conjunctivitis. Pneumonia caused by oculogenital *C trachomatis* is not known after six months of age. Otitis media, vaginitis, and proctitis in neonates are relatively rare complications or intrapartum infection by these organisms.

Manifestations

The scant information available suggests that fetal manifestations of *C psittaci* infection are limited to fetal death or psittacosis. Trachoma and LGV apparently do not manifest in the fetus.

As noted, conjunctivitis is the most common of the neonatal chlamydial infections. Onset of this illness occurs 5 days after birth (range, 3–20 days), 2 days after the mean day of onset of gonococcal ophthalmia. The infant acutely develops a mucopurulent ocular discharge, prominent blepharoedema, papillary hypertrophy, and, occasionally, pseudomembrane formation. Untreated clinical illness resolves in about one month, although shedding of the organism persists for many months. Although generally a benign illness, neonatal chlamydial conjunctivitis can result in corneal damage. Micropannus formation or conjunctival scarring has been shown on follow up in up to half of these children. Preliminary data suggest that early treatment eliminates such scarring.

Neonatal chlamydial pneumonia begins at 4–6 weeks (range, 5 days to 6 months) of age as a gradually progressive pertussislike cough, a series of closely spaced staccato coughs without the inspiratory "whoop" of pertussis. Fever is rare. Cyanosis and vomiting are uncommon complications. Auscultatory findings are often absent, although fine rales may be heard. Chest x-ray shows a focal or diffuse interstitial pattern and hyperinflation, and pleural effusion may be seen. Leukocytosis is mild, but eosinophilia may be striking. Immunoglobulin levels are elevated, most constantly IgM; IgG levels may exceed 500 mg/dL. However, antichlamydial antibodies account for very little of the total immunoglobulin rise. Sequelae of chlamydial pneumonia are not known; whether the excess of adolescent respiratory infections and early onset of chronic obstructive pulmonary disease associated with infantile pneumonia in general will hold for chlamydial disease remains to be seen.

The little available information addressing chlamydial otitis media, vaginitis, and proctitis in the neonate reveals no specific features. Neonatologists must remain alert to the increasing likelihood that oculogenital strains of *C trachomatis* must be considered in the diagnosis and treatment of these diseases, and in this regard that maternal age, sexual behavior, and cervical findings are important diagnostic clues.

Diagnosis

Diagnosis of psittacosis, trachoma, and LGV in the neonate is as described for these diseases in the adult.

The diagnosis of oculogenital *C trachomatis* infections in the neonate is based on an understanding of the limitations of the cytologic, serologic, and culture modalities available (see Table 87–1). In conjunctivitis, there is minimal antibody response, especially at the time of the infection. The diagnosis is made by taking a scraping or firm swabbing from the lower eyelid. Half of this specimen is spread on a clear glass microscopy slide, stained with Giemsa or fluorescein-labeled antibodies (direct or indirect), and examined for typical cytoplasmic inclusions. A slide must be evaluated for 20 minutes by the clock before being declared negative. The other half of the specimen is placed in appropriate cold transport medium and submitted for culture, if available.

In neonatal chlamydial pneumonia, a more invasive infection is operative, and serologic response is more pronounced. Cytologic preparations of lung or tracheal aspirates are not useful. Isolation of the organism from nasopharyngeal swabbings, tracheal aspirates, or lung aspirate or biopsy, but not oropharyngeal swabbings, is highly reliable. Thus, the diagnosis is made by the clinical characteristics of the illness (including maternal epidemiologic considerations) and culture of the organism from an appropriate specimen. In the absence of availability of culture, a fourfold rise in chlamydial antibodies or a single titer of 1024 or greater is adequate for diagnosis. It has been shown that the site most frequently yielding a positive culture in infants is the nasopharynx, and 78% of infants with chlamydial infection at any site are positive in the nasopharynx. Infants with otitis media whose mothers are young, unwed women with a history of sexually transmitted disease should undergo nasopharyngeal swabbing for *Chlamydia* culture and chlamydial serology by the micro-IF test if available. Infants with vaginitis or proctitis whose mothers carry such epidemiologic features should also undergo swabbing of the affected orifice and serologic testing.

The differential diagnosis of neonatal chlamydial conjunctivitis includes gonococcal ophthalmia and other bacterial causes, chemical irritation by silver nitrate prophylaxis, and lacrimal duct stenosis. In chlamydial pneumonia, viral infection and other bacterial causes of pneumonia must be considered, especially cytomegalovirus, which is a common companion to *C trachomatis*. In neonatal vaginitis, gonococcus, group B β-hemolytic streptococci, foreign body, *Trichomonas vaginalis*, and fungi must also be considered. In proctitis, viral, bacterial, and parasitic infections form the differential diagnosis.

Treatment

The treatment of neonatal chlamydial infections is uniform regardless of the site of infection. Specifically, the use of topical therapy in conjunctivitis is effective for that illness, but it leaves the infant at high risk for persistent nasopharyngeal colonization and subsequent pneumonia, otitis media, recurrent ocular infection, and probably transmission of the organism to others in the household. Thus, any manifestations of chlamydial infection in the neonate requires systemic therapy with oral erythromycin, 50 mg/kg per day in four divided doses, for at least 2 weeks; in pneumonia, treatment should be continued for at least 3 weeks. Almost all therapeutic failures are the result of lack of compliance, and when failure occurs, the course of erythromycin should be repeated. Sulfisoxazole, 150 mg/kg per day for 2 weeks, has shown excellent efficacy in a small number of infants with chlamydial pneumonia, but carries the risk of induction of kernicterus and hemolysis in those infants with glucose-6-phosphate dehydrogenase deficiency. Physicians treating neonatal chlamydial infections must be prepared to provide or arrange for treatment of the mother and her sexual partner(s). Siblings born 2–4 years apart to untreated mothers have developed chlamydial conjunctivitis.

Prevention

Application of 0.5% erythromycin ointment in a single dose to the eyes of newborns is highly effective prophylaxis against chlamydial conjunctivitis[33]; topical 1% tetracycline ointment is less effective. However, neither therapy reliably prevents nasopharyngeal colonization and subsequent pulmonary, otic, or ophthalmic infection. The key to prevention of neonatal chlamydial infection lies in the identification and treatment of adults who harbor these organisms in the genital tract. It has been estimated by cost-benefit analysis that a prevalence of more than 5–10% of chlamydial cervicitis in an obstetric population justifies routine screening cultures for all patients.

REFERENCES

1. Becker Y. The Chlamydia: molecular biology of procaryotic obligate parasites of eucaryocytes. *Microbiol Rev.* 1978;42:274.
2. Bird BR, Forrester FT. *Laboratory Diagnosis of Chlamydia Trachomatis Infections.* Atlanta, GA: Centers for Disease Control; 1980. US Dept of Health, Education, and Welfare, Public Health Service, Laboratory Training and Consultation Division, Virology Training Branch, Development.
3. Schaffner W. Psittacosis. In: Mandell GL, Douglass RG, Bennett JE, eds. *Principles and Practice of Infectious Diseases.* New York, NY: John Wiley & Sons; 1979:1476.
4. Hare MJ, Toone E, Taylor-Robinson E, et al. Follicular cervicitis: colposcopic appearances and association with *Chlamydia trachomatis. Br J Obstet Gynaecol.* 1980;88:174.
5. Mardh PA, Ripa T, Svensson L, et al. *Chlamydia trachomatis* infection in patients with acute salpingitis. *N Engl J Med.* 1977;296:1377.
6. Hutchinson GR, Taylor-Robinson D, Dourmashkin RR. Growth and effect of chlamydiae in human and bovine oviduct organ cultures. *Br J Vener Dis.* 1979;55:194.
7. Bowie W, Holmes K. *Chlamydia trachomatis.* In: Mandell GL, Douglas RG, Bennett JE, eds. *Principles and Practice of Infectious Disease.* New York, NY: John Wiley & Sons; 1979:1464.
8. McCormak WM, Evrard JR, Laughlin CF, et al. Sexually transmitted conditions among women college students. *Am J Obstet Gynecol.* 1981; 139:130.
9. Schaffner W, Drutz DJ, Duncan GW, et al. The clinical spectrum of endemic psittacosis. *Arch Intern Med.* 1967;119:433.
10. Schachter J. Lymphogranuloma venereum and other non-ocular *Chlamydia trachomatis* infections. In: Hodson D, Holmes KK, eds. *Nongonococcal Urethritis and Related Infections.* Washington, DC: American Society for Microbiology; 1976:91.
11. Thorsteinsson SB. Lymphogranuloma venereum: review of clinical manifestations, epidemiology, diagnosis, and treatment. *Scand J Infect Dis.* 1983;32(suppl):127.
12. Arya OP, Mallison H, Pareek SS, et al. Post-gonococcal cervicitis and post-gonococcal urethritis. *Br J Vener Dis.* 1981;57:395.
13. McCormack WM, Alpert S, McComb DE, et al. Fifteen-month followup study of women infected with *Chlamydia trachomatis. N Engl J Med.* 1979; 300:123.
14. Wager GP, Martin DH, Koutsky L, et al. Puerperal infectious morbidity: relationship to route of delivery and to antepartum *Chlamydia trachomatis* infection. *Am J Obstet Gynecol.* 1980;138:1028.
15. Moller BR, Ahrons S, Laurin J, et al. Pelvic infection after elective abortion associated with *Chlamydia trachomatis. Obstet Gynecol.* 1982;59:210.
16. Henry-Suchet J, Catalan F, Loffredo V, et al. *Chlamydia trachomatis* associated with chronic inflammation in abdominal specimens from women selected for tuboplasty. *Fertil Steril.* 1981;36:599.
17. Mardh PA, Zeeberg B. Toxic effect of sampling swabs and transportation test tubes on the formation of intracytoplasmic inclusions of *Chlamydia trachomatis* in McCoy cell cultures. *Br J Vener Dis.* 1981;57:268–272.
18. Purola E, Paavonen J. Routine cytology as a diagnostic aid in *Chlamydia* cervicitis. *Scan J Infect Dis.* 1982;32(suppl):55.
19. Schachter J, Cles L, Ray R, et al. Failure of serology in diagnosing *Chlamydia* infections of the female genital tract. *J Clin Microbiol.* 1979; 10:647.
20. Beer RJS, Bradford WP, Hart RJC. Pregnancy complicated by psittacosis acquired from sheep. *Br Med J.* 1982; 284:1156.
21. Centers for Disease Control. Sexually transmitted disease treatment guidelines. *MMWR.* 1982;31(suppl):35S.
22. Bowie WR, Manzon LM, Borrie-Hume CJ, et al. Efficacy of treatment regimens for lower urogenital *Chlamydia trachomatis* infection in women. *Am J Obstet Gynecol.* 1982;142:125.
23. Driscoll SG. Genitourinary opportunists: mycoplasmae and chlamydiae. *Perspect Pediatr Pathol.* 1981;6:167.
24. Martin DH, Koutsky L, Eschenbach DA, et al. Prematurity and perinatal mortality in pregnancies complicated by maternal *Chlamydia trachomatis* infections. *JAMA.* 1982;247:1585.
25. Heggie D, Lumicao GG, Stuart LA, et al. *Chlamydia trachomatis* infection in mothers and infants. *Am J Dis Child.* 1981;135:507.
26. Gravett MG, Nelson HP, DeRouen T, et al: Independent association of bacterial vaginosis and *Chlamydia trachomatis* infection with adverse pregnancy outcome. *JAMA.* 1986;256:1899.
27. Sweet RL, Landers DV, Walker C, et al. *Chlamydia trachomatis* infection and pregnancy outcome. *Am J Obstet Gynecol.* 1987;156:824.
28. Martius J, Krohn MA, Hillier SL, et al. Relationships of vaginal *Lactobacillus* species, cervical *Chlamydia trachomatis,* and bacterial vaginosis to preterm birth. *Obstet Gynecol.* 1988;71:89.
29. Alger LS, Lovchik JC, Hebel JR, et al. The association of *Chlamydia trachomatis, Neisseria gonorrhoeae,* and group B streptococci with preterm rupture of the membranes and pregnancy outcome. *Am J Obstet Gynecol.* 1988;159:397.
30. Hammerschlag MR. Chandler JW, Alexander ER, et al. Longitudinal studies on *Chlamydia* infections in the first year of life. *Pediatr Infect Dis.* 1982;1:395.
31. Beem MO, Saxon E, Tipple MA. Treatment of chlamydial pneumonia of infancy. *Pediatrics.* 1979;63:198.
32. Schachter J, Holt J, Goodner, et al. Prospective study of *Chlamydia* infection in neonates. *Lancet.* 1979;2:377.
33. Hammerschlag MR, Chandler, JW, Alexander ER, et al. Erythromycin ointment for ocular prophylaxis of neonatal chlamydial infection. *JAMA.* 1980;244:2291.

H
TORCH INFECTIONS

Chapter Eighty-Eight
Toxoplasmosis

Katharine D. Wenstrom

88

Toxoplasmosis is a parasitic infection caused by the protozoon *Toxoplasma gondii.* It occurs worldwide, with infection rates ranging from 5–95% among adults living in different geographic areas.[1] Among pregnant women in the United States, approximately 38.7% (range 12–41%) show serologic evidence of past *Toxoplasma* infection.[2] The fetuses of such women are not at risk for congenital toxoplasmosis. If a woman becomes infected for the first time during gestation, however, the fetus is at high risk of acquiring the parasite transplacentally. Several large studies suggest that 2–8/1000 pregnant women seroconvert during pregnancy.[3] The risk of transmission to the fetus is related to the gestational age at the time of infection, and increases during gestation from 25% in the first trimester to 65% in the third trimester. The severity of the consequences to the fetus, however, decrease steadily toward term. Virtually none of the infants exposed in the third trimester demonstrate problems related to congenital infection, while 75% of those exposed in the first trimester are severely affected.

The poor prognosis for those infants infected early in pregnancy has provided the impetus to develop reliable antenatal screening methods, accurate diagnostic tests, and effective therapy. Some knowledge of the life cycle of the organism and the immunologic response it provokes is necessary to understand the sometimes confusing data available on this subject.

BIOLOGY OF THE PARASITE

There are three infective stages during the life cycle of *T gondii:* the *trophozoite,* the *tissue cyst,* and the *oocyst.* Although trophozoite can invade many different mammalian cells, they enter the sexual phase of their cycle only in felines, their definitive hosts.

Domestic cats and various species of wild felines become infected after ingesting raw meat containing *Toxoplasma* oocysts or tissue cysts. During passage through the gastrointestinal tract, the oocysts invade the epithelium and release trophozoite, which begin an asexual cycle called schizogony. This is followed by a sexual cycle called gametogony, which results in the development of a noninfectious, unsporulated oocyst. These oocysts are excreted in the feces of the cat for approximately two weeks, contaminating the soil or cat box. Within 1–5 days, sporogeny occurs, and an infectious oocyst is produced. These oocysts may remain viable and infectious for more than a year if kept warm and moist, or they may be rendered noninfectious by boiling or desiccation. If a farm animal eats contaminated grass, or a human being inadvertently puts soil- or cat box-contaminated fingers in his or her mouth, the oocyst enters the gastrointestinal epithelium and releases trophozoites, which multiply by endodyogeny (two daughter cells formed from each parent). These trophozoites travel throughout the body in the bloodstream and lymphatics and produce a parasitemia that stimulates antibody production in an immunocompetent host. In the first 2–6 months of infection, high levels of *Toxoplasma*-specific IgM antibody are produced, followed by high and then steady low levels of IgG. The parasite survives, however, by encysting in muscle and other tissues. These tissue cysts maintain their ability to become infectious unless they are desiccated, heated to 66°C, or frozen and thawed. Thus, the ingestion of raw or undercooked, contaminated meat (pork, lamb, beef, or goat) provides another source of infection of human beings. This accounts for the high prevalence rate of toxoplasmosis in France, where eating raw meat is popular.

In addition to transmission by way of cat litter and ingestion of raw meat, two other rare methods of infection have been reported. Toxoplasmosis has occurred as the result of whole blood transfusions[4] (via white cells) and after organ transplantation.[5]

MATERNAL INFECTION

The response to primary infection varies over a wide range, but is usually mild. The most common manifestation is asymptomatic lymphadenopathy, usually in the cervical area. The nodes are usually discrete, nontender, and of variable consistency. Occasionally, lymphadenopathy may be accompanied by fever, malaise, sore throat, headache, maculopapular rash, or hepatosplenomegaly. Atypical lymphocytosis may occur, and can contribute to a clinical picture similar to infectious mononucleosis or cytomegalovirus infection. Although the lymphocytosis usually resolves quickly, lymphadenopathy may persist for months. Rarely, a more severe form of the disease occurs, in which a major organ system may be seriously affected. Myocarditis, pericarditis, hepatitis, polymyositis, pneumonitis, and encephalitis secondary to toxoplasmosis have all been reported.

If the host is immunodeficient (that is, secondary to human immunodeficiency virus [HIV] infection, immunosuppressive drugs, or malignancy), the initial infection or even the reactivation of a latent infection may result in more severe problems. Necrotizing encephalitis, pneumonitis, and myocarditis are the most frequent findings at autopsy in such cases. More than half of these patients exhibit signs and symptoms referrable to the central nervous system, including seizures, clouding of consciousness, motor impairment, and headaches.

Primary infection during pregnancy is very similar to infection during the nonpregnant state. Pregnant women who become infected, however, are at increased risk of pregnancy complications compared to those who are not infected. The incidence of spontaneous abortion and stillbirth is increased. In addition, a study by the Collaborative Perinatal Project (which monitored 22,845 pregnant women for toxoplasmosis) has shown that women who seroconverted during pregnancy had an increased incidence of both thrombophlebitis and asthma compared to pregnant women with low or negative titers.[2] The explanation for these findings is unknown.

The woman who has recovered from her primary infection before conception and begins pregnancy seropositive for antitoxoplasma IgG is not at risk. Prospective studies have shown no increase in spontaneous abortion or congenital infection in the infants of these otherwise healthy mothers. Because a primary infection may be asymptomatic or very mild, however, it may be difficult to distinguish a primary from a chronic infection by performing serologic tests for the first time during the pregnancy. For this reason, many authors have advocated that all women of childbearing age be screened to determine exposure to toxoplasmosis before conception.

FETAL INFECTION

When a primary *Toxoplasma* infection occurs during pregnancy, approximately 40% of the fetuses will be infected. As noted earlier, the timing of the exposure in gestation correlates with the severity of fetal infection. Of all infected offspring, 15% have severe clinical damage and another 19% will exhibit mild manifestations of the disease.[2]

The most severe fetal infections result from maternal parasitemia occurring in the first trimester. The most frequent postnatal clinical manifestations in such fetuses are chorioretinitis, blindness, and low intelligence quotient (IQ). Ocular involvement has been estimated to occur in over 70% of neonates with known infection, and possibly over 80% of subclinical cases.[6] Other findings include deafness, convulsions, hydrocephalus, fever, lymphadenopathy, jaundice, hepatosplenomegaly, vomiting, microcephalus, diarrhea, cataracts, abnormal bleeding, hypothermia, rash, and pneumonitis. The majority of infected children are asymptomatic at birth, as the above signs or symptoms of damage may not manifest until months or even years later. A prospective study of congenitally infected infants conducted in Amsterdam originally concluded that seropositive children who were asymptomatic from birth to age five years were not at risk to develop serious manifestations of their disease.[7] However, when these children were followed until age 20, the authors had to reverse their conclusions. Four of six infected children who were asymptomatic until age 5 developed new scars in the eyes before age 20; 2 of these had severe visual impairment. Three of five symptomatic children who were treated at birth had normal eye exams until age five but then developed new retinal lesions before 20 years of age.[8] All had severe impairment of vision.

At present, there is no reliable method to predict the outcome in neonates with asymptomatic or subclinical infection at birth. Some data, however, suggests that women with high antitoxoplasma antibody titers are at greatest risk to have children who eventually display manifestations of their infection. The Collaborative Perinatal Project followed children at risk to age seven and found that the incidence of microcephaly, IQ <70, and deafness at that age correlated with high maternal antibody titers (256–512) during gestation.[2]

Diagnosis

The diagnosis of primary toxoplasmosis in a pregnant patient is usually based on serial antibody titers and symptomatology if present. In France, where the seroprevalence rate among reproductive-age women approaches 90%[9], serologic screening to detect primary infection during gestation is compulsory. Pregnant women are screened at their first prenatal visit, and tests are repeated monthly if necessary to detect seroconversion. Comparison of serial antibody titers and, ultimately, direct serologic evaluation of the fetus may be the only way to definitively make the diagnosis of maternal and congenital infection. For the French, who experience a 1.5–6% incidence of congenital toxoplasmosis, the considerable investment of time and money required by such a screening protocol is worthwhile. The prevalence rate of congenital infection in the United States, however, is currently estimated to be 1–2/1000 live births. In certain parts of the country (that is, Colorado, where only 3% of gravidas are seropositive[10]; or Alabama, with a 0.06% seroprevalence rate[11]), the incidence is even lower. Accordingly, debate continues regarding the utility of widespread screening in North America. In addition, choosing the best tests and correctly interpreting the results can be very difficult.

Various serologic techniques are available to verify the presence of antitoxoplasma antibodies in maternal serum. The *Sabin-Feldman dye test* (DT) and the *indirect fluorescent antibody test* (IFA) primarily detect the presence of IgG antibodies. Although the titers of DT and IFA antibodies may be expected to rise acutely one to two weeks after a primary infection, they decline fairly slowly over months to years and remain positive for life. If such tests were performed for the first time during pregnancy, it would be difficult to distinguish an acute from a chronic infection based on these results.

Since IgM antibodies typically appear before IgG antibodies (within five days of infection) and disappear after recovery from acute infection, the sudden presence of a high antitoxoplasma IgM antibody titer in a previously negative individual correlates most closely with recent infection. IgM antibodies are typically measured by the *IgM fluorescent antibody test* (IgM-IFA) or by *Enzyme-Linked Immunosorbent Assay* (ELISA). Both tests are rated highly by the Centers for Disease Control for qualitative test performance. These tests have slightly different sensitivities, however. The ELISA IgM titers tend to be much higher and persist longer than those measured by IgM-IFA. For this reason, it is important that serial samples be quantified using the same test in the same laboratory, and that previous samples be saved and retested in parallel with all new samples.

Some authors have suggested that a single IgM titer, if high enough, is diagnostic of acute infection. An ELISA IgM titer above 1:256[12] or an IgM-IFA titer of 1:512[13] or greater have been reported to correlate well with recent exposure to toxoplasmosis. Others report that a DT or IFA titer (which primarily measure IgG) of ≥1:1000 is diagnostic.[4] A diagnosis based on a single serologic titer, however, may be made in error, because several confounding factors may affect a single result. IgM development can be quite variable from individual to individual. Titers may therefore be low when acute infection has occurred, or may remain high for months or even years after the initial exposure.[14] IgM-IFA titers have been reported to be persistently elevated for up to one year. False-negative IgM antibody tests may occur in the presence of rheumatoid factor or in sera containing competing levels of other TORCH-specific IgG or IgM antibodies (rubella, cytomegalovirus, or herpes simplex virus), while false-positive tests have been associated with antinuclear antibody.[14]

The ideal testing scheme would involve testing only those women at high risk for toxoplasmosis (that is, those who recently acquired cats, who handle cat litter, who eat raw or undercooked meat, or who have had a recent mononucleosislike syndrome) by DT or IFA before conception. The presence of low titers (1:4–1:64) would be most consistent with past infection and would signify immunity. The presence of a high titer ($\geq$1:256) might indicate recent (within 12 months) infection and should be followed by a repeat DT or IFA and IgM quantification. If the IgM-IFA titer is <1:128, the patient either has had an infection in the past (with persistent high DT or IFA titers) or has only recently been exposed and has not yet produced high levels of IgM. Such a patient should have all titers repeated in 2–3 weeks in order to detect rising or falling levels. In addition, a complement fixation (CF) test, if available, may be useful in identifying the recently exposed patient. Since CF antibodies appear several weeks after DT antibodies, demonstration of a rising CF titer in a patient who already has high DT and IgM titers would be consistent with acute infection. Documentation of such an acute infection in a nonpregnant immunocompetent individual is important in terms of future pregnancies, but requires no specific therapy or supportive care.

If such testing were done in high risk patients before conception, the question of immunity versus susceptibility could be answered before a fetus was placed at risk. Unfortunately, the more typical situation is one in which a pregnant patient, usually during or after the period of organogenesis, raises the issue of exposure to toxoplasmosis. Although the same diagnostic steps apply, the ultimate question becomes whether or not the fetus is infected, as congenital toxoplasmosis infection does mandate specific therapeutic intervention. If serial IgG, IgM, and CF titers indicate that the patient is likely to have an acute infection, the fetus should be directly evaluated.

Fetal evaluation should begin with a thorough ultrasound. Congenital toxoplasmosis may produce several anatomic malformations clearly identifiable by sonogram. Abnormalities of intracranial structures are most commonly reported. Hydrocephalus, aqueductal stenosis, and agenesis of the corpus callosum are all suggestive of fetal *Toxoplasma* infection[15], as are microcephalus and cerebral calcifications. Toxoplasmosis should also be considered when nonimmune hydrops is detected. Failure to identify any of these abnormalities, however, does not rule out congenital infection since many affected fetuses have appeared sonographically normal throughout gestation. More invasive testing may be necessary to demonstrate fetal parasitism definitively.

Both fetal blood and amniotic fluid have been shown to be useful for diagnosis. In a study of 278 women at risk of having a child with congenital toxoplasmosis, Desmonts et al[16] combined the results of several tests performed on fetal blood and amniotic fluid with ultrasound evaluation to diagnose congenital infection in nine fetuses correctly. Blood was useful to determine specific IgM antibody titers (present in 4 of 9) and to measure levels of gammaglutamyl transpeptidase, lactate dehydrogenase, and eosinophils (abnormal in 9 of 9). Inoculation of both blood and amniotic fluid into mice resulted in successful *Toxoplasma* isolation in 9 of 9 and 7 of 9 cases, respectively. Six of the nine infected fetuses also had an increased ventricle/hemisphere ratio on ultrasound exam. Of the eight placentas examined, all were parasite-positive.

The authors of this study suggested that a detailed ultrasound exam, combined with fetal IgG and IgM titers, liver function tests, and complete blood count, would greatly improve the accuracy of fetal diagnosis. Because of the technical limitations of cordocentesis, such direct evaluation of fetal blood is probably not possible much before 16–18 weeks' gestation.

The authors also felt that the most important test was inoculation of fetal blood and amniotic fluid into mice, and stated that "no group should undertake the diagnosis of fetal *Toxoplasma* infection without the help of a laboratory where the methods of isolation of parasites have been mastered."[15] The mouse inoculation test, however, takes 4–6 weeks to complete and would therefore not be optimal for the patient who was considering pregnancy termination pending results. Another group has recently suggested that inoculation of human embryonic fibroblast tissue culture may produce similar results in only four days.[17] If this procedure proves to be accurate and reproducible, definitive diagnoses of toxoplasmosis may be greatly simplified.

Treatment

Therapy in the United States has consisted of pyrimethamine (a diaminopyrimidine) together with a sulfonamide. These drugs affect different points in the synthesis of nucleic acids, and thus are synergistic when used in combination. Although the optimal dosage regimen has not been firmly established, a 28-day course of pyrimethamine, 25 mg orally every day, along with sulfadiazine, 1 g orally four times daily, has been recommended.[18] Because pyrimethamine is a folic acid antagonist, it should be withheld during the first trimester. When it is prescribed, folinic acid should be given concurrently (6 mg orally three times a week or intramuscularly once). Sulfadiazine should be withheld near term, because it competes with bilirubin for binding sites on albumin and may increase the risk of kernicterus in the neonate. Patients on this regimen should be evaluated with weekly peripheral blood cell and platelet counts, as pyrimethamine may cause bone marrow depression.

Another effective agent, spiramycin, has been widely used in Europe for over 27 years. It has recently become available in the United States by special application to the Food and Drug Administration. Spiramycin is a macrolide antibiotic that has been shown to reduce the incidence of congenital toxoplasmosis in animal studies and in nonrandomized trials of infected pregnant women. It may not be as effective as the combination of pyrimethamine and sulfadiazine, but it has fewer side effects and is less toxic. A recent study, in which 223 placentas from acutely infected women were carefully examined for infectivity, showed that when patients received no or inadequate therapy, 90% of the placentas were infected. When patients received 3 g of spiramycin a day for more than 15 days, only 75% were infected. The best treatment, however, appeared to be spiramycin in combination with pyrimethamine and a sulfonamide, because only 50% of the placentas from women undergoing this treatment contained parasites.[19]

Because the pharmacologic therapy described is not 100% effective and entails some risk to the patient, the decision to begin treatment should be arrived at only after thorough evaluation and patient counseling. Most would agree that any patient with a well diagnosed acute infection during pregnancy should be offered termination if possible. Immunocompetent patients who choose this route do not need to undergo treatment of their own condition. Some patients, however, may be unwilling to make this decision or may request more information about the fetal condition.

Cordocentesis should then be offered. Patients under 16–18 weeks' gestation (or in whom cordocentesis is not technically feasible) should be placed on 3 g of spiramycin per day until the procedure can be performed. Spiramycin is the drug of choice in this situation if available because it is effective, yet produces minimal side effects. When cordocentesis is performed, fetal blood should be sent for complete blood count, liver function tests, serology, and tissue culture or mouse inoculation. All results should be evaluated together to confirm or disprove congenital infection. If the fetus is not considered to have an active infection, the mother should be continued on spiramycin alone until delivery. If the fetus is infected, and the patient elects to continue the pregnancy, aggressive therapy with pyrimethamine, sulfadiazine, and spiramycin should be initiated for fetuses under 28 weeks' gestation. For fetuses at a more advanced gestational age, consideration can be given to treatment with spiramycin alone. In order to avoid toxicity, triple therapy prescribed daily for three weeks can be alternated with spiramycin alone for three weeks until delivery. All fetuses should be followed with serial ultrasounds every two weeks. Daffos et al[20] described this protocol in a prospective study of 746 gravidas with documented acute *Toxoplasma* infection. All were treated with spiramycin as soon as their diagnosis was made, and underwent cordocentesis when possible (usually >20 weeks). Seven hundred four women carried fetuses who appeared to be uninfected and continued to receive spiramycin alone until delivery. All but three infants born to these mothers were unaffected at birth. The authors attributed this very low infection rate to initiation of spiramycin therapy early in pregnancy. Of 42 women whose fetuses were considered to be infected, 24 elected to terminate the pregnancy. The 15 who chose to continue were treated aggressively with triple agents until delivery. Eleven of these infants appeared clinically unaffected at birth, while four had intracranial calcifications. Two of the apparently healthy fetuses developed chorioretinitis during follow up (4–18 months). A total of 9 of 15 infants in this treatment group apparently responded to therapy and were unaffected, although long-term follow up is pending.

Prevention

Many authors have suggested that the complicated and imperfect treatment protocol outlined above could be avoided by actively employing prevention strategies. Ideally, all women contemplating pregnancy should be tested for infection, and those who remain seronegative should actively avoid exposure. They should be persuaded to wash their hands thoroughly after contact with raw meat, cats, cat-box litter, or soil. All meat must be cooked adequately, and tasting of undercooked meat during preparation should be avoided. It has been estimated that these simple measures could decrease the incidence of maternal infection by at least 50%, and could save millions of dollars in treatment and long-term care.[21] In practice, however, prevention measures alone may not be sufficient to eliminate the problem. When such an aggressive prevention protocol was undertaken in Brussels, and 6549 pregnant women were studied prospectively over a six-year period, no significant reduction in either the rate of maternal seroconversion or in the percentage of patients with high initial antibody titers could be demonstrated.[22]

Ultimately, immunization of susceptible women may become the treatment of choice. Although the wild type *Toxoplasma* would make an almost perfect vaccine (the initial infection is usually asymptomatic, yet immunity is produced), it cannot be used because it could lead to recrudescence of the disease if the patient became immunocompromised at a later date. Vaccine might be made from a nonpersisting strain (that is, strain ts-4), from a related organism, or a subunit vaccine may be developed.[3] Some consideration has been given to immunizing house cats as well. Until such a vaccine can be developed, and as long as pregnant patients continue to be exposed to *T gondii*, however, perinatologists must continue their efforts to design better methods of diagnosis and more effective treatment strategies.

REFERENCES

1. Alford CA, Pass RF. Epidemiology of chronic congenital and perinatal infections of man. *Clin Perinatol.* 1981;8:397.
2. Sever J, Ellenberg J, Ley A, et al. Toxoplasmosis: maternal and pediatric findings in 23,000 pregnancies. *Pediatr.* 1988;82:181.
3. Carter AO, Frank JW. Congenital toxoplasmosis: epidemiologic features and control. *CMAJ.* 1988;135:618.
4. Anderson SE, Remington JS. Toxoplasmosis. In: Hoeprich PE, ed. *Infectious Diseases.* 2nd ed. New York, NY: Harper and Row; 1977:970.
5. Hakim M, Wreghitt T, English T, et al. Significance of donor transmitted disease in cardiac transplantation. *Heart Transp.* 1985;IV:302.
6. Plotkin SA, Starr SE. Congenital toxoplasmosis. *Clin Perinatol.* 1981;3:426.
7. Koppe JG, Kloosterman GJ, deRoever-Bonnet H, et al. Toxoplasmosis and pregnancy, with a longterm follow up of the children. *Eur J Obstet Gynecol Reprod Biol.* 1974;4:101.
8. Koppe JG, Loewer-Sieger DH, deRoever-Bonnet H. Results of 20 year follow up of congenital toxoplasmosis. *Lancet.* 1986;254.
9. McLabe R, Remington TS. Toxoplasmosis: the time has come. *N Engl J Med.* 1988;318:313.
10. Hershey DW, McGregor JA. Low prevalence of toxoplasma infection in a Rocky Mountain prenatal population. *Obstet Gynecol.* 1987;70:900.
11. Hunter K, Stagno S, Capps E, Smith RJ. Prenatal screening of pregnant women for infections caused by cytomegalovirus, Epstein-Barr Virus, herpes virus, rubella, and *Toxoplasma gondii. Am J Obstet Gynecol.* 1983;145:269.
12. Sever JL. TORCH infections: the list keeps growing. *Contemp OB-GYN.* 1989;65.
13. Lee RV. Protozoan infections in pregnancy. In: *Principles of Medical Therapy in Pregnancy.* New York, NY: Plenum Medical Book Co; 1985:612.
14. Fung JC, Tilton RC. TORCH serologies and specific IgM antibody determination in acquired and congenital infections. *Am Clin Lab Sci.* 1985;15:204.
15. Romero R, et al. *Prenatal Diagnosis of Congenital Anomalies.* Norwalk, CT: Appleton and Lange; 1988:23,25,67.
16. Desmonts G, Daffos F, Forestier F, et al. Prenatal diagnosis of congenital toxoplasmosis. *Lancet.* 1985;500.
17. Derouin F. Early prenatal diagnosis of congenital toxoplasmosis using amniotic fluid samples and tissue culture. *Eur J Clin Microbiol Infect Dis.* 1988;7:423.
18. Sever JL, Larsen JW, Grossman JH. *Handbook of Perinatal Infections.* Boston, MA: Little Brown and Co; 1979:160.
19. Courreur J, Desmont G, Thulliez P. Prophylaxis of congenital toxoplasmosis. Effects of spiramycin on placental infection. *J Antimicrob Chemo.* 1988;22:193.
20. Daffos F, Forestier F, Capella-Pavlovsky M, et al. Prenatal management of 746 pregnancies at risk for congenital toxoplasmosis. *N Engl J Med.* 1988;318:271.
21. Frenkel JK. Congenital toxoplasmosis: prevention or palliation? *Am J Obstet Gynecol.* 1981;141:359.
22. Foulon W, Naessens A, Lauwers S, et al. Impact of primary prevention on the incidence of toxoplasmosis during pregnancy. *Obstet Gynecol.* 1988;72:363.

Chapter Eighty-Nine
Rubella

Marvin S. Amstey

89

Rubella, also known as *German measles* or three-day measles, is a mild, exanthematous, viral infection that affects children primarily. Young adults also can be infected by this virus; therefore, the most important problem associated with rubella is its occurrence during pregnancy. Except for rubella infecting pregnant women, there are practically no complications of note. Prior to the knowledge that rubella could cause congenital anomalies if acquired during pregnancy, the only real importance of the infection was that it needed to be differentiated from more important, and potentially more serious, exanthems such as rubeola and scarlet fever. German investigators, in the early 19th century, succeeded in making this differential diagnosis; this fact probably accounts for its popular appellation, "German measles."

ETIOLOGY

Rubella virus is a small, RNA-containing virus measuring approximately 50–80 μm. Its characterization is not clear enough to place it into a specific virus classification, although most evidence suggests that rubella should be considered a togavirus. It can be isolated in human, monkey, rabbit, hamster, chick, duck, and many other cell culture systems. It is interesting to note that even with the availability of all these culture systems, rubella virus was not isolated until 1962.

Rubella virus-infected cells will produce complement-fixing and hemagglutinating antigens, depending upon which cell system is used to grow the virus. The virus also will infect several laboratory animals, including primates. However, there is no satisfactory laboratory model for studying rubella infection in pregnancy because the virus will not cross the placenta of any of these animals in the same manner as in a human, nor will it cause the embryopathy seen in humans.[1,2]

PATHOGENESIS

The virus enters the body by way of aerosols and infection of the upper respiratory tract. Following this, a viremia occurs with dissemination of the virus. The incubation period is approximately 10–14 days, at which time the characteristic rash and other manifestations of the infection become apparent. Rubella can be isolated from the oropharynx and from the blood approximately 4–6 days after initial infection. Virus will continue to be shed from the oropharynx up to 24 days after infection or up to 10 days after the rash has disappeared.

In pregnancy, the viremia leads to placental infection. Small vessel damage is apparent in the placental vasculature and is characterized by endothelial necrosis. This same picture is apparent in the fetus. In addition, cell destruction occurs by a direct viral effect in the placenta and fetus. However, cell lysis is not the only pathologic result of rubella virus infection. More importantly, placental and fetal cells become chronically infected without cell destruction. This results in viral shedding for many weeks to years after the initial infection. The pathologic mechanism of this chronic infection is not understood well; however, the subtle changes that occur in these cells (and some not so subtle, such as chromosome breaks) probably account for the great variety of fetal or neonatal effects.

EPIDEMIOLOGY

The incidence of rubella in this country has changed dramatically since the advent of vaccination. Whereas the last epidemic of rubella in the United States (1964–1965) resulted in 20,000 infants with a diagnosis of congenital rubella syndrome, only 2290 cases were reported to the Centers for Disease Control (CDC) in 1982.[3] However, even with current vaccination procedures, nearly 15–20% of the young adult population is susceptible to rubella infection. This figure suggests that we will continue to see cases of rubella infection during pregnancy, and we will continue to see cases of congenital rubella syndrome.

The true attack rate for rubella infection is unknown. This is true partially because of the mildness of the infection and also because of inapparent or subclinical infection. In fact, there are at least two cases of subclinical infection (using a serologic response as the criterion for infection) for every obvious case.

The risk of fetal infection is not known precisely, but the best epidemiological studies, using proper prospective serologic techniques for diagnosis, suggest that as many as 80% will be infected if maternal infection occurs during the first trimester. More than 25% of fetuses will be infected if maternal rubella occurs during the second trimester. This data, however, does not mean that all of these infants will have congenital rubella syndrome—only that the fetuses are shedding virus. It is estimated that the overall chance of the syndrome occurring is 20% if maternal infection occurs in the first trimester.[4]

MANIFESTATIONS

The hallmarks of rubella infection include a maculopapular rash that spreads from the thorax and face distally to the extremities; postauricular lymphadenopathy, often preceding the rash by several days; and low grade fever. The rash begins to fade from the central parts often before it appears on the extremities, and the total duration of rash is close to three days. In adults, there often are arthralgia symptoms, which may occasionally stem from arthritis. These are usually transient, but the arthralgias occur in up to 20% of adults.

The infection in the newborn may range from no symptoms to multiorgan system involvement to the congenital rubella syndrome. The latter is characterized by a growth-retarded infant who has chronic cellular infection with this virus, and who has fewer total cells in each organ involved. Many infants infected *in utero* who have no apparent organ damage at birth may manifest auditory, ocular, or central nervous system (CNS) damage later in life. There is virtually no organ system in the fetus or neonate that can escape possible involvement by this virtue. The most important factor that determines the extent of fetal or neonatal involvement is the gestational age at which maternal infection first occurs. The frequency of defects detected at four years of age drops from 85% if maternal infection occurred at less than eight weeks' gestation to nearly 10% if maternal infection occurred at 20 weeks' gestation. This information mirrors the incidence of chronic infection of the fetus, which is near 50% if maternal rubella occurred at 8 weeks' gestation and near 5% if maternal rubella occurred at 16 weeks gestation.

DIAGNOSIS

The clinical diagnosis of rubella is frequently wrong. An interesting study demonstrated that 35% of illnesses characterized by low-grade fever and rash that were called rubella by pediatricians were, in fact, other viral illnesses. With this in mind, it is not difficult to understand how a history of previous rubella infection may be unrealiable when obtaining a medical history. Therefore, the only useful method to determine whether an individual has ever had rubella is to look for a specific antibody. It is believed that previous infection confers lifetime immunity; this is easily detected by measuring either neutralizing antibody (a cumbersome and expensive procedure) or hemagglutinating antibody (HA) (a simple, reliable, and inexpensive procedure).

The difficult problem is detecting an active new infection in the pregnant woman. Demonstrating a fourfold rise in any antibody responding to rubella infection will diagnose the infection clearly. However, if the woman presents at a time when the rash already has appeared or is fading, or she presents with a history of exposure two to three weeks earlier, it requires consideration of which antibody will provide the most reliable information. The single, most useful measure of a recent rubella infection, when paired sera are not available to look for a fourfold rise in HA, is rubella-specific IgM antibody. This antibody persists for only about 30 days after infection. One other antibody measure that may have some clinical usefulness is complement fixation (CF). This antibody appears soon after infection and may persist for about one year, after which it declines to undetectable levels. A woman with a significant HA antibody titer, but a negative CF antibody, probably is immune from a long-forgotten or subclinical childhood infection.

Isolation of the virus will also confirm the diagnosis of rubella. This is done rarely in the mother. However, it may be an important measure in the newborn suspected of having congenital rubella. As mentioned above, some infants will continue to shed virus for many months after birth. Such an infant poses a risk for any pregnant woman who may come into contact with this baby. The presence of rubella-specific antibody in the cord blood will diagnose *in utero* infection, but will not allow one to know if the baby is a danger to pregnant women.

PREVENTION

Rubella vaccine has been available since 1968. Its use is credited with the absence of a major epidemic of rubella that was predicted for 1971–1972. Prior to vaccination, rubella seemed to appear in 6- to 9-year cycles, the last of which was in 1964. The vaccinations were directed at preschool children with the thought that the amount of virus circulating in the general population would be reduced. This seems to have occurred, because the frequency of congenital rubella and congenital rubella syndrome has been reduced substantially. However, the vaccination program has not been a total success because the number of susceptible individuals over the age of 15 years has not changed appreciably. This has led to several small epidemics and infection of pregnant women.

The vaccine is known as the RA 27/3 strain of rubella. It is a live, attenuated virus strain grown on human diploid cells. Antibody response to this vaccine virus closely resembles that from natural infection and persists for more than 15 years (and probably for a lifetime). The vaccine is indicated for preschool children and for women of childbearing age who will not become pregnant for at least three months after vaccination. It is incumbent upon the physician to ensure that the woman is not pregnant at the time of vaccination. Too many such cases have occurred, suggesting that women are not questioned closely enough or are not using adequate contraception prior to vaccination. Although the recommendation had been made to test women for susceptibility prior to vaccination, this practice is an unnecessary expense that probably is not warranted. There is no harm in vaccinating an immune individual; the practice should be the same as for any other immunization such as for polio or tetanus—infections for which prior antibody testing is not done.[5]

A practical time to vaccinate women is immediately postpartum. This is a time period in which the likelihood of pregnancy within three months is low. Although one study has demonstrated a greater number of failures at this time, perhaps because of some immunologic suppression from remaining high levels of progesterone, most authors believe the practicality outweighs the risk of failure. If one waited until 48–72 hours after delivery to vaccinate the woman, the risk of failure would be very small. It is known that the vaccine virus will appear in breast milk and will occasionally immunize the infant; however, this is of no clinical significance. The vaccine virus, while excreted, is not communicable to others, so that pregnant women should have no fear of coming into contact with a recently-vaccinated adult or child.

For those women receiving Rh immune globulin postpartum, no additional concerns are necessary when considering rubella vaccination. The globulin has too little rubella antibody and will not interfere with immunization. This information also points out the fact that passive immunization with pooled gamma globulin is not effective in preventing rubella infection or the transmission of virus to the fetus.

Even with all the stated precautions, there are some women who will be vaccinated close to the time of conception. It is known that the vaccine virus will infect the placenta; it is not known whether the vaccine virus will infect the fetus. Nevertheless, the CDC follow up of more than 700 women has demonstrated no instances of the congenital rubella syndrome occurring in infants born to mothers inadvertently vaccinated within three months of conception. This data should ease the concern that a woman and her physician might have, and it should argue against the vaccination as an indication for abortion. Any instance of vaccination within three months of conception (before or after) should be reported to the state health department or to the CDC.[6]

Because the only real concern with rubella as an infectious disease is the possibility of infecting the fetus, our attention must be turned to preventing the infection in postpubertal females. This requires that all primary care physicians, internists, pediatricians, obstetricians, family physicians, and others such as outpatient clinic staffs must encourage a vigorous vaccination program. In addition, anyone working in a hospital should be vaccinated, male and female alike. With attention to these areas, rubella probably could be eliminated from the United States.

REFERENCES

1. Alford CA. Rubella. In: Remington J, Klein J, eds. *Infectious Diseases of the Fetus and Newborn Infant.* Philadelphia, PA: WB Saunders Co; 1976:71.
2. Monif G. *Infectious Diseases in Obstetrics and Gynecology.* Philadelphia, PA: Harper and Row; 1982:89.
3. Centers for Disease Control. Rubella—United States, 1979–1982. *MMWR.* 1982;31:568.
4. Mann J, Preblud S, Hoffman R, et al. Assessing risks of rubella infection during pregnancy. *JAMA.* 1981;245:1647.
5. Parkman P, Meyer H, Kirschstein R, et al. Attenuated rubella virus. I. Development and laboratory characterization. *N Engl J Med.* 1966;275:569.
6. Preblud S, Serdula M, Frank J, et al. Rubella vaccination in the United States: a ten year review. *Epidemiol Rev.* 1980;2:170.

Chapter Ninety
Cytomegalovirus

Kenneth F. Trofatter, Jr.

90

In 1904, Jesionek and Kiolemenoglou noted protozoanlike cells in lungs, liver, and kidneys of an 8-month-old fetus. Goodpasture and Talbot in 1921 coined the term *cytomegalia* to describe similar findings in autopsy material from a 6-week-old neonate. During the same year, a viral etiology for these findings was suggested by Lipshutz, who noted the similarity of the intranuclear inclusions to those found in herpesvirus infections. In 1950, Wyatt defined the clinical entity *cytomegalic inclusion disease* as generalized congenital infection associated with cytomegalic cells and typical intranuclear inclusions found in multiple organ sites. Smith reported growing human cytomegalovirus (CMV) in cultured human cells in 1956. Since then, CMV has become recognized as the most common congenitally and perinatally acquired virus disease known in humans and the single most important infectious cause of mental retardation and congenital deafness in the United States.[1,2]

Morphologically, CMV is a member of the herpes family. It is an enveloped virus with an icosahedral capsid containing 162 capsomeres. The virus is approximately 180 nm in diameter. It contains a linear double-stranded DNA (150 $\times$ 10^6 mol wt; 56% guanosine plus cytosine), which can exist in four isomers. The envelope is generally required for infection and makes the virus ether-soluble. CMV is heat-labile at 37°C, heat-inactivated at 56°C, poorly tolerates freezing, and is most stable in urine at 4°C. CMV does not encode its own DNA polymerase or thymidine kinase. It can be cultured readily only in diploid human fibroblasts, although major targets *in vivo* appear to be epithelial cells, and requires a high particle-to-infectivity ratio. Replication occurs in the cell nucleus to intermediate titers (10^4–10^5 particles/mL). Like other herpesviruses, CMV induces Fc receptors on the cell surface, but the significance of these is unknown.

Human CMV is restricted to humans and there are no animal reservoirs known. It is ubiquitous, with infection more common than overt disease. By serology, 80–90% of individuals are exposed to the virus during their lifetime.[3] Exposure tends to occur at earlier ages in lower socioeconomic groups and among promiscuous individuals. Seropositivity among women in the common childbearing years (18–35) is on the order of 50% for middle and upper socioeconomic groups and 90% for lower socioeconomic groups.[4,5] Specific factors correlated with seropositivity include an ethnic racial background, being breast-fed as an infant, over 30 years of age, and the presence of young children in the living group.

Transmission of CMV most often occurs by way of the venereal route, respiratory route, or by contact with infected urine and saliva. There is no apparent change in susceptibility to primary infection with CMV in normal individuals throughout their lives. Major risks for primary infection among seronegative women include age less than 25 years, promiscuity, and exposure to young children at home and possibly in the work place.[6,7] Among seronegative women, the chance of seroconversion ranges between 1–3% per year, depending on the various risk factors detailed above. Congenital infections occur in 1–3% of all pregnancies and indicate that CMV can cross the placenta with relative ease compared to other herpesvirus. Neonatal infections are most commonly acquired by exposure to an infected genitourinary tract and by breast milk. Organ transplants and blood transfusions are other sources of infection. The spread of CMV among the general population is facilitated by asymptomatic primary and recurrent infections, multiple sites of excretion, prolonged excretion, and excretion of infectious virus despite the presence of specific immunity. No cross-reactive immunity is afforded by previous infections with other herpesviruses.

PATHOPHYSIOLOGY

Development of a cytopathologic effect *in vitro* is relatively slow. By 24 hours, a juxtanuclear inclusion in the cytoplasm can be found; by 48 hours, an intranuclear inclusion, often surrounded by a halo, giving an "owl-eye" appearance, develops; and by 72 hours, the virus can be isolated from fluid and infected cells. Concomitantly, cells enlarge to 25–40 μm. As in other herpesvirus infections, productively infected cells generally go on to die.

Viral-specific changes consistent with the above are

found *in vivo*. In addition to the typical cytomegalic cells containing large, basophilic nuclear inclusions, lesions characteristically show focal necrosis and inflammatory infiltrates. Healing may range from fibrosis and calcification to complete restoration of apparently normal tissue architecture. Secondary infections can occur by reinfection with the same or different strains of CMV despite cross-reactive immunity. More often, recurrences are the result of reactivation of latent infections. The sites of latency are unknown, but leukocytes, nerve cells, and chronically infected cells in affected organs are all possible sources. Persistent low-grade infection, reinfections, and intermittent exacerbation by reactivation may contribute to the chronic tissue destruction typical of the long-term progressive sequelae of CMV infections. In addition to the primary cytopathic effect of the virus, a role of immune complexes in this process has been hypothesized, but their significance is unclear.

Congenital CMV infections are usually the result of transplacental acquisition of the virus during primary or recurrent maternal infections. Invasive procedures, such as amniocentesis or intrauterine transfusion, are other potential sources of transmission. By virtue of its slow growth, CMV has a far greater teratogenic potential than the rapidly replicating and typically destructive herpes simplex virus (HSV). CMV-related congenital anomalies and late-occurring sequelae are characterized by relative hypoplasia and disruption of normal architecture in affected organs, and by attrition of productively infected cells. At autopsy, findings include typical inclusion-bearing cells, most commonly in the salivary glands, kidneys, liver, lungs, and central nervous system (CNS), with inflammatory infiltrate, focal necrosis, granulomatous lesions, and calcification present.

EFFECTS OF PREGNANCY ON DISEASE

There appears to be a relatively constant percentage (5–15%) of seropositive individuals excreting CMV from the genitourinary tract at a given time. Reactivation of CMV generally diminishes as time from seroconversion increases. However, the incidence of excretion during pregnancy tends to increase throughout gestation. In one study, 35% of women aged 21 or younger were found to be excreting CMV at some time during the third trimester.[8] Pregnancy does not by itself appear to increase the risk of contracting CMV, nor is it associated with a greater risk for more severe maternal infections. Immunocompetent pregnant women demonstrate the same spectrum of symptomatic and asymptomatic disease, and have primary infections followed by specific immunologic responses comparable, at least qualitatively, to nonpregnant women. However, there is some evidence that women who develop CMV mononucleosis and those asymptomatic women who are at greatest risk for transmitting the virus to the fetus do differ quantitatively in their antibody responses to CMV. The disease course in these women is characterized by more intense IgG antibody responses to CMV cytoplasmic proteins and longer virus excretion than asymptomatic women who do not infect their children.[9] There may be differences also in the cellular immune responses among women who are at increased risk for intrauterine infection. In one small study, lymphocytes from pregnant women with primary infections were used in transformation assays to CMV antigen, with findings that positive responses were much less likely to be associated with intrauterine infection than negative responses.[10]

Overall, among seronegative women, there is approximately 0.5–1% risk of a primary CMV infection in each pregnancy. This risk is somewhat higher in seronegative women from lower socioeconomic groups and with the risk factors detailed previously.[11] The incubation period from the time of exposure to the onset of virus excretion, with or without symptoms, is usually 4–12 weeks. At least 50% of the primary and the vast majority of the recurrent infections are entirely asymptomatic. When symptomatic infections occur, these characteristically present as mononucleosislike syndromes with fever, often high, spiking, and prolonged (3–5 weeks); malaise; myalgia; arthralgia; hepatosplenomegaly; pharyngitis; and lymphadenopathy. Rarer manifestations include pneumonitis, a transient rubellilike rash on the trunk and extremities, hemolytic anemia, thrombocytopenia, myocarditis, pericarditis, cholestatic hepatitis, intestinal ulcerations, aseptic meningitis, encephalitis, and Guillain-Barré syndrome. There does not appear to be an increase in the severity of maternal disease contracted during pregnancy. Milder primary cases often are missed because the symptomatic complaints are confused with those commonly attributed to the pregnancy itself; however, these infections may be no less significant with regard to fetal outcome.

Severe maternal infections generally are limited to immunocompromised individuals. In the past, these were most often the consequence of immunosuppressive therapy, organ transplantation, cancer chemotherapy, underlying malignancy, lymphoma, or leukemia. In recent years, patients infected with human immunodeficiency virus (HIV) have become a major reservoir for active CMV infections. These conditions have confirmed the evidence that complete recovery from CMV infections is dependent on the normal function of various populations of cytotoxic lymphocytes, including both specific cytotoxic lymphocytes and nonspecific effectors of natural killer (NK) and antibody-dependent cell-mediated cytotoxic (ADCC) activities.[12] Failure to develop cytotoxic activity has been correlated with more severe acute and chronic infections, prolonged CMV viremia and excretion, and depressed lymphokine production. Interestingly, there is now evidence that CMV can infect and adversely influence the function of these same lymphocyte subpopulations.

By definition, congenital CMV infections are those acquired *in utero* as indicated by clinical features of disease, virus excretion, or serologic evidence found within the first two weeks of life. Transmission of CMV to the fetus can occur during both primary and recurrent infections despite maternal antibody and has been documented in consecutive pregnancies. Although maternal immunity is incompletely protective against intrauterine or perinatal transmission of CMV, it plays a major role in reducing the virulence of infection in the fetus and newborn.[13] Congenital infections occur in about 1–2% of all pregnancies, accounting for an estimated 50,000 infected infants per year. The frequency of congenitally infected infants among seropositive women is approximately 2–3% and appears to be relatively constant. Primary maternal CMV infections, however, carry an overall risk of congenital or perinatal transmission in the range of 25–50%.[5,11,14] Ninety percent or more of congenitally infected infants will shed virus at birth and may do so continuously for six years or longer afterwards, even in the presence of specific antibody.[4]

Congenital infections range from asymptomatic and unrecognized in approximately 90% of cases to multiple organ system involvement incompatible with life. Although most of the asymptomatic infections pose no immediate life threat, 10–15% of these infants are at risk for long-term sequelae, usually evident by two years of age, such as progressive sensorineural hearing loss, chorioretinitis, and dental abnormalities. Of the late-appearing sequelae, the sensorineural hearing loss is by far the most significant because delay in its early detection contributes to psychomotor retardation.[15,16]

About 5–10% of congenitally infected infants will have significant stigmata of infection evident at birth.[17] Approximately one half of these will have classic cytomegalic inclusion disease and one half will have atypical involvement. Virtually 100% of these infants will excrete CMV at birth and may continue to do so for years. Infants in this group have a 20–30% chance of eventual mortality and account for 90% of the significant mental and psychomotor retardation associated with CMV infections. Although case reports have described cytomegalic inclusion disease in infants born to women proven to be seropositive prior to pregnancy, the most severely infected children are almost exclusively the result of primary maternal infections.[4] Overall, primary infections during pregnancy are associated with a 30–40% incidence of intrauterine growth retarded and small-for-gestational-age infants and a greater risk for intrauterine death beyond 20 weeks' gestation.[7] An association between early spontaneous abortion and primary CMV infection probably exists, but reports have conflicted on this issue.

On physical examination, the most common abnormalities in congenital cytomegalic infection syndromes include petechiae (70–80%), hepatosplenomegaly (75%), jaundice (60%), microcephaly (50%), abnormality of the dental enamel (40%), and chorioretinitis (10–15%). Associated defects include hydrocephaly, dolichocephaly, micrognathia, cleft or high-arched palate, encephalomalacia, cerebellar aplasia, microphthalmia, cataracts, seizures, cerebral calcifications, abnormalities of endochondral bone formation with decreased density of the femoral metaphyses without periosteal changes (celery stalking), abnormal dermatoglyphics, pneumonitis, and a variety of cardiovascular, gastrointestinal, and genitourinary abnormalities. Long-term consequences are characterized by progression of abnormalities that may not necessarily be detected at birth, including microcephaly, sensorineural hearing loss, mental and psychomotor retardation, optic atrophy, chorioretinitis, hypotonia, spasticity, and dental defects.

Among women actively excreting CMV, transmission to the baby at the time of delivery or in the neonatal period, particularly when the woman is breast-feeding, is quite common. However, the consequences of perinatally acquired disease are considerably less than congenital infection. As in the adult, the incubation period from time of exposure to symptoms or asymptomatic excretion of the virus is on the order of 4–12 weeks. At least half of these infections are asymptomatic or go unrecognized. When symptomatic infections occur during early infancy, they often present as bilateral diffuse pneumonitis, most commonly found in premature or small-for-gestational-age infants. Approximately 80% of these infants will be afebrile, 70% will develop an elevated serum IgM, and 50% or more will require oxygen or more intensive respiratory support.[18] Hearing loss usually does not develop in infants acquiring CMV perinatally.

DIAGNOSIS

As a general statement, primary CMV infections during pregnancy are usually only identified when there is high clinical suspicion. The differential diagnosis includes infections with other TORCH organisms, Epstein–Barr virus, hepatitis viruses, enteroviruses, and the multiple organisms commonly associated with respiratory disease. When CMV is involved, nonspecific laboratory findings often include variably abnormal liver function tests with an elevated SGOT common even in asymptomatic patients. Alkaline phosphatase is often elevated as well, but this is not a useful indicator during pregnancy because of the normal placental contribution to circulating levels. The serum bilirubin is rarely significantly elevated. Among the hematologic findings, a relative lymphocytosis occurs in 50–60%, atypical lymphocytes in 20–40%, a left shift in 20%, and thrombocytopenia in 10–15%. Serologic studies typically reveal a heterophil-negative status, which usually differentiates CMV mononucleosis from Epstein–Barr virus mononucleosis. Nonspecific elevations of cold agglutinins are found in 40–60%, rheumatoid factor in 30–50%, antinuclear antibodies in 20–40%, and cryoglobulins in 10–40%. In immunocompetent individuals, it is rare for any of these laboratory studies to be abnormal during recurrent CMV infections.

The differential diagnosis of congenital CMV infections includes the organisms noted above as well as various syndromes, chromosomal abnormalities, environmental teratogens, and inborn errors of metabolism. Congenitally infected infants with the full-blown stigmata of cytomegalic inclusion disease are not easily missed. More difficult to identify are the relatively asymptomatic congenitally infected infants who will, nevertheless, go on to develop the significant sequelae associated with their infection. Certainly, in situations in which it is known that the mother has CMV during the current or in a previous pregnancy, extra efforts should be made within the first two weeks of life to identify the congenitally infected infant.

A variety of laboratory procedures are now available to ascertain the diagnosis of CMV in mother and newborn. The standard against which each of these techniques is measured is still the virus culture. Cultures are the most sensitive and specific means of detecting CMV, but they are not by themselves sufficient to differentiate primary, secondary, or recurrent infections.[19] Standard culture techniques also suffer the disadvantages of potential delay in diagnosis and a reliable diagnostic laboratory capable of prolonged maintenance of the specimen is needed. Although a cytopathologic effect of CMV on diploid human fibroblasts can be found as early as 48–72 hours after inoculation, cultures cannot be considered negative until six weeks. To circumvent this delay, many laboratories have turned to a shell vial tissue culture technique with the detection of CMV-induced antigens by monoclonal antibodies, allowing identification of the virus within 24 hours.[20] Specimens for culture can be taken from sources of body fluids such as urine, cervix, throat, saliva, tears, amniotic fluid, and blood buffy coat. The best results seem to be obtained from urine. If the specimens cannot be cultured immediately, they are best stored at 4°C or on wet ice.

At times, cytology and even histology are useful adjuncts to the diagnosis of CMV infection. As diagnostic tools, both techniques are rapid and highly specific when the typical inclusion-bearing cytomegalic cells, described previously, are found. However, the practical value of these techniques is compromised by sampling error, which results in a relatively low sensitivity on the order of 50–70%, even under the best of circumstances. Immunofluorescent techniques, particularly those which employ CMV-specific monoclonal antibodies, have raised the sensitivity of CMV detection in certain histologic specimens to a level comparable to viral cultures.[21] The highest yield specimens for cytologic evaluation include urine sediment, gastric washings, and cerebrospinal fluid. The highest yields for histopathologic evaluation are from biopsies of liver, lung, and kidneys.

Serology is useful in establishing the diagnosis of a primary CMV infection; however, one must be aware of certain pitfalls that can confound the interpretation of serologic profiles. During well-documented primary infections, first IgM and then high titer IgG antibodies can be found within 1–2 weeks of the onset of clinical disease. Unlike most common viral infections, however, IgM may persist for as long as six to nine months following its appearance. Furthermore, IgM has been found to reappear on occasion with reactivation of latent CMV infection. Despite these pitfalls, the finding of CMV-specific IgM is of clinical importance in documenting primary maternal and fetal infections and should be sought. In the past, the indirect fluorescent antibody test has been commonly used to detect IgM antibody to CMV; however, this test is subject to inaccurate interpretation because CMV-specific IgG can compete with IgM, thereby giving an apparent reduction in IgM titers, and also because CMV infections are associated with a high incidence of rheumatoid factor (IgM anti-IgG) production. Currently, IgM-specific enzyme-linked immunosorbent assay (ELISA) tests provide the most sensitive, specific, and reliable means of detecting CMV-specific IgM.[22]

Generally, it is safe to assume primary infection in the individual who seroconverts; that is, an individual who develops IgM or has at least a fourfold rise in paired serum antibody titers in the face of an acute viral syndrome. However, serologic profiles must be interpreted more cautiously in asymptomatic individuals and in those in whom seronegative status has not been found previously. For example, longitudinal follow up of seropositive individuals has shown that complement-fixing antibodies, which are generally IgG with a high specificity for antigens produced late in the replicative cycle and shared by different CMV strains, may fluctuate widely between detectable ($\geq$1:8) and undetectable ($\leq$1:4) levels and may at times exceed the fourfold threshold ordinarily used to indicate recent exposure.[23]

When primary maternal CMV infection is suspected during pregnancy, amniocentesis and even percutaneous umbilical blood sampling have been used to help confirm congenital infection by culture and serology, although results must be interpreted with caution. If cultures are negative, they do not rule out congenital infection, and if they are positive they do not indicate the severity of the disease. In addition, there is the small possibility of introducing CMV infection as a consequence of these procedures. As an alternative to intrauterine sampling, the diagnosis of congenital infection can be made if virus is culturable from body fluids of a newborn infant obtained within two weeks of life. Cytologic evaluation can be performed on these same body fluids and is valuable if positive. Serologic evidence of congenital infection is more difficult to interpret. Complement-fixing antibody, predominantly IgG, is transmitted across the placenta and is therefore not useful in documenting congenital infections during the neonatal period. Indeed, maternal IgG may obscure the identification of CMV-specific fetal IgM for reasons indicated above. When CMV-specific IgM is found in cord blood, it is highly suggestive of congenital infection but even then infection should be corroborated by viral cultures.[24] From the practical standpoint of counseling, if neither IgG nor IgM is found in cord blood, then *in utero* infection can be excluded.

TREATMENT

There is no safe specific therapy for the management of CMV infections during pregnancy. Treatment regimens with antiviral agents and adjunctive immunotherapy have been relegated mostly to immunosuppressed or congenitally infected individuals and, until recently, have met with limited success. Adenine arabinoside (ara-A), cytosine arabinoside (ara-C), idoxuridine (IUDR), floxuridine (FUDR), and phosphonoformic acid (PFA) have at times been correlated with clinical improvement in these individuals, but often have only been found to reduce virus shedding and not alter the course of disease.[25] Unfortunately, even though several of these agents have shown efficacy, they also exhibit cytotoxic and immunosuppressive properties that make them undesirable as antiviral agents and contraindicated in otherwise healthy pregnant women. Acyclovir, despite its popularity and success in the treatment of herpes simplex virus infections, is both theoretically and practically not useful because CMV does not induce its own thymidine kinase. Interferon therapy, alone or in combination with various antiviral agents, has also been shown on occasion to reduce virus shedding but does not alter the course of an established infection.[26] Currently, interferons and other immunomodulatory agents are absolutely contraindicated during pregnancy.

In recent years, one of the more promising antiviral agents to be evaluated has been ganciclovir (2′-deoxyguanosine, 9-[(1,3-dihydroxy-2-propoxy) methyl] guanine), or DHPG. Although the mechanism of action in CMV-infected cells is not completely understood, ganciclovir does appear to selectively inhibit the CMV DNA polymerase. Ganciclovir has shown great promise in the management of chronic CMV infections in immunocompromised patients and, specifically, has proven itself to be the first agent to have a significant impact on the unrelenting course of chorioretinitis in these individuals.[27,28] Unfortunately, ganciclovir, too, has toxicity that would preclude its use in otherwise healthy pregnant women, but perhaps it will set the standard for the development of similar, more specific and safer agents that could be used in the management of primary maternal disease, congenital infections, and progressive sensorineural hearing loss.

Since the best defense for the fetus appears to be acquired maternal immunity, probably the most practical means of preventing severe infections, which take the greatest toll on both the patient and society, would be the widespread use of a vaccine administered prior to the childbearing years. Elek and Stern were the first to describe the use of a live human tissue culture attenuated CMV strain that successfully stimulated neutralizing and complement-fixing antibodies when inoculated subcutaneously.[29] As yet, neither live, killed, nor subunit virus vaccines have completed clinical trials, and none is available for routine use in the United States.

The prevention of primary infections in seronegative women during pregnancy would be more valuable than any of the current treatment regimens. However, realizing this goal is nearly impossible simply because the virus is endemic and there are so many asymptomatically infected individuals. Routine serologic screening in all pregnant patients is probably not yet practical, but it might be considered in women of childbearing age who work in certain high-risk settings, such as day care centers, intensive care nurseries, dialysis units, and institutions for the mentally retarded, to ascertain those individuals who are seronegative and therefore at risk. Until a safe and efficacious vaccine is available, women who are known to be seronegative and anticipating pregnancy or currently pregnant should minimize contact with known chronic CMV excreters and observe strict handwashing regimens if exposed on a regular basis to body fluids. If there is an option to transfer these women to a different work environment, this can be considered, but it is not clear whether such action would have any real impact on reducing their risk for primary infections. Repeat serologic studies during pregnancy may be offered, and in those who seroconvert, active counseling should begin.[30]

When CMV is included in the differential diagnosis during pregnancy or in the postpartum period for either maternal or fetal indications, it is important to confirm the diagnosis and ascertain if the infection is a primary or a recurrent one. For counseling purposes, very few severely affected children are born to women who are seropositive prior to pregnancy, and a woman who has delivered a severely affected child in the past is at low risk for repeating this at a subsequent pregnancy, though milder congenital infection can occur. If primary infection during pregnancy is documented, the patient should be given current information regarding the risks for congenital infection, for an infant being severely affected ($\leq$5%), and for a child who will develop sequelae of chronic infection such as sensorineural hearing loss. It is important that she understand that sequelae can occur following infection at any stage of gestation. Although a high percentage of infants delivering through an infected genitourinary tract will contract the disease, CMV infection outside the uterus is generally mild, and prophylactic cesarean section is certainly not indicated. By the same token, breast-feeding, at least in the term infant, despite being a major source of neonatally-acquired infection, is not contraindicated.[31] The position on breast-feeding is not so clear in the case of the preterm infant when any major infection might be detrimental to survival. In instances where premature infants require transfusion, a reduction in acquired CMV infection and subsequent complications have been found when blood products from seronegative donors are used.

There is little doubt that when an obvious congenital infection is confirmed, abnormalities should be detailed carefully, and plans for ongoing neurologic evaluation begun. The real challenge, however, is identifying those asymptomatically infected infants who are at risk for the long-term sequelae, such as progressive sensorineural hearing defects and chorioretinitis, so that potentially reversible causes of perceptual and psychomotor retardation are identified and corrective measures are taken. Ideally, routine screening for congenital CMV infection could be done at birth, but cost-effectiveness and impact on long-term outcome will have to be demonstrated before this is widely accepted.

REFERENCES

1. Ho M. *Cytomegalovirus: Biology and Infection.* New York, NY: Plenum Press; 1982.
2. Hanshaw JB. On deafness, cytomegalovirus and neonatal screening. *Am J Dis Child.* 1982;126:886.
3. Betts RF. Cytomegalovirus infection epidemiology and biology in adults. *Semin Perinatol.* 1983;7:22.
4. Stagno S, Pass R, Dworsky M, et al. Congenital and perinatal cytomegalovirus infections. *Semin Perinatol.* 1983;7:31.
5. Griffiths PD, Baboonian C. A prospective study of primary cytomegalovirus infection during pregnancy: a final report. *Br J Obstet Gynaecol.* 1984;91:307.
6. Stagno S, Cloud G, Pass RF, et al. Factors associated with primary cytomegalovirus infection during pregnancy. *J Med Virol.* 1984;13:347.
7. Yow MD, Williamson DW, Leeds LJ, et al. Epidemiologic characteristics of cytomegalovirus infection in mothers and their infants. *Am J Obstet Gynecol.* 1988;158:1189.
8. Chandler SH, Alexander ER, Holmes KK. Epidemiology of cytomegaloviral infection in a heterogeneous population of pregnant women. *J Infect Dis.* 1985;152:249.
9. Alford CA, Hayes K, Britt W. Primary cytomegalovirus infection in pregnancy: comparison of antibody responses to virus-encoded proteins between women with and without intrauterine infection. *J Infect Dis.* 1988;158:917.
10. Stern H, Hannington G, Booth J, et al. An early marker of fetal infection after primary cytomegalovirus infection in pregnancy. *Br Med J.* 1986;292:718.
11. Stagno S, Pass RF, Cloud G, et al. Primary cytomegalovirus infection in pregnancy: incidence, transmission to fetus and clinical outcome. *JAMA.* 1986;256:1904.
12. Rook AH. Interactions of cytomegalovirus with the human immune system. *Rev Infect Dis.* 1988;10(suppl 3):S460.
13. Stagno S, Pass R, Dworsky M, et al. Congenital cytomegalovirus infection: the relative importance of primary and recurrent maternal infection. *N Engl J Med.* 1982;306:945.
14. Grant S, Edmond E, Syme J. A prospective study of cytomegalovirus infection in pregnancy: laboratory evidence of congenital infection following maternal primary and reactivated infection. *J Infect.* 1981;3:24.
15. Pass R, Stagno S, Myers G. Outcome of symptomatic congenital cytomegalovirus infection: results of long-term longitudinal follow-up. *Pediatrics.* 1980;66:758.
16. Stagno S, Reynolds D, Amos C, et al. Auditory and visual defects resulting from symptomatic and subclinical congenital cytomegaloviral and toxoplasma infections. *Pediatrics.* 1977;59:669.
17. Hanshaw J. Congenital cytomegalovirus infection: a fifteen year prospective. *J Infect Dis.* 1971;123:555.
18. Pass RF. Cytomegalovirus in the surgical patient. *Infect Surg.* 1983;2:571.
19. Stagno S, Pass R, Reynolds D, et al. Comparative study of diagnostic procedure for congenital cytomegalovirus infection. *Pediatrics.* 1980; 65:251.
20. Gleaves CA, Smith TF, Shuster EA, et al. Comparison of standard tube and shell vial cell culture techniques for the detection of cytomegalovirus in clinical specimens. *J Clin Microbiol.* 1985;21:217.
21. Hackman RC, Myerson D, Meyers JD, et al. Rapid diagnosis of cytomegaloviral pneumonia by tissue immunofluorescence with a murine monoclonal antibody. *J Infect Dis.* 1985;151:325.
22. Schaefer L, Cesario A, Demmler G, et al. Evaluation of CMV-M enzyme immunoassay for detection of cytomegalovirus immunoglobulin M antibody. *J Clin Microbiol.* 1988;26:2041.
23. Waner JL, Weller TH, Kevy SV. Patterns of cytomegaloviral complement-fixing antibody activity: a longitudinal study of blood donors. *J Infect Dis.* 1973;127:538.
24. Reynolds D, Stagno S, Stubbs K, et al. Inapparent congenital cytomegalovirus infection with elevated cord IgM levels: causal relationship with auditory and mental deficiency. *N Engl J Med.* 1974;290:291.
25. Verheyden JPH. Evolution of therapy for cytomegalovirus infection. *Rev Infect Dis.* 1988;10(suppl 3):S477.
26. Hirsch MS, Schooley RT, Cosimi AB, et al. Effects of interferon-alpha on cytomegalovirus reactivation syndromes in renal transplant recipients. *N Engl J Med.* 1983;308:1489.
27. Snydman DR. Ganciclovir therapy for cytomegalovirus disease associated with renal transplants. *Rev Infect Dis.* 1988;10(suppl 3):S554.
28. Buhles WC, Mastre BJ, Tinker AJ, et al. Ganciclovir treatment of life- or sight-threatening cytomegalovirus infection: experience in 314 immunocompromised patients. *Rev Infect Dis.* 1988;10(suppl 3):S495.
29. Elek S, Stern J. Development of a vaccine against mental retardation caused by cytomegalovirus infection in utero. *Lancet.* 1974;1:1.
30. Knox G. Cytomegalovirus: patient counseling. *Semin Perinatol.* 1983;7:43.
31. Stagno S, Reynolds D, Pass R, et al. Breast milk and the risk of cytomegalovirus infection. *N Engl J Med.* 1980;302:1073.

Chapter Ninety-One
Herpes Simplex Viruses
Kenneth F. Trofatter, Jr.

91

The term *herpes,* derived from the Greek "to creep," was introduced to the medical literature 2500 years ago and has been used to describe a multitude of skin disorders.[1] Cooke in 1676 and Turner in 1714 provided the first descriptions of skin lesions that were clearly the result of infection with herpes simplex virus (HSV). Astruc in 1736 suggested a venereal means of transmission in his description of a disease, different from syhpilis, which probably was HSV. In 1814, Bateman restricted the term *herpes* to a limited number of conditions characterized by localized groups of vesicles and a short, self-limited course. Among these were the entities *Herpes labialis* (fever blisters) and *Herpes praeputialis* (genital herpes), which we commonly associate today with HSV infection.

Gruter in 1920 confirmed the infectious nature of herpes when he produced keratitis in rabbits with material taken from human herpetic lesions. Ten years later, Andrewes and Carmichael established the ubiquity of HSV when they found specific neutralizing antibodies in 75% of randomly sampled individuals. Hass in 1935 described premature infants with hepatoadrenal necrosis and intranuclear inclusions resulting from perinatally acquired HSV infection.[2] Since then, HSV has become recognized as a major venereal disease with signficiant short- and long-term sequelae for infected individuals and their offspring.

There are two major types of HSV, *HSV-1* and *HSV-2,* and multiple strains of each. The types are structurally similar, with icosahedral nucleocapsids comprised of 162 caposomeres sheathed by a lipid envelope acquired by budding through the cell membrane. The virus has a linear, double-stranded DNA of 100×10^6 molecular weight containing 68–69% guanosine plus cytosine. Each strand of DNA is composed of covalently linked long (L) and short (S) components, with four isomeric forms possible. HSV-1 and HSV-2 share about 50% of their DNA sequences. Virus replication occurs in the cell nucleus with the production of virus within 10–14 hours after infection.

Humans are the sole natural host of HSV, and 70–90% of childbearing-age individuals have serologic evidence of prior exposure. In the United States alone, an estimated 160,000,000–180,000,000 people have antibody to one or both HSV types. Of these, 20,000,000–25,000,000 have four or more recurrences per year. Although the highest prevalence rates for genital HSV originally reported were found among patients from lower socioeconomic groups, the recent epidemic of genital HSV affects all socioeconomic levels, and in some reports the highest incidence of new disease is present in caucasian middle class women. Transmission of HSV occurs by intimate contact, most often by oral–oral, genital–genital, and oral–genital routes. Although rare, transmission by fomites freshly contaminated with body fluids has been documented. Commonly, exposure to HSV-1 occurs in early childhood, and exposure to HSV-2 occurs after becoming sexually active, with the peak incidence being from ages 14–39. Although either type can cause infection at any body site, approximately 80% of infections above the waist are caused by HSV-1, and 80% of those below the waist by HSV-2.

PATHOPHYSIOLOGY OF DISEASE

HSV replicates in human tissues derived from all three embryonic layers. Usually, the virus enters through disruption of the superficial epithelium and first replicates in parabasal and intermediate cells. As infectious virus is produced, it spreads to adjacent cells with or without an extracellular phase. HSV is neurotropic and, early in the course of infection, associates with nerve cell endings in the epithelium, along which it ascends to the local ganglia.

Productively infected epithelial cells develop intranuclear inclusions, may develop syncytia, undergo ballooning degeneration, and inevitably die. Accompanying cell necrosis, an infiltrate of polymorphonuclear leukocytes and mononuclear leukocytes can be found within and at the periphery of the lesion. Macroscopically, the typical fluid-filled vesicles on an erythematous base are seen. Both humoral and cellular immunity help to limit the spread of the infection.

After invasion and replication at the portal of entry, dissemination of the infection can occur by local spread, by hematogenous routes, by viremia and within infected leukocytes, and by ascension along peripheral nerves to the ganglia. Replication can then occur at these secondary sites. In the ganglia, some cells that do not support productive infections immediately are able to harbor the virus in a latent state. The actual mechanism of latency is unknown, but no detectable viral antigens are expressed by these infected cells.

Despite cross-reactive immunity, secondary infections with the same or a different HSV type may occur.[3] More commonly, however, recurrent infections occur by reactivation of latent virus in the ganglia. Once reactivated, infectious virus can spread by peripheral axonal transport to the site served by the ganglion, by replication and extension within the ganglion, or by hematogenous routes. Discrete and localized vesicular lesions typify reactivation recurrences; however, at times infectious virus can be cultured from sites of previous infection even in the absence of visible lesions.

The mechanism of reactivation remains a mystery, but numerous factors have been correlated with this, including exposure to UV light, fever, trauma, and nerve stimulation, fever therapy, menstruation, stress, and immunosuppressive therapy. Although prostaglandins have been proposed as a common factor to many of these stimuli because of their immunosuppressive capabilities, particularly with regard to cell-mediated immunity, their role *in vivo* remains to be proven.[4]

Primary infections can be defined as those occurring in individuals with no prior antibody to HSV-1 or HSV-2. After the first month of life, primary infections are commonly divided into two major forms, gingivostomatitis and genital herpes. Gingivostomatitis often occurs in early childhood, is usually the result of HSV-1 infection, may be asymptomatic, or may go unrecognized. As a primary event during pregnancy, gingivostomatitis has minimal consequences for the mother or fetus. On the other hand, primary genital infections during pregnancy, particularly those with HSV-2, are reason for considerable concern.

The natural history of primary genital HSV infections has been well documented.[5] The incubation period from the time of exposure to the onset of disease is approximately 3–9 days. Prodromal tingling, burning, or itching may occur, and infectious virus may be isolated 1–2 days prior to the outbreak of vesicles. Vesicles then ulcerate and may coalesce, frequently involving multiple sites. During primary infections, lesions in various stages of development are common, with new lesions occurring for 3–6 weeks. Individual ulcers persist up to two weeks before crusting over on cutaneous surfaces or reepithelializing on mucosal surfaces. In most instances, healing is complete. Systemic symptoms, including fever, headaches, malaise, and myalgias, occur in about 70% of women. The symptoms worsen over the course of the first 7–10 days and gradually resolve. During overt primary infections, virtually 100% of women experience pain, 80% experience dysuria, and 80% experience tender lymphadenopathy. Ten to twenty percent of women will have clinical evidence of HSV pharyngitis. HSV can be isolated from the cervix and urethra in 80–90% of women. Extensive ulcerative necrotic cervical lesions can occur and are usually associated with a profuse watery discharge.

Following a primary genital infection, the recurrence rates from reactivation of latent virus approach 50% for HSV-1 and 90% for HSV-2.[6] Primary infections during pregnancy are associated with a greater incidence of genitourinary tract recurrences throughout pregnancy and an increased likelihood of virus excretion at delivery, probably reflecting an incompletely developed maternal immune response.[7-9] Recurrent infections are more likely to be asymptomatic and localized but may occur with more than one site of excretion. When symptoms do occur with recurrences, about 50% of individuals will have prodromal tingling or itching 1–2 days prior to the outbreak of vesicles. Interestingly, about one fourth of women with recurrences at delivery will experience fever not associated with proven bacterial infection.[10] Vesicles tend to occur in discrete patches and ulcerate within 24–48 hours. Pain will develop in 80–90% of women, and 10–15% will have systemic complaints. External dysuria occurs in about 25%. The duration of pain, viral shedding, and time until healing is generally shorter than in primary infections, usually with complete resolution in 7–10 days. During external genital recurrences, 10–15% of women will also shed virus from their cervix. Recurrent infections alone during pregnancy probably do not contribute significantly to the incidence of maternal morbidity, spontaneous abortion, intrauterine growth retardation, or prematurity; however, they are a silent and deadly reservoir for neonatal infections.

EFFECT OF PREGNANCY ON DISEASE

In various studies, the presence of HSV in the genitourinary tract at some time during pregnancy has been documented in 0.4–7.4% of all obstetric patients.[11] Isolation of HSV from asymptomatic women on the day of delivery reportedly ranges from 0.2–4.0%. Recurrences tend to increase in frequency during each trimester of pregnancy, a finding that suggests the development of a subtle progressive immunodeficiency toward HSV throughout gestation. Antibody responses to primary infections during pregnancy are comparable to those in nonpregnant women. HSV-specific IgM can be found within the first 7–10 days, followed by IgG within three weeks. Permanent humoral immunity is maintained with the IgG response, and titers fluctuate very little over time. The presence of certain HSV-specific antibodies has been correlated with differences in natural history of HSV infections in different individuals.[6,12] For example, the presence of high-titer complement-independent neutralizing antibodies after a primary genital infection is associated with a greater risk of subsequent recurrences.

Primary genital HSV infections have been found in about 1.5 of 10,000 pregnancies. Although more than 80% of recurrent genital infections are due to HSV-2, 20–50% of primary genital infections during pregnancy can be expected to be the result of infection with HSV-1. Maternal complications of primary genital HSV infections most often include dysuria, urinary retention, dyspareunia, aseptic meningitis, and extragenital mucocutaneous lesions (fingers, buttocks, groin, thighs, eyes). On rare occasions, dissemination and death have occurred in the noncompromised host, including several reports of maternal death secondary to primary HSV infection during pregnancy.[13] Although maternal HSV infections generally follow a self-limited course, this is the exception rather than the rule in the overtly infected fetus or neonate.[14] For this reason, the overriding concern with maternal HSV infections is that the virus will be transmitted to the baby.

True congenital infections prior to the rupture of the chorioamnionic membranes are uncommon but have been the subject of case reports. These are almost exclusively the consequence of primary maternal infections. Transmission of HSV under these circumstances probably occurs by hematogenous routes, with maternal viremia in the absence of maternal antibody resulting in placentitis or the direct transfer of infectious virus or infected leukocytes across the placenta. The contribution of ascending infection from the cervix is unknown in these instances. Congenital infection, when it occurs early in gestation is usually incompatible with life, most often resulting in fetal demise and spontaneous abortion rather than congenital anomalies. For this reason, primary infection in early pregnancy is not considered to be an indication for abortion. Later in gestation, congenital infection is associated with significant fetal mortality, premature labor and delivery, intrauterine growth retardation, and major multiorgan system sequelae should the infant survive.[2,14-16]

Perinatally acquired infections are much more common than congenital infections. Transmission to the baby can occur by ascending cervical infection following rupture of membranes, by delivery through an infected genitourinary tract, and by contact after delivery with active lesions or infected secretions from parents, visitors, or nursery personnel. Although 1% or more of women may be excreting HSV at delivery, and as many as 4% of infants born vaginally to women with recurrences will have culture-proven colonization with HSV, only 1 in 5,000 to 1 in 20,000 infants develop clinical infection. However, this attack rate approaches 40% when typical cytologic changes are detectable.[8] True primary infections in the peripartum period are associated with a 50% incidence of neonatal disease.[15,17] Overall, it is estimated that 3000–7500 infants born annually will develop clinical evidence of HSV infection.

Unfortunately, maternal symptoms do not necessarily correlate with the extent of maternal disease.[5] Indeed, 50–75% of women who have infants with neonatal HSV are asymptomatic and only about one-third will have any history of HSV infection. In many instances, the mothers are young, with little or no prenatal care, and the infants are firstborn. About 50% of affected infants are the product of a preterm delivery.

The incubation period from exposure until the onset of overt disease in the neonate is about 4–12 days, and the infant appears to be at increased risk for the first month of life. The portal of entry may be obvious, such as a scalp electrode site or a skin abrasion, but more often it goes unrecognized, involving the eye, umbilicus, or mucous membranes. In many instances, the primary site of infection is never found, and the infant presents with disseminated multiorgan system involvement. Although type-specific antibodies, particularly those indicating prior maternal infection, such as anti-HSV-2 glycoprotein G, which may not appear for a month or more after primary infection, are associated with a smaller risk of disseminated infection, widespread disease can occur even in the presence of transplacentally acquired antibody.[12] The exact mechanisms for this are unknown, but subtle defects in specific and nonspecific cellular immunity and lymphokine production, and even infected mononuclear leukocytes, may be involved.[18]

Neonatal disease may be mild and localized (5–15%) or limited to the central nervous system (CNS) (5–15%) but is most often widely disseminated (70–90%).[14] Neurologic signs typically predominate and comprise the spectrum of seizures, lethargy, poor feeding, irritability, vomiting, poor temperature control, and coma. Multiorgan system involvement is common in disseminated infection, with massive hepatic and adrenal necrosis described classically.[2] Meningoencephalitis can be rapid, devastating, and poorly responsive to therapy. Bleeding diathesis, jaundice, respiratory distress, and shock are generally the terminal events. Fifty percent or more of infants recognized as having neonatal infection will die, usually within 6–10 days.[14] Of those infants surviving, greater than 50% will have permanent ocular or neurologic sequelae. Even newborns who survive apparently localized superifical lesions have a 40–50% chance of these sequelae. Although the frequency of CNS involvement is comparable between HSV-1 and HSV-2, the latter tends to result in more destructive lesions and a greater likelihood of permanent neurologic sequelae, even among those infants surviving with antiviral chemotherapy.[16]

DIAGNOSIS OF DISEASE

The initial diagnosis of maternal HSV infection is usually suspected on clinical grounds or from historical accounts of typical lesions, especially if these are recurrent. A history of exposure to a consort with documented or suspected HSV is extremely useful and should be sought.[10] The differential diagnosis includes syphilis, chancroid, lymphogranuloma venereum, granuloma inguinale, herpes zoster, Behçet's disease, Crohn's disease, carcinoma, and excoriation, but all of these are much less common than HSV. In general, a high index of suspicion accompanied by a low threshold for obtaining confirmatory studies in pregnant patients with complaints of unusual discharge, pruritis, dysesthesia, and vulvar or cervical lesions may help to pick up previously undiagnosed maternal HSV infections.

When possible, and especially during pregnancy, the diagnosis should be confirmed by appropriate laboratory studies. Among these, virus culture remains the most sensitive, specific, and widely available diagnostic tool. HSV grows in a variety of human and animal cell lines, and when significant virus is present, a culture-proven diagnosis can be made in 90–95% of instances within 48–72 hours. Best results are obtained by collecting fluid from fresh, unruptured vesicles. When cultures are indicated during pregnancy in the absence of visible lesions, sampling sites of previous lesions, areas with prodromal symptoms, and the cervix give the highest yields. HSV is labile to drying; therefore, it is beneficial to moisten the swab with the transport medium prior to culturing an area of suspected involvement. For best results, swabs then should be placed immediately in an appropriate medium containing antibiotics, transported on ice, and inoculated as soon as possible after being obtained. If storage is necessary, this is best done at −70°C.

Although not yet widely available, the detection of specific HSV antigens in exfoliated infected cells is now possible by immunofluorescence and enzyme-linked immunoadsorbent assays (ELISA).[19] The use of monoclonal antibodies has made these relatively rapid procedures comparable in sensitivity and specificity to culture techniques; however, their role in the evaluation and management of the obstetric patient has yet to be defined.

Under selected circumstances, cytology is also useful in establishing a diagnosis. This procedure has the advantages of simplicity, rapidity, and relatively high specificity, but suffers from the disadvantages of low sensitivity and sampling error. Use of cytology is only practical when vesicular lesions are present and should never be used alone to exclude the diagnosis. When sampling for cytology is done, fresh vesicles should be unroofed and the margins scraped. If the lesions are crusted over, they can be covered for 15–20 minutes with sterile saline-soaked dressing before proceeding. Slide specimens should be placed immediately in fixative solution before they dry. When present, multinucleated giant cells and cells with typical intranuclear inclusions confirm the diagnosis. Cytology always should be backed up by culture.

Because of the convenience, accuracy, and widespread availability of other techniques, serology usually plays a small role in the diagnosis of HSV infections. For suspected primary infections, however, a fourfold increase in complement-fixing or neutralizing antibodies on paired sera 2–3 weeks apart or the detection of HSV-specific IgM is diagnostic. Serology is of little practical use in documenting recurrent infections, but, theoretically, it could be used to confirm secondary infections with a different HSV type or strain.

Early diagnosis is critical to the management of neonatal HSV infections but is still, unfortunately, the exception rather than the rule. The 4- to 12-day incubation period often means the infant is discharged from the hospital prior to onset of symptoms. By the time parents recognize an abnormality and bring this to the physician's attention, the delay has allowed time for viral dissemination and its attendant high morbidity and mortality, even with aggressive antiviral chemotherapy.

HSV infection should be included in the differential diagnosis of any infant with hepatosplenomegaly, skin vesicles, seizures, irritability, temperature instability, lethargy, or poor feeding.[14,16] Although infrequently associated with congenital anomalies, HSV should be considered with the other TORCH organisms when etiologic agents are sought. Certainly, any infant born with or developing typical herpetic lesions at any site should be evaluated thoroughly and rapidly. Under these circumstances, ELISA, immunofluorescence, and cytology can help to determine if HSV is the cause, but cultures always should be done to support the diagnosis. Although serology is of little immediate benefit compared to these other diagnostic techniques, the presence of HSV-specific IgM confirms primary neonatal infection. Adjunctive evaluation often includes complete blood count with differential liver function tests, assessment of cerebral spinal fluid, electroencephalogram, and computerized tomography. Due to the poorer prognosis of CNS HSV-2 infections, type-specific serology or cultures may aid counseling with regard to expectations for long-term outcome. In any case, if HSV is suspected, antiviral chemotherapy should be started even prior to disease confirmation.[20]

Cooperation between obstetrician and pediatrician can be vital to the diagnosis of a neonatal HSV infection. Mothers with past documented HSV should be evaluated at the time of presentation in labor, as detailed below, even in the absence of lesions. When suspicious lesions are present, or if the woman complains of prodromal symptoms, specimens for culture, ELISA, or in some instances, cytology, should be obtained, and the pediatrician alerted that the infant was delivered through or was exposed to a potentially infected genitourinary tract. Parents should be instructed in the signs and symptoms of HSV infection when there has been any question of neonatal exposure, and they should be encouraged to seek immediate medical attention with the earliest evidence of skin lesions or alteration in neurologic status. Under some circumstances, daily evaluation by trained medical personnel during the first two weeks of life is not unreasonable.

TREATMENT OF DISEASE

The goals of management during pregnancy are to prevent primary and secondary infections, to minimize maternal and fetal morbidity, and to prevent perinatal transmission of HSV to the baby. Realizing these goals begins with a careful history from patient and partner regarding proven or suspected sexually transmitted diseases. Pregnant women with no prior history of HSV should avoid sexual contact with males who have obvious genital lesions or prodromal symptoms typical of recurrent HSV infection. If HSV is suspected, the diagnosis should be confirmed, preferably by culture, at the time of an outbreak. In addition, any patient presenting with preterm labor or premature rupture of membranes, who also has suspicious vulvar or cervical lesions or unexplained fever, should be considered for HSV culture. Primary HSV infections have been implicated in these pregnancy complications, and the preterm infant is unusually susceptible to its most serious complications.

After the diagnosis has been established, current guidelines from the Infectious Disease Society for Obstetrics–Gynecology should be followed. These are listed below:

> *In women with history of genital herpes, but without lesions: 1) Weekly prenatal cultures should be abandoned. 2) In the absence of genital herpetic lesions, vaginal delivery should be expected. 3) In order to identify potentially exposed neonates, a culture for herpes virus may be obtained from either the mother on the day of delivery or from the neonate. 4) Isolation is not necessary for the mother. 5) It is recognized that with such a policy, there is a small risk (approximately one per thousand) of neonatal infection.*
>
> *In women with herpetic lesions of the genital tract when either labor or membrane rupture occurs: 1) Cesarean delivery is a technique that can reduce the risk of neonatal herpes virus infection. 2) Ideally, cesarean section should be performed before or within four to six hours of membrane rupture, but cesarean delivery may be of benefit in preventing neonatal herpes regardless of duration of membrane rupture.*
>
> *In women with genital herpetic lesions at or near term, but before labor or membrane rupture: Cultures collected at three- to five-day intervals may be performed to assure the absence of virus at the time of birth and to increase the likelihood of vaginal delivery.*[21]

The author's approach paraphrases the Society's recommendations. When a patient with known or suspected HSV presents in labor, a careful history is obtained with attention to recent outbreaks and prodromal symptoms. The patient is then examined and cultures are obtained from the sites of previous recurrences and from the cervix. If prodromal symptoms or suspicious lesions are absent, vaginal delivery is anticipated; if they are present, cesarean section is recommended. If the patient has a history of frequent recurrences, induction is considered at term during a disease-free period. During labor, an attempt is made to minimize vaginal examinations, internal monitoring, fetal scalp sampling, and forceps delivery, although none of these is absolutely contraindicated. During the postpartum period, patients and visitors with active oral or genital lesions should keep affected areas covered and should wash their hands before handling the baby. Kissing the infant is best avoided with active oral lesions and primary genital infections in view of the high incidence of associated pharyngitis in the latter.

When a woman develops primary, or severe, recurrent disease during pregnancy, aggressive symptomatic and chemotherapeutic management should be considered. Because patients often present relatively late in the course of disease, a treatment regimen should be instituted when indicated even while confirmatory studies are pending.[18] Due to the potentially serious maternal and fetal complications of severe cases, a liberal policy for hospitalization and parenteral antiviral therapy is warranted. Conditions that can justify hospitalization include high fever, severe pain, urinary retention, mental status changes, seizures, focal neurologic signs, premature labor or suspected premature rupture of membranes, and liver function or hematologic abnormalities. Fever should be aggressively managed with acetominophen and even prostaglandin inhibitors, if necessary. Pain management frequently requires the use of narcotics. External genital lesions can be washed with plain soap and water three or four times daily followed by drying with a blow dryer or heat lamp. Urinary retention may necessitate catheterization.

If antiviral chemotherapy is to be used, this should be added to the above regimen as early in the course of disease as possible. Acyclovir (Zovirax) is the most reasonable choice for treatment of genital HSV infections by virtue of its high specificity, efficacy, and low toxicity to mother and, theoretically, fetus.[22,23] It is a synthetic acyclic purine nucleoside that is converted to its monophosphate form significantly only by the HSV thymidine kinase. The monophosphate is then converted to the triphosphate predominantly by cellular guanydylate synthetase. The triphosphate selectively inhibits the HSV DNA polymerase. It also competes with guanosine triphosphate and, if incorporated into DNA, interrupts DNA synthesis. The result is the concentration of the drug predominantly in cells actively involved in HSV replication, cells already destined to be destroyed having been committed to this process. As a side benefit, acyclovir probably has minimal carcinogenic and teratogenic potential at the dosages currently recommended. For these reasons, although not approved for use in pregnancy, it should be considered under circumstances that threaten maternal or fetal well-being.

When used during primary infections, acyclovir can reduce the length of virus shedding, shorten healing times, and decrease symptoms.[24] It is most effective if begun early during a primary infection and generally is not needed for treatment of most recurrent infections. Although long-term use of oral acyclovir in patients with frequent recurrences can reduce the number and severity of these outbreaks, the efficacy of prophylactic use in pregnancy has not been established.[25] Forms and regimens for using acyclovir are as follows. (1) Intravenous: 5 mg/kg body weight over 45–60 minutes every 8 hours for 5–7 days. In nonpregnant adults, this regimen shortens the median course of first episodes by about a week. At present, this should be reserved for the most severe infections during pregnancy.[23,24] (2) Oral: 200 mg five times per day for 7–10 days begun within one week of onset of primary infections or severe recurrent infections may shorten the course of disease up to five days. Orally, 200 mg two to five times per day (or 400 mg two times per day) has been found to be effective for prophylaxis against frequent recurrences and for management of minor recurrences. Again, prophylactic use in pregnancy has not been reported. Generally, the oral form is well absorbed and comparable in efficacy to the intravenous form. In the postpartum woman, acyclovir is concentrated in breast milk, but even at the maximum recommended oral doses, the baby would be expected to receive <1 mg/day.[26] (3) Topical: 5% ointment applied every 3–4 hours to external lesions. This form is minimally absorbed, and therefore would be most acceptable; however, it has minimal benefit in decreasing viral shedding and has no significant effect on symptoms or healing time. Therefore, it is never indicated for use alone during severe primary or recurrent infections, and probably has little practical use during pregnancy.

In addition to providing symptomatic relief and specific antiviral therapy, a critical role of the physician in managing the patient diagnosed with genital HSV is to provide up-to-date information, psychological support, and the opportunity for ongoing counseling. Basic information should include descriptions of the disease course in primary and recurrent infections, the concept of latency, and the realistic risks and planned management of pregnancy. One can expect patient responses of guilt, anger, anxiety, helplessness, and sexual dysfunction. These should be managed in a concerned, uncritical, informed, and, justifiably, reassuring manner. To assist in the counseling process, the patient can be directed to a number of community and national support groups that are a source of timely information and the first-hand experiences of others with genital HSV.

While aggressive chemotherapeutic management of maternal disease can be debated, specific antiviral therapy should be started in the neonate as soon as the diagnosis of HSV infection is suspected.[20,27] Without treatment, mortality due to disseminated HSV infection in neonates exceeds 80%, and less than 10% of survivors will have normal neurologic development. In some institutions, prophylactic therapy is employed whenever the infant is inadvertently delivered through an infected birth canal, particularly if the infant is the result of a preterm delivery. Open to more debate is the role of prophylactic therapy versus careful observation under circumstances where viral cultures obtained at the time of delivery in the absence of obvious lesions return positive for HSV within 48–72 hours.[17]

Again, acyclovir is the drug of choice for antiviral therapy because of its high specificity and relatively low toxicity. No matter how localized the disease appears, HSV infection in the newborn should always be considered a systemic disease, and therapy should be administered by intravenous infusion. Oral therapy in the neonate is probably impractical and there is absolutely no role for topical therapy under these circumstances. Delay in therapy can only worsen the outcome, and the potential benefits of acyclovir far outweigh its risks.

Although not widely used nor proven effective, adjuncts to specific antiviral chemotherapy can be considered. Hyperimmunoglobulins, interferons, and other immunomodulators, such as interleukins, are experimental forms of therapy, but could be beneficial in the setting of primary maternal infection at delivery and suspected or confirmed disseminated neonatal infection.

REFERENCES

1. Beswick TSL. The origin and use of the word herpes. *Med Hist.* 1962;6:214.
2. Hass GM. Hepato-adrenal necrosis with intranuclear inclusion bodies: report of a case. *Am J Pathol.* 1935;11:127.
3. Landry ML, Zibello TA. Ability of herpes simplex virus (HSV) types 1 and 2 to induce clinical disease and establish latency following previous genital infection with the heterologous type. *J Infect Dis.* 1988;158:1220.
4. Trofatter KF, Daniels CA. Interactions of human cells with prostaglandins and cyclic AMP modulators: effects on complement-mediated lysis and antibody-dependent cell-mediated cytolysis of herpes simplex virus infected human fibroblasts. *J Immunol.* 1979;122:1363.
5. Corey L, Adams H, Brown Z, et al. Genital herpes simplex virus infections: clinical manifestations, course, and complications. *Ann Intern Med.* 1983;98:958.
6. Reeves W, Corey L, Adams H, et al. Risk of recurrence after first episodes of genital herpes: relation to HSV type and antibody response. *N Engl J Med.* 1981;305:315.
7. Scher J, Bottone E, Desmond E, et al. The incidence and outcome of asymptomatic herpes simplex genitalis in an obstetric population. *Am J Obstet Gynecol.* 1982;144:906.
8. Nahmias AJ, Josey WE, Naib ZM, et al. Perinatal risk associated with maternal genital herpes simplex virus infection. *Am J Obstet Gynecol.* 1971;110:825.
9. Harger JH, Amortegui AJ, Meyer MP, et al. Characteristics of recurrent genital herpes simplex infections in pregnant women. *Obstet Gynecol.* 1989;73:367.
10. Whitley RJ, Corey L, Arvin A, et al. Changing presentation of herpes simplex virus infection in neonates. *J Infect Dis.* 1988;158:109.
11. Nerurkar LS, Jensen LP, McCallum P, et al. Frequency of asymptomatic genital herpes in pregnant women at term. *Obstet Gynecol Surv.* 1988;43:132.
12. Sullender WM, Yasukawa LL, Schwartz M, et al. Type-specific antibodies to herpes simplex virus type 2 (HSV-2) glycoprotein G in pregnant women, infants exposed to maternal HSV-2 infection at delivery, and infants with neonatal herpes. *J Infect Dis.* 1988;157:164.
13. Young EJ, Killam AP, Greene JF. Disseminated herpes-virus infection. Association with primary genital herpes in pregnancy. *JAMA.* 1976;235:2731.
14. Hanshaw JB, Dudgeon JA. Herpes simplex virus of the fetus and newborn. In: *Viral Diseases of the Fetus and Newborn.* Philadelphia, PA: WB Saunders, 1978;153.
15. Brown ZA, Vontver LA, Benedetti J, et al. Effects on infants of a first episode of genital herpes during pregnancy. *N Engl J Med.* 1987;317:1246.
16. Corey L, Stone EF, Whitley RJ, et al. Difference between herpes simplex virus type 1 and type 2 neonatal encephalitis and neurological outcome. *Lancet.* 1988;1:1.
17. Prober CG, Hensleigh PA, Boucher FD, et al. Use of routine viral cultures at delivery to identify neonates exposed to herpes simplex virus. *N Engl J Med.* 1988;318:887.
18. Trofatter KF, Williams RJ, Gall SA, et al. Growth of type II herpes simplex virus in newborn and adult mononuclear leukocytes. *Intervirology.* 1979;11:117.
19. Baker DA, Gonik B, Milch PO, et al. Clinical evaluation of a new herpes simplex virus ELISA: a rapid diagnostic test for herpes simplex virus. *Obstet Gynecol.* 1989;73:322.

20. Corey L, Holmes K. Genital herpes simplex virus infections: current concepts in diagnosis, therapy and prevention. *Ann Intern Med.* 1983;98:973.
21. Biggs RS, Amstey MS, Sweet RL, et al. Management of genital herpes infection in pregnancy. *Obstet Gynecol.* 1988;71:779.
22. Elion G, Furman P, Fyfe J, et al. Selectivity of action of an antiherpetic agent, 9-(2-hydroxyethoxymethyl) guanine. *Proc Natl Acad Sci.* 1977;74:5716.
23. Brown ZA, Baker DA. Acyclovir therapy during pregnancy. *Obstet Gyencol.* 1989;73:526.
24. Corey L, Fyfe K, Benedetti J, et al. Intravenous acyclovir for the treatment of primary genital herpes. *Ann Intern Med.* 1983;98:914.
25. Baker DA, Blythe JG, Kaufman R, et al. One-year suppression of frequent recurrences of genital herpes with oral acyclovir. *Obstet Gynecol.* 1989;73:84.
26. Meyer LJ, de Miranda P, Sheth N, et al. Acyclovir in human breast milk. *Am J Obstet Gynecol.* 1988;158:586.
27. Arvin AM. Antiviral treatment of herpes simplex infection in neonates and pregnant women. *J Amer Acad Dermatol.* 1988;18:200.

I
VIRAL INFECTIONS

Chapter Ninety-Two
Introduction to Viral Infections

Marvin S. Amstey

92

CLASSIFICATION

Attempts have been made to classify viruses in the same manner that has been used to classify bacteria. In recent times, this has succeeded to a limited extent. However, the ability to assign a species classification is not possible in most instances, nor has isolation of all viruses been accomplished, so that even a genus category is tentative for many viruses. Nevertheless, great strides have been made to classify more than 400 viruses known to infect man. In general, viruses share the following characteristics: they all have a nucleic acid or genome surrounded by a protein shell, and they can multiply only within living cell because they have no synthetic or energy-producing systems of their own.

The major criteria for assigning any virus to a particular category or family are the morphologic, genetic, physical, and chemical properties of the virus particle or virion. Various combinations of these criteria will produce the same categorical breakdown of viruses; therefore, it is not clear whether all of these criteria are needed or which system is better than another. For example, a system of classification using just the structure and size of the viral genome will result in a listing that is the same as a classification based simply on electron microscopic morphology.

The major families of viruses that infect man are listed in Table 92–1. They are divided into groups by the type of nucleic acid found in the nucleocapsid. Many other morphologic factors, such as whether the nucleic acid is single or double stranded, whether an envelope is present, and the molecular weight, can be found in a text on basic virology.[1-3]

PATHOGENESIS

In order for any virus to produce an effect or cause disease, it must enter the cell. This process is referred to as *adsorption*. On a cellular level, all viruses produce a cytopathic effect that may be easily recognized or that may be very subtle and measured only with sophisticated biochemical or immunologic means. Adsorption occurs because of the presence of specific receptors on the cell surface. There are usually a large number of viral receptors on a cell, so that a large number of viral particles may be adsorbed. The next steps necessary for the virus particle to reproduce within the cell and achieve the characteristic cytopathology are *penetration* and *uncoating*. Penetration is obvious, as the virus particle can be seen entering the cytoplasm. The uncoating of the viral genome is a process by which the protective protein coat is stripped away from the nucleic acid, so that the genome becomes available for the next, or *synthetic*, step in viral reproduction.

The synthetic phase of viral–cell interaction utilizes the cell's own machinery to accomplish genome replication, synthesis of viral proteins, and completion of progeny virus. These processes take place either in the cell nucleus or the cytoplasm, depending upon the particular family of viruses. In addition, part of the synthetic phase may occur in the nucleus and part in the cytoplasm; however, viral protein is sythesized in the cellular cytoplasm because that is the location of the ribosomes, messenger RNA, and transfer RNA that the virus must use.

The last step in the process of viral multiplication is *release* of viral progeny. In some viruses, this process may result in the coating of the nucleocapsid by host cell membrane protein. However, most viruses are simply released from the cell. Both coated and uncoated viruses are released from the cell as the cell dies. This is known as a *lytic* effect. The reason lytic viruses destroy their cells is not clear. The most obvious effect of cell lysis is the cytopathic effect that can be observed in cell culture—or individual cells—by microscopy. After the cell dies, it releases large amounts of virus (unless the virus buds from the cell membrane, in which case the virus remains attached to the cellular debris from the dying cell). This sequence of events probably occurs in the intact host (compared to a cell culture system), with the added possibility that the phagocytosis of lysed cells causes dissemination of the virus throughout the host.

Lytic viruses are not the only ones that produce a pathogenic effect in humans. Some viruses establish a stable relationship with premissive cells such that cell growth and viral multiplication occur together. This results in a chronic or persistent viral infection. The best example of this is the *in utero* infection of the fetus with rubella, wherein virus continues to be shed—without causing cell death—for many months after delivery. Other possible examples of persistent virus infection with pathologic effects are subacute sclerosing panencephalitis by a virus similar to or identical to measles virus (rubeola) and progressive multifocal leukoencephalopathy by a papovavirus.

Another form of persistent virus infection without cell death is the latent phase of several viruses that cause recurrent lytic infection in some other cell. Examples of these are the viruses in the Herpesviridae family, herpes simplex, varicella zoster, and cytomegalovirus.

After the cellular events described above occur, the resultant pathology in the host is due to the usual changes that are seen with any infectious disease, that is, inflammation, tissue destruction, and immunologically mediated cellular and tissue destruction.

TABLE 92–1. MAJOR FAMILIES OF VIRUSES INFECTING HUMANS

Family	Size (nm)	Examples of Viruses in A Family
DNA Viruses		
Adenoviridae	70–90	31 different serotypes
Herpesviridae	150–200	Simplex, varicella, CMV, EB
Papovaviridae	45–55	Papilloma, polyoma
Parvoviridae	18–26	Adeno-associated viruses
Poxviridae	200–300	Variola, molluscum
Unknown	40–50	Hepatitis B
RNA Viruses		
Arenaviridae	80–130	LCM, Tacaribe, Lassa
Bunyaviridae	100	Arbor, Calif. encephalitis
Coronaviridae	80–130	Infectious bronchitis virus
Orthomyxoviridae	80–120	Influenza viruses
Paramyxoviridae	150–300	Parainfluenza, mumps, measles
Picornaviridae	20–30	ECHO, polio, coxsackie, rhino
Reoviridae	60–80	Respiratory-enteric-orphan
Retroviridae	150	Leukemia viruses
Rhabdoviridae	75–80	Rabies, Marburg, Ebola fever
Togaviridae	40–60	Rubella, EEE, yellow fever, dengue, St. Louis encephalitis
Unknown	25–30	Hepatitis A

DIAGNOSIS

Virus infections, like bacterial infections, are diagnosed most appropriately by isolating the organism from the site of infection.[4] However, this is not always possible. The virus may be producing a systemic infection, so that no one site is available (for example, rubella); the virus may not be a lytic one, so that no virus is available outside the cell (for example, some of the encephalitis viruses); the virus may be a latent one, so that there is no virus available anywhere (only its genetic material is present in some cells) (for example, the herpesviruses); or techniques may be not yet available for isolating that particular virus (for example, human papillomaviruses). The term *isolation* when applied to viruses refers to the changes that one can observe in a host cell (cytopathic effect) or whole organism. One does not usually see the virus, because of its size. However, one can see the effect of the virus in an appropriate cell culture system or the effect of the virus on an animal.

The clinical virology laboratory can provide the standard systems for isolation of many viruses. The cell culture systems include primary monkey kidney cells, primary human embryonic kidney cells, human diploid cells, and human heteroploid cells. The usual animal systems include suckling mice and embryonated chick eggs. Beyond these, there are a number of other cell and animal models available which only specialized laboratories have access to. Certain viruses (Epstein–Barr virus, coronaviruses, and some of those viruses associated with chronic degenerative brain diseases) can be isolated only in specialized laboratories. Because of the risk of epidemics and the potential economic loss, viruses for hoof and mouth disease, for example, are restricted to certain laboratories.

Unlike most bacterial infections, viral infections also can be diagnosed by serologic techniques. A greater than fourfold rise in an antibody titer to a particular virus is satisfactory evidence of a recent viral infection. The type of antibody to be measured (neutralizing, complement-fixing, hemagglutinating, fluorescing) varies with the particular virus under investigation. In addition to detecting the antibody to a virus, one may be able to detect the antigen of a virus present in the tissues of the individual under investigation. This has been done with immunofluorescence, immunoperoxidase assays, and counterimmunoelectrophoresis.

Lastly, the presence of a virus may be detected by observing it, as is true with most bacteria. This is done infrequently in the clinical setting because of the requirement for electron microscopy. However, for organisms such as papilloma virus or human wart virus, this is the only means available.

Given the large number of viruses, the multitude of isolation techniques, and the antigen and antibody detection techniques available, it is in the clinician's best interest to work closely with the clinical virologist in order to determine the most efficient and reliable means to diagnose a suspected viral infection.

CONTROL

There are numerous ways to control the spread of viral infections. These vary from specific antiviral therapy to removing the vectors of virus transmission to actively immunizing individuals. To some degree, all of these are currently used.

Perhaps the oldest standard control method for viral infection is attention to the vectors of transmission. This idea is taken directly from methods used for controlling certain bacterial diseases, such as plague and brucellosis. Removing the mosquito hosts for the encephalitis viruses reduces the incidence of infection. Removing the rabid animal—or avoiding animals known to harbor rabies—reduces the chance of this virus infection.

The newest control measure for viral infection is the use of antiviral therapy—analogous to antibiotics. This procedure began in the middle 1960s with the development of amantadine hydrochloride, which works against influenza virus by inhibiting its uncoating. It is most effective when used prophylactically, and it has no beneficial effects against any other human virus infection.

Another class of antiviral drug is that which inhibits viral replication by interfering with nucleic acid production or its incorporation into nucleotides. Idoxuridine (Stoxil, Herplex) was the first compound to be used and was used for herpesvirus infections of the eye, for which it is still used. Vidarabine is used for the same indication. In addition, it is used for the systemic treatment of disseminated herpesvirus infections. Both of these compounds are useful *in vitro* against DNA-containing viruses only. The former is incorporated into DNA in the place of thymidine after phosphorylation, and the latter inhibits viral and cellular DNA polymerase after it is phosphorylated. Neither drug has any effect on any other family of DNA virus *in vivo*.

The latest class of antiviral drug to be approved for use in man is acycloguanosine (acyclovir). This drug is unique in that it is effective against herpesvirus-infected cells because it requires the activity of a virus-specified thymidine kinase in order to be phosphorylated. In the latter form it becomes a competitive inhibitor of DNA polymerase (more so of viral than host DNA polymerase).[5]

Unfortunately, none of these compounds approaches the effectiveness of antibiotics for many reasons, and none of these compounds may be used in pregnancy because of their effect on cellular nucleic acid metabolism. A large number of other drug classes are being used experimentally in cell culture and animal models, many of which show promise for clinical trials. Some of these, such as interferon and its inducers, are currently undergoing clinical testing. The era of antiviral therapy is only beginning, and in the future we should see a whole new spectrum of therapeutic compounds so that one can reach for the specific drug just as one reaches for the specific antibiotic.[6]

Lastly, the most successful control measures for viral infection in humans have been the use of vaccines for active immunization. This was demonstrated first for smallpox in the 18th century by Jenner, but was not used for any other virus until the early 20th century when Pasteur successfully immunized people with live, attenuated rabies vaccine. Next came killed and live attenuated poliovirus vaccines in the 1950s and attenuated measles virus vaccine and killed influenza vaccines in the early 1960s. These were followed by live, attenuated rubella and mumps vaccines. The latest vaccines developed for clinical use are an improved rabies vaccine and a killed vaccine against hepatitis B. In addition to active immunization against viral infection as illustrated by the vaccines mentioned here, there have been a number of hyperimmune globulins developed for such virus infections as hepatitis B, varicella zoster, and rabies. These globulins provide effective passive immunization.

Future activity in the control of viral infections will be a continuation of these same three measures—prevention of vector transmission, improved antiviral drugs, and new and improved vaccines for active and passive immunization.

REFERENCES

1. Hayden FG, Douglas RG. Antiviral agents. In: Mandell GL, Douglas RG, Bennett JE, eds. *Principles and Practice of Infectious Diseases*. New York, NY: John Wiley and Sons; 1979:353.
2. Hughes SS. *The Virus: A History of the Concept*. New York, NY: Neale Watson Academic Pub; 1977.
3. Joklik WK. The structure, components, and classification of viruses. In: Joklik W, Willett H, Amos D, eds. *Zinsser's Microbiology*. 17th ed. New York, NY: Appleton-Century-Crofts; 1980:980.
4. Menegus MA, Douglas RG. Viruses, rickettsiae, chlamydia and mycoplasmas. In: Mandell GL, Douglas RG, Bennett JE, eds. *Principles and Practice of Infectious Diseases*. New York, NY: John Wiley and Sons; 1979:175.
5. Whitely RJ, Alford CA Jr. Towards therapy and prevention of herpetic infections. *Sem Perinatol*. 1983;7:64.
6. Wishnow RN, Steinfeld JL. The conquest of the major infectious diseases in the United States: a bicentennial retrospective. *Ann Rev Microbiol*. 1976;30:427.

Chapter Ninety-Three
Chemotherapy of Viral Infections

Marvin S. Amstey

93

The use of antiviral chemotherapy in pregnancy is limited by the fear of using this therapy for what is usually a localized, self-limited infection. There is little data about the effects of this therapy on the fetus and neonate. The opportunity to use antiviral chemotherapy is limited significantly by the very few cases of severe viral infection in pregnant women, where the benefit–risk ratio of using this therapy outweighs initial fears. Perhaps anecdotal reports and reviews such as this will enable us to make more rapid and informed decisions about antiviral chemotherapy in pregnancy.

There is a relatively short history about antiviral drugs, with most changes and progress occurring in the past decade. The first clinically used antiviral drug, 5-iodo-2-deoxyuridine—developed for herpes keratitis—appeared in 1961,[1] with fairly rapid development of other nucleoside analogues over the next decade. A summary of this history appears in the first two conferences on antiviral substances.[2,3] In this first decade it was learned that some if not all of these nucleoside analogues are teratogenic in animal models.[4]

Even the latest and more commonly used nucleoside analogue, 9-B-D-arabinofuranosyladenine (ara-A) is cytotoxic.[5] The last ten years, however, have provided some data on the use of the newer antiviral drugs, acyclovir,[6] ribavirin, and amantadine[7] which will be discussed below.

MECHANISM OF DRUG ACTION

Before discussing the specifics of the currently available antiviral drugs, it is important to keep in mind the special changes of pregnancy that modify drug distribution, dosage, and effectiveness. Figure 93–1 illustrates most of the

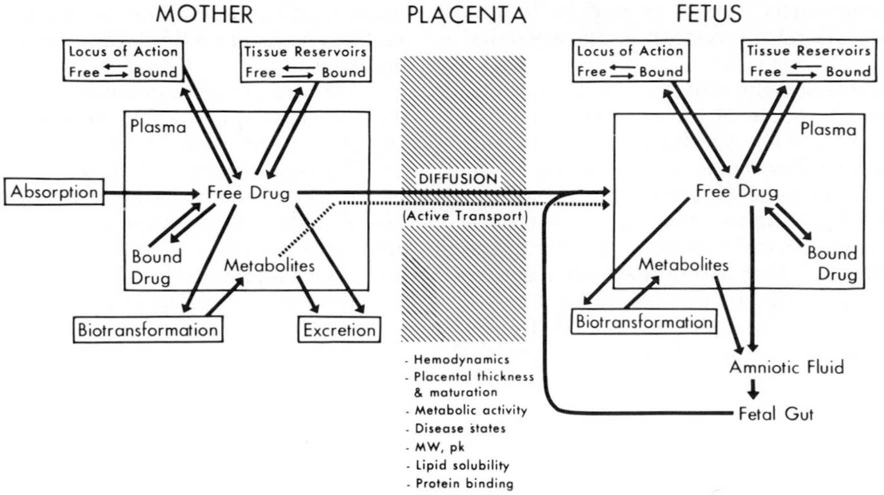

Figure 93–1. The multiple interactions of mother, placenta, and fetus on the pharmacokinetics of drugs in pregnancy. (*From Chow A, Jewesson P. Antimicrobiol drug use in pregnancy.* Rev Inf Dis. *1985;7:287.*

factors that play a role in pregnancy. Clearly, there are a multitude of effects contributed by the mother, placenta, and fetus. Some or all of these factors may change not only how much drug to use but whether to use it at all.

Table 93–1 lists antiviral drugs currently available and their respective uses. The mechanisms of action for each of these is different.

Acyclovir (Zovirax) is 9-(2-hydroxyethoxymethyl) guanine and acts as substrate for virus-specified thymidine kinase. This enzyme phosphorylates acyclovir to the monophosphate form that, in turn, is converted to the triphosphate form by cellular enzymes. Acyclovir triphosphate then becomes the substrate for the DNA polymerases of herpes simplex type 1 and type 2 and, to a lesser extent, of varicella zoster virus and Epstein–Barr virus. The viral DNA polymerases incorporate the acyclovir monophosphate into the DNA primer templates, thereby providing a false message for replication of virus and inactivating the viral DNA polymerases. Because the virus-specified polymerases utilize the acyclovir triphosphate so effectively and completely, there is little left for cellular DNA polymerase, and therefore, there are little or no false templates for normal cell division. This behavior, plus the need for virus-specified thymidine kinase for activation of acyclovir builds in a remarkable safety factor such that there is little toxicity to nonvirus infected cells.[8]

TABLE 93–1. ANTIVIRAL DRUGS AND THEIR INDICATED USES

Drug	Indication
Acyclovir	Genital herpes simplex infections
Amantadine	Influenza A prophylaxis and treatment
Interferon (alpha)	Human papilloma virus; hairy cell leukemia (HTLV-II virus)
Ribavirin	Acute respiratory syncytial virus infection of infants and children
Trifluridine	Keratoconjunctivitis due to herpes simplex
Vidarabine	Disseminated herpes simplex infections; herpes zoster (shingles) infections in immunosuppressed patients
Zidovudine	Human immunodeficiency virus (HIV) infections

The thymidine kinases specified by varicella zoster, Epstein–Barr, and cytomegaloviruses also phosphorylate acyclovir, but only weakly. Therefore, one would predict significantly less clinical benefit in treating such infections with acyclovir. Currently, acyclovir is approved only for therapy of herpes simplex virus infections.

Acyclovir is bound minimally to protein, is not metabolized to any extent in the face of normal renal function, and is excreted primarily by glomerular filtration.[9] There have been no reports of fetal or neonatal toxicity to date.

Amantadine (Symmetrel) is a synthetic, primary amine, first approved for the treatment and prevention of H_2N_2 subtype of influenza A in 1966. Ten years later, it was approved for all types of influenza A. It has no effect on influenza B or any other virus. The mechanism of action of this drug is unknown. It appears that amantadine prevents the release of infectious viral nucleic acid into the cell. This may occur by interfering with uncoating of virus or transcription of viral RNA. The drug does not interfere with the immunogenicity of inactivated influenza A vaccines.

Like acyclovir, amantadine is excreted almost unchanged in the urine. Its excretion is affected significantly by age and decreased renal clearance.

Amantadine's primary effect is in prophylaxis against influenza A infections. While it is also an effective therapy, it must be given within 48 hours of infection or it loses its therapeutic ability. This is probably due to the proposed mechanisms of action.

In contrast to acyclovir, amantadine is both embryotoxic and teratogenic when tested in a rat pregnancy model. These effects are not seen in pregnant rabbits using twice the toxic rat dose.

Interferon (alpha) (Roferon-A, Intron-A) is a human protein that is induced by a host of viruses. The commercially available products are the result of recombinant DNA technology; they first appeared in 1987 for the treatment of hairy cell leukemia. This disease is believed to be caused by human T-lymphocyte virus, type 2 (HTLV-2). It was approved for use by injection into warts (human papilloma virus—HPV) in 1988.

Interferon is species-specific but not virus-specific; hence, the need to use a source of human interferon for its manufacture. Recombinant DNA technology has enabled this to be possible using an *Escherichia coli* containing DNA that codes for this human protein. This interferon is biologically closest in activity to human leukocyte interferon, which is produced in response to a viral infection. This contrasts with "immune" interferon, which is produced when sensitized lymphocytes are stimulated by their specific antigens. There is no commercially available product similar to immune interferon currently available. Interferon undergoes enzymatic degradation during tubular readsorption after being totally filtered by the glomeruli.

As with amantadine, the exact mode of action of this protein is unknown. It appears that the interference of viral replication is caused by another, as yet unidentified, protein, which is induced by interferon. It appears that the interfering protein inhibits translation of early viral messanger RNA because no virus-specified proteins are synthesized, resulting in no progeny viral genomes. At high doses, interferon also modifies the immune response and inhibits the multiplication of both normal and tumor cells.[10]

Interferon alpha has an abortifacient activity in rhesus monkeys at extremely high doses. However, this effect is not seen at 25 million Iu/kg/day. There is no data about this in humans, although one study showed decreases in serum estradiol and progesterone in nonpregnant women treated with human leukocyte interferon.[11]

Ribavirin (Virazole) is a unique drug that appears to be an analogue of guanosine. It works by interfering with guanosine synthesis and interferes with some viral polymerases. It has a wide range of antiviral activity, including herpes viruses, influenza virus, and respiratory syncytial virus (RSV). It is approved for use only as an aerosol (aerosolization in a SPAG-2 nebulizer only) for the treatment of children hospitalized with severe RSV disease. However, it is being used in experimental human studies of human immunodeficiency virus (HIV) infection and in patients with acquired immune deficiency syndrome (AIDS) superinfected with other virus infections. Therefore, its use in the future may be extended.

The pharmacokinetics and metabolism of this drug are not understood completely. It is known that the drug accumulates in red blood cells (RBC) during use, with a half-life of 40 days in RBCs.

Ribavirin is embryotoxic and teratogenic in all lower species tested, but not in pregnant baboons.[12]

Trifluridine (Viroptic) is used topically only for herpes virus-induced keratoconjunctivitis. It has a number of mechanisms of action, all of which interfere with DNA synthesis. It is basically a cellular poison. However, systemic absorption following therapeutic use in the eyes appears to be negligible. No drug was found in the sera of subjects using trifluridine seven times daily for 14 days. There are fetal toxic effects in animal models when injected systemically but none when used topically in the eye.[13]

Vidarabine (Vira-A) is adenine arabinoside, a purine nucleoside analogue. Its chemical name is 9-B-D-arabinofuranosyladenine monohydrate. Although this antiviral drug is one of the oldest, its exact mechanism of action is not clear. The drug is first converted to a nucleotide that is known to inhibit herpes simplex type 1 and type 2 viral DNA polymerases. It also inhibits the viral DNA polymerase of varicella zoster virus. Vidarabine is indicated for use in disseminated herpes simplex viral infections and for herpes zoster (shingles) viral infections in immunosuppressed patients.

This drug is teratogenic in rats and rabbits.[14] However, it has been used in the third trimester of pregnancy without any harm to the fetus or neonate.[15]

Zidovudine (Retrovir) or *AZT* is the newest of the antiviral drugs currently available. Like the others, it is not approved for use in pregnancy. Nonetheless, as with the others, there may be a time and place for using this antiviral drug in a pregnant woman.

The only indication for this drug currently is in a patient with AIDS who has had one episode of *Pneumocystis carini* pneumonia or an absolute CD_4 (T_4 helper) lymphocyte count of less than 200. However, there are many ongoing trials of this drug in less advanced cases of AIDS and in asymptomatic HIV-infected individuals.

AZT is a thymidine analogue that is converted by cellular thymidine kinases to the triphosphate derivative. The AZT triphosphate interferes with HIV viral, RNA-dependent, DNA polymerase (the reverse transcriptase), thereby inhibiting viral replication. This inhibition occurs because the AZT triphosphate is incorporated into viral DNA chains by the reverse transcriptase, resulting in termination of the DNA chain. The drug has several other *in vitro* mechanisms of action, all of which are less significant than this one. The amount of drug necessary to inhibit virus reproduction in chronically infected cells (presumably those in which HIV DNA is incorporated into cellular DNA) is 100-fold greater than in acutely infected cells. The drug's effects, major and minor, are not limited to virus-infected cells, and AZT is quite toxic to a variety of normal cells. Severe hematologic effects such as anemia and granulocytopenia are common; nausea, edema, tremor, muscular spasms, hearing loss, and mucous membrane ulceration, among other effects, also occur. The drug is not teratogenic in rats at 20 times the usual adult dose; it has not been tested in other species. AZT, like all other antiviral drugs, is excreted by renal clearance.

USES IN PREGNANCY

None of the drugs described above is approved for use in pregnancy. However, the use of any drug for any purpose is a decision solely based upon benefit–risk considerations. All of the earlier described antiviral drugs have been shown to be effective for one or more viral infections. One must weigh their benefit in the pregnant woman against any risk to either mother or fetus from normal cellular toxicity and adverse reactions.

Of all the drugs listed in Table 93–1, the least toxic for normal cells and the one with the greatest clinical experience for use in pregnancy is acyclovir. A large body of anecdotal data has accumulated that illustrates that acyclovir has an identical antiviral benefit in pregnant women. Moreover, no ill effects have been found in offspring.[16] This review emphasizes that the most reasonable uses for parenteral acyclovir in pregnancy are with disseminated herpes simplex infection, varicella pneumonia, and severe primary genital herpes virus infections. Whether acyclovir has a use in eliminating asymptomatic or mildly symptomatic recurrent genital herpes virus infections and viral shedding near term is not yet determined. The potential benefits of such a strategy include the possible reduction in incidence of neonatal infections with a reduction in cesarean section rates. These concepts require further testing, and a registry of acyclovir use in pregnancy is being kept.[17] Because acyclovir is relatively nontoxic compared to vidarabine, which has the same indications for use, there may never be data or a need to use vidarabine in pregnancy. There is, however, a concern by the Food and Drug Administration (FDA) about the concentrations of acyclovir in amniotic fluid and acyclovir-induced nephropathy in the fetus.[18]

The increasing incidence of HIV-infected women and of women with AIDS will increase the experience with the use of AZT in pregnancy. It should not be long, therefore, before the benefit–risk ratio of AZT use in pregnancy can be established.

REFERENCES

1. Kaufman H, Martola E, Dohlman C. Use of 5-iodo-2-deoxyuridine in treatment of herpes simplex keratitis. *Arch Ophthalmol*. 1962;68:235.
2. Conference on Antiviral Substances. *Ann NY Acad Sci*. 1965;130.
3. Conference on Antiviral Substances. *Ann NY Acad Sci*. 1970;173.
4. Chaube S, Murphy ML. The teratogenic effects of cytosine arabinoside on the rat fetus. *Proc Am Assoc Cancer Res*. 1965;6:11.
5. Schardein J, Hentz D, Petrere J, et al. The effect of vidarabine on the development of the offspring of rats, rabbits and monkeys. *Teratology*. 1977;15:231.
6. Proceedings of a symposium on acyclovir. *Amer J Med*. 1982;73.
7. Johnson DC. Antiviral drugs for common respiratory diseases. *Post Grad Med*. 1988;83:136.
8. Elion G. Mechanism of action and selectivity of acyclovir. *Amer J Med*. 1982; (acyclovir symposium);7.
9. Lietman P. Acyclovir clinical pharmacology. *Amer J Med*. 1982; (acylcovir symposium);193.
10. Joklik W. Antiviral chemotherapy, interferon and vaccines. In: Joklik W, Willett H, Amos D, eds. *Zinsser's Microbiology*. (17th ed). New York, NY: Appleton-Century-Crofts; 1980;1117.
11. Kauppila A, Cantell K. Serum sex steroid in peptide hormone concentrations and endometrial estrogen and progestin receptor levels during administration of human leukocyte interferon. *Intl J Ca*. 1982;29:291.
12. Nicholson K. Properties of antiviral agents 2. *Lancet*. 1984;2:562.
13. Itori M, Getter J, Kaneko N, et al. Teratogenicities of ophthalmic drugs. I. Antiviral ophthalmic drugs. *Arch Ophthalmol*. 1975;93:46.
14. Hirsch M, Swartz M. Antiviral agents. *N Engl J Med*. 1980;302:903.
15. Young E, Killam A, Greene J. Disseminated herpes virus infection. Association with primary, gential herpes in pregnancy. *JAMA*. 1976;235:2731.
16. Brown Z, Baker D. Acyclovir therapy during pregnancy. *Obstet Gynecol*. 1989;73:526.
17. Andrews E, Tilson H, Hurn B, et al. Acyclovir in pregnancy registry. *Am J Med*. 1988;85:123.
18. Arvin A. Antiviral treatment of herpes simplex infection in neonates and pregnant women. *J Am Acad Dermat*. 1988;18:200.

Chapter Ninety-Four
Viral Respiratory Diseases: An Overview

Richard V. Lee

94

Viral respiratory infections are ubiquitous in human populations. The clinical illnesses they cause range from mild coryza to fatal primary influenza pneumonia. Most respiratory viruses are a nuisance, but pregnancy alters both maternal anxiety and clinical illness so that questions about the effects of colds and medications for colds are common obstetric concerns.

ETIOLOGY

A confusing, large array of viruses can cause acute respiratory illness. Their taxonomy often seems clinically irrelevent because viral diagnostic procedures for such common complaints are not often pursued, and when they are, they usually are not useful for clinical management because the patient has recovered by the time reports are complete. The most common groups of viruses and their most important illness patterns are given in Table 94–1. Some, like influenza and adenoviruses, cause distinct syndromes, which allow clinical diagnosis.

PATHOGENESIS

Respiratory viruses replicate in the nasopharyngeal mucosa, which is infected when the patient inhales virus containing droplet nuclei produced by sneezing and coughing by infected individuals or when the patient transmits virus-containing secretions by skin-to-skin contact. Most respiratory viruses do not disseminate systemically, but some contiguous spread to the larynx and trachea is common. Coryza, scratchy throat and voice, myalgias, headache, and cough are universal symptoms of the common cold. Contiguous spread to the lower respiratory tract by inhalation or aspiration is a feature of influenza and respiratory syncytial virus infections. Except for influenza, viremia is rare, and there is little risk for intrauterine fetal infection.

Pregnancy is associated with an increase in nasal secretions and vascularity of the nasal mucosa. Many women complain of nasal stuffiness during gestation. Additional edema and inflammation of the nasopharyngeal mucosa caused by a cold may predispose the patient to secondary bacterial sinusitis and otitis. Because the pregnant woman has come to accept her stuffy nose and nasal drainage, these more serious consequences of a viral upper respiratory infection (URI) may be overlooked.

Pregnancy also changes patterns of breathing. Minute ventilation, work of breathing, and dyspnea are increased, especially in the latter half of pregnancy as the uterus extends out of the pelvis into the abdominal cavity. After 28–30 weeks' gestation, many women find that they cannot cough effectively, especially in the supine position. A URI may be more keenly felt by the pregnant patient and may have a protracted course because of superimposed bronchitis or sinusitis.

Because most respiratory viruses do not cause viremia and systemic disease, subtle, pregnancy-induced changes in cell-mediated immunity do not alter the clinical course of the infection. Influenza is the only possible exception.

Fever, especially sustained fever, is a potential hazard to the fetus and for premature labor. Fortunately, most URIs are unaccompanied by prolonged high temperatures. However, secondary bacterial infection, influenza, and

TABLE 94–1. VIRUSES CAUSING ACUTE RESPIRATORY ILLNESSES

Virus	Nucleic Acid	Virus Subgroups	Serotypes	Important Clinical Syndromes
Orthomyxovirus	RNA	Influenza	3, with frequent antigen variation	Fever, tracheitis, primary influenza, pneumonia
Paramyxovirus pneumovirus	RNA	Respiratory syncytial virus	Antigenic polymorphism with frequent strain variation	Fever, bronchiolitis, pneumonia: infants and children in particular
Paramyxovirus	RNA	Parainfluenza virus	4	"Cold"
Picornavirus	RNA	Rhinovirus	over 100	"Cold"
		Enterovirus		
		Coxsackie A	24	Herpangina, hand-foot-mouth syndrome
		Coxsackie B	6	Pleurodynia, myocarditis
		Echovirus	over 30	Bronchiolitis, pneumonia, aseptic meningitis
Coronavirus	RNA	Coronavirus	4	"Cold"
Adenovirus	DNA	Adenovirus	75	Pharyngoconjunctival fever, epidemic teratoconjunctivitis

some adenoviruses can produce substantial, sustained fever.

EPIDEMIOLOGY

The large number of serotypes and the antigenic liability of the respiratory viruses contribute to cycles of epidemic URI. Partial or waning immunity and frequent antigenic alterations mean that even adults can be susceptible to the colds that circulate among school children. In the United States, adults average two to four colds per year and children six to eight. Transmission by droplet aerosols, skin, and fomites is abetted by placing groups of people indoors and in close contact. In North America, conglomeration of children in school in the autumn is followed by late autumn and winter time outbreaks of respiratory illness among susceptible students, who then bring home the virus to their family. The larger the pool of susceptibles, the larger the epidemic.

DIAGNOSIS

Determining specific viral etiology is usually impossible on clinical grounds alone. Identification of respiratory viruses requires demonstration of virus or viral antigens in nasopharyngeal secretions, blood, or stool, by isolation in tissue culture, immunologic identification of viral antigens, or by rising titers of antibody for the specific virus. A variety of immunofluorescent, radioimmunoassay, and enzyme-linked immunosorbent assay (ELISA) techniques are available. The problem is that the costs are high, the turnaround time for results is slow, and clinical management is not altered by specific virus identification in an individual patient. However, when an epidemic situation is present, identification of the causative virus is important for public health measures and to provide appropriate advice to the community.

Other than isolation of the infecting virus or identification of viral antigens in secretions or documentation of rising titers of virus-specific antibody, there are no distinctive laboratory features of viral respiratory infection. Except when bacterial superinfection occurs, there is no consistent alteration in total and differential leukocyte count. Pregnancy by itself may elevate the white blood cell count and the erythrocyte sedimentation rate.

PREVENTION

Except for influenza, there are no reliable vaccines for respiratory viruses. Prevention is principally common sense, and good public health information greatly enhances common sense. Pregnant women should avoid contact with infected people. Assiduous attention to handwashing reduces risk, expecially for mothers of infected children. When respiratory viral infections are epidemic, pregnant patients should take extra care, avoiding crowded places, especially groups of children. Complete isolation is impossible, and upper respiratory infections in pregnant women are common. Patients need to be alerted to the risks of bacterial superinfection and indiscriminate use of over-the-counter medication.

MANAGEMENT

Respiratory viral diseases pose a significant risk to pregnancy, not because the viruses are teratogenic or cause life-threatening disease, but because they are common, they cause misery, and the afflicted are likely to take a vast variety of medications. The use of antihistamines and decongestants should be eschewed because they tend to thicken secretion and exaggerate the already increased risks of superimposed bacterial sinusitis, bronchitis, and otitis. The increased incidence of congenital malformations following the 1957–1958 Asian influenza epidemic has been related to the use of cold remedies.

Treatment of acute respiratory viral illness during pregnancy is supportive. Reassurance and specific instruction to avoid over-the-counter remedies are essential. Smokers should be admonished. Acetaminophen is safe for relief of fever, myalgias, and headache. Increased hydration, both internal and external, is useful and comforting. Our patients are advised that watery secretions that drain easily are desirable even though they are messy. Increased humidity, frequent steaming showers, and increased oral fluids are the best and safest decongestants.

Specific antiviral chemotherapy, like amantadine and ribavirin, is not generally recommended during pregnancy. Patients at high risk because of underlying medical conditions combined with pregnancy may be candidates for such therapy.

REFERENCES

1. Andrewes CH. Adventures among viruses: the puzzle of the common cold. *N Engl J Med*. 1950;242:235.
2. Evans AS. *Viral Infections of Humans*. 3rd ed. New York, NY: Plenum Medical; 1989.
3. Incaudo GA. Diagnosis and treatment of rhinitis during pregnancy and lactation. *Clin Rev Allergy*. 1987;5:325.
4. Korones SB. Uncommon virus infections of the mother, fetus, and newborn: influenza, mumps and measles. *Clin Perinatol*. 1988;15:259.
5. Lee RV. Olfaction—and the smell of summer. *J Chron Dis*. 1987;40:819.
6. Lee RV. The aches and pains of pregnancy. *Med N Am*. 1989;38:6796.
7. Leontic EA. Respiratory disease in pregnancy. *Med Clin N Am*. 1977;61:111.
8. Schoenbaum SC, Weinstein L. Respiratory infections in pregnancy. *Clin Obstet Gynecol*. 1979;22:293.

Chapter Ninety-Five

Important Clinical Syndromes in Adults Caused by Respiratory Viruses

Richard V. Lee

95

Despite the multitude of viral respiratory pathogens, there are only a few distinct clinical syndromes that result from infection (Table 95–1). Clinical diagnosis of a specific causative virus is virtually impossible; only a virus diagnostic laboratory can provide an accurate etiologic diagnosis. Practically, a clinical diagnosis is sufficient almost all of the time. The majority of these viruses, with a few exceptions, pose no special threat to pregnancy. Antiviral chemotherapy has only limited utility in the management of respiratory viral infections during pregnancy; ribavirin, amantadine, and rimantadine are embryotoxic and teratogenic in rodents.[1] Unless there is compelling benefit to the use of these drugs and accurate identification of the causative virus, antiviral drugs for respiratory infections should not be given to pregnant women.

About half of all episodes of pneumonia in pregnant women are preceded by an acute upper respiratory infection (URI).[2] An association between the presence of maternal acute URIs and hemolytic streptococcal puerperal infections was recognized in the past.[3] Although these are usually mild infections, they must be regarded as markers for potentially serious complications of pregnancy and the puerperium.[4]

THE COMMON COLD

Over 100 different virus types can be associated with the common cold (Table 95–2). Colds are principally an infection of the nasal mucosae. After an incubation period of 2–5 days, mild constitutional symptoms and chilly sensations followed within a few hours by nasal obstruction, sneezing, and rhinorrhea are noted. There is edema and hyperemia of the mucosa and submucosa and an increase in the number

TABLE 95–1. CLINICAL SYNDROMES ASSOCIATED WITH VIRUSES INFECTING THE RESPIRATORY TRACT

				Lower Airway Disease				
Agent	Rhinitis	Pharyngitis	Laryngitis	Tracheobronchitis	Bronchiolitis	Pneumonia	Fever	Secondary Bacterial Infection
Rhinoviruses	+++[c]	+[a]	+	+	±[d]	Rare	±	Rare
Coronaviruses	++-+++	+	+	±	±	Rare	±	Rare
Parainfluenza viruses	+	++-+++	++-+++	++	+	Rare	±	Occasional
Respiratory syncytial viruses	++[b]	+	++	++	+++	Occasional	±	Occasional
Influenza virus, A and B	+	+	++	+++	++	Occasional severe	++	Not rare
Adenoviruses	+	++	++	++	±	Occasional severe	++	Occasional
Enteroviruses, (eg coxsackie, echoviruses)	+	++-+++	++	+	+	Rare	++	Occasional

[a]+ = Occasional
[b]++ = Often
[c]+++ = Common
[d]± = Unusual

TABLE 95–2. ETIOLOGIC AGENTS ASSOCIATED WITH THE COMMON COLD

Agent	
Rhinoviruses (>100 serotypes)	15–40%
Coronaviruses (≥3 serotypes)	10–20%
Influenza viruses (A,B) Parainfluenza viruses (4 serotypes) Respiratory syncytial virus (1 serotype) Adenoviruses (several serotypes)	5–10%
Group A β-hemolytic streptococci	2–10%
Enteroviruses (various serotypes of coxsackie and echoviruses)	1–2%
No specific agent, but presumed to be viral	30–50%

Modified from Kapikian AZ. The Common Cold. In: Wyngaarden JB, Smith LH Jr, eds. Cecil Textbook of Medicine. *Philadelphia, PA: WB Saunders; 1988:1753.*

and mucous production of goblet cells. These are appropriately labeled *catarrhal states.* Rhinorrhea may be profuse, up to 15 g per day, and may require 20–40 disposable handkerchiefs for collection and disposal.

Scratchy throat, mild headache, and nonproductive cough may develop in a quarter to half of patients.[5] Low-grade fever is unusual; myalgias and malaise are common. Occasionally, tracheobronchitis supervenes. Some viruses, like rhinovirus, seem to precipitate wheezing in children and adults with reactive airway disease or chronic bronchitis. These symptoms peak after 3–4 days and then progressively resolve.

Not only are there a large number of different viruses causing colds, immunity to each can be variable and evanescent so that reinfection commonly occurs. No clinically useful vaccines are available.

Management of colds during pregnancy is supportive and directed at excluding treatable, nonviral infections, like *Mycoplasma pneumoniae* and group A β-hemolytic streptococci. Throat culture and serologic tests for *Mycoplasma* are helpful if fever, persistent cough, and pharyngeal exudates complicate a cold.

Nasal congestion associated with pregnancy is common because of normal vasodilatation and increased blood volume.[6] Recognition of bacterial sinusitis is important, especially for those women who develop bothersome, persisting nasal congestion following a URI and who have no history of rhinitis preceding the pregnancy.[7] Pregnant women with purulent sinusitis may not present with the classic history and findings of acute sinusitis. Continuing nasal obstruction with purulent discharge even without pain, epistaxis, or fever may indicate the need for imaging examinations of the paranasal sinuses and specialist examination.[6]

Antihistamines, decongestants, and nasal sprays should be avoided. Antihistamines cause thickening of secretions and predispose to diminished clearance of secretions from the nose and sinuses.[8,9] A variety of fetal anomalies have been attributed to antihistamines. Neonatal withdrawal has been attributed to regular maternal use of antihistamines.[7] Of all the decongestants, only pseudoephedrine has shown no association with adverse fetal effects. However, topical and systemic vasoconstrictors should not be used during pregnancy, especially for women with labile or elevated blood pressure.

Patients should be instructed that watery nasal secretions, which enhance clearance from the nasopharynx and sinuses, are desirable. Local steam, hot showers, gargles, and increased oral intake of liquids are useful and do not generate doctor–patient anxiety about fetal well-being.

FEBRILE PHARYNGITIS

Sore throat, fever, pharyngeal or faucial erythema, exudate, or vesicopustules, and cervical lymphadenopathy are the hallmarks of viral febrile pharyngitis (Table 95–3). Throat culture for streptococci is essential because there are no sure clinical clues to the etiology of this syndrome. Fever greater than 38°C and lasting more than a few hours and pharyngeal lesions clearly separate this syndrome from the benign common cold.

Infectious mononucleosis caused by Epstein–Barr virus is characterized by debility and generalized lymphadenopathy, including splenomegaly, in addition to exudative pharyngitis. In many adenovirus infections, pharyngitis is accompanied by moderate to severe conjunctivitis, or *pharyngoconjunctival fever.* Coxsackieviruses have a predilection for causing vesiculopustular lesions (herpangina) of the palate, fauces, and pharynx. Although these are childhood diseases in clinical thinking, it is important to remember that there is a growing proportion of youthful mothers and that adults are not entirely spared from infections with these usual childhood viruses. Orogenital sexual behavior may increase during pregnancy. The clinician must be alert to the possibility that febrile pharyngitis could be a sexually transmitted infection. The evaluation of pharyngitis during pregnancy includes consideration of genital symptoms or findings, including appropriate cultures. Except for bacterial infection, there is no acceptable antimicrobial therapy. Risk to the pregnancy is small. However, intrapartum maternal herpes simplex or coxsackievirus infection can be followed by severe, occasionally fatal, neonatal infection.

LARYNGOTRACHEOBRONCHITIS AND BRONCHIOLITIS

Cough, hoarse voice, croup, stridor, and wheezing can be produced by a diverse array of viruses (Table 95–4). Bronchiolitis is the dominant feature of respiratory syncytial virus infection in infants, and croup is the dominant feature of parainfluenza infection in children. There is a tendency to regard viral etiologies for exacerbation of asthma and tracheobronchitis as a condition exclusively of childhood, and to downplay the role of viruses in the lower respiratory diseases of adults.

Chronic bronchitis associated with smoking tobacco clearly dominates the panoply of adult respiratory diseases.

TABLE 95–3. FEBRILE PHARYNGITIS

Common Etiologic Agents
Group A β-hemolytic streptococci
Mycoplasma pneumoniae
Adenoviruses
Coxsackieviruses
Epstein–Barr virus
Less Common Etiologic Agents
Neisseria gonorrhoeae
Corynebacterium
Herpes simplex virus

TABLE 95–4. ETIOLOGIC AGENTS IN LARYNGOTRACHEOBRONCHITIS AND BRONCHITIS

Etiologic Viruses
Influenza viruses
Parainfluenza viruses
Respiratory syncytial virus
Other Etiologic Agents Important for Differential Diagnosis
Mycoplasma pneumoniae
Haemophilus influenzae species

It has been extraordinarily difficult to document a causal role of respiratory virus infection in the progression of chronic bronchitis. No one questions the pathogenesis of influenzal tracheobronchitis, and there is no doubt about the fundamental importance of mucociliary clearance in the genesis of bronchial disease.

The characteristic cough of viral tracheobronchitis in a nonsmoking patient is nonproductive and paroxysmal. There may be tracheal tenderness, and patients often complain of burning substernal discomfort with coughing. In a smoker or patient with chronic bronchitis, viral tracheobronchitis may produce a change in sputum color and consistency as well as an increase in frequency of cough and coughing paroxysms. Unless pneumonia or ventilation-perfusion mismatching caused by bronchiolar obstruction or reactive bronchospasm supervene, most patients do not have changes in ventilation or oxygenation.

Immunity against viruses that infect the lower respiratory tract is not so long lasting or solid that future infections with a particular virus will be prevented. Epidemiologic evidence suggests that secretory IgA and circulating IgG and IgM-mediated immunity are boosted by repetitive exposure. Extended intervals between "boosts" set the stage for clinical illness as opposed to inapparent infection. Parainfluenza and respiratory syncytial virus respiratory tract infection occurs in adults with some frequency. Previous experience with the infecting virus modulates but may not obviate clinical expression of the infection. Teachers, nurses, and mothers of young and school-age children have frequent contact with respiratory viruses and over time have diminishing severity of the resulting clinical illness.

Viremia is not a feature of respiratory viral infections, except for severe influenza. Pregnancy may exacerbate symptoms but does not intrude upon the usual benign outcome of these viral diseases. Dyspnea, nasal congestion, and coughing may be more noticeable and bothersome during pregnancy. A pregnant smoker is at risk for protracted illness because of bacterial superinfection. A unique bacterial superinfection complication of influenza was reported in 1987: toxic shock syndrome.[10,11] Exotoxin-producing *Staphylococcus aureus* was recovered from eight out of ten patients suffering a toxic shocklike syndrome following influenzalike illness. Six of these ten patients died.

Ribavirin by aerosol is used to treat infants with severe respiratory syncytial virus bronchiolitis.[12] Pregnant pediatric nurses are a special problem because of the risk of inhalation and surface contact with ribavirin.[1] No proven adverse fetal effects in humans have been recorded. It seems eminently reasonable to interdict exposure to ribavirin therapy for pregnant nurses.

PNEUMONIA

Invasion of the lung parenchyma is unusual for most respiratory viruses except for the adenoviruses, enteroviruses, and influenza viruses (Table 95–5). Infection extending beyond the bronchial mucosa causes alveolar and bronchial filling with consequent ventilation perfusion mismatch and hypoxemia. Pregnancy-related pulmonary vascular plethora and decline in serum colloid osmotic pressure may exacerbate the density and extent of pulmonary infiltrates.[4] Because maternal oxygen consumption is accelerated by fetoplacental metabolism, even modest maternal hypoxia may be poorly tolerated.

Containment and elimination of the viral pathogen requires cell-mediated as well as humoral immunity and phagocytic host defenses. Alterations in cell-mediated immunity by gestation may diminish the pregnant patient's capacity to contain viral pathogens once they have intruded into the lung parenchyma. The combination of the physiologic and immunologic circumstances of pregnancy seems to predispose pregnant women, especially late in pregnancy when the physiologic and anatomic alterations are at their greatest, to a greater risk for and a more severe course with viral pneumonia. In contrast, pregnancy does not really alter the risk or course of bacterial pneumonia for which phagocytic cells and antibody are the principal host defenses.

The course of primary viral pneumonia during pregnancy can be dramatic. A woman in the latter half of pregnancy develops the acute clinical symptoms of influenza or pharyngoconjunctival fever. Her illness follows the usual

TABLE 95–5. PNEUMONIA

Viral Pneumonia
Influenza virus, A and B
Adenoviruses
Enteroviruses
Coxsackievirus
Echoviruses
Nonviral Pathogen Causing a Similar Syndrome
Mycoplasma pneumoniae
Pneumocystis carinii
Bacterial bronchopneumonia

TABLE 95–6. INFLUENZA VACCINE DURING PREGNANCY

Comorbid conditions that make a pregnant woman at high risk during influenza epidemics:
Heart Disease
Rheumatic valvular disease
Congestive heart failure
Chronic Lung Diseases
Asthma
Chronic bronchitis
Ephysema
Bronchiectasis
Cystic fibrosis
Restrictive of infiltrative pulmonary disease
1) Tuberculosis
2) Sarcoidosis
Chronic Renal Failure
Metabolic Disorders
Diabetes
Chronic corticosteroid therapy

course for 2–3 days, when increasing nonproductive cough and dyspnea ensue and become progressive over the next 24–36 hours. The patient then presents as a pale, frightened, tachypneic woman with cyanosis and diffuse rales without consolidation. Chest x-ray shows patchy, scattered infiltrates, which progress to confluent infiltrates as the patient's clinical condition deteriorates with progressive hypoxia and ultimately ventilator-dependent respiratory failure. Comorbid conditions, like pulmonary vascular hypertension or congestion associated with valvular or congenital heart disease, increase the risk for a more severe course of viral pneumonia.

Primary prevention by immunization or isolation are the only effective prophylactic measures (Table 95–6). After the patient is infected and the pneumonic process is started, there is little to be done except to provide ventilatory support, prevent or treat superimposed bacterial infection, and monitor fetal status in order to rescue the fetus in time should the mother's demise become imminent. There is little positive benefit from premature operative delivery in this setting. The use of amantadine or rimantadine for influenza prophylaxis or treatment of active infection may be justified when a pregnant patient is at especially high risk.

REFERENCES

1. Jin A, Guglielmo J, Bernard BB. Assessing exposures of health care personnel to aerosols of ribavirin: california. *MMWR*. 1988;37:560.
2. Hopwood HG. Pneumonia in pregnancy. *Obstet Gynecol*. 1965;25:875.
3. Schaefer G. Pulmonary infections in pregnancy. *Clin Obstet Gynecol*. 1959;2:639.
4. Leontic EA. Respiratory disease in pregnancy. *Med Clin N Am*. 1977;61:111.
5. Curley FJ, Irwin RS, Pratter MR, et al. Cough and the common cold. *Am Rev Respir Dis*. 1988;138:305.
6. Incaudo GA. Diagnosis and treatment of rhinitis during pregnancy and lactation. *Clin Rev Allergy*. 1987;5:325.
7. Lee RV. The aches and pains of pregnancy. *Med N Am*. 1989;38:6796.
8. Gaffey MJ, Gwaltney JM, Sastre A, et al. Intranasally and orally administered antihistamine treatment of experimental rhinovirus colds. *Am Rev Respir Dis*. 1987;136:556.
9. Gaffey MJ, Kaiser DL, Hayden FG. Ineffectiveness of oral terfenadine in natural colds: evidence against histamine as a mediator of common cold symptoms. *Pediatr Infect Dis J*. 1988;7:223.
10. Sperber SJ, Francis JB. Toxic shock syndrome during an influenza outbreak. *JAMA*. 1987;257:1086.
11. MacDonald KL, Osterholm MT, Hedberg CW, et al. Toxic shock syndrome: a newly recognized complication of influenza and influenza like illness. *JAMA*. 1987;257:1053.
12. Hall CB, McBride JT, Walsh EE, et al. Aerosolized ribavirin treatment of infants with respiratory syncytial viral infection. *N Engl J Med*. 1983;308:1443.

Chapter Ninety-Six
Common Respiratory Viruses

Richard V. Lee

96

RHINOVIRUSES

Rhinoviruses, as their name indicates, affect the nose. They are the most common virus causing the common cold, and they are responsible for the majority of acute respiratory infections of humankind. It is something of a paradox that the most common of human viral pathogens is one of the more difficult viruses to study in the clinical and laboratory setting. Rhinoviruses thrive at temperatures of 33–34°C and are ideally adapted to the nasal mucosa, which maintains a surface temperature of approximately 34°C. Viral diagnostic studies using tissue culture must therefore be carried out at lower temperatures than those used in most clinical viral diagnostic laboratories. There are over 100 rhinovirus serotypes. Infection by one serotype does not produce immunity to infection by heterologous serotypes.[1,2]

Rhinovirus infections begin during infancy and continue throughout adult life at a rate of about 0.5 infections per person per year. Specific antibody responses develop in pregnancy and peak in young adulthood, presumably because of repetitive natural boosting. Antibody titers decline among older people without frequent exposures to children.

Rhinoviruses are easily and efficiently transmitted by inoculation of mucosal surfaces by way of hands and fomites carrying virus-containing secretions. Rhinoviruses are not efficiently transmitted by aerosol. Close personal contact among family and in nursing homes and schools is an easy way to transmit rhinovirus colds. There are no available, clearly efficacious vaccines or chemotherapeutic agents for rhinovirus infections.

CORONAVIRUSES

The coronaviruses were identified as a new RNA virus group recovered from patients suffering from common colds in several centers between 1965 and 1968. Coronaviruses are fastidious, growing only in human respiratory epithelial or embryonic kidney cell cultures. Their unique cell culture requirements restrict clinical virus diagnostic laboratories from routine isolation and work with coronaviruses. Several serotypes are known, and more probably exist. Seroepidemiologic surveys have shown wide distribution with about half of the adult population possessing antibody against coronaviruses. The clinical disease produced following nasal inoculation is mild; about half of the volunteers will have asymptomatic infection. It is estimated that after rhinoviruses, coronaviruses are the second most common virus group causing the common cold.[3]

Related animal viruses can infect the gastrointestinal tract and cause gastroenteritis. The majority of human coronavirus infections involve the upper respiratory tract. However, gastroenteritis may be a feature of the colds caused by coronavirus in adults. In infants, coronaviruses have caused pneumonia and necrotizing enterocolitis.

Infection during pregnancy is not dangerous for the fetus.[4] Intrapartum and postpartum maternal infection may be a risk for the neonate.

PARAINFLUENZA VIRUSES

There are four serotypes of parainfluenza virus, a member of the paramyxovirus group. They are common serious pathogens in children, causing croup, bronchiolitis, and pneumonia. Repetitive exposure results in substantial differences between childhood and adult illness. Most adults have antibody to all four types of parainfluenza virus and, when infected, develop common cold or laryngotracheobronchitis symptoms. Primary infections in children and in adults are almost always symptomatic. Types 1 and 2 are associated with laryngeal and subglottic infection, especially in children, which must be distinguished from epiglottitis caused by *Haemophilus influenzae* type B. Type III parainfluenza virus is most often associated with bronchiolitis and pneumonia and must be distinguished from respiratory syncytial virus and *Mycoplasma pneumoniae* infection.

Experimental killed and live virus vaccines have been developed but have not been widely employed, possibly because even with wild virus infection the immunity produced is not completely protective. Ribavirin has been successfully used to treat severe childhood disease. Whether ribavirin should be used during pregnancy is debatable.[5]

RESPIRATORY SYNCYTIAL VIRUS

Respiratory syncytial virus (RSV) is another member of the RNA paramyxovirus group. There is only one serotype. Although antigenic variations occur, human neutralizing antibodies specific for RSV neutralize all variants. Virtually 100% of adults have neutralizing antibodies, which are passively transferred to all infants. After six to eight months of age, after passively transferred antibody has disappeared, infants develop neutralizing antibodies because of natural infection. At age 5, 95% of children have antibody.[6]

Primary infection in children can be fatal. The most severe clinical illness occurs in infants with passively-acquired antibodies or with antibodies induced by killed virus vaccine, suggesting that at least part of the pathogenesis of RSV bronchiolar inflammation is immunologically mediated, a type of Arthus reaction.[7]

The virus is acquired through the upper respiratory tract, with the nose and eye being equally efficacious routes of inoculation. The virus is spread through the bronchial tree by cell-to-cell passage of virions. The peribronchiolar and lung parenchymal infiltrates are composed principally of mononuclear cells. Virus shedding may persist for long periods following clinical improvement and recovery. Reinfection by RSV is common. Most adults will develop common colds. Nosocomial RSV outbreaks including medical and nursing staff are common. Infection by RSV during pregnancy is not usually a serious problem. Exposure to ribavirin may be a problem. It seems reasonable to segregate pregnant women from children with RSV infection receiving ribavirin therapy.[8]

ENTEROVIRUSES

In addition to the rhinoviruses, the picornavirus group contains the enteroviruses: echoviruses, coxsackieviruses, polio viruses, and hepatitis A virus. The echoviruses and coxsackieviruses regularly produce clinical illness of the respiratory tract. In contrast to rhinovirus infection, infections by the enteroviruses are often serious and involve other viscera, especially the gastrointestinal tract.[9,10] Aseptic meningitis, carditis, hepatitis, septic shock syndrome, intrauterine fetal death, and infant death have been caused by echoviruses and coxsackieviruses.[11,12] Maternal enterovirus infections early in pregnancy have been reported to be associated with fetal anomalies. However, there is no consistent association or pattern of teratogenesis.

Several reports over the past 15 years have documented the dangers to the neonate of intrapartum maternal echovirus infection.[11-16] The mother's clinical illness in some instances includes both respiratory and abdominal symptoms. In one series, two women had sufficiently severe abdominal pain to cause their obstetricians to suspect placental abruption and carry out premature cesarean section.[15] As with many enteroviruses, patients may continue to excrete virus despite the appearance of circulating neutralizing antibodies and clinical recovery. Infants of mothers with antibodies are protected from clinical illness but may have transient, asymptomatic infection.[17] Asymptomatic mothers and infants shedding virus pose risks to nonimmune nursery and maternity patients.

Coxsackieviruses are noted for the syndromes of herpangina and pleurodynia, but echoviruses can also cause these conditions. Coxsackieviruses are increasingly recognized as the causative agents of myocarditis and progressive cardiomyopathy. Their role in the rare syndrome of peripartum cardiomyopathy is unexamined. Intrapartum maternal infection with coxsackie B viruses has been associated with fatal myocarditis in neonates.

Immunization is not available for enteroviruses, except for active immunization with polio virus and passive immunization for hepatitis A virus.

There are 23 serotypes of coxsackie A virus, 6 serotypes of coxsackie B virus, 31 serotypes of echoviruses, and 4 serotypes of enteroviruses. Some cross immunity within each group occurs, but coxsackie A viruses do not confer immunity to coxsackie B or echoviruses. While these are principally infections of childhood, there are substantial numbers of susceptible adults.

The severity of enteroviral disease in neonates dramatizes the need to make appropriate diagnosis of maternal infection. Most viral diagnostic laboratories can promptly isolate the virus from fecal and nasopharyngeal samples. Modlin et al recommend that delivery should be delayed for mothers suspected of having enteroviral infections to allow for the production and transfer of maternal antibodies in order to protect the neonate.[18]

ADENOVIRUSES

There are 41 recognized serotypes or species of human adenoviruses. They are DNA viruses with a predilection for respiratory, gastrointestinal, and conjunctival infection. Some possess oncogenic potential in animals. Like most DNA viruses, the adenoviruses can establish a prolonged intracellular latency.

The common adenoviruses (types 1, 2, 5, and 6) are prevalent among young children. Adenoviruses 4, 7, 8, 14, and 21 tend to occur later in life, especially among military recruits and college students. Adenoviruses 8, 19, and 37 are associated with epidemic keratoconjunctivitis.[19] Pharyngoconjunctival fever is most commonly caused by adenoviruses 3 and 7 and is usually an epidemic disease in summer camps with small lakes. Acute respiratory disease with febrile pharyngitis and patchy viral pneumonia has been most frequently caused by adenoviruses 4, 7, and 21.

Most infections by adenoviruses are acute and self-limited. Species-specific neutralizing antibodies protect against symptomatic reinfection. Asymptomatic viral shedding may be prolonged despite the presence of neutralizing antibody. Adenoviruses can probably cause persistent latent infection that can, under appropriate circumstances, reactivate.[20]

Adenoviruses may invade the blood stream in some instances. Presumably, destruction of local or systemic host response predisposes to viremia. For example, in rare fatal cases, virus has been recovered from most viscera, and the viremia appears to have extended from areas of necrotizing bronchiolitis. Diminution or loss of cell-mediated immunity may contribute to dissemination of the virus. Adenovirus infections in acquired immune deficiency syndrome (AIDS) patients are particularly aggressive.

Pregnancy has not been reported to be a special risk for enhanced virulence. However, the immunologic events of pregnancy suggest caution. Pregnant women should not swim in lakes or pools where epidemic keratoconjunctivitis is known to be present. Special concern is needed for neonates of mothers suffering active intrapartum adenoviral disease.

Both killed and live virus vaccines have been developed and used successfully, principally for epidemic disease among military recruits.[17] The safety and utility of these vaccines for obstetric and neonatal cases are unexamined.

REFERENCES

1. Andrewes CH. Adventures among viruses: the puzzle of the common cold. *N Engl J Med*.1950;242:235.
2. Gwaltney JM Jr. Rhinoviruses. In: Evans AS, ed. *Viral Infections of Humans. Epidemiology and Control.* New York, NY: Plenum Medical Book Company; 1989:593.
3. Monto AS. Coronaviruses. In: Evans AS, ed. *Viral Infections of Humans. Epidemiology and Control.* New York, NY: Plenum Medical Book Company; 1989:153.
4. Chany C, Moscovici O, Lebon P, et al. Association of coronavirus infection with neonatal necrotizing enterocolitis. *Pediatrics.* 1982;69:209.
5. Glezen WP, Loda FA, Denny FW. Parainfluenza viruses. In: Evans AS, ed. *Viral Infections of Humans. Epidemiology and Control.* New York, NY: Plenum Medical Book Company; 1989:493.
6. Hall CB, Kopelman AE, Douglas RG Jr, et al. Neonatal respiratory syncytial virus infection. *New Engl J Med.* 1979;300:393.
7. Chanock RM, McIntosh K, Murphy BR, Parrott RH. Respiratory syncytial virus. In: Evans AS, ed. *Viral Infections of Humans. Epidemiology and Control.* New York, NY: Plenum Medical Book Company; 1989:525.
8. Englund JA, Sullivan CJ, Jordan MC, et al. Respiratory syncytial virus infection in immunocompromised adults. *Ann Intern Med.* 1988;109:203.
9. Hanshaw JB, Dudgeon JA, Marshall WC. *Viral Diseases of the Fetus and Newborn.* 2nd ed. Philadelphia, PA: WB Saunders; 1985:1,154.
10. Melnick JM. Enteroviruses. In: Evans AS, ed. *Viral Infections of Humans. Epidemiology and Control.* New York, NY: Plenum Medical Book Company; 1989:191.
11. Modlin JF. Perinatal echovirus infection: insights from a literature review of 61 cases of serious infection and 16 outbreaks in nurseries. *Rev Infect Dis.* 1986;8:918.
12. Freedman PS. Echovirus 11 infection and intrauterine death. *Lancet.* 1979;1:96.
13. Nagington J, Wrighitt TG, Gandy G, et al. Fatal echovirus 11 infections in outbreak in special care baby unit. *Lancet.* 1978;2:725.
14. Davies DP, Hughes CA, MacVicar J, et al. Echovirus 11 infection in a special care baby unit. *Lancet.* 1979;1:96.
15. Modlin JF. Fatal echovirus 11 disease in premature neonates. *Pediatrics.* 1980;66:775.
16. Chow CB, Chan KY, Tam A, et al. Outbreak of Echo virus type 11 infection in newborn infants in a maternity ward: clinical presentation. *J Trop Pediatr.* 1987;33:305.
17. Insel RA. Maternal immunization to prevent neonatal infections. *N Engl J Med.* 1988;319:1219.
18. Modlin JE, Polk BF, Horton P, et al. Perinatal echovirus infection. Risk of transmission during a community outbreak. *N Engl J Med.* 1981;305:368.
19. Foy HM. Adenoviruses. In: Evans AS, ed. *Viral Infections of Humans. Epidemiogy and Control.* New York, NY: Plenum Medical Book Company; 1989:77.
20. Zahradnik JM, Spencer MJ, Porter DD. Adenovirus infection in the immunocompromised patient. *Am J Med.* 1980;68:725.

Chapter Ninety-Seven

Influenza

Richard V. Lee

97

Influenza is an acute febrile respiratory illness clinically characterized by myalgias, laryngotracheobronchitis causing a brassy, nonproductive cough; acute and chronic debilitation; and periodic epidemics and pandemics. Pandemic disease with striking attack rates, severe morbidity, and excess mortality such as occurred in the great influenza epidemics of 1918, 1957–1958, and 1968–1969 has made influenza one of the most dramatic and feared ills of humankind. One 19th century physician described the 1836–1837 epidemic thus: "Influenza is not by any means so severe or so rapidly fatal a disease as cholera, but the mortality which it has produced is greater as it affects almost every person in society, while the ravages of cholera were comparatively limited."[1]

ETIOLOGY AND EPIDEMIOLOGY

Influenza virus is an orthomyxovirus. The virus is composed of an RNA-containing capsid surrounded by a glycoprotein envelope. The three major serotypes of influenza virus are determined by capsid antigens.Type A causes most epidemics and the most severe clinical illnesses. Type C is of little clinical importance. The two principal surface glycoprotein antigens, hemagglutinin and neuraminidase, determine the strain identity. Influenza A virus, unlike influenza B and C viruses, is capable of substantially altering these two surface antigens so that major changes in the virus allow it to elude previously established humoral immunity. Influenza A virus possesses the capacity to generate several distinct hemagglutinins and two distinct neuraminidases (Table 97–1).

Influenza A viruses are classified according to their hemaglutinin (H) and neuraminidase (N) antigens. Minor antigen variations occur as well, so that there are several variants of influenza AH3N2 and of influenza B viruses (see Table 97–1). Minor antigenic variants are identified by the geographic locations of the laboratory, the culture sample number, and the year of isolation. For example, the 1968–1969 Hong Kong "flu" was caused by a H3N2 virus, A/Hong Kong/1/68.

TABLE 97–1. HUMAN INFLUENZA VIRUSES

Type	Subtype	Variants
A	H1N1	A/New Jersey/8/76
		A/USSR/90/77
		A/Brazil/11/78
		A/England/333/80
		A/Chile/1/83
	H2N2	A/Japan/305/57
	H3N2	A/Hong Kong/1/68
		A/Port Chalmers/3/75
		A/Texas/1/77
		A/Bangkok/1/79
		A/Philippines/2/82
B	None	B/Hong Kong/5/72
		B/Singapore/222/79
		B/USSR/100/82

The minor variations, antigenic drifts, occur from year to year, possibly related to selective pressures produced by a progressively immune population. Major changes in antigenic constituents, so called antigenic shifts, occur every 2–4 years, resulting in large epidemics. The appearance of new antigenic determinants or the reappearance of old but not currently circulating antigenic determinants are presumably the origin of pandemic influenza.

Influenza pandemics have a 10 to 12 year periodicity. Attack rates may vary from 25–60%, and there is a spectrum of clinical illness varying from asymptomatic seroconversion to severe fatal disease. The attack rate and pattern of morbidity are determined by the distribution of older immune and younger susceptible people. The longer the interval between pandemics, the larger the pool of susceptibles and the more dramatic the clinical impact of the disease. The shorter interval influenza outbreaks associated with antigenic drift and shift are more likely to affect younger children and to spare adults.

Like all respiratory viruses, influenza is spread by aerosol and by direct contact. Spread of the infection is proportional to crowding and close contact: classrooms, barracks, nursing homes, aircraft, and ships provide optimum conditions for transmission.[2-6]

PATHOGENESIS AND IMMUNITY

There is an equal chance of deposition of virus on the nasopharyngeal mucosa or on the lower bronchial tree following inhalation of influenza virus in a droplet nuclei aerosol. Direct contact transmission leads only to nasopharyngeal deposition. The incubation period, from inoculation to onset of clinical illness and virus shedding, is 1–5 days. Virus shedding lasts for another 3–5 days, longer in children and in patients with severe illness.

Influenza is an infection of the respiratory epithelium. Viral replication in ciliated columnar epithelial cells produces local inflammation, cell death, and contiguous spread. Denudation of the tracheobronchial tree results in decreased ciliary clearance, decreased mucus production, edema, and debris obstructing small airways, and decreased ventilation and diffusion capacity. The brassy, nonproductive cough often causes central mediastinal and tracheal pain or burning. Coughing is precipitated by cold air and otherwise innocuous irritants. Dyspnea and a sense of incomplete inspiration are common subjective complaints. Wheezing, especially fine end expiratory wheezes, as with bronchiolitis, may occur.

Viremia does occur.[7] It seems to be remarkably transient and rare: the virus is extraordinarily difficult to isolate from blood. However, well documented virus isolation from placenta, muscles, liver, heart, cerebrospinal fluid, and urine confirms systemic dissemination. The rate of occurrence of viremia is not defined. Isolation of virus from sites other than the respiratory tract has been reported only from patients with intense or complicated clinical illness.

Immunity to influenza follows naturally occurring infection and experimental challenge with live virus. Secretory IgA and circulating IgM and IgG are produced, and immunity to reinfection and illness with homologous virus persists for decades. Immunity to heterologous but serologically related viruses also develops and is long lasting. However, as epidemic variants become progressively less serologically cross-reactive with established antibody, immunity progressively declines.

Cell-mediated immunity (CMI) has been shown to play a role in the recovery from influenza infection. T-lymphocyte-mediated cytotoxicity develops following infection with influenza virus and reaches a peak before antibody is detectable. Passive transfer of activated T-lymphocytes to infected mice produces a reduction in viral concentration in the lungs and the severity of pneumonia. Diminished CMI is likely to be associated with aggressive influenza virus infection.

The severity of influenza is determined in part by the immune status of the patient and the coexistence of underlying medical illness. The most severe illness follows the emergence of new strains of virus for which the host has little or no cross reactive immunity. Patients most seriously affected, regardless of the prevalent viral strain causing infection, are those with preexisting lung disease and heart disease causing congestive heart failure or pulmonary congestion. A nonimmune patient with compensated congestive heart failure and chronic bronchitis is at greatest risk for complicated, possibly fatal influenza.

There are two categories of complications. The first and most common category is bacterial superinfections: sinusitis, otitis, and pneumonia. Disruption of mucociliary clearance and impaired macrophage and polymorphonuclear leukocyte function produced by influenza virus infection sets the stage for infection by *Streptococcus pneumoniae*, *Staphylococcus aureus*, *Haemophilus influenzae*, and *Klebsiella pneumoniae*. The second category of complications follows dissemination of the virus and infection of tissues other than respiratory epithelium: primary influenza pneumonia, myositis, myocarditis, encephalitis, and transplacental fetal infection.

Impaired mucociliary clearance mechanisms and phagocytic function to preexisting influenza infection increase the likelihood of superimposed bacterial infection. Altered cell-mediated immunity may contribute to failure to contain the virus to respiratory epithelium, allowing for hematogenous spread. Diminished cardiopulmonary function and reserve would then predispose to severe illness.

THE CLINICAL DIAGNOSIS OF INFLUENZA

The spectrum of clinical illness caused by influenza virus ranges from inapparent infection to fulminant viral pneumonia. When a large portion of the population has at least partial immunity, about 20% of the infections will be inapparent and another 30% will have only coryza without fever.

Febrile flu will occur in about 50% of the infected, and about 5% of these patients will have lower respiratory tract involvement.

The classic picture of influenza is unmistakable: sudden onset of chills and fever, myalgias including extraocular muscle pain and photophobia, headache, profound malaise, sore throat, and a brassy, painful nonproductive cough. The acute phase lasts for 3–7 days and is often followed by prolonged convalescence.

The clinical diagnosis is easy during influenza outbreaks, but sporadic infection may resemble the illnesses caused by other respiratory pathogens. Virologic confirmation of influenza infection is desirable when increases in respiratory illnesses occur in the community.

Nasal washes and throat swabs are the best specimens. Virus culture in eggs or tissue culture remain the standard procedure. However, rapid methods for detecting virus or viral antigens, including immunofluorescence and radioimmunoassay, may be available in some laboratories. Serologic confirmation by demonstrating rising antibody titers is helpful for epidemiologic surveys.

MATERNAL INFLUENZA

The impact of influenza on pregnant women has been most dramatic during major pandemics. In 1918, the mortality for all pregnant women was 27%; among women contracting influenza in the last month of gestation, mortality was in excess of 60%.[15] During the same pandemic, nonpregnant patients with influenza complicated by pneumonia suffered a 30% mortality; over 50% of pregnant patients with pneumonia died. Similar but less depressing trends were present in the 1957–1958 Asian flu epidemic.[16,17] There was an increase in the incidence of death from primary influenza pneumonia among pregnant patients. In New York City, half the young women dying from influenza were pregnant.[16] Throughout the United States, there was a sharp increase in maternal mortality associated with the 1957–1958 influenza outbreak, but not as marked as in the 1918 pandemic. Women with preexisting heart disease and women in the last few weeks of gestation were at greatest risk. In all major epidemics, severe maternal disease has been associated with intrauterine fetal death, premature labor, and premature delivery (see also Chapter 121).

It seems likely that the alterations in cell-mediated immunity induced by pregnancy contribute to some of the excess risk. Increased blood volume and decreased serum albumin predispose pregnant women to pulmonary edema. Diffuse injury to the lung, as with hematogenous spread of a pathogenlike influenza virus to the pulmonary parenchyma, can produce progressive, refractory pulmonary infiltrates and acute respiratory failure.

It is important to remember, however, that the majority of pregnant women, even during an influenza epidemic, will not suffer serious disease. Pregnant patients at greatest risk are those that have heart disease (especially rheumatic valvular disease), type I insulin-dependent diabetes, chronic lung disease including smoking, and altered host defense mechanisms (mucociliary disorders, phagocyte dysfunction, hemoglobinopathies, and immunodeficiency states.[8-14]

MATERNAL INFECTION AND THE FETUS

There has been an increase in stillbirths, prematurity, and congenital anomalies associated with maternal influenza during every major influenza epidemic of the 20th century.[18-28] No consistent pattern of congenital anomalies or fetal injury are discernible suggesting that the fetal effects of influenza virus infection are multifactorial. Severity of maternal illness clearly contributes to excess fetal mortality.

Transplacental fetal infections have been clearly documented. McGregor et al[29] reported a woman suffering acute A/Bangkok (H3N2) influenza with uterine tenderness suggesting chorioamnionitis, from whom the virus was isolated from nasal washings and amniotic fluid. The healthy infant delivered three weeks after maternal recovery had no virus isolated from the placenta, amniotic fluid, or nasal washings. Cord blood contained IgM and IgA antibodies against the infecting virus. Fetal influenza infection with recovery does occur, as long as the mother eventually eliminates the virus. In some fatal maternal cases, influenza virus has been recovered from both maternal and fetal tissue.[30,31] But fetal infection has not been found in most of the reports.[32,33]

The clinical data suggests that maternal viremia is unusual and that transplacental infection is rare. Moreover, viremia with metastatic visceral infection is associated with serious maternal illness. Asymptomatic viremia capable of causing fetal infection and teratogenesis would seem highly improbable.

Nevertheless, maternal influenza virus infection has been claimed as the cause of fetal anomalies and childhood disease. Congenital anomalies, including neural tube defects, cleft lip and palate, and limb reduction, have occurred in the infants of women reporting influenzalike illness during pregnancy.[18-25] An increased incidence of neoplasms has been reported in children born during and following influenza epidemics.[34-36]

Unfortunately, the majority of studies reporting an increase in congenital anomalies and childhood neoplasms have not included specific viral diagnostic studies. Hardy et al[27] reported increased malformations without any consistent pattern among women whose serologic tests indicated gestational influenza, especially when infection occurred early in pregnancy. There are virus serotype, epidemic year, and geographic differences in the pattern of congenital anomalies associated with maternal influenza. During the 1957–1958 Asian influenza pandemic, Ireland reported anencephaly as the most common anomaly[19], but cardiac lesions were predominant in the United States.[20] During the 1968–1969 Hong Kong influenza pandemic, neural tube defects, not including anencephaly, were common.[25] In Scandinavia, the association between maternal influenza and cold remedy use and oral clefts was found following the Hong Kong influenza epidemic.[37] The role of fever in the genesis of fetal anomalies during influenza outbreaks has been unexplored.

The impact of severe maternal disease on fetal well being is obvious. There is no convincing evidence that influenza virus, by itself, is a teratogen or carcinogen for the fetus.

TREATMENT AND PREVENTION

Supportive care is the sole solace for pregnant patients with influenza: rest, fluids, humidity, acetaminophen, and frequent reassurance. Antibiotics are indicated only for secondary bacterial infection. Patients should be observed for changes in chest examination, dyspnea, and changes in secretions that might indicate superimposed bacterial infection or aggressive viral disease. Pneumonia warrants admission and closer observation.

Amantadine and rimantadine block replication of influenza A, but not type B influenza virus. They have been used prophylactically and to treat infected, high-risk patients. Amantadine is an effective prophylactic agent in crowded settings like nursing homes and appears to dampen and shorten the clinical course of acute influenza. Unfortunately, these agents are embryotoxic and teratogenic in rodents and cannot be recommended for general use during pregnancy. During epidemics, however, some pregnant patients with valvular heart disease and chronic lung disease should be offered amantadine prophylaxis if they are susceptible and in the third trimester. In this circumstance, the benefits probably outweigh the risks.

A better solution is to immunize such high risk patients with multivalent influenza vaccine before conception or if necessary during pregnancy. The only real contraindication to influenza immunization is allergy to eggs, which are used for propagating the virus. New split antigen vaccines have proved even safer. Women have been immunized safely during gestation and have provided good titers of transplacentally transmitted protective influenza-specific antibody.[38] Whether all pregnant women should receive influenza vaccine is debatable.

REFERENCES

1. Graves RJ. Influenza. In: *System of Clinical Medicine*. Graves RJ, Gerhard WW, eds. Philadelphia, PA: E Barrington and GD Haswell; 1848:462.
2. Glezen WP, Couch RB. Influenza viruses. In: *Viral Infections of Humans*, 3rd edition. Evans AS, ed. New York, NY: Plenum; 1989:419.
3. Hers JF, Mulder J. Broad aspects of the pathology and pathogenesis of human influenza. *Am Rev Respir Dis*. 1961;83:84.
4. Sweet C, Smith H. Pathogenicity of influenza virus. *Microbiol Rev*. 1980;44:303.
5. Noble GR. Epidemiological and clinical aspects of influenza. In: *Basic and Applied Influenza Research*. Beare AS, ed. Boca Raton, FL: CRC Press; 1982:11.
6. Frost WH. The epidemiology of influenza. *JAMA*. 1919;73:313.
7. Naficy K. Human influenza infection with proved viremia: report of a case. *N Engl J Med*. 1963;269:964.
8. Walker WM, McKee AP. Asian influenza in pregnancy. *Obstet Gynecol*. 1959;13:394.
9. Leontic EA. Respiratory disease in pregnancy. *Med Clin N Am*. 1977;61:111.
10. Griffiths PD, Ronalds CJ, Heath RB. A prospective study of influenza infections during pregnancy. *J Epidemiol Commun Health*. 1980;34:124.
11. Larsen JW Jr. Influenza and pregnancy. *Clin Obstet Gynecol*. 1982;25:599.
12. Korones SB. Uncommon virus infections of the mother, fetus, and newborn: influenza, mumps, and measles. *Clin Perinatol*. 1988;15:259.
13. Martin CM, Junin CM, Gottlieb LS, et al. Asian influenza A in Boston, 1957–1958. *Arch Intern Med*. 1959;103:515.
14. Widelock D, Csizmas L, Klein S. Influenza, pregnancy, and fetal outcome. *Public Health*. 1963;78:1.
15. Harris JW. Influenza occurring in pregnant women. *JAMA*. 1919;72:978.
16. Greenberg M, Jacobziner H, Pakter J, et al. Maternal mortality in the epidemic of asian influenza, New York City, 1957. *Am J Obstet Gynecol*. 1958;76:897.
17. Freeman DW, Barno A. Deaths from Asian influenza associated with pregnancy. *Am J Obstet*. 1959;78:1172.
18. Campbell WAB. Influenza in early pregnancy. Effects of the fetus. *Lancet*. 1953;1:173.
19. Coffey VP, Jessop WJE. Maternal influenza and congenital deformities: a progressive study. *Lancet*. 1959;2:935.
20. Wilson MG, Heins HL, Imagawa DT, et al. Teratogenic effects of Asian influenza. *JAMA*. 1959;171:638.
21. Doll R, Hill AB, Jakula J. Asian influenza in pregnancy and congenital defects. *Br J Prev Soc Med*. 1960;14:167.
22. Leck I. Incidence of malformations following influenza epidemics. *Br J Prev Soc Med*. 1963;17:70.
23. Coffey VP, Jessop WJ. Maternal influenza and congenital deformities: a follow-up study. *Lancet*. 1963;1:748.
24. Wilson MG, Stein AM. Teratogenic effects of Asian influenza. *JAMA*. 1969;210:336.
25. Hakosalo J, Saxen L. Influenza epidemic and congenital defects. *Lancet*. 1971;2:1346.
26. MacKenzie JS, Houghton M. Influenza infections during pregnancy: association with congenital malformations and with subsequent neoplasms in children, and potential hazards of live virus vaccines. *Bacteriol Rev*. 1974;38:356.
27. Hardy JB, Azarowicz EN, Mannini A, et al. The effect of Asian influenza on the outcome of pregnancy. Baltimore, 1957–1958. *Am J Public Health*. 1961;51:1182.
28. Walker WM, McKee AM. 633 women with Asian flu antibodies. No congenital malformations (retrospective study). *Obstet Gynecol*. 1959;13:394.
29. McGregor JA, Burns JC, Levin MJ, et al. Transplacental passage of influenza A/Bangkok (H3N2) mimicking amniotic fluid infection syndrome. *Am J Obstet Gynecol*. 1984;149:856.
30. Yawn DH, Pyeatte JC, Joseph JM, et al. Transplacental transfer of influenza virus. *JAMA*. 1971;216:1022.
31. Ruben FL, Thompson DS. Cord blood lymphocyte in vitro responses to influenza A antigens after an epidemic of influenza A/Port Chalmers/73 (H3N2). *Am J Obstet Gynecol*. 1981;141:443.
32. Monif GRG, Sowards DL, Eitzman DV. Serologic and immunologic evaluation of neonates following maternal influenza infection during the second and third trimesters of gestation. *Am J Obstet Gynecol*. 1972;114:239.
33. Ramphal R, Donnelly WH, Small PA Jr. Fatal influenzal pneumonia in pregnancy: failure to demonstrate transplacental transmission of influenza virus. *Am J Obstet Gynecol*. 1980;138:347.
34. Leck I, Steward JK. Incidence of neoplasms in children born after influenza epidemics. *Br Med J*. 1972;4:631.
35. Fedrick J, Alberman ED. Reported influenza in pregnancy and subsequent cancer in the child. *Br Med J* 1972;2:485.
36. Austin DF, Karp S, Dworsky R, et al. Excess leukemia in cohorts of children born following influenza epidemics. *Am J Epidemiol*. 1975;101:77.
37. Saxen I. The association between maternal influenza, drug consumption, and oral clefts. *Acta Odontol Scand*. 1975;33:259.
38. Puck JM, Glezen WP, Frank AL, et al. Immunoprophylaxis: protection of infants from infection with influenza A virus by transplacentally acquired antibody. *J Infect Dis*. 1980;142:844.

Chapter Ninety-Eight
Measles

Marvin S. Amstey

98

Measles or rubeola is a disease seen in humans characterized by a generalized rash and high fever. It has been known as a clinical entity since at least the 7th century AD. Although measles has generally been thought to be a minor exanthematous viral infection, it is a generalized infectious disease that in adults can be severe, with death resulting from pneumonia or encephalitis.

ETIOLOGY

Measles is caused by a paramyxovirus that was first grown in tissue culture by Enders and Peebles. This was the beginning of successful attempts to modify the virus in tissue culture, thereby making a vaccine possible for active immunization. The current vaccine is a live, attenuated virus grown in chick embryo cell cultures.[1]

PATHOGENESIS

The virus is acquired from contaminated aerosols that infect the respiratory mucosa initially. Following an incubation period of 10–14 days, at which time a viremia occurs, the initial symptoms of an upper respiratory infection (URI) appear. Along with the reddened mucous membranes and conjunctivae, a high fever occurs before the appearance of the characteristic maculopapular rash that begins on the face and neck. Prior to the rash, Koplik's spots appear on the mucous membranes of the pharynx. At its peak, the rash seems to be concentrated on the face and trunk. These spots are inflammatory lesions of the submucosal glands. Epithelial giant cells and syncytial cells can be demonstrated in bronchial mucosa. If pneumonia occurs, there is a bronchiolitis and interstitial bronchopneumonia. The peribronchial infiltration is characterized by mononuclear and giant cells.

EPIDEMIOLOGY

The incidence of measles today is quite low because of widespread vaccination. Historically, when the infection was introduced into an isolated community or population, the frequency of severe disease and death was high. However, in most Western populations, prior to vaccination, the disease had a low complication rate, with 97% occurring in people under the age of 15. The attack rate in susceptible populations was extremely high, reaching more than 90 out of 100 susceptible children between four and eight years of age. This makes measles one of the most infectious diseases known.

Prior to vaccination, the attack rate among pregnant women was very low—approximately 6–40 cases in 100,000 pregnancies. This is in part due to the fact that pregnant women are not in the susceptible age group. However, the proportion of measles cases has shifted since widespread vaccination began, so that children under age 5 and adults over age 20 account for the greatest proportion of all measles cases.

MANIFESTATIONS

Measles in pregnancy follows the same course as in nonpregnant women and is described above. Following the incubation period, the course of the infection runs for about eight days, ending with a break in the fever curve, some desquamation of the erupted skin, and some brown staining of other parts of the skin, which may persist for a few weeks. The patient is contagious from 1–4 days before the coryza to seven days after the appearance of rash.

A severe form of the infection, which has been called *atypical measles*, occurs in those adults who received an older, formalin-inactivated, killed measles vaccine. Atypical measles results from reinfection of these individuals with wild virus. They experience a high fever; pneumonitis; pneumonia; and a coarse, hemorrhagic, or urticarial rash. These individuals are not contagious; however, whether a pregnant woman could transmit atypical measles to her fetus is unknown. The disease is self-limiting and treatment is supportive.[2]

A third form of measles is called *modified measles* and occurs in those individuals who have received gamma globulin during the incubation period of measles. This is a mild disease, and the patient may not become ill at all. This form of the infection may occur in infants who received passively transferred maternal antibody.

DIAGNOSIS

Any patient with a clinical picture of measles should be reported to the local or state health authorities. The case definition includes fever (>101°F), rash for more than 3 days, and cough, coryza, or conjunctivitis. This clinical picture is measles, until proven otherwise. Hemagglutination inhibition (HI) serologic tests are the most widely used for diagnosis; a fourfold rise in antititers between acute serum (within 3 days of rash) and convalescent serum (drawn 10–20 days later) is diagnostic. The HI antibody persists for years, and therefore is a useful means of detecting immunity, also. A complement fixation (CF) antibody is also measurable, and a fourfold rise in this antibody is also diagnostic of recent measles. The presence of an IgM-HI specific antibody will also diagnose a new case of measles. Ideally, this should be drawn 5–10 days after the onset of rash.

The differential diagnosis includes a long list of diseases with mobilliform rashes and fever. They vary from serum sickness from drug reactions to rubella and exanthem subitum. The timing of the onset of fever, rash, upper respiratory symptoms, and conjunctivitis help eliminate many of these exanthems.

TREATMENT

There is no specific treatment for measles, whether the patient is pregnant or not. However, immune globulin will effectively modify the infection to make the illness much less intense if it can be given during the incubation period. Therefore, it is important to document the case to which the pregnant patient became exposed. Any adult should be observed carefully for the development of viral specific or secondary pneumonias. The dose of immune globulin is 0.25mL/kg body weight. It is unknown whether this will modify disease in the fetus.

PREVENTION

Vaccination with the live, attentuated measles vaccine is more than 95% effective. Appropriate use of this vaccine could eliminate measles as a disease in our lifetime, as smallpox vaccination has eliminated that disease. The vaccine is not for pregnant women or for women who plan to be pregnant within three months. Vaccines should not be given to anyone who has received gamma globulin within three months.[3]

FETAL ASPECTS

Abortions and premature deliveries were much higher during epidemics of measles than would otherwise be expected. However, whether this was due to the infection is not known. The high fevers and generalized illness also could have accounted for the increased abortion and prematurity rates. Fortunately, immunization has eliminated the large epidemics that were seen in the past. In one study, measles infection during pregnancy was associated with a fivefold increased risk of low birth weight but not with an increase in perinatal mortality. Although numerous reports of congenital anomalies following measles in pregnancy have appeared, there has been no consistent pattern of abnormality.[4] Case-controlled studies have failed to demonstrate any increase in congenital anomalies. Rare cases of congenital measles have occurred in newborns. As in the adult, pneumonia is a serious complication of measles in newborns. To date, there have been no reported infections or anomalies among newborns of susceptible mothers who have been vaccinated inadvertently during or within three months of pregnancy.

Pregnant patients infected with measles or vaccinated with measles vaccine should be reported to the Centers for Disease Control in Atlanta (Telephone 404–639–3311).

REFERENCES

1. Krugman S, Katz S. Measles. In: *Infectious Diseases of Children.* 7th ed. St. Louis, MO: CV Mosby Co.; 1981:144.
2. Hinman A, Koplan J. Public health policy toward atypical measles syndrome in the United States. *Med Decision Making.* 1982;2:71.
3. Immunization Practices Advisory Committee. Measles prevention. *MMWR.* 1982;31:217.
4. Dyer I. Measles complicating pregnancy. *Southern Med J.* 1940;33:601.

Chapter Ninety-Nine

Varicella and Herpes Zoster Infections: Chickenpox and Shingles

Marvin S. Amstey

99

Varicella and herpes zoster are different manifestations of the same virus infection. The virus, varicella-zoster, will produce an infection called *chickenpox* when it first infects humans, that is, a primary infection. Like all members of this virus group, it will remain latent within the body. When varicella-zoster is reactivated, it will manifest itself as *shingles* or a *herpes zoster* infection.

Varicella-zoster (V-Z) virus is a member of the human herpes viruses. The infectious particle is a large virus measuring approximately 180–200 nm. It contains a linear double-stranded DNA surrounded by a capsid and a lipid and protein envelope. This outer envelope is composed of the inner nuclear membrane of the host cell. The V-Z virus can be isolated readily on a variety of tissue culture preparations of both human and simian origin. The best source of material for virus solation is vesicular fluid from the skin lesions of this infection. Cytologically, this virus produces large multinucleated giant cells, which contain eosinophilic intranuclear inclusions.

Although the first signs of this infection are fever followed quickly by a rash, the initial site of viral entrance or the initial site of viral replication is unknown. However, once the virus does gain entrance to the body, it is disseminated rapidly by viremia. It is believed that the appearance of skin lesions in crops is related to intermittent viremias. Antibody begins to appear on about the fourth day after the appearance of skin lesions, after which the infection begins to subside.

The skin reaction begins as a papule, which quickly fills with edema fluid, forming a vesicle. The base of the vesicle contains the multinucleated giant cells containing intranuclear inclusions.

Next, the vesciles begin to dry, forming pustules, which finally crust and are shed, leaving newly regenerated epithelium. Characteristically, the lesions are in various stages of healing (hence, the idea of crops), which distinguish these lesions from those of smallpox or variola. Unlike those of smallpox, the crusts are not infectious.

Varicella pneumonia is a diffuse interstitial and peribronchiolar reaction with consolidation and hemorrhage. The same intranuclear inclusions can be seen in the alveolar cells, endothelial cells, and elsewhere in the respiratory epithelium.

Chickenpox is very contagious and may be second only to measles in this regard. It is a disease primarily of children and occurs worldwide. Humans are the only source of the infection and are undoubtedly the only reservoir for varicella. Because the initial site of viral replication is unknown, the mode of spread is also unknown; however, spread is believed to occur by droplet and direct contact with infected lesions. The infection is contagious from about one day before the outbreak of rash until the lesions have dried.

Because this is a disease of children, infection during pregnancy should be relatively uncommon. Approximately 5 cases per 100,000 pregnancies might be expected, based on the admittedly poor data from the Collaborative Perinatal Research Study of 1958–1964. Other sources of data have estimated that only 1–2 cases per 100,000 pregnancies are to be expected. On the other hand, zoster infection or shingles is most commonly seen in adults. However, this manifestation is directly related to age, so that it is less common during the childbearing years than in older age. The true incidence of zoster in pregnancy is unknown, but it seems to be less frequent than chickenpox.

DIAGNOSIS

After an incubation period that varies from 12–18 days, fever is followed within 24 hours by rash that begins on the face and scalp. The rash spreads quickly to the trunk with less effect on the extremities. New crops of lesions continue to appear for about five days. These are usually associated with an intense pruritus, and pregnancy does not seem to alter this picture. The total number of skin lesions may vary from only one or two to almost confluence.

The former picture has led many adults to deny that they ever had chickenpox, which raises some anxiety when such an individual is pregnant and comes into contact with an obvious case of chickenpox. Only serologic testing will alleviate these concerns.

Chickenpox pneumonia is the most common complication of this exanthem and may be expected to occur in 15–50% of adults. Controversy has continued for a long time as to whether this complication is more severe during pregnancy.[1] It is clear that uncomplicated chickenpox is the same whether the woman is pregnant or not. However, varicella pneumonia in pregnancy has been reported to result in a maternal mortality rate of 41%, compared to a mortality rate of 11% in nonpregnant individuals. Another report has shown a maternal mortality rate of 46% among 22 pregnant women with this complication.

The reactivation of latent V-Z virus infection is manifested as a localized skin eruption that is usually limited to the skin area of the distribution of one sensory ganglion. Pain and paresthesias occur in the involved dermatome several days prior to the outbreak of the vesicular lesions. As in chickenpox, new crops of lesions may continue to appear for several days, but in contrast, these lesions usually are not pruritic but are associated with moderate to severe neuralgia. Unfortunately, this neuralgia persists for weeks to months after the disappearance of lesions. This picture is not different in the pregnant woman. Because these individuals usually have substantial circulating antibodies, the fetuses and neonates of women with herpes zoster are at very little risk for becoming infected.[2]

The well known presentation of chickenpox and shingles makes the clinical diagnosis relatively easy. Uncommonly, disseminated herpes simplex infection, impetigo, contact dermatitis, and, historically, smallpox and disseminated vaccinia were included in the differential diagnosis.

More specifically, scrapings from a vesicle may demonstrate multinucleated giant cells with intranuclear inclusions when stained with Giemsa or Wright's stain (Tzanck smear). Virus can be isolated from these vesicles relatively easily. In addition, viral antigen has been demonstrated by direct fluorescent staining of cellular material from fresh vesicles.

Most commonly, antibody can be demonstrated by complement fixation (CF), by direct immunoflourescence of V-Z membrance antigen (FAMA), or by enzyme-linked immunosorbent assays (ELISA). The latter two tests are becoming available widely and have several advantages over CF tests. They are more sensitive, and these antibodies persist for years if not a lifetime. Therefore, either the FAMA or ELISA test must be done in order to determine whether a woman has ever had V-Z virus infection. The CF antibody declines rapidly after infection, so that it may be undetectable after one year.[3]

TREATMENT AND PREVENTION

There is no specific treatment for this viral infection to date. However, a number of anecdotal reports have suggested acyclovir in a dose of 10–18 mg/kg every 8 hours. None of these were controlled studies. One randomized, placebo-controlled study of intravenous acyclovir at 10 mg/kg every 8 hours for 5 days in nonpregnant, adult varicella infection showed no effect on the disease course.[4] This is not too surprising because the effectiveness of this drug relates to the availability of a specific (herpes simplex), viral-specified thymidine kinase. Normal cellular thymidine kinases (or other viral-specified enzymes) are not nearly as good at activating acyclovir by a factor of several hundred. Because of the accumulation of anecdotes about acyclovir's benefit in varicella infections, it is important to consider its use in a truly life-threatening adult varicella infection. On the positive side, one study did show that a daily dose of 1500 mg/m^2 reduced dissemination of V-Z virus and hastened healing even in compromised hosts.[5]

Passive immunotherapy is available in the form of varicella-zoster immune globulin (VZIG). This immunoglobulin is distributed through the American Red Cross blood services. It is intended primarily for use by those patients who are exposed to the infection less than three days prior to administration and who are known to be susceptible (that is, nonimmune) to this virus infection. While the use of VZIG was restricted in the past to immunocompromised individuals and infants under the age of three months, there may be another group who should be considered for therapy. This group is otherwise healthy susceptible pregnant women. If one accepts the argument that varicella infection is worse in pregnant women, then use of VZIG follows logically. Even without this argument, it can be stated categorically that a pregnant woman who is very ill with varicella pneumonia not only has a high mortality rate, but the severe illness alone will compromise the fetus and result in intrauterine death, or in premature delivery. All of these reasons argue strongly for the use of VZIG in susceptible pregnant women.

Demonstration of susceptibility should follow these logical steps. If the pregnant woman or her family knows that she had chickenpox as a child, she is immune. The correlation with history is very high. Without a history, measurement of the FAMA or ELISA antibody will determine the need for VZIG. The absence of antibody is a clear indication of susceptibility.

FETAL ASPECTS

Fetal death is the result of severe maternal varicella infection, usually with pneumonia. However, this is a secondary result because of the severe maternal infection. It has not been shown that the virus directly affects the fetus, leading to intrauterine death, nor does there appear to be an increase in fetal wastage after first trimester maternal infection by varicella.[6]

There is a constellation of abnormalities in neonates born to mothers who experience first trimester varicella infections. This constellation of malformations includes fetal growth retardation, aplasia of a single limb, cicatrization of the skin, neurologic damage, and ocular abnormalities. Some or all of these malformations may occur. In no reported case has the virus been isolated from the affected neonate. Fewer than 20 such cases have been reported, but the combination of abnormalities has been so consistent that little doubt remains that this syndrome is an example of varicella embryopathy.[7]

In addition to the first trimester effects of varicella in pregnancy, the fetus or neonate may be at risk for developing varicella (the infection, not the malformations) if the mother acquires the infection late in pregnancy. The newborn who develops varicella within ten days of birth is considered to have acquired the infection *in utero*. This is deduced from the fact that the incubation period for varicella is almost always more than 12 days. This congenital varicella infection has been distinguished from neonatal varicella by this magical 10-day period and the fact that the most severe illness occurred in those infants with congenital infection. However, there has been sufficient overlap between these two entities (congenital varicella and neonatal varicella) in severity and prognosis that one should think of them together simply as varicella of the newborn. The severity of the infection seems to relate to the amount of passively transferred antibody and therefore to the duration of the mother's infection. Thus, an infant born to a mother whose onset of symptoms is less than five days before delivery or two days after delivery is at the greatest risk for developing varicella of the newborn. In the past, VZIG was in such short supply that only these infants were eligible to receive this immunoprophylaxis. However, today all infants exposed to varicella in the first three months of life should receive VZIG.

One should remember that fewer than 10% of women who deny having had varicella as a child are truly susceptible to this virus. They either forgot about the infection or their infection was so mild that it was not recognized as chickenpox.

REFERENCES

1. Amstey MS. Varicella in pregnancy. *J Reprod Med.* 1978;21:89.
2. Brunell PA. Fetal and neonatal varicella-zoster infections. *Semin Perinatol.* 1983;7:47.
3. Gold E. Serologic and virus isolation studies of patients with varicella or herpes-zoster infection. *N Engl J Med.* 1966;274:181.
4. Al-Nakib W, Al-Kandari S, El-Kholik M, et al. A randomized controlled study of intravenous acyclovir, Zovirax R, against placebo in adults with chickenpox. *J Infect.* 1983;6:49.
5. Gershon A, Chickenpox: how dangerous is it? *Contemp Obstet Gynecol.* 1988;31:41.
6. Laforet EG, Lynch CL. Multiple congenital defects following maternal varicella. *N Engl J Med.* 1947;236:534.
7. Young NA. Chickenpox, measles, and mumps. In: Remington J, Klein J, eds. *Infectious Diseases of the Fetus and Newborn Infant.* Philadelphia, PA: WB Saunders; 1976:521.

Chapter One Hundred

Other Viral Exanthematous Diseases

Stanley A. Gall

100

A number of microorganisms, in addition to such common viral diseases as measles, rubella, and varicella, are associated with skin manifestations of disease. A partial listing is included in Table 100–1. Each disease entity has its own importance and is discussed in a separate chapter. However, some of the viruses, especially the enteroviruses, have particular obstetric significance and will be discussed in more detail.

Many individual enteroviruses cause a variety of exanthems as well as enanthems.[1,2] As with most viral exanthematous diseases, these occur more commonly in children than in adults and the rashes are not diagnostic. More commonly implicated serotypes include echovirus serotypes 1–7, 9, 11, 12, 14, 16, 18, 19, 20, 25, 30, and coxsackievirus serotypes A4, A5, A6, A9, A10, A16, and B2, B3, and B5. Direct virus isolation from the maculopapular lesion has not been accomplished; therefore, the laboratory evidence to support an enteroviral exanthem must come from the culture virus from vesicles, blood, feces, or throat secretions.

Enterovirus exanthems cause little morbidity but have to be used as a guide to the prevalence of coxsackievirus and echovirus infection in the community.

Fine maculopapular rashes resembling rubella but occurring during summer epidemics have been reported most often with echoviruses. The highest attack rates occur with echovirus 9, the serotype most commonly associated with rash. The rash characteristically occurs simultaneously with fever and begins on the face (100%) and neck (75%), then spreads to the trunk (64%) and extremities (56%) and may involve the palms or soles, and persists 3–5 days. The rash can be confused with rubella but there is an absence of posterior cervical and postauricular lymphadenopathy. In 30% of patients, an enanthem on the buccal mucosa occurs, and this can be confused with Koplik's spots; however, no coryza or conjunctivitis is present.

Fine maculopapular rashes may be seen with other echovirus serotypes such as 2, 4, 11, 19, and 25. Coxsackievirus A9 causes eruptions on the trunk and face, with lesions most numerous on distal parts of the limbs. There is generally a fever of 38°–40°C with posterior cervical lymphadenopathy in half of the patients.[3]

Echovirus 16 produces a rash that does not appear until there is defervescence of the fever. The prototype is the Boston exanthem first described in 1951. Most cases occur sequentially in families, with children usually affected. Symptoms include fever 38–39°C, coryza, and pharyngitis. The fever lasts 24–36 hours. The salmon pink macules on the face are discrete, nonpruritic, and about 0.5–1.5 cm in diameter. The rash lasts 1–5 days.[4]

Coxsackievirus and echovirus infections during pregnancy have not been associated with early pregnancy losses. However, transplacental transmission has been demonstrated, but there have been too few reports to make a judgment. A critical time for these infections during pregnancy is at term because cases of neonatally acquired disease resulting in fetal demise from hepatic failure and disseminated intravascular coagulation (DIC) have been reported. It is recommended that a careful history be obtained from all patients who are scheduled to undergo elective repeat cesarean section as to the presence of fever or exanthem. If either is present, it is highly advisable to delay the cesarean section until the patient has recovered clinically and has developed antibodies that can protect the neonate.

A newer virus, parvovirus B19, discovered in 1975, has been determined to be the causative agent of erythema infectiosum, also known as fifth disease, a common childhood illness.[5] The obstetrician's concern is that this virus has a predilection for infection of red blood cell precursors in the fetus, leading to transient aplastic crisis, severe anemia, high output failure, generalized edema, and death.

TABLE 100–1. CAUSES OF MACULOPAPULAR ERUPTIONS

Viral	Other
Adenoviruses	Bacterial toxins
Arboviruses	Streptococci
Enteroviruses: Coxsackievirus	Staphylococci
Echovirus	Drug eruptions
Erythema infectiosum	Live-virus vaccines
Exanthem subitum	*Mycoplasma pneumoniae*
Infectious mononucleosis	Rat-bite fever
Measles	Rickettsial diseases
Reoviruses	Syphilis
Rubella	Typhoid fever

The incubation period for parvovirus B19 is short, generally lasting 4–14 days. B19 virus is efficiently transmitted by way of respiratory secretions after close contact. The period of infectivity is almost over by the time the rash has occurred. Transmission will occur in 10–60% of school contacts.

This viral infection is characterized by a facial rash that resembles the cheek having been slapped. The lacelike rash is often present on the trunk and extremities, also. Approximately 20–25% may have asymptomatic infection. In some outbreaks, arthralgias have been common. The virus can be transmitted by transfusions and from mother to fetus by transplacental vertical transmission.

B19 infection can be diagnosed by B19 IgM after the third day of the rash. The IgM titers decline after 30–60 days. B19 IgG is usually present after seven days and remains positive for years. The most sensitive technique is the detection of B19 DNA by nucleic acid hybridization. This test can identify B19 DNA in serum, leukocytes, respiratory secretions, urine, and tissue specimens.

The major effect of maternal B19 infection is fetal death. The estimated likelihood of fetal death following maternal B19 infection is less than 10%.[6] For the pregnant woman who has a documentated infection, an elevated alpha fetoprotein may indicate early fetal hydrops. Diagnostic ultrasound examination is probably the most widely available test to detect fetal hydrops. Intrauterine vascular transfusion is likely to be effective therapy.[7]

REFERENCES

1. Lerner AM, Klein JO, Cherry JD. New viral exanthems. *N Engl J Med.* 1963;269:678.
2. Lerner AM. Exanthems caused by coxsackieviruses, echovirus and reovirus infections. In: Demis DJ, Dobson RL, McGuire J, eds. *Clinical Dermatology.* Vol 3, Unit 14–19. Hagerstown, MD: Harper and Row; 1976:1.
3. Lerner AM, Klein JO, Levin HS, Finland M. Infections due to coxsackie virus group A, type 9, in Boston, 1959, with special reference to exanthems and pneumonia. *N Engl J Med.* 1960;263:1265.
4. Wenner HA. Virus diseases associated with cutaneous eruptions. *Prog Med Virol.* 1973;16:269.
5. Mortimer PP, Cohen BJ, Buckley MM, et al. Human parvovirus and the fetus. *Lancet.* 1985;2:1012. Letter.
6. Risks associated with human parvovirus B19 infection. *MMWR.* 1989;38:81.
7. Naides SJ, Weiner CP. Antenatal diagnosis and palliative treatment of nonimmune hydrops fetalis secondary to fetal parvovirus B19 infection. *Prenat Diagn.* 1989;9:105.

Chapter One Hundred and One

Epstein–Barr Virus Infections Including Infectious Mononucleosis

Kenneth F. Trofatter, Jr.

101

Epstein and colleagues discovered the virus that now bears their names growing in cultured lymphoblasts derived from Burkitt's lymphoma biopsies.[1] Morphologically, Epstein–Barr virus (EBV) is a member of the herpes family (see also Chapters 90 and 91). It contains a linear double-stranded DNA with approximately 170 $\times$ 10^3 base pairs and a guanosine-plus-cytosine content of 57%. Variability exists in EBV DNA isolated from different individuals, but different strains have similar, cross-reactive antigenic profiles and do not account for differences in the epidemiology of EBV-associated diseases.

EBV infection is ubiquitous, with a worldwide distribution and 95% or more of adults having serologic evidence of prior exposure.[2] Humans are the only natural hosts. Transmission occurs by oral–oral contact, fomites contaminated with blood, oropharyngeal or salivary gland secretions, and as a consequence of blood transfusion. The incubation period is unknown but has been estimated to be between two weeks and two months. Although intimacy promulgates disease, and infection of the genitourinary tract has been described in association with chronic infection[3], sexual transmission has not been proven. Epidemics do not occur, but case clustering is commonly seen on college campuses and military bases. An estimated 15–20% of all seropositive individuals excrete virus at any given time.

Worldwide, two peaks of primary infection are recognized. In underdeveloped nations, the major peak occurs during infancy and early childhood. This has been demonstrated by following, prospectively, the evolution of seroconversion of EBV viral capsid antigen (VCA) among African newborns.[4] In an area endemic for Burkitt's lymphoma, virtually 100% of the adults had serologic evidence of prior exposure to EBV. All of the neonates studied had maternal anti-VCA at birth, which declined with a half-life of about five weeks. Depending on the initial titers, all infants were seronegative within 2–8 months. Infection by EBV occurred as early as the third month after anti-VCA was undetectable, and by 21 months, 81% had seroconverted. Generally, seroconversion occurred without clinical evidence of disease.

In contrast, contact with EBV in the United States and

other Western societies is generally delayed until puberty. Among higher socioeconomic groups, the peak of exposure is between the ages of 15 and 25, with females encountering the virus slightly earlier than males.[5] Among lower socioeconomic groups, the early childhood and adolescent peaks are replaced by a progressive increase in seropositivity beginning at about age 4–5 years. Serial epidemiologic data would indicate that earlier infection occurs among lower socioeconomic groups, regardless of racial background, and may be the result of increased intimacy related to cultural habits, overcrowding, poor hygiene, or poor nutrition. There does not appear to be a genetic susceptibility to infection by EBV, although this has been proposed as an etiology for unusual and severe manifestations of the disease.

EBV has been implicated in a wide range of clinical entities, from the characteristically self-limited asymptomatic or unrecognized infections of early childhood and the symptomatic infectious mononucleosis of adolescence, to the associated sequelae of Burkitt's lymphoma and nasopharyngeal carcinoma.[6] As a general rule, the serologic profile at any given time can be used to classify EBV infections as primary, latent, or recurrent, and to predict outcome of associated malignancies.[7] Because of the rarity of these latter conditions in Western societies and the complex nature of their association with EBV, they are generally excluded from the discussions that follow. Our major concerns herein are the primary and recurrent EBV infections occurring in women during the childbearing years and the impact these have on pregnancy and intrauterine fetal development.

PATHOPHYSIOLOGY OF DISEASE

EBV has a restricted host and host–cell specificity with a tropism for human lymphoreticular tissues. Despite this limited host range, EBV displays a broad spectrum of cell–virus interactions.[8] Permissive infection with EBV results in the production of infectious virus and, ultimately, cell degeneration and death. During primary or recurrent infections *in vivo*, permissive infection appears to be limited only to a small percentage of the infected cell population. This situation is reflected *in vitro* by certain EBV-transformed cell lines in which only a small proportion of infected cells become producers of infectious virus with each passage.

The majority of cells that become infected both *in vivo* and *in vitro* are nonpermissive. In nonpermissive infections, a complex cell–virus relationship is established, which has been described as a proliferation-stimulating interaction. Under these circumstances, cells can be shown to contain EBV DNA qualitatively, by the presence of EBV nuclear antigen (EBNA), and quantitatively, by DNA hybridization studies. Other EBV antigens, such as early antigen (EA) and VCA, are variably present, suggesting multiple levels of control over the viral genome expression. These nonproducer cells characteristically proliferate more quickly than uninfected cells and in the process transmit the viral genome to their progeny. Probably, it is this population from which latent virus is reactivated *in vivo*.

Pathologic changes associated with primary symptomatic EBV infections, such as infectious mononucleosis, characteristically reflect the host cell–virus interactions described above. There is usually a generalized polyclonal, reticuloendothelial, proliferative response accompanied by a lymphocytic perivascular infiltrate in multiple nonlymphoid organs. Lymph nodes generally maintain their normal architecture but display prominent follicles secondary to proliferation of atypical lymphocytes. The spleen is often enlarged twofold to threefold and is hyperemic, with the normal architecture obscured by follicular prominence. The liver is only slightly enlarged and may have an infiltrate and focal necrosis similar to that found in infectious hepatitis. Hematologic changes reflect the systemic disease and are described subsequently. If the central nervous system (CNS) and heart are involved, findings are usually only nonspecific, with perivascular infiltration and edema present. When viremia occurs, it is buffy-coat cell-associated.

EFFECT OF PREGNANCY ON DISEASE

The incidence of clinical disease ranges from approximately 40–50 in 100,000 in the general population and 150–250 in 100,000 in the armed forces to 500–1000 in 100,000 among college students. Overall, the incidence of seroconversion among seronegative young adults is estimated at 12% per year. Seroconversion rates among seronegative pregnant women appear to parallel those of the general population.[2,9] Therefore, pregnancy does not seem to increase susceptibility to primary infection with EBV. However, among seropositive pregnant women, it has been shown that 55% will demonstrate a rise in anti-EA, consistent with recurrent infections at some time during their pregnancies.[10,11] This is double the rate of recurrent infections in nonpregnant patients derived from the same population base. Interestingly, the majority of women develop the rise in anti-EA during the first trimester of pregnancy. Thus, pregnancy may not only predispose individuals to reactivation of latent EBV, but when this occurs, it is usually coincident with organogenesis.

EFFECT OF DISEASE ON PREGNANCY

The effects on pregnancy outcome of active EBV infections are not entirely clear. Fleisher and Bolognese found no significant difference between seropositive individuals with recurrences (that is, anti-EA positive) and without recurrences (that is, anti-EA negative) during pregnancy with regard to fetal outcome, anomalies, or hyperbilirubinemia.[10] Furthermore, they found six women with serologically proven primary EBV infections in early pregnancy who had uncomplicated outcomes and no evidence of fetal infection by serologic and virologic evaluations of their offspring.[12] Similarly, Chang and Seto demonstrated the presence of EBV-transformed cells, indicative of congenital infection, in only one of 2696 (0.037%) umbilical cord blood specimens, and this infant demonstrated no abnormalities.[13] On the other hand, Icart and colleagues, in their analysis of more than 700 women with serologic profiles consistent with active EBV infections, demonstrated a positive correlation of active infection with abnormal births.[14] Of particular interest were the outcomes in six patients whose profiles indicated primary infections during pregnancy: Four had premature labor and delivery at 32 weeks or less, one had an infant with multiple anomalies, one had a stillborn, and two of the infants died in the neonatal period. EBV was not proven to be etiologic in any of these cases; however, in support of its possible role, pathologic changes have been observed in placental and fetal tissues in abortuses from five women with documented primary EBV infections during the first two months of pregnancy.[15] Major findings included necrotizing deciduitis, chorioamnionitis, and villitis, as well as one fetus with congenital abnormalities and two with evidence of myocarditis. Summarizing these data, it is probably reasonable to conclude that significant congenital disease rarely occurs in the face of adequate maternal immunity, and primary infections, even though uncommon, could be implicated in the full range of adverse pregnancy outcomes (for example, spontaneous abortion, congenital malformations, intrauterine growth retardation, premature delivery, and intrauterine demise) characteristic of the classical TORCH organisms.

Transmission of the virus to the fetus during maternal infection probably occurs by the hematogenous route, specifically by the transplacental spread of infected maternal lymphocytes. Theoretically, congenital infection also could occur as a consequence of invasive procedures such as amniocentesis or intrauterine transfusion. Documented significant congenital infections with EBV are exceedingly rare. Intrapartum infection is probably equally uncommon. EBV has been found in genitourinary tract secretions[3], but even if the infant was exposed during the birth process, transmission of disease would be unlikely in the presence of passively-acquired maternal antibody. Perinatal infection might occur in the rare instance the fetus or neonate is exposed to infected blood or oropharyngeal secretions during an acute primary maternal infection when IgG antibodies have not accumulated sufficiently prior to delivery to provide passive immunity. Seronegative newborns have developed documented infections as a result of blood transfusions during the neonatal period.

When significant congenital infections occur, they are probably limited to instances of primary maternal infection acquired during the first trimester of pregnancy. Although anomalies associated with EBV under these circumstances have been described, whether the virus by itself is teratogenic has yet to be firmly established.[15-18] Certainly, the potential for teratogenesis exists. Chromosomal aberrations have been detected in EBV-infected lymphocytes, and EBV is clearly associated with both Burkitt's lymphoma and nasopharyngeal carcinoma.[8] Pathologic changes occurring in the fetus as the result of primary maternal infection during the second and third trimesters are not well documented. Presumably, they would run a rather self-limited course; however, the long-term consequences of such infections are not known. Extrahepatic bile duct atresia has been described in association with neonatal EBV infections.[19]

DIAGNOSIS

More than 50% of primary EBV infections and the vast majority of secondary or recurrent infections are entirely asymptomatic. The primary infection-to-disease ratio during the childbearing years is probably on the order of two or three to one. The diagnosis of acute symptomatic EBV infection is based on clinical features of the disease and is confirmed by laboratory studies detailed below. A high index of suspicion helps to make the diagnosis in the pregnant patient. Although the differential diagnosis is extensive, common pathogens to be excluded because of their potential for adverse maternal and fetal outcome are cytomegalovirus (CMV), human immunodeficiency virus (HIV), herpes simplex virus (HSV), and rubella. Other diseases that can be considered in the differential diagnosis include acute streptococcal pharyngitis, *Neisseria gonorrhoeae,* mumps, rubeola, and other viral agents (for example, adenovirus, enterovirus, hepatitis virus), as well as toxoplasmosis, diphtheria, pertussis, brucellolis, syphilis, *Mycoplasma, Staphylococcus aureus,* drug fever, serum sickness, lymphoproliferative diseases, and collagen vascular disorders.

When symptomatic infection occurs, this typically presents as a mononucleosis syndrome. The hallmarks of infectious mononucleosis include the classic complex of fever, malaise, sore throat, and lymphadenopathy. Fever occurs in 80–90% of cases, is usually high (39–40°C), intermittently spiking, and peaks during the first 7–10 days of illness. Pharyngitis is present in 80% or more, coincides with the onset of fever, and may persist two weeks or longer. Lymphadenopathy occurs in virtually 100% of cases, usually precedes the fever and pharyngitis by 1–2 days, and may persist a month or more. Although the lymphadenopathy is generalized, the anterior and posterior cervical nodes are most prominently involved. In patients with infectious mononucleosis, virus excretion from the oropharynx can be documented in about 90% during the acute phase of the disease, with intermittent shedding in 70–80% over subsequent months.

Frequent accompanying signs and symptoms of acute EBV infection include sweats, chills, headaches, anorexia, nausea, myalgias, and periorbital edema. If present, a palatal enanthem consisting of petechial lesions at the junction of the hard and soft palates is useful, though not pathognomonic, in making the diagnosis in 25–30% of patients. Splenomegaly occurs in 50% or more of cases, but hepatomegaly is much less common (10–15%). A mild macular skin rash has been described but is usually associated with coinciding ampicillin therapy.

Although the duration of symptoms varies, the usual course of infection is benign and self-limited, with complete recovery in 1–4 weeks. Occasionally, the disease does persist for months with prolonged malaise, fatigue, and laboratory abnormalities. Chronic, active EBV infections which have been described are characterized, most commonly, by neuromyasthenia (profound fatigue, recurrent fever and sore throat, musculoskeletal discomfort, lymphadenopathy, headaches, and difficulty concentrating). The more severe cases may be accompanied by persistent thrombocytopenia, anemia, leukopenia, hepatosplenomegaly, pneumonitis, and uveitis. A selective antibody deficiency to a component of EBNA and high titers (>1:5000) of antibody to VCA and EA, antigens associated with EBV replication, have been correlated with chronic active EBV infections.[20,21]

It appears that primary EBV infection during pregnancy does not increase maternal morbidity; however, this is a subject that has not been well addressed in the literature and will require further study. Atypical presentations and complications of acute EBV infections include splenic rupture, airway obstruction, pneumonitis, myocarditis, pericarditis, hepatic necrosis, Reye's syndrome, Guillain-Barré syndrome, Bell's palsy, aseptic meningitis, meningoencephalitis, transverse myelitis, acute cerebellar ataxia, metamorphopsia (Alice-in-Wonderland syndrome)[22], hemolytic anemia, pancytopenia, and agranulocytosis. At least 15–20 deaths each year in the United States can be directly attributed to one of these complications. It is obvious that pregnancy could, at least theoretically, delay or confuse the diagnosis when EBV presents in an atypical fashion. Chronic active EBV infections in particular could be easily masked by symptoms typically attributed to normal pregnancy.

Major laboratory findings in adults with infectious mononucleosis are rather nonspecific, except for the serologic changes. Varying degrees of liver function test abnormalities occur in 95% of individuals, but fewer than 50%

develop hyperbilirubinemia, and fewer than 10% develop clinical jaundice. In hepatitis associated with EBV infections, peak levels of SGOT and SGPT are usually less than 200 IU and generally occur 2–3 weeks after disease onset, with complete resolution by 5–6 weeks. Leukopenia and granulocytopenia during the earliest phase of illness have been described in 75% or more of individuals; however, total white blood count then rises and frequently peaks during the first 7–10 days of illness in the range of 10,000–20,000/mm^3. In general, this represents both a relative and absolute lymphocytosis with a 50–95% (≥4500/mm^3) lymphocytes plus monocytes, including 10–60% atypical forms. The vast majority of atypical lymphocytes appear to be uninfected activated T cells, whereas the acutely infected lymphocytes, and presumed reservoir for relapsing infections, are predominantly B cells. The white blood cell elevation and atypical forms may persist 1–2 months. Interestingly, the erythrocyte sedimentation rate is generally not increased.

Serologic changes occurring with EBV infections are diverse and have a broad range of specificity.[7,23] These remain, however, the key to establishing EBV as the infectious agent and to differentiating primary and recurrent infections. The cornerstone of serologic diagnosis in acute disease still rests in the assays for heterophil antibodies. Heterophil antibodies are of the IgM class, are frequently detectable during the first week of illness, and, although nonspecific, are diagnostic of EBV infection. They are found in at least 80–90% of adults with primary EBV infections. Heterophil antibodies can be measured by titering serum agglutination of sheep red blood cells. Titers ≤1:56 are not unusual in normal individuals and in patients with other illnesses, and titers ≥1:224 provide presumptive evidence of infectious mononucleosis. During acute EBV infections, differential adsorption of the serum with guinea pig red blood cells should not reduce the titer to less than 25% of the original value. Interestingly, adsorption with beef red blood cells completely removes EBV-associated heterophil antibodies, and this is the opposite of what occurs in normal patients and in patients with serum sickness. Heterophil antibodies peak 2–3 weeks after disease onset and may persist 3–6 months or longer after a primary infection. Although titers of heterophil antibody are not correlated completely with the severity of disease, those with the highest titers during acute illness tend to have more persistent infections. Another nonspecific antibody that develops in about two thirds of individuals within the first 12 months following primary infection is rheumatoid arthritis nuclear antigen (RANA). Its diagnostic and prognostic significance at this point is unclear.

Assays for antibodies to specific EBV antigens are less widely used for routine diagnosis but may be of value when the heterophil antibody screen is negative or equivocal or when pregnancy counseling is indicated. EBV-specific IgM can be detected 1–3 weeks after disease onset, is predominantly directed against VCA, is short-lived, and generally disappears prior to the disappearance of heterophil antibodies. The presence of EBV-specific IgM indicates infection within three months. Recently, a rapid anti-EBV IgM-enzyme-linked immunosorbent assay (ELISA) has been described that employs the antibody capture-principle.[24] The sensitivity and specificity of this assay approaches 99%, and it has been proven useful in the early diagnosis of infectious mononucleosis, even prior to detection of heterophil antibodies.

Following a rise in IgM, a host of EBV-specific IgG antibodies appear. These include antibodies to EBV membrane antigen (MA), EBNA, and two forms of EA, EA(R) (restricted) and EA(D) (diffuse), as defined by differential sensitivity to alcohol. IgG antibodies to VCA, MA, and EBNA tend to persist with time, whereas anti-EA usually disappears and then reappears with recurrent infections. Anti-EA is useful, therefore, in monitoring asymptomatic reactivation of latent EBV.

Any pregnant woman presenting with the syndrome complex of fever, sore throat, malaise, and adenopathy should probably be evaluated by complete blood count with differential and smear tests, pharyngeal culture for *Streptococcus*, and some assessment of heterophil antibody status, such as the monospot test. If the patient is acutely ill, and has a positive monospot test and a peripheral blood smear consistent with EBV infection, then the diagnosis is established, and no further diagnostic study is indicated. If jaundice ensues, liver function tests should be obtained as well as serologic studies to rule out hepatitis viruses. If the initial monospot test is negative but the clinical picture and peripheral smear are consistent with acute EBV infection, one has the option of performing EBV-specific serodiagnostic studies, if available, and repeating the monospot test in 2–3 weeks. However, under these circumstances, other diagnostic studies that should be considered, if not done previously, include a TORCH screen, HIV screen, pharyngeal viral cultures, and even lymph node biopsy.

Because EBV may not be suspected until late in the course of a primary infection, serum antibody profiles may be more useful in establishing the diagnosis than absolute titers. If assays for specific EBV antibodies are performed, recent primary infection is indicated by the serologic findings of EBV-specific IgM in high titers and IgG anti-VCA in the absence of anti-EBNA. Transient elevations of anti-EA, generally anti-EA(D), can be found in 70% or more of primary infections in adults, and this tends to appear later in the course of the disease. Previous, but not current, infection with EBV is indicated by modest and stable titers of anti-VCA and anti-EBNA in the absence of anti-EA. Recurrent infections are suggested by the addition of detectable levels (≥1:20) of anti-EA, generally anti-EA(R). If the specific serologic profile is found to be inconsistent with the typical clinical patterns of EBV infections, one should consider the possibilities of collagen vascular disease, immunosuppression, or the presence of an associated malignancy, specifically nasopharyngeal carcinoma or Burkitt's lymphoma.

Virus cultures for EBV are rarely practical because of the expense, high percentage of asymptomatic excreters in the general population, length of time required for results (15–90 days), and technical difficulty in setting up and interpreting the culture assay. When such cultures are performed, throat washings are inoculated into human umbilical cord lymphocytes over a monolayer of feeder fibroblasts.[25] The presence of EBV is suggested by cell clumping and confirmed using fluorescent-labeled anti-EBNA. Recently, specific viral diagnosis using DNA-based probes and enzymatic amplification of target DNA has been described and may prove more practical than any culture technique currently available.[26]

No specific syndrome attributable to congenital EBV infection has been described. In the absence of specific anomalies associated with congenital EBV infection, it should be considered in infants with multiple congenital defects or intrauterine growth retardation, especially in the presence of a persistent atypical lymphocytosis and in the absence of evidence for more common pathogens. The index of suspicion should be raised when any mother suffers a documented primary EBV infection just prior to conception or during the first trimester. The diagnosis in the infant would be confirmed by serologic studies (IgM anti-EBV) performed on umbilical cord blood and by serial evaluation of changes in the serologic profile at intervals postdelivery. The other, more common pathogens noted above should be ruled out by appropriate diagnostic studies.

In the well documented report of congenital anomalies associated with EBV infection, Goldberg and colleagues described a low-birth weight infant with hypotonia, micrognathia, bilateral central cataracts, cryptorchidism, and metaphyseal radiolucencies with diametaphyseal striation (celery stalking).[17] At birth, there was no evidence of organomegaly, congenital heart disease, skin rash, or adenopathy. Laboratory findings were significant for thrombocytopenia (55,000–110,000/mm^3), lymphocytosis (55–77%), atypical lymphocytosis (10–19%), anti-VCA (IgM, then IgG), anti-EBNA, and anti-EA. In addition, total serum IgM was elevated. Heterophil antibody was not detected, and liver function tests were normal. Cultures were negative for rubella, HSV, CMV, enterovirus, and adenovirus. Findings were consistent with congenital insult at 5–6 weeks' gestation. Developmental assessment at 20 months placed the infant at 8–9 months and audiologic studies were normal.

Other, less clearly demonstrated, presumed congenital EBV infections were reviewed by these same authors.[16,18] Findings of note included congenital heart disease, microcephaly, myositis, microphthalmia, low-set ears, biliary atresia, cleft lip and palate, hypertelorism, simian creases, digital abnormalities, skin laxity, CNS malformations, hip dysplasia, and clubbed feet. It would appear, therefore, that the degree and type of congenital anomalies related to EBV infection are dependent on the state of organogenesis at the time of infectious insult.

TREATMENT

No specific therapy for EBV infections is currently available; however, aggressive symptomatic management is indicated in the pregnant patient. High fever should be controlled with acetaminophen and even prostaglandin inhibitors, if indicated. A cooling blanket may be appropriate if antipyretics alone are ineffective. Fluids should be encouraged, and if anorexia or pharyngitis prevents adequate oral intake, intravenous hydration should be employed. Topical anesthetic agents can be helpful in relieving the discomfort of the pharyngitis. Corticosteroids may be necessary when complications such as airway obstruction, thrombocytopenia, and hemolytic anemia develop. Acyclovir has been shown to inhibit oropharyngeal shedding of EBV, may shorten total time to recovery, and may prove useful in the management of unusually severe or protracted infections.[27] Modified bed rest should be encouraged, and exertion should be avoided. In addition, patients should be counseled in the recognition of the signs and symptoms of acute complications of infectious mononucleosis.

Counseling is also indicated for patients who have a documented primary infection during the first trimester of pregnancy. Although these infections fortunately are rare, reports noted previously have implicated EBV in congenital anomalies associated with primary EBV infections. In the absence of much hard data to the contrary, these anecdotal reports should be considered seriously. Although abortion cannot be recommended based on these cases, if it is requested at an appropriate time in gestation, the request should not be taken lightly. By the same token, recurrent infections during pregnancy are a common phenomenon and seem to pose little risk to the fetus. Parents should be reassured in this regard.

If their immune status is unknown, pregnant women should probably avoid intimate contact with individuals suffering from acute infectious mononucleosis. Fortunately, because so many women in the childbearing years have prior immunity, even when such contact occurs, transmission of infection is not common. Casual contact alone does not result in the spread of EBV in the absence of contamination by infected oropharyngeal secretions or exchange of blood. If a pregnant woman is clearly exposed to an infected individual and has no documented prior history of infectious mononucleosis, assessment of her immune status should be offered. Although not generally indicated, hyperimmune globulin might be considered in seronegative women exposed to infectious mononucleosis during pregnancy, particularly during the first trimester. This also might be of value in the prevention of neonatal infection in infants born of mothers with primary infection at the time of delivery. At present, there seems to be no rationale for routine EBV screening during pregnancy from standpoints of either practicality or cost-effectiveness.

There is hope that in the near future an attenuated or subunit EBV vaccine will be available. A vaccine that could be administered prior to the childbearing years might completely eliminate EBV as a potential source of significant congenital infection. Other possible advantages include decreasing the severity and complications of primary infections as well as the prolonged morbidity associated with infectious mononucleosis. In Africa and Southeast Asia, where Burkitt's lymphoma and nasopharyngeal carcinoma, respectively, are endemic health problems, such a vaccine might also reduce the incidence of these conditions.

Infants suspected of congenital EBV infection should have anomalies carefully categorized at birth. Correctable lesions should be addressed as indicated. Close supervision of psychological and motor development should be performed. Periodic ophthalmologic and at least one audiologic assessment should be made. Otherwise, at present, conservative symptomatic management is the only therapeutic intervention that can be recommended. When considering the long-term sequelae, one should keep in mind that these infants, at least theoretically, might be at higher risk for malignant sequelae of EBV infections. When intrauterine or neonatal transfusion is required, the use of blood from a seronegative donor might be considered.

REFERENCES

1. Epstein M, Achong B, Barr Y. Virus particles in cultured lymphoblasts from Burkitt's lymphoma. *Lancet.* 1964;1:702.
2. Le CT, Chang RS, Lipson MH. Epstein-Barr virus infections during pregnancy: a prospective study and review of the literature. *Am J Dis Child.* 1983;137:466.
3. Sixbey JW, Lemon SW, Pagano JS. A second site for Epstein-Barr virus shedding: the uterine cervix. *Lancet.* 1986;2:1122.
4. Biggar R, Henle W, Fleisher G, et al. Primary Epstein-Barr virus infections in African infants. I. Decline of maternal antibodies and time of infection. *Int J Cancer.* 1978;22:239.
5. de-The G. Epidemiology of Epstein-Barr virus and associated diseases in man. In: Roizman B, ed. *The Herpesviruses.* Vol 1. New York, NY: Plenum Press; 1982:25.
6. Purtilo DT. Epstein-Barr virus: the spectrum of its manifestations in human beings. *South Med J.* 1987;80:943.
7. Henle W, Henle G. Immunology of Epstein-Barr virus. In: Roizman B, ed. *The Herpesviruses.* Vol 1. New York, NY: Plenum Press; 1982:209.
8. Robinson JE, Miller G. Biology of lymphoid cells transformed by Epstein-Barr virus. In: Roizman B, ed. *The Herpesviruses.* Vol 1. New York, NY: Plenum Press; 1982:151.

9. Fleisher G, Bolognese R. Seroepidemiology of Epstein-Barr virus in pregnant women. *J Infect Dis.* 1982;145:537.
10. Fleisher G, Bolognese R. Persistent Epstein-Barr virus infection and pregnancy. *J Infect Dis.* 1983;147:982.
11. Costa S, Barrasso R, Terzano P, et al. Detection of active Epstein-Barr infection in pregnancy. *Eur J Clin Microbiol.* 1985;4:335.
12. Fleisher G, Bolognese R. Epstein-Barr virus infections in pregnancy: a prospective study. *J Pediatr.* 1984;104:374.
13. Chang RS, Seto DSY. Perinatal infection by Epstein-Barr virus. *Lancet.* 1979;2:201.
14. Icart J, Didier J, Dalens M, et al. Prospective study of Epstein-Barr virus (EBV) infection during pregnancy. *Biomedicine.* 1981;34:160.
15. Ornoy A, Dudai M, Sadovsky E. Placental and fetal pathology in infectious mononucleosis: a possible indicator for Epstein-Barr virus teratogenicity. *Diagn Gynecol Obstet.* 1982;4:11.
16. Brown Z, Stenchever M. Infectious mononucleosis and congenital anomalies. *Am J Obstet Gynecol.* 1978;131:108.
17. Goldberg G, Fulginiti V, Ray C, et al. In utero Epstein-Barr virus infectious mononucleosis infection. *JAMA.* 1981;246:1579.
18. Zane A, Brown M, Morton A, et al. Infectious mononucleosis and congenital anomalies. *Am J Obstet Gynecol.* 1978;131:108.
19. Weaver LT, Nelson R, Bell TM. The association of extrahepatic bile duct atresia and neonatal Epstein-Barr virus infection. *Acta Paediatr Scand.* 1984;73:155.
20. Miller G, Grogan E, Rowe D, et al. Selective lack of antibody to a component of EB nuclear antigen in patients with chronic active Epstein-Barr virus infection. *J Infect Dis.* 1987;156:26.
21. Schooley RT, Carey RW, Miller G, et al. Chronic Epstein-Barr virus infection associated with fever and interstitial pneumonitis. Clinical and serological features and response to antiviral chemotherapy. *Ann Intern Med.* 1986;104:636.
22. Sanguineti G, Crovato F, DeManchi R, et al. "Alice in Wonderland" syndrome in a patient with infectious mononucleosis. *J Infect Dis.* 1983;147:782.
23. Sumaya C. Endogenous reactivation of Epstein-Barr virus infections. *J Infect Dis.* 1977;135:374.
24. Wielaard F, Scherders J, Dagelinckx C, et al. Development of an antibody-capture IgM-enzyme-linked immunosorbent assay for diagnosis of acute Epstein-Barr virus infections. *J Virol Methods.* 1988;21:105.
25. Visintine AM, Gerber P, Nahmias AJ. Leukocyte transforming agent (Epstein-Barr virus) in newborn infants and older individuals. *J Pediatr.* 1976;89:571.
26. Sixbey JW, Shirley PS. Viral diagnosis using DNA-based probes. Enzymatic amplification of target DNA. *Ann NY Acad Sci.* 1988;549:158.
27. Andersson J, Britton S, Ernberg I, et al. Effect of acyclovir on infectious mononucleosis: a double-blind, placebo-controlled study. *J Infect Dis.* 1986;153:283.

J

Central Nervous System Viruses

Chapter One Hundred and Two

Aseptic Meningitis and Encephalitis

David A. Baker

102

Numerous viral infections can affect the central nervous system (CNS), causing a spectrum of disease entities. Viruses shown to cause CNS infections are both RNA and DNA viruses that infect the patient, multiply in specific organs, and then are transferred into the CNS secondary to a viremia.

Depending on the specific structure affected within the CNS, the clinical entity is an *encephalitis*, a *meningitis*, or a *myelitis*. Viral involvement of the substance of brain tissue, within either the cerebrum, cerebellum, or medulla, is viral encephalitis. Meningitis is the viral infiltration that causes inflammation of the membranes of the brain or spinal cord. When the substance of the spinal cord is involved in a viral infection with subsequent inflammation, it is myelitis.[1]

ETIOLOGY AND PATHOGENESIS

Viral infections that invade the CNS usually result from previous infection in another body site. A varied and long list of viruses has been implicated in CNS infection, including viruses that contain RNA as well as those with DNA. The most common viral entities producing CNS infections are herpesvirus (see Chapter 91), viruses in the enterovirus group, mumps, and adenovirus (see Chapters 103, 104).[2]

The pathogenesis of these viral infections differs markedly, depending on the viral agent involved. Usually, there is primary multiplication of virus in the gastrointestinal tract, lymph nodes, or respiratory tract, with possible secondary sites of multiplication in the liver or spleen. There can be subsequent seeding into the bloodstream and viral entrance into the CNS, a process that is still poorly understood. Neural spread into the CNS, as well as spread by olfactory pathways, has been demonstrated for specific viruses. The amount of virus that gets to the CNS, the specific virus, and the extent of nerve cell involvement and destruction will determine the specific outcome in the disease. After a virus reaches the CNS, there can be nerve cell infection with cell lysis and viral spread to adjacent cells, or there can be contamination of the entire ventricular fluid with involvement of the numerous ependymal surfaces, suggesting rapid viral spread.[2]

EPIDEMIOLOGY

Although exact statistics for viral CNS infections are difficult to establish, the Centers for Disease Control Surveillance[3] suggests that the major organisms involved in encephalitis and meningitis are mumps, enterovirus, and arboviruses. The specific epidemiology is related to the region within the United States, and approximately three fourths of the reported cases do not have an identifiable etiology. It appears that the major incidence for acute viral meningitis is within a population under the age of 30. Enterovirus infections have been shown to occur more commonly during the summer, whereas for mumps, the highest prevalence is during the winter. The mode of transmission with enterovirus infections is by the oral-fecal route, and insect transmission has been clearly documented for the arboviruses. Figure 102–1 shows the incidence of encephalitis within the United States between 1970 and 1979. The increase in reports during the summer months appears to reflect arbovirus and enterovirus infections. Figure 102–2 shows the reported cases of aseptic meningitis in the United States from 1983–1988.

DIAGNOSIS

The clinical presentation of acute viral CNS infections may either be subtle or may show significant organ involvement. The onset is usually that of an acute illness, and the presentation can include fever, headache, irritability, and neck rigidity. Clinical manifestations of disease entity outside the CNSD may provide specific diagnostic clues, including parotitis (mumps) and rash (enteric viruses). In viral meningitis, Kernig's and Brudzinski's signs are often positive. Within the clinical manifestations of encephalitis, the initial presentation can be followed by stupor, confusion, convulsion, coma, and death. Depending on the etiologic agent, there can be severe sequelae, including mental and motor retardation, deafness, and blindness.

The cerebrospinal fluid (CSF) findings are similar in viral encephalitis and meningitis. The CSF pressure is normal or elevated in viral encephalitis. With parenchymatous CNS involvement, few white cells can be found (5–10/mm^3); however, when there are predominant signs of meningeal irritation, the white count is markedly increased, with predominance of lymphocytes. The protein in the CSF is slightly increased, and the glucose level is normal in the majority of cases.[4]

A specific agent responsible for this viral entity can be demonstrated either by isolation from the CSF or blood or by elevation of antibody titers to a specific virus. It must be emphasized that it is extremely difficult to specifically incriminate one virus without viral isolation and demonstration of antibody rise. Not only does the CSF need to be cultured, but cultures of stool and throat are excellent sources of viral isolation. The specific diagnosis of an acute CNS infection and its causative agents become important

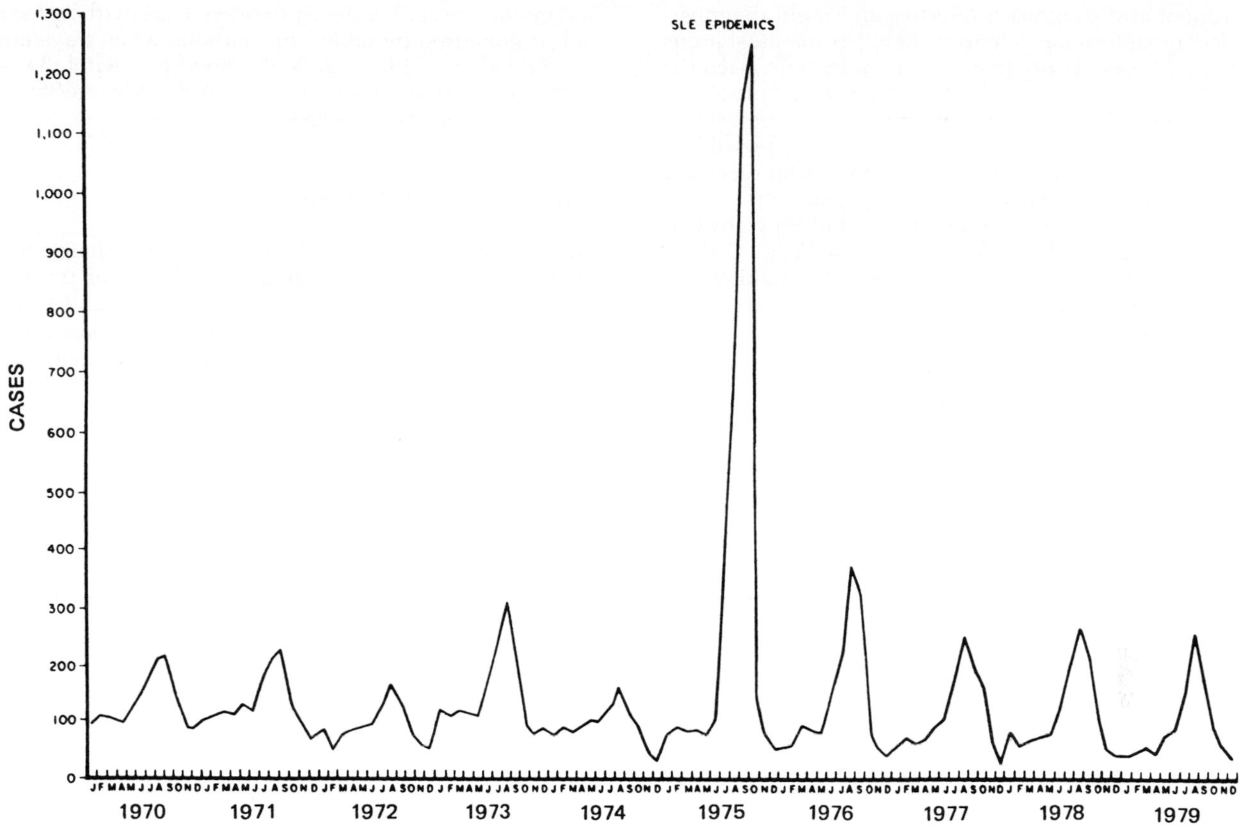

Figure 102–1. Encephalitis, reported cases by month of onset, United States, 1970–1979. Encephalitis reporting for 1979 was typical of nonepidemic years (1975 was an epidemic year). The increase in reports during the warmer months probably reflects a composite of arboviral and enteroviral activity. (*From Centers for Disease Control.*[3])

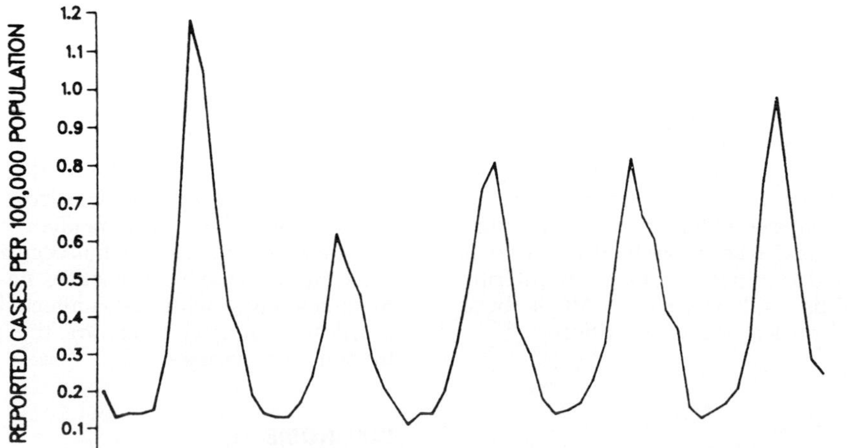

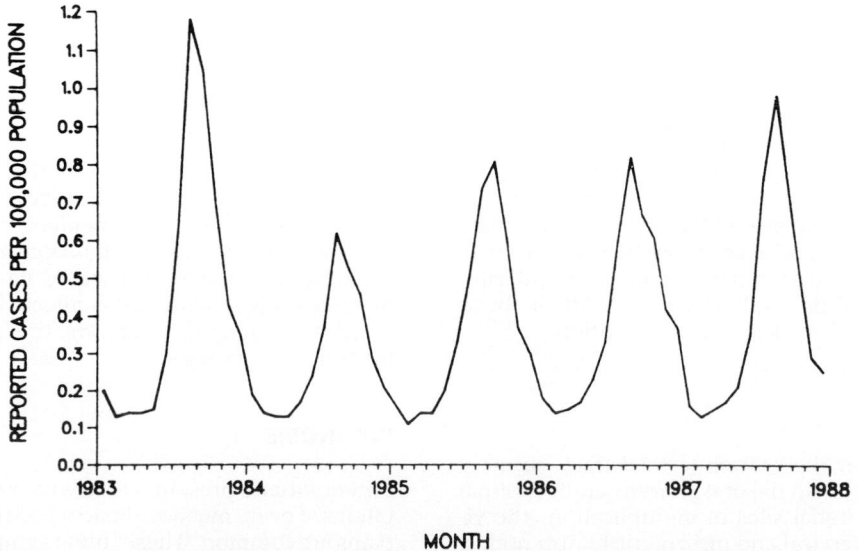

Figure 102–2. Aseptic meningitis—by month, United States, 1983–1988. (*From Centers for Disease Control.*[6])

for treatment and prognosis. Effective and rapid diagnosis is needed to determine whether the CNS manifestations are caused by organisms that are treatable as in bacterial meningitis, infections from fungi, rickettsia, or protozoa. In such patients, CNS lesions, either benign or metastatic, need to be investigated, keeping in mind the possibility of systemic manifestations from collagen vascular diseases, which can produce similar clinical manifestations. Other disease entities of the CNS that are rare but may present as a viral meningitis include Behçet's disease, Vogt–Koyanagi and Harada's syndromes, and Mollaret's meningitis.[1] Rapid diagnosis is required to prevent morbidity and mortality by treatable causative agents.

TREATMENT AND PREVENTION

A majority of viral agents causing CNS infections do not have specific therapies at the present time. Acute viral meningitis is a self-limiting disease, and patients usually recover without short-term or long-term sequelae. Antiviral chemotherapy is available for the treatment of CNS infections caused by herpes simplex and varicella-zoster viruses (see also Chapters 91 and 93).

Among the numerous agents responsible for viral CNS infection, there are several vaccines that have been highly effective in preventing disease, most notably those of polio and mumps virus. The ability to prevent arbovirus infections can be enhanced by taking precautions when travelling in an endemic area. It is difficult, however, with the wide variety of viral agents that can cause CNS infections, to prevent the majority of cases.

PREGNANCY CONCERNS

The pregnant patient is subjected to a risk similar to that of the rest of the adult population. Many of these viral infections are uncommon during pregnancy, and there are only a few case reports to define the pathogenesis in pregnant women, the fetus, and the newborn. In the following chapters, specific viral infections of the CNS are discussed and the effects on mother and fetus are described.

REFERENCES

1. Kennard C, Swash M. Acute viral encephalitis, its diagnosis and outcome. *Brain*. 1981;104:129.
2. Koskiniemi M, Vaheri A. Acute encephalitis of viral origin. *Scand J Infect Dis*. 1982;14:181.
3. Centers for Disease Control. Annual Summary 1980. *MMWR*. 1981;29:31.
4. Fishman RA, ed. *Cerebrospinal Fluid in Diseases of the Nervous System*. Philadelphia, PA: WB Saunders; 1980:269.
5. Centers for Disease Control. *MMWR*. 1988;36:19.

Chapter One Hundred and Three

Enteric Viruses

David A. Baker

103

The enteric viruses, a varied group of infectious agents exhibiting similar characteristics and infecting the human gastrointestinal tract, are small, RNA-containing viruses without a lipid coat.[1] Although the original classification of enteroviruses included poliovirus, coxsackievirus, and echoviruses, this has been extended to some new and recently-isolated viruses.

Numerous viruses infect the human gastrointestinal tract. Polio virus occurs in three distinct types. Coxsackie A occurs in 23 types, and coxsackie B occurs in six types. Echovirus makes up 31 antigenically distinct viruses. Some new isolations have been labeled enteroviruses 68 through 71. Recently, hepatitis A has also been classified as enterovirus 72. Other viruses linked to epidemic acute gastroenteritis include reovirus, rotavirus, and parvovirus. All of these viruses differ in size and nucleic acid composition.

PATHOGENESIS

After viral agents enter the gastrointestinal tract, primary viral multiplication occurs in the oral pharynx and intestinal mucosa.[2] From these initial sites of multiplication, the viruses extend into the cervical and mesenteric lymph nodes, from where seeding into the blood stream with a short-lived viremia occurs. In a majority of viral infections, the virus is limited to the lymphatic stage. Through viremia, virus may, however, spread into the central nervous sytem (CNS) with the potential of subsequent paralytic disease.[3] The classic lesion in poliomyelitis is destruction of anterior horn cells. Similar damage may also be seen in the substance of medulla, brainstem, and motor cortex.

EPIDEMIOLOGY

Enteroviruses are widely distributed throughout the world. The epidemiology of poliovirus, coxsackievirus, and echovirus are similar, with peak incidences of disease in the summer months. Summer or fall occurrence, with an August peak, of nonpolio enteroviruses has been reported in numerous studies, with males affected at a greater rate than females.[4] Young children are the principal reservoirs of human enteroviruses.

DIAGNOSIS

Enteric viruses present with a wide range of clinical manifestations. Fever, malaise, headache, nausea, and abdominal pains are common. These initial symptoms may be followed in approximately three days by the onset of meningeal signs, although it must be emphasized that the majority of infections do not progress to meningitis or encephalitis.[3] One of the predominant clinical features is diarrhea.[5] Other clinical manifestations can include pleurodynia, respiratory illness, eye disease, and cardiac disease. Laboratory studies are not very helpful in the diagnosis, although there may be mild elevations of total white blood cell count and erythrocyte sedimentation rate. Depending on the specific organ involved, there can be liver function abnormalities and alterations in electrolytes secondary to diarrhea.

The specific diagnosis must rest with viral isolation and identification. In addition, specific antibody responses to infection can be helpful. Manifestations and CNS ramifications will also depend on the specific virus involved. CNS infections are usually self-limited. Therefore, they must be differentiated from those conditions that produce encephalitis with significant mortality and morbidity and from individuals with collagen vascular diseases who have CNS involvement.

TREATMENT AND PREVENTION

Polio

Because there are no specific treatments for enteroviral infections, the major emphasis has to be on prevention. With the advent of effective live and killed poliovirus vaccines, polio has been significantly limited, and the CNS manifestations of this entity have been almost eradicated in industrialized countries. The Centers for Disease Control suggest that all children be vaccinated with the oral polio vaccine and that adults 18 years or older be vaccinated if they are traveling to areas where polio is endemic or if they are health care or laboratory workers in contact with poliovirus.[6] Because the risks of vaccine-associated paralysis following oral polio vaccine is higher in adults than in children, the inactivated vaccine is recommended for adults at risk. Adverse reactions of either mother or fetus after either oral or inactivated polio vaccine administration during pregnancy do not appear to occur. On theoretical grounds, it has been suggested that pregnant women should not be vaccinated. The Centers for Disease Control nevertheless recommend that if immediate protection against poliomyelitis is needed, oral polio vaccine should be given.[6]

Other Enteroviruses

No preventative measures are presently available for other enteroviruses. Pooled human gamma globulin may contain specific antibodies against those viruses; however, after infection has been established, its use would probably be ineffective. During an outbreak of enteroviral infections, increased physical activity apparently makes individuals more susceptible to infection. Therefore, this should be discouraged. Trauma and operative procedures such as tonsillectomy have a similar effect and should, therefore, also be avoided. Susceptibility to infections may also be increased by ingestion of alcohol and by malnourishment.

PREGNANCY CONSIDERATIONS

Polio

Several reports suggest that there is an enhanced susceptibility to poliovirus in pregnancy. This may also be true for other enteric viruses. Weinstein et al[7] suggested the effect of pregnancy in increasing susceptibility to clinical poliomyelitis. Siegel and Greenberg[8], in a prospective study, indicated a 60% increase in incidence of poliomyelitis in women who were pregnant. The difference in attack rate affecting pregnant and nonpregnant women also rises progressively with age and becomes quite marked between 25 and 39 years of age. It appears that congenital poliomyelitis is a rare phenomenon; however, subclinical or inapparent disease may go unnoticed, producing long-term sequelae. With utilization of poliovirus vaccine, cases of neonatal or congenital infection with poliovirus have been markedly reduced.

Although there have been studies of other enteroviral infections in different pregnant populations[9-12], there is little current information as to whether these infections are more severe in pregnant women. It has been suggested that the majority of these infections is asymptomatic. Case reports[13,14] suggest that infections with coxsackievirus may be common during pregnancy. In pregnant women with aseptic meningitis or with an undifferentiated febrile illness, coxsackievirus B5 was cultured from the cervix in five out of seven patients.[14] All these women recovered, however, without problem.

During maternal viremia with an enterovirus, the fetus may become secondarily infected by virus crossing the placenta. Fetal risk after a maternal infection has not been well documented, but association of fetal congenital anomalies after enteroviral infections has been reported. With regard to other enteric viruses, such as coxsackie and echoviruses, various reports documenting congenital or neonatal infection with fulminant and fatal disease within the newborn have appeared in the literature.

The epidemiology of neonatal enterovirus infection is not presently known. One collaborative study suggests serologic evidence of coxsackievirus infection during pregnancy in 9% of 198 women. There has also been sufficient documentation that types 3, 6, 9, and 14 of echoviruses have caused congenital and neonatal infections. Apparently, epidemic outbreaks with enteric viruses can occur. Within the past 20 years, at least 10 outbreaks of perinatal and neonatal epidemic infections with echovirus have been reported.[12,15] The frequency of neonatal rotavirus infection varies from 0–52%, with wide geographic and seasonal variations in incidence.[5]

A wide spectrum of disease can be found in infants infected with these viruses. For example, an infant may be asymptomatic or, if documented with coxsackievirus[10] and echovirus infections[11,12], may present severely ill and die within a few days. The initial presentation may be vague, with irritability and lethargy, or there may be signs of respiratory distress, leading rapidly to severe jaundice and the presentation of a generalized septicemia. Involvement of organ systems depends on the specific viral disease. The hematologic system is frequently affected, with disseminated intravascular coagulopathy reported. There can also be hepatic necrosis, adrenal necrosis, and especially CNS involvement. With coxsackie B viruses, myocarditis and encephalomyocarditis have been reported, with fulminant infection and death within the first few days of life. *In utero* infection with these viruses has been associated with intrauterine growth retardation, prematurity, a higher incidence of stillbirth and spontaneous abortion. Coxsackie A16, B 1 to 5, and echovirus 7, 9, and 11 have been reported to produce problems in fetuses and newborns of infected mothers.[16] Older information suggests that coxsackievirus A9, B3, and B4 are associated with congenital cardiac, urological, and gastrointestinal tract anomalies.[17]

The diagnosis of neonatal disease relies on the viral isolation and serologic evidence (demonstration of group-specific IgM antibody within the cord serum).

It appears that the transfer of maternal antibody into

the fetal compartment offers some level of protection to the newborn. Two thirds of non-nosocomially echovirus-infected infants came from mothers who had an acute illness within one week before delivery.[15] Use of pooled immunoglobulin may be effective in the therapy of newborns, who contract these viral infections.[16]

REFERENCES

1. Dolin R. Viral infections of the gastrointestinal tract. In: Galasso CJ, Morgan TC, Buchanan RA, eds. *Antiviral Agents and Viral Diseases of Man*. New York, NY: Raven Press; 1979:461.
2. Ginsberg HS. Picornaviruses. In: Davis BD, Dulbecco R, Eisen HN, et al, eds. *Microbiology*. 3rd ed. Philadelphia, PA: Harper & Row; 1980:1095.
3. Griffith JF, Ch'ien LT. Viral infections of the central nervous system. In: Galasso GJ, Morgan TC, Buchanan RA, eds. *Antiviral Agents and Viral Diseases of Man*. New York, NY: Raven Press; 1979:491.
4. Moore M. Enteroviral disease in the United States, 1970–1979. *J Infect Dis*. 1982;146:103.
5. Gurwith M, Wensman W, Hinde D, et al. A prospective study of rotavirus infection in infants and young children. *J Infect Dis*. 1981;144:224.
6. Centers for Disease Control. Poliomyelitis prevention. *MMWR*. 1982;31:22.
7. Weinstein L, Asycock L, Feemster RF. The relation of sex, pregnancy and menstruation to susceptibility in poliomyelitis. *N Engl J Med*. 1951;245:54.
8. Siegel M, Greenberg M. Incidence of poliomyelitis pregnancy. *N Engl J Med*. 1955;253:841.
9. Jemista JA, Menegus MA. Enteroviruses: coxsackie, ECHO and poliovirus. In: Amstey MA, ed. *Virus Infection in Pregnancy*. New York, NY: Grune & Stratton; 1984:1.
10. Baker DA, Phillips CA. Maternal and neonatal infection with coxsackievirus. *Obstet Gynecol*. 1980;55:125.
11. Modlin JF, Polk BF, Horton P, et al. Perinatal echovirus infection: risk of transmission during a community outbreak. *N Engl J Med*. 1981;305:368.
12. Piraino FF, Sedmak G, Raab K. Echovirus 11 infections of newborns with mortality during the 1979 enterovirus season in Milwaukee. *Wis Public Health Rep*. 1982;97:346.
13. McKernan PD, Schare MB. Type B2 coxsackievirus meningitis in pregnancy. *J Rep Med*. 1988;33:667.
14. Reyes MP, Zalenski D, Smith F, et al. Coxsackievirus-positive cervixes in women with febrile illness during the third trimester in pregnancy. *Am J Obstet Gynecol*. 1986;155:159.
15. Modlin JF. Perinatal echovirus infection: insights from a literature review of 61 cases of serious infection and 16 outbreaks in nurseries. *Rev Infect Dis*. 1986;8:918.
16. Christie AB. Enterovirus infections. In: *Infectious Diseases: Epidemiology and Clinical Practice*. Vol. 2. London: Churchill Livingstone; 1987:753.
17. Brown GC, Karunas RS. Relationship to congenital anomalies and maternal infection with selected enteroviruses. *Am J Epidemiol*. 1972;95:207.

Chapter One Hundred and Four

Mumps

David A. Baker

104

Mumps is an acute viral illness primarily of childhood, characterized by parotitis that can also present with significant complications, such as meningoencephalitis, within an adult population.

Mumps is an RNA virus with a nuclear protein core surrounded by a lipid-containing outer membrane. The outer surface contains neuraminidase and hemagglutinin and induces an immune response, producing protective antibody.

This viral, highly contagious infection is spread by way of the respiratory route.[1] The incubation period of between 2 and 3 weeks starts with viral multiplication, initially within the upper respiratory tract, with subsequent dissemination of virus to the regional lymph nodes. Following this, there is a viremia, with seeding of target organs such as the meninges, pancreas, breasts, thyroid, heart, liver, and gonads. With this viral disease, a viremia can last up to five days, and a significant percentage (one third) of these infections apparently are asymptomatic.

With the introduction of a successful mumps vaccine in the mid 1970s, the incidence of mumps has significantly fallen (Figure 104–1). The Centers for Disease Control estimated in 1977 that the disease incidence was 8.5 per 100,000 and the incidence of mumps, encephalitis, aseptic meningitis, and deaths associated with mumps, a disease more common in the spring months, has fallen significantly as well. The incidence of mumps cases is directly related to the school immunization laws of that state. States with strict immunization laws had lower rates (1.1 mumps cases/100,000 population) than states with no immunization laws (11.5 cases/100,000 population).

DIAGNOSIS

Mumps is usually a general systemic viral infection during which the patient will present with fever and enlargement of the parotid glands, either unilateral or bilateral. Signs of central nervous system (CNS) involvement may appear, especially eighth nerve involvement. It must be emphasized, however, that parotitis may not be present. For example, one half of patients with meningoencephalitis do not present in such a fashion. In females, approximately 30% of those over the age of 15 had mastitis. Mumps, which can cause meningitis, meningoencephalitis, or encephalitis, has been one of the more common causes of these syndromes in the United States.[2] According to the Centers for Disease Control, in a 10-year period between the mid-1960s and 1970s, 0.3% of all encephalitis was caused by mumps.[3] Most patients appear to recover from CNS infections with mumps without long-term sequelae, but there have been reported deaths and numerous reports of rare CNS complications associated with this disease entity. Hearing loss postinfection of the CNS with mumps has been well documented.[4]

In addition to a clinical syndrome suggestive of mumps, isolation of the virus from blood, throat, and cerebrospinal fluid (CSF) will definitively diagnose the condition. Paired sera can be used to look at a rise in antibody titers or at seroconversion in order to document acute mumps infection.[4]

Other viral diseases can also cause parotitis. In addition, it also can be caused by bacteria, especially in those patients who are immunosuppressed or severe diabetics.

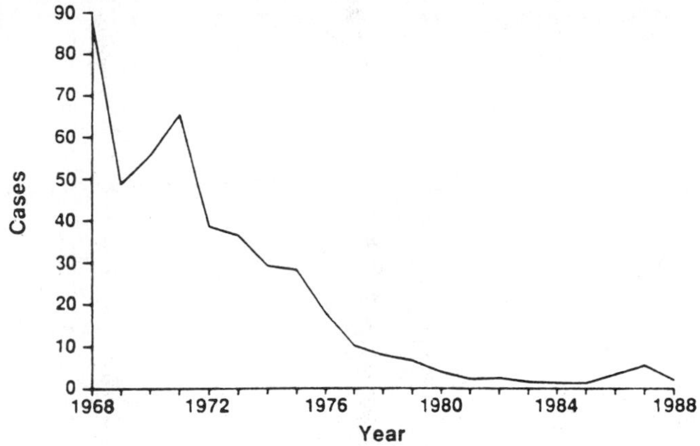

Figure 104–1. Reported mumps cases per 100,000 population by year—United States, 1968–1988. (*From Centers for Disease Control.*[9])

Other etiologies of parotitis can include blocked ducts, drug reactions, tumors of the parotid gland, malignancies such as Hodgkin's disease, as well as manifestations of collagen vascular diseases. All can be confused with mumps.

TREATMENT AND PREVENTION

At the present time, no specific treatment for this viral infection is available aside from symptomatic therapy. A live attenuated mumps virus vaccine has been shown to be highly effective and affords protection to 95% of receiving individuals. It is without serious side effects and confers long-term protection.[3]

MATERNAL AND FETAL ASPECTS

Although relevant data are limited, it appears that pregnancy does not enhance mumps.[5]

Mumps virus enters the placental-fetal unit through a maternal viremia, with seeding of the placenta. It appears that virus is then seeded into specific organs of the fetus, including the CNS. The basic outcome of mumps infection probably relates to the gestational age of the fetus and the length of exposure time as well as to the amount of virus that penetrates into the fetal-placental compartment.

It seems that mumps infection with fetal involvement is a rare event, with the Collaborative Perinatal Study estimating an attack rate of 15 maternal cases per 10,000 deliveries. The advent of an effective vaccination program should further reduce the incidence of infection in pregnancy and fetal involvement.

There is a continuing controversy concerning clinical presentations and manifestations of mumps in the fetus. Reports have documented intrauterine transmission with resultant congenital mumps. Experimental models in animals suggest that mumps can cause CNS and cardiac abnormalities. In addition, there has been some evidence to associate intrauterine mumps infection with endocardial fibroelastosis[6] and aqueductal stenosis.[7] During the first trimester, acute maternal mumps infection will, if the mother has CNS involvement, lead to a twofold increase in the spontaneous abortion rate.[8] It also appears that the mother with acute mumps infection around time of delivery can transmit mumps to her infant, who will demonstrate signs of mumps, including parotitis and pneumonia.

To diagnose mumps infection in a newborn is difficult unless parotitis is present. Viral isolation and demonstration of IgM antibodies in cord blood will confirm the diagnosis of intrauterine mumps infection.

Because there is no specific treatment for mumps, the major emphasis has to be on prevention through vaccination. It has been shown that mumps vaccine virus can infect the placenta; however, the virus used in the vaccine has not been isolated from fetal tissues. It has been suggested that, because this is a live attenuated vaccine, vaccination in pregnancy should be avoided.

REFERENCES

1. Feldman HA. Mumps. In: Evans AS, ed. *Viral Infections of Humans*. New York, NY: Plenum Press; 1982:419.
2. Ray CG. Mumps. In: Retersdorf RG, Adams RD, Braunwald E, et al. *Harrison's Principles of Internal Medicine*. 10th ed. New York, NY: McGraw-Hill; 1983:1132.
3. Centers for Disease Control. Mumps vaccine. *Ann Intern Med*. 1980;92:803.
4. Jones JF, Ray CG, Fulginiti VA. Brief clinical and laboratory observations—perinatal mumps infection. *J Pediatr*. 1980;96:912.
5. Kim-Farley RJ. Mumps in pregnancy. In: Amstey MA, ed. *Virus Infection in Pregnancy*. New York, NY: Grune & Stratton; 1984:169.
6. Overall JC. Intrauterine virus infections and congenital heart disease. *Am Heart J*. 1972;84:823.
7. Baumann B, Danon I, Weitz R, et al. Unilateral hydrocephalus due to obstruction of the foramen of monro: another complication of intrauterine mumps infection? *Eur J Pediatr*. 1982;139:156.
8. Siegel MS, Fuerst HT, Peress NS. Comparative fetal mortality in maternal virus diseases: a prospective study on rubella, measles, mumps, chicken-pox and hepatitis. *N Engl J Med*. 1966;274:768.
9. Centers for Disease Control. *MMWR*. 1989;38:101.

Chapter One Hundred and Five

Rabies

David A. Baker

105

Rabies is an acute central nervous viral disease with a high incidence of mortality.

The virus contains RNA, is bullet-shaped when viewed with the electron microscope, and is enveloped with a lipid bilayer. It appears that there are antigenically distinct strains of rabies virus.

Virus is usually introduced into the host by a contaminated animal bite. The animal's saliva contains the infectious rabies virus. A long variation in incubation period, from days to months, has been documented. Local multiplication of virus at the site of contamination occurs. Neuronal degeneration within the central nervous system (CNS) is the con-

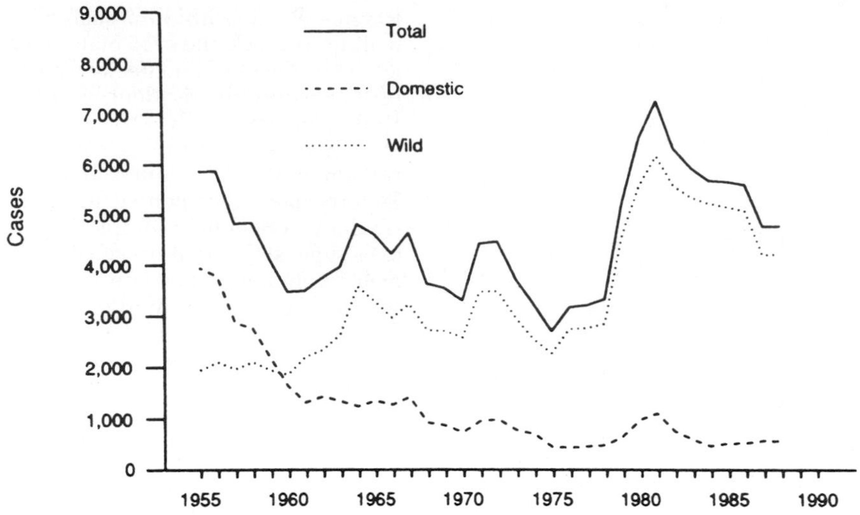

Figure 105–1. Source of rabies virus—domestic versus wild animals.

sequence of infection. Rabies virus is neurotrophic. It apparently seeks out nerves and travels by way of the peripheral nerves into the CNS. The major area of viral replication is within the gray matter. After it reaches the CNS, the virus produces severe encephalitis. It seems that the specific inoculation dose is directly related to the incubation period.[1]

The major reservoir for rabies within the population is in mammals. Animals in the wild, especially bats and skunks, are reported to be major sources of rabies (Figure 105–1).[2] The United States has fewer cases reported per year (Figure 105–2) than other areas of the world.[2] At the present time, wild mammals account for three fourths of reported cases, whereas domestic animals are rarely infected with rabies. It has been demonstrated that rabies can also be transmitted from organ transplants and through aerosol inoculation.

DIAGNOSIS

A high degree of mortality occurs with this CNS viral infection. Several days of symptomatology, including fever, headache, nausea, vomiting and irritability precede the onset of CNS manifestations. This is followed by signs of CNS involvement and an encephalitic process in which there is excessive motor activity. There is subsequent progression to confusion, hallucinations, and other signs of a degenerative CNS process. Not only is the cerebrum affected, but the brainstem and cranial nerves are also involved. The apparent cause of death is usually brainstem involvement, leading to respiratory and cardiac arrest, making recovery from this CNS viral infection indeed rare.[1]

The diagnosis requires a proper history and clinical presentation of the disease, viral isolation, and serologic

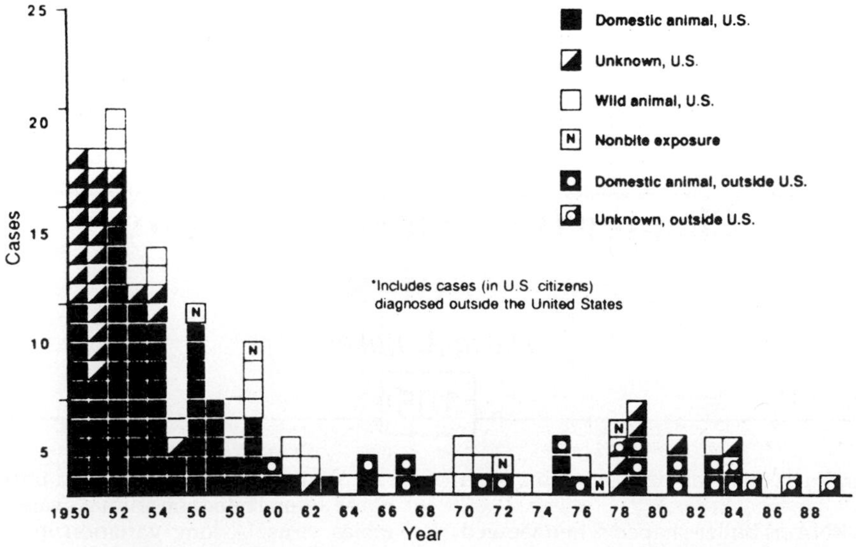

Figure 105–2. Rabies cases—worldwide versus United States.

evidence of infection. Tissue samples can be used for viral inoculation. Direct staining techniques are available for the identification of viral antigens and examination of tissue for Negri bodies can also be employed.

TREATMENT AND PREVENTION

The major emphasis in the prevention of rabies is prophylaxis and the use of rabies vaccine in those individuals who are at high risk. This disease, once established, has no specific therapy aside from supportive measures. Although the number of cases of rabies reported in the United States is extremely low, the incidence of animal bites and subsequent rabies prophylaxis is considerable. One million Americans are bitten by animals each year.[3,4] Those who have a high risk of contracting rabies, such as laboratory workers or animal handlers, should have pre-exposure immunization with rabies vaccine.

Initial therapy after the bite of an animal should consist of local therapy to the wound. A 20% soap solution should be used to scrub the wound, followed by large-volume water irrigation. Treating the wound with a quaternary ammonium compound (1–4% benzalkonium chloride) should follow.

The Centers for Disease Control[5] advocates the use of the human diploid cell vaccine (HDCV) of rabies vaccine, with a required three-dose regimen. If there is an animal bite, the animal should be captured and assessed for rabies with appropriate laboratory tests. If rabies is present within the wildlife community or if there is documentation that an animal is rabid, it is recommended that a combination of passive and active immunization be performed. Inoculations with rabies immune globulin (human rabies immune globulin is preferred) should be given by administering half the dose by local infiltration at the wound site and the remainder of the dose intramuscularly. Active immunization should be performed with HDCV. Either the intramuscular or intradermal route of injection can be used. Numerous injections over many days are required to obtain active production of rabies antibodies. It has been demonstrated that the human diploid cell vaccine, originally licensed in the United States in 1980, is by far more immunogenic than other available vaccines and also has lower toxicity.

PREGNANCY CONSIDERATIONS

An insufficient number of rabies cases in pregnancy prohibits the delineation of the pathogenesis of this disease entity. In experimental animals, rabies virus has been demonstrated to cross the placenta. It appears that the pathogenesis would be different from that in the adult, with virus producing a systemic disease viremia with CNS involvement in the fetus as the result of the viremia.[6]

Data concerning fetal problems are derived from animal experiences. In some such reports, the rabies virus has been proposed as a teratogen in chick embryos and humans, although other reports suggest that this is not the case.

The diagnosis in the newborn comes from a maternal history of animal bite together with the development of clinical signs and symptoms of disease.

Basic prevention includes avoidance of wild animals and the vaccination of domestic animals with rabies. Women of reproductive age who are laboratory or research workers with the possibility of exposure to rabies should be immunized prior to conception.[7] Cases of postexposure rabies prophylaxis in pregnancy have been reported without detrimental effects to the mother or newborn. The pregnant woman is to receive 20 IU/kg of rabies immune globulin and begin a course of vaccination with the HCDV to prevent maternal or fetal disease.[8] Adverse side effects in the mother can include abdominal discomfort, anorexia, and fatigue. No detrimental effects have been reported in the fetus after rabies prophylaxis.

REFERENCES

1. Lindtjorn B. Clinical features of rabies in man. *Trop Doctor.* 1982;12:9.
2. Centers for Disease Control. Cases of rabies in animals by year—United States, 1955–1988. *MMWR.* 1989;38:10.
3. Centers for Disease Control. Cases of rabies in human by year and exposure category. United States 1955–1988. *MMWR.* 1989;38:10.
4. Corey L. Rabies and rhabdoviruses. In: Braunwald E, Isselbacher KJ, Petersdorf RG, et al, eds. *Harrison's Principles of Internal Medicine.* 11th ed. New York, NY: McGraw-Hill; 1987:142.
5. Centers for Disease Control. Recommendations of the immunizations practices committee. Rabies prevention. *MMWR. 1980;29:265.*
6. Shope, RE. Rabies. In: Evans AS, ed. *Viral Infections of Humans.* New York, NY: Plenum Press; 1982:455.
7. Varner MW, McGuiness GA, Galask RP. Rabies vaccination in pregnancy. *Am J Obstet Gynecol.* 1982;143:717.
8. Horstman DM. Viral infections. In: Burrow GN, Ferris RF, eds. *Medical Complications During Pregnancy.* 2nd ed. Philadelphia, PA: WB Saunders; 1982:347.

Chapter One Hundred and Six
Arboviruses

David A. Baker

106

Arboviruses are termed arthropodborne viruses because they replicate in arthropods and are transmitted to humans or other vertebrate hosts by insects, usually after a blood meal from the host.

These viruses are diverse and numerous (over 350 arthropodborne viruses isolated), and their mode of transmission, rather than specific viral characteristics, identifies them as belonging to this viral classification. Recently, numerous viruses were reclassified, and the arbovirus group was placed into the family of Togaviridae, Bunyaviridae, and Reoviridae, with additional subgroups within each family. These viruses possess RNA nucleic acids and have lipid envelopes. It appears that at least 80 distinct arboviruses are capable of infecting man, and the presentation of clinical symptomatology is varied.

In the United States, approximately 10% of cases of

encephalitis each year are caused by arboviruses. St. Louis encephalitis virus, eastern equine encephalitis virus, western equine encephalitis virus, and the California serogroup viruses produce the most cases of encephalitis in the country.

Because viruses in these families present with numerous clinical symptomatologies, only those viruses that present chiefly with central nervous system (CNS) ramifications are covered in great detail. These infections are transmitted by a bite, and the skin represents the sole portal of entry. The virus is inoculated directly into the blood stream or lymph, with dissemination and seeding to target organs. The reticuloendothelial system may be a site of viral multiplication, but this has not yet been clarified. After initial seeding and multiplication in organs, there is a viremia which lasts from a few days to a week. With seeding into the CNS, encephalitis is produced. It appears that there is an initial phase of virus multiplication and spread, giving systemic symptomatology, followed by viremia and seeding into the CNS. Major pathology occurs through the direct invasion into nerve cells, with viral replication and cell death secondary to lysis. The replication phase of these viruses is short, and the viruses multiply in the cytoplasm of infected cells.[1]

EPIDEMIOLOGY

Many mosquitoes, sand flies, and ticks transmit these viruses, which are endemic in tropical and subtropical areas, although epidemics can also occur in temperate zones. Numerous factors seem to be related to the epidemiology of these infections, including the behavior of the arthropod vector. The proximity of humans who may get infected by bites, the antibody status of the population, insect control measures, and the availability of other vertebrate hosts are all important. The distribution of these infections is worldwide. Outbreaks of arboviral infections in the United States occur periodically and most often unpredictably, with western and southern areas of the United States having the highest incidence. In the United States, infection occurs primarily in late summer and fall, and socioeconomic factors, such as a greater possibility of exposure and possibly decreased host resistance, play a role in infection. Within the United States, the specific incidence of encephalitis caused by arboviruses is small, with approximately 50 cases reported by the Centers for Disease Control per year.

DIAGNOSES

The clinical manifestation of these viral entities depends on the age at infection. Adult symptomatology is acute, with fever, nausea, vomiting, and severe headaches. In a short period of time, other CNS aberrations occur with disturbances in mentation the marked clinical feature. Lethargy, tremor, and cranial nerve abnormalities are common. Like the abrupt onset, there is an abrupt cessation of clinical symptomatology, which usually occurs within 14 days from the initial episode. There is generally good clinical improvement, unless specific anatomic damage from virus has been present to disrupt cell function. Depending on the specific viral encephalitis, case fatality ratios can range from 1–2% to greater than 20%. Significant sequelae occur within a range of 5–30%. Most are long-term neurologic or motor problems.[1]

A specific clinical diagnosis is difficult. A high degree of clinical suspicion, the association of epidemiologic factors, and perhaps previous documentation of an epidemic tend to support a clinical diagnosis. Arbovirus infection constitutes, however, only a small fraction of encephalitis cases seen in the United States. The mainstay of diagnosis is laboratory isolation of virus or a signficant rise in antibody titer to a specific virus.

TREATMENT AND PREVENTION

No specific treatment modalities exist except for symptomatic and supportive measures. The mainstay of prevention takes two approaches: vector control and immunization with vaccines. The use of insecticides and the reduction of breeding grounds have also sometimes been successful tools. Resistance of arthropods to these insecticides may, however, prove a potential problem. Protective clothing and insect repellents and the avoidance of areas that may have a high number of ticks or insects are appropriate during the months when these disease entities occur. Immunization has been limited to yellow fever and dengue encephalitis in endemic areas, but experimental vaccines are now being produced and tested.[2]

MATERNAL AND FETAL ASPECTS

A number of reports have demonstrated that arboviruses can infect the placenta and lead to fetal or neonatal infection. A maternal viremia directly extends into the fetal placental compartment, with inoculation of virus directly into the blood stream of the fetus.[3] Major disease entities shown to affect pregnant women include those that are generally more prevalent in the normal population: western equine encephalitis, Venezuelan equine encephalitis, St. Louis encephalitis, and Japanese encephalitis.

The incidence of infection in pregnancy and of resulting fetal problems is unknown. Epidemic reports of arboviral infections indicate that a small number of pregnant women will be infected along with the remainder of the population.[4]

Sporadic information has been compiled concerning these infections in the fetus. For example, in one episode of transplacental infection with Japanese encephalitis virus, two out of five women had spontaneous abortions, two delivered normal infants, and one patient was lost to follow up.[3] Disease entities can present as congenital infection early in pregnancy, leading to early spontaneous abortion or stillbirth. Some reports also suggest the possibility of congenital neurologic abnormalities. If the agent infects the mother within a few weeks prior to delivery, infants can be born with congenital infection and develop such signs of systemic viral infections as fever, lethargy, and CNS malformations.[5] Numerous viruses within the arbovirus group have been shown to produce congenital anomalies in animals. For example, viruses within the Bunyaviridae family (California encephalitis) have been shown to produce abortion, stillbirth, and premature birth in cattle, and these agents have also been used in experimental models that have produced developmental defects. It has also been demonstrated that attenuated live vaccines of the arbovirus group (Rif Valley fever vaccine, blue tongue virus vaccine) produce congenital anomalies in cattle and sheep after maternal inoculation. These congenital anomalies include microcephaly, porencephaly, and hydrocephaly.[6]

The diagnosis of fetal infection has to rely on the maternal clinical presentation and on the epidemiologic patterns of viruses within the community. It is also important to observe the incidence of congenital disease and fetal infection in asymptomatic mothers. Prevention includes the use of live attenuated virus vaccines in epidemic areas with the realization that these vaccines may cross the placenta and produce significant fetal problems. Prevention also includes eradication of vector breeding and grounds. The pregnant woman is well advised to limit her exposure and to use insect repellents.

REFERENCES

1. Downs WG. Arboviruses. In: Evans AS, ed. *Viral Infections of Humans.* New York, NY: Plenum Press; 1982:95.
2. NIAID Task Force. Advances in cell biology through virus research. *HIH Rep.* 1979;2:147.
3. Chaturvedi UC, Mathur A, Chandra A, et al. Transplacental infection with Japanese encephalitis virus. *J Infect Dis.* 1980;141:712.
4. Parsonson IM, Della-Porta AJ, Snowdon WA. Developmental disorders of the fetus in some arthropod-borne virus infections. *Am J Trop Med Hyg.* 1981;30:660.
5. Wenger F. Venezuelan equine encephalitis. *Teratology.* 1977;16:359.
6. London WT, Levitt NH, Kent SG. Congenital cerebral and ocular malformations induced in rhesus monkeys by Venezuelan equine encephalitis virus. *Teratology.* 1977;16:285.

Chapter One Hundred and Seven

Arenaviruses

David A. Baker

107

Arenaviruses are characterized by the distinctive electron microscopic appearance of the virions. Members of the group include *lymphocytic choriomeningitis virus* (LCM), *Lassa virus,* and the *Tacaribe viruses,* all important agents in producing human disease entities.

The viruses are RNA-containing viruses that are unique in containing host–cell lysosome within the virion envelope. Infection may not kill cells, and chronic arenavirus infection may be established with no changes in intracellular functions. This virus causes persistent infection in cells in culture.[1-3]

The specific modes of transmission of arenaviruses to the human are not clear, but it appears that the virus enters the human through the oral cavity or the respiratory tract, multiplies locally, and then produces a viremia with dissemination into target organs. In humans, clinical disease is apparently directly related to viral cell destruction and does not mimic disease in mice, which is an immunologic reaction to viral infection. The virus produces lymphadenopathy together with involvement of endothelial linings of capillaries and arterioles, and the disease entity may cause disseminated intravascular coagulopathy. Postmortem examinations in patients with Lassa fever suggest that direct viral destruction of cells is the major pathologic finding. It appears that invasion of the reticuloendothelial system results in effects on cells involved in humoral and cellular immunity. Capillary damage leads to hypovolemic shock. The major virus of this group, causing meningitis and meningoencephalitis, is LCM.[1-4]

Central nervous system (CNS) problems associated with the viruses in this group appear to be rare, and the incidence of LCM infection has declined over the last few years. For example, the CNS illness produced by this virus had an apparent prevalence rate of approximately 8% of those diagnosed with aseptic meningitis in the 20-year period between 1940 and 1960. This incidence has since markedly decreased, with reports of only a few confirmed cases each year. Only 1% of the population of the United States has antibody to this virus. A seasonal fluctuation, with more cases being reported in the winter than in the summer, has been suggested. The main reservoir of this virus is within rodents, particularly mice. Mouse urine, excretions, and secretions contain the virus, which may be transmitted to humans either through contamination of food or water or through evaporation, with aerosol contamination of the human upper respiratory tract. The virus is maintained mainly in the house mouse, but it seems that other species, such as hamsters and guinea pigs, can be infected as well.

DIAGNOSIS

Specific infection with LCM suggests that there may be numerous clinical presentations, and this virus has been implicated in meningitis and meningoencephalitis; however, an influenzalike illness, as well as a disease entity not involving the CNS, may also be experienced. Incubation is between one and two weeks, with the onset of fever, malaise, arthralgia, and perhaps bronchitis common. These symptoms are followed by definite signs of meningeal irritation, such as headache, nausea, and stiff neck, which may persist for upwards of two weeks or which may be very short-lived. The prognosis is good, because there are only a few reports of fatalities associated with this infection.[4]

Diagnosis is mainly confirmed through virus isolation, either from blood or cerebrospinal fluid. Some serologic and indirect fluorescent tests can also be used.

TREATMENT AND PREVENTION

There are no specific therapeutic modalities that can be offered, and the only preventive aspect of the disease is rodent control. Treatment is mainly supportive and symptomatic.

MATERNAL AND FETAL ASPECTS

The fate of these viruses within the fetal-placental unit is unknown. Only few reports of infected cases have appeared in the literature. It appears, however, that the virus can get into the fetal-placental unit secondary to maternal viremia.

Specific manifestations in the newborn are poorly described and not well understood.[5] Whether the disease occurs in the newborn as in the mother, with viral infection and lytic cell destruction, or whether it causes an infection, as has been demonstrated in mice, in which the immune response is the etiology of specific manifestations of CNS problems, is unknown.

In the presence of maternal infection, viral isolation and serologic evidence of infection should be obtained from the newborn.

REFERENCES

1. Andrews C, Pereira HG, Wilde P, eds. *Viruses of Vertebrates*. 4th ed. London: Bailliere Tindall; 1978:166.
2. Casals J. Arenaviruses. In: Evans AS, ed. *Viral Infections of Humans*. New York, NY: Plenum Press, 1982:127.
3. NIAID Task Force Report. Persistent viral infections. *NIH Rep*. 1979;3:116.
4. Sanford JP. Arenavirus infections. In: Petersdorf RG, Adams RD, Braunwald E, et al, eds. *Harrison's Principles of Internal Medicine*. 10th ed. New York, NY: McGraw-Hill; 1983:1156.
5. Sheinbergas MM. Hydrocephalus due to prenatal infection with lymphocytic choriomeningitis virus. *Infection*. 1976;4:1.

Chapter One Hundred and Eight

Diseases Caused by Slow Viruses

David A. Baker

108

The disease entities reviewed here are grouped together because of their association with viral agents and their long-term, slow, degenerative processes. There appear to be four distinct characteristics of these disease entities: an incubation period of many months or years, a degenerative course ending in death, a site usually localized to the central nervous system (CNS), and limitation to a single host species. Some specific disease entities that fall into slow viral diseases of the CNS and that affect humans are subacute sclerosing panencephalitis (SSPE), progressive rubella panencephalitis (PRP), progressive multifocal leukoencephalopathy (PML), kuru, and Creutzfeldt–Jakob disease (CJD).

The immunologic agents differ depending on the specific disease state, and they may be related to initial infection with a specific virus and subsequent long-term problems associated with the host's handling of the viral disease, or they may be related to differences within the virus itself. These entities include: SSPE, which has been associated with measles; PRP, associated with rubella; and PML, associated with a virus labeled JC, probably a papovavirus. The specific etiologic agents for kuru and CJD have not been identified or characterized at the present time.

SUBACUTE SCLEROSING PANENCEPHALITIS

The specific pathogenesis of SSPE is not fully understood, but it appears that there is either an abnormal response of the host to a previous measles virus infection or that specific viruses have been altered. Pathologic lesions occur throughout the substance of the brain, including the medulla, cerebellum, and cerebral hemispheres. There are infiltrates containing lymphocytes and monocytes around small arteries and veins, as well as Cowdry type A inclusion bodies in brain cells and eosinophilic intranuclear inclusions. The basic process seems to be that of cellular destruction leading to clinical change. There also appears to be astrocyte proliferation in the white matter, and virions have been identified on electron microscopic studies.[1]

This disease entity, rare in the United States, primarily affects children, with a higher incidence in males, and with the past history showing prior measles infection. There are approximately 15 new cases reported each year, indicating a decline since measles vaccine has been introduced. The disease appears to exist worldwide, and the age of peak incidence of the disease is within the early 20s. Therefore, women in the childbearing years can be exposed to this disease entity, although this would be extremely uncommon. It seems that the attack rate of this disease in children with wild-type measles is ten times that of those children vaccinated with the attenuated live virus.[2]

Diagnosis

The disease presents with the slow onset of mental involvement, usually detected by the initial decline in the ability to perform adequate work. There is subsequent involvement of the CNS with initial focal neurologic signs and involuntary movements. In addition, there are visual abnormalities and the possibility of numerous types of seizure activity. The late stages of the disease include stupor, and myoclonus heralds the last stages of the disease. Death is usually secondary to infection.[3]

The clinical presentation may lead to a diagnosis. It can be confirmed by finding high levels of antibody to the measles virus in the serum and cerebrospinal fluid (CSF). IgG complexes have been found in numerous organs, and viral particles can be seen with electron microscopy in brain tissue and in biopsies from lymph nodes. Electroencephalograms show specific patterns in this disease.

Treatment and Prevention

No specific treatment exists for this disease. Once the disease ensues, there is progressive deterioration toward death. The best prevention presently is the use of live attenuated vaccine. The number of new cases has indeed been markedly reduced in the United States since 1973, when this vaccination program was initiated on a wide scale.

Specific pregnancy-related information is sparse. Case reports suggest that SSPE when associated with pregnancy may demonstrate an unusually rapid neurologic deterioration.[4-6] Some authors have suggested that pregnancy may have played a crucial role in the appearance of the disease and in the rapid (within one month) CNS deterioration of affected patients.

PROGRESSIVE RUBELLA PANENCEPHALITIS

This disorder is characterized by destruction of white matter with subsequent neuronal deterioration. There is significant cerebellar atrophy, and amorphous vascular deposits have been observed in the white matter.

This disease entity usually occurs during the second decade of life and has been described in patients with acute congenital rubella. There is most often a delay of at least 10 years after rubella infection before manifestations of disease are evident.[7]

Diagnosis

Manifestations are similar to those of SSPE. Antibody levels to rubella virus are very high in both serum and CSF. Again, there are also elevated IgG levels of antibody in the CSF.

Treatment and Prevention

No treatment is currently available. Prevention includes the use of rubella vaccine.

It appears that this is one disease that occurs as a consequence of the congenital rubella syndrome. The specific pathogenesis may lie in the host's inability to recognize this virus as foreign. The affected newborn excretes rubella virus for many years. This disease then develops with progressive mental and motor deterioration in the second decade.[7,8]

PROGRESSIVE MULTIFOCAL LEUKOENCEPHALOPATHY

PML is a rare disease caused by a member of the papovavirus group. Approximately 100 cases have been reported; PML usually affects the immunosuppressed patient and causes a chronic inflammatory disease of the CNS. There is focal destruction of the myelin sheath, which forms plaquelike lesions. Inclusion bodies filled with papovavirus, may be viewed under the electron microscope. As opposed to the other diseases in this section, there is little perivascular infiltration.[2]

This virus appears to be an opportunistic organism, and usually affects adults in the fifth to seventh decades of life.

Diagnosis

Apparently, this is a markedly degenerative CNS disease with hemiparesis and dementia as the most common manifestations. Symptoms of cerebellar involvement and seizures are frequent, along with visual disturbances, progressive mental degeneration, dysplasia, and, perhaps, ataxia. Systemic manifestations, aside from CNS involvement, are not present, and remissions have been reported.[1]

The specific diagnosis relies on clinical suspicion as well as on examination of tissue with electron microscopy. Also, computed tomography and an electroencephalogram (EEG) may aid in the diagnosis.

Treatment and Prevention

No specific treatment or preventive measures have been found successful. Antiviral agents have not been useful.

Little has been reported concerning this disease in pregnancy.

KURU AND CREUTZFELDT–JAKOB DISEASE

Unlike the other diseases discussed, kuru and CJD involve the gray matter of the CNS. Specific pathologic changes occur, including spongiform degeneration and destruction of neurons with proliferation and hypertrophy of astrocytes. There is also swelling and vacuolization of neurons without signs of inflammation.[2]

Because kuru is limited to New Guinea, it is not discussed further in this section. CJD has a prevalence of approximately one to two cases per million per year. The possibility of direct contact transmission of this disease has been raised, but this is yet to be proven. This disease may also show a pattern of autosomal dominant transmission and may be an example of a virus-induced disease that is genetically determined. The bulk of cases have been reported in North America and Europe, although there is a worldwide distribution. The age groups most commonly affected are between 40 to 69 years, with the mean age of death being approximately 60 years. Males and females are equally affected.

Diagnosis

The cerebellum and cerebrum are the major targets of this disease and there is a loss of gray matter. CJD mimics changes of presenile dementia with presentation of bizarre behavior, memory loss, and inability to use reason as well as judgment. The presentation can include hallucinations and confusion with deterioration to the point at which the patient becomes stuporous; this is followed by rapid progression to death.[3]

A specific diagnosis of these diseases is based on clinical grounds; EEG abnormalities can be found, and a computerized tomography (CT) scan can differentiate other specific disease entities. The final diagnosis of CJD relies on the examination of biopsy or autopsy materials.

Little information is known concerning either maternal or fetal aspects of CJD. No maternal transmission has been reported in humans or experimentally in animal models.

REFERENCES

1. Gilden DH. Slow virus diseases of CNS. *Postgrad Med.* 1983;73:99,113.
2. Brody JA, Gibbs CJ. Chronic neurologic diseases. In: Evans AS, ed. *Viral Infections of Humans.* 2nd ed. New York, NY: Plenum Press; 1982:675.
3. Matthews WB. Slow virus infections. *J R Coll Phys Lond.* 1981;15:109.
4. Wirguin I, Steiner I, Kidron D, et al. Fulminant subacute sclerosing panencephalitis in association with pregnancy. *Arch Neurol.* 1988;45:1324.
5. Nelson RF, Dennery JM, Montpetit V. SSPE and Pregnancy. *Lancet.* 1972;1:1289.
6. Gaines KJ, Jabbour JT, Whitaker JN, et al. Subacute sclerosing panencephalitis during pregnancy. *Arch Neurol.* 1979;36:314.
7. Stroop WGH, Baringer JR. Persistent slow and latent viral infections. *Prog Med Virol.* 1982;28:1.
8. NIAID Task Force. Persistent viral infections. *NIH Rep.* 1979;3:75.

K
MISCELLANEOUS AND PRESUMPTIVE VIRAL INFECTIONS

Chapter One Hundred and Nine
Human Papilloma Virus Infection and Molluscum Contagiosum

Stanley A. Gall

109

PAPILLOMA VIRUS INFECTION

Warts are benign epithelial or fibro-epithelial tumors of the skin or contiguous mucous membranes caused by the human papilloma virus (HPV).

The papilloma viruses are a subgroup of the Papovaviridae family exhibiting a naked icosahedral capsid of 55 nm and a supercoiled, covalent, closed, circular, double-stranded DNA molecule. The molecular weight is approximately 5×10^6 d. These viruses are found in animals and humans and are highly host- and tissue-specific.[1] Viruses included in the papovavirus group of agents include the papilloma viruses of humans and animals, human wart virus, shope papillomavirus of rabbits, polyomaviruses of mice, and vacuolating viruses of monkeys (SV40). Although the human wart virus has never been convincingly cultured *in vitro,* it can be demonstrated by electron microscopy in extracts and thin sections of warts.[1] Studies using restriction endonuclease analysis of HPV DNA indicate that many subtypes exist and that the strain differences vary according to the anatomic site from which the warts are recovered. HPV types 1 and 2 are found in plantar or common warts. HPV-3 is associated with flat or plain warts but has been seen in patients with vulvar and cervical carcinoma.[2,3] HPV-4 seems to be antigenically distinct from HPV-1 and 3 but is occasionally seen in plantar warts. HPV-5 is associated with epidermodysplasia-verruciformlike syndromes with skin cancers. HPV-6 is commonly found in genital warts in 60% of cases, with HPV-11 found in 30%. In the remainder of patients, HPV types 1, 2, 11, 16, and 18 are found. HPV types 16, 18, and 31 are predominantly found in lesions in the upper one third of the cervix and in the cervix. Lesions with these HPV DNA types are more likely to demonstrate malignant transformation.[4,5] Patients with these higher risk HPV DNA types are also more likely to show more frequent recurrences of HPV infection and more recurrences of malignant disease after primary therapy.

Pathogenesis, Pathology, and Epidemiology

Experimentally, after direct inoculation through abrasions in the skin, virus appears to infect single epithelial cells, which are stimulated to divide. Formation of lesions at the site of experimental infections in human volunteers indicated an incubation period of up to six months (average 3–4 months). The incubation period in natural infection may be much longer. The infection is due to proliferation of epithelial cells with mitotic figures seen in layers beyond the basal layer. There is a marked proliferation of the prickle cells with large vacuolated cells in the upper stratum malpight and granular layer. These vacuolated cells are an important distinguishing characteristic in differentiating viral from nonviral papillomas. Hematoxylin-eosin (H & E) staining of warty lesions may show cells that contain both nuclear and cytoplasmic inclusions. The cytoplasmic inclusions are eosinophilic and represent deranged keratohyalin development, while the nuclear inclusions stain basophilic and represent aggregates of virus particles.

Warts occur as a single lesion or in multiple clusters and are widely dispersed over the body. Genital warts usually occur in clusters, with progression of lesions over the vulva, perineum, and anorectal areas. Warts have a significant rate of spontaneous remission and it is estimated that one third of warts disappear spontaneously within a six-month period. The reasons for the spontaneous remission are unknown, but alterations in the host's immune system and a limited life span of infected cells have been proposed as explanations. A mononuclear cellular infiltrate has been observed in the area of receding warts, thereby giving strength to the importance of cellular immunity. Warts may become much larger and more extensive in pregnancy and in immunosuppressed patients.

HPV disease is very common, with approximately 20% of the population affected. Genital warts, condyloma acuminata, are thought to be sexually transmitted, although other direct person-to-person contact may allow inoculation to occur. Autoinoculation of virus to adjacent or distant sites is common. The incidence of warts is much higher in teenagers than in adults. The incidence of HPV infection has dramatically increased in the past 10 years, with a 1000% increase noted in private office consultations and sexually transmitted disease (STD) clinics.

Manifestations

HPV may manifest itself as overt or subclinical infection in the cervix, vagina, vulva, perineal body, or perianal area, or as abnormal genital cytology or Bowen's disease. HPV is present in cervical intraepithelial neoplasia (CIN), vaginal intraepithelial neoplasia (VaIN), vulvar intraepithelial neoplasia (VIN), as well as in virtually all invasive squamous cell carcinomas of the genital tract.

Condyloma acuminata tend to occur as multiple, polymorphic lesions that may coalesce to form large masses in the vulvar, perineal, or anal areas. Frequently, condylomata are found within the vagina and on occasion grow to the extent that vaginal delivery is precluded. Warts are commonly found on the urethral meatus and clitoris.

Condyloma acuminata are commonly found on the cervix and appear either as mucus lesions or as white spots with fine punctuation on colposcopic examination. Cytologic abnormalities such as multinucleated cells and koilocytosis are evidence of condylomata and occur in about 1–2% of routine Papanicolaou smears. Recent reports on the use of a peroxidase–antiperoxidase technique indicate the presence of condyloma antigens in patients with condyloma of the cervix, condyloma of the cervix with nuclear atypia, but not in patients with invasive carcinoma of the cervix or carcinoma *in situ* of the cervix or moderate dysplasia. In other studies, cells suggestive of condyloma were described in one third of patients with cervical dysplasia, carcinoma *in situ,* and invasive carcinoma.

The differential diagnosis of condyloma acuminata includes condylomata lata of secondary syphilis (serologic testing will differentiate between the two entities), granuloma inguinale, and carcinoma of the vulva. In addition, condyloma must be differentiated from fibroepitheliomas and seborrheic keratosis (biopsy) and molluscum contagiosum.

Generally, the diagnosis can be made by inspection. However, should the lesion be noted to increase in size, degenerate to cause bleeding, or cause pain, biopsy is indicated. During pregnancy, biopsy can be accompanied by brisk bleeding. Excisional biopsy is preferred. Malignant transformation of condyloma acuminata in the childbearing years is very rare.

Treatment

There is no specific treatment for warts, but a variety of chemical and physical agents have been used. These methods include application of 25% podophyllin in tincture of benzoin, 85% trichloroacetic acid or 5-fluorouracil cream, the use of electrodesiccation and curettage, application of liquid nitrogen, CO_2 cryotherapy, or laser ablation. Surgical excision may be attempted, but the warts frequently recur. More recent therapy includes use of the laser, immunotherapy with autologous vaccine, or levamisole and the use of interferon.

Podophyllin may be toxic, teratogenic, and carcinogenic and is contraindicated during pregnancy. Adequate therapy for condyloma acuminata during pregnancy has not been established, but a recent study suggests therapeutic effectiveness using CO_2 laser.[6] Topical 85% trichloroacetic acid can be safely used in pregnancy in the vagina or vulva. Radical therapy should be avoided because the overt warts frequently resolve spontaneously in the postpartum period. However, if the condyloma become severely painful, cause bleeding, or degenerate, surgical excision is indicated. Autologous vaccine injections have been used on a limited scale with some success. Trials with interferon administration to nonpregnant patients with condyloma acuminata have been encouraging, but trials in pregnant patients have not begun.

Fetal Aspects

The presence of condyloma acuminata during pregnancy have never been shown to cause an adverse outcome of the fetus. The human papilloma virus is not transmitted to the fetus. However, concern has been raised as to the development of juvenile laryngeal papillomatosis (JLP) in infants born to mothers infected with HPV at the time of delivery. A retrospective study indicated that 5 of 9 children who developed JLP were delivered by mothers who had genital condyloma acuminata. However, the same authors subsequently reported a prospective study of 31 children born of mothers with condyloma acuminata, and no child developed JLP.[7,8] Juvenile laryngeal papillomas have been examined for the presence of HPV genoma and capsid antigens.[9] The viral DNA found in JLP were found to be HPV-6 with four different subtypes designated HPV-6c to HPV-6f. HPV-6c was detected in over 50% of the juvenile laryngeal papillomas examined. Therefore, it seems likely that the same virus, HPV-6, may cause condyloma acuminata and JLP. Management of the pregnant woman with overt condyloma acuminata at the time of delivery should be determined by obstetric factors. The evidence that the presence of condyloma acuminata in the laboring patient predisposes the infant to JLP is not strong enough to warrant routine cesarean section. Further studies must be done to determine the relationship between condyloma acuminata, vaginal delivery, and JLP.

MOLLUSCUM CONTAGIOSUM

Molluscum contagiosum is a human disease, distributed worldwide and caused by a member of the poxvirus group.[10] The virus is one of the largest viruses to cause human disease measuring 250–320 nm in diameter. It can be demonstrated in direct touch preparations of lesions using oil immersion light microscopy.

The disease is characterized by a long incubation period from two weeks to two months. The development of the disease is heralded by firm, shiny, flesh-colored lesions that become pearly white and umbilicated and discharge a caseous material. The lesions are characterized by proliferation, hyperplasia, thickening, and degeneration of the epidermis. The infected epithelial cells become enlarged and develop large, intracytoplasmic, eosinophilic, hyaline inclusion bodies. The lesions are usually not pruritic and measure 1–5 mm in diameter but may form larger clusters.

The infection can be transmitted directly by sexual intercourse or by fomites. Epidemics have been seen in boarding schools with closed populations.

The principal sites of involvement include the eyelids, face, trunk, and anogenital areas. Molluscum lesions evolve over a period of 1–2 months and are frequently traumatized, with autoinoculation resulting. Secondary bacterial infection may occur. The lesions may persist for periods up to 1 year but have persisted 3–4 years. Spontaneous regression without scarring usually occurs, and recurrences are rare. Patients who are immunosuppressed may develop extensive involvement.[11,12]

The diagnosis of molluscum contagiosum is usually made by inspection of the characteristic umbilicated white papule. Differential diagnosis includes lichen planus, verrucous papules, basal cell epithelioma, and pyogenic granuloma. If the diagnosis is in doubt, the caseous material should be examined for intracytoplasmic inclusions. Treatment by sharp curettage or expression of porous material will facilitate healing without scarring.

REFERENCES

1. Faras AJ, Kryzek RA, Ostrow RS, et al. Genetic variation among papillomaviruses. *NY Acad Sci.* 1980;77:60.

2. Gissman L, DeVilliers EM, Zur Hausen H. Analysis of human genital warts (condyloma acuminata) and other genital tumors of human papillomavirus type 6 DNA. *Int J Cancer*. 1982;29:143.
3. Smotkin D. Virology of human papillomavirus. *Clin Obstet Gynecol*. 1989;32:117.
4. Ferenczy A. HPV-associated lesions in pregnancy and their clinical implications. *Clinical Obstet Gynecol*. 1989;32:191.
5. Durst M, Gissman L, Ikenberg H, et al. A papillomavirus DNA from a cervical carcinoma and its prevalence in cancer biopsy samples from different geographic regions. *Proc Natl Acad Sci USA*. 1983;80:3812.
6. Ferenczy A. Treating genital condyloma during pregnancy with the carbon dioxide laser. *Am J Obstet Gynecol*. 1984;148:9.
7. Cook TA, Brunschwig JP, Butel JS, et al. Laryngeal papilloma: etiologic and therapeutic considerations. *Ann Otol*. 1973;82:649.
8. Cohn AM, Kos JT, Taber LH, et al. Recurring laryngeal papilloma. *Am J Otol*. 1981;2:129.
9. Mounts P, Shah KV, Kashima H. Viral etiology of juvenile and adult onset squamous papilloma of the larynx. *Proc Natl Acad Sci*. 1982;79:5425.
10. Davis BD, Dulbecco R, Elsen HN. Other poxviruses that infect man. In: *Microbiology*. 2nd ed. Hagerstown, MD: Harper and Row; 1973:1275.
11. Lynch PJ, Menkin W. Molluscum contagiosum of the adult: probable venereal transmission. *Arch Dermatol*. 1968;98:141.
12. Brown ST, Weinberger J. Molluscum contagiosum: sexually transmitted disease in 17 cases. *J Am Vener Dis Assoc*. 1974;1:35.

Chapter One Hundred and Ten
Cat-Scratch Disease

Stanley A. Gall

110

Cat-scratch disease is characterized by an indolent, usually self-limiting infection in an immunocompetent host, primarily a child or adolescent with lymphadenitis. The cutaneous lesion at the site of inoculation may look like an insect bite. In 90% of the cases, however, cat scratches or close contact with cats are reported.

ETIOLOGY

A long-suspected infectious etiologic agent has been isolated, cultivated, and recently described.[1] These gram-negative bacteria have a delicate, pleomorphic form and are slightly curved or rodlike with bulbous ends. Flat or slightly elevated transparent colonies 0.2 mm wide and 0.1 mm deep develop on biphasic brain–heart infusion media in 2–9 days. Staining lymph node sections with Warthin–Starry silver impregnation reveals pleomorphic, gram-negative bacilli, not acid-fast, ranging from 0.3–1.0 μm in diameter and 0.6 to 3.0 μm in length. The bacteria are located in the walls of capillaries and in macrophages lining the sinuses in or near germinal centers. The bacilli appear as single organisms or in chains or clumps. They also are found in thrombosed vessels and in necrotic foci, where they are clustered in histiocytes, suggesting intracellular multiplication.

Ultrastructure descriptions of the bacilli have been reported.[2] The bacilli are intracellular, irregularly shaped, slightly curved, and slightly clubbed on one end, and are found in clumps adjacent to mammalian cell nuclei. They measure 0.2 μm in diameter and 1.0 to 2.5 μm in length. The ultrastructure of the bacillary wall consists of an outer glycocalyx, that is, a thin peptidoglycanlike layer bounding the bacillary protoplasm.

EPIDEMIOLOGY

In temperate climates, cat-scratch disease is a seasonal illness; 75% of cases occur in the fall and early winter, with a peak in December. The disease occurs in children and young adults; 80% of the cases involve patients less than 20 years of age. Approximately 90% of people with cat-scratch disease have had contact with a cat, and 75% report having been scratched by an apparently healthy cat.[3]

PATHOLOGY

The histologic appearance of the lymph nodes is not specific for cat-scratch disease. The histopathologic features are nodular and diffuse lymphoid hyperplasia, tingible histiocytes forming a starry sky pattern in reactive follicles and interfollicular spaces, and microabscesses beginning in the germinal centers. The microabscesses are composed of necrotic cells, with karyorrhectic nuclei and acidophilic debris or combinations of necrosis with polymorphs and epithelioid histiocytes or palisaded epithelioid histiocytes or both. Peripheral sinuses are dilated and filled with lymphocytes, and there is a perinodal inflammation. All stages, from abscesses to granulomas, can be seen in the same node. The histologic changes are not unlike those seen with atypical mycobacterial infection, lymphogranuloma venereum, toxoplasmosis, sarcoidosis, and brucellosis.

MANIFESTATIONS

The disease usually has a slow, mild course. The primary inoculation lesion is present in two thirds of patients when a physician is contacted.[4] The primary lesion is frequently a raised, tender, nonpruritic papule with a small, vesicular crown or eschar present. This papule develops in about 10 days (range, 3–30 days) after the scratch. The physician is rarely consulted at this stage. Regional lymphadenopathy occurs in all patients in 5–50 days (usually 10–14 days) after the disappearance of the papule. No intervening lymphangitis is noted. The adenopathy is usually unilateral and asymmetric and involves only one lymph node. The axillary, cervical, preauricular, and other lymph nodes (upper extremities, 65%; head and neck, 25.6%; lower extremities, 10%) become visibly enlarged and painful with erythema of the overlying skin. Occasionally, the lymph nodes will suppurate (12%) but will heal spontaneously in 85% of the patients within six weeks. Systemic symptoms will occur in 65% of patients, malaise in 40%, and fever in 25%. Usually, the systemic symptoms are mild, but on occasion, temperatures as high as 40°C may occur, as well as erythema nodosum, erythema multiforme, and thrombocytopenic purpura.

Atypical presentations occur in approximately 10% of patients. The most common is a unilateral swelling of a preauricular lymph node with fever (Parinaud's oculoglandular syndrome). Other clinical forms include transverse myelitis presenting as a Brown–Sequard lesion; encephalitis characterized by fever, convulsions, alterations in the conscious state, or mild cerebrospinal pleocytosis with elevation of protein; mesenteric lymphadenitis; and osteolytic bone lesions.

DIAGNOSIS

A clinical diagnosis of cat-scratch disease requires the presence of three or four criteria: (1) a history of animal (usually a cat) contact with the presence of a scratch or primary dermal or eye lesion; (2) positive cat-scratch disease skin test; (3) negative laboratory studies for other causes of lymphadenopathy; and (4) characteristic histopathology of a biopsied lymph node.

The specific diagnosis is made by a skin test, and the cat-scratch antigen may be obtained from HA Carithers, MD, 1661 Riverside Avenue, Jacksonville, FL 32204, or from Andrew M. Margileth, MD, Department of Pediatrics, Uniformed Services University of the Health Sciences, 4301 Jones Bridge Road, Bethesda, MD 20814–4799. The skin test antigen (0.1 cc) is injected intradermally on the flexor surface of the forearm. The site is inspected in 72 hours; 5 mm or greater of induration is a positive reaction. The size of the reaction does not correspond with the severity of illness.[5]

Other laboratory abnormalities may include a leukocytosis up to 15,000 cell/mm^3, an eosinophilia, and an elevated erythrocyte sedimentation rate (≥20 mm) during the first two weeks of adenitis.

Cat-scratch disease is a benign disease with uniformly good prognosis. The main area of concern is its confusion with other more serious diseases. These include lymphogranuloma venereum, tularemia, atypical mycobacterial infection, tuberculosis, brucellosis, toxoplasmosis, pyogenic adenitis, sarcoidosis, lymphoma, and systemic fungal disease.

TREATMENT

The course of the disease is benign and self-limited in immunocompetent patients. Most recover within two months, but lymphadenopathy may persist for one year (2%). Antibiotics and steroids have not been successful; however, recent reports suggest that the use of aminoglycosides was efficacious in shortening the course of cat-scratch disease in immunocompetent[6] and in immunocompromised hosts.[7]

EFFECT OF DISEASE ON PREGNANCY AND FETUS

No reports of the disease in pregnancy have been published. The pregnant patient should be treated symptomatically while the medical evaluation including lymph node biopsy is being accomplished. The major goals of therapy are to rule out the more serious diseases listed in the differential diagnosis and not to overtreat the patient with potentially dangerous or teratogenic drugs.

REFERENCES

1. English CK, Wear DJ, Margileth AM, et al. Cat-scratch disease. Isolation and culture of the bacterial agent. *JAMA*. 1988;259:1347.
2. Hadfield TL, Malaty RH, Van Dellen A, et al. Electron microscopy of the bacillus causing cat-scratch disease. *J Infect Dis*. 1985;152:643.
3. Carithers HA, Carithers CM, Edwards RO Jr. Cat-scratch disease: its natural history. *JAMA*. 1969;207:312.
4. Margileth AM. Dermatologic manifestations and update of cat-scratch disease. *Pediatr Dermatol*. 1988;5:1.
5. Moriarity RA, Margileth AM. Cat-scratch disease. *Infect Dis Clin North Am*. 1987;1:575.
6. Bogue CW, Wise JD, Gray GF, Edwards KM. Antibiotic therapy for cat-scratch disease? *JAMA*. 1989;262:813.
7. Black JR, Herrington DA, Hadfield TL, et al. Life-threatening cat-scratch disease in an immunocompromised host. *Arch Intern Med*. 1986;146:394.

L

PROTOZOAN AND HELMINTHIC INFECTIONS

Chapter One Hundred and Eleven

Protozoan Infections

Richard V. Lee

111

Protozoa, unique single-cell organisms, are distributed throughout nature. They are hardy, adaptable, and evolutionarily successful. Only a fraction of the present day species of protozoans are pathogens; the vast majority of protozoans are free living or symbiotic creatures.

Familiarity with the biology and life cycles of pathogenic protozoans provides the clinician with an understanding of the diseases caused by protozoa and the risks to and manifestations in pregnant women. The usefulness of this familiarity is illustrated by the prevalence of malaria and intestinal protozoa in immigrants to the United States and travelers from the United States. Each year there are more than 20 million international travelers to and from the United States. The rapidity of air travel allows for travelers to acquire so-called exotic parasitic infections during a trip, but suffer clinical illness from the infection only after returning home.

Pathogenic protozoa are adapted to, and dependent upon, life in or on other living creatures. Most pathogenic species have evolved life cycles that ensure survival of the species despite the death of the host (Table 111–1). The remarkably tough cysts, *Entamoeba histolytica,* and the extraordinary life cycles of plasmodia and trypanosomes, which allow for the transmission by arthropods of parasites from infected to uninfected hosts, are examples. Protozoan diversity and adaptability, the changing environment, and host responses resulting from human living practices, agriculture, animal husbandry, and industry have led to the regular discovery of new protozoan diseases of humankind.[1-3] The recognition of the important role of *Cryptosporidium* species in diarrheal disease, first among patients with acquired immune deficiency syndrome (AIDS), then among healthy people, is an example.

Many pathogenic protozoans can persist in one or more morphologic or antigenic configurations for a long time within or on the same host. The clinical expression of the infection is determined by the location of the infecting organisms and the host response. Surface dwellers may never or rarely penetrate integumentary or mucosal barriers. Tissue-invasive protozoa have the potential to infect the placenta and the fetus. Asymptomatic or nonspecifically ill individuals harboring a protozoan parasite serve as an important reservoir and a potential vector. They may develop illnesses different from the early clinical manifestations of the infection at a time remote from the acquisition of the parasite. Silent parasitemia may result in unsuspected intrauterine fetal infection. The life cycles of tissue-invasive protozoa usually involve nonhuman vectors or intermediate hosts, which result in circumscribed geographic distribution.[4] In contrast, asexually reproducing luminal protozoa of humans are found worldwide, wherever human beings go.

Pregnancy alters cell-mediated immune responses.[5] Immune surveillance of parasitized cells and containment of tissue dwelling parasites may be muted during gestation, setting the stage for activation of latent infection or for transient parasitemia, with risks to both maternal and fetal well-being. Alterations in host parasite interaction may produce amelioration of clinical symptoms despite persistence or dissemination of the parasite during pregnancy. The return of normal immune function in the postpartum period may be accompanied by another transformation in the clinical appearance of the mother's protozoan infection.

Protozoan parasitic infections can adversely influence a woman's reproductive capacity in six ways (Table 111–2).[6-12] First, the disease may impair fertility by causing local damage to the reproductive organs or by causing serious constitutional illness. Second, infection by protozoans may injure the mother's health, causing spontaneous interruption of pregnancy or forcing medical intervention that seriously jeopardizes the fetus or necessitates premature termination of the pregnancy. Third, protozoan infections may respond to changes in host defenses produced by pregnancy and parturition by local or systemic spread and more aggressive clinical disease during the puerperium. Fourth, some protozoan pathogens are capable of traversing the placenta and producing congenital infection or fetal loss because of placental failure or fetal infection. Fifth, the neonate may acquire infection during delivery through a parasitized birth canal or after delivery from contact with infected maternal secretions of skin. Sixth, treatment of serious protozoan infection may expose the mother and fetus to potentially toxic or teratogenic chemicals.

INTESTINAL PROTOZOA

Intestinal protozoa (Table 111–3) reproducing asexually have a simple life cycle. The infective cyst is ingested by the host. On reaching the appropriate intestinal site, excystation takes place and the trophozoites take up residence in or on the mucosa. During passage through the gut lumen, some of the trophozoites encyst, ensuring survival after passage in the stool.

The evolution of intracellular sexual reproduction in the gastrointestinal epithelia increased the complexity of the life cycle of some intestinal protozoa by increasing the number of infective stages. Species specificity for the sexual reproductive phase and the capacity to produce intracellular infection and cell death characterize these organisms. Infection may follow ingestion of viable organisms in flesh, and ingestion of asexually and sexually produced cysts.

The epidemiology of intestinal protozoa is generally governed by the "rule of Fs": fingers, feces, fluids, food,

TABLE 111–1. LIFE CYCLES OF PATHOGENIC PROTOZOANS

Organism	Site(s) of Infection in Humans	Environmental Form	Insect Vector or Route of Infection	Alternate and Intermediate Animal Hosts
Entamoeba histolytica	GI tract: colon, extraintestinal spread of trophozoites: liver	Cyst	Fecal-oral, direct inoculation	
Giardia lamblia	GI tract: duodenum, jejunum	Cyst	Fecal-oral	Beavers
Toxoplasma gondii	Lymph nodes, striated muscle, CNS, eyes	Oocyst (shed in cat feces)	Ingestion of cyst or oocyst	Cats (sexual cycle), rodents, sheep, pigs, beef
Malaria	Hepatocytes, RE cells, RBCs		Anopheline mosquitoes	
Leishmania donovani	RE cells of liver, spleen, and lymph nodes		Sandfly (*Phlebotomus*)	Dogs, rodents
Leishmania braziliensis and *mexicana*	Skin and mucosae		Sandfly (*Phlebotomus*)	Rodents
Trypanosoma brucei	RE cells, lymph nodes, and spleen; central nervous system		Tsetse fly (*Glossina*)	Wild bovidae: bush buck, gazelles, domestic cattle
Trypanosoma cruzi	RE cells, striated muscle, myocardium		Reduviid bugs (*Triatoma*)	Rodents, other wild animals
Pneumocystis carinii	Lungs	Cyst	Inhalation of infective cysts	Numerous mammals

flies, fomites, and fornication. Parasites transmitted by the fecal-oral route often coexist with other pathogens acquired in similar fashion. *Salmonella, Shigella, Campylobacter, Yersinia,* and enterotoxigenic bacteria may cause illness that obscures or complicates intestinal protozoan infections.

Protozoan Parasites Asexually Reproducing in the Gastrointestinal Tract

Protozoans residing and dividing asexually in the human gastrointestinal tract (Figure 111–1) (Table 111–4) are ubiquitous human companions, found wherever human beings live, from the polar ice caps to the equator. The majority are not pathogenic: *Endolimax nana, Dientamoeba fragilis, Lodamoeba buetschlii, Entamoeba coli, Entamoeba hartmanni, Chilomastix mesnili, Trichomonas hominis. E histolytica* and *Giardia lamblia* are the principal pathogens in this group of organisms. *Balantidium coli,* a large ciliated protozoan, is a rare cause of diarrhea in humans.

Amebiasis. The trophozoite or motile form of *E histolytica* lives in the lumen of the human large intestine, where it divides and differentiates into the cyst, which is responsible for the transmission of the infection.[13-15] The spectrum of disease ranges from asymptomatic intestinal infection to fatal colitis or extraintestinal infection. When the parasite exists as a commensal, the host has no evidence of tissue invasion, has few symptoms, and is detected only by the finding of cysts in stool examination. Asymptomatic cyst passers are a major reservoir for the organism for transmission.

The myth that amebiasis is exclusively a tropical disease should be eliminated from medical teaching. Accurate statistics defining incidence and prevalence of amebiasis are unavailable because of inability to examine all of the asymptomatic population, confusion in identification of nonpathogenic amebas, and the recognition that some varieties of *E histolytica,* the so-called Laredo strains, have rela-

TABLE 111–2. EFFECTS OF PROTOZOAN INFECTIONS ON REPRODUCTION

	Impaired Fertility	Prematurity	Transplacental or Congenital Infection	Puerperal Exacerbation	Neonatal Infection
Amebiasis	X	X		X	Rare
Giardiasis	X	?		X	Rare
Leishmaniasis	X	X	X		
Malaria	X	X	X		
Trypanosomiasis	X	X	X		
Toxoplasmosis		?	X		
Pneumocystosis			X		X

TABLE 111–3. INTESTINAL PROTOZOA OF IMPORTANCE DURING PREGNANCY

Asexual Reproduction
Entamoeba histolytica
Giardia lamblia
Balantidium coli
Sexual Reproduction
Toxoplasma gondii
Other *Coccidia species*
Cryptosporidia
Isospora
Sarcocystis

tively low or even no pathogenicity. Rough estimates of prevalence, ranging from 40% or more in some tropical countries to 2–5% in the United States, suggest that a substantial portion of the world's population (5–10%) harbor *E histolytica*. The vast majority of these folk have no symptoms of their infection.

E histolytica is spread through the fecal pollution of drinking water or from person-to-person by cyst-contaminated hands, food, or utensils. Infection is more common among populations where poor sanitation, low hygienic standards, and certain agricultural and food preparation practices are prevalent. Where human excreta are used as fertilizer (night soil), fruit and vegetables are a common source of infection. Lack of water and attention to hand and utensil washing contribute to spread of the infection by food and eating equipment. Human behavior is the major factor in the maintenance of endemic infection at high levels,

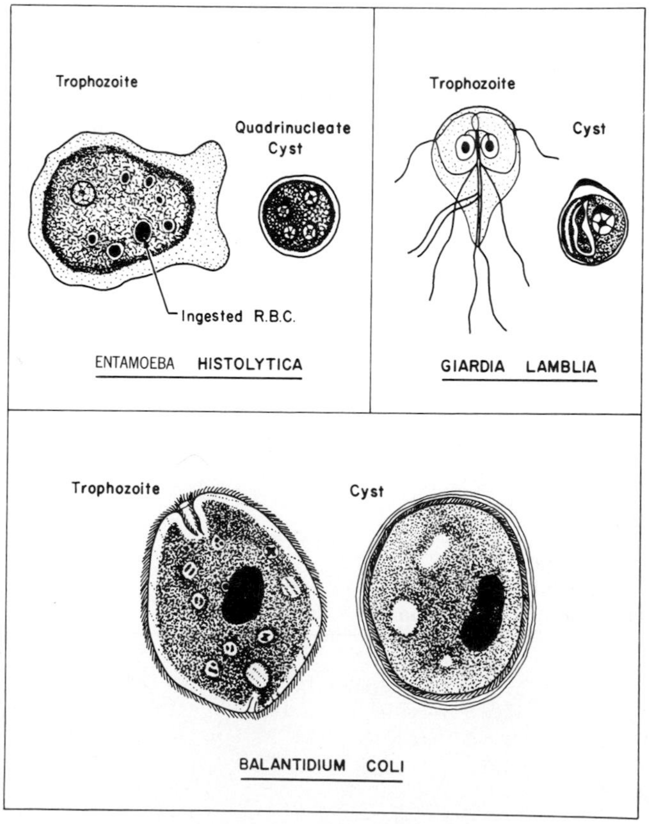

Figure 111–1. Intestinal protozoa.

which allows for the emergence and maintenance of more virulent strains of *E histolytica*. In tropical areas of Africa, Asia, and Latin America, invasive intestinal and extraintestinal amebiasis are major health and social problems in contrast to populations living in temperate climates. Epidemics of amebic dysentery such as the famous Chicago epidemic of 1933 are infrequent and usually water-borne.

Direct inoculation of invasive trophozoites into the skin and mucosa can produce infection. *E histolytica* can be transmitted by sexual practices involving anogenital or oro-anal contact. In the United States, intestinal amebiasis and cutaneous or genital amebiasis have become a problem among homosexual and bisexual men and their female sexual contacts.

E histolytica has two forms. The trophozoite is motile, ingests erythrocytes, and is invasive. The cyst is nonmotile. Cysts are hardy: usual concentrations of chlorine in drinking water, gastric acid, and mild desiccation fail to destroy them. However, prolonged freezing and desiccation and temperatures greater than 68°C will kill them. Cysts are never produced by trophozoites invading tissue. Trophozoites die rapidly when removed from the colon or from tissue.

After ingestion, cysts reach the distal ileum where the cyst capsule is disrupted by intestinal enzymes working in an alkaline environment. The quadrinucleated metacyst divides into four uninucleated trophozoites. They persist as commensals, ingesting bacteria and debris; some undergo encystment. This commensal condition, luminal amebiasis, may persist for extended periods. Most cyst passers are asymptomatic. A variety of complaints has been associated with the presence of cysts in the stool of nondysenteric patients: flatulence, constipation, weight loss, malaise, and even sexual impotence. Transient, limited invasion of the mucosal surface may cause episodic changes in bowel habit.

Conditions that alter the balance among the ameba, the microenvironment of the colonic lumen, and the host favor the emergence of invasive amebiasis. The nature of these conditions is, as yet, poorly understood. Changes in diet and intestinal flora are associated with the development of virulence and invasive disease in experimental animals and humans. Malnutrition and immunosuppression may predispose to severe clinical illness and transform the asymptomatic commensal state into aggressive invasive disease. Some strains of *E histolytica* have greater virulence, possibly through the production of cytotoxic substances that injure host tissues.

Invasive trophozoites produce submucous abscesses. As the trophozoites undermine the colonic mucosa, thrombosis of mucosal and submucosal blood vessels develops, resulting in necrosis and ulceration. Bacterial superinfection causes acute inflammation and the appearance of pus in the stool. Amebic dysentery follows submucosal invasion and mucosal disruption. Despite rectal urgency, cramps, flatulence, low-grade fever, and the passage of five to 15 purulent, bloody, or blood-tinged, mucousal stools, patients with amebic dysentery may not seem as ill-appearing as patients with bacillary dysentery.

Transmural involvement of the colon produces amebic colitis. Peritonitis may follow extrusion of trophozoites from transmural infections or from localized colonic perforation. When trophozoite invasion becomes transmural, patients become abruptly and critically ill. Abdominal distention and signs of peritonitis are present. Fever is usually greater than 103°F and the patient appears toxic. Severe abdominal cramps and tenesmus accompany the profuse diarrhea—up to 30 bloody, mucoid stools per day. Large areas of bowel surface may be sloughed as mucosal casts. The clinical

TABLE 111–4. PATHOPHYSIOLOGY OF INTESTINAL PROTOZOAN INFECTION

Site	Clinical Syndromes	Organisms
Luminal Infections	Asymptomatic carriage	*Entamoeba histolytica* *Giardia lamblia* *Balantidium coli*
Infection Confined to Epithelium of Mucosa		
Superficial mucositis	Diarrheal syndromes	*E histolytica* *G lamblia* *B coli*
Erosive mucositis	Dysentery	*E histolytica* *B coli*
Infection Extended Beyond Mucosa		*E histolytica* *B coli*
Ulceration		
Abscess formation	Ameboma Typhlitis	
Perforation with local and/or metastatic spread	Peritonitis Liver abscess	

picture may be confused with toxic megacolon from ulcerative colitis or serious postpartum pelvic infection with peritonitis or septic pelvic thrombophlebitis. Fatalities are common, especially if the diagnosis of *E histolytica* infection is missed and the patient is operated on for suspected obstruction or toxic megacolon. Fulminant amebic colitis may have no prodrome of amebic dysentery. This appears to be especially true in term pregnant patients living in areas of highly prevalent endemic infection.

Localization of trophozoites through an exuberant fibroplastic and granulomatous response can produce mucosal thickening of the bowel wall, the so-called ameboma. Amebomas present clinically with fever, weight loss, cramps, signs of partial bowel obstruction, and a firm painful mass often palpable on an abdominal or rectal examination. Amebomas may be confused with tuberculosis, regional enteritis, or carcinoma. Rarely, ameboma may mimic the findings of acute pelvic inflammatory disease with tubo-ovarian abscess and symptoms of perirectal irritation with urgency and tenesmus. As with amebic colitis, patients with undiagnosed ameboma brought to operation fare poorly.

Entrance of trophozoites from colonic foci into the portal circulation presumably is not an infrequent occurrence. Most of the time, the reticuloendothelial cells and cellular immune response eliminate these metastatic organisms. Occasionally, trophozoites may successfully infect the liver, producing an abscess and a focus from which bloodborne metastasis of trophozoites to other viscera may occur. Amebic liver abscess is characterized by septic fever, hepatic tenderness and enlargement, and referred pain to the back or shoulder. Jaundice is not common.

Metastasis of trophozoites to the liver is more likely to occur in the relatively asymptomatic patient before vigorous host immune and inflammatory responses confine the organism to the colonic mucosa. Liver abscess follows symptomatic dysentery in only one of 50 patients. Amebic abscess is predominantly a male illness: males are affected seven times more frequently than women. Liver abscess originating during pregnancy is unusual.[16,17]

Effects of Pregnancy. The biology of pregnancy does not influence the acquisition of amebic infection. However, food, hygienic, or sexual practices associated with pregnancy may expose the woman to cyst-contaminated food or drink or to infective trophozoites. Pregnancy is capable of magnifying the severity of amebiasis. Corticosteroids and progesterone have been shown to exacerbate experimental infections in animals. Increased concentrations of serum cholesterol may favor the growth of the parasite. Diminished gastrointestinal tone and motility may allow greater concentrations of trophozoites to accumulate in and to migrate away from the colonic lumen.

There is an association between invasive amebic infection (dysentery and colitis) and pregnancy. Compared to nonpregnant West African females of similar age, amebiasis is a more frequent cause of death during pregnancy and during the first postpartum week. During pregnancy and the immediate postpartum period, asymptomatic or clinically subacute amebiasis can erupt into fulminant, sometimes fatal, colitis with peritonitis.[18-22]

E histolytica is not known to cause intrauterine and fetal infection because it rarely escapes from the colon and from the portal circulation. However, there is evidence that invasive amebiasis during pregnancy may have an adverse effect on the fetus and the successful completion of the pregnancy.[18] Amebic dysentery and colitis, especially when accompanied by subserosal infection or localized bowel perforation, may produce pelvic peritoneal scarring and adhesions that may adversely affect fertility or predispose to ectopic pregnancy.

Neonates are at risk for acquiring the organism by ingesting cysts on maternal skin or from contaminated food. Amebic infections in children under the age of six months are not common, suggesting that some protecting factors, possibly passively transferred maternal antibodies or secretory antibodies in breast milk, are present.[23]

Diagnosis. The clinician's suspicion should be heightened when seeing a history of residence in or visitation to areas of endemic infection with *E histolytica*. Episodic diarrhea with mucous, pus, blood, and rectal urgency or tenesmus suggests amebiasis.

Asymptomatic patients with suspicious illness history and travel background should have stool, even normally formed stool, examined for cysts by appropriate flotation and concentration techniques. For symptomatic patients, it is best to examine the mucus from a fresh stool for motile, hematophagous trophozoites. Identification of *E histolytica* cysts and trophozoites can be difficult for the inexperienced observer. Always have the specimen examined by an experienced physician, parasitologist, or technician.

Invasive colonic and extracolonic infection is accompanied by an antibody response. Serologic tests—immunodiffusion, indirect hemagglutination, and gel precipitation—are positive in over 90% of patients with invasive disease. Asymptomatic cyst passers have positive serologic tests if they have had episodes of invasive disease in the past. Antibody titers may remain elevated for years.

Management of the Pregnant Patient. Optimum management during pregnancy includes early diagnosis and treatment. Special attention needs to be given to nutrition and hygiene. In areas of high prevalence and endemicity, treatment is promptly followed by reinfection. Without adequate nutrition and sanitation, drug therapy of asymptomatic cyst passage or mildly symptomatic dysentery is often futile. In some settings, it may be useful to remove the gravid patient from the unsafe environment.

E histolytica can multiply at three sites: the lumen of the colon, the submucosa of the colon, and extraintestinal tissues. Drug therapy must be aimed to the site of infection and parasite reproduction (Tables 111–4, 111–5, and 111–6). Poorly absorbed drugs will be effective only in the lumen of the colon. Well-absorbed, tissue-active drugs may be ineffective against luminal infections because of the inadequate concentrations in the contents of the gut lumen. Some experts, therefore, recommend that a minimum of two drugs be used for any patient with amebiasis: a luminally active and a tissue-active agent. Because well-absorbed, tissue-active drugs have potential risk to the fetus, drug treatment of the pregnant patient must be carefully individualized.

Every pregnant patient with amebiasis warrants careful consideration for treatment, regardless of paucity of symptoms or adverse clinical effects. Some agents such as the tetracyclines are contraindicated during pregnancy. Other agents such as metronidazole, emetine, dehydroemetine, and chloroquine should be used with great caution and only when serous invasive disease threatens the health of the mother and the success of the pregnancy.

If the risk of reinfection can be minimized, luminal amebiasis and mild dysentery in pregnant patients should be treated with paromomycin. Paromomycin is a poorly absorbed aminoglycoside antibiotic that is active against the gut bacteria necessary for *E histolytica* to persist and against luminal amebae. The dose is 500 mg three times a day for 7 to 10 days. Other luminally active drugs include diiodohydroxyquin and diloxanide furorate. Both have been used successfully during pregnancy, but neither is recommended as first-choice agents for treating amebiasis in the pregnant patient.

TABLE 111–5. MANAGEMENT OF AMEBIASIS DURING PREGNANCY

For Luminal or Mild (afebrile, fewer than five stools per day) Dysentery
- Luminally active agents only—paromomycin, erythromycin, diiodohydroxyquin
- Careful follow-up stool examination for the remainder of pregnancy

For Amebic Dysentery (more than five stools with blood and/or mucous per day, constitutional symptoms)
- Luminally active agent
- Tissue-active agents—chloroquine
- Careful follow-up stool examination for the remainder of pregnancy

For Serious Invasive Disease—amebic colitis, ameboma, extraintestinal infection
- Luminally active agent, especially if dysentery is present
- Tissue-active agent—metronidazole
- Careful follow-up stool examination for the remainder of pregnancy

TABLE 111–6. RECOMMENDED DRUGS FOR AMEBIASIS DURING PREGNANCY

Luminal and mild dysentery	Paromomycin 30 mg/kg per day in 3 doses for 5–10 days
Dysentery (greater than five stools/day)	Paromomycin 30 mg/kg per day in 3 doses for 5–10 days Chloroquine phosphate 1 g daily for 2 days, then 0.5 g daily for 10–14 days
Colitis, ameboma, visceral abscess	Paromomycin 30 mg/kg per day in 3 doses for 5–10 days Metronidazole 750 mg TID for 7–10 days (or another nitroimidazole)

The pregnant patient with amebic dysentery passing mucus and blood in excess of five movements a day and with fever and constitutional symptoms should be treated with at least two drugs: one active against trophozoites in the lumen and superficial mucosa, and the other active against the trophozoites invading the deeper layers of the colon and possibly other viscera. The luminal agent can be paromomycin, erythromycin, or diiodohydroxyquin. Many experts recommend metronidazole or other nitroimidazoles as the tissue-active or extraluminal drug. Although metronidazole has been used without ill effect in a large number of pregnancies, it has been shown to be mutagenic. The carcinogenic and teratogenic risks, although hypothetical in humans[24], are sufficient to warrant cautious deliberation before using metronidazole to treat moderate amebic dysentery during pregnancy. Chloroquine phosphate in a dose of 1 g daily for two days and then 0.5 g daily for two to three weeks can be used instead of metronidazole. Because pregnancy has been associated with acceleration and exacerbation of amebic dysentery, it is wisest to treat the patient even though the treatment has risks. After completion of therapy, the physician should reevaluate the patient's condition. In the absence of persistent or metastatic infection, additional therapy can be withheld. The patient should then be monitored at frequent intervals for evidence of recurrent metastatic amebic infection.

Patients with ameboma, hepatitis, hepatic abscess, or amebic colitis are seriously ill. Therapy even with potentially harmful drugs is mandatory. Metronidazole is used in a dose of 750 mg three times a day for seven to 10 days. Chloroquine phosphate can also be used. A third group of tissue-active drugs, emetine and dehydroemetine, possess considerable cardiac toxicity. Under certain circumstances, however, their use is justified. Visceral abscesses often require drainage, as well as chemotherapy for maximally effective treatment. This should be carried out by needle aspiration. Many patients with extraintestinal amebiasis will have persistent cyst passage consistent with luminal amebiasis. It has been the author's practice to treat all pregnant patients with serious extraintestinal disease or ameboma and colitis with both a tissue-active and a luminally-active drug.

Giardiasis. Infection of the proximal small intestine by the flagellate *G lamblia* produces an illness spectrum ranging from no symptoms to severe diarrhea with malabsorption and weight loss.[25,26] *G lamblia* is transmitted by the fecal-oral route. The cysts may be spread by water and by direct contact. The organism can be maintained in rodents, dogs, and beavers. It causes human infection on all five continents and almost all islands habited by humans. Epidemics are usually waterborne. Acquisition of the parasite has been particularly common in some cities in Europe and North America and in areas with poor sanitation. The importance of direct person-to-person transmission of *Giardia* is illustrated by outbreaks of the disease in daycare centers and among homosexual men. About one quarter of healthy people exposed to *G lamblia* by visiting an endemic area will become infected. The risk of infection is directly proportional to the duration of exposure and the number of cysts ingested. Achlorhydria and immunodeficiency enhance the risk of acquiring infection.

In the United States, *G lamblia* is the most commonly detected intestinal parasite, occurring in 3–9% of stool specimens sent for parasitologic examination. Infection of pregnant women is, therefore, not uncommon. Serious clinical illness among pregnant women with *Giardia* infection has heretofore been rarely diagnosed. Recognition of giardiasis as a widespread clinical problem for practicing physicians is a recent event. Case reports and the author's personal experience since 1970 indicate an upward trend in the diagnosis of giardiasis as a cause of gastrointestinal disease in pregnant patients from the United States.

The geographic ubiquity of *Giardia* and the focality of human disease suggests that there is variation in virulence of various isolates of *Giardia*. Host factors play an important role in clinical manifestations and epidemiology. Experimental human infections have demonstrated a protective immune response. Cellular immunity, circulating immunoglobulins, and secretory immunoglobulins have been described. Breast milk contains protective factors, which may help explain the rarity of *Giardia* infection in infants under six months of age.[27] Among Southeast Asian refugees in Thailand, maternal giardiasis is common; however, cases of giardiasis in infants were not seen until four to seven months of age when weaning usually took place.[8]

The trophozoites reside in the small intestine, where they may attach to the epithelial surface by a ventral disk-shaped structure. The trophozoite may detach itself from the epithelial microvilli and insert itself between epithelial cells. It does not penetrate beyond the lamina propria. As trophozoites move caudally, they undergo encystation and are passed in the feces.

There is considerable evidence for malfunction of the small intestinal epithelium in giardiasis.[26] Temporary disaccharidase deficiency and fat and vitamin B_{12} malabsorption have been described in both human and animal infections. The mechanisms of injury to the epithelial cell are not clearly defined. Cultured *Giardia* trophozoites produce cytotoxic substances. The attachment of the trophozoite to the epithelial cell surface produces morphologic abnormalities of the microvilli, which may result in digestive dysfunction. A mononuclear cell inflammatory response proportional to the intensity of the infection and the quantity of organisms present is elicited in the submucosa. The association of giardiasis with nodular lymphoid hyperplasia of the small intestine and IgA immunoglobulin deficiency is well documented. Persistent and resistant *Giardia* infection should serve as the stimulus to search for underlying immunologic or gastrointestinal disarray.

The symptoms of giardiasis are preeminently abdominal (Table 111–7); however, a surprisingly large number of adult patients complain bitterly about malaise, fatigue, and lassitude. Illness beginning within a week or two after infection may present suddenly with flatulence; nausea; anorexia; abdominal distention; and explosive, watery, odoriferous diarrhea. Blood, pus, and mucus in the stools are rarely found. The white blood cell count is usually not elevated or shifted to the left. Most patients with early onset disease complain of cramps, borborygmi, and malaise even in the absence of diarrhea. Fever is unusual and never more than low grade. Febrile diarrhea suggests amebiasis or bacterial disease.

TABLE 111–7. COMMON SYMPTOMS OF PARASITOLOGICALLY DOCUMENTED GIARDIASIS

	Frequency of Symptoms (%)
Diarrhea	50–80
Abdominal pain	40–70
Flatulence	45–65
Nausea	20–55
Anorexia	15–70
Weight loss	30–60
Vomiting	15–30
Weakness	10–75

Most patients resolve the acute, early onset episode in a few days or a week. A few patients may continue to have serious gastrointestinal and constitutional symptoms with progressive weight loss, dehydration, and electrolyte imbalance. In the usual case, the infection proceeds to a subacute or chronic state in which asymptomatic periods are interspersed with episodes of belching, embarrassingly foul flatulence, borborygmi, abdominal cramps, and loose bulky stools. These episodes may recur for years with minimal adverse effects on the health of a relatively asymptomatic cyst passer.

The immunologic perturbations of pregnancy, theoretically, are capable of allowing a stable asymptomatic carrier state to convert into more injurious clinical disease. This has not been unequivocally demonstrated in human or animal infections. Giardiasis has not been shown to be injurious during pregnancy beyond causing adverse nutritional and constitutional impact on the mother.

Acute *Giardia* infection during pregnancy can have serious adverse effects on maternal nutrition. A heavy parasite burden may compete for essential micronutrients, such as folic acid and vitamin B_{12}, as well as interfere with digestion and absorption of essential nutrients, such as disaccharides, essential fatty acids, fat-soluble vitamins, and amino acids. Continuation of severe acute disease beyond a few days with weight loss, malabsorption, ketosis, and fluid and electrolyte imbalance necessitates not only vigorous supportive therapy but also antiparasitic chemotherapy during pregnancy.

Subacute or chronic disease may plague the pregnant patient and her obstetrician. Recurrent bouts of vague gastrointestinal distress and lassitude may be attributed to morning sickness or psychosomatic problems. Subacute, chronic, or recurrent infection may prevent adequate weight gain and may exaggerate the nutritional effects of pregnancy, amplifying iron and folic acid needs and, thus, enhancing the appearance of anemia. Persistent nausea and vomiting with weight loss and ketosis may be mistakenly attributed to hyperemesis gravidarum.

Giardiasis should be suspected in all cases of prolonged abdominal illness, especially during pregnancy when nutritional demands are increased. In acute early infection or recrudescent chronic infection, motile trophozoites and cysts may be seen in the stool. Fixation and concentration techniques may be necessary, particularly in asymptomatic cases. Because cyst passage in chronic infection is usually intermittent, several stool examinations over several weeks should be obtained. Patients with abdominal complaints, but without parasites demonstrable in stool, should have small bowel or duodenal samples, obtained by aspiration through a nasogastric tube, by small intestinal biopsy, or by use of a string, examined for trophozoites. There are no widely available, reliable serologic tests for *G lamblia* infection.

Difficulties in providing safe, effective therapy for intestinal protozoan infections during pregnancy have reawakened interest in the aminoglycoside antibiotic paromomycin, first used to treat amebiasis in 1959. Clinical reports since the early 1960s indicate that this agent is effective against both *E histolytica* and *G lamblia,* as well as tapeworms and a wide array of anaerobic and aerobic bacteria. It is poorly absorbed. Early studies failed to demonstrate any antibacterial activity in the plasma of subjects receiving 2 g per day for as long as 50 days. Paromomycin should be the first drug selected to treat the pregnant patient with giardiasis (Table 111–8).[25] If possible, and always in the asymptomatic or mildly ill patient, the clinician is advised to delay drug treatment until after the completion of the first trimester.

In the nonpregnant patient, metronidazole or other nitroimidazoles are the treatment of choice. Quinacrine and furazolidone are alternate agents. All are effective in 80–90% or more of patients. They are absorbed from the gastrointestinal tract and cross the placenta in varying proportions. None of these agents is without potential hazard during pregnancy. Furazolidone is associated with mammary neoplasia in rats. Quinacrine often causes gastrointestinal upset. It is slowly metabolized and excreted and may accumulate in tissues. Despite widespread, apparently safe usage in pregnancy during the 1940s and 1950s prior to the advent of safer antimalarial compounds, quinacrine should not be used during pregnancy without compelling indications.

As with quinacrine, metronidazole has been used widely and safely during pregnancy. However, it is mutagenic in bacteria, has been associated with carcinogenesis in laboratory rodents, and is presumed to be teratogenic. Despite the uniform success of metronidazole in low doses for giardiasis, it should be used during pregnancy with cautious deliberation only after the first trimester, only when less potentially toxic therapy has failed, and only when the pregnancy is in jeopardy. Metronidazole is remarkably effective against a variety of protozoan parasites, and single session treatment for trichomoniasis has become increasingly popular. Such a therapeutic approach minimizes some of the adverse effects of the drug. Single session metronidazole treatment with a 2 g oral dose has eradicated symptomatic giardiasis in a small, uncontrolled trial among Laotian and Cambodian refugees in two Thailand refugee camps.

TABLE 111–8. RECOMMENDED DRUGS FOR GIARDIASIS DURING PREGNANCY

First-line agent	Paromomycin, 30 mg/kg per day divided into 3 doses for 5–10 days
Agents of last resort	Metronidazole, 250 mg TID for 5–10 days
	Quinacrine, 100 mg TID for 3–10 days

Treatment of the asymptomatic cyst passer can be delayed until after delivery, if careful observation of the mother can be maintained. Whether such patients require therapy at all is, in part, determined by the living conditions of the family. In endemic areas with poor sanitation and hygiene, treatment of asymptomatic chronic infection is of little lasting value because reinfection is the rule.

Because of nutritional and direct effects of *G lamblia* on the intestinal epithelial cells, recovery of normal digestive function may lag behind eradication of the parasite. Lactose and fat intolerance may persist for months. Continuing attention to diet is, therefore, essential even in the treated patient. Because the patient may continue to have gastrointestinal symptoms, it is wise to repeat stool examinations for trophozoites and cysts on several occasions following therapy.

Balantidium Coli. *B coli* is the only ciliate and the largest protozoan parasite pathogenic for man. Swine are regarded as the principal reservoir and the most common source of human infection. However, it is a cosmopolitan organism inhabiting the gastrointestinal tract of a large number of mammals, birds, and some arthropods, including the cockroach.[28]

Among residents of communities with poor sanitation and hygiene in the western hemisphere, asymptomatic infection is common. Symptoms and pathology indistinguishable from those of amebic dysentery are seen in individuals with primary infection or recrudescent chronic infection. Balantidial peritonitis following perforation of colonic ulcers and balantidial vaginitis have been reported. Typhlitis and partial intestinal obstruction may supervene upon the asymptomatic carrier state. No cases in pregnancy have been described; however, in endemic areas, *B coli* is one of the organisms to be considered as a cause of dysentery symptoms in pregnant patients. Trophozoites and cysts are unmistakable because of their size. Paromomycin is effective and should be used to treat the pregnant patient. Metronidazole is also effective.

Protozoan Parasites Sexually Reproducing in the Gastrointestinal Tract

In contrast to the organisms asexually reproducing in the gastrointestinal tract, protozoa sexually reproducing in gastrointestinal epithelium, such as *Toxoplasma gondii,* are a threat to both mother and fetus. These parasites are transmitted by ingestion of oocysts or tissue cysts, which liberate invasive trophozoites that may circulate in the blood and penetrate numerous organs, including the placenta and fetus. They can infect herbivorous, carnivorous, and omnivorous animals including all orders of mammals and some birds. They are common wherever human beings live in close contact with their domestic animals. Some species are capable of sexually reproducing only in a specific definitive host. Others are less rigorous in their requirements for the sexual phase of their life. Most can infect many other animals, the intermediate hosts, for the asexual phase.

Toxoplasmosis. There are three infective stages in the life cycle of *T gondii:* the tachyzoite, the tissue cyst, and the oocyst.[29]

Tachyzoites are the agents of the acute stages of infection and can invade many kinds of mammalian cells. Once within a cell, the tachyzoite multiplies until the cell lyses and releases the invasive daughter tachyzoites. These may infect other cells and may remain viable in extracellular secretions such as peritoneal fluid, milk, urine, saliva, and tears for many hours. They may be transmitted by blood transfusion and needle sticks. Tachyzoites are not able to survive freezing and thawing, desiccation, or digestive juices.

The tissue cyst is formed within host cells, which for reasons as yet unclear, are not disrupted by the growing parasite. Tissue cysts may be found as soon as the eighth day of infection and are presumed to persist, containing viable parasites, throughout the life of the host. Brain and striated muscle are the most frequent sites of tissue cyst persistence, although they can be found in virtually every organ. Freezing and thawing, desiccation, and cooking destroy the tissue cyst. Following ingestion of viable tissue cysts, the cyst wall is destroyed by peptic digestion. The liberated parasite may be viable for several hours of exposure to digestive juices, long enough to allow invasion of the host by way of the digestive tract.

The sexual cycle of the organism takes place only in felines, the definitive hosts. Following invasion of the gastrointestinal epithelium by trophozoites liberated from oocysts of tissue cysts, the parasite goes through an enteroepithelial asexual cycle (schizogony), followed by the sexual cycle (gametogony). Oocysts are not infectious until they undergo sporogony, which takes place outside the body after the oocysts are shed in the feces. Oocysts do not sporulate below 4°C or above 37°C. They are remarkably resistant to a variety of biochemical and physical agents and, under favorable conditions, may remain infectious for as long as one year. The sporozoites formed in the oocysts are infective for man and a wide array of domestic animals.

Early infection is almost always accompanied by parasitemia. In immunocompetent hosts, acquired infection is usually not obvious clinically. The most commonly recognized illness is lymphadenopathy, which may be accompanied by fever, malaise, splenomegaly, and skin rash. The adenopathy may be localized or generalized; characteristically, the posterior cervical chain is involved. The lymph nodes are not usually tender and do not suppurate. Atypical lymphocytosis may occur, indistinguishable from that found in patients with mononucleosis caused by Epstein–Barr virus or cytomegalovirus. The atypical lymphocytosis is usually transient but the lymphadenopathy may persist for months. As the acute illness subsides, host responses confine the parasite to tissue cysts. Intrauterine infection is possible only when the mother has active toxoplasmosis with circulating tachyzoites. The risk of intrauterine fetal infection is confined to nonimmune mothers experiencing their primary infection and, rarely, to latently infected immunoincompetent mothers experiencing reactivation.

Immunodeficiency may alter the balance between host and parasite, which allows for the disruption of tissue cysts and release of infective trophozoites into the circulation. Reactivation of latent infection requires serious disruption of immune function. Pregnancy is not known to cause reactivation of latent *Toxoplasma* infection.

T gondii infection is common; clinical disease is uncommon. The clinical manifestations of infection are determined by the size of the inoculum, by the immune status of the host, and possibly by differences in virulence among strains of *Toxoplasma*. The most severe acute disease occurs in immunosuppressed or immunoimmature hosts such as patients with AIDS, malignancies or transplants, and fetuses of less than five or six months of gestation.

The importance of toxoplasmosis to obstetricians resides in the ability of the organism to produce parasitemia and intrauterine infection while causing clinically vague or silent infection in the mother.

Epidemiology. *T gondii* is a global zoonotic parasite of felines. All species of cat may be infected. The domestic cat is the greatest source of human infection; however, tribal hunters of wild cats (jaguars, lions, leopards) that do not keep domestic cats also have a high incidence of infection. *T gondii* infection occurs in all mammals and some avian species, especially ground-feeding birds.

The prevalence of *Toxoplasma* specific antibodies varies around the world.[30] The prevalence of antibodies to *Toxoplasma* in pregnant women ranges from 84% in Paris, France, to 12.5% in Oslo, Norway. In New York, London, and Finland, 22–32% of pregnant women have positive serologic tests for *Toxoplasma*.

In the United States, the prevalence of toxoplasmosis ranges from 20% to 70%, depending on the area of the country and style of living, especially the keeping of pets. There is increasing frequency of positive serologic tests with increasing age, regardless of sex. In one national survey, 38% of women of childbearing age had antibodies to *Toxoplasma*.[31] Practitioners can expect that 50–60% of their female patients reaching childbearing status could be susceptible to primary *Toxoplasma* infection.

Several recent studies suggest that common source outbreaks, especially in family and residential groups, are not unusual[32] and that clinical and serologic examination to identify subclinical infection in women of reproductive age in the exposed group is of value. Identification of primary infection can be of importance, even for nonpregnant women, by defining their susceptibility status. For example, we detected acute asymptomatic toxoplasmosis in early pregnancy in a woman without cats, who was riding at a stable that had infected cats associated with several other infections in nonpregnant women.[33]

The incidence of congenital toxoplasmosis is approximately one in 1000 live births in the United States. About 10% of congenitally infected newborns with toxoplasmosis have signs and symptoms of complications of their transplacentally acquired disease. The risk of infection for the fetus and the severity of disease produced by such infection appear to be related to the time during pregnancy when maternal infection occurs.[34] Presumably, the differences in severity of clinical disease in the fetus and neonate depend on the immune capacity of the fetus at the time parasitemia occurs.

Careful studies in France have followed pregnant women who acquired toxoplasmosis before and during pregnancy.[35] Abortion, stillbirth, or severe congenital infection occurred almost exclusively when women had been infected early in pregnancy. However, such severe clinical disease occurred in only 10–15% of such pregnancies. Women infected before conception had no evidence of abortions, stillbirth, or congenital infection caused by *Toxoplasma* species. Among the offspring of 542 women acquiring toxoplasmosis during pregnancy, 61% had evidence of congenital infection.[36] In the affected infants, 6% suffered perinatal death, 5% had severe clinical disease, 9% had mild clinical disease, and 41% had subclinical disease. Abortion, perinatal death, or severe congenital infection occurred almost exclusively in the offspring of women infected early in preg-

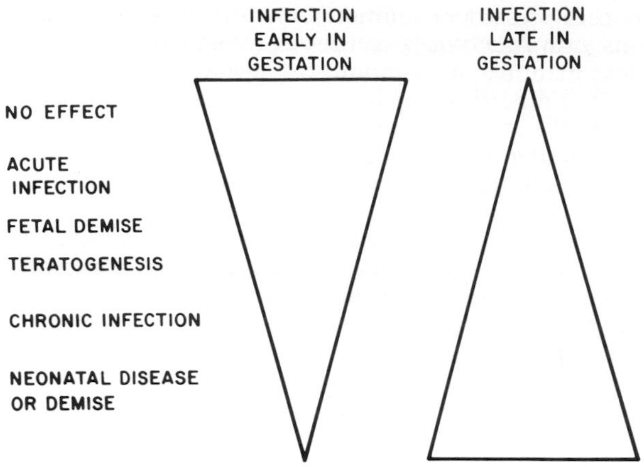

Figure 111–2. The small, developing placenta of early pregnancy is an effective barrier to the transmission of pathogenic microbes from the maternal circulation to the fetus. During early pregnancy, the fetus commonly escapes infection but when infection does occur, the effects are almost always devastating: fetal demise, abortion, dysmorphic growth, and chronic infection with severe residual effects.

As the maternal-placental interface expands and matures, the placental barrier becomes less effective and transplacental infection during maternal parasitemia is more common. The maturing fetal immune response modulates the effects of intrauterine fetal infection so that subclinical infection is more common than with infections in early pregnancy. More neonates are likely to be infected but with less drastic impact when maternal infection occurs in late pregnancy. *From Lee RV[33] with permission.*

nancy. As with other intrauterine infections, the risk of infection for the fetus and the severity of the disease produced are related to the time during pregnancy when maternal and transplacental infection occur (Figure 111–2). If the mother is infected early in pregnancy, transmission to the fetus is uncommon, but the disease produced is severe: abortion, severe congenital infection with teratogenesis, abnormal growth, or disabling residual. Survivors of intrauterine infection early in pregnancy have the most severe residual effects of congenital infection: cerebral calcifications, hydrocephaly or microcephaly, abnormal cerebral spinal fluid, chorioretinitis, seizures, fever, hepatosplenomegaly, and jaundice. Transmission of *Toxoplasma* is most likely when maternal infection is acquired during the last trimester but the illness in the child is more likely to be subclinical. Two thirds of congenitally infected infants have no symptoms and the infection is recognized only by use of serologic tests. The most common finding in the overtly infected neonate is bilateral chorioretinitis. The manifestations of toxoplasmosis in the newborn can mimic infection by virtually any pathogen producing intrauterine disease, especially syphilis, cytomegalovirus, and rubella. Because so many maternal infections are asymptomatic and do not produce obvious clinical manifestations in the neonate, no reliable data have been assembled to predict the outcome of infants with subclinical or asymptomatic congenital *Toxoplasma* infection.

There is evidence that some chronically infected mothers may have foci of *Toxoplasma* in the uterus. Whether this may result in congenital infection of the fetus or abortion is not clear. There is no conclusive evidence from animal or human studies that *Toxoplasma* can cause abortion in chronically infected females.

Diagnosis. Isolation of the organism from blood or biopsy tissue by animal inoculation or by direct microscopic identification is the most direct diagnostic method. Animal inoculation techniques are not readily available except in hospitals with active research laboratories.

Because of the difficulties in demonstrating the organism directly, serologic techniques (Table 111–9) have become the mainstay of clinical diagnosis.[37] The most commonly used serologic tests are the Sabin–Feldman dye test, the complement fixation (CF) test, the indirect fluorescent antibody (IFA) test, and enzyme-linked immunosorbent assays (ELISA). They measure antibodies that begin to rise within one to three weeks after infection. Complement-fixing antibodies appear later than those demonstrated by the dye test and IFA test; complement fixation tests become positive three to six weeks after infection.

The indirect fluorescent antibody test can be modified to demonstrate IgM antibodies, which begin to increase within the first week of infection. Antitoxoplasma IgM can also be demonstrated by the recently developed ELISA. Antitoxoplasma IgG may persist in titers of 1:16 to 1:256 for the lifetime of an infected individual. IgM levels usually begin to decline several months after the resolution of the acute infection.

The diagnosis of acute acquired toxoplasmosis is established by the demonstration of rising serologic titers. A single measurement of antitoxoplasma IgG does not confirm the diagnosis. The absence of IgM *Toxoplasma* antibody probably excludes the diagnosis of acute toxoplasmosis in an immunologically healthy patient. A rising IgM fluorescent antibody titer or a titer of 1:512 or more appears to correlate well with recent onset of infection. Rheumatoid factors and antinuclear antibodies may cause false-positive indirect immunofluorescence tests for IgM.

T gondii was isolated by mouse inoculation from amniotic fluid obtained by amniocentesis and from placenta obtained later after prostaglandin-induced abortion in one

TABLE 111–9. DIAGNOSTIC METHODS FOR TOXOPLASMOSIS

Serologic Tests
- Sabin–Feldman dye test (DT)
  - Measures IgG antibodies which appear within 1–2 weeks of illness onset, increase for six to eight weeks, and then persist in slowly declining titer for years. Titer does not correlate with severity of illness or risk to pregnancy.
  - Specific and sensitive
  - Indirect immunofluorescence (IFA)
  - Measures IgG and IgM antibodies.
  - False positive IgM results from antinuclear antibodies and rheumatoid factors.
  - IgG lasts for years. IgM slowly declines.
  - Complement fixation (CF)
  - Measures IgG antibodies.
  - Becomes positive several weeks later than DT or IFA, variable duration of positive test.
  - Enzyme-linked immunosorbent assay (ELISA)
  - Measures both IgG and IgM antibodies.
  - Similar time course as IFA.
- Demonstration of Antigens
  - Isolation of *Toxoplasmosis gondii* in mice or tissue culture.
  - ELISA tests for membrane antigens.

case report.[38] No organisms were seen in cytologic or histologic preparations. The patient was one of 37 people in a common source epidemic and was shown by serologic tests to have acute toxoplasmosis. The French Toxoplasmosis Research Group was able to isolate *Toxoplasma* from fetal blood obtained by chordocentesis or amniotic fluid or both in nine women with serologic evidence of recent primary toxoplasmosis.[39] Amniocentesis and chordocentesis may be useful in identifying fetal infection if parasitologic studies, including animal inoculation, are carefully done.

The fetus born of an infected mother is likely to have passively transferred IgG antibodies producing positive indirect fluorescent antibody tests, Sabin–Feldman dye tests, and complement fixation tests. If the fetus has been infected *in utero,* it will produce IgM antibodies measured by the IgM IFA and may have an elevation of the total IgM. The presence of antitoxoplasma IgM and the persistence of positive IgG tests, indicating that the fetus has begun to produce antitoxoplasma IgG, is diagnostic for congenital toxoplasmosis.

Management. Otherwise healthy nonpregnant immunocompetent adults are not given antibiotics unless symptoms or organ involvement are severe. Progressive illness, cerebritis, or ocular infection suggest immune compromise and can be treated with sulfonamides, pyrimethamine, trimethoprim, clindamycin, or a combination.[30]

The clinician has three questions to ask about each pregnant patient: (1) is the patient susceptible and not infected?, (2) does the patient have an inactive, latent infection?, and (3) does the patient have a recent, active infection potentially hazardous to the fetus? Diagnosis usually depends on serologic tests, chiefly the indirect fluorescent antibody tests for antitoxoplasma IgG and IgM. The Sabin–Feldman dye test and newer ELISA tests may be used but most contemporary protocols for serodiagnosis emphasize the IgG and IgM IFA tests. Because the rise and fall of antitoxoplasma antibodies vary from case to case, it is best to follow the results of two or more sets of tests. The probability of recent infection is high if the IgM titer is high (200 IU/ml or 1:512 or more). The probability of recent infection is highest if the IgG titer is 1:1024 (1000 IU/mL) or more and the IgM titer is 1:256 or more. Table 111–10 provides the author's recommendations for obtaining and interpreting *Toxoplasma* serologies in the pregnant patient.

When recent or active infection is documented, the patient and her physicians have three options. First, if infection occurs early in pregnancy and obstetric and ethical circumstances permit, the patient may elect to terminate the pregnancy. Second, careful evaluation of the fetus, including amniocentesis and chordocentesis, can be established. If the fetus is thriving and no evidence of infection is found, therapy could be withheld. If infection is demonstrated, therapy or termination would be indicated. The third option is to treat presumptively with or without attempts to document fetal infection.

The macrolide antibiotic, spiramycin, has been widely used in Europe and has reduced the risk of fetal infection by as much as 50%.[30,40,41] Spiramycin reaches high concentrations in the placenta and has not proven to be teratogenic in humans. Some centers have added pyrimethamine, a sulfonamide, and folinic acid supplements when fetal infection has been proven. The standard dose of spiramycin is 3 g per day. It can be given in an interrupted course: three weeks of therapy alternating with two weeks off therapy. It can be given continuously until delivery.

Preconception toxoplasmosis testing and counseling are useful components of routine health care for childbearing women. A nonpregnant woman found to have antibody to *Toxoplasma* can be reassured about the rarity of intrauterine fetal infection when she does conceive. A woman found to be susceptible should be advised to avoid cats, cat litter, and uncooked meat, and urged to have repeat serologic tests performed during pregnancy (Table 111–11). As with rubella, all physicians share an obligation to alert women to the risks of toxoplasmosis and to pursue epidemiologic detection of cases. The purpose of preconception and prenatal screening of susceptible women is to reduce the risk of acute maternal infection with the attendant risk of congenital infection and to identify the acutely infected mother soon enough to choose acceptable management options.

TABLE 111–10. MANAGEMENT STRATEGY FOR TOXOPLASMA SEROLOGIC TESTING DURING PREGNANCY[33]

1	Serologic testing preferably before conception of the first prenatal visit.	2
2a	If negative IgG, retest at 18–22 weeks.	6
2b	If positive IgG, immediately repeat tests including IgG and IgM.	3
3a	If IgG positive, stable, or low titer, IgM negative, suspect old or preconception exposure. Repeat tests in 2–4 weeks.	4
3b	If IgG positive, any titer, IgM positive, suspect recent exposure. Repeat tests in 2–4 weeks.	5
4a	If repeat IgG positive, titer stable, IgM negative, confirm old exposure. No further testing necessary.	—
4b	If repeat IgG positive, titer rising, IgM positive, suspect recent exposure. Repeat tests in 2–4 weeks.	5
5a	If repeat IgG and IgM positive (stable or declining titer), suspect recent exposure 2–6 months before tests obtained. Treat according to gestational age at time of presumed infection and according to patient wishes.	—
5b	If repeat IgG and IgM positive with rising titers, suspect active recent infection. Treat according to gestational age and patient wishes.	—
6a	If repeat serologic tests negative, repeat tests at 36 weeks.	—
6b	If repeat serologic tests positive, retest as in 3.	3

From Lee RV.[33]

Other Protozoa Sexually Reproducing in the Gastrointestinal Mucosa

Species of *Isospora, Sarcocystis,* and Cryptosporidia can infect the human intestinal epithelium. Most of these organisms infect domestic animals or other creatures residing in human habitations: rats, mice, cattle, sheep, swine, dogs, and cats.

TABLE 111–11. PREVENTING *TOXOPLASMA* INFECTION DURING PREGNANCY

Avoid contact with cats, cat feces, cat litter boxes, and bedding, or sandboxes used by cats.

Avoid travel to areas with endemic toxoplasmosis.

Use gloves when gardening or cleaning.

Cook meat thoroughly (minimum 66°C).

Avoid handling raw meat; do not touch mucous membranes or eyes if handling raw meat.

Keep kitchen and cooking areas scrupulously clean, especially after processing raw meat.

In humans, these infections are characterized primarily by self-limited diarrheal disease in immunocompetent hosts and protracted, disabling diarrhea in immunocompromised patients. However, tissue cysts of Cryptosporidia and *Sarcocystis* have been identified in human tissues, suggesting the potential for intrauterine infection if the infection is acquired during pregnancy. Increasing awareness of this group of organisms because of their serious effects in immunodeficiency disorders, especially AIDS, will surely be followed by more clinical reports including infections in gravid women.

Cryptosporidiosis

Cryptosporidium is a common cause of diarrhea around the world. Animal-to-human and human-to-human transmissions occur. The fecal-oral route of transmission is well documented and direct inoculation by way of anogenital and orogenital sexual activity is presumed. Diagnosis is best accomplished by direct examination of wet preparations of fresh stool. A variety of staining procedures have been used to identify *Cryptosporidium* oocysts.

In immunocompetent adults, the clinical manifestations range from asymptomatic infection to explosive watery diarrhea and constitutional symptoms which resolve after 10–14 days. Fever and leukocytosis are uncommon: eosinophilia suggests the coexistence of metazoan intestinal parasites. Transient lactose and fat malabsorption may occur.

The immunocompromised patients' clinical manifestations usually have an insidious onset with escalation of severity as the immune defect progresses. Inanition and voluminous diarrhea are common in AIDS patients. Patients receiving immunosuppressive drugs will improve with deduction or cessation of treatment. Pregnancy, by itself, has not yet been identified as an immunologic risk for progressive or severe cryptosporidiosis.

There is, as yet, no reliable therapy.

Isosporidiosis

Isospora belli, like *Cryptosporidium*, can cause self-limited diarrheal disease in immunocompetent patients and protracted illness in immunocompromised patients. Unlike *Cryptosporidium*, *Isospora* responds to sulfonamides and pyrimethamine, or the combination.[42]

BLOOD AND TISSUE PROTOZOA

Diseases caused by infections with species of Plasmodia, *Leishmania*, and *Trypanosoma* (Figure 111–3) have special importance to the obstetrician because of their capacity to produce intrauterine infection, as well as to disable the mother and to destroy her reproductive potential. Their life cycle includes arthropod vectors and the capacity to persist in the human host for long periods of time. The distribution and prevalence of human disease is determined by the availability of suitable vectors. In the United States, these infections are considered exotic and rare, whereas across much of the earth, they are common causes of serious illness.

Pneumocystis carinii has emerged as an epidemic pathogen in the immunologically impaired. It does not require an arthropod vector but is found in many mammalian species. Whether the increase in human immunodeficiency virus (HIV) infected women on obstetrical services will impact on obstetrical and neonatal care because of *P carinii* infections in mothers and newborn intensive care units is problematic.

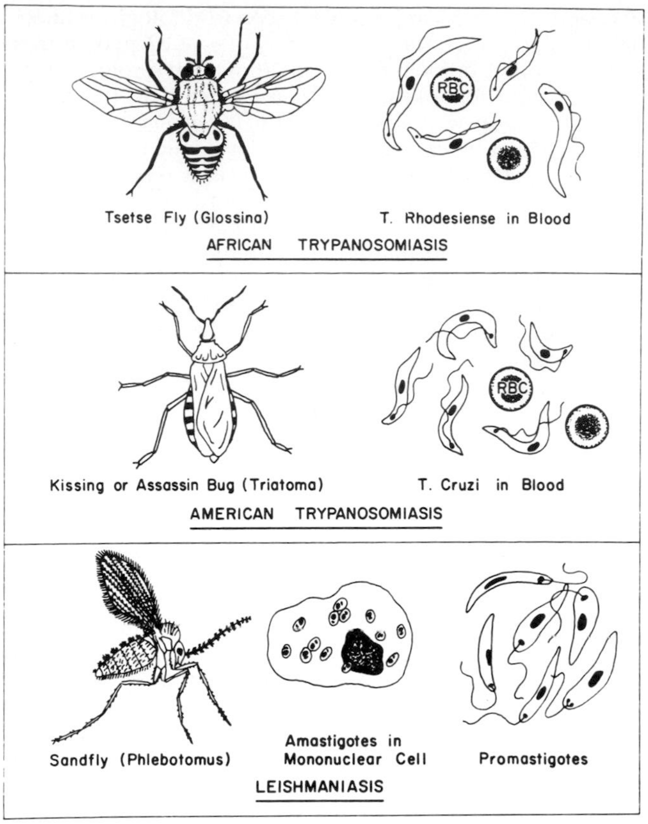

Figure 111–3. Blood and tissue protozoa.

Fever, lymphadenopathy, and splenomegaly are common manifestations of many infectious diseases endemic to the Tropics. The clinician must, therefore, exclude the possibility of multiple infections including roundworm (filariasis), flukes (schistosomiasis), and bacteria (brucellosis, tuberculosis, and others) in every resident or traveling pregnant patient with fever and reticuloendothelial system hypertrophy.

The treatment of blood and tissue protozoa requires drugs that penetrate tissue, including the placenta and fetus, and that have serious potential toxicity (Table 111–12).[12]

Tissue Parasites Not Requiring Arthropod Vectors

Pneumocystis Carinii. *P carinii* (a protozoan organism) is worldwide in distribution and found in the otherwise healthy lungs of virtually every mammalian species.[43-45] Recently antigenic differences have been found among *P carinii* obtained in different mammalian hosts, suggesting that the organism has host specificity.[46] Although many animals may carry the organism, there is no clear-cut evidence that animals are a reservoir and a source of human infection.

The life cycle is not completely understood. A thick-walled cyst and a thin-walled trophozoite have been described. Both of these forms are always found extracellularly in the pulmonary alveoli. The cyst contains six to eight sporozoites, which develop into trophozoites when released from the cyst. Trophozoites transform into cysts under, as yet, poorly defined conditions.

TABLE 111–12. RECOMMENDED DRUGS FOR TREATING BLOOD AND TISSUE PROTOZOA DURING PREGNANCY

Disease	Drug	Principal Adverse Effects	Special Precautions in Pregnancy	Dose
Malaria	Chloroquine PO4	Generally safe; retinal, VIII nerve injury rare	Generally safe; VIII nerve injury of fetus	1.0 g, then 500 mg in 6 h, then 500 mg QD for two days For prophylaxis: 500 mg weekly
	Quinine SO4	Cinchonism, hemolysis	Hypoglycemia; VIII nerve injury of fetus; oxytocic	650 mg t.i.d. for three days 600 mg/300 mL intravenous over one hr; repeat q 8 h
	Fansidar (pyrimethamine + sulfadoxine)	Folic acid deficiency, bone marrow suspension	Folic acid deficiency, teratogenic (?)	One tablet (25 mg pyrimethamine, 500 mg sulfadoxine) weekly for prophylaxis
African trypanosomiasis	Suramin	Collapse, fever, hepatic and renal toxicity, rash, pruritus, anaphylaxis, peripheral neuropathy	Excreted slowly; teratogenicity not clear, hepatic and renal toxicity	1.0 g IV on days 1,3,7,14,21 for non-central nervous system infection, start with 100 mg intravenous as test dose
	Melarsoprol	Myocardial and renal toxicity, encephalopathy, Herxheimer reaction	Same; teratogenicity not clear	2–3 mg/kg per day intravenous for three doses; repeat one week and three weeks later
	Pentamidine	Hypotension, hypoglycemia, renal toxicity, diabetogenic, pancreatitis	Hypoglycemia, diabetogenic	4 mg/kg per day intramuscular for 10 days
American trypanosomiasis	Nifurtimox	Anorexia, vomiting, weight loss, paresthesias	Hypoglycemia, anorexia, vomiting, weight loss; teratogenicity not clear	5 mg/kg per day in 4 divided doses, increase by 2 mg/kg per day every 2 weeks until daily dose reaches 15–17 mg/kg
Leishmaniasis: visceral and Old World cutaneous disease	Pentostam (stibogluconate, sodium antimony)	Myocardial toxicity, muscle pain	Myocardial toxicity, hepatic and renal toxicity; not teratogenic	20 mg/kg/day IM or IV for 6–10 days (maximum 800 mg/day)
	Pentamidine	Same as African trypanosomiasis	Same as African trypanosomiasis	2–4 mg/kg per day intramuscular for 10–15 days
American mucocutaneous leishmaniasis	Pentostam	Same as above	Same as above	Same as above
	Amphotericin B	Renal toxicity, electrolyte imbalance	Renal and hepatic toxicity, hypokalemia with exacerbation of pregnancy-induced glucose intolerance, anemia	0.25–1.0 mg/kg slow intravenous QD for 40–48 days
Pneumocystis	Pentamidine	Same as African trypanosomiasis	Same as African trypanosomiasis	4 mg/kg day intramuscular for 12–14 days
	Trimethoprimsulfamethoxizole	Folic acid deficiency	Folic acid deficiency	

The vast majority of creatures harboring *Pneumocystis* are not ill and the lung tissue contains occasional groups of cysts without alveolar exudate. Seroepidemiologic studies indicate that acquisition of *P carinii* is common: one third of children have antibodies to *P carinii* by one year of age and three quarters are seropositive by the age of four. In humans, corticosteroids, cancer chemotherapy, alterations in cellular immunity associated with lymphoma, AIDS, and immunologic immaturity, as seen in malnourished or premature infants, are associated with the emergence of active pulmonary inflammation and multiplication of *Pneumocystis* trophozoites.

The epidemiology of human infection suggests that the transmission is by the respiratory route by way of droplets. The organism is presumably present in the pulmonary secretions of many asymptomatic humans who are the reservoir and source of human disease. Epidemics of *Pneumocystis* pneumonia in nurseries have resulted from airborne spread of the organism from an asymptomatic carrier. Although the organism is almost always confined to the lung, *Pneumocystis* may be found in lymph nodes, spleen, or bone marrow, suggesting that bloodborne dissemination can occur. This may explain the rare occurrence of congenital infection, presumably resulting from transplacental transmission.

The characteristic picture of *Pneumocystis* infection is an alveolar and interstitial pneumonia with progressive hypoxemia. The alveoli fill with proteinaceous fluid containing both trophozoites and cysts. Nonproductive cough, tachypnea, dyspnea, and cyanosis are the dominant clinical features. Rales, rhonchi, and wheezing are occasional findings. At the onset of clinical symptoms, chest x-ray reveals a perihilar interstitial or reticulogranular pattern with sparing of the periphery. Arterial blood gases demonstrate decreased PO_2, oxygen saturation, and PCO_2 consistent with hyperventilation and intrapulmonary shunting. Oxygen therapy may fail to correct the hypoxemia because of progressive pulmonary consolidation. Chest x-ray in advanced disease shows diffuse alveolar infiltrates with air bronchograms involving the entire lung. Pleural reaction and effusion or asymmetric or nodular infiltrates are usually caused by coinfections.

Because *Pneumocystis* is a pathogen in the immunocompromised, it is often only one among several pathogens isolated from secretions or tissue. Not infrequently, the clinical and pathologic findings in such patients are those of a fungal, viral, or bacterial infection, and the presence or role of *Pneumocystis* in the clinical progression of the illness is obscured.

The diagnosis should be considered in the clinical setting of immunodeficiency and progressive pulmonary symptoms. The organism can be identified in pulmonary secretions or lung tissue by methenamine silver, Giemsa, or Gram–Weigert stains. Coughed, suctioned, or transtracheally aspirated sputum contains the organism in such a small percentage of cases (fewer than 20%) that bronchoscopy with bronchial brushing or transbronchial biopsy should be given high priority. Open-lung biopsy provides the optimum opportunity for the diagnosis of hypoxemic diffuse pulmonary infiltrates in the immunologically crippled. Reliable serologic and immunofluorescent techniques are not widely available.

Early diagnosis is important because the disease is eminently treatable when therapy is started before the underlying immune-disrupting disease or overwhelming respiratory failure precludes success, despite effective antipneumocystic drugs. Trimethoprim-sulfamethoxazole (cotrimoxazole) has supplanted pentamidine isethionate as the agent of first choice. Both antimicrobial drugs have risks for pregnancy but the circumstances and inexorable course of the infection mandate treatment. There should be no hesitation to treat the pregnant patient with *P carinii* pneumonia.

For the obstetrician, the importance of *P carinii* resides in its potential to produce epidemic pneumonia in the premature nursery. Pregnancy does not cause activation of the parasite. However, clinicians and hospital staff managing high risk pregnancies need to recognize the rising incidence of AIDS and its associated infections, such as pneumocystosis, among the young adult women automatically considered high obstetric risks: intravenous drug users, prostitutes, and the sexually promiscuous. There is no reliable or cost-effective way to screen pregnant patients or clinical staff for asymptomatic carriage of the parasite.

Tissue Parasites Requiring Arthropod Vectors

Leishmaniasis. *Leishmania* (Table 111–13) are intracellular protozoan parasites transmitted among mammalian hosts by the bite of phlebotomine sandfly vectors. *Leishmania* infections are zoonoses of wild and domestic animals, especially edentates, rodents and canines, with humans as incidental hosts. The clinical manifestations of human infection range from visceral disease with hepatosplenomegaly to one of several cutaneous or mucocutaneous syndromes. Clinical disease patterns are determined by the species of *Leishmania* and host immune responses.[47,48]

Over the past decade, biochemical and immunologic methodologies have established a leishmanial taxonomy that is independent of host and environmental factors. These studies indicate that many *Leishmania* can produce a wide spectrum of human disease, not a single clinical entity as previously thought, and that some new *Leishmania* species are parasites of nonhuman mammals, but are not pathogenic for humans.[49,50]

The leishmanial cycle has two distinct forms. In the sandfly (*Phlebotomus* species and *Lutzomyia* species), the parasite propagates as a flagellated extracellular promastigote. Sandflies are small, relatively weak fliers that breed in cool, moist places: burrows and crevices in walls. They may pass through standard mosquito netting. They stay close to the ground and they bite in the evenings.

When the mammalian host is bitten, the injected promastigotes are ingested by mononuclear phagocytes and transform into amastigotes lacking the free flagellum. Within the macrophage, amastigotes divide until the cell is so heavily parasitized that it ruptures. The released amastigotes circulate and are ingested by other macrophages. Sandflies become infected when they feed on an infected mammalian host and take up parasites from the blood or skin.

The severity and extent of the infection are modulated by host immune responses. Widespread visceral, mucocutaneous, and reticuloendothelial invasion by copious numbers of parasites is associated with a diminution in T-lymphocyte-mediated immune responses and an exaggeration of humoral, β-lymphocyte immune response. Localized mucocutaneous disease is characterized by vigorous cell-mediated immunity and well-defined granuloma formation. Infection does not always progress to local or disseminated disease. Presumably, asymptomatic and self-limited infections are not uncommon. The ability of the host to contain and eradicate the parasite is related, in part, to genetic and acquired immune response determinants, the size of the inoculum, and the virulence and tropism of the *Leishmania* species inoculated. Recovery from leishmanial infection confers lifelong immunity against infection by the same strain or species of *Leishmania.*

The immunologic aberrations induced by pregnancy may interfere with the generation of protective cellular immunity in a nonimmune woman or may predispose to disseminated infection in immune women. Diminution in the clearance and containment of amastigotes by the reticuloendothelial system permits the intrusion of the parasite into the placental and fetal circulation. Although rarely reported, intrauterine infection does occur.

Visceral Leishmaniasis. Visceral leishmaniasis or kala-azar is a zoonotic with several epidemiologic patterns involving canines, rodents, and humans. The incubation period is usually two to six months. The first symptom is fever, usually gradual in onset and accompanied by sweats. The fever progresses from intermittent episodes to a characteristic pattern of twice daily elevations. Generalized lymphadenopathy and splenomegaly are common physical findings. Hepatomegaly is found in one fifth of patients. In the absence of infarcts, neither the spleen nor liver is tender; the patient, however, may complain of heaviness or discomfort in the hypochondrium. Hyperpigmentation of the hands, feet, and abdomen is responsible for the name, kala-azar, the black sickness.

The organism occupies increasing amounts of bone marrow, resulting in anemia. Splenomegaly is often accompanied by hypersplenism. Hypoalbuminemia, caused by

TABLE 111–13. DISTRIBUTION OF CLINICAL SYNDROMES CAUSED BY *LEISHMANIA*

Clinical Syndrome	*Leishmania* Species	Geographic Distribution	Usual Vector	Usual Reservoir/Host
Visceral leishmaniasis (kala-azar)	*Leishmania donovani*	"Old World": East and sub-Saharan Africa, south Asia (India, Iran), China	*Phlebotomus orientalis, Phlebotomus martini, Phlebotomus argentipes*	Canines: wild and domestic
	Leishmania infantum (? separate species)	"Old World": North Africa, southern Europe, Near East	*Phlebotomus orientalis*	Canines: wild and domestic
	Leishmania chagasi	"New World": Brazil, Venezuela, Colombia, Central America	*Lutzomyia longipalpis*	Canines: wild and domestic
Cutaneous and mucocutaneous leishmaniasis				
Cutaneous ulcers	*Leishmania major*	"Old World": North and Central Africa, Middle East, South Asia	*Phlebotomus papatasii*	Rodents
	Leishmania aethiopica	Ethiopia, Kenya	*Phlebotomus longipes*	Hyrax
Cutaneous ulcers; chronic relapsing cutaneous disease	*Leishmania tropica*	Middle East, South Asia	*Phlebotomus sergenti*	Domestic canines
Cutaneous ulcers; some patients develop diffuse cutaneous or mucocutaneous disease	*Leishmania mexicana* complex (*L mexicana, amazonensis, venezuelansis* and others)	"New World": southern USA, Central America, North and South America	Various *Lutzomyia* species	Rodents, canines, nonhuman primates
	Leishmania braziliensis complex (*L braziliensis, lainsoni, panamensis, peruviana* and others)	"New World": Central America, South America to northern Argentina	Various *Lutzomyia* species	Armadillos, canines, rodents, marsupials

increasingly profound malnutrition and liver involvement, contrasts with the elevation of immunoglobulins. The total serum protein exceeds 10 g/dL. Bleeding is not unusual as the disease runs its course; this is a result of thrombocytopenia and hepatic dysfunction with prolonged prothrombin and clotting times. After months or years, the patient, emaciated and exhausted, dies from massive gastrointestinal hemorrhage or, more commonly, from serious intercurrent infection.

Pregnancy is unusual in women with established, untreated visceral leishmaniasis. Pregnant women, especially nonimmune nonresidents of the endemic area, may have a more rapid and aggressive progression of the infection with the risk of intrauterine infection of the fetus.

The diagnosis can be made by needle aspiration of spleen, bone marrow, liver, or lymph nodes. The material obtained should be made into a thin film and inoculated into NNN medium for culture. Antileishmanial antibodies can be demonstrated by a number of serologic tests. The leishmanin (Montenegro) skin test is negative in active visceral leishmaniasis, but becomes positive after recovery.

Chemotherapy is effective. Pentavalent antimony is still the drug of choice. Pentamidine isethionate and amphotericin B are reliable alternatives. Pentamidine is not recommended during pregnancy because about 10% of patients receiving this drug develop diabetes. Pentamidine may exaggerate the fasting hypoglycemia and diabetogenic effects of pregnancy. Pregnant patients with untreated infection are often so ill that they cannot sustain the nutritional, physiological, and emotional demands of pregnancy. Nutritional repair of inanition and vitamin deficiencies is essential. Visceral leishmaniasis acquired during pregnancy should be treated despite the risks. The best course would seem to be to initiate or maintain chemotherapy, which may take as long as four to six weeks, and to terminate the pregnancy if the patient's clinical condition warrants.

Cutaneous Leishmaniasis. Infections by *Leishmania* species preferring the skin have a worldwide distribution not unlike that of visceral leishmaniasis, reflecting the climatic and ecologic conditions suitable for the *Phlebotomus* vectors and a mammalian population of suitable reservoirs and susceptibles. The organisms appear to have thermal requirements for growth that foster localization in the skin. At the site of inoculation, the parasite elicits a vigorous mononuclear cell response. As the infection progresses, necrosis with ulceration occurs, followed by gradual reduction in the quantity of amastigotes and eventual healing with scar formation. The leishmanin skin test becomes strongly positive as the nodular lesion progresses to ulceration. Healing is accompanied by the appearance of protective immunity, which usually lasts for life.

In rare individuals, protective immunity fails to develop so that the primary nodule does not progress to ulceration and the leishmanin skin test does not become positive. In these patients, after some months, the lesion begins to expand locally and the disease disseminates to other areas, producing nodular or infiltrative lesions, especially on the skin of the face and the extensor surfaces of the extremities. The route of spread is not clearly documented but is probably by way of lymphatics and the bloodstream. There is considerable variation in the clinical progression of cutaneous leishmaniasis, which is related, in part, to geographic and genetic differences in host response and to alterations in host defense induced by concurrent or intercurrent conditions. Pregnancy has been said to delay the healing of cutaneous leishmaniasis. It is possible for pregnancy to allow more extensive spread and metastasis of the organism. Intrauterine infection has not been reported in cutaneous leishmaniasis.

Leishmania can be identified in material from the base or indurated edges of the lesion by stains and culture of animal inoculation. *Leishmania braziliensis,* however, may be remarkably difficult to find in smears or tissue sections.

In many parts of the Old World, prophylactic inoculation of children is practiced. In endemic areas, virtually all adults bear the scars of earlier, immunity-producing infection. Almost all cutaneous lesions caused by *Leishmaniasis tropica* heal without therapy. For indolent lesions, local heat may be useful. Pregnant women with Old World cutaneous leishmaniasis need not be treated until after delivery, if at all.

The New World *Leishmania* cause more persistent and aggressive disease and usually require long term chemotherapy with pentavalent antimony. Amphotericin B can also be used if antimonials are not effective. Pregnant women with New World cutaneous leishmaniasis can be carefully observed during pregnancy. Treatment may be withheld during pregnancy unless there is progression of the infection with the appearance of new distant metastasis or progressive destruction of nasopharyngeal structures. In this instance, termination of pregnancy to restore full immune competence and to permit aggressive antimonial chemotherapy could be considered. Alternatively, the pregnant patient with progressive mucocutaneous leishmaniasis can be treated with amphotericin B, which may be safer to use during pregnancy than repetitive, large doses of stibogluconate.

Trypanosomiasis. All three of the trypanosomes[51] pathogenic for man undergo a developmental cycle in a bloodsucking insect. Infective, flagellated trypanomastigotes in the arthropod gut are transmitted by injection or abrasion into the host with the saliva of the tsetse fly or the feces released by the triatoma bug during feedings. Trypanosomiasis can be transmitted by blood transfusion, by direct inoculation of trypanomastigotes from laboratory accidents, needle sticks, or through open wounds, and by transplacental passage, causing intrauterine and congenital infection.

There are three phases in the human infection. Initially, the organisms multiply at the site of inoculation. A secondary phase of bloodstream dissemination follows with involvement of the reticuloendothelial system and seeding of target organs. Trypanomastigotes are found in blood films during the secondary phase. The tertiary stage is marked by target organ damage. The development of immune responses contributes to the inflammatory and destructive process and to the reduction of circulating trypanosomes. Unsuspected and undetected parasitemia occurs episodically, possibly explaining the occasional infant with congenital infection from a not very ill mother.

The rate of disease progression is determined by the virulence and tropisms of the infecting species of trypanosome, the size of the inoculum, and host immune factors. A minimum of 350 trypanosomes is necessary to produce experimental infections through human skin. Presumably a smaller number would be needed to produce intrauterine infection or to infect by way of a blood transfusion.

Trypanosomes elicit both humoral and cell-mediated immune responses. The organism is able to persist in the host by variation of surface antigens in the case of the African trypanosomes and by invasion of the cells of heart and smooth muscle in the case of Chagas' disease. The ability of these organisms to persist in the host for long periods elicits host immune responses, which are the major determinants of the clinical findings of tertiary disease.

African Trypanosomiasis (Sleeping Sickness). *Trypanosoma brucei* has influenced human settlements and reproduction in subsaharan Africa by causing human and domestic cattle infections. *T brucei* is noninfectious from humans, but causes a chronic wasting disease of cattle (Nagana) and wild bovine species. About four million square miles of Africa are unpopulated because of inability to maintain cattle.

T brucei has two subspecies which are the cause of human trypanosomiasis in Africa. *Trypanosoma brucei gambiense* is a human parasite. It is transmitted by riverine tsetse flies, *Glossina palpalis* group, that breed in forests and feed in the clearings that border rivers and streams. In the well-watered parts of tropical Africa, Gambian sleeping sickness is a continuing problem among villagers, pastoralists, and farmers. *Trypanosoma brucei rhodesiense* is primarily a parasite of wild game and is transmitted by tsetse flies of the *Glossina morsitans* group. The vector breeds in woods and brush and feeds in open grassland. In the dry savannah country, Rhodesian sleeping sickness is a sporadic problem among pastoralists, tourists, hunters, and wardens.

About 10,000 new cases of African trypanosomiasis are reported annually. Approximately 45 million people are at risk, but only six million are under routine surveillance. More than 30 cases of congenital infection have been reported in the literature, but the actual impact of African trypanosomiasis on pregnancy is underestimated because of inadequate surveillance and reporting.

Infection by *T brucei gambiense* begins eight to 14 days following a bite by an infected tsetse fly. The nodular primary lesion is not especially large or painful and often goes unnoted. Host factors influence the rate at which the organism extends locally and spreads to regional lymph nodes. It may be months or years before the second stage of infection becomes clinically apparent. Fever and nontender lymphadenopathy, including splenomegaly, are the main clinical features. The organism can be demonstrated in aspirates of lymph nodes and in thick or thin blood films. Hyperglobulinemia is characteristic.

During the secondary phase, the organism invades the central nervous system. Meningoencephalitis and meningomyelitis with a predominance of lymphocytes and plasma cells are associated with mononuclear pleocytosis and elevated cerebrospinal fluid protein, especially IgM. Rarely, trypanosomes can be seen in the cerebrospinal fluid. As the tertiary stage emerges, the patient complains of headache and backache and becomes increasingly listless and drowsy. Chorea, athetosis, and stupor are more common manifestations than cranial nerve or pyramidal tract signs. Obesity, amenorrhea, and impotence are common, possibly reflecting both hypothalamic involvement and the effects of chronic disease.

Infection by *T brucei rhodesiense* has a more accelerated

clinical course. Secondary or disseminated infection is often marked by involvement of the heart and the liver with congestive heart failure, jaundice, hypoglycemia, anemia, thrombocytopenia, and disseminated intravascular coagulopathy.[52] Death may intervene even before lymphadenopathy or central nervous system disease becomes manifest.

In the absence of treatment, most women infected with *T brucei rhodesiense* will die before conception or the completion of pregnancy. Intrauterine infection occurs with both African trypanosomes.[53] However, maternal survival, completion of pregnancy, and delivery of a congenitally infected infant is more likely with *T brucei gambiense* infection.

Abortion and prematurity are reported in pregnancies complicated by infections with both trypanosomes. The placenta can be heavily parasitized, which may contribute to the frequency of hydramnios, intrauterine growth retardation, and prematurity. In the neonate, congenital infection presents as fever, anemia, and meningoencephalitis. Lymphadenopathy is absent and parasites may be difficult to detect in the blood. Indeed, the cerebrospinal fluid (CSF) may contain trypanosomes when none are found in the cord blood. Congenital infection is likely if the parasite is found in blood or the CSF during the first week of life or if the diseased neonate of a mother infected with trypanosomiasis has never been in the endemic region.

In residents of endemic areas, the diagnosis is not difficult. The diagnosis may be elusive in travelers to tropical Africa. Clinicians must consider trypanosomiasis in the differential diagnosis of unexplained fever and lymphadenopathy in any patient who has traveled in an endemic area, even for only a brief visit. Examination of thick and thin blood smears and of material aspirated from lymph nodes is essential. Serologic tests are available but have limited usefulness in managing an acutely ill patient. Lumbar puncture is an essential component of the management of the patient with documented infection in order to guide therapy. Occasionally, the diagnosis of trypanosomiasis is made by examination of the CSF.

Treatment must be directed toward both the circulating and central nervous system trypanosomes. Suramin and pentamidine isethionate can be used in early stages, before invasion of the central nervous system has occurred, because they do not cross the blood-brain barrier. Melarsoprol, an arsenical, is used in concert with suramin or pentamidine for late disease with active central nervous system involvement. Courses of therapy are long and should be carried out in hospital wherever and whenever possible. Attention must be given to nutrition and concurrent infection. Relapses are not infrequent and increase in frequency the later treatment is started in the course of the infection.

All of the agents used in the treatment of trypanosomiasis are toxic and have potentially serious adverse effects on gestation. Herxheimer reactions can occur. However, despite the risks of treatment, the serious impact of African trypanosomiasis on the mother necessitates treatment without regard to the stage of gestation.

American Trypanosomiasis (Chagas' Disease). In Central and South America, more than 15 million people are infected with *Trypanosoma cruzi.* A variety of mammals, including rodents and canines, can be infected. The vector triatomid bugs thrive in the shantytown shacks that surround cities. They usually bite at night around the face, hence the common name "kissing bug." The bite site initially may have some swelling and erythema as a result of local reactions to the bite. After 10 to 14 days, proliferation of trypanomastigotes produces local swelling and regional adenopathy. Dissemination of the organism is accompanied by fever, lymphadenopathy, and hepatosplenomegaly. Trypanomastigotes can be seen in thick and thin blood films and aspirates of lymph nodes. The parasite penetrates myocardial and smooth muscle cells and phagocytic reticuloendothelial cells and transforms into the amastigote or leishmanial form. Myocarditis, myositis, and meningoencephalitis may develop during the acute stage of dissemination. Mortality in early disease is high among young children and immunocompromised hosts. Healthy individuals may have few or no symptoms despite the presence and dissemination of the organism. Only 1–2% of infected people develop symptoms that lead to the diagnosis of acute disease.

In nonfatal and asymptomatic infections, the acute stage resolves with the emergence of effective host responses and the clearance of trypanomastigotes from the bloodstream. The organism persists intracellularly. Episodic parasitemia continues to occur, presumably originating from intracellular foci. The location and quantity of amastigotes determine the clinical picture and severity of the chronic stage of the illness. The majority of patients do not progress to serious chronic disease, and the latent or indeterminant phase lasts for their lifetime. They may be unwitting reservoirs and transmitters of infection through blood donation or during pregnancy.[54]

Usually, chronic Chagas' disease develops insidiously in patients with no history of acute disease. Cardiac and gastrointestinal manifestations predominate. Involvement of myocardial cells may produce myocarditis, conduction abnormalities, arrhythmias, and congestive heart failure. A Brazilian longitudinal study demonstrated that, each year, the chronic disease progresses in 5–6% of patients.[55] The mortality was about 1% per year. Sudden deaths from conduction defects occurred in 38% and cardiac failure was the cause of death in 58%. Megacolon and megaesophagus result from injury to the smooth muscle and autonomic nerve cells of the gut wall. The affected segment of gut has focal myositis and occasional muscle cells contain amastigotes. Injury to the autonomic nerve cells may be caused by toxic or "autoimmune" factors produced by the presence of the organism.

Congenital infection is well known.[56,57] Over 100 cases have been reported in the literature. The true incidence of congenital infection and adverse effects on pregnancy is not known because of inadequate surveillance and reporting. In endemic areas, the estimated incidence of congenital disease in newborns weighing less than 2 kg is about 2%. It is assumed that Chagas' disease contributes to intrauterine growth retardation; however, the prevalence of serious nutritional and socioeconomic distress in the infected population makes the association difficult to document.

Transplacental passage may occur during any stage of the disease. In the majority of cases, the mother has been asymptomatic.[58] The organism produces a chronic placentitis with focal necrosis. Amastigotes may be found in placental macrophages. Clinical findings in the neonate are related to the time during pregnancy that transplacental parasitemia occurred. The earlier in gestation the fetus is infected, the more likely it will have evidence of infection at birth. Hepatosplenomegaly, anemia, jaundice, meningoencephalitis, and gastrointestinal symptoms including impaired esophageal motility are the principal problems. Parasites may not be present in the blood or cerebrospinal fluid and xenodiagnosis may be required to establish the diagnosis. The indirect IgM immunofluorescence test may be helpful. The prognosis is poor, even with treatment. Twenty-seven of 60 documented cases of congenital infection died, the majority before reaching the age of four months. It is not known whether the asymptomatic, congenitally infected infant will develop late manifestations.

Transmission of the trypanosomes through breast milk has been shown in animals. The role of this route of infection in human disease is not clear.

Finding the trypanomastigote in thick or thin blood smears is the most reliable test for diagnosis. During the acute phase, parasitemia is frequent and, at times, intense. During the later stages of infection, parasitemia is infrequent and in small concentration, making serologic, xenodiagnostic, and histologic methods more important. Xenodiagnosis, using laboratory-raised triatoma bugs, may isolate the organism in as many as 50% of cases. In addition to serologic techniques such as complement fixation, immunofluorescence, and hemagglutination, there is a nonspecific increase in immunoglobulins, which may cause positive syphilis and heterophil antibody tests.

Pregnancy may be associated with breathlessness, palpitations, and symptoms of altered gastrointestinal motility: constipation and esophageal reflux. The early manifestations of chronic Chagas' disease may, therefore, be confused with common problems of pregnancy. Women living or traveling in endemic areas should have careful investigation of their cardiac and gastrointestinal symptoms, including serologic and xenodiagnostic tests for *T cruzi*, if the history, physical examination, or electrocardiogram suggests the possibility of Chagas' disease. The appearance of ventricular extrasystoles, supraventricular tachyarrhythmias, and intraventricular conduction defects in infected women is a cause for concern. Patients with chronic myocarditis caused by *T cruzi*, even without symptoms, are remarkably susceptible to arrhythmias induced by β-adrenergic agents, β-adrenergic blocking agents, and digitalis. Premature labor and abortion occur with increased incidence in patients with Chagas' disease. In these patients, the use of cardioactive drugs to treat premature labor and toxemia is hazardous. Studies on infected experimental animals suggests that calcium channel blockers, like verapamil, may have a beneficial effect upon the chagasic myocarditis.[59] Improved microcirculation in areas adjacent to infected lesions appear to improve myocardial function and reduce ectopy and arrhythmias.

Chemotherapy of *T cruzi* infection is not entirely satisfactory. Two drugs appear to kill circulating trypanomastigotes: nifurtimox and benznidazole. Patients with acute disease and parasitemia given either of these agents will clear the agents from the bloodstream. Some of these patients, however, may have relapses and may progress to chronic disease. Antiparasite chemotherapy does not reverse the lesions in the gastrointestinal tract and myocardium. Because of the risk of congenital infection, prematurity, miscarriage, and progression to serious chronic disease, pregnant women with parasitemia and acute disease should be treated, despite the toxicity of the drugs and their, as yet, undetermined effects on the fetus. Whether a pregnant patient with chronic or latent infection should be treated is not clear. The author recommends careful observation for activity of the infection during pregnancy, including examination of blood films for parasites and serial serologic tests. If parasitemia occurs, or if there are rising titers of antibody, chemotherapy should be considered. The role of amniocentesis and examination of amniotic fluid for parasites in the diagnosis and management of the pregnant patient with Chagas' disease is unexplored.

Malaria. Malaria is an infection characterized by relapsing fever, rigors, splenomegaly, and anemia caused by four *Plasmodium* species transmitted from human to human by the bite of female anopheline mosquitoes. It has been, and continues to be, a worldwide health problem.[60] Both the organism and the vector have the capacity to develop resistance to naturally occurring and synthetic insecticides, repellents, and chemotherapy. Malaria is an endemic disease in many parts of tropical and subtropical Africa, Asia, and Central and South America, where environmental features, including temperature, humidity, bodies of water, and agriculture, support the breeding of the mosquito vectors and encourage frequent contact between mosquitoes and man.

Epidemic malaria may be produced when the parasite is introduced or reintroduced into a region with a large nonimmune population and the appropriate vectors. In countries such as Sri Lanka, the combination of insecticide spraying and widespread surveillance and medical treatment during the 1950s and 1960s had reduced the number of cases dramatically. Reduction in malaria control measures and the development of insecticide resistance during the decade of the 1960s was followed, in a few years, by a malaria epidemic affecting more than one million people.

Vectors for transmission of *Plasmodium* persist in North America. Several small outbreaks of introduced malaria, transmitted by local mosquitoes, serve to remind us that indigenous malaria was a continuing problem in the United States until 50 years ago. In 1988, 1023 cases of malaria were reported from the United States and its territories.[61] Thirty-two of these patients acquired the infection in the United States. One infant suffered from congenital malaria. In 1980–1981, 13 cases of congenital malaria were reported to the Centers for Disease Control (CDC).[62] Over half of the cases occurred in U.S. citizens. *Plasmodium falciparum* was the organism in 45% and *Plasmodium vivax* was found in 43%.

When an anopheline female bites an infected human, male and female malarial gametocytes in the blood are taken into the mosquito's stomach. A sexual reproductive cycle, taking about two weeks, ensues, producing sporozoites that accumulate in the salivary gland and are infective for the human being. When the mosquito bites, sporozoites are injected into the bloodstream and infect hepatic parenchymal cells. The parasite multiplies in the liver during this preerythrocyte or exoerythrocytic phase, which is usually not clinically apparent. Within 5 to 15 days, merozoites are released into the bloodstream. Invasion of red blood cells by merozoites begins the cycle of multiplication (schizogony) that results in the destruction of the parasitized erythrocyte. This cycle takes 36–48 hours for *Plasmodium falciparum*, 48 hours for *Plasmodium vivax* and *Plasmodium ovale*, and 72 hours for *Plasmodium malariae.* When a sufficient concentration of parasites in the blood is in synchrony, the clinical cycle of periodic fever begins. The symptoms of chills and fever coincide with the rupture of red cells and the release of merozoites.

Merozoites attach to specific receptors on the red blood cell surface. The Duffy blood group substance is important for the entrance of *Plasmodium vivax* into erythrocytes. Individuals and populations lacking the Duffy antigen are relatively resistant to *P vivax* malaria.

The morphology of the parasite in the infected erythrocyte is characteristic and helpful in identification of the infecting species. Diagnosis of active infection depends on careful examination of thick and thin blood films for the parasite. The organism may elude the unpracticed eye even when present in large quantities. Serologic tests are of help in chronically infected patients with fever and splenomegaly but few or no parasites in the peripheral blood.

The severity of a clinical attack is related, in part, to the concentration of parasites. The merozoites of *Plasmodium falciparum* will invade erythrocytes of any age, whereas *Plasmodium vivax* infects young red cells and *Plasmodium malariae* infects older red cells. *Plasmodium falciparum* is capable of increasing the concentration of parasitized erythrocytes rapidly and to high concentrations. All species of *Plasmodia* diminish the deformability of the parasitized red blood cells.[63] However, in *P falciparum* infection, the erythrocytes develop knobby projections, assume unusual shapes, and become more "sticky." High parasite concentrations and diminished red blood cell compliance produce reduction in capillary flow with resulting tissue hypoxia. The brain, kidneys, and placenta are especially vulnerable to the accumulation of parasitized erythrocytes. Severe hemolysis, renal failure, coma, pulmonary edema, and intrauterine fetal death are features almost exclusively of *P falciparum* malaria.[64-66]

In malarious areas, infection first occurs in early childhood. Persistence of the parasite and repeated inoculation of parasites with bites by infected mosquitoes produce humoral and cell-mediated immune responses. After five to 10 years of residence in an endemic area, the youth has sufficient immunity to reduce the severity and duration of repetitive clinical attacks. Circulating antibodies are important in the control of the acute infection. Maternal antibody has been shown to protect the newborn from mosquito-transmitted infection. Antimalarial IgG given to infected patients reduces the severity of the illness. As time passes, the parasite disappears from the blood and the infection may be clinically manifest by splenomegaly, hyperglobulinemia, elevated antimalarial antibodies, and transient episodes of low-concentration parasitemia. Disruption of the host-parasite balance by malnutrition, pregnancy, or introduction of new strains of parasite may precipitate recrudescent or more severe clinical attacks.

As the infection continues, antibody- and cell-mediated immunity contribute to the pathogenesis of some of the clinical features of malaria, as well as to the abatement of the erythrocyte cycle.[67] Immune complexes, Coombs'-positive hemolytic anemia, and accelerated hemolysis of parasitized red cells may exacerbate the clinical course of the acute disease. The nephrotic syndrome is a well-documented complication of chronic infection by *Plasmodium malariae*. Tropical splenomegaly is marked by enlargement of the reticuloendothelial system and polyclonal hyperglobulinemia.

The interaction of pregnancy and malaria is influenced by the nature of the organism and the immune status of the host. Life-threatening acute disease is caused by *Plasmodium falciparum*.[68] The majority of malaria infections during pregnancy are *P falciparum*, especially in Africa. Among Cambodian refugees in Thailand, chloroquine-resistant *P falciparum* malaria has caused severe maternal disease and fetal wastage without regard to the mother's nutritional or immune status. Nonimmune women have more severe acute disease from any of the human *Plasmodia* than immune residents of a malarious region. A large body of clinical observations indicates that pregnancy exerts a dampening effect on the immunity to malaria.[69-71] In endemic areas, clinical attacks are more frequent during pregnancy than in the nonpregnant state. Asymptomatic or latent malaria may recrudesce during pregnancy and the puerperium. Parasitemia and parasitization of the placenta are more likely and more intense in primiparous mothers.

In addition to the fever, chills, and splenomegaly of the clinical attack, malaria in the mother can cause profound anemia, predispose toward serious intercurrent illness, cause intrauterine infection and placental insufficiency, and contribute to intrauterine growth retardation, prematurity, low birth weight, abortion, and stillbirth.[70,72,73] Preexisting maternal and malaria immunity and the immune effects of pregnancy appear to modulate both the clinical expression of the infection in the mother and the effectiveness of the placenta as a barrier against fetal infection.[74] Congenital malaria may occur in the absence of any clinical evidence for malaria in the mother. Parasites are found in the placenta in the majority of patients with malaria during pregnancy.[75-77] In one study from a malaria-endemic region in West Africa, 40% of mothers had demonstrable parasitemia, but 16% had parasites found only in the placenta, not in the maternal or cord blood.[70] The incidence of congenital malaria in immune mothers residing in malarious areas is about 0.3% but 1–4% in nonimmune mothers living in the same region. *P falciparum* is the most common organism causing congenital infection, reflecting its predominance as the most common cause of serious maternal infection.

In the neonate, congenital malarial infection usually becomes evident 48–72 hours after birth. Parasitemia, fever, hepatosplenomegaly, jaundice, anemia, seizures, and occasionally pulmonary edema may occur. Occasionally, there may be a prolonged latent phase with clinical signs developing several weeks after delivery, even though parasites are present in the placenta and cord blood. Spontaneous clearance of *P falciparum* in congenitally infected infants may be common. Indeed a series of recent studies from Malawi, Southeast Africa, suggest that once the placenta is removed, both mother and infant can spontaneously clear parasites from the peripheral blood.[78]

There is striking disparity between the common finding of placental parasitization and the rarity of fetal or neonatal infection. Several factors seem to explain this observation. Maternal antibody coating the merozoites may favor their rapid clearance by the fetal reticuloendothelial system. Soluble malaria antigens crossing into the fetus may elicit protective IgM and cellular fetal immune responses. The nondeformable, sticky parasitized red cell may be unable to migrate through the placental circulation into the fetal circulation. *P falciparum* does not thrive in erythrocytes containing fetal hemoglobin.

As a general rule, clinicians working in areas of endemic malaria can expect a high proportion of pregnant women to have the infection. Young, primiparous women will have more severe clinical attacks and more intense placental infection than older, multiparous women who are more likely to have subclinical infection. Congenital infection will be unusual. Women given malaria prophylaxis throughout pregnancy have larger placentas, larger babies, and less anemia than nontreated women.

The physicians of pregnant travelers or migrants to endemic areas should regard the onset of any febrile illness within two months of exposure with grave suspicion. Nonimmune mothers may be expected to have severe clinical attacks, intense parasitemia, and dense parasitization of the placenta with the risk of intrauterine infection and fetal death.

Management. Clinical attacks of malaria during pregnancy should be treated promptly (Table 111–14); maternal infection with *P falciparum* should always be considered a life-threatening problem. Except for drug-resistant *P falciparum*, the recommended treatment during pregnancy is chloroquine phosphate, 1 g initially followed by 0.5 g after six hours and then once a day for two days. Because all species of human malaria except *P falciparum* have a prolonged exoerythrocytic phase, primaquine phosphate, 26.3 mg by mouth daily for 14 days, should be given to prevent relapses of malaria from *Plasmodium vivax*, *Plasmodium malariae*, and

TABLE 111–14. CHEMOPROPHYLAXIS AND CHEMOTHERAPY OF MALARIA DURING PREGNANCY

Plasmodium vivax *Plasmodium malariae* *Plasmodium ovale*	*Plasmodium falciparum*
Prophylaxis: Chloroquine phosphate 500 mg Q week beginning 1 week before departure and for 6 weeks after departure	Mefloquine 250 mg Q week beginning 1 week before departure and for 6 weeks after departure
Therapy: Chloroquine phosphate 1.0 gm initially, 0.5 gm in 6 hours, then 0.5 gm QD for 2 days	Mefloquine 1.0 gm PO as single dose
Continue chloroquine 500 mg Q week until delivery, then treat with primaquine 26.3 mg QD for 2 weeks for radical care	Quinine phosphate 600 mg PO Q 8 hours for three to seven days
	Combination therapy may also include tetracyclines, clindamycin
	Quinine or quinidine can be given intravenously

Plasmodium ovale. However, primaquine should be used with caution, preferably after delivery. Pregnant patients with drug-resistant *Plasmodium falciparum* should be treated with a regimen of multiple drugs including quinine.[79]

Many clinical reports document the safety of antimalarial drugs given during pregnancy for appropriate medical indications.[80,81] However, all antimalarial agents have potentially adverse effects on the fetus. Chloroquine can cause retinal and cochleovestibular damage in both mother and fetus. Quinine is ototoxic, mildly oxytocic, and can produce profound maternal hypoglycemia.[82,83] Primaquine causes methemoglobinemia and hemolysis in susceptible individuals. Other recommended drugs include sulfonamides, sulfones, tetracycline, pyrimethamine, and trimethoprim-sulfamethoxazole combinations. None are without serious potential hazard.[84] Tetracycline is contraindicated during pregnancy because of maternal liver toxicity and fetal bone and tooth defects. Pyrimethamine is teratogenic in laboratory animals. Pyrimethamine, sulfonamides, and trimethoprim-sulfamethoxazole have adverse effects on folic acid metabolism in mother and fetus. Sulfonamides interfere with the neonatal bilirubin metabolism.

Chloroquine-resistant *P falciparum* is now found in Southeast Asia, Africa, the northern areas of the Amazon Basin, and in some Pacific islands. Fansidar, a combination of sulfadoxine and pyrimethamine, has been used for many years as an alternative for treatment and prophylaxis against resistant *P falciparum* malaria. Among Cambodian refugees in Southeast Asia, however, strains of *P falciparum* resistant to sulfadoxine and pyrimethamine have now emerged. Indeed, there are now cases of *P falciparum* malaria in Southeast Asia that have failed to respond to quinine and tetracycline. In these areas, the treatment of *P falciparum* malaria is a major clinical dilemma. Mefloquine has been used in the treatment of multiply drug resistant *P falciparum* during pregnancy with good results.[85] Considering the desperate circumstances of a pregnant patient unfortunate enough to have acquired multiply drug-resistant *P falciparum,* it is probably wisest to elect to treat the patient with quinine and mefloquine. Liberal supplementation with folic acid and meticulous attention to the maternal blood sugar are essential.

Conscientious chemoprophylaxis during and after travel to endemic malarious areas is mandatory if traveling cannot be postponed until after delivery. The standard chemoprophylactic regimen is 500 mg of chloroquine phosphate by mouth once a week beginning one week before departure to an endemic area and continued for eight weeks after departing from the endemic area. Chloroquine alone suppresses the erythrocytic phase of infection but does not affect the liver or tissue phase, hence the necessity for continuing chloroquine for two months after leaving a malarious area.

The best prophylaxis is not to go to malarious places. Pregnancy is a contraindication to travel or residence in areas known to have drug-resistant *P falciparum.* However, should such travel be unavoidable, it is probably best for the patient to take mefloquine 25 mg weekly or 500 mg every two weeks, recognizing that there are potential risks.[85] The risk of acquiring chloroquine-resistant *P falciparum* malaria, however, far outweighs the problems associated with effective chemotherapy.

For pregnant patients living in holoendemic areas, it is probably best to treat the mother prophylactically, especially an expatriate woman without the opportunity to develop immunity to infections during childhood and early adulthood. Any person traveling or residing in a malarious area should not be allowed to overlook the need for taking precautions against mosquitoes: insect repellent and mosquito netting.

Babesiosis. Babesiosis is a worldwide zoonotic disease caused by species of intraerythrocytic protozoan *Babesia* transmitted by infected ticks. The illness is characterized by hemolytic anemia, splenomegaly, and fever. The clinical course and parasitized red blood cells may cause confusion with malaria. There is a wide spectrum of infection from asymptomatic parasitemia to disseminated intravascular coagulopathy, renal failure, and death. The illness is more severe in splenectomized or immunocompromised individuals. The virulence of the infecting species of *Babesia* also determines the clinical course. Treatment with clindamycin and quinine is indicated for the seriously ill.

Babesia infect many mammalian species. The recent outbreak of babesiosis in the northeastern United States has been caused by the rodent species, *Babesia microti.* The tick vector, *Ixodes dammini,* is also the vector for the causative spirochete of Lyme disease. Simultaneous infection with *Babesia* and *Borrelia burgdorferi,* the spirochete causing Lyme disease, has been reported in a small number of patients.[86] About half of patients with babesiosis acquired in endemic areas have antibodies against *B burgdorferi.*

Infection during pregnancy is rarely reported. One woman, not asplenic, recovered without specific chemotherapy following a clinically mild, low parasitemic *Babesia* infection, which began during the fifth month of gestation. The neonate had no clinical or hematologic evidence of babesiosis and no IgM antibody to *Babesia microti.* Babesiosis during pregnancy should be expected in endemic areas where as many as 6% of susceptibles may acquire the infection.

Advice for the Pregnant Traveler

Adventurous visits to exotic places have become a commonplace event. The rapidity and ease of air travel for the well-off of the world entice even the cautious gravid woman. A Pandora's box of ills awaits the unsuspecting and unprepared traveler (Table 111–15). Travelers often mimic the inhabitants of the places they visit, failing to consider that

TABLE 111–15. IMPORTANT ADVICE TO PROTECT PREGNANT TRAVELERS

Water:	Only boiled, sterilized, or bottled
Food:	No raw foods (meat, shellfish, vegetables)
Dress:	Protect against insects; wear long sleeves, pants Use insect repellant
Sleeping:	Mosquito nets. Spray for bedbugs, Triatoma bugs. Only with someone you know and know well.
Other Health Precautions:	Be wary of injections, transfusions, intimate contacts; AIDS kills both mothers and babies; Take malaria prophylaxis
Specific Advice About:	Chagas' disease, African trypanosomiasis, Toxoplasmosis, Giardiasis and amebiasis, Other arthropodborne pathogens
Specific instructions and referrals for obstetrical care including a doctor's letter giving specifics of prenatal care	
Specific instructions and plans for medical/obstetrical evacuation	

the resident population has usually acquired immunity to indigenous infectious diseases. If the native population looks healthy to the tourist, it is often because the people with fevers, deformities, and disabilities are not on display.

The patient should be given practical common sense advice about water, food, and protection from insects. Water can be purified quickly with tincture of iodine, one or two drops per pint, which sterilizes bacteria and the cysts of all intestinal protozoa. Mosquito netting with a fine mesh should be used even during the day and in the city. Insect repellant should be applied on the ankles and legs first because sandflies, trombiculid mites, and ticks all cluster close to the ground. Exposing a great deal of skin is an invitation to biting insects. Skipping doses of malaria prophylaxis, not using mosquito netting, and drinking unsafe water because the inhabitants do not seem ill are foolhardy.

Travel to areas with endemic diseases transmitted by arthropod vectors should be discouraged during pregnancy. Although malaria, trypanosomiasis, and leishmaniasis are not as common a problem among travelers as enterotoxigenic travelers' diarrhea, giardiasis, and sunburn, they have far more serious effects on the health of the mother and the success of the pregnancy. Moreover, the usual methods of protection such as chemoprophylaxis and the use of insecticides and repellants carry some risks for the pregnant woman and her fetus. Treatment for any of the protozoan infections travelers may acquire is not without hazard. It is a good general rule that there is no antiparasitic drug entirely safe to use during pregnancy.

REFERENCES

1. Mahmoud AA. Parasitic protozoa and helminths: biological and immunological challenges. *Science*. 1989;246:1015.
2. Manson-Bahr PEC, Bell DR. *Manson's Tropical Diseases*. 19th ed. London: Balliere Tindall; 1987.
3. Marcial-Rojas RA, ed. *Pathology of Protozoal and Helminthic Diseases*. Baltimore, MD: Williams & Williams; 1971.
4. Snow KR. *Insects and Disease*. London: Routledge and Kegan Paul; 1974.
5. Gall SA. Maternal adjustments in the immune system. *Clin Obstet Gynecol*. 1983:26:521.
6. Reinhardt MC. Effects of parasitic infections in pregnant women. *Ciba Found Symp*. 1980;77:149.
7. Loke YW. Transmission of parasites across the placenta. In: Baker JR, Muller R; eds. *Advances in Parasitology*. London: Academic Press Inc.; 1982;21:155.
8. D'Alauro FD, Lee RV, Pao-In K, et al. Intestinal parasites and pregnancy. *Obstet Gynecol*. 1985;66:639.
9. MacLeod CL, Lee RV. Parasitic infections. In: Burrow GN, Ferris TF, eds. *Medical Complications During Pregnancy*. Philadelphia: WB Saunders Company; 1988:425.
10. MacLeod CL, ed. *Parasitic Infections in Pregnancy and the Newborn*. Oxford: Oxford University Press; 1988.
11. Keusch GT, ed. The biology of parasitic infection: workshop on interactions of nutrition and parasitic diseases. *Rev Infect Dis*. 1982;4:735.
12. Drugs for Parasitic Infections. *Medical Letter*. 1990;32:23.
13. Lewis EA, Antia AV. Amoebic colitis: review of 195 cases. *Trans R Soc Trop Med Hyg*. 1969;63:633.
14. Martinez-Palomo A, Martinez-Baeq M. Amebiasis in selective primary health care: strategies for control of disease in the developing world. *Rev Infect Dis*. 1983;5:1093.
15. Ravdin JI. *Entamoeba histolytica:* from adherence to enteropathy. *J Infect Dis*. 1989;159:420.
16. Wagner VP, Smale LE, Lischke JH. Amebic abscess of the liver and spleen in pregnancy and the puerperium. *Obstet Gynecol*. 1975;45:562.
17. Cowan DB, Houlton MC. Rupture of an amoebic liver abscess in pregnancy. *S Afr Med J*. 1978;53:460.
18. Czeizel E, Hancsok M, Palkovich I, et al. Possible relation between fetal death and *E. histolytica* infection of the mother. *Am J Obstet Gynecol*. 1966;96:264.
19. Rivera RA. Fatal postpartum amoebic colitis with trophozoites in peritoneal fluid. *Gastroenterology*. 1972;62:314.
20. Abioye AA. Fatal amoebic colitis in pregnancy and puerperium: a new clinico pathological entity. *J Trop Med Hyg*. 1973;76:97.
21. Armon PJ. Amoebiasis in pregnancy and puerperium. *Br J Obstet Gynaecol*. 1978;85:264.
22. Constantine G, Menon V, Luisley D. Amoebic peritonitis in pregnancy in the United Kingdom. *Post Grad Med J*. 1987;63:495.
23. Gillon FD, Reiner DS, Wang C. Human milk kills parasitic intestinal protozoa. *Science*. 1983;221:1290.
24. Beard CM, Noller KL, O'Fallon WM, et al. Cancer after exposure to metronidazole. *Mayo Clin Proc*. 1988;63:147.
25. Kreutner NK, Del Bene VE, Amstey MS. Giardiasis in pregnancy. *Am J Obstet Gynecol*. 1981;140:895.
26. Jokipii L, Jokipii AMM. Giardiasis and balantidiasis. In: Braude AI, ed. *Medical Microbiology and Infectious Diseases*. Philadelphia: WB Saunders; 1981:1075.
27. Nayak N, Ganguly NIC, Walia BNS, et al. Specific secretory IgA in the milk of *Giardia lamblia*–infected and uninfected women. *J Infect Dis*. 1987;155:724.
28. Lee RV, Prowten AW, Anthone S, et al. *Balantidium coli* typhlitis in captive lowland gorillas. *Rev Infect Dis*. 1990;12:1052.
29. Dubey JP, Beattie CP. *Toxoplasmosis of Animals and Man*. Boca Raton: CRC Press; 1988.
30. Koskiniemi M, Lappalainen M, Hedman K. Toxoplasmosis needs evaluation. *Amer J Dis Child*. 1989;143:724.
31. Sever JL. Perinatal infections affecting the developing fetus and newborn. In: Eichenwald H, ed. *The Prevention of Mental Retardation Through Control of Infectious Diseases*. Washington D.C.: U.S. Government Printing Office; 1968. Public Health Service Publication #1692:37.
32. Luft BJ, Remington JS. Acute *Toxoplasma* infection among family members of patients with acute lymphadenopathic toxoplasmosis. *Arch Intern Med*. 1984;144:53.
33. Lee RV. Parasites and pregnancy: the problems of malaria and toxoplasmosis. *Clin Perinatol*. 1988;15:351.
34. Desmonts G, Couvreur J. Congenital toxoplasmosis: a prospective study of 378 pregnancies. *N Engl J Med*. 1974;290:1110.
35. Daffos F, Forestier F, Capella-Pavlovsky M, et al. Prenatal management of 746 pregnancies at risk for congenital toxoplasmosis. *N Engl J Med*. 1988;318:271.
36. Desmonts G, Couvreur J. Congenital toxoplasmosis: a prospective study of the offspring of 542 women who acquired toxoplasmosis during pregnancy—pathophysiology of congenital disease. In: Thalhammer O, Baumgarden K, Pollak A, eds. *Perinatal Medicine*. Stuttgart: Georg Thieme; 1979:51.
37. Brooks RG, McCabe RE, Remington JS. Role of serology in the diagnosis of toxoplasmic lymphadenopathy. *J Infect Dis*. 1987;9:1055.
38. Tetusch SM, Sulzer AJ, Ramsey JE, et al. *Toxoplasma gondii* isolated from amniotic fluid. *Obstet Gynecol*. 1980;55:2.
39. Desmonts G, Forestier F, Thulliez PH, et al. Prenatal diagnosis of congenital toxoplasmosis. *Lancet*. 1985;1:500.
40. Couvreur J, Desmonts G, Thulliez PH. Prophylaxis of congenital toxo-

plasmosis. Effects of spiramycin on placental infection. *J Antimicrob Chemother.* 1988;22:193.
41. Hohlfeld P, Daffos F, Thulliez P, et al. Fetal toxoplasmosis: outcome of pregnancy and infant follow up after in utero treatment. *J Pediatrics.* 1989;115:765.
42. Weiss LM, Perlman DC, Sherman J, et al. *Isospora belli* infection: treatment with pyrimethamine. *Ann Intern Med.* 1988;109:474.
43. Burke VA, Good RA. *Pneumocystis carinii* infection. *Medicine.* 1973;52:23.
44. Walzer PD, Perl DP. Krogstad DJ, et al. *Pneumocystis carinii* pneumonia in the United States. *Arch Intern Med.* 1974;80:83.
45. Stagno S, Pifer LL, Hughes WT, et al. *Pneumocystis carinii* pneumonitis in young immunocompetent infants. *Pediatrics.* 1980;66:56.
46. Hughes WT, Giglio HiF. Nomenclature for *Pneumocystis carinii. J Infect Dis.* 1988;157:432.
47. Pearson RD, Wheeler DK, Harrison LH, et al. The immunobiology of leishmaniasis. *Rev Infect Dis.* 1983;5:907.
48. Fernandez-Guerero ML, Aguado JM, Buzon L, et al. Visceral leishmaniasis in immunocompromised hosts. *Am J Med.* 1987;83:1098.
49. Grimaldi G, Tesh RB, McMahon-Pratt D. A review of the geographic distribution and epidemiology of leishmaniasis in the New World. *Am J Trop Med Hyg.* 1989;41:687.
50. Corredor A, Kreutzer RD, Tesh RB, et al. Distribution and etiology of leishmaniasis in Colombia. *Am J Trop Med Hyg.* 1990;42:206.
51. Molyneux DH. African trypanosomiasis in selective primary care: strategies for control of disease in the developing world. *Rev Infect Dis.* 1983;5:945.
52. Nieman RE, Kelly JJ, Waskin HA. Severe African trypanosomiasis with spurious hypoglycemia. *J Infect Dis.* 1989;159:360.
53. Olowe SA. A case of congenital trypanosomiasis in Lagos. *Trans R Soc Trop Med Hyg.* 1975;69:57.
54. Grant IH, Gold JWM, Wittner M, et al. Transfusion associated acute Chagas' disease acquired in the United States. *Ann Intern Med.* 1989; 111:849.
55. Laraja FS, Dias E, Nobrega G, et al. Chagas' disease: a clinical, epidemiologic, and pathologic study. *Circulation.* 1956;14:1035.
56. Szarfman A, Cossio PM, Arana RM, et al. Immunologic and immunopathologic studies in congenital Chagas' disease. *Clin Immunol Immunopathol.* 1975;4:489.
57. Bittencourt AL. Congenital Chagas' disease. *Am J Dis Child.* 1976;130:97.
58. Carlier Y, Rivera MT, Truyens C, et al. Pregnancy and humoral immune response in mice chronically infected by *Trypanosoma cruzi. Infect Immun.* 1987;55:2496.
59. Tanowitz HB, Morris SA, Weiss LM, et al. Effect of verapamil on the development of chronic experimental Chagas' disease. *Am J Trop Med Hyg.* 1989;41:643.
60. Wyler DJ. Malaria—resurgence, resistance, and research. *N Engl J Med.* 1983;308:875,934.
61. Centers for Disease Control. *Malaria Surveillance Annual Summary 1988.* (issued November, 1989).
62. Lobel HO, Campbell CC. *Trends in Imported Malaria, United States.* CDC Surveillance Summaries. *MMWR.* 1983;32:1555.
63. Lee MV, Ambrus JL, DeSouza JM, et al. Diminished red blood cell deformability in uncomplicated human malaria. *Medicine.* 1982;13:479.
64. Strang A, Lachman E, Piesoe SB, et al. Malaria in pregnancy with fatal complications—case report. *Br J Obstet Gynecol.* 1984;91:399.
65. Feldman RM, Singer C. Noncardiogenic pulmonary edema and pulmonary fibrosis in *falciparum* malaria. *Rev Infect Dis.* 1987;9:134.
66. Currier JS, Maguire JH. Problems in the management of *falciparum* malaria. *Rev Infect Dis.* 1989;11:988.
67. Clark IA. Cell-mediated immunity in protection and pathology of malaria. *Parasitol Today.* 1987;3:300.
68. Moran JS, Bernard KW. The spread of chloroquine-resistant malaria in Africa. *JAMA.* 1989;262:245.
69. Taufa T. Malaria and pregnancy. *Papua New Guinea Med J.* 1978;21:197.
70. McGregor IA, Wilson ME, Billewicz WZ. Malaria infection of the placenta in the Gambia, West Africa: its incidence and relationship to stillbirth, birthweight, and placental weight. *Trans R Soc Trop Med Hyg.* 1983;77:232.
71. Riley EM, Schneider G, Sambou I, Greenwood BM. Suppression of cell-mediated immune responses to malaria antigens in pregnancy Gambian women. *Am J Trop Med Hyg.* 1989;40:141.
72. Breman JG, Steketee RW, Wirima JJ, et al. Fetal wastage in Malawi, an area of high malaria endemicity. *Proc Ann Mtg Amer Soc Trop Med Hyg.* December 1989; abstract #271.
73. Slutsker L, Wirima J, Khoroman CO, Steketee RW. Neonatal mortality associated with low birth weight in Malawi. *Proc Annu Meet Am Soc Trop Med Hyg.* December 1989; abstract #269.
74. Yamada M, Steketee R, Abramivksy C, et al. *Plasmodium falciparum* associated placental pathology: a light and electron microscopic and immunohistologic study. *Am J Trop Med Hyg.* 1989;41:161.
75. Reinhardt MC, Ambriose-Thomas P, Cavallo-Sera R, et al. Malaria at delivery in Abidjan. *Helv Paediatr Acta.* 1978;33:65.
76. Hindi RD, Azimi PH. Congenital malaria due to *Plasmodium falciparum. Pediatrics.* 1980;66:977.
77. Quinn TC, Jacobs RF, Mertz GI, et al. Congenital malaria: a report of four cases and a review. *J Pediatr.* 1982;101:229.
78. Wirima JJ, Heymann DL, Steketee RW. Congenital malaria: spontaneous postpartum clearance, Malawi. *Proc Annu Meet Am Soc Trop Med Hyg.* December 1989; abstract #272.
79. Main EM, Main DM, Krogstad DJ. Treatment of chloroquine-resistant malaria during pregnancy. *JAMA.* 1983;249:3207.
80. Wolfe MS, Cordero JF. Safety of chloroquine in chemosuppression of malaria during pregnancy. *Br Med J.* 1985;290:1466.
81. Parke A. Antimalarial drugs and pregnancy. *Am J Med.* 1988;85:30.
82. White NJ, Warrell DA, Chanthavanich P, et al. Severe hypoglycemia and hyperinsulinemia in *falciparum* malaria. *N Engl J Med.* 1983;309:61.
83. Okitolonda W, Delacollette C, Malengreau M, Henquin JC. High incidence of hypoglycemia in African patients treated with intravenous quinine for severe malaria. *Br Med J.* 1987;295:716.
84. Zitelli BJ, Alexander J, Taylor S, et al. Fatal hepatic necrosis due to pyrimethamine-sulfadoxine (Fansdiar). *Ann Intern Med.* 1987;106:393.
85. Steketee RW, Wirima J, Heymann DL, et al. Efficacy of mefloquin and chloroquine prophylaxis in pregnancy. *Proc Annu Meet Am Soc Trop Med Hyg.* December 1989; abstract #283.
86. Gadbaw JJ, et al. Babesiosis—Connecticut. *MMWR.* 1989;38:649.

Chapter One Hundred and Twelve
Helminthic Infections

Robert L. Murphy

112

Helminthic infections occur in over 54 million individuals in the United States. In some developing countries, helminths may infect up to 90% of the population within certain geographic areas. Helminths or worms are unique pathogens, not only in their high prevalence rates, but also by their relatively large size—up to 50 feet in the case of *Diphyllobothrium latum*, the fish tapeworm. Their presence within the human host often induces eosinophilia as part of the immune response, a phenomenon associated with protozoal infections and hypersensitivity reactions to certain drugs as well.[1,2]

One of the most unusual features of these infections is that the majority of helminths cannot multiply within the human host. With the notable exception of strongyloides and the echinococcus, a complex life cycle exists within the environment or within intermediate hosts. Typically, an adult worm residing in the gut will shed thousands of eggs per day. The eggs will then pass with the feces, embryonate in the environment or within another host, and get ingested by a human in whose gut the larvae will mature to an adult worm; then, the cycle begins again. The other common scenario involves skin penetration by infectious larvae followed by migration by way of the blood stream to the lungs with continued migration up the bronchial tree and then on toward the gut where the maturation phase is completed and the cycle begins again.

Most helminthic infections are asymptomatic or associated with mild or moderate symptoms. Heavy worm burdens may be associated with abdominal pain, diarrhea, anemia, and rarely, abdominal obstruction. Therapeutic indications during pregnancy should focus more on worm burden than on total eradication since many of the anthelminthic therapies are dangerous when administered during this time. The risk-benefit ratio in treating pregnant patients with significant helminthic infections continues to be a clinical dilemma.

Helminths can be categorized into three main groups. The first are nematodes or round worms, which can be further subclassified into those causing primarily intestinal or tissue infection. The second group are the trematodes or flukes, and the third are the tapeworms.

NEMATODES, INTESTINAL ROUND WORMS

Intestinal nematodes account for the largest group of helminthic infections in humans. Three such infections, trichuriasis, ascariasis, and ancylostoma or hookworm occur in approximately 1 billion persons each year. Additionally, this is the second largest phylum in the animal kingdom. Serologic detection assays are essentially useless in these infections since replication occurs outside the human host in most helminthic infections.

Trichuriasis (Whipworm)

Trichuris trichira infects over 800 million people worldwide. In the United States, it is estimated that there are 2.2 million infected individuals, mostly in the rural southeastern areas of the country and in Puerto Rico where conditions are warm and moist. The adult worms anchor themselves to the mucosa of the cecum and ascending colon where they ingest 0.005 mL of blood per day. The mean length of the adult worm is 40 mm. Life expectancy is one year. Females produce up to 20,000 egg per day. Soil pollution by humans and animals determines the major factor in the spread of the infection, predominantly within poor rural communities. Clinical conditions associated with infection are usually mild and many are completely asymptomatic. Mild anemia, bloody diarrhea, growth retardation, and rectal prolapse may occur. Eosinophilia is not usually present. Diagnosis is easily made on stool exam by the presence of the typical lemon-shaped eggs.

Treatment recommendations call for mebendazole 100 mg twice daily for three days. Mebendazole is associated with embryotoxic and teratogenic effects in pregnant rats and is, therefore, contraindicated during pregnancy.[3]

Enterobiasis (Pinworm)

Enterobius vermicularis is a 1 cm, thread-like worm that lives in the cecum. Adult females migrate to the perianal region to lay their eggs at night. The eggs embryonate within six hours and are, then, transferred to clothing and bed linens. The most common mode of transmission is by way of the patient's hands. Familial and institutional infections are common. There appears to be no predilection to socioeconomic class and whites tend to have higher prevalence rates than blacks. Eggs may remain infective for up to 20 days. The life span of the adult worm is 35 days. Many patients are asymptomatic but the most common symptom is pruritus ani. Rarely, worm migration may cause appendicitis, salpingitis, or ulcerative lesions in the colon. Eosinophilia is not a feature of this infection. Diagnosis can be made by the naked eye or adhesive tape test.

Treatment recommendations are the same as for trichuriasis.[3]

Ascariasis

Ascaris lumbricoides is the most common helminthic infection worldwide, occurring in over one billion people; four million of them are in the southeastern United States. These worms grow to 35 cm and live primarily in the small intestine. Worms live 10–24 months and produce 200,000 eggs per day. Ingested eggs hatch in the bowel where the embryo penetrates the bowel wall and migrates by way of the blood stream to the lungs. Here, the embryonate breaks out into the alveoli, passes up through the bronchus and trachea, and are swallowed. They mature to adult worms in the intestines. Transmission is primarily from hand to mouth. The eggs are sturdy and may withstand significant environmental insult. Although overt disease is rare, bowel obstruction, pneumonitis, nutritional disorders, and even blockage of the fallopian tubes has been observed. Eosinophilia is common. Diagnosis is made by seeing the typical eggs on stool examination.

Treatment recommendations include mebendazole, which is contraindicated in pregnancy. However, piperazine citrate 150 mg/kg, followed by 65 mg/kg, twice daily for three days, has been proven relatively safe in pregnancy.[4,5]

Hookworm

Ancylostoma duodenal and *Necator americans* are 1-cm worms that infect the upper intestines in 25% of the world's population. There is a low degree of infection in the southeastern United States. Ancylostoma duodenal is capable of ingesting 0.2 mL of blood per day. Females pass 7000 eggs per day. Worms live two to five years. Eggs pass in the stool and hatch in moist soil. Larvae can penetrate the skin if contact for five to 10 minutes is made. They, then, are carried by way of the blood stream to the lung, break out through the alveoli and migrate up the bronchial tree, and are swallowed. They mature to adulthood in the intestine. Ground itch at the site of penetration is common. A Löffler's type pneumonitis is common and eosinophilia is noted in sputum, as well as blood. Iron deficiency anemia, hypoalbuminemia, abdominal pain, diarrhea, malabsorption, and weight loss can be seen. Diagnosis is made by finding the characteristic eggs on stool examination.

Treatment is with mebendazole, as in trichuriasis, and is contraindicated during pregnancy.

Strongyloidiasis

Strongyloides stercoralis is a potentially lethal infection, especially in the immunocompromised human host. Unlike most other helminthic infections, autoinfection is possible, leading to potentially enormous worm burdens on the host. Prevalence rates within the United States range from 0.4–4.0% in southern portions of the country. Infective larvae penetrate skin and travel by way of the blood stream to the lung with eventual migration to the gut, where they bore into the mucosa. The larvae hatch in the mucosa and bore to the lumen where they may transform to the infective form. Clinically, one third of all infections are asymptomatic. The skin and pulmonary symptoms are similar to hookworm. Abdominal pain, diarrhea, nausea, vomiting, weight loss, and malabsorption are not uncommon. Urticarial rash beginning perianally may be seen. Massive tissue invasion can occur, especially in the immunocompromised hosts. Gram-negative bacteremia may also be seen. Diagnosis is made on stool examination or duodenal aspirate.

Treatment is with thiabendazole 25 mg twice daily for two days. Thiabendazole is associated with cleft palate and axial skeletal defects in mice given 10 times the human dose and, therefore, should be avoided during pregnancy. Piperazine can be substituted during pregnancy (see ascariasis).[6]

TISSUE NEMATODES

Trichinosis

Trichinella spiralis infects humans who have ingested encysted larvae present in undercooked meat that break out of their cyst in the stomach and migrate to the small intestine where they mature into adult worms. Five hundred larvae are produced every two weeks. The larvae seed the skeletal muscle, encyst, and live there for several years. One hundred to two hundred cases are reported in the United States per year, primarily in the northeast and western portions of the country. Autopsy series have demonstrated a prevalence rate as high as 4%. Most infections are thought to be related to eating undercooked pork. As demonstrated by the autopsy data, most cases are subclinical. Diarrhea, abdominal pain, vomiting, and enteritis characterize the intestinal phase of the infection. Fever, periorbital edema, myositis, cough, extraocular palsies, shortness of breath, dysphagia, and rash peak in frequency at two to four weeks after exposure, then subside. Death is rare. Diagnosis is made on clinical grounds, particularly the periorbital edema, myositis, fever, and eosinophilia. An antibody test (bentonite flocculation) is available. Sedimentation rate is usually normal.

Treatment is with thiabendazole 25 mg/kg per day for seven days if given within 24 hours after exposure. This drug is contraindicated in pregnancy. The mainstay of therapy is bed rest.

Dracunculiasis (Guinea Worm)

Dracunculus medinensis infects 140 million people worldwide, mostly in tropical areas where people bathe in water that is used for drinking. Infection starts when water infested with infected crustaceans is ingested. Larvae are then released in the intestine where they penetrate the mucosa and reach the retroperitoneum where they mature and mate. The female migrates to subcutaneous tissues, usually in the lower extremities where the worm protrudes. The overlying skin ulcerates and, when exposed to water, larvae are released and crustaceans ingest them. Patients are asymptomatic until the worm protrudes. Urticaria, nausea, vomiting, diarrhea, and dyspnea can occur. The worm is absorbed or discharged over several weeks. Adult females reach 1 m in length. Diagnosis is made clinically.

Treatment is with thiabendazole (see strongyloides) or metronidazole 5 mg/kg twice daily for one week. This helps with the inflammatory reaction only and does not kill the worm. Metronidazole is carcinogenic in rodents and since no good studies have been performed on pregnant women, the drug should be avoided during pregnancy. The worm should be rolled out onto a stick and progressively rolled daily until it is completely removed.

Bancroftian and Brugian Filariasis

Wuchereria bancrofti, Brugia malayi, and *Brugia timori* are transmitted to humans by way of mosquitoes. Infective larvae then travel by way of the lymph channel to the nodes where they mature to adult worms up to 40 mm in length. The adults discharge microfilariae into the blood stream where biting mosquitoes ingest and transform to infective larvae. Symptoms, when present, are usually related to lymphatic obstruction. Chronic hydrocele is common. Diagnosis is made by examination of blood smear, chylous or hydrocele fluid, tissue analysis, or on clinical grounds.

Treatments are unsatisfactory. Diethylcarbamazine citrate 3 mg/kg three times daily for 21 days is known to reduce the filarial form. Its safety in pregnancy is undetermined.

Loiasis

Loa loa is transmitted to humans by thetabanid flies (Chrysops species) that live in the canopy of the tropical rain forest. They are attracted to people moving through the jungle. These are white thread-like worms that cause transient subcutaneous swellings. Microfilariae are released into the blood. Biting horse flies can take up the microfilariae while feeding. Eosinophilia, Calabar swellings, pruritus, urticaria, subconjunctival passing, renal disease, endomyocardial fibrosis, retinopathy, encephalopathy, peripheral neuropathy, and arthritis may occur. Diagnosis is made by blood examination, on clinical grounds or by eye worm extraction.

Treatment is with diethylcarbamazine.[7]

Onchocerciasis (River Blindness)

Onchocerca volvulus is transmitted by blackflies (Simulium) in Africa and Central and South America. These flies are usually found near running streams. After contact, itchy dermatitis, subcutaneous nodules, and keratitis may appear. Eosinophilia is common. Diagnosis is made by examination of skin snips, slit lamp exam, or nodule biopsy.

Treatment is with diethylcarbamazine, as in loiasis, in gradually increasing doses to 3 mg/kg per day for 21 days. Invermectin 150 μg/kg in a single dose has also been used. These treatments kill only the microfilariae. Suramin kills adult worms but is very toxic. None of these drugs has been proven to be safe during pregnancy. Surgical removal of nodules should be done whenever practical.[7]

TREMATODES (FLUKES)

Schistosomiasis

Schistosoma mansoni, Schistosoma japonica, Schistosoma mekongi, Schistosoma haematobia, and *Schistosoma intercalatum* are the five human blood flukes that currently infect more than 200 million people. It is estimated that 400,000 persons are infected in the United States, mainly immigrants from Puerto Rico, Brazil, the Middle East, and the Philippines. In the Great Lakes region, infection may occur following exposure to avian schistosomes. Overall, worldwide prevalence is on the increase. Mature flukes pass eggs in the stool where they, in the presence of fresh water, hatch into motile ciliated miracidia that penetrate into the body of the snail. Once in the snail, cercariae are formed which emerge to penetrate the skin of humans. Inside the human host, the cercariae loses its tail to become a schistosomulae which migrates to the lung and liver. There they mature to adult worms and move to the venous system of the intestines where they may live for up to 10 years. Clinical presentations relate to the dermatitis, febrile illness, or fibro-obstructive sequelae that occurs with chronic infection. Eosinophilia, fatigue, abdominal pain, and diarrhea are common. In *S haematobia,* bladder and ureter invasion is common and infection is associated with bladder cancer and salmonella carrier states. Diagnosis is made by stool or urine examination or rectal biopsy.

Treatment with praziquantel 40 mg/kg in one dose is effective in treating *S mansoni* and *S haematobia* infection. *S japonica* dosing is 20 mg/kg three times in one day. Praziquantel is associated with increased abortion rates in rats. No studies in pregnant women have been performed. Other agents, such as metrifonate and oxamniquine, can also be used. Oxamniquine is associated with embryocidal effects in rabbits and mice. No studies of the drug have been done in pregnant women and safety data are limited or nonexistent.[8]

Clonorchiasis

Clonorchis sinensis is a parasite of fish-eating mammals that infects millions of Asians. Adult flukes in the biliary tract lay eggs that pass by way of the feces to water where they are picked up by snails and hatch into miracidia. The miracidia transform into cercariae that pass into fresh water where they penetrate fish and encyst. When eaten either raw or undercooked by mammals, the metacercariae encyst in the duodenum and pass through the ampulla of Vater where the adult worms mature inside of the bile ducts. The clinical symptoms, if any, are associated with biliary obstruction and cholangiocarcinoma. Diagnosis is made on stool exam.

Treatment is with praziquantel as in schistosomiasis.

Fascioliasis

Fasciola hepatica is a common fluke in sheep-raising areas of the world. The snail is the intermediate host.

Treatment is with praziquantel as in schistosomiasis.

Fasciolopsiasis

Frasiolopsis buski is endemic in the Far East and Southeast Asia. The infectious miracidia invade the snail where they multiply and encyst on almost any aquatic plant which, subsequently, may be ingested by the human host. Adult worms mature and reside in the intestines. Treatment is with praziquantel as in schistosomiasis.

Heterophiliasis

Heterophyes heterophyes is a common fluke in the Nile Delta where they encyst in freshwater fish. In the human, adult worms live in the small intestines. Treatment is with praziquantel as in schistosomiasis.

Paragonimiasis

Paragonimus westermani, the lung fluke, inhabits parts of West Africa, the Far East, India, Central America, and South America. Adult worms encapsulate in the lungs. Eggs are coughed up and some are swallowed and passed in the stool to fresh water where they hatch and penetrate snails. After a three to five month maturation phase in the snail, cercariae emerge and encyst in the crayfish and freshwater crabs which are then eaten by humans. Once in the human, they penetrate the intestinal wall, enter the peritoneum, and migrate through the diaphragm and into the pleural space and lung where they lodge and lay eggs. Diagnosis is made by examination of sputum or stool.

Treatment is with praziquantel 25 mg/kg three times daily for three days.[8]

TAPEWORMS

Taenia saginata (the Beef Tapeworm)

Infection occurs when poorly cooked muscle of diseased cattle are ingested. Within two months, mature adult worms are formed. Eggs are passed in the stool and ingested by cattle. Worms can grow to 30 feet. Symptoms are usually minimal consisting of cramps, weight loss, and, rarely, obstruction. Eosinophilia is common. Diagnosis is made by examination of the stool.

Treatment is with niclosamide 2 g in one dose. Toxicity studies in animals have been negative. Little information is available regarding its use in pregnancy. Other treatments include praziquantel 10 mg/kg in one dose (see schistosomiasis) and paromomycin sulfate 1 g every four hours for four doses. Paromomycin is very poorly absorbed and is essentially 100% eliminated in the stool. Studies in pregnant women have not been published.

Taenia solium (the Pork Tapeworm)

This is similar to *Taenia saginata* except for pork being the intermediate host.

Cysticercosis

Contact with human feces containing the eggs of *Taenia solium* causes the disease cysticercosis. The larvae can develop in any tissue of the body, but the most common clinical problem relates to the presence of cysts occurring in the brain. Infection is common in Mexico, South America, and parts of Africa. Seizures are often the presenting sign. Diagnosis can be made by computerized tomography (CT) or magnetic resonance imaging (MRI) of the brain. Serology can be useful as well.

Treatment consists of surgery, if accessible. Praziquantel 50 mg in three divided doses for two weeks may be helpful. Steroids may be required as adjuvant therapy because of the often intense inflammatory reaction that occurs when the organisms die.

Diphyllobothriasis (the Fish Tapeworm)

D latum is spread by eating raw or undercooked fish. Adult worms may reach 50 feet in length. Eggs hatch in the intestine and pass in the feces to fresh water, where they are eaten by crustaceans that are eaten by fish. Infections are seen in Finland, Sweden, Japan, the Baltics, as well as in Eskimos and Jewish cooks who sample gefilte fish during its preparation. Vitamin B_{12} deficiency and bowel obstruction may occur. Diagnosis is made on examination of the stool or by characteristic lower gastrointestinal x-rays.

Treatment is with praziquantel as in schistosomiasis.

Hymenolepiasis

Hymenolepis nana or dwarf tapeworm is spread by human-to-human contact and occurs worldwide. Clinical features include abdominal cramps, diarrhea, dizziness, and seizures. Diagnosis is made by stool examination.

Treatment is with niclosamide 2 g per day for five to seven days (see *T saginata*).

Echinococcosis

Echinococcus granulosus exists when dogs eat infected beef or lamb and pass infectious eggs in their stool, which are taken up by humans. Once in the intestines, the oncospheres invade the mesenteric vessels and travel to the lungs and liver and form hydatid cysts. The cysts grow approximately 1 cm per year. Infections are common in sheep-raising areas of the world, particularly in Greece and Lebanon. Sixty percent of the cysts occur in the right lobe of the liver. Cysts commonly have a smooth rim of calcification. Eosinophilia is common. Disgnosis is made by clinical evaluation and serology.

Treatment is primarily surgical although mebendazole (see trichuriasis) or albendazole is usually given preoperatively. Praziquantel may also be effective (see schistosomiasis). The effects of albendazole in pregnant women is unknown. Only enlarging cysts need removal.[9]

OTHER HELMINTHIC INFECTIONS

Visceral Larvae Migrans

Toxocara canis and *Toxocara cati* occur when dogs ingest viable eggs or encapsulated cysts in rodents. Humans get infected because of their exposure to dogs. United States prevalence rates range from 2.8% to 54%.[10] Infection is more common among blacks, children under six years old, pica, and those exposed to young puppies. Clinical features include cough, fever, wheezing, eosinophilia, and hepatomegaly. The diagnosis is made by clinical history and demonstration of larvae in the tissues. Serology may be useful.

Treatment is usually not required because most patients recover uneventfully. Thiabendazole (see strongyloides), diethylcarbamazine, and mebendazole (see trichuriasis) have been used.

Cutaneous Larvae Migrans

Ancylostoma braziliense is the dog and cat hookworm found mostly in the southeast United States in sandy, shady beach areas. Larvae are able to penetrate the human skin, causing itching, vessicle formation, and serpiginous tracts. Only rarely does systemic involvement occur. Diagnosis is made on clinical grounds.

Treatment is usually not required and most symptoms resolve within four weeks. Topical or oral thiabendazole 25 mg/kg twice daily for two days has been employed and may shorten the clinical course to one week[11] (see strongyloides).

REFERENCES

1. Strickland GT. Helminthic infections. In: Strickland GT, ed. *Tropical Medicine*. 6th ed. Philadelphia; WB Saunders; 1984;616.
2. Warren KS. Diseases due to Helminths. In: Mandel GL, Douglas RG, Bennett JE, eds. *Principles and Practices of Infectious Diseases*. 3rd ed. New York; Churchill Livingstone; 1990:2134.
3. Mahmoud AAF. Intestinal nematodes. In: Mandel GL, Douglas RG, Bennett JE, eds. *Principles and Practices of Infectious Diseases*. 3rd ed. New York; Churchill Livingstone; 1990:2135.
4. World Health Organization. Prevention and Control of Intestinal Parasitic Infections: Report of a Who Expert Committee. *WHO Tech Rep Ser*. 749. Geneva; World Health Organization, 1987.
5. Swartwelder JC, Miller JH, Sappenfield RW. The use of piperazine for the treatment of human helminthiasis. *Gastroenterology*. 1957;33:87.
6. Young RL, Zund G, Mason BA, Faro S. Pelvic inflammatory disease complicated by massive helminthic hyperinfection. *Obstet Gynecol*. 1989;74:484.
7. Grove DF. Tissue nematodes. In: Mandel GL, Douglas RG, Bennett JE, eds. *Principles and Practices of Infectious Diseases*. 3rd ed. New York: Churchill Livingstone; 1990:2140.
8. Mahmoud AAF. Trematodes. In: Mandel GL, Douglas RG, Bennett JE, eds. *The Principal and Practice of Infectious Diseases*. 3rd ed. New York: Churchill Livingstone; 1990:2145.
9. Jones TC. Cestodes. In: Mandel GL, Douglas RG, Bennett JE, eds. *Principles and Practices of Infectious Diseases*. 3rd ed. New York: Churchill Livingstone; 1990:2151.
10. Nash TE. Visceral larva migrans and other unusual helminthic infections. In: Mandel GL, Douglas RG, Bennett JE, eds. *Principles and Practices of Infectious Diseases*. 3rd ed. New York: Churchill Livingstone; 1990:2157.
11. Katz R, Ziegler J, Blank H. The natural course of creeping eruption and treatment with thiabendazole. *Arch Dermatol*. 1965;91:420.
12. Safety of antimicrobial drugs in pregnancy. *Med Lett Drugs Ther*. 1987;29:61.

Appendix 112–1

Antihelminthic Agents and Their Use in Pregnancy

Drug	Comments
Albendazole	Albendazole is not approved for use in the United States, but it is used in other areas of the world. No information is available about its use in pregnancy. It is related to mebendazole.
Diethylcarbamazine	Not available in the United States. No information available.
Ivermectin	Ivermectin is a veterinary parasiticide marketed as Ivomec in the UK. No information is available about its use in pregnancy.
Mebendazole	Embryotoxic and teratogenic in rats when given at low doses. No adequate and controlled studies have been done in humans. In a limited number of women who received the drug during the first trimester of pregnancy, no teratogenic risk was associated with the mebendazole therapy in 170 full term deliveries. Recommendation: use only when benefits outweigh the risks.
Metrifonate	Metrifonate is an organophosphorus insecticide used in agriculture and as a veterinary anthelminthic. It has been used for human helminth infections in various parts of the world, but it is not marketed in the United States. No information is available about its use in pregnancy.
Metronidazole	Studies in rats and rabbits using metronidazole up to 5 times the human dose have revealed no harm to the fetus. No adequate or controlled studies have been done in pregnant women. Recommendation: use in pregnancy only when clearly needed. Its use in the first trimester is contraindicated.
Niclosamide	Reproduction studies in rats and rabbits using doses up to 25 times the usual human dose and in mice up to 12 times the usual human dose have shown no harm to the fetus. There are no adequate or controlled studies in humans. Recommendation: use in pregnancy only when clearly needed.
Paromomycin Sulfate	Literature suggests that the use of paromomycin in pregnant women is safe. However, there are no controlled studies and no animal data available. The Centers for Disease Control recommends that paromomycin be used in pregnancy when necessary. Its use should be delayed until the woman is past the first trimester if possible. (Recommendation of Parke-Davis Corporation)
Oxamniquine	Available in the United States. When given to rabbits and mice at doses 10 times the human dose, oxamniquine was embryocidal. There are no adequate and well-controlled studies in pregnant women, so it is recommended that it be used only when the benefits outweigh the potential hazards.
Piperazine Citrate	Safe use in pregnancy has not been established, but the drug has been reported to have been used in pregnant women with no adverse effects.
Praziquantel	Reproduction studies in rats and rabbits using doses up to 40 times the usual human dose have not shown any harm to the fetus. An increase in the rate of spontaneous abortion occurred in rats following doses 3 times the usual human dose. No adequate and controlled studies have been conducted in humans. Recommendation: use in pregnancy only when the potential benefits outweigh the risks.
Thiabendazole	Reproduction and teratogenicity studies in rats receiving thiabendazole doses equivalent to the human dose, in mice receiving doses 2.5 times the usual human dose, and in rabbits receiving doses up to 15 times the usual human dose have not revealed any harm to the fetus. Other studies in mice receiving an aqueous solution at a dose 10 times the usual human dose showed no harm to the fetus, but cleft palate and axial skeletal defects were observed when the same dose was given in an oil suspension. No adequate and controlled studies have been conducted in humans. Recommendation: use only when benefits outweigh the risks.

From reference 12.

M

Obstetrics and Gynecologic Infections

Chapter One Hundred and Thirteen

Intra-Amniotic Infections

Jorge D. Blanco

113

To the pathologist, chorioamnionitis is the leukocytic infiltration of the placenta, while, to the clinician, chorioamnionitis refers to the clinically evident infection of the mother, fetus, and amniotic cavity. The two entities are not synonymous. There can be histologic evidence of placental inflammation with no evidence of clinical infection. Because of the confusing usage of the term chorioamnionitis—throughout this chapter, the term intra-amniotic infection (IAI) will be used to refer to the clinically evident infection of the mother, baby, and amniotic cavity.

IAI occurs in approximately 0.5–1% of all pregnancies.[1,2] This rate rises with length of rupture of membranes (ROM). IAI may cause significant morbidity in the fetus and mother. The perinatal mortality rate is also increased, but maternal mortality is rare.

PATHOGENESIS

The most common pathogenic mechanism for IAI is an ascending infection with the vaginal, the cervical flora, or both after ROM. Prior to ROM, the physical and chemical barriers formed by the intact membranes and the cervical mucus prevent the entry of bacteria into the amniotic cavity. Therefore, it is rare to see IAI in patients with unruptured membranes. These barriers result in sterile amniotic fluid (AF). Whenever labor or ROM occurs, these barriers are breached. Once this occurs, genital microorganisms may ascend into the uterine cavity and cause IAI. In the rare patient with intact membranes and IAI, the common mechanism of infection is transplacental transmission of an organism from the maternal circulation. *Listeria monocytogenes* and the group A streptococcus are organisms that are transplacentally transmitted to the fetus.[3] IAI due to *Listeria* is very difficult to diagnose. The patients usually have high fever and a history of an upper respiratory infection but few localizing signs. Delays in diagnosis may result in late treatment with subsequent fetal demise.

For the majority of patients, the common risk factors for IAI are: number of vaginal exams, duration of ruptured membranes, use of internal monitors, and the duration of total labor.[4] Other special situations also increase the risk of IAI. The risk of IAI increases with a cervical cerclage.[5] Charles and Edwards reported that 11 of 115 (9.6%) patients developed chorioamnionitis within the first four weeks of cerclage placement.[5] Another 14.8% of the patients developed an infection after the first four weeks. These rates are higher than in the overall population. Although it is not clear what the specific mechanism of infection is in these patients, it is likely that the manipulation of the cervix, the presence of the foreign body, and, possibly, the exposure of the amniotic membranes to bacteria from the vagina at surgery may all play a role in the development of infection.

HOST DEFENSE MECHANISMS

Host defense mechanisms must play an important role in the prevention of IAI. There are few patients who develop this infection, despite many patients with long labors and long intervals of ROM. A variety of factors in the AF have been reported that may prevent infection in these patients. Some of these factors include: polymorphonuclear leukocytes, lysozyme, beta-lysin, transferrin, immunoglobulins, and the bacterial growth inhibitory factor. Amniotic fluid inhibits bacterial growth. While several of the above-mentioned factors may play a role in this inhibition, Galask and coworkers studied the bacterial growth inhibitory factor, a polypeptide-zinc complex in amniotic fluid that appears to inhibit bacterial replication.[6-12] The exact mechanism of bacterial inhibition is unclear, but electromicroscopic studies demonstrated that exposure of bacteria to amniotic fluid results in the microorganisms growing and elongating, but not dividing.[13,14] These organisms become aberrant and eventually die.

Regardless of the exact mechanism of inhibition, the inhibitory activity of AF is an important clinical entity. Studies by Blanco and colleagues demonstrated that the majority of AF from patients with IAI did not inhibit bacteria, whereas the majority of AF from uninfected patients inhibited bacteria.[15,16] These studies, however, do not investigate the source of the inhibitory activity, nor do they describe whether the numbers, virulence, or other properties of the bacteria alter the inhibitory activity of amniotic fluid. The authors postulate two possible mechanisms for the development of IAI. In some patients, the amniotic fluid may not have any inhibitory activity and any invasion of the amniotic cavity by microorganisms from the vaginal flora results in clinical infection. In other patients, the inhibitory activity may be initially present, but as more bacteria gain entry into the AF and are neutralized, the inhibitor is inactivated or consumed. Any subsequent bacterial contamination then results in sufficient microorganisms to create a clinically recognized infection. With either mechanism, it appears likely that the types and quantities of microorganisms are important.

Although not surprising, it is interesting that the inhibitory activity of AF appears to vary by the test microorganism used.[17,18] This variability may be due to differences in the inhibitory factor itself, differences in specific bacteria, differences in the assay technique, or the presence of multiple factors preventing bacterial growth.

MICROBIOLOGY

As expected from the mechanism of infection, the bacteria isolated in IAI mirrors the polymicrobial genital flora. In a study of 52 patients with IAI and 52 matched, uninfected controls, Gibbs and colleagues described the bacterial isolates from the AF.[2] Table 113–1 shows the common AF isolates in IAI. Most patients with IAI had two or more isolates in the amniotic fluid. Forty-eight percent had aerobes and anaerobes isolated, 38% had aerobes only, 8% had anaerobes only, and 6% had no aerobic or anaerobic bacteria in the AF. The study concludes that patients with IAI are more likely to have greater than 10^2 colony-forming units (CFU) of any bacterial isolate per milliliter (mL) in the AF, any number of high virulence isolates in the AF, and greater than 10^2 CFU of a high virulence isolate per mL of AF. Isolation rates for Lactobacillus, *Staphylococcus epidermidis*, and diptheroids (thought to be low virulence organisms) were similar in the infected and uninfected groups.

The role of other common genital organisms in IAI is unclear. *Chlamydia trachomatis* grows in untreated amniotic cell monolayers; however, the clinical significance of this finding is unknown.[19] Few studies have looked at chlamydia in IAI. In a prospective study of perinatal mortality in pregnancies complicated by maternal chlamydial infection, two of six (33.3%) fetal deaths in the chlamydia-positive group were associated with chorioamnionitis versus one of eight (12.5%) in the control group.[20] Another study showed that patients with chlamydia in the cervix antepartum have a higher rate of intrapartum fever than patients without antepartum chlamydial infection.[21] With so little data, however, the role of chlamydia in IAI is still unclear.

TABLE 113–1. RATE OF ISOLATION OF SELECTED MICROORGANISMS IN PATIENTS WITH INTRA-AMNIOTIC INFECTION

Microorganism	Percent of Patients (N = 52)
High Virulence	
Bacteroides species	33%
Group B streptococcus	15%
Escherichia coli	13%
Clostridium species	12%
Alpha streptococci	12%
Peptococcus species	10%
Klebsiella species	8%
Fusobacterium species	8%
Low Virulence	
Lactobacillus	38%
Diphtheroids	19%
Eubacterium lentum	12%
Staphylococcus epidermidis	8%

From Barclay DK.[2]

More data exists for the genital mycoplasmas in IAI. There is a case report of a patient with chorioamnionitis who had genital mycoplasma isolated from the amniotic fluid; however, the cultures were obtained after the initiation of antibiotic therapy, and this might have altered the microbiologic flora.[22] Another study reported an association between the genital mycoplasmas and placental inflammation, but this study did not correlate the isolation of *Mycoplasma hominis* and *Ureaplasma urealyticum* with clinically evident infection.[23] A study by Blanco and colleagues describes a high isolation rate of *M hominis* from the AF of infected patients (35%) when compared to matched, uninfected patients (8%).[24] However, the authors caution that the majority of AF (84%) that were positive for *M hominis* also contained greater than 10^2 CFU of a high virulence bacterial isolate per mL of AF. It is unclear, therefore, whether the *Mycoplasma* caused the IAI or whether the other high virulence organisms were the cause of the infection. The role of the mycoplasmas is further suspect because the patients responded to antibiotic therapy not specific for these organisms. Further, the same study describes uninfected patients with *M hominis* in the AF and no sequelae. *U urealyticum* appears to be a part of the genital flora and does not appear to cause IAI. In the same study, 50% of the infected and uninfected patients had this organism in the AF.[24] Therefore, it appears that the pathogenic potential of *U urealyticum* in patients with IAI is limited while that of *hominis* may still be unclear.

DIAGNOSIS

IAI is difficult to diagnose. The common clinical signs and symptoms are not specific or sensitive. This leads to delays in diagnosis. To avoid diagnostic delay, the clinician should think of IAI whenever the mother develops a fever or tachycardia, or there is a fetal tachycardia. Other antepartum or intrapartum complications, however, may result in these findings. An infection at another site or dehydration may result in a low grade maternal fever. Maternal tachycardia may be seen in patients with hypotension, dehydration, anxiety, medications, or fever from another source. Likewise, fetal tachycardia may be the result of drugs, a fetal arrhythmia, or prematurity. The more specific signs of IAI, such as uterine tenderness or malodorous AF, usually do not develop until late in the infection and may not develop at all. Table 113–2 shows the percent of patients who had certain specific diagnostic signs for IAI in a large study of IAI.[25] Because of the lack of specificity and sensitivity of

TABLE 113–2. PERCENT OF PATIENTS WITH EACH DIAGNOSTIC CRITERIA FOR INTRA-AMNIOTIC INFECTION

Criteria	(N = 171)
Rupture of membranes	98.2%
Peripheral leukocytosis	86.1%
Maternal fever	85.3%
Fetal tachycardia	36.8%
Maternal tachycardia	32.9%
Foul-smelling amniotic fluid	21.6%
Uterine tenderness	12.9%
Foul odor to neonate	9.4%

From Gibbs RS, Gastillo MS, Rodgers PJ.[25]

TABLE 113–3. DIAGNOSTIC CRITERIA FOR INTRA-AMNIOTIC INFECTION

1. Fever (>37.8°C)
2. Rupture of membranes
3. Two or more of the following:
   Maternal tachycardia (pulse >100)
   Fetal tachycardia (FHT >160)
   Uterine tenderness
   Malodorous amniotic fluid
   Peripheral leukocytosis (WBC >15,000)
4. No other site of infection

the diagnostic criteria, IAI should always be considered in any febrile pregnant woman, especially if the membranes are ruptured. Table 113–3 lists the clinical criteria to diagnose IAI.

The laboratory findings in IAI are also nonspecific and nonsensitive. The peripheral leukocyte count is commonly elevated in IAI; however, laboring patients may also normally have an elevation in the white blood cell count. Blood cultures are positive in approximately 10% of patients with IAI. Commonly, the bacteremia will be with a single microorganism. However, the infection is still likely to be polymicrobial.

Microscopic examination of the AF assists in the diagnosis of IAI. In patients with an intrauterine pressure catheter, AF may be easily obtained by aspiration through the catheter. One should discard the first 7–10 mL of the fluid collected, since this is a mixture of AF and irrigating solution. After the initial quantity is discarded, the aspirated AF should be sent for culture, Gram's stain, and cell count. In some patients, it may be impossible to obtain free flow of the AF. Before ROM, amniocentesis may also be used to obtain an AF sample. However, after ROM, transabdominal amniocentesis may be unsuccessful in 50% of patients and the procedure may be more hazardous.[26]

All pregnant patients with a fever should be evaluated for a source of infection. Whenever an obvious source of infection is lacking, an amniocentesis should be considered for diagnostic purposes, even if there is no history of ruptured membranes. If the AF is free of white blood cells and bacteria, then there is some reassurance that the source of the fever is not in the amniotic cavity. However, a positive AF culture and Gram's stain may point to an intrauterine infection.

Interpretation of the amniotic fluid Gram's stain must be done with care. While there is an association between finding bacteria, white blood cells, or both in the AF and IAI, not all patients with white blood cells and bacteria in the AF necessarily have IAI. In a study of patients with IAI, Gibbs and colleagues found that 29% of uninfected patients with ROM had leukocytes in the AF and another 11% had bacteria. Once ROM has occurred, a significant number of patients may have white blood cells, bacteria, or both in the AF. Therefore, this finding by itself is not diagnostic of IAI. However, the absence of white blood cells or bacteria usually excludes IAI. Since vaginal pool aspirates contain contaminants from the vagina, they are of little use for Gram's stain or culture. AF sampling should be performed through the intrauterine pressure catheter or, if obtainable and indicated, through amniocentesis. Unfortunately, amniocentesis carries with it some risks and may not be successful in all patients.[26] If possible, the isolates from the AF culture should be quantitated to assist with the interpretation of the culture and to minimize the effects of any contamination of the cervical-vaginal flora.

The laboratory evaluation of the neonate born to a mother with IAI is also important. The evaluation should include blood cultures, peripheral leukocyte count, and a chest radiograph. Other tests may be performed as indicated. Frequently, spinal taps are performed on these neonates. However, a recent study shows that with appropriate treatment and progression to delivery, neonates born of mothers with IAI are unlikely to have positive cerebrospinal fluid cultures.[27] In this study, none of the 49 neonates born to mothers receiving appropriate treatment for IAI had positive cerebrospinal fluid cultures. Therefore, the performance of this invasive test may be questioned. Other sites commonly cultured, such as the gastric contents or external ear canals, are probably of little use since they are contaminated by passage through the vagina. Placental cultures are also of limited value as they are exposed to the same type of contamination. While histologic examination of the placenta may yield some information, the finding of a leukocytic infiltrate is not specific for IAI and may not assist with the diagnosis.

TREATMENT

The keys to the treatment of IAI are the prompt administration of antibiotics at the time of diagnosis and promot progression to delivery. Obviously, the patients also needs to be monitored for vital signs, urine output, fetal heart rate, and progression of labor.

Antibiotic Usage

Antibiotics should be administered to patients with IAI as soon as the diagnosis is made and appropriate cultures obtained. Prompt initiation will limit the spread of infection to the mother and neonate. Because of the polymicrobial etiology and the severity of the infection, a potent broad-spectrum antibiotic or combination of antibiotics should be used. There are no large comparative studies of the effectiveness of various antibiotic therapies in IAI; however, many regimens are used on an empiric basis. There are studies to support the use of a combination of intravenous penicillin G 5 million units q 6 h and intravenous gentamicin 1.5 mg/kg intravenously q 8 h at the time of diagnosis.[2,27] Some clinicians prefer to use an ampicillin–gentamicin combination. Ampicillin appears to penetrate into the fetal compartment better than penicillin; therefore, treatment of the fetus may be improved with the ampicillin–gentamicin combination. These combinations do not have appropriate coverage for anaerobes, specifically, the Bacteroides species. In the patient who delivers vaginally, either combination is adequate and results in a high cure rate. However, if the patient is delivered by way of cesarean section, clindamycin should be added because of the importance of resistant Bacteroides in postcesarean section infection, and the high failure rate of penicillin-gentamicin or ampicillin-gentamicin in endometritis after cesarean section. Because of the weakness in these regimens, some clinicians recommended the use of the newer third generation cephalosporins or extended-spectrum penicillins. However, there are little clinical data to support their use at this time. It is known that many of the newer third generation cephalosporins enter the fetal compartment well, and this should be of some benefit in IAI. Likewise, these antibiotics provide broad-spectrum coverage for the polymicrobial flora. However, further published clinical experience with these antibiotics is required prior to widespread use.

Regardless of the antibiotic used, they should be instituted as soon as possible after the diagnosis of IAI is made. Any delay in antibiotic therapy increases the neonatal morbidity. A recent study showed that delay of antibiotic therapy until after delivery (to avoid alterations in the neonatal flora) resulted in higher rates of neonatal sepsis (19.6% versus 2.8%, $P < 0.001$).[28] Furthermore, this delay may subject the mother to the unnecessary risk of disseminated infection. In a small prospective study of intrapartum versus postpartum treatment of IAI, there was a lower rate of neonatal sepsis (0% versus 21%, $P < 0.003$) with intrapartum treatment.[29] It is, therefore, clear that antibiotics should not be delayed in patients with IAI. Cultures may be obtained from the AF and these should be useful for the fetus. Further, cultures of the neonate are also useful despite the initial transplacentally-transmitted antibiotics. It is clear that antibiotics should be initiated immediately after the diagnosis is made even if delivery is eminent.

Timing and Route of Delivery

In IAI, evacuation of the infected contents, ie, delivery of the fetus, is part of the treatment. Delivery allows drainage of the infected site and also allows direct treatment of the neonate with antibiotics. With aggressive antibiotic therapy, studies demonstrate that there is no preset time limit by which delivery must occur to prevent major maternal/fetal complication.[25,27] These studies show that there is no correlation between the time interval from the diagnosis of IAI to delivery and subsequent maternal or neonatal outcome.

No critical diagnosis-to-delivery interval has been demonstrated when aggressive, prompt antibiotic treatment and quick progression to delivery has occurred. However, the majority of patients in these reports delivered within 12 hours of diagnosis. Therefore, little data exists for diagnosis-to-delivery intervals longer than 12 hours, and it is prudent to deliver patients with IAI prior to 12 hours after the diagnosis is made.

In IAI, the maternal morbidity is less with a vaginal delivery. Women with IAI who deliver vaginally have shorter hospital stays, as well as a lower fever index.[27] IAI is not an indication for cesarean section, and abdominal deliveries should be reserved for the usual obstetrical indications. However, abdominal delivery is more common in patients with IAI. This is due to a higher rate of dysfunctional labor. It is likely that the infected intrauterine environment results in altered uterine contractility. Silver and coworkers compared the labors of patients with high virulence organisms in the AF to patients with low virulence organisms only.[30] Patients with high virulence organisms in the AF had a lower cervical dilatation rate (despite higher levels of oxytocin administration) and a higher cesarean section rate.

In patients who require an abdominal delivery, the surgical technique of choice is a transperitoneal cesarean section. There are reports of the extraperitoneal approach to avoid contamination of the peritoneal cavity by the infected AF; however, the extraperitoneal approach is more difficult and time-consuming than the transperitoneal approach. Inadvertent entry into the peritoneal cavity or bladder is not infrequent with the extraperitoneal approach. Also, a recent study showed that patients delivered by way of the transperitoneal approach versus the extraperitoneal approach did not have a statistically significant difference in outcome.[31] Since the teaching of this technique has declined to the extent that many practitioners have little familiarity with it, because the extraperitoneal approach may be more difficult to perform, and since it appears that the transperitoneal approach yields excellent results, there is no benefit to performing an extraperitoneal cesarean section in patients with IAI when appropriate antibiotics have been administered.

Although most patients with IAI do well with delivery and antibiotic therapy, an occasional patient may require a cesarean hysterectomy because of extensive myometrial infection and necrosis or from intractable uterine bleeding due to atony.

In patients with a nonviable fetus and IAI, maternal interests are the prime concern. Since there is a nonviable fetus, vaginal delivery is certainly preferred for these patients and can usually be obtained by induction or augmentation with oxytocin. Cesarean section in these circumstances should be reserved for the unusual case of an unresponsive uterus or in selected cases of maternal septicemia.

MATERNAL OUTCOME

Most recent studies of patients with IAI do not report maternal deaths as a consequence of infection.[25,26,29,32] Maternal morbidity, however, is increased with IAI. Patients with IAI are more likely to have a cesarean delivery due to dysfunctional labor and to have a complicated postpartum course. They commonly have longer postdelivery hospital stays and a larger fever index than uninfected controls.[27] Approximately 10–12% of mothers with IAI will develop a bacteremia. Aggressive antibiotic therapy and delivery of the fetus, however, results in resolution of the infection without catastrophic consequences.

Perinatal Outcome in the Term Gestation

Few major complications are reported in the term neonates born to mothers with IAI. The prospective matched study of Yoder and colleagues showed one perinatal death in 67 patients with IAI.[27] This intrauterine death was unrelated to the infection. In that study, none of the term neonates delivered of mothers with IAI had clinical evidence of meningitis or enterocolitis. Approximately 20% of neonates had chest radiographs that were interpreted as possible pneumonia, but only 4% had clear radiological evidence of pneumonia. Eight percent of the neonates had a documented bacteremia. Other measures of morbidity did not appear to be significantly different in the infected and uninfected groups. Other retrospective studies support the low rate of infectious complications and perinatal deaths due to IAI in term neonates.[32]

Perinatal Outcome in the Preterm Gestation

Unlike the outcome in the term neonate, the preterm neonate appears to suffer an increased rate of mortality and morbidity secondary to IAI. While many of the problems in these neonates are related to prematurity and its complications, the risk from the infection does appear to be increased. In a study of 47 preterm neonates born of mothers with IAI compared to 204 uninfected preterm neonates, the perinatal death rate was higher in the infected versus the uninfected group, and the rate of respiratory distress syndrome or any diagnosis of infection was higher in the neonates from mothers with IAI.[26] Another study of low birth weight neonates with IAI showed that the less than 2500-g neonate born to a mother with IAI had a higher rate of sepsis (16.2% versus 4.1%, $P = 0.005$), and a higher rate of death from sepsis (10.8% versus 0%, $P < 0.001$) than the over-2500 g neonate born to mothers with IAI.[33]

CONCLUSIONS

It appears that IAI has a significant adverse affect on mother and neonate, but a good outcome can be obtained with vigorous antibiotic therapy and prompt progression to delivery. An excellent prognosis can be expected for the mother and for the term neonate; however, the combination of prematurity and infection still results in significant perinatal morbidity.

REFERENCES

1. Gibbs RS, Blanco JD. Premature rupture of the membranes. *Obstet Gynecol.* 1982;60:671.
2. Gibbs RS, Blanco JD, St. Clair PJ, et al. Quantitative bacteriology of amniotic fluid from patients with clinical intraamniotic infection at term. *J Infect Dis.* 1982;145:1.
3. Petrilli ES, D'Ablaing G, Ledger WJ. *Listeria monocytogenes* chorioamnionitis: diagnosis by transabdominal amniocentesis. *Obstet Gynecol.* 1980;55:5S.
4. Soper DE, Mayhall CG, Dalton HP. Risk factors for intraamniotic infection: a prospective epidemiologic study. *Am J Obstet Gynecol.* 1989;161:562.
5. Charles D, Edwards WR. Infectious complications of cervical cerclage. *Am J Obstet Gynecol.* 1981;141:1065.
6. Galask RP, Snyder IS. Bacterial inhibition by amniotic fluid. *Am J Obstet Gynecol.* 1968;1092:949.
7. Larsen B, Snyder IS, Galask RP. Bacterial growth inhibition by amniotic fluid: I. In vitro evidence for bacterial growth inhibiting activity. *Am J Obstet Gynecol.* 1974;119:492.
8. Larsen B, Snyder IS, Galask RP. Bacterial growth inhibition by amniotic fluid: II. Reversal of amniotic fluid bacterial growth inhibition by addition of a chemically defined medium. *Am J Obstet Gynecol.* 1974;119:497.
9. Schlievert P,Larsen B, Johnson W, et al. Bacterial growth inhibition by amniotic fluid: IV. Studies on the nature of bacterial inhibition with the use of plate-count determinations. *Am J Obstet Gynecol.* 1975;122:814.
10. Schlievert P, Johnson W, Galask RP. Bacterial growth inhibition by amniotic fluid: V. Phosphate-to-zinc ratio as a predictor of bacterial growth inhibitory activity. *Am J Obstet Gynceol.* 1976;125:899.
11. Schlievert P, Johnson W, Galask RP. Bacterial growth inhibition by amniotic fluid: VI. Evidence for a zinc-peptide antibacterial system. *Am J Obstet Gynecol.* 1976;125:906.
12. Schlievert P, Johnson W, Galask RP. Isolation of a low molecular weight antibacterial system from human amniotic fluid. *Infect Immun.* 1976;14:1156.
13. Galask RP, Larsen B, Snyder IS. Amniotic fluid-induced surface ultramicrocytopathology of *Eschericia coli. Am J Obstet Gynecol.* 1974;118:921.
14. Larsen B, Schlievert P, Galask RP. The spectrum of bacterial activity of human amniotic fluid determined by scanning electron microscopy. *Am J Obstet Gynecol.* 1974;119:895.
15. Blanco JD, Gibbs RS, Krebs LF, et al. The association between the absence of amniotic fluid bacterial inhibitory activity and intra-amniotic infection. *Am J Obstet Gynecol.* 1982;143:749.
16. Blanco JD, Gibbs RS, Krebs LF. Inhibition of Group B streptococci by amniotic fluid from patients with intraamniotic infection and from control subjects. *Am J Obstet Gynecol.* 1983;147:247.
17. Miller J, Michel J, Bercovici B, et al. Studies on the antimicrobial activity of amniotic fluid. *Am J Obstet Gynecol.* 1976;125:212.
18. Appelbaum PC, Holloway Y, Ross SM, et al. The effect of amniotic fluid on bacterial growth in three population groups. *Am J Obstet Gynecol.* 1977;128:868.
19. Harrison HR, Riggin RT. Infection of untreated primary human amnion monolayers with *Chlamydia trachomatis. J Infect Dis.* 1979;140:968.
20. Martin DH, Koutsky L, Eschenbach DA, et al. Prematurity and perinatal mortality in pregnancies complicated by maternal *Chlamydia trachomatis* infections. *JAMA.* 1982;247:1585.
21. Wager GP, Martin DH, Koutsky L, et al. Puerperal infectious morbidity: relationship to route of delivery and antipartum *Chlamydia trachomatis* infection. *Am J Obstet Gynecol.* 1980;138:1028.
22. Brunnel PA, Dische RM, Walker MB. Mycoplasma, amnionitis, and respiratory distress syndrome. *JAMA.* 1969;207:2097.
23. Shurin PA, Alpert S, Rosner B, et al. Chorioamnionitis and colonization of the newborn infant with genital mycoplasmas. *N Engl J Med.* 1975;293:5.
24. Blanco JD, Gibbs RS, Malherbe H, et al. A controlled study of genital mycoplasmas in amniotic fluid from patients with intra-amniotic infection. *J Infect Dis.* 1983;147:650.
25. Gibbs RS, Gastillo MS, Rodgers PJ. Management of acute chorioamnionitis. *Am J Obstet Gynecol.* 1980;136:709.
26. Garite TJ, Freeman RK. Chorioamnionitis in the preterm gestation. *Obstet Gynecol.* 1982;59:539.
27. Yoder PR, Gibbs RS, Blanco JD, et al. A prospective controlled study of maternal and perinatal outcome after intra-amniotic infection at term. *Am J Obstet Gynecol.* 1983;145:695.
28. Sperling RS, Ramamurthy RS, Gibbs RS. A comparison of intrapartum versus immediate post partum treatment of intraamniotic infection. *Obstet Gynecol.* 1987;70:861.
29. Gibbs RS, Dinsmoor MJ, Newton ER, Ramamurthy RS. A randomized trial of intrapartum versus immediate post partum treatment of women with intraamniotic infection. *Obstet Gynecol.* 1988;72:823.
30. Silver RK, Gibbs RS, Castillo M. Effect of amniotic fluid bacteria on the course of labor in nulliparous women at term. *Obstet Gynecol.* 1986;68:587.
31. Yonekura ML, Wallace R, Eglinton G. Amnionitis-optimal operative management: extraperitoneal cesarean section versus low cervical transperitoneal cesarean section. Annual Meeting, Society of Perinatal Obstetricians, Abstract 24A, San Antonio, TX. January 1983.
32. Koh KS, Chan FH, Monfared AH, et al. The changing perinatal and maternal outcome in chorioamnionitis. *Obstet Gynecol.* 1979;53:730.
33. Sperling RS, Newton E, Gibbs RS. Intraamniotic infection in low-birthweight infants. *J Infect Dis.* 1988;157:113.

Chapter One Hundred and Fourteen
Vulvitis

Mark C. Maberry, Susan M. Ramin, and Larry C. Gilstrap III

114

Vulvitis, especially that associated with vaginitis, is relatively common in young women. The vulvar skin is especially sensitive and vulvitis may occur in association with a variety of conditions such as infection, allergies, or various medical illnesses such as systemic lupus erythematosus or diabetes mellitus (Table 114–1).

MATERNAL ASPECTS

Fungal Infections

Fungal infections are probably the most common cause of vulvitis during pregnancy, especially those associated with vaginitis. In fact, the vagina is the most likely reservoir

TABLE 114–1. ETIOLOGY OF VULVITIS DURING PREGNANCY

Infections	
	Fungal
	Bacterial
	Parasitic
	Viral
Dermatologic Conditions	
	Neurodermatitis
	Contact dermatitis
	Psoriasis
	Vulvar dystrophy
Medical Conditions	
	Lupus erythematosus
	Diabetes

for the most common fungi, *Candida albicans,* which accounts for 95% of such infections. Fungal vulvitis may also be caused by other species of *Candida,* as well as *Torulopis glabrata.* Garner and Kaufman reported that candidal infections are 10–20 times more common in pregnant women.[1] The preponderance of candida is felt to result from an increase in estrogen levels normally associated with pregnancy and an increase in vaginal glycogen. In addition, pregnancy results in depressed cellular immunity, and much like diabetes mellitus, produces a propensity for fungal overgrowth.

Pruritus is the most common symptom. Pelvic exam may reveal a thick, white, "cottage cheese" discharge and physical exam of the external regions may reveal marked erythema and edema of the perineum, buttock, and intertriginous regions with chafing and cracking of the involved skin areas. The diagnosis can be confirmed by placing the discharge or skin scrapings on a microscopic slide and adding 10% potassium hydroxide. In the majority of cases, the potassium hydroxide preparation will reveal the branched and budding pseudohyphae of the candidal organisms when viewed under low power.

There are numerous treatment regimens for candidal vulvovaginitis. A commonly used antifungal agent, nystatin, is available in vaginal suppositories, cream, or ointment with a usual dose of either one suppository or 1 g of the cream intravaginally two times a day for seven days. The newer imidazoles (miconazole and clotrimazole) may be more effective in eradicating fungal infection. The usual dose for both agents is one suppository or applicator of cream intravaginally every night for seven days. The cream may also be applied to the vulva to relieve the pruritus associated with candidal infections. Terconazole is a relatively new triazole antifungal reported to be effective for the treatment of *C albicans.* The usual dose is one applicator of cream intravaginally once daily for seven days or one vaginal suppository once daily for three days. Gentian violet, a topical 1% aqueous dye, has also been reported to be effective when painted on the vaginal and vulvar surfaces of patients with candidal infection.

All antifungal medications above are FDA category B except for terconazole and gentian violet which are FDA category C drugs. Treatment of fungal vaginitis is discussed in more detail in Chapter 115.

Dermatophytoses such as tinea cruris may also occur in the vulvar region. The two most common organisms recovered in these infections are *Trichophyton mentagrophytos* and *Trichophyton rubrum.*[2] The primary symptom is pruritis and the main physical finding is an erythematous, circumscribed, often scaly lesion on the vulva and inner thigh. The diagnosis is relatively easy to make clinically and can be confirmed by way of microscopic examination or culture. Treatment in the pregnant and nonpregnant patient is primarily with tolnaftate (tinactin) cream or ointment.

Bacterial Infections

Bacteria such as staphylococci and streptococci may cause superficial infection of the vulva or vulvitis.[2] For example, staphylococcal infection may cause impetigo, folliculitis, or hidradenitis. Streptococcal infection may cause impetigo, erysipelas, or hidradenitis. Impetigo is a superficial skin infection more common in children than adults and generally presents as vesicles or bulli which rupture and crust over.[2] Treatment generally consists of locally applied antibiotics. Erysipelas is an erythematous lesion of the superficial skin caused by β-hemolytic streptococci and may be associated with systemic symptoms such as fever and chills.[2] Treatment is primarily with parenteral penicillin or erythromycin. Hidradenitis suppurativa is a chronic infection of the skin, subcutaneous tissue, and apocrine glands. Antibiotics may be beneficial in early, minor disease but surgical excision is often necessary. This is generally best accomplished in the nonpregnant state.

Bacterial vaginosis is primarily limited to the vagina (vaginitis) and does not generally cause vulvitis, although patients may occasionally experience irritation and pruritis from associated discharge.

Parasitic Infections

Pregnant women may develop vulvar edema and erythema in association with trichomonal vaginitis. Although trichomonas is commonly seen in pregnancy, severe infection involving the vulva is rare. The mainstay of treatment for trichomonal vulvovaginitis is metronidazole (Flagyl) given as a single 2 g oral dose. Although metronidazole is a FDA category B drug, it is generally not recommended for use in the first trimester unless the patient has severe symptoms. Patients with asymptomatic trichomonal infection in the first trimester generally require no therapy (see Chapter 115 on vaginitis).

Pediculosis pubis is a parasitic infection of the external genital tract caused by the crab louse, *Phthirus pubis.* Pediculosis pubis particularly affects the pubic and perianal area and is the most contagious of all sexually transmitted diseases with a 95% attack rate with each sexual encounter.[3] Typically the patients will present with intense pruritus of the external genitalia. Examination of the pubic and vulvar regions with a magnifying glass will help identify the larvae, nits, and lice forms of the parasite.

The treatment for crab lice consists of the topical application of 1% lindane (Kwell) cream or lotion. Lindane should be used with caution in pregnant women because increased skin absorption with central nervous system toxicity has been reported. Pyrethrins and piperonyl butoxide (Rid; A-200) applied to the affected area may be a reasonable alternative to 1% lindane.[3] Lindane is listed as a category B drug by two of its manufacturers and has not been shown to be teratogenic in various laboratory animals.[4]

Scabies is caused by the ectoparasite or mite, *Sarcoptes scabiei,* and may cause severe pruritis and an eczematous rash on the vulva. The diagnosis is based primarily on the characteristic skin lesions or burrows and by microscopic identification of mites.[5] In the pregnant patient with scabies, initial therapy should be with crotamiton (Eurax) or sulfur in petrolatum with lindane being reserved for more serious infections for reasons mentioned above.

Viral Infections

Genital herpes simplex is a sexually transmitted disease caused most commonly by the herpes simplex type II virus (see also Chapter 91). Occasionally, genital herpes is asymptomatic, but most often presents as a primary infection with characteristic lesions consisting of painful groups of vesicles in varying states of progression, usually accompanied by fever and regional lymphadenopathy. The lesions in primary herpes simplex generally last about two to three weeks and approximately 50% of women with the initial infection will have recurrences. The vulvar lesions in recurrent herpes simplex are fewer in number, less painful, and, generally, of shorter duration.

Diagnosis is based on the typical vesicular lesions characteristic of herpes simplex. The most reliable confirmatory test is a viral culture of the lesion. Cytologic methods of detecting herpes simplex such as Tzanck preparations and Pap smears are much less reliable and have an unacceptably high false-negative rate.

The treatment of herpes simplex vulvitis in pregnancy is primarily symptomatic. Analgesics and topical emollients such as Burrows' solution are useful for relief of discomfort associated with both primary and recurrent infections. Although acyclovir (Zovirax) given orally has been shown to decrease viral shedding, as well as the number of recurrences, it is currently not recommended for use during pregnancy except in life-threatening infections. The use of topical acyclovir is controversial and not currently recommended for use during pregnancy.

Other viral infections that may infect the vulva such as *Molluscum contagiosum* and *Condyloma accuminata* are discussed in other chapters.

Neurodermatitis

Neurodermatitis, also called *lichen simplex chronicus,* is a chronic skin condition resulting from continued scratching. It frequently involves the groin area, as well as neck, legs, and trunk. The lesions are pruritic, lichenified eczematous areas[6] which are often preceded by pruritis setting up a cycle of continued scratching. The best treatment is to convince the patient of the cause; topical and injected steroids may be helpful in decreasing the pruritis, as well as systemic antihistamines.

Contact Dermatitis

Contact dermatitis may result from a variety of chemicals or irritants and basically represents a hypersensitivity reaction. Common agents associated with this type of vulvar dermatitis include deodorants, perfumes, douches, lubricants, and soaps. The vulvitis usually consists of erythematous and edematous lesions. In severe cases, actual vesicles may occur. The diagnosis is based primarily on a high degree of suspicion and the characteristic lesions. The mainstay of treatment is removing the causative factor. In addition, Burrow's soaks may provide relief as well as topical steroids.

Psoriasis

This particular dermatitis may affect virtually all parts of the body surface including the vulvar area. Lesions may appear red and inflamed, similar to that seen with fungal infections. Scaling may or may not be present in this region. Diagnosis is based primarily on history and by ruling out other causes such as fungal infections. Treatment is primarily with topical steroids.

Other Conditions

Dermatitis or vulvitis may also be associated with systemic disease such as lupus erythematosus. In this condition, the dermatitis is characterized by ulcers and inflammation. Diagnosis is usually confirmed by biopsy and treatment consists of steroids.

A rare disorder of unknown etiology is *Behçet's syndrome* which may present as recurrent ulcers in both the oral and genital regions. Diagnosis is basically one of exclusion and by the characteristic lesions. Steroids may be of benefit in some patients.

Lichen sclerosis et atrophicus is a relatively common vulvar dystrophy which may be confused with vulvitis. It is found in women of reproductive age. This lesion generally appears whitish and the patient often presents with pruritis. Diagnosis can be confirmed by biopsy. Topical testosterone is the therapy of choice in the nonpregnant patient but is not recommended for use during pregnancy. Pregnant women generally require no therapy, although topical corticosteroids may relieve itching.

The hypertrophic vulvar dystrophies generally are found in women after the age of 40 and are rarely encountered during pregnancy. If it were to occur during pregnancy, therapy could generally be delayed until after pregnancy.

FETAL ASPECTS

In the majority of cases, maternal vulvitis has very little effect on the fetus. Obvious exceptions include *herpes vulvitis, Group B β-hemolytic streptococcal infections,* and occasionally *fungal infections.* Both herpes and Group B streptococcal infections can obviously cause serious infection in the newborn. Fungal infections such as *C albicans* may result in newborn thrush.

REFERENCES

1. Garner HL, Kaufman RH. Candidiasis. In: *Benign Diseases of the Vulva and Vagina.* 2nd ed. St. Louis, MO: C.V. Mosby; 1981:218.
2. Barclay DK. Benign disorders of the vulva and vagina. In: Pernoll ML, Benson RL, eds. *Current Obstetric and Gynecologic Diagnosis and Treatment.* Norwalk, CT: Appleton & Lange; 1987:636.
3. Gibbs RS, Sweet RL. Sexually transmitted diseases. In: *Infectious Diseases of the Female Genital Tract.* Baltimore: Williams & Wilkins; 1985:38.
4. Barnhart ER. *Physicians Desk Reference.* 43rd ed. Oradell, NJ: Medical Economics Co; 1989:2670.
5. Orkin M, Maibach HI. Current views of scabies and *Pediculosis pubis. Cutis.* 1984;33:85.
6. Parker F. Skin diseases. In: Wyngaarden JG, Smith LA, eds. *Cecil Textbook of Medicine,* 18th ed. Philadelphia: W.B. Saunders; 1988:2300.

Chapter One Hundred and Fifteen
Vaginitis

Susan M. Ramin, Mark C. Maberry, and Larry C. Gilstrap III

115

Vaginitis is a frequent disorder of pregnancy. The most common symptom, vaginal discharge, is also seen in pregnant women without infection, thereby making the diagnosis of vaginitis sometimes difficult. The normal vaginal discharge or leukorrhea associated with pregnancy is usually white and profuse in nature. The marked changes in the hormonal milieu that occur during pregnancy are responsible for the leukorrhea. This increase in vaginal discharge is usually not bothersome to the patient and is clinically insignificant except when confused with vaginal infection or rupture of the fetal membranes. In contrast, vaginitis may be quite troublesome to the pregnant woman and is often difficult to eradicate and recurrences are common. Treatment presents a therapeutic dilemma to the clinician and may have to be altered or delayed because of fetal considerations.

ETIOLOGY AND PATHOPHYSIOLOGY

The three most common types of vaginitis during pregnancy are candidiasis, trichomoniasis, and nonspecific vaginitis. The actual incidence of symptomatic infection is difficult to ascertain and is influenced to a certain extent by the population studied. It is reported that *Candida* and *Trichomonas* can be recovered from in 25–30% of pregnant patients.[1-4] Furthermore, Garner and Kaufman[5] have reported that candidal vaginitis is 10–20 times more common during pregnancy. The increased estrogen production, along with the increased glycogen content of the vagina during pregnancy, probably account for this increased incidence.[1,4] Candidiasis may remain an asymptomatic infection in numerous pregnant women.[5]

The gram-negative bacillus associated with nonspecific vaginitis, *Gardnerella vaginalis* (formerly *Hemophilus vaginalis* or *Corynebacterium vaginale*) can be recovered from 44% of pregnant women with symptomatic vaginitis compared to 10% of women without symptoms.[6] McCormack et al[7] recovered this organism from 32% of 466 unselected women presenting to a gynecologist. Moreover, in a five-year survey of over 25,000 women presenting with vaginal infection or discharge, Fleury[4] found that *Gardnerella* contributed to 33% of cases of vaginal infections, while *Candida* and *Trichomonas* accounted for approximately 20% and 10%, respectively.

The majority of cases of fungal vaginitis are those caused by the genus *Candida*, with *Candida albicans* being the species most commonly isolated. *C albicans* may generally be found in the gastrointestinal tract and the oral cavity, as well as the vagina. Other species of this genus, as well as *Torulopis glabrata*, are pathogenic and may be responsible for fungal vaginitis.[5-8] Additionally, these other organisms may be accountable for either recurrent infection or failures.[9] It is not entirely clear why *Candida* is pathogenic in some women and not in others, but *Candida* vaginitis is more common in patients with decreased cellular immunity and in conditions of elevated blood glucose[9], which are seen more frequently during pregnancy. Moreover, the growth of *Candida* is usually inhibited by the various lactobacilli and corynebacteria normally present in the vagina but because of the hormonal fluctuations during pregnancy, there is an alteration in the vaginal microflora which permits *C albicans* to flourish.

Trichomonas vaginalis, a flagellated parasite, is the etiologic agent of trichomonas vaginitis. This anaerobic protozoan is most often sexually transmitted and frequently coexists with other sexually transmitted organisms.[9] Moreover, this parasite commonly exists in vaginal and cervical secretions in females and in the seminal fluid in males.[10] Thus, the reservoir for *T vaginalis* may be either male or female, although the male is more apt to be asymptomatic than the female and mainly serves as a vector for transmission. The human is the only known host for *T vaginalis*.

Controversy still remains as to the etiologic agent of nonspecific vaginitis, although the consensus of opinion is that it is associated with *G vaginalis*. As Eschenbach[9] has demonstrated, women with nonspecific vaginitis have an increase in the mean concentration of anaerobic gram-negative bacilli and gram-positive cocci, and these organisms, along with others, may, in fact, play a significant role in the pathogenesis of nonspecific vaginal infections. *Polymicrobial vaginitis* may be a more appropriate term for this entity.

Other etiologic agents associated with the production of an inflammatory vaginal discharge include *Chlamydia trachomatis*, herpes simplex, or *Neisseria gonorrhoeae*. The vaginal discharge produced by these organisms is secondary to cervicitis and does not usually cause vaginitis per se.

EFFECT OF PREGNANCY

As mentioned previously, candidal infections are significantly more common during pregnancy and are often difficult to eradicate. It has been demonstrated that progesterone enhances the adherence of *C albicans* to vaginal epithelial cells. Sobel[11] reported the greater affinity of intermediate vaginal cells to bind yeast cells than that of superficial epithelial cells. Pregnancy is associated with increased levels of progesterone and, thus, a predominance of intermediate vaginal epithelial cells. There is no evidence that pregnancy predisposes to the acquisition of either *G vaginalis* or trichomonal infections or alters their course.

The major clinical manifestation of these vaginal infections is discharge. Women with *Candida* vaginitis usually complain of a thick white discharge ("cottage cheese"). Pruritis may be present in women with significant infections, as well as pain, chafing, and even dysuria in cases of coexisting vulvitis.

Depending on the severity of inflammation and secondary infection, the discharge associated with trichomoniasis will vary in appearance. Classically, the characteristic discharge is frothy and yellow. However, the discharge may range from white and watery to thick and green. Trichomonal infections are usually associated with a malodorous discharge which may result in pruritis, burning, or dysuria. The *"strawberry cervix"* describes the characteristic red punctate lesions which may be seen upon examining the cervix, although this may be difficult to discern from the normal cervical changes encountered during pregnancy and is seen in less than 5% of women with active trichomonal infection. Vaginal and vulvar erythema may be present when the infection is severe.

The discharge associated with nonspecific vaginitis is usually grayish-white in color and very malodorous. Unlike fungal or trichomonal infections, there are few, if any, signs or symptoms of inflammation such as erythema, swelling, pruritis, or burning.

FETAL ASPECTS

The actual incidence of adverse fetal effects from maternal vaginitis is unknown, but they are rare.

Neonatal thrush associated with maternal monilial vulvovaginitis is the most common fetal manifestation of maternal vaginal infection. The distinctive lesions of thrush are aphthae or whitish spots on the tongue and oral mucosa. *In utero* infection resulting in congenital moniliasis is rare with only 15 reported cases in the literature up to 1974.[12] There is no substantial evidence that maternal monilial vaginitis is associated with increased incidence of fetal wastage.

Maternal trichomoniasis is not known to be associated with any adverse fetal effects. Moreover, there is no clear association between nonspecific vaginitis and adverse fetal effects. Reports of abortion and puerperal infections resulting from *G vaginalis* have been described but the association is not strong.[13,14]

Neonatal thrush is typically a self-limited process. If treatment is necessary, the lesions can be treated with a nystatin solution (100,000 units/mL) in a dose of 1 mL once or twice daily.

The best way to prevent potential fetal effects is to detect and eradicate maternal infection.

DIAGNOSIS

Diagnosis of vaginal infection is usually established by both history and physical examination and simple office laboratory tests (Table 115–1). Monilial infections can be confirmed by placing the discharge on a microscopic slide and adding 10% potassium hydroxide (KOH) which lyses the vaginal epithelial cells. The characteristic microscopic finding is the presence of mycelia—the branched and budding pseudohyphae of the candidal organisms. The KOH preparation will detect *Candida* in approximately 80% of infected patients.[10] Occasionally, it may be necessary to culture the discharge using Nickerson's media to confirm the diagnosis of *Candida*.

By using the wet preparation of vaginal secretions with a drop of saline, the motile flagellated trichomonads can be easily demonstrated on microscopic examination in 80–90% of infected patients.[1,10] *T vaginalis* can also be cultured and is clearly the most sensitive diagnostic method, although this is not a practical tool for the clinician. Trichomonads can also be identified on Papanicolaou-stained smears but not as reliably as with the wet saline preparation.[10] Krieger et al[15] recently compared the diagnostic accuracy of two culture media against wet preparations, cytologic studies, and a rapid immunodiagnostic method for the diagnosis of trichomoniasis in 600 high-risk women. Of the 88 positive cases, the Feinberg–Whittington and Diamond's culture medium yielded the diagnosis in 82 and 78 cases, respectively. In comparison, wet-mount examination and cytologic smears were relatively insensitive identifying 60% and 56% of the 88 cases, respectively. Papanicolaou smears were the least specific method for diagnosis. Finally, direct immunofluorescence with monoclonal antibodies identified 86% of the 88 cases and is promising as an adjunct to our present diagnostic tests.

The diagnosis of nonspecific vaginitis is frequently a clinical one after excluding all other causes. When a small drop of 10% potassium hydroxide is added to the vaginal secretions, a "fishy" odor is often released ("positive whiff test").[4,9,16] This odor is caused by the amines released by metabolism of anaerobic organisms associated with *G vaginalis*.[16] Patients with trichomoniasis may have a positive amine test, although the odor is not as strong.[9] Some clinicians use the presence of clue cells, which are desquamated epithelial cells with clusters of bacteria attached to their surfaces, on microscopic examination to confirm the diagnosis of nonspecific vaginitis. However, up to 40% of women with *G vaginalis* will not have clue cells.[9]

As previously mentioned, cervicitis must be considered in the differential diagnosis of vaginal discharge and may be due to *N gonorrhoeae, C trachomatis,* or herpes simplex infection. One should consider the diagnosis of cervicitis in any woman with persistent discharge and no apparent etiology. Appropriate cultures should be performed for suspected gonococcal, chlamydial, or herpetic cervical or vaginal infections.

TREATMENT

Possible adverse fetal effects of medications administered to a patient during pregnancy must always be considered. Fortunately, many of the drugs for treatment of vaginitis have been extensively used during pregnancy without obvious adverse effects. The basic principle is to treat only symptomatic women.

There are numerous antifungal regimens available for the treatment of monilial vaginitis with little-to-no vaginal

TABLE 115–1. SIGNS, SYMPTOMS AND MICROSCOPIC FINDINGS IN WOMEN WITH VAGINITIS

	Vaginal Discharge	Microscopic Findings	Symptoms
Monilial	Thick white	Pseudohyphae	Pruritis
Trichomonas	Thin, copious, yellow	Motile trichomonads	Copious discharge, pruritis
Nonspecific	Scant, gray	Clue cells	Fishy odor, discharge

TABLE 115–2. TREATMENT REGIMENS FOR CANDIDIASIS[a]

Agent	Dose
Nystatin	One vaginal suppository or 1 g cream bid × 7 days
Miconazole or clotrimazole	One vaginal suppository or one applicatorful of cream × 7 days
Terconazole	One vaginal suppository qhs × 3 days or one applicatorful of cream qhs × 7 days

[a] Refer to manufacturer's recommendations.

absorption (Table 115–2). The most commonly used antifungal agent is nystatin, obtained from cultures of *Streptomyces noursei*. It is available in vaginal suppositories, cream or ointment, with the usual dose of either one suppository (100,000 units) or 1 g (100,000 units per gram) of the cream applied intravaginally twice daily for seven days. There is a high failure rate reported during pregnancy with nystatin, and recurrent infections are common.[17-19] The newer imidazoles, including miconazole and clotrimazole, have been shown to be more effective in eradicating infection.[4] In two relatively recent studies comparing nystatin and miconazole for the treatment of candidal vulvovaginitis during pregnancy, the cure rates were significantly higher with miconazole.[18,19] Furthermore, there was no evidence of adverse fetal effects with either regimen. The usual dose for both miconazole and clotrimazole is one suppository or applicatorful intravaginally every night for seven days. The cream may also be applied to the vulva to relieve the pruritis associated with candidal infection. A relatively new triazole antifungal, terconazole, is reported to be effective in the treatment of *C albicans*. The usual dose is one applicatorful of cream intravaginally once daily for seven days or one vaginal suppository once daily for three days. Terconazole is an FDA Category C drug and was not found to be teratogenic in laboratory animals. However, it should probably be avoided during the first trimester. More recently, Van Slyke et al[20] have reported on the efficacy of boric acid capsules containing 600 mg of boric acid powder intravaginally for candidiasis, but only in nonpregnant women. The safety of its use in pregnancy remains unknown.

The only effective medication for the treatment of *T vaginalis* is metronidazole (Flagyl), usually administered as a single dose of 2 g orally (Table 115–3). This dosage may be divided into two 1 g administrations, usually one in the morning and one at bedtime, to minimize gastrointestinal disturbance. It may be necessary to treat women with frequent recurrences for a longer time period, such as 250 mg tid for seven days. A side effect of metronidazole therapy, especially with longer duration, is the development of candidiasis, probably due to the eradication of specific vaginal flora.

Significant controversy exists concerning whether to treat the male consort of a patient with trichomonas vaginitis.[4,9] Because the organism has a short survival time in the male genital tract and the potential anti-alcohol effect of metronidazole, treatment of the partner is probably not warranted. The female patient should be advised to refrain from intercourse during treatment or use a condom to prevent reinfection. There is also controversy concerning the possible oncogenicity, mutagenicity, and teratogenicity of metronidazole.[4,9,21-26] Although metronidazole is an FDA Category B drug (that is, relatively safe), it is generally recommended that metronidazole not be used during the first trimester. Even though there are no available studies that would implicate metronidazole as a teratogenic agent, because of the fear of litigation, most clinicians use clotrimazole for symptomatic relief of trichomoniasis during the first trimester. Both clotrimazole and miconazole are FDA Category B drugs, and are safe for use during pregnancy, as are ampicillin and cephalosporins (Table 115–4). It is also recommended that metronidazole not be used during breast-feeding because it is excreted in breast milk.[4] Women who are breast-feeding can be given a single dose of metronidazole, pump their breasts for 24 hours, and then resume breast feeding.

Numerous agents have been used for the treatment of nonspecific vaginitis including local agents such as sulfa vaginal creams and tetracycline vaginal tablets, as well as systemic agents such as tetracycline, ampicillin, cephalosporins, and most recently, metronidazole (Table 115–3).[4,9,27,28] Vaginal sulfa creams have been shown not to be effective against *Gardnerella* and tetracyclines are contraindicated during pregnancy due to potential adverse fetal effects. The therapy of choice is metronidazole which has been found to be the most effective treatment for nonspecific vaginitis.[4,9,27] However, ampicillin or a cephalosporin should be used first during pregnancy, especially in the first trimester. Thus, metronidazole should be reserved for use in symptomatic women after the first trimester who fail to respond to initial treatment or who are penicillin allergic. As with metronidazole, protracted therapy with either ampicillin or a cephalosporin may be associated with candidal overgrowth.

PREVENTION

Prevention of vaginal infections during pregnancy may be difficult, if not impossible, to achieve. The use of condoms by infected males may be of some benefit in the prevention of trichomonal infections in the female. However, the role

TABLE 115–3. RECOMMENDED TREATMENT REGIMENS FOR *TRICHOMONAS* AND NONSPECIFIC VAGINITIS

	Agent	Dose
Trichomonas	Metronidazole	2 g single oral dose 250 mg p.o. tid × 5–7 days
	Clotrimazole[a]	One vaginal suppository QD
Nonspecific Vaginitis	Metronidazole	250 mg p.o. tid × 5–7 days
	Ampicillin	250 mg qid × 5–7 days
	Cephalosporin	250 mg p.o. qid × 5–7 days

[a] Symptomatic therapy only (see text).

TABLE 115–4. FDA DRUG CATEGORY OF AGENTS USED IN THE TREATMENT OF VAGINITIS DURING PREGNANCY

Agent	Category
Ampicillin	B
Clotrimazole	B
First generation cephalosporin	B
Metronidazole[a]	B
Miconazole	B
Pyrantel pamoate	C
Terconazole	C

[a] First trimester use not recommended.

of the male in both monilial and nonspecific vaginitis is not clear. Some uncircumcised men will harbor *Candida* beneath the foreskin; this may represent a possible reservoir for infection. Antifungal prophylaxis should be considered for women on protracted broad-spectrum antibiotics to prevent monilial infections.

REFERENCES

1. Penza J, Rankin JS. Infectious vaginopathies during pregnancy. *Clin Obstet Gynecol.* 1970;13:223.
2. Catterall RD. Trichomonal infections of the genital tract. *Med Clin North Am.* 1972;56:1203.
3. Pritchard JA, MacDonald PC. Prenatal care. In: *Williams Obstetrics,* 16th ed. New York: Appleton-Century-Crofts; 1980:325.
4. Fleury FJ. Adult vaginitis. *Clin Obstet Gynecol.* 1981;24:407.
5. Gardner HL, Kaufman RH. Candidiasis. In: *Benign Diseases of the Vulva and Vagina.* 2nd ed. St. Louis: CV Mosby; 1981:218.
6. Lewis JF, O'Brien SM, Ural UM, et al. *Corynebacterium vaginale* vaginitis in pregnant women. *Am J Clin Pathol.* 1971;56:580.
7. McCormack WM, Hayes CH, Rosner B, et al. Vaginal colonization with *Corynebacterium vaginale (Haemophilus vaginalis). J Infect Dis.* 1977;136:740.
8. Oriel JD, Patridge BM, Denny MJ, et al. Genital yeast infections. *Br Med J.* 1972;4:761.
9. Eschenbach DA. Vaginal infection. *Clin Obstet Gynecol.* 1983;26:186.
10. McLennan MT, Smith JM, McLennan CE. Diagnosis of vaginal mycosis and trichomoniasis: reliability of cytologic smear, wet smear, and culture. *Obstet Gynecol.* 1972;40:231.
11. Sobel JD. Epidemiology and pathogenesis of recurrent vulvovaginal candidiasis. *Am J Obstet Gynecol.* 1985;152:924.
12. Schirar A, Rendu C, Vielh JP, et al. Congenital mycosis (*Candida albicans*). *Biol Neonate.* 1974;24:273.
13. Delaha EC, Curtin JA, Stevens G, et al. Incidence and significance of *Hemophilus vaginalis* in nonspecific vaginitis. *Am J Obstet Gynecol.* 1964; 98:996.
14. Monif GRG, Bear H. *Hemophilus* (*Corynebacterium*) *vaginalis* septicemia. *Am J Obstet Gynecol.* 1974;120:1041.
15. Krieger JN, Tam MR, Stevens CE, et al. Diagnosis of trichomoniasis. Comparison of conventional wet-mount examination with cytologic studies, cultures, and monoclonal antibody staining of direct specimens. *JAMA.* 1988;259:1223.
16. Chen KCS, Forsyth PS, Buchanan TM, et al. Amine content of vaginal fluid from untreated patients with nonspecific vaginitis. *J Clin Invest.* 1979;63:828.
17. Long WE, Stella JG, Benchakan V. Nystatin, vaginal tablets in treatment of candidal vulvovaginitis. *Obstet Gynecol.* 1956;8:364.
18. Wallenburg HCS, Wladimiroff JW. Recurrence of vulvovaginal candidosis during pregnancy: comparison of miconazole versus nystatin treatment. *Obstet Gynecol.* 1976;48:491.
19. McNellis D, McLeod M, Lawson J, et al. Treatment of vulvovaginal candidiasis in pregnancy: a comparative study. *Obstet Gynecol.* 1977; 50:674.
20. Van Slyke KK, Michel VP, Rein MF. Treatment of vulvovaginal candidiasis with boric acid powder. *Am J Obstet Gynecol.* 1981;141:145.
21. Beard C, Noller K, O'Fallon W, et al. Lack of evidence for cancer due to use of metronidazole. *N Engl J Med.* 1979;301:519.
22. Peterson WF, Stauch JE, Ryder CD. Metronidazole in pregnancy. *Am J Obstet Gynecol.* 1966;94:343.
23. Cantu JM, Garcia-Cruz D. Midline facial defects as a teratogenic effect of metronidazole. *Birth Defects.* 1982;18:84.
24. Robinson SC, Mirchandani G. *Trichomonas vaginalis* V. Further observations on metronidazole (including infant follow-up). *Am J Obstet Gynecol.* 1965;93:502.
25. Morgan I. Metronidazole treatment in pregnancy. *Int J Gynecol Obstet.* 1978;15:501.
26. Goldman P. Metronidazole: Proven benefits and potential risks. *Johns Hopkins Med J.* 1980;147:1.
27. Pheifer TA, Forsyth PS, Durfee MA, et al. Nonspecific vaginitis: Role of *Hemophilus vaginalis* and treatment with metronidazole. *N Engl J Med.* 1978;298:1429.
28. Smith RF, Dunkelberg WE. Inhibition of *Corynebacterium vaginale* by metronidazole. *Sex Transm Dis.* 1977;4:20.

Chapter One Hundred and Sixteen

Pelvic Inflammatory Disease

Jack M. Graham and Jorge D. Blanco

116

Acute pelvic inflammatory disease, the symptomatic infection of the fallopian tubes, is usually attributed to ascending spread of microorganisms from the vagina and endocervix to the endometrium, fallopian tubes, or contiguous structures. It predominantly occurs in the nonpregnant state, without preceding surgical entry of the abdomen or endometrial cavity. Rarely, salpingitis has been described in pregnancy.

HISTORY

In the beginning of the 20th century, pelvic inflammatory disease in pregnancy was not thought to occur. Holtz, in 1930, reported that only nine of 1262 cases of pelvic inflammatory disease occurred in pregnancy.[1] In 1949, Lennon reported two cases in the English literature with all previous references in the French literature.[2] Acosta and colleagues reviewed 5124 admissions from 1/1/66 to 12/31/69 and found 12 cases listed as acute gonococcal pelvic inflammatory disease during pregnancy.[3] These reports described pelvic inflammatory disease in pregnancy as a real entity that was more common than expected, and was under or misdiagnosed.

ETIOLOGY AND PATHOPHYSIOLOGY

There are several risk factors for acute pelvic inflammatory disease. Most have been described for nonpregnant women, but there is little likelihood that they are different for the pregnant patient. A prior history of gonococcal salpingitis predisposes to recurrent infections, and while the exact process is not clear, possible loss of maternal protective mechanisms or toxin mediated destruction of fallopian tube cilia has been suggested as the cause for recurrences.[4-6] Multiple sexual partners are also a risk factor. Women with multiple partners have a 4.6 times increased risk of developing acute pelvic inflammatory disease compared to monogamous women.[5]

In nonpregnant women, the intrauterine device (IUD) is a clear risk factor.[5,7-13] Women with IUDs have an estimated three to five times increased risk of developing acute pelvic inflammatory disease. The adolescent female is at significant risk to develop acute salpingitis. In a report of Westrom, nearly 70% of women with acute pelvic inflammatory disease were less than 25 years of age, 33% experienced their first infection before 19 years of age, and 75% were nulliparous.[14] Westrom estimated that by the year 2000, 50% of the women who turned 15-years-old in 1970 will have a history of at least one episode of acute salpingitis.[14]

Pregnancy complicated by an IUD is at risk for abortion, sepsis, and prematurity. The abortion rate in 54% with the device left in, compared to 25% if removed. The abortion is likely to be septic, with significant effect on maternal morbidity and mortality.[15]

Little is known of risk factors that may specifically apply in pregnancy; however, there is little reason to think that they would be different from the nonpregnant. Likewise, the pathogenesis of infection is probably the same in pregnant and nonpregnant patients, although the exact mechanisms may have to be modified by the presence of the gestational sac. In 1939, Metzger proposed several mechanisms of infection in pregnancy, and since that time, other possibilities have arisen (Table 116–1).[16]

One mechanism of infection in pregnancy may result from the direct spread of microorganisms from the cervix to the fallopian tubes. The usual route of spread of the gonococcus is thought to be direct canalicular spread of the organism from the endocervix, along the endometrial surface to the tubal mucosa, resulting in endosalpingitis. Chlamydia may also spread from the endocervix to the endometrium to the fallopian tube.[17,18] Approximately 10% of women with endocervical chlamydia trachomatis develop chlamydia salpingitis.[19] In theory, a pregnant woman could develop acute pelvic inflammatory disease if the uterine cavity has not been obliterated by the gestational sac. There is little data to support the lymphatic or hematologic spread of microorganisms from the cervix or vagina to the adnexa.

Since the reactivation of chronic salpingitis appears to occur, flare-up of infection may be another possible explanation for pelvic inflammatory disease in pregnancy. A nidus of old infection harbored in the fallopian tube could be reactivated. Bleeding with a threatened abortion or bleeding after conception may provide an ideal culture medium for any organisms harbored in old disease.

TABLE 116–1. POSSIBLE MECHANISMS IN THE PATHOPHYSIOLOGY OF ACUTE SALPINGITIS IN PREGNANCY

Infection at time of fertilization
Infection after fertilization, but before fusion of decidua capsularis and parietalis
Lymphatic spread from cervix or vagina
Vascular spread from cervix or vagina
Reactivation of chronic pelvic inflammatory disease
Instrumentation
Ascending infection during abortion or bleeding
Contiguous spread from adjacent organs

Modified from Metzger M.[16]

Since the gonococcus is able to attach to sperm, sperm may transport the bacteria into the fallopian tube.[20] Carney and Taylor–Robinson demonstrated that as gonococci reach the endosalpinx, they become attached to mucosal epithelial cells, penetrate the cells, and cause cell destruction.[21] Within two to seven days of infection, ciliary motility is lost. Another mechanism for tubal damage may involve the gonococcus producing an endotoxin that directly damages ciliated cells in the fallopian tube. The destruction of the endosalpinx results in the production of purulent exudate. In the early stages of pelvic inflammatory disease, the tubal lumina are open, and purulent material exudes out the fimbriated ends of the tubes, resulting in pelvic peritonitis. As a result of the peritoneal inflammation, contiguous pelvic structures such as the ovary, omentum, sigmoid colon, small intestine, broad ligament, and appendix may become involved in the process. In pregnancy, the above initiating mechanism of infection may occur any time after conception, but before fusion of the decidua capsularis, and parietalis. This fusion occurs by approximately the fourth month of gestation.

Instrumentation breaks the natural barriers to infection and may result in acute pelvic inflammatory disease. These barriers include the mucus plug and the fetal membranes. Also, disruption of the endometrium, which may offer local protection, can occur with foreign body insertion.

Ascending infection during abortion is another possible mechanism. This possibility would involve refluxed blood from the endometrial cavity, which is an excellent culture medium.

Finally, acute salpingitis in pregnancy could result from contiguous spread of infection from adjacent organs. Infections such as acute appendicitis or ruptured diverticuli may spread to the adnexa. This type of salpingitis should be unilateral and most probably diagnosed at the time of laparotomy for the instigating condition.

DIAGNOSIS

In 1969, Jacobson and Westrom found that only 65% of women with the clinical diagnosis of pelvic inflammatory disease had laparoscopically proven acute pelvic inflammatory disease, 23% had normal pelvic findings, and 12% had other pelvic pathology such as appendicitis, endometriosis, ruptured ovarian cysts, or ectopic pregnancies.[22] These errors in diagnosis, proven by way of laparoscopy, led to the development of standard diagnostic criteria. In 1983, Hager and colleagues established the criteria for the diagnosis of acute salpingitis.[23] This criteria based the diagnosis of acute pelvic inflammatory disease on findings of pain and tenderness with the presence of acute inflammation. Ideally, laparoscopy should be used to confirm the diagnosis of salpingitis; however, it may be impractical and not cost-effective to use the laparoscope in all patients. Therefore, the clinical criteria are commonly used.

In pregnancy, the reported signs, symptoms, and physical examination of a patient with acute pelvic inflammatory disease are extremely variable. Abdominal pain can vary from mild tenderness to significant guarding with rebound. The patient may have nausea and vomiting, a low grade temperature, or symptoms of a urinary tract infection. The white blood cell count is usually elevated with a left shift. A purulent vaginal discharge is very common. The diagnostic criteria of Hager et al, with modification for the pregnant state, should be used when the diagnosis of pelvic inflammatory disease in pregnancy is a possibility (Table 116–2). The erythrocyte sedimentation rate is normally elevated in pregnancy, and the white blood cell count can be 10–15K, so elevations of these two criteria must be interpreted with caution.

The varying reports in the literature concerning signs, symptoms, and physical exam result in a difficult clinical situation. If the diagnostic criteria have been met and a septic abortion, chorioamnionitis or both have been excluded, then the diagnosis may be that of pelvic inflammatory disease in pregnancy. If an intrauterine infection is discovered, the salpingitis likely is secondary to this, not vice versa. Most of the cases of acute pelvic inflammatory disease in pregnancy have occurred in the first trimester and are associated with significant fetal wastage. Cases of salpingitis in the second trimester have also been reported with the same increased risk of fetal wastage. Whether the salpingitis results in septic abortion, chorioamionitis, or an undiagnosed or misdiagnosed intra-amniotic infection results in acute salpingitis is not certain. Intact fetal membranes have not been well documented in reported cases and intrauterine or intra-amniotic infection have not been excluded in most cases reported in the literature.[2,3,24-26] The increased fetal wastage regardless of trimester suggests infected uterine contents.

TABLE 116–2. CRITERIA FOR THE DIAGNOSIS OF PELVIC INFLAMMATORY DISEASE IN PREGNANCY

All Three Must Be Present
History of lower abdominal pain and the presence of lower abdominal tenderness, with or without evidence of rebound
Cervical motion tenderness
Adnexal tenderness
One of These Must Be Present
Temperature >38°C
Leukocytosis >15,000 per mm^3
A culdocentesis which yields peritoneal fluid containing white blood cells and bacteria
Presence of an inflammatory mass noted on pelvic examination or sonography
Gram's stain from the endocervix revealing gram-negative intracellular diplococci suggestive of *Neisseria gonorrhoeae* or a monoclonal directed smear from endocervical secretions revealing *Chlamydia trachomatis*

Modified from Hager et al.[23]

The differential diagnostic list covers most causes of acute and chronic pelvic pain such as: 1) appendicitis; 2) urinary tract infection/pyelonephritis; 3) renal stone; 4) adnexal torsion; 5) threatened or incomplete abortion; 6) ectopic pregnancy; 7) abruption; 8) bowel obstruction; 9) pancreatitis; 10) degenerating uterine fibroid; and 11) medical illnesses such as sickle cell crisis or porphyria. The diagnosis in the above list can be excluded by using appropriate radiographic exams, sonography, and biochemical testing.

DIAGNOSIS IN PREGNANCY

When the diagnosis of acute pelvic inflammatory disease in pregnancy is entertained, specific steps are needed to assure the diagnosis. The following evaluation is recommended: clinical symptoms should meet the modified Hager et al criteria, and in a pregnancy less than 16 weeks, fetal viability should be ensured by way of sonography and, if possible, an amniocentesis performed to exclude intra-amniotic infection. If bacteria are present in the amniotic fluid, then septic abortion is the diagnosis. If the criteria of Hager and colleagues are met, the fetus is viable with

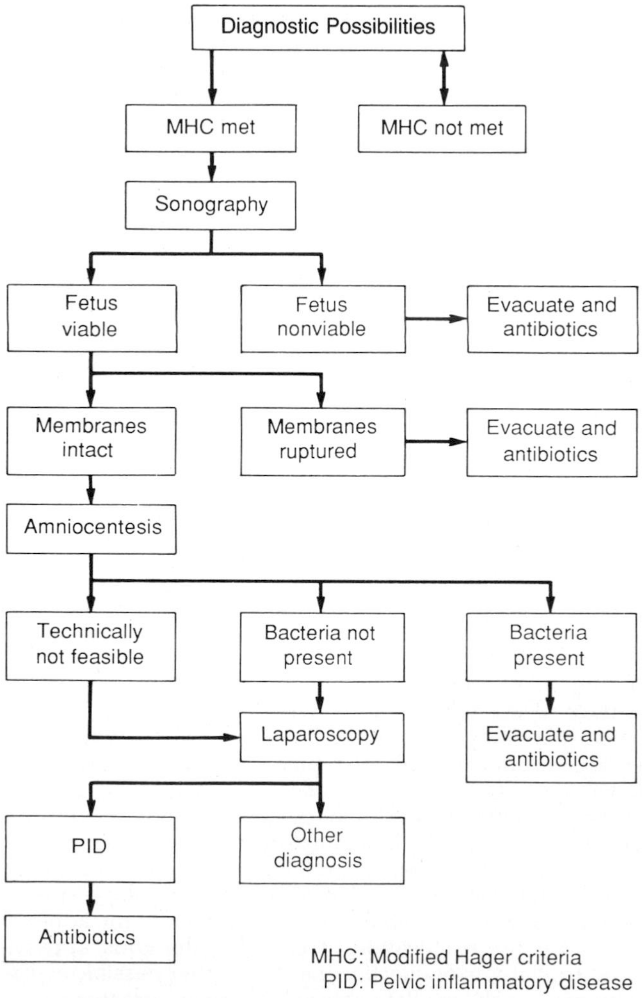

Figure 116–1. Diagnostic and treatment schema recommended in the evaluation of patients with possible acute salpingitis in pregnancy before 16 weeks.

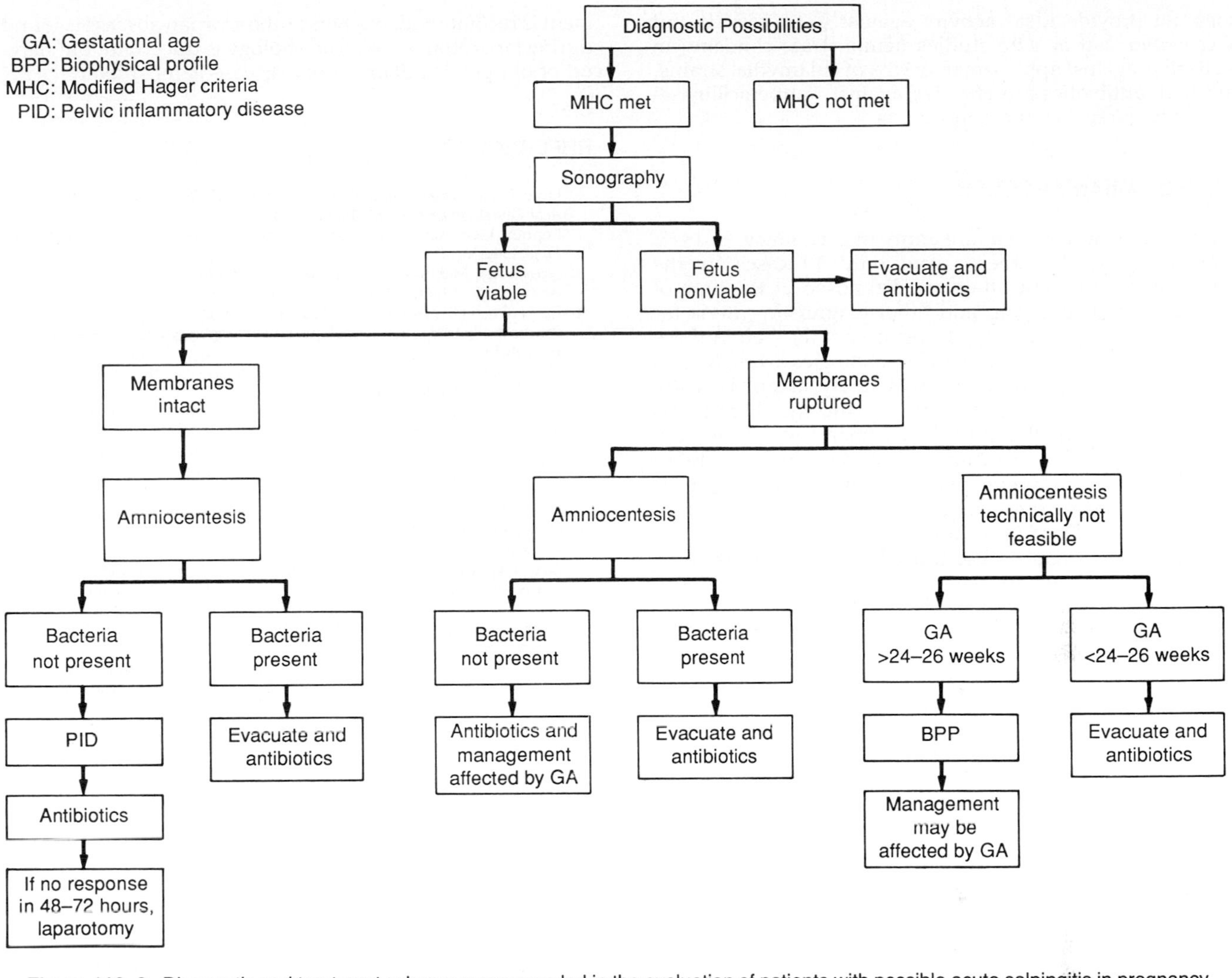

Figure 116–2. Diagnostic and treatment schema recommended in the evaluation of patients with possible acute salpingitis in pregnancy after 16 weeks.

intact membranes, and an intra-amniotic infection is excluded, a laparoscopy should be performed to confirm the diagnosis. After 16 weeks, the same criteria should be met. However, laparoscopy may not be a practical diagnostic procedure. If the evaluation reveals no other source of infection, and the diagnostic criteria are met, treatment should be initiated. If the diagnosis is uncertain or the patient does not respond to therapy, immediate laparotomy should be performed to confirm the diagnosis and to exclude other sources of infection. Figure 116–1 summarizes the diagnostic and treatment schema for pregnancies before 16 weeks while Figure 116–2 summarizes the diagnostic and treatment schema for pregnancy after 16 weeks.

MICROBIOLOGY

The reported microbiology of this infection in pregnancy may have changed over the years; however, it is uncertain if the change is due to a true alteration in flora or to improvements in culture and isolation techniques. Lancet, in 1959, reported *Escherichia coli* as the most common offender while the gonococci was rarely present.[24] However, today the *Neisseria gonorrhea, Chlamydia trachomatis* and nongonococcal, nonchlamydial aerobic and anaerobic bacteria are the major organisms involved in the pathogenesis of pelvic inflammatory disease. Older reports did not have the availability of modern aerobic and anaerobic culture techniques or collecting methods, especially through the laparoscope. In summary, the microbiology involved in the genesis of pelvic inflammatory disease in pregnancy must be assumed to be the same as in nonpregnant pelvic inflammatory disease.

TREATMENT

If pelvic inflammatory disease in pregnancy is diagnosed with the steps previously mentioned, only one of the treatment schedules recommended by the Centers for Disease Control (CDC) is appropriate. Cefoxitin plus doxycycline should not be used because tetracycline is contraindicated in pregnancy. Therefore, the treatment of choice should be clindamycin 900 mg q 8 hours plus gentamicin 2 mg/kg intravenously followed by 1.5 mg/kg intravenously q 8 hours in patients with normal renal function. This regimen does not provide ideal activity against *C trachomatis* and *N gonorrhea*, but *in vitro* studies demonstrate clindamycin is effective against approximately 90% of chlamydial strains, and both antibiotics are effective against nonpenicillinase-producing strains of the gonococcus.[27]

TUBO-OVARIAN ABSCESS

Tubo-ovarian abscess is a rare entity in pregnancy. In 1977, Jafari reported that there were only 19 cases in the literature.[28] All except one were diagnosed at the time of laparotomy.[29] Pelvic pain and other diagnostic criteria for pelvic inflammatory disease were commonly seen in these patients. However, other possible etiologies were considered and a medical approach was rarely taken. Usually, these patients underwent laparotomy and the abscess was discovered incidentally. In 1959, Friedman and Bobrow suggested the possible mechanisms of developing a tubo-ovarian abscess in pregnancy as hematogenous spread, lymphatic spread from contiguous organs, infection of an ovarian cyst, or flare-up of an old postabortal infection.[30] Critical review suggests the most likely etiology is flare-up of preexisting pelvic inflammatory disease, but evidence is lacking. Most tubo-ovarian abscesses are unilateral with only one of 14 being bilateral as reported by Jafari.[28]

In contrast to acute pelvic inflammatory disease in pregnancy, tubo-ovarian abscesses in pregnancy were evenly distributed throughout pregnancy with six diagnosed in the first trimester, eight in the second trimester, and five in the third trimester.[28] Only two were found at term. The symptoms of tubo-ovarian abscess in pregnancy were variable. Pain was the most frequent complaint, but two patients were asymptomatic. Temperature elevation usually was low grade and the temperature was only elevated in approximately 50% of patients. Cultures of peritoneal fluid at laparotomy grew streptococcus, anaerobic streptococcus, or were sterile. In Jafari's report, the pregnancy outcome was eight surviving infants, two neonatal deaths, and seven abortions.[28] There were three maternal deaths, but two occurred prior to the antibiotic era. The management of tubo-ovarian abscess in pregnancy should not vary from management in a nonpregnant patient. Although there is no consensus, it is recommended that conservative surgery be performed (oophorectomy/salpingo-oophorectomy) since pregnancies can remain intact and carry to term.[28] Antibiotic coverage with penicillin, clindamycin, and an aminoglycoside is also recommended for adequate bacterial coverage.

CONCLUSIONS

In summary, pelvic inflammatory disease in pregnancy is rare. Initial review of the reported cases may raise doubt about the true existence of this entity. A compilation of the reported cases show approximately 80% occurred at 16 weeks or less and were associated with abortion 70% of the time.[2,3,24-26] The probability that septic abortion precedes the salpingitis and not the opposite should be seriously considered.

Tubo-ovarian abscess in pregnancy is an even rarer diagnosis and is usually not found until laparotomy. Pregnancies complicated with tubo-ovarian abscess can result in term fetuses; therefore, conservative surgical management is recommended when a tubo-ovarian abscess is found during laparotomy. The true etiology is uncertain, but flare-up of old pelvic inflammatory disease is most likely.

REFERENCES

1. Holtz F. Klinsche studien uber die nicht tuberkulose salpingo-oophoritis. *Acta Obstet Gynecol Scand.* 1930;Suppl:10.
2. Lennon GG. Acute salpingitis during pregnancy. *J Obstet Gynaec Br Emp.* 1949;56:1035.
3. Acosta AA, Mabray RC, Kaufman RH. Intrauterine pregnancy and coexistent pelvic inflammatory disease. *Obstet Gynecol.* 1971;37:282.
4. Eschenbach DA, Holmes KK. Acute pelvic inflammatory disease: current concepts of pathogenesis, etiology, and management. *Clin Obstet Gynecol.* 1975;18:35.
5. Eschenbach DA. Epidemiology and diagnosis of acute pelvic inflammatory disease. *Obstet Gynecol.* 1980;55:142.
6. Gregg CR, Melly MA, McGee ZA. Gonococcal lipopolysaccharide: a toxin for human fallopian tube mucosa. *Am J Obstet Gynecol.* 1980;138:981.
7. Eschenbach DA, Harpisch JP, Holmes KK. Pathogenesis of acute pelvic inflammatory disease: role of contraception and other risk factors. *Am J Obstet Gynecol.* 1977;128:838.
8. Kaufman DW, Shapiro S, Rosenberg L, et al. Intrauterine contraceptive device use and pelvic inflammatory disease. *Am J Obstet Gynecol.* 1980; 136:159.
9. Ory HW. A review of the association between intrauterine devices and acute pelvic inflammatory disease. *J Reprod Med.* 1978;20:200.
10. Osser S, Gullberg B, Lieholm P, Sjoberg NO. Risk of pelvic inflammatory disease among intrauterine device users irrespective of previous pregnancy. *Lancet.* 1980;1:386.
11. Senanayake P, Kramer DG. Contraception and the etiology of pelvic inflammatory disease: New perspectives. *Am J Obstet Gynecol.* 1980; 138:852.
12. Westrom L, Bengtsson LP, Mardh PA. The risk of pelvic inflammatory disease in women using intrauterine contraceptive devices as compared to non-users. *Lancet.* 1976;2:221.
13. Lee NC, Rubin GL, Ory AW, Burkman RT. Type of intrauterine device and the risk of pelvic inflammatory disease. *Obstet Gynecol.* 1983;62:1.
14. Westrom L. Incidence, prevalence, and trends of acute pelvic inflammatory disease and its consequences in industrialized countries. *Am J Obstet Gynecol.* 1980;138:880.
15. Tatum HJ, Schmidt FH, Jain AK. Management and outcome of pregnancies associated with Copper-T intrauterine contraceptive device. *Am J Obstet Gynecol.* 1976;126:869.
16. Metzger M. Salpingitis et grossesse. *Bull Soc OB Gyn Paris.* 1939;28:470.
17. Sweet RL, Schachter J, Robbie MO. Failure of beta-lactam antibiotics to eradicate *Chlamydia trachomatis* in the endometrium despite apparent clinical care of acute salpingitis. *JAMA.* 1983;250:2641.
18. Mardh PA, Moller BR, Paavonen J. Chlamydial infection of the female genital tract with emphasis on pelvic inflammatory disease. A review of Scandanavian studies. *Sex Transm Dis.* 1981;8(s):140.
19. Sweet RL, Gibbs RS. *Infectious Diseases of the Female Genital Tract.* Baltimore: Williams & Wilkins; 1985:62.
20. Toth A, O'Leary WM, Ledger WJ. Evidence for microbial transfer by spermatozoa. *Obstet Gynecol.* 1982;59:556.
21. Carney FE, Taylor-Robinson D. Growth and effect of *Neisseria gonorrhea* in organ cultures. *Br J Vener Dis.* 1973;49:435.
22. Jacobson L, Westrom L. Objectivized diagnosis of acute pelvic inflammatory disease. *Am J Obstet Gynecol.* 1969;105:1088.
23. Hager WD, Eschenbach DA, Spence MR, Sweet RL. Criteria for diagnosis and grading of salpingitis. *Obstet Gynecol.* 1983;61:113.
24. Lancet M, Cohen A. Acute purulent salpingitis in late pregnancy. *Obstet Gynecol.* 1959;14:426.
25. McCord JM, Simmons CM. Acute purulent salpingitis during pregnancy. *Am J Ob Gyn.* 1953;65:1136.
26. Blanchard AC, Pastorek JG, Weeks T. Pelvic inflammatory disease during pregnancy. *South Med J.* 1987;80(11):1363.
27. Draper DL, James JF, Hadley WK, Sweet RL. Auxotypes and antibiotic susceptibilities of *Neisseria gonorrhea* from women with acute salpingitis. Comparison with gonococci causing uncomplicated genital tract infections in women. *Sex Transm Dis.* 1981;8:43.
28. Jafari K, Vilovic-Kos J, Webster A, Stepto RC. Tubo-ovarian abscess in pregnancy. *Acta Obstet Gynecol Scand.* 1977;56:1.
29. Dudley AG, Lee F, Barclay D. Ovarian and tubo-ovarian abscess in pregnancy: report of the cause and review of the literature. *Milit Med.* 1970;135:403.
30. Friedman S, Bobrow ML. Pelvic inflammatory disease in pregnancy. *Obstet Gynecol.* 1959;14:417.

Chapter One Hundred and Seventeen

Postpartum Endometritis

Jorge D. Blanco

117

Even with the current advances in microbiologic technique, diagnostic criteria and antibiotic development, postpartum infections continue to pose a threat to the puerperal woman. Older texts describe general definitions of postpartum febrile morbidity; however, in today's environment, such descriptions are of little benefit. Specific diagnoses should be formulated for appropriate treatment.

The most common puerperal infection is genital tract infection. Various authors have described this infection as endometritis, endoparametritis, and endomyometritis. Except where there is clear extension into the adnexa or spread into the pelvis, most investigators are describing similar infections. For consistency, we will use the term endometritis.

DIAGNOSIS

Criteria for the diagnosis of endometritis vary, but fever, uterine tenderness, and exclusion of another infected site are common findings.[1] Tachycardia and peritoneal irritation may also be seen. Nonspecific signs and symptoms such as malaise, abdominal pain, and chills are also commonly present.

Laboratory evaluation of the patient suspected of endometritis should include hematocrit, white blood cell count, and differential, as well as endometrial, and blood cultures. Often, the diagnosis of endometritis relies on excluding another source for the fever, such as atelectasis, pneumonia, viral syndrome, or pyelonephritis.

Endometrial cultures are important to treat the patient appropriately. Care must be exercised to avoid cervical or vaginal contamination since the bacteria in the cervix, vagina, or both may not be identical to those in the endometrial cavity. For endometritis, anaerobic cultures are necessary; therefore, swabbing of the lower genital tract is of limited value. A single or double-lumen catheter results in a less contaminated sample of the microbiologic flora of the endometrium and culture material suitable for both aerobic and anaerobic cultures.[2] Ideally, the endometrial sample should be obtained through sterile, protected catheters and cultured for aerobic and anaerobic bacteria. If appropriate endometrial specimens are unobtainable or adequate laboratory facilities are unavailable, an aerobic cervical culture may be of some use. Such a culture will identify certain aerobic pathogens that require specific action. Some of these organisms include group A Streptococcus, group B Streptococcus, *Staphylococcus aureus, Neisseria gonorrhoeae,* chlamydia, or enterococcus. These isolates require special treatment or precautions by the clinician. Therefore, knowledge of their isolation is important. Unfortunately, a simple aerobic swab culture does not identify all pathogens involved in the infection, and will usually not be helpful in patients who do not respond to initial therapy.

Blood cultures are important to obtain. They will be positive in 10–20% of patients.[3] Isolation of an organism from the blood does not imply that the isolated organism is, by itself, responsible for the infection. Endometritis is a polymicrobial infection; antibiotic therapy directed solely against a blood isolate would be inadequate treatment.

In some circumstances, abdominal radiography, ultrasonography, or computed tomographic (CT) scan may be helpful in delineating a mass, abscess, or pelvic thrombophlebitis.

RISK FACTORS

The major predisposing risk factor for pelvic infection is cesarean delivery. Both the frequency and severity of infection are greater following an abdominal delivery. With a different study design but in the same population, Gibbs and colleagues report that the incidence of endometritis following vaginal delivery is 1.2% versus 38.5% after a cesarean.[4,5] Other investigators report similar findings.[6] Serious complication and failure of initial therapy are also higher for the cesarean section group.[4,5]

The type of uterine incision does not appear to alter the infectious morbidity. In a retrospective, controlled study of 89 patients, Blanco and Gibbs did not show a higher rate of infectious morbidity in patients with a classical cesarean section compared to low cervical transverse cesareans.[7] However, the majority of their patients had short periods of labor and rupture of membranes.

The exact cause for the increased incidence of infection after cesarean section has not been systematically studied, but common reasons cited include: increased intrauterine manipulation, foreign body (suture) reactions, tissue necrosis at the suture line, hematoma-seroma formation, wound infections, and spillage of contaminated amniotic fluid into the peritoneal cavity.

In patients undergoing an abdominal delivery, the duration of labor is the most important determinant of infection. With a discriminant analysis technique to eliminate confounding variables, D'Angelo and Sokol reported that duration of labor was the most significant factor related to postpartum infectious morbidity.[8] Other studies confirm this result.[9,10]

There is also an association between the duration of rupture of membranes (ROM) and the rate of intrauterine infection.[9] The study by D'Angelo and Sokol did not find this relationship but few patients in their study had prolonged rupture of membranes.[8] Since bacterial contamination of the amniotic cavity occurs after ROM, it seems logical to anticipate that ROM may play a role in postpartum endometritis. Bobitt and Ledger showed that no amniotic fluid (AF) specimen was sterile after 12 hours of ROM and many patients had high colony counts.[11] Gilstrap and Cunningham reported that at cesarean section all the amniotic fluids in 56 women with ROM greater than or equal to six hours contained some microorganisms.[12] Further, 95% of these women developed endometritis. Amniotic fluid cultures at cesarean are predictive of postpartum infection with bacterial quantitation and analysis of the virulence of the microorganisms. Blanco and coworkers showed that none of the patients in a study of 24 women undergoing cesarean section without labor or ROM had greater than or equal to 10^2 colony forming units (cfu) of a high virulence organism per milliliter of amniotic fluid (a positive culture).[13] Only 25% of these patients developed endometritis. However, of 36 patients with ROM, labor, or both ROM and labor, 13 (36%) patients had positive cultures. Ninety-two percent of the positive group developed endometritis compared with 39% of the group without a positive culture—a statistically significant difference. Therefore, quantitation and evaluation of bacterial virulence at cesarean identifies a group at high risk for postpartum infection. The pathogenesis of infection for the groups without or with ROM and labor is probably different. There was a significantly shorter time interval from surgery to diagnosis of endometritis in the patients with a positive culture (18.1 versus 45 hours).[13] Most likely, patients with a positive culture at cesarean section have subclinical infection and soon, thereafter, manifest signs and symptoms. In the group without positive cultures at abdominal delivery, the uterine infection may occur after delivery by another mechanism.

While quantitative cultures of AF may be helpful in understanding the pathogenesis of endometritis after cesarean section, the cultures are not practical for predicting infection. In most postpartum patients, clinical infection is evident before culture results become available. Other more rapid techniques need to be developed. A technique such as gas liquid chromatography might be helpful in predicting infection and also in identifying the organisms. This would enable an improved selection of the appropriate antibiotic therapy.

The socioeconomic status of the patient is also an important determinant of infection. Indigent patients, independent of race, have higher puerperal infection rates than do middle-class patients. The cause is unclear but differences in flora, hygiene, nutrition, and amniotic fluid bacterial inhibitor activity have all been postulated as reasons. While vaginal examinations do not increase infection risk over rectal examinations in labor, published studies are contradictory on whether the number of vaginal examinations correlates with risk for infection. Because the internal fetal monitor (IFM) is a foreign body, concern exists that its use may increase intrauterine infection. Since they are commonly used in patients with abnormal labor, prolonged ROM, and at increased risk for infection, it is difficult to separate the effect of IFM from these other risk factors. Most of the evidence shows no increase in infection with the use of the IFM. Some studies associate anemia with postpartum infection. Anemia probably represents a marker for poor nutrition or lower socioeconomic class instead of being a cause of infection. Obesity has not been a consistent risk factor for genital infection, although it has been implicated in wound infection. Recent data demonstrates that young age may also be a risk factor for postcesarean endometritis.[14] It is unclear why youth should be a risk factor but differences in microbiologic flora, host-immune defenses, or other factors have been postulated as causes.

MICROBIOLOGY

Endometritis is a polymicrobial infection with both aerobic and anaerobic bacteria. With properly performed cultures, two to three microorganisms can be recovered from the endometrial cavity. Many more may be isolated in some patients. A study of 198 patients with endometritis after cesarean section reported that 53.5% of the endometrial isolates were aerobes while 46.5% were anaerobes.[15]

Anaerobic organisms have a major role in postpartum infection. They are isolated in 80% of properly collected and handled genital cultures. The most common isolate is often of the Bacteroides species. Because of its role in intraperitoneal abscess formation and its pattern of resistance to antibiotics, this anaerobic gram-negative bacilli is very important. *Bacteroides fragilis* is a common isolate in genital tract infections. Some centers, however, report *Bacteroides bivius* as the predominant anaerobic isolate from the genital tract.[15] Both of these microorganisms are resistant to many antibiotics, especially penicillin. Many of the newer penicillins and cephalosporins were developed to be active against these organisms. Clindamycin and metronidazole also have good activity against the *Bacteroides* species. Other common anaerobic isolates are *Peptococcus, Peptostreptococcus, Fusobacterium,* and *Clostridium.* These organisms are usually sensitive to many antibiotics, including penicillin, clindamycin, and the newer cephalosporins and penicillins. Patients with *Clostridium perfringens* infection (even bacteremia) do well with antibiotic therapy alone. Therefore, isolation of *C perfringens,* even from the bloodstream should not, by itself, prompt surgical intervention. Hysterectomy should be reserved for cases with evidence of myonecrosis.

The next most common family of isolates are the aerobic gram-negative bacilli.[15] *Escherichia coli* is the most common of these. Other organisms that are often isolated are the gram-positive cocci such as the streptococci.

Even though all isolated organisms are important in each patient's endometritis, there are certain microorganisms that require special management if found. One of these is the Group B streptococcus. Colonization of the neonate by this organism may result in fulminant neonatal sepsis. Therefore, whenever Group B streptococci is isolated from a mother with endometritis, the nursery should be notified. The Group A streptococcus is also of concern. Patients with this organism need to be isolated and promptly treated to prevent the nosocomial spread of this infection. *S aureus* is rarely isolated in endometritis (less than 5% of cases), but it is commonly resistant to penicillin and may spread to other sites. Prompt, appropriate treatment is required. Recently, the enterococcus has gained prominence. This organism is resistant to the new cephalosporins and the clindamycin aminoglycoside combinations commonly used to treat endometritis. Recent reports show that the enterococcus is commonly isolated in patients with endometritis.[16] Isolation of this organism in a patient not responding to initial therapy should prompt the addition of an antibiotic effective against the enterococcus (ampicillin, penicillin-gentamicin, or one of the new, extended spectrum penicillins).

Both *Mycoplasma hominis* and *Ureaplasma urealyticum* have been associated with postpartum infection. McCormack and coworkers and Wallace and colleagues recovered *M hominis* from the blood-stream of postpartum women while Lamey and associates isolated genital mycoplasmas in 16 of 125 (12.8%) blood cultures from febrile puerperal women.[17-19] Further, Platt and coworkers showed an association between a fourfold rise in mycoplasmacidal antibody titer and fever after vaginal delivery.[20] Because of the small number of studies with a relatively small number of patients, systematic studies of the genital mycoplasmas are needed to better delineate their role in puerperal infection.

Few studies have investigated the role of *Chlamydia trachomatis* in postpartum infection. Wager and colleagues described an association between the antepartum presence of *C trachomatis* in the cervix and late endometritis after a vaginal delivery.[21] However, Blanco and coworkers did not show an association between chlamydia isolation and early postpartum endometritis.[22] It would appear that patients developing endometritis shortly after the cesarean do not have chlamydia as an etiologic agent, but in those patients who develop the infection late (more than seven days after delivery) chlamydia infection should be considered and treated. Patients readmitted after discharge with late postpartum endometritis should be cultured for chlamydia and the antibiotic regime should include antichlamydial coverage.

MANAGEMENT

Clinical experience and the animal model of bacterial peritonitis have altered the antibiotic therapy of severe puerperal infection. In 1974, Weinstein and colleagues developed a rat model of intra-abdominal infection.[23] Contamination of the peritoneum with bowel flora (which is similar to genital flora) resulted in a biphasic infection. In the initial phase, 100% of the animals developed peritonitis and 37–43% died (probably from sepsis). This stage lasted four to five days. When the peritonitis resolved and death did not occur, 100% of the survivors developed intraperitoneal abscesses (second phase). The peritonitis phase resulted from infection with gram-negative aerobic bacilli, such as *E coli,* while the abscess stage was the result of anaerobes, especially Bacteroides. Treatment with gentamicin, an antibiotic specific for gram-negative bacilli, reduced the mortality rate to 4%, but 98% of the survivors still developed abscesses. Conversely, treatment with an antibiotic active against anaerobes, such as clindamycin, did not decrease the mortality rate. However, only 5% of the survivors developed abscesses. Administration of both clindamycin and gentamicin resulted in a 9% mortality rate and a 6% rate of abscess formation.[24]

These and other studies demonstrated the need to use broad-spectrum antibiotics with anti-anaerobic coverage initially in postpartum, infected patients. Before 1979, most investigators did not initially use antibiotics with specific activity against the bacteroides. Commonly, a penicillin-aminoglycoside combination was used for postpartum endometritis. Since then, several clinical trials show excellent results with clindamycin-gentamicin (Cl-Gm) over penicillin-gentamicin (Pn-Gm) for serious pelvic infection. In patients with endometritis after cesarean section, diZerega and colleagues treated 100 people with Pn-Gm and another 100 with Cl-Gm.[25] The rate of clinical cure was significantly higher in the Cl-Gm group (86%) compared to the Pn-Gm group (64%) ($P < 0.001$), but more importantly no serious complications occurred in the Cl-Gm group, while in the Pn-Gm group, one patient developed an abscess, two required heparin for presumed septic pelvic thrombophlebitis, and one had a wound evisceration. Measures of morbidity, such as length of hospital stay and fever index, were improved in the Cl-Gm group. In some studies, failure rates of 20% are reported in patients with endometritis after a cesarean treated with penicillin-gentamicin. Four percent of these patients develop abscesses or septic pelvic thrombophlebitis.[4] Failure rates for Cl-Gm as low as 6% with no abscesses or septic pelvic thrombophlebitis are reported.

The improved outcome with the Cl-Gm combination most likely results from the susceptibility of *Bacteroides fragilis* and *Bacteroides bivius* to clindamycin, whereas these organisms are usually resistant to penicillin. Therefore, to reduce the serious sequelae of endometritis after cesarean, initial therapy should consist of broad-spectrum antibiotics with activity against the anaerobes, especially the Bacteroides species, as well as the gram-negative and gram-positive aerobes. Ampicillin, penicillin-gentamicin, ampicillin-gentamicin, and cephalothin-gentamicin do not provide this spectrum, and should not be used for treatment of this infection. In controlled studies, penicillin-gentamicin has not been as effective as clindamycin-gentamicin for the treatment of endometritis after cesarean section.[25] Because of its broad-spectrum coverage, its excellent cure rate, and its reduction of serious infection-related complications, the combination of clindamycin-gentamicin is the standard of therapy for severe endometritis after cesarean.

The Cl-Gm combination is not without problems. Both drugs have serious side effects. Clindamycin has been associated with diarrhea and pseudomembranous colitis. Aminoglycoside therapy may lead to nephrotoxicity or ototoxicity. Further, adequate aminoglycoside levels are difficult to achieve in the postpartum patient with the common treatment regimens.[26] Because the administration of two agents may be more expensive and time-consuming than a single drug and because of the possible toxic side effects, the pharmaceutical industry developed a multitude of broad-spectrum single agents for postpartum endometritis.

Most of the single, broad-spectrum agents are extended spectrum penicillins and second and third generation cephalosporins. No single agent provides activity against the entire bacterial spectrum, but most have sufficient aerobic and anaerobic activity to merit clinical trials for pelvic infections. A recent review by Duff compares the spectrum of activity of many of these agents and their results in clinic trials.[3] Results with many of these agents are good. Therefore, some of these antibiotics may have a role in the treatment of postpartum endometritis. However, the clinical trials have been with small numbers of patients. Because serious complications (for example, abscess, septic pelvic thrombophlebitis) occur rarely, the limited scope of the trials prevents any firm conclusions about the prevention of serious complications by these single agents. Also, their usefulness in more serious infections (like septic shock) is unclear, and few studies include severely ill patients. For mild to moderate obstetric infections, single agent therapy with the newer penicillins and cephalosporins may be useful. Some of these single agents include cefoxitin, moxalactam, cefoperazone, cefotaxime, ceftizoxime, piperacillin, and mezlocillin. Some agents such as cefamandole, ceforanide, and cefonicide have relatively limited activity against anaerobic gram-negative bacilli and are not ideal drugs for single use in endometritis. Others exist and many others are being and will be developed that yield equivalent results. Some of these agents have an *in vitro* broader spectrum of coverage than others, but the clinical significance of small differences in bacterial inhibition is unclear. Larger trials and greater clinical experience with the single agents may show one to be superior to the others but at present, there is insufficient data to arrive at a conclusion. The new single agents are usually well-tolerated and have few side effects. However, the broad-spectrum of these agents may alter bowel flora and result in diarrhea in a small percentage of patients. Patients on any broad-spectrum antibiotic or combination of antibiotics should be closely monitored for diarrhea.

Administration of a single agent is thought to be less costly. With combination therapy, more containers, tubing, and nursing time may be needed. However, most newer agents are more expensive than the combinations and their cost may outweigh any decreased administration cost. A recent report of the cost of moxalactam versus clindamycin-gentamicin found no differences in total hospital costs or patient charges.[27]

Besides the tremendous proliferation of new agents,

other older agents are appearing that have different therapeutic indications. Metronidazole, has excellent anaerobic activity and it is now available in parenteral form. It has little activity against aerobes so it should not be used alone. In postpartum endometritis, it may be used in combination with agents that provide gram-positive and gram-negative aerobic activity. A combination of cefazolin and metronidazole or penicillin, gentamicin, and metronidazole would provide theoretically appropriate coverage. However, these combinations have not been extensively studied. For postpartum infections, the role of metronidazole may be to replace clindamycin, not as initial therapy, but in patients who develop significant diarrhea.

New cephalosporin derivatives, the monobactams, have exquisite gram-negative activity, but little activity in the rest of the bacterial spectrum. These agents may be able to replace gentamicin. Clinical trials of one of these monobactams (aztreonam) show equivalent clinical response in a limited number of patients.[28]

Endometritis after vaginal delivery is usually mild and responds to many antibiotic regimens. Few antibiotic trials for this infection exist. Because of the limited information, rational recommendations are more difficult. In a study of 188 patients with endometritis after vaginal delivery, over 90% responded to therapy—usually a penicillin aminoglycoside combination. All patients responded rapidly and a pelvic abscess developed in only one.[5] However, with all the single agent, broad-spectrum therapies available, this combination may no longer be ideal. Although it is unclear if the new extended spectrum penicillins or second and third generation antibiotics might improve the outcome, their success in more serious postcesarean infections and their ease of administration as a single agent supports their usefulness in endometritis after vaginal delivery.

TREATMENT FAILURES

With use of broad-spectrum agents (whether in combination or alone), the overwhelming majority of patients with endometritis will respond promptly. However, an occasional patient will continue to be ill and have fever 48 hours after the initiation of therapy.

Patients who do not show a resolution of the infection and fever or at least have a trend to resolution within 48 hours after treatment should be reevaluated. A repeat abdominal and pelvic exam and protected aerobic and anaerobic endometrial cultures should be performed. The physical exam should specifically look for any evidence of wound infection, such as erythema, edema, or induration. If any signs of wound infection are found, the abdominal wound should be probed. The release of any serosanguinous or purulent material should prompt the opening of the entire wound. The fascia should be checked for integrity and the wound cleaned. The wound will need further cleaning and care to heal by secondary intention. The pelvic exam should reveal any obvious large abscess or hematoma which may require drainage. A likely cause of failure to respond to antibiotics will be a resistant organism, and the change or addition of antibiotics should help. If there is no evidence of wound infection, abscess, or hematoma, and if there is no other source of infection and the uterus is still tender, the antibiotic regimen should be altered. If a single agent was initially used, the patient should be placed on clindamycin-gentamicin. If Cl-Gm was initially used, penicillin or ampicillin should be added. Failure to respond after 48 hours should again prompt investigation. Sources of a continuing infection such as wound abscess, retained products, or pelvic abscess should be excluded. A CT scan of the pelvis is usually helpful. Uncommonly, a patient may require surgical intervention. Curettage may be necessary for retained, infected placental fragments in a rare patient while drainage of an abscess or hematoma may be required in another. Hysterectomy is rarely needed, but may be lifesaving for the patient with gas gangrene of the uterus or with septic shock that fails to respond to vigorous antibiotic and supportive therapy. Patients who continue to be febrile after antibiotic changes but have no obvious source may have septic pelvic thrombophlebitis.

Classically, septic pelvic thrombophlebitis presents as a protracted, spiking fever that persists despite appropriate antibiotic therapy.[29] Physical findings are often absent, and there is no evidence of an abscess or hematoma. When septic pelvic thrombophlebitis is suspected, a diagnostic and therapeutic trial of intravenous heparin should be instituted. If the patient defervesces within 48 to 72 hours, the diagnosis is confirmed. A CT scan of the pelvis may also be useful. Heparin therapy should be continued for 10 days, but long-term oral anticoagulant therapy is not necessary unless there have been pulmonary emboli. The mechanism of action of heparin in this entity is unclear.

Rarely, paracervical or pudendal blocks will result in infections beneath the gluteus or behind the psoas muscle. These infections are often severe and characterized by persistent, spiking temperature elevations and hip or poorly localized pelvic pain. In one half the cases, a radiograph documented gas in the soft tissues of the hip. Vigorous antibiotic therapy and drainage are required for treatment. These patients often have extensive hospitalizations, and deaths have also been reported.[30]

Antibiotic Prophylaxis

One clear advance in the prevention of postpartum endometritis has been the use of perioperative antibiotics in patients at risk for infection after cesarean section. Prophylactic antibiotics are important in cesarean section because of the increased rate and severity of infection, and the high cesarean rate in the United States. Prophylactic antibiotics are not needed in vaginal deliveries because of the low rate of endometritis, the rarity of severe complications, and the possibility of side effects from the antibiotics. In 1981, Swartz and Grolle reviewed 26 published studies of antibiotic prophylaxis in cesarean section.[31] From theirs and more recent studies, several conclusions emerge. First, perioperative antibiotics significantly decrease the overall incidence of postoperative pelvic infections. This difference is most pronounced in populations with infection rates higher than 20–25%. With infection rates below 20%, the decrease in the rate of infection is not impressive. Second, many studies show excellent results with a three dose, 24-hour regimen; however, more recent studies show similar results with a single dose. Third, inexpensive antibiotics, with a narrow spectrum, such as ampicillin, cephalothin, or cefazolin, yield results comparable to other more expensive and more broad-spectrum regimens.[32] Fourth, to avoid fetal antibiotic exposure, the initial dose should be administered after cord clamping. The maternal outcome appears to be the same as if administered prior to the cesarean and the fetus avoids antibiotic exposure.[33]

Most studies administer the prophylactic antibiotic either intramuscularly or intravenously. Some reports describe a method of rinsing the uterus, peritoneum, and wound with antibiotics.[34] While initial reports described failure rates below those attained with prophylaxis by the intramuscular or intravenous route, more recent reports show no difference.[35] Further, systemic antibiotic absorption occurs. With a similar lavage technique, Duff and coworkers showed significant serum antibiotic levels.[36] The lavage technique, therefore, appears to offer little benefit.

Although widely used, there are concerns with widespread use of prophylactic antibiotics. First, even in populations with a 50% infection rate, prophylaxis exposes many patients to antibiotics needlessly (since 50% would not have become infected). Second, simple measures of infection control are important to decrease the rate of endometritis. Iffy and colleagues reported that the rate of postpartum infection in their population dropped from 83% to 16% when strict aseptic technique was emphasized.[37] Third, prophylactic antibiotics do not appear to decrease the rate of serious complications (eg, abscess, septic pelvic thrombophlebitis) after cesarean section. Fourth, the frequency of resistant organisms increases after prophylaxis. Fifth, widespread use of antibiotics for prophylaxis may sensitize or result in allergic reactions in some patients.

REFERENCES

1. Duff WP, Gibbs RS, Blanco JD, et al. Endometrial culture techniques in puerperal patients. *Obstet Gynecol.* 1983;61:217.
2. Blanco JD, Gibbs RS, Castaneda YS. Bacteremia in obstetrics: clinical course. *Obstet Gynecol.* 1982;58:621.
3. Duff WP. Pathophysiology and management of post cesarean endomyometritis. *Obstet Gynecol.* 1986;67:269.
4. Gibbs RS, Jones PM, Wilder CJ. Antibiotic therapy of endometritis following cesarean section: treatment successes and failures. *Obstet Gynecol.* 1978;52:31.
5. Gibbs RS, Rodgers PJ, Castaneda YS, et al. Endometritis following vaginal delivery. *Obstet Gynecol* 1980;56:555.
6. Sweet RL, Ledger WJ. Puerperal infectious morbidity. *Am J Obstet Gynecol.* 1973;117:1093.
7. Blanco JD, Gibbs RS. Infections following classical cesarean section. *Obstet Gynecol.* 1980;55:167.
8. D'Angelo LJ, Sokol RJ. Time-related peripartum determinants of postpartum morbidity. *Obstet Gynecol.* 1980;55:319.
9. Gibbs RS. Clinical risk factors for puerperal infection. *Obstet Gynecol.* 1980;55:178S.
10. Gibbs RS, Listwa HM, Read JA. The effect of internal fetal monitoring on maternal infection following cesarean section. *Obstet Gynecol.* 1976; 48:653.
11. Bobitt JR, Ledger WJ. Amniotic fluid analysis: its role in maternal and neonatal infection. *Obstet Gynecol.* 1978;51:56.
12. Gilstrap LC, Cunningham FG. The bacterial pathogenesis of infection following cesarean section. *Obstet Gynecol.* 1979;53:545.
13. Blanco JD, Gibbs RS, Castaneda YS, et al. Correlation of quantitative amniotic fluid cultures with endometritis after cesarean section. *Am J Obstet Gynecol.* 1982;143:897.
14. Magee KP, Blanco JD, Rayburn C, Prien S. Endometritis after cesarean: effect of age. Annual Meeting of the Infectious Disease Society for Obstetrics-Gynecology. Quebec, Canada. 1989, abstract #11.
15. Gibbs RS, Blanco JD, Castaneda YS, et al. A double-blind, randomized comparison of clindamycin-gentamicin versus cefamandole for treatment of post-cesarean endomyometritis. *Am J Obstet Gynecol.* 1982;144:261.
16. Walmer D, Walmer KR, Gibbs RS. Enterococci in post cesarean endometritis. *Obstet Gynecol.* 1988;71:159.
17. McCormack WM, Lee Y, Lin J, et al. Genital mycoplasmas in postpartum fever. *J Infect Dis.* 1973;127:193.
18. Wallace RJ, Alpert S, Browne K, et al. Isolation of *Mycoplasma hominis* from blood cultures in patients with post-partum fever. *Obstet Gynecol.* 1978;51:181.
19. Lamey JR, Eschenbach DA, Mitchell SH, et al. Isolation of mycoplasmas and bacteria from the blood of postpartum women. *Am J Obstet Gynecol.* 1982;143:104.
20. Platt R, Lin JL, Warren JW, et al. Infection with *Mycoplasma hominis* in postpartum fever. *Lancet.* 1980;2:1217.
21. Wager GP, Martin DH, Koutsky L, et al. Puerperal infectious morbidity: relationship to route of delivery and to antepartum *Chlamydia trachomatis* infection. *Am J Obstet Gynecol.* 1980;138:1028.
22. Blanco JD, Diaz KC, Lipscomb KA, et al. *Chlamydia trachomatis* isolation in patients with endometritis after cesarean section. *Am J Obstet Gynecol.* 1985;152:278.
23. Weinstein WM, Onderdonk AB, Bartlett JG, et al. Experimental intraabdominal abscesses in rats: development of an experimental model. *Infect Immun.* 1974;10:1250.
24. Weinstein WM, Onderdonk AB, Bartlett JG, et al. Antimicrobial therapy of experimental intraabdominal sepsis. *J Infect Dis.* 1975;132:282.
25. diZerega G, Yonekura L, Roy S, et al. A comparison of clindamycin-gentamicin and penicillin-gentamicin in the treatment of post-cesarean section endomyometritis. *Am J Obstet Gynecol.* 1979;134:238.
26. Blanco JD, Gibbs RS, Duff P, et al. Serum tobramycin levels in puerperal women. *Am J Obstet Gynecol.* 1983;147:466.
27. Knodel LC, Goldspiel BR, Gibbs RS. Prospective cost analysis of moxalactam versus clindamycin plus gentamicin for endomyometritis after cesarean section. *Antimicrob Agents Chemother.* 1988;32:853.
28. Gibbs RS, Blanco JD, Lipscomb KA, et al. Aztreonam versus gentamicin, each with clindamycin, in the treatment of endometritis. *Obstet Gynecol.* 1985;65:825.
29. Duff P, Gibbs RS. Pelvic vein thrombophlebitis: diagnostic dilemma and therapeutic challenge. *Obstet Gynecol Surv.* 1983;38:365.
30. Shy KK, Eschenbach DA. Fatal perineal cellulitis from an episiotomy site. *Obstet Gynecol.* 1979;54:292.
31. Swartz WH, Grolle K. The use of prophylactic antibiotics in cesarean section: a review of the literature. *J Reprod Med.* 1981;26:595.
32. Stiver HG, Forward KR, Livingstone RA, et al. Multicenter comparison of cefoxitin versus cefazolin for prevention of infectious morbidity after non-elective cesarean section. *Am J Obstet Gynecol.* 1983;145:158.
33. Cunningham FG, Leveno KJ, DePalma RT, et al. Perioperative antimicrobials for cesarean delivery: before or after cord clamping? *Obstet Gynecol.* 1983;62:151.
34. Rudd EG, Cobey EA, Long WH, et al. Prevention of endomyometritis using antibiotic irrigation during cesarean section. *Obstet Gynecol.* 1982; 60:413.
35. Leveno KJ, Quirk JC Jr., Cunningham FG, et al. Perioperative antimicrobials at cesarean section: lavage versus three intravenous doses. *Am J Obstet Gynecol.* 1984;149:463.
36. Duff P, Gibbs RS, Jorgensen JH, et al. The pharmacokinetics of prophylactic antibiotics administered by intraoperative irrigation at the time of cesarean section. *Obstet Gynecol.* 1982;60:409.
37. Iffy L, Kaminetzky HA, Maidman JE, et al. Control of perinatal infection by traditional preventive measures. *Obstet Gynecol.* 1979;54:403.

PART IX | Pulmonary Diseases

Uri Elkayam, Section Editor

Chapter One Hundred and Eighteen

Pulmonary Physiology

Joseph Rosman

118

Over the span of a woman's pregnancy, an array of physiologic changes occurs that impact on the respiratory system. The uterus enlarges and raises the diaphragm, hormonal changes cause hyperventilation, and increased maternal and fetal weight gain causes increased metabolic demands. Yet, unless there is marked pulmonary insufficiency, these changes are well tolerated. This is due to the lungs' extraordinary reserves. They have the capacity to quickly change from rest to sustained exertion and are well equipped to handle increased ventilatory and circulatory loads. It is, therefore, not surprising that during pregnancy the lungs are quite capable of maintaining physiologic homeostasis.

LUNG VOLUMES

Measurements of lung volumes can be divided into *volumes*, which are basic subdivisions and *capacities*, which are sums of various lung volumes (Figure 118–1). Important definitions are:

Tidal Volume (V_t)—The amount of air exhaled during a quiet breath. This is normally about 6–8 cc/kg in the nonpregnant individual.

Expiratory Reserve Volume (*ERV*)—the maximum amount of air that can be exhaled after the end of a normal breath.

Residual Volume (*RV*)—The amount of air that remains in the lung at the end of a maximum exhalation. This is usually 20–25% of the total lung capacity.

Vital Capacity (*VC*)—the amount of air that can be exhaled after a maximum inspiration. Normally, this is about 65 cc/kg in the nonpregnant female.

Total Lung Capacity (*TLC*)—the amount of air in the lung after a maximum inhalation. This is residual volume plus vital capacity.

Inspiratory Capacity (*IC*)—the amount of air that can be inspired starting at the end of a normal breath.

Functional Residual Capacity (*FRC*)—the amount of air in the lung at the end of a normal quiet breath. The lung is at FRC at the end of a quiet expiration. The *FRC = RV + ERV*

The FRC represents the equilibrium point between the chest wall's outward pull and the lungs' inner pull. Anything that changes this dynamic tension, such as pregnancy, will affect the FRC. Chronic obstructive lung disease, pulmonary fibrosis, obesity, and chest wall disease are other examples.

Measuring lung volumes in pregnancy has been attempted since the 1830s. The first serial measurements, however, were only done in 1953 by Cugell.[1] Since then, a number of similar studies have led to the following observations concerning pulmonary physiology in pregnancy.[2-6]

A reduction in both the ERV and RV (and, therefore, the FRC) becomes apparent between the fifth and sixth month of pregnancy and they continue to decrease during the last trimester (Figure 118–1). At term, the FRC has thus dropped by about 18%, the ERV has dropped by about 15%, and the RV has decreased about 20%.

The IC increases as pregnancy progresses. This increase preserves the VC and indicates that the diaphragm does not lose its ability to descend on inspiration.

TLC and VC appear unchanged, although some studies have reported either small increases or decreases in the VC.

A striking increase of the (V_t) occurs. Cugell[1] found a 33% increase and other studies have reported similar values.

The respiratory rate does not change significantly.

Several factors explain these changes. First, the enlarging uterus elevates the diaphragm in late pregnancy up to 4 cm.[7] This will reduce the FRC or resting volume of the lung. Diaphragm excursion is, however, preserved and, since the diaphragm is the main muscle of inspiration, the IC is increased. The fact that the VC is not reduced suggests that the stretched abdominal muscles may be at better mechanical advantage for exhalation.[4]

Another cause of volume reduction is increased pulmonary blood flow which takes up space that would otherwise be air.[8] Chest wall changes, such as breast enlargement, also contribute to lung volume reduction. These reductions are counterbalanced by an increase in the anterior-posterior and transverse diameter of the chest, which increases chest circumference 5–7 cm and causes a flare-out of the lower rib cage.[9]

Prowse and Gaensler[5] have likened these mechanical

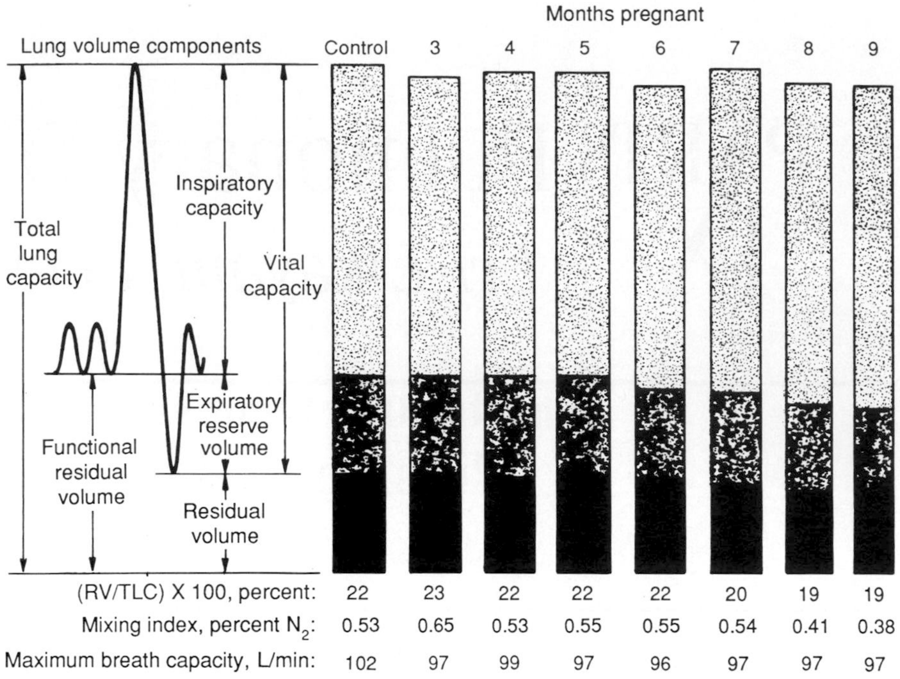

Figure 118–1. Monthly measurements of lung volumes during pregnancy. (*From Prowse CM, Gaensler EA[5]—from data of Cugell with permission.*)

changes of pregnancy to those seen in a pneumoperitoneum and also to changes seen when one assumes the supine position. All result in increased intraabdominal pressure, a higher resting diaphragm with preserved excursion, and reduced FRC. This is in contrast to other abdominal problems, such as abdominal binding, ascites, or severe obesity. The latter group will also elevate the diaphragm, but motion is not preserved on inspiration.

The reduced resting lung volume (FRC) has several clinical implications. A decreased FRC results in quicker induction with general anesthesia and in quicker reversal.[8] Second, a low FRC can cause small airway closure, especially toward the end of pregnancy when lung volumes are at their lowest, although this appears to happen only in the supine position.[10-12] Third, a reduced FRC, combined with increased minute consumption of oxygen, results in oxygen stores being used up quicker when there is apnea.[13] This would be relevant in a woman with any sort of apnea, and it has been demonstrated in pregnant women who have received succinylcholine for tracheal intubation.[14]

While it is tempting to explain the dyspnea commonly seen in pregnancy on FRC reduction, investigators have not been able to correlate a change in lung volumes with clinical symptoms. Moreover, the dyspnea begins before there is a noticeable change in lung volumes.[2]

In summary, pregnancy reduces resting lung volume (FRC), reduces ERV and RV, increases IC, and preserves TLC and VC.

LUNG MECHANICS

Chest wall and abdominal circumstances change during pregnancy. But, do the lungs[7] mechanical properties change? And if so, how does pregnancy affect stiffness (or compliance) of lungs and resistance of airways?

Gee[15] measured *compliance* ($\Delta V/\Delta P$) during the last trimester of pregnancy and could not show a change in *lung compliance* [C_L]. He also found *airway resistance* (ΔP/*flow*) actually decreased as pregnancy progressed. This is surprising since decreased lung volumes and hypocarbia usually increase airway resistance. The causes for these observations is unclear. Perhaps, the effects of elevated progesterone, cortisol, or cyclic AMP during pregnancy counterbalance any reduction in airway resistance caused by the drop in lung volumes. It should be noted, however, that other reports suggest either no change or a very slight increase in airway resistance during pregnancy.[11]

FLOWS

Spirometry is used to measure flow in the large airways. Important terms used to quantify airflow are the following.

Forced Vital Capacity (*FVC*)—the amount of air that can be forcefully exhaled after a maximal inhalation (going from TLC to RV) (Figure 118–2).

Forced Expiratory Volume in One Second [FEV_1]—the amount of air that can be forcefully exhaled in the first second of expiration. The FEV_1 is lowered with obstruction.

FEV_1/FVC *ratio* helps correct for differences in lung volume. Like the FEV_1, it is reduced with obstruction.

Mid-maximal expiratory flow [*MMEF or* $FEF_{25-75\%}$]—a slope connecting two points on the spirometry curve. The two points are at 25% and 75% of the vital capacity. This is often the earliest value to change as significant obstruction develops.

Several studies using spirometry during pregnancy show little change of flow.[3,8,11] This is consistent with earlier mentioned studies that showed no decrease in airway resistance.

SMALL AIRWAYS

Small airways are defined as less than 2 mm in diameter. They are thought to be the earliest site of airway obstruction in chronic obstructive lung disease. Small airways are prone

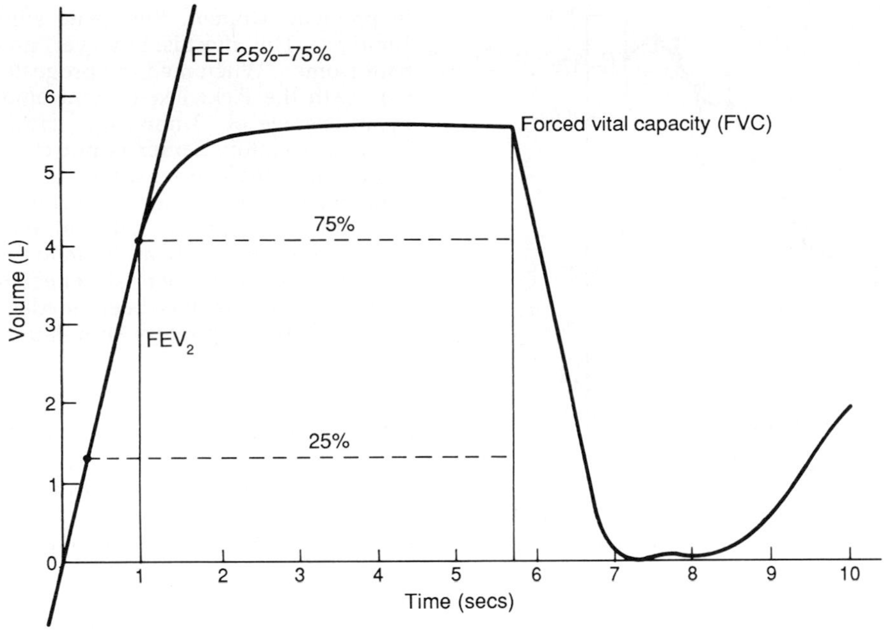

Figure 118–2. Normal spirometry.

to collapse when the outside pleural pressure becomes greater than the inside airway pressure. This usually happens at end-expiration in the lower lobes under conditions of low lung volumes (low FRC). The volume threshold below which small airway closure is seen is called the *closing volume.*

Russell[12] used the *single breath nitrogen test* to test for small airway closure in 10 nonsmoking women. If the test was performed in the sitting position, no significant airway closure at any stage of pregnancy was noted. In contrast, in the supine position, FRC dropped below closing volume in 50% of subjects. This usually occurred during the seventh month of pregnancy. Despite this change, there was not a strong correlation between a drop in FRC below closing capacity and a decrease in pO_2.

DIFFUSION CAPACITY

Diffusion capacity is the ability of a marker gas (usually carbon monoxide) to cross the alveolar-capillary membrane. It is a function of available alveolar surface area, pulmonary capillary blood volume, and the ability of carbon monoxide to combine with hemoglobin. Milne[16] performed monthly diffusing capacities during pregnancy and found the highest values in the first trimester. This was followed by a gradual decline that leveled off at the sixth month [Figure 118–3]. These values were controlled for hemoglobin and alveolar ventilation and could not be accounted for by changes in pulmonary blood flow or cardiac output. Other studies during the last trimester have shown no change in diffusion capacity.[17,18]

CONTROL OF BREATHING

The usual stimuli to hyperventilate are hypoxia, acidosis, and hypercarbia. Hypoxia (less than 50 mm Hg) causes increased ventilation and hypercarbia will usually do the same. The elevated P_{CO_2} causes increases in hydrogen ion in the cerebral spinal fluid which, in turn, stimulates chemoreceptors located in the medulla.

In pregnancy, the respiratory center responds to rising progesterone levels. In fact, hyperventilation can be seen

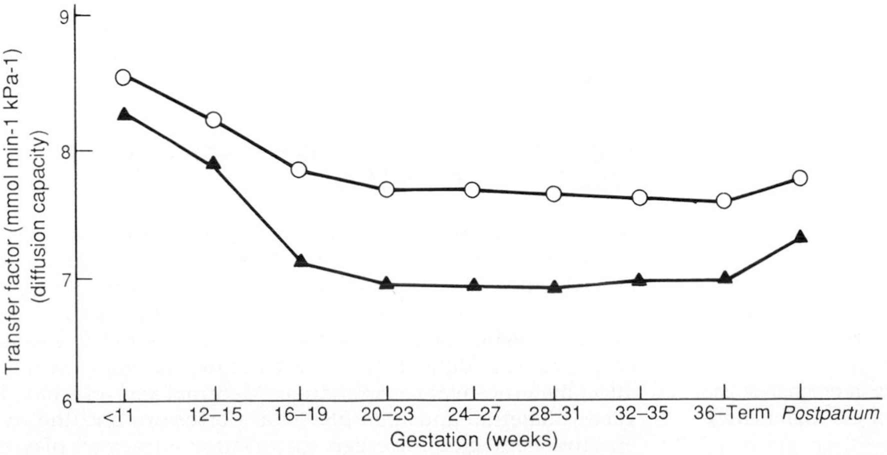

Figure 118–3. Serial diffusion measurements during pregnancy. (*From Milne JA, Mills RJ, Coutts JRT, et al[16] with permission.*)

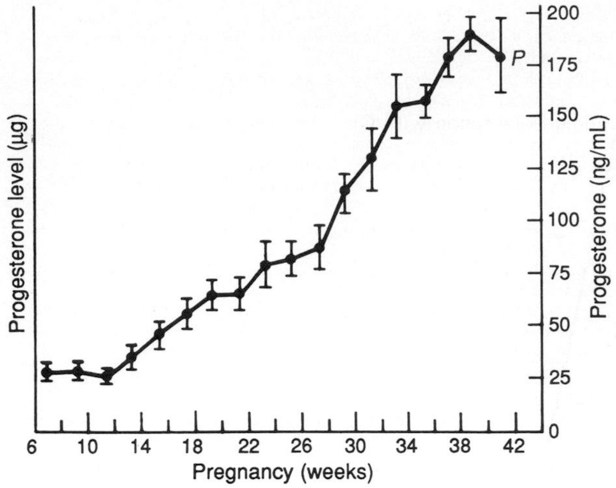

Figure 118–4. Progesterone levels during pregnancy. (*From Tullchinsky D, Hobel CJ, Yeager E et al*[38] *with permission.*)

in the progesterone-dominated luteal phase of a normal menstrual cycle.[19] In early pregnancy, a progressive rise in progesterone occurs[20] (Figure 118–4) while tidal volume (V_t) and *minute ventilation* (V_e) rise in parallel to up to 50% by term.[21]

The ventilatory response to progesterone is measured by looking at the V_e response to inhaled CO_2 (Figure 118–5). Lyons and Antonia[22] have shown a striking CO_2 sensitivity in pregnant women. Normally, a 1 mm Hg rise in alveolar PCO_2 will produce a 1.5 l/min increase in minute ventilation.

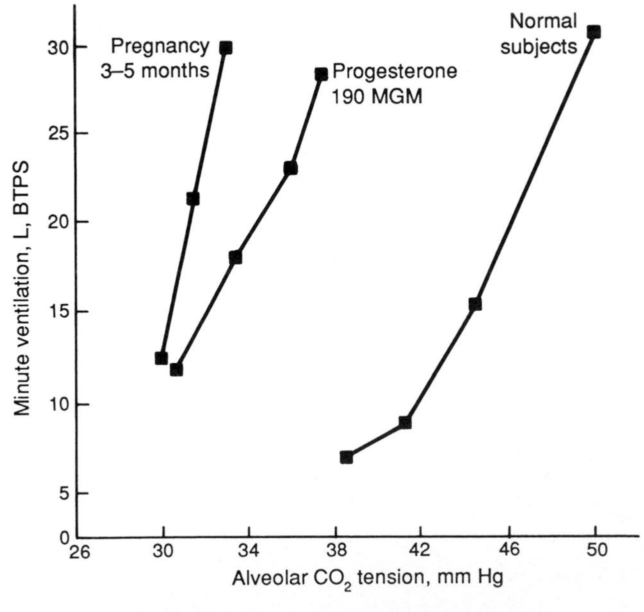

Figure 118–5. Carbon dioxide sensitivity curves in pregnancy and in normal subjects. (*From Prowse CM, Gaensler EA*[5] *with permission.*)

In pregnant women, this same stimulus will cause a 6 l/min rise. This effect is, however, not only limited to pregnant women. When medroxyprogesterone is used in obese men with the Pickwickian syndrome, the PCO_2 will drop by an average of 13 mm Hg.[23] How progesterone works on the respiratory center is not clear. Proposals have included an increase in sensitivity to CO_2 or, perhaps, a direct stimulation of the respiratory center. Progesterone can be found in the cerebral spinal fluid and appears to cross the blood-brain barrier.[24] In addition to the progesterone effect, there may be some synergistic effect of estrogen.[4] An interesting observation has been made by Hellegers[75], who found that the respiratory stimulation of high altitude and pregnancy are additive.

pH AND PCO_2

The PCO_2 is dependent on two factors: how much CO_2 is produced ($\dot{V}CO_2$) and how much is ventilated. As might be expected, the hyperventilation of pregnancy produces a chronic respiratory alkalosis. Most investigators have found about a 10 mm Hg drop in the PCO_2.[26,27]

In response to hyperventilation, an increased renal excretion of bicarbonate takes place. The average HCO_3^- is 19 meq. and the average pH ranges from 7.40 to 7.45.

Increased dead space can raise PCO_2 because it lowers effective alveolar ventilation. Templeton[28] studied 20 pregnant patients and could not show any increase in dead space. Pernoll[21] demonstrated, however, an average increase of 61 cc in dead space, which is presumed to be the result of the increase in airway caliber. He also measured effective alveolar ventilation and found it also increased. This would indicate that increased dead space is not a driving force in hyperventilation.

PO_2

Unlike PCO_2 , PO_2 can be affected in many ways. Shunts, ventilation-perfusion mismatches, changes in ventilaton, and cardiac output can all effect PO_2. In pregnancy, there are several important variables. First, hyperventilation should raise PO_2 as PCO_2 falls. Templeton[28] found an average PO_2 ranged from 101 to 106 mm Hg in the semirecumbent position. Going from sitting to a supine position, however, lowers oxygen tension. In late pregnancy, the supine position can cause small airway closure and can also reduce cardiac output by vena caval compression. Together, these effects can reduce oxygenation by approximately five to eight mm Hg.[29,30] Since the slope of the hemoglobin-oxygen dissociation curve is flat at these values, these changes do not affect either oxygen saturation or content significantly.

LABOR AND THE EFFECT OF MATERNAL BLOOD GAS CHANGES ON THE FETUS

The normal hyperventilation of pregnancy does not have any harmful effect on the fetus. In labor, hyperventilation exceeds often what is even normal for pregnancy.[31,32] One report noted a mean maternal pH of 7.55 with a high value of 7.68.[31] Whether this alkalosis has any harmful effects on the fetus is difficult to answer because so many factors affect materno-fetal gas exchange. Maternal and fetal blood gases, maternal and fetal placental perfusion, and the respective hemoglobin-oxygen dissociation curves all play a role in oxygen transport to the fetus. Most reports suggest no suspected signs of fetal distress or acidosis during normal labor, even in the presence of active hyperventilation.[33] An exception may occur with passive hyperventilation, such as in mechanical ventilation where the effect may be due to a reduction in cardiac output.[33]

O_2 CONSUMPTION, CO_2 PRODUCTION DURING PREGNANCY

The increasing fetal and maternal weight gain during pregnancy dictate an increased *minute consumption of oxygen* ($\dot{V}O_2$) and increased *production of* CO_2 ($\dot{V}CO_2$). Pernoll[34] found a 33% increase at term in resting minute consumption of oxygen. Others have reported a somewhat lower rise in $\dot{V}O_2$, but generally the rise corresponds to the increase in tissue mass, although the overall metabolic rate does not change.[35] This increase in $\dot{V}O_2$ is still not enough to account for the large increase in minute ventilation. As stated before, most of the increased respiratory drive appears to be due to a progesterone effect.

RESPONSE TO EXERCISE IN PREGNANCY

Exercise intolerance is a frequent complaint in pregnancy. This is due, in part, to increased body weight, which makes exercise, especially weight-bearing exercise, inefficient. For nonweight bearing exercise, such as cycling, there is conflicting data, but most reports suggest that pregnant women have a greater minute ventilation and oxygen consumption compared to their nonpregnant peers of similar weight and fitness. Part of this is due to an increased respiratory drive. During vigorous exercise, pregnant women are not able to reach as high a maximum $\dot{V}O_2$ consumption as nonpregnant controls. Perhaps, this is due to the lungs' smaller FRC being unable to meet the high O_2 demands of the body and consequently may indicate a decreased ability to exercise anaerobically.[36]

The effect of maternal exercise on the fetus has remained controversial due to a relative lack of invasive measurements. In animals, a reduction in uterine blood flow has been observed.[35] This does not necessarily indicate there is any adverse effect on the fetus. Uterine blood flow is just one of several variables that affect fetal oxygen transport. Noninvasive measurements suggest that mild-to-moderate exercise has no adverse effect on the fetus.[36]

DYSPNEA OF PREGNANCY

Dyspnea is a very common complaint during pregnancy, often occurring before a change in pulmonary function tests is evident. Milne[37] found that in the fourth month of pregnancy most women first notice the sensation of dyspnea. By 20 weeks, 50% complain of dyspnea and by 30 weeks, 76%. The severity of dyspnea seems to level off after 30 weeks. There has been speculation by Milne and others that those who notice dyspnea may be only responding to the increased ventilation of pregnancy.[37]

REFERENCES

1. Cugell DW, Frank NR, Gaensler EA, et al. Pulmonary function in pregnancy: serial observations in normal women. *Am Rev Tuberc.* 1953;67:568.
2. Alaily AB, Carrol KB. Pulmonary ventilation in pregnancy. *Br J Obstet Gynecol.* 1978;85:518.
3. Gazioglu K, Kaltrider NL, Rosen M, et al. Pulmonary function during pregnancy in normal women and in patients with cardiopulmonary disease. *Thorax.* 1970;25:445.
4. Knuttgen HG, Emerson K. Physiological response to pregnancy at rest and exercise. *J Appl Physiol.* 1970;36:549.
5. Prowse CM, Gaensler EA. Respiratory and acid-base changes during pregnancy. *Anesthesiology.* 1965;26:381.
6. Rubin A, Russo N, Gaucher D, et al. The effect of pregnancy upon pulmonary function in normal women. *Am J Obstet Gynecol.* 1956;72:963.
7. Ginty AP. Comparative effects of pregnancy and phrenic nerve interruption on the diaphragm and their relation to pulmonary tuberculosis. *Am J Obstet Gynecol.* 1938;35:237.
8. Fishburne JI. Physiology and disease of the respiratory system in pregnancy. A review. *J Reprod Med.* 1979;22:177.
9. Thomson KJ, Cohen ME. Studies on the circulation in pregnancy. II. Vital capacity observations in normal pregnant women. *Surg Gynecol Obstet.* 1938;66:591.
10. Holdcroft A, Bevan DR, O'Sullivan JC, Sykes M. Airway closure during pregnancy. *Anesthesiology.* 1977;32:517.
11. Milne JA, Mills RJ, Howie AD, Pack AL. Large airways function during normal pregnancy. *Br J Anaesth.* 1977;84:448.
12. Russell IF, Chambers WA. Closing volume in normal pregnancy. *Br J Anaesth.* 1981;53:1043.
13. Brownwell LG, West P, Kryger MH. Breathing during sleep in normal pregnant women. *Am Rev Resp Dis.* 1986;133:38.
14. Archer GW, Marx GF. Arterial oxygen tension during apnea in parturient women. *Br J Anaesth.* 1974;46:358.
15. Gee JBL, Packer BS, Millen JE, Robin ED. Pulmonary mechanics during pregnancy. *J Clin Invest.* 1967;46:945.
16. Milne JA, MIlls RJ, Coutts JRT, MacNaughton MC, Maron F, Pack AI. The effect of human pregnancy on pulmonary transfer factor for carbon monoxide as measured by the single-breath method. *Clin Sci Mol Med.* 1977;53:271.
17. Bedell GN, Adams RW. Pulmonary diffusing capacity during rest and exercise. A study of normal persons and persons with atrial septal defect, pregnancy and pulmonary disease. *J Clin Invest.* 1962;41:1908.
18. Krumholz RA, Echt CR, Ross JC. Pulmonary diffusing capacity, capillary blood volume, lung volumes and mechanics of ventilation in early and late pregnancy. *J Lab Clin Med.* 1964;63:648.
19. England SJ, Farhi LE. Fluctuations in alveolar CO_2 and in base excess during the menstrual cycle. *Respir Physiol.* 1976;26:157.
20. Yannone ME, McCundy JR, Goldfien A. Plasma progesterone levels in normal pregnancy, labor and puerperium. *Am J Obstet Gynecol.* 1968;101:1058.
21. Pernoll ML, Metcalfe J, Kovach PA, Wachtel R. Ventilation during rest and exercise in pregnancy and postpartum. *Respir Physiol.* 1975;25:295.
22. Lyons MA, Antonia R. The sensitivity of the respiratory center in pregnancy and after the administration of progesterone. *Trans Assoc Am Phys.* 1959;72:173.
23. Sutton FD, Zwillich CW, Creagh C, et al. Progesterone for out-patient treatment of Pickwickian syndrome. *Ann Int Med.* 1975;83:476.
24. Skatrud JB, Dempsey JA, Kaiser DG. Ventilatory response to medroxyprogesterone acetate in normal subjects: time course and mechanism. *J Appl Phsiol Respir.* 1978;44:939.
25. Hellegars A, Metcalfe J, Huckabee W, et al. The alveolar pCO_2 in pregnancy and in non-pregnant women at altitude. *J Clin Invest.* 1959;38:1010.
26. Blechner JN, Cotter JR, Stenger VG, Hinkley CM, et al. Oxygen, carbon dioxide and hydrogen ion concentrations in arterial blood during pregnancy. *Am J Obstet Gynecol.* 1968;100:1.
27. Lim VS, Katz AI, Lindheimer MD. Acid-base regulation in pregnancy. *Am J Physiol.* 1976;231:1764.
28. Templeton A, Kelman GR. Maternal blood gases, [$pA_o2-p_aO_2$], physiologic shunt, and V_d/V_t in normal pregnancy. *Br J Anesthesiol.* 1976;48:1001.
29. Ag CK, Tan TH, Walters WAW, Wood C. Postural influence on maternal capillary oxygen and carbon dioxide tension. *Br J Med.* 1969;4:201.
30. Awe RJ, Nicotra B, Newsome TD, Viles R. Arterial oxygenation and alveolar-arterial gradients in term pregnancy. *Obstet Gynecol.* 1979;53:182.
31. Miller FC, Petrie RH, Arce JJ, Paul RH, et al. Hyperventilation during labor. *Am J Obstet Gynecol.* 1974;489.
32. Reid DHS. Respiratory changes during labor. *Lancet.* 1966;1:784.
33. Novy MJ, Edwards MJ. Respiratory problems during pregnancy. *Am J Obstet Gynecol.* 1967;99:1024.
34. Pernoll ML, Metcalfe JL, Schlenker TL, Welch JE, et al. Oxygen consumption at rest and during exercise in pregnancy. *Respir Physiol.* 1975;25:285.
35. Lotgering FK, Gilbert RD, Longo LD. Maternal and fetal responses to exercise during pregnancy. *Physiol Rev.* 1985;65:1.
36. Artell R, Wiswell R, Romem Y, Dorey F. Pulmonary responses to exercise in pregnancy. *Am J Obstet Gynecol.* 1988;154:378.
37. Milne JA, Howie AD, Pack AI. Dyspnoea during normal pregnancy. *Br J Obstet Gynecol.* 1978;85:260.
38. Tullchinsky D, Hobel CJ, Yeager E et al. Plasma estrone, estradiol, estriol, progesterone and 17-hydroxyprogesterone in human pregnancy. I. Normal pregnancy. *Am J Obstet Gynecol* 1972;112:1095.

Chapter One Hundred and Nineteen

Pulmonary Embolism and Thrombophlebitic Disorders

F. Susan Cowchock and Geno J. Merli

119

The reported prevalence of deep venous thrombosis (DVT) ranges widely because a variety of diagnostic methods with different degrees of sensitivity and specificity were used for diagnosis. DVT of the lower extremities occurs in 0.2–3.0% of deliveries.[1] DVT is three to five times more common postpartum than antepartum and three to 16 times more common after delivery by cesarean section. Pulmonary embolism (PE) has been reported to occur in 15–24% of DVT cases with a 12–15% mortality.[2] PE is diagnosed in about one out of 2000 deliveries and has been cited as the major single cause of maternal death. Venous or arterial thrombosis can occur in any site, but cerebral thrombosis or infarction and septic pelvic or ovarian vein thrombophlebitis pose exceptional risks for pregnant women. The risk for cerebral thrombosis was estimated to be 13 times higher during pregnancy.[3] Like DVT, cerebral thrombosis is most frequent during the second and third trimesters or the postpartum period. Ovarian or pelvic vein thrombophlebitis is often associated with puerperal infection and occurs in about one out of 1000 pregnancies.[4] A combination of mechanical factors which promote stasis, and progressive changes in the complex balances of the coagulation system explain both the increased risk for thrombosis associated with pregnancy and its timing (see also Chapter 210).

Clinical factors which increase the risk for thrombosis include trauma, infection, dehydration, sickle cell anemia, shock, obesity, lower extremity varicosities, and edema.[5] Many of these are commonly observed in pregnant women, and even uncomplicated pregnancy is associated with progressive venous distensibility and mechanical obstruction of venous drainage by the enlarging uterus. All of these contribute to intimal injury (distended vessels) and stasis (mechanical obstruction). These mechanical factors, together with the profound changes in the coagulation system described below, fulfill *Virchow's Triad* for the development of thrombosis.

During pregnancy, the delicate balances of the coagulation system are subject to progressive and profound changes. These probably evolved to protect women from severe hemorrhage during placental separation. Levels of all the procoagulant plasma factors except factors XI and XIII increase during pregnancy. Levels of anticoagulant factor protein S decrease during pregnancy, but levels of protein C and C-4b-binding protein actually increase, while antithrombin III levels are unchanged.[6-8] Women with hereditary or acquired deficiencies of these coagulation factors or their inhibitors and women with antibodies to phospholipid antigens intimately involved in coagulation pathways (lupus anticoagulants, anticardiolipin antibodies, and so on) are at special hazard for thrombosis during pregnancy because of these physiologic changes. Inherited or acquired deficiencies in anticoagulant pathways have been diagnosed in up to 15% of nonobstetric patients with thrombosis.[9] There is growing recognition of a similar frequency in obstetric patients. Pregnant women whose thrombotic episode leads to the diagnosis of a coagulation abnormality may constitute the greater part of the obstetric population actually in need of prophylaxis for recurrent thrombosis in subsequent pregnancies.[10] Because of the importance of these coagulation abnormalities in the diagnosis and management of thrombotic episodes during pregnancy, the physiologic pathways involving protein C will be reviewed (Figure 119–1). The balances of the protein C system are, in turn, dependent on other coagulation factors such as tissue plasminogen activators (t-PA), as well as circulating binding proteins and inhibitors. Unfortunately, information on normal levels of these proteins in pregnant women or documentation of an association between changes in measured levels and thrombosis in pregnancy is scanty.[11-13] Thrombin generated by activation of the coagulation cascade is inactivated by circulating antithrombin III, which also inactivates procoagulant factors IXa, Xa, XIa, and XIIa.

Thrombin is also bound to its endothelial cell receptor, thrombomodulin, and in the process rapidly activates large quantities of protein C. Protein C(a) acts directly to slow coagulation by inactivating factors Va and VIIIa. It promotes fibrinolysis by both increasing tissue plasminogen activator (t-PA) activity and inactivating t-PA inhibitor. Activated protein S is a cofactor for the anticoagulant activity of protein C(a).[14] Acquired or inherited deficiencies in levels of protein C or S, or their activated forms, will result in an increased risk for thrombosis. The protein C system may also play an important role in thrombosis secondary to antiphospholipid antibodies. Lupus anticoagulants are antiphospholipid antibodies that block *in vitro* conversion of prothrombin to thrombin. The activation of protein C on the thrombomodulin receptor occurs in intimate association with phospholipids, just as the conversion of prothrombin to thrombin is associated with phospholipids of the platelet membrane. Purified IgG fractions from lupus anticoagulant patients have been demonstrated to block the activation of protein C by endothelial cells.[15] The effects of phospholipid antibodies on the protein C pathway provide both an explanation for the observed fetal wastage and thrombosis in women with antibodies to phospholipids and a rationale for the use of heparin in treatment of these patients. There is growing recognition that proteins C and S, in association with t-PA and t-PA inhibitors, serve as a bridge between normal and abnormal immune responses and the coagulation system.

DIAGNOSIS OF DVT/PE IN PREGNANCY

The diagnosis of DVT depends on radiographic visualization, because even in nonpregnant patients physical examination has a reliability of only 50%. The traditional physical signs are pain, tenderness, swelling, edema, and Homans'

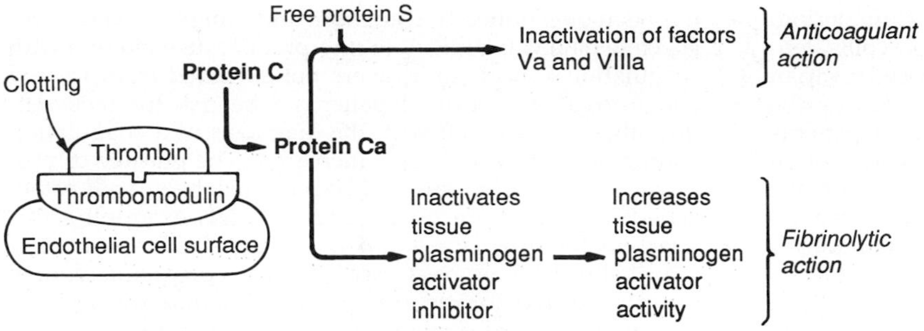

Figure 119–1. Diagram of protein C metabolic pathways. (*Data taken from Clouse, LH.*[14])

sign. Noninvasive testing has been used extensively for diagnosis and evaluation of DVT in other patient populations. The choice of noninvasive tests is altered in pregnant women: I125-fibrinogen scanning is a sensitive test for distal DVT, but is contraindicated during pregnancy because I125 crosses the placenta. In addition, the isotope has a 60-day half-life and is excreted in breast milk, limiting its use in the postpartum period. Impedance plethysmography (IPG) uses electrical resistance to measure changes in blood volume in the lower extremities. The sensitivity of IPG for diagnosis of DVT compared to venography is in the range of 71–96% in nongravid populations.[16-18] However, compression of the inferior vena cava by the gravid uterus may give false-positive results in this test or in Doppler flow studies. Duplex ultrasound scanning has even better diagnostic sensitivity for proximal lower extremity thrombosis (91–100%).[19-21] These tests are not as reliable in the diagnosis of DVT of the calf veins. Invasive testing may be indicated to confirm an equivocal noninvasive test or when intervention such as embolectomy or caval interruption is planned. Venography can be performed in the pregnant patient with relative safety since the field of radiation can be specifically directed and the fetus shielded. The estimated radiation exposure for the fetus is 21 millirads, well within accepted radiation dose levels of less than 10 rads.[22] Further assessment of the extent of clot into the iliac veins or above and below the renal veins for filter placement requires additional venography of the vena cava.

Occult pulmonary embolism is not uncommon in patients with proximal DVT.[23] Even in the absence of known DVT, the diagnosis of pulmonary embolism should still be a first priority for obstetric patients with tachypnea, dyspnea, or chest pain.[24] Ventilation perfusion (VP) lung scanning has high sensitivity, but variable specificity for pulmonary embolism. Lung scans should always be interpreted together with a chest x-ray. Fetal radiation exposure from a lung scan is about 50 mrem. Scans demonstrating multiple segmental or lobar perfusion defects with normal ventilation and no corresponding defects on chest x-ray yield the highest probability for PE. Table 119–1, from data published by Hull and coworkers, gives probabilities for a confirmed pulmonary embolus based on VP lung scan findings.[25]

Patients with clinical findings suggesting pulmonary embolus in whom lung scan findings are indeterminate or which demonstrate matching ventilation and perfusion defects, should undergo pulmonary angiography. Pulmonary angiography produces the highest fetal radiation exposures (about 850 millirads with appropriate shielding) compared to the other radiologic tests reviewed here.[22] Other indications for pulmonary angiography include:

1. A high probability lung scan in a patient with a relative contraindication to anticoagulation (for example, active bleeding).
2. Suspected pulmonary embolus in a patient with another pulmonary disease resulting in an abnormal chest x-ray (for example, cystic fibrosis).
3. Massive pulmonary embolus requiring suction embolectomy.

DIAGNOSIS OF THROMBOSIS IN OTHER SITES

The diagnosis and management of cerebrovascular thrombosis in pregnancy is discussed elsewhere (see Chapter 199). Pelvic thrombophlebitis is intimately related to endometritis, but ovarian vein thrombosis can occur in the absence of an obvious source for infection. Recent case reports have documented the diagnosis of ovarian vein thrombosis by computed tomography (CT) and sonography with duplex Doppler scanning.[26,27] Women with pelvic or ovarian vein

TABLE 119–1. PROBABILITY OF EMBOLUS DIAGNOSED BY PULMONARY ANGIOGRAPHY BASED ON VENTILATION-PERFUSION SCAN RESULTS[a]

Perfusion Abnormality	Ventilation Scan Results	Embolism by Angiography
One or more segmental or greater defects	Mismatch	86%
	Match	23%
One or more subsegmental defects	Mismatch	27%
	Match	13%
Indeterminate		17%
None		2%

[a] Taken from Hull and coworkers.[25]

thrombophlebitis usually present in the peripartum period, often with severe abdominal pain, sepsis, fever, chills, leukocytosis, nausea, and vomiting. A thrombosed ovarian vein is usually tender, palpable (50%), and located on the right (90%).[4] Physical findings can be sparse in patients with septic pelvic thrombophlebitis. The diagnosis is often suspected when fever persists despite adequate antibiotic therapy.[1] Treatment includes both intravenous anticoagulation and appropriate antibiotics. The risk for pulmonary embolus is high.

DIAGNOSIS OF COAGULATION ABNORMALITIES IN OBSTETRIC PATIENTS WITH THROMBOSIS

Women with recurrent thromboses, thrombosis at an unusual site (cerebral thrombosis), or in whom thrombosis is associated with fetal wastage or fetal growth retardation should be evaluated for the most common associated coagulation abnormalities. Based on the known etiologies for recurrent thrombosis in pregnant and nonpregnant populations, the evaluation should include tests for antiphospholipid antibodies, levels of protein C and protein S, and antithrombin III, fibrinogen, and plasminogen activity as well as a platelet count to exclude thrombocythemias.[28,29] The laboratory diagnosis of each of these may be modified by pregnancy, anticoagulant therapy, consumption of clotting factors, and inflammatory reactions. Tests for antiphospholipid antibodies should include both lupus anticoagulant (LA) and enzyme-linked immunosorbent assay (ELISA) tests. The most specific LA tests are either an activated partial thromboplastin time performed with a sensitive thromboplastin or dilute Russell's viper venom time—both confirmed by mixing with normal plasma or platelet neutralization.[30] Interpretation of LA testing is difficult when patients are treated with heparin, and serum antibody-binding in ELISA testing is altered by pregnancy or elevated levels of polyclonal immunoglobulins (particularly IgM class) consequent to an inflammatory response.[31] The diagnosis of a phospholipid antibody under these circumstances should be confirmed by multiple tests (see also Chapter 50). Platelet counts may or may not be decreased in normal late pregnancy, compared to the nonpregnant state. The suspicion of thrombocythemias based on total platelet count (usually greater than 500,000 mm^3) may be subject to some modification in the third trimester.[32-34] As discussed in the previous section, levels of anticoagulant factors may vary with pregnancy or the presence of active clotting. Confirmation of protein S deficiency, in particular, may need to be postponed until pregnancy is completed. The absence of a family history of thrombosis, however, does not make a hereditary coagulation defect unlikely because these autosomal dominantly inherited disorders have a low penetrance.[28] A strong suspicion of an underlying coagulation disorder may require more extensive and sophisticated evaluation by a specialist. The confirmation of one of these diagnoses suggests that anticoagulation should be continued throughout pregnancy into the postpartum period and that the patient is at high risk for recurrent thromboses in future pregnancies.

PROPHYLAXIS FOR DVT/PE IN PREGNANT PATIENTS

Prophylactic treatment with subcutaneous heparin has been recommended for pregnant women at high risk or for those with a prior history of thrombosis. Recently, this policy has been questioned by Tengborn and others.[10] Their retrospective data was difficult to interpret because women with coagulation abnormalities were not excluded from treated and untreated groups of patients. The risk for recurrent thrombosis in women with the diagnosis of a coagulation abnormality appeared to be increased. The efficacy of prophylactic heparin in surgical patients has been well established, but there are no comparable trials examining this question for pregnant women. The expected benefits are not likely to be as great, because most pregnant women are at lower risk for recurrent thrombosis than the selected groups of surgical patients studied. Furthermore, heparin treatment will be required for a long time, compared to perioperative periods, and risks of therapy increase with treatment times. A prospective trial would have been difficult to design because sensitive noninvasive tests for the diagnosis of DVT suitable for pregnant women have just been developed. Furthermore, it is likely that pregnant women with inherited or acquired thrombotic disorders are at above average risk for thrombosis or recurrent thrombosis and should be considered separately. Either risk or benefit considerations for prophylactic anticoagulation will be more favorable when low molecular weight heparin is generally available because the morbidity associated with heparin antibodies is likely to be significantly reduced or abolished.

No consensus on this issue is possible at this time, but it has been suggested that pregnant or obese women require higher doses of subcutaneous heparin for prophylaxis than nonpregnant or slimmer women. Weiner has recommended a dose of 5000 units every 12 hours in the first trimester which is increased to 7500 units in the second trimester, and 10,000 in the third trimester.[1] The midinterval APTT was not usually prolonged at these gestational ages. For prophylactic treatment of pregnant women at higher risk with phospholipid antibodies, we have recommended 10,000 units every 12 hours, adjusted downward until the midinterval APTT falls within or at the top of the normal range. Table 119–2 gives suggested heparin dose adjustments based on a top normal APTT of 45 seconds. Duplex ultrasound scanning should be employed when patients at risk have signs or symptoms of acute thrombophlebitis. Duplex scanning at three month intervals may also be suggested for women at risk who are not given heparin prophylaxis.

TREATMENT OF DVT/PE

Standard regimens for heparin therapy are generally used for antepartum DVT/PE. We agree that there is little place for coumarins in treatment of pregnant women.[1] Because coumarins are excreted in breast milk, their use is contraindicated for postpartum nursing women as well. Recent pro-

TABLE 119–2. SUBCUTANEOUS HEPARIN DOSE ADJUSTMENTS FOR PROPHYLAXIS

Six-Hour APTT	Change in q 12-Hour Heparin Dose
Less than 36 seconds	+1000 units
36–40 seconds	+ 500
41–45 seconds	0
46–50 seconds	− 500
Greater than 50 seconds	−1000

spective randomized trials comparing intravenous heparin regimens to subcutaneous injection have indicated that adjusted dose subcutaneous injections were equally effective in treatment of distal DVT in nonobstetric patients, and less costly.[35-37] Intravenous regimens may be more effective for proximal vein thrombosis and are recommended in the presence of PE.[38] Subcutaneous heparin is usually started for this purpose at a dose of 15,000 units every 12 hours and adjusted (Table 119–2) until the midinterval APTT is 1.5–2.0 times baseline.[39] The usual initial dose of heparin for intravenous infusion is 1000 units per hour. Intravenous infusions are usually changed to subcutaneous injections after seven days. A baseline complete blood count, including platelet count and APTT, are obtained before subcutaneous or intravenous treatment is started. Therapeutic treatment is continued for at least three months in early pregnancy then replaced by prophylactic doses, or until the sixth week postpartum. One method for adjustment of intravenous heparin infusion by measurement of APTT is given in Table 119–3.

RISKS OF PROPHYLACTIC OR THERAPEUTIC ANTICOAGULATION

The most important maternal risks associated with heparin treatment include manifestations of heparin antibodies, osteopenia, and increased risk for bleeding. Heparin antibodies may result in heparin-associated thrombocytopenia (HAT), white clot syndrome, and cutaneous or fat necrosis. Since heparin does not cross the placenta, direct fetal risks are not a consideration. The incidence of these associated risks is generally related to heparin dose, duration of therapy, and, in the case of heparin antibodies, repeated exposure.

Heparin-induced antibody complexes of high molecular weight cause platelet aggregation, leading to thrombocytopenia and thrombosis. Platelet aggregates in small vessels are responsible for both cutaneous and fat necrosis, as well as disseminated intravascular coagulation (white clot syndrome). Even the small amounts of heparin used to flush arterial lines have been associated with this complication when patients were previously exposed to the drug.[40] Simple thrombocytopenia (platelet count less than 100,000/mm^3) may occur in 10% of treated patients, but manifestations of the white clot syndrome are fortunately rare in pregnant women.[41,42] Although uncommon, the white clot syndrome is associated with significant morbidity and mortality.[43] A history of previous heparin exposure should be sought before treatment. Prior heparin-associated thrombocytopenia mandates the substitution of low molecular weight heparins. Low molecular weight heparin is not associated with platelet aggregation because the antibody complexes formed are much smaller. Serial platelet counts should be obtained for two weeks after heparin therapy is initiated.[44] Thrombosis associated with heparin antibodies has been treated or prevented with aspirin or low molecular weight heparin.[45,46] We add 80 mg aspirin daily to prophylactic heparin when treating obstetric patients with phospholipid antibodies to reduce the risk of platelet aggregation. Addition of even low dose aspirin or aspirin-like drugs to full anticoagulant doses of heparin would not be advised because the risk for bleeding may be increased. When possible, aspirin can be discontinued two weeks before delivery.

Osteopenia is usually manifest radiographically by vertebral collapse and heralded by back pain. Although similar osteopenia occurs in uncomplicated pregnancies, heparin-associated osteopenia has not been reported in obstetric patients receiving prophylactic dosages less than 15,000 units per day. The frequency of this complication is unknown—estimates range from one out of 20 women to zero out of 75.[1,47] One of the authors has treated 50 women with either unexplained fetal demise or pregnancy wastage associated with phospholipid antibodies with an average of 15,000–16,000 units of heparin daily throughout pregnancy without observing symptomatic osteopenia. From these figures, an estimate of the prevalence of this complication is one out of 145 or less. Because heparin inhibits 1-alpha hydroxylation of 25-hydroxyvitamin D, supplemental calcium or vitamin D may prevent clinical osteopenia, but the low frequency of this complication precludes a meaningful clinical trial.[48]

The risk for bleeding complications associated with anticoagulant treatment of obstetric patients is dependent on both duration and intensity of therapy.[49] Other medical factors such as liver dysfunction, severe anemia, or malignancy are unlikely in this group of patients. There are few reports from which the prevalence of bleeding complications, associated with prophylactic or with therapeutic anticoagulation, in obstetric patients can be estimated. Since heparin is discontinued before delivery, or reversible in an emergency with protamine, and because uterine hemostasis is unaffected, major hemorrhage is unlikely in otherwise uncomplicated vaginal deliveries. Women delivered by cesarean section may be at greater risk. An increased incidence of wound hematomas was noted in surgical patients receiving prophylactic heparin.[50] Hall's review noted that 10% of 135 complicated obstetric cases treated with intravenous heparin were complicated by hemorrhage.[51] Minor bleeding problems have been associated with both therapeutic and prophylactic treatment. Rosove and others reported minor hematuria and nosebleeds in women with phospholipid antibodies on therapeutic doses of heparin.[52] One of the authors has observed one case with nosebleeds, one episiotomy hematoma, and one episode of microscopic hematuria among 50 women given low dose aspirin and prophylactic heparin throughout pregnancy.[53]

The choice of epidural anesthesia for labor and delivery

TABLE 119–3. ADJUSTMENT OF HEPARIN INFUSION RATES TO ACHIEVE THERAPEUTIC RANGE OF 55–75 SECONDS (NORMAL RANGE 35–45 SECONDS) OR APTT 1.5–2.0 TIMES BASELINE MEASUREMENT

First APTT Six Hours after Beginning Infusion at 1000 Units/Hour	
APTT	**Response**
Less than 55 seconds	Increase infusion rate to 1200 units/hour.
55–75 seconds	Maintain infusion rate.
Greater than 75 seconds	Decrease infusion rate to 800 units/hour.
Second APTT Six Hours after First Adjustment	
Less than 45 seconds	Add bolus 2000 units to infusion rate.
55–75 seconds	Maintain adjusted rate.
Greater than 75 seconds	Decrease infusion rate to 600 units/hour.
Third APTT Six Hours after Second Adjustment	
Less than 45 seconds	Add bolus 2000 units to infusion rate.
55–75 seconds	Maintain adjusted rate.
greater than 75 seconds	Decrease infusion rate to 400 units/hour.

Subsequent adjustments: If APTT consistently less than 55 seconds, increase infusion rates by 200 units/hour to a maximum of 2000 units/hour.

requires careful consideration in women receiving anticoagulants. The incidence of epidural hematoma could be as high as 0.35% in anticoagulated patients and often results in permanent paraplegia.[54] Anticoagulation before catheter insertion does not appear to be a problem if the patient's clotting tests have returned to the normal range. Most epidural hematomas have been reported when anticoagulation is initiated or resumed after lumbar puncture. Epidural anesthesia was safely performed in two reports surveying 4164 patients given heparin after epidural catheter insertion.[55,56] In each series, great care was taken to minimize the risk of hematoma; epidural anesthesia was not given if blood was aspirated at lumbar puncture. Maintenance doses of heparin were not given until at least one hour after catheter removal. Last, intravenous heparin was given in small increments with careful monitoring of coagulation studies to avoid any period of overcoagulation. Epidural hematoma has rarely been reported in patients receiving only aspirin, but discontinuation of aspirin or other antiplatelet agents at least two weeks before delivery is a reasonable recommendation. When these precautions have been taken, the risk of epidural hematoma in anticoagulated women appears to be lower than the risks associated with general anesthesia in most cases.[57]

OTHER TREATMENTS FOR ACUTE THROMBOSIS IN PREGNANCY

Thrombolytic therapy should be considered when ischemia threatens survival of a limb or severe cardiopulmonary compromise places a mother and fetus at risk from hypoxia.[58,59] The use of the approved agents urokinase and streptokinase is relatively contraindicated in pregnant patients because hemorrhage into the placenta and abortion can occur (see Table 119–3).[60] Tissue plasminogen activator (t-PA) of recombinant origin will soon be released for thrombolytic treatment. The information summarized in Table 119–4 should be reviewed before thrombolytic therapy is instituted.

TABLE 119–4. CONTRAINDICATIONS FOR THROMBOLYTIC THERAPY

Absolute
1. Active internal bleeding
2. Central nervous system vascular disease or procedure within two months
3. Severe preeclampsia[a]

Relative, major
1. Major surgery within 10 days[a]
2. Obstetrical delivery within five days[a]
3. Organ biopsy
4. Previous puncture of a noncompressible vessel (such as, supraclavicular catheter placement)[a]
5. Recent gastrointestinal bleeding
6. Hypertension[a]
7. Thrombolytic therapy (streptokinase) within the last three months

Relative, minor
1. Minor trauma
2. Mitral valve disease with atrial fibrillation
3. Bacterial endocarditis
4. Hepatic/renal disease
5. Pregnancy or menstrual bleeding[a]
6. Diabetic hemorrhagic retinopathy

[a] Of particular importance in obstetric patients.

Transvenous caval interruption has been used in pregnant patients at high risk for pulmonary embolus for whom anticoagulation is contraindicated or as an adjunct to anticoagulation in severe thromboembolic disease. Hux and others reported on the successful placement of Greenfield filters in six pregnant patients.[61] Pulmonary embolectomy is an appropriate emergency procedure in the presence of massive pulmonary embolus. These patients are near or in cardiovascular collapse, so immediate mortality is high. The survival rate following pulmonary embolectomy was 56% using the transvenous approach.[62]

Specific treatments are available for prophylactic or adjunctive treatment of thrombosis in patients with a known coagulation disorder. Protein C and S and antithrombin III concentrates are available for patients with known deficiency disorders and pure protein C will soon be produced through recombinant technology. Heparin requires antithrombin III for its anticoagulant activity. Intravenous gamma globulin infusions have been used for the prevention of fetal wastage in selected women with phospholipid antibodies and are likely to be useful as well in the adjunctive care of such patients with acute thromboses.[63]

PRECONCEPTIONAL COUNSELING OF WOMEN WITH A HISTORY OF THROMBOSIS

In general, a history of thrombosis is a contraindication to the use of oral contraceptives. Estrogens should be avoided by women with the diagnosis of an autoimmune or hereditary clotting disorder. Androgenic progestins may not be contraindicated in treatment of such patients. In fact, the androgens stanozolol and danazol have been used to treat nonpregnant patients with hereditary protein C deficiency. Danazol has been used in the treatment of systemic lupus erythematosus. Women with a history of thrombosis are not at increased risk for pregnancy wastage unless an underlying coagulation disorder has been diagnosed. In particular, women with antiphospholipid antibodies, thrombocytosis, and protein C deficiency are at increased risk for preeclampsia, fetal growth retardation, miscarriage, or fetal demise. Counseling in each case would depend on the specific diagnosis. Coumarins have been recommended for long-term treatment of patients with a coagulation disorder and even for the midtrimester treatment of ATIII-deficient patients resistant to heparin.[64] Coumarins cross the placenta and may result in early miscarriage from hemorrhage or late fetal bleeding, in addition to significant teratogenesis. The fetal warfarin syndrome is associated with first trimester use, while midline defects of the central nervous system have been described with exposure in later pregnancy.[51] For these reasons, coumarins should be discontinued or another anticoagulant substituted before planned conception. With this important exception, none of the drugs used in the treatment of thrombosis is known to be teratogenic and women with thrombotic disorders are not at increased risk for fetal abnormalities. The only exception might be the few cases of fetal thrombosis reported in pregnancies complicated by the lupus anticoagulant.

REFERENCES

1. Weiner CP. Diagnosis and management of thromboembolic disease during pregnancy. *Clin Obstet Gynecol.* 1985;28:107.
2. Rutherford SE. Thromboembolic disease in pregnancy. *Clin Perinatol.* 1986;13:719.

3. Weibers DO. Ischemic cerebrovascular complications of pregnancy. *Arch Neurol.* 1985;42:1106.
4. Munsick RA, Gillanders LA. A review of the syndrome of puerperal ovarian vein thrombophlebitis. *Obstet Gynecol Survey.* 1981;36:57.
5. Clarke-Pearson DL, DeLong ER, Synan IS, et al. Variables associated with postoperative deep venous thrombosis: a prospective study of 411 gynecology patients and creation of a prognostic model. *Obstet Gynecol.* 1987;69:146.
6. Malm J, Laurel M, Dahlback B. Changes in the plasma levels of vitamin K-dependent proteins C and S and of C4-b-binding protein during pregnancy and oral contraception. *Br J Haematol.* 1988;68:437.
7. Boer K, tenCate JW, Sturk A, et al. Enhanced thrombin generation in normal and hypertensive pregnancy. *Am J Obstet Gynecol.* 1989;160:95.
8. Comp PC, Thurnau GR, Welsh J, Esmon CT. Functional and immunologic protein S levels are decreased during pregnancy. *Blood.* 1986;68:881.
9. Gladson CL, Scharrer I, Hach V, et al. The frequency of type I heterozygous protein S and protein C deficiency in 141 unrelated young patients with venous thrombosis. *Throm Haemost.* 1988;59:18.
10. Tengborn L, Bergqvist D, Matzsch T, et al. Recurrent thromboembolism in pregnancy and puerperium. Is there a need for prophylaxis? *Am J Obstet Gynecol.* 1989;160:90.
11. Nilsson IM, Ljungn'er H, Tengborn L. Two different mechanisms in patients with venous thrombosis and defective fibrinolysis: low concentration of plaminogen activator or increased concentration of plasminogen activator inhibitor. *Br Med J.* 1985;290:1453.
12. Juhan-Vague I, Valadier J, Alessi MC, et al. Deficient t-PA release and elevated PA inhibitor levels in patients with spontaneous or recurrent deep venous thrombosis. *Thromb Haemost.* 1987;57:67.
13. Han P, Koay ES, Tsakok M, et al. Altered fibrinolysis in DVT: influence of site of sampling. *Thromb Haemost.* 1988;60:50.
14. Clouse LH, Comp PC. The regulation of hemostasis: the protein C system. *N Engl J Med.* 1986;314:1298.
15. Cariou R, Tobelem G, Bellucci S, et al. Effect of lupus anticoagulant on antithrombogenic properties of endothelial cells—inhibition of thrombomodulin-dependent protein C activation. *Thromb Haemost.* 1988;60:54.
16. Naidich JB, Feiberg AW, Karp-Harman H, et al. Contrast venography: reassessment of its role. *Radiology.* 1988;168:97.
17. Cardella JF, Young AT, Smith TP, et al. Lower-extremity venous thrombosis: comparison of venography, impedance plethysmography, and intravenous manometry. *Radiology.* 1988;168:109.
18. Comerota AJ, Katz ML, Grossi RJ, et al. The comparative value of noninvasive testing for diagnosis and surveillance of deep vein thrombosis. *Vasc Surg.* 1988;7:40.
19. Aitken AF, Godden DJ. Real time ultrasound diagnosis of deep vein thrombosis: a comparison with venography. *Clin Radiol.* 1987;38:309.
20. Rollins DL, Semrow CM, Friedell ML, et al. Progress in the diagnosis of deep venous thrombosis: the efficacy of real-time B-mode ultrasonic imaging. *J Vasc Surg.* 1988;7:638.
21. Vogel P, Laing FC, Jeffrey RB Jr, Wing VW. Deep venous thrombosis of the lower extremity: US evaluation. *Radiology.* 1987;163:747.
22. Personal communication. Robert Boone, Department of Radiology, Jefferson Medical College, Philadelphia, PA.
23. Dorfman GS, Cronan JJ, Tupper TB, et al. Occult pulmonary embolism: a common occurrence in deep venous thrombosis. *Am J Radiol.* 1987;146:263.
24. Fulkerson WJ, Coleman RE, Ravin CE, Saltzman HA. Diagnosis of pulmonary embolism. *Arch Intern Med.* 1986;146:961.
25. Hull R, Hirsh J, Carter C, et al. Pulmonary angiography, ventilation lung scanning, and venography for clinically suspected pulmonary embolism with abnormal perfusion lung scan. *Ann Int Med.* 1983;98:891.
26. Rozier JC, Brown EH, Freeman AF. Diagnosis of puerperal ovarian vein thrombophlebitis by computed tomography. *J Obstet Gynecol.* 1988;159:737.
27. Baka IJ, Lev-Toaff AS, Friedman AC, et al. Ovarian vein thrombosis with atypical presentation: role of sonography and duplex doppler. *Obstet Gynecol.* 1989;73:887.
28. Mannucci PM, Tripodi A. Laboratory screening of inherited thrombotic syndromes. *Thromb Haemost.* 1987;57:247.
29. Rodgers GM, Shuman MA. Congenital thrombotic disorders. *Am J Hematol.* 1986;21:419.
30. Exner T, Triplett DA, Taberner D, et al. Comparison of test methods for the lupus anticoagulant: International survey on lupus anticoagulants-I (ISLA-1) *Thromb Haemost.* 1990;64:478.
31. Cowchock S, Fort J, Munoz S, et al. False positive ELISA tests for anticardiolipin antibodies in sera from patients with repeated abortion, rheumatologic disorders and primary biliary cirrhosis: correlation with elevated polyclonal IgM and implications for patients with repeated abortion. *Clin Exp Immunol.* 1988;73:289.
32. Still PR, Lind T, Walker W. Platelet values during normal pregnancy. *Br J Obstet Gynaecol.* 1985;92:480.
33. O'Brien WF, Saba HI, Knuppel RA, et al. Alterations in platelet concentration and aggregation in normal pregnancy and preeclampsia. *Am J Obstet Gynecol.* 1986;155:486.
34. Nagy DA, Alger LS, Edelman BB, et al. Reacting appropriately to thrombocytopenia in pregnancy. *South Med J.* 1986;79:1385.
35. Doyle DJ, Turpie AF, Hirsh J, et al. Adjusted subcutaneous heparin or continuous intravenous heparin in patients with acute deep vein thrombosis. A randomized trial. *Ann Intern Med.* 1987;107:441.
36. Walker MG, Shaw JW, Thomson GJ, et al. Subcutaneous calcium heparin versus intravenous sodium heparin in treatment of established acute deep vein thrombosis of the legs: a multicentre prospective randomised trial. *Br Med J.* 1987;294:1189.
37. Rooke TW, Osmundson PJ. Heparin and the in-hospital management of deep venous thrombosis: cost considerations. *Mayo Clin Proc.* 1986;61:198.
38. Hull RD, Raskob GE, Hirsh J, et al. Continuous intravenous heparin compared with intermittent subcutaneous heparin in the initial treatment of proximal-vein thrombosis. *N Engl J Med.* 1986;315:1109.
39. Hull R, Delmore T, Carter C, et al. Adjusted subcutaneous heparin versus warfarin sodium in the long term treatment of venous thrombosis. *N Engl J Med.* 1982;306:189.
40. Cines DB, Tomaski A, Tannenbaum S. Endothelial-cell injury in heparin-associated thrombocytopenia. *N Engl J Med.* 1987;316:581.
41. Ansell JE, Price JM, Shah S, Beckner RR. Heparin-induced thrombocytopenia. What is its real frequency? *Chest.* 1985;88:878.
42. Calhoun BC, Hesser JW. Heparin-associated antibody with pregnancy: discussion of two cases. *Am J Obstet Gynecol.* 1987;156:964.
43. Cohen GR, Hall JC, Yeast JD, Field-Dreise D. Heparin-induced cutaneous necrosis in a post-partum patient. *Obstet Gynecol.* 1988;72:498.
44. Silver D, Kapsch DN, Tsoi EKM. Heparin-induced thrombocytopenia, thrombosis, and hemorrhage. *Ann Surg.* 1983;198:301.
45. Leroy J, Leclerc MH, Delahousse B, et al. Treatment of heparin-associated thrombocytopenia and thrombosis with low molecular weight heparin (CY216) *Semin Thromb Hemost.* 1985;11:326.
46. Janson PA, Moake JL, Carpinito G. Aspirin prevents heparin-induced platelet aggregation in vivo. *Br J Haematol.* 1983;53:166.
47. Howell R, Fidler J, Letsky E, DeSwiet M. The risks of antenatal subcutaneous heparin prophylaxis: a controlled trial. *Br J Obstet Gynaecol.* 1983;90:1124.
48. Aarskog D, Aksnes L, Lehmann V. Low 1,25-dihydroxyvitamin D in heparin-induced osteopenia. *Lancet.* 1980;2:650.
49. Landefeld CS, Cook EF, Flatley M, et al. Identification and preliminary validation of predictors of major bleeding in hospitalized patients starting anticoagulant therapy. *Am J Med.* 1987;82:703.
50. van Ooijen B. Subcutaneous heparin and postoperative wound hematomas. A prospective, double-blind, randomized study. *Arch Surg.* 1986;121:937.
51. Hall JG, Pauli RM, Wilson KM. Maternal and fetal sequelae of anticoagulation during pregnancy. *Am J Med.* 1980,68:122.
52. Rosove MH, Tabsh K, Howard P, et al. Heparin therapy for prevention of fetal wastage in women with anticardiolipin antibodies and lupus anticoagulant. *Blood.* 1987;70:379.
53. Personal communication. FS Cowchock (1989), Jefferson Medical College, Philadelphia, PA.
54. Owens EL, Kasten GW, Hessel EA, II. Spinal subarachnoid hematoma after lumbar puncture and heparinization. *Anesth Analg.* 1986;65:1201.
55. Rao TLK, El-Etr AA. Anticoagulation following placement of epidural and subarachnoid catheters: an evaluation of neurologic sequelae. *Anesthesiol.* 1981;55:618.
56. Odoom JA, Sih IL. Epidural analgesia and anticoagulant therapy. Experience with one thousand cases of continuous epidurals. *Anaesthesia.* 1983;38:254.
57. Ramus KT, Rottman RL, Kotelko DM, et al. Unrecognized thrombocytopenia and regional anesthesia in parturients: A retrospective review. *Obstet Gynecol.* 1989;73:943.
58. Ludwig H. Results of streptokinase therapy in deep venous thrombosis during pregnancy. *Postgrad Med J.* 1973;49:65.
59. Declos GL, Davila F. Thrombolytic therapy for pulmonary embolism in pregnancy: a case report. *Am J Obstet Gynecol.* 1986;155:375.
60. Sharma GRV, Cella G, Parisi AF, Sasahara AA. Thrombolytic therapy. *N Engl J Med.* 1982;306:1268.
61. Hux CH, Wapner RJ, Chayen B, et al. Use of the Greenfield filter for thromboembolic disease in pregnancy. *Am J Obstet Gynecol.* 1986;155:734.
62. Greenfield L, Dirnmanl C, McCurdy W. Transvenous removal of pulmonary embolae by vacuum-cup catheter technique. *J Surg Res.* 1969;9:347.
63. Wapner RJ, Cowchock FS, Shapiro SS. Successful treatment of two women with antiphospholipid antibodies and refractory pregnancy losses with intravenous immunoglobulin infusions (IVIG). *Am J Obstet Gynecol.* 1989;161:1271.
64. DeStefano V, Leione G, DeCarolis S, et al. Management of pregnancy in women with Antithrombin III congenital defect: report of four cases. *Thromb Haemost.* 1988;59:193.

Chapter One Hundred and Twenty

Amniotic Fluid Embolism

William C. Mabie

120

Amniotic fluid embolism was first described by Meyer in 1926.[1] The importance of amniotic fluid embolism was first emphasized by Steiner and Lushbaugh in 1941 when they reported eight autopsied cases.[2] Since that time, over 300 cases have been published. The incidence varies from one in 27,000 deliveries in Southeast Asia to one in 80,000 deliveries in England and Wales. The incidence in the United States is one in 20,000–30,000 deliveries.[3] The typical patient is a multipara having a rapid, tumultuous labor who has sudden onset of dyspnea, cyanosis, hypotension, and cardiovascular collapse. One third of patients die in the first hour after onset of symptoms. Amniotic fluid embolism has been reported in a variety of settings including: first trimester suction abortion, second trimester abortion via saline, prostaglandin, urea, or hysterotomy. It has occurred during uncomplicated second trimester pregnancy, during cesarean section, and following abdominal trauma, amniocentesis, normal labor and delivery, and even postpartum.[4] Predisposing factors are strong uterine contractions, meconium, intrauterine fetal demise, fetal macrosomia, multiparity, and advanced maternal age.[2] Oxytocin has been incriminated as a cause of amniotic fluid embolism, although this is not likely because oxytocin is widely used and amniotic fluid embolism is rare.[4] In a 1979 review of 272 cases, maternal mortality was 86%.[1]

PATHOPHYSIOLOGY

Some authors have questioned whether clinically recognized amniotic fluid embolism is just the tip of the iceberg, and that subclinical embolism occurs frequently.[3] We do not yet know the answer to this question. An interesting study by Sparr and Pritchard[5] indicates that this is unlikely. They injected radioactive chromium-labeled maternal red blood cells into the amniotic sacs of patients having repeat cesarean section, spontaneous labor, or induction of labor. All delivered within a few days. Serial maternal blood samples revealed no radioactivity above background levels indicating that no more than a trace amount of amniotic fluid entered the maternal circulation. They concluded that amniotic fluid embolism is not a simple exaggeration of a physiologic phenomenon but is a pathologic process. An autopsy study by Roche and Norris[6] reached a similar conclusion. Nevertheless, a few authors have reported finding amniotic fluid detritus in blood drawn from Swan–Ganz catheters in women undergoing hemodynamic monitoring for various indications during the peripartum period.[7,8]

The components of the embolism are as follows: (1) epithelial squames from the fetal skin, (2) lanugo hairs, (3) fat from the vernix caseosa, (4) mucin from the fetal gut, and (5) bile containing meconium.[1] There have been several attempts to develop an animal model of amniotic fluid embolism using rabbits, dogs, cats, sheep, and cattle. Filtered amniotic fluid, unfiltered fluid, meconium-stained fluid, and meconium enriched fluid have been used. Problems with interpretation of the studies include crossed species of amniotic fluid (eg, injecting human amniotic fluid into rabbits), abnormal concentrations of fetal debris in the fluid, species differences, storage of the fluid, and use of general anesthesia in the experimental animals.[8] In some of the animal studies, infusion of amniotic fluid into the circulation caused a marked increase in pulmonary artery pressure, central venous pressure, and pulmonary vascular resistance without a concomitant rise in wedge pressure. However, pulmonary hypertension resolved within 10–30 minutes after injection and pulmonary edema was not observed.[9,10]

Amniotic fluid obtained from humans in labor has increased toxicity compared to amniotic fluid from nonlaboring patients. Presumably this is because metabolites of arachidonic acid, such as prostaglandins and leukotrienes, have hemodynamic and hematologic effects.[4,11,12] Amniotic fluid embolism is thought to involve three pathophysiologic mechanisms: pulmonary hypertension with acute cor pulmonale, left ventricular failure, and disseminated intravascular coagulation (DIC).[1,3,4]

There are three proposed mechanisms for pulmonary hypertension. The first involves pulmonary vascular occlusion by embolic material. The pulmonary circulation is characterized as a high-flow, low resistance circuit. One may cross-clamp a main pulmonary artery and remove an entire lung in a patient with lung cancer and not increase pulmonary artery pressures. Therefore, it would take extensive embolization to explain the pulmonary hypertension on the basis of embolic occlusion alone. Autopsy studies have shown that there is no relationship between symptoms and the extent of embolic occlusion.[8] Furthermore, in two case reports, pulmonary angiograms done four and 34 hours after delivery were entirely normal.[13,14] A second explanation of the pulmonary hypertension is vasoconstriction due to humoral mediators (eg, prostaglandins, leukotrienes, serotonin, and probably many other vasoactive substances) either present in the amniotic fluid or released by activation of the clotting cascade.[4,11,12] The third mechanism is hypoxic pulmonary vasoconstriction secondary to ventilation-perfusion mismatch and dead space ventilation.[3,4]

Left ventricular failure is a new finding which has been emphasized by Clark et al.[15] In contrast to the animal studies, all published hemodynamic data in human cases of amniotic fluid have shown a high wedge pressure and low cardiac output.[8,14-19] Pulmonary artery pressures were only mildly to moderately elevated; however, the earliest data obtained was 70 minutes after the initial event. In order to unify the animal and human data, Clark postulated a biphasic hemodynamic response. First, a transient period of pulmonary artery vasospasm leads to acute cor pulmonale, which may account for the 50% of patients who die within the first hour. Subsequently, a picture of left ventricular failure predominates. He also suggests that there is a component of noncardiogenic pulmonary edema because the degree of pulmonary edema on chest x-ray is out of proportion to the elevation in pulmonary capillary wedge pressure. The cause of the left ventricular failure is unclear at this time. It is probably related to profound hypoxia during the acute event. Other possibilities are an effect of amniotic fluid on the myocardium, coronary artery emboli, or increased right ventricular afterload and decreased left ventricular preload due to pulmonary vascular obstruction.

About 40% of patients with amniotic fluid embolism develop DIC.[1] This is often accompanied by uterine atony and massive hemorrhage. Normal amniotic fluid contains an activator of factor X, and amniotic fluid obtained greater than two weeks after intrauterine fetal demise exhibits true thromboplastin activity. Shock with endothelial damage and tissue thromboplastin release probably also contributes to the development of DIC, as does platelet aggregation on the embolic material.[3]

CLINICAL FINDINGS

Amniotic fluid embolism is a spectrum from patients who die within an hour to patients who recover within three days with minimal supportive care. In the review of 272 cases by Morgan, the presenting symptoms were respiratory distress with cyanosis in 51%, cardiovascular symptoms in 27%, seizures in 10%, and bleeding in 12%.[1]

LABORATORY FINDINGS

The arterial blood gas usually demonstrates hypoxemia, hypocapnea, and metabolic acidosis. Disseminated intravascular coagulation will be confirmed by fragmented red cells on the peripheral smear, prolonged prothrombin time, and partial thromboplastin time, reduced platelet count and fibrinogen, and elevated fibrin degradation products. Anemia is often present. The electrocardiogram may show only sinus tachycardia or it may show S_1 Q_3 T_3 with right-axis deviation, ST segment depression or both. The chest x-ray shows pulmonary edema in 25–70% of cases.[1,15] The lung scan reveals multiple filling defects. Pulmonary angiography has rarely been reported.

DIAGNOSIS

It used to be said that definitive diagnosis of amniotic fluid embolism was based only on autopsy findings; if the patient survived, the diagnosis was uncertain. In 1947, Gross and Benz[20] found that blood from the right ventricle in an amniotic fluid embolism can yield three layers if centrifuged with amniotic fluid forming a zone on top of the buffy coat. It was not until 1976[21] that a direct, clinical application was discovered when mucin and squamous cells were identified in maternal blood taken from a central venous catheter. In a few cases of amniotic fluid embolism, lanugo hairs and squamous cells are found in the sputum, presumably because amniotic fluid debris extravasated into the alveoli. Sputum examination is of limited value because of the inconsistency of the finding and the presence of morphologically similar cellular contamination from the maternal respiratory tree.[3] Currently, it is recommended that maternal blood be withdrawn from the pulmonary artery through a Swan–Ganz catheter and examined with special stains (eg, Wright's stain, oil red O, Papanicolaou stain, and alcian blue) looking for fetal squames, lanugo, and mucin. It has been emphasized that finding this debris in the maternal blood is necessary, but not sufficient, for the diagnosis of amniotic fluid embolism.[8] Recent studies of pregnant women undergoing pulmonary artery catheterization for various indications have shown squamous cells in the maternal pulmonary circulation. It is unclear whether these squamous cells represent fetal debris, contamination by maternal epithelial cells from the skin site of central catheterization, or both. It is difficult to differentiate maternal from fetal squames.[8] Nevertheless, a typical history, physical, laboratory findings, and evidence of fetal debris in the maternal blood are sufficient evidence on which to base patient management. The differential diagnosis includes other causes of shock such as hemorrhagic shock from uterine atony, inversion, rupture, or placental abruption, cardiogenic shock due to myocardial infarction, septic shock, obstructive shock due to massive thromboembolism, aspiration pneumonia, eclampsia, and epidural anesthetic accidents such as total spinal or intravascular injection of local anesthetic.

TREATMENT

Since amniotic fluid embolism is such a rare complication, there are no preventive measures. Supportive care involves oxygenation, maintaining cardiac output, and combating the coagulopathy.[4] Endotracheal intubation and mechanical ventilation may be required within minutes after the onset of symptoms. Positive end expiratory pressure is usually required to prevent alveolar collapse and to recruit atelectatic alveoli for gas exchange, thus, permitting a lower inhaled oxygen fraction. The patient should be transferred to an intensive care unit for close observation. Invasive hemodynamic monitoring should be instituted and blood withdrawn from the pulmonary artery to be examined with special stains. Fluids, dopamine, and furosemide are administered based on hemodynamic parameters. Before hemodynamic monitoring is in place, hypotension should be treated with volume expansion in order to increase right-sided filling pressures to offset the high right ventricular afterload. Dopamine is added if hypotension is not corrected with volume expansion. Blood products such as fresh frozen plasma, cryoprecipitate, packed red blood cells, and platelets are given as needed. Heparin and epsilon aminocaproic acid are controversial but they have been used successfully in patients whose DIC would not correct with blood products.[22] Their value is not proven and their safety is not established, but they may be used with careful hematologic monitoring. Renal failure is likely to develop in surviving patients due to acute tubular necrosis and may require dialysis.[1,13,18] Line sepsis, nosocomial pneumonia, gastrointestinal bleeding, and multiple organ system failure must be guarded against if prolonged intensive care is required.

REFERENCES

1. Morgan M. Amniotic fluid embolism. *Anesthesia*. 1979;34:20.
2. Steiner PE, Lushbaugh BS. Maternal pulmonary embolism by amniotic fluid. *JAMA*. 1986;255:2187.
3. Sperry K. Amniotic fluid embolism. *JAMA*. 1986;255:2183.
4. Clark SL. Amniotic fluid embolism. *Female Patient*. 1989;14:49.
5. Sparr RA, Pritchard JA. Studies to detect the escape of amniotic fluid into the maternal circulation during parturition. *Surg Gynecol Obstet*. 1958;107:560.
6. Roche WD, Norris HJ. Detection and significance of maternal amniotic fluid embolism. *Obstet Gynecol*. 1974;43:729.
7. Plauche WC. Amniotic fluid embolism. *Am J Obstet Gynecol*. 1983;147:982.
8. Clark SL. New concepts of amniotic fluid embolism. *Contemp Obstet Gynecol*. 1986;27:93.
9. Reis RL, Pierce WS, Behrendt DM. Hemodynamic effects of amniotic fluid embolism. *Surg Gynecol Obstet*. 1969;129:45.
10. Attwood HD, Downing SE. Experimental amniotic fluid and meconium embolism. *Surg Gynecol Obstet*. 1965;120:255.
11. Azegami M, Mavi N. Amniotic fluid embolism and leukotrienes. *Am J Obstet Gynecol*. 1986;155:1119.

12. Clark SL. Amniotic fluid embolism and leukotrienes. *Am J Obstet Gynecol.* 1988;158:681.
13. Lumley J, Owen J, Morgan M. Amniotic fluid embolism. A report of three cases. *Anesthesia.* 1979;34:33.
14. Dolynuik M, Orfei E, Vania H, et al. Rapid diagnosis of amniotic fluid embolism. *Obstet Gynecol.* 1983;61:28S.
15. Clark SL, Mantz FJ, Phelan JP. Hemodynamic alterations associated with amniotic fluid embolism: a reappraisal. *Am J Obstet Gynecol.* 1985;151:617.
16. Schaerf RHM, Campo TD, Civetta JM. Hemodynamic alterations and rapid diagnosis in a case of amniotic fluid embolus. *Anesthesiology.* 1977;46:155.
17. Duff P, Engelsgjerd B, Zingery LW, et al. Hemodynamic observations in a patient with intrapartum amniotic fluid embolism. *Am J Obstet Gynecol.* 1983;146:112.
18. Moore PG, James OF, Saltors N. Severe amniotic fluid embolism: case report with hemodynamic findings. *Anesth Intensive Care.* 1982;10:40.
19. Masson RG, Ruggieri J, Siddiqui MM. Amniotic fluid embolism: definite diagnosis in a survivor. *Am Rev Resp Dis.* 1979;120:187.
20. Gross P, Benz EJ. Pulmonary embolism by amniotic fluid: report of three cases with a new diagnostic procedure. *Surg Gynecol Obstet.* 1947;85:315.
21. Resnik R, Swartz WH, Plumer MH, et al. Amniotic fluid embolism with survival. *Obstet Gynecol.* 1976;47:295.
22. Bates ME, Verma UL, Tejani NA, Ditroia DJ. Amniotic fluid embolism. *N Y State J Med.* 1985;85:265.

Chapter One Hundred and Twenty-One

The Pneumonias

Norbert Gleicher

121

Pneumonias are not uncommon in pregnancy. Whether, in fact, pregnancy increases the risk to develop pneumonias and whether pregnancy will cause a more severe form of the disease has remained controversial, although a majority opinion today would argue against both of these suppositions. The notion of pregnancy as a risk factor for pneumonias stems from historical observations. Maternal mortality was exceedingly high during the influenza pandemics of 1917 and 1957.[1] More recent investigations of smaller influenza epidemics do not demonstrate a similar risk for pregnant women, even though the human correlation between advancing age and influenza mortality can also be observed in pregnancy.[2]

Historic investigations also suggested that the incidence of pregnancy loss, fetal malformations, and childhood leukemias may be increased following influenza pandemics. However, this association has also been called into question twice.[1,2]

The incidence of pneumonia in pregnancy has been reported as 0.6–2.3%.[3] Pneumonias can be categorized by causative agent as bacterial, viral, or fungal.

BACTERIAL PNEUMONIAS

Pneumococcal Pneumonia

Among bacterial pneumonias, Mycoplasma and pneumococcal infection are most frequent (see also Chapter 61), sometimes in association with Hemophilus influenza. It often presents with a single episode of shaking, chills, and chest pains, followed by high fever, headache, malaise, at times severe pleuritic pain, dyspnea, and cough. The cough is often productive of purulent discharge and results at times in blood-tinged sputum. The patient usually appears acutely ill and findings on physical exam are compatible with a lobar pneumonia.

In properly treated cases, the incidence of maternal, as well as fetal, complications should be low.[1,3] However, especially older mothers still appear at significant risk of maternal death, primarily when age is also associated with a debilitating disease, immunodeficiency disorder, or both. Perinatal mortality may be slightly increased due to an associated increase in prematurity.[4]

The diagnosis should be based on the reliable identification of the organism as discussed in detail in Chapter 61.

Treatment of choice is penicillin (600,000 units every six hours) either by oral or intravenous route, depending on severity of the disease. Patients who are allergic to penicillin can be treated with a first generation cephalosporin or with erythromycin. For more detail see also Chapter 61.

A polyvalent vaccine is presently available for individuals at risk to develop pneumococcal pneumonia (Table 61–1).

Mycoplasma Pneumonia

This form of pneumonia is caused by *Mycoplasma pneumoniae,* an organism described in more detail in Chapter 86.

The pneumonia caused by this agent differs from pneumococcal pneumonia in that it usually presents in a more insidious way, as it slowly spreads through families. Fever and cough are classic presenting symptoms, although the clinical presentation usually does not suggest the severity of the pulmonary infiltrate noted on the chest x-ray. The diagnosis should be suspected whenever upper respiratory tract symptoms persist over two weeks or rales are heard on auscultation.

M pneumoniae infections are spread through infected respiratory secretions and, therefore, affect population groups in crowded conditions, such as college students and the military.[5,6] The incidence in pregnancy is not well defined but has been suggested to match that in the general population.[7] The limited number of reported cases in pregnancy also precludes any definite conclusion about fetal impact from the infection. From published reports, no significant adverse effects have been reported (for more detail, see Chapter 86).

Erythromycin is the drug of choice during pregnancy (500 mg orally four times daily for 14–21 days).[1] While tetracyclines are also effective against *M pneumoniae,* they are contraindicated in pregnancy because of their effect on developing teeth.

Meningococcal Pneumonia

This is a much rarer bacterial pneumonia than either pneumococcal or Mycoplasma pneumonia. It is usually acquired through the inhalation of infected respiratory particles. The causative organism is *Neisseria meningitidis,* a rare, but potentially very dangerous, agent.

Chest pain, because of pleuritis and pleural effusions, is common (for more detail, see chapter 64).

The specific diagnosis is made by identifying the organism, one of the very few gram-negative agents that cause pneumonia. As most other gram-negative pneumonias, meningococcal pneumonias are seen in pregnancy primarily in situations of chronic illness such as cystic fibrosis.

The antibiotic therapy of choice is penicillin (600,000 units) either intramuscularly or intravenously every 8–12 hours for five to seven days. Intravenous ampicillin (200–400 mg/kg) every day is equally effective. Prevention of meningococcal infection is usually achieved with rifampin (600 mg twice daily for two days) in case of contact. This drug is, however, a category C drug and its use in pregnancy should, therefore, be considered with caution (see Chapter 64).

No specific effects on the fetus have been reported that can be directly attributed to the organism. The severity of maternal disease will, however, obviously affect perinatal outcome in an indirect way.

Staphylococcal Pneumonia

The organism responsible for this form of pneumonia is *Staphylococcus aureus.* While this organism is a rare cause of pneumonia in the general population, it occurs more frequently among debilitated individuals, especially if hospitalized. The pneumonia occurs due to hematogenous spread from another location. This form of pneumonia is usually characterized by an abrupt onset, by high fever accompanied by chills, cough, and often pleuritic pain. The sputum can be purulent and blood-stained.[8]

The diagnosis is confirmed by isolation of the responsible organism in culture.

Treatment should be instigated with penicillinase-resistant antibiotics since most strains of staphylococci produce β-lactamase enzymes (for more details, see Chapter 62).

Legionnaires' Disease

This disease represents a relatively newly recognized clinical entity, caused by a gram-negative bacillus named *Legionella pneumophila,* which classically presents with a fulminant pulmonary syndrome. It is described in more detail in Chapter 75.

VIRAL PNEUMONIAS

Viral pneumonias occur quite commonly in pregnancy and may, in fact, represent the primary infection which is then superinfected with bacterial organisms such as pneumococci or staphylococci.

Influenza Pneumonia

The causative agent of this pneumonia is the influenza virus. The classification of influenza viruses is described in detail in Chapter 97. This is the most frequent viral pneumonia in pregnancy and usually represents a self-limited problem, requiring only supportive care.

Influenza pandemics occur every 10–12 years. As previously noted, early influenza pandemics resulted in significant maternal mortality, an observation not made in more recent times.

As a respiratory virus, influenza is spread by aerosol and through direct contact. The incubation period has been reported to lie between one and five days. Influenza pneumonia is often superinfected with bacterial organisms.

Pneumonia represents one of the most severe complications of maternal influenza infection and occurs in only a small minority of infected individuals. The severity of the disease has been shown to correlate with the host's immune status, and it has been suggested that changes in the maternal immune system, brought on by pregnancy, result in an excessive risk of pregnant women to succumb to the disease.[9,10] During the Asian flu epidemics of 1957 and 1958, half of the deaths attributed to the virus among young females in New York City occurred in pregnancy.[11] The risk appears the greatest in chronically debilitated individuals and women with heart disease.

While no direct effect of the virus on the fetus has been reported, severe maternal disease has been uniformly associated with an increase in intrauterine death and premature delivery. Moreover, the general incidence of congenital anomalies has been reported to increase during pandemics, though no specific congenital anomaly has been identified in association with influenza infection (for details, see Chapter 97). More recent reports have questioned the association.[1,2]

Treatment is solely based on supportive care and should be provided in a hospital setting. Two drugs—amantadine and rimantadine—have been shown to block replication of some strains of influenza virus. The safety of these agents has, however, not been determined in pregnancy and they should, therefore, not be used (see also Chapter 97).

Prophylactic immunization of high-risk patients represents a safer approach. While immunization with multivalent influenza vaccine prior to conception is preferable for high-risk patients, this immunization can apparently also safely be performed during pregnancy.

Not infrequently, patients with influenza pneumonia appear to recover, only to deteriorate once again. Such a clinical presentation should always raise the possibility of a secondary bacterial pneumonia.

Parainfluenza Pneumonia

Parainfluenza viruses can cause pneumonia and can be differentiated from respiratory syncytial virus and *M pneumoniae* infections. Adults usually have antibodies to all four types of virus; consequently, this type of pneumonia is usually restricted to children. As an increasing number of very young females have children, one has to consider this etiology in the differential diagnosis (see Chapter 96).

Varicella Pneumonia

Varicella pneumonia is a not uncommon complication of varicella infection. The diagnosis is simple in view of the concurrent skin condition. Nevertheless, maternal mortality has been reported to be quite high and, in fact, even higher than in the nonpregnant state (45% versus 15–20%).[1]

Once again, the severity of maternal disease will reflect the mother's immune status. For more detail, see Chapter 99 and the following discussion of the acquired immune deficiency syndrome (AIDS).

FUNGAL PNEUMONIAS

Fungal pneumonias are rare during pregnancy and occur primarily in immune-compromised hosts. An exception to this rule are the mycoses caused by dimorphic (pathogenic) fungi, which are obligate pathogens. They will cause disease even in healthy and immunocompetent individuals if the inoculum is sufficiently large. These fungi are discussed in detail in Chapter 84. The resultant pneumonias usually disappear without any sequelae. In a small minority, however, dissemination and serious disease may follow. This appears especially often to be the case among Orientals and Filipinos.[12] If dissemination occurs, which in pregnancy seems to be the case more often than in the nonpregnant state, exceedingly high rates of maternal, as well as fetal, mortality have been reported.[2,13]

A detailed review of fungal infections, inclusive of treatment recommendations, is presented in Chapter 84.

ACQUIRED IMMUNE DEFICIENCY SYNDROME (AIDS)

The topic of pneumonias cannot be reviewed without mentioning that pneumonias can often be the presenting symptoms for an infection with the human immunodeficiency virus (HIV). The occurrence of *Pneumocystis carinii* pneumonia has to be considered almost pathognomonic for the infection. For more detail, see Chapter 46.

REFERENCES

1. Schoenbaum SC, Weinstein L. Respiratory infections in pregnancy. *Clin Obstet Gynecol*. 1979;22:293.
2. Weinberger SE, Weiss ST, Cohen WR, et al. Pregnancy and the lung. *Am Rev Respir Dis*. 1980;121:559.
3. Benedetti TJ, Valle R, Ledger WJ. Antepartum pneumonia in pregnancy. *Am J Obstet Gynecol*. 1982;144:413.
4. Gransder WR, Eykyu S, Philips I. Pneumococcal bacteremia: 325 episodes diagnosed at St. Thomas Hospital. *Br Med J*. 1985;290:505.
5. Foy HM, Grayston JT, Kenny GE, et al. Epidemiology of *Mycoplasma pneumoniae* infection in families. *JAMA*. 1966;197:859.
6. Mogabgab WJ. *Mycoplasma pneumoniae* and adenovirus respiratory illnesses in military and university personnel 1959–1966. *Am Rev Respir Dis*. 1968;97:345.
7. Balassanian N, Robbins FC. *Mycoplasma pneumoniae* infection in families. *N Engl J Med*. 1967;277:719.
8. Sheagren JN. *Staphylococcus aureus*. The persistent pathogen. *N Engl J Med*. 1984;310:1368.
9. Larsen John W Jr. Influenza and pregnancy. *Clin Obstet Gynecol*. 1982;25:599.
10. Korones SB. Uncommon virus infections of the mother, fetus and newborn: influenza, mumps and measles. *Clin Perinatol*. 1988;15:259.
11. Greenberg M, Jacobziner H, Pakter J, et al. Maternal mortality in the epidemic of asian influenza, New York City, 1957. *Am J Obstet Gynecol*. 1958;76:897.
12. Drutz DJ, Cantanzano A. Coccidiomycosis. *Am Rev Respir Dis*. 1978;117:559.
13. McCoy MJ, Ellenberg JF, Killam AP. Coccidiomycocis complicating pregnancy. *Am J Obstet Gynecol*. 1980;137:739.

Chapter One Hundred and Twenty-Two
Asthma

Leonard Schreier

122

Asthma has been recognized as a distinct entity since ancient times. Early in this century, Sir William Osler believed that spasm of bronchial muscles, swelling of the bronchial mucous membranes, and an exudative bronchiolitis were the major causes of asthmatic symptoms.[1] A definition of asthma which satisfies most people has, however, been difficult to achieve. A joint committee of the American Thoracic Society section of the American College of Chest Physicians proposed the following definition: "asthma—a disease characterized by an increased responsiveness of the airways to various stimuli and manifested by prolongation of forced expiration, which changes in severity either spontaneously or with treatment."[2] More recently, with the recognition of the importance of the inflammatory component in asthma, defining it as a desquamative eosinophilic bronchitis has been proposed. Regardless, it is a reversible airway disease. The older classification of asthma into extrinsic and intrinsic is not clinically appropriate now. A more expressive classification is listed in Table 122–1.

EPIDEMIOLOGY

The overall incidence of asthma in the population is 4–8%. The incidence in pregnant women is believed to be 1.0%, but it is probably higher.[3] Asthma is the leading cause of time lost from school in children and a highly significant cause of lost work time in adults. Hospital admissions for asthma are increasing and the current death rate from asthma is 1.6 out of 100,000 people in the United States. The death rate of blacks is twice that of whites and it is increasing.

CLINICAL PICTURE AND PHYSICAL FINDINGS

The classic symptoms of cough, wheezing, and dyspnea are well known. However, approximately 20% of asthmatics have a cough with or without dyspnea or chest tightness as their presenting symptom.[4] The cough may wake them up or be worse either with exertion or after laughing and talking. A response to asthma therapy may be necessary to establish that the cough is asthma. On rare occasions, vomiting is a dominant symptom of asthma.[5] The classical physical findings are bilateral expiratory wheezing on auscultation of the lungs. At times, forced expiration may be necessary to elicit wheezing and may also produce post-expiratory coughing. The nasal passages should be examined. Usually this will reveal a pale, boggy nasal mucosa and in a small percentage, polyps.

TABLE 122–1. PROPOSED CLASSIFICATIONS OF ASTHMA

I. Antigen-(allergen) induced or atopic asthma (formerly extrinsic)
II. Episodic severe asthma without a known cause (formerly intrinsic)
III. Asthma induced by viral infections
IV. Asthma from ambient air pollution
V. Exercise-induced asthma. May be part of I & II or by itself
VI. Medication-induced asthma—aspirin and beta blockers for example. Can be rapidly life-threatening
VII. Occupational asthma—may be irritant- or allergen-mediated
VIII. Asthma superimposed on chronic obstructive pulmonary disease
IX. Asthma induced by food and drug additives—metabisulfites for example.
X. Patients exhibiting components of any combination of the above; it is possible to experience all the above causes in a single patient.

LABORATORY EVALUATION

Peripheral blood eosinophilia in the range of 250–2500 mm is found in a majority of, but not in all, adult asthmatics untreated with corticosteroids, and correlates with disease severity, as measured by the *forced expiratory volume 1* (FEV1) (see also Chapter 118).[6] A greater percentage of eosinophils in asthmatics than in normal individuals are hypodense, reflecting activation with release of mediators and the eosinophilic major basic protein.[7,9] Skin tests are still the most sensitive method for evaluating IgE-mediated (allergen-induced) asthma. They are less costly than the radio allergosorbant (RAST) and other similar serum tests for specific IgE allergens. Properly done, a prick with supplemental intradermal tests, if necessary, is also safe. Among thousands of patients who were tested in our practice in over 21 years, we observed only two mild systemic reactions. Both responded to one injection of epinephrine. Total serum IgE adds no significant information to skin testing unless bronchopulmonary aspergillosis is suspected and a positive aspergillus fumigatus skin test has been obtained. Unless the asthma is severe, a chest x-ray in a non-smoking asthmatic is usually not necessary. This applies to pregnant women as well. A sinus x-ray should be done only if there is resistant rhino-sinus disease or asthma. Sinus computerized tomography yields far more information than regular sinus x-rays and may now be the procedure of choice.[10]

Pulmonary function tests should be given to all asthmatics, even if they are completely asymptomatic when seen. If the result of the test is normal, it will be a good baseline for future comparison. Early changes (Fig. 122–1) are a fall in the FEV1 (which measures larger airway disease), or in the force expiratory flow 25–75% (FEF 25–75, which measures changes more in the smaller airways), or in both. During severe asthma both parameters can fall to 20% or less of the predicted range. The hallmark of asthma is its reversibility with either bronchodilators, steroids, or both. This results in improvement of at least 15–20% and frequently functions will approach normal with prolonged therapy. Pulmonary functions during severe asthma can resemble pulmonary emphysema, but the latter disease is virtually not a consideration in the childbearing age group.

PATHOPHYSIOLOGY OF ASTHMA

Cross-sectional views of the bronchial wall in asthma can vary from normal, in very mild asthma, to a violent inflammatory response in which all semblance of the normal architecture is drastically altered, as seen in fetal asthma. Figures

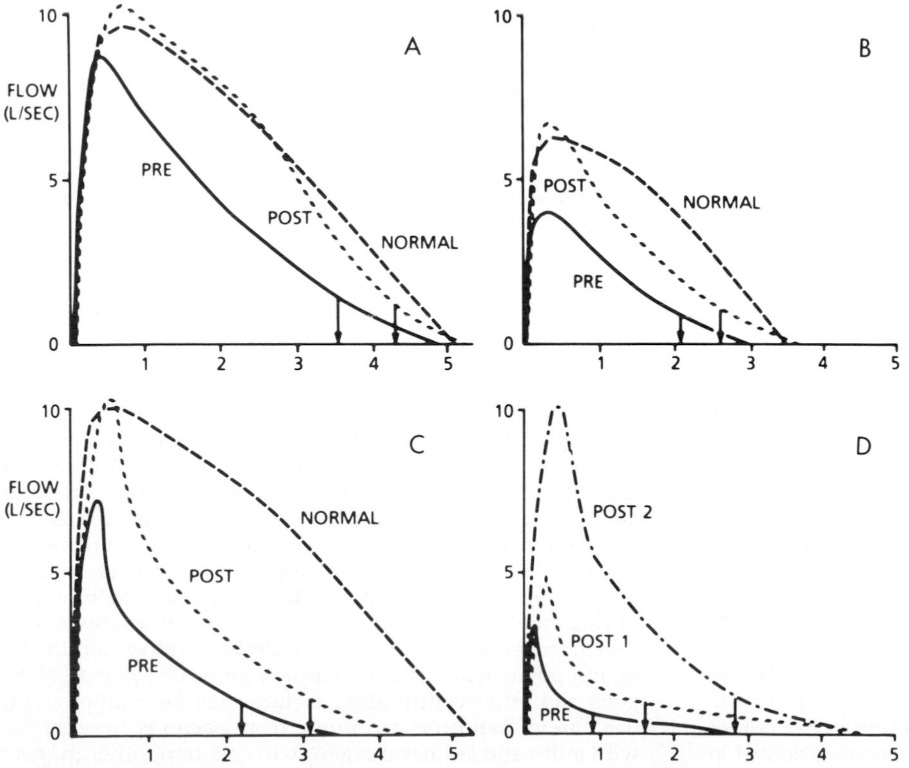

Figure 122–1. Flow-volume spirometric measurements of patients with respiratory symptoms. **A.** full, **B, C,** and **D.** partial reversal of airway obstruction in separate patients *POST* - - - - following inhalation of aerosol of metaproterenol as compared with baseline *PRE* ——— *and 95% predicted for NORMAL* ----- subjects of comparable age and height. For patient **D,** *POST 2* —·—·— following three-week course of daily high-dose corticosteroid and bronchopulmonary toilet regimen. *(From Mathison DA. Asthma in adults. In Middleton E, Jr et al, eds.* Allergy: Principles and Practice. *3rd ed. St. Louis: CV Mosby; 1988: 1070 with permission.)*

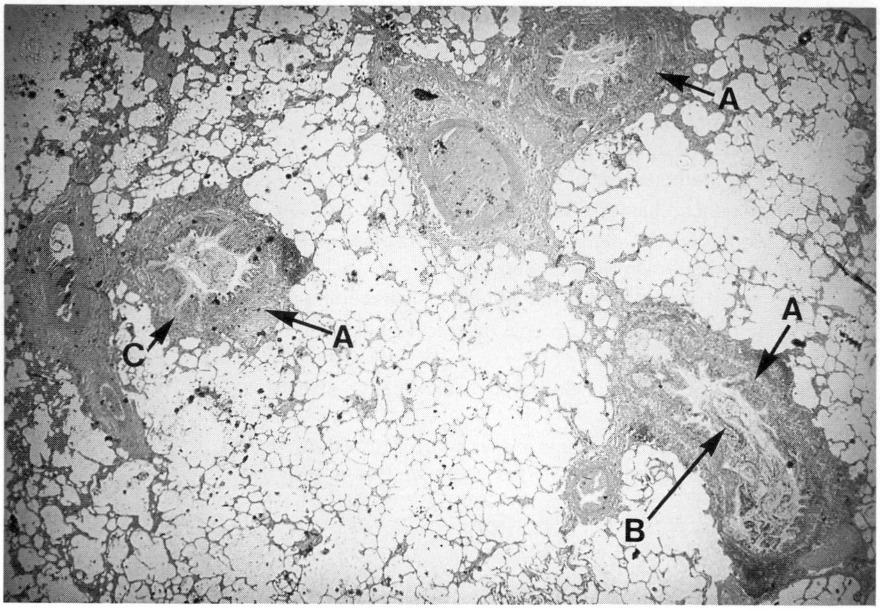

Figure 122–2. Three medium sized bronchioles: (A) all occluded by mucous plugs (B) and very thick hyalinized basement membrane (BM) (C).

122–2, 122–3, and 122–4 are slides from a fatal asthma attack in a 9-year-old girl. The airways here are completely blocked with tenacious, viscid mucous plugs that are filled with numerous eosinophils and polymorpho-nuclear neutrophils (PMNS). The eosinophilic response is striking. The bronchial epithelium is markedly hyperplastic with three layers or more of stratified columnar epithelium and numerous mucous secreting goblet cells. In some areas, the epithelium has sloughed off the basement membrane, which is significantly thickened (hyalinized). The bronchial wall is markedly edematous with hypertrophied smooth muscles, numerous mucous glands, and walls which have numerous villous-like invaginations. Although this is the end (fatal) stage of the inflammatory process in asthma, it will be present to an increasing degree as asthma worsens. Most of this inflammation is related to presence of the eosinophil and its byproducts, the degree of which correlates with the severity of the asthma.[11]

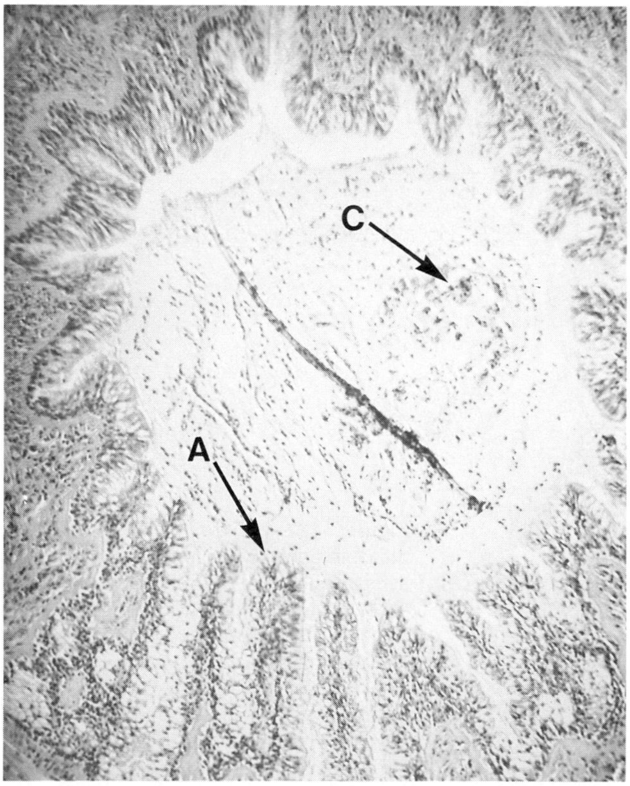

Figure 122–3. Higher power of bronchioles demonstrating: (A) markedly hyperplastic epithelium with villous pseudo intestinal pattern; (B) very thick hyalinized basement membrane with intense cellular infiltrate (mostly eosinophils) and (C) in the mucous plug and in the submucosa.

Pulmonary mast cells and other cells are responsible for the increasing eosinophilic infiltrate with increasing asthma. The most powerful eosinophilic chemotactic factor for tissue infiltration is platelet activating factor (PAF), which also is released by eosinophils. It is enhanced by interleukin 5 (IL5), which stimulates the bone marrow production of eosinophils and also activates them.[9] Some eosinophilic chemotactic factors, such as PAF, also attract neotrophils. The intensity of the eosinophilic response is abetted by factors such as IL3, IL5, and others which selectively prolong the survival of eosinophils. The deposition of the eosinophilic major basic protein and of other eosinophilic substances seems to occur where most of the pathologic bronchial changes in asthma take place.

An allergen cross-linking with at least two mast cell surface IgE molecules and releasing mediators from mast cells is the usual situation in allergic asthma. Other factors (Fig 122–5) may cause mast cell degranulation, although not all, such as anaphylatoxins, are important in asthma. The degree of mast cell response is dependent on the number of allergens, amount of specific IgE on its surface, amount and variety of other factors, and the length of time during which all of this takes place. Allergen reactions with specific mast cell IgE under controlled laboratory conditions do not reflect what usually happens clinically. *In vivo*, allergens and other contributing factors may be multiple, and the time of exposure can range from seconds to years (as with mites and animal allergens). In addition, other triggers (viral infections, aspirin, and other irritants) can initiate

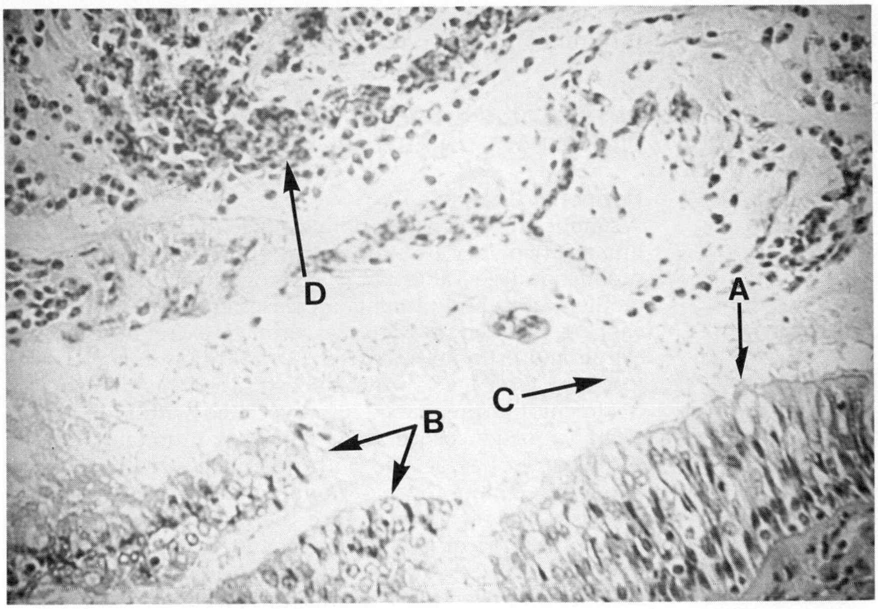

Figure 122–4. Even higher power view demonstrating: (A) markedly hyperplastic epithelium; (B) a strip of epithelium sloughed from elsewhere in the mucous plug; (C) tenacous mucous filling the entire lumen which is filled with inflammatory cells; (D) almost all being eosinophils. The possible series of events that could lead to this horror is discussed in the text.

or aggravate asthma through nonmast cell mechanisms that are still poorly understood; perhaps through non IgE or mast cell-mediated helper (CD4) T cell activation.[12] CD4 + T lymphocytes are a significant source of lymphokines that recruit and activate eosinophils. Finally, the inflammatory cells themselves (eosinophils, neutrophils, and the like) can release factors that recruit more inflammatory cells. The full number of such substances and their roles in the inflammatory asthmatic response are still yet to be discovered. Depending on amount, duration, and a combination of these factors, the inflammatory asthmatic response may be minimal (mild asthma) to intense (potentially fatal asthma).

Table 122–2 lists mast cell-derived mediators. Table 122–3 summarizes the pathologic changes in asthma and the possible responsible mediators. Approximately half of the mast cells in the human lung are found beneath the basement membrane of the bronchi and bronchioles. The other half are in the intra-alveolar septa. Both locations are immediately adjacent to capillaries.[13] Exposing lung mast cells to antigen for 15 minutes begins the degranulation process, which is completed in 30 minutes.[13]

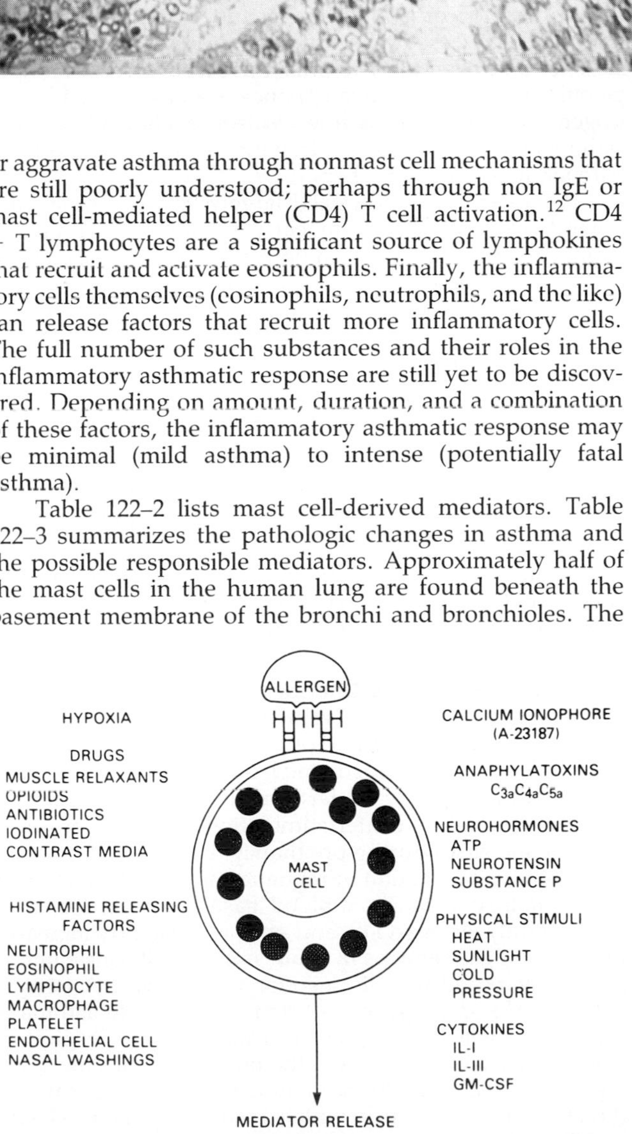

Figure 122–5. Mast cell secretagogues. Listed around the mast cell are the currently recognized factors that can cause mast cell degranulation. GM-CSF, granulocyte and macrophage colony-stimulating factor. (*From Kaliner*[13] *with permission.*)

ASTHMATIC RESPONSES

In recent years, the differentiation between an early and late asthmatic response to various stimuli has been well

TABLE 122–2. MAST CELL-DERIVED MEDIATORS

Performed and Rapidly Released under Physiologic Conditions
Histamine
Eosinophil chemotactic factors of anaphylaxis
Neutrophil chemotactic factors
Kininogenase
Arylsulfatase A
Exoglycosidases (–hexosaminidase, –D–galactosidase, –glucuronidase)
Secondary or Newly Generated Mediators
Superoxide and other reactive oxygen species
Leukotrienes C, D, E (previously known as SRS-A)
Prostaglandins
Monohydroxyeicosatetraenoic acids
HETES
Thomboxanes
Prostaglandin-generating factor of anaphylaxis
Adenosine
Bradykinin
PAF
Granule-associated Mediators
Heparin or other proteoglycans
Tryptase
Chymotryptic proteinase
Inflammatory factors of anaphylaxis
Peroxidase
Superoxide dismutase
Arylsulfatase B

From Kaliner MA, Eggleston PA, Mathews KP et al[59] *with permission.*

TABLE 122–3. PATHOLOGIC CHANGES IN ASTHMA AND THE MEDIATORS POSSIBLY RESPONSIBLE

Bronchial smooth muscle contraction	Histamine (H, response) Leukotrienes C, D, E Prostaglandins and thromboxane A Bradykinin PAF
Mucosal edema	Histamine (H, response) Leukotrienes C, D, E Prostaglandin E Bradykinin PAF
Cellular infiltration (airway hyperreactivity)	Inflammatory factors of anaphylaxis Eosinophil chemotactic factors Neutrophil chemotactic factors Monohydroxyeicosatetraenoic acids IL5 Leukotriene B IL3 PAF
Mucus secretion	Histamine (H, response) Prostaglandins Monohydroxyeicosatetraenoic acids Leukotrienes C, D, E

Modified from Kaliner MA[60] with permission.

delineated. In a patient with asthma, an inhalation challenge with an allergen usually leads to an early asthmatic response within 10 minutes that peaks in 10 to 30 minutes and resolves in one to three hours. In at least half of these cases a late response, beginning as early as three to four hours postchallenge that peaks in the next few hours and lasts 24 hours or more, is seen. Occasionally, a late response is seen without an early one. Features of a late response are that it is more severe and prolonged than the early response and that it is characterized by an inflammatory response, usually associated with increased airway irritability, which can last for weeks to months after a single exposure. With persistent exposure to an allergen or sensitizers, the asthmatic inflammatory response, and therefore symptoms, can become persistent even when the exposure finally ceases.[14] The process has the ability to feed on itself. At times, direct T cell activation (as discussed above) may play a role here. Asthma that responds readily to bronchodilators is probably because of an early response. Severe allergic asthma, postinfectious asthma, idiopathic (intrinsic) asthma, chemical sensitizer-induced asthma (toluene diisocyanate), and almost all fatal asthma cases are probably caused by a late inflammatory response or its equivalent.

The mast cell is responsible for the early response. The basophil, mast, and other cells are probably responsible for initiating the late response. The early response can be prevented and treated by sympathomimetics, theophylline, and cromolyn sodium, but not by steroids. The late response is usually only prevented by cromolyn sodium and steroids and is treated by steroids only. Recent evidence indicates a role for theophylline and beta agonists in some patients with the late response.[15] Understanding the critical role of the late or inflammatory response in asthma is vital to the understanding of changing concepts of primary therapy in asthma, something which even applies to pregnancy.

PHYSIOLOGIC CHANGES IN PREGNANCY WITH IMPACT ON ASTHMA

Hormonal Changes

A significant portion of the physiologic changes seen during human pregnancy are effected through increasing hormonal production (see Table 122–4). Estrogen production by the mother, fetus, and placenta increases enormously with advancing pregnancy. Maternal urinary excretion rates for estron and estradiol increases 100-fold between preovalatory and term levels, and for estriol 1000-fold. Estrogen treatment and pregnancy are associated with a decreased clearance of glucocorticoids, which may account for the rise in cortisol associated with pregnancy, reaching levels two to three times those of nonpregnant women.[16] Hypercorticism is rarely found since there is some receptor refractoriness to cortisol, perhaps due to receptor competition with increased levels of progesterone, deoxycorticosterone, and even aldosterone. Increased cortisol-binding globulin (CBG) levels in pregnancy are also caused by estrogen. Any increase in free cortisol levels could benefit asthma by increasing beta-adrenergic responsive and beta-adrenergic receptor numbers.[17]

Progesterone, synthesized largely from maternal cholesterol, rises steadily from early gestation reaching 160 mg/mL at term. It relaxes smooth muscles throughout the body, including the gastroesophageal sphincter, leading to reflux and pyrosis (heartburn), which by themselves can aggravate asthma.[18] Progesterone should theoretically relax bronchial smooth muscle thereby leading to less asthma as pregnancy proceeds. However, there is no correlation with changes in bronchial activity and progesterone level.[19] Theophylline, a primary drug for asthma, also causes gastroesophageal reflux and this side effect can be further increased by progesterone. Progesterone also facilitates the gestational increase in minute ventilation,[20] and competes with cortisol for binding to CBG and specific glucocorticoid receptors.[16] The effects of human chorionic gonadotropin and placental lactogen, two other important placental hormones, on asthma are unknown.

Pulmonary Physiology Changes

A 50% increase in minute ventilation total over non-pregnant levels is seen by the end of pregnancy (see also Chapter 118).[21] This is perhaps mediated by a progesterone-induced increase in respiratory center sensitivity to carbon dioxide or direct respiratory center stimulation. Oxygen consumption also increases during pregnancy, but to a lesser degree than minute ventilation. Pregnancy is also characterized by respiratory alkalosis.[22] Blood gases show a decreased P_{CO_2} slightly elevated P_{O_2} and normal to slightly increased pH.[22] Blood gas changes in acute asthma will consequently be superimposed on this respiratory alkalosis. A P_{CO_2} of >35 mm Hg or a P_{O_2} of <70 mm Hg, in acute asthma of pregnancy, will thus represent a more severe respiratory distress than similar values in the non-pregnant state. Closing volume (CV) is closer to functional residual capacity (FRC) in late pregnancy which results in airway closure in 50% of supine pregnant women at term. This decreases ventilation, especially in the dependent portions of the lung, and can lead to an increase in the alveolar-arterial P_{O_2} gradient. The latter, in turn, can enhance the resting hypoxemia that occurs if asthma flairs during late pregnancy.

TABLE 122–4. MAJOR PLACENTAL HORMONES OF PREGNANCY

Hormone	Proposed Pregnancy Functions	Effects of Potential Relevance to Allergic Disease and Asthma
Estrogen	Maintain increased uteroplacental blood flow. Softening of cervical/lower uterine segment connective tissue.	Decreased pulmonary diffusing capacity for carbon monoxide. Increased alpha-adrenergic receptors (?). Decreased metabolic clearance rate of glucocorticosteroids. Increased cortisol-binding globulin.
Progesterone	Uterine muscle quiescence Increased maternal ventilation to provide oxygen needs of the fetus.	Bronchial smooth muscle relaxation. Decreased gastroesophageal sphincter tone. Increased minute ventilation. Competition with cortisol for binding to cortisol-binding globulin and to glucocorticosteroid receptors.
Human chorionic gonadotropin	Maintenance and stimulation of the corpus luteum cyst of early pregnancy. Regulation of steroid production by the fetal adrenal gland and testis. Thyroid-stimulating activity.	
Human placental lactogen	Maintenance of supply of glucose and amino acids to the fetus. Maintenance of maternal hyperlipidemia for maternal fuel source.	Unknown.

Fetal Oxygenation

The fetus has four major compensatory mechanisms for the low oxygen tension of fetal blood: there is up to 2.5 times greater blood flow to fetal tissues than to adult tissues; fetal hemoglobin has a higher affinity for oxygen than adult hemoglobin; increased fetal hemoglobin levels of 15–20 g/100 mL by term increase the oxygen carrying capacity of fetal blood; and specific fetal vascular shunts direct oxygenated blood to high priority tissues such as liver, heart, and brain and divert deoxygenated blood back to the placenta for gas exchange. There is evidence that maternal hypoxia, hypocapnia, and alkalosis, as seen early in acute asthma, may impair fetal oxygen delivery.[23] This reinforces the need for good asthma control and optimal oxygen therapy for acute asthma in pregnancy.

ASTHMA IN PREGNANCY

A review of asthma studies through the decades reveals a change in outcome which, in turn, is reflected in changing opinions on the effect of asthma upon pregnancy. Early studies reported lower preterm and term birth weights, and an increase in fetal mortality and maternal complications. These studies were, however, retrospective and the control of the maternal asthma was not up to current standards.[24] Recently, prospective studies have shown no difference between asthmatic and control patients with regard to length of gestation, birth weight, incidence of perinatal deaths, mean Apgar scores, neonatal respiratory difficulties, hyperbilirubinemia, congenital malformations, and respiratory distress syndrome in the infant.[25,26] Although not prospective, a recent report of pregnant adolescents with severe asthma revealed no maternal or fetal deaths and no intrauterine growth retardation.[27] A slight increase in maternal hypertension and mild preeclampsia may occur, especially in severe asthmatic patients.[28] The number of women worsening, improving, or staying the same in their asthma, varied among the studies.[25,26,28] This variability may reflect the severity of asthma in a chosen population.[29] The more severe the asthma is before pregnancy, the more likely it will exacerbate during pregnancy.[30]

Good control of asthma during pregnancy is the most likely explanation for lack of any difference in pregnancy outcome between asthmatic and control groups in these newer studies.[25,28] In two very recent series, the great majority of women experienced no symptoms of asthma during labor and delivery.[25,28] The symptoms that did occur during labor and delivery were easy to control.[25,28] Moreover, women also had fewer asthmatic symptoms during weeks 37–40 of pregnancy.[28] The generally reported peak incidence of symptoms occurred between the 24th and 36th week of gestation.[28]

In a very recent article, lower maternal gestational FEV1 was related to intrauterine growth retardation.[31]

Management of Asthma

Certain basic issues need to be emphasized:

1. A physician skilled in the treatment of asthma is essential to insure optimal results in pregnancy.
2. Frequent and regular prenatal follow up is needed monthly or even more often if the patient is steroid-dependent or requires daily asthma medication.
3. Twenty-four-hour accessibility to competent specialty care is essential. The patient should not need to worry about bothering the doctor when she makes a call.
4. Patient education about the possibility that the effectiveness of the patient's regular medications may lessen during pregnancy is essential, and should include advice to call her physician under such a circumstance.
5. The daily use of a peak flow meter, particularly in patients on regular medication, will allow earlier detection of deterioration in the patient's asthma.

During pregnancy, both mother and fetus are exposed to all pharmacologic interventions. To reduce the medicolegal risk, two points should be emphasized with the expectant parents and should be documented in the patient's medical record:

1. Good asthma control during pregnancy is the single most important factor in insuring good maternal and fetal outcome.
2. While nothing in medicine is certain, medicines discussed below help to ensure good asthma control and have shown no increased fetal risk.

Table 122–5 is a summary of current safety evaluations of the most commonly used drugs in asthma.

Pharmacologic Protocols

Since asthma is a chronic disease, women frequently are on regular medication when they become aware that they are pregnant. Any unfavorable fetal effect of a drug easily could have occurred by then. A review of the literature reveals disagreement among writers regarding preferred medications in pregnancy. For example, Chung and Barnes said ephedrine should not be used[32], while Greenberger and Patterson do use it.[33] Similar controversy exists with epinephrine with Mawhinney and Spector[34] against its use and Greenberger and Patterson for its use.[33] Albuterol is the most widely used inhalational beta 2 agonist in the world in nonpregnant individuals. (Salbutamol is the same drug as albuterol; in the United States it is known as albuterol. In all future mention of it in the text, albuterol will be used even when quoting foreign authors.) Because of one mouse study, most authorities are, however, reluctant to recommend its use in pregnancy, even though many asthmatic women are on this therapy when they find out that they are pregnant. In a recent prospective study involving 198 pregnant asthmatics, albuterol was used as the major beta 2 agonist and no adverse effects were experienced.[25] Desgrange et al used oral albuterol, 4 mg q 4 h, from the 26th to the 34th gestational week to delay labor. No fetal or neonatal problems other than an increased growth hormone level were noted.[35] There is now general agreement that inhaled and systemic corticosteroids are safe during gestation.[36] Their use in asthma is, therefore, recommended when other medications have failed.

Chronic Symptom Patterns

MILD INTERMITTENT DISEASE. No medication other than the use of metaproterenol or albuterol by metered dose inhaler (MDI), 1–2 sprays q 4 h prn.

MORE CONTINUOUS AND MODERATE SYMPTOMS. These patients are more likely to have more of the late asthmatic inflammatory response than patients with mild intermittent disease. Add cromolyn MDI, two puffs, q 4 h, preceded by two

TABLE 122–5. SAFETY OF PREFERRED MEDICATIONS FOR ASTHMA DURING PREGNANCY AND POSTPARTUM

Agent	Year Introduced in US	FDA Category	First Trimester	Second Trimester	Third Trimester	Breast Feeding
Sympathomatic						
a. Subcutaneous						
Epinephrine	Pre 1910	—	variable	yes	yes	yes
Terbutaline	1974	B	yes	yes	yes (may delay labor)	yes
b. Inhalational						
Albuterol (salbutamol)	1981	C	yes	yes	yes	yes
Metaproterenol	1973	C	yes	yes	yes	yes
Terbutaline	1974	B	yes	yes	yes	yes
c. Oral						
Ephedrine	Pre 1930	—	variable	yes	yes	yes
Others in group b above inhalational route now preferred		C except	yes	yes	yes (may delay labor)	yes
		Terbutaline B	yes	yes	yes	yes
Theophylline	Pre 1938					
a. Oral (delayed release)		—	yes	yes	yes (may slow labor)	yes
b. Intravenous		—	yes	yes	yes	yes
Corticosteroids						
a. Inhaled (beclomethasone)	1976	C	yes	yes	yes	yes
b. Oral (prednisone)	1955	—	yes	yes	yes	yes
c. Intravenous (methylprednisolone)	Pre 1960	—	yes	yes	yes	yes
Cromolyn Sodium	1973	B	yes	yes	yes	yes
Ipratropium	1987	B	yes	yes	yes	yes

sprays of their beta 2 agonist. Since cromolyn's primary role is that of a mast cell stabilizer, it may not handle the inflammatory response that is already present. Cromolyn may, therefore, take 4–6 weeks to become effective and a corticosteroid burst (see below) will frequently allow it to be effective sooner. The use of a spacing device, such as the aerochamber or inspirease device, is also recommended with all MDI to facilitate a proper inhalational technique and reduce the side effects.[37,38] The spray from the MDI is squirted into the device and the patient then inhales the medication from the device.

SYMPTOMS NOT CONTROLLED WITH THE FIRST TWO REGIMENS. In such a situation, we use a 4-day steroid burst (without taper) of 50 mg prednisone daily, (50 mg tablet q d × 4), followed by beclomethasone MDI 4 sprays qid, preceded by their beta agonist MDI. Once the patient is stable on beclomethasone MDI, we reduce the dose to two to four sprays bid as a maintenance.[38] The beclomethasone spray frequently obviates the need for chronic systemic steroids, or at least, reduces the daily maintenance dose for those asthmatics who require systemic maintenance with steroids. This effect is achieved without causing any systemic steroid side effects of its own.

PATIENT RELAPSE OR NONRESPONSE TO THE FIRST THREE REGIMENS. We recommend 60 mg prednisone daily until symptoms clear, and then tapering slowly to a maintenance dose of either daily or alternate-day prednisone. The dose will depend on the asthma response to the steroid taper. While on prednisone, beclomethasone MDI should be stopped until the prednisone dose is below the daily equivalent of 30 mg. This will minimize any risk of oral thrush from the beclomethasone aerosol. The addition of a sustained release theophylline product in more severe asthma may help in some cases.[39] Even though a recent study demonstrated that sustained release theophylline preparations did not aggravate reflux symptoms in non-pregnant patients[40], caution is indicated with this product in pregnant asthmatics with reflux. Of interest is a report of a lowered incidence of preeclampsia in asthmatics on theophylline.[41]

Patients who are on any combination of the aforementioned drugs when pregnancy is diagnosed, should continue the regimen. If the patients are on other drugs, a vigorous attempt should be made to switch to the previously recommended protocol in reference to the inhalational drugs.

Acute Asthma. In cases of acute asthma, initial treatment is the following. Arterial blood gases are to be performed and if the Pa_{O_2} is less than 75 mm Hg, oxygen is indicated. Inhaled metaproterenol, 0.3 cc, or albuterol, 0.5 cc in 3 cc saline, by handheld nebulizer, up to three doses, 20–30 minutes apart is the immediate therapy. If there is poor to partial response to the initial dose of metaproterenol, prednisone, 75—150 mg, or intravenous methylprednisolone, 60–125 mg, is to be added right away. Moreover, if the patient should be admitted, she should receive this dose of methylprednisolone, q 6 h, for the first two to three days.[42] If the patient is already on inhaled or oral steroids, then she should be given the initial dose of prednisone or methylprednisolone, regardless of her response. If there is good response to this regimen, then the patient should be sent home on a four-day burst of prednisone, 50–75 mg to prevent relapse and reduce the future need for hospitalization.[43]

The addition of theophylline to any emergency treatment is debatable. Some believe it only adds to the side effects of intensive beta 2 agonist therapy.[44] When arterial blood gases reveal a Pa_{CO_2} of 36 mm Hg or greater or a Pa_{O_2} of 60 or less, the patient will invariably need admission to the hospital. One recent report to the contrary notwithstanding[45], once admitted, aminophylline may be added. If not already on oral theophylline, 4–5 mg/kg of aminophylline to true body weight over 30 minutes as loading dose is given intravenously, with maintenance of 0.5 mg/kg per hour. The dose is then adjusted depending on the blood theophylline level. We prefer theophylline levels between 7 and 10 μg/mL. The therapeutic response to a higher level is not enough to warrant the increased risk of side effects.

For patients who do not respond well to any of the above, the addition of terbutaline injections, 0.25 mg q 1 h × 2, or even aqueous epinephrine, 0.3 cc subq, q 1 h × 3, may give better results. If the therapeutic response is still poor, the patient should be transferred to the intensive care unit and repeat arterial blood gases must be obtained. If the Pa_{CO_2} rises above 45 mm Hg, in spite of the above therapy, then intubation is indicated. Although intravenous $NaHCO_3$ has been recommended in nonpregnant asthmatics whose pH is falling, it is best avoided in pregnancy.[46]

For inpatient care, a pregnant asthmatic who requires admission to the hospital should be under the care of an allergist, or pulmologist, or a perinatologist experienced in the management of pregnant asthmatics. If intubation is necessary, the maintenance of an adequate Pa_{O_2} is vital (>70mm Hg).[47] Warm metaproterenol saline irrigation and suction through the endotracheal tube are very effective in mobilizing secretions.[48]

Prevention of Fatal Bronchial Asthma. Strunk recently reviewed asthmatics who were more likely to die during a subsequent attack.[49] In general, these patients are more noncompliant, have more personal and family problems of a psychological nature, and often refuse proper doses of steroids. Patients who actually become frightened and not just anxious during an asthma attack, are more likely to die. Since the 1960s, it has been suggested that underuse of corticosteroids may be the major reason for asthmatics' deaths.[50] Referral to a psychotherapist is advisable in a noncompliant pregnant asthmatic, but getting the patient to agree or to stay in psychotherapy is difficult.

Asthma Management During Labor. With the patient's asthma under good control, obstetric management in labor is no different than in nonasthmatics. Even though halogenated anesthetics have bronchodilator properties, they should be avoided, because of increased blood loss with cesarean section, secondary to their muscle relaxing effect on the uterine musculature.[51] Patients on inhaled medication should continue these into labor and those on oral theophylline should receive intravenous theophylline or aminophylline. In the 10% of patients whose asthma exacerbates during labor[28], an inhalation treatment, as previously described for acute asthma, should be given. In the rare instance where this is not effective, the rest of acute asthma therapy should be followed, including intravenous methyl prednisolone. Steroid-dependent asthmatics need supplemental corticosteroids during labor and delivery. Hydrocortisone 100 mg IVP immediately and q 8 h should be given until the mother delivers and is stable. Corticosteroid prophylaxis of the newborn is rarely necessary.[52]

ALLERGY EVALUATION AND ENVIRONMENTAL CONTROL

The majority of asthmatic women in the childbearing age group have contributing allergies.[13] Pregnant women requiring daily asthma medication should be referred to an allergist in an attempt to eliminate or reduce the amount of identified antigens, such as dust, mites, and animals. This may lessen the severity of the patient's asthma and, therefore, the risk to the fetus.

IMMUNOTHERAPY

A pregnant woman who was receiving immunotherapy before conception, should continue to receive it. Continuation of immunotherapy in pregnancy has been shown to be both safe and effective.[53] Whether immunotherapy should be begun during pregnancy is controversial. Probably, it should be considered only in those women in whom the elimination or reduction of antigens and irritants has not been sufficiently effective and, therefore, still requires systemic corticosteroids. Effective immunotherapies for dust, mite, grass, and ragweed antigens are available. Elimination of the family cat(s) or dog(s) is frequently a major problem because of very powerful and deeply rooted psychological attachments. Cat immunotherapy has also been shown to be both safe and effective.[54] Starting immunotherapy in the last trimester of pregnancy is not a good idea logistically. The pregnancy will end before the treatment becomes effective. In case immunotherapy is started during pregnancy, it should be discontinued immediately if any large local or systemic reaction occurs. It can be resumed following parturition.

Influenza Vaccine

Influenza vaccine has been shown to be both safe and effective in pregnancy and should be given to all pregnant asthmatics who are not allergic to eggs.

GENETIC AND OTHER COUNSELING BEFORE AND DURING PREGNANCY

Asthma and other atopic diseases (allergic rhinitis and excema) are extremely common and treatable diseases. The avoidance of pregnancy or the performance of such diagnostic tests as amniocentesis is usually not indicated. Although asthma is thought to be polygenetic in nature, the exact genetic mode of transmission is not clear.[55] An asthmatic mother is more likely to have an asthmatic child. This likelihood is further increased if a previous child is an asthmatic. In our experience, if both parents are asthmatics, almost all of their children will be as well. Age of onset and severity of disease can, however, vary considerably. Avoidance of more pregnancies should be based on the emotional and financial impact of previous asthmatic children on the family. This impact can be quite severe.

Whether breast-feeding will prevent or delay the development of respiratory allergies in the infant is controversial.[56] Consequently, the decision to breast-feed should be based on the mother's personal desires. Eliminating milk and eggs in the last trimester does not alter the incidence of atopy, including asthma, in the subsequent offspring.[57] A recent study employing maternal elimination of cow's milk, egg, and peanut, during the third trimester and lactation, coupled with a strict dietary manipulation in the infant, resulted in a lower incidence of food-associated atopic dermatitis, urticaria, and gastrointestinal disease.[58] The incidence of asthma and rhinitis was unaffected.[58] Maternal dietary restriction in the last trimester is not warranted, unless it can be adhered to postpartum and coupled with a strict infant dietary avoidance program.

REFERENCES

1. Osler W, McCrae T. *Principles and Practice of Medicine*. 8th ed. New York: Appleton and Co; 1916:196.
2. ACCP-AIS. Joint Committee on Pulmonary Nomenclature: Pulmonary Terms and Symbols. *Chest*. 1975;67:583.
3. Schaefer G, Silverman F. Pregnancy Complicated by Asthma. *Am J Obstet Gynecol*. 1961;106:182.
4. Caroo W, Brannan SS, Irwin RS. Chronic Cough as the Sole Presenting Manifestation of Bronchial Asthma. *N Engl J Med*. 1979;300:633.
5. Schreier L, Cutler RM, Saigal VJ. Vomiting as a Dominant Symptom of Asthma. *Ann Allergy*. 1987;58:118.
6. Baigelman W, Chodosh S, Pizzuto D, et al. Sputum and Blood Eosinophils During Corticosteroid Treatment of Acute Exacerbation of Asthma. *Am J Med*. 1983;75:929.
7. Fukuda T, Dunnette SL, Reed CE, et al. Increased Numbers of Hypodense Eosinophils in the Blood of Patients With Bronchial Asthma. *Am Rev Respir Dis*. 1985;132:981.
8. Rothenberg ME, Owens WF Jr, Silberstein DS, et al. Human Eosinphils Have Prolonged Survival, Enhanced Functional Properties, and Become Hypodense, Exposed to Human Interleukin 3. *J Clin Invest*. 1988;81:1986.
9. Gleich GJ, Abu-Ghazaleh R. Editorial: Update on Eosinophils. *Allergy Proc*. 1989;10:71.
10. Zimerch J, Kennedy DW, Rosenbaum AE. Paranasal Sinuses: CT Imaging Requirements for Endoscopic Surgery. *Radiology*. 1987;163:769.
11. Bousguet J, Chanez P, Lacoste JY, et al. Eosinophilic Inflammation in Asthma. *N Engl J Med*. 1990;323:1033.
12. Corrigan CJ, Kay AB. CD4 T-Lymphocyte Activation in Acute Severe Asthma. *Am Rev Respir Dis*. 1990;141:970.
13. Kaliner Michael. Asthma and Mast Cell Activation. *J Allergy Clin Immunol*. 1989;83:510.
14. Chan-Yeung M, Lam S, Koerner S. Clinical Features and Natural History Occupational Asthma Due to Western Red Cedar. *Am J Med*. 1982;70:411.
15. Nielson CP, Crowley JJ, Morgan ME, et al. Polymorphonuclear Leukocyte Inhibition by Therapeutic Concentrations of Theophylline Is Mediated by Cyclic 3′–5′-adenosine monophosphate. *Am Rev Respir Dis*. 1988;137:25.
16. Demey-Ponsart EL, Foidart JM, Sulon J, et al. Serum CBG, Free and Total Cortisol and Circadian Patterns of Adrenal Functions in Normal Pregnancy. *J Steroid Biochem*. 1982;16:165.
17. Stiles GL, Caron MC, Lefkowitz RJ. Beta Adrenergic Receptors: Biochemical Mechanisms of Physiological Regulations. *Physiol. Rev*. 1984;64:661.
18. Mansfield LE. Gastroesophageal Reflux and Respiratory Disorders: A Review. *Ann Allergy*. 1989;62:158.
19. Juniper EF, Daniel EE, Roberts RS. Improvement in Airway Responsiveness and Asthma Severity During Pregnancy. *Am Rev Respir Dis*. 1989;140:924.
20. Huch R. Maternal Hyperventilation and the Fetus. *J Perinatal Med*. 1986;14:3.
21. Knuttgen HG, Emersork JR. Physiological Response to Pregnancy at Rest and During Exercise. *J Appl Physiol*. 1974;36:549.
22. Fadel EF, Northrup G, Misenhimer R, et al. Normal Pregnancy: A Model of Sustained Respiratory Alkalosis. *J Perinatal Med*. 1979;7:195.
23. Middleton E Jr., ed. *Allergy Principles and Practice*. 3rd ed. St. Louis, MO: CV Mosby Co; 1988;2:1100.
24. Bahna SL, Bzerkedal T. The Course and Outcome of Pregnancy in Women With Bronchial Asthma. *Acta Allergol*. 1972;27:397.
25. Aarniala BS, Piirila P, Teramo K. Asthma and Pregnancy: A Prospective Study of 198 Pregnancies. *Thorax*. 1988;43:12.
26. Schatz M, Zieger RS, Harden KM, et al. The Safety of Inhaled Beta-Agonist Bronchodilators During Pregnancy. *J Allergy Clin Immunol*. 1988;82:686.
27. Opter AJ, Greenberger PA, Patterson R. Outcome of Pregnancy in Adolescents with Severe Asthma. *Arch Intern Med*. 1989;149:2571.
28. Schatz M, Harden K, Forsythe A. The Course of Asthma During Pregnancy, Post Partum with Successive Pregnancies, Prospective Analysis. *J Allergy Clin Immunol*. 1988;81:509.
29. White RJ, Coutts IS, Gibbs CJ, et al. Prospective Study of Asthma During Pregnancy and the Puerperium. *Resp Med*. 1989;83:103.
30. Gluck JC, Gluck PA. The Effects of Pregnancy on Asthma: A Prospective Study. *Ann Allergy*. 1976;37:164.
31. Schatz M, Zieger RS, Hoffman CP. Intrauterine Growth is Related to Gestational Pulmonary Function in Pregnant Asthmatic Women. *Chest*. 1990;98:389.

32. Chung KF, Barnes PJ. Prescribing in Pregnancy. Treatment of Asthma. *Br Med J*. 1987;294:103.
33. Greenberger PA, Patterson R, Frederiksen MC. Asthma and Pregnancy: Responsibility of Physicians and Patients. Ann Allergy. 1990;65:469.
34. Mawhinney H, Spector SL. Optimum Management of Asthma in Pregnancy. *Drugs*. 1986;32:178.
35. Desgrange MF, Montguin JM, Piloquin A. Effects of Maternal Oral Salbutamol Therapy on Neonatal Endocrine Status at Birth. *Obstet Gynecol*. 1987;69:582.
36. Fitzsimons R, Greenberger PA, Patterson R. Outcome of Pregnancy in Women Requiring Corticosteroids for Severe Asthma. *J Allergy Clin Immunol*. 1986;78:349.
37. Prahl P, Jensen T. Decreased Adreno-Cortical Suppression Utilizing the Nebuhaler for inhalation of Steroid Aerosols. *Clin Allergy*. 1987;17:393.
38. Li JTC, Reed CE. Proper Use of Aerosol Corticosteroids to Control Asthma. *Mayo Clin Proc*. 1989;64:205.
39. Paumell RA. New Aspects of the Therapeutic Potential of Theophylline in Asthma. *J Allergy Clin Immunol*. 1989;83:548.
40. Hubert D, Gaudrio M, Guerre J, et al. Effect of Theophylline of Gastroesophageal Reflux in Patients With Asthma. *J Allergy Clin Immunol*. 1988;81:1168.
41. Dombrowski MP, Bottoms SF, Boike GM, et al. Incidence of Preeclampsia Among Asthmatic Patients Lower With Theophylline. *Am J Obstet Gynecol*. 1986;155:265.
42. Haskell RJ, Wang BM, Hansen JE. A Double Blind Randomized Clinical Trial of Methylprednisolone in Status Asthmaticus. *Arch Intern Med*. 1983;43:1324.
43. Littenberg B, Cluck EH. A Controlled Trial of Methylprednisolone in the Emergency Treatment of Acute Asthma. *N Engl J Med*. 1986;314:150.
44. Siegel D, Sheppard D, Gill A, et al. Aminophylline Increases the Toxicity but not the Efficacy of an Inhaled Beta Adrenergic Agonist in the Treatment of Acute Exacerbation of Asthma. *Am Rev Respir Dis*. 1985;132:283.
45. Self TH, Abou-Shala N, Burns R, et al. Inhaled Albuterol and Oral Prednisone Therapy in Hospitalized Adult Asthmatics. Does Aminophylline add any Benefit. *Chest*. 1990;98:1317.
46. Sachs BP, Brown RS, Yeh J. Is Maternal Alkalosis Harmful to the Fetus? *Int J Gynecol Obst*. 1987;25:65.
47. Gordon M, Niswander KR, Berendes H, et al. Fetal Morbidity Following Potentially Anoxegenic Obstetric Conditions VII. Bronchial Asthma. *Am J Obstet Gynecol*. 1970;106:421.
48. Schreier L, Cutler RM, Saigal VJ. Respiratory Failure in Asthma During the Third Trimester: Report of 2 Cases. *Am J Obstet Gynecol*. 1989;160:80.
49. Strunk RC. Identification of the Fatality-Prone Subject With Asthma. *J Allergy Clin Immunol*. 1989;83:477.
50. Ghannam RD, Schreier L, Vanselow NA. Fatal Bronchial Asthma: An Analysis of Terminal Treatment in Twenty Cases. *Ann Allergy*. 1968;24:194.
51. Gilstrap LC, Hauth JC, Henkins GDV, et al. Effect of Type of Anesthesia on Blood Loss at Caesarean Section. *Obstet Gynecol*. 1987;69:328.
52. Sidhu RK, Hawkins DP. Corticosteroids. *Clin Obstet Gynecol*. 1981;8:383.
53. Metzger WJ, Turner E, Patterson R. The Safety of Immunotherapy During Pregnancy. *J Allergy Clin Immunol*. 1978;61:268.
54. Van Metre TE Jr, Marsh DG, Adkinson NF. Immunotherapy for Cat Asthma. *J Allergy Clin Immunol*. 1988;82:1055.
55. Blumenthal MN, Yunis E, Mendell N, et al. Preventive Allergy: Genetics of IgE-Mediated Diseases. *J Allergy Clin Immunol*. 1986;78:962.
56. Middleton E Jr, ed. Pulmonary function. *Allergy Principles and Practice*. 3rd ed. St Louis, MO: CV Mosby Co; 1988;961.
57. Magnusson KF, Kjellman NIM. Development of Atopic Disease in Babies Whose Mothers Were Receiving Exclusion Diet During Pregnancy: A Randomized Study. *J Allergy Clin Immunol*. 1987;12:869.
58. Zieger RS, Heller S, Mellon MH, et al. Effect of Combined Maternal and Infant Food-Allergen Avoidance on Development of Atopy in Early Infancy: A Randomized Study. *J Allergy Clin Immunol*. 1989;84:72.
59. Kaliner MA, Eggleston PA, Mathews KP, et al. Rhinitis and asthma. *JAMA*. 1987;258:2851.
60. Kaliner MA. *Chest*. 1987;91:171.

PART X | Cardiovascular Diseases

Uri Elkayam, Section Editor

Chapter One Hundred and Twenty-Three

The Evaluation of the Cardiac Patient

Uri Elkayam and Norbert Gleicher

123

The evaluation of cardiac disease during pregnancy can be complicated by anatomic, as well as functional, changes of the cardiovascular system which are associated with the normal pregnant state. They can give rise to signs and symptoms which can either simulate the existence of, or obscure the presence of, heart disease (also see Chapter 124). In addition, the diagnostic approach to cardiac disease in pregnancy is also substantially influenced by potential fetal risks of diagnostic modalities and, at times, even by very specific risks to the mother. The understanding of signs and symptoms associated with the normal cardiocirculatory adaptation to pregnancy and of the potential risks of some of the commonly used diagnostic tools are, therefore, essential for the management of the cardiac patient during pregnancy.

HISTORY AND PHYSICAL EXAMINATION

Normal pregnancy is often accompanied by symptoms of fatigue, decreased exercise capacity, and shortness of breath.[1] Lightheadedness and even syncope can be seen as part of the supine hypotensive syndrome of pregnancy, which has been associated with occlusion of the inferior vena cava due to pressure exerted by the pregnant uterus.[2,3] Shallow, rapid ventilation is commonly noted in pregnancy and may be erroneously interpreted as dyspnea. Distention of jugular veins, as a result of increased blood volume[14], and edema of legs and ankles are also commonly found in late pregnancy[5], and may lead to overestimation of the degree of existing heart failure. Systemic arterial pulses are full and collapsing and are very similar to those palpated in patients with aortic regurgitation and hyperthyroidism.[1] A left ventricular impulse in late pregnancy is easily palpated in most women. It is usually hyperactive, brisk, and unsustained, and may be displaced to the left. The quality of the impulse of the left ventricle may simulate a volume overload state, such as seen in aortic or mitral valve regurgitation. In many cases, the pulmonary trunk is palpable, which erroneously supports the diagnosis of pulmonary hypertension.

During cardiac auscultation, the first heart sound is loud, especially after the end of the first trimester, and demonstrates an exaggerated splitting. The wide split of the first sound may be misinterpreted as a fourth heart sound or early systolic click. The physiologic increase in amplitude of the second element of the first heart sound during inspiration should, however, help to differentiate this sound from other abnormal auscultatory events. The second heart sound (S_2) is often increased in late pregnancy and may exhibit persistent expiratory splitting when the patient is examined in the lateral position. These changes in S_2 may be wrongly interpreted as signs of pulmonary hypertension (loud S_2) or of an atrial septal defect (fixed splitting of S_2). A third heart sound, which is a specific sign for ventricular dysfunction in the nonpregnant patient, has been reported to be extremely common in late pregnancy and to diminish or disappear within several days after delivery.[6] In our experience, however, the auscultatory finding of a S_3 has been rare in normal pregnancy. Consequently, its presence should lead to further evaluation of the patient to rule out underlying heart disease. Similarly to the S_3, a fourth heart sound is also heard infrequently in normal pregnant women.

Innocent systolic murmurs can be found in most pregnant women.[6] These murmurs are the result of the hyperkinetic circulation of pregnancy. They are heard best at the lower left sternal edge and over the pulmonary auscultatory area, radiating to the suprasternal notch and the left side and, less frequently, to the right side of the neck. The murmurs can often sound like those of an atrial septal defect or of a stenosis of one of the semilunar valves (pulmonic and aortic). The cervical venous hum and the mammary souffle are two benign continuous murmurs frequently heard during gestation. The venous hum is usually maximal over the right supraclavicular fossa but can radiate to the contralateral area and sometimes to the areas below the clavicle.[7] The mammary souffle, which is a result of increased flow in the mammary vessels, can be either continuous or heard only in systole. It is maximal at the second left and/or right intercostal space, but can also be heard over the breast in late gestation and in the postpartum period in the lactating woman. Characteristically, the murmur decreases or vanishes when pressure is applied on the stethoscope or when the patient moves to the upright position.[8] These continuous murmurs can easily be misinterpreted as caused by a patent ductus arteriosus or an arterial venous fistula. They can also be misinterpreted as either systolic or diastolic murmurs.

Diastolic murmurs have been described during normal pregnancy at the lower left sternal edge and over the pulmonary area. They can simulate the murmurs of aortic and pulmonic regurgitation or stenosis. It is important to note, however, that the incidence of diastolic murmurs during normal pregnancy is low and the presence of such a murmur always requires an adequate diagnostic workup to rule out organic disease.

The pregnancy-related increase in blood volume and flow across the various cardiac valves may result in an increase in intensity of systolic murmurs of aortic and pulmonic stenosis and the diastolic murmur of mitral stenosis.[4] In contrast, murmurs of mitral or aortic regurgitation may be softer due to the decrease in systemic vascular resistance during pregnancy.[9] The increase in blood volume during pregnancy may also affect auscultatory findings in other volume-dependent cardiac abnormalities, such as mitral valve prolapse and obstructive hypertrophic cardiomyopathy. The increase in left ventricular volume may abolish the systolic click and murmur, which is commonly heard in patients with mitral valve prolapse[10], and decrease the systolic murmur heard in patients with hypertrophic cardiomyopathy.[11]

ELECTROCARDIOGRAPHY

The electrocardiogram (ECG) is an important diagnostic tool that can suggest abnormalities, such as enlargement of cardiac chambers, increased myocardial mass, myocardial ischemia and infraction, pericarditis and myocarditis, conduction abnormalities, and cardiac arrhythmias. In normal pregnancy, a shift of the QRS axis to either the left or right can be seen.[1] Transient ST segment depressions and T wave changes are common. A small Q wave and an inverted P in lead III are frequently seen and usually disappear during inspiration. In addition, there is a high incidence of increased R wave amplitude in lead V_2. A possible increased susceptibility to arrhythmias during pregnancy can also be manifested by the ECG.[12] Atrial and ventricular premature beats are frequent in the normal pregnant patient and a benign paroxysmal supraventricular tachycardia is not uncommon, even without underlying cardiac disease. A high incidence of such arrhythmias as atrial, ventricular, and atrioventricular nodal premature beats, sinus arrhythmia, sinus bradycardia, wandering atrial pacemaker, sinus arrest with nodal escape rhythm, supraventricular tachycardia, aberrant ventricular conduction, and sinus tachycardia have been described during labor and delivery. Although most cardiac arrhythmias during pregnancy are benign and require no therapy, conduction or rhythm irregularities can be the first manifestation of organic heart disease. If a cardiac arrhythmia seems significant, a continuous ECG recording (Holter) for 24 hours should be performed.

CHEST X-RAY

The use of chest x-rays during pregnancy is restricted due to the potential hazard of radiation to the fetus (Chapter 5). Although the radiation dose associated with a routine chest x-ray is minimal (average skin dose in primary beam is between 0.07 and 0.15 rad and the estimated dose to the uterus is between 0.2 and 44.3 milirad)[13,14], the possibility of an adverse biologic effect has to be considered. Consequently, the pelvic area should be shielded from accidental direct exposure by the use of protective lead material whenever an x-ray is indicated in pregnancy. The traditional use of chest x-rays for the assessment of cardiac anatomy and function has been largely replaced by newer, more accurate methods such as echocardiography and Doppler flow techniques. However, normal pregnancy changes seen on chest x-rays may simulate cardiac disease and should, therefore, be interpreted with caution.[1,15] The straightening of the left upper cardiac border, due to prominence of the pulmonary conus, can simulate left atrial enlargement, commonly associated with rheumatic mitral valve disease. Many pregnant women demonstrate an apparently enlarged heart due to horizontal positioning secondary to an elevated diaphragm. Increases in lung markings may simulate flow redistribution usually seen with increased pressures in the pulmonary venous bed due to left ventricular failure or mitral valve disease. Recent reports have suggested the frequent occurrence of pleural effusions during the early postpartum period.[16] They are usually small and resorb one to two weeks after delivery.[17,18]

ECHOCARDIOGRAPHY

M-mode and two-dimensional echocardiography are of great value in the evaluation of anatomy and function of cardiac chambers, valves, the pericardial sac, and the great vessels, such as aorta, pulmonary artery, and inferior vena cava. Echocardiography involves the use of ultrasound for the evaluation of the heart. Although some concerns have been expressed regarding the use of ultrasound during pregnancy, no hazard has been identified in humans and both maternal and fetal echocardiography should be considered safe during gestation.[19,20] The normal changes of the cardiovascular system during pregnancy are reflected echocardiographically and should be taken into consideration when an echocardiogram of a pregnant patient is interpreted. When the patient is examined in the left lateral position, an increase in left and right ventricular end-diastolic dimensions, due to the volume load of pregnancy, is expected.[21-23] This change progresses with the state of pregnancy and returns to a nonpregnant baseline postpartum. Left ventricular systolic dimensions and function are either unchanged or increased during pregnancy. Left atrial size and right atrial dimension may show a mild increase during gestation. A pericardial effusion of mostly small size, has been reported in approximately 40% of healthy pregnant women in late pregnancy.[24]

Doppler Echocardiography

The technique of Doppler echocardiography can provide accurate qualitative and quantitative information regarding regurgitation and stenosis of valves, malfunction of prosthetic valves, intracardiac shunts, cardiac function, cardiac output, and hemodynamic changes during various interventions.[25,26] Since it may provide accurate and sufficient diagnostic information in some cases, it may obviate the need for cardiac catheterization. This technique is, therefore, extremely important during pregnancy when the use of radiation needs to be minimized. Recent studies using Doppler echocardiography, have shown a high incidence of tricuspid and pulmonary regurgitation during pregnancy. This finding seems to be related to dilatation of right-sided chambers and valve annulus.[27,28]

PULMONARY ARTERY CATHETERIZATION

The introduction of the balloon-tipped pulmonary catheter by Swan, Ganz and their associates[29] provided the clinician with an excellent bedside tool for hemodynamic monitoring. The inflatable balloon at the tip of the catheter allows flotation of the tip with the blood flow into the pulmonary artery. In a majority of patients, the insertion of such a catheter can be performed successfully using pressure monitoring without need for fluoroscopy. The pulmonary catheter allows the measurements of right atrial, right ventricular, and pulmonary artery pressures, and when the inflated balloon totally occludes the small pulmonary artery branch in which it is placed, a pulmonary artery wedge pressure is obtained. This pressure correlates well, in most cases, with left ventricular end diastolic pressure, an important determinant of left ventricular function.

In addition to pressure monitoring, the Swan-Ganz catheter also allows the determination of cardiac output by the thermodilution technique. This technique is the most widely used method for the measurement of cardiac output. In the absence of an intracardiac shunt, it is accurate and reproducible and correlates well with other standard methods, such as the Fick or dye dilution method.[30] The use of the pulmonary artery catheter has become routine in the management of critically ill patients[31], and should be used without hesitation at any stage of pregnancy if conclusive information cannot be obtained by a noninvasive cardiac workup.[32]

We recommend the insertion of a Swan-Ganz catheter in early labor in any patient with cardiac disease who has been symptomatic during pregnancy. The availability of continuous hemodynamic monitoring allows early recognition and treatment of problems associated with the stress of labor and delivery. It is important to remember that significant hemodynamic changes occur after delivery in the early postpartum stage.[1] The most important changes are an increase in stroke volume, cardiac output, and systemic vascular resistance. In patients with high risk cardiac disease, hemodynamic monitoring should be continued for 24–48 hours postdelivery to assure hemodynamic stability.

RADIONUCLIDE TECHNIQUES

In the last several years a number of radionuclide techniques have been developed. They provide a relatively atraumatic and safe approach to the assessment of a variety of cardiac conditions.[33] In the pregnant patient, radionuclide cardiac imaging may be of value in the assessment of cardiac function, in the qualitative and quantitative evaluation of cardiac shunts, and in the detection of coronary artery disease in the rare cases where this problem may be suspected. A potential limitation of this technique during pregnancy is, however, the radiation exposure to the fetus. Although any radiation to the fetus should be avoided if possible, the risk of radionuclide imaging of the heart in pregnancy is relatively low. The dose, estimated to reach the fetus from radiopharmaceuticals generally used for radionuclide cardiac imaging, is less than or equal to 0.8 rad.[34]Although fetal malformation is unlikely with doses of less than 5 rad, even when received at the critical period for induction of maldevelopments[35], when one considers the use of radionuclide cardiac imaging, the following considerations should be made:

1. Use of these techniques should be avoided, if possible, during the first trimester of pregnancy.
2. One should first try to obtain the necessary diagnostic information using other noninvasive tests, such as echocardiography and Doppler echocardiography. Radionuclide imaging should be performed only when the desirable information cannot be obtained by other techniques.

MAGNETIC RESONANCE IMAGING

Magnetic Resonance Imaging (MRI) has been used in cardiology mainly in the evaluation of pericardial disease, neoplastic disease, congenital heart disease, and thoracic aortic disease.[36] The safety of MRI and its effect on the fetus have not been established. For that reason, exclusion of pregnant women from MRI has been recommended during their first trimester.[37] Colletti and Platt[38] recently recommended the use of MRI during pregnancy for the following situations: (1) MRI is known to be efficacious; (2) evaluation cannot be delayed until after pregnancy; (3) ultrasound cannot provide definitive imaging of the area in question; and (4) computed tomography would ordinarily be performed.

CARDIAC CATHETERIZATION

In some cases of cardiac decompensation during pregnancy, particularly where surgical intervention is considered and sufficient information cannot be obtained by other approaches, cardiac catheterization should be performed during pregnancy. This technique, although providing high quality information, is associated with a high dose of radiation (medial value of skin dose = 47 rads per examination).[13] The potentially deleterious effect of ionizing radiation is linearly proportional to the absorbed dose and exists at all times after fertilization. Its effect and likelihood to occur varies with the stage of fetal development. Radiation during the first week of pregnancy may result in absorption or resorption of the preimplanted blastocyst, while the risk of teratogenic effects is predominant during the second to sixth week of pregnancy. Developing brain cells can be affected by radiation during the seventh to fifteenth week, which may lead to alterations in neurological function or behavior. Irradiation throughout pregnancy has been associated with an increased risk of childhood cancers.[39] This risk seems to be higher when radiation is taking place during the first trimester. Because of the risk to the fetus, cardiac catheterization during gestation should only be performed if information cannot be obtained by alternative noninvasive methods. Moreover, it may be performed by the brachial[40], rather than the femoral, approach in order to prevent radiation to the pelvic area. The pelvic area should be appropriately shielded and the x-ray exposure should be kept to a minimum. In order to minimize the use of ionizing radiation, one should combine techniques such as echocardiography and Doppler with cardiac catheterization for the complete cardiac evaluation.[41,42]

REFERENCES

1. Elkayam U, Gleicher N. Changes in cardiac findings during normal pregnancy. In: Elkayam U, Gleicher N, ed. *Cardiac Problems in Pregnancy Diagnosis and Management of Maternal and Fetal Disease*. 2nd ed. New York: Alan R. Liss; 1990:31.
2. Elkayam U, Gleicher. Hemodynamics and cardiac function during normal pregnancy and the puerperium. In: Elkayam U, Gleicher N eds. *Cardiac Problems in Pregnancy Diagnosis and Management of Maternal and Fetal Disease*. 2nd ed. New York: Alan R. Liss; 1990:5.
3. Kjeldsen J. Hemodynamic investigators during labor and delivery. *Acta Obstet Gynecol Scand*. 1979;Suppl 89.
4. Perloff JK. Pregnancy and cardiovascular disease. In: Braunwald E, ed. *Heart Disease*. 3rd ed. Philadelphia: WB Saunders Company; 1988:1848.
5. Hytten EF, Thomson AM, Taggart N. Total body water in normal pregnancy. *J Obstet Gyneacol Br Commonw*. 1966;73:553.
6. Cutforth R, MacDonald CB. Heart sounds and murmurs in pregnancy. *Am Heart J*. 1966;71:741.
7. Perloff, JK. *The Clinical Recognition of Congenital Heart Disease*, 3rd ed. Philadelphia: WB Saunders Company; 1987;11.
8. Tabatznik B, Randall TW, Hersch C. The mammary souffle of pregnancy and lactation. *Circulation*. 1960;22:1069.
9. Marcus FI, Ewy FA, O'Rourke RA, et al. The effect of pregnancy on murmurs of mitral and aortic regurgitation. *Circulation*. 1970;41:795.
10. Haas JM. The effect of pregnancy on the midsystolic click and murmur of the prolapsing posterior leaflet of the mitral valve. *Am Heart J*. 1976;92:407.
11. Kumar A, Elkayam U. Hypertrophic cardiomyopathy in pregnancy. In: Elkayam U, Gleicher N, eds. *Cardiac Problems in Pregnancy Diagnosis and Management of Maternal and Fetal Disease*. 2nd ed. New York: Alan R. Liss; 1990:129.
12. Upshaw CB Jr. A study of maternal electrocardiograms recorded during labor and delivery. *Am J Obstet Gynecol*. 1970;107:17.
13. Syllabus on diagnostic x-ray radiation protection for certified x-ray supervisors and operators. Department of Health Services, Sacramento, CA, 1982, 71.
14. Wagner LK, Lester RG, Saldana LR. Exposure of the Pregnant Patient to Diagnostic Radiations. A Guide to Medical Management. Philadelphia: J.B. Lippincott Co.; 1985:52.
15. Turner AF. The chest radiograph in pregnancy. *Clin Obstet Gynecol*. 1975;18:65.
16. Hughson WG, Friedman PJ, Feigin DS, et al. Postpartum pleural effusion: A common radiologic finding. *Ann Int Med*. 1982;97:856.
17. Hessen I. Roentgen examination of pleural fluid. A study of the localization of free effusions, the potentialities of diagnosing minimal quantities of fluid and its existence under physiological conditions. *Acta Radiologica*. 1951;86(suppl)1.
18. Austin JHM. Postpartum pleural effusions. *Ann Int Med*. 1983;98:555.
19. Gardin JM, Askenazi J, Lesch M. Assessment of cardiovascular function. In: Sciarra J, Depp R, eds. *Maternal and Fetal Medicine. Volume III. Gynecology and Obstetrics*. Hagerstown, MD: Harper & Row; 1979:1.
20. Kremkau FW. Biological effects and possible hazards. Ultrasound in obstetrics and gynecology; recent advances. *Clin Obstet Gynecol*. 1983;10:395.
21. Rubler S, Prabodhumar MD, Pinto ER. Cardiac size and performance during pregnancy estimated with echocardiography. *Clin Obstet Gynecol*. 1977;40:534.
22. Katz R, Karliner JS, Resnik R. Effects of a natural volume overload state (pregnancy) on left ventricular performance in normal human subjects. *Curculation*. 1978;58:434.
23. Robson SC, Hunter S, Boys RJ, Dunlop W. Serial study of factors influencing changes in cardiac output during human pregnancy. *Am J Physiol*. 1989;256:H1060.
24. Enein M, Aziz A, Zina A, et al. Echocardiography of the pericardium in pregnancy. *Obstet Gynecol*. 1987;69:851.
25. Feigenbaum H. Echocardiography. In: Braunwald E, ed. *Heart Disease*. Philadelphia: WB Saunders Co.; 1988:83.
26. Lee W, Rokey R, Cotton DB. Noninvasive maternal stroke volume and cardiac output determinations by Doppler echocardiography. *Am J Obstet Gynecol*. 1988;158:505.
27. Limacher MC, Ware JA, O'Meara ME, et al. Tricuspid regurgitation during pregnancy: Two-dimensional and pulsed Doppler echocardiographic observations. *Am J Cardiol*. 1985;55:1059.
28. Campos O, Martinez E, Andrade JL, et al. Detection of right-sided valve regurgitation during normal pregnancy by Doppler echocardiography. *J Am Coll Cardiol*. 1990;15:139A.
29. Swan HJC, Ganz W, Forrester JS, et al. Catheterization of the heart in man with the use of a flow-directed balloon-tipped catheter. *N Engl J Med*. 1970;283:447.
30. Elkayam U, Berkley R, Azan S, et al. Cardiac output by thermodilution technique effect of injectate's volume and temperature on accuracy and reproducibility in the critically ill patient. *Chest*. 1983;84:418.
31. Wiedemann HP, Matthay MA, Matthay RA. Cardiovascular pulmonary monitoring in the intensive care unit (Part I). *Chest*. 1984;85:537.
32. Lee W, Shak PK, Amin DK, Elkayam U. Hemodynamic monitoring of cardiac patients during pregnancy. In: Elkayam U, Gleicher N, eds. *Cardiac Problems in Pregnancy Diagnosis and Management of Maternal and Fetal Disease*. 2nd ed. New York, NY: Alan R. Liss; 1990:47.
33. Holman BL. Nuclear cardiology. In: Braunwald E, ed. *Heart Disease*, 3rd ed. Philadelphia, PA: WB Saunders Co.; 1988:311.
34. Kereiakes JJ, Rosenstein M. *Handbook of Radiation Doses in Nuclear Medicine and Diagnostic X-Ray*. Boca Raton, Fl: CRC Press; 1980:170.
35. Medical radiation exposure of pregnant and potentially pregnant women: recommendations of the National Council on Radiation Protection and Measurements. Washington, DC: National Council on Radiation Protection and Measurements, 1977, 13.
36. Higgins CB. Newer cardiac imaging techniques: digital subtraction angiography; computed tomography; magnetic resonance imaging. In: Braunwald E, ed. *Heart Disease*. Philadelphia, PA: WB Saunders Co.; 1988:356.
37. National Radiological Protection Board: Revised guidance on acceptable limits of exposure during nuclear magnetic clinical imaging. *Br J Radiol*. 1983;56:974.
38. Colletti PM, Platt LD. Obstetric MRI acceptable under specific criteria. *Diag Radiol*. 1989;11:84.
39. Bithell JM, Stewart AM. Prenatal irradiation and childhood malignancy: a review of British data from the Oxford survey. *Br J Cancer*. 1975;31:271.
40. Grossman W. Cardiac catheterization by direct exposure of artery and vein. In: Grossman W, ed. *Cardiac Catheterization and Angiography*. 3rd ed. Philadelphia: Lea & Febiger; 1986:45.
41. Elkayam U, Kawanishi D, Reid CL, et al. Contrast echocardiography to reduce ionizing radiation associated with cardiac catheterization during pregnancy. *Am J Cardiol*. 1983;52:213.
42. Vidalliet HJ Jr, Skelton TN, Kisslo KB, et al. Echocardiographic guidance of cardiac catheterization for atrial septal defect in pregnancy. *Am J Cardiol*. 1986;58:1133.

Chapter One Hundred and Twenty-Four

Cardiovascular Physiology of the Normal Pregnancy

Thomas R. Easterling

124

Pregnancy is a time of significant cardiovascular adaptation. Teleologically, these changes are presumed to prepare the mother for the support of a growing fetus and the demands of parturition. The uterus and its contents have rapidly increasing needs; significant reserves in intravascular volume and red cell mass may be required to insure the survival of a peripartum hemorrhage. The hemodynamic changes of pregnancy are well tolerated by healthy women and, therefore, represent a survival advantage to the individual and the species. However, these same changes that benefit a healthy woman may lead to a dramatic decompensation during medically complicated pregnancies. Fortunately, the physiological parameters which regulate the system are well-described and can usually be directly measured. An understanding of basic cardiovascular physiology and the changes associated with pregnancy, coupled with the appropriate collection of data from an individual patient, can then lead to a rational management plan whose effectiveness can be directly assessed and subsequently adapted to the individual needs of the patient.

Hemodynamics is the study of the mechanics of the movement of fluid and blood cells within the vascular tree. Three basic physiological principles govern the system. The relationship of pressure, flow, and resistance is described by *Ohm's Law*. In a cardiovascular system, the relationship between mean arterial pressure (MAP), cardiac output (CO), and total peripheral resistance (TPR) is:

$$\text{MAP} = 80(\text{TPR})(\text{CO}).$$

Mean arterial pressure is directly proportional to cardiac output and vascular resistance. Resistance is always calculated and represents the slope of the linear relationship between pressure and output.

The heart is the pump of the hemodynamic system. It is uniquely adapted to increase its pumping capacity in response to an increase in return of blood from the systemic circulation. As myocardial fibers are stretched by increased venous return, they contract more vigorously to increase cardiac output. The relationship between left ventricular end diastolic volume and cardiac output is expressed by *Starling's Law* of the heart. In clinical practice, end diastolic volume is difficult to approximate; therefore, end diastolic pressure is used instead. When myometrial contractility is altered by physiological conditions, the slope of the relationship between these two variables will be altered so that at a given pressure, cardiac output may be elevated or depressed.

Finally, fluid must remain within the cardiovascular system to maintain hemodynamic stability and to insure that pulmonary spaces remain dry. Hydrostatic pressure within vessels works to force fluid out of vessels into the low pressure interstitium. Resisting this flow is an oncotic gradient generated by the concentration of proteins within the plasma. The semipermeable capillary wall maintains the oncotic gradient while permitting a flux of fluid across the vessel wall. The relationship between these variables is expressed by *Starling's Law of Capillary Fluids:*

$$Q_f = K_f[(P_c - P_i) - R(\pi_c - \pi_i)]$$

where

Q_f = net flow of fluid across capillary membrane
K_f = fluid filtration coefficient
P_c = capillary hydrostatic pressure
P_i = interstitial hydrostatic pressure
R = reflection coefficient
π_c = capillary oncotic pressure
π_i = interstitial oncotic pressure.

Hemodynamic adaptations to pregnancy do not alter the fundamental relationships expressed by these principles. Pregnancy does, however, change the point of baseline equilibrium. Although the baseline changes are well-tolerated in normal pregnancies, they are of much greater clinical significance when medical complications are superimposed on the pregnant condition. The goal of this chapter is to review the hemodynamic changes that are associated with normal pregnancy.

OHM'S LAW

Measurement of blood pressure in pregnancy is usually done manually with a stethoscope and sphygmomanometer. Reproducible measurement of the diastolic pressure is complicated by the absence of a fifth Korotkoff sound in many women. The pulse can be heard over the brachial artery after the cuff has been completely deflated. Therefore, the fourth sound is frequently used. Measurement of blood pressure by auscultation is subject to multiple sources of bias and can, therefore, be misleading when used for research or clinical purposes unless a rigorous protocol is followed. Ideally, a random zero cuff is used but it is impractical in most clinical conditions.[1] Automated cuffs are widely available and avoid many operator-dependent biases associated with auscultated pressures. This method has been evaluated against pressures measured directly with an intra-arterial catheter and has been found to be accurate.[2]

The position in which blood pressure is measured in pregnancy is of critical importance. In the sitting position, systolic and diastolic blood pressure are approximately 10 mm Hg higher than in the recumbent position.[3] After mid-pregnancy, women in the recumbent position are prone to caval occlusion due to compression from the gravid uterus. Pressures are usually measured in the left lateral position. In this position, significant differences are found between the upper and lower arm due to hydrostatic forces.[4]

Most longitudinal studies of blood pressure in pregnancy have not gathered data prior to the first trimester.[3,5,6] Blood pressures measured six weeks postpartum are used to represent a nonpregnant baseline. While the assumption that postpartum pressures are the same as antepartum pressures is reasonable, little data exists to support this position. Systolic blood pressure in the first trimester is approximately 12 mm Hg lower than postpartum values. Diastolic pressures are approximately 10–20 mm Hg lower, creating a modest elevation in pulse pressure. In some studies, a modest rise in blood pressure is reported in the late third trimester. In others, no change in blood pressure is reported.

Diastolic blood pressures greater than 90 mm Hg in pregnancy are clearly abnormal. If they occur prior to 20 weeks, the patient is said to have chronic hypertension. If the blood pressure rises in the second half of pregnancy, the patient is said to have gestational hypertension, which may progress to preeclampsia if proteinuria ensues. Diastolic blood pressures in the 80s are not clearly normal. They may represent latent hypertension which has been masked by the physiological reduction of blood pressure in pregnancy or incipient hypertensive disease of pregnancy. Clinically, modest elevations in blood pressure such as this must be followed closely due to the potential for rapid exacerbation of hypertension in pregnancy. (For more detail, see Chapters 138–141).

The most widely accepted techniques for measuring cardiac output are invasive, requiring arterial and central venous access. All of these methods are similar in that they are dilutional. Oxygen, an inert dye, or cold saline may be used as the dilutional agents. Use of the *Fick technique*, with oxygen or dye dilution, requires special equipment and expertise. Thermodilution is used most frequently in clinical practice. Recirculation of the dilutional agent is avoided permitting multiple sequential measurements. Cardiac output can be measured noninvasively with M-mode echocardiography, Doppler echocardiography, or with impedance technique. The validations of M-mode in nonpregnant patients are limited. Given the significant remodeling of cardiac architecture that occurs in pregnancy[7,8], rigorous validation of this method in pregnancy is needed. The Doppler technique has been validated in pregnancy by several operators.[9-11] In experienced hands, this method may be considered as accurate as thermodilution.

Several investigators have reported a good correlation between impedance technique and thermodilution in pregnancy.[12,13] These studies have been marred by the use of statistical methods which overestimate the correlation between methods.

In addition, longitudinal studies using impedance technique have produced results which are physiologically improbable.[14] The weaknesses of this method during pregnancy have been extensively reviewed.[15] In severely ill hypertensive patients, it has been found to underestimate cardiac output by as much as 50%.[16]

Cardiac output increases 30–50% during pregnancy.[17-21] Much of the increase has occurred in the first trimester prior to the time that earliest measurements have been made. A modest, but steady, increase in cardiac output continues until at least 32 weeks of pregnancy. In the supine position, cardiac output falls in the third trimester, probably due to caval compression by the gravid uterus. In the lateral position, some studies have reported that cardiac output is maintained[18] while others describe a fall in output toward term.[17] Our recent lontigudinal study of normotensive women in pregnancy has confirmed a fall in mean cardiac output from 32 weeks to term.[22] The performance of individual patients is less predictable. Cardiac output falls in the majority of patients, but rises in a significant minority of others. The individual variability probably explains the differences in findings between previous small studies.[17,18]

Cardiac output is the product of stroke volume and heart rate. Each is elevated in pregnancy. While stroke volume falls near term, heart rate continues to rise.[17] The relative tachycardia of pregnancy is clinically significant when superimposed on conditions such as mitral stenosis where ventricular filling is dependent on adequate diastolic filling times. The elevation in cardiac output in pregnancy is more than adequate to meet the associated increase in metabolic needs as demonstrated by a narrowing of the difference in arterial and central venous oxygen saturation.[23]

Cardiac output can be corrected for the size of the individual by dividing output by body surface area to get the cardiac index. This correction assumes that cardiac output is related to the size of the individual. In pregnancy, body surface area and cardiac output are not related. We have previously reported a correlation of 0.04 for normotensive pregnant women.[9] If the assumption is valid for non-pregnant individuals, the magnitude of the increase in cardiac output associated with pregnancy seems to obscure the relationship. We, therefore, use the cardiac output rather than the cardiac index in pregnancy.

Vascular resistance is directly proportional to mean arterial pressure and inversely proportional to cardiac output. Resistance is not measured directly but is calculated from mean arterial pressure and cardiac output. Given a fall in blood pressure and a rise in cardiac output, vascular resistance must, therefore, fall. As blood pressure rises toward term and cardiac output falls, vascular resistance rises. In our lab, where cardiac output is measured by Doppler technique, total vascular resistances of greater than 1200 dyne-sec-cm^{-5} are usually considered abnormal. Those that are less than 700–800 dyne-sec-cm^{-5} may also be abnormal.

STARLING'S LAW OF THE HEART

The etiology of the rise in cardiac output is unclear. Blood volume increases by approximately 40%[24], but to a large extent fills an increased vascular capacitance on the venous side.

Increased blood volume could augment cardiac output by the Starling mechanism of increased preload. However, the elevation in left ventricular end diastolic pressure required to increase cardiac output by 40% would be large and in some individuals pathological. In studies of normal subjects[25], hypertensives[26-30] and patients with cardiac disease[31], cardiac output has been found to be elevated despite normal pulmonary artery wedge pressures. In addition, a primary increase in cardiac output, driven by preload, would be expected to result in a modest increase in blood pressure rather than the observed reduction.

The observed fall in vascular resistance represents a fall in afterload and would, therefore, be expected to increase cardiac output due to an associated increase in ejection fraction. It would result in the observed fall in blood pressure but would require an ejection fraction of more than 90%.[32] An additional mechanism must also be at work.

During pregnancy, the architecture of the heart is remodeled such that end diastolic volume is increased without an increase in end diastolic pressure.[7,8] The heart becomes more compliant. Although echocardiographic studies suggest that fractional shortening is unchanged in pregnancy[7,8], total shortening is increased since ejection fraction is maintained in the face of a dilated heart. In the sense that at a given preload stroke volume is increased, functional contractility is increased. Studies of systolic time intervals support a modest increase in contractility.[33,34]

A primary increase in cardiac output would increase blood pressure and activate compensatory mechanisms to reduce pressure toward normal. Since physiological compensatory mechanisms do not return a parameter to the original set point, one would expect blood pressure in pregnancy to be elevated if increased cardiac output was due to increased contractility alone. On the contrary, blood pressure is lower in pregnancy. More than one mechanism seems to be operating to increase cardiac output in pregnancy. The available data suggests that given a physiologically dilated heart, ejection fraction is maintained with a small increase in contractile forces and a large reduction in afterload.

STARLING'S LAW OF CAPILLARY FLUIDS

Edema is ubiquitous in pregnancy. The accumulation of fluid in the interstitium indicates that the balance of forces across capillary membranes has been disrupted. A net flux of fluid into the interstitium must be accounted for by four possible mechanisms: (1) increased capillary hydrostatic pressure; (2) decreased capillary oncotic pressure; (3) disruption of capillary membrane integrity; or (4) obstruction of lymphatic flow of fluid out to the interstitium.

Blood pressure is decreased in pregnancy. Therefore, increased pressure distal to the terminal arteriole is not likely to cause edema. As vascular volume expands in pregnancy, red cell mass expands more slowly creating the well-described physiological anemia of pregnancy. In a similar fashion, the concentration of plasma proteins are reduced in pregnancy by the dilution effect of plasma volume expansion. Albumin concentration and colloid osmotic pressure are reduced by approximately 18% by term.[35,36] Although the reduction in oncotic pressure is modest, the propensity toward edema formation is increased.

There is growing evidence to suggest that a loss of membrane integrity is associated with the hemodynamic changes of pregnancy. In hypertensive pregnancies, increasing levels of protein are found in the edema fluid as the disease becomes more severe.[37] Data is not available from normotensive pregnancies. In normotensive pregnancies, microalbumenuria does increase significantly throughout pregnancy indicating a loss of membrane integrity in the glomerulus.[38] Women with preeclampsia develop pulmonary edema at lower pulmonary artery wedge pressures than would be expected in the nonpregnant population.[27] Our experience suggests that this tendency may be present to some degree in pregnant patients who do not have preeclampsia.

In the third trimester, the gravid uterus obstructs the vena cava increasing venous and lymphatic pressure distal to the obstruction. Edema formation is, therefore, encouraged in the lower extremities.

The source of edema formation in pregnancy is clearly multifactorial. Clinically, edema of pregnancy complicates the evaluation of medical conditions characterized by edema. The physician cannot easily determine if an increase in edema is the result of worsening condition or merely a normal change of pregnancy. Of more critical importance is the ease with which pregnant women under certain conditions develop pulmonary edema in the face of filling pressures that would otherwise be well tolerated.[27]

EXERCISE

Pregnant women are known to tolerate clinically most forms of mild to moderate exercise without adverse effect on the mother or fetus.[39,40] Women who have trained prior to pregnancy are usually limited in late pregnancy by the awkwardness associated with their weight gain and gravid abdomen rather than by compromised cardiovascular performance.

Most exercise is carried out in an upright position. Therefore, hemodynamic changes associated with position are experienced during exercise. The hemodynamic effects of orthostatic stress in pregnancy are well described.[41] Standing is associated with a reduction in cardiac output of approximately 1.8 L/min in early and late pregnancy. Sitting is associated with a somewhat smaller reduction. These changes are not different from those seen in the nonpregnant condition. Mean arterial pressure is maintained by a rise in vascular resistance. The increase in vascular resistance required to maintain blood pressure is approximately 50% less in late pregnancy than when not pregnant. The smaller rise in vascular resistance is associated with a proportionally smaller increase in circulating norepinephrine.[42]

Exercise in pregnancy is associated with expected hemodynamic changes. In a longitudinal study of moderate exercise, (200 kpm), on a bicycle ergometer, Ueland et al reported elevations in cardiac output and heart rate prior to term that were comparable in absolute magnitude to those seen postpartum.[17] Near term, the increases in cardiac output and heart rate were somewhat less than observed earlier in pregnancy and postpartum.

Guzman and Caplan in a similar study also reported augmentation of heart rate and cardiac output at three levels of exercise that were similar in magnitude to those seen postpartum.[23] They did not find differences near term.

Clinically, one wonders if the hemodynamic response to exercise is adequate in the face of the increased hemodynamic requirements of pregnancy. At rest, pregnancy is associated with a decreased arterio-venous O_2 difference, (a-v O_2 difference). If the metabolic requirements of exercise in pregnancy were incompletely met by the hemodynamic response, one would expect to see a fall in central venous O_2 saturation and a widening of a-v O_2 difference due to increased oxygen extraction in the periphery. This is not the case. Guzman and Caplan found that the a-v O_2 difference at all gestional ages and all levels of exercise remained substantially less than postpartum values.[23] These findings are reassuring in the context of total maternal adaptation to exercise. They do not, in and of themselves, indicate that adequate perfusion of the uteroplacental unit is preserved. Several studies of maternal and fetal adaptation to exercise in pregnancy have reported transient bradycardias in the fetus.[43,44] In these studies and in others where no bradycardia was reported[45,46], the fetal outcome was uniformly good.

Healthy women with normal pregnancies tolerate exercise in pregnancy well. This is not true for women whose pregnancies are compromised by cardiac disease. No data exists regarding the maternal or fetal response to exercise or orthostatic stress in the face of hypertension of uteroplacental compromise. For more details concerning exercise in pregnancy, the reader is referred to Chapters 4 and 11.

LABOR AND DELIVERY

Labor and delivery is the period in pregnancy of maximal hemodynamic stress. Although these stresses are tolerated well by normal women, those with preexisting limitations may decompensate. Pain and anxiety in labor create a state of high catecholamine release, tachycardia, and additional augmentation of cardiac output. These changes are particularly important in cardiac conditions such as mitral and aortic stenosis when adequate diastolic or systolic time intervals are required for the passage of blood across a stenosed orifice.

Baseline cardiac output in labor increases by approximately 13% by 8 cm cervical dilation. These changes are largely due to increased stroke volume.[11] Uterine contractions are estimated to return acutely approximately 500 mL of blood to the systemic circulation. Associated with this autotransfusion is an increase in preload and an augmentation in cardiac output by approximately 34% above labor baseline. The total increase in cardiac output during a contraction in late labor is, therefore, 50% above a prelabor baseline.[11] In the face of an obstructive cardiac lesion or a failing heart, uterine contractions produce abrupt elevations of pulmonary artery wedge pressure and contribute to the development of pulmonary edema.[31]

Epidural and general anesthesia are associated with a 37% and 26% increase in cardiac output above preinduction levels.[47] The increase is associated with elevations of heart rate and stroke volume. Within 60–90 minutes hemodynamic parameters have returned to baseline levels. By two weeks postpartum, cardiac output falls 26% and is only 10% above values measured at 24 weeks postpartum.[48]

Within hours of delivery, a marked diuresis begins. This is presumably due to a mobilization of fluid from the expanded extravascular space and a contraction of the intravascular space. Little data exists on the impact of this fluid mobilization on cardiac filling pressures. However, in pregnancies complicated by mitral stenosis with limited capacity to increase cardiac output, pulmonary artery wedge pressure rises dramatically after delivery.[49]

Pregnancy creates a hyperdynamic condition characterized by elevations in cardiac output, heart rate and stroke volume, and a reduction in vascular resistance and mean arterial pressure. The combined effect of increased stroke volume and reduced resistance maintains stroke work within a normal range. The hemodynamic changes of pregnancy begin in the early weeks of gestation and are out of proportion to the needs of the early conceptus. Immediately after delivery, hemodynamic parameters begin to normalize. The hyperdynamic state of pregnancy is certainly associated with associated changes in hormonal milieu but, to date, the precise etiology is unknown.

REFERENCES

1. de Swiet M. The cardiovascular system. In: Hytten FaC G, ed. *Clinical Physiology in Obstetrics*. Boston, MA: Blackwell/Year Book Medical Publishers; 1980:10.
2. Kirshon B, Rossavik I, Giebel R, Cotton D. Direct versus indirect blood pressure monitoring in pregnancy. Seventh Annual Meeting, Society of Perinatal Obstetricians. Lake Buena Vista, FL: 1978:177.
3. Gallery E, Ross M, Hunyor S, Gyory A. Predicting the development of pregnancy-associated hypertension: the place of standardized blood pressure measurement. *Lancet*. 1977;1:1273.
4. Benedetti T, Read J. The effect of hydrostatic pressure on interpretation of the supine pressor test. *J Reprod Med*. 1982;27:161.
5. Moutquin J, Rainville C, Giroux L. A prospective study of blood pressure in pregnancy: prediction of preeclampsia. *Am J Obstet Gynecol*. 1985;151:191.
6. Reiss R, O'Shaughnessy R, Quilligan T, Zuspan F. Retrospective comparison of blood pressure course during preeclamptic and matched control pregnancies. *Am J Obstet Gynecol*. 1987;156:894.
7. Lard-Meeter K, van de Ley G, Bom T, et al. Cardiocirculatory adjustments during pregnancy: an echocardiographic study. *Clin Cardiol*. 1979;2:328.
8. Rubler S, Damani P, Pinto E. Cardiac size and performance during pregnancy estimated with echocardiography. *Am J Cardiol*. 1977;49:534.
9. Easterling T, Watts D, Schmucker B, Benedetti T. Measurement of cardiac output during pregnancy: validation of Doppler technique and clinical observations in preeclampsia. *Obstet Gynecol*. 1987;69:845.
10. Lee W, Rokey R, Cotton D. Noninvasive maternal stroke volume and cardiac output determinations by pulsed Doppler echocardiography. *Am J Obstet Gynecol*. 1988;158:505.
11. Robson S, Dunlop W, Boys R, Hunter S. Cardiac output during labour. *Br Med J*. 1987;295:1169.
12. Secher N, Thomsen A, Arnsbo P. Measurement of rapid changes in cardiac stroke volume: an evaluation of the impedance cardiography method. *Acta Anaesthesiol Scand*. 1977;21:353.
13. Milsom I, Forssman L, Sivertsson R, Dottori O. Measurement of cardiac stroke volume in the last trimester of pregnancy. *Acta Obstet Gynecol Scand*. 1983;62:473.
14. Atkins A, Watt J, Milan P, et al. A longitudinal study of cardiovascular dynamic changes throughout pregnancy. *Eur J Obstet Gynecol Reprod Biol*. 1981;12:215.
15. de Swiet M, Talbert D. The measurement of cardiac output by electrical impedance plethysmography in pregnancy: are the assumptions valid? *Br J Obstet Gynaecol*. 1986;93:721.
16. Easterling T, Benedetti T, Carlson K, Watts D. Measurement of cardiac output in pregnancy: impedance vs thermodilution techniques. *Br J Obstet Gynaecol*. 1989;96:67.
17. Ueland K, Novy M, Peterson E, Metcalfe J. Maternal cardiovascular dynamics. IV. The influence of gestational age on the maternal cardiovascular response to posture and exercise. *Am J Obstet Gynecol*. 1969;104:856.
18. Lees M, Taylor S, Scott D, Kerr M. A study of cardiac output at rest throughout pregnancy. *J Obstet Gynecol Br Commonwealth*. 1967;74:319.
19. Roy S, Malkani P, Virik R. Circulatory effects of pregnancy. *Am J Obstet Gynecol*. 1966;96:221.
20. Bader R, Bader M, Rose D. Hemodynamics at rest and during exercise in normal pregnancy as studied by cardiac catheterization. *Eur J Clin Invest*. 1955;34:1524.
21. Werko L. Pregnancy and heart disease. *Acta Obstet Gynecol Scand*. 1954;33:162.
22. Easterling TR, Benedetti TJ, Schmucker BC, Millard SP. Maternal hemodynamics in normal and preeclamptic pregnancies: a longitudinal study. *Obstet Gynecol*. 1990;76.
23. Guzman C, Caplan R. Cardiorespiratory response to exercise during pregnancy. *Am J Obstet Gynecol*. 1970;108:600.
24. Hytten F, Paintin D. Increase in plasma volume during normal pregnancy. *J Obstet Gynaecol Br Commonw*. 1963;70:402.
25. Groenendijk R, Wallenburg H. Hemodynamic measurements in preeclampsia: preliminary observations. *Am J Obstet Gynecol*. 1984;150:232.
26. Benedetti T, Cotton D, Read J, Miller F. Hemodynamic observations in severe preeclampsia with a flow-directed pulmonary artery catheter. *Am J Obstet Gynecol*. 1980;136:465.
27. Benedetti T, Kates R, Williams V. Hemodynamic observations in severe preeclampsia complicated by pulmonary edema. *Am J Obstet Gynecol*. 1985;152:330.
28. Henderson D, Vilow G, Milne K, Nichol P. The role of Swan-Ganz catheterization in severe pregnancy-induced hypertension. *Am J Obstet Gynecol*. 1984;148:570.
29. Strauss R, Keefer J, Burke T, Civetta J. Hemodynamic monitoring of cardiogenic pulmonary edema complicating toxemia of pregnancy. *Obstet Gynecol*. 1980;55:170.
30. Phelan J, Yurth D. Severe preeclampsia. Peripartum hemodynamic observations. *Am J Obstet Gynecol*. 1982;144:17.
31. Easterling T, Chadwick H, Otto C, Benedetti T. Aortic stenosis in pregnancy. *Obstet Gynecol*. 1988;72:113.
32. Morton M, Metcalfe J. Changes in maternal hemodynamics during pregnancy. In: Artal (Mittelmark) R, Wiswell R, eds. *Exercise in Pregnancy*. Baltimore, MD: Williams & Wilkins; 1986:113.
33. Burg J, Dodek A, Kloster F, Metcalfe J. Alterations of systolic time intervals during pregnancy. *Circulation*. 1974;49:560.
34. Rubler S, Hammer N, Schneebaum R. Systolic time intervals in pregnancy and the postpartum period. *Am Heart J*. 1973;86:182.
35. Wu P, Udani V, Chan L. Colloid osmotic pressure: variations in normal pregnancy. *J Perinatol Med*. 1983;11:193.
36. Robertson E, Cheyne G. Plasma biochemistry in relation to oedema of pregnancy. *J Obstet Gynecol Br Commonw*. 1972;79:769.
37. Oian P, Maltau J, Noddeland H, Fadnes H. Transcapillary fluid balance in pre-eclampsia. *Br J Obstet Gynaecol*. 1986;93:235.
38. Lopez-Espinoza I, Dhar H, Humphreys S, Redman C. Urinary albumin excretion in pregnancy. *Br J Obstet Gynaecol*. 1986;93:176.
39. Kulpa PJ, White BM, Visscher R. Aerobic exercise in pregnancy. *Am J Obstet Gynecol*. 1987;156:1395.
40. Hall DC, Kaufmann DA. Effects of aerobic and strength conditioning on pregnancy outcomes. *Am J Obstet Gynecol*. 1987;157:1199.
41. Easterling T, Schmucker B, Benedetti T. The hemodynamic effects of orthostatic stress during pregnancy. *Obstet Gynecol*. 1988;75:550.
42. Barron W, Mujais S, Zinaman M, et al. Plasma catecholamine responses to physiologic stimuli in normal human pregnancy. *Am J Obstet Gynecol*. 1986;154:8.
43. Veille JC, Bacevice AE, Wilson B, et al. Umbilical artery waveform during bicycle exercise in normal pregnancy. *Obstet Gynecol*. 1989;73:957.
44. Artal R, Paul RH, Romem Y, Wiswell R. Fetal bradycardia induced by maternal exercise. *Lancet*. 1984;2:258.
45. Sorensen KE, Borlum KG, Fetal heart function in response to short-term maternal exercise. *Br J Obstet Gynecol*. 1986;93:310.
46. Clapp JF III. Fetal heart rate response to running in midpregnancy and late pregnancy. *Am J Obstet Gynecol*. 1985;153:251.
47. James C, and Banner T, Caton D. Cardiac output in women undergoing cesarean section with epidural or general anesthesia. *Am J Obstet Gynecol*. 1989;160:1178.
48. Robson S, Dunlop W. Haemodynamic changes during early pregnancy loss. *Br J Obstet Gynaecol*. 1988;95:1334.
49. Clark S, Phelan J, Greenspoon J, et al. Labor and delivery in the presence of mitral stenosis: central hemodynamic observations. *Am J Obstet Gynecol*. 1985;152:384.

Chapter One Hundred and Twenty-Five
Cardiovascular Pharmacotherapy in Pregnancy and Lactation

Josef Widerhorn, Arie L.M. Widerhorn, and Uri Elkayam

125

Cardiovascular drugs are often used in pregnancy for the treatment of maternal and fetal conditions. The complex physiologic changes occurring during pregnancy may significantly affect the pharmacokinetics of many drugs and, consequently, the toxicity and therapeutic response. Of special concern are the effects of maternal therapy on the fetus and the undesired translactal passage of drugs to newborns. Although the body of information regarding cardiovascular therapy in pregnancy is incomplete, some of the available data are summarized in this chapter (see also Chapter 7).

CARDIAC GLYCOSIDES

Cardiac glycosides have been known to humanity since the ancient Egyptian and Roman era. Used for centuries for different purposes, digitalis emerged as one of the major drugs in the therapy of congestive heart failure, as well as in terminating paroxysmal supraventricular tachycardia and controlling ventricular rate in patients with atrial fibrillation and flutter.

Among various digitalis preparations, digoxin is the most accepted and widely used. During pregnancy, the most common maternal and fetal indications are congestive heart failure or supraventricular tachyarrhythmias.[1-16]

Only 60–80% of an oral dose is absorbed, mostly in the proximal small intestine. As with other drugs, the presence of food or delayed gastric emptying that may occur in pregnancy may retard its absorption. Digoxin is only 20–25% bound to proteins; therefore, the decreased albumin level seen during pregnancy should not affect its serum concentration significantly. Peak level and maximal effect following oral administration are reached after two to three hours and four to six hours, respectively. The intravenous (IV) preparation has a rapid onset of action (within five to twenty minutes) and a maximal effect within one and a half to three hours. The half-life of digoxin is 36–40 hours. The volume of distribution (V_D) is significantly increased during pregnancy.[17] For rapid digitalization, the dosage is similar to that in the nonpregnant state, ie 0.75–1.5 mg IV. Digoxin is excreted primarily by the kidneys. During pregnancy, there is a linear correlation between digoxin and creatinine clearance; therefore, the dosage has to be adjusted with impaired renal function. The maintenance dose has to be approximately 35% of total body stores; it may need adjustments throughout pregnancy in order to obtain optimal therapeutic effect.

In 1972, Rogers et al[1] reported that serum digoxin level at term was lower than four weeks postdelivery in mothers treated with the same maintenance dose. However, this data could not be confirmed by other authors[2,4,6] who found digoxin concentration in the therapeutic range at the time of delivery. Luxford et al[2] demonstrated that despite increased digoxin and creatinine clearance and increased 24 hours urinary digoxin elimination, serum digoxin level was higher during the third trimester of pregnancy than during the postpartum period.

Recently, several studies[18-26] have demonstrated the existence of endogenous digoxin-like substances (DLIS) in pregnant women and neonates. These substances interfere with the radioimmunoassay for exogenous digoxin leading to reading errors ranging from 0.1 μg/L to more than 2 μg/L. To complicate the situation further, the degree of interference caused by DLIS varies significantly with different commercially available digoxin immunoassay kits.[21] This variability probably results from differences among various immunoassay kits with different binding activities for DLIS. Knowing the type of immunoassay kit, the degree of DLIS interference in certain population groups assessed with the respective kit (a list of interferences may be obtained from kit manufacturer) and measuring the DLIS concentration prior to digoxin treatment may be helpful in management of pregnant patients. Unfortunately, the DLIS serum concentration changes with gestational age making it difficult to interpret the digoxin levels over extended periods of time.[20] Due to the serious inaccuracies in digoxin level measurements during pregnancy, the assessment of digoxin dosing with electrocardiographic and clinical criteria becomes of paramount importance and should prevail over plasma concentration monitoring.

Treatment of fetal conditions is based on the ability of digoxin to cross the placenta. Although this property was well documented by numerous authors[1-16,24-26], the magnitude of digoxin transfer to the fetus assessed with immunoassay methods is somewhat conflicting. Rogers et al[1] found similar concentrations of digoxin in both maternal and fetal blood at the time of delivery. Chan et al[4] found lower levels in fetal blood and postulated the existence of a placental barrier for digoxin. Allonen et al[6] noted lower digoxin concentration in fetuses but at a different gestational age (12–16 weeks). Significant dissociation of fetomaternal serum digoxin concentration has also been found by Mimura et al[24] and Younis et al.[25] They attributed the inability to control the fetal tachyarrhythmias to lower fetal levels of digoxin and hypothesized an altered transplacental passage of digoxin in fetuses with hydrope fetalis because of high intravascular hydrostatic pressure and placental edema. However, the variability of fetomaternal serum digoxin ratio may be due to DLIS interference. Weiner et al[26] reported that the digoxin concentration in sick fetuses whose mothers received digoxin did not differ from DLIS measured in those fetuses with similar problems whose mothers had not received digoxin. Healthy control fetuses had significantly less DLIS measured than was found in ill fetuses. In the light of these reports on endogenous digoxin-like substances and their effect on digoxin measurements, it is difficult to interpret the above data.

In a different study using radioisotopes, Saarikosky et al[5] demonstrated that placental transfer of digoxin occurs fairly rapidly. Five minutes following the injection of H^3-digoxin in maternal blood, radioactivity was demonstrated in umbilical cord blood, and by 30 minutes, fetal and maternal blood concentration of radioisotopes were approximately equal. He also demonstrated that the fetal heart binds digoxin much less avidly than the infant heart. Based on the above reports the fetomaternal digoxin concentration ratio probably ranges from 0.5 to 1.0.

During the last decade, digoxin has become the drug of choice for treatment of fetal supraventricular tachycardia and congestive heart failure.[7-16] Although digoxin alone often is effective[9,10], in some cases, it may be necessary to add a second drug, such as verapamil[8] or quinidine.[12] As in the nonpregnant state, the addition of quinidine or verapamil may significantly increase the digoxin level. Therefore, the same precaution regarding drug interactions apply during pregnancy as in the nonpregnant state. For treatment of fetal tachyarrhythmia, higher-than-normal maternal doses of digoxin may be necessary.[7,8] In refractory cases, digitalization by direct intramuscular injection[14] or direct intraperitoneal administration to the fetus[15] have been attempted.

To date, few adverse effects have been observed in fetuses of mothers treated chronically with digoxin. Occasionally, low birth weight infants have been born of mothers with cardiac conditions treated with digitalis. It has been postulated that digoxin may affect amino acid transport through placenta with consequent growth retardation.[27] However, the duration of pregnancy and labor has been noted to be shorter in mothers on long-term digoxin therapy.[28] It is, therefore, conceivable that the low birth weight reported with digoxin treatment is secondary to prematurity rather than to intrauterine growth retardation.

Despite the above concerns, digoxin is considered a safe drug during pregnancy and, to date, there are no reports of teratogenesis in humans. However, caution is advised in digitalis administration, because overdose can be detrimental to the mother and may be lethal to the fetus.[3]

Digoxin is excreted in the breast milk and the milk plasma ratio ranged from 0.59 to 0.9.[4,29] The total amount of digoxin ingested daily by the infant has been estimated to be approximately one out of 100 of pediatric recommend doses of 12.5 μg/kg for one day.[29] No apparent clinical effects were demonstrated in newborns. Therefore, digoxin therapy of the mother should not affect breast-feeding decisions.

QUINIDINE

Quinidine, a class IA antiarrhythmic drug, is effective in suppressing both supraventricular and ventricular arrhythmias. It is used for cardioversion, as well as prophylaxis against recurrences of paroxysmal supraventricular tachycardia, atrial flutter, atrial fibrillation, and reciprocating tachycardias associated with Wolff–Parkinson–White syndrome. It is frequently employed in suppressing ventricular premature beats and ventricular tachycardia.

Quinidine has no significant direct depressant effect on the myocardium unless large doses are given rapidly intravenously.[30] It decreases myocardial automaticity, excitability, and conduction velocity and increases the fibrillation threshold. The diminished conduction velocity and the increased effective refractory period induced by quinidine are very useful in terminating reentry.[31] Due to its vagolytic effects, the atrioventricular conduction may be enhanced in some patients. Quinidine also has alpha-adrenergic blocking effects which may result in vasodilation.

Approximately 70–80% of an oral dose of quinidine is absorbed.[32] Food and antacid may delay the absorption. In patients with congestive heart failure, the decreased volume of distribution (V_D) may lead to higher drug levels despite diminished absorption.[33] Maximum serum levels are attained within 60–90 minutes and the half-life is five to nine hours. Eighty percent is bound to protein; therefore, the unbound fraction increases during hypoalbuminemic conditions such as gestation. Quinidine is metabolized primarily in the liver and some of the metabolites are active. Ten to 20% is eliminated unchanged by the kidney[34] and alkalinization of the urine may decrease urinary excretion.[35] The therapeutic level is 3–6 μg/mL; levels greater than 7–8 μg/mL are associated with increased toxicity.

Unfortunately, quinidine has many adverse effects. Nausea, vomiting, and diarrhea can be disabling. Some patients may develop skin rashes, thrombocytopenia, hemolytic anemia, or fever. In 2–4% of patients, quinidine may produce syncope, most often due to polymorphic ventricular tachycardia ("torsade de pointes").[36,37] Among interactions with other drugs, of particular importance is the potentiation of warfarin effects and the elevation of digoxin blood concentration. The latter effect is due to a decrease in the volume of distribution, renal clearance, and afinity of tissue receptors for digoxin.[38,39] In up to 30% of the patients, the side effects are serious enough to discontinue therapy.

Quinidine has been used in pregnancy since 1930.[40] Several recent reports documented its transplacental transfer.[12,41,42] Hill et al[41] reported a case of quinidine treatment throughout the pregnancy to prevent maternal ventricular tachycardia. During pregnancy, maternal quinidine levels were fairly constant and ranged between 5.1 to 7.8 μg/mL. At delivery, the serum level in the neonate was 2.3 μg/mL and in amniotic fluid 9.3 μg/mL. Five days postpartum, maternal level rose to 9.0 μg/mL. The authors hypothesized that the high levels found in the amniotic fluid may have been due to fetal voiding or to a technical error in measurement of quinidine metabolites.

Spinnato et al[12] described three cases of fetal supraventricular tachycardia treated with digoxin and quinidine. In all three cases, the addition of quinidine to digoxin was successful in controlling fetal arrhythmia and in two of these fetuses, ascites as well. At delivery, maternal quinidine serum levels were 0.7–2.1 μg/mL, cord blood levels 0.5–1.6 μg/mL, and amniotic fluid level, 0.9 μg/mL. The low levels may be explained by the fact that quinidine was discontinued 24 hours prior to delivery. No side effects were noted; fetal development was normal and the labor was uneventful.

Guntheroth et al[43] described a successful case of quinidine cardioversion of fetal supraventricular tachycardia resistant to digoxin and propranolol. On a dose of 1600 mg/day, the maternal quinidine level was 4.5 μg/mL and cord blood level was 0.8 μg/mL (feto-maternal ratio 0.18). However, the drug levels were not collected simultaneously and the last maternal dose was given 18 hours prior to delivery. Killeen and Bowers[44] reported a case of 3-hydroxyquinidine (a metabolite of quinidine with antiarrhythmic activity) toxicity in a 33-week pregnant patient who was given very large doses of quinidine (up to 4500 mg/day) to treat fetal supraventricular tachycardia. The quinidine blood level was within low to midtherapeutic level but 3-hydroxyquinidine levels were substantially elevated. This patient demonstrated an unusually fast metabolism of quinidine to 3-hydroxyquinidine with subsequent quinidine toxicity despite low to midtherapeutic levels of quinidine. Simultaneous blood and amniotic fluid sampling revealed similar quinidine concentrations, 2.6 μg/mL and 2.2 μg/mL, respectively. At delivery (two days after discontinuation of quinidine), the cord blood quinidine level was only 37% of maternal level. The infant, who later was diagnosed to have an accessory atrioventricular bypass tract, tolerated the delivery well (Apgar score 8–9) and had no signs of quinidine toxicity. From the above reports, it appears that fetal quinidine blood levels are lower than maternal levels. However, the fetomaternal ratio is variable. The quinidine dosage for treatment of fetal tachyarrhythmias should be adjusted according to clinical response and careful monitoring of quinidine and its metabolites is recommended. Combination therapy with digoxin and quinidine should be considered in cases not responding to usual dosage of quinidine or digoxin.[12]

Quinidine has a minimal oxytoxic effect[40,45] which manifests mostly after the onset of spontaneous uterine contraction.[45] Fetal thrombocytopenia was also associated with quinidine treatment.[46] Toxic doses may cause premature labor[47], abortion[48], or damage to the fetal eighth cranial nerve.[49] Quinidine in therapeutic concentrations depresses pseudocholinesterase activity by 60–70%.[50] This additional effect on the already low level of pseudocholinesterase activity induced by gestation may affect the hydrolysis of esther-type anesthetics (procaine, tetracaine, chloroprocaine) and the duration of action of succinylcholine, with potential toxicity during epidural or general anesthesia.[50-52]

However, large clinical experience with the use of this drug in pregnancy has shown low incidence of side effects and no known teratogenic effects. Prudent quinidine use appears to be safe for both maternal and fetal indications. Quinidine is secreted in the breast milk and the milk plasma ratio is 0.71.[41]

PROCAINAMIDE

Procainamide, synthesized from procaine by substituting an esther linkage with an amide group, was introduced as an antiarrhythmic agent in 1951.[53] The drug is very effective in abolishing premature ventricular contractions, ventricular tachycardia, and reciprocating tachycardias associated with Wolff–Parkinson–White syndrome.[54]

It has a depressant effect on the heart, and similar to quinidine, it decreases automaticity, excitability, conduction velocity, and contractility. The effective refractory period is prolonged and the fibrillation threshold increased. Its anticholinergic activity is less than that of quinidine.

Procainamide can be given orally and parenterally. Following oral administration, approximately 75–95% of the dose is absorbed. The absorption may be retarded with delayed gastric emptying, decreased intestinal motility, or intestinal changes.[55] Only 10–20% is bound to plasma proteins. Peak levels are reached in 45–75 minutes after an oral capsule dose. Half-life is about three to five hours in patients with no evidence of heart or kidney failure. Therapeutic levels are 4–10 μg/mL. Approximately 40–70% of a procainamide dose is eliminated unchanged by the kidneys. Therefore, renal impairment may markedly decrease the elimination with consequent increase in serum levels. Ten to 34% of the drug is metabolized in the liver to N-acetylprocainamide (NAPA)[56] at a variable rate depending on acetylator status. NAPA has less antiarrhythmic potency and its efficacy is limited. However, the treatment with NAPA does not induce antinuclear antibody formation or lupus syndrome[57], as does procainamide. NAPA is 85% eliminated by the kidneys; its therapeutic range is 9.4–19.5 μg/mL. Congestive heart failure and renal impairment prolong both procainamide and NAPA half-lives.[58] In order to avoid toxicity, both procainamide and NAPA levels have to be closely monitored.

Procainamide may be administrated intravenously as a loading dose of 15 mg/kg of body weight at a rate of 25–50 mg/min, followed by continuous maintenance infusion of 2–4 mg/min. Intravenous administration may produce hypotension, QT interval prolongation, and serious arrhythmias.[59] Nausea, vomiting, and diarrhea are noted more frequently with the oral route but are less pronounced than with quinidine. Central nervous system (CNS) toxicity may manifest as mental depression, hallucinations, and psychosis. Hypersensitivity reactions such as drug fever, agranulocytosis, and skin rashes may occur and drug-induced lupus may develop in 20–40% of the patients.[59]

Transplacental transfer of procainamide is well documented in two reports of treatment of fetal supraventricular tachycardia.[60,61] Dumesic et al[60] reported successful control of fetal supraventricular tachycardia and heart failure when procainamide was administrated to the mother in addition to digoxin. The fetal arrhythmia was refractory to previous treatment with digoxin alone or in combination with propranolol. After four weeks of treatment, the arrhythmia recurred and became more difficult to control despite increased dose of digoxin and procainamide. At delivery, while digoxin levels were equal in the mother and neonate blood (0.8 μg/mL), procainamide level was higher in maternal blood (15.6 μg/mL versus 4.3 μg/mL in fetus). A similar therapeutic approach was also reported by Given et al.[61] Fetal supraventricular tachycardia resistant to the combination of digoxin and propranolol converted with digoxin and procainamide. Also in this case, fetal tachyarrhythmia recurred. However, the digoxin and procainamide levels at delivery were discordant with those found by Dumesic. Fetal levels were 30% higher for procainamide and 50% lower for digoxin. NAPA levels in the maternal and fetal blood were 3.0 μg/mL and 3.7 μg/mL, respectively. At the present time, there is no evidence of teratogenic effects[62,63] and the drug appears to be safe in pregnancy.[40,64,65] However, due to limited information available and serious potential maternal side effects, procainamide should be used as a second line antiarrhythmic drug.

Translactal passage of procainamide was reported by Pittard and Glazier.[66] They found a milk plasma ratio of 4.3 ± 2.4 for procainamide and of 3.8 ± 1.8 for NAPA. Although the high ratio milk plasma may suggest accumulation in the milk of both procainamide and NAPA, the amount daily ingested by the infant is not expected to produce a significant plasma levels.[66]

DISOPYRAMIDE

Disopyramide, structurally different from quinidine and procainamide class IA antiarrhythmic drugs, was approved in 1977 for the treatment of ventricular arrhythmias in the United States. For suppression of premature ventricular contractions (PVCs), it appears equal to or better than quinidine or procainamide.[67] During myocardial infarction, it is useful in reducing PVCs and the frequency of ventricular tachycardia. However, it is not clear if it can prevent ventricular fibrillation.[68] In Europe, it was found to be equal to quinidine in the treatment and prophylaxis of supraventricular arrhythmias.[69,70]

Disopyramide has similar electrophysiologic properties to other class IA antiarrhythmic agents. It decreases excitability, conduction velocity, automaticity, and contractility. It also prolongs effective refractory period and action potential duration. It has marked negative inotropic effect and increases the systemic vascular resistance.[71,72] These hemodynamic effects, while not clinically evident in patients with normal ventricular function, may be deleterious in patients with limited cardiac function.[73] Disopyramide has 10% of the anticholinergic effects of atropine.[74] Approximately 80–90% of an oral dose is absorbed; peak plasma levels are reached by one to two hours, and the half-life is about six to nine hours. Approximately 30% was found to be bound to plasma proteins at a concentration of 3 μg/mL; however, the binding varies directly with serum concentration and may be as high as 90%.[59] Forty to 90% is eliminated in the urine unchanged, therefore, the dosage has to be adjusted in renal failure. The remainder of the drug is metabolized in the liver via dealkylation.[75] Therapeutic levels are 2–5 μg/mL. The oral dose is 400–1200 mg/day. This dose has to be reduced to hepatic, cardiac, or renal insufficiency.

The most common untoward effects of disopyramide are due to its anticholinergic activity and include dry mouth, constipation, blurred vision, and urinary retention. It may precipitate congestive heart failure in patients with ventricular dysfunction[73] and, similar to quinidine, can induce QT prolongation, ventricular tachycardia, and "torsade de pointes."[76,77]

There is very little information regarding disopyramide treatment in pregnant women. Shaxted et al[78] described a 26-week pregnant patient treated with 600 mg/day for symptomatic ventricular tachycardia. At delivery, the maternal and fetal levels were 2.3 μg/mL and 0.9 μg/mL, respectively (feto-maternal ratio of 0.39). No adverse effects were noted and the delivery was normal. Ellsworth et al[79] reported a 27-year-old woman with a history of exertional ventricular fibrillation treated throughout the pregnancy with disopyramide. The pregnancy course was uneventful. At delivery, on a dose of 1350 mg/day, the maternal and fetal blood levels were 2.7 μg/mL and 0.7 μg/mL, respectively (feto-maternal ratio of 0.26). The neonate had no evidence of congenital abnormalities or intrauterine growth retardation. However, Leonard et al[80] reported the treatment of refractory supraventricular tachycardia in a pregnant woman with mitral valve prolapse in which the administration of disopyramide initiated uterine contractions that resolved when the drug was discontinued.

Disopyramide is secreted in the breast milk in similar concentrations to plasma; no adverse effects were noted in the infant.[79,81-83]

Due to the limited information, the use of disopyramide in pregnancy should be limited to patients with arrhythmias refractory to alternative safer drug therapy.

LIDOCAINE

Lidocaine is a local anesthetic of the amide type which has been used as an antiarrhythmic agent since 1950. It is one of the most common drugs used in the intensive cardiac care unit. Lidocaine is effective in suppressing ventricular premature beats and ventricular tachyarrhythmias, particularly during acute myocardial infarction, cardiac surgery, and digitalis toxicity.[84] Lidocaine depresses automaticity in Purkinje fibers and increases the threshold for ventricular fibrillation.[85] Action potential duration is decreased significantly, and to a lesser extent, also effective refractory period (ERP) in both Purkinje fibers and ventricular muscle. The effect on the ERP of atrioventricular node is variable. Lidocaine effectively decreases conduction velocity and suppresses ventricular reentry in ischemic myocardium. There is no apparent effect on blood pressure or contractility.[86] Lidocaine is administrated parenterally; oral administration is ineffective because of extensive metabolism during first pass through the liver. It has immediate onset of action and its half-life is appproximately 100 minutes. A loading dose of 1–1.5 μg/kg of body weight is followed by continuous infusion. A second dose, usually half of the first dose, may be necessary. Lidocaine is 70% bound to proteins, principally to alpha$_1$-acid glycoprotein and its clearance approximates hepatic blood flow. Therefore, any condition or drug that decreases hepatic blood flow, such as liver disease, congestive heart failure, propranolol[87], or cimetidine[88] may decrease lidocaine clearance. Prolonged infusion of lidocaine for several days may also decrease its hepatic clearance; therefore, the dose should be adjusted after 24, 48, and 72 hours.[89,90]

Lidocaine is metabolized in the liver to two compounds: glycinexylidide and monoethylglycinexylidide. Both metabolites are less active than lidocaine[91]; however, they may contribute to its antiarrhythmic activity and CNS toxicity.[92] About 10% of lidocaine undergoes kidney excretion unchanged.

Lidocaine in toxic doses may produce myocardial depression and hypotensions; however, the main target is CNS. Paresthesias, blurred vision, dizziness, drowsiness, hallucination, tremor, and seizures may manifest when levels are 5 μg/mL or above.[59]

Lidocaine has mainly been used during pregnancy for epidural or local anesthesia. Stokes et al[93] reported the use of lidocaine as an antiarrhythmic agent in an 18-week pregnant woman who suffered an acute myocardial infarction and cardiac arrest. The infant was delivered at 38 weeks' gestation with some growth retardation but had normal neurological examination at birth and at 17 months. Menon et al[94] described a 15-year-old pregnant patient successfully treated with intravenous lidocaine for paroxysmal ventricular tachycardia. Juneja et al[95] reported a 20-year-old patient with frequent ventricular ectopy and runs of nonsustained ventricular tachycardia which increased in frequency during uterine contractions. The ventricular arrhythmia was controlled with continuous epidural infusion of 0.375% lidocaine. The plasma lidocaine concentration ranged between 1.2–3 μg/mL. Subsequently, fetal heart rate showed late deceleration and the scalp blood pH was 7.27. Cesarean section was performed and a 3680-g neonate with an Apgar score of 8 was delivered.

The drug crosses the placenta rapidly.[96,97] Following maternal administration, it can be detected in the umbilical cord in two minutes[98] and fetomaternal plasma concentration ratio is 0.5–0.7. The lower fetal concentrations of lidocaine may be due to lower fetal concentration of alpha$_1$-acid glycoprotein, which is approximately one third of maternal levels.[12] This hypothesis is supported by Tucker[98] who has found a lower binding capacity of fetal plasma for lidocaine. However, Shnider et al[96], using ultrafiltration techniques, demonstrated similar binding capacities of both fetal and maternal plasma. Lidocaine's metabolism in the fetus is also hepatic.

Shnider et al[99], in a study of 57 mothers treated with lidocaine, observed five infants with CNS depression at birth. Three of these infants had a lidocaine level greater than 3 μg/mL. No apparent evidence of CNS toxicity was noted when the fetal level was below 2.5 μg/mL. The therapeutic range of lidocaine in the nonpregnant state is 1–5 μg/mL. If the fetal plasma concentration is 50–60% of the maternal level, it is probably safe to have maternal levels below 4 μg/mL in order to avoid maternofetal toxicity.

As a weak base, lidocaine may be trapped by the slightly acidic environment of amniotic fluid. Several studies[97,100,101] have shown higher fetal drug concentration during fetal acidosis. In addition, acidosis may increase the unbound fraction of lidocaine facilitating further fetal trapping.[102]

Most reports of lidocaine toxicity in fetuses are associated with maternal paracervical, caudal, and pudendal anesthesia. Bozynski et al[103] described a neonate with severe lidocaine toxicity delivered 20 minutes after administration of 20 cc of 1% lidocaine for pudendal block. The neonate developed apnea and bradycardia soon after birth, requiring mechanical ventilation and intensive supportive therapy. Fetal lidocaine level was 2–3 μg/mL. The infant recovered completely within a few days. At two months follow up, his physical examination was normal. Kim et al[104] described a case of accidental lidocaine injection of the fetal scalp during local anesthesia for episiotomy. Fifteen minutes after birth, the newborn manifested severe toxicity, evidenced by apnea, hypotonia, and fixed dilated pupils, and then, at one hour, seizures. Fetal lidocaine level was 14 μg/mL. With appropriate treatment, the neonate recovered completely with normal neurological and behavioral examinations at three days and at seven months of age. The Collaborative Perinatal Project surveyed 50,282 mothers, of whom 293 had exposure to lidocaine during their first trimester.[62] Lidocaine administration could not be associated with increased risk of any major group of malformations. However, anomalies of the respiratory system (three cases), tumors (two cases), and inguinal hernias (eight cases) had greater frequency than expected. Several studies showed that lidocaine does not have deleterious neurobehavioral effects on neonates.[105,106] Despite the paucity of information on lidocaine's use as an antiarrhythmic agent during pregnancy, the data illustrated above indicate that lidocaine is safe as long as blood levels are closely monitored.

MEXILETINE

Mexiletine, a class Ib antiarrhythmic drug, is structurally very similar to lidocaine. Initially studied as an anticonvulsant drug, it soon became evident that mexiletine possesses antiarrhythmic properties resembling those of lidocaine. It is effective in suppressing ventricular premature beats and ventricular tachycardia. Its antiarrhythmic activity seems to be independent of the nature of underlying cardiac condition, that is, it has equal effectiveness in acute and chronic ischemic heart disease, as well as cardiomyopathy.[107,108] Mexiletine has a membrane stabilizing effect, a manifestation of its local anesthetic properties. It slows maximal rate of depolarization of the action potential and shortens the action potential duration in Purkinje fibers.[107-117] In patients with a compromised atrioventricular node or His–Purkinje systems the conduction velocities are decreased and the effective refractory periods may be increased. It has no effect on the normal sinus node. However, patients with diseased sinus nodes may develop sinus arrest.[108] Mexiletine has no apparent hemodynamic effects[108,117], and does not significantly affect the ejection fraction in patients with left ventricular dysfunction.[118]

Mexiletine is almost completely absorbed in the proximal small bowel. The delayed gastric emptying that occurs in pregnancy may retard the absorption. The peak level is reached after 1.5 hours.[113] Seventy-five percent of the drug is protein-bound. First pass hepatic metabolism is only 10%, with bioavailability of 90% following oral administration. The drug is metabolized in the liver. The renal clearance of the unchanged drug is highly dependent on urinary pH, varying from 35% in the acid urine to 1% in alkaline urine.[114] The half-life is eight to ten hours in the normal subject, but it may be prolonged to 15 hours in patients with myocardial infarction.[115] The therapeutic range is 0.75–2 μg/mL, and it has a narrow toxic-therapeutic window. Following a loading oral dose of 400 mg, a daily dose of 450–1200 mg should be sufficient to achieve therapeutic levels. The dosage has to be reduced in chronic liver disease.[116]

The adverse effects of mexiletine may occur in 30–40% of the patients and are related to plasma concentration. Tremor, diplopia, dizziness, paresthesia, nausea, and vomiting are particularly frequent. Ataxia, sleep disturbances, fatigue, headache, psychosis, seizures, fever, and rashes have also been reported. Thrombocytopenia and hepatitis are rare complications. Mexiletine is also arrhythmogenic; some authors reported induction of "torsade de pointes."[117,119]

In 1980, Timis et al[109] reported a case of successfully treated ventricular tachycardia in a 32-week pregnant patient given a daily dose of propranolol 120 mg and mexiletine 600 mg. On this regimen, the trough plasma concentration of mexiletine was 0.3–0.6 μg/l. At 39 weeks of pregnancy, the patient went into spontaneous labor and delivered a normal child. At delivery, the maternal and fetal mexiletine levels were equal (0.3 μg/mL). For six hours postdelivery, the infant heart rate was only 90 beats per minute. Thereafter, it rose to 120 beats per minute and remained stable throughout puerperium. In another report[110], mexiletine and propranolol were used to suppress ventricular tachycardia resistant to procainamide in a 14-week pregnant woman. The patient gave birth to a healthy boy and no maternal or fetal adverse effects could be noted. Lownes and Ives[111] described a 26-year-old woman with a history of mitral valve prolapse, ventricular ectopy, and ventricular tachycardia treated with mexiletine 750 mg/day and atenolol 50 mg/day throughout her conception, pregnancy, and postnatal course. During prenatal evaluations, the fetus was thought to be small-for-gestational-age. At 39 weeks, she delivered vaginally a healthy male infant weighing 2600 g with an Apgar score of 9 and 10 at one and five minutes, respectively. Serum mexiletine levels of the mother on admission and of the child nine hours postpartum were < 0.2 and 0.4 μg/mL, respectively. During the immediate postpartum period, the infant had failure to feed and at eight months was reevaluated for seizurelike episodes. He had normal neurologic examination and normal electroencephalogram, but was found to have gastroesophageal reflux. Subsequently, the baby developed normally. Gregg and Tomich[112] described another patient with mitral valve prolapse and symptomatic premature ventricular contractions treated with mexiletine prior to conception and throughout the pregnancy. The dose of mexiletine was increased throughout the pregnancy from 300 mg/day at the time of conception to 800 mg/day at delivery. During cesarean section delivery (done at 38 weeks' gestation), lidocaine was added to control her ventricular ectopy. A male infant weighing 3750 g with an Apgar score of 4 and 9 was delivered. Subsequently, hypoglycemia in the newborn period was noted and corrected. At delivery, the maternal and cord blood mexiletine levels were 0.6 and 0.4 μg/mL, respectively. In summary, mexiletine appears to freely cross the placenta, and fetomaternal ratio ranges from 0.7 to 1.[109,112] Although the use of mexiletine during pregnancy was initially thought to be safe[109], the reported fetal bradycardia, small-for-gestational-age[111], low Apgar score, and neonatal hypoglycemia[112] were particularly bothersome. Despite these concerns, no teratogenic or long-term adverse consequences have been reported.

Mexiletine is secreted in breast milk. Both Timis et al[109] and Lewis et al[110] found higher concentrations of mexiletine in the breast milk than in mothers' plasma; the milk-plasma ratio varied between 0.78 and 1.89.[109] However, the calculated daily quantity ingested by the infant appears to be way below therapeutic range[110] and mexiletine levels were undetectable in the infant blood.[109] Due to very limited experience with this drug, no recommendation can be made until its safety in pregnancy and lactation is further documented.

AMIODARONE

Amiodarone, a benzofuran derivative, is a very effective class III antiarrhythmic agent. It has been widely employed in Europe in the management of various supraventricular and ventricular arrhythmias. The US Food and Drug Administration has approved the drug for oral treatment of life-threatening ventricular tachycardia and fibrillation refractory to other drugs.

Amiodarone prolongs the duration of action potential and reduces the maximum rate of depolarization.[120] It increases refractory period and prolongs repolarization.[121] It does not affect resting membrane potential. It depresses the sinus node and prolongs PR, QRS, and QTc intervals.[122,123] In patients with Wolff–Parkinson–White syndrome, it increases the antegrade and retrograde refractory periods of accessory pathways.[124]

Amiodarone has noncompetitive alpha-adrenergic and beta-adrenergic blocking activity, and it is a potent coronary and systemic vasodilator.[125] It also reduces myocardial contractility and heart rate and may lower the blood pressure.

Absorption of amiodarone following oral administration is variable and unpredictable. However, it is estimated to be approximately 40%. Its oral bioavailability ranges from 22 to 86%.[126,127] Peak plasma concentration is reached within two to 10 hours, but a therapeutic effect may take up to 21 days to occur. The metabolism of amiodarone is not fully elucidated. After absorption, the drug is widely distributed into various tissues. Being lipophilic, it accumulates mostly in adipose tissues but is also extensively taken up by the lung, the liver, and cardiac and skeletal muscle.[126] The drug undergoes hepatic metabolism and of its metabolites, the desethylamiodarone (DEA) accumulates in plasma during chronic therapy. Only 1% of the dose is excreted unchanged in the urine. Biliary excretion probably plays an important role.[126] Protein binding is about 96%.[127] The elimination half-life ranges from 13 to 100 days, with an average of 40–50 days.[126] Amiodarone and DEA are not dialysable. Doses do not need to be reduced in patients with renal insufficiency. To initiate oral treatment, a loading dose of 800–1600 mg per day is given for one to three weeks, then the dose decreases to 800 mg per day for two to four weeks, then 600 mg daily for four to eight weeks, and, thereafter, to a maintenance dose of 400 mg per day. The therapeutic plasma levels are 1–2.5 μg/mL.[128]

Amiodarone has numerous adverse effects.[129] The most severe is pulmonary fibrosis that carries a 10% mortality and may be reversible if the drug is discontinued. Amiodarone may produce sinus bradycardia, AV block, QT prolongation, and "torsade de pointes." Anorexia, nausea, vomiting, and elevation of transaminases are common. Amiodarone has high iodine content, ie, 75 mg of elemental iodine in a 200 mg dose of drug; both hypo- and hyperthroidism may occur. Corneal microdeposits might affect the patient's vision. Photosensitivity and bluish gray discoloration of the skin develop frequently. CNS toxicity (tremor, ataxia, and dizziness) or peripheral neuropathy are uncommon, but reported.

Amiodarone interacts with numerous drugs.[130] It potentiates the effects of warfarin and increases serum concentration of digoxin, diltiazem, quinidine, procainamide, and phenytoin.

The adverse effects may persist months after discontinuation of the drug.

The use of amiodarone during pregnancy has been documented in several reports.[128,131-138] McKenna et al[131] treated a 34-week pregnant woman who had paroxysms of atrial flutter-fibrillation associated with Wolff–Parkinson–White syndrome and resistant to quinidine. A loading dose of 800 mg per day for one week was followed by a maintenance dose of 400 mg per day. At 41 weeks, the patient delivered a normal child that was slightly bradycardic for 48 hours (104–120 beats/min). Amiodarone and desethylamiodarone plasma levels in the infant at birth were approximately 25% of the mother's levels.

Pitcher et al[128] also reported a case of successful treatment with amiodarone of atrial tachycardia resistant to propranolol, digoxin, and verapamil during the last three weeks of pregnancy. Transplacental transfer of amiodarone and DEA was 10% and 25%, respectively. Neither the mother nor the child had untoward effects.

Robson et al[132] described two additional cases in which amiodarone was administrated during pregnancy for longer periods. In the first case, amiodarone was given at a dose of 200 mg per day to control atrial fibrillation associated with mitral stenosis. The patient became pregnant while on treatment and the drug was continued through the pregnancy. At 34 weeks, she delivered a healthy baby. Maternal levels through pregnancy were 0.5–0.7 mg/mL. Cord level was 0.05 mg/mL and amniotic fluid level was 0.02 mg/mL. Desethylamiodarone levels in maternal plasma, cord blood, and amniotic fluid were 0.8 mg/l, 0.15 mg/l, and 0.11 mg/l, respectively. In the second case, amiodarone (400 mg/day) was given in addition to metoprolol (50 mg/day) to control atrial tachycardia in a 22-week pregnant patient. At 39 weeks, she delivered a healthy child. Again, amiodarone and DEA levels in cord blood were 10% and 20% of maternal levels, respectively.

Rey et al[133] reported a 19-year-old pregnant patient treated with propranolol 80 mg/day and amiodarone 400 mg/day four days a week for recurrent ventricular tachycardia. Throughout the pregnancy, the patient developed diffuse thyroid enlargement but she was clinically euthyroid and thyroid function tests were normal. The patient delivered a healthy 2670 g baby with no signs of amiodarone toxicity. At delivery, despite a high iodine content, maternal and fetal thyroid function tests were normal. Foster and Love[134] described a 32-week pregnant patient treated with amiodarone 400 mg/day for ventricular ectopy and self-limiting ventricular tachycardia. A healthy neonate was delivered at 37 weeks by cesarean section. The infant's heart rate varied from 40 to 163 beats/minute during the following four days postdelivery, and the corrected QT interval was 58 seconds. Amiodarone and DEA levels in the fetal cord blood were 0.1 mg/l and 0.2 mg/l, respectively. Although these initial reports showing no fetal adverse effects were encouraging, other authors reported a less favorable neonatal outcome.[135,136] DeWolf et al[135] reported a severe case of congenital hypothyroidism with goiter, associated with maternal ingestion of 200 mg daily from the 13th week of pregnancy. The baby also had persistent hypotonia and bradycardia, large anterior and posterior fontanels and macroglossia. Cord blood TSH was >100 mU/l (normal range: 10–20), T_4 was 35.9 μg/l (normal range: 60–170), and thyroid antibody were absent. Iodine content in the fetal urine was 144 μg/DL (normal value: <15). Amiodarone and DEA levels drawn on the fifth day postdelivery were 0.65 μg/mL and 0.45 μg/mL, respectively. Bone maturation was 28 weeks. The infant required substitution therapy with levothyroxine up to 20 months of age. At that time, its thyroid function tests were normal, but his psychomotor development revealed four months retardation and a bone age of 12 months. Laurent et al[136] reported another case of neonatal hypothyroidism following treatment with digoxin 0.5 mg/day and amiodarone 1200 mg/day for three days and 600 mg/day for three weeks, for control of fetal supraventricular tachycardia and congestive heart failure. At 35 weeks, a 2960 g infant was delivered. The infant had a heart rate of 200 beats/min; mild heart failure and goiter thyroid function tests revealed hypothyroidism. With proper thyroxine replacements, the infant recovered completely by three months of age.

The use of amiodarone for the treatment of fetal supraventricular tachycardia was attempted in several cases.[137-139] Arnoux et al[137] described a case of fetal supraventricular tachycardia and congestive heart failure resistant to digoxin alone or in combination with either sotalol or verapamil that was successfully treated with digoxin and amiodarone. Amiodarone was started at 31 weeks of pregnancy and continued until term (38 weeks). A normal infant was delivered with amiodarone level of 12.7% of maternal level. The comparison of doses and fetomaternal levels showed a linear concentration-dosage relation. Therefore, maternal levels may be used as an indicator for fetal levels. Rey et al[139] described a case of fetal supraventricular tachycardia resistant to digoxin alone and in combination with propranolol successfully treated with verapamil and amiodarone. The patient delivered spontaneously, at 33 weeks of gestation, a male infant weighing 2700 g with an Apgar score of 8 and 9. No drug levels were obtained.

In summary, amiodarone crosses the placenta and fetal levels reach approximately 10–25% of maternal levels. The concentration of amiodarone in the placenta is higher than in adipose tissue, but the significance of this finding is not clear. Plasma iodine concentrations were found to be elevated in both maternal and fetal cord blood.[133,135] Maternal amiodarone toxicity is similar to that in nonpregnant patients. Potential problems may arise, however, if epidural or general anesthesia is required during cesarean or vaginal delivery.[140] General anesthesia in patients receiving amiodarone has been associated with increased morbidity and mortality. Interaction between amiodarone and anesthetics have been observed during anesthesia for both cardiac and noncardiac surgery. Sinus arrest, junctional rhythms, heart block, atropine resistant bradycardias, persistent hypotension, and a blunted response to phenylephrine are some of the complications reported. Epidural anesthesia is safer, but maximum precautions should be taken to avoid any alteration of patient's hemodynamics.

The reports of neonatal hypothyroidism[135,136], premature birth[136,139], and other adverse effects described above, cast doubts on aminodarone safety during pregnancy. Pending further studies, amiodarone should be used with extreme caution in life-threatening, refractory maternal or fetal tachyarrhythmias. Close monitoring of maternal and neonate thyroid function tests and thyroid size are of paramount importance to avoid the consequences of neonatal hypothyroidism.

Amiodarone is secreted in breast milk in quantities significant enough to be detected in infant blood.[131] The effect of chronic amiodarone exposure in neonates is unknown; therefore, breast feeding is not recommended to women who are treated with amiodarone.

VERAPAMIL

Verapamil, a papaverine derivative and a calcium entry blocking agent, was initially used in the 1960s as an antianginal agent. The drug was approved in the United States in 1981 for angina pectoris and supraventricular tachyarrhythmias. It is very effective in terminating atrioventricular nodal and reciprocating tachycardias.[141] In patients with atrial flutter or fibrillation and multifocal atrial tachycardia, verapamil slows the ventricular response and sometimes causes conversion in sinus rhythm.[141] Generally, it is not used for ventricular arrhythmias unless they are precipitated by coronary spasm or triggered activity. Other indications are angina, hypertension, and hypertrophic cardiomyopathy.

Verapamil blocks the slow influx of calcium and probably of sodium in the sinus and atrioventricular nodes.[142] It decreases the conduction velocity and increases the refractory period in nodal tissue. The direct effect of slowing the sinus node could, however, be partially offset by sympathetic activation secondary to peripheral vasodilation.

Oral verapamil is absorbed quite completely, is 90% bound to proteins, and peak levels are reached in one to two hours. However, during first pass through the liver, it is extensively eliminated. Therefore, the drug has a bioavailability of only 10–35%. In the liver, the drug is metabolized to several compounds, of which norverapamil is most active. The elimination half-lives of verapamil and norverapamil are two to five hours and eight to ten hours, respectively. The hepatic metabolism of verapamil may decrease with chronic administration. In the patient with advanced liver disease (ie, cirrhosis), the half-life of verapamil may increase dramatically up to 14–16 hours or more.[143] The onset of action with intravenous (IV) preparation is five to fifteen minutes and its duration is approximately six hours.[144] The usual dose employed is 0.15 mg/kg given intravenously at 1 mg/min.

In patients with compromised sinus or AV node, verapamil may precipitate bradycardia, asystole, or AV block because of the vasodilatory effect of the drug or it may cause hypotension. The most frequent noncardiac side effects are headache, dizziness, nausea, constipation, and peripheral edema. It may induce galactorrhea and hyperprolactinemia.[145] The drug reduces renal clearance of digoxin and, therefore, results in a substantial increase in serum digoxin concentration.

The majority of reports regarding verapamil administration during pregnancy are from Europe. The drug has been used for various indications: maternal and fetal supraventricular arrhythmia[146-148], premature labor[149,150], severe preeclampsia[151], or severe postpartum gestational proteinuric hypertension.[152]

Klein et al[146] described a 38-year-old hyperthyroid pregnant patient treated with verapamil for supraventricular tachycardia resistant to digoxin and propranolol. The arrhythmia converted to sinus rhythm after 5 mg of intravenous verapamil. The fetal monitoring tracing showed a transient decrease in fetal heart rate but no decelerations. One month later, she delivered uneventfully. In an attempt to investigate the pharmacokinetics of verapamil during pregnancy, Wolff et al[148] administered a single 80 mg oral dose to six women during the first state of labor. The infants were born 49–564 minutes after drug administration and their umbilical-vein verapamil levels were 17–26% of maternal levels. However, during chronic administration of oral verapamil, the fetal levels may reach 30–40% of maternal levels.[153]

Transplacental passage of verapamil forms the basis for *in utero* treatment of fetal tachycardias. The experience with use of verapamil for fetal supraventricular tachycardia has been steadily growing[14-16,139,141,147,148,153-155] and many authors consider verapamil alone or in combination with digoxin the second choice after digoxin.[14,16] In a series of hydropic fetuses due to fetal tachyarrhythmias, the combination therapy with verapamil and digoxin was successful in achieving cardioversion in approximately two thirds of the patients.[16] In another series of 14 cases[153], six were controlled on digoxin alone, six on combination with digoxin and verapamil, and the remaining two cases with digoxin and propranolol. Maternal adverse effects from verapamil resemble those seen in nonpregnant patients. Although dysfunctional labor or postpartum hemorrhage attributable to verapamil have not been reported, some authors prefer to discontinue the drug at the onset of labor.[153] To date, no teratogenic effects have been described and verapamil appears to be safe for acute managment of maternal and fetal arrhythmias. More data is necessary to establish the safety of chronic therapy during pregnancy. Verapamil lowers digoxin renal clearance and consequently increases digoxin serum concentration. Therefore, close monitoring of therapy is necessary in patients receiving concomitant therapy with these two drugs.

Verapamil is excreted in breast milk[156-158]; its concentration ranges from 23 to 94% of maternal blood concentration.[156,158] The estimated total amount of verapamil secreted in milk is less than 0.01–0.04% of the administered dose. The amount of verapamil ingested by infants is minimal and no pharmacological effects have been observed in neonates.

PROPRANOLOL

Propranolol, a nonselective beta-blocker, has been extensively used in the treatment of various conditions occurring during pregnancy, such as dysfunctional labor[159], hypertension[160-165], thyrotoxicosis[160,166,167], hypertrophic cardiomyopathy[168,169], and maternal[160,170,171] and fetal[60,61,147,148,153,171] supraventricular tachyarrhythmias. However, with some exceptions[172], the treatment of fetal tachyarrhythmias was rather disappointing.[147] Propranolol is a class II antiarrhythmic drug and beta-adrenergic receptor blockade appears to be the main mechanism for its antiarrhythmic effect.[59] However, a membrane-stabilizing effect may also be involved, particularly at higher concentrations.[84,173]

Propranolol decreases automaticity in the sinus node and the Purkinje fibers and increases the effective refractory period of atrial and AV nodal tissue. This latter effect is the main mechanism in abolishing paroxysmal supraventricular tachycardia due to AV nodal reentry. The responsiveness in Purkinje fibers is decreased at concentrations of propranolol much higher than those required to obtain beta adrenergic blockade (1000–3000 ng/mL versus 100–300 ng/mL).[173]

Propranolol lowers blood pressure by several mechanisms including a decrease in myocardial contractility and heart rate[84,162], inhibition of renin secretion, and blockade of peripheral presynaptic beta-adrenoreceptors.

Propranolol is almost completely absorbed from the gastrointestinal tract but due to extensive metabolism during first pass through the liver, only one third enters into systemic circulation. Its estimated bioavailability is 20–50%. Peak plasma concentrations are reached within 60–90 minutes and the half-life is three to six hours. The drug is 90–95% bound to proteins, mostly to $alpha_1$ acid glycoproteins.

The hepatic metabolism is probably dependent on saturable mechanisms[174] and is highly variable in different patients. Propranolol clearance approximates that of hepatic blood flow. Chronic administration of propranolol may decrease its hepatic extraction and may lead to an increase in its half-life.[175] Among various propranolol metabolites, the 4-hydroxypropranolol appears to have beta-blocking activity but has a short half-life.

Due to individual variation, there is a wide therapeutic range. A serum concentration of 40–80 μg/mL is probably sufficient to control premature ventricular beats. However, for ventricular tachycardia, levels of more than 1000 ng/mL may be necessary.[176] In the management of hypertension, 20–80 mg orally four times per day is usually sufficient. However, doses up to 640 mg/day may be required. Intravenous administration is used mostly to control tachyarrhythmias and ischemia. Doses up to 0.15–0.2 mg/kg can be given very slowly with frequent monitoring of blood pressure and cardiac function. Propranolol may precipitate heart failure in the patient with systolic ventricular dysfunction. In patients with diseased AV node or who are treated concomitantly with digitalis, propranolol may cause complete AV block. It may increase airway resistance and is contraindicated in patients with bronchospastic conditions. The penetration into the CNS may cause depression, insomnia, vivid dreams, and hallucinations. Fatigue and decreased exercise tolerance may also occur. It increases serum triglycerides and decreases HDL cholesterol. Allergic disorders and rare and blood dyscrasias are infrequently reported. Sudden withdrawal may be dangerous, especially in the patient with ischemic heart disease. The drug masks sympathetically mediated recovery of hypoglycemia and delays recovery of blood glucose in this condition and, therefore, caution is recommended in patients with diabetes mellitus.

During pregnancy, propranolol may affect uterine contractility. In the myometrium, the alpha and $beta_2$ receptors mediate opposite effects; alpha-receptor stimulation induces smooth muscle contraction and, consequently, increases uterine tone, whereas, beta-receptor stimulation produces relaxation. Barden et al[177] has demonstrated that propranolol given to pregnant women blocks the inhibitory effects of epinephrine on myometrial activity. Therefore, its administration may facilitate an increase in uterine activity. The clinical importance of these findings and the potential risk for premature labor is not clear.

The pharmacokinetics of propranolol during pregnancy is similar to the nonpregnant state. O'Hare et al[178] administered propranolol to six healthy pregnant volunteers between 32 and 36 weeks of gestation. There were no significant changes in elimination half-life, clearance, volume of distribution (V_D), and bioavailability. However, Perruca et al[179] found that protein binding of propranolol is decreased during pregnancy.

Propranolol readily crosses the placenta[160,167,170,172,180,181], and at delivery, the fetal serum concentration is equal[160,170] or less[172] than maternal concentration. The unbound fraction of propranolol is higher in fetal plasma, probably because of low concentration of alpha$_1$-acid glycoprotein. Because of decreased hepatic metabolism and altered protein binding, the serum concentration and the half-life of propranolol may be increased in the neonate during the first days of life.[160,180]

Several fetal and neonatal adverse effects were reported.[160-163, 169,181-184] Pruyn et al[160] noted that 10 of 11 neonates from mothers treated chronically with propranolol had intrauterine growth retardation. Extrapolating data from an animal study[185], they suggested that propranolol may decrease umbilical blood flow and consequently, fetal nutrition. While reported by many other authors[161-163,169,183,186], the true incidence of intrauterine growth retardation is unclear. In some prospective studies[161-163,169] the incidence of intrauterine growth retardation was only 3–4% (four of 94 pregnancies). Furthermore, two of these four mothers who had small babies delivered normal babies in subsequent pregnancies despite continuous treatment with propranolol.[169] There are many hypothetical mechanisms by which propranolol may induce growth retardation. A decrease in cardiac output, combined with plasma volume contraction and increased systemic vascular resistance occurring during hypertension in pregnancy, may decrease uterine blood flow.[186] Propranolol has been shown to reduce umbilical blood flow in pregnant ewes.[185] Other postulated mechanisms may involve a decreased peripheral conversion of T_4 to T_3 and a theoretical effect on neurotransmitters which may affect the brain's influence on fetal growth.[186] In spite of these theoretical considerations, Redmond[186] in an extensive review of human and animal literature, concluded that the evidence implicating propranolol in growth retardation is suggestive but inconclusive.

Turnstall et al[182] described a delay in the onset of respiration of newborns when propranolol was administrated to the mother prior to cesarean section. Another major source of concern is the effects of propranolol and of beta-blockade therapy, in general, on the fetal response to hypoxia. During asphyxia, several hormonal, metabolic, and circulatory adaptive mechanisms are activated. Most responses are mediated through catecholamines and beta receptors. As has been demonstrated in experimental animal studies[187,188], propranolol therapy may be particularly deleterious during these circumstances of fetal distress. Beta-blockade may also be responsible for lack of fetal heart acceleration provoked by sound stimulation[184] and persistently nonreactive nonstress test and contraction stress test.[183]

To date, propranolol was not demonstrated to be teratogenic. However, three cases of congenital malformations have been associated with propranolol therapy during pregnancy, for example, pyloric stenosis, crepitus of the hip, and tracheoesophageal fistula.[165,189,190] It is not clear at all if this is a coincidental occurrence or a true teratogenic effect of propranolol. In any case, if the last hypothesis is correct, these malformations are probably very rare.

Although the information concerning use of propranolol during pregnancy has expanded steadily, its safety is still somewhat controversial. Despite favorable reviews[165,191], there is a potential for the side effects[160,186,189,192] which should be anticipated by the clinician.

Propranolol is excreted in breast milk.[193-195] Karlberg et al[193] showed that propranolol is secreted into the breast milk in a dose-dependent manner and the milk-plasma ratio is approximately 1.0. Bauer et al[194] found a milk-plasma ratio of 0.4–0.6; they estimated that the daily dose ingested by the infant is probably 1% of the recommended pediatric daily dose. No adverse effects were observed in infants breast-fed by mothers treated with propranolol. However, the newborn hepatic microsomal enzyme systems are immature and propranolol may accumulate. Therefore, careful observation of these infants is recommended.

METOPROLOL

Metoprolol is a beta$_1$-selective adrenoreceptor-blocking agent. It is similar in its effectiveness to other nonselective beta-adrenoreceptor blocking drugs used in the treatment of angina pectoris and essential hypertension.

Metoprolol has negative inotropic and chronotropic activity and reduces plasma renin activity. It has no intrinsic beta agonist activity. Beta-adrenergic blockade is the main antiarrhythmic-mechanism. It has no membrane stabilizing properties.[173]

Metoprolol is absorbed completely from the gastrointestinal tract. After the first pass through the liver, only 40–50% of an oral dose is available to the systemic circulation.[196] Peak plasma concentration is reached between one and three hours after oral administration. Protein binding is only 10%. The drug is extensively metabolized in the liver and only 3–10% is excreted unchanged in the urine. Hepatic cirrhosis decreases the clearance and increases the availability. Hyperthyroidism has the opposite effect, increasing the clearance. Metoprolol may also reduce FEV_1 in asthmatic patients but less than propranolol and does not oppose bronchodilatation induced by beta$_2$ agonist drugs. Like other beta-blockers, metoprolol may impair glucose tolerance and mask the reaction to hypoglycemia in diabetic patients. Other side effects are fatigue, headaches, drowsiness, and insomnia.

Metoprolol is available in oral and intravenous preparations. An oral dose of 50–300 mg per day is adequate in controlling angina or mild to moderate hypertension. However, sometimes doses up to 450 mg per day may be necessary.[196] The intravenous-preparation is used mainly during the acute phase of myocardial infarction.

In pregnancy, metoprolol has been primarily used to control hypertension[197-200] or tachyarrhythmias.[201] Its metabolism during pregnancy is increased and, therefore, half-life, serum concentration, and bioavailability is decreased.[202] The most plausible explanation is that steroid hormones increases the activity of the hepatic monooxygenase system, which is involved in metoprolol metabolism.[202] Protein binding is not altered during pregnancy.

Metoprolol crosses the placenta and the fetomaternal serum concentration ratio is approximately 1.0.[199,203] Because of redistribution, relative immaturity of hepatic enzymatic systems, or both, in the newborn, the serum concentration of metoprolol increases fourfold during the first hours of life, but then declines over five to 20 hours.[203]

Metoprolol alone or combined with hydralazine was studied in 101 hypertensive pregnant patients.[199] The metoprolol group experienced lower perinatal mortality (2% versus 8%) and a lower incidence of intrauterine growth retardation (11.7 versus 16.3%). Theoretically, this might be explained by metoprolol's lack of action on uterine tone (beta$_2$ effect) and beta-mediated vasodilation. No differences in Apgar score, gestational age, or birth weight were noted. Högstedt et al[197], in a recent controlled trial, compared the combination of metoprolol and hydralazine with nonpharmacologic management of hypertension in 161 pregnant patients. The outcome for the neonates with respect to birth weight, head circumference, Apgar score, incidence of respiratory distress, bradycardia, and hypoglycemia was similar in both groups, confirming the results previously reported.[204] There was one case of fetal malformation in each group. This may be an unrelated event because the combination metoprolol-hydralazine was started during the second and third trimesters. Sandstrom[200] has shown the combination of metoprolol and hydralazine to be superior to hydralazine and thiazide for the treatment of pregnant hypertensive patients with regard to maternal well being, fetal infrauterine growth, 10-minute Apgar scores, and perinatal mortality. To date, no cases of fetal malformation induced by metoprolol have been reported, but experience during the first trimester is lacking.

Despite encouraging data, caution is recommended. Kjellmer et al[205] in an animal study showed that beta$_1$ adrenoreceptor blockade is potentially dangerous in cases of fetal asphyxia. This data is in agreement with previous experimental results obtained with the nonselective beta blocker propranolol.[187,188]

Metoprolol is secreted in breast milk.[206] However, the daily fetal quantity ingested by the neonate is very small. Unless hepatic function in the newborn is markedly impaired, breast-feeding should not be discouraged.

In summary, although metoprolol appears to be safe in pregnancy, the information available is somewhat limited and caution is recommended.

ATENOLOL

Atenolol is another relatively selective beta$_1$ adrenergic-blocking agent used to treat hypertension during pregnancy.[204,207-212]

Like metropolol, it has negative inotropic and chronotropic activity. It has insignificant partial beta$_1$ mimetic activity and weak membrane stabilizing properties.

Only 50–60% of an oral dose is absorbed and five to 15% is protein bound. Elimination half-life is six to eight hours. Very little is metabolized in the liver and 40–50% is eliminated unchanged in the urine. Therefore, in severe renal insufficiency, the dosage has to be decreased. The daily dose is 50–100 mg/day. Although CNS penetration is poor, fatigue and depression may occur. Other side effects are similar to metoprolol except that atenolol is less likely to potentiate insulin-induced hypoglycemia.[84]

Transplacental transfer of atenolol is well documented.[210,211] Although there is a threefold to sixfold individual variation in plasma-atenolol concentration in each patient studied, its concentration was found to be equal in maternal and fetal blood (ratio 1.0).[210] Rubin et al[207] reported a prospective double-blind randomized trial involving 120 pregnant women with hypertension diagnosed in the third trimester treated with atenolol (100–200 mg/day) or placebo. Atenolol was effective in lowering maternal blood pressure and allowed the pregnancy to continue longer than the placebo group. No significant differences were noted in regard to birth weight (3017 g in the placebo group versus 2961 g in the treated group) and Apgar score. Respiratory distress syndrome developed in three neonates in the placebo group. Bradycardia was more common in the atenolol group while hypoglycemia was slightly more frequent in the placebo group. There were two stillbirths in the placebo group and one in the atenolol group. Thorely et al[208] adminstrated atenolol in 13 pregnant patients with pregnancy-induced hypertension. He also noticed a slight drop in heart rate (137–130 beats/minute). However, the response of fetal heart rate to stress was not blunted. One baby was born prematurely. Lunell et al[209] reported another five cases of hypertension during pregnancy treated with atenolol. No adverse effects on neonates were observed. However, the data reported by other authors[204,211,213] is less favorable. Lardoux et al[211] compared atenolol with labetolol in 56 hypertensive pregnant women. The two groups were well-matched. Blood pressure was well controlled in both groups. However, the birth weight was lower in the atenolol group. There were also two stillbirths in the atenolol group.

Another large study[204] reported an incidence of lower birth weight of 12% in the atenolol group. Dubois et al[213] compared acetobutol, pindolol, and atenolol in 56, 38, and 31 hypertensive pregnant patients, respectively. Again, the birth weight was low in the atenolol group. However, no differences were noted in Apgar score, bradycardia, or hypotension. One infant from the acetobutol group had hypoglycemia. No malformations were observed in the atenolol group.

In summary, several studies have demonstrated the safety of the use of atenolol for the treatment of hypertension during pregnancy. However, similar to other beta-blocking agents, low birth weight is often associated with atenolol exposure. Atenolol is secreted in breast milk, and no adverse effects have been noted in atenolol exposed babies. Therefore, breast-feeding does not need to be discontinued.[206]

PINDOLOL

Pindolol is a nonselective beta-adrenergic blocking agent that has an intrinsic sympathetic activity. It has also some membrane stabilizing effects but many fewer than propranolol.

The advantage of intrinsic agonist activity is that the decrease in heart rate and cardiac output at rest is not as pronounced as with nonagonistic beta-blocking drugs. However, the exercise-induced increase in heart rate and cardiac output are blunted.[214,215] This may be of particular benefit in patients with cardiac dysfunction or those prone to bradycardia.[84] Pindolol is almost completely absorbed. Due to insignificant hepatic metabolism during the first pass, 90% of an oral dose is available systemically. Interpatient plasma level variation is about fourfold. Beta blocking concentration is 5–15 ng/mL. Pindolol is 95% protein-bound and has moderate lipid solubility. Forty to 50% of an oral dose is excreted unchanged in the urine. Elimination half-life is three to four hours. However, antihypertensive effects persist for longer periods of time.

Adverse effects are similar to other beta-blocking drugs. The recommended dose is 15–20 mg per day and increments of 10 mg per day every three weeks up to 60 mg per day may be necessary.

Theoretically, pindolol may be particularly advantageous in pregnancy because the lack of effects on resting heart rate and cardiac output combined with a direct vasodilator effect are not expected to compromise uterine blood flow[216] or to decrease basal fetal heart rate.[217]

Pindodol crosses the placenta and the fetomaternal concentration ratio is less than 1.0.[218] Elimination half-lives in fetus and mother are 1.6 and 2.2 hours, respectively. Dubois et al[213] compared acetobutol, pindolol, and atenolol in 56, 38, and 31 hypertensive pregnant patients, respectively. In the pindolol group, the birth weight was significantly higher than in the atenolol group (3345 grams versus 2745 grams). Apgar score, gestational age, fetal heart rate, and frequency of hypoglycemia were not affected by pindolol treatment. However, two cases of malformation were reported in the pindolol group—cleft palate (pindolol started at 29 weeks' gestation) and vesicoureteral reflux (second full pregnancy on pindolol in a mother with asymmetrical segmental renal hypoplasia).

In another study[219], pindolol was compared with methyldopa in 32 consecutive patients with pregnancy induced hypertension. Maternal blood pressure was better controlled in the pindolol group. Furthermore, a drop in creatinine levels and an increase in creatinine clearance were noted in mothers treated with pindolol. No difference was observed between the two groups in regard to intrauterine growth, Apgar score, or fetal morbidity. The birth weight was the same in the two groups (2850 grams). Nonstress tests were normal and no bradycardia was observed in pindolol group.

Rosenfeld et al[216] randomly assigned 44 consecutive hypertensive pregnant patients to two treatment groups: hydralazine alone (21 patients) or hydralazine and pindolol (23 patients). These investigators found a lower incidence of maternal side effects such as dizziness or headaches in the combination therapy group. No differences were noted in the two groups concerning birth weight, gestational age, hypothermia, hypoglycemia, Apgar score, or mode of delivery. Two major malformations were noted in the hydralazine alone group. However, thrombocytopenia was noted only in the hydralazine-pindolol group.

Although those preliminary reports are favorable for use of pindolol in pregnancy, the information available is limited. Therefore, further research is necessary to confirm its safety during pregnancy.

LABETOLOL

Labetolol is a peculiar antihypertensive agent with selective $alpha_1$ and nonselective beta-adrenergic blocking activity. It has intrinsic $beta_2$ agonist activity, but less than pindolol; similarly, its membrane stabilizing effects are fewer than those of propranolol. It also has direct vasodilator properties.[220] The drug is employed in the treatment of hypertension, ischemic heart disease, and arrythmias. However, in the United States, it is approved for hypertension only. Its potency in blocking alpha and beta receptors is approximately one out of 10 and one out of three of those of phentolamine and propranolol, respectively.[84] Hemodynamic responses to labetolol are similar to those produced by concomitant administration of propranolol with hydralazine or prazosin, for example, a decrease in blood pressure and systemic vascular resistances, slight decrease or no change in resting heart rate, and no change in cardiac output. The drug blunts the heart rate response to exercise and decreases plasma renin activity.[220]

Following oral administration, labetolol is almost completely absorbed. Due to extensive metabolism during the first pass through the liver, only 30% is systemically available.[220,221] The drug is extensively metabolized in the liver and only trace amounts can be recovered unchanged from urine. Hepatic clearance of labetolol approximates that of hepatic blood flow. Cimetidine and food appear to increase its bioavailability. Protein-binding is almost 50% and the elimination half-life is three to four hours.

Labetolol may induce bronchospasm in asthmatic patients; however, it is less active than propranolol. Other side effects are fatigue, lethargy, postural hypotension, central nervous system disturbances, gastrointestinal disturbances, impotence, and dry mouth. Approximately 15% of the patients may develop antinuclear and antimitochondrial antibodies.[222] However, systemic lupus erythematosuslike syndrome is very rare.[223]

Labetolol is a very versatile drug. Oral dose varies from 200 mg to 320 mg per day. In order to avoid excessive hypotension, the initial dose should be low, ie, 100 mg twice daily.[221] The intravenous preparation is used mainly to control hypertensive emergencies. A dose of 0.5–2 mg/kg given in slow incremental boluses of 10–15 mg is followed by an infusion of 0.5–1 mg/kg per hour which can be doubled hourly if necessary. The most common side effects following intravenous administration are nausea, vomiting, paresthesia, and sweating.

Labetolol crosses the placenta.[224,225] The fetomaternal concentration ratio is 0.5.[225] Its clearance and volume of distribution are not altered during pregnancy.[226]

There have been a number of favorable reports describing the safe use of labetolol in pregnancy. Lamming et al[227] randomized 26 patients with pregnancy-induced hypertension in two groups: one treated with labetolol (n = 14 patients) and one treated with methyldopa (n = 12 patients). Improvement of renal function and a better control of blood pressure were observed in the labetolol group. The incidence of spontaneous labor and Bishop score were also higher in the labetolol group. Theoretically, the higher incidence of spontaneous labor could be due to myometrial relaxation induced by $alpha_1$ blocking and the $beta_2$ mimetic activity of labetolol. Furthermore, Nylund et al[228] and Jouppilla et al[225] demonstrated that despite significant reduction in blood pressure, uterine blood flow was not affected. Labetolol was again compared with methyldopa in a larger randomized control trial involving 176 pregnant women with mild-to-moderate hypertension.[229] Both drugs were equally effective in lowering the diastolic blood pressure. There were four intrauterine deaths in the methyldopa group, as compared with only one in the labetolol group. The average birth weight and the proportion of preterm or small-for-gestational-age babies were similar in both groups. There is also evidence that labetolol may promote fetal lung maturation; Michael[230] observed higher-than-expected lecithin-sphingomyelin ratio in amniotic fluid as early as 31 weeks' gestation in patients treated with labetolol. This effect is probably mediated by $beta_2$-mimetic activity because salbutamol, a $beta_2$-mimetic drug, has similar effects.[231] Several studies[232,233] showed that no fetal adverse effects were associated with labetolol treatment.

Labetolol is also useful in the acute management of severe hypertension with or without superimposed eclampsia.[234-237] Michael[234] randomly assigned 90 patients with severe hypertension (diastolic blood pressure greater than 105 mm Hg) to receive intravenous labetolol (45 patients) or intravenous diazoxide (45 patients). The control of blood pressure was better in the labetolol group. A precipitous fall of blood pressure (60/40 mm Hg) was noted only in the diazoxide group (eight patients). No fetal bradycardia, hypoglycemia, hypothermia, and malformations were noted. There was a higher operative delivery rate in the diazoxide group. Mabie et al[237] randomized 60 peripartum patients with diastolic blood pressure of 110 mm Hg or higher to receive repeated intravenous injections of labetolol (20–80 mg) or hydralazine (5 mg). There were four treatment failures in the labetolol group and none in the hydralazine group. Labetolol lowered the blood pressure more than hydralazine in the first five to 15 minutes, but this effect reversed between 45 and 120 minutes, with hydralazine achieving better blood pressure control than labetolol. Labetolol decreased the maternal heart rate by 7.1 ± 13.6 beats/min, while hydralazine increased it by 19.7 ± 8.8 beats/min. There was considerable interpatient variability in the dose of labetolol required to control blood pressure. Although labetolol had a rapid effect on blood pressure, the duration of action is variable with the shortest duration occurring in those patients who required the highest dosage for blood pressure control. Fetal distress occurred in two of six cases involving antenatal hydralazine but did not in any of 13 cases given antenatal labetolol.

The results obtained in several studies regarding the use of labetolol for all types of hypertension during pregnancy, including hypertensive emergencies, are very encouraging. Labetolol appears to be safe and an effective alternative to hydralazine or methyldopa.[227,236,237]

Labetolol is secreted in breast milk and no adverse effects were noted in neonates.[238] However, the nursing babies should be closely monitored.

SODIUM NITROPRUSSIDE

Sodium nitroprusside (SN) is one of the most potent drugs available for treatment of hypertensive emergencies. It was approved in the United States in 1974. Chemically, sodium nitroprusside is disodium pentacyanonitrosylferrate. The hypotensive component of sodium nitroprusside is the free nitroso (NO) group which by way of the formation of cyclic guanosine monophosphate interferes with calcium influx leading to relaxation of vascular smooth muscle, but not of uterine smooth muscle. SN directly relaxes arteriolar and venous smooth muscle, decreasing preload and afterload. Blood pressure decreases and heart rate slightly increases. Renal blood flow and glomerular filtration rate is preserved; plasma renin activity is increased. Nitroprusside rapidly reacts with hemoglobin yielding methemoglobin and cyanide. The latter compound undergoes metabolism in the liver or kidney to thiocyanate, which is excreted in the urine. Cyanide may also be eliminated as cyanomethemoglobin or cyanocobalamine. In case of liver disease, hepatic immaturity or excessive administration, cyanide ions may poison the cytochrome oxidase system which leads to anaerobic metabolism and, clinically, metabolic acidosis.

SN is given intravenously in light protected tubing. The initial rate of infusion should be initially 0.1–0.2 μg/kg per minute and slowly increased (5–10 μg every five to ten minutes), until the desired effect is obtained or a dose of 10 μg/kg per minute is reached. Cyanide, thiocyanate, methemoglobin level, and arterial pH should be periodically monitored.

Prolonged use of SN, renal failure, or both, may result in excessive thiocyanate formation, accumulation, or both, which manifests initially with CNS symptoms (tinitus, blurred vision, confusion, psychosis, and so on). Plasma thiocyanate above 10 mg/100 mL are toxic and above 20 mg/100 mL, fatal. Other adverse effects are methamoglobinemia, increased intracranial pressure, headache, rash, nausea, abdominal pain, and muscle twitching.

During pregnancy, SN has been used to control blood pressure during intracranial aneurysm surgery[239-241] or severe gestational hypertension.[242] SN was demonstrated to cross the placenta in both human[243,244] and animal studies.[245-249]

The experimental data concerning the pharmacodynamic effects of SN in pregnant animals is still conflicting.[245-249] Ring et al[245] compared SN with hydralazine in phenylephrine-induced hypertension in near-term pregnant ewes. Both agents were equally effective in lowering the blood pressure. However, only hydralazine counteracted the effects of phenylephrine, ie, increasing uterine blood flow, heart rate, and cardiac output. Wheeler et al[246] found that nitroglycerin and nitroprusside have similar effects on uterine flow, ie, mostly increased or in a few cases unchanged. Ellis et al[248] found that SN increases uterine blood flow in pregnant ewes, whereas Lieb et al[249] noted a significant (25–35%) decrement. Naulty et al[247] observed a decrease in blood pressure without any changes in uterine blood flow.

There is very little information regarding the use of SN in pregnant women. Donchin et al[239] and Willoughby[240,241] reported successful use of SN during surgery for intracranial aneurysms. No fetal adverse effects were noted.

Paull et al[242] described four severe preeclamptic patients with hypertension resistant to diazoxide and other conventional methods treated successfully with nitroprusside. The only fetus alive at the onset of therapy was delivered uneventfully. Four other patients with severe pregnancy-induced hypertension and refractory congestive heart failure were successfully treated with SN.[244] One premature infant expired. The other infants were free of side effects or malformations. The infusion rate varied from 0.013 μg/kg per minute to 2.75 μg/kg per minute. Measurements made in one case showed equal, but negligible (0.1 μg/mL), concentration of cyanide in maternal and fetal blood. Shoemaker et al[243] described a 24 week pregnant patient with severe preeclampsia not controlled by hydralazine and magnesium sulfate. Blood pressure was controlled with AN and labor was induced with pitocin. Fifteen hours after the onset of SN therapy, the patient delivered a 478-g stillborn infant. The nitroprusside dose was 3.9 μg/kg per mL. The level of cyanide in the fetal liver was less than 10 μg/mL, with toxic levels reported to be 30–40 μg/mL. The authors speculated that fetal death was due to severe eclampsia.

In summary, nitroprusside is a very effective, but toxic, drug. It has been used mostly in desperate cases and the data available are minimal. Until further studies clarify its pharmacodynamics, kinetics, and safety during pregnancy, caution is recommended.

NITRATES

Organic nitrates, esthers of nitric acid, have been extensively used for more than a century for the treatment of the symptoms of ischemic heart disease. More recently, their use was extended to congestive heart failure. Nitrates are very potent dilators predominantly of venous vessels; arterial dilatation becomes evident at high doses. Nitrates' effects lead to a decrease in venous return and, consequently, to lower right and left ventricular end diastolic pressures. Systemic vascular resistance is not significantly changed, heart rate is unchanged or increased, and cardiac output is usually unchanged. In higher doses, nitrates may lower the blood pressure and cardiac output which triggers a compensatory sympathetic activation with reflex tachycardia and vasoconstriction. Nitroglycerin also decreases pulmonary vascular resistance. The antianginal effects are mostly due to a decrease in myocardial oxygen requirements by reducing preload and afterload. Nitrates are metabolized in the liver. Nitroglycerin metabolites have only 10% of nitroglycerin's potency and their half-life is approximately 40 minutes. Following sublingual administration, the peak plasma concentration is reduced in four minutes and the half-life is one to three minutes. Intravenous administration is used mostly in acute ischemic syndromes and congestive heart failure.[250] It is also used to control systemic hypertension after and during coronary artery bypass surgery.

Continuous exposure to nitrates may lead to early development of tolerance.[251-255] These problems probably may be avoided by increasing the dosing interval and allowing nitrate-free intervals of at least 10 hours over 24 hours.[254,255] The most common side effects are headache, dizziness, and postural hypotension; syncopal episodes are not common.

During pregnancy, intravenous nitroglycerin was used to control severe pregnancy-induced hypertension and for uterine relaxation in the postpartum patient with retained placenta.[256-258] Having a very small molecular weight and being uncharged, nitroglycerin easily crosses the placenta.[259] Experimental data in pregnant ewes[260] showed a fetomaternal arterial blood concentration ratio of 0.15. The authors advanced the hypothesis that the low fetal levels are probably due to rapid metabolism, poor placental transfer, or widespread binding. Snyder et al[256] and Hood et al[257] used nitroglycerin to control the elevation of blood pressure that occurs during tracheal intubation in preeclamptic patients. Nitroglycerin not only successfully lowered the basal blood pressure, but also blunted the hypertensive response to intubation. No evidence of fetal compromise was noted. Cotton et al[259] studied the hemodynamic effect of intravenous nitroglycerin, coupled with blood volume expansion, in six preeclamptic patients. The mean gestational age was 37.3 ± 3.6 weeks. Nitroglycerin, alone, effectively reduced the mean arterial blood pressure by 27.5%. The hypotensive effect was blunted by volume expansion. In two patients in whom blood pressure was suddenly lowered, fetal deceleration and bradycardia were observed. In the other three patients, a flat fetal heart rate with an average beat-to-beat variability of less than five beats per minute was noted. The authors suggested that this is probably due to a loss of cerebral autoregulation and increased intracranial pressure induced by nitroglycerin.

In summary, it appears that nitrates' treatment is not free of side effects, and the information available regarding their use during pregnancy is very limited. Of particular concern are the effects on uterine blood flow, oxygen delivery, and fetal hemodynamics. Further studies are needed to fully clarify its effects and safety during pregnancy. Therefore, no recommendation can be made at this time.

CONCLUSIONS

There are many clinical situations that require the use of cardiovascular medications in pregnancy. It is hard to evaluate drugs during pregnancy, so the available information on the safety of many medications is limited. However, certain drugs (digoxin, quinidine, beta-blockers, alphamethyldopa, hydralazine) have been used with relative safety to both mother and fetus. It always is best to avoid medications in pregnancy but, when necessary, drugs for cardiovascular disease may be used when the risk-benefit ratio is favorable.

REFERENCES

1. Rogers MC, Willerson JT, Goldblatt A, Smith TW. Serum digoxin concentrations in the human fetus, neonate and infant. *N Engl J Med.* 1972;287:1010.
2. Luxford AME, Kellaway GSM. Pharmacokinetics of digoxin in pregnancy. *Eur J Clin Pharmacol.* 1983;25:117.
3. Sherman JL, Locke RV. Transplacental neonatal digitalis intoxication. *Am J Cardiol.* 1960;6:834.
4. Chan V, Tse TF, Wong V. Transfer of digoxin across the placenta and into breast milk. *Br J Obstet Gynecol.* 1978;85:605.
5. Saarikoski S. Placental transfer and fetal uptake of ^{3}H-digoxin in humans. *Br J Obstet Gynecol.* 1976;83:879.
6. Allonen H, Kanto J, Iisalo E. The feto-maternal distribution of digoxin in early human pregnancy. *Acta Pharmacol Toxicol.* 1976;39:477.
7. Heaton FC, Vaughan R. Intrauterine supraventricular tachycardia: cardioversion with maternal digoxin. *Obstet Gynecol.* 1982;60:749.
8. Lilja H, Karlsson K, Lindecrantz K, Sabel KG. Treatment of intrauterine supraventricular tachycardia with digoxin and verapamil. *J Perinatol Med.* 1984;12:151.
9. Hirata K, Kato H, Yoshioka F, Matsunaga T. Successful treatment of fetal atrial flutter and congestive heart failure. *Arch Dis Child.* 1985;60:158.
10. Golichowski AM, Caldwell R, Hartsough A, Peleg D. Pharmacologic cardioversion of intrauterine supraventricular tachycardia. *J Reprod Med.* 1985;30:139.
11. Repke JT, Steibach G. Fetal supraventricular tachycardia refractory to digoxin cardioversion. *J Reprod Med.* 1986;31:195.
12. Spinnato JA, Shaver DC, Flinn GS, et al. Fetal supraventricular tachycardia: in utero therapy with digoxin and quinidine. *Obstet Gynecol.* 1984;64:730.
13. Nagashima M, Asai T, Suzuki C, et al. Intrauterine supraventricular tachyarrhythmias and transplacental digitalization. *Arch Dis Child.* 1986;61:996.
14. Weiner CP, Thompsom MIB. Direct treatment of fetal supraventricular tachycardia after failed transplacental therapy. *Am J Obstet Gynecol.* 1988;158:570.
15. Gembruch U, Hansman M, Pedel DA, Bold R. Intrauterine therapy of fetal tachyarrhythmias: intraperitoneal administration of antiarrhythmic drugs to the fetus in fetal tachyarrhythmias with severe hydrops fetalis. *J Perinatol Med.* 1988;16:39.
16. Maxwell DJ, Crawford DC, Curry PVM, et al. Obstetric importance, diagnosis and management of fetal tachycardias. *Br Heart J.* 1988;297:107.
17. Marzo A. Dati preliminari sulla farmacocinetica della digossina in gravidanza. *Boll Soc Ital Biol Sper.* 1980;56:219.
18. Koren G, Farine D, Maresky D, et al. Significance of the endogenous digoxin-like substance in infants and mothers. *Clin Pharmacol Ther.* 1984;36:759.
19. Hicks JM, Brett EM. Falsely increased digoxin concentrations in samples from neonates and infants. *Ther Drug Monit.* 1984;6:461
20. Valdes R, Jr. Endogenous digoxin-like immunoreactive factors: impact

on digoxin measurements and potential physiological implications. *Clin Chem.* 1985;31:1525.
21. Cook JD, Koch TR, Cook MS, Knoblock EC. Inaccuracies in digoxin measurements. *Clin Biochem.* 1988;21:353.
22. Fitzsimmons WE. Influence of assay methodologies and interferences on the interpretation of digoxin concentrations. *Drug Intell Clin Pharm.* 1986;20:538.
23. Witherspoon L, Shiller S, Alyea K, et al. Digoxin-like substances in term pregnancy, newborns, and renal failure. *J Nucl Med.* 1986;27:1418.
24. Mimura S, Suzuki C, Yamazaki T. Transplacental passage of digoxin in the case of nonimmune hydrops fetalis. *Clin Cardiol.* 1987;10:63.
25. Younis JS, Granat M. Insufficient transplacental digoxin transfer in severe hydrops fetalis. *Am J Obstet Gynecol.* 1987;157:1268.
26. Weiner CP, Landos S, Persoon TJ. Digoxon-like immunoreactive substances in fetuses with and without cardiac pathology. *Am J Obstet Gynecol.* 1987;157:368.
27. Whitsett AJ, Wallick ET. Ouabain binding and Na^+-K^+-ATPase activity in human placenta. *Am J Physiol.* 1980;238:E38.
28. Weaver JB, Pearson JF. Influence of digitalis on time of onset and duration of labour in women with cardiac disease. *Br Med J.* 1973;3:519.
29. Loughnan PM. Digoxin excretion in human breast milk. *J Pediatr.* 1978;92:1019.
30. Zipes PD. Management of cardiac arrhythmias: pharmacological, electrical, and surgical techniques. In: Braunwald E, ed. *Heart Disease,* 3rd ed. Philadelphia: WB Saunders 1988:621.
31. Federman J, Vliestra R. Antiarrhythmic drug therapy. *Mayo Clin Proc.* 1979;54:531.
32. Conn HL, Jr, Luchi RJ. Some cellular and metabolic considerations relating to the action of quinidine as a prototype antiarrhythmic agent. *Am J Med.* 1964;37:685.
33. Crouthamel WG. The effect of congestive heart failure on quinidine pharmacokinetics. *Am Heart J.* 1975;90:335.
34. Winkle RA, Glantz SA, Harrison DC. Pharmacological therapy for ventricular arrhythmia. *Am J Cardiol.* 1975;36:629.
35. Kelliher GJ, Kowey P, Engel T, Wetstein L. Clinical pharmacology of antiarrhythmic agents. *Cardiovasc Clin.* 1985;16:287.
36. DiSegni E, Klein HO, David D, et al. Overdrive pacing in quinidine syncope and other long QT interval syndromes. *Arch Int Med.* 1980;140:1036.
37. Smith WM, Gallagher JJ. "Les torsades des pointes": an unusual ventricular arrhythmia. *Ann Int Med.* 1980;93:578.
38. Doerig W. Quinidine-digoxin interaction. *N Engl J Med.* 1979;301:400.
39. Ball WJ, Tse-Eng D, Walick ET, et al. Effect of quinidine on the digoxin receptor in vitro. *J Clin Invest.* 1981;68:1065.
40. Meyer J, Lackner JE, Schochet SS. Paroxysmal tachycardia in pregnancy. *JAMA.* 1930;94:1901.
41. Hill LM, Malkasian GD. The use of quinidine sulfate throughout pregnancy. *Obstet Gynecol.* 1979;54:366.
42. Colin A, Lambotte R. Influence teratogene des medicaments adminstres a la femme enceinte. *Rev Med Liege.* 1972;27:39.
43. Guntheroth WG, Cyr DR, Mack LA, et al. Hydrops from reciprocating atrioventricular tachycardia in a 27-week fetus requiring quinidine for conversion. *Obstet Gynecol.* 1985;66:29S.
44. Killeen AA, Bowers A. Fetal supraventricular tachycardia treated with high dose quinidine: Toxicity associated with marked elevation of the metabolites 3(s)-3-hydroxyquinidine. *Obstet Gynecol.* 1987;70:445.
45. Szekely P, Snaith L. *Heart Disease and Pregnancy.* Edinburgh: Churchill-Livingstone; 1974.
46. Mauer AM, Devaux LO, Lahey ME. Neonatal and maternal thrombocytopeic purpura due to quinine. *Pediatrics.* 1957;19:84.
47. Bellett S. Essentials of cardiac arrhythmias. *Diagnosis & Management.* Philadelphia, PA: W.B. Saunders Co, 1972.
48. Merx W. Herzrhythmusstörungen in der schwangershaft. *Dtsch Med Wochenschr.* 1972;97:1987.
49. Mendelson CL. Disorders of heart beat during pregnancy. *Am J Obstet Gynecol.* 1956;72:1268.
50. Kambam JR, Franks JJ, Smith BE. Inhibitory effect of quinidine on plasma pseudocholinesterase activity in pregnant women. *Am J Obstet Gynecol.* 1987;157:897.
51. Miller RD, Walter LW, Katzning BG. The potentiation of neuromuscular blocking agents by quinidine. *Anesthesiology.* 1967;26:1036.
52. Foldes FF, Foldes VM, Smith JC, Zsigmond EK. The relation between plasma cholinesterase and prolonged apnea caused by succinylcholine. *Anesthesiology.* 1963;24:208.
53. Mark LC, Kayden HJ, Steele JM, et al. The physiological disposition and cardiac effects of procainamide. *J Pharmacol Exp Ther.* 1951;102:5.
54. Hoffman BF, Rosen MR, Wit AL. Electrophysiology and pharmacology of cardiac arrhythmias: VII. Cardiac effects of quinidine and procainamide. *Am Heart J.* 1975;90:117.
55. Bigger JT, Giardina EGV. Drug interaction in antiarrhythmic therapy. *Ann NY Acad Sci.* 1984;427:140.
56. Giardina EGV, Dreyfuss J, Bigger JT Jr, et al. Metabolism of procainamide in normal and cardiac subjects. *Clin Pharm Ther.* 1976;19:339.
57. Stec GP, Lertora JJL, Atkinson AJJ, et al. Remission of procainamide-induced lupus erythematosus with N-acetylprocainamide therapy. *Ann Int Med.* 1979;90:799.
58. Kessler KM, Lowenthal DT, Werner H, et al. Quinidine elimination in patients with congestive heart failure or poor renal function. *N Engl J Med.* 1974;290:706.
59. Nestico PF, DePace NL, Morganroth J. Therapy with conventional antiarrhythmic drugs for ventricular arrhythmias. *Med Clin North Am.* 1984;58:5, 1295.
60. Dumesic DA, Silverman NH, Tobias S, Golbus MS. Transplacental cardioversion of fetal supraventricular tachycardia with procainamide. *N Engl J Med.* 1982;307:1128.
61. Given BD, Phillippe M, Sanders SP, Dzau V. Procainamide cardioversion of fetal supraventricular tachyarrhythmia. *Am J Cardiol.* 1984;53:1460.
62. Heinonen OP, Slone D, Shapiro S. *Birth Defects and Drugs in Pregnancy.* Littleton, MA: Publishing Sciences Group; 1977:358.
63. Merx W, Effert S, Heinrich KW. Heart disease in pregnancy, intra- and postpartum. *Z Geburtshilfe Perinatol* 1974;178:317.
64. Metcalfe J, Ueland K. The heart and pregnancy. In: Hurst JW, ed. *The Heart,* 4th ed. New York, NY: McGraw-Hill; 1978;1721.
65. Condemi JJ, Blomgren SE, Vaughan JH. The procainamide-induced lupus syndrome. *Bull Rheum Dis.* 1970;20:604.
66. Pittard III WB, Glazier H. Procainamide excretion in human milk. *J Pediatr.* 1983;102(4):631.
67. Heel RC, Brogden RN, Speight TM, et al. Disopyramide: a review of its pharmacologic properties and therapeutic use in treating cardiac arrhythmias. *Drugs.* 1978;15:331.
68. Jennings G, Jones M, Besterman EM, et al. Oral disopyramide in prophylaxis of arrhythmias following myocardial infarction. *Lancet.* 1976;1:51.
69. Hartel G, Louhija A, Konttinen A. Disopyramide in the prevention of recurrence of atrial fibrillation after electroconversion. *Clin Pharmacol Ther.* 1974;15:551.
70. Luoma PV, et al. Efficacy of intravenous disopyramide in the termination of supraventricular arrhythmias. *J Clin Pharmacol.* 1978;18:293.
71. Kotter V, Linderer T, Schroder R. Effects of disopyramide on systemic and coronary hemodynamics and myocardial metabolism in patients with coronary artery disease: comparison with lidocaine. *Am J Cardiol.* 1980;46:469.
72. Naqvi N, Thompson DS, Morgan WE, et al. Hemodynamic effects of disopyramide in patients after open-heart surgery. *Br Heart J.* 1979;42:587.
73. Podrid PJ, Schoeneberger A, Lown B. Congestive heart failure caused by oral disopyramide. *N Engl J Med.* 1980;302:614.
74. Mirro MJ, Watanabe AN, Bailey JC. Electrophysiological effects of disopyramide and quinidine on guinea-pig atria and canin cardiac Purkinje fibers: dependence on underlying cholinergic tone. *Circ Res.* 1980;46:660.
75. Grant AM, Marshall RJ, Ankier SI. Some effects of disopyramide and its N-dealkylated metabolite on isolated nerve and cardiac muscle. *Eur J Pharmacol.* 1978;49:389.
76. Meltzer RS, McMorrow M, Robert EW, et al. Atypical ventricular tachycardia as a manifestation of disopyramide toxicity. *Am J Cardiol.* 1978;42:1049.
77. Nicholson WJ, Martin CE, Gracey JG, et al. Disopyramide induced ventricular fibrillation. *Am J Cardiol.* 1979;43:1053.
78. Shaxted EJ, Milton PJ. Disopyramide in pregnancy: a case report. *Curr Med Res Opin.* 1979;6:70–72.
79. Ellsworth AJ, Horn JR, Raisys VA, et al. Disopyramide and N-monodesalkyl disopyramide in serum and breast milk. *DICP.* 1989;23:56.
80. Leonard RF, Braun TE, Levy AM. Intiation of uterine contractions by disopyramide during pregnancy. *N Engl J Med.* 1978;299:84.
81. Barnett DB, Hudson SA, McBurney A. Disopyramide and its N-monodesalkyl metabolite in breast milk. *Br J Clin Pharmacol.* 1982;14:310.
82. Mackintosh D, Buchanan N. Excretion of disopyramide in human breast milk. *Br J Clin Pharmacol.* 1985;19:856.
83. Hoppu K, Neuvonen PJ, Korte T. Disopyramide and breast feedings. *Br J Clin Pharmac.* 1986;21:553.
84. Gilman AG, Goodman LS, Rall TW, Murad F. *The Pharmacological Basis of Therapeutics,* 7th ed. New York: MacMillan Publishing, 1985.
85. Bigger JT, Mandel WJ. Effects of lidocaine on the electrophysiological properties of ventricular muscle and Purkinje fibers. *J Clin Invest.* 1970;49:63.
86. Rahimtoola SH, Sinno MZ, Loeb HS, et al. Lidocaine infusion in acute myocardial infarction. *Arch Int Med.* 1971;128:416.
87. Branch RA, Shand DG, Wilkinson GR, et al. The reduction of lidocaine clearance by d-propranolol: an example of a hemodynamic drug interaction. *J Pharmacol Exp Ther.* 1973;184:515.
88. Knapp AB, Maguire W, Keren G, et al. The cimetidine-lidocaine interaction. *Ann Int Med.* 1983;98:174.
89. Wong BYS, Hurwitz A. Simple method for maintaining serum lidocaine levels in therapeutic range. *Arch Int Med.* 1985;145:1588.

90. Bauer LA, Brown T, Gibaldi M, et al. Influence of long term infusions on lidocaine kinetics. *Clin Pharmacol Ther.* 1982;31:433.
91. Warang PK, Crouthamel WG, Carliner NH. Lidocaine and its active metabolites. *Clin Pharmacol Ther.* 1978;24:654.
92. Blumer J, Strong JM, Atkinson AJ. The convulsant potency of lidocaine and its N-dealkylated metabolites. *J Pharmacol Exp Ther.* 1973;186:31.
93. Stokes IM, Evans J, Stone M. Myocardial infarction and cardiac arrest in the second trimester followed by assisted vaginal delivery under epidural analgesia at 38 weeks gestation. *Br J Obstet Gynecol.* 1983;91:197.
94. Menon KPS, Mahpatra RK. Paroxysmal ventricular tachycardia associated with Bell's palsy in a teenager at late pregnancy. *Angiology.* 1984;35:534.
95. Juneja MM, Ackerman WE, Kaczorowski DM, et al. Continuous epidural lidocaine infusion in the pasturient with paroxysmal ventricular tachycardia. *Anesthesiology.* 1989;71:305.
96. Shnider SM, Way EL. The kinetics of transfer of lidocaine across the human placenta. *Anesthesiology.* 1968;29:944.
97. Biehl D, Shnider SM, Levinson G, et al. Placental transfer of lidocaine: effects of fetal acidosis. *Anesthesiology.* 1978;48:409.
98. Tucker GT, Boyes RN, Bridenbaugh PO, Moore DC. Binding of anilide-type local anesthetics in human plasma. *Anesthesiology.* 1970;33:304.
99. Shnider SM, Way EL. Plasma levels of lidocaine in mother and newborn following obstetrical conduction anesthesia: clinical applications. *Anesthesiology.* 1968;29:951.
100. Brown WU, Bell GC, Alper MH. Acidosis, local anesthetics, and the newborn. *Obstet Gynecol.* 1976;48:27.
101. Petrie RH, Paul WL, Miller FC, et al. Placental transfer of lidocaine following paracervical block. *Obstet Gynecol.* 1974;120:791.
102. Burney RG, DiFazio CA, Foster JH. Effects of pH on protein binding of lidocaine. *Anesth Analg.* 1978;57:478.
103. Bozynski ME, Ruberth LB, Patel JA. Lidocaine toxicity after maternal prudential anesthesia in a term infant with fetal distress. *Am J Perinat.* 1987;4:164.
104. Kim WY, Pomerance JJ, Miller AA. Lidocaine intoxication in a newborn following local anesthesia for episiotomy. *Pediatrics.* 1979;64:643.
105. Kileff MB, James FM, Dewan D, et al. Neonatal neurobehavioral responses after epidural anethesia for cesarean section with lidocaine and buipvacaine. (abstract) *Anesthesiology.* 1982;57:A403.
106. Abboud TK, Sarkis F, Blikian A, Varadian L. Lack of adverse neurobehavioral effects of lidocaine. (abstract) *Anesthesiology.* 1982;57:A404.
107. Symllie HC, Doar JWH, Head CD, Leggett RJE. A trial of intravenous and oral mexiletine in acute myocardial infarction. *Eur J Clin Pharmacol.* 1984;26:537.
108. Campbell RWF. Mexiletine. *N Engl J Med.* 1987;316:29.
109. Timis AD, Jackson G, Holt DW. Mexiletine for control of ventricular dysrhythmias in pregnancy. *Lancet.* 1980;647.
110. Lewis AM, Johnston A, Patel L, Turner P. Mexiletine in human blood and breast milk. *Postgrad Med J.* 1981;57:546.
111. Lownes HE, Ives TJ. Mexiletine use during pregnancy and lactation. *Am J Obstet Gynecol.* 1987;157:446.
112. Gregg AR, Tomich PG. Mexiletine use in pregnancy. *J Perinat.* 1988;8:33.
113. Woosely RL, Wang T, Stone W, et al. Pharmacology, electrophysiology and pharmokinetics of mexiletine. Am Heart J. 1984;107:1058.
114. Mitchell BG, Clements JA, Pottage A, Prescott LF. Mexiletine disposition: individual variation in response to urine acidification and alkalinisation. *Br J Clin Pharmacol.* 1983;16:281.
115. Pentikainen PJ, Halinen MO, Helin MJ. Pharmacokinetics of oral mexiletine in patients with acute myocardial infarction. *Eur J Clin Pharmacol.* 1983;25:773.
116. Nitsch J, Steinbeck G, Luderitz B. Increase of mexiletine plasma levels due to delayed hepatic metabolism in patients with chronic liver disease. *Eur Heart J.* 1983;4:810.
117. Podrid PJ, Lown B. Mexiletine for ventricular arrhythmias. *Am J Cardiol.* 1981;47:895.
118. Stein J, Podrid P, Lown B. Effects of oral mexiletine on left and right ventricular function. *Am J Cardiol.* 1984;54:575.
119. Cocco G, Strozzi, C, Chu D, Pansini R. Torsades de pointes as a manifestation of mexiletine toxocity. *Am Heart J.* 1980;100:878.
120. Sloskey GE: Amiodarone. A unique antiarrhythmic agent. *Clin Pharm.* 1983;2:330.
121. Singh BN, Vaughan Williams EM. The effects of amiodarone, a new antianginal drug on cardiac muscle. *Br J Pharmacol.* 1970;39:657.
122. Nademanee K, et al. Antiarrhythmic efficacy and electrophysiologic actions of amiodarone in patients with life-threatening ventricular arrhythmias: potent suppression of spontaneously occurring tachyarrhythmias versus inconsistent abolition of induced ventricular tachycardia. *Am Heart J.* 1982;103:950.
123. Finerman WB, Hamer A, Peter T, et al. Electrophysiologic effects of chronic amiodarone therapy in patients with ventricular arrhythmias. *Am Heart J.* 1982;104:987.
124. Wellens HJJ, Lie KI, Bar FW, et al. Effect of amiodarone in the Wolff–Parkinson–White syndrome. *Am J Cardiol.* 1976;38:189.
125. Charlier R, Deltour G, Bandine A, Chailet F. Pharmacology of amiodarone, an antiangina drug with a new biological profile. *Arzneimittelforschung.* 1968;18:1408.
126. Latini R, Tognoni G, Kates RE. Clinical pharmokinetics of amiodarone. *Clin Pharmacokinet.* 1984;9:136.
127. Riva E, Gerna M, Latini R, et al. Pharmokinetics of amiodarone in man. *J Cardiovasc Pharmacol.* 1982;4:270.
128. Pitcher D, Leather HM, Storey GCA, Holt DW. Amiodarone in pregnancy. *Lancet.* 1983;1:597.
129. Greene HL, Graham EL, Werner JA, et al. Toxic and therapeutic effects of amiodarone in the treatment of cardiac arrhythmias. *J Am Coll Cardiol.* 1983;2:1114.
130. Marcus FI. Drug interactions with amiodarone. *Am Heart J.* 1983;106:924.
131. McKenna WJ, Harris L, Rowland E, et al. Amiodarone therapy during pregnancy. *Am J Cardiol.* 1983;51:1231.
132. Robson D, Jeeva Raj MV, Storey GCA, Holt DW. Use of amiodarone during pregnancy. *Post Grad Med J.* 1985;61:75.
133. Rey E, Bachrach LK, Buttow GN. Effects of amiodarone during pregnancy. *Can Med Assoc J.* 1987;136:959.
134. Foster CJ, Love HG. Amiodarone in pregnancy: case report and review of literature. *Int J Cardiol.* 1988;20:307.
135. DeWolf D, De Schepper, Verhaaren H, et al. Congenital hypothyroid goiter and amiodarone. *Acta Paediatr Scand.* 1988;77:616.
136. Laurent M, Betremieux P, Biron Y, Lellelloco A. Neonatal hypothyroidism after treatment by amiodarone during pregnancy. *Am J Cardiol.* 1987;60:142.
137. Arnoux P, Seyral P, Llurens M, et al. Amiodarone and digoxin for refractory fetal tachycardia. *Am J Cardiol.* 1987;59:166.
138. Lusson JR, Beytout M, Jacquetin B, et al. Traitement d'une tachycardie supraventriculaire foetale: Association digoxine-amiodarone. *Coeur.* 1985;15:315.
139. Rey E, Duperron L, Gautheir R, et al. Transplacental treatment of tachycardia-induced fetal heart failure with verapamil and amiodarone. *Am J Obstet Gynecol.* 1985;153:311.
140. Koblin DD, Romanoff ME, Martin DE, et al. Anesthetic management of the parturient receiving amiodarone. *Anesthesiology.* 1987;66:551.
141. Waxman HL, Myerburg RJ, Appel R, et al. Verapamil for control of ventricular rate in paroxysmal supraventricular tachycardia and atrial fibrillation or flutter. *Ann Int Med.* 1981;94:1.
142. Kohlhardt M, Bauer B, Krause H. New selective inhibitors of the Ca conductivity in mammalian-myocardial fibers. *Experientia.* 1972;15:288.
143. Somogyi A, Albrecht M, Kliems G, et al. Pharmacokinetics, bioavailability and ECG response of verapamil in patients with liver cirrhosis. *Br J Clin Pharmacol.* 1981;12:51.
144. Singh BN, Collett JT, Chew CYC. New perspectives in the pharmacologic therapy of cardiac arrhythmias. *Prog Cardiovasc Dis.* 1980;22:243.
145. Fearrinton EL, Rand CH Jr, Rose JD. Hyperprolactinemia-galactorrhea induced by verapamil. *Am J Cardiol.* 1983;51:1466.
146. Klein V, Repke JT. Supraventricular tachycardia in pregnancy: cardioversion with verapamil. *Obstet Gynecol.* 1984;63:16S.
147. Wladimiroff JW, Stewart PA. Fetal therapy: treatment of fetal cardiac arrhythmias. *Br J Hosp Med.* 1985;34:134.
148. Wolff F, Breuker KH, Schlensker KH, et al. Prenatal diagnosis and therapy of fetal heart rate anomalies: with a contribution on the placental transfer of verapamil. *J Perinat Med.* 1980;8:203.
149. Mosler KH, Jung H. Methoden der pharmakologischen geburtserleichterung und uterus-relaxation. Internationales Symposion, Bad-Aachen. Stuttgart, Germany: Thieme; 1972:170.
150. Strigl R, Pfeiffer U, Erhardt W, et al. Does the administration of the calcium antagonist verapamil in tocolysis with beta sympathromimetics still make sense? *J Perinat Med.* 1981;9:235.
151. Serafini PC, Petracco AL, Vicosa HN Jr., et al. Arterial hyposensitive effect of verapamil in severe preeclampsia: preliminary study. *Arq Bras Cardiol.* 1979;32:57.
152. Belfort MA, Moore PJ. Verapamil in the treatment of severe post partum hypertension. *S Afr Med J.* 1988;74:265.
153. Kleineman CS, Copel JA, Weinstein EML, et al. Treatment of fetal supraventricular tachyarrhythmias. *J Clin Ultrasound.* 1985;13:265.
154. Allan LD, Crawford DC, Anderson RH. Evaluation and treatment of fetal arrhythmia. *Clin Cardiol.* 1984;7:467.
155. Bergmans MGM, Jonker GJ, Kock HCLV. Fetal supraventricular tachycardia: review of the literature. *Obstet Gynecol Surv.* 1985;40:61.
156. Miller MR, Withers R, Bhamra R, Holt DW. Verapamil and breast feeding. *Eur J Clin Pharmacol.* 1986;30:125.
157. Inoue H, Unno N, Ou MC, et al. Level of verapamil in human milk. *Eur J Clin Pharmacol.* 1984;26:657.
158. Andersen JH. Excretion of verapamil in human milk. *Eur J Clin Pharmacol.* 1984;26:657.
159. Mitrani A, Oettinger M, Abinader EG, et al. Use of propranolol in dysfunctional labour. *Br J Obstet Gynecol.* 1975;82:651.
160. Pruyn SC, Phelan JP, Buchanan GC. Long-term propranolol therapy in pregnancy: maternal and fetal outcome. *Am J Obstet Gynecol.* 1979;135:485.

161. Eliahou HE, Silverberg DS, Reisin E, et al. Propranolol for the treatment of hypertension in pregnancy. *Br J Obstet Gynecol.* 1978;85:431.
162. Tcherdakoff PH, Colliard M, Berrard E, et al. Propranolol in hypertension during pregnancy. *Br Med J.* 1978;2:670.
163. Bott-Kanner G, Schweitzer A, Reisher SH, et al. Propranolol and hydralazine in the management of essential hypertension in pregnancy. *Br J Obstet Gynecol.* 1980;87:110.
164. Livingstone I, Braswell PW, Bevan EB, et al. Propranolol in pregnancy: three year prospective study. *Clin Exper Hyper-Hyper Pregnancy.* 1983;B2:341.
165. Bott-Kanner G, Schweitzer A, Schoenfeld A, et al. Treatment with propranolol and hydralazine throughout pregnancy in a hypertensive patient: a case report. *Isr J Med Sci.* 1978;14:466.
166. Bullock JL, Harris RE, Young R. Treatment of thyrotoxicosis during pregnancy and propranolol. *Am J Obstet Gynecol.* 1975;121:242.
167. Langer A, Hung CT, McA'Nulty JA, et al. Adrenergic blockade: a new appraoch to hyperthyroidism in pregnancy. *Obstet Gynecol.* 1974;44:181.
168. Turner GM, Oakley CM, Dixon HG. Management of pregnancy complicated by hypertrophic obstructive cardiomyopathy. *Br Med J.* 1968;4:281.
169. Oakley GDG, McGarry K, Limb DG, Oakley CM. Management of pregnancy in patients with hypertrophic cardiomyopathy. *Br Med J.* 1979;1:1749.
170. Cottrill CM, McAllister RG Jr., Gettes L, Noonan JA. Propranolol therapy during pregnancy, labor and delivery: evidence for transplacental drug transfer and imparied neonatal drug disposition. *J Pediatr.* 1977;91:812.
171. Schroeder JS, Harrison DC. Repeated cardioversion during pregnancy: treatment of refractory paroxysmal atrial tachycardia during three successive pregnancies. *Am J Cardiol.* 1971;27:445.
172. Teuscher A, Bossi E, Imhof P, et al. Effect of propranolol on fetal tachycardia in diabetic pregnancy. *Am J Cardiol.* 1978;42:304.
173. Davis LD, Temte JV. Effects of propranolol on the transmembrane potentials of ventricular muscle and Purkinje fibers of the dog. *Circulation.* 1968;22:661.
174. Evans GH, Wilkinson GR, Shand DG. The disposition of propranolol IV: a dominant role for tissue uptake in the dose-dependent extraction of propranolol by the perfused rat liver. *J Pharmacol Exp Ther.* 1973;186:447.
175. Shand DG. Drug therapy: propranolol. *N Engl J Med.* 1975;293:280.
176. Woosley RL, Shand D, Kornhauser D, et al. Relation of plasma concentration and dose of propranolol to its effect on resistant ventricular arrhythmias. (abstract) *Clin Res.* 1977;25:262A.
177. Barden TP, Stauder RW. Effects of adrenergic blocking agents and catecholamines in human pregnancy. *Am J Obstet Gynecol.* 1968;102:225.
178. O'Hare MF, Kinney CD, Murnaghan GA, McDevitt DG. Pharmacokinetics of propranolol during pregnancy. *Eur J Clin Pharmacol.* 1984;27:583.
179. Perucca E, Crema A. Plasma protein binding of drugs in pregnancy. *Clin. Pharmacokinet.* 1982;7:336.
180. Gladstone GR, Horolof A, Gersony WM. Propranolol administration during pregnancy: effects on the fetus. *J Pediatr.* 1975;86:962.
181. Datta S, Kitzmiller JL, Ostheimer GW. Propranolol and parturition. *Am J Obstet Gynecol.* 1968;101:91.
182. Turnstall MB. The effects of propranolol on the onset of breathing at birth. *Br J Anaesthesia.* 1969;41:792.
183. Margulis E, Binder D, Cohen AW. The effects of propranolol on the nonstress test. *Am J Obstet Gynecol.* 1984;148:340.
184. Jensen OH. Fetal heart rate response to a controlled sound stimulus after propranolol administration to the mother. *Acta Obstet Gynecol Scand.* 1984;63:199.
185. Oakes GK, Walker AD, Ehrenkrauz RA, Chez RA. Effect of propranolol infusion on the umbilical and uterine circulations of pregnant sheep. *Am J Obstet Gynecol.* 1976;126:1038.
186. Redmond GP. Propranolol and fetal growth retardation. *Semin Perinatal.* 1982;6:142.
187. Joelson I, Barton MD. The effect of blockade of the beta receptors of the sympathetic nervous system of the fetus. *Acta Obstet Gynecol Scand.* 1969;3(suppl)48:75.
188. Hokegard KH, Karlsson K, Kjellmer I, Rosen KG. ECG changes in the fetal lamb during asphyxia in relation to beta-adrenoreceptor stimulation and blockade. *Acta Physiol Scand.* 1979;105:195.
189. Campbell JW. A possible teratogenic effect of propranolol. *N Engl J Med.* 1986;313:518.
190. O'Connor PC, Jick H, Hunter JR, et al. Propranolol and pregnancy outcome. *Lancet.* 1981;2:1168.
191. Rubin PC. Beta-blockers in pregnancy. *N Engl J Med.* 1981;305:1323.
192. Sanstrom B. Clinical trials of adrenergic antagonists in pregnancy hypertension. *Acta Obstet Gynecol Scand.* 1984;(suppl)118:57.
193. Karlberg B, Luudberg D, Aberg H. Excretion of propranolol in human breast milk. *Acta Pharmacol Toxicol.* 1974;34:222.
194. Bauer JH, Pape B, Zajicek J, Groshong T. Propranolol in human plasma and breast milk. *Am J Cardiol.* 1979;43:860.
195. Levitan A, Manion J. Propranolol therapy during pregnancy and lactation. *Am J Cardiol.* 1973;32:247.
196. Regardh CG, Johnsson G. Clinical pharmacokinetics of metoprolol. *Clin Pharmacokinet.* 1980;5:557.
197. Högstedt S, Lindeberg S, Axelsson O, et al. A prospective controlled trial of metoprolol—hydralazine treatment in hypertension during pregnancy. *Acta Obstet Gynecol Scand.* 1985;64:505.
198. Finnestrom O, Ezitis J, Rydeu G, Wichman K. Neonatal effects of beta-blocking drugs in pregnancy. *Acta Obstet Gynecol Scand.* 1984;118:91.
199. Sandstrom B. Antihypertensive treatment with the adrenergic beta receptor blocker metoprolol during pregnancy. *Gynecol Obstet Invest.* 1978;9:195.
200. Sandstrom B. Adrenergic beta-receptor blockers in hypertension of pregnancy. *Clin Exp Hypertens.* 1982;B1:127.
201. Brodsky MA, Sato DA, Oster PD, et al. Paroxysmal ventricular tachycardia with syncope during pregnancy. *Am J Cardiol.* 1986;58:563.
202. Hogstedt S, Lindberg B, Perig DR, et al. Pregnancy-induced increase in metoprolol metabolism. *Clin Pharmacol Ther.* 1985;37:688.
203. Lindeberg S, Sandstrom B, Lundborg P, Regard CG. Disposition of the adrenergic blocker metoprolol in the late pregnant woman, the amniotic fluid, the cord blood and the neonate. *Acta Obstet Gynecol Scand.* 1984;118:61.
204. Solum T, Montan S, Sjoberg NO. Treatment of pregnancy induced hypertension with a beta-specific blocker. *Clin Exp Hypertens* 1982;B1(2–3):259.
205. Kjellmer I, Dagbjartsson A, Hrbek A, et al. Maternal beta-adrenergic blockade reduces fetal tolerance to asphyxia. *Acta Obstet Gynecol Scand.* 1984;118:75.
206. Liedholm H, Melander A, Bitzeu PO, et al. Accumulation of atenolol and metaprolol in human breast milk. *Eur J Clin Pharmacol.* 1981;20:229.
207. Rubin PC, Bulters L, Clark DM, et al. Placebo-controlled trial of atenolol in treatment of pregnancy-associated hypertension. *Lancet.* 1983;1:431.
208. Thorley KJ, McAinsh J, Cruickshank JM. Atenolol in the treatment of pregnancy-induced hypertension. *Br J Clin Pharmacol.* 1981;12:725.
209. Lunell NO, Persson B, Aragon G, et al. Circulatory and metabolic effects of acute beta-blockade in severe pre-eclampsia. *Acta Obstet Gynecol Scand.* 1979;58:443.
210. Melander A, Niklasson B, Ingemarsson I, et al. Transplacental passage of atenolol in man. *Eur J Clin Phamacol.* 1978;14:93.
211. Lardoux H, Gerard J, Blazquez G, et al. Hypertension in pregnancy: evaluation of two beta blockers, atenolol and labetolol. *Eur Heart J.* 1983;4:(suppl G)35.
212. Liedholm H. Atenolol in treatment of hypertension in pregnancy. *Drugs.* 1983;25:206S.
213. Dubois D, Petiteolas J, Temperville B, et al. Beta blocker therapy in 125 cases of hypertension during pregnancy. *Clin Exper Hyper-Hyper Pregnancy.* 1983;B2:41.
214. Kostis JB, Frishman W, Hosler MH, et al. Treatment of angina pectoris with pindolol: the significance of intrinsic sympathomimetic activity of beta-blockers. *Am Heart J.* 1982;104:496.
215. Man in't Veld AJ, Schalekamp MADH. How intrinsic sympathomimetic activity modulates the hemodynamic responses to beta-adrenoceptor antagonists: a clue to the nature of their antihypertensive mechanism. *Br J Clin Pharmacol* 1982;13:245S.
216. Rosenfeld J, Bott-Kauner G, Boner G, et al. Treatment of hypertension during pregnancy with hydralazine monotherapy or with combined therapy with hydralazine and pindolol. *Eur J Obstet Gynecol Reprod Biol.* 1986;22:197.
217. Ingermarsson I, Liedholm H, Montan S, et al. Fetal heart rate during treatment of maternal hypertension with beta-adrenergic antagonists. *Acta Obstet Gynecol Scand.* 1984;118(suppl):95.
218. Grunstein S, Ellenbogen A, Anderman S, et al. Transfer of pindolol across the placenta in hypertensive pregnant woman. *Curr Ther Res.* 1985;37:587.
219. Ellenbogen A, Jasehervatzky O, Davidson A. Management of pregnancy-induced hypertension with pindolol—comparative study with methyldopa. *Int J Gynaecol Obstet.* 1986;24:3.
220. MacCarty EP, Bloomfield SS. Labetolol: a review of its pharmacology, pharmacokinetic-clinical uses and side effects. *Pharmacotherapy.* 1983;3:193.
221. Kanto JH. Current status of labetolol, the first alpha and beta-blocking agent. *Int J Clin Pharm Ther Toxicol.* 1985;23:617.
222. Waal-Manning HJ, Simpson FO. Review of long-term treatment with labetolol. *Br J Clin Pharmacol.* 1982;B:64S.
223. Griffiths ID, Richardson J. Lupus-type illness associated with labetolol. *Br Med J.* 1979;2:495.
224. Riley AJ. Clinical pharmacology of labetolol in pregnancy. *J Cardiovasc Pharmacol.* 1981;3:S53.
225. Jouppila P, Kirkinen P, Koirula A, Ylikorkala O. Labetolol does not alter the placental and fetal blood flow or maternal prostanoids in preeclampsia. *Br J Obstet Gynecol.* 1986;93:543.
226. Rubin PC, Butters L, Kelman AW. Labetolol disposition and concentra-

tion-effect relationships during pregnancy. *Br J Clin Pharmacol.* 1983;15:465.
227. Lamming GD, Broughton, Pipkin, Symonds EM. Comparison of the alpha and beta blocking drug, labetolol and methyldopa in the treatment of moderate and severe pregnancy-induced hypertension. *Clin Exp Hypertens.* 1980;B2:865.
228. Nylund L, Lunell NO, Lewander R, et al. Labetolol for the treatment of hypertension in pregnancy. *Acta Obstet Gynecol Scand.* 1984;118:71.
229. Plouin P, Breart G, The Labetolol Methyldopa Study Group, et al. Comparison of antihypertensive efficacy and perinatal safety of labetolol and methyldopa in the treatment of hypertension in pregnancy: a randomized, controlled trial. *Br J Obstet Gynecol.* 1988;95:868.
230. Michael CA. Use of labetolol in the treatment of severe hypertension during pregnancy. *Br J Clin Pharmacol.* 1979;8(suppl 2):2115.
231. Nicholas TE, Lugg AM, Johnson RG. Maternal administration of salbutamol and labetolol increases the amount of alveolar surfactant in lung of the dog, 27 foetal rabbit. *Proc Aust Physiol Pharmacol Soc.* 1978;9:146P.
232. Michael CA. The evaluation of labetolol in the treatment of hypertension complicating pregnancy. *Br J Clin Pharmacol.* 1982;B:127S.
233. Symonds EM, Lamming GD, Jadoul F, et al. Clinical and biochemical aspects of the use of labetolol in the treatment of hypertension in pregnancy: comparison with methyldopa. In: Riley A, Symonds EM, eds. *The Investigation of Labetolol in the Management of Hypertension in Pregnancy.* Princeton, NJ: Excerpta Medica;1982:62.
234. Michael CA. Intravenous labetolol and intravenous diazoxide in severe hypertension complicating pregnancy. *Aust N Z J Obstet Gynecol.* 1986;26:26.
235. Garden A, Dommisse J, Davey DA. Intravenous labetolol and dihydralazine in severe hypertension in pregnancy. *Clin Exp Hypertens.* 1982;B1:371.
236. Ache RG, Moodlex J, Richards AM, Philpott RH. Comparision of labetolol and dihydralazine in hypertensive emergencies of pregnancy. *S Afr Med J.* 1987;71:354.
237. Mabie WC, Gonzales AR, Sibai BM, Amon E. A comparative trial of labetolol and hydralazine in the acute management of severe hypertension complicating pregnancy. *Obstet Gynecol.* 1987;70:328.
238. Lunell NO, Kulas J, Rane A. Transfer of labetolol into amniotic fluid and breast milk in lactating women. *Eur J Clin Pharmacol.* 1985;28:597.
239. Donchin Y, Amirav B, Sahar A, et al. Sodium nitroprusside for aneurysm surgery in pregnancy. *Br J Anaesth.* 1978;50:849.
240. Willoughby JS. Sodium nitroprusside, pregnancy and multiple intracranial aneurysms. *Anaesth Int Care.* 1984;12:351.
241. Willoughby JS. Sodium nitroprusside, pregnancy and multiple intracranial aneurysms. *Anaesth Int Care.* 1984;12:358.
242. Paull J. Clinical report of the use of sodium nitroprusside in severe preeclampsia. *Anaesth Int Care.* 1975;3:72.
243. Shoemaker CT, Meyers M. Sodium nitroprusside for control of severe hypertensive disease of pregnancy: a case report and discussion of potential toxicity. *Am J Obstet Gynecol.* 1984;149:171.
244. Sterupel JE, O'Grady JP, Morton MJ, et al. Use of sodium nitroprusside in complications of gestational hypertension. *Obstet Gynecol.* 1982;60:533.
245. Ring G, Krawes E, Shnider S, et al. Comparison of nitroprusside and hydralazine in hypertensive pregnant ewes. *Obstet Gynecol.* 1977;50:598.
246. Wheeler AS, James FM, Greiss FC, Meis PJ, et al. Effects of nitroglycerin to control severe hypertension of pregnancy during cesarean section. (abstract) *Anesthesiology.* 1979;51:563.
247. Naulty J, Cefalo RC, Levis PE. Fetal toxicity of nitroprusside in the pregnant ewe. *Am J Obstet Gynecol.* 1981;139:708.
248. Ellis SC, Wheeler AS, James FM III, et al. Fetal and maternal effects of sodium nitroprusside used to counteract hypertension in gravid ewes. *Am J Obstet Gynecol.* 1982;143:766.
249. Lieb SM, Zugain M, Huwauhid B, et al. Nitroprusside induced hemodynamic alteration in normotensive and hypertensive pregnant sheep. *Am J Obstet Gynecol.* 1981;139:925.
250. Jaffe AS, Roberts R. The use of intravenous nitroglycerin in cardiovascular disease. *Pharmacotherapy.* 1982;2:273.
251. Abrams J. Nitrates tolerance and dependence. *Am Heart J.* 1980;99:113.
252. Reichek N, Priest C, Zimrin D, et al. Antianginal effects of nitroglycerin patches. *Am J Cardiol.* 1984;54:1.
253. Thadani U, Fung HL, Darke CA, Parker OJ. Oral isosorbide dinitrate in angina pectoris: comparison of duration of action and dose-response relation during acute and sustained therapy. *Am J Cardiol.* 1982;49:411.
254. Parker OJ, Vankoughnett K, Farrell B. Comparison of buccal nitroglycerin and oral isosorbide dinitrate for nitrate tolerance in stable angina pectoris. *Am J Cardiol.* 1985;56:724.
255. Parker OJ, Farrell B, Lahey AK, et al. Effect of intervals between doses on the development of tolerance to isosorbide dinitrate. *N Engl J Med.* 1987;316:1440.
256. Snyder SW, Wheeler AS, James FM. The use of nitroglycerin to control severe hypertension of pregnancy during caesarean section. *Anesthesiology.* 1979;51:563.
257. Hood DD, Dewan DM, James FM, et al. The use of nitroglycerin in preventing the hypertensive response to tracheal intubation in severe preeclamptics. (abstract) *Anesthesiology.* 1983;59(3):A423.
258. Peng ATC, Gorman RS, Shulam SM, et al. Intravenous nitroglycerin for uterine relaxation in the post partum patient with retained placenta. *Anesthesiology.* 1989;71:172.
259. Cotton DB, Longmire S, Jones MM, et al. Cardiovascular alterations in severe pregnancy-induced hypertension: effects of intravenous nitroglycerin coupled with blood volume expension. *Am J Obstet Gynecol.* 1986;154:1053.
260. DeRosayro M, Nahrwold ML, Hill AB, et al. Nitroglycerin: plasma levels and effects in pregnant ewes. (abstract) *Anesthesiology.* 1979;51:S312.

Chapter One Hundred and Twenty-Six
Rheumatic Heart Disease

John H. McAnulty

126

"How many cases of acute rheumatic fever have you seen?" It is a question often asked doctors, and one that doctors ask students and residents. While recognized rheumatic fever is uncommon in developed countries, this is not true for most of the world. It continues to be the most important cause of heart disease in many less developed areas of the world.[1] Even in the United States there have been demonstrated areas of resurgence after a decline in incidence[2], and much rheumatic fever may go unrecognized—possibly because the disease is changing.[3] Additionally, immigration into the United States from less developed countries brings some rheumatic fever and rheumatic heart disease. Although rheumatic fever causes rheumatic heart disease, each has a different relationship to pregnancy. They, therefore, will be discussed separately.

RHEUMATIC FEVER

Rheumatic fever can affect pregnancy. This is particularly true in those with previous recognized rheumatic cardiac involvement. It is a disease of the young. Women appear to be affected more often than men. Caused by the *Group*

A β-hemolytic streptococcus, it is more common in persons repeatedly exposed to the infection—school children, parents of school children, teachers, medical personnel, and young people in group activities, such as military recruits. It occurs in 0.3% of children after they have had a streptococcal infection and as many as 2% of people who have been part of an epidemic of streptococcal throat infection.[4,5]

While the Group A β-hemolytic streptococcus appears to be "the sole agent causing initial and recurrent attacks of rheumatic fever[6]," the mechanism by which it does this is not clear. It is noteworthy that rheumatic fever occurs only when this organism affects the throat. Skin infections do not result in subsequent rheumatic fever. They are more likely to increase the risk of subsequent glomerulonephritis. It appears that the streptococcus that affects the throat is unique. It possibly affects the heart based on immunologic characteristics. It has been suggested that one may have a congenital susceptibility to the infection.[7] The mechanism by which rheumatic fever causes heart disease remains, however, uncertain. Since it is not due to direct infection by the streptococcus, an immunologic reaction is thought most likely to be the underlying process.

The diagnosis of rheumatic fever can be difficult. At greatest risk are those who have had a previous episode. Suspicion should, therefore, be the greatest in individuals who have had the problem in the past. Patients with rheumatic heart involvement are at highest risk among those who have a history of rheumatic fever. It should also be suspected in those with findings meeting the revised Jones criteria (Table 126–1).[8] The existence of two major criteria or one major and two minor criteria, along with evidence of a recent streptococcal infection (documented by an elevated anti-streptolysin–O titer), are necessary to make the diagnosis. Not surprisingly, this can be difficult. Although the most common manifestation is polyarthritis, it is nonspecific, tending to be migratory and lasting only a few days to weeks with no residual. The recognition of myocarditis generally makes physicians more likely to think of rheumatic fever. Myocarditis occurs in 40% of patients during their initial attack and in 70% with recurrence. Chest pain, congestive heart failure symptoms, and electrocardiogram changes can help make the diagnosis. Occasionally, patients with acute rheumatic fever also develop a heart murmur; but it is usually transient (chronic valve changes do not generally become manifest until 5–20 years after the acute episode). Rheumatic fever is too uncommon to be listed on the top of a differential diagnosis in young patients with either cardiopathy, myocarditis, or both.

Associated *chorea* (purposeless, writhing motions with jerking, occasionally severe enough to make a patient completely helpless), *erythema marginatum* (an evanescent migratory erythematous rash with well demarcated borders and central clearing), and *subcutaneous nodules* (nontender extensor surface extremity nodules) may lead to the diagnosis.

Rheumatic fever can alter pregnancy. Since it is young women who most frequently get rheumatic fever, an association between the two is not surprising. If a woman has had rheumatic fever in the past, a recurrence can occur with pregnancy and, if so, it is more likely to occur early in the pregnancy. Rheumatic fever with one pregnancy leads to a tendency towards recurrence with subsequent pregnancies.[9] Many maternal deaths from rheumatic fever were reported prior to 1960.[10] If a woman develops rheumatic fever with chorea during pregnancy, maternal morbidity, and maternal and fetal mortality may be high. This *chorea gravidarum* was at one time associated with a 10% maternal death rate and a 50% fetal mortality.[11] In the past 30 years reports of maternal mortality as the direct result of acute rheumatic myocarditis are rare.[12]

Treatment of rheumatic fever should start with prevention. Antibiotic prophylaxis has been proven effective. In the United States, rheumatic fever is so uncommon that there is controversy about who should receive antibiotic treatment. Young women who previously had rheumatic fever are at increased risk, especially if they experienced cardiac involvement. In such patients, antibiotic prophylaxis is required. The American Heart Association (AHA) recommends life-long antibiotic prophylaxis.[13] While this recommendation may be controversial, it seems appropriate to continue this approach for at least five years after the last documented episode. Prophylaxis is also recommended through the childbearing years. Benzathine penicillin, 1.2 million units intramuscularly every four weeks, or oral penicillin G, 200 thousand units, twice daily, are most effective. In case of penicillin allergy, sulfadiazine, 1.0 g daily or erythromycin 250 mg, twice daily, are acceptable alternatives. The use of sulfa dosages in pregnancy is controversial, however (see also Chapter 125).

There is no clear evidence that antibiotic treatment will alter the disease or prevent subsequent chronic valve deformity. However, antibiotics are often given and this may be the reason the disease is less severe than previously reported.[3] If rheumatic fever is diagnosed, a course of penicillin therapy is recommended, even if throat cultures are negative. Arthritis symptoms should be treated with aspirin, 2–4 g per day. Aspirin therapy in pregnancy should be given for significant symptoms only and the effects of the drug on pregnancy should be considered. Aspirin should be stopped, if possible, at least seven days prior to delivery to minimize the risk of bleeding. Other nonsteroidal anti-inflammatory drugs have not been studied adequately during pregnancy and are, therefore, not recommended.[14] A course of systemic steroids should be used if arthritis symptoms are severe despite aspirin therapy.

Debilitating chorea can be treated with muscle relaxants, such as diazepam. Fetal monitoring, particularly at the time of delivery, is essential. Congestive heart failure

TABLE 126–1. REVISED JONES CRITERIA FOR RHEUMATIC FEVER[a]

Major
Carditis
Arthritis
Sydenham's chorea
Erythema marginatum
Subcutaneous nodules
Minor
Previous history of rheumatic fever
Fever
Elevated acute phase reactants (ESR, CRP)
Prolonged PR interval
Arthralgia

[a] To make the diagnosis of rheumatic fever, two major criteria or one major and two minor criteria have to be present in combination with evidence of a Group A streptococcal infection (positive throat culture, history of scarlet fever or a raised or rising streptococcal antibody titer).[8]

should be treated with digitalis and diuretics (Chapter 125).

A history of previous rheumatic fever should not influence recommendations about pregnancy, unless significant rheumatic heart disease persists. The importance of antibiotic prophylaxis against any recurrence in women of childbearing age who have had rheumatic fever is worth a final reemphasis.

RHEUMATIC HEART DISEASE

Recognition of rheumatic heart disease may be difficult. A history of previous rheumatic fever can be used as a clue, but given the difficulty with that diagnosis, it can be misleading. Evidence for valve disease is most helpful in making the diagnosis. *Mitral stenosis* is almost always rheumatic in origin. Thus, mitral stenosis by itself, or in combination with any other valve abnormality, suggests the diagnosis of chronic rheumatic heart disease. Pure *mitral regurgitation* can be the result of rheumatic fever but is more often due to other causes. The same is true for isolated *aortic regurgitation.* A rheumatic etiology for isolated mitral or aortic regurgitation has probably been underestimated in series where the diagnosis was solely based on clinical evaluation. In some patients, echocardiography may show the typical rheumatic mitral valve changes (commissure closure, tip tethering) in patients who on examination otherwise do not demonstrate any clues for mitral stenosis. Isolated *aortic stenosis* is rarely (if ever) caused by rheumatic fever.

The prevalence of rheumatic heart disease during pregnancy varies in different populations. In Western countries it is probably decreasing.[1] In one large obstetrical series in the late 1960s, it was detected in 0.7% of women[9]; 90% had mitral stenosis and only 7% mitral regurgitation. Treatment of the primary disease and of complications has significantly decreased the severity of rheumatic heart disease.[3] Still, this large study reported 14 maternal deaths from rheumatic heart disease over a three year period.[9] In California, heart disease was the dominant nonobstetric cause of maternal death between 1960 and 1968, with rheumatic heart disease being the most common, causing 28 maternal deaths (see also Chapter 125).[12]

Treatment During Pregnancy

Each form of rheumatic heart disease can result in complications. As a rule, complications of rheumatic heart disease should be managed as they are in nonpregnant women. Because almost all cardiovascular drugs cross the placenta and potentially have an adverse effect on the fetus, activity and diet alterations are a preferable form of treatment. However, maternal safety remains the highest priority, and if drugs or cardiovascular procedures are necessary, they should be used.[15]

Recurrence. Rheumatic heart disease increases the chance of recurrent rheumatic fever, which, in turn, will cause further heart damage. If possible, a recurrence should be prevented. Antibiotic prophylaxis against rheumatic fever is effective and should be used in all women of childbearing age with rheumatic heart disease.[13]

Congestive Heart Failure. Dyspnea, fatigue, pedal edema, and an S_3 gallop may occur with normal pregnancies. This makes the diagnosis of congestive heart failure at times more difficult. Severe symptoms, rales, and an elevation of the central venous pressure support the diagnosis. If heart failure is present, treatment begins with limiting activity and control of sodium intake. If these fail to control symptoms, pharmacologic therapy should be used. Digitalis and diuretics alone can be effective. If required, vasodilators can be added, though some may reduce uterine blood flow (Chapter 125). Hydralazine has been shown to be safe and efficacious. The angiotensin-converting enzyme inhibitors should probably be avoided until their teratogenicity is better defined. If congestive heart failure cannot be controlled with strict activity limitation, dietary control, and medications, a surgical approach to the valve lesions can be considered during pregnancy, although the need for this is rare.

Hypotension and Low Perfusion Syndromes. These conditions put women with mitral stenosis and aortic stenosis, and particularly women with pulmonary hypertension, at increased risk of death. When recognized, positioning the woman on her left side to minimize obstruction by the uterus to inferior vena cava blood flow should be the first therapy. If this does not resolve the problem, fluid administration should be initiated and a careful clinical evaluation performed to determine the cause. Invasive monitoring may be required. In patients with severe valve stenosis or pulmonary hypertension, pulmonary capillary wedge and arterial pressure measuring lines should be in place during labor, delivery, and for the first few postpartum days (see Chapter 123).

Arrhythmias. Treatment of arrhythmias should mostly be the same as in a nonpregnant woman.[17] While it is preferable to avoid most antiarrhythmic drugs, dangerous rhythms or those compromising maternal hemodynamics, and thus uterine blood flow, require treatment (see Chapter 135). All antiarrhythmic drugs cross the placenta and the effect of most on the fetus has not been well defined. Each of the atrioventricular (AV) node blocking agents can be used. Digoxin does not advesely affect the fetus at therapeutic levels. The β-blockers have been reported to have some potentially adverse effects on the fetus but have been extensively and safely used in pregnant women for the treatment of hypertension (see Chapters 125 and 141). If required, β-1 selective drugs are preferable. The calcium-channel blockers have not been shown to have adverse fetal effects. Verapamil, given parenterally or orally, can be effective in treatment of supraventricular tachycardias. Adenosine has not been well studied, but its short half-life suggests that it could be used to treat maternal paroxysmal supraventricular tachycardia. Among the more frequently used arrhythmia drugs, quinidine is used most often in pregnancy. It does not appear to cause adverse fetal effects. There is little or no experience with some newer Class IA, IB, IC or Class III agents during pregnancy, and they should be used only when required for maternal safety. Cardioversion can also be performed in the pregnant woman, if medically indicated.

Symptomatic bradyarrhythmias should be treated. Atropine and isoproterenol can be used in emergency situations. If a pacemaker is required, it should be inserted, using techniques that minimize radiation exposure. For more detail, see Chapter 135.

Thromboembolic Complications. Warfarin crosses the placenta and has a 5–25% chance of causing fetal abnormalities. It is contraindicated during parts of pregnancy. Since its risk is highest in the first trimester[19], some suggest that it should be avoided during that time and used subsequently up until the time of delivery. However, heparin therapy throughout pregnancy seems preferable. Heparin has the inherent advantage of not crossing the placenta and thus does not have the teratogenicity of warfarin. Long-term subcutaneous heparin use has been shown to be well tolerated during pregnancy.[20] Antiplatelet agents, other than aspirin, have not been well evaluated. As noted previously, if aspirin is used, it is preferable to stop the drug seven days prior to delivery.

Bacterial Endocarditis. This complication, like rheumatic fever, is more easily prevented than treated. Antibiotic prophylaxis for dental or surgical procedures in women with valve abnormalities should be the same during pregnancy as at other times.[21] While the AHA does not recommend antibiotic prophylaxis at the time of labor and delivery, many would disagree. Occasional bacteremia during pregnancy, the severity of endocarditis itself, and the relatively low risk of antibiotics make us recommend that antibiotics be started with labor and continued for 24 hours after delivery. Admittedly, this may lead to some difficulty if false labor occurs. Ampicillin, gentamycin, and amoxicillin should be used for prophylaxis unless an allergy is present. If endocarditis occurs, standard treatment is essential, including valve surgery if necessary to protect the mother. For more detail, see Chapter 128.

Valve Surgery. In a sense, the need for valve surgery can be considered a complication of rheumatic valve disease. If surgery is required in the woman of childbearing age, a commissurotomy of a stenotic valve or the rapair of a regurgitant valve is preferable to the insertion of a prosthesis. The complications from a prothesis—*prosthetic heart valve disease*—can be severe and occur at a rate of 3–5% per year. These include systemic emboli, bleeding from anticoagulation, endocarditis, and death. On occasion, rheumatic valve disease is sufficiently severe to accept these risks, especially when a repair is not possible.

The experience with prosthetic valves during pregnancy has been reported in over 300 women. Results have not been consistent, and it is often not clear whether a mechanical or tissue valve is preferable.[22-24] Risks to the mother during pregnancy are about the same with either type.[24] The risk of death is 0–5%, and 5–40% of patients develop worsening heart failure, embolic events, or endocarditis. Tissue valve dysfunction in young women is common, and pregnancy may accelerate the process. Up to one third of pregnant women require valve replacement within two years of delivery.[21]

The risk to the fetus is also great in a woman with a prosthetic heart valve. The spontaneous abortion rate can exceed 50% in those with mechanical prostheses (some have wondered whether this is due to the warfarin therapy), and 20% of pregnancies in women with tissue prostheses end in abortion. Warfarin use with mechanical valves has resulted in the fetal embryopathy syndrome in up to 25% of live-born infants (see also Chapter 137).

The selection of a prosthesis for a woman who could become pregnant has to be individualized. A tissue valve eliminates the need for anticoagulation during pregnancy but results in a high likelihood for subsequent reoperation. A mechanical valve is potentially more durable but it means the woman will have to be instructed in home heparin administration during pregnancy.

RHEUMATIC HEART LESIONS AND PREGNANCY

The three most commonly encountered rheumatic heart lesions during pregnancy are mitral stenosis, mitral regurgitation, and aortic regurgitation. Each has to be considered separately and in the context of major hemodynamic and volume changes that occur during a normal pregnancy (see also Chapter 124).[25]

Mitral Stenosis

Mitral stenosis is still the leading cause of cardiac death during pregnancy.[10,12] It is also a frequent cause of symptoms.

Considering the pathophysiology of mitral stenosis, it is not surprising that the hemodynamic changes of pregnancy are not well tolerated. The stenotic valve impedes blood flow to the left ventricle and, as a consequence, left atrial pressure rises. The normal 40% increase in cardiac output and 50% increase in blood volume put the pregnant woman at risk for pulmonary edema. This is the most alarming and dangerous complication of mitral stenosis. Associated hemoptysis may be more common during pregnancy, possibly because of the increased tendency toward vascular rupture due to structural alterations caused by hormonal changes. Pulmonary artery or arteriolar vasoconstriction follows the rise in left atrial pressure. This results in pulmonary hypertension. If chronic, a subsequent increase in right heart diastolic pressures can cause fluid retention in legs, abdomen, and neck.

Hypovolemia can also be a problem in mitral stenosis patients. It can result in a significant reduction in left atrial pressure and a fall in left ventricular filling, sufficient to decrease cardiac output. The rapid volume shifts of pregnancy, often exacerbated by obstruction of the inferior vena cava by the gravid uterus, make this particularly likely to occur. Sudden deaths have been reported in mitral stenosis patients during pregnancy, with no previous recognized heart failure—possibly the result of this hypovolemic state.[10]

An already precarious situation from either volume extreme can be exacerbated by the development of *atrial fibrillation.* The rapid ventricular response compromises diastole. Consequently, there is less time for blood to flow from the left atrium to the left ventricle—already a problem without tachycardia. This can cause or worsen pulmonary edema and may result in a fall in cardiac output. Atrial fibrillation, in combination with the dilated left atrium, also increases the risk of thrombus development with the occurrence of subsequent systemic emboli.

Pregnancy can make the diagnosis of mitral stenosis more difficult. Hemoptysis or a systemic embolism are occasionally alarming presenting symptoms; fatigue, dyspnea, orthopnea, and dizziness are more common. A loud first heart sound, an opening snap, and a diastolic rumble may confirm the diagnosis. The chest x-ray can support the diagnosis by demonstrating left atrial enlargement. The electrocardiogram may also show this, atrial fibrillation, or both. An echocardiogram with Doppler flow measurements can confirm the diagnosis and help quantitate the degree of stenosis. An echocardiogram will also exclude the diagnosis of an atrial myxoma which, although rare, can mimic the presentation and examination findings of mitral stenosis.

Management of Mitral Stenosis. The woman with symptoms from recognized mitral stenosis prior to pregnancy is at increased risk during the pregnancy. If hemodynamic evaluation confirms significant stenosis, a mechanical approach to relieve the stenosis prior to conception is indicated. Balloon valvuloplasty or surgical mitral commissurotomy is preferable to valve replacement.

Once pregnancy occurs, digoxin therapy is indicated—not because it prevents atrial fibrillation, but because it will slow the ventricular response rate should that rhythm develop. If signs of congestive heart failure cannot be controlled with diet, activity, and medication, a mechanical approach can be utilized. There is only limited information about the use of balloon valvuloplasty in pregnancy, although it would seem appropriate for consideration, particularly late in pregnancy, when the danger of radiation exposure to the fetus has decreased. In our experience, the need to proceed to mitral valve surgey is rare, although it can be done.[26]

If the woman has adapted to the volume and hemodynamic changes of the pregnancy, labor and delivery are generally tolerated well. A vaginal delivery is appropriate, unless there are obstetrical contraindications.

Mitral Regurgitation

When present in women of childbearing age, mitral regurgitation is commonly due to rheumatic fever. The symptoms and physical examination findings are not greatly altered by pregnancy. An echocardiogram with Doppler flow evaluation can confirm the etiology, define the severity of the mitral regurgitation, and provide an assessment of ventricular function.

The fall in peripheral vascular resistance that occurs with pregnancy should decrease the amount of mitral regurgitation and assist a poorly functioning ventricle. These may be reasons why pregnancy is generally well tolerated in women with mitral regurgitation. Pregnant women with mitral regurgitation need not be discouraged unless there is severe ventricular dysfunction or clinical evident congestive heart failure. If either is present, or if mitral regurgitation is severe, mechanical correction of the valve, preferably a mitral valve repair, will make pregnancy safer. Persistence of severe ventricular dysfunction, despite treatment of mitral regurgitation, may increase the risk of maternal death, perhaps to as high as 5–10%[24], and will also increase fetal loss.

When mitral regurgitation is first recognized during pregnancy, no specific treatment is required unless the woman develops symptoms. Congestive heart failure and other complications can be treated as described earlier. The need for surgical treatment of mitral regurgitation during pregnancy is exceptionally rare. Successful valve replacement has been achieved when bacterial endocarditis threatens the mother and does not quickly respond to antibiotics.

Aortic Regurgitation

Pregnancy does not ease the difficulty of selecting optimum therapy for young women with aortic regurgitation. While the goals of preventing symptoms, minimizing complications, and optimizing life span are clear, the treatment is not. It has been suggested that medical therapy may preserve left ventricular function in the patient with asymptomatic or minimally symptomatic aortic regurgitation. It is not clear that this treatment will decrease subsequent symptoms, events, or death. Surgery for aortic insufficiency, due to uncontrolled bacterial endocarditis, can improve survival but optimal timing for surgical intervention in other aortic insufficiency patients is unclear. This uncertainty makes recommendations about pregnancy difficult. Still, when women with aortic regurgitation have been followed during pregnancy, the pregnancy has not worsened the hemodynamic condition of the mother and the valve regurgitation has rarely compromised the pregnancy. The normal fall in peripheral vascular resistance with pregnancy, with its expected beneficial effect on aortic regurgitation, may be one explanation for this.

Aortic regurgitation that is recognized before pregnancy is not a reason to discourage a pregnancy, unless a woman is significantly symptomatic or has severely compromised left ventricular function. While surgical correction may not always improve either, it should be considered before a woman becomes pregnant.

When first recognized during pregnancy, aortic insufficiency does not require treatment unless the woman is severely symptomatic or develops the complications of valve disease. These should be treated as described previously.

Other Abnormalities

Right-sided valve disease can occur with rheumatic heart disease, although it is usually seen in association with left-sided disease. Occasionally, tricuspid stenosis is sufficiently severe to require mechanical intervention, but this has not been reported during pregnancy. Tricuspid regurgitation is well tolerated during pregnancy.

REFERENCES

1. Padmaviti S. Rheumatic fever and rheumatic heart disease in developing countries. *Bull Who.* 1978;56:543.
2. Veasy LG, Widemeier SE, Orsmond GS, Ruttenberg HD, et al. Resurgence of acute rheumatic fever in the intermountain area of the United States. *N Engl J Med.* 1987;316:421.
3. Masseli BF, Chute CG, Walker AM, Kurland GS. Penicillin and the marked decrease in morbidity and mortality from rheumatic fever in the United States. *N Engl J Med.* 1988;318:280.
4. Mortimer EA, Rammelkamp CH, Jr. Prophylaxis of rheumatic fever. *Circulation.* 1956;14:1144.
5. Siegel AC, Johnson EE, Stollerman GH. Controlled studies of streptococcal pharyngitis in a pediatric population: I. Factors related to the attack rate of rheumatic fever. *N Engl J Med.* 1961;265:559.
6. Stollerman GH. Etiology and Pathogenesis of Rheumatic Fever. In Hurst JW, Logue RB, Schlant RC, Wenger NK, eds., *The Heart*, 4th ed. New York:McGraw-Hill. 1978;947.
7. Gray ED, Regelmann EW, Abdin Z, Kholy A, et al. Compartmentalization of cells bearing "rheumatic" cell surface antigens in peripheral blood and tonsils in rheumatic heart disease. *J Infec Dis.* 1987;155:247.
8. Committee on the Prevention of Rheumatic Fever and Bacterial Endocarditis of the American Heart Association: The Jones Critera (Revised). *Circulation.* 1984;70:893A.
9. Zagala JG, Feinstein AR. The preceding illness of acute rheumatic fever. *JAMA.* 1962;179:863.
10. Szekely P, Turner R, Snaith L. Pregnancy and the changing pattern of rheumatic heart disease. *Br Heart J.* 1978;35:1293.
11. Lewis BV, Parsons M. Chorea gravidarum. *Lancet.* 1966;1:284.
12. Hibbard LT. Maternal mortality due to cardiac disease. *Clin Obstet Gynecol.* 1975;18:27.
13. Committee on the Prevention of Rheumatic Fever and Bacterial Endocarditis of the American Heart Association: Prevention of rheumatic fever. *Circulation.* 1988;78:1083.
14. Urowitz MB, Gladman DD. Rheumatic disease in pregnancy. In: Burrow GN, Ferris TF, eds. Philadelphia: WR Saunders Co.; 1988.
15. Ueland K, McAnulty JH, Ueland FR, Metcalfe J. Special consideration in the use of cardiovascular drugs. In Ueland K, ed., *Cardiovascular Disease in Pregnancy.* Hagerstown: Harper and Row; 1981.
16. Metcalfe J, McAnulty JH, Ueland K. *Burwell and Metcalfe's Heart Disease and Pregnancy, Physiology and Management.* Boston: Little Brown: 1986;367.

17. Rotmensch HH, Elkayam U, Frishman W. Antiarrhythmic drug therapy during pregnancy. *Ann Intern Med.* 1983;98:487.
18. Hall JT, Pauli RM, Wilson KM. Maternal and fetal sequelae of anticoagulation during pregnancy. *Am J Med.* 1980;68:122.
19. Iturbe-Alessio I, Fonseca MC, Mutchinik O, Santos MA, et al. Risks of anticoagulant therapy in pregnant women with artificial heart valves. *N Engl J Med.* 1986;315:139.
20. Brabeck MC. Ambulatory management of thromboembolic diseases during pregnancy with continuous infusion of heparin. *JAMA.* 1987; 257:1790.
21. Dajari AS, Bisno AL, Chung KJ, Freed M, et al. Prevention of bacterial endocarditis. *JAMA.* 1990;264:2919.
22. Lutz DJ, Noller KL, Spittell JA Jr., Danielson GK, et al. Pregnancy and its complications following cardiac valve prostheses. *Am J Obstet Gynecol.* 1978;131:460.
23. Deviri E, Levinsky L, Yechezkel M, Levy MJ. Pregnancy after valve replacement with porcine xenograft prothesis. *Surg Gynecol Obstet.* 1985; 160:437.
24. McAnulty JH, Blair N, Walance C, Ueland K. Prosthetic heart valves and pregnancy: maternal and infant outcome. *J Am Coll Cardiol.* 1986; 7:171A.
25. Metcalfe J, McAnulty JH, Ueland K. In: Burwell CS and Metcalfe J, eds., *Heart Disease and Pregnancy, Physiology and Management.* Boston: Little Brown; 1986:11.
26. Becker RM. Intracardiac surgery in pregnant women. *Ann Thorac Surg.* 1983;36:453.
27. Walsh JJ, Burch GE, Black WC, et al. Idiopathic myocardiopathy of the puerperium (postpartal heart disease). *Circulation.* 1965;32:19.

Chapter One Hundred and Twenty-Seven

Congenital Heart Diseases

Joseph K. Perloff

127

For much of the 20th century, upward of 4% of pregnancies in the United States and Western Europe were complicated by cardiac disease.[1,2] Overall, prevalence has decreased somewhat in the last several decades, but the principal change has been less in prevalence than in the relative incidence of the various types of cardiac disorders in pregnant women.[3] Congenital heart disease is encountered more often, while the frequency of rheumatic heart disease has declined.[4]

Survival to childbearing age of women with congenital malformations of the heart and circulation is the result of natural selection or the benefits of surgery. Reparative surgery not only increases the life span of women with anomalies that have inherent tendencies for long survival, but also permits increasing numbers of women with disorders that were previously fatal in early life to reach reproductive age.[5] This chapter deals with pregnancy in women with either unoperated or operated congenital heart disease. Central to the topic is the complex interplay between maternal circulatory and respiratory physiology and congenital heart disease and the effects of this interplay on the fetus that is exposed to immediate risks that threaten its viability and to remote risks that express themselves as transmitted congenital anomalies or developmental defects.

TABLE 127–1. COMMON MALFORMATION WITH EXPECTED ADULT SURVIVAL IN APPROXIMATE ORDER OF PREVALENCE AMONG WOMEN

Acyanotic	Cyanotic
Atrial septal defect (secundum)	Fallot's tetralogy
Patent ductus arteriosus	
Pulmonic valve stenosis	
Coarctation of the aorta	
Aortic valve disease	

ETIOLOGY AND PATHOPHYSIOLOGY

The common *acyanotic* congenital malformations of the heart and circulation in which unoperated (natural) survival into childbearing age can be anticipated are (Table 127–1): ostium secundum atrial septal defect, patent ductus arteriosus, pulmonic valve stenosis, coarctation of the aorta, and aortic valve disease.[3,6] The most common *cyanotic* malformation is Fallot's tetralogy.[3,6] However, the *postoperative* cardiac female now constitutes one of the most important aspects of pregnancy and heart disease, and represents a new, growing patient population.[5] Successful cardiac surgery improves fertility and stabilizes the pregnancy in women whose congenital cardiac malformations had appreciably reduced sexual and ovarian function. Accordingly, women who were physiologically ill-equipped to bear children or who previously would not have reached reproductive age are now presenting for obstetric and cardiologic care after successful reparative surgery for congenital heart disease.

PHYSIOLOGIC RESPONSE TO THE NORMAL GRAVID STATE

An understanding of the relationship between heart disease and pregnancy presupposes knowledge of the maternal circulatory and respiratory adaptations to the normal gravid state (see Chapter 124). These adaptations are represented by four important variables: (1) the time of onset of the response, (2) the magnitude of the change, (3) the time when the change reaches its peak, and (4) the behavior of the adaptive response when it reaches its maximum deviation from the nonpregnant state.[2] The circulatory and respiratory changes during normal pregnancy provide a basis for understanding symptoms and physical signs that are sometimes erroneously attributed to heart disease.[3] Breathlessness (hyperpnea), easy fatigability, a decrease in exercise tolerance, basal rales, and peripheral edema are often misconstrued. The systemic arterial pulse during normal pregnancy exhibits a brisk rise and collapse beginning in the first trimester. The jugular venous pulse becomes more conspicuous after the 20th week, with enhanced X and Y descents making the A and V waves more obvious. Mean jugular venous pressure, estimated from the superficial jugular vein, remains normal, however. Precordial palpation discloses relatively hyperdynamic, but nonsustained, impulses, over the left and right ventricles and over the pulmonary trunk because both ventricles handle larger volumes ejected against relatively low resistances. As pregnancy progresses, enlargement of the breasts and abdomen makes accurate palpation difficult, if not impossible. Auscultatory changes accompanying normal gestation include variations in the heart sounds, and the presence of both systolic and continuous murmurs.[3] The first heart sound becomes louder because of the increase in heart rate and left ventricular contractility. The second heart sound tends to exhibit persistent expiratory splitting toward the end of pregnancy, especially when patients are examined in the lateral decubitus position. Third heart sounds are common because of the increased rate and volume of atrioventricular flow, but fourth heart sounds do not occur in normal pregnancy. Innocent pulmonic midsystolic murmurs and normal supraclavicular systolic murmurs are augmented by the gestational increase in cardiac output and stroke volume.[6] The mammary souffle—systolic or continuous—is peculiar to pregnancy and is heard over the breasts in late gestation, but especially in the postpartum period in lactating women. A far more common continuous murmur is the venous hum which is virtually universal during gestation. Certain organic murmurs associated with congenital heart disease may either increase or decrease during the course of pregnancy.[3] The augmented gestational cardiac output and stroke volume reinforce systolic murmurs across outflow valves. The decline in systemic vascular resistance reduces the intensity of systolic murmurs across incompetent systemic atrioventricular valves and reduces the intensity of diastolic murmurs across incompetent systemic outflow valves.

Pregnancy affects maternal congenital heart disease and congenital heart disease affects the gravid female and her fetus. In light of the physiologic responses during normal gestation, it is necessary to examine the interplay between maternal congenital heart disease and pregnancy in the unoperated patient and then in the gravida who has undergone reparative cardiac surgery.

THE EFFECT OF PREGNANCY ON MATERNAL CONGENITAL HEART DISEASE

In a practical clinical sense, the most important category of unoperated patients are those with common congenital cardiac anomalies likely to be found in adult women (see above). *Ostium secundum atrial septal defect* is especially important becaue its natural history spans the reproductive years, and because the majority of these patients are female.[2,6,7] Despite the gestational increase in cardiac output and stroke volume, young women with uncomplicated ostium secundum atrial septal defects generally tolerate pregnancy with no tangible ill effects. After the fourth decade, however, patients with otherwise uncomplicated secundum defects experience an increased incidence of supraventricular arrhythmias that may cause right ventricular failure and peripheral edema.[6] Varicose veins, in addition to, and apart from, peripheral edema, increase the risk of venous stasis and paradoxic embolization. Thrombi are carried by the inferior vena cava through the atrial septal defect into the systemic circulation.[6,8] Meticulous leg care minimizes venous stasis. Also important, but less well known, is the potentially deleterious effect of acute blood loss in patients with unoperated ostium secundum atrial septal defects. Hemorrhage results in a rise in systemic vascular resistance and in a decline in systemic venous return, a combination that augments the left-to-right shunt, sometimes appreciably. Pulmonary hypertension is relatively uncommon in ostium secundum atrial septal defect and occurs, if at all, relatively late in the natural history.[6] An elevation in pulmonary vascular resistance significantly increases the risk of pregnancy.[3]

An asymptomatic young woman with a small or moderate size *patent ductus arteriosus* and normal pulmonary arterial pressure can anticipate an uneventful pregnancy apart from the risk of infective endocarditis during delivery.[3,7] If there is a relatively large patent ductus with a sizeable left-to-right shunt, the gestational fall in systemic vascular resistance tends to decrease ductal flow, but the benefit is not likely to outweigh the augmented hemodynamic burden of pregnancy. The patient with a nonrestrictive patent ductus, suprasystemic pulmonary vascular resistance, and a reversed shunt is at highest risk. The gestational decline in systemic vascular resistance reinforces the right-to-left shunt through the ductus, so intrauterine oxygen saturation is further reduced.

In isolated *pulmonic valve stenosis*, 50% of patients are female.[6] The natural history typically permits adult survival, even in the presence of significant obstruction to right ventricular outflow.[6] Mild-to-moderate pulmonic stenosis is little or no threat to the mother, and occasionally even severe obstruction is well tolerated despite the gestational volume overload imposed upon an already excessively pressure-loaded right ventricle.[7] Infective endocarditis prophylaxis is required during delivery irrespective of the degree of stenosis.

Coarctation of the aorta predominates in males, but is dealt with here because maternal morbidity—cardiovascular complications without death—is high.[6,9-11] The risk of aortic rupture or dissection and of cerebral hemorrhage from rupture of an aneurysm of the circle of Willis increases during pregnancy.[3,6,10] Blood pressure variations in pregnant women with coarctation of the aorta are similar in direction to the variations in normal pregnancy, but from an initially higher level.[3] Importantly, the incidence of toxemia is lower with the hypertension of coarcation than in pregnant women with other forms of hypertension.[3] Left ventricular failure is exceptional despite the increased volume load imposed upon the already pressure-loaded left ventricle. The risk of infective endocarditis is much higher on a coexisting bicuspid aortic valve than at the site of coarctation.[6]

An isolated *functionally normal bicuspid aortic valve* often goes unrecognized in young women because of the low clinical index of suspicion (predominant occurrence in males and inconspicuous auscultatory signs).[6] The anomaly may first announce itself after delivery because of acute aortic regurgitation caused by infective endocarditis.[6]

Chronic bicuspid *aortic regurgitation* is generally well tolerated during pregnancy, provided the adaptive response of the left ventricle permits normal function, which is generally the case. The gestational decline in systemic vascular resistance, together with the increase in cardiac output, result in a reduction in regurgitant flow. Infective endocarditis prophylaxis at delivery goes without saying.

Asymptomatic women entering pregnancy with mild-to-moderate congenital bicuspid *aortic stenosis* generally do well, but if the obstruction is severe, circulatory reserve is limited.[12] Dyspnea, angina pectoris, or cerebral symptoms prior to conception or during early gestation predict serious sequelae.[12] The stenotic valve is at risk of infective endocarditis.

The most common cyanotic malformation that permits natural survival to reproductive age is *Fallot's tetralogy,* and the sex distribution is nearly equal.[6,13,14] Relative absence of symptoms before conception does not assure an uncomplicated course. The gestational decline in systemic vascular resistance, together with the augmented cardiac output and the increased venous return to an obstructed right ventricle, result in an increase in right-to-left shunt and a parallel fall in systemic arterial oxygen saturation. Labile hemodynamics during labor delivery and the puerperium incur additional risks. A sudden fall in systemic vascular resistance may precipitate intense cyanosis, syncope, and death. Conversely, bearing down during labor may abruptly and dangerously reduce systemic blood flow. Infective endocarditis during delivery is an additional concern.

Ventricular septal defects are seldom seen in women of reproductive age.[6] The occasional adult female with a small-to-moderate size defect confronts pregnancy with a comparatively low risk determined by the magnitude of the left-to-right shunt and the adaptation of her left ventricle to the accompanying volume overload. However, nonrestrictive ventricular septal defects that permit survival into adulthood generally do so because a progressive rise in pulmonary vascular resistance reduces left ventricular volume overload, but culminates in a reversed shunt.[6] The gestational risk of pulmonary vascular disease is emphasized once again.[3] Maternal death in Eisenmenger's complex can occur during pregnancy, labor, delivery, or the puerperium, with the cumulative risk estimated at 30–70%.[15-17] The gestational decline in systemic vascular resistance increases the right-to-left shunt, further reducing systemic arterial oxygen saturation. The fixed pulmonary vascular resistance precludes adaptive responses to the volatile fluctuations in systemic resistance, cardiac output, and blood volume during labor, delivery, and the puerperium. A sudden fall in systemic resistance may precipitate intense cyanosis, and bearing down during labor suddenly elevates systemic vascular resistance, depresses systemic blood flow, and may provoke fatal syncope.[6]

Certain congenital heart diseases are uncommon in infancy and childhood, but are relevant here because they permit high probabilities of survival into reproductive age. Among the most important is *primary pulmonary hypertension,* which typically becomes clinically overt in young women (sex ratio approaching 5:1), and poses formidable risks during pregnancy.[3,6,18] The high, fixed pulmonary vascular resistance blunts or precludes adaptive responses to the hemodynamic variations during gestation, labor, delivery, and the puerperium. Maternal mortality is approximately 50%.[6]

An uncommon disorder that permits survival to child-bearing age is *congenital complete heart block.*[6] Approximately half of these patients are female. Asymptomatic young women with congenital complete heart block generally tolerate pregnancy uneventfully provided the QRS duration is not prolonged.[19-22] The narrow QRS indicates that the pacemaker is *above* the bifurcation of the His bundle, so the ventricular rate is more likely to be within an acceptable physiologic range. Stokes–Adams attacks occasionally occur during gestation, however, and the heart does not always respond adequately to the volatile circulatory demands of labor and delivery.[19,20,22]

The majority of patients with *Ebstein's anomaly of the tricuspid valve* reach adulthood, and half are female.[6] The functionally inadequate right ventricle, already volume-overloaded by tricuspid regurgitation, copes poorly with the gestational increase in cardiac output and blood volume.[23,24] Paroxysmal atrial arrhythmias, which occur in about one third of nongravid patients with Ebstein's anomaly, are potential hazards during pregnancy.[6] Wolff–Parkinson–White bypass tracts set the stage for excessive ventricular rates in response to atrial fibrillation or flutter. The consequences can be catastrophic. Cyanosis in Ebstein's anomaly (right-to-left shunt at atrial level) may first become manifest during pregnancy because of a rise in right ventricular filling pressure. The right-to-left interatrial shunt increases the risk of paradoxical embolization[8] (see earlier discussion).

The Postoperative Congenital Cardiac Patient

Pregnancy after cardiac surgery is now one of the most important aspects of gestation and heart disease.[5] A prime objective of reparative surgery is to increase the safety and success of pregnancy and the subsequent health of mother and child.[25] Operation should, therefore, be anticipatory. With few exceptions, however, cardiac surgery or interventional catheterization leaves behind residua and sequelae of varying degrees of significance.[5] The risk of pregnancy to the mother is then determined principally by the presence, type, and magnitude of these cardiac and vascular residua and sequelae. Nevertheless, there is a uniform consensus that a successful operation prior to gestation can be pivotal in reducing maternal risk. The postoperative benefits will now be underscored by commenting on the anomalies discussed above. It goes without saying that an operation has no bearing on genetic transmission of maternal congenital heart disease.

An asymptomatic woman of reproductive age who has undergone closure of her ostium secundum atrial septal defect in childhood or young adulthood can anticipate pregnancy virtually devoid of maternal cardiac risk.[7] Successful closure of the defect also eliminates the risk of paradoxic embolization. There are usually few or no significant postoperative residua or sequelae, except occasional atrial flutter years after successful repair.

Surgical closure of a small, nonpulmonary hypertensive *patent ductus arteriosus* in childhood represents one of the few unqualified cures of congenital heart disease. Such patients are then normal in the literal sense. Closure of a nonrestrictive patent ductus, however, may be followed by an incomplete decline in pulmonary vascular resistance.[5] The presence of postoperative pulmonary vascular disease is an important residuum depending upon its degree (see above).

When surgical repair or balloon dilatation of congenital *pulmonic valve stenosis* leaves behind little or no gradient, the mother can anticipate a normal pregnancy except for the risk of infective endocarditis, which is reduced, if not eliminated. Mild-to-moderate low pressure pulmonary regurgitation is not an important sequel.

Surgical correction of *coarctation of the aorta* with complete relief of obstruction, especially in early childhood, materially increases the prospect of long-term normalization of blood pressure, and significantly reduces the risk of gestational aortic dissection or rupture.[7,26] Balloon dilatation of previously *unoperated* (native) coarctation may appreciably decrease the gradient, but the risk of aortic rupture or dissection can be no less than in mild coarctation without prior intervention. After successful operation, susceptibility to infective endocarditis at the site of the coarctation repair is, for all practical purposes, absent, but the risk of infection on a coexisting bicuspid aortic valve is necessarily unaffected. To what extent successful correction of coarctation of the aorta diminishes the hazard of gestational rupture of an aneurysm of the circle of Willis is unknown, but the incidence of death caused by postoperative intercranial hemorrhage is reassuringly low.[26]

When congenital *aortic valve stenosis* is accompanied by a gradient of 50 mm Hg or more in a young woman, surgical relief appreciably lowers the risk of pregnancy except for susceptibility to infective endocarditis.[7] Every attempt should be made to avoid aortic valve replacement, especially with a rigid prosthesis that requires anticoagulants[27] (see below). If a woman with *aortic regurgitation,* even moderate-to-marked, wishes to become pregnant, it is generally better for her to do so without aortic valve replacement, provided the left ventricle is functioning normally. If an aortic valve prosthesis is required in a female of reproductive age, a tissue valve should be used.[27]

Successful intracardiac repair of Fallot's tetralogy justifies an air of optimism regarding pregnancy, especially if there is little or no outflow gradient and only mild postoperative pulmonary regurgitation.[28] Relief of cyanosis increases the likelihood of successful conception and improves stability of the pregnancy and the prospect of normal fetal growth and development (see below). Electrophysiologic sequelae, including bifascicular block, high degree heart block, or right ventricular ectopic rhythms cannot be ignored, however.[29]

If a moderately restrictive or nonrestrictive *ventricular septal defect* is closed early enough in its natural course to preclude the development of pulmonary vascular disease, pregnancy can be anticipated with impunity. Significant postoperative electrophysiologic sequelae are few and far between.[29]

An occasional female with *congenital complete heart block* requires a pacemaker, but pregnancy can, nevertheless, proceed with relative confidence. Ventricular function is usually normal, so an artificial fixed-rate pacemaker provides satisfactory physiologic support.[30]

Surgical repair of Ebstein's anomaly of the tricuspid valve ideally takes the form of reconstruction rather than replacement. A large, mobile anterior tricuspid leaflet sets the stage for reconstruction into a relatively competent unicuspid atrioventricular valve. Surgical dissociation between right atrium and right ventricle eliminates potential or active bypass tracts. The risk of pregnancy to the mother is then appreciably reduced, but not eliminated.[7]

Pregnancy after repair of certain types of *complex cyanotic congenital heart disease* is now a practical clinical issue. The Fontan operation for tricuspid atresia or univentricular heart with pulmonic stenosis creates an atrial-dependent pulmonary circulation without a subpulmonic ventricle. After operation, patients can achieve approximately twofold increments in cardiac index in response to isotonic exercise, and the physiologic response to isolated increments in heart rate by atrial pacing is similar to normal.[31] These hemodynamic observations suggest that women who have had successful Fontan repairs confront the physiologic load of pregnancy with circulations that potentially possess adequate functional reserve.

Medical Management of the Gravida

The expectant mother's *cardiac reserve* is encroached upon by the hemodynamic burdens of pregnancy, but this challenge can usually be met by minimizing the factors that aggravate maternal heart disease (Table 127–2).[3] These factors include anxiety, the tendency to retain sodium and water, strenuous or isometric exercise, heat and humidity, anemia, infection (especially pyelonephritis and lower respiratory), arrhythmias, and thromboembolic predispositions.[3] Anxiety is a source of stress, especially in the prima gravida as she confronts the new experience of pregnancy. The expectant mother should be told what to anticipate during each stage of gestation, labor, delivery, and the puerperium. Certitude that the pain of labor and delivery will be ameliorated is an important element in reducing anxiety as term approaches. The tendency for an increase in body water and total exchangeable sodium in the gravid state is addressed by sodium restriction, not diuretics. Diuretics should be used judiciously, if at all (see below), notably for the edema of cardiac failure, not for the edema of normal pregnancy. Excessive weight gain is controlled by restriction of calories. Exercise is an additional physiologic imposition, so the pregnant congenital cardiac patient should avoid sudden, strenuous, or isometric effort. Heat and humidity add to the hemodynamic burden and may aggravate heart failure in otherwise stable pregnant women with heart disease. A cool, dry environment promotes dissipation of heat and improves regulation of body temperature.

Noncardiac diseases also exert undesirable circulatory effects. The physiological anemia of pregnancy must be distinguished from pathologic anemia. An increase in plasma volume during the first trimester is normally accompanied by a fall in hematocrit that reaches its lowest level at 32–34 weeks. Oral iron is legitimately used to minimize the physiological anemia, but should be used highly selectively in cyanotic patients.[32] Infection, especially pyelonephritis, is relatively common during pregnancy and the postpartum period, and can add to the cardiac burden. Lower respiratory infections pose special problems for the pregnant cardiac patient when pulmonary venous or pulmonary arterial pressure is elevated. Arrhythmias can be

TABLE 127–2. MEDICAL MANAGEMENT OF THE GRAVIDA

Factors that encroach upon cardiac reserve and aggravate maternal heart disease
Major cardiac risks to the mother
Labor, delivery, and the puerperium
Infective endocarditis prophylaxis
Cardiovascular drugs during pregnancy
Beneficial effects of cardiac surgery
Long-term effects of gestation on maternal congenital heart disease

matters of concern especially, but not exclusively, in patients who have had right ventriculotomies or right atrial incisions. The gestational tendency for stasis in lower extremity veins and the attendant risk of thromboembolism are reduced by meticulous leg care and early ambulation after delivery.

Brief comment is made here on the use of oxygen during gestation in cyanotic women. Suffice to say that there is no convincing evidence that oxygen administration benefits the mother, and no evidence that a favorable effect is exerted on a growth-retarded fetus.[7,32,33]

Maternal mortality generally varies directly with functional class (Table 127–3). In the presence of certain congenital cardiac malformations, however, childbearing imposes such a formidable threat to maternal survival that pregnancy is proscribed or should be interrupted irrespective of functional class. The two major *maternal cardiac risks* are pulmonary hypertension (more specifically pulmonary vascular disease) and pulmonary edema.[3] Pulmonary vascular disease limits or precludes appropriate adaptive responses to the circulatory changes of pregnancy and to the volatile changes during labor, delivery, and the puerperium. Primary pulmonary hypertension (see above) is emblematic, and Eisenmenger's complex combines the maternal risk of pulmonary vascular disease with the fetal risk of cyanosis (see below). It is worth reemphasizing that a sudden fall in systemic vascular resistance in Eisenmenger's complex may precipitate intense cyanosis, and the sudden rise in systemic resistance prompted by bearing down during labor may abruptly depress cardiac output and provoke fatal syncope (see above). Similar risks confront the patient with Fallot's tetralogy.

Pulmonary edema is a second major maternal cardiac risk. Although a less common occurrence in pregnant women with congenital heart disease than in those with acquired heart disease[34], pulmonary edema is usually due to left ventricular failure (pressure or volume overload), responds poorly to medical management, and with few exceptions, is beyond rational surgical options.

Medical management extends into labor, delivery, and the puerperium. In women with functionally mild unoperated congenital cardiac lesions and in those after successful intracardiac repair (see below), management of labor and delivery is essentially the same as for normal women. Otherwise, labor in the lateral decubitus position attenuates the undesirable hemodynamic fluctuations associated with major supine uterine contractions.[35] Analgesia (generally meperidine) is effective for relief of pain and apprehension. A strong consensus favors spontaneous vaginal delivery. It is best to have the fetus pass through the pelvis under the force of uterine contractions unassisted by straining in order to minimize, if not avoid, the undesirable effects of the Valsalva maneuver. Cesarean section, with few exceptions (see later), is reserved for obstetric indications, especially cephalopelvic disproportion. Selection of anesthesia is based upon the anticipated hemodynamic response to a given agent.[36] Women with greater functional impairment

TABLE 127–3. MATERNAL AND FETAL MORTALITY ACCORDING TO FUNCTIONAL CLASS

Maternal Mortality		Fetal Mortality	
Classes I and II	0.4%	Class I	
Classes III and IV	6.8%	Class IV	30.0%

benefit from the circulatory stability offered by conduction anesthesia.[7] Injection into the epidural space of narcotics is preferred during labor for patients whose cardiac function is particularly sensitive to changes in preload and afterload, but pudendal block is then necessary for delivery. Lumbar epidural anesthesia effectively controls pain during labor *and* delivery, but care must be taken to avoid hypotension caused by loss of sympathetic tone. Oxygen inhalation is often intuitively administered during labor, especially in cyanotic women, but without proven efficacy.[33]

In patients who require invasive monitoring, elective induction of labor can be employed to time its onset. A flotation catheter offers the security of meticulous hemodynamic surveillance, not only during labor and delivery, but also in the immediate postpartum period. Individual judgment is required, however. In Eisenmenger's complex, for example, the risks of a Swan–Ganz catheter outweigh the benefits.[37]

After expulsion of the placenta, it is important to minimize blood loss, especially in patients with pulmonary vascular disease or Fallot's tetralogy, but also in women with unoperated ostium secundum atrial septal defect (see earlier). The probability of thromboembolism increases during the postpartum period, so patients with lesions susceptible to paradoxical embolization are at particular risk.[8,38] Ostium secundum atrial septal defect is such a lesion because pelvic or lower extremity emboli are carried through the inferior vena cava across the atrial septum into the systemic circulation. Meticulous leg care, the use of elastic support stockings, and early ambulation are essential.

Breast-feeding, commonly practiced today, should be advised selectively in patients with congenital heart disease. Limited circulatory reserve may be encroached upon by the demands of breast-feeding and the risk of mastitis and bacteremia is not to be ignored. Bromocriptine is commonly used to suppress lactation, but should be administered cautiously because of potential hypotension.[7]

Prophylaxis for *infective endocarditis* is an important part of the medical management of susceptible patients.[3,39] During gestation, the gravida should be instructed on oral hygiene, and a dental examination carried out at least once during pregnancy, with the visit preceded and immediately followed by antibiotic prophylaxis as recommended by the guidelines of the Committee on Rheumatic Fever and Infective Endocarditis of the American Heart Association.[40] The incidence of bacteremia after a normal uncomplicated vaginal delivery varies from 0–5%.[39] Accordingly, it has been argued that prophylaxis is unnecessary in uncomplicated vaginal deliveries because bacteremia is neither a natural nor inevitable sequel. It is not prudent to assume, however, that delivery will be uncomplicated so that pregnant women with susceptible cardiac lesions should receive antibiotics from the onset of labor through the third or fourth postpartal day.[3]

Cardiovascular drugs in the gravida with congenital heart disease fall into two major categories—antiarrhythmics and anticoagulants.[2,41] Anticoagulants will be dealt with later in the section on risks to the fetus. The efficacy of antiarrhythmic agents during pregnancy is similar in principle to their use in nongravid patients except for placental transfer of the pharmacologic agent and the effect of gestation on dosage. Details on specific cardiovascular drugs are provided elsewhere (see Chapter 125).

The chief beneficial effects of reparative cardiac surgery are to increase the safety and success of pregnancy and the subsequent health of mother and child. One of the most effective ways of simplifying medical management is for operation to precede conception. Cardiac surgery during pregnancy is seldom an issue, even less so in the context of congenital heart disease (see also Chapter 136).[3,42]

What are the long term effects of pregnancy in maternal congenital heart disease? Is a woman's impaired cardiac reserve "like a bank account that is irreversibly depleted by the cost of pregnancy"?[34] With few exceptions, current opinion does not support this view. Women with congenital heart disease may be at a higher risk during pregnancy but if they survive, no long term harmful cardiac effects have been confidently identified.[3]

Risk to the Fetus

Maternal congenital heart disease exposes the fetus to immediate risks that threaten its intrauterine viability and to remote risks that express themselves after birth as congenital and developmental malformations. Immediate risks are determined principally by the functional class of the mother, maternal cyanosis, and anticoagulants. Extracorporeal circulation is associated with a high incidence of fetal wastage, but cardiac surgery is rarely employed during pregnancy, especially in patients with congenital heart disease.[3,42] The hypertension of coarctation of the aorta does not threaten the fetus as do other forms of hypertension.[3] Remote risks to the fetus take the form of genetic transmission,[43-46] teratogenic effects of certain cardiac drugs[47,48], and the harmful effects of certain environmental toxins and environmental exposures.[49,50]

The risk to the fetus of maternal functional class is shown in Table 127–3. The incremental fetal risk varies from virtually zero in asymptomatic gravida (Class I) to nearly 30% in gravid women who are symptomatic at rest (Class IV).

Maternal cyanosis threatens the growth, development, and viability of the fetus and materially increases fetal wastage.[3,6] Infants born to cyanotic mothers are typically dysmature or premature. The high rate of spontaneous abortion increases roughly in parallel with the mother's hypoxemia. However, even when maternal cyanosis is initially mild, the rate of spontaneous abortion is not low because the right-to-left shunt tends to increase during the course of pregnancy owing to the fall in systemic vascular resistance. Surgical correction of congenital heart disease eliminates the cyanosis and materially improves maternal functional class, underscoring the desirability of anticipatory operative intervention.

Anticoagulants are, with few exceptions, obligatory in gravida with mechanical valve prostheses, especially because of the hypercoagulable state of pregnancy.[51-55] Antiplatelet drugs (aspirin) are unacceptable alternatives to anticoagulants because of the potential for closing the fetal ductus and because of low efficacy.[56] There is presently no consensus regarding the best method for administering anticoagulants to pregnant women. Anticoagulants expose the fetus to risks, but no benfits, except indirectly by protecting the mother from the morbidity and potential mortality of thromboembolic complications. Warfarin, which is a coumarin derivative, is the oral anticoagulant of choice and heparin is the only currently employed parenteral anticoagulant. Warfarin is a low molecular weight compound that freely crosses the placental barrier, while heparin is a high molecular weight compound that does not cross the placental barrier. Warfarin is potentially teratogenic, and during the second and third trimesters has been linked to nonteratogenic fetal abnormalities especially of the central nervous system. Heparin is not teratogenic, but the 30% risk of fetal wastage is about the same as with warfarin.[51] In deciding between warfarin, heparin, or a combination of the two drugs, the variables include the risk of warfarin embryopathy and of warfarin developmental injury[57], the risk of warfarin-induced fetal hemorrhage associated with preterm labor, and the side effects of chronic heparin usage in addition to the maternal inconvenience of long-term subcutaneous administration. Therapeutic recommendations broadly include four options: (1) maintenance of the warfarin that was begun before conception, and continued use of warfarin through the 36th week of pregnancy when heparin is substituted in anticipation of labor; (2) replacement of the warfarin begun before conception with subcutaneous heparin as soon as pregnancy is established, returning to warfarin administration in the second and third trimesters until the 36th week; (3) replacing warfarin with heparin prior to conception, continuing the heparin through the first trimester, then returning to warfarin during the second and third trimesters; and (4) replacing warfarin with heparin before conception and continuing heparin throughout gestation. Whatever regimen is selected, it is best to advise the patient of her options before she becomes pregnant. My own preference is option four, with option three as the fallback position. If preterm labor develops in a patient on subcutaneous heparin, only the mother is anticoagulated, and protamine sulphate reverses maternal heparinization. If preterm labor develops in a patient on warfarin, management is more complex because both the mother *and* the fetus are anticoagulated. Fetal levels of coagulation factors do not correlate with maternal levels[58,59], so infusion of fresh frozen plasma into the mother cannot be depended upon to reverse the fetal anticoagulation. An emergency cesarean section may circumvent hemorrhagic fetal death during labor and delivery, and should be followed by infusion of fresh frozen plasma into the salvaged newborn.

Let us now turn to remote risks to the fetus. The risk of genetic transmission is greater if a parent, rather than a sibling, has congenital heart disease, and greater if the mother, rather than the father, has the congenital malformation.[43-46] The significantly greater risk of transmission of congenital heart disease from the mother, rather than the father, is ascribed to maternal vulnerability to teratogens and cytoplasmic inheritance. There is apparent non-Mendelian behavior of certain autosomal genes, the expression of which depends upon the sex of the parent from which the gene is inherited. A tendency for inheritance to occur predominatly through the female line is a distinguishing feature of cytoplasmic material, such as mitochondria that are inherited from the mother.

It is now appropriate to discuss certain noncardiac agents to which the pregnant woman may be exposed and which may produce congenital heart disease in her offspring. Recall that in the first trimester, especially the 2nd to 9th weeks, the risk of exposure is teratogenicity. In the second and third trimesters, the risks are represented by adverse effects on fetal growth and development, especially the central nervous system which continues to mature throughout gestation.[47,48] Most relevant to this discussion of heart disease and pregnancy is exposure of the fetus to maternal agents that may cause cardiac malformations. Ethyl alcohol is an example.[48,49] The teratogenic effects of the fetal alcohol syndrome include congenital anomalies of the heart, generally isolated defects in the ventricular septum, less commonly Fallot's tetralogy, or atrial septal defect. Another example is lithium carbonate. Use of the drug in the first trimester is accompanied by a risk of congenital malformations of the heart and great arteries, especially Ebstein's anomaly of the tricuspid valve.[48,60-62]

Certain environmental exposures, unrelated to drugs or toxins, increase the probability of congenital heart disease in the fetus. Patent ductus arteriosus is approximately six times as frequent in offspring of women who bear children at high altitudes, as in offspring of women who are pregnant at sea level.[6] There is also a predilection for increased pulmonary vascular resistance in such offspring, even if the ductus is restrictive. Atrial septal defect is more likely to be associated with pulmonary hypertension in children living at high altitude than in those at sea level.[50]

REFERENCES

1. Szekely P, Snaith L. *Heart Disease and Pregnancy*. Edinburgh: Churchill Livingstone:1974.
2. Metcalfe J, McAnulty JH, Ueland K. *Burwell & Metcalfe's Heart Disease and Pregnancy*. 2nd ed. Boston: Little, Brown & Co:1986.
3. Perloff JK. Pregnancy and cardiovascular disease. In: Braunwald E, ed. *Heart Disease*. Philadelphia: W. B. Saunders Co; 1988:1848.
4. McFaul PB, Dornan JC, Lamki H, Boyle D. Pregnancy complicated by maternal heart disease. A review of 519 women. *Br J Obstet Gynaecol*. 1988;95:861.
5. Engle MA, Perloff JK. *Congenital Heart Disease after Surgery*. New York: Yorke Medical Books: 1983.
6. Perloff JK. *The Clinical Recognition of Cong. Heart Disease*. Philadelphia; W.B. Saunders Co:1987.
7. Pitkin RM, Perloff JK, Koos BJ, Beall MH. Pregnancy and congenital heart disease. *Ann Int Med*. 1990;112:445.
8. Loscalzo J. Paradoxical embolization: clinical presentation, diagnostic strategies, and therapeutic options. *Am Heart J*. 1986;112:141.
9. Mortensen JD, Joelsson I. Coarctation of the aorta in pregnancy. *JAMA*. 1965;191:596.
10. Deal K, Wooley CF. Coarctation of aorta and pregnancy. *Ann Int Med*. 1973;78:706.
11. Bjork VO, Bergdahl L, Jonasson R. Coarctation of the aorta. The world's longest follow-up. *Adv Cardiol*. 1978;22:205.
12. Easterling TR, Chadwich HS, Otto CM, Benedetti TJ. Aortic stenosis in pregnancy. *Obstet Gynecol*. 1988;72:113.
13. Meyer EC, Tulsky AS, Sigmann P, et al. Pregnancy in the presence of tetralogy of Fallot. *Am J Cardiol*. 1964;14:874.
14. Jacoby WJ. Pregnancy with tetralogy and pentalogy of Fallot. *Am J Cardiol*. 1964;14:866.
15. Gleicher N, Midwall J, Hochberger D, Jaffin H. Eisenmenger's syndrome and pregnancy. *Obstet Gynecol Surv*. 1979;34:721.
16. Bitsch M, Johansen C, Wennevold A, Osler M. Eisenmenger's syndrome and pregnancy. *Eur J Obstet Gynecol Reprod Biol*. 1988;28:69.
17. Spinnato JA, Kraynak BJ, Cooper MW. Eisenmenger's syndrome in pregnancy. *N Engl J Med*. 1981;304:1215.
18. Nielsen NC, Fabricius J. Primary pulmonary hypertension with special reference to prognosis. *Acta Med Scand*. 1961;170:731.
19. Esscher EB. Congenital complete heart block (Review). *Acta Paedriatr Scand*. 1981;70:131.
20. Mowbray R, Bowley C. Congenital complete heart block complicating pregnancy. *J Obstet Gynaecol Br Emp*. 1948;55:438.
21. Michaelsson M, Engle MA. Congenital complete heart block—an international study of the natural history. *Cardiovasc Clin*. 1972;4:85.
22. Kenmure ACF, Cameron AJV. Congenital complete heart block in pregnancy. *Br. Heart J*. 1967;29:910.
23. Waickman LA, Skorton DJ, Varner MW, et al. Ebstein's anomaly and pregnancy. *Am J Cardiol*. 1984;53:357.
24. Littler WA. Successful pregnancy in a patient with Ebstein's anomaly. *Br Heart J*. 1970;32:711.
25. Shime J, Mocarski EJM, Hastings D, et al. Congenital heart disease in pregnancy: short- and long-term implications. *Am J Obstet Gynecol*. 1987; 156:313.
26. Steele PM, Fuster V, Ritter DG, McGoon DC. Isolated coarctation of the aorta—long term operative results. In: Engle MA, Perloff JK, eds. *Congenital Heart Disease after Surgery*. New York: Yorke Medical Books: 1983.
27. Denbow CE, Matadial L, Sivapragasman S, Spencer H. Pregnancy in patients after homograft cardiac valve replacement. *Chest*. 1983;83:540.
28. Ralstin JH, Dunn M. Pregnancies after surgical correction of tetralogy of Fallot. *JAMA*. 1976;235:2627.
29. Vetter VL, Horowitz LN. Electrophysiologic residua and sequelae of surgery for congenital heart disease. In: Engle MA, Perloff JK, eds. *Congenital Heart Disease after Surgery*. New York, NY: Yorke Medical Books; 1983:261.
30. Shouse EE, Acker GA. Pregnancy and delivery in a patient with external-internal cardiac pacemaker. *Obstet Gynecol*. 1964;24:817.
31. Barber G, Di Sessa T, Child J et al. Hemodynamic responses to isolated increments in heart rate by atrial pacing after a Fontan procedure. *Am Heart J*. 1988;115:837.
32. Perloff JK, Rosove M, Child JS, Wright GB. Adults with cyanotic congenital heart disease: hematologic management. *Ann Int Med*. 1988;109:406.
33. Wilcourt RJ, King JC, Queenan JT. Maternal oxygen administration and fetal transcutaneous PO_2. *Am J Obstet Gynecol*. 1983;146:714.
34. Chesley LC. Rheumatic heart disease in pregnancy. *Obstet Gynecol*. 1975; 46:699.
35. Van Donsen PW, Eskes TK, Martin CB, Van Hof MH. Postural blood pressure differences in pregnancy. *Am J Obstet Gynecol*. 1980;138:1.
36. Roberts SL, Chestnut DH. Anesthesia for the obstetric patient with cardiac disease. *Clin Obstet Gynecol*. 1987;30:601.
37. Devitt JH, Noble WH, Byrick RJ. A Swan-Ganz catheter related complication in a patient with Eisenmenger's syndrome. *Anesthesiology*. 1982; 57:335.
38. Rutherford SE, Phelan JP. Thromboembolic disease in pregnancy. *Clin Perinat*. 1986;13:719.
39. Sugrue D, Blake S, Troy P, McDonald D. Antibiotic prophylaxis against infective endocarditis after normal delivery—is it necessary? *Br Heart J*. 1980;44:499.
40. Shulman ST, Amren DP, Bisno AL. Prevention of bacterial endocarditis. *Circulation*. 1984;70:1123A.
41. Briggs GG, Bodendorfer TW, Freeman RK, Yaffe SJ. *Drugs in Pregnancy and Lactation*. Baltimore, MD: William and Wilkins:1983.
42. Bernal JM, Miralles PJ. Cardiac surgery with cardiopulmonary bypass during pregnancy. *Obstet Gynecol Surv*. 1986;41:1.
43. Nora JJ, Nora AH. Update on counseling the family with a first-degree relative with a congenital heart defect. *Am J Med Genet*. 1988;29:137.
44. Nora JJ, Nora AH. Maternal transmission of congenital heart diseases: new recurrence risk figures and the questions of cytoplasmic inheritance and vulnerability to teratogens. *Am J Cardiol*. 1987;59:459.
45. Nora JJ, Nora AH. Familial risk of congenital heart defect. *Am J Med Genet*. 1988;29:231.
46. Pyeritz RE, Murphy EA. Genetics and congenital heart disease: perspectives and prospects. *J Am Coll Cardiol*. 1988;13:1458.
47. Beeley L. Adverse effects of drugs in the first trimester of pregnancy. *Clin Obstet Gynecol*. 1986;13:177.
48. Beeley L. Adverse effects of drugs in later pregnancy. *Clin Obstet Gynecol*. 1986;13:197.
49. Mills JL, Graubard BI. Is moderate drinking during pregnancy associated with an increased risk for malformations? *Pediatrics*. 1987;80:309.
50. Khoury GH, Hawes CR. Atrial septal defect associated with pulmonary hypertension in children living at high altitudes. *J Pediatr*. 1967;70:432.
51. Howie PW. Anticoagulants in pregnancy. *Clin Obstet Gynecol*. 1986; 13:349.
52. Iturbe-Alessio I, Fonseca M, del C, et al. Risks of anticoagulant therapy in pregnant women with artificial heart valves. *N Engl J Med*. 1986; 315:1390.
53. Ben Ismail M, Abid F, Trabelsi S, et al. Cardiac valve prostheses, anticoagulation, and pregnancy. *Br Heart J*. 1986;55:101.
54. Lee P, Wang RYC, Chow JSF, et al. Combined use of warfarin and adjusted subcutaneous heparin during pregnancy in patients with an artificial heart valve. *J Am Coll Cardiol*. 1986;8:221.
55. Chesebro JH, Adams PC, Fuster VV. Antithrombotic therapy in patients with valvular heart disease and prosthetic heart valves. *J Am Coll Cardiol*. 1986;8:41B.
56. Rudolph AM. Effects of aspirin and acetaminophen in pregnancy and in the newborn. *Arch Int Med*. 1981; 141:358.
57. Pauli RM, Lain JB, Mosher DF, Stuttie JW. Association of congenital deficiency of multiple vitamin K-dependent coagulation factors and the phenotype of warfarin embryopathy. *Am J Hum Genet*. 1987; 41:566.
58. Forestier F, Dafos F, Sole Y, Rainaut M. Prenatal diagnosis of hemophilia by fetal blood sampling under ultrasound guidance. *Haemostasis*. 1986; 16:346.
59. Daffos F, Forestier F, Kaplan C, Cox W. Prenatal diagnosis and management of bleeding disorders with fetal blood sampling. *Am J Obstet Gynecol*. 1988; 158:939.
60. Weinstein MR, Goldfield MD. Cardiovascular malformations with lithium use during pregnancy. *Am J Psych*. 1975; 132:529.
61. Long WA, Willis RW. Maternal lithium and neonatal Ebstein's anomaly. *Am J Perinat*. 1984; 1:182.
62. Nora JJ, Nora AH, Toews WH. Lithium, Ebstein's anomaly, and other congenital heart defects. *Lancet*. 1974; 2:594.

Chapter One Hundred and Twenty-Eight

Infective Endocarditis

Cheryl L. Reid, Uri Elkayam, and Shahbudin H. Rahimtoola

128

Heart disease, most frequently valvular or congenital defects, has been reported to occur in 1% to 4% of pregnancies.[1,2] Infective endocarditis during pregnancy is estimated to occur in 0.005% to 1.0% of all pregnancies.[3-6] Although rare, its occurrence during pregnancy may have devastating consequences on both the mother and the fetus. The maternal mortality rate is approximately 20% and fetal death has been reported in 23%.[7,8] Early diagnosis of this disease in pregnancy is, therefore, critical. Pregnancy affects the cardiovascular system resulting in increases in cardiac output, blood volume, heart rate, and the common presence of heart murmurs (see Chapter 124). These normal pregnancy changes can complicate the clinical assessment of patients with infective endocarditis. The management of pregnant patients with infective endocarditis involves the same general principles as in the nonpregnant patient. However, special considerations should be made in the diagnostic and therapeutic approach to this disease when it occurs during gestation in order to reduce the risks to the fetus.

PREDISPOSING FACTORS

Underlying structural abnormalities of the heart have long been recognized as a predisposing factor for the development of infective endocarditis. Rheumatic heart disease, although declining in incidence, still accounts for the majority of the cases.[6,9] The successful correction of many of the congenital heart abnormalities now allows more women to reach childbearing age and results in altering the pattern of cardiac disease during pregnancy.[10]

Mitral valve prolapse has been estimated to occur in 2% to 17% of the young adult population with a female to male predominance of 2:1.[11] The risk of developing infective endocarditis in these patients is increased five times and is highest in those patients with associated mitral regurgitation.[12] The prevalence of mitral valve prolapse in series of infective endocarditis is 12% to 15%.[10] Thus, it would be expected that mitral valve prolapse would be an underlying abnormality increasing the risk of infective endocarditis during pregnancy.[13]

Although pre-existing cardiac, especially valvular, abnormalities are typical of patients with infective endocarditis, infection occurring on functionally normal cardiac valves is increasingly being recognized.[14] There are numerous case reports in the literature of infective endocarditis during pregnancy without a previous history of cardiac disease.[15-20] These cases may result from a more virulent organism or an inadequate host response. Systemic diseases such as diabetes mellitus[18] or collagen vascular disease can suppress host defenses. In addition, intravenous drug usage can lead to infective endocarditis with common tricuspid valve involvement in patients with normal valves.

A variety of diagnostic and therapeutic procedures may result in bacteremia and can lead to infective endocarditis. Dental procedures are common predisposing events; in addition, surgery and diagnostic procedures, particularly those involving the genitourinary and gastrointestinal tract, may result in significant transient bacteremia.[21] Intravenous drug usage is increasing in frequency and has also been associated with acute baterial endocarditis during pregnancy.[22] Obstetric and gynecologic procedures have been reported as causing 26% of the cases of infective endocarditis in females.[8,23] Bacteremia may occur following abortion, vaginal delivery with manual removal of the placenta, curettage, infected intrauterine contraception devices, and pelvic infections.[17,23] Although infective endocarditis has been reported to occur following a normal vaginal delivery, it is rare.[2,5]

MICROBIOLOGY

The most common organism to cause infective endocarditis during pregnancy is *Streptococcus viridans*.[4,8] Infection with this organism is often a subacute form with symptoms present for several months before diagnosis. The patient may present, however, with an acute, fulminant picture due to the development of a complication of infective endocarditis such as valvular rupture and the occurrence of congestive heart failure.[24] Acute bacterial endocarditis, with symptoms present for only a few weeks, however, is often due to *Staphylococcus aureus*[3], *Streptococcus pneumoniae,* and *Streptococcus pyogenes*.[15] Isolated case reports have described a variety of organisms causing infective endocarditis including *Pseudomonas aeruginosa,* nonhemolytic streptococci, *Hemophilus aphrophilus*[25], *Listeria monocytogenes*[18], *Chlamydia trachomatis*[26], salmonella[27], and *Mycobacterium tortuitum*.[28] Any organism capable of causing infective endocarditis in the nonpregnant state would also be expected to be a potential pathogen during pregnancy. In patients with a history of intravenous drug usage, *S aureus* is the predominant organism although polymicrobial infections may also occur.

Many of the organisms reported to cause infective endocarditis during pregnancy have also been cultured from the normal vagina and postpartum uterus.[29,31] Blood cultures taken immediately after delivery in 101 patients were positive for *S aureus* in one.[32] A larger series of women studied less than an hour following delivery showed a 5% incidence of positive blood cultures with mostly streptococci, including anaerobic, microaerophilic, and alpha hemolytic streptococci.[33] Bacteremia occurs in 10% of obstetrical patients who develop complications including endoparametritis and pyelonephritis.[34] Organisms predominantly isolated in these patients include Group B streptococcus and *Escherichia coli.*

CLINICAL FEATURES

Infective endocarditis may have a variety of clinical manifestations which may mimic many other disease states. The clinical features are related to the infectious process itself, the cardiovascular complications, and the noncardiac complications. The onset of the disease may be acute with symptoms present for only a few days or weeks or subacute with signs and symptoms present for months before diagnosis. The classic triad of fever, murmur, and anemia should certainly raise the suspicion of infective endocarditis. Fever is present in almost 100% of patients, but it may be absent in patients taking antipyretics, steroids, or who have had previous antibiotic therapy.[35] General manifestations also include headaches, malaise, fatigue, and musculoskeletal pain.[36] Patients who present with an acute form of the disease may be extremely ill with chills, sweats, nausea, vomiting, chest pain, peripheral emboli, or dyspnea.

The development of a cardiac murmur or a change in character or intensity of a preexisting murmur has been considered to be an important characteristic feature of the disease. However, neither the presence nor a change in character of a murmur are invariable findings. The hemodynamic changes during pregnancy make the occurrence of cardiac murmurs common (see Chapter 124).[2,10] New murmurs may develop or previously existing murmurs may diminish in intensity. These changes in murmurs or the appearance of new murmurs may be misinterpreted as the presence of infective endocarditis. Both systolic and diastolic murmurs may appear during the course of the pregnancy which are related to the normal physiologic changes (see Chapter 124). Furthermore, a mammary souffle due to increased flow in the mammary vessels may be misinterpreted as cardiac in origin. Conversely, murmurs of mitral or tricuspid stenosis may be detected first during pregnancy because of the increased flow across the valves. Aortic and mitral regurgitation murmurs may actually decrease in intensity presumably from the decreased peripheral resistance during pregnancy.[37] Thus, the evaluation of cardiac murmurs may be extremely difficult during pregnancy.

Peripheral Manifestations

Clinical manifestations of infective endocarditis can occur in almost any organ due to the bacteremia, septic or nonseptic emboli, or immunologic responses of the host to the infection.

Cutaneous Manifestations. Four lesions involving the skin has classically been described for infective endocarditis: petechiae, subungual hemorrhages, Osler nodes, and Janeway lesions. The frequency of these peripheral manifestations has been decreasing during the antibiotic era. Petechiae (most commonly involving the conjunctival or oral mucosa), are the most frequent finding and are reported to occur in 26% of patients.[36] Subungual splinter hemorrhages are most often the result of trauma and, therefore, have less diagnostic value. Osler nodes are tender, erythematous lesions noted on the palms and terminal phalanges of the hand or soles of the feet and are considered to be due to a hypersensitivity reaction.[36] Janeway lesions are small, nontender, macular nodular hemorrhagic spots which are present on the palms and soles.[38] Both Osler nodes and Janeway lesions are uncommon today.

Renal Manifestations. Involvement of the kidney is relatively common in both acute and subacute infective endocarditis. Three distinct types of renal abnormalities occur: (1) renal infarctions; (2) focal, embolic glomerulonephritis; and (3) diffuse, proliferative glomerulonephritis. Renal infarction due to emboli occurs in approximately 60% of patients with left-sided infective endocarditis.[35] The infarcts are usually sterile and generally do not result in renal failure; septic infarcts may result in abscess formation. The two types of glomerulonephritis are due to immune-complex glomerular injury. Renal insufficiency may result from either of these lesions, although control of the infection frequently reverses the serologic abnormalities and azotemia; cure of the infection may be achieved by antibiotics with or without surgery.

Careful monitoring of renal function during therapy for infective endocarditis is important to detect abnormalities early. Since many of the drugs used to treat infective endocarditis are excreted by the kidneys and may cause nephrotoxicity, appropriate reductions in dosages must be made, depending on the degree of renal insufficiency. If renal failure develops during the course of antibiotic therapy for infective endocarditis, differentiation between immune-complex injury and nephrotoxicity from drug therapy can be difficult. Recovery from nephrotoxicity from drugs usually occurs following discontinuation of the antibiotics. If the infection is controlled but renal abnormalities persist, renal biopsy may become necessary to differentiate immune-complex injury from the nephrotoxicity caused by the antibiotics.

Neurologic Manifestations. Neurologic or psychiatric symptoms occur in approximately one third of patients with infective endocarditis.[39,40] The central nervous system manifestations are due to (1) embolization, (2) rupture of mycotic aneurysms, and (3) meningitis or meningo-cerebritis. The occurrence of hemiplegia in a young female should raise the suspicion of infective endocarditis. Aphasia, ataxia, cortical sensory loss, and homonymous hemianopsia may also develop due to emboli or rupture of a mycotic aneurysm. Embolic cerebral infarction is the commonest neurologic complication of infective endocarditis occurring in approximately 20% of patients usually within the first two weeks of therapy.[40] Meningitis is most often aseptic; cerebrospinal fluid cultures may be positive in acute bacterial endocarditis particularly when due to *S aureus*.[41] A variety of neurologic manifestations may occur including headaches, seizures, or mental aberrancy.

Cardiac and Noncardiac Complications

Infective endocarditis is a highly destructive process which may result in a variety of cardiac abnormalities (Table 128–1). The most common cause of death (60%) in patients with infective endocarditis is congestive heart failure.[35] Valvular regurgitation, particularly of the aortic valve, is the most frequent cause of the congestive heart failure. Eighty percent of patients with aortic valve endocarditis and 50% of patients with mitral valve endocarditis develop congestive heart failure.[42] Valve disruption from the infection may result from erosion of valve edges, total destruction of the valves by highly invasive organisms, perforation or prolapse of a leaflet, or rupture of chordae tendinea. Stenosis of a valve may occur rarely when the vegetations are very large such as with fungal endocarditis. The most frequent valve involved in infective endocarditis is the aortic valve (55%), followed by the mitral valve (28%), and less frequently, multiple valves, or the tricuspid or pulmonic valves.

Extension of the infection into the myocardium can lead to the development of left-to-right shunts. The most common are sinus of Valsalva aneurysm rupture, septal

TABLE 128–1. CARDIOVASCULAR COMPLICATIONS OF ENDOCARDITIS

Valve destruction with resultant regurgitation
Localized suppuration
Perivalvular or myocardial abscesses
Creation of left-to-right shunts (sinus of Valsalva rupture, ventricular septal defects, aortopulmonary fistula, ventriculoatrial fistula)
Emboli
Systemic
Coronary artery with myocardial infarction
Mycotic aneurysms
Conduction abnormalities; rhythm disturbances
Pericarditis

From O'Rourke R, ed. The Heart and Renal Disease. 1984:189 *with permission.*

perforation with the development of a ventricular septal defect, the creation of an aortopulmonary fistula, or ventriculoatrial fistula. Congestive heart failure due to the left-to-right shunt can result from these defects.

Systemic emboli occur in one third of cases of infective endocarditis. Major central nervous system embolization has been reported in 6–31% of patients.[38] Hemiplegia, aphasia, and sensory loss are the usual clinical manifestations due to a cerebral embolus. Pulmonary emboli are commonly seen with infections of the tricuspid valve. Other sites of emboli include the coronary arteries, spleen, and kidney. Myocardial infarction may result from a coronary artery embolus, particularly when the aortic valve is involved. Frequently, the infarction may not be detected electrocardiographically, but it may contribute to the development of congestive heart failure.

Myocardial abscesses have been noted in 20% of patients with infective endocarditis at autopsy.[35] Abscesses can result from direct extension of the infection or from bacteremia. Myocardial abscesses are difficult to detect clinically but may be suspected when conduction abnormalities or arrhythmias occur. Other complications of abscesses include intracardiac fistula which may precipitate congestive heart failure and antibiotic failure.

Suppurative pericarditis may occur with extension into the pericardial space. Pericarditis occurring during infective endocarditis may also develop as a result of an immunologic reaction, uremia, or congestive heart failure. By two-dimensional echocardiography, pericardial effusions occur in 54% of patients but are generally associated with a benign clinical course.[43]

New conduction abnormalities in the absence of other known causes are generally associated with myocardial abscesses and virulent organisms and are an indication for surgery. Temporary pacing should be initiated if mobitz II or higher degrees of block are present; subsequently, a permanent pacemaker implantation may be needed.

Mycotic aneurysms may develop due to direct invasion of bacteria into the arterial wall, embolic occlusion of the vasa vasorum, or deposition of immune complexes. The areas in which aneurysms develop are the brain, abdominal aorta, superior mesenteric, splenic, coronary, and pulmonary arteries, sinus of Valsalva, and ligated ductus arteriosus. Mycotic aneurysms that have not ruptured are associated with few or no symptoms; they can be the cause of persistent sepsis, fever, pain, and neurologic symptoms. Diagnosis is difficult but is best made by angiography. Since rupture and hemorrhage can occur at any time during or after therapy, surgery is recommended if the aneurysm is recognized and is in a surgically accessible site.

DIAGNOSIS

The main reason for not diagnosing infective endocarditis is not thinking of it; therefore, a high index of suspicion is needed.[34] The most useful clinical findings suggestive of infective endocarditis in these patients are fever, cardiac murmur or history of preexisting cardiac disease, and positive blood cultures.

The majority of cases of infective endocarditis can be diagnosed by three paired blood cultures (six bottles: three vented, three unvented drawn over a two-hour period). Bacteremia associated with infective endocarditis is continuous. Blood cultures are usually positive in over 80% of cases.[29] In approximately 16% of patients with infective endocarditis, blood cultures will be negative.[35] Blood cultures are most likely to be negative in patients who have received prior inadequate antibiotic therapy or when the causative agent cannot be easily cultured with standard techniques. In patients who have received antibiotic therapy within two weeks, the antibiotics should be discontinued if clinically possible, and cultures redrawn beginning 24 to 48 hours later. The patient should have blood cultures repeated twice during a seven-day interval, and if the cultures remain negative, then a diagnosis other than infective endocarditis such as collagen vascular disease, atrial myxoma, or marantic endocarditis should be considered. Blood for serologic studies for Q-fever, psittacosis, and tularemia should also be obtained in patients with negative blood cultures.

The erythrocyte sedimentation rate, although nonspecific, is elevated in over 90% of patients with infective endocarditis.[36] Anemia is common but may also be related to the pregnancy.[2] Elevation of the white blood cell count frequently occurs in acute endocarditis but may be normal with the exception of a leftward shift in cases of subacute infective endocarditis. Examination of the urine may be helpful when the presence of an active sediment suggests renal involvement because of glomerulonephritis or renal infarction.

Chest x-ray is helpful in the diagnosis of pulmonary complications such as embolization and congestion (Fig. 128–1). Echocardiography is useful to detect vegetations of the cardiac valves and intracardiac complications. M-mode and two-dimensional echocardiography demonstrate vegetations in 80% or more of patients with infective endocarditis.[44] Contrast two-dimensional echocardiography can be used to detect complications of infective endocarditis such as tricuspid insufficiency or intracardiac shunts. In pregnant patients undergoing cardiac catheterization prior to valve replacement, contrast two-dimensional echocardiography can be used to evaluate the presence and severity of valvular regurgitation.[45,46] This technique decreases the requirement for radiation during cardiac catheterization and, thus, reduces the risk to the fetus.[45] Furthermore, the adverse hemdynamic consequences of contrast medium can be avoided in patients who are in moderate-to-severe heart failure. Doppler echocardiography has been shown to be a reliable noninvasive assessment of the severity of valvular stenosis, pressure gradients, and valvular regurgitation.[47-49] Color Doppler echocardiography may

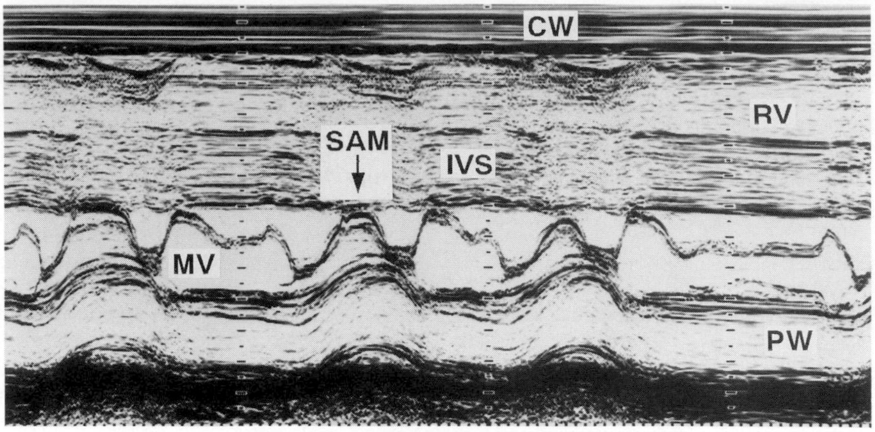

Figure 128–1. Patchy infiltrates in both lung fields representing septic embolization in a 22-year-old patient at 33-weeks' gestation. The patient had *Staphylococcus aureus* endocarditis of the tricuspid valve due to intravenous drug abuse.

also provide a clinically useful estimate of the presence and severity of valvular regurgitation.[50]

MANAGEMENT OF INFECTIVE ENDOCARDITIS

Antibiotic Therapy of Infective Endocarditis

The choice of antibiotics for infective endocarditis depends upon proper microbiological identification of isolated organisms or blood cultures and susceptibility testing. In pregnancy, the choice of antibiotics must also be based upon consideration of the possible adverse effects upon the fetus.[51]

Proper microbiologic identification and susceptibility testing is important because of the increasing incidence of infective endocarditis caused by uncommon organisms, including gram-negative organisms and fungi, and of antibiotic resistance. Usually, in subacute infective endocarditis, treatment does not need to be instituted before the two to three days required for microbiologic testing. In contrast, acute infective endocarditis is often caused by highly destructive organisms; therefore, it is imperative that there be no delay in starting antibiotic therapy beyond the time needed to obtain the blood cultures. In such patients, the etiology of infective endocarditis can be suspected on the basis of the clinical setting—for example, infected skin lesions, urinary tract infection, intravenous drug abuse, or antibiotic therapy initiated against the most likely causative organism. Initial therapy should consist of a penicillin, a penicillinase-resistant penicillin, and an aminoglycoside. Subsequently, if the results of microbiologic isolation dictates a different antibiotic therapy, substitution can be made at that time.

Antibiotic therapy is given intravenously in intermittent doses at four-to-six hour intervals in patients with normal renal function or by continuous infusion. The duration of antibiotic therapy is still debated; however, it is generally accepted that therapy should be continued for at least four, and preferably six weeks.

The management of patients with culture-negative infective endocarditis depends on the clinical situation. Acute illnesses should be handled as discussed earlier. If cultures remain negative but there has been a clinical response, the antibiotics should be continued. If the infection is subacute, it is reasonable to start antibiotics using penicillin, a penicillinase-resistant penicillin, and an aminoglycoside. Therapy is continued for at least one or two weeks. If there is a clinical response, antibiotics should be continued; if not, they should be stopped and the patient re-evaluated.

Prosthetic valve endocarditis is usually divided into early and late. Early infections, occurring within two months of surgery, are felt to be due to contamination of the implant site, often by staphylococcus or gram-negative organisms. Late prosthetic infections are caused by the same organisms that are found in native valve endocarditis. About half the patients can be treated successfully with antibiotics alone while the rest also require surgical treatment for cure of infection, heart failure, or both.

The antibiotics chosen should be bactericidal. The easiest way to assess adequacy of chemotherapy is a serum dilution test for bactericidal activity.[52] Ideally, the patient's serum should show lethal activity against the isolated organism at a dilution of 1:8 at all times. Serial blood cultures should be repeated at 48 hours and frequently throughout the course of therapy despite defervescence and clinical improvement to assure sterility of the blood.[53]

Congestive Heart Failure

As previously stated, the most common cause of death in patients with infective endocarditis is congestive heart failure. If the mortality of infective endocarditis is to be reduced, early aggressive diagnosis and treatment of congestive heart failure is essential.[53]

In patients with infective endocarditis who have moderate-to-severe congestive heart failure, admission to an acute care unit and hemodynamic monitoring with a balloon flotation catheter in the right side of the heart is mandatory. If congestive heart failure is present, medical therapy should then be promptly instituted with digoxin and diuretics. Digitalis preparations have been used extensively during pregnancy and are considered safe for both the fetus and mother.[54] Dosing adjustments may need to be made during pregnancy. Diuretics, either thiazide or furosemide, may also be used during pregnancy to treat congestive heart failure. Care must be taken to avoid dehydration of the patient which might compromise uterine blood flow. Vasodilators (arteriolar and venous dilators) are also usually needed. Arteriolar dilators reduce aortic and mitral regurgitation, increase forward cardiac output, and may reduce left ventricular filling pressure. Hydralazine and prazosin are vasodilators which have been used safely during pregnancy for the treatment of hypertension and should be used if indicated for the treatment of heart failure.[55,56] Venodilators, such as nitroglycerin or isosorbide dinitrate, may also be required to reduce left ventricular volumes and filling pressures. Nitrate preparations have been incompletely studied during pregnancy and should probably only be used if the potential benefits outweigh the possible risks to the fetus. Nitroprusside during pregnancy is not generally recommended since it crosses the placenta and its toxic byproduct, cyanide, may cause fetal death.[57] The use of vasodilators during pregnancy should be performed only with the benefit of hemodynamic monitoring because of the potential adverse hemodynamic effects upon the mother and fetus. After the congestive heart failure has been controlled with aggressive medical therapy, cardiac catheterization may be performed with contrast echocardiography to define the presence of any correctable lesion.[46] Valve replacement or repair of any correctable lesion can then be performed on a nonemergent basis once the congestive heart failure is controlled regardless of the duration of antibiotic therapy.

The clinical diagnosis and assessment of mild congestive heart failure can often be wrong. If there is any doubt, hemodynamic monitoring should be performed for accurate diagnosis and optimal care. If congestive heart failure is not easily controlled by medical therapy, urgent surgery should be recommended. In medically controlled cases, antibiotics and medical therapy should be continued with reassessment in four to six weeks.

Surgical Therapy

Surgical intervention, especially valve replacement, has had a dramatic impact on the mortality of patients with moderate-to-severe congestive heart failure. With valve replacement, survival rates of 73–86% in these patients have been reported.[58] Successful cardiac surgery during pregnancy has been reported and should be performed in patients with infective endocarditis in whom medical therapy fails. Zitnik et al, in 1969, reported on 21 patients who had open heart surgery during pregnancy.[59] The maternal mortality was 5% and the fetal mortality 33%. Since that review, many other patients have had successful cardiac surgery during pregnancy.[60] It would appear that pregnant patients can have cardiac surgery at a risk no greater than to a nonpregnant patient. Although fetal mortality is high, it is acceptable and can probably be improved with newer techniques for fetal monitoring and greater attention to maternal hemodynamics during cardiopulmonary bypass.[61] Cardiac surgery is theoretically best performed after the twenty-fourth to twenty-eighth week when organogenesis is complete. Good perfusion of the placenta must be maintained during cardiopulmonary bypass and, therefore, invasive hemodynamic monitoring of the mother seems indicated during surgery.

The indications for surgical intervention are listed in Table 128–2. Infections that are uncontrolled despite good antibiotic therapy are best managed with surgical debridement and the replacement of the infected valve.[62] Persistently positive blood cultures may result from infection elsewhere in the body; therefore, noncardiac sources of persistent infection must be excluded before undertaking cardiac surgery. Infective endocarditis with *S aureus* is associated with a high mortality ranging from 45–73% and replacement of the infected valve has been recommended within two to seven days of diagnosis.[58] However, staphylococcal infections of the tricuspid and pulmonic valves respond reasonably well to medical therapy alone.[63] Therefore, it would seem more appropriate to employ aggressive medical treatment for the infection and congestive heart failure and reserve surgical therapy for those patients with staphylococcal infections of the aortic or mitral valve who fail to respond.[64] Gram-negative infections are frequently resistant to antibiotic therapy and surgical treatment may be necessary. Schondelmeyer et al have recently reported the need for a tricuspid valvulectomy during pregnancy in a patient with *Enterobacter cloacae* enterococcus endocarditis due to recurrent episodes at septic embolization despite antibiotic therapy.[65] Medical therapy in fungal endocarditis is associated with mortality rates of 80–100% and, therefore, urgent surgical therapy is indicated in almost all cases.[66]

TABLE 128–2. INDICATIONS FOR SURGERY IN THE TREATMENT OF INFECTIVE ENDOCARDITIS

Congestive heart failure
Infections
- Uncontrolled by antibiotic therapy
- Fungal, usually with staphylococal infections of aortic and mitral valves, Serratia, and gram-negative bacillary infections

Recurrent systemic emboli despite adequate antibiotic therapy
Acquired heart block
Others
- Acquired intraventricular conduction defects
- Pericarditis, suppurative
- Mycotic aneurysm of coronary artery
- Mycotic aneurysm of sinus of Valsalva
- Rupture of sinus of Valsalva, rupture of ventricular or atrial septa, or others (eg, development of arteriovenous and ventriculoatrial shunts)

From Reid CL, et al[53] with permission.

Other complications of infective endocarditis are also amenable to surgical correction. New conduction abnormalities and arrhythmias often suggest an uncontrolled infection and abscess formation for which surgery may be required. The development of a sinus of Valsalva aneurysm with rupture into a cardiac chamber, ventricular septal defects, or other structural abnormalities are usually an indication for surgery because they are associated with congestive heart failure and uncontrolled infection.

Recurrent systemic emboli despite optimal antibiotic therapy are another indication for surgery. Because patients with infective endocarditis often have structural abnormalities or arrhythmias which increase the risk for nonseptic emboli, an attempt should be made to determine the nature of the embolus prior to recommending surgery. A reasonable guideline is that if emboli reoccur despite 48 to 72 hours of appropriate antibiotic therapy, surgery should be considered.

PREVENTION

Chemoprophylaxis is appropriate whenever patients with increased susceptibility to the development of infective endocarditis undergo manipulation or surgical procedures likely to result in bacteremia. The severe consequences of this disease emphasize the importance of this preventive measure. Prophylaxis is appropriate when these patients undergo manipulations or surgical procedures likely to be associated with bacteremia. These include chemoprophy-

TABLE 128–3. CHEMOPROPHYLAXIS OF INFECTIVE ENDOCARDITIS

Cardiac Abnormalities Requiring Prophylaxis
- Prosthetic heart valves
- Congenital heart disease
- Rheumatic or other acquired valvular heart disease
- Hypertrophic cardiomyopathy
- Mitral valve prolapse syndrome with mitral insufficiency
- Previous episode of infective endocarditis

Prophylaxis Not Required
- Uncomplicated secundum atrial septal defect
- Previous coronary artery bypass surgery
- Six months after cardiac surgery for:
  - Uncomplicated secundum atrial septal defect, ventricular septal defect or patent ductus arteriosus
- Mitral valve prolapse without valvular regurgitation
- Physiologic, functional, or innocent heart murmurs
- Cardiac pacemakers and implanted defibrillators
- Previous rheuamtic fever without valvular dysfunction

Adapted from the recommendations of the American Heart Association.[67]

TABLE 128–4. PROCEDURES FOR WHICH PROPHYLAXIS IS INDICATED

- All dental procedures likely to induce gingival or mucosal bleeding
- Tonsillectomy/adenoidectomy
- Surgical procedures or biopsy involving intestinal or respiratory mucosa
- Bronchoscopy with rigid bronchoscope
- Sclerotherapy for esophageal varices
- Incision and drainage of infected tissue
- Esophageal dilatation
- Gallbladder surgery
- Cystoscopy
- Urethral dilatation
- Urethral catheterization and urinary tract surgery in patients with urinary tract infection
- Vaginal hysterectomy
- Vaginal delivery in the presence of infection

Adapted from the recommendations of the American Heart Association.[67]

laxis for most dental and upper respiratory tract procedures; lower gastrointestinal, gallbladder, and genitourinary surgery or instrumentation; and surgical procedures involving infected or contaminated tissues. The prophylaxis for procedures in the mouth is directed mainly against strains of *S viridans*. Prophylaxis for procedures involving instrumentation of the genitourinary or gastrointestinal tract should be directed against the enterococcus. Cardiac lesions likely to be encountered during pregnancy which should be covered with prophylactic antibiotics are listed in Table 128–3. Procedures likely to result in significant bacteremia are shown in Table 128–4. Recommendations for antibiotic prophylaxis (Table 128–5) are based upon those made by the American Heart Association.[67]

The need for antibiotic prophylaxis during routine delivery in patients with underlying cardiac abnormalities is controversial. Recent reviews of the subject would seem to indicate that routine prophylaxis is not necessary in uncomplicated deliveries.[5,68] The American Heart Association recommends that in patients with prosthetic valves, a previous history of endocarditis, or surgically constructed systemic-pulmonary shunts or conduits, physicians may choose to administer prophylactic antibiotics during uncomplicated vaginal delivery.[67] Endocarditis prophylaxis is recommended for vaginal deliveries in the presence of infection in patients with cardiac lesions at risk (see Table 128–3).[67] However, because of the small risk of bacteremia even after uncomplicated vaginal delivery, the relatively low risk and cost of therapy and the potentially devastating effect of endocarditis, prophylactic antibiotic treatment is given routinely in our medical center to all patients who are susceptible to bacterial endocarditis.

TABLE 128–5. INITIAL AND SUBSEQUENT THERAPY FOR PROPHYLAXIS OF INFECTIVE ENDOCARDITIS (ADULTS)

	Initially	Subsequently
Dental Oral or Upper Respiratory Tract	Amoxicillin 3 q orally	1.5 q 6 h after initial dose
	Allergic patients	
	Erythromycin 1.0 g orally 2 h before procedure	0.5 g 6 h after initial dose
	Clindamycin 300 mg orally 1 h before procedure	150 mg 6 h after initial dose
Genitourinary/ Gastrointestinal	Ampicillin 2 g IV or IM and Gentamicin 1.5 mg/kg (not to exceed 80 mg) 30 min before procedure	Amoxicillin 1.5 orally 6 h after initial dose
	Allergic patients	
	Vancomycin 1.0 g IV (over 1 h) +IV Gentamicin 1.5 mg/kg (not to exceed 80 mg) 1 h before procedure	Repeat 8 h after initial dose
	Low-Risk patients	
	Amoxicillin 3.0 g orally 1 h before procedure; then 1.5 g 6 h after initial dose	

From the recommendations of the American Heart Association.[67]

REFERENCES

1. McFaul PB, Dornan JC, Lamki H, Boyle D. Pregnancy complicated by maternal heart disease: A review of 519 women. *Br J Obstet Gynecol.* 1988;95:861.
2. Szekely P, Snaith L. Heart disease and pregnancy. Edinburgh and London: Churchill Livingston; 1974:29.
3. Ward H, Hickman RC. Bacterial endocarditis in pregnancy. *Aust NZ Obstet Gynecol.* 1971;11:189.
4. Payne DG, Fishburne JI, Rufty AJ, Johnston FR. Bacterial endocarditis in pregnancy. *Obstet Gynecol.* 1982;60:247.
5. Sugrue D, Blake S, Troy P, McDonald D. Antibiotic prophylaxis against infective endocarditis after normal delivery—is it necessary? *Br Heart J.* 1980;44:599.
6. Sugrue D, Blake S, MacDonald D. Pregnancy complicated by maternal heart disease at the National Maternity Hospital, Dublin, Ireland. *Am J Obstet Gynecol.* 1981;139:1.
7. Hamilton BE. Report from the Cardiac Clinic of Boston Lying-in Hospital for the first twenty-five years. *Am Heart J.* 1947;33:663.
8. Seaworth BJ, Durack DT. Infective endocarditis in obstetric and gynecologic practice. *Am J Obstet Gynecol.* 1986;154:180.
9. Szekely P, Turner R, Snaith L. Pregnancy and the changing pattern of rheumatic heart disease. *Br Heart J.* 1973;35:1293.
10. Conradsson T, Werko L. Management of heart disease in pregnancy. *Prog Card Dis.* 1974;16:407.
11. Levy D, Savage D. Prevalence and clinical features of mitral valve prolapse. *Am Heart J.* 1987;113:1281.
12. MacMahon SW, Roberts JK, Kramer-Fox R, Zucker DM, et al. Mitral valve prolapse and infective endocarditis. *Am Heart J.* 1987;113:1291.
13. Strasberg GD. Postpartum group B streptococcal endocarditis associated with mitral valve prolapse. *Obstet Gynecol.* 1987;70:485.
14. Roberts WC. Characteristics and consequences of infective endocarditis (active or healed or both) learned from morphologic studies. In: Rahimtoola SH, ed. *Infective Endocarditis.* New York: Grune & Stratton; 1978:55.
15. Holt S, Hicks DA, Charles RG, Coulshed N. Acute staphylococcal endocarditis in pregnancy. *Practitioner.* 1978;220:619.
16. Hanson GC, Philiss J. A fatal case of subacute bacterial endocarditis in pregnancy. *J Obstet Gynecol Br Commonw.* 1965;72:781.
17. Jemsek JC, Layne OG, Greenberg SB. Malignant group B streptococcal endocarditis associated with saline-induced abortion. *Chest.* 1979;76:695.
18. Hofshouser CA, Amsbacher R, McNitt T, Steele R. Bacterial endocarditis due to *Listeria monocytogenes* in a pregnant diabetic. *Obstet Gynecol.* 1978;51:9.
19. Sexton DJ, Rockson SG, Hempling RE, Cathey CW. Pregnancy-associated group B streptococcal endocarditis: A report of two fetal cases. *Obstet Gynecol.* 1985;66:44S.
20. Burstein H, Sampson MB, Kohler JP, Levitsky S. Gonococcal endocarditis during pregnancy: Simultaneous cesarean section and aortic valve surgery. *Obstet Gynecol.* 1985;66:48S.
21. Everett ED, Hirschmann JV. Transient bacteremia and endocarditis. A review. *Medicine (Baltimore).* 1977;56:61.
22. Pastorek JG, Plauche WC, Faro S. Acute bacterial endocarditis in pregnancy: A report of three cases. *J Reprod Med.* 1983;28:611.
23. Lein JN, Stander RW. Subacute bacterial endocarditis following obstetric and gynecologic procedures: Report of eight cases. *Obstet Gynecol.* 1959;13:568.
24. Castillo RA, Llado I, Adamsons J. Ruptured chordae tendineae complicating pregnancy: A case report. *J Reprod Med.* 1987;32:137.
25. Anand CM, MacKay AD, Evans JI. *Haemophilus aphrophilus* endocarditis in pregnancy. *J Clin Pathol.* 1976;29:812.
26. Bel-Kahn JM, Watanakunakorn C, Menefee MG, Long H, et al. *Chlaymdia trachomatis* endocarditis. *Am Heart J.* 1978;95:627.
27. Gill GV. Endocarditis caused by salmonella enteritis. *Br Heart J.* 1978;42:353.
28. Alvarez-Elcordo S, Mateos-Mora M, Zajarias A. *Mycobacterium tortuitum* endocarditis after mitral valve replacement with a bovine prosthesis. *South Med J.* 1985;78:865.
29. Hunter CA, Long KR. A study of the microbiological flora of the vagina. *Am J Obstet Gynecol.* 1958;75:865.
30. Hesseltine HC, Kite KE. Bacteriology of the gynecologic and involuting puerpheral uterus. *Am J Obstet Gynecol.* 1949;57:143.
31. Rabe LK, Winterscheid KK, Hillier SL. Association of viridans group streptococci from pregnant women with bacterial vaginosis and upper genital tract infection. *J Clinc Micro.* 1988;26:1156.
32. Redleaf PD, Fadell EJ. Bacteremia during parturition. *JAMA.* 1959;94:1285.
33. McCormack WM, Rosner B, Lee YH, Rankin JS, et al. Isolation of genital mycoplasmas from blood obtained shortly after vaginal delivery. *Lancet.* 1975;1:596.
34. Blanco JD, Gibbs RS, Castaneda YS. Bacteremia in obstetrics: Clinical course. *Obstet Gynecol.* 1981;58:621.
35. Weinstein L, Rubin RH. Infective endocarditis—1973. *Prog Cardiovasc Dis.* 1973;16:239.
36. Lerner PI, Weinstein L. Infective endocarditis in the antibiotic era. *New Eng J Med.* 1966;274:199.
37. Marcus FI, Ervy GA, O'Rourke RA, Walsh B, et al. The effect of pregnancy on the murmurs of mitral and aortic regurgitation. *Circulation.* 1970;41:795.
38. McAnulty JH, Rahimtoola SH, DeMots H, Griswold HE. Clinical features of infective endocarditis. In: Rahimtoola SH, ed. *Infective Endocarditis.* New York: Grune & Stratton; 1978:125.
39. Ziment I. Nervous system complications in bacterial endocarditis. *Am J Med.* 1969;47:593.
40. Pruitt AA, Rubin RH, Karchner AW, Duncan GW. Neurologic complications of bacterial endocarditis. *Medicine (Baltimore).* 1978;57:329.
41. McComb JM, McNamee PT, Sinnamon DG, Adgey AAJ. Staphylococcal endocarditis presenting as meningitis in pregnancy. *Int J Card.* 1982;1:325.
42. Mills J, Utley J, Abbott J. Heart failure in infective endocarditis: Predisposing factors, course, and treatment. *Chest.* 1974;66:151.
43. Reid CI, Rahimtoola SH, Chandraratna PAN. Frequency and significance of pericardial effusion detected by two-dimensional echocardiography in infective endocarditis. *Am J Cardiol.* 1987;60:394.
44. Melvin ET, Berger M, Lutzker LG, Goldberg E, et al. Noninvasive methods for detection of valve vegetations in infective endocarditis. *Am J Cardiol* 1981;47:271.
45. Elkayam U, Kawanishi D, Reid CL, Chandraratna PAN, et al. Contrast echocardiography to reduce ionizing radiation associated with cardiac catheterization during pregnancy. *Am J Cardiol.* 1983;52:213.
46. Reid CL, Kawanishi DT, McKay CR, Elkayam U, et al. Accuracy of evaluation of presence and severity of aortic and mitral regurgitation by contrast 2-dimensional echocardiographic technique. *Am J Cardiol.* 1983;52:519.
47. Stamm B, Martin RP. Quantification of pressure gradients across stenotic valves by Doppler ultrasound. *JACC.* 1983;2:707.
48. Pearlman AS, Scoblionko DP, Saal AK. Assessment of valvular heart disease by Doppler echocardiography. *Clin Cardiol.* 1983;6:573.
49. Smith MD, Handshoe R, Handshoe S, Kivan OL, et al. Comparative accuracy of two-dimensional echocardiography and Doppler pressure half-time methods in assessing seventy of mitral stenosis in patients with and without prior commissurotomy. *Circulation.* 1986;73:100.
50. Helmcke F, Nanda NC, Hsiung MC, Soto B, et al. Color Doppler assessment of mitral regurgitation with orthogonal planes. *Circulation.* 1987;75:175.
51. Cesario TC. Antibiotic therapy in pregnancy. In: Elkayam U, Gleicher N, eds. *Cardiac Problems in Pregnancy, Diagnosis and Management of Maternal and Fetal Disease.* New York: Alan R. Liss; 1990;137.
52. Wilson WR, Guiliani ER, Danielson GK, Geraci JE. General considerations in the diagnosis and treatment of infective endocarditis. *Mayo Clin. Proc.* 1982;57:81.
53. Reid CL, Leedom JM, Rahimtoola SH. Infective endocarditis. In: Conn HF, ed. *Current Therapy.* 28th ed. Philadelphia: WB Saunders Co; 1983.
54. Rotmensch HH, Elkayam U, Frishman W. Antiarrhythmic drug therapy during pregnancy. *Ann Intern. Med.* 1983;98:487.
55. Curet LB, Olson RW. Evaluation of a program of bedrest in the treatment of chronic hypertension in pregnancy. *Obstet Gynecol.* 1979;53:336.
56. Dommissee J, Davey DA, Roos PJ. Prazosin and oxprenolol therapy in pregnancy hypertension. *S Afr Med J.* 1983;13:231.
57. Naulty J, Cefalo RC, Lewis PE. Fetal toxicity of nitroprusside in the pregnant ewe. *Am J Obstet Gynecol.* 1981;139:708.
58. Richardson JV, Karp RB, Kirklin JW, Dismukes WE. Treatment of infective endocarditis: A 10-year comparative analysis. *Circulation.* 1978;58:589.
59. Zitnik RS, Brandelburg RO, Sheldon R, Wallace RB. Pregnancy and openheart surgery. *Circulation.* 1969;39(Suppl):257.
60. Gazzaniga AB. Cardiac surgery during pregnancy. In: Elkayam U, Gleicher N, eds. *Cardiac Problems in Pregnancy, Diagnosis and Management of Maternal and Fetal Disease.* New York: Alan R. Liss; 1990;259.
61. Nazarian M, McCullough GH, Fielder DL. Bacterial endocarditis in pregnancy: Successful surgical correction. *J Thorac Cardiovasc Surg.* 1976;71:880.
62. Black S, O'Rourke RA, Karliner JS. Role of surgery in the treatment of primary infective endocarditis. *Am J Med.* 1974;56:357.
63. Hubbell G, Cheitlen MD, Rapaport E. Presentation, management and follow-up evaluation of infective endocarditis in drug addicts. *Am Heart J.* 1981;102:85.
64. Rapaport E. The changing role of surgery in the management of infective endocarditis. *Circulation.* 1978;58:598.
65. Schondelmeyer RW, Sunderrajan EV, Atay AE, Strickland JL, et al. Successful tricuspid valvulectomy without replacement for endocarditis during pregnancy. *Am Heart J.* 1986;112:859.
66. McLeod R, Remington JS. Fungal endocarditis. In: Rahimtoola SH, ed. *Infective Endocarditis.* New York: Grune and Stratton; 1978;211.
67. Dajani AS, Bisno AL, Chung KJ, Durack DT, et al. Prevention of bacterial endocarditis: Recommendations by the American Heart Association. *JAMA.* 1990;264:2919.
68. Fleming HA. Antibiotic prophylaxis against infective endocarditis after delivery. *Lancet.* 1977;1:144.

Chapter One Hundred and Twenty-Nine
Myocarditis

Avraham Shotan, Anil O. Mehra, and Uri Elkayam

129

Myocarditis is a focal or diffuse inflammatory process involving the heart muscle. It may be caused by virtually any bacterial, viral, rickettsial, mycotic, or parasitic organism, as well as by several noninfectious processes.[1-11] Viral infection appears to be the most common cause of myocarditis in North America and Europe with coxsackie B accounting for nearly 50% of all cases[9]; coxsackie A, and echo and polio viruses accounting for most of the remainder. Influenza A and B, rubeola, rubella, mumps, cytomegalic, rabies, herpes simplex, herpes zoster, varicella, Epstein–Barr, yellow fever, and adenovirus may also cause the disease.[1-8] In animals, there is an initial phase of active viral replication in the heart and direct myocardial damage modified by the humoral immune system. The virus is then cleared by the monocyte-macrophage system. This phase is followed by a T-cell-mediated cytotoxic reaction, probably in response to antigenic alterations in the myocardium.[6,10] Recent reports have demonstrated the association of myocarditis with acquired immune deficiency syndrome (AIDS) due to opportunistic infection by a variety of organisms, metastatic involvement by Kaposi's sarcoma, or the human immunodeficiency virus (HIV), itself.[12,13] Bacterial myocarditis is uncommon and is usually a complication of bacterial endocarditis.[4] In certain regions of Central America and South America, Chagas' disease, which is caused by *Trypanosoma cruzi*, is the most common cause of acute or chronic myocarditis.[14]

Noninfectious inflammation of the myocardium occurs with hypersensitivity states such as acute rheumatic fever or autoimmune diseases such as systemic lupus erythmatosus. Myocarditis can also result from radiation, chemicals (for example, lead), pharmacological agents (for example, doxorubicin, cocaine, catecholamines excess, cyclophosphamide, emetine) and metabolic disorders (for example, uremia).[3,5,11]

Although any of the above-mentioned causes may produce myocardial inflammation during pregnancy, none is known to produce it with any frequency or regularity. The majority of cases of myocarditis in pregnancy have been documented in the peripartum period.[8,15] Only a few cases of specific myocarditis have been reported to occur in pregnancy; these include luetic myocarditis and rheumatic fever.[16] Gumes and Gates[17] noted a unique myocarditis associated with abortion in four cases, all of them ended fatally within several days of the procedure and had autopsy evidence of myocardial inflammation. Farber and Glasgow[18] found that pregnant mice, infected with encephalomyocarditis virus, had higher titers of cardiac virus than did pregnant controls, despite the fact that brain titers were equal between the two groups. This finding may suggest increased susceptibility for myocarditis during pregnancy. Cesario[8] suggested that at least two factors may enhance the development of viral myocarditis during pregnancy: increased physiological stresses and hemodynamic load that may lead to some myocardial hypoxia, and excessive amounts of circulatory steroids. These suggestions are supported by animal experimentations demonstrating worsening of myocardial necrosis in mice infected with coxsackie B or A viruses and high incidence and severity of viral cardiac lesions after reducing myocardial oxygen supply or increasing physical stress.[19,20]

Recent reports have demonstrated histological evidence for myocarditis in patients with peripartum cardiomyopathy[15] (see Chapter 131). Several authors have, therefore, suggested myocarditis as an important etiological factor in patients with peripartum cardiomyopathy. The incidence of active myocardial inflammation in this patient population, however, has varied significantly among different reports. Additional data, collected in a systematic, prospective fashion, is required to establish the relationship between acute myocarditis and peripartum cardiomyopathy.

CLINICAL FEATURES

The clinical manifestations of myocarditis may vary with the extent and location of the inflammatory process in the myocardium and the associated systemic illness. Myocarditis may be clinically silent, and has been reported as an incidental finding in one to seven percent of autopsies.[2] Sometimes electrocardiographic or chest film abnormalities are detected during a routine evaluation in an infectious disease. The disease often presents initially as a systemic illness with viral symptomatology, such as fever, sore throat, cough, arthralgia, myalgia, abdominal pain, nausea, vomiting, diarrhea, and skin rash. Cardiac manifestations usually become apparent only a few days to a few weeks later and are usually manifested as fatigue, decreased exercise tolerance, dyspnea, palpitations, and, occasionally, precordial discomfort. Pleuropericardial chest pain may occur due to associated pericarditis. Focal myocarditis may present with localized electrocardiographic changes and wall motion abnormalities and can mimic acute myocardial infarction.[21,22] Hemodynamic instability and even circulatory collapse may result secondary to a high degree atrioventricular block, ventricular arrhythmias, or associated cardiac tamponade. Myocarditis may result in unexpected sudden death, presumed to be due to fatal tachyarrhythmia or complete atrioventricular block.[7] Systemic and pulmonary emboli have been reported in myocarditis and may be the presenting feature.[1,5,7]

Changes in physical examination will depend on the severity of the disease and while no abnormal findings can be found in mild cases, persistent fever and excessive tachycardia, both at rest and during exercise, are common. Tachycardia is often disproportionate to the degree of fever. Hypotension is not infrequent with a narrow pulse pressure. Clinical findings of congestive heart failure with mitral and tricuspid regurgitation may occur in the more severe cases. A pericardial friction rub may be audible in patients with associated pericarditis. In patients with severe cardiac involvement, dilatation of cardiac chambers will result in a diffuse and displaced point of maximal impulse and right ventricular heave. A third heart sound and murmurs due to mitral and tricuspid regurgitation can be heard. Neck veins may be distended in patients with heart failure, pericardial effusion, or both. Auscultation of the lungs can reveal bilateral rales.

LABORATORY TESTS

Electrocardiogram

In the acute stage, the electrocardiogram is always abnormal, demonstrating ST-segment elevation with inversion or flattening of the T wave. The QTc interval may be prolonged. The ST-segment changes usually return to baselne in a few days, while the T-wave changes may persist for several weeks or months. Abnormal Q waves may sometimes develop and mimic acute myocardial infarction.[22] Ventricular premature beats are commonly seen and atrial and ventricular tachyarrhythmias are present in about one third of the patients. Bundle branch and atrioventricular blocks of varying degress may occur and are usually transient, although permanent complete atrioventricular block has been reported.[7]

Chest X-ray

Chest roentgenogram may show cardiac enlargement due to chamber dilatation, pericardial effusion, or both. Additional findings may include pulmonary venous congestion, interstitial and, even, alveolar edema, mild atrial enlargement, prominence of superior vena cava or azygos vein, patchy pulmonary infiltrates, and pleural effusion.

Laboratory Data

The erythrocyte sedimentation rate is elevated in about 70% of the cases but rarely exceeds 80 mm/hr. White blood cell count may be slightly to moderately elevated with a neutrophil response in about half of the patients. Eosinophilia may indicate an underlying parasitic etiology. Myocardial necrosis usually results in an increase in cardiac enzymes—creatine phosphokinase (CPK), lactic dehydrogenase (LDH) and glutamic oxaloacetic transaminase (GOT).[5,7,11]

Virus recovery is usually possible during the first few days of the illness.[5,6] Recent viral infection may be diagnosed in the acute and convalescent (two to six weeks after illness) phases of the illness by a fourfold or greater rise in virus antibody titers.[11] Antibodies are usually not found until about one week after the onset of the illness. The immunoglobulin class may help in determining the duration of the disease process, since IgM antibody levels peak in two to three weeks and are later undetectable and IgG antibody levels peak later and may remain elevated for months or years. Newer radioimmunoassay and enzyme linked immunosorbent assay (ELISA) are useful in rapid identification and polyvalent reagents can be used.[7]

Echocardiography

Echocardiogram helps in evaluating chambers' size and their global and regional function which may vary from normal to substantial enlargement with focal or diffused hypokinesia.[22-24] Transient asymmetric septal hypertrophy and transient wall thickening may result, presumably from inhomogeneous edematous inflammation. Mural thrombi are not infrequently found.[23,24] Use of the Doppler technique enables the detection and assessment of the severity of the mitral and tricuspid valve's regurgitation.

Nuclear Imaging

Radionuclide ventriculography may reveal biventricular global dysfunction and enlargement, or regional hypokinesis or dyskinesis, especially at the apex.[5] Myocardial imaging with technetium-99 pyrophosphate[25], galium-67 citrate[26] or indium-111-labeled leukocyte[27] scans may show

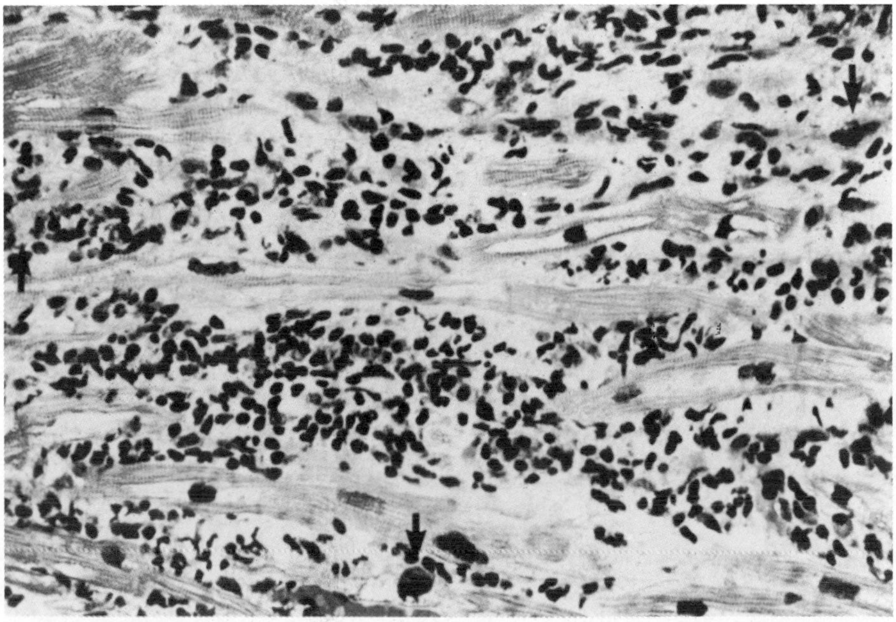

Figure 129–1. Severe diffuse lymphocytic myocarditis. There is extensive interstitial lymphocytic infiltrate and myocyte necrosis (arrows) is readily seen. No fibrosis is present (hematoxylin and eosin: magnification × 350). *(From Aretz et al.* Am J Cardiovasc Path *1987;1:3.)*

uptake as evidence of diffuse or focal myocardial inflammation or necrosis. The clinical usage of these procedures in pregnancy is limited due to expected radiation to the fetus (see Chapter 5).

Endomyocardial Biopsy

During the last decade, endomyocardial biopsy has become the "gold standard" for the diagnosis of myocarditis. Recently established Dallas Criteria[28] for the histological diagnosis of myocarditis include findings of inflammatory infiltrate associated with adjacent myocyte necrosis or degeneration (Figure 129–1). It should be noted that although a positive biopsy is of diagnostic value, a negative biopsy does not rule out myocarditis. In severe cases in which a definite diagnosis has therapeutic implications, a repeat endomyocardial biopsy may be indicated.[29,30]

The ability to perform endomyocardial biopsy during pregnancy is somewhat limited by the need to use fluoroscopy and, therefore, ionizing radiation. In such cases, the procedure can be done by trained individuals under echocardiographic guidance (Figure 129–2).[31]

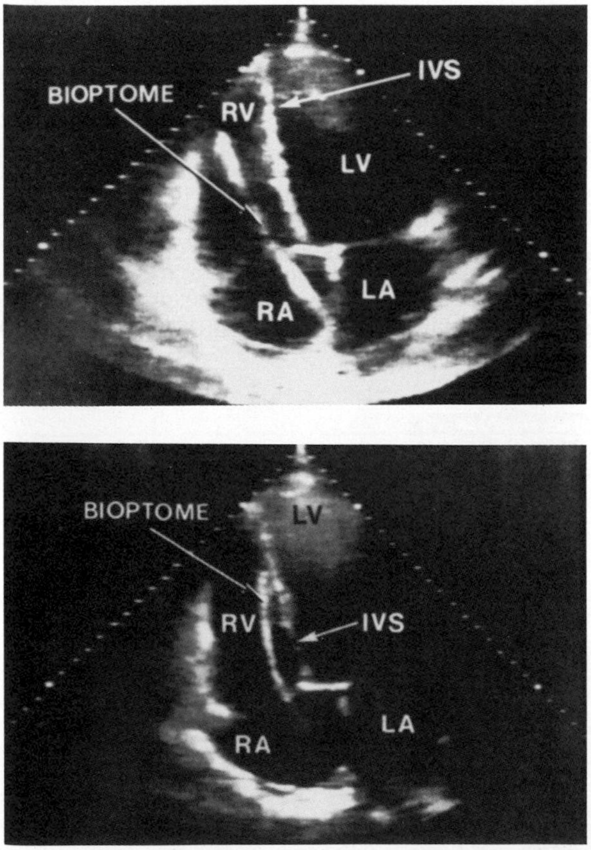

A

B

Figure 129–2. Echocardiogram showing the apical four-chamber view of the heart and demonstrating the guidance of the bioptome (black and white arrow) with a sample being obtained at the right ventricular (RV) free wall (A) and a sample being obtained at the interventricular septum (IVS) (B). LV-left ventricle; RA-right atrium; and LA-left atrium. (*From: Miller et al.*[31])

TREATMENT

All pregnant women with suspected myocarditis should be hospitalized. Patients with hemodynamic instability, heart failure, significant pericardial effusion at risk of tamponade, and serious arrhythmias should be adequately monitored in an intensive cardiac care unit.[5,7] Therapy is often supportive and includes rest and adequate oxygenation. Congestive heart failure should be treated with diuretics, digoxin, and vasodilators. Safety and potential side effects of the various drugs available for the treatment of heart failure are discussed in Chapter 131. Important arrhythmias should be treated with lidocaine, quinidine or procainamide which are relatively safe in gestation (see Chapter 125).[32] The use of corticosteroids with or without immunosuppressive drugs is controversial. During the acute tissue invasive stage, immunosuppressive agents may provoke viral replication and should, therefore, not be used. However, the majority of patients with myocarditis present at the postinvasive stage, when inflammation is due to immune response toward the altered myocardial antigenicity.[3,6,7] Although several reports have demonstrated marked improvement following immunosuppression and relapses after discontinuation of the therapy[2,3,7], comprehensive review of the literature reveals conflicting reports and insufficient evidence for the role of immunosuppression in patients with myocarditis.[6,33]

REFERENCES

1. Wynne J, Braunwald E. The cardiomyopathies and myocarditis. In: Braunwald E, ed. *Heart Disease: A Textbook of Cardiovascular Medicine.* 3rd ed. Philadelphia: WB Saunders; 1987:1440.
2. Shah PM. Cardiomyopathies. In: Stein JH, ed. *Internal Medicine.* 3rd ed. Boston, MA: Little, Brown; 1990:177.
3. Perloff JK, Stevenson LW. Diseases of the myocardium. In: Wyngaarden JB, Smith LH, eds. *Cecil Textbook of Medicine.* Philadelphia: WB Saunders; 1988:352.
4. Wynne J, Braunwald E. The cardiomyopathies and myocarditis. In: Wilson JD, Braunwald E, Isselbacher KD, et al. eds. *Harrison's Principles of Internal Medicine.* 12th ed. New York: McGraw-Hill; 1990:975.
5. Wenger NK, Abelman WH, Roberts WC. Myocarditis. In: Hurst JW, Schlant RC eds. *The Heart.* 7th ed. New York: McGraw-Hill; 1990:1256.
6. Maze SS, Adolph RJ. Myocarditis: unresolved issues in diagnosis and treatment. *Clin Cardiol.* 1990;13:69.
7. Cherian C, Abraham MT. Myocarditis. In: Parmley WW, Chatterjee K, eds. *Cardiology: Cardiovascular Disease.* Philadelphia, PA: J.B. Lippincott; 1989:1.
8. Cesario TC. Myocarditis and pregnancy. In: Elkayam U, Gleicher N, eds. *Cardiac Problems in Pregnancy: Diagnosis and Management of Maternal and Fetal Disease.* 2nd ed. New York: Alan R. Liss; 1990:109.
9. Reyes MP, Lerner AM. Coxsackie virus and myocarditis—with special reference to acute and chronic effects. *Prog Cardiovasc Dis.* 1985;27:373.
10. Woodruff JF. Viral myocarditis: a review. *Am J Pathol.* 1980;101:427.
11. Kopecky SL, Gersh BJ. Dilated cardiomyopathy and myocarditis: natural history, etiology, clinical manifestations, and management. *Curr Probl Cardiol.* 1987;12:571.
12. Cohen IS, Anderson DW, Virmani R, et al. Congestive cardiomyopathy in association with the acquired immunodeficiency syndrome. *N Engl J Med.* 1986;35:628.
13. Baroldi G, Corallo S, Moroni M, et al. Lymphocytic myocarditis in acquired immunodeficiency syndrome (AIDS): a correlative morphologic and clinical study in 26 consecutive fatal cases. *J Am Coll Cardiol.* 1988;12:463.
14. Acosta AM, Santos-Buch CA. Autoimmune myocarditis induced by *Trypanosoma cruzi. Circulation.* 1985;71:1255.
15. Midei MG, DeMent SH, Feldman AM, et al. Peripartum myocarditis and cardiomyopathy. *Circulation.* 1990;81:922.
16. Ueland K, Metcalfe J. Acute rheumatic fever in pregnancy. *Am J Obstet Gynecol.* 1966;95:586.
17. Gumes D, Gates C. Fatal myocarditis associated with abortion in early pregnancy. *South Med J.* 1980;73:236.

18. Farber P, Glasgow L. Viral myocarditis during pregnancy: encephalomyocarditis virus infection in mice. *Am Heart J*. 1970;80:96.
19. Tilles J, Elson S, Shaka J, et al. Effects of exercise on Coxsackie A_9 myocarditis in adult mice. *Proc Soc Exp Biol Med*. 1964;117:777.
20. Pearce J. Heart disease and filtrable viruses. *Circulation*. 1960;21:448.
21. Chandraratna PAN, Nimalasuria A, Reid CL, et al. Left ventricular asynergy in acute myocarditis: simulation of acute myocardial infarction. *JAMA*. 1983;250:1428.
22. Spodick DH. Infection and infarction: acute viral (and other) infection in the onset, pathologesis and mimicry of acute myocardial infarction. *Am J Med*. 1986;81:661.
23. Nieminen MS, Heikkila J, Karjalainen J. Echocardiography in acute infectious myocarditis: relation to clinical and electrocardiographic findings. *Am J Cardiol*. 1984;53:1331.
24. Weinhouse E, Wanderman KL, Safer S, et al. Viral myocarditis simulating dilated cardiomyopathy in early childhood: evaluation by serial echocardiography. *Br Heart J*. 1986;56:94.
25. Mitsutake A, Nakamura M, Inou T, et al. Intense, persistent myocardial avid technetium 99M pyrophosphate scintigraphy in acute myocarditis. *Am Heart J*. 1981;101:683.
26. O'Connel JB, Henkin RE, Robinson JA, et al. Galium-67 imaging in patients with dilated cardiomyopathy and biopsy-proven myocarditis. *Circulation*. 1984;70:58.
27. Yasuda T, Palacios IF, Dec GW, et al. Indium 111-monoclonal antimyosin antibody imaging in the diagnosis of acute myocarditis. *Circulation*. 1987;76:306.
28. Aretz HT, Billingham ME, Edwards WD, et al. Myocarditis: a histopathologic definition and classification. *Am J Cardiovasc Pathol*. 1987;1:1.
29. Dec GW, Fallon JT, Southern JF, Palacios I. "Borderline" myocarditis: an indication for repeat endomyocardial biopsy. *J Am Coll Cardiol*. 1990;15:283.
30. Factor SM. Borderline myocarditis on initial endomyocardial biopsy: No man's land no more? *J Am Coll Cardiol*. 1990;15:290.
31. Miller LW, Labovitz AJ, McBride LA, et al. Echocardiographic-guided endomyocardial biopsy. A 5-year experience. *Circulation*. 1988;78(Suppl III):99.
32. Rotmensch HH, Pines A, Donchin V. Antiarrhythmic drugs in pregnancy. In: Elkayam U, Gleicher N, eds. *Cardiac Problems in Pregnancy: Diagnosis and Management of Maternal and Fetal Disease*, 2nd ed. New York: Alan R. Liss; 1990:361.
33. Mason JW, O'Conner JB. A model of myocarditis in humans. *Circulation*. 1990;81:1154.

Chapter One Hundred and Thirty

Diseases of the Pericardium

Anil O. Mehra, Avraham Shotan, and Uri Elkayam

130

This chapter describes common pericardial disorders and the approach to them during pregnancy.

ACUTE PERICARDITIS

Although there are several reported cases of acute pericarditis during pregnancy, pregnancy does not appear to predispose to development of this disease. Acute pericarditis is often clinically inapparent and may be overlooked, even if symptomatic, because of its varied and atypical manifestations.[1] Most cases are self-limited and show a mild course; however, some patients are at risk for serious involvement including myocarditis and cardiac tamponade.

Idiopathic or viral pericarditis during pregnancy has been reported with a benign course and normal fetal outcome in the majority of cases[2-4]; pregnancies complicated by pyogenic pericarditis or pericarditis secondary to systemic lupus erythematosus have been reported to be associated with premature labor and occasional fetal death.[5-8]

Etiology

Idiopathic or presumed viral pericarditis is the most common cause. Common viruses implicated are coxsackie group B and echovirus. Others are the coxsackie A, adenovirus, mumps, varicella, infectious mononucleosis and rubella viruses.

Bacterial pericarditis is rare and is usually secondary to pneumonia or empyema. The most common organisms are pneumococci, staphylococci, and streptococci; however gram-negative organisms should be considered in the immunocompromised host. Tuberculous pericarditis should be considered in a patient with a positive tuberculin skin test, history of weight loss, nonproductive cough, night sweats, anorexia, arthralgias, low-grade fever, and a large serosanguinous pericardial effusion.[10] Other etiologies for pericarditis that may be seen during childbearing age include collagen vascular disease, especially systemic lupus erythematosus[10], chest trauma, and drug-related pericarditis (hydralazine, procainamide). A more complete list of common causes of pericarditis is presented in Table 130–1.

Clinical Findings

Acute pericarditis is a clinical entity characterized by three major features including chest pain, friction rub, and fever. Chest pain, sharp or dull, is frequently the chief complaint.[1] The pain is usually localized to the retrosternal and left precordial regions, aggravated by lying in a supine position, coughing, deep inspiration, and swallowing. It is relieved by sitting up and leaning forward. It frequently radiates to the trapezial ridge and the neck. Some patients have acute pericarditis without pain; in others, the pain mimics ischemic disease. Acute pericarditis may be associated with rapid and shallow breathing forced by the chest pain which may present as dyspnea. A history suggestive of upper respiratory tract infection frequently precedes the development of acute idiopathic and viral pericarditis. Frequently, because of an accompanying myocarditis, fatigue and malaise persist for weeks after the pain has subsided.

The pericardial friction rub is the most important characteristic physical sign, although often transient and variable. This is a leathery, scratching, or grating noise, best

TABLE 130–1. COMMON CAUSES OF ACUTE PERICARDITIS

Inflammatory
Idiopathic
Infections
Bacterial
Viral
Tubercular
Mycotic
Miscellaneous (protozoal, mycoplasmal and spirochetal) associated with acute transmural infection
Acquired Immune Deficiency Syndrome (AIDS)
Acute myocardial infarction
Postmyocardial infarction syndrome (Dressler's syndrome)
Postpericardiotomy syndrome
Traumatic
Metabolic disorders (uremia, myxedemia, gout)
Connective tissue diseases (systemic lupus erythematosus, progressive systemic sclerosis, rheumatoid arthritis, rheumatic fever)
Allergic and hypersensitivity diseases (serum sickness, drugs; ie, procainamide, minoxidil, hydralazine, isoniazid, and so on).
Neoplastic disorder
Postirradiation
Postanticoagulation
Chylopericardium
Cholesterol pericarditis
Rupture of dissecting aorting aneurysm

heard during expiration along the lower left sternal border by the diaphragm of the stethoscope applied firmly and the patient sitting and leaning forward. Classically, it has three components for each cardiac cycle: presystolic, systolic and protodiastolic. All three components are not always heard in any one patient. Absence of a friction rub does not rule out acute pericarditis, and presence of a friction rub does not rule out pericardial effusion.

Other common signs of acute pericarditis are fever and tachycardia. The presence of a large pericardial effusion may result in distant heart sounds and dullness to percussion at the area below the left scapula because of lung compression (Ewart's sign).

Laboratory Evaluation

Diagnosis of acute pericarditis is usually based on the clinical history (chest pain), physical examination (friction rub), and laboratory evidence of nonspecific acute inflammatory process such as leukocytosis and increased sedimentation rate. Electrocardiogram, chest x-ray, and echocardiogram may provide the supportive evidence of acute pericardial inflammation. Additional diagnostic tests, such as tuberculin skin test, blood urea nitrogen and serum creatinine, antinuclease antibody titer (ANA) and rheumatoid factors, ASO titer as well as bacterial, viral and fungal cultures may define the underlying etiologies for acute pericarditis.

Electrocardiogram

The electrocardiogram characteristically shows sinus tachycardia and diffuse ST-segment elevation in multiple leads without Q-wave formation or reciprocal ST depression.[11] Sequential electrocardiograms are useful in distinguishing acute pericarditis from acute myocardial infarction and early repolarization changes. Depression of PR segment (below the TP segment) is common in acute pericarditis. Electrocardiographic changes occur in 90% of patients with acute pericarditis and progress in the following stages.

Stage 1 is a generalized concave ST-segment elevation with upright T waves and depression of PR segment (Fig. 130–1) usually seen at the time of chest pain. Stage 2 is return of ST segments to baseline with T wave flattening. Stage 3 is T-wave inversion without appearance of Q waves or loss of R waves as seen in acute myocardial infarction. Stage 4 is reversion to normal, which usually occurs within weeks to months after the onset of chest pain.

Arrhythmias are common, occurring in one fifth of patients with pericarditis and include intermittent atrial fibrillation, paroxysmal supraventricular tachycardia and atrial flutter. In the presence of a large pericardial effusion, low-voltage QRS complexes and voltage alternation (electrical alternans) may occur.

Chest Roentgenogram

The chest x-ray is usually not useful in the diagnosis of pericarditis, but may be of great value in determination of the pulmonary processes causing the involvement of the pericardium. The cardiac silhouette is usually normal in size but may be enlarged in cases of more than 250–300 mL of pericardial effusion. Echocardiography has practically replaced chest x-ray film for the diagnosis and quantification of pericardial effusion.

Echocardiogram

Echocardiography allows a rapid and noninvasive diagnosis of pericardial effusion (Fig. 130–2). The procedure has high sensitivity and high specificity for this indication and can detect as little as 20 cc of fluid.[12] Two-dimensional echocardiography is superior to M-mode echocardiography in the detection of localized pericardial effusion which may be seen in postoperative, postradiation, or pyogenic pericarditis. In addition, echocardiography may provide useful information regarding pericardial thickness, cardiac chambers' size and function, and early signs of cardiac tamponade. Assessment of valvular and myocardial function as well as cardiac chambers' size allow differentiation between cardiac enlargement secondary to associated myocardial involvement (myocarditis) and large pericardial effusion with or without cardiac tamponade.

A band of echoes in the vicinity of posterior left ventricular visceral pericardium and parietal pericardium may suggest thickened pericardium. Diagnostic accuracy of echocardiography in detecting thickened pericardium is approximately 75%.[13]

Differential Diagnosis

Differential diagnosis should include conditions associated with chest pain such as pleurisy, pneumonia, acute myocardial infarction, pulmonary embolism, and dissecting aneurysm.

MANAGEMENT

Most pregnant patients suspected of having acute pericarditis should be hospitalized for observation and initial diagnostic work up. Initial management of acute pericarditis

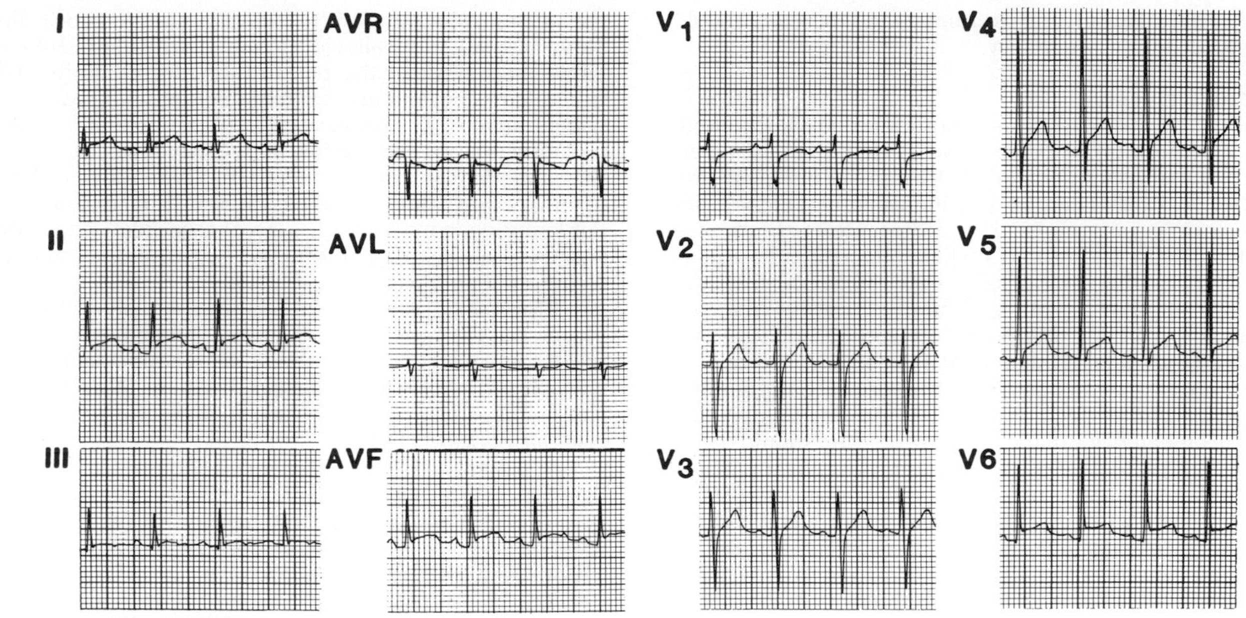

Figure 130–1. Electrocardiogram of a patient with acute pericarditis. Notice the diffuse concave ST segment elevations with upright T waves and depression of PR segments.

includes observation for signs of cardiac tamponade; symptomatic therapy with analgesics and anti-inflammatory agents, and determination and treatment of the underlying etiology. Most patients with viral or idiopathic pericarditis recover rapidly with symptomatic therapy, such as aspirin, within a few days. However, patients with associated myocardial dysfunction due to myocarditis may develop heart failure. Heart failure, if it occurs, should be promptly managed with digitalis, diuretics, and vasodilator agents.

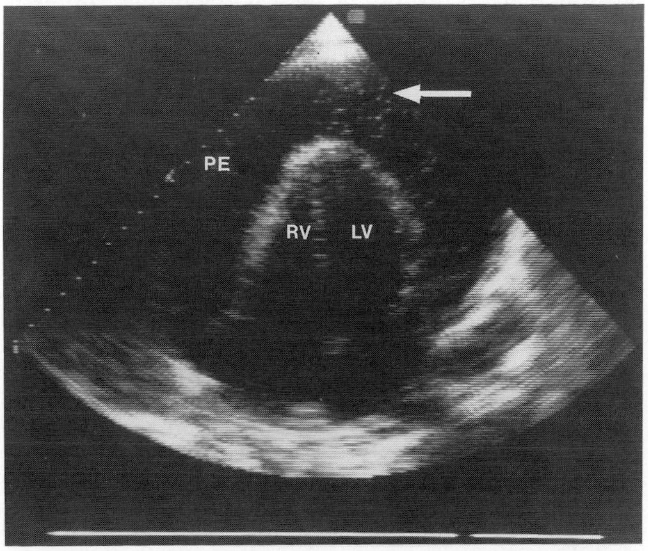

Figure 130–2. Two-dimensional echocardiogram for the apical four chambers view. Large circumferential effusion is seen (PE). RV = right ventricular cavity. LV = left ventricular cavity. Arrow shows echogenic contrast used during pericardiocentesis to verify needle position in the pericardial space.

Among vasodilator agents, hydralazine and prazosin have shown to be safe in pregnancy when used for the treatment of hypertension.[14,15] In contrast, nitroprusside and angiotensin-converting enzyme inhibitors should be avoided because of potential fetal toxicity.[16,17]

Arrhythmias

Hemodynamically significant, symptomatic persistent arrhythmia can be treated with drug therapy in most cases. Guidelines for antiarrhythmic therapy in pregnancy is described in Chapter 125. Direct current cardioversion may be utilized in cases of hemodynamic embarrassment.[18]

Analgesia

Analgesia may be readily accomplished with aspirin or nonsteroidal anti-inflammatory drugs (NSAIDS) with reasonable safety within 48 hours. NSAIDS probably have little advantage over aspirin. If pain is severe, persistent, and unresponsive to NSAIDS, and tuberculosis or infection is not suspected, then prednisone may be used (60–80 mg per day) in divided doses. The dose should then be decreased in two to three days and tapered within two weeks. Exacerbation of symptoms is not uncommon after withdrawal of steroids which may have to be reinstituted. Left-stellate ganglion blockade for severe recurrent pain may be considered.[1]

Antibiotics

Antibiotic therapy should be used only to treat documented bacterial pericarditis or suspected tuberculous pericarditis. Antibiotic therapy should be given according to the identified organism and the effects of various antibiotic agents on the fetus.[19] A triple-drug antituberculous regimen should be used for tuberculosis with close follow up for early detection of the development of constrictive pericarditis. Antituberculous drugs, including isoniazid, para-aminosalicyclic acid, ethambutol and streptomycin, have been shown to be safe for use during pregnancy. Rifampin has been shown to cause fetal malformations in animals and therefore should be avoided during pregnancy.[20]

Pericardiocentesis

Diagnostic pericardiocentesis is not indicated in uncomplicated acute pericarditis except in suspected bacterial, tuberculous, or malignant pericardial effusion.[21] Therapeutic removal of pericardial fluid is only indicated in patients with hemodynamic compromise. Pericardiocentesis can provide definitive diagnosis in 15% of patients with tuberculous pericarditis, in almost all cases of bacterial pericarditis, and in 50–75% of patients with malignant pericardial effusion. In pregnant patients, this procedure can be safely accomplished by the subxiphoid approach. Complications of pericardiocentesis include damage to the coronary arteries and hemopericardium which may lead to cardiac tamponade. Except in emergency situations, the procedure should therefore be performed only by experienced persons in patients with moderate-to-large pericardial effusion detected both anteriorly and posteriorly. The use of contrast is very helpful in guiding the needle to the pericardial space and in avoiding the cardiac chambers.[22] (See Figure 130–2.) Risk of developing life-threatening complications, if the procedure is done under the above-mentioned conditions, is only 0% to 5%. Pericardiocentesis is likely to be complicated or unsuccessful in patients with small pericardial effusion (less than 200 cc) with no anterior effusion on the echocardiogram, loculated effusion, fibrin and clot in the pericardial sac, or acute traumatic hemopericardium.

Pericardiotomy

Under local anesthesia, through a subxiphoid approach, removal of a small piece of pericardium allows excellent drainage of pericardial fluid and an excellent pericardial biopsy specimen. The technique has a higher yield than pericardiocentesis for the diagnosis of tuberculous or malignant pericardial effusions.[23]

Pericardiectomy

Partial pericardiectomy by way of the left hemithorax offers no advantage over subxiphoid pericardiotomy and is associated with higher mortality.[23] Therefore, complete pericardiectomy is the procedure of choice in definitive treatment of bacterial pericarditis, malignant pericardial effusion in patients with good life-expectancy and intractable chest pain in viral or idiopathic pericarditis.[24]

PERICARDIAL EFFUSION AND CARDIAC TAMPONADE

Etiology

Most conditions which may be associated with accumulation of effusion in the pericardial sac are listed in Table 130-1. The most common causes for pericardial effusion in women during the childbearing age are idiopathic pericarditis, tuberculosis, collagen vascular disease, myxedema, uremia, malignancy, and radiation to the chest. Recent reports indicate that 20–43% of normal pregnant women are found to have pericardial effusion of varying size during the last trimester.[25] This finding is clinically inapparent, is detectable only by echocardiography, and resolves during the first two months postpartum. The exact mechanism of this phenomenon remains unclear.

Signs and Symptoms

In general, hemodynamic effect of pericardial effusion depends upon the rate of fluid accumulation, the volume of the effusion, and physical characteristics of the pericardium. Slow accumulation allows gradual pericardial stretching while thickening of the pericardium decreases its ability to stretch. The amount of fluid required for tamponade will be smaller. The primary effect of pericardial fluid accumulation is restricted diastolic filling. Most pericardial effusions are silent and do not cause hemodynamic compromise or tamponade. Clinical findings of pericardial effusion without tamponade may include pain of associated pericarditis, shortness of breath, orthropnea, cough, fatigue, and anorexia in patients with large effusions.

Physical signs of pericardial effusion include tachycardia, elevated central venous pressure, hepatic enlargement, weak apical cardiac impulse, faint heart sounds and Ewart's sign. The friction rub of pericarditis may disappear with large effusions; however, presence of friction rub does not rule out pericardial effusion.

In patients with hemodynamic compromise due to cardiac tamponade, complaints of lightheadedness and dizziness are common. Further progression of cardiac tamponade may lead to a state of shock with signs and symptoms of peripheral hypoperfusion. Physical signs show neck vein distention with prominent X descent but diminution of Y descent, tachycardia, pulsus paradoxus (more than 10 mm Hg drop in arterial systolic blood pressure with inspiration), narrow pulse pressure, systemic hypotension, Kussmaul's sign and enlargement of the liver in some cases.[1]

Laboratory Findings

Electrocardiogram. Pericardial effusion may be accompanied by reduction in QRS voltage and flattening of T waves. In cases with massive effusion electrical alternans (alternation of the QRS amplitude on every other beat) can be found.[1]

Chest X-ray. Accumulation of more than 200–300 cc of pericardial fluid is usually associated with symmetrically enlarged, water-bottle shaped, cardiac silhouette with clear lung fields. Epicardial fat lines can be seen within the cardiac shadow. Chest x-ray may be normal in patients with rapid accumulation of fluid where cardiac tamponade may be caused by a relatively small amount of effusion. Fluoroscopy reveals diminished cardiac pulsations. Although the sensitivity of chest x-ray for the detection of pericardial effusion is far inferior to that of echocardiography, it may provide information regarding the etiology of the underlying disease (tuberculous, malignancy, and so on).

Echocardiogram. Echocardiography plays an important supportive role in the diagnosis as well as therapy of pericardial effusion. In patients with suspected cardiac tamponade, echocardiogram helps to document the presence and assess the magnitude of pericardial effusion as well as to differentiate it from constrictive pericarditis, right ventricular infarction, or extrinsic cardiac compression by tumor or hematoma.

The most commonly used two-dimensional and M-mode echocardiographic signs of tamponade are continued diastolic collapse of the right ventricular free wall after systolic contraction and continued collapse of the right atrial wall (Fig. 130–3). The longer the collapse lasts, the greater the certainty of tamponade. Right ventricular collapse appears earlier and is more predictive of cardiac tamponade than pulses paradoxus. In various studies, the sensitivity and specificity of right ventricular collapse in the diagnosis of tamponade have been 79–92% and 90–100%, respectively.[26]

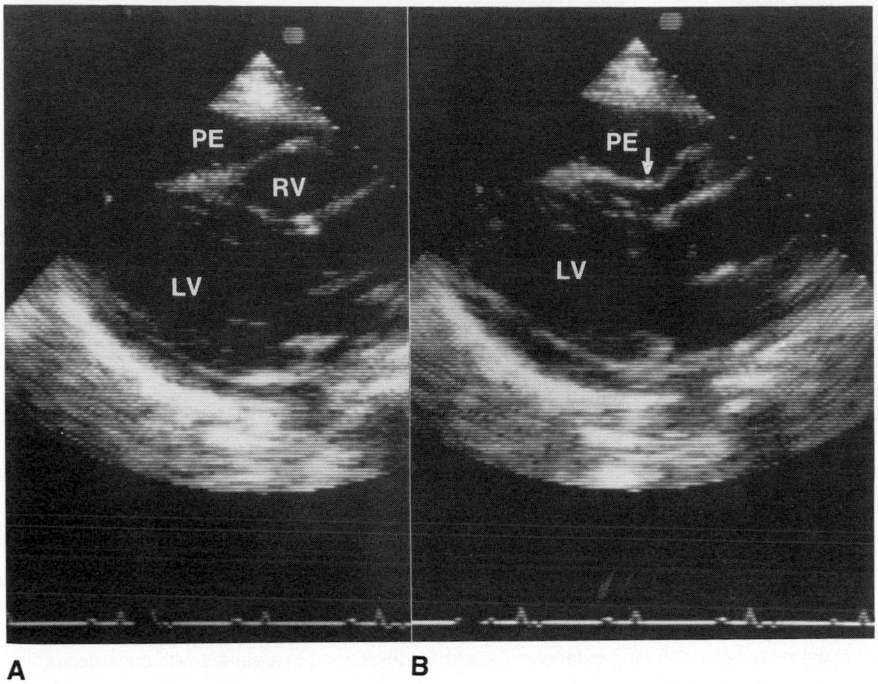

Figure 130–3. Long axis two-dimensional echocardiogram of a patient with pericardial effusion (PE) and cardiac tamponade during systole (A) and end-diastole (B). The anterior wall of the right ventricle (RV) is collapsed during diastole (arrow) and normal during systole. LV = left ventricle.

Hemodynamic Evaluation

The insertion of a balloon flotation catheter into the pulmonary artery is helpful in the assessment of hemodynamic consequences of the pericardial fluid and the effects of its removal by pericardiocentesis. Persistence of hemodynamic compromise following removal of the effusion strongly suggests an element of pericardial constriction. This procedure can be performed at the bedside, under pressure monitoring without the use of fluoroscopy.[27] In pericardial tamponade, the right atrial, right ventricular end-diastolic, pulmonary diastolic, and pulmonary artery wedge pressures will be equal (within 5 mm Hg). The recording of the right atrial pressure usually shows the absence of Y descent. In addition, the limited filling of cardiac chambers will result in a fall in cardiac output and pressure with reflex tachycardia.

CONSTRICTIVE PERICARDITIS

This is a situation in which the pericardium is heavily fibrosed or calcified (Fig. 130–4) and usually restricts the filling of all four cardiac chambers.[1]

Etiology

Tuberculosis is a common cause for constrictive pericarditis; however, as the incidence of this disease has significantly decreased in many countries, most cases of constrictive pericarditis are now idiopathic. Other identifiable causes for this disease include connective tissue disorders, chronic renal failure, mediastinal irradiation, cardiac trauma, pyogenic infection, and neoplasm.

Signs and Symptoms

The characteristic pathophysiologic abnormality of constrictive pericarditis is the restriction of diastolic filling by a fibrous or calcified pericardium. In some patients, myocardial fibrosis associated with pericardial disease may also lead to systolic left ventricular dysfunction. As in cardiac tamponade, the symptoms are mostly related to low cardiac output, elevated right atrial and central venous pressures, congestion of the liver, and the presence of ascites. Patients complain of weakness, malaise, edema, abdominal swelling, postprandial fullness, dyspepsia, flatulence, and anorexia. If left ventricular filling pressure is also elevated, exertional dyspnea, orthopnea, and paroxysmal nocturnal dyspnea are seen. Physical examination reveals distention of the neck veins; however, in contrast to patients with cardiac tamponade, both X and Y descents are present, Y descent being more prominent. Venous distention often demonstrates an augmentation during inspiration (Kussmaul's sign). Tachycardia is commonly seen and paradoxical pulse is present but rarely exceeds 15 mm Hg. By inspection and palpation of the chest, a systolic retraction of the apical impulse can be noted. In auscultation, a diastolic pericardial knock may be heard. This is an early diastolic sound which occurs 0.09–0.12 seconds after A_2, corresponding to the sudden cessation of ventricular filling and Y descent on the jugular venous wave form.

Abdominal examination can reveal hepatomegaly and ascites, which may be accompanied by leg edema; dependent edema being less common than ascites. Constrictive pericarditis is a frequently missed diagnosis and a careful examination of jugular venous pulse would usually avoid diagnostic errors.

Electrocardiogram. The electrocardiographic findings in constrictive pericarditis are nonspecific and include reduction of the QRS voltage, diffuse T wave changes, and notching of the P waves in the inferior leads. Atrial fibrillation is often seen in patients with constrictive pericarditis. Myocardial fibrosis in these patients may result in conduction abnormalities and deep, wide Q waves simulating myocardial infarction.

Chest X-ray. Chest x-ray usually shows normal or slightly enlarged cardiac silhouette with clear lung fields. Pericardial calcification may be seen in some patients, especially with tuberculosis. (See Fig. 130–4.) A lateral chest x-ray increases

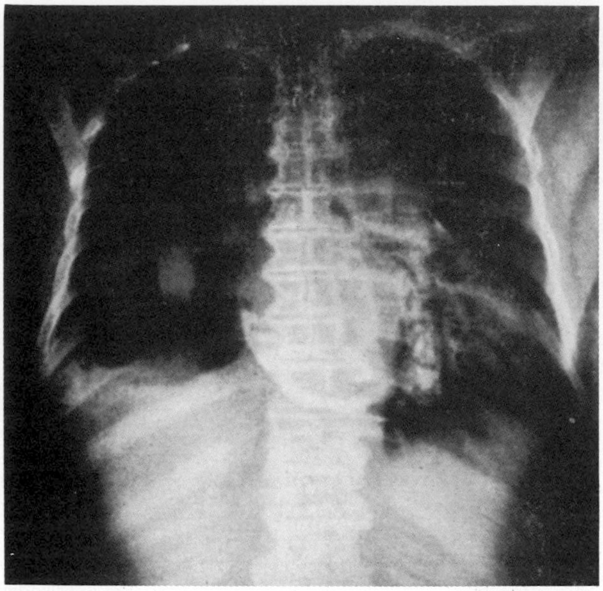

A

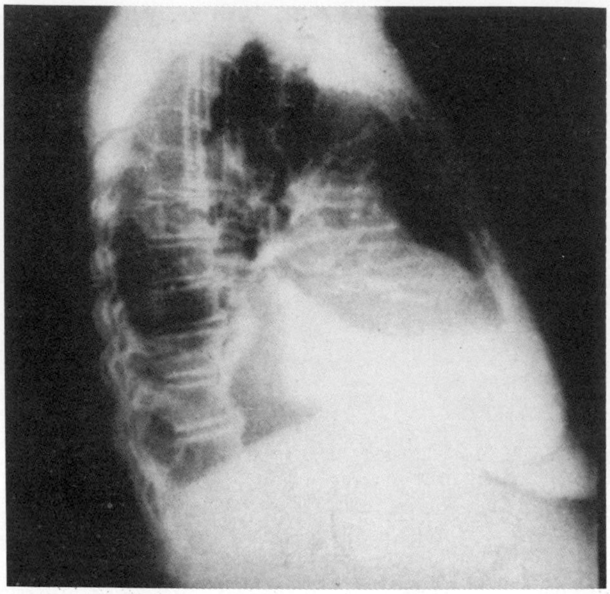

B

Figure 130–4. Posteroanterior (A) and lateral (B) chest x-ray demonstrating extensive pericardial thickening in a patient with constrictive calcified pericarditis. (*From Lorell and Braunwald*[1] *with permission.*)

the sensitivity for the detection of calcification. The superior vena cava is enlarged and can cause a prominence of the right superior mediastinum.

Echocardiogram. This technique may show pericardial thickening, flattening of the mid-diastolic and late diastolic motion of the left ventricular wall, a rapid E-to-F slope of the mitral valve, abnormal septal motion, and a premature opening of the pulmonic valve.[12] Two-dimensional echocardiography may demonstrate dilated inferior vena cava and hepatic veins without normal respiratory variations, dilated atria with small ventricles, and leftward bulging of both interventricular and interatrial septa during inspiration. Echocardiographic signs of constrictive pericarditis are neither sensitive nor specific, but they may be helpful in conjunction with clinical and hemodynamic findings. Computed-assisted digitization of M-mode echocardiogram may be useful in differentiating early diastolic filling of constrictive pericarditis from a more delayed filling pattern seen in restrictive cardiomyopathy.[28] Comparison of respiratory changes in transvalvular flow velocities can also differentiate constrictive pericarditis from restrictive cardiomyopathy.[29]

Computed Tomography

Documentation of pericardial thickening by computed tomography (CT) scan, defined as pericardial thickness greater than 4 mm, helps greatly in the diagnosis of constrictive pericarditis and the differentiation from restrictive cardiomyopathy. However, thickened pericardium itself is not diagnostic of constrictive pericarditis because it can be seen in the early postoperative period, in rheumatic heart disease, and in rheumatoid arthritis without constriction. CT may also show dilatation of inferior vena cava; hepatic veins; enlargement of atria, especially right atrium; and small-volume, narrow, tubular ventricles. It is the most sensitive technique for identifying pericardial calcification by density resolution. Extensive calcification in the visceral pericardium along the atrioventricular and interventricular grooves suggests the presence of constrictive pericarditis. The use of CT scanning is limited during pregnancy because of the potential risk of radiation to the fetus.[30]

Magnetic Resonance Imaging

Gated magnetic resonance imaging (MRI) has been useful for demonstrating pericardial thickness as well as other findings commonly seen in constrictive pericarditis such as dilatation of venae cavae and hepatic veins and narrowing of the right ventricle. Gated MRI is superior to echocardiography in differentiating pericardial hemotoma from other types of effusions. Although there are a number of reports of using MRI in pregnancy for obstetric and nonobstetric reasons, the safety of this technique in pregnancy is not yet established.[31]

Hemodynamic Evaluation

Similar to what has previously been described in patients with cardiac tamponade, pericardial constriction will also result in equalization of right atrial, right ventricular end-diastolic, pulmonary artery diastolic and pulmonary artery wedge pressures. The right ventricular pressure shows the typical square-root sign, characterized by an early diastolic dip followed by rapid rise of pressure and a plateau.[32] Right atrial pressure is usually elevated and demonstrates prominent X and Y descents. In contrast to restrictive cardiomyopathy, the pulmonary artery systolic pressure in constrictive pericarditis rarely exceeds 50 mm Hg, and the right ventricular pulse pressure is normally narrowed with a ratio of systolic-to-diastolic pressure of less than 3.5.

EFFUSIVE CONSTRICTIVE PERICARDITIS

This is a condition where constrictive pericarditis is found concomitantly with pericardial effusion.[32] The constriction is often caused by visceral pericarditis rather than parietal pericarditis. In this condition, cardiac compression will persist even after the removal of pericardial effusion. The most common causes for this condition are tuberculosis, mediastinal radiation, connective tissue disease, trauma, and relapse of idiopathic pericarditis.

MANAGEMENT

Diagnosis and assessment of the hemodynamic significance of the disease is important prior to pregnancy or early in pregnancy. The restriction of left ventricular filling can prevent the physiologic increase in cardiac output seen during pregnancy and jeopardize a normal fetal development and growth. On the other hand, signs and symptoms which may be seen in a normal pregnancy, such as dyspnea, neck vein distention, and leg edema, may be misleading when the severity of the disease is assessed. It is, therefore, important to perform a thorough evaluation including noninvasive and invasive studies, if needed, to guide the correct course of action. Although benign pericardial effusion is commonly seen during normal pregnancy, there is only one case reported in the literature of cardiac tamponade during pregnancy requiring pericardiocentesis. Simpson et al in 1988[33] described a case of acute idiopathic pericarditis presenting as cardiac tamponade at 32 weeks' gestation. After successful pericardiocentesis, a viable infant was delivered by cesarean section. The only treatment for cardiac tamponade is, however, removal of the pericardial fluid by emergency pericardiocentesis or surgical drainage. To maintain left ventricular filling volumes and to increase cardiac output and blood pressure until these procedures are performed, rapid volume expansion with intravenous fluids (300–500 cc/15 minutes) and increase of heart rate with isoproterenol should be used.[34]

The treatment of pericardial constriction is a surgical removal of the pericardium. Patients with mild to moderate symptoms may be carried through the pregnancy without surgery.[35,36] However, surgery has been performed during pregnancy[24,37] with good results, and it should be utilized in symptomatic patients and in patients where hemodynamic effect may compromise placental blood flow. Operative mortality has been reported to be as high as 15% in patients with constrictive pericarditis. Recurrence of constriction postsurgery is rare and long-term results are satisfactory although improvement may be gradual. Myocardial fibrosis or incomplete resection should be suspected if no hemodynamic improvement is noted.

Congenital partial absence of the left pericardium is a rare occurrence (3 out of 27,000 autopsy patients).[38] Savage and Nolan[39] recently reported a case of a 22-year-old pregnant Malaysian woman with partial absence of left pericardium. Patient presented at 28 weeks' gestation with chest wall pain. A prominent left atrial appendage seen on chest x-ray suggested the diagnosis. She had an uncomplicated vaginal delivery at 41 weeks' gestation.

REFERENCES

1. Lorell BH, Braunwald E: Pericardial disease. In: Braunwald E ed. *Heart Disease*, 3rd ed. Philadelphia: WB Saunders Company; 1988:1484.
2. Krausz Y, Naparstek E, Eliakim M. Idiopathic pericarditis and pregnancy. *Aust NZ J Obstet Gynaecol.* 1978;18:86.
3. Probst R, Mier T. Acute pericarditis complicating pregnancy. *Obstet Gynecol.* 1963;22:393.
4. Adams CW. Postviral myopericarditis associated with the influenza virus. *Am J Cardiol.* 1959;4:56.
5. Valenzuela GJ, Koos B, Mejias A. An unusual presentation of a case of staphyloccal pericarditis during pregnancy. *Am J Obstet Gynecol.* 1985;151:752.
6. Braester A, Nuusem D, Horn Y. Primary meningococcal pericarditis in a pregnant woman. *Int J Cardiol.* 1986;11:355.
7. Quismorio FP. Immune complexes in pericardial fluid in systemic lupus erythematosus. *Arch Intern Med.* 1980;140:112.
8. Averbuch M, Bojko A, Levo Y. Cardiac tamponade in the early postpartum period as the presenting and predominant manifestation of systemic lupus erythematosus. *J Rheumatol.* 1986;13:444.
9. Strang JIG. Tuberculous pericarditis in Transkei. *Clin Cardiol.* 1984;5:667.
10. Elkayam U, Weiss S, Laniado S. Pericardial effusion and mitral valve involvement in systemic lupus erythematosus. *Ann Rheum Dis.* 1977;36:349.
11. Surawicz B, Lassiter KC. Electrocardiogram in pericarditis. *Am J Cardiol.* 1970;26:471.
12. Feigenbaum H. *Echocardiography.* 4th ed. Philadelphia: Lea & Febiger; 1986:548.
13. Schnittger I, Bowden RE, Abrams J and Popp RL. Echocardiography: pericardial thickening and constrictive pericarditis. *Am J Cardiol.* 1978;42(3):388.
14. Dommissee J, Darey DA, Roos PJ. Prazosin and oxaprenolol therapy in pregnancy hypertension. *S Afr Med J.* 1983;13:231.
15. Pritchard JA, MacDonald PC, Grant NF, eds. *Obstetrics*, 17th ed. Norwalk, CT: Appleton-Crofts; 1985:548.
16. Naulty J, Cefalo RC, Lewis PE. Fetal toxicity of nitroprusside in the pregnant ewe. *Am J Obstet Gynecol.* 1981;139:708.
17. Lubbe WF. The use of captopril in pregnancy (Letter). *NZ Med J.* 1983;94:1029.
18. Rotmensch HH, Elkayam U, Frishman W. Antiarrhythmic drug therapy during pregnancy. *Ann Int Med.* 1983;98:487.
19. Cesario TC. Antibiotic therapy in pregnancy. In: Elkayam U, Gleicher N, eds. *Cardiac Problems in Pregnancy: Diagnostic and Management of Maternal and Fetal Disease.* New York: Alan R. Liss; 1990:437.
20. Berkowitz RL, Constan DR, Mochizuki TK. *Handbook for Prescribing Medications During Pregnancy.* 2nd ed. Boston/Toronto: Little, Brown and Company. 1986:260.
21. Permanyer-Miralda G, Sagrista-Sauleda J, Soler-Soler J. Primary acute pericardial disease: a prospective series of 231 consecutive patients. *Am J Cardiol.* 1985;56(10):623.
22. Callahan JA, Seward JB, Nishimura RA, Miller FA Jr, et al. Two-dimensional echocardiography guided pericardiocentesis: experience in 117 consecutive patients. *Am J Cardiol.* 1985;55:476.
23. Palatianos GM, Thurer RJ, Kaiser GA. Comparison of effectiveness and safety of operations on the pericardium. *Chest.* 1985;88:30.
24. Miller JI, Mansour KA, Hatcher CR Jr. Pericardiectomy: current indications, concepts and results in a university center. *Ann Thorac Surg.* 1982;34(1):40.
25. Haiat R, Halphen C, Clement F, Michelon B. Silent pericardial effusion in late pregnancy. *Chest.* 1981;79:717.
26. Singh S, Wann LS, Schychard GH, Klopfenstein HS, et al. Right ventricular and right atrial collapse in patients with cardiac tamponade—a combined echocardiographic and hemodynamic study. *Circulation.* 1984;70:966.
27. Lee W, Shaw PK, Amin DK, Elkayam U. Hemodynamic monitoring in cardiac patients during pregnancy. In: Elkayam U and Gleicher N eds. 2nd ed. New York: Alan R. Liss; 1990:47.
28. Janos GG, Argunan K, Meyer RA, Engel P, et al. Differentiation of constrictive pericarditis and restrictive cardiomyopathy using digitized echocardiography. *J Am Coll Cardiol.* 1983;6:471.
29. Hattle LR, Appelton CP, Popp RL. Differentiation of constrictive pericarditis and restrictive cardiomyopathy by Doppler echocardiography. *Circulation.* 1989;79(2):357.
30. Powell MC, Worthington BJ, Buckley JM, Symonds EM. MRI in obstetrics: maternal anatomy. *Br J Obstet Gynecol.* 1988;95(1):31.
31. Yoshizymi TT, Suneja SK, Teal JS. Practical CT dosimetry. *Radiol Technol.* 1989;60(6):505.
32. Lorrell BH, Grossman W. Profiles in constrictive pericarditis, restrictive cardiomyopathy, and cardiac tamponade. In: Grossman W ed. *Cardiac Catheterization and Angiography.* 3rd ed. Philadelphia: Lea & Febiger; 1986: 427.
33. Simpson WG, Depriest PD, Conover WB. Acute pericarditis complicated by cardiac tamponade during pregnancy. *Am J Obstet Gynecol.* 1989;160(2):415.
34. Fowler NO, Holmes JC. Hemodynamic effects of isoproterenol and nonepinephrine in acute cardiac tamponade. *J Clin Invest.* 1969;48:502.
35. Mendelson CL. *Cardiac Disease in Pregnancy.* Philadelphia: F.A. Davis; 1966:297.
36. Szekely P, Snaith L. *Heart Disease and Pregnancy.* London: Churchill Livingstone; 1974:195.
37. Watson PJ, Harelda CJ, Sorosky J, Kochenoyz NK. Irradiation-induced constrictive pericarditis requiring pericardiectomy during pregnancy. *J Reprod Med.* 1980;24:127.
38. Morgan J, Rogers A, Forker A. Congenital absence of the left pericardium. *Ann Intern Med.* 1971;74:370.
39. Savage RW, Nolan TE. Pregnancy in a woman with partial absence of the left pericardium. A case report. *J Reprod Med.* 1988;33:385.

Chapter One Hundred and Thirty-One

Peripartum Cardiomyopathy

Uri Elkayam, Enrique L. Ostrzega, and Avraham Shotan

131

Peripartum cardiomyopathy (PPCM) is a form of dilated congestive cardiomyopathy leading to the development of congestive heart failure in the peripartum period. Symptoms occur in the majority of patients during the last two months of gestation or the immediate postpartum period, although presentation delayed up to six months postpartum may occur.[1,2] The incidence of the disease was reported to be between one in 1300 to one in 4000 live births.[1] More recent information and our own experience, however, have suggested a lower incidence of PPCM of approximately one in 15,000 or less live births.[3]

PPCM usually presents with symptoms of congestive heart failure including fatigue, shortness of breath, paroxysmal nocturnal dyspnea, cough which worsens in the supine position, chest pain, and palpitations. Physical examination may reveal jugular venous distention, right and left ventricular enlargement manifested by parasternal heave, and diffuse and displaced point of maximum impulse. Auscultation of the heart may reveal somewhat diminished first sound (S_1), increased pulmonary component of the second heart sound (P_2) due to pulmonary hypertension and the presence of a third heart sound (S_3). An apical holosystolic murmur of mitral regurgitation and a systolic murmur over the tricuspid area increasing with inspiration due to tricuspid valve incompetence may be present. Auscultation of the lungs usually reveal pulmonary rales. Hepatomegaly is often found as well as peripheral edema. Because of increased incidence of intracardiac thrombosis, embolic phenomena are not uncommon.[1]

Electrocardiogram usually demonstrates abnormalities consisting of left ventricular hypertrophy, left atrial enlargement and T-wave and ST-segment changes. Conduction abnormalities and arrhythmias may also occur. Chest x-ray may show cardiac enlargement, pulmonary venous congestion with interstitial or alveolar edema, and pleural effusion. The echocardiogram usually reveals enlargement of all four cardiac chambers with diffuse hypokinesis of both ventricles and reduced fractional shortening of the left ventricle (Fig. 131–1). Small-to-moderate pericardial effusion may be found.[2,4] Doppler echocardiography often reveals mild-to-moderate mitral valve and tricuspid valve regurgitation and, occasionally, pulmonary regurgitation. Poor right-and-left ventricular systolic function can be also demonstrated by radionuclide ventriculography which reveals enlarged and poorly contractiled ventricles with reduced ejection fraction. All these findings are not specific to peripartum cardiomyopathy and may be found in patients with dilated cardiomyopathy of any type, however, when other causes for the disease can be ruled out and symptoms are present in the peripartum period, the diagnosis of peripartum cardiomyopathy is highly likely.[5]

Hemodynamic evaluation reveals data indistinguishable from other forms of dilated cardiomyopathy with markedly elevated mean right atrial, mean pulmonary arterial, and mean pulmonary artery wedge pressures. There is a decrease in cardiac output, stroke volume and left ventricular stroke work index, and a significant increase in pulmonary and systemic vascular resistance.[2] Coronary angiography usually reveals normal coronary arteries.

Endomyocardial biopsy may demonstrate inflamma-

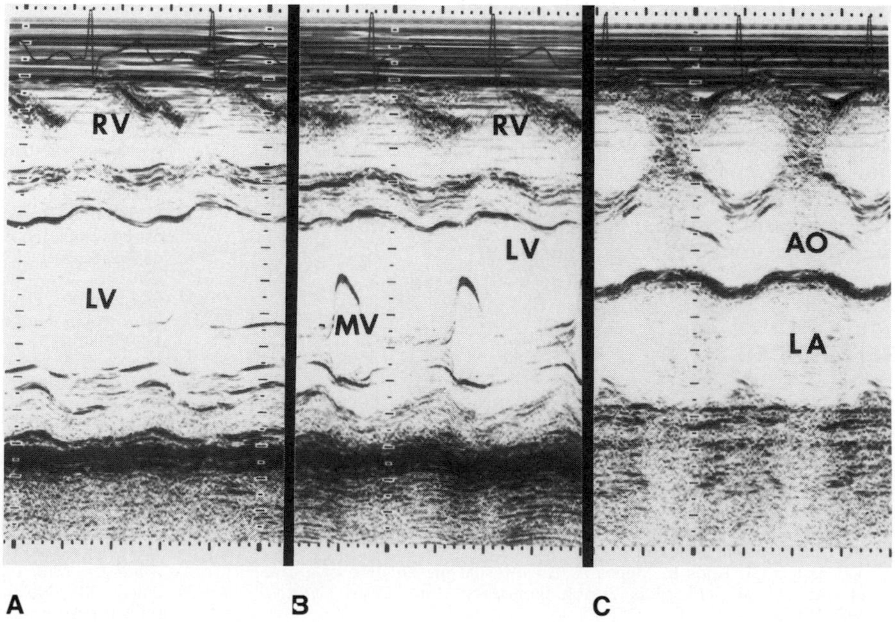

Figure 131–1. M-mode echocardiogram of an 18-year-old female with mild form of peripartum cardiomyopathy. The patient presented in the 38th week of pregnancy with pulmonary edema. The echocardiogram shows moderate increase in the size of the left ventricle and dysfunction of the left ventricle. (A = Echocardiogram just below level of mitral valve; B = Echocardiogram at level of mitral valve; C = Echocardiogram at level of aortic valve; RV = right ventricle; LV = left ventricle; MV = mitral valve; AO = aorta; LA = left atrium.)

tory changes consisting of myocarditis with mononuclear infiltrate and myocardial damage consisting of necrosis, degeneration of adjacent myocytes, or both.[2,6,7]

In spite of a number of potential etiologies, the precise cause of PPCM is still unknown. Although exacerbation of preexisting congestive cardiomyopathy due to the increased hemodynamic load of pregnancy has been suggested as a potential cause for the peripartum development of heart failure[5], there are various features to this syndrome which suggest its unique nature and distinguish it from other forms of cardiac dysfunction. In contrast to PPCM, other forms of congestive cardiomyopathy rarely occur in patients, especially females below middle age.[8] Complete recovery of cardiac size and function as well as symptoms is seen in approximately one half of patients with PPCM and is less common in other forms of cardiomyopathy.[8] In addition, PPCM may recur during subsequent pregnancies even in patients who demonstrate recovery from the first episode, suggesting pregnancy-mediated cardiac dysfunction. Several etiologies have been suggested by various authors but could not be confirmed by others. Such etiologies include malnutrition, toxemia, and exacerbation of chronic hypertension.[5,9] Recent reports have demonstrated high incidence of endomyocardial biopsy-proven myocarditis in patients with PPCM.[6,7,10] These findings may suggest an etiological role for myocarditis in patients with PPCM. The reported incidence of active myocardial inflammation, however, has varied greatly in the literature ranging from 29% to 100%.[1,2,6,7,10] Cole et al[4] have recently reported histological findings of myocarditis in none of five patients with PPCM.

PROGNOSIS

The course of PPCM varies among patients.[1,5] Approximately 50% of the cases demonstrate complete or near complete recovery of cardiac size and function as well as clinical status with favorable long-term prognosis. The other 50% of the cases demonstrate either continuous clinical deterioration and early death or persistent left ventricular depression and chronic heart failure with high morbidity and mortality. Demakis and Rahimtoola[11] reported 54% 5-year mortality in 13 patients who continued to have cardiomyopathy and gallop rhythms at the end of 6 months postpartum.

MANAGEMENT

The acute treatment of heart failure patients with PPCM include oxygen, inotropic support with digitalis and, if indicated, with intravenous dobutamine. Digitalis should be used with caution because of reported sensitivity and high incidence of digitalis toxicity in these patients.[5] Diuretics should be used in order to correct increased blood volume and to prevent sodium and fluid retention. Vasodilators may be useful in unloading the failing ventricles. The use of arterial dilation with hydralazine has been shown to be safe during pregnancy and may be used to augment cardiac output in patients with PPCM. Venodilation with nitrates may further improve the hemodynamic profile of patients with PPCM and may cause reduction of right and left ventricular filling pressures, pulmonary arterial pressures, and vascular resistance. The use of organic nitrates during pregnancy, however, has been limited and in one report, reduction of blood pressure with nitroglycerin in patients with pregnancy-induced hypertension was associated with fetal rate deceleration and bradycardia.[12] There is only limited experience with these agents during gestation. Nitroprusside is useful for reduction of both left ventricular preload and afterload but may be toxic to the fetus and should therefore be used antepartum only when other drugs fail.[13] Angiotensin-converting enzyme inhibitors (ACEI) have been shown to improve hemodynamic, symptomatic, and functional status of patients with heart failure. In addition, ACEI have been shown to improve survival in patients with chronic heart failure. These drugs, however, have been associated with deleterious effects on fetal blood pressure control and renal function and are not recommended for use during pregnancy.[14] Because of the increased incidence of thromboembolic events in patients with PPCM, anticoagulation therapy is strongly recommended.

Since PPCM may be reversible, the temporary use of an intra-aortic balloon pump helps to stabilize patients until improvement occurs.[15] The use of a left ventricular assist device has been reported as a bridge to cardiac transplantation in a patient who demonstrated continued deterioration in spite of maximal medical therapy.[16] Because of common association of peripartum myocarditis and cardiomyopathy, immunosuppressive therapy has been recommended in patients with PPCM and myocarditis proven by endomyocardial biopsy.[7] However, the evidence that PPCM improves with immunosuppression is conflicting and insufficient.[4,17] For this reason, we recommend immunosuppressive therapy only to patients with biopsy-proven myocarditis who continue to demonstrate clinical deterioration on conventional therapy of congestive heart failure. Because of the high mortality seen in patients with continued clinical deterioration, cardiac transplantation should be considered as a therapeutic option in such patients.

After hemodynamic optimization prior to delivery, and under careful hemodynamic monitoring, most women with peripartum cardiomyopathy should be able to tolerate labor induction and vaginal delivery under regional anesthesia. Cesarean section should be reserved primarily for obstetric indications and for patients in severe distress or hemodynamic instability.

Treatment of chronic heart failure in patients recovering from the acute phase of the disease should include digitalis, diuretics, and vasodilators. Chronic anticoagulation is recommended because of the high incidence of intracardiac thrombus formation and peripheral embolization. Because of the increased risk of thromboembolic events, oral contraceptives should be avoided.

RECOMMENDATIONS FOR SUBSEQUENT PREGNANCIES

Review of the literature published from 1957 revealed 61 subsequent pregnancies in 49 PPCM patients.[7,11,18-25] Eleven relapses and ten deaths were reported in 17 pregnancies in women with persistently abnormal left ventricular function, increased cardiac size, or both. Because of the high risk of morbidity and mortality, such patients should be advised against recurrent pregnancy. A favorable outcome of subsequent pregnancies in four women who showed recovery of left ventricular function after presentation with PPCM has recently been published. Review of all published data in similar patients, however, reveals ten relapses and four deaths in 46 subsequent pregnancies. These data suggest, therefore, that subsequent pregnancy in patients recovering from PPCM is not risk-free and may be associated with recurrent disease associated with cardiac deterioration and even death for PPCM patients with normal cardiac size.

REFERENCES

1. Homans DC. Peripartum cardiomyopathy. *N Engl J Med*. 1985;312:1432.
2. O'Connell JB, Costanzo-Nordin MR, Subramanian R, Robinson JA. Peripartum cardiomyopathy: clinical, hemodynamic, histologic and prognostic characteristics. *J Am Coll Cardiol*. 1986;8:52.
3. Cunningham FG, Pritchard JA, Hankins GDV, Anderson PL. Peripartum heart failure: idiopathic cardiomyopathy or compounding cardiovascular events? *Obstet Gynecol*. 1986;67:157.
4. Cole P, Cook F, Plappert T, Saltzman D. Longitudinal changes in left ventricular architecture and function in peripartum cardiomyopathy. *Am J Cardiol*. 1987;60:871.
5. Ribner HS, Silverman RI. Peripartal cardiomyopathy. In: Elkayam U, Gleicher N eds.: *Cardiac Problems in Pregnancy Diagnosis and Management of Maternal and Fetal Disease*. 2nd ed. New York: Alan R. Liss; 1990;115.
6. Sanderson JE, Olsen EGJ, Gate D. Peripartum heart disease: an endomyocardial biopsy study. *Br Heart J*. 1986;56:285.
7. Midei MG, DeMent SH, Feldman AM, Hutchins GM. Peripartum myocarditis and cardiomyopathy. *Circulation*. 1990;81:922.
8. Fuster V, Gersh BJ, Giuliani ER, Tajik AJ. The natural history of idiopathic dilated cardiomyopathy. *Am J Cardiol*. 1981;47:525.
9. Demakis JF, Rahimtoola SH, Sutton GC, Meadows WR. Natural course of peripartum cardiomyopathy. *Circulation*. 1971;44:1053.
10. Melvin KR, Richardson PJ, Olsen EGJ, Daly K. Peripartum cardiomyopathy due to myocarditis. *N Engl J Med*. 1982;307:731.
11. Demakis JG, Rahimtoola SH. Peripartum cardiomyopathy. *Circulation*. 1971;44:964.
12. Cotton DB, Longmire S, Jones MM, et al. Cardiovascular alterations in severe pregnancy-induced hypertension: effects of intravenous nitroglycerin coupled with blood volume expansion. *Am J Obstet Gynecol*. 1986;154:1053.
13. Widerhorn J, Rubin JN, Frishman WH, Elkayam UE. Cardiovascular drugs in pregnancy. *Cardiol Clin*. 1987;5:651.
14. Editorial. Are ACE inhibitors safe in pregnancy? *Lancet*. 1989;2:482.
15. Brantigan CO, Grow JB Sr, Schoonmaker FW. Extended use of intraaortic balloon pumping in peripartum cardiomyopathy. *Ann Surg*. 1976;183:1.
16. Hovsepian PG, Ganzel B, Sohi GS, Kupersmith J. Peripartum cardiomyopathy treated with a left ventricular assist device as a bridge to cardiac transplantation. *South Med J*. 1989;82:527.
17. Mason JW, O'Connell JB. A model of myocarditis in humans. *Circulation*. 1990;81:1154.
18. Meadows WR. Idiopathic myocardial failure in the last trimester of pregnancy and the puerperium. *Circulation*. 1957;15:903.
19. Seftel H, Susser M. Maternity and myocardial failure in African women. *Br Heart J*. 1961;23:43.
20. Wilmer G. Postpartal heart disease. *South Med J*. 1963;56:803.
21. Walsh JJ, Burch GE, Black WC, Ferrans VJ. Idiopathic myocardiopathy of the puerperium (postpartal heart disease). *Circulation*. 1965;32:19.
22. Brockington JF. Postpartum hypertensive heart failure. *Am J Cardiol*. 1971;27:650.
23. Lee W, Cotton DB. Peripartum cardiomyopathy: current concepts and clinical management. *Clin Obstet Gynecol*. 1989;32:54.
24. Stuart KL. Cardiomyopathy of pregnancy and the puerperium. *Quarterly J Med*. 1968;37:463.
25. St. John Sutton M, Cole P, Saltzman D, Goldhaber S. Risks of cardiac dysfunction in peripartum cardiomyopathy (PPCM) with subsequent pregnancy. *Circulation*. 1989;80:Supplement II 320.

Chapter One Hundred and Thirty-Two
Hypertrophic Cardiomyopathy

Anil Kumar and Uri Elkayam

132

Synonymous with idiopathic hypertrophic subaortic stenosis (IHSS) and muscular subaortic stenosis, hypertrophic cardiomyopathy is a disease of unknown etiology characterized by a hypertrophy of the left ventricular myocardium. In some patients with this disorder, the hypertrophy of the cardiac muscle is associated with a pressure gradient between the left ventricular cavity and the left ventricular outflow tract. In contrast to aortic stenosis, the pressure gradient seen in hypertrophic cardiomyopathy is dynamic; it may vary in the same patient from one time to another or may be provoked only by physical exertion or maneuvers. The presence of a pressure gradient in the left ventricle has led to the use of terms such as IHSS or muscular subaortic stenosis. However, in a large proportion of patients, no pressure gradient is measurable at rest or on provocation. Although the etiology of hypertrophic cardiomyopathy is not known, the disease tends to occur both sporadically and in clusters in families. The mode of inheritance is probably autosomal dominant. The wide spectrum of its clinical presentation extends from the asymptomatic relative of a known sufferer to severe illness often leading to poor effort tolerance, heart failure, or sudden death.[1,2]

PATHOLOGY AND PATHOGENESIS

As the name indicates, hypertrophy of the myocardium is the hallmark of the disease. It mainly involves the left ventricle, although other cardiac chambers may also experience hypertrophy to a lesser degree. In the majority of patients, the hypertrophy is diffuse and involves all of the left ventricular myocardium. In some patients, myocardial hypertrophy is characterized by a disproportionate thickening of the interventricular septum close to the base of the heart. This is manifested on echocardiography and pathologic study by asymmetric septal hypertrophy (ASH). On histopathologic examination, the involved myocardium shows a lesion characterized by *myocardial fiber disarray*. The normal myocardial architecture is lost in the involved areas, and histologically distinct hypertrophied myocardial cells are noticed interspersed between normal-looking myocytes. This pathologic picture is not unique to hypertrophic cardiomyopathy and may also be seen in coronary artery disease and ventricular hypertrophy from pressure overload.

Pathophysiological features of the illness include a dynamic gradient across the left ventricular outflow tract in some patients and the presence of a small ventricular cavity with thickened walls in most patients. The latter disorder leads to impaired filling of the ventricle and thus to elevation of the left atrial and pulmonary pressures.

A large proportion of patients with hypertrophic cardiomyopathy, are asymptomatic. The disease which occurs in a wide spectrum of ages most frequently manifests clinically in the young adult. Well defined cases of hypertrophic cardiomyopathy have been reported in the elderly, and in the newborn—especially to diabetic mothers.[3] Women tend to present more often with symptomatic disease. Dyspnea is the predominant presenting symptom. Chest pain, anginal or atypical; syncope; and palpitations because of arrhythmias and symptoms of heart failure such as exertional dyspnea, orthopnea, and paroxysmal nocturnal dyspnea all may occur during the course of the illness. Sudden death may be the first clinical manifestation of the disease in an occasional young patient. Most symptoms are worsened on exertion, and poor effort tolerance is a frequent presenting complaint.

Physical examination may be entirely normal in the patient who does not have a left ventricular outflow tract gradient. A fourth heart sound may be the only finding on physical examination. In patients with a large pressure gradient across the left ventricular outflow tract, the apical precordial impulse is forceful, and a prominent apical presystolic impulse may be palpable. In consonance with vigorous atrial activity, prominent A waves are seen in the jugular venous pulse. The carotid pulse in the patient with a pressure gradient shows a brisk upstroke followed by a short decline at midsystole and a secondary rise. A systolic thrill can often be palpated along the lower left sternal border and the apex. On auscultation, the diagnostic hallmark is a diamond-shaped systolic murmur along the left sternal border. The murmur is increased in intensity during the strain phase of the Valsalva maneuver and during exercise or tachycardia. Standing also increases the intensity of the murmur. On squatting, isometric hand grip, and during the overshoot phase of the Valsalva maneuver, the murmur is decreased in intensity. The murmur should be differentiated from other systolic murmurs of valvular stenosis and mitral regurgitation.

Electrocardiographic features include left ventricular hypertrophy, ST- and T-wave abnormalities, and presence of abnormal Q waves in inferior or lateral leads. In some patients with asymptomatic disease, the electrocardiogram may be normal. On ambulatory electrocardiography (Holter), ventricular tachyarrhythmias are frequently seen.[4] Echocardiography is the test most frequently used to make a definitive diagnosis of hypertrophic cardiomyopathy. Echocardiographic features of the disease include an asymmetric septal hypertrophy (ASH), generalized left ventricular hypertrophy, hypertrophy localized to a small segment of the ventricle such as the apex or the septum, systolic anterior motion (SAM) of the anterior mitral leaflet, decreased septal motion, and a decreased size of the ventricular cavity.

DIAGNOSIS, PROGNOSIS AND MANAGEMENT OF HYPERTROPHIC CARDIOMYOPATHY IN PREGNANCY

Care must be taken in making the diagnosis of hypertrophic cardiomyopathy in pregnancy. This is important because systolic murmurs are frequent in pregnancy, and thus the likelihood of making a wrong diagnosis is increased.

Echocardiography—M-mode or two-dimensional—is a definitive test for the diagnosis of hypertrophic cardiomyopathy and should be done in symptomatic patients in whom the clinical suspicion is high. In the presence of classic echocardiographic findings, the diagnosis is secure. The presence and severity of pressure gradient across the left ventricular outflow tract and mitral regurgitation can be assessed with the aid of the Doppler technique.[5] Cardiac catheterization, which is associated with a large dose of ionizing radiation, is, therefore, not needed in most cases during pregnancy.

In a recent review of the literature[6], information was reported on 82 pregnancies in 35 patients since 1967. The reports showed favorable outcome of pregnancy in most cases, although new onset or worsening of cardiac symptoms, including congestive heart failure, chest pain, palpitations, dizziness and syncope, occurred in many patients. Two patients had ventricular arrhythmias which led to mortality in one of them. Fetal outcome did not seem to be influenced by the disease. Spontaneous abortion was reported in 20% and low birth weight in 10% of the pregnancies. Fifteen percent of pregnancies were delivered by cesarean section and forceps delivery was reported in 6% of the cases. Premature delivery was reported in 7% of the pregnancies. Three infants had respiratory problems either at birth or shortly thereafter, and one case had fetal death secondary to maternal mortality from ventricular arrhythmia.[7]

The management of pregnancy in the patient with hypertrophic cardiomyopathy should start with prepregnancy consultation with the patient and her family regarding the potential risk of pregnancy to the patient and the fetus. The likelihood of transmission of the disease to the child may be as high as 50% in families with high gene penetrance and an autosomal dominant inheritance and less than 25% in sporadic cases.[8]

In the asymptomatic patient with mild disease, no treatment is necessary, and the outcome of pregnancy is almost uniformly good. In general, interventions that decrease left ventricular size by reducing venous return or those that decrease afterload and thus increase the outflow gradient in the left ventricle should be studiously avoided, especially in the patient with documented resting or provocable pressure gradient across the left ventricular outflow tract. These include hypovolemia from diuretics, vasodilation from drugs or anesthesia, use of cardiostimulants such as digoxin and isoproterenol, and recurrent Valsalva maneuvers associated with straining. It is important to note, however, that the strain of vaginal delivery is well tolerated by women with hypertrophic cardiomyopathy.[9]

Since the main cause of mortality in hypertrophic cardiomyopathy is arrhythmia rather than hemodynamic decompensation[10], an attempt should be made to identify patients who have complex ventricular arrhythmias and are therefore at an increased risk of sudden death. Ambulatory electrocardiographic monitoring (Holter) is the best means to detect the presence of arrhythmias and should be done in all patients. If complex ventricular arrhythmias are present, appropriate antiarrhythmic medications should be started[8], and the response to these medications, that is, suppression of arrhythmias, should be assessed by repeat Holter monitoring. The considerations regarding selection of antiarrhythmic therapy during pregnancy are discussed in Chapters 125 and 135. The fact that a patient is on β blockers and shows symptomatic improvement does not automatically mean that β blockers are effective in suppressing arrhythmias, and repeat Holter monitoring should be carried out in all patients to demonstrate decreased arrhythmic activity.[4]

Specific indications for drug therapy in the symptomatic patient include the presence of angina, dyspnea, and arrhythmias. Even in the presence of dyspnea, digoxin is likely to worsen symptoms by increasing outflow gradient and should be avoided. The β blockers have been traditionally used in the management of most symptomatic patients with hypertrophic cardiomyopathy. Propranolol increases myocardial compliance, decreases oxygen consumption, and has an antiarrhythmic effect. Anginal chest pain responds better to this therapy than does dyspnea, and in many patients larger doses of propranolol than those conventionally used for angina pectoris are required. The use of propranolol during pregnancy has been shown to be relatively safe. It is important, however, to note that complications such as bradycardia, hypoglycemia, and apnea have been described in the newborn of women treated with propranolol[11-13], and although their incidence seems to be very small, they should be anticipated.

Calcium-channel blocking agents, particularly verapamil, have shown a beneficial effect on patients with hypertrophic cardiomyopathy. Several large studies have shown a beneficial effect of verapamil in symptomatic patients.[14,15] However, vasodilator properties of the drug have the potential of increasing the pressure gradient in patients with hypertrophic cardiomyopathy. The therapy is associated with a variety of serious side effects[16] and should be used with particular caution in the patient with symptoms of overt congestive heart failure such as orthopnea and paroxysmal nocturnal dyspnea. It may lead to conduction disturbances, and in an occasional patient, severe hypotension, at times fatal, may develop. Verapamil has been used in pregnancy for the treatment of maternal and fetal arrhythmias, premature labor, and severe preeclampsia. However, because of the limited information available at the present time, the safety of verapamil for chronic treatment during pregnancy is not known.

Atrial fibrillation has been associated with increased risk of thromboembolic events in patients with hypertrophic cardiomyopathy.[17] Anticoagulant therapy should therefore be given to such patients.

Since sudden death in hypertrophic cardiomyopathy is frequently associated with strenuous activity[10], it would be useful to advise patients to avoid overexertion. In addition, patients with hypertrophic obstructive cardiomyopathy are at an increased risk of developing infective endocarditis and should be given appropriate antibiotic prophylaxis.[18,19] Indications for antibiotic prophylaxis for the prevention of bacterial endocarditis in pregnancy and during childbirth are discussed in Chapter 128.

The limited experience of investigators in this field has shown that the outcome of pregnancy in patients with hypertrophic cardiomyopathy is good.[20] On the basis of this experience, it can be said that the average patient with hypertrophic cardiomyopathy would go through pregnancy and childbirth with either no or only mild-to-moderate worsening of symptoms. In the patient with no obstetric complications, a normal vaginal delivery can be accomplished without increased risk to the mother or the fetus. Left uterine displacement is advisable during labor and delivery in order to increase venous return to the heart.

Because of potentia vasodilatory effect, the use of prostaglandins to augment uterine contractions should be avoided. The use of oxytocin has been done safely in patients with hypertrophic cardiomyopathy.[7,20] Hypovolemia should be avoided during pregnancy. Blood loss should be replaced with intravenous fluids and cross-matched blood should be available for potential need.

Because of potential aggravation of pressure gradient across the left ventricular outflow tract, the use of beta mimetic drugs for tocolysis should be avoided. In symptomatic patients and those with left ventricular outflow obstruction, hemodynamic monitoring should be used for labor and delivery.[21]

Spinal and epidural anesthesia should be avoided or performed with great caution in patients with obstructive hypertrophic cardiomyopathy because of their vasodilatory effect.[22] Systemic medications, inhalation analgesia, or paracervical and pudendal blocks are recommended for labor and delivery in such patients.[23]

REFERENCES

1. Wynne J, Braunwald E. The cardiomyopathies and myocarditides. In: Braunwald E, ed: *Heart Disease,* 3rd ed. Philadelphia: WB Saunders. 1988;1410.
2. Wigle ED. Hypertrophic cardiomyopathy: 1987 viewpoint. *Circulation.* 1987;75:311.
3. Lusson JR, Gaulme J, Raynaud EJ, Cheynel J. Asymmetrical hypertrophic cardiomyopathy in neonates of diabetic mothers. *Arch Fr Pediatr.* 1982;39:433.
4. McKenna WJ, Chetty S, Oakley CM, Goodwin JF. Arrhythmia in hypertrophic cardiomyopathy: exercise and 48-hour ambulatory electrocardiographic assessment with and without β-adrenergic blocking therapy. *Am J Cardiol.* 1980;45:1.
5. Maron BJ, Gottdiener JS, Arce J, Rosing DR, et al. Dynamic subaortic obstruction in hypertrophic cardiomyopathy: pulsed Doppler echocardiography. *J Am Col Cardiol.* 1985;6:1.
6. Kumar A, Elkayam U. Hypertrophic cardiomyopathy in pregnancy. In: Elkayam U, Gleicher N, eds. *Cardiac Problems in Pregnancy, Diagnosis and Management of Maternal and Fetal Disease.* 2nd ed. New York: Alan R. Liss, 1990;129.
7. Shah DM, Sunderji SG. Hypertrophic cardiomyopathy and pregnancy: report of a maternal mortality and review of the literature. *Obstet Gynecol Surv.* 1985;40:444.
8. Maron BJ, Mulvihill JJ. The genetics of hypertrophic cardiomyopathy. *Ann Intern Med.* 1986;105:610.
9. Oakley GDG, McGarry K, Limb DG, Oakley CM. Management of pregnancy in patients with hypertrophic cardiomyopathy. *Br Med J.* 1979;1:1749.
10. Maron BJ, Roberts WC, Epstein SE. Sudden death in hypertrophic cardiomyopathy: a profile of 78 patients. *Circulation.* 1982;65:1388.
11. Tunstall ME. The effect of propranolol on the onset of breathing at birth. *Br J Anaesthesiol.* 1969;41:792.
12. Habib A, McCarthy JS. Effects on the neonate of propranolol administered during pregnancy. *J Pediatr.* 1977;91:808.
13. Gladstone GR, Hordof A, Gersony WM. Propranolol administration during pregnancy: effects on the fetus. *J Pediatr.* 1975;86:962.
14. Rosing DR, Kent KM, Maron BJ, Epstein SE. Verapamil therapy: a new approach to the pharmacologic treatment of hypertrophic cardiomyopathy. II. Effects of exercise capacity and symptomatic status. *Circulation.* 1979;60:1208.
15. Rosing DR, Condit JR, Maron BJ, Kent KM, et al. Verapamil therapy: a new approach to the pharmacologic treatment of hypertrophic cardiomyopathy. III. Effects of long-term administration. *Am J Cardiol.* 1981;48:545.
16. Epstein SE, Rosing DR. Verapamil: its potential for causing serious complications in patients with hypertrophic cardiomyopathy. *Circulation.* 1981;64:437.
17. Furlan AJ, Craciun AR, Raju NR, Hart N. Cerebrovascular complications associated with idiopathic hypertrophic subaortic stenosis. *Stroke.* 1984;15:282.
18. Vecht RJ, Oakley CM: Infective endocarditis in three patients with hypertrophic obstructive cardiomyopathy. *Br Med J.* 1968;2:455.
19. Chagnac A, Rudniki C, Loebel, Zahavi I. Infectious endocarditis in idiopathic hypertrophic subaortic stenosis: report of three cases and a review of the literature. *Chest.* 1982;81:346.
20. Kolibash AJ, Ruiz DE, Lewis RP. Idiopathic hypertrophic subaortic stenosis in pregnancy. *Ann Intern Med.* 1975;82:791.
21. Lee W, Shah PK, Amin DK, Elkayam U. Hemodynamic monitoring of cardiac patients during pregnancy. In Elkayam U, Gleicher N, eds.

Cardiac Problems in Pregnancy, Diagnosis and Management of Maternal and Fetal Disease. 2nd ed. New York: Alan R. Liss. 1990;47.
22. Thompson RC, Liberthson RR, Lowenstein E. Perioperative anesthetic risk of noncardiac surgery in hypertrophic obstructive cardiomyopathy. *JAMA*. 1985;254:2419.
23. Geller E, Rudick V, Niv D. Analgesia and anesthesia during pregnancy. In: Elkayam U, Gleicher N, eds. *Cardiac Problems in Pregnancy, Diagnosis and Management of Maternal and Fetal Disease*. 2nd ed. New York: Alan R. Liss. 1990;283.

Chapter One Hundred and Thirty-Three

Coronary Artery Disease

E. Albert Reece and Efstratios A. Assimakopoulos

133

Coronary artery disease (CAD) in young women is uncommon and is found even less frequently during pregnancy.[1] However, myocardial infarctions have been documented and can occur during pregnancy or in the postpartum period. The overall incidence of myocardial infarction during pregnancy is estimated to be less than 1 in 10,000 pregnancies; however, since the disease is rare, accurate estimation is difficult.[2] Myocardial infarction during pregnancy was first described by Katz in 1921.[3] Since then, fewer than 100 cases have been reported in the world literature. Cortis et al reported 76 cases from 1922–1979, and 12 more cases were added subsequently.[4]

The incidence of ischemic heart disease from different causes has been estimated to be 0.4% to 4.1%. Ischemic heart disease is one of the most common causes of death in the United States, resulting in about 500,000 deaths of women, annually, related to cardiovascular disease.[5] Despite the popular belief that women in the reproductive years essentially do not develop cardiovascular disease, statistics reveal that women die of heart attacks as frequently as men, only about 10 years later in life.[5] It is true, however, that very few women die of CAD before menopause. In the Framingham Heart Study, only 6 of 1600 premenopausal women died of CAD. However, other atherosclerotic lesions were found in autopsied adolescent girls.

In a review article, Hankins et al[6] reported on 68 women with documented myocardial infarction during pregnancy or delivery between 1922 and 1983. In this report, the mean maternal age was 33.8 years, ranging from 16 to 45 years. Of the overall death rate, 37% occurred during pregnancy or shortly after delivery as a direct consequence of the infarction or of complications thereof. For women 35 years or younger, the maternal mortality rate was 43%; and for women 36 years or older, it was 34%. Of major importance is the observation that two thirds of the women experienced myocardial infarction during the third trimester of pregnancy and only one third during the first and second trimesters. In the same series, fetal loss occurred in 34%.

Since CAD exists among premenopausal women and contemporary trends point toward women delaying marriage and childbearing until later in life, it is possible that the incidence of ischemic heart disease during pregnancy may increase. In this light, the high incidence of reported mortality, a discussion on etiology, early diagnosis, and management are of fundamental importance to this subject.

ETIOLOGY AND PATHOPHYSIOLOGY

Pathogenesis of cardiovascular disease involves atherosclerosis of the medium and large coronary arteries that causes most of the cases of myocardial infarction and ischemic heart disease.[7] Furthermore, other less common etiologies have been reported, such as coronary artery spasm, coronary artery emboli of different types, structural cardiac diseases, trauma, hemoglobinopathies, clotting abnormalities, and metabolic diseases. Major coronary risk factors are considered to be high cholesterol levels, diabetes mellitus, hypertension, obesity, stress, cigarette smoking, positive family history of premature CAD, and oral contraceptives, especially in women over age 35 who are smokers. Direct correlation between high levels of serum cholesterol and the risk for atherosclerotic disease has been well established. For every 1% increase in the total serum cholesterol level above normal, a 2% increase in the incidence of CAD is reported in young women (Figure 133–1).[8,9]

Cholesterol is transferred into the blood as lipoprotein molecules. There are three types of these lipoprotines: very low-density lipoprotein (VLDL) which carries triglycerides; low-density lipoprotein (LDL) which contains mainly cholesterol; and high-density lipoprotein (HDL) which transfers cholesterol to the liver. High levels of LDL are considered to be an independent risk factor for CAD in both men and women, whereas HDL has a protective effect against CAD. Thus, the higher the level of HDL, the lower the risk for CAD. Conversely, if the total cholesterol : HDL ratio is $\geq$4.5 or if the LDL concentration is $>$150 mg/dL, the patient is at high risk for heart disease.[10]

In theory, mechanisms of plaque formation include platelet adhesion after endothelial damage, smooth-muscle cell proliferation as a response to stimulation from platelet-derived growth factors, dietary hypercholesteremia, inflammation and macrophage activity, defective utilization of LDL by way of deficient receptors, and deficiency in cellular lysosomal enzymes.[7] Data indicate that lowering the cholesterol levels may result in the reversal or improvement of atherosclerotic lesions. To reduce the risk of CAD, the goal is to maintain total serum cholesterol below 200 mg/dL. Diet and drug therapy are also effective agents in reducing the incidence of cardiovascular disease by reducing cholesterol levels.[11]

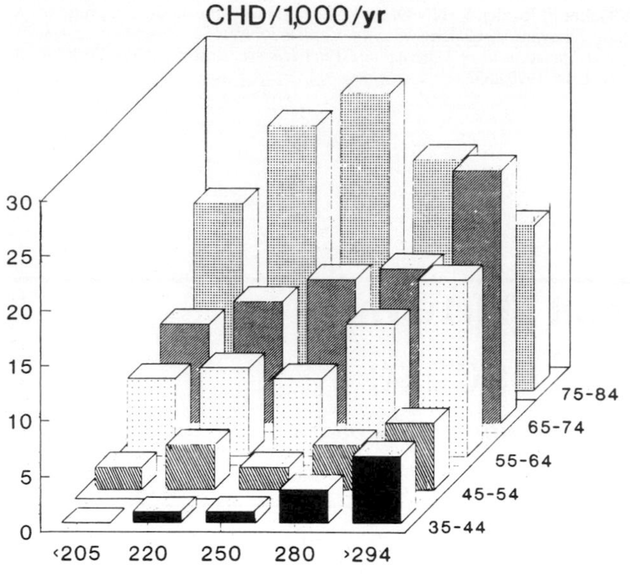

Figure 133–1. Associated risk of coronary heart disease with increasing cholesterol levels. (*From Castelli et al* [9] *with permission.*)

Diabetes mellitus, either insulin-dependent or noninsulin-dependent, is associated with high risk for the development of CAD. Young women are felt to be protected from clinical arteriosclerotic disease, but this protection seems to be absent if long-term diabetes is present.[1] The risk of myocardial infarction is twice as high in patients with diabetes as in those without.[2] In these patients, the arterial age equals the chronologic age plus the number of years of diabetes. For example, a young woman, 30 years old, who has had diabetes for 20 years may have arteries that are effectively 50 years old.[1] The precise mechanism by which glucose intolerance leads to an increased risk of cardiovascular disease is not entirely understood. Several mechanisms are proposed: (1) carbohydrate-induced elevation in VLDL and glycosaminoglycan, (2) hyperinsulinemia-induced stimulation of smooth-muscle cell proliferation, (3) sorbitol-induced cellular damage, and (4) diabetes-induced abnormalities in cells, platelets, or lipoprotein metabolism (Figure 133–2).[12]

In a recent study, Zovaroni et al[13] found that even patients with only abnormal oral glucose tolerance tests were hypercholesterolemic and hypertriglyceridemic and had significantly elevated systolic blood pressure and heart rates. They suggested that even mild degrees of diabetes pose a risk factor for CAD. Class H diabetes is defined as the presence of diabetes of any duration associated with ischemic myocardial disease.[14] These patients are at high risk for maternal mortality in pregnancy. Hence, if pregnancy occurs, pregnancy termination may be considered. If pregnancy is continued, meticulous control of the glycemic state and intensive fetal and maternal monitoring are necessary. Hypoglycemia (below 60 mg/dL) in these patients may also be a stimulus for myocardial ischemia. Gast et al[14] suggested that a glycemic goal at the upper limits of normal be attained for this group of patients. Therefore, levels of greater than 70 mg/dL for fasting and close to 120 mg/dL for postprandial glucose levels should be sought.

Elevated systolic or diastolic blood pressure is also a contributing factor to CAD. Once again, hyperinsulinemia has been shown to be responsible for high plasma catecholamine levels[15] and may possibly cause elevated blood pressure and increased heart rates in patients with abnormal glucose tolerance. In addition, hyperinsulinemia also increases renal tubular sodium reabsorption that may enhance blood pressure elevation. Obesity (greater than 20% ideal body weight) has been found to be an independent but weak risk factor for CAD.[16] Potential links between obesity and CAD in some studies have given conflicting results. It has been suggested that the distribution of fat in the body may be a better indicator of CAD risk than the overall obesity. A somewhat controversial area is the notion that emotional stress and personality type seem to be moderate risk factors for CAD in both women and men. Persons who can be described as aggressive, hostile, ambitious, competitive or driven by a sense of time urgency (Type A) have been found to experience twice as many CAD events when compared to so-called Type B (calm, less impulsive, and less emotional) personalities.[16] In contrast, employment or type of labor do not appear to be risk factors for CAD but have proven beneficial for general health.[17]

Cigarette smoking is also a risk factor for CAD, especially in young women, and the higher the number of cigarettes smoked, the greater the risk for disease. In a recent study[18], it has been observed that women who smoked even one to four cigarettes daily had a twofold to fourfold greater relative risk for CAD than nonsmokers. If they smoked 45 or more cigarettes per day, the risk was 10.8 compared with nonsmokers. In the United States, it has been estimated that 30% to 40% of deaths from CAD are attributable to smoking. The responsible mechanism is not clear, and its role in atherosclerosis has not been proved; however, both nicotine and carbon monoxide are known to affect cardiac contractility and irritability.[19,20]

The possibility that immunological mechanisms are involved in the pathogenesis of CAD has been investigated by Bjorkholm et al.[21] They found low IgG levels in patients with myocardial infarction, suggesting that immunological mechanisms may play a role in the pathogenesis of CAD.

Stone et al[22] attempted to define independent genetic risk factors for CAD and investigated whether isolated ge-

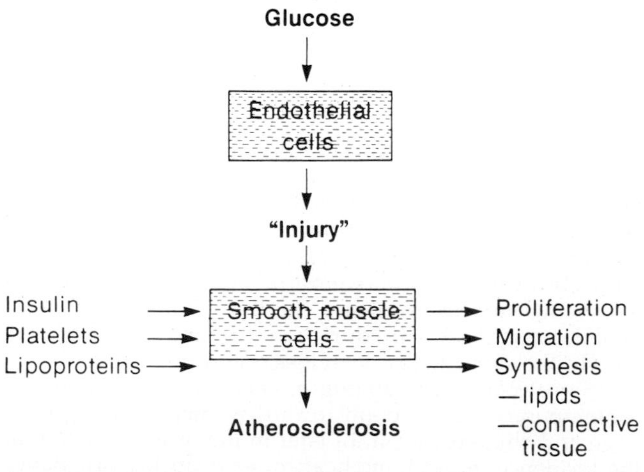

Figure 133–2. Proposed mechanism whereby glucose intolerance leads to an increased risk of cardiovascular disease. (*From Stout RW*[12] *with permission.*)

netic factors controlled by genes in the human leukocyte antigen (HLA) chromosomal region might have any role in the pathogenesis of "premature" CAD. They found a statistically significant association between the presence of HLA-BW38 and premature CAD, suggesting that HLA-tissue antigens are involved in the pathogenesis of the disease.

Another study[23] showed that eclampsia may play a role in CAD. In eclampsia, vascular spasm is an important component of the syndrome. Thus, in autopsies of women who died from eclampsia, the presence of myocardial necrosis in 35% of the cases suggested that arterial spasm may be a contributing factor for myocardial infarction. Coronary artery spasm is believed to play an important role in angina and myocardial infarction, which occur during pregnancy or puerperium, in women who have had normal coronary arteries on a prior angiogram.

Factors implicated in causing arterial spasm include drugs such as ritodrine, ergonovine maleate, and even bromocriptine.[24] Ergonovine, as intravenous infusion, is the standard provocative test for coronary vasospasm. Myocardial infarction has been reported after ergonovine stress testing. Tocolytic agents such as ritodrine are potent sympathomimetic drugs capable of increasing myocardial work. Some investigators have recommended electrocardiographic monitoring of patients receiving these agents.

Coronary emboli may cause myocardial infarction in a background of mitral stenosis, atrial fibrillation, prosthetic valves, bacterial endocarditis, mural thrombi, and paradoxical emboli. The term *paradoxical embolism* is used to describe the condition in which emboli derived from the systemic venous system pass to the arterial circulation by way of an intracardiac shunt. Coronary emboli during pregnancy is a rare diagnosis, with only 27 cases reported in the literature including a recent case diagnosed in a 24-year-old primigravid woman four days postpartum.[25]

THE EFFECT OF CAD ON PREGNANCY

Acute myocardial infarction has been reported to carry a high incidence of maternal mortality. In cases where myocardial infarctions occurred during the third trimester, approximately two thirds of the patients died. Premature delivery is also increased among these patients.

In pregnancy, the total plasma triglyceride concentration increases 2.5-fold over the nonpregnant level. LDL cholesterol increases linearly to a maximum of 1.6-fold over nonpregnant values at term. HDL cholesterol also increases to a maximum value about 1.45 times the nonpregnant level in midgestation and then declines but remains 1.15-fold above baseline at term.[26] The pregnant woman experiences significant hemodynamic alterations during the antepartum, intrapartum, and postpartum periods. It is well known that during normal pregnancy, blood volume and cardiac output increase up to 50%. Labor and delivery pose an additional load on the maternal cardiovascular system.[27] Multifetal gestations increase blood volume up to 60–70%. These changes may relate directly to the risk of a myocardial infarction in pregnancy since the majority of ischemic episodes occur in the third trimester or during the peripartum period.[6]

Salem et al[28] noted that there is a relationship between gravidity and the time of infarction. Primigravid women tend to develop infarctions postpartum, whereas multiparous women experience infarctions antepartum. Maternal age does not seem to have any positive influence on survival since the mortality rate observed was higher for women 36 years or younger.

Another report reviewed 54 well documented cases of myocardial infarctions in pregnancy. Of these, it was revealed that the majority of patients experienced transmural and anterior wall infarctions, while the remainder had primarily subendocardial and inferior wall lesions.

Pregnancy seems to pose an increased risk of infarction in patients who have underlying disease, and obstetric factors may influence the timing or site of infarction.

Women with diabetes and CAD carry a poor prognosis for both mother and fetus.[29] However, there are some reports of patients with class H diabetes having successful pregnancies. The factors associated with poor or satisfactory outcome are unclear. It appears that meticulous attention to the cardiac status, glycemic control and, in a few cases, coronary artery bypass graft prior to pregnancy resulted in improved pregnancy outcome.[14] Table 135–1 outlines all reported cases and outcomes of pregnancies complicated by diabetes-associated CAD.[29] Fetal mortality is also high and is due to maternal death. If the mother survives, then the pregnancy is usually associated with normal fetal outcome.[6]

Concern should be raised also for fetal effects due to cardiovascular drugs administered during pregnancy. A number of antiischemic drugs are categorized as category C (little or no information available regarding safety during pregnancy) or as category D (drugs that may have some adverse effects on the fetus, but the benefits may outweigh their risks). An attempt should be made to use drugs with established safety during pregnancy.[31] (see Chapter 125)

DIAGNOSIS

The major problem in diagnosing angina or myocardial infarction during pregnancy is the lack of a clinical suspicion that the disease may, in fact, occur.[2] Obstetricians do not face this disease frequently; hence, dysrhythmia or subtle electrocardiographic changes may go unnoticed. Classic symptoms for CAD in the presence of myocardial infarction or ischemia include the experiencing of precordial chest pain with radiation of pain to the left arm, neck or jaw. It is noteworthy that nausea, vomiting, dyspnea, or syncope may also accompany chest pain. Factors that trigger pain, ischemia, or both, include exposure to cold weather or cold water; emotional stress; large meals; hyperactivity; and in pregnancy, the induction of labor or the administration of anesthetic agents to achieve general anesthesia.

Chest pain in a pregnant woman may result from noncardiac causes such as esophageal reflux, gastritis, hiatal hernia, or psychosomatic disorders. Many other physiologic changes in pregnancy mimic signs and symptoms of cardiac disease.[2] Since the prognosis of the disease and the pregnancy outcome are dependent on early diagnosis, the aforementioned symptoms in diabetic patients with other risk factors for CAD (heavy smokers, over 40 years old, and high blood pressure) should raise the suspicion of heart disease. A low threshold should exist for performing electrocardiographic evaluation and serial cardiac enzyme studies to rule out myocardial infarction. An initial ECG may or may not suggest myocardial infarction or ischemia; however, follow-up ECGs will be necessary to fully exclude that possibility.[31]

It should be noted that a number of factors other than coronary artery spasm, myocardial infarction, or ischemia can cause ECG changes—for example, drugs or electrolyte

TABLE 133–1. REPORTED CASES OF DIABETES-ASSOCIATED CORONARY ARTERY DISEASE

Case No.	Author	Gravidity/ Parity	Age (yr)	White's classification	Type of coronary disease	Time of Occurrence	Outcome	
							Maternal	Fetal
1	Brock et al (*JAMA.* 1953;152:1030)	4/4	34	B	MI[c]	1st Trimester	Survived	Survived
2	Siegler et al (Obstet Gynecol. 1956;7:306)	1/1	38	B	MI	1st Trimester	Survived	Survived
3	Delaney & Ptacek (*Am J Obstet Gynecol.* 1970;160:550)	–	32	B	MI	3rd Trimester	Died	–
4	White (*J Am Med Women's Assoc.* 1972;27:293)	–	35+	B	MI	1st Trimester	Died	Aborted
5		–	35+	B	MI	1st Trimester	Died	Aborted
6		–	35+	B	MI	1st Trimester	Died	Aborted
7	Hubbard (*Clin Obstet Gynecol.* 1975;18:27)	1/1	36	R	MI	1st Trimester	Died	Aborted
8	Hare and White (*Diabetes.* 1977;26:953)	–[a]	–	–	MI	Prior to Pregnancy	Survived[d]	Survived
9		–	–	–	MI	3rd Trimester	Died	Survived
10		–	–	–	MI	4 week post-partum	Died	Survived
11		–	–	–	MI	4 week post-partum	Died	Died
12	Silfen (*Obstet Gynecol.* 1980;55:749)	1/1	23	D	MI	Prior to Pregnancy	Survived	Survived
13	Reece et al[30]	1/1	32	HFR	Severe Angina; occlusion of LAD[b] artery	Prior to Pregnancy	Survived[b]	Survived

[a] – = Information not reported. [b] LAD = Left anterior descending. [c] MI = Myocardial infarction. [d] Coronary artery bypass procedure prior to pregnancy. *From Reece et al[29] with permission.*

imbalance. It should be emphasized that minor ST-segment depression and T-wave inversion occur commonly in pregnancy in patients without heart disease.

Determination of abnormal cardiac enzymes helps in the diagnosis of acute myocardial infarction. Serum creatine kinase (CK) exceeds normal within six to eight hours, peaks at 24 hours, and returns to baseline in three to four days. The CPK MB isoenzyme is the most sensitive and specific enzyme for detecting myocardial infarction. Serum glutamic oxaloacetic (SGOT) levels may also be elevated within 8–12 hours following an episode of chest pain, peaking after 18–36 hours, and returning to normal after three to four days. Serum lactic dehydrogenase (LDH) is elevated within 24–48 hours, peaks in three to six days, and returns to normal levels after 8–14 days following the infarction. The heart contains mainly LDH I, an isoenzyme of LDH, which is a useful parameter in the detection of myocardial infarction since it is elevated in 95% of patients when myocardial damage occurs, and remains elevated after CPK and SGOT enzyme levels have normalized.

Echocardiography with Doppler is a noninvasive method and is not contraindicated in pregnancy. This technique permits the assessment of cardiac wall motion, thickness, and valvular competency.[32] The submaximal exercise tolerance test is recommended and can be performed in the select group of at-risk patients for diagnostic and prognostic reasons.

Radionuclide or radiographic studies may be helpful in the diagnosis of ischemic heart disease and the assessment of cardiac function but are associated with radiation exposure to the fetus. It has been estimated that for each 200 mrad of dosage to the fetus, the risk of cancer increases by 10%.[33] Thus, these methods are reserved, if possible, for the nonpregnant state. CINF angiography is the best method to reveal arterial stenosis but is associated with a large dose of radiation and should be delayed until after pregnancy, if possible.[34]

MANAGEMENT

Acute Myocardial Infarction

If myocardial infarction occurs during pregnancy, patient care should be done in collaboration with a perinatologist and cardiologist. There is general agreement that once an infarction has occurred, either in early pregnancy in which therapeutic abortion is often elected or in advanced pregnancy in which delivery is affected, surgical procedures are contraindicated for the next three to six months. Anesthesia and surgery carry an increased mortality risk in such patients. As current knowledge is limited, decisions in cases of acute myocardial infarction should be made based on the clinical judgment of the physicians (cardiologist, anesthesiologist, and perinatologist) and the medical status of the patient.

When patients experience persistent or recurrent chest pain, a diagnosis of heart disease should be excluded. An electrocardiogram, preferably a 12-lead, may show evidence of an acute myocardial infarction. The possibility of sudden ventricular fibrillation has to be kept in mind; and for this reason, continuous EKG monitoring may be necessary. After the diagnosis is made, the patient should be transferred to the hospital's intensive care unit where acute management care can be effected. In the case of cardiac arrest, external cardiac massage should be started immediately and then direct electrical shock therapy initiated if necessary. Ventricular fibrillation is the most common cause of early death associated with myocardial infarction in the unmonitored outpatient. The treatment of choice is unsynchronized defibrillation, starting with an energy level of 200 joules. If the first attempt fails, a second and third shock should be given to a maximum of 320 to 400 joules. If electric shock is not successful, then intravenous lidocaine should be administered and the defibrillation process repeated.[35]

Fetal surveillance with continuous electronic fetal monitoring is recommended. Drugs like atropine may be required to manage bradycardia and lidocaine to control ventricular extrasystoles. In addition, monitoring of central pressures, direct intra-arterial pressure, and hourly urine output are also recommended. If the clinical situation is less dramatic than described above but the diagnosis of myocardial infarction is certain, the following should be addressed: an intravenous line should be inserted immediately and 5% dextrose solution at low infusions should be started. Intramuscular injection should be avoided in order to prevent false elevation of muscle enzymes. Blood should be drawn for laboratory examinations including cardiac enzymes. Initial values will be compared with subsequent levels. Oxygen administration, two liters/minute via nasal prongs, is particularly useful. Subsequently, patient anxiety should be eliminated in an attempt to control the release of catecholamines. Morphine sulfate, up to 10 mg, can be administered over a 30-minute period, in two to four mg increments every five minutes.[2] For angina, nitroglycerin in sublingual tablets may be given during the first 30 minutes of chest pain. Drugs such as morphine and nitroglycerin induce hypotension as a side effect; therefore, increased saline infusion may be necessary. The Swan–Ganz catheters have been used successfully in both pregnant and puerperal women after myocardial infarction, and such monitoring is believed to be associated with a decrease in maternal mortality.

The most frequently used parameters are central venous pressure and pulmonary capillary wedge pressure, which reflect the filling pressure of the right and left ventricles.[2] Preload can be reduced by agents such as furosemide and nitroglycerin or increased by the use of fluids. The pulmonary capillary wedge pressure can be regulated at a level of about 18–24 mm Hg in cases of myocardial infarction and mild cardiac failure.[36] The management goal is to maximize myocardial oxygen delivery and minimize the oxygen requirements; avoidance of aggravating factors, such as smoking and excessive physical activity, and regulation of hypertension or anemia, if present.

Refractory Angina

Therapy for angina includes sublingual nitroglycerin for the phase of the acute attack of angina followed by transdermal, oral, or intravenous nitroglycerin preparations. Side effects of nitrates such as headaches, flushing, and hypertension are expected due to the vasodilatory effect of the drug. β-adrenergic blocking agents are used to reduce oxygen consumption by decreasing heart rate, blood pressure, and myocardial contractility. Hypoglycemia and bronchospasm are known side effects from these agents. Propranolol reduces the frequency of anginal episodes by reducing myocardial oxygen demands and has been found to be a safe drug for the fetus; hence, it can be used during pregnancy. However, side effects such as hypoglycemia, bradycardia, and fetal depression have been reported with propranolol therapy.

Finally, calcium-entry blocking agents are relatively new drugs which influence favorably the myocardial oxygen supply–demand ratio.[30] More data, however, are needed regarding safety of these drugs before in chronic therapy during pregnancy. Postpartum heart examination to estimate the status of myocardial injury and cardiac functions is recommended.[29,37]

Obstetric Management

For a woman with angina during the first trimester of pregnancy, management is dependent on the status of the disease. If angina is not well controlled despite maximum medical therapy, termination of pregnancy should be advised. With well controlled disease, pregnancy can continue to fetal maturity.

The second trimester does not present any major problems, and management of the pregnant woman with myocardial infarction does not differ from nonpregnant patients.

Problems begin to arise when the pregnancy enters the third trimester, during labor, delivery, and particularly the postpartum period where major redistribution of body fluids occurs. In the case of spontaneous induction of labor, which is not unusual in these patients, tocolytic agents must not be used.[14] It has to be emphasized that the later in pregnancy an episode of myocardial infarction occurs, the worse the prognosis for both mother and fetus.[6]

The optimum delivery route is controversial. Proponents argue as forcefully as opponents. Cesarean section has been considered by some to be advantageous because patients can avoid labor and its stress. In 1966, Listo and Bjorkenheim[39] reported a rapid improvement in pulmonary edema after cesarean section in a woman who experienced acute anterior wall myocardial infarction and cardiogenic shock during labor. Ostheimer and Alper[40] suggest that all these patients should have elective cesarean sections because there is less hemodynamic disturbance than with vaginal delivery and the patient is exposed to a shorter duration of stress on the myocardium.[41] These authors also thought that cesarean section had the added advantage of providing an immediate opportunity for tubal sterilization. Recently, Mabie et al[42] found cesarean section beneficial in managing a 42-year-old woman with acute transmural infarction and multiple associated applications such as ventricular fibrillation, congestive heart failure, left ventricular thrombosis, and pulmonary edema. According to the authors, cesarean section ten hours after induction dramatically improved the patient's congestive heart failure. In a review by Hawkins et al[6], the maternal mortality rate was 14% when women delivered vaginally, 23% when delivered by cesarean section. Acute hemodynamic stress with severe blood loss, increased metabolic demands, and increased postpartum morbidity were associated with cesarean section. Risks from general anesthesia such as the cardiac stress from tracheal intubation are also additional factors associated with cesarean section.

Short-term vaginal delivery with proper epidural anesthesia is advocated by many authors[4,37], citing the reduced risk of hemodynamic changes and the potential for fewer postoperative morbidities. Furthermore, good analgesia may minimize endogenous catecholamine release and decrease cardiac work.[43]

It also has been recommended that oxytocin should not be used in women with ischemic heart disease. This natural hormone is known to have antidiuretic activity which may reduce coronary artery flow; however, synthetic oxytocin does not cause such effects.[6] Diluted oxytocin solutions have been used without adverse hemodynamic effects or coronary vasoconstriction. Judicious use of diluted oxytocin under continuous ECG, pulmonary artery monitoring, and cardiotocographic surveillance of the fetus may lead to a successful outcome.[2,4,6,34]

In case of maternal death during labor or delivery, an emergency postmortem cesarean section should be performed. Weber[45] reported on 153 cases of successful infant survival after postmortem cesarean sections.

REFERENCES

1. Hare NJ. Diabetic neuropathy and coronary heart disease. In: Reece EA, Coustan DR, eds, *Diabetes Mellitus in Pregnancy: Principles and Practice*. New York: Churchill Livingstone; 1988:515.
2. Nolan ET, Hankins DVG. Myocardial infarction in pregnancy. *Clin Obstet Gynecol*. 1989;32:68.
3. Katz H. Ueber den plotzlichen naturlichen Tod in Schwangerschast, Geburt und Wochenbett. *Archiv fur Gynakolgie*. 1921;115:2.
4. Dawson PJ, Ross AW. Pre-eclampsia in a parturient with a history of myocardial infarction. A case report and literature review. *Anesthesia*. 1988;43:659.
5. Castelli PW. Cardiovascular disease in women. *Am J Obstet Gynecol*. 1988;158:1553.
6. Hankins DVG, Vendel DG, Leveno KJ, et al. Myocardial infarction during pregnancy: a review. *Obstet Gynecol*. 1985;65:139.
7. Lobo AR. Lipids, clotting factors and diabetes: endogenous risk factors for cardiovascular disease. *Am J Obstet Gynecol*. 1988;158:1584.
8. Lipid Research Clinics Program. The Lipid Research Clinics Coronary Primary Prevention Trial Results: II. The relationship of reduction in incidence of coronary heart disease to cholesterol lowering. *JAMA*. 1984;251:365.
9. Castelli WP, Garrison RJ, Wilson PWF, et al. Incidence of coronary heart disease and lipoprotein cholesterol levels: the Framingham Study. *JAMA*. 1986;256:2835.
10. Castelli WP. The triglyceride issue: a view from Framingham. *Am Heart J*. 1986;112:432.
11. National Cholesterol Education Program. Report of the National Education Program Expert Panel on Detection, Evaluation, and Treatment of High Blood Cholesterol in Adults. *Arch Intern Med*. 1988;148:36.
12. Stout RW. Insulin and atheroma—An update. *Lancet*. 1987;1:1077.
13. Zavaroni I, Dall'aglio E, Bonora E, et al. Evidence that multiple risk factors for coronary artery disease exist in pregnancy with abnormal glucose tolerance. *Am J Med*. 1987;83:609.
14. Gast JM, Rigg AL. Class H diabetes and pregnancy. *Obstet Gynecol*. 1985;66:5S.
15. Rowe JW, Young JB, Minaker KL, et al. Effect of insulin and glucose infusions on sympathetic nervous system activity in normal man. *Diabetes*. 1981;30:219.
16. Burkman TR. Obesity, stress and smoking: their role as cardiovascular risk factors in women. *Am J Obstet Gynecol*. 1988;158:1592.
17. La Rosa HJ. Women, work and health: Employment as a risk factor for coronary heart disease. *Am J Obstet Gynecol*. 1988;158:1597.
18. Willett WC, Green A, Stampfer MJ, et al. Relative and absolute excess risks of coronary heart disease among women who smoke cigarettes. *N Engl J Med*. 1987;317:1303.
19. Fuchs R, Scheidt SS. Prevention of coronary atherosclerosis. I. *Cardiovasc Rev Rep*. 1983;4:671.
20. Krauss RM, Perlman AJ, Ray R, et al. Effects of estrogen dose and smoking on lipid and lipoprotein levels in postmenopausal women. *Am J Obstet Gynecol*. 1988;158:1606.
21. Bjorkholm M, De Faire V, Golin G. Immunologic evaluation of patients with ischemic heart disease. Genetic determination and relation to disease. *Atherosclerosis*. 1980;36:195.
22. Stone PH, Cherrid MV, Cohn KE. Correlation of HLA types in premature coronary artery disease: our attempt to define independent genetic risk factors. *Chest*. 1981;79:381.
23. Bower TW, Moore GW, Hutchins GM. Morphologic evidence for coronary artery spasm in eclampsia. *Circulation*. 1982;65:255.
24. Taylor GJ, Cohey B. Ergomorine-induced coronary artery spasm and myocardial infarction alter normal delivery. *Obstet Gynecol*. 1985;66:821.
25. Jungbluth A, Erbel R, Darius H, et al. Paradoxical coronary embolism: case report and review of the literature. *Am Heart J*. 1988;116:879.
26. Knopp HR. Cardiovascular effects of endogenous and exogenous sex hormones over a woman's lifetime. *Am J Obstet Gynecol*. 1988;158:1630.
27. Clark LS. Labor and delivery in the patient with structural cardiac disease. *Clin Perinatal*. 1986;13:695.
28. Salem DN, Isner JM, Hopkins P, et al. Ergonovine provactation in postpartum myocardial infarction. *Angiology*. 1984;35:110.
29. Reece EA, Egan JFX, Coustan DR, et al. Coronary artery disease in diabetic pregnancies. *Am J Obstet Gynecol*. 1986;154:150.
30. Little BB, Gilstrap CL III. Cardiovascular drugs during pregnancy. *Clin Obstet Gynecol*. 1989;32:13.
31. Fenstermacher K. *Dysrhythmia Recognition and Management*. Philadelphia: W.B. Saunders Company; 1989:106.
32. Easton LW, Weiss JL, Bulkley BH, et al. Regional cardiac dilatation after acute myocardial infarction. Recognition by 2-D echocardiography. *N Engl J Med*. 1979;300:57.
33. Campbell JA. Antenatal radiation hazards in obstetric diagnosis by radiographic, ultrasonic and nuclear methods. Baltimore: Williams & Wilkins, 1977;10:1.
34. Bembridge M, Lyons G. Myocardial infarction in the third trimester of pregnancy. *Anesthesia*. 1988;43:202.
35. Brown ELC, Wendel GD. Cardiac arrhythmias during pregnancy. *Clin Obstet Gynecol*. 1989;32:89.
36. Yeomans RE, Hankins DVG. Cardiovascular physiology and invasive cardiac monitoring. *Clin Obstet Gynecol*. 1989;32:2.
37. Chestnut DH, Zlatnik FJ, Pittun RM, et al. Pregnancy in a patient with a history of myocardial infarction and coronary artery bypass grafting. *Am J Obstet Gynecol*. 1986;155:372.
38. Gordon S. Pregnancy following percutaneous transluminal angioplasty. *Am J Cardiol*. 1988;62:1152.
39. Listo M, Bjorkenheim G. Myocardial infarction during delivery. *Acta Obstet Gynecol Scand*. 1966;45:268.
40. Ostheimer GW, Alper MH. Intrapartum anesthetic management of the pregnant patient with heart disease. *Clin Obstet Gynecol*. 1975;18:81.
41. Metcalfe J, McAnulty JH, Ueland K. *Heart Disease and Pregnancy: Physiology and Management*. Boston: Little, Brown, and Co; 1986:119.
42. Mabie CW, Anderson DG, Addington MB, et al. The benefit of cesarean section in acute myocardial infarction complicated by premature labor. *Obstet Gynecol*. 1988;71:503.
43. Jouppila R, Jouppila P, Hollmen A, et al. Lumbar epidural analgesia to improve intervillous blood flow during labor in severe pre-eclampsia. *Obstet Gynecol*. 1982;59:158.
44. Weber CE. Postmortem cesarean section: a review of the literature and case reports. *Am J Obstet Gynecol*. 1971;110:158.

Chapter One Hundred and Thirty-Four

Aortic Dissection

Uri Elkayam and Avraham Shotan

134

In the usual case, a tear in the aortic intima marks the beginning of aortic dissection, which is followed by separation of the media in a course parallel to the flow of blood.[1,2] The dissecting channel is in the outer part of the aortic media, and its containment is nearly adventitial, explaining the high frequency of extravasation of blood outside the aorta, rather than rerupture into the true aortic lumen. Manifestations of the disease, therefore, relate to the specific anatomic structures involved.

ETIOLOGY

The etiology of the aortic intimal tear and propensity for medial dissection is unknown. Pregnancy is just one of several clinical settings that have been described in association with aortic dissection. If intimal disruption is not related to direct trauma, then it may represent an aberration of a more or less continuous process of vascular endothelial injury and repair. This process may be compromised by the pregnant state or by an associated condition not specifically related to pregnancy.[3] Conditions that are associated with aortic dissection include congenital abnormalities, either of collagen, such as Marfan's syndrome or Ehlers–Danlos syndrome, or of morphologic development, such as coarctation of the aorta or bicuspid aortic valve. Other conditions such as atherosclerosis, syphilis, inflammatory disease, and mycotic infection, although commonly associated with arterial aneurysm formation, probably play a small role in the syndrome of acute aortic dissection.

The exact cause of aortic dissection has remained elusive, but a common denominator noted in nearly three fourths of general adult patients has been hypertension.[4-6] In the reported cases occurring in coincidence with pregnancy[6-24], the level of systemic blood pressure has not always been recorded. There is no evidence to associate eclampsia and aortic dissection, although in the nonpregnant adult population, there is some reason to believe that the frequency of aortic dissection may be higher with the syndrome of malignant hypertension.

Dissection of the aorta is uncommon in young people, yet Hirst, Schnitker, and others[4,6] have found that up to 50% of dissections in women less than 40 years of age occurred during or shortly after pregnancy. Investigators have tried to link the physiological change of pregnancy as a causal factor in aortic dissection. The fact that dissection occurs infrequently during or after labor effectively dismisses the stress of labor as relevant.[7] Changes in blood volume and cardiac output similarly seem unimportant, as cirulatory overload is not unique to pregnancy.

Histopathologic studies have attempted to show a causal relationship between morphologic changes in the human aorta and the pregnant state. A natural conclusion to this type of investigation would be that these changes are in some way related to the development of aortic disease. Unfortunately, there is no consistency in these studies. For example, Manolo–Estrella and Barker[25] looked at the aortic histology of 15 pregnant women dying of nonvascular causes and found only various nonspecific findings. Cavanzo and Taylor[26] found normal aortas at necropsy in 43 pregnant women.

Histochemical work has been unable to present a unifying pathogenetic mechanism. In rats, the turnover of collagen has been shown to be increased during both pregnancy and renal hypertension, and further increased if both conditions exist concurrently.[27] Additional information comes from a rat model in which estrogens have been shown to inhibit collagen and elastin deposition in the aorta and progestogens to minimally accelerate the deposition of aortic noncollagenous proteins.[28] Hartman and Eptychiadis[29] recently suggested a genetic predisposition for dissection of the aorta and muscular arteries. They believe that smooth muscle proliferation with areas of vacuolar degeneration and coagulation necrosis, elastin fragmentation, fibrosis, and collagen degeneration are unrelated to pregnancy and, in fact, are qualitatively similar, but quantitatively greater in reported cases of dissection than in controls.

A study of hormonal influences on connective tissue provides a potential explanation for the development of arterial aneurysms; however, the exact role of these factors is still unclear.[28,30,31] It has been found that pregnancy-related change in the microscopic appearance of arteries in rabbits is also induced by the administration of norethynodrel and ethynyl estradiol. Intimal hyperplasia, which is seen in pregnant or hypertensive women, has also been found in women treated with oral contraceptives.

PATHOLOGY

In most cases, a continuous intimal tear is identified in addition to the disruption of the aortic media.[1,2] This tear, which marks the beginning of the dissection, occurs about 2 cm above the aortic valve cusps in 70% of patients and at the descending thoracic aorta just beyond the origin of the left subclavian artery in 20% of patients.[1] The entrance tear will sometimes be located in the aortic arch but this is uncommon. An entrance tear below the diaphragm is rarely seen in a pregnant women, as well as in the general population. The entrance tear involves about one half of the circumference of the aorta or much less. In contrast to the entrance tear, a reentry tear is found in about 10% of patients, producing the so-called "double-barrel" aorta. Although dissection is a longitudinal separation of the media, the percent of aortic circumference involved by the dissection at any particular level is variable. Usually half of the aortic circumference is dissected; the other half is left intact.[1] Dissections beginning in the ascending portion usually involve the right lateral aortic wall and course downstream along the greater curvature of the ascending, transverse, and descending thoracic aorta. Because of their location, involvement of the right coronary, innominate, left common carotid, and left subclavian arteries is common. The aortic dissection, once initiated, progresses unchecked unless limited by extensive atherosclerotic plaquing, aortic isthmus coarctation, or inflammatory fibrosis, all of which are uncommon in women of childbearing age.

EPIDEMIOLOGY

There are probably no more than 200 reported cases of pregnancy-related aortic dissections. In the nonpregnant population, increasing age, male sex, hypertension, aortic coarctation, bicuspid aortic valve, and Marfan's syndrome all seem to indicate an increased risk for aortic dissection.[1,4,32] In pregnancy, it is much more difficult to weigh risk factors by examining published clinical reports. Konishi et al[12] showed that 60% of their 52 cases were over age 30 and 77% occurred in multiparous women; 20% had coarctation of the aorta, and a few were marfanoid. Others had not demonstrated increasing maternal parity to be important.

The most frequent time of occurrence is the third trimester. Pedowitz and Perell[8] described 47 patients with dissection of the aorta or its major branches. Two percent of these patients dissected in the first trimester, 17% in the second, 49% in the third, 13% in labor or the first 24 postpartum hours, and 19% two days or more after delivery.

CLINICAL MANIFESTATIONS

Most dissections are associated with a sudden onset of severe pain, typically in the chest, which may radiate to the back, shoulders, and abdomen.[32] Other symptoms are related to complications of the dissection. The most catastrophic and immediate complication is through-and-through rupture of the aorta with extravasation of blood into the pericardial space, pleural space, mediastinum, retroperitoneum, wall of the pulmonary trunk, atrial or ventricular cardiac septum (involvement of the atrioventricular conduction system), lung, or esophagus.[1] In addition, the partial or complete obstruction by the medial hematoma of any artery arising from the aorta can occur, including the coronary (sudden death or myocardial infarction), innominate or common carotid (syncope, confusion, stroke, coma), innominate or subclavian (upper limb ischemia or paralysis), intercostal or lumbar (spinal cord ischemia), celiac, renal, mesenteric, or common iliac arteries. Acute and severe aortic regurgitation can result from dilatation of the aorta or extension of the dissection to the level of the valve and may produce pulmonary edema. Obstruction of the aorta or pulmonary artery may produce circulatory collapse.

DIAGNOSIS

Aortic dissection is a life-threatening condition to the mother as well as to the fetus. Proper treatment requires a prompt diagnosis and a precise identification of the location and extent of the dissection. Attention to the details of history and clinical examination is of first priority. Radiographs of the chest, particularly those showing widening of the mediastinum, are most helpful in diagnosing thoracic dissections.

Various diagnostic methods are currently at our disposal. Which procedure should a pregnant woman with suspected acute dissection have as a definite study? Aortography is still considered by many physicians and surgeons as the most reliable technique and may be done from the femoral, brachial, or axillary approach, depending on the condition of the patient and skill of the angiographer. However, there are a few limiting factors that include the invasive nature of the technique, the use of contrast injection, and the fetal exposure to irradiation. An attempt should, therefore, be made to limit radiation by providing an appropriate shield to the abdomen. Computed tomography (CT) scanning may be useful for diagnosis in stable cases[32-34]; however, it is also associated with irradiation to the fetus. Magnetic resonance imaging (MRI), including cine-MRI, is highly sensitive and specific in the diagnosis of aortic dissection (Figure 134–1). Its main disadvantages are the length of the study and the inability to use it with unstable cases or patients on a ventilator or on those who have a pacemaker.[32,34,35] Transthoracic Doppler–echocardiography has only a limited role in the diagnosis of aortic dissection[36], but is an excellent tool for diagnosing some of its complications, such as cardiac tamponade and aortic regurgitation. The recent introduction of transesophageal echo technique, when combined with transthoracic echocardiography, is becoming, in many centers, the procedure of choice in view of its safety, high sensitivity and specificity, and ease of attainment (Figure 134–2).[34,37,38] However, the diagnostic workup should be tailored in each center according to the prompt availability and the local expertise in each of the above-mentioned techniques. One has to realize that each of the available diagnostic techniques may infrequently yield a false negative result.[32,35,38] For this reason, if the diagnosis of dissection is still clinically suspected, another technique should be used.

Nonspecific laboratory findings that are seen in patients with aortic dissection include anemia and evidence of mild hemolysis. The electrocardiogram is of limited value in the diagnosis of aortic dissection; however, it may help to reveal an acute myocardial infarction, a possible complication of the disease.

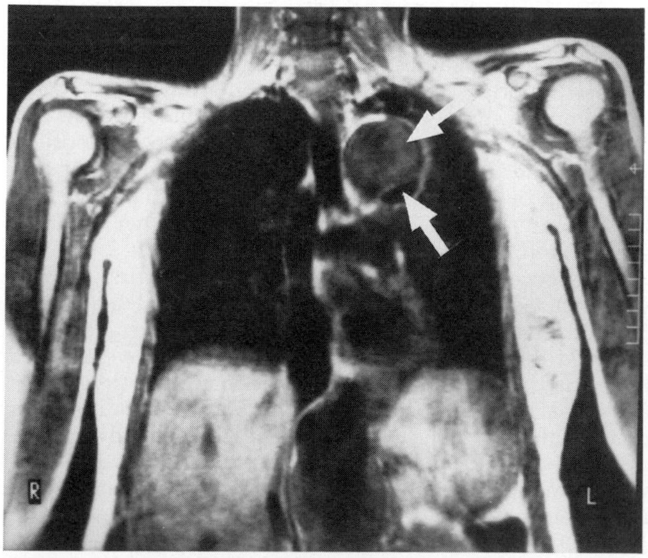

Figure 134–1: Coronal view spin echo MRI demonstrating aortic dissection. A flap is separating a thin lumen (lower arrow) from a false lumen (upper arrow). The patient is a woman with Marfan's syndrome in her 18th week gestation.

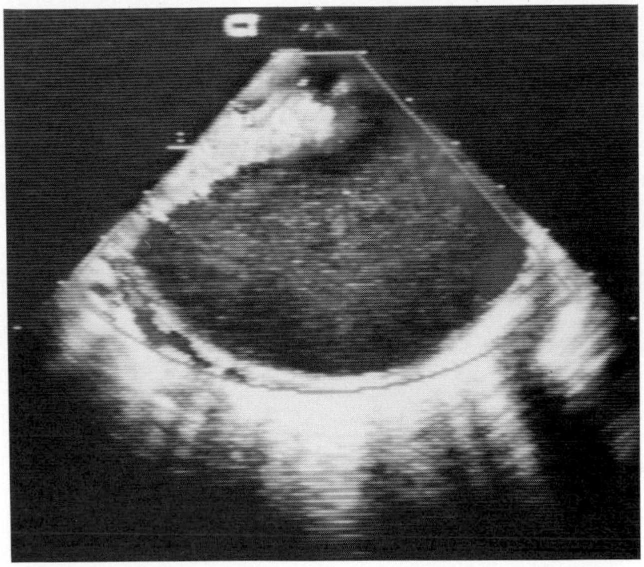

Figure 134–2: Transesophageal echo of the descending aorta demonstrating aortic dissection. Doppler signal indicating flow in the true lumen while mild echogenicity in the false lumen indicating a presence of blood clot. (Patient as in Figure 134–1.)

TREATMENT

Once the diagnosis is made, an aggressive approach to management is mandatory and may be lifesaving. The patient should be moved to an intensive care setting, preferably with the capability for hemodynamic monitoring. Invasive measurement of systemic arterial pressures will facilitate optimal care. Continuous clinical assessment is necessary to avoid misleading data brought about by changing anatomic involvement of the arterial system. Medical therapy involves controlling the blood pressure and decreasing the force and velocity of myocardial contraction, thus lowering the likelihood of progression of the dissection.[32] Current recommendations are the use of an intravenous beta-blocking drug at a dose required to lower heart rate 10–20 beats/minute, followed by a maintenance intravenous or oral dose. The blood pressure should be maintained by nitroprusside infusion at minimally acceptable levels of mean arterial pressure (controlled hypotension). Because of the potential fetal toxicity of nitroprusside (see chapter 125), hydralazine may be preferred antepartum. This drug can be given either orally (25–50 mg tid or qid) or intravenously (2.5–5.0 mg intravenous push over one minute followed by 2.5–5.0 mg q 10 minutes to achieve desired effect). Treatment of aortic regurgitation and cardiac tamponade are discussed elsewhere in this section.

Cardiac surgery with the use of extracorporeal circulation has been performed safely during pregnancy.[39] Surgical treatment, however, must be individualized to the patient and to the expertise of the available surgical team. This surgery might include excision of the intimal tear, oversewing the aortic layers, and reapproximation of the aorta, often with synthetic material. Replacement of the aortic valve is not necessary in every case with aortic regurgitation and should be avoided if possible.

The obstetric management of patients with aortic dissection occurring in the third trimester should include, whenever possible, cesarean section prior to repair of the aorta.[16] Although cardiopulmonary bypass for replacement of heart valves and correction of congenital cardiac malformations during the first and second trimesters has produced viable pregnancies[39], there have been only two reports of successful pregnancies following repair of an aortic dissection or disruption.[40]

REFERENCES

1. Roberts WC. Aortic dissection: anatomy, consequences, and causes. *Am Heart J*. 1981;101:195.
2. Wilson SK, Hutchins GM. Aortic dissection aneurysms: causative factors in 204 subjects. *Arch Pathol Lab Med*. 1982;106:175.
3. Schlatmann TJM, Becker AE. Pathogenesis of dissecting aneurysm of the aorta. Comparative histopathologic study of significance of medical changes. *Am J Cardiol*. 1977;39:21.
4. Hirst AE, Johns VJ, Kime SW. Dissecting aneurysms of the aorta: a review of 505 cases. *Medicine*. 1958;37:217.
5. Erb BD, Tullis F. Dissecting aneurysm of the aorta. The clinical features of thirty autopsied cases. *Circulation*. 1960;22:315.
6. Schnitker MA, Bayer CA. Dissecting aneurysm of the aorta in young individuals particularly in association with pregnancy with report of a case. *Ann Int Med*. 1944;20:486.
7. Mandel W, Evans EW, Walford RL. Dissecting aortic aneurysm during pregnancy. *N Engl J Med*. 1954;251:1059.
8. Pedowitz P, Perell A. Aneurysms complicated by pregnancy, Part I: Aneurysms of the aorta and its major branches. *Am J Obstet Gynecol*. 1957;73:720.
9. Hume M, Krosnick G. Dissecting aneurysm in pregnancy associated with aortic insufficiency. *N Engl J Med*. 1963;286:174.
10. Sutinen S, Piiroinen D. Marfan's syndrome, pregnancy and fetal dissection of the aorta. *Acta Obstet Gynecol Scand*. 1971;50:295.
11. Parkes JR, Hendry DT, Hellberg BW, Theron LL. Postpartum ruptured abdominal aortic aneurysm: a case report. *S Afr Med J*. 1977;51:926.
12. Konishi Y, Tatsuta N, Kumada K, et al. Dissecting aneurysms during pregnancy and the puerperium. *Jpn Circ J*. 1980;44:726.
13. Barrett JM, Van Hooydonk JE, Boehm FH. Pregnancy related rupture of arterial aneurysms. *Obstet Gynecol Surv*. 1982;37(9):557.
14. Ferguson JE, Ueland K, Stinson EB, Maly RP. Marfan's syndrome: acute aortic dissection during labor, resulting in fetal distress and cesarian section, followed by successful surgical repair. *Am J Obstet Gynecol*. 1983;147:759.
15. Rosenblum NG, Grossman AR, Gabbe SG, et al. Failure of serial echocardiographic studies to predict aortic dissection in a pregnant patient with Marfan's syndrome. *Am J Obstet Gynecol*. 1983;146:470.
16. Katz NM, Coles JV, Moront MG, et al. Aortic dissection during pregnancy: treatment by emergency cessarean section immediately followed by operative repair of the aortic dissection. *Am J Cardiol*. 1984;54:699.
17. Cola LM, Lavin JP Jr. Pregnancy complicated by Marfan's syndrome with aortic arch dissection, subsequent aortic arch replacement and triple coronary artery bypass grafts. *J Reprod Med*. 1985;30:685.
18. Pumphrey CW, Fay T, Weir I. Aortic dissection during pregnancy. *Br Heart J*. 1986;55:106.
19. Shemin RI, Phillippe M, Dzan V. Acute thrombosis of a composite ascending aortic conduit containing a Bjork-Shiley valve during pregnancy. Successful emergency cesarean section and operative repair. *Clin Cardiol*. 1986;9:299.
20. Diehl FT, Moon B, LeClerc V, et al. Acute type A dissection of the aorta: surgical management with the sutureless intraluminal prosthesis. *Ann Throac Surg*. 1987;43:502.
21. William GH, Bott VL, Brawley RK, et al. Aortic disease associated with pregnancy. *J Vasc Surg*. 1988;8:470.
22. Snir E, Levinsky L, Solomon J, et al. Dissecting aortic aneurysm in pregnant women without Marfan disease. *Surg Gynecol Obstet*. 1988;167:463.
23. Smith VC, Eckinbrecht PD. Marfan's syndrome, pregnancy and the cardiac surgeon. *Milit Med*. 1989;154:404.
24. Barker SC, Burnard KG. Retrograde illiac dissection in Marfan's syndrome. A case report. *J Cardiovasc Surg–Torino*. 1989;30:953.
25. Manalo-Estrella P, Barker A. Histopathologic findings in human aortic media associated with pregnancy. *Arch Pathol*. 1967;83:336.
26. Cavanzo FJ, Taylor HB. Effect of pregnancy on the human aorta and its relationship to dissecting aneurysms. *Am J Obstet Gynecol*. 1969;105(4):567.
27. Foidart JM, Rorive G, Nusgens B. Aortic collagen biosynthesis during renal hypertension, pregnancy and hypertension during pregnancy in the rat. *Biomedicine*. 1978;28(4):215.

28. Wolinsky H. Effects of estrogen and progestogen treatment on the response of the aorta of male rats to hypertension. *Circ Res*. 1972;30:341.
29. Hartman JD, Eptychiadis AS. Medial smooth muscle cell lesions and dissection of the aorta and muscular arteries. *Arch Pathol Lab Med*. 1990;114:50.
30. Danforth DN, Manolo-Estrella P, Buckingham JC. Effect of pregnancy and of enovid on the rabbit vasculature. *Am J Obstet Gynecol*. 1964;88:962.
31. Irey NS, Norri HJ. Intimal vascular lesions associated with female reproductive steroids. *Arch Pathol*. 1973;96:227.
32. Eagle KA, Desanctis RW. Aortic dissection. *Curr Probl Cardiol*. 1989;14:225.
33. Heibey E, Wolverson MK, Sundaram M, Shields JB. CT in aortic trauma. *Am J Radiol*. 1983;140:1119.
34. Laas J, Schlueter G, Daniel W, et al. Acute type-A dissection of the aorta: which diagnostic modes remain for surgical indication? *Eur J Cardiovasc Surg*. 1987;1:169.
35. Freuhwald FX, Neuhold A, Fezoulicks J, et al. Cine MR in dissection of the thoracic aorta. *Eur J Radiol*. 1989;9:37.
36. Khandheria BK, Tajik AJ, Taylor AJ, et al. Aortic dissection: review of value and limitations of two-dimensional echocardiography in a six year experience. *J Am Soc Echocardiogr*. 1989;2:17.
37. Hashimoto S, Kumada T, Osakada G, et al. Assessment of transesophageal Doppler echography in dissecting aortic aneurysm. *J Am Col Cardiol*. 1989;14:1253.
38. Kotler MN. Is transesophageal echocardiography the new standard for diagnosing dissecting aortic aneurysms? *J Am Coll Cardiol*. 1989;14:1263.
39. Becker RM. Intracardiac surgery in pregnant women. *Ann Thorac Surg*. 1983;36:453.
40. Merin G, Bitran D, Donchin V, et al. Traumatic rupture of the thoracic aorta during pregnancy. Surgical considerations. *Chest*. 1981;79:99.

Chapter One Hundred and Thirty-Five
Cardiac Rhythm Disorders

Josef Widerhorn, Shahbudin H. Rahimtoola, and Uri Elkayam

135

Most arrhythmias occurring during pregnancy are benign, and hemodynamically significant dysrhythmias are uncommon.[1] Some authors[2-4] have suggested that the frequency of tachyarrhythmias (mainly supraventricular) is increased during pregnancy. Several hypothetical mechanisms have been invoked to explain this increased propensity for arrhythmias in pregnancy. These include hormonal, autonomic, and hemodynamic changes.[2,5] Even though clinically overt underlying heart disease may not be readily evident in the obstetric population, cardiac arrhythmias are often a manifestation of congenital or acquired structural heart abnormalities, which provide the substrate for abnormal impulse generation, conduction, or both. In fact, the arrhythmia may be the initial manifestation of an underlying heart disease and its appearance may create an additional risk for the mother and the fetus.

The assessment of a pregnant patient presenting with cardiac arrhythmias is similar to that of the nonpregnant patient. An intense effort should be made to diagnose any possible underlying heart disease or any other organ system dysfunction which may cause or precipitate the arrhythmias. A detailed history and careful physical examination are very important. Noninvasive evaluation should include 12-lead electrocardiography, 24-hour Holter monitoring, and assessment of cardiac anatomy and function with two-dimensional echocardiography–Doppler. Signal-averaged electrocardiography may also be helpful in an occasional pregnant patient, presenting with wide-QRS complex tachycardia or with syncope of unknown origin. In these patients, the presence of late potentials, documented with signal average techniques, is very suggestive of ventricular tachycardia as a cause for wide-QRS complex tachycardia or syncope. Even more important, the absence of late potentials has a high negative predictive accuracy and, therefore, usually rules out ventricular tachycardia as a cause of the patient's symptoms.[6] The clinician should be aware of certain electrocardiographic changes that occur during normal pregnancy. The QRS axis may shift in any direction, and a small Q wave and inverted T wave may be seen in lead III.[7] Transient ST-T wave changes are common. Among the noninvasive tests, 24-hour Holter monitoring is the most useful method to document and quantitate the frequency and complexity of arrhythmia, correlate the arrhythmia with the patient's symptoms, and evaluate the efficacy of antiarrhythmic therapy.

Most arrhythmias occurring during pregnancy are benign and do not require pharmacologic treatment. Often, patient reassurance, removal of stimulants such as caffeine, alcohol, tobacco, stimulant drugs, and anxiety controls is all that is required. Antiarrhythmic drugs should be used mostly for the hemodynamically significant arrhythmias, where the risk–benefit ratio is evident. Almost all antiarrhythmic drugs cross the placenta and the effects of these agents on the fetus should be carefully assessed. In choosing a drug, toxicity, metabolism, and gestational age are of crucial importance in order to avoid serious adverse effects. The pharmacokinetics of drugs may be modified during pregnancy; because of a multitude of factors, these changes cannot always be predicted and close monitoring of therapy is of utmost importance.

SINUS NODE ARRHYTHMIAS

Normal Sinus Rhythm

Normal sinus rate at rest ranges between 60 to 100 beats per minute. The sinus impulse originates in the highly specialized group of cells located at the junction between the superior vena cava and right atrium. The sinus node rate is the result of the two opposing autonomic influences—sympathetic and parasympathetic—on the intrinsic discharge rate of the pacemaker cells. Sinus node rate may vary significantly depending on many factors such as age, sex, activity, and endocrine status.

Sinus Arrhythmia

Sinus arrhythmia is characterized by a phasic variation in sinus cycle length of more than 10% of baseline cycle length and is commonly related to the respiratory cycle. The nonrespiratory type of sinus arrhythmia may be the result of digitalis excess. The respiratory type of sinus arrhythmia is a normal phenomenon and does not require treatment.

Sinus Tachycardia

Sinus tachycardia is diagnosed when the rate exceeds 100 beats per minute. With extreme exertion, sinus node rate may reach rates of 180–200 beats per minute. Sinus tachycardia is due to an acceleration of phase 4 diastolic depolarization of pacemaker cells and has a gradual onset and termination. During pregnancy, the heart rate increases steadily and reaches a peak of 10–20 beats above baseline during the third trimester and at term.[8] Sinus tachycardia may be seen in normal pregnant women mainly during the third trimester (or even earlier in twin pregnancy) and at delivery and has no pathologic significance. However, persistent sinus tachycardia may be associated with various pathologic states such as fever, congestive heart failure, myocardial disease, and endocrine and metabolic abnormalities. Often sinus tachycardia may be related to intake of stimulants such as caffeine, nicotine, antiasthmatic drugs, or rithodrine therapy. Treatment should focus on removal of stimulants and correction of any underlying pathologic state responsible for sinus tachycardia.

Sinus Bradycardia

Sinus bradycardia is diagnosed when sinus node rate is below 60 beats per minute. Sinus bradycardia may occur normally in healthy young adults, in athletes, and during sleep when rates of 35–40 beats per minute and pauses of two seconds or longer have been observed.[9] Transient sinus bradycardia may occur after delivery and during the postpartum period.[8] Commonly, sinus bradycardia is asymptomatic and treatment is rarely required. If symptoms due to hemodynamic impairment are present, atropine (0.5–2 mg intravenous) or isoproterenol (1–2 μg/min intravenous) may be effective. Permanent pacing may on rare occasions be necessary for long-term management of severe symptomatic sinus bradycardia when the underlying cause of the sinus bradycardia cannot be corrected.

Wandering Pacemaker

Wandering pacemaker is the result of passive shifting of the dominant pacemaker from the sinus node to latent pacemakers located in the atria or atrioventricular (AV) junction. Wandering pacemaker, similar to the respiratory variant of sinus arrhythmia, is a normal phenomenon occurring in young adults and rarely requires treatment. Therapy is similar to that of sinus bradycardia.

Sinus Node Dysfunction

Sinus node dysfunction or sick sinus syndrome (SSS) is manifested by a wide range of abnormalities of sinus node impulse formation and conduction and includes persistent spontaneous sinus bradycardia, inappropriate for the physiological circumstances; sinus arrest; sinus exit block; sinoatrial and atrioventricular conduction disorders; and alternation of paroxysm of rapid regular or irregular atrial tachyarrhythmias with bradyarrhythmias.[10,11] Although the vast majority of patients afflicted by this syndrome are above 50 years of age, a substantial number of patients are below the age of 30 with an equal distribution between males and females.[12] The exact incidence of SSS during pregnancy is not known, but due to the biomodal distribution of the syndrome, it may occur in women of childbearing age. Schatz et al[13] have described a 21-year-old primigravida with severe bradycardia–junctional tachycardia syndrome associated with Ebstein's anomaly, requiring multiple drug treatments and temporary transvenous pacing during delivery. Mendelson[2] described a 32-year-old pregnant woman with sinus exit block that caused occasional fainting. She had three pregnancies with normal term deliveries without receiving any therapy. The frequency of syncopal episodes was not affected by pregnancy.

The treatment depends upon the type of rhythm disturbance; permanent pacing may be necessary for bradyarrhythmia and drug therapy may be required for the tachyarrhythmias.

SUPRAVENTRICULAR ARRHYTHMIAS

Atrial Premature Complexes

Atrial premature complexes (APCs) are frequently found in the young population. Twenty-four hour Holter monitor recordings performed in 50 young women with no evidence of heart disease revealed APCs in 64% of the study population.[14] APCs may occur in normal hearts but are more frequent in patients with underlying heart disease. Their frequency may be increased by infection, myocardial diseases, anxiety, stimulants, and labor. In general, pharmacologic treatment of APCs should be avoided. Removal of stimulants, reassurance, and correction of precipitating factors may be sufficient to decrease or abolish symptoms. In severely symptomatic patients and in patients in whom APCs may trigger sustained supraventricular or ventricular tachyarrhythmias, treatment with beta-adrenergic blocking drugs, verapamil, or Class IA antiarrhythmic drugs may be indicated.

Supraventricular Tachycardias

Supraventricular tachycardias (SVTs) are characterized by a narrow QRS complex (except for cases of preexisting bundle branch block or aberrant conduction), regular R-R interval and rates ranging from 150 beats/minute to 250 beats/minute. Supraventricular tachycardias encompass a variety of tachycardias originating in the sinus node, atria, and AV junction. Included in this group are also the reciprocating tachycardias using anomalous (*accessory*) AV or nodoventricular pathways even though these arrhythmias require the participation of both atria and ventricle in the reentrant circuit, and the premature beat starting the tachycardia may originate in the ventricle and not necessarily above the ventricles.

A variety of electophysiologic mechanisms are involved in the genesis of SVT. Abnormal automaticity and triggered activity are responsible for a minority of SVT cases. More than 90% of SVTs are produced as a result of reentry which may occur at the level of the sinus node, atria, or AV junction.[15] Approximately 60% of paroxysmal SVTs are due to reentry in the AV node. This requires dual AV nodal pathways.[16] In the majority of patients, during AV nodal reentrant tachycardia, the antegrade conduction occurs over a slow (*alpha*) pathway and retrograde conduction over a fast (*beta*) pathway. The reentrant mechanism is set when a premature impulse blocks the fast pathway, which is still refractory and conducts with delay over the slow pathway. In five to ten percent of the patients with AV nodal reentry, the antegrade conduction occurs over the fast pathway and retrograde conduction over the slow pathway. This type of SVT is called the atypical form of AV nodal reentrant tachycardia. On surface electrocardiogram (ECG), the P wave appears long after QRS (RP greater than PR interval). In contrast, during the typical AV nodal reentrant tachycardia, the P wave is mostly buried within the QRS complex. Fifteen to 20% of reentrant SVTs occur over a "*concealed*" bypass tract. These tachycardias use a macroreentrant circuit which includes both atria and ventricles. In the orthodromic-AV reciprocating tachycardia, the antegrade conduction occurs over the AV node and His-Purkinje system and the retrograde conduction over the accessory pathway. On surface ECG, the P waves may be buried within the QRS or closely follow it. In the remaining paroxysmal SVTs, the reentrant circuit may occur in the atria or sinus node. Automatic tachycardias are responsible for four to eight percent of SVTs and may arise in the atria or AV junction. Automatic atrial tachycardia has rates below 200 beats/minute and commonly cannot be initiated by premature atrial stimulation. The rate may accelerate after initiation (*warm up* phenomenon) and cannot be terminated by pacing. If the automatic focus arises from the AV junction, the rate is much slower (70–130 beats/minute) and the SVT is named nonparoxysmal AV junctional tachycardia. This tachycardia occurs in patients with underlying heart disease or digitalis intoxication.

The incidence of paroxysmal SVTs during pregnancy has been estimated to be as high as 2.6%.[17] In the obstetric literature, SVTs are often called paroxysmal auricular, atrial, or supraventricular tachycardia. However, the underlying electrophysiologic mechanism has rarely been defined. Therefore, the nomenclature refers to the supraventricular origin of tachycardia and has no electrophysiologic implications. Mendelson[2] summarized 82 cases of SVT published in 12 articles before 1956. Most authors mentioned in the review noted an increase in susceptibility to SVT episodes during pregnancy. In patients with a previous history of SVT, the frequency, duration, and severity of episodes appeared to be increased during pregnancy. More recently, Panja et al[18] observed four cases of atrial tachycardia in a study of 239 consecutive pregnancies. All four cases were associated with rheumatic heart disease and the tachycardias developed during pregnancy. Hubbard et al[19] reported another case of atrial tachycardia which occurred only during pregnancy. McFaul et al[20] observed 10 cases of SVT in a review of 519 pregnancies; however, there is no information about whether the arrhythmias occurred only during pregnancy or if pregnancy had any effect on it. Whittemore et al[21] observed paroxysms of SVT in four women who had undergone surgery for atrial septal defect closure. These episodes of SVT persisted postpartum. In one woman, the arrhythmia was probably present before pregnancy.

In general, the clinical manifestations and the management of SVTs occurring during pregnancy are similar in the nonpregnant patient. Although the hemodynamic consequences of SVT on fetal well-being are of concern, there is no evidence of increased fetal morbidity or mortality in these patients. Vagal stimulation or pharmacologic agents are frequently effective in terminating the attacks. Verapamil, digoxin, beta-adrenergic blocking drugs, and Class IA antiarrhythmic drugs have been shown to be effective and safe during pregnancy.[22-25] Direct current cardioversion should be reserved for drug refractory, hemodynamically significant SVTs, or both, and is rarely necessary. The same drugs used to terminate the acute episode are also effective for long-term treatment. In patients with frequent and severe attacks of SVT, long-term antiarrhythmic prophylaxis is necessary. Nonpharmacologic measures, such as avoidance of stimulants, should be routinely instituted in these patients.

Atrial Flutter

Atrial flutter is less common than atrial fibrillation, and even though its paroxysmal forms may manifest in patients without structural heart disease, its chronic form is almost always found in patients with underlying heart disease (rheumatic, ischemic, or cardiomyopathy). It is frequently unstable, reverting to sinus rhythm or degenerating into atrial fibrillation.[26]

On ECG, atrial flutter frequently has a *sawtooth* morphology. The atrial rate ranges from 250 to 350 beats/minute; however, there is usually 2:1 conduction, and the ventricular rate is commonly 150 beats/minute. The electrophysiologic mechanism responsible for atrial flutter is believed to be reentry, and prolonged atrial conduction appears to be a predisposing factor for its genesis.[27]

Atrial flutter occurs uncommonly during pregnancy. Mendelson[2] found only four reported cases in addition to his personal observation in a pregnant patient with Graves' disease. Two other cases associated with rheumatic heart disease have been reported by Panja et al.[18] Among 233 pregnancies in mothers with congenital heart disease, atrial flutter was observed only in two patients; one had three ventriculotomies for repair of ventricular septal defect and the other was a woman with aortic regurgitation after aortic valvotomy.[21]

The therapeutic approach in patients with atrial flutter is dictated by the hemodynamic status. In hemodynamically stable patients, verapamil, digoxin and beta-adrenergic blocking agents may control the ventricular rate and occasionally terminate the dysrhythmia. Sodium channel-blocking drugs such as quinidine, procainamide, and disopyramide may successfully achieve cardioversion in 10–20% of the patients. In order to avoid 1:1 conduction and hemodynamic compromise, Class IA antiarrhythmic drugs should be administered only after the ventricular rate has been controlled. Electrical cardioversion is required in hemodynamically unstable patients and in nonresponders to drug therapy and should be started at low energy levels. Prevention of atrial flutter is similar to prevention of SVT. Digoxin alone or in combination with quinidine appears to be safe and effective. Monotherapy with verapamil, digoxin, beta-adrenergic blocking agents, and Class IA antiarrhythmic drugs may be equally effective.

Atrial Fibrillation

Atrial fibrillation is characterized by totally disorganized atrial depolarization at a rate of 350–600 beats/minute without effective atrial contraction. Most atrial impulses are blocked due to concealed conduction within the AV node and consequently, the ventricular rate is irregular and slower than atrial rates (100–200 beats/minute). Similar to atrial flutter, atrial fibrillation occurs in a paroxysmal or chronic form; the former may occur in normal hearts, while the latter is associated with myocardial or systemic diseases. The arrhythmia is common in patients with rheumatic heart disease, cardiomyopathy, ischemic heart disease, atrial septal defect, hypertensive heart disease, pericarditis, and thyrotoxicosis. While atrial fibrillation does not appear to increase mortality in patients without cardiac disease, in patients with cardiovascular diseases, it is associated with doubling the mortality and morbidity.[28] In patients with chronic atrial fibrillation and underlying heart disease, especially in patients with mitral stenosis, there is a significant increase in the frequency of embolic stroke and peripheral embolization.[29] In the absence of underlying heart disease, the risk of embolization is much lower.

During pregnancy, atrial fibrillation is associated mainly with rheumatic heart disease. Mendelson[2] in a review of 92,315 pregnancies, identified 3252 patients with organic heart disease. Among them, he observed 31 cases of atrial fibrillation of which 29 had rheumatic heart disease. Nineteen of these patients were in NYHA Class III and IV; the maternal and fetal mortality were 19% and 58%, respectively. Five patients (23%) had embolic complications.

In another review of 8843 pregnancies[30], 99 of 112 patients with organic heart disease had rheumatic heart disease. Only two patients with severe rheumatic heart disease had atrial fibrillation and both patients died.

Among 15 cases of cardiac arrhythmia seen in 118 pregnant patients with rheumatic heart disease, nine patients had atrial fibrillation.[18] Six of these patients were known to have atrial fibrillation before pregnancy and in the remaining patients, the arrhythmia developed during pregnancy. Atrial fibrillation was also observed in three of 24 patients with congenital heart disease.[18]

The hemodynamic consequences of atrial fibrillation during pregnancy are dependent on the severity of underlying heart disease and on the ventricular rate. In patients with mitral stensis (MS), an increase in heart rate shortens the diastolic filling period and increases the transvalvular pressure gradient. Therefore, the sudden onset of atrial fibrillation with rapid ventricular rate elevates left atrial pressure and causes rapid onset of dyspnea and even of pulmonary edema. Atrial contraction contributes up to 30% of presystolic transvalvular gradient; sudden cessation of atrial transport may decrease the cardiac output by 20% and result in hypotension and peripheral hypoperfusion. Therefore, in patients with significant MS, an effort should be made to restore and preserve normal sinus rhythm and to control the ventricular rate. This may be achieved with digoxin, beta-adrenergic blocking agents, and verapamil. The decision to proceed with cardioversion should be made after careful consideration has been given to underlying heart disease, the duration of atrial fibrillation, left atrial size, and the condition of the patient and fetus. Prior to electrical cardioversion, quinidine sulfate should be administered for a few days. In 10–15% of the patients, sinus rhythm may be restored during this period. In addition, quinidine is necessary to prevent recurrences of atrial fibrillation. Direct current (DC) cardioversion has been performed safely during pregnancy.[31,32] If elective cardioversion is contemplated, a special consideration should be given to anticoagulation. This may be indicated in patients with mitral stenosis, atrial fibrillation of recent onset, recurrent or recent emboli, prosthetic mitral valve, and dilated cardiomyopathy. The incidence of embolization during cardioversion is one to three percent. In patients without contraindications, anticoagulation given for two weeks prior to and several weeks post cardioversion may decrease the incidence of embolic events.[26] After successful cardioversion, long term therapy with digoxin and quinidine may be indicated to prevent recurrences of atrial fibrillation.

In patients with "lone" atrial fibrillation, anticoagulation is probably not necessary; drug therapy is indicated in symptomatic patients and is often successful in controlling the arrhythmias. When the atrial fibrillation is part of tachycardia–bradycardia syndrome, pacing may be required in addition to drug therapy.

Preexcitation syndrome

Preexcitation occurs as a result of an anomalous myocardial muscular connection between atria and ventricles outside of normal specialized conducting tissue. These muscular bridges are named accessory atrioventricular pathways and may be located anywhere around the atrioventricular rings. Left-sided pathways are more common than right-sided ones.[33] In addition to atrioventricular bypass tracts directly connecting atria to ventricles (Kent bundle), *Wolff–Parkinson–White* (WPW) syndrome may be due to nodoventricular and fasciculoventricular connections (Mahaim fibers). Preexcitation occurs when the supraventricular impulse depolarizes part of or the entire ventricle earlier than if the impulse is conducted through the normal conduction system.

Electrocardiographically, the syndrome is characterized by a PR interval shorter than 120 ms, the QRS complex exceeding 120 ms with a slurred onset (delta wave), and the ST-T waves directed in the opposite direction of the QRS vector.

The incidence of preexcitation in the normal population ranges from 0.01% to 0.3%.[26] The frequency of the syndrome is increased in certain conditions, such as Ebstein's anomaly and mitral valve prolapse. However, the majority of patients with preexcitation have no evidence of underlying heart disease. Ten percent of the patients with preexcitation may have multiple accessory pathways.

The WPW syndrome is clinically important because some of the tachyarrhythmias may be life-threatening. Approximately 80% of patients with tachyarrhythmias have reciprocating orthodromic or antidromic tachycardias. In the orthodromic variety, the antegrade conduction occurs over the normal conduction system and the retrograde conduction through the bypass tract. In the antidromic variety, the antegrade conduction is over the bypass tract and the retrograde conduction over the AV node. Fifteen to 30% of the patients may have atrial fibrillation. These patients are at higher risk because of the possibility of very rapid conduction over the accessory pathway and, consequently, may have very rapid ventricular rates that lead to ventricular fibrillation.

The incidence of paroxysmal tachycardias in the young adult population (20–39-years old) with preexcitation is approximately 10%.[33] The exact incidence of WPW syndrome during pregnancy is not known and it is not clear if pregnancy may facilitate the onset of tachyarrythmia in patients with previous asymptomatic preexcitation. Gleicher et al[34], in a report of three patients, suggested that pregnancy may predispose asymptomatic patients with preexcitation to tachyarrythmias.

McKenna et al[35] described a 27-year-old pregnant woman with WPW syndrome who had her attacks of tachyarrhythmias (atrial fibrillation and reentrant atrioventricular tachycardia) during two subsequent pregnancies. Prior to her first pregnancy and during the interval between the pregnancies, she was asymptomatic. The other reports of

WPW syndrome during pregnancy[36-38], did not address the issue of whether the pregnancy predisposed to arrhythmias in asymptomatic patients with preexcitation.

Asymptomatic patients with electrocardiographic evidence of preexcitation do not require therapy. The treatment of symptomatic atrioventricular tachycardia is similar to that described for SVT (see above) with the exception of digitalis preparations and intravenous verapamil or lidocaine. Digitalis preparations may shorten the refractory period of the accessory pathway and, therefore, accelerate the ventricular rates of patients with atrial fibrillation. Both intravenous verapamil and lidocaine may increase the ventricular rate and precipitate ventricular fibrillation. For symptomatic hemodynamically stable patients, class IA antiarrhythmic drugs are preferable. Intravenous procainamide appears to be the drug of choice. In the hemodynamically unstable patients, DC cardioversion should be immediately performed. For long term prophylaxis, oral Class IA antiarrhythmic drugs alone or the combination with β-adrenergic blocking drugs or verapamil are recommended. In some drug-refractory cases, amiodarone has been successful in controlling the arrhythmia[34-37], however, in one report the fetal side effects were devastating.[37] After pregnancy, patients with preexcitation and symptomatic, hemodynamically significant, tachyarrhythmias should undergo extensive electrophysiologic evaluation and eventually may need surgical or radiofrequency catheter ablation of the bypass tracts.

VENTRICULAR ARRHYTHMIAS

Premature Ventricular Complexes

Premature ventricular complexes (PVCs) appear to be common in a young population and their prevalence increases with age.[39,40] In a study of 50 healthy women undergoing 24-hour Holter monitoring, 54% of the patients had PVCs with 6% having more than 50 beats/24 hour.[14] The prognosis of patients with frequent and complex ventricular ectopy with no apparent underlying heart disease is similar to that of a healthy US population.[41,42] During pregnancy, PVCs may be commonly detected with 24-hour Holter monitoring in women complaining of palpitations. The majority of pregnant women with PVCs have no evidence of underlying heart disease and their prognosis is excellent. In some patients, PVCs are associated with systemic infections, hypoxia, a variety of medications, anxiety, electrolyte abnormalities, and intake of stimulants (caffeine, tobacco, alcohol). Reassurance, sedation, and avoidance of stimulants are often sufficient to abolish symptoms.

For patients with underlying heart disease and frequent simple or complex ventricular ectopy the prognosis may be worse. However, there is considerable debate whether the PVCs are actively playing a role in precipitating sudden cardiac death or are a simple marker of the arrhythmogenic substrate and underlying heart disease. Also, there is insufficient evidence that antiarrhythmic drug therapy, which effectively suppresses the ventricular ectopy, prevents sudden cardiac death.[42,43] The incidence of proarrhythmic effects appear to be higher in patients with ventricular dysfunction.[44]

Therefore, the decision about whether to treat should be weighed carefully and should be made only after complete assessment of the arrhythmia, underlying cardiac status, and the potential risks to mother and fetus. As a general rule, pharmacologic therapy should be avoided. However, in some severely symptomatic patients, antiarrhythmic drugs may be required. All Class IA antiarrhythmic drugs are effective in suppressing ventricular ectopy. Among them, quinidine has been most extensively used in pregnancy and has a good safety track record.[2,25] Among Class IB antiarrhythmic agents, the safest appears to be lidocaine as long as the blood levels are closely monitored.[25] Mexiletine has been used in pregnancy; however, the data regarding its safety is limited.[25] The patients treated with antiarrhythmic drugs should be carefully followed with frequent serum drug levels and 24-hour electrocardiographic monitoring.

Ventricular Tachycardia

A diagnosis of ventricular tachycardia (VT) has been made when three or more ventricular complexes occur in rapid succession (rate more than 100 beats/min). However, recent data revealed a bimodal distribution of repetitive ventricular form length, suggesting a natural break point between five and six ventricular complexes.[45] This information supports the classification of arrhythmias based on a hierarchy of forms which separates the salvos (three to five repetitive forms) from ventricular tachycardia (runs of more than six ventricular repetitive forms).[46] VT may be sustained or nonsustained. Nonsustained VT is self-terminating in less than 30 seconds while sustained VT lasts more than 30 seconds or causes hemodynamic decompensation requiring electrical cardioversion in less than 30 seconds.

On routine electrocardiogram, the ventricular origin of the tachycardia is suggested by a bizarre morphology of QRS complex, QRS duration greater than 120 ms, superior axis, fusion beats, capture beats, and AV dissocation. It must be remembered that 50% of the VTs may have retrograde conduction to the atria. However, occasionally, the differentiation from wide-QRS tachycardia of supraventricular origin may be difficult and may require more sophisticated electrophysiologic testing. The R-R interval of VT may be regular or may vary. However, grossly irregular wide-QRS tachycardia with a fast rate (200–300 beats/min) may be the result of atrial fibrillation with conduction over a bypass tract. At times, vagal maneuvers or pharmacologic interventions acting on slowing the conduction over the AV node are helpful in revealing the supraventricular origin of wide-QRS tachycardia.

The three mechanisms involved in the genesis of VT are reentry, abnormal automaticity, and triggered activity. These various mechanisms are typically associated with certain clinical settings. However, in individual patients, different mechanisms may be involved despite the same underlying pathologic process.

The majority of VTs encountered in clinical practice are due to reentry. The conditions necessary for reentry are: (1) unidirectional block; (2) slow conduction in an adjacent pathway; and (3) recirculation of the impulse to the original point due to complete recovery of the area of unidirectional block. The anatomic and functional substrate for reentry occurs commonly in ischemic heart disease, post-myocardial infarction, and various cardiomyopathies.

Automaticity is a normal property of the nodal and specialized conduction system cells. Abnormal automaticity may occur in pathologic states when the cell membrane is partially depolarized leading to spontaneous firing. Abnormal automaticity is probably the cause of accelerated idioventricular rhythms but, with the exception of repetitive monomorphic VT, is rarely a cause for recurrent sustained VT.[47]

Triggered activity occurs when the impulse is the result of early or delayed after-depolarizations.[48] In abnormal automaticity, the impulse is initiated spontaneously, while the triggered activity mechanism requires a prior impulse or a train of impulses which is followed by after-depolarizations. The after-depolarizations are oscillation of the resting membrane potential following an action potential. These oscillations may have enough amplitude to reach the membrane threshold and cause another action potential. Calcium ions and slow, inward calcium channels are believed to be involved in the genesis of triggered activity. In fact, calcium-channel blocking drugs like verapamil are effective in suppression of triggered arrhythmias. After-depolarizations are enhanced by catecholamines. Consequently, beta-adrenergic blocking agents may be a helpful additional treatment. *In vivo,* the arrhythmias produced by digitalis toxicity are believed to be due to triggered activity mechanisms. Triggered activity may be also involved in arrhythmias associated with acquired or congenital long-QT syndrome.[49]

The hemodynamic consequences of VT and, therefore, the symptomatology depend on the rate of VT and underlying heart disease. VTs commonly arise in patients with structural heart disease. The most common underlying heart disease is ischemic heart disease, closely followed by cardiomyopathy (dilated and hypertrophic) and less commonly, mitral valve prolapse, and valvular and congenital diseases. Some VTs arise in the heart with no clinical evidence of structural abnormalities. These patients are classified in the group of primary electrical disease.[50] However, in some of these patients, endomyocardial biopsy may reveal myocardial abnormalities.[51,52]

During pregnancy, VT is a rare occurrence. The first case was published by McMillan and Bellet in 1931.[53] Since then, more than 26 other cases have been reported.[21,54-78] The majority of patients with paroxysmal VT had no evidence of underlying heart disease (primary electrical disease). However, in some reports, the patients had mitral valve prolapse[69], valvular disease[76], and cardiomyopathy.[77,78] Maternal outcome was good except for two cases of sudden cardiac death.[57,78] The first case was a 19-year-old pregnant woman who died during her sixth month of pregnancy, three weeks after treatment with procainamide was administered.[57] The second case was a pregnant woman with hypertrophic cardiomyopathy who died from VT in her 39th gestational week.[78]

Several factors have been noted to precipitate the attacks of paroxysmal VT including emotional upset, fear, exercise, caffeine, smoking, alcohol, trauma, changes in posture, hypokalemia, and imbalance of the autonomic system.[56,68,69] With the exception of one report of a patient who had short runs of VT during pregnancy which were not present for several months after delivery, it is not clear from the information available if pregnancy increases the frequency of paroxysmal VT episodes, nor is there a clear pattern of variability during various trimesters of pregnancy.

The prognosis in patients with nonsustained VT and no structural disease is essentially good, although sudden death may occur.[42,79] Some of these VTs are catecholamine-sensitive; in this subset of patients, exercise should be avoided and therapy with beta-adrenergic blocking drugs is indicated.

The prognosis of patients with nonsustained VT and underlying heart disease is less favorable than the prognosis of patients with primary electrical disease.[79] The risk for sudden death, even though it may vary according to the type and degree of underlying heart disease, is increased in these patients and antiarrhythmic therapy may be indicated.[79] Patients with untreated sustained VT and structural heart disease have a dismal prognosis. This high-risk subgroup of patients should be aggressively evaluated and treated.

If the VT causes hemodynamic decompensation, immediate DC cardioversion should be performed. Low-energy synchronized shock (20–50 joules) are often successful in restoring sinus rhythm. If the VT is well tolerated, pharmacologic treatment should be administered initially. Intravenous lidocaine or procainamide are the first line drugs. If VT does not respond to drug therapy, DC cardioversion is indicated.

After the acute episode has been controlled, the patients should undergo a careful evaluation of their cardiac status, and precipitating factors such as myocardial ischemia, electrolyte imbalance, congestive heart failure, offending drugs, hypoxemia, and stimulants should be corrected.

Long-term antiarrhythmic drug therapy to prevent recurrences may be successful in 20–50% of the cases, depending on the mechanism of VT and underlying heart disease. During pregnancy, several Class IA and IB antiarrhythmic drugs have been safely used.[64,65,72,73,77] For VT that is refractory to standard drugs, amiodarone has been successfully used.[70,74]

During pregnancy, the majority of VTs occur in patients without clinically evident structural heart disease (primary electrical disease). In some of these patients, verapamil[80] or beta-adrenergic blocking drugs (preferably β_1 selective drugs) may be effective, especially when the precipitating factors are emotional stress or exercise.[81] Treatment of VT associated with digitalis toxicity should be pharmacologic (potassium, lidocaine, propanolol, phenytoin).

AV BLOCKS

First Degree AV Block

PR-interval represents the time taken by the impulse to travel from the sinus node to the ventricle and, normally, is 0.12–0.20 seconds. First-degree AV block is diagnosed when PR-interval is prolonged. The delay commonly occurs in the AV node but rarely may be intra-atrial or infranodal. PR-interval may vary with sinus rate: shorter at faster rates and longer at slower rates. Prolonged PR-interval may be found in 0.52% of the normal population.[82] PR prolongation may be a manifestation of increased vagal tone, drug effect, or ischemia or rheumatic heart disease.

During pregnancy, first-degree heart block has been associated mainly with rheumatic heart disease.[2] If no underlying pathology can be identified, first-degree AV block has no clinical significance.

Second-Degree AV Block

Second-degree AV block is divided into two types: Mobitz type I (Wenckebach) and Mobitz type II. Mobitz type I AV block is characterized by a progressive lengthening of PR-interval until an impulse is blocked; therefore, no QRS follows the blocked P wave. In Mobitz type II AV block, an impulse suddenly blocks without previous prolongation of PR-Interval.

Mobitz type I (Wenckebach) is a relatively benign block and may occur normally in athletes during sleep or any other situation in which vagal tone is increased. Mobitz type I AV block generally occurs in AV node and often is transient and reversible. It is commonly associated with rheumatic fever, ischemia, inferior wall myocardial infarction, or is a manifestation of drug effects and seldom progresses to complete AV block.

Mobitz type II often heralds the development of symptomatic complete heart block. When the block occurs in the setting of acute myocardial infarction, it is associated with larger infarcts, higher morbidity, and requires temporary, permanent, or temporary and permanent pacing. On surface ECG, the block is often accompanied by bundle branch block and the location of the block is mainly infranodal (His–Purkinje system).

During pregnancy, the incidence of second-degree AV block is very low.[2] Among 26 cases of acquired heart block, six cases had second-degree AV block. In comparison, only one of 21 patients with congenital heart block had second-degree AV block. Therefore, second-degree AV block was mainly acquired and occurred in association with rheumatic heart disease or infections.[2] Treatment with permanent pacing in patients with Mobitz Type I is indicated only in seriously symptomatic patients. For pregnant patients with Mobitz type II, permanent pacing is indicated in symptomatic patients.

Third-Degree AV Block

Third-degree AV block occurs when no supraventricular impulses are conducted to the ventricles. Therefore, the atrial and ventricular rates are determined by their own independent pacemakers with complete AV dissociation. The ventricular rate is usually low (45–50 beats/min and 35–45 beats/min for junctional and idioventricular rhythms, respectively) and the atrial rate is greater than the ventricular rate. A diagnosis of complete heart block should not be made when the AV dissociation occurs with high ventricular or with very low sinus/atrial rates. In these cases, the AV dissociation may be due to an escape mechanism or to an accelerated junctional or idioventricular rhythm. Complete heart block may be acquired or congenital. The site of the block is mainly infranodal (His–Purkinje system) in acquired and nodal in the congenital type. The congenital complete AV block is often the result of immunologic offense by maternal antibodies against the fetal AV node.[83,84]

Mendelson[2] reviewed 40 cases of complete heart block occurring in pregnancy. Half of these patients had acquired AV block and the etiologies were rheumatic in 11 patients, myocarditis in two patients, infections in six patients, and coronary artery disease in one patient. Half of the cases of congenital block were associated with ventricular septal defect. The patients with congenital heart block had a more favorable course and outcome of the pregnancy.

The onset of complete heart block occurred almost always prior to pregnancy, and pregnancy does not appear to affect its frequency. Heart block by itself rarely affects the course or outcome of pregnancy if the ventricular rate remains in the range of 50–60 beats/min. If the rate suddenly slows, syncope may occur.[2,85,86,87] In some patients, the Morgagni–Adams–Stokes syndrome occurred during delivery and required temporary pacing.[85,88]

The treatment of symptomatic complete heart block is permanent pacemaker implantation. Due to possible tension and skin ulceration over the generator unit during pregnancy, pacemaker implantation in childbearing age women should not be performed in the abdominal area. Pregnancy in patients with electronic pacemakers is usually well tolerated and safe.[89,90] In a review of 20 reported cases, the most frequent complication was skin ulceration at the site of implant; battery failure and its successful replacement during pregnancy was described in another two cases.[89]

In summary, the majority of patients with third-degree AV block may have a benign course during pregnancy. This is particularly true for patients with congenital heart block. Due to increased hemodynamic burden during delivery, temporary pacemaker insertion may be necessary. Permanent pacing during pregnancy is a desirable option in symptomatic patients.

REFERENCES

1. Spritzer RC, Seldon M, Mattes LM, et al. Serious arrhythmias during labor and delivery in women with heart disease. *JAMA.* 1970;211:1005.
2. Mendelson CL. Disorder of the heart beat during pregnancy. *Am J Obstet Gynecol.* 1956;72:1268.
3. Vander Veer JB, Kuo PT. Cardiac disease in pregnancy. *Am Heart J.* 1950;39:2.
4. Szekely P, Snaith L. Paroxysmal tachycardia in pregnancy. *Br Heart J.* 1953;15:195.
5. McAnulty JH, Metcalfe J, Ueland K. General guidelines in the management of cardiac disease. *Clin Obstet Gynecol.* 1981;24:773.
6. Vatterott PJ, Hamill SC, Bailey KR, et al. Signal-averaged electrocardiography: a new noninvasive test to identify patients at risk for ventricular arrhythmias. *Mayo Clin Proc.* 1988;63:931.
7. Carruth JE, Mirris SB, Brogan DR, et al. The electrocardiogram during normal pregnancy. *Am Heart J.* 1981;102:1075.
8. Elkayam U, Gleicher N. Hemodynamics and cardiac function during normal pregnancy and puerperium. In: Elkayam U, Gleicher N, eds. *Cardiac Problems in Pregnancy.* 2nd ed. New York: Alan R. Liss; 1990:5.
9. Hilgard J, Ezri MD, Denes P. Significance of ventricular pauses of three seconds or more detected on twenty-four hour Holter recording. *Am J Cardiol.* 1985;55:1005.
10. Surawicz B, Reddy CP. Tachycardia-bradycardic syndrome. In: Surawicz B, et al, eds. *Tachycardias.* Boston, MA: Martinus Nijhoff; 1984:199.
11. Ferrer MI. The sick sinus syndrome. *Circulation.* 1973;47:635.
12. Rubinstein JJ, et al. Clinical spectrum of sick sinus syndrome. *Circulation.* 1972;46:5.
13. Schatz JW, Fisher JA, Lee RF, Lampe RM. Pacemaker therapy in pregnancy for managment of sinus bradycardia—junctional tachycardia syndrome. *Chest.* 1974;65:461.
14. Sobotka PA, Mayer JH, Bauerfeind RA, et al. Arrhythmias documented by 24-hour continuous ambulatory electrocardiographic monitoring in young women without apparent heart disease. *Am Heart J.* 1981;101:753.
15. Josephson ME. Paroxysmal supraventricular tachycardia: an electrophysiologic approach. *Am J Cardiol.* 1978;41:1123.
16. Wu D, Denes P, Amat-Y-Leon F, et al. Clinical electrocardiographic and electrophysiologic observations in patients with paroxysmal supraventricular tachycardia. *Am J Cardiol.* 1973;41:1045.
17. Hayes DM. *Medical Complication of Pregnancy.* New York, NY: McGraw-Hill; 1969:151.
18. Panja M, Mitra K, Kar AK, et al. A clinical profile of heart disease in pregnancy. *Ind Heart J.* 1986;38:392.
19. Hubbard WN, Jenkins BA, Word DF. Persistent atrial tachycardia in pregnancy. *Br Med J.* 1983;287:327.
20. McFaul PB, Dornan JC, Lamki H, Boyle D. Pregnancy complicated by maternal heart disease. A review of 519 women. *Br J Obstet Gynecol.* 1988;95:861.
21. Whittemore R, Hobbins JC, Engle MA. Pregnancy and its outcome in women with and without surgical treatment of congenital heart disease. *Am J Cardiol.* 1982;50:641.
22. Klein V, Repke JT. Supraventricular tachycardia in pregnancy: cardioversion with verapamil. *Obstet Gynecol.* 1984;63:165.
23. Pruin SC, Phelan JP, Buchanan GC. Long-term propranolol therapy in pregnancy: maternal and fetal outcome. *Am J Obstet Gynecol.* 1979;135:485.
24. Finley JP, Waxman MB, Wong PY, Lickrish GM. Digoxin excretion in human breast milk. *J Pediatr.* 1979;94:339.
25. Widerhorn J, Rubin NJ, Frishman WH, Elkayam U. Cardiovascular drugs in pregnancy. *Cardiol Clin.* 1987;5(4):651.
26. Zipes D. Specific arrhythmias: diagnosis and treatment. In: Braunwald E, ed. *Heart Disease.* Philadelphia, PA: WB Saunders; 1988:658.
27. Simpson RJ, Foster JR, Gettes LS. Atrial excitability and conduction in patients with interatrial conduction defects. *Am J Cardiol.* 1982;50:1331.
28. Kannel WB, Abbott RD, Savage DD, McNamara PM. Epidemiologic feature of chronic atrial fibrillation: the Framingham study. *N Engl J Med.* 1982;306:1018.
29. Olshansky B, Waldo AL. Atrial fibrillation: update on mechanism, diagnosis and management. *Mod Concepts Cardiovasc Dis.* 1987;56:23.
30. Jensen J, Wegner C, Keys EH, Smith HR. Pregnancy and heart disease—an 8-year experience. *Obstet Gynecol.* 1940;39:443.
31. Schroeder JS, Harrison DC: Repeated cardioversion during pregnancy. *Am J Cardiol.* 1971;27:445.

32. Finlay AY, Edmunds V. DC cardioversion in pregnancy. *Br J Clin Pract.* 1979;33:88.
33. Guize L, Soria R, Chaouat JC, et al. Prevalence and course of Wolff-Parkinson-White syndrome in a population of 138,048 subjects. *Ann Med Interne.* (Paris) 1985;136:474.
34. Gleicher N, Meller J, Sandler RZ, Sullum S. Wolff-Parkinson-White syndrome in pregnancy. *Obstet Gynecol.* 1961;58:748.
35. McKenna WJ, Harris I, Rowland E, et al. Amiodaron therapy during pregnancy. *Am J Cardiol.* 1983;51:1231.
36. Penn IM, Barrett PA, Pannikote V, et al. Amiodarone in pregnancy. *Am J Cardiol.* 1985;56:196.
37. DeWolf D, DeSchepper J, Verharen H, et al. Congenital hypothyroid goiter and amiodarone. *Acta Paediatr Scand.* 1988;77:616.
38. Wittry MD, Zimmerman TJ, Janosik DL, Williams GA. Postpartum myocardial infarction in a patient with intermittent ventricular preexcitation. *Am Heart J.* 1989;117:191.
39. Moss AJ. Clinical significance of ventricular arrhythmias in patients with and without coronary artery disease. *Prog Cardiovasc Dis.* 1980;23:33.
40. Kostis JB, McCrone K, Moreyra AE, et al. Premature ventricular complexes in absence of heart disease. *Circulation.* 1981;63:1351.
41. Kennedy HL, Whitlock JA, Sprague MR, et al. Long-term follow-up of asymptomatic healthy subjects with frequent and complex ventricular ectopy. *N Engl J Med.* 1985;312:193.
42. Surawicz B. Prognosis of ventricular arrhythmia in relation to sudden cardiac death: therapeutic implications. *J Am Coll Cardiol.* 1987;10:435.
43. McGovern BA, Garan H, Ruskin JN. Treatment of ventricular arrhythmias. *Curr Probl Cardiol.* 1988;13(12):785.
44. Slater W, Lampert S, Podrid PJ, Lown B. Clinical predictors of arrhythmia worsening by antiarrhythmic drugs. *Am J Cardiol.* 1988;61:349.
45. Lowery M, Marchena EJ, Castellanos A, et al. Interrelationship of variable coupling, multiformity and repetitive forms: implications for classification of ventricular arrhythmias. *Am Heart J.* 1990;119:301.
46. Meyerburg RJ, Kessler KM, Luceri RM, et al. Classification of ventricular arrhythmias based on parallel hierarchies of frequency and form. *Am J Cardiol.* 1984;59:1355.
47. Bigger JT Jr, Dresdale RJ, Heissenbuttel RH, et al. Ventricular arrhythmias in ischemic heart disease: mechanism, prevalence, significance and management. *Prog Cardiovasc Dis.* 1977;19:255.
48. Wit AL, Cranefield PF, Gadsby DC. Triggered activity. In: Zipes DP, Bailey JC, Elhaffar V, eds. *The Slow Inward Current and Cardiac Arrhythmias.* The Hague: Martinus Nijhoff; 1980.
49. Schechter E, Freeman CC, Lazzara R. After depolarizatons on mechanism for long QT syndrome: electrophysiologic studies of a case. *J Am Coll Cardiol.* 1984;3:1556.
50. Naccarelli GV, Prystowsky EN, Jackman WM, et al. Role of electrophysiologic testing in managing patients who have ventricular tachycardia unrelated to coronary artery disease. *Am J Cardiol.* 1982;50:165.
51. Strain JE, Grose RM, Factor SM, Fisher JD. Results of endomyocardial biopsy in patients with spontaneous ventricular tachycardia but without apparent structural heart disease. *Circulation.* 1983;68:1171.
52. Sugrue DD, Holmes DR Jr, Gersh BJ, et al. Cardiac histologic findings in patients with life-threatening ventricular arrhythmias of unknown origin. *J Am Coll Cardiol.* 1984;4:952.
53. McMillan TM, Bellet S. Ventricular paroxysmal tachycardia: report of a case in a pregnant girl of sixteen years with an apparently normal heart. *Am Heart J.* 1931;7:70.
54. Peters CM, Penner SL. Orthostatic paroxysmal ventricular tachycardia. *Am Heart J.* 1946;32:645.
55. Hair TE, Eagan JT, Orgain ES. Paroxysmal ventricular tachycardia in the absence of demonstrable heart disease. *Am J Cardiol.* 1962;9:209.
56. Adams CW. Functional paroxysmal ventricular tachycardia. *Am J Cardiol.* 1962;9:215.
57. Rally CR, Walters MB. Paroxysmal ventricular tachycardia without evident heart disease. *Can Med Assoc J.* 1962;86:268.
58. Pine HL, Fox L, Shook D, McK. Paroxysmal ventricular tachycardia complicating pregnancy. *Am J Cardiol.* 1965;15:732.
59. Gettes LS, Surawicz B. Long-term prevention of paroxysmal arrhythmias with propranolol therapy. *Am J Med Sci.* 1967;254:257.
60. Ledwich JR, Fay JE. Idiopathic recurrent ventricular fibrillation. *Am J Cardiol.* 1969;24:255.
61. Russell RO. Paroxysmal ventricular tachycardia associated with pregnancy. *Am J Med Sci.* 1969;6:111.
62. Reed RL, Cheney CB, Fearon RE, et al. Propranolol therapy throughout pregnancy: a case report. *Anesth Anal.* 1974;53:214.
63. Shaxted EJ, Milton PJ. Disopyramide in pregnancy: a case report. *Curr Med Res Opin.* 1979;6:70.
64. Hill LM, Malkasian Jr GD. The use of quinidine sulfate throughout pregnancy. *Obstet Gynecol.* 1979;54:366.
65. Timmis AD, Jackson G, Holt DW. Mexiletine for control of ventricular dysrhythmias in pregnancy. *Lancet.* 1980;2:647.
66. O'Callaghan AC, Normandale JP, Morgan M. The prolonged QT syndrome: a review with anesthetic implication and a report of two cases. *Anaesth Int Care.* 1982;10:50.
67. Menon KPS, Mahapatra RK. Paroxysmal ventricular tachycardia associated with Bell's palsy in a teenager at late pregnancy. *Angiology.* 1984;35:534.
68. Brodsky MA, Sato DA, Oster PD, et al. Paroxysmal ventricular tachycardia with syncope during pregnancy. *Am J Cardiol.* 1986;58:563.
69. Lownes HE, Ives TJ. Mexiletine use in pregnancy and lactation. *Am J Obstet Gynecol.* 1987;157:446.
70. Rey E, Bachrach LK, Burrow GN. Effects of amiodaron during pregnancy. *Can Med Assoc J.* 1987;136:959.
71. Vlay SC. Catecholamine-sensitive ventricular tachycardia. *Am Heart J.* 1987;114:455.
72. Juneja MM, Ackerman WE, Kaczorowski DM, et al. Continous epidural lidocaine infusion in the parturient with paroxysmal ventricular tachycardia. *Anesthesiology.* 1989;71:305.
73. Kimigawa T, Fujimoto Y, Miyakoda H, et al. A case of paroxysmal ventricular tachycardia in pregnancy. *Jpn Circ J.* 1989;53:807.
74. Foster CJ, Love HG. Amiodaron in pregnancy. Case report and review of literature. *Int J Cardiol.* 1988;20:307.
75. Lewis AM, Patel L, Johnston A, Turner P. Mexiletine in human blood and breast milk. *Postgrad Med J.* 1981;57:546.
76. Brunozzi LT, Meniconi L, Chiocchi P, et al. Propafenone in the treatment of chronic ventricular arrhythmias in a pregnant patient. *Br J Clin Pharmacol.* 1988;26:489.
77. Barnett DD, Hudson SA, McBurney A. Disopyramide and its N-monodesalkyl metabolite in breast milk. *Br J Clinic Pharmacol.* 1982;14:310.
78. Shah DM, Sunderji SG. Hypertrophic cardiomyopathy and pregnancy: report of a maternal mortality and review of literature. *Obstet Gynecol Surv.* 1985;40:444.
79. Prystowsky EN. Antiarrhythmic therapy for asymptomatic ventricular arrhythmias. *Am J Cardiol.* 1988;61:102A.
80. Sung RJ, Shapiro WA, Shen EN, et al. Effects of verapamil in ventricular tachycardias possibly caused by reentry, automaticity and triggered activity. *J Clin Invest.* 1983;72:350.
81. Coumel P, Rosengarten MD, Ledereg JF, Attuel P. Role of sympathetic nervous system in non-ischemic ventricular arrhythmias. *Br Heart J.* 1982;47:137.
82. Johnson RL, Averill KH, Lamb L. Electrocardiographic findings in 67,375 asymptomatic individuals. Part VII A-V block. *Am J Cardiol.* 1960;6:153.
83. Ho SY, Esscher E, Anderson RH, Michaelsson M. Anatomy of congenital heart block and relation to maternal anti-RO antibodies. *Am J Cardiol.* 1986;58:291.
84. Chameides L, Truex RC, Vetter V, et al. Association of natural systemic lupus erythematosus with congenital heart block. *N Engl J Med.* 1977;297:1204.
85. Schobrun M, Rowland W, Quiroz AC. Complete heart block in pregnancy. *Am J Obstet Gynecol.* 1966;27:243.
86. Eddy W, Frankenfeld R. Congenital complete heart block in pregnancy. *Am J Obstet Gynecol.* 1977;128:223.
87. Abramovici H, Faktor JH, Gonen Y, et al. Maternal permanent bradycardia: pregnancy and delivery. *Obstet Gynecol.* 1984;63:381.
88. Ginns HM, Hollinrake K. Complete heart block in pregnancy treated with internal pacemaker. *J Obstet Gynaecol Br Commonw.* 1970;77:710.
89. Jaffe R, Gruber A, Fejgin M, et al. Pregnancy with an artificial pacemaker. *Obstet Gynecol Surv.* 1987;42:137.
90. Andersen C, Oxhoj H, Arnsbo P, Lybecker H. Pregnancy and cesarean section in a patient with a late-responsive pacemaker. *PACE* 1989;12:386.

Chapter One Hundred and Thirty-Six

Cardiac Surgery

Kenneth L. Noller and Paul J. Weinbaum

136

It is most interesting to read the obstetrics textbooks of the late 1940s. Puerperal sepsis had been largely eliminated by the introduction of antibiotics, the treatment of the toxemias of pregnancy was becoming standardized and modern, and cesarean sections were no longer considered an obstetric failure. But few inroads had been made into the problem of correcting cardiac disease in women of reproductive age. Therefore, these textbooks contain long and detailed chapters on the management of cardiac disease during pregnancy. Cardiac disease was becoming (as it remains today) the most common nonobstetric cause of maternal mortality.

Modern textbooks of obstetrics still contain large sections on cardiac disease in pregnancy. However, the emphasis has changed remarkably. No longer is it sufficient to categorize disease solely by functional categories, such as the New York Heart Association groups I–IV (though this system is still useful). Today, it is important to determine the exact cause of the cardiac deficiency so that specific intervention may be instituted.

And, in fact, cardiac disease first diagnosed in a pregnant woman is rapidly becoming an anachronism. It is rare to see a major congenital defect that has not been corrected by surgery. Rheumatic heart disease is now most often prevented but managed surgically when it occurs. Since 1952, it is estimated, more than 200,000 mechanical valves have been implanted in humans.[1] Several hundred pregnancies with artificial valves and even cardiac transplantation have been reported in the literature.[2-4]

These advances in the treatment of cardiac disease in young women have changed the practicing obstetrician's management of the pregnant patient with cardiac disease. The obstetrician must now be concerned with the care of the woman who has already undergone extensive cardiac evaluation and, often, open-heart surgery, which may have involved placement of artificial valves and membranes or relocation of major vessels. Therefore, this chapter is devoted mainly to a description of the management of pregnant women who have undergone open-heart surgery.

However, some cardiac disease remains undiagnosed until the first prenatal examination. The obstetrician must still be an astute diagnostician and may have a major part in the detection of cardiac disease. Therefore, the second part of the chapter is devoted to identification of those cardiac problems that may require surgical intervention during pregnancy.

PREGNANCY FOLLOWING CARDIAC SURGERY

Congenital Heart Disease

Prior to the availability of open-heart surgery, persons with significant congenital heart disease [New York Heart Association (NYHA) Classes III and IV] rarely lived to reproductive age, and the women, if they survived to their 20s, were often so debilitated that ovulation was unlikely. Consequently, the older obstetric textbooks stated that congenital heart disease was rarely associated with intrauterine pregnancy. Among pregnant women today, over 30% of all cardiac disease causing a significant lowering of functional class is of the congenital type (see also Chapter 127).[5]

Most texts state that congenital heart lesions affect approximately 1% of all live born infants in the United States.[6,7] However, this figure underestimates true disease frequency because congenital heart lesions are often missed on neonatal examinations, and may even be missed during the first few years of life. A mother who has a congenital heart lesion is at increased risk for delivering an infant with cardiac problems. Although the risk has been stated as 3–5%[8], a recent study by Whittemore et al of a large cohort of such mothers found the rate of congenital heart disease in their offspring to be 16.2%.[9] In two thirds of these cases, the lesion in the child was concordant with the mother's diagnosis. In addition, mothers with obstructive lesions were more likely than women with shunting abnormalities to deliver children with heart defects. Since many of these infants may now live a normally active life into the reproductive years, obstetricians are seeing an increase in the number of pregnant women with corrected congenital heart disease.

The frequency of congenital cardiac disease is also increased by maternal ingestion of drugs, such as phenytoin, alcohol, or lithium, and certain maternal biochemical disease states such as phenylketonuria.[10] However, the majority of cases of congenital heart lesions result from incompletely understood interaction between an individual's genes and the environment (multifactorial inheritance).

Types of Defects. There has been no change in the relative frequency of individual congenital cardiac defects during this century. Thus, atrial and ventricular septal defects and patent ductus arterisus account for a majority of the disease. Various single-valve disorders, especially pulmonic and aortic stenosis, and tetralogy of Fallot account for most of the rest.[11] Coarctation of the aorta is also seen wth some frequency.

Recently, the disorder termed mitral valve prolapse (MVP) has been recognized. If this is accepted as a form of congenital heart disease, it clearly is the most common lesion, occurring in approximately 6% of the general population.[12] MVP seems to be asymptomatic in most cases, and thus is omitted from further consideration in this section.

It is useful to classify those lesions with septal defects in a general way based on the direction in which blood is shunted. Atrial septal defect (ASD), ventricular septal defect (VSD), and patent ductus arteriosus (PDA) permit left-to-right shunts, whereas tetralogy of Fallot is, by far, the most common defect allowing right-to-left shunt. A right-to-left shunt causes obvious cyanosis and rarely goes undiagnosed into the reproductive years. However, a small left-to-right shunt may become the cause of cyanosis in the third decade if pulmonary hypertension occurs, and this is the type of case where the diagnosis is more likely to await the obstetrician.

Left-to-Right Shunts.

ATRIAL SEPTAL DEFECT. Defects of the atrial septum are the most common form of congenital heart disease.[11,13] Three major defects are identified: ostium primum, ostium secundum, and sinus venosus. Usually it is not important for the obstetrician to know which type is present in a pregnant woman.

Most women with ASDs are totally asymptomatic and may not suspect that they have a cardiac lesion. The first sign that there is a problem is often a systolic ejection murmur heard at the base of the heart with wide, fixed splitting of the second heart sound. This murmur is caused by the increased flow of blood across the pulmonic valve. If the defect is large and the right ventricle has hypertrophied, there may be a left parasternal systolic lift on physical examination.

Most ASDs causing functional changes will have been identified and repaired in childhood. The surgical procedure is common and carries minimal risk. The patch used to cover the defect is usually small and often becomes completely covered by the endocardiac epithelium. Patients in such cases rarely have problems. They are virtually all NYHA functional class I, and their lifestyle has not been impaired by the previously corrected defect.

A pregnant woman with an ASD satisfactorily corrected may be treated as any other pregnant woman. Although the initial physical examination must be thorough, it is not necessary to order additional tests or plan extraordinary management during labor and delivery. However, most authorities believe in prophylaxis against bacterial endocarditis and suggest that such a woman receive this preventative therapy just prior to and after delivery.

VENTRICULAR SEPTAL DEFECT. Defects of the ventricular septum may be the most common form of congenital heart disease at birth, but most of the small defects close spontaneously during infancy and early childhood. Those that persist are usually identified and corrected in later childhood.

The major clinical finding with an uncorrected VSD is a holosystolic murmur heard best along the left sternal border in the third and fourth intercostal spaces. The size of the defect and the resultant damage to the cardiac musculature are the cause of the physical findings that may be associated. A thrill may be palpated in some cases if the murmur is very loud, and signs of left ventricular hypertrophy and enlargement may be present. However, most women who become pregnant with an untreated VSD are asymptomatic because of the very small size of the lesion.

Those women who have had correction of a VSD during early childhood and who have remained functionally free from signs of cardiac disease are at little, if any, increased risk for problems during pregnancy. They may be treated as other pregnant women except for prophylaxis to prevent bacterial endocarditis.

PATENT DUCTUS ARTERIOSUS. Although not strictly a cardiac anomaly, patent ductus arteriosus is one of the most common congenital abnormalities of the cardiovascular system. Because it is so easily diagnosed in neonates, virtually all patients with this anomaly have been treated before their reproductive years. In women who have had such correction, pregnancy presents no increased risk, and they may be managed in the usual manner.

Right-to-Left Shunts.

TETRALOGY OF FALLOT. Among infants and young children, tetralogy of Fallot is the most common cause of cyanotic heart disease.[13] Right-to-left shunting of blood occurs from a combination of ventricular septal defect, pulmonary valve stenosis, right ventricular hypertrophy, and displacement of the base of the aorta. Most cases of this syndrome are detected at or shortly after birth, but it is now recognized that the clinical spectrum of the disease is wide because of the varied severity of the component lesions. Nevertheless, it is unusual for this combination of defects to go undiagnosed beyond the age of five. In fact, very few persons with tetralogy of Fallot live beyond age 25 unless it is surgically corrected. Although many procedures have been performed in the past, total correction is now the usual choice. Many persons who have had this complete procedure are now entering their reproductive years, and reports of pregnancy in women so treated have been published.[14]

It is difficult to know exactly how to best care for these persons. Many of them have led relatively normal lives if the correction was accomplished in early childhood. They may not have dyspnea on exertion, which is the hallmark of the disease in untreated persons.

The initial prenatal evaluation should include a thorough physical examination with particular attention to signs of cyanosis or cardiac hypertrophy. A chest roentgenogram and electrocardiogram should be obtained. Because pregnancy increases cardiac work approximately 50% and labor also will add 50%, cardiac stress testing is recommended. If the patient tolerates a doubling of the cardiac work load without compromise, the pregnancy should progress with little risk.

Still, one should bear in mind that experience with pregnancy in women with total correction of the tetralogy is limited. A cardiologist should always be consulted in these cases, and frequent examinations are essential.

Women with total correction should be instructed to limit physical activity, although ordinary work, that is not of a strenuous physical nature, may be continued. All such patients should be encouraged to obtain several hours of rest per day. Labor and delivery may pass uneventfully, but problems may arise if hypotension is allowed to occur. Close evaluation of maternal cardiac status and electronic fetal monitoring is essential. Maternal blood gases should be drawn at the onset of labor and repeated as necessary during the intrapartum and postpartum periods. Invasive hemodynamic monitoring may be helpful to monitor accurately maternal volume status and to determine the need for intrapartum pharmacologic therapy.

Beta-mimetic agents should be used with caution in patients with uncorrected or partly corrected fixed or cyanotic lesions who experience preterm labor. However, magnesium sulfate or oral indomethacin are potentially effective and safer agents in these patients and do not cause the significant tachycardia and acute volume shifts seen with the beta-agonists.

Congenital Valvular Defects. Isolated congenital valvular defects—except for prolapse of the mitral valve—are relatively rare. Congenital aortic stenosis is the most common, yet occurs much less frequently in females than in males. If this condition is severe, the treatment is usually surgical and usually involves replacement of the valve. If replacement is completed successfully and the patient is in NYHA class I, pregnancy should be tolerated well. (A complete discussion of pregnancy subsequent to insertion of mechanical valves is contained below in the section on acquired heart disease.)

Abnormalities of each of the other cardiac valves are much less frequent than aortic valve abnormalities. These may be managed by valvuloplasty or replacement of the defective valve with a mechanical or porcine valve.

Acquired Cardiac Disease

Rheumatic Heart Disease. Although congenital heart disease has become a more frequent cause of cardiac disease in pregnancy, rheumatic heart disease remains several times more common in the general population. Indeed, recently there have been several outbreaks of acute rheumatic fever in young populations. Women are much more likely to have cardiac sequelae from the acute disease process than are men, and the mitral valve is the most commonly affected. In fact, the single entity mitral stenosis may still account for nearly one third of all cardiac disease associated with pregnancy. Therefore, this single lesion is the most important for the obstetrician to understand in detail. Mitral stenosis is also one of the most easily corrected lesions, and cardiac surgeons have considerable experience with its repair.

However, any of the cardiac valves may be diseased following acute rheumatic fever. The mitral valve is the most commonly involved, and mitral stenosis is much more frequent than mitral regurgitation. The aortic valve is the second most common site for disease, and again, stenosis is more frequent than regurgitation. This lesion is rarely present without mitral involvement. The tricuspid valve also is involved in some cases, and both stenosis and regurgitation are reported. The pulmonary valve is rarely involved, but it certainly should be examined whenever evaluation of a case of rheumatic heart disease is undertaken.

The treatment of disease of any of these valves by the cardiac surgeon involves either valvulotomy—forceful opening of the valve with a finger or a dilator—or valve replacement with either a glutaraldehyde-preserved porcine valve or a mechanical valve. The management of subsequent pregnancy is greatly affected by the type of valve that is inserted (see below).

Bacterial Endocarditis Prophylaxis

It has long been recognized that bacterial endocarditis, either acute or subacute, may follow episodes of bacteremia. The most common organisms are the streptococci. Dental surgery, vaginal delivery, cosmetic surgery, and several other procedures have been implicated as initiating events in some cases, presumably by the showering of the bloodstream with bacteria at the time of these minor operative interventions. Although the host defense mechanisms normally clear the offending organism from the blood in a short time, the bacteria can potentially lodge at the site of a cardiac valvular abnormality.

Bacterial endocarditis is only rarely associated with pregnancy.[15] Whether this is a result of the widespread use of antibiotic prophylaxis or of a true rarity of the disease in association with pregnancy is not known with any certainty. Recently, some authors have suggested that routine use of such prophylaxis in women with valvular disease is unwarranted.[13] Others, however, argue for continued use in women with cardiac disease.[16,17]

In view of the dramatic and tragic effects of bacterial endocarditis most authorities continue to recommend that all women with cardiac abnormalities be given antibiotic prophylaxis just before, during, and after delivery. Coverage should be given for both gram-positive and gram-negative organisms. Current recommendations of the American Heart Association include a synthetic penicillin or cephalosporin for gram-positive and an aminoglycoside for gram-negative bacteria. If an anaerobic infection is feared, then an additional agent should be added, but this is not commonly done in the United States. In patients who are allergic to penicillin, vancomycin may be substituted.

Pregnancy Following Valvulotomy

One of the earliest and greatest advances in cardiac surgery was the demonstration that some patients with life-threatening mitral stenosis could be salvaged by incision into the left atrium and passage of the surgeon's finger through the mitral valve. This simple procedure broke down calcifications and usually resulted in clinical improvement, although very often with some degree of mitral regurgitation. The procedure has been refined, and dilators and flow meters have been developed which can predict the area of the valve opening after the procedure.

Large series of pregnant women who have had this procedure are reported in the literature.[15-20] When the procedure is performed before pregnancy, and the woman has attained functional class I or II, maternal mortality is very low. The increased work load of the heart that results from pregnancy usually is well tolerated.[20] However, the amount of damage done to the cardiac muscle before the procedure is most important. The fortunate concurrence between the amount of permanent damage and the functional classification makes prediction of pregnancy outcome relatively simple.

Women who are of functional class I or II after valvulotomy and become pregnant should be cautioned in the usual manner for cardiac disease in pregnancy. They should be instructed to obtain an increased amount of rest, to avoid very strenuous physical activity, and to take their pulse several times a day to detect the occurrence of any arrhythmia (usually atrial fibrillation). Consultation with an internist or cardiologist should be obtained early in pregnancy. It is also wise to obtain a baseline electrocardiogram (ECG) and an echocardiogram. Then, should the functional status or physical findings become a concern, the change can be considered in perspective. Any evidence of congestive heart failure must be treated aggressively.

The most common cause of sudden cardiac failure in women with mitral stenosis is the development of atrial fibrillation. This may cause very rapid cardiac failure that is difficult to treat.[11] Women in chronic atrial fibrillation do not have the same tendency to acute failure; it is only those who suddenly develop this arrhythmia who tend to decompensate rapidly.

Treatment of cardiac failure in women who have undergone valvulotomy depends on the cause. If atrial fibrillation is the initiating event, it may be necessary to convert the maternal rhythm to sinus. This should be attempted by employing drugs or DC electroversion in the same manner as in the nonpregnant state.[21,22]

In any case, if medical management of the disease does not improve the condition remarkably in just a few days, or if the patient's condition worsens, consideration should be given to valve replacement even in the pregnant state. (This is covered below in the second portion of this chapter.)

Pregnancy Following Valve Replacement

Many young women have undergone replacement of one or more cardiac valves with mechanical devices, and the literature is filled with case reports, but very few series of any size have been reported. A Mayo Clinic series containing only 40 pregnancies in 23 women is the largest reported from the United States.[2]

The most important challenge facing a physician caring for a pregnant woman who has undergone mechanical valve replacement appears to be related to those problems associated with the chronic anticoagulated state such patients must maintain. All of these women are at high risk for maternal and fetal complications. They should be prepared carefully for pregnancy and its complications and should be informed of the risks. Unfortunately, a review of pregnancies following valve replacement done at the Mayo Clinic disclosed that the pregnant women frequently received incomplete or incorrect advice from their attending physicians.

All women with mechanical heart valves should be seen by their obstetrician before attempting pregnancy. Unfortunately, many are not, but for all who do seek advice beforehand, certain concerns should be addressed.

First, the pregnant woman should have a clear idea of her chances for long term survival. This should be discussed fully with her by her cardiologist and cardiac surgeon. If it has not been done, the obstetrician should arrange for such a discussion. The obstetrician may add the information that studies by Chesley[23] and by Estafanous and Buckley[24] have shown convincingly that pregnancy does not shorten the lives of women with rheumatic heart disease. Even with the best of care, however, some women die from their cardiac disease despite valve replacement. The woman contemplating pregnancy must consider the possibility that she might die before her child becomes an adult.

The ability of the woman with a mechanical valve to undergo successful pregnancy is based largely on her NYHA functional classification prior to pregnancy and her compliance with the medical instructions she is given. This latter consideration must be emphasized to the patient. Many of the problems that have been encountered in pregnant women with mechanical valves have been results, ultimately, of patient noncompliance.

Mechanical heart valves cause a large number of pregnancy losses.[2,3,25-28] Few publications include information on very early pregnancy losses, but in the Mayo Clinic series, nearly half of all of the pregnancies in women who had mechanical valves and were taking coumarin resulted in spontaneous abortion.[2]

Women should also be cautioned that certain congenital anomalies seem to be associated wtih chronic use of coumarin derivatives during early pregnancy.[2,3,28,29] Although these generally are not life-threatening, they may cause facial disfiguration and developmental problems of the long bones. Certainly, most infants born after chronic coumarin exposure are normal, but anomalies are reported in approximately 10% of cases.

Prenatal evaluation should also consider a patient's fertility status. Since avoidance of coumarin derivatives during the first trimester of pregnancy will be recommended, some information concerning a patient's likelihood of conception should be obtained. For example, the woman who has menstrual bleeding only every 10 or 12 weeks may be pregnant for a considerable time before this fact is ascertained.

A woman taking coumarin derivatives who is attempting pregnancy should have the fact of conception confirmed as early as possible. With the availability of quantitative assays for human chorionic β-gonadotropin (hCG), it is possible to document pregnancy at approximately the time of implantation. Every woman taking coumarin drugs who is attempting to become pregnant should maintain a basal body temperature chart and, once ovulation has occurred, obtain an hCG assay if temperature remains elevated for five days.

Because of the expense involved in multiple pregnancy tests, it may be desirable to determine whether the fallopian tubes are patent before attempting pregnancy. For this, hysterosalpingography is recommended. Also recommended is a semen analysis to ascertain the likely fertility of the male sexual partner. With these evidences of potential fertility, it should be expected that conception will occur during the first few months, and only limited expense will be incurred by repeated testing for pregnancy.

Anticoagulant Therapy During Pregnancy

The use of anticoagulants in pregnancy is covered in great detail in Chapters 119 and 125. However, certain aspects relate particularly to those women who have mechanical valves.

Virtually all women who have had mechanical cardiac valves inserted are continuously anticoagulated.[2,3,28,30,31] In the United States, the drugs most commonly used for this purpose are the coumarin derivatives. These compounds have the advantage of being effective orally, and they maintain a fairly stable anticoagulated state over long periods. Their two disadvantages in pregnancy are that they have been associated with intrauterine fetal anomalies (the warfarin syndrome) and massive fetal hemorrhages even with close monitoring of the prothrombin time. As previously mentioned, there is some uncertainty about the frequency with which anomalies are associated with fetal exposure to coumarin derivatives in early pregnancy. However, it appears that this risk is significant enough that coumarin drugs should be withheld from pregnant women during the first trimester.

Once it is likely that conception has occurred, heparin should be substituted for the coumarin derivative. (Because of its molecular weight and charge, heparin does not cross the placenta and, therefore, does not reach the fetus.) The change from coumarin derivatives to heparin therapy is very critical. It is important that this be accomplished quickly to avoid a significant period during which the blood resumes its normal coagulable state. Should that occur, significant cerebral, coronary, and systemic embolization may develop.

The conversion to heparin may be attempted with the patient in or out of the hospital, depending on local circumstances. After the last dose of the long-acting anticoagulant, subcutaneous or intravenous administration of heparin should be started immediately.

There are two routes of administration of heparin: intravenous and subcutaneous.[32] The latter route has been used more often in an outpatient setting to maintain the activated partial thromplastin time (APTT) at 1.5–2 x normal control values, when checked six hours after a dose has been administered.

However, recent improvements in technology have simplified the long-term administration of intravenous heparin. Heparin may now be administered by way of a portable infusion pump through a centrally placed catheter (Hickman or Broivac type) in an outpatient situation.[33] The intravenous infusion rate may be adjusted up or down as necessary depending on the APTT value. Although heparin may also be administered by way of a peripheral vein, frequent site changes are mandatory to reduce infectious morbidity.

If the subcutaneous route of administration is chosen, heparin injections are generally administered in the subcutaneous tissues of the lower abdomen. Care must be taken not to inject the drug into abdominal muscles, which may result in bleeding or significant pain. Approximately 10,000 units of heparin must be given every 12 hours to achieve a significant anticoagulated state. The APTT or clotting time should be checked approximately six hours after the first dose, so the next dose may be adjusted up or down. It is necessary to obtain at least daily values for the clotting parameter for the first two weeks and then weekly. Unfortunately, even with seemingly adequate anticoagulation, there have been reported cases with life-threatening valve compromise.[28] A few of the newest mechanical valves are reported to have a much lower frequency of fatal valve clots with subcutaneous heparin administration.

Subcutaneous injection of heparin has the advantages of low risk and ease of patient self-administration. Sterile abscesses in the abdominal wall and hematomas can occur, but they usually are not more than nuisances. Thrombocytopenia may be striking in a few cases; platelets should be checked at least biweekly. Osteoporosis may also develop during pregnancy during long-term use of heparin. The patient should be counseled against the use of aspirin while on heparin therapy. Heparin therapy is also discussed in Chapters 119 and 125.

After the 16th week of gestation, the patient may be either changed back to coumarin derivatives or maintained with heparin throughout the pregnancy. The choice is not easy: heparin therapy avoids fetal risk but is somewhat difficult to manage; warfarin therapy is easy but there is concern about possible abnormalities of fetal eye and central nervous system (CNS) development even after the period of organogenesis. If return to coumarin is chosen, it is most important to continue the heparinization until an adequate response to coumarin has been obtained as demonstrated by prolongation of the prothrombin time to approximately two and a half times the normal value. After adequate anticoagulation is attained, prothrombin times should be checked weekly. It is rather common for the patient to require varying dosages of coumarin to maintain adequate anticoagulation as pregnancy approaches the third trimester.

Labor and Delivery. The patient with a mechanical heart valve must be prepared carefully for labor and delivery. The first, and perhaps most important, consideration is the anticogulated state. If the patient is on a warfarin derivative it is necessary to change to intravenous heparin. The pregnant woman will exhibit a normal prothrombin time approximately 72 hours after discontinuing the coumarin drug. However, it is well-documented that the fetus may continue to be anticoagulated for seven to 10 days after maternal discontinuance of the drug.

Gestational age should be known with considerable certainty in these cases. If there is any question about it, ultrasonography should be performed early in pregnancy and serially thereafter. At approximately the 37th week of gestation, the patient should be admitted to the hospital, and intravenous heparin therapy should be begun while coumarin therapy is discontinued. The patient should be maintained with intravenous heparin for at least seven days to allow for normal fetal coagulation factors to accumulate. At the end of seven days, the fetus may be considered to be at minimal or no risk from the forces of labor. Intravenous heparin therapy should be continued, and labor may be induced, or the patient may be watched until labor begins spontaneously. A more controlled situation will exist if induction is performed.

Heparin therapy should be continued during early labor if the patient is a primigravida but discontinued at the start of active labor if she has previously had vaginal deliveries. Heparin administered by continuous intravenous infusion has a half-life of approximately 30 minutes, so the APTT and clotting time should become nearly normal within four hours. Delivery should be timed to occur when the patient has just regained normal clotting values.

LABOR. It is most helpful if the patient has attended childbirth education classes for training in relaxation techniques. Often anesthesia and analgesia can be minimized or completely avoided in correctly prepared patients. This is most useful, since certain types of pain relief are best avoided in these cases. For example, epidural anesthesia is best avoided because the patient will be anticoagulated almost immediately after delivery, and bleeding into the epidural and subarachnoid space may occur.[34]

DELIVERY. Normal vaginal delivery may be allowed to occur if close attention is paid to avoiding techniques that may cause hematoma formation. For this reason, pudendal anesthesia is best avoided because of the frequency with which the pudendal vein and artery are punctured when the drug is administered. If episiotomy and repair require anesthesia, local anesthesia is best. When episiotomy is performed in a patient who will be anticoagulated in a few hours, great care should be taken that hemostatic stitches are placed. Use of several layers in the closure and deep figure-of-eight stitches in the perineal tissues is recommended. The uterus should be liberally massaged to encourage uterine contraction, and pitocin or ergot derivatives should be given to cause prolonged uterine contraction.

Intravenous heparin therapy should be restarted within four hours after delivery. Oral administration of coumarin derivatives may be started also, but a sufficient level of anticoagulation from these compounds will not be achieved for three or four days. It is important to restart the anticoagulants very soon after delivery. The chance of hematoma is increased by this, but a hematoma is a far less important problem than an embolism.

Pregnancy after Porcine Valve Placement

In recent years, glutaraldehyde-preserved porcine valves have been inserted in many patients with diseased valves. A review of the long-term results with these valves has indicated that they are capable of prolonged function.[3,35]

Women who have porcine valves in place, are in NYHA functional class I, and have no other cardiac disease usually require little, if any, special care during pregnancy. The major advantage of the porcine valve in pregnancy is the lack of need for anticoagulant therapy.

However, it is important that women with porcine valves have cardiac auscultation performed at each prenatal visit. Any difference in cardiac rhythm or a new murmur suggests possible developments that might be of great importance. A change in rhythm from sinus to atrial fibrillation or the development of a murmur suggesting either stenosis or regurgitation should be reported immediately to the patient's cardiologist. Additionally, any sign of cardiac decompensation should be investigated thoroughly.

Women with porcine valves should receive prophylaxis against bacterial endocarditis.

CARDIAC SURGERY DURING PREGNANCY

Cardiac disease should be diagnosed before pregnancy begins so that medical or surgical correction can be accomplished before the stress of pregnancy is added. Despite the logic of this statement, some cases of cardiac disease in young women await diagnosis by the obstetrician. The lesions may be either congenital or acquired. Except for peripartum cardiomyopathy, it is very rare for cardiac disease to develop for the first time during pregnancy.

Cardiac disease may present with different signs and symptoms in pregnancy than in the nonpregnant state. Cardiac auscultation during pregnancy usually reveals the presence of a systolic murmur, which probably is related to the increase of blood flow across the pulmonic and aortic valves. Additionally, the mammary vessels become dilated, and flow murmurs from these vessels, often extending into the carotid arteries, are common. A third heart sound may be detected, and, in some cases, a very soft diastolic murmur may be heard. For more detail on the diagnosis of cardiac disease, see Chapter 123.

Congenital Heart Disease

It is extremely rare for a pregnant woman to have significant congenital heart disease, discovered for the first time in pregnancy. With the multiple examinations that are routinely performed on children in the United States, most disease is diagnosed by age 12. Some anomalies, however—particularly small atrial and ventricular septal defects—may persist into adulthood and be detected late. The patient in such cases is often of functional class I, and usually her pregnancy may be allowed to continue and correction be delayed until several months postpartum. Nevertheless, cardiac consultation should always be obtained when there is any question concerning these defects.

Congenital cyanotic heart disease would not be detected for the first time during pregnancy. Patients with such severe problems have a short life span unless correction is performed early. However, "palliative" operations were often performed for tetralogy of Fallot in the past, and complete correction may never have been achieved. Certainly, prior cardiac surgery in any pregnant woman should be made known to a cardiologist, and the operative notes should be obtained.

Pulmonary hypertension occasionally becomes evident for the first time when a woman in her 20s becomes pregnant. Typically, its development in such cases has been insidious and slow, but some signs of compromise should have become noticeable before the start of pregnancy. These worsen progressively during the first few weeks. Pulmonary hypertension is an extremely serious and life-threatening abnormality when associated with pregnancy. Maternal mortality rates have been very high in all reported series.[11,13,16]

Some congenital disorders of the cardiac valve may be extremely mild and, consequently, may not have been detected during childhood. In general, management of such congenital lesions—if they are single—is much like management of acquired lesions, as described below. However, complete cardiac evaluation should be performed because there might be multiple defects. The safest and most informative procedure that may be performed during pregnancy is echocardiography (see also Chapter 127).

Acquired Heart Disease

Nearly all women who will require cardiac surgery during pregnancy have valvular disease from either rheumatic heart disease or bacterial endocarditis. The most prevalent single lesion is mitral stenosis, with aortic stenosis and regurgitation ranking next.

The woman with known cardiac disease should be followed very closely during pregnancy. If signs of cardiac decompensation become evident, medical management must be very aggressive. If overt congestive heart failure is noted, the patient should be admitted immediately to an intensive care unit and monitored carefully. Many of the usual clinical signs of congestive failure that are followed in the nonpregnant state become confusing during pregnancy. To monitor pregnant women with suspected heart failure, it is necessary to use Swan-Ganz catheterization.[36] This procedure is not entirely without complications; it must be used carefully and judiciously.[37] Maternal positioning also is important, since it may have much effect on the hemodynamic parameters. When the pregnant woman in the third trimester is lying supine, the enlarged uterus—particularly if the fetal head is engaged—markedly decreases venous return to the heart. This may result in an incorrect assessment of the cardiac status and reserve. The left lateral recumbent position is preferred for hemodynamic measurements during the latter part of pregnancy. Additionally, the supine position will often cause a decrease in utero-placental perfusion.

If aggressive medical management cannot stabilize the pregnant woman in congestive heart failure, delivery should be accomplished. While it is preferable to attain a fetal gestational age of at least 32 weeks before delivery, in severe maternal cardiac failure, it is occasionally necessary to deliver sooner. Although neonatal intensive care units generally can assure the survival of an infant weighing more than 750 g, prolonged hospitalization and possible long term sequelae are still common.

If it appears that delivery may improve the maternal condition, amniocentesis should be performed, and a sample sent for determination of the lecithin-sphingomyelin ratio and the presence of phosphatidyl-glycerol. These determinations may be made rapidly and are quite accurate in predicting the maturity of the fetal lungs. When the maternal condition continues to deteriorate despite delivery of the fetus, or when this may not be accomplished with safety, open-heart surgical correction of the cardiac defect must be employed.

Cardiopulmonary Bypass in Pregnancy

Maternal Considerations. There are now many reported cases of open-heart surgery during pregnancy. In general, the patients have done well during and after the procedure. At operation, the patient should be in a slightly levorotated position, if possible, to allow the uterus to move off the inferior vena cava.[36] Many obstetric suites have operating tables that allow a lateral tilt for cesarean sections. Although such tables are not generally available in the cardiac surgical areas, it may be useful to inquire whether one is available. If not, towels, sheets, or a wooden wedge may be placed under the right side of the maternal thorax and abdomen to effect a slight rotation into the left lateral position. Median sternotomy may still be carried out with ease in this position.

Recently, valve replacement has become the standard procedure for pregnant women with congestive heart failure not controlled by medical management. The patients have done well whether the procedure was necessitated by rheumatic heart disease or by bacterial endocarditis.[17] Usually a mechanical prosthesis must be employed, and this requires immediate institution of continuous anticoagulation. The considerations assessed above must be taken into account.

Valvulotomy also has been performed on large numbers of pregnant women with mitral valve disease, and although this is an older procedure, not often considered at the present time, the results may be quite good. One recent series of 42 cases showed excellent survival.[19]

Coronary artery disease, although uncommon in young females, can also be the indication for bypass surgery during pregnancy. Coronary artery disease is often manifested as an acute myocardial infarction during pregnancy, and has been treated successfully with coronary bypass grafting with good outcomes for both mother and fetus.[38] Percutaneous transcoronary angioplasty has also been performed during pregnancy to relieve significant angina following an acute myocardial infarction.[39] Using a short screening time and appropriate fetal shielding, fetal exposure to radiation is minimal.

Fetal Considerations. Continuous electronic fetal monitoring must be done throughout all cardiac surgery during pregnancy. Earlier reports of cardiopulmonary bypass during pregnancy did not include data from fetal monitoring[40], but more recent reports suggest that fetal distress during the procedure may result largely from inadequacy of the flow rate.[41] The personnel calculating the correct pump flow rate should be well informed regarding the altered hemodynamic status of a pregnant woman. Cardiac output may be increased 30–50% in a normal pregnant woman, and blood flow to the uterus alone may be 500 mL/min.

It is recommended that an obstetrician be present to observe the fetal heart-rate patterns during any open-heart operation performed during pregnancy. If abnormalities of the fetal heart tracing are noticed, the pump flow rate should be increased. This response has corrected the fetal heart-rate abnormality in some cases.[41]

REFERENCES

1. Harrison EC, Roschke EJ. Pregnancy in patients with cardiac valve prostheses. *Clin Obstet Gynecol.* 1975;18:107.
2. Lutz DJ, Noller KL, Spittell JA Jr, et al. Pregnancy and its complications following cardiac valve prostheses. *Am J Obstet Gynecol.* 1978;131:460.
3. Salazar E, Zajarias A, Gutierrez N, Iturbe I. The problem of cardiac valve protheses, anticoagulants, and pregnancy. *Circulation.* 1984;70:F-169.
4. Key TC, Resnik R, Dittrich HC, Reigner LS. Successful pregnancy after cardiac transplantation. *Am J Obstet Gynecol.* 1989;160:367.
5. Messer JV. Heart disease in pregnancy. *J Reprod Med* 1973;10:102.
6. Hoffman JIE, Christianson R. Congenital heart disease in a cohort of 19,502 births with long-term follow-up. *Am J Cardiol.* 1978;42:641.
7. Feldt RH, Avasthey P, Yoshimasu F, et al. Incidence of congenital heart disease in children born to residents of Olmsted County, Minnesota, 1950–1969. *Mayo Clin Proc.* 1971;16:794.
8. Nora JJ, Nora AH. The evolution of specific genetic and environmental counseling in congenital heart diseases. *Circulation* 1978;57:205.
9. Whittemore R, Hobbins JC. Pregnancy and genetics in congenital heart disease. Proceedings of the Society of Perinatal Obstetricians, Las Vegas, NV. February 1985.
10. Annegers JF, Elveback LR, Hauser WA, et al. Do anticonvulsants have a teratogenic effect? *Arch Neurol.* 1974;31:364.
11. Etheridge MJ, Pepperell RJ. Heart disease and pregnancy at the Royal Women's Hospital. *Med J Aust.* 1977;2:277.
12. Rayburn WF, Fontana ME. Mitral valve prolapse and pregnancy. *Am J Obstet Gynecol.* 1981;141:9.
13. Sugrue D, Blake S, MacDonald D. Pregnancy complicated by maternal heart disease at the National Maternity Hospital, Dublin, Ireland, 1969 to 1978. *Am J Obstet Gynecol.* 1981;139:1.
14. Loh TF, Tan NC. Fallot's tetralogy and pregnancy: a report of a successful pregnancy after complete correction. *Med J Aust.* 1971;2:141.
15. Cavalieri RL, Watkins L Jr, Abraham RA, et al. Acute bacterial endocarditis with postpartum aortic valve replacement. *Obstet Gynecol.* 1982;59:124.
16. De Swiet M, Fidler J. Heart disease in pregnancy: some controversies. *J R Coll Physicians Lond* 1981;15:183.
17. Payne DG, Fishburne JI Jr, Rufty AJ, et al. Bacterial endocarditis in pregnancy. *Obstet Gynecol.* 1982;60:247.
18. Szekely P, Turner R, Snaith L. Pregnancy and the changing pattern of rheumatic heart disease. *Br Heart J.* 1973;35:1293.
19. El-Maraghy M, Senna IA, El-Tehewy F, et al. Mitral valvotomy in pregnancy. *Am J Obstet Gynecol.* 1983;145:708.
20. Commerford PJ, Hastie T, Beck W. Closed mitral valvotomy: actuarial analysis of results in 654 patients over 12 years and analysis of preoperative predictors of long-term survival. *Ann Thorac Surg.* 1982;33:473.
21. Ogburn PL Jr, Schmidt G, Linman J, et al. Paroxysmal tachycardia and cardioversion during pregnancy. *J Reprod Med.* 1982;27:359.
22. DeSilva RA, Graboys TB, Podrid PJ, et al. Cardioversion and defibrillation. *Am Heart J.* 1980;100:881.
23. Chesley LC. Severe rheumatic cardiac disease and pregnancy: the ultimate prognosis. *Am J Obstet Gynecol.* 1980;136:552.
24. Estafanous FG, Buckley S. Management of anesthesia for open heart surgery during pregnancy. *Cleve Clin Q.* 1976;43:121.
25. Casanegra P, Aviles G, Maturana G, et al. Cardiovascular management of pregnant women with a heart valve prosthesis. *Ann J Cardiol.* 1975;36:802.
26. Oakley C, Doherty P. Pregnancy in patients after valve replacement. *Br Heart J.* 1976;38:1140.
27. Limet R, Grondin CM. Cardiac valve prostheses, anticoagulation, and pregnancy. *Ann Thorac Surg.* 1977;23:337.
28. Iturbe I, Fonseca M, Mutchink O, et al. Risks of anticoagulant therapy in pregnant women with artificial heart valves. *N Engl J Med.* 1986;315:1390.
29. DiSaia PJ. Pregnancy and delivery of a patient with a Starr-Edwards mitral valve prosthesis: Report of a case. *Obstet Gynecol.* 1966;28:469.
30. Chesebro JH, Fuster V. Thromboembolism in heart valve replacement. In: Kwaan HC, ed. *Textbook of Thrombosis.* Philadelphia, PA: WB Saunders; 1982:146.
31. Fuster V, Chesebro JH. Series on pharmacology in practice. 10. Antithrombotic therapy: Role of platelet-inhibitor drugs Ill. Management of arterial thromboembolic and atherosclerotic disease (third of three parts). *Mayo Clin Proc.* 1981;56:265.
32. Spearing G, Fraser I, Turner G, et al. Long-term self-administered subcutaneous heparin in pregnancy. *Br Med J.* 1978;1:1457.
33. Brabeck MC. Ambulatory management of thromboembolic disease during pregnancy with continuous infusion of heparin. *JAMA.* 1987;257:1790.
34. Pedersen H, Finster M. Anesthetic risk in the pregnant surgical patient. *Anesthesiology.* 1979;51:439.
35. Cohn LH, Mudge GH, Pratter F, et al. Five to eight-year follow-up of patients undergoing porcine heart-valve replacement. *N Engl J Med.* 1981;304:258.
36. Ueland K. Intrapartum management of the cardiac patient. *Clin Perinatol.* 1981;8:155.
37. Devitt JH, Noble WH, Byrick RJ. A Swan-Ganz catheter related complication in a patient with Eisenmengers syndrome. *Anesthesiology.* 1982;57:335.
38. Majdan JF, Walinsky Pt, Lowchoele SF, et al. Coronary artery bypass surgery during pregnancy. *Am J Cardiol.* 1983;52:1145.
39. Cowan NC, Belder MA, Rothman MT. Coronary angioplasty in pregnancy. *Br Heart J.* 1988;59:588.
40. Zitnik RS, Brandenburg RO, Sheldon R, et al. Pregnancy and open-heart surgery. *Circulation* 1969;39(suppl 1):257.
41. Levy DL, Warriner RA, Burgess GE Ill. Fetal response to cardiopulmonary bypass. *Obstet Gynecol.* 1980;56:112.

Chapter One Hundred and Thirty-Seven
Pregnancy After Cardiac Transplantation

Marla A. Mendelson

137

Cardiac transplantation for chronic end stage cardiac disease, congenital heart disease, and, more recently, primary pulmonary hypertension has increased over the past 20 years. Survival of these patients has increased due to improved immunosuppressive therapy with cyclosporine. In 1987, one year survival was greater than 80% and adult actuarial survival at five years was approximately 60%.[1] Quality of life is improved due to marked reduction of symptoms, decreased incidence of rejection, and better tolerance of medical regimens. As survival and quality of life improve, patients have been able to resume relatively normal lifestyles including return to work, as well as normal physical and sexual activities and this includes women of childbearing age who are now able to consider pregnancy. Pregnancy for the transplant patient raises complex medical and ethical issues that the physician, the patient, and her family must address prior to conception.

The physiologic and functional changes following cardiac transplantation create an altered and complex environment for both the mother and the developing fetus. Although the transplanted denervated heart usually demonstrates normal contractility and contractile reserve[2], chronotropic responses to exercise may be abnormal. In addition, the majority of patients treated with cyclosporine therapy may have increases in arterial blood pressure, which may cause alterations in cardiac hemodynamic measurements.[3] Pregnancy places increased demands on the cardiovascular system, because of increases in blood volume, changes in heart rate, and changes in vascular resistance. The anticipated physiologic changes rarely result in permanent impairment of a normal ventricle. The pregnant patient who has had cardiac transplantation cannot be expected to have a normal uncomplicated pregnancy. There may be complications unique to this group of patients, despite apparent restoration of health.

Table 137–1 demonstrates that four cases of pregnancy after cardiac transplantation have been reported in the literature[4-7], and two patients have become pregnant after heart-lung transplantation.[8] These cases illustrate some of the potential problems that may occur in this unique patient population. The patients reported were clinically stable with normal exercise capacity, under age 30, and became pregnant at least one year after surgery. One patient underwent an extensive work up prior to conception[6], whereas the other patients presented pregnant to their physicians. All of the patients became pregnant while taking immunosuppressive drugs on various regimens, including cyclosporine, azothiaprine, and corticosteroids, which were continued throughout pregnancy. Cesarean section was performed either for obstetric indications or the development of hypertension prior to term. There were no adverse fetal outcomes in these reported cases except that three[5,6,8] of the six babies were born premature and another pregnancy was complicated by preterm labor which resolved.[4] The only maternal death occurred five months postpartum due to poor compliance with the recommended medical regimen and subsequent transplant rejection.[4] As with renal transplant patients, the outcome of pregnancy after cardiac transplants appears to be encouraging, although the available data are still quite limited.

CARDIAC PATHOPHYSIOLOGY

Hemodynamic changes, which occur during normal pregnancy, may impact upon the transplanted heart, which may have altered intercardiac pressures, valvular abnormalities, abnormal physiologic responses, and accelerated atherosclerosis. Patients maintained on cyclosporine usually develop elevations in systolic and mean arterial blood pressure.[9] There are elevations in right atrial pressure, pulmonary artery, pulmonary capillary wedge, and end diastolic ventricular pressures. When compared to normal controls, ejection fraction, cardiac index, and stroke volume index are slightly lower, although myocardial biopsy in the posttransplant patients reveals either abnormal fibrosis or inflammation.[3] The transplanted denervated heart is subject to inherent physiologic changes, as well as to the effects of immunosuppressive agents. Hemodynamic alterations have been documented in asymptomatic cardiac transplant patients who almost uniformly have elevations in their systolic and mean arterial blood pressures when studied on cyclosporine. In a small subset of patients, restudied at two years, these changes improved or resolved.

Tricuspid regurgitation was present in two thirds of the patients during the first year after transplantation, but in only one third at the end of one year.[9] This was associated with enlargement of the right ventricle. Normal pregnancy has been associated with right ventricular enlargement with tricuspid regurgitation as a result of increased blood volume and, theoretically, these patients may have worsening of tricuspid regurgitation. Physiologic responses of the transplanted heart have been studied with pharmacologic challenge[3] and during exercise.[10] Ventricular contractile characteristics and cardiac reserve in transplanted hearts without evidence of rejection are essentially normal. However, an exaggerated chronotrophic response to catecholamine challenge has been demonstrated.[2] After cardiac transplantation, patients can tolerate exercise and usually become New York Heart Association functional class I or II, although the transplanted heart is a denervated heart and responds differently to stress and exercise. The heart rate increase with exercise may be delayed and initial adaptation occurs by use of the Frank-Starling mechanism.[10] The usual decrease in heart rate during recovery is attenuated in the transplant patient. However, cardiac output does rise appropriately.[10]

The cardiac transplant patient is also at an increased risk for the development of coronary atherosclerosis and she has to be followed closely for development of myocardial ischemia, infarction, and congestive heart failure, or complex ventricular ectopy. The development of atherosclerosis occurs in up to 50% of patients at five years.[9] It is poorly understood and may be due to chronic rejection. Therefore, the definitive treatment would be retransplantation.[9]

TABLE 137–1. SUMMARY OF REPORTED CASES OF PREGNANCY AFTER CARDIAC AND HEART-LUNG TRANSPLANTATION

Patients	Age (Months)	Post-operative (Months)	Immunosuppression	Medications	Outcome Fetal	Outcome Maternal
Heart Transplant						
#1 (Inoperable cardiac tumor)[4]	23	60	Prednisone, azathioprine	Dipyridamole, trimethaphan, sulfumeth-oxazole	39 wks normal infant	Died at five months—rejection of trans-plant
#2 (Cardiomyopathy)[5]	19	14	Cyclosporine	Furosemide	31 wks	
#3 (Postpartum cardiomyopathy)[6]	29	60	Prednisone, azathioprine	Aspirin	36 wks	34 wks—Listeria infection
#4 (Cardiomyopathy)[7]	28	20	Cyclosporine, prednisone	Aspirin	38 wks	
Heart-Lung Transplant						
#5 (Pulmonary arteriopathy)[8]	19	22	Cyclosporine, azathioprine		34 wks normal infant	
#6 (Eisenmenger's—VSD)[8]	20	24	Cyclosporine, azathioprine		Term, normal infant	

IMMUNOSUPPRESSION

The patient who has received a cardiac transplant is continually at risk of rejection. She must be maintained lifelong on immunosuppressive medications, which usually include a regimen of prednisone with either cyclosporine or azathioprine. Patients are continually monitored for clinical signs and symptoms of rejection, which include fever, weight gain, edema, and dyspnea. The electrocardiographic signs of rejection include arrhythmia and decreased QRS voltage. Patients are also monitored periodically with myocardial biopsies to diagnose definitively rejection. Fertility does not appear to be affected by immunosuppressive therapy.[11] Immunosuppressive agents pose risks not only to the patient, but also to a developing fetus. Many of those complications of immunosuppressive agents have been studied in renal transplant patients who have become pregnant.[12] In that population, fetal growth retardation has been ascribed to immunosuppressive therapy. Other factors may, however, also influence fetal growth, such as impaired renal function, persistent hypertension, and the effects of antihypertensive medications.[13]

Cyclosporine has been shown to improve survival in renal and cardiac transplant patients. In pregnancy, it has been studied in the renal transplant population. Cyclosporine acts upon T-lymphocytes, thereby inhibiting aspects of cellular immunity. Almost uniformly, patients develop hypertension[10] and medications to control hypertension are required. Other maternal risks of cyclosporine include nephrotoxicity, hepatotoxicity, tremor, hirsutism, paresthesias, seizures, tremor, gout, and gingival hypertrophy.[14] During pregnancy, radioimmunoassays can be performed to maintain 24 hour serum levels of cyclosporine at 50–150 mg/mL[12,14] and immunosuppressive activity can be assessed using a mixed lymphocyte culture assay of suppression.[8] Although body weight may increase in pregnancy, the doses of cyclosporine do not have to be increased accordingly. In fact, in some studies of renal transplant patients, it has been found that the doses have to be lowered during later stages of pregnancy.[12] Blood levels will decline by 50% at 48 hours postpartum and be undetectable in the baby at one week.[14] Levels of cyclosporine have been documented in breast milk, therefore, breast-feeding is contraindicated for patients who remain on cyclosporine.[12] Cyclosporine crosses the placenta and levels have been found in the fetus. They may have immunosuppressive properties throughout the first week of life. Chromosomal abnormalities have, however, not been identified in animal studies.[12] Cyclosporine has been shown to be embryogenic and fetotoxic in some animal studies[15] at toxic doses, although lethal or teratogenic effects were not seen at clinical doses. A study of two infants' cord lymphocytes demonstrated no evidence of chronic immunosupperssion.[8] The drug may also be associated with growth retardation[12] and neonatal thrombocytopenia.[14]

Most immunosuppressive regimens include prednisone, which decreases the number of circulating monocytes and lymphocytes, blocks antigen sensitization, and inhibits the response of monocyte chemotactic factors. The side effects of prednisone include weight gain, fluid retention, electrolyte abnormalities, glucose intolerance, peptic ulceration, increased risk of infection, elevated blood pressure, and osteoporosis.[16] Long-term use puts the patient at risk for pancreatitis, myopathy, elevated intraocular pressure, psychosis, cataracts, striae, acne, and aseptic bone necrosis. There is no known teratogenicity. However, some studies in pregnancy have suggested an increased incidence of spontaneous abortions, placental insufficiency, exophthalmos, and cleft palate.[11] Fetal lymphocytes may be resistant to glucocorticoid medications administered during pregnancy.[17] Numerous studies, which document the use of steroids during pregnancy for many other medical illnesses, suggest that corticosteroids in general are safe during gestation.

The third drug that has been used for immunosuppression is azathioprine. It is a derivative of 6-mercaptopurine and suppresses T-lymphocytes and cell-mediated immunity.[18] The side effects of this drug are dose-dependent and include bone marrow suppression, increased susceptibility to infection, rash, alopecia, gastrointestinal upset, arthralgias, hypersensitivity pancreatitis, and toxic hepatitis. Long-term use may be associated with risk of tumors.[18] Active metabolites cross the placenta.[19] Again, most of the experience in the use of this drug in pregnancy has been gleaned from experience with renal transplant patients. There is no confirmed teratogenicity of azathioprine to humans, although there have been reports in animal studies.[18] There have also been reports of chromosomal aberrations.[18]

In mothers taking immunosuppressants after renal transplants, the incidence of small-for-gestational-age babies is as high as 60–70% in patients who had an otherwise uncomplicated neonatal course.[20] It may, however, be difficult to distinguish the effects of the drug from the effects of the underlying maternal illness.

A monoclonal antibody (OKT3) to T cells is now also being used to reverse acute rejection and as a prophylactic agent. OKT3 eliminates circulating T cells within hours of administration. The adverse reactions associated with this agent include susceptibility to infection and neoplasm, tremor, headache, anaphylactic shock, chest pain, hypotension, neurospasm, pulmonary edema, gastrointestinal upset, rash, and allograft vascular thrombosis.[21] There have been no reports of the use of this agent in pregnancy.

RISK OF INFECTION

The chronically immunosuppressed patient is at an increased risk of infections. Bacterial, viral, and protozoal infection occur early after surgery. Listeria or cryptococcal infections may occur at any time after transplantation, whereas cytomegalovirus (CMV), toxoplasmosis, and opportunistic infection usually occur in the first six months.[22] The incidence of infection falls after the first year. Both the mother and fetus are at risk for the development of CMV infections[22,23], although the incidence has not been documented. Rubella is another risk, and it has been recommended that mothers be immunized three months prior to a transplant and prior to being placed on immunosuppressive agents.

ANTENATAL RISK ASSESSMENT AND PRENATAL MANAGEMENT

The cardiac transplant patient desiring pregnancy faces a difficult decision involving multiple medical, social, and ethical issues that impact not only on the patient, but also on her family and the developing fetus. The reported cases of pregnancy after cardiac transplantation are limited but pregnancy was usually undertaken in patients who were asymptomatic and were New York Heart Association functional class I.[4-8] The patient with normal cardiac function, documented by echocardiography, and cardiac catheterization without evidence of rejection by myocardial biopsy, or evidence of coronary atherosclerosis by angiography, would be expected to tolerate best the hemodynamic changes of pregnancy. Therefore, ideally, patients should undergo assessment prior to conception, including hemodynamic parameters, functional capacity, angiography, and myocardial biopsy. The patient should be evaluated by the transplant physician, along with a cardiologist and obstetrician specializing in high risk obstetrical care. Evaluation of cardiac function throughout the pregnancy can be performed with echocardiography to follow cardiac chamber size, ventricular wall motion, and tricuspid regurgitation. Immunosuppressive therapy is maintained and cyclosporine serum trough levels should be monitored closely by radioimmunoassay throughout pregnancy and doses adjusted accordingly. Cyclosporine will concentrate in placental tissue and levels have, as noted earlier, been reported to abruptly increase postpartum, thus requiring that doses be decreased.[12] Patients may also be on antihypertensive drugs and the specific risks of these drugs to the fetus need also be considered. Infections unique to this patient population may occur and must be treated promptly and aggressively. These patients require close monitoring throughout pregnancy by the obstetrician, cardiologist, and transplant physician. Also, prenatal consultation during the third trimester with the anesthesiologist is strongly encouraged to anticipate anesthetic management and potential complications of delivery.

MANAGEMENT OF LABOR AND DELIVERY

The management of delivery should be planned well in advance, as these patients may deliver early. The mode of delivery is usually determined by obstetric indications. Hemodynamic monitoring to assess ventricular filling pressures may be of use if the patient requires a cesarean section or if there are abnormal baseline hemodynamics. It is recommended that the cardiac transplant patient receive antibiotic prophylaxis with penicillin and gentamycin for cesarean section or forceps delivery.[11] The selection of antibiotics for the patient allergic to penicillin may be complicated, as some antibiotics, such as erythromycin, trimethoprim, sulfamethoxazole, and ciprofloxacin, may interact adversely with cyclosporine.

The increased sensitivity of the denervated heart to catecholamines must be considered in the anesthetic management of the patient, as these patients may have arrhythmias, which are possibly due to the increased sensitivity to catecholamines[24], but may also be a manifestation of rejection. These patients also have a lack of normal vagal tone and vagal reflex activity.[6] Therefore, only direct-acting agents will exert inotropic or chronotropic effects.[24] There may also be a blunted chronotropic response to stress. Elective cesarean section after cardiac transplantation was performed using epidural anesthesia.[4,6] This allows a controlled administration of anesthetics with respect to balancing peripheral vasodilatation and volume loading.[6]

LONG-TERM CONSIDERATIONS

Breast-feeding is not recommended for the mother on immunosuppression.[12,20] Cyclosporine has been found to be present in breast milk in concentrations as high as in maternal blood.[12,14] Azathioprine and prednisone have also been found in breast milk, though in small quantities.

The patient and her family must be aware of her actuarial survival as a cardiac transplant patient, her risk of atherosclerosis, and how her state of health may impact the baby's future development and care. Any permanent effects of pregnancy upon the transplanted heart have not been elucidated.

CONTRACEPTION

Contraception is a complex problem in the patients who do not desire pregnancy after cardiac transplantation, as options for birth control are limited. Immunosuppressive drugs may interfere with the function of intrauterine devices and, therefore, with their effectiveness. The intrauterine device also poses the risk of infection and is, thus, an unpreferred mode of contraception.[11] Birth control pills carry the risk of myocardial infarction, hypertension, thromboembolic events, or stroke and may interact with steroids and antibiotics. The progestins may adversely affect lipids which may be problematic in the patient already at risk for accelerated atherosclerosis. For these reasons, birth control pills are not recommended in the cardiac transplant patient. Data has, however, remained limited.[11] In summary, barrier methods are probably the safest temporary method for birth control with the least effect upon the health of the patient. However, decreased efficacy needs to be considered in any decision about its use. Many centers counsel patients to undergo tubal ligation.

REFERENCES

1. Schroeder JS, Hunt SA. Cardiac transplantation: where are we? *N Engl J Med.* 1986;315:961.
2. Borow KM, Neumann A, Frederick BS, et al. Left ventricular contractility and reserve in humans after cardiac transplantation. *Circulation.* 1985;71:866.
3. Greenberg ML, Uretsky BF, Reddy PS, et al. Long-term hemodynamic follow-up of cardiac transplant patients treated with cyclosporine and prednisone. *Circulation.* 1985;71:487.
4. Key TC, Resnik R, Dittrich HC, Reisner LS. Successful pregnancy after cardiac transplantation. *Am J Obstet Gynecol.* 1989;160:367.
5. Lowenstein BR, Vain NW, Perrone SV, et al. Successful pregnancy and vaginal delivery after heart transplantation. *Am J Obstet Gynecol.* 1988;158:589.
6. Camann WR, Goldman GA, Johnson MD, et al. Cesarean delivery in a patient with a transplanted heart. *Anesthesiology.* 1989;71:618.
7. Lopes P, Petit T, Quentin M, et al. Grossesse et accouchement chez une transplantic cardiaque. *La Presse Medical.* 1988;17:869.
8. Rose ML, Dominguez M, Leaver N, et al. Analysis of T-cell subpopulations and cyclosporine levels in the blood of two neonates born to immunosuppressed heart-lung transplant recipients. *Transplantation.* 1989;48:223.
9. Thompson JA, Rider-Katz S, Hess ML, et al. Management and long-term following of outpatient care in the cardiac transplant recipiant. In: Thompson ME, ed. *Cardiac Transplantation.* Philadelphia, PA: F.A. Davis Company; 1990:213.
10. Pope SE, Stinson EB, Daughters GT, et al. Exercise response of the denervated heart in long term cardiac transplant recipients. *Am J Cardiol.* 1980;46:213.
11. Kossoy LR, Herbert CM III, Colston Wentz A. Management of heart transplant recipients: guidelines for the obstetrician-gynecologist. *Am J Obstet Gynecol.* 1988;159:490.
12. Flechner SM, Katz AR, Rogers AJ, et al. The presence of cyclosporine in body tissues and fluids during pregnancy. *Am J Kid Dis.* 1985;5:60.
13. Hou S. Pregnancy in women with chronic renal disease. *N Engl J Med.* 1985;312:836.
14. Berkowitz RL, Coustam DR, Mochizuk TK, eds. *Handbook for Prescribing Medications During Pregnancy.* 2nd ed. Boston: Little, Brown, and Company; 1986:94.
15. Mason RJ, Thomson AW, Whiting PH, et al. Cyclosporine induced fetotoxicity in the rat. *Transplantation.* 1985;39:9.
16. Berkowitz RL, Coustam DR, Mochizuk TK, eds. *Handbook for Prescribing Medications During Pregnancy,* 2nd ed. Boston: Little, Brown, and Company; 1986:85.
17. Kauppila A, Hartikainen-Sorri AL, Koivisto M, Ryhanen P. Cell-mediated immunocompetence of children exposed in utero to short- or long-term action of glucocorticoids. *Gynecol Obstet Invest.* 1983;15:41.
18. Berkowitz RL, Coustam DR, Mochizuk TK, eds. *Handbook for Prescribing Medications During Pregnancy,* 2nd ed. Boston: Little, Brown, and Company; 1986:33.
19. Saarikoski S, Seppala M. Immunosuppression during pregnancy: transmission of azothioprione and its metabolites from the mother to the fetus. *Am J Obstet Gynecol.* 1973;115:1100.
20. Lau RJ, Scott JR. Pregnancy following renal transplantation. *Clin Obstet Gynecol.* 1985;28:339.
21. Cameron DE, Traill TA. Complications of immunosuppressive therapy. In: Baumgartner WA, Reitz BA, Achuff SC, eds. *Heart and Heart-Lung Transplantation.* Philadelphia: WB Saunders Co; 1990:237.
22. Dummer JS, Bahnson HT, Griffith BP, et al. Infections in patients on cyclosporine and prednisone following cardiac transplantation. *Tranplant Proc.* 1983;15:2779.
23. Onorato IM, Morens DM, Martone WJ, Stansfield SK. Epidemiology of cytomegaloviral infections: recommendations for prevention and control. Rev Infect Dis. 1985;7:479.
24. Kanter SF, Samuels SI. Anesthesia for major operations on patients who have transplanted hearts, a review of 29 cases. *Anesthesiology.* 1977;46:65.

PART XI | Hypertensive Disease

Baha M. Sibai, Section Editor

Chapter One Hundred and Thirty-Eight

Pathophysiology of Hypertensive Disorders

Gustaaf Albert Dekker and Baha M. Sibai

138

NORMOTENSIVE PREGNANCY

Impressive physiologic changes take place in pregnancy in the uteroplacental vasculature in general and in the cardiovascular system in particular, most likely induced by the interaction of the fetal (paternal) allograft with maternal tissue. The development of mutual immunologic tolerance[1] in the first trimester is thought to lead to important morphologic and biochemical changes in the systemic and uteroplacental maternal circulation.

The human placenta receives its blood supply from numerous uteroplacental arteries that are developed by the action of migratory interstitial and endovascular trophoblast on the spiral arteries in the placental bed. Morphologic changes due to invasion of migratory trophoblast into the walls of the spiral arteries transform the uteroplacental arterial bed into a low resistance, low pressure, high flow system. The conversion of the spiral arteries of the nonpregnant uterus to the uteroplacental arteries has been termed *physiological changes* by Brosens and others.[2] In a normal pregnancy, these trophoblast-induced vascular changes extend from the intervillous space to the origin of the spiral arteries from the radial arteries in the inner one-third of the myometrium. It is suggested that these vascular changes are effected in two stages: "the conversion of the decidual segments of the spiral arteries by a wave of endovascular trophoblast migration in the first trimester and the myometrial segments by a subsequent wave in the second trimester."[3]

During the first trimester blood volume begins to increase, reaching a level of about 40% above nonpregnant values at week 30 of gestation. Part of the rise in blood volume results from an increase in the number of erythrocytes. A much larger portion of the increase is caused by expansion of plasma volume, which rises to a level about 50% above nonpregnant values by week 32 of pregnancy. The increase in plasma volume is believed to be subsequent to changes in the eicosanoid and renin-angiotensin-aldosterone system (RAAS), possibly following the rise in blood progesterone and estrogen levels seen in normal pregnancy.[4] Release of renin initiates a sequence of events that results in salt and water retention, thus expanding plasma volume.

The large increases in plasma volume and interstitial space are accompanied by a gradual retention of 800–1000 mEq of sodium. This gain, distributed between the products of conception (40%) and the maternal compartment (60%), accumulates gradually over a 9-month period.[5] During pregnancy, effective renal plasma flow and glomerular filtration rate (GFR) increase to levels of 30–50% above those measured in nonpregnant women. Increments in GFR are observed already during the initial weeks following conception. They peak by the early second trimester and are sustained through the 36th gestational week, after which a small decrease may occur. The increment in GFR means that the filtered load of sodium also will increase by 30–50% as compared with nonpregnant levels, or from about 20,000 mEq/day to as much as 30,000 mEq/day. Such increments in filtered load obviously must be accompanied by parallel increments in tubular reabsorption. The adaptive incremental tubular reabsorption of sodium accommodates the large increase in filtered load in pregnancy, and an additional 2–6 mEq of sodium is reabsorbed daily for fetal and maternal stores. This increase in tubular reabsorption represents the largest renal adjustment during pregnancy.[5,6]

The RAAS plays an important role in the control of vascular tone and blood pressure. In this system, angiotensinogen secreted by the liver is cleared by renin to produce angiotensin I. Inactive angiotensin I then is converted into biologically active angiotensin II by angiotensin-converting enzyme that is bound to vascular endothelium. Circulating angiotensin II interacts with specific receptors to induce smooth muscle contraction, stimulates aldosterone production and sodium retention, facilitates norepinephrine release and inhibits norepinephrine reuptake by sympathetic nerve terminals, and thus potentiates vascular smooth muscle reactivity to norepinephrine. In normal pregnancy, concentrations of all components of the RAAS are increased.[7] However, the vascular response to most pressor substances is impaired.[8]

Biochemical adaptations in the maternal vasculature

also include changes in the prostaglandin system, leading to an increasing dominance of the vasodilator and platelet-aggregation of PGI_2 over the vasoconstrictor and platelet-aggregation–promoting effects of platelet-derived TXA_2. The physiologic inhibition of platelet aggregation in the uteroplacental vascular bed, as well as the vasodilatation and low vascular resistance to flow, and the vascular refractoriness to vasoconstrictors, such as angiotensin II and norepinephrine, may depend on production of biologically balanced amounts of vasodilator prostaglandins and vasoconstrictor TXA_2 (Fig. 138–1).

The mechanisms underlying the increase in production of vasodilator prostaglandins, the interrelationships with adaptational changes in vasoconstrictor systems, and the possible links to fetal-maternal immunologic interaction are still obscure. Recently, a number of these adaptational changes have been summarized by Wallenburg[9] (Fig. 138–2).

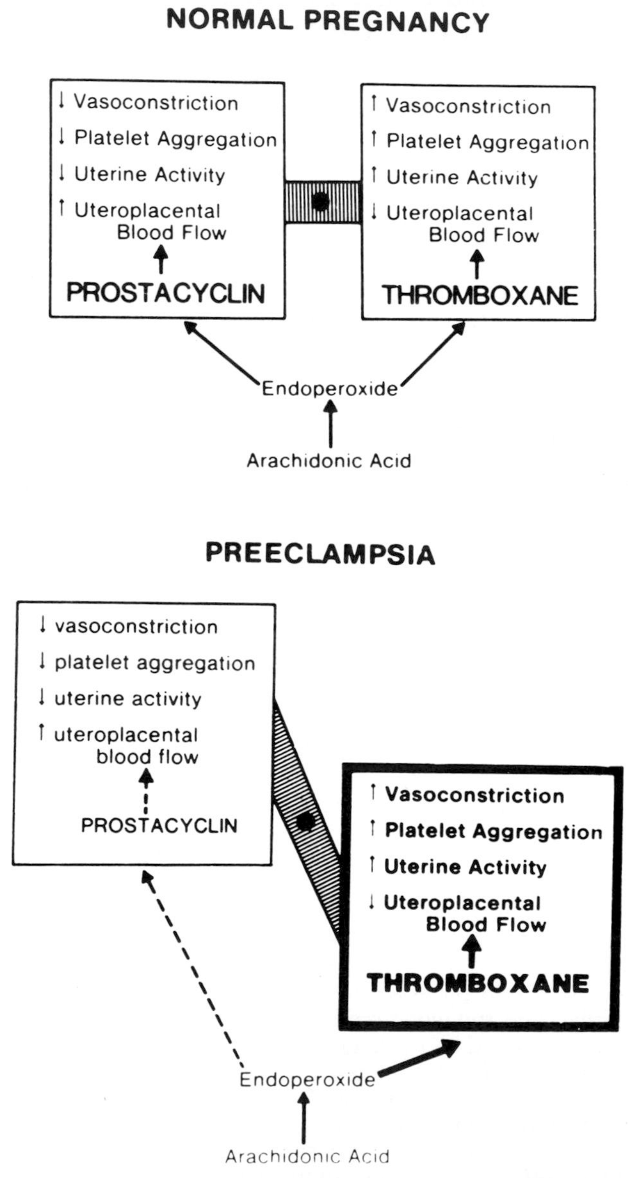

Figure 138–1. Comparison of the balance in the biologic actions of prostacyclin and thromboxane in normal pregnancy with the imbalance of increased thromboxane and decreased prostacyclin in preeclamptic pregnancy. The heavy type and box for thromboxane suggest an exacerbation of its actions in preeclampsia, whereas the lighter type and box for prostacyclin suggest a diminution of its actions. *(From Walsh[44] with permission.)*

HYPERTENSIVE PREGNANCY

Hypertensive disorders in pregnancy constitute a syndrome, that is, a collection of signs and, to a lesser extent, symptoms which have been observed clinically to occur together and to form a characteristic pattern, but are not necessarily due to the same pathologic cause. The central signs by which the hypertensive syndrome in pregnancy is recognized are an elevated arterial blood pressure and a pregnant or early postpartum state. Other classic signs of the syndrome are edema, proteinuria, and convulsions.

The terminology and definitions used to describe the hypertensive disorders of pregnancy have been, and still are, inconsistent and confusing.[10] More than 60 names in English and over 40 in German have been applied to the condition; *toxemia, toxicosis,* and *gestosis* are still used in many countries. Most definitions of the syndrome emphasize four features, occurring alone or in combination: hypertension, edema, proteinuria, and convulsions. Of these, an elevation of blood pressure is essential to define the disorder as hypertensive. However, the threshold between normotension and hypertension has been defined using various and mostly arbitrarily chosen levels; the same is true for the definitions of pathologic proteinuria. The diagnosis of convulsions causes little difficulty, but the recognition and assessment of edema is very subjective.

Another and perhaps even more important source of confusion is the fact that the hypertensive syndrome in pregnancy comprises two different etiologic entities. One is pregnancy-induced hypertensive disease, a disorder induced by pregnancy, the cause of which lies within the gravid uterus. It is a disease mainly, but not exclusively, of the nullipara. It appears in the course of pregnancy and is reversed by delivery. The other condition is preexisting chronic hypertension or proteinuria, unrelated to, but coinciding with pregnancy, which may be detected for the first time in pregnancy and will not regress after delivery. To complicate matters further, the two conditions may occur together in one patient.

This review of the pathophysiology of hypertensive pregnancy will focus on pregnancy-induced hypertensive disorders that, as a group, will be designated PIH.

VOLUME OF BLOOD AND WATER

Many investigators agree that pregnancies complicated by a pregnancy-induced hypertensive disorder, at least in its more severe forms, are associated with a reduction in plasma volume, roughly in proportion to the severity of the disease. Chesley[11] reported that the average plasma volume in women with preeclampsia was 9% below expected values and was as much as 30–40% below normal in those with severe disease. It is not clear whether the reduction in maternal plasma volume is a cause or a result of the vasoconstriction. Some investigators have demonstrated that inadequate plasma volume expansion occurs before any clinical signs of PIH are present.[12] On the other hand, Sibai et al[13] found no difference in mean plasma volumes between normotensive pregnant women and women with mild pregnancy-

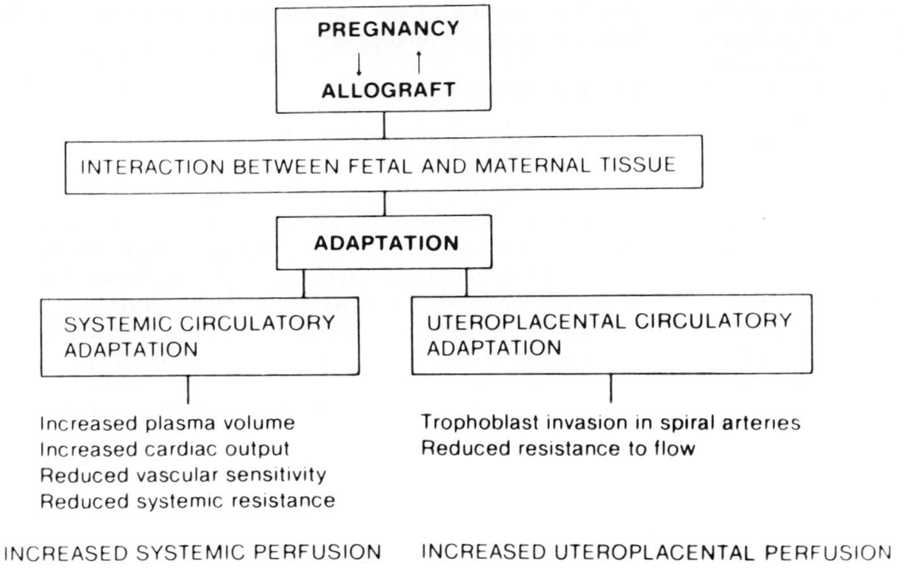

Figure 138–2. Concept of physiologic adaptational circulatory changes in pregnancy. *(From Wallenberg[9] with permission.)*

induced hypertension. Plasma volume in this study was reduced only in pregnancies with mild pregnancy-induced hypertension and delivery of small-for-gestational-age infants. In this study, no patient showed a reduction of plasma volume antedating the development of hypertension.

Even if a reduction in plasma volume antedates the development of hypertension, that is no proof that the contraction of plasma volume causes the vasoconstriction. In normotensive pregnancy, vasodilatation precedes any alteration in circulating blood volume. Gant et al[14] showed that the increase in pressor response to angiotensin II, which precedes the clinical development of PIH, antedates all other cardiovascular changes, including the decrease in circulating blood volume. These observations are consistent with the concept that the development of PIH begins with a loss of vascular refractoriness to vasoactive agents, followed by vasoconstriction. This results in a decrease in intravascular volume, and intravascular water is shunted to extravascular spaces.

The decrease in plasma volume results in hemoconcentration. With increasing hemoconcentration, the circulatory properties of the blood will change. In preeclampsia, Buchan[15] found a mean increase of 30% in whole blood viscosity. This increased viscosity is caused by increased hematocrit, reduced red cell deformability, and increased plasma viscosity. Hyperviscosity reduces the oxygenation of the tissues with a fall in the local pH, which in turn causes an increasing rigidity of the erythrocyte wall. The rigid red cell in PIH may fragment during capillary passage, causing the hemolysis that is a clinical sign of severe preeclampsia.[16] The reduced flow qualities of the blood during severe PIH also may be of pathophysiologic importance in causing (coupled with a disturbance in platelet-vessel wall interaction) thrombosis in the uteroplacental arteries. The frequency of large placental infarcts, leading to fetal growth retardation and perinatal death, is correlated positively with the hematocrit of the mother, and in preeclampsia maternal hemoglobin concentration is inversely correlated with the weight percentile of the newborn.[17]

In preeclamptic gravidae, GFR and effective renal plasma flow are, on the average, 30% and 20% lower, respectively, than in normotensive pregnant women, and usually fall in ranges that would be normal in nonpregnant women. Preeclamptic women have lower urinary sodium concentration or excretory rates, and they also excrete a smaller percentage of an infused sodium load as compared with normotensive pregnant women. A salt tolerance test was used once as a means of distinguishing PIH from other hypertensive disorders during pregnancy. However, the degree of impairment in the ability to excrete sodium varies considerably.[18]

In contrast to what might be expected, plasma atrial natriuretic peptide (ANP) levels in PIH are raised, the highest values found in severe preeclampsia.[19] ANP levels also are elevated in patients with essential hypertension who usually have an increased central venous pressure and pulmonary capillary wedge pressure. This may explain the increased production of ANP in this condition. In contrast, preeclamptic patients have a low central venous pressure and a low or normal pulmonary capillary wedge pressure. It currently is not known why preeclampsia is associated with increased plasma ANP concentrations.

HEMODYNAMICS

Systemic Blood Pressure

By definition, arterial blood pressure is elevated in hypertensive pregnant women, whether they have pregnancy-induced hypertensive disease or chronic hypertension. Also, blood pressure behavior appears to be altered in hypertensive pregnant women. Women with PIH may have a reversal of the normal diurnal blood-pressure rhythm, so that the highest levels occur during the night. Hypertension in PIH is characteristically labile, probably reflecting the intense sensitivity of the vasculature to the endogenous vasoconstrictor substances, angiotensin II, TXA_2, and catecholamines. In women with PIH, blood pressure usually returns rapidly to normal following parturition, but in 10–20% of cases hypertension may continue or even increase during the puerperium. This may be followed by a slow fall, with blood pressure returning to normal only after weeks of observation.

Cardiac Output

The cardiovascular hemodynamics of preeclampsia have been reported to range from a low-output, high-resistance state to a high-output, low-resistance state. Hankins et al[20] reviewed the six published studies and classified them according to therapy prior to insertion of the Swan-Ganz catheter. Proposed explanations for the differences in the various hemodynamic studies are as follows: (1) small number of patients in each series (usually 10 or less), (2) variable severity and duration of preeclampsia, (3) underlying medical problems such as cardiac or renal disease, (4) therapeutic interventions prior to invasive monitoring, and (5) the dynamic fluctuation of the cardiovascular system. This sensitivity makes it difficult to control for all the variables that can affect hemodynamics, for example, gestational age, labor, pain, anxiety, hydralazine, intravenous fluids, analgesics, and anesthesia. For practical reasons, patients often are transferred to a tertiary care center several hours after initial therapy has been started. In addition, the clinical diagnosis of preeclampsia often is suspect, particularly in patients remote from term when underlying renal disease is likely. Most reports in the literature concern uncontrolled studies and describe only a few patients studied during childbirth, lying on their back, or receiving parenteral fluids, antihypertensive treatment, or magnesium sulfate. An important exception is the report by Wallenburg.[9] In this report, the author compared the hemodynamic findings in preeclamptic women before treatment, during and after treatment, and in normotensive patients. The cardiac index was significantly lower in the untreated preeclamptic group with a median of 3 L/min/m^2 (range 2.0–4.7) as compared to the treated group with a median of 3.8 L/min/m^2 (range 2.2–7.1) and to the normotensive group, with a median of 4 L/min/m^2 (range 3.9–5.0).[21]

Recently, Easterling et al[22] measured cardiac output by Doppler technique longitudinally in 120 nulliparous women throughout pregnancy. Six women (5%) became preeclamptic, 43 (36%) developed PIH, and 71 (59%) remained normotensive. In pregnancies complicated by preeclampsia, cardiac output was significantly elevated prior to onset of hypertension and remained higher than that found in normotensives throughout pregnancy. There were no differences among the groups in calculated systemic vascular resistance. They concluded that preeclampsia is a hyperdynamic condition characterized by elevated cardiac output rather than increased systemic vascular resistance.

Peripheral Vascular Resistance

Since systemic arterial blood pressure is elevated in PIH and cardiac output is said to be decreased in the untreated patient, the calculated peripheral vascular resistance must be elevated. The calculated increase in peripheral vascular resistance may be expected because vasoconstriction is fundamental to the disease process of PIH. The vasoconstriction imposes a resistance to blood flow and accounts for the development of arterial hypertension. Alternatively, the increased blood pressure may be due to increased cardiac output. The issue remains unresolved.

VASOCONSTRICTOR AND VASODILATOR SYSTEMS

There is evidence that the vasoconstriction that occurs in pregnant women who develop PIH results from a breakdown of the normally benign interaction between vasoconstrictor and vasodilator systems. A brief overview is presented of the changes that have been reported to occur in the vasoconstrictor and vasodilator systems of pregnant women with a pregnancy-induced hypertensive disorder. Of the vasoconstrictor systems, most emphasis will be placed on the RAAS; for the vasodilator systems, we will focus on the eicosanoid system.

Vasoconstrictor Systems

Renin-Angiotensin-Aldosterone System. The majority of studies on plasma renin activity (PRA) and plasma renin concentration (PRC) found lower levels in patients with PIH in comparison with normotensive pregnancy.[23] Levels of active renin may be even lower than those of nonpregnant women. The levels of angiotensin II in plasma of preeclamptic women have been reported as severely depressed, normal, and considerably elevated in comparison with those in normal pregnancy.[24] However, more recent studies show a similar pattern to that of PRC and PRA, with suppression of plasma angiotensin II levels in severe preeclampsia.[23] The plasma aldosterone concentration also is suppressed in PIH, although not to the extent that might be expected from the suppressed PRA.[23]

Proposed causes of the decreased activity of the RAAS in pregnancy-induced hypertensive disorders include:

1. A loss of vascular refractoriness to angiotensin II, thus an increased effectiveness of angiotensin II negative feedback on the juxtaglomerular apparatus[25]
2. Lower blood ionized calcium level[25]
3. Deficient production of vasodilator prostaglandins.[23] Prostacyclin could be the main determinant of the stimulation of the RAAS that is physiologic in pregnancy. For that reason, a deficient production of prostacyclin may be the central mechanism in the reduction in RAAS activity in women with pregnancy-induced hypertensive disorders.[26]

The Adrenergic System. Different results and opinions about the role of the sympatho-adrenal system in PIH have been published. Differences in methodology and varying criteria for patient selection might explain some of the contradictions. Venous plasma norepinephrine concentrations have been observed to be reduced[27], normal[28], or elevated.[29] Results from venous plasma epinephrine measurements also have shown reduced[27], unaltered[28], or elevated levels.[29] In urine, increased excretion of both norepinephrine and epinephrine in PIH has been observed.[30] Arterial levels of norepinephrine have been observed to be similar or elevated[31] in PIH as compared to the levels found in normotensive pregnancy.

Nisell[31] concluded that normal adrenomedullary suppression during pregnancy is absent in PIH but that there are no indications of an altered sympathetic nerve activity in the body as a whole in PIH. This, however, does not exclude the possibility of a neurogenic contribution to blood pressure elevation in PIH since sympathetic nerve activity occurs in a differentiated fashion. In addition, several vascular and sympatho-adrenal responses in preeclamptic patients are similar to those observed in the nonpregnant state, implying an inadequate adaptation of the autonomic nervous system in PIH.[31]

The reduction in vasodilator prostaglandin production said to be present in PIH could be one of the mechanisms involved in the increased production of catecholamines and the increase in pressor responses to their exogenous administration.

Natriuretic Hormone. Beyers et al[32] found higher levels of *digoxinlike substance* (DLS) in cord blood of infants born to preeclamptic mothers than in cord blood of infants born to normotensive women. Recently Graves et al[33] found higher levels of DLS in serum of preeclamptic women. They also found a significant correlation between DLS levels and diastolic blood pressure. The increased levels of DLS in postpartum preeclamptic women were found to normalize rapidly. Recently, however, Gonzales et al[34] found no differences between DLS levels in preeclampsia compared to normotensive pregnancy. They also found a poor correlation between DLS levels and plasma volume in preeclampsia. From a theoretical point of view, endogenous DLS could contribute to the increased vascular tone and vascular sensitivity to angiotensin II in PIH. However, these findings require further study, particularly concerning the exact molecular structure of this still hypothetical circulating vasoconstrictor. DLS may represent a previously unrecognized vasoactive compound, but identification is needed to determine its exact pathophysiologic role in the development of PIH. The recent findings of Gonzales et al[34] suggest that DLS does not play any major role in regulating plasma volume or the degree of vasoconstriction in preeclampsia.

The Vascular Responsiveness to Vasoconstrictor Substances. A considerable body of evidence confirms the view that women with PIH have a markedly greater pressor response to several vasoconstrictor hormones than normotensive pregnant women.

Gant et al[14] demonstrated that pressor responsiveness to angiotensin II can be significantly increased already at 22 weeks' gestation in women who are destined to develop PIH, well before the onset of hypertension and other abnormalities such as a reduction in plasma volume. It is this observation, probably more than any other, that led to the concept of PIH as a chronic disease, albeit one confined by definition to pregnancy. This progressive loss of angiotensin II refractoriness that develops even before PIH is clinically manifest may be a consequence of a vasodilator prostaglandin deficiency.

In comparison to the blunted pressor response in normotensive pregnant women, norepinephrine infusion in hypertensive pregnant women causes an increased pressor response comparable to that in normotensive nonpregnant women.[31] The pressor response during infusion of norepinephrine in PIH is caused mainly by vasoconstriction and essentially is similar to the degree of vasoconstriction and pressor response in the nonpregnant state. Again, an insufficient action of vasodilator prostaglandins may be the main mechanism causing the increase in vascular responsiveness to catecholamines in PIH.

Some 50 years ago it was found that the vascular reactivity to the pressor effects of vasopressin is enhanced in preeclamptic women in comparison to normotensive pregnant women.[35] The increased pressor response to vasopressin in PIH also may be due to a deficiency in vasodilator prostaglandins.

Tulenko et al[37] recently developed an *in vitro* model to identify the serum factors responsible for the changes in vascular sensitivity to vasoconstrictor substances that occur in PIH. Sensitivity of isolated segments of the rabbit carotid artery to vasoconstrictor substances and endothelium-mediated relaxation was studied. Tulenko and his coworkers found that arteries exposed to serum from preeclamptic women developed a 2.9-fold increase in sensitivity to angiotensin II, and a 1.6-fold increase in sensitivity to norepinephrine. Endothelium-mediated relaxation was not affected by serum from preeclamptic women. This study supports the concept that a mechanism proximal to the intracellular vasoconstrictor pathways is altered in PIH; a likely site would be the smooth muscle cell membrane and its angiotensin II and norepinephrine receptor excitation-coupling mechanism.[37]

Vasodilator Systems

The Eicosanoid System. Changes in prostaglandin production or catabolism in uteroplacental and fetal tissues have been reported to be associated with PIH, although the reports are often conflicting.[26] These discrepancies may reflect some of the known problems inherent in the assessment of prostaglandin action. Recent evidence suggests that PIH is a state of relative PGI_2 deficiency and TXA_2 dominance.[38]

Prostacyclin and Thromboxane: Several groups have supplied evidence for a deficiency of PGI_2 production at the tissue level by measuring reduced plasma levels[39] and urinary PGI_2 metabolites.[40] In addition, Moodley et al[41] found significantly lower levels of 6-keto-PGF_1 alpha and PGE_2 in central venous blood in 21 primigravid women with eclampsia.

The normal gestational increment in urinary excretion of PGI_2 metabolites is diminished in PIH. Fitzgerald[40] found a 5- to 10-fold increase in urinary metabolites of PGI_2 during normotensive pregnancy; by contrast, in patients who subsequently developed PIH, the increase in urinary metabolites of PGI_2 was only 2- to 3-fold. However, they found no relation between vascular angiotensin II sensitivity and urinary excretion of prostaglandin metabolites. In PIH, reduction in the urinary excretion of 2,3-dinor-6-keto-PGF_1 alpha precedes the development of clinical disease and is detectable already in the first trimester. As PGI_2 is a local rather than a circulating hormone and all tissues studied in PIH show reduced PGI_2 production, PIH may be considered a state of generalized PGI_2 deficiency. A deficiency already occurs at an early stage in the development of PIH.

In addition to a PGI_2 deficiency, a relatively or absolutely increased TXA_2 generation could cause the hemodynamic changes and changes in platelet behavior occurring in PIH.[42] Maternal plasma levels of TXB_2 in PIH were increased in some studies but were normal in others.[26] The production of malondialdehyde by platelets, a stable byproduct of platelet TXA_2 synthesis, is enhanced in hypertensive pregnancies complicated by fetal growth retardation.[42]

Placental production of PGI_2 is decreased significantly in PIH. Remuzzi et al[43] found umbilical PGI_2 production more impaired than that of the maternal vasculature in PIH. Walsh[44] found the production of TXA_2 by placentas from preeclamptic patients to be three times as high as TXA_2 production in placentas from normotensive women. This author suggests that the increased placental production of TXA_2 is secreted into the fetal circulation as well as into the maternal circulation. Because prostaglandins and thromboxanes do not readily cross the placenta, a more logical explanation for this finding is an increase in maternal placental TXA_2 production, caused by increased uteroplacental platelet activation and consumption.

A physiologic balance between PGI_2 and TXA_2 and other vasoconstrictor substances, rather than either agent alone, may be of major importance in maintaining a vasodilated state in pregnancy. The impairment in uteroplacental blood flow that is known to occur in PIH may be caused by a relative dominance of vasoconstrictor TXA_2 leading to vasoconstriction. Wallenburg studied the ratio between the two eicosanoids in uterine venous blood in preeclamptic patients, finding increased TXA_2 and decreased PGI_2 levels in uterine venous blood with a TXB_2/6-keto-PGF1 alpha ratio of 5:6 as compared to a ratio of 2:0 in normotensive pregnancy. In this study umbilical cord values showed a TXB_2/6-keto-PGF1 alpha ratio of 6:9 in PIH and 2:0 in normotensive pregnancy.[45]

The decrease in uteroplacental blood flow in PIH may be caused by uteroplacental vasoconstriction as well as by more permanent changes in the uteroplacental arteries. The elevated uteroplacental levels of PGI_2 in normotensive pregnancy may be important for an unimpaired development of the trophoblast-induced physiologic changes in the spiral arteries. In women with PIH the physiologic changes in the uteroplacental arteries are confined to the decidual portions of the arteries. The myometrial segments remain anatomically intact and do not dilate, and the adrenergic nerve supply remains intact.[3] This observation implies failure or inhibition of the second wave of endovascular trophoblast migration into the myometrial segments of the uteroplacental arteries. This may have the effect of curtailing the increased blood supply required by the fetoplacental unit in the later stages of pregnancy. The imbalance between PGI_2 and TXA_2 that may exist in PIH may be important in causing this impairment of normal development of uteroplacental arteries. Also, secondary lesions involving the spiral arteries in PIH, such as acute atherosis and thrombosis, may be caused by an imbalance between PGI_2 and TXA_2. On the virtually nonendothelialized surface of the spiral arteries in the absence of an adequate production of antiaggregatory PGI_2 by the uteroplacental vasculature or endovascular trophoblast, surface-mediated platelet activation may occur.[45] Platelets will adhere and release their alpha and dense granule constituents. TXA_2 will be generated and more circulating platelets will be recruited. Coagulation will be triggered and thrombin will be generated locally, contributing to platelet aggregation and inducing the formation of fibrin to stabilize the platelet thrombus that may occlude maternal blood flow to a placental cotyledon, thus leading to placental infarction. Thrombin will be inactivated by ATIII; in this reaction ATIII is consumed. This concept of surface-mediated platelet activation and consumption in the uteroplacental vasculature fully explains the platelet and coagulation changes observed in PIH.[45]

Because the platelet is the principal source of circulating serotonin, the increased platelet aggregation in PIH may be the cause of the higher levels of serotonin reported in blood and placentae of women with hypertensive pregnancies as compared to women with normotensive pregnancies.[46] The increased level of free circulating, platelet-derived serotonin facilitates further platelet aggregation, but also may amplify the vasoconstrictor action of certain neurohumoral mediators, in particular catecholamines and angiotensin II, and may cause direct contraction of vascular smooth muscle itself.

Defective PGI_2 generation in the uteroplacental vascular bed and elsewhere in the maternal vasculature also could explain the microangiopathy that is associated with PIH. Such a microangiopathy also is observed in other syndromes in which a defective PGI_2 generation is said to exist, including the hemolytic uremic syndrome (HUS), thrombotic thrombocytopenic purpura (TTP) and the lupus anticoagulant syndrome. The pathologic pictures of TTP, HUS, and PIH are remarkably similar; a strong argument can be made for a common pathogenesis that results in disease localized in the renal circulation in HUS or manifest in multiple organs in TTP and PIH.

In pregnancy-induced hypertensive disease, reduced vascular PGI_2 synthesis may be linked, by way of a decrease in platelet cAMP and a redirection of prostaglandin endoperoxides, to increased platelet TXA_2 production and the increased peripheral plasma levels of its stable hydrolysis product TXB_2 found in PIH. The production of MDA, a stable byproduct of platelet TXA_2 synthesis, is enhanced in PIH complicated by fetal growth retardation.[42]

Platelets from normotensive pregnant women are less sensitive to the inhibitory effect on platelet aggregation induced by PGI_2 than platelets from nonpregnant women.[47] In patients with fetal growth retardation and PIH, platelet sensitivity to PGI_2 is decreased still further, probably caused by a post-receptor defect, because platelet PGI_2 receptors have the same affinity and binding capacity in normotensive and hypertensive pregnancies.[47]

There is an ongoing debate concerning whether the kidney is the culprit or victim in many of the hypertensive disorders in nonpregnant individuals. The same holds true for the increase in vascular tone and hypertension seen in PIH. The primary pathology in PIH is in the spiral arteries. However, it is impossible to induce sustained hypertension without some change in renal function. Although the changes in kidney function and morphology in PIH are part of the so-called secondary pathology of PIH, these changes are essential in the pathogenesis of the rise in blood pressure.[18]

In PIH, the intrarenal production of PGE_2 and PGI_2 is decreased.[24] Renal failure to produce vasodilator prostaglandins in this condition may be the cause of the decrease in effective renal plasma flow, GFR, urate clearance, and the development of proteinuria.[18]

The deficiency in intrarenal vasodilator prostaglandins may result in unopposed intrarenal vascular effects of angiotensin II, in this way causing an impaired ability to excrete sodium. The impaired ability to excrete sodium causes a shift to the right in the renal-pressure-natriuresis curve and thus causes an increase in vascular tone and blood pressure.

Free-radical activity increases during normal pregnancy. This may be due to increased cell turnover or to decreased antioxidant free-radical scavenging mechanisms. Plasma concentrations of free-radical oxidation products are said to be higher in PIH. Wickens et al[48] found a correlation between rising blood pressure and increased free-radical activity. Because of the effects of free-radical oxidation products on vascular PGI_2 synthesis, platelet aggregation, and clotting, it is possible that in the pathogenesis of PIH, free-radical activity contributes to the prostacyclin deficiency. Erskine et al[49], found a significantly higher ratio of 18:2 (9,11) to 18:2 (9,12) linoleic acid at 28 weeks' gestation in 6 women who subsequently developed PIH, compared with the ratio in normotensive pregnant women. Erskine and colleagues postulated that these findings reflect increased free-radical activity occurring before the onset of symptoms and signs of PIH. Rogers et al[50] found serum from preeclamptic women to be cytotoxic to endothelial cells *in vitro*. Consistent with the reversal of the clinical condition after delivery, cytotoxic activity in the serum of preeclamptic women is reduced after 24–48 hours postpartum. This cytotoxic activity may be the cause of endothelial cell dysfunction in preeclampsia and thus cause a decrease in endothelial prostaglandin production. The authors speculated that possible mediators of such endothelial injury might include peptide factors or other metabolic products generated by abnormally perfused trophoblast. They also mentioned the possibility of antiendothelial cell antibodies. Because the women in this study all had well established preeclampsia, it is not known whether this cytotoxic factor is primary rather than secondary to some other pathophysiologic event.

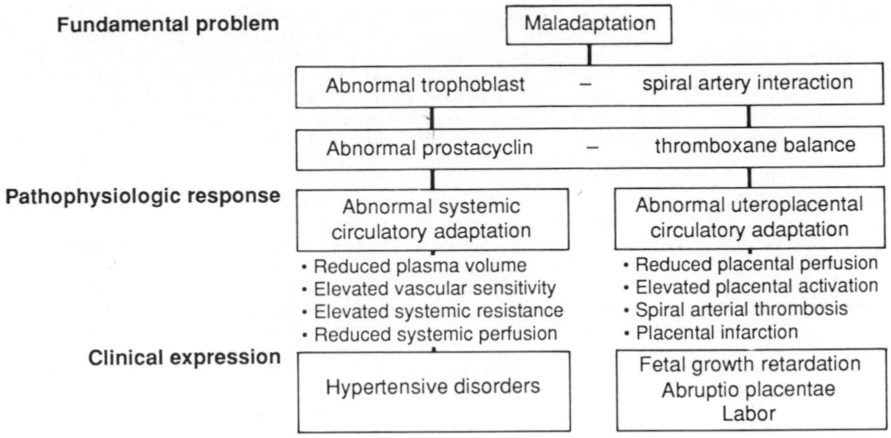

Figure 138–3. Concept of circulatory maladaptation in pregnancy, leading to MAD disease, of which PIH-PE is one of the clinical expressions. *(From Wallenberg[9] with permission.)*

Kallikrein-Kinin System. In a normotensive pregnancy, maximal levels of active urinary kallikrein are found around the end of the first trimester with progressively lower levels later on in pregnancy. The same pattern was found in studies of women who later in pregnancy developed hypertension, but the active urinary kallikrein levels in these hypertensive pregnant women were significantly lower as compared with those in a normotensive group.[51] Inactive urinary kallikrein levels are lower in preeclamptic women as compared to normotensive pregnant women; this difference is present already in the first trimester, long before hypertension develops.[51] Amniotic fluid from PIH patients has significantly lower kallikrein levels than that from normotensive pregnant women.[52]

A direct link between kallikrein and the prostaglandins is formed by bradykinin, the peptide that stimulates blood vessels to synthesize vasodilator prostaglandins, as has been demonstrated to occur in the kidney and in the umbilical cord vessels.[53] Bradykinin reduces vasoconstrictor responses to norepinephrine, sympathetic nerve stimulation, and angiotensin II by an action that is prostaglandin-dependent and that is abolished by endomethacin. Thus a decrease in the activity of the kallikrein-kinin system in PIH may contribute to prostacyclin deficiency and vasoconstriction.

Atrial Natriuretic Peptide. ANP levels in PIH are elevated. The highest values are found in severe PIH. The cause of the increase in plasma ANP levels in PIH has yet to be clarified, but the phenomenon may contribute to some of the abnormalities occurring in PIH, such as reduced plasma volume, increased capillary permeability, and suppression of the RAAS.[54]

Calcitonin Gene-Related Peptide. No data about calcitonin gene-related peptide (CGRP) in PIH are available. Taufield et al[55] recently demonstrated the occurrence of hypocalciuria in PIH. Theoretically, if CGRP concentrations in PIH were lower, and this was associated with lower plasma concentrations of calcitonin, these lower levels of calcitonin could be a cause of the hypocalciuria in PIH, because calcitonin inhibits tubular reabsorption of calcium. In PIH, hypocalciuria is said to be caused by increased distal tubular reabsorption of calcium.[55] However, Pedersen et al[56] found no difference in levels of calcitonin in preeclampsia as compared to normal pregnancy. The abnormal urinary calcium excretion in preeclampsia probably is not related to parathyroid hormone or calcitonin but is, if it really exists, caused by intrarenal hemodynamic changes.[57]

CONCLUSION

Some healthy and usually nulliparous women apparently fail to exhibit or maintain proper adaptational responses to the presence of fetal trophoblasts. Trophoblast invasion into the walls of the uteroplacental arteries is incomplete or even absent. The spiral arteries are left with a nonpregnant architecture and fail to dilate. Prostacyclin dominance fails to develop, leading to an increase in TXA_2 action. Abnormal adaptational changes also have been demonstrated in various other systems, for example, the RAAS.

Recently, Wallenburg[9] developed the concept of circulatory *maladaptation disease* (MAD disease) of pregnancy, of which PIH may be regarded as one of the clinical expressions. Fetal growth retardation, *abruptio placentae* and, perhaps, premature labor could be other clinical signs of a MAD disease, occurring alone or in combination with PIH (Fig. 138–3). The causative factor(s) of a failure to respond adequately to fetal-maternal immunologic interaction remain unknown, although a lack of (or a defective) gene product has been postulated.[58]

The data presented above suggest that the pathogenesis of pregnancy-induced hypertensive disorders could be a consequence of a deficiency in vasodilator prostaglandins, especially prostacyclin, resulting from a deficiency of precursors, reduced synthetic capacity, or defective action. The balance between vasodilator prostaglandins and vasoconstrictors such as TXA_2 and angiotensin II, especially in the uteroplacental circulation and the kidney, may be pivotal in the development of pregnancy-induced hypertensive disease. The absence of the normal stimulation of the renin-angiotensin system, despite significant hypovolemia, and the increased vascular sensitivity to angiotensin II and norepinephrine can be explained by a single mechanism: a deficiency in production or activity of vasodilator prostaglandins, particularly prostacyclin. The increased thromboxane-A_2 to prostacyclin ratio, observed by investigators in many maternal and fetal tissues, may be the cause of hemolysis as well as the reduced uteroplacental blood flow with arterial thrombosis and placental infarction.

REFERENCES

1. Stirrat GM. The immunology of hypertension in pregnancy. In: Sharp F, Symonds EM, eds. *Hypertension in Pregnancy*. Ithaca, New York: 1987;249.
2. Brosens J, Robertson WB, Dixon HG. The physiological response of

the vessels of the placental bed to normal pregnancy. *J Pathol Bacteriol* 1967;569.
3. Khong TY, Dewolf F, Robertson WB, et al. Inadequate maternal vascular response to placentation in pregnancies complicated by preeclampsia and small-for-gestational age infants. *Br J Obstet Gynaecol* 1986;93:1049.
4. de Sweit M. The physiology of normal pregnancy. In: Rubin PC, ed. *Handbook of Hypertension, Vol 10: Hypertension in Pregnancy*. B.V. Amsterdam: Elsevier Science Publishers; 1988;1.
5. Barron WM, Lindheimer MD. Renal sodium and water handling in pregnancy. In: Wynn RM, ed. *Obstet Gynecol Annual*. Norwalk, CT: Appleton-Century-Crofts, 1984;13:36.
6. Lindheimer MD, Katz AI: The kidney in pregnancy. In: Benner BM, Rector FC, eds. *The Kidney*, 3rd ed. Philadelphia, Pa: WB Saunders; 1986;1253.
7. Nolten WE and Ehrlich EN. Sodium and mineralocorticoids in normal pregnancy. *Kidney Int* 1980;18:162.
8. Talledo OE, Chesley LC, Zuspan FP. Renin, angiotensin system in normal and toxemic pregnancies, differential sensitivity to angiotensin II and norepinephrine in toxemia of pregnancy. *Am J Obstet Gynecol* 1968;100:218.
9. Wallenberg HC. Prevention of hypertension disorders. In: *Clinical Experimental Hypertension in Pregnancy*. New York: Dekker; 1988:121.
10. Sibai BM. Pitfalls in the diagnosis and management of preeclampsia. *Am J Obstet Gynecol* 1988;159:1.
11. Chesley LC. Plasma and red cell volumes during pregnancy. *Am J Obstet Gynecol* 1972;112:440.
12. Gallery EDM, Hunyor SN, Gyary AZ. Plasma volume contraction: a significant factor in both pregnancy associated hypertension (preeclampsia) and chronic hypertension in pregnancy. *QJ Med* 1979;48:593.
13. Sibai BM, Anderson GD, Spinnato JA, Shaver DC. Plasma volume findings in patients with mild pregnancy induced hypertension. *Am J Obstet Gynecol* 1983;147:16.
14. Gant NF, Chand S, Whalley PJ, MacDonald PC. The nature of pressor responsiveness to angiotensin II in human pregnancy. *Obstet Gynecol* 1974;43:854.
15. Buchan PC. Preeclampsia—A hyperviscosity syndrome. *Am J Obstet Gynecol* 1982;142:111.
16. Sibai BM, Taslimi M, El-Nazer A, et al. Maternal-perinatal outcome associated with the syndrome of hemolysis, elevated liver enzymes, and low platelets in severe preeclampsia-eclampsia. *Am J Obstet Gynecol* 1986;155:501.
17. Koller O. The clinical significance of hemodilution during pregnancy. *Obstet Gynecol Survey* 1982;37:649.
18. Lindheimer MD, Chesley LC, Taylor JR, et al. Renal function and morphology in the hypertensive disorders of pregnancy. In: Sharp F, Symonds EM, eds. *Hypertension in Pregnancy*. Ithaca, New York: Perinatology Press; 1987;73.
19. Thomsen JK, Storm TL, Thamsborg G, et al. Atrial natriuretic peptide concentrations in preeclampsia. *Br Med J* 1987;294:1508.
20. Hankins GDV, Wendel GD, Cunningham FC, Leveno KL. Longitudinal evaluation of hemodynamic changes in eclampsia. *Am J Obstet Gynecol* 1984;150:506.
21. Wallenburg HCS: Hemodynamics in hypertensive pregnancy. In: Rubin PC, ed. *Handbook of Hypertension, Volume 10*. Amsterdam: Elsevier Science BV; 1988;66.
22. Easterling TR, Benedetti TJ, Schmucker BC. Maternal cardiac output in preeclamptic pregnancies: A longitudinal study. Proceedings of the 9th Annual Meeting of the Society of Perinatal Obstetricians, New Orleans, LA, Feb. 1989;4.
23. Broughton Pipkin F. The renin-angiotensin system in normal and hypertensive pregnancies. In: Rubin PC, ed. *Handbook of Hypertension, Volume 10: Hypertension in Pregnancy*. Amsterdam: Elsevier Science BV; 1988;118.
24. Pedersen EB, Aakjaer C, Christensen NJ, et al. Renin, angiotensin II, aldosterone, catecholamines, prostaglandins and vasopressin: the importance of pressor and depressor factors for hypertension in pregnancy. *Scand J Clin Lab Invest* 1984;44(Suppl 169):48.
25. Churchill PC. Second messengers in renin secretion. *Am J Physiol* 1985;249:F175.
26. Friedman SA. Preeclampsia: A review of the role of prostaglandins. *Obstet Gynecol* 1988;71:122.
27. Tunbridge RDG. Pregnancy-associated hypertension, a comparison of its prediction by "roll-over test" and plasma noradrenaline measurement in 100 primigravidae. *Br J Obstet Gynecol* 1983;90:1207.
28. Pedersen EB, Rasmussen AB, Christensen NJ, et al. Plasma noradrenaline and adrenaline in preeclampsia, essential hypertension in pregnancy and normotensive control subjects. *Acta Endocrinologica* 1982;99:594.
29. Davey DA, MacNab MF. Plasma adrenaline, noradrenaline and dopamine in pregnancy hypertension. *Br J Obstet Gynaecol* 1981;88:611–615.
30. Zuspan FP, O'Shaugnessy RW, Iams JD. The role of the adrenal gland and sympathetic nervous system in pregnancy. *J Reprod Med* 1981;26:483.
31. Nisell H, Lunell NO, Hjemdahl P, Linde B. Catecholamines in pregnancy-induced hypertension. In: Sharp F, Symonds EM, eds. *Hypertension in Pregnancy*. Ithaca, New York: Perinatology Press; 1987;187.
32. Beyers AD, Odendaal HJ, Spruyt LL. The possible role of endogenous digitalis like substance in the causation of preeclampsia. *S Afr Med J* 1984;65:883.
33. Graves SW: The possible role of digitalis-like factors in pregnancy-induced hypertension. *Hypertension* 1987;10(Suppl 1):84.
34. Gonzalez AR, Sibai BM, Phelps S, et al. Digoxin-like immunoreactive substance in pregnancy. *Am J Obstet Gynecol* 1987;157:660.
35. Dieckmann WJ, Michel HL. Vascular-renal effects of posterior pituitary extracts in pregnant women. *Am J Obstet Gynecol* 1937;33:131.
36. Paller MS: Mechanism of decreased pressor responsiveness to Ang II, NE, and vasopressin in pregnant rats. *Am J Physiol* 1984;247:H100.
37. Tulenko T, Schneider J, Floro C, Sicilla M. The in vitro effect on arterial wall function of serum from patients with pregnancy induced hypertension. *Am J Obstet Gynecol* 1987;156:817.
38. Ylikorkala O, Makila UM. Prostacyclin and thromboxane in gynecology and obstetrics. *Am J Obstet Gynecol* 1985;152:318.
39. Lewis PJ, Shepherd J, Ritter J, et al. Prostacyclin and preeclampsia. *Lancet* 1981;1:559.
40. Fitzgerald DJ, Entmann SS, Mulloy K, Fitzgerald GA. Decreased prostaglandin biosynthesis preceding the clinical manifestation of pregnancy-induced hypertension. *Circulation* 1987;75:956.
41. Moodley J, Reddi K, Norman RJ. Decreased central venous concentrations of immunoreactive prostaglandins, E, F, and 6-keto-F1a, in eclampsia. *Br Med J* 1984;288:1487.
42. Wallenburg HCS, Rotmans N. Enhanced reactivity of the platelet thromboxane pathway in normotensive and hypertensive pregnancies with insufficient fetal growth. *Am J Obstet Gynecol* 1982;144:323.
43. Remuzzi G, Marchesi D, Zoja C, et al. Reduced umbilical and placental prostacyclin in severe preeclampsia. *Prostaglandin* 1980;20:105.
44. Walsh SW: Preeclampsia: An imbalance in placental prostacyclin and thromboxane production. *Am J Obstet Gynecol* 1985;152:335.
45. Wallenburg HCS. Changes in the coagulation system and platelets in pregnancy-induced hypertension and preeclampsia. In: Sharp F, Symonds EM, eds. *Hypertension in Pregnancy*. Ithaca, New York: Perinatology Press; 1987;227.
46. Weiner CP. The role of serotonin in the genesis of hypertension in preeclampsia. *Am J Obstet Gynecol* 1987;156:885.
47. Shepherd GL, Lewis PJ, de May C, et al. Platelet prostacyclin receptors in pregnancy. In: Lewis PJ, Moncada S, O'Grady J, eds. *Prostacyclin in Pregnancy*. New York: Raven Press; 1983;199.
48. Wickens D, Wilkins MH, Luney J, et al. Free-radical oxidation (peroxidation) products in plasma in normal and abnormal pregnancy. *Ann Clin Biochem* 1981;18:158.
49. Erskine KJ, Iversen SA, Davies R. An altered ratio of 18:2 (9,11) to 18:2 (9,12) linoleic acid in plasma phospholipids as a possible predictor of preeclampsia. *Lancet* 1985;1:554.
50. Rodgers GM, Taylor RN, Roberts JM. Preeclampsia is associated with a serum factor cytotoxic to human endothelial cells. *Am J Obstet Gynecol* 1988;159:908.
51. Kovatz S, Arber I, Korzets Z, et al. Urinary kallikrein in normal pregnancy, pregnancy with hypertension and toxemia. *Nephron* 1985;40:48.
52. Bodzenta A, Thomden JM, Paller L, et al. Prostacyclin-like and kallikrein activity of amniotic fluid in preeclampsia. *Br J Obstet Gynaecol* 1981;88:1217.
53. Hong SL. Effect of bradykinin and thrombin on prostacyclin synthesis in endothelial cells from calf and pig aorta and human umbilical vein. *Thromb Res* 1980;18:787.
54. Visser W, Vanden Dorpen MA, Derkx FHM, et al. Atrial natriuretic peptide and haemodynamics in untreated preeclampsia. *J Hypertension* 1987;5(Suppl 5):S33.
55. Taufield PA, Alex KL, Resnick L, et al. Hypocalciuria in preeclampsia. *N Eng J Med* 1987;316:715.
56. Pedersen EB, Johannesen P, Kristensen S, et al. Calcium, parathyroid hormone and calcitonin in normal pregnancy and preeclampsia. *Gynecol Obstet Invest* 1984;18:156.
57. Roelofsen JMT, Berkel JM. Urinary excretion rate of calcium and magnesium in normal and complicated pregnancies. *Eur J Obstet Gynecol Reprod Biol* 1988;27:227.
58. Cooper DW. Immunological relationships between mother and conceptus in man. In: Hearn JP, ed. *Immunological Aspects of Reproduction and Fertility Control*. Lancaster, PA: MTP Press;1980;33.

Appendix 138–1

Consensus Report

National High Blood Pressure Education Program Working Group Report on High Blood Pressure in Pregnancy*

FOREWORD

This statement on high blood pressure in pregnancy represents a consensus between obstetricians and internists on a controversial topic in which no consensus existed previously.

The National High Blood Pressure Education Program of the National Heart, Lung, and Blood Institute, working with the American College of Obstetricians and Gynecologists, appointed a working group of physicians and scientists with expertise and experience in either hypertension or pregnancy or both. The group met five times between September 1988 and May 1989, and between the regular meetings members corresponded with each other by telephone, fax, and US mail, exchanging ideas and drafts of chapters. The resulting document has been reviewed and approved by both the Coordinating Committee of the National High Blood Pressure Educational Program and the Committee on Obstetrics: Maternal and Fetal Medicine of the American College of Obstetricians and Gynecologists.

The members of the Working Group were conscientious in carrying out their assignments and faithful in attending the meetings. Special citation goes to Leon Chesley, PhD, who devoted a distinguished career to this subject and whose perspective, knowledge, and good humor added immeasurably to our deliberations.

- *Claude Lenfant, MD*
  Chairman, National High Blood Pressure Education Program Coordinating Committee
  Director, National Heart, Lung, and Blood Institute

- *Ray W. Gifford, Jr., MD*
  Chairman of the Working Group
  American Medical Association Representative to the National High Blood Pressure Education Program Coordinating Committee

- *Frederick P. Zuspan, MD*
  Member of the Working Group
  Editor, *American Journal of Obstetrics and Gynecology*

Members of the Working Group on High Blood Pressure in Pregnancy

Ray W. Gifford, Jr., MD
Vice Chairman, Division of Medicine
Senior Physician, Department of Hypertension and Nephrology
Cleveland Clinic Foundation
Cleveland, Ohio

Phyllis August, MD
Assistant Professor of Medicine and Obstetrics and Gynecology
Cornell University Medical College
New York Hospital
New York, New York

Leon C. Chesley, PhD
State University of New York
Brooklyn, New York

Gary Cunningham, MD
Professor and Chairman
Department of Obstetrics and Gynecology
University of Texas Southwestern Medical Center
Dallas, Texas

Thomas F. Ferris, MD
Nesbitt Professor and Chairman
Department of Medicine
University of Minnesota Medical School
Minneapolis, Minnesota

Marshall D. Lindheimer, MD
Professor of Medicine and Obstetrics and Gynecology
University of Chicago
Pritzker School of Medicine
Chicago, Illinois

C. W. G. Redman, FRCP
Reader in Obstetric Medicine and Gynecology
Department of Obstetrics and Gynecology
John Radcliff Hospital
Headington, Oxford, United Kingdom

James M. Roberts, MD
Professor of Obstetrics, Gynecology, and Reproductive Sciences
Senior Staff, Cardiovascular Research Institute
University of California, San Francisco
San Francisco, California

Frederick P. Zuspan, MD
Professor, Richard L. Meiling Chair
Department of Obstetrics and Gynecology
Ohio State University
Columbus, Ohio

Ex Officio Members

Michael J. Horan, MD, ScM
Associate Director for Cardiology
Division of Heart and Vascular Diseases
National Heart, Lung, and Blood Institute
Bethesda, Maryland

Donald McNellis, MD
Special Assistant for Obstetrics
Pregnancy and Perinatology Branch
National Institute of Child Health and Human Development
Bethesda, Maryland

* The following paper represents a consensus by the Working Group on High Blood Pressure in Pregnancy, convened in 1988, by the National High Blood Pressure Education Program, National Heart, Lung, and Blood Institute, Bethesda, Maryland.

Edward J. Roccella, PhD, MPH
Coordinator, National High Blood Pressure Education Program
National Heart, Lung, and Blood Institute
Bethesda, Maryland

Staff
Mary McDonald, RN, MS
University Research Corporation
Bethesda, Maryland

The members of the Working Group on High Blood Pressure and Pregnancy also gratefully acknowledge the contributions of Kathleen Auerbach, PhD, IBCLC, Ray Borzanian, Jane Rusche, RN, BS, and William B. White, MD.

Member Organizations of the National High Blood Pressure Education Program Coordinating Committee

American Academy of Family Physicians
American Academy of Ophthalmology
American Academy of Physician Assistants
American Association of Occupational Health Nurses
American College of Cardiology
American College of Chest Physicians
American College of Physicians
American College of Preventive Medicine
American Dental Association
American Diabetes Association, Inc.
American Dietetic Association
American Heart Association
American Hospital Association
American Medical Association
American Nurses' Association, Inc.
American Occupational Medical Association
American Optometric Association
American Osteopathic Association
American Pharmaceutical Association
American Podiatric Medical Association
American Public Health Association
American Red Cross
American Society of Hospital Pharmacists
American Society of Hypertension
Association of Life Insurance Medical Directors of America
Citizens for the Treatment of High Blood Pressure, Inc.
National Black Nurses' Association, Inc.
National Heart, Lung, and Blood Institute
National Heart, Lung, and Blood Institute Ad Hoc Committee on Minority Populations
National Hypertension Association, Inc.
National Kidney Foundation
National Medical Association
National Optometric Association
Society for Nutrition Education

EXECUTIVE SUMMARY

High blood pressure complicates almost 10% of all pregnancies, and the incidence is higher if the women are nulliparous or carrying multiple fetuses. Causes of hypertension in pregnancy are multiple, and many current and previously used classification systems are elaborate and confusing, in part because of difficulty in making an etiologic diagnosis by clinical criteria alone. The consensus group recommends the schema proposed by the American College of Obstetrics and Gynecologists (ACOG) in 1972, which has been in wide use for some time, is practical and concise, and considers hypertension associated with gestation in only four categories: (1) chronic hypertension (of whatever cause but mainly essential), (2) preeclampsia, (3) preeclampsia superimposed on chronic hypertension, and (4) transient hypertension.

Preeclampsia (pure or superimposed) represents the greatest danger for the fetus and is associated with life-threatening maternal syndromes, whereas transient hypertension is a fairly benign disorder characterized by mild to moderate elevations of blood pressure late in pregnancy that return to normal postpartum. Essential hypertension, also, is usually well tolerated if elevations remain (with or without therapy) below diastolic levels (In this document diastolic blood pressure is defined as the onset of Korotkoff phase V [disappearance of sound].) of 100 mm Hg (Korotkoff phase V), but complications such as midtrimester loss, growth retardation, and abruptio placentae may occur more frequently. Because the preeclamptic syndromes and essential hypertension constitute more than three quarters of the hypertensive disorders in pregnancy, this document focuses on the presentation, pathophysiology, and management of these diseases.

Preeclampsia, a disease peculiar to pregnancy, mainly in nulliparous women, occurs primarily after gestational week 20, most frequently near term. Signs helpful in its diagnosis are presence of proteinuria, edema (especially if of recent and rapid onset), and any of the following: hemoconcentration, hypoalbuminemia, hepatic function or coagulation abnormalities, and increased urate levels. The predictive value of raised serum iron and low antithrombin III levels and hypocalciuria is under investigation.

A major pathophysiologic feature of this disease is a marked increase in peripheral resistance. This vasospasm is, in part, the result of exaggerated vascular responsiveness to circulating angiotensin II and catecholamines (and possibly an imbalance between thromboxane and prostacyclin production). Before intervention, cardiac output is often decreased, pulmonary capillary wedge pressure is normal or low, and intravascular volume is below that of normal pregnant women. Renal hemodynamics also decrease in part because of a characteristic morphologic lesion in the glomerulus, and there may be increased vascular permeability leading to albumin loss from the intravascular space. Uteroplacental perfusion is often compromised, which may lead to fetal growth retardation.

Preeclampsia can lead to two life-threatening complications. The first is a rapidly developing syndrome characterized by microangiopathic hemolytic anemia and marked signs of liver dysfunction, as well as coagulation changes. This variant, termed HELLP (hemolysis, elevated liver enzymes, low platelet count), constitutes an emergency requiring prompt termination of pregnancy. The second complication is progression of preeclampsia to a convulsive phase termed eclampsia, at one time the major cause of cerebral bleeding and maternal death in this disorder. Pending or frank eclampsia also requires immediate termination of gestation.

Therapy for preeclampsia when gestation is advanced is delivery. Severe intrapartum hypertension is controlled with intravenous hydralazine, which is successful in most instances. Favorable results have been recorded with parenteral diazoxide, labetalol, and clonidine as well as oral nifedipine. Nitroprusside should be avoided unless maternal jeopardy is extreme. Magnesium sulfate remains the drug of choice to prevent or treat eclamptic convulsions.

Women with essential hypertension often have reductions in blood pressure during the first two trimesters; failure for this to occur is an unfavorable prognostic sign. When pharmacologic intervention is required, α-methyldopa, because of its long history of safe use and a trial including a 7-year follow-up of the neonate, remains the drug of choice to treat chronic hypertension in pregnancy. Data relevant to β-blocking agents and combined β- and α-adrenergic receptor antagonists demonstrate their usefulness with little or no evidence of fetal jeopardy. Thiazide diuretics, which have been used safely in normotensive gravid women, may be used in hypertensive pregnant women, especially those who are sensitive to salt. Preliminary information concerning calcium channel antagonists is also encouraging, but angiotensin-converting enzyme inhibitors are contraindicated in pregnant women.

Finally, like all pregnant women, those with hypertension should refrain from alcohol and tobacco. The roles of calcium supplementation and low-dose aspirin (which decreases thromboxane synthesis while sparing prostacyclin production) to prevent preeclampsia and chronic and transient hypertension are under investigation.

INTRODUCTION

The hypertensive disorders during pregnancy are important causes of maternal death throughout the world, and most of these deaths are attributed to eclampsia. The hypertensive disorders also contribute extensively to stillbirths and neonatal morbidity and death. Hypertensive expectant mothers (or gravidas) are predisposed to the development of potentially lethal complications, notably abruptio placentae, disseminated intravascular coagulation, cerebral hemorrhage, hepatic failure, and acute renal failure.

The prevalence of chronic hypertension in pregnancy (that is, in those hypertensive women who become pregnant) is not known. It differs widely in different geographic areas but is probably present in 1% to 5% of all pregnancies.[1] The number of women who become hypertensive during pregnancy (preeclamptic) is also unclear, but one estimate from an indigent population is calculated to be about 13%[2], and incidences ranging from 10% to 20% have been noted in nulliparous women.[3-6]

The purpose of this report is to provide guidance to the practicing physician in (1) managing hypertensive patients who become pregnant (hypertension that is present and observable before pregnancy or diagnosed before the twentieth week of gestation) and (2) managing pregnant patients who become hypertensive (the pregnancy-specific condition termed preeclampsia). This report expands on the recommendations of The 1988 Report of the Joint National Committee on Detection, Evaluation, and Treatment of High Blood Pressure.[7]

CLASSIFICATION OF HYPERTENSIVE DISORDERS OF PREGNANCY

The most important consideration in the classification of increased blood pressure during pregnancy is the differentiation of hypertension that antedates pregnancy from a pregnancy-specific condition, which is characterized by poor perfusion of many organs and usually has increased blood pressure as one of its features. In the former condition, elevated blood pressure is the cardinal pathophysiologic feature, whereas in the latter increased blood pressure is important primarily as a sign of the underlying disorder. As might be expected, the impact of these two conditions on mother and fetus is quite different, as is their management. Unfortunately, attempts to differentiate these two classes of patients have led to confusion in terminology worldwide. The system proposed by the ACOG in 1972[8], although imperfect, has been in wide use for some time and has the advantage of clarity and simplicity.* According to this terminology, women with increased blood pressure are divided into the following groups:

- Chronic hypertension
- Preeclampsia-eclampsia
- Preeclampsia superimposed on chronic hypertension
- Transient hypertension

Chronic Hypertension

Chronic hypertension is defined as hypertension that is present and observable before pregnancy or that is diagnosed before the twentieth week of gestation. Hypertension is defined as a blood pressure equal to or greater than 140/90 mm Hg. Hypertension that is diagnosed for the first time during pregnancy and persists beyond the forty-second day post partum is also classified as chronic hypertension.

Preeclampsia-Eclampsia

The pregnancy-specific condition is termed preeclampsia in the ACOG classification[8] and usually occurs after 20 weeks' gestation (or earlier with trophoblastic diseases such as hydatidiform mole or hydrops). It is determined by increased blood pressure accompanied by proteinuria, edema, or both. Either of the following criteria suffice for the diagnosis of hypertension in this situation: (1) systolic blood pressure increases of 30 mm Hg or greater or (2) diastolic blood pressure increases of 15 mm Hg or greater from early values (average of values before 20 weeks' gestation). If prior blood pressure is not known, readings of 140/90 mm Hg or greater after 20 weeks' gestation are considered sufficiently elevated to satisfy the blood pressure criteria of preeclampsia. Note, however, that many young pregnant women will show the blood pressure increase required for the diagnosis of preeclampsia without increasing their pressure to 140/90 mm Hg.

In preeclampsia and eclampsia the blood pressure often is widely variable from moment to moment, and two observers measuring the blood pressure successively may obtain very different readings.

Proteinuria is defined as the excretion of 0.3 g or greater in a 24-hour specimen. This will usually correlate with 30 mg/dL ("1 + dipstick") or greater in a random urine determination. Proteinuria usually is a late sign in the course of preeclampsia; although it is nonspecific, its appearance greatly bolsters the diagnosis of preeclampsia. Edema is diagnosed as clinically evident swelling, but fluid retention may also be manifested as a rapid increase of weight without evident swelling.

Preeclampsia always presents potential danger to mother and infant. However, certain signs are particularly ominous:

- Blood pressure of 160 mm Hg or more systolic or 110 mm Hg or more diastolic
- Proteinuria of 2.0 gm or more in 24 hours (2+ or 3+ on qualitative examination); *the proteinuria should occur for the first time in pregnancy and regress after delivery*

---

* More recent classifications are available from the ACOG[9], World Health Organization (WHO)[10], and the International Society for the Study of Hypertension.[11] This working group elected to use this earlier classification scheme for purposes of clarity.

- Increased serum creatinine values (>1.2 mg/dL unless known to be elevated previously)
- Platelet count less than 100,000 µl or evidence of microangiopathic hemolytic anemia (with increased lactic acid dehydrogenase)
- Elevated hepatic enzymes (alanine aminotransferase or aspartate aminotransferase)
- Headache or other cerebral or visual disturbances
- Epigastric pain
- Retinal hemorrhage, exudates, or papilledema; *these are extremely rare and it is most unlikely that they would occur in the absence of other major signs of severe disease; when present, these signs almost always denote underlying chronic hypertension*
- Pulmonary edema

Eclampsia is the occurrence of seizures in a patient with preeclampsia that cannot be attributed to other causes.

Preeclampsia Superimposed on Chronic Hypertension

There is ample evidence that preeclampsia may occur in women already hypertensive (ie, who have chronic hypertension), and the prognosis for mother and fetus is much worse than with either condition alone. The Committee on Terminology[8] recommended that the diagnosis be made on the basis of increases of blood pressure (30 mm Hg systolic or 15 mm Hg diastolic or 20 mm Hg mean arterial pressure) together with the appearance of proteinuria or generalized edema.

Transient Hypertension

Transient hypertension is the development of elevated blood pressure during pregnancy or in the first 24 hours postpartum without other signs of preeclampsia or preexisting hypertension. This condition is often predictive of the eventual development of essential hypertension. This is obviously a retrospective diagnosis, and if any uncertainty regarding the diagnosis exists, these patients should be managed as if they had preeclampsia.

Problems with Classification

Problems are inherent in the use of blood pressures measured in early pregnancy to diagnose chronic hypertension or to define basal blood pressure for the diagnosis of preeclampsia. Blood pressure usually decreases early in pregnancy, reaching its nadir at about the stage of pregnancy at which women usually seek obstetric care. The decrease averages 7 to 10 mm Hg for diastolic readings. In some women, obviously, blood pressure decreases more than 7 to 10 mm Hg, and the early decline and subsequent return of blood pressure to or toward prepregnant levels in late gestation will be sufficient to diagnose preeclampsia. Because women who are hypertensive before pregnancy have a greater decrease in blood pressure in early pregnancy than do normotensive women,[12] they are even more likely to be erroneously diagnosed as having preeclampsia according to blood pressure criteria.

It is well established that seizures as a result of eclampsia may occur when the blood pressure is only mildly increased.[13,14] Therefore any rise in blood pressure in a pregnant woman is potentially dangerous, and the final diagnosis of "mild" or "severe" preeclampsia should not be made until after the patient is delivered and returns home.

Even the triad of proteinuria, edema, and hypertension is nonspecific; each sign could be the result of conditions other than preeclampsia. Edema is a physiologic finding present in many normal pregnant women. There is no reason to believe that the normal physiologic edema of pregnancy should not occur in women with transient hypertension, but when it does the clinically oriented classification calls for the diagnosis of preeclampsia (almost always "mild preeclampsia"). Transient hypertension is sometimes the preproteinuric phase of preeclampsia and sometimes the recurrence of chronic hypertension abates in midpregnancy, but more often it seems to be a manifestation of latent essential hypertension brought to light by pregnancy, as several follow-up studies have shown.[15-17] Transient hypertension has a high rate of recurrence in later pregnancies (up to 88%) and probably is the usual basis for the erroneous diagnosis of preeclampsia in multiparous women.

The diagnosis of superimposed preeclampsia is especially difficult. Women fulfilling diagnostic criteria for superimposed preeclampsia may indeed have preeclampsia, but in some of these women the origin of signs may instead be renal disease, either causing the hypertension or caused by it, that may coincidentally worsen during pregnancy. Conversely, many women who actually have preeclampsia may not have been diagnosed. This is a special problem in women receiving antihypertensive therapy, in whom early stages of superimposed preeclampsia without proteinuria may be masked by therapeutic lowering of blood pressure. Superimposed preeclampsia is especially difficult to diagnose in the hypertensive woman with proteinuria at the onset of pregnancy. To aid in diagnosis, investigators have suggested using criteria such as increasing levels of serum uric acid and decreasing platelet counts.[18]

Preeclampsia has a clinical spectrum ranging from mild to severe forms and then potentially to eclampsia. Affected patients do not "catch" eclampsia but progress through this spectrum. In most cases progression will be slow and the disorder may never proceed beyond mild preeclampsia. In others the disease may progress more rapidly, changing from mild to severe in days to weeks. In the most serious cases, progression may be fulminant, with mild preeclampsia evolving to severe preeclampsia or eclampsia within days or even hours. *Thus for clinical management, preeclampsia should be overdiagnosed, because a major goal in managing preeclampsia is the prevention of eclampsia, primarily through timing of delivery.*

More stringent criteria must be used in the selection of cases for research studies of preeclampsia. No classification is accurate or verifiable in the absence of a good understanding of the cause of preeclampsia to permit the development of a specific diagnostic test. Definitions that depend on a numeric threshold arbitrarily imposed on a continuous spectrum of changes (eg, rising blood pressure) create artifacts around the chosen threshold. This is particularly true of the definitions for hypertension in pregnancy and preeclampsia. A major obstacle to the advancement of our knowledge of preeclampsia-eclampsia is the publication of studies of "mild preeclampsia," because the diagnosis is likely to be erroneous in half the cases; the women may have preeclampsia, transient hypertension, or chronic hypertension that abated during much of pregnancy or any of a wide variety of renal diseases.[19]

Another problem pertinent to clinical management is that some women with pregnancy-specific pathophysiologic changes identical to those present in preeclampsia, including coagulation and liver function abnormalities, will not have the specific signs of preeclampsia sufficient to satisfy the ACOG definition.[20] These women are nonetheless at increased risk, as are their infants, and should be managed like the more typical patient with preeclampsia.

In spite of the difficulties in making the clinical diagnosis, there is no question that a pregnancy-specific condition (preeclampsia in the ACOG Committee's classification)[8] in which reduced perfusion to many organs, including the placenta, results in increased maternal and fetal morbidity and death. Unlike chronic hypertension, in which hypertension is the important pathogenic factor, in preeclampsia blood pressure is usually important primarily as a marker of disease. Also unlike chronic hypertension, which progresses slowly over the years, preeclampsia can proceed rapidly, with attendant increased risk to mother and infant. Thus it is mandatory to attempt to differentiate these disorders to appropriately manage the pregnant woman with increased blood pressure. *If a diagnosis of preeclampsia cannot be excluded, it is most appropriate to manage the woman as though she had preeclampsia.*

BLOOD PRESSURE IN NORMAL PREGNANCY AND THE EPIDEMIOLOGY OF HYPERTENSIVE DISORDERS

As noted previously, diastolic pressure decreases by an average of about 7 to 10 mm Hg early in gestation, with a rise to or toward the (assumed) prepregnancy levels in the third trimester. Only minimal changes in the systolic pressure seem to occur, which is reasonable because the increase of 30% to 40% in the cardiac output largely offsets the decrease in total peripheral resistance.

The following factors predispose to preeclampsia-eclampsia:

- Primigravid women are from six to eight times more susceptible than are multiparous women.[21]
- About one third of primigravid women who have had eclampsia have hypertension in about 20% of later pregnancies, but generally they have mere rises in blood pressure alone (transient hypertension) rather than preeclampsia. Only 10% to 15% have proteinuric hypertension.[1] Transient hypertension, usually miscalled mild preeclampsia in the past as well as in some current classifications, recurs in 80%[16] to 88%[15] of women pregnant again and often portends ultimate chronic hypertension.
- Multiparous women who have had preeclampsia or eclampsia usually have some predisposing factor, often chronic hypertension; in these women the recurrence of superimposed preeclampsia may be as high as 70%.[1]
- The tendency for preeclampsia is inherited.[22]
- Twin pregnancy increases the risk five times.[21]
- Diabetes is a potent factor, but relative risk cannot be specified because diabetic persons often have other forms of hypertension that confuse the diagnosis.[23]
- Large, rapidly growing hydatidiform moles increase the risk 10 times in both primigravid and multiparous women.[24]
- Fetal hydrops increases the risk 10 times in both primigravid and multiparous women.[25]

Relative risk of chronic hypertension cannot be estimated because the incidence of superimposed preeclampsia varies greatly as diagnosed and is greatly overdiagnosed from one center to another.

Contrary to popular belief, hydramnios alone[26] and social class[27] do not predispose to preeclampsia, which has the same incidence in white and black American women. Lack of prenatal care may lead to failure to recognize this condition in its early stages. Black women in the childbearing age have two to three times the prevalence of essential hypertension than white women. In black women frank and latent chronic hypertension and transient hypertension often are misdiagnosed as preeclampsia.

Pregnancy can be considered a screening test for ultimate chronic hypertension because women with normotensive pregnancies, especially after age 25 years, have a low likelihood of developing later chronic hypertension; women with transient hypertension have a high probability of ultimate essential hypertension. Preeclamptic and eclamptic hypertension predict nothing, because the disorder does not permit the screening. Had it not been for the intercurrent and unrelated preeclampsia, the pregnancy could have been either normotensive or complicated by transient hypertension.

THE PATHOLOGY AND PATHOPHYSIOLOGY OF HYPERTENSION IN PREGNANCY FOCUSING ON PREECLAMPSIA

Vasospasm

Vasospasm is presumed basic to the pathophysiology of preeclampsia-eclampsia. Vascular constriction causes resistance to blood flow and subsequent arterial hypertension. In some presentations the cardiac output is not maintained, and the resulting absent or mild hypertension underestimates the severity of the disorder. In this context it should be noted that there is good evidence for the condition of "normotensive preeclampsia."[28] Vasospasm and associated vascular damage that cause endothelial cell leaks, together with local hypoxia of surrounding tissues, presumably lead to hemorrhage, necrosis, and other end-organ disturbances of severe preeclampsia.

Vascular reactivity to infused angiotensin II and catecholamines is decreased in normal pregnancy. There is an increased pressor response to some vasoactive hormones in early preeclampsia[29], and this increased response clearly precedes the onset of hypertension.[30] Angiotensin II refractoriness, observed in normal pregnancy, may be mediated by vascular endothelial synthesis of vasodilatory prostaglandins (eg, prostacyclin or prostaglandin E_2 or a prostaglandin-like substance). There are data suggestive that preeclampsia may be associated with inappropriately increased production of a prostaglandin with vasoconstrictor properties or either increased inactivation or diminished synthesis or release of another with vasodilator properties or a combination of these events.

Cardiovascular Changes

Values obtained by invasive cardiovascular monitoring in women with severe preeclampsia and eclampsia have helped to define cardiovascular status. At least five general observations can be made[31-33]: (1) Before treatment, myocardial contractility is rarely impaired. (2) Cardiac afterload is elevated in the absence of therapeutic interventions. (3) Cardiac output varies inversely with vascular resistance. (4) Medications that reduce vascular resistance (e.g., hydralazine) result in increased cardiac output. (5) Ventricular preload, measured by central venous and pulmonary capillary wedge pressures, is usually normal or even low in severe preeclampsia and eclampsia, unless substantial volumes of fluids are administered.

Hemoconcentration is common in women with severe preeclampsia or eclampsia, and the intravascular volume expansion that is normal for pregnancy is not present or is reduced significantly.[34] The woman of average size usually has a blood volume of nearly 5000 mL during the last several weeks of a normal pregnancy, compared with about 3500 mL when nonpregnant. With preeclampsia or eclampsia, however, pregnancy-induced hypervolemia either never develops or is reduced significantly after vasospasm ensues. In the absence of hemorrhage, the intravascular compartment in these women usually is not "underfilled," because vasospasm has contracted the space to be filled. Hemoconcentration usually persists a few hours to a few days after delivery when typically the vascular system dilates, the blood volume increases, and the hematocrit level falls. *In the woman with severe preeclampsia or eclampsia, therefore, hypertension may be exacerbated and the risk of pulmonary edema increased as the result of vigorous fluid therapy administered in an attempt to expand the contracted blood volume to normal pregnancy levels. Likewise hypovolemia can develop even with normal blood loss at delivery.*

Hematologic Changes

Thrombocytopenia, although infrequently severe, is the most commonly found hematologic aberration (by routine clinical testing) associated with hypertension in pregnancy. Fibrin degradation products in serum are elevated only occasionally. Unless there is some degree of abruptio placentae, plasma fibrinogen levels do not differ remarkably from levels found late in normal pregnancy.[35]

Antithrombin III levels are lower and fibronectin levels higher in women with preeclampsia compared with normal pregnant women; these levels are consistent with those in vascular endothelial injury.[36,37] The clinical utility of serial antithrombin III or fibronectin measurements for the diagnosis and management of preeclampsia awaits further evaluation.

The development of overt thrombocytopenia (ie, a platelet count $<100{,}000/\mu l$) is an ominous sign in women with preeclampsia. Without delivery, the platelet count most often continues to decrease and may reach levels that can result in cerebral or subcapsular hepatic bleeding, as well as excessive blood loss during and after delivery, especially by cesarean section. *Maternal thrombocytopenia is not an indication for cesarean delivery.*

The cause of the thrombocytopenia is not firmly established. It has been ascribed to platelet deposition at sites of endothelial damage[35] or to an immunologic process.[38] There is no firm evidence that the fetuses-infants born to women with severe preeclampsia-eclampsia will have thrombocytopenia, despite severe maternal thrombocytopenia.[39]

Renal Changes

The majority of women with preeclampsia have mild to moderately diminished renal perfusion and glomerular filtration with correspondingly elevated plasma creatinine and uric acid levels. An elevated plasma creatinine level is a late development in the evolution of preeclampsia and is often discerned only in the range that would be considered healthy for nonpregnant individuals (eg, 0.8 to 1.0 mg/dL). In some cases of severe preeclampsia, renal involvement may be profound and plasma creatinine levels may be elevated twofold to threefold over normal values in nonpregnant women. This probably is caused by intrinsic renal changes.[40] In unusual instances, preeclampsia may lead to acute tubular, and even cortical, necrosis.

Although some degree of proteinuria should be found for the diagnosis of preeclampsia-eclampsia to be reliable[41], proteinuria usually develops late in the course of the disease, so some women may be delivered before it appears. Thus they may have "true preeclampsia" without proteinuria. This type of proteinuria is nonselective; the increased permeability includes proportionally more of larger molecular weight proteins such as transferrin and several globulins than in renal diseases with selective proteinuria. Thus abnormal albumin excretion is accompanied by increased quantities of many other proteins. Proteinuria usually recedes within 1 week after delivery and resolution of hypertension, but in exceptional cases the protein leak may take more than 1 month to heal.

Renal changes identifiable by light and electron microscopy include those in the capillary loops, which are variably dilated and contracted. The endothelial cells are swollen; deposited within and beneath these cells are fibrils, which have been mistaken for thickening and reduplication of the basement membrane. Electron microscopic studies are consistent with the view that the characteristic changes are caused by swelling of *intraglomerular* cells, primarily endothelial cells but on occasion mesangial cells. These changes, which may be accompanied by subendothelial deposits of a fibrinlike protein material, are termed *glomerular capillary endotheliosis.*[40,42]

Hepatic Changes

Severe preeclampsia may result in alterations in tests of hepatic function and integrity, including elevation of serum aspartate aminotransferase levels. The lesion most likely to account for hepatic impairment is *periportal hemorrhagic necrosis.* Bleeding from these lesions may extend beneath the hepatic capsule to form a *subcapsular hematoma.* Hepatic involvement in preeclampsia-eclampsia is serious, and it frequently is accompanied by evidence of involvement of other organs, especially the kidney and brain, along with hemolysis and thrombocytopenia.[43]

Changes in the Brain

The principal postmortem lesions described in the brains of women who died of eclampsia are hyperemia, focal anemia, thrombosis, and hemorrhage.[44] Cerebral blood flow, oxygen consumption, and vascular resistance were reported as not altered in women with preeclampsia[45], but the possibility of focal blood flow changes could not be excluded. However, cerebral oxygen consumption is reported to be decreased by 20% in eclampsia with normal blood flow, such that McCall[45] alluded to it as "histotoxic hypoxia." Nonspecific abnormalities in the electroencephalogram are common in women with eclampsia within 48 hours of seizures, but the tracings are usually normal by 3 months.[46]

Until recently, cranial computed tomographic scans usually were reported to be normal in women with otherwise uncomplicated eclampsia. However, with more advanced equipment, nearly half of women with eclampsia have abnormal radiographic findings.[47] The most common of these findings are hypodense areas, frequently seen in the cortical areas, that correspond to areas of petechial hemorrhage and infarction.[48]

Although visual disturbances are common with severe preeclampsia, blindness, either alone or accompanying convulsions, is uncommon. Women with *amaurosis* of varying degrees usually have computerized tomographic evidence of extensive occipital lobe hypodensities. These women completely recover within 1 week. *Retinal detachment* also may cause altered vision, although it is usually one-sided and seldom causes total loss of vision. Even without surgical treatment, vision usually returns to normal within approximately 1 week.

Uteroplacental Perfusion

Compromised placental perfusion caused by placental disease (failure of trophoblastic invasion of spiral arteries) and vasospasm is almost certainly a major culprit in the genesis of increased perinatal morbidity and death associated with preeclampsia. However, there are formidable problems to measuring uteroplacental blood flow in humans with preeclampsia. In an earlier study[49] it was observed that ^{24}Na injected into the intervillous space was cleared two to three times more rapidly in normotensive pregnant women than in women with preeclampsia, implying decreased uteroplacental perfusion.

These findings are supported indirectly by studies of the clearance rate of dehydroisoandrosterone sulfate through placental conversion to estradiol-17β. More recently, measurement of the velocity of blood flowing through the uterine arteries has been used to estimate uteroplacental blood flow. Using arterial velocity waveforms obtained by Doppler ultrasonography, vascular resistance is estimated by comparing systolic and diastolic waveforms. Normally the uterine vascular bed is a low-resistance circuit and flow continues throughout diastole. As resistance increases, diastolic velocity diminishes in relation to systolic velocity, and this relationship is used to estimate decreased flow. Some investigators report an increased systolic-diastolic ratio in uterine arteries of women with preeclampsia.[50,51] It should be emphasized that the aforementioned methods do not measure perfusion.

DIFFERENTIAL DIAGNOSIS OF HYPERTENSION IN PREGNANCY

Discussions concerning the clinical spectrum of the hypertensive disorders in pregnancy relate to those symptoms, signs, and laboratory aberrations that permit differentiation of preeclampsia (pure or superimposed) from the more benign forms of high blood pressure, mainly essential and gestational (or transient) hypertension.

The need to distinguish preeclampsia from other disorders is particularly important in the management of women in midpregnancy (before gestational week 28) and in counseling about future pregnancies. With respect to the former, patients with midterm elevations in blood pressure caused by essential hypertension may be managed conservatively even when they have moderate to severe degrees of hypertension. However, attempts to temporize in the presence of severe preeclampsia can be disastrous, as shown by Sibai et al.[52] These authors attempted conservative therapy in 60 consecutive gravida women with severe preeclampsia between the eighteenth and twenty-seventh gestational weeks. The perinatal mortality rate was 87%. Ten mothers had convulsions, two had hypertensive encephalopathy, and one had an intracerebral hemorrhage. In addition, there were five instances of severe coagulopathy, one resulting in a ruptured capsular hematoma of the liver, and three women had acute renal failure. Although there are still dissenting opinions, most authorities consider temporization of *severe* midterm preeclampsia too risky, and interruption of gestation is usually in the mother's best interest.

The second reason for establishing a correct diagnosis relates to counseling. Subsequent pregnancies are often apt to be normotensive when preeclampsia-eclampsia develops in nulliparous women, whereas preeclampsia (or high blood pressure as a result of other causes) in a multiparous woman is associated with a greater likelihood of hypertension in subsequent gestations. In summary, when hypertension complicates pregnancy, establishing an accurate diagnosis may be useful both to help clinicians assess the immediate well-being of mother and fetus and to counsel her when she seeks advice on future pregnancies.

Results from renal biopsy studies underscore the difficulty in distinguishing clinically between preeclampsia (pure or superimposed) and other causes of high blood pressure in pregnancy. Investigators continue to seek sensitive and specific tests with which to make this differentiation.[1,19] Some tests now of historic interest only include demonstration of decreased fractional urate clearance, reduced sodium excretory capacity after infusions of hypertonic saline solution, and exaggerated pressor responses to vasopressin or after changing from lateral recumbency to a supine posture (the "roll-over" maneuver). These tests have proved unreliable or have insufficient specificity to make them clinically useful.[1]

Several additional approaches that might help in the correct diagnosis of pure or superimposed preeclampsia have been proposed recently. These include measurements of plasma antithrombin III[53], serum iron and carboxyhemoglobin[54], and urinary excretion of calcium.[55] Currently, however, the validity of these approaches has not been proved* and some have been challenged.[56] Other tests under study are detection of antibodies to laminin[57] and identification of serum factors that increase mitogenic activity in fibroblasts or are toxic to endothelial cells in culture.[57,58]

Recommended Laboratory Tests

Laboratory tests may aid in the diagnosis and management of hypertension during pregnancy. They also provide reference data when high-risk patients are first seen for prenatal care.

High-Risk Patients with Normal Blood Pressure. Gestations in women with normal blood pressure but at high risk include women with a history of increased blood pressure when not pregnant, those who have had hypertension in a previous pregnancy other than the first, and those with diabetes, collagen vascular disease, or underlying renal vascular or renal parenchymal disease (see section on Blood Pressure in Normal Pregnancy and the Epidemiology of Hypertensive Disorders). Certain baseline data, when compared with results obtained in later gestations, will assist in the early diagnosis of preeclampsia. Baseline data in such women should include hematocrit, hemoglobin, and platelet count, as well as serum creatinine and uric acid levels. If routine urinalysis demonstrates qualitative proteinuria of 1+ or greater, a 24-hour collection should be obtained, including determination of creatinine content to check for accuracy of measurement and to permit calculation of the creatinine clearance. Some might include serum albumin and serum oxaloacetic transaminase determinations in the baseline assessment, whereas others would seek these tests only in the presence of frank hypertension. These patients should also undergo ultrasonography at the initial visit for accurate dating and as a baseline for evaluating subsequent fetal growth.[59]

* Studies designed to detect preeclampsia are currently hampered by the fact that renal biopsies are rarely indicated today, and absence of morphologic correlations makes it difficult to assess the true sensitivity and specificity of test results.

Patients with Hypertension before Gestational Week 20. Most women with hypertension before gestational week 20 have (or will have) essential hypertension, and their management is discussed in the next section. Some of these patients will be under the care of primary physicians and will have been screened for signs of secondary hypertension. If not, we recommend the approach to evaluation and diagnosis of hypertension suggested in The 1988 Report of the Joint National Committee on Detection, Evaluation, and Treatment of High Blood Pressure.[7] Finally, gravid women with preexisting or early gestational hypertension are among the population in whom secondary hypertension is more apt to be found (eg, renal disease, renovascular hypertension, primary aldosteronism, Cushing's syndrome, and pheochromocytoma). Thus further evaluation is warranted even for minimal suspicion. For example, pheochromocytoma, although rare, has a propensity to manifest or be activated by pregnancy, and it is associated with high maternal mortality rates when undiagnosed.[60,61] Thus suspicion warrants performance of a screening test to detect pheochromocytoma (eg, 24-hour excretion rate of vanillylmandelic acid or metanephrines or plasma norepinephrine and epinephrine levels).

Baseline determinations of renal function (serum creatinine and uric acid levels) and platelet count can be compared with values in later pregnancy to help determine if increases in blood pressure at this time are the usual physiologic increases in blood pressure or the onset of preeclampsia. Because these fetuses are at high risk for the development of intrauterine growth retardation, baseline ultrasonography for dating and fetal size are indicated before 20 weeks' gestation.

Patients with Hypertension after Midpregnancy. Table 1 summarizes the laboratory evaluation of women with hypertension after midpregnancy and the rationale for testing them biweekly or more often if clinical circumstances lead to hospitalization of the patient. It is important to recognize that one or more of these abnormalities may be present even when blood pressure elevation is minimal. If there is a life-threatening abnormality such as coagulopathy or abnormal hepatic or renal function, it may be necessary to terminate the pregnancy despite only mild hypertension (see section of Management of Preeclampsia).

TABLE 1. LABORATORY EVALUATION OF WOMEN WHO DEVELOP HYPERTENSION AFTER MIDPREGNANCY

Test	Rationale
Hemoglobin and hematocrit	Hemoconcentration supports diagnosis of preeclampsia and is an indicator of severity. Values may be decreased, however, if hemolysis accompanies the disease.
Blood smear	Signs of microangiopathic hemolytic anemia (eg, schistocytes) favor diagnosis of preeclampsia and may be present when blood pressure is only mildly elevated.
Platelet count	Decreased levels suggest severe preeclampsia.
Urinalysis	If qualitative dipstick is 1 + or greater, a quantitative measurement of protein excretion should be done. Hypertensive gravid women with proteinuria should be considered to have preeclampsia (pure or superimposed) until proved otherwise.
Serum creatinine level	Abnormal or rising levels, especially when associated with oliguria, suggest severe preeclampsia.
Serum uric acid level	Increased levels aid in the differential diagnosis of preeclampsia and are an indicator of disease severity.
Serum oxaloacetic transaminase	Abnormal values suggest severe preeclampsia with hepatic involvement.
Lactic acid dehydrogenase	Elevated levels are associated with both hemolysis and hepatic involvement and suggest severe preeclampsia.
Serum albumin	Values may be decreased even in the absence of heavy proteinuria and may relate to "capillary leak" or hepatic involvement in preeclampsia.

MANAGEMENT OF HYPERTENSION IN PREGNANCY

Management of Preexisting Chronic Hypertension in Pregnancy

Counseling. Hypertensive women considering pregnancy should be counseled before conception. They should be informed of the high likelihood of a favorable outcome in most cases of mild to moderate essential hypertension. They should be aware of the increased risk of superimposed preeclampsia and the possible complications if preexisting renal disease or systemic illness is present.

It is helpful to inform women before pregnancy of possible adjustments in life-style that may be necessary during pregnancy if the blood pressure is elevated, specifically, the possibility that restricted activity, bed rest, or even hospitalization may be advisable.

Patients with intrinsic renal disease who are normotensive and have minimal renal dysfunction usually do well in pregnancy. However, those with azotemia (creatinine >2 mg/dL or, some say, 1.5 mg/dL) and hypertension should be advised of a number of risks.[62,63] These include a high incidence of superimposed preeclampsia, increased risk of perinatal morbidity and death, and the possibility that maternal renal function may deteriorate further as a result of the pregnancy.[63,64] These concerns are especially applicable to women with renal transplants, in whom pregnancy should be undertaken only after consultation with a nephrologist with expertise in this area.

Nonpharmacologic Treatment. Close medical supervision is the mainstay of management of pregnant women with chronic hypertension. It is preferable to control the blood pressure without medication when possible. In patients with diastolic blood pressure from 90 to 99 mm Hg, this goal is not difficult to attain, because blood pressure falls in most pregnant women during the first and second trimesters.

The strategies for nonpharmacologic treatment of hypertension during pregnancy differ from those in nonpregnant individuals. Whereas weight reduction and exercise might benefit a nonpregnant individual, these measures are not encouraged during pregnancy. Although there are no studies that address the issue of exercise in hypertensive pregnancy, given the theoretic concerns regarding the role of the uteroplacental blood flow in the pathogenesis of preeclampsia, women with chronic hypertension should not be encouraged to participate in vigorous exercise.

Restriction of Activity. Bed rest is a good means of maximizing uteroplacental blood flow during pregnancy and is considered established therapy in preeclampsia. In chronic hypertension its effectiveness has not been well studied, but it is an integral feature of management. Rest has been shown to reduce premature labor, lower blood pressure, and promote diuresis.[65] Strict bed rest is rarely necessary. However, all pregnant women with elevated blood pressure, whatever the cause, should be advised to limit their activities when possible and set aside time during the day when they can be "off their feet." Although many women may find it difficult to restrict their activity, it is helpful to explain the benefits to the patient before pregnancy so she can make adjustments in child care, her job, and other responsibilities. In patients with mild to moderate hypertension, restriction of activity may be effective in lowering blood pressure and antihypertensive medications may be avoided. It is usually advisable to hospitalize patients with severe hypertension for bed rest and medication when necessary.

Diet. Weight reduction may be helpful in reducing blood pressure in nonpregnant individuals, but it cannot be recommended during pregnancy. If a hypertensive woman is overweight and planning a pregnancy, weight reduction before pregnancy is advisable.

Pregnant women with hypertension have lower plasma volume than do normotensive women, and some studies suggest that the severity of hypertension correlates with the degree of plasma volume contraction.[66] For this reason, sodium restriction is generally not recommended during pregnancy.[67] If, however, a pregnant woman with chronic hypertension is known to have salt-sensitive hypertension and has been treated successfully with a low-salt diet before pregnancy, it is reasonable to continue some sodium restriction during pregnancy. Patients with renal disease and reduced creatinine clearances are more likely to require sodium restriction for blood pressure control, and this should be continued during pregnancy. The amounts of weight gained during the pregnancy may be an indication of whether salt intake is appropriate.

Preliminary studies have shown that dietary calcium supplementation lowers blood pressure in pregnant and nonpregnant individuals.[68,69] However, there are insufficient data to recommend its use for treatment of hypertension.

Home Blood Pressure Monitoring. The rationale for close observation of the pregnant woman with hypertension is that changes in clinical status (such as development of superimposed preeclampsia) can be recognized before they become severe. This is easier to accomplish if patients are instructed to take their blood pressures at home and keep a record of the readings. They can then contact medical personnel if the blood pressure rises significantly before a scheduled visit. Home monitoring of blood pressure is often helpful because it will enable the patient to determine how much limitation of activity is necessary to keep her blood pressure controlled. This technique also helps discriminate truly elevated blood pressure from labile blood pressure increases common in young patients. Patients who are candidates for home blood pressure monitoring should have formal instruction on the correct technique for determination of blood pressure. In addition, their equipment should be checked periodically for accuracy. Preliminary data on home blood pressure monitoring during pregnancy suggest that it is a useful adjunct to the care of the pregnant woman.[70]

Alcohol and Tobacco. The use of alcohol and tobacco during pregnancy should be discouraged strongly. Both have a deleterious effect on the fetus and mother. Excessive consumption of alcohol can aggravate hypertension or raise blood pressure in the mother de novo.

Rationale for Pharmacologic Treatment. The majority of women with chronic hypertension in pregnancy have mild to moderate elevations in blood pressure, and therefore the risk of acute cardiovascular complications is extremely low. In the small percentage of women who have severe hypertension, the increased risk of cerebral hemorrhage, cardiac failure, and myocardial infarction necessitates close monitoring and aggressive treatment during pregnancy.

Although there is increased risk of perinatal morbidity and death when the mother has chronic hypertension[1,71,72], most pregnancies in these women result in healthy, full-term infants. Women with chronic hypertension are at increased risk of development of superimposed preeclampsia, and there is evidence that most, if not all, of the increased perinatal morbidity and death associated with chronic hypertension is attributable to this complication.[73] However, the literature is conflicting. Some studies have shown that infants born to women with chronic hypertension in pregnancy who do *not* have superimposed preeclampsia do as well as those born to normotensive women.[73] Other studies report a higher perinatal loss in uncomplicated pregnancy in hypertensive women (compared with normotensive women), especially with higher levels of blood pressure.[1]

The objective in treating a pregnant woman with chronic hypertension is to minimize the short-term risks to the mother of elevated blood pressure while avoiding therapeutic maneuvers that compromise fetal well-being. The specific goals for the mother are to prevent cardiovascular complications of severe hypertension and, if possible, preeclampsia. When maternal blood pressure reaches diastolic levels of 100 mm Hg or more, treatment should be instituted to avoid hypertensive vascular damage. Some experts believe at least nonpharmacologic treatment is warranted at diastolic blood pressures of 90 mm Hg or greater.

The indications for treatment of hypertension (at diastolic blood pressures of 90 to 99 mm Hg) during pregnancy are less clear. In the nonpregnant individual, treatment of mild to moderate hypertension is recommended for prevention of long-term cardiovascular consequences of elevated blood pressure.[7]

To date, clinical trials and clinical experience have not given us a conclusive answer to the question, "Does treatment of chronic hypertension prevent preeclampsia?" Many of the clinical trials of antihypertensive therapy in chronic hypertension have evaluated treatment begun in the third trimester.[74-76] This is largely a consequence of the fact that blood pressure falls in most women during the first trimester, reaching its nadir by midpregnancy. This phenomenon occurs in patients with chronic hypertension as well, and because most patients have only mild hypertension to begin with, by midpregnancy the majority will be normotensive. Therefore it is frequently not until the third trimester, when the blood pressure rises, that treatment is begun. If superimposed preeclampsia in the patient with chronic hypertension is associated with the same placental disease as in pure preeclampsia, then the definitive morphologic changes are already present by 20 weeks. Thus, one would not expect antihypertensive medication begun in the third trimester to alter these changes. To complicate matters, patients enrolled in clinical trials that have started treatment in the third trimester are frequently a heterogeneous population and include patients with transient hypertension, preeclampsia, and chronic hypertension.

There are almost no data available that would either support or dispute the notion that early treatment of chronic hypertension (in the first half of pregnancy) prevents superimposed preeclampsia. Carefully conducted clinical trials are needed to resolve this issue.

It is not uncommon for a pregnant woman with chronic hypertension to be hospitalized because of elevated blood pressure. Early treatment of hypertension in pregnancy may reduce the need for such hospitalization, but it may obscure the diagnosis of superimposed preeclampsia, because a rise in blood pressure may be the first sign of this condition.[77] It is particularly important to monitor women being treated for hypertension during pregnancy for signs of preeclampsia, because this condition is associated with adverse fetal outcome.

With regard to fetal well-being, several studies suggest, but do not conclusively demonstrate, benefits of treating mild to moderate hypertension during pregnancy.[78] In the largest published clinical trial demonstrating a reduction in perinatal deaths in mothers treated with methyldopa, the major intake of patients was during the second trimester, with a significant proportion entering earlier in the first half of pregnancy.[79] Because the beneficial outcome was the result of a decrease in midtrimester pregnancy losses, it is not clear whether lowering blood pressure was responsible for the improved outcome. Given the potential hazards of antihypertensive treatment during pregnancy (the possibility that medication may reduce placental blood flow or adversely affect the fetus), treatment of hypertension (at diastolic levels of 90 to 99 mm Hg) must be undertaken cautiously, weighing the risks and benefits of treatment for both mother and child at all times. Excessive reduction in blood pressure is to be avoided, and a conservative approach is recommended.

Drug Treatment of Chronic Preexisting Hypertension. The goal of treating chronic hypertension during pregnancy is the reduction of maternal risk and perhaps that of the fetus (see section on Management of Preexisting Chronic Hypertension in Pregnancy). With this goal in mind it is mandatory to establish not only the efficacy of drugs to reduce blood pressure but also the acute and long-range effects of these drugs on fetal well-being, especially (based on the mechanism of action of many antihypertensive drugs) long-range neurologic effects. So far only one drug, methyldopa, meets these criteria. Thus if feasible, methyldopa therapy should be chosen in pregnancy. If this drug is ineffective or cannot be tolerated (which happens not infrequently), alternative therapy is determined by guidelines based on limited clinical experience and rational choices based on the mechanisms by which the drugs act. It is important to point out that, in spite of theoretic concerns, none of the drugs currently used to treat hypertension other than the angiotensin-converting enzyme inhibitors have been demonstrated to increase the risk in perinatal morbidity or death within the limits of acute follow-up. The following categories of antihypertensive agents are addressed alphabetically.

ANGIOTENSIN-CONVERTING ENZYME INHIBITORS. This new class of antihypertensive agents, which act in part by inhibiting conversion of angiotensin I to angiotensin II, has become popular in the treatment of essential hypertension and hypertension associated with renal disease in nonpregnant patients because of its minimal side effects. Although no teratogenic effects have been observed in animals using these drugs, they do lower uterine blood flow and reduce fetal survival in pregnant rabbits and sheep, perhaps by decreasing uterine prostaglandin E_2 and I_2 synthesis.[80] Acute renal failure with lethal consequences has also been described in the neonates of women treated with angiotensin-converting enzyme inhibitors in the last trimester.[81-84] Because other antihypertensive agents are available, it is recommended that angiotensin-converting enzyme inhibitors be avoided during pregnancy.

β-ADRENERGIC BLOCKING AGENTS. Evidence is accumulating that β-adrenergic blocking drugs are useful and sufficiently safe in treating preexisting hypertension during pregnancy.[78,85] There is also evidence that the combined α- and β-blocking agent labetalol (α and β antagonism ratio 1:4) is relatively safe and effective in pregnancy.[85-88] Most studies to date demonstrate equal effectiveness when β-adrenoreceptor antagonists and the combined α- and β-blocker labetalol are compared with methyldopa.[85]

Finally, despite a growing and reassuring literature of controlled trials with β- and combined β- and α-adrenoreceptor agents, we must interject a note of caution. Most studies were relatively small and gestational age at entry was usually 29 to 33 weeks, leaving unanswered the possibility that treatment of larger numbers of patients or a longer duration of drug administration may reveal adverse effects.[87,89] For instance, Butters et al[89] suggest that the long-term use of β-blockers predisposes to major growth retardation. Finally, although some prefer β-adrenergic blockers because they cause less somnolence than methyldopa, others continue to favor the α-agonists because of concern that β-blocking agents, which cross the placenta, may interfere with interpretation of fetal heart rate, as well as because of the theoretic possibility that β-blockers compromise the ability of the fetus to withstand hypoxic stress.

CALCIUM CHANNEL BLOCKERS. Calcium channel blockers have been used to treat essential hypertension for many years in Europe and recently have been introduced into the United States. Nifedipine, which has a greater effect on vascular smooth muscle than on the myocardium, has proved promising in treating hypertension. However, it is teratogenic in rats when given in doses 30 times the maximum recommended human dose. There are very few studies of its use throughout human pregnancy, although these drugs are used in later pregnancy as treatment for preterm labor, without adverse consequences.[90,91]

CENTRALLY ACTING ADRENERGIC INHIBITORS. Methyldopa and clonidine are the two most commonly used central adrenergic antagonists and both are used during pregnancy.[92-94] Clonidine is a centrally acting adrenergic inhibitor that inhibits sympathetic output from the central nervous system. The effect of methyldopa is more complex, but it also inhibits central sympathetic discharge. Methyldopa was the first antihypertensive agent used in the treatment of hypertension during pregnancy, so the experience with it is the longest. Follow-up studies of children born to mothers taking methyldopa throughout pregnancy have revealed normal mental and physical development in these children at 10 years of age.[95] Methyldopa given to women with essential hypertension has been demonstrated to reduce the number of midtrimester abortions without affecting neonatal survival or fetal growth.[79]

Methyldopa causes somnolence in many individuals. However, its demonstrated safety for the fetus in long-term follow-up[95] makes this the initial drug of choice in the management of chronic hypertension in pregnant women and the benchmark against which other antihypertensive agents must be tested.

DIURETICS. The use of diuretic agents in pregnancy is controversial. The primary concern is theoretic. It is known that preeclampsia is associated with a reduction of plasma volume[96], and fetal outcome is worse in women with chronic hypertension who do not have expanded plasma volume.[97] Whether this is a cause-and-effect relationship is not clearly established. Nonetheless, women who use diuretics from early pregnancy do not have increased blood volume to the degree that usually occurs in normal pregnancy.[98] This theoretic concern must be tempered by extensive experience in several well-controlled studies with the prophylactic use of diuretics in normotensive gravid women, in whom no excess of perinatal death or morbidity was evident.[99] A metaanalysis of nine randomized trials comprised of more than 7000 subjects revealed a decrease in the tendency of these women to have edema or hypertension[100] and confirmed no increased incidence of adverse fetal effects. Based on the theoretic concerns, diuretics are usually not used as first-line drugs. However, if their use is indicated, they are safe and efficacious agents, can markedly potentiate the response to other antihypertensive agents, and are not contraindicated in pregnancy except in settings in which uteroplacental perfusion is already reduced (preeclampsia and intrauterine growth retardation).

Although data concerning the use of diuretics in pregnant women with essential hypertension are sparse, this Committee concluded that gestation does not preclude use of saluretic drugs to reduce or control blood pressure in women whose hypertension predated conception or manifested before midpregnancy. (The Joint National Committee IV recommended smaller doses of diuretics than were used previously, thus minimizing metabolic effects.[7])

VASODILATORS. Hydralazine is a vasodilator that is relatively ineffective when used alone because of the reflex tachycardia with increased cardiac output that occurs with its use. However, when hydralazine is combined with a β-adrenergic blocking agent, the reflex tachycardia is prevented, and the combination is quite effective in reducing blood pressure. Hydralazine is used extensively, usually with methyldopa, in treating preexisting hypertension in pregnancy and is considered to be safe for mother and fetus by most obstetricians. Still, one survey in Scandinavia has reported fetal thrombocytopenia.[101] Therefore its use as a first-line drug in treating pregnant women with chronic preexisting hypertension should be limited.

In summary, although this working group endorses judicious antihypertensive therapy for pregnant women with preexisting essential (chronic) hypertension (diastolic blood pressures greater than or equal to 90 mm Hg), there is no good existing evidence that the use of antihypertensive therapy improves fetal survival. Methyldopa may prevent midgestational losses.

Maternal-Fetal Surveillance. Whether the patient has acute or chronic hypertension, fetal surveillance is indicated. The methods for fetal surveillance are the same in both cases and the interpretation is similar. If the fetus is compromised, decision making and judgment are necessary. If intrauterine growth retardation is identified by fundal measurements and documented by ultrasonography, biophysical testing should be implemented. The amount of amniotic fluid is significant, because a decreased amount of fluid may be associated with cord problems during labor.

Nonstress testing, oxytocin challenge testing, ultrasonography, and fetal movement counts constitute the most common fetal surveillance techniques. If determination of pulmonary maturity would influence management, amniocentesis should be done to determine this before the interruption of pregnancy.

Fetal surveillance involves determining if the fetus is growing appropriately. When fundal height measurements are inappropriate, other investigative avenues such as ultrasound biophysical testing should be pursued. As long as the fetus continues to grow in an appropriate manner, it can be inferred that the placenta and uterine blood flow is appropriate.

Management of Preeclampsia

Prevention of Preeclampsia. Our ability to prevent preeclampsia is limited by lack of knowledge regarding its cause. The cornerstone of "prevention" in patients with preeclampsia has been identification of the high-risk individual (see section on Blood Pressure in Normal Pregnancy and the Epidemiology of Hypertensive Disorders), followed by close clinical and laboratory monitoring so that the disease process can be recognized in its early stages. Women can then be hospitalized for more intensive monitoring or delivery. Although these measures do not enable us to prevent preeclampsia, they do help to prevent its catastrophic maternal and fetal sequelae.

Although various dietary and pharmacologic strategies (low-salt and high- or low-protein diet and diuretics) have been employed with the hope of preventing preeclampsia or minimizing its severity, none have proved effective so far. Many obstetricians consider daily rest to be effective in preventing preeclampsia or minimizing its severity in high-risk individuals, although this has not been proved.

One preventive strategy that is currently receiving a great deal of attention is the use of low-dose aspirin. At the present time many centers around the world are investigating the ability of low-dose aspirin to prevent preeclampsia. These clinical trials have been prompted by two initial encouraging reports.[102,103] In both trials, low-dose aspirin[103] or low-dose aspirin plus dipyridamole[102] was successful in reducing the incidence of preeclampsia in the groups studied. There were no fetal or maternal complications attributable to aspirin in either study; however, the total number of women who received aspirin was fewer than 100. Two recently published trials of low-dose aspirin in moderate- and high-risk pregnant women support these earlier encouraging reports and provide evidence that the beneficial effects of aspirin are associated with selective inhibition of platelet thromboxane A_2 generation, with preservation of vascular prostacyclin generation.[104,105] However, because aspirin in large doses is associated with hemorrhagic complications in the newborn[106], and prostaglandins play a major role in maternal-fetal physiology, we do not recommend treatment of women at risk for preeclampsia with low-dose aspirin until large clinical trials have conclusively documented the safety and efficacy of this therapy.

Rationale for Treatment. The objectives of therapy for preeclampsia are based on a philosophy of management arising from the knowledge of the pathology and pathophysiology and the prognosis of the disorder for mother and infant.

- *Delivery is always appropriate therapy for the mother but may not be so for the fetus.* For maternal health, the goal of therapy is to prevent eclampsia, *as well as other severe complications of preeclampsia.* Preeclampsia is the precursor of eclampsia, and careful antepartum observation can identify the woman at risk. Preeclampsia is completely reversible and begins to abate with delivery. Thus if only maternal well-being were considered, the delivery of all women with preeclampsia, regardless of severity of the process or stage of gestation, would be appropriate. Considering the fetus, however, one should not induce delivery in mildly preeclamptic women whose fetuses are immature but have no signs of fetal compromise. There are two important corollaries of this statement. First, any therapy for preeclampsia other than delivery must have as its successful end point the reduction of perinatal death and morbidity. Second, the cornerstone of obstetric management of preeclampsia is based on a decision as to whether the infant is more likely to survive in utero or in the nursery.
- *The signs and symptoms of preeclampsia are not of pathogenetic importance.* The pathologic and pathophysiologic changes of preeclampsia indicate that poor perfusion is the major factor leading to the derangement of maternal physiologic function and to increased perinatal mortality and morbidity rates.

  Attempts to treat preeclampsia by natriuresis or the lowering of blood pressure do not alleviate the important pathophysiologic changes. In fact, natriuresis may be counterproductive and may adversely affect fetal outcome, because plasma volume is already reduced in women with preeclampsia.
- *The pathogenetic changes of preeclampsia are present long before clinical criteria leading to the diagnosis are manifest.* Several studies indicate that changes in vascular reactivity, plasma volume, and renal function antedate, in some cases by months, the increases in blood pressure, protein excretion, and sodium retention. These findings suggest that irreversible changes affecting fetal well-being may be present before the clinical diagnosis. This possibility probably explains why dietary, pharmacologic, and postural therapy is not successful when avoidance of perinatal morbidity and death is taken as the end point. If a rationale for modes of therapy other than delivery of the fetus exists, it would be to palliate the maternal condition to allow fetal maturation. However, even this rationale is controversial.

Accelerated and severe hypertension can complicate any phase of gestation. Fortunately, most of these crises occur late in pregnancy and are associated with preeclampsia; the challenge to the physician is to maintain maternal blood pressure at safe levels while effecting a delivery.

Nonpharmacologic Management

MATERNAL EVALUATION. Antepartum monitoring of the mother has two goals. The first is the early recognition of the condition, because infants of mothers with even mild preeclampsia are at increased risk, and the second is to gauge the rate of progression of the condition, both to prevent eclampsia by delivery and to determine whether fetal well-being can be monitored safely by the usual intermittent observations. Ideally, identification of early changes would allow intervention before the advent of clinical symptoms. At present, other than the early increased sensitivity to angiotensin II, which is not practical for application to widespread screening, no test has a predictive value sufficient to use clinically. Notably unsuccessful are the "rollover test" and elevated second-trimester blood pressures.

At present, clinical management is dictated by the overt clinical signs of preeclampsia. Unfortunately, proteinuria, the most valid clinical indicator of preeclampsia, is often a late change, sometimes even preceded by seizures, and so is not a useful sign for early recognition. Although rapid weight increase and facial and digital edema indicate the fluid and sodium retention characteristic of preeclampsia, they are neither universally present nor uniquely characteristic of preeclampsia. These signs are, at most, a reason for closer observation of blood pressure and monitoring of urinary protein levels. Early recognition of preeclampsia is based primarily on diagnostic blood pressure increases in the late second and early third trimesters relative to early pregnancy. Use of blood pressure changes without evidence of proteinuria as an indicator does, undoubtedly, result in the diagnosis of preeclampsia in some normal women, as well as in some with underlying renal or vascular disease. Because the goal of early diagnosis is to identify patients requiring more careful observation, however, overdiagnosis is preferable to underdiagnosis.

Once the blood pressure changes suggestive of preeclampsia appear, an office examination within 24 to 48 hours is strongly recommended or, with selected patients, blood pressure and urinary protein values must be checked at home. These measures are directed at determining how fast the condition is progressing to ensure that it is not following a fulminant course. Frequency of subsequent observations is determined by these initial observations and the ensuing clinical progression. If the condition appears stable, weekly observations may be appropriate. If it appears to be accelerating, more frequent observations, usually in the hospital, are required. The initial appearance of proteinuria is an especially important sign of progression and dictates frequent observations, which is best accomplished in the hospital.

If an increasing rate of deterioration is noted, as determined by laboratory findings, symptoms, and clinical signs, the decision to continue the pregnancy is determined day by day. Important clinical signs are blood pressure, urinary output, and fluid retention as evidenced by daily weight increase. Laboratory studies are performed at intervals of no more than 48 hours. These include examination for possible activation of the coagulation system as determined by platelet count and evaluation of renal function as measured by urinary protein excretion and serum creatinine and urate levels. In addition, subjective evidence of central nervous system involvement, such as headache, disorientation, and visual symptoms, and the presence of hepatic distention, as indicated by abdominal pain and hepatic tenderness, are equally important indicators of worsening preeclampsia.

ANTEPARTUM MANAGEMENT OF PREECLAMPSIA. There is little to suggest that therapeutic efforts alter the underlying pathophysiology of preeclampsia. Therapeutic intervention is palliative. At best it may slow the progression of the condition, but more likely it merely allows continuation of the pregnancy. Bed rest is a usual and reasonable recommendation for the woman with mild preeclampsia, although its efficacy is not clearly established. Strict sodium restriction or diuretic therapy has no role in the prevention or treatment of preeclampsia. In women with marked sodium retention as manifested by significant edema, modest sodium restriction may not alter the course of the disease but may reduce discomfort.

INDICATIONS FOR DELIVERY. Prolonged antepartum management of women with severe preeclampsia is not practiced in most centers. With improvements in neonatal care, many investigators regard delivery of women with rapidly progressing preeclampsia beyond 30 weeks' gestation to be in the best interest of not only the mother but also the fetus. When gestational age is critical (between 25 and 30 weeks), one might consider controlling maternal blood pressure along with meticulous observation of the maternal and fetal condition. Delivery is then indicated by worsening maternal symptoms, laboratory evidence of end-organ dysfunction, or deterioration of fetal condition. Whether this plan of action can effect a decrease in perinatal morbidity and mortality rates is not clear. The use of this approach with even very immature fetuses may only replace a nonviable neonate with an extremely premature one, with the attendant risk of long-range neurologic disability. Such an approach should therefore be attempted only in centers equipped to provide meticulous maternal observation and daily assessment of fetal and maternal condition.

FETAL INDICATIONS. The major consideration in decisions for delivery should usually be fetal well-being, for the reasons cited. Thus if the maternal condition is stable, delivery is indicated by signs of abnormal fetal function. If fetal growth and well-being remain normal, pregnancy should proceed to spontaneous labor. If the maternal condition is deteriorating rapidly, however, delivery is indicated for fetal well-being. With maternal deterioration, a reflection of increasingly poor perfusion of brain, kidney, and liver, uteroplacental blood flow is also likely to be compromised. In addition, the predictive value of all tests of fetal well-being is invalidated by rapid changes in the maternal and, hence, fetal condition.

MATERNAL INDICATIONS. Although fetal considerations usually dictate the timing of delivery, there are important exceptions. In the rare case in which a choice is made to palliate maternal signs and symptoms to allow fetal growth or maturation, such efforts must be abandoned if the maternal condition worsens. Also, a potentially lethal complication of preeclampsia, hepatic rupture, cannot be prevented by any mode of therapy other than delivery. It has a mortality rate of 65%. Thus the woman with hepatic capsular distention manifested by hepatomegaly, tenderness of the liver, and abnormal hepatic function values should be delivered regardless of fetal well-being or maturity.

ROUTE OF DELIVERY. Vaginal delivery is preferable to cesarean delivery for women with preeclampsia. It is desirable, if possible, to avoid the added stress of surgery because of multiple physiologic abnormalities. Palliation for several hours should not increase maternal risk if performed appropriately. Induction should be carried out aggressively and expeditiously once the decision for delivery is made. In gestation remote from term in which delivery is indicated but fetal and maternal condition are stable enough to permit pregnancy to be prolonged 36 hours, glucocorticoids can be administered safely to accelerate fetal pulmonary maturity.

The aggressive approach to induction indicates that amniotomy be performed as soon as possible and a clear end point be formulated at the initiation of therapy, usually within 8 to 12 hours of the decision to induce delivery. A trial of induction is warranted regardless of cervical condition. Obviously, if vaginal delivery cannot be effected within the predetermined time frame, cesarean delivery should be considered. Likewise, cesarean delivery is performed for other usual obstetric indications.

A regional anesthetic such as epidural analgesia offers its usual advantages for vaginal and cesarean delivery *but does carry the possibility of extensive sympatholysis, with consequent decreased cardiac output, hypotension, and impairment of already-compromised uteroplacental perfusion. This is a common problem with a spinal anesthetic, which is believed by most experts to be contraindicated in the woman with preeclampsia.* This problem can be avoided by meticulous attention to anesthetic technique and volume expansion. A regional anesthetic is not a rational means to lower blood pressure because it does so at the expense of cardiac output. Likewise, although analgesia with narcotics is not contraindicated and should be used when necessary, there is abundant evidence that attempting to manage or prevent eclampsia with profound maternal sedation is dangerous and ineffective.

Drug Treatment of Hypertension Related to Preeclampsia. Disagreement exists on whether, and how efficiently, the uteroplacental blood flow is autoregulated. Those who liken the uterine circulation to a rigid conduit incapable of autoregulation caution against precipitous decrements in mean arterial pressure, because placental perfusion is already compromised in preeclampsia.[1,2,107] Others[108] prefer a more aggressive approach when treating hypertension. Resolution of this problem awaits perfection of reliable and safe methods to measure placental perfusion, followed by appropriately designed therapeutic trials. In the interim the following guidelines are recommended.

TREATMENT OF HYPERTENSION REMOTE FROM DELIVERY. As cited in several sections of this report, the palliative management of preeclampsia remote from delivery is controversial. The sole rationale is to allow maturation of the fetus and, if attempted, it must not subject the mother to undue risk. An important part of safe management is control of elevated blood pressure. In the woman with diastolic blood pressure 100 mm Hg or greater, risk is sufficient to warrant pharmacologic therapy. The therapy is solely for maternal benefit; there is neither theoretic basis nor empiric evidence that such therapy is beneficial to the fetus. If therapy is elected, methyldopa is the drug of choice. If this is not tolerated or is unsuccessful, calcium channel blockers, β-blockers, and hydralazine are reasonable additions or alternatives. Successful control of blood pressure should not be interpreted as eliminating risk for mother or infant. No evidence indicates that therapy improves fetal well-being or reduces the risk of abruptio placentae, disseminated intravascular coagulation, seizures, or other maternal risk. Both maternal

TABLE 2. GUIDELINES FOR DRUG TREATMENT OF SEVERE HYPERTENSION NEAR TERM OR DURING LABOR[a]

- Hydralazine administered intravenously is the drug of choice. Use low doses (start with a 5 mg intravenous bolus and then give 5 to 10 mg every 20 to 30 minutes to avoid precipitous decreases. Side effects include tachycardia and headache. Neonatal thrombocytopenia has been reported.
- Diazoxide is recommended for the occasional patient whose hypertension is refractory to hydralazine. Use 30 mg miniboluses, because maternal vascular collapse and death have been associated with the customary 300 mg dose. Side effects include arrest of labor and neonatal hyperglycemia.
- Experience with parenteral labetalol is growing, and this drug may replace diazoxide as the second-line drug.
- Favorable results have been reported with calcium channel blockers. However, if magnesium sulfate is being infused, the magnesium ion may potentiate the effect of calcium channel blockers, resulting in precipitous and severe hypotension.
- Do not use sodium nitroprusside (fetal cyanide poisoning has been reported in animal models) or diuretics (e.g., furosemide; see text). However, in the final analysis, maternal well-being will dictate the choice of therapy.

[a] The degree to which blood pressure should be decreased is disputed. Levels from 90 to 104 mm Hg diastolic are recommended (see text).

and fetal assessment must be carried out meticulously regardless of the degree of blood pressure control.

TREATMENT OF ACUTE HYPERTENSION DURING DELIVERY. In the more usual situation, antihypertensive therapy occasionally may be indicated as acute palliative therapy in the woman in whom delivery is indicated. Antihypertensive agents can be withheld as long as maternal pressure is only mildly elevated. However, persistent diastolic levels of 105 mm Hg or higher should be treated.[a] When treatment is required, the ideal drug that reduces pressures to a safe level should:

- Act quickly
- Reduce pressure in a controlled manner
- Not lower cardiac output
- Reverse uteroplacental vascular constriction
- Result in no adverse maternal or fetal effects

The medications used to treat hypertensive crises in pregnancy are summarized in Table 2. Details of their pharmacology and safety are discussed elsewhere.[85,107,109]

The current drug of first choice is intravenous hydralazine, which if given cautiously is successful in most instances. It has been shown to be effective against preeclamptic hypertension.[34] Although this is sometimes used as an intravenous infusion, the pharmacokinetics (maximal effect at 20 minutes; duration of action 6 to 8 hours) indicate that intermittent bolus injections are more sensible. A 5 mg bolus is given intravenously for 1 to 2 minutes. Twenty minutes later, subsequent doses are dictated by the initial response. Once the desired effect is obtained, the drug is repeated as necessary (frequently in several hours). If a total of 20 mg is administered without therapeutic response, other agents should be considered.

Diazoxide is restricted to the occasional resistant case and should be administered in small doses (30 mg boluses). Preliminary successes have been recorded when calcium channel blockers (eg, nifedipine) have been used, and in 1989 this group of drugs was undergoing testing.[107,110] One concern about calcium channel blockers, however, is that most patients with acute hypertension during delivery will also be receiving magnesium sulfate (see below). Magnesium may potentiate the effects of calcium channel blockers and lead to precipitous decreases in blood pressure. Nifedipine acts rapidly, causing significant reduction in arterial blood pressure within 10 to 20 minutes of oral administration. The onset of antihypertensive activity can possibly be shortened by chewing the capsule or puncturing it with several needle holes before it is swallowed. The principal side effects are headache and cutaneous flushing, but minimal reflex tachycardia may occur. Like vasodilators, calcium channel blockers may cause cessation of uterine contractions. They are used to stop premature labor without maternal or fetal side effects.

Limited data are available on the use of parenteral labetalol (which some advocate as a second-line drug), starting with 10 mg and not to exceed 1 mg/kg, or clonidine. Neither labetalol nor clonidine appears to be more effective than hydralazine. Sodium nitroprusside is chosen only after the failure of hydralazine, diazoxide, calcium channel blockers, labetalol, and clonidine because of cyanide poisoning and fetal death reported in laboratory animals.[111]

Finally, the use of potent saluretic agents such as furosemide in treating hypertensive crises at term, as adjunct therapy to the vasodilators just discussed, is condemned by most authorities but still has its advocates.[108] Given the hemoconcentration and cardiovascular hemodynamics of preeclampsia and the susceptibility of some women with this disease to either intraportal hypotension or puerperal vascular collapse, many counsel against the use of potent loop diuretics and care must be taken with all antihypertensive agents. In the last analysis, however, the mother's well-being should take precedence, even if the therapy necessary to control pressure may potentially harm the fetus.

ANTIECLAMPTIC THERAPY. The pathophysiology of eclampsia is discussed in the section on Pathology and Pathophysiology of Hypertension in Pregnancy Focusing on Preeclampsia. It is a mistake to equate the eclamptic convulsion with hypertensive encephalopathy, because *the convulsion* can arise in a seemingly stable patient manifesting only minimal elevation in blood pressure. For this reason many clinicians initiate prophylactic therapy when women with suspected preeclampsia are in labor, even if premonitory signs are absent.

Because the pathogenesis of the eclamptic convulsion is still poorly understood[107], it is not surprising to find disagreements on how to treat women with impending convulsions or frank eclampsia.[2,107,112-114] Most authorities, especially in North America, use parenterally administered magnesium sulfate[34]; others prefer conventional anticonvulsant drugs such as diazepam and phenytoin. Critics of the use of magnesium sulfate stress that it crosses the blood-brain barrier very slowly[115] and has no effect on electroencephalographic abnormalities.[116] Defense of magnesium sulfate therapy has been mainly empiric, but of interest are recent observations of the effect of magnesium ions on prostaglandin metabolism. For example, Watson et al[117] have demonstrated that magnesium at levels measured in

[a] It may, however, be prudent to treat lower levels in certain situations (e.g., the young gravid woman whose recent diastolic levels were below 75 mm Hg or the woman with chronic hypertension for many years and in whom hypertensive heart disease may be present).

treated patients with preeclampsia increases prostacyclin release by cultured endothelial cells from human umbilical veins and plasma from women with preeclampsia treated with magnesium sulfate had similar actions. The preference for magnesium sulfate, especially in the United States, is documented by its successful use in several large series[1,34,108,117,118], but it has never undergone a definitive controlled trial. Similarly, there is a need for more extensive data regarding the effect of both magnesium and standard anticonvulsant drugs on the neonate. Preliminary data on the effects of magnesium sulfate on fetuses are encouraging.[119]

VOLUME EXPANSION THERAPY. Just as there are advocates of saluretic agents, there are claims that volume expansion may reduce blood pressure in selected patients with preeclampsia. This approach derives from observations that plasma volume, cardiac output, and pulmonary capillary wedge pressure may be decreased in this condition, as well as from reports that infusion of colloids decreased blood pressure[33,120] and peripheral vascular resistance[33], despite increments in intravascular volume. However, the effects of colloid infusion are usually transient, probably because the vasculature in preeclampsia is "leaky,"[121] whereas infusion of crystalloids alone decreases oncotic pressure, which is already depressed in preeclampsia.[122] Such decrements can lead to pulmonary or cerebral edema, especially in the immediate puerperium, when oncotic pressure levels decrease further, whereas central volume and pulmonary capillary wedge pressure tend to rise.[31,122] Thus one should be cautious concerning crystalloid infusions into women with preeclampsia during labor and until a postpartum diuresis is established. Signs suggesting poor renal perfusion (i.e., oliguria) resolve quickly after delivery, and acute renal failure is an unusual complication, even in severe preeclampsia.

OTHER CONSIDERATIONS. Invasive cardiovascular monitoring may be required in severe or complicated cases, especially during operative procedures. Criteria have recently been proposed for pulmonary artery catheterization in the patient with severe preeclampsia.[123] Many experts, however, believe that these criteria are too broad and find the indications for use of Swan-Ganz catheters (a procedure associated with a certain morbidity) relatively uncommon.[124]

Treating Hypertension Persisting Postpartum

The potential problems of serious compromise of placental perfusion and, in turn, fetal well-being that can be induced by antihypertensive agents are obviated by delivery. If there is a problem after delivery controlling persisting severe hypertension, intermittent intravenous hydralazine can be used repeatedly early in the puerperium to control it. Once repeated blood pressure readings remain near normal, the hydralazine is stopped and treatment with standard oral regimens should be started.

Several other regimens are effective for control of severe postpartum hypertension. These have been discussed in the Joint National Committee Report[7] and include infusion of nitroprusside (0.5 to 10 mg/kg a minute). Labetalol, 20 to 80 mg by intravenous bolus, lowers blood pressure in 5 to 10 minutes and may be repeated at 10-minute intervals.

Acute hypertensive changes induced by pregnancy usually dissipate rapidly after delivery, certainly within the first several days. If severe hypertension persists more than 3 to 5 days, the likelihood of underlying chronic hypertension is greatly increased. In these cases oral antihypertensive therapy is begun before discharge and the woman is evaluated in 1 week. For women who were hypertensive before pregnancy, chronic treatment is likely to be necessary. If prepregnancy blood pressure was normal or unknown, it is reasonable to stop oral medication after 3 to 4 weeks and observe the blood pressure at weekly intervals for 1 month and at monthly intervals for 1 year. If hypertension recurs, treatment should be resumed.

Lactation. Many women who have been chronically hypertensive during pregnancy will have the desire to breastfeed their infants for a period of several weeks to 1 year. The concentrations of most of the antihypertensive drugs have been assessed in human breast milk and plasma[125] after single or multiple dosings and all agents studied have been detectable in the milk. However, only a few reports have evaluated whether the drug is detectable in the plasma of the breast-fed infant[126–128] or if there is any hemodynamic or adverse effect of the agent on the infant. Furthermore, there have been no clinical trials involving several subjects that have studied the cardiovascular effects of any antihypertensive agent on the breast-fed infant.

In mothers with mild hypertension who wish to breastfeed for a few months, the clinician may consider withholding medication with close observation of the maternal blood pressure. After discontinuation of the nursing period, the antihypertensive therapy should be reinstituted as appropriate. For those patients with more severe elevation of blood pressure taking a single antihypertensive agent, the clinician may consider reducing antihypertensive drug dosage with close observation of both the mother and breastfed infant. If the mother requires multiple agents for controlling the hypertension, breast-feeding is not advisable.

REMOTE PROGNOSIS

Eclampsia

The weighted average prevalence of hypertension after eclampsia is 23.8%, as derived from 53 articles reporting follow-up studies of 2637 women.[1] There are only two studies of large series with long-term follow up, and they agree that the prevalence of remote hypertension is not increased over that in unselected women matched for age and race. Bryans[129] at the Medical College of Georgia followed up 335 women for 1 to 44 years (average 14). The average age-specific blood pressures of 168 white women at follow-up fell in the middle of averages for unselected women in three epidemiologic studies of blood pressure, and there was no excess of women with diastolic pressures of 90 mm Hg or higher. The average age-specific blood pressures of 167 black women were higher than in white women but were within the range of such pressures in unselected black women.

For an average of 33 years, Chesley et al[130] followed up 99% of the 270 women who survived eclampsia between 1931 and 1951 in the Margaret Hague Maternity Hospital in New Jersey, with all but 3 traced to 1974. Remote deaths among the 206 women who had eclampsia when primiparous did not exceed the number expected, as derived from age-specific death rates for American women matched for age and race. Only 29% of the remote deaths were associated with hypertensive vascular disease. In contrast, three times the expected number of deaths occurred among the 64 women who had had eclampsia when multiparous, and 80% of the deaths were caused by cardiovascular-renal complications. Chronic hypertension had been known to antedate the eclampsia in several of the women. The lowest expected prevalence of hypertension among 11 epidemiologic studies of blood pressure was reported in the study by Hamilton et al[131]; therefore their study was used as the most rigid control. The distributions of diastolic and systolic pressures at an average of 33 years after eclampsia in primiparous women were virtually identical to those of the control subjects matched for age, and there was no excess of patients with hypertension among the women with posteclampsia, whatever blood pressure might be taken as the dividing line. There was an excess of cases of hypertension among the multiparous women.

Preeclampsia

Many of the numerous articles describing follow-up studies of women thought to have had preeclampsia have found high prevalences of hypertension, and some authors have believed that preeclampsia may cause chronic hypertension in women who otherwise never would have had it. It is significant that such "residual" hypertension is more common after multiparous than after primiparous pregnancies, more common after mild than severe preeclampsia, and lowest of all after eclampsia. In a word, the more secure the diagnosis, the lower the rate of ultimate hypertension. In the past, and still in most classifications, the diagnosis of mild preeclampsia is made in women with transient hypertension (see the following section). In the unique study by Fisher et al[19] the diagnosis of preeclampsia was confirmed by renal biopsy. The prevalence of hypertension at follow-up was about 10%, almost identical to the expected rate as derived from women in the National Health Survey when matched for age and race.

Thus the prevalance of chronic hypertension after eclampsia[129,130] or preeclampsia[19] in primigravid women is the same as in unselected women matched for age and race. Preeclampsia-eclampsia is an intercurrent event, unrelated to chronic hypertension (except that chronic hypertension may predispose to it).

Transient Hypertension

Also called gestational or late hypertension, transient hypertension is the diagnosis for mere rises in blood pressure without significant edema or proteinuria, with a return of the blood pressure to normal within 10 days after delivery. Follow-up studies by Berman[16], Herrick and Tillman[15], Chesley et al.[130], Adams and MacGillivray[17], and others indicate that transient hypertension usually recurs in later pregnancies and often predicts ultimate chronic hypertension. It probably most often is latent essential hypertension unmasked by pregnancy.

REFERENCES

1. Chesley LC. *Hypertensive Disorders in Pregnancy.* New York: Appleton-Century-Crofts, 1978.
2. Cunningham FG, Leveno KJ. Management of pregnancy-induced hypertension. In: Rubin PC, ed. *Handbook of Hypertension, vol 10.* Hypertension in pregnancy. Amsterdam: Elsevier, 1988:290.
3. Pollak VE. Pre-eclampsia and kidney disease. In: Coggins CH, Cummings NB, eds. *Prevention of Kidney and Urinary Tract Diseases.* DHEW Publication No. (NIH)78–855, 1978:95.
4. Robinson N. Salt in pregnancy. *Lancet.* 1958;1:178–81.
5. MacGillivray I. Some observations on the incidence of preeclampsia. *J Obstet Gynaecol Br Empire.* 1958;65:536.
6. Thompson AM, Chun D, Baird D. Perinatal mortality in Hong Kong and in Aberdeen, Scotland. *J Obstet Gynaecol Br Commonw.* 1963;70:871.
7. The 1988 Joint National Committee. The 1988 report of the Joint Committee on Detection, Evaluation, and Treatment of High Blood Pressure. *Arch Intern Med.* 1988;148:1023.
8. Hughes EC, ed. *Obstetric-gynecologic terminology.* Philadelphia: Davis, 1972:422.
9. American College of Obstetricians and Gynecologists. Management of preeclampsia. *ACOG Technical Bulletin.* No. 91. February 1986.
10. World Health Organization Study Group. The hypertensive disorders of pregnancy. *WHO Technical Report Series No. 758.* Geneva: World Health Organization, 1987.
11. Davey DA, MacGillivray I. The classification and definition of the hypertensive disorders of pregnancy. *Clin Exp Hypertens Pregnancy.* 1986;B5:97.
12. Chesley LC, Annitto JE. Pregnancy in the patient with hypertensive disease. *Am J Obstet Gynecol.* 1947;53:372.
13. Dieckmann WJ. *The Toxemias of Pregnancy.* 2nd ed. St. Louis: CV Mosby, 1952:422.
14. Sibai BM, McCubbin JH, Anderson GD, Lipshitz J, Dilts PV Jr. Eclampsia. I. Observations from sixty-seven recent cases. *Obstet Gynecol.* 1981;58:609.
15. Herrick WW, Tillman AJB. The mild toxemias of late pregnancy: their relation to cardiovascular and renal disease. *Am J Obstet Gynecol.* 1936;31:832.
16. Berman S. Observations in the toxemia clinic, Boston Lying-in Hospital, 1923–1930. *N Engl J Med.* 1930;203:361.
17. Adams EM, MacGillivray I. Long-term effect of preeclampsia on blood pressure. *Lancet.* 1961;2:1373.
18. Redman CW, Beilin LJ, Bonnar J, et al. Plasma urate measurements in predicting fetal death in hypertensive pregnancy. *Lancet.* 1976;1:1370–3.
19. Fisher KA, Luger A, Spargo BH, Lindheimer MD. Hypertension in pregnancy: clinical-pathological correlations and remote prognosis. *Medicine.* 1981;60:267.
20. Aarnoudse JG, Houthoff HJ, Weits J, Vellenga E, Huisjes HJ. A syndrome of liver damage and intravascular coagulation in the last trimester of normotensive pregnancy: a clinical and histopathological study. *Br J Obstet Gynaecol.* 1986;93:145.
21. Hinselmann H. Allgemeine Krankheitslehre. In: Hinselmann H, ed. *Die Eklampsie.* Bonn: Cohen, 1924:1.
22. Chesley LC, Cooper DW. Genetics of hypertension in pregnancy: possible single gene control of pre-eclampsia and eclampsia in the descendants of eclamptic women. *Br J Obstet Gynaecol.* 1986;93:898.
23. White P. Pregnancy complicating diabetes. *Surg Gynecol Obstet.* 1935;61:324.
24. Page EW. The relation between hydatid moles, relative ischemia of the gravid uterus, and the placental origin of eclampsia. *Am J Obstet Gynecol.* 1939;37:291.
25. Jann R. Spätgestosen bei Hydrops fetus et placentae infolge Rhesus-Inkompatibilität. *Arch Gynaekol.* 1954;184:731.
26. Scott JS. Pregnancy toxaemia associated with hydrops foetalis, hydatidiform mole, and hydramnios. *J Obstet Gynaecol Br Empire.* 1958;65:689.
27. Nelson TR. A clinical study of pre-eclampsia, pts I and II. *J Obstet Gynaecol Br Empire.* 1955;62:48.
28. Redman CW. Eclampsia still kills. *Br Med J.* 1988;296:1209.
29. Talledo OE, Chesley LC, Zuspan FP. Renin-angiotensin system in normal and toxemic pregnancies. III. Differential sensitivity to angiotensin II and norepinephrine in toxemia of pregnancy. *Am J Obstet Gynecol.* 1968;100:218.
30. Gant NF, Daley GL, Chand S, Whalley PJ, MacDonald PC. A study of angiotensin II pressor response throughout primigravid pregnancy. *J Clin Invest.* 1973;52:2682.
31. Hankins GD, Wendel GD Jr, Cunningham FG, Leveno KJ. Longitudinal evaluation of hemodynamic changes in eclampsia. *Am J Obstet Gynecol.* 1984;150:506.
32. Groenendijk R, Trimbros JB, Wallenburg HC. Hemodynamic measurements in preeclampsia: preliminary observations. *Am J Obstet Gynecol.* 1984;150:232.
33. Wallenburg HCS. Hemodynamics in hypertensive pregnancy. In: Ruben PC, ed. *Handbook of Hypertension, vol 10. Hypertension in Pregnancy.* Amsterdam: Elsevier, 1988:66.
34. Pritchard JA, Cunningham FG, Pritchard SA. The Parkland Memorial Hospital protocol for treatment of eclampsia: evaluation of 245 cases. *Am J Obstet Gynecol.* 1984;148:951.
35. Pritchard JA, Cunningham FG, Mason RA. Coagulation changes in eclampsia: their frequency and pathogenesis. *Am J Obstet Gynecol.* 1976;124:855.
36. Roberts JM, Taylor RN, Musci TJ, Rodgers GM, Hubel CA, McLaughlin MK. Preeclampsia: an endothelial cell disorder. *Am J Obstet Gynecol.* 1989;161:1200.
37. Saleh AA, Bottoms SF, Welch RA, Ali AM, Mariona FG, Mammen EF. Preeclampsia, delivery and the hemostatic system. *Am J Obstet Gynecol.* 1987;157:331.
38. Burrows RF, Hunter DJ, Andrew M, Kelton JG. A prospective study investigating the mechanism of thrombocytopenia in preeclampsia. *Obstet Gynecol.* 1987;70:334.
39. Pritchard JA, Cunningham FG, Pritchard SA, Mason RA. How often does maternal preeclampsia-eclampsia incite thrombocytopenia in the fetus? *Obstet Gynecol.* 1987;69:292.

40. Gaber LW, Spargo BH, Lindheimer MD. Renal pathology in preeclampsia. *Clin Obstet Gynaecol.* (Bailliere) 1987;1:971.
41. Chesley LC. Diagnosis of preeclampsia. *Obstet Gynecol.* 1985;65:423.
42. Spargo B, McCartney CP, Winemiller R. Glomerular capillary endotheliosis in toxemia of pregnancy. *Arch Pathol.* 1959;68:593.
43. Sibai BM, Taslimi MM, el Nazer A, Amon E, Mabie BC, Ryan GM. Maternal-perinatal outcome associated with the syndrome of hemolysis, elevated liver enzymes and low platelets in severe preeclampsia-eclampsia. *Am J Obstet Gynecol.* 1986;155:501.
44. Sheehan HL. Pathologic lesions in the hypertensive toxemias of pregnancy. In: Hammond J, Browne FJ, Wolstenholm GEW, eds. *Toxemias of Pregnancy: Human and Veterinary.* Philadelphia: Blakiston, 1950:16.
45. McCall ML. Cerebral circulation and metabolism in toxemia of pregnancy: observations on the effects of Veratrum viride and Apresoline (1-hydrazinophthalazine). *Am J Obstet Gynecol.* 1953;66:1015.
46. Sibai BM, Spinnato JA, Watson DL, Lewis JA, Anderson GD. Eclampsia. IV. Neurological findings and future outcome. *Am J Obstet Gynecol.* 1985;152:184.
47. Brown CE, Purdy P, Cunningham FG. Head computed tomographic scans in women with eclampsia. *Am J Obstet Gynecol.* 1988;159:915.
48. Sheehan HL, Lynch JB, eds. Cerebral lesions. In: *Pathology of Toxaemia of Pregnancy.* Baltimore: Williams & Wilkins, 1973:524.
49. Browne JCM, Veall N. The maternal placental blood flow in normotensive and hypertensive women. *J Obstet Gynaecol Br Empire.* 1953;60:141.
50. Fleischer A, Schulman H, Farmakides G, et al. Uterine artery Doppler velocimetry in pregnant women with hypertension. *Am J Obstet Gynecol.* 1986;154:806.
51. Trudinger BJ, Giles WB, Cook CM. Flow velocity waveforms in the maternal uteroplacental and fetal umbilical placental circulations. *Am J Obstet Gynecol.* 1985;152:155.
52. Sibai BM, Taslimi M, Abdella TN, Brooks TF, Spinnato JA, Anderson GD. Maternal and perinatal outcome of conservative management of severe preeclampsia in midtrimester. *Am J Obstet Gynecol.* 1985;152:32.
53. Weiner CP, Kwaan HC, Xu C, Paul M, Burmeister L, Hauck W. Antithrombin III activity in women with hypertension during pregnancy. *Obstet Gynecol.* 1985;65:301.
54. Entman SS, Kambam JR, Bradley CA, Cousar JB. Increased levels of carboxyhemoglobin and serum iron as an indicator of increased red cell turnover in preeclampsia. *Am J Obstet Gynecol.* 1987;156:1169.
55. Taufield PA, Ales KL, Resnick LM, Druzin ML, Gertner JM, Laragh JH. Hypocalciuria in preeclampsia. *N Engl J Med.* 1987;316:715.
56. Lindheimer MD, Katz AI. Preeclampsia: pathophysiology, diagnosis, and management. *Annu Rev Med.* 1989;40:233.
57. Foidart JM, Hunt J, Lapiere CM, et al. Antibodies to laminin in preeclampsia. *Kidney Int.* 1986;29:1050.
58. Rodgers GM, Taylor RN, Roberts JM. Preeclampsia is associated with a serum factor cytotoxic to human endothelial cells. *Am J Obstet Gynecol.* 1988;159:908.
59. Musci TJ, Roberts JM, Rodgers GM, Taylor RN. Mitogenic activity is increased in the sera of preeclamptic women before delivery. *Am J Obstet Gynecol.* 1988;159:1446.
60. Ellison GT, Mansberger JA, Mansberger AR Jr. Malignant recurrent pheochromocytoma during pregnancy: case report and review of the literature. *Surgery.* 1988;103:484.
61. Schenker JG, Chowers I. Pheochromocytoma and pregnancy: review of eighty-nine cases. *Obstet Gynecol Surv.* 1971;26:739.
62. Packham DK, Fairley KF, Ihle BU, Whitworth JA, Kincaid-Smith P. Comparison of pregnancy outcome between normotensive and hypertensive women with primary glomerulonephritis. *Clin Exp Hypertens [A].* 1987–1988;B6:387.
63. Hou SH, Grossman SD, Madias NE. Pregnancy in women with renal disease and moderate renal insufficiency. *Am J Med.* 1985;78:185.
64. Lindheimer MD, Katz AI. Gestation in women with kidney disease: prognosis and management. *Clin Obstet Gynaecol (Bailliere).* 1987;1:921.
65. Papiernik E, Kaminski M. Multifactorial study of the risk of prematurity at thirty-two weeks of gestation. I. A study of the frequency of thirty predictive characteristics. *J Perinat Med.* 1974;2:30.
66. Gallery ED, Hunyor SN, Györy AZ. Plasma volume contraction: a significant factor in both pregnancy-associated hypertension (preeclampsia) and chronic hypertension in pregnancy. *Q J Med.* 1979; 48:593.
67. Palomaki JF, Lindheimer MD. Sodium depletion simulating deterioration in a toxemic pregnancy. *N Engl J Med.* 1970;282:88.
68. Kawasaki N, Matsui K, Ito M, et al. Effect of calcium supplementation on the vascular sensitivity to angiotensin II in pregnant women. *Am J Obstet Gynecol.* 1985;153:576.
69. Villar J, Repke J, Belizan JM, Pareja G. Calcium supplementation reduces blood pressure during pregnancy: results of a randomized controlled clinical trial. *Obstet Gynecol.* 1987;70:317.
70. Rayburn WF, Zuspan FP, Piehl EJ. Self-monitoring of blood pressuring during pregnancy. *Am J Obstet Gynecol.* 1984;148:159.
71. Page EW, Christianson R. The impact of mean arterial blood pressure in the middle trimester upon the outcome of pregnancy. *Am J Obstet Gynecol.* 1976;125:740.
72. Friedman EA, Neff RK. *Pregnancy Hypertension: a Systematic Evaluation of Clinical Diagnostic Criteria.* Littleton, MA: PSG, 1977.
73. Dunlop JCH. Chronic hypertension and perinatal mortality. *Proc R Soc Med.* 1966;59:838.
74. Leather HM, Humphreys DM, Baker P, Chadd MA. A controlled trial of hypotensive agents in hypertension in pregnancy. *Lancet.* 1968;2:488.
75. Rubin PC, Butters L, Clark DM, et al. Placebo-controlled trial of atenolol in treatment of pregnancy-associated hypertension. *Lancet.* 1983; 1:431.
76. Wichman K, Ryden G, Karlberg BE. A placebo-controlled trial of metoprolol in the treatment of hypertension in pregnancy. *Scand J Clin Lab Invest.* 1984;169:90.
77. Landesman R, McLarn WD, Ollstein RN, Mendelsohn B. Reserpine in toxemia of pregnancy. *Obstet Gynecol.* 1957;9:377.
78. Fletcher AE, Bulpitt CJ. A review of clinical trials in pregnancy. In: Rubin PC, ed. *Hypertension in Pregnancy.* New York: Elsevier, 1988:186.
79. Redman CW, Beilin LJ, Bonnar J, Ounsted MK. Fetal outcome in trial of antihypertensive treatment in pregnancy. *Lancet.* 1976;2:753.
80. Ferris TF, Weir EK. Effect of captopril on uterine blood flow and prostaglandin E synthesis in the pregnant rabbit. *J Clin Invest.* 1983;71:809.
81. Schubiger G, Flury G, Nussberger J. Enalapril for pregnancy-induced hypertension: acute renal failure in a neonate. *Ann Intern Med.* 1988;108:777.
82. Rosa FW, Bosco LA, Graham CF, Milstien JB, Dreis M, Creamer J. Neonatal anuria with maternal angiotensin-converting enzyme inhibition. *Obstet Gynecol.* 1989;74:371.
83. Scott AA, Purohit DM. Neonatal renal failure: a complication of maternal antihypertensive therapy. *Am J Obstet Gynecol.* 1989;160:1223.
84. Knott PD, Thorpe SS, Lamont CAR. Congenital renal dysgenesis possibly due to captopril. *Lancet.* 1989;1:451.
85. Barron WM, Murphy MD, Lindheimer MD. Management of hypertension during pregnancy. In: Laragh JH, Brenner BM, eds. *Hypertension, Diagnosis and Management.* New York: Raven Press, 1990:1809.
86. Redman CW. A controlled trial of the treatment of hypertension in pregnancy: labetalol compared with methyldopa. In: Riley A, Symonds EM, eds. *Investigation of labetalol in the Management of Hypertension in Pregnancy.* International Congress series 591. Amsterdam: Excerpta Medica, 1981:101.
87. Sibai BM, Gonzalez AR, Mabie WC, Moretti M. A comparison of labetalol plus hospitalization versus hospitalization alone in the management of preeclampsia remote from term. *Obstet Gynecol.* 1987;70:323.
88. Sibai BM, Mabie WC, Villar M, Shamsa F, et al. A comparison of no medication versus methyldopa or labetalol in chronic hypertension during pregnancy. *Am J Obstet Gynecol.* 1990;162:960.
89. Butters L, Kennedy S, Rubin P. Atenolol and fetal weight in chronic hypertension [Abstract]. *Clin Exp Hypertens [A].* 1989;B8:468.
90. Constantine G, Beevers DG, Reynolds AL, Luesley DM. Nifedipine as a second-line antihypertensive drug in pregnancy. *Br J Obstet Gynaecol.* 1987;94:1136.
91. Ulmsten U. Treatment of normotensive and hypertensive patients with preterm labor using oral nifedipine, a calcium antagonist. *Arch Gynecol.* 1984;236:69.
92. Fidler J, Smith V, Fayers P, DeSwiet M. Randomized controlled comparative study of methyldopa and oxprenolol in treatment of hypertension in pregnancy. *Br Med J.* 1983;286:1927.
93. Kincaid-Smith P, Bullen M, Mills J. Prolonged use of methyldopa in severe hypertension in pregnancy. *Br Med J.* 1966;1:274.
94. Redman CW. Treatment of hypertension in pregnancy. *Kidney Int.* 1980;18:267.
95. Ounsted M, Cockburn J, Moar VA, Redman CW. Maternal hypertension with superimposed pre-eclampsia: effects of child development at 7-½ years. *Br J Obstet Gynaecol.* 1983;90:644.
96. Hays PM, Cruikshank DP, Dunn LJ. Plasma volume determination in normal and preeclamptic pregnancies. *Am J Obstet Gynecol.* 1985;151:958.
97. Arias F, Zamora J. Antihypertensive treatment and pregnancy outcome in patients with mild chronic hypertension. *Obstet Gynecol.* 1979;53:489.
98. Sibai BM, Grossman RA, Grossman HG. Effects of diuretics on plasma volume in pregnancies with long-term hypertension. *Am J Obstet Gynecol.* 1984;150:831.
99. Kraus GW, Marchese JR, Yen SSC. Prophylactic use of hydrochlorothiazide in pregnancy. *JAMA.* 1966;198:1150.
100. Collins R, Yusuf S, Peto R. Overview of randomised trials of diuretics in pregnancy. *Br Med J.* 1985;290:17.
101. Widerlov E, Karlman I, Storsater J. Hydralazine-induced neonatal thrombocytopenia (letter). *N Engl J Med.* 1980;301:1235.
102. Beaufils M, Uzan S, Donsimoni R, Colau JC. Prevention of pre-eclampsia by early antiplatelet therapy. *Lancet.* 1985;1:840.
103. Wallenburg HC, Dekker GA, Makovitz JW, Rotmans P. Low-dose aspirin prevents pregnancy-induced hypertension and pre-eclampsia in angiotensin-sensitive primigravidae. *Lancet.* 1986;1:1.
104. Schiff E, Peleg E, Goldenberg M, et al. The use of aspirin to prevent pregnancy-induced hypertension and lower the ratio of thromboxane

A_2 to prostacyclin in relatively high-risk pregnancies. *N Engl J Med.* 1989;321:351.
105. Benigni A, Gregorini G, Frusca T, et al. Effect of low-dose aspirin on fetal and maternal generation of thromboxane by platelets in women at risk for pregnancy-induced hypertension. *N Engl J Med.* 1989;321:357.
106. Stuart MJ, Gross SJ, Elrad H, Graeber JE. Effects of acetylsalicylic-acid ingestion on maternal and neonatal hemostasis. *N Engl J Med.* 1982;307:909.
107. Davison JM, Lindheimer MD. Hypertension and pregnancy. In: Schrier RW, Gottschalk CW, eds. *Diseases of the Kidney, vol 2.* 4th ed. Boston: Little Brown & Co, 1988:1653.
108. Ferris TF. How should hypertension during pregnancy be managed? An internist's approach. *Med Clin North Am.* 1984;68:491.
109. Naden RP, Redman CW. Antihypertensive drugs in pregnancy. *Clin Perinatol.* 1985;12:521.
110. Walters BN, Redman CW. Treatment of severe pregnancy-associated hypertension with the calcium antagonist nifedipine. *Br J Obstet Gynaecol.* 1984;91:330.
111. Naulty J, Cefalo RC, Lewis PE. Fetal toxicity of nitroprusside in the pregnant ewe. *Am J Obstet Gynecol.* 1981;139:708.
112. Ferris TF. Prostanoids in normal and hypertensive pregnancy. In: Rubin PC, ed. *Hypertension in Pregnancy.* New York: Elsevier, 1988:102.
113. Dinsdale HB. Does magnesium sulfate treat eclamptic seizures? Yes. *Arch Neurol.* 1988;45:1360.
114. Kaplan PW, Lesser RP, Fisher RS, Repke JT, Hanley DF. No, magnesium sulfate should not be used in treating eclamptic seizures. *Arch Neurol.* 1988;45:1361.
115. Thurnau GR, Kemp DB, Jarvis A. Cerebrospinal fluid levels of magnesium in patients with preeclampsia after treatment with intravenous magnesium sulfate: a preliminary report. *Am J Obstet Gynecol.* 1987;157:1435.
116. Sibai BM, Spinnato JA, Watson DL, Lewis JA, Anderson GD. Effect of magnesium sulfate on electroencephalographic findings in pre-eclampsia-eclampsia. *Obstet Gynecol.* 1984;64:261.
117. Watson KV, Moldow CF, Ogburn PL, Jacob HS. Magnesium sulfate: rationale for its use in preeclampsia. *Proc Natl Acad Sci USA.* 1986;83:1075.
118. Sibai BM, Anderson GD. Pregnancy outcome of intensive therapy in severe hypertension in first trimester. *Obstet Gynecol.* 1986;67:517.
119. Pruett KM, Kirshon B, Cotton DB, Adam K, Doody KJ. The effects of magnesium sulfate therapy on Apgar scores. *Am J Obstet Gynecol.* 1988;159:1047.
120. Gallery ED, Delprado W, Györy AZ. Antihypertensive effect of plasma volume expansion in pregnancy-associated hypertension. *Aust NZ J Med.* 1981;11:20.
121. Øian P, Maltau JM, Noddeland H, Fadnes HO. Transcapillary fluid balance in pre-eclampsia. *Br J Obstet Gynaecol.* 1986;93:235.
122. Zinaman M, Rubin J, Lindheimer MD. Serial plasma oncotic pressure levels and echoencephalography during and after delivery in severe pre-eclampsia. *Lancet.* 1985;1:1245.
123. Clark SL, Cotton DB. Clinical indications for pulmonary artery catheterization in the patient with severe preeclampsia. *Am J Obstet Gynecol.* 1988;158:453.
124. American College of Obstetricians and Gynecologists. Invasive hemodynamic monitoring in obstetrics and gynecology. *ACOG Technical Bulletin.* October 1988, No. 121.
125. White WB. Management of hypertension during lactation. *Hypertension.* 1984;6:297.
126. White WB, Andreoli JW, Cohn RD. Alpha-methyldopa disposition in mothers with hypertension and in their breast-fed infants. *Clin Pharmacol Ther.* 1985;37:387.
127. Miller ME, Cohn RD, Burghart PH. Hydrochlorothiazide disposition in a mother and her breast-fed infant. *J Pediatr.* 1982;101:789.
128. Krause W, Stoppelli I, Milia S, Rainer E. Transfer of mepindolol to newborns by breast-feeding mothers after single and repeated daily doses. *Eur J Clin Pharmacol.* 1982;22:53.
129. Bryans CI Jr. The remote prognosis in toxemia of pregnancy. *Clin Obstet Gynecol.* 1966;9:973.
130. Chesley LC, Annitto JE, Cosgrove RA. The remote prognosis of eclamptic women: sixth periodic report. *Am J Obstet Gynecol.* 1976;124:446.
131. Hamilton M, Pickering GW, Roberts JAF, Sowry GSC. The aetiology of essential hypertension: the arterial blood pressure in the general population. *Clin Sci.* 1954;13:11.
132. Frohlich ED, Grim C, Labarthe DR, Maxwell MH, Perloff D, Weidman W. Recommendations for human blood pressure determination by sphygmomanometers: report of a special task force appointed by the Steering Committee, American Heart Association. *Hypertension.* 1988;11:209A.

APPENDIX

Blood Pressure Measurement Protocol

Accurate and consistent blood pressure measurements are essential to establish a baseline and monitor subtle changes throughout the duration of the pregnancy. Blood pressures should be taken in a standardized fashion by all personnel who see the pregnant woman during her antepartum, intrapartum, and postpartum care. In 1987 the American Heart Association (AHA) updated its standards for the fifth time since 1939 in its Recommendations for Human Blood Pressure Determination by Sphygmomanometers.[132] Although this document focuses primarily on nonpregnant populations, many of its paradigms relate to the gestational period as well.

For accurate blood pressure measurements in all clinical situations, the AHA document recommends a standardized measurement technique. This includes:

- Have the patient sit* for 5 minutes before blood pressure measurement with the arm resting on a table at heart level (using the same arm on each measurement occasion for consistency).
- Measure the bared arm for proper cuff size and have available commonly used cuff sizes for adults, notably regular and large adult cuffs with respective bladder widths of 12 and 15 cm (or in general, a bladder width of 40% of the arm circumference, ensuring a bladder length that encircles 80% of the upper arm).
- Assess for approximate systolic blood pressure level before measurement by finding where the radial pulse disappears with simultaneous palpation and inflation to disappearance.
- Maintain a slow, steady deflation rate of 2 to 3 mm Hg per second or per heartbeat when doing a reading.
- Take the average of the two readings (also recommended by the Joint National Committee) to help minimize variations in recorded blood pressure across time caused by blood pressure's inherent variability (reflected in isolated readings).
- Use accurate equipment (mercury sphygmomanometer or calibrated aneroid).

It is important to remember that blood pressure measurements are influenced by the relationship of the cuff to the level of the heart (caused by hydrostatic pressure, the effect of gravity on the column of blood). Blood pressure with the cuff higher than the level of the heart will be lower; blood pressure with the cuff lower than the level of the heart will be higher. For example, the practice of taking the blood pressure in the upper arm with the woman on her side will give falsely lower readings. Each centimeter above or below heart level translates to an 0.8 mm Hg change. Thus these readings will naturally differ from those taken when the arm is appropriately at heart level (ie, woman in supine position with the arm at her side or preferably seated with the arm resting on a standard table top).

In listening to blood pressure readings, the first of at least two consecutive beats should be recorded as phase I, the systolic pressure. The AHA recommends that the onset of phase V (disappearance of sound), marked by the last sound heard, be used for defining diastolic pressure in adults. The onset of phase IV or muffling, sometimes used in the past, is harder to recognize and is subject to greater interobserver and intraobserver variability. The vast body of epidemiologic evidence from clinical trials in nonpregnant populations, linking levels of diastolic pressure

---

* The WHO Study Group[10] notes that it probably does not matter whether the patient sits or lies slightly on the left side (15- to 30-degree tilt), provided the same position is used. For practical purposes the seated position with the arm resting at heart level is the procedure used in virtually all prenatal clinics.

to increased cardiovascular disease risk, is based on the phase V criterion. In pregnancy phase V seems to correlate best with intraarterial pressure.[33]

However, the AHA recognized certain conditions in which phase V is absent (ie, the Korotkoff sounds do not disappear but may be heard until the pressure in the cuff falls to near 0 mm Hg). Among these conditions are high cardiac output states including pregnancy. Also, the WHO has noted that in approximately 15% of pregnant women the diastolic pressure falls to zero before the last sound is heard. Under these conditions, phase IV is a better index of diastolic pressure than is phase V. Both the AHA and WHO advise that if the phase IV (muffled) sounds are heard to zero (absent phase V), both phase IV and phase V readings should be recorded (eg, 148/84/0 mm Hg). It seems prudent, given that the AHA recommends recording the onset of phase V as the diastolic blood pressure in adults, coupled with the probability of an absent phase V in a certain percentage of pregnant women in whom the onset of phase IV should then be recorded, that personnel should record both readings throughout the duration of the woman's pregnancy starting at the woman's initial prenatal visit. This will help ensure that no information will be lost (eg, baseline phase IV and V readings) and that subtle changes will be detected.

Chapter One Hundred and Thirty-Nine
Preeclampsia: Diagnosis and Management

Baha M. Sibai and Jaime J. Rodriguez

139

Hypertensive disorders are the most common medical complication of pregnancy. Approximately 7–10% of all pregnancies are complicated by hypertension. The two most common forms of hypertension are pregnancy-induced hypertensive disease (PIH), which accounts for 70% of hypertension during pregnancy, and preexisting chronic hypertension, which is responsible for the remaining cases.[1] Hypertensive disorders are associated with significant maternal and perinatal mortality and present as a wide spectrum of disorders, ranging from minimal elevation of blood pressure only to severe hypertension with multiple organ dysfunction.

TERMINOLOGY

Pregnancy-induced hypertension is unique to human pregnancy. The terminology used to describe the condition has been confusing and inconsistent. More than 60 names in English have been applied to the condition. The American College of Obstetricians and Gynecologists' committee on terminology defines hypertension in pregnancy as either a systolic pressure of ≥140 mm Hg or an increment of ≥30 mm Hg (from a baseline in the first half of pregnancy), or a diastolic pressure of ≥90 mm Hg or an increment of ≥15 mm Hg. The absolute level of blood pressure or increments in pressure must be observed on at least two occasions six hours apart.[2] The committee also considers a mean arterial pressure of 105 mm Hg, or an increment of 20 mm Hg, as diagnostic of pregnancy-induced hypertension. The diagnosis of preeclampsia is based on hypertension with proteinuria, edema, or both. This definition differs from others used by some European countries, making comparisons of studies very difficult.

CLASSIFICATIONS

Multiple classifications have been proposed to classify the hypertensive disorders of pregnancy. In 1972, the committee on terminology suggested five categories:

1. Gestational hypertension, defined as hypertension appearing in the second half of pregnancy or in the first 24 hours postpartum without edema or proteinuria, and with a return to normotension within 10 days after delivery
2. Preeclampsia, defined as hypertension together with abnormal edema or proteinuria
3. Eclampsia, defined as the development of convulsions or coma in patients with signs and symptoms of preeclampsia in the absence of other causes of convulsions
4. Chronic hypertensive disease, defined as chronic hypertension of any cause. This group includes patients with preexisting hypertension, patients with preexistent elevation of blood pressure to at least 140/90 mm Hg on two occasions before 20 weeks, and patients with hypertension that persists for more than 42 days postpartum.
5. Superimposed preeclampsia or eclampsia, defined as the development of preeclampsia or eclampsia in patients with diagnosed chronic hypertension. About 15–30% of chronically hypertensive women will develop preeclampsia.

Preeclampsia also is classified as either mild or severe. Severe preeclampsia is diagnosed when any of the criteria listed in Table 139–1 is present. These criteria for severe preeclampsia do not include other findings that also indicate severe disease such as abnormal hepatic function, low platelets, and fetal growth retardation. The classifications and definitions of the hypertensive disorders of pregnancy are

TABLE 139–1. CRITERIA FOR THE DIAGNOSIS OF SEVERE PREECLAMPSIA

Blood pressure ≥160 mm Hg systolic or ≥110 mm Hg diastolic on two occasions at least six hours apart with the patient at bed rest
Proteinuria ≥5 g in a 24-hour urine collection or ≥3 on dipstick in at least two random clean-catch samples at least four hours apart
Oliguria (≤400 ml in 24 hours)
Cerebral or visual disturbances
Epigastric pain
Pulmonary edema or cyanosis
Thrombocytopenia

Adapted from ACOG Technical Bulletin.[2]

TABLE 139–3. PREECLAMPSIA IN SINGLETON VERSUS TWIN GESTATIONS

	Singleton (n = 2434) %	Twin (n = 166) %
Primiparas (incidence)	14.1	35.2
Multiparas (incidence)	5.7	20.4
Total (incidence)	9.3	25.9
Early onset	24.4	68.7
Severe hypertension	20.9	45.2
Proteinuria	48.4	60.4
Eclampsia	0.7	3.6

Modified from Long and Oats.[4]

confusing. It frequently is difficult to differentiate between preeclampsia, chronic hypertension, and chronic hypertension with superimposed preeclampsia. The normal midtrimester fall in blood pressure may conceal the presence of underlying chronic hypertension; unless the patient presents in the first trimester or has a well documented history of chronic hypertension, accurate classification is impossible.

This review will focus on diagnosis and management of pregnancy-induced hypertensive disorders which will include PIH, preeclampsia and superimposed preeclampsia.

PREECLAMPSIA

Preeclampsia is a disorder peculiar to human pregnancy. Reported incidences range from 2% to 35% depending on the diagnostic criteria and the population studied. It is principally a disease of young primigravidas. The incidence is about 6–7% of all pregnancies in the United States; however, it is 19.6% among young primigravidas at our institution.[3]

Although geographic and racial differences in incidence have been reported, several risk factors have been identified as predisposing to the development of preeclampsia in different populations (Table 139–2). The incidence is significantly increased in patients with multiple gestation and in those with previous preeclampsia. For patients with twin gestation, both the incidence and severity are higher than in those with singleton pregnancy (Table 139–3).[4] In addition, the incidence is significantly higher in patients with previous preeclampsia and in those with previous preeclampsia remote from term.[5] Patients over 35 years of age also have an increased incidence of preeclampsia, mainly due to increased undiagnosed chronic hypertension in this group of patients.

TABLE 139–2. RISK FACTORS FOR PREECLAMPSIA

Nulliparity
Multiple gestation
Family history of preeclampsia-eclampsia
Preexisting hypertension/renal disease
Previous preeclampsia-eclampsia
Diabetes
Nonimmune hydrops fetalis
Molar pregnancy

DIAGNOSIS

Preeclampsia traditionally has been described as a triad of edema, proteinuria, and hypertension. However, a spectrum of clinical signs and symptoms, presenting either alone or in combination, makes the diagnosis of preeclampsia a subject of great controversy. Abnormal blood pressure elevation is the traditional hallmark for the diagnosis of the disease. The measurement of blood pressure is subject to many errors; several variants may influence the readings—faulty equipment, race, obesity, smoking, position, patient anxiety, or duration of the resting period.[6]

There also is controversy regarding which Korotkoff phase should be used to measure the diastolic blood pressure. Both Korotkoff Phase 4 (muffling of sound) and Phase 5 (disappearance of sound) had been used for diagnosis and clinical trials. Phase 4 measures about 5–10 mm Hg higher than Phase 5. It has been suggested that Phase 4 be used for diagnosis and clinical trials.[6]

The diagnosis of PIH requires the presence of increased blood pressure criteria only (without proteinuria). The elevation in blood pressure could be an absolute value of 140/90 mm Hg or a relative value, in which blood pressure must increase ≥15 mm Hg diastolic from a previous recording prior to 20 weeks' gestation (see section on terminology). The use of blood pressure increments to define hypertension during pregnancy has been the subject of great controversy.[3] It requires a baseline reading that may not be available, and there is a gradual increase in blood pressure from the second to the third trimester seen in most normotensive pregnancies. MacGillivray et al[7] reported that 73% of primigravid patients with normotensive pregnancies demonstrate an increase in diastolic pressure of >15 mm Hg at some stage during the course of their pregnancies. In addition, 57% of these patients demonstrated an increase of >20 mm Hg during the course of their gestation. Redman and Jeffries[8] analyzed different thresholds of raised diastolic blood pressure in 16,211 singleton pregnancies to determine the best blood pressure criteria to diagnose preeclampsia. They found that elevations in diastolic blood pressure of at least 25 mm Hg and a maximum reading of at least 90 mm Hg gave the best acceptable criteria.

Villar and Sibai[3] studied blood pressure changes during the course of pregnancy in 700 young primigravidas. They found that a threshold increase in diastolic pressure of ≥15 mm Hg on two occasions was present in 68% of normotensive pregnancies and a threshold increase in systolic pressure was present in 67% of these patients. The sensitivity and positive predictive values for preeclampsia were 39% and 32%, respectively, for a threshold increase in diastolic pressure. The respective values for a threshold increase in systolic pressure were 22% and 33%. In addition to the fact that at least two observations of elevated blood pressure are required for the diagnosis of PIH, these observations will be influenced by at least three factors: gestational age at first observation, frequency of blood pressure measurements, and the two observations to be selected. Thus the increments in blood pressure criteria should not be used, especially for research purposes or clinical trials.

The diagnosis of preeclampsia requires the presence of elevated blood pressure with proteinuria, edema, or both. The presence of proteinuria usually is determined by the use of dipsticks or the sulfosalicylic acid test on random urine samples. The concentration of urinary protein is highly variable. It is influenced by several factors including contamination with vaginal secretions, blood or bacteria, urine specific gravity and pH, exercise, and posture. The definitive test for diagnosing proteinuria thus should be quantitative measurement of total protein excretion over a 24-hour period. Significant proteinuria should be defined as >300 mg per 24-hour urine sample. For making the diagnosis of severe preeclampsia based on proteinuria only, it is recommended that a 24-hour urine excretion of protein >5 g be documented. The diagnosis of severe preeclampsia based on dipstick measurements in urine samples (≥3) is not adequate for such a diagnosis.

EDEMA

The assessment of edema is highly subjective. Moderate edema is present in 80% of normal pregnancies. In addition, 40% of patients with eclampsia at our institution had no edema before the onset of convulsions. Edema should be considered pathologic only if generalized, involving the hands, face, and legs. Consequently, it is now accepted that the presence of edema is not required for the diagnosis of preeclampsia.

PREDICTION OF PREECLAMPSIA

The fact that the etiology of preeclampsia remains unknown has made the prediction of preeclampsia very difficult, and numerous clinical and biochemical tests have been reported as predicting preeclampsia. Some of the recommended clinical tests are summarized in Table 139–4. Several reports suggested using the average mean arterial blood pressure in the second trimester (MAP-2) to identify patients destined to develop PIH. MAP-2 can be calculated as follows:

$$\text{MAP} = \frac{\text{SYSTOLIC BP} + \text{DIASTOLIC BP} \times 2}{3}$$

The average readings of MAP during the second trimester can be expressed as MAP-2.

Chesley and Sibai[9] summarized several reports that included 39,876 cases of preeclampsia and 207 cases of eclampsia and investigated the predictive value of elevated mean arterial pressure in the second trimester. The sensitivity in these reports ranged from 0% to 92%, and the specificity varied from 53% to 97%. They concluded that if increased second trimester mean arterial blood pressure predicts anything, it is transient hypertension rather than preeclampsia or eclampsia. Villar and Sibai[3] evaluated the predictive value of MAP-2 in 700 young primigravidas that were followed throughout pregnancy. The sensitivity of MAP-2 ≥90 mm Hg was 8% and the positive predictive value was 23%. The authors concluded that this test was not predictive of future preeclampsia.

The *rollover test* was first described by Gant et al.[10] It usually is performed in primigravidas between 28 and 32 weeks' gestation. The patient initially is placed in the left lateral recumbent position until a stable diastolic blood pressure is recorded. The patient then is turned to a supine position five minutes later, and the blood pressure is measured again. A rise in diastolic pressure >20 mm Hg on change of position is considered positive. The authors reported that 15 of 16 (93%) primigravid women with a positive test subsequently developed PIH. Conversely, 20 of 22 (91%) with a negative test remained normotensive. Contrary to Gant et al, other investigators have reported a significant incidence of false-negative and false-positive results. To date, the value of this test in predicting PIH was evaluated in 14 reports. Sensitivity ranged from 0% to 93% and the specificity ranged from 54% to 91%. In summary, none of these clinical tests seems sufficiently reliable for use as a screening test for PIH.[6] At our institution, none of these tests are used for screening purposes.

The *angiotensin II* (A-II) *test* is an invasive procedure that requires infusions of the potent vasopressor A-II at 26–30 weeks and subsequent measurement of diastolic blood pressure. Whether the test is positive or negative depends on the amount of A-II required to elicit an increase in diastolic pressure of ≥20 mm Hg. The value of the A-II infusion test for the prediction of PIH has been studied by several investigators. It has a specificity of 90–95%, but the sensitivity is very variable with a high incidence of false positive results.

TABLE 139–4. CLINICAL TESTS TO PREDICT PREECLAMPSIA

Average MAP-2 ≥ 90 mm Hg
Average MAP-2 ≥ 85 mm Hg
Maximal MAP-2 ≥ 90 mm Hg
MAP at 20 weeks ≥ 90 mm Hg
Diastolic in mid-trimester ≥ 80 mm Hg
Rollover test at 28–32 weeks
Combination of the above
A-II infusion test at 26–30 weeks
Isometric exercise test

MAP-2 = mean arterial pressure in second trimester
A-II = Angiotensin II

PREVENTION OF PREECLAMPSIA

There are numerous reports and clinical trials describing the use of various methods to prevent or reduce the incidence of preeclampsia. Since the etiology of the disease is unknown, these methods were used to correct the pathophysiologic abnormalities in the hopes of ameliorating the course of, or preventing, the disease. Some of the methods used are summarized in Table 139–5. To date, none of these methods have been shown conclusively effective in preventing the disease.

Diets low in salt and high in protein, as well as restricted caloric intake, have been suggested to prevent preeclampsia. In addition, the use of diuretics has been recommended

TABLE 139–5. PREVENTION OF PREECLAMPSIA

Dietary Manipulation
Low-caloric diet
High-protein diet
Low-salt diet
Nutritional supplementation
Calcium, magnesium, zinc
Fish oil and evening primrose oil
Pharmacologic Manipulation
Diuretics
Antihypertensives
B-Sympathomimetics
Antithrombic agents
Low-dose aspirin
Dipyridamole
Dazoxiben
Heparin
Vitamin E
Personal Habit Changes
Frequent prenatal care
Daily rest in lateral position
Keep same partner
Avoid or reduce smoking
Avoid or reduce coffee

to prevent preeclampsia.[11] However, the efficacy of these measures has never been proven.

Several epidemiologic studies and few clinical supplementation trials have suggested a relationship between calcium, magnesium, zinc intake, and pregnancy-induced hypertension. These studies are reviewed in the section on nutritional supplementation during pregnancy (see Chapter 22) and will not be discussed here.

As stated in Chapter 138, enhanced platelet activation with resultant abnormalities in the thromboxane/prostacyclin balance appears to play a central role in the pathogenesis of preeclampsia and its manifestations. Several authors thus used antithrombotic agents to alter these pathologic changes in an attempt to prevent or ameliorate the course of preeclampsia.

There is some evidence from case reports and a few clinical trials that low-dose aspirin (60–150 mg/d) with or without dipyridamole may reduce the incidence of preeclampsia.[12] The majority of these studies had a small sample size and included patients with previous poor obstetric outcome who were considered at risk for preeclampsia. Some of these studies used aspirin empirically early in pregnancy[13,14], while others[15,16] randomized patients who had positive screening tests (A-II infusion or rollover test) at 28–29 weeks.

Beaufils and associates[13] studied 102 patients at risk for preeclampsia, fetal growth retardation, or fetal demise. A total of 52 women were treated with aspirin 150 mg/d plus dipyridamole 300 mg/d from 12 weeks' gestation until delivery. The other 50 patients served as controls. The authors reported absent preeclampsia and fetal deaths in the treatment group, while there were six cases of preeclampsia and five fetal deaths in the control group. The incidence of fetal growth retardation was 8.3% among the treated group and 28.8% among the controls. However, the study results are questionable in that the two groups were not randomized and that they deferred in parity and degree of preexisting chronic hypertension or renal disease.

Benigni et al[14] studied the effect of long-term daily administration of 60 mg of aspirin or placebo on maternal and neonatal prostanoid production in women at risk for pregnancy-induced hypertension. The authors reported absent preeclampsia, lower incidence of fetal growth retardation and higher neonatal birth weights in the aspirin-treated group. They also found significant inhibition of maternal platelet thromboxane production with minimal effects on prostacyclin production in the aspirin-treated group. However, the sample size was too small and one third of the women studied received antihypertensive medications for chronic hypertension. The diagnosis of pregnancy-induced hypertension thus is questionable in this study.

Wallenburg et al[15] studied 207 primigravidas that were screened by A-II infusions at 28 weeks' gestation. A total of 46 patients had positive tests and thus were judged to be at increased risk for preeclampsia. These 46 patients were randomized to receive a placebo or aspirin 60 mg/d. Two patients in the aspirin group were later excluded for poor compliance. At 33–35 weeks' gestation, a venous blood sample was drawn for determination of thrombin-induced production of malondialdehyde (MDA) by platelets. This dose caused 90% inhibition of platelet MDA synthesis. The aspirin-treated group had no preeclampsia or severe PIH, while the placebo-treated group had three cases with severe PIH, seven with preeclampsia, and one woman developed eclampsia. The incidence of fetal growth retardation was 19% in the aspirin group and 39% in the control group. Although this is an interesting finding, the small sample size makes it difficult to draw any conclusions.

Schiff et al[16] studied 791 women at risk for preeclampsia who were screened by the rollover test at 28–29 weeks' gestation. A total of 69 patients had positive tests and thus were judged to be at high risk for subsequent preeclampsia. Of these women, 65 were randomized to receive a placebo or aspirin 100 mg/d. The incidence of pregnancy-induced hypertension was 35.5% in the placebo-treated group and 11.8% in the aspirin-treated group. The mean ratio of maternal serum levels of thromboxane A_2 to serum levels of prostacyclin metabolites was significantly lower in the aspirin-treated group. The authors concluded that low daily doses of aspirin in the third trimester of pregnancy reduces the incidence of pregnancy-induced hypertension in women at risk for this disorder.

Currently, large clinical trials are underway in the United States and worldwide to assess the safety and efficacy of low-dose aspirin in preventing preeclampsia and its complications. The value of such therapy should await the results of these clinical trials.

LABORATORY FINDINGS

There are considerable differences regarding the incidence, etiology, clinical significance, and management of most of the laboratory abnormalities reported in patients with preeclampsia. All laboratory tests studied tend to reflect the pathophysiologic abnormalities associated with the development of the disease process (see Chapter 138 on pathophysiology). Some tests were suggested to predict the development of preeclampsia, some were diagnostic of preeclampsia, and others were recommended to predict perinatal outcome. Numerous reports have evaluated the value of every biochemical substance that can be measured in maternal blood or urine during the diagnosis and management of preeclampsia. Results of these studies have been inconsistent and contradictory. In addition, results of the pooled data suggest that no single laboratory test is sufficiently reliable, sensitive, or specific for use in clinical management of these patients. However, some of these tests (such as platelet count and liver enzymes) may be useful in association with other clinical parameters in monitoring the clinical course of the disease process.

In general, the frequency, nature, and degree of laboratory abnormalities usually correlate with the organ system involved as well as the severity of the disease process. Patients with preeclampsia may have normal laboratory findings or a wide spectrum of abnormalities in renal function, liver function, and hemostasis tests. Creatinine clearance and serum creatinine usually are normal in patients with mild pregnancy-induced hypertension, while they are significantly abnormal in patients with severe preeclampsia remote from term. Serum uric acid usually is abnormal in most patients with preeclampsia and the levels tend to correlate with the severity of the disease process. However, the levels do not correlate with perinatal outcome.[17]

Liver function tests usually are normal in most patients with mild disease, and abnormal in about 20–30% of patients with severe disease. Again, the levels of these tests do not correlate with perinatal outcome. Thrombocytopenia (platelet count $<100 \times 10^3/mm^3$) is found in about 10% of pregnancies with severe preeclampsia; its presence makes the diagnosis of severe disease regardless of the level of blood pressure or amount of proteinuria. Prothrombin time, activated partial thromboplastin time, and fibrinogen levels are normal in most patients with preeclampsia. These tests usually are abnormal in preeclampsia complicated by severe *abruptio placentae* or fetal demise.

HELLP SYNDROME

Hemolysis, abnormal liver function tests, and thrombocytopenia have been recognized as complications of preeclampsia for many years.[18] In 1982, Weinstein[19] coined the term *HELLP syndrome* to describe the presence of these abnormalities: *H* for *hemolysis*, *EL* for *elevated liver enzymes*, and *LP* for *low platelets*. Since then, several articles and case reports claiming to describe this syndrome have appeared in the medical literature. A review of the literature by Sibai et al[20] revealed considerable differences concerning the terminology, incidence, cause, diagnosis, and management of this syndrome. This syndrome has been labelled as an early form of severe preeclampsia, unique variant of preeclampsia, EPH gestosis, and misdiagnosed preeclampsia. The reported incidence of this syndrome ranges from 2% to 12%, which reflects the different diagnostic criteria and different methods used in studies claiming to describe this syndrome.[20] In addition, there are considerable differences regarding the time of onset, type, and degree of laboratory abnormalities used to make the diagnosis of this syndrome. Some studies included patients who had the abnormalities on admission, some included patients who developed the abnormalities during conservative management of patients with preeclampsia, and others included patients who developed the abnormalities in the postpartum period.

A significant percentage of the reports included patients who had no hemolysis; other reports included patients whose platelet count was $>100 \times 10^3/mm^3$. There is no consensus in the literature regarding which liver function test abnormalities should be used to diagnose this syndrome. Our criteria for the diagnosis of this syndrome requires the presence of the following laboratory findings:[20]

- Hemolysis defined by abnormal peripheral smear, increased bilirubin ($\geq$1.2 mg/dl), and increased lactic dehydrogenase ($\geq$600 U/L)
- Elevated liver enzymes defined as increased SGOT ($\geq$70 U/L), and increased LDH
- Low platelets defined as platelet count $<100 \times 10^3/mm^3$.

The typical clinical presentation is that of a white, multiparous patient with a history of poor pregnancy outcome. The patient classically presents remote from term complaining of epigastric or right upper quadrant pain (90%), some will have nausea or vomiting (50%) and others will have nonspecific viral syndromelike symptoms. The majority of patients (90%) will give a history of malaise for the past few days prior to presentation. Hypertension or proteinuria may be absent or slightly abnormal.[21] Some of these patients thus may present with a variety of signs and symptoms, none of which are diagnostic of classic severe preeclampsia.

Upon physical examination, the patient will have right upper quadrant tenderness (80%) and significant weight gain with generalized edema (60%). Hypertension may be absent (20%), mild (30%), or severe (50%), depending on the duration of signs and symptoms.[22] In some cases, the patient may present with gastrointestinal bleeding, hematuria, flank or shoulder pain, and jaundice. As a result, these patients are often misdiagnosed as having various medical and surgical disorders (Table 139–6).

MANAGEMENT OF PREECLAMPSIA

Once the diagnosis of preeclampsia is well established, definitive therapy in the form of delivery is the desired goal, since it is the only cure for the disease. The decision for immediate delivery versus expectant management is usually dependent on one or more of the following: severity of the disease process, fetal gestational age, maternal condition, fetal condition, and cervical Bishop score.

MILD PREECLAMPSIA

All patients with diagnosed preeclampsia should be hospitalized at the time of diagnosis. These pregnancies usually are associated with reduced uteroplacental blood flow as measured by functional placental scintigraphy.[23] The uteroplacental blood flow is already reduced by about 50% by the time the patient develops the clinical signs of preeclampsia. The mother also is at slightly increased risk for the

TABLE 139–6. DIFFERENTIAL DIAGNOSIS OF PATIENTS WITH HELLP SYNDROME

Viral hepatitis
Gastroenteritis
Gallbladder disease
Kidney stones
Pyelonephritis
Peptic ulcer
Idiopathic thrombocytopenia
Thrombotic thrombocytopenic purpura
Hemolytic uremic syndrome
Acute glomerulonephritis
Encephalopathy of various etiologies

development of *abruptio placentae* (1%) or convulsions (0.2%). Thus, women with mild disease who have a favorable cervix for induction (Bishop score ≥7) should receive intravenous magnesium sulfate to prevent convulsions and undergo induction of labor for delivery. Similar management is indicated for all patients at ≥40 weeks' gestation irrespective of cervical status.

Management of mild disease remote from term is highly controversial. A review of the literature indicates disagreement regarding one, or more, of the following: ambulatory management versus hospitalization for the duration of pregnancy; use of salt restriction; need for antihypertensive therapy; and use of sedatives and anticonvulsive prophylaxis during labor. Bed rest is generally recommended by all physicians. European and Australian physicians are more likely to use antihypertensive drugs than American physicians. On the other hand, American obstetricians are more likely to use anticonvulsive prophylaxis during labor than Europeans, who do not use intrapartum prophylaxis for patients with mild disease.

In the United States, management of these patients usually involves hospitalization for the duration of pregnancy since this approach enhances fetal survival and reduces the frequency of progression to severe disease. This approach usually arrests the clinical course of the disease or at least improves it long enough to achieve fetal maturity without jeopardizing maternal safety.[24,25] The success rate of expectant management depends on fetal gestational age and on maternal status at the time of hospitalization. In general, patients hospitalized with mild elevations of hypertension only (diastolic pressure <100 mm Hg, absent proteinuria) and gestational age ≥32 weeks have a better pregnancy outcome than those hospitalized with earlier gestational age and higher diastolic pressures in association with proteinuria.

Gilstrap et al[24], studied 545 nulliparous women with mild pregnancy-induced hypertension, who were managed with bed rest in the hospital for the duration of pregnancy. These women were allowed to ambulate as desired, were given a general hospital diet, and none received antihypertensive drugs. Gestational age at time of hospitalization ranged from 25 to 38 weeks, and 373 (69%) were less than 37 weeks' gestation. The majority of the patients had hypertension and only 8% of the women had proteinuria of ≥100 mg/dL at time of hospitalization. Duration of pregnancy prolongation ranged from 2 to 120 days (average of 24 days) and 87% were delivered at ≥37 weeks. The overall perinatal mortality was 9/1000, and only 8.4% of the infants were small-for-gestational-age.

Sibai et al[25] reported on 200 women with mild preeclampsia at 26–35 weeks' gestation who were randomized to treatment with bed rest alone in the hospital or in combination with antihypertensive treatment with labetalol. All patients had hypertension with proteinuria. The average duration of pregnancy prolongation was 21 days, the overall perinatal mortality was 5/10,000, and 13.5% of the infants were small-for-gestational-age. The pregnancy outcome for the above two studies is summarized in Table 139–7.

The antepartum use of antihypertensive drugs for mild preeclampsia remote from term is highly controversial. There are numerous clinical reports (controlled and uncontrolled) describing the use of various drugs in an attempt to prolong gestation and improve perinatal outcome in these pregnancies. A detailed description of these reports and the drugs used is mentioned elsewhere (see Chapter 111 on antihypertensive drugs). It is important to note that these drugs are used overseas and are rarely used in this

TABLE 139–7. PREGNANCY OUTCOME IN HOSPITALIZED PATIENTS WITH MILD PREECLAMPSIA

	Gilatrapetal[24] N = 545	Sibai, et al[25] N = 200
GA[a] at hospitalization (wk)	25–38	26–35
Average prolongation (days)	24	21
Mean birth weight (g)	2824	2258
Small for gestation (%)	46 (8.4)	27 (13.5)
Perinatal deaths (%)	5 (0.9)	1 (0.5)
Abruptio placentae (%)	5 (1)	2 (1)
Eclampsia (%)	1 (0.5)	0

[a]GA = gestational age

country for such purposes. In addition, none of these studies has reported a better perinatal outcome than studies that used hospitalization only for preeclampsia.

All patients with mild preeclampsia are hospitalized at the time of diagnosis at this institution. Patients are allowed to eat a regular hospital diet without salt restriction and their activity is not restricted to complete bed rest. Diuretics and antihypertensives are not prescribed and sedatives are not used. All patients undergo serial evaluation of maternal and fetal well-being until delivery. The frequency of testing usually depends on the fetal gestational age and maternal response following hospitalization. Fetal evaluation should include serial ultrasonography for evaluation of fetal growth every two weeks, daily fetal movement count, nonstress testing (NST) every week, and biophysical profile if needed. Maternal evaluation should include frequent blood pressure monitoring (q 4 hours during the day), checking of patellar reflexes, and maternal weight, and presence of edema daily. In addition, all patients should be questioned regarding symptoms of impending eclampsia (persistent headaches, visual disturbances, or epigastric pain). Laboratory evaluation should include measurements of urine protein, hematocrit and platelet count (every two days), and liver function tests (1–2 times/wk). This evaluation is extremely important since patients may develop thrombocytopenia and elevated liver enzymes with minimal blood pressure elevations.

If the patient becomes normotensive in the absence of significant proteinuria, outpatient observation may be considered in a select group of patients. This form of management is appropriate in a reliable patient only during the early stages of the disease and in the absence of any evidence of fetal jeopardy. These patients should be instructed to have bed rest at home, and to have daily urine dipstick measurements of proteinuria, and have blood pressure monitoring (self or by nurse). The patient should be instructed to keep fetal movement counts and to report any symptoms of impending eclampsia. The patient then is evaluated in the antepartum testing area for maternal and fetal well-being at least two times per week. If there is any evidence of disease progression or if acute hypertension or proteinuria develop, then prompt hospitalization is indicated. If there are any signs of worsening maternal or fetal conditions at any time during hospitalization, then delivery is indicated.

SEVERE PREECLAMPSIA

The clinical course of severe preeclampsia is usually characterized by progressive deterioration in both maternal and fetal status. These pregnancies usually are associated with increased rates of perinatal mortality and morbidity.[26] Most of the fetal-neonatal complications are related to intrauterine fetal growth retardation and prematurity.[27] In addition, such pregnancies are associated with increased rates of maternal mortality and morbidity. The ultimate goals of therapy always must be safety of the mother first and then consideration for optimum perinatal outcome. Since the only cure for severe preeclampsia is delivery, there is universal agreement to deliver all patients if the disease develops beyond 34 weeks' gestation or if there is evidence of fetal lung maturity or fetal jeopardy prior to that time. In this situation, appropriate management should include parenteral medications to prevent convulsions (magnesium sulfate in the United States), control of maternal blood pressure within a safe range, and then induction of labor to initiate delivery.

On the other hand, management of patients with severe disease remote from term (≤34 weeks) is highly controversial. Some institutions consider delivery as the definitive therapy for all cases, regardless of gestational age, while others recommend prolonging pregnancy in all patients remote from term until one or more of the following is achieved:

- Fetal lung maturity
- Fetal jeopardy
- Gestational age ≥36 weeks
- Maternal jeopardy

Sibai et al[26] reported on 303 pregnancies complicated by severe preeclampsia that were delivered within 48 hours of admission. The overall perinatal mortality was 13.5%, and 20.0% of the births were small-for-gestational-age. Ninety-one of the 303 patients had superimposed preeclampsia and these patients had a significantly high incidence of perinatal complications: perinatal deaths (32%), fetal growth retardation (33%), and *abruptio placentae* (10%). In addition, the authors found a perinatal survival of zero for patients delivered before 28 weeks, a neonatal survival of 94% for infants delivered between 29 and 32 weeks' gestastion, and 100% for those delivered after 32 weeks. However, neonatal morbidity was still significant especially in those delivered before 32 weeks (Table 139–8).

At this institution, all patients with severe preeclampsia are admitted to labor and delivery area for close observation of maternal and fetal condition. All patients receive intravenous magnesium sulfate to prevent convulsions and bolus doses of hydralazine (5–10 mg) intravenously as needed to keep diastolic pressure below 110 mm Hg. All patients with persistent severe hypertension or other signs of maternal or fetal deterioration usually are delivered within 24 hours irrespective of gestational age or fetal lung maturity. Women with gestational age beyond 35 weeks and those with evidence of fetal lung maturity at 33–35 weeks usually are delivered within 24 hours. Patients at 33–35 weeks with immature fluid receive steroids to accelerate fetal lung maturity and then are delivered.

For pregnancies at 28–32 weeks, the management is dependent on their clinical response during the observation period. Some of these women will demonstrate marked diuresis and improvement in blood pressure during observation. If the blood pressure remains below 100 mm Hg diastolic (without antihypertensive therapy) after the observation period, magnesium sulfate is discontinued and the patients are followed closely in the hospital until fetal maturity is achieved. During hospitalization, they undergo frequent evaluation of maternal and fetal well-being. Steroids usually are used as indicated. The authors' experience has been that the majority of these patients will require delivery within two weeks after hospitalization. However, some patients may continue with their pregnancy for more than two weeks. It is important to note that such pregnancies should be managed at tertiary care centers.

TABLE 139–8. NEONATAL COMPLICATIONS IN SEVERE PREECLAMPSIA

GA[a] at Delivery	Respiratory Distress %	Cerebral Hemorrhage %	Renal Failure %
≤28	40	100	100
29–30	25	45	5
31–32	25	20	7
33–36	2	1	0
>36	0	0	0

[a] GA = gestational age
Modified from Sibai, et al[26]

SEVERE PREECLAMPSIA IN MIDTRIMESTER

Occasionally, a patient may develop severe preeclampsia at ≤28 weeks' gestation. These pregnancies are associated with high maternal and perinatal mortality.[28,29] These pregnancies cause a difficult management decision for every obstetrician. Immediate delivery will result in extremely high perinatal mortality and morbidity, whereas an aggressive attempt to delay delivery may expose the mother to severe morbidity. No single institution has enough patients to compare conservative management versus immediate delivery. Sibai et al[28] reviewed pregnancy outcome in 60 such patients that had conservative management over a seven-year period. The perinatal outcome for these pregnancies was exceptionally poor, with 31 of the 60 resulting in fetal demise, and 21 resulting in a neonatal death, for a total perinatal mortality rate of 87%. In addition, maternal morbidity was significantly high. This study was retrospective, the majority of the pregnancies were managed at level I hospitals, and a few of these pregnancies had antepartum fetal evaluation. The perinatal survival was 3% for those developing severe disease before 25 weeks compared with 24% in those developing disease at ≥25 weeks.

Odendaal et al[29] described the results of conservative management in 45 patients with severe preeclampsia before 28 weeks. Eleven were <24 weeks at time of diagnosis with all of them resulting in perinatal deaths. The remaining 34 were between 24 and 28 weeks' gestation with 14 (41%) resulting in a surviving infant.

During the past five years, we have managed about 100 pregnancies with severe preeclampsia in the midtrimester. Based on this recent experience and a review of the literature, we recommend the following management. If the gestation is ≤24 weeks, we recommend termination of pregnancy with prostaglandin E_2 vaginal suppositories. If the gestation is more than 24 weeks, the patients are counseled regarding the risks and benefits of continuing the pregnancy. If they elect to continue with the pregnancy, they are given intravenous magnesium sulfate for at least 24 hours, and blood pressure then is controlled aggressively with antihypertensive medications such as methyldopa, labetalol or nifedipine. These patients should undergo intensive evaluation of maternal and fetal status on a daily basis. Pregnancy then is continued until the development of either maternal or fetal jeopardy.

DEFINITIVE THERAPY

Delivery of the fetus and placenta is the definitive treatment of preeclampsia. All patients should have continuous fetal heart rate and uterine activity monitoring during labor. If labor is not well established and no fetal malpresentation or distress is noted, intravenous oxytocin may be used to induce labor in all patients at ≥32 weeks' gestation irrespective of the extent of cervical dilation or effacement. A similar approach is used for patients at less than 32 weeks, if the cervix is favorable for induction. In patients with severe disease at <32 weeks and unripe cervix, elective cesarean section is the method of choice for delivery in these patients. This approach is based on our previous experience of a high incidence of complications such as *abruptio placentae*, fetal growth retardation, and fetal distress in women developing the disease before 32 weeks.

Maternal analgesia can be provided by the intermittent use of small intravenous doses (25–50 mg) of meperidine. Local infiltration anesthesia with pudendal block may be used in most cases for vaginal delivery. Epidural analgesia may be used in all patients with mild disease and most patients with severe preeclampsia. The use of epidural anesthesia for patients with severe disease is highly controversial. Some authors[30] caution against its use in this situation because of the potential maternal hypotension and reduced uteroplacental blood flow in an already compromised maternal intravascular volume. However, others believe that epidural anesthesia not only controls pain but aids in stabilizing blood pressure and improves uterine perfusion. It is important to note that this approach requires the availability of personnel with special expertise in obstetric anesthesia. It also requires the availability of central hemodynamic monitoring in some patients, since infusions of large amounts of crystalloids usually are used as precautionary measures before epidural is used.[31] The use of conduction anesthesia is contraindicated in the presence of fetal distress, in the presence of coagulopathy, if the platelet count is less than $100 \times 10^3/mm^3$, or if the bleeding time is prolonged (see Chapter 202 on anesthesia for high-risk pregnancies).

For patients with the *HELLP syndrome,* the use of pudendal block or epidural anesthesia is contraindicated, since these patients are at risk of bleeding into these areas. In the case of cesarean section, platelet transfusions usually are indicated to correct severe thrombocytopenia prior to surgery. Our policy is to transfuse 10 buttons of platelets in all patients with a platelet count less than $50 \times 10^3/mm^3$ prior to intubation in the operating room. Generalized oozing from the operative site is very common; to minimize the risk of hematoma formation, we recommend that a subfascial drain be used, the bladder flap be left open, and the wound left open with sutures *in situ* from the level of the fascia. All these wounds can be successfully closed within 72 hours. Failure to adhere to these recommendations will result in 25% incidence of hematoma formation.

All patients must be monitored very closely during labor and delivery, with special attention to fluid intake and output. Patients with severe preeclampsia, especially those in early pregnancy or with HELLP Syndrome, are at increased risk for the development of pulmonary edema from fluid overload.[32] Urinary output should be monitored every hour, and fluid administration should not exceed 150 mL/h. If the patient has oliguria (less than 100 mL/4 h), the rate of both fluid administration and dose of magnesium sulfate should be reduced accordingly. At the time of delivery, a pediatrician skilled in neonatal resuscitation should be present in the delivery room.

PREVENTION OF CONVULSIONS

Parenteral magnesium sulfate ($mgSO_4{\cdot}7H_20USP$) is the drug of choice against convulsions due to eclampsia in the United States.[33] Its major advantages include its relative maternal and fetal safety when used properly. All women who are diagnosed to have preeclampsia (irrespective of severity or presence or absence of proteinuria) should receive magnesium sulfate during labor, delivery, and postpartum. This recommendation is based on the observation that about 20% of eclamptic women develop convulsions, with minimal elevations of blood pressure, and without proteinuria.[34] At our institution, magnesium sulfate is administered by controlled intravenous infusion with a loading dose of 6 g over 15–20 minutes followed by a maintenance infusion of 2 g/h. This regimen gives adequate serum magnesium levels in the majority of patients. Alternative regimens may include the use of an intramuscular regimen, as suggested by Pritchard.[35] It is important to note that about 0.3% of preeclamptic patients may develop a seizure while receiving standard doses of magnesium sulfate.

All patients receiving magnesium sulfate should have patellar reflexes, urine output, and respiratory rate checked hourly. Loss of patellar reflexes is the first sign of magnesium intoxication, hence, absent reflexes should be an indication for discontinuation of magnesium administration. A serum magnesium level should then be obtained and magnesium sulfate administration should then be resumed accordingly. Magnesium sulfate should be reduced or discontinued in the presence of oliguria. It is important to keep an ampule containing 1 g of calcium gluconate at the bedside for intravenous administration as an antidote, in case of magnesium toxicity (magnesium level >15mg/dL or respiratory difficulty).

In many centers outside the United States, drugs such as diazepam, barbiturates, chlormethiazole, and phenytoin usually are used to prevent or treat eclamptic convulsions.[36] However, none of these drugs has proven to be safer than or as effective as magnesium sulfate. In addition, their use is associated with significant maternal and neonatal complications.

CONTROL OF SEVERE HYPERTENSION

The objectives of treating severe hypertension are to prevent maternal complications without compromising uteroplacental blood flow, which is already reduced in severe preeclampsia. Hydralazine is a safe and effective drug for this purpose. If the diastolic blood pressure is ≥110 mm Hg, we give bolus doses of hydralazine of 5–10 mg every 20 minutes to keep diastolic pressure between 90 and 100 mm Hg. This requires monitoring of blood pressure every 5 minutes for at least 30 minutes after the drug is given. An alternative regimen is to use bolus injections of labetalol hydrochloride 20–40 mg every 10 minutes.[37] Unlike hydralazine, labetalol does not cause maternal tachycardia, flushing, or headaches. Diuretics are not used, except in the presence of pulmonary edema.

POSTPARTUM MANAGEMENT

Following delivery, the patient should be monitored in the recovery room for 12–24 hours, during which time maternal vital signs including reflexes, and intake and output should be monitored hourly. Twenty-five percent of cases of eclampsia are reported to occur postpartum; thus, close observation is mandatory. Salt restriction and diuretics are not needed. Most patients will show evidence of resolution of the disease process within 24 hours. Some, however, mainly those with severe disease in the midtrimester, and those with HELLP syndrome require intensive monitoring for 2–4 days. In such patients, magnesium sulfate may be needed for more than 24 hours. In addition, these patients are at increased risk for development of pulmonary edema from fluid overload, fluid mobilization, and compromised renal function.[32]

Most patients will be normotensive at the time of discharge from the hospital. In these patients, birth control pills may be prescribed without problems. A few patients may continue to have severe hypertension that can be controlled with either methyldopa or labetalol. Prophylactic anticonvulsive drugs such as phenobarbital are not needed. The patient is then seen at weekly intervals until her blood pressure is in the normal range without the use of medications. If this change does not occur by six weeks, a workup to assess hypertension should be performed.

REFERENCES

1. Sibai BM. Chronic hypertension during pregnancy. In: Sciarra, J, ed. *Gynecology and Obstetrics*. Philadelphia, PA: JB Lippincott Company; vol 2:1.
2. American College of Obstetricians and Gynecologists Technical Bulletin, #91, February 1986.
3. Villar MA, Sibai BM. Clinical significance of elevated mean arterial pressure in second trimester and threshold increase in systolic or diastolic blood pressure during third trimester. *Am J Obstet Gynecol* 1989;160:419.
4. Long P, Oats J. Preeclampsia in twin pregnancy—severity and pathogenesis. *Aust NZ J Obstet Gynaecol* 1987;27:1.
5. Sibai BM, El-Nazer A, Gonzalez-Ruiz A. Severe preeclampsia-eclampsia in young primigravidas: subsequent pregnancy outcome and remote prognosis. *Am J Obstet Gynecol* 1986;1555:1011.
6. Sibai BM. Pitfalls in diagnosis and management of preeclampsia. *Am J Obstet Gynecol* 1988;159:1.
7. MacGillivray I, Rose GA, Rowe D. Blood pressure survey in pregnancy. *Clin Sci* 1969;73:395.
8. Redman CWE, Jeffries M. Revised definition of preeclampsia. *Lancet* 1988;1:809.
9. Chesley LC, Sibai BM. Clinical significance of elevated mean arterial pressure in the second trimester. *Am J Obstet Gynecol* 1988;159:275.
10. Gant NF, Chand S, Worley RJ, et al. A clinical test useful for predicting the development of acute hypertension of pregnancy. *Am J Obstet Gynecol* 1974;120:1.
11. Collins R, Yusuf S, Peto R. Overview of randomized trials of diuretics in pregnancy. *Br Med J* 1985;190:17.
12. Sibai BM, Mirro R, Chesney CM, Leffler C. Low dose aspirin in pregnancy. *Obstet Gynecol* 1989;74:551.
13. Beaufils M, Donsimoni R, Uzan S, et al. Prevention of preeclampsia by early antiplatelet therapy. *Lancet* 1985;2:840.
14. Benigni A, Gregorini G, Frusca T, et al. Effect of low-dose aspirin on fetal and maternal generation of thromboxane by platelets in women at risk for pregnancy-induced hypertension. *N Eng J Med* 1989;321:357.
15. Wallenburg HC, Dekker GA, Makowitz JW. Low-dose aspirin prevents pregnancy-induced hypertension and preeclampsia in angiotensin-sensitive primigravidae. *Lancet* 1986;1:1.
16. Schiff E, Peleg E, Goldenberg M, et al. The use of aspirin to prevent pregnancy-induced hypertension and lower the ratio of thromboxane A_2 to prostacyclin in relatively high-risk pregnancies. *N Eng J Med* 1989;321:351.
17. Sibai BM, Anderson GD, McCubbin JH. Eclampsia II: Clinical significance of laboratory findings. *Obstet Gynecol* 1982;59:153.
18. Chesley LC. Disseminated intravascular coagulation. In: Chesley LC, ed. *Hypertensive disorders of pregnancy*. New York, NY: Appleton-Century-Crofts; 1978;88.
19. Weinstein L. Syndrome of hemolysis, elevated livery enzymes, and low platelet count: A severe consequence of hypertension in pregnancy. *Am J Obstet Gynecol* 1982;142:159.
20. Sibai BM, Taslimi MM, El-Nazer A, et al. Maternal-perinatal outcome associated with the syndrome of hemolysis, elevated livery enzymes, and low platelets in severe preeclampsia-eclampsia. *Am J Obstet Gynecol* 1986;155:501.
21. Schwartz ML, Brenner WE. Pregnancy-induced hypertension presenting with life-threatening thrombocytopenia. *Am J Obstet Gynecol* 1983;146:756.
22. Sibai BM. The HELLP Syndrome. Much ado about nothing? *Am J Obstet Gynecol* 1989, in press.
23. Lunell NO, Nylund L, Lewwander R, et al. Uteroplacental blood flow in preeclampsia: measurements with indium-113m and a computer-linked gamma camera. *Clin Exp Hypertens in Pregnancy* 1982;B1:105.
24. Gilstrap LC, Cunningham GF, Whalley PJ. Management of pregnancy-induced hypertension in the nulliparous patient remote from term. *Semin Perinatol* 1978;2:73.
25. Sibai BM, Gonzalez AR, Mabie WC, Morrctti M. A comparison of labetalol plus hospitalization versus hospitalization alone in the management of preeclampsia remote from term. *Obstet Gynecol* 1987;70:323.
26. Sibai BM, Spinnato JA, Watson DL, et al. Pregnancy outcome in 303 cases with severe preeclampsia. *Obstet Gynecol* 1984;64:319.
27. Long PA, Abell DA, Beischer NA. Parity and preeclampsia. *Aust NZ J Obstet Gynaecol* 1979;19:203.
28. Sibai BM, Taslimi M, Abdella TN, et al. Maternal perinatal outcome of conservative management of severe preeclampsia in mid-trimester. *Am J Obstet Gynecol* 1985;152:32.
29. Odendall JH, Pattinson RC, Dutoit R. Fetal and neonatal outcome in patients with severe preeclampsia before 34 weeks. *S Afr Med J* 1987;71:555.
30. Lindheimer MD, Katz AI. Hypertension in pregnancy. *N Eng J Med* 1985;313:675.
31. Jones MM, Joyce TH. Anesthesia for the parturient with pregnancy-induced hypertension. *Clin Obstet Gynecol* 1987;30:591.
32. Sibai BM, Mabie BC, Harvey CJ, Gonzalez AR. Pulmonary edema in severe preeclampsia-eclampsia: Analysis of 37 consecutive cases. *Am J Obstet Gynecol* 1987;156:1174.
33. Sibai BM, Graham JM, McCubbin JH. A comparison of intravenous and intramuscular magnesium sulfate regimens in preeclampsia. *Am J Obstet Gynecol* 1984;150:728.
34. Sibai BM, McCubbin JH, Anderson GD, et al. Eclampsia I. Observations from 67 recent cases. *Obstet Gynecol* 1981;58:609.
35. Pritchard JA. The use of magnesium sulfate in preeclampsia-eclampsia. *J Reprod Med* 1979;23:107.
36. Slater RM, Wilcox FL, Smith WD, et al. Phenytoin infusion in severe preeclampsia. *Lancet* 1987;1:1417.
37. Mabie WC, Gonzalez AR, Sibai BM, Amon E. A comparative trial of labetalol and hydralazine in the acute management of severe hypertension complicating pregnancy. *Obstet Gynecol* 1987;70:328.

Chapter One Hundred and Forty

Eclampsia

Baha M. Sibai and Fiona M. Fairlie

140

Eclampsia is defined as the onset of seizures or coma in a pregnant woman who has signs and symptoms of preeclampsia. The hazards of convulsions in pregnancy have been documented for centuries. Hippocrates observed that headaches, drowsiness, and seizures were serious complications of pregnancy.[1,2] De la Motte in 1772 noted that pregnant women with convulsions were more likely to recover if promptly delivered. In 1900, Stroganoff advocated a combination of chloroform, chloral hydrate, and morphine to treat eclampsia and reported this regimen was associated with significantly lower maternal mortality when compared with European and American treatments of the same period.[1,2]

The published incidence of eclampsia ranges from 1 in 100 to 1 in 3448 pregnancies.[3,4] Occurrence rate is highest among nonwhite nulliparous women of low socioeconomic status. Peak incidence occurs in the teenage years and early twenties. The incidence also is increased in women over 35 years of age. In Memphis, a tertiary referral center for this condition, the incidence has remained stable at 1 in 300 for the last 25 years.

PATHOPHYSIOLOGY

The pathophysiology of preeclampsia and eclampsia is unknown. The incidence of the disorder is increased in the presence of a large placental mass, notably multiple gestation, hydatidiform mole and nonimmune hydrops fetalis. This suggests an etiologic role for the placenta. In normal pregnancy, the placental production of prostacyclin and thromboxane is balanced. In preeclampsia, the prostacyclin and thromboxane balance is altered in favor of thromboxane production.[5] Severe preeclampsia is associated with vasoconstriction, thrombocytopenia and placental infarction, features compatible with a predominance of thromboxane activity.[6] Although an imbalance of thromboxane/prostacyclin may explain some of the histologic and hematologic changes of preeclampsia, it does not indicate the underlying etiology of the disorder.

Compared with normal pregnancy, preeclampsia and eclampsia are associated with a deficiency of vasodilator prostaglandins and an increased responsiveness to certain vasoconstricting hormones. Studies of the renin-angiotensin-aldosterone system (RAAS) in preeclampsia have produced conflicting results, but the majority favor decreased activity of this system. It has been suggested that prostacyclin is the main stimulator of the renin-angiotensin system in normal pregnancy; a deficiency of this agent could explain the reduced activity of RAAS in preeclampsia.[7] Prostacyclin deficiency also has been proposed as one mechanism involved in the increased production of catecholamines and increased pressor response to their exogenous administration seen in preeclampsia.[8,9]

Kinin is a vasodilator synthesized by the action of an enzyme kallikrein. Urinary kallikrein rises significantly during normal pregnancy while in pregnancies complicated by preeclampsia, activity of the kallikrein-kinin system usually is decreased.[10] This may render the individual more susceptible to vasoconstrictors. A genetic predisposition to preeclampsia and eclampsia has been recognized for many years. Elliot[11] in 1883 described eclampsia in a mother and her four daughters.[11] More recently, a high incidence of eclampsia in the daughters of eclamptic mothers was reported by Cooper et al.[12] Daughters who were themselves a product of an eclamptic pregnancy showed the highest frequency of eclampsia. Genetic studies over three and four generations suggested a dominant or multifactorial inheritance in contrast to previous reports which favored an autosomal recessive mechanism.[11,13] There appears to be little doubt that genetic factors are involved in the etiology of eclampsia and preeclampsia, but their precise role has yet to be elucidated.

The relationship between preeclampsia and eclampsia is complex. A number of mechanisms for the onset of convulsions have been postulated ranging from cerebral vasospasm, hemorrhage or edema, to disseminated intravascular coagulation in the cerebral microcirculation.[14] However, evidence to support these theories is scanty. Sheehan observed that cerebral edema was not associated with eclampsia if autopsy was performed within 2–3 hours of death. Further evidence to suggest that cerebral edema may be postmortum change was provided by Sibai et al[15] who reported the absence of demonstrable cerebral edema on computerized axial tomographic scans of eclamptic patients.

The blood pressure level does not closely correlate with the development of eclamptic seizures. However, autoregulation of cerebral perfusion varies from person to person. A level of 170/110 in a chronically hypertensive patient may have no adverse effect, while this level may be associated with convulsions or cerebral hemorrhage in a patient who normally has a blood pressure of 110/70. Eclamptic seizures should not be confused with hypertensive encephalopathy. The features of this condition (retinal hemorrhages, exudates and papilledema) are very uncommon in eclampsia. Metabolic derangements have been suggested as a possible cause for eclampsia but without convincing evidence.

HISTOPATHOLOGY

The classic hepatic lesion associated with severe preeclampsia/eclampsia is periportal hemorrhage with fibrin deposition.[16] This lesion has been found throughout the livers of women dying from eclampsia, and Sheehan and Lynch[17] thought it was specific to fatal eclampsia. However, periportal fibrin deposition has been observed in the livers of women dying from infections, *abruptio placentae* or postpartum hemorrhage[18] and is probably associated with any disorder resulting in vasospasm and intravascular coagulation. Areas in liver necrosis have been found in fatal cases of eclampsia.[17] The necrosis usually involves centilobular and midzonal portions of lobules and is thought to be due to hypoxia. Identical necrotic lesions have been seen in the livers of patients dying from shock of any cause.

Cerebral hemorrhage or edema are common autopsy findings in patients dying from eclampsia.[17,19,20] Multiple petechial hemorrhages or infarcts in the cortex and subcortical areas are more common than massive hemorrhage. Less is known about the incidence and characteristics of cerebral hemorrhage in nonfatal eclampsia. In the large series of Sheehan and Lynch[17], hemorrhages were seen only in about 20% of women who survived for more than 2 days. Govan[21] observed a high incidence of fibrinoid changes in the walls of the cerebral vessels of eclamptic patients. The renal and placental histologic abnormalities associated with eclampsia are identical to those found in preeclampsia.[22]

CLINICAL FEATURES

Multiple organ dysfunction is common, particularly if there has been a delay in diagnosis and treatment of preeclampsia or if there are coexistent obstetric or medical complications. The hallmark of eclampsia is hypertension. The latter may be mild (90–100 mm Hg diastolic or 140–150 mm Hg systolic), moderate (100–110 mm Hg diastolic or 150–160 mm Hg systolic), or severe (>110 mm Hg diastolic or >160 mm Hg systolic). Recorded blood pressure levels in some eclamptic patients never rise above 90 mm Hg diastolic or 140 mm Hg systolic, but there is a relative rise from baseline recordings earlier in pregnancy. In 200 eclamptic patients in Memphis, severe hypertension was present in 40%, while 20% had blood pressure levels below 140 mm Hg systolic or 90 mm Hg diastolic. The onset of convulsions or coma is probably more closely related to the increment of blood pressure rise or the rate of rise rather than the absolute level.

Almost 150 years ago, Sir James Young Simpson of Edinburgh taught that patients with puerperal convulsions almost always had albuminuria. Proteinuria associated with preeclampsia and eclampsia is usually nonselective in nature. In normal pregnancy urinary protein increases from approximately 5 mg per 100 mL in the first and second trimesters to 15 mg per 100 mL in late pregnancy. Screening for proteinuria by random dipstick testing will not detect these low levels. Eclampsia usually is associated with significant proteinuria (>2+ on dipstick). The degree of proteinuria may fluctuate widely over a 24-hour period and 24-hour urinalysis is a more accurate quantitative assessment of protein excretion. Moller and Lindmark[4] found proteinuria in 97% of patients with eclampsia presenting before 37 weeks' gestation, while only 71% of patients who developed eclampsia at or beyond 37 weeks had proteinuria. Ninety-eight (49%) out of 200 eclamptic patients studied in Memphis had significant proteinuria (> 2+ on dipstick), 29% had ≤2+ and 22% had no proteinuria. Most eclamptic patients have impaired renal function with reduced glomerular filtration rate, decreased renal plasma flow and reduced creatinine clearance.[23] Generalized edema is not a consistent characteristic of eclampsia. A recent review of 200 eclamptic patients managed in Memphis revealed a 32% incidence of convulsions without edema, and only 22% had generalized edema.

The onset of eclampsia usually is preceded by signs and symptoms of preeclampsia. However, in 15–20% of cases a prodromal phase is not apparent.[4,24] Classical premonitory signs and symptoms include severe and persistent headache, photophobia or blurred vision, epigastric or right upper quadrant pain, and hyperactive deep tendon reflexes with clonus. The most frequent symptoms preceding convulsions in 67 cases studied by Sibai et al[25] were headache (82.5%), visual disturbances (44.4%), and upper abdominal pain (19%). Plasma volume usually is reduced significantly in severe preeclampsia and eclampsia with hemoconcentration and increased blood viscosity. Hankins et al[26] performed hemodynamic monitoring in 8 eclamptic patients. They found low right and left ventricular filling pressures and increased left ventricular stroke work index. The average initial central venous pressure was low (1 ± 1 mm Hg), as was the average initial capillary wedge pressure (3.9 ± 2.3 mm Hg). These findings are compatible with a high-output-high-resistance state with low ventricular filling pressures.

Right upper quadrant or epigastric pain is thought to result from obstruction of blood flow in the hepatic sinusoids which are occluded by intravascular fibrin deposition. The pathologic changes observed in eclampsia with liver involvement include subcapsular and intrahepatic hemorrhages, capsular rupture, and focal or diffuse necrosis.[27] Although usually focal, these changes sometimes affect extensive areas of liver and result in a large capsular tear with profuse bleeding into the peritoneal or pleural cavities.[28] Hepatic rupture complicating eclampsia typically occurs in the older primigravida.[29]

Visual disturbances are reported to occur in 30–50% of eclamptics. Shulka and Prasad[30] described 4 grades of retinal changes in preeclampsia and eclampsia and drew attention to the correlation between the severity of ocular abnormalities and the severity of the hypertensive disease. Serous exudative retinal detachments have been reported to occur in 10% of patients with eclampsia.[31] They are usually bilateral and bullous. Detachment is thought to be a consequence of nonperfusion and infarction of the choroid. In most cases, retinal detachments completely resolve within a few weeks postpartum and normal vision returns. Transient cortical blindness is a well recognized complication of eclampsia. Cerebral edema of the occipital lobes has been demonstrated by computerized axial tomography (CT scan) with a return to normal appearances within a few weeks after delivery. Occasionally, blindness may be caused by retinal artery and vein occulsion.

LABORATORY INVESTIGATION

There are no biochemical or hematologic abnormalities specific to eclampsia, and laboratory parameters may range from almost normal to grossly abnormal depending on the presence or absence of obstetric and medical complications. Hematocrit usually is raised, reflecting hemoconcentration. The mean hematocrit in 67 eclamptic women studied by Sibai et al[32] was 35%, which was significantly higher than the mean value for normotensive controls (29%).

Lopez-Llera et al[33] reported abnormal coagulation and fibrinolysis in 18 patients with eclampsia. Most of these patients were severely ill and death occurred in 5 cases. In contrast, the average platelet count in 95 eclamptic patients studied by Pritchard et al[34] was 202,000 mm^2 and the incidence of hypofibroginemia and abnormal fibrin split products was low. Thrombocytopenia (platelet count <150,000 mm^2 was found in 15% of 200 eclamptic patients studied by Sibai. Only 9 (4.5%) showed evidence of disseminated intravascular coagulopathy. Apparently, significant coagulation abnormalities are uncommon in eclampsia unless treatment is delayed or *abruptio placentae* occurs.[35]

The incidence of abnormal liver function tests in eclampsia ranges between 11 and 74%. Abnormalities are particularly likely in the presence of upper abdominal pain. Sibai et al[32] and Shukla et al[36] reported elevated serum transaminases, lactic dehydrogenases, and bilirubin. Clinical jaundice is rare. About 10% of eclamptic patients develop the syndrome of hemolysis, elevated liver enzymes, and thrombocytopenia *(HELLP syndrome)* described by Weinstein.[37] The presence of HELLP increases the risk of subcapsular hematoma of the liver. Cunningham et al[38] studied red cell morphology in 9 eclamptic patients. Compared with normal pregnancies, the patients with eclampsia had significantly more schistocytes and echinocytes but not spherocytes. Echinocytes are characteristic of cell membrane changes, while schistocytes reflect microangiopathic hemolysis. Cunningham et al[38] speculated that alterations in membrane composition may lead to echinocytosis and increased susceptibility to microangiopathic hemolysis, resulting in the formation of schistocytes.

Renal function tests are abnormal in about 50–70% of eclamptic patients. Sibai found an elevated serum creatinine (≥ 0.9 mg/dL) in 51% of 200 cases of eclampsia, while the average creatinine clearance in a study of 152 eclamptic patients was 79 ± 33 mL/min (range 9–186 mL/min). Uric acid is usually above the normal range (>6.2 mg per dL).

Cerebral pathology is common in fatal cases of eclampsia but less is known about the incidence and etiology of cerebral dysfunction in survivors. Table 140-1 summarizes the literature relating to the incidence of cerebral pathology in eclampsia. The term *cerebral damage* includes cerebral edema, hemorrhage and infarction. Table 140-2 shows the neurologic abnormalities encountered among 254 eclamptic patients managed in Memphis. The overall incidence of abnormalities was low (8%), and there was only 1 maternal death. The electroencephalogram (EEG) indirectly measures electrical activity of the brain. However, only cortical phenomena that simultaneously activate large areas of cortex will be recorded on an EEG. Rosenbaum and Maltby[39] reported 13 of 20 eclamptic patients with abnormal EEG findings one week to five years after the pregnancy episode. They observed a strong family history of seizures in these patients and suggested that a positive family history for convulsive disorders plus abnormal EEG findings in pregnancy may indicate individuals at increased risk from eclampsia. However, the women they studied were attending a psychiatric-neurology clinic and probably had a high incidence of seizure disorder compared with the general population.

Jost[40] studied EEG recordings in 9 eclamptic women and reported a correlation between EEG abnormalities and the severity of maternal hypertension. EEG appearances improved when maternal blood pressure was lowered to the normal range. However, Kolstad[41] found no relationship between blood pressure and EEG recordings in 17 patients with preeclampsia or eclampsia. Sibai et al[15] reported EEG findings within the first 48 hours after hospitalization in 65 eclamptic patients. The EEG was acutely abnormal in 49 (75%). The abnormalities were similar to patterns reported in association with hypoxia and metabolic derangements, such as water intoxication and hypocalcemia. There was no relationship between the degree of EEG abnormality and the severity of maternal hypertension. Abnormalities persisted for up to 6 weeks postpartum in 7 patients but returned to normal in all patients by 6 months. None of the patients in the study group had permanent neurologic deficits. The authors concluded that EEG is rarely helpful in the management of eclamptic seizures.

The advent of the CT scan has provided an opportunity to investigate the nature of cerebral abnormalities in living eclamptic patients. This technique is considered safe in pregnancy after 7 weeks' gestation. Table 140-3 summarizes the reported findings in the literature of CT scans in eclampsia. An early CT study of eclampsia[42] showed cerebral edema and reduction in lateral ventricular size. The patient's condition improved after treatment with dexamethasone and fluid restriction. Beeson and Duda[43] reported loss of

TABLE 140–1. INCIDENCE OF CEREBRAL PATHOLOGY IN ECLAMPSIA

Authors	Number of Cases	Cerebral Damage		Intracranial Hemorrhage	
		n	%	n	%
Donnelly and Lock 1946–1953	533[a]	180	33.8	89	16.7
Hibbard 1957–1972	67[a]	34	50.7	21	31.4
Lopez-Llera 1963–1979	86[a] 498[b]	62 37	72.1 7.4	— —	— —
Pritchard et al 1955–1983	245 1[a]	N/A		0	—
Sibai et al 1977–1989	254 1[a]	1	0.4	0	—
Richards et al 1983–1984	192 5[a]	5	2.6	2	1.0

[a] Deaths
[b] Survivors
N/A = not analyzed

TABLE 140–2. NEUROLOGIC ABNORMALITIES AMONG 232 CASES OF ECLAMPSIA

	n	%
Transient deficit	7	3.0
Transient cortical blindness	6	2.6
Retinal detachment	2	0.9
Comatosed state	2	0.9
Cerebral death	1	0.4

TABLE 140–3. REPORTED CT FINDINGS IN ECLAMPSIA

- Cerebral Edema
  - Low-density pattern diffusely distributed throughout the white matter
  - Patchy areas of low density
  - Occipital white matter edema
  - Loss of normal cortical sulci
  - Reduced ventricular size
  - Acute hydrocephalus
- Cerebral Hemorrhage
  - Intraventricular hemorrhage
  - Parenchymal hemorrhage (high density)
- Cerebral Infarction
  - Low attenuation areas
  - Basal ganglia infarcts

occipital lobe density in an eclamptic patient with acute onset blindness. The CT findings were consistent with cerebral edema, and a repeat scan after treatment with mannitol and dexamethasone showed resolution of the inital abnormalities. Other authors[44,45] have reported similar findings and recommended using mannitol or dexamethasone to treat such patients. Brown et al[46] performed CT scans in 49 patients with eclampsia over a 6-year period. Overall, only 14 scans (29%) were abnormal. However, the incidence of abnormal findings significantly increased when high resolution equipment became available, suggesting that some of the early scans were falsely read as negative. In the final year of the study, half the eclamptic women had abnormal findings ranging from occipital hypodensities to diffuse cerebral edema. CT scan findings altered clinical management in only 1 patient, and none of the patients studied had long-term neurologic sequelae. Brown et al[46] concluded that although CT scan may be abnormal in eclampsia, its routine use is not warranted, particularly in uncomplicated cases, which show prompt response to standard treatment. Sibai et al[15] obtained CT scans in 20 eclamptic patients with neurologic deficits or an atypical clinical course. None of the scans were abnormal. The authors concluded that CT scanning is rarely helpful in the management of eclampsia and should be restricted to patients with late-onset postpartum convulsions or patients with associated neurologic deficits in whom there is a higher risk of cerebrovascular pathology.

Nuclear magnetic resonance (NMR) has been widely employed for neuroradiologic studies in the nonpregnant population. It is suitable for use in pregnancy since it does not require ionizing radiation. Crawford et al[47] described NMR appearances in an eclamptic patient 48 hours postpartum which were consistent with the distribution of cortical petechiae described by Sheehan and Lynch.[17] They thought that the NMR findings probably represented edema in response to injury rather than hemorrhage. Interestingly, the patient's CT scan was normal. Although more studies are required, NMR holds promise as a useful diagnostic technique in eclampsia, particularly when the diagnosis is in doubt. Figure 140-1 is a NMR of a patient managed in Memphis. It shows areas of increased density compatible with cerebral ischemia.

DIFFERENTIAL DIAGNOSIS

Eclamptic convulsions are *grand mal* in type and may be isolated or multiple. The duration of coma is variable. Rarely convulsions become continuous and can be controlled only by muscular paralysis, intubation, and assisted ventilation. Patients usually have no memory of events preceding the onset of eclampsia.

Traditionally, eclampsia has been defined as the development of convulsions in a preeclamptic patient after 20 weeks' gestation or within 48 hours postpartum. Approximately 50% of eclampsia develops antepartum, 25% intrapartum and 25% postpartum. The timing of postpartum eclampsia has aroused controversy. Chesley[48] stated that convulsions beginning more than 24 hours after delivery are rarely, if ever, caused by eclampsia. However, Bernard[49] described 19 cases of eclampsia that occurred 3 or more days after delivery and Lopez-Llera[20], in a study of 704 cases of eclampsia, reported cases occurring up to 2 weeks postdelivery. Sibai et al[50] reviewed the late postpartum eclampsia controversy and presented 6 cases of eclampsia occurring 3–11 days postdelivery. The authors concluded that eclampsia can occur more than 3 days postdelivery. Seizure control is the first priority. Once the patient is stable, a complete neurologic and metabolic investigation is indicated to exclude other causes of seizures. In the past decade, 33 cases of late postpartum eclampsia have been managed by the Memphis Perinatal Center. All patients reported headaches or visual disturbances for 1–4 days' duration prior to the onset of convulsions; laboratory and clinical findings immediately postseizure were consistent with eclampsia. A marked diuresis (>4 L per day) lasting for about 48 hours occurred in all cases. There was no incidence of neurologic deficits or seizures on followup. Eclampsia before 20 weeks' gestation is uncommon and usually is associated with hydatidiform changes in the placenta. Sibai et al[51] described 3 patients with convulsions beginning at 18–20 weeks' gestation without molar degeneration of the placenta. In each case, the clinical and laboratory findings were consistent with eclampsia, and there was no history of a seizure disorder. Since this publication, three additional cases with a similar presentation have been managed in Memphis (Table 140-4). Convulsions associated with hypertension, proteinuria, and hyperuricemia presenting in the first half of pregnancy should be treated as eclampsia until proven otherwise.

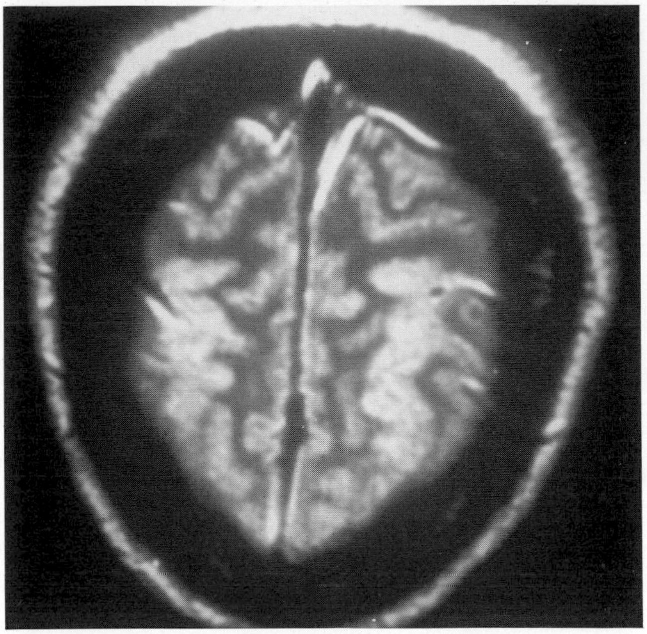

Figure 140–1. A magnetic resonance imaging of the brain in a patient with eclampsia. The abnormal areas probably represent ischemic changes.

TABLE 140–4. GESTATIONAL AGE AT THE ONSET OF CONVULSIONS (n = 232)

Weeks' gestation	n	%
<20	6	2.6
21–26	8	3.4
27–36	109	47.0
37–41	109	47.0

Eclampsia is associated with a wide spectrum of signs and symptoms which may present diagnostic difficulties. The conditions most commonly confused with eclampsia include:

1. Cerebrovascular accidents (eg, intracerebral hemorrhage, cerebral thrombosis)
2. Space-occupying central nervous system lesions (eg, brain tumor or abscess)
3. Hypertensive diseases (eg, hypertensive encephalopathy, pheochromocytoma)
4. Epilepsy
5. Metabolic diseases (eg, hypoglycemia, water intoxication)
6. Infectious diseases (eg, meningitis, encephalitis)
7. Thrombotic thrombocytopenic purpura

MANAGEMENT

Eclampsia is a life-threatening complication of pregnancy. Prompt action is required to minimize maternal and perinatal mortality and morbidity. The goals of management are outlined in Table 140-5. The first steps are to prevent maternal injury, ensure adequate oxygenation, and minimize the risk of aspiration. The patient should be placed in the left lateral position and gently restrained from falling out of bed. A padded tongue blade should be used to prevent the patient from biting her tongue. Suction should be available to prevent aspiration of excessive oral secretions and promote adequate oxgenation. Usually, the convulsion is self-limiting, and once the patient begins active spontaneous respirations, an intravenous line should be secured to administer magnesium sulfate. Different regimens have been recommended for the administration of magnesium sulfate. All are based on a loading dose followed by a smaller maintenance dose. Based on experience of managing more than 250 eclamptic patients, Sibai recommends a loading dose of 6 g intravenously given slowly over 10–15 minutes. This is followed by a maintenance regime of 2–3 g per hour. Approximately 10–15% of patients will suffer recurrent convulsions after a loading dose of magnesium sulfate. However, most of these will respond to a bolus of 2 g magnesium sulfate given over a 3-minute period. Should convulsions persist, sodium amobarbital 250 mg intravenously over 3–5 minutes should be administered. Occasionally, a patient will fail to respond to this protocol; in this case, muscular paralysis and intubation will be required.

Some believe that the anticonvulsant effect of magnesium sulfate is mainly peripheral and mediated by inhibition of acetylcholine. However, anticonvulsant effects are present well below the concentrations required to produce neuromuscular blockade, suggesting the possibility of a central anticonvulsant action. Certain properties of magnesium sulfate provide a theoretical basis for an antihypertensive effect. Its administration is associated with increased prostacyclin production by vascular endothelium. It is also a calcium antagonist and theoretically could block vasoconstriction.[52] These mechanisms have not been fully elucidated and the mode of action of magnesium sulfate remains unclear.

Magnesium excretion is controlled over a wide range by the kidney, thus hypermagnesemia is uncommon. Serum magnesium levels normally fall during pregnancy. To minimize the risks of magnesium toxicity, it is recommended that magnesium sulfate therapy should be titrated to maintain a serum level between 4.8 and 8.4 mg per dL. Magnesium usually has no maternal sedative effects if plasma concentration remains below 8.4 per dL, but the therapeutic level is unknown. The signs and symptoms of maternal hypermagnesemia are shown in Table 140-6. Magnesium crosses the placenta and reported neonatal effects include absent cry, flaccidity, hyporeflexia, and respiratory distress.[53] Sibai et al[54] studied the EEG recordings in eclamptic patients before and during the administration of magnesium sulfate. There was local and diffuse slowing of activity with varying degrees of severity. The most consistent change was diffuse slowing of alpha-wave rhythms and more prominent delta-wave rhythms. These abnormalities were not altered by magnesium therapy despite adequate serum magnesium levels.

In Europe, intravenous diazepam or chlormethiazole have been the drugs of choice for preventing and controlling eclampsia. Although effective as anticonvulsants, it is often difficult to achieve a maternal plasma concentration that is anticonvulsant without the unwanted side effects of respiratory and cardiovascular depression. Both drugs cross the placenta and significant neonatal depression has been reported.[55-57] Recently, phenytoin has been advocated for the prevention of eclampsia in patients with severe preeclampsia. This drug does not impair consciousness level. In a study of 24 preeclamptic and 2 eclamptic patients, intravenous administration was associated with therapeutic levels at 30 minutes, and there were no maternal or neonatal side effects. Further studies are required to evaluate the potential of this drug in preeclampsia and eclampsia.

Maternal hypoxemia or acidemia increases the risk of toxic effects from anticonvulsant medication and anesthetic agents. Once convulsions have been controlled, arterial blood gases should be measured and a chest x-ray obtained to ensure adequate maternal oxygenation and exclude aspiration.

The next step is to correct maternal hypertension. The main dangers of hypertension are maternal cerebrovascular accidents and congestive heart failure from increased afterload. Care must be taken not to lower blood pressure excessively since this may exacerbate maternal cerebral ischemia and hypoxia by lowering cerebral perfusion[3] or endanger fetal well-being by impairing placental perfusion. Blood pressure levels should be maintained within the range of

TABLE 140–5. GOALS IN THE MANAGEMENT OF ECLAMPSIA

Maintain maternal vital functions
Control convulsions
Stabilize maternal blood pressure
Correct maternal hypoxemia and acidemia
Evaluate the patient for delivery

TABLE 140–6. SIGNS OF MAGNESIUM TOXICITY AND APPROXIMATE PLASMA CONCENTRATIONS

Sign	Plasma magnesium concentration (mg/dL)
Loss of patellar reflex	10–12
Respiratory arrest	14.6
Paralysis	15.0
Cardiac arrest	30

From Villar and Sibai[83] with permission.

140–150 mm Hg systolic and 90–100 mm Hg diastolic. This level appears to be adequate to avoid maternal cerebral complications. In the United States, hydralazine is the preferred antihypertensive agent. It is administered as intermittent boluses of 5 mg every 20 minutes.

Following stabilization of maternal condition, measures must be taken to procure delivery. Continuous monitoring of the fetal heart and uterine activity is indicated. Transient changes in both of these parameters are commonly observed during and after an eclamptic convulsion. There is an increase in baseline uterine tone and contraction frequency which may last up to 15 minutes. Reported fetal heart rate changes include severe bradycardias and late decelerations that may last for up to 9 minutes.[58] Persistent hypertonic uterine activity or fetal bradycardia suggest *abruptio placentae,* a well recognized complication of eclampsia. The method of delivery is dictated by gestational age, fetal presentation, presence or absence of fetal or maternal distress, and state of the cervix. Sibai et al[59] reported a high incidence of *abruptio placentae,* fetal growth retardation, and intrapartum fetal distress in most patients with eclampsia before 32 weeks' gestation. In the light of this experience, elective cesarean section is advised before 32 weeks. For gestations ≥32 weeks, induction of labor may be attempted with intravenous oxytocin. Induction may be considered in some patients less than 32 weeks if the cervix is favorable and there is no evidence of fetal distress.

Maternal analgesia in labor can be achieved successfully with intermittent boluses of intravenous meperidine (25–50 mg) or administration of epidural anesthesia. Cesarean section may be performed under general or epidural analgesia. There has been some controversy over the use of epidural blockade for preeclamptic or eclamptic patients. Although this procedure is associated with a fall in maternal blood pressure, it should not be selected on the basis of its hypotensive effect; there are more effective methods of controlling maternal blood pressure. Theoretically, it may improve placental perfusion, although this is difficult to quantify. Those who caution its use point out the potential hazards of sudden maternal hypotension secondary to sympathetic blockade and the risk of hemorrhage into the epidural space if the patient has a coagulopathy.[60] Epidural analgesia should not be used in the presence of thrombocytopenia or a prolonged bleeding time (>12 minutes) or if there is evidence of fetal distress.

During labor and postpartum, the eclamptic patient should be kept in a well illuminated room and closely supervised. Urine output must be carefully monitored and if hourly volumes fall below 25 mL, both fluid and magnesium sulfate administration should be reduced accordingly.

Most patients show signs of recovery by 24 hours postpartum. A minority will require magnesium sulfate therapy and close observation for two to four days. These cases are at particular risk for delayed mobilization of extracellular fluid and pulmonary edema. Antihypertensive therapy may be required in the postpartum period. Patients may be discharged on oral antihypertensive therapy once their blood pressure level has stabilized but should be checked within the first week. Usually, blood pressure normalizes within one or two weeks and therapy can be discontinued. If hypertension persists for more than six weeks, detailed evaluation of renal function is indicated.

There have been several reports describing the use of Swan–Ganz catheters for the management of severe preeclampsia and eclampsia.[26,61] The combined experience of these authors suggest that hemodynamic monitoring is indicated rarely in uncomplicated cases of eclampsia but may be helpful in the presence of pulmonary edema or renal failure. The Memphis experience of hemodynamic monitoring in eclampsia concurs with this conclusion.

Eclampsia should be managed in a tertiary care center. Sibai recommends the following guidelines for the transport of eclamptic patients:

1. Consultation with the physician at the perinatal center prior to transport.
2. The patient should be accompanied by her medical records.
3. Maternal hypertension must be stabilized and convulsions controlled before transfer.
4. Magnesium sulfate should be administered prior to transport: 4 g IV and 10 g IM simultaneously, or 6 g IV and 4 g in 250 mL; Ringer lactate infused at 125 mL per hour.
5. A medical practitioner should accompany the patient at all times.

MATERNAL COMPLICATIONS AND OUTCOME

Eclampsia is still one of the most frequent causes of maternal death throughout the world. The reported maternal mortality varies from 0 to 14%. Complicated eclampsia and mismanaged cases account for most of the maternal deaths. Although improvements in antenatal care have been associated with a fall in incidence in Western countries, it is difficult to prove cause and effect. However, once eclampsia has occurred, prompt hospitalization and appropriate intensive care will increase the likelihood of a good maternal outcome.[25,62,63]

The most common terminal events in women dying from eclampsia are cerebral dysfunction (usually cerebral hemorrhage)[64] pulmonary edema, renal, hepatic, or respiratory failure. In developing countries, the onset of maternal infection plays a significant role in maternal mortality.[65] Table 140-7 shows the maternal mortality rates from various regions of the world. The highest incidences are found in

TABLE 140–7. MATERNAL MORTALITY IN ECLAMPSIA

Author	Cases	n	%
Lopez-Llera[20]			
1963–1971	704	98	13.9
1973–1979			
Ekwempu[65]			
1978–1979	100	9	9
Akinkugbe and Coker[66]			
1967–1976	273	29	10.6
Zuspan[74]			
1956–1965	69	2	2.9
Gedekoh et al[62]			
1970–1980	52	3	5.8
Pritchard et al[63]			
1955–1983	245	1	0.4
Sibai[68]			
1977–1989	254	1	0.4
Moller and Lindmark[4]			
1976–1980	74	1	1.4

TABLE 140–8. MATERNAL COMPLICATIONS IN 232 CASES OF ECLAMPSIA

	n	%
Abruptio placentae	23	10
Acute renal failure	9	3.9
Pulmonary edema	10	4.3
Cardiorespiratory arrest	8	3.4
Aspiration	5	2.2
Maternal death	1	0.4

the least privileged populations.[66] The only maternal death in Memphis was a patient who was moribund on admission.

Table 140-8 lists the maternal complications among 254 cases of eclampsia managed in Memphis. *Abruptio placentae* is one of the most frequent complications associated with eclampsia worldwide. Lopez-Llera et al[35] analyzed 46 cases of *abruptio placentae*-complicating eclampsia which were referred to the high-risk pregnancy unit in Mexico City. There were 10 maternal deaths and a total perinatal mortality of 44.7%. Older and multiparous women had more complications, larger placental separations, and higher mortality. Pritchard et al[34] reported a 5.5% incidence of *abruptio placentae* in association with antepartum eclampsia. This sequence of events contributed to 3 stillbirths. There were no maternal deaths. *Abruptio placentae* complicating eclampsia occurred in 13 of 55 cases in Memphis reviewed by Abdella et al.[67] There were 3 stillbirths and 3 neonatal deaths (perinatal mortality of 46%).

Richards et al[3] recently considered the management of the unconscious eclamptic patient. This report came from Durban, South Africa, where there is a high incidence of eclampsia. There were 192 cases in the 15-month study period (incidence of 1% total deliveries). Five patients died. Twenty unconscious patients had CT scans. In 15 cases (75%) there were changes compatible with cerebral edema. Cerebral hemorrhage occurred in 9%. The authors described a protocol of intensive neurologic management that was associated with a reduction in mortality rate for unconscious eclamptics from 50% to 17%. The aims of this regimen were to optimize cerebral perfusion and control intracranial pressure.

PERINATAL COMPLICATIONS AND OUTCOME

Eclampsia continues to be a major cause of perinatal mortality and morbidity worldwide. Sibai[68] recently reviewed the perinatal outcome of 254 cases of eclampsia managed in Memphis. Among 263 total births (9 sets of twins) there were 16 stillbirths and 15 neonatal deaths, giving a perinatal mortality rate of 11.8%. This compares well with reported incidences worldwide that range between 10% and 28%. The main causes of perinatal mortality and neonatal morbidity are preterm delivery[68], fetal growth retardation[69], and *abruptio placentae*. The latter accounts for most of the stillbirths in eclampsia. In a study of 72 eclamptic pregnancies resulting in live-born infants, Sibai et al[58] recorded a neonatal mortality of 4%. Forty infants were ≤36 weeks' gestation and 12 of the 40 were small-for-gestational-age. Long-term follow up for a maximum of 4 years revealed normal growth and neurologic development for infants of mothers with uncomplicated eclampsia. Neurologic abnormalities were associated with *abruptio placentae* or severe fetal growth retardation. Neonatal complications were common but were similar in nature and incidence to those encountered in a matched group of preterm infants delivered by normotensive women.

PREDICTION AND PREVENTION OF ECLAMPSIA

Blood pressure level is not a useful predictor of eclampsia. Almost all Swedish women have regular and frequent antenatal care and deliver in the hospital. Despite this close monitoring, less than 40% of 74 eclamptic patients in a study from Sweden[4] were diagnosed as being hypertensive 4 or more days before the first convulsion.

Redman et al[70] and Wood[71] reported an association between hyperuricemia in preeclampsia and adverse perinatal outcome. Friedman and Neff[72] and MacGillivray[18] concluded that the development of significant proteinuria in pregnancy-induced hypertension was associated with an increased risk of eclampsia and perinatal death. Romero et al[73] recently proposed thrombocytopenia as an important risk factor in the occurrence of maternal and fetal complications in pregnancy-induced hypertension. In contrast to these studies, Sibai et al[32] found no correlation between the level of serum uric acid, serum albumin or blood urea nitrogen, and maternal or fetal outcome in 67 eclamptic patients.

It has been suggested that eclampsia is a preventable condition and its occurrence is the result of inadequate antenatal care or failure to recognize the onset of preeclampsia or inadequate treatment of preeclampsia.[74] Although attention to these factors lowers the incidence of eclampsia, there is a core of patients who develop the condition without warning signs and despite regular antenatal surveillance. Table 140-9 shows the factors responsible for 99 cases of eclampsia managed in Memphis and classified as unavoidable. Unavoidable cases comprised 39% of all eclampsia presenting to the perinatal center.

Two recent studies suggested that low-dose aspirin may lower the incidence of preeclampsia and by inference eclampsia.[75,76] Conclusive evidence to recommend this therapy is lacking and the results of ongoing multicenter studies in the United States and Europe are anticipated.

LONG-TERM PROGNOSIS AFTER ECLAMPSIA

Studies relating to the reproductive performance after eclampsia were summarized by Chesley.[77] The incidence of recurrent eclampsia ranged from 0% to 21% (mean

TABLE 140–9. FACTORS RESPONSIBLE FOR THE ATYPICAL ONSET OF ECLAMPSIA

	All Cases (n = 254)	Unavoidable Cases (n = 99)
Abrupt onset	50	41
Late postpartum onset	40	29
Convulsions during magnesium sulfate therapy	33	15
Mild preeclampsia with good response	10	10
Early onset (<20 weeks)	6	4

10.3%). Hypertensive disorders in subsequent pregnancies ranged from 12–51% (average 33%). Chesley[77] investigated the outcome of subsequent pregnancies in 158 women who suffered eclampsia in their first pregnancy. There were 409 subsequent pregnancies. Recurrent eclampsia occurred in 0.9% and hypertension affected 19.5%. The incidences of abruptio placentae and perinatal mortality were higher in subsequent pregnancies (2.1% and 4.6%, respectively). Adelusi and Ojengbede[78] reported a recurrence rate of eclampsia of 15.6% despite optimal antenatal care.

Sibai et al[79] studied subsequent pregnancy outcome and remote prognosis among 287 women who had either preeclampsia (n = 287) or eclampsia (n = 119) in their first pregnancy. Outcome was compared with 409 well matched controls who were normotensive throughout their first pregnancy. *Abruptio placentae* (2.5%), perinatal mortality (5.9%), fetal growth retardation, and preterm delivery (15%) all occurred more frequently in the subsequent pregnancies of the preeclamptic/eclamptic group. The incidence of preeclampsia in a subsequent pregnancy was significantly higher in patients who developed preeclampsia and eclampsia in their first pregnancy before 30 weeks' gestation compared with those who developed preeclampsia and eclampsia after 30 weeks' gestation.

Chesley et al[80] reported the average incidence of chronic hypertension to be 23.8% among 2637 eclamptic women followed from 6 weeks to 44 years. Sibai et al[79] followed up 409 preeclamptic and eclamptic first pregnancies for an average of 6.6 years and found an overall incidence of chronic hypertension of 14.8%. For those followed less than 10 years, the mean incidence was 4.4%. This compared with an incidence of 1.5% in matched normotensive pregnancies. The difference was even more marked with a mean incidence of 51% in those followed for 10 years or longer (51% among preeclamptic and eclamptic pregnancies compared with 14% among normotensive controls).

Sexton[81] suggested a correlation between eclampsia and future development of epilepsy. A more recent study by Sibai et al[15] did not confirm this finding.

The familial incidence of eclampsia and preeclampsia in relatives of eclamptic women was reviewed by Chesley et al.[82] Table 140-10 summarizes the risk of eclampsia and preeclampsia in relatives of eclamptic women.

Eclampsia remains a major cause of maternal and perinatal mortality and morbidity. It is not always preventable. Optimum outcome is associated with prompt hospitalization in a tertiary care center, prevention of further seizures, judicious control of maternal blood pressure, prevention of hypoxia, and early delivery.

TABLE 140–10. THE RISK OF ECLAMPSIA IN RELATIVES OF WOMEN WITH ECLAMPSIA

Relationship to eclamptic woman	Number with pregnancies >20 weeks	Preeclampsia n	Preeclampsia %	Eclampsia n	Eclampsia %
Eclampsia women (all future pregnancies)	340	70	20.6	3	0.9
Sister (all future pregnancies)	147	54	37.6	6	4.1
Daughter (first pregnancy)	257	63	24.9	7	2.7
Daughter-in-law (first pregnancy)	75	6	8.0	—	—

Modified from Chesley LC, Annitto JE, Cosgrove RA. The familial factor in toxemia of pregnancy. Obstet Gynecol. *1968;32:303.*

REFERENCES

1. Chesley LC. History. In: Chesley LC, ed. *Hypertensive Disorders in Pregnancy*. New York: Appleton-Century-Crofts; 1978:17.
2. Dieckmann WJ. *The Toxemias of Pregnancy*. 2nd ed. St. Louis, MO: CV Mosby; 1954.
3. Richards AM, Moodley J, Graham DI, Bullock MRR. Active management of the unconscious eclamptic patient. *Br J Obstet Gynaecol*. 1986;93:554.
4. Moller B, Lindmark G. Eclampsia in Sweden, 1976–1980. *Acta Obstet Gynecol Scand*. 1986;65:307.
5. Walsh SW. Preeclampsia: An imbalance in placental prostacyclin and thromboxane production. *Am J Obstet Gynecol*. 1985;152:335.
6. Moncada S, Vane JR. Pharmacology and endogenous roles of prostaglandin endoperoxides, thromboxane A_2, and prostacyclin. *Pharmacol Rev*. 1979;30:293.
7. Friedman SA. Preeclampsia: A review of the role of prostaglandins. *Obstet Gynecol*. 1988;71:122.
8. Broughton-Pipkin F. Hypertension in pregnancy—physiology or pathology. In: *The Physiological Development of the Fetus and Newborn*. London: Academic Press; 1985:699.
9. Pedersen EB. Autonomic nervous system and vascular reactivity in normal and hypertensive pregnancy. In: Rubin PC, ed. *Handbook of Hypertension Vol 10: Hypertension in Pregnancy*. New York, NY: Elsevier Science Publishers, 1988:152.
10. Campbell SK, Farrer A, Albano JDM, Steel PJ, et al. The renal kallikrein system in pregnancy. In: Sharp F, Symonds EM, eds. *Hypertension in Pregnancy*. Ithaca, NY: Perinatology Press, 1987:201.
11. Chesley LC, Cooper DW. Genetics of hypertension: possible single gene control of pre-eclampsia and eclampsia in the descendants of eclamptic women. *Br J Obstet Gynaecol*. 1986;93:898.
12. Cooper DW, Hill JA, Chesley L, Bryans C. Genetic control of susceptibility to eclampsia and miscarriage. *Br J Obstet Gynaecol*. 1988:95:644.
13. Cooper DW, Liston WA. Genetic control of severe pre-eclampsia. *J Med Genet*. 1979;16:409.
14. McKay DG. Chronic intravascular coagulation in normal pregnancy and preeclampsia. *Contrib Nephrol*. 1981;25:108.
15. Sibai BM, Spinnato JA, Watson DL, et al. Eclampsia IV. Neurological findings and future outcome. *Am J Obstet Gynecol*. 1985;152:184.
16. Rolfes DB, Ishak KG. Liver diseases in toxemia of pregnancy. *Am J Gastroenterol*. 1986;81:1138.
17. Sheehan HL, Lynch JB. *Pathology of Toxaemia of Pregnancy*. London: Churchill Livingstone:1973.
18. MacGillivray I. *Pre-eclampsia. The Hypertensive Disease of Pregnancy*. London: Saunders; 1983.
19. Hibbard LT. Maternal mortality due to acute toxemia. *Obstet Gynecol* 1973;42:263.
20. Lopez-Llera MM. Complicated eclampsia. Fifteen years' experience in a referral medical center. *Am J Obstet Gynecol*. 1982;142:28.
21. Govan ADT. The pathogenesis of eclamptic lesions. *Pathol Microbiol*. 1961;24:561.
22. Fox H. Histopathology of pre-eclampsia and eclampsia. In: Sharp F, Symonds EM, eds. *Hypertension in Pregnancy*. Ithaca, NY: Perinatology Press;1987:119.
23. Altchek A. Liver-kidney interrelation in pregnancy and toxemia. *Clin Obstet Gynecol*. 1968;11:487.
24. Campbell DM, Templeton AA. Is eclampsia preventable? In: Bonnar J, MacGillivray I, Symonds EM, eds. *Pregnancy Hypertension*. Baltimore, MD: University Park Press;1980:483.
25. Sibai BM, McCubbin JH, Anderson GD, Lipshitz J, et al. Eclampsia I. Observations from 67 recent cases. *Obstet Gynecol*. 1981;58:609.
26. Hankins GDV, Wendel GD, Cunningham FG, et al. Longitudinal evaluation of hemodynamic changes in eclampsia. *Am J Obstet Gynecol*. 1984;150:506.
27. Steven MM. Progress report: Pregnancy and liver disease. *Gut*. 1981;22:592.
28. Browne CH, Hanson GC, de Jode LR, Roberts PA. Rupture of subcapsular haematoma of the liver in a case of eclampsia. *Br J Surg*. 1975;62:237.
29. Manas KJ, Welsh JD, Rankin RA, Miller DD. Hepatic hemorrhage without rupture in preeclampsia. *N Eng J Med*. 1985;312:424.
30. Shukla BK, Prasad GN. Retinal changes in eclampsia and preeclampsia. *J Indian M A*. 1978;66:8.
31. Sunness J. The pregnant woman's eye. *Surv Opthalmol*. 1988;32(4):219.
32. Sibai BM, Anderson GD, McCubbin JH. Eclampsia II. Clinical significance of laboratory findings. *Obstet Gynecol*. 1982;59:153.

33. Lopez-Llera M, de la Luz Espinosa MM, Diaz de Leon PM, Rubio Linares G. Abnormal coagulation and fibrinolysis in eclampsia. *Am J Obstet Gynecol*. 1976;124:681.
34. Pritchard JA, Cunningham FG, Mason RA. Coagulation changes in eclampsia—their frequency and pathogenesis. *Am J Obstet Gynecol*. 1976;142:855.
35. Lopez-Llera MM, de la Luz Espinosa MM, Arratia SC. Eclampsia and placental abruption: basic patterns, management and morbidity. *Int J Gynecol Obstet*. 1988;27:335.
36. Shulka PK, Sharma D, Mandal RK. Serum lactate dehydrogenase in detecting liver damage associated with preeclampsia. *Br J Obstet Gynaecol*. 1978;85:40.
37. Weinstein L. Syndrome of hemolysis, elevated liver enzymes, and low platelet count: A severe consequence of hypertension in pregnancy. *Am J Obstet Gynecol*. 1982;142:159.
38. Cunningham FG, Lowe T, Guss S, Mason R. Erythrocyte morphology in women with severe pre-eclampsia and eclampsia. Preliminary observations with scanning electron microscopy. *Am J Obstet Gynecol*. 1985;153:358.
39. Rosenbaum M, Maltby GL. Cerebral dysrhythmia in relation to eclampsia. *Arch Neurol Psych*. 1943;49:204.
40. Jost H. Electroencephalographic records in relation to blood pressure changes in eclampsia. *Am J Med Sci*. 1948;57:216.
41. Kolstad P. The practical value of electroencephalography in preeclampsia and eclampsia. *Acta Obstet Gynecol*. 1961;40:127.
42. Benedetti TJ, Quilligan EJ. Cerebral edema in severe pregnancy-induced hypertension. *Am J Obstet Gynecol*. 1980;137:860.
43. Beeson JH, Duda EE. Computed axial tomography scan demonstration of cerebral edema in eclampsia preceded by blindness. *Obstet Gynecol*. 1981;60:529.
44. Dunn R, Lee W, Cotton DB. Evaluation of computerized axial tomography of eclamptic women with seizures refractory to magnesium sulfate therapy. *Am J Obstet Gynecol*. 1986;155:267.
45. Kirby JC, Jaindl JJ. Cerebral CT scan findings in toxemia of pregnancy. *Radiology*. 1984:151:114.
46. Brown CEL, Purdy P, Cunningham FG. Head computed tomographic scans in women with eclampsia. *Am J Obstet Gynecol*. 1988;159:915.
47. Crawford S, Varner MW, Digre KB, et al. Cranial magnetic resonance imaging in eclampsia. *Obstet Gynecol*. 1987;70:474.
48. Chesley LC. *Hypertensive Disorders in Pregnancy*. New York, NY: Appleton-Century-Crofts; 1978:1.
49. Bernard S. Postpartum eclampsia. *Obstet Gynecol*. 1960;15:748.
50. Sibai BM, Schneider JM, Morrison JC, et al. The late postpartum eclampsia controversy. *Obstet Gynecol*. 1980;55:74.
51. Sibai BM, Abdella TH, Taylor HA. Eclampsia in the first half of pregnancy. A report of three cases and a review of the literature. *J Rep Med*. 1982;27:706.
52. Zavet GM. Possible treatment of preeclampsia with calcium channel blocking agents. *Med Hypotheses*. 1983;12:303.
53. Lipsitz PJ, English IC. Hypermagnesemia in the newborn infant. *Pediatrics*. 1967;40:856.
54. Sibai BM, Spinnato JA, Watson DL, et al. Effects of magnesium sulfate on electroencephalographic findings in pre-eclampsia-eclampsia. *Obstet Gynecol*. 1984;64:261.
55. McCarthy GT, O'Connell B, Robinson AE. Blood levels of diazepam in infants of two mothers given large doses of diazepam in labour. *J Obstet Gynaecol Brit Commonw*. 1973;80:349.
56. Cree JE, Meyer J, Hailey DM. Diazepam in labour: its metabolism and effect on the clinical condition and thermogenesis of the newborn. *Br Med J*. 1973;4:251.
57. Johnson RA. Adverse neonatal reaction to maternal administration of intravenous chloromethiazole and diazoxide. *Br Med J*. 1976;1:943.
58. Paul RH, Koh SK, Bernstein SG. Changes in fetal heart rate uterine contraction patterns associated with eclampsia. *Am J Obstet Gynecol*. 1978;130:165.
59. Sibai BM, Anderson GD, Abdella TN, et al. Eclampsia III. Neonatal outcome, growth, and development. *Am J Obstet Gynecol*. 1983;146:307.
60. Wright JP. Anesthetic considerations in preeclampsia-eclampsia. *Anesth Analog*. 1983;63:590.
61. Clark SL, Divon MY, Phelen JP. Preeclampsia/eclampsia. Hemodynamic and neurologic correlations. *Obstet Gynecol*. 1985;66:337.
62. Gedekoh R, Hayashi T, MacDonald H. Eclampsia at Magee Women's Hospital, 1970–1980. *Am J Obstet Gynecol*. 1981;140:860.
63. Pritchard J, Pritchard S. Standardized treatment of 154 consecutive cases of eclampsia. *Am J Obstet Gynecol*. 1975;123:543.
64. Melrose EB. Maternal deaths at King Edward VIII Hospital, Durban. *S Afr Med J*. 1984;65:161.
65. Ekwempu CC. Maternal mortality in eclampsia in the Guinea Savannah region of Nigeria. *Clin Exper Hyper in Pregnancy*. 1982;B1(4):531.
66. Akinkugbe A, Coker OO. Mortality in eclampsia in relation to treatment modalities: 10-year review. In: Bonnar J, MacGillvray I, Symonds EM, eds. *Pregnancy Hypertension*. Baltimore, MD: University Park Press; 1980:475.
67. Abdella TN, Sibai BM, Hays JM, et al. Relationship of hypertensive disease to abruptio placentae. *Obstet Gynecol*. 1984;63:365.
68. Sibai BM. Eclampsia VI. Maternal-perinatal outcome in 254 consecutive cases. *Am J Obstet*. 1990;163:1049.
69. Wightman H, Hibbard BM, Rosen M, Perinatal mortality and morbidity associated with eclampsia. *Br Med J*. 1978;2:235.
70. Redman CW, Beilin L, Bonnar J, et al. Plasma-urate measurements in predicting fetal death in hypertensive pregnancy. *Lancet*. 1976;1:1370.
71. Wood SM. Assessment of renal functions in hypertensive pregnancies. *Clin Obstet Gynecol*. 1977;4:747.
72. Friedman EA, Neff RK. Pregnancy outcome as related to hypertension, edema and proteinuria. In: Lindheimer MD, Katz AI, Zuspan FP, eds. *Hypertension in Pregnancy*. New York, NY: John Wiley and Sons; 1976:13.
73. Romero R, Mazor M, Lockwood CJ, et al. Clinical significance, prevalence, and natural history of thrombocytopenia in pregnancy induced hypertension. *Am J Perinatol*. 1989;6:32.
74. Zuspan FP. Problems encountered in the treatment of pregnancy-induced hypertension. *Am J Obstet Gynecol*. 1978;131:591.
75. Beaufils M, Uzan S, Donsimoni R, Colau JC. Prevention of pre-eclampsia by early platelet therapy. *Lancet*. 1985;1:840.
76. Wallenberg HCS, Dekker GA, Makovitz JW, Rotmans P. Low dose aspirin prevents pregnancy induced hypertension and pre-eclampsia in angiotensin sensitive primigravidae. *Lancet*. 1986;1:1.
77. Chesley LC. Remote prognosis. In: Chesley LC, ed. *Hypertensive Disorders in Pregnancy*. New York, NY: Appleton-Century-Crofts; 1978;421.
78. Adelusi B, Ojengbede OA. Reproductive performance after eclampsia. *Int J Gynecol Obstet*. 1986;24:183.
79. Sibai BM, El-Nazer A, Gonzalez A. Severe preeclampsia/eclampsia in young primigravida; subsequent pregnancy outcome and remote prognosis. *Am J Obstet Gynecol*. 1986;155:1011.
80. Chesley LC, Annitto JE, Cosgrove RA. The remote prognosis of eclamptic women; sixth periodic report. *Am J Obstet Gynecol*. 1976;124:446.
81. Sexton JA. Epilepsy as a sequel of obstetrical complications. *J Ky Med Assoc*. 1976;74:595.
82. Chesley LC, Annitto JE, Cosgrove RA. The familial factor in toxemia of pregnancy. *Obstet Gynecol*. 1968;32:303.
83. Villar MA, Sibai BM. Eclampsia. *Obstet. Gynecol. Clin. N. Amer*. 1988;15:364.

Chapter One Hundred and Forty-One

Chronic Hypertension and Antihypertensive Drugs

William C. Mabie and Baha M. Sibai

141

The most widely agreed upon definition of hypertension is a blood pressure equal to or exceeding 140/90 mm Hg. There is controversy about whether the fourth (muffling) or fifth (disappearance) Korotkoff sound is used to determine the diastolic blood pressure. The Joint National Committee on the Detection, Evaluation, and Treatment of High Blood Pressure recommends using the fifth Korotkoff sound. The blood pressure should be taken in the sitting position after 5 minutes of quiet rest. Since hypertension is labile, the average of two or more measurements should be taken. If the first two readings differ by more than 5 mm Hg, additional readings should be obtained. If the bladder of the blood pressure cuff does not encircle at least two-thirds of the arm, an artificially high pressure may be obtained; a thigh cuff is useful in obese patients.[1] Home blood pressure monitoring improves compliance with antihypertensive drugs and gives a more accurate reflection of blood pressure during daily living by eliminating the *white-coat* response when blood pressure is measured in the physician's office.

The prevalence of hypertension in the United States in the National Center for Health Statistics National Health and Nutrition Examination Survey performed in 1976–1980 was 30,762,000 or 21.7% of the US population. Fifty-five percent of the hypertensive population was not on treatment. Of the 45% of hypertensives on treatment, 54% were controlled and 46% were not controlled.[2]

The level of diastolic blood pressure is used to grade severity of hypertension: mild (90–104 mm Hg), moderate (105–114 mm Hg), and severe (115 mm Hg and above). Eighty percent of all hypertensives have mild hypertension, 15% moderate, and 5% severe. Hypertension is a powerful risk factor for atherosclerotic cardiovascular disease along with age, sex, total cholesterol, positive family history, obesity, smoking, diabetes, peripheral or cerebral vascular disease, and ECG evidence of left ventricular hypertrophy with strain.[2]

Over 90% of hypertension is primary, or essential, or idiopathic. Genetic factors probably play a role. Hypertension is considered a polygenic, multifactorial disease. Increased genetic sensitivity predisposes to a series of environmental influences including salt intake, obesity, occupation, family size, and crowding.[3]

The mechanism of essential hypertension is not well understood. There are several explanations for the hypertension. One is that hypertensives have an inherited defect in renal sodium excretion. About 15% of the population is salt sensitive. These patients retain sodium and expand their extracellular fluid volume. This produces hypertension. It also produces an increase in circulating natriuretic factors, one of which is the digoxin-like immunoreactive substance. This substance inhibits the sodium-potassium-ATPase pump and leads to increased intracellular calcium and hyperactive vascular smooth muscle. Another postulated explanation of hypertension is a generalized membrane defect. Red cells from about 35–50% of patients with essential hypertension have abnormalities of sodium transport across the cell membrane. This defect is assumed to occur in all cells of the body, particularly the vascular smooth muscle. This would allow an abnormal accumulation of calcium within vascular smooth muscle resulting in heightened vascular responsiveness to vasoconstrictor agents.[3]

HEMODYNAMICS OF ESSENTIAL HYPERTENSION

Blood pressure = cardiac output × total peripheral resistance. Thus, blood pressure can go up if cardiac output increases, if peripheral vascular resistance increases, or if both increase. Blood pressure and cardiac output are measured directly and peripheral vascular resistance is derived from these values. While it is difficult to find subjects with early essential hypertension, invasive hemodynamic monitoring in patients with borderline hypertension (ie, some readings exceeding 90 mm Hg) have shown that cardiac index (cardiac output divided by body surface area) is increased above normal. This is due to an increase in heart rate while stroke index (stroke volume divided by body surface area) is usually normal. The calculated peripheral vascular resistance is not significantly different from normal. Tachycardia and elevated cardiac index have been demonstrated in a large proportion of adolescents and children with borderline hypertension. This has given rise to the concept of a hyperkinetic circulatory system in the initial phase of essential hypertension. As the hypertension becomes moderate several years later, the cardiac output is usually lower than in normotensive controls. The heart rate is usually higher than in controls and the stroke volume is normal or low. In patients with severe hypertension, systemic vascular resistance is markedly increased and cardiac output and stroke volume are markedly decreased. When heart failure is present, cardiac output is low and peripheral resistance is very high together with increased pressures in the pulmonary circulation and reduced left ventricular ejection fraction. As long as heart failure is not present, the pulmonary circulation is normal in essential hypertension.[4,5]

Longstanding hypertension results in structural changes in the left ventricle and in the resistance vessels. It produces concentric left ventricular hypertrophy. The increased thickness of the myocardium may interfere with coronary artery perfusion. Angina pectoris may occur because of accelerated coronary artery disease and increased myocardial oxygen requirements as a consequence of the increased myocardial mass. Ventricular hypertrophy results in diastolic dysfunction or impaired ventricular relaxation, requiring increased left atrial filling pressures with resulting left atrial hypertrophy.[6] Ultimately, systolic function deteriorates, the ventricle dilates, and signs and symptoms of heart failure appear. Longstanding hypertension also increases the thickness of the arterial walls, reducing the arterial lumen. An interesting finding in some experimental animals and in human studies is that certain antihypertensive drugs cause regression of left ventricular hypertrophy. Some of these drugs are methyldopa, calcium-channel blockers, beta blockers, and the angiotensin-converting enzyme inhibitors. On the other hand, vasodilators (eg, hydralazine or minoxidil), peripheral adrenergic inhibitors (eg, prazosin), and diuretics do not seem to cause a reduction in left ventricular hypertrophy.[7]

ETIOLOGY

The causes of hypertension in the nonpregnant state are many and will not be discussed here.

COMPLICATIONS OF HYPERTENSION

In addition to the cardiac changes described above, there is endothelial denudation and smooth muscle proliferation in the arterial wall. Atherosclerosis is accelerated. Cerebral arteriolar microaneurysms form. Coronary artery disease, angina, myocardial infarction, congestive heart failure, aortic aneurysm dissection, lacunar infarcts and intracerebral hemorrhage are all linked to hypertension. Renal damage is both structural and functional, ie, arterial nephrosclerosis, proteinuria, accelerated malignant hypertension, azotemia, and end-stage renal disease. Ocular complications include two types of retinopathy—neuroretinitis, which is associated with hemorrhages and exudates, and arteriosclerosis, which is associated with arteriovenous (AV) crossing changes, copper or silver wiring, and focal or diffuse vessel narrowing.[10]

BENEFITS OF TREATMENT

A summary of clinical trials of treating hypertension can be found elsewhere.[8] It is fairly clear that patients with moderate to severe hypertension (diastolic blood pressure greater than 105 mm Hg) should receive active treatment. For example, in the Veterans Administration trial of patients with diastolic blood pressure of 115–129 mm Hg, morbidity rate was reduced from 30% to 2% in one year.[9] In those with diastolic blood pressure in the range of 105–114 mm Hg, the reduction was from 9.6% to 2.5% in one year.[9] Six clinical trials have examined the benefits of drug therapy for mild hypertension, ie, diastolic blood pressure between 90 and 104 mm Hg. Antihypertensive therapy significantly reduces morbidity and mortality from hypertensive complications such as stroke, heart failure, left ventricular hypertrophy, and progression to more severe hypertension, but provides inconsistent protection from atherosclerotic complications such as coronary artery disease and may even increase mortality from coronary disease.[8,9]

The most glaring example of treatment worsening prognosis is the Multiple Risk Factor Intervention Trial (MRFIT). In this trial, half of the patients received standard care in the community and the other half were randomized to specialty clinics in which aggressive treatment of cigarette smoking, hypercholesterolemia, and hypertension was given over a period of 6 years. Coronary mortality was 7.1% lower in the specialty clinic group, which was not statistically significant. However, in the specialty clinic group there was an excess of sudden deaths after two years of therapy in a subgroup of hypertensive men with nonspecific ECG changes. It was hypothesized that the patients in the specialty clinic group were given a higher dose of diuretic (usually 100 mg of hydrochlorothiazide or chlorthalidone daily), which resulted in a greater prevalence of hypokalemia with resultant ventricular arrhythmias and sudden death. The MRFIT study also revealed that antihypertensive treatment adversely affects blood lipids. Diuretic treatment is associated with a rise in total cholesterol and low-density lipoprotein cholesterol. There may be a fall in high-density lipoprotein cholesterol and a rise in triglycerides. Some beta blockers have similar effects on HDL and triglycerides.[8-10]

These disturbing findings have raised the possibility that the side effects of therapy may undermine the benefit of blood pressure control on ischemic heart disease. A middle ground view of the treatment of mild hypertension would be to treat patients with diastolic blood pressure greater than 95 mm Hg as well as patients at high risk for cardiovascular disease with target organ damage already. Treatment of mild hypertension would be expected to reduce left ventricular mass and to slow the decline of renal function in diabetic patients with renal involvement. Patients with diastolic blood pressure of 90–94 mm Hg who are otherwise at low risk probably do not need pharmacologic therapy. Nonpharmacologic therapy including weight reduction, low-salt diet, dynamic exercise, and cessation of cigarette smoking and alcohol consumption should be pursued.[2,3,8-10] The oral drugs currently available for the treatment of hypertension in the United States are listed in Table 141–1.

TABLE 141–1. ORAL ANTIHYPERTENSIVE DRUGS CURRENTLY AVAILABLE IN THE UNITED STATES

Diuretics	Adrenergic Inhibitors	Vasodilators	Ace Inhibitors	Calcium Antagonists
	Beta-adrenergic blockers			
Bendroflumethiazide	Acebutolol	Hydralazine	Captopril	Diltiazem
Benzthiazide	Atenolol	Minoxidil	Enalapril	Nicardipine
Chlorothiazide	Metoprolol		Lisinopril	Nifedipine XL
Chlorthalidone	Nadolol			Verapamil
Cyclothiazide	Penbutolol			Verapamil SR (long-acting)
Hydrochlorothiazide	Pindolol			
Hydroflumethiazide	Propranolol			
Indapamide	Propranolol, long-acting			
Methyclothiazide	Timolol			
Metolazone	**Centrally acting alpha-blockers**			
Polythiazide	Clonidine			
Quinethazone	Clonidine TTS (patch)			
Trichlormethiazide	Guanabenz			
Loop diuretics	Guanfacine			
Bumetanide	Methyldopa			
Ethacrynic acid	**Peripheral-acting adrenergic antagonists**			
Furosemide	Guanadrel			
Potassium-sparing agents	Guanethidine			
Amiloride	*Rauwolfia* alkaloids			
Spironolactone	*Rauwolfia* (whole root)			
Triamterene	Reserpine			
	Alpha$_1$-adrenergic blockers			
	Prazosin			
	Terazosin			
	Combined alpha- and beta-adrenergic blockers			
	Labetalol			

TABLE 141–2. DRUGS RECOMMENDED FOR HYPERTENSIVE EMERGENCIES AND URGENCIES

Emergencies	Urgencies
Parenteral Therapy Required	**Oral Therapy Preferred**
Sodium nitroprusside	Clonidine
Diazoxide	Nifedipine
Trimethaphan	Captopril
Nitroglycerin	Labetalol
Labetalol	
Hydralazine	
Captopril (only available orally)	

HYPERTENSIVE EMERGENCIES AND URGENCIES

In the 1984 report of the Joint National Committee on Detection, Evaluation, and Treatment of High Blood Pressure, the classification of hypertensive emergencies and urgencies was proposed.[10] The group suggested that emergencies were situations with greatly elevated blood pressure that must be lowered in one hour to reduce patient risk. Urgencies were situations in which severe elevations in blood pressure were not causing immediate end organ damage but should be controlled within 24 hours. Based on actuarial data, the committee had previously defined a diastolic blood pressure of 115 mm Hg or greater as a hypertensive emergency. They now felt that this was arbitrary and confusing. They stressed the concept that the rate of change of blood pressure may be more important than the absolute level. For example, a woman with preeclampsia may be seen initially with a clinically emergent state from acute but only modest elevations of blood pressure. By contrast, a patient may present with 150 mm Hg diastolic without complaints or evidence of end organ dysfunction. The association of elevated blood pressure with evidence of new or progressive end organ damage determines the seriousness of the clinical situation. Examples of hypertensive emergencies include hypertensive encephalopathy, intracranial hemorrhage, acute left ventricular failure with pulmonary edema, dissecting aortic aneurysm, and severe hypertension associated with preeclampsia, head trauma, extensive burns, unstable angina, or myocardial infarction. Hypertensive urgencies were considered to be marked elevations in blood pressure without evidence of new or worsening end organ dysfunction. Examples were accelerated or malignant hypertension without impending complications and perioperative hypertension, including patients requiring emergency surgery. A clear distinction between emergencies and urgencies is not always possible.[11]

The drugs recommended in Table 141–2 are those suggested by Ferguson and Vlasses[11] in an excellent review of hypertensive emergencies and urgencies. There are risks associated with too rapid or excessive reduction of elevated blood pressure. Although the cerebral blood flow is maintained constant over a wide range of blood pressures, there is a lower level as well as an upper limit to autoregulation. In chronic hypertensives who have a rightward shift of the cerebral autoregulation curve (Fig. 141–1) secondary to medial hypertrophy of the cerebral vasculature, lowering blood pressure too rapidly may produce cerebral ischemia. Coronary blood flow and renal perfusion also may deteriorate initially. Treatment of hypertensive emergencies requires hospitalization and intravenous medication. Frequently, hypertensive urgencies can be treated with oral medications. Sodium nitroprusside is the primary agent for true emergencies. Trimethaphan is the agent of choice in dissecting aortic aneurysm or intracranial hemorrhage. In situations in which careful monitoring is not possible, intravenous diazoxide, labetalol, or hydralazine or sublingual or oral nifedipine may be used. Intravenous furosemide is a useful adjunct in the therapy of hypertensive emergencies.[2,11] A more complete discussion of the rationale of drug selection, mechanism of action, complications, and safety in pregnancy will be included under the discussion of chronic hypertension in pregnancy.

CHRONIC HYPERTENSION IN PREGNANCY

The incidence of chronic hypertension varies among different populations, ranging from 0.5 to 4.0% and averaging 1.5%. Chronic hypertension is usually idiopathic (80%) or due to renal disease (20%), although the figures may reflect insufficient investigation. A number of renal diseases may be causative, the most common being chronic glomerulonephritis, interstitial nephritis, diabetic glomerulosclerosis, IGA nephropathy, and renal artery stenosis.

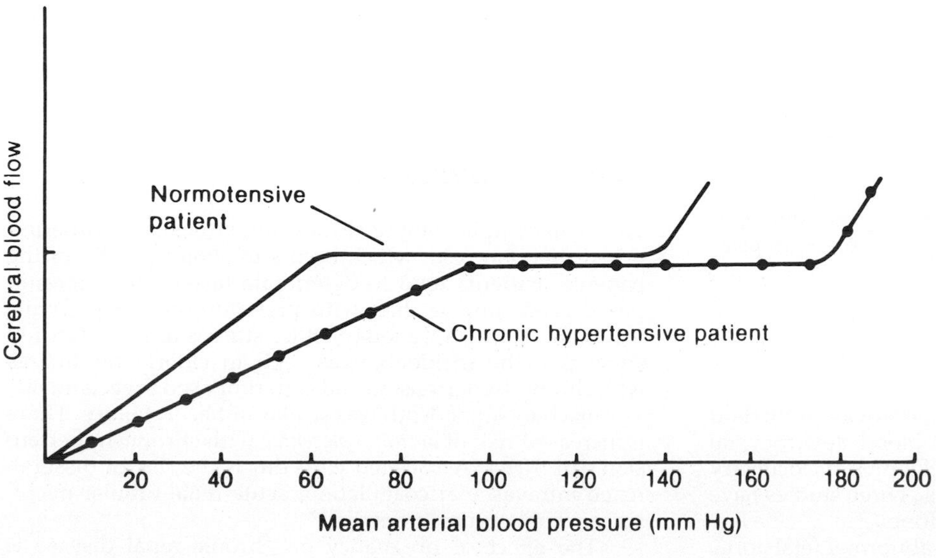

Figure 141–1. Representation of the relationship between cerebral blood flow and mean arterial blood pressure. Blood flow is kept constant within a wide range of mean blood pressure in both normotensive and hypertensive patients. However, patients with chronic hypertension have the lower and upper limits of autoregulation shifted to higher blood pressure values. (*From Donaldson[115] with permission.*)

SIGNS AND SYMPTOMS

Patients tend to be over 30 years of age, obese, and multiparous, with associated medical problems such as diabetes or renal disease. The incidence is higher in black women and in women with a family history of hypertension.[12] A woman who has delivered one or more infants and has hypertension in this pregnancy most likely has chronic hypertension. The typical patient has hypertension without other signs of preeclampsia (eg, proteinuria or nondependent edema). The diagnosis is made on the basis of documented hypertension before conception, or before 20 weeks' gestation, or persistence of hypertension after the puerperium (6 weeks). Whether worsening hypertension represents superimposed preeclampsia or hypertension associated with renal disease is sometimes difficult to determine. Preexisting renal disease alone may have all the manifestations of preeclampsia (hypertension, edema, proteinuria, and hyperuricemia). A diagnosis could be made with renal biopsy, but it is rarely necessary because the decision to deliver can be based on difficulty of blood pressure control, renal function, and fetal well-being. For the same reasons, renal biopsy usually is not performed for the work-up of proteinuria or elevated serum creatinine in pregnancy.

LABORATORY, X-RAY, ECG, AND ECHOCARDIOGRAPHY

The ECG may show left ventricular hypertrophy in 5–10% of patients with chronic hypertension in pregnancy.[12] Echocardiography is more sensitive in diagnosing left ventricular hypertrophy. When ECG and echocardiography are compared with autopsy findings, ECG has a sensitivity of diagnosing left ventricular hypertrophy of 35% versus 85% for echocardiography.[13] Thompson et al[14] attempted to differentiate preeclampsia from chronic hypertension by measuring left ventricular mass serially during pregnancy. Normal patients and patients with preeclampsia had a left ventricular mass less than 200 g, whereas patients with chronic hypertension had a left ventricular mass greater than 200 g. No change was noted in left ventricular mass in any group during the course of pregnancy. Left ventricular mass was not altered by superimposed preeclampsia in the chronic hypertensive group. If confirmed, this technique may be useful in differentiating preeclampsia from chronic hypertension.

Elevated serum creatinine, decreased creatinine clearance, and proteinuria are present in about 5–10% of patients with chronic hypertension. The chest x-ray is usually normal, although it may reveal cardiomegaly. Patients with left ventricular hypertrophy or elevated serum creatinine are at increased risk for developing superimposed preeclampsia. Patients with cardiomegaly due to either hypertensive cardiovascular disease or congestive cardiomyopathy are at increased risk for superimposed preeclampsia, pulmonary edema, and arrhythmias.[12]

DOPPLER FLOW STUDIES

Doppler ultrasound examination is a noninvasive method of measuring uteroplacental and fetal blood flow. Several studies have investigated the value of Doppler velocimetry in a variety of pregnancy complications. Three studies have focused on hypertensive pregnancy alone.

Jouppila and Kirkinen[15] reported abnormal fetal aortic blood flow velocity waveforms in hypertensive pregnancies complicated by fetal growth retardation. Cameron et al[16] measured Doppler waveforms in the fetal aorta and umbilical artery in 41 patients with hypertension in pregnancy. Fourteen had chronic hypertension, 17 had mild preeclampsia, and 10 had severe preeclampsia. Doppler abnormalities were seen in 2 patients with chronic hypertension, both of whom delivered growth-retarded infants. The highest number of abnormal Doppler waveforms in both the fetal aorta and umbilical artery were found in patients with severe preeclampsia. Abnormalities were detected in the fetal aorta more frequently than in the umbilical artery. Doppler assessment was often abnormal before a nonstress test or biophysical profile became abnormal. Three healthy fetuses with no Doppler abnormalities were delivered by preeclamptic mothers with uncontrollable hypertension, supporting the concept that some fetuses can tolerate the consequences of maternal hypertension for a long time without any hemodynamic alteration.

Ducey et al[17] studied 136 pregnant women with hypertension with Doppler velocimetry of the uterine and umbilical arteries. The patients were classified into 4 groups according to values of the systolic/diastolic (S/D) ratios. The first group had normal ratios in both the umbilical and the uterine arteries. The second group had elevated umbilical artery ratios and normal ratios in the uterine arteries. The third group had elevated uterine artery ratios with normal umbilical S/D ratios, and the fourth group had elevated ratios in both vessels. Women in the group with normal ratios in both vessels gave birth to infants with normal birth weight at term. The values for the 3 groups with abnormal velocimetry were abnormal umbilical–normal uterine: birth weight 2098 ± 811 g, gestational age 35.7 ± 3.2 wk; elevated uterine–normal umbilical: birth weight 2464 ± 722 g, gestational age 36.3 ± 3 wk; and elevated ratios in both vessels: birth weight 1627 ± 697 g, gestational age 33.3 ± 2.7 wk. There were 27 growth-retarded infants, 26 of whom had abnormal Dopplers (96%). The authors suggested that Doppler evaluation of the uterine and umbilical S/D ratios should be part of the clinical evaluation of all pregnant women with hypertension. The authors hypothesized that women with reduced flow velocity in both vessels have abnormal trophoblastic invasion of the myometrial segments of the spiral arteries, which normally occurs at 14–16 weeks' gestation. Those with normal uterine but reduced umbilical flow have a high resistance placenta possibly related to failure of angiogenesis, acute vasospasm, or thrombosis in the placenta. Based on these hypotheses, antihypertensive therapy may have adverse effects on fetuses in both groups of patients.

MATERNAL COMPLICATIONS

The main complication of chronic hypertension is superimposed preeclampsia, which occurs in about 20–30% of the patients. Patients tend to deteriorate faster with superimposed preeclampsia than with preeclampsia alone. While maternal death is rare today, older studies of hypertension show that the incidence was high in elderly multiparas with chronic hypertension and superimposed preeclampsia. The mechanism of death was stroke and heart failure. There is increased risk of *abruptio placentae* with chronic hypertension (0.4–10%). Associated with this is the risk of disseminated intravascular coagulation, acute renal tubular necrosis, or renal cortical necrosis.[18]

The effect of pregnancy on chronic renal disease is

uncertain. Although there are few data for patients with severe disease, limited evidence suggests that if renal function is well preserved (serum creatinine less than 1.5 mg/dL) pregnancy does not change the course of renal disease; but if renal insufficiency exists prior to pregnancy (serum creatinine greater than 1.5 mg/dL), the decline in renal function may be more rapid than expected.[19]

FETAL COMPLICATIONS

The fetus has a 25–30% risk of prematurity and a 10–15% risk of being growth-retarded. Preeclampsia tends to occur after 34 weeks' gestation, so that prematurity is not a great concern. Preeclampsia superimposed on chronic hypertension frequently occurs earlier (25–34 weeks), and in such cases, fetuses are at double jeopardy for prematurity and intrauterine growth retardation. In addition, there is a risk of stillbirth or intrapartum fetal distress due to *abruptio placentae* or chronic intrauterine asphyxia.[12,18]

PREVENTION

There are no absolute criteria for blood pressure or renal function on which to base recommendations for therapeutic abortion or sterilization in patients with chronic hypertension. At a 1986 international symposium on renal disease in pregnancy sponsored by the National Kidney Foundation, there was uniform agreement that pregnancy in patients with a serum creatinine greater than 4.0 mg/dL was contraindicated. Patients who attempt pregnancy with the serum creatinine greater than 2.0 mg/dL are at considerable risk. Still, there have been occasional reports of successful pregnancies in patients on dialysis,[20] and over 1500 patients have had successful pregnancies after renal transplantation.[21] Although data are few in patients with severe hypertension, in one group there was a maternal survival of 100% and a perinatal survival of 75% in 44 patients with diastolic blood pressure greater than 110 mm Hg in the first trimester.[22]

CONTROL OF HYPERTENSION

There is general agreement among most authorities that antihypertensive therapy will decrease the incidence of stroke and heart failure in pregnant patients with diastolic blood pressure exceeding 110 mm Hg. The controversy concerns the value of antihypertensive therapy of mild hypertension (approximately 95% of pregnant patients with chronic hypertension have mild hypertension). The Veterans Administration Cooperative Study demonstrated that treatment of diastolic blood pressure 105–114 mm Hg in men decreased cardiovascular morbidity in just 10 months. Patients with diastolic blood pressure of 95–104 mm Hg showed benefits of therapy only after 5 years had elapsed. Therefore, no benefits of antihypertensive therapy for mild chronic hypertension could be expected during the 9 months of pregnancy. Therapy cannot be justified with the same arguments used in general internal medicine. Some authors claim that antihypertensive therapy for mild chronic hypertension will decrease the incidence or delay the onset of superimposed preeclampsia, thus lowering perinatal mortality and morbidity. Others claim there is no benefit and considerable risk. Since this issue is still unresolved, a review of some of the recent clinical studies is helpful.

ANTIHYPERTENSIVE DRUGS FOR CHRONIC HYPERTENSION DURING PREGNANCY

There have been many clinical trials of antihypertensive therapy in chronic hypertension since the first one was published by Hans and Kopelman in 1964.[23] They are of two types: American studies that use strict criteria for the diagnosis of chronic hypertension; and European and Australian studies of pregnancy-associated hypertension, which include preeclampsia, chronic hypertension, and chronic hypertension with superimposed preeclampsia.

Among the American studies, Arias and Zamora[24] looked at 58 patients with mild chronic hypertension. A total of 29 were treated with various antihypertensive agents and 29 served as control subjects. Antihypertensive therapy decreased the incidence of superimposed preeclampsia (13.8 versus 44.8%). Perinatal outcome was similar in both groups.

Curet and Olson[25] studied 66 patients with mild chronic hypertension treated with bed rest alone unless the diastolic blood pressure exceeded 100 mm Hg, in which case hydralazine was added. They found that an average diastolic blood pressure greater than 100 mm Hg constituted a very high risk group with a 56% incidence of preeclampsia and intrauterine growth retardation and a 33% incidence of a positive oxytocin challenge test. They concluded that bed rest, avoidance of diuretics, and judicious use of hydralazine results in the best perinatal outcome.

Sibai et al[26] studied 211 patients with mild chronic hypertension. All antihypertensive medications were discontinued on the first visit and only reinstituted if blood pressure exceeded 160/110 mm Hg. This became necessary in 13% of the patients. The incidence of intrauterine growth retardation was 7.9%. Abnormal antepartum fetal heart rate testing was found in 6% of the patients. The perinatal mortality was 28.1 per 1,000.

Mabie et al[12] studied 169 cases of chronic hypertension in pregnancy. Antihypertensive medications were given if the diastolic blood pressure exceeded 90 mm Hg. The goal of the therapy was to keep the diastolic blood pressure less than 90 mm Hg. Methyldopa was the first drug used up to a dose of 2000 mg per day. If blood pressure was not controlled, hydrochlorothiazide (50 mg per day) was added. If the combination of methyldopa and hydrochlorothiazide did not control blood pressure, then propranolol (40–240 mg per day) was added. A spectrum of medical problems complicated management in 51% of the patients. The most common medical problems were obesity in 36% and diabetes in 22%. The overall perinatal mortality was 28.4 per 1000. One-third of the patients developed superimposed preeclampsia. The poorest outcome occurred in patients with early-onset superimposed preeclampsia, requiring delivery at 27–34 weeks' gestation. Antepartum fetal heart rate testing was abnormal in 10% of the patients with intrauterine growth retardation occurring in 15%. The perinatal outcome in this study was similar to the outcome of studies in which antihypertensive therapy was withheld. This indicates that controlling blood pressure is merely one aspect of the management of chronic hypertension. Accurate dating, attention to associated medical problems, antepartum fetal assessment by ultrasound and heart rate monitoring, and carefully timed delivery are additional important factors.

There have been many reasonably large European and Australian antihypertensive trials, some examples of which follow. Redman et al[27] studied 242 patients with a blood pressure exceeding 140/90 mm Hg in pregnancy. A total of 117 were treated with methyldopa; 125 served as controls.

There were nine pregnancy losses in the control group versus one in the treated group, but this was primarily due to a decrease in mid-trimester abortions.

Gallery et al[28] compared methyldopa (27 patients) with oxprenolol (26 patients) for the treatment of pregnancy-associated hypertension. Oxprenolol is a β_1-selective blocker. They found improved maternal blood volume expansion, fetal birth weight, and perinatal mortality in the oxprenolol group. No harmful fetal side effects of the beta blocker were seen.

Fiddler et al[29] repeated the Gallery study in a larger number of patients with nearly opposite findings. There was no significant difference in fetal weight or perinatal mortality. Methyldopa seemed to be better than oxprenolol in controlling blood pressure; there was a higher incidence of abnormal fetal heart rate tracings in labor in patients treated with oxprenolol.

Sandstrom et al[30] studied patients with sustained hypertension after two weeks of a thiazide diuretic and a week of bed rest in the hospital. A total of 101 patients received the beta blocker metoprolol, and 97 received hydralazine. A lower incidence of intrauterine growth retardation (11.7% versus 16.3%) and a lower perinatal mortality (2% versus 8%) in the beta blocker group were found. No fetal side effects were noted.

Rubin et al[31] compared atenolol, a long-acting, β_1-selective drug, with placebo in 120 patients with mild-to-moderate, pregnancy-associated hypertension. Atenolol decreased the incidence of superimposed preeclampsia and of respiratory distress syndrome, reduced the number of hospital admissions, and improved perinatal mortality. Most of the difference in pregnancy outcome could be ascribed to women who entered the study between 27 and 32 weeks' gestation with mild hypertension. The placebo-treated patients had a higher rate of disease progression with subsequent spontaneous or obstetrically determined preterm delivery and all the associated neonatal complications of prematurity. In women who entered after 32 weeks' gestation, there was no difference in pregnancy outcome, but blood pressure was substantially lower in the treated group. Bradycardia was common in the atenolol-exposed fetuses but was not clinically significant.

In the study of Redman et al[32], children born to hypertensive women were followed from birth and examined up to the age of 7.5 years. Physical and mental problems were the same in children of treated and untreated women. Sons of untreated mothers were heavier and taller than those of treated mothers. Among children of women who entered the trial between 16 and 20 weeks' gestation, sons of treated mothers had slightly larger heads than sons of untreated mothers. There was no difference in mean intelligence quotient. Therefore, methyldopa seems safe to use in pregnancy. A similar follow-up study was performed on the infants in Rubin's beta blocker study.[33] The placebo group had a worse pregnancy outcome and this difference was still detectable in the children at one year of age, in that the only child with permanent disability was in the placebo group.

Pickles et al[34] compared labetalol and placebo in a multicenter, randomized, double-blind study of 152 patients with blood pressure 140–160 mm Hg systolic and 90–105 mm Hg diastolic. The patients had pregnancy-induced hypertension without proteinuria. Mean gestational age at onset of treatment was 34 weeks and at delivery was 38 weeks. Labetalol dosage ranged from 300–600 mg per day. No additional antihypertensive therapy was needed in either the placebo or the labetalol group, indicating rather mild disease. Maternal mean arterial pressure was lowered approximately 8 mm Hg in the labetalol-treated group. There were no perinatal deaths or congenital malformations, and the maternal and fetal outcomes in the two groups were similar. Labetalol was tolerated well by the mothers, and there was no increase in neonatal bradycardia, hypotension, or hypoglycemia in their infants. The incidence of respiratory distress syndrome and jaundice was slightly lower in the labetalol-treated group.

A partial summary of clinical trials comparing antihypertensive therapy to no treatment is found in Table 141–3. Other than the study of Rubin et al, the evidence of maternal or fetal benefit is unimpressive. One problem with virtually all antihypertensive trials in pregnancy is that they include only patients with mild hypertension. Patients with more severe hypertension (diastolic blood pressure >100 or 110 mm Hg) are excluded for ethical reasons. Further-

TABLE 141–3. A PARTIAL LISTING OF CONTROLLED TRIALS OF ANTIHYPERTENSIVE THERAPY IN PREGNANCY

Author	Number of Subjects	Treatment	Control	Maternal Benefit	Fetal Benefit
Leather et al (1968)	100	Methyldopa, diuretic	No treatment	None	Reduced mid-trimester abortions, prolonged gestation, heavier babies
Redman et al (1976)	242	Methyldopa	No treatment	None	Reduced mid-trimester abortions
Arias et al (1978)	59	Methyldopa, hydralazine, hydrochlorothiazide	No treatment	Decreased frequency of pregnancy aggravated hypertension	None
Rubin et al (1983)	120	Atenolol	Placebo, double-blind	Lowered blood pressure prevented proteinuria, reduced hospital admission rate	Reduced RDS
Sibai et al (1988)	200	Labetalol plus hospitalization	Hospitalization alone	Reduced incidence of delivery for severe hypertension	None
Pickles et al (1989)	152	Labetalol	Placebo, double-blind	None	None

more, patients in the placebo group usually are treated with hydralazine or another agent if the hypertension becomes severe remote from term so that, in effect, there is no untreated group. Finally, the duration of antihypertensive treatment is often short (2–3 weeks) making conclusions about drug effects on fetal growth or intelligence quotient at follow up of dubious significance.

Many drugs have been used in the treatment of hypertension during pregnancy. Only the major ones will be considered in the following discussion, which will emphasize newer agents such as labetalol, nifedipine, captopril, and ketanserin.

Oral Agents

Thiazide Diuretics. Thiazide diuretics have been reported to cause a number of harmful maternal and fetal side effects, the main one being plasma volume contraction.[35] Studies in nonpregnant patients show that thiazides have acute and chronic effects.[36,37] Acutely, they cause a 5–10% decrease in plasma volume, which lowers cardiac output and blood pressure in the first 3–5 days of treatment. Over the next 4–6 weeks, renal compensatory mechanisms return the plasma volume toward normal but not to pretreatment levels. At the same time cardiac output returns to pretreatment levels, but total peripheral resistance stays low. Thus, the acute blood pressure lowering effect of thiazides is due to volume contraction. The sustained antihypertensive effect is thought to involve mobilization of excess sodium from the arterial wall. This leads to widening of the vascular lumen and possibly to decreased vascular responsiveness to endogenous catecholamines. Sibai et al[38] showed that plasma volume contraction occurs in early pregnancy in hypertensive patients on chronic thiazide therapy. When the therapy was stopped, normal physiologic volume expansion occurred. If the thiazide was continued, plasma volume expansion was minimal (18% mean increase in patients taking thiazide versus 52% mean increase in patients in whom diuretics were discontinued early in pregnancy). Perinatal outcome was the same in both groups, however. Another consideration is the volume expansion caused by antihypertensive therapy. It may be that the sodium and water retention produced by antihypertensive agents offsets the volume contraction caused by the thiazide.

In 1985, Collins et al[39] reviewed 9 randomized trials of diuretics in pregnancy involving nearly 7000 women. Diuretic therapy significantly decreased the incidence of preeclampsia when all trials were taken together; however, in 4 of the 9 separate trials the benefit had not been statistically significant. The incidence of stillbirth was one-third less in the diuretic-treated patients, but this was not statistically significant. They concluded that future randomized trials would require extremely large numbers of patients to detect a difference in perinatal mortality since perinatal mortality is now less than 1%.

Because the initiation of diuretic therapy causes a fall in blood volume and cardiac output and a rise in vascular resistance, adding a diuretic late in pregnancy is probably contraindicated, unless it is needed for treatment of pulmonary edema. On the other hand, continuing a diuretic as part of a therapeutic program in patients with chronic hypertension who become pregnant remains an unresolved issue. Our policy is to discontinue thiazide diuretics in such patients at the time of first visit.

Methyldopa. Methyldopa, a central α_2-adrenergic agonist, was first marketed in 1964 and is the only antihypertensive drug whose long-term safety for the mother and fetus has been adequately assessed. It is the most frequently used antihypertensive drug in pregnancy and is the standard to which other drugs are compared. Alpha$_2$-receptor stimulation in the brain stem causes decreased efferent sympathetic activity. Methyldopa reduces systemic vascular resistance without causing physiologically significant changes in heart rate or cardiac output, and renal blood flow is maintained. If methyldopa is used alone, fluid retention, and loss of antihypertensive control is frequent. For this reason, methyldopa usually is combined with a diuretic for treatment of nonpregnant patients. It usually is started at a dose of 250 mg three times a day and increased to 2 g per day. Peak plasma levels occur 2–3 hours after oral administration; the plasma half-life is about 2 hours, and the maximum effect occurs 4–6 hours after an oral dose. Most of the agent is excreted by the kidney. The most common side effects are sedation, postural hypotension, and impotence. With prolonged therapy, 10–20% of patients develop a positive direct Coombs test, usually after 6–12 months of therapy. Hemolytic anemia occurs in fewer than 5% of these patients and is an indication to stop the drug. Fever, liver function abnormalities, granulocytopenia, and thrombocytopenia have occurred rarely.[40]

Clonidine. Clonidine is another central α_2-adrenergic agonist. Treatment usually is started at 0.1 mg twice daily and increased in increments of 0.1–0.2 mg per day up to 2.4 mg per day. A transdermal preparation of clonidine designed to deliver the drug continuously over a week causes fewer side effects than oral therapy and may improve compliance. Blood pressure declines 30–60 mm Hg with use of clonidine, with a maximal effect in 2–4 hours and a duration of action of 6–8 hours. Renal blood flow and glomerular filtration rate are preserved, but cardiac output falls. This is attributable to a decrease in venous return secondary to systemic vasodilatation and bradycardia. Cardiac output responds normally to exercise. Xerostomia and sedation are the most frequently encountered side effects. Withdrawal of clonidine produces a hypertensive crisis that responds well to reinstitution of the drug.[40] Horvath et al[41] performed a randomized double-blind study in 100 pregnant women, comparing oral clonidine and methyldopa. They found no significant difference in blood pressure control or maternal and fetal outcome. There was one neonatal death with each drug (98% survival). Clonidine was as well tolerated as methyldopa.

Guanabenz. Guanabenz is a third centrally quanethidine-like α_2-adrenergic agonist that also has a guanethidinelike neuronal blocking action. It has two distinct advantages: it produces a 20% decrease in serum cholesterol with long-term use, and it does not cause significant salt and water retention. Nevertheless, guanabenz is not recommended for pregnant or nursing mothers because it causes skeletal abnormalities in mice and fetal loss in rats and rabbits in doses 3–6 times the maximum recommended human dose.[40]

Prazosin. Prazosin is a postsynaptic α_1-adrenergic blocker that causes vasodilatation equally in the resistance and capacitance vessels, thus reducing cardiac preload and afterload. Hemodynamic studies show that the fall in blood pressure is not accompanied by a significant change in heart rate, cardiac output, renal blood flow, or glomerular filtration rate. Prazosin is used in the treatment of hypertension and heart failure. It is only a mild to moderately potent antihypertensive agent and therefore is used most commonly in combination with a diuretic, beta blocker, or central α_2-agonist. Dosage range is 6–15 mg per day in 2–3 divided doses. Postural hypotension can occur following the first dose of the drug. Animal studies have demonstrated no teratogenic effects.[40] Lubbe and Hodge[42] used prazosin alone or in combination with oxprenolol in 44 pregnant women. No fetal abnormalities or adverse effects were noted. Dommisse et al[43] used prazosin with or without oxprenolol to treat pregnancy hypertension beginning before 34 weeks' gestation. None of the 22 patients had significant maternal or fetal side effects attributable to drug therapy. Although available since 1976, prazosin has not been widely used in pregnancy.

Hydralazine. Hydralazine is a direct arteriolar vasodilator that causes a secondary baroreceptor-mediated sympathetic discharge, increasing heart rate and cardiac output. It is an excellent drug for intravenous therapy of hypertension in pregnancy; however, it is not tolerated well taken orally as a single agent. Hydralazine is absorbed mostly from the gastrointestinal tract but undergoes "first pass" acetylation in the gut wall as well as in the liver. Bioavailability is thus only 26–50% of an oral dose. Hydralazine is 85% protein-bound. Peak serum concentrations occur between 0.5–2.0 hours after oral administration. Plasma half-life is 2–4 hours. The half-life of hydralazine's antihypertensive action is longer than its serum half-life because hydralazine is concentrated in the walls of muscular arteries. Thus, it is detectable there long after it has been cleared from the blood. About 50% of the US population are genetically determined *slow-acetylators* and are at higher risk for hypotension and other side effects. Prominent side effects with hydralazine include: headache, tachycardia, palpitations, fluid retention, and a lupus-like syndrome when chronic dosage exceeds 200 mg per day. Many of the unwanted side effects are minimized when it is used with a diuretic, methyldopa, or a beta blocker; however, use of multiple agents is discouraged in pregnancy. Dosage is initiated at 10 mg 4 times daily and increased to 200 mg per day.[40]

Minoxidil. This is the most powerful orally active antihypertensive agent available in the United States. It is an arteriolar vasodilator primarily used in patients with severe hypertension and renal disease. It usually must be given with a diuretic and a beta blocker because it tends to cause salt and water retention and tachycardia. Pericardial effusion is seen occasionally. Right atrial fibrosis is found in beagle dogs treated with minoxidil, but autopsy studies have shown no evidence of this in humans. The most common adverse effect is hypertrichosis, especially involving the face and extremities, which occurs after 3–6 weeks of therapy. This can be controlled with depilatories or shaving; however, many female patients discontinue minoxidil because of this cosmetic disturbance. The hypertrichosis disappears after the drug is stopped. Minoxidil has been shown to reduce conception in rats and to increase fetal resorption in rabbits when administered at five times the human dose.[40] There have been only 2 case reports of its use in pregnancy. One was associated with fetal malformation and hypertrichosis, but captopril was used in the patient as well.[44] In the other case, the newborn was normal.[45] Dosage is started at 5 mg once daily and is increased by 5 to 10 mg per day every two to three days up to 100 mg per day. The usual dosage ranges from 10 to 40 mg per day given as a once or twice daily dose.

Beta Blockers. Beta blockers were introduced for clinical use in 1964 and have been used in pregnancy to treat migraine headaches, hypertrophic cardiomyopathy, mitral valve prolapse, Graves' disease, and hypertension.[46] Beta blockers usually are not adequate to control severe hypertension and frequently are combined with a diuretic or a vasodilator or both. Beta blockers have been associated with neonatal bradycardia, hypoglycemia, hyperbilirubinemia, intrauterine growth retardation, respiratory depression, blocking the tachycardic response to hypoxia, and an increase in uterine muscle tone causing decreased uterine blood flow.[46-49] Extensive clinical experience with various beta blockers indicates that the frequency of these side effects is low and that they are considered to be relatively safe for use in pregnancy. Infants of mothers receiving beta blockers should be monitored after delivery for side effects.[46]

The mechanism of action, despite extensive research, has not been established. It is likely that a variety of mechanisms contribute to a greater or lesser extent. There is a fall in cardiac output, resulting from a negative inotropic and chronotropic effect. All beta blockers suppress renin levels, but this probably plays a minor role in the antihypertensive action of beta blockers. Beta blockers reduce sympathetic activity of the heart. They therefore reduce the transient rises in systolic and diastolic blood pressure as well as cardiac output that occur in hypertensives in response to stimuli such as exercise. It has been proposed that this reduction in peak levels of sympathetic activity on the heart may recondition the baroreceptors to produce their vasomotor inhibitory impulses at lower levels of blood pressure. Still other central effects are postulated.[40]

Some beta-blocking agents (eg, atenolol and metoprolol) preferentially bind to β_1-receptors and are termed β_1-specific or cardioselective. They are less likely to cause bronchospasm, disturbances in lipid and carbohydrate metabolism, and interfere less with the response to hypoglycemia in insulin-dependent diabetics. However, β_1-specific blocking agents also block β_2-receptors at larger doses such as may be employed in antihypertensive therapy. Some beta-blockers have intrinsic sympathomimetic activity (ISA). Pindolol, oxprenolol, and acebutolol have ISA and are less likely to produce bradycardia and decreased cardiac output. Beta blockers are contraindicated in patients with cardiac failure and are relatively contraindicated in patients with chronic obstructive pulmonary disease and diabetes mellitus. Most beta blockers are excreted primarily by the kidney so that a reduced dose is necessary in renal failure.

The main beta blockers which have been used in pregnancy are propranolol, metoprolol, oxprenolol, and atenolol. Propranolol was the first beta blocker used in the United States beginning in 1976. It is a nonselective beta blocker possessing no ISA. The major disadvantage of propranolol is that it is more lipid soluble than the other beta blockers; therefore, it readily penetrates the blood-brain barrier and probably causes more central nervous system (CNS) side effects such as drowsiness, fatigue, and confusion. Eliahou et al[50] treated 25 hypertensive pregnant patients with propranolol and noted a reduction of predicted fetal wastage. Tcherdakoff[51] studied nine patients treated with propranolol in combination with other agents and noted good blood pressure control with no increase in fetal mortality. Bott-Kanner et al[52] used combination therapy with propranolol and hydralazine in the management of long-standing hypertension in 13 patients during 15 pregnancies. They found that patients tolerated the regimen without difficulty and blood pressure remained below 140/90 mm Hg in all cases. None of the patients developed superimposed preeclampsia; however, there was one unexplained stillbirth and two cases of hypoglycemia.

Atenolol is the least lipid soluble beta blocker and therefore produces fewer CNS side effects. It is a β_1-selective agent, requires one daily dosing, and has no ISA. Rubin et al used atenolol 100–200 mg daily compared to placebo in a prospective, randomized, double-blind trial that was described previously. Easterling and Benedetti advocate the use of atenolol to control the hyperdynamic circulation in preeclampsia.[53,54]

Metoprolol is another cardioselective beta blocker. It may be used with caution in patients with chronic obstructive pulmonary disease, diabetes, and Raynaud's phenomenon. It has no ISA. It requires multiple daily dosing and is only moderately lipid soluble. Studies by Sandstrom et al[30] and Hogstedt et al[55] have revealed no significant maternal or fetal complications with metoprolol.

Gallery et al[28] and Fiddler et al[29] studied oxprenolol versus methyldopa. Gallery et al concluded that both drugs controlled blood pressure but oxprenolol resulted in a better pregnancy outcome because of greater fetal growth. Fiddler et al came to the opposite conclusions.

Pindolol is a beta blocker with ISA. It has been reported to lower blood pressure without a reduction in uteroplacental blood flow measured by IN scintigraphy.[56] Pindolol has no effect on fetal heart rate.[57]

Labetalol. Labetalol is an antihypertensive agent, available for both oral and intravenous use, that produces nonselective beta blockade and postsynaptic α_1-blockade, combining the effects of propranolol and prazosin. The beta blockade is more potent than the alpha-blockade, with a beta or alpha ratio of 3:1 for oral administration and 7:1 for intravenous administration. Recent reports suggest that the drug also may have a vasodilator action mediated by β_2-receptor stimulation. Hemodynamic studies conflict, but overall it appears that labetalol decreases systemic vascular resistance with little or no change in heart rate or cardiac output.[58-61]

The drug was introduced in Europe in 1975 but did not receive FDA approval in the United States until 1984. Labetalol is readily absorbed after oral administration but undergoes considerable "first pass" hepatic metabolism, resulting in a bioavailability of only about 25%. There are no active metabolites and the elimination half-life is approximately 6 hours. Labetalol has been found useful in the treatment of essential hypertension, renal hypertension, pheochromocytoma, hypertensive emergencies, controlled hypotension during surgery, ischemic heart disease, and pregnancy hypertension.[62] Side effects are mild and transient and include posture-related dizziness, scalp tingling, tiredness, headache, skin rash, fever, impotence, and upper gastrointestinal disturbances. Labetalol is contraindicated in patients with greater than first degree heart block. Oral therapy begins at 200 mg 2–3 times per day and increases to a maximum of 2400 mg per day.[40,58] Most pregnant hypertensive patients are controlled on 1600 mg per day or less. Intravenous therapy can be given in escalating dosages of 20, 40, 80, 80, and 80 mg every 10 minutes to a maximum cumulative dosage of 300 mg.[63] An alternative regimen is a constant infusion beginning at 0.5 mg/kg per hour and increasing the dosage every 30 minutes by 0.5 mg/kg per hour to a maximum of 3 mg/kg per hour.[64]

Many studies now have been done using labetalol in pregnancy. The drug crosses the placental barrier with fetal-to-maternal plasma concentration ratios of 0.5–1.0. Nevertheless, most authors emphasize that the neonatal side effects associated with beta blockers (eg, bradycardia, hypoglycemia, respiratory depression, or growth retardation) are seen rarely with labetalol. During chronic treatment with labetalol, drug levels in breast milk ranged from 22% to 45% of maternal blood labetalol concentration. Only very small amounts of labetalol are secreted into breast milk (approximately 0.004% of the dose) after oral administration of the drug. No adverse effects have been noted in neonates of patients who breast feed during labetalol therapy.[58]

Nylund et al[65] studied the effects of labetalol 1 mg/kg intravenously on uteroplacental blood flow in 8 preeclamptic patients using a radioactive indium clearance technique. Despite a significant drop in maternal blood pressure, no change in uteroplacental blood flow or fetal heart rate was found.

The drug has been widely used intravenously for severe hypertension in the nonpregnant state; 3 series have been published concerning its intravenous use during pregnancy. Davey et al[66] compared a continuous intravenous infusion of labetalol with a continuous infusion of dihydralazine in 12 patients with severe preeclampsia or eclampsia. Five of the 6 labetalol-treated patients achieved satisfactory control of blood pressure. Two of the 6 dihydralazine-treated patients had satisfactory blood pressure control, and 4 had hypotension. Three labetalol-exposed infants had bradycardia at birth.

Michael[64] compared intravenous labetalol with intravenous diazoxide in 90 patients with diastolic blood pressure exceeding 105 mm Hg. Forty-two of 45 in the labetalol group and 31 of 45 in the diazoxide group had satisfactory blood pressure control. Three labetalol patients had no response. Six in the diazoxide group had no response, and 8 had a precipitous fall in blood pressure. No bradycardia, hypotension, or hypoglycemia were seen in the labetalol-exposed infants. Michael suggested that smaller infants had less risk with labetalol because there was a smoother reduction in blood pressure.

Mabie et al[63] compared bolus labetalol to bolus hydralazine in a randomized trial involving 60 peripartum patients. Hydralazine lowered mean arterial pressure more than did labetalol (33.3 ± 13.2 versus 25.5 ± 11.2 mm Hg, mean ± SD), but labetalol had a more rapid onset of action. There was considerable interpatient variability in the dosage of labetalol required to control blood pressure. The duration of antihypertensive action also varied in the labetalol group, with the shortest duration occurring in those patients who required the highest dosage for blood pressure control. No fetal or neonatal problems ascribable to drug treatment were noted in the 13 instances in which labetalol was given before delivery. However, fetal distress due to overshoot hypotension occurred in 2 of the 6 cases involving antenatal hydralazine.

There have been several clinical trials using oral labetalol for hypertension in pregnancy. Michael[67] evaluated the effects of labetalol in 85 women with various types of pregnancy-associated hypertension. Effective blood pressure control was achieved in all but 6 patients using dosages up to 1200 mg per day. Perinatal mortality was 4.4%, which he felt was excellent considering the severity of the disease. Of the 89 infants born alive, 24 were growth-retarded. Only 11 infants had respiratory distress syndrome, which suggested to the author that labetalol promotes fetal lung maturity—a speculation that has not been confirmed.

Walker et al[68] reported 70 patients with mild to moderate hypertension treated with either labetalol or bed rest. Labetalol treatment resulted in significant reductions in severe hypertension, proteinuria, and platelet consumption. There were no adverse side effects in either the mothers receiving labetalol or their infants. In a subsequent report Walker[69] stated that labetalol directly inhibited platelet aggregation *in vitro* by stimulating prostacyclin production.

Sibai et al[70] studied the effects of labetalol and bed

rest in the hospital versus bed rest alone in 200 primigravidas with mild preeclampsia. The drug was tolerated well in a dosage that ranged up to 2400 mg per day. The only benefit of labetalol treatment was a reduced incidence of delivery for severe hypertension. There were no stillbirths but one neonatal death in the labetalol group. Gestational age at delivery, birth weight, number of neonatal ICU admissions, and cord blood gas measurements were not different between the 2 groups. However, intrauterine growth retardation was higher in the labetalol group (19% versus 9%).

Plouin et al[71] compared labetalol and methyldopa in a randomized trial involving 176 pregnant women with mild to moderate hypertension. Four stillbirths occurred in women treated with methyldopa and 1 neonatal death occurred in the labetalol group. Blood pressure control was better with labetalol (supplementary therapy was needed in 21% of the methyldopa group versus 13% of the labetalol group). Mean birth weight, gestational age at delivery, and newborn parameters in the nursery were similar.

Labetalol was compared with methyldopa in two other randomized trials. Lamming et al[72] compared 39 patients treated with labetalol with 35 treated with methyldopa and observed better blood pressure control, a lower frequency of proteinuria, and more frequent spontaneous labor in the group treated with labetalol. Redman et al[73] found no difference in blood pressure control or proteinuria. Induced labor was more frequent with labetalol. There was no difference in birth weight, gestational age, or Apgar score between the 2 groups in either trial.

In summary, labetalol is a well tolerated, moderately powerful antihypertensive agent that seems to be relatively safe for the fetus. With oral administration it is slightly more potent than methyldopa but has no great advantage over it. The intravenous form of labetalol has a rapid onset of action and produces a smooth reduction of blood pressure with little risk of overshoot hypertension. However, dosage requirements are very variable, and in patients requiring high dosages the duration of action is short.

Calcium-Channel Blockers. Calcium-channel blockers are a structurally and pharmacologically diverse class of drugs that have been available in Europe since 1962, but which have been introduced only recently in the United States. Currently available calcium blockers include verapamil, nifedipine, diltiazem, and nicardipine. Calcium-channel blockers may be divided into 2 pharmacologic classes: those resembling verapamil (eg, verapamil, diltiazem, and bepridil) and those resembling nifedipine (eg, nifedipine, nicardipine, and nitrendipine).[40]

The drugs act by inhibiting transmembrane calcium ion flux from the extracellular space into the cytoplasm, thus blocking excitation-contraction coupling in muscle fibers. The concentration of free calcium ions in the cell determines the interaction between actin and myosin. Intracellular calcium ions come from two sources: intracellular stores in the sarcoplasmic reticulum and through the calcium slow channels in the plasma membrane. Because intracellular stores of calcium are greater in skeletal muscle than in cardiac or smooth muscle, skeletal muscle is affected less by shifts of extracellular calcium into the cell and is less affected by calcium-channel blocker therapy.[74]

Since calcium-channel blockers affect such a fundamental cellular response, they have activity in many tissues. Therapeutic applications thus have been wide-ranging: angina pectoris, Prinzmetal's angina, supraventricular tachycardia, hypertrophic cardiomyopathy, hypertension, cardiac failure due to diastolic dysfunction, Raynaud's phenomenon, myocardial preservation during surgery, migraine prophylaxis, neurologic recovery following hypoxia, subarachnoid hemorrhage, asthma, premature labor, dysmenorrhea, fetal supraventricular tachycardia, achalasia, inhibition of platelet aggregation, adjunctive treatment in cancer therapy, and management of hypoglycemia.[74]

Calcium-channel blockers have been used extensively in the treatment of hypertensive emergencies and urgencies as monotherapy or as part of combination therapy with diuretics, beta blockers, alpha and beta blockers, and central alpha-adrenergic agonists. They may be considered to be direct-acting vasodilators like hydralazine, diazoxide, and minoxidil. Older patients and those with low renin hypertension respond better to calcium-channel blockers. Nifedipine has the most potent vasodilating properties and is the calcium-channel blocker most frequently used to treat hypertension during pregnancy; therefore, it will be considered in detail.

Ninety percent of oral nifedipine is absorbed from the gastrointestinal tract; after moderate first-pass liver metabolism, the bioavailability is 65–70%. Onset of action is less than 20 minutes with oral administration and about 3 minutes after sublingual administration. The drug has an initial fast half-life of 2.5–3.0 hours and a terminal slow half-life of 5 hours. It is almost completely metabolized by the liver and is excreted 90% by the kidney and 10% in the feces.[40] In contrast to verapamil, in which the negative inotropic and chronotropic effects cause a decrease in cardiac output, nifedipine causes an increase in cardiac output. The decrease in systemic vascular resistance and the increase in heart rate more than offset the depressant effects on myocardial contractility. Nifedipine also lacks the depressant effects on AV nodal conduction seen with verapamil. Common nuisance side-effects include headache, flushing, cough, tachycardia, edema, nausea, and fatigue. More troublesome side-effects include overshoot hypotension, stroke, angina pectoris, acute myocardial infarction, and worsening renal function.[40,75] Since magnesium sulfate is a calcium-channel blocker, the use of both nifedipine and magnesium sulfate together could be potentially hazardous (eg, hypotension). Nifedipine has been shown to be teratogenic in rats when given in 30 times the normal human dose.[40] The effects of nifedipine on fetuses have been studied in pregnant animals.

Golichowski et al[76] studied the tocolytic and hemodynamic effects of nifedipine compared to ritodrine in the pregnant ewe. Nifedipine was found to be more potent as a tocolytic than ritodrine and caused less maternal hemodynamic disturbance. Fetal heart rate was increased more by nifedipine than by ritodrine. Veille et al[77] studied the effects of bolus nifedipine in dosages ranging from 2.5–45 μg/kg on the maternal uterine blood flow, arterial pressure, and heart rate in the pregnant pygmy goat. Uterine blood flow did not fall significantly. A transient fall in maternal blood pressure occurred but returned to normal after 5 minutes. Maternal heart rate increased immediately after the bolus of nifedipine, but returned toward the control value by 30 minutes. Harake et al[78] investigated the effect of intravenous nifedipine on the fetal and maternal circulation of sheep. Nifedipine produced a significant fall in maternal blood perssure and heart rate increased. Uterine blood flow fell by 21% and fetal arterial oxygen content decreased by 15%. Fetal cerebral blood flow increased 30–50%, raising concerns about increasing the risk of intracerebral hemorrhage. Ducsay et al[79] reported a dramatic decrease in fetal arterial pH and partial 0_2 pressure during continuous nifedipine infusion in pregnant rhesus monkeys. Ahokas et al[80] studied the short-term effects of nifedipine on maternal hemodynamics and organ perfusion in 12 hypertensive, term-pregnant, spontaneously hypertensive rats using a radioactive-labeled microsphere technique. Nifedipine caused a 25% decrease in mean arterial pressure by decreasing total peripheral resistance 38%. Cardiac output was increased 15%. Blood flow to nearly all vascular beds increased except blood flow to the skin, which remained unchanged. Blood flow increased to the reproductive organs, primarily the ovaries and the uterine wall. Placental blood flow was not significantly changed, but resistance decreased. Thus, in the rat, nifedipine can lower maternal blood pressure in pregnancy complicated by extreme hypertension without decreasing uteroplacental perfusion. In summary, the effect of nifedipine on uteroplacental blood flow is controversial. The differences in results among the studies may be related to hypertensive versus normotensive animals, to differences in the uteroplacental vasculature of the various animal species, or to the dosage of nifedipine and whether maternal hypotension occurred.

Using Indium-113 scintigraphy, Lindow et al[81] found no change in uteroplacental blood flow after reduction of blood pressure in 10 women with pregnancy-induced hypertension. Nifedipine has been used successfully in two studies for the treatment of premature labor.

Walters and Redman[82] gave nifedipine to 21 women with severe hypertension during pregnancy or the puerperium. Blood pressure fell by an average of 26/20 mm Hg at 20 minutes after oral administration. The principal side effects were headache and flushing. No adverse effects to the fetus were detected.

Constantine et al[83] used slow-release nifedipine as part of combination therapy in 23 pregnant hypertensive women. Good control of blood pressure was achieved in 20. Perinatal mortality was 130/1000 with a high cesarean section rate, a high rate of abnormal fetal heart rate tracings, and a high rate of intrauterine growth retardation (IUGR). Whether this was due to the disease or the medication was uncertain. The authors concluded that combination therapy with nifedipine should be used only in severe hypertension or in the context of a controlled, clinical trial.

Rubin[84] reported preliminary results using a combination of nifedipine and atenolol in 7 patients with severe preeclampsia. Other calcium blockers have been used to treat pregnancy hypertension.

Intravenous verapamil was used for severe postpartum hypertension in 10 patients with severe preeclampsia. Blood pressure decreased by 30%. The main side effects were headache and flushing.[85]

Allen et al[86] studied the acute affects of a single 20 mg oral dose of nitrendipine in 10 women with pregnancy-induced hypertension. Maternal blood pressure fell significantly and remained under control for at least four hours. Maternal heart rate increased by 10%; fetal heart rate was unchanged. Interestingly, plasma levels of norepinephrine, epinephrine, renin, and vasopressin did not change after reduction of maternal blood pressure with nitrendipine indicating that reflex counter-regulatory effects are not a problem with this drug.

Angiotensin-Converting Enzyme Inhibitors. Three agents are available in the United States: captopril, enalapril, and lisinopril. They induce vasodilatation by inhibiting the enzyme that converts angiotensin I to angiotensin II. Since angiotensin-converting enzyme (ACE) is identical to kininase II, which inactivates bradykinin, an additional antihypertensive effect may be from increased bradykinin levels.[87] Finally, certain ACE inhibitors increase the synthesis of vasodilating prostaglandins. Little change in heart rate, wedge pressure, cardiac output, or response to exercise is observed. Total peripheral resistance is lowered. Renal blood flow and glomerular filtration rate increase. The low side-effect profile makes ACE inhibitors acceptable for first-line therapy in nonpregnant patients.[87-89]

Captopril was the first of these agents introduced and was associated with 4 major side effects: neutropenia, proteinuria, rash, and taste disturbances. Early experience with very high doses (up to 900 mg per day) resulted in considerable toxicity. Substantially lower toxicity is seen with currently employed dosages that rarely exceed 200 mg per day. Patients with bilateral renovascular stenosis and patients with stenosis in a solitary functioning kidney or a transplanted kidney may develop renal failure when treated with ACE inhibitors. Hyperkalemia also may occur with these drugs, which inhibit angiotensin-II mediated aldosterone secretion. Nonproductive cough has been reported in 0.2–4.4% of patients and appears to be seen with all ACE inhibitors.[87-89]

Captopril causes abortions and fetal death in rabbits by reducing uteroplacental blood flow, probably by interfering with the renin-angiotensin system and prostaglandins.[90] In a study of pregnant ewes, it appeared to increase the stillbirth rate.[91] In human pregnancy, ACE inhibitor therapy has been associated with several fetal and neonatal complications including hypotension, growth retardation, oligohydramnios, anuria, renal failure, malformations (2 with captopril, 1 with enalapril), stillbirth, and neonatal death.[91-94] Although they have been used in pregnancy, it has been recommended that ACE inhibitors not be used. The prescription either preceded conception or was justified by severe maternal hypertension unresponsive to regular treatment. Coen et al[95] treated a patient with chronic glomerulonephritis throughout a twin pregnancy with a combination of captopril, hydralazine, and metoprolol. At term she delivered growth-retarded twins at 2250 g and 2020 g whose subsequent course to 10 months of age was unremarkable. Mochizuki et al[96] reported good results with captopril as part of combination therapy in late pregnancy in 3 patients. Kreft-Jais et al[97] reported the results of a French survey of pregnancies exposed to ACE inhibitors between June, 1985 and December, 1986. Twenty-two women received captopril and 9 enalapril. Most women had renal disease or chronic essential hypertension. Two stillbirths occurred in the captopril group and 1 in the enalapril group. Preterm delivery occurred in 11 women given captopril and in 1 given enalapril. Six of the 26 live-born babies were growth retarded: 4 in the captopril-treated group and 2 in the enalapril-treated group.

Since many other antihypertensive drugs may be used in pregnancy and since there is considerable doubt about the safety of ACE inhibitors, they should probably be avoided in pregnancy until long-term evaluation of offspring in human drug trials have established their safety.

Ketanserin. Ketanserin is a selective S_2-serotoninergic receptor antagonist with additional α_1-adrenergic blocking properties. The mechanism of its antihypertensive effect is unclear. It cannot be attributed to either the S_2-serotoninergic or α_1-adrenergic blockade alone, but an interaction between the two effects appears to be required. The major source of serotonin is the intestinal enterochromaffin cells. When released into the circulation serotonin is rapidly cleared by the pulmonary and hepatic beds or it is taken up by platelets.[98] Four serotonin receptors have been identified, but specific physiologic responses have been characterized only for the type 2 serotonin receptor. These receptors are located on platelets and vascular and bronchial smooth muscle. Serotonin stimulation of the type 2 receptor facilitates platelet aggregation, produces vasoconstriction in peripheral vessels, and amplifies the vasoconstrictive effect of other neurohumoral mediators. Platelet dysfunction and decreased platelet serotonin have been reported in women with preeclampsia.[99] Although serotonin has vascular effects, it has no well-defined role in the pathogenesis of hypertension.[98]

The hemodynamic profile of the drug is that of a vasodilator that acts on both resistance and capacitance vessels. The main hemodynamic effect is a fall in systemic vascular resistance. Heart rate increases transiently with intravenous injection but falls by about 4 beats per min during long-term oral therapy. Exercise capacity and renal function are preserved.[98]

Weiner et al[99] studied the effect of ketanserin using a randomized, double-blind, placebo-controlled study design in 20 hypertensive postpartum women. Dosage was a 10 mg bolus intravenously followed by 4 mg per hour with increases as necessary to maintain diastolic blood pressure below 95 mm Hg. Eleven patients had preeclampsia and 9 had chronic hypertension with superimposed preeclampsia. All patients responded to ketanserin with a wide range of dosage requirement. Patients with chronic hypertension and superimposed preeclampsia were more refractory to therapy. Side effects were confined to blurred vision in 3 and hypotension in 1.

Hulme and Odendaal[100] administered 10 or 20 mg boluses of ketanserin to 16 patients with severe preeclampsia in labor. They found that ketanserin satisfactorily lowered blood pressure. Maternal heart rate was unchanged. Mean fetal heart rate increased 4.6 beats per min. Variability was not affected. Frequency of contractions was reduced from 3.6 to 2.4 per 10 minutes. The mechanism of the reduction in uterine contractions is unknown since serotonin receptors have not been described in the uterus. No serious adverse effects occurred.

Voto et al[101] reported preliminary results of an open, randomized trial of oral ketanserin versus methyldopa for the treatment of pregnancy-associated hypertension. There were only 10 patients in each treatment group. Ketanserin controlled maternal blood pressure as well as methyldopa; however, it was associated with a fetal morbidity of 40% versus 10% for methyldopa. The morbidity (respiratory distress syndrome, respiratory depression, and sepsis) may not have been caused by the ketanserin.

Experience with ketanserin in the control of severe hypertension in nonpregnant patients has been less favorable. Four studies including 100 patients revealed a high failure rate which makes it unsuitable for routine use in hypertensive emergencies. It also produced sedation and dizziness.[98]

Studies of its chronic antihypertensive effect show that it works best in patients over 60 years of age, that it lowers blood pressure on the order of 14/12 mm Hg, and that it has additive effects when combined with a beta blocker or a diuretic. Other uses for ketanserin are for intermittent claudication, Raynaud's phenomenon, intraoperative and postoperative hypertension, and carcinoid syndrome. A 1988 review stated that nearly 19,000 patients had been treated with parenteral or oral ketanserin up to September, 1986.[98] Nevertheless, its usefulness in the treatment of pregnancy-associated hypertension is just beginning to be studied.

PARENTERAL AGENTS

Parenteral agents used for treatment of severe hypertension in pregnancy are usually vasodilators that can be classified as balanced or equal arterial and venular vasodilators (eg, sodium nitroprusside, trimethaphan), predominately arterial vasodilators (eg, hydralazine, diazoxide), and predominately venular vasodilators (eg, nitroglycerin). Labetalol, and alpha and beta blocker, also is being used more frequently in pregnancy because it is well tolerated and the patient may be easily switched from parenteral to oral therapy with the same drug. Oral and sublingual nifedipine are being used with increasing frequency for hypertensive emergencies and urgencies in pregnancy as well. The latter two drugs were discussed in detail previously. Finally, intravenous methyldopa, while less potent and having a slower onset of action, is still useful in hypertensive urgencies of moderate severity.

Hydralazine is the agent most commonly used for parenteral therapy in pregnant patients with diastolic blood pressure exceeding 110 mm Hg. Introduced in 1951, it has a long record of safety in pregnancy. It is a moderately powerful, dependable agent that will control hypertension in at least 95% of cases of pregnancy-associated hypertension. Hydralazine failure is seen most commonly in patients with renal insufficiency.

Hydralazine is an arterial vasodilator that causes a baroreceptor-mediated sympathetic discharge, resulting in tachycardia and increased cardiac output. A 10 mg intravenous dose produces an approximately 13 beat per min increase in heart rate and a 0.9 L per min/m^2 increase in cardiac index.[102]

Adverse effects include hypotension in the mother or fetus, fetal distress in labor, reflex tachycardia with flushing and chest pain, and a lupus-like syndrome when chronic dosage exceeds 200 mg per day. Intravenous hydralazine has an onset of action in 10–20 minutes with a peak effect in 60 minutes and a duration of action of 4–6 hours. Some studies have shown the drug to have a somewhat erratic onset of action and peak effect. The lack of immediate effect and the long duration of action make it unsuitable for titration of maternal blood pressure by continuous infusion. Hydralazine has been shown to increase uterine blood flow.[40,103]

Diazoxide, introduced in 1973, is now used infrequently for severe pregnancy hypertension in the United States. The major problem with the drug was with fetal distress when the drug was given as a 300 mg bolus. The dosage has since been reduced to 30–75 mg boluses administered every 10–15 minutes, and the problem with hypotension has diminished. Other adverse effects are hyperglycemia in the mother and fetus, retention of salt and water, cessation of labor, and burning at the injection site because of the alkaline pH (11.6).[40,104]

Sodium nitroprusside (1974) is the most powerful antihypertensive agent on the market. It is an equal arterial and venular vasodilator that can be used for minute-to-minute titration of maternal blood pressure. It should be given in an intensive care unit setting with an infusion pump and an arterial line for continuous blood pressure measurement. Onset of action is immediate and duration of action is 1.5–2.0 minutes. Photoinstability of the drug mandates frequent changes of solutions and use of light-protected containers and tubing. It is metabolized hepatically and excreted renally. Adverse effects include hypotension, a hyperdynamic cardiac response to afterload reduction, undesired vasodilation (eg, increasing cerebral

TABLE 141–4. ANTIHYPERTENSIVE AGENTS ADMINISTERED BY CONSTANT INFUSION

Drug	Infusion (mg/mL)	Concentration (μg/mL)	Dosage (μg/kg/min)
Nitroprusside	50/250	200	0.5–4
Trimethaphan	500/250	2000	5–30
Nitroglycerin	50/250	200	0.5–5

edema, causing coronary artery steal, increasing intrapulmonary shunting), hypothyroidism, and fetal thiocyanate and cyanide toxicity.[40,105] Nitroprusside's effect on uterine blood flow is controversial.[103,106,107] It has been recommended that nitroprusside not be used for longer than 30 minutes during pregnancy; however, longer usage has been reported.[108,109]

Trimethaphan (Arfonad) is a ganglionic blocker with equal arterial and venular vasodilating effects. It may be used like nitroprusside for minute-to-minute titration of maternal blood pressure and should be administered by infusion pump. Adverse effects are indiscriminate ganglionic blockade, paralytic ileus in the mother or fetus, urinary retention, and hypotension.[40] It also may interact with succinylcholine, causing prolonged neuromuscular blockade during cesarean section under general anesthesia.[110]

Nitroglycerin is a moderately powerful hypotensive agent when used as an intravenous drug. It is a predominately venular vasodilator. Adverse effects are hypotension, headache, tachycardia, and undesired venodilation. It crosses the placenta but no adverse effects to the fetus have been noted.[40,111] In pregnant ewes uterine blood flow is unchanged by nitroglycerin.[107,112]

Tables 141–4 and 141–5 summarize the administration of the parenteral antihypertensive agents described above.

MANAGEMENT OF CHRONIC HYPERTENSION IN PREGNANCY

The patient is encouraged to have her blood pressure checked several times before pregnancy to establish the severity of her hypertension in the nonpregnant state. She should then come in for her first exam at less than 12 weeks' gestation to establish gestational age correctly and to determine the severity of her hypertension in the first trimester. A careful history and physical is done. In taking the history, particular attention should be paid to the duration of hypertension, use of antihypertensive medications, history of cardiac or renal disease, and the outcome of previous pregnancies. The physical examination should include a careful examination of the optic fundi, listening for a renal artery bruit, and checking the dorsalis pedis pulses for coarctation of the aorta. At the first prenatal visit, baseline laboratory studies should be obtained for the organ systems that are likely to be affected by chronic hypertension or are likely to deteriorate during pregnancy. These tests include: urinalysis, complete blood count, blood urea nitrogen, creatinine, electrolytes, uric acid, calcium, phosphorus, liver function tests, electrocardiogram, 24-hour urine for creatinine clearance and total protein, and a 50 g glucola screening test. If hyperglycemia or wide blood pressure swings are evident, a 24-hour urine for vanillylmandelic acid and metanephrines is recommended to rule out pheochromocytoma. An antinuclear antibody and serum complement are done if the patient has significant proteinuria. The patient is seen by a dietician and instructed on a 4 g sodium diet and advised to stop smoking. If the patient is likely to have left ventricular hypertrophy from severe or longstanding hypertension, or if she has signs or symptoms of heart failure, an echocardiogram should be done. The first obstetric ultrasound usually is done at approximately 18 weeks' gestation and is repeated in 4–6 weeks. If these two studies are consistent, no further ultrasounds are done unless the patient has severe hypertension, growth retardation, or another indication, in which case the ultrasounds are continued at 4- to 6-week intervals. Weekly antepartum fetal testing using the biophysical profile is started at 34 weeks' gestation or whenever the patient develops superimposed preeclampsia. Doppler assessment of the systolic-diastolic ratio in the midportion of the fetal umbilical artery is useful as a screening test. The role of Doppler in the management of pregnancy hypertension is unclear at this time, as it is a relatively new technology. We would not deliver a patient based on Doppler findings alone, but look for reassurance from the Doppler. If it is abnormal, we look closely at other parameters for an indication to deliver.

As stated previously, the use of antihypertensive drugs for mild to moderate chronic hypertension in pregnancy (less than 110 mm Hg diastolic) is controversial. The following regimen is used by the authors.[113,114] Antihypertensive drugs are given if the diastolic blood pressure exceeds 105 mm Hg. The goal of antihypertensive therapy is to keep the blood pressure less than 150 mm Hg systolic and 100 mm Hg diastolic. Methyldopa is the first drug used in a dosage of 750 mg up to 4000 mg per day. The second drug added is hydralazine in a dosage ranging from 40 to 200 mg per day. If maternal blood pressure is not controlled with a combination of methyldopa and hydralazine and the pregnancy is less than 32 weeks' gestation, other agents should be used. Adding another antihypertensive agent may control the blood pressure, but the disease process may lead to fetal growth retardation, *abruptio placentae*, or fetal death. Thus, these pregnancies should be monitored very closely in the hospital.

If the patient has mild chronic hypertension and presents on a diuretic alone, the drug is stopped and the blood pressure is observed. If it becomes elevated, methyldopa is started. On the other hand, if the patient has severe hypertension and is on a combination of drugs, one of which is a thiazide diuretic, the drug combination may be continued. Ganglionic blockers, reserpine, and ACE inhibitors are not used in pregnancy because of undesirable maternal and fetal side effects.

Other agents that are useful as monotherapy in severe hypertension are labetalol up to 2400 mg per day, nifedipine up to 120 mg per day, and clonidine up to 2.4 mg per day. Combination therapy with atenolol-nifedipine or labetalol-nifedipine may be useful, as are other combinations of beta blockers, central alpha-agonists, vasodilators, and diuretics. Many drugs will work to control hypertension, but there is no panacea. The choice of antihypertensive

TABLE 141–5. ANTIHYPERTENSIVE AGENTS ADMINISTERED BY BOLUS INJECTION

Drug	Dosage (mg)	Interval (min)
Hydralazine	5	15
Diazoxide	30–75	10–15
Labetalol	20, 40, 80, 80, 80	10

agent is not as important to pregnancy outcome as other factors such as timing of the delivery, attention to associated medical problems, and compulsive antenatal fetal assessment.

Antepartum Evaluation

These pregnancies should be followed with serial ultrasonography for fetal growth and amniotic fluid evaluation. Antepartum testing with nonstress test (NST) or biophysical profile should start at 34 weeks' gestation and repeated weekly or earlier if needed. In cases with severe hypertension (those who develop superimposed preeclampsia and those with associated medical disorders such as class F diabetes and lupus), testing should be started as early as 26 weeks to be repeated twice weekly.

Particular difficulty is encountered in interpreting antenatal testing at less than 30 weeks' gestation. In the extreme case, one may have a nonreactive NST with spontaneous decelerations, oligohydramnios, and reverse diastolic flow on Doppler. At the other extreme, one may have a reactive NST, normal fluid, and a normal Doppler. Unfortunately, most of the patients with severe hypertension at less than 30 weeks do not have either of these profiles, and one must make a judgment based on the overall pattern of findings including the NST, amniotic fluid volume, biophysical profile, gestational age, L/S ratio, fetal growth, degree of maternal blood pressure control, associated medical problems, past obstetric history, and other factors.

Superimposed preeclampsia is diagnosed on the basis of worsening hypertension (30 mm Hg systolic or 15 mm Hg diastolic rise) plus elevated uric acid (>6 mg/dL) and proteinuria (> 300 mg per day). Some of the more frequent indications for early delivery include superimposed preeclampsia, underlying medical problems such as diabetes or renal insufficiency, abnormal antepartum fetal heart rate testing, and intrauterine growth retardation. A patient with worsening hypertension may be given betamethasone to accelerate fetal lung maturity if the L/S ratio is less than 2:1 and if delivery can be delayed for 48 hours after the first dose of steroid. The fetal heart rate is monitored closely during this 48–72 hour period and delivery is accomplished if signs of fetal distress develop. Patients usually are given epidural anesthesia for labor or cesarean section. If the cervix is unfavorable and the gestational age is less than 32 weeks, a primary cesarean section is done without a trial of labor, especially if fetal growth retardation is suspected.

Severe Chronic Hypertension

All patients with severe hypertension should receive antihypertensive drugs as described previously to keep systolic and diastolic blood pressures below 150 mm Hg and 100 mm Hg, respectively. These pregnancies are at increased risk for superimposed preeclampsia (30–50%) and *abruptio placentae* (2–10%).[22] Patients with severe hypertension in the first trimester are a very high risk group, but this should not be considered an indication for termination. With recent advances in obstetrics and neonatal care, the perinatal survival in this group is about 75%. However, the patients should be counseled regarding the need for frequent and prolonged hospitalization during pregnancy and the potential maternal risks from continuing pregnancy.[22] It is important to emphasize that superimposed preeclampsia is responsible for nearly all maternal and perinatal morbidities in these patients. Hence, patients that do not develop superimposed preeclampsia will have excellent maternal and perinatal outcome.

CONCLUSIONS

Pregnancies complicated by essential chronic hypertension should be treated as high-risk pregnancies. Most patients will have good perinatal outcome with proper obstetric and neonatal management. The use of antihypertensive drugs in patients with mild disease is not necessary to achieve the desired perinatal outcome. Most of the maternal and perinatal complications associated with these pregnancies are due to superimposed preeclampsia and the presence of medical complications other than hypertension.

REFERENCES

1. The 1988 report of the Joint National Committee on Detection, Evaluation, and Treatment of High Blood Pressure. *Arch Intern Med.* 1988;148(5):1023.
2. Kaplan NM. *Clinical Hypertension.* 4th ed. Baltimore, MD: Williams and Wilkins; 1986.
3. Williams GH, Braunwald E. Hypertensive vascular disease. In: Braunwald E, Isselbacher KJ, Petersdorf RG, et al, eds. *Harrison's Principles of Internal Medicine.* 11th ed. New York, NY: McGraw-Hill; 1987:1024.
4. Lund-Johnsen P. Hemodynamics in essential hypertension. *Clin Sci.* 1980;59:343.
5. Messerli FH, Schmieder RE, Nunez BD. Heterogenous pathophysiology of essential hypertension: implications for therapy. *Am Heart J.* 1986;112:886.
6. Harizi RC, Blanco JA, Alpert JS. Diastolic function of the heart in clinical cardiology. *Arch Int Med.* 1988;148:99.
7. Frohlich ED. Hemodynamic considerations in clinical hypertension. *Med Clin NA.* 1987;71:803.
8. Moser M. Treating hypertension: a review of clinical trials. *Am J Med.* 1986;81(Suppl 6 C):25.
9. Shoenberger JA. Mild hypertension: the rationale for treatment. *Am Heart J.* 1986;112:872.
10. The 1984 report of the Joint National Committee on Detection, Evaluation and Treatment of High Blood Pressure. *Arch Intern Med.* 1984;144:1043.
11. Ferguson RK, Vlasses PH. Hypertensive emergencies and urgencies. *JAMA.* 1986;255:1607.
12. Mabie WC, Pernoll MK, Biswas MK. Chronic hypertension in pregnancy. *Obstet Gynecol.* 1986;67:197.
13. Devereaux RB. Cardiac involvement in essential hypertension: Prevalence, pathophysiology, and prognostic implications. *Med Clin NA.* 1987;71:813.
14. Thompson JA, Hays PM, Sagar KB, Giulshanks DP. Echocardiographic left ventricular mass to differentiate chronic hypertension from preeclampsia during pregnancy. *Am J Obstet Gynecol.* 1986;155:994.
15. Jouppila P, Kirkinen P. Blood velocity waveforms of the fetal aorta in normal and hypertensive pregnancies. *Obstet Gynecol.* 1986;67:856.
16. Cameron AD, Nicholson SF, Nimrod CA, et al. Doppler waveforms in the fetal aorta and umbilical artery in patients with hypertension in pregnancy. *Am J Obstet Gynecol.* 1988;158:339.
17. Ducey J, Schulman H, Farmakides G, et al. A classification of hypertension in pregnancy based on Doppler velocimetry. *Am J Obstet Gynecol.* 1987;157:680.
18. Zuspan FP, O'Shaughnessy RW. Maternal physiology and diseases: Chronic hypertension in pregnancy. In: Pitkin RM, Zlatnik FJ, eds. *Yearbook of Obstetrics and Gynecology.* Chicago, IL: Yearbook Medical Publishers; 1979:11.
19. Kincaid-Smith P, Fairley KF. Renal disease in pregnancy. Three controversial areas: mesangial IgA nephropathy, focal glomerular sclerosis (focal and segmental hyalinosis and sclerosis), and reflex nephropathy. *Am J Kidney Dis.* 1987;9:328.
20. Hou S. Pregnancy in women requiring dialysis for renal failure. *Am J Kidney Dis.* 1987;9:368.
21. Davison JM. Renal transplantation and pregnancy. *Am J Kidney Dis.* 1987;9:374.
22. Sibai BM, Anderson GD. Pregnancy outcome of intensive therapy in severe hypertension in first trimester. *Obstet Gynecol.* 1986;67:517.
23. Hans SF, Kopelman H. Methyldopa in the treatment of severe toxemia of pregnancy. *Brit Med J.* 1964;1:736.
24. Arias F, Zamora J. Antihypertensive treatment and pregnancy outcome in patients with mild chronic hypertension. *Obstet Gynecol.* 1979;53:489.
25. Curet LB, Olson RW. Evaluation of a program of bed rest in the treatment of chronic hypertension in pregnancy. *Obstet Gynecol.* 1979;53:336.
26. Sibai BM, Abdella TN, Anderson GD. Pregnancy outcome in 211 patients with mild chronic hypertension. *Obstet Gynecol.* 1983;61:571.

27. Redman CWG, Beilin LJ, Bonnar J, Ounsted MK. Fetal outcome in trial of antihypertensive treatment in pregnancy. *Lancet*. 1976;2:753.
28. Gallery EDM, Saunders DM, Hunyor SN, Gyory AZ. Randomized comparison of methyldopa and oxprenolol for treatment of hypertension in pregnancy. *Brit Med J*. 1979;1:591.
29. Fiddler J, Smith V, Fayers P, DeSwiet M. Randomized controlled comparative trial of methyldopa and oxprenolol in treatment of hypertension in pregnancy. *Brit Med J*. 1983;286:1927.
30. Sandstrom B. Antihypertensive treatment with the adrenergic beta-receptor blocker metoprolol during pregnancy. *Gynecol Obstet Invest*. 1978;9:195.
31. Rubin PC, Butters R, Clark DM, et al. Placebo-controlled trial of atenolol in treatment of pregnancy-associated hypertension. *Lancet*. 1983;1:431.
32. Cockburn J, Moar VA, Ounsted M, Redman CWG. Final report of study on hypertension during pregnancy: The effects of specific treatment on the growth and development of the children. *Lancet*. 1982;1:647.
33. Reynolds B, Butters L, Evans J, et al. The first year of life after the use of atenolol in pregnancy associated hypertension. *Arch Dis Child*. 1984;59:1061.
34. Pickles CJ, Symonds EM, Broughton-Pipkin F. The fetal outcome in a randomized double-blind controlled trial of labetalol versus placebo in pregnancy-induced hypertension. *Brit J Obstet Gynecol*. 1989;96:38.
35. Lindheimer MD, Katz AI. Sodium and diuretics in pregnancy. *N Engl J Med*. 1973;288:891.
36. Hansen J. Hydrochlorothiazide in the treatment of hypertension. *Acta Med Scand*. 1968;183:317.
37. Tarazi RC, et al. Long term thiazide therapy in essential hypertension. *Circulation*. 1970;41:709.
38. Sibai BM, Grossman RA, Grossman HG. Effects of diuretics on plasma volume in pregnancies with long-term hypertension. *Am J Obstet Gynecol*. 1984;150:831.
39. Collins R, Yusuf S, Peto R. Overview of randomized trials of diuretics in pregnancy. *Brit Med J*. 1983;290:17.
40. McMahon FG. *Management of Essential Hypertension: the New Low-Dose Era*. 2nd ed. Mount Kisco, NY: Futura Publishing; 1984.
41. Horvath JS, Phippard A, Korda A, et al. Clonidine hydrochloride—A safe and effective antihypertensive agent in pregnancy. *Obstet Gynecol*. 1985;66:634.
42. Lubbe WF, Hodge JV. Combined alpha and beta adrenoceptor antagonism with prazosin and oxprenolol in control of severe hypertension in pregnancy. *NZ Med J*. 1981;94:169.
43. Dommisse J, Davey DA, Roos PJ. Prazosin and oxprenolol therapy in pregnancy hypertension. *SA Med J*. 1983;64:231.
44. Kaler SG, Patrinas ME, Lambert GH, et al. Hypertrichosis and congenital anomalies associated with maternal use of minoxidil. *Pediatrics*. 1987;79:434.
45. Valdiveso A, Valdes G, Spiro TE, Westerman RL. Minoxidil in breast milk. *Ann Intern Med*. 1985;102:135.
46. Rubin PC. Beta-blockers in pregnancy. *N Engl J Med*. 1981;305:1323.
47. Habib A, McCarthy JS. Effects on the neonate of propranolol administered during pregnancy. *J Pediatr*. 1977;91:808.
48. Pruyn SC, Phelan JP, Buchanan GC. Long-term propranolol therapy in pregnancy: Maternal and fetal outcome. *Am J Obstet Gynecol*. 1979;135:485.
49. Gladstone GR, Hordof A, Gersony WM. Propranolol administration during pregnancy: Effects on the fetus. *J Pediatr*. 1975;86:962.
50. Eliahou HE, Silverberg DS, Reisin E, et al. Propranolol for the treatment of hypertension in pregnancy. *Brit J Obstet Gynecol*. 1978;85:431.
51. Tcherdakoff PH, Colliard M, Berrard E, et al. Propranolol in hypertension during pregnancy. *Br Med J*. 1978;2:670.
52. Bott-Kanner G, Schweitzer A, Reisner SH, et al. Propranolol and hydralazine in the management of essential hypertension in pregnancy. *Br J Obstet Gynecol*. 1980;87:110.
53. Easterling TR, Benedetti TJ, Schmucker BC, Carlson KL. Antihypertensive therapy in pregnancy directed by noninvasive hemodynamic monitoring. *Am J Perinatol*. 1989;6:86.
54. Easterling TR, Benedetti TJ. Preeclampsia: a hyperdynamic disease model. *Am J Obstet Gynecol*. 1989;160:1447.
55. Hogstedt S, Lindberg B, Peng DR, et al. Pregnancy-induced increase in metoprolol metabolism. *Clin Pharmacol Ther*. 1985;37(6):688.
56. Lunell NO, Nylund L, Lewander A, et al. Uteroplacental blood flow in pregnancy hypertension after the administration of a beta-adrenoceptor blocker, pindolol. *Gynecol Obstet Invest*. 1984;18(5):269.
57. Ingemarsson S, Liedholm H, Montan S, et al. Fetal heart rate during treatment of maternal hypertension with beta-adrenergic antagonists. A preliminary report. *Acta Obstet Gynecol Scand*. 1984;118(suppl):95.
58. MacCarthy EP, Bloomfield SS. Labetalol: A review of its pharmacology, pharmacokinetics, clinical uses, and adverse effects. *Pharmacotherapy*. 1983;3:193.
59. Gagnon RM, Morissette M, Presant S, et al. Hemodynamic and coronary effects of intravenous labetalol in coronary artery disease. *Am J Cardiol*. 1982;49:1267.
60. Mehta J, Feldman RL, Marx JD, Kelly GA. Systemic, pulmonary and coronary hemodynamics effects of labetalol in hypertensive subjects. *Am J Med*. 1983;75(suppl):32.
61. Koch G. Hemodynamic changes after acute and long-term combined alpha-beta adrenoceptor blockade with labetalol as compared with beta-receptor blockade. *J Cardiovasc Pharmacol*. 1981;3(suppl 1):30.
62. Cohn JN, Mehta J, Francis GS. A review of the hemodynamic effects of labetalol in man. *Br J Clin Pharmacol*. 1982;13(suppl 1):19.
63. Mabie WC, Gonzalez AR, Sibai BM, Amon E. A comparative treat of labetalol and hydralazine in the acute management of severe hypertension complicating pregnancy. *Obstet Gynecol*. 1987;70:328.
64. Michael CA. Intravenous labetalol and intravenous diazoxide in severe hypertension complication in pregnancy. *Aust NZ J Obstet Gynecol*. 1986;26:26.
65. Nylund L, Lunnell NO, Lewander R. Labetalol for the treatment of hypertension in pregnancy. Pharmacokinetics and effects on the uteroplacental blood flow. *Acta Obstet Gynecol Scand*. 1984;118(suppl):71.
66. Davey DA, Dommissee J, Garden A. Intravenous labetalol and intravenous dihydralazine in severe hypertension in pregnancy. Excerpt Med Int Congr Ser. 1982;59:51.
67. Michael CA. The evaluation of labetalol in the treatment of hypertension during pregnancy. *Br J Clin Pharmacol*. 1982;113(Suppl):127.
68. Walker JJ, Crooks A, Erwin L, et al. Labetalol in pregnancy-induced hypertension: Fetal and maternal effects. In: Riley A, Symonds EM, eds. *The Investigation of Labetalol in the Management of Hypertension in Pregnancy*. Amsterdam: Excerpta Medica International Congress Series; 1982:591.
69. Walker JJ, Erwin L, Lang E. Labetalol and platelet function in preeclampsia. *Lancet*. 1982;2:279.
70. Sibai BM, Gonzalez AR, Mabie WC, Moretti M. A comparison of labetalol plus hospitalization versus hospitalization alone in the management of preeclampsia remote from term. *Obstet Gynecol*. 1987;70:323.
71. Plouin PF, Breat G, Milard F, et al. Comparison of antihypertensive efficacy and perinatal safety of labetalol and methyldopa in the treatment of hypertension in pregnancy: a randomized controlled trial. *Br J Obstet Gynecol*. 1988;95:868.
72. Lamming GD, Broughton-Pipkin F, Symonds EM. Comparison of the alpha and beta blocking drug, labetalol, and methyldopa in the treatment of moderate and severe pregnancy-induced hypertension. *Clin Exp Hypertens B*. 1980;2:865.
73. Redman CWG. A controlled trial of treatment of hypertension in pregnancy: labetalol compared with methyldopa. In: Riley A, Symonds EM, eds. *The Investigation of Labetalol in the Management of Hypertension in Pregnancy*. Amsterdam: Excerpta Medica; 1982:101.
74. Cho C, Pruitt AW. Therapeutic uses of calcium channel-blocking drug in the young. *Am J Dis Child*. 1986;140:360.
75. Henry PD. Comparative pharmacology of calcium antagonists: nifedipine, verapamil, and diltragena. *Am J Cardiol*. 1980;46:1047.
76. Golichowski AM, Hathaway DR, Fineberg N, Peleg D. Tocolytic and hemodynamic effects of nifedipine in the ewe. *Am J Obstet Gynecol*. 1985;151:1134.
77. Veille JC, Bissonnette JM, Hohimer AR. The effect of calcium channel blockers. 1986;154:1160.
78. Harake B, Gilbert RE, Ashwal S, Power GC. Nifedipine: Effects on fetal and maternal hemodynamics in pregnant sheep. *Am J Obstet Gynecol*. 1987;157:1003.
79. Ducsay CA, Cook MJ, Veille JC, et al. Cardiorespiratory effects of calcium channel blocker tocolysis in pregnant rhesus monkeys. In: Jones CT, Nathanielsz PW, eds. *The Physiological Development of the Fetus and Newborn*. London: Academic Press; 1985;423.
80. Ahokas RA, Sibai BM, Mabie WC, Anderson GD. Nifedipine does not adversely affect uteroplacental blood flow in the hypertensive pregnant rat. *Am J Obstet Gynecol*. 1988;159:1440.
81. Lindow SW, Davies N, Davey DA, Smith JA. The effect of sublingual nifedipine on uteroplacental blood flow in hypertensive pregnancy. *Br J Obstet Gynecol*. 1988;95:1276.
82. Walters NJ, Redman CWG. Treatment of severe pregnancy-associated hypertension with the calcium antagonist nifedipine. *Br J Obstet Gynecol*. 1984;91:330.
83. Constantine G, Beevers DG, Reynolds AL, Luesley DM. Nifedipine as a second line antihypertensive drug in pregnancy. *Br J Obstet Gynecol*. 1987;94:1136.
84. Rubin PC, McCabe R, Low RA. Calcium channel blockade with nifedipine combined with atenolol in the management of severe preeclampsia. *Clin Exp Hypertens B*. 1984;B3:379.
85. Belfort MA, Moore PJ. Verapamil in the treatment of severe postpartum hypertension. *SA Med J*. 1988;74:265.
86. Allen J, Maigaard S, Forman A, et al. Acute effects of nitrendipine in pregnancy-induced hypertension. *Br J Obstet Gynecol*. 1987;94:222.
87. Mimran A, Taghetta R, Laroche B. The antihypertensive effect of captopril: evidence for an influence of kinins. *Hypertension*. 1980;2:732.
88. Brogden RN, Todd PA, Sorkin EM. Captopril: An update of its pharmacodynamic and pharmacokinetic properties, and therapeutic use in hypertension and congestive heart failure. *Drugs*. 1988;36:540.

89. Williams G. Converting enzyme inhibitors in the treatment of hypertension. *N Engl J Med*. 1988;319:1517.
90. Ferris TF, Weir E. Effect of captopril on uterine blood flow and prostaglandin E synthesis in the pregnant rabbit. *J Clin Invest*. 1983;71:809.
91. Broughton-Pipkin F, Symonds EM, Turner SR. The effect of captopril (SQ 14,225) upon mother and fetus in the chronically cannulated ewe and in the pregnant rabbit. *J Physiol*. 1982;323:415.
92. Broughton-Pipkin F, Baker PN, Symonds EM. ACE inhibitors in pregnancy. *Lancet*. 1989;2:96.
93. Duminy PC, Burger P du T. Fetal abnormality associated with the use of captopril during pregnancy. *S Afr Med J*. 1981;60:805.
94. Guignard JP, Gouyon JB. Adverse effect of drugs on the immature kidney. *Biol Neonat*. 1988;53:243.
95. Coen G, Cugini P, Gerlini G, et al. Successful treatment of long-lasting severe hypertension with captopril during a twin pregnancy. *Nephron*. 1985;40:498.
96. Mochizuki M. Treatment of hypertension in pregnancy by a combined drug regimen including captopril. *Clin Exp Hypertens*. 1986;B5(1):69.
97. Kreft-Jais C, Plouin PF, Tchobroutsky C, et al. Angiotensin converting enzyme inhibitors in pregnancy: a survey of 22 patients given captopril and 9 given enalapril. *Br J Obstet Gynecol*. 1988;95:420.
98. Vanhoutte P, Oney A, Birkenhager W, et al. Serotoninergic mechanisms in hypertension: Focus on the effects of ketanserin. *Hypertension*. 1988;11:111.
99. Weiner CP, Socol ML, Vaisrub N. Control of preeclamptic hypertension by ketanserin, a new serotonic receptor antagonist. *Am J Obstet Gynecol*. 1984;149:496.
100. Hulme VA, Odendaal HJ. Intrapartum treatment of preeclamptic hypertension by ketanserin. *Am J Obstet Gynecol*. 1988;155:260.
101. Voto LS, Zin C, Neira J, et al. Ketanserin versus alpha-methyldopa in the treatment of hypertension during pregnancy. A preliminary report. *J Cardiovasc Pharmaco*. 1987;10(suppl 3):101.
102. Cotton DB, Gonik B, Dorman KF. Cardiovascular alterations in severe pregnancy induced hypertension seen with an intravenously given hydralazine bolus. *Surg Gynecol Obstet*. 1985;161:240.
103. Ring G, Krames E, Shnider SM, et al. Comparison of nitroprusside and hydralazine in hypertensive pregnant ewes. *Obstet Gynecol*. 1977;50:598.
104. Morris JA, Acre JJ, Hamilton CJ, et al. The management of severe preeclampsia and eclampsia with intravenous diazoxide. *Obstet Gynecol*. 1977;49:675.
105. Naulty J, Cefalo RC, Lewis PE. Fetal toxicity of nitroprusside in the pregnant ewe. *Am J Obstet Gynecol*. 1981;139:708.
106. Lieb SM, Zugaib M, Nuwayhid B, et al. Nitroprusside-induced hemodynamic alterations in normotensive and hypertensive pregnant sheep. *Am J Obstet Gynecol*. 1981;139:925.
107. Wheeler AS, James FM III, Meis PJ, et al. Effect of nitroglycerin and nitroprusside on the uterine vasculative of gravid ewes. *Anesthesiology*. 1980;52:390.
108. Stempel JE, O'Grady JP, Martin MJ, Johnson KA. Use of sodium nitroprusside in complications of gestational hypertension. *Obstet Gynecol*. 1982;60:533.
109. Rigg D, McDonogh LA. Use of sodium nitroprusside for deliberate hypotension during pregnancy. *Br J Anesth*. 1981;53:985.
110. Poulton TJ, James FM III, Lockridge O. Prolonged apnea following trimethophan and succinylcholine. *Anesthesiology*. 1979;50:54.
111. Cotton DB, Longmire S, Jones M, et al. Cardiovascular alterations in severe pregnancy-induced hypertension: Effects of intravenous nitroglycerin coupled with blood volume expansion. *Am J Obstet Gynecol*. 1986;154:1053.
112. Craft JB, Co EG, Yonekura ML, Gilman RM. Nitroglycerin therapy for phenylephrine-induced hypertension in pregnant ewes. *Anesth Analg*. 1980;59:494.
113. Ricke PS, Elliott JP, Freeman RK. Use of corticosteroids in pregnancy-induced hypertension. *Obstet Gynecol*. 1980;55:206.
114. Lamont RF, Dunlap PDM, Levene MI, Elder MG. Use of glucocorticoids in pregnancies complicated by severe hypertension and proteinuria. *Brit J Obstet Gynecol*. 1983;90:199.
115. Donaldson JO. *Neurology of Pregnancy*. Philadelphia: WB Saunders; 1978:216.

PART XII Renal and Urinary Tract Diseases

Baha M. Sibai, Section Editor

Chapter One Hundred and Forty-Two

Renal Function and Volume Homeostasis

William M. Barron and Marshall D. Lindheimer

142

This section focuses on the striking alterations in renal function and body fluid composition that take place during normal pregnancy. Such alterations have a number of important implications for the physician caring for pregnant women.

CHANGES IN URINARY TRACT STRUCTURE AND FUNCTION

Kidney Size and Ureteral Dilatation

Although data in humans are scarce, it appears that kidney weight and size increase during pregnancy, mainly because of increments in renal interstitial and vascular volumes. Kidney length, as estimated by intravenous pyelography, increases approximately 1 cm.[1] The most striking changes, however, occur in the urinary collecting system (Table 142–1), where dilatation of the renal calyces, pelves, and ureters is observed as early as the first trimester and may persist for 3 to 4 months postpartum (Fig. 142–1).[2,3] The cause of this dilatation is controversial and has been ascribed to both humoral and mechanical factors.[4,5] For instance, increased progesterone levels may have a direct relaxant effect on the smooth muscle of the ureters. In addition, the ureter, particularly the right, is compressed between the enlarged uterus and the iliac artery as the latter crosses the pelvic brim[2], and some investigators believe that enlargement of the uterine veins during pregnancy may cause ureteral obstruction. These anatomic changes have several important clinical implications:

1. Timed urinary collection is made more difficult because large volumes of urine may remain in the dilated collecting system. This may be minimized by establishing high urine flow rates and having the patient avoid lying supine for 30 minutes before the beginning and before the end of the collection period.
2. Urinary stasis may help to explain why so many gravidas with asymptomatic bacteriuria develop pyelonephritis.
3. Urinary tract obstruction is more difficult to diagnose.
4. Because physiologic dilatation persists postpartum, elective radiologic examination of the urinary tract should be deferred for approximately 4 months after delivery.

Finally, there is also a *distention syndrome* in late pregnancy characterized by abdominal pain and demonstration of marked hydronephrosis as well as occasionally slight increments in creatinine levels managed by the placement of ureteral stents.[5,6] It is unclear, however, whether this syndrome is an extreme case of the dilatation that normally occurs in gestation or reflects underlying pathology.

Functional Alterations

Renal Hemodynamics. During gestation, both glomerular filtration rate (GFR), estimated by either inulin or creatinine clearance, and effective renal plasma flow (ERPF) increase 30–50% above those measured in nonpregnant women.[7] The rise in GFR starts with a first missed menstrual period, and substantial increments in creatinine clearance are observed during the initial weeks following conception. Increases in GFR peak by the second trimester and remain elevated until term as long as measurements are made with the woman lying on her side. According to some investigators, these increments are sustained until term, whereas others have observed a decline in creatinine clearance during the last weeks of pregnancy. These latter observations may reflect the marked reductions in GFR and ERPF that occur when pregnant women assume the upright or supine position, particularly during the latter half of pregnancy. Because renal perfusion is maximal when the pregnant woman lies on her side, this position is recommended for gravidas with preeclampsia and other disorders associated with renal dysfunction.

The reasons why renal hemodynamics increase during pregnancy are obscure, and several hypotheses are detailed elsewhere.[4,7] Of interest are data derived from animal studies that indicate the stimulus is maternal in origin.[8] Also,

TABLE 142–1. RENAL CHANGES IN NORMAL GESTATION

Alteration	Manifestation	Clinical Relevance
Increased kidney size	Kidney length ≃1 cm greater on x-ray	Postpartum reduction in size should not be mistaken for parenchymal loss
Dilatation of pelves, calyces, and ureters	Resembles hydronephrosis on intravenous pyelography and is more marked on the right	Not to be mistaken for obstructive uropathy; elective pyelography should be deferred until the 12th postpartum week; urinary tract infections are more frequent; retained urine leads to collection errors
Increased real hemodynamics	Glomerular filtration rate and renal plasma flow increase 25–40%	Serum creatinine and urea nitrogen values decrease during gestation (values >0.8 mg/dL creatinine and >13 mg/dL urea nitrogen are suspect); albumin, amino acid, and glucose excretion increase
Changes in acid-base metabolism (primary respiratory alkalosis)	Renal bicarbonate threshold decreases	Serum bicarbonate is 4–5 mEq/L lower in normal gestation
Renal water handling	Osmoregulation altered in gestation	Serum osmolality lower by ≃10 mosm/liter; serum sodium decreases ≃5 mEq/L during normal gestation

micropuncture experiments have demonstrated that gestational vasodilatation in rats involves an even reduction in the tone of the pre- and postglomerular arterioles so that intraglomerular blood pressure is maintained constant.[8] Thus, hyperfiltration in the rat has no adverse effect on the animal's kidney.

The changes in renal hemodynamics during gestation have additional important clinical implications. Because

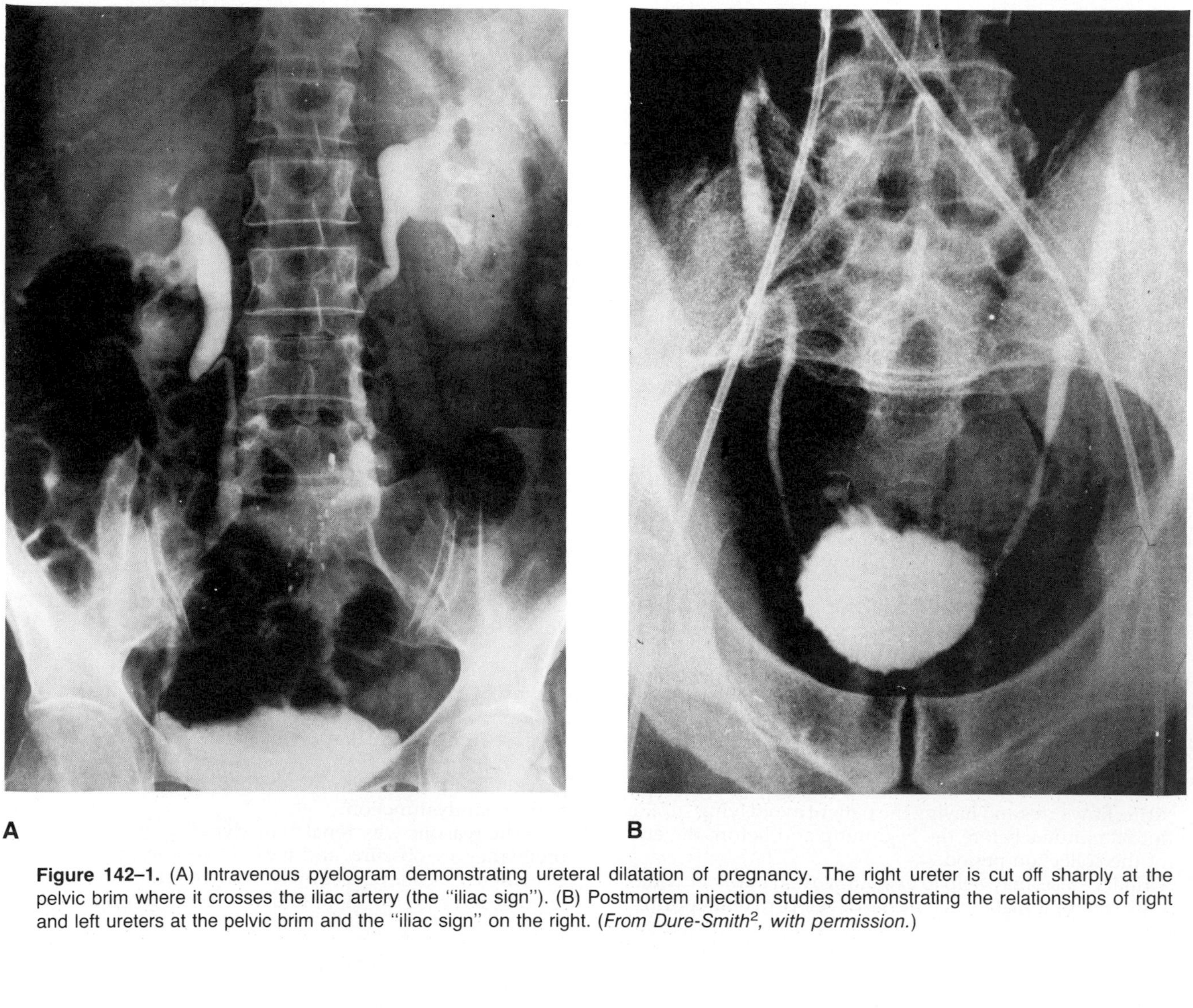

A B

Figure 142–1. (A) Intravenous pyelogram demonstrating ureteral dilatation of pregnancy. The right ureter is cut off sharply at the pelvic brim where it crosses the iliac artery (the "iliac sign"). (B) Postmortem injection studies demonstrating the relationships of right and left ureters at the pelvic brim and the "iliac sign" on the right. (*From Dure-Smith[2], with permission.*)

GFR increases without substantial alterations in the production of creatinine or urea nitrogen, levels of these solutes decrease from nonpregnant values of approximately 0.7 and 12.0 mg/dL, respectively, to 0.5 and 9.0 mg/dL, respectively. Therefore, values considered normal in nongravid women may reflect substantially impaired renal function during pregnancy. Concentrations of serum creatinine and urea nitrogen greater than 0.8 and 13 mg/dL, respectively, indicate underlying renal disease and need further evaluation.

Increases in GFR and ERPF also may help to explain the enhanced excretion of protein, amino acids, and water-soluble vitamins during pregnancy.[7] For instance, protein excretion up to 300–500 mg per day may be considered normal, a value approximately double that acceptable in nongravid patients. For this reason, increasing urinary protein excretion in a pregnant woman with known renal disease does not necessarily signify deteriorating renal function. Also, during normal pregnancy the filtered load of amino acids rises, whereas tubular reabsorption may decrease. These changes result in excretion of up to 2 g per day of amino acids during normal pregnancy, amounts that become significant in underdeveloped areas of the world, where nutrition is already marginal. Such nutritional problems may be compounded further, as the clearance of several water-soluble vitamins including nicotinic acid, ascorbic acid, and folate also increases in normal gestation.

Renal Tubular Function

Glucose. There is a major change in renal glucose handling during pregnancy as a result of increases in GFR and decrements in the renal tubular reabsorption of this solute.[7] Nonpregnant women excrete less than 100 mg of glucose daily, whereas almost 90% of gravidas excrete more. Many pregnant women with normal carbohydrate metabolism excrete over 1 g per day and some as much as 10 g per day, becoming nonglycosuric postpartum. Because this glycosuria is intermittent and bears no consistent relationship to blood glucose levels or stage of pregnancy, urine glucose measures are unreliable for managing diabetic gravidas. This increased excretion of glucose, as well as of amino acids and protein, may be one reason that pregnant women are susceptible to urinary tract infection.

Uric Acid. Plasma urate levels decrease early in pregnancy, and values in mid trimester average 2.5–4.0 mg/dL, compared with 4–6 mg/dL in nonpregnant women. This fall is caused by increases in GFR as well as by decreases in the fractional reabsorption of urate by the renal tubule.[7] Uric acid production appears unaltered. In late pregnancy, however, levels often return to near nonpregnant values.

Measurement of plasma urate is most useful during the third trimester in patients with hypertension of unclear etiology. Elevated levels support a diagnosis of pure or superimposed preeclampsia, while women with other forms of hypertension are more likely to have normal values. The magnitude of the elevation appears to be correlated with the severity of the preeclamptic renal lesion and with fetal jeopardy.

Acid Excretion. Renal bicarbonate reabsorption and hydrogen ion secretion are intact during normal pregnancy. However, a mild alkalemia of respiratory origin is routinely observed; arterial P_{CO_2} decreases from a mean nonpregnant value of 39 to 31 mm Hg during gestation, and arterial pH rises slightly, from an average of 7.40 to 7.44.[9] Since plasma bicarbonate levels concomitantly decrease about 4 mEq/L, values of 18–22 mEq/L should be considered normal. Because there is already a decrement in P_{CO_2}, the gravida is less able to defend blood pH in the face of acute metabolic acidosis.

Potassium. The pregnant woman retains approximately 350 mEq of potassium, primarily in the tissues of the enlarging fetus as well as in the breast, uterus, and placenta (Table 142–2). This retention occurs despite two conditions that enhance potassium excretion: the tendency to develop bicarbonaturia at lower serum bicarbonate levels and, more important, increased levels of aldosterone and other potent mineralocorticoids. Potassium conservation, despite these factors, appears to result in part from increased blood levels of progesterone, a hormone that antagonizes the renal tubular effect of the mineralocorticoids. For example, the renal potassium loss and hypokalemia characteristic of primary aldosteronism may be ameliorated by gestation.[7]

Control of Body Tonicity

Plasma osmolality (P_{osm}) decreases during normal gestation to values that average 8–10 mosm/kg below those of nonpregnant women (Figure 142–2).[10] This decrement starts shortly after conception, becomes significant during the fifth week of gestation, and reaches a nadir by the tenth week of pregnancy, after which the decreased osmolality is sustained until term. Only about 1.5 mosm/kg of this decrement represents a decrease in urea levels, and most of the change results from a decline in the concentration of plasma sodium and its attendant anions. Thus, pregnancy is characterized by a true decrease in effective plasma osmolality.

If similar decreases in the tonicity of body fluids were to occur in a nonpregnant subject, secretion of antidiuretic hormone (vasopressin) would cease, and a large and continuous water diuresis similar to that in patients with *diabetes insipidus* would ensue. However, pregnant women maintain their new P_{osm}, and water loading or fluid restriction leads to appropriate dilution and concentration of their urine.[10] Such data suggest that osmoregulation is altered during pregnancy; it has been demonstrated that osmotic thresholds for both vasopressin secretion and thirst are decreased approximately 10 mosm/kg during gestation in both humans and rodents.[10] It should be stressed that parallel declines in the osmotic thresholds for both vasopressin release and thirst are required to maintain the new steady-state P_{osm}

TABLE 142–2. STORAGE OF ELECTROLYTES AND MINERALS DURING PREGNANCY

Storage Site	Sodium (meq)	Potassium (meq)	Calcium (g)
Fetus	290	154	28.00
Placenta	57	42	0.65
Amniotic fluid	100	3	Negligible
Uterus	80	50	0.22
Breasts	35	35	0.06
Plasma	140	4	0.12
Red cells	5	24	0.38
Edema fluid	240	8	0.25
Total	947	320	29.68

From Hytten and Leitch[27] with permission.

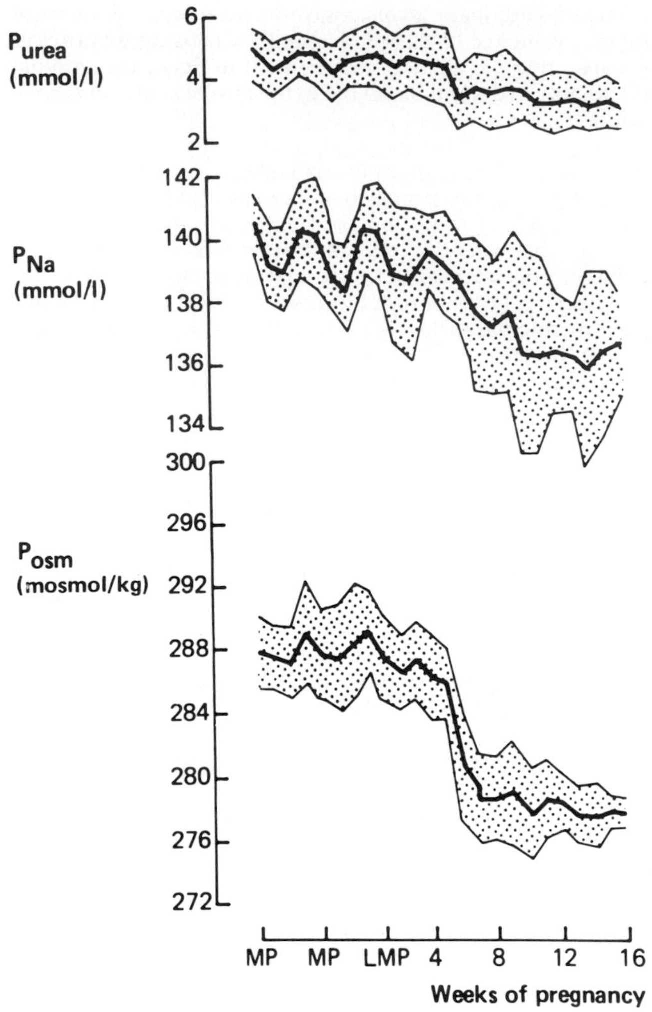

Figure 142–2. Mean values (±SD) for plasma urea (P_{urea}), sodium (P_{NI}) and osmolality (P_{osm}) measured weekly starting prior to conception and through the first trimester in 9 healthy women with a normal gestational outcome. MP and LMP are menstrual and last menstrual periods, respectively. (*From Davison et al* [28] *with permission.*)

within a narrow range. For example, P_{osm} will rise despite maximal antidiuretic hormone secretion if the subject is not stimulated to drink at a lower level of body tonicity; conversely, considerable polydipsia would be required to maintain any P_{osm} in the absence of vasopressin.

Little is known about nonosmotic factors controlling vasopressin secretion in pregnancy, but in nongravid humans, volume is an important determinant of antidiuretic hormone release. Hypovolemia stimulates and increments in intravascular volume may blunt hormone secretion. In gestation, absolute blood volume increases markedly, but how the effective volume is sensed is a subject of considerable speculation. In this regard, it is of interest that the gravid rat, which also experiences a 40–50% increase in blood volume near term, alters its volume-sensing vasopressin-secretory mechanism such that its expanded circulating volume is recognized as normal.[10]

The ability to excrete a water load appears to be impaired in late gestation.[11] Studies suggesting this phenomenon were performed with gravidas either seated or supine; therefore, these observations have been attributed to posturally induced hemodynamic alterations caused by the progressively enlarging uterus. In fact, in late gestation, merely changing from a lateral recumbent to a supine position markedly decreases urine flow, and quiet standing is progressively more antidiuretic as pregnancy advances. Furthermore, administration of hypotonic fluid to pregnant women placed in the lateral recumbent position results in a minimal urinary osmolality comparable to that of similarly treated nonpregnant individuals.[7] Although the mechanisms responsible for posture-induced decrements in water excretion remain unclear, antidiuretic hormone does not appear to be the central cause, since the phenomenon has been observed in a gravida with diabetes insipidus.

Reasons for the fascinating osmoregulatory changes described are obscure, although recent studies suggest human chorionic gonadotropin may play a role.[12] The gravida's osmoregulatory ability also may be influenced by changes in the metabolism of arginine vasopressin (AVP) evident after midpregnancy when the metabolic clearance of this hormone increases fourfold.[13] Reasons for this increment appear to relate to two phenomena peculiar to gestation: The blood of gravidas contains large quantities of a cystine aminopeptidase enzyme (vasopressinase) of placental origin. This enzyme inactivates large quantities of both vasopressin and oxytocin *in vitro*.[10,13] The second factor is the placenta itself, which may be responsible for at least one third of the increased hormonal disposal rate in pregnancy.[14]

Finally, there are problems in water handling that complicate human gestation which may relate to the increased metabolic clearance of vasopressin or the vasopressinase enzyme. For instance, women with central diabetes insipidus (DI) may require more replacement therapy. There is also a syndrome, *transient DI of pregnancy*, which usually presents later in gestation. Some of these women have inapparent central DI, which manifests because of gestation. Others have extremely high levels of vasopressinase and fail to respond to large doses of vasopressin, but are cured with 1-deamino-8-d-arginine vasopressin (DDAVP), an analogue of vasopressin resistant to the cystine aminopeptidase enzyme.[10]

VOLUME REGULATION

Weight Gain in Normal Pregnancy

The ideal study measuring body weight prior to conception and serially throughout pregnancy in a large cohort of healthy women has not been done. The best data available are from Great Britain[15] where the studied populations were recruited in the first trimester. They indicate that healthy primigravidas gain an average of 12 kg during gestation, whereas multiparous women gain about 11 kg. It should be emphasized that such figures are not maximum limits of acceptable weight gain but rather averages, which are accompanied by large standard deviations. Thus, physiologically normal weight gain during pregnancy varies widely; normal outcomes may be accompanied by little or no weight gain, or by more than 20 kg. This point is stressed because many physicians have ignored these data, restricting calories and salt or prescribing diuretics to their pregnant patients in an attempt to limit excessive weight gain. There is no evidence that such an approach is beneficial to mother or fetus, and it may actually be harmful.

The components of weight gain in pregnancy have been discussed in detail by Hytten[15], who notes that in gravid subjects who are edema-free or have leg swelling only (approximately 80% of normal gravidas), about 60% of the total weight increment is attributable to water, and less than 10% can be attributed to increases in protein. The remainder is accumulation of fat, which accounts for a weight gain of about 3 kg in the average subject.

Alteration in Fluid Volumes

The best estimates of body water in pregnancy are those in which deuterium oxide was used as a tracer.[15] Results from serial investigations suggest that body water increases 7–8 L, but since the last antepartum measurements in these studies are usually between gestational weeks 36 and 38, the total accumulation is probably underestimated by 0.5–1.0 liters (see also Chapter 4).

The extracellular component of water gain during pregnancy remains uncertain, largely because of the lack of an acceptable tracer. Published estimates vary widely, and there is often little data on those subjects in whom both extracellular and total body water were measured simultaneously. Several investigators using thiocyanate as a tracer have calculated a gain of 6–7 L in the extracellular space during gestation.[15,16] Such values appear reasonable, because when thiocyanate is added to the 1.8–2.5 liters of intracellular water gained during gestation, the total approximates that measured directly with deuterium oxide. Nonetheless, considerably more research in this area will be needed before definitive conclusions can be reached.

The extracellular fluid includes both plasma and interstitial volumes. Only the former can be measured with any degree of accuracy; the latter must be measured indirectly. Both Evans' blue dye (T-1824) and radioactive iodinated serum albumin have been used to measure plasma volume in pregnancy.[15,16] Initially, it was claimed that plasma volume reached a peak by the middle of the third trimester and then declined slowly towards term. It is now evident that such determinations were incorrect, because in late pregnancy the tracer may not attain complete mixing if the subject is in the supine or sitting position. More recent investigations, in which women were studied in the lateral recumbent position, have shown that plasma volume increments start in the first trimester, accelerate in the second, peak near gestational week 32, and remain elevated until term. The maximum gain averages 1100–1300 mL, although larger increments may occur when there are multiple fetuses. The physiologic significance of this plasma volume expansion and the attendant "hemodilution" remains ill-defined, but a number of investigators have found that smaller increments in plasma volume during pregnancy are associated with lower birth weight, poor pregnancy outcome, or both.

Since expansion of the plasma volume accounts for only 20–25% of the increase in the extracellular space, increments in interstitial fluid must be substantial.[15,16] There appears to be remarkably good agreement between the estimated and measured increases in total body water at midpregnancy, but at term there is a discrepancy of about 2.5 L in women with no edema or edema of the legs only, an increase that is presumed to accumulate in the maternal interstitium. For women with generalized edema (approximately 10–20% of normal gravidas), an excess of water, also presumed to be in the interstitium, is apparent at all stages of pregnancy and reaches approximately 5 L at term. In normal gravidas with and without edema, the greatest increase in interstitial fluid occurs in the third trimester, contrasting with the increment in plasma volume that takes place primarily in the first two trimesters.

The increments in interstitial fluid result in part from decreases in plasma albumin (oncotic pressure), but it also has been speculated that some of this gain may be caused by alterations in the properties of connective tissue ground substance. Such "complexed" fluid may be poorly mobilized by diuretics, and alterations in interstitial compliance, which conceivably can influence blood pressure, possibly may be mediated through humorally induced changes in mucopolysaccharides.

During pregnancy, substantial quantities of fluid thus are stored in the products of conception as well as in the maternal plasma and interstitial compartments. This physiologic "hypervolemia" is sensed as normal, and when salt restriction or diuretic therapy limits such volume expansion, the maternal response is similar to that of salt-depleted, nonpregnant subjects.

SODIUM HOMEOSTASIS

Approximately 950 mEq of sodium are gained during pregnancy, over 60% of which is in the maternal compartment (Table 142–2). Since renal sodium handling is the prime determinant of volume homeostasis, it is worthwhile to consider how the hormonal and hemodynamic changes that occur during gestation might influence urinary sodium excretion.

Factors Tending to Promote Sodium Excretion

Increased Glomerular Filtration. As noted previously, GFR increases during gestation to levels 30–50% above those measured in nonpregnant women. The filtered load of sodium thus will also increase 30–50%, from nonpregnant levels of approximately 20,000 mEq per day to as much as 30,000 mEq per day. These changes must be accompanied by parallel increments in tubular reabsorption of sodium to prevent rapid onset of massive sodium depletion and shock. The ability of the kidney to adjust tubular reabsorption to match increments in filtration, a phenomenon known as glomerulotubular balance, is not peculiar to pregnancy, for it occurs in both humans and experimental animals when GFR is acutely or chronically increased by a variety of maneuvers. In the case of the gravida, the adaptive tubular reabsorption not only equals the large increase in filtered load, but an additional 2–5 mEq of sodium are reabsorbed daily for fetal and maternal stores. This increase in sodium reabsorption represents the largest renal adjustment during pregnancy.

Hormonal Alterations. Plasma progesterone increases during gestation to levels that average 5- to 20-fold higher than those measured during the luteal phase of the menstrual cycle.[4,7,11] This hormone is natriuretic in normal man and inhibits the sodium-retaining effect of exogenous mineralocorticoids in adrenalectomized nonpregnant humans and animals.[7,11] Although such data have been interpreted to indicate that progesterone is a competitive inhibitor of aldosterone, it has been suggested that this hormone inhibits sodium reabsorption at proximal as well as distal sites in the nephron. Also, progesterone, which inhibits smooth muscle contraction, produces renal vasodilatation, an effect that would promote natriuresis.

The vasodilatory prostaglandins (eg, PGE, PGI_2), plasma and urinary levels of which may increase during pregnancy, could augment sodium excretion through effects on renal blood flow, GFR, and tubular solute handling.

Complex interactions of the prostaglandins with the renin-angiotensin system, catecholamines, and bradykinin also may have important effects on intrarenal sodium handling, but such physiologic actions have not been investigated in gravid human subjects. Similarly, the effects of oxytocin, circulating neurophysins, melanocyte-stimulating hormone, and bradykinin on sodium excretion during gestation remain unclear.[7] Urinary levels of dopamine, a catecholamine that may increase both GFR and sodium excretion, have been reported to be markedly increased during pregnancy.

Finally, the role of natriuretic factors in pregnancy are obscure. For instance, activity of two cellular membrane cation pump systems, Na-K-ATPase and Na-Li counter transport are increased in the red blood cells of normal pregnant women, but so are levels of ouabain-like inhibitors of Na-K-ATPase in plasma.[7] Immunoreactive atrial peptides also may increase in human gestations, but increments described are small in relation to the marked expansion of intravascular volume.

Physical Factors. Decrements in renal vascular resistance and an increase in renal plasma flow during pregnancy are factors that could enhance sodium excretion. In most studies, renal plasma flow increases more than GFR so that filtration fraction decreases. This should lead to decrements in postglomerular plasma oncotic pressure, which may decrease the reabsorption of filtrate (and thus sodium) from the proximal tubule. The normal decrement in plasma albumin levels in pregnancy would have similar oncotic effects. All of these potentially natriuretic factors, however, may be opposed by the small decrease in arterial blood pressure that is observed during normal gestation.

Factors Tending to Promote Reabsorption

Hormonal Alterations. Production of several antinatriuretic hormones also increases substantially during pregnancy. Those studied in greatest detail are aldosterone and deoxycorticosterone.

ALDOSTERONE. The secretory rate, plasma concentration, and urinary excretion of aldosterone and its metabolites all are elevated in normal gestation, often to levels exceeding those measured in patients with primary aldosteronism.[7,11] These changes have been viewed by some as balancing the increases in natriuretic influences described above, but others have regarded the augmented aldosterone levels as excessive. In the latter formulation, volume homeostasis in gravidas is considered similar to that of volunteers with experimentally induced chronic volume expansion or of patients with primary hyperaldosteronism.

The view that aldosterone secretion increases to balance the increments in glomerular filtration rate, progesterone production, or both is based on the following reasoning: filtration rate increases 30–50%, and if glomerulotubular balance is maintained in the proximal tubule, more sodium will reach aldosterone-sensitive parts of the distal nephron. Compensatory increments in mineralocorticoid levels occur and prevent sodium wasting. Since progesterone is a competitive inhibitor of aldosterone at these nephron sites, even greater amounts of hormone must be secreted to avoid excessive diuresis.

The above view may explain some of the aldosterone increment but is probably too simplistic for several reasons. In nonpregnant subjects, aldosterone-dependent sodium reabsorption amounts to less than 2% of the filtered load. By contrast, the daily increment in filtered sodium in pregnancy ranges from 5000 to 10,000 mEq. Aldosterone-stimulated sodium retention clearly is inadequate to balance this load appreciably. There is no consistent correlation between creatinine clearance and aldosterone secretory rates in pregnant subjects.

The hypothesis that the aldosterone increase is secondary to that of progesterone has been explored by several investigators with conflicting results. In some reports, pregnanediol excretion correlates with that of aldosterone, whereas others have been unable to demonstrate such a correlation. More recently, attempts have been made to correlate plasma concentrations of progesterone and aldosterone, but the results are inconsistent. Finally, although progesterone administered to normal nonpregnant volunteers and women with intact placentas but dead fetuses increases aldosterone excretion, even when administered doses resemble secretion in pregnancy, the increments are less than those observed during normal gestation.

In contrast to the above, some have suggested that the increased aldosterone production in pregnancy exceeds physiologic requirements. Such a view was derived from the following observations: in nonpregnant subjects, the sodium retention induced by the continued administration of mineralocorticoids usually ceases within 1 week after approximately 400 mEq of sodium has been retained, weight has increased 2–3 kg, and sodium balance has been regained. After this new steady state is achieved, additional doses of the hormone do not cause sodium retention, an adaptation termed the *renal escape* phenomenon. Results from earlier studies seemed to demonstrate that mineralocorticoids and ACTH do not induce sodium retention in pregnant women. Such data were compatible with the view that the increased secretion of aldosterone during pregnancy actually exceeds physiologic requirements and the escape mechanism was already operative. In addition, the degree of maternal physiologic hypervolemia approximates (and at times exceeds) that observed in subjects whose fluid volume has been expanded by mineralocorticoids.

Data contrary to this formulation are the following: (1) Secretion, excretion, and blood levels of aldosterone change appropriately and in a manner similar to that seen in nonpregnant subjects when extracellular fluid volume is altered by variations in sodium intake and postural maneuvers as well as by administration of diuretics or deoxycorticosterone.[7,11] In fact, although basal levels are already high, sodium restriction leads to maked increases in both aldosterone production and plasma levels, and these increments surpass those seen when nonpregnant subjects are similarly restricted. (2) Patterns of solute and water excretion in gravidas resemble those of normal nonpregnant subjects and differ from those observed in volunteers with chronically expanded volume and in patients with primary aldosteronism. (3) In contrast to earlier observations in the literature (described above) that suggested that the renal tubule was relatively insensitive to aldosterone during pregnancy, it has been reported that relatively small doses of deoxycorticosterone (DOC) produce sodium retention and weight gain in pregnant subjects ingesting carefully supervised diets. In such studies aldosterone excretion decreased when salt was retained during DOC administration, an expected result if the aldosterone secretory mechanism is not autonomous but is volume sensitive. After DOC was stopped, a natriuresis ensued that did not subside until aldosterone excretion had returned to its high pretreatment value. (4) In other studies, aldosterone excretion was decreased in normal pregnant subjects without concomitant volume expansion by administration of heparinoid (RO1–8307), a compound that inhibits aldosterone secretion by undefined mechanisms. It was observed that natriuresis and weight loss commenced during day 3 of therapy, while aldosterone excretion, although reduced, was still well above normal nonpregnant values. After the drug was discontinued, sodium loss abated as urinary aldosterone increased toward control values. Such results indicate that sodium conservation during gestation is dependent on the augmented secretion of aldosterone.

In summary, it appears that changes in aldosterone production during normal pregnancy are not excessive but serve a homeostatic function, as they do in nonpregnant individuals. Although circulating levels of the hormone are high, production remains responsive to physiologic demands. In the presence of sodium depletion, the increase in aldosterone secretion can be striking, whereas with volume expansion, hormonal levels decrease, albeit sluggishly. Elevated aldosterone, far from being a factor that causes excessive sodium retention, thus could even represent a compensatory response to suboptimal increases in sodium content and extracellular volume.

Deoxycorticosterone. Levels of DOC, its plasma free index, and urinary-free DOC are markedly increased in pregnancy.[7,11] Plasma levels of this potent mineralocorticoid are significantly increased in the first trimester and rise gradually to levels that at term are 10–20 times higher than those measured in nonpregnant women.

Previously, the fetal-placental unit was thought to be the source of the increased DOC secretion in pregnancy. More recent studies, however, suggest that circulating DOC in the mother is produced primarily within the maternal compartment. In this regard, one group of investigators[18] has demonstrated that DOC is formed by extra-adrenal 21-hydroxylation of plasma progesterone in men and nonpregnant and pregnant women and that the rate of formation of DOC by this pathway is proportional to the plasma concentration of progesterone. Furthermore, 21-hydroxylase activity, which has been identified in both adult and fetal kidney, has been found to be high in the kidney of a pregnant woman. Pregnancy thus may be characterized by the production of large amounts of potent mineralocorticoid in the vicinity of its renal receptor.

The physiologic role of augmented free DOC levels in pregnancy is obscure, although in certain pathologic circumstances abnormal DOC metabolism could lead to disturbances in sodium homeostasis. For example, it has been suggested that renal conversion of progesterone to DOC may be increased in preeclampsia. Also, DOC-SO_4, a major, presumably inactive metabolite of DOC, is almost undetectable in nonpregnant subjects but is markedly elevated in pregnancy. Since DOC sulfurylated in the liver, at least in nongravid subjects, is immediately excreted into the bile, plasma DOC-SO_4 in gravidas presumably is formed elsewhere. It has been suggested[19] that sulfurylation of DOC occurs in the maternal kidney, on the hypothesis that C-21 hydroxysteroid sulfotransferase activity, which has not been identified in renal tissue of nonpregnant adults, is induced in the kidneys of pregnant women, perhaps by the high levels of estrogen. It is also speculated[19] that failure of sulfurylation (and hence inactivation) of DOC formed in the kidneys of primigravidas would lead to increased levels of DOC within renal cells to act *in situ* to effect the salt retention characteristic of preeclampsia. If these theories are confirmed, DOC could have an important role in volume regulation during pregnancy (see also Chapter 37).

Other Hormones. Plasma concentrations of 18-hydroxycorticosterone, a biosynthetic precursor of aldosterone, are unchanged during normal pregnancy, but urinary levels of this hormone are elevated significantly in third-trimester gravidas.[7,11] This apparent discrepancy requires confirmation but could be explained by displacement of the steroid from protein-binding sites, thus increasing the amount of free hormone available for both biologic activity and urinary excretion. However, whether 18-hydroxycorticosterone has significant salt-retaining effects remains controversial.

Plasma estrogens, the levels of which increase progressively throughout pregnancy[7,11], are well known to induce sodium retention[7,11] although the mechanism(s) remain obscure. Some authors suggest that the sodium-retaining effect of the hormone is mediated through stimulation of the renin-angiotensin-aldosterone system. In this regard, much of the marked increase in renin activity during gestation has been attributed to estrogen-induced increments in renin substrate. Also, high levels of estrogen may enhance extra-adrenal 21-hydroxylase activity and thus increase the conversion of the natriuretic progesterone to the salt-retaining hormone DOC.

The role during pregnancy of several other potentially antinatriuretic hormones remains to be elucidated. These include prolactin, placental lactogen, growth hormone, ACTH, and cortisol.[7,11] Cortisol, total and free levels of which increase in pregnancy, has generally been considered only mildly antinatriuretic, but as noted previously, when elevated, cortisol will displace the potent mineralocorticoid DOC from cortisolbinding globulin. However, under certain conditions urinary-free cortisol is directly correlated with sodium excretion, suggesting that cortisol may be involved in the natriuretic system. Epinephrine and norepinephrine may also affect sodium excretion either directly by way of sympathetic innervation of the kidney or indirectly by their hemodynamic effects. Basal plasma and urinary levels of these catecholamines are, however, not different from those of nongravid women.

The Renin-Angiotensin System. The role of angiotensin II in the natriuretic system is poorly understood, but at physiologic circulating levels its initial renal effect is probably antinatriuretic. Angiotensin's major contribution to volume homeostasis, however, relates mainly to its role in the control of aldosterone secretion. Plasma renin activity, concentration (primarily in the form of big or inactive renin), and substrate, as well as angiotensin II levels increase substantially in pregnancy, and normal pregnant women are resistant to the pressor and renal effects of infused angiotensin.[7,11,20,21] Whether these changes result from or cause alterations in volume homeostasis is unclear. For example, the consistent correlation between the renin and aldosterone systems in most studies on nongravid subjects are not always present when pregnant populations are investigated. Nevertheless, basal renin activity, initally high despite increases in circulatory volume and renal blood flow in pregnancy, increases further in response to both postural maneuvers and decreases in dietary sodium.[7,11,20,21] Such data are consistent with a new set point in the system.

In contrast to the above is the theory that enhanced renin secretion is secondary to increases in the production of vasodilating prostaglandins during pregnancy.[7,17] It is suggested that systemic vasodilation leads to decrements in mean arterial pressure and a dilated vascular volume. This vasodilation, or perhaps the increased prostinoid levels themselves, leads to *compensatory* stimulation of the renin-angiotensin system. Such a theory explains why angiotensin II and aldosterone levels are increased in the face of the absolute hypervolemia that occurs in gestation (eg, the "effective volume" is still *sensed* as suboptimal) as well as increased renal perfusion (a direct prostaglandin action). In favor of this view all data that in early pregnancy infusion of an angiotensin-converting enzyme inhibitor causes exaggerated decreases in blood pressures[7], while graded infusion of angiotensin II leads to greater increments in aldosterone than in nonpregnant women (the expected response with salt depletion).[22]

Physical Factors. Upright posture decreases sodium excretion in nonpregnant subjects, and the antinatriuretic effects of this position may be exaggerated in pregnancy.[7,11] In addition, in late gestation, merely turning from a lateral to a supine position results in decreased sodium excretion, which has been shown to occur despite placement of thick-walled catheters in the ureters, presumably excluding ureteral compression by the enlarged uterus as an explanation. The potent antinatriuretic effects of supine posture have been characterized further. Sodium retention will occur even if the gravida is acutely volume loaded prior to the maneuver, and the effect is independent of mineralocorticoid activity or changes in glomerular filtration rate. There are also data to suggest that the antinatriuretic effect of the supine position is mediated in part by increased fractional reabsorption in the proximal nephron.[7]

Of interest are studies delineating the chronic effects of posture. One group of investigators performed metabolic balance studies[7,11] in which gravidas eating a constant diet were kept in bed positioned in lateral recumbency for 2 or 3 days; subsequently were mobile or sitting during the day; and slept supine on a head-up tilted bed at night. The women, all in their third trimester of pregnancy, remained in positive sodium balance for 48 to 72 hours, excreting the retained salt during a final recovery day when they were positioned again in lateral recumbency. The same phenomenon occurred in volunteers pretreated with DOC, but no increment in aldosterone occurred when these subjects assumed an upright posture. Such data underscore the potent antinatriuretic effects of posture during pregnancy and suggest that it occurs by mechanisms other than the renin-aldosterone system.

It also is important to note that despite the considerable sodium retention and weight gain provoked in these studies, no gravida developed hypertension or proteinuria. Some physicians may attribute such rapid increments in weight to a pathologic condition such as imminent preeclampsia, but changes in a gravida's activity pattern and posture may lead to readily reversible weight gains and do not necessarily signal disease. Prescription of the lateral recumbent position may be helpful in mobilizing excessive fluid and is preferable in the rare circumstances in which a diuretic is indicated.

Postural influences may help to explain alterations in urinary water and solute excretion observed in some gravidas. In nonpregnant subjects, urinary volume and sodium excretion diminish substantially during noctural recumbency. In many pregnant women, there is an increase in urine flow and sodium excretion at night, frequently exceeding values observed during the day. This may be related in part to the potent antinatriuretic effects of upright posture, an influence operative during a large portion of daytime hours. However, such an explanation may be insufficient, because nighttime excretion of sodium and solute-free water has been claimed to be greatest in the first trimester, when postural effects of pregnancy are minimal, suggesting that hormonal rather than mechanical causes are responsbile for the changes.[27]

Maternal posture also may play a role in determining salt excretion by its influence on ureteral pressure. A marked increase in intraureteral pressure may occur when third-trimester gravidas assume a supine or standing position; this pressure decreases significantly when the obstructive influence of the gravid uterus is eliminated by placing subjects in the lateral decubitus or knee-chest position. Graded ureteral obstruction will decrease sodium excretion in dogs, an effect that appears to be a direct function of the elevated pressure, since the decrement in urinary sodium can occur in the absence of discernible decreases in glomerular filtration rate. The same phenomenon could be operative in pregnant women. Thus, during pregnancy, a part of the antinatriuretic effect of the supine and upright positions may be mediated by increments in ureteral pressure.

The uteroplacental circulation has been likened to an arteriovenous shunt. In both humans and experimental animals, the creation of such vascular communications causes sodium retention, which is reversed when the shunt is closed.

Effects of Acute and Chronic Sodium Loads

Questions concerning the predominance of sodium-retaining or salt-losing factors during gestation may be clarified experimentally by testing the ability of pregnant and nonpregnant subjects to excrete infused saline. Results in the literature are conflicting.[7,11,23] In one study, 3% saline (410 mEq of sodium in 30 minutes) was infused into test subjects; pregnant women excreted the administered sodium as well as their nonpregnant counterparts, despite the fact that the former were in the supine position and had been moderately sodium restricted prior to the test. However, others have observed that gravid subjects given 2 L of isotonic saline over 4 hours secreted significantly less sodium than did similarly treated nonpregnant controls. More recently, Brown et al[23,24] have published a study in which dietary sodium was controlled carefully and the subjects were studied serially during the second and third trimester as well as postpartum. Their results confirm those cited above, which noted that gravidas and nonpregnant women excreted salt similarly.

The above considerations do not necessarily apply to homeostatic mechanisms occurring more slowly, and several investigators have performed metabolic balance studies in an attempt to study salt handling over a more prolonged period. Some authors suggest that gravidas have difficulty conserving sodium and may manifest signs of volume depletion when dietary salt content is too low. One group even noted that normal third-trimester gravidas had difficulty conserving salt and required at least 100 mEq of sodium daily for 10 days to avoid negative balance. The authors of another report[25] concluded that pregnant women achieved balance as quickly as nonpregnant controls while consuming diets containing as little as 10 mEq sodium daily. During this study, urinary sodium excretion in third-trimester gravidas and nonpregnant controls decreased to similar values 5–7 days after the low-salt diet was instituted. Such data, however, may lead to conclusions very different from those of the authors when the following factors are considered. Normally, the small daily positive sodium balance of 3–6 mEq in late gestation is too small to measure during routine metabolic studies, and gravidas appear to excrete all their ingested sodium. However, when such subjects are salt restricted, maternal-fetal requirements should cause the pregnant woman to resemble certain patients with cirrhosis or severe congestive heart failure, who virtually eliminate sodium from their urine. In this regard, dietary restriction to 10 mEq daily should have revealed discernible differences between pregnant and control subjects. Furthermore, gravidas in this study did not gain the usual approximate one pound of weight expected during a seven-day period in late pregnancy but actually lost over two pounds. Also, plasma aldosterone increased to levels that are very high even for pregnant women. The data thus do not demonstrate convincingly the conclusion that salt balance in pregnant and nonpregnant subjects is similar but may actually support the concept that some gravidas have a slow renal leak and may cope with rigid salt restriction poorly. When they do, however, balance is achieved by stressing compensatory mechanisms such as steroid production.

Another way to assess sodium handling during gestation is to increase dietary sodium intake over a prolonged period and observe the clinical effects. One investigator studied over 2000 gavidas in a prospective trial, advising alternate subjects to add extra salt to their diets and eat more salty foods or to reduce dietary sodium as much as possible. Mean weekly weight gain as well as the incidence of edema, hypertension, and a wide variety of obstetric complications were no greater and actually tended to be lower in the group advised to take more salt. Unfortunately, urinary sodium was not measured, so that salt intake could not be quantitated. Nevertheless, in view of the large number of patients studied, it is reasonable to conclude that normal pregnant women handle liberal dietary salt intake without significant adverse clinical effects.

Our understanding of volume homeostasis and sodium handling during gestation remains incomplete. Although some maintain that salt balance is similar in pregnant and nonpregnant women, there are data that indicate that some gravidas cope with rigid salt restriction poorly. In this regard, it appears that the accumulation of sodium and the concomitant volume expansion that occur during gestation may be important for optimal pregnancy outcome. Thus, restriction of dietary sodium and use of prophylactic diuretics should be avoided. Most gravid women seem to tolerate considerable variation in dietary salt, and if the physician feels compelled to treat asymptomatic edema, bed rest with the patient positioned in lateral recumbency usually results in effective diuresis.

REFERENCES

1. Bailey RR, Rolleston GL. Kidney length and ureteric dilatation in the puerperium. *J Obstet Gynaecol Br Commonw.* 1971;78:55.
2. Dure-Smith P: Pregnancy dilatation of the urinary tract. The iliac sign and its significance. *Radiology.* 1970;96:545.
3. Fried AM. Hydronephrosis of pregnancy: Ultrasonographic study and classification of asymptomatic women. *Am J Obstet Gynecol.* 1979;135:1066.
4. Lindheimer MD, Katz AL. *Renal Function and Disease in Pregnancy.* Philadelphia, PA: Lea & Febiger; 1977.
5. Rasmussen PE, Nielsen FR. Hydronephrosis in pregnancy: A literature survey. *Eur J Obstet Gynecol Reprod Biol.* 1988;27:249.
6. Nielsen FR, Rasmussen PE. Hydronephrosis during pregnancy: four cases of hydronephrosis causing symptoms during pregnancy. *Eur J Obstet Gynecol Reproduc Biol.* 1988;27:245.
7. Lindheimer MD, Katz AL. The kidney in pregnancy. In: Brenner BM, Rector FC Jr, eds. *The Kidney.* 3rd ed. Philadelphia, PA: WB Saunders; 1986:1253.
8. Baylis C. Glomerular filtration and volume regulation in gravid animal models. *Clin Obstet Gynaecol (Balliere).* 1987;1:789.
9. Lim VS, Katz AL, Lindheimer MD. Acid-base regulation in pregnancy. *Am J Physiol.* 1976;231:1764.
10. Lindheimer MD, Barron WM, Davison JM. Osmoregulation of thirst and vasopressin release in pregnancy (editorial review). *Am J Physiol.* in press, Aug, 1989.
11. Barron WM, Lindheimer MD. Renal sodium and water handling in pregnancy. *Obstet Gynecol Annu.* 1984;13:35.
12. Davison JM, Shiells EA, Philips PR, Lindheimer MD. Serial evaluation of vasopressin release and thirst in human pregnancy: Role of human chorionic gonadotrophin in the osmoregulatory changes of gestation. *J Clin Invest.* 1988;81:798.
13. Davison JM, Shiells EA, Barron WM, et al. Changes in the metabolic clearance of vasopressin and in plasma vasopressinase throughout human pregnancy. *J Clin Invest.* 1989;83:1313.
14. Landon MJ, Copas OK, Shiells EA, Davison JM. Degradation of radio labelled arginine vasopressin (^{125}I AVP) by the human placenta perfused *in vitro. Br J Obstet Gynecol.* 1988;95:488.
15. Hytten FE. Weight gain in pregnancy. In: Hytten F, Chamberlain G, eds. *Clinical Physiology in Obstetrics.* Oxford: Blackwell Scientific Publications; 1981:193.
16. Chesley LC. *Hypertensive Disorders of Pregnancy.* New York, NY: Appleton-Century-Crofts; 1978:190.
17. Ferris TF. Prostenoids in normal and hypertensive pregnancy. In: Rubin PC, ed. *Handbook of Hypertension, Vol 10 Hypertension in Pregnancy.* Amsterdam: Elsevier; 1988:102.
18. Winkel C, Milewich L, Parker R Jr, et al. Conversion of plasma progesterone to deoxycorticosterone in men, nonpregnant and pregnant women and adrenalectomized subjects: evidence for steroid 21-hydroxylase activity in nonadrenal tissues. *J Clin Invest.* 1980;66:803.
19. Casey ML, MacDonald PC. Metabolism of deoxycorticosterone and deoxycorticosterone sulfate in men and women. *J Clin Invest.* 1982;70:312.
20. Hsueh WA, Luetscher JA, Carlson EJ, et al. Changes in active and inactive renin throughout pregnancy. *J Clin Endocrinol Metab.* 1982;54:1010.
21. Broughton-Pipkin F. The renin-angiotensin system. In: Rubin PC, ed. *Handbook of Hypertension, Vol. 10.* Amsterdam: Elsevier; 1988:118.
22. Brown MA, Broughton-Pipkin F, Symonds EM. The effects of intravenous angiotensin II upon sodium and urate excretion in human pregnancy. *J Hypertens.* 1988;6:457.
23. Brown MA. Sodium and plasma volume regulation in normal and hypertensive pregnancy: a review of physiology and clinical implications. *Clin Exper Hypertens.* 1988;B7:265.
24. Brown MA, Gallery EDM, Ross MR, Esker RP. Sodium excretion in normal and hypertensive pregnancy: a prospective study. *Am J Obstet Gynecol.* 1988;159:297.
25. Bay WH, Ferris TF. Factors controlling plasma renin and aldosterone in pregnancy. *Hypertension.* 1979;1:410.
26. Robinson M. Salt in pregnancy. *Lancet.* 1958;1:178.
27. Hytten FE, Leitch I. *The Physiology of Human Pregnancy.* 2nd ed. Oxford: Blackwell Scientific Publications; 1971.
28. Davison JM, Vallaton MB, Lindheimer MD. Plasma osmolality and urinary concentration and dilution during and after pregnancy: evidence that lateral recumbancy inhibits maximal urinary concentrating ability. *Br J Obstet Gynaecol.* 1981;88:472.

Chapter One Hundred and Forty-Three

Urinary Tract Infections

William W. Andrews and Larry C. Gilstrap III

143

Urinary tract infections are common in young women and represent the most frequent medical complication encountered during pregnancy. Infection of the urinary tract is most often asymptomatic during pregnancy; however, the physiologic changes of pregnancy predispose the bacteremic patient to an increased risk for development of acute pyelonephritis, which has been associated with considerable morbidity and even mortality. The presence of urinary tract infection during pregnancy also may impact adversely on the fetus. Therefore, an understanding of the etiology, evaluation and treatment of these infections is essential to the management of pregnant patients. Infections that will be discussed in detail include asymptomatic bacteriuria, cystitis, and acute pyelonephritis.

ETIOLOGY

The etiology of urinary tract infections during pregnancy is similar to that in the nonpregnant patient. It has been estimated that approximately 15% of all women will experience at least one episode of urinary tract infection during their lifetime.[1,2] Several anatomic differences explain the increased frequency of urinary tract infections in women compared to men. The female urethra is relatively short (approximately 3–4 cm in length) and is very close to the vaginal canal, which in turn borders the anus and rectum. The vagina is richly colonized with organisms from the lower gastrointestinal tract such as *Escherichia coli, Klebsiella pneumoniae, Enterobacter*, and *Proteus* species, all of which are common pathogens isolated from women with urinary tract infections. Urethral trauma resulting from intercourse also may play a role in the colonization of the lower urinary tract. Development of acute cystitis has been reported to be associated with recent sexual intercourse.[3] Regardless of the specific etiology of urinary tract colonization, it is well known that women acquire bacteriuria early in life. For example, 5% of teenage girls[4] and 8% of nulliparous married women[5] have bacteriuria.

The most common bacterial isolates recovered in pregnant women with urinary tract infections, including asymptomatic bacteriuria, are summarized in Table 143–1. The *Enterobacteriaceae*, especially *E coli* and *Klebsiella-Enterobacter* species account for 85–90% of urinary tract infections during pregnancy. *E coli* also is responsible for the majority of recurrent urinary tract infections in young women, and it has been shown that these women are likely to have introital colonization with bacteria manifesting bacterial adherence.[6]

It is important to note that Group B Streptococcus may be associated with asymptomatic bacteriuria in a significant number of pregnant women.[7,8] *Staphylococcus saprophyticus* also has been reported to cause urinary tract infections in women.[9] Other organisms such as *Citrobacter, Proteus*, and *Pseudomonas* species are uncommon pathogens in urinary tract infections during pregnancy. Anaerobic bacteria probably play little or no role in the etiology of asymptomatic bacteriuria during pregnancy.

TABLE 143–1. MICROBIOLOGY OF URINARY TRACT INFECTIONS ENCOUNTERED DURING PREGNANCY

Escherichia coli[a]
Klebsiella-Enterobacter[a]
Enterococcus
Streptococcus
Staphylococcus
Proteus
Pseudomonas
Citrobacter

[a] Account for 85–90% of infections.

PATHOGENESIS

The pathogenesis of asymptomatic bacteriuria is probably the same in pregnant and nonpregnant women. The majority of these infections are felt to represent ascending contamination as a result of one or a combination of factors described above. The pathogenesis of acute symptomatic urinary tract infection is less clear, although it is presumed that the majority of these infections also are related in part to ascending bacterial contamination.

Another important component in the pathogenesis of symptomatic urinary tract infection, as in any bacterial infection, is the concept of bacterial virulence. The presence or absence of certain virulence factors may explain why some women with asymptomatic urinary tract infections go on to develop symptomatic infections while others do not. The capacity of certain pathogens to adhere to the uroepithelium has long been considered an important factor related to bacterial virulence. This adhesive capacity is mediated by the presence of "adhesins" that are located on the bacterial cell surface. The considerable progress that has been made in the characterization of these adhesins in strains of *E coli* recently has been reviewed.[10] Different strains of uropathogenic *E coli* express combinations of several different surface adhesins known as pili or fimbriae. These adhesins reversibly bind to oligosaccharide receptors on the surface of numerous different cell types, including red blood cells and uroepithelial cells. Most *E coli* strains express so-called type 1 pili that bind to mannose-containing receptors in the mucin of uroepithelial cells.[11,12] However, such binding results in only poor attachment, and these bacteria are effectively washed out of the urinary tract along with the mucin. As a result, type 1 pili have not been strongly associated as a virulence factor for urinary tract infection. More recently, other adhesins known as P-fimbriae have been described that specifically bind to the disaccharide galactose-$\alpha(1\text{–}4)$galactose-β component of globoseries glycolipids.[13,14] These glycolipids serve as receptors on the surface of uroepithelial cells.

The presence of P-fimbriae has been suggested by many[15-21] to be a virulence marker for urinary tract infection. While P-fimbriae are expressed on 10–20% of *E coli* strains isolated from patients with cystitis or asymptomatic bacteriuria[15,16], over 80–90% of strains isolated from acute nonobstructive pyelonephritis patients express P-fimbriae.[15-20] The exact role bacterial adherence may play in the pathogenesis of urinary tract infections in pregnant women is unclear at this time. However, a preponderance of P-fimbriated *E coli* strains in pregnant patients with acute pyelonephritis compared to *E coli* isolated from patients with asymptomatic bacteriuria has been reported.[22]

ASYMPTOMATIC BACTERIURIA

Asymptomatic bacteriuria (ASB) is defined as the presence of a urinary tract infection in the absence of specific urinary tract symptoms. Since pregnancy does not predispose a patient to the acquisition of bacteriuria, the prevalence of this condition is essentially the same in both pregnant and nonpregnant women. The incidence of ASB is approximately 5–6% in pregnant women with some reports as high as 10% in certain high-risk populations.[23] Interestingly, only 1% of women actually will acquire bacteriuria during pregnancy if it is not already present at the time of the initial screening culture.

Several factors have been associated with an increased

frequency of bacteriuria, which probably apply to both pregnant and nonpregnant women. Socioeconomic status is the strongest associated risk factor for ASB, with the incidence being higher in indigent patients compared to nonindigent patients.[24] Neither race nor ethnic background has been linked to the presence of ASB. In fact, most studies have failed to demonstrate a significant difference in the incidence of ASB between black and white women when controlled for socioeconomic status.[23,24] The association of age and parity with ASB during pregnancy is unclear. It has been established that pregnant women with sickle cell trait have a two-fold increased frequency of ASB compared to pregnant women without this condition.[25]

Clinical Significance

Asymptomatic bacteriuria in the nonpregnant patient probably carries little or no significant health risk. For this reason, it is neither necessary nor cost-effective to perform routine screening for bacteriuria in asymptomatic nongravid women. This is certainly *not* true in the pregnant patient, in whom the presence of ASB clearly represents a signficiant health risk. Although pregnancy itself does not predispose to the acquisition of ASB, it does predispose to the acquisition of symptomatic urinary tract infections such as acute pyelonephritis. This increased risk is compounded by the presence of bacteriuria. It is now well established that as many as 28% of pregnant women with ASB will develop acute pyelonephritis if untreated.[23] Acute pyelonephritis in turn carries a significantly increased risk for both the mother and the fetus. Treatment of ASB in pregnancy has been shown to reduce the incidence of progression to acute pyelonephritis to approximately 3–4%.[23]

Other adverse effects that have been attributed to ASB in pregnancy include maternal anemia, maternal hypertension, increased incidence of preterm labor and birth, and an increased frequency of low birth weight infants.[26] In 1960, Kass[27] was the first to report an association between bacteriuria and prematurity and, more important, that eradication of bacteriuria during pregnancy would result in a decreased frequency of premature births. While there have been additional reports supporting Kass's initial observation regarding bacteriuria and prematurity[28,29], others have failed to demonstrate such an association.[30,31] As a result, significant controversy remains regarding the association of bacteriuria and prematurity. A potential explanation for the discrepancy in the results of these reports may lie in the different means by which these investigators defined prematurity. The earlier reports considered prematurity using the classic 1935 American Academy of Pediatrics definition of a liveborn infant weighing less than 2500 g. We now know that as many as one third of these babies are actually growth-retarded and not premature. As pointed out by Cunningham and Whalley[31], it is nearly impossible "to determine from early reports whether infants born to mothers with bacteriuria were premature, dysmature, or both." Another potential explanation for the diversity of opinion is the possibility that subgroups of pregnant women may have greater risk factors for complications. For example, certain subgroups of women may be colonized with P-fimbriated *E coli*, a potentially more virulent infection. Also, it is now well established that approximately 50% of women with ASB have bacteriuria of renal origin[26] and this group may be at increased risk for having premature or low birthweight infants.[32] This hypothesis was tested by Gilstrap et al[26] who evaluated the presence or absence of antibody-coated bacteria to localize the site of bacteriuria, that is, upper or lower tract, in 250 pregnant women with ASB. No association was found between the presence of bacteriuria and hypertension, anemia, prematurity, or low birth weight when compared to 250 pregnant women without bacteriuria. These investigators were unable to identify a subgroup of pregnant women, that is, those with renal bacteriuria, at increased risk for various complications. For ethical reasons, this study suffered from the lack of a control group of untreated patients with ASB. From a pragmatic point of view, however, whether ASB is associated with prematurity or low birth weight is probably a moot point because *all* pregnant women with this condition should be treated to prevent the development of acute pyelonephritis.

Diagnosis

Since these women by definition have no symptoms of urinary tract infection, the diagnosis of asymptomatic bacteriuria is based solely on demonstrating the presence of significant bacteriuria. The most commonly accepted definition of *significant bacteriuria* is the presence of ≥100,000 colonies of a single uropathogen per mL of urine. The most common method of collection is via the clean-voided technique. Unless obtained by catheterization, counts of less than 100,000 organisms/mL, or specimens containing more than one organism, generally represent contamination and not urinary tract infection. The accuracy of a single culture obtained by way of the clean-voided technique is approximately 85% compared to 96% when obtained by catheterization.[26,33] When bacteriuria is confirmed on a repeat specimen obtained by the clean-voided technique, the accuracy approaches that of catheterization. The presence of any bacteria obtained by suprapubic aspiration probably is clinically significant and indicative of urinary tract infection. However, this latter technique generally is unacceptable to patients, unnecessary, and should be utilized only in very unusual circumstances. From a practical and cost-effective standpoint, a single specimen obtained by the clean-voided technique should be used for screening in the majority of pregnant women. Although there may be a 15% false-positive rate, false negatives are extremely uncommon.

Various other methods used to screen for the presence of bacteriuria during pregnancy are summarized in Table 143–2. Of these, routine urinalysis is grossly inaccurate and should not be used as the sole screening tool to detect the presence or absence of bacteriuria. The presence of white blood cells or *pyuria,* on urinalysis, is not always indicative of urinary tract infection, especially asymptomatic

TABLE 143–2. SCREENING TECHNIQUES USED FOR THE DETECTION OF BACTERIURIA DURING PREGNANCY

Urinalysis
Leukocyte esterase activity
Drop of unspun urine
Nitrite (Griess) test
Urine culture
Pour plate dilution
Calibrated loop
Urine culture kits
Testuria (Ayerst)
Bactercult (Wampole)
Uricult (Bristol)
Microstix-3 (Ames)
Bac-T-Screen (Marion)

TABLE 143–3. ANTIMICROBIAL REGIMENS FOR THE TREATMENT OF ASYMPTOMATIC BACTERIURIA DURING PREGNANCY

Antimicrobial (or Drug) Agent	Dose[a]
Sulfonamides	500 mg to 1 g qid
Nitrofurantoin	50–100 mg qid
Cephalosporins	250 mg qid
Ampicillin	250 mg qid

[a] Oral dose given for 5 to 7 days

bacteriuria, and is often found in pregnant women without infection. However, the presence of bacteria in a drop of unspun urine has been shown to correlate with the presence of signficant bacteriuria as demonstrated by urine culture.[34] The sensitivity and specificity of the other tests listed in Table 143–1 vary depending on the source. A urine culture remains the most accurate (although more expensive) screening method for detecting the presence of bacteriuria during pregnancy. Most hospital laboratories use the pour plate or calibrated loop technique in performing quantitative urine cultures. Alternatively, several commercial kits that are easy to use, relatively inexpensive, and amazingly accurate, have been marketed for performing quantitative urine cultures.[35]

Treatment

Numerous antimicrobial agents can be successfully used to treat asymptomatic bacteriuria during pregnancy as outlined in Table 143–3. All of these are FDA category B drugs. Although no one regimen has proven satisfactory in all patients, one particular regimen that has been found to be especially successful in the majority of patients is nitrofurantoin macrocrystals (100 mg given once a day at bed time for 10 days). Various single-dose regimens also have been used during pregnancy for the treatment of asymptomatic bacteriuria with reasonable success.[36-39] These regimens are outlined in Table 143–4. For patients with frequently recurrent or persistent infections following therapy, continuous antimicrobial suppression for the remainder of pregnancy should be considered. A useful agent for continuous suppression is nitrofurantoin macrocrystals (100 mg given at bed time) for the remainder of the pregnancy. The frequent use of antimicrobials such as ampicillin or cephalosporins intermittently or for suppression may be associated with significant side effects, including the development of chronic vulvovaginitis secondary to an overgrowth of *Candida albicans.*

The combination of a sulfonamide and trimethoprim is a popular and efficacious regimen used to treat bacteriuria in the nonpregnant patient. Although this combination has been used in Europe successfully and without apparent adverse maternal or fetal effects, it is not recommended currently for use in pregnant women in the United States. The major reason for this is largely theoretical and based on the fact that trimethoprim is an antifolate. Other antifolates such as methotrexate and aminoptherin have been associated with fetal anomalies. However, according to available data, it is unlikely that the combination of a sulfonamide and trimethoprim results in fetal anomalies.

A new group of antimicrobials, the quinolones, has proven especially successful in the treatment of urinary tract infections; the FDA has approved one of these, norfloxacin, for the treatment of urinary tract infections. Although this antimicrobial is effective against the majority of pathogens isolated from the urinary tract and is useful especially in resistant infections, there is little information available regarding its safety and efficacy during pregnancy. It is listed as a category C drug by its manufacturer and as such should not be used to treat asymptomatic bacteriuria during pregnancy unless other antimicrobial agents have proven unsuccessful.

Amoxicillin has recently been combined with the β-lactamase inhibitor clavulanic acid to provide better coverage against a variety of organisms. Although amoxicillin is an FDA category B drug, its combination with clavulanic acid should be reserved for patients who demonstrate resistant organisms or have persistent infections. This combination is relatively expensive compared to ampicillin, sulfonamides, or nitrofurantoin.

Tetracycline has been reported to cause yellow-brown discoloration of the deciduous teeth of the fetus[40] and generally should be avoided during pregnancy. This is also true for the newer tetracyclines. As a group, the tetracyclines are listed as category D drugs.

Some antibiotics may cause adverse effects in the mother or fetus such as hemolytic anemia or hyperbilirubinemia. A thorough understanding of the potential of each specific antimicrobial agent to cause such effects is a prerequisite to the use of these drugs in pregnancy.

Follow Up

Regardless of the antimicrobial agent selected or the duration of therapy, approximately one third of women with asymptomatic bacteriuria will experience persistence or recurrence of infection during pregnancy. Following the initial treatment of bacteriuria, it is important to evaluate these patients with frequent surveillance urine cultures. For women with persistent or recurrent episodes of bacteriuria, suppressive therapy can be used as outlined above.

A significant number of women with bacteriuria during pregnancy will have bacteriuria when studied 10–14 years later.[41] Zinner and Kass[41] reported that approximately 38% of women who had bacteriuria during pregnancy also had

TABLE 143–4. SINGLE-DOSE ANTIMICROBIAL THERAPY IN PREGNANT WOMEN WITH ASYMPTOMATIC BACTERIURIA

Reference	# Patients	Antibiotic	Cure Rate
Bailey (1984)[36]	24	Co-trimoxazole	88%
Jakobi et al (1987)[37]	50	Amoxicillin or cephalexin	84%
Harris et al (1982)[38]	86	Ampicillin or cephalexin plus probenecid Nitrofurantoin Sulfisoxazole	69%
McFadyen et al (1987)[39]	86	Cephalexin	65%

bacteriuria many years later. On the other hand, only 5% of women without bacteriuria during pregnancy had bacteriuria 10–14 years later.[41] Although a significant number of women with bacteriuria during pregnancy will have urinary tract infections on subsequent followup, there is little evidence to suggest that this poses a significant increased risk to their health or quality of life.[42]

CYSTITIS

Surprisingly, cystitis is not a commonly reported complication of pregnancy, and the exact incidence of this complication is not known. However, it has been reported that cystitis occurs in approximately 0.3–2.0% of pregnant women.[22,43] While pregnancy itself does not appear to increase the risk of acquiring this infection, one third of the patients who develop cystitis have a positive screening culture for bacteriuria at their initial visit. The remaining two thirds of the patients have a negative screening culture or present initially with cystitis during pregnancy.[43]

CLINICAL SIGNIFICANCE

The primary morbidity of acute cystitis during pregnancy relates largely to the extreme discomfort experienced by the patient. Whether acute cystitis is associated with an increased risk of acute pyelonephritis or certain adverse effects during pregnancy such as hypertension, anemia, or prematurity is unclear at this time. Although one might logically expect that the risk and complications (including pyelonephritis) of acute cystitis would be similar to that of ASB during pregnancy, this may not be true. In 95% of the cases of acute cystitis, the infection is limited to the bladder, whereas in asymptomatic bacteriuria 50% of the patients have been shown to have bacteriuria of renal origin (Table 143–5).

Diagnosis

In contrast to pregnant women with ASB, pregnant women with cystitis usually present to the physician because of symptoms outlined in Table 143–6. Frequent complaints such as urgency, frequency, and nocturia do not indicate cystitis during pregnancy since many pregnant women without urinary tract infections also experience these symptoms. Suprapubic pressure or pain, a common symptom in nonpregnant women with cystitis, also is nonspecific in making this diagnosis during pregnancy since many pregnant women will have this symptom as a result of pressure from the presenting fetal part, especially in the late second or third trimesters of pregnancy. Dysuria is the most reliable symptom of cystitis in pregnant patients.

TABLE 143–5. LOCALIZATION OF THE SITE OF INFECTION IN 224 WOMEN WITH URINARY TRACT INFECTIONS DURING PREGNANCY

	Site of Infection	
	Renal	Bladder
Asymptomatic Bacteriuria (n = 152)	45%	55%
Acute Cystitis (n = 35)	5%	95%
Acute Pyelonephritis (n = 37)	65%	35%

Adapted from Harris and Gilstrap.[43]

TABLE 143–6. CLINICAL AND LABORATORY FINDINGS IN PREGNANT WOMEN WITH ACUTE CYSTITIS

- Urgency
- Frequency
- Suprapubic discomfort
- Dysuria[a]
- No fever or costovertebral angle tenderness
- Positive urine culture
- Occasional hematuria or pyuria

[a] Most reliable symptom

Common laboratory findings include a positive urine culture, pyuria, and occasionally gross hematuria. The presence of pyuria or microscopic hematuria in the absence of a positive culture usually is not indicative of acute cystitis because as many as 10–15% of normal uninfected pregnant women have these findings.[44]

Unlike patients with ASB, most women (95%) with acute cystitis during pregnancy will have bacteria localized to the bladder (Table 143–5). The bacterial etiology of acute cystitis during pregnancy is similar to that for ASB and acute pyelonephritis as summarzied in Table 143–1.

Treatment

The treatment of pregnant women with acute cystitis is similar to that of pregnant women with ASB except that single-dose regimens generally are ineffective and not recommended for use during pregnancy. Patients may be treated as outpatients with an oral preparation such as ampicillin or a cephalosporin (250–500 mg qid), a sulfonamide (1 g qid), or nitrofurantoin macrocrystals (100 mg qid) for 5–7 days. Since these patients are symptomatic, therapy usually is empiric and should be initiated before the results of the culture and sensitivity are known.

Follow Up

Approximately 25% of patients with acute cystitis during pregnancy will experience another infection of the urinary tract sometime during the pregnancy.[43] Thus, it is important to follow these patients with frequent surveillance cultures coinciding with their normal prenatal visits. There are no long-term follow-up studies of pregnant women with acute cystitis, but there is little reason to think that their course would be any different from those with ASB.

ACUTE PYELONEPHRITIS

Acute pyelonephritis is one of the most common serious medical complications of pregnancy and occurs in approximately 1–2% of all pregnant women.[42] About two thirds of the cases arise from women with preexisting bacteriuria, while approximately one third arise in women who have not had bacteriuria documented during pregnancy.[42] Unlike bacteriuria or acute cystitis, pregnancy significantly increases the risk of acquiring acute pyelonephritis. The major reason for this predisposition is that pregnancy results in a relative obstruction of the urinary tract with resultant stasis of urine and bacteriuria as outlined in Figure 143–1. The etiology of this relative obstruction is two fold. First, there is dilatation of the ureters secondary to the hormonal influences of pregnancy, especially progesterone, which

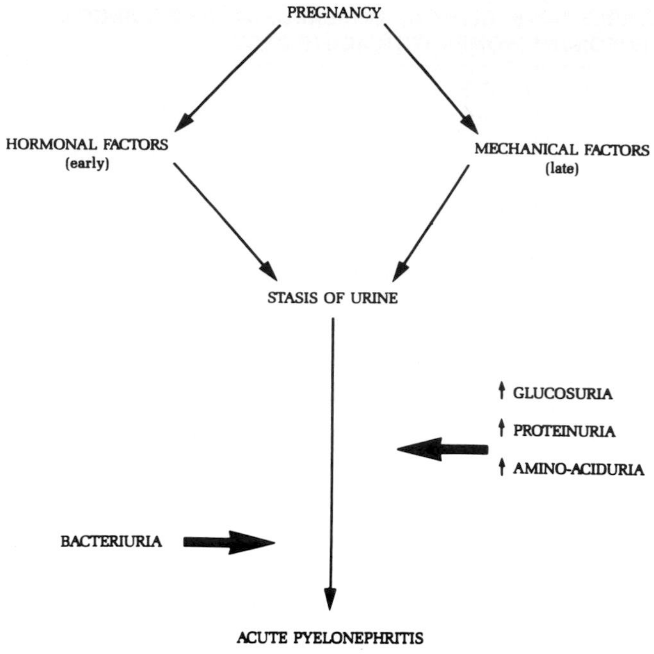

Figure 143–1. Pathogenesis of acute pyelonephritis during pregnancy. Note: Bacteriuria is present in two thirds of cases on initial urine screen. (*From Gilstrap et al* [45] *with permission.*)

is known to be a smooth muscle relaxant. Second, there is actual mechanical obstruction from the pregnant uterus and its contents, which results in a pressure gradient of approximately 15 mL of water between the lower and upper ureter.[45] An additional contributing factor to the pathogenesis of acute pyelonephritis in pregnancy is the presence of glucosuria and aminoaciduria, which favor the proliferation of bacteria. Acute pyelonephritis during pregnancy is associated with several predisposing factors identical to those for ASB, which were reviewed earlier in this chapter.

The majority of cases of acute pyelonephritis occur in the second and third trimesters. In one review of 656 women with acute pyelonephritis[42], 482 cases (73%) occurred during the antepartum period. Of these, 9% occurred in the first trimester, 46% in the second trimester, and 45% in the third trimester. This is probably because of the increase in relative obstruction and stasis of urine as pregnancy progresses.

Adverse Maternal Effects

As outlined in Table 143–7, acute pyelonephritis may result in multisystem dysfunction.[45] Dysfunction of the hypothalamic temperature-regulating center is evident in many patients and is characterized by extremes of temperature ranging from high spiking temperatures (≥40°C) to very low temperatures or hypothermia (≤35°C).

Renal dysfunction is manifested by both an elevated serum creatinine and a significant decrease in creatinine clearance. In a study by Gilstrap et al[42], 20% of pregnant women with acute pyelonephritis had a serum creatinine of greater than 1 mg/dL. Approximately one fourth of the patients will have a 24-hour creatinine clearance of less than 80 cm^3/minute corrected for body surface area.[46] This renal dysfunction is transient and the creatinine clearance usually returns to normal within 3–6 weeks after an episode of acute pyelonephritis.

TABLE 143–7. MULTIPLE ORGAN SYSTEM DYSFUNCTION IN PREGNANT WOMEN WITH ACUTE PYELONEPHRITIS

Thermoregulatory Instability
Hyperthermia
Hypothermia
Hematologic Dysfunction
Anemia
Leukocytosis
Thrombocytopenia
Renal Dysfunction
Elevated serum creatinine
Decreased creatinine clearance
Pulmonary Dysfunction
Adult respiratory distress syndrome (ARDS)

Data are based on studies discussed in references 34 and 35.

Hematologic abnormalities also may occur and the most common manifestations are anemia (hematocrit <30%) or a significant drop in the patient's hematocrit.[42,45] In extreme cases, the patient may show drops in the hematocrit of 10 points or greater. Although dehydration followed by rehydration can certainly affect the patient's hematocrit, the drop in the majority of patients is not secondary to fluid changes as evidenced by the fact that the hematocrit is generally still very low several days after the acute episode of pyelonephritis. In one study of pregnant women with acute pyelonephritis[45], 24 out of 36 women (66%) had a hematocrit of <30 volumes percent and 36% had a decrease in the hematocrit of ≥6 volumes percent. Although the platelet count may be low in a few patients, overt thrombocytopenia is an uncommon manifestation. However, when thrombocytopenia does occur, it is usually an ominous sign.[34]

Pulmonary dysfunction, ranging from a few opacifications suggestive of infiltrates and mild respiratory distress to overt pulmonary failure and adult respiratory distress syndrome (ARDS), may occur in one out of every 50 pregnant women with acute pyelonephritis.[47] First described by Cunningham and associates in 1984[48], respiratory insufficiency may be manifested by dyspnea, tachypnea, hypoxia, and x-ray findings of pulmonary infiltrates occurring on the first or second day following admission (Figure 143–2).[47] These patients also may manifest renal dysfunction (serum creatinine >1.2 mg/dL), evidence of red cell hemolysis, platelet counts of <100,000/mm^3, white blood cell counts >14,000/mm^3, and evidence of intravascular coagulation.[47] Scanning electron microscopy of the red cells of these patients has revealed evidence of red cell membrane damage and abnormal morphologic forms such as schizocytes or echinocytes.[49]

It has been postulated that the multisystem dysfunction seen in pregnant women with acute pyelonephritis is secondary to the effects of endotoxin[47], which is the lipopolysaccharide cell wall component of gram-negative organisms. Endotoxin is a logical common denominator in the explanation of many complications of pyelonephritis including ARDS, transient renal dysfunction, red cell hemolysis, thrombocytopenia, and intravascular coagulation.

Acute pyelonephritis also results in overt septic shock in about 1–2% of women.[50] This is obviously a life-threatening complication. Fortunately, appropriate treatment of pregnant women with acute pyelonephritis results in only transient organ dysfunction, and these patients usually do not experience life-threatening complications.

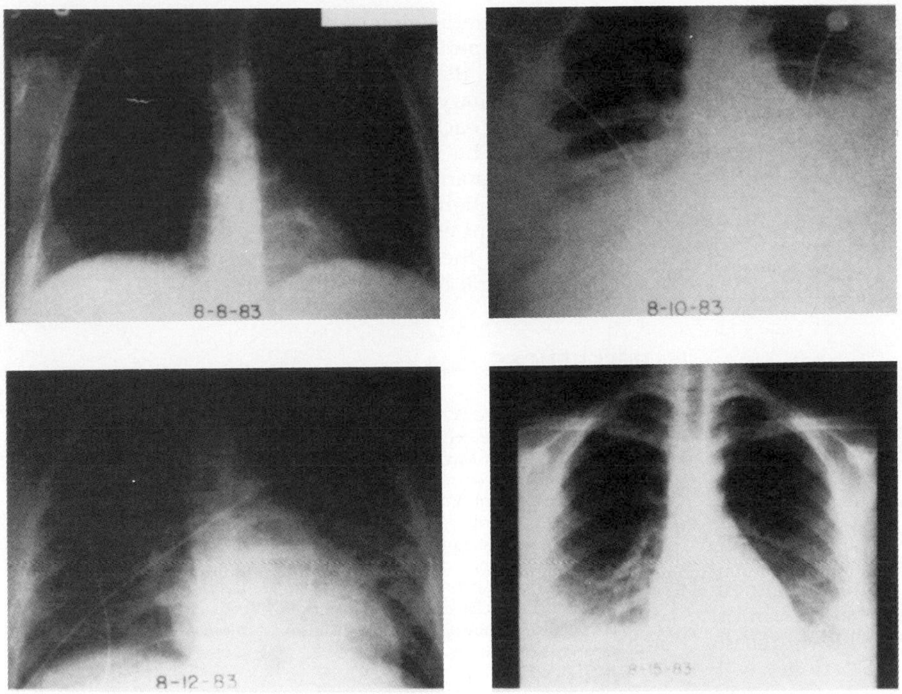

Figure 143–2. Radiographic findings in pregnant women with acute pyelonephritis and ARDS. *(From Cunningham et al[47] with permission.)*

Long-Term Prognosis

Women with acute pyelonephritis or frequent urinary tract infections during pregnancy ultimately may be shown to have urinary tract abnormalities. As many as 27–37% of these women will have either recurrent infection or radiographic anomalies.[23,51] In an 8–13 year follow up of 208 women with acute pyelonephritis[42], 41% were treated for one or more episodes of symptomatic urinary tract infections when not pregnant, and 38% of those with subsequent pregnancies had another episode of infection during pregnancy. Despite risks of frequent recurrences and the presence of urinary tract abnormalities, it is uncommon for these women to develop end-stage renal insufficiency.[52]

Adverse Fetal and Newborn Effects

Acute pyelonephritis has been reported to be associated with an increase in both low birth weight and premature infants. This, in turn, is secondary to an increased incidence of premature labor in patients with acute pyelonephritis. In one large series[26], approximately 15% of neonates born to mothers with acute pyelonephritis weighed less than 2500 grams. However, the mean birth weight of infants born to mothers with acute pyelonephritis was not significantly different from that of infants born to women without pyelonephritis (Table 143–8).

TABLE 143–8. NEONATAL OUTCOME IN 487 WOMEN WITH ACUTE PYELONEPHRITIS VERSUS CONTROLS

	Women with Pyelonephritis	Controls
Birth weight <2500 g	71 (15%)[a]	50 (10%)[a]
Mean birth weight	3044	3059
Perinatal losses	13 (2.7%)	12 (2.5%)

[a] $p < 0.05$

Adapted from Gilstrap et al.[26]

Diagnosis

The diagnosis of acute pyelonephritis is based primarily on systemic signs and symptoms in the presence of a positive urine culture. Specific signs and symptoms include fever, chills, nausea and vomiting, and costovertebral angle (CVA) or flank tenderness. The fever may be very high, reaching 40°C in many patients and is generally spiking in nature. In one series[42], 85% of 656 women had a temperature of ≥38°C (100.4°F) and 12% ≥40°C (104°F). One patient had a temperature of 107°F. Moreover, 54% had right CVA tenderness, 27% had bilateral CVA tenderness, and 16% had left CVA tenderness. In such cases, urinalysis reveals clumps of white blood cells and many bacteria, and the urine culture will invariably be positive for one of the pathogens listed in Table 143–1. If the urine culture is negative, the patient should be questioned as to whether she is taking antibiotics. Many patients with pyelonephritis have had previous urinary tract infections and may have started antibiotics on their own. Even a single oral dose of an antibiotic may render the urine sterile.

The peripheral blood white cell count may vary from normal to as high as 17,000 or greater. A number of patients also will exhibit a significant drop in their hematocrit. The serum creatinine may also be elevated in approximately 20% of the patients with a concomitant decrease in the 24-hour urine creatinine clearance.[46]

Treatment

General guidelines for the management of pregnant women with acute pyelonephritis are summarized in Table 143–9.[53] First, and most important, all pregnant women with acute pyelonephritis should be hospitalized for close observation. Many of these women have nausea and vomiting, are dehydrated, and are unable to tolerate oral fluids or medications. Patients with acute pyelonephritis should receive parenteral hydration and antibiotics. Vital signs should be monitored frequently, as should urine output. Initial antimicrobial therapy is empiric since the results of

TABLE 143–9. GUIDELINES FOR THE MANAGEMENT OF ACUTE PYELONEPHRITIS IN PREGNANT WOMEN

Hospitalization
Hydration
Intravenous antibiotics
Frequent monitoring of urine output and vital signs
Urine and blood cultures
Complete blood count and serum creatinine
Clinic follow up with frequent surveillance cultures

Adapted from Gilstrap and Wendel.[53]

the urine culture and sensitivity are not known, and a wide variety of agents may be used as summarized in Table 143–10.[53] Ampicillin alone is no longer recommended for acute pyelonephritis since in most hospitals many common uropathogens, such as *E coli*, are resistant to it. Gentamicin or other aminoglycosides should be used with caution in these patients, since a significant number of them experience transient renal dysfunction. The risk to the fetus when an aminoglycoside is included in this treatment regimen appears to be very low. Therapy with a cephalosporin or one of the newer extended penicillins generally will result in a cure rate of 85–90%.[54] The majority of patients will be afebrile and asymptomatic within 24–48 hours after initiation of therapy. Other factors must be excluded in those patients who fail to respond during this time frame. Reasons for failure include resistant organisms, nephrolithiasis, segmental infection (*lobar nephronia*), perinephric abscess, or obstruction secondary to the pregnancy itself.

Follow Up

Following discharge from the hospital, patients should be followed in the clinic with frequent urine culture surveillance. Recurrent infection is common and occurs in at least 25% of patients following an initial episode of acute pyelonephritis.[42] When frequent clinic visits are not feasible, an alternative is to use continuous antibiotic suppressive therapy throughout pregnancy. In one review of suppressive therapy[55], the incidence of recurrence in women not receiving suppression was 60% compared to approximately 3% of those receiving suppression. Continuous suppression with nitrofurantoin macrocrystals, 100 mg orally every night, has proven to be a satisfactory regimen.[31]

CONCLUSIONS

Urinary tract infection is a common complication encountered during pregnancy, occurring in 2–10% of such women.

TABLE 143–10. ANTIMICROBIAL REGIMENS FOR THE TREATMENT OF PREGNANT WOMEN WITH ACUTE PYELONEPHRITIS

Single-Agent Therapy
Ampicillin 500 mg to 1 g IV q6h
First generation cephalosporin 500 mg to 1 g IV q6h
Cefoxitin 1–2 g IV q6h
Mezlocillin or piperacillin 3–4 g IV q6h
Combination Therapy
(Aminoglycoside plus antibiotic listed above)
Gentamicin 3 mg/kg per day IV in divided doses
Tobramycin 3 mg/kg per day IV in divided doses

Adapted from Gilstrap and Wendel.[53]

Detection and eradication of bacteriuria at the first prenatal visit are of paramount importance in preventing acute pyelonephritis and its attendant maternal and fetal risks. The majority of urinary tract infections are caused by gram-negative enteric bacteria, with *E coli* the most common single uropathogen. The urine culture remains the mainstay in diagnosis. Pregnant women with ASB or cystitis can be treated as outpatients with oral antimicrobial agents. However, all pregnant women with acute pyelonephritis should be admitted to the hospital for close observation and to receive parenteral hydration and antibiotics.

REFERENCES

1. Kass EH, Savage W, Santamarina BAG. The significance of bacteriuria in preventive medicine. In: Kass EH, ed. *Progress in Pyelonephritis*. Philadelphia, PA: FA Davis; 1965:3.
2. Schaeffer AJ. Recurrent urinary tract infections in women: Pathogenesis and management. *Postgrad Med*. 1987;81:51.
3. Nicolle LE, Harding GK, Preiksaitis J, Ronald AR. The association of urinary tract infection with sexual intercourse *J Infect Dis*. 1982;146:579.
4. Kunin CM. Urinary tract infections in children. *Hosp Pract*. 1976;11:91.
5. Sleigh JD, Robertson JG, Isdale MH. Asymptomatic bacteriuria in pregnancy. *J Obstet Gynaecol Br Commonw*. 964;71:74.
6. Fowler JE, Stamey TA. Studies of introital colonization in women with recurrent infections. VII. The role of bacterial adherence. *J Urol*. 1977;117:472.
7. Wood EG, Dillon HC. A prospective study of Group B streptococcal bacteriuria in pregnancy. *Am J Obstet Gynecol*. 1981;140:515.
8. Mead PJ, Harris RE. The incidence of group B beta hemolytic streptococcus in antepartum urinary tract infections. *Obstet Gynecol*. 1978;51:412.
9. Latham RH, Running K, Stamm WE. Urinary tract infections in young adult women caused by *Staphylococcus saprophyticus*. *Jama*. 1983;250:3063.
10. Svanborg-Eden C. Bacterial adherence in urinary tract infections caused by *Escherichia coli*. *Scand J Urol Nephrol*. 1986;20:81.
11. Duguid JP, Gilles RR. Fimbriae and adhesive properties in dysentery bacilli. *J Pathol Bact*. 1957;74:397.
12. Ofek I, Mirelman D, Sharon N. Adherence of *Escherichia coli* to human mucosal cells mediated by mannose receptors. *Nature*. 1977;265:623.
13. Källenius G, Möllby R, Svensson B, et al. The P^k antigen as receptor for the haemagglutinin of pyelonephritic *Escherichia coli*. *FEMS Microbiol Lett*. 1980;7:297.
14. Leffler H, Svanborg-Edén C. Chemical identification of a glycosphingolipid receptor for *Escherichia coli* attaching to human urinary tract epithelial cells and agglutinating human erythrocytes. *FEMS Microbiol Lett*. 1980;8:127.
15. Väisänen V, Tallgren LG, Makela PH, et al. Mannose-resistant haemagglutination and P antigen recognition are characteristic of *Escherichia coli* causing primary pyelonephritis. *Lancet*. 1981;2:1366.
16. Källenius G, Svenson SB, Hultberg H, et al. Occurrence of P-fimbriated *Escherichia coli* in urinary tract infections. *Lancet*. 1981;2:1369.
17. Lomberg H, Hanson LA, Jacobsson B, et al. Correlation of P blood group, vesicoureteral reflux and bacterial attachement in patients with recurrent pyelonephritis. *N Engl J Med*. 1983;308:1189.
18. Elo J, Tallgren LG, Väisänen V, et al. Association of P and other fimbriae with clinical pyelonephritis in children. *Scand J Urol Nephrol*. 1985;19:281.
19. Dowling K, Roberts JA, Kaack MB. P-fimbriated *Escherichia coli* urinary tract infection: A clinical correlation. *South Med J*. 1987;80:1533.
20. Lidfelt KJ, Bollgren I, Källenius G, Svenson SB. P-fimbriated *Escherichia coli* in children with acute cystitis. *Acta Paediatr Scand*. 1987;76:775.
21. Svanborg Edén C, Hagberg L, Leffler H, Lomberg H. Recent progress in the understanding of the role of bacterial adhesion in the pathogenesis of urinary tract infection. *Infection*. 1982;10:327.
22. Stenquist K, Sanberg G, Lidin-Janson F, et al. Virulence factors of *Escherichia coli* in urinary isolates from pregnant women. *J Infect Dis*. 1987;156:870.
23. Whalley P. Bacteriuria of pregnancy. *Am J Obstet Gynecol*. 1967;97:723.
24. Turck M, Goff BS, Petersdorf RG. Bacteriuria in pregnancy: relation to socioeconomic factors. *N Engl J Med*. 1962;266:857.
25. Whalley PJ, Martin RG, Pritchard JA. Sickle cell trait and urinary tract infection during pregnancy. *JAMA*. 1964;189:903.
26. Gilstrap LC, Leveno KJ, Cunningham FG, et al. Renal infection and pregnancy outcome. *Am J Obstet Gynecol*. 1981;141:709.
27. Kass EH. In: Quinn EL, Kass EH, eds. *Biology of Pyelonephritis*. Boston: Little, Brown & Co; 1960:399.
28. Stuart KL, Cummins GTM, Chin WA. Bacteriuria, prematurity and hypertensive disorders of pregnancy. *Br Med J*. 1965;1:554.
29. Brumfitt W. The effects of bacteriuria in pregnancy on maternal and fetal health. *Kidney Int*. 1975;8(suppl):113.

30. Whalley PJ, Cunningham FG. Short-term versus continuous antimicrobial therapy for asymptomatic bacteriuria in pregnancy. *Obstet Gynecol.* 1977;49:262.
31. Cunningham FG, Whalley PJ. Asymptomatic bacteriuria during pregnancy. In: Buchsbaum HJ, Schmidt JD, eds. *Gynecologic and Obstetric Urology.* 2nd ed. Philadelphia, PA: WB Saunders; 1982;519.
32. Zinner SH. Bacteriuria and babies revisited. *N Engl J Med.* 1979;300:853.
33. Kass EH. Asymptomatic infections of the urinary tract. *Trans Assoc AM Physicians.* 1956;69:56.
34. Kunin CM: Initial significance of bacteriuria visualized in the unstrained urinary sediment. *N Engl J Med.* 1961;265:589.
35. Hankins GDV, Whalley PJ. Acute urinary tract infection in pregnancy. *Clin Obstet Gynecol.* 1985;28:266.
36. Bailey RR: Single-dose antibacterial treatment for bacteriuria in pregnancy. *Drugs.* 1984;27:183.
37. Jakobi P, Neiger R, Merzbach D, Paldi E. Single-dose antimicrobial therapy in the treatment of asymptomatic bacteriuria in pregnancy. *Am J Obstet Gynecol.* 1987;156:1148.
38. Harris RE, Gilstrap LC, Pretty A. Single-dose antimicrobial therapy for asymptomatic bacteriuria during pregnancy. *Obstet Gynecol.* 1982;59:546.
39. McFadyen IR, Campbell-Brown M, Stephenson M, Seal DV. Single dose treatment of bacteriuria in pregnancy. *Eur Urol.* 1987;13:22.
40. Kutscher AH, Zegarelli EV, Tovell HM, et al. Discoloration of deciduous teeth induced by administration of tetracycline antepartum. *Am J Obstet Gynecol.* 1966;96:291.
41. Zinner SH, Kass EH. Long-term (10 to 14 years) follow-up of bacteriuria of pregnancy. *N Engl J Med.* 1971;285:820.
42. Gilstrap LC, Cunningham FG, Whalley PJ. Acute pyelonephritis in pregnancy: An anterospective study. *Obstet Gynecol.* 1981;57:409.
43. Harris RE, Gilstrap LC. Cystitis during pregnancy: A distinct clinical entity. *Obstet Gynecol.* 1981;57:578.
44. Lacy SS. Urinary tract infections. In: Buchsbaum HJ, Schmidt JD, eds. *Gynecologic and Obstetric Urology.* Philadelphia, PA: WB Saunders; 1978:301.
45. Gilstrap LC, Hankins GDV, Snyder RR, Greenberg RT. Acute pyelonephritis in pregnancy. *Comprehensive Therapy.* 1986;12:38.
46. Whalley PJ, Cunningham FG, Martin FG. Transient renal dysfunction associated with acute pyelonephritis of pregnancy. *Obstet Gynecol.* 1974;46:174.
47. Cunningham FG, Lucas MJ, Hankins GDV. Pulmonary injury complicating antepartum pyelonephritis. *Am J Obstet Gynecol.* 1987;156:797.
48. Cunningham FG, Leveno KJ, Hankins GDV, Whalley PJ. Respiratory insufficiency associated with pyelonephritis during pregnancy. *Obstet Gynecol.* 1984;63:121.
49. Cox SM, Shelburne P, Mason RA, Cunningham FG. Erythrocyte morphology in women with acute antepartum pyelonephritis. Infectious Disease Society for Obstetrics & Gynecology. Snowmass, CO. August 1988;Abstract.
50. Cunningham FG, Morris GB, Mickal A. Acute pyelonephritis of pregnancy: A clinical review. *Obstet Gynecol.* 1973;42:112.
51. Leigh DA, Gruneberg RN, Brumfitt W. Long-term follow-up of bacteriuria of pregnancy. *Lancet.* 1968;1:603.
52. Freedman LR. Chronic pyelonephritis at autopsy. *Ann Int Med.* 1967;66:697.
53. Gilstrap LC, Wendel GD. Urinary tract infections in pregnancy. *The Female Patient.* 1988;13:57.
54. Cox SM, Cunningham FG. Ureidopenicillin therapy for acute antepartum pyelonephritis. *Curr Ther Res.* 1989;44:1029.
55. Harris RE, Gilstrap LG. Prevention of recurrent pyelonephritis during pregnancy. *Obstet Gynecol.* 1974;44:637.

Chapter One Hundred and Forty-Four

Acute Renal Failure

Marshall D. Lindheimer and Adrian I. Katz

144

Thirty years ago the incidence of acute renal failure (ARF) in pregnancy was estimated at 1 in 2000 to 1 in 5000 gestations and represented a considerable portion of cases reported in large series. More recently, the number of patients with renal failure from obstetric causes has declined markedly, and the incidence is now estimated to be less than one in 10,000 pregnancies.[1,2] This trend, attributed to liberalization of abortion laws and improvement of prenatal care, has not been shared by the poorer and less industrialized nations, where such patients still account for up to 25% of referrals to dialysis centers and where renal failure in pregnancy continues to be a significant cause of maternal and fetal mortality. This chapter reviews the causes, pathophysiology, and treatment of ARF in pregnant women, focusing on several diseases peculiar to this population.

PERSPECTIVE

Definitions and Etiology

Acute renal failure is a dramatic syndrome characterized by a sudden decrease in renal function accompanied by rapidly progressing azotemia and often, but not always, by oliguria. (In about one fifth of all cases urine volume is maintained; these are called *nonoliguric acute renal failure.*) Clinical appreciation of what constitutes a rapid rise in creatinine and urea nitrogen levels or the definition of true oliguria may be difficult, but the more commonly accepted values are increments of plasma creatinine and urea nitrogen levels of at least 0.5 mg/dL and 10 mg/dL daily, respectively, and a reduction of urinary volume to below 400 mL/per day.[3] The causes of such deterioration may be *prerenal* (causing kidney hypoperfusion), renal parenchymal, or *postrenal* (obstructive) in origin, and include renal ischemia (the most common offender), nephrotoxins, obstructive uropathy, intrinsic renal disease such as acute nephritis, and coagulation disorders.

Diagnosis

The causes of ARF include rapidly reversible and specifically treatable entities such as hypoperfusion, obstruction, and certain intrarenal parenchymal and vascular diseases. These must be differentiated from the more common acute tubular necrosis. A more ominous condition, acute cortical necrosis, is less common. Diagnosis, often apparent from clinical circumstances as well as a careful history and physical examination, may be very difficult because these diseases all lead to an identical syndrome of deteriorating renal function. In such circumstances, the chemical composition and tonicity of the urine as well as microscopic examination may be helpful. For example, urine sediment containing few formed elements or only hyaline casts suggests prerenal azotemia or obstructive uropathy; brownish pigmented casts and increased numbers of tubular cells, acute tubular necrosis; red blood cells and casts, glomerular nephritis or a vascular inflammatory disease; and clumps of polymorphonuclear leukocytes or their presence in casts, acute pyelonephritis. On the other hand, acute tubular necrosis may occur with minimal urinary findings. In acute cortical necrosis, the patient is often anuric.

Urine osmolality, specific gravity, and the concentrations of sodium, creatinine, and urea also are helpful in differentiating causes of ARF. Urine tonicity tends to be high in prerenal failure, whereas isosthenuria suggests acute tubular necrosis. The urine to plasma (U/P) osmolality ratio is a sensitive index, values <1.1 being characteristic of acute tubular necrosis.

In prerenal failure, sodium is avidly reabsorbed, and its concentration decreases below 10 mEq/L in random samples, whereas reabsorptive capacity is impaired in tubular necrosis so that urine sodium concentration is at least 25 mEq/L in patients with the latter form of oliguric failure. This index, however, may be misleading in differentiating nonoliguric causes of renal failure. A helpful way of ascertaining the capacity of the kidney to handle sodium is to calculate fractional sodium excretion $[(U/P_{Na}/(U/P)_{creatinine}]$ or its index $[U_{Na}/(U/P)_{creatinine}]$. In prerenal failure, these indices rarely exceed a value of 1.[3,4]

The $(U/P)_{urea}$ and $(U/P)_{creatinine}$ ratios also are valuable in distinguishing prerenal failure from acute tubular necrosis: $(U/P)_{urea}$ usually is greater than 20 in prerenal failure but below 3 in tubular necrosis, and $(U/P)_{creatinine}$ is often ≈ 40 (at least >10) when failure is prerenal and always below 15 in acute tubular necrosis.

Table 144–1 summarizes means of differentiating rapidly reversible prerenal failure from acute tubular necrosis. An important clinical requirement is to ensure that these tests are performed prior to the institution of therapeutic maneuvers such as volume replacement, the infusion of mannitol, or the administration of "loop" diuretics. Finally, the pattern of urinary flow is another aid to ascertaining the cause of rapidly declining renal function. Complete anuria is unusual in acute tubular necrosis but occurs in cortical necrosis, certain forms of rapidy progressive nephritis, disseminated or intrarenal coagulopathy, and bilateral ureteral obstruction. Wide fluctuations in daily urinary volume suggest intermittent obstructive uropathy, and normal urine volume or polyuria can occur when the obstruction is partial.

Course and Management

The course and management of ARF in general are detailed elsewhere.[2,3,5] Briefly, acute tubular necrosis is divided classically into an oliguric, polyuric, and recovery phase. Death during the oliguric period from uremia, hyperkalemia, and volume overload may be avoided by scrupulous and conservative management, with attention to fluid restriction and with diets devoid of protein or containing only essential amino acids, as well as use of hemodialysis or peritoneal dialysis. Dehydration, hypokalemia, and other forms of electrolyte imbalance may complicate the polyuric phase; ARF patients in general are highly susceptible to bacterial infections, which must be promptly treated.

Prognosis is related to the underlying cause and the health of the patient prior to renal failure. Nevertheless, despite decades of improved understanding of the pathophysiology and treatment of ARF, mortality remains high, varying between 20% and 70% of all cases.

ACUTE RENAL FAILURE IN OBSTETRICS

As noted in the introduction, the incidence of ARF in pregnancy has declined more than fourfold from values reported 20 years ago and is now below 0.01%. For instance, in 11 reports of ARF occurring mainly during the 1950s and 1960s, 22% of 5725 cases were related to obstetrics.[1] During this same period renal failure was a substantial cause of maternal mortality; 18% of gravidas with this complication died. More recently, a striking decrease in admission for renal failure complicating obstetrics has been noted, mainly in the industrialized countries, primarily because of liberalized abortion laws and improved perinatal care. For example, in France, obstetrics-related cases constituted 40% of all instances of ARF in 1966 but declined to 4.5% in 1978 because of the virtual disappearance of cases caused by septic abortion. Data from one center are shown in Fig. 144–1. Similarly, maternal mortality from ARF seems to have declined substantially[1,2], but some authorities have noted that women currently presenting with ARF in gestation still have a guarded prognosis, for a greater proportion of these cases are now the result of more ominous diseases such as idiopathic postpartum renal failure and acute cortical necrosis.

In contrast to the situation in developed nations, there are still parts of the world in which the incidence of severe

TABLE 144–1. DIFFERENTIAL DIAGNOSIS OF OLIGURIA

	Prerenal Failure	Acute Tubular Necrosis
History	Vomiting, diarrhea, and other causes of dehydration	Dehydration, ischemic insult, or ingestion of nephrotoxin; however, no specific history in 50% of cases.
Physical examination	Decreased blood pressure, increased pulse, poor skin turgor.	May also have signs of dehydration, but physical examination often normal.
Urine analysis	Concentrated urine, few formed elements in sediment, but many hyalin casts	Isosthenuria; sediment contains renal tubular cells and pigmented casts but may be normal.
Urinary sodium	<20 mEq/L, most <10 mEq/L	At least 25 mEq/L; usually >60 mEq/L
Urine/plasma ratios		
Osmolality	Often 1.5 or greater	<1.1
Urea	>20	<3
Creatinine	>40	<15
Fractional Na excretion	$<1\%$	$>1\%$
Renal failure index $[U_{Na}/(U/P)_{creatinine}]$	<1	>1

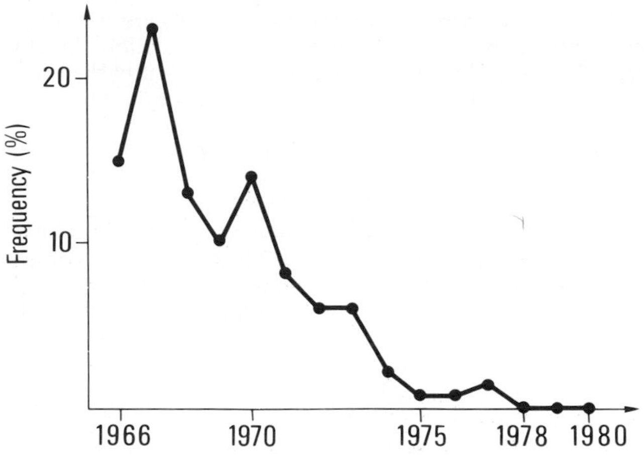

Figure 144–1. Incidence of acute renal failure following septic abortion among all patients with acute renal failure referred to the Nephrology Service at the Necker Hospital (Paris) from 1966 through 1980. (*From Lindheimer et al*[1] *with permission.*)

ARF in pregnancy remains high. In northern India, for example, 22% of the patients referred for dialysis have disease related to pregnancy, and their mortality approaches 55%.[1,6]

The frequency distribution of ARF during pregnancy was at one time bimodal: an initial peak early in gestation comprising most of the cases associated with septic abortion and a second peak between gestational weeks 35 and the puerpuerium, primarily because of preeclampsia and bleeding complications, especially abruptio placentae. Where liberalized abortion laws exist, the initial peak has declined markedly or disappeared.

Renal Failure in Septic Abortion

Prior to the legalization of abortion, it was estimated that there were between 200,000 and 1,000,000 illegal abortions annually in the United States alone; up to 5% of these women became critically ill. Although there has been a marked decline and even apparent disappearance of these severe syndromes, one should remain alert to this complication in view of the increasing likelihood that some countries may repeal their existing laws permitting clinic-based abortion.

Clinical Presentation. Septic abortions, especially those infected with clostridia and *Escherichia coli*, may cause striking clinical syndromes. Onset may be sudden, from several hours to 2 days after attempted abortion. One may be misled by a seemingly asymptomatic patient, admitted because of an incomplete abortion, who rapidly develops shock by the next morning. The disease is characterized by an abrupt rise in temperature (40°C or above) and the presence of myalgia; vomiting; and diarrhea, occasionally bloody. Muscular pain is generalized but most intense in the proximal limbs, thorax, and abdomen. The clinical picture may be confused with intra-abdominal inflammatory disease, especially when a history of provoked abortion is denied or not sought, and vaginal bleeding is surprisingly absent in a significant number of patients. Once signs and symptoms develop, hypotension, dyspnea, and progression to frank shock occur rapidly. The patient usually is jaundiced and has a peculiar bronze color ascribed to the association of jaundice with cutaneous vasodilation, cyanosis, and pallor. Despite fever, the extremeties often are cold, and purplish areas, the precursors of small patches of necrosis on toes, fingers, or nose, may be present.

Characteristic laboratory findings include severe anemia as a result of hemolysis, and direct bilirubin levels are markedly elevated, usually above 10 mg/dL. There also may be evidence of disseminated intravascular coagulation. A striking leukocytosis ($\approx$25,000/mm^3) with a marked shift to the left and thrombocytopenia below 50,000/mm^3 are often noted. Hypocalcemia, severe enough to provoke tetany, has been described. The urine is scanty, and both hemoglobin and qualitative proteinuria (4+) are present. Red blood cells and pigmented casts are seen in the sediment. An abdominal x-ray may demonstrate air in the uterus or abdomen caused by gas-forming organisms or perforation.

Despite the toxic and septicemic picture described above, the identification of bacteria is difficult. The situation is confused further by the normal presence of clostridia in the female genital tract.

Death occurs only hours after the attempted abortion in approximately 7% of these cases; in most others, fever and symptoms usually respond to antibiotic treatment and volume replacement, leaving a patient who requires management of her renal failure. The role of surgical intervention, including hysterectomy, is discussed below. Persistence of fever beyond 48 hours suggests a mixed infection, which should be identified and treated.

There is another group of patients whose symptoms develop more insidiously and in whom fever persists longer. On occasion, a toxic hemolytic syndrome develops only after 2 or 3 days, but muscle pain, gross hemolysis, and hemoglobinuria are absent or minimal.

The clinical course of the renal failure is usually that of acute tubular necrosis in general, although bilateral or patchy cortical necrosis may occur. The latter diseases result in irreversible total or almost total renal failure. The oliguric phase in patients with septic abortion often is prolonged to three or more weeks, and anuria may occur during this period. Often, it is just when one suspects that the patient has cortical rather than tubular necrosis that the diuretic phase begins.

Etiology. The ARF associated with septic abortion may have multiple causes. Vomiting leads to volume depletion, and sepsis may aggravate the hypotension, a combination that leads to severe renal ischemia. Hemoglobuinuria also is present. The agents used to provoke abortion, such as Lysol, may be nephrotoxic. It also is of interest that whereas sepsis in pregnancy usually is caused by gram-negative bacteria, clostridia, which are responsible for 0.5% or fewer of the cases developing shock, frequently are associated with renal failure. This has led some to postulate that these organisms produce a specific nephrotoxin. It also is claimed that gravidas are more susceptible to syndromes resembling a generalized Shwartzman-like reaction and that endotoxemia precipitating such a syndrome may be responsible for the occasional case of cortical necrosis that occurs after septic abortion. However, the incidence of cortical necrosis in early pregnancy (when most septic abortion occurs) is no different from that in nonpregnant women.

Treatment. The initial steps should include vigorous supportive therapy and antibiotics (usually high-dose penicillin, an aminoglycoside or another drug with broad-spectrum coverage for gram-negative organisms, and often a third agent such as clindamycin. Use of antitoxin when clostridia are present and treatment of these organisms with hyperbaric oxygen and exchange transfusion remain controversial. The greatest controversy, however, exists over the role of a surgical intervention. Some who believe the uterus is a huge culture medium for bacterial growth and toxin formation state that rapid removal of this organ is crucial if the mother is to survive. The picture of a necrotic and grossly infected uterus that often accompanies chemically produced abortions is sufficient to convince many that hysterectomy is necessary. Others, however, note that modern-day antibiotics are sufficient and that surgery when the patient is so critically ill may be too risky. Data have been reported supporting both the radical and conservative approaches.[1,7,8]

Acute Pyelonephritis and Renal Failure

Acute pyelonephritis, the most common infectious complication of gestation, is more likely to lead to ARF in gravidas than in nonpregnant women.[1,9] The reason is obscure, but a report by Whalley et al[10] on the effect of acute pyelonephritis on kidney function is revealing. These authors noted that such infections in pregnant women were accompanied by marked decrements in glomerular filtration rates and significant increases in their serum creatinine levels. This contrasts with the situation in nongravid women, in whom acute pyelonephritis is said to have little effect on renal function. Whalley and colleagues[10] suggest that the vasculature of gravidas may be more sensitive to the vasoactive effects of bacterial endotoxins. Acute pyelonephritis during pregnancy has been associated with hypotension[11] and on occasion renal vein thrombosis.[9] Thus, the potential gravity of pyelonephritis in pregnancy should not be underestimated, and such patients should always be hospitalized, observed closely, and treated aggressively with antibiotics and appropriate supportive measures.

Volume Contraction from Bleeding and Dehydration

Uterine hemorrhage is a major cause of ARF in late pregnancy and the puerperium. Antepartum bleeding can be more difficult to diagnose than that which occurs postpartum because it may not be observed externally ("concealed hemorrhage"). Uterine hemorrhage most often leads to acute tubular necrosis, but in certain women with abruption or coinciding preeclampsia, cortical necrosis occasionally ensues.

Volume depletion is probably the precipitating cause of acute tubular necrosis complicating hyperemesis gravidarum or when severe vomiting occurs with pyelonephritis. In the former disease, dietary deficiency and renal potassium loss lead to hypokalemia, another factor contributing to the decrease in glomerular filtration rate. In many of the cases in which hyperemesis gravidarum was associated with ARF, vomiting occurred or continued until late in pregnancy. Functional vomiting beyond the first trimester is uncommon and should prompt the clinician to search for organic causes.

Preeclampsia and Eclampsia

Preeclampsia is accompanied by a number of renal changes (see also Chapter 139). The glomerulus increases in size because of swelling of cells. This and the generalized vasoconstriction characteristic of the disease leads to renal ischemia, proteinuria, and a reduction in glomerular filtration, which averages 25% below values in normal pregnancy but is comparable to that in nonpregnant women. In most instances, therefore, serum creatinine levels are usually at or slightly above values for the general population. At Chicago Lying-in Hospital, for example, severe preeclamptics are frequently delivered when serum creatinine levels are only minimally greater than 1 mg/dL. In a group of patients in whom preeclampsia was confirmed by renal biopsy (the biopsied women are primarily those with the most severe disease), the mean was 1.1 mg/dL (SE ± 0.3).[12] Surprisingly, in several of the biopsies that showed ultrastructural evidence of preeclampsia, there were light microscopic changes suggesting acute tubular necrosis, which had not been suspected clinically because serum creatinine levels had hardly increased and renal function improved rapidly after delivery. Such data underscore the fact that even at these creatinine levels (normal in nongravid terms), the preeclamptic gravida, having lost 50% of her normal function for pregnancy with a relatively ischemic kidney, already may be in an early phase of acute tubular necrosis.

In view of the above changes, it is not surprising that on occasion preeclampsia will progress to frank ARF; it is listed as an important cause of this complication in late pregnancy.[1,6,9] This is true especially in the older literature when the disease often was not diagnosed or, if it was detected, the patient often was observed for considerable periods of time prior to intervention. Because of the increased survival of low-weight babies, obstetricians currently intervene early, thus avoiding such complications as eclampsia and progression of the renal lesion.

Some preeclamptic women manifest signs of consumption coagulopathy and on occasion develop marked intravascular hemolysis. Thus, decrements in their renal function also may be ascribed to disseminated intravascular coagulation and hemoglobinuria. In the past, 20% of the kidneys of eclamptic women who had autopsies contained intratubular hemoglobin casts. Finally, intravascular volume is decreased in the vasoconstricted, hemoconcentrated, preeclamptic patients, and the susceptibility of hypertensive gravidas to the development of prerenal azotemia when salt is restricted or when they are treated with diuretics has been amply demonstrated.[13,14] Such patients, who also have an increased incidence of *abruptio placentae,* may be more susceptible to the adverse renal effects of antepartum or intrapartum blood loss than are normal gravidas.

Acute renal failure accompanying preeclampsia usually is caused by tubular necrosis. However, preeclampsia has been known to progress to cortical necrosis, and in some series preeclamptics account for a surprisingly large number of patients with this complication.[6] (See also Chapter 139.)

Renal Cortical Necrosis

Renal cortical necrosis, a morphologic diagnosis, is characterized by tissue death throughout the cortex with sparing of the medullary portions of the kidney.[1,2,6,9,15-17] Fortunately, this complication is not common in general, but when it occurs, it is found more in obstetric than in nonpregnant patients. Acute cortical necrosis may develop in patients with intravascular coagulation that sometimes complicates septic abortion, but cortical necrosis is actually more common in late pregnancy or the puerperium, when septic complications occur less often.

Cortical necrosis is more likely to occur in multigravidas who are beyond 30 years of age and tends to be associated with certain obstetric complications. Most of the cases occur in association with *abruptio placentae* and less commonly with prolonged intrauterine death. At one time it was estimated that cortical necrosis occurred in one of every 200 instances of *abruptio placentae* with unrecognized retroplacental bleeding, but currently the incidence is much lower.[1,2] Still, *abruptio placentae* should be suspected when ARF develops between gestational weeks 26 and 30, because 45% of the cases in one series[17] had concealed hemorrhage. It is of interest that similar blood losses in nonpregnant patients do not lead to cortical necrosis. The incidence of cortical necrosis associated with preeclampsia is disputed. Some find little evidence of an association, whereas others report it in as many as 11% of the patients described.[1]

Although cortical necrosis may involve the entire renal cortex, resulting in irreversible renal failure, it is the incomplete or patchy variety that occurs more often in pregnancy.[1,17] The latter condition is characterized by an initial episode of severe oliguria and even anuria, the duration of which is considerably longer than that of uncomplicated acute tubular necrosis. This is followed by a variable return of function and a stable period of moderate renal insufficiency. Years later, renal function decreases again, at times leading to end-stage renal failure.[9] The reason for this course is obscure.

Diagnosis of cortical necrosis is based on renal biopsy or selective angiography.[17] Both methods may provide information about the extent of the lesion. Cortical calcification is a late sign, appearing six weeks or later after the onset of the disease. It is obvious that the biopsy needle may miss the lesion in women with patchy necrosis. Thus, the diagnosis should still be considered in women with incomplete functional recovery even if the tissue sample reveals no necrosis. By arteriography one notes lack of a cortical nephrogram in complete necrosis (Fig. 144–2A) and a heterogeneous appearance in the patchy variety (Fig. 144–2B).

Renal blood flow measured with the ^{133}Xe washout technique has been found to be profoundly decreased in patients with cortical necrosis. Flows are usually less than 50 mL/100 g per minute, compared with values above 100 mL/100 g per minute in pregnant women with acute tubular necrosis, even though the clinical picture of the two conditions can be very similar.[17] Unfortunately, ^{133}Xe washout methodology is a research tool that usually is unavailable to the clinician.

Why pregnant women develop cortical necrosis more readily than nonpregnant patients is obscure. Many of these patients are older multiparas, and in some cases arteriolar nephrosclerosis is present in the biopsy, suggesting that their kidneys were more vulnerable to the inciting factor (ie, ischemia or coagulation). Some authors attribute the pathogenesis to severe and prolonged selective renal vasospasm, which may be followed by local activation of coagu-

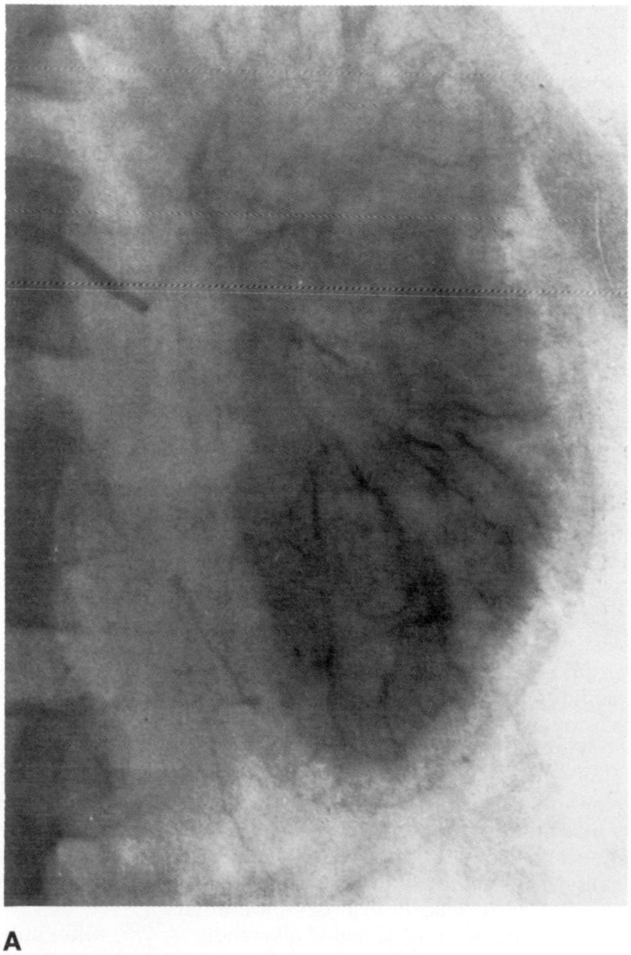

A

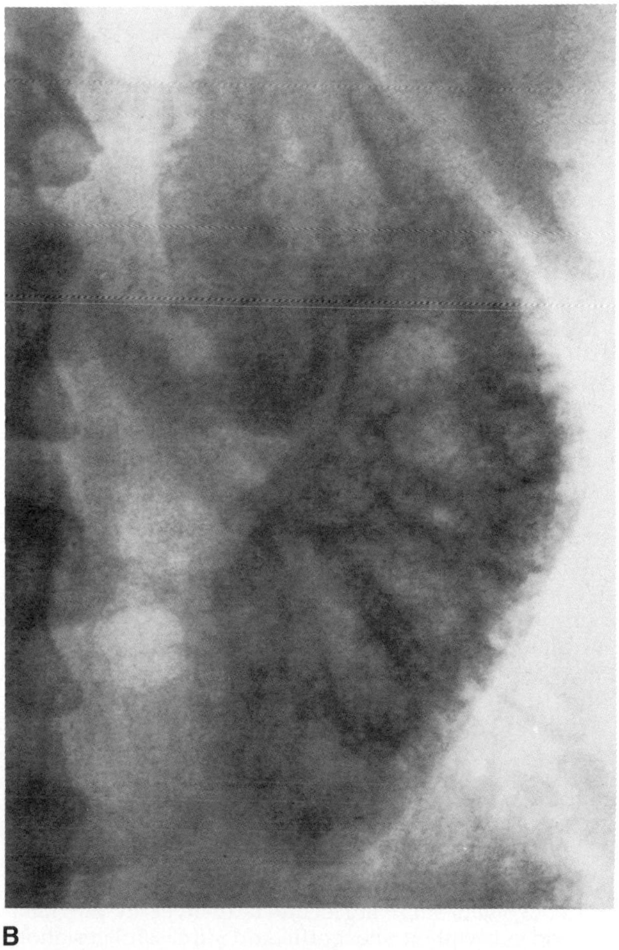

B

Figure 144–2. (A) Selective left renal arteriogram in total cortical necrosis. Cortical nephrogram is absent. The outer edge of the cortex is poorly outlined and is separated from the inner by a clear, nonvascularized area. (B) Selective left renal arteriogram demonstrating partial (patchy) cortical necrosis. The cortical nephrogram is nonhomogeneous with alternating clear (necrotic) areas and densely striped perfused regions. An appreciable amount of the inner cortex also was spared. This patient had partial recovery of function. (*From Kleinknecht et al*[17] *with permission.*)

lation; others attribute a primary role to the coagulopathies. The Sanarelli–Shwartzman reaction can be produced more easily in pregnant animals than in nongravid controls.[18]

Acute Fatty Liver of Pregnancy

Fatty infiltration of the liver (see also Chapter 151), a complication of pregnancy that affects primarily primigravidas, is characterized by jaundice and severe hepatic dysfunction in late pregnancy or the immediate puerperium and is often complicated by renal failure. Until 1980, this disease was considered a rare but lethal disorder. Fewer than 100 cases had been described, and the estimated incidence was one per million gestations, while both fetal and maternal mortality approached 85%.[1,19] Subsequently, many more cases of varying severity have been described, and the incidence is now believed to be 1 in 13,000, with >90% of the women and >75% of the fetuses surviving.[1] The typical patient presents with fever, abdominal pain, and nausea; vomiting as an early clue may be overlooked and considered functional because the patient is pregnant. She then develops jaundice and hepatic encephalopathy. Laboratory tests often reveal evidence of disseminated intravascular coagulopathy, including decreases in antithrombin III. Some authors note a high incidence of hypertension accompanying the coagulation changes and suggest that acute fatty liver is a variant of preeclampsia.[20] Other abnormalities include marked hyperbilirubinemia with only minimally elevated transaminases. Alkaline phosphatase and amylase levels also may be elevated and hyperammonemia may be present. Serum urate levels may be elevated out of proportion to the degree of renal dysfunction, another similarity to preeclampsia.

The hepatic lesion is characterized by the deposition of fat microdroplets within the hepatocytes, most prominently in the central portion of the lobule. Inflammation and necrosis usually are absent but there are exceptions[20,21] and some cases of acute fatty liver may be misdiagnosed as hepatitis. Ultrastructural changes in the mitochondria resembling those in livers of children with Reye's syndrome have been described.[22] The renal lesion is variable: The kidney may be morphologically normal or may manifest fatty vacuolization of tubular cells, focal tubular cell necrosis, or nonspecific changes consistent with tubular regeneration. In addition, light microscopic and ultrastructural changes similar to those seen in the hemolytic-uremic syndrome also have been described.

The cause of acute fatty liver in pregnancy is unknown, as is why it is often complicated by renal failure. Tetracycline toxicity was implicated in the past, but this disease predated the antibiotic era, and cases continue to appear even though tetracycline is used very rarely in obstetric practice. It recently has been suggested that this disease is an adult form of Reye's syndrome provoked by the metabolic stress of pregnancy. Consistent with this hypothesis is the description of urea cycle enzyme deficiencies similar to those seen in Reye's syndrome.[22] Treatment of acute fatty liver in pregnancy consists of rapid termination of the gestation and supportive therapy for hepatic and renal failure. The efficacy of pregnancy termination, however, has not been proved. Finally, women surviving acute fatty liver in pregnancy have had subsequent uneventful and successful gestations, a fact that does not support the hypothesis that these patients have hepatic enzyme deficiencies such as those expected in an adult form of Reye's syndrome.

Obstruction

Urinary tract obstruction secondary to stones is discussed elsewhere in this text (see Chapter 146). In addition, in describing the physiologic changes that occur in the ureter during gestation (see Chapter 142), the authors note that ureteral dilatation may be obstructive in origin. Whether the enlarging uterus is ever associated with ARF in pregnancy was long debated but rarely substantiated, and the very fact that glomerular filtration rate in gravidas remains elevated despite ureteral dilatation argued against this possibility. Nevertheless, cases have been described in which ARF in late pregnancy caused by obstruction from an enlarging uterus seems to have been adequately documented[1,23,24], and severe oligoanuria in a woman with a single kidney has been reported.[1]

When renal dysfunction secondary to obstruction is suspected, the pregnant patient should be placed in lateral recumbency or asked to assume a knee-chest position because both of these postures should relieve the obstruction if it is caused by the enlarged uterus.

Idiopathic Postpartum Renal Failure

Idiopathic postpartum renal failure[1,9], characterized by the onset of renal failure in the puerperium after an uneventful gestation, was first delineated as a specific clinical entity during the 1960s.[22-24] By 1983, fewer than 100 cases had been reported under a variety of names such as postpartum malignant nephrosclerosis, accelerated nephrosclerosis and postpartum acute renal failure in normotensive women, irreversible postpartum renal failure, late postpartum intravascular coagulation with acute renal failure, and postpartum hemolytic-uremic syndrome.

Idiopathic postpartum renal failure may occur one day to several weeks after delivery. A typical patient presented with oliguria or at times anuria, rapidly progressing azotemia, and frequently with evidence of microangiopathic hemolytic anemia or consumption coagulopathy. Blood pressure on admission was normal or only minimally elevated in early descriptions of this disease, although severe accelerated hypertension has been reported in the more recent literature. Some patients exhibited extrarenal manifestations involving the cardiovascular (cardiac dilatation and congestive heart failure) and central nervous systems (lethargy, convulsions) that appeared disproportionate to the degree of uremia, hypertension, or volume overload present.

The etiology of this syndrome is obscure, and suggestions include a viral illness prior to the onset of the disease, retained placental fragments, or drugs such as ergotamine compounds, oxytocic agents, or oral contraceptives prescribed shortly after delivery. Several patients manifested hypocomplementemia, suggesting a possible immunologic cause. Deficiencies in prostaglandin production and antithrombin III levels akin to those described in the hemolytic-uremic syndrome have been ascribed to idiopathic postpartum renal failure as well.

The pathophysiology of idiopathic postpartum renal failure has been compared with that of thrombotic thrombocytopenic purpura as well as other diseases characterized by disseminated intravascular coagulation such as the adult hemolytic-uremic syndrome. This disease also has been compared with the generalized Shwartzman reaction, which develops more readily in pregnant animals.

The renal lesions, detailed elsewhere[1,9,28-30], differ substantially in various reports but fall into two general categories: changes in the glomerular capillaries resembling those seen in the hemolytic-uremic syndrome and arteriolar lesions reminiscent of malignant nephrosclerosis or scleroderma. Immunofluorescent staining is nonspecific; fibrin-like material often is present in the mesangium, glomerular capillary walls, and arterioles, and C_3 deposits also are commonly seen. The presence of other immunoglobulins has been rare and inconsistent.

The prognosis is guarded. Most women have succumbed, required chronic dialysis, or have survived with severely reduced renal function; only a few have recovered. Of interest is a patient reported to have a mild form of *postpartum hemolytic syndrome* whose disease occurred in two successive gestations.[31]

Treatment is aimed primarily at reduction of high blood pressure, when present, and general supportive measures are used for all patients with ARF. In the past[6], bilateral nephrectomy was used as a lifesaving measure in a few women with accelerated hypertension unresponsive to treatment. This should be unnecessary today when potent vasodilators, converting enzyme blockers, and calcium-channel blocking agents are available.

Some investigators have claimed that the early use of anticoagulant therapy such as heparin and fibrinolytic agents may reverse renal failure. To date, these data are not convincing, and such drugs are not harmless. In view of the possible contributing role of retained placental fragments, dilatation and curettage should be considered for women in whom this syndrome occurs close to delivery. Other regimens, such as antiplatelet therapy, infusion of blood products including concentrates of antithrombin III, or exchange transfusions, have been advocated on the basis of their alleged success in patients with thrombotic thrombocytopenic purpura or the adult hemolytic-uremic syndrome. However, proof of efficacy in this condition is lacking, and these treatments are not recommended. Finally, several of these patients have received kidney allografts, and most have done well after transplantation.

Miscellaneous Causes of Renal Failure in Pregnancy

Acute renal failure of pregnancy has followed amniotic fluid embolism, intra-amniotic saline administration, and accidents or illnesses unrelated to gestation. The latter include drug ingestion, incompatible blood transfusions, and bacterial endocarditis complicating valvular rheumatic heart disease. Sudden renal failure during gestation has been associated with acute poststreptococcal glomerulonephritis and various collagen diseases, and even with sarcoidosis (the latter of interest as it was reversed with steroids[32]). Finally, gravidas with underlying renal disease but with good or adequate renal function prior to pregnancy may be more susceptible to acute tubular necrosis when their gestations are complicated by superimposed preeclampsia.[33]

DIALYTIC THERAPY IN PREGNANCY

Peritoneal dialysis and hemodialysis both have been used in patients with obstetric renal failure, and neither pelvic peritonitis nor the enlarged uterus is a contraindication to the former method.[1,34] When the peritoneal route is used, the catheter is inserted best high in the abdomen under direct vision. Since both peritoneal dialysis and hemodialysis are safe, choice of procedure should be determined by the underlying clinical situation. For example, the peritoneal route is preferable in the patient with septic shock or any other hypotensive complication and has the advantage that antibiotics can be instilled directly into the peritoneal cavity when peritonitis is present. On the other hand, this method may be difficult in patients who have undergone previous abdominal surgery or in whom traumatic tears in the peritoneum may be evident or suspected. When possible, however, peritoneal dialysis is preferred because it causes more gradual changes in fluid and solute levels, and is less likely to be associated with precipitous hypotension or premature contractions. The above problems can be minimized in hemodialysis patients by using daily treatments for shorter time periods and avoiding high flux technology.

Since urea, creatinine, and probably other metabolites that accumulate in uremia cross the placenta, dialysis should be undertaken early in pregnant women. The aim of the treatment should be to maintain urea nitrogen levels at or below 50 mg/dL. The advantages of early dialysis proposed for nonpregnant patients become more germane for gravidas, making the argument for prophylactic dialysis compelling. During the dialysis, fluid balance should be monitored carefully with caution taken to avoid excessive shifts that might lead to decreased uteroplacental perfusion. If the conceptus is near maturity or at a weight at which nursery treatment carries a high probability of survival, it should be delivered as soon as the mother's condition has stabilized. Of importance, however, is alerting pediatric physicians to the fact that the neonate may have a high urea level, and may become dehydrated quickly by the solute diuresis that occurs shortly after delivery.

Prognosis for survival is considerably better in obstetric ARF than in patients whose disease has a surgical or medical cause[1], and maternal mortality has declined sharply in the past 20 years.[1] Prognosis for the fetus, however, is worse than that for the mother, and many pregnancies end in abortion or stillbirth. However, the outlook for the fetus is also improving, as increasing fetal survival is being reported.[9] Finally, there are few data concerning the effects of ARF on subsequent maternal reproductive performance. However, sporadic reports suggest that once patients have recovered, many have no difficulty conceiving or carrying their gestations to term.

REFERENCES

1. Lindheimer MD, Katz AI, Ganeval D, et al. Acute renal failure in pregnancy. In: Brenner BM, Lazarus JM, eds. *Acute Renal Failure.* 2nd ed. New York, NY: Churchill Livingstone; 1988:597.
2. Madias NE, Donohoe JF, Harrington JT. Postischemic acute renal failure. In: Brenner BM, Lazarus JM, eds. *Acute Renal Failure.* 2nd ed. New York, NY: Churchill Livingstone; 1988:251.
3. Brezis M, Rosen S, Epstein FH. Acute renal failure. In: Brenner BM, Rector FC Jr, eds. *The Kidney.* 3rd ed. Philadelphia, PA: WB Saunders; 1986:735.
4. Espinal CH, Gregory AW: Differential diagnosis of acute renal failure. *Clin Nephrol.* 1980;13:73.
5. Brenner BM, Lazarus JM, eds. *Acute Renal Failure, Section IV.* 2nd ed. New York, NY: Churchill Livingstone; 1988:743.
6. Chugh KS, Singhal PC, Shamra BK, et al. Acute renal failure of obstetric origin. *Obstet Gynecol.* 1976;48:642.
7. Bartlett RH, Yahia C. Management of septic abortion with renal failure: report of five consecutive cases with five survivors. *N Engl J Med.* 1969;281:747.
8. Hawkins OF, Sevitt LH, Fairbrother DF, et al. Management of chemical septic abortion with renal failure: use of a conservative regimen. *N Engl J Med.* 1975;292:722.
9. Grünfeld JP, Ganeval D, Bournerias F. Acute renal failure in pregnancy. *Kidney Int.* 1980;18:179.
10. Whalley PJ, Cunningham FG, Martin FG. Transient renal dysfunction associated with acute pyelonephritis of pregnancy. *Obstet Gynecol.* 1975;46:174.
11. Cunningham FG. Urinary tract infections in pregnancy. *Clin Obstet Gynaecol (Ballière).* 1987;1:891.
12. Fisher K, Luger A, Spargo BH, et al. Hypertension in pregnancy: Clinicalpathological correlations and remote prognosis. *Medicine.* 1981; 60:267.
13. Mulé JG, Tatum H, Sawyer RE. "Nitrogenous retention" in patients with toxemia of pregnancy—an unusual complication of salt restriction. *Am J Obstet Gynecol.* 1957;74:526.
14. Palomaki J, Lindheimer MD. Sodium depletion simulating deterioration in a toxemic pregnancy. *N Engl J Med.* 1970;282:88.
15. Sheehan HL, Moore HC. *Renal Cortical Necrosis and The Kidney of Concealed Accidental Hemorrhage.* Springfield, IL: Charles C. Thomas; 1953.

16. Williams TF. Renal cortical necrosis, renal infarction, and hypertension due to renal disease. In: Strauss MB, Welt LG, eds. *Disease of the Kidney*. Boston, MA: Little, Brown; 1963:526.
17. Kleinknecht D, Grunfeld J-P, Gorney PC, et al. Diagnostic procedures and long term prognosis in bilateral renal cortical necrosis. *Kidney Int*. 1973;4:390.
18. Conger JD, Falk S, Guggenheim SJ. Glomerular dynamics and morphologic changes in the generalized Shwartzman reaction in postpartum rats. *J Clin Invest*. 1981;67:1334.
19. Kaplan ML: Acute fatty liver of pregnancy. *N Eng J Med*. 1985;313:367.
20. Reily CA, Latham PS, Romero R, et al. Acute fatty liver of pregnancy. A reassessment based on observations in 9 patients. *Am Int Med*. 1987;106:703.
21. Rolfes DB, Ishak KG. Acute fatty liver of pregnancy: A clinicopathologic study of 35 cases. *Hepatology*. 1985;5:1149.
22. Weber FL, Snodgrass PJ, Powell DE, et al. Abnormalities of hepatic mitochondrial urea-cycle enzyme activities and hepatic ultrastructure in acute fatty liver of pregnancy. *J Lab Clin Med*. 1979;94:27.
23. Homas DC, Blake GD, Harrington JT, et al. Acute renal failure caused by ureteral obstruction of a gravid uterus. *JAMA*. 1981;246:1230.
24. Rasmussen PE, Nielsen FR. Hydronephrosis in pregnancy: A literature survey. *Eur J Obstet Gynecol Reprod Biol*. 1988;27:249.
25. Scheer RL, Jones DB. Malignant nephrosclerosis in women postpartum. *JAMA*. 1967;201:600.
26. Wagoner RD, Holley KE, Johnson WJ. Accelerated nephrosclerosis and postpartum acute renal failure. *Ann Intern Med*. 1968;69:237.
27. Robson JS, Martin AM, Ruckley VA, et al. Irreversible pospartum renal failure: a new syndrome. *QJ Med*. 1968;37:423.
28. Sun NC, Johnson WJ, Sung DTW, et al. Idiopathic postpartum renal failure: Review and report of a successful renal transplantation. *Mayo Clin Proc*. 1975;59:395.
29. Schoolwerth AC, Sandler RC, Klahr S, et al. Postpartum nephrosclerosis and nephrosclerosis in women taking oral contraceptives. A report of two cases. *Arch Intern Med*. 1976;136:178.
30. Segonds A, Louradour N, Suc JM, et al. Postpartum hemolytic uremic syndrome: A study of three cases and a review of the literature. *Clin Nephrol*. 1979;12:229.
31. Gomperts ED, Sessel L, DuPlesis V, et al. Recurrent postpartum haemolytic syndrome. *Lancet*. 1978;1:48.
32. Warren GV, Sprague SM, Corwin HC. Sarcoidosis presenting as acute renal failure in pregnancy. *Am J Kid Dis*. 1988;12:161.
33. Katz AI, Davison JM, Hayslett JP, et al. Pregnancy in women with renal disease. *Kidney Int*. 1980;18:192.
34. Hou S. Peritoneal dialysis and haemodialysis in pregnancy. *Clin Obstet Gynaecol (Ballière)*. 1987;1:1009.

Chapter One Hundred and Forty-Five
Chronic Renal Disease

John M. Davison and Marshall D. Lindheimer

145

DISTURBANCES OF RENAL FUNCTION

Familiarity with the anatomic and physiologic changes in the urinary system of normal gravidas is important in the detection and management of renal problems during pregnancy. These conditions have already been discussed in this section (Chapter 142), and it is against this background that pregnancy in women with various renal problems is discussed.

PREGNANCY IN WOMEN WITH CHRONIC RENAL DISEASE

The majority view is that with the exception of certain specific disease entities such as systemic lupus erythematosus (SLE), renal polyarteritis nodosa, and scleroderma, outcome usually is successful provided that renal function is at most moderately compromised and hypertension is minimal or absent. Furthermore, pregnancy does not adversely affect the natural history of the renal disease; however, there are four entities that are controversial: IgA nephropathy, membranous proliferative glomerulonephritis, reflux nephropathy, and focal glomerular sclerosis (FGS). Some believe that pregnancy adversely affects the course of these diseases. Others believe that the outcome is similar to that of most other renal disorders (Figures 145–1 and 145–2 and Table 145–1).[1-4]

In women with chronic renal disease, the pathology may be both chemically and clinically silent. Most individuals remain symptom-free until their glomerular filtration rate (GFR) falls to approximately 25% of its original level. Many plasma constituents frequently are normal until a late stage of the disease. As renal function declines, the ability to conceive, let alone to sustain a viable pregnancy, decreases.[1-6] Degrees of functional impairment that do not cause symptoms or do not appear to disrupt homeostasis in nonpregnant individuals can jeopardize pregnancy.

Normal pregnancy is very unusual when renal function decreases to a degree that nonpregnant creatinine and urea nitrogen levels exceed 3 mg/dL and 30 mg/dL, respectively. These increments above normal nonpregnant levels are moderate but represent considerable loss of function. The basic question for a woman with renal disease is whether pregnancy is advisable. If it is, the sooner she starts to plan a family the better, since in many cases renal function will continue to decline with time. Women are not always counseled prior to pregnancy and may therefore present as a *fait accompli* with suspected or known renal disease. And then the question must be: Should the pregnancy continue?

Renal Impairment and the Impact of Pregnancy

Obstetric and renal prognoses differ in women with different degrees of renal insufficiency. The impact of pregnancy is best considered by categories of functional renal status prior to conception (Table 145–2).[1,4,6-8]

Preserved or Mildly Impaired Renal Function. Women with chronic renal disease, but normal or mildly decreased prepregnancy renal function (plasma creatinine ≤1.4 mg/dL or 124 umol/L), usually have a successful obstetric outcome and pregnancy does not adversely affect the course of their disease.[7-9] Although true for most patients, some suggest that this statement be tempered for focal glomerular sclerosis, IgA and reflux nephropathies, and perhaps membranoproliferative glomerulonephritis, which appear to be more sensitive to intercurrent pregnancy.[1] Prognosis is more guarded with SLE, but most of these women do well. However, pregnancy should probably be contraindicated or ter-

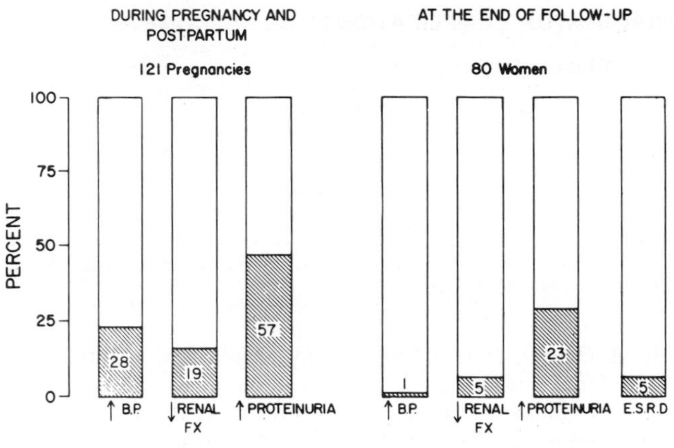

Figure 145–1. The course of renal disease in 89 women during 121 pregnancies and immediately after delivery (three bars on left) and 80 of those women followed up after pregnancy (four bars on right). The numbers within bars are individual pregnancies (on left) and individual women (on right). FX, function; ESRD, end-stage renal disease.

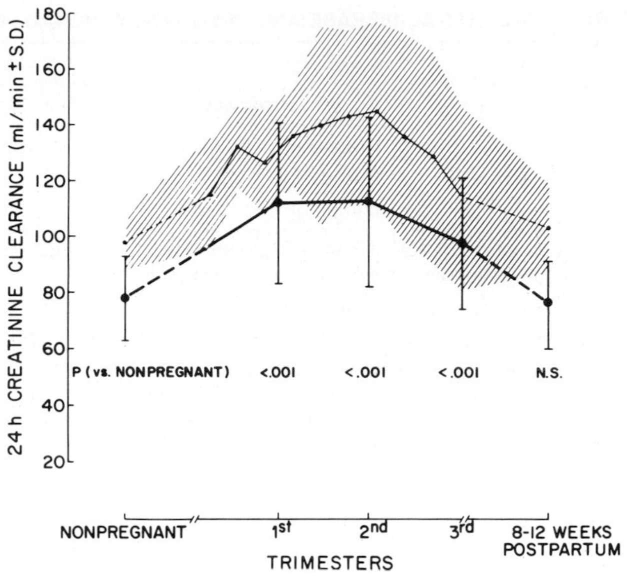

Figure 145–2. Serial 24-hour creatinine clearances (mean ± 1 SD) during pregnancy complicated by chronic renal disease (solid line). Thirty-three pregnancies of 26 women were studied preconception, in each trimester, and 8–12 weeks after delivery. Measurements are from 10 healthy women (mean ± 1 SD) shown by hatched area. (*From Katz et al*[9] *with permission of the authors and publisher.*)

minated in women with periarteritis or scleroderma even when function is preserved.

Most women with mild underlying renal disease show increments in GFR during pregnancy, although the magnitude is less than seen in normal pregnant women. Increased proteinuria is common, occurring in 50% of pregnancies (although rarely in women with chronic pyelonephritis), and it can be massive (often exceeding 3 g in 24 hours).[9] The prevalence of hypertension, renal functional abnormalities and proteinuria, as well as their severity, are considerably lower between pregnancies and during long-term follow up. When renal failure does occur, it usually reflects the inexorable course of a particular renal disease.

TABLE 145–1. OUTCOME OF PREGNANCY IN RELATION TO TYPE OF RENAL DISEASE

Diagnosis	Gravidas	Pregnancies	Fetal Deaths[a]	Neonatal Deaths	Preterm Deliveries	Small-for-gestational-age Infants	Birth Weight of Live Infants[b] 1500 g	1500–2000 g	2000–2500 g	>2500 g
Diffuse glomerulonephritis	26	33	3	3	13	9	6	3	6	13
Focal glomerulonephritis	12	26	2	2	1	6	0	1	7	18
Membranoproliferative glomerulonephritis	4	4	0	0	0	1	0	0	1	3
Membranous nephropathy	7	10	0	0	1	1	0	0	2	5
Lipoid nephrosis	3	6	0	0	1	4	0	0	4	2
Focal glomerulosclerosis	1	1	0	0	0	0	0	0	0	1
Interstitial nephritis (pyelonephritis)	21	26	1	1	4	2	0	1	4	20
Arteriolar nephrosclerosis	8	8	0	0	3	3	2	2	0	4
Others[d]	7	7	1	0	1	1	1	0	1	4
Totals	89	121[c]	7	6	24	27	9	7	25	70
Percent			5.7%	4.9%	20.0%	24.3%	8.1%	6.3%	22.5%	63.1%

[a] Stillbirths and second-trimester spontaneous abortions.
[b] Birth weight available for only 111 of the 116 live infants.
[c] Two sets of twins.
[d] Includes sickle cell nephropathy (two patients) and polycystic disease, IgA nephropathy, diabetic glomerulosclerosis, renal amyloidosis, and bilateral renal artery stenosis (one case of each).

TABLE 145–2. RENAL DISEASE AND PREGNANCY: RENAL FUNCTIONAL STATUS, COMPLICATIONS AND OUTCOME

	Disease Severity		
Prospects	**Mild**	**Moderate**	**Severe**
Pregnancy complications	20%	44%	84%
Successful obstetric outcome	95% (82%)	90% (56%)	47% (8%)
Long-term sequelae	<5%	25% (77%)	58% (92%)

Estimates based on 1069 women/1413 pregnancies (1973–1988) which attained at least 28 weeks gestation (SLE not included). Figures in brackets refer to prospects when pregnancy complications developed prior to 28 gestational weeks. *Adapted from references 1 and 11.*

Moderate Renal Insufficiency. Prognosis is poorer when renal function is moderately impaired before pregnancy (plasma creatinine 1.5–2.5 mg/dL or 133–265 umol/L). It is difficult to draw firm conclusions about pregnancy in these women, chiefly because the number of cases surveyed is still relatively small. Reviews have appeared elsewhere outlining the major problems in this condition as accelerated renal deterioration, uncontrolled hypertension, variable obstetric outcome, and accelerated postdelivery decline in renal function.[1,6,10]

Severe Renal Insufficiency. Most women in this category (plasma creatinine ≥ 3 mg/dL or 265 umol/L) are amenorrheic or anovulatory. The likelihood of conception and having a normal pregnancy and delivery are decreased but are not, as some have thought, impossible. The risk of severe maternal complications is much greater than the probability of a successful obstetric outcome. Realistically, these patients should not take additional health risks, thus pregnancy should be vigorously discouraged. The aim should be to preserve what little renal function remains in these patients or to achieve renal rehabilitation by way of dialysis and a transplant program. The question of pregnancy then can be reconsidered, if appropriate.[11]

PRINCIPLES OF MANAGEMENT

Is Pregnancy Advisable? (Assessment Before Pregnancy)

We prefer to restrict pregnancy to women whose plasma creatinine levels are 2 mg/dL (177 umol/L) or less and who have a diastolic blood pressure of 90 mm Hg or lower (preferably below 80 mm Hg). Others are more strict, recommending that pregnancy should not be undertaken when plasma creatinine concentrations exceed 1.5 mg/100 ml/dL (133 umol/L).[1] Guidelines for assessing advisability of pregnancy should consider that degrees of impairment that do not cause symptoms or appear to disrupt homeostasis in nonpregnancy individuals can still jeopardize pregnancy.[10,11]

Should Pregnancy Continue? (Assessment During Pregnancy)

Occasionally, renal disease is first suspected or noted during pregnancy. It then is essential to establish a diagnosis. If a patient presents with hypertension, proteinuria, or abnormal renal function, it is difficult to distinguish parenchymal renal disease from preeclampsia. A prior history of renal disorders, abnormal urine analysis, a family history of renal disease, or a history of systemic illness known to involve the kidneys obviously is helpful, but in the last analysis, renal disease and preeclampsia may coexist. Assessment of the patient is similar to that of nonpregnant patients, but a definitive diagnosis usually has to be postponed until further assessment after delivery.

Renal Biopsy During Pregnancy—Role and Indications

Experience with renal biopsy in pregnancy is sparse, mainly because clinical circumstances rarely justify the risks. Biopsy therefore is usually deferred until postpartum.[12,13] Reports of excessive bleeding and other complications in pregnant women have led some to consider pregnancy as a relative contraindication of renal biopsy[14], although others have not observed this morbidity.[12,13] When biopsy is undertaken in the immediate postdelivery phase in women with well controlled blood pressure and normal coagulation screen, the morbidity is no different from that reported in the nonpregnant population.[13]

A recent report[15] on 111 biopsies in pregnant women, all preterm, confirms and extends the impression that risks of the procedure resemble those in the nonpregnant population. The incidence of transient gross hematuria (0.9%) [all patients undergoing biopsy have microscopic hematuria unless the kidney has been missed)], was considerably lower than in nonpregnant patients, in which it is 3–5%. Such excellent statistics reflect the experience and technical skills of the unit; statistics also have been improved by refinement of the prebiopsy evaluation.

It is still important, however, to have specific indications for renal biopsy in pregnancy. Packham and Fairley[15] have suggested that closed (percutaneous) needle biopsy should be undertaken very often, because they believe that certain glomerular disorders are adversely influenced by pregnancy and that specific therapy, such as antiplatelet agents, might be beneficial. The consensus, however, goes against such broad indications and reiterates that renal biopsy should be performed infrequently during pregnancy.[13] Even in nonpregnant populations, the reasons for renal biopsy are not clearly defined and experts categorize indications as "most useful," "possibly useful," or "of little or no use."

The few widely agreed upon indications for antepartum biopsy are as follows: (1) Sudden deterioration of renal function prior to 30–32 weeks' gestation with no obvious cause. Certain forms of rapidly progressive glomerulonephritis may respond to aggressive treatment with steroid "pulses," chemotherapy, and perhaps plasma exchange, when diagnosed early. (2) Symptomatic nephrotic syndrome prior to 30–32 weeks' gestation. While some suggest a therapeutic trial of steroids in such cases, it is best to determine beforehand whether the lesion is likely to respond to steroids, because pregnancy is itself a hypercoagulable state prone to worsening by such treatment. A patient with well preserved renal function who has neither marked hypoalbuminemia nor intolerable edema should be examined at more frequent intervals and biopsy deferred until postdelivery. This is because the consensus of most investigators[1,2,5,7-9] is that prognosis is determined mainly by the level of renal function and the presence of hypertension. A similar approach is applied when managing pregnancies with asymptomatic microscopic hematuria alone, when neither stone nor tumor is suggested on sonar. (3) A presentation characterized by "active urinary sediment" (red and white blood cells and casts) with proteinuria and borderline renal function, in a gravida who has not been evaluated in the past. This is a controversial area: It could be argued that diagnosis of a collagen disorder such as scleroderma or periarteritis justifies termination of the pregnancy, or that classification of the type of lesion in a woman with SLE would determine the type and intensity of therapy. The first two diseases are diagnosed infrequently by renal biopsy, and a normotensive woman with stable renal function who has neither systemic involvement nor laboratory evidence of these collagen disorders is watched closely without intervening. Biopsy may be indicated, however, in the latter condition, that is, in selected patients with SLE and lupus nephropathy of uncertain histopathology.

ANTENATAL CARE

Patients with known renal disease should be seen every 2 weeks until 32 weeks' gestation, after which assessment should be weekly. Routine serial antenatal observations should be supplemented with the following:

1. Assessment of renal function, preferably by 24-hour creatinine clearance and protein excretion.
2. Early detection of asymptomatic bacteriuria or confirmation of urinary tract infection.
3. Careful monitoring of blood pressure for early detection of hypertension and assessment of its severity.
4. Early detection of preeclampsia (pregnancy-induced hypertension).
5. Assessment of fetal size, development, and well-being.

Renal Function

If renal function deteriorates at any stage of pregnancy, treatable causes should be sought, such as urinary tract infection; subtle dehydration; or electrolyte imbalance, occasionally precipitated by inadvertent diuretic therapy. Near term, a 15% decrease in function that affects plasma creatinine minimally is permissible. When proteinuria occurs and persists, but blood pressure is normal and renal function is preserved, the pregnancy should be allowed to continue.

Blood Pressure

Most of the specific risks of moderate hypertension appear to be mediated through superimposed preeclampsia. There still is controversy about the incidence of preeclampsia in those women who have preexisting renal disease. This is because the diagnosis cannot be made with certainty on clinical grounds alone, since hypertension and proteinuria may be manifestations of the underlying disease.[4,9] Whereas women with essential hypertension are often not treated until their diastolic levels reach 100 mm Hg. Those with chronic renal disease should be treated more aggressively, aiming to keep diastolic levels between 80–85 mm Hg.

Fetal Surveillance

Assessment of fetal well-being is important because renal disease is associated with intrauterine growth retardation[9] and when complications arise, the judicious moment for intervention is influenced by fetal status. All current antenatal treatments should be used: sonar, antenatal cardiotocography, and amniotic fluid assessment of fetal pulmonary maturity.

Decisions Regarding Delivery

If pregnancy proceeds satisfactorily, it may be advisable to induce labor at 38 weeks because beyond this time, there can be a greater risk of placental failure and intrauterine death. Deliberate preterm delivery is necessary: if renal function deteriorates markedly, if there are signs of impending intrauterine death, if uncontrollable hypertension develops, or if eclampsia occurs. Regardless of gestational age, most babies weighing 1500 g or more survive better in a special care nursery than in a hostile intrauterine environment. Patients should be delivered where full facilities and personnel are available for fetal monitoring, operative delivery, and neonatal resuscitation.

Main Considerations When Counseling Patients

The patient's expectation is usually high. A patient may ask whether pregnancy is advisable or may be harmful to the mother and to the child. Consequently, a balance must be struck between pregnancy outcome and the long-term impact of the pregnancy on the patient.[1,8,11] The crucial determinants are prepregnancy renal function, presence of hypertension (and its management), and the renal disease itself. Other factors are optimal fetal surveillance, more timely delivery, and recent neonatology advances.

Pregnancy does not adversely affect the natural history of the renal lesion if kidney dysfunction is minimal and hypertension is absent before pregnancy, with the exception of a few disorders (see above). An important factor in remote prognosis may be the sclerotic effects that hyperfiltration and increased glomerular capillary pressure may already have had in the residual (intact) glomeruli of these patients.[16,17] Because GFR increases in pregnancy, there is a theoretical possibility that further progressive loss of function could occur; however, this does not seem to be the case in animals during normal pregnancy or when gestation is superimposed on experimental glomerulonephritis.[18,19] Similarly, the superimposition of pregnancy hyperfiltration on the compensatory changes already present in a single kidney could lessen the life span of that kidney. It is theorized that increases in single nephron filtration or glomerular pressure can cause sclerosis[16] within the glomerulus and that in pregnancy further physiological hyperfiltration augments the damage. This does not appear to be the case with rats[18,19], and it also it seems unlikely that women with mild dysfunction have long term sequelae[20], but more data are needed. This especially is true for women with moderately severe renal disease in whom we know that there can be unpredicted accelerated and, at times, irreversible loss of function during or immediately following pregnancy.[1-6]

SPECIFIC DISEASE STATES

Asymptomatic or Covert Bacteriuria

This is a condition in which true bacteriuria exists but in which there are no symptoms or signs of acute urinary tract infection (See also Chapter 143).

Diagnostic Criteria

Pregnant women often present with symptoms of frequency of urination, dysuria, urgency, or nocturia—singly or in combination. Such symptoms are not in themselves diagnostic of urinary tract infection and can be elicited from women with sterile urine.

The growth of bacteria from culture of urine may represent true bacteriuria (the multiplication of bacteria within the urinary tract) or contamination of the urine with urethral or perineal organisms at the time of collection. True bacteriuria can be separated from contamination on the basis of colony counts from a freshly obtained midstream urine specimen (MSU), with 100,000 colonies/mL of urine as the dividing line. Recent evidence, however, indicates that lower colony counts may represent active infection.[21] Two consecutive clean-voided specimens containing the same organism in numbers greater than 100,000 colonies/mL of urine represent true bacteriuria, as does a single suprapubic aspiration with any bacterial growth.[22] A number of presumptive tests based on changes in chemical indicators are available, but they are not reliable for clinical practice.

Asymptomatic bacteriuria is a heterogeneous condition.[23] Several different techniques have been used to try to differentiate between upper and lower urinary tract bacteriuria: ureteral catheterization, bladder washout tests, renal biopsy, urinary concentration tests, and measurement of serum antibody titers. However, none of these techniques is sufficiently precise to localize infections. The identification of antibody-coated bacteria in the urine as a predictor of the presence and site of a urinary tract infection remains controversial.[24]

Epidemiology and Clinical Considerations

It is estimated that 5% of young women develop asymptomatic bacteriuria during childhood, but only 1.2% are infected at any one time.[25] The increased incidence after puberty coincides with sexual activity and varies from 2% to 10% depending on the techniques used for testing and the socioeconomic status of the patients.[23,25]

In pregnancy, true asymptomatic bacteriuria is diagnosed at the first antenatal visit, and fewer than 1.5% subsequently acquire bacteriuria in late pregnancy. Up to 40% of the infected group will develop acute symptomatic urinary tract infection[26,27], and treating this group should prevent approximately 60–70% of all cases of acute urinary tract infection. Nevertheless, about 2% of those with negative cultures will develop acute infections. This means that of the 90–98% that do not have asymptomatic bacteriuria at the initial visit (and therefore are not treated), the number actually at risk of developing acute urinary tract infection is significant, accounting for about 30–40% of all cases of acute urinary tract infection during pregnancy. The available data suggest that the association of asymptomatic bacteriuria with increased fetal loss, prematurity, preeclampsia, and anemia is unproven.[28] Several of these correlations may have resulted from inaccuracies in matching cases and controls, and none appears to be supported by more recent studies.[25,29]

It has been suggested that some 30–40% of pregnant women with asymptomatic bacteriuria have upper urinary tract infection. These women may be a population at greater risk for complications of pregnancy and acute urinary tract infections. Even this assumption has been questioned[30] because there is no difference in pregnancy outcome in women with treated asymptomatic bacteriuria of renal origin (diagnosed by antibody-coated bacteria technique, with a 20% false-positive rate) and those with treated bladder bacteriuria as well as noninfected control subjects. It can be argued that screening for asymptomatic bacteriuria is not justified because bacteriuric patients do not necessarily develop urinary tract infection, and the majority of patients with infection do not have bacteriuria on routine screening.[31] It has been shown that the combination of bacteriuria during pregnancy and a history of urinary tract infection signifies the biggest risk of infection. In such women, the likelihood of developing symptomatic urinary infection is ten times greater than in those with neither feature and four times greater than in those with asymptomatic bacteriuria alone.[32] While the above data are provocative, most authorities still recommend routine screening of all gravidas and prompt treatment when cultures are positive.

Views on Management

Eradicating the Bacteriuria. The choice of antibiotics to be dispensed to gravidas with asymptomatic bacteriuria is based on sensitivity of the isolated organism(s), with attention paid to the limitations on use of certain drugs during pregnancy. At least 60% of patients have bladder involvement alone, and short-term therapy (2 weeks) should be satisfactory.

Relapse is the recurrence of bacteriuria caused by the same organism, usually within 6 weeks of the initial infection. *Reinfection* is the recurrence of bacteriuria involving a different strain of bacteria after successful eradication of the initial infection, limited to the bladder and occurring at least 6 weeks after therapy.[34] Approximately 25% of patients will have a recurrence during pregnancy and need a second course of treatment. Of the patients who relapse or who are resistant to the first course of therapy, only about 40% will have asymptomatic bacteriuria cleared with subsequent therapy.

Long-Term Assessment. As the interval between treatment and bacteriuria in pregnancy and post-delivery follow up increases, the influence of the initial course of treatment on the incidence of bacteriuria becomes less noticeable.[35] Ten or more years after an initial episode of bacteriuria during pregnancy, the prevalence of bacteriuria in women not treated during pregnancy is 25%. Women who were never bacteriuric during pregnancy have rates of bacteriuria of about 5%.

The use of postpartum intravenous urography is controversial. About 20% of all patients with asymptomatic bacteriuria have urographic abnormalities; this percentage is increased among patient with acute infections during pregnancy or with infections that are difficult to eradicate.[36] The significance of roentgenographic abnormality is not certain, however, because it may signify predisposition to infection, may result from infection, or it may be unrelated to infection.[37] In order to detect nine out of ten of the 20% of women with major urinary tract abnormalities or to document a nonobstructed urinary tract, an intravenous pyelogram should be performed in women with the following additional criteria: (1) difficulty in eradicating the bacteriuria during pregnancy; (2) episode(s) of acute symptomatic urinary tract infection during pregnancy; (3) history of acute infections before the index pregnancy; (4) persistence or recurrence of asymptomatic bacteriuria or acute infection postpartum.

Symptomatic Urinary Tract Infection

Acute pyelonephritis is the most common urinary tract complication of pregnancy, occurring in about 2% of all pregnancies. There is controversy about its role in the etiology of intrauterine growth retardation, congenital abnormalities, and sudden intrauterine death, but there is little doubt that it can mimic or precipitate premature labor.[25,28] Gravidas are more vulnerable to endotoxins than nonpregnant women, which is one reason why they tolerate pyelonephritis poorly. Some even develop septic shock (usually in association with instrumentation of the infected urinary tract) or adult respiratory distress syndrome.[38]

There is controversy about the type and duration of antimicrobial therapy. In patients showing clinical deterioration or in those whose urine cultures reveal bacteria resistant to the selected antibiotic, repeated urine cultures are mandatory, and antibiotic therapy should be reviewed. After the completion of the course of treatment (usually 3–6 weeks), urine cultures should be obtained at every visit for the rest of the pregnancy. Regular assessment of renal function should be performed; although the infectious attack is said to have little effect on renal hemodynamics in nonpregnant patients, such attacks during pregnancy have been observed to cause transient but marked decreases in GFR.

In severely ill patients, blood specimens should be obtained for culture to exclude bacteremia. Gram-negative sepsis can occur with acute pyelonephritis, but the situation is commonly associated with instrumentation of an infected urinary tract.

Urolithiasis

The prevalence of urolithiasis in pregnancy is 0.03–0.35%.[39] Renal and ureteric calculi are among the most common causes of nonuterine-related abdominal pain severe enough to require inpatient management during pregnancy. When there are complications that indicate the need for surgical intervention, pregnancy should not be a deterrent to intravenous urography, even though there is a valid reluctance on the part of the obstetrician to consider radiologic investigation. Recently, it has been proposed that a set of specific clinical criteria be met before x-ray evaluation is undertaken. These are: (1) microscopic hematuria, (2) recurrent urinary tract symptoms, and (3) sterile urine culture when pyelonephritis is suspected.[40] If two of these are present, they point to a diagnosis of calculi in approximately 50% of gravidas; if echography is inconclusive, an intravenous pyelogram (limited to fewer than three exposures) can be undertaken.

Management should be conservative in the first instance, consisting primarily of adequate hydration, appropriate antibiotic therapy, and pain relief. Although pain usually may be relieved by systemic analgesics, continuous segmental epidural block (T11 to L2) has been used successfully.[41] This approach has been applied for many years in nonpregnant patients with ureteric colic and may even favorably influence spontaneous passage of the calculi. When the block is carefully confined to the relevant segments for pain relief, the patient can urinate without difficulty, can move without assistance, and is at lower risk of thromboembolic problems than one who is immobilized in bed with drowsiness, pain, nausea, and vomiting.

Alternative management to using x-rays during pregnancy that involves the cystoscopic placement of an internal ureteral tube or stent, between bladder and kidney, under local anesthesia recently has been proposed.[41] The stent retains its position because it has a pigtail or J-like curve at each end (double-J); to prevent encrustation it can be changed every eight weeks. Early empirical use for presumed stone obstruction in pregnant women with flank pain could be helpful, especially when hydration, analgesia, and antibiotics do not reduce pain or fever. When pregnancy is over, the usual radiology should be undertaken and standard management resumed.

Acute Hydronephrosis and Hydroureter

There is a broad spectrum of so-called *overdistention syndrome*.[42] Obstruction may occur at varying levels at or above the pelvic brim. Some women only have mild loin pain, while others have recurrent episodes of severe loin or lower abdominal pain that spreads to the groin. Urinanalysis reveals few or no red cells and repeat midstream urine cultures are sterile. The variation in symptoms with changes in posture and position are standard indications of the condition. Diagnosis can be confirmed using limited excretory urography or sonar scanning. Positioning of the gravida in lateral recumbency or the knee-chest position often gives relief, but if this fails, uretheral catheterization or nephrostomy may be needed. It is best to delay corrective surgery until the postpartum period.

Nontraumatic Rupture of the Urinary Tract

The intrusion of unremitting pain and hematuria upon the onset of pyelonephritis or the *overdistention syndrome* suggests rupture of the urinary tract. This complication can masquerade as other obstetric and surgical abdominal catastrophes, including appendicitis, pelvic abscess, cholecystitis, urolithiasis or *abruptio placentae*. Prompt recognition may prevent a small tear or urine leak, treatable by posture or tube drainage from extending or expanding. Rupture of the renal parenchyma, with hemorrhagic shock formation of frank mass or dissection of urinary tract contents intraperitoneally requires prompt surgical intervention, usually with nephrectomy.[42]

Hematuria During Pregnancy

Spontaneous gross or microscopic hematuria can be due to a variety of causes.[43] If associated with congenital anomalies, then urinary tract infection (UTI) can be difficult to eradicate and can predispose to hematuria. Rupture of small veins about the dilated renal pelvis also may cause bleeding. Very rarely, hematuria may be due to acute glomerulonephritis, primary or metastatic neoplasm, hemangioma(s), calculi, or fungal diseases.[44] Endometriosis, inflammatory bowel lesions, leukoplakia, amyloidosis and granulomata may invade the renal tract and also produce hematuria. A bleeding ureteral stump after a nephrectomy (for either benign or malignant disease) should not be forgotten.

Investigation may be deferred until postpartum, but the clinician should assess all the circumstances to decide whether it takes absolute priority. In the absence of any demonstrable cause, hematuria should be classified as idiopathic and recurrence unlikely in the current or subsequent pregnancy.

Specific Parenchymal Disease

The critical factors are always the effect of a particular disease on the pregnancy and the effect of the pregnancy on that disease. A summary of the various problems is given in Table 145–3.

Acute and Chronic Glomerulonephritis. Acute poststreptococcal glomerulonephritis complicating pregnancy is very rare and has been mistaken for preeclampsia when it does occur. The prognosis of chronic glomerulonephritis during pregnancy is hard to evaluate, primarily because most reports are poorly documented, often failing to list the degrees of functional impairment, blood pressure prior to conception, and the histology of the "glomerulonephritis."

TABLE 145–3. EFFECTS OF PREGNANCY ON PRE-EXISTING RENAL DISEASE

Renal Disease	Effects
Chronic pyelonephritis (infectious tubulointerstitial disease)	Bacteriuria in pregnancy can lead to exacerbation.
Nephrolithiasis	Infections can be more frequent, but ureteral dilatation and stasis do not seem to affect natural history.
Permanent urinary diversion	Might be associated with other malformations of the urogenital tract. Urinary tract infection common during pregnancy. Renal function may undergo reversible decrease. No significant obstructive problem but caesarean section often needed for abnormal presentation.
Chronic glomerulonephritis and noninfectious tubulointerstitial disease	Usually no adverse effect in the absence of hypertension. One view is that glomerulonephritis is adversely affected by the coagulation changes of pregnancy. Urinary tract infections may occur more frequently.
Systemic lupus erythematosus (SLE)	Controversial; prognosis most favorable if disease in remission >6 months prior to conception. Steroid dosage should be increased postpartum. Fetal prognosis is dismal and maternal death often occurs. If onset during pregnancy there can be rapid overall deterioration. Reactivation of quiescent scleroderma may occur postpartum.
Diabetic nephropathy	No adverse effect on the renal lesion, but there is increased frequency of infection, edema and/or pre-eclampsia.
Polycystic disease	Functional impairment and hypertension usually minimal in childbearing years.
After nephrectomy, solitary and pelvic kidneys	Might be associated with other malformations of urogenital tract. Pregnancy well tolerated. Dystocia rarely occurs with a pelvic kidney.

Some investigators[3,4] have stated that pregnancy tends to aggravate most glomerular diseases because of the hypercoagulable state that accompanies pregnancy, claiming that crescentric glomerular lesions occur most readily. They also indicate that such patients are more susceptible to superimposed preeclampsia or hypertensive crises earlier in pregnancy. Our experience is that renal function decreases most often in patients with diffuse glomerulonephritis in whom hypertension is both more common and severe; nonetheless, most of the pregnancies are successful.

The course of pregnancy in women with IgA nephropathy is controversial. On the one hand, substantial and occasionally irreversible declines in renal functions are emphasized, while on the other hand, others emphasize that pregnancy outcome and remote renal prognosis are excellent when hypertension is absent before pregnancy and GFR is well preserved.[2,5,8]

Hereditary nephritis is an uncommon disorder that first may be manifested or exacerbated during pregnancy.[1] There is a variant of hereditary nephritis in which the patients have disordered platelet shape and function. Pregnancy in these women has been successful from a renal viewpoint, but their pregnancies can be complicated by bleeding problems.

Systemic Lupus Erythematosus

There are differing opinions regarding the effects of pregnancy on lupus nephropathy (see Chapter 51). Transient improvements, no change, and a tendency to relapse all have been reported. Some patients have a definite tendency to relapse (occasionally severe) in the puerperium; therefore, it is prudent to prescribe or increase the use of steroids at this time. This does not, however, seem to have been confirmed in a carefully performed case-controlled study.[45]

The majority of pregnancies reach full term[46,47], especially if the maternal disease is in sustained, complete clinical remission for at least 6 months prior to conception. This applies even if the patient had heavy proteinuria in the early stages of her disease and severe pathologic changes in the original renal biopsy. However, continued signs of disease or increasing renal dysfunction reduce the likelihood of an uncomplicated pregnancy.

Lupus nephropathy sometimes may become manifest during pregnancy, and when accompanied by hypertension and renal dysfunction in late pregnancy, it may be mistaken for preeclampsia. Placental transmission of lupus serum factors (perhaps the so-called lupus anticoagulant [LA], as well as antiphospholipid antibodies) also occurs, which may relate to the high frequency of spontaneous abortions in these women.[48] Although the LA was first described in patients with SLE, it since has been observed in patients with other conditions and even in patients without any identifiable disorder. Intrauterine death is common in gravidas with circulating LA (and certain other antibodies; eg, antiphospholipids); the placentas in such cases show extensive thrombotic and arteriosclerotic changes.[49] Since treatment with steroids and aspirin may lead to successful pregnancies, it is important to screen for LA and related antiphospholipid antibodies in all women with SLE to identify this SLE subgroup as well as other women with a history of recurrent intrauterine deaths or thrombotic episodes.[47]

An increased incidence of congenital cardiac anomalies has been described in the offspring of women with SLE and other maternal connective-tissue disease, even when maternal disease appears quiescent.[50] This association appears to be related to the transplacental passage of a maternal antibody to soluble tissue ribonucleoprotein. This maternal antibody [anti-Ro(SS-A)] is detectable in almost all cases of isolated congenital complete heartblock.[51] The prevalence of anti Ro(SS-A) in patients with SLE is 25–30%, where it may also have other untoward associations, particularly recurrent abortion. Paradoxically, the mother's heart usually is unaffected even though the antibody is present in her system at a higher concentration than in the fetus. The fetal heart therefore may be more vulnerable to antibody-mediated damage than the mature heart, or it may have phase-specific antigens. Alternatively, blocking maternal antibodies of the IgA or IgM class (not transferred to the fetus) could stop an IgG antibody from causing maternal damage. There are controversies about prospective attempts to reduce the effect of anti-Ro antibody in the fetus (and possibly the mother) using high-dose steroid regimens (prednisone 1 mg/kg per day) supplemented with plasmapheresis. Success is rare and when it has been achieved, it is interesting that anti-Ro antibody was never absent from the maternal serum and was detected in cord blood.

Other Connective-Tissue Disorders

In contrast to lupus nephropathy, the outcome of pregnancy in women with renal involvement caused by periarteritis nodosa and scleroderma is very poor, largely because of the associated hypertension, which is frequently malignant. Fetal prognosis is dismal, and many of the cases reported ended with maternal deaths[47] (see also Chapter 51).

Diabetic Nephropathy

Since many patients are juvenile diabetics, they probably already harbor microscopic changes in their kidneys (see also Chapter 43). During pregnancy, diabetic women have an increased prevalence of bacteriuria and may be more susceptible to symptomatic urinary tract infection. They also have an increased frequency of peripheral edema and preeclampsia. Most women with diabetic nephropathy demonstrate normal increases in renal function, and pregnancy does not accelerate deterioration of diabetic nephropathy.[52] However, up to 50–60% of patients with prepregnancy proteinuria manifest increases in protein excretion to the nephrotic range as well as frank hypertension late in pregnancy.[52]

Tubulointerstitial Disease

The prognosis of pregnancy in women with "chronic pyelonephritis" seems similar to that of patients with glomerular disease in that its outcome is most favorable in normotensive patients with adequate renal function.[8,9] Diseases of infectious origin in women tend to exacerbate during pregnancy; adverse effects may be minimized if patients are well hydrated and rest frequently in lateral recumbency. (Ureteral obstruction by the enlarged uterus does not occur in this position.) It had been suggested that these patients are more susceptible to hypertensive complications during pregnancy, but more recent reports indicate that they have a more benign antenatal course than do women with glomerular disease.

Polycystic Renal Disease

This entity may remain undetected during pregnancy, but careful questioning of pregnant women for a history of familial problems and the use of ultrasonography may lead to earlier detection. These patients do well when functional impairment is minimal and hypertension is absent, which is often the case during childbearing years. They do, however, have an increased incidence of hypertension late in pregnancy and a higher perinatal mortality compared to the pregnancies of sisters unaffected by this autosomal-dominant disease. If a parent has polycystic renal disease, he or she should seek genetic counseling. There will be a 50% chance of transmitting the disease to the offspring. DNA probe techniques now are being developed so that antenatal diagnosis may be possible by chorionic villus biopsy, allowing women to undergo selective termination of pregnancy.[53]

Reflux Nephropathy

This term is used to describe renal morphological and functional changes that relate to past (and usually present) vesicoureteric reflux (VUR), often complicated by recurrent infection. It usually begins in childhood and is present in a significant number of women of childbearing age. One view[3] is that pregnancy has an adverse effect on the cause of the disease, but careful analysis of the literature indicates that women who do poorly are those who had moderate renal dysfunction or hypertension from the outset.[2] Specific problems during pregnancy include frequent urinary tract infections (which need prompt treatment), severe fetal intrauterine growth retardation, and the risk of sudden rapid worsening of hypertension and renal function with accelerated progression to renal failure.

Solitary Kidney of Congenital Origin or after Nephrectomy

Some patients have a congenital absence of one kidney or marked unilateral hypoplasia. The majority, however, have had a prior nephrectomy because of pyelonephritis with abscess, hydronephrosis, unilateral tuberculosis, congenital abnormalities, or tumor.

When counseling women with a single kidney, it is important to know the indication for and the time since the nephrectomy.[44] In patients who had an infectious or structural renal problem, sequential prepregnancy investigation is needed to detect any persistent infection. There is no difference if the right or left kidney remains as long as it is located in the normal anatomic position. If function is normal and stable, all such women seem to tolerate pregnancy well.

Ectopic kidneys (usually pelvic) are more vulnerable to infection and are associated with decreased fetal salvage, probably because of an association with other malformations of the urogenital tract. If infection occurs in a solitary kidney during pregnancy and does not respond quickly to antibiotics, termination of pregnancy may have to be considered to preserve renal function.

Permanent Urinary Diversion

This procedure is still used in the management of young patients with congenital lower urinary tract defects but its use has declined for neurogenic bladders since the invention of self-catheterization. The most common complication is UTI. Premature labor occurs in 20%, and the use of prophylactic antibiotics throughout pregnancy may reduce its incidence. Declines in renal function are related to infection or intermittent obstruction. With an ileal conduit, elevation and compression by the enlarging uterus can cause outflow obstruction, whereas with a ureterosigmoid anastomesis obstruction of the ureter may occur.[54] The changes usually reverse postdelivery.

The mode of delivery is dictated by obstetric factors. Abnormal presentation accounts for a cesarean section rate approaching 30%, related to other genital abnormalities. Vaginal delivery is safe, but if an episiotomy is needed, the anal sphincter must be kept intact at all costs.

Chronic Renal Disease: Conclusions

With few exceptions, pregnancy does not adversely affect the natural history of underlying chronic renal disease if kidney function is preserved and hypertension is absent at conception.[1] Although the fetal prognosis is less favorable than in healthy women, it does not justify discouraging pregnancy in women with renal disease.

As mentioned earlier, it has been suggested that the hyperfiltration of residual (intact) nephrons in the kidneys of patients with moderate renal insufficiency might cause further progressive loss of renal function.[18] This hypothesis is controversial and relevant to pregnancy in women with underlying renal disorders, since such patients, like healthy women, experience physiologic hyperfiltration during pregnancy.[17] At present, this caution is theoretical and is an area for further study.

Nephrotic Syndrome

The most common cause of nephrotic syndrome in late pregnancy is preeclampsia.[55] This results in a poorer fetal prognosis than preeclampsia with less heavy proteinuria, but maternal prognosis is similar. Other causes of nephrotic syndrome in pregnancy include membranous nephropathy, proliferative or membranoproliferative glomerulonephritis, lipid nephrosis, lupus nephropathy, hereditary nephritis, diabetic nephropathy, renal vein thrombosis, amyloidosis, and secondary syphilis. Some of these conditions do not respond to, and may even be seriously aggravated by, steroid therapy. The clinician therefore must be aware of the importance of establishing a tissue diagnosis before initiating steroids.

If renal function is adequate and hypertension is absent, there should be few complications during pregnancy. Several of the physiologic changes occurring during pregnancy may, however, simulate aggravation or exacerbation of the disease. For example, increases in renal hemodynamics as well as increase in renal vein pressure may enhance protein excretion. Levels of serum albumin usually decrease by 0.5 g/dL ml in normal pregnancy, and the further decreases that can occur in the nephrotic syndrome may enhance the tendency to fluid retention. Despite edema, diuretics should be avoided, because these patients have a decreased intravascular volume, and this therapy could compromise further uteroplacental perfusion or aggravate the increased tendency to thrombotic episodes. Nevertheless, some of these subjects have such a high tendency to retain sodium that diuretics have to be used (although judiciously) to avoid tissue breakdown and blood pressure problems.

Although the majority of these pregnancies are maintained to term, there is evidence that hypoalbuminemia and the associated decreased intravascular volume may cause small-for-date infants. Furthermore, there is a report that infants of normotensive mothers who had heavy proteinuria during pregnancy manifested impaired neurologic and mental development. Finally, there is a tendency to restrict protein intake in nonpregnant nephrotics. This appears to be paradoxical, but it results in a rise in serum albumin, as a low-protein diet decreases the catabolism of albumin. We caution against protein restriction during pregnancy, however, until more is known about the effects of such diets on the fetus, especially on brain development.

Hemodialysis and Pregnancy

Counseling Hemodialysis Patients. Chronic renal failure requiring hemodialysis usually is preceded by relative infertility and decreased libido potency. Despite this, women on dialysis can conceive and should always use contraception if they wish to avoid pregnancy.[56] The substantial arguments against pregnancy must be brought to the patient's attention, and any optimism in the lay or medical press must be judged in the context of clinicians' reluctance to publish their failures. There is an alarming lack of data on the true incidence of unsuccessful pregnancies as well as the complication rate and sequelae of pregnancies in women on hemodialysis. The high therapeutic abortion rate in these patients, however, does indicate that those who become pregnant do so accidentally, probably because they are unaware that pregnancy is possible.[57,58]

Diagnosis of Pregnancy and Antenatal Assessment. Early diagnosis of pregnancy can be difficult. Irregular menstruation is common and a missed period usually will be ignored, thus the possibility of pregnancy may not be considered. Because urine pregnancy tests are unreliable even if there is any urine available, early diagnosis of pregnancy and estimation of gestational age are accomplished best by blood tests and sonar.

For any chance of a successful outcome, scrupulous attention must be paid to fluid balance, blood pressure control, nutritional status, treatment of anemia, increased hours and frequency of dialysis, and fetal surveillance. Because progressive anemia is always evident in these patients and is most marked in those who have undergone nephrectomy[57], an elective predelivery blood transfusion may be advisable as a safeguard against obstetric complications. Cesarean sections should be necessary only for purely obstetric reasons, but it may be argued that elective section in all cases would eliminate the potential problems of labor. Interestingly, preterm labor is generally the rule, and the use of cesarean section in these circumstances might be considered beneficial, but again this is open to argument.

Little is known about the long-term aftermath of pregnancy. In most of the cases reported in the literature, the women remained reasonably healthy after pregnancy, with little or no change in their hemodialysis regimens.[57,58]

Reports now are appearing of pregnancy in women with chronic ambulatory peritoneal dialysis, as ovulatory cycles and menses may occur more often in such patients. These cases should be reviewed carefully when the number of such cases increases. Finally, erythropoetin, too, may increase fertility.

RENAL TRANSPLANTATION AND PREGNANCY

Counseling Renal Transplant Patients

Following transplantation, there is a rapid restoration of renal and endocrine function, and normal sexual activity usually follows. It has been estimated that 2% of women of childbearing age with a functioning renal transplant become pregnant. Spontaneous abortion, therapeutic termination of pregnancy, and ectopic pregnancy account for about 40% of all conceptions. Of the pregnancies that continue past the first trimester, however, 90% deliver successfully. To date, over 2000 pregnancies are on record in women who have received a renal allograft (Tables 145-4 and 145-5).[59-61] The possibility of conception in female transplant recipients of childbearing age raises the need for appropriate counseling in these patients. All women should be advised routinely about contraception, and couples who want a child should be encouraged to discuss all the implications. Whether a woman should be advised against pregnancy must be decided on the basis of strict guidelines[59,60], which should include:

TABLE 145–4. RENAL TRANSPLANTATION AND PREGNANCY: COMPLICATIONS AND OUTCOME

Problems in Pregnancy	Successful Obstetric Outcome	Long-term Sequelae
46%	92% (73%)	11% (24%)

Estimates based on 819 women in 1025 pregnancies which attained at least 28 weeks gestation (1961–1987). Figures in brackets refer to prospects when pregnancy complications developed prior to 28 gestational weeks. *Adapted from references 60 and 61.*

1. Good general health for 2 years after transplantation
2. Stature compatible with good obstetric outcome
3. No proteinuria
4. No significant hypertension
5. No evidence of graft rejection
6. No evidence of pelvicalyceal distention on a recent excretory urogram
7. Stable glomerular filtration rate; plasma creatinine of 2 mg/dL 177 umol/L or less (and preferably less than 1.5 mg/dL 133 umol/L)
8. Drug therapy; prednisone, 15 mg/day or less, and azathioprine, 2 mg/kg body weight per day or less. A safe dose of cyclosporin A has not been established yet because of limited experience, but quoted anecdotally is 5 mg/kg body weight (or less) daily, or even a change from cyclosporin A to azathioprine before or in early pregnancy

Antenatal Assessment

A gravida with a renal allograft must be monitored as a high-risk patient.[59] Management requires fetal surveillance as well as monitoring and controlling renal function, blood pressure, bone disease, anemia, and any infections (however trivial).[59,61] The better the renal function before pregnancy, the more satisfactory will be the obstetric outcome. Meticulous assessment of fetal growth and well-being is needed; this is performed best by serial sonar assessment.

Permanent impairment of renal function is seen occasionally, especially where renal function is already compromised prior to conception. In patients with satisfactory renal function before pregnancy, there may be some deterioration as well as proteinuria during the third trimester, but usually this is transient, with normal function returning postpartum. Renal transplant patients have a 30% chance of developing preeclampsia. Plasma uric acid levels and 24-hour urinary protein excretion are occasionally well above the physiologic norm for pregnancy, but this does not necessarily indicate the onset of preeclampsia.

Other maternal complications include graft rejection, serious infection, septicemia, steroid-induced hyperglycemia, and uterine rupture.

TABLE 145–5. RENAL TRANSPLANTATION AND PREGNANCY: EFFECTS OF PREPREGNANCY RENAL STATUS

Plasma Creatinine (mg/DL)	Problems in Pregnancy	Successful Obstetric Outcome	Long-term Sequelae
<1.5	31%	96%	7%
>1.5	82%	63%	27%

Estimates based on 819 women in 1025 pregnancies which attained at least 28 weeks gestation (1961–1987).[60,61]

Management of Delivery and Neonatal Problems

The transplanted kidney very rarely produces mechanical dystocia during labor, and it does not sustain apparent mechanical injury during vaginal delivery. Cesarean section is usually necessary only for purely obstetric reasons. Regardless of the route of delivery, steroids must be used at this time.

There is some hazard to the neonate. Preterm delivery occurs in 50% and intrauterine growth retardation in at least 20%. Although there are no frequent or predominant congenital abnormalities, one or more complications occur in about 35%, including respiratory distress syndrome, leukopenia, thrombocytopenia, adrenocortical insufficiency, infection, and presence of HBsAg. Obviously, some of these problems are related to immunosuppressive drugs, particularly azathioprine. With the introduction of the new immunosuppressive agent cyclosporin A, which supposedly is more effective than conventional immunosuppression (azathioprine or steroids), new evaluations will be needed. Since the first report of pregnancy in a transplant patient taking cyclosporin A[62] more data have accrued[61,63,64], but it still is not known whether this agent should be used routinely in recipients contemplating pregnancy. Whatever the immunosuppression regimen the offspring has been exposed to *in utero*, long-term surveillance is essential.

Long-Term Considerations

Long-term effects, both in terms of renal prognosis and patient well-being, are difficult to qualify. Our experience and that reported in the literature indicate that to wait two years after transplantation before becoming pregnant is safe; pregnancy does not seem to cause any irreversible decline in renal function.[59] On the basis of comparison of very small groups of renal cadaver transplant recipients (those who became pregnant and those who did not), one group of investigators concluded that pregnancy had no effect on graft function or survival.[65] This clearly is an area in which long-term studies are needed.

Another long-term consideration is that female renal allograft recipients may have any gynecologic disorder that affects the general population, and symptoms secondary to pelvic disease must not be attributed to failing renal function or to the transplant itself because of its location near the pelvis.[59] Last, but not least, there is an increased risk of malignancy in this group of patients.[66]

REFERENCES

1. Lindheimer MD, Katz AI. Gestation in women with kidney disease: prognosis and management. *Clin Obstet Gynaecol (Baillière)*. 1987;1:921.
2. Jungers P, Houiller P, Forget D. Reflux nephropathy and Pregnancy. *Clin Obstet Gynaecol (Baillière)*. 1987;1:955.
3. Kincaid-Smith P, Fairley KF. Renal disease in pregnancy. Three controversial areas: Mesangial IgA nephropathy, focal glomerular sclerosis (focal and segmental hyalinosis and sclerosis) and reflux nephropathy. *Amer J Kid Dis*. 1987;9:328.
4. Packham DK, North RA, Fairley KF, et al. Primary glomerulonephritis and pregnancy. *Q J Med*. 1989;266:537.
5. Abe S, Amagasaki Y, Konishi K, et al. The influence of antecedent renal disease on pregnancy. *Am J Obstet*. 1985;94:145.
6. Hou SH, Grossman SD, Madias NE. Pregnancy in women with renal disease and moderate renal insufficiency. *Am J Med*. 1985;78:185.
7. Surian M, Imbasciati E, Cosci P, et al. Glomerular disease and pregnancy: a study of 123 pregnancies in patients with primary and secondary glomerular disease. *Nephrology*. 1984;36:101.
8. Barcelo P, Lopez-Lillo J, Caberto L, et al. Successful pregnancy in primary glomerular disease. *Kidney Int*. 1986;30:914.
9. Katz AI, Davison JM, Hayslett JP, et al. Pregnancy in women with kidney disease. *Kidney Int*. 1980;18:192.
10. Bear RA. Pregnancy in patients with renal disease: a study of 44 cases. *Obstet Gynecol*. 1976;48:13.

11. Davison JM, Katz AI, Lindheimer MD. Pregnancy in women with renal disease and renal transplantation. Proc EDTA-ERA 22, 1985:439.
12. Lindheimer MD, Katz AI. *Kidney Function and Disease in Pregnancy*. Philadelphia, PA: Lea and Febiger; 1977:
13. Lindheimer MD, Davison JM. Renal biopsy during pregnancy: "To be or not to be." *Brit J Obstet Gynaecol*. 1987;94:932.
14. Schewitz LJ, Friedman EA, Pollak VE. Bleeding after renal in pregnancy. *Obstet Gynecol*. 1965;26:295.
15. Packham D, Fairley KF. Renal biopsy: indications and complications in pregnancy. *Brit J Obstet Gynaecol*. 1987;94:935.
16. Anderson S. Progression of chronic renal disease: role of systemic and glomerular hypertension. *Am J Kid Dis*. 1989;6(suppl 1):8.
17. Brenner BM, Meyer TW, Hosteter TH. Dietary protein intake and the progressive nature of kidney disease: The role of hemodynamically medicated glomerular injury in the pathogenesis of progressive glomerular sclerosis in aging, renal ablation and intrinsic renal disease. *N Engl J Med*. 1982;307:652.
18. Baylis C. Glomerular filtration and volume regulation in gravida animal models. *Clin Obstet Gynaecol (Baillière)*. 1987;1:789.
19. Baylis C, Rennke HG. Renal hemodynamics and glomerular morphology in repetitively pregnant aging rats. *Kidney Int*. 1985;28:140.
20. Davison JM. The effect of pregnancy on long-term renal function in women with chronic renal disease and single kidneys. *Clin Exp Hypertens*. 1989;B8:226. Abstract.
21. Stamm WE, County GW, Running UR, et al. Diagnosis of coliform infection in acutely dysuric women. *N Engl J Med*. 1982;307:463.
22. McFadyen IR, Eykyn SJ, Gardner NHN, et al. Bacteriuria of pregnancy. *J Obstet Gynaecol Br Common*. 1973;80:385.
23. Urinary tract infection during pregnancy. *Lancet*. 1985;2:190. Editorial.
24. Gargan RA, Brumfitt W, Hamilton-Miller JMT. Antibody-coated bacteria in urine: Criterion for a positive test and its value in defining a higher risk of treatment failure. *Lancet*. 1983;2:704.
25. Cunningham FG. Urinary tract infections complicating pregnancy. *Clin Obstet Gynaecol (Baillière)*. 1987;1:821.
26. Whalley PJ. Bacteriuria of pregnancy. *Am J Obstet Gynecol*. 1967;97:723.
27. Williams JD, Reeves DS, Condie AP, et al. Significance of bacteriuria in pregnancy. In: Kass EH, Brumfitt W, eds. *Infections of the Urinary Tract*. Chicago, IL: University of Chicago Press; 1978:8.
28. Lindheimer MD, Katz AI. The kidney in pregnancy. In: Brenner BM, Rector FC Jr, eds. *The Kidney*. 3rd ed. Philadelphia, PA: WB Saunders; 1986:1253.
29. Davison JM, Sprott MS, Selkon JB. The effect of covert bacteriuria in schoolgirls on renal function at 18 years and during pregnancy. *Lancet*. 1984;2:651.
30. Gilstrap LC, Leveno KJ, Cunningham FG, et al. Renal infection and pregnancy outcome. *Am J Obstet Gynecol*. 1981;1441:709.
31. Lawson DH, Miller AWF. Screening for bacteriuria in pregnancy: A critical reappraisal. *Arch Intern Med*. 1973;132:925.
32. Chang PK, Hall MH. Antenatal prediction of urinary tract infection in pregnancy. *Br J Obstet Gynaecol*. 1982;89:8.
33. Campbell-Brown M, McFadyen IR, Seal DV, et al. Is screening for bacteriuria in pregnancy worthwhile? *Brit Med J*. 1987;294:1579.
34. Turck M, Ronald AR, Petersdorf RG. Relapse and reinfection in chronic bacteriuria. II. The correlation between site of infection and pattern of recurrence in chronic bacteriuria. *N Engl J Med*. 1968;278:422.
35. Mead PB, Gump DW. Asymptomatic bacteriuria in pregnancy. In: de Alvarez RR, ed. *The Kidney*. New York, NY: John Wiley & Sons; 1976:45.
36. Gower PE, Haswell B, Sidaway ME, et al. Follow-up of 164 patients with bacteriuria. *Lancet*. 1968;1:990.
37. Fowler JE, Pulaski ET. Excretion urography, cystography and cystoscopy in the evaluation of women with urinary tract infection. *N Engl J Med*. 1982;304:462.
38. Cunningham FG, Lucas MJ, Hankins GDV. Pulmonary injury complicating antepartum pyelonephritis. *Am J Obstet Gynecol*. 1987;156:797.
39. Miller DR, Kakkis J. Prognosis, management and outcome: obstructive renal disease in pregnancy. *J Reprod Med*. 1982;27:199.
40. Marikranz P, Coe FL, Parks J, et al. Nephrolithiasis and gestation. *Clin Obstet Gynaecol (Baillière)*. 1987;1:909.
41. Loughlin KR, Bailey RB. Internal ureteral stents for conservative management of ureteral calculi during pregnancy. *N Engl J Med*. 1986;315:1647.
42. Meyers SJ, Lee RV, Munschauer RW. Dilatation and nontraumatic rupture of the urinary tract during pregnancy: a review. *Obstet Gynecol*. 1983;66:809.
43. Danielli L, Korchazak D, Beyar H, et al. Recurrent hematuria during pregnancies. *Obstet Gynecol*. 1987;69:446.
44. Klein EA. Urologic problems of pregnancy. *Obstet Gynecol Surv*. 1983;39:605.
45. Lockshin MD, Reiutz E, Druzen NZ, et al. Case control perspective study demonstrating absence of lupus exacerbation during or after pregnancy. *Am J Med*. 1984;77:893.
46. Babie G, Liote F, Huiller P, et al. Pregnancy in lupus nephritis and related disorders. *Am J Kidney Dis*. 1987;9:337.
47. Mor-Josef S, Navot D, Rabinowitz R, et al. Collagen disease in pregnancy. *Obstet Gynecol Surv*. 1984;39:67.
48. Lupus anticoagulant. *Lancet*. 1984;1:1157. Editorial.
49. Abromowsky CR, Vegas ME, Swinehar G, et al. Decidual pathology of the placenta in lupus erythematosus. *N Engl J Med*. 1980;303:668.
50. Scott JS, Maddison PJ, Taylor PV, et al. Connective-tissue disease, antibodies to ribonucleoprotein and congenital heart block. *N Engl J Med*. 1983;309.
51. Taylor PV, Scott JS, Gerlis LM, et al. Maternal antibodies against fetal cardiac antigens in congenital complete heart block. *N Engl J Med*. 1986;315:667.
52. Reece EA, Coustan DL, Hayslett JP, et al. Diabetic nephropathy. Prepregnancy performance and fetal-maternal outcome. *Am J Obstet Gynecol*. 1988;159:56.
53. Reeders ST, Zerres K, Gal A, et al. Prenatal diagnosis of autosomal dominant polycystic kidney disease with a DNA probe. *Lancet*. 1986;2:6.
54. Baral RJ, Peters WA. Pregnancy following urinary diversion. *Obstet Gynecol*. 1983;62:582.
55. Fisher K, Luger A, Spargo BH, et al. Hypertension in pregnancy: Clinical-pathological correlations and remote prognosis. *Medicine*. 1981;60:267.
56. Lim VS. Reproductive endocrinology in uremia. *Clin Obstet Gynaecol (Baillière)*. 1987;1:997.
57. Hou S. Peritoneal and hemodialysis in pregnancy. *Clin Obstet Gynaecol (Baillière)*. 1987;1:1009.
58. Redraw M, Cherem L, Elliot J, et al. Dialysis and management of pregnant patients with renal insufficiency. *Medicine*. 1988;67:199.
59. Davison JM. Pregnancy in renal allograft recipients. Prognosis and Management. *Clin Obstet Gynaecol (Baillière)*. 1987;1:1027.
60. Davison JM, Lindheimer MD. Pregnancy and renal transplantation: Look before you leap. *Int J Artif Org*. 1989;12:144.
61. Hou S. Pregnancy in organ transplant recipients. *Med Clin N Am*. 1989;73:667.
62. Calne RY. Cyclosporin in cadaveric renal transplantation: 3 years follow-up of a multicenter trial. *Lancet*. 1987;2:506.
63. Derfler K, Schaller A, Harold C, et al. Successful outcome of a complicated pregnancy in a renal transplant recipient taking cyclosporine-A. *Clin Nephrol*. 1988;29:96.
64. Lewis GJ, Lamont CAR, Lee HA, et al. Successful pregnancy in a renal transplant recipient taking cyclosporin A. *Br Med J*. 1983;286:603.
65. Whetam JCG, Cardelle C, Harding M. Effect of pregnant graft function and graft survival in renal cadaver transplant patients. *Am J Obstet Gynecol*. 1983;145:193.
66. Allons M, Barr BBB, McLaen KM, et al. Human papillome virus infection and cervical intraepithelial neoplasia in women with renal allographs. *Br Med J*. 1989;288:153.

Chapter One Hundred and Forty-Six

Urolithiasis

M. Amanda Skoll

146

Stones form in the urinary tract when the balance between solute excretion and water conservation in the kidney is disturbed. Normally, protective mechanisms exist to maintain excretory products in solution. However, when these are overwhelmed by such factors as diet, exercise and excessive solute load, crystals may form and precipitate onto a skeletal matrix to produce stones.[1]

Both in pregnancy and in the nonpregnant state, the

vast majority of calculi formed within the urinary tract are composed of calcium crystals. The crystalline component often is mixed, with calcium oxalate and mixed calcium oxalate and calcium phosphate stones being the most common forms encountered.[1] Other forms include uric acid stones, most commonly found in males; struvite stones, related to infection; and cystine stones secondary to homozygous cystinuria. In the few reports in which stone analysis has been performed in pregnant patients, the breakdown of type of stones appears to parallel that of the general population.[2-5]

A number of etiologic factors predispose to stone formation. These include: metabolic disorders such as enzyme disorders and hypercalciuric states; ion transport disturbances within the intestinal tract and kidney, including renal tubular acidosis; and dietary abnormalities such as reduced intake of fluid. Secondary urolithiasis may occur in association with infection, obstruction, urinary diversion or medullary sponge kidney.

There appear to be no etiologic factors unique to pregnancy. Although the physiologic hydronephrosis of pregnancy has been postulated to contribute to urinary stasis, this mechanism would tend to result in a majority of right-sided stones. Review of the literature, however, reveals an equal distribution of stones on both sides.[4-8] Most series report approximately twice as many multigravid as primigravid patients. However, this association is not significant when corrected for the recognized increase in incidence of nephrolithiasis with increasing age.

The incidence of renal calculi in pregnancy ranges from 0.03% to 0.53% with a mean of 0.24%.[2,4-9] As in the nonpregnant state, there is an increased incidence in the so-called "stone belt" in the southeastern United States. The incidence of stones presenting in pregnancy does appear to change with gestational age. Lattanzi and Cook[6], in a review of six reports detailing trimester of presentation, found only 12% of stones presenting in the first trimester, with 45% and 43% in the second and third trimesters, respectively.

Pregnancy itself does not appear to have an effect on the progression or severity of nephrolithiasis. In 1978, Coe et al[3] reported on a group of 78 women with documented stone disease during the reproductive years. Within this group, 148 pregnancies were recorded, 90 before and 58 after the diagnosis of stone formation. Stones were passed during 20 of these pregnancies. Calculations of predicted rates of stone passage in a nonpregnant population revealed that the incidence in pregnancy is not elevated over the expected incidence in the nonpregnant state.

Coe[3] examined the occurrence of pregnancy complications in women with a history of stone disease, as well as in those presenting with their first calculus during pregnancy. There was no difference in the incidence of abortion, prematurity, hypertension, or cesarean section between groups, or between this population and a group of pregnant patients without stone disease. The only significant difference found was an increased incidence of symptomatic urinary tract infection, occurring in 20% of patients manifesting stone disease before or during pregnancy, and in 6.5% of patients diagnosed after their last pregnancy.

The presentation of renal calculi in pregnant patients may be obscure compared to that in nonpregnant individuals. Although severe flank pain is a common presenting complaint, abdominal and visceral complaints may predominate. Nausea and vomiting also may be prominent symptoms, as may dysuria and urgency.[8] Renal colic is rare, particularly after the first trimester. Not surprisingly, premature labor, appendicitis and pyelonephritis all may be considered in the differential diagnosis.[8] Premature labor has been reported in association with acute manifestations of stone disease with contractions subsiding following treatment of the underlying urologic disorder.

The history is extremely important in suggesting a diagnosis of urolithiasis. Jones et al[11] reported six of 20 patients having had previous episodes of stone disease prior to their presentation in pregnancy. In a group of 11 patients reported by Lattanzi and Cook[6], three had had a previous calculus, one of which occurred during a previous pregnancy, and one patient had a positive family history. In addition, a history of recurrent urinary tract infection may be significant. In the series of Jones,[11] ten patients had urinary tract infections documented prior to pregnancy, and seven during the index pregnancy. A history of previous surgery on the urinary tract also is important.

Gross hematuria is present less often with stone disease in pregnancy, although microscopic hematuria reportedly is present in 63–89% of cases.[2-9] However, the finding of hematuria in pregnancy is not necessarily a reliable indicator of the presence of calculi. Hormonal influences and dilatation of the collecting system cause vascular dilatation, which may result in spontaneous bleeding into the urinary tract.[12]

One of the most difficult aspects of the diagnosis of stone disease in pregnancy is its differentiation from uncomplicated acute pyelonephritis. The latter is relatively common, occurring in almost 2% of pregnancies.[13] Thus, the presence of fever and leukocytosis, with or without bacteriuria, associated with flank pain often prompts a diagnosis of acute pyelonephritis. Persistence of fever and pain despite 48 hours of parenteral antibiotics suggests calculus complicating the infection.

In the nonpregnant patient, the mainstay of diagnosis of stones anywhere in the urinary tract is an intravenous pyelogram (IVP). This investigation is relatively easy to perform, and provides information regarding the size and location of calculi, as well as the extent of obstruction present. Unfortuantely, concern about the effects of ionizing radiation on the developing fetus means that this examination must be used judiciously in pregnancy. This is further supported by a report in which the early use of IVP in all pregnant patients with symptoms suggesting calculi revealed stones in only one of 23 examinations.[14] Horowitz and Schmidt[2] recommend the following criteria for performance of an IVP: (1) persistent fever or persistent positive urine culture despite 48 hours of parenteral antibiotics; (2) persistent obstruction as manifested by increasing levels of blood urea nitrogen (BUN) and serum creatinine; (3) massive hydronephrosis on abdominal ultrasonography; or (4) protracted pain or hydration problems from continuing emesis. Using these criteria, the diagnostic yield in their series was approximately 60%, and many patients were able to avoid radiologic studies.

It also should be noted that when an IVP is indicated in pregnancy, it is important to tailor the timing of exposures to minimize the radiation dose. A protocol using a scout film, and a second film no sooner than 20 minutes after injection of contrast, plus a delayed film at one hour if evidence of delayed excretion is present, will limit the radiation dose to approximately 0.4–0.6 roentgen.[15]

Most centers now use ultrasonography as the first-line screening test for the presence of stones in a symptomatic pregnant patient. This modality has the advantage of being safe, and it can delineate the presence of hydronephrosis with reliability. However, it is unreliable in distinguishing between physiologic dilatation of the upper tract that occurs in normal pregnancy[16] from the pathologic dilatation secondary to calculi. It also is not helpful in diagnosing ureteral stones. On the other hand, ultrasound is the primary imaging modality for placement of percutaneous nephrostomy drainage in the rare situations in which this is necessary.[17]

Although radionuclide imaging (with only 10% of the radiation dose of an IVP) has been studied in pregnancy[18], it has not been shown to be able to localize well the site of obstruction.

A review of series published since 1980 reveals a 70% rate of spontaneous stone passage during pregnancy.[2,6-10,19] It is thought that the physiologic dilatation of the ureters accounts for this increased rate of spontaneous passage compared with nonpregnant patients. Clearly, conservative management is the first step in the treatment of the gravida with acute manifestations of urinary calculi. This includes bed rest with intravenous hydration and analgesics. Narcotics may be required for adequate pain control. Parenteral antibiotics are indicated in those cases in which concomitant infection is likely.

In those patients in whom conservative management is unsuccessful (that is, those with complete obstruction, persistent pain or sepsis, or evidence of decreasing renal function), surgical intervention is indicated. The specific surgical procedure depends on the size and location of the stone. Generally, the procedure of choice for ureteral calculi is basket extraction or retrograde stent placement at cystoscopy. Stents placed to relieve obstruction may be left in place for months at a time, to allow passage of the stone or postponement of an open surgical procedure to the postpartum period. Placement of the stents is easiest in the first and second trimesters. Distortion of the pelvic floor anatomy by the enlarged uterus during the third trimester may prevent their use later in gestation. Successful percutaneous nephrostomy for complete obstruction during the third trimester has been reported to relieve obstruction temporarily.[2,20] The disadvantage of both these approaches is that they involve the use of an indwelling foreign body, with consequent increased risk of urinary tract infection. The use of flexible ureteroscopes under local anesthesia to directly visualize stones for removal for proximal placement of a drainage stent has been reported.[21] The authors cite the avoidance of fluoroscopy as an advantage of this method during pregnancy.

Rarely, open procedures including ureterolithotomy, pyelolithotomy, or even partial nephrectomy may be required, primarily for stones located in the upper tract, or those that cannot be managed by the cystoscopic or percutaneous approach.

Regardless of the surgical procedure required, treatment of urinary calculi appears to be relatively safe for both mother and fetus. Lattanzi and Cook[6] reviewed a series of 31 surgical procedures reported by a number of different groups, with no fetal complications and only one case of maternal septic shock. Historical reports of universal surgical intervention for stones in pregnancy did not reveal nearly as good an outcome.[22]

Although extracorporeal lithotripsy is used increasingly for management of calculi outside of pregnancy, its safety during pregnancy has not been studied yet. For that reason, it is currently not indicated in pregnancy.

Following delivery, patients with recurrent stone disease should undergo a metabolic workup to determine any underlying etiology. Patients presenting with a history of stone disease can be counseled that they are no more likely to form stones during a future pregnancy than during any other nine-month period. They also do not appear to be at increased risk of any pregnancy complications aside from urinary tract infections. It seems prudent, therefore, to follow these patients with periodic urine cultures throughout gestation.

REFERENCES

1. Smith LH. The medical aspects of urolithiasis: an overview. *J Urol.* 1988;141:707.
2. Horowitz E, Schmidt JD. Renal calculi in pregnancy. *Clin Obstet Gynecol.* 1985;28:324.
3. Coe FL, Parks JH, Lindheimer MD. Nephrolithiasis during pregnancy. *N Engl J Med.* 1978;298:324.
4. Cass AS, Smith CS, Gleich P. Management of urinary calculi in pregnancy. *Urology.* 1986;28:370.
5. Harris RE, Dunnihoo DR. The incidence and significance of urinary calculi in pregnancy. *Am J Obstet Gynecol.* 1967;99:237.
6. Lattanzi DR, Cook WA. Urinary calculi in pregnancy. *Obstet Gynecol.* 1980;56:462.
7. Boes D. Urinary calculi in pregnancy: diagnosis and management. *Am Osteo Assoc J.* 1982;81:697.
8. Drago JR, Rohner TJ Jr, Chez RA. Management of urinary calculi in pregnancy. *Urology.* 1982;20:578.
9. Miller RD, Kakkis J. Prognosis, management and outcome of obstructive renal disease in pregnancy. *J Reprod Med.* 1982;27:199.
10. Gregory MC, Mansell MA. Pregnancy and cystinuria. *Lancet.* 1983;19:1158.
11. Jones WA, Correa RJ Jr, Ansell JS. Urolithiasis associated with pregnancy. *J Urol.* 1979;122:333.
12. Walter WC. The urinary tract in pregnancy. *J Urol.* 1981;125:271.
13. Gilstrap LC III, Cunningham FG, Whalley PJ. Acute pyelonephritis in pregnancy: an antero-spective study. *Obstet Gynecol.* 1981;57:409.
14. Rigby MR, MacEwan DW. Urography during pregnancy. *J Can Assoc Radiol.* 1976;27:227.
15. Strong DW, Murchison RJ, Lynch DF. The management of ureteral calculi during pregnancy. *Surg Gynecol Obstet.* 1978;146:604.
16. Fried AM, Woodring JH, Thompson DJ. Hydronephrosis of pregnancy: a prospective sequential study of the course of dilatation. *J Ultrasound Med.* 1983;2:255.
17. Reznek RH, Talner LB. Percutaneous nephrostomy. *Radiol Clin North Am.* 1984;22:232.
18. Voigt R, Toll W, Arndt J. The value of radio-isotope investigations of the urinary tract for the diagnosis of urinary tract calculi during pregnancy. *Geburtshilfe Frauenheilkd.* 1980;40:863.
19. Perreault JP, Paquin JM, Faucher R, Maufee F. Urinary calculi in pregnancy. *Can J Surg.* 1982;25:453.
20. Hedegaard CK, Wallace D. Percutaneous nephrostomy: current indications and potential uses in obstetrics and gynecology. *Obstet Gynecol Surv.* 1987;42:671.
21. Rittenbery MH, Bagley DH. Ureteroscopic diagnosis and treatment of urinary calculi during pregnancy. *Urology.* 1988;32:427.
22. Arnell RE, Getzoff PL. Renal and ureteral calculi in pregnancy. *Am J Obstet Gynecol.* 1942;44:34.

PART XIII Gastrointestinal Tract

Robert M. Galbraith, Section Editor

Chapter One Hundred and Forty-Seven

Upper Gastrointestinal Tract Disease

John T. Cunningham

147

The approach to upper gastrointestinal disease during pregnancy presents some unique problems in that pregnancy itself produces certain physiologic changes that may increase or decrease the incidence of some disorders, although others are unaffected. The presence of the fetus and its gestational age have a profound influence on the diagnostic and therapeutic options that are available. Individual risk/and benefit ratios must be assessed, although very little or no objective data exist as to the safety or efficacy of many agents or procedures in pregnancy.

PREGNANCY: PHYSIOLOGIC AND ANATOMIC CHANGES

Diminished lower esophageal sphincter (LES) tone has been demonstrated well during later pregnancy.[1-3] For example, at the beginning of the second trimester, baseline LES tone may be unchanged, but there is a marked diminution in the normal rise of LES pressure in response to a series of stimuli, including pentagastrin and protein meal ingestion.[4] This blunted response may represent the first change in LES function and represents the loss of an important protective reflex. Elevated estrogen and progesterone levels are present and have been implicated in the pathogenesis of this change, but a direct correlation with absolute estrogen levels has not been demonstrated. Patients on sequential oral contraceptives may demonstrate a decrease in LES pressure that coincides with the progestational phase of the cycle, a finding suggesting that estrogen plays a "priming" role for the progesterone effect on smooth muscle.[5] Delivery of the fetus or discontinuing the contraceptive agents results in a return of LES pressure to normal. Other reported changes in esophageal motility during pregnancy include an increase in secondary peristalsis and nonpropulsive peristalsis.[1] There is also an increased incidence of hiatus hernia, especially in multiparous patients.[6] Increased intragastric pressure with flattening of the hemidiaphragms causes a loss of the normal acute esophagogastric angle.

Physiologic changes within the upper tract have been less well defined but include: decreased gastric and small bowel motility with delayed transit times[7], pyloric sphincter incompetence, and reflux of bile salts and alkaline duodenal contents back into the stomach.[8,9] In the stomach there is no apparent change in gastrin physiology, but a small though statistically significant decrease in basal and stimulated acid output has been observed. This has been attributed to the effects of progesterone.[10] Mucus output is increased, presumably secondary to both estrogen and progesterone.[11] How these changes might be related and what pathogenic role they play are discussed later in the chapter (see also Chapter 4).

SYMPTOMS IN UPPER GASTROINTESTINAL DISEASES

Dysphagia implies the impairment of passage of a bolus from the hypopharynx to the stomach and can be caused by a variety of disorders. When it is present, either physiologic (neuromuscular) or anatomic obstruction can be demonstrated in a high percentage of patients. The level at which the patient perceives the blockage correlates well with the true level of dysfunction, although a small proportion (approximately 10%) of patients with obstruction at the gastroesophageal junction will refer to the suprasternal notch in describing their symptoms. Dysphagia is a specific symptom, and an organic etiology can be found in 95% of patients.

Odynophagia is the perception of pain as a bolus passes down the lumen and implies a severely inflamed esophagus. It is common in infectious and caustic esophagitis and can be localized to the cervical esophagus in acute thyroiditis but is uncommon in reflux esophagitis, which causes a retrosternal burning (heartburn) sensation, usually postprandially. Heartburn implies irritation of the esophagus from a variety of irritant stimuli and is not specific for acid reflux. Conversely, the complaint of a "lump" in the throat that is perceived continuously, localized to the hypopharynx, and does not interfere with deglutition is almost always functional and referred to as the *globus reaction* or *globus hystericus*.

DIAGNOSTIC PROCEDURES: IMPLICATIONS OF PREGNANCY

Investigation of the gastrointestinal (GI) tract during pregnancy is hampered by the potential hazards of several procedures to both patient and fetus. Many radiographic procedures are not recommended during pregnancy, particularly if the fetus might be in the exposure field, as in upper GI series or barium enema examinations.[12] If a specific procedure is indicated, appropriate shielding of the fetus can be undertaken. Dosimeters should be placed under the shield over the uterus to document the lack of exposure to the fetus. The need for radiography in the diagnosis of esophageal and gastric disorders is reduced, as it does not provide specific additional information that could not be provided by other procedures: for example, the source of an upper intestinal hemorrhage or the etiology of an inflammatory esophagitis. Other procedures may yield similar or better information at less risk. Esophageal manometry has provided important information about the pathogenesis of various disorders in pregnancy[1,2,13], but in the evaluation of the individual patient it does not often yield information of significant therapeutic benefit. Some uncommon indications do exist, such as in achalasia and esophageal spasm, where manometry may be particularly helpful. Upper endoscopy with the more recently developed flexible fiberoptic endoscope allows for excellent visualization of the esophagus, stomach, and proximal duodenum with relative ease and safety and is well tolerated by the pregnant patient.[2,14] The procedure can be performed with only topical hypopharyngeal anesthesia, since several studies have demonstrated that systemic sedatives or analgesics are not often required for routine diagnostic upper endoscopy, and patient acceptance is good.[15,16]

ESOPHAGUS

Ptyalism

Ptyalism is a very rare complication of pregnancy in which there is a markedly increased output of saliva from the major glands with expectorated volumes of 1–2 L per day.[17] The quality of the salivary juice and swallowing mechanism are normal. Onset usually occurs within several weeks of the first missed menstrual period, and ptyalism abates spontaneously with delivery. Some cases are sufficiently severe to require hospitalization because of weight loss and volume depletion. Patients frequently present with a history of nausea and vomiting when they attempt to swallow their saliva. Physical examination is usually normal, although patients are drooling or constantly expectorating saliva and evidence of volume depletion may be present. It is of interest to note, however, that such patients do not generally manifest any difficulties during sleep.

The pathogenesis of ptyalism is unknown, but most authors suggest a psychosomatic origin for which many forms of therapy have been recommended, including anticholinergics and bromides. Unfortunately, none has been consistently effective. The problem in assessing this disorder is that total daily volumes of saliva produced often do not exceed the normal.[18] This finding, combined with a lack of biochemical or physical changes, has indicated a neuropsychiatric origin. Good emotional support and reassurance that the condition is self-limited are paramount in management of this condition, which is very distressing to the patient.

Infectious Diseases

Monilial Esophagitis. Infection with *Candida albicans* usually presents with severe odynophagia; the diagnosis can be suspected by the finding of typical satellite lesions in the oropharynx. However, in 70% of cases only the esophagus is involved, and the diagnosis is established by endoscopy with the finding of white plaque-like lesions lining the mucosa. Examination of wet preparations obtained by brushing demonstrate the admixture of mycelial elements and budding yeasts.[19] Biopsy or culture is not needed unless unusual circumstances are present or typical lesions fail to respond to conventional therapy. Therapy consists of the oral, nonabsorbed antifungal mycostatin in a dose of 100,000 U qid for 10–14 days.[20]

Herpes Esophagitis. Herpes simplex virus is now being recognized in healthy young patients who are neither debilitated nor immunocompromised.[21] It usually presents with fever and severe odynophagia. Some cases have fever blisters in the oral cavity or vesicular eruptions on the genitalia. The diagnosis can be suspected when these typical mucocutaneous lesions are evident, but confirmation with a rise in viral titers by complement fixation requires 2–3 weeks, by which time the syndrome has usually resolved. Diagnosis can be established more definitively by endoscopy. Early lesions are small, clear vesicles that erupt to form shallow ulcerations. Biopsy may reveal acute and chronic inflammatory reaction with eosinophilic, intranuclear Cowdry type A inclusion bodies within the epithelial cells.[22] Culture in appropriate media may grow herpes virus; however, the later the biopsy or culture is obtained from the onset of symptoms, the lower is the yield.[21] Therapy usually is not indicated, as the disease is self-limiting and will resolve in 1–2 weeks. Symptomatic treatment with antacids may alleviate some symptoms. Acyclovir has no known fetal toxicity but is recommended only with caution for resistant cases.

Heartburn in Pregnancy

Symptoms of heartburn are extremely common in pregnancy, occurring in excess of 50% of patients.[23] Heartburn usually occurs during the second and third trimesters and in most instances disappears after pregnancy. A major stumbling block to determining the cause is that reflux of both acid and alkaline gastric contents can elicit identical symptoms.[24] The pathogenesis is multifactorial, but generally decreased lower esophageal sphincter pressure is combined with increased intragastric pressure as the uterus rises out of the pelvis. These combine to decrease the normal pressure gradient between the stomach and the esophagus, thereby promoting reflux of gastric contents. It is not surprising, therefore, that the pressure across this barrier is significantly lower in pregnant than nonpregnant controls, with a tendency towards even lower pressure in symptomatic pregnant patients than in their asymptomatic counterparts.

The role of other anatomic factors such as hiatus hernia and flattening of the hemidiaphragms, which decreases the insertion angle at the esophagogastric junction, is controversial. The nature of the refluxed material may be important as well. For example, it is generally agreed that hyperacidity is not always present and that significant esophagitis can occur with prolonged reflux of material of "physiologic" pH or even alkaline duodenal contents containing bile salts. Pyloric incompetence and gastric stasis are considered important in setting the stage for alkaline damage to the esophagus.

The clinical presentation is typically a complaint of an epigastric or substernal warmth or burning sensation that becomes worse with bending, sitting, and recumbency. The correlation between symptoms and definite pathology is very variable and depends on the thoroughness of the investigation. For example, in one series, 22 of 25 pregnant patients with heartburn had endoscopic biopsy evidence of esophagitis.[25] However, it is definitely uncommon for the clinical complications of stricture or hemorrhage to occur.

The clinical features usually are sufficient to suggest the diagnosis, and additional testing usually is not indicated in the absence of dysphagia, bleeding, or other complications. Endoscopy, biopsy, and the Bernstein test, in which dilute acid is instilled into the esophagus, offer little additional useful information in these patients, and they should be treated symptomatically. Initial therapy should be aimed at reducing the duration and frequency of reflux of gastric contents back into the esophagus. This is accomplished by taking frequent small meals during the day, avoiding food for two hours prior to bedtime, and avoiding recumbency for 30 minutes to one hour after meals. The head of the bed may be elevated on 4- to 6-inch blocks. Additionally, conventional antacid therapy with standard aluminum and magnesium hydroxide gels are given 30 to 60 minutes postprandially in a dose sufficient to neutralize 80 mEq of acid. Most antacid preparations are a combination of magnesium and aluminum hydroxide, and diarrhea is a common side effect. The pure aluminum hydroxide antacids have a theoretical advantage as they also bind bile salts, but their clinical efficacy in bile-induced injury is unproven, and the side-effect of severe constipation is not tolerated well. They can be alternated with magnesium-containing antacids when diarrhea is a problem. Sodium bicarbonate and magnesium trisilicate should be avoided. Particular attention should be given to the sodium content, which varies greatly among various preparations[26], and low-sodium preparations should be administered when clinically indicated.

An alternative or complementary mode of therapy involves the nonabsorbable alginic acid preparations, which are formulated with weak acid-neutralizing properties. Their primary mode of action is to float in a raft-like manner on the gastric contents; they are therefore the first material to enter the esophagus when reflux occurs. There are reports of more subjective symptomatic improvement as compared with conventional antacids[27]; however, biopsy or endoscopic improvement is not as well documented. Perhaps the increased subjective relief may be explained by a mucosal coating action that is protective against both acid and alkaline reflux. Again, studies in pregnancy are lacking, and safety is not established. The idea that heartburn during pregnancy can be secondary to either acid or alkaline reflux has led several authors[28,29] to resort to a therapeutic regimen in which either a standard antacid or a dilute 0.1 N HCl mixture is administered. If a positive response is not obtained with the first, then the patient is switched to the other mode of therapy. However, this therapy should be considered controversial, and more controlled experience is necessary.

In general, the above methods produce subjective improvement in 95% of patients; more aggressive measures should be reserved for unresponsive patients or those with complications of their reflux disease. H_2-receptor blockers such as cimetidine, ranitidine, or famotidine produce significant reduction in hydrogen ion secretion and are efficacious in reflux esophagitis.[30] No controlled trials have been published in pregnancy, and anecdotal reports of safe short-term usage[31,32] are limited and do not allow applications for widespread use. Nevertheless, when significant maternal morbidity is present, the use of H_2-receptor blockers may be warranted.

The above modalities are aimed at neutralizing or reducing the secretion of the injurious agent and not at what is considered to be the primary pathogenic problem, loss of the LES barrier. Metoclopramide, a compound of the phenothiazine family, has been demonstrated to increase the LES pressure in nonpregnant patients with reflux esophagitis[33,34] and to reduce the number of reflux episodes.[33] In symptomatic patients during their third trimester, metoclopramide produced subjective improvement in 16 of 17 cases, but manometric improvement with increased barrier pressure occurred in only four of ten cases.[35] What roles possible augmentation of gastric emptying[36] or centrally mediated antiemetic effect[37] play is conjectural, but these considerations suggest that heartburn during pregnancy may involve different pathophysiologic processes from the similar, subjective disease in the nonpregnant patient. The exact mechanism of action of this compound is unknown. It has cholinergic agonist properties in that it stimulates smooth muscle contraction but does not stimulate gastric secretion.[37] Many of its undesirable effects are caused by dopaminergic antagonist properties in the central nervous system, and side effects occur in up to 10% of patients.[38] Somnolence and weakness are common, but the most significant complications are the extrapyramidal reactions including oculogyric crisis, opisthotonos, and trismus. Most reactions disappear with drug withdrawal, but intravenous diphenhydramine, 50–100 mg, will rapidly reverse the more severe neuromuscular reactions.

The use of these more aggressive modes of therapy should be reserved for the patient in whom the disease itself represents a significant risk to the viability of the fetus and therefore justifies their use; in most patients the symptoms abate after delivery. Esophageal stricture[31] and hemorrhage[39] represent the most severe manifestations of the disease. When symptoms suggest these complications, upper endoscopy is indicated to assess the severity of the disease, establish the benign nature of the stricture, and possibly dilate the stricture by passing hydrostatic dilators over a guidewire and dilating under direct vision. Maloney or Hurst dilators also can be passed by experienced personnel if the stricture is interfering with adequate nutrition.

Esophageal Motor Disorders

Motor disorders of the esophagus are uncommon in pregnancy, but when dysphagia is present in the face of an inconclusive or normal endoscopy, these diagnoses should be considered. Esophageal motility studies are most helpful at this point in the differential diagnosis. Transfer dysphagia occurs when there is difficulty in movement of a bolus from the oropharynx through the hypopharynx into the esophagus. These patients commonly have more problems with liquids than solids and may have nasal regurgitation as an important clinical symptom. Two main groups of disorders must be considered, muscular and neural. Primary skeletal muscle diseases of the upper third of the esophagus include myasthenia gravis, dermatomyositis, polymyositis, and the muscular dystrophies. Esophageal manometry may provide a valuable clue to the diagnosis by demonstrating a hypotonic upper sphincter and diminished motility. Neural disorders that would affect the pharynx or hypopharynx, including amyotrophic lateral sclerosis, bulbar and pseudobulbar palsy, as well as brainstem infarction, can present similarly. Usually, concomitant physical findings will help determine the diagnosis.[40] For both categories, therapy is directed at the primary disorder, with dietary manipulation to provide maximum calories in a form that can be readily ingested.

In the lower esophagus, dysphagia can be caused by achalasia and diffuse esophageal spasm, the latter being both intermittent and usually accompanied by substernal pain. Manometry is the method of choice to establish the diagnosis. Therapy is dependent on the severity of the symptoms. In achalasia, if nutritional support can be maintained until delivery, then therapy with forceful dilation of the esophagus can be delayed until a more suitable time.[41] If malnutrition becomes a problem, enteral or parenteral nutrition may be required. It is the nutritional status of the mother that determines fetal outcome and not the disease itself. Potential risk–benefit ratios must be assessed before more dramatic forms of therapy are considered.

UPPER GASTROINTESTINAL HEMORRHAGE

Despite the rather common occurrence of upper gastrointestinal symptoms during pregnancy, complications including acute intestinal hemorrhage are by contrast remarkably uncommon. In those rare cases in which complications occur, the bleeding has been reported to be secondary to esophagitis in 41%, to esophageal varices in 25%, to acute gastritis in 17%, and to Mallory-Weiss lacerations (which usually occur in conjunction with pernicious vomiting) in the remaining 17%.[39] Initial management is directed at basic support with IV fluids, transfusion as needed, and early endoscopy after stabilization to establish the origin of bleeding, and where appropriate, injection therapy with 98% ethyl alcohol at the bleeding site to establish hemostasis and prevent surgical intervention.[42] The volume of injection is low and systemic absorption negligible.

Esophagitis can be managed as outlined earlier with particular attention directed to control of the recurrent vomiting. Careful attention must be paid to this group of patients, as a significant number will develop stricture in the immediate postpartum period.[39] The therapy of vomiting in pregnancy is discussed below.

Variceal hemorrhage in the pregnant patient can occur in established cirrhosis with portal hypertension[43], secondary to hepatic venous obstruction[44] (Budd-Chiari syndrome), or as a sequel to extrahepatic (noncirrhotic) portal hypertension.[45] Transient portal hypertension that resolves postpartum also has been reported[46], but this was poorly characterized and may have been related to multiple hepatic adenomata or focal nodular hyperplasia. Overall, these patients have a more benign course with survival of 82% for cirrhotics and 95% for noncirrhotics.[43] Therapy is always individualized. For most patients, basic support with fluid replacement and transfusion will be sufficient, with more aggressive management with surgical shunts or sclerotherapy reserved for the unusual patient who cannot be managed conservatively. The risk of rebleeding once the pregnancy is terminated is unaltered in the cirrhotic and decreases in the noncirrhotic.[46]

Hemorrhage secondary to mucosal laceration in the region of the esophagogastric junction (Mallory-Weiss syndrome) resolves with conservative therapy in 90% of patients.[47] The most important factor is prevention of rebleeding by control of the underlying cause, generally nausea and vomiting during pregnancy. Therapy is directed at fluid maintenance, transfusion, and control of emesis with chlorpromazine or metoclopramide. Other methods for control short of surgery may include endoscopy with monopolar electrocoagulation[48], bipolar coagulation[49], endoscopic laser photocoagulation[50], and injection of 1:10,000 epinephrine or 98% ethyl alcohol.[42] The latter two techniques carry a lower risk of penetration or perforation of the bowel and do not involve passage of any potential of injury to the fetus, which could possibly be damaging.

Hemorrhagic gastritis can be managed best with conventional antacid regimens with administration of seven doses per day (15–30 mL) given one and three hours after meals and at bedtime. Despite a wealth of controversial literature, the efficacy of pharmacologic agents in bringing an established active hemorrhage under control has yet to be demonstrated. Few studies have demonstrated adequate prevention of rebleeding once hemostasis has been achieved. These statements are true for both H_2 receptor blockers and mucosal barrier protectors. Antacids and sucralfate probably are best for prevention of stress ulcers in the acutely ill patient, since multiple trials in nonpregnant patients have demonstrated superiority over placebo[51] or cimetidine.[52] Antacids should be administered in sufficient amounts to keep the gastric pH greater than 3.5.[51] Intragastric pH should be monitored in severely ill patients by placement of a nasogastric tube and aspirating gastric fluid prior to the next dose.[52] Continuous infusion of H_2 blocker may be superior to intermittent bolus therapy, but in severely stressed patients pH must be monitored.[53] Sucralfate has the benefit of providing protection from stress bleeding, and this is derived independent of gastric pH.[54] The synthetic prostaglandin E_2, misoprostil, recently has been approved for treatment of nonsteroidal-induced gastric mucosal damage. The agents have an abortifactant potential and have been used to induce therapeutic abortions.[55]

Peptic ulcers, rarely with bleeding, are noticeable by their relative absence during pregnancy (one in 70,000).[56] The relevant symptoms and complications seem to show a predilection for the latter portion of the third trimester or puerperium.

PEPTIC ULCER DISEASE

Many authors have emphasized the beneficial effects of pregnancy on the incidence of peptic ulcer disease.[56,57] In one study, 88% of women with dyspeptic symptoms reported improvement during pregnancy[58], and in 50% the symptoms recurred within three months of delivery. This correlates with the reported incidence of ulcer in females; there is a bimodal distribution with peaks occurring during the latter portion of the second decade of life (menarcheal spike) and again during the fourth decade (postmenopausal spike), with a steady lower plateau during the childbearing years. The possibility that the true incidence of ulcer is higher[59] has been argued on the grounds that ulcer symptoms may be obscured by symptomatic reflux and its subsequent treatment. There is a correlation with the recurrence of symptoms and rise in gastric acid and pepsin output during the latter portion of the third trimester.

The pathogenesis of these beneficial effects is still debated. Hormonal changes in estrogen and progesterone may have the effect of decreasing acid secretion and increasing mucin production. Placental histaminase production during pregnancy also has been implicated in reducing acid pepsin secretion by reducing the parietal cell response to endogenous histamine.[60] However, the precise role of these factors are conjectural.

Diagnosis

A careful assessment of the history is important to plan therapy and anticipate potential complications. When the pain or burning is localized to the epigastrium and is relieved by food, only to recur two to three hours later, pyloric channel or duodenal ulcer is likely. Invasive or more aggressive diagnostic procedures should be withheld, and a carefully observed therapeutic trial instituted (see below). If no relief is achieved, endoscopy should be considered. The introduction of smaller, more flexible, optically improved instruments has allowed the experienced endoscopist to perform a competent examination of the upper tract in 5–10 minutes with no premedication other than hypopharyngeal anesthesia. The procedure should be performed only when the information gained would be expected to produce a significant change in management. If the patient fails to respond to therapy, or if gastric ulcer is suspected, endoscopy with biopsy and brushing are indicated to exclude an ulcerating malignancy.[61]

Treatment

The dictum "no acid, no ulcer" continues to maintain its clinical relevance. Most methods of therapy, both medical or surgical, are directed toward reduction of the effects of acid and pepsin on the gastric mucosa, either by neutralization, decreasing secretion, or enhancing mucosal defense. Antacids continue to be the standard against which all ulcer therapies are compared, although there is little good objective data to prove their efficacy.[62] Their safety, although generally assumed, has not been rigorously established. In one retrospective study, a small increase in major and minor fetal abnormalities was demonstrated when antacids as a group were given in the first trimester, but no single preparation could be implicated directly.[63] Doses sufficient to neutralize 80 mEq of HCl are given one and three hours after meals and at bedtime. Treatment should be continued for 4–6 weeks regardless of improvement in symptoms, since the latter correlate poorly with ulcer healing.[62]

Other available modalities that have proven beneficial in healing ulcer, but are not proven safe in pregnancy, include the histamine (H_2) blockers[64] and surface protective agents.[65] Cimetidine, ranitidine, famotidine and nizatidine are four of the currently available H_2 blockers. They differ in relative potency, but all are now approved as once-a-day therapy. There may be fewer problems with drug interaction with the newer compounds. Sucralfate is an aluminum salt of a sulfated disaccharide that has unique properties in that it is a weak antacid, a potent inhibitor of pepsin, and binds to the denatured protein in the ulcer crater.[66] It has been demonstrated to be only minimally absorbed, with <5% being excreted in the urine[65,67], and thus should have a theoretical advantage. Moreover, extensive tests in animals have failed to demonstrate any teratogenicity.[68] However, like so many other useful therapeutic agents, no studies have been carried out to demonstrate safety in pregnancy. The standard regimen is 1 g given 1 hour prior to meals and at bedtime. Even though this agent has chemical similarities to heparin, no anticoagulant activity has been demonstrated despite extensive clinical use.[65]

All of the above regimens should be withheld until there is a clear lack of response to standard antacid therapy or it is apparent that the disease is a significant hazard to the mother or fetus. Once complications such as hemorrhage occur and endoscopic therapy fails, surgical intervention must be considered. Since complications usually occur in the third trimester, fetal development is such that cesarean section also may be considered, particularly since spontaneous vaginal delivery frequently occurs in the perioperative period after intestinal surgery.[69] Uncontrolled hemorrhage, perforation, and gastric outlet obstruction should be considered surgical indications. The maternal outcome is good and fetal survival acceptable under these dire circumstances.[69]

NAUSEA AND VOMITING

Pathogenesis

Nausea and vomiting during pregnancy are best considered as a syndrome that occurs during the first trimester and for which no underlying disorder can be found. It is reported to occur in approximately 50% of pregnancies, and is associated with younger age, heavier maternal weight, primigravidas, and a history of previous emesis if multiparous.[70] Hyperemesis gravidarum is the most severe extreme of this disorder, occurring in 1–2% of cases, and is accompanied by weight loss, ketonemia, acetonuria, and profound volume depletion.[71] The incidence is said to be decreasing with the advent of chemotherapy for this disorder. Nausea and vomiting with an onset after the first trimester should be considered as indications of other disorders, especially genitourinary and hepatic disease and preeclampsia.[72]

Despite a wealth of literature and controversy, very little incontrovertible evidence exists about the etiology of this syndrome, and a psychogenic basis is considered most important.[71] One popular hormonal theory, elevation of human chorionic gonadotropin, has been challenged.[73] Another study implicated elevated estradiol and low progesterone levels when compared to nonemetic controls.[74] A recent study has reported an elevated free T_4 in 73% of patients in the face of a failure to respond to TRH, indicating autologous T_4 production. This phenomenon is self-limiting; the level of hormone abnormality correlates with the severity of the emesis and resolves spontaneously at delivery.[75] It is thought to be a physiologic response to the emesis and not a pathologic state. Multiple other etiologies have been suggested, including vitamin deficiency, disturbed carbohydrate metabolism, and other endocrine abnormalities.

Management

The majority of patients can be reassured of the transient and benign nature of this disorder and can be managed with simple maneuvers such as avoidance of offending foods or situations that evoke symptoms. Sitting up in bed and ingesting dry crackers may suffice to alleviate symptoms. A recent rash of litigation has produced some reluctance to use pharmacologic agents. However, there is a wealth of information indicating a lack of teratogenicity of many antinauseant compounds[71,76], and phenothiazine, proclorperazine, dimenhydrinate, and meclizine[76] all have been demonstrated to be safe. The latter agent is thought to carry the lowest risk. Of interest is the demonstration of an apparent favorable association of nausea and vomiting with a lower perinatal mortality.[70]

Metoclopramide, because of its central antiemetic effect[37], recently has been used clinically for hyperemesis gravidarum. Few controlled clinical studies have been published[77], and its use is recommended for more clinically severe cases. This compound readily crosses the placenta into the fetal circulation, and although increases in maternal serum prolactin have been demonstrated, no concomitant hormone increases have occurred in the fetus. Efficacy is superior to placebo and equivalent to that of other antiemetic agents in a dose of 10 mg three times a day. Thus far, no harmful effects have been reported in the fetus.[78] Side effects have been reviewed above.

If symptoms persist, hospital admission with IV fluid support and electrolyte replacement is indicated. The support of nutritional or dietary services with manipulation of the diet may be valuable in formulation of a plan by which nutrients can be reintroduced to the patient.[79] Elimination of all regular food may be required, followed by gradual reintroduction of normal dietary constituents. If this cannot be tolerated, then standard nutritional supplements can be given as multiple small feedings in dilute form. Only rarely will a patient need a more aggressive approach such as enteral alimentation via a small-bore duodenal tube[80] or parenteral intravenous supplemenmentation.[81] Markers of nutritional status, including albumin, prealbumin, and serum transferrin concentrations, should be followed closely, although it should be noted that levels of these components are altered during pregnancy (see Chapter 4). During this period of support, attempts should be made to reintroduce oral feedings. With current advances in nutritional support, fetal mortality is now infrequent.

REFERENCES

1. Nagler R, Spiro HM. Heartburn in late pregnancy. Manometric studies of esophageal motor function. *J Clin Invest*. 1961;40:954.
2. Castro L de P. Reflux esophagitis as the cause of heartburn in pregnancy. *Am J Obstet Gynecol*. 1967;98:1.
3. Hey VM, Crowley DJ, Ganguli PC, et al. Gastroesophageal reflux in late pregnancy. *Anesthesia*. 1977;32:372.
4. Fisher RS, Roberts GS, Grabowski CJ, et al. Altered lower esophageal sphincter function during early pregnancy. *Am J Physiol*. 1978;74:1233.
5. Van Thiel DH, Gavaler JS, Stremple J. Lower esophageal sphincter pressure in women using sequential oral contraceptives. *Gastroenterology*. 1976;71:232.
6. Mixson WT, Woloshin HJ. Hiatus hernia in pregnancy. *Obstet Gynecol*. 1956;8:249.
7. Wald A, Van Thiel DH, Noechstetter L, et al. Gastrointestinal transit: The effect of the menstrual cycle. *Gastroenterology*. 1981;80:1497.
8. Gillison EW, Nyhus LM. Bile reflux, gastric secretion and heartburn. *Br J Surg*. 1971;56:864.
9. Atley RD, Gillison EW, Horton AL. A fresh look at pregnancy heartburn. *J Obstet Gynaecol Br Commonw*. 1973;80:63.
10. Murray FA, Erskine JP, Fielding J. Gastric secretion in pregnancy. *J Obstet Gynaecol Br Emp*. 1957;64:373.
11. Parbhoo SP, Johnston IDA. Effects of oestrogens and progestogens on gastric secretion in patients with duodenal ulcer. *Gut*. 1966;7:612.
12. Doust BD, Doust V. Ultrasound, roentgenography, and radionuclide imaging in obstetric diagnosis. In: Danfort DN, ed. *Obstetrics and Gynecology*. 3rd ed. Hagerstown, MD: Harper & Row, 1981;517.
13. Lind JF, Smith AM, McIver DK, et al. Heartburn in pregnancy—a manometric study. *Can Med Assoc J*. 1968;98:571.
14. Palmer ED. Upper gastrointestinal hemorrhage during pregnancy. *Am J Med Sci*. 1961;242:223.
15. Jackson FD. Office endoscopy without sedation. *Gastrointest Endosc*. 1981;27:123.
16. Nichols AM, Cunningham JT. Upper endoscopy without sedation. *Gastrointest Endosc*. 1982;28:140.
17. Cooper SB. Ptyalism complicating pregnancy. *J Obstet Gynaecol Br Emp*. 1956;63:582.
18. Texter CE, Chou CC, Laureta HC, et al. *Physiology of the gastrointestinal tract*. St Louis, MO: CV Mosby; 1968:143.
19. Kodsi BE, Wickremesunghe PC, Kozinn PJ, et al. Candida esophagitis: A prospective study of 27 cases. *Gastroenterology*. 1976;71:715.
20. Gilman AG, Goodman S, Gilman A. *The Pharmacological Basis of Therapeutics*. 6th ed. New York, NY: Macmillan; 1980:1232.
21. Solammadevi SV, Patwardhan R. Herpes esophagitis. *Am J Gastroenterol*. 1982;77:48.
22. Springer DJ, DaCosta LR, Beck JT. A syndrome of acute self-limiting ulcerative esophagitis in young adults probably due to herpes simplex virus. *Dig Dis Sci* 1979;24:535.
23. Nebel OT, Fornes MF, Castell DO. Symptomatic gastroesophageal reflux: incidence and precipitating factors. *Am J Dig Dis*. 1976;21:953.
24. Castro L de P. Reflux esophagitis as the cause of heartburn in pregnancy. *Am J Obstet Gynecol*. 1967;98:1.
25. Pellegrini CA, DeMeester TR, Wernly JA, et al. Alkaline gastroesophageal reflux. *Am J Surg*. 1978;135:177.
26. Drake D, Hollander D. Neutralizing capacity and cost effectiveness of antacids. *Ann Intern Med*. 1981;94:215.
27. Chevrel B. A comparative crossover study on the treatment of heartburn and epigastric pain: liquid Gaviscon and a magnesium-aluminum antacid gel. *Intern Med Res*. 1980;8:300.
28. Atlay RD, Weekes ARL, Entwistle GD, et al. Treating heartburn in pregnancy: Comparison of acid and alkali mixtures. *Br Med J*. 1978;1:919.
29. Hart DM. Heartburn in pregnancy. *J Intern Med*. 1978;6(suppl 1):1.
30. Wesdorp E, Bartelsman H, Pape K, et al. Oral cimetidine in reflux esophagitis: a double blind controlled trial. *Gastroenterology*. 1978;74:821.
31. Zulli P, Dinisio Q. Cimetidine treatment during pregnancy. *Lancet*. 1978;2:925.
32. Swinhoe JR, Cochrane GW, Wisharl R. Oesophageal stricture due to reflux oesophagitis in pregnancy. *Br J Obstet Gynaecol*. 1981;88:1249.
33. Cohen S, Morris DW, Schoen HJ, et al. The effect of oral and intravenous metoclopramide on human lower esophageal sphincter pressure. *Gastroenterology*. 1976;70:484.
34. Stanciu C, Bennett JR. Metoclopramide in gastroesophageal reflux. *Gut*. 1973;14:275.
35. Hey VMF, Ostick DG. Metoclopramide in gastroesophageal sphincter: a study in pregnant women with heartburn. *Anesthesia*. 1978;33:462.
36. Connell AM, George JD. Effect of metoclopramide on gastric function in man. *Gut*. 1969;10:678.
37. Pinder RM, Brogden RN, Sawyer PR, et al. Metoclopramide: a review of its pharmacologic properties and clinical use. *Drugs*. 1976;12:81.
38. Malagelada JR, Rees WDW, Mazzotta LJ, et al. Gastrin motor abnormalities in diabetic and post vagotomy gastroparesis: effect of metoclopramide and bethanechol. *Gastroenterology*. 1980;78:286.
39. Palmer ED. Upper gastrointestinal hemorrhage during pregnancy. *Am J Med Sci*. 1961;242:223.
40. Kilman WJ, Goyal RK. Disorders of pharyngeal and upper esophageal sphincter motor function. *Arch Intern Med*. 1976;136:592.
41. Stroup RE. Achalasia of the esophagus during pregnancy. *Obstet Gynecol*. 1961;18:236.
42. Sugawa C, Fujita Y, Ikedo T, et al. Endoscopic hemostasis of upper gastrointestinal bleeding by local injection of dehydrated (98%) ethanol. *Surg Gynecol Obstet*. 1986;162:159.
43. Britton RC. Pregnancy and esophageal varices. *Am J Surg*. 1982;143:421.
44. Khuroo MS, Datta DV. Budd-Chiari syndrome following pregnancy. Report of 16 cases with roentgenologic, hemodynamic and histologic studies of the hepatic out-flow tract. *Am J Med*. 1980;68:113.
45. Gheng Y-S. Pregnancy in liver cirrhosis and/or portal hypertension. *Am J Obstet Gynecol*. 1977;128:812.
46. Palmer ED, Brick IB. Esophageal varices: causes other than cirrhosis and portal vein block. *Am J Geriatr Soc*. 1955;3:681.
47. Knauer CM. Mallory-Weiss syndrome: Characterization of 75 Mallory-Weiss lacerations in 528 patients with upper gastrointestinal hemorrhage. *Gastroenterology*. 1976;71:5.
48. Papp JP. Endoscopic electrocoagulation of upper gastrointestinal hemorrhage. *JAMA*. 1976;236:2076.
49. Gilbert DA, Verhoeven T, Jessen K, et al. A multicenter clinical trial of the Bicap probe for upper gastrointestinal bleeding. *Gastrointest Endosc*. 1982;28:150.
50. Rutgeerts P, Van Trappen G, Broeckaert L, et al. Controlled trial of YAG laser treatment of upper digestive bleeding. *Gastroenterology*. 1982;83:410.
51. Hastings PK, Skillman JJ, Bushnell LS, et al. Antacid titration in the prevention of acute gastrointestinal bleeding. *N Engl J Med*. 1978;298:1041.
52. Priebe HJ, Skillman JJ, Bushnell LS, et al. Antacid versus cimetidine in preventing acute gastrointestinal bleeding. *N Engl J Med*. 1980;302:426.
53. Ostro MJ, Russell JA, Soldin SJ, et al. Control of gastric pH with cimetidine: boluses versus primed infusions. *Gastroenterology*. 1985;89:532.
54. Borrero E, Bank M, Margolis I, et al. Comparison of antacid and sucralfate in the prevention of gastrointestinal bleeding in patients who are critically ill. *Am J Med*. 1985;79:62.
55. Shaler E, Tsabar A, Edelstein S, et al. Intracervical administration of prostaglandin E_2-gel prior to therapeutic abortion: a prospective randomized double-blind study. *Int J Gynaecol Obst*. 1988;27:119.
56. Sandweiss DJ, Podolsky MB, Saltzstein HC, et al. Deaths from perforation and hemorrhage of gastroduodenal ulcer during pregnancy and puerperium. *Am J Obstet Gynecol*. 1943;45:131.
57. Vasicka A, Lin TJ, Bright RH. Peptic ulcer and pregnancy. Review of

hormonal relationships and a report of one case of massive hemorrhage. *Obstet Gynecol Surv.* 1957;12:1.
58. Clark DH. Peptic ulcer in women. *Br Med J.* 1953;1:1254.
59. Rider AJ, Kirsner JB, Palmer WL. Active duodenal ulcer in pregnancy. *Gastroenterology.* 1953;14:357.
60. Tornquist A. The effects of exogenous histamine on the forearm blood flow in pregnant and nonpregnant women before and after inhibition of histamine. *Acta Obstet Gynecol Scand.* 1968;47:391.
61. Duckler L, Cohen HR. Hyperemesis gravidarum with gastric carcinoma. *Obstet Gynecol.* 1975;45:348.
62. Peterson WL, Sturdevant RA, Frankl HD, et al. Healing duodenal ulcer with an antacid regimen. *N Engl J Med.* 1977;297:341.
63. Nelson MM, Forfar JO. Association between drug administered during pregnancy and congenital abnormalities. *Br Med J.* 1971;1:523.
64. Ippolitis AF, Sturdevant RAL, Iseberg JI, et al. Cimetidine versus intensive antacid therapy for duodenal ulcer. *Gastroenterology.* 1978;74:393.
65. McHardy GG. A multicenter, double-blind trial of sucralfate and placebo in duodenal ulcer. *J Clin Gastroenterol.* 1981;3:147.
66. Nagashima R. Development and characteristics of sucralfate. *J Clin Gastroenterol.* 1981;3:103.
67. Steiner K, Buhring KU, Faro HP, et al. Sucralfate: pharmacokinetics, metabolism and selective binding to experimental gastric and duodenal ulcers in animals. *Arzneim Forsch.* 1982;32:512.
68. Shioda S, Matsuoka A, Fukaya T, et al. Effects of basic aluminum sucrose sulfate on the fetal development and growth in small laboratory animals. Report on Ulcerlmin 9. Tokyo: Chugai Pharmaceutical Co, Ltd 1966.
69. Becker-Anderson H, Husfeldt V. Peptic ulcer in pregnancy. *Acta Obstet Gynecol Scand.* 1971;50:391.
70. Klebanoff MA, Koslowe PA, Kaslow R, et al. Epidemiology of vomiting in early pregnancy. *Obstet & Gyn.* 1985;66:612.
71. Semmens JP. Female sexuality and life situations. *Obstet Gynecol.* 1971;38:555.
72. Biggs JSG. Vomiting pregnancy: causes and management. *Drugs.* 1975;9:299.
73. Depue RH, Bernstein L, Ross RK, et al. Hyperemesis gravidarum in relation to estradiol levels, pregnancy outcome, and other maternal factors: a seroepidemiologic study. *Am J Obstet Gynecol.* 1987;156:1137.
74. Jarnfelt-Samsioe, Bremme K, Eneroth P. Steroid hormones in emetic and nonemetic pregnancy. *Eur J Obstet Gynecol Reprod Biol.* 1986;21:87.
75. Mori M, Amino N, Tamaki H, et al. Morning sickness and thyroid function in normal pregnancy. *Obstet Gynecol.* 1988;72:355.
76. Leathem AM. Safety and efficacy of antiemetics used to treat nausea and vomiting in pregnancy. *Clin Pharm.* 1986;5:660.
77. Singh MS, Lean TH. The use of metoclopramide and hyperemesis gravidarum. *Proc Obstet Gynecol Soc Singapore.* 1970;1:43.
78. Harrington A, Hamilton CW, Brogden RN, et al. Metoclopramide: an updated review of its pharmacological properties and clinical use. *Drugs.* 1983;25:477.
79. Schulman PK. Hyperemesis gravidarum: an approach to the nutritional aspects of care. *J Am Diet Assoc.* 1982;80:577.
80. Smith CV, Rufleth P, Phelan JP, et al. Long-term enteral hyperalimentation in the pregnant woman with insulin dependent diabetes: a report of two cases. *Am J Obstet Gynecol.* 1981;141:180.
81. Hew LR, Deitel M. Total parenteral nutrition in gynecology and obstetrics. *Obstet Gynecol.* 1980;55:464.

Chapter One Hundred and Forty-Eight

Dental Diseases

David J. Mishkin and Tariq Javed

148

There are no signs or changes in the oral cavity that are pathognomonic for pregnancy. No specific lesions of the teeth, salivary glands, tongue, or oral mucous membranes occur. However, while pregnancy does not cause gingivitis, it accentuates the gingival response to local irritants. Pregnancy also necessitates treatment planning modifications when the gravid woman seeks dental care.

Since 50% of the American population do not seek regular dental care, the obstetrician or internist may be the primary source of information for a significant number of pregnant women with diseases of the oral cavity.

Many people are convinced that pregnancy causes tooth loss. They base this concept on the mistaken premise that the developing fetus causes calcium to be removed from the teeth. Calcium is present in the teeth in a very stable crystalline form and as such is not available to the systemic circulation to supply fetal calcium demand.[1] Therefore, calcium supplementation to prevent "soft teeth" is unwarranted. Supplemental prenatal fluorides also are not indicated. The placenta acts as a barrier to most systemic fluoride.[1]

GINGIVAL DISEASE IN PREGNANCY

Etiology and Pathophysiology

The primary etiologic factor in gingivitis is dental plaque, an adherent bacterial mass that attaches to the teeth within 24 hours after tooth cleaning. Plaque formation occurs in the absence of food intake. Plaque causes gingivitis in 9–21 days if not removed.[2] No notable changes occur in the gingiva during pregnancy in the absence of plaque or other local irritants (Fig. 148–1). Pregnancy does not initiate gingivitis, but is a modifying factor.

A preexisting gingivitis will become worse during pregnancy. Gingival areas with slight inflammation before pregnancy may become excessively erythematous (fiery red), edematous, and enlarged during the course of the pregnancy (Fig. 148–2). Areas with a slight amount of gingival bleeding before pregnancy may now bleed profusely upon the slightest provocation. This exaggerated response to local irritants is sometimes referred to as *pregnancy gingivitis*. Also increased in pregnancy are tooth mobility (the teeth may get loose), pocket depth (deepening of the space between the gingiva and the tooth), and gingival fluid flow.

These gingival changes are noticeable in pregnant women from the second month of gestation, peak in the eighth month, and decrease slightly in the ninth month.[3] There is partial reduction in the severity of gingivitis by 2 months postpartum, and after one year the gingival condition is comparable to that seen before conception.[4] The gingiva, however, does not return to health unless the microbial plaque is removed.

Apart from the generalized gingival changes associated with pregnancy, discrete, single, tumor-like masses occasionally may develop in the gingiva between the teeth as a result of local minor trauma or irritation (Fig. 148–3). These tumor-like growths, sometimes called *pregnancy tumors*, are reported to occur with a frequency of 0–5% and are histologically identical with the pyogenic granuloma.[5]

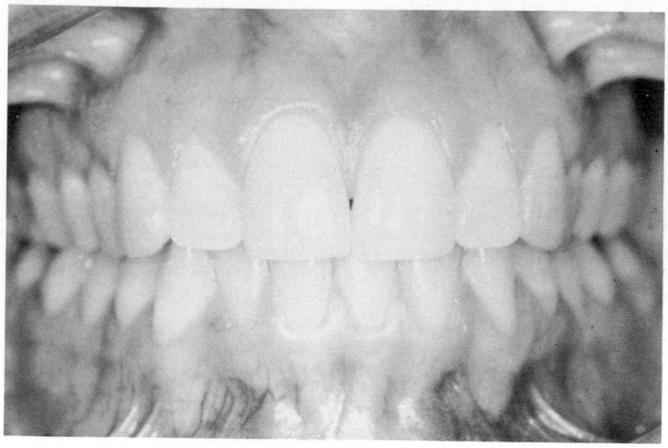

Figure 148–1. Normal gingiva in a pregnant woman with excellent oral hygiene. (*From Robert G. Gellin D.M.D. with permission.*)

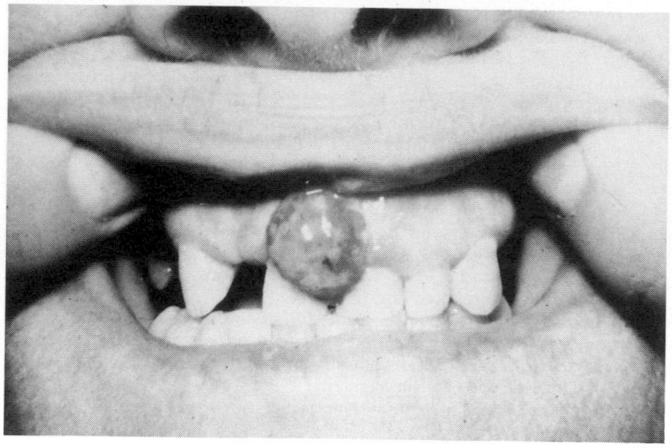

Figure 148–3. Pregnancy tumor. Pyogenic granuloma in pregnant woman as a result of localized trauma. (*From William O. Engler D.D.S. with permission.*)

A pregnancy tumor is not a true neoplasia. It is mostly a pedunculated, fiery red soft growth, often with small fibrin-covered areas, and seldom gets larger than $2mm^2$. It appears in the third month of pregnancy or later. It gradually increases in size, and may or may not regress after delivery. If surgically removed during pregnancy, it frequently recurs.

There appears to be no justification for retaining the term pregnancy tumor, since lesions of identical clinical and histologic nature are seen in men and nonpregnant women.[5]

Several studies have suggested that the exaggerated inflammatory response seen during pregnancy is a result of increased levels of progesterone, which produce vasodilation and tortuosity of the gingival microvasculature, circulatory stasis, and increased susceptibility to mechanical irritation.[6,7]

Bacteroides intermedius, a putative periodontopathogen, and other anerobes increase in number during pregnancy. It is reported that the increase in *B intermedius* occurs in association with an increase in gingivitis and elevated serum levels of estradiol and progesterone during pregnancy.[8]

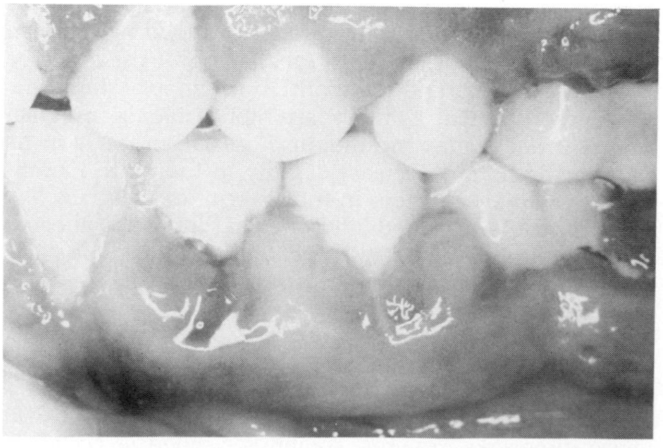

Figure 148–2. Pregnancy gingivitis. Exaggerated inflammatory response to local irritants in a pregnant woman with poor oral hygiene.

Histopathology of Gingival Disease in Pregnancy

The microscopic picture of gingival disease in pregnancy presents itself as a nonspecific, vascularizing, proliferative, inflammatory reaction.[9] The most prominent features are the proliferation of engorged capillaries and intra- and extracellular edema.

Gingival disease does not affect pregnancy. Despite the fact that there are 100 million bacteria in only 1 mm^2 of plaque (1mg. wet wt.)[10], and bacteremias occur during mastication and oral hygiene procedures, there is no evidence that gingival disease affects the fetus in any way. However, since the delivery of dental care involves some potentially harmful elements including ionizing radiation, drug administration, and stress, gingival disease and dental caries should be prevented.

TREATMENT OF DENTAL DISEASES ALTERED BY PREGNANCY

Dental treatment of pregnant patients differs from treatment of nonpregnant patients in its timing, scope, and methodology. While routine dental care probably is safe, it must be modified to avoid the possible teratogenic effects of acute infection, x-rays, drugs, or the stress and anxiety produced by (1) painful dental disease, (2) the impending dental appointment, or (3) the dental treatment itself. The condition of pregnancy also will necessitate modifications in the management of the dental patient because of the discomfort, fatigue, and tendency for blood pressure alterations.

All patients should be seen by their dentist as early as possible in pregnancy, so that the emphasis of dental therapy can be upon preventing gingival disease and pulpal infections, and treating existing gingival disease before it progresses.

Other than oral hygiene instruction and oral prophylaxis, only emergency dental care should be rendered during the first trimester, because of the vulnerability of the fetus. The second trimester is the safest period for routine dental care. Extensive reconstructive procedures such as crowns, bridges, and partial dentures should not be performed at any time during the pregnancy.

The early part of the third trimester is still a relatively good time to provide routine dental care. However, no elective dental treatment is advisable late in the third trimester because of the discomfort of the mother and the occurrence of supine hypotensive syndrome in about 10% of patients.[1]

Supine hypotensive syndrome involves an abrupt drop in blood pressure and loss of consciousness while the pregnant woman is in the standard supine position in which dental treatment is delivered today. It is caused by impairment of venous return to the heart by a gravid uterus compressing the inferior vena cava. This causes the sudden fall in blood pressure, decreased cardiac output, and syncope that characterize the syndrome. Emergency care consists of rolling the patient onto her left side to lift the uterus off the vena cava and administering 100% oxygen.

Appointments should be kept short. The patient should be positioned in a semi-reclining position and should be encouraged to change her position frequently.

The decision to remove pyogenic granulomas associated with pregnancy should be made by the dentist after consultation with the patient's obstetrician.

DENTAL RADIOGRAPHS IN PREGNANCY

Due to modern features of high speed film, filtration, collimation and lead aprons, dental radiography is very safe. With the leaded aprons currently used to protect the patient's torso and pelvic regions, there is no exposure of the reproductive organs, embryo, or fetus.[11] Nevertheless, x-rays should only be taken during pregnancy when dental treatment is necessary to treat an acute condition or an accurate diagnosis cannot be made without them. The Food and Drug Administration Panel[12] considered the appropriateness of dental radiographic examinations for patients who are or may be pregnant. It concluded that there appears to be no rationale to preclude a properly justified dental radiographic examination because of pregnancy. Radiography may be deferred during pregnancy in some cases for purely psychological reasons.[12]

DRUG ADMINISTRATION IN THE PREGNANT DENTAL PATIENT

Ideally, no drugs should be administered during pregnancy, especially during the first trimester. However, should it become necessary to provide acute or nonelective dental care at any time during pregnancy, the dentist should not hesitate to render whatever treatment is necessary. The stress and effects resulting from dental pain or acute infection could be detrimental to the mother or fetus, and thus should be treated.

The most commonly used drugs in dentistry are relatively safe. Lidocaine (or mepivacaine) and epinephrine for local anesthesia, penicillin or erythromycin for infection, and aspirin and codeine for pain should be used only when absolutely necessary. Tetracycline, phenacetin, sedatives and hypnotics, and nitrous oxide should not be used.[1]

Seldom is more than 0.036 mg of epinephrine used for dental procedures. The advantages of achieving more profound and prolonged anesthesia when epinephrine is used as a vasoconstrictor far outweigh the risks. The vasoconstriction epinephrine produces results in a slower entrance of the local anesthetic into the systemic circulation, thus decreasing the chance of a toxic reaction.

PRECONCEPTIONAL COUNSELING RELATIVE TO DENTAL DISEASES

Since 80–100% of American adults have gingivitis, the obstetrician may assume the patient is afflicted, particularly if the patient reports any gingival bleeding during oral hygiene procedures or mastication. Healthy gingiva does not spontaneously bleed in a patient unless she has a blood dyscrasia, is on certain medications, or has advanced liver, kidney or bone marrow disease. Preconceptional counseling should emphasize to the patient the importance of seeking dental care and achieving gingival health and caries control prior to becoming pregnant. While dental care is probably safe, there are risks; therefore the need for dental treatment should be prevented.

Patients should be advised not to take the antibiotic tetracycline or its synthetic analogues, that is, minocycline and doxycycline. These drugs cause staining of the developing primary (deciduous) teeth of the fetus. Patients should be advised that the developing fetus does not extract calcium from their teeth and make them soft. Acid production by dental plaque causes dental caries.

It should be emphasized that pregnancy does not cause any dental disease, but it will intensify plaque-induced or trauma-induced inflammatory gingival disease.

Patients should be informed that the stress and infection caused by acute dental disease are potentially more harmful than the dental treatment itself.

REFERENCES

1. Little JW, Falace DA. *Dental Management of the Medically Compromised Patient*. St Louis, MO: CV Mosby; 1980:127.
2. Loe H, Theilade E, Jensen SB. Experimental gingivitis in man. *J Periodontol*. 1965;36:177.
3. Loe H. Periodontal changes in pregnancy. *J Periodontol*. 1965;36:209.
4. Cohen DW, Shapiro J, Friedman L, et al. A longitudinal investigation of the periodontal changes during pregnancy and fifteen months postpartum. II. *J Periodontol*. 1971;42:653.
5. Shafer WG, Hine MK, Levy BM, Tomich CE. *A Textbook of Oral Pathology*. Philadelphia, PA: WB Saunders; 1983:361, 774.
6. Hugoson A. Gingival inflammation and female sex hormones: a clinical investigation of pregnant women and experimental studies in dogs. *J Periodont Res*. 1970;5(suppl):7.
7. Mohamed AH, Waterhouse JP, Friederici HH. The microvasculature of the rat gingiva as affected by progesterone: an ultrastructural study. *J Periodontol*. 1974;45:50.
8. Kornman KS, Loesche WJ. The subgingival microbial flora during pregnancy. *J Periodont Res*. 1980;15:111.
9. Ziskin DE, Blackberg SN, Stout A. The gingivae during pregnancy: an experimental study and a histopathologic interpretation. *Surg Gynecol Obstet*. 1933;57:719.
10. Lindhe J. *Textbook of Clinical Periodontology*. Philadelphia, PA: Munksgaard; 1983:87.
11. Richards AG, Colquitt WN. Reduction in dental x-ray exposures during the past 60 years. *JADA*. 1981;103:713.
12. *Dental Radiographic Examinations*. Rockville, MD: Food and Drug Administration; 1987. Center for Devices and Radiological Health, HHS Publication FDA 88–8273.

Chapter One Hundred and Forty-Nine
Small and Large Bowel Diseases

Daniel J. Adler and Burton I. Korelitz

149

Gastrointestinal (GI) symptoms attributable to the small and large bowel occur commonly during pregnancy. Constipation is the most frequent of these and its causes are many, including alterations in dietary habits, lack of exercise, compression of the sigmoid colon by the expanding uterus, decreased intestinal transit time and the oral use of ferrous sulfate as contained in prenatal vitamin preparations. Diarrhea is less commonly seen and is usually self-limited. When diarrhea presents with blood, pus, and mucus, however, it usually is indicative of an invasive bacterial infection or inflammatory bowel disease. Abdominal pain may be a difficult problem to assess in the pregnant patient. The acute abdomen in the clinically toxic patient is managed as in the nonpregnant patient. In evaluating less severe cases, the physician must weigh the potential risks versus gains of diagnostic procedures to the pregnant women and the fetus.

This chapter considers the clinical presentation, methods of diagnosis, and therapeutic considerations for diseases of the small and large intestine that may occur in association with pregnancy.

GASTROINTESTINAL HEMORRHAGE

The most common causes of upper gastrointestinal bleeding during pregnancy are the *Mallory-Weiss tear* secondary to frequent and protracted emesis, and acute gastritis. Bleeding from peptic ulcer disease also is seen despite the decreased incidence of this disease during pregnancy. GI bleeding from a small bowel source, however, is rare. When it occurs, the differential diagnosis should include malignant neoplasms, that is, carcinoma, lymphoma and sarcoma, and benign tumors such as the adenomatous polyp and leiomyoma. Intestinal carcinoid and the familial polyposis may be either benign or malignant in nature. Polyps, cancer, arteriovenous malformations, and diverticulosis are common causes of intestinal bleeding in the elderly, but are rare in the pregnant population. *Meckel's diverticulum,* arteriovenous malformations as seen in the Olser–Weber–Rendu syndrome, pseudoxanthoma elasticum, and inflammatory bowel disease, of which *Crohn's disease* is the most common, are the most likely small bowel lesions to present with first time bleeding in the young adult population.

In the lower GI tract, hemorrhoids and fissures remain the most common cause of rectal bleeding. These tend to respond to conservative management such as a high fiber diet, stool softeners, anti-inflammatory suppositories, and sitz baths. If bleeding from internal hemorrhoids persists, rubber band ligation and injection sclerotherapy are useful. The efficacy and safety of newer methods of treating hemorrhoids such as IR photocoagulation or direct current obliteration has not been evaluated in the pregnant patient.

Bleeding from *ulcerative colitis* or Crohn's disease may worsen or have its initial presentation during pregnancy.[1] The bleeding can be massive and require emergency surgery. Fortunately, aggressive medical management with blood transfusion and colloid replacement along with vigorous intravenous treatment of the underlying disease with hydrocortisone or adrenocorticotrophic hormone (ACTH) usually will quiet the inflammation.

Whatever the cause of gastrointestinal bleeding, initial supportive therapy is essential. Blood and fluid should be replaced aggressively to avoid maternal and fetal hypoxia. Blood pressure, central venous pressure, urine output, serial blood counts and electrolytes should be monitored carefully. In all cases, a nasogastric tube should be passed to detect a bleeding site proximal to the ligament of Treitz. The presence of bright blood (indicating recent or active bleeding) or older "coffee grounds" should be noted. The presence or absence of bile also should be noted in aspirates indicating sampling of duodenal contents. If an upper GI source is suspected, fiberoptic gastroscopy under mild sedation with diazepam and meperidine is the method of choice. It is safe, fast, avoids fetal exposure to ionizing radiation, and provides the option for therapeutic cauterization of bleeding sites if warranted. In all instances of suspected small bowel bleeding, a nuclear bleeding scan and a nuclear Meckel's scan may be performed. If lower GI bleeding is suspected, sigmoidoscopy is essential to rule out hemorrhoids, anal fissure, and colitis. If further diagnostic studies are needed, a barium enema or colonoscopy may be performed according to clinical judgment. If the bleeding is vigorous, the presence of blood in the colon may negate the value of colonoscopy. Angiography may be the best diagnostic option; it allows for therapeutic embolization or use of intra-arterial vasoconstrictors. Any contraindication to these procedures because of the pregnancy must be considered relative under conditions of a life-threatening gastrointestinal hemorrhage.

INTESTINAL OBSTRUCTION

Intestinal obstruction in the pregnant patient is a rare occurrence, but it is being seen with increasing incidence at a rate of one in 2500–3000 deliveries.[2] This trend is attributable directly to the increasing number of laparotomies being performed in young women with predisposition for later adhesion formation. It is essential to recognize that obstruction as a delay in diagnosis and treatment will have dire consequences for both the mother and fetus.

Approximately 60% of all obstructions are secondary to adhesions; appendectomies and prior gynecologic surgery are the most frequent preceding operations.[3] Other causes include inflammatory strictures most often due to Crohn's disease, volvulus, intersusception, colonic pseudo-obstruction, and neoplasms. Hernias account for only about 3% of cases of intestinal obstruction in pregnancy since the enlarging uterus displaces the bowel up and away from the inguinal and femoral rings. Neither age nor parity have been found to correlate with risk of intestinal obstruction. However, women in their first pregnancy, following abdominal surgery, are the highest risk group. Some 80% of obstructions caused by adhesions have been found in the primigravida after appendectomy.[4]

The diagnosis of intestinal obstruction may be suspected by the onset of crampy abdominal pain, distention, and vomiting. When the obstruction is complete, the patient is unable to pass gas or defecate. The differential diagnosis initially must include all intra-abdominal pathology, complications of pregnancy, and exaggerated symptoms of normal pregnancy. If the diagnosis of obstruction is suspected, it should be confirmed with plain films of the abdomen in the supine and erect position, looking for multiple air fluid levels or a trapped loop of bowel. The contraindication to x-rays during the first trimester must be weighed against the clinical urgency of the situation. Initial therapy should include nasal passage of a small bowel tube with intermittent suction to decompress the proximal intestine and intravenous fluid replacement. For the patient with adhesions, surgical intervention for lysis of adhesions will be needed in most cases.

In the case of obstruction caused by Crohn's disease, most patients can be managed with nonoperative therapy including small bowel tube, parenteral ACTH or corticosteroids and antibiotics in some.[5] If, however, there is no improvement, surgical intervention is warranted to prevent perforation or vascular compromise of the bowel.

Volvulus may involve either the cecum or the sigmoid colon and may occur either during pregnancy or in the postpartum period. In the absence of adhesive bands, volvulus often can be treated by detorsion with a rigid sigmoidoscope or fiberoptic colonoscope. If vascular compromise of the bowel has occurred, colonic resection or multistage procedures will be necessary.

APPENDICITIS

Acute appendicitis is the most common nonobstetric complication requiring surgery during pregnancy, with a reported incidence of one case in 1500 pregnancies.[6] The occurrence of appendicitis is neither increased nor decreased in pregnancy. The pregnancy can alter many of the usual signs and symptoms of appendicitis, and physicians are often reluctant to explore surgically the pregnant patient when the diagnosis is suspected. Balber[7] stated over 75 years ago that "the mortality of appendicitis complicating pregnancy is the mortality of delay." The wisdom of this statement holds equally true today.

During pregnancy, the enlarging uterus displaces the appendix upward and to the right. Appendicitis early in pregnancy will present with typical right lower quadrant symptoms. However, in the second and third trimester, right upper quadrant and flank pain are more common and may mimic acute cholecystitis, peptic ulcer disease, pancreatitis, or urinary tract disease. When appendicitis is suspected, the treatment is surgical. In a recent series of 12 patients with appendicitis, one maternal death and three fetal losses occurred in six patients with perforated appendix.[8] There were, however, no such complications in the absence of perforation. Pregnancy is not a reason to delay surgery.

Meckel's diverticulum, a congenital anomaly, may present with hemorrhage, intestinal obstruction, diverticulitis, and perforation with peritonitis. This entity may have a presentation similar to that of appendicitis, and its management also is usually surgical.

TUMORS OF THE SMALL AND LARGE BOWEL

Neoplasms of the small bowel comprise 1–5% of all GI tumors. Benign tumors include adenoma, leiomyoma and lipoma. Although they are most prevalent among patients more than 50 years old, they have been found in persons as young as nine years old. Clinically, these tumors may be responsible for obstruction and occult or gross bleeding. Therapy is determined by documentation of diagnosis and whether the tumors are symptomatic.

Malignant neoplasms of the small bowel make up about 1–2% of all malignant GI tumors. Histologically, they include adenocarcinoma, lymphoma, and leiomyosarcoma. Most symptomatic patients are older than 50, except those with lymphoma, who generally are 10 years younger. Malignant neoplasms of the small bowel have rarely been diagnosed during pregnancy. When present, however, they may cause obstruction, bleeding, and with lymphoma, malabsorption.

In the large bowel, rectal and colonic polyps should be considered in the differential diagnosis of rectal bleeding during pregnancy, particularly when there is a family history. Carcinoma of the colon is diagnosed rarely during pregnancy; only 19 cases of this association have been reported.[9] The age range was 23–39. Four of the 19 had predisposing factors including ulcerative colitis, familial polyposis, Gardner's syndrome, and a villous tumor. Delay in diagnosis during pregnancy can be a significant problem. Symptoms of rectal bleeding, change in bowel habits, and weight loss should be investigated with digital rectal examination and flexible fiberoptic sigmoidoscopy. Many cancers of the large bowel will be found with these tests. If the results are negative and suspicion remains high, an examination of the more proximal colon by fiberoptic colonoscopy can be performed.

As in the nonpregnant patient, the prognosis for symptomatic colon cancer in pregnant women is poor. It appears, however, that pregnancy does not adversely affect the course of the cancer nor does the cancer adversely affect the pregnancy. Fifteen of 19 infants born to mothers with carcinoma of the colon were reported to be alive and well.[10] Therapy depends on the operability of the tumor and the period of gestation. If the lesion is advanced, the surgery should be palliative and the pregnancy, if possible, should be continued until the fetus has matured. If the lesion is contained, and the gestational age permits pregnancy termination, immediate treatment involving appropriate colon resection and adjuvant therapy can be performed. During the third trimester, elective cesarean section might be carried out coincident with colon resection.

IRRITABLE BOWEL SYNDROME

Irritable bowel syndrome may be defined as a functional disorder in which the normal activity of the large bowel is exaggerated or distorted, leading to constipation, diarrhea, or abdominal pain.[11] This entity has been referred to in the past as *spastic colon, spastic colitis, mucus colitis,* and *nervous diarrhea.* It is very common and is not an inflammatory lesion, as the term *colitis* would dictate. The etiology of this condition is unknown, but altered intestinal motility by way of hormonal or myoelectrical mechanisms have been implicated. The major presenting symptoms include diarrhea, constipation, constipation alternating with diarrhea, mucus, and crampy abdominal pain. The diarrhea may vary from 1–2 movements per day to greater than 20. A functional diarrhea never awakens the patient from sleep, and it is important to ascertain this information during the history. The abdominal discomfort is often left-sided, along the sigmoid colon, worse after several days of constipation, and relieved by passage of stool. Symptoms tend to be subjectively worse during periods of emotional stress or altered diet. Constipation often has been a problem for years and laxatives may have been used by these patients as a matter of routine.

During pregnancy, constipation is very common. Decreased transit time through the intestine has been described and is probably hormonally mediated.[12] In the third trimester, the expanding uterus will extrinsically compress the sigmoid colon and retard normal passage of stool. Change in diet, lack of exercise, and oral ferrous sulfate preparations also may be contributing factors.

The diagnosis of irritable bowel syndrome is most often clinical. A careful history usually can date the onset of symptoms well before pregnancy. If, however, the diagnosis is in doubt, an evaluation consisting of routine physical examination, blood counts, serum chemistries, proctosigmoidoscopy and stool studies for culture, ova and parasites, leukocytes, and occult blood should be performed. X-ray studies should be avoided. If visualization of the proximal colon is warranted, fiberoptic colonoscopy is the procedure of choice. When diarrhea is the predominant symptom, lactose intolerance should be suspected since many women increase their daily consumption of milk products during pregnancy. This diagnosis can be confirmed safely and easily with a 2-hour lactose tolerance test or an empiric trial of a lactose-free diet for several days.

Treatment of irritable bowel syndrome is supportive and depends on the presenting symptom. For constipation, increasing the fiber content of the diet will provide stool bulk and improve the muscular function of the colon. Intake of adequate amounts of water and fresh, canned, or dried fruits also should be encouraged. Increased fiber intake is most reliably achieved with a once-a-day pharmacologic preparation such as Metamucil or natural unprocessed bran (1–6 tablespoons per day). An increase in exercise also is helpful. Laxatives and enemas should be avoided as their use will lead to dependence and atony of the colon.

For diarrhea, restricting fruit and fiber in the diet may reduce symptoms. A lactose-free diet can be initiated if lactase deficiency is suspected. Of all the antidiarrheals, Kaolin is the safest in pregnancy. All others such as lomotil, loperamide, and the bismuth preparations have not been studied adequately. Paragoric is an opium alkaloid that crosses the placenta and is excreted in breast milk. Its use can cause fetal addiction and withdrawal states. It is contraindicated in pregnancy and lactation.[13] The safety of anticholinergic agents to decrease intestinal motility has not been adequately studied in pregnancy and should be avoided.

INFECTIOUS DIARRHEA

Infectious diarrheas usually present with a rather sudden onset in patients with previously normal intestinal function. The *viral enteridites* are by far the most common. They usually are preceded by a short prodrome of myalgias, joint aches, and fever before the onset of profuse watery diarrhea, often accompanied by nausea and vomiting. A mild leukocytosis is common usually with lymphocytosis and the presence of atypical lymphocytes as well. A viral enteritis usually will clear spontaneously within 24–48 hours. Therapy should be directed to avoid dehydration with either oral or intravenous fluids. Antiemetics should be used only when absolutely necessary. Among those available, only meclizine (Antivert) and promethazine (Phenergan) are thought to be without adverse fetal effects in humans.[13] Antidiarrheals should be avoided, as their use might retard rapid recovery.

Staphylococcal food poisoning can mimic a viral enteritis. Distinguishing features include a very abrupt onset of intestinal symptoms without the flulike prodrome, multiple cases linked to a common contaminant, and recovery in less than 24 hours. Therapy is the same as outlined above.

Infectious diarrhea from either bacteria or protozoa may be acquired from exposure to contaminated food or water, often during travel. Nonbloody diarrhea is characteristic of *Escherichia coli*, salmonella, and giardiasis. Pathogens such as *Shigella, Yersinia, Campylobacter,* and amebae typically cause bloody diarrhea and can clinically, radiographically, and endoscopically mimic idiopathic inflammatory bowel disease. Diagnostic evaluation should include a careful travel history, physical examination, and stool studies. Sigmoidoscopic examination with rectal biopsy will occasionally reveal characteristic gross or histologic findings. Increased yield for giardiasis can be obtained from an endoscopic duodenal aspirate or small bowel biopsy. Therapy should include fluid and electrolyte replacement as well as appropriate antimicrobial treatment of the underlying infection. Stool cultures often take many days to grow out pathogenic isolates, and empiric use of antibiotics is justified in the setting of clinical toxicity after appropriate cultures have been obtained.

If the patient presenting with diarrhea is using or has used antibiotics within the preceding three months, a diagnosis of *Clostridium difficile,* antibiotic-associated pseudomembranous colitis, should be suspected. Diagnostic evaluation should include a stool sample for *C difficile* toxin assay, and proctosigmoidoscopy looking for the characteristic pseudomembrane. If the diagnosis is confirmed, treatment with the nonabsorbable oral vancomycin (250 mg qid) should be initiated for a seven-day course and all other antibiotics withdrawn. A 20% failure rate is expected from a single course of such treatment.

INFLAMMATORY BOWEL DISEASE

Estimates of the prevalence of inflammatory bowel disease (IBD) in the United States range between one and two million people.[14] A total of 20,000–25,000 new cases are diagnosed each year. Since ulcerative colitis and Crohn's disease are predominantly diseases of young persons with peak incidence at 15–30 years for Crohn's disease and 20–35 years for ulcerative colitis, both diseases coincide with the most fruitful childbearing years.

Many issues arise for the female patient with IBD who is pregnant or contemplating pregnancy, such as fertility, the effect of the gestational period on IBD and vice versa, the risk of inheritance of IBD by offspring, the safety of drugs to control the disease on the developing fetus and nursing newborn, and the surgical options for treatment. Issues regarding fertility and potential teratogenicity of medications to control the disease also concern couples when the male is the one afflicted with IBD.

Much of the data available regarding pregnancy in the IBD patient has been based on studies and observations from the 1940s and 1950s, prior to the advent of the modalities with which we now treat these diseases. Although more recent studies have served to supplement these earlier observations, many questions still remain unanswered.

Despite decades of research, the etiology of Crohn's disease or ulcerative colitis has not been determined. The major theories of pathogenesis have centered on mucosal injury from ingested toxins or infectious agents, including those producing "self-limited" enteritis and colitis, *C difficile*, cell wall defective bacteria (L-forms), and mycobacteria. Many abnormalities of humoral and cell-mediated immune function have been observed in the IBD patient, but which ones are primary and therfore possibly etiologic and which ones are secondary to some initiating event is not known. Finally, the role of genetic and psychologic factors in these patients remains to be clarified.

Fertility in women with ulcerative colitis was thought to be subnormal when compared to the general population.[15] However, when adjusted for patient age and the desire for pregnancy, their fertility rate probably is normal.[16] The situation for Crohn's disease, however, is different; fertility is reduced.[17] Reduction in fertility is proportional to the activity of Crohn's disease and is reversed when appropriate drug therapy results in remission. The ovaries and fallopian tubes may be involved in the inflammatory process, especially on the right side due to their proximity to the terminal ileum.[18] One study showed that fertility is less when the colon is involved compared to ileal involvement.[18] Perhaps this is due to the higher incidence of perianal, perineal, and rectovaginal abscesses and fistulas seen in this distribution, and the resulting poor hygiene, dyspareunia, and decreased libido for the patient or her husband. The overall toxicity of Crohn's disease with its attendant fever, abdominal pain, diarrhea, and suboptimal nutrition also had been implicated.[19]

Although far more difficult to quantify, it is our opinion that fear of pregnancy is also a major factor reducing fertility in young women with Crohn's disease. This fear often is introduced by either the obstetrician or gastroenterologist who may overemphasize to the patient the potentially negative course of the disease during pregnancy or suggest an unfavorable outcome for the fetus.

The chance of having a child who will eventually develop IBD is for Crohn's disease approximately 30%. This estimate is based on the fact that approximately 30% of affected patients have at least one blood relative who also has Crohn's disease. Familial Crohn's disease occurs in both Jews and non-Jews, but most familial groupings have been documented among Jews. The most common relationships have been father-daughter, father-son, brother-sister and first cousins.

Familial ulcerative colitis appears to be somewhat less frequent. Farmer et al[20] at the Cleveland Clinic reported 29% of ulcerative colitis patients had a family history of IBD, in contrast to approximately 35% with Crohn's disease.

Despite these observations, geneticists have not been willing to establish either Crohn's disease or ulcerative colitis as inheritable diseases. In giving advice to patients, the above statistics and a polygenic type of influence with varying degrees of penetration should be acknowledged.

Many studies have examined the effects of ulcerative colitis on pregnancy. The largest reports, examining more than 100 patients, have suggested normal healthy offspring in 76–97%, congenital abnormalities in 0–3%, spontaneous abortions in 1–13%, and stillbirths in 0–3%.[21] Each of these figures approximates that of a normal population. Among most recent data, Baiocco and Korelitz[22] reported that 83% of mothers with ulcerative colitis delivered normal healthy newborns. Premature delivery was seen in 2.5% and spontaneous abortion in 12%, but no stillbirths or congenital abnormalities were observed. Another study found that babies born to mothers with ulcerative colitis were lower in birth weight than normal, but this study did not achieve statistical significance. In addition, the presence of the ulcerative colitis did not affect mode of delivery or the incidence of preeclampsia and eclampsia during the gestational period.[23]

A few large studies exist that focus on the pregnant patient with Crohn's disease. Those involving greater than 100 cases cite normal offspring in 70–93%, congenital abnormalities in 0–1%, stillbirths in 1–4%, and spontaneous abortion in 3–9%, all approximating that of the non-IBD population.[21] A recent study found that among patients with Crohn's disease whose pregnancies resulted in developmental defects, stillbirth, or spontaneous abortions, active disease was present in 62%. Case analysis suggested that disease activity and not the drug treatment was primarily responsible for the increase in complications.[22]

The effects of drug therapy in treating IBD also should be considered. Most drugs used in the treatment of the pregnant IBD patient are the same as those used in the nonpregnant patient. These include corticosteroids, sulfasalazine and its derivative 5-aminosalicylic acid (5-ASA), and antibiotics.

The sulfonamides generally have been considered safe medications during all stages of pregnancy and lactation. Sulfasalazine reaches the breast milk at a level equal to 45% of those in the maternal serum. These medications will cross the placenta and can displace unconjugated bilirubin from albumin, introducing the theoretical risk of drug-induced neonatal jaundice and kernicterus. However, this has recently been quantified, and the amount of sulfasalazine transferred to neonates in breast milk is negligible with regard to the risk of kernicterus for the full-term infant without hemolytic disease.[24] Neither sulfasalazine nor its split products, sulfapyridine or 5-ASA, have been shown to cause harm to the neonate.[25] These drugs are effective for inducing and maintaining remission in both ulcerative colitis and Crohn's disease, especially with colonic involvement.

Animal studies have suggested that corticosteroids may be associated with low birth weights, decreased litter size and may result in the occurrence of cleft palate and spontaneous abortion.[26] Human studies, however, suggest that steroids are tolerated well.[27]

Metronidazole has been associated with at least two infants born with craniofacial abnormalities to mothers treated for amebiasis in the first trimester of pregnancy, but a causal relation has not been established.[28] There has been no evidence of fetal complications in a report on over 800 pregnancies in which metronidazole was given to over 300 patients during the first trimester.[29]

Immunosuppressive therapy with either azathioprine or 6-mercaptopurine (6-MP) is being used with increasing frequency in refractory patients with Crohn's disease and ulcerative colitis. Therapeutic advantages include its ability to eliminate steroids and induce remission in both diseases.[30,31] Experimental studies have implicated these agents in causing low fetal birth weights and congenital abnormalities.[32] Human renal transplant recipients, taking azathioprine (at higher doses than used in IBD) demonstrated, however, birth defects in only 7 of 103 births.[33] While this issue has been studied insufficiently to date, lack of Food and Drug Administration approval for the use of immunosuppressive agents in pregnancy has made most physicians hesitant to use them. In light of medicolegal implications, the authors have considered pregnancy a frank contraindication to their use. We consequently have recommended conscientious birth control for couples when either the male or female is on 6-MP therapy. We also recommend three months off the drug before attempting conception. Whether therapeutic abortion should be performed if accidental conception occurs while a patient is on the drug has remained controversial and should remain the patient's choice after appropriate counseling is given.

The effect of pregnancy on IBD appears to depend on the disease activity at the time of conception. Relatively quiescent ulcerative colitis will exacerbate in about one third of patients during gestation, will improve in one third of cases, and in one third will demonstrate no change in disease activity. Three out of 4 patients who have active disease at the time of conception will, however, continue to experience active disease throughout the gestational period.

Patients with Crohn's disease have shown a 15–40% relapse rate during pregnancy if in remission at the time of conception. This rate is not markedly different from that of the nonpregnant population with Crohn's disease. Cesarean section often may be the preferred route of delivery in the Crohn's disease patient with perianal disease. This avoids the possibility of involving the episiotomy scar in a fistulous tract.

Patients who have undergone total proctocolectomy with ileostomy are very capable of pregnancy and delivery of healthy children. Prolapse of the ileal stoma has been a reported complication of labor, but this is without long-term consequence. A total of 84–95% of women who have undergone subtotal colectomy with ileoanal anastomosis or Kock pouch have reported a postoperative increase in frequency of intercourse, most attributable to increased general health.[34] Both types of procedures have also led to a decreased incidence of dyspareunia. Approximately 80% of women were able to conceive after such surgery, and then delivered with vaginal and cesarean rates comparable to those of the normal population.

Surgical intervention in the pregnant patient with IBD is appropriate for unequivocal indications such as severe hemorrhage, perforation, and megacolon refractory to medical therapy and nonoperative decompression. Total colectomy and ileostomy with its attendant manipulation of the uterus at the time of surgery carries, however, a 60% overall risk of postoperative spontaneous abortion. The clinician thus should administer aggressive medical management of the IBD patient to induce remission as early as possible if a patient contemplates pregnancy or is already pregnant.

Treatment also should include general supportive measures such as control of diarrhea and perinatal vitamin supplementation. The use of total parenteral nutrition in the pregnant IBD patient has been studied well. At present, it should be reserved for similar maternal indications, such as those in the nonpregnant state. Fetal indications are present only rarely to warrant total parenteral nutrition.

CONTRACEPTION AND INFLAMMATORY BOWEL DISEASE

Two recent studies examined the absorption and bioavailability of oral contraceptives in ulcerative colitis patients who had undergone proctocolectomy and ileostomy. The first study examined the serum concentrations of ethinylestradiol and levonorgestrel (L-norgestrel) after oral administration.[35] The mean serum concentrations in the patients were equivalent to those in a noncolitis control group. A second study examined plasma concentrations of L-norgestrel in colitis patients before and after colectomy and found that the postoperative patients had a slight decrease in serum levels that was statistically significant when compared to controls.[36] This suggests that patients with active colitis or an ileostomy may rely on oral contraceptives, though not on low-dose "mini-pills."

REFERENCES

1. Rubin MR, Herrington JL, Schneider R. Regional enteritis with major gastrointestinal hemorrhage as the initial manifestation. *Arch Intern Med.* 1980;140:217.
2. Lewis G. Intestinal obstruction complicating pregnancy. *JAMA.* 1974;74:113.
3. Anderson GV, Ball A. Acute abdominal problems in pregnancy. *Contemp OB-GYN.* 1981;18:27.
4. Davis MR, Bohon CJ. Intestinal obstruction in pregnancy. *Clin Obstet Gynecol.* 1983;26(4):832.
5. Yaffe BH, Korelitz BI. Prognosis for non-operative management of small bowel obstruction in Crohn's disease. *J Clin Gastroenterol.* 1983;5:211.
6. Babakina A, Parsa H, Woodruff JD. Appendicitis during pregnancy. *Obstet Gynecol.* 1977;50:40.
7. Balber EA. Perforative appendicitis complicating pregnancy. *JAMA.* 1980;51:1310.
8. Horowitz MD, Gomez GA, Santiesteban R, et al. Acute appendicitis during pregnancy. *Arch Surg.* 1985;120:1362.
9. Girard RM, Lamarche J, Baillot R. Carcinoma of the colon associated with pregnancy: Report of a case. *Dis Col Rect.* 1981;24:473.
10. O'Leary JA, Bepko FJ Jr. Rectal carcinoma and pregnancy. *Am J Obstet Gynecol.* 1962;84:459.
11. Spiro HM. The irritable bowel. In: Spiro HM, ed. *Clinical Gastroenterology.* 3rd ed. New York: Macmillan; 1983:713.
12. Wald A, Van Thiel DH, Hochsletter L, et al. Effect of pregnancy on gastrointestinal transit. *Dig Dis Sci.* 1982;27:1015.
13. Lewis JH, Weingold AB. The use of gastrointestinal drugs during pregnancy and lactation. *Am J Gastroenterol.* 1985;80:912.
14. Kirsner JB, Shorter RG. Recent developments in non-specific inflammatory bowel disease. *N Eng J Med.* 1982;306:837.
15. deDombal FT, Watts JM, Watkinson G, et al. Ulcerative colitis and pregnancy. *Lancet.* 1965;2:599.
16. Willoughby CP, Truelove SC. Ulcerative colitis and pregnancy. *Gut.* 1980;21:469.
17. Mayberry JF, Weterman IT. European survey of fertility in women with Crohn's disease: a case controlled study by a European collaborative group. *Gut.* 1986;27:821.
18. Fielding JF, Cooke WT. Pregnancy and Crohn's disease. *Br Med J.* 1970;2:76.
19. Khosla R, Willoughby CP, Jewell DP. Crohn's disease and pregnancy. *Gut.* 1984;25:52.
20. Farmer RG, Michner WM, Mortimer EA. Studies of family history among patients with inflammatory bowel disease. *Clin Gastroenterol.* 1980;9:271.
21. Hanan IM, Kirsner JB. Inflammatory bowel disease in the pregnant woman. *Clin Perinatol.* 1985;12(3):682.
22. Baiocco PJ, Korelitz BI. The influence of inflammatory bowel disease and its treatment on pregnancy and fetal outcome. *J Clin Gastroenterol.* 1984;6:211.
23. Porter RJ, Stirrat GM. The effects of inflammatory bowel disease on pregnancy: a case-controlled retrospective analysis. *Br J Obstet and Gynecol.* 1986;93:1124.
24. Esbjorner E, Janerot G. Sulphasalazine and sulphapyradine serum levels in children to mothers treated with sulphasalazine during pregnancy and lactation. *ACTA Ped Scan.* 1987;76(1):124.
25. Khan AKA, Truelove SC. Placental and mammary transfer of sulphasalazine. *Br Med J.* 1979;2:1553.
26. Fraser FC, Fainstat TD. Production of congenital defects in offspring of pregnant mice treated with cortisone: Progress Report. *Pediatrics.* 1951;8:527.
27. Bongiovanni AM, McPadden AJ. Steroids during pregnancy and possible fetal complications. *Fertil Steril.* 1960;11:181.
28. Cantu JM, Garcia-Cruz D. Midline facial defects as a teratogenic effect of metronidazole. *Birth Defects.* 1982;18:85.
29. Briggs GG, Bodendorfer TW, Freeman RK, et al. *Drugs in Pregnancy and Lactation: a Reference Guide to Fetal and Neonatal Risk.* Baltimore, MD: Williams & Wilkins; 1983:
30. Present DH, Korelitz BI, Wisch N, et al. Treatment of Crohn's disease with 6-Mercaptopurine: a long-term randomized, double blind study. *N Eng J Med.* 1980;302:981.

31. Adler DJ, Korelitz BI. The therapeutic efficacy of 6-Mercaptopurine in refractory ulcerative colitis. *Am J Gastroenterol.* 1988;83:1042.
32. Rosenkranz JC, Githens JH. Azathioprine (Imuran) and pregnancy. *Am J Obstet Gynecol.* 1967;97:387.
33. Davison JM, Lindheimer MD. Pregnancy in women with renal allografts. *Semin Nephrol.* 1984;4:244.
34. Metcalf AM, Dozios RR, Kelly KA. Sexual function in women after proctocolectomy. *Ann Surg.* 1986;204(6):624.
35. Grimmer SF, Black DJ, Orme ML, et al. The bioavailability of ethinyloestradiol and levonorgestrel in patients with an ileostomy. *Contraception.* 1986;33:151.
36. Nilsson LO, Victor A, Kral JG, et al. Absorption of an oral contraceptive gestagen in ulcerative colitis before and after proctocolectomy and construction of a continent ileostomy. *Contraception.* 1985;31(2):195.

PART XIV Liver and Pancreas

Robert M. Galbraith, Section Editor

Chapter One Hundred and Fifty

Liver Disease: General Considerations

Robert M. Galbraith

150

A wide variety of disorders can cause jaundice in pregnancy.[1-9] Although important from a historical perspective, jaundice related to infections such as pyelonephritis and clostridial septicemia declined rapidly following the introduction of antibiotics. Jaundice following self-induced abortion as a result of infection or quinine is now a rarity. The current incidence of jaundice is between one in 500 and one in 5000 pregnancies; the vast majority of cases (75% or more) are caused by acute viral hepatitis or intrahepatic cholestasis during pregnancy.

From a practical viewpoint, the greatest diagnostic difficulty is determining the causes in the remaining 20–25% of cases. In fact, the association of chronic liver disease and pregnancy is rare simply because the chances of such patients being fertile and becoming pregnant are greatly reduced. These factors simplify the differential diagnosis of jaundice during pregnancy. However a small number of cases remain in which elucidation of the etiology can be difficult; this problem is compounded by the fact that some, but not all, standard tests of liver function undergo dramatic changes during normal pregnancy.

This chapter therefore emphasizes alterations in liver function in normal pregnancy, and summarizes the more commonly used approaches for diagnosis and differential diagnosis. Some general points also are made concerning the management of liver disease during pregnancy and its effects on the fetus.

LIVER FUNCTION DURING PREGNANCY

Clinical Features

Angiomata (spider nevi) and palmer erythema occur in 60–70% of normal pregnant women and apparently are related to increased levels of circulating estrogen. Since they are so frequent in the absence of liver disease, these findings cannot be assumed to indicate chronic parenchymal disease and are of low diagnostic specificity. Conversely, although liver blood flow and size do not change significantly during pregnancy, the liver tends to become displaced superiorly and posteriorly by the enlarging uterus. This may result in masking of mild to moderate hepatomegaly. As a general rule, a palpable liver thus is a helpful sign of abnormality, particularly in the third trimester. Certain other potentially helpful physical findings may be unchanged; for example, ascites that antedates pregnancy points strongly to the presence of cirrhosis, and signs of longstanding cholestasis such as scratch marks, xanthomata, xanthelasmata, and pigmentation suggest primary biliary cirrhosis.

Biochemical Parameters Generally Unchanged

Several standard liver function tests are essentially unchanged during normal pregnancy and thus retain their diagnostic usefulness. Serum transaminases (SGOT and SGPT or AST and ALT), γ-glutamyl transpeptidase, and lactic acid dehydrogenase are unaltered, and serum bilirubin is elevated only occasionally. Total serum alkaline phosphatase is an inaccurate index of cholestasis, since levels usually are elevated (see below), but levels of the hepatic isoenzyme and of 5′-nucleotidase are unchanged. Such measurements therefore are reliable. Prothrombin time also is normal and can be used as an index of hepatic synthetic capacity though serum albumin levels may be reduced.

Biochemical Parameters That May Change

Several other plasma components are altered, reflecting increased plasma volume and effects of the fetoplacental unit. Detailed accounts of these have been published by several authors[1-9] and they are given here in outline form. Total alkaline phosphatase activity is elevated consistently, mostly as a reflection of placental isoenzyme, which, in contrast to liver and bone enzymes, is unusually heat stable and remains active after heating to 60°C for 5 minutes.[10,11] Although the function of this isoenzyme is unclear, it is known to be produced in large amounts by the trophoblast, which is in direct anatomic contact with maternal blood in the intervillous spaces.[10-12] Fragments of syncytiotrophoblast also are known to embolize by way of the uterine veins into the maternal circulation in large numbers even during normal pregnancy.[13] In addition, although heat-stable isoenzyme in the serum originally was thought to be derived exclusively from the placenta, other tissues, such as endocervix and peripheral blood lymphocytes after activation[12,14], now are known to contain heat-stable isoenzyme and therefore could contribute to the circulating pool. In view of these considerations, it is not surprising that total serum levels of alkaline phosphatase become considerably elevated (twice normal or even greater) in pregnancy.

Levels of albumin generally are decreased. This occurs in part as a result of the expanded plasma volume and also may reflect decreased gene expression. Decreased albumin levels therefore do not necessarily indicate impaired synthetic reserve of the liver, particularly in the absence of a lengthened prothrombin time.

The hormonal changes in normal pregnancy appear to contribute to decreased excretory capacity with decreased bile-salt–independent flow and increased retention of Bromsulphalein (BSP). Although the BSP test is not now a routine measure of liver function, the importance of this observation lies in the recognition that serum triglyceride and cholesterol levels are increased, bile is more lithogenic, and gallbladder contractility is impaired. The practical effect therefore may be to heighten the propensity to gallstone formation in susceptible individuals.

A number of plasma proteins that have been loosely termed acute-phase reactants—α_1-antitrypsin, α_2-macroglobulin, C-reactive protein, ceruloplasmin, hemopexin, haptoglobin, orosomucoid (α_1-acid glycoprotein), serum amyloid protein, group-specific protein (G_c), and some coagulation components including fibrinogen—also increase during normal pregnancy. Some of these serve important carrier functions, eg, ceruloplasmin for copper and G_c for vitamin D metabolites, and may provide the developing fetus with vital nutrients. In this context, transferrin, which is a carrier protein for iron and numerous divalent cations and for which the syncytiotrophoblast membrane expresses large numbers of high-affinity specific receptors,[15,16] is similarly increased.

Several relevant changes occur in hematologic parameters. Although these are detailed elsewhere (Chapter 4), it is stressed that leukocyte count normally increases to 10,000–15,000/mm^3 and the erythrocyte sedimentation rate may be somewhat elevated (20–50 mm/hour). In addition, in view of the hemodilution that occurs, the label of anemia probably is reserved best for hemoglobin levels <10 g/100 mL. Generally, the alterations noted above all tend to progress throughout pregnancy. Some may increase transiently during delivery, and all should revert to normal within four to six weeks following delivery. For these reasons, it is difficult to give accurate cut-off levels that will define normality for these components reliably. However, it is safe to assume that levels of the relevant components during uncomplicated pregnancy lie at or about the outer limits of normal.

DIAGNOSTIC APPROACHES

The liver function tests described above can, with appropriate allowances, provide a useful indication of whether the abnormalities in a jaundiced patient are primarily hepatocellular or cholestatic as well as whether the underlying liver disease is acute or chronic. These can be supplemented with other serologic tests, for example, the mitochondrial antibodies typical of primary biliary cirrhosis and the antinuclear antibodies found in many women with "lupoid" chronic active hepatitis (see Chapter 153). Tests also may be performed for the smooth muscle antibodies present in chronic active hepatitis and more transiently in acute viral hepatitis, although it should be stressed that these antibodies may be found in pregnant women in the absence of liver disease.[17]

In contrast, there is rarely a strong indication for performance of x-ray procedures, including computer-assisted tomography (CT). Visualization of suspected esophageal or gastric varices and distinction from other potential sources of upper gastrointestinal hemorrhage can be achieved as easily by endoscopy. Similarly, abdominal ultrasound often provides information of equal or greater value than do biliary tract x-rays and can be used as a substitute for radioisotopic liver-spleen scanning. Liver biopsy probably presents no greater risk to the pregnant patient than to the nonpregnant patient and, because appearances are not altered noticeably during normal pregnancy, it often is helpful. On the other hand, biopsy may be somewhat more difficult technically because of displacement of the liver. Although this procedure may provide useful diagnostic information in a difficult case, it may add little to determination of prognosis or appropriate therapy.

DIFFERENTIAL DIAGNOSIS

The differential diagnosis often is considered in three main groups: acute hepatitis, liver disease of pregnancy (disorders that present during pregnancy and essentially are unique to pregnancy), and chronic liver disease that may antedate conception. More detailed discussions of these categories are given in other chapters, but the major points in the differential diagnosis are summarized here.

When liver disease arises during pregnancy, the most important distinction is between two clear-cut syndromes. If the picture is predominantly one of hepatocellular jaundice with elevations in serum bilirubin and transaminases and prolongation of the prothrombin time, the diagnosis is likely to be *acute viral hepatitis*. Although the degree of abnormality and the severity of the prodrome are variable, an acute onset and the appearance or presence of serum markers of hepatitis virus infection (Chapter 152) usually confirm the diagnosis. On the other hand, if the patient complains of itching and presents a predominantly cholestatic picture, the cause is generally *intrahepatic cholestasis of pregnancy*. This disorder nearly always occurs in the third trimester, whereas acute viral hepatitis can present at any point during pregnancy, and bilirubin levels in intrahepatic cholestasis almost never exceed 5 mg/100 ml. There also may be a positive family history or indications of a similar syndrome related to use of oral contraceptives. As noted above, these two disorders account for some 75–80% of cases of jaundice arising during pregnancy.

Potentially useful distinguishing features often are found in other relevant disorders. For example, *hyperemesis gravidarum* is a disease of the first trimester, whereas preeclampsia and acute fatty liver of pregnancy occur typically in the third trimester. The characteristic presentation of fatty liver is an acute onset of hepatocellular damage that may lead rapidly to fulminant hepatic failure and renal insufficiency, a picture that must be differentiated mainly from that of acute viral hepatitis. In contrast, the onset of preeclampsia is usually more insidious and often is obvious from the occurrence of the typical features of hypertension, proteinuria, and edema, although occasionally distinction from acute fatty liver is more difficult. In view of the importance of terminating the pregnancy if acute fatty liver is present (see below), this is one situation in which a liver biopsy for diagnostic purposes may, if feasible, be strongly justified.

When chronic liver disease is present, and in particular antedates pregnancy, the diagnosis often is known. Although spider nevi and palmar erythema are unreliable as signs of chronic liver disease, other cutaneous stigmata of liver disease and the presence of ascites or other signs of portal hypertension and of chronic portosystemic encephalopathy (alterations in mentation, mood, or conscious level; asterixis; and fetor) will usually indicate chronic parenchymal or biliary disease. If fulminant hepatic failure does not develop, it is often more informative and safer to observe the progression of the clinical picture than to perform more aggressive investigations.

EFFECTS ON FETUS AND MANAGEMENT

General Considerations

The management of liver disease during pregnancy generally is determined by the likely effects on the fetus. The effects are usually and perhaps surprisingly mild. The major risk is prematurity, particularly in the rare patient with chronic liver disease antedating pregnancy, and there probably is little that can be done to prevent this from happening. In acute viral hepatitis, there is a risk that the fetus may develop hepatitis or, in the case of the B virus, become a carrier. However, transmission cannot be recognized reliably antenatally. The carriage rate for hepatitis B approaches 20% in some areas of the world, so that early induction of labor is not justified (see Chapter 152). The beneficial effects of terminating the pregnancy of the mother, even in the minority who develop fulminant hepatic failure, is small in comparison with the potential risks. However, there are two disorders in which induction may be justified, namely, acute fatty liver of pregnancy and severe preeclampsia. Under these circumstances, evacuation of the uterus may be lifesaving for the mother and may permit survival of the fetus. Therapeutic termination is also a reasonable approach during the first trimester in cirrhotics with life-threatening complications such as variceal bleeding, and also in patients with severe hemoglobinopathies such as sickle cell disease and homozygous hemoglobin C disease.

Fetal Alcohol Syndrome

The assumption frequently is made that alcoholic liver disease in pregnancy other than fatty degeneration is unusual. Although the apparently increasing scale of alcohol abuse casts some uncertainty on this contention, it is clear that certain fetal effects of alcohol consumption during pregnancy are being increasingly recognized. These effects have become known informally as the *fetal alcohol syndrome*[18-21] (see Chapter 8). The common factor is prolonged heavy consumption or binge drinking, and although the precise number of pregnancies at risk is not known, it has been estimated that fetal alcohol syndrome may occur in as many as 20–40% of chronic alcoholics who are pregnant. Unmarried mothers and those of limited means appear to be at particular risk, and alcohol consumption may be combined with other risk factors such as heavy smoking, malnutrition, and drug abuse.

There are a wide variety of abnormalities. The facies appear to be characteristic, with hypoplastic facial bones, small palpebral fissures, epicanthic folds, an underdeveloped philtrum, thin upper lip, and cleft palate. Affected neonates frequently are small-for-age at birth and may exhibit failure to thrive. They also display several major abnormalities of the cardiovascular system, including ventricular septal defects, patent ductus arteriosus, pulmonic stenosis, Fallot's tetralogy, and transposition of the great vessels. The central nervous system also is affected, with epilepsy, hypotonia, spastic diplegia or quadriplegia, retarded psychomotor development, and myopia. However, thus far fetal liver damage does not seem to be a major manifestation. Several of these disorders may exist in a given infant, and although the precise cause of the syndrome is unclear, it appears likely that alcohol may cause greatest damage during the crucial period of organogenesis between approximately 15–60 days' gestation. The management of the syndrome depends on the particular abnormalities, and therapy is discussed in the appropriate chapters. In general, however, the damage already has been done by the time of presentation, and the main thrust for the future is in prevention through identification and counseling of pregnant mothers at high risk (see also Chapter 8).

REFERENCES

1. Thorling L. Jaundice in pregnancy: A clinical study. *Acta Med Scand.* 1955;302(suppl):1.
2. Ikonen E. Jaundice in late pregnancy. *Acta Obstet Gynecol Scand.* 1964;5(suppl):1.
3. Iber FL. Jaundice in pregnancy—a review. *Am J Obstet Gynecol.* 1965;91:721.
4. Haemmerli UP. Jaundice during pregnancy, with special emphasis on recurrent jaundice during pregnancy and its differential diagnosis. *Acta Med Scand.* 1966;444(suppl):1.
5. Sherlock S. Jaundice in pregnancy. *Br Med Bull.* 1968;24:39.
6. Bergstein NAM. *Liver and Pregnancy.* Amsterdam: Excerpta Medica. 1973.
7. Furhoff AK, Hellstrom J. Jaundice in pregnancy: a followup study of the series of women originally reported by L. Thorling. Present health of the women. *Acta Med Scand.* 1974;196:181.
8. Sherlock S. *Diseases of the Liver and Biliary System.* 6th ed. Oxford: Blackwell Scientific; 1981:400.
9. Krejs GJ, Haemmerli UP. Jaundice during pregnancy. In: Shiff L, Schiff ER, eds. *Diseases of the Liver.* 5th ed. Philadelphia, PA: JB Lippincott; 1982:1561.
10. Fishman WH. Perspectives on alkaline phosphatase isoenzymes. *Am J Med.* 1974;56:617.
11. Badger KS, Sussman HH. Structural evidence that human liver and placental alkaline phosphatase isoenzymes are coded by different genes. *Proc Natl Acad Sci USA.* 1976;73:2201.
12. Kantor RRS, Galbraith RM, Emerson DL, et al. Placental alkaline phosphatase is a major specificity in antisera raised to human trophoblast membranes. *Am J Reprod Immunol.* 1981;1:336.
13. Douglas GW, Thomas L, Carr M, et al. Trophoblast in the circulating blood during pregnancy. *Am J Obstet Gynecol.* 1959;78:960.
14. Goldstein DJ, Rogers C, Harris H. A search for trace expression of placental-like alkaline phosphatase in non-malignant human tissues: demonstration of its occurrence in lung, cervix, testis and thymus. *Clin Chim Acta.* 1982;125:63.
15. Wada HG, Hass PE, Sussman HH. Transferrin receptor in human placental brush border membranes: studies on the binding of transferrin to placental membrane vesicles and the identification of a placental brush border glycoprotein with high affinity for transferrin. *J Biol Chem.* 1979;254:12,629.
16. Galbraith GMP, Galbraith RM, Faulk WP. Immunological studies of transferrin and transferrin receptors of human placental trophoblast. *Placenta.* 1980;1:33.
17. Pietarinen I, Hartikainen-Sorri AL, Makitalo R, et al. Smooth muscle antibodies in complicated pregnancies. *Am J Reprod Immunol.* 1983;3:43.
18. Clarren SK, Smith DW: The fetal alcohol syndrome. *N Engl J Med.* 1978;298:1063.
19. Sokol RS, Miller SI, Reed G. Alcohol abuse during pregnancy: an epidemiology study. *Alcoholism (NY).* 1980;4:135.
20. Streissguth AP, Landesman-Dwyer S, Martin JC, et al. Teratogenic effects of alcohol in human and laboratory animals. *Science.* 1980;209:353.
21. Lipson AH, Walsh DA, Webster WS. Fetal alcohol syndrome: a great pediatric imitator. *Med J Aust.* 1983;1:266.

Chapter One Hundred and Fifty-One
Liver Diseases

Patricia S. Latham

151

Liver dysfunction and jaundice during pregnancy may be the result of etiologic factors occurring coincidentally with pregnancy, such as hepatitis (see Chapter 150), or the direct result of conditions unique to pregnancy itself, so-called *jaundice of pregnancy*, or *liver disease of pregnancy*. This latter subgroup includes cholestasis of pregnancy, preeclampsia and eclampsia, hematoma and rupture of the liver, acute fatty liver of pregnancy, and hyperemesis gravidarum.

INTRAHEPATIC CHOLESTASIS OF PREGNANCY

Intrahepatic cholestasis of pregnancy (*recurrent jaundice of pregnancy, benign cholestasis of pregnancy, obstetric cholestasis, pruritus gravidarum*) was first described in a publication by Svanborg.[1] The disease follows viral hepatitis as the second most common cause of jaundice during pregnancy, occurring in approximately 20% of cases.[2] The diagnosis, however, is still infrequent, occurring in only one of 100–10,000 pregnancies.[3] The highest incidences are in reports from Chile and Scandinavia, but the syndrome is also documented well in the United States.[4] The syndrome has not been described in blacks with the exception of one questionable recent case report.[5] Generally, it is accepted that pruritus gravidarum and intrahepatic cholestasis of pregnancy, by their similar laboratory abnormalities and occurrence of symptoms, are the same disease.[3] Patients with jaundice, however, tend to have more severe biochemical parameters of liver disease than patients with pruritus alone.[3,6] The symptoms tend to recur in subsequent pregnancies. Each pregnancy in an affected woman may be associated with a range of variations in clinical and laboratory expression of the syndrome complex.[2]

Clinical Description

Jaundice occurs in approximately 75% of patients after the 22nd week of pregnancy, but has been reported as early as the sixth week.[7] Before the patient notices icterus, however, she has usually presented with complaint of itching. Pruritus often precedes jaundice by one to two weeks but may occur as early as 22 weeks prior to the onset of icterus.[7] Pruritus is concurrent with jaundice in over 90% of cases[8] but may occur as the only symptom of liver dysfunction in as many as 50%.[6,9] The urine usually darkens with or without change in stool color, as the hyperbilirubinemia usually is mild and plateaus at less than 5.0 mg% (Table 151–1). A largely asymptomatic steatorrhea can be documented in the majority of icteric patients, which resolves 3–9 weeks after delivery.[10] However, the steatorrhea does not appear to correlate with the decrease in weight or height ratio and the fetal distress that is seen with increased incidence in these cases.[10] Premature labor may occur in as many as 35% of cases with evidence of fetal distress during labor and at delivery.[2,6,9]

Approximately 70% of patients with intrahepatic cholestasis of pregnancy have a recurrence in a subsequent pregnancy[8], which may feature either jaundice, pruritus, or both. These two symptoms are usually the only manifestations of intrahepatic cholestasis and will continue until delivery, at which time they begin to subside over one to two weeks or even within the first day.[2] Mild alkaline phosphatase elevation or icterus, however, may persist for several months.[2,3,7]

The physical exam typically shows no abnormalities except for icterus, dark urine, and possible excoriations from scratching. The liver and spleen usually are not enlarged, and generally, no other signs of prolonged cholestasis are present with exception of a tendency for postpartum hemorrhage, which may occur rarely if prothrombin is not adequately synthesized because of bile salt-deficient malabsorption of fat-soluble vitamin K.[11]

Laboratory Evaluation and Diagnosis

Laboratory evaluation of liver function suggests an obstructive pattern. Serum bilirubin in such patients is predominantly direct, with a total value that is usually 5 mg/dL or less. Serum alkaline phosphatase activity is increased moderately in the majority of women to a much greater extent than in normal pregnancy.[2,8] This increase in alkaline phosphatase during intrahepatic cholestasis of pregnancy is predominantly of liver origin, as opposed to the normal increase during pregnancy of placental alkaline phosphatase (Table 151–1). The hepatic nature of this enzyme rise is suggested by increased 5′-nucleotidase activity.[12] The level of serum alkaline phosphatase may not peak until after delivery, although other laboratory parameters usually are improving at that time.[2] The serum transaminase enzyme activity generally is normal or less than 250 IU. If transaminase activity is increased, it is frequently the earliest evidence of liver dysfunction.[7] A rarely prolonged prothrombin time, as discussed above, should return briskly to normal with administration of vitamin K intramuscularly. The albumin and globulin levels are normal for the pregnant state, as are other laboratory parameters. The typical features of this disorder are compared and contrasted with those of preeclampsia and eclampsia of pregnancy, fatty liver of pregnancy, and hyperemesis gravidarum in Table 151–1.

Although a liver biopsy is rarely necessary in the diagnosis of intrahepatic cholestasis of pregnancy, the histology shows a bland, predominantly centrilobular, cholestasis in hepatocytes and canaliculi.[2] Focal Kupffer cell activation also may appear. There is no other significant inflammation beyond a nonspecific, minimal, mononuclear portal infiltrate as seen in normal pregnancy.[13] The changes have been observed to regress after delivery.[2]

The diagnosis of intrahepatic cholestasis of pregnancy rests on the typical history of pruritus or jaundice in the third trimester and the laboratory evidence of a nonprogressive, mild cholestasis with little elevation of transaminase enzyme.

Etiology and Pathophysiology

Etiology. Considerable evidence indicates that intrahepatic cholestasis of pregnancy is the result of an inherited metabolic disorder that becomes manifest under conditions of

TABLE 151–1. LIVER DISEASES OF PREGNANCY

	Hyperemesis Gravidarum	Intrahepatic Cholestasis	Preeclampsia and Eclampsia	Fatty Liver	Normal
Onset (trimester)[a]	I	III	III	III	—
Major sign and symptoms	Vomiting	Pruritis Jaundice	Hypertension Edema Albuminuria Jaundice ± Convulsions	Nausea/vomiting Abdominal pain Confusion/coma Jaundice ± Fever ± Preeclampsia ± Hemorrhage	—
Laboratory signs[b]					
Transaminase	3× ↑	5× ↑	5× ↑	10× ↑	Normal
Alkaline phosphatase	2× ↑	7–10× ↑	2–3× ↑	3× ↑	2× ↑
Bilirubin (mg/100 mL)	3.5	<5.0	10.0 (unconjugated)	10.0	1.0
Prothrombin time	Normal	2×	± ↑	2× ↑	Normal
Other		bile acids 10–100×		WBC ↑ (20–30,000)	WBC ↑ (10–15,000)
Liver biopsy	Normal	Centrilobular Cholestasis	Periportal Fibrin deposits, and hemorrhagic necrosis	Centrilobular Microvesicular fat and cholestasis	Normal

[a] Trimester most frequently represented.
[b] Usual peak values.

pregnancy. The frequency of reports from Scandinavia and Chile suggests that these populations have a 10- to 20-fold increased risk for developing this syndrome during pregnancy.[3] In Chile, there is a particularly high prevalence in the subpopulation of Araucanian Indians.[3] In this subpopulation, the disease has a prevalence of 5.5% with jaundice and 22.1% with pruritus alone versus an incidence of 2.4% and 13.2%, respectively, in the general Chilean population of pregnant females. Similar findings are described in the United States, with transmission of the trait over three generations.[4] The genotype HLA-B8 appears in the affected family members in this U.S. study group, but statistical analysis to link the trait to any HLA haplotype is inconclusive.[4] The relationship of this syndrome to another cause of jaundice, benign recurrent intrahepatic cholestasis, is unclear, but they show similar clinical features. The simultaneous appearance of benign recurrent intrahepatic cholestasis and intrahepatic cholestasis of pregnancy in a similar study group has been reported.[14]

Clinical symptoms tend to parallel increases in serum estrogen and progesterone hormone levels as they fluctuate in normal pregnancy. Thus the syndrome tends to recur in subsequent pregnancies and may be induced in some patients by oral contraceptives, which can induce an exogenous estrogen and progesterone effect.[15,16] Steroid hormones in forms such as the C17-alkyl-substituted ethinylestradiol are known cholestatic agents.[15,17,18] Experimentally, exogenous estrogens can induce cholestasis and biochemical abnormalities of liver function similar to those seen in intrahepatic cholestasis of pregnancy.[18] In addition, ethinylestradiol can produce the clinical symptoms of nausea, pruritus, and jaundice in women with a previous history of intrahepatic cholestasis of pregnancy.[18] The response of these women to ethinylestradiol suggests a constitutional hypersensitivity to estrogen or an increased synthesis or decreased ability to metabolize it. Evidence suggests that synthesis of estrogen and progesterone hormones is normal in intrahepatic cholestasis of pregnancy, but a decrease in the biliary excretion of estrogen and progesterone has been documented.[19]

Pathophysiology. The mechanism by which the two major symptoms of jaundice and pruritus occur is not entirely understood.[20,21] Pruritus is an integral part of the syndrome. It may occur alone, with, or before the appearance of jaundice. Increased serum bile acids as a result of cholestasis have been linked to the symptom of pruritus by their irritation of sensory receptors in the skin[22] and serum bile acids are increased in virtually all cases of intrahepatic cholestasis of pregnancy.[20,21] Although the degree of itching does not have an absolute correlation with the level of bile acids in serum or skin[23] it is likely that the bile acids themselves, or an as yet unmeasured bile acid associate, is responsible for the symptom of itch.

The cholestasis is entirely intrahepatic, as demonstrated by liver biopsy and the appearance of normal bile ducts in those cases studied by biliary imaging.[2] The mechanism of the cholestasis appears to be a defect in bilirubin excretion from the hepatocytes. In uncomplicated pregnancy, the serum bromsulphalein (BSP) clearance generally is normal, but there is a decrease in BSP transport maximum (Tm) and an increase in storage capacity (S).[24] In intrahepatic cholestasis of pregnancy, the condition of pregnancy results in a decrease in both aspects of BSP excretion and a 10–25% decrease in BSP clearance from the serum of these patients.[25] This finding suggests that entry of bilirubin into the cell probably is normal, but conjugation or exit from the cell is blocked. There is evidence that this metabolic defect is independent of the pregnancy, since an abnormal increase in BSP (S) has been found in nonpregnant patients with a history of intrahepatic cholestasis of pregnancy.[26] The high levels of estrogen and progesterone seen during pregnancy may stress this metabolic pathway to result in an inadequate excretion of bilirubin from the liver cells.

This idea is supported by the observations that high dose ethinylestradiol rechallenge in these patients can result in abnormal BSP clearance.[27] The increase in estrogen and progesterone hormones also has other effects that can contribute to biliary stasis, such as an inhibition of Na+, K+-ATPase activity, which is in turn linked to bile salt independent flow from hepatocytes; estradiol may cause alterations in plasma membrane rigidity.[28]

An increase in fetal prematurity and death are common complications of this syndrome, but the cause is not clear. Abnormal uterine contractions have been noted in response to oxytocin in one study of these patients.[29] The authors suggest that a hypersensitivity of uterine muscle may exist in response to increased serum bile acids and a changed calcium balance, but there is as yet no data to support or refute this idea. It is noteworthy that serum bile acids do cross the placenta. Laatikainen[30] has suggested that the increase in serum bile acids, seen in this disorder, may itself be the source of fetal distress, but the involved mechanism is still unclear.

Medical Care

Treatment of Symptoms. The patient with intrahepatic cholestasis of pregnancy usually is in overall good health and has a sense of general well-being. Management of the syndrome is, therefore, aimed at controlling the pruritus. Cholestyramine is the only proven effective treatment for itching. In most cases, 7–14 days are required as response time. Antihistamines usually are ineffective. Cholestyramine at doses of 12–16 g per day is standard treatment, but up to 27 g per day may be necessary to control itching.[31] Even at these doses, however, a remarkable proportion of patients do not respond, with clinical loss of pruritus, despite a decrease in bile acids.[30] Phenobarbital also may decrease bilirubin, but is generally not clinically efficacious in this syndrome.[30] An investigational drug, which offers some hope for future therapy, is S-adenosyl-L-methionine (SAMe).[32] In one report, this drug resulted in improved liver chemistries, some decrease of itching, and no significant side effects in six symptomatic women treated for 10–20 days. However, further studies are needed before this drug can be recommended for therapy in this disorder.

Management of Pregnancy. There is no evidence that jaundice and increased bile acids are hazardous to the mother.[2,8] There is some evidence, however, that the presence of the syndrome may be hazardous to the fetus. Haemmerli's complete review[2] of available reports on the course of intrahepatic cholestasis of pregnancy showed a cumulative increase in fetal prematurity and mortality, but it showed no correlation between the severity of hyperbilirubinemia and complications to the fetus. Two more recent reports[6,9] of case series have demonstrated premature delivery in approximately 35% of patients with a 10% fetal mortality. In Reid's study of 56 cases, including 27 with pruritus alone, fetal complications correlated with the presence of hyperbilirubinemia of greater than 2 mg/dL. There was, however, no relationship between the severity of jaundice and the incidence of either fetal prematurity or death.[6] None of the infants in published reports have been jaundiced. Since there is no specific factor which has been identified as responsible for the morbidity to the fetus, the standard management of the patient approaching delivery is still used. Supportive management includes prophylactic administration of vitamin K for jaundice of greater than two weeks' duration and antepartum testing of the fetus. Induced delivery at greater than 37 weeks had been recommended by some investigators of this syndrome before the concept of antepartum testing became routine practice.[6] A majority of the patients will reach spontaneous labor and delivery. The physician, however, should be prepared for evidence of fetal distress before and during delivery.

Counseling. A woman with a family history of intrahepatic cholestasis of pregnancy has an enhanced likelihood of developing the syndrome during her pregnancy. The risk, however, cannot be quantified in the general population and varies in different parts of the world. After a previous pregnancy, complicated by this syndrome, a women has a 70% chance for a recurrence in a subsequent pregnancy. Symptoms then may include jaundice, pruritus, or both.[8] She also may experience cholestasis with the use of oral contraceptives containing synthetic estrogens and progesterones.[15,16] The syndrome is not associated with an increased risk to the survival of the mother, but there is an increased risk to the fetus. There is no contraindication to future pregnancy. At present, there is no generally accepted sign or biochemical marker which can predict future occurrence of the syndrome or the outcome of a pregnancy.

THE HEPATIC PRESENTATION OF PREECLAMPSIA AND ECLAMPSIA

Clinical Description

Preeclampsia is a syndrome of unknown etiology occurring in approximately 5% of pregnancies (see also Chapter 139). It is characterized by hypertension, proteinuria, and edema of variable severity. Eclampsia is the expression of these same signs in conjunction with convulsions. The syndrome may occur in any age, but is most common at the extremes of childbearing, the ages below 20 and above 35 years. It has no clear genetic basis, but there appears to be some familial predisposition.[33] Although mortality has been decreasing, it continues to be the leading cause of maternal death during pregnancy.[33]

Evidence of liver dysfunction is an unusual manifestation of mild preeclampsia. The liver usually is unaffected by early disease. However, the liver becomes a target organ of injury as a complication of severe disease. Evidence of liver dysfunction in these cases may be present in upwards to 50% of cases.[2,34] Liver disease occurs mostly in the young primigravid female, but severe disease also is seen in some multiparous patients.[35] It tends to present in the third trimester or the last half of pregnancy. The degree of liver abnormality roughly parallels the severity of the clinical syndrome. Jaundice occurs in only 20% of all cases.[2] In more severe preeclampsia and eclampsia, however, jaundice may be accompanied by signs of severe liver disease, upper mid- or right-sided abdominal pain, and nausea with vomiting in 40% of cases. The liver may be tender on examination and possibly enlarged. Such enlargement of the liver is difficult to diagnose in the last trimester of pregnancy.[35] In 10% of patients with such a severe course of disease, a clinical presentation has been described including hemolysis (H), elevated serum level of liver enzymes (EL), and low platelets (LP), the so-called *HELLP syndrome*[36] (see also Chapter 139). Patients with preeclampsia and eclampsia may present first with signs of liver disease in 10% of cases. In the series studies by Rolfes and Ishak et al[35], delay in the correct diagnosis was evident in 22% of these cases.

Delay in correct diagnosis and therapy appeared to contribute to maternal mortality in 50% of fatal cases.[35] In this series, hepatic complications alone accounted for up to 16% of maternal mortality related to preeclampsia and eclampsia.[35] Since liver dysfunction is associated with the more severe grades of the disease, its presence should prompt close observation and attention to supportive care. Rupture of the liver is one of the most dramatic and urgent of these complications. It is discussed in detail in a later section of this chapter.

Laboratory Evaluation and Diagnosis

Laboratory examination of liver function in preeclampsia and eclampsia usually reveals a serum transaminase activity of less than 250 IU. In a majority of patients with severe disease and significant liver dysfunction, this value is substantially higher (>1000 IU).[33] Serum alkaline phosphatase is increased in a greater percentage of patients than in normal gestation, but ranges are not beyond those accepted in normal pregnancy. The prothrombin time is rarely increased and tends to correlate with the severity and duration of liver dysfunction. An elevation of bilirubin may be clinically apparent in as many as 20% of cases.[2] It usually is mild and rarely exceeds a fivefold elevation. In approximately 10% of cases with eclampsia or severe preeclampsia, laboratory or clinical evidence of diffuse intravascular coagulation (DIC) is present.[37,38] During pregnancy, one study suggested that marked thrombocytopenia may be the earliest and most reliable sign of DIC.[39] In addition, serial platelet counts indicated that a decrease in platelet count may represent an early indication of the onset of preeclampsia and is associated with elevated urate levels as well as a severe and complicated clinical course.[40,41] Intravascular hemolysis associated with DIC can contribute to the occurrence of jaundice.[42]

In patients with the HELLP syndrome, a distinctive coagulopathy occurs that in nearly all cases is associated with a drop in hematocrit, a blood smear compatible with microangiopathic hemolysis, and a significant thrombocytopenia (platelets <100,000/mm^3). Prothrombin time, partial thromboplastin time, and fibrinogen level, however, are normal.[36] The severity of laboratory findings does not always correlate with the severity of the clinical condition, and the clinical findings are not consistent with classic diffuse intravascular coagulation.[36,37,39]

Histology of the liver shows few tissue changes in mild cases of preeclampsia. Nonspecific features of increased lipofuscin in hepatocytes, increased activation of Kupffer's cells in sinusoids, and an increase in binucleated hepatocytes have been described.[34] In more severe cases of preeclampsia and with eclampsia, the liver and kidney may demonstrate histopathologic changes. In both organs, hyaline deposits are seen in the capillary network associated with variable necrosis and hemorrhage of involved tissues.[43-45] In the kidney, electron-dense deposits occur in the mesangium composed of fibrin and fibrinogen, IgG, IgM, and C3. In the liver, similar deposits of bland fibrin and fibrinogen are seen in portal arterioles and in the sinusoids. There is, however, little inflammation associated with these conditions.[35] Surrounding these focal collections are variable zones of dilated sinusoids, necrosis, hemorrhage, and infarction, characteristically in the periportal region (Figures 151–1 and 151–2). These foci are particularly marked in severe preeclampsia and eclampsia and are seen in 90% of patients with fatal disease, but in only 28% of surviving patients.[43]

Typical preeclampsia and eclampsia do not present a difficult differential diagnosis; however, other considerations for diagnosis include biliary tract obstruction, hepatitis, and fatty liver of pregnancy. Hepatitis should be excluded in such cases by appropriate serology including antibody to hepatitis A (IgM), HBsAg, anti-HB core (IgM) hepatitis, and antibody to delta virus (IgM) in patients who are known to be HBsAg-positive. Hepatobiliary imaging should be done to identify gallstones or obstruction when these diagnoses are possible. A sonogram usually is sufficient for this purpose, however, computerized axial tomography (CAT) also can help to identify sites of significant

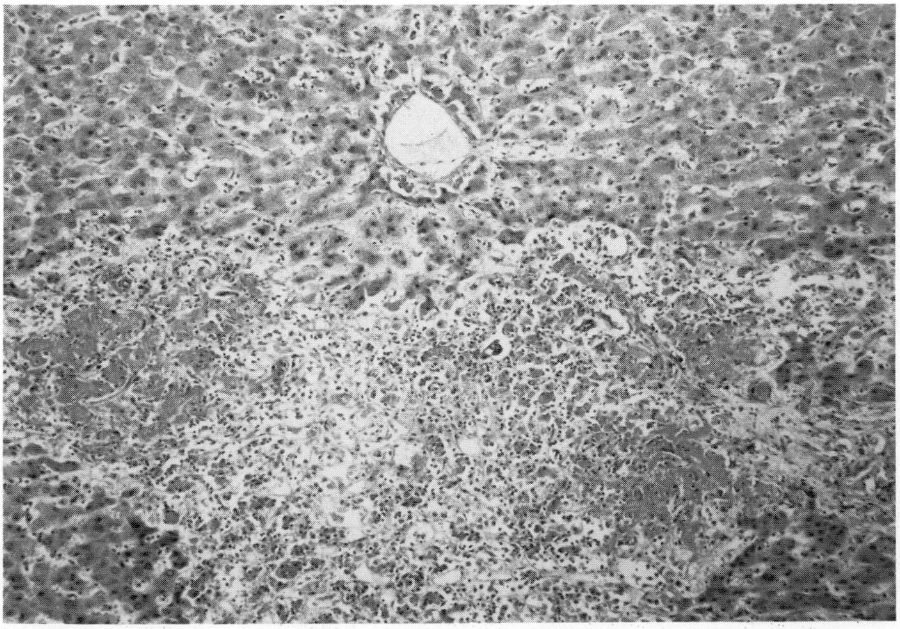

Figure 151–1. Liver section from a patient dying with preeclamptic-eclamptic liver failure. The centrilobular area is intact with a normal appearance. Large fibrin deposits are present in the periportal area with portal edema and necrosis of the adjacent parenchyma. (×63)

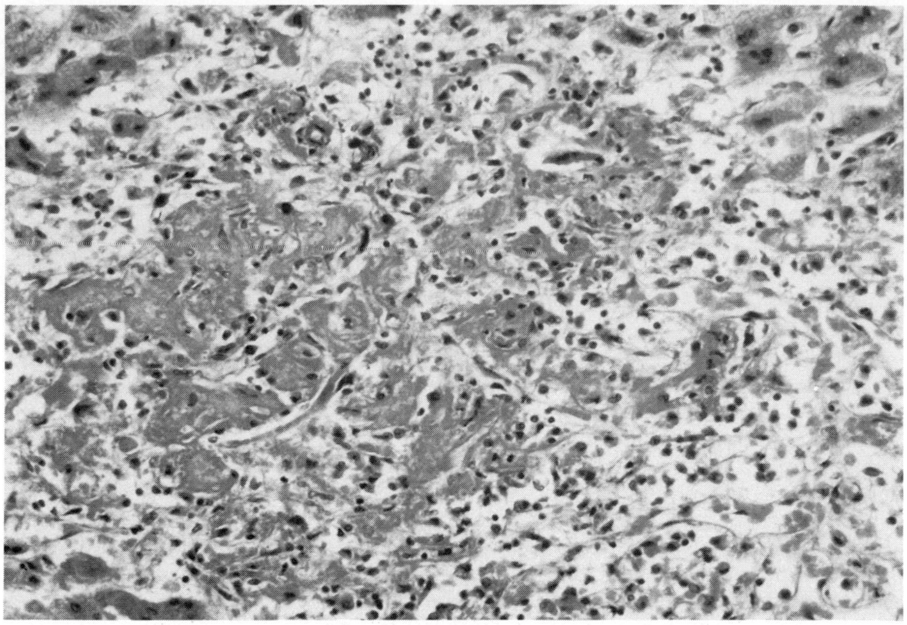

Figure 151–2. Greater detail of the periportal area and fibrin in Fig. 151–1. (×160)

hemorrhage and infarction. Liver biopsy rarely is necessary to diagnose liver disease due to preeclampsia and eclampsia and often is contraindicated by the accompanying coagulopathy. Liver biopsy, however, may be more urgent in cases in which the clinical pattern is not typical and hepatitis cannot be excluded. It generally is considered safe during pregnancy in the absence of other contraindications.

It is still unknown whether the HELLP syndrome represents a more severe form of preeclampsia and eclampsia or a specific and distinct entity. An autoimmune mechanism for this syndrome has been suggested because of its similarities to thrombotic thrombocytopenia purpura, including an increase in peripheral platelet destruction, microangiopathic hemolytic anemia, and systemic involvement with kidney and liver as target organs. There also is evidence that an effector can be passively transferred to the fetus to induce some of the clinical manifestations.[36] In 25–50% of cases, offspring of mothers with the HELLP syndrome may show a transient thrombocytopenia and leukopenia.[36]

Medical Care

Treatment of Symptoms. The most important aspect of managing liver disease in preeclampsia and eclampsia is the recognition that it is a manifestation of a systemic disease process. In general, it will improve when the underlying disease is treated appropriately. Specific therapy for clinical manifestations of liver failure are supportive, as in other settings of liver dysfunction, with special attention to the management of intravascular fluid balance and coagulopathy.[8,46] This is discussed in more detail below.

Management of the Pregnancy. Liver disease with mild preeclampsia requires careful observation and appropriate therapy to prevent progression of disease and complications. The fetus generally is delivered as soon as it is feasible obstetrically. Morbidity to mother and infant increase dramatically when the disease is severe. Under such circumstances, the child should be delivered promptly in the most expedient manner. The complication of hepatic rupture constitutes a surgical emergency, and the fetus should be delivered at operation as discussed below.

HEMATOMA AND RUPTURE OF THE LIVER

Rupture of the liver during pregnancy was reported first by Abercrombie in 1844 and well over 100 cases have been reported since that time.[35,47] The underlying etiology in the vast majority of cases is preeclampsia and eclampsia, especially with accompanying DIC or HELLP syndrome.[48] The disease also may be seen with fatty liver of pregnancy, intrahepatic tumors, or trauma.

Clinical Description

The patient with preeclampsia and eclampsia who develops hematoma or rupture is usually in the older age range for this syndrome. Although nulliparous women are more likely than multiparous women to develop preeclampsia and eclampsia, the opposite is true of hepatic hematoma and rupture.[49] The presence of coagulopathy and tendency toward hemorrhagic necrosis increases the likelihood of developing this complication.[48-50] Hematoma and subcapsular hemorrhage are obvious predisposing factors in the development of rupture.

The clinical symptoms associated with the occurrence of a hematoma typically are the onset of persistent right upper quadrant pain, which may radiate to the back or right shoulder. In the case of rupture, there is an associated precipitous drop in blood pressure, accompanied by peritoneal signs. Physical examination at first may demonstrate only right upper quadrant tenderness and hepatomegaly, but the clinical cause usually progresses to include abdominal distention, pain, and peritoneal symptoms. Rupture is very often a catastrophic event.

Laboratory Evaluation and Diagnosis

No laboratory biochemistries will confirm the diagnosis of hepatic hematoma and rupture, although a sudden drop in hematocrit or a sudden rise in serum transaminase activity, if available in time, is very suggestive. The differential diagnosis must include *abruptio placentae,* rupture of the uterus, and uterine torsion. Other diagnoses that have to be considered include ovarian tumor, acute cholecystitis or pancreatitis, perforation of gastric or duodenal ulcers, appendicitis with perforation, myocardial infarction, pulmonary embolus, and acute pyelonephritis. Hepatic and abdominal imaging may identify successfully hepatic infarctions, hematoma, and subcapsular hemorrhage in this setting.[49,51-53] The CAT scan is likely to be more useful given this differential diagnosis, since it is less operator-dependent and can visualize the entire abdomen. A sonogram, however, may be more practical to perform, since the equipment is often on-hand in the obstetrical unit. These procedures may demonstrate a collection of blood, or a clot, most commonly in the anterior, superior right upper lobe with involvement of the left lobe in less than 11%.[48,49] A right pleural effusion may occur in some cases. A peritoneal tap may be used to confirm the presence of peritoneal blood in the case of rupture, but the source of the bleeding is ultimately identified further by angiography or surgery.[54]

Etiology and Pathophysiology

The pathogenesis of hepatic hematoma and rupture is attributed to the same factors that are thought to result in local deposition of fibrin in the liver of patients with preeclampsia and eclampsia.[35,47] These factors then might predispose to focal ischemia and intimal tears in the liver with hemorrhage and infarction.

Treatment and Management of Pregnancy

The diagnosis of hepatic rupture in pregnancy will result in virtually 100% mortality to the mother and fetus if surgery is not performed promptly. Delay in diagnosis and surgery or misdiagnosis has been considered responsible for a significant percentage of fatal cases.[48] Immediate surgery and delivery of the fetus has been considered responsible for the decrease in maternal and fetal mortality from 100% to approximately 65% in more recently reported series.[47,48] Immediate therapy should be directed at vascular instability and coagulopathy to improve the patient's operative risk and to control continued bleeding.[49] Surgery must be performed immediately to stop further bleeding. The surgery may include resection of a hepatic lobe or temporary packing.[55] Hepatic artery ligation also has been used successfully to control hepatic bleeding.[56]

Hepatic hematoma, without evidence of vascular instability or bleeding, may be managed conservatively, but careful follow up with imaging is necessary to confirm resolution of the hematoma and to assure that complications such as abscess formation or bleeding do not occur.[51] Rupture of a hematoma has been reported to occur days and even weeks after delivery.

There is no need to interrupt a pregnancy for a nonprogressive hematoma of the liver. However, surgery to control bleeding during hepatic rupture should be accompanied by cesarean section, which has been shown to reduce maternal and fetal operative mortality markedly.[49]

FATTY LIVER OF PREGNANCY

The earliest description of fatty liver of pregnancy (*acute obstetric yellow atrophy, fatty metamorphosis of pregnancy*) in the English language is attributed to a case reported by Stander and Cadden in 1934[57], but the earliest description of fatty liver of pregnancy as a syndrome is largely attributed to Sheehan in 1940.[58] Although more than 125 cases have been reported since that time, fatty liver of pregnancy remains the rarest of the diseases causing jaundice in pregnancy. Along with severe preeclampsia and eclampsia it is, however, associated with a devastating incidence of maternal and fetal mortality.[2,59,60]

More recent series of cases with fatty liver of pregnancy indicate a significant decrease in maternal and fetal mortality from a high of 75–85% before 1980[2,59,60] to a low of approximately 20% maternal and 20% fetal mortality.[59,61-63] Survival in fatty liver of pregnancy now is considered the rule rather than the exception.[64] The decrease in mortality is attributed to the early diagnosis of a significant proportion of still mild cases that previously went undetected.[60,62] Improved recognition allows timely institution of appropriate therapy.

Clinical Description

The patient is most frequently in the third trimester of her first pregnancy.[64] Symptoms are often those of preeclampsia, such as hypertension, edema, coagulopathy, or proteinuria and renal insufficiency. They occur in approximately 47% of cases.[2,8,64] The fetus involved in fatty liver of pregnancy is male in upwards to 75% of cases[65], and twins are noted in 14% of involved pregnancies.[64] The syndrome usually presents as the sudden occurrence of nausea and vomiting in approximately 75% of cases, associated with right upper quadrant pain in 50–60%.[65-67] Jaundice occurs at some time in greater than 70% of cases.[67] Other symptoms and signs may include pyrexia and tachycardia in approximately 50%, oliguria in approximately 40%, and gastrointestinal bleeding in approximately 60%.[67] These symptoms occur most frequently at 36–40 weeks, but they have been noted at 30 weeks of pregnancy. Jaundice follows shortly after the early signs of gastrointestinal distress, and the condition of the patient then may deteriorate rapidly to include confusion, coma, and other signs of liver decompensation such as ascites.[61,66] The early course is marked more often by tachycardia in the absence of fever, which may occur later.[2] After the onset of jaundice, the patient frequently goes into spontaneous labor, which may be premature. The patient may worsen or improve at that time; this syndrome may even have its onset at the time of delivery.[2,68] The delivery may be associated with excessive hemorrhage. Other sources of bleeding may arise, particularly from the stomach in the form of hematemesis. A hemorrhagic diathesis is a prominent part of the syndrome in the majority of patients[66], and significant postpartum bleeding may be a problem. A pattern of DIC often is present and may be associated with profound deficiency in antithrombin III, which may persist when other coagulation factors have normalized.[69,70] Hepatic rupture has been described. Gastrointestinal bleeding, hypoglycemia and renal failure also are manifestations of the deterioration associated with progressive liver failure.[66,71] Renal failure usually is manifest as oliguria, but *diabetes insipidus* with profuse urine output also has been described.[72] These complications ultimately may be responsible for the patient's death. The duration of symptoms leading to death or recovery has been reported to span 3 days to 6 weeks, but averages 1–2 weeks.[59] It is important to note that jaundice and hyperbilirubinemia may continue to increase for several days after delivery has occurred and the liver injury has peaked, before it begins to resolve.

Laboratory Evaluation and Diagnosis

Laboratory evaluation of patients with fatty liver of pregnancy shows evidence of liver dysfunction by an increase in serum transaminase activity, alkaline phosphatase and bilirubin. These increases generally are very mild in comparison to the acute hepatic inflammation of viral hepatitis. The syndrome, however, can be confused with acute viral hepatitis when an atypical course and biopsy are present.[73] The serum transaminase activity in fatty liver of pregnancy averages less than 300–500 IU and bilirubin is usually less than 10 mg/dL but may be as high as 25 mg/dL.[66] The hyperbilirubinemia appears to be the result of liver dysfunction, since the elevation cannot be explained by hemolysis, as is the usual case in preeclampsia and eclampsia.[74] The abnormal liver function tests seem to result in modest alterations when compared with those of a patient with clinical evidence of fulminant failure, often including hypoglycemia and hyperammonemia. Other characteristic laboratory test results found in fatty liver of pregnancy include an elevated white blood cell count in the range of 20,000–30,000 and prolonged prothrombin time.[2] Laboratory evidence of DIC may be associated with a clinical hemorrhagic diathesis characterized by thrombocytopenia, an increase in fibrin split products, and hypofibrinogemia.[75] A profound deficiency of antithrombin III is described in several reported cases that may persist after other coagulation factors have returned to normal.[69,70] Evidence of renal insufficiency often is present in the form of an elevation in BUN or creatinine and an increase in serum uric acid.

As in preeclampsia and eclampsia, hyperuricemia may be one of the earliest signs of progressive disease.[76] Clinical signs of diabetes insipidus have been described in rare cases.[72] In a case reported by Cammu et al[72], the diabetes insipidus was presumed to be of transient nephrogenic type, since normal serum levels of vasopressin and neurophysin were found and the urine output could be controlled by exogenous vasopressin and saline loading.

Hepatic imaging by ultrasound or CAT scan can help diagnose fatty liver of pregnancy by the identification of a decreased attenuation due to fatty infiltrate in the liver.[77,78] However, false negative results are obtained in greater than 20% of cases studied by ultrasound and the diagnosis by CAT scan, also may be missed perhaps because of the diffuse, variable, and transient nature of the intracellular microvesicular fatty infiltrate.[77,78] Hepatic imaging, however, is advisable in the evaluation of fatty liver of pregnancy, since it also is used to rule out other hepatobiliary causes of jaundice such as biliary obstruction. It also rules out the presence of such complications as hematoma or hepatic rupture.

Liver biopsy may be helpful in the differential diagnosis of fatty liver of pregnancy since it has a distinctive pathology.[2,68,79-82] Biopsy should be done when an atypical course cannot exclude the diagnosis of hepatitis. Biopsy generally is not required to differentiate fatty liver of pregnancy from severe preeclampsia and eclampsia, since the management of advanced disease in these two entities is similar. If a liver biopsy is deemed necessary, special processing of tissue for frozen section or electron microscopy will be required to diagnose the characteristic lipid deposits seen in this disorder. Biopsies and autopsies obtained within approximately two weeks of symptom onset show, in most cases, a typical pattern of microvesicular fatty infiltrate in hepatocytes, predominantly in centrilobular zone 3 (Figures 151–3 and 151–4). In cases of fatty liver, fatty infiltration also has been described in the proximal convoluted tubule of the kidney and in the pancreas, brain, and bone marrow.[2,68,81] On routine light microscopy, the hepatocytes have a pale, swollen appearance with, on closer inspection, a finely vacuolated cytosol. The vacuoles are seen by oil red O stain of frozen section or by electron microscopy to be lipid droplets. This microvesicular fat in hepatocytes characteristically surrounds a centrally located nucleus instead of displacing it to one side, as do the more common macrovesicles of fat. The nature of this intracellular fat often is difficult to diagnose by light micriscopy. Sparing of a periportal rim free of fatty infiltrate in liver tissue has been considered a helpful histopathologic characteristic.[8] Cholestasis in canaliculi and in hepatocytes may be present in the centrilobular area. In the classic description of fatty liver of pregnancy, there is no cellular necrosis and only minimal diffuse mononuclear inflammation. There are several case reports, however, in which significant hepatocellular necrosis is noted with variable collapse of trabeculi and mild-to-moderate, mixed inflammatory infiltrate in portal areas and parenchyma.[79-81] These latter cases may be confused with hepatitis.[63,64,82] Some investigators have attributed the findings of necrosis and inflammation in fatty liver of pregnancy to superimposed preeclampsia and eclampsia or ischemic shock.[65,68] In those patients who survive, serial studies of liver histology show gradual resolution of pathology to normal with loss of fat proceeding from centrilobular to periportal areas.[71,80,83] Several months to

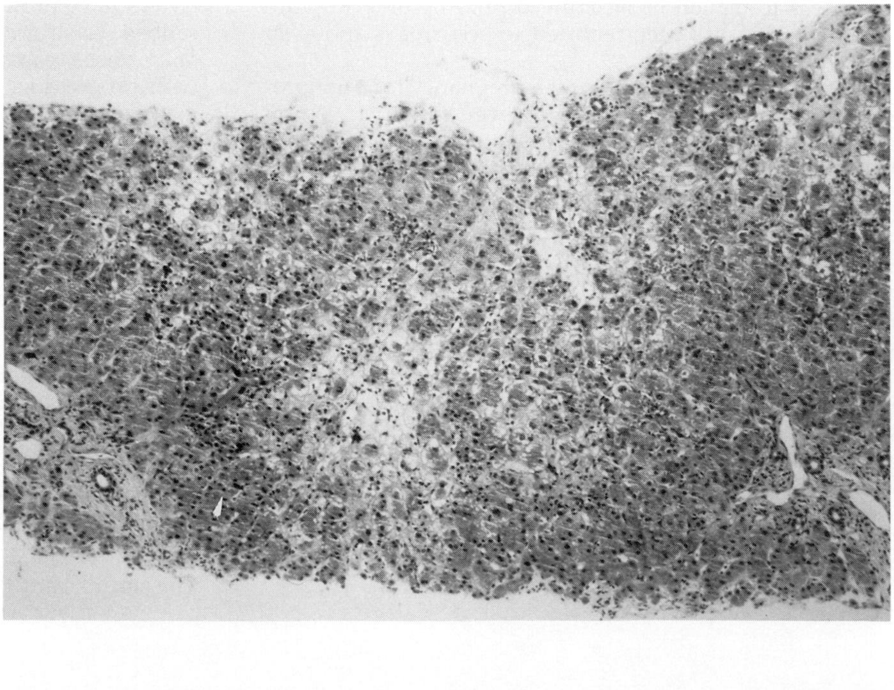

Figure 151–3. Needle biopsy from a surviving patient with fatty liver of pregnancy. The centrilobular area shows swollen, finely vacuolated hepatocytes (×63). Mild diffuse mononuclear infiltrate can be observed, as well as a suggestion of centrilobular hepatocellular dropout. This is a typical biopsy of fatty liver of pregnancy as seen by the author.

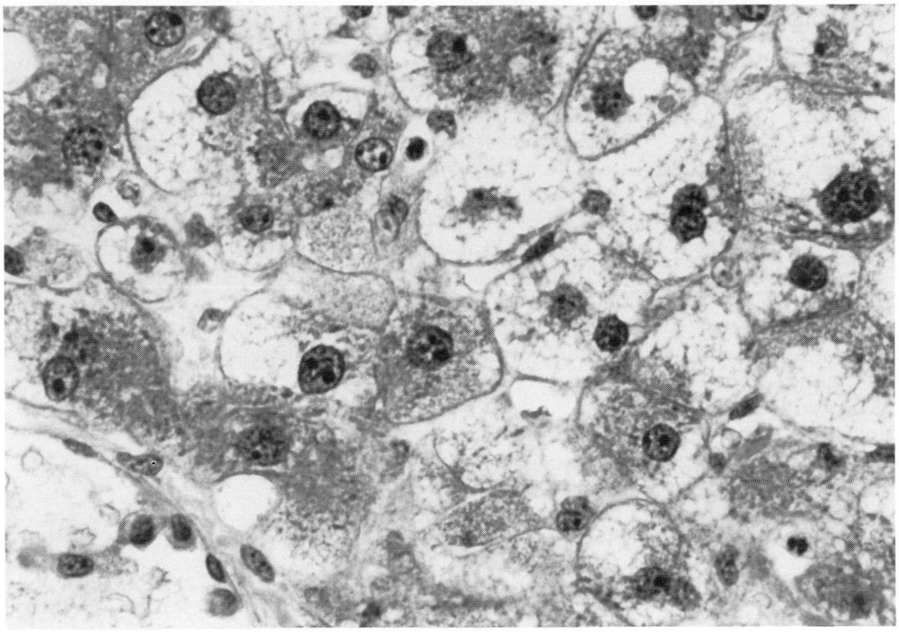

Figure 151–4. Swollen hepatocytes seen in the centrilobular area of Fig. 151–1. The foamy appearance of the cells is caused by numerous droplets of microvesicular fat. (×400)

a year may be necessary for histologic resolution, whereas clinical improvement is more rapid. There have been no reports of jaundice or liver pathology in the fetus.

Etiology and Pathophysiology

Fatty liver of pregnancy appears to be a unique complication of pregnancy without any genetic basis. It has not yet been reported to occur in a subsequent pregnancy or in other family members.[71,84] The pathogenesis of fatty liver of pregnancy is enigmatic, but the typical pattern of microvesicular fatty infiltration of hepatocytes in fatty liver of pregnancy is distinctive and provides the basis for considering this etiology. The histologic "gold standard" for diagnosis of fatty liver of pregnancy has been blurred recently by reports describing frequent symptoms and signs of preeclampsia in cases with the histologic microvesicular fat of fatty liver of pregnancy[64], and by reports of microvesicular fat in a large number of cases having the typical clinical features of preeclampsia.[85] These observations suggest that etiologies of liver disease during pregnancy may overlap in pathogenesis and etiology.

The distinctive finding of diffuse microvesicular fat in the liver is known to occur in only a few conditions besides fatty liver of pregnancy. Efforts have been directed at finding possible pathogenetic links between the few etiologies known to produce the characteristic liver pathology and fatty liver of pregnancy. A role for toxins has been suggested by the knowledge that tetracycline, in particular, can result in a microvesicular fatty infiltrate in liver. Tetracycline can be implicated in many early cases reported in the literature.[8,81,86] Valproate, an antiepileptic drug, also may produce a similar steatosis and liver injury.[87] These drugs, however, are no longer used during pregnancy, and another toxin has not been identified.

Nutritional deficiencies also have been suggested as predisposing factors for fatty liver of pregnancy when the needs of the fetus increase the nutritional demand in advanced pregnancy.[68] The fat-infiltrated cells, resulting from insufficient protein synthesis and lack of protein mobilization, could become sufficiently numerous and swollen so that hepatic blood flow or canalicular bile flow could be compromised, particularly in the centrilobular area. Diets characterized by specific amino acid deficiencies have been noted to produce similar microvesicular fat deposits in the livers of female, but not male, rats. The lipid found on analysis of liver in nutritional steatoses, however, was triglyceride[88], not the fatty acid that has been described in fatty liver of pregnancy.[89] Carnitine also has been suggested as a possible etiologic factor, since diseases producing carnitine deficiency can result in a microvesicular fatty acid deposition in liver.[64] Carnitine is synthesized in liver and functions as an essential cofactor in the transport of fatty acid into the mitochondria for fatty acid oxidation. A similar effect of mitochondrial fatty acid transport is presumed to be caused by hypoglycin toxin in unripe Ackee fruit, which is believed to result in the liver failure and microvesicular fatty infiltrate seen in fatal Jamaican Vomiting Sickness.[64] Feller et al[90] suggest that carnitine deficiency might be a factor in fatty liver and liver dysfunction during pregnancy, since levels of carnitine are found to be low in this condition. However, no studies have tested this hypothesis.

Reye's syndrome in children has a similar liver pathology, presentation, and clinical course to that seen in fatty liver of pregnancy. The profound effects on the mitochondria in fatty liver of pregnancy are similar to those in Reye's syndrome.[83] The urea cycle enzymes ornithine transcarbamylase and carbamylphosphate synthetase may be depressed, and the ultrastructure of the mitochondria may be abnormal, showing pleomorphic forms and laminar crystalline deposits. The abnormal mitochondrial function can explain the hyperammonemia seen in fatty liver of pregnancy, as it does in Reye's syndrome. The morphologic changes of mitochondria in fatty liver of pregnancy differ from Reye's syndrome, however, in their appearance on electron microscopy and in the prolonged time (months) required for histologic and enzymatic recovery. It also is noted that in fatty liver of pregnancy, the amino acid profile shows a decrease in serum levels of most amino acids, whereas these same amino acids tend to be increased in most cases of Reye's syndrome. The etiology of Reye's syndrome also is unknown at this time. However, there is an increased incidence of preceding viral illness, such as influenza and varicella. Viral and bacterial infections, in the form of circulating endotoxins, also have been suggested as potentially important in fatty liver of pregnancy. Hague et al[67] reported a 39% incidence of preceding infection in 128 cases of fatty liver of pregnancy. However, no controlled data investigating this issue have been reported.

Fibrin deposits and multifocal infarcts in the placenta of patients with fatty liver of pregnancy, especially in those with DIC, is likely to contribute to the placental insufficiency and fetal distress that is evident in many cases.[80,91]

Medical Care

Treatment of Symptoms. Management of patients with fatty liver of pregnancy is supportive, with particular attention to potential complications. A particularly distressing complication that is a frequent cause of death is coagulopathy. Often, evidence of bleeding from the gastrointestinal tract or in the liver can be observed.[92] The hemorrhagic diathesis should be treated by administration of vitamin K, fresh frozen plasma, and platelets as required. Fresh plasma may be particularly necessary, even when coagulation is largely returned to normal, because of a profound and persistent deficiency of antithrombin III in many cases.[69,70] The use of factor concentrates in fatty liver of pregnancy generally is avoided since they have the potential to transmit hepatitis. In addition, they may contain activated coagulation factors that may not be cleared adequately in liver disease, resulting in further thrombosis and progression of DIC.[92]

The treatment should be supportive and usually conservative, since the disease generally will improve when the pregnancy is terminated. Manifestations of liver failure, such as coagulopathy, gastrointestinal bleeding, hypoglycemia, ascites, and encephalopathy are frequent in severe disease and should be treated as other etiologies of liver failure. Care must be taken to avoid intravascular depletion. The use of diuretics and cathartics must be balanced carefully with the renal insufficiency, which frequently accompanies fatty liver or severe preeclampsia and eclampsia. General anesthesia and narcotics must be avoided or used sparingly in fatty liver of pregnancy, since extreme central nervous system (CNS) depression may occur when potentially toxic levels of drug, as a result of poor liver metabolism, combine with the CNS depression of hepatic encephalopathy.

Management of Pregnancy. Generally, it is recommended that diagnosis of fatty liver of pregnancy be followed as soon as possible by immediate delivery of the fetus.[8,68,93] The liver disease generally will continue to worsen with increasing risk to mother and child until delivery occurs. The improved maternal survival recently described with this disease is largely attributed to early diagnosis and prompt delivery.[93] Induced delivery is advised if the mother and fetus are stable, but cesarean section is recommended otherwise. Spinal anesthesia should be used to avoid the complication of CNS depression caused by systemic narcotics that require metabolism in the liver. Fetal monitoring is necessary for this high-risk situation, in which uteroplacental insufficiency is likely to occur.[91]

Counseling. Fortunately, the mother and infant who survive fatty liver of pregnancy do so with no lasting sequelae and the disease usually does not recur in future pregnancies.

HYPEREMESIS GRAVIDARUM

This subcategory of jaundice of pregnancy is distinguished from the others by occurring most frequently in the first trimester. It is manifested clinically by protracted nausea and vomiting, which may result in a state of dehydration and relative malnutrition. Patients requiring hospitalization may demonstrate icterus and abnormal liver function tests.[94] The bilirubin is generally less than 3.5 mg/dL, and serum transaminase activity is mildly elevated (less than threefold). In addition, a delay in BSP clearance may occur, which is not seen in normal pregnancy. The course in the majority of cases is a return to normal when the patient is provided with nutrition and rehydrated. Malnutrition with calorie-to-protein imbalance as a result of persistent vomiting is the presumed etiology of the abnormal liver function tests. Generally, no specific therapy beyond hydration, antiemetics and assurance of adequate nutrition is necessary.

REFERENCES

1. Svanborg A. A study of recurrent jaundice in pregnancy. *Acta Obstet Gynecol Scand.* 1954;33:434.
2. Haemmerli UP. Jaundice during pregnancy. *Acta Med Scand.* 1966;44(suppl):1.
3. Reyes H. The enigma of intrahepatic cholestasis of pregnancy: lessons from Chile. *Hepatology.* 1982;2:87.
4. Holzbach RT, Sivak DA, Braun WE. Familiar recurrent intrahepatic cholestasis of pregnancy: a genetic study providing evidence for transmission of a sex-limited, dominant trait. *Gastroenterology.* 1983;85:175.
5. Wilson JAP. Intrahepatic cholestasis of pregnancy with marked elevation of transaminases in a black American. *Dig Dis Sci.* 1987;32:665.
6. Reid R, Ivey KJ, Rencoret RH, et al. Fetal complications of obstetric cholestasis. *Br Med J.* 1976;1:870.
7. Haemmerli UP, Wyss HI. Recurrent intrahepatic cholestasis of pregnancy: report of six cases and review of the literature. *Medicine.* 1967;46:299.
8. Iber FL. Jaundice in pregnancy—a review. *Am J Obstet Gynecol.* 1965;91:721.
9. Friedlander P, Osler M. Icterus and pregnancy. *Am J Obstet Gynecol.* 1967;97:894.
10. Reyes H, Radrigan ME, Gonzales MC, et al. Steatorrhea in patients with intrahepatic cholestasis of pregnancy. *Gastroenterol.* 1987;93:584.
11. Johnston WG, Baskett TF. Obstetric cholestasis: a 14 year review. *Am J Obstet Gynecol.* 1979;133:299.
12. Fallon HJ. Liver diseases. In: Burrow GN, Ferris TF, eds. *Medical Complications during Pregnancy, Vol 14.* Philadelphia, PA: WB Saunders; 1975:351.
13. Ingerslev M, Teilum G. Biopsy studies on the liver in pregnancy. *Acta Obstet Gynecol Scand.* 1945;35:339.
14. de Pagter AFG, van Berge Henegouwen GP, ten Bokkel Huinink, et al. Familial benign recurrent intrahepatic cholestasis. Interrelation with intrahepatic cholestasis of pregnancy and from oral contraceptives? *Gastroenterology.* 1976;71:202.
15. Adelcreutz H, Tenhunen R. Some aspects of the interaction between natural and synthetic female sex hormones and liver. *Am J Med.* 1970;49:630.
16. Kleiner GJ, Kresch L, Arias IM. Studies of hepatic excretory function. II. The effect of norethynodrel and mestranol on bromsulpthalein sodium metabolism in women of childbearing age. *N Engl J Med.* 1965;273:420.
17. Gallagher JF, Mueller MN, Kappas A. Estrogen pharmacology. IV. Studies on structural basis for estrogen-induced impairment of liver function. *Medicine.* 1966;45:471.
18. Kreek MJ, Weser F, Sleisenger MH, et al. Idiopathic cholestasis of pregnancy. The response to challenge with the synthetic estrogen, ethinyl estradiol. *N Engl J Med.* 1967;277:1391.
19. Adelcreutz H, Tikkamen MJ, Wichmann K, et al. Recurrent jaundice in pregnancy. IV. Quantitative determination of urinary and biliary estrogens, including studies in pruritus gravidarum. *J Clin Endocrinol Metab.* 1974;38:51.
20. Sjovall K, Sjovall J. Serum bile acids in pregnancy with pruritus. *Clin Chim Acta.* 1966;13:207.
21. Laatikainen T, Ikonen E. Serum bile in cholestasis of pregnancy. *Obstet Gynecol.* 1977;50:313.
22. Schoenfield LJ, Sjovall J, Perman E. Bile acids on the skin of patients with pruritus hepatobiliary disease. *Nature.* 1967;213:93.
23. Ghent CN, Bloomer JR, Klatskin G. Elevations in skin tissue bile acid levels in human cholestasis: relation to serum levels and pruritus. *Gastroenterology.* 1977;73:1125.
24. Combes B, Shibata H, Adams R, et al. Alterations in sulfobromphthalein sodium removal mechanisms from blood during normal pregnancy. *J Clin Invest.* 1963;42:1431.
25. Kater RM, Harrison DD, Mistilis SP. Alterations in sulfobromophthalein

sodium removal from blood in patients with pruritus of pregnancy. *Gastroenterology*. 1967;53:941.
26. Frezza M, Chiesa L, Pozzato G, et al. Alteration in sulfobrompthalein hepatic storage capacity (S) in non-pregnant women previously affected with intrahepatic cholestasis of pregnancy (ICP). *Acta Obstet Gynecol Scand*. 1986;65:577.
27. Reyes H, Ribalta, Gonzales MC, et al. Sulfobromphthalein clearance tests before and after ethinyl estradiol administration in women and men with familial history of intrahepatic cholestasis of pregnancy. *Gastroenterology*. 1981;81:226.
28. Davis RA, Kern F, Schowalter R, et al. Alterations of hepatic Na+, K+-ATPase and bile flow by estrogen: effects on liver surface membrane lipid structure and function. *Proc Natl Acad Sci USA*. 1978;75:4130.
29. Israel EJ, Guzman ML, Campos GA. Maximal response to oxytocin of the isolated myometrium from pregnant patients with intrahepatic cholestasis. *Acta Obstet Gynecol Scand*. 1986;65:581.
30. Laatikainen T. Effect of cholestyramine and phenobarbital on pruritus and serum bile acid levels in cholestasis of pregnancy. *Am J Obstet Gynecol*. 1978;132:501.
31. Seymour CA, Chadwick VS. Liver and gastrointestinal function in pregnancy. *Postgrad Med*. 1979;55:343.
32. Frezza M, Pozzato G, Stramentinoli G, Di Padova C. Reversal of intrahepatic cholestasis of pregnancy in women after high dose S-adenosyl-L-methionine administration. *Hepatology*. 1984;4:274.
33. Chelsay LC. History and epidemiology of preeclampsia-eclampsia. *Clin Obstet Gynecol*. 1984;27:801.
34. Antia FP, Watsa MC, Master J. Liver in normal pregnancy, pre-eclampsia and eclampsia. *Lancet*. 1958;2:776.
35. Rolfes DB, Ishak KG. Liver disease in toxemia of pregnancy. *Am J Gastroenterol*. 1986;81:1138.
36. Weinstein L. Syndrome of hemolysis, elevated liver enzyme, and low platelet count: A severe consequence of hypertension in pregnancy. *Am J Obstet Gynecol*. 1982;142:159.
37. Roberts JM, May WJ. Consumptive coagulopathy in severe pre-eclampsia. *Obstet Gynecol*. 1976;48:163.
38. Pritchard JA, Cunningham FG, Mason RA. Coagulation changes in eclampsia: their frequency and pathogenesis. *Am J Obstet Gynecol*. 1976;124:855.
39. Beecham JB, Watson W, Clapp JF. Eclampsia, preeclampsia and DIC. *Obstet Gynecol*. 1974;43:576.
40. Redman CWG, Bonnar J, Beilin LJ. Early platelet consumption in preeclampsia. *Br Med J*. 1978;1:467.
41. Redman CWG, Beilin LJ, Bonnar J, et al. Plasma-urate measurements in predicting fetal death in hypertensive pregnancy. *Lancet*. 1976;1:1370.
42. Long RG, Scheuer PJ, Sherlock S. Pre-eclampsia presenting with deep jaundice. *J Clin Pathol*. 1977;30:212.
43. Arias F, Mancilla-Jimenez R. Hepatic fibrinogen deposits in preeclampsia. Immunofluorescent evidence. *N Engl J Med*. 1976;295:578.
44. Sheehan HL, Lynch JB. *Pathology of Toxemia in Pregnancy*. London: Churchill Livingstone; 1973.
45. Rakoczi I, Tallian F, Bagdany S, et al. Platelet life span in normal pregnancy and preeclampsia as determined by a non-radioisotope technique. *Thromb Res*. 1979;15:553.
46. Perkins RP. The conservative management of toxemia: a brief report of effect perinatal concepts. *Obstet Gynecol*. 1977;44:498.
47. Heller TD, Goldfarb JP. Spontaneous rupture of the liver during pregnancy. A case report and review of the literature. *NY State J Med*. 1986;86:314.
48. Bis KA, Waxman B. Rupture of the liver associated with pregnancy: a review of the literature and report of 2 cases. *Obstet Gynecol Surv*. 1976;31:763.
49. Henney CP, Lim AE, Brummelkamp WH, et al. A review of the importance of acute multidisciplinary treatment following spontaneous rupture of the liver capsule during pregnancy. *Surg Gynecol Obstet*. 1983;156:593.
50. Nelson EW, Archibald L, Albo D. Spontaneous hepatic rupture in pregnancy. *Am J Surg*. 1977;134:817.
51. Manas KJ, Walsh JD, Rankin RA, Miller DD. Hepatic hemorrhage without rupture in preeclampsia. *N Eng J Med*. 1985;312:424.
52. Greca FH, Coelho JCU, Fillho ODB, Wallbach A. Ultrasonographic diagnosis of spontaneous rupture of the liver in pregnancy. *J Clin Ultrasound*. 1984;12:516.
53. Winer-Muram HT, Muram D, Salazar J, Massie JD. Hepatic rupture in preeclampsia: the role of diagnostic imaging. *J Assoc Can Radiol*. 1985;36:34.
54. Sommer DG, Greenway GD, Bookstein JJ, et al. Hepatic rupture with toxemia of pregnancy: angiographic diagnosis. *Am J Roentgenol*. 1979;132:455.
55. Herbert WNP. Hepatic rupture and pregnancy. *NY State J Med*. 1986;86:286.
56. Naraysingh V, Gopeesingh TB. Hepatic artery ligation for spontaneous hepatic rupture in pregnancy. *WI Med J*. 1984;33:198.
57. Stander HJ, Cadden JF. Acute yellow atrophy of the liver in pregnancy. *Am J Obstet Gynecol*. 1934;28:61.
58. Sheehan HL. The pathology of acute yellow atrophy and delayed chloroform poisoning. *J Obstet Gynaecol Br Emp*. 1940;47:49.
59. Varmer M, Ronderknecht NK. Acute fatty metamorphosis of pregnancy: a maternal mortality and literature review. *J Reprod Med*. 1980;24:177.
60. Hatfield AK, Stein JH, Greenberger NK, et al. Idiopathic acute fatty liver of pregnancy: death from extrahepatic manifestations. *Dig Dis Sci*. 1972;17:167.
61. Bernuau J, Degott C, Nouel O, et al. Non-fatal acute fatty liver of pregnancy. *Gut*. 1983;24:340.
62. Pockros PJ, Peters RL, Reynolds TB. Idiopathic fatty liver of pregnancy: findings in ten cases. *Med (Balt)*. 1984;63:1.
63. Rolfes DB, Ishak KG. Acute fatty liver of pregnancy: a clinicopathologic study of 35 cases. *Hepatol*. 1985;5:1149.
64. Riely CA. Acute fatty liver of pregnancy. *Sem in Liver Dis*. 1987;7:47.
65. Burroughs AK, Seong NH, Dojcinov DM. Idiopathic acute fatty liver of pregnancy in 12 patients. *QJ Med*. 1982;204:481.
66. Nash DT, Dale JT. Acute yellow atrophy of liver in pregnancy. *NY State Med J*. 1971;71:458.
67. Hague WM, Fenton DW, Duncan SLB, Slater DN. Acute fatty liver of pregnancy. *J R Soc Med*. 1983;76:652.
68. Ober WB, Le Compte PM. Acute fatty metamorphosis of the liver associated with pregnancy. *Am J Med*. 1955;19:743.
69. Liebman HA, McGehee WG, Patch MJ, Feinstein DI. Severe depression of antithrombin III associated with disseminated intravascular coagulation in women with fatty liver of pregnancy. *Ann Int Med*. 1983;98:330.
70. Laursen B, Frost F, Mortensen JZ, Hansen KB, et al. Acute fatty liver of pregnancy with complicating disseminated intravascular coagulation. *Acta Obstet Gynecol Scand*. 1983;62:403.
71. Breen KJ, Perkins KW, Mistitis SP, et al. Idiopathic acute fatty liver of pregnancy. *Gut*. 1970;11:822.
72. Cammu H, Velkeniers B, Charels K, et al. Idiopathic acute fatty liver of pregnancy associated with transient diabetes insipidus: case report. *Br J Obstet Gynecol*. 1987;94:173.
73. Brown MS, Reddy KR, Hensley GT, et al. The initial presentation of fatty liver of pregnancy mimicking acute viral hepatitis. *Am J Gastroenterol*. 1987;82:554.
74. Sherlock S. Acute fatty liver of pregnancy: Etiology of fetal distress and fetal wasting. *Obstet Gynecol*. 1987;69:482.
75. Cano RI, Delman MR, Pitchumoni CS, et al. Acute fatty liver of pregnancy: complication of disseminated intravascular coagulation. *JAMA*. 1975;231:159.
76. Quigley MM. Acute obstetric yellow atrophy presenting as idiopathic hyperuricemia. *So Med J*. 1974;67:142.
77. Campillo B, Bernaua J, Witz MO, et al. Ultrasonography in acute fatty liver of pregnancy. *Ann Int Med*. 1986;105:383.
78. Mabie WC, Dacus JV, Sibai BM, et al. Computed tomography in acute fatty liver of pregnancy. *Am J Obstet Gynecol*. 1988;158:142.
79. Czernobilsky B, Bergnes MA. Acute fatty metamorphosis of the liver in pregnancy with associated liver cell necrosis. *Obstet Gynecol*. 1965;26:791.
80. Davies MH, Wilkinson SP, Hanid MA, et al. Acute liver disease with encephalopathy and renal failure in late pregnancy and the early puerperium: a study of fourteen patients. *Br J Obstet Gynecol*. 1980;87:1005.
81. Kunelis CT, Peters JL, Edmondson HA. Fatty liver of pregnancy and its relationship to tetracycline therapy. *Am J Med*. 1965;38:359.
82. Riely CA, Latham PS, Romero R, Duffy TP. Acute fatty liver of pregnancy: a reassessment based on observations in nine patients. *Ann Int Med*. 1987;106:703.
83. Weber FL, Snodgrass PJ, Powell DE, et al. Abnormalities of hepatic mitochondrial urea cycle enzyme activities and hepatic ultra-structure in acute fatty liver of pregnancy. *J Lab Clin Med*. 1979;94:27.
84. MacKenna J, Pupkin M, Crenshaw C, et al. Acute fatty metamorphosis of the liver: a report of two patients who survived. *Am J Obstet Gynecol*. 1977;127:400.
85. Minakami H, Oka N, Sato T, et al. Preeclampsia: a microvesicular fat disease of the liver? *Am J Obstet Gynecol*. 1988;159:1043.
86. Peters RL, Edmonson HA, Mikkelsen WP, et al. Tetracycline-induced fatty liver in nonpregnant patients: a report of six cases. *Am J Surg*. 1967;113:622.
87. Gerber N, Dickinson RG, Harland RC, et al. Reye-like syndromes associated with valproic acid therapy. *J Pediatr*. 1979;95:142.
88. Dick F, Hall WK, Sydenstricker VP, et al. Accumulation of fat in the liver with deficiencies of threonine and of lysine. *Arch Pathol*. 1952;53:154.
89. Eisele JW, Barker EA, Smuckler EA. Lipid content in the liver of fatty metamorphosis of pregnancy. *Am J Pathol*. 1975;81:545.
90. Feller A, Ugarte G, Pino ME, et al. Acute fatty liver of pregnancy: a possible disorder of carnitine metabolism. *Gastroenterol*. 1983;84:1150A.
91. Moise KJ, and Shah DM. Acute fatty liver of pregnancy: etiology of fetal distress and fetal wasting. *Obstet Gynecol*. 1987;69:482.
92. Gillespie P, Hunter C. Idiopathic fatty liver of pregnancy with maternal and fetal survival. *Aust NZ J Obstet Gynecol*. 1978;18:90.
93. Ebert EC, Sun EA, Wright SH, et al. Does early diagnosis and delivery in acute fatty liver of pregnancy lead to improvement in maternal and infant survival? *Dig Dis Sci*. 1984;29:453.
94. Adams RH, Gordon J, Combes B. Hyperemesis gravidarum. I. Evidence of hepatic dysfunction. *Obstet Gynecol*. 1968;31:659.

Chapter One Hundred and Fifty-Two
Viral Hepatitis

Raymond S. Koff

152

Viral hepatitis is a major cause of morbidity throughout the world; each known form of the disease (hepatitis A, B, D, and bloodborne and enterically transmitted non-A, non-B hepatitis) has been identified in almost all regions and populations. It therefore is not surprising that viral hepatitis is the most common cause of jaundice during pregnancy. Because many episodes of viral hepatitis are anicteric, inapparent, or entirely subclinical, the actual frequency of infection has been underestimated in pregnancy as well as in the general population. Recognition requires documentation of serum enzyme abnormalities and specific serologic testing. Unfortunately, even when clinically silent, viral hepatitis is not a trivial disease; the future health of the pregnant woman and her infant may be jeopardized. As a result, the pregnant woman with viral hepatitis causes special problems for her health care providers. Coordination of care among the obstetrician, primary-care physician, and pediatrician is necessary to provide optimal management and to institute appropriate preventive measures.

ETIOLOGIC AGENTS

Pregnant women are susceptible to the same agents that cause viral hepatitis in the general population, that is, the viruses of hepatitis A, hepatitis B, hepatitis D, and the three putative viruses of non-A, non-B hepatitis.[1] Hepatitis A virus (HAV) is an enterovirus that contains single-stranded RNA; the HAV particle has a diameter of 27 nm and demonstrates cubic symmetry.[2,3]

Hepatitis B virus (HBV) is a DNA virus.[4] The HBV particle is a spherical structure with a diameter of 42 nm; it is comprised of a 27-nm diameter, electron-dense core surrounded by an outer envelope with a thickness of 7 nm. The core of the HBV particle contains circular, partially double-stranded DNA, and DNA polymerase with reverse transcriptase activity.[5] The surface of the core harbors specific antigenic material known as the hepatitis B core antigen (HBcAg) and its derivative—the hepatitis B "e" antigen (HBeAg).[6] The outer envelope of the HBV contains a specific hepatitis B surface antigen (HBsAg), comprising three envelope proteins: the major protein, a large protein, and a middle protein, as well as lipid and carbohydrate components. HBsAg also is found on two other particles that circulate in the sera of patients infected with HBV: a spherical particle with a diameter of 22nm and a tubular particle also 22 nm in diameter but of variable length. These DNA-free, noninfectious particles are HBV envelope materials synthesized in infected hepatocytes in excess of intact HBV particles.

Hepatitis D virus (HDV) is a defective RNA virus that requires the helper function of HBV for its expression and replication.[7] It has a diameter of 36 nm and an envelope composed of HBsAg. HDV infection is limited to individuals with coprimary acquisition of HBV/HDV or HDV superinfection of HBV carriers.

The antigens of HAV, HBV, and HDV induce the formation of specific antibodies by their hosts. These serologic markers are used to establish the diagnosis of hepatitis A, B, or D (see below). Although several candidate antigen-antibody systems have been described in bloodborne and enterically transmitted non-A, non-B hepatitis, isolation of a cDNA cloned from the genome of the major bloodborne agent, tentatively labeled the hepatitis C virus (HCV), has been reported recently[8], and a serologic test for antibody to this flaviviruslike agent also has been described.[9] Clinical and experimental evidence suggests that there may be two agents responsible for bloodborne non-A, non-B hepatitis and at least one agent responsible for enterically transmitted disease.[10] Presently, the diagnosis of acute non-A, non-B hepatitis is made in patients who have no serologic evidence of acute HAV, HBV, of HDV infection and in whom clinical circumstances suggest viral hepatitis rather than other disorders. Serologic diagnosis of acute HCV is problematic. The enterically transmitted form may be available in the near future.[11]

EPIDEMIOLOGY AND RISK FACTORS

Hepatitis A

HAV is excreted in the stools of infected persons, and fecal-oral transmission is the predominant mode of spread. Parental transmission of hepatitis A appears to be a rare event, probably because the viremic phase of HAV infection is so short-lived. Since there is no evidence of a prolonged fecal carrier state in hepatitis A, infection is generally the result of a susceptible individual's contact with the feces of an acutely infected person. Such contact commonly occurs by fecal contamination of fingers, eating utensils, crockery, food (including bivalve mollusks), or water.[12] Not surprisingly, attack rates vary inversely with the quality of the population's hygienic conditions. The pregnant woman, like members of the general population, is particularly at risk for HAV infection if there is an infected household member, if she has close contact with an infected person, or if she works in a setting where poor toilet habits are common, such as day-care centers for preschool children or institutions for the mentally retarded. The incubation period of hepatitis A is 15–50 days with a mean of 30 days.

Hepatitis B

In contrast to hepatitis A, HBV infection commonly results in a viremia that lasts for weeks to months, and as few as 1% or as many as 5% of adult patients develop chronic infection and persistent viremia.[13] Thus, HBV infection traditionally has been a hazard to persons who are exposed to infected blood and blood products. This mode of transmission explains the high rate of HBV infection in parenteral drug abusers, in dialysis patients, and in health care workers and others who have frequent contact with blood and blood products (eg, dentists, surgeons, dialysis unit staff, laboratory and blood bank technicians, morticians). Unlike HAV, HBV is not spread by the fecal-oral route. Parenteral exposure is not necessary for transmission of HBV; however, contact transmission of HBV is now recognized as an important mode of spread.[14] HBsAg and HBV have been found in semen, vaginal secretions, and other body fluids of infected individuals. Thus, transmission may occur during sexual intercourse or may follow inadvertent inoculation through the use of shared razors, toothbrushes, or other vehicles of infection. It follows that household and particularly sexual contracts of HBV carriers are at high risk for HBV infection. Maternal-neonatal and maternal-infant transmission are also key epidemiologic entities (see below). The incubation period of hepatitis B ranges from 15–210 days, with an average of 60–90 days.

Hepatitis D

HDV infections occur solely in individuals at risk for HBV infection, including parenteral drug abusers, homosexual men, and recipients of high-risk blood products. Percutaneous transmission is the predominant mode of spread; contact transmission and maternal-neonatal transmission also occur.[15] The incubation period of hepatitis D is estimated to be several weeks.

Bloodborne Non-A, Non-B Hepatitis

Elucidation of the epidemiology of non-A, non-B hepatitis has been confounded by the lack of a reliable serologic marker of non-A, non-B infection. However, it appears that bloodborne non-A, non-B hepatitis closely resembles hepatitis B in its epidemiologic characteristics.[16] Clearly, non-A, non-B hepatitis is spread by the parenteral route. Now that blood donors are screened routinely for HBsAg, non-A, non-B hepatitis is responsible for more than 95% of transfusion-associated hepatitis. Screening of the blood supply of the United States with indirect, nonspecific, "surrogate" tests has been undertaken in an attempt to reduce the frequency of non-A, non-B hepatitis in blood recipients. Screening of donor blood for anti-HCV was introduced in the United States in May 1990. Its effectiveness has not yet been determined. Circumstantial evidence suggests that contact transmission of bloodborne non-A, non-B hepatitis occurs, but the importance of this mode of transmission is unclear. The risk of developing chronic infection, that is, a carrier state, with the bloodborne non-A, non-B agents is even higher than that with HBV infection. The incubation period of bloodborne non-A, non-B hepatitis generally ranges from 15–160 days, with a major peak at about 50 days. An earlier peak at two to four weeks also has been described.

Enterically Transmitted Non-A, Non-B Hepatitis

Enterically transmitted non-A, non-B hepatitis is a largely waterborne, epidemic disease that also occurs in endemic forms.[10] Outbreaks have been reported in the Indian subcontinent, Asia, Africa, North America, and in Mexico.[17] Imported cases in the United States have been recognized in returning travelers and in immigrants from endemic regions. This etiologic form of viral hepatitis is important particularly in pregnancy because susceptibility to fatal, fulminant hepatitis is increased dramatically.

CLINICAL, LABORATORY, AND HISTOLOGIC FEATURES

Clinical Features

The clinical manifestations of viral hepatitis range from asymptomatic, inapparent infection, detectable only as serologic abnormalities, to fulminant disease terminating in hepatic coma and death. Symptomatic illness exhibits a typical pattern in most patients, however. Infections with HAV, HBV, HDV, and the non-A, non-B hepatitis viruses produce similar clinical syndromes; these infections are not distinguished reliably by clinical criteria alone. Specific serologic tests are required to make that distinction (see below).

Viral hepatitis results in a variety of nonspecific constitutional and gastrointestinal symptoms that may be confused with those of pregnancy. These symptoms include fatigue, malaise, anorexia, nausea, and vomiting. Flulike symptoms of pharyngitis, cough, coryza, photophobia, headache, and myalgias may be prominent in the early phase of the acute illness. In hepatitis A, the onset of these symptoms tends to be abrupt. In the other forms, the onset usually is insidious. Fever is uncommon in viral hepatitis, except in hepatitis A, in which a low-grade fever is seen in 70% of patients. Arthritis and other manifestations of an immune-complex–mediated, serum-sicknesslike syndrome occur in less than 10% of patients with hepatitis B and, rarely, in the other etiologic forms. Most of the abovementioned symptoms tend to abate or disappear with the onset of jaundice, although the anorexia, malaise, and weakness may increase transiently. Jaundice usually is indicated by the appearance of dark urine. Pruritus commonly occurs as the jaundice increases but usually is mild and of short duration.

Physical examination of the patient with viral hepatitis commonly reveals a mildly enlarged and slightly tender liver. The liver does not increase in size during normal pregnancy and in fact becomes more difficult to palpate as it is displaced upwards and backwards by the enlarging uterus. Thus, an easily palpable and tender liver in a pregnant woman usually has pathologic importance, particularly in the third trimester. Fifteen to 20% of patients with viral hepatitis will have an enlarged spleen and posterior cervical lymphadenopathy. Spider angiomata and palmar erythema are not reliable signs of liver disease in pregnancy, since each is found in at least two thirds of normal gestations.

Laboratory Features

In typical viral hepatitis, the most prominent biochemical abnormality is a marked elevation of the serum aminotransferase (transaminase) levels. Peak aminotransferase levels vary from 500 to 5000 mμ/mL. Although peak levels may be somewhat lower in viral hepatitis in pregnancy, normal pregnancy is not characterized by any elevation in serum aminotransferase levels. The serum bilirubin level rarely rises above 10 mg/dL in viral hepatitis. Since the serum bilirubin level may rise to between 1 and 2 mg/dL in 2–6% of normal pregnancies, isolated slight bilirubin elevations should be interpreted with caution. Mild elevations of the serum alkaline phosphatase levels are common in viral hepatitis, but caution also is warranted in their interpretation since elevations of serum alkaline phosphatase levels may occur in normal pregnancy as a result of the contribution of placental alkaline phosphatase. In interpreting the serum albumin level, the clinician should consider that serum albumin normally declines by about 20% at midpregnancy.

Histologic Features

Uncomplicated pregnancy results in only minor nonspecific changes in liver histology, which should not be confused with the changes of hepatitis. Liver biopsy examination in acute viral hepatitis reveals a combination of hepatic cell necrosis and regeneration, diffuse infiltration with mononuclear inflammatory cells, hyperplasia of Kupffer's cells, and variable amounts of bile stasis. Liver biopsy examination will not identify specific etiologic agents of hepatitis, however, and is not required often.

SEROLOGIC STUDIES

HAV Infection

HAV usually is undetectable in serum by the time the infected patient becomes symptomatic and seeks medical attention. Testing for HAV in serum thus is not recommended. The serologic diagnosis of hepatitis A usually is established by the detection of antibody to HAV (anti-HAV) of the IgM class. Since IgM anti-HAV is strongly positive only during acute HAV infection, a single serum specimen obtained during the acute illness establishes the diagnosis. Detection of anti-HAV only of the IgG class indicates remote infection with HAV.

HBV Infection

The serologic diagnosis of acute hepatitis B often is established by the detection of circulating HBsAg, which is the first serologic marker of HBV infection to appear, usually within one to three months after exposure (see Figure 152–1). The most reliable serologic test is the presence of anti-HBc of the IgM class, which usually appears at about the time the patient develops symptoms. HBeAg is detectable shortly after the appearance of HBsAg and before or at the time that aminotransferase levels begin to rise, but HBeAg disappears after a period of days to weeks. The risk of transmitting HBV infection with HBsAg-positive material is higher if that material is also HBeAg positive. In resolving HBV infection, IgM anti-HBc is replaced by IgG anti-HBc, which decreases in titer over many years. Neither IgM nor IgG anti-HBc are neutralizing antibodies. Antibody to HBsAg (anti-HBs) is the last antibody to appear; it is a neutralizing antibody. Its appearance indicates recovery from HBV infection and immunity to re-infection. Chronically infected carriers of HBV can be identified by the persistent presence of HBsAg (with or without HBeAg), with anti-HBc (predominantly of the IgG class), and absent or low-level anti-HBs (see below).

HDV Infection

The serologic diagnosis of acute hepatitis D requires the demonstration of antibody to HDV (anti-HDV) of the IgM class in an HBsAg-positive individual.[18] Past infection with HDV may be detected by identification of IgG anti-HDV.

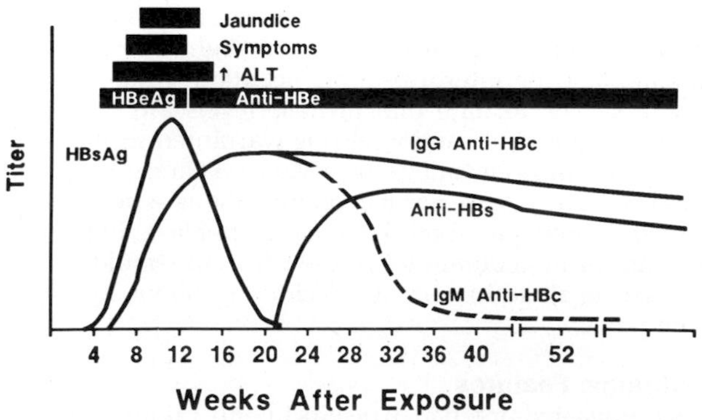

Figure 152–1. Schematic diagram of the serologic events and clinical and laboratory features of acute hepatitis B. *(From the Clinical Teaching Project of the American Gastroenterological Association with permission.)*

In many instances, anti-HDV titers fall to undetectable levels with resolution of infection.

Non-A, Non-B Hepatitis

Presently, the available assays for non-A, non-B hepatitis are not useful in diagnosis of HCV infection because the measured antibodies develop slowly. Ordinarily, the diagnosis of acute non-A, non-B hepatitis is made in the patient in whom serologic tests for IgM anti-HAV, HBsAg, and anti-HBc are negative and in whom clinical circumstances suggest acute viral hepatitis.

OTHER CAUSES OF LIVER DISEASE IN PREGNANCY

Since HAV, HBV, and HBV/HDV infections usually are readily diagnosed with appropriate serologic tests, most diagnostic confusion involves distinguishing non-A, non-B hepatitis from other hepatic disorders. Virtually any hepatic disorder that affects the general population can occur during pregnancy. One important group of disorders includes intrahepatic cholestasis, acute fatty liver, preeclampsia, toxemia, and hyperemesis gravidarum, disorders that are either peculiar to or particularly common in pregnancy; these are discussed in Chapters 138, 139, and 140. Another major consideration is drug-induced liver disease.

A wide variety of drugs can induce hepatic dysfunction that mimics viral hepatitis. Chlorpromazine, which has been used in the treatment of hyperemesis gravidarum, is notorious for causing jaundice in a small percentage of patients. Intravenous tetracycline may induce a fatal hepatic disorder that clinically and histologically resembles acute fatty liver of pregnancy. When possible, nonessential medications should be withdrawn in patients who develop signs of hepatitis; prompt resolution of the hepatic dysfunction strongly implicates the drugs.

Symptomatic cholelithiasis is uncommon during pregnancy. Pregnancy itself is unusual in patients with cirrhosis but may result in a symptomatic deterioration of already compromised liver function. Other uncommon causes of hepatic dysfunction in pregnancy include sickle-cell disease, hydatidiform mole, pyelonephritis, and Dubin–Johnson syndrome.

NATURAL HISTORY

The majority of patients with acute viral hepatitis will experience complete clinical, histologic, and biochemical recovery within three to six months. The frequency of complete recovery varies with the specific etiologic agent. Hepatitis A appears to be an acute, self-limited disease that does not result in either chronic liver injury or carriage of HAV. In contrast, some 1–5% of adult patients with hepatitis B develop evidence of chronic HBV infection with persistence of circulating HBsAg for months to years. The risk of persistent infection is age-dependent; as many as 90% of infected neonates may become carriers. All true HBsAg carriers have detectable anti-HBc; the frequency of circulating HBeAg and anti-HBe is variable, and low-level anti-HBs is detectable in 10–40%. Carriers of HBsAg may or may not have symptoms of liver disease; liver biopsy examination reveals a spectrum of findings ranging from normal histology to chronic active hepatitis with cirrhosis. A dreaded but late complication of chronic HBV infection is the development of primary hepatocellular carcinoma. Malignant transformation of hepatocytes appears to be etiologically related to the integration of HBV DNA into the host liver cell DNA.[19] In addition to liver disease, HBV infection has been associated with membranous glomerulonephritis and nephrosis in children. Glomerular deposition of HBV-associated immune complexes may play a pathogenetic role.

HDV superinfection of HBV carriers may lead to chronic HDV infection superimposed on chronic HBV infection with chronic hepatitis and cirrhosis. Chronic bloodborne non-A, non-B hepatitis, predominantly HCV, has been reported in 20–70% of infected patients (based on circumstantial evidence), and a viremic carrier state has been established by transmission experiments. As many as 20% of patients with bloodborne chronic non-A, non-B hepatitis may develop cirrhosis. In contrast, no sequelae have been recognized in enterically transmitted non-A, non-B hepatitis.

MATERNAL COMPLICATIONS

The major maternal complication of viral hepatitis is the development of fulminant hepatitis. This catastrophic complication of viral hepatitis is characterized by rapidly progressive hepatic failure that terminates in coma and death in 70–95% of patients. Cerebral edema is common, and neurologic complications are the most frequent cause of death. Other life-threatening features of fulminant hepatitis include gastrointestinal bleeding in 50%, adult respiratory distress syndrome in 30%, cardiac arrhythmias in 40%, and sepsis in 10–20% of patients. Serial examinations characteristically reveal a rapidly shrinking liver. Leukocytosis, hyponatremia, and hypokalemia are common. Hypoglycemia occurs in fewer than 10%, but may be severe. Marked elevations of the serum bilirubin and aminotransferase levels are typical. Liver biopsy examination, although usually precluded by coagulopathy, reveals extensive "drop-out" (disappearance) of hepatocytes, collapse of the reticulin framework, and inflammation. Although there is no specific therapy for fulminant hepatitis, complete recovery is possible with meticulous supportive care or hepatic replacement by liver transplantation.

The reported incidence of fulminant-viral hepatitis in pregnancy varies widely. Extraordinarily high rates of fulminant hepatitis in pregnant women, particularly during the third trimester, have been reported in outbreaks of enterically transmitted non-A, non-B hepatitis. In the United States and other developed countries, viral hepatitis during pregnancy is typically a mild disease, with the risk of fulminant hepatitis well below 2%. The mechanisms responsible for the increased susceptibility to fulminant hepatitis in pregnant women with enterically transmitted non-A, non-B hepatitis remain unknown.

FETAL COMPLICATIONS

From both a clinical and epidemiologic point of view, the major complication of maternal viral hepatitis is transmission of infection to the newborn infant (see section below). Fetal wastage rates (defined as intrauterine and neonatal deaths) in viral hepatitis during pregnancy generally parallel the incidence of fulminant hepatitis. In fulminant hepatitis the fetal wastage rate may exceed 70% and is largely a consequence of maternal death.[20,21] In uncomplicated viral hepatitis in pregnancy, fetal wastage rates are not increased above background rates.

Prematurity, as defined by a gestational age of less than 37 weeks, appears to be two to three times more common in maternal viral hepatitis, regardless of etiology, than in the general pregnant population.[22] Premature delivery is largely a complication of hepatitis in the third trimester. The average interval between onset of clinical hepatitis and onset of premature labor is about 4 weeks. Although prematurity is associated with maternal viral hepatitis, the incidence of small-for-gestational-age infants is not increased, and the spontaneous abortion rate is not enhanced in women with uncomplicated viral hepatitis.

Maternal viral hepatitis has no influence on the incidence or nature of congenital malformations. Although chromosomal abnormalities have been identified occasionally in the leukocytes of newborn infants of HBV carrier women, no specific chromosomal syndrome has been identified in these infants.

TREATMENT

Uncomplicated Hepatitis

The treatment of maternal viral hepatitis is similar to that in the nonpregnant patient. Unless there is evidence of persistent vomiting or severe anorexia leading to dehydration or symptoms, signs, or laboratory features of fulminant hepatitis, the patient is managed at home. Other than maintenance of adequate caloric and fluid intake, no specific dietary recommendations are made. Because the anorexia, nausea, and vomiting associated with viral hepatitis often worsen during the day, resulting in a progressive decline in oral intake, a large breakfast may be the best tolerated meal of the day. Vigorous or prolonged physical activity is best avoided during the acute illness and the need for limitation of daily activities and institution of rest periods are best determined by the severity of the patient's fatigue and malaise. No specific drug treatment is available; corticosteroids are of no value. Prohibition of alcohol ingestion is reemphasized. All nonessential drugs are discontinued. In uncomplicated viral hepatitis in the pregnant woman, a conservative course of obstetric management is indicated, since the outcome for both the mother and newborn should be favorable.

Fulminant Hepatitis

The management of fulminant hepatitis is exceedingly difficult. Hospitalization is required as soon as this severe variant of viral hepatitis is recognized. Management is best undertaken in the intensive care unit of an institution experienced in the management of fulminant hepatic failure. The goal of therapy is early recognition, maintenance of vital functions, and treatment of life-threatening complications. As indicated above, high-risk and frequent complications include bacterial infection, respiratory and renal failure, cerebral edema, gastrointestinal or generalized bleeding, hypoglycemia, and acid-base and electrolyte disturbances. Continuous monitoring with supportive measures may permit resolution of the infection and restoration of hepatic function. Although some clinicians have recommended immediate delivery by caesarean section, there are no convincing data that induction of delivery or early termination of pregnancy affects the prognosis for the woman with fulminant hepatitis or that for her fetus. For patients in whom the likelihood of recovery seems small, hepatic transplantation may be performed.Whether the risk of fetal wastage is further increased or reduced by hepatic transplantation in this setting is not clear.

MATERNAL-INFANT TRANSMISSION

HAV Transmission

Transmission of HAV from the acutely infected woman to her fetus or neonate has yet to be established as an epidemiologic entity.[23] The short-lived viremic phase of HAV infection and the absence of a HAV carrier state probably are responsible for the absence of maternal-fetal or maternal-neonatal transmission.

HBV Transmission

Transmission of HBV from HBsAg-positive pregnant women to their newborn infants has been documented in diverse areas of the world. Transmission from carrier mothers to their newborns appears to be an exceedingly important factor in the perpetuation of HBV infection in certain parts of the world, particularly those regions in which the reservoir of HBsAg carriers is large, exceeding 5% of the general population.[24] In these areas, as many as 90% of neonatal infections will become persistent, that is, the HBV-infected infants become carriers. Acute HBV infection in the second half of pregnancy also is associated with transmission of HBV to the infant. The risk is highest when acute HBV infection occurs in the third trimester or in the immediate postpartum period. In both the carrier and the acutely infected HBsAg-positive pregnant woman, the risk of transmission to the infant is highly correlated with the presence of HBeAg in maternal sera; HBeAg-negative, HBsAg-positive women also may infect their infants, but the risk is lower.

Several mechanisms appear to be responsible for HBV transmission from mother to infant.[25] *In utero*, transplacental, and early postnatal infection have been implicated, but the bulk of available data indicate that transfer of HBV is most likely during labor and delivery. Maternal-fetal transfusion during labor or contamination of the infant during delivery appears to be responsible. The newborn of the HBV-infected woman is born contaminated with maternal blood and secretions containing HBV and HBsAg; these can be recovered from the infant's skin, conjunctiva, mucous membranes, and gastrointestinal tract. Whether cesarean section reduces the risk of transmission remains undetermined.[26]

HDV Transmission

Coprimary transmission of HBV and HDV from infected mothers to their newborn infants has been described, but the frequency of this event is low.

Non-A, Non-B Transmission

Information about the transmission of bloodborne and enterically transmitted non-A, non-B viral hepatitis from pregnant women to their infants is very limited at present. Available data suggest that acute non-A, non-B hepatitis infections in the second trimester (and, by inference, probably in the first trimester) do not produce biochemical evidence of hepatic injury in neonates. In contrast, acute sporadic (presumably bloodborne) non-A, non-B hepatitis in the third trimester has been reported to result in serum aminotransferase elevations without jaundice or clinical manifestations of hepatitis in newborn infants. In some affected infants, aminotransferase abnormalities persisted for three months or longer. It seems likely that these represent maternal-infant transmission episodes with development of the non-A, non-B carrier state in the infant. Proof of the latter is not yet available in the absence of specific serologic tests for non-A, non-B infections. By analogy to HBV infection, it is thought that transmission of bloodborne non-A, non-B infection from carrier mothers to their newborns may occur; serologic documentation of this phenomenon suggests that maternal-neo-natal spread of HCV is not an efficient mode of transmission.

POSTPARTUM TRANSMISSION

Mothers with acute HAV infection in the postpartum period may transmit infection by the fecal-oral route to their infants and young children. Acute HBV infection in the postpartum period also may be transmitted from mother to infant or young child, but in this instance the mode of spread is predominantly an oral-oral one. Exchange of saliva through kissing, premastication of baby food, and utensils shared by mother and child appear to be responsible.[27] This mechanism also has been implicated in the postnatal acquisition of HBV infection by susceptible young children of HBeAg-positive HBsAg carrier mothers. Since HBsAg has been detected rarely in unconcentrated breast milk samples and no evidence of an increased risk of HBV infection has been found in breast-fed infants of carrier mothers when compared to infants who were not breast-fed, breast-feeding does not appear to play an important role in postpartum HBV transmission. HDV/HBV dual transmission presumably occurs by mechanisms identical to those responsible for transmission of HBV alone. Intrafamilial postpartum transmission of non-A, non-B hepatitis from carrier mothers or mothers with acute infection to their infants and young children is possible, presumably through mechanisms similar to those described for HBV transmission. Documentation of such transmission is not yet available.

CONSEQUENCES OF MATERNAL-INFANT AND MATERNAL-CHILD TRANSMISSION

HAV Transmission

HAV infections in infants and young children usually are not apparent clinically, are recognized infrequently, and produce no important sequelae.

HBV Transmission

Although severe and even fatal hepatitis have been observed, serious liver disease caused by HBV infection in infancy and childhood is distinctly uncommon. The majority of HBV infections of early life are asymptomatic and anicteric, but in contrast to HAV infection, HBV may persist for years, and the infected infant or child is identified as a HBsAg carrier. In addition to the prolonged infectivity of carriers who acquire infection early in life, persistent HBV infection early in life may be accompanied by evidence of chronic hepatitis as reflected by elevation of serum aminotransferase levels or the subsequent development of chronic hepatitis on follow up. Chronic active hepatitis, postnecrotic cirrhosis, and primary hepatocellular carcinoma are the major sequelae of persistent HBV infection acquired in early life.[24] The latent period between the onset of HBV infection and the recognition of primary hepatocellular carcinoma varies between 20 and 50 years in most series, but a latent period as short as three to four years from perinatal infection has been described. The importance of the relationship among early HBV infection, persistent infection, and primary hepatocellular carcinoma cannot be overemphasized, since there is abundant evidence that the lifetime risk of hepatocellular carcinoma in male HBsAg carriers approaches 40–50% in some populations.

HDV Transmission

The consequences of chronic HBV/HDV infection in early life are poorly understood. Whether the sequelae of dual infection are more frequent or more serious than those of HBV alone remains to be determined in infected infants.

Non-A, Non-B Transmission

Clinical sequelae of acute or persistent non-A, non-B hepatitis virus infections in infancy and childhood will remain poorly understood until confirmed serologic markers are identified. Rarely, aplastic anemia is seen in the convalescent phase of clinically recognized infection. Very rarely, aplastic anemia may follow HAV or HBV infections. Chronic hepatitis, cirrhosis, and primary hepatocellular carcinoma are possible outcomes of bloodborne non-A, non-B hepatitis acquired early in life.

PREVENTION

Prevention of Maternal Hepatitis

HAV Immunoprophylaxis. The cornerstone of prevention of maternal HAV infection is the administration of immunoglobulin to exposed contacts of infective cases. Pregnant women who are household or intimate contacts of individuals with acute HAV infection should receive immunoglobulin in an intramuscular dose of 0.02 mL/kg body weight as soon as possible. Casual contact in the office, school, or factory is not an indication for immunoprophylaxis unless extensive fecal contamination of the environment is suspected, for example, in day-care centers for preschool children that accept non-toilet-trained infants or toddlers. Inactivated HAV vaccines currently are being developed.[28]

HBV Immunoprophylaxis. Prevention of acute HBV infection in the pregnant woman may be difficult since contact or inapparent permucosal or percutaneous exposure leading to infection may not be recognized and the infective source may be asymptomatic and not identified. For women in high HBV risk categories, for example, health care and hospital workers regularly exposed to blood such as surgeons, pathologists, medical technicians, blood bank technologists, dialysis staff, operating-room, intensive-care, and emergency-room nurses, dentists and dental professionals, parenteral drug users, workers in institutions for the mentally retarded, recipients of high-risk blood products on multiple occasions, and inmates of prisons in which parenteral drug use may continue, preexposure prophylaxis with the HBV vaccine is recommended. In the United States, two recombinant yeast-derived vaccines are available. One mL of the selected vaccine (containing either 20 or 10 μg of HBsAg protein) are given intramuscularly (deltoid injection only) initially and repeated one and six months later. Gluteal injection sites should not be used since the immune response following gluteal injection is reduced. Prevaccination screening to determine susceptibility (absence of either anti-HBs or anti-HBc) is warranted in high-risk groups if exposure has been prolonged, but is usually unnecessary for individuals beginning their careers. Susceptible women who are sexual contacts of HBsAg carriers also are candidates for vaccination.

The vaccines are highly immunogenic, inducing protective levels of anti-HBs in well over 90% of healthy young (under 40 years of age) recipients who receive all three doses. They are 85–95% effective in preventing HBV infection or clinical hepatitis B.[29] HBV vaccine may be administered safely to pregnant women, although experience with this population is still limited. Major side effects are transient pain at the deltoid injection site in 10% to 25% of recipients and short-lived, mild fever in fewer than 3%. For prolonged protection, a booster 1-mL dose may be needed five to eight years after initial vaccination. HBV vaccine has no efficacy in the individual with established infection.

Postexposure prophylaxis for susceptible pregnant women who are inadvertently exposed to HBV is dependent on the intramuscular administration of hepatitis B immunoglobulin (HBIG), a preparation of immunoglobulin containing high titers of anti-HBs, and a course of HBV vaccine. Between 0.04–0.07 mL/kg is given as early as possible after exposure and the first of three 1-mL doses of HBV vaccine are given at another site (deltoid) at the same time or within several days. The second and third vaccine doses are given one and six months later. Earlier administration of the second and third vaccine doses is under study.[30]

HDV Immunoprophylaxis. Because neither specific anti-HDV immunoglobulins nor HDV vaccines are available, immunoprophylaxis is dependent on the prevention of HBV by the appropriate use of HBV vaccine or HBIG. For patients with established HBV infection, immunoprophylaxis has no role and other prevention strategies are required.

Non-A, Non-B Immunoprophylaxis. Immunoprophylaxis of both bloodborne and enterically transmitted non-A, non-B viral hepatitis is an unsettled issue. Although evidence of efficacy is lacking, immunoglobulin (not HBIG) is used by some clinicians when contact exposure with an index case of non-A, non-B hepatitis is suspected in the pregnant woman or when the pregnant woman must travel to areas in which non-A, non-B hepatitis is endemic. The dose may be the same as or larger than that used in the prophylaxis of HAV infection and may be repeated one or more months after the first injection.

Prevention of Maternal-Infant and Maternal-Child Transmission

If acute HAV infection is recognized in the mother or other household members, infants and young children should receive immunoglobulin prophylaxis (0.02 mL/kg body weight) by intramuscular injection.

Prevention of HBV transmission currently is dependent on identification of HBsAg carriers among pregnant women and recognition of acute HBV infection in the latter half of pregnancy or postpartum period. All pregnant women should be screened by the obstetrician at the first or another early visit to determine carrier status.[31] For newborns of HBsAg-positive women, a combination of passive immunization with HBIG and active immunization with HBV vaccine is recommended.[31,32,33] In some parts of the world in which HBV infection is highly prevalent, universal immunization of neonates may be undertaken. The United States is likely to adopt such a policy in the near future. Immunization currently is recommended only for the neonates of HBsAg-positive mothers. Because optimal dose schedules are not yet established, the following suggested protocol may require revision as new information becomes available. A dose of 0.5 mL of HBIG is given within a few hours of birth (preferably within 1 hour) into the anterolateral muscle of the thigh of the neonate. HBV vaccine is given in a dose of 0.5 mL within a week of birth (at another site in the anterolateral muscle) and repeated at one and six months. Protective efficacy exceeds 95%. Treated infants should be tested at about 12 months of age for HBsAg, anti-HBs, and anti-HBc. The presence of HBsAg, with or without IgM anti-HBc, indicates treatment failure, since the infant is actively infected.[34] The presence of both anti-HBs and anti-HBc suggests that infection occurred but was modified by immunoprophylaxis. In this case, immunity is likely to be prolonged. Presence of anti-HBs alone suggests vaccine-induced immunity that can be expected to persist for about five years.[35] Booster injections at five-year intervals may be needed for continuing protection. Although it may be that immunoprophylaxis of the neonate can be accomplished with HBV vaccine alone (without HBIG), data supporting this concept are limited at present.[36] Successful immunoprophylaxis against HBV also will provide protection against HDV transmission.

Immunoglobulin prophylaxis for newborns or infants of mothers with non-A, non-B infection is of uncertain value. If used, a dose similar to or larger than that used in the prophylaxis of HAV may be tried and repeated at one-month and three-month intervals.

REFERENCES

1. Tabor E. The three viruses of non-A, non-B viral hepatitis. *Lancet.* 1985;1:743.
2. Gust ID, Coulepis AG, Feinstone SM, et al. Taxonomic classification of hepatitis A virus. *Intervirology.* 1983;20:1.
3. Lemon SM. Type A viral hepatitis. New developments in an old disease. *N Engl J Med.* 1985;313:1059.
4. Tiollais P, Pourcel C, Dejean A. The hepatitis B virus. *Nature.* 1985;317:489.
5. Mack DH, Bloch W, Nath N, et al. Hepatitis B virus particles contain a polypeptide encoded by the largest open reading frame: a putative reverse transcriptase. *J Virol.* 1988;62:4786.
6. Miller RH. Proteolytic self-cleavage of hepatitis B virus core protein may generate serum e antigen. *Science.* 1987;236:722.
7. Wang KS, Choo QL, Weiner AJ, et al. Structure, sequence and expression of the hepatitis delta viral genome. *Nature.* 1986;323:508.
8. Choo Q-L, Kuo G, Weiner AJ, et al. Isolation of cDNA clone derived from a blood-borne non-A, non-B viral hepatitis genome. *Science.* 1989;244:359.
9. Kuo G, Choo Q-L, Alter HJ, et al. An assay for circulating antibodies to a major etiologic virus of human non-A, non-B hepatitis. *Science.* 1989;244:362.
10. Bradley DW, Maynard JE. Etiology and natural history of post-transfusion and enterically-transmitted non-A, non-B hepatitis. *Sem Liver Dis.* 1986;6:56.
11. Panda SK, Datta R, Kaur J, et al. Enterically transmitted non-A, non-B hepatitis: recovery of virus-like particles from an epidemic in South Delhi and transmission studies in rhesus monkeys. *Hepatology.* 1989;10:466.
12. Lowry PW, Levine R, Stroup DF, et al. Hepatitis A outbreak on a floating restaurant in Florida, 1986. *Am J Epidemiol.* 1989;129:155.
13. Koff RS. Natural history of acute hepatitis B in adults re-examined. *Gastroenterology.* 1987;92:2035.
14. Koff RS, Slavin MM, Connelly LJD, et al. Contagiousness of acute hepatitis B. *Gastroenterology.* 1977;72:297.
15. Bonino F, Smedile A. Delta agent (type D) hepatitis. *Sem Liver Dis.* 1986;6:28.
16. Dienstag JL. Non-A, non-B hepatitis. I. Recognition, epidemiology, and clinical features. *Gastroenterol.* 1983;85:439.
17. Centers for Disease Control. Enterically transmitted non-A, non-B hepatitis - Mexico. *MMWR.* 1987;36:597.
18. Aragona M, Mecagno S, Caredda F, et al. Seriological response to the hepatitis delta virus in hepatitis D. *Lancet.* 1987;1:478.
19. Yaginuma K, Kabayashi H, Kobayashi M, et al. Multiple integration site of hepatitis B virus DNA in hepatocellular carcinoma and chronic active hepatitis tissues from children. *J Virol.* 1988;61:1808.
20. Borhanmanesh F, Haghighi P, Hekmet K, et al. Viral hepatitis during pregnancy. Severity and effect on gestation. *Gastroenterol.* 1973;64:304.
21. Khuroo MS, Teli MR, Skidmore S, et al. Incidence and severity of viral hepatitis in pregnancy. *Am J Med.* 1981;70:252.
22. Hieber JP, Dalton D, Shorey J, et al. Hepatitis and pregnancy. *J Pediatr.* 1977;91:545.
23. Tong MJ, Thursby M, Rakela J, et al. Studies on the maternal-infant transmission of the viruses which cause acute hepatitis. *Gastroenterol.* 1981;80:999.
24. Seeff LB, Koff RS. Evolving concepts of the clinical and serologic consequences of hepatitis B virus infection. *Sem Liver Dis.* 1986;6:11.
25. Lee AKY, Ip HMH, Wong WCW. Mechanisms of maternal-fetal transmission of hepatitis B virus. *J Infect Dis.* 1978;138:668.
26. Lee SD, Tsai YT, Wu TC, et al. Role of cesarean section in prevention of mother-infant transmission of hepatitis B virus. *Lancet.* 1988;2:833.
27. Beasley RP, Hwang LY. Postnatal infectivity of hepatitis B surface antigen carrier mothers. *J Infect Dis.* 1983;147:185.
28. Binn LN, Bancroft WJ, Lemon SM, et al. Preparation of a prototype inactivated hepatitis A virus vaccine from infected cell culture. *J Infect Dis.* 1986;153:749.
29. Szmuness W, Stevens CE, Zang EA, et al. A controlled clinical trial of the efficacy of the hepatitis B vaccine (heptavax-B): a final report. *Hepatology.* 1981;1:377.
30. Wahl M, Hermodsson S, Iwarson S. Hepatitis B vaccination with short dose intervals—a possible alternative for post-exposure prophylaxis. *Infection.* 1988;16:229.
31. Centers for Disease Control. Immunization Practices Advisory Committee. Prevention of perinatal transmission of hepatitis B virus: prenatal screening of all pregnant women for hepatitis B surface antigen. *MMWR.* 1988;37:341.
32. Arevalo JA, Washington AE. Cost-effectiveness of prenatal screening and immunization for hepatitis B virus. *JAMA.* 1988;259:365.
33. Stevens CE, Taylor PE, Tong MJ, et al. Yeast-recombinant hepatitis B vaccine: efficacy with hepatitis B immune globulin in prevention of perinatal hepatitis B virus transmission. *JAMA.* 1987;257:2612.
34. Panda SK, Bhan MK, Guha DK, et al. Significance of maternal and infant serum antibodies to hepatitis B core antigen in hepatitis B virus infection of infancy. *J Med Virol.* 1988;24:343.
35. Lo KJ, Lee SD, Tsai YT, et al. Long-term immunogenicity and efficacy of hepatitis B vaccine in infants born to HBeAg-positive HBsAg-carrier mothers. *Hepatology.* 1988;8:1647.
36. Poovorawan Y, Sanpavat S, Pongpunlert W, et al. Protective efficacy of a recombinant DNA hepatitis B vaccine in neonates of HBe antigen-positive mothers. *JAMA.* 1989;261:3278.

Chapter One Hundred and Fifty-Three

Chronic Liver Disease

William M. Lee

153

Pregnancy in patients with chronic liver disease is infrequent because cirrhosis primarily affects postmenopausal women. Although younger women may have cirrhosis, they frequently are amenorrheic and anovulatory as well. Nevertheless, pregnancy may occur in all stages of chronic liver disease and a careful assessment of the risk to mother and fetus is necessary in each case. A favorable outcome for the pregnancy frequently is possible but is dependent on the type and severity of the underlying condition. As a general rule, pregnancy does not worsen the concomitant liver disease, except in certain cholestatic diseases such as primary biliary cirrhosis. In these patients, improvement in the cholestasis can be expected to occur following delivery. Liver blood flow is thought to be unaltered in pregnancy, although significant increases in blood volume, fluid retention, and intra-abdominal pressure characterize the third trimester. The presence of esophageal varices has been noted by one author to occur in normal pregnancy[1], and portal pressures during labor are markedly increased. Despite these theoretical hazards, earlier recommendations of termination of pregnancy and sterilization of young women with chronic liver disease have given way to a more conservative and expectant approach judged on a case-by-case basis. Although the natural history of the chronic liver disease may not be altered by the pregnancy, it should be borne in mind that many mothers with advanced liver disease may not live to see their children mature; this may merit consideration when making recommendations to these patients. Liver transplantation has become commonplace and carries an approximately 80% chance for long-term survival with good quality of life (and improved fertility). Counseling of the patient with cirrhosis in the childbearing years should include consideration of liver transplantation prior to planning a family, if there is already any evidence of hepatic failure.

THE HYPERBILIRUBINEMIAS

Congenital hyperbilirubinemias such as *Gilbert's syndrome* (asymptomatic unconjugated hyperbilirubinemia) usually do not significantly alter the outcome of pregnancy for mother or fetus. Pregnancy has been said to improve the mild increase in unconjugated bilirubin seen in patients with Gilbert's syndrome, although this has not been thoroughly studied. In *Dubin–Johnson syndrome,* a further increase in conjugated bilirubin has been noted in association with pregnancy and oral contraceptives, with maximal levels reached in the third trimester. One study suggests an increased incidence of fetal wastage in such patients.[2] Jaundice may lessen in patients with *Rotor's syndrome* during pregnancy. The rare patient with familial benign recurrent intraheptic cholestasis may sustain an exacerbation of disease characterized by intense pruritus and jaundice during pregnancy or with oral contraceptive therapy. This would be difficult to distinguish from intrahepatic cholestasis of pregnancy except by examining the history of the patient or other family members having previous attacks of pruritus and jaundice lasting weeks or months and occurring while neither pregnant nor receiving contraceptive medication.

BILIARY TRACT DISEASE

Cholesterol gallstones are more common in women than men in all populations. One explanation for this may involve the effects of pregnancy. Pregnancy and oral contraceptives are considered risk factors for cholelithiasis, although a strong correlation with multiparity is not evident. Gallbladder volume is increased twofold in pregnancy, and contraction following a meal is sluggish so that incomplete emptying occurs.[3] This has been suggested as the reason for the increased frequency of cholesterol cholelithiasis in previously pregnant women; however, hormonal factors also may be involved. Despite these facts, no increased incidence of cholecystitis or cholangitis is apparent in pregnancy. In one large series, only 27 of 456 patients with jaundice during pregnancy were found to have biliary obstruction by stones as the cause of their disease.[4] In any case, the diagnosis and management of biliary tract disease occurring during pregnancy is that accorded the nonpregnant patient. Immediate surgery may be required on occasion for cholangitis or acute cholecystitis, while diagnostic studies requiring standard x-ray techniques are to be avoided when possible. Endoscopic retrograde cholangiopancreatography may be performed with proper shielding for diagnosis and for removal of common bile duct stones or bypass of strictures.

INFECTIOUS DISEASES

In general, treatment of suspected chronic liver infections such as tuberculosis or other granulomatous diseases is not altered by pregnancy, and a liver biopsy may be performed during pregnancy if indicated. Several infections have received particular attention, including amebiasis and herpes virus infection, because the course of the disease appears to be more severe in the pregnant patient.

Amebiasis

Chronic infection with *Entamoeba histolytica* frequently causes diarrhea, but even asymptomatic infection may become more active during pregnancy due to altered immunity, humoral factors or direct pressure on the liver by the gravid uterus. Experimental evidence suggests that progesterone may promote amebic growth. Immunoglobulin levels that are diminished during pregnancy may be responsible for an altered immune response, leading to abscess enlargement. Rupture of amebic liver abscesses does occur in pregnancy, usually near term or in the puerperium, and seems to occur more often than in males and nonpregnant females, although this has been debated.[5]

The clinical presentation begins with the syndrome of "prerupture," characterized by a period of local peritoneal irritation in the right upper quadrant followed by frank spillage of abscess contents into the peritoneal cavity. Liver scan, serum immune hemagglutination assay, and aspiration of the cavity under ultrasound guidance may establish the diagnosis in the prerupture period; however, frank peritonitis demands surgical exploration and drainage as well as antibiotic therapy, usually with metronidazole plus a second broad spectrum agent. Prognosis for the mother is generally good with prompt diagnosis, but some instances of stillbirth or spontaneous abortion have occurred.[6] Treatment of the unruptured amebic abscess is with metronidazole.

Herpes Virus Infection

Fulminant hepatitis due to *Herpesvirus hominis* is a rare occurrence in the healthy adult and usually occurs in the setting of severe immune deficiency due to high-dose immunosuppressive therapy or leukemia. Several instances of fulminant *Herpesvirus* infection have occurred in pregnant women, suggesting a role for altered immune defenses during pregnancy in this disease as well. The patient initially presents with a sore throat, lip ulceration, and signs of systemic toxicity. Cowdry Type A intranuclear inclusions can be seen on liver biopsy or at autopsy. Consideration of liver biopsy and appropriate culture should be made in patients who develop a hepatitic picture with antecedent sore throat or lip lesions in view of the generally fatal outcome and the possibility that acyclovir may be effective once a specific diagnosis is made (see also Chapter 91).

Leptospirosis

Leptospirosis or Weil's disease is characterized by the sudden onset of nausea, vomiting, fever, and cholestatic jaundice. Hemorrhagic manifestations occur in many organs. Renal failure, cardiac and central nervous system involvement also may be present. Although cases initially were seen primarily in miners, and sewer and abattoir workers, exposure to leptospires is now ubiquitous and housewives and children are also exposed, usually by contact with contaminated water. Immunosuppression is also a predisposing factor. Cases occurring in pregnant women have been reported and appear to result in increased fetal wastage. Too few cases have been recorded to know whether increased maternal mortality occurs. Differential diagnosis includes staphylococcal septicemia (which also has been associated with cholestatic jaundice), meningitis, viral hepatitis, and acetaminophen overdose. The diagnosis is made by a variety of serologic tests involving agglutination of live leptospires by patient serum. Acute and convalescent samples are needed. Transaminase levels are not elevated greatly, a differentiating point from viral hepatitis or acetaminophen toxicity. Jaundice appears to be due to both intrahepatic cholestasis and hemolysis, as well as failure to excrete conjugated bilirubin by the kidneys, if renal failure is present. Although tetracycline has been used, penicillin G (intramuscularly) is the drug of choice for the pregnant patient in view of the suggested association of tetracycline with acute fatty liver of pregnancy.

THE HEPATIC PORPHYRIAS

Acute intermittent porphyria (AIP) is characterized by periodic attacks of abdominal pain, vomiting, seizures, and personality change. The diagnosis frequently is missed in the initial examination. Drugs including barbiturates and estrogens have been implicated in initiation of the attacks, and hypertension is a frequent concomitant finding. Thus, it is not surprising that this form of porphyria may go unrecognized or be mistaken for toxemia in the pregnant patient. The diagnosis of AIP is made by use of the Watson–Schwartz test, which identifies the presence of porphobilinogen in the urine. Whether AIP attacks are precipitated more frequently by pregnancy is debatable. Likewise, the increased maternal mortality suggested by early studies has recently been questioned. In one recent study, only 32% of patients with AIP had attacks during pregnancy. Fetal wastage was 16%, which approximates that for the normal population, and no maternal deaths were recorded.[7] The disease does not remit with delivery and, if undiagnosed, may lead to continued symptoms and more extensive use of barbiturates and other sedatives leading to further acute attacks. Sedative use during pregnancy may be responsible for the increased frequency of attacks in such patients. Treatment is mainly symptomatic after removal of any offending agents. Patients with the rarer hereditary coproporphyria have been found to experience a similar frequency (16%) of attacks during pregnancy, a figure probably not higher than that expected for the disease in the nonpregnant woman.

WILSON'S DISEASE

Much has been written concerning Wilson's disease and pregnancy since patients frequently manifest this disease in the reproductive years. The disease is characterized by two defects relating to copper metabolism: diminished levels of ceruloplasmin, a plasma copper transport protein; and abnormal sequestration of copper in the liver due to ineffective biliary copper excretion. Characteristically, the disease initially is recognized when signs of acute or chronic hepatitis or cirrhosis appear in adolescence or in young adults. Mental deterioration and dystonic movements due to damage to the basal ganglia indicate disease progression as copper begins to accumulate secondarily in the brain as well as the liver. Kayser–Fleischer corneal rings are evident in those with significant CNS copper accumulation but are not evident in many with advanced liver disease. The liver may not be enlarged, but the spleen is usually very prominent, and ascites and variceal hemorrhage are common complications. The use of penicillamine, which increases urinary copper excretion, has altered significantly the outcome for Wilson's disease patients; the neurologic manifestations are reversible for the most part. The cirrhosis does not progress further, and improvement in portal pressures may occur with decreasing inflammation once treatment is administered.

Ceruloplasmin levels increase in pregnancy and with oral contraceptives in Wilson's disease patients as well as in normal women.[8] Patients not on therapy with penicillamine have been said to show improvement in symptoms during pregnancy, presumably due to the fetus removing significant quantities of maternal copper. Since penicillamine therapy is lifesaving and is generally tolerated well by Wilson's disease patients, it seems logical to continue such therapy during pregnancy. However, many drugs are contraindicated for use during pregnancy, and penicillamine came under suspicion following the birth of an abnormal infant to a mother with cystinuria who was on penicillamine therapy. The baby was found to have a "connective-tissue defect." Since penicillamine is believed to alter collagen formation, the drug was implicated. Two series, that combined total 28 mothers and 44 pregnancies, failed to demonstrate any increased maternal or fetal morbidity or mortality related to penicillamine therapy.[9,10] In all, two children were born prematurely and one apparently normal child died secondary to prematurity. One mother died at seven months postpartum due to progression of her liver disease.

Recommendations based on these observations would include therapeutic abortion for the mother with severe liver disease or documented variceal hemorrhage. Penicillamine should be continued in the usual dose throughout the pregnancy unless cesarean section is contemplated, in which case the dose is reduced to 0.25 g in the third trimester so as not to hinder postoperative wound healing. No clear risk to the fetus can be attributed to penicillamine at the present time and prevention of relapse in this condition is a reasonable goal. Maternal mortality in treated or untreated Wilson's disease appears to be a function of the severity of the hepatic injury, which may not at all times be fully appreciated. Nevertheless, pregnancy is tolerated well by the well-treated and compensated patient and should be viewed optimistically in light of the nearly normal lifespan for most treated patients.

CHRONIC HEPATITIS

Young women make up the largest single group of patients with chronic hepatitis and nonalcoholic cirrhosis. The pathogenesis of the liver damage is unknown in most instances. Although viruses such as those causing hepatitis B and non-A, non-B hepatitis (see Chapter 152) may trigger the initial damage to the liver, the development of a state of chronic liver damage is thought to involve altered recognition of self-antigens or "*autoimmunity*." Such patients have been noted to have autoantibodies such as those directed against smooth muscle, and frequently display extrahepatic manifestations, such as rash, arthritis, colitis, amenorrhea and Cushingoid body habitus. Since the term *chronic hepatitis* is applied to a wide variety of conditions, it is helpful to classify such patients on the basis of severity and presumed etiology—the group as a whole being referred to as *chronic active liver disease (CALD)*.

Chronic Persistent Hepatitis

Chronic persistent hepatitis (CPH) is a term that characterizes a milder form of chronic liver injury, detectable as slight elevations in transaminase levels in serum and a characteristic biopsy picture. Such patients have a favorable prognosis for remission of their hepatitis, although it may take months or years. Corticosteroid therapy seldom is used. As might be expected, pregnancy is tolerated well by such patients, and no increase in fetal or maternal morbidity or mortality or disease activity should be seen.[11] Exacerbation of disease during pregnancy, should it occur, might make the diagnosis questionable.

Chronic Active Hepatitis

Chronic active hepatitis (CAH) is more common and severe than CPH. In the initial descriptions in the 1950s, the most obvious forms of the disease were recognized: the patients were typically young women, with multiple autoantibodies positive as well as high gamma globulin levels. We now realize that these cases represent the autoimmune variety. More subtle forms occurring in the absence of autoantibodies have become evident and an association with hepatitis B and non-A, non-B hepatitis (NANB) has been made. The latter represents, in most instances, post-transfusion hepatitis, which appears in a chronic low-grade form leading to cirrhosis and in which markers for hepatitis B and hepatitis A are notably absent. As with hepatitis B, sporadic cases may occur and a carrier state is thought to be present. An antibody test for one of the putative NANB viruses will be available soon. However, NANB hepatitis and hepatitis B are relatively uncommon in pregnancy. Accurate diagnosis is an important consideration, since in contrast to "autoimmune" CAH, these forms generally are not considered to be as amenable to treatment with corticosteroid therapy as is the autoimmune type. Interferon therapy may be curative in chronic NANB hepatitis, but has not been used during pregnancy.

Most typically, the young nonpregnant female patient with autoimmune CAH presents with several weeks of fatigue, anorexia, and mild jaundice. Amenorrhea may antecede all other symptoms and suggests chronicity. This often is confirmed by the finding of established cirrhosis in addition to portal tract inflammation at the initial liver biopsy. Most disease manifestations will respond promptly to prednisone in doses of from 20–60 mg per day, although the cirrhotic features do not improve. In nonpregnant women, azathioprine often is added in a dose of 50–100 mg per day since it appears to be steroid sparing though ineffective by itself. With remission, normal menstrual cycles and improved fertility return. Despite treatment, cirrhosis often progresses, although complete remissions are sometimes seen in early cases without established fibrosis and prednisone sometimes may be discontinued without subsequent relapse.

Since conception is unlikely in patients with severe CAH, most pregnant patients with CAH have milder disease. Pregnancy does not appear to result in worsening of the hepatitis, nor does it significantly improve it. Maternal mortality is increased in patients with chronic active hepatitis when cirrhosis is present, but not above that expected for the disease in the nonpregnant woman. Spontaneous abortion rates (less than 20 weeks) approximate those of the normal population; however, increased fetal wastage and prematurity occurs as with other forms of cirrhosis.[12,13] Based on these considerations, the use of prednisone should be dictated by the need to control the liver disease and otherwise should remain unaltered throughout the pregnancy. Generally, doses of 15–20 mg daily can be tolerated during pregnancy without any difficulty. Although some evidence of teratogenicity has been noted with azathioprine in experimental animals, none has been reported in humans. Nevertheless, its use in pregnancy is discouraged since the disease generally is mild, and increased doses of corticosteroid may be substituted if necessary for the limited duration of the pregnancy.

As with Wilson's disease, termination of pregnancy seldom is indicated. The one exception is for cases with evidence of severe hepatic decompensation (encephalopathy, ascites, variceal hemorrhage, jaundice), but such patients infrequently become pregnant. Portacaval shunts have been performed in pregnant cirrhotic patients successfully. The prognosis for a full life is probably somewhat less than the treated patient with Wilson's disease, though very variable in this condition; transplantation remains an option if hepatic failure becomes refractory to management.

CIRRHOSIS

Most series describing the outcome of pregnancy in cirrhosis include all forms of cirrhosis together without regard to the probable causes. Patients with *Laennec's cirrhosis* are likely to fare worse than those with inactive *cryptogenic cirrhosis* or *primary biliary cirrhosis*, but accurate figures are not available. Maternal health generally will be well preserved through most pregnancies if the cirrhosis is reasonably compensated. However, increased fetal mortality (as high as 30–40%) characterizes all forms of cirrhosis.

The most dreaded complication in all cirrhotic patients is variceal hemorrhage. This probably does not occur with increased frequency in pregnancy, although it would intuitively seem likely. The current therapy for acute variceal hemorrhage includes stabilization with blood and blood products, early endoscopy, and intravenous pitressin therapy. The latter might be prohibited because of the possibility of inducing labor, but the alternative, Sengstaken–Blakemore balloon tamponade, also is dangerous in view of its frequent association with aspiration and poor results in inexperienced hands. When these measures are needed to stem the massive hemorrhage typical of such patients, one or the other must be used. Esophageal injection sclerotherapy by way of a flexible endoscope currently is being used in most centers instead of portacaval anastomotic surgery; however, reports of its use in pregnant patients have not appeared thus far. Sclerotherapy generally is accepted as the first line of treatment both for acutely bleeding varices and for documented variceal bleeding following initial stabilization.[14] Ascites does not occur with greater frequency in pregnancy despite the tendency to increased fluid accumulation. Development of abdominal fluid probably is limited by the already increased intra-abdominal pressure, at least during the latter stages of pregnancy. Diuretics may be used, the most satisfactory of which is spironolactone. Hepatic encephalopathy usually is engendered in the cirrhotic patient not by worsening liver function but by injudicious use of sedatives, or by gastrointestinal hemorrhage, infection, constipation or diuretic therapy, all of which are manageable. Lactulose or neomycin may be used to diminish gut absorption of nitrogenous components, but attention to the cause of the decompensation is equally important.

EXTRAHEPATIC PORTAL VEIN OBSTRUCTION (EHPVO)

This uncommon condition may be due to omphalitis and umbilical vein thrombosis leading to portal vein thrombosis in the neonatal period.[15] Intermittent variceal hemorrhage, usually beginning in the second decade of life, may continue over many years with relatively good preservation of liver function. While the cause of the portal vein occlusion may be apparent in those with known umbilical vein infections or abdominal trauma, the majority of cases of EHPVO are idiopathic. Portal vein block also may occur in the setting of advanced cirrhosis of any cause; the prognosis for such patients is poor. Other causes of extrahepatic portal vein occlusion include schistomiasis, which produces a portal fibrosis and "prehepatic" portal hypertension with splenomegaly and variceal bleeding. Except for the cirrhotic patient, those with EHPVO typically have nearly normal liver function tests and tolerate surgery very well. These patients are good candidates for portacaval anastomoses except that technical difficulties will be encountered in finding a suitable vessel if the main portal channels are thrombosed.

Fertility of patients with EHPVO is near normal unless cirrhosis is present and the number of expected spontaneous abortions and stillbirths approaches that for the general population. Variceal hemorrhage is the common complication of this condition but does not appear with increased frequency during pregnancy. Management is similar to that for such patients in the nonpregnant state.

HEPATIC VEIN THROMBOSIS (BUDD–CHIARI SYNDROME)

Acute hepatic vein thrombosis is characterized by right upper quadrant pain due to relatively sudden hepatic enlargement and rapid onset of ascites in previously healthy individuals. A strong association has been established between hepatic vein thrombosis and oral contraceptive medication, and a weaker one between this condition and pregnancy. When the Budd–Chiari syndrome occurs, it is usually in the immediate postpartum period.[16,17] The diagnosis is established by liver biopsy and by hepatic venous angiographic studies demonstrating the occlusion. Treatment with anticoagulation and diuretics are used initially and may be all that is needed for mild cases. Portacaval shunt operations are reasonably successful for moderately severe disease; transplantation is also an option for severe cases.

HEPATIC TUMORS

Focal Nodular Hyperplasia and Liver Cell Adenoma

Two benign lesions in the liver have been associated with oral contraceptive medication and have been reported to occur in pregnancy: liver cell adenoma (LCA) and focal nodular hyperplasia (FNH). Although there has been some confusion surrounding the differences between these tumors, they are morphologically distinct and carry a different prognosis.[18] Both tumors are almost exclusively seen in women, but liver cell adenoma is a true neoplasm and is strongly associated with oral contraceptives. Although focal nodular hyperplasia is a hypervascular lesion and adenomas are only poorly vascularized, it is the adenomas that are associated with intraperitoneal hemorrhage, which occurs in approximately 25% of reported cases. Liver function tests for both are typically normal. Like hepatocellular carcinoma, both FNH and LCA may be multifocal. Their angiographic appearances are different, reflecting their distinct vascular patterns. Neither appears to have significant malignant potential and there is no association with preexisting liver disease as there is with hepatocellular carcinoma.

Several reports have indicated that adenomas can cause high maternal and fetal mortality secondary to acute rupture. Whether bleeding and rupture is more frequent in pregnancy is unclear, and it is not known whether the increased estrogen levels of pregnancy might stimulate growth of previously established tumors.

Hepatocellular Carcinoma

Primary hepatocellular carcinoma (HCC) is distinctly unusual in young women without antecedent liver cirrhosis. Rare instances of HCC in association with oral contraceptive medication have been reported. It is of note that human chorionic gonadotropin is occasionally synthesized by primary hepatocellular carcinomas. Serum alpha-fetoprotein levels provide a useful tumor marker in the normal or cirrhotic patient with HCC. These levels also are elevated in normal pregnancy and are particularly high with twinning or with fetal demise, but are of still greater magnitude in HCC than any of the above conditions of pregnancy. Intraperitoneal hemorrhage also occurs with HCC, and it may be difficult to distinguish LCA and HCC without careful histologic study. This is important in view of the radically different prognosis of these conditions. Chemotherapy in HCC has not proved helpful and should be avoided in pregnancy. Occasionally, resection of an hepatic lobe will cure a localized HCC. Careful diagnostic distinctions need to be made, particularly in patients with hepatic neoplasms, since the prognosis is so different for each condition.

REFERENCES

1. Palmer ED. *Clinical Gastroenterology*. New York, NY: Hoeber; 1963:514.
2. Friedlander P, Osler M: Icterus and pregnancy. *Am J Obstet Gynecol*. 1967;97:894.
3. Everson GI, McKinley C, Lawson M, et al. Gallbladder function in the human female: effect of the ovulatory cycle, pregnancy, and contraceptive steroids. *Gastroenterology*. 1982;82:711.
4. Haemmerli UP. Jaundice in pregnancy with special reference on recurrent jaudice during pregnancy and its differential diagnosis. *Acta Med Scand*. 1966;444:(suppl):1.
5. Cowan DB, Houlton MC. Rupture of an amoebic liver abscess in pregnancy. A case report. *S Afr Med J*. 1978;53:460.
6. Wagner VP, Smale LE, Lischke JH. Amebic abscess of the liver and spleen in pregnancy and the puerperium. *Obstet Gynecol*. 1974;43:191.
7. Brodie MJ, Beattie AD, Moore MR, et al. Pregnancy and hereditary Hepatic Porphyria. In: Doass H, ed. *Porphyrins in Human Diseases*. Basel: Karger; 1976:251.
8. Kaushansky A, Fryduran M, Kaufman H, Homburg R. Endocrine studies of the ovulatory disturbances of Wilson's Disease (hepatolenticular degeneration). *Fertil Steril*. 1987;47:270.
9. Scheinberg IH, Sternleib I. Pregnancy in Penicillamine-treated patients with Wilson's Disease. *N Engl J Med*. 1975;293:1300.
10. Walshe JM. Pregnancy in Wilson's Disease. *Q J Med*. 1977;181:73.
11. Infeld DS, Borkowf HI, Varma RR. Chronic-persistent hepatitis and pregnancy. *Gastroenterology*. 1979;77:524.
12. Borhanmanesh F, Haghighi P. Pregnancy in patients with cirrhosis of the liver. *Obstet Gynecol*. 1970;36:315.
13. Cheng Y-S. Pregnancy in liver cirrhosis and/or portal hypertension. *Am J Obstet Gynecol*. 1977;128:812.
14. Britton RC. Pregnancy and Esophageal Varices. *Am J Surg*. 1982;142:421.

15. Maddrey WC, Basu Mallik KC, Iber FL, et al. Extra-hepatic obstruction of the portal venous system. *Surg Gynecol Obstet*. 1968;127:989.
16. Khuroo MS, Datta DV. Budd-Chiari syndrome following pregnancy. Report of 16 cases with roentgenologic, hemodynamic and histologic studies of the hepatic outflow tract. *Am J Med*. 1980;68:113.
17. Tiliacos M, Tsantoulas D, Tsoulias A, et al. The Budd-Chiari syndrome in pregnancy. *Postgrad Med J*. 1978;54:686.
18. Knowles DM, Casarella WJ, Johnson P, et al. The clinical, radiologic and pathologic characterization of benign hepatic neoplasms: alleged associations with oral contraceptives. *Medicine (Baltimore)*. 1978;57:223.

Chapter One Hundred and Fifty-Four

Pancreatic Disease

Shakir A. Hyder and Jamie S. Barkin

154

PANCREATITIS

Pancreatic disease in pregnancy is mostly restricted to the occurrence of acute pancreatitis. The incidence of pancreatitis during pregnancy ranges from 0.01% to 0.1%, therefore those physicians caring for pregnant patients must be aware of its existence. Acute pancreatitis in pregnancy initially was reviewed by Langmade and Edmondson[1], who reported its occurrence during pregnancy or within six weeks postpartum. More than 150 cases now have been reported, although the actual number is higher as many cases are not reported.

The incidence of pancreatitis increases in the late stages of pregnancy and in the puerperium.[2] The most frequent etiologic factors are cholelithiasis and hyperlipidemia. Overall, however, coexisting cholelithiasis is present in approximately 35–90% of these patients[3-5] (Table 154–1).

The development of acute pancreatitis during pregnancy increases the maternal mortality rate. Wilkinson reported a maternal mortality rate of 37%, which is five to ten times greater than that of nonpregnant individuals. The series, however, included at least 22 patients with acute fatty liver of pregnancy; when these cases were excluded, the mortality rate was reduced to 20%. This is still an increase over the mortality for nonpregnant patients under 50 years of age, which varies between 3.1% to 6.6%.[3] Parity does not predispose to pancreatitis, as there is no difference in parity between those patients who develop pancreatitis and obstetric patients in general.[3,6] Primigravidas, however, have a higher maternal mortality rate (39.8%) than the multiparous patient (30.8%).[6-8] In addition to this increased maternal mortality, the perinatal mortality is 13.5% higher in the primigravida than the multiparous woman. Thus, although pancreatitis does not occur more frequently in the primigravida, it is associated with a higher maternal and perinatal mortality.[3]

Etiology and Pathophysiology

Pregnancy-related gastrointestinal disorders are due mostly to a decrease in gut motility. This is secondary to the effects of increased sex hormone levels as well as to the displacing effect on the bowel of the gravid uterus.[9]

The decreased motility that affects the gallbladder predisposes to the occurrence of cholelithiasis. The usual pathogenic events involved in cholesterol gallstone formation are hepatic secretion of lithogenic bile[10-13], followed by physiochemical changes including nucleation[14] and the formation of crystals[15-17], then the adherence of crystals in the gallbladder, which occurs over a mean nucleation time of 3 days.[14,15] These changes require retention of lithogenic bile in the gallbladder. They would not occur if emptying were prompt, as the lithogenic bile and formed cholesterol crystals would pass uneventfully into the duodenum, interrupting the sequence that leads to gallstone formation.[10] Thus gallbladder hypomotility predisposes to gallstone formation. Evidence supporting this theory is that in pregnant women, the volume of the gallbladder is increased and its contraction is sluggish.[18-21] This hypomotility is secondary to effects of progesterone that inhibit intestinal smooth muscle activity as well as gallbladder emptying.[9] In pregnant women, the gallbladder has a slower, late rate of emptying. While this is felt to be hormonal, it is not supported by studies in women taking contraceptive steroids who have gallbladder emptying rates similar to controls. Studies in patients taking birth control pills have shown that the phase of an ovulation cycle does not affect gallbladder function, but rather that pregnancy caused retention of bile in the gallbladder throughout the day and night. Prolonged use of contraceptive steroids in these groups induces an increase in bile retention after an overnight fast, but not

TABLE 154–1. UNDERLYING ETIOLOGIC OR ASSOCIATED CONDITIONS IN 98 PREGNANT PATIENTS WITH ACUTE PANCREATITIS

Condition	Incidence
Gallstones[a]	17
Preeclampsia	9
Acute fatty metamorphosis of liver[b]	22
Drugs	
Tetracycline[c]	9
Thiazide diuretics	8
Hyperlipidemia	3
Hyperparathyroidism	1
Alcoholism	1
No associated condition	28

[a] Only 47 patients underwent gallbladder evaluation; thus, 17 patients represent a 36% incidence of gallstones.
[b] Eighteen of these patients received tetracycline.
[c] Excluding patients with tetracycline-associated fatty metamorphosis of liver.
Based on Wilkinson.[3]

during the day. These changes in gallbladder function may contribute to the pathogenesis of cholesterol cholelithiasis.[10] In addition, bile acid output by the liver is decreased by estrogen.[9] These changes result in decreased cholesterol solubility and, as expected, an increase in the incidence of gallstones during pregnancy. Pancreatitis during pregnancy is caused most often by these gallstones. Overall, 70–80% of cases of pancreatitis in pregnancy are related to alcohol abuse and gallstone disease, which is similar to the rate in the nonpregnant population.[22]

Pregnant patients, in addition to being predisposed to gallstones, are predisposed to hypertriglyceridemia-induced pancreatitis.[23] The usual level of triglycerides required for the induction of acute pancreatitis is 750–1000 mg%.[24] Acute pancreatitis is especially likely to occur in patients with Frederickson types I, IV, and V. The common denominator seems to be the level of triglycerides.[25] The diagnosis of hypertriglyceridemia may be suspected by examining a specimen of fasting plasma, which, on inspection will be markedly turbid. This plasma, upon standing for 24 hours, will settle into a thick, creamy layer made up of chylomicrons above a turbid infranatant. This chylomicronemia reflects an increase in plasma cholesterol and triglyceride level. Type I hyperlipoproteinemia occurs in most instances because of the absence of lipoprotein lipase (LPL) activity and rarely because of absent or defective apolipoprotein-C11(apoC11). The latter is the co-factor needed for the hydrolysis of lipoprotein triglyceride by LPL. The biochemical changes mentioned above are greatly enhanced during pregnancy.[26,27] Defective lipolysis probably also plays a role in causing the adult form of hyperlipoproteinemia. All chylomicronemic disorders, regardless of their origin, are complicated by an increased rate of acute pancreatitis. Conversely, pancreatitis by itself may cause hyperlipidemia[27] or the lipid and clinical disorder may both be secondary consequences of an independent factor such as alcoholism.

In summary, hyperlipidemia is a major precipitating factor in many instances of pancreatitis in pregnancy. Its mechanism is that pregnancy enhances plasma triglyceride levels, although other changes in the lipoprotein profile also occur. Hyperlipidemia of pregnancy may be due to decreased levels of apo-C11 or to an estrogen-induced increase in triglyceride synthesis and very low density lipoprotein (VLDL) secretion.[23,28] In normal pregnancy, at term, these physiologic factors result in the elevation of neutral fat to 100% above normal, which may lead to the occurrence of pancreatitis.[29-31]

In view of the potential morbidity and mortality of acute pancreatitis during pregnancy, as well as the potential for its prevention, fasting plasma samples of all patients should be examined in early pregnancy. Inspection will reveal a milky, opalescent appearance when the total plasma triglyceride concentration exceeds 600 mg/dL; when levels exceed 1500 mg/dL, a creamy layer often can be observed floating over this milky layer.[24] It is especially important to check for hyperlipidemia in a patient whose pregnancy appears normal, but in whom there is an increased suspicion of covert familial hypertriglyceridemia. The latter is suggested by a prior medical history of pancreatitis or recurrent episodes of unexplained abdominal pain. The treatment for hyperlipidemic pancreatitis in pregnancy is prolonged bowel rest and intravenous hydration.[32] This will not pose nutritional problems if the patient presents near or at term. When oral feedings can be tolerated, they should be fat free. In situations where prolonged bowel rest is required, total parenteral nutrition should be initiated, as with other causes of pancreatitis. The published experience of the use of total parenteral nutrition in pregnancy, while scanty, suggests that this form of nutritional support is tolerated well by the mother, does not present any risk to the fetus, and can effectively support fetal growth.[33-35]

Antibiotics and diuretics may be taken by women of childbearing age, and may cause acute pancreatitis[36] (Table 154–2). The antibiotics include those containing sulfur as well as metronidazole (Flagyl).[37] Intravenous tetracycline may result in fatty liver, and although pancreatitis is found as part of the symptom complex, hepatic and renal failure are the most dominant presentations.[38] Diuretics such as hydrochlorothiazide and Lasix may cause pancreatitis.

Preeclampsia is an uncommon cause of pancreatitis. Its mechanism is thought to result from small vessel thrombosis with pancreatic ischemia. There is presumptive evidence of a relationship between hypercalcemia and pancreatitis. Pancreatitis occurs more frequently, approximately 2%, in patients with primary hyperparathyroidism and other hypercalcemic conditions; however, its pathogenesis is unclear.[39] Pregnancy often exacerbates hyperparathyroidism, therefore any patient with a history of renal calculi, osteoporosis, peptic ulcer, pancreatitis, or prolonged nausea and vomiting during pregnancy should be screened for hypercalcemia. In addition to the maternal morbidity that may result from hypercalcemia, perinatal complications also may result. These include stillbirth and neonatal hypocalcemic tetany.[39-41] A total serum calcium value above 10 mg/dL should be investigated because serum calcium normally falls as gestation progresses. Neck exploration should be considered in the pregnant patient with rising serum calcium levels and worsening symptomatology or hyperparathyroid crises, which is unresponsive to medical treatment. Pregnancy does not protect the patient from the other causes of acute pancreatitis that are found in the nonpregnant patient.[42] Therefore, while we need to focus on certain etiologies, other causes of pancreatitis should be considered; for example, infections which may affect the pregnant as well as the nonpregnant woman.

Diagnosis

Elevated serum amylase levels occurs in approximately 90% of patients with acute pancreatitis. Amylase is found in the pancreas and other organs such as salivary glands, small bowel, fallopian tubes, and liver. Therefore, any pathologic conditions that affect these organs may result in an elevation of serum amylase. These states include intestinal ischemia, salivary gland disease, malignant tumors, and ovarian cyst, as well as a ruptured ectopic pregnancy.[43] It is especially important to consider these states in the differential diagnosis of patients with abdominal pain and elevated amylase levels (Table 154–3). Amylase elevation occurs in situations of prolonged acidosis, that is, diabetic

TABLE 154–2. DRUGS IMPLICATED IN THE ETIOLOGY OF ACUTE PANCREATITIS

Azathioprine	Steroids
Thiazides	Phenformin
Furosemide	L-asparaginase
Sulfonamides	Methyldopa
Tetracyclines	Ethacrynic acid
Estrogens	Valproic acid
	Clonidine

From Mallory and Kern[73] with permission.

TABLE 154–3. DISORDERS ASSOCIATED WITH AN ELEVATED TOTAL SERUM AMYLASE LEVEL

Intra-abdominal Disorders	Extra-abdominal Disorders
Pancreatic Disorders	Salivary Gland Disorders
Acute pancreatitis	Mumps
Chronic pancreatitis	Parotitis
Trauma	Trauma
Carcinoma	Impaired Amylase Excretion
Abscess	Renal failure
Pseudocyst	Macroamylasemia
Pancreatic ascites	Miscellaneous
Nonpancreatic Disorders	Cerebral trauma
Biliary tract disease	Severe burns
Intestinal obstruction	Diabetic ketoacidosis
Mesenteric infarction	Pregnancy
Ruptured aortic aneurysm	Drugs
Perforated peptic ulcer	Pneumonia
Peritonitis	
Acute appendicitis	
Ruptured ectopic pregnancy	
Salpingitis	

From Crist and Cameron[74] with permission.

ketoacidosis or ingestion of methyl alcohol, or when there is decreased clearance of amylase as in patients with renal failure.[44] The effect of healthy pregnancy on serum amylase levels is controversial. Most likely it does not affect amylase levels; therefore, if an increased level is found, its source should be investigated.[45]

The tests that are more specific for determining the presence of pancreatitis are pancreatic isoamylase levels and lipase. Two large components of amylase are the P-type that originates from the pancreas and the S-type that orginates from the salivary glands.[46] In pancreatitis and other disorders of the pancreas, P-type amylase predominates, whereas S-amylase elevation is present in patients with salivary gland disorders. Lipase, although more specific for pancreatic disease, is not pathognomic for pancreatitis and may be elevated in other pathologic conditions such as intestinal ischemia.[47] Lipase levels remain elevated longer in patients with acute pancreatitis than either amylase or isoamylase. Therefore, their determination may be helpful in patients who have abdominal pain of several days duration and who have a normal amylase. Lipase levels remain normal during normal pregnancy. The amylase/creatinine clearance ratio (cam/CCR%) requires determination of serum amylase and creatinine and urine amylase and creatinine. The ratio is normally between 1% and 4%, whereas if acute pancreatitis is present, it is increased. The ratio is unaltered in acute intestinal obstruction and cholelithiasis but may be elevated in patients with perforated duodenal ulcers, severe burns, diabetic ketoacidosis or severe renal insufficiency. During normal pregnancy, the ratio is generally lower and ranges from 2.35% at 12 weeks to 2.8% at 40 weeks of gestation. This is thought to be secondary to increased clearance. In pregnant patients with pancreatitis, the ratio remains elevated even when the serum amylase decreases. This makes the determination of the amylase/creatinine clearance very useful in evaluating patients who present with abdominal pain of several days duration and who have normal serum amylase levels. Overall, it has a diagnostic accuracy of 94% in cases of pancreatitis in pregnancy, although its use is declining as serum lipase determinations become common.[43]

Clinical Features and Complications of Acute Pancreatitis

The pregnant patient with abdominal pain can be one of the most difficult diagnostic challenges to both the obstetrically and nonobstetrically oriented physician. This is secondary to the maternal physiologic and anatomic changes that may alter the symptoms as well as the normal response to intra-abdominal disease.

However, the clinical presentation of acute pancreatitis is similar in pregnant and nonpregnant patients. The major symptom is abdominal pain, which is constant, epigastric in location, boring in nature, and often radiating to the back.[3,49] Nausea and vomiting frequently are present and may be confused with that occurring in pregnancy. Abdominal distention may not be appreciated as it is found frequently in the pregnant patient without pancreatitis. Therefore, these early findings may not be considered significant. Physical examination in most instances reveals direct abdominal tenderness. Bowel sounds may be decreased or absent because of secondary ileus. The finding of peritoneal signs is unusual and if found in association with greater than 101°, should suggest a complicating infection of the pancreas or an intra-abdominal process other than pancreatitis, such as perforated peptic ulcer. Cullen's sign, a bluish discoloration around the umbilicus, or Grey Turner's sign, a bluish or brown discoloration of the flank, are not found often, but when seen suggest necrotizing pancreatitis.[50,51]

Jaundice occurs in 10% of patients with acute pancreatitis. This can be secondary to choledocholithiasis or compression of the common bile duct by an edematous, inflamed head of the pancreas or a pseudocyst.[22,48]

Imaging

The development of noninvasive imaging of the pancreas with ultrasonography or computerized tomography (CT) allows visualization of the local complications of pancreatitis. They also may be used to guide percutaneous needle aspiration of pancreatic fluid collections. CT can delineate more clearly the pancreas and its complications; however, it will expose the pregnant patient to radiation. Therefore, ultrasonography using high resolution, real-time scanners is the diagnostic imaging modality of choice in pregnant patients. Ultrasound findings in patients with pancreatitis range from the pancreas that appears normal to pancreatic enlargement or pancreatic or peripancreatic fluid collection(s). A normal pancreatic scan does not preclude the presence of mild-to-moderate pancreatitis; however, patients with severe pancreatitis have abnormal pancreatic anatomy. Ultrasound is an excellent modality to visualize the presence of cholelithiasis or sludge, both of which suggest a biliary origin of the pancreatitis. Magnetic resonance imaging (MRI), like ultrasound, is noninvasive, involves no radiation, and is thought to be safe in pregnancy.[52,53] Overall, its imaging of the pancreas can demonstrate many of the abnormalities found with CT and ultrasound. However, respiratory variation may result in bothersome artifacts with MRI, and spatial resolution is not clear. Pancreatic fluid collections have prolonged, half-resolution times. Their T_1 relaxation times are variable, and there is overlap in many of the pancreatic inflammatory complications as well as with non-pancreatic fluid collections.[54,55]

Prognosis

Complications of acute pancreatitis are classified as systemic and local. We will focus on the common systemic manifestations. Hypotension and ileus usually improve with supportive therapy. The mechanism of hypovolemia is vomiting, third space losses of fluid, and retroperitoneal hemorrhage, contributing to depletion of intravascular volume with hypotension. Occasionally, hypovolemia may proceed to shock and acute renal failure.

Pulmonary complications range from mild hypoxemia to adult respiratory distress syndrome (ARDS); its pathogenesis is unclear. It is imperative to determine PO_2 in all patients with pancreatitis. Pulmonary effusions are usually left-sided, transitory, and do not cause significant consequences.[22]

There is a tendency for low calcium values to occur as a sequella of normal pregnancy. Therefore, hypocalcemia associated with pancreatitis in pregnancy is very common, occurring in 50% of pregnant patients.[3,56] Its presence reflects more severe disease; management with supplementation is similar to that of the nonpregnant patient.

In most cases the disease is relatively mild, self-limited and does not become complicated by lasting tissue injury or infection. However, in up to 20% of patients, there is a prolonged clinical course, which is characterized by pancreatic swelling, peripancreatic inflammation, and may be complicated by necrosis of tissue.

Ranson has delineated prognostic criteria that are determined on admission and within 48 hours after admission (Table 154–4). Patients with three or more signs have an increased morbidity and mortality. Unfortunately, the validity of these risk factors has not been assessed in pregnant patients. In general, patients with respiratory or renal disease or acidosis have a poor prognosis. Maternal mortality from acute pancreatitis is very difficult to assess. Wilkinson, in a retrospective review, found a mortality rate of 20%. Fetal salvage is similarly difficult to assess, but in most cases fetal death is due to extreme prematurity. This was evidenced by two first trimester abortions and one intrauterine death at 24 weeks' gestation, after which the pancreatitis rapidly subsided.[57] Premature labor may occur in as many as 60% of patients when the onset of pancreatitis is in late pregnancy.[58]

BILIARY DISEASE

The goal of early diagnosis and therapy of biliary disease is to ensure maternal and fetal survival during pregnancy.

TABLE 154–4. SIGNS FOR CLASSIFICATION OF SEVERITY OF ACUTE PANCREATITIS

At time of admission or diagnosis
Age >55 years
White blood cell count >16,000/mm
Blood glucose >200 mg/dL
Serum lactate dehydrogenase more than twice normal
Serum glutamic-oxaloacetic transaminase more than six times normal
During initial 48 hours
Decrease in hematocrit of >10%
Serum calcium <8 mg/dL
Increase in blood urea nitrogen of >5 mg/dL
Arterial PO_2 <60 mm Hg
Base deficit >4 mEq/L
Estimated fluid sequestration >6,000 mL

Adapted from Ranson JHC, et al.[75]

The entire spectrum of biliary disease may be encountered any time during pregnancy as reported by Hiatt et al.[59] In 26 patients, symptoms initially appeared in the first trimester in 7 patients, second trimester in 5, third trimester in 12, and in the early postpartum period in 2 patients. No severe cases of pancreatitis occurred in this group in which CT scanning was not done.

Ultrasonography demonstrated cholelithiasis in 18 patients and dilated intrahepatic ducts in one of two patients with surgically proven choledocholithiasis. Therefore, true positives were found in 19 of 26. Nineteen of 26 patients underwent cholecystectomy and cholangiography, nine of whom had surgery during pregnancy. Surgery for the remaining 10 was delayed until delivery; seven were not explored within the period of follow up, up to postpartum. Two of the seven patients who presented in their first trimester had term pregnancies, whereas five had abortions, three at the request of the mother and two spontaneously. Conversely, all patients who presented in their third trimester had premature labor and there were no maternal deaths. In general, definitive biliary surgery should be delayed until after delivery whenever possible, unless the patient's symptoms do not resolve with medical measures.

Treatment

The medical management of patients with acute pancreatitis is the same for the pregnant patient as for the nonpregnant patient. The guiding principle is the early institution of vigorous supportive measures including volume replacement, oxygen supplementation and early recognition of necrotizing pancreatitis. In 10–20% of patients with necrotizing pancreatitis, cardiac, pulmonary and renal monitoring is mandatory as the appropriate supportive measures can be instituted to prevent organ failure. Management also should consist of the administration of adequate analgesia, nasogastric aspiration if there is protracted vomiting or ileus, and replacement of calcium and magnesium if these become depleted.[60] There is no recognized medical therapy that has been proven to inhibit or suppress necrosis or the systemic inflammatory consequences of this disease.

If prolonged periods of bowel rest are required, patients should receive total parenteral nutrition.[61] Fat emulsion solutions can be utilized as long as the acute pancreatitis is not caused by hypertriglyceridemia. The indications for immediate surgery in patients with acute pancreatitis are (1) clinical deterioration, depsite supportive medical therapy; (2) unclear diagnosis (these criteria should not be used frequently as abdominal CT imaging enables visualization of an abnormal pancreas in patients with necrotizing pancreatitis); and (3) emergent decompression of the biliary tree in severely ill patients. Surgical or endoscopic removal of common bile duct or impacted stones in patients with severe necrotizing biliary pancreatitis results in improved survival.[62,63]

Sterile pancreatic pseudocysts and infected pancreatic necrosis and abscesses are the most frequent local complications of acute pancreatitis. Pancreatic pseudocyst results from leakage of pancreatic enzymes into the lesser sac and surrounding tissue. Pseudocysts occur in 10–20% of patients with acute pancreatitis and most often are associated with pancreatic inflammatory diseases that are caused by alcohol and biliary disease.[64] Most pseudocysts will resolve spontaneously, usually within several weeks after the acute episode. Conversely, cysts larger than 5 cm in diameter, or which persist for 6 or more weeks, are unlikely to resolve spontaneously. At this point they are prone to develop complications such as infection and bleeding. Therefore, they should be drained surgically, percutaneously or endoscopically.[65-67]

The local septic complications of pancreatitis include infected necrosis that occurs early in the patient's course and pancreatic abscess that occurs later in the course and may evolve from an area of infected necrosis. In addition, a pseudocyst may become secondarily infected. These infectious complications should be suspected when the patient with acute pancreatitis has a temperature of >101°F or severe disease. There are no clinical features that allow us to clearly distinguish those patients with septic complications from those with severe diseases. Therefore, we must utilize abdominal imaging. If nonhomogeneous areas or pancreatic or peripancreatic fluid collections are identified, percutaneous needle aspiration should be performed.[68] The aspirate should be gram-stained for bacteria that, if present, will enable differentiation between sterile and infectious fluid collection. This is our usual approach to nonpregnant patients; although we have not utilized this technique in pregnant patients, the only precautionary measure would be a safe path for the needle placement. If an infected fluid collection such as infected pseudocyst is identified, our initial approach is percutaneous drainage; if the infected lesion is a primary, solid lesion, that is, infected necrosis, surgical drainage is our preferred therapeutic modality.

Recurrent or intractable pancreatitis during pregnancy may necessitate cholecystectomy, because the mortality rate of untreated pancreatitis approaches 15% during pregnancy and is responsible for both an increase in spontaneous abortion and premature delivery.[57,69] Therefore, cholecystectomy, other than appendectomy, may be the most common surgical procedure performed during pregnancy.[58] This is performed between one and six times per 10,000 pregnancies. Hill et al[70] reported the results of cholecystectomy performed in 20 pregnant women. Four were performed between 0–9 weeks' gestation, 13 between 10–20 weeks', 2 between 21–33 weeks' and only one between 34–40 weeks'.

Overall, cholecystectomy was performed on the majority of patients during the second trimester of pregnancy. The four cholecystectomy cases during the first nine weeks of gestation included one patient with biliary colic that was associated with jaundice, one patient who was not known to be pregnant, and two with severe, repeated attacks of biliary colic. If cholecystectomy is to be performed during pregnancy, the second trimester is believed to be the optimal time since the peak period for spontaneous abortion has passed and the uterus is not large enough to impinge on the operating field.

Block et al[71] evaluated the timing of surgical therapy in pregnant patients with biliary pancreatitis in a long-term study over 22 years. A total of 21 women with gallstone pancreatitis were included. In 11 of these patients, pancreatitis occurred during pregnancy and in 10 within six weeks postpartum. During the acute episode, only two patients underwent surgical intervention, while the other 19 were successfully managed with conservative medical therapy. After the acute episode had subsided, however, these 19 patients underwent elective cholecystectomy during the second trimester or early postpartum period. This approach had no associated maternal morbidity or fetal mortality, nor did pancreatitis recur.

The risks of elective cholecystectomy during pregnancy most likely are not increased significantly over the nonpregnant patient. Corbett and Michell[6] report three pregnant patients and Jouppila, et al[54] also reported three patients who underwent cholecystectomy with no maternal deaths. McKay and co-workers[5] reported seven pregnant patients with acute pancreatitis. Two developed pancreatitis in their first pregnancy, two during their second pregnancy, two during their third pregnancy and one patient during her fourth pregnancy. The episodes usually occurred in the third trimester in four of seven patients; however, in two patients it occurred in their first trimester and in one, the second trimester. Overall, there were no maternal deaths, but one fetal death occurred following emergency laparotomy and drainage procedure at 25 weeks' gestation. Apart from the risk of death from the effects of premature delivery, surgery does not seem to have any influence on fetal loss, whereas maternal mortality may well be influenced.[58] Patients with severe gallstone pancreatitis who are unresponsive to conventional therapy may benefit from surgical intervention or endoscopic sphincterotomy with stone extraction. Surgery for gallstone pancreatitis may pose a risk to both mother and fetus; therefore, there is increasing interest in endoscopic sphincterotomy. This recently has been shown to reduce the incidence of complications in nonpregnant patients with severe biliary pancreatitis. Neoptoleomos et al[62] conducted a randomized trial of endoscopic retrograde cholangiopancreatography (ERCP) and endoscopic sphincterotomy versus conventional therapy in patients with gallstone pancreatitis. They found that early ERCP and sphincterotomy is not hazardous in the presence of acute gallstone pancreatitis. Although there was reduction in the overall mortality from 8% to 2% in patients undergoing endoscopic sphincterotomy, this was not statistically significant but obtained significance in the severe group. The overall incidence of complication, however, was reduced in the group undergoing endoscopic sphincterotomy. This approach has shown that the progression of pancreatitis can be interrupted and its effects are most evident in severely ill patients. Two pregnant patients in their 3rd trimester with pancreatitis that was unresponsive to medical therapy were successfully treated with endoscopic sphincterotomy and common bile duct stone removal.[72] Endoscopic sphincterotomy was performed with fetal shielding and external monitoring. Elective cholecystectomy was performed postpartum but during their hospitalization. These case reports emphasize that endoscopic sphincterotomy with fetal shielding and monitoring could be safely performed and result in rapid resolution of biliary pancreatitis in pregnant patients who are unresponsive to conventional therapy.

In summary, elective surgical treatment for gallstone pancreatitis, when possible, should be delayed until the postpartum period, or if necessary, can be performed safely in the second trimester. Patients with severe biliary pancreatitis can be successfully managed with endoscopic sphincterotomy with common bile duct extraction.

REFERENCES

1. Langmade CF, Edmondson HA. Acute pancreatitis during pregnancy and the post-partum period: a report of 9 cases. *Surg Gynecol Obstet.* 1951;92:43.
2. Dreiling DA, Bordalo O, Rosenberg V, Rudick J. Pregnancy and pancreatitis. *Am J Gastro.* 1975;64:23.
3. Wilkinson EJ. Acute pancreatitis in pregnancy. A review of 98 cases and a report of 8 new cases. *Obstet Gynecol Surg.* 1973;28:281.
4. Berk JE, Smith BH, Akrawi MM. Pregnancy pancreatitis. *Am J Gastro.* 1971,56:216.
5. McKay AJ, O'Neill J, Imrie CW. Pancreatitis pregnancy and gallstones. *Br J Obstet Gynecol.* 1980;87:47.
6. Coblett RC, Michell DR. Pancreatitis in pregnancy. *Am J Obstet Gynecol.* 1972;113:281.
7. Becker WF. Acute pancreatitis: clinical study of one hundred cases. *J Louisiana M Soc.* 1954;106:166.

8. Romer JF, Carey LC. Pancreatitis: a clinical review. *Am J Surg.* 1966;111:795.
9. Bynum TE. Hepatic and gastrointestinal disorders in pregnancy. *Med Clin N Am.* 1979;61:129.
10. Everson GT, McKinley C, Lawson M, Johnson M, Kern F Jr. Gallbladder function in the human female: effect of the ovulatory cycle, pregnancy, and contraceptive steroids. *Gastroenterology.* 1982;82(8):711.
11. Small DM. Cholesterol nucleation and growth formation in gallstone formation. *N Engl J Med.* 1980;302:1305.
12. Small DM. Management of gallstones, particularly the silent variety: advantages of a varied and individualized approach. In: Ingelfinger FJ, Ebert RB, Finland M, Relman AS, eds. *Controversies in Internal Medicine II.* Philadelphia: WB Saunders; 1974;545.
13. Shaffer A, Small DM. Gallstone disease pathogenesis and management. *Curr Probl Surg.* 1976;13(7):1.
14. Holan KR, Holzbach RT, Hermann RE, et al. Nucleation time: a key factor in the pathogenesis of cholesterol gallstone disase. *Gastroenterology.* 1979;77:611.
15. Sedaghat A, Grundy SM. Cholesterol crystals and the formation of cholesterol gallstones. *N Engl J Med.* 1980;302:1274.
16. Walton AG. *The Formation and Properties of Precipitates.* New York: Interscience; 1967;23.
17. Craven BM. Crystal structure of cholesterol monohydrate. *Nature.* 1967;260:727.
18. Shaffer EA, Taylor PJ, Logan K, et al. The effect of a progestin on gallbladder function in young women. *Am J Obstet Gynecol.* 1984;148:504.
19. Braverman OZ, Johnson ML, Kern F Jr. Effects of pregnancy and contraceptive steroids on gallbladder function. *N Engl J Med.* 1980;302:362.
20. Potter MG. Observation of the gallbladder and bile during pregnancy at term. *JAMA.* 1938;106:1070.
21. Gerdes MM, Boyden EA. The rate of emptying of the human gallbladder in pregnancy. *Surg Gynecol Obstet.* 1938;66:145.
22. Toskes PP, Greenberger NJ. Acute and chronic pancreatitis. *Disease a Month.* 1983;29:1.
23. Glueck CJ, Christopher C, Mishkel MA, et al. Pancreatitis familial hypertriglyceridemia and pregnancy. *Am J Obstet Gynecol.* 1980;136:755.
24. Cameron JL, Capuzzi DM, Zuidema GD, Margolis S. Acute pancreatitis with hyperlipidemia: evidence for a persistent defect in lipid metabolism. *Am J Med.* 1974;56:482.
25. Frederickson DS, Goldstein JL, Brown MS. The familial hyperlipoproteinemias. In: Stanbury JB, Wyngaarden JB, Frederickson DS, eds. *The Metabolic Basis of Inherited Disease.* 4th ed. New York, NY: McGraw-Hill; 1978:604–655.
26. Nikkila EA. Familial lipoprotein lipase deficiency and related disorders of chylomicron metabolism. In: Stanbury JB, Fredrickson DS, Goldstein JL, Brown MS, eds. *The Metabolic Basic of Inherited Disease.* New York: McGraw-Hill; 1983.
27. De Chalain TMB, Michell WL, Berger GMB. Hyperlipidemia, pregnancy and pancreatitis. *Surg Gynecol Obstet.* 1988;167:469.
28. Glueck CJ, Christopher C, Tsang RC. Cholesterol-free diet and the physiologic hyperlipidaemia of pregnancy in familial hypercholesterolaemia. *Metabolism.* 1980;29:949.
29. Boyd EM. The lipemia of pregnancy. *J Clin Invest.* 1934;13:347.
30. de Alvarez RR, Gaiser DF, Simkins DM, et al. Serial studies of serum lipids in normal human pregnancy. *Am J Obstet Gynecol.* 1959;77:743.
31. Millen RS, Russ EM, Eder HA, Barr DP. Pregnancy complicated by hyperlipemia. *Am J Obstet Gynecol.* 1956;71:326.
32. Glueck CJ, Christopher C, Miskel MA, et al. Pancreatitis, familial hypertriglyceridemia and pregnancy. *Metabolism.* 1980;136:755.
33. Benny PS, Legge M, Aickin DR. The biochemical effects of maternal hyperalimentation during pregnancy. *NZ Med J.* 1978;88:282.
34. Loludice TA, Chandkrakaar C. Pregnancy and jejunoileal bypass: treatment of complications with total parenteral nutrition. *So Med J.* 1980;73:256.
35. Webb GA. The use of hyperalimentation and chemotherapy in pregnancy: a case report. *Am J Obstet Gynecol.* 1980;137:263.
36. Ances IG, McClain CA. Acute pancreatitis following the use of thiazide in pregnancy. *South Med J.* 1971;64:267.
37. Sandford KA, Mayle JE, Dean HA, Greenbaum DS. Metronidazole associated pancreatitis. *Ann Int Med.* 1988;109(9):756.
38. Schiffer MA. Fatty liver associated with administration of tetracycline in pregnant and nonpregnant women. *Am J Obstet Gynecol.* 1966;86:326.
39. Rajala B, Abbasi RA, Hutchinson HT, Taylor T. Acute pancreatitis and primary hyperparathyroidism in pregnancy: treatment of hypercalcemia with magnesium sulfate. *Obstet Gynecol.* 1987;70:460.
40. Levine G, Tsin D, Risk A. Acute pancreatitis and hyperparathyroidism in pregnancy. *Obstet Gynecol.* 1979;54(2):246.
41. Delmonico FL, Neer RM, Cosimi AB, et al. Hyperparathyroidism during pregnancy. *Am J Surg.* 1976;131:328.
42. Thomason JL, Sampson MB, Farb HF, Spellacy WN. Pregnancy complicated by concurrent primary hyperparathyroidism and pancreatitis. *Obstet Gynecol.* 1981;57(suppl):34.
43. De Vore G, Bracken M, Berkowitz RL. The amylase/creatinine clearance ratio in normal pregnancy and pregnancies complicated by pancreatitis, hyperemesis gravidarum, and toxemia. *Am J Obstet Gynecol.* 1980;136:747.
44. Johnson SG, Ellis CJ, Levitt MD. Mechanism of increased renal clearance of amylase/creatinine in acute pancreatitis. *N Engl J Med.* 1976;295:1214.
45. Kaiser R, Berk JE, Fridhandler L, et al. Serum amylase changes during pregnancy. *Am J Obstet Gynecol.* 1975;122:283.
46. Koehler DF, Eckfeldt JH, Levitt MD. Diagnostic valve of routine isoamylase assay of hyperamylasemic serum. *Gastroenterology.* 1982;82:887.
47. Fitzgerald O. Pancreatitis following pregnancy. *Br Med J.* 1955;1:349.
48. Herfort K, Fialova V, Srp B. Acute pancreatitis in pregnancy. *Mat Med Pol.* 1981;13:15.
49. Harary AM, Barkin JS. Acute pancreatitis. In: Gleicher N, Galbraith RM, eds. *Principles of Medical Therapy in Pregnancy.* 1st ed. Norwalk, CT: Appleton & Lange; 1985:853.
50. Montgomery WH, Miller FC. Pancreatitis and pregnancy. *Obstet Gynecol.* 1970;35:658.
51. Meyers MA, Feldberg MAM, Oliphant M. Grey Turner's sign and Cullen's sign in acute pancreatitis. *Gastrointest Radiol.* 1989;14:31.
52. Jeffrey RB Jr. Sonography in acute pancreatitis. *Radiol Clin NA.* 1988;27:5.
53. Anderson JM, Lee TG, Nagel N. Ultrasound diagnosis of nonobstetric disease during pregnancy. *Obstet Gynecol.* 1976;48:359.
54. Stark DD, Moss AA, Goldberg HI, et al. Magnetic resonance and CT of the normal and diseased pancreas: a comparative study. *Radiology.* 1984;150:153.
55. Stark DS, Bradley WS. *Biliary System, Pancreas, Spleen and Alimentary Tract in Magnetic Resonance Imaging.* St. Louis, MO: CV Mosby; 1988;1060.
56. Berk JE, Smith BH, Akrawi MM. Pregnancy pancreatitis. *Am J Gastroenterol.* 1971;56:216.
57. Jouppila P, Mokka R, Larmi TKI. Acute pancreatitis in pregnancy. *Surg Gynecol Obstet.* 1974;139:879.
58. Young KR. Acute pancreatitis in pregnancy. Two case reports. *Obstet Gynecol.* 1982;139:69.
59. Hiatt JR, Hiatt JCG, Williams RA, Klein SR. Biliary disease in pregnancy: strategy for surgical management. *Am J Surg.* 1986;151:263.
60. Geokas MC, Baltaxe HA, Banks PA, et al. Acute pancreatitis. *Ann Int Med.* 1985;103:86.
61. Weinberg RB, Sitrin MD, Adkins GM, Lin CC. Treatment of hyperlipidemic pancreatitis in pregnancy with total parenteral nutrition. *Gastroenterol.* 1982;83:1300.
62. Neoptolemos JP, Carr-Locke DL, London NJ, et al. Controlled trial of urgent endoscopic retrograde cholangiopancreatography and endoscopic sphincterotomy versus conservative treatment for acute pancreatitis due to gallstones. *Lancet.* 1988;8618:979.
63. Neoptolemos JP, London N, Slater ND, et al. A prospective study of ERCP and endoscopic sphincterotomy in the diagnosis and treatment of gallstone acute pancreatitis. *Surgery.* 1986;121:697.
64. Rattner DW, Warshaw AL. Surgical intervention in acute pancreatitis. *Crit Care Med.* 1988;16:89.
65. Cremer M. Endoscopic cystoduodenostomy. *Proceedings of the 3rd Symposium of Digestive Endoscopy.* 1981:29.
66. Hiatt JR, Fink AS, King W III, Pitt HA. Percutaneous aspiration of peripancreatic fluid collection. *Dig Dis Sci.* 1985;30:974.
67. Barkin JS, Smith FR, Pereiras R, et al. Therapeutic percutaneous aspiration of pancreatic pseudocysts. *Dig Dis Sci.* 1981;26:585.
68. Hill MC, Dach JL, Barkin JS, et al. The role of percutaneous aspiration in the diagnosis of pancreatic abscesses. *AJR.* 1984;141:1305.
69. Printen KJ, Ott RA. Cholecystectomy during pregnancy. *Amer Surg.* 1978;44:432.
70. Hill LM, Johnson CE, Lee RA. Cholecystectomy in pregnancy. *Obstet Gynecol.* 1975;46(3):291.
71. Block P, Kelly TR. Management of gallstone pancreatitis during pregnancy and the postpartum period. *Surg Gynec Obstet.* 1989;168:426.
72. Buchner WF Jr, Stoltenberg PH, Kirtley DW. Endoscopic management of severe gallstone pancreatitis during pregnancy. *Am J Gastroenterol.* 1988;83(9):1073.
73. Mallory A, Kern F. Drug-induced pancreatitis: a critical review. *Gastroenterology.* 1980;78:813.
74. Crist DW, Cameron JL. The current management of acute pancreatitis. *Adv Surg.* 1970;20:69.
75. Ranson JHC, et al. *Surg Gynecol Obstet.* 1976;143:209.

PART XV | Hematologic Diseases

Stanley A. Gall, Section Editor

A

GENERAL ASPECTS

Chapter One Hundred and Fifty-Five

Anemia

Walter E. Davis

155

Decrease in the red cell mass defines the condition known as anemia. As anemia develops, there is a minor increase in the oxygen-carrying ability of each red cell, but this internal compensatory mechanism is soon overwhelmed. To maintain adequate oxygen delivery to tissues, cardiac output must increase. All is well for the period that increasing cardiac output compensates for the lowered ability to carry oxygen, but as the maximum cardiac output is reached, tissue hypoxia and injury to mother and fetus appear.

DEFINITION OF ANEMIA

Hemoglobin varies with age, sex, and the altitude at which we live. In the nonpregnant female of childbearing age living at sea level, a hemoglobin value between 12 and 16 is considered normal. During pregnancy the hemoglobin normally falls 10–15% below the nonpregnant value. In pregnancy this does not represent a pathologic condition, but rather reflects one of the rare instances in which an individual's blood volume increases. This increase in blood volume compensates for the decrease in hematocrit, so that oxygen delivery to the tissues is not compromised.

The number of careful studies, such as that by Low et al[1], defining the parameters of blood volume in the pregnant patient is small because of the reluctance to use radioactive tracers to accurately measure blood volume. Pritchard's studies[2] using more accurate labeling techniques demonstrate that early in pregnancy the plasma volume and red cell mass remain within the normal nonpregnant range. Between the sixth and 24th week of gestation, however, there is a significant increase in the plasma volume, a mild increase in the total red cell mass, and the resulting increase in total blood volume. This "dilution" effect is maximum at the 24th week in an uncomplicated pregnancy, leading to the lowest normal hemoglobin at that point. Near the end of the third trimester, plasma volume decreases slightly without any significant change in the red cell mass. This results in a mild increase in hemoglobin and hematocrit as delivery nears.

There is considerable variation in the magnitude of plasma volume changes among individuals, thus the variation of hemoglobin levels seen in pregnancy is wider than in the nonpregnant population. The maxim that the hemoglobin should remain above 10 g/dL and hematocrit above 30 is most useful clinically. One must be aware that some women during pregnancy will have hemoglobin and hematocrit values somewhat below this, and despite extensive hematologic evaluation, no defined cause of anemia will be found. They probably represent patients in whom the degree of increase in the plasma volume is greater than average. They appear to suffer no ill effects on their pregnancy and return to normal hematologic status following delivery.

NORMAL HEMATOPOIESIS

During the first trimester of pregnancy, fetal erythropoiesis begins in the liver with cells that migrated from the yolk sac.[3] Shortly thereafter, erythropoiesis is seen in thymus, lymph nodes, and spleen. By the eighth month gestation, the hemoglobin concentration has risen to 14 g/dL, and the primary site of red cell production is the bone marrow.

ERYTHROPOIESIS

Red cells, like white cells and megakaryocytes, arise from multi-potential stem cells in the bone marrow.[4] These stem cells reproduce themselves and also mature in a stepwise fashion to develop into differentiated elements.[5] At an unidentified point in its life span, the stem cell loses its pleuripotential ability and is said to be committed to development into only one cell line, for example, erythropoiesis. Stem cells are present in the marrow in small number. Thought to have the characteristic of a lymphocyte, they are morphologically unrecognizable and can be identified only by culture of the marrow. In soft agar marrow cultures, there are three types of erythroid-forming elements, presumably identifiying three progressively more mature stages of development in the committed stem cell. The most mature is CFU-E, which leads to small colonies of red cells after seven days of culture; the next younger is BTU-E, which produces large colonies of cells in approximately two weeks of culture; and the least mature is DFU-E, which produces very large colonies with multiple subcolonies after three weeks of incubation.

The first morphologically recognizable red cell precursor is the pronormoblast, a deeply basophilic mononuclear cell with large amounts of endoplasmic reticulum. In the normal marrow, this cell undergoes a sequence of four divisions resulting in 16 mature erythrocytes. During maturation there is rapid synthesis of hemoglobin within the cell with loss of basophilia, extrusion of the nucleus, and then release into the circulation as a reticulocyte whose inclusions are residual polyribosomes. Reticulocytes released into the circulation spend a brief period sequestered in the spleen where inclusions are removed.[6] The cell then is released into the general circulation to complete its approximate 120-day life span.

REGULATORY MECHANISMS

Erythropoietin, a circulating glycoprotein hormone, is the primary regulator of red cell production. Its level in the blood varies with the adequacy of oxygen delivery to the tissues. The primary monitor of oxygen delivery is located in the kidney, probably in the area of the juxtaglomerular apparatus. Erythropoietin is synthesized predominantly in the kidney, and levels rise with falling oxygen delivery to the peripheral tissues.[7] Erythropoietin acts by increasing the rate of maturation of uncommitted stem cells to normoblasts. Many other effects of erythropoietin include reduced intermitotic time in normoblast division, increased rate of hemoglobin synthesis, and shorter intramedullary retention of reticulocytes. With intense stimulation, normal bone marrow can increase red cell production from sixfold to tenfold.

HEMOGLOBIN STRUCTURE

Approximately 90% of the dry weight of each red cell is made up of this oxygen-carrying protein. The other components of the red cell, which do not carry oxygen, facilitate the primary red cell function of oxygen binding and transfer. Hemoglobin is a tetramer with two pairs of identical polypeptide chains. An iron-containing pyrrole ring (heme) is bound to each chain, and is the specific structure that binds and transports the oxygen molecule. Hemoglobin is one of the best characterized proteins present in the body, and all of its primary structure (amino acid sequence) is known. There is considerable knowledge of its secondary and tertiary structure, which allows understanding of defects in oxygen transport caused by amino acid deletion and substitution.

RED CELL DESTRUCTION

Red cells newly released into the circulation have a finite life span. Some red cell destruction occurs in the marrow, where defective cells are eliminated before release to the circulation. Red cells spend a short period following their release in the spleen, where inclusions are removed or "pitted," and other as yet unidentified metabolic conditioning may occur. The cell then is released into the circulation, and survives for an average of 120 days. It then is removed from the circulation and replaced by a new cell from the bone marrow.

During its life span, the red cell progressively ages, leading to a senescent cell that is removed by the reticuloendothelial system, phagocytized, and catabolized. The key change that occurs in the cell signaling its impending demise is not known. Several enzyme systems progressively deteriorate in the older cell, and their assay can be used as a marker for the process of senescence. Generally, they protect the cell from internal and external oxidants, changes in shape, and maintain elastic deformability. The capacity of these enzyme systems progressively declines, and defects in one of these functions mark the cell for elimination.[8]

Senescent red cells are removed by the reticuloendothelial (RE) system, mostly in the spleen. Splenectomy does not lead to prolongation of normal red cell survival, demonstrating that other parts of the RE system can assume this role when the spleen is absent or nonfunctioning. After the red cell is engulfed by a phagocyte, the iron is removed from the heme ring and recycled to the bone marrow for incorporation into new normoblasts. The pyrrole ring is cleaved, transported to the liver as bilirubin, conjugated, and excreted in the bile. The protein is catabolized by proteases and returned to the general amino acid pool.

The life span of red cells can be measured by pulse labeling of cells and serial observation of their disappearance from the circulation.[9] A second method of determining red cell life span is to measure the carbon monoxide produced by cleavage of the pyrrole ring.[10] There is a linear relationship between endogenous carbon monoxide production and the rate of red cell destruction. Quantitation of the carbon monoxide production allows calculation of the red cell life span.

EVALUATION OF THE ANEMIC PATIENT

Faced with a patient whose hemoglobin is less than normal, the physician should review the medical history, physical examination, and laboratory data, obtain further information as needed, and determine the single diagnosis that fits the available data. The difficulty with this process is that there are few symptoms or physical findings that are pathognomonic; thus, one depends extensively on laboratory data that are both expensive and time consuming to collect. Laboratory studies must be chosen such that the number of tests is minimized and the results are available quickly. A useful approach for streamlining evaluation eliminates groups of diagnoses with a single simple test, and progressively decreases the possibilities in the differential diagnosis. Initially, blood loss should be eliminated as the cause of anemia by history and testing the stool for occult blood. The physician then should follow one of two major approaches to classifying anemia. The first separates anemias into those caused by decreased red cell production, or those caused by a decreased red cell survivial as shown in Tables 155–1 and 155–2. The second divides anemia on

TABLE 155–1. ANEMIA DUE TO DECREASED PRODUCTION OF RED CELLS

Deficiency of Required Substance
Iron deficiency
Folate deficiency
B_{12} deficiency
Marrow Suppression by Systemic Disease
Chronic infection
Malignancy
Chronic inflammatory disease
Chronic renal failure
Endocrine diseases
Marrow Infiltration
Infection
Malignancy
Miscellaneous
Sideroblastic anemia
Myelodysplastic syndrome
Aplasia
Toxins

the basis of red cell size, as demonstrated in Table 155–3.

The first approach, which depends on the reticulocyte count as the pivotal laboratory study, is favored; either, however, provides an appropriate template for evaluation. Each has its shortcomings because available laboratory studies are not absolutely specific. One must be aware of this lack of specificity, and be flexible in the interpretation of certain tests or incorrect conclusions will be drawn. The reticulocyte count, for example, may be elevated falsely in patients with abnormalities of bone marrow structure where developing cells are released prematurely, in patients following splenectomy, and in patients in whom blood loss has not been adequately excluded. Failure to consider these possible false positives will lead to the incorrect diagnosis of anemia due to red cell destruction. Likewise, the reticulocyte count may be low in the setting of a hemolytic anemia complicated by deficiency of a required hematemic and again lead to the wrong diagnosis. The elevated reticulocyte count is not the only way to demonstrate hemolysis, it is the most simple. Low serum haptoglobin levels, elevated LDH levels, elevated bilirubin levels, and declining hematocrits in the absence of bleeding all suggest the presence

TABLE 155–2. ANEMIA DUE TO INCREASED RED CELL DESTRUCTION

Hemolysis Due to Acquired Abnormalities
Autoimmune hemolytic anemia
Fragmentation hemolytic anemia
Hypersplenism
Paroxysmal nocturnal hemoglobinuria
Hemolysis with infection, and chemical agents
Hemolysis Due to Inherited Abnormalities
Eliptocytosis and stomatocytosis
Hereditary spherocytosis
Hemoglobinopathies
Thalassemia
Methemoglobinemia
Glycolytic enzyme defects
Pentose shunt enzyme defects

TABLE 155–3. CLASSIFICATION OF ANEMIA BY RED CELL SIZE

Microcytic Anemia
Iron deficiency
Thalassemia
Sideroblastic anemia
Anemia due to systemic disease
Macrocytic Anemia
Folic acid deficiency
B_{12} deficiency
Hemoglobin C disease
Liver disease and alcohol use
Hypothyroidism
Some myelodysplastic syndromes

of red cell destruction. In complicated situations, the following may be needed to make the distinction between the two types of anemia. When necessary, red cell survival measurement using the technique of carbon monoxide production rates may be used. The more commonly available red cell survival study using radioactive chromium should be avoided in pregnancy.

An example of the initial processes in evaluating anemia follows. For a patient with anemia, a reticulocyte count is ordered. If the reticulocyte count is low, the disorders listed in Table 155–1 (those associated with decreased red cell synthesis) are considered. If the reticulocyte count is elevated and blood loss externally or into body tissues is eliminated, the group of disorders listed in Table 155–2 is considered. Once this initial separation has been made, the next discriminant test is red cell size. The current instruments used for the routine complete blood count (CBC) provide the mean corpuscular volume (MCV). These values are reproducible and generally are more reliable in evaluating cell size than is the inexperienced or out-of-practice physician studying an often poorly prepared blood film. Using these two tests, reticulocyte count and red cell size measurement, the physician usually can reduce the number of diagnostic possibilities to a small number (Table 155–3). Applying the more specific or diagnostic test eliminates the few remaining elements in the differential diagnosis, pinpointing the cause of the anemia, and treatment is begun.

EFFECT OF ANEMIA ON THE FETUS

During most of the fetal growth period, the fetus has a different type of hemoglobin than the adult. Fetal hemoglobin allows the fetus to remove oxygen bound to maternal hemoglobin preferentially because of the greater affinity of fetal hemoglobin for oxygen. When the hemoglobin reaches very low levels, this protective mechanism fails; fetal tissues suffer from ischemia with resulting delayed or faulty maturation, and in its extreme, fetal death. There is not a single value above which the fetus suffers no adverse effects and below which damage always occurs. Individual circumstances of cardiac reserve, local blood flow to the uterus, adequacy of the placental transfer mechanism, and very likely a large number of other unidentified factors govern the degree of fetal injury. But in general, there is an inverse relationship between the degree of anemia during pregnancy and the frequency of miscarriage, stillbirth, APGAR scores, and birth weight.

TREATMENT OF ANEMIA IN PREGNANCY

If anemia occurs during pregnancy, it should be evaluated and treated. In many instances there is not a specific treatment, and one must consider whether to treat the anemia with transfusion to assure normal fetal development. Unfortunately, there is not a single hemoglobin level below which transfusion is mandatory. Cunningham et al[11] and Ricks[12] showed, predominantly with the hemoglobinopathies, that transfusion increases the frequency of successful conclusion of the pregnancy. A recent extensive study by Koshy et al[13], which randomizes pregnant women with sickle cell disease to be treated with prophylactic transfusion or to be followed carefully and transfused for standard indications, shows no difference in fetal or maternal loss. If transfusion is chosen, the hemoglobin should be kept above the 8–9 g/dL range. In other anemias, a hemoglobin in this range seems to be the point below which fetal and pregnancy complications increase.

Most physicians recommend transfusion to maintain hemoglobin at or above 8 g/dL if no other treatment is available. The last decade has complicated this decision, as the human immunodeficiency virus (HIV) has contaminated more of the blood supply. Although the frequency of acquired immune deficiency syndrome (AIDS) transmission from single donor units of standard sources is low, transmission of this always fatal illness to a pregnant woman is devastating. It is likely that transfusion will be used less frequently because of this problem. With deterioration of either the mother's or fetus's health because of anemia, there may not be available alternatives.

REFERENCES

1. Low JA, Johnston EE, McBride RL. Blood volume adjustments in the normal obstetric patient with particular reference to the third trimester of pregnancy. *Am J Obstet Gynecol.* 1965;91:356.
2. Pritchard JA. Changes in the blood volume during pregnancy and delivery. *Anesthesiology.* 1965;26:393.
3. Hesseldahl H, Falck LJ. Hematopoiesis and blood vessels in human yolk sac: an electron microscopic study. *Acta Anat.* 1971;78:274.
4. Till JE, McCulloch EA. A direct measurement of the radiation sensitivity of normal mouse bone marrow cells. *Radiation Res.* 1961;14:213.
5. Gregory CJ, Eaves AC. Human marrow cells capable of erythropoietic differentiation in vitro: definition of three erythroid colony responses. *Blood.* 1977;49:855.
6. Crosby WH. Normal functions of the spleen relative to red blood cells: a review. *Blood.* 1959;14:399.
7. Erslev AJ. The role of erythropoietin in the control of red cell production. *Medicine.* 1964;43:661.
8. Kadlubowski M, Agutter PS. Changes in the activities of some membrane-associated enzymes during the in vivo aging of the normal human erythrocyte. *Br J Haematol.* 1977;37:111.
9. International Committee for Standardization in Hematology. Recommended methods for radioisotope red cell survival studies. *Blood.* 1971;38:378.
10. Lundh B, Cavallin-Stahl E, Mercke C. Heme catabolism, carbon monoxide production and red cell survival in anemia. *Acta Med Scand.* 1975;197:161.
11. Cunningham FG, Prtichard JA, Mason R. Pregnancy and sickle cell hemoglobinopathies: results with and without prophylactic transfusions. *Obstet Gynecol.* 1983;62:419.
12. Ricks P Jr. Further experience with exchange transfusion in sickle cell anemia and pregnancy. *Am J Obstet Gynecol.* 1968;100:1087.
13. Koshy M, Burd L, Wallace D, et al. Prophylactic red-cell transfusions in pregnant patients with sickle cell disease: A randomized cooperative study. *N Eng J Med.* 1988;319:1447.

Chapter One Hundred and Fifty-Six

Bleeding

Walter E. Davis

156

Bleeding is a normal response to trauma, but in excess it becomes a life-threatening emergency. Only a few events are as difficult to manage rationally as the development of major bleeding in pregnancy. While some patients may have known bleeding disorders, most report no prior history and present acutely, often with disastrous consequences. Knowledge of the coagulation mechanisms and of the many disorders that may affect them gives physicians the best basis to face emergencies in a pregnant woman and to bring the mother and her fetus unscathed through pregnancy.

NORMAL HEMOSTASIS

Clotting mechanisms allow the blood to flow freely in vessels, but do not permit excessive blood loss with injury. This involves complex interactions of at least four distinct components: vasoconstriction and maintenance of endothelial integrity; platelet adhesiveness and aggregation; fibrin formation; and fibrinolysis. Despite much recent new information on hemostatic mechanisms, the knowledge of control mechanisms and interactions among those four major components remains incomplete. Although one can detail with considerable biochemical sophistication the *in vitro* interactions of individual elements, it is difficult to convey the dynamic interplay among them, proceeding simultaneously, that stops bleeding.

Vascular Component

Probably the least understood component among normal hemostatic mechanisms is the role played by the blood vessels themselves. For many years, one of the classic teachings was that circumferential contraction of a severed vessel with resulting decrease in blood flow represented a major factor in hemostasis. To date, however, no acquired or congenital bleeding disorders attributed to defects in this function have been reported. Although vasoconstriction appears important by decreasing blood flow to a bleeding area, it rarely is adequate to staunch severe bleeding.

Normal intact vascular endothelium is basically a nonthrombogenic surface. Alteration of this surface by disease or trauma will lead promptly to thrombus formation. The subendothelial portion of vessels consists of the basement membrane, elastin, and microfibrils. Thrombus formation occurs in close association with the subendothelial area.

This subendothelial portion of the vessel wall contains collagen as well as a sizable number of other poorly characterized noncollagen glycoproteins. It seems likely that the major contribution of these substances to hemostasis is the induction of platelet adhesion to sites of injury, the initiation and facilitation of platelet aggregation, and directly activating one or more of the contact-phase procoagulants.[1] By providing a catalytic surface, the vessel walls accelerate later phases of fibrin generation. Research in the past decade, using labeling techniques and *in vitro* culture, has demonstrated that endothelial cells have the ability to produce both factor VIII antigen, and Von Willebrand factor.[2] At this time, the functional implications of this are not clear. These observations suggest, however, a complex interdependence of the components of hemostasis.

Platelets

Platelet contributions to hemostasis appear to depend on three processes: the ability to adhere to abnormal vascular surfaces (adhesion); the ability to form firm gel-like plugs (aggregation); and extrusion of intracellular components (secretion). If endothelial surfaces are disrupted, the adhesion of circulating platelets to the area within a few seconds of the injury can be observed. Platelets appear to change shape, form pseudopodia, and adhere to these surfaces. Changes occur in the membranes of adherent platelets that induce further accumulation and formation of small platelet clumps in the area of injury. The aggregate functions as a physical barrier to continued blood loss. During aggregation, secretion of intracellular particles occurs, which is important in amplifying the process of platelet aggregation. This, however, also releases several components of the intrinsic fibrin-generating pathway. The quantitative importance in fibrin generation, relative to circulating components, is not known.[3]

Fibrin Formation

The third and final component of the hemostatic mechanism, fibrin formation, is probably the best understood of the three components. In its most simple form, it can be considered a series of enzymatic steps, sequentially converting circulating zymogens to active enzymes, and resulting in the conversion of fibrinogen to fibrin monomer. Fibrin monomer polymerizes, forming what we recognize macroscopically as a fibrin clot. This stepwise process may begin in two ways: first, an enzyme can be released from damaged tissue and initiate clot formation through interaction with circulating procoagulant proteins; second, activation of clotting can be initiated entirely within the vascular space from contact of circulating procoagulants with subendothelial surfaces. Although the stimulus for fibrin formation usually involves both intrinsic and extrinsic stimuli occurring together, it is easier to detail the mechanism by considering each individually.

The intrinsic pathway of fibrin formation is initiated by the association of factor XII with an, as yet, unidentified component of the subendothelial portion of the vessel wall. The basement membrane is believed to be the most likely anatomic structure involved, but the specific biochemistry of this event is not known.[4] Contact with the basement membrane leads to cleavage of the factor XII molecule to two major products, both of which have enzymatic activity. These activation products (factor XIIa) have the ability to cleave other factor XII molecules and plasma prekallikrein. Plasma prekallikrein, once cleaved or activated by factor XIIa, gains the enzymatic ability to activate further factor XII zymogen. A third participant in the contact stage of intrinsic coagulation is high-molecular-weight kininogen (HMW kininogen). This material functions not enzymatically but catalytically on both of the above reactions. It works as a ligand, binding reactants and facilitating conversion.

The result of the above reactions, termed *contact activation,* is the localized intravascular production of a serine protease, factor XIIa. Factor XIIa, largely bound to HMW kininogen, interacts with factor XI, splitting a peptide, and changing the molecule from two identical peptide chains to two dimers. Each of these dimers, through change in tertiary structure, now has acquired a protease activity that is termed factor XIa. Activated factor XI (factor XIa) produces an enzymatic cleavage of factor IX. Factor IX, a circulating single-chain glycoprotein, is activated by factor XIa, resulting in an active serine protease named factor IXa. This protease conjugates with factor VIII, a phospholipid (supplied at least in part by the platelet membrane), and calcium into a macromolecular complex that has the enzymatic activity needed to activate the next zymogen, factor X. This macromolecular complex is called intrinsic thromboplastin. The steps leading to its production have been termed the first stage of coagulation.

Conceptually, the formation of intrinsic thromboplastin is a branch point. The activation of factor X can occur by way of this stepwise production of intrinsic thromboplastin or through the production of another macromolecular activator, extrinsic thromboplastin. The extrinisic pathway includes Factor VII, a circulating single chain glycoprotein, that complexes with tissue factor (a membrane lipoprotein thought to be released from damaged tissue), and functions as a thromboplastin capable of activating factor X. Thus, there are two pathways leading to activation of factor X: the intrinsic pathway, involving factor XII, XI, prekallikrein, HMW kininogen, factor IX, and factor VIII; and an extrinsic pathway with factor VII and tissue factor. The two pathways converge at the point where factor X is activated and subsequently are identical.

The activation of factor X by either intrinsic or extrinsic thromboplastin complexes involves a stepwise binding of components, and peptide cleavage of factor X from a single to a double chain, with concomitant exposure of its active proteolytic site. The physiology of factor X activation is complex because of autocatalytic and feedback loops associated with both intrinsic and extrinsic pathways, and similar interactions between the two thromboplastin complexes themselves. They result in the formation of activated factor X (factor Xa), a small glycopeptide serine protease. Factor Xa then complexes with a lipoprotein (again thought to be supplied *in vivo* by platelet membranes), circulating factor V, and calcium, forming an enzyme activity capable of cleaving prothrombin (factor II) to thrombin. These two steps, the activation of factor X and its complex formation, with development of prothrombin conversion activity, are termed the second stage of coagulation.

The remainder of the coagulation mechanism involves the cleavage of fibrinogen by thrombin. Thrombin acts on fibrinogen by cleaving stepwise two small peptide fragments called fibrinopeptide A and B. Following release, the resulting fibrin monomer polymerizes, forming chains that make up the macroscopic fibrin clot. Concomitant with its activity on fibrinogen, thrombin splits the alpha chain of fibrin-stabilizing factor (factor XIII), converting it to an active transglutaminase that binds the side chains of lysine and glutamine residues on neighboring fibrin monomers into covalent bonds. This process cross-links the developing fibrin clot and makes it mechanically stable.

Although the sequential activation of circulating zymogen, leading to fibrin formation, is complex, the process is more complicated than outlined above because of the existence of multiple positive and negative feedback loops. In addition to the interaction of product and substrate, there are two other regulatory mechanisms: the antithrombin system, consisting of several components that function to inhibit the activity of procoagulants, and the plasmin system, which fragments fibrin once formed.

DIAGNOSTIC APPROACH TO BLEEDING DISORDERS

As with other medical disorders, the approach to the bleeding patient requires the three basic tools of history, physical examination, and laboratory evaluation. Evaluating bleeding disorders proceeds at two levels: first, it is important to determine when bleeding is inappropriately severe, thus suggesting an underlying defect in hemostasis; second, the cause of the hemostatic defect must be determined.

History

The medical history is focused on three major areas: family history of excessive or abnormal bleeding, a personal history of spontaneous bleeding, and a personal history of excessive bleeding following major or minor trauma. A difficulty in evaluating a patient's history is the inability to quantitate the stimulus that produced the bleeding. Epistaxis, hemoptysis, hematemesis, hematuria, and melena are abnormal but usually are not spontaneous or occur in response to either local trauma or specific local disease. The evaluation of these symptoms requires the search for local factors or diseases. Only in their absence, or the presence of an apparent excessive amount of bleeding, does the consequence suggest an underlying hemostatic defect.

The development of multiple petechiae, usually located on dependent body parts, rarely is caused by trauma or normal stimuli and strongly suggests a bleeding diathesis. Bruises of the skin, whether they are small purpuric lesions or larger ecchymotic lesions, are more difficult to classify as normal or abnormal. As these lesions are nearly always the result of direct trauma, the amount of trauma involved must be considered. Typically, bruises occurring on the arms and legs or small, infrequent lesions represent the result of mild and often forgotten events. Bruises on the trunk and face, if not associated with known trauma, are more likely to represent pathologic events.

Excessive bleeding following surgery (a form of controlled trauma) is easier to evaluate. Intraoperative blood loss can be quantitated roughly, and a general notion as to what is excessive exists. As the patient rarely is aware of the extent of previous intraoperative blood loss, the history regarding surgical blood loss is probably most valuable in regard to the need for blood transfusion following surgery or delivery, or the need to return to the operating room to control bleeding. This history is often most impressive with relatively minor surgery. Examples are: bleeding for several days following tooth extractions, the need to reoperate following tonsillectomy to stop bleeding, or days of bleeding following transurethral resections. The above considerations apply to the individual, but the same line of questioning and evaluation is applied to the patient's family history. As several of the coagulation abnormalities show distinct inheritance patterns, the relationships of affected family members is often more useful than the general knowledge that a single family member was a "bleeder."

Physical Examination

The physical examination is of little assistance in evaluating bleeding diatheses. It can help when petechiae or ecchymoses are visible, and the physical finding of chronic liver disease, malnutrition, or uremia may aid in the evaluation of etiology. Unfortunately, patients with severe disorders may have normal physical findings, giving no clue to the underlying problems to come with surgery or delivery.

Laboratory Studies

Laboratory evaluation of hemostasis is time consuming, expensive, and often inaccurate. Ideally, one would like to have available a small group of inexpensive tests that, if normal, would exclude any bleeding disorder; and another group, sensitive enough to define the etiology of any abnormalities found during screening. The most frequently used group of tests for screening includes platelet count, prothrombin time, partial thromboplastin time (PTT), and the Ivy bleeding time. The four tests together provide what is best termed a reasonable but not entirely satisfactory screening panel. The major argument in favor of using this panel is that at least the initial three tests are widely available at moderate cost. The bleeding time is less frequently used, mostly because it is labor intensive and not a test that can be batched to fit a laboratory work schedule. The major shortcoming of this panel is that, although it is effective in detecting severe abnormalities, it is often normal in less severe but nonetheless significant coagulation abnormalities.

Thrombocytopenia, the most common acquired bleeding diathesis, is detected reliably. Severe or moderate deficiencies and development of inhibitors of the intrinsic coagulation system also are screened reliably. Platelet function disorders and Von Willebrand's disease may or may not be detected, but abnormalities of fibrinolysis and of vascular components usually remain occult. In the current economic environment, it is difficult to advocate that the pregnant patient be screened for every abnormality that may affect the course or outcome of her pregnancy. Given the potential risk bleeding disorders can cause for mother and fetus, it seems good judgment to screen each patient for these disorders when history or physical examination suggests the possibility of a bleeding disorder.

A more detailed evaluation of hemostasis requires a dedicated laboratory. Interpretation of results also requires an understanding of the pitfalls of coagulation tests and of the variations often seen in coagulation disorders.

Abnormalities of the vascular components of hemostasis are identified by demonstrating a normal platelet number and function, normal procoagulant zymogens, and the presence of abnormalities associated with connective tissue disorders, vasculitis, or other systemic illnesses. Competence of the platelet contribution to hemostasis is measured by platelet number and by testing of platelet function with the bleeding time, platelet aggregation, platelet adhesion to synthetic surfaces, and quantitation of products extruded during the platelet release reaction. Abnormalities of the fibrin generating system are detected through quantitation of the individual coagulation factors and functional assays of isolated portions of the coagulation sequence.

The clinical and laboratory tools available to evaluate and treat the patient with a bleeding diathesis thus are extensive, however, they are also imperfect. It is not unusual to encounter a patient whose evaluation suggests no hemostatic abnormalities but who bleeds extensively following trauma, surgery, or delivery. An underlying disorder can elude detection by history or screening studies. One also will encounter patients with a striking history of abnormal bleeding in whom a very extensive laboratory evaluation defines no specific disorder, and yet excessive bleeding occurs or continues. Both situations frustrate the physician but at the same time emphasize the fragmentary knowledge of this field.

MATERNAL CONSIDERATION

By and large, the above discussion of the normal coagulation mechanism and evaluation of bleeding problems applies to both the pregnant and nonpregnant woman. There are, however, several aspects of the hemostatic process that are altered by pregnancy. Late in the first trimester and throughout the remainder of pregnancy, several of the normal circulating procoagulants increase above their usual concentration. Increases in the concentration of the following factors have been described: factor X, VIII, VII, fibrinogen, and plasminogen.[5-7] Factor XIII[7] and antithrombin III[8] have been assayed nonsystematically and found to decrease to some extent. Data concerning changes in factor IX are conflicting, with reports of both increase and decrease during pregnancy.[5,6] The mechanism by which this occurs seems to be an increase in synthesis rather than any change in half-life; most observers have suggested that the change is triggered by increasing estrogen levels. This phenomenon is poorly documented and is thought not to fill any defined physiologic need.

Very rarely, one sees the development of a circulating anticoagulant directed against factor VIII during pregnancy, which may be the cause of a significant bleeding diathesis postpartum.[9] Disseminated intravascular coagulation has many causes, but several are complications of pregnancy. *Abruptio placentae,* retained dead fetus, amniotic fluid embolization, saline-induced or septic abortion, and toxemia all have been associated with the development of this complex coagulation disorder.

FETAL CONSIDERATIONS

It appears that there is no measurable transplacental passage of coagulation factors or platelets.[10] The presence of the procoagulants and elements of the fibrinolytic system in the fetus can be demonstrated by the tenth week of gestation. By 20 weeks' gestation, all but the vitamin K-dependent coagulation factors (II, VII, IX, X) are present in the fetal circulation at nearly the normal adult concentration.[10] In the immediate postpartum period, the concentrations of the vitamin K-dependent factors fall slowly depending on the exogenous provision of vitamin K in the diet.[11] From the midportion of gestation until delivery, the platelet count is maintained at approximately normal adult values and rises slightly following normal delivery.[12] There is evidence of mildly abnormal platelet function immediately following delivery.[13] Whether this abnormality is present during a significant portion of the fetal existence is unknown.

There is little evidence to suggest abnormal bleeding because of coagulation abnormalities in the fetus. The cause of spontaneous abortion and intrauterine death is often unclear, and at times evidence of fetal hemorrhage is found. Whether this intrafetal hemorrhage is related to a coagulation abnormality or is the result of other fetal abnormalities is not known. The incidence of miscarriage in pregnancies in which the fetus ultimately is found to have one of the congenital coagulation factor deficiencies is not significantly different from that in the population at large. This suggests that intrauterine fetal hemorrhage is not usually the result of a congenital bleeding diathesis.[14]

It is in the immediate newborn period that coagulation abnormalities are more likely to be seen as a result of the trauma associated with passage through the birth canal. One may see considerable bruising associated with traumatic delivery in the fetus with coagulation factor deficiencies or thrombocytopenia. Surprisingly, prolonged bleeding from the severed umbilical stump is not very frequent and is seen most commonly with the extremely rare factor XIII deficiency.[15] For reasons that are unclear, the severe congenital coagulation factor deficiencies usually do not manifest in the immediate postpartum period unless there is an extraordinary amount of trauma associated with the birth itself.

REFERENCES

1. Tschopp TB, Baumgartner HR, Silberauer K, et al. Platelet adhesion and platelet thrombus formation on subendothelium of human arteries and veins exposed to flowing blood in vitro: a comparison with rabbit aorta. *Haemostasis.* 1979;8:19.
2. Jaffe EA, Hoyer LW, Nachmann RL. Synthesis of von Willebrand factor by cultured human endothelial cells. *Proc Nat Acad Sci.* 1974;71:1906.
3. Mann KG. Membrane-bound enzyme complexes in blood coagulation. *Prog Hemost Thromb.* 1984;7:1.
4. Griffin JH. The role of surface in the surface-dependent activation of Hageman factor (blood coagulation factor XII). *Proc Nat Acad Sci.* 1978;75:1998.
5. Beller FK, Ebert. The coagulation and fibrinolytic enzyme system in pregnancy and in the puerperium. *Eur J Obstet Gynecol Reprod Biol.* 1982;13:177.
6. Hellgren M, Blomback M. Studies on blood coagulation and fibrinolysis in pregnancy, during delivery and in the puerperium. *Gynecol Obstet Invest.* 1981;12:141.
7. Gjonnaess H, Fagorhol MK. Studies on coagulation and fibrinolysis in pregnancy. *Acta Obstet Gynecol Scand.* 1975;54:363.
8. Weenink GH, Treffers PE, Kahle LH, Ten Cate W. Antithrombin III in normal pregnancy. *Thromb Res.* 1982;26:281.
9. Voke J, Letsky E. Pregnancy and antibody to Factor VIII. *J Clin Pathol.* 1977;30:928.
10. Terwiel J. Veltkamp JJ, Bernina RM, Muller HP. Coagulation factors in the human fetus of about 20 weeks gestational age. *Br J Haematol.* 1980;45:641.
11. Muntean W. Petek, Rosanelli K, Mutz ID. Immunologic studies of prothrombin in newborns. *Pediatr Res.* 1979;13:1262.
12. Sell EJ, Corrigan JJ. Platelet counts, fibrinogen concentrations, and factor V and VIII levels in healthy infants according to gestational age. *J Pediatr.* 1973;82:1028.
13. Stuart MJ, Dusse J, Clark DA, Walenga RW. Differences in thromboxane production between neonatal and adult platelets in response to arachidonic acid and epinephrine. *Pediatric Res.* 1984;18:823.
14. Mammen EF. Factor V deficiency. *Seminars in Thromb Hemostasis.* 1983;9:17.
15. Hathaway WE, Bonnar J. *Perinatal Coagulation.* New York: Grune & Stratton; 1978:53.

Chapter One Hundred and Fifty-Seven

Conditions of Lymph Nodes and Spleen

Walter E. Davis

157

Lymph nodes and spleen often are considered together because of their structural and functional similarities. Although both can be thought of as filters of either blood or lymph, they are complex structures whose general functions are to remove foreign or damaged elements from the blood or lymph. They also provide a structural framework for a major portion of the body's immunologic response.

NORMAL ANATOMY AND PHYSIOLOGY

Lymph nodes are encapsulated and interrupt lymphatic vessels at various sites. There the lymph flow is directed through a series of channels where it is in contact with immunologically competent cells and phagocytic cells. Lymph nodes can range in size from several millimeters to 2 cm, are bean-shaped; and arteries, veins, and the efferent lymphatic channels exit from their substance at the hilum. Afferent lymphatic channels discharge their contents around the periphery of the node into a prominent subcapsular sinus.

The majority of the node itself consists of a network of branching reticulin fibers where large numbers of macrophages and lymphocytes attach. Lymphocytes reach the node from the peripheral blood. It also is believed that macrophages arise elsewhere and are transported to the node as blood monocytes.[1] Radial sinuses carry the afferent lymph toward the hilum of the node, where the sinuses coalesce and form the efferent vessel.

Lymph nodes are not homogeneous but show a functional organization of their lymphatic components.[2] B lymphocytes, with their predominant function of antibody production, are clustered into nodules or germinal centers located in the cortex of the node. T lymphocytes, which mediate cellular immunity and modulate B cell function, are found circumferentially adjacent to the germinal centers. Phagocytes and macrophages are scattered at random throughout the cortex and medulla of the node.

The spleen filters blood through a large capillary bed that is lined with lymphatic tissue. Blood enters the capsule and is carried by a series of arterioles through a rich lymphatic tissue called white pulp. It then is discharged near the periphery into a large series of sinuses that collect at the hilum and discharge their content into the portal circulation by way of the splenic vein. Thus, the spleen, like lymph nodes, functions to bring blood-borne foreign material and potential antigens into contact with these phagocytic and immunocompetent effector cells.

In addition to its role as a site of intense immunologic and phagocytic function, the spleen also functions as a major site for the removal of senescent or abnormal red blood cells.[3] This function is complex and involves peculiar characteristics of vascular endothelium in the splenic arterioles and sinusoids that the red cell must traverse to reenter the circulation. These areas have a relatively low oxygen concentration and thus require the red cells to expend energy reserves to maintain their internal environment. This also requires considerable deformability and flexibility of the red cell membranes to traverse these small and irregular spaces. As the red cell ages, its capacity to tolerate such an inhospitable environment and to undergo deformation without rupture of the membrane decreases. If the cell is unable to traverse the splenic sinuses, it is phagocytized and removed permanently from the circulation.

EVALUATION OF SPLENIC ENLARGEMENT

Splenic enlargement usually is detected with physical examination by palpating the lower pole below the left costal margin. About 3% of the normal population will have a palpable spleen.[4-6] Members of the group with minimal splenic enlargement usually have tall and thin body structure, and mostly represent people with slightly larger-than-average spleens which are often more anteriorly placed than usual. In patients who are obese, pregnant, or have ascites, the spleen may be two to four times normal size before it is palpated. Splenomegaly often is detected by x-ray or ultrasound. It is best defined by nuclear scanning, but its configuration and the presence or absence of abnormal tissue is seen best with computerized tomography (CT) scanning.

CAUSES OF SPLENIC ENLARGEMENT

There are several mechanisms that cause splenic enlargement. Disorders that impair venous outflow cause congestion and consequent enlargement. Thrombosis or compression of the splenic vein are obvious causes, but most frequently enlargement by congestion is caused by disease of the liver with subsequent development of portal hypertension. The spleen can enlarge because a disease stimulates normal splenic function, be it an immunologic response to infection or an increase in phagocytosis, as with hemolytic anemia. Enlargement also may occur because of infiltration of the spleen with benign tissue, such as granulomata or with malignant cells.

The syndrome of hypersplenism may develop as a complication of any disease that results in splenomegaly. Hypersplenism is primarily a hematologic syndrome characterized by any combination of granulocytopenia, thrombocytopenia, and anemia—associated with splenic enlargement. It resolves with the return of the spleen to normal size or its removal. This syndrome is associated with increased production of cellular elements of the blood and their sequestration or destruction by the enlarged spleen. The anemia is usually mild to moderate. Thrombocytopenia and granulocytopenia may, however, become severe, and bleeding from thrombocytopenia is probably the most common severe consequence. Granulocytopenia rarely leads to frequent or overwhelming infection except in the case of Felty's syndrome (hypersplenism caused by rheumatoid arthritis), in which some degree of immunologic granulocyte injury appears to exist in addition to hypersplenism.[7]

The cause of splenomegaly is established by first seeking evidence of the more common systemic illnesses with which it is associated. Liver disease, infectious diseases,

TABLE 157–1. CAUSES OF SPLENIC ENLARGEMENT

Infections
Viral (mononucleosis, hepatitis, CMV, Toxo)
Bacterial (typhoid, SBE)
Granulomatous (TB, coccidiomycosis, histoplasmosis)
Parasitic (malaria, trypanosomiasis, schistosomiasis)
Vascular Congestion
Splenic or portal vein thrombosis
Liver disease
Collagen Vascular Disease
Rheumatoid arthritis
Systemic lupus erythematosus
Hemolytic Anemia
Congenital
Acquired
Infiltrative Diseases
Sarcoidosis
Lipidoses
Neoplastic Diseases
Lymphoma
Myeloproliferative disorders
Histiocytosis
Metastatic carcinoma and sarcoma

and hematologic disorders are the most common causes in nontropical areas. Thus, evaluation of blood counts and film, liver function studies, serologic evaluation for viral illness, and search for enlarged lymph nodes usually lead to the diagnosis. If this approach does not yield a diagnosis, ultrasound or CT scanning may help. The last option is diagnosis by pathologic study after splenectomy. Although most treatable diseases are diagnosed without splenectomy, a splenic neoplasm may be found only with surgical removal. If a cause for splenomegaly can not be found, it is wise to observe the patient carefully during the remainder of her pregnancy and proceed to splenic removal at the termination of the pregnancy. Common causes of splenic enlargement are shown in Table 157–1.

TREATMENT OF SPLENIC ENLARGEMENT

Since splenic enlargement is not a disease process in itself but rather a manifestation of systemic disease, there is no specific treatment. Treatment is directed at the underlying disease process, with appropriate caution based on the coexisting pregnancy. Following splenectomy, vaccination with a pneumococcal preparation is recommended to prevent the potentially fatal overwhelming pneumococcal sepsis that is a rare sequella of splenic removal. This is seen most commonly in children with sickle cell disease whose spleen is nonfunctioning because of multiple infarcts. It can occur, however, with surgical removal of the spleen.[8]

EVALUATION OF LYMPH NODE ENLARGEMENT

Lymph node enlargement is a normal response to antigenic stimulation, and thus may be a normal finding. It is normal for regional lymph nodes to enlarge following inflammation, infection, or foreign body introduction into the area that normally drains to the involved lymph nodes. Patients with localized lymph node enlargement should first be carefully examined to determine if there is local infection or inflammation. Lymph nodes enlarged from such a cause should resolve slowly with treatment of the local problem, but the rate of resolution may be measured in weeks. If lymph nodes are resolving gradually, observation alone is sufficient.

Determining the cause of enlarged nodes in the absence of a local condition requires the identification of a systemic disease that may cause lymph node enlargement. Diagnosis may be only possible through surgical removal and pathologic study. Recently, the cytologic study of material, removed by needle aspirate, is becoming more accurate and useful. It is always difficult to determine how quickly after its appearance an enlarged lymph gland should be biopsied. Large or rapidly enlarging nodes without evident etiology should be biopsied promptly. Small nodes or fluctuating node size often can be watched safely for several weeks before biopsy.

TABLE 157–2. CAUSES OF LYMPH NODE ENLARGEMENT

Reaction to Immunologic Stimuli
Local infection (cellulitis, abscess)
Systemic infection (mononucleosis, AIDS, TB)
Foreign substance (serum sickness)
Neoplastic Infiltration
Lymphoma
Leukemia
Metastatic carcinoma and sarcoma
Idiopathic Disorders
Collagen vascular disease
Sarcoidosis
Drug reactions
Hyperthyroidism

CAUSES OF LYMPH NODE ENLARGEMENT

The lymph nodes enlarge when the number of lymphocytes contained in the nodes increases. This occurs when the lymphocytes in the lymph node respond to antigenic stimulation. This mechanism accounts for the lymph node enlargement that is seen when bacteria or foreign material is carried into the lymph node from disruption of the skin or development of a local infection. Most infections result in attempts at an immunologic response, but not all infections cause generalized lymph node enlargement. It is not clear what characteristic of the infecting organism leads to this generalized enlargement. In some infections, such as infectious mononucleosis, the organism can be identified in the nodes, but in others, this is not demonstrated.

The reason that lymph nodes enlarge in collagen vascular disease presumably represents hypertrophy of lymphoid tissue in response to some unidentified antigen. Enlargement in several of the idiopathic causes shown in Table 157–2 is unexplained.

REFERENCES

1. Brooks DA, et al. Membrane antigens of human cell of the monocyte/macrophage lineage studied with monoclonal antibodies. *Pathology.* 1983;15:45.
2. Galton DA, MacLennan IC. Clinical patterns in B lymphoid malignancy. *Clin Haematol.* 1982;11:561.
3. Wagner HN Jr, et al. Removal of erythrocytes from the circulation. *Arch Intern Med.* 1962;110:90.

4. Schloesser LL. The diagnostic significance of splenomegaly. *Am J Med Sci.* 1963;245:84.
5. McIntyre OR, Ebaugh FG Jr. Palpable spleens in college freshmen. *Ann Int Med.* 1967;66:301.
6. Ebaugh FG Jr, McIntyre OR. Palpable spleens: ten-year follow-up. *Ann Int Med.* 1979;90:130.
7. Brunner CM, Davis JS. Characteristics of antinuclear factors in Felty's Syndrome. *Arthritis Rheum.* 1970;13:33.
8. Ammann AJ. Polyvalent pneumococcal-polysaccharide immunization of patients with sickle-cell anemia and patients with splenectomy. *N Eng J Med.* 1977;297:897.

B

RED BLOOD CELL DISORDERS

Chapter One Hundred and Fifty-Eight
Red Blood Cell Disorders

John C. Morrison

158

Hemoglobin is contained in all red blood cells and is a complex protein composed of four prosthetic groups called heme, each bound to a polypeptide chain. Proper function of hemoglobin in the red blood cell is critical for oxygen transport. The heme portion of the molecule is synthesized in most tissues. The globin chains are produced in reticuloendothelial sites and in the bone marrow. Human red blood cells contain at least three different types of hemoglobin, all having two α chains and a pair of β ($HbA\text{-}\alpha_2\beta_2$), α ($HbF\text{-}\alpha_2\gamma_2$), or δ ($HbA_2\text{-}\alpha_2\delta_2$) chains. These protein chains are differentiated from one another by their combinations and numbers of amino acids.[1]

Red blood cell disorders may be divided into those associated with diminished red cell production, increased blood loss, or increased erythrocyte destruction (Table 158–1). The direct effects of red blood cell abnormalities on the mother and fetus and neonate are determined mostly by the severity of the effect of the erythrocyte disorder on oxygenation. Indirectly, these abnormalities may drastically effect maternal homeostasis, which will adversely affect the progeny. The following chapters define the etiologic categories of erythrocyte disorders as well as their diagnosis and management.

TABLE 158–1. RED BLOOD CELL DISORDERS DURING PREGNANCY

Decreased Erythrocyte Production	Increased Erythrocyte Loss	Increased Erythrocyte Destruction
Iron deficiency	Hemorrhage	Hemoglobinopathies
Thalassemia	Parasites	Hemolytic anemias
Chronic disease	Hemorrhoids	Chemical toxicity
Bone marrow failure		
Folate deficiency		
Inflammatory processes		
Malignancy		

REFERENCE

1. Kaplan BH, Hunt T, London IM. The synthesis of heme and protein (globin). In: Williams WJ, Buetler E, Ersler AJ, et al, eds. *Hematology*. New York: McGraw-Hill; 1977:149.

Chapter One Hundred and Fifty-Nine
Iron Deficiency Anemia

G. Rodney Meeks, Kathy Gookin, and John C. Morrison

159

ETIOLOGY

Anemia is the most frequent maternal complication diagnosed during pregnancy. By World Health Organization (WHO) standards, anemia during pregnancy is defined as a hemoglobin (Hb) concentration ≤13.0 g/dL. Using this definition, anemia complicates over 50% of all gestations in the United States.[1] Although a combination of etiologies may cause anemia during pregnancy, iron deficiency is by far the most common. Of pregnant women with an abnormally low Hb concentration and packed cell volume (PCV), 75–85% have iron deficiency anemia (IDA).[2] Increased requirements, as with pregnancy, or inadequate dietary intake of iron may lead to varying degrees of iron depletion. If iron depletion is profound, IDA occurs. Some degree of iron depletion appears to be almost universal during pregnancy. The problem is compounded by multiple gestations, successive short-pregnancy intervals (<2–3 years apart), adolescent pregnancy, chronic blood loss, intravascular hemolysis, and poor iron absorption associated with certain medical conditions.

PATHOPHYSIOLOGY

Several iron compartments have been described based on anatomic distribution, chemical characteristics, and physiologic function. The largest compartment is Hb in the red blood cell mass.[3] In the iron-sufficient gravida, Hb iron expands by approximately 500 mg as the red cell mass enlarges to meet the increased metabolic demands of pregnancy. Storage iron is divided equally between ferritin and hemosiderin; the former represents iron absorption, the latter iron balance.[3] The transport iron is the smallest but kinetically the most active compartment.[3] Transport iron is bound to transferrin, which increases during pregnancy and is estrogen-dependent. Myoglobin (muscle protein) iron, parenchymal (enzyme and tissue) iron, and the labile iron pool are not altered significantly by pregnancy. During pregnancy two additional compartments exist: the fetus and the placenta. These compartments contain approximately 275 mg and 25 mg of iron, respectively, at term.[1]

Approximately 1 mg of iron each day is lost through desquamation of intestinal villus cells, perspiration, and desquamation of skin. This basal loss and the requirements for normal pregnancy approximate 1.2 g of elemental iron and must be met by iron absorption. A North American diet of 1800–2000 kcal ordinarily provides 11–14 mg of iron, which compensates basal losses.[4] Elemental ferrous iron salts, hemoglobin from animal food sources, and ferric iron (Fe^{3+}) from vegetable complexes are often present in the diet. As much as 20–40% of heme iron may be absorbed; however, meat forms only a small fraction of the normal diet, especially in disadvantaged populations.[3] Relatively small amounts of iron are available in cereal grain, and ordinarily <5% of cereal grain iron is absorbed. It may be increased, however, to 30% in the presence of ascorbic acid or meat.[3] Because iron can be absorbed only in the ferrous form (Fe^{2+}), a diet rich in Fe^{2+} is best, since no alteration is necessary for absorption. However, once Fe^{2+} is incorporated into the intestinal cells, it must be oxidized to Fe^{3+} for utilization.

EFFECTS OF PREGNANCY ON DISEASE

During the first 20 weeks of pregnancy, iron requirements are elevated slightly. However, during the second half of pregnancy, iron requirements rise dramatically as maternal red cell mass increases, fetal needs accelerate, and placental demand intensifies. Dietary iron absorption increases each trimester to meet the demand. During the first trimester, approximately 10% of iron is absorbed; this increases to 25% and 30% in the second and third trimesters, respectively.[5] The demands of pregnancy cannot be met by dietary iron alone, even with the increased efficiency of absorption or by using iron stores, which are at best 300 mg in most young women.[6] Therefore, pregnant women must have iron supplementation. If IDA is present during gestation, the demands of pregnancy worsen the clinical picture. In cases where iron depletion is present, without signs of deficiency, frank IDA may develop during or after the gestation (Figure 159–1).

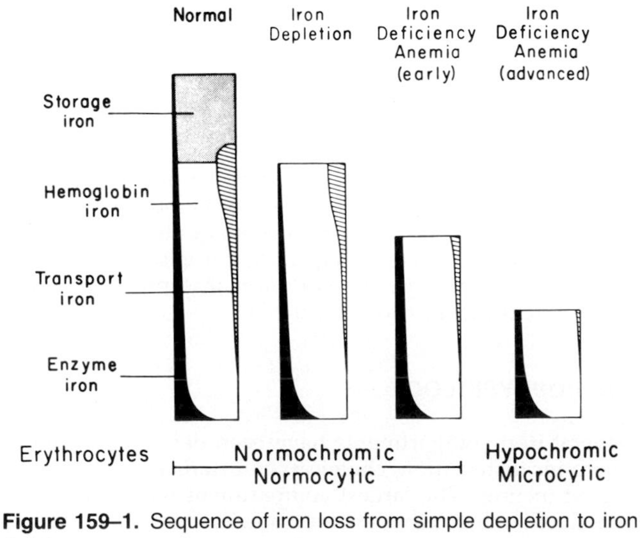

Figure 159–1. Sequence of iron loss from simple depletion to iron deficiency.

EFFECTS OF DISEASE ON PREGNANCY

Maternal Effects

As iron deficiency develops, fatigue, irritability, and malaise appear and, in many cases, precede hematologic laboratory signs. Since pregnancy is associated with some of the same generalized complaints as anemia, patients may note no additional symptoms when anemia develops slowly. Severity of symptoms correlates poorly with Hb concentration in patients with IDA. As iron deficiency worsens, headache, parathesias, burning of the tongue, and pica may develop, probably because tissue iron is lost. Pallor, glossitis, stomatitis, cheilitis, koilonychia, retinal hemorrhages, splenomegaly, and shortness of breath may be encountered if the Hb is <5 g/dL.[2] Decreased oxygenation of tissues and high output congestive heart failure may be life-threatening.

Iron deficiency anemia has been associated with postpartum hemorrhage, increased incidence of operative delivery, *abruptio placenta*, and *placenta praevia*. However, a causal relationship cannot be made because of confounding variables such as poor nutritional status, smoking, inadequate prenatal care, and socioeconomically disadvantaged background. Severe anemia is associated with placenta hypertrophy and pregnancy-induced hypertension.

Fetal Effects

Fetal iron deficiency is seen rarely if ever because iron is preferentially transferred to the placenta and the fetus even in severe maternal deficiency states. No detrimental fetal effects of mild to moderate maternal iron deficiency have been documented. However, severe IDA (Hb <6.5 g/dL) has been associated with fetal growth retardation and stillbirths as well as hypertension.[7] The fetus ordinarily stores enough iron to meet requirements for three to six months of extrauterine life. Following this time, the infant needs to have iron supplementation to avoid iron depletion.[8] Iron deprivation, even to a mild degree, in the first two years of life has been associated with poor attention span and cooperativeness during mental/developmental testing.[9]

DIAGNOSIS OF IRON DEFICIENCY ANEMIA DURING PREGNANCY

Hemoglobin concentration <13 G/dL or PCV <35% should alert the clinician to the possibility of IDA.[1] The reticulocyte count normally averages 1–2% during pregnancy, and values <1% characteristically are seen with iron deficiency.[1] Peripheral blood smears may show poikilocytosis (pear-shaped cells), schistocytes (red cell fragments), basophilic stippling, and hypochromic, microcytic erythrocytes (Figure 159–2). The mean corpuscular hemoglobin concentration

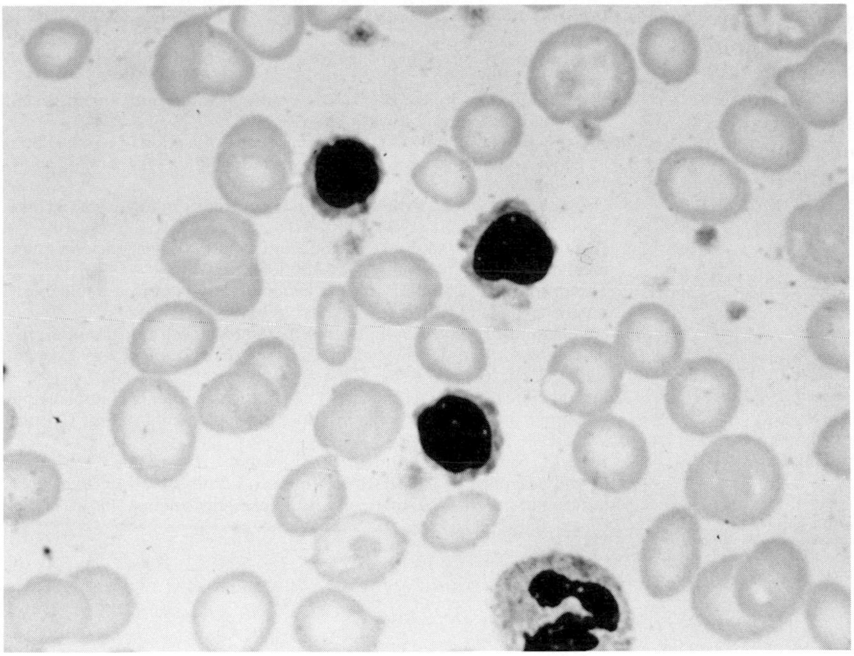

Figure 159–2. Smear revealing hypochromic red blood cells.

(MCHC) is a reliable index, and values <30% usually indicate IDA.[4] However, use of mean corpuscular volume (MCV) and mean corpuscular hemoglobin (MCH) to diagnosis IDA are negated because of disproportionate changes in plasma volume and red cell mass during pregnancy. Serum iron normally decreases with advancing gestational age in relation to increased iron requirements of the fetus, exhausted iron stores in the mother, and increased maternal iron utilization. However, values <60 μg/dL indicate IDA, and values <30 μg/dL are virtually diagnostic.[1] An increase in transferrin, as measured by the unsaturated iron binding capacity (UIBC), can be seen as early as the third month of gestation and ranges from 280 to 400 μg/dL.[2] A UIBC >400 μg/dL suggests iron deficiency. Increased iron utilization leads to a decrease in transferrin saturation from 25–35% in the nonpregnant state to 15–30% during pregnancy. A transferrin saturation <15% indicates iron deficiency.[9] Serum ferritin, which reflects iron stores, is normally 55–70 μg/L during pregnancy, and values <10 μg/L are diagnostic of iron deficiency.[9] Zinc may replace iron in the protoporphyrin ring. Measurement of red cell zinc protoporphyrin is a rapid, low cost, and accurate predictor of IDA.[11] Normal levels of serum iron, UIBC, transferrin saturation, and serum ferritin eliminate iron deficiency as the cause of anemia.

TREATMENT

Treatment of IDA during pregnancy is not appreciably different than in the nonpregnant state. Iron requirements are, however, significantly higher during pregnancy. Eighty percent of normal pregnant women, if not given supplemental iron, have Hb values <11.0 g/dL at term.[1] Prophylactic iron supplementation and proper diet during pregnancy can preclude IDA. In the iron-sufficient gravida, administration of 30–60 mg of elemental iron as ferrous sulfate is adequate, but 200–300 mg is necessary in iron deficiency states.[3] Nausea, vomiting, abdominal cramps, and constipation may be associated with ferrous salts, although they are also common complaints of pregnancy. Absorption can be enhanced by taking iron with meals because postprandial stomach acidity, vitamin C, and meat increase absorption. In addition, gastrointestinal (GI) side effects may be decreased with prandial administration.

The newer iron preparations demonstrate no definite advantage over traditional ferrous sulfate. Iron preparations combined with vitamins are no more effective.[11] When GI side effects from oral tablets or capsules are severe, ferrous sulfate syrups may be substituted. Previously enteric-coated capsules were thought to be poorly absorbed because they release iron into the jejunum and ileum where it is not absorbed efficiently.[3] However, it has now been shown that approximately 80% of the iron in these preparations is absorbed even though the lower small bowel is less efficient than the duodenum in absorbing iron. These compounds may have a role in those women who have significant gastrointestinal side effects from the traditional iron preparations. Elemental iron complexed with carbohydrates may be given intramuscularly or intravascularly but is indicated in very few patients. These include the noncompliant woman, the patient with severe IDA, those with severe GI side effects, and parturients with absorptive disorders. Pruritis, malaise, or a metallic taste occurs in approximately 10% of patients receiving parenteral therapy, and severe reactions such as fetal growth abnormalities, renal toxicity, bronchospasm, anaphylaxis, hemolysis or disseminated intravascular coagulation may occur.[13] Occasionally, PCV <24% or Hb <8 g/dL is treated best by transfusion. This is especially true when rapid anemia correction is necessary, such as in a patient who must undergo a cesarean birth or other surgical procedure. It must be emphasized, however, that most women can be treated adequately with oral iron supplementation. Iron supplementation appears to be safe for the fetus when given during the entire course of gestation, just prior to delivery, or during lactation.

A therapeutic trial of iron for those with mild-to-moderate anemia should be instituted unless a more severe hematologic disease is suspected. It is an inexpensive, noninvasive method of diagnosis and also safe during pregnancy. An increase in the corrected reticulocyte count occurs within 7–10 days after initiation of therapy. Within 3–5 weeks, changes in the blood smear occur with a return of chromicity and normal size. By 6–8 weeks, PCV and Hb concentration begin to increase, and by 7–9 weeks, red blood cell indices return to normal. If these changes do not occur, the patient should be reexamined and another cause of anemia considered.

REFERENCES

1. Gookin K, Morrison JC. Anemia associated with pregnancy. In: Depp R, Eschenbach DA, eds. *Gynecology and Obstetrics: Maternal and Fetal Medicine, Vol. 3 (16)*. New York: Harper & Row; 1989:1.
2. Fairbanks VF, Beutler E. Iron deficiency. In: Williams WJ, Beutler E, Ersler AJ, et al, eds. *Hematology*. New York, NY: McGraw-Hill; 1977:366.
3. Finch CA, Huebers H. Perspectives in iron metabolism. *N Engl J Med*. 1982;306:1520.
4. Gookin KS, Morrison JC. Nutritional anemias complicating pregnancy. In: Laros RK Jr, ed. *Blood Disorders in Pregnancy*. Philadelphia: Lea & Febiger; 1986:19.
5. Bjorn-Rasmussen E. Iron absorption: present knowledge and controversies. *Lancet*. 1983;1:914.
6. Pritchard JA, Mason RA. Iron stores of normal adults and replenishment with oral iron therapy. *JAMA*. 1964;190:897.
7. Murphy JF, Newcombe RG, O'Riordan J, et al. Relation of haemoglobin levels in first and second trimesters to outcome of pregnancy. *Lancet*. 1986;1:992.
8. Dallman PR, Siimes MA, Stekel A. Iron deficiency in infancy and childhood. *Am J Clin Nutr*. 1980;33:86.
9. Walter T, Kovalskys J, Stekel A. Effect of mild iron deficiency on infant mental development scores. *J Pediatr*. 1983;102:519.
10. Thompson WG. Comparison of tests for diagnosis of iron depletion in pregnancy. *Am J Obstet Gynecol*. 1988;159:1132.
11. Schifman RB, Thomasson JE, Evers JM. Red blood cell zinc protoporphyrin testing for iron-deficiency anemia in pregnancy. *Am J Obstet Gynecol*. 1987;157:304.
12. Seligman PA, Caskey JH, Frazier JL, et al. Measurements of iron absorption from prenatal multivitamin-mineral supplements. *Obstet Gynecol*. 1983;61:356.
13. Kaisi M, Ngwalle EW, Runyoro DE, Rogers J. Evaluation of tolerance of and response to iron dextran (inferon) administered by total dose infusion to pregnant women with iron deficiency anemia. *Int J Gynaecol Obstet*. 1988;26:235.

Chapter One Hundred and Sixty

Megaloblastic Anemias

James N. Martin, Jr. and Joe C. Files

160

ETIOLOGY

The megaloblastic anemias are a group of disorders associated with a common characteristic morphology, ineffective hematopoiesis, and moderate hemolysis of circulating red cells. The underlying biochemical defect is impaired thymidylate formation, an essential rate-limiting preliminary step in the deoxyribonucleic acid (DNA) synthesis of all body cells that require tetrahydrofolic acid as a coenzyme. The incidence of folic acid deficiency varies considerably among obstetric populations. Late in gestation, it may be as frequent as 95% in some English populations, 60% in one Australian study, and 30–69% in several socioeconomically depressed populations in the United States. World Health Organization (WHO) studies suggest that one in three women worldwide suffers from folic acid deficiency.[1] Less frequent in all populations is the occurrence of frank megaloblastic anemia, which is estimated to occur variably in approximately 1 in 70 to 1 in 250 pregnancies.

FOLIC ACID DEFICIENCY

Physiology and Pathophysiology

The folates are a group of related pteridine (pterin) compounds in the water-soluble vitamin B complex family. They are essential nutrients for human growth and reproduction and must be acquired from dietary sources such as leafy green vegetables, peanuts, yeast, and meats. Folate in food is in the form of folic acid (pteryolglutamic acid), which is conjugated to a number of glutamic acid residues. These must be cleaved from the folic molecule prior to absorption in the proximal third of the intestine. Folic acid is heat labile, and extensive cooking of foods, especially in large volumes of water, will extract or destroy up to 90% of it. Most of the limited body stores are contained in the liver and normally are sufficient for four to six weeks. Tissue folate stores are homeostatically maintained in excess of minimum body requirements. The daily requirement of 50 μg folate for the nonpregnant individual is increased to 150–350 μg per day during pregnancy.

In a folate- or vitamin B_{12}-deficient state, nuclear maturation and mitotic activity are delayed, although cytoplasmic development progresses normally. Cell division is decreased, and enlarged cells are produced with an increased cytoplasmic RNA-to-nuclear-DNA ratio. Hence, red cell precursors are retarded in formation, and intramedullary and extramedullary hemolysis ensues with the development of anemia. Although erythrocyte formation is most obviously impaired, dysplastic maturation of leukocytes and platelets also occurs, leading to leukopenia and thrombocytopenia in cases of severe disease. The cause of most megaloblastic anemia in pregnancy is chronic deficiency of metabolically active folate (MA-folate), as vitamin B_{12} deficiency (MA-B_{12}) is extremely rare in gestation.[2-8]

Effects of Pregnancy on the Disease

Pregnancy aggravates folic acid depletion. This finding is attributable to several factors.[1-8] Most important is an increased demand for the vitamin by the trophoblast, the rapidly developing fetus, and the expanding maternal red cell mass. Inadequate nutrition from poor eating habits or a compromised socioeconomic condition are also major factors. Complications of pregnancy such as prolonged hyperemesis, persistent gastroenteritis, unusual diets, prior upper gastrointestinal tract surgery, and malabsorption states will limit absorption. Slowed gastrointestinal absorption of folate during gestation may be secondary to increased circulating levels of estrogen and progesterone. Concomitant infection of any type, a coexisting chronic hemolytic anemia, the presence of multiple fetuses, or several recent closely spaced pregnancies can substantially increase maternal requirements. Usage by the pregnant patient of any of several drugs including the anticonvulsant phenytoin, ethanol, or certain antibiotics such as nitrofuradantoin and trimethoprim is associated with impaired absorption, utilization, or metabolism of folate. Finally, prolonged lactation following pregnancy can be a contributing factor in puerperal women on folate-poor diets.

The folate-deficient gravida develops overt megaloblastic anemia in an insidious manner over an extended period of time. Roughly 50% of cases of megaloblastic anemia in pregnancy develop prior to delivery, and the remainder are detected in the puerperal period. During pregnancy, most folate deficiency presents in the third trimester unless there is an associated medical disorder with unusually high folate requirements. The primary direct consequences of severe gestational folate deficiency are megaloblastic anemia, an increased risk of transfusion therapy, and possibly an increased risk of hemorrhage secondary to thrombocytopenia.

Effects on the Mother, Fetus, and Newborn

Although severe folate deficiency in experimental animals has been associated with a greater than expected frequency of pregnancy abnormalities and pregnancy wastage, extensive human studies have not revealed a definite cause-and-effect relationship between maternal folate deficiency and fetal malformation, prematurity, *abruptio placenta*, preeclampsia, or other fetal or perinatal morbidity or mortality.

Despite even severe degrees of maternal folate deficiency (MA-folate), the human fetus maintains normal hemoglobin and folate levels by selective transfer of needed nutrients and vitamins at the mother's expense. Thus, at birth the infant of a mother suffering from a prolonged and severe state of folate deficiency usually is not anemic and appears unaffected. Nevertheless, maintenance of optimal maternal folate stores may be of unmeasurable quantitative as well as qualitative benefit to the developing fetus. Pritchard's finding[9] that severe megaloblastic anemia during pregnancy frequently is accompanied by a smaller blood volume than that of a normal pregnancy may be related to a purportedly slower fetal growth rate observed in some folate-deficient gestations.[10]

Diagnosis

Gestational megaloblastic anemia caused by MA-folate usually is suspected from history and clinical presentation, but can be confused with preeclampsia complicated by thrombocytopenia and increased LDH concentrations as seen with severe preeclampsia and HELLP syndrome (see also Chapter 139). Folic acid deficiency can be associated with pancytopenia or just thrombocytopenia or leukopenia.[11,12] Life-threatening thrombocytopenia rarely occurs.[13] The typical affected parturient is socioeconomically and nutritionally deprived, multiparous, severely anemic, and late in gestation without antecedent prenatal care. There are no firmly established, universally accepted laboratory criteria defining this type of gestational anemia. In the absence of concomitant iron deficiency, mild MA-folate is characterized by low-fasting serum folate (<3 ng/mL by radioassay) and neutrophilic nuclear hypersegmentation (average lobe value of $\geq$ 3.27 or more than 4% with 5 lobes or one with 6 lobes in 100 consecutive polymorphonuclear neutrophils). Serum folate values in pregnant women generally are considerably lower than those in nonpregnant women and progressively decrease toward term; neutrophilic hypersegmentation is the more sensitive indicator of folate deficiency.

In more severe deficiency states, red cell macrocytosis, elevated serum iron concentration, elevated LDH (particularly LDH-1 and LDH-2 isoenzyme fractions), and elevated transferrin saturation are noted. Assay of a very low erythrocyte folate activity (<20 ng/mL) has been suggested to be the best biochemical index of folic acid deficiency. Anemia, changes in red cell indices, and aberrant red cell morphology generally are poor diagnostic tests because they represent late changes and do not accurately reflect the current degree of folate deficiency. The peripheral blood smear (Figure 160–1) is suggestive but not diagnostic, revealing hypersegmented neutrophils, a dimorphic red cell population with many macrocytes, as well as a relative scarcity of neutrophils and platelets. Because it does not distinguish between MA-folate and MA-B_{12}, bone marrow aspiration for differential diagnosis of MA-disorders is not performed routinely in pregnancy. Gastrointestinal, vaginal and cervical epithelium also reflect megaloblastic changes and can be misread, for instance, as cervical dysplasia on pap smear. The diagnosis of MA-folate also can be confirmed by demonstrating a rapid and predictable response to orally administered folate.

Treatment

Effective treatment should include the administration of enough folic acid to produce a maximal hematologic response, replenish body stores, and provide the minimal daily requirement. An overall treatment plan does not differ from that used in the nonpregnant state and should include adequate folic acid to accomplish these objectives, a well balanced diet, and usually iron. Maximal folate absorption, even in deficiency states, is only 10–20 μg every 6–8 hours. Daily oral consumption of 0.5 mg supplemental folate (one half of a 500 μg scored tablet bid) has been demonstrated to be adequate for both prophylaxis and correction of overt gestation MA-folate.[12] Decreased hypersegmentation and a distinct elevation in the reticulocyte count after two to four days of therapy are the earliest morphologic signs of remission. Indirect bilirubin and serum LDH values, usually elevated in moderate-to-severe, folate-deficient states secondary to intramedullary hemolysis of abnormal red cell precursors, decrease early in treatment in parallel with a rising reticulocyte count. The serum potassium level should be followed closely since it may fall dramatically as potassium is incorporated into reticulocytes. After one week of therapy the hematocrit and hemoglobin usually begin to rise. Complete correction of all aberrant indices requires several weeks of therapy.

Pregnant patients treated for MA-folate should be followed closely in order to verify a satisfactory hematologic response and to rule out MA-B_{12} concomitant iron deficiency, or any other cause of megaloblastosis. Very often a mixed anemia of iron and folate deficiency is present, which may be difficult to detect because laboratory data and red cell changes are not diagnostic. Supplemental iron

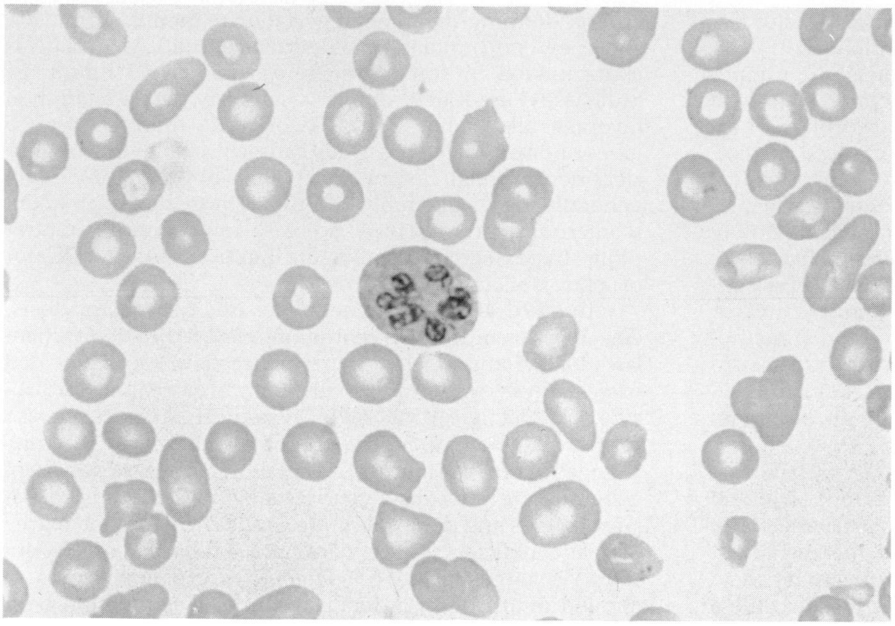

Figure 160–1. Blood smear of a patient with megaloblastic anemia.

administration, therefore, is recommended as an integral part of therapy for the folate-deficient parturient. If treatment is incomplete late in gestation and transfusion is indicated for operative delivery, cautious transfusion of packed red cells with frequent reassessment is recommended.

Routine dietary supplementation generally is recommended for populations whose diet is relatively poor in folate. Gravidas with overt, chronic hemolytic anemia, a hemoglobinopathy, a malabsorption syndrome, multiple fetuses, closely spaced pregnancies, previous treatment for megaloblastic anemia, or those who have previously undergone an upper small intestinal resection should be supplemented from early in gestation. Also, gravidas who are receiving anticonvulsant medications routinely should receive supplementation. Concern that a rare pregnant patient with undiagnosed pernicious anemia could be masked and harmed by the routine administration of folate in the recommended dose of 250 μg twice a day appears highly unlikely. Inclusion of at least 500 μg of folic acid in any prenatal vitamin supplement prescribed for most obstetric patients is recommended.

VITAMIN B_{12} DEFICIENCY

Physiology and Pathophysiology

The two metabolically active forms of vitamin B_{12} (adenosylcobalamin and methylcobalamin) are essential cofactors required in the conversion of methymalonyl coenzyme A (CoA) to succinyl CoA and homocysteine to methionine, respectively. The normal developing fetus requires only 50 μg of vitamin B_{12}, a very small fraction and drain on the normal maternal stores of 3000 μg.[5] For this reason, and because patients with pernicious anemia often have infertility, vitamin B_{12} deficiency as a cause for megaloblastic anemia (MA-B_{12}) is rarely encountered during pregnancy (1 in 6000 to 1 in 8000). Its rare gestational occurrences usually are related to a longstanding strict vegetarian diet, tropical sprue, or incipient pernicious anemia in parturients over 30 years of age. Recently, giardiasis infection with diarrhea and steatorrhea during pregnancy has been identified as a disorder potentially responsible for megaloblastic anemia due to vitamin B_{12} and folate malabsorption.[14]

Effects of Disease on Mother, Fetus, and Newborn

There are no adverse effects of pregnancy itself on vitamin B_{12} deficiency. However, secondary to physiologic transfer of vitamin B_{12} to the fetus, maternal serum levels fall progressively during gestation to intermediate levels (80–120 pg/mL). Low fetal stores and low vitamin B_{12} content in maternal milk are the consequences of maternal vitamin B_{12} deficiency. Breast-fed neonates whose mothers are suffering with this disorder themselves may develop a severe deficiency syndrome characterized by apathy, involuntary movements, developmental regression, pigmentation, and anemia appearing 4–12 months after birth. The reported association between maternal folate and B_{12} deficiency and neural tube defects requires further study.[15,16] By six weeks postpartum, they have returned to normal.

Diagnosis

Megaloblastic anemia with vitamin B_{12} levels below 50 pg/ml (MA-B_{12}) requires therapy and is suggestive of pernicious anemia. Fetuses deficient in transcobalamin 2 (TC2) by genetic defect are asymptomatic at birth, but they can rapidly develop clinical B_{12} deficiency. In a subsequent pregnancy, the mother of such a child can undergo antenatal diagnostic testing at midgestation by amniocentesis and amniocyte culture.[17] Prenatal maternal treatment in affected pregnancies with B_{12} injection to be continued in the neonate postpartum offers hope for normal infant growth and development.[18]

Treatment

Appropriate therapy includes six weekly injections of 100 μg hydroxycobalamin as well as standard prophylactic iron plus folic acid supplementation. Augmented histamine and Schilling testing usually are deferred until after the postpartum period.

REFERENCES

1. Herbert V. The nutritional anemias. *Fem Patient*. 1978;Dec:43.
2. Beck WS. Metabolic aspects of vitamin B_{12} and folic acid (chapter 34); and the megaloblastic anemias (chapter 47). In: Williams WJ, Beutler E, Erslev AJ, Lichtman MA, eds. *Hematology*. 3rd ed. New York: McGraw-Hill; 1983:311–331, 434.
3. Herbert V. Biology of Disease: megaloblastic anemias. *Laboratory Invest*. 1985;52:3.
4. Kitay DZ: Folic acid deficiency in pregnancy. *Am J Obstet Gynecol*. 1969;104:1067.
5. Bitran JN, Miller JB, Golomb HM. Megaloblastic anemia during pregnancy. *J Reprod Med*. 1977;19:186.
6. Kitay DZ. Folic acid and reproduction. *Clin Obstet Gynecol*. 1979;22:809.
7. Shojania AM. Folic acid and vitamin B_{12} deficiency in pregnancy and in the neonatal period. *Clin Perinatol*. 1984;11:433.
8. Davis RE. Clinical chemistry of folic acid. *Advances in Clin Chem*. 1986; 25:233
9. Poelmann AM, Aarnoudse JG. A pregnant woman with severe epistaxis—a rare manifestation of folic acid deficiency. *Eur J Obstet Gynecol Reprod Biol*. 1986;23:249.
10. Solano FX Jr, Councell RB. Folate deficiency presenting as pancytopenia in pregnancy. *Am J Obstet Gynecol*. 1986;154:1117.
11. Pritchard JA, Mason RA, Wright MR. Megaloblastic anemia during pregnancy and the puerperium. *Am J Obstet Gynecol*. 1962;83:1004.
12. Pritchard JA, MacDonald PC. Megaloblastic anemia. In: Williams *Obstetrics*. 16th ed. New York: Appleton-Century-Crofts; 1980:717.
13. Rolschau J, Date J, Kristoffersen K. Folic acid supplement and intrauterine growth. *Acta Obstet Gynecol Scand*. 1979;58:343.
14. Heazlewood VJ, Kasan PN. Giardiasis and vitamin B_{12} deficiency. *Aust NZ J Med*. 1987;17:261.
15. Yates JRW, Ferguson-Smith MA, Shenkin A, et al. Is disordered folate metabolism the basis for the genetic predispostion of neural tube defects? *Clin Genetics*. 1987;31:279.
16. Rhoads GG, Mills JL. Can vitamin supplements prevent neural tube defects? Current evidence and ongoing investigations. *Clin Obstet Gynecol*. 1986;29:569.
17. Rosenblatt DS, Hosack A, Matiaszuk N. Expression of transcobalamin II by amniocytes. *Prenatal Diag*. 1987;7:35.
18. Rosenblatt DS, Cooper BA, Schmutz SM. Prenatal vitamin B_{12} therapy of a fetus with methylcobalamin deficiency (cobalamin E disease) *Lancet*. 1985;I:1127.

Chapter One Hundred and Sixty-One
Disorders of Bone Marrow

James F. McCaul IV and John C. Morrison

161

Bone marrow disorders are a rare occurrence in the practice of obstetrics and gynecology. However, once failure of the multipotential hematopoietic stem cell occurs, the resulting pancytopenia (anemia, neutropenia, and thrombocytopenia) can be devastating. A hypocellular bone marrow with fatty degenerative changes is called *aplastic anemia*.[1,2] On the other hand, the rare selective aplasia of the erythropoietic cell line is designated as *pure red cell aplasia*. When the bone marrow is replaced with tumor or granulomatous changes, *myelophthistic anemia* is the diagnosis. Finally, *paroxysmal nocturnal hemoglobinuria* is thought to be caused by the bone marrow production of an abnormal clone of defective red cells, platelets, and granulocytes.

APLASTIC ANEMIA

The development of a fatty, hypocellular bone marrow with pancytopenia may be produced by a variety of drugs and chemicals as well as exposure to radiation and several diseases. Industrialization and increasing medical technology have exposed humans to more solvents, insecticides, food additives, and pharmaceuticals than ever before. A few agents that are believed to cause this disease include acetylsalicylic acid, benzene, chloramphenicol, chlorpromazine, gold salts, ibuprophen, indomethacin, phenanthrene, phenylbutazone, sulfonamides, and tolbutamide. Both hepatitis A and B have been associated with severe aplastic anemia. There may be a genetic predisposition to aplastic anemia based on studies in mice, and an immunologic role has been proposed in some patients. About 50% of cases are classified as idiopathic without a clear etiologic mechanism.

The exact pathophysiologic mechanism for failure of the pluripotential stem cells followed by a decline in the hemopoietic precursor cells has remained elusive in most cases of aplastic anemia. Genetic, chemical, and immunologic changes in the microenvironment of the stem cell all have been postulated. A genetic pattern of aplastic anemia has been produced in two inbred strains of mice. In one, there is a failure of multipotential stem cell development and in the other, an alteration in the bone marrow itself. This suggests the possibility of both a constitutional and a genetic susceptibility in some humans. These individuals may not be able to detoxify chemicals as efficiently as others or their stem cells may be less resistant to damage.

The hepatitis virus may interfere with stem cell replication, perhaps by chromosomal damage. Radiation exposure produces aplastic anemia only after whole-body exposure to a lethal or sublethal dose that results in extensive cellular death in the bone marrow. The erythroid cell type is most sensitive to acute radiation exposure followed by the myeloid cells, and finally, the megakaryocytes.

Effects of Disease on Pregnancy

In general, the course of aplastic anemia does not seem to be significantly altered by pregnancy. However, the normal progression of pregnancy may be altered dramatically by the presence of this disease. There have been over 80 reported cases of aplastic anemia associated with pregnancy since the original description in 1888 by Eilich. In the Japanese literature, an incidence of approximately one case per year is reported. The exact incidence is obviously extremely low.

Cases of aplastic anemia for clinical management and prognosis should be divided into two groups. Those with aplastic anemia diagnosed prior to pregnancy generally present in a stable disease state. A second group discovered during pregnancy commonly presents for evaluation of petechial bleeding and hemorrhagic symptoms. In contrast, a few are discovered on routine blood analysis. A diagnosis of aplastic anemia prior to pregnancy is associated with an improved maternal survival and a successful outcome for the pregnancy. A higher hemoglobin concentration on initial visit generally is felt to be associated with a better maternal survival, with the literature revealing successful pregnancy in only two out of nine with a hemoglobin <6 g/dL and no successful cases if the hemoglobin was <3.5 g/dL. The initial leukocyte count, platelet count, and gestational age at the time of diagnosis did not appear to correlate with clinical outcome. Prognosis was also evaluated over time. A significant improvement was noted during the years 1959–1969, but no additional amelioration has been observed after that time. The major causes of maternal demise remain consistent, with hemorrhage and sepsis being responsible for 90% of the deaths. The hemorrhagic diathesis usually is generalized, and only two patients were noted to have genital bleeding during delivery or in the puerperium. In general, the course of aplastic anemia may be extremely short, lasting three to four months, or a smoldering disease lasting several years.[3,4] When hepatitis A or B is associated with severe aplastic anemia, the outcome usually is fatal.

Hematologic abnormalities have been reported in at least six infants of parturients with aplastic anemia. These neonates were anemic at birth, including two with pancytopenia. In both cases of neonatal pancytopenia, the presence of an antiplatelet antibody was described in the maternal and fetal blood. In general, after 1959, the survival rate of the neonate has exceeded 75% in reported cases. Prematurity is the major morbidity associated with maternal aplastic anemia. Neonatal bleeding complications secondary to parturition theoretically might be diminished by analysis of the fetal platelet count and utilization of cesarean delivery if thrombocytopenia is found. Fetal thrombocytopenia can be diagnosed *in utero* by cordocentesis.

Diagnosis

A thorough physical examination and laboratory evaluation are necessary to rule out other causes of pancytopenia (Table 161–1). Splenomegaly or lymphadenopathy generally excludes the diagnosis of aplastic anemia. Pancytopenia on peripheral blood count may show variable depression of any cell line. Total white blood count may be low or normal, but the absolute number of granulocytes is decreased, with normal lymphocytes composing the majority of the cells. The magnitude of granulocytopenia, which is always present, is important as an immediate prognostic guide since an absolute granulocytic count less than 200 per mm^3 correlates with susceptibility to infections. The red blood cells usually are normochromic and normocytic, but occasionally may be macrocytic. The absolute number of reticulocytes is low, with an index usually under 1.0%. The peripheral smear should be examined closely for nucleated red cells, which, if present, would be more physiologically compatible with bone marrow dysfunction than hypoplasia. Thrombocytopenia to some degree is invariably present. Hemorrhagic studies involving platelet function (bleeding time) will be prolonged variably. Serum iron is elevated because of the low-iron turnover rate, but the iron-binding capacity is normal. Serum folate and vitamin B_{12} levels are normal, as is red blood cell life span.

TABLE 161–1. CAUSES OF PANCYTOPENIA ASSOCIATED WITH ABNORMAL BONE MARROW

- Aplastic Anemia
  - Constitutional (Fanconi's)
  - Acquired
    - Idiopathic
    - Chemical and physical agents
    - Infectious hepatitis
    - Metabolic: pancreatitis
- Pure Red Cell Aplasia—erythroid component only
  - Thymomas
  - Pregnancy
- Paroxysmal Nocturnal Hemoglobinuria
- Myelophthisic Anemia—bone marrow replacement
  - Hematologic malignancy: leukemia, lymphoma, or myeloma
  - Metastatic tumor: breast, lung, and thyroid
  - Storage cell disorders: Gaucher's, Neiman–Pick
  - Granulomatous disease: tuberculosis

Bone marrow evaluation is necessary for diagnosis. Bone marrow aspiration may result in a "dry tap" and necessitate a bone marrow biopsy. The marrow will reveal a severely hypocellular or aplastic appearance with a variable degree of fatty replacement. Occasionally, the marrow will show a clustering effect of cellular elements, particularly lymphoid. Predominance of erythroid or myeloid cells is more compatible with refractory normoblastic anemia, Di Guglielmo syndrome, or aleukemia leukemia. Further bone marrow sampling and iron metabolism studies should clarify the diagnosis. Although the diagnosis of idiopathic aplastic anemia is made 50–70% of the time, a careful search for causative, external agents must be performed.

Treatment

The basic goal is to remove the causative agent if present or to obtain supportive therapy to attain a possible spontaneous remission. Transfusion with washed, packed red cells is indicated when the hemoglobin concentration approaches 8 g/dL, dependent on the disease course or if symptoms occur. Platelet transfusion is an important tool in the prevention and treatment of hemorrhage in patients with aplastic anemia. When available, the use of HLA-compatible platelets may decrease the incidence of platelet antibody formation. Platelet transfusion is recommended prior to delivery or surgical procedures. A variable effect is noted with steroid administration; therefore, it is justified to initiate a therapeutic trial for two to four weeks. The risk of gastrointestinal hemorrhage and disseminated infections is increased with steroid dosages above 20 mg per day. A critical evaluation of steroid benefits is advised before this level is exceeded, particularly beyond 2 weeks. Several patients have benefited from the bone marrow stimulatory action of certain androgens. A therapeutic trial of a synthetic oral testosterone preparation such as oxymetholone (3–5 mg/kg per day) is indicated after pregnancy is completed. A definitive response may be slow, but when a response is noted, androgen treatment should be continued for at least 4 months. Bone marrow transplantation may be a therapeutic option depending on the severity of the disease and the HLA compatibility of sibling donors. Graft versus host disease may occur in 50% of transplantations despite HLA comparability. Successful bone marrow transplants have been reported in 2 of 4 pregnant patients in the third trimester.[5] The use of antithymocyte globulin may be an option postpartum but has not been utilized in pregnancy because of the unknown effect on the fetus. The transplantation of fetal liver hematopoietic stem cells to the adult with aplastic anemia may be a future method of treatment. Fetal liver stem cells have not been associated with graft versus host disease in humans, but sustained engraftment has been a problem to date.[6]

Infections in patients with aplastic anemia are serious and necessitate early aggressive antibiotic therapy. As soon as fever or local signs of infection appear, appropriate cultures should be obtained, and the patient started on bactericidal, broad-spectrum antibiotics. Antibiotic prophylaxis for delivery or operative procedures is recommended, particularly if steroids are being given. All patients with aplastic anemia should avoid environmental routes for transmission of pathogens and exposure to infected persons. In the hospital, reverse isolation is advised only when the granulocyte count is less than 200/mm^3.

PURE RED CELL APLASIA

A selective failure of the erythroid elements in bone marrow occurs in this disease, with normal granulopoiesis and megakaryocytopoiesis. Acquired pure red cell aplasia is an uncommon disease associated with thymic tumors in 30–50% of the cases. Its association with systemic lupus erythematosus and the report of relapsing pure red cell aplasia during pregnancy strongly suggests an immunologic basis for this disease.[7,8] Circulating antibodies directed against nucleated red cells are found in 50% of patients and the favorable response of some patients to corticosteroid therapy lends further credence to this hypothesis.

A toxic mechanism also has been postulated in those patients with pure red cell aplasia apparently secondary to a specific drug. Carbamazepine and diphenylhydantoin have been implicated in case reports and the disease resolved with cessation of therapy.[9,10] A rare chronic constitutional red blood cell aplasia known as Diamond–Blackfan syndrome may appear in infants at time of birth and persists until the age of 2 years. Minor congenital anomalies may be present in 25% of the offspring.

Although case reports are few, pregnancy outcome in patients with pure red cell aplasia is usually good. However, complications associated with untreated anemia might be postulated (intrauterine growth retardation, prematurity, and *abruptio placentae*).

A normochromic, normocytic anemia with an absolute reticulocytopenia and with normal leukocyte and platelet counts is the hallmark of this disorder. Bone marrow examination is normal except for profound erythroid hypoplasia.

Transfusion with packed red blood cells is the primary therapy. This may become difficult over time because of the development of red blood cell antibodies or hypersplenism. If the thymus is enlarged, removal is the usual treatment. Corticosteroids are often helpful, but high doses may be necessary with their inherent risks. The use of intravenous immunoglobins to block antibodies against erythrocytes and plasma exchange also have been reported successful in some cases of pure red cell aplasia.[11,12] The use of immunosuppressive agents generally is avoided during pregnancy, as is the supplemental use of androgens. Interruption of pregnancy is rarely necessary.

PAROXYSMAL NOCTURNAL HEMOGLOBINURIA

This is a rare disorder of unknown etiology in which an abnormal clone of bone marrow stem cells produces defective red cells that are extremely sensitive to complement-mediated intravascular hemolysis. This anemic state is associated with marked hypercoagulability, occasional granulocytopenia, and thrombocytopenia without antiplatelet antibodies. The fertility rate is believed to be decreased in these patients, although the number of reported cases is small.

These patients have a higher incidence of spontaneous abortion. If early termination does not occur, a successful fetal outcome is the rule, but high maternal morbidity associated with thromboembolic events is common. The major life-threatening events are hepatic vein or cerebral venous thrombosis.[13,14]

During a hemolytic episode, the patient may experience headaches, abdominal pain, and myalgias. Laboratory evaluation generally reveals a mild pancytopenia with an elevated corrected reticulocyte count. The urine contains hemosiderin, and the sucrose lysis test is positive. Hyperbilirubinemia also may be present depending on the frequency of hemolytic episodes.

The recommended treatment during pregnancy is intermittent prophylactic transfusions with washed, packed red blood cells during the first trimester to maintain the packed cell volume between 25% and 30%. This seems to decrease severe hemolytic episodes, risk of spontaneous abortion, and serious thrombotic episodes. Anticoagulation therapy with heparin during any antepartum thrombotic episode and prophylactically in the puerperium may be helpful. As in all bone marrow dysplasias, the patient must be monitored closely at all times for signs of infection. Corticosteroid therapy may be helpful in some patients with paroxysmal nocturnal hemoglobinuria.[1,5] Patients often are evaluated for possible antiplatelet antibody, although this occurs infrequently with this disease.

MYELOPHTHISIC ANEMIA

Infiltration of the bone marrow with tumor or granulomatous cells resulting in severe normochromic, normocytic anemia is the hallmark of myelophthisic anemia. Peripheral smear evaluation usually demonstrates a high percentage of abnormal red cells such as tear drops and fragmented cells with basophilic stippling. The absolute reticulocyte count is reduced and the white blood cell count is elevated with a left shift in the differential count. This combination of immature myeloid cells and normoblasts in the peripheral smear is characteristic of this anemia.

Treatment consists of therapies appropriate to eradicate or palliate the primary disease process. Pregnancy among those with myelophthisic anemia is rare and may alter therapy used because of the fetal risk from chemotherapy, immunosuppressive agents, or radiation therapy. Premature delivery may be indicated as soon as viability is reached, or the patient may choose to terminate the pregnancy early in gestation so that conventional treatment can be initiated. Fetal and maternal outcome will be dependent on the specific primary disease and its course.

REFERENCES

1. Erslev AJ. Hemopoietic stem cell disorders—aplastic. In: Williams WJ, Beutler E, Erslev AJ, et al, eds. *Hematology*. 3rd ed. New York: McGraw-Hill; 1983:151.
2. Rappeport JM, Bunn HF. Bone marrow failure: Aplastic anemia and other primary bone marrow disorders. In: Braunwald E, Isselbacher KJ, Petersdorf RG, et al, eds. *Principles of Internal Medicine*. 11th ed. New York: McGraw-Hill; 1987:1533.

3. Suda T, Omine M, Tsuchija J, et al. Prognostic aspects of aplastic anemia in pregnancy. *Blut.* 1978;36:285.
4. Issaragrisil S, Vanachivanavin V, Piankijagum A, et al. Aplastic anemia with pregnancy. *J Med Assoc Thailand.* 1982;65:111.
5. Doney K, Storb R, Buckner CD, et al. Marrow transplantation for treatment of pregnancy-associated aplastic anemia. *Exp Hematol.* 1985; 13:1080.
6. Gale RP: Fetal liver transplantation in hematologic disorders. In: Gale RP, Touraine JL, Lucarellie G, eds. *Fetal Liver Transplantation.* New York: Alan R. Liss; 1985;193:293.
7. Lehman G: Reversible pure red cell hypoplasia in pregnancy. *JAMA.* 1982;247:1170.
8. Picot C, Tiadou P, Lacombe C, et al: Relapsing pure red cell aplasia during pregnancy. *N Engl J Med.* 1984;311:196.
9. Medberry CA, Pappas AA, Ackerman BH. Carbamazepine and erythroid arrest. *Drug Intell Clin Pharm.* 1987;21:439.
10. Dessypris EN, Redline S, Harris JW, et al. Diphenyhydantoin-induced pure red cell aplasia. *Blood.* 1985;65:789.
11. Katakkar SB. Pure red blood cell aplasia: response to intravenous immunoglobins, a blocking antibody. *Arch Intern Med.* 1986;146:2288.
12. Khelif A, Van HV, Tremisi JP, et al. Remission of acquired pure red cell aplasia following plasma exchanges. *Scand J Haematol.* 1985;34:13.
13. Hurd W, Meodovnik M, Step S. Pregnancy associated with paroxysmal nocturnal hemoglobinuria. *Obstet Gynecol.* 1982;60:742.
14. Solal-Celigny P, Tertian G, Fernandez H, et al. Pregnancy and paroxysmal nocturnal hemoglobinuria. *Arch Intern Med.* 1988;148:593.
15. Issaragrisil S, Piankijagum A, Tang-Naitrisorana Y. Corticosteroids therapy in paroxysmal nocturnal hemoglobinuria. *Am J Hematol.* 1987;25:77.

Chapter One Hundred and Sixty-Two

Anemia Associated With Chronic Systemic Disorders

Sterling W. McColgin and John C. Morrison

162

Anemia associated with chronic systemic disorders is the third most common type behind iron deficiency anemia and the thalassemias. The illnesses most often implicated in the past with these anemias include alcoholism, chronic liver and renal disease, longstanding infections, chronic inflammatory conditions, endocrine deficiency diseases, and malignancy. More recently, acquired immune deficiency syndrome (AIDS) has been added to this list and is often a more severe anemia. The anemias that follow these diseases are generally mild to moderate and nonprogressive. The anemia tends to correct as the chronic disorder improves but may worsen if the disease state deteriorates. They most frequently are manifested by low ferritin levels despite iron stores that range from adequate to increased. They do not improve with iron supplementation unless there is a concomitant improvement in the disease state. The anemia is typically normochromatic and normocytic but may become hypochromic and even microcytic with a more severe or longstanding process. An exception to the characteristic abnormalities of iron metabolism are the anemias of chronic endocrinologic disease. Hypoferremia does not accompany the anemias of hypothyroidism or panhypopituitarism, for example, unless there is complicating iron deficiency.[1]

These anemias may result from secretion of endogenous pyrogen (EP), leukocyte endogenous mediator (LEM), or interleukin-1 (IL-1).[1] Lactoferrin is a protein produced by leukocytes in copious quantities during inflammatory states and may interfere with iron transport in these patients.[2] The etiology of most anemias of chronic disease, however, remains unproven.

PATHOPHYSIOLOGY

The anemia associated with chronic systemic disorders stems from a combination of moderately increased red blood cell (RBC) destruction and a failure to evoke compensatory RBC production. RBCs continue to be synthesized at a normal rate, which in itself is abnormal since production should rise to correct the anemia. There are two reasons why the marrow fails to increase erythropoiesis. First, despite tissue hypoxia secondary to anemia, production of erythropoietin apparently is not increased. Also, the release of iron from the reticuloendothelial cells to plasma transferrin is impaired.[3] In general, it is evident that the life span of RBC's is shortened and the bone marrow response for increased erythropoiesis is inadequate.

EFFECT OF PREGNANCY ON DISEASE

Pregnancy appears to have no harmful effect on the anemia of chronic systemic disorders. Although there is an increase in maternal-fetal morbidity and mortality with anemia of chronic systemic disorders, it is directly related to the disease process rather than the anemia itself.

DIAGNOSIS

Anemia associated with chronic systemic disorders remains a diagnosis of exclusion. Patients should undergo a complete anemia work up to exclude correctable causes of anemia.[2] The hematocrit rarely falls below 30%. The anemia generally is fully developed during the work up and thereafter does not worsen.[1] The symptoms in these patients tend to be those of the underlying disease with few manifestations of the anemia itself.[1] An exception to this can occur in AIDS patients in whom the packed cell volume (PCV) may fall <20% and is often progressive.[4] There is some evidence that red cell autoantibodies may play a role in AIDS patients.[5]

Infections most commonly seen with these anemias are less frequently encountered today than in the past but include untreated tuberculosis, bacterial endocarditis, chronic pyelonephritis, and osteomyelitis. Common inflammatory disorders with associated anemia include rheumatoid arthritis and systemic lupus erythematosus. Endocrine deficiency diseases include hypopituitarism and hypothyroidism, which may be complicated by an anemia. All neoplasias may produce this type of anemia, but it is most prevalent especially in patients with solid tumors, lymphomas, and AIDS patients.

Anemias found in patients with chronic illness that are secondary to the systemic disorder demonstrate RBCs that are normochromic to slightly hypochromic, and normocytic to slightly microcytic. The reticulocyte count is usually normal but the serum iron level and total iron binding capacity are reduced, with a resultant reduced transferrin saturation value. In contrast, iron stores in reticuloendothelial cells in the bone marrow are increased, while serum ferritin levels are normal to increased. In contrast, iron deficiency anemia is marked by low serum iron accompanied by an increase in total iron binding capacity and a low serum ferritin level (<12 ng/mL). In addition, patients with iron deficiency anemia also exhibit decreased iron stores in their reticuloendothelial cells in the bone marrow.

TREATMENT

The mainstay of treatment of the anemia of chronic disorders is therapy for the underlying disease process. Fortunately, the anemia is usually mild-to-moderate in degree and only rarely is it life-threatening. Iron supplementation, nutritional support, or vitamin preparations does not correct the underlying anemia. Blood transfusions can be utilized in patients who are overtly symptomatic as a result of the anemia and in whom the cause is not imminently remedial. In the vast majority of cases, physician reassurance is the best treatment.

REFERENCES

1. Lee GR. The anemia of chronic disease. *Sem Hematol.* 1983;20:61.
2. Beutler E. The common anemias. *JAMA.* 1988;259:2433.
3. Rapaport SI. Secondary anemias in nonhematological disorders. In: *Introduction to Hematology.* 2nd ed. Philadelphia: JB Lippincott; 1987;185.
4. Frontiera M, Myers AM. Peripheral blood and bone marrow abnormalities in the acquired immunodeficiency syndrome. *West J Med.* 1987;147:157.
5. McGinniss MH, Macher AM, Rook AH, et al. Red cell autoantibodies in patients with acquired immune deficiency syndrome. *Transfusion.* 1986;26:405.

Chapter One Hundred and Sixty-Three

Disorders of Hemoglobin Structure, Function, and Synthesis

Kenneth G. Perry, Jr. and John C. Morrison

163

Disorders of hemoglobin integrity most commonly involve abnormal globin structure in the erythrocyte. Fortunately, most of these abnormal hemoglobins are very rare. By 1989, there had been more than 325 hemoglobinopathies reported, although only a few are clinically significant, and none are extremely common. In most of these disorders, there are single amino acid substitutions (300), additions (8), deletions (11), or fusions (12) in either the α or β globin chains. Clinically significant hemoglobinopathies rarely affect the δ or γ chains, which are present in hemoglobin A_2 (HbA_2) or fetal hemoglobin (HbF), respectively. Occasionally, the globin is structurally normal, but the synthesis of the α or β chain is diminished, as in the thalassemia syndromes. Abnormal hemoglobins may be classified by several different schemes. The hemoglobinopathies usually deal with a mutation point at the heme or globin contact region, whereas the more rare disorders have either internally or externally directed amino acid substitutions in the globin chain. The clinically important variants include the sickle hemoglobinopathies, unstable hemoglobins, those with abnormal oxygen affinity, methemoglobins (cyanotic), as well as miscellaneous categories that include hemoglobins C, D, E. G, and O.[1]

UNSTABLE HEMOGLOBIN

The unstable hemoglobins result from substitutions and deletions of amino acids in the α or β chains; over 70 varieties have been identified.[2] Hemoglobin Koln is the most common, yet only 50 cases have been reported in the world literature. The trait for unstable hemoglobin is inherited by autosomal dominant means, although well documented cases of spontaneous mutations have been reported. Pathophysiologically, it is characterized by a hemolytic anemia of variable severity, usually with signs of pallor, jaundice, and splenomegaly, that may be present at any time during life. These hemoglobinopathies are not thought to be adversely affected by pregnancy. Nevertheless, certain drugs such as sulfas and furantoin derivatives should be avoided since they may increase hemolysis. Increased susceptibility to infection, particularly the *pneumococcus*, is common. The effect on the mother as well as the fetus is mediated by the degree of anemia, although no increase in morbidity or mortality in the progeny has been ascribed to these disorders. The diagnosis is suggested by a hematologic picture of a normocytic, hypochromic anemia with Heinz body inclusions in the red blood cells. The electrophoretic mobility of these hemoglobins is determined by their electrical charge, and it is different with each variety, thus allowing confirmation. The mainstays of therapy usually revolve around transfusion and splenectomy, but these are not often necessary as most episodes are self-limiting.

METHEMOGLOBINEMIA

Hemoglobin M, or methemoglobin, is formed when iron atoms are oxidized to the ferric state and thus are unable to combine with molecular oxygen.[3] Methemoglobin anemia is transmitted by a Mendelian dominant mechanism, and only heterozygotes are reported, since homozygosity would be incompatible with life. On the other hand, methemoglobin reductase deficiency results from the autosomal recessive error. Although this condition may result from treatment with various drugs and chemicals or from a deficiency of the enzyme methemoglobin reductase, it usually occurs from a single amino acid substitution in one of the globin chains. Of the five varieties known, in two the substitution is in the α chain, which causes cyanosis in infants at birth. Three types involve the β chains, and cyanosis does not appear until the third or fourth month of life. Methemoglobin usually constitutes 15–30% of the total hemoglobin in α chain disease and 40–50% in β-chain defects.

Although the patients and progeny are cyanotic, they are entirely asymptomatic. Pregnancy does not affect the disease. There is no adverse effect of these disorders on the mother or fetus during pregnancy, and the percentage of hemoglobin M does not change during pregnancy. The diagnosis is established in a comparison of hemoglobins using the absorption spectral characteristics of the cyanmethemoglobin. More recently, electron paramagnetic resonance and agar gel electrophoresis using electrofocusing techniques have permitted a clear separation of normal hemoglobin from different varieties of methemoglobin. The M-hemoglobin reductase deficiency is revealed as normal in spectral analysis and hemoglobin electrophoresis but has the same symptomatology noted in the structural abnormality type disorders. Although methylene blue and ascorbic acid are useful in the treatment of the enzyme-deficient and drug-induced types of methemoglobinemia, structural hemoglobin M disorders are unaffected by such therapy, and simple reassurance is the treatment of choice.

ABNORMAL OXYGEN AFFINITY

Nearly 50 disorders with abnormal oxygen affinity have been reported. They represent both high-affinity (32 varieties) and low-affinity (15 varieties) abnormalities.[4] The inheritance pattern for both types of altered oxygen affinity disorders is autosomal dominant. The disease alters normal physiology and results in compensatory polycythemia and increased red cell mass without leukocytosis in those with increased affinity (familial erythrocytosis) because oxygen is delivered to the tissue less readily. In contrast, mild cyanosis is the pathophysiologic consequence among those with decreased oxygen affinity. The cyanotic varieties, which are extremely rare during pregnancy, have not been reported to affect adversely the gestation or vice versa. Those with increased erythrocytosis may be more susceptible to coagulation disorders during pregnancy, but adverse outcomes in the mother and fetus have been reported only on rare occasions.

Most patients are asymptomatic except for lethargy and easy fatigability, although more severe disease processes associated with cyanosis and polycythemia must be ruled out during the diagnostic process. Hemoglobin electrophoresis utilizing starch or agar gel will identify most hemoglobin variants with altered oxygen affinity. Additional hematologic assessment that may prove helpful in these cases includes measurements of the red blood cell (RBC) mass and blood volume, particularly in low-affinity disorders. Erythropoietin levels may be useful in detecting the high-affinity hemoglobinopathies. Cautious phlebotomy can be utilized in symptomatic patients with polycythemia. For those with low oxygen affinity and cyanosis, no therapy is necessary.

THALASSEMIAS

Etiology

Thalassemia disorders are characterized by decreased production of the β-globin chains or α-globin chains, which are structurally normal.[5] It is felt that most α-thalassemias result from a gene deletion with decreased production of messenger RNA (mRNA) and subsequent limit in α-chain synthesis. The β-thalassemias, unlike the α-thalassemias, do not attribute their decreased production of the β-globin to a gene deletion. A decreased rate in transcription of mRNA or a diminished rate of translation at the level of the ribosome, due to instability of mRNA, have been described as possible etiologies. The mode of inheritance in thalassemic disorders is autosomal dominant. The defect in globin synthesis usually is expressed in both the heterozygous and homozygous states, but is more pronounced in the latter.

Pathophysiology

In the homozygous state, α-thalassemia (α-Thal) is incompatible with life because all four genes are deleted and no α-chains are produced. Subsequently, there is continued formation of hemoglobin Bart's (Hb Bart's) (γ^4). Because of its high oxygen affinity, the fetus develops a high output cardiac failure resulting in hydrops and dies *in utero* or shortly after birth. Hemoglobin H (Hb H) disease is another form of the α-Thal that results from the deletion of three genes and is the most severe type that allows survival. It is characterized by moderately severe hemolytic anemia in childhood with association of Hb H (β^4) and Hb Bart's (γ^4). α-Thal minor where two genes are deleted usually evinces a mild hypochromic, microcytic anemia similar to iron deficiency anemia, whereas those with only one deletion clinically are undetectable. Patients with homozygous β-Thal or Cooley's anemia produce no β-chain and rarely become pregnant because they expire early in life from severe hemolysis. In the heterozygous state, β-Thal is denoted at β^+, where β-chain production is diminished or β^0 when production of the chain is absent. Mild-to-moderate anemia and variable symptomatology are the hallmark of these two disorders.

Effect of Pregnancy on Disease

Patients who become pregnant with heterozygous α-thalassemia note little to no change in their disease except a mild lowering of the packed cell volume (PCV). Similarly, those with β^+ or β^0-thalassemia notice little or no change associated with the pregnancy. On the other hand, those with homozygous β-thalassemia (Cooley's anemia) may note an increase in hemolytic episodes and a marked lowering of their already reduced PCV and hemoglobin content.

In many cases, this disorder has been considered justification for termination of pregnancy.

Effect of Disease on Pregnancy and Fetus

In patients with Cooley's anemia the effect on the parturient depends on the severity of oxygen deprivation from chronic anemia. If transfusion therapy can be given without iron overload, these maternal effects usually can be reversed. Similarly, if the mother's oxygen content drops below 70 mm Hg, abortion, growth retardation, preterm labor, and stillbirth can result. These patients also are susceptible to cardiovascular failure, particularly from midpregnancy on; thus, careful assessment and bed rest should be the rule. In contrast, patients with heterozygous β or α-thalassemia usually suffer no ill effects during pregnancy and can be treated as normal parturients. As will be discussed later, however, when β^0-thalassemia is combined with other disorders, such as sickle hemoglobinopathy, significant maternal and fetal morbidity may result.

Diagnosis

The diagnosis of thalassemia is difficult because the hemoglobin is structurally normal. A complete reticulocyte count, red blood indices, and iron studies as well as free erythrocyte protoporphyrin usually reveal an iron-sufficient microcytic, hypochromic pattern.[6] Hemoglobin electrophoresis will reveal increased HbF and HbA_2 in those with heterozygous β-Thal. A bone marrow aspirate stain (methyl violet) for inclusions may be helpful. In α-Thal, globin synthesis rate, pedigree studies, and radioactive α-chain pool measurements may be necessary.

Treatment

Treatment of patients with thalassemia syndromes varies from no therapy in the "silent carriers," to folate supplementation in the heterozygous state, to blood transfusion and possibly splenectomy in those affected by the more severe disease.

SICKLE CELL ANEMIA

Etiology

The most common hemoglobinopathies involve single amino-acid substitutions in the β-chain. Sickle hemoglobin is the most common example of this variety and is caused by substitution of valine for glutamic acid in the sixth position from the N terminus of both β-chains. The etiology of sickle hemoglobin appears to be related to a genetic point mutation clinically enabling sickle heterozygotes to better withstand infestation by the parasite *Falciparum malaria* in endemic areas. The incidence of homozygous sickle cell anemia (HbS-S) is 1 in 708 in Black Americans, whereas other clinically significant sickling disorders are less common (HbS-C, 1 in 757; HbS-β-Thal, 1 in 1672).[7] All these disorders are known collectively as sickle cell disease. The sickle cell trait (HbA-S) is very common (one per 12 Black Americans). This hemoglobinopathy is inherited in an autosomal dominant pattern. The manifestations in patients with sickle hemoglobin also range from a serious disease, which is responsible for some 80,000 deaths annually throughout the world, to no symptoms, as noted in those with sickle cell trait.

Pathophysiology

While sickle hemoglobin functions normally while oxygenated, during deoxygenation there is a tendency for the neutral valine to form hydrophobic bonds with similar positions in the helical structure of the globin chain. This aggregation causes tetramers of hemoglobin molecules to form inside the red blood cells, which then coalesce into strands or microcables. When several of these microcables within the erythrocyte bind together, tactoids are formed and this distorts the cell into the characteristic sickle shape (Figure 163–1).[8] The capacity of oxygen transfer by such a cell is reduced dramatically, and these abnormal red blood cells tend to block the microcirculation (Figure 163–2). This stagnation causes further deoxygenation and compensatory sickling. This vicious cycle leads to tissue deoxygenation and eventually infarction of the affected area, which is associated with clinical symptoms (pain) known as vaso-occlusive crisis.[9] These sickle cells also become irreversibly damaged when the corpuscular membrane is altered permanently during the sickling process, and they are destroyed prematurely by the reticuloendothelial system, thus causing the constant anemia seen in these patients. Patients also may have hemolytic, aplastic, or megaloblastic types of crisis or splenic sequestration, all of which are rare in adult females.[10]

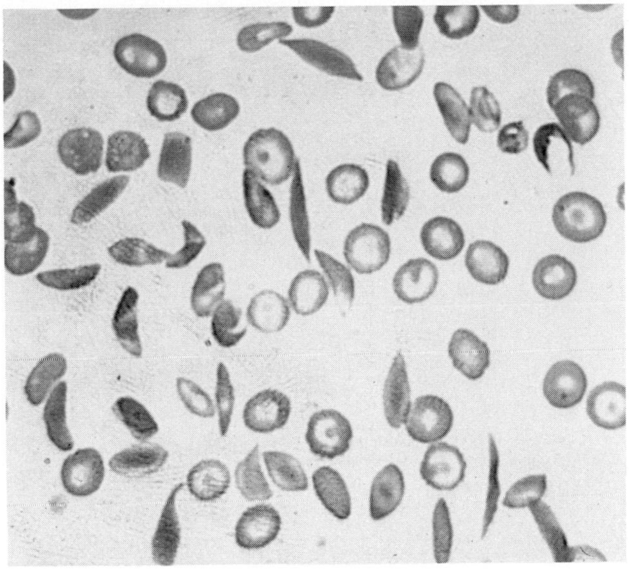

Figure 163–1. Sickled red blood cells during crisis—peripheral smear.

Effects of Pregnancy on Disease

Patients with sickle cell disease appear to be susceptible to exacerbations of their clinical disease during pregnancy. This most likely is due to the increase in metabolic demands during pregnancy, increase in vascular stasis in the pelvic organs, and the hypercoagulable state associated with pregnancy. Painful crisis occurs more commonly during pregnancy and particularly during labor and delivery when the demands for oxygen are increased. Pregnancy may also exacerbate chronic leg ulcers and subsequent bone infection because of stasis in the lower extremity and pelvic veins. Because of changes in the gastrointestinal system, patients with sickle hemoglobinopathies have a higher likelihood of being symptomatic from cholelithiasis (25% compared to 10% during the nonpregnant state). The renal system is also more prone to infection during pregnancy because of stasis and the effect of progesterone on the ureteral collecting system. This, combined with the altered immune

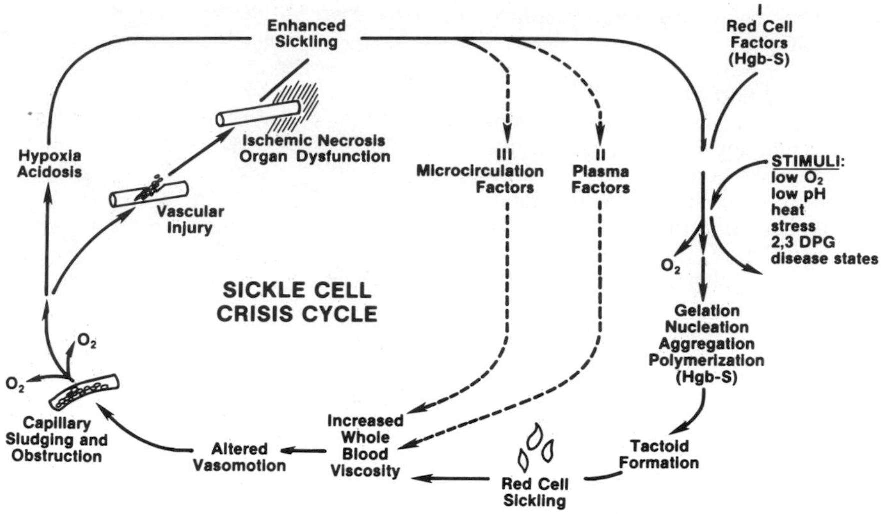

Figure 163–2. Vicious cycle during sickle cell crisis.

state present in patients with sickle cell disease, frequently results in an increased infectious morbidity for these patients.

Effect of Disease on Pregnancy and Fetus

Overall, there is an increase in maternal morbidity and mortality during pregnancy in those with sickle cell disease. With improvements in obstetric and prenatal care there has been a marked decrease in maternal and perinatal morbidity over the past 15 years.[11,12] This has not always been the case since several series prior to 1970 reported maternal mortality as high as 10–12% with maternal morbidity being up to 80–90%.[8] Significant fetal loss rates during that time period of 50–60% were common.[5] Nevertheless, the constant anemia and concomitant association of pregnancy-induced hypertension continue to complicate gestations in patients who have sickle cell disease. In general, the anemias differ dependent on which type of sickle hemoglobinopathy is present.

Anemia is a constant feature, and usually the PCV averages 18–20% in HbS-S to 25–28% in HbS-C and 28–32% in HbS-β-Thal. Nonhematologic manifestations include bone abnormalities; small vessel damage in the kidney and eye from obstruction and hypoxia; integument ulcers, particularly in the lower extremities; and central nervous system accidents such as strokes. Jaundice and hepatomegaly are common, and cardiovascular signs of hyperdynamic flow are often present. Patients with severe sickling disorders frequently display a lack of immune response because of deficient complement production. In addition, they exhibit defective opsonization. This leads to frequent and unusual infections in these patients such as osteomyelitis, pneumococcal and atypical pneumonia, cholecystitis, and pyelonephritis. Diagnosis of the vaso-occlusive crisis in patients known to have sickling disorders, however, frequently may be difficult.[9] This is the case because various areas of the body (such as the chest, abdomen, and extremities) may be involved, and the crisis may be confused with surgical causes of an acute abdomen, lung or heart disease, or arthritis. Modifications in treatment regimen usually allow the physician to make this distinction.

The effects on the fetus of maternal sickle hemoglobinopathies closely parallel the symptomatology seen in the parturient. As long as maternal oxygenation is not threatened, the fetus generally fares very well. However, there have been reports of infertility, increased abortion, and stillbirths as well as an increase in intrauterine growth retardation and preterm labor among offspring of women with sickle cell hemoglobinopathies. In general, if the parturient has a benign course during pregnancy regardless of treatment, the baby does very well. Nevertheless, fetal health assessment tests, including the nonstress or contraction stress tests as well as biophysical profiles, are recommended. Serial ultrasound examinations to rule out growth retardation are also helpful.

Diagnosis

The diagnosis of sickle hemoglobin can be made by screening tests, which should be offered to all black parturients. This assessment usually involves the use of hemoglobin electrophoresis on cellulose acetate for preliminary identification of the abnormal hemoglobin. Starch gel electrophoresis and citrate agar gel electrophoresis may be used to differentiate HbS from those others that migrate with HbS. The starch gel electrophoresis is also useful for identification of patients with S-thalassemia.

Treatment

The treatment of patients with sickling disorders is variable. Patients with sickle cell disease require early and frequent prenatal assessments. Supplemental folic acid is a useful adjunct to promote erythrocyte production. Iron therapy is controversial. Most agree that routine use during pregnancy is not justified but testing should be carried out to identify those who need supplementation.[13] Pain crises are treated similarly in the pregnant and nonpregnant state with supplemental oxygen, hydration, analgesia, and blood transfusions.

During pregnancy, many favor prophylactic exchange transfusions by manual or erythrocytophoresis techniques so that the parturients may be protected against infections and crises, which adversely affect the mother, fetus, or newborn (Table 163–1).[14,15] Others feel that with intense perinatal risk assessment, early treatment of infection, and good nutrition, infusions of blood can be withheld until specific crisis or severe anemia processes make such treatment mandatory.[12,16,17] Both forms of treatment seem to

TABLE 163–1. METHODS OF TRANSFUSION

Simple Transfusion
Hypertransfusion
Partial Exchange Transfusion
  Manual (discontinous)
  Automated
    Haemonetics (discontinuous)
    IBM 2977 (continuous)

yield good results during pregnancies, particularly in series from developed countries after 1970.

The main advantage of prophylactic transfusions is that they decrease the fraction of S-containing cells while increasing the oxygen-carrying capacity of the individual by elevating the level of HbA. The disadvantage of this regimen is that it increases the risk of hepatitis, human immunodeficient virus (HIV) infection, transfusion reaction, and allosensitization.[11,12,18] Nevertheless, those who have used prophylactic blood infusions routinely suggest that by the use of all black donors, preferably from family members, careful screening for infectious products, assiduous typing of blood, and the administration of buffy-coat, poor-washed red cells, these risks can be reduced substantially. If blood infusions are used, they usually are begun early in pregnancy to treat the adverse effects occurring prior to 20 weeks. The transfusions are performed to raise the HbA percentage above 50% and the PCV to 28–30%. Retransfusions are performed at 6- to 10-week intervals when the level of HbA falls below 20%. These transfusions also may be administered during crisis or during labor and can be performed by erythrocytophoresis within one to two hours. It is important to recognize that even if prophylactic transfusions are not used, up to 75% of patients receiving conservative management techniques will require infusion of blood products at some time during gestation.

Other forms of treatment such as hydration, anticoagulation, and alkalinization have had little success. Future means of treatment using desickling agents appear promising. However, most of the compounds that have been investigated, such as urea, cyanate, and adipamate, are too toxic to be employed except on an extracorporeal basis. On the other hand, the benign desickling substances such as amino acids and peptides cannot currently be infused in large enough quantities to be effective *in vivo,* although they do work *in vitro.* Therapeutic manipulation of globin gene expression in the form of increased HbF production with 5-azacytidine and hydroxyurea has been proposed, but the concerns over its toxicity limit their value during pregnancy. The levels of increased HbF produced with these agents are not likely to alleviate the symptoms of the disease state.[19] High doses of recombinant human erythropoietin when given to primates results in a significant increase in the fetal hemoglobin, but awaits human experimentation.[20]

At the present time, the interest of all patients is served through education and appropriate family counseling. *In utero* genetic diagnosis by amniocentesis, cordocentesis, or chorionic villus sampling using restriction endonuclease analysis offers detection of homozygous infants early enough in gestation so that pregnancy termination is an option.[21] It is also advantageous to know the type of hemoglobinopathy in the mother and father. Cord blood assessment is recommended for infants of mothers with sickle hemoglobinopathies so that education of the family as well as the parents may begin as early as possible. Usually, no neonatal treatment of affected infants is necessary because there is no manifestation of the hemoglobinopathies other than the abundance of fetal hemoglobin, which prevents any significant sickling because of its increased affinity of oxygen. This benign condition continues through 4–5 months of age, when the first signs of compromise occur in those infants with significant sickling disorders.

In summary, the severe sickle cell disorders comprising sickle cell disease are known to have adverse effects on the parturient as well as on the fetus or newborn; these should be treated intensively during pregnancy. On the other hand, patients with potentially adverse sickling disorders such as SD and SE are rare and usually not clinically significant. Those patients with sickle cell trait should experience no difficulty in successful childbearing. Those with C, D, E, G, and O hemoglobinopathies should have a benign course, even in the homozygous state.

REFERENCES

1. Adachi I, Kelleher JF. Human hemoglobin variants. In: Schwartz E, ed. *Hemoglobinopathies in Children*. Littleton, MA: PSG Publishing Company; 1980:25.
2. White JM. The unstable haemoglobin disorders. *Clin Haematol.* 1974;3:333.
3. Lehman H, Huntsman RG. *Man's Hemoglobins*. Philadelphia: JB Lippincott; 1974:156.
4. Charache S. Haemoglobins with altered oxygen affinity. *Clin Haematol.* 1974;3:357.
5. Laros RJ Jr. The hemoglobinopathies. In: Laros RJ Jr, ed. *Blood Disorders in Pregnancy*. Philadelphia: Lea & Febiger; 1986:37.
6. Roberts WE, Blake PG, Morrison JC. Evaluation of anemia in pregnancy. In: Kitay DZ, ed. *Hematologic Problems in Pregnancy*. Boston; GK Hall; 1984:137.
7. Schneider RG, Hightower B, Hasty TS, et al. Abnormal hemoglobins in a quarter million people. *Blood*. 1976;48:629.
8. Gookin KS, Morrison JC. Anemia associated with pregnancy. In: Depp R, Eschenback DA, eds. *Gynecology and Obstetrics: Maternal and Fetal Medicine, vol 3*. New York: Harper & Row; 1984:1.
9. Martin JN, Morrison JC. Sickle cell crisis: Recognizing it and treating it. *Contemp Ob/Gyn*. 1982;20:171.
10. Martin JN, Morrison JC. Managing the parturient with sickle cell crisis. In: Huddleston JF, ed. *Sickle-Cell Crisis in the Gravid Woman*. New York; Harper & Row; 1984:39.
11. Powars DR, Sandhu M, Niland-Weiss J, et al. Pregnancy in sickle cell disease. *Obstet Gynecol*. 1986;67A:271.
12. Charache S, Niebyl JR. Pregnancy in sickle cell disease. *Clin Haematol*. 1985;14:729.
13. Akinyanju OO, Nnatu SNN, Ogedengbe OK. Antenatal iron supplementation in sickle cell disease. *Int J Gynaecol Obstet*. 1987;25:433.
14. Morrison JC, Schneider JM, Whybrew WD, et al. Prophylactic transfusion in pregnant patients with sickle hemoglobinopathies: benefit versus risk. *Obstet Gynecol*. 1980;56:274.
15. Cunningham FG, Pritchard JA. Prophylactic transfusion of normal red blood cells during pregnancies complicated by sickle cell hemoglobinopathies. *Am J Obstet Gynecol*. 1979;135:994.
16. Koshy M, Burd L, Wallace D, et al. Prophylactic red cell transfusion in pregnant patients with sickle cell disease: a randomized cooperative study. *N Engl J Med*. 1988;319:1447.
17. Poddar D, Maude GH, Plant MJ, et al. Pregnancy in Jamaican women with homozygous sickle cell disease: fetal and maternal outcome. *Br J Obstet Gynaecol*. 1986;93:727.
18. Miller JM, Horger EO, Key TC, et al. Management of sickle hemoglobinopathies in pregnant patients. *Am J Obstet Gynecol*. 1981;141:237.
19. Noguchi CT, Rogers GP, Sergeant G, et al. Levels of fetal hemoglobin necessary for treatment of sickle cell disease. *N Engl J Med*. 1988;318:96.
20. Al-Kahtti A, Veith RW, Papayannopoulou T, et al. Stimulation of fetal hemoglobin synthesis by erythropoietin in baboons. *N Engl J Med*. 1987;317:415.
21. Old JM, Fitches A, Heath C, et al. First-trimester fetal diagnosis for haemoglobinopathies: report on 200 cases. *Lancet*. 1986;1:763.

Chapter One Hundred and Sixty-Four
Hemolytic Anemias

William E. Roberts and John C. Morrison

164

Occasionally, the obstetrician may encounter a parturient with anemia whose hematologic profile is characterized by persistent reticulocytosis, a finding that indicates that the anemia is the result of erythrocyte destruction in excess of compensatory erythropoiesis in the bone marrow. This type of anemia is termed *hemolytic anemia* and is categorized further into intrinsic hemolytic anemia, in which the hemolysis is caused by a defect in the red blood cell (RBC), or extrinsic hemolytic anemia, in which a mechanical, infectious, or immune factor is responsible for decreased red cell survival.

PATHOPHYSIOLOGY

Effects of Pregnancy on Disease

Studies indicate that pregnancy has no ameliorating or detrimental effects on hemolytic anemia. Although hemoglobin (Hb) and packed cell volume (PCV) values fall during gestation secondary to maternal blood volume expansion, the reticulocyte count remains unchanged, and the pregnant state does not alter the values of the specific laboratory assessments used to diagnose the various types of hemolytic anemias.

Effect of Disease on Pregnancy and Fetus

There is an increased incidence of maternal and fetal morbidity and mortality associated with hemolytic anemia. This appears to be correlated with both the severity of anemia and the inability of the provider to correct the anemic state. Also, because some forms of hemolytic anemias are genetically transmitted, an obstetrician may be consulted by patients prior to pregnancy regarding the overall prognosis of pregnancy and the likelihood of transmission of the disorder to offspring. Specific adverse effects of such disorders are well documented and therapeutic regimens are dependent on the type of hemolytic anemia and its severity.

INTRINSIC HEMOLYTIC ANEMIA

Intrinsic hemolytic anemias, also termed *hereditary hemolytic anemias,* frequently are discovered in childhood. Included in this group are hereditary spherocytosis and RBC (red blood cell) enzyme deficiencies.

Hereditary spherocytosis is an autosomal-dominant inherited disorder in which the erythrocyte membrane is abnormally permeable to sodium.[1] To prevent influx of water and subsequent cell rupture, increased metabolic work is required by the erythrocyte cell membrane. This leads to glucose deprivation and premature cell death. The disease usually is not adversely affected by pregnancy and there are no specific maternal or fetal abnormalities. The diagnosis of hereditary spherocytosis is confirmed by the *in vitro* demonstration of increased osmotic fragility or by the newer and more specific acidified glycerol lysis test.[2] Because the principal site for spherocyte destruction is the spleen, splenectomy frequently is employed, with subsequent improvement in the hematologic profile.

Enzymatic defects in various metabolic pathways within the erythrocyte can lead to shortened erythrocyte survival. The two most common disorders of this type are glucose-6-phosphate dehydrogenase (G6PD) deficiency and pyruvate kinase deficiency. Glucose-6-phosphate dehydrogenase deficiency is transmitted on the X chromosome with full expression in the hemizygous male and partial expression in the heterozygous female.[3,4] The disorder is found more commonly in blacks, with 13% of American black males being affected and 25% of black women being carriers for this disorder. When a patient with G6PD deficiency is exposed to an oxidizing drug such as primaquine or nitrofurantoin, an acute hemolysis occurs with accompanying hemoglobinuria. In addition, viral or bacterial infections can precipitate a hemolytic episode. The methemoglobin and dye reduction tests are readily available laboratory assessments used to confirm the diagnosis of G6PD deficiency but are unreliable in detecting the carrier state. Because of the variable expression of the enzyme deficiency in the heterozygote, carrier state detection is presently difficult and probably not cost-effective.

Pyruvate kinase deficiency is an autosomal recessive disorder and is most commonly noted in people of northern European extraction. It usually is diagnosed in childhood in the presence of persistent anemia and jaundice. The fluorescent spot test for pyruvate deficiency is available from most laboratories as a confirmatory test. Pregnancy does not exacerbate either of these hemolytic anemias, but effects on the mother and the fetus are dependent on the severity of hemoglobin and length of time the process is not corrected.

EXTRINSIC HEMOLYTIC ANEMIA

In contrast to intrinsic hemolytic anemia, erythrocytes produced by the bone marrow in acquired or extrinsic hemolytic anemia are structurally and metabolically normal, but suffer early destruction from environmental causes. The most frequent types of extrinsic hemolytic anemias are hypersplenism, microangiopathic hemolytic anemia, and Coombs-positive hemolytic anemia.

An enlargement of the spleen from any cause can lead to excessive red cell sequestration and destruction in addition to varying degrees of leukopenia and thrombocytopenia.[5] The degree of anemia is generally mild, with reticulocyte counts rarely exceeding 6%. Effective treatment and overall prognosis for the mother and fetus in an anemia caused by hypersplenism is dependent on the underlying disorder.

In microangiopathic hemolytic anemia (MHA), schistocytes (red cell fragments) are seen in large numbers in the

TABLE 164–1. DISORDERS ASSOCIATED WITH MICROANGIOPATHIC HEMOLYTIC ANEMIA

Systemic lupus erythematosus (SLE)
Eclampsia
Disseminated intravascular coagulation (DIC)
Thrombotic thrombocytopenia purpura (TTP)
Acute glomerulonephritis
Renal cortical necrosis
Polyarteritis
Malignant hypertension

peripheral blood smear (Figure 164–1). Although a variety of diseases can cause MHA, all involve disease of small blood vessels.[6] Table 164–1 lists some of the disorders that have been associated with MHA. In these disorders, which are caused by coagulation or small vessel damage, fibrin strands are deposited in capillaries and occlude the microcirculation. This obstruction causes fragmentation and lysis of the erythrocytes. Therapy of MHA involves diagnosis and treatment of the underlying disorder with attempts to reestablish the microcirculation.

Some patients with hemolytic anemia will have a positive direct Coombs test, which indicates the presence of IgG antibody or complement that is irreversibly fixed to the erythrocyte membrane, resulting in cell lysis.[7] The Coombs-positive hemolytic anemias can be categorized further into warm- and cold-antibody hemolytic anemias. Warm-antibody hemolytic anemias are associated with IgG antibody attachment to the erythrocyte surface. The disorder is associated with collagen vascular diseases, lymphomas, and drug reactions, most notable to α-methyldopa. The majority of patients, however, will have no discernible cause for the autoimmune process. Cold autoantibodies associated with hemolytic anemia are usually of the IgM class. They are usually idiopathic but may develop after a viral or mycoplasmal infection. The IgM antibody does not become fixed to the RBC membrane but may stimulate complement formation, which is responsible for the positive Coombs test.

Therapy for all Coombs-positive hemolytic anemias is affected best by treatment of the underlying disorder. If a drug-induced hemolytic anemia is suspected, the medication should be discontinued. Although the direct Coombs test may remain positive for up to one year, hemolysis usually will cease in two to three weeks. Transfusions are used only for emergent situations, since transfused cells also suffer a shortened life span. Corticosteroids are frequently beneficial, especially in patients with warm-antibody hemolytic anemia. If corticosteroids fail, splenectomy has proven effective in some cases. The prognosis of patients with Coombs-positive hemolytic anemia is mainly that of the underlying disease process and response to medical or surgical treatment.

THE HELLP SYNDROME

On occasion, the obstetrician may encounter a preeclamptic or eclamptic patient who has clinical findings and laboratory assessments consistent with the HELLP syndrome (see also Chapter 139). This multiple organ dysfunction syndrome has been so named because of the findings of *hemolysis* (*H*) (MHA type), *elevated liver functions* (*EL*), and *thrombocytopenia* (*LP*).[8] Although the hemolysis usually is not severe enough to require transfusion therapy, because the HELLP syndrome is a variant of a severe form of preeclampsia, steps should be taken to expedite delivery.[9] After delivery, the hemolytic process usually quickly abates. In some patients, plasmapheresis and fresh frozen plasma may be necessary to assist in the reversal of this hemolytic process.[10]

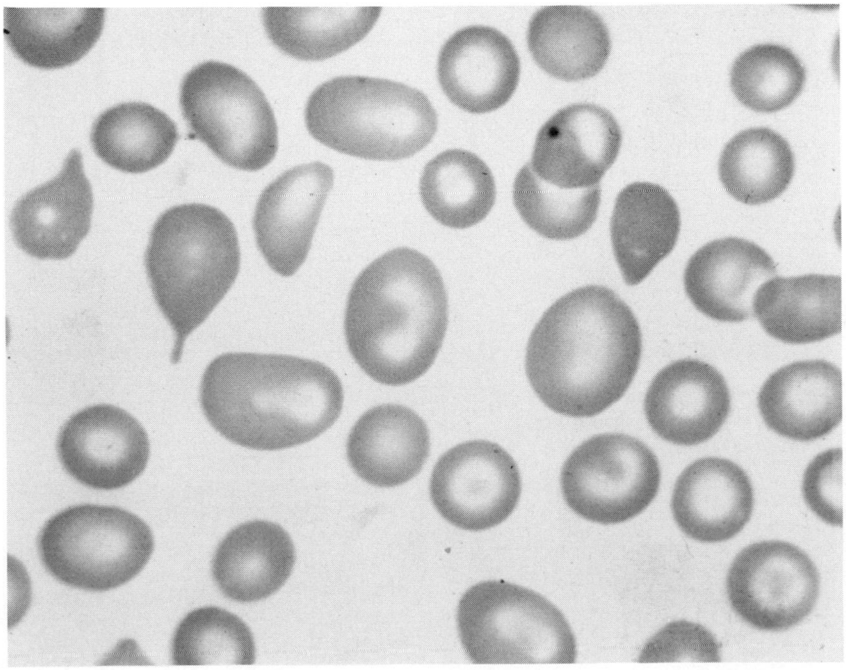

Figure 164–1. Marked poikilocytosis seen with schistocytes.

ADULT RESPIRATORY DISTRESS SYNDROME

Extrinsic hemolytic anemia also is seen frequently in the adult respiratory distress syndrome (ARDS). This poorly understood clinical entity occurs in association with massive trauma, severe infection, hypovolemic shock, viral pneumonia, aspiration pneumonitis, and pancreatitis.[11] Appropriate treatment of ARDS involves respiratory support and treatment of the underlying disorder. The hemolytic anemia that accompanies ARDS is most likely a result of the condition rather than a cause.

REFERENCES

1. Weed R. Hereditary spherocytosis: a review. *Arch Intern Med.* 1975;135:1316.
2. Zanella A, Izzo C, Rebulla P, et al. Acidified glycerol lysis test: a screening test of spherocytosis. *Br J Haematol.* 1980;45:481.
3. Destorges JF. Genetic implication of G6PD deficiency. *N Engl J Med.* 1976;294:1438.
4. Schrier SL. Human erythrocyte G6PD deficiency: pathophysiology, prevalence, diagnosis and management. *Comp Ther.* 1980;6:41.
5. Eichner ER. Splenic function: Normal, too much and too little. *Am J Med.* 1979;66:311.
6. Brain ML. Microangiopathic hemolytic anemia. *N Engl J Med.* 1969;281:833.
7. Dalie JV. Autoimmune hemolytic anemia. *Arch Intern Med.* 1975;135:1293.
8. Weinstein L. Preeclampsia/eclampsia with hemolysis, elevated liver enzymes, and thrombocytopenia. *Obstet Gynecol.* 1985;66:657.
9. Sibai BM, Taslimi MM, El-Nazer A, et al. Maternal-perinatal outcome associated with syndrome of hemolysis, elevated liver enzymes, and low platelets in severe preeclampsia-eclampsia. *Am J Obstet Gynecol.* 1986;155:501.
10. Martin JN Jr, Files JC, Blake PG, Norman PH, et al. Plasma exchange for preeclampsia I: Postpartum use for persistently severe preeclampsia-ecampsia with HEELP syndrome. *Am J Obstet Gynecol.* 1990; 162:126.
11. Martin JN, Sessums NC, Norman PF, et al. Sepsis-associated acute adult respiratory distress syndrome (ARDS) in pregnancy. *Obstet Gynecol.* (in press), 1991.

C

CLOTTING DISORDERS

Chapter One Hundred and Sixty-Five

Platelet Disorders

Robert A. Welch and Robert D. Eden

165

Interpreting platelet disturbances occupies a considerable portion of time in a busy obstetric service. Although their significance often is downplayed, the clinical entities associated with platelet abnormalities may represent a substantial threat to the well-being of both mother and fetus.

The peripheral blood platelet count for both nonpregnant and pregnant adults normally ranges from 150,000 to 400,000/mm^3. Platelets develop as a result of bone marrow stimulation by thrombopoietin, which promotes stem cell activation and maturation to megakaryocytes. Once mature, platelets are released from this source into the systemic circulation, where they remain viable from eight to nine days. Platelet viability is unaffected by pregnancy. A subtle, progressive decline in number occasionally may be noted with advancing gestation. This decrease may result from physiologic hemodilution or placental sequestration. While platelet counts of less than 150,000/mm^3 are considered thrombocytopenia in nonpregnant adults, platelet counts of less than 100,000/mm^3 constitutes thrombocytopenia in pregnancy.[2-4]

Several conditions account for thrombocytopenia (Table 165–1).[1] Bone marrow stem cell failure generally affects all blood elements produced in this organ, and thrombocytopenia may be representative of this underlying phenomenon. Cytotoxic agents such as gold, sulfonamides, ethanol, and radiation may result in destruction and underproduction of stem cells. Similarly, stem cells may be replaced with infiltration by fibrosis, leukemia, or metastatic carcinoma.

Defective platelet maturation occurs with vitamin B_{12} or folate deficiency, myeloproliferative disorders, paroxysmal nocturnal hemoglobulinuria, and some inherited disorders. Abnormal platelet distribution or sequestration occurs in clinical disorders accompanied with massive splenomegaly. Platelet survival may be reduced to as short as one day in antibody-mediated disorders, disseminated intravascular coagulation, and pregnancy-induced hypertension. Gram-negative and viral sepsis can cause peripheral platelet consumption and suppression of production. Thrombocytopenia may result from massive maternal hemorrhage.

PATHOPHYSIOLOGY

Platelet disorders initially are characterized by petechiae of the skin and mucosal membranes. These small, nonblanching, relatively fine petechiae result from extravasation of erythrocytes through small blood vessel walls and are not found often with other coagulation disturbances. Nonthrombocytopenic purpura petechiae are larger, symmetrical, palpable discrete lesions. In the presence of petechiae, a blood smear or a platelet count accurately distinguishes thrombocytopenic and nonthrombocytopenic purpura. Prolonged bleeding times, decreased clot retraction, and a positive tourniquet test (Trousseau's sign) occur in both types of disorders.[1,2,4]

A platelet count of greater than 50,000/mm^3 usually is associated with normal platelet hemostasis. This level usually is considered adequate for urgent surgical interventions. Spontaneous bleeding may be associated with platelet counts of less than 20,000/mm^3. Intracranial hemorrhage is the leading cause of death in this circumstance and is particularly likely with platelet counts below 5,000/mm^3.

Bone marrow evaluation is helpful in differentiating the etiology of thrombocytopenia. The presence of adequate or even abundant numbers of megakarocytes suggests that the thrombocytopenia is secondary to peripheral destruction or sequestration of platelets. Decreased platelet production occurs when diminished numbers of functionally suppressed megakaryocytes are present in the marrow. Hypersegmentation of polymorphonuclear white blood cells occurs with a megaloblastic bone marrow process. Erythrocyte morphology also may provide clues to the etiology of thrombocytopenia. Traumatic hemolysis occurs with pregnancy-induced hypertension, disseminated intravascular coagulation, and thrombotic thrombocytopenic purpura. Fragmentation of red blood cells suggest a microangiopathic process as the cause of thrombocytopenia. Immunologic mechanisms of thrombocytopenia are characterized by normal red cell morphology. A normal prothrombin time, partial thromboplastin time, thrombin time, fibrinogen level, and fibrin split products exclude disseminated intravascular coagulation as the cause of thrombocytopenia.[1,2,4]

In general, evaluation of hemorrhagic disorders requires a thorough history and physical examination to determine whether a disorder of blood coagulation, platelets, or blood vessels is present. A drug history is particularly important if the bleeding disorder is of recent or sudden onset. Elimination of the causative agent in drug-induced thrombocytopenia will result in remission in the majority of patients. With immune causes, steroid administration, high dose immunoglobulins, and platelet transfusions are the most widely used forms of initial therapy and usually effect remission in the majority of patients. Thrombocytopenia unresponsive to these treatment modalities may require splenectomy. Splenectomy during pregnancy is reserved for life-threatening cases and carries a high maternal-fetal morbidity and mortality.[1,2,4]

TABLE 165–1. CAUSES OF THROMBOCYTOPENIA

Defective Platelet Production
Reduced thrombopoiesis
Marrow injury, failure, invasion
Thrombopoietin deficiency
Defective maturation
Vitamin B_{12} deficiency
Folic acid deficiency
Hereditary
Sequestration
Splenomegaly
Hypothermic anesthesia
Accelerated Destruction
Immunologic
Systemic lupus erythematosus
Lymphoproliferative diseases
Autoimmune thrombocytopenic purpura
Isoimmune thrombocytopenic purpura
Nonimmunologic
Thrombotic thrombocytopenic purpura
Septicemia
Chronic hepatitis
Hypergammaglobulinemic states

IMMUNE THROMBOCYTOPENIC PURPURA

Immune thrombocytopenic purpura (ITP) is a syndrome characterized by persistent thrombocytopenia resulting from a circulating IgG antibody directed against a platelet-associated antigen leading to platelet destruction by the reticuloendothelial system (see also Chapter 51).[4-7] IgG antibodies occur either alone (72%) or in combination with IgM, IgA, or both in 95% of the ITP patients; IgM is the only antibody present in 5% of ITP patients. The majority of the IgG in patients having ITP consists of the IgG_1 subclass, although IgG_2, IgG_3, and IgG_4 subclasses may be present in conjunction with IgG_1. Rarely, IgG_3 or IgG_4 subclasses are present in the absence of IgG_1. This has important fetal implications since only certain IgG subclasses are able to cross the placenta. Since there is shared antigenicity between human platelets and megakaryocytes, it is not surprising to find that the antiplatelet IgG antibody binds to the megakaryocyte, markedly altering thrombopoiesis.[4,5,7] Circulating immune complexes are demonstrable in most patients with ITP. An alternative pathogenesis of ITP may involve antibody binding to soluble platelet antigens with subsequent platelet Fc receptor binding, thus accentuating the thrombocytopenia.[4]

The spleen, a major site of antibody production in patients with ITP, produces daily amounts of platelet-specific IgG that could easily saturate the daily production of platelet antigen binding sites. In addition to the splenic production of antibody, bone marrow cells produce IgG antibody.[7] Platelet-associated antigen appears to be a native platelet membrane molecule, as the antigen is manifest on both megakaryocytes and platelets. The antigen appears to differ among patients and may involve platelet glycoproteins IIb and IIIa.[4,7]

Immunocompetent cells of the spleen respond to platelet antigens while bone marrow cells respond to antigenic determinants on the megakaryocyte or intramedullary platelets. The spleen predominates in the early immunologic response followed by bone marrow response later. Following the initial splenic response, circulating B- and T-lymphocyte memory cells develop and initiate the bone marrow response. Early splenectomy appears to inhibit the response to intravascular antigens, but once recirculating B- and T-lymphocyte memory cells develop, splenectomy appears to have little effect. It is not surprising that patients with longstanding disease experience weaker responses to splenectomy.[4,5,7]

The autoimmune phenomenon of ITP remains an enigma. Autoimmune disease may result from a breakdown in the immunoregulatory network that involves helper and suppressor T cells and the antibody-producing B cells.[4,7]

The diagnosis of immune thrombocytopenia can be established by a radiolabeled Coombs test for detection of platelet-associated IgG and C3. The test is a very sensitive indicator of platelet-associated IgG and C3 and plasma antiplatelet antibody in autoimmune and isoimmune platelet disorders. Positive results are obtained in essentially all patients with thrombocytopenia, and titers tend to correlate with clinical presentation.[4]

Serum antiplatelet antibody assays are considered to have less than adequate reliability because antiplatelet antibody titers may be low or absent when the majority of the antibody is platelet bound. Other humoral factors, immune complexes, or isoantibodies may result in false-positive findings. Most important, the results of serum assays do not correlate with clinical status.[4,5,7] The development of a radiolabeled monoclonal antibody to the Fc portion of the human IgG allows measurement of platelet-bound IgG in patients with ITP. The assay appears to be very sensitive and specific for discriminating patients with ITP. It offers future promise after its reliability and accuracy have been investigated more thoroughly.[8]

Patients with ITP complain of easy bruising. Severe thrombocytopenia is associated with mucosal and upper respiratory tract bleeding, with epistaxis, or with gingival bleeding. Hematuria, menorrhagia, or gastrointestinal bleeding may occur. Hemorrhagic vesicles or bullae of the oral mucosa are associated with very low platelet counts, usually less than $5000/mm^3$. Conjunctival or retinal hemorrhage usually indicates impending or imminent central nervous system bleeding. The resulting intracranial hemorrhage usually is fatal. Physical examination reveals bruising, petechiae, or mucosal bleeding. Adenopathy and splenomegaly are unusual. Peripheral blood counts demonstrate thrombocytopenia with increased percentages of large platelets. Bone marrow examination reveals normal granulocytic and erythrocytic elements. However, a marked increase in the number and degree of immature megakaryocytes is seen in the bone marrow smears.[2,4,5,7]

Effects of Pregnancy on Disease

ITP is approximately three times more common in females than in males; the incidence is greater in whites than blacks. The syndrome usually first occurs prior to 30 years of age and may be coincident with pregnancy. Symptoms tend to worsen during pregnancy but treatment of ITP has improved outcomes through the use of adrenal corticosteroids, immunoglobulins, blood platelet transfusions, and the infrequent use of splenectomy.[2,4,5,7]

Infertility does not complicate the clinical course of ITP, although the incidence of spontaneous abortion varies between 5% and 33%. Reproductive counseling should include proper patient advice that pregnancy should be postponed until disease remission is achieved. Ideally, the patient should not require steroids or immunosuppressive agents to maintain remission. All patients should be informed that a cesarean section for hemorrhagic maternal and fetal complications may be required.[4]

The crucial question concerning delivery of the patient with ITP is whether cesarean section is less traumatic than vaginal delivery for both mother and fetus. In the past, elective cesarean section for all mothers with platelet counts less than 100,000/mm^3 at the time of delivery was recommended to avoid both maternal hemorrhage caused by expulsive efforts of labor and cerebral trauma to the fetus. The recommendation was based on a high incidence of neonatal thrombocytopenia and an increased risk of neonatal intracerebral hemorrhage from vaginal delivery in infants born to mothers with platelet counts less than 100,000/mm^3 at the time of delivery. Cesarean section also has been recommended for delivery following splenectomy regardless of platelet count. In addition, abdominal delivery was recommended when the spleen was present if the maternal platelet count was less than 100,000/mm^3.[2,4,5,7,8]

More recent investigations demonstrate no consistent correlation between infant platelet count and maternal platelet count, previous maternal splenectomy, or maternal corticosteroid treatment.[8] Maternal serum antiplatelet antibody titers were not found to be clinically useful in patient management. However, direct measurement of fetal platelet count by fetal scalp blood sampling proved to be reliable in assessing the degree of fetal thrombocytopenia and in selecting the appropriate route of delivery.[9]

The diagnostic tests available for prediction of fetal platelet count prior to delivery fail to provide adequate direction in choosing the appropriate route of delivery. Although initial evidence suggested that maternal platelet counts correlate well with neonatal platelet counts, some evidence suggests that a poor correlation exists.[6-12] Fetal scalp blood sampling, although accurate in estimating fetal platelet counts, is associated with trauma to the fetal head and requires adequate cervical dilatation for successful scalp sampling. This requires that fetal scalp blood sampling be performed only after labor has progressed to adequate cervical dilatation. The test has little impact on the management of significant numbers of patients early in or prior to the onset of labor. Recent evidence suggests that fetal scalp sampling can be performed in only approximately 25–50% of patients.[12] The introduction of percutaneous umbilical blood sampling (cordocentesis) has contributed substantially to the successful management of many ITP pregnancies in tertiary care centers. This technique generally is performed prior to the onset of labor and provides an accurate assessment of fetal platelet status. Levels of anti-platelet antibodies can also be ascertained from the specimen.

The use of cesarean section is reserved for obstetric indications. Critical review of pregnancies complicated by ITP reveals that although the incidence of intracranial hemorrhage is increased in thrombocytopenic infants, the use of cesarean section has not been demonstrated to be of protective value.[5] This view is supported further by the fact that half of the fetal deaths in ITP pregnancies occur prior to the onset of labor from etiologies distinct from intracranial hemorrhage.[13] Therefore, the choice of route of delivery should be based on a host of clinical, obstetric, and laboratory factors and not on a single laboratory value.

A high incidence of maternal postpartum hemorrhage in patients with ITP with platelet counts less than 100,000/mm^3 exists. Myometrial contraction and retraction effectively controls bleeding from the placental site and is relatively independent of platelet count. However, cervical and vaginal lacerations, episiotomy, and trauma require an adequate number and function of platelets for effective hemostasis. Therefore, these complications should be avoided whenever possible and should be repaired meticulously to avoid hematoma formation.[2,5]

Although marked improvements in the diagnosis and treatment of ITP have been made in recent years, there has been little change in the fetal mortality rate. The overall fetal mortality rate for infants born to ITP mothers ranges between 15% and 25%. The most common causes of mortality are stillbirth, spontaneous second-trimester abortion, and hemorrhage. Improved surgical technique in recent years has significantly lowered the fetal mortality rate for splenectomy during pregnancy.[2,4,5,7]

In pregnancy, corticosteroids should be used at the lowest dose possible to attain safe platelet counts because of the association between steroid administration and eclampsia, hypertension, adrenal insufficiency, and psychosis.[14] Steroid administration can cause glucose intolerance during pregnancy with subsequent neonatal hypoglycemia. Estriol production is decreased by the steroidal depression of fetal adrenal estriol precursor production.[2] A recent report of a successful intravenous IgG infusion (Sandoglobulin) of 0.4 g/kg in a patient with ITP who was nonresponsive to steroid administration raises the possibility that IgG infusion may block Fc-receptor-mediated endocytosis by the placenta, thus reducing placental transfer of maternal antibody. This treatment may prove successful in pregnancies having low platelet counts prior to delivery.[15]

Experimental evidence in nonpregnant ITP patients suggests that treatment with high-dose intravenous polyvalent intact immunoglobulin leads to a rapid reversal of thrombocytopenia and that the effect of the immunoglobulin might be attributable to transient blockade of the reticuloendothelial system.[15] This may be accomplished by interference with phagocyte Fc-receptor-mediated immune clearance. This form of therapy, a noninvasive temporary chemical splenectomy, appears to be safe and may be clinically indicated for control of acute hemorrhage, for preparation of corticosteroid-resistant patients for splenectomy, or for safer performance of other surgical procedures in the nonpregnant patient with life-threatening disease.

PLATELET DISORDERS WITH PREGNANCY-INDUCED HYPERTENSION

Pregnancy-induced hypertension (*preeclampsia and eclampsia syndrome*) is characterized by hypertension, proteinuria, and edema and usually occurs in primigravidas after the 20th week of gestation (see Chapters 139 and 140). It also may occur in multigravidas and chronic hypertensive patients.[16] The hypertensive disorders of pregnancy remain major causes of maternal and fetal morbidity and mortality. The clinical manifestations are varied and may present difficulties in diagnosis because of their wide spectrum of clinical presentations. The severity of thrombocytopenia often correlates with the severity of clinical disease in patients with pregnancy-induced hypertension. Although thrombocytopenia is more likely to be present in association with eclampsia, thrombocytopenia is most frequently found in patients remote from term or having underlying vascular disease.

Thrombocytopenia in association with acute liver disease, DIC, and hypertension may occur prior to eclamptic episodes. These patients often cause problems in diagnosis because the initial signs and symptoms often are misinterpreted. Subsequent liver dysfunction results in jaundice and painful hepatomegaly and may occur despite minimal changes in fibrinogen levels and prothrombin times.[17]

A unique group of pregnancy-induced hypertension patients having laboratory evidence of hemolysis (H), elevated liver enzymes (EL), and a low platelet count (LP) has been identified recently; this is referred to as the *HELLP syndrome*. This triad of laboratory abnormalities has been noted to occur in the absence of more common signs and symptoms of severe pregnancy-induced hypertension.[18]

The clinical appearance of HELLP syndrome may occur remote from term, following hospitalization and observation, or early in the postpartum period. In rare patients, the classically described signs and symptoms of pregnancy-induced hypertension may be absent, often leading to misdiagnosis. If this syndrome remains undiagnosed, significant maternal and neonatal mortality may occur.

Little attention has been directed to the deterioration of various renal function tests that occurs in patients having the HELLP syndrome. Recent evidence strongly suggests that renal function should be included in the definition of the HELLP syndrome. Decreases in renal creatinine clearance and urine output occur in the majority of, if not all, patients.[19]

HUS–TTP

Hemolytic uremic syndrome (HUS) is a disorder with microvascular lesions limited to the renal glomeruli.[20] Similar to the HELLP syndrome, it also is manifested by hemolytic anemia of the microangiopathic type and thrombocytopenia. It is extremely uncommon in obstetric patients although when it is found, it may be seen most frequently in the postpartum period. This has earned it the term *postpartum nephrosclerosis*. It deserves special mention since early recognition and supportive therapy may be life saving.

Thrombotic thrombocytopenic purpura (TTP) is an unusual disease of unknown etiology that most frequently afflicts women in their third and fourth decades of life.[21] The clinical features of TTP are characterized by a combination of hematologic and neurologic findings. Other manifestations include ecchymoses, malaise, abdominal pain, fever, jaundice, and pallor. The development of seizures and coma are considered unfavorable prognostic signs. Diagnosis of TTP is based on hemolytic anemia with microangiopathic features and thrombocytopenia in a patient with fever and neurologic manifestations. Gingival or skin biopsy have been suggested previously as methods to establish the diagnosis, although their interpretation is difficult and frequently of no benefit.

Past approaches to treatment for TTP have included various combinations of steroids, immunosuppressive agents, platelet suppressors, and supportive therapy, including dialysis for renal failure. Despite these treatments, mortality from TTP ranged from 50–90%. The recent introductions of plasma infusion, plasma exchange, and whole blood exchange have resulted in response rates ranging up to 90%. Platelet transfusions alone in these patients may lead to massive aggregation in the microvasculature, underscoring the need to make an early diagnosis.

Differentiating pregnancy-induced hypertension from HUS–TTP may prove difficult in the patient presenting with hypertension, proteinuria, and renal failure, especially when there are neurologic signs and laboratory features of microangiopathic hemolytic anemia (fragmented red blood cells).[22] Distinctive features to be considered include the degree of thrombocytopenia, which is frequently more severe in HUS–TTP, and the degree of hemolysis leading to a marked fall in the hemoglobin, serum haptoglobin, and elevated plasma LDH levels, also more characteristic of HUS–TTP. This is one of the few situations in which a skin biopsy may help differentiate the disorders. Readers are referred to two excellent reviews that may be beneficial in helping to establish a differential diagnosis when confronted by these entities.[23,24]

REFERENCES

1. Nossel HL. Platelet disorders, in Petersdorf RG, Adams RD, Braunwald E, et al, eds. *Harrison's Principles of Internal Medicine*, 10. New York: McGraw-Hill; 1983:1900.
2. Levin J. Hematologic disorders of pregnancy. In: Burrows GN, Ferris TF, eds. *Medical Complications during Pregnancy*, 2nd ed. Philadelphia: WB Saunders; 1982:70.
3. Pitkin RM, Witte DL. Platelet and leukocyte counts in pregnancy. *JAMA*. 1979;242:2696.
4. Romero R, Duffy T. Platelet disorders in pregnancy. *Clin Perinatol*. 1980;7:327.
5. Kagan R, Laros RK. Immune thrombocytopenia. *Clin Obstet Gynecol*. 1983;26:537.
6. Cines DB, Dusak B, Tomaski A, et al. Immune thrombocytopenic purpura and pregnancy. *N Engl J Med*. 1982;306:827.
7. McMillan R. Chronic idiopathic thrombocytopenic purpura. *N Engl J Med*. 1981;304:1135.
8. Scott JR, Cruikshank DP, Kochenour NK, et al. Fetal platelet counts in the obstetric management of immunologic thrombocytopenic purpura. *Am J Obstet Gynecol*. 1980;136:495.
9. Ayromlooi J. A new approach to the management of immunologic thrombocytopenic purpura in pregnancy. *Am J Obstet Gynecol*. 1978;130:235.
10. LoBuglio AF, Court WS, Binocur L, et al. Use of a (125)I-labeled antihuman IgG monoclonal antibody to quantify platelet-bound IgG. *N Engl J Med*. 1983;309:459.
11. Fehr J, Hofmann V, Kappeler U. Transient reversal of thrombocytopenia in idiopathic thrombocytopenic purpura by high-dose intravenous gamma globulin. *N Engl J Med*. 1982;306:1254.
12. Territo M, Finklestein J, Oh W, et al. Management of autoimmune thrombocytopenia in pregnancy and in the neonate. *Obstet Gynecol*. 1973;41:579.
13. Noriega Guerra L, Aviles Miranda A, de la Cadena OA, et al. Pregnancy in patients with autoimmune thrombocytopenic purpura. *Am J Obstet Gynecol*. 1979;133:439.
14. Karpatkin M, Porges RF, Karpatkin S. Platelet counts in infants of women with autoimmune thrombocytopenia: effect of steroid administration to the mother. *N Engl J Med*. 1981;305:936.
15. Wahbeh CJ, Eden RD, Killam AP, et al. ITP and pregnancy. *Am J Obstet Gynecol*. 1984;149:238.
16. Jones RW, Asher MI, Rutherford CJ, et al. Autoimmune (idiopathic) thrombocytopenic purpura in pregnancy and the newborn. *Br J Obstet Gynaecol*. 1977;84:679.
17. Newland AC, Boots MA, Patterson KG. Intravenous IgG for autoimmune thrombocytopenia in pregnancy. *N Engl J Med*. 1984;301:261.
18. Gant NF, Worley RJ. *Hypertension in Pregnancy*. New York, NY: Appleton-Century-Crofts; 1980:5, 49.
19. Killam AP, Dillard SH, Patton RC, et al. Pregnancy-induced hypertension complicated by acute liver disease and disseminated intravascular coagulation. *Am J Obstet Gynecol*. 1975;123:823.
20. Weinstein L. Syndrome of hemolysis, elevated liver enzymes and low platelet count: a severe consequence of hypertension in pregnancy. *Am J Obstet Gynecol*. 1982;142:159.
21. MacKenna J, Dorer NL, Brame RG. Pre-eclampsia associated with hemolysis, elevated liver enzymes, and low platelets—an obstetric emergency? *Obstet Gynecol*. 1983;62:751.
22. Moschcowitz E. An acute febrile pleiochromic anemia with hyaline thrombosis of the terminal arterioles and capillaries: an undescribed disease. *Arch Int Med*. 1925;36:89.
23. Kennedy SS, Zacharski LR, Beck JR. Thrombotic thrombocytopenic purpura: analysis of 48 unselected cases. *Semin Thromb Hemost*. 1980;6:341.
24. Petitt RM. Thrombotic thrombocytopenic purpura: a 30-year review. *Semin Thromb Hemost*. 1981;7:1.

Chapter One Hundred and Sixty-Six

Bleeding Disorders Caused by Vessel Wall Abnormalities

Robert D. Eden and Robert A. Welch

166

Bleeding caused by *vessel wall abnormalities* (*nonthrombocytopenic purpuras*) are uncommon during pregnancy. These abnormalities are of two types: those related to vascular endothelial cell disruption and those related to vascular fragility (Table 166–1).

Blood vessels contribute to hemostasis to a limited extent through contraction and spasm of vascular smooth muscle. In contrast, vascular endothelium performs a number of vital roles. Normal endothelium neither activates the soluble component coagulation system nor attracts platelets. Endothelium is the major source of prostacyclin, a potent inhibitor of platelet adhesion and aggregation[1], and binds or synthesizes Von Willebrand factor, which is essential to platelet adhesion. Vascular endothelium is the major source of tissue plasminogen activator, which is essential in preventing venous thrombosis.[2]

Endothelial cell disruption may occur as a consequence of severe systemic infections, as an allergic response to certain medications, and as hypersensitivity reactions, including the Schoenlein–Henoch syndrome. Structural protein depletion resulting in fragile blood vessels is the common etiology for some severe systemic illnesses. Of these, scurvy, Cushing's syndrome, hereditary hemorrhagic telangiectasia, and hyperglobulinemic purpuras are the most common.

A number of severe systemic infections that have been associated with vessel wall endothelial damage and capillary fragility include meningococcal sepsis, typhoid fever, subacute bacterial endocarditis, rickettsiae and some childhood viral infections. Bleeding from these infections represents local endothelial damage from bacterial toxins resulting in extravasation of blood into the subvascular space.

Allergies to commonly employed medications, such as penicillins, sulfonamides and allopurinol, have been implicated as a cause of purpura, although urticarial or maculopapular rashes are generally the more common manifestation of allergic response.

Hypersensitivity Angiitis (Schoenlein–Henoch Purpura)

A variety of drugs, food, and bacteria have been implicated in "hypersensitivity angiitis." Schoenlein–Henoch syndromes or *anaphylactoid purpura* is a distinct, self-limited type of vasculitis that occurs in children and young adults. It may be related to acute nephritis and rheumatic fever after a streptococcal sore throat. Hypersensitivity angiitis is characterized by acute inflammatory reaction of the capillaries and mesangial tissues of the small arterioles, resulting in increased vascular permeability, exudation, and hemorrhage into surrounding tissues.[3] Immunoglobulin A and alternate pathway complement components have been identified in the capillaries of these patients.

Scurvy

Scurvy (vitamin C deficiency) is rarely encountered in industrialized nations (see also Chapter 19). This disease may present with painful episodes of perifollicular skin bleeding, bleeding into muscles, gingival swelling, skin hyperkeratosis, and urinary or gastrointestinal tract hemorrhage. The etiology of bleeding from ascorbic acid deficiency appears to be from defective hydroxyproline biosynthesis leading to reduced collagen formation in intracellular capillary cell walls.[2]

Cushing's Syndrome

Although not completely understood, bleeding associated with Cushing's syndrome in the nonpregnant patient has many similarities to bleeding from protein-wasting syndromes (see also Chapter 42). In this disease, vessel walls sustain loss of perivascular supporting tissues, leading to vascular fragility. These supporting tissues appear to be lost as a result of the protein-wasting effects of high endogenous glucocorticoids.

Hereditary Hemorrhagic Telangiectasia (Osler–Rendu Syndrome)

This disease is inherited as a simple dominant trait. Although the sexes are affected equally, bleeding appears to be less severe in females.[4] The resulting developmental structural abnormality of the vasculature, characterized by the local dilatation and convolution of the capillaries, causes distinct telangiectasias. Telangiectasias may appear throughout the life span of the patient but are most commonly found during the fourth and fifth decades of life. At autopsy, telangiectasias have been found in all major organ systems. Hemorrhagic manifestations result from capillary friability of the widely disseminated lesions.[4]

Hyperglobulinemic Purpura

Vascular nonthrombocytopenic purpura may occur in disorders causing "hyperglobulinemic purpura" such as macroglobulinemia, multiple myeloma, or cryoglobulinemia. In contrast to blood vessel fragility resulting from loss of protein in the integument, these syndromes are characterized by damage to vessel walls and capillary proteins from the anoxia of hyperviscosity. Platelet and blood coagulation function also may be abnormal. A maculopapular purpura occurs in association with a mixed cryoglobulinemia from immune complex damage to the vessel wall and usually is associated with arthralgia, weakness, and nephritis. Plasmapheresis may result in short-term clinical improvement, but the long-term management of these patients includes identification and treatment of the underlying disease.[4]

EFFECTS OF PREGNANCY ON DISEASE

There is little evidence that pregnancy is related directly to the bleeding manifestations of these vessel wall abnormalities. Physiologic changes in pregnancy, however, may increase susceptibility to some of the underlying conditions leading to nonthrombocytopenic purpura. Pregnancy alters nutritional requirements, down-regulates some aspects of immune function, and increases vascular compliance and blood volume.

TABLE 166–1. ETIOLOGIES OF BLEEDING CAUSED BY VESSEL WALL ABNORMALITIES

Endothelial Disruption
Infection
Drug ingestion
Schoenlein–Henoch syndrome
Vascular Fragility
Scurvy
Cushing's syndrome
Hereditary hemorrhagic telangiectasia
Hyperglobulinemic purpura

Purpura related to vessel wall abnormalities in pregnancy are extremely uncommon. Generally, maternal mucous membrane or skin bleeding from capillary endothelium damage ceases within 48 hours. This maternal bleeding has virtually no effect on the fetus. One cannot ignore, however, the potential effects of the underlying etiology for maternal purpura on the fetus. Caregivers must be cognizant of the potential impact of maternal therapy on the fetus. Operative interventions during pregnancy may become necessary to control disease, but should be considered with great care since anesthetic and surgical complications may compromise fetal well-being. Corticosteroids, which may be required to alleviate some of the symptoms of hypersensitivity angiitis and similar conditions in pregnancy, should be used with caution even though they have not been shown to be teratogenic in humans.

Nonthrombocytopenic purpura is a manifestation of underlying disease. At times it may be difficult to differentiate this type of bleeding from the bleeding of an obstetric coagulopathy. Serious infection is an example of a clinical condition confounded by coexistent coagulopathies. Except in the most extreme cases, diagnostic differentiation may be made based on the laboratory findings. The consumptive coagulopathy and disseminated intravascular coagulation of obstetric hemorrhage usually are associated with low platelets and coagulation factors.

Patients suspected of having bleeding related to scurvy may have this diagnosis confirmed by obtaining an ascorbic acid level on white blood cells. This extreme hypovitaminosis suggests serious nutritional deprivation; diagnostic consideration of fetal growth may be part of the evaluation during pregnancy.

The clinical presentation of *hypersensitivity angiitis* (*Schoenlein–Henoch syndrome*) includes a purpuric rash and urticaria on the extensor surfaces of the arms, legs, and buttocks. Abdominal pain resulting from extravasation of fluid and blood into the intestinal wall may occur; this must be differentiated from uterine activity. Polyarthralgia and polyarthritis are common. Characteristically, platelet function and coagulation tests are unremarkable. Hematuria, albuminuria, and casts reflect a transient focal glomerulonephritis. Progression of hypersensitivity angiitis from acute diffuse glomerulonephritis to acute renal failure, edema, and hypertension occasionally occurs.

Fewer than 50 cases of Cushing's syndrome have been reported in pregnancy.[3] This disease is associated with high maternal and fetal morbidity and mortality. Although bleeding from this disease is rare, the diagnosis must be suspected if "Cushingoid features" are present. Laboratory tests may reveal hypokalemia, high serum and urine cortisol and 17-ketosteroid levels. The dexamethasone suppression test has been employed to make this diagnosis during pregnancy and may help to diagnose adrenal tumors. Ultrasound of the maternal adrenal glands may visualize larger tumors. Cushing's syndrome often is associated with diabetes, which may require intensive prenatal surveillance.

Hereditary hemorrhagic telangiectasia (Osler–Rendu syndrome) is associated with recurrent hemorrhage and anemia from recurrent rupture of small, nonpulsatile blood vessels. These violaceous lesions blanch with finger pressure and are found over a variety of areas including nasal and buccal mucous membranes, skin, and viscera.[2,4] Recurrent epistaxis occurs in approximately 80% of these patients. Vascular malformations associated with pulmonary arterial venous fistulas may result in shunting of blood and lead to clubbing of the digits, mild hypoxemia, or secondary polycythemia. Although rarely encountered, two patients with hereditary hemorrhagic telangiectasia during pregnancy were recently reported to develop heart failure from angiography-confirmed arteriovenous hepatic shunts. Both recovered spontaneously after delivery and signs of congestive failure disappeared within six months.[5] Recurrent cerebral embolism and brain abscess may occur as a consequence of pulmonary shunting of blood. Arteriovenous fistula of the cerebral or retinal vessels and aneurysms of the hepatic and splenic arteries and aorta have occurred.

Hepatosplenomegaly may be found in patients with telangiectasia involving this organ. Cirrhosis and portal hypertension may result.[4] Laboratory findings are related to the severity of the hemorrhagic manifestations and a hypochromic, microcytic anemia is common. The degree of reticulocytosis and depletion of total body iron stores are proportional to the degree of blood loss. Iron replacement therapy and blood transfusions are effective support measures when employed for recurrent bleeding episodes. Therapy for the control of hemorrhage includes pressure to the bleeding point, application of absorbable topical hemostatic agents such as oxidase cellulose, and electrocoagulation for recurrent lesions. Sophisticated surgical interventions may be required to control severe epistaxis or visceral hemorrhage. This is often unrewarding since repeated surgeries become necessary to control the multiple telangiectasias.[4]

REFERENCES

1. Dusting GJ, Moncada S, Varne JR. Prostacyclin: its biosynthesis, actions and chemical potential. *Adv Prostaglandin Thromboxane Leukotriene Res.* 1982;10:59.
2. Handin HL. Bleeding and Thrombosis. In: Braunwald E, Isselbacher KJ, Petersdorf RF, et al, eds. *Harrison's Principles of Internal Medicine.* 11th ed. New York, NY: McGraw-Hill; 1987:266.
3. Casson IF, Davis JC, Jeffreys RV, et al. Successful management of Cushing's disease during pregnancy by transsphenoidal adenectomy. *Clin Endocrinol.* 1987;27:423.
4. Handin RI. Disorders of the Platelet and Vessel Wall. In: Braunwald E, Isselbacher KJ, Petersdorf RF, et al, eds. *Harrison's Principles of Internal Medicine.* 11th ed. New York, NY: McGraw-Hill; 1987:1471.
5. Livneh A, Langevitz P, Morag B, et al. Functionally reversible hepatic arteriovenous fistulas during pregnancy in patients with hereditary hemorrhagic telangiectasis. *S Med J.* 1988;81:1047.

Chapter One Hundred and Sixty-Seven
Disorders of Blood Coagulation Factors

Robert A. Welch and Robert D. Eden

167

Coagulation is the process of clot formation.[1] This enzymatic mechanism is a vital part of the process of hemostasis, which involves the blood vessel wall, platelets, and plasma proteins. Normally, this phenomenon relies on two phases that must occur harmoniously. The first of these, primary hemostasis, involves platelet aggregation at the site of vascular injury. This initial seal slows further hemorrhage and may be assayed with a bleeding time. Formation of a fibrin clot that serves to stabilize the initial platelet plug constitutes the second phase of hemostasis. This process depends on activation of a series of coagulation factors, the individual importance of each being emphasized by clot breakdown and further bleeding should a deficiency or defect occur.[2-4]

Birth is a physiologic event that relies heavily on maternal and fetal coagulation system homeostasis. Abnormalities of this system, either congenital or acquired (Table 167–1), may result in dramatic and sometimes disastrous consequences for the parturient and offspring. This chapter reviews some of these disturbances and their relevance in human reproduction. Since pregnancy-induced hypertension, immune thrombocytopenic purpura, thrombotic thrombocytopenic purpura, and hemolytic uremic syndrome are discussed elsewhere (see Chapter 165), these disorders will not be reviewed here.

CONGENITAL DISORDERS OF COAGULATION

Von Willebrand's Disease

Von Willebrand's disease most frequently is inherited as an autosomal dominant trait, although a recently described, less common mode of inheritance is autosomal recessive.[5] The disease is characterized by an abnormality of the von Willebrand factor portion of the factor VIII complex. It accounts for approximately 10% of all inherited disorders of blood coagulation and is found in 1 in 10,000 persons, making it the most common hereditary coagulopathy seen by obstetricians.[6]

Pathophysiology. There are three basic types of von Willebrand's disease. *Type I* or *classic* von Willebrand's disease consists of a quantitative decrease of von Willebrand's factor. *Type IIA* is characterized by the absence of large and intermediate-sized multimers of von Willebrand's factor from both plasma and platelets. *Type IIB* consists of absence of multimers from plasma only.[7] Patients with this disease may present with a variety of bleeding complaints depending on the severity of the factor VIII abnormality. Menorrhagia and postpartum hemorrhage are perhaps the most frequent manifestations of von Willebrand's disease seen by the obstetrician-gynecologist.[8] Excessive bleeding during surgery is another frequently encountered complication leading to discovery of this disease, while post-trauma hemorrhage, gastrointestinal bleeding, epistaxis and gingival bleeding may arouse suspicion.

The diagnosis of von Willebrand's disease is made through laboratory demonstration of platelet function abnormalities. Abnormal platelet adhesion owing to absent or nonfunctional von Willebrand factor may cause a prolongation of the bleeding time. The level of factor VIII:C also may modify the PTT. Platelet aggregation may fail with the antibiotic ristocetin. Defective platelet adhesion to subendothelial collagen of the capillary wall results from the absence of the Von Willebrand protein, leading to delayed hemostatic formation and a prolonged bleeding time. Patients with von Willebrand's disease demonstrate a concordant decrease in the level of the antihemophilic factor VIII:C, von Willebrand's factor, and factor VIIIR:Ag. In contrast, only factor VIII:C is decreased in hemophilia A. Von Willebrand's disease may result from an impaired synthesis of the entire factor VIII protein complex responsible for coagulation and platelet function. However, the exact nature of the molecular abnormality remains to be determined.[8–11] Hemostatic and platelet defects associated with von Willebrand's disease are corrected by infusion of concentrated factor VIII, cryoprecipitate, or fresh frozen plasma.

Effect of Disease on Pregnancy. Complications from von Willebrand's disease are infrequent during pregnancy. As with the other coagulation factors, there is a rise in both factor VIII:C and von Willebrand factor during pregnancy. In the majority of patients, factor VIII levels almost reach or achieve normality at the time of delivery.[12] Postpartum hemorrhage may not occur in the presence of low factor VIII:C levels as long as they are greater than 50% of expected levels.[8,11-13] Early pregnancy loss, however, from spontaneous miscarriage or abortion before the physiologic elevation of coagulation factors may increase the likelihood for bleeding. Following delivery, factor VIII:C falls to prepregnancy levels within two to three days, increasing the risk for late postpartum hemorrhage.[14-15]

For the occasional patient who experiences postpartum hemorrhage related to this disease, cryoprecipitate is the treatment of choice. Cryoprecipitate generally is readily available and contains all forms of the factor VIII macromolecular complex.[16] As previously noted, most women with known von Willebrand's disease will have factor VIII:C levels above 50% by term. Treatment of those who fall under these levels or those who require cesarean delivery consists of prophylactic transfusion with cryoprecipitate or fresh frozen plasma.[17-18] Delayed postpartum hemorrhage requires similar transfusion therapy. A recommended dosage of cryoprecipitate in these patients consists of 15–20 units twice daily for at least one week.[5] While this therapy achieves coagulation, it may cause a delay in the natural production of factor VIII:C.

Hemophilia A

Hemophilia A is inherited as an X-linked recessive disease affecting 10–15 per 100,000 males in the United States.[19] It is limited almost exclusively to men having normal sons and obligatory carrier daughters. Hemophilia may occur rarely in a homozygous female offspring of a paternal hemophiliac and maternal carrier. In addition, a few accounts of women carriers of this disease experiencing bleeding

TABLE 167–1. CONGENITAL AND ACQUIRED DISORDERS OF COAGULATION

Congenital
Von Willebrand's disease
Hemophilia A and B
Antithrombin III deficiency
Factor deficiencies
Acquired
Abruptio placentae
Dead fetus syndrome
Amniotic fluid embolus
Sepsis
Pregnancy-induced hypertension
Immune thrombocytopenic purpura
Thrombotic thrombocytopenic purpura
Hemolytic uremic syndrome

manifestations secondary to "extreme lyonization" have been reported.[20-21] These rare reports do not supercede the major significance of this disease in pregnancy—its inheritance pattern.

Pathophysiology. Hemophilia A results from a deficiency of factor VIII activity. Immunologic studies of this disease suggest a heterogeneous disorder. Plasma from the majority of patients with hemophilia A is incapable of neutralizing naturally occurring human antibodies to factor VIII. Conversely, a small portion of these patients are capable of neutralizing these antibodies. Regardless, the fundamental abnormality in hemophilia A is a qualitative defect rather than a quantitative defect in factor VIII. The immunologically active clotting component is designated factor VIII-related antigen (VIIIR:Ag).[2,10]

The clinical severity of hemophilia is characterized by the patient's tendency to bleed. Severe hemophiliacs may experience spontaneous bleeding into skin, viscera, and joints. Moderate cases have fewer spontaneous bleeding episodes, but may have significant bleeding from minor trauma, while minor hemophiliacs may have serious bleeding from injury or surgery.

A common symptom for all forms of hemophilia is excessive and persistent bleeding following dental extraction. Subcutaneous or intramuscular hematomas are found most often on the legs, and severe anemia and shock may result from hemorrhage dissecting along fascial planes. Although dramatic, bleeding episodes are rarely fatal, but are associated with permanent debilitation through deformities in the calves, thighs, buttocks, and forearms. Compression of peripheral nerves leads to peripheral neuropathies, excruciating pain, paresthesia, and muscle atrophy.

Death is usually a result of hemorrhage within the intracranial cavity; up to ten percent of these patients develop evidence of intracranial hemorrhage. However, hemarthrosis is the most frequent indication for hospital admission. Trauma or unusual exertion results in painful, tender, and swollen joints. Extensive joint destruction and reactive changes in the adjacent bone and tissues result in deformity and pain. The joint becomes stiff and unstable, and movement is greatly restricted. Joint deformity results in muscle wasting and soft tissue contractures. Osteoporosis with complete loss of articular surfaces and flattening of bone ends is a frequent sequela. Hematuria, epistaxis, and mucous membrane bleeding occur frequently.[2,10-11,22]

Laboratory identification of this disease is based on quantitation of circulating factor VIII:C. These levels are less than 1% in severe hemophiliacs (factor VIII:C $<1\%$, <0.01 U/mL). Levels of 1–5 are considered moderate, and those with $>5\%$ factor VIII:C are classified as mild.

The diagnosis of hemophilia is confirmed with laboratory findings of a prolonged partial thromboplastin time (PTT), normal TCT, PT, and low factor VII:C level. Factor VIIIR:Ag levels are usually normal in carriers and affected individuals with hemophilia A. Laboratory diagnosis may be confounded by the wide fluctuations in factor VIII:C normally and in response to physiologic and pathophysiologic conditions (eg, exercise, fever). Thus, carrier status cannot be determined merely by ascertaining factor VIII:C levels.[23-24] In general, carriers are expected to have 50% factor VIII:C plasma levels, producing a 1:2 plasma ratio of factor VIII:C to factor VIIIR:Ag. This allows for up to 90% identification of carriers when serum factor VIII laboratory data and pedigree are combined into the determination.[23-25]

Effect of Disease on Pregnancy. Counseling of patients at risk for delivering male offspring with hemophilia A should be performed early enough in pregnancy to allow for informed decisions. Women who are offspring of a hemophiliac are obligate carriers and those with a family history of hemophilia should be given genetic counseling. Fetal sex determination must be determined through chorionic villus sampling or genetic amniocentesis.[26-27] Percutaneous umbilical blood sampling now has supplanted fetoscopy as a means for obtaining fetal blood[28-29]; this technique is the preferred method for obtaining fetal blood for factor VIII:C and VIIIR:Ag ratios.[30] Restriction fragment length polymorphisms obtained through chorionic villus sampling are an even newer technique offered in a few laboratories (see Chapter 14).[31,32]

In general, coagulation factors have been noted to increase during pregnancy, including factors VIII:C and VIIIR:Ag.[13] Reflecting the rarity of homozygous females with this disease, there have been only four affected women reported to deliver and one did have abnormal postpartum hemorrhage. Curiously, the medical literature is devoid of case reports of hemorrhagic fetal death before or during labor and natural childbirth has not been reported as unsafe for the affected male infant. Whether a fetal scalp electrode is safe to use during labor has not been determined, but it would appear prudent to avoid one unless there are strong obstetric considerations. Upon delivery of a male infant known to be at risk for hemophilia A, cord blood should be obtained to determine PTT and factor VIII:C activity. Neonatal interventions and circumcision should be avoided until coagulation status of the newborn is known.[4]

Since pregnancies of only four women with hemophilia A have been reported, the necessity for controlling hemorrhage from a hemophiliac obstetric patient is rare. Still, if treatment becomes necessary, cryoprecipitate, fresh frozen plasma, or factor VIII concentrate should be given. Factor VIII concentrate carries a considerable risk for hepatitis B since it is obtained from pooled donors.

Hemophilia B (Factor IX)

Hemophilia B is also known as *Christmas disease* and is due to congenital deficiency of factor IX.[33] This rare coagulation disorder (1–3 per 100,000) is inherited as a sex-linked recessive, and females are rarely affected. Affected males display clinical features very similar to hemophilia A, with levels of severity ranging from mild to severe.

Pathophysiology. Mild cases of hemophilia B have more than 5% factor IX levels, those with moderate disease have 1–5%, and those with severe disease have less than 1%.[5] Laboratory evaluation usually demonstrates normal coagulation studies except for an abnormally long PTT, and occasionally the PT may be prolonged. The diagnosis is confirmed by demonstrating low factor IX levels. Carriers are suspected when factor IX levels are only 25% of expected levels.[34]

Effect of Disease on Pregnancy

Prenatal diagnosis of factor IX deficiency has been accomplished.[3] Fetal blood may be obtained through percutaneous blood sampling or fetoscopy, although factor IX in amniotic fluid may increase the risk for incorrect diagnosis.[35]

Factor IX levels are thought to increase with pregnancy. This would appear to be protective of the rare parturient affected with this disorder. The three cases of this entity reported during pregnancy do not confirm this speculation.[20,36] While one delivered without complications, another required plasmapheresis and plasma transfusions for excessive bleeding because of factor IX deficiency.

Plasma transfusion is used to replace factor IX, usually in combination with plasmapheresis to prevent fluid overload. Cryoprecipitate lacks substantial quantities of factor IX. Factor IX concentrate is available commercially, but carries a risk of hepatitis B.[37]

Other Factor Deficiencies

Deficiencies of factors V, VII, X and XIII are not encountered often, but may be considered when unexplained bleeding occurs with the laboratory observation of a prolonged PTT. These disorders are inherited in an autosomal recessive fashion and are prevalent in from 1 in 500,000 to 1 in 1,000,000 individuals.[5] While the majority of clotting factors increase during pregnancy, factor V does not appear to rise above normal. Factor XIII deficiency causes umbilical cord bleeding in nearly all of affected individuals within the first days of life.[38] Bleeding from this disorder may be lifelong and mimic severe hemophilia A. Recurrent miscarriage with remarkable uterine bleeding has been described with factor XIII deficiency[39], and male patients are sterile.[40]

Antithrombin III Deficiency

Antithrombin III deficiency (AT III) is relatively common, with an estimated prevalence of 1 in 2000 people.[41] This anticoagulant factor is a principle inhibitor of thrombin, factor Xa, and other serine proteases. Its deficiency markedly increases the risk of deep vein thrombosis.

Pathophysiology. Symptomatic deep vein thrombosis occurs in 40–70% of individuals with AT III deficiency, and the majority express this condition by age 35.[42] Laboratory diagnosis is made by determining AT III activity in the patient's plasma. Levels of 25–50% are considered deficient.

Prophylactic heparin (5000 units subcutaneously every 12 hours) may be beneficial in preventing recurrent thrombosis in these individuals.[43] Fresh frozen plasma is the only source for AT III available and may be combined with heparin administration in severe cases. If thrombosis occurs, full heparinization is required to elevate the PT to 1.5–2.0 times normal baseline.

Effect of Disease on Pregnancy. As many as 70% of women with AT III deficiency will experience a thrombotic event during pregnancy.[44] Women with known AT III deficiency may benefit from prophylactic heparin administration. Those experiencing their first thrombotic episode during pregnancy need to have AT III levels evaluated, as pregnancy does not appear to impact these values.[5]

ACQUIRED DISORDERS OF COAGULATION

Abruptio Placentae

Abruptio placentae occurs in 0.4–3.5% of pregnancies and is defined as premature separation of the normally located placenta from the uterus before birth of the infant.[45-48] Although maternal hemorrhage from this condition can be dramatic, maternal mortality is rare. In contrast, perinatal death ranges between 5 and 15%.

Pathophysiology

Abruptio placentae appears to be more common in older gravidas in association with higher parity. Hypertension appears to be a contributing factor[47], as does trauma.[49] Consumption of cocaine also has been recognized recently to cause *abruptio placentae* through the intense vasospasm and hypertension associated with this illicit drug.[50]

With separation of the placenta during abruptio, coagulation and fibrinolysis commence without the usual physiologic modifying cofactors. Myometrial contraction increases and labor accelerates. While this process is occurring, there is a corresponding reduction in available placental surface exposed to the uterus. This may result in fetal hypoxia and is the principle etiology for perinatal morbidity and mortality in these cases. Intramyometrial extravasation of blood (Couvelaire uterus) prevents myometrial contraction and allows for ongoing hemorrhage.

Consumption of plasma fibrinogen and production of fibrin degradation products are a consistent laboratory finding with *abruptio placentae.*[51] Release of tissue thromboplastins as the placenta tears from the uterine wall triggers the coagulation cascade, resulting in consumption of clotting factors, including fibrinogen, factor V, factor VII, factor VIII, and antithrombin III. With the consumption of these factors, disseminated intravascular coagulation (DIC) ensues. There is controversy as to the exact mechanism of DIC in *abruptio placentae.* Pritchard et al[52] suggest that thromboplastin is released systemically and is a direct cause of DIC. Bonnar et al[53] have calculated the total decrease in fibrinogen versus clot size and note that only through systemic intravascular coagulation could the dramatic falls in fibrinogen occur.

For the purposes of treatment, *abruptio placentae* has been categorized into three grades.[47] Grade I consists of mild hemorrhages of uncertain etiology. This grade usually is diagnosed after delivery with retrospective examination of the placenta and discovery of an attached clot. Grade II includes cases with classic features of *abruptio placentae* (ie, uterine hypertonicity) in which the fetus is still living. Grade III is severe and the fetus is always dead. This grade is subdivided further into grade IIIA when coagulopathy is not present and IIIB when coagulopathy is present.

Management of severe *abruptio placentae* consists of rapid assessment of clinical condition, initiation of supportive care, and correction of electrolyte and hematologic abnormalities. Estimation of blood loss in these cases frequently may be erroneous because of a large retroplacental clot ("concealed abruptio"). Blood component therapy consists of replacement of coagulation factors and oxygen-carrying capacity. Fresh frozen plasma provides essential clotting components, while packed red blood cells replace oxygen-carrying capacity. Ten milliliters of 10% calcium gluconate should be given for every 4 units of packed cells or fresh frozen plasma. Platelet transfusion may be considered when total platelet count drops below 50,000/mL, especially if this value is encountered and emergency surgery is considered.[54]

Dead Fetus Syndrome

An association between obstetric coagulopathy and fetal demise was first made by Weiner et al in 1950.[55] Since this initial report, there have been a variety of reports proposing various mechanisms for development of DIC related to fetal demise.[56]

Pathophysiology. Popular theory concerning the mechanism of DIC in the dead fetus syndrome recognizes the release of tissue thromboplastin from the fetoplacental unit, causing activation of the extrinsic clotting pathway.[55] Support for this theory comes from animal experiments demonstrating the development of DIC after infusion of placental tissues.

The bleeding diathesis associated with this syndrome stems from intense fibrinolytic activity.[57] Laboratory findings verifying this process consist of a low fibrinogen concentration, the presence of fibrin degradation products, prolongation of the PT and PTT, and a normal platelet count.[58] Other laboratory evidence consists of an increase in clot lysis, decreased plasminogen concentration, and prolonged euglobulin lysis time.[56-58]

Although this clinical entity is not encountered often in modern obstetrics, the occasional case deserves aggressive management. Induction of labor with oxytocin or prostaglandins should be accomplished with the usual obstetric considerations. Hemostatic factors need to be corrected in uncompensated cases. Frequently, this consists of fibrinogen replacement since this factor is most often affected. For every 10 units of cryoprecipitate the fibrinogen concentration will rise approximately 50 mg/dL.[59] Heparin therapy has been used with varying success to reverse DIC in patients not in labor and with multifetal gestations in which one fetus is premature and still alive.[60-61]

Amniotic Fluid Embolus

Amniotic fluid embolus is a serious obstetric event that often leads to catastrophe (see also Chapter 120). Its frequency is difficult to determine since the diagnosis often is not determined until after maternal death, but estimates of one in 20,000–30,000 deliveries seem realistic.[62]

Pathophysiology. Several factors have been associated with amniotic fluid embolus. These patients generally have tumultuous labors or labors stimulated with oxytocin. Meconium in the fluid or fetal death are more frequent in this group, and these patients are generally older and multiparous. *Abruptio placentae,* amniotomy, operative delivery by the vaginal route and cesarean birth also are commonly associated with amniotic fluid embolus.[63]

Typically, these patients develop respiratory distress, shock, hemorrhage, and coma in a rapid sequence. These initial findings may be accompanied by cyanosis, pulmonary edema, and convulsions. Attempts to increase oxygenation often are unsuccessful, but if the patient manages to survive the initial event, coagulation abnormalities, renal failure, and persistent hypoxemia may ensue.[64] Differentiation from pulmonary embolus, ruptured uterus, drug reaction, and myocardial infarct initially may prove difficult. Other clinical syndromes, such as aspiration of gastric contents, pneumothorax, septicemia, drug overdose, eclampsia, cerebral vascular accidents, air embolism, and severe supine hypotension syndrome must be considered among the differential diagnoses.[65]

Demonstration of amniotic fluid within the pulmonary artery confirms the diagnosis of amniotic fluid embolus. If the clinical situation allows for introduction of a Swan–Ganz catheter, it may be possible to collect heparinized blood to examine the buffy coat for fetal squamous cells, lanugo hair, or vernix. A Swan–Ganz catheter may be used to determine the presence of pulmonary hypertension, which also may suggest an embolic phenomenon. The coagulopathy associated with amniotic fluid embolus consists of rapid evolution of DIC.

Treatment of amniotic fluid embolism requires full cardiopulmonary resuscitation with subsequent ventilatory and hemodynamic monitoring and intensive care support. Delivery of the fetus should be considered even during cardiopulmonary resuscitation.[62]

Sepsis

Bacterial shock causes abnormal activation of the coagulation system. Gram-positive bacteria are seen in 5% of cases compared to gram-negative strains, which cause 95% of cases.[66] It appears that coagulation in septic shock is activated by endotoxins released from cell wall lysis of gram-negative bacteria.[67] In contrast, *Staphylococcus aureus* causes coagulation abnormalities by elaborating exotoxins that induce adenosine triphosphate (ATP) release from human endothelium.

Pathophysiology. When gram-negative bacteria are destroyed by the host, the outer cell wall is metabolized to endotoxins. These high-molecular weight lipopolysaccharide complexes are the principle etiologic factor behind activation of the coagulation system.[66-68] They also destroy vascular endothelium; this may be responsible for development of acute lung injury (shock lung) in some of these patients. Commonly isolated bacteria associated with this disorder include *Escherichia coli, Klebsiella enterobacter, Proteus,* and *Pseudomonas.*

In the small animal model, the pathologic events of septic shock have been reproduced through injection of bacterial endotoxins.[69] It has been noted that death is associated with organ necrosis secondary to fibrin deposition in the microvasculature. This phenomenon was termed the *generalized Shwartzman reaction* (GSR).[70]

Effects of Disease on Pregnancy. In pregnancy, gram-negative sepsis has been noted to be accentuated.[71] Various authors have observed that pregnant animals need lower doses of endotoxin to produce the GSR.[70] Endotoxin also produces lesions in the placenta, but the etiology is uncertain and may reflect the consequences of DIC.

Diagnosis of septic coagulopathy should be considered in patients with known or suspected infection with a drastic drop in platelet number, fibrinogen concentrations, and leukocytes, often in association with hypothermia. Following the initial phase, leukocytosis and fever usually occur.[72] Treatment consists of antibiotic therapy directed at the underlying organism and intravenous heparin.[73] High-dose glucocorticoids have not been found beneficial in management of septic shock.

REFERENCES

1. *Dorland's Illustrated Medical Dictionary*. 26th ed. Philadelphia: WB Saunders; 1985:281.
2. Jackson CM, Nemerson Y. Blood coagulation. *Ann Rev Biochem*. 1980;49:765.
3. Gallop PM, Lian JB, Hauschka PV. Carboxylated calcium-binding proteins and vitamin K. *New Engl J Med*. 1980;302:1460.
4. Hoyer L. The factor VIII complex: structure and function. *Blood*. 1981;58:1.
5. Caldwell DC, Williamson RA, Goldsmith JC. Hereditary coagulopathies in pregnancy. *Clin Obstet Gynecol*. 1985;28:53.
6. Silwer J. Von Willebrand's disease in Sweden. *Acta Paediatr Scand*. 1973;238(suppl):1.
7. Zimmerman TS, Ruggeri ZM. von Willebrand's disease. *Prog Hemost Thromb*. 1982;6:203.
8. Weiss HJ. Von Willebrand's disease. In: Williams WJ, Beutter E, Erslev AJ, et al, eds. *Hematology*. 2nd ed. New York: McGraw-Hill; 1973:1434.
9. Nossel HL. Disorders of blood coagulation factors. In: Petersdorf RF, Adams RD, Braunwald E, et al, eds. *Harrison's Principles of Internal Medicine*. 10th ed. New York: McGraw-Hill; 1983:1900.
10. Horger ED. Disorders of hemostatis. In: Sciarra JJ, ed. *Gynecology and Obstetrics, Vol III*. Philadelphia: Harper & Row; 1983.
11. Houge C. Hemophilia and related conditions—congenital deficiencies of prothrombin (factor II), factor V, and factors VII to XII. In: Williams WJ, Beutter E, Erslev AJ, et al, eds. *Hematology*. 2nd ed. New York, NY: McGraw-Hill; 1978:1402.
12. Conti M, Mari D, Conti E, et al. Pregnancy in women with different types of von Willebrand's disease. *Obstet Gynecol*. 1986;68:282.
13. Telfer MC, Chediak J. Factor VIII-related disorders and their relationship to pregnancy. *J Reprod Med*. 1977;19:211.
14. Bennett B, Ratnoff OD. Changes in anti-hemophilic factor (AHF, Factor VIII) procoagulant activity and AHF-like antigen in normal pregnancy, and following exercise and pneumoencephalography. *J Lab Clin Med*. 1972;80:256.
15. Mannucci PM, Cagnatelli G, d'Alonzo P. Stress and blood coagulation. In: Brinkhous KM, ed. *Thrombosis Risk Factors and Diagnostic Approaches*. Stuttgart: Schatlauer; 1972.
16. Chediak JR, Alban GM, Maxey B. von Willebrand's disease and pregnancy: management during delivery and outcome of offspring. *Am J Obstet Gynecol*. 1986;155:618.
17. Evans P. Obstetric and gynecologic patients with von Willebrand's disease. *Obstet Gynecol*. 1971;38:37.
18. Lipton RA, Ayromlooi J, Coller BS. Severe von Willebrand's disease during labor and delivery. *JAMA*. 1982;248:1355.
19. *Pilot Study of Hemophilia Treatment in the United States*. National Heart and Lung Institute's Blood Resource Studies. Vol. 3. Department of Health, Education and Welfare. U.S. Government Printing Office, Washington, DC, 1972.
20. Lusher JM, McMillan CW. Severe factor VII and factor IX deficiency in females. *Am J Med*. 1978;65:637.
21. Graham JB. Mode of inheritance and current research. In: Brinkhous KM, Hemker HC, eds. *Handbook of Hemophilia*. Amsterdam: Excerpta Medica; 1975:175.
22. DePalma AF. Hemophilic arthropathy. *Clin Orthop*. 1967;52:145.
23. Klein HG, Aledort LM, Bouma BN, et al. A cooperative study for the detection of the carrier state of classical hemophilia. *New Engl J Med*. 1977;296:959.
24. Ratnoff OD, Steinberg AG. Recent advances in hemophilia. Part II: Detection of the carrier state of classic hemophilia. *Ann NY Acad Sci*. 1975;240(Jan 20):95.
25. Graham JB. Genotype assignment (carrier detection) in the haemophilias. *Clin Haematol*. 1979;8:115.
26. Birnholz JC. Determination of fetal sex. *New Engl J Med*. 1983;309:942.
27. Daffos F, Forestier F, Kaplan C, et al. Prenatal diagnosis and management of bleeding disorders with fetal blood sampling. *Am J Obstet Gynecol*. 1988;158:939.
28. Rodeck CH, Campbell S. Umbilical cord insertion as source of pure fetal blood for prenatal diagnosis. *Lancet*. 1979;1:1244.
29. Forestier F, Daffos F, Solie Y. Prenatal diagnosis of hemophilia by fetal blood sampling under ultrasound guidance. *Haemostasis*. 1986;16:346.
30. Ljing R, Tedgard U, McNeil T, et al. How do carriers of hemophilia experience prenatal diagnosis by fetal blood sampling? *Clin Genet*. 1987;31:297.
31. Pecorara M, Casarino L, Mori PG, et al. Hemophilia A: carrier detection and prenatal diagnosis by DNA analysis. *Blood*. 1987;70:531.
32. Kogan SC, Doherty M, Gisshier J. An improved method for prenatal diagnosis of genetic diseases by analysis of amplified DNA sequences: application to hemophilia A. *New Engl J Med*. 1987;317:985.
33. Oosterud B, Bouma BN, Griffin JH. Human blood coagulation factor IX: purification properties and mechanism of activation by activated factor XI. *J Biol Chem*. 1978;253:5946.
34. Thompson AR. Factor IX antigen by radioimmunoassay in heterozygotes for hemophilia B. *Thromb Res*. 1977;11:193.
35. Holmberg L, Gustavii B, Cordesius E, et al. Prenatal diagnosis of hemophilia B by an immunoradiometric assay of factor IX. *Blood*. 1980;56:397.
36. Briet E, Reisner HM, Blatt PM. Factor IX levels during pregnancy in a woman with hemophilia B. *Haemostasis*. 1982;11(2):87.
37. White GC, Roberts HR, Kingdon HS, et al. Prothrombin complex concentrates: potentially thrombogenic materials and clues to the mechanism of thrombosis in vivo. *Blood*. 1977;49:159.
38. Britten AFH. Congenital deficiency of factor XIII (fibrin-stabilizing factor): report on a case and review of the literature. *Am J Med*. 1967;43:751.
39. Fisher S, Rikover M, Naor S. Factor 13 deficiency with severe hemorrhagic diathesis. *Blood*. 1966;28:34.
40. Kitchens CS, Newcomb TF. Factor XIII. *Medicine*. 1978;58:413.
41. Rosenberg RD. Actions and interactions of antithrombin and heparin. *New Engl J Med*. 1975;292:146.
42. Thaler E, Lechner K. Antithrombin III deficiency and thromboembolism. *Clin Haematol*. 1981;10:369.
43. De Stefano V, Leone G, De Carolis S, et al. Management of pregnancy in women with antithrombin III congenital defect: report of 4 cases. *Thromb Haemost*. 1988;59:193.
44. Hellgren M, Tengborn L, Abildgaard V. Pregnancy in women with congenital anti-thrombin III deficiency: experience of treatment with heparin and antithrombin. *Gynecol Obstet Invest*. 1982;14:127.
45. Lunan GB. The management of abruptio placentae. *J Obstet Gynaecol Br Commonw*. 1973;80:120.
46. Pritchard JA, Brekkan AL. Clinical and laboratory studies on severe abruptio placentae. Am J Obstet Gynecol. 1967;97:681.
47. Sher G. A rational basis for the management of abruptio placentae. *J Reprod Med*. 1978;21:123.
48. Golditch IM, Boyce NE. Management of abruptio placentae. *JAMA*. 1970;212:288.
49. Kettel LM, Branch DW, Scott JR. Occult placental abruption after maternal trauma. *Obstet Gynecol*. 1988;71:449.
50. Chasnoff IJ, Burns WJ, Schnoll SH, et al. Cocaine use in pregnancy. *New Engl J Med*. 1985;313:666.
51. Graeff H, Von Hugo R. Fibrinogen derivatives in a case of abruptio placentae. *Am J Obstet Gynecol*. 1974;120:335.
52. Pritchard JA. Abruptio placentae and fibrinogen consumption. *Am J Obstet Gynecol*. 1958;76:365.
53. Bonnar J, McNicol GP, Douglas AS. The behavior of the coagulation fibrinolytic systems in abruptio placentae. *J Obstet Gynaecol Br Commonw*. 1968;76:799.
54. Sher G, Statland BE. Abruptio placentae with coagulopathy: a rational basis for management. *Clin Obstet Gynecol*. 1985;28:15.
55. Weiner AE, Reid DE, Roby CC, et al. Coagulation defects with intrauterine death from Rh isosensitization. *Am J Obstet Gynecol*. 1950;60:1015.
56. Jimenez JM, Pritchard JA. Pathogenesis and treatment of coagulation defects resulting from fetal death. *Obstet Gynecol*. 1968;32:449.
57. Pfeffer RI. Hypofibrinogenemia in the dead fetus syndrome treated with aminocaproic acid. *Am J Obstet Gynecol*. 1966;95:1095.
58. Attar S, Rosenstein PF, Rimer BA. Fibrinolysis in the dead fetus syndrome: report of a case. *Obstet Gynecol*. 1967;29:662.
59. Romero R, Copel J, Hobbins JC. Intrauterine fetal demise and hemostatic failure: the fetal death syndrome. *Clin Obstet Gynecol*. 1985;28:24.
60. Skelly H, Marivate M, Normal R, et al. Consumptive coagulopathy following fetal death in triplet pregnancy. *Am J Obstet Gynecol*. 1982;142:595.
61. Romero R, Duffy TP, Berkowitz RL, et al. Prolongation of a preterm multiple gestation complicated with DIC due to the death of a single twin: effects of heparin. *New Engl J Med*. 1984;310:772.
62. Killam A. Amniotic fluid embolism. *Clin Obstet Gynecol*. 1985;28:32.
63. Courtney LD. Amniotic fluid embolism. *Obstet Gynecol Surv*. 1974;29:169.
64. Duff P, Engelsgjerd B, Zingery LW, et al. Hemodynamic observations in a patient with intrapartum amniotic fluid embolism. *Am J Obstet Gynecol*. 1983;146:112.
65. Guidotti RJ, Grimes DA, Cates W. Fatal amniotic fluid embolism during legally induced abortion, United States, 1972 to 1978. *Am J Obstet Gynecol*. 1981;141:257.
66. Beller FK. Pathophysiologic aspects of endotoxin in septic abortion. *Int J Obstet Gynecol*. 1970;8:617.
67. Orskov F. Virulence factors of the bacterial cell surface. *J Infect Dis*. 1978;137:630.
68. Graeff H, Kuhn W. *Coagulation Disorders in Obstetrics*. Stuttgart, New York: Thieme; 1980.
69. Beller FK, Graeff H. Deposition of glomerular fibrin in the rabbit after infusion with endotoxin. *Nature*. 1967;215:295.
70. Selye AH. *Thrombo-hemorrhagic Phenomena*. Springfield, IL: Charles C. Thomas; 1966:44.
71. Beck Jansen P, Brinkmann CR, Johnson CH, et al. Circulatory shock in pregnant sheep. I. Effects of endotoxin on uteroplacental and fetal umbilical circulation. *Am J Obstet Gynecol*. 1972;112:1084.
72. Beller FK. Sepsis and coagulation. *Clin Obstet Gynecol*. 1985;28:46.
73. Blick RL, Bick MD. Antithrombin III patterns in disseminated intravascular coagulation. *Am J Clin Pathol*. 1980;73:577.

D

OTHER HEMATOLOGIC DISORDERS

Chapter One Hundred and Sixty-Eight

Transfusion Therapy

James T. Perkins

168

The histories of transfusion medicine and obstetrics intersect at a number of important points. It was obstetrician James Blundell who revived the practice of transfusion in 1818, 150 years after a false start with infusion of animal blood into humans.[1] Blundell acted on experimental evidence that transfusion should be performed with homologous blood (blood from the same species), and, after only temporary success with transfusion of a gastric carcinoma patient, he used transfusion to revive several women suffering from postpartum hemorrhage. The second major point of intersection was the fight by obstetricians, pediatricians, and blood group serologists against hemolytic disease of the newborn (HDN), which played a critical part in the development of blood grouping methods and compatibility testing, as well as the development of transfusion techniques and the recognition of certain transfusion hazards. These historical examples, showing that transfusion may be a life-saving emergency procedure in the pregnant patient and that blood compatibility problems are inherent in some of the most important obstetrical disorders, illlustrate the obstetrician's need to understand transfusion medicine.

The premise of transfusion medicine education is that each physician who prescribes blood must have a working knowledge of pretransfusion tests and their interpretation, the nature of the blood components to be transfused, the potential adverse consequences of such transfusion, and its demonstrated benefits. It is the general experience that blood components often are transfused unnecessarily in situations in which the risks outweigh the potential benefits. In addition, unnecessary delays in patient care often result from a lack of understanding of pretransfusion tests; immunohematologic consultation should be available but it is not a substitute for a basic knowledge of blood compatibility. Transfusion medicine is an area that should be, and is, receiving increasing attention. In the age of transfusion-associated-acquired immune deficiency syndrome (AIDS), strict evaluation of the risks and benefits of transfusion is mandatory.

IMMUNOHEMATOLOGY

Immune-mediated Destruction of Red Blood Cells

Table 168–1 shows the spectrum of disorders that entail immune-mediated red blood cell (RBC) destruction, which is generally considered to occur by one of two mechanisms, termed *intravascular* and *extravascular hemolysis*. Intravascular hemolysis refers to an entirely humoral mechanism that begins with the binding of a potentially complement-fixing antibody to a red blood cell (RBC) antigen. Activation of the complete complement sequence yields a membrane attack complex that creates a channel for salt and water through the membrane and results in lysis of the cell. This form of RBC destruction is characteristic of antibodies directed against the ABO blood group system. Because lysis is within the circulation, it is characterized by hemoglobinemia and, once the renal threshold of hemoglobin is exceeded, hemoglobinuria. Activation of the complete complement sequence leads to the release of several anaphylatoxins, which, directly and indirectly, cause vasodilatation and an increase in vascular permeability, activation of the coagulation cascade, and other systemic effects. These, in turn, produce the much feared clinical consequences of intravascular hemolysis: shock, disseminated intravascular coagulation (DIC), and renal failure.

Extravascular hemolysis also is initiated by antibody, but in this case, the effector mechanisms are cellular. The best documented cellular mechanism is complete or partial phagocytosis by macrophages, but extracellular lysis by monocytes or lymphocytes also may play a role. The destruction of RBCs by cellular mechanisms is enhanced by the fixation of early complement components to the RBCs, and monocytes have receptors both for the Fc portion of IgG and for C3b. Extravascular hemolysis is characteristic of antibodies directed against antigens of the Rh blood group system—antibodies that, as a rule, do not fix complement. In general, such hemolysis has relatively mild clinical consequences.

If complete phagocytosis were the only cell-mediated mechanism of hemolysis, one would not expect hemoglobinuria to accompany extravascular hemolysis. In fact, hemoglobinuria may accompany such hemolysis, even that caused by Rh antibodies.[2] The concepts of intravascular and extravascular destruction are useful ways to think about hemolysis, but, in actual practice many different, incompletely characterized factors determine the outcome when a given antiserum is combined *in vivo* with its corresponding antigen. Because of the multiplicity of such factors, the clinical consequences of hemolysis form a continuum.

Blood Groups and Blood Group Antibodies

The term *blood group* refers to an RBC antigen, and, like all antigens, a blood group is defined by its corresponding antibody. Blood groups are organized into systems by virtue of their allelic relationships, genetic linkage, and biochemical relationships. The antigenic activity of blood groups is carried by oligosaccharides that form part of complex mem-

TABLE 168–1. DISORDERS OF IMMUNE-MEDIATED RBC DESTRUCTION

RBC Destruction by Alloantibody
- Hemolytic transfusion reactions
  - Immediate hemolytic reactions
  - Delayed hemolytic reactions
- Hemolytic disease of the newborn

RBC Destruction by Autoantibody
- Warm autoimmune hemolytic anemia
  - Primary
  - Secondary (SLE, rheumatoid arthritis)
- Cold autoimmune hemolytic anemia
  - Paroxysmal cold hemoglobinuria
  - Cold agglutinin disease
    - Primary
    - Secondary (CLL, infectious mononucleosis)

RBC Destruction by Drug-related Antibodies

brane lipids (as in the ABO, Lewis, P, and I systems) or by peptides or oligosaccharides of membrane proteins (as in the Rh, Kell, MN, Duffy, and Kidd systems).

Blood groups may stimulate formation of autoantibodies, alloantibodies, or heterologous antibodies, that is, antibodies directed against self antigen, or against RBC antigens of individuals of the same species or different species, respectively. Blood group alloantibodies may be present in individuals who have never been exposed to foreign RBCs by transfusion or pregnancy. Such naturally occurring antibodies are made in response to the presentation of the same or similar antigens in the form of bacteria or other exogenous agents. ABO antibodies are of this type and, because such exposure appears to be universal, are found in all normal individuals who lack the corresponding antigen. Alloantibodies of other specificities, including most Rh system antibodies, may be found only in individuals who have been exposed to foreign RBCs; such antibodies are termed *immune*. The term *unexpected antibody* is reserved for all non-ABO antibodies, whether naturally occurring or immune.

Different blood groups are not equally immunogenic. The Rh antigen (more specifically, the Rh_o or D antigen) is the most immunogenic of non-ABO blood groups, with the Kell antigen, which is just one-tenth as immunogenic, being next.

Blood groups are clinically significant if they stimulate formation of antibodies that destroy RBCs *in vivo*, are relatively common, or that cause HDN. Although over 600 blood group antibody specificities have been defined, only 5% of these specificities are significant in ordinary clinical practice. A number of factors, such as the class (IgG versus IgM) or subclass (IgG1, IgG2, IgG3, IgG4) of blood group antibodies, their thermal optima and complement-fixing abilities, the quantity and equilibrium constant of antisera, and the characteristics of the antigen (eg, its density or mobility), have been demonstrated to determine the clinical significance of blood group antibodies. However, even with a knowledge of these factors, clinical significance is difficult to predict in a given case. Demonstration of the specificity of an antiserum and the comparison of that specificity with past clinical outcomes remain the most important predictors of significance for a specific individual. The transfusion of ABO-compatible RBCs provides adequate safety in the vast majority of first transfusions, and ensuring Rh specificity for Rh-negative individuals ensures the safety of most subsequent transfusions.

The ABO Blood Group System

ABO antigencity is determined by terminal sugars of oligosaccharides, which are part of the complex lipids of the RBC membrane and are present in relatively large numbers. The presence of these antigens is coded by structural genes of glycoseal transferases that add sugar moieties to a precursor substance. For this reason, the A and B genes are codominant alleles, the oligosaccharide product being detectable whenever the corresponding transferase is present. Group O individuals do not make an active transferase. A and B antigens are present on all cells; therefore, they are significant not only in transfusion, but also in the transplantation of solid organs. Although ABO antigens are present on platelets, when ABO-incompatible platelets are transfused, only a minor fraction is destroyed.

ABO alloantibodies appear within the first 6–8 months of life in all individuals with normal immune systems who lack the corresponding antigen. Because of this, individuals can be ABO typed by tests of their RBCs for antigen (so-called *forward typing*) or their serum for antibody (*reverse typing*). A or B antisera invariably contain IgM antibodies, but IgG with ABO specificity also occurs, particularly in group O individuals, and can cross the placenta to cause relatively mild HDN (see Chapter 170). Group O individuals make an antibody that reacts with both group A and group B RBCs, termed *anti-A,B*. These relationships are summarized in Table 168–2.

ABO antibodies typically cause intravascular hemolysis with severe clinical consequences. For this reason, and because of their common presence as expected antibodies, the ABO group is highly significant by the criteria cited above.

The Rh Blood Group System

The term *Rh positive* and *Rh negative* refer to the presence or absence of an antigen, Rh_o or D (the designation Rh here is used interchangeably with D). Eighty-five percent of individuals are Rh positive. No antibody has ever been found to define a blood group that is antithetical to D. The D antigen is highly immunogenic: 80% of Rh-negative recipients of a single unit of Rh-positive RBCs will form anti-D. Two other pairs of alleles—designated C and c, and E and e—are closely linked genetically to D. The clinical

TABLE 168–2. THE ABO BLOOD GROUP SYSTEM

Phenotype	Antigens	Antibodies	Gene Product	Genotypes
O	Precursor (H)	Anti-A, -B, -A,B	Inactive transferase	OO
A	A (H)	Anti-B	A-transferase	AO, AA
B	B (H)	Anti-A	B-transferase	BO, BB
AB	A&B (H)	None	A- and B-transferases	AB

TABLE 168–3. APPLICATIONS OF THE INDIRECT ANTIGLOBULIN TEST

Procedure	Serum	Cells
Antibody screen	Unknown antibodies (Recipient or donor)	Known antigens
Antigen typing	Known antibody	Unknown antigen (patient or donor)
Crossmatch (major)	Recipient	Donor
Antibody identification	Unknown antibody	Known antigens (panel)
Crossmatch (minor)	Donor	Recipient

significance of these alleles is proportionate to their lesser immunogenicity.

Occasional Rh-positive individuals express a weakened form of the antigen, termed D^u. Such individuals may be misclassified as Rh negative if less sensitive tests are used (see below). This is significant for blood donors, as the RBCs of a D^u phenotype donor, misclassified as Rh negative, could immunize a truly Rh-negative recipient. Conversely, such misclassification of a D^u phenotype recipient is of no significance. The misclassification of an Rh-positive, D^u phenotype gravida as Rh negative is of moderate significance: Such a woman unnecessarily might receive Rh immunoglobulin (RhIG). Very rare individuals with the D^u phenotype have only a portion of the Rh antigen and can make an antibody against the remainder that appears to represent anti-D; in a few instances this antibody has caused HDN. This occurrence would be prevented by the administration of Rh immune globulin (RhIG), but few D^u individuals would benefit. This is not a standard recommendation.

Rh system antibodies virtually always are formed in response to foreign RBCs and cause RBC destruction *in vivo*. As mentioned above, because such destruction does not involve complement, its clinical manifestations are relatively mild. However, anti-Rh causes the most severe form of HDN, and its clinical significance derives, in large part, from this fact as well as from the high immunogenicity of the D antigen.

Pretransfusion Testing

Pretransfusion testing asks two questions: (1) Does this recipient have an antibody against this donor's RBCs? and (2) Could this recipient make an antibody against this donor's RBCs? The former question is investigated by the antibody screening test, the major crossmatch, and ABO typing of donor and recipient. The latter question necessitates Rh typing of the recipient and donor. Both questions focus on the incompatibility of recipient antibody with donor RBCs, termed *major-side incompatibility*. The minor-side reactions of donor antibodies against recipient antigens are of lesser importance and are ignored except for whole blood or plasma transfusion.

TABLE 168–4. A STANDARD PRETRANSFUSION TESTING PROTOCOL

Donor	Recipient
ABO type Forward Reverse	ABO type Forward Reverse
Rh type including D^u	Rh type
Antibody screen	Antibody screen
Major Crossmatch	

Routine pretransfusion tests are based on the ability of antibody in a given serum to agglutinate RBCs containing the corresponding antigen. In the case of ABO typing, agglutination will occur after the simple admixture of serum containing anti-A or anti-B with dilute suspensions of RBCs containing the corresponding antigens. Such tests can be performed very rapidly. However, some blood group antibodies are able to bind to or sensitize RBCs, but not to agglutinate them. In such cases, the addition of Coombs' serum or anti-human globulin (AHG), an antiserum directed against human immunoglobulin or complement, may crosslink the RBC-bound blood group antibody and achieve agglutination, thus demonstrating the presence of blood group antibody in the test serum. In immunohematology, the latter sequence is termed an *indirect antiglobulin test* (IAT), and it detects *in vitro* sensitization of RBCs. Hemagglutination tests can be used for several purposes, depending on the RBCs and antisera selected in the first step, as shown in Table 168–3. In each case, the IAT methodology has the greatest sensitivity, although important information, particularly about ABO incompatibility, can be gained without the addition of AHG.

AHG also is used to detect the *in vivo* sensitization of RBCs by antibody or complement in the disorders listed in Table 168–1. In such cases, a patient's RBCs are washed to remove unbound antibody, mixed with AHG, and examined for agglutination; this is a direct Coombs' or *direct antiglobulin test* (DAT).

The above hemagglutination tests are combined into a pretransfusion testing protocol as shown in Table 168–4. Although the major crossmatch often is referred to as the compatibility test, it should be emphasized that no one test ensures compatibility. Compatibility is determined by a battery of tests, of which correct ABO typing is the most important. In fact, it has been shown that if no serologic problems are detected in blood typing and the antibody screen, the antiglobulin phase of the major crossmatch can be omitted. This is the basis for the *type-and-screen* protocol used at many hospitals; if the recipient's antibody screen is negative, the crossmatch is abbreviated to a quick test that checks for ABO typing errors before issuing RBCs. This form of abbreviated pretransfusion testing offers many logistic advantages, since blood can be made rapidly available without reserving it for a specific patient in advance. A complete AHG-crossmatch occasionally will detect incompatibility in sera with a negative antibody screen, but mild, clinically evident hemolysis occurs very rarely—one in 250,000 crossmatches in the study of Shulman.[3]

The type-and-screen test, whether followed by an abbreviated crossmatch or a complete AHG crossmatch, is applicable particularly to obstetric practice, in which many patients are at a relatively low risk of hemorrhage, but those who need blood must have it on an emergency basis. A recent, negative type-and-screen assures the clinician relatively safe transfusion in an emergency, "recent" referring to the Food and Drug Administration regulation that the sample must be less than 48 hours old. A positive type-and-screen prompts the laboratory to begin immediate antibody identification should transfusion be needed. A type-and-screen test should be ordered for all women entering the hospital for delivery.

Compatibility testing for neonatal patients can be abbreviated because the formation of new RBC alloantibodies is rare in the first 4 months of life and the relevant RBC alloantibodies are derived maternally, in a process that ceases at parturition. Therefore, the mother's serum is preferable for compatibility testing; if her antibody screen is negative and all components transfused during the neonatal period are compatible, no crossmatches or other compatibility tests need be done. Any RBCs transfused must be ABO compatible with the mother's and infant's sera, and transfused plasma must be compatible with the infant's ABO group. Cellular blood components should be Rh specific.

The Safe Transfusion of "Incompatible" Blood

It is important for all physicians, particularly those who take care of surgical or obstetric emergencies, to understand that, at times, transfusion must be performed in spite of certain blood group incompatibilities. For example, in platelet transfusion, ABO incompatibility of donor plasma (platelet units contain 50–60 mL of plasma) and recipient RBCs frequently is ignored. Hemolysis due to such minor incompatibility is very rare, and the risk often is overridden by the need to transfuse whatever platelets are available. Similarly, it may be necessary to transfuse RH-positive platelets to an Rh-negative individual. The small amount of RBCs contaminating the platelets carries a low risk of immunizing the recipient, and such immunization can be prevented by subsequent administration of RhIG.

Another circumstance in which incompatibility is ignored is that of patients with RBC autoantibodies. *Auto*antibodies may cause positive crossmatches with all donor RBCs. In such a circumstance, it is important to rule out concomitant blood group *allo*antibodies, the presence of which may be masked by autoantibody and which can cause significant transfusion reactions. However, once this is done, donor RBCs that react with the recipient's autoantibody are expected to survive no differently than the recipient's own RBCs. As long as ABO-compatible blood products are available, no patient should be allowed to exsanguinate for lack of completely compatible blood components. In such a situation, the physician should consult with an experienced immunohematologist.

BLOOD COMPONENTS AND PLASMA DERIVATIVES

The adoption in the early 1960s of plastic bags for blood collection and subsequent transfusion made it possible to separate whole blood into its components by differential centrifugation in a closed system. This technologically simple procedure accomplishes two powerful and related ends: it allows the physician to treat the individual patient's deficiency of a blood element, such as platelets, RBCs, or coagulation factors, with that specific element, rather than "shotgunning" all deficiencies with whole blood, and it allows the storage of the separated components to be optimized, rather than sacrificing platelets and factor VIII (FVIII) for the optimization of RBC survival, as is the case when blood is stored whole.

Blood component safety begins with a donor who, in the United States, is typically a volunteer, that is, a person for whom there is no financial incentive to donate in spite of personal knowledge of potentially transmissible disease. The donor is screened for conditions that might compromise his or her own safety or that of the recipient. Blood, generally 450 mL (±10%), then is drawn into a primary bag containing citrate for anticoagulation, dextrose as a glycolytic energy source, and phosphate and adenine to supplement adenosine triphosphate (ATP) generation. If components are to be made, the unit of whole blood is centrifuged at a relatively low speed to separate the RBCs from platelet-rich plasma, and the latter is expressed into an integrally connected secondary bag. The connecting tubing is heat-sealed and cut, and the platelet-rich plasma is centrifuged at a higher rate that results in a platelet pellet and plasma supernatant. Most of the plasma is expressed into another secondary bag and immediately frozen, yielding fresh-frozen plasma (FFP); 50–60 mL of the plasma is used to resuspend the platelet pellet. The resulting unit of RBCs is stored at 4°C, the FFP at −18°C or lower, and the platelets at room temperature with continuous agitation. Three variations on this sequence are used frequently. In the first, an additive solution is combined with the separated RBCs, which extends their shelf life from 35 to 42 days. Second, the FFP may be thawed slowly, a procedure that precipitates coagulation factors VIII and XIII and fibrinogen; this *cryoprecipitate* then is pelleted, resuspended in a reduced volume of plasma, and refrozen. Third, the RBCs may be frozen after addition of glycerol. The properties of the blood components resulting from these manipulations are summarized in Table 168–5.

Other manipulations can be performed at the time of issue. RBCs frequently are washed in saline to remove plasma, anticoagulant, and leukocytes. More efficient leukocyte removal can be achieved by filtration, either in the blood bank or at the bedside. This procedure is applicable to units of platelets more readily than is washing. Multiple units of platelets or cryoprecipitate frequently are pooled into one bag for transfusion. FFP and cryoprecipitate, of course, must be thawed before issue. Each of these maneuvers confers a short expiration time on the blood component, so terminal preparation steps should only be ordered immediately before the intended transfusion. Wastage often results when such blood components are ordered before the clinician has made a definite determination to transfuse.

The above sequences are employed by blood centers and hospital-based donor services. Further fractionation of plasma is performed on an industrial scale to yield the products listed in Table 168–6. These include the colloid agents albumin or plasma protein fraction (PPF); FVIII (antihemophilic factor) concentrate; coagulation factor IX (FIX) concentrate; FIX complex, a concentrate containing FIX; and variable levels of factors II, VII, and X, antithrombin III concentrate, and the various preparations of immunoglobulins such as RhIG or intravenous immunoglobulin (IVIG). In the past, the coagulation factor concentrates listed above carried high risks of transmission of the hepatitis and AIDS

TABLE 168–5. PROPERTIES OF BLOOD COMPONENTS

Component[a]	Contents	Storage	Blood Group Selection: Recipient	Blood Group Selection: Donor
RBCs	170–210 mL RBCs 50 mL plasma 10 mL anticoagulant	35 days 1–6°C	O A B AB	O A or O B or O AB or A,B,O
FFP	170–225 mL plasma 43 mL anticoagulant 1 unit/mL all factors	1 year below −18°C	O A B AB	O or A,B,AB A or AB B or AB AB
Platelets	5.5–8.0 × 10^{10} platelets 50–60 mL plasma 10 mL anticoagulant	5 days Room temperature	Type specific preferred; otherwise as available	
Cryoprecipitate	80–100U FVIII:c 40–70% original FVIII:vwf 10 mL plasma	1 year below −18°C	Type specific preferred; otherwise as available	

[a] Alternatives to type specific components are in order of priority.

viruses, but new methods of isolation or heat treatment have reduced or eliminated these risks.

The reader is referred to the convenient handbook on blood transfusion therapy[4] published by the American Association of Blood Banks for a more complete discussion of the specifics of each of these blood components and plasma derivatives.

AUTOLOGOUS TRANSFUSION

Autologous transfusion refers to three different procedures: the deposit of blood before anticipated losses, such as those at surgery or delivery, followed by storage and subsequent transfusion; hemodilution immediately before surgery with reinfusion of the removed blood during the operation; and intraoperative salvage of shed blood followed by washing and reinfusion of the RBCs. Advance deposit of blood allows the form of autologous transfusion most often applied to obstetric practice, and its safety in this circumstance has been demonstrated.[5] Absolute contraindications to this procedure include bacteremia and the inability of the patient to replace the removed RBCs; certain forms of cardiac disease constitute relative contraindications. Because liquid storage of whole blood is limited to 35 days and second-trimester or early third-trimester deposit generally would be preferred to donation late in pregnancy, most blood donated by obstetric patients must be stored frozen, which somewhat limits its availability and increases the cost. These limitations must be weighed against the low frequency with which obstetric patients must be transfused; in one study[6], only 1.1% of obstetric patients were transfused. To improve their cost–benefit ratio, the authors of that study attempted to predict who might need peripartum transfusion, but only *placenta previa* was predictive. The options for pregnant patients in regard to autologous transfusion have been reviewed recently.[5,7]

TABLE 168–6. AVAILABLE PLASMA DERIVATIVES

Oncotic Agents
Albumin
Plasma protein fraction
Coagulation Factor Concentrates
Factor VIII concentrate
Factor IX concentrate
Anti-inhibitor concentrate
Immunoglobulins
Rh immune globulin
Intravenous immunoglobulin
Gamma globulin (intramuscular)

ADVERSE CONSEQUENCES OF TRANSFUSION

Adverse reactions to transfusion are common, and they may have long-term negative consequences for the recipient. The transfusing physician must be able to recognize such transfusion reactions so that they are treated appropriately and are reported to the transfusion service (to prevent future reactions). In addition, the physician must know the magnitude of these risks, so that they may be balanced appropriately against the potential benefits of transfusion. A high index of suspicion is required so that transfusion reactions can be identified. Any adverse reaction occurring at the time of transfusion is considered to be due to transfusion until proven otherwise, and the safest course is to stop the transfusion until the cause is identified. In cases of uncertainty, consultation should be sought.

Adverse reactions to transfusion can be classified in different ways. Although they often are listed as immediate versus delayed reactions, we prefer a pathogenetic classification that begins by distinguishing immune-mediated and nonimmune reactions. Because of their importance, infectious complications are treated separately.

Immune-mediated Transfusion Reactions

All of the basic elements of blood can act as immunogens, and each element has a corresponding transfusion reaction, as shown in Table 168–7. With the exception of *graft-versus-host disease* (GVHD), the well-characterized reactions are all antibody-mediated. Transfusion also may cause immune suppression, but since this is still controversial, it is discussed separately.

Immunization itself is listed as a transfusion reaction, because it frequently results from transfusion and eventually may lead to such adverse consequences as HDN, transfusion reactions, or platelet refractoriness. For example, because immunization to platelets may cause later platelet refractoriness, prophylactic platelet transfusion generally is not indicated in patients with congenital thrombocytopathy or long-term thrombocytopenic states such as aplastic anemia; in such patients, platelets are reserved for treatment of significant hemorrhage.

Hemolytic Transfusion Reactions. Hemolytic reactions may occur immediately upon the transfusion of donor RBCs, or they may be delayed. Hemolysis in *immediate hemolytic transfusion reactions* (IHTRs) may be intravascular or extravascular, or it may occur by a combination of these mechanisms. The clinical consequences of the reaction are determined largely by the degree and rapidity of complement fixation and its resulting generation of anaphylotoxins. The most common manifestation of an IHTR is fever, which often is preceded by a rigor. The rapid lysis of RBCs is manifested by hemoglobinemia and hemoglobinuria and, within 5–7 hours, by icterus. The other manifestations classically associated with IHTR usually are limited to reactions due to ABO antibodies. Such reactions may be heralded by phlebitis, which is followed by flank pain and a general sense of discomfort. There also may be pain in the chest or abdomen, as well as nausea, vomiting, and diarrhea. The release of anaphylatoxins is the presumed cause of urticaria, flushing, bronchospasm, and hypotension. DIC may occur, both because the membranes (*stroma*) of lysed RBCs are thromboplastic and because complement fixation may activate the coagulation cascade. Renal failure occurs because of DIC and hyptension, but it typically resolves if the patient can be supported by fluid and electrolyte management or dialysis. Because the anesthetized patient cannot complain of the early, subjective symptoms of an IHTR, the initial manifestation during operations may be DIC-related oozing or other severe complications.

Several studies suggested an IHTR rate of 1 per 10,000–20,000 RBC transfusions and a mortality of approximately 10%[8], which is in general agreement with the estimate by an NIH consensus statement[9] of 1 fatal IHTR per 100,000 RBC transfusion. Most fatal IHTRs are due to ABO mismatches between donor and recipient, and 89% of these are due to clerical error in specimen labeling, transcription of results, or identification of the recipient.[10] For this reason, hospital blood banks tend to be very exacting about specimen labeling, and emergency situations should not be considered an exception to required identification practices.

Delayed hemolytic transfusion reactions (DHTRs) occur in previously immunized recipients in whom the strength of the resulting blood group antibody has declined to a point at which it cannot be detected by the antibody screening test or crossmatches. Memory lymphocytes are present, however, and are able to generate an anamnestic antibody response with subsequent lysis of the donor RBCs carrying the corresponding antigen. RBC destruction generally is extravascular with mild clinical consequences. DHTRs typically are detected when a patient is found to have a declining hematocrit (Hct) about a week after transfusion and RBCs are ordered; pretransfusion followed by testing reveals a new RBC antibody. Review of the patient's record often will show that the patient had fever since transfusion, and the patient occasionally develops icterus, but the DHTR seldom is suspected on clinical grounds alone. Renal failure is uncommon in the absence of other causes. DHTRs are not uncommon, occurring after 1 in 1600 RBC transfusions according to various studies[8], and they cannot be prevented.

TABLE 168-7. IMMUNE-MEDIATED TRANSFUSION REACTIONS

Type of Reaction	Blood Element With Antigen
Immunization	
Hemolytic	Donor RBCs
Immediate	(Minor side reactions rare)
Delayed	
Febrile	Donor WBCs
Allergic	Donor plasma proteins
Anaphylactic	(Minor side reactions
Anaphylactoid	reported)
Urticarial	
Transfusion-related acute lung injury	Recipient WBCs
Post-transfusion purpura	Donor platelets
Graft-versus-host disease	All recipient tissues

Reactions Due to Antibodies Directed Against Leukocytes. Febrile transfusion reactions are analogous to hemolytic reactions, but the causative antibody is directed against donor leukocyte antigens, including HLA antigens. The lysis of leukocytes in units of RBCs or platelets releases endogenous pyrogen that causes fever, which often is preceded by a rigor. Because leukocyte antigens are highly immunogenic, such reactions are common in the parous or previously transfused patient, occurring in one case per each 100–200 transfusions of cellular blood components. Reactions can be prevented by the provision of blood components made leukocyte-poor by filtration or washing, but because reactions recur in only one of eight patients, such components generally are used only after there have been two reactions. Although febrile reactions can be very uncomfortable, their major importance is in their differential diagnosis: that is, fever at the time of transfusion may represent a hemolytic reaction or bacterial contamination of the unit, both of which can be devastating. For this reason, transfusion always should be stopped when fever occurs, and the reaction should be reported and investigated.

Transfusion-related acute lung injury (TRALI) is thought to represent the minor-side equivalent of the febrile reaction; that is, donors have been found to have potent antibodies against leukocytes of recipients developing respiratory failure during or soon after the transfusion of plasma-containing blood components.[11] In this syndrome, severe hypoxemia is associated with fever, hypotension and the bilateral infiltrates characteristic of pulmonary edema. The last is thought to be due to a capillary leak syndrome, which perhaps is initiated by pulmonary leukocyte sequestration and degranulation. Most cases require mechanical ventilation, but if the patient can be supported successfully, the problem can resolve without sequelae.

Allergic Transfusion Reactions. Allergic transfusion reactions include a spectrum of findings, from urticaria to anaphylactic shock. It generally is thought that allergic reactions represent recipient allergy to antigens in donor plasma, but this has been documented only at the severe end of the spectrum, in patients with IgA deficiency who react to donor IgA as a foreign antigen and make anti-IgA. At the mild end of the spectrum, the responsible antigen specificities are unknown; an urticarial reaction is found occasionally in a transfusion recipient with severe food allergy, perhaps triggered by something the donor had eaten. Hypotension and anaphylactoid symptoms also are associated with the infusion of solutions containing immunoglobulin aggregates and would occur if immunoglobulin preparations, such as RhIG, intended for intramuscular use were given intravenously.

The frequency of urticaria generally is given as 1–3% or more, as attested by the regularity with which antihistamines are prescribed before transfusion. Urticarial reactions constitute the only transfusion reaction after which transfusion with the same unit can be restarted safely; this is acceptable if the patient has a history of urticaria and if the symptoms have resolved after antihistamine administration (25–50 mg of intravenous diphenhydramine). Urticaria generally is prevented easily with pretransfusion antihistamines.

Anaphylactic reactions are rare, occurring in one recipient per 20,000 or more transfusions, and are characterized by flushing, hypotension, dyspnea, and gastrointestinal symptoms that begin soon after initiation of transfusion. A chill may occur, but fever characteristically is absent. The differential diagnosis of hypotension associated with transfusion includes an IHTR and the transfusion of a unit contaminated with bacteria. Treatment is with epinephrine and supportive measures. Severe reactions generally can be prevented by repeatedly washing RBCs before transfusion. If plasma-containing components must be given, they can be obtained from IgA-deficient blood donors.

Post-transfusion Purpura. Post-transfusion purpura (PTP) is a rare reaction in which the recipient, usually a multiparous woman, develops thrombocytopenic purpura 5–10 days after the transfusion of RBCs or whole blood. Serologic investigation reveals the presence of an alloantibody in the patient's serum directed against platelet antigens, but the reason that this leads to the destruction of both donor (allogeneic) and recipient (autogeneic) platelets is unknown. Without treatment, severe thrombocytopenia may last for 1–4 weeks, but most cases will respond to plasma exchange or IVIG.

Graft-Versus-Host Disease. Graft-versus-host disease (GVHD) can occur after the transfusion of blood components, containing viable donor lymphocytes, into recipients who are severely immunodeficient or into individuals tolerant of the donor lymphocyte antigens. The former type of patient includes bone marrow transplant recipients and patients with congenital cellular immunodeficiency; the latter group includes fetuses who receive intrauterine transfusion (IUT), or exchange transfusion subsequent to IUT and to recipients who share HLA haplotypes with the donor. Transfusion-related GVHD differs from GVHD occurring after bone marrow transplantation in that the transfusion recipient's marrow is *histoincompatible* with the engrafted lymphocytes, and death almost invariably results from the ensuing bone marrow failure. Transfusion-related GVHD can be prevented by the irradiation of cellular blood components intended for at-risk patients, a process that does not interfere with the function of the transfused cells but which prevents lymphocyte engraftment.

Transfusion-related Immunosuppression

It is well accepted that transfusion prior to renal transplantation improves graft survival, and this effect may be due to some form of immunosuppression. A number of studies also have suggested that transfusion promotes postoperative wound infection or increases the risk of tumor recurrence after cancer surgery[12], but these observations are controversial. The question remains whether transfusion is an independent variable promoting these adverse outcomes or is correlated because of patient variables such as a more advanced cancer, which, in addition to producing the adverse outcome, makes transfusion more likely. Many immune function tests change after transfusion, but the direction of such changes reported by various studies differs[13], and the relevance of these changes is unknown. This is an area of active investigation, and transfusion-mediated immunosuppression may prove to be numerically one of the most important adverse consequences of transfusion.

Nonimmune-mediated Transfusion Reactions

Although blood banks tend to identify themselves most closely with immunohematologic investigation, no less effort is expended in preventing adverse reactions to transfusion that are not mediated by immune mechanisms. The recent focus on AIDS and other forms of virus transmission has, of course, greatly increased the latter role. Table 168–8 lists the important categories of such reactions.

The term *storage lesion* refers to those changes in a unit of blood, particularly whole blood, that are consequences of storage conditions optimized for the preservation of RBCs. These changes may have clinical consequences for the recipient. For example, the citrate used as an anticoagulant chelates ionized calcium when infused. Lower concentrations of ionized calcium may produce a tingling sensation (typically, in the face), muscle tremors, and, if very severe, myocardial depression and arrhythmias. In practice, however, the liver metabolism of citrate is fast enough that symptomatic depression of the ionized calcium level occurs only when whole blood or plasma is being transfused at a rate above 1 unit every 4–5 minutes, and life-threatening cardiac events are not expected unless even higher rates are obtained. Citrate toxicity typically is a problem only in patients with very severe liver disease, during liver transplant surgery, or in rapid-exchange transfusions of infants.

Other potential toxins accumulating in liquid-stored whole blood and RBCs include organic acids and potassium,

TABLE 168–8. ADVERSE CONSEQUENCES OF TRANSFUSION NOT IMMUNE-MEDIATED

Clinical Consequences of the Storage Lesion
Accumulation of toxins
Decline in function
Cold
Intravascular Volume Overload
Iron Overload
Non-alloimmune Hemolysis
Transfusion of Infected Blood
Transmission of infection
Viruses (Hepatitis, HIV, CMV, others)
Bacteria (Gram-negative bacilli, treponemes, others)
Parasites (Malaria, *T. cruzi*, others)
Reaction to preformed endotoxin (shock)

both of which have potential cardiac toxicity. In actual massive transfusion cases, however, metabolic alkylosis and hypokalemia are observed more often, probably as consequences of citrate metabolism. Concern also has focused on the adenine used to extend storage and the plasticizers that accumulate in stored blood, but problems involving these elements have not materialized. Microaggregates that form unavoidably after a few days of storage were once thought to promote the pulmonary toxicity sometimes seen after massive transfusion, but the current concept is that this is caused by the patient's underlying problem, typically trauma and shock.

With storage, RBCs become progressively less viable and their level of diphosphoglycerate (2,3 DPG) declines, which increases their oxygen affinity. This increased oxygen affinity might be expected to affect the ability of transfused RBCs to deliver oxygen in massively transfused patients, but, here again, real problems have not been documented, largely because 2,3 DPG is repleted within 24 hours after infusion. In spite of this, RBCs less than five days old, which maintain their 2,3 DPG levels, are commonly used for neonatal patients and IUT.

Of more concern is the dilutional coagulopathy that has been attributed to massive transfusion with stored whole blood that is deficient in platelets and, to a variable degree, clotting factors VIII and V. This coagulopathy was studied in Vietnam battle casualties by Miller and coworkers[14], who demonstrated a progressive increase in the incidence of microvascular bleeding that is characteristic of a coagulopathy, beginning after approximately two blood volumes had been replaced and affecting all patients after replacement of a third blood volume. This clinical finding was paralleled by a decline in platelet counts and an increase in clotting times; both trends tended to progress with larger transfusion volumes in a fashion that suggested that the patients' own hemostatically effective blood was being diluted by the platelet-deficient and coagulation factor-deficient whole blood. When Miller et al examined the coagulation variables, they discerned a clear relationship between the onset of bleeding and fall in the platelet count below 60,000. On the other hand, no such relationship could be determined between a patient's clotting times and the onset of bleeding. In addition, when patients with pathologic bleeding were treated with fresh whole blood—the only available source of active platelets—all stopped bleeding. In contrast, when similar patients were treated with FFP, none stopped bleeding.

Subsequent studies have refined these observations. Significant platelet dysfunction has been demonstrated in massively transfused trauma patients.[15,16] Counts and coworkers[17,18] demonstrated the dilution of platelets and clotting factors V and VII but emphasized the variability of coagulation parameters in different patients. In their studies, the prothrombin time (PT) are partial thromboplastin time (PTT) predicted pathologic bleeding only when they were 1.5–1.8 times control. Better predictors of hemostatic failure were a fibrinogen level below 50 mg per dL and a platelet count below 50,000; consumption (DIC) was thought to be the major cause of these abnormalities. In a group of patients receiving similar numbers of transfusions, Harke and Rahman[19] correlated the degree of platelet and clotting abnormalities with the length of time the patient was hypotensive. Taking these data together, Collins[20] concluded that ". . . coagulopathy in heavily transfused patients was due to hypoperfusion, not transfusion."

A final effect of storage is that RBCs or whole blood will be cold (4°C) when transfused, and hypothermia and even cold cardioplegia can result from their rapid transfusion. Again, cardiac arrest is likely to occur only when cold blood components are being transfused very rapidly, on the order of 50 mL or more per minute. However, hypothermia may impair platelet function and increase oxygen demand, so that a blood warmer should be used in massive transfusion.

Intravascular volume overload is a common complication of transfusion. Patients with chronic anemia are particularly at risk, as they may be compensating for their anemia with a hyperdynamic, hypervolemic circulation and may have myocardial damage as well. Volume overload can be prevented to some degree by prior treatment with diuretics. RBCs can be administered over four hours, or RBC units can be split in two, with one half left in the blood bank refrigerator and transfused 12 hours later.

Iron overload is a major problem in thalassemia-major patients or any other patients who are completely dependent on transfused RBCs. Each milliliter of RBCs contains 1 mg of iron, or approximately the amount absorbed or lost in one day. Because the excretion of iron cannot be increased, a positive iron balance is inevitable in the chronically transfused. The manifestations of chronic iron overload include cirrhosis, heart failure, and diabetes. Transfusion hemochromatosis can be prevented by chelation therapy with desferoxamine.

Units of RBCs can be hemolyzed by nonimmune mechanisms, in particular by contact with dextrose or hypotonic solutions, or by contact with drugs such as furosemide. For this reason, blood components should come in contact with normal saline only in IV lines, and no drugs should be added to the unit.

Transfusion-transmitted Infection

Transfusion is one of the most efficient vectors for the transmission of an infectious agent to the bloodstream. In 1937, Ottenberg, the first individual to apply blood typing and crossmatching to actual transfusions, stated: "Today transfusion has become so safe . . . the chief problem it presents is the finding of large sums of money needed for the professional donors who now provide most of the blood."[21] The irony of this statement is obvious to us, in this era of transfusion-associated AIDS (TA-AIDS), but it highlights an important principle. The morbidity and mortality of transfusion-associated infections typically are delayed, which has resulted in a delay in the recognition that infection with agents such as *human immunodeficiency virus* (HIV) and *hepatitis C virus* (HCV, an agent causing parenterally transmitted *non-A, non-B hepatitis* [NANBH]) is related to transfusion. Second-guessing blood banks as to when transfusion-associated transmission of AIDS should have been recognized has become an industry upon which the outcome of many malpractice suits will hinge. The prolonged incubation periods of HIV and HCV infections also may explain much of the overuse of blood components. For example, the vast majority of transfusion-associated hepatitis cases are occult, in spite of which there is a high rate of chronic infection, often with progression to cirrhosis. Because this manifestation does not soon become evident, the transfusing physician is seldom reinforced negatively for having ordered the transfusion and is not prompted to reexamine whether the transfusion was really needed. Recently developed tests have largely eliminated the transmission of HIV by transfusion and promise to reduce greatly the transmission of HCV. Thus, the medical community may become complacent about the infectious risks of transfusion. The examples of HIV and HCV should warn us that such complacency is not warranted. Other agents undoubtedly are being transmitted by transfusion; we cannot surmise what diseases they may cause.

Essentially, all of the viral agents known to cause hepatitis have been found to be transmitted by transfusion. Although hepatitis A (HAV) has the highest incidence of hepatitis viruses in North America, because it does not have a chronic carrier state, it causes only occasional cases of post-transfusion hepatits (PTH). When the test for hepatitis B surface antigen (HBsAg) was introduced in the early 1970s, it was discovered that most PTH cases were NANBH, caused by another agent(s) that, until recently, defied serologic detection. Nonetheless, the introduction of routine testing of donated blood for HBsAg, coupled with a concomitant shift in the nation's blood supply from commercial to volunteer donors, led to a drop in PTH incidence from as high as one third of all blood recipients to approximately one tenth by the end of the 1970s. A number of changes in blood donor recruiting and testing, initiated during the 1980s, have led to further reductions in PTH incidence, although the magnitude of their net effect is unknown; these changes include progressively intensified donor screening for AIDS risk factors, HIV antibody testing, and alanine aminotransferase (ALT, syn. SGPT) and hepatitis B core antibody (HBcAb) testing of donated units (the latter two are surrogate tests for NANBH). The development of tests for a newly identified NANBH virus, HCV, promises to decrease the risk of PTH to below 1%.

The PTH risk posed by different blood components (RBCs, FFP, platelets, cryoprecipitate) generally is assumed to be the same, but that of frozen deglycerolized units may be somewhat less. Hepatitis transmission by plasma derivatives, which are prepared in large batches, has been almost invariable in the past. However, methods developed to inactive HIV may considerably reduce this risk.

The high rates of infection cited above conflict with the common experience of physicians, because most patients with PTH are anicteric and asymptomatic; such high rates are found only in prospective studies in which NANBH is defined by elevations of the ALT level on two occasions separated by a week or more, within 2–26 weeks after exposure. Such studies also demonstrate a 50% rate of chronicity in NANBH with 20% or more of the chronic cases progressing to cirrhosis.[22]

TA-AIDS has focused the public's attention on the risks of transfusion as never before and has led to an increased scrutiny of the indications for transfusion, an increased use of autologous transfusion, public demand for *directed-donor* transfusion, the use of consent forms specifically for transfusion, and a heightened sensitivity within the blood banking community to the prevention of transfusion-transmitted disease. These changes have occurred in spite of the fact that HIV antibody testing has reduced the risk of TA-AIDS to very low levels. The risk is not zero; however, the transmission of HIV from seronegative individuals can occur early in the course of their infection. Studies have suggested that HIV is transmitted by 1 of 38,000[23] to 153,000[24] seronegative units of blood components, or approximately 130–460 components per year. In a layman's comparison, this roughly corresponds to the number of individuals per year who are struck by lightning in the United States. The rate of such HIV transmission does not appear to be reduced by tests for circulating HIV p24 antigen.[25,26]

Cytomegalovirus (CMV) commonly establishes latent infections in leukocytes, making transmission by transfusion likely; in recent studies[27], approximately 1% of CMV-seronegative blood recipients became infected. Although most primary CMV infections are mild, intrauterine infections can have devastating sequelae, as can the infection of low birth weight (< 1250 g) infants of seronegative mothers and other immunosuppressed individuals. The reactivation of latent infection can occur after transfusion from either seropositive or seronegative donors, and therefore it cannot be prevented. Transmission of CMV can be lessened by providing CMV-seronegative blood components, or by leukocyte reduction procedures such as the freezing and deglycerolization of RBCs or leukocyte filtration. CMV-seronegative blood components are indicated for seronegative pregnant women, seronegative newborn infants weighing less than 1500 g, and seronegative bone marrow or organ transplant recipients whose transplant donor is seronegative.

INDICATIONS FOR TRANSFUSION

Risk-benefit Ratios in Transfusion

The decision to transfuse, like any other therapeutic decision, must be based on a comparison of the relevant risks and benefits. Although this is a simple truism, it often is neglected. Studies of the use of blood components invariably demonstrate overuse. Decision making in transfusion therapy has been studied. Avorn and coworkers[28] determined that transfusing physicians could estimate relatively accurately the risk of transfusion, but there was wide variation in their experimental subjects' estimation of the benefit of receiving blood components, or, as it was phrased in the study, the "risk of not transfusing." This deficit of knowledge appears not to reflect a specific blind spot on the part of physicians. Instead, there simply appears to be a dearth of hard data in this area. This impression is bolstered by inspection of the National Institutes of Health (NIH) Consensus Conference statements on the use of FFP[29], platelets[30], and RBCs[9], in which repeated reference is made to the need for further study of the purported indications for transfusion.

In most instances, the uncertainty or controversy regarding the use of blood components centers on prophylactic rather than therapeutic indications. Therapeutic indications include transfusion for clearcut clinical problems, such as hemorrhagic shock or pathologic bleeding, and the success of the transfusion often is readily seen in the reversal of the problem. Prophylactic indications generally relate to specific laboratory findings, such as thrombocytopenia in the absence of bleeding or anemia in the absence of symptoms. The rationale for such prophylactic transfusions is based on the assumption that the abnormal laboratory finding is predictive of an adverse consequence for the patient. However, this is not the case for many laboratory findings, since the limits of normalcy are established from population statistics, not on the test's predictive value for specific clinical outcomes. Thus, the rationale for prophylactic modes of transfusion should not be simply to correct an abnormal laboratory value that might predict a given adverse outcome. Instead, prophylactic transfusion should be based either on a demonstrated efficacy in decreasing the rate of the relevant occurrence or, at the very least, on a demonstration that the laboratory value to be corrected truly is predictive of the occurrence to be prevented.

Red Blood Cells

Red blood cells (RBCs) are prescribed most often to treat hypovolemia or anemia (decreased oxygen-carrying capacity); they also may be used to replace abnormal RBCs, such as antibody-sensitized RBCs in HDN or RBCs affected by sickling hemoglobinopathies. Because anemia and hypovolemia are relatively commonplace in clinical practice, the appropriate use of RBCs may appear to be a simple matter; however, RBCs are subject to overuse for both indications.

A loss of 20% of the patient's total blood volume is frequently cited as an indication for transfusion. Loss of blood, of course, produces a deficit of RBCs as well as total volume, although the latter clearly has primacy. In fact, if perfusion can be maintained with volume expanders other than blood components and blood loss can be stopped, many obstetric patients can tolerate a volume loss of more than 20% without requiring transfusion. The crucial issue is usually whether there are occult or ongoing losses. In this regard, it is well known that the Hct may be an unreliable guide to the extent of acute blood loss. In massive hemorrhage, whole blood is the most appropriate form of transfusion. However, most donor blood drawn today is separated into components, and many transfusion services do not routinely stock whole blood units. This has led to the addition of FFP administration to the management of patients with hemorrhage, to prevent the development of dilutional coagulopathy, with the unfortunate result of increased donor exposures for the patient. In fact (as discussed above), dilutional coagulopathy is an uncommon cause for bleeding, and this use of FFP generally is unnecessary.

A major therapeutic indication for RBCs can be stated simply as the treatment of symptomatic anemia. Although this criterion seems easy to apply, a number of factors must be considered, in particular, whether the development of anemia is acute or chronic and, if chronic, whether it is due to a deficiency of iron, vitamin B_{12}, or folate. When nutrient deficiencies contribute to the anemia, treatment of the specific deficiency without transfusion is the safest course, unless life-threatening symptoms such as unstable angina are present. The patient with chronic anemia has considerable compensatory resources available, the power of which was demonstrated in the elegant studies of Elwood and coworkers[31], who showed that at Hcts as low as 24%, the symptoms one classically associates with anemia, such as fatigue, decreased exercise tolerance, and palpitations, do not correlate with the degree of anemia. Instead, the best predictors of the presence of such nonspecific symptoms were personality factors. Correction of the anemia by iron administration did not improve these symptoms to any greater degree than did placebo. These data should prompt the physician electing to transfuse an anemic patient to consider whether the reported symptoms are severe enough to limit the patient's lifestyle and, if so, to follow the course of the symptoms after transfusion to ensure that they are reversed.

The initial compensation for anemia is by increased RBC levels of 2,3 DPG, which promote increased oxygen unloading by hemoglobin; this change occurs over the course of several days. If arterial oxygenation is normal, this mechanism can normalize oxygen delivery in the presence of Hcts as low as 24–25%[32], but compensatory increases also occur in the increments in cardiac output in response to work, so patients with lesser degrees of anemia and cardiac or pulmonary disease may require transfusion. Cardiac output at rest begins to increase at an Hct of approximately 21%, but many patients with the anemia of chronic renal failure or sickle cell anemia tolerate Hct below this level. In a recent study directed at defining a transfusion trigger for the patient with normal cardiovascular pathology, baboons were hemodiluted rapidly to an Hct of 15%, their hemodynamic variables were measured, and the animals were simply released back into the colony and observed: No deleterious effects were evident.[33]

In many cases when transfusion is used for anemia, the physician's intent is prophylactic; that is, anemia is being reversed to prevent an adverse event, particularly a cardiovascular or other ischemic event that might be potentiated by a decrease in oxygen-carrying capacity. The rule that the preoperative Hct must be 30% for a patient to receive general anesthesia is an example of such a prophylactic indication. Because of a decreased physiologic reserve in the event of hypoxia or ischemia, a lower Hct is thought to promote an increased rate of adverse outcomes, such as perioperative cardiovascular events, but there are few data proving that this is the case. For example, it is well documented that patients with renal failure and Hcts as low as 13% do not have an increased incidence of complications in spite of their increased risk of coronary artery disease.[34] On the basis of such experiences, the NIH[9] recommended that the "hematocrit 30 rule" be dropped and be replaced by clinical judgment based on multiple patient factors. The NIH panel concluded that there is no evidence that postoperative anemia impairs wound healing. Because of the magnitude of the risk from transfusions, the panel emphasized that transfusions be kept to a minimum and that alternatives be explored in the form of autologous transfusion, aggressive use of volume expanders to support perfusion, and pharmacologic approaches, such as desmopressin to enhance hemostasis and erythropoietin to enhance hematopoiesis.

Sickle cell disease in pregnancy also has been considered an indication for the prophylactic transfusion of RBCs. A recent study[35] compared two randomly assigned groups of pregnant patients with sickle cell disease; one group was transfused prophylactically to maintain an Hct of approximately 33% and a hemoglobin S level less than 35%; the other was transfused therapeutically for standard medical or obstetric indications, including an Hct below 18 or reticulocyte count below 3%. In the latter group, 16 of 36 patients required transfusion at some time during the study. Although the prophylactic transfusion group had a lower rate of painful crises, there were no other differences in the rate of adverse maternal or fetal outcomes.

The use of RBCs for IUT is discussed in the chapters on HDN (Chapters 170 and 171).

FFP and Cryoprecipitate

FFP is the blood component that probably is overused most frequently and the use of which most often generates controversy in blood utilization review committees. Again, a focus on whether a presumed indication for use of this component is therapeutic or prophylactic often will help resolve the issue: Evidence for the prophylactic use of FFP is almost entirely lacking. The appropriate use of FFP has been considered by NIH Consensus Development Conference[29]; the panel's conclusions are summarized in Table 168–9, and several of them deserve comment.

Differences in physicians' practice for the most part involve the treatment of deficiencies of multiple coagulation factors, as found in patients with liver disease, DIC, or dilutional coagulopathy, or in patients receiving warfarin therapy. In such cases, if the patient is bleeding from multiple sites (such as needle punctures), if sites where hemostasis was established previously bleed again, or if the surgeon finds that there is poor clot formation by shed blood, it is reasonable to conclude that the patient would benefit from the replacement of clotting factors. The grounds for such replacement are less strong when there is bleeding from a specific site in the presence of coagulopathy, but if surgical hemostasis has been attempted and coagulation times are elevated to more than 1.5 to 1.8 times the prothrombin time (PT) or partial thromboplastin time (PTT) control value,

TABLE 168–9. NIH CONSENSUS CONFERENCE RECOMMENDATIONS FOR USE OF FFP

FFP is not recommended for
- Volume expansion
- Nutritional source
- Routine management of massive hemorrhage (prophylaxis against dilutional coagulopathy)

Indications for FFP
- Isolated deficiencies of factor II, V, VII, IX, X, and XI when more specific components are unavailable or inappropriate.
- TTP
- Reversal of coumadin effects in bleeding patients or before emergency surgery
- Massive transfusion (>1 blood vol) and pathological hemorrhage if factor deficiencies are presumed to be the sole or principal derangement.
- Bleeding patients with multiple coagulation factor deficiencies (such as those with liver disease)

Adapted from the NIH consensus statement on the use of FFP.[39] Note: Indications that have become obsolete since the original publication of this statement have been omitted.

it may be efficacious to attempt to correct the coagulopathy. When dilution is the presumed cause of the coagulopathy, thrombocytopenia or platelet dysfunction must be ruled out first, because, as discussed above, platelet problems more commonly limit hemostasis in this circumstance, and the correction of clotting times often does not lead to a cessation of bleeding.[14] Consumption coagulopathy also must be ruled out, as FFP replacement will not adequately replete fibrinogen, and cryoprecipitate generally is required in DIC.

Studies of massive transfusion generally have concluded that prophylactic formulas for FFP supplementation are not appropriate.[14,18,20,36] The major controversy centers on the need for prophylactic coagulation factor replacement in patients with abnormal clotting times who are to have invasive procedures. There is little evidence that mildly to moderately elevated coagulation times predict bleeding complications of invasive procedures. In a particularly well executed study, Ewe[37] was unable to show any relationship between PT or platelet count and the extent of bleeding from liver biopsy sites under direct laparoscopic visualization. Similarly, a study[38] of patients undergoing paracentesis or thoracentesis failed to show any relation of excess bleeding to coagulation times that were as much as twice the control level. In the face of such data, the generally low rate of bleeding complications after biopsy, and the known risks of transfusion, the principle of *primum non nocere* would seem to preclude FFP prophylaxis in most cases. Nonetheless, many texts advocate advance FFP treatment of patients with mild coagulopathies who are scheduled for biopsies, and, for some levels of coagulopathy, either such treatment or avoidance of the procedure appears rational. But the question is: At what level of coagulopathy is prophylactic coagulation factor replacement appropriate? In the absence of better data, coagulation times 1.5-fold those of the control are a frequently cited indication for FFP transfusion.[39]

When factor replacement is elected, the next issue is the appropriate dose. Coagulation abnormalities in patients with liver disease are notoriously resistant to correction, particularly if the patient has not responded to vitamin K supplementation. In one study[40], only 20% of patients' PT values decreased after the infusion of 600 mL of FFP; 8 of 11 patients treated in another study[41] achieved parital correction with volumes from 600 to 1800 mL of FFP, but the PT returned toward baseline two to four hours after cessation of infusion. The infusion of volumes of plasma large enough to correct coagulopathies in such patients often leads to volume overload and pulmonary edema. For these reasons, the ability to correct and then demonstrate the correction of a coagulopathy in patients with liver disease prior to a procedure often proves to be impossible. Instead, if prophylaxis is to be attempted, we have suggested rapid infusion of two units of FFP immediately before the procedure and additional supplementation during the procedure, particularly if excessive bleeding occurs.

DIC often accompanies trauma or other circumstances leading to hemorrhagic shock, such as *abruptio placentae*. It is important to perform an appropriate work up for this condition, since the treatment for simple dilutional coagulopathy will not be sufficient. Bleeding due to DIC reflects the consumption of platelets and labile clotting factors, particularly fibrinogen and FVIII, so that initial therapy should be a platelet transfusion (6–8 units for an adult) and a cryoprecipitate transfusion (generally 10 units). As factors V and II also may be consumed, additional supplementation with two units of FFP can be employed. Subsequently, therapy should be guided by laboratory values, with the goal being to maintain a fibrinogen level greater than 100 units per dL and a platelet count greater than 50,000 per uL.

Thrombotic thrombocytopenic purpura (TTP) may be associated with pregnancy and may share some features with the hemolysis-elevated liver enzymes–low platelets (HELLP) syndrome in severe toxemia (see Chapter 139). The most effective form of therapy for TTP is plasma exchange using FFP as replacement for the plasma removed; the HELLP syndrome also has responded to plasma exchange.

Cryoprecipitate is used for the treatment of von Willebrand's disease, hemophilia A (deficiency of FVIIIc), and fibrinogen deficiencies or abnormalities. Discussion of the treatment of congenital deficiencies of individual coagulation factors is beyond the scope of this chapter (see Chapter 167).

Platelets

The therapeutic and prophylactic indications for platelet transfusion are much better understood than are those for FFP; this form of treatment has had a major impact on the survival of many patients, particularly those with hematologic malignancies. Severely thrombocytopenic patients typically develop skin or mucosal bleeding that is manifest as petichiae, epistaxis, oral bleeding, hematuria, gastrointestinal blood loss, and delayed hemostasis after instrumentation. Intracerebral bleeding is the most feared complication of thrombocytopenia and in the past was a common cause of death in leukemia patients. In thrombocytopenic patients, once bleeding stops, it rarely starts again unless there is associated coagulopathy. The frequency and gravity of such bleeding is directly related to the platelet count:[42] major visible hemorrhage occurs in some patients at platelet counts of 20,000 per uL and becomes frequent at counts below 5,000. The bleeding time also is related directly to platelet count at levels below 100,000.

The appropriate indications for platelet transfusion as outlined by an NIH consensus conference panel[30] are shown in Table 168–10. Therapeutic indications for platelet transfusions are relatively clearcut. When the platelet count is less than 50,000 and active bleeding is present in the absence

TABLE 168–10. NIH CONSENSUS CONFERENCE RECOMMENDATIONS FOR THE USE OF PLATELETS

Platelets generally are not indicated for
- Aplastic anemia patients
- ITP patients in the absence of severe bleeding
- Prophylactic treatment before or following cardiopulmonary bypass

Indications for the use of platelets
- Actively bleeding patients with
  - Platelet count less than 50,000
  - Platelet function abnormality and bleeding time greater than twice normal
  - Massive transfusion and documented thrombocytopenia
- Prophylaxis
  - Temporary thrombocytopenia with platelet count less than 20,000
  - Before invasive procedure to correct bleeding time (especially if hemostasis cannot be observed)

Adapted from the NIH consensus statement on the use of platelets.[30]

of a lesion requiring surgical correction, elevation of the platelet count by 40,000 or more is expected to resolve bleeding.[43] If the platelet count cannot be increased because of immunologic or other factors, a response is not expected. The same is true of patients with normal numbers of platelets but with congenital or acquired platelet function abnormalities sufficient to elevate the bleeding time to more than twice normal. If pathologic bleeding develops in the setting of massive transfusion and thrombocytopenia, platelet replacement is expected to stop the bleeding.[14]

Prophylactic indications for platelet transfusion have a rationale based on the data cited above, and prophylactic platelet transfusion in prospective controlled trials has been effective in preventing hemorrhage but not in prolonging survival, probably because the trials have not been large enough.[44] In the study by Murphy and coworkers[45], a disturbing finding was that, during the last month of life, there was an increase in the duration of hemorrhage experienced by patients who had been transfused prophylactically, presumably because these patients had had a greater exposure to donor units and had become alloimmunized—and therefore refractory—to further platelet transfusion. This observation raises the belief that such prophylactic transfusion protocols are relevant only to patients in whom thrombocytopenia is expected to be a temporary condition; if thrombocytopenia or platelet dysfunction will be prolonged, the development of refractoriness eventually can be expected to limit the response to platelets, particularly if immune function is normal as in patients with aplastic anemia or congenital thrombocytopathies.

Patients with severe preoperative thrombocytopenia generally are assumed to benefit from prophylactic platelet transfusion, but this has not been demonstrated in experimental studies. In the utilization criteria of various hospitals, the threshold for such prophylaxis typically is set at platelet counts between 50,000 and 70,000. Prophylactic transfusion of platelets has been investigated in circumstances in which thrombocytopenia is expected to develop intraoperatively, either because of dilution[46] or cardiopulmonary bypass[47]; in both cases, prophylaxis was ineffective. Although it endorsed the logic of prophylactic platelet transfusion for thrombocytopenic patients undergoing surgery, the NIH consensus panel[30] suggested that such transfusions made the most sense for patients in whom hemorrhage could not be observed or when it occurred where it could be critical in small amounts, as in the central nervous system (CNS). In this regard, it may be more important to infuse platelets prior to closing wounds, rather than prior to incision.

Patients with idiopathic thrombocytopenic purpura generally are not considered to be candidates for platelet transfusion for two reason. The first is that, in spite of very low platelet counts, their bleeding times are often relatively normal, and life-threatening hemorrhage is rare. The second is that, as rapid destruction of transfused platelets is the rule, transfusion, particularly for prophylaxis, exposes the patient to a risk with little potential benefit. The same logic applies to patients with TTP. In addition to the usual transfusion reactions, the TTP patient may have an increased risk of complications of microvascular thrombosis when transfused with platelets; this should be avoided particularly if there are CNS signs.

Poor responses to platelet transfusion are relatively common, either because of immune-mediated platelet destruction, or because of nonimmune-mediated destruction/consumption. The former may be due to HLA antibodies, platelet antigen-specific antibodies, or drug-related antibodies. Clinical factors leading to destruction or consumption include fever, infection, DIC, splenomegaly, and bleeding. The approaches to these two groups of problems are quite different. In the former case, compatible platelets must be sought; in the latter, the dose must be increased if platelets are truly required. A poor response to platelets, as measured at 0.5–1 hour after transfusion, tends to favor immune-mediated causes of refractoriness, while nonimmune-mediated refractoriness is often manifest as an adequate response at 1 hour, with a return to baseline by 18–24 hours.[48] This generalization has recently been challenged[49], but in combination with the patient's history and a screen for HLA antibodies, it generally allows a decision to be made as to the efficacy of providing HLA-matched platelets.

REFERENCES

1. Oberman HA. The history of transfusion medicine. In: Petz LD, Swisher SN, eds. *Clinical Practice of Transfusion Medicine*. 2nd ed. New York: Churchill Livingstone; 1989:9.
2. Mollison PL, Engelfriet CP, Contreras M. *Blood Transfusions in Clinical Medicine*. 8th ed. Oxford: Blackwell Scientific Publications, 1987.
3. Shulman I. The risk of overt hemolytic transfusion reaction following the use of an immediate spin crossmatch. *Arch Pathol Lab Med*. 1990;114:112.
4. Pisciotto PT, ed. *Blood Transfusion Therapy: A Physician's Handbook*. 3rd ed. Arlington, VA: American Association of Blood Banks, 1989.
5. Kruskall MS. The safety and utility of autologous donations by pregnant patients: Pro. *Transfusion*. 1990;30:168.
6. Cannon DL, Pepkowitz SH, Jacobs A, et al. Autologous predeposit for obstetrical patients: multiple risk factors do not identify potential transfusion candidates. *Transfusion*. 1989;29(suppl):47S. Abstract.
7. Sayers MW. Autologous blood donation in pregnancy: Con. *Transfusion*. 1990;30:172.
8. Popovsky MA. Immune-mediated transfusion reactions. In: Nance SJ, ed. *Immune Destruction of Red Blood Cells*. Arlington, VA: American Association of Blood Banks, 1989:201.
9. NIH Consensus Conference. Perioperative red cell transfusion. *JAMA*. 1988;260:2700.
10. Honig CL, Bove RJ. Transfusion-associated fatalities: Review of Bureau of Biologics reports 1976–1978. *Transfusion*. 1980;20:653.
11. Popovsky MA, Moore SB. Diagnostic and pathogenetic considerations in transfusion-related acute lung injury. *Transfusion*. 1985;25:573.
12. George CD, Morello PJ. Immunologic effects of blood transfusion upon renal transplantation, tumor operations, and bacterial infections. *Am J Surg*. 1986;152:329.
13. Blumberg N. Heal JM. Transfusion and recipient immune function. *Arch Pathol Lab Med*. 1989;113:246.
14. Miller RD, Robbins TO, Tong MJ, Barton SL. Coagulation defects associated with massive blood transfusions. *Ann Surg*. 1971;174:794.

15. Lim RC, Olcott C, Robinson AJ, Blaisdell FW. Platelet response and coagulation changes following massive blood replacement. *J Trauma.* 1973;13:577.
16. Harrigan C, Lucas CE, Ledgerwood AM, et al. Serial changes in primary hemostasis after massive transfusion. *Surgery.* 1985;98:836.
17. Counts RB, Haisch C, Simon TL, et al. Hemostasis in massively transfused trauma patients. *Ann Surg.* 1979;190:91.
18. Ciavarella D, Reed RL, Counts RB, et al. Clotting factor levels and the risk of microvascular bleeding in the massively transfused patient. *Br J Haematol.* 1987;67:365.
19. Harke H, Rahman S. Haemostatic disorders in massive transfusion. *Bibl Haematol.* 1980;46:179.
20. Collins JA. Recent developments in the area of massive transfusion. *World J Surg.* 1987;11:75.
21. Ottenberg R. Reminiscences of the history of blood transfusion. *J Mt Sinai Hosp NY.* 1937;4:264.
22. Alter HJ. You'll wonder where the yellow went: a 15-year retrospective of posttransfusion hepatitis. In: Moore SB, ed. *Transfusion-transmitted Viral Diseases.* Arlington, VA: American Association of Blood Banks; 1987:53.
23. Ward JW, Holmberg SD, Allen JR, et al. Transmission of human immunodeficiency virus (HIV) by blood transfusions screened as negative for HIV antibody. *N Engl J Med.* 1988;318:473.
24. Cumming PD, Wallace EL, Schorr JB, Dodd RY. Exposure of patients to human immunodeficiency virus through the transfusion of blood components that test antibody-negative. *N Engl J Med.* 1989;321:941.
25. Alter HJ, Epstein JS, Swenson SG, et al. Collaborative study to evaluate HIV-antigen (HIV-ag) screening of blood donors. *Transfusion.* 1989;29(suppl):56S. Abstract.
26. Transfusion Safety Study Group. HIV-1 P-24 antigen screening of male blood donors from high anti-HIV prevalence areas. *Transfusion.* 1989; 29(suppl):56S. Abstract.
27. Tegtmeier GE. Posttransfusion cytomegalovirus infections. *Arch Pathol Lab Med.* 1989;113:236.
28. Avorn J, Soumerai SB, Salem SR, Popovsky M. Documenting and correcting inappropriate use of blood components. In: Kurtz SR, Summers S, eds. *Improving Transfusion Practice: The Role of Quality Assurance.* Arlington, VA: American Association of Blood Banks; 1989:21.
29. Willis JL, ed. *Use of Blood Components.* FDA Drug Bull, July 1989.
30. Consensus Development Panel. Platelet Transfusion Therapy. *Transfus Med Rev.* 1987;1:195.
31. Elwood PC, Waters WE, Creene WJW, et al. Symptoms and circulating haemoglobin level. *J Chronic Dis.* 1969;21:615.
32. Hogman CR. Oxygen affinity of stored blood. *Acta Anaesth Scand.* 1971;45(suppl):53.
33. Levine E, Rosen A, Sehgal L, et al. Physiologic effects of acute anemia: implications for a reduced transfusion trigger. *Transfusion.* 1990;30:11.
34. Graves CL, Allen RM. Anaesthesia in the presence of severe anemia. *Rocky Mt Med J.* 1970;000:35.
35. Koshy M, Burd L, Wallace D, et al. Prophylactic red-cell transfusions in pregnant patients with sickel cell disease: a randomized cooperative study. *N Engl J Med.* 1988;319:1447.
36. Mannucci PM, Federici AB, Sirchia G. Hemostasis testing during massive blood replacement. *Vox Sang.* 1982;42:113.
37. Ewe K. Bleeding after liver biopsy does not correlate with indices of peripheral coagulation. *Dig Dis Sci.* 1981;26:388.
38. McVay PA, Toy P. Lack of increased bleeding after paracentesis and thoracentesis in patients with mild coagulopathy. *Transfusion.* 1989; 29(suppl):37S. Abstract.
39. Consensus Development Panel, National Institutes of Health. Fresh frozen plasma. Indications and risks. *JAMA.* 1985;253:551.
40. Gazzard BG, Henderson IM, Williams R. The use of fresh frozen plasma or a concentrate of factor IX as a replacement therapy before liver biopsy. *Gut.* 1975;16:621.
41. Spector I, Corn M, Ticktin HE. Effect of plasma transfusion on the prothrombin time and clotting factors in liver disease. *N Engl J Med.* 1966;275:1032.
42. Gaydos LA, Freireich EJ, Mantel N. The quantitative relationship between platelet count and hemorrhage in patients with acute leukemia. *N Engl J Med.* 1962;266:905.
43. Djerassi I, Farber S, Evans AE. Transfusions of fresh platelet concentrates to patients with secondary thrombocytopenia. *N Engl J Med.* 1963;268:221.
44. Kelton JG, Ali AM. Platelet transfusions—a critical appraisal. *Clin Oncol.* 1983;2:549.
45. Murphy S, Litwin S, Herring LM, et al. Indications for platelet transfusion in children with acute leukemia. *Am J Hematol.* 1982;12:347.
46. Reed RL, Ciaruella D, Heimbach DM, et al. Prophylactic platelet administration during massive transfusion: a prospective, randomized, double-blind clinical study. Ann Surg. 1986;203:40.
47. Simon TL, Akl BF, Murphy W. Controlled trial of routine administration of platelet concentrates in cardiopulmonary bypass surgery. *Ann Thorac Surg.* 1984;37:359.
48. Daly PA, Schiffer CA, Aisner J, Wiernik PH. Platelet transfusion therapy: one-hour posttransfusion increments are valuable in predicting the need for HLA-matched preparations. *JAMA.* 1980;243:435.
49. McFarland JG, Anderson AJ, Slichter SJ. Factors influencing the transfusion response to HLA-selected apheresis donor platelets in patients refractory to random platelet concentrates. *Br J Haematol.* 1989;73:380.

Chapter One Hundred and Sixty-Nine

Polycythemia Vera

Camille J. Wahbeh

169

Polycythemia vera (PV) is a chronic panmyelosis resulting in the excessive proliferation of all marrow elements with a preponderance of the erythroid series. This leads to the characteristic increase in the red cell mass and often to an elevation in the peripheral white blood cell and platelet counts. Polycythemia vera belongs to the spectrum of myeloproliferative disorders that include chronic myelocytic leukemia, agnogenic myeloid metaplasia, primary hemorrhagic thrombocythemia, and erythroleukemia.

Polycythemia vera usually begins in late middle age with a peak incidence in the fifth decade. There is a slightly higher incidence in males. No clear familial tendency exists, but there are a few reports of PV in monozygotic twins.[1] An accurate incidence is not available; however, Modan estimates a prevalence of five per million population in the Baltimore area.[2] Some report a low incidence in blacks and a slightly higher than expected incidence in Jews of European origin.

ETIOLOGY AND PATHOPHYSIOLOGY

Recent evidence indicates that the proliferation of all cellular elements originates from a single abnormal clone, most likely at the level of the pluripotent stem cell. *In vitro* culture data suggest the presence of two populations of erythroid precursors. The abnormal clone appears to be autonomous, but the other behaves like cells from normal individuals requiring erythropoietin for proliferation.[3] There is a decline in the proportion of normal elements as the disease progresses.

Plasma and urinary levels of erythropoietin are markedly reduced to absent in polycythemia vera, presumably secondary to negative feedback from the overproduction of red cells. This is in distinction to secondary polycythemia, which results from increased erythropoietin production. However, the ability to produce erythropoietin is intact, as demonstrated in the response to phlebotomy. The plasma volume usually is normal in polycythemia vera as opposed to individuals with relative polycythemia secondary to a reduced plasma volume. Increased red cell production is apparent in radioisotope studies.

Several hematopoietic stimuli, including a viral stimulus, have been considered, but no factor capable of producing a panmyelosis has been demonstrated yet. As such, the etiology of PV remains unknown.

The symptoms of PV are nonspecific. They are mostly secondary to the increased RBC mass and hemoglobin concentration. This results in an increase in the total volume and viscosity of blood and an increased peripheral vascular resistance. Consequently, perfusion of vital organs is poor, and tissue hypoxia may result. Thus, there is decreased exercise tolerance. Disturbance in the cerebral circulation explains such complaints as headache, dizziness, and auditory and visual alterations. Symptoms of coronary insufficiency (angina) and peripheral vascular insufficiency (intermittent claudication) may be present. Thrombotic phenomena are seen, and there is a tendency to increased bleeding (epistaxis, peptic ulcer bleeds). This bleeding tendency is caused by a combination of an intrinsic platelet dysfunction and the distention of the vasculature resulting from the increased blood volume.

Peptic ulcer is at least four times more prevalent in PV than in the general population. Abdominal fullness, early satiety, and left upper quadrant pain are present when marked enlargement of the spleen leads to stretching and infarction of its capsule. Pruritus occurs in nearly half of these patients and may be related to altered histamine metabolism. With extensive cell proliferation, hyperuricemia is found; however, secondary gout and uric acid nephropathy are not common. Arterial hypertension may be present; however, the advanced age at onset makes the possibility of worsening of preexisting hypertension likely.

The disease is gradual in onset and runs a slowly progressive course. Manifestations other than the increased RBC production (ie, leukocytosis, thrombocytosis, splenomegaly, and myelofibrosis) are present to a variable degree at the onset and progress variably during the course of the disease. One fifth of patients progress to the "spent" phase with marrow fibrosis and may require transfusions. Some believe that this process is hastened by radiotherapy and chemotherapy. Without therapy, most patients die within 2 years of vascular complications or unrelated causes. Patients with PV have a slightly higher than expected incidence of hematologic neoplasms (acute and chronic leukemias, lymphomas, and multiple myeloma).

Pregnancy Effects

Reports of PV in pregnancy are rare. Only 5.2% of patients are below age 40 and with a slightly higher male preponderance (ratio 1.3:1)[4], there is a rare occurrence in women of the reproductive age group. The available reports indicate that pregnancy has no adverse effects on the disease.[5-8] Hochman and Stein reported a gradual normalization of RBC counts and a decreased need for phlebotomy as pregnancy progressed in three pregnancies in a single patient.[5] Others have reported decreased erythrocytosis during the first two trimesters with a return to the elevated hemoglobin concentrations in late pregnancy or postpartum.[8] The physiologic plasma volume expansion in the first two trimesters of gestation is probably contributory. Wasserman, however, found an actual lowering of RBC mass in a few pregnant patients with PV.[9] He also noted suppression of RBC production in a few male patients treated with estrogen and concluded that estrogen output of the placenta may be enough to suppress erythrocyte production. However, the erythropoietin-augmenting action of human placental lactogen and prolactin also must be considered in evaluating the net effect of pregnancy on hematopoiesis.

All reports of PV in pregnancy indicate that the disease apparently has an adverse effect on fertility and pregnancy outcome. Poor uteroplacental perfusion may be the underlying factor. A tendency for postpartum hemorrhage also has been reported. In the few reported pregnancies in the literature, the fetal salvage rate was 53%.[7] No hematologic abnormalities in these infants were reported. Decreased uterine blood flow and feto-placental perfusion may be responsible for the increased rate of spontaneous abortion, intrauterine fetal death, and premature delivery that is reported. The tendency to manifest arterial hypertension in PV may result in an increased incidence of superimposed pregnancy-induced hypertension.[5] The adverse effects of failure of plasma volume expansion on pregnancy outcome in gravidas with chronic and pregnancy-induced hypertension are established.

Koller et al[10] reported on the association between elevated hemoglobin concentrations in the last two trimesters of pregnancy (with no apparent underlying cause) and growth retardation and death of the fetus. Causal considerations such as increased blood viscosity and interference with placental circulation were cited.

DIAGNOSIS

Few patients present with the typical syndrome of splenomegaly, increased red cell mass, and pancytosis in the marrow. Those that do are discovered on routine evaluation. Hematocrits at or above 60% most likely represent true erythrocytosis. The peripheral smear reveals normochromic, normocytic RBCs when the iron stores are adequate. Late in the disease, when extramedullary hematopoiesis sets in, nucleated RBCs may be seen in the periphery. The erythrocyte sedimentation rate is, not surprisingly, very low. Leukocytosis is found in 70% of patients (> 12,000/mL without evidence of infection).[4] The leukocyte alkaline phosphatase is often elevated. Thrombocytosis (platelet count > 500,000) is seen in more than half of these patients. *In vitro* platelet function studies reveal defective platelet adhesiveness. The bone marrow shows erythroid or panhyperplasia. When thrombocytosis is present, there is increased megakaryocytic nuclear ploidy. Chromosomal abnormalities occasionally have been reported.

In the less obvious case, determination of RBC mass by isotope dilution using ^{51}Cr may be critical in distinguishing true and relative erythrocytosis. Radioactive isotopes should be avoided in pregnancy. Arterial blood gases with a normal arterial O_2 saturation distinguish PV from erythrocytosis secondary to hypoxia. Leukocytosis with an absolute basophil count over $65/mm^3$ aids in the diagnosis if found.[4] If the diagnosis is still questionable, plasma erythropoietin and urinary excretion levels may resolve the uncertainty. In the obese patient, an abdominal computerized tomography (CT) scan may be indicated in the face of inability to demonstrate splenomegaly clinically.

TREATMENT

Optimal therapy for polycythemia vera requires a clear understanding of the pathophysiology and currently is not completely settled. Individualization of therapy is stressed.

Phlebotomy remains the most widely used, the safest, and the least controversial form of treatment. It can be used repeatedly and is preferred in the young patient with mild disease.[9] Exchange phlebotomy with plasma expanders being replaced avoids acute shifts in blood volume. The goal of therapy with repeated phlebotomy should be a normal hemoglobin concentration. This mode of therapy alone results in a 10-year survival. It is extremely useful in reducing bleeding and mortality in the patient requiring emergency surgery.

Marrow suppression may be achieved with radioisotope or chemotherapy. Radioactive ^{32}P was used widely in the past for marrow suppression. However, the finding of an increased incidence of acute leukemic transformation has limited its use greatly.[11] The Polycythemia Vera Study Group found no difference in survival in a prospective randomized trial between radioactive phosphorus or chemotherapy in conjunction with phlebotomy and phlebotomy alone.[12] Myelosuppression with hydroxyurea may be indicated in the patient at high risk for thrombotic complications or a history of such events. Experience with this form of therapy in pregnancy is lacking and its long-term effects, particularly its mutagenic potential, are not known.[13] Splenectomy with or without prior radiation carries a high morbidity and mortality and is very rarely employed. Allopurinol is useful in decreasing the frequency of gouty attacks when significant hyperuricemia is present.

For the pregnant patient with PV, some investigators maintain that careful observation is all that is needed because of the tendency to normalization of RBC counts.[9] This is probably the result of the plasma volume expansion and the relative dilutional anemia of pregnancy. If worsening occurs, exchange phlebotomy should be attempted first and can be repeated to maintain the hematocrit below 50%.[7] If phlebotomy fails and the need is extreme, low-dose busulfan therapy (4–6 mg daily) may be attempted after the first trimester of gestation. This agent has been used with apparent safety in the pregnant patient with chronic myelocytic leukemia. Busulfan suppresses erythropoiesis less effectively than it suppresses leukocyte and platelet production, and its prolonged use may result in pulmonary fibrosis. Other alkylating agents were found to result in a greater than 10% incidence of acute leukemia, and their use is not recommended by the Polycythemia Vera Study Group.[12]

Regional anesthesia is said to be preferable for delivery in a pregnant patient with PV. A bleeding time should be performed prior to administration of epidural anesthesia as some patients will demonstrate a bleeding tendency. Alteration of lung compliance and abnormal ventilation-perfusion distribution can result in respiratory acidosis if general anesthesia is used.[14]

The prevention of pregnancy complications in PV entails careful and frequent prenatal follow up. Exchange phlebotomy should be utilized to decrease RBC mass and normalize the hemoglobin concentration.[7] Early recognition of signs of preterm labor and pregnancy-induced hypertension is important in reducing morbidity. Serial ultrasonographic evaluation to screen for intrauterine growth retardation with appropriate antenatal biophysical monitoring is essential for a successful pregnancy outcome. Umbilical and uterine artery Doppler flow studies may prove to be of value in managing the pregnant patient with PV.

REFERENCES

1. Friedland MC, Wittels EG, Robinson RF. Polycythemia vera in identical twins. *Am J Hematol.* 1981;10:101.
2. Modan B. An epidemiological study of polycythemia vera. *Blood.* 1965;26:657.
3. Porchal JF, Axelrad AA. Bone marrow response in polycythemia vera. *N Engl J Med.* 1974;290:1382.
4. Berlin NI. Diagnosis and classification of the polycythemias. *Semin Hematol.* 1975;12:339.
5. Hochmann A, Stein JA. Polycythemia and pregnancy. *Obstet Gynecol.* 1961;18:230.
6. Ruch WA, Klein RL. Polycythemia vera and pregnancy. Report of a case. *Obstet Gynecol.* 1964;23:107.
7. Cantrone A, Freda RN, McGowan L. Polycythemia rubra vera in pregnancy. *Obstet Gynecol.* 1967;30:657.
8. Ferguson JE, Ueland K, Aronson WJ. Polycythemia rubra vera and pregnancy. *Obstet Gynecol.* 1983;62:16S.
9. Hoffman R, Wasserman LR. Natural history and management of polycythemia vera. *Adv Intern Med.* 1979;24:255.
10. Koller O, Sandrei R, Sagen N. High hemoglobin levels during pregnancy and fetal risk. *Int J Gynaecol Obstet.* 1980;18:53.
11. Landaw SA. Acute leukemia in polycythemia vera. *Semin Hematol.* 1976;13:33.
12. Wasserman LR. The treatment of polycythemia vera. *Semin Hematol.* 1976;13:57.
13. Berk PD, Goldberg JD, Donovan PB, et al. Therapeutic recommendations in polycythemia vera based on Polycythemia Vera Study Group protocols. *Semin Hematol.* 1986;23:132.
14. Giliberti BJ. Clinical anesthesia conference: Polycythemia vera and anesthesia. *NY State J Med.* 1962;62:400.

Chapter One Hundred and Seventy

Hemolytic Disease of the Newborn

James T. Perkins

170

The term *hemolytic disease of the newborn* (HDN), or, more properly, hemolytic disease of the fetus and newborn, encompasses a number of manifestations once thought to represent separate diseases, namely erythroblastosis fetalis, icterus gravis neonatorum, icterus praecox, congenital anemia, and hydrops fetalis. The elucidation of the underlying unity of these problems and of their cause, treatment, and prevention is one of the more fascinating and successful chapters in the history of medicine.[1] Figure 170–1 depicts this success as a decline in the HDN mortality rate in relation to a series of therapeutic discoveries, beginning with exchange transfusion and culminating in the development of Rh immunoglobulin (RhIG). It is easy for a younger physician to take Rh immunoprophylaxis for granted and to forget that at the time most of us were born, HDN constituted the most frequent cause of perinatal mortality.

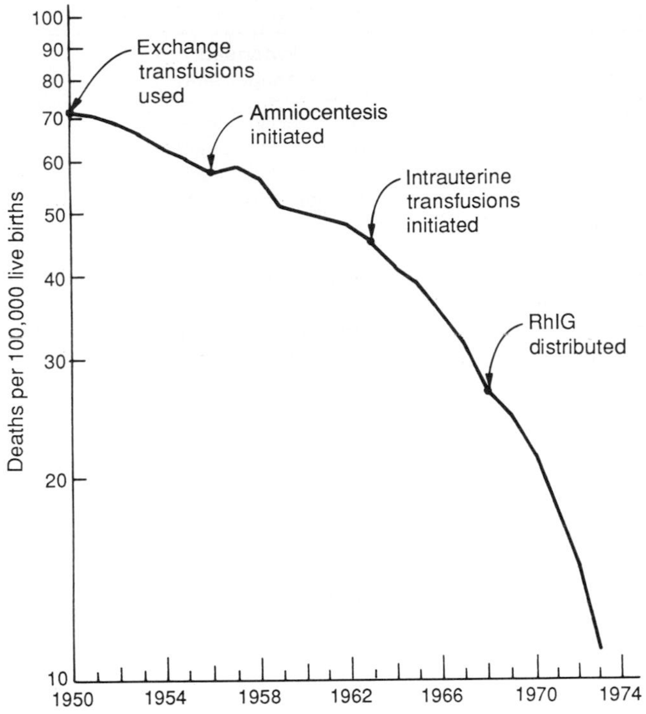

Figure 170–1. Decline in HDN mortality with new developments in management and prevention. (*From Centers for Disease Control[42] with permission.*)

PATHOGENESIS

HDN is a disorder in which maternal *alloantibody* (antibody against "not-self" components of the members of the same species, previously "isoantibody") destroys fetal red blood cells (RBCs). In the classic and most severe forms of this disease, the responsible alloantibody is directed against the Rh blood group (more specifically, the D or Rh_o antigen). Milder disease frequently is caused by ABO antibodies, and other blood groups are occasionally involved. The pathogenesis HDN can be broken down into several steps, each of which may provide insight into the available means of diagnosis, prevention, and treatment. Maternal antibody also may be directed against other fetal blood elements; this chapter will briefly consider the states initiated by such antibodies.

Immunizing Stimulus

The first event in the pathogenesis of HDN is the antigen stimulus. In HDN mediated by the Rh blood group (Rh HDN), the stimulus is fetal RBCs in the form of small *feto-maternal hemorrhages* (FMHs). FMH measurable by the Kleihauer–Betke test occurs in approximately 50% of pregnancies and most often is detectable at the time of delivery[2], but minute FMHs probably occur during all pregnancies as shown by flow cytometry.[3] The average FMH revealed by flow cytometry was 0.156 mL.[3] When immunization is caused by such small volumes of RBCs, several months and repeated stimulation typically are required before significant levels of antibody are formed.[4] Because of this, the first pregnancy is affected only rarely in Rh HDN.

Fetal RBCs have been identified in the maternal circulation as early as 8 weeks' gestation, and 20% of maternal exposure to fetal RBCs occurs before parturition (by Kleihauer–Betke test). Although these events usually do not result in antibody formation during the current pregnancy, lymphocyte memory cells can be generated in a process termed *sensibilization*. For this reason, RhIG prophylaxis is more complete if delivered antepartum as well as postpartum.

The mother can be exposed to fetal RBCs in the course of other events, including amniocentesis, abortion, ectopic pregnancy, maternal trauma, and other manipulations such as external version, which thus become indications for immunoprophylaxis. Transfusion also may cause blood group immunization; an old adage in blood banking says, "Never transfuse a woman with her husband's blood," because paternal blood groups are those which the mother, in future pregnancies, treats as not-self.

FMH can be massive, causing fetal anemia, stillbirth, and occasionally hydrops on a nonimmunologic basis.[5] FMH of more than 30 mL occurs in 0.3–0.4% of pregnancies[2] and necessitates an increased dose of RhIG to prevent immunization; therefore, all Rh-negative women should be screened after delivery for FMH of this magnitude. In cases of cesarean section, the spillage of fetal cells into the peritoneum may occur in a delayed fashion. When this is suspected, quantitation of FMH should be delayed correspondingly.

RBCs are not the only form of blood group antigen presentation. ABO antigens are encountered in the form of bacteria early in life, and normal individuals form antibodies to whatever ABO antigens they lack. Thus, HDN mediated by ABO antibodies (ABO HDN) is as likely to affect the first infant as subsequent ones.

Antibody Formation

Once there has been an antigen stimulus, the mother may respond by producing antibody. The Rh antigen is the blood group primarily associated with HDN because it is the most immunogenic of blood groups for which the antigenic stimulus is RBCs themselves (excluding ABO antigens). Anti-Rh (this term is used in place of the more specific "anti-D") has been formed after the experimental injection of as little as 0.03 mL of Rh-positive RBCs in divided doses.[4] An Rh-negative mother having an Rh-positive baby has a risk of immunization of about 16% for the first pregnancy.[6] In about half of the cases in which immunization occurs, Rh antibody is not detectable after delivery; instead sensibilization becomes evident only during a subsequent pregnancy when there is an anamnestic reaction. The immunization rate plateaus at about 50% by the fifth at-risk pregnancy. Rising titers of blood group antibody during pregnancy suggest the presence of ongoing stimulation by antigen-positive fetal RBCs.

With respect to ABO antigens, antibody production does not require prior pregnancy or transfusion. Overall, 20% of pregnancies are incompatible; that is, the mother makes an ABO antibody directed against a fetal antigen. However, only 2% of infants have detectable ABO-mediated hemolysis, and severe ABO HDN is uncommon.[7]

There is an interesting interaction between ABO and Rh incompatibility. If the mother and the fetus are both Rh and ABO incompatible, the frequency of immunization by the first pregnancy drops from 16 to 2%[6], presumably because maternal anti-A or anti-B destroys Rh-positive fetal RBCs before they can immunize the mother. This fact was an important clue to the possibility of Rh immunoprophylaxis[1], as passively administered anti-Rh might achieve the same effect.

TABLE 170–1. BLOOD GROUP ALLOANTIBODIES CAUSING HDN

Blood Group System	Specific Antigen	Severity	Proposed Management
Rh (non-D)	C	Mild to moderate	Amniotic fluid studies
	c	Mild to severe	Amniotic fluid studies
	E	Mild to severe	Amniotic fluid studies
	e	Mild to moderate	Amniotic fluid studies
Lewis		Not a proven cause of HDN	
I		Not a proven cause of HDN	
Kell	K	Mild to severe with hydrops fetalis	Amniotic fluid studies
	k	Mild to severe	Amniotic fluid studies
Duffy	Fy^a	Mild to severe with hydrops fetalis	Amniotic fluid studies
	Fy^b	Not a proven cause of HDN	
Kidd	Jk^a	Mild to severe	Amniotic fluid studies
	Jk^b	Mild to severe	Amniotic fluid studies
MNSs	M	Mild to severe	Amniotic fluid studies when IgG titer is high
	N	Mild	Expectant
	S	Mild to severe	Amniotic fluid studies
	s	Mild to severe	Amniotic fluid studies
Lutheran	Lu^a	Mild	Expectant
	Lu^b	Mild	Expectant
Diego	Di^a	Mild to severe	Amniotic fluid studies
	Di^b	Mild to severe	Amniotic fluid studies
Xg	Xg^a	Mild	Expectant
P	P_1	Not a proven cause of HDN	
	PP_1P^k (Tj^a)	Mild to severe	Amniotic fluid studies
Wright	$Wright^a$	Severe	Amniotic fluid studies
	$Wright^b$	Mild	Expectant

Adapted from Weinstein L.[43]

Blood groups other than Rh and ABO, particularly Kell and c, can give rise to HDN (Table 170–1). Many antibodies defining blood group specificities were detected first in such cases, and the antigen specificity was named for the antibody-forming mother. Disease due to such antibodies was responsibile for 12% of HDN deaths in England and Wales from 1983 to 1985.[8] Mothers of infants with non-Rh, non-ABO HDN are nine times more likely to have been transfused in the past; such immunization could be regarded as a delayed transfusion reaction.

Transplacental Antibody Transfer

Once a mother has made antibody, it must traverse the placenta into the fetus to do its damage. This active process, mediated through the Fc portion of IgG, concentrates antibody in the fetal circulation[9], presumably enhancing neonatal disease resistance. IgM antibodies are not transferred, which partly explains why many ABO-incompatible pregnancies are not at risk for hemolysis. Group O individuals usually have anti-A and anit-B of the IgG class, however, and ABO HDN is limited mostly to group A or B babies of group O mothers, which is the case in 15% of gestations.

Although sensitization of fetal RBCs by potent maternal anti-Rh has been demonstrated as early as 6–10 weeks, pregnancies severely affected before 20 weeks are uncommon. Maternal IgG in the fetal circulation reaches a concentration of about 15% of the adult level by the beginning of the third trimester and rises exponentially thereafter to 120% of the maternal level.[9] Thus, the severity of fetal hemolysis progresses in affected pregnancies.

Sensitization of Fetal RBCs

Once a mother has made transportable antibody, the next pathogenic step is the sensitization of fetal RBCs by this antibody. For this to occur, the red cell must express the corresponding antigen at the fetal stage of life. Since ABO antigens do not develop to their full strength until after birth, ABO HDN is less severe than that mediated by Rh. The number of A antigen sites on neonatal RBCs correlates with the severity of hemolysis in affected infants.[10] This principle can be generalized to other blood groups, such as those of the Lewis system, that do not cause HDN or for which the disease is generally mild. A second modifier may be soluble fetal A or B antigen, which can neutralize maternal anti-A and anti-B.

Antibody-mediated Hemolysis

The Rh antibodies causing most cases of severe HDN do not fix complement and therefore do not cause intravascular hemolysis. Instead, hemolysis probably occurs by way of cell-mediated destruction of antibody-opsonized RBCs, which largely takes place in the spleen. Although we think of such RBC destruction as occurring by phagocytosis, other cell-mediated mechanisms exist, including the "antibody-dependent cellular cytotoxicity" mediated by natural killer cells.

Sensitization does not result invariably in clinically significant RBC destruction. For example, 40% of Rh-positive infants born to mothers with anti-Rh will not require treatment[11], and anti-Rh–sensitized fetal RBCs may survive normally. Likewise, 38% of group A or B infants of group O mothers in one study[7] had a positive direct antiglobulin test (DAT) at birth, but only 30% of DAT-positive infants had detectable hemolysis.

A number of immunohematologic factors that influence the occurrence of hemolysis have been identified, but this knowledge does not allow us to predict this occurrence with accuracy. For example, the titer of maternal antibody is a poor predictor. For non-ABO antibodies known to cause HDN, a titer of 16–32 generally is considered to represent the threshold at which hemolysis may occur. However, titration tests are nonspecific and are used only as a trigger for the performance of direct tests of hemolysis, such as amniocentesis. Anti-Rh can be quantitated in μg, and such quantitation may have a better predictive value than titration. IgG subclasses vary in the efficiency with which they fix complement or opsonize RBCs, and there may be variation from one individual to another in the subclass of antibody formed; these facts may account for some of the variation in the hemolytic potential of different maternal sera.[12] Factors relating to the specific blood group are important, and characterization of the maternal antibody specificity is essential to the planning of a course of investigation and treatment. Finally, there is unexplained individual variation due to unmeasurable factors, including the activity of the fetal reticuloendothelial system.

Amniocentesis has been the standard method for predicting a degree of antepartum hemolysis that requires treatment, but it has two major drawbacks: it cannot be employed until about 20 weeks' gestation, and amniocentesis itself may cause FMH. FMH stimulates maternal anti-Rh production and has been observed to worsen the severity of the very problem being studied.[13] Percutaneous umbilical blood sampling (PUBS) predicts fetal hemolysis with increased sensitivity and specificity, but it suffers from the same drawbacks as amniocentesis. Thus, a noninvasive test based on characterization of the maternal serum would be useful in predicting fetal hemolysis, particularly if the fetus does not require intervention, or if modes of therapy other than intrauterine transfusion (IUT), that do not replace fetal RBCs with compatible cells, are to be employed.

Clinical Consequences of Hemolysis

The final step in the pathogenesis of HDN is the mechanism by which fetal hemolysis gives rise to clinical problems. Hemolysis itself, of course, can cause anemia. Fetal anemia was probably the cause of the 29% incidence of stillbirth in second-affected fetuses seen before the development of effective therapy.[9] The second direct result of hemolysis is icterus. Bilirubin released from RBCs destroyed *in utero* is eliminated through the placenta, but a small amount of bilirubin accumulates in the amniotic fluid by processes not completely understood. Quantitation of this bilirubin and of other hemoglobin breakdown pigments in amniotic fluid is useful in predicting the severity of HDN. Because of the relative immaturity of the neonatal liver's bilirubin uptake and conjugation mechanism, even mildly increased rates of neonatal hemolysis may result in marked jaundice. In classic HDN, jaundice appears on the first day of life (*icterus praecox*), unlike physiologic jaundice of the newborn, which tends to appear on the third day. Unconjugated bilirubin is lipid soluble and is able to cross the immature blood-brain barrier causing kernicterus, the staining of the basal ganglia, and cerebellum. The resulting neuronal toxicity manifests most often as motor deficits, hearing loss, and mental retardation.

The fetus attempts to compensate for hemolysis; many of the characteristic clinical manifestations of HDN reflect this compensation. Compensatory erythropoiesis gives rise to erythroblastosis fetalis, an increased number of reticulocytes and nucleated RBCs in the fetal circulation. Expanded erythropoiesis can occur only at extramedullary sites, where it in turn causes hepatosplenomegaly.

Compensation may not be sufficient. Congestive heart failure and anasarca, or hydrops fetalis, once thought to be due to anemia and compensatory volume expansion, probably are caused by reduced fetal plasma oncotic pressure and high output failure. In newborns, some of whom had been transfused *in utero*, cord blood concentration of albumin correlated better with the degree of hydrops fetalis than did hematocrit or estimated blood volume.[14] In another study[15], fetoscopic blood sampling revealed that 10 of 14 infants with hemoglobin <4 g/dL (normal 9.7–13.3) were hydropic, whereas none with higher hemoglobin levels had hydrops. Hypoalbuminemia was present in six of seven hydropic fetuses but in only two of ten nonhydropic, affected fetuses.[16] Although decreased synthesis was the presumed cause of hypoalbuminemia, increased capillary permeability due to chronic hypoxia may have contributed as well, as suggested by elevated levels of ascitic fluid albumin. The placenta is affected by hydrops and is described classically as enlarged and edematous.

Hemorrhagic phenomena occur, and thrombocytopenia is well documented in fetuses[17] and newborns[18] with HDN. Other potentiating factors may include decreased hepatic synthesis of coagulation factors and DIC.[19] Hemorrhage was the most common cause of death in a large series of infants with Rh HDN treated in the era of exchange transfusion.[20] Of 4315 live births, 197 (4.5%) infants died within four weeks. A total of 58 (29%) of these deaths were due to hemorrhage; of these, 49 were judged to be a direct consequence of HDN. Bleeding occurred in the lungs in 35 infants, in the subarachnoid space in six, and in both sites in seven. Most infants with fatal hemorrhage due to HDN had a cord blood hemoglobin of <8 g/dL. Left ventricular failure may have been an important precipitating event in the pulmonary hemorrhage. The other frequent causes of death were hydrops alone (35 in 197), hyaline membrane disease (27 in 197), congenital malformations alone (18 in 197), sudden death during exchange transfusion (17 in 197), and kernicterus alone (12 in 197).

In their comprehensive studies, Phibbs and coworkers[14,21,22] have emphasized the importance of intrapartum asphyxia, prematurity and other factors in producing respiratory distress syndrome in HDN. They also documented that a significant minority of newborns with HDN are hypovolemic after resuscitation. Other clinical problems in newborns with HDN include hypoglycemia and benign cholestasis.[23]

In predicting the clinical severity of HDN, the obstetric history is of great value in disease caused by anti-Rh, but is not of use in predicting ABO antibody-mediated disease. For untreated Rh HDN, two generalizations have been made.[24] First, the disease tends to be less severe overall in first-affected infants than in subsequent Rh-positive infants; second, within a family, the severity tends to remain constant. The stillbirth rate increased from 6% in first-affected pregnancies to 26% in all subsequent pregnancies, and the fraction requiring treatment increased from 57% to 75%. However, if a previous affected infant did not require treatment, 60% of subsequent infants did not need treatment and only 2% of subsequent pregnancies resulted in a stillbirth, a prognosis significantly better than for first-affected pregnancies. Conversely, if there was a previous history of stillbirth due to HDN, only 20% of subsequent affected fetuses were born alive if allowed to go to term. ABO incompatibility between mother and fetus did not alter the severity of Rh HDN once the mother was immunized, nor did a prolonged interval between pregnancies.

In contrast to Rh KDN, disease caused by ABO antibodies occurs in the first infant in 50% of affected families, and severely affected infants may be followed by infants with mild or no disease. As mentioned before, clinically significant hemolysis by ABO antibodies is uncommon. In one series of 665 group A or B infants of group O mothers, 31% had a positive DAT, but only 4% developed icterus severe enough to require therapy and only 1.6% needed exchange transfusion.[25] ABO HDN, measured as the incidence of a positive DAT, jaundice on the first day, or an indirect bilirubin level over 10 mg/dL, is two to six times more common in black infants than in white, despite a similar incidence of ABO-incompatible pregnancies.[26]

Antibody-mediated Immunosuppression

Although the prevention or augmentation of immunization by passive administration of specific antibody had been known for a long time to immunologists involved in vaccine research, its application to Rh HDN was delayed, in part because of fear of causing fetal hemolysis, the very problem that was to be prevented.[27] The efficacy of human-derived antibody to the RH factor (RhIG) in preventing active Rh immunization when passively administered around the time of antigen exposure was demonstrated first in volunteers by experimental exposure to Rh-positive RBCs, and subsequently seen in postpartum mothers. It is relatively well established that 20 μg of RhIG is required to neutralize the immunizing stimulus of 1 mL of Rh-positive RBCs. The period within which administration must occur is not well established, however; the standard 72-hour interval is a historic accident.[1] A 50% reduction in the rate of experimental immunization was observed when RhIG was given 13 days after the RBC stimulus.[28] Postpartum RhIG prophylaxis reduces the incidence of immunization from 16 to 1–2%.[9,29] This 1% to 2% failure rate reflects antepartum Rh immunization or immunization occurring because of an insufficient dose of RhIG. The addition of an antepartum dose of RhIg results in further reduction as high as tenfold in the incidence of immunization.[30,31]

Antepartum prophylaxis frequently results in a positive maternal antibody screen at the time of delivery or in a positive DAT in the newborn, but it does not cause clinically evident hemolysis. Both events should be recognized as passive immunization, so that the mother is not denied further prophylaxis postpartum and the newborn is not exposed to unnecessary testing.

Three hypotheses regarding the mechanism of antibody-mediated immune suppression have been proposed, namely antigen deviation, antigen blocking, and central inhibition. The antigen deviation hypothesis suggests that passive administration of blood group antibody achieves the elimination of fetal RBCs expressing the corresponding antigen in a fashion such that the antigen is not presented to the maternal cells that initiate the immune response. This mechanism seems to explain the difference in the incidence of Rh immunization in ABO-compatible and ABO-incompatible pregnancies. However, the mechanism of RBC elimination by antibodies directed against ABO and Rh antigens is very different, so the mechanism of immunosuppression might differ as well. In experiments using various ratios of RhIG to Rh-positive RBCs, the failure of immunosuppression appears to be related to the rate of clearance; this has been cited as evidence that clearance is the mechanism of suppression.[4] However, when RhIG is given before very large doses of Rh-positive RBCs at an Ig:RBC ratio known to be immunosuppressive, suppression has been observed despite the survival of the transfused RBCs for as long as 1 month.[32] Similarly, in a rabbit model using a blood group system analogous to Rh, immunosuppression was achieved with a level of passive antibody administration that resulted in only 30% reduction in the half-life of the stimulating RBCs.[33]

The antigen deviation hypothesis also predicts that immunosuppression should not be antigen specific. That is, if RhIG works by removing Rh-positive fetal RBCs before immunization can occur, maternal immunization by blood group antigens on fetal RBCs other than Rh also should be prevented. This was not the case in the rabbit model[33] or in a model using multiple haptenic antigens.[34] In contrast, the one experiment in humans demonstrated nonspecificity[35]; that is, volunteers negative for Rh and Kell blood groups were given RBCs positive for both antigens along with anti-Kell. The response to both antigens was suppressed.

The second hypothesis, antigen blocking, suggests that the Rh antigen is rendered nonimmunogenic by the binding of passively administered anti-Rh. However, at a suppressive dose of RhIG, only a fraction of Rh antigen sites are bound by antibody. In addition, suppression by F(ab) fragments can be achieved only at very high doses.[36]

The central inhibition hypothesis suggests that antibody-mediated immunosuppression is a manifestation of the basic control mechanisms of antibody synthesis and that the mechanisms affect the immunologically active cells themselves, rather than preventing the antigen's access to those cells.[34] Because these control mechanisms are not well understood, it is difficult to develop hypotheses that can be tested from this statement. However, the fact that augmentation of the immune response can be achieved with low doses of RhIG or with IgM anti-Rh is taken as evidence for this mechanism. Augmentation occurs at ratios of 1–2 μg of RhIG to 1 mL of Rh-positive RBCs, or one tenth of the dose that is suppressive.[4] In such circumstances, it is of interest that antibody administered passively at nonsuppressive doses may enhance the affinity of the antibody that is produced actively, thus mimicking the usual course of the primary immune response toward the development of a higher-affinity antibody with time and demonstrating central immune modulation by passive antibody.[34] Specificity of suppression, as discussed above, is taken as evidence for central inhibition. This is an area of ongoing controversy.

OTHER IMMUNE-MEDIATED NEONATAL CYTOPENIAS

A fetus may immunize its mother to antigens on other formed elements of blood besides RBCs, specifically, platelets and granulocytes. *Neonatal alloimmune thrombocytopenia* (NAT) results from maternal antiplatelet antibody that is most commonly directed against the $P1^{A1}$ antigen, but involvement of most platelet antigen systems has been described. One in 2000 pregnancies may be affected, including first pregnancies. The rate of recurrence in subsequent infants is more than 75% and can be predicted by studying the father's zygosity. Neonatal patients typically present in the first 24 h of life with severe thrombocytopenia and signs of bleeding ranging from petechiae to overt hemorrhage. Intracranial hemorrhage is the most feared complication, affecting up to 30% of cases[37], and often occurs antenatally or during delivery. Maternal autoimmune thrombocytopenia should be ruled out by a blood count, as should infection in the thrombocytopenic newborn. Diagnostic platelet antibody studies generally are available only at specialized centers including larger blood centers, and the availability of antigen typing sera is considerably more restricted. Untreated, thrombocytopenia may last for 2–3 weeks, but it can last longer.[38] Mortality is approximately 10%.

As recurrence of NAT can be expected after one infant has been affected, cesarean section delivery of subsequent infants is indicated. Specific therapy until recently has been available only after delivery, in the form of compatible platelet transfusion. Because most of the responsible antibodies are directed against high-frequency antigens, maternal platelets are the most accessible and can be procured by whole blood donation or apheresis techniques. Such platelets must be pelleted and resuspended in compatible plasma to remove maternal antibody. Since up to 25% of intracranial hemorrhages due to NAT occur antenatally and can occur as early as 20 weeks[39], therapy prior to delivery is needed. IUT of washed maternal platelets was accomplished by Daffos[40] to prepare the neonatal patient for delivery, but that procedure cannot be extended realistically to prevent early hemorrhage. Initial results show that IVIG administered to the mother can correct fetal thrombocytopenia. Bussel and coworkers[87] treated seven fetuses with weekly doses of 1 g per kg of IVIG. All of the infants were delivered with platelet counts above 30,000 per uL, and none experienced hemorrhage. In six of the seven, serial umbilical blood sampling showed initial thrombocytopenia that improved with treatment. Since therapy is costly, a demonstration that the fetus is affected would be economical.

Alloimmune neonatal neutropenia is not as well characterized as NAT, in part because granulocyte serology is even less generally available than platelet antibody testing. Affected infants are born with neutropenia and present with infection.[41] Although infections are often mild, a 5% mortality is reported. Treatment is with antibiotics.

Maternal autoantibodies against formed elements of fetal blood can cross the placenta to cause fetal cytopenias, as in maternal autoimmune thrombocytopenia and occasionally in warm autoimmune hemolytic anemia. These conditions are discussed in Chapters 164 and 165.

REFERENCES

1. Zimmerman DR. *Rh: The Intimate History of a Disease and its Conquest.* New York: Macmillan, 1973.
2. Sebring ES. Fetomaternal hemorrhage—incidence and methods of detection and quantitation. In: Garratty G, ed. *Hemoloytic Disease of the Newborn.* Arlington, VA: American Association of Blood Banks; 1984:87.
3. Medearis AL, et al. Detection of fetal erythrocytes in maternal blood post partum with the fluorescence-activated cell sorter. *Am J Obstet Gynecol.* 1984;148:290.
4. Mollison PL. Some aspects of Rh hemolytic disease and its prevention. In: Garratty, G, ed. *Hemolytic Disease of the Newborn.* Arlington, VA: American Association of Blood Banks; 1984:1.
5. Pai MKR, Bedritis I, Zipursky A. Massive transplacental hemorrhage: clinical manifestations in the newborn. *Can Med Assoc J.* 1975;112:585.
6. Bowman JM. Controversies in Rh prophylaxis. In: Garratty G, ed. *Hemolytic Disease of the Newborn.* Arlington, VA: American Association of Blood Banks; 1984:67.
7. Walker RH. Relevancy in the selection of serologic tests for the obstetric patient. In Garratty G, ed. *Hemoloytic Disease of the Newborn.* Arlington, VA: American Association of Blood Banks; 1984:173.
8. Clarke CA, Whitfield ABW, Mollison PL. Deaths from Rh haemoloytic disease in England and Wales in 1984 and 1985. *Br Med J.* 1987;294:1001.
9. Mollison PL, Engelfriet CP, Contreras M. *Blood Transfusion in Clinical Medicine.* 8th ed. Oxford: Blackwell Scientific Publications; 1987.
10. Brouwers HAA, et al. Maternal antibodies against fetal blood group antigens A or B: lytic activity of IgG subclasses in monocyte-driven cytotoxicity and correlation with ABO haemolytic disease of the newborn. *Br J Haematol.* 1988;70:465.
11. Walker W. The changing pattern of haemolytic disease of the newborn (1948–1957). *Vox Sang.* 1958;3:225.
12. Zupanska B, et al. Serological and immunological characteristics of maternal anti-Rh(D) antibodies in predicting the severity of haemolytic disease of the newborn. *Vox Sang.* 1989;56:247.
13. Grant CJ, Hamblin TJ, Smith DS, Wellstead L. Plasmapheresis in Rh hemolytic disease: the danger of amniocentesis. *Int J Artif Organs.* 1983;5:83.
14. Phibbs RH, et al. Cardiorespiratory status of erythroblastotic newborn infants: II. Blood volume, hematocrit, and serum albumin concentration in relation to hydrops fetalis. *Pediatrics.* 1974;53:13.
15. Nicolaides KH, et al. Fetal haematology in rhesus isoimmunization. *Br Med J.* 1985;290:661.
16. Nicolaides KH, Warenski JC, Rodeck CH. The relationship of fetal plasma protein concentration and hemoglobin level to the development of hydrops in rhesus isoimmunization. *Am J Obstet Gynecol.* 1985;152:341.
17. Harman CR, et al. Profound fetal thrombocytopenia in rhesus disease: serious hazard at intravascular transfusion. *Lancet.* 1988;2:741.
18. Koenig JM, Christensen RD. Neutropenia and thrombocytopenia in infants with Rh hemolytic disease. *J Pediatr.* 1989;114:625.
19. Chessels JM, Wigglesworth JS. Haemostatic failure in babies with rhesus isoimmunization. *Arch Dis Child.* 1971;46:38.
20. Ellis MI, Hey EN, Walker W. Neonatal death in babies with rhesus isoimmunization. *Q J Med.* 1979;190:211.
21. Phibbs RH, et al. Cardiorespiratory status of erythroblastotic infants: II. Relationship of gestational age, severity of hemolytic disease, and birth asphyxia to idiopathic respiratory distress syndrome and survival. *Pediatrics.* 1972;49:5.
22. Phibbs RH, et al. Cardiorespiratory status of erythroblastotic newborn infants: III. Intravascular pressures during the first hours of life. *Pediatrics.* 1976;58:484.
23. Dunn PM. Obstructive jaundice and haemolytic disease of the newborn. *Arch Dis Child.* 1963;38:54.
24. Walker W, Murray S. Haemolytic disease of the newborn as a family problem. *Br Med J.* 1956;1:187.
25. Dufour DR, Monoghan WP. ABO hemolytic disease of the newborn: a retrospective analysis of 254 cases. *Am J Clin Path.* 1980;73:369.
26. Kirkman HN. Further evidence for a racial difference in frequency of ABO hemolytic disease. *J Pediatr.* 1977;90:717.
27. Pollack W, Gorman JG, Freda VJ. Rh immune suppression: past, present, and future. In: Frigoletto FD, Jewett JF, Konugres AA, eds. *Rh Hemolytic Disease: New Strategy for Eradication.* Boston: G.K. Hall Medical Publishers; 1982:9.
28. Samson D, Mollison PL. Effect on primary Rh immunization of delayed administration of anti-Rh. *Immunology.* 1975;28:349.
29. Davey MG, Zipursky A. McMaster conference on prevention of Rh immunization. *Vox Sang.* 1979;36:50.
30. Bowman JM, Pollock JM. Failures of intravenous Rh immune globulin prophylaxis: an analysis of the reasons for such failures. *Transfus Med Rev.* 1987;1:101.
31. Tovey LAD, Townley A, Stevenson BJ, Taverner J. The Yorkshire antenatal anti-D immunoglobulin trial in primigravidae. *Lancet.* 1983;2:244.
32. Pollack W, et al. Studies on Rh prophylaxis II; Rh immune prophylaxis after transfusion with Rh-positive blood. *Transfusion.* 1971;11:340.
33. Pollack W, et al. Antibody-mediated immune suppression to the Rh factor: Animal models suggesting mechanism of action. *Transfusion.* 1968;8:134.
34. Siskind GW. The role of circulating antibody in the control of antibody synthesis: mechanism for the suppressive effect of passive antibody on active antibody synthesis. *Transfusion.* 1968;8:127.
35. Woodrow JC, et al. Mechanism of Rh prophylaxis: an experimental study on specificity of immunosuppression. *Br Med J.* 1975;2:57.
36. Pollack W. Mechanisms of Rh immune suppression by Rh immune globulin. In Garratty G, ed. *Hemolytic Disease of the Newborn.* Arlington, VA: American Association of Blood Banks; 1984:53.
37. Deaver JE, Leppert PC, Zaroulis CG. Neonatal alloimmune thrombocytopenic purpura. *Am J Perinatol.* 1986;3:127.
38. Miller D, Etzel R, McFarland JG, et al. Prolonged neonatal alloimmune thrombocytopenic purpura associated with anti-Bak[a]. *Am J Perinatol.* 1987;4:55.
39. Herman JH, Jumbelic MI, Ancona RJ, Kickler TS. In utero cerebral hemorrhage in alloimmune thrombocytopenia. *Am J Pediatr Hematol Oncol.* 1986;8:312.
40. Daffos F. Technical aspects of prenatal samplings and fetal transfusion. *Curr Stud Hematol Blood Transfus.* 1988;55:127.
41. McCullough J, Clay M, Press C, Kline W. *Granulocyte Serology: a Clinical and Laboratory Guide.* Chicago: American Society of Clinical Pathologists, 1988.
42. Centers for Disease Control. *Rh Hemolytic Disease Surveillance-Annual Report.* June 1975.
43. Weinstein L. Irregular antibodies causing hemolytic disease in the newborn. *Obstet Gynecol Surv.* 1976; 31:581.

Chapter One Hundred and Seventy-One

Management of Blood Group Isoimmunization

Michael L. Socol

171

The introduction and proper use of Rh immunoglobulin is a prototype example of the effectiveness of preventive medicine. As a result, the incidence of maternal rhesus sensitization has decreased dramatically. It therefore is not surprising that many obstetricians now find themselves unfamiliar with the principles of managing blood group isoimmunization.

PREVENTION OF SENSITIZATION

Transplacental hemorrhage into the maternal circulation of as little as 0.1 mL of fetal red blood cells may stimulate antibody formation.[1] Most fetal-maternal bleeding occurs peripartum, but the Rh antigen is present on the fetal red blood cell by 6 completed weeks of pregnancy.[2] The importance of this observation is that maternal sensitization can occur throughout pregnancy.

Prior to the institution of Rh prophylaxis, antibody production was observed within 6 months of delivery in approximately 8% of Rh-negative women following Rh-positive, ABO-compatible pregnancies. Another 8% were identified early in the course of the next pregnancy. This latter group was thought to reflect a secondary immune response, and this phenomenon was termed *sensibilization.* ABO incompatibility between mother and fetus confers partial protection against Rh immunization, the risk dropping to 1.5–2%.[3]

The institution of postpartum prophylaxis with 300 μg of Rh immunoglobulin for all Rh-negative women who delivered a D- or D^u-positive fetus decreased the incidence of isoimmunization to 1.5–2%.[4] Because many of these antibodies were discovered in the second or third trimester, antepartum prophylactic trials were undertaken. These trials reduced the incidence of maternal sensitization to 0.2%[5] and have led to the current recommendations.[6]

All Rh-negative patients, unless the father of the baby also is known to be Rh negative, should have an indirect Coombs' test performed at the initial prenatal visit to detect circulating anti-D antibodies. If this is negative then and when repeated in the late second trimester, 300 μg of Rh immunoglobulin should be administered intramuscularly at 28 weeks' gestation. The likelihood of maternal sensitization occurring during the remainder of pregnancy is negligible, therefore repeat antibody testing prior to delivery is unnecessary. Sufficient data do not exist to recommend another dose of Rh immunoglobulin should the pregnancy continue past 40 weeks. After the birth of a D- or D^u-positive infant, a second dose of Rh immunoglobulin should be administered, preferably within 72 hours of delivery. It is important to remember that the half-life of Rh immunoglobulin is 25 days. Consequently, 15% to 20% of women will have low titers, that is, 1:4, of passive antibody in their serum at delivery. Occasionally, a newborn may have a weakly positive direct Coombs' test. These patients are still candidates for postpartum Rh immunoglobulin. On the other hand, once a patient is known to be isoimmunized, Rh immunoglobulin is ineffective therapy.[7]

Clinical conditions potentially associated with larger fetal to maternal bleeding include *abruptio placentae, placenta previa,* manual removal of the placenta, and cesarean section. Fortunately, only 0.2% of patients experience a transplacental hemorrhage greater than 30 mL of fetal blood (15 mL of fetal red cells), the amount which is effectively neutralized by the standard 300 μg dose of Rh immunoglobulin.[8] The slide rosette test can screen for these large bleeds, which then can be quantitated with the Kleihauer–Betke acid elution test.[9]

Other important sources of maternal sensitization are abortion, ectopic pregnancy, chorionic villus sampling, and amniocentesis. For CVS or a first trimester pregnancy loss, whether it is an ectopic pregnancy, spontaneous, or induced abortion, the minidose of 50 μg of Rh immunoglobulin is sufficient prophylaxis. Failure to treat appropriately has been associated with the development of antibodies in approximately 4% of patients. Following second trimester losses the standard 300 μg dose of Rh immunoglobulin is required. This dose also is recommended for either second or third trimester amniocentesis. Even after genetic amniocentesis, as many as 3% of patients may become sensitized.[10] Patients who receive Rh immunoglobulin after CVS or second trimester amniocentesis also should be treated prophylactically at 28 weeks' gestation. For those patients in whom delivery is planned within 48 hours of third trimester amniocentesis, Rh immunoglobulin can be withheld until the newborn is confirmed to be Rh positive.

PATHOGENESIS OF FETAL DISEASE

The pathogenesis of fetal hydrops has been a matter of debate. The prevailing school of thought contends that extramedullary hematopoiesis secondary to severe hemolysis leads to disordered hepatic parenchyma and an increase in portal pressure.[2] Portal hypertension is accompanied by hypoproteinemia related to liver dysfunction and a decrease in colloid osmotic pressure. As hypoproteinemia worsens, generalized edema, or fetal hydrops, ensues (Figure 171–1). Support for this hypothesis includes pathologic findings at autopsy, the documentation of fetal hypoproteinemia by fetoscopic blood sampling[11], and the apparent absence of increased intravascular volume.[12]

With the advent of percutaneous umbilical blood sampling, it has become apparent that profound anemia is a prerequisite for the development of hydrops fetalis. Fetal hemoglobin was noted to be 7–10 g/dL below the normal mean for gestation in 48 fetuses with ultrasound features of hydrops.[13] It also has been observed that the fetal reticulocyte count increases linearly with anemia in contrast to the erythroblast count, which increases exponentially.[14] Significant erythroblastosis was observed only when the hemoglobin deficit exceeded 7 g/dL. Reticulocytes are the product of both medullary and extramedullary erythropoiesis, whereas erythroblasts are released by extramedullary sites only.[15] Consequently, it appears that medullary hematopoiesis is stimulated by mild anemia and that recruitment of extramedullary sites occurs when anemia is severe.

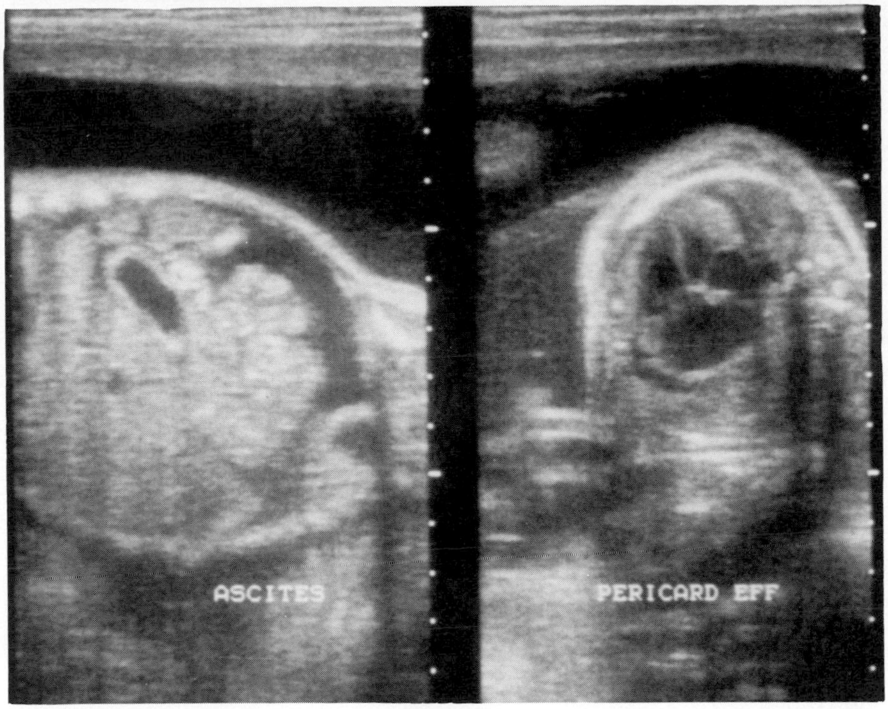

Figure 171–1. Abdominal ascites (left) and pericardial effusion (right) are present at 24 weeks' and 6 days of gestation. (*From Socol ML et al*[38] *with permission.*)

Fetal hypoproteinemia thereby would result from decreased protein production by the liver due to extensive infiltration by erythropoietic tissue and is probably further contributed to by hypoxia-induced endothelial leakage secondary to the drop in pH that accompanies a hemoglobin deficit greater than 8 g/dL.[16]

A contrary opinion is that the primary pathologic process in fetal hydrops is fetal heart failure. Improved perinatal outcome reported with adjunctive therapy using digoxin or lasix is consistent with this premise.[17] Additionally, arginine vasopressin is reduced in the anemic fetus before transfusion[18] and fetuses with immune hydrops have very high atrial natriuretic factor levels.[19] These observations suggest that the severely anemic fetus is in a state of relative hypervolemia. Further support is generated by the intriguing observation in two hydropic fetuses of the rapid decline of elevated umbilical venous pressure to normal levels during or immediately after intravascular transfusion.[20] The initial elevation of umbilical venous pressure very likely was contributed to by portal hypertension and liver dysfunction, but the rapid return to normal suggests a component of myocardial dysfunction and high output cardiac failure.

MANAGEMENT OF A SENSITIZED PREGNANCY

The severity of Rh hemolytic disease tends to remain the same or become progressively worse in subsequent pregnancies.[21] Occasionally, a patient with previously mildly affected pregnancies may present with early onset fetal hydrops. To the contrary, although unusual, disease may sometimes be less severe than in a prior pregnancy. This is important to keep in mind when critically evaluating trials of immunosuppression to ameliorate severe isoimmunization. For the most part, experience has not been encouraging.[7]

Antibody Titers

Maternal serum antibody titers can be measured by a variety of techniques.[2] Agglutination of Rh-positive red blood cells in saline measures only maternal IgM antibody; this is too large a molecule to cross the placenta. Albumin is a more viscous media; therefore the smaller IgG molecules are capable of agglutinating Rh-positive cells, but the contribution by IgM is not eliminated. The most sensitive and accurate barometer for clinical practice is the indirect Coombs' test.

The usefulness of maternal serum antibody titers is dictated by past reproductive history. If a patient has had a prior severely affected pregnancy (neonatal exchange transfusion, early delivery, or intrauterine transfusion), antibody titers are not helpful because amniocentesis still will be required. On the other hand, for a patient never experiencing a prior pregnancy complicated by Rh-related neonatal morbidity other than phototherapy, antibody titers are the initial step of management. An antibody titer should be determined at the first prenatal visit, 20 weeks' gestation, and approximately every four weeks thereafter. Once the antibody titer, whether directed to D or another paternal antigen capable of causing severe erythroblastosis, is equal to or greater than 1:16 in albumin or 1:32 by indirect antiglobulin (indirect Coombs') amniocentesis becomes necessary.[22]

Amniocentesis/Percutaneous Umbilical Blood Sampling

Amniotic fluid bilirubin most likely is derived from fetal tracheal and pulmonary secretions. It can be quantitated by spectrophotometrically measuring absorbance at the 450-nm wave length in a specimen of amniotic fluid that has been shielded from light. The deviation from linearity (ΔOD_{450}) is determined by measuring the difference between this absorbance and a straight line drawn from points 365 nm to 550 nm on the spectrophotometric curve. Heme pigment also will generate a peak at the 405-nm wavelength; in the absence of blood contamination this may be indicative of severe hemolysis.[2]

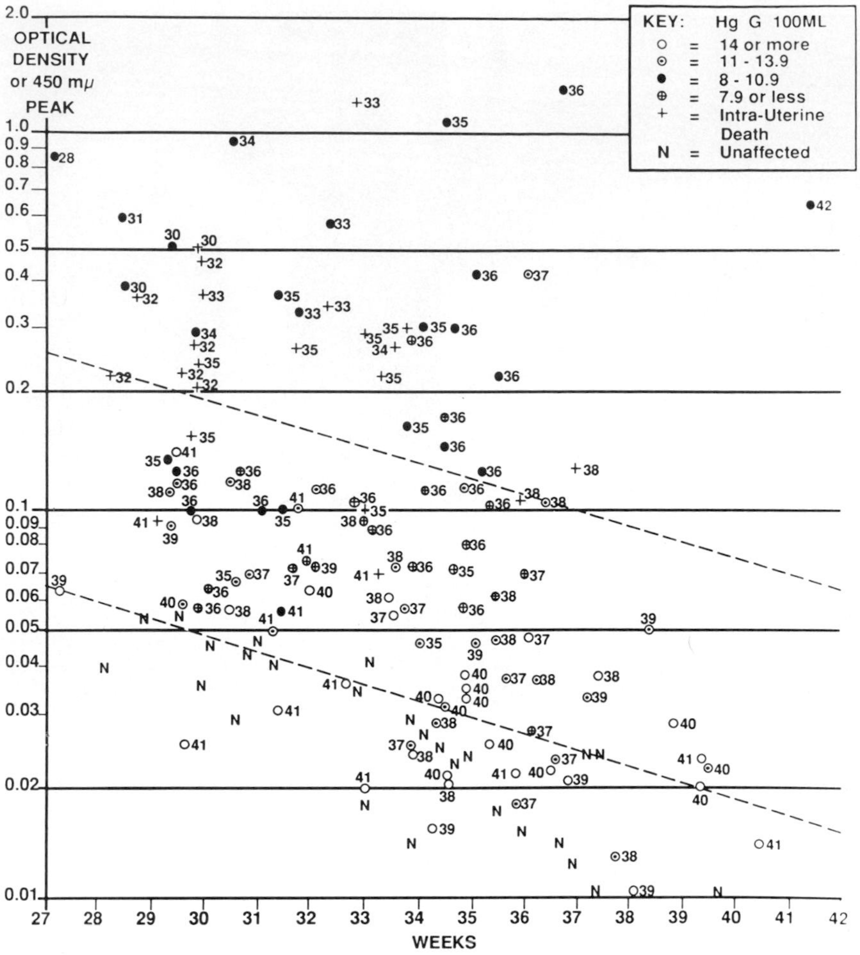

Figure 171–2. Spectrophotometric measurements of the ΔOD_{450} peaks plotted versus gestational age. The symbols represent the ultimate condition or fate of the fetuses, and the attendant numbers represent the week in which delivery or intrauterine death occurred. *(From Liley AW[23] with permission.)*

Fetal status is determined by plotting the ΔOD_{450} measurement on a Liley graph[23] (Figure 171–2). Readings in zone III (upper zone) suggest severe hemolytic disease with a high probability of fetal death within seven to ten days. Readings in zone I (lowest zone) are reassuring, although neonatal exchange transfusion occasionally may be necessary. Traditional teaching has been that amniocentesis should be repeated every one to two weeks if the ΔOD_{450} measurements are in zone II (middle zone) and every three weeks if they have dropped into zone I. Declining values are encouraging although they do not preclude mild hemolytic disease. Stable or rising ΔOD_{450} measurements should be interpreted as worrisome. In general, patients in zone I or low zone II can be carried to term, at which point they should have labor induced. Patients in midzone II most often can be carried to 36 to 38 weeks' gestation, at which time delivery should be accomplished by induction of labor if possible. Those patients in upper zone II or zone III, depending on gestational age, should be delivered or receive intrauterine fetal transfusion. Often these patients are delivered by cesarean section because of an unfavorable cervix, but a trial of labor is not contraindicated.

Percutaneous umbilical blood sampling, or cordocentesis, has improved the obstetric care for the isoimmunized patient because of the ability to precisely evaluate fetal status (Figure 171–3). This is particularly true in the middle trimester when amniotic fluid from unaffected fetuses also will contain bilirubin, peak values being present between 20 and 24 weeks' gestation. Historically, obstetricians have extrapolated backwards the Liley curve that was generated from pregnancies of at least 28 weeks' gestation, but this may be inappropriate.[24] In the second or third trimester, knowledge of the specific fetal hematocrit enables a more rational approach to the need, volume, and timing of fetal transfusions. In some instances, the fetus may even be shown to not have the blood group antigen in question and therefore require no further evaluation. Perhaps, most important, the use of amniocentesis in conjunction with percutaneous umbilical blood sampling allows a more aggressive approach at an earlier gestational age. Most often, the initial amniocentesis now will be performed around 20 weeks' gestation or even earlier.

Ancillary Testing

Ultrasonography is an integral component of modern obstetric management. In the severely isoimmunized patient, ultrasonographic signs of early hydrops may facilitate timely intervention. More problematic and controversial is the ability of ultrasound to detect a deteriorating fetus prior to the onset of hydrops. Reported early signs of worsening fetal anemia include an increase in the size of the fetal liver[25,26], increase in placental thickness[27], pericardial effusion[28], polyhydramnios[29], visualization of both sides of the fetal bowel[30], and abnormalities of pulsed Doppler flow-velocity waveforms.[31,32] However, it still remains highly questionable whether ultrasonographic markers can

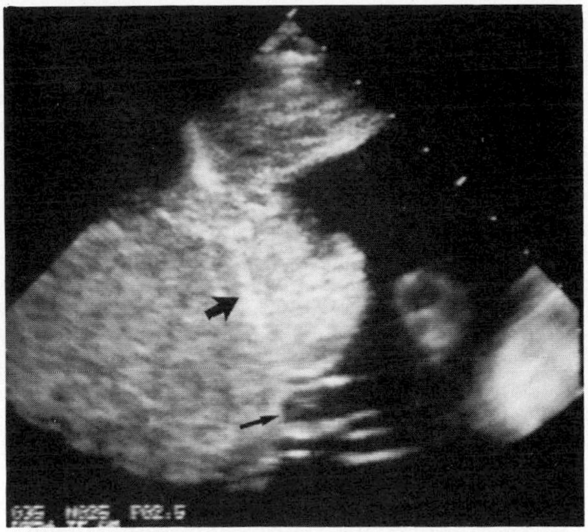

Figure 171–3. The needle (*large arrow*) can be seen traversing the anterior placenta and entering the umbilical cord at its placental insertion (*small arrow*). (*From Socol ML et al*[38] *with permission.*)

reliably distinguish mild from severe hemolytic disease in the absence of fetal hydrops.[33]

Electronic fetal heart rate monitoring enables dynamic evaluation of fetal well-being and central nervous system reactivity. Some severely anemic fetuses will exhibit a sinusoidal heart rate pattern that has been attributed to the absence of autonomic nervous system control over the heart[34], high output cardiac failure[35], or tissue hypoxia of the fetal heart and central nervous system.[36] Nonreactive, suboptimal, or pathologic fetal heart rate patterns also have been reported more often in sensitized fetuses that were hypoxic and anemic than in those that were normoxemic and nonanemic.[37] Pathologic features were more closely related to fetal oxygenation than to hemoglobin concentration. Characteristics of the fetal heart rate pattern, however, did not accurately predict the degree of anemia or oxygenation.[16]

Intrauterine Fetal Transfusion

Prior to the capability of gaining direct access to the fetal circulation, intraperitoneal fetal transfusion was indicated if serial spectrophotometric measurements rose into upper zone II before 30 weeks' gestation or into zone III between 30 and 34 weeks of pregnancy. The infused blood was absorbed into the fetal circulation through the subdiaphragmatic lymphatics. In the nonhydropic fetus, the rate of absorption was estimated to be 10–15% per 24 hours, probably somewhat slower if hydrops was already evident. The volume of transfusion was calculated by the formula:

$$\text{Volume} = (\text{weeks' gestation} - 20) \times 10 \text{ mL}$$

A second transfusion was administered in approximately 10 days with any subsequent transfusions performed at 4-week intervals. Delivery was accomplished approximately 4 weeks after the last transfusion, which was rarely attempted after 33 weeks' gestation.[2]

Intravascular fetal transfusion[38] generally has replaced the intraperitoneal technique, although some investigators advocate a combined intravascular and intraperitoneal approach under select circumstances.[39] The technique we have adapted for intravascular transfusion is similar to that of fetal blood sampling with a few modifications (Figure 171–4). The placental insertion of the umbilical cord is identified, often by both linear-array and sector real-time ultrasonography, inasmuch as use of both transducers sometimes facilitates appreciation of spatial relationships. The abdomen then is aseptically prepared before local infiltration with lidocaine. A complete surgical scrub is not performed, although the operators wear a cap, mask, and gloves. A 22-gauge, 5-inch disposable spinal needle then is guided

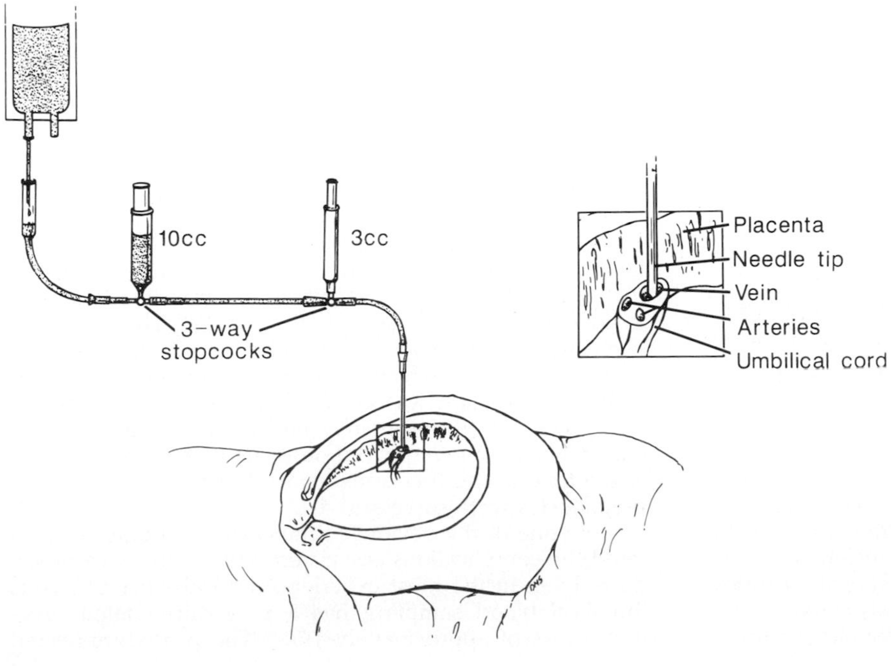

Figure 171–4. Graphic depiction of the setup for an intrauterine intravascular transfusion. The volume of the distal connector tubing is 0.3 mL.

toward the umbilical cord (preferably the umbilical vein at the placental insertion site) with the 5-mHz sector transducer. Upon placement of the needle tip into an umbilical vessel, fetal blood is aspirated for immediate hematocrit determination and complete blood count (the MCV of fetal red blood cells should be greater than 100 μm^3), blood type and Rh factor, and Kleihauer–Betke test as deemed necessary. Prior to beginning the transfusion, pancuronium bromide, a nondepolarizing neuromuscular blocking agent, is administered as an intravascular bolus at the dose of 0.05–0.10 mg/kg of ultrasonographically estimated fetal weight.[40] Throughout the transfusion, the fetal heart rate is visualized intermittently, as is turbulence in the umbilical cord to assure continued proper needle placement. By incorporating connector tubing and two 3-way stopcocks, both fetal transfusion and aspiration of fetal blood samples to assess hematocrit can be performed without disconnecting the system. We do not utilize prophylactic antibiotics or tocolytic drugs, although several authors have recommended these agents particularly for prolonged procedures.

The fetal hematocrit at which to initiate transfusion is somewhat arbitrary, but the value of 25% seems most reasonable.[41] Transfusions are performed using type O, Rh-negative, CMV-negative, washed, irradiated packed cells cross-matched against maternal blood. With knowledge of the fetal blood type, it occasionally may be possible to use maternal blood or a targeted donor whose blood is compatible with both mother and fetus. The simplest method to estimate transfusion volume is by the following formula:[42]

$$V_2 = \frac{(\text{Hctf} - \text{Hcti})}{\text{Hctd}} \times \text{EFW} \times V_1$$

where V_2 is the transfusion volume, Hctf is the desired final hematocrit (approximately 45%), Hcti is the initial or pretransfusion fetal hematocrit, Hctd is the hematocrit of donor blood (usually about 80%), EFW is the ultrasonographically estimated fetal weight in kilograms for nonhydropic fetuses or mean birth weight for gestational age for hydropic fetuses, and V_2 is the fetoplacental blood volume (150 mL/kg).[43] It is important to note that the assumption of a fetoplacental blood volume of 150 mL/kg throughout gestation may be incorrect as there is now evidence to suggest that 110 mL/kg[39,44,45] may be a more accurate figure and that fetoplacental blood volume/kg decreases with advancing gestational age.[45,46] Nonetheless, clinically the formula appears to be reliable, with transfusion volumes usually ranging between 30 and 100 mL. The donor blood is infused at 3–5 mL/min and fetal blood is aspirated at the conclusion of the transfusion to determine adequacy of therapy.

Repeat transfusions are planned when the fetal hematocrit is predicted to be between 20 and 25%. This may be approximated by assuming a 1% decline per day or may be calculated based on the following equations:[47]

$$\text{Hct pred} = \text{Hctf} - \text{i} \times (\text{EFW}_1/\text{EFW}_2) \times (120 - \text{days})/120$$

or

$$\text{Hct pred} = \text{Hctf} \times (\text{EFW}_1/\text{EFW}_2) \times (120 - \text{days})/120$$

where Hct pred is the predicted hematocrit at the subsequent transfusion or birth, Hctf–i is the final hematocrit minus the initial hematocrit at the index transfusion, Hctf is the final hematocrit at the index transfusion, EFW_1 is the ultrasonographically estimated fetal weight at the index transfusion, EFW_2 is the ultrasonographically estimated fetal weight at the subsequent transfusion or birth, days is the number of days between the index and subsequent transfusion or birth, and it is assumed that the life span of donor red cells in the fetal circulation is 120 days. (This may be somewhat overestimated as 50% of transfused red blood cells have been calculated to be present 43 days after intravascular transfusion compared to 33 days following an intraperitoneal procedure.[39]) The first equation applies to the interval between first and second transfusion, which is more problematic because of the unpredictable hemolysis of the remaining fetal red blood cells. In those fetuses with more severe hemolytic anemia, few fetal red blood cells will survive the transfusion interval. The second equation applies to the interval between subsequent transfusions or birth when fetal blood has essentially all been replaced by adult donor red blood cells. The interval between first and second transfusions is usually 7–14 days, whereas between subsequent transfusions or birth the interval is 21–28 days.

The theoretical risk of cardiovascular compromise from fluid overload with simple transfusions as opposed to exchange transfusions has been raised.[48] However, the fetal circulation is in continuity with the placental vasculature, which is a low resistance, large volume vascular bed. Further, experimental evidence from sheep suggests that packed cell transfusions increase fetal blood volume by only 50% of the transfused volume because of the loss of plasma from the circulation.[44] Whereas exchange transfusion removes the endogenous fetal red blood cells and reduces hemolysis, by the time of the second transfusion relatively few fetal red blood cells usually remain.[49] Consequently, any significant advantage of exchange transfusion would seem to be limited to the initial transfusion. This has to be weighed against the increase in time required to perform the procedure with the propensity for an increase in complications.

Perinatal Outcome

With the advent of ultrasonography to guide placement of the intraperitoneal catheter, the prognosis for the severely isoimmunized fetus improved dramatically. Survival rates approaching 75% were reported following intraperitoneal transfusions for nonhydropic fetuses during the 1970s[17], and two centers reported 100% survival in the 1980s.[17,50] However, for hydropic fetuses or those requiring early therapy, the outcome was considerably more dismal. As an example, in one report only 2 of 11 hydropic fetuses first transfused prior to 26 weeks' gestation survived.[51]

Direct intravascular transfusion eliminates the erratic and incomplete absorption of red blood cells inherent with the intraperitoneal approach. In addition, the intravascular technique enables more precise evaluation of the need and adequacy of therapy by measurements of the initial and final fetal hematocrit. Consequently, it is not surprising that perinatal survival for severely isoimmunized fetuses is now reported in excess of 80%.[49,52,53,54] The improved survival is especially noteworthy when considering the early gestational ages at which therapy is being attempted. Our earliest transfusion was at 17 weeks' gestation, although that pregnancy unfortunately ended in fetal death. Also encouraging is the improved outcome for hydropic fetuses at the time of the first transfusion. In one series, 16 of 20 pregnancies were successful.[55]

In spite of the obvious enthusiasm, one must keep in mind the complications associated with an invasive procedure. Even in the most experienced hands, percutaneous umbilical blood sampling has a procedure-related pregnancy loss of approximately 1%.[56] The procedure-related

TABLE 171–1. ISOIMMUNIZATION DUE TO IRREGULAR ANTIBODIES

Blood Group System	Antigen
Rh	c*, C*, e*, E*
Kell	K*, k, Ko, Kp^a, Kp^b Js^a, Js^b
Duffy	Fy^{a*}, Fy^b, Fy^3
Kidd	Jk^{a*}, Jk^{b*}, Jk^3
MNSs	M*, N, S*, s*, U*, Mi^{a*}, Mt^{a*}, Vw, Mur, Hil, Hut
Lutheran	Lu^a, Lu^b
Diego	Di^{a*}, Di^{b*}
Xg	Xg^a
P	PP$_1$p^k (Tj^a)*
Public antigens	Yt^{a*}, Yt^b, Lan, En^{a*}, Ge, Jr^a, Co^{a*}, Co^{a-b-}
Private antigens	Batty, Becker, Berrens, Biles*, Evans, Gonzazles, Good*, Heibel*, Hunt, Jobbins, Radin*, Rm, Ven, Wright^{a*}, Wright^{b*}, Zd*

* Antigens most likely to be associated with moderate or severe hemolytic disease; Lewis (Le^a, Le^b) and I antigens are not causes of hemolytic disease of the newborn.

mortality for intravascular transfusion has been reported between 4% to 9%.[49,52,53,55] Additional significant morbidity has included nonremediable prolonged fetal heart rate decelerations that required emergent cesarean section[57] and increases in maternal antibody titer, presumably secondary to fetal-maternal hemorrhage.[58] When weighing the procedure-related risks against those for the neonate in the nursery, serious thought should be given to the performance of an intravascular transfusion after 34 completed weeks of pregnancy.

Atypical Blood Group Isoimmunization

Antibodies to atypical blood group antigens are present in 0.5–2% of all pregnancies. If these antibodies are of the IgG class, particularly IgG_1 and IgG_3, they may cross the placenta and have the same severe implications for the fetus as in Rh isoimmunization.[59] Consequently, all pregnant patients should have an indirect Coombs' test performed at the initial prenatal visit in addition to ABO and Rh typing. In contrast to Rh sensitization, most atypical blood group isoimmunization follows maternal transfusion because crossmatching is not performed routinely for the minor antigens. Atypical blood group antigens implicated in fetal disease are listed in Table 171–1.[60]

Management of pregnancies complicated by atypical blood group isoimmunization generally is accepted to be similar to Rh disease. There is some controversy, however, as severe fetal disease has been reported with a maternal anti-Kell titer of 1:4[61] and fetal death has occurred in a Kell sensitized pregnancy without excessive elevation of the amniotic fluid ΔOD_{450}.[62] Of particular importance in Kell sensitization is determination of the father's blood type because 90% of individuals are Kell negative.

REFERENCES

1. Zipursky A, Israels LG. The pathogenesis and prevention of Rh immunization. *Can Med Assoc J*. 1967;97:1245.
2. Bowman JM. Maternal blood group isoimmunization. In: Creasy RK, Resnik R, eds. *Maternal-Fetal Medicine: Principles and Practice*. Philadelphia. WB Saunders; 1984:561.
3. Woodrow JC. Rh immunization and its prevention. *Series Hematologia*. Copenhagen: Munksgaard; 1970;3:34.
4. Bowman JM, Chown B, Lewis M, Pollock JM. Rh isoimmunization during pregnancy: antenatal prophylaxis. *Can Med Assoc J*. 1978;118:623.
5. Bowman JM, Pollock JM. Antenatal prophylaxis of Rh isoimmunization: 28 weeks' gestation service program. *Can Med Assoc J*. 1978;118:627.
6. The American College of Obstetricians and Gynecologists. Prevention of Rho (D) isoimmunization. *ACOG Technical Bulletin #147*, October 1990, Washington, DC.
7. Bowman JM. Suppression of Rh isoimmunization. *Obstet Gynecol*. 1978;52:385.
8. Pollack W, Ascari WQ, Kochesky RJ, et al. Studies on Rh prophylaxis. 1. Relationship between doses of anti-Rh and size of antigenic stimulus. *Transfusion*. 1971;11:333.
9. Stedman CM, Baudin JC, White CW, Cooper ES. Use of the erythrocyte rosette test to screen for excessive fetomaternal hemorrhage in Rh-negative women. *Am J Obstet Gynecol*. 1986;154:1363.
10. Murray JC, Karl LE, Williamson RA, et al. Rh isoimmunization related to amniocentesis. *Am J Med Genet*. 1983;16:527.
11. Nicolaides KH, Warenski JC, Rodeck CH. The relationship of fetal plasma protein concentration and hemoglobin level to the development of hydrops in rhesus isoimmunization. *Am J Obstet Gynecol*. 1985;152:341.
12. Phibbs RH, Johnson P, Tooley W. Cardio-respiratory status of erythroblastotic infants. II. Blood volume, hematocrit and serum albumin concentration in relation to hydrops fetalis. *Pediatrics*. 1974;53:13.
13. Nicolaides KH, Clewell WH, Mibashan RS, et al. Fetal haemoglobin measurement in the assessment of red cell isoimmunization. *Lancet*. 1988;1:1073.
14. Nicolaides KH, Thilaganathan B, Rodeck CH, Mibashan RS. Erythroblastosis and reticulocytosis in anemic fetuses. *Am J Obstet Gynecol*. 1988;159:1063.
15. Nicolaides KH, Thilaganathan B, Mibashan RS. Cordocentesis in the investigation of fetal erythropoiesis. *Am J Obstet Gynecol*. 1989;161:1197.
16. Nicolaides KH. Studies on fetal physiology and pathophysiology in rhesus disease. *Sem Perinatol*. 1989;13:328.
17. Harman CR, Manning FA, Bowman JM, Lange IR. Severe Rh disease—poor outcome is not inevitable. *Am J Obstet Gynecol*. 1983;145:823.
18. Robillard JE, Weiner CP, Smith F. Human fetal arginine vasopressin (AVP) and acute, intravascular volume expansion. *Fetal Ther*. in press, 1991.
19. Robillard JE, Weiner CP. Atrial natriuretic factor in the human fetus—effect of volume expansion. *J Pediatr*. 1988;113:552.
20. Weiner CP, Heilskov J, Pelzer G, et al. Normal values for human umbilical venous and amniotic fluid pressures and their alteration by fetal disease. *Am J Obstet Gynecol*. 1989;161:714.
21. Bowman JM. The management of Rh isoimmunization. *Obstet Gynecol*. 1978;52:1.
22. Bowman JM, Pollock JM. Transplacental fetal hemorrhage after amniocentesis. *Obstet Gynecol*. 1985;66:749.
23. Liley AW. Liquor amnii analyses in the management of pregnancy complicated by rhesus sensitization. *Am J Obstet Gynecol*. 1961;82:1359.
24. Nicolaides KH, Rodeck CH, Mibashan RS. Have Liley charts outlived their usefulness? *Am J Obstet Gynecol*. 1986;155:90.
25. Vintzileos AM, Campbell WA, Storlazzi E, et al. Fetal liver ultrasound measurements in isoimmunized pregnancies. *Obstet Gynecol*. 1986;68:162.
26. Roberts AS, Mitchell JM, Pattison NS. Fetal liver length in normal and isoimmunized pregnancies. *Am J Obstet Gynecol*. 1989;161:42.
27. Grannum PA. Ultrasound examination of the placenta. *Clin Obstet Gynaecol*. 1983;10:459.
28. DeVore GR, Donnerstein RL, Kleinman CS, et al. Fetal echocardiography II. The diagnosis and significance of a pericardial effusion in the fetus using real-time–directed M-mode ultrasound. *Am J Obstet Gynecol*. 1982;144:693.
29. Chitkara U, Wilkins I, Lynch L, et al. The role of sonography in assessing severity of fetal anemia in Rh- and Kell-isoimmunized pregnancies. *Obstet Gynecol*. 1988;71:393.
30. Benacerraf BR, Frigoletto FD. Sonographic sign for the detection of early fetal ascites in the management of severe isoimmune disease without intrauterine transfusion. *Am J Obstet Gynecol*. 1985;152:1039.
31. Rightmire DA, Nicolaides KH, Rodeck CH, Campbell S. Fetal blood velocities in rhesus isoimmunization: relationship to gestational age and to fetal hematocrit. *Obstet Gynecol*. 1986;68:233.
32. Copel JA, Grannum PA, Green JJ, et al. Pulsed Doppler flow-velocity waveforms in the prediction of fetal hematocrit of the severely isoimmunized pregnancy. *Am J Obstet Gynecol*. 1989;161:341.
33. Nicolaides KH, Fontanarosa M, Gabbe SG, Rodeck CH. Failure of ultrasonographic parameters to predict the severity of fetal anemia in rhesus isoimmunization. *Am J Obstet Gynecol*. 1988;158:920.
34. Rochard F, Schifrin B, Goupil F, et al. Nonstressed fetal heart rate monitoring in the antepartum period. *Am J Obstet Gynecol*. 1976;126:699.

35. Modanlou HD, Freeman RK, Ortiz O, et al. Sinusoidal fetal heart rate pattern and severe fetal anemia. *Obstet Gynecol.* 1977;49:537.
36. Elliott JP, Modanlou HD, O'Keefe DF, Freeman RK. Significance of fetal and neonatal sinusoidal heart rate pattern: further clinical observations in Rh incompatibility. *Am J Obstet Gynecol.* 1980;138:227.
37. Nicolaides KH, Sadovsky G, Cetin E. Fetal heart rate patterns in red blood cell isoimmunized pregnancies. *Am J Obstet Gynecol.* 1989;161:351.
38. Socol ML, MacGregor SN, Pielet BW, et al. Percutaneous umbilical transfusion in severe rhesus isoimmunization: resolution of fetal hydrops. *Am J Obstet Gynecol.* 1987;157:1369.
39. Pattison N, Roberts A. The management of severe erythroblastosis fetalis by fetal transfusion: survival of transfused adult erythrocytes in the fetus. *Obstet Gynecol.* 1989;74:901.
40. Pielet BW, Socol ML, MacGregor SN, et al. Fetal heart rate changes after intravascular treatment with pancuronium bromide. *Am J Obstet Gynecol.* 1988;159:640.
41. Reece EA, Copel JA, Scioscia AL, et al. Diagnostic fetal umbilical blood sampling in the management of isoimmunization. *Am J Obstet Gynecol.* 1988;159:1057.
42. Rodeck CH, Nicolaides KH, Warsof SL, et al. The management of severe rhesus isoimmunization by fetoscopic intravascular transfusions. *Am J Obstet Gynecol.* 1984;150:769.
43. Morris JA, Hustead RF, Robinson RG, Haswell GL, et al. Measurement of fetoplacental blood volume in the human previable fetus. *Am J Obstet Gynecol.* 1973;118:927.
44. Brace RA. Ovine fetal cardiovascular responses to packed red blood cell transfusions. *Am J Obstet Gynecol.* 1989;161:1367.
45. Nicolaides KH, Clewell WH, Rodeck CH. Measurement of human fetoplacental blood volume in erythroblastosis fetalis. *Am J Obstet Gynecol.* 1987;157:50.
46. MacGregor SN, Socol ML, Pielet BW, et al. Prediction of fetoplacental blood volume in isoimmunized pregnancy. *Am J Obstet Gynecol.* 1988;159:1493.
47. MacGregor SN, Socol ML, Pielet BW, Sholl J. Prediction of hematocrit decline after intravascular fetal transfusion. *Am J Obstet Gynecol.* 1989;161:1491.
48. Grannum PA, Copel JA, Plaxe SC, et al. *In utero* exchange transfusion by direct intravascular injection in severe erythroblastosis fetalis. *N Engl J Med.* 1986;314:1431.
49. Ney JA, Socol ML, Dooley SL, et al. Perinatal outcome following intravascular transfusion in severely isoimmunized fetuses. *Intl J Gynecol Obstet.* (in press, 1991).
50. Watts DH, Luthy DA, Benedetti TJ, et al. Intraperitoneal fetal transfusion under direct ultrasound guidance. *Obstet Gynecol.* 1988;71:84.
51. Frigoletto FD, Umansky I, Birnholz J, et al. Intrauterine fetal transfusion in 365 fetuses during fifteen years. *Am J Obstet Gynecol.* 1981;139:781.
52. Berkowitz RL, Chitkara U, Wilkins IA, et al. Intravascular monitoring and management of erythroblastosis fetalis. *Am J Obstet Gynecol.* 1988;158:783.
53. Barss VA, Benacerraf BR, Frigoletto FD, et al. Management of isoimmunized pregnancy by use of intravascular techniques. *Am J Obstet Gynecol.* 1988;159:932.
54. Parer JT. Severe Rh isoimmunization—current methods of *in utero* diagnosis and treatment. *Am J Obstet Gynecol.* 1988;158:1323.
55. Grannum PAT, Copel JA, Moya FR, et al. The reversal of hydrops fetalis by intravascular intrauterine transfusion in severe isoimmune fetal anemia. *Am J Obstet Gynecol.* 1988;158:914.
56. Daffos F, Capella-Pavlovsky M, Forestier F. Fetal blood sampling during pregnancy with use of a needle guided by ultrasound: a study of 606 consecutive cases. *Am J Obstet Gynecol.* 1985;153:655.
57. Pielet BW, Socol ML, MacGregor SN, et al. Cordocentesis: an appraisal of risks. *Am J Obstet Gynecol.* 1988;159:1497.
58. Nicolini U, Kochenour NK, Green P, et al. Consequences of fetomaternal haemorrhage after intrauterine transfusion. *Br Med J.* 1988;297:1379.
59. Taslimi MM, Sabai BM, Mason JM, Dacus JV. Immunoglobulin G subclasses and isoimmunized pregnancy outcome. *Am J Obstet Gynecol.* 1986;154:1327.
60. Weinstein L. Irregular antibodies causing hemolytic disease of the newborn: a continuing medical problem. *Clin Obstet Gynecol.* 1982;25:321.
61. Copel JA, Scioscia A, Grannum PA, et al. Percutaneous umbilical blood sampling in the management of Kell isoimmunization. *Obstet Gynecol.* 1986;67:288.
62. Berkowitz RL, Beyth Y, Sadovsky E. Death *in utero* due to Kell sensitization without excessive elevation of the ΔOD_{450} value in amniotic fluid. *Obstet Gynecol.* 1982;60:746.

PART XVI | Malignant Diseases

Stanley A. Gall, Section Editor

Chapter One Hundred and Seventy-Two

Neoplasia

Gunter Deppe, John M. Malone, Jr., and Pamela E. Smith

172

Vital statistics reports from the Department of Health and Human Services estimate that about one of every 118 female patients who are found to have cancer will be pregnant at the time of diagnosis.[1,2] Pregnant women develop the same types of cancer as nonpregnant women. Their evaluation and therapy, however, are complicated by the altered physiology expectations and emotional status of pregnancy.

Ironically, pregnancy serves as an ideal biological model for the study of the development of malignancy. Both states represent biological conditions in which antigenic tissue is tolerated by the host's immune system. Several immunologic factors may be responsible for such tolerance, including depression of aspects of cellular immunity, circulating blocking factors, immunosuppressive effects of various hormones, suppressor T-cells, leukocyte migration enhancement factors, and decreased red blood cell immune adherence.[3]

Despite concerns regarding maternal fetal well-being, the evaluation of pregnant women with cancer is, with few exceptions, similar to that of the nonpregnant woman. These exceptions revolve around the fetus, specifically the use of radiodiagnostic materials and maternal anxiety over fetal viability in the presence of life-threatening disease.

Preventive and screening measures aimed at the general population remain essentially unchanged when dealing with the pregnant patient. The obstetrician has a unique opportunity to screen pregnant women at the time of their first prenatal visit. The physiologic adaptations of pregnancy may hamper the significance of various signs and symptoms. Nevertheless, a thorough history and physical examination are the first steps in the investigation of any patient and, if done properly, can lead to the detection of most cancers, even those concurrent with pregnancy.

Early warning signs (including changes in bowel or bladder habits, unusual bleeding, development of a breast lump, or a change in size and color of a mole) are equally applicable in pregnancy and the nonpregnant state.

The American Cancer Society has recommended guidelines for cancer screening in asymptomatic women.[4] (Table 172–1). Most can be performed, if indicated, in pregnancy; others must be postponed or done only if the information gained exceeds the potential risks to mother and fetus.

RADIODIAGNOSTIC PROCEDURES AND TERATOGENICITY

Radiodiagnostic procedures should be employed with due caution. Diagnostic tests may lead to spontaneous abortion or a congenitally malformed infant, although cause and effect are sometimes difficult to prove (see Chapter 5). Consequently, they should be performed only if the results justify the risks. Patients should be carefully counseled and testing should be limited and selective.

Adequately ascertaining the effect of radiation to the developing fetus is a difficult task. The patient should be advised that there is a 3% rate of spontaneous congenital anomalies and that there is limited knowledge regarding the cause of such defects.[5,7] Depending on the gestational age, radiation effects may lead to cell death, embryonic death, or teratogenesis, as extrapolated from animal data (Table 172–2). Based on the atomic experience in Japan in 1945, Hall has reached the following conclusions:[8]

1. The dose required for a doubling in the mutation rate is 10–1000 rad (15–30 for acute exposure). The dose delivered to the fetus or maternal gonads is shown in Table 172–3.
2. The safe cutoff for fetal exposure appears to be approximately 10 rads.

TABLE 172–1. EARLY DETECTION OF CANCER IN ASYMPTOMATIC WOMEN

Test or Procedure	Age	Frequency
Sigmoidoscopy	>50	Every 3–5 years; after two negative exams 1 year apart.
Stool guaiac slide test	>50	Every year
Digital rectal examination	>40	Every year
Pap smear	20–65; under 20 if sexually active	At least every 3 years; after 2 negative exams 1 year apart[a]
Pelvic examination	20–40	Every 3 years
	Over 40	Every year
Endometrial tissue sample	At menopause	At menopause
	Women at high risk[b]	
Breast self-examination	Over 20	Every month
Breast physical examination	20–40	Every 3 years
	Over 40	Every year
Mammography	35–40	Baseline
	Under 50	Consult personal physician[c]
	Over 50	Every year

[a] The American College of Obstetricians and Gynecologists recommends annual smears for all sexually active women because of their substantially higher risk for development of cervical neoplasia.

[b] History of infertility, obesity, failure of ovulation, abnormal uterine bleeding, or estrogen therapy.

[c] History of personal or family history of breast cancer will determine frequency of mammography.

3. An exposure of 50 rads any time during pregnancy will have a deleterious effect.
4. The relationship between gestational age at exposure and effects are summarized in Table 172–4.

Radiation may kill the fertilized egg. Prior to the blastocyst stage, the embryo is a multicellular organism. The embryo is most sensitive, however, during the period of organogenesis (14–70 days). The foundation of each fetal organ system is established at 10 weeks' gestation. Each system has a specific period of maximum sensitivity to the damaging effects of ionizing radiation or to other toxic agents.

The period of teratogenic susceptibility of most organ systems remains limited; however, the central nervous system, eye, genital, and hematopoietic systems remain sensitive throughout the pregnancy. Radiation administered in the second trimester may be responsible for growth retardation and microcephaly. Growth retardation may be the most sensitive indicator of intrauterine exposure.[6,7] Recent studies suggest that the developing fetus is relatively safe when exposed to most diagnostic radiographic procedures (Table 172–3).

Procedures such as computerized tomography and lymphangiography expose the fetus to high doses of radiation and therefore have potentially substantial teratogenic and carcinogenic effects. Increased risks of leukemia and of other childhood malignancies have been reported in children exposed *in utero* to even low-dose (2 rad) diagnostic radiation.[9,10] This issue, however, has remained controversial.

Diagnostic ultrasonography avoids the damaging effects of ionizing radiation and has been found to accurately display size and position of internal tumor masses. It also can be useful in the detection of ascites and intraperitoneal metastasis. Ultrasonography also allows us to follow the response of tumors to therapy and is an effective adjunct in diagnostic and follow-up phases of various malignancies.[7,11]

Magnetic resonance imaging (MRI) is a rapidly evolving technique that is safe to use in pregnancy and allows for high resolution imaging of the pelvis. Its use is limited by lack of availability. Weinreb[12,13] has reported on its use in

TABLE 172–2. ESTIMATION OF MINIMAL LETHAL AND MALFORMING DOSES OF RADIATION FOR THE HUMAN EMBRYO[a]

Age	Approximate Minimal Lethal Dose	Minimum Dose for Nonrecuperable Growth Retardation	Minimum Dose for Recognizable Gross Malformations
Day 1	10 R	a	b
Day 14	25 R	25 R	
Day 18	50 R	50–100 R	25 R
Day 28	>50 R	>50 R	25–50 R
Day 50	>100 R	>50 R	50 R
Late fetus to term		>50 R	>50 R

[a] Surviving embryos do not exhibit growth retardation even after high exposure.

[b] Malformation incidence is low even after high doses of radiation.

Modified from Brent[8]

TABLE 172–3. ESTIMATED AVERAGE FETAL DOSE

Procedure	Dose to Fetus (mrad)
Barium enema	800
Upper GI series	560
IVP	400
Hip	300
Abdomen	290
Lumbar spine	275
Cholecystography	200
Pelvis	40
Chest x-ray	8
Skull	4
Cervical spine	2
Shoulder	1
Extremity (upper or lower)	1

16 pregnant women. These women all had pelvic masses detected by ultrasound; in seven instances, MRI contributed additional information.

TUMOR MARKERS

Cancer cells may elaborate a variety of substances that can be quantitated and potentially may be used as tumor markers. Many of these are not specific for a particular cell line and can be elevated by a number of conditions, including pregnancy. Tumor markers, nevertheless, can help with the diagnosis of malignancy and also can be used to follow the effect of treatment.[14]

Many tumor markers have been described (a selected group of tumor markers are listed in Table 172–5). Except for the use of human chorionic gonadotropin (hCG) in gestational trophoblastic disease, none are adequate for screening. Pregnancy itself causes the elevation of hCG, fetoprotein (FP), and cancer antigen 125 (CA125).[15,16] The clinician must remember that there are a large number of benign conditions that also may cause elevation of tumor markers.

TABLE 172–5. BIOCHEMICAL MARKERS FOR MALIGNANT DISEASE

Marker	Tumor
Oncofetal antigens	
Carcinoembryonic antigen (CEA) α-Fetoprotein (α-FP)	Highest in gastrointestinal cancer Hepatoma, teratoma, endodermal sinus tumor
Oncofetal carbohydrate antigens	
CA-125	Epithelial ovarian cancer
Hormones	
Choriogonadotropic hormone	Choriocarcinoma
Adrenocorticotropic hormone	Bronchial carcinoma
Antidiuretic hormone (ADH)	Pancreatic carcinoma
Parathormone	Parathyroid tumors Bronchial and pancreatic cancer
Erythropoietin hepatoma	Hypernephroma Testicular neoplasms Cerebellar hemangioblastoma
Insulin	Insulinoma
Thyroid-stimulating hormone (TSH)	Choriocarcinoma
Follicle-stimulating hormone (FSH)	Hepatoma, teratoma
Luteinizing hormone (LH)	Hepatoma, teratoma
5-Hydroxyindoleacetic acid (5HIAP)	Carcinoid
Norepinephrine metabolites	Pheochromocytoma Neuroblastoma
Enzymes	
Histaminase	Medullary carcinoma Thyroid tumor
Acid phosphatase	Prostatic cancer
Amylase	Pancreatic cancer
Immunoglobulins	
IgA, G, D, E	Lymphoid
Light chains	Tumors, including myeloma

PROGNOSTIC FACTORS

Factors that affect prognosis include stage of disease, presence or absence of metastasis, host performance status, immunocompetence of the host, patient's age and the presence of concomitant diseases. The effects of pregnancy on survival vary[2,17], and the effects of malignancy and its treatment on the fetus also differ greatly between tumors.

The risk of maternal cancer metastasizing to the fetus is small. Fewer than 50 case reports of metastasis to the placenta of a pregnant woman are described in the literature.[18-20] A wide variety of malignancies has been implicated, including carcinomas and sarcomas. Metastatic melanoma, breast cancer, and the leukemia-lymphoma group are those most frequently cited. In only two patients were both placenta and fetus involved, and the pregnant mother had disseminated disease in both cases. Intervillous sequestration, transvillous passage of tumor cell, fetal dissemination and the fetal host response may determine placental-fetal involvement. Although involvement of placenta and fetus by maternal cancer appears to be rare, careful examination of the placenta and observation of the infant after birth nevertheless are necessary.

TABLE 172–4. RELATIONSHIP BETWEEN GESTATIONAL AGE AT EXPOSURE AND FETAL EFFECTS

≥200 rad before 2–3 weeks' gestation: no abnormalities, some deaths.
Between 4 and 11 weeks, irradiation leads to severe abnormalities.
Between 11 and 16 weeks, will see stunted growth, microcephaly, and mental retardation.
Between 16 and 30 weeks, microcephaly, mental retardation, growth retardation.
After 30 weeks: functional disabilities.

CLASSIFICATION OF NEOPLASIA

Complete and accurate classification of malignant tumors is necessary for the planning of treatment, estimation of prognosis, evaluation of treatment results, exchange of information between treatment centers and the continuing clinical investigation of human cancer. The TNM system of staging is recommended by the American Joint Committee on Cancer and the International Union Against Cancer. It is based on the assessment of the extent of the primary tumor (T), the status of the regional lymph nodes (N), and the absence or presence of distant metastasis (M). The addition of numbers (eg, T1, N0, M1) indicates the extent of the tumor. Confirmation of malignancy by histologic examination is obligatory: T, N, and M categories must be determined prior to definitive treatment. They may be qualified by additional histopathologic and surgical information.

Cancer is usually a progressive disease, and it may encompass different anatomic boundaries subsequent to a phase of growth. The original stage assignment, however, should not be changed.

EVALUATION OF RESPONSE

Objective evaluation of response to treatment often can be difficult. Attempts can be made clinically, radiologically, biochemically, or by surgical means.[21,22] The method used to determine such a response always should be specified. In general, four weeks should be used as the minimum duration of a reported response.

If measurable tumor is present in a given patient, the following definitions of objective response are used:

1. *Complete response (CR):* The disappearance of all known disease, determined by two observations not less than four weeks apart.
2. *Partial response (PR):* A 50% or more decrease in total tumor size by two observations not less than four weeks apart. There should be no appearance of new lesions or progression of any lesion.
3. *No change (NC):* A 50% decrease in total tumor size cannot be established, nor has a 25% increase in the size of one or more measurable lesions been demonstrated.
4. *Progressive disease (PD):* A 25% or more increase in the size of one or more measurable lesions or the appearance of new lesions.

In summary, the diagnostic workup of the pregnant woman varies little from that of her nonpregnant counterpart. Special consideration must be given to possible consequences of radiologic exposure to the developing fetus. The most formidable issue to tackle is, however, the anxiety of patient and physician when a neoplasm coexists with pregnancy. What to do and when to do it therefore must be an individual decision, taking into account prognosis, gestational age, and the effect of therapy on the fetus. As in nonpregnant patients, a delay of diagnosis strongly influences the ultimate prognosis. Just because a person is pregnant does not preclude the existence of a malignancy. The obstetrician must remain vigilant and be alert to the possibility of cancer during the gestational period.

REFERENCES

1. *Vital Statistics Report, No. 28. Annual summary for the United States, 1979.* Washington, DC: US Department of Health and Human Services, 1980:1.
2. Barber HRK. Malignant disease in the pregnant woman. In: Coppleston M, ed. *Gynecologic Oncology: Fundamental Principles and Clinical Practice.* Edinburgh: Churchill Livingstone; 1981:795.
3. Gleicher N, Deppe G, Cohen CJ. Common aspects of immunologic tolerance in pregnancy and malignancy. *Obstet Gynecol.* 1979;54:335.
4. American Cancer Society. Guidelines for the cancer related check-up: Recommendations and rationale. *Cancer.* 1980;30:194.
5. Boice JD. Cancer following medical irradiation. *Cancer.* 1981;47:1081.
6. Brent RL. Irradiation in pregnancy. In: Sciarra J, ed. *Gynecology and Obstetrics, vol. 2.* New York: Harper & Row; 1980:1.
7. Brent RL. The effects of embryonic and fetal exposure to x-ray, microwaves, and ultrasound. *Clin Obstet Gynecol.* 1983;26:484.
8. DiSaia PJ, Creasman WT. *Clinical Gynecologic Oncology.* 2nd ed. St. Louis, MO: 1984:551.
9. Shiono PG, Chung CS, Myrianthopoulos NC. Preconception radiation, intrauterine diagnostic radiation and childhood neoplasia. *J Natl Cancer Inst.* 1980;65:681.
10. Court-Brown WM, Sole R, Hill RG. Incidence of leukemia after exposure to diagnostic radiation in utero. *Br Med J.* 1960;2:1539.
11. Lurain JR. Newer diagnostic approaches to the evaluation of gynecologic malignancies. *Obstet Gynecol Surv.* 1983;37:437.
12. Weinreb JC, Lowe TW, Santos-Ramos R, et al. Magnetic resonance imaging in obstetric diagnosis. *Radiology.* 1985;154:157.
13. Weinreb JC, Brown CE, Lowe TW, et al. Pelvic masses in pregnant patients: MR and US imaging. *Radiology.* 1986;159:717.
14. Berlin NI. Tumor markers in cancer prevention and detection. *Cancer.* 1981;47:1151.
15. Barbati A, Anceschi MM, Alberti P, et al. Ontogeny of CA 125 antigen in pregnancy: immunoradiometric determination in amniotic fluid and immunohistochemical localization in fetal membranes. *Am J Obstet Gynecol.* 1989;160:514.
16. Itahashi K, Inaba N, Fukazawa I, Takamizawa H. Immunoradiometrical measurement of tissue polypeptide antigen (TPA) and cancer antigen 125 (CA125) in pregnancy and at delivery. *Arch Gynecol & Obstet.* 1988;143:191.
17. Mitchell MS, Capizzi RL. Neoplastic diseases. In: Barber HRK, Graver EA, eds. *Surgical Diseases in Pregnancy.* Philadelphia: WB Saunders; 1974:510.
18. Rothman LA, Cohen CJ, Astarloa J. Placental and fetal involvement by maternal malignancy: A report of rectal carcinoma and review of the literature. *Am J Obstet Gynecol.* 1973;116:1023.
19. Smythe AR II, Underwood PB, Kreutner A Jr. Metastatic placental tumors: Report of three cases. *Am J Obstet Gynecol.* 1976;125:1149.
20. Read EJ, Platzer PB. Placental metastasis from maternal carcinoma of the lung. *Obstet Gynecol.* 1981;58:387.
21. Beahrs OH, Henson DE, Hutter RVP, Myers MH, eds. *Manual for Staging of Cancer.* 3rd ed. Philadelphia: JB Lippincott; 1988.
22. Carr DT. Is staging of cancer of value? *Cancer.* 1983;51:2503.

Chapter One Hundred and Seventy-Three
Principles of Cancer Therapy

Carl W. Christensen, Pamela E. Smith, and Gunter Deppe

173

When considering the treatment of the pregnant patient with cancer, it is important to consider (1) the underlying principles of cancer therapy, including surgery, radiation therapy, and chemotherapy; (2) modifications of pregnancy on the patient's survival of cancer (ie, the "increased vascularity" of the malignant breast in pregnancy); (3) the risk of malignancy to the fetus (ie, melanoma); and (4) the effects of cancer treatment on the fetus, with emphasis on the period of organogenesis. As will be shown in the following chapters, treatment actually varies little between the gravid and nongravid patient.[1-5] There are a number of special considerations to be taken into account when choosing and designing a therapeutic regimen for the pregnant patient with cancer.

More than 250 different types of cancer have been recognized; therefore, it is imperative that a specialist be consulted to ensure optimum patient care. However, the primary-care physician should be pivotal in coordinating the care of the patient since that physician is probably more familiar with the patient and probably will continue to attend to the medical needs of the patient subsequent to the termination of the pregnancy and treatment of her current disorder.

Another important factor to be considered and discussed at length with the patient is the timing of therapeutic intervention in regard to fetal growth, development, and viability. The patients must understand clearly that the mere presence of a cancer does not adversely affect the fetus but that the major risks to fetal survival originate from the toxicities of the various treatment modalities. Also, the presence of a fetus has not been shown conclusively to accelerate cancerous growth and, in this regard, elective abortion offers no therapeutic advantage to the mother. Intuitively, however, any cancer left untreated is being given an optimal opportunity to metastasize and grow, therefore it becomes a therapeutic challenge for the attending physician to evaluate the necessity of immediate intervention for maternal indications versus awaiting fetal viability or administering potentially toxic or teratogenic agents concurrent with intrauterine growth and development.

Although much research remains to be done, several authors have identified commonly recognized and preferred therapies for most malignancies during pregnancy[3-5] (Tables 173–1 and 173–2).

SURGICAL TREATMENT

The presence of the fetus does not prohibit the general surgical techniques utilized in gynecologic oncology. These principles include the use of surgical procedures to diagnose preinvasive and microinvasive disease of the cervix and vulva (cervical conization), surgical staging of early malignancies to determine the need for additional therapy (staging laparotomy in early ovarian cancer), the use of modified radical techniques to lessen the morbidity of radical surgery (Type II hysterectomies for early cervical carcinomas) with *en bloc* dissection of larger malignant lesions (radical hysterectomy). The presence of the fetus, however, does mandate certain modifications. Some examples are discussed below:

Diagnosis of Malignant Disease in the Pregnant Patient

It has been suggested that the poorer prognosis of breast carcinoma in pregnancy is due not to the changes from pregnancy but to delay in diagnosis by postponing biopsies. The same theory holds true for cervical and vulvar disease where a physician may be unwilling to biopsy a vascular, cervical, or vulvar lesion with resultant hemorrhage. In preinvasive cervical disease, the majority of lesions can be followed by colposcopic observation, due to the natural extroversion of the cervix during pregnancy. Cervical conization usually is limited to its only absolute indication, the diagnosis of microinvasive carcinoma. The cone is modified to a coin shape to spare the endocervix and limit hemorrhage.

Staging Laparotomy

The diagnosis of a unilateral ovarian cystadenocarcinoma or malignant germ cell tumor mandates a staging laparotomy for rational therapeutic management. This would include peritoneal cytology (including smears or biopsies of the diaphragm), omentectomy, peritoneal biopsies of suspicious areas, and selective lymphadenectomy. Lymphadenectomy normally includes both pelvic and para-aortic lymph nodes, including the external iliac and obturator nodes. In the pregnant patient, sampling of the obturator nodes may be avoided because of the manipulation of the uterus that is required. The remainder of the staging procedure can be carried out as planned. Failure to perform adequate surgical staging requires additional surgery or risks of over- or undertreatment.

Radical Hysterectomy and Modified Radical Hysterectomy

Historically, a diagnosis of invasive cervical carcinoma made before 24 weeks' gestation was treated without regard to the fetus with delay in therapy if diagnosed after 24 weeks. With larger fetuses, radical hysterectomy may be preceded by cesarean section or hysterotomy to facilitate surgery. The historical cutoff of 24 weeks' gestation, formerly used to disregard the fetus, may be individualized as neonatologists improve the survival of very low birth weight infants.

RADIATION THERAPY

Definitions

1. *Gamma Rays*—electromagnetic radiation produced by the decay of radioactive nuclei (*intra*nuclear production), which is a naturally occurring process.
2. *X-rays*—electromagnetic radiation created by electrons passed through a potential difference (*extra*nuclear pro-

TABLE 173–1. TREATMENT OF GYNECOLOGIC MALIGNANCIES COMPLICATING PREGNANCY

Type of Cancer	Status of Pregnancy	Treatment
Vagina	Fetus viable	Abdominal delivery prior to treatment
	Fetus nonviable	Start external radiotherapy, followed by intracavitary therapy
Adenocarcinoma (DES)	Fetus viable	Cesarean section prior to radical hysterectomy, vaginectomy, pelvic node dissection
Vulva	First and second trimesters	Radical vulvectomy, groin dissection
	Third trimester (small lesion)	Vaginal delivery followed by surgery
	Third trimester (large lesion)	Abdominal delivery followed by surgery
Cervix	First and early second trimester	Radical hysterectomy, pelvic lymphadenectomy with fetus *in utero*
	Late second trimester	Await viability of fetus, classical cesarean section followed by radical hysterectomy, pelvic lymphadenectomy
	Third trimester	Classical cesarean section followed by radical hysterectomy, pelvic lymphadenectomy
	Nonviable fetus	Radiation therapy as if not pregnant, spontaneous abortion is preferred to intervention
	Viable fetus	Classical cesarean section followed by external radiotherapy and then intracavitary therapy
Endometrium	First trimester	Total abdominal hysterectomy, bilateral salpingo-oophorectomy, assessment of pelvic and aortic nodes, adjunctive radiotherapy for deep myometrial invasion, and poorly differentiated tumors.
Ovary and tube		Treatment as if pregnancy were not present; if extraovarian implants are present, total hysterectomy, bilateral salpingo-oophorectomy, debulking of tumor; chemotherapy as indicated; unilateral salpingo-oophorectomy only in low-grade, unilateral, and encapsulated tumors.

duction). Both x-rays and gamma rays consist of photons.

3. *Ionization*—the removal of orbital electrons, resulting in the production of ion pairs. This process is believed to be the direct cause of injury to normal and neoplastic cells.
4. *Oxygen Enhancement Ratio (OER)*—A measurement of the increased radiosensitivity of oxygenated versus hypoxic cells. The OER is usually 2.5–3.0.
5. *Linear Energy Transfer (LET)*—refers to the rate at which an ionizing particle loses energy to the medium surrounding its path. High-LET radiation contact (ie, fast neutron) is densely ionizing and, when contact is made with a cell, it invariably results in lethal damage.

Physical and Radiobiological Principles

Photons interact with the atoms of the medium through which they travel, resulting in ionization. Ionization, in turn, leads to a sequence of chemical changes in the surrounding environment that may destroy the cell (lethal damage) or damage biologically important cell molecules (sublethal damage). For example, malignant tissue is composed of cells that differ in radiosensitivity according to variations in oxygen concentration and according to where they are in the cell cycle (Table 173–3). The interaction between a cell and an ionizing particle, however, may circumvent these crucial factors depending on the linear energy transfer (LET) properties of the particle.

High-LET radiation contact (ie, fast neutrons) is densely ionizing, and when contact is made with a cell, it invariably results in lethal damage. High-LET radiation, therefore, is capable of producing its effect independent of oxygen or cycle variation. In contrast, low-LET radiation more often leads to sublethal damage and intracycle variations in tumor sensitivity and requires free oxygen to kill a cell.[6,7] Thus, high-LET particles (ie, alpha particles) offer the advantage of being independent of the OER and are effective at killing hypoxic cells.

Tumor mass is another important factor to consider when implementing radiation therapy. Hypoxic cells are known to be relatively radioresistant, and large tumor masses frequently establish anoxic environments. One method of overcoming tumor hypoxia is the administration of chemical sensitizers (ie, misonidazole) that selectively increase the radiosensitivity of hypoxic cells without changing the response of oxygenated cells.[8] Furthermore, clinical experience has shown that increasing doses of radiation are required to kill an increasing volume of tumor cells[7,8] and for a given dose of irradiation, a constant percentage of cells is destroyed (ie, fractional cell kill). With these factors in mind, clinical radiation therapy generally is administered in fractionated doses with daily increments. By administering the dose in this manner, it is less likely that any cell or group of cells will remain in a radioresistant phase of the cell cycle throughout the entire therapeutic course.

TABLE 173–2. TREATMENT OF NONGYNECOLOGIC MALIGNANCIES COMPLICATING PREGNANCY

Type of Cancer	Status of Pregnancy	Treatment
Rectum	First and second trimesters	Abdominal-perineal resection or anterior resection
	Late second trimester or third trimester	If possible, delay treatment until baby is viable; cesarean section followed by abdominal-perineal resection.
Breast	First trimester	Mastectomy with or without adjuvant chemotherapy; same treatment as if not pregnant; abortion should be considered only if chemotherapy is administered.
	Second and third trimester	Await viability of fetus, if possible, prior to treatment
Melanoma		*En bloc* excision with regional lymph node dissection; possible adverse effect of pregnancy-controversial reports, abortion is not considered therapeutic
Liver		Hepatomas should be resected; pregnancy may increase vascularity of liver and predispose to tumor rupture; abortion may be indicated in a patient with either unresectable or only partially resectable hepatoma
Brain		Same treatment as if not pregnant. If fetus is viable, delivery should be done prior to treatment; vaginal delivery is preferred; use forceps to avoid increase in intra-abdominal pressure in the second stage of labor.
Hodgkin's disease		Avoid staging laparotomy before 12 weeks' and beyond 18 weeks' gestation; pregnancy does not affect the disease, chemotherapy and radiotherapy are used; both modalities can endanger the growing fetus.
Leukemia (acute and chronic)		Combination chemotherapy; pregnancy does not affect the disease.
	First trimester	Chemotherapy causes fetal malformations and abortion.
	Second and third trimesters	Chemotherapy has little effect on fetus.
Thyroid	Second and third trimesters	Is stimulated by pregnancy; total thyroidectomy, unilateral or bilateral neck dissection; radioactive iodine is contraindicated in pregnancy.

Ideally, the goal is to direct high-LET radiation towards the abnormal cells, obtaining the desired therapeutic effect, while sparing the normal tissue environment. Such specificity, at this time, is difficult to achieve, and frequently destruction of normal surrounding and supporting tissue structures occurs. Acute radiation damage is most promptly observed in those organ systems, characterized by rapid cellular proliferation (eg, skin, oropharyngeal mucosa, large intestine). Side effects include necrosis, fibrosis, fistula formation, and nonhealing ulcerations.

Long-Term Effects of Radiation Therapy

The long-term effects of radiation therapy may be quite varied. For example, consequences of localized radiation appear to be less harmful if the irradiated volume is small. Low doses of radiation, however, may increase the incidence of malignancies over a period of time.[9] High-dose whole body irradiation has been demonstrated to have a profound effect on the immune response system[7], however, a long-term study of patients with cervical cancer who received high therapeutic radiation doses did not show an increase in tumor incidence.[10]

The effects of radiation on the fetus are discussed in Chapter 5.

TABLE 173–3. FACTORS AFFECTING RADIOSENSITIVITY

Increased Sensitivity
Cell cycle: mitosis (M phase), postsynaptic phase (G_2)
Oxygenated tumors
Chemotherapeutic agents: Actinomycin D, doxorubicin, 5FU, methotrexate
Hyperthermia
Decreased Sensitivity
Cell cycle: DNA synthesis (S phase), presynthetic G_1 phase (variable)
Poorly oxygenated tumors

CHEMOTHERAPY: GENERAL PRINCIPLES

Chemotherapy may be given for the following reasons:

1. With curative intent (choriocarcinoma, Hodgkin's lymphoma, ovarian carcinoma)
2. As adjunctive therapy following surgery or radiation therapy (head and neck tumors)
3. As an inductive therapy to shrink tumors before definitive therapy
4. As palliative therapy without expectation of cure (recurrent ovarian carcinoma, cervical carcinoma)
5. As experimental therapy to determine toxicity (Phase 1) or efficacy (Phase II)

Rational implementation of chemotherapeutic agents, however, requires basic knowledge of cellular kinetics, as well as familiarity with anticipated organ system toxicities.

Cellular Kinetics

Cancer is characterized by uncontrolled proliferations with the capacity for local invasion and metastasis. Tumor cells, like normal cells, go through the various phases of the cell cycle as they divide. The M (mitosis) phase is the period of cell division, lasting 0.5–1.0 hour. The G_1 (Gap 1) phase is the most variable period of the cell cycle. Slowly growing populations may remain in G_1 for several days in contrast to rapidly growing cells, whose G_1 phase may last only several hours. The primary function in G_1 is synthesis of protein and RNA. As the G_1 phase starts to last longer, the cell is considered to enter the G_0 (Gap 0) phase, where it may rest in a nondividing state for an indefinite period of time (cells in G_0, however, may reenter the cell cycle if they are appropriately stimulated). The S (synthesis) phase is the period during which the cellular content of DNA doubles, lasting on the average 6–20 hours. In the G_2 (Gap 2) phase, with a duration between 2 and 10 hours, RNA and protein synthesis proceed in preparation for mitosis.[11]

Cancer cell growth, however, is not just a function of the length of the cell cycle. It is related to the availability of oxygen, adequate amounts of glucose, amino acids, and other nutrient factors. A tumor will continue to grow as long as more cells are produced than are killed. During early stages of tumor growth, tumor doubling time is rapid, and growth is characteristically logarithmic. As the tumor cell population increases, however, the growth rate slows and then plateaus. This growth pattern is known as the Gompertzian growth curve (after Benjamin Gompertz, an English insurance actuary who described a mathematical model that illustrates the relationship of an individual's age to expected time of death).[12]

Categories of Therapeutic Agents

Categories of chemotherapeutic agents used in the pregnant patient (Table 173–4)[12,13] include alkylating agents, the antimetabolites, plant alkaloids, and miscellaneous agents. Cancer cell populations, however, have different sensitivities to antineoplastic agents depending on the particular phase of the cell cycle. In this regard, the agents may be subdivided further into cell-cycle, specific and cell-cycle, nonspecific agents (Table 173–5). Cell-cycle, specific agents are more effective against rapidly growing tumors (because a larger portion of cells are actively engaged in cell division) than they are against the slower growing tumors, which have fewer actively dividing cells. The cell-cycle, nonspecific agents act independently of the cell cycle.

Just as the fractional cell kill theory applies to radiation therapy, similar principles are applicable to chemotherapy. Anticancer drugs are believed to kill a constant fraction of the total number of cancer cells present regardless of tumor size. In this regard, tumor volume becomes important in determining the number of courses necessary to effect cure. It is readily apparent that a small tumor cell population can be eradicated with fewer treatment courses and thus with less patient toxicity.

Devising a Therapeutic Regimen

A number of variables must be considered when devising a chemotherapeutic regimen for a patient. The choice of the agent, dose, and scheduling of administration should depend on the pharmacology of the drug, the kinetics of the tumor, and toxicity to the patient. Drugs that are metabolized rapidly may require continuous intravenous infusion (eg, cytosine arabinoside), whereas an agent that binds tightly to a target molecule may be administered more infrequently (eg, doxorubicin). Bone marrow toxicity is a common side effect of most antineoplastic agents. If the patient has undergone radiotherapy with concomitant bone marrow damage, the dose of the chemotherapeutic agent must be appropriately reduced. The general condition of the patient also plays an important role in the effectiveness of chemotherapy and overall prognosis. Patients with immunologic deficiencies, chronic illnesses, and malnourished states are difficult to treat adequately even if maximum chemotherapy is administered.

Delivery of the drug to the tumor is another absolute requirement. Large cancers or tumors with inadequate

TABLE 173–4. CLASSIFICATION OF CHEMOTHERAPEUTIC AGENTS BY MECHANISM OF ACTION

- I. Alkylating Agents
  - Classic alkylating agents
    - Bis (chlorethyl) amines
      - Chorambucil
      - Melphalan
    - Ethyleneimines
      - Triethylene thiophosphoramide
    - Alkyl sulfonates
      - Busulfan
  - Nitrosoureas
    - Carmustine (BCNU)
    - Semusitine (Me-CCNU)
    - Streptozocin
  - Antitumor antibiotics
    - Anthracyclines
      - Daunorubicin
      - Doxorubicin
    - Other antitumor antibiotics
      - Dactinomycin
      - Mithramycin
      - Mitomycin
      - Bleomycin
  - Miscellaneous alkylator-like agents
    - Cisplatin
    - Galactiol
    - Hexamethylmelamine
- II. Antimetabolites
  - Folate antagonists
    - Methotrexate
  - Purine antagonists
    - Mercaptopurine
    - Thioguanine
  - Pyrimidine antagonists
    - 5-Azacytidine
    - Cytarabine
    - Fluorouracil
- III. Plant Alkaloids
  - Vinblastine
  - Vincristine
  - Vindesine
  - Etoposide
- IV. Miscellaneous Agents
  - Hydroxyurea
  - Asparaginase
  - Procarbazine

TABLE 173–5. CLASSIFICATION OF CHEMOTHERAPEUTIC AGENTS ACCORDING TO THEIR EFFECT ON THE CELL CYCLE

Cell-cycle Phase-specific Agents
- G_1-phase dependent
  - Asparaginase
- S-phase dependent
  - Antifolates
    - Methotrexate
  - Antipyrimidines
    - Azacytidine
    - Cytarabine
    - Fluorouracil
  - Antipurine
    - Mercaptopurine
  - Miscellaneous
    - Hydroxyurea
    - Procarbazine
- G_2-phase dependent
  - Bleomycin
- M-phase dependent
  - Vinca alkaloids
    - Vincristine
    - Vinblastine
  - Etoposide (VP-16)

Cell-cycle Phase-nonspecific Agents
- Alkylating agents
  - Busulfan
  - Chlorambucil (Leukeran)
  - Cyclophosphamide (Cytoxan)
  - Melphalan (Alkeran)
  - Nitrogen mustard
- Nitrosoureas
  - Carmustine (BCNU)
  - Lomustine (CCNU)
- Antitumor Antibiotics
  - Daunorubicin
  - Doxorubicin
  - Dactinomycin
  - Mithramycin
- Miscellaneous
  - Cisplatin
  - Dacarbazine
  - Streptozocin
  - Chlorozotocin

blood supply secondary to previous surgery or radiation are less likely to respond to chemotherapy because it will be difficult to deliver adequate drug levels to the core of the tumor nidus. Also, certain chemotherapeutic drugs may be metabolized and degraded before reaching the tumor mass.

Finally, tumor cell populations may develop resistance to therapy. In this regard, the concept of combination chemotherapy has been most helpful in subduing the problem of emergence of resistant strains by employing agents that work at different stages of the cell cycle.[12] The principles of such therapy are outlined below.

Combination Chemotherapy. An effective treatment for many cancers is a combination of chemotherapeutic agents that have been used effectively as single agents. When combined, these drugs often have varied rather than cumulative toxicity and may have a synergistic antitumor effect. The principles below should be followed in the development of such regimens:

1. Administer agents that are active when used alone.
2. Administer drugs that have a biochemical basis for suspected synergism.
3. Administer drugs with different mechanisms of action.
4. Administer drugs that produce toxicity in different organ systems.
5. Use drugs with which toxicity occurs at different times following drug administration.
6. Administer drugs in repeated brief courses to minimize the immunosuppressive effects that might occur otherwise.

The treating physician must know the incidence, predictability, severity, and reversibility of potential side effects of the chemotherapeutic agents employed. They differ with the drug, dose, route of administration, simultaneous use of other drugs, and with the patient's age, nutrition, and preexisting organ damage. Side effects are classified as *immediate* (onset in hours to days), *early* (onset in days to weeks),

TABLE 173–6. CLASSIFICATION OF CHEMOTHERAPEUTIC SIDE EFFECTS

	Common to Many Agents	Predominantly Seen With One or Two Agents
Immediate Side Effects	Nausea, vomiting Local tissue necrosis Phlebitis Hyperuricemia Renal failure Anaphylaxis Skin rash	Hemorrhagic cystitis (cyclophosphamide) Hypocalcemia, flushing (mithramycin) Fever, chills (bleomycin) Radiation recall (Act D)
Early Side Effects	Leukopenia Thrombocytopenia Alopecia Stomatitis Diarrhea Megaloblastosis	Ileus (vincristine) DIC, pancreatitis (asparaginase) Pulmonary infiltrates (methotrexate, bleomycin) Cerebellar ataxia (5-fluorouracil) Ototoxicity (cisplatin)
Delayed Side Effects	Anemia Aspermia Hepatocellular damage Hyperpigmentation Pulmonary fibrosis	Peripheral neuropathy (vincristine) Cardiac necrosis (daunorubicin, cytoxan) Constipation (vincristine) Addisonian-like syndrome (busulfan)
Late Side Effects	Sterility Hypogonadism Acute leukemia Lymphoma Solid tumors Other second malignancies	Hepatic fibrosis, encephalopathy (methotrexate) Bladder carcinoma (cyclophosphamide)

Modified from Perry.[14]

TABLE 173–7. GYNECOLOGIC ONCOLOGY GROUP ADVERSE EFFECTS CRITERIA (ABBREVIATED)

System	1 (Mild)	4 (Life Threatening, Most Severe)
Hematologic		
HGB (g/dL)	9.5–10.9	6.5
WBC (per mm^3)	3000–3999	≤1000
Platelets (per mm^3)	100,000–149,999	≤25,000
Anemia/blood loss (cumulative)	Transfusion required	Reexploration to control bleeding, transfusion 5 units, or hypovolemic shock
Gastrointestinal		
Nausea and vomiting	Nausea only	Life threatening dehydration or bleeding
Diarrhea	Watery/semisolid; no therapy needed	Hemorrhagic, severe dehydration/electrolyte loss
Mechanical problems	Temporary ileus of 3 days or fewer duration	Fistula, performation, chronic bleeding requiring diversion
Stomatitis	Erythema or enanthema	Life-threatening dehydration, hemorrhage, ulceration, sepsis, aspiration
Esophagus	Transient, no therapy required	
SGOT/SGPT, bilirubin, alkaline phosphatase	Up to 2.5 N	≥10 N
Genitourinary		
Renal		
BUN	≤40 mg/dL	Irreversible without dialysis
Creatine	≤2.5 N	≥10 N
Bladder and ureter, acute	Dysuria, frequency or microscopic hematuria, injury of bladder with primary repair	Life-threatening hematuria; septic shock; obstruction of both kidneys; vesicovaginal fistula requiring diversion
Bladder and ureter, chronic	Dysuria, frequency, minimal changes on cystoscopy	Decreased bladder volume requiring diversion or catheter drainage; fistula; necrosis; permanent bilateral obstruction or loss of renal function requiring dialysis
Infection	Minor infection responding to oral antibiotics	Fulminant; local or visceral infection with sepsis, shock, or other system failure
Allergic	Dermatitis or urticaria	Anaphylaxis
Cutaneous		
Skin	Erythema, pigmentation	Exfoliative dermatitis, necrosis; requires grafting
Hair	Minimal hair loss	Total nonreversible
Wound	Wound seroma/hematoma	Necrotizing fasciitis
Cardiovascular	Asymptomatic	Dysfunction not responsive to therapy
Venous problems	Superficial phlebitis	Pulmonary embolus requiring embolectomy or caval ligation
Arterial problems	Spasm	Myocardial infarction; resection of organ (bowel, limb, etc.)
Lymphatics	Mild lymphedema	Severe edema limiting function with ulceration

delayed (onset in weeks to months), and *late* (onset in months to years)[14] (Table 173–6).

The Gynecologic Oncology Group (GOG) has established a comprehensive list of laboratory and clinical criteria by which side effects of the various chemotherapeutic agents may be ascertained (Table 173–7). The clinician should find such a list valuable in considering the immediate and long-term follow up of these patients.

Effects of Chemotherapy on the Fetus

All antineoplastic agents affect rapidly proliferating cell populations, and therefore are potentially dangerous to the growing fetus.[15-16] Their administration may lead to fetal death, congenital malformations, and growth retardation. The danger to the fetus, however, is influenced primarily by the dosage and gestational age at the time of exposure. Most of the available data in the literature seem to illustrate less danger than that anticipated from theoretical considerations or from data derived from experiments in laboratory animals.[16] Nevertheless, the consensus is that the fetus is most sensitive during the first trimester (Table 173–8). Also, single-agent chemotherapy appears to cause few problems when administered in the second and third trimesters. Caution must be exercised when any therapeutic agent is given to a pregnant woman, however, because the long-term effects of cytotoxic agents on the fetus essentially are unknown. The development of clear-cell adenocarcinoma in young women exposed *in utero* to diethylstilbestrol emphasizes the potentially dangerous long-term effect of any drug exposure during pregnancy.

Placental metabolism also may offer some form of fetal protection. Roboz[17] reported the absence of doxorubicin in the amniotic fluid at 20 weeks' gestation in a patient treated for metastatic granular cell myoblastoma.

TABLE 173–8. REPORTED MALFORMATIONS FOLLOWING FIRST-TRIMESTER SINGLE-AGENT CHEMOTHERAPY

Chemotherapeutic Agents	Malformations
Cyclophosphamide	Hemangioma of thigh Umbilical hernia
Busulfan	Bilobar spleen, anomalous deviation of liver
Aminopterin	Cranial anomalies Cleft palate Anencephaly Micrognathia
Methotrexate	Cranial anomalies
Cytarabine	Digital anomalies Micrognathia

Modified from Gililland.[18]

Sokal[16] reviewed 50 pregnant patients who were treated with antineoplastic agents. There were no obvious fetal malformations when chemotherapy was administered only in the second and third trimesters. Eight patients had fetal abnormalities, 16 had spontaneous abortions, and seven had therapeutic abortions. Nicholson[15] collected 1985 reports of pregnant women who received chemotherapy prior to 1967. One hundred and ten patients were treated during the first trimester. The infants' status was described in 68 instances. Fifteen obvious fetal malformations were found. No infants were congenitally malformed when the drugs were administered during the second and third trimesters.

From a survey of the literature, basic conclusions may be drawn regarding the effects of antineoplastic agents used in pregnancy:

1. Aminopterin, busulfan, chlorambucil, 5-fluorouracil, cyclophosphamide, methotrexate, and thioguanine should not be used during the first trimester.
2. Avoid first-trimester exposure to any agent unless the patient's life is threatened.
3. If first-trimester use of anticancer agents does not lead to spontaneous abortion, the advisability and effect of therapeutic abortion must be individualized for each pregnant patient's situation.
4. Second- and third-trimester exposure causes less teratogenic and mutagenic problems. Possible dangers to the fetus must be compared to the possible damaging effect on the mother of not administering the antineoplastic agents.
5. Possible damages to the fetus must be balanced against the possible adverse effects to the mother from not receiving antineoplastic agents during pregnancy.

CONCLUSIONS

In summary, the goals of cancer therapy in the pregnant patient should be to cure the mother and to limit the side effects of therapy to the fetus as much as possible. Although there are justified concerns regarding the potential toxicities of chemotherapy, radiation therapy, and surgery on the fetus in many instances, neither mother nor fetus would survive without treatment. As the efficiency of the various treatments does not appear to be affected adversely by pregnancy, the timing of intervention should be determined primarily by maternal indications with secondary fetal consideration except, perhaps, when the fetus has reached a stage of extrauterine viability. In most centers this may be realized at approximately 28 weeks' gestation.

Thus, with aggressive obstetric and antineoplastic management, cure rates similar to those in nonpregnant patients and excellent fetal survival are realistic, obtainable goals.

REFERENCES

1. Boronow RC. Extrapelvic malignancy and pregnancy. *Obstet Gynecol Surv.* 1964;19:1.
2. DiSaia PJ, Creasman WT. Cancer in pregnancy. In: DiSaia PJ, Creasman WT, eds. *Clinical Gynecologic Oncology.* St. Louis, MO: CV Mosby; 1981:376.
3. Roberts JA. Management of gynecologic tumors during pregnancy. *Clin Perinatol.* 1983;10:369.
4. Boronow RC. Extrapelvic malignancy in pregnancy. In: Barber HRK, Graber EA, eds. *Surgical Disease in Pregnancy.* Philadelphia: WB Saunders; 1974:691.
5. Barber HRK. Malignant disease in the pregnant woman. In: Coppleson M, ed. *Gynecologic Oncology: Fundamental Principles and Clinical Practice.* Edinburgh: Churchill Livingstone; 1981:795.
6. Wharton JT, Fletcher GH. The principle of radiation therapy for malignant pelvic lesions. *Surg Clin North Am.* 1978;48:181.
7. Hellman S. Principles of radiation therapy. In: DeVita VT Jr, Hellman S, Rosenberg SA, eds. *Cancer—Principles and Practice in Oncology.* Philadelphia: JB Lippincott; 1982:103.
8. Ritter MA. The radiobiology of mammalian cells. *Semin Oncol.* 1982;8:3.
9. Smith PG, Doll R. Late effects of X-irridiation in patients healed for metropathica hemorrhagica. *Br J Radiol.* 1976;49:224.
10. Boice JD, Hutchinson GB. Leukemia in women following radiotherapy for cervical cancer: ten-year follow up of an international study. *J Natl Cancer Inst.* 1980;65:115.
11. Baserga R. The cell cycles. *N Engl J Med.* 1981.304:453.
12. DeVita VT Jr. Principles of radiation therapy. In DeVita VT Jr, Hellman S, Rosenberg SA, eds. *Cancer—Principles and Practice in Oncology.* Philadelphia: JB Lippincott; 1982:132.
13. Krakoff IH. *Cancer Chemotherapeutic Agents.* Washington: American Cancer Society, 1977.
14. Perry MC. Chemotherapy, toxicity and the clinician. *Semin Oncol.* 1982;9:1.
15. Nicholson HO. Cytotoxic drugs in pregnancy. *J Obstet Gynaecol Br Commonw.* 1968;75:307.
16. Sokal JE, Lessmann EM. Effects of cancer chemotherapeutic agents on the human fetus. *JAMA.* 1960;172:1765.
17. Roboz J, Gleicher N, Wu K, et al. Does doxorubicin cross the placenta? *Lancet.* 1979;2:1382.
18. Gililland J, Weinstein L. The effects of cancer chemotherapeutic agents on the developing fetus. *Obstet Gynecol Surv.* 1983;38:6.

Chapter One Hundred and Seventy-Four

Acute Leukemia

Susan H. McDunn and Jane N. Winter

174

The acute leukemias are malignant disorders resulting from the neoplastic transformation of hematopoietic precursor cells. They are characterized by the proliferation of immature cells called *blasts* in the bone marrow and peripheral blood and are associated with cytopenias including anemia, granulocytopenia, and thrombocytopenia. The overall incidence of acute leukemia is roughly 5 per 100,000 in the general population per year; the median survival of untreated patients is less than two to three months.[1] Advances in chemotherapy and the supportive care of leukemic patients have led to a 1- to 2-year median survival with 20% to 40% of patients surviving long-term.[2] Currently, very intensive therapies including bone marrow transplantation are under investigation and may result in greater numbers of long-term survivors in the future. Fortunately, the incidence of acute leukemia occurring in pregnancy has been estimated at only one per 75,000 pregnancies.[3] There have been approximately 400 cases reported in the literature thus far.[4] The management of acute leukemia in pregnancy presents the challenge of optimizing chances for prolonged remission and cure in the mother while minimizing toxicity to the unborn fetus. The management of this subset of pregnant patients requires a team approach consisting of the hematologist-oncologist, obstetrician, patient, and family.

ETIOLOGY

Most cases of acute leukemia develop *de novo* and are not related to any known cause. There are, however, a number of genetic factors that may play a role in the development of leukemia; certain conditions resulting from chromosomal abnormalities such as Down's, Klinefelter's, and Turner's syndromes are associated with an increased incidence of leukemia.[1] Hereditary conditions in which there is chromosomal breakage or faulty repair of genetic damage such as Fanconi's anemia and Bloom's syndrome and conditions associated with immune deficiency such as ataxia telangiectasia (defective cell-mediated immunity) or X-linked agammaglobulinemia (defective humoral immunity) also are associated with a higher incidence of leukemia.[1] The chronic myeloproliferative disorders (eg, chronic myelogenous leukemia) and the myelodysplastic syndromes may evolve into acute leukemia after a variable period of time. Exposure to benzene and other solvents has been causally linked to the development of acute leukemia. Ionizing irradiation and chemotherapy, particularly the alkylating agents, also are known to be leukemogenic. Therapy-related leukemias may be seen in young patients treated previously for Hodgkin's disease, especially those treated sequentially with irradiation and chemotherapy. The secondary leukemias often prove very resistant to therapy.[1]

Pregnancy may be, in some limited ways, an immunosuppressed state in which the mother's immune system tolerates the foreign paternal antigens of the fetus. However, pregnancy does not predispose patients to the development of leukemia. In fact, some authors have speculated that the incidence of pregnancy occurring with leukemia is lower than expected for this age group because the leukemia itself may predispose the patient to infertility.[5]

DIAGNOSIS

Pathology

Acute leukemia is categorized according to the cell of origin. *Acute myeloid leukemia* (AML) is derived from a malignant myeloid precursor, whereas *acute lymphoblastic leukemia* (ALL) is the result of malignant transformation occurring at the level of a lymphoid progenitor. On occasion, the leukemic process originates in a more primitive hematopoietic cell, in which case the leukemic blasts may lack the phenotype of either myeloid or lymphoid lineage or, in rare instances, may bear both myeloid and lymphoid markers. AML is seen most commonly in adults, whereas ALL affects children predominantly.

The leukemias are classified according to the French, American, and British (FAB) system, which is based on the histologic appearance of the peripheral blood, bone marrow aspirate, and biopsy. Special stains and enzymatic reactions are used to differentiate further the various subtypes of leukemia. In general, the blasts seen in AML tend to be larger in size than those of ALL. The cytoplasm is more generous and granules often are detectable. Auer rods, which on Wright-Giemsa stain are red-purple staining cytoplasmic inclusions, are present in approximately 50% of cases of AML. Well-defined nucleoli are characteristic of myeloid leukemias, whereas the lymphoblasts of childhood ALL tend to be smaller and more rounded with a central round nucleus and faint nucleoli. The blasts of adult ALL may be more irregular in size and shape, but the nucleoli also are indistinct. It is important to distinguish between acute myeloid and acute lymphoid leukemia as the treatments and prognoses differ. Enzymatic reactions and special stains such as myeloperoxidase, Sudan Black, nonspecific esterase, and periodic-acid–Schiff (PAS) are helpful in this regard. Electron microscopy also may prove helpful if cytoplasmic granules are seen.

Monoclonal antibody reagents that identify lineage-specific cell surface antigens may be used to establish an immunologic phenotype, thereby differentiating myeloid from lymphoid leukemia.[1] These reagents also can help to distinguish the various subtypes of AML and ALL. Immunophenotypic analysis is useful especially in ALL because the different immunologic subsets respond differently to therapy, and treatment must be planned accordingly. In children, ALL with T cell markers has an unfavorable prognosis characterized by rapid progression, poor response to therapy, and early relapse. Most non-T cell ALL is of B cell lineage; although the majority of cases do not bear surface immunoglobulin and were once classified as "non-T, non-B cell" ALL, they are derived from an immature B cell and, in most cases, express the common ALL antigen (CALLA).[1] CALLA-positive ALL is common in children, the majority of whom are cured with chemotherapy.

Chromosomal analysis of the leukemic cells also is helpful in making a diagnosis of acute leukemia and in establishing the prognosis. For example, the presence of the Philadelphia chromosome in ALL indicates a poor outcome.[1] Patients with AML in whom karyotyping of the leukemic blasts reveals an exchange of genetic material between chromosomes 8 and 21 [t(8,21)] have a good prognosis and are likely to have sustained remission.[1]

Clinical Manifestations of Acute Leukemia

The diagnosis of acute leukemia is made by examination of the peripheral blood and the bone marrow aspirate and biopsy. Patients may present with unexplained anemia, thrombocytopenia, or pancytopenia. Blasts are often present on the peripheral smear. Patients may present initially with unexplained cytopenias and be asymptomatic, or they may present with easy bruising, fatigue, bleeding, fever, dyspnea or bone pain. Physical examination may reveal pallor of the skin or a petechial rash. Gingival hypertrophy is sometimes present. Hepatosplenomegaly, if present, is usually mild and may not be clinically evident. Lymphadenopathy can be seen in AML but is more common in ALL. The differential diagnosis may include viral infection, chronic leukemia, or a leukemoid reaction, but these diagnoses may be excluded by evaluation of the bone marrow.

PATHOPHYSIOLOGY

Acute leukemia is evident in the bone marrow only when there are at least 10^9 leukemic cells present. From the time of malignant transformation, it takes roughly 120 days to accumulate this many neoplastic cells. The process of malignant transformation is the subject of a considerable research effort today. Retroviruses have been implicated in the pathogenesis of leukemia, and avian, murine, and cat leukemia viruses have been associated with the development of leukemia in animals.[2] Only one virus, HTLV-I, has been found to be associated with the development of leukemia in man.[1,2] HTLV-I infection is endemic in Japan and the Caribbean but also has been demonstrated in patients from the United States. HTLV-I is a unique retrovirus with characteristics similar to the AIDS virus, HTLV-III, and is transmitted through blood transfusion. HTLV-I-associated adult T cell leukemia is characterized by adenopathy, splenomegaly, lytic bone lesions, skin involvement, and hypercalcemia. Antibodies to HTLV-I have been identified in asymptomatic relatives of patients with HTLV-I-associated leukemia.

Oncogenes also have been implicated in the pathogenesis of various malignancies, including leukemia. It has been shown that their expression is increased in certain solid tumors and some leukemic cell lines.[1] Although there is no proven causative link between oncogene amplification and malignant transformation, there is data to suggest that oncogenes may play a part in the process of leukemogenesis. For example, there is evidence that structural rearrangements in recurring chromosomal abnormalities specific for leukemias involve oncogenes such as MYC.[1]

The manifestations and complications of acute leukemia are the result of the proliferation of leukemic cells and the associated anemia, granulocytopenia, and thrombocytopenia. Infection and bleeding are common and are frequently the cause of death in those patients who die from leukemia. Infection may be bacterial or fungal or secondary to other opportunistic organisms. Bleeding complications are usually secondary to thrombocytopenia, but may be exacerbated by disseminated intravascular coagulation (DIC) in AML. DIC is most common in acute promyelocytic leukemia (APL); the malignant promyelocytes release cytoplasmic granules containing procoagulants, especially during cytotoxic therapy. Although it is controversial, some authors advocate the use of prophylactic anticoagulation with heparin when DIC is present in patients with APL.[6]

Leukemic cells also may infiltrate normal tissues directly. Infiltration of the liver and spleen results in hepatosplenomegaly. Gingival infiltration causes spongy gum enlargement seen frequently in leukemias with monocytic features. Leukemic cells also may infiltrate skin, mucosal membranes, lymph nodes, or meninges. The central nervous system (CNS) is a sanctuary site for leukemia. Involvement of the cerebrospinal fluid may be demonstrated in any type of acute leukemia, but it is most common in ALL.

The hyperleukocytic syndrome is another complication of the uncontrolled proliferation of leukemic cells. It is more common in AML than ALL and is seen when blast counts are in excess of 50,000–100,000/mm^3. Myeloblasts are larger and stickier than lymphoblasts. Perivascular infiltration of myeloblasts and plugging of the microvasculature of the lung and brain can lead to bleeding or thrombosis. Symptoms of the hyperleukocytic syndrome include dyspnea, blurred vision, dizziness, ataxia, delirium, and coma.[6] If left untreated, it may result in cerebral hemorrhage and death. Rapid cytoreduction is indicated and is accomplished by emergency leukapheresis and brain irradiation. Leukapheresis has been performed safely in some cases of leukemia during pregnancy with good results.[7,8]

EFFECTS OF PREGNANCY ON LEUKEMIA

Although pregnancy may be a state of altered immune function, it does not appear to affect the natural history of leukemia adversely.[9-12] The overall complete remission rate after standard induction chemotherapy should be comparable to that seen in the general population (50–80%) as long as chemotherapy doses and other treatment are not compromised during pregnancy.[3,13] However, pregnancy may affect adversely the chances for remission or cure in the mother if suboptimal treatment is administered or treatment is delayed in an attempt to protect the fetus.[11]

EFFECT OF LEUKEMIA ON PREGNANCY

Leukemia can make obstetric management difficult. Spontaneous abortion occurring in the presence of thrombocytopenia may result in life-threatening hemorrhage.[14] Therapeutic abortion, cesarean section, or vaginal delivery also may be dangerous if platelet support cannot be maintained. Similarly, obstetric infectious complications can be fatal in the setting of neutropenia.[10] If therapeutic abortion is planned, some authors have argued that the best approach is to treat the mother with cytotoxic therapy prior to the procedure. These authors contend that termination of pregnancy is safest when performed after a remission is obtained and peripheral counts have recovered to normal levels.[9,13,15,16] Others argue that abortion can be performed safely prior to induction chemotherapy as long as blood product support and antibiotic therapy is provided.[17] Similarly, when acute leukemia occurs late in pregnancy, some argue that labor should be induced prior to treatment to avoid fetal exposure to chemotherapy.[18] Others contend that it is safer to induce labor after remission is obtained with chemotherapy.[16,19-21]

TABLE 174–1. SUMMARY OF RESULTS OF TREATMENT OF ACUTE LEUKEMIA OCCURRING DURING PREGNANCY[a]

	Earliest Trimester Treated	Number of Cases	Fetal Outcome		Maternal Outcome		
			Alive	Dead	Unknown	CR[d]	No CR
AML	1st	4	4	0	3	1	0
	2nd	20	18	2[b]	8	8	4
	3rd	6	6	0	3	1	2
ALL	1st	3	2	1[c]	0	1	2
	2nd	5	5	0	0	5	0
	3rd	4	4	0	0	4	0

[a] Standard induction for AML is defined here as a chemotherapy regimen containing an anthracycline + cytarabine. Induction therapy for adults with ALL is defined as a regimen containing an anthracycline + vincristine ± steroids.
[b] One patient presented at 16 weeks of pregnancy and suffered a spontaneous abortion at 18 weeks. The other presented at 15 weeks; intrauterine fetal death occurred at 20 weeks.
[c] Mother died of sepsis in the 5th month of pregnancy. Placenta and fetus were normal at autopsy.
[d] CR = complete remission
Based on reference numbers 3, 10, 12, 13, 19-22, 25, 29-33

Many authors advocate prenatal monitoring of fetal development to plan delivery as soon as the fetus is viable.[15] Delivery also may be planned to coincide with a recovering maternal blood count after chemotherapy.[9,13,22] Until more data are available, the timing of obstetric intervention in relation to the treatment of acute leukemia must be individualized.

The treatment approach to acute leukemia occurring during pregnancy has been variable. Over the past several decades the overall fetal survival has improved. Recent literature suggests that with aggressive hematologic and obstetric management the overall fetal survival rate is 80–95% when leukemia occurs during pregnancy.[15] This is most likely attributable to improvements in obstetric management, advances in blood product support, better control of infectious complications, and the development of effective chemotherapy. (See Table 174-1 for a summary of cases treated with induction chemotherapy during pregnancy.)

The literature suggests that there is a higher incidence of prematurity and low birth weight in infants born to mothers with acute leukemia occurring during pregnancy.[3,4,13,22] The earlier in pregnancy that a diagnosis of leukemia is made, the greater the risk is for prematurity and low birth weight.[19] It is not clear whether the administration of chemotherapy during pregnancy increases this risk.[23] Most authors agree that it is relatively safe to administer chemotherapy during the second or third trimester.[3,12,19,21,22,24,25] Transient myelosuppression has been reported in neonates when chemotherapy was prescribed late in pregnancy[4,10,22] yet all have had full recovery of their peripheral blood counts over time. The safety of cytotoxic therapy during early pregnancy is not established. Nicholson and others reported a 10% incidence of congenital malformations when patients received chemotherapy and radiation during the first trimester.[26] Yet even in early pregnancy, chemotherapy has been administered without apparent harm to the fetus.[4,11,13,15,19,22] Reynoso et al summarized 49 cases of leukemia occurring during pregnancy that resulted in 50 live births.[19] All received chemotherapy during various stages of pregnancy, except for 4 patients, who did not receive chemotherapy until after delivery. Of those 50 live births, there was only one infant with congenital malformations (esophageal atresia, an anomalous vena cava, undescended testis, duplicated urinary collection system, and a clubbed hand). His mother had received maintenance chemotherapy with cyclophosphamide and prednisone throughout pregnancy. At age 11 years he had learning problems. At the time of the report he had undergone treatment for both neuroblastoma and papillary thyroid cancer. His twin sister was alive and well at 17 years without abnormalities. One other infant in Reynoso's series was found to have congenital adherence of the iris to the cornea.[19] Schafer reported a mother who received maintenance cytarabine and thioguanine during the first trimester of two separate pregnancies. Both pregnancies produced viable infants with normal karyotypes. However, one infant had distal limb defects while the other was completely normal.[27]

In addition to the risks of congenital malformation or secondary malignancies, chemotherapy also may cause karyotypic abnormalities in the fetus when administered during pregnancy. Mauer et al found an abnormal karyotype in an aborted fetus after *in utero* exposure to cytarabine and 6-thioguanine.[28] Schleuning found chromosomal gaps and rings in a clinically normal infant exposed to chemotherapy *in utero*.[29]

There are only a few series that report the long-term follow up on infants exposed *in utero* to chemotherapy. Aviles reported follow up of 4–22 years on 17 children exposed to chemotherapy *in utero*. Reynoso reported 1–17 years follow up on 7 patients. There were no significant abnormalities in growth or development reported in these two series.[4,19] Nonetheless, the data are insufficient to predict the frequency of long-term sequelae such as sterility, secondary malignancies, or other effects in children exposed to chemotherapy *in utero*.

TREATMENT OF LEUKEMIA DURING PREGNANCY

Once the diagnosis of acute leukemia is made, treatment should not be delayed. The patient should be admitted to a private room and neutropenic precautions should be maintained. The examining physician should pay close attention to signs and symptoms of bleeding or infection. Supportive care guidelines for leukemic patients include platelet transfusions for counts below 20,000/mm^3 or below 50,000/mm^3 if there is bleeding. Red cell transfusions should be provided to maintain a hemoglobin of 9 g/mm^3. If the patient becomes febrile while the granulocyte count is less than 500/mm^3, it is a medical emergency. The patient should be cultured extensively, and a careful physical examination performed with attention to possible sources of infection such as indwelling catheters. Intravenous antibiotics should be prescribed regardless of whether a source of infection is identified. The initial antibiotic therapy should be designed to cover a broad spectrum of bacterial organisms. Most clinicians begin with a semisynthetic penicillin and an aminoglycoside. Amphotericin B usually is added empirically for possible fungal infection if fever persists despite adequate antibacterial coverage.

In general, chemotherapy should be started as soon as the diagnosis of acute leukemia is confirmed. The initial course of chemotherapy is called *induction* and is designed to reduce the total number of neoplastic cells to a level at which they are undetectable by bone marrow examination. This is termed a *remission*. Following the attainment of a remission, an additional course of therapy (*consolidation*) may be administered to further eradicate remaining leukemic cells. This is sometimes an additional course of the induction regimen, or an alternative combination of agents designed to eliminate cells that may have been resistant to the induction treatment. Intermittent or continuous low-dose chemotherapy may be prescribed subsequently for one or more years to further reduce the tumor burden. This is called *maintenance therapy*, and is routine for patients with ALL. Its role in the treatment of patients with AML is still controversial. Allogeneic or autologous bone marrow transplantation is an alternative to consolidation therapy for patients who attain a complete remission.

For patients with AML, induction chemotherapy usually includes cytarabine (ara-C), an antimetabolite, and daunorubicin, an anthracycline. During induction chemotherapy, there is rapid cell lysis that can cause electrolyte imbalances or kidney damage if adequate hydration and urine output are not maintained. A bone marrow aspirate is performed approximately one week following therapy to assess the response.

For adults with ALL, induction therapy commonly includes vincristine, a mitotic spindle inhibitor, prednisone and daunorubicin and may include L-asparaginase, a protein synthesis inhibitor. Patients with ALL are at high risk for central nervous system (CNS) involvement and therefore receive therapy designed to eliminate subclinical CNS infiltration. Maintenance chemotherapy usually consists of methotrexate, an antimetabolite, and 6-mercaptopurine, a purine analogue, vincristine and prednisone.

CONCLUSIONS

Once the diagnosis of acute leukemia during pregnancy is established, appropriate treatment should proceed without delay. If the decision is made to continue the pregnancy, chemotherapy doses should not be reduced in an effort to protect the fetus.[3,9,11] There is an ill-defined risk to the fetus when chemotherapy is administered during pregnancy. The literature suggests that the risk for fetal damage is low when chemotherapy is prescribed during the second or third trimester, but may be slightly higher during the first trimester (see Table 174-1). The overall fetal survival actually may be better when mothers are treated with appropriate chemotherapy than when only supportive treatment or suboptimal chemotherapy is administered.[13] If the leukemia is left untreated or if treatment is suboptimal, the mother may not survive long enough for the fetus to mature to a viable state.[15] Also, delivery in the presence of uncontrolled leukemia may carry greater risk for both mother and fetus.[11]

In general, aggressive chemotherapy is indicated in all cases of acute leukemia during pregnancy. The decision to attempt to complete or terminate the pregnancy must be made on an individual basis. With the use of effective cytotoxic therapy and obstetric management, successful outcome for both mother and fetus is a realistic goal.

REFERENCES

1. Wiernik PH, Canellos GP, Kyle RA, Schiffer CA, eds. *Neoplastic Diseases of the Blood*. New York: Churchill Livingstone; 1985.
2. Bachner T, Schellong G, Hiddemann W, et al, eds. *Acute Leukemias: Prognostic factors and treatment strategies. Hematology and Blood Transfusion Vol 30*. Berlin: Springer-Verlag; 1987.
3. Bartsch HH, Meyer D, Teichmann AT, Speer CP. Treatment of Promyelocytic leukemia during pregnancy. *Blut* 1988;57:51–4.
4. Aviles A, Niz J. Long-term follow up of children born to mothers with acute leukemia during pregnancy. *Med and Pediatr Oncol*. 1988;16:3.
5. Nicholson HO. Leukemia in Pregnancy. *J Obstet Gynaecol Br Commonw*. 1968;75:512.
6. Jandl JH, *Blood: Textbook of Hematology*. Boston, MA: Little Brown; 1987.
7. Meyer RJ, Cuttner J, Truog P, et al. Therapeutic leukapheresis of acute myelo-monocytic leukemia in pregnancy. *Med and Pediatr Oncol*. 1978;4:77.
8. Fitzgerald D, Rowe JM, Heal J. Leukapheresis for control of chronic myelogenous leukemia during pregnancy. *Am J Hematol*. 1986;22:213.
9. DeSouza JJ, Bezwoda WR, Jetham D, Sonnendecker EW. Acute leukemia in pregnancy. *S Afr Med J*. 1982;62:295.
10. Juarez S, Cuadrado Pasto JM, Feliu J, et al. Association of leukemia and pregnancy: clinical and obstetric aspects. *Am J Clin Oncol*. 1988;11:159.
11. Pizutto J, Aviles A, Noriega L, et al. Treatment of acute leukemia during pregnancy: presentation of nine cases. *Cancer Treat Rep*. 1980;64:679.
12. Cantini F, Yanes B. Acute myelogenous leukemia in pregnancy. *South Med J*. 1984;77:1050.
13. Catanzarite VA, Ferguson JE. Acute leukemia and pregnancy: A review of management and outcome, 1972–1982. *Obstet and Gynecol Surv*. 1984;39:663.
14. Katagiri S, Tsubakio T, Minami G, et al. Successful embolization for uterine hemorrhage in a patient with acute promyelocytic leukemia. *Acta Haematol*. 1983;70:119.
15. Catanzarite VA, McHargue A. Leukemia and pregnancy (letter). *Am J Obstet Gynecol*. 1983;145:384.
16. Volkenandt M, Buchner T, Hiddemann W, Van De Loo J: Acute leukemia during pregnancy (letter). *Lancet*. 1988;1:1404.
17. Murray JA, Gee H. Acute leukemia during pregnancy (letter). *Lancet*. 1988;1:243.
18. Griffiths M. Acute leukemia during pregnancy (letter). *Lancet*. 1988;1:586.
19. Reynoso EE, Shepherd FA, Messner HA, et al. Acute leukemia during pregnancy: The Toronto Leukemia Study Group Experience with Long Term Follow-Up of Children Exposed In Utero to Chemotherapeutic Agents. *J Clin Oncol*. 1987;5:1098.
20. Volkenandt M, Buchner T, Hiddemann W, Van De Loo J: Acute leukemia during pregnancy (letter). *Lancet*. 1987;2:1521.
21. Sigler E, Vavon D, Lugassy G, et al. Favorable outcome in T-cell acute lymphoblastic leukemia with mediastinal mass during pregnancy. *Am J Med*. 1988;85:125.
22. Okun DB, Groncy PK, Sieger L, Tanaka KR. Acute leukemia in pregnancy: transient neonatal myelosuppression after combination chemotherapy in the mother. *Med and Pediatr Oncol*. 1979;7:315.
23. Mulvihill JJ, Mckeen EA, Rosner F, Zarrabi MA. Pregnancy outcome in cancer patients. *Cancer*. 1987;60:1143.
24. Lilleyman JS, Hill AS, Anderton KJ. Consequences of acute myelogenous leukemia in early pregnancy. *Cancer*. 1977;40:1300.
25. Awidi AS, Tarawneh MS, Shubair KS, et al. Acute leukemia in pregnancy: report of five cases treated with a combination which included a low dose of Adriamycin. *Eur J Cancer Clin Oncol*. 1983;19:881.
26. Nicholson HO. Cytotoxic drugs in pregnancy. *J Obstet Gynecol Br Commonw*. 1968;75:307.
27. Schafer AI. Teratogenic effects of antileukemia chemotherapy. *Arch Intern Med*. 1981;141:514.
28. Maurer LH, Forcier RJ, McIntyre OR. Fetal Group C trisomy after cytosine arabinoside and 6-thioguanine. *Ann Intern Med*. 1971;75:809.
29. Schleuning M, Clemm C. Chromosomal aberrations in a newborn whose mother received cytotoxic treatment during pregnancy (letter). *N Engl J Med*. 1987;317:1666.
30. Karp GI, Von Oeyen P, Valone P, et al. Doxorubicin in pregnancy: possible transplacental passage. *Cancer Treat Rep*. 1983;67:773.
31. Feliu J, Juarez S, Ordonez A, et al. Acute leukemia and pregnancy. *Cancer*. 1988;6:580.
32. Fassas A, Kartalis G, Klearchou N, et al. Chemotherapy for acute leukemia during pregnancy. *Nouv Rev Fr Hematol*. 1984;26:19.
33. Turchi J, Villasis C. Anthracyclines in the treatment of malignancy in pregnancy. *Cancer*. 1988;61:435.

Chapter One Hundred and Seventy-Five
Chronic Leukemia

Kevin S. Weibel and Martin S. Tallman

175

Chronic myelogenous leukemia (CML) and *chronic lymphocytic leukemia* (CLL) are acquired malignant diseases of white blood cells characterized by overproduction and accumulation of predominantly myeloid cells and lymphocytes, respectively. Both diseases arise from a single cell and are thus clonal in origin. Chronic myelogenous leukemia originates in a pluripotent hematopoietic stem cell. Chronic lymphocytic leukemia arises from a single clone of lymphocytes. Almost all cases of CLL are derived from a B-lymphoid clone, as indicated by the expression of a single type of immunoglobulin light chain, either kappa or lambda, on the cell surface.[1,2] Recently described nonrandom chromosome abnormalities[3] as well as glucose-6-phosphate dehydrogenous (G6PD) isoenzyme studies[4] also support the clonal nature of the disease. T-cell CLL occurs in approximately 5% of cases and may be identified by specific T-cell surface markers.[5]

Chronic myelogenous leukemia is one of the myeloproliferative disorders that also include polycythemia rubra vera, agnogenic myeloid metaplasia (myelofibrosis), and essential thrombocythemia. Although each manifests itself in predominantly one cell line, all three cell lines—myeloid, erythroid, and megakaryocytic—are involved. In CML, leukocytosis is usually the most striking finding, but erythrocytosis and thrombocytosis occur as well. Thrombocytosis is seen in 30–50%[6], and increased numbers of eosinophils and basophils are present characteristically in the marrow and peripheral blood (Figure 175–1). The peripheral blood of patients with CLL shows predominantly mature-appearing lymphocytes and often numerous smudge cells, reflecting the fragile nature of these cells, which become distorted as the peripheral blood smear is prepared (Figure 175–2).

Leukemia complicates approximately 1 in 75,000 pregnancies, with a slight predominance (4:3) of acute compared to chronic forms.[7] Chronic myelogenous leukemia comprises 90% of all cases of chronic leukemia during pregnancy.[8] Although the median age at diagnosis is 50 years, approximately 7% of patients with CML are of childbearing age.[8] Chronic lymphocytic leukemia is a rare complication of pregnancy since it is very uncommon in individuals less than 40 years old.[7,9]

ETIOLOGY

Although the incidence of CML is slightly higher than expected among patients treated with ionizing radiation for ankylosing spondylitis and among atomic bomb survivors[10,11], most cases cannot be attributed to known physical or chemical leukemogens. The disease is not an inherited disorder.

Chronic myelogenous leukemia is the first human malignancy identified to be associated with a specific chromosomal abnormality, the *Philadelphia chromosome,* which has become the diagnostic hallmark.[12,13] The Philadelphia chromosome is a shortened chromosome 22 that results from a reciprocal translocation of portions of the long arms of chromosomes 9 and 22. Occasionally, patients have complex translocations involving other chromosomes in addition to 9 and 22.[14]

The breakpoint on chromosome 22 occurs in a limited region, termed the *breakpoint cluster region* (bcr). The breaks on chromosome 9 occur in a large region near a cellular oncogene. Also called proto-oncogenes, these genes can cause malignant transformation of normal cells. The cellular oncogene on chromosome 9 is called c-abl and is very similar in amino acid sequence to the v-abl oncogene associated with the Abelson strain of murine leukemia virus.[15,16] During formation of the Philadelphia chromosome, the c-abl oncogene is translocated to the bcr region of chromosome 22, creating a fusion gene (bcr/abl), which codes for a new c-abl related protein (p210) unique to CML.[17] This protein has increased tyrosine kinase activity, which is associated with the ability of several oncogenic retroviruses to transform nonmalignant cells to malignant ones. Although this evidence strongly suggests that the bcr/abl fusion gene is involved in the pathogenesis of CML, its precise role has not been determined.

The cause of CLL also is unknown. There are no known associated leukemogens. In contrast to CML, CLL is not associated with radiation exposure. Familial cases have been reported, suggesting predisposing factors that have not yet been identified.[18] Nonrandom chromosomal abnormalities are found in approximately 40% of the cases[3] and the most common finding is trisomy 12.[19] The exact role of this specific chromosomal abnormality in the pathogenesis of the disease is unknown. Other chromosomal abnormalities are seen occasionally and appear to have prognostic value.[3,20]

PATHOPHYSIOLOGY

The clonal nature of CML has been demonstrated with G6PD isoenzyme studies in heterozygous women.[21] The single type of G6PD found in granulocytes also is present in red cells, platelets, and monocyte-macrophages. Certain populations of lymphoid cells also are derived from the stem cell clone and express the single G6PD isoenzyme.[22] In contrast, marrow fibroblasts do not arise from the same stem cell clone.

In CML, the malignant clone of myeloid cells expands the total stem cell pool, which results in a markedly hypercellular bone marrow. Granulocyte life span and turnover time are relatively normal and the peripheral leukocytosis is primarily due to the overproduction of cells. In contrast, CLL involves lymphocytes with a greatly increased life span that typically accumulate in the peripheral blood, bone marrow, lymph nodes, spleen, and liver.

The natural history of CML is characterized by three stages: the chronic, accelerated, and terminal or blast crisis phase. These phases are usually sequential beginning with the chronic phase; however, occasionally patients present in blast crisis. The chronic phase may be insidious at onset and often discovered incidentally when routine blood studies are obtained. The white blood cell count is elevated

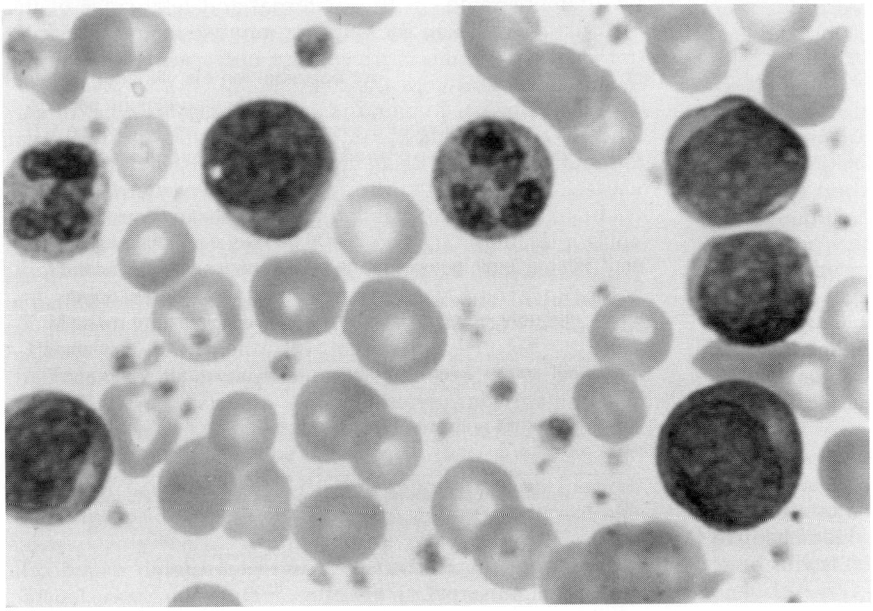

Figure 175–1. Peripheral blood smear of a patient with chronic myelogenous leukemia showing both mature and immature myeloid cells, an increased number of platelets, and large platelets. (Wright Stain × 2000).

and granulocytes in the peripheral blood show the complete spectrum of development from blasts and promyelocytes to mature granulocytes. The median duration of the chronic phase is 42 months; however, patients occasionally remain in the chronic phase for a considerably longer period of time.[23] Chemotherapy during the chronic phase does not prolong survival.

The accelerated phase is a somewhat ill-defined transitional phase between the chronic phase and blast crisis. It may be indicated by symptoms such as malaise, fatigue, bone pain, fever, and weight loss, or by a change in the number and types of cells in the peripheral blood. Approximately 80% of patients develop new chromosomal abnormalities, which mark the transition of the disease to the accelerated phase.[24] In general, higher doses of chemotherapeutic agents are needed to control peripheral counts and symptoms than in the chronic phase.

The majority of patients with CML will die in blast crisis, which clinically and morphologically resembles acute leukemia. A rapid rise in the peripheral white blood count, caused by the proliferation of blasts rather than more mature forms, is the precursor of this phase. The malignant cells in the blast crisis show evidence of differentiation along one of several hematopoietic pathways. The cells are of myeloid origin in two-thirds of the cases and lymphoid in one-third.[25,26] The lymphoid characteristics include terminal deoxynucleotidyl transferase (TdT) activity, common acute lymphoblastic leukemia antigen (CALLA) expression, and immunoglobulin gene rearrangements. The Philadelphia chromosome persists in blast cells, usually together with

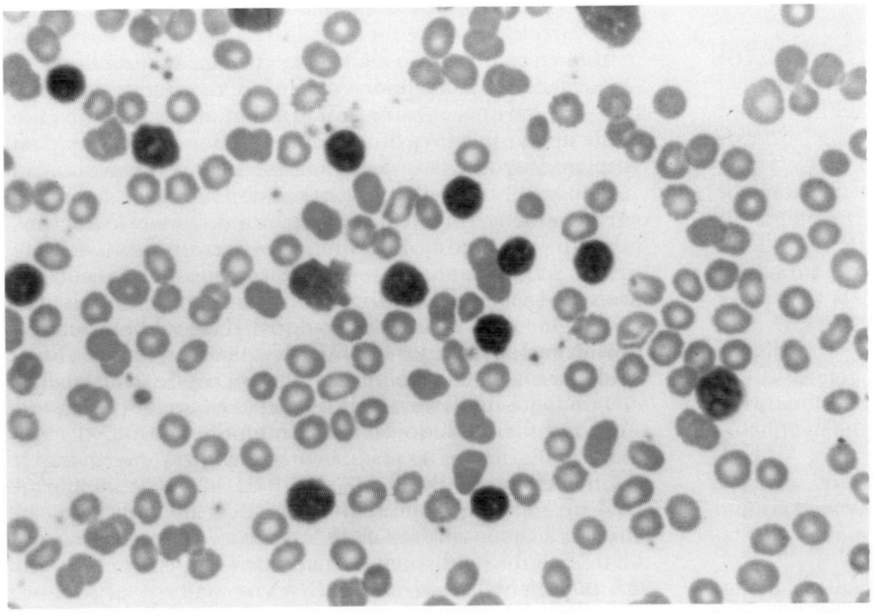

Figure 175–2. Peripheral blood smear of a patient with chronic lymphocytic leukemia showing numerous mature-appearing lymphocytes and a smudge cell in the center of the field. (Wright Stain × 700).

TABLE 175–1. STAGING OF CHRONIC LYMPHOCYTIC LEUKEMIA

Stage 0: Blood lymphocytosis, >15,000/mm^3; marrow, >40% lymphocytes

Stage I: Lymphocytosis with lymphadenopathy

Stage II: Lymphocytosis with splenomegaly or hepatomegaly; lymphadenopathy not necessarily present

Stage III: Lymphocytosis with anemia. Lymph nodes, liver and spleen may or may not be enlarged.

Stage IV: Lymphocytosis with thrombocytopenia <100,000/mm^3: anemia and lymphadenopathy. Hepatic and splenic enlargement may be present.

Adapted from Rai et al.[30]

additional nonrandom chromosomal abnormalities such as a second Philadelphia chromosome, trisomy 8 or isochrome 17.[27,28] Prompt intensive therapy is required as in acute leukemia. However, sustained remissions in this phase are rare and the median survival after the onset of the blast crisis is 2 months.[29]

Chronic lymphocytic leukemia most often presents with asymptomatic lymphocytosis. As the disease progresses, lymphadenopathy, splenomegaly, and cytopenias develop. The disease is staged most frequently according to the Rai classification[30] as outlined in Table 175–1. Patients with stages 0–2 generally survive more than 6 years, while those with stage 3 or 4 usually survive less than 2 years. The disease most often is indolent with a mean interval of 5.3 years from diagnosis to the time when treatment is required. As in CML, treatment is palliative and does not prolong survival.

EFFECT OF PREGNANCY ON DISEASE

Multiple series show that pregnancy does not alter the course of leukemia.[7,8,31-35] Median survival for pregnant patients with CML is 38 months, not significantly different from the expected survival for nonpregnant patients.[7,8,31,33,35,36]

EFFECT OF DISEASE ON PREGNANCY AND THE FETUS

During the chronic phase of CML, the probability of completing the pregnancy with a healthy neonate is good. In most cases the disease does not seem to have a deleterious effect on the offspring. One child born to a mother with CML has been followed for 20 years without evidence of the disease.[31] In another case, the children and grandchildren of a patient were followed for over 30 years without evidence of leukemia.[31]

Fetal and neonatal mortality is estimated to be 16–38% in CML.[7,8,32,37] Fetal health is generally better when leukemia develops late in pregnancy. Decreased fetal viability may be due to anoxia caused by the mother's low hemoglobin, maternal-fetal interference from placental leukemic infiltrates, and to complications such as infection. Splenomegaly may make uterine growth difficult and may be responsible for premature births. Prematurity is common among pregnant patients with CML and the average gestation time is 32 weeks.[7,8,37]

Rothman and colleagues cite 35 cases of maternal malignancies with either placental or fetal involvement.[38] Tumor was demonstrated on the maternal and fetal sides of the placenta as well as in the fetus in only two instances. Violation of the placental barrier is not necessarily followed by fetal involvement with the disease.[7,38]

The placental barrier and relative immunologic competence of the fetus, acquired after the first trimester, seem to diminish the risk of maternal-fetal transfer of malignant disease.[38] Studies with murine leukemia have demonstrated the inability of maternal leukemic cells to penetrate the mouse placenta.[39]

Three cases of possible leukemic transmission from mother to fetus have been reported.[7] All three cases involved acute lymphocytic leukemia diagnosed in the children prior to one year of age. In none of these cases was the placenta studied, so it is impossible to prove maternal-fetal transmission. There are no reports of transmission of CML or CLL from mother to fetus.

DIAGNOSIS

In the chronic phase of CML, the mean white blood cell count at diagnosis is 225,000/mm^3.[40] Thrombocytosis, eosinophilia, and basophilia often are present. The peripheral blood smear resembles normal bone marrow since virtually all myeloid precursors are present in abundant numbers. In the chronic phase, blast forms represent less than 5% of the cells present. Mild normochromic, normocytic anemia is common. Platelets frequently are increased in number and often are functionally abnormal.

Occasionally, patients will present with symptoms of malaise, fatigue, pallor, fever, weight loss, bone pain, abdominal fullness, and early satiety. Some patients complain of pruritis especially after a bath or shower, which usually is associated with an increase in the number of circulating basophils. Gout, resulting from increased cell turnover or end organ dysfunction due to leukostasis, may be presenting signs. Bleeding or bruising occasionally are seen due to qualitative platelet defects.

Mild-to-moderate splenomegaly usually is present. Hepatomegaly and peripheral lymphadenopathy may be present, but are uncommon. Extramedullary leukemic nodules called chloromas or granulocytic sarcomas are unusual until late in the course of the disease and denote a poor prognosis.[41]

Other poor prognostic factors include basophilia (over 20% of the total white blood count), platelet counts greater than 700,000/mm^3, rising leukocyte alkaline phosphatase (LAP) in the face of clinical deterioration, fever, marked lymphadenopathy, the development of myelofibrosis, and chromosomal abnormalities in addition to the Philadelphia chromosome.[42] The most important independent variables indicating a poor prognosis are splenic enlargement of more than 6 cm below the costal margin, and the presence of more than 1% blasts in the peripheral blood.[43]

Examination of the bone marrow reveals hypercellularity with a greatly increased myeloid to erythroid ratio. Marrow fibrosis is rare at diagnosis but is common in the accelerated phase. Leukocyte alkaline phosphatase (LAP) activity is characteristically low in the chronic phase of CML. The LAP may normalize or may become elevated after therapy, with infections, or during the blast crisis.

Currently, the definitive diagnostic test for CML is a karyotype analysis of peripheral blood or bone marrow cells. The Philadelphia chromosome is found in more than 90% of patients at presentation.[44] The majority of patients with Philadelphia chromosome-negative disease demonstrate the presence of a bcr rearrangement on chromosome 22 and have a clinical course similar to Philadelphia chromosome-positive disease.[45] Patients without evidence of the bcr rearrangement who are Philadelphia chromosome-negative probably do not have CML and usually have a poorer prognosis.[46] It is likely that tests with the bcr probe will replace chromosome analysis as the best diagnostic test for CML.

The differential diagnosis of leukocytosis in pregnancy includes infections, pregnancy itself, inflammatory conditions, and other myeloproliferative disorders.

The diagnosis of CLL is made by finding persistent and otherwise unexplained lymphocytosis. The absolute lymphocyte count ranges from 15,000 to 150,000/mm^3. The lymphocytes usually appear mature with scanty cytoplasm and clumped nuclear chromatin. When blood smears are made, the cells are distorted easily, producing typical smudge cells.

The differential diagnosis of lymphocytosis in pregnancy includes benign causes such as viral infections, particularly hepatitis, cytomegalovirus, and Epstein–Barr virus; autoimmune diseases, drug and allergic reactions, thyrotoxicosis, and the postsplenectomy state. Malignant etiologies include hairy cell leukemia, cutaneous T-cell lymphoma, prolymphocytic leukemia, and the leukemic phase of a non-Hodgkin's lymphoma. These conditions usually can be excluded by the morphologic appearance of the cells in peripheral blood.

TREATMENT

Therapy of CML in the chronic phase is directed at controlling splenomegaly, peripheral blood counts, and constitutional symptoms related to a hypermetabolic state. Therapy may be avoided during the entire pregnancy if peripheral blood counts are satisfactory and the patient remains asymptomatic. Treatment is required when the white blood cell count increases rapidly, when massive splenomegaly develops, or when constitutional symptoms are troublesome. There is general agreement that specific therapy should be delayed as long as practical in early pregnancy to avoid potential risks to the developing fetus.

Splenic irradiation with pelvic shielding has been advocated for the control of CML in early pregnancy.[8,47] However, a trial comparing splenic irradiation and busulfan versus busulfan alone in patients with CML showed a clear advantage to using busulfan alone.[48] Median survival with radiation was 2.4 years as compared with 3.3 years with busulfan alone.[48] Although splenic irradiation with pelvic shielding has been reported in several series without apparent deleterious effects on the fetus,[8,47] ionizing radiation *in utero* may have late carcinogenic effects.[32,49] Children exposed to radiation *in utero* may have an increased incidence of leukemia.[32,49]

Chemotherapy traditionally has included busulfan and more recently hydroxyurea, as single oral agents.[8,9,31,32,34,50,51] Busulfan is an alkylating agent presumed to react with DNA, causing antimitotic, mutagenic, and cytotoxic effects.[34] Busulfan may cause fairly prolonged myelosuppression and so may be taken intermittently. Treatment usually is started at 6 mg/day and discontinued when white count falls to 20,000–50,000/mm^3.[23,34] Thereafter, the leukocyte count continues to fall for several weeks. Maternal side effects include pulmonary fibrosis, an Addison's-like illness, and irreversible gonadal failure.[23,52] Cumulative marrow toxicity of busulfan may increase the complications associated with subsequent marrow transplantation[53]; therefore, it seems prudent to avoid busulfan in patients likely to undergo bone marrow transplantation.

In adult rats, busulfan produces gonadal atrophy, amenorrhea, and endometrial hypoplasia.[34,50] It passes the placental barrier in rats, causing abortion and severe stunting and sterility of surviving offspring.[34,50]

Boros reported congenital malformations in an infant exposed to busulfan and allopurinol after the 20th week of pregnancy.[51] Seven of 11 infants exposed to busulfan *in utero* were small-for-gestational-age at delivery. Infants born to mothers with untreated CML were average for gestational age at delivery, suggesting that busulfan given during the third trimester may adversely affect fetal growth.

Maloney[33] reported 12 women who were treated with busulfan during the course of their pregnancies. Among 6 patients, this was the only drug administered. A single patient gave birth to a malformed child. However, this mother also received splenic irradiation and 6-mercaptopurine during the first trimester.

Another series reported that newborns of 12 women treated with busulfan during pregnancy were all normal even though 10 of the mothers received the drug in the first trimester.[34,37]

Hydroxyurea, an antimetabolite, is now the drug most commonly used to control the leukocytosis and symptoms during the chronic phase of CML. It inhibits the enzyme ribonucleotide reductase, thus blocking DNA synthesis and causing cells to accumulate in the S-phase of the cell cycle. Its duration of action is shorter than busulfan, therefore the dose may be adjusted easily to control the blood counts. It has fewer long-term side effects and has not been associated with second malignancies. It is generally less toxic than busulfan. Most patients are controlled easily with 1–3 grams per day.[54,55] The drug is tolerated well. Maternal side effects include mild gastrointestinal symptoms, skin rash, and headaches.[23] Chemotherapeutic agents used in pregnancy may suppress fetal bone marrow function and result in decreased blood counts at birth.[50]

Hydroxyurea has been used extensively in studies of teratogenicity to produce craniofacial, limb, and trunk defects in several animal models.[56] Embryotoxicity with hydroxyurea is due to at least 2 mechanisms: the immediate production of severe pathologic cardiovascular conditions in the embryo that result from a decreased uterine blood flow, and the subsequent cytotoxicity and inhibition of DNA synthesis that reduce the embryo's ability to recover from the initial vascular event.[56] The use of hydroxyurea in human pregnancy has not been studied thoroughly.

The management of pregnant patients with CML may be difficult because of the need to control the mother's symptoms as well as the desire to avoid potentially harmful fetal exposure to cytotoxic drugs or ionizing radiation. Therapeutic leukapheresis can be used in patients to decrease leukocyte and platelet counts, prevent progressive splenic enlargement, and occasionally improve anemia.[57-61] The effects of leukapheresis can be long-acting, and the patient may require no further therapy once the leukocytosis has been controlled.[58,59,61] Leukapheresis has no teratogenic potential.

There have been several anecdotal reports of leukapheresis used to control CML in pregnancy.[57-61] Plasmapheresis has been used frequently in the treatment of Rh sensitization in pregnancy[59] without fetal deaths or complications. For these reasons this treatment is preferred over chemotherapy or splenic irradiation to control CML during pregnancy.

Although bone marrow transplantation has no role in

the treatment of CML during pregnancy, it is the only potentially curative therapy and may be considered once the pregnancy has been completed if a suitable donor is available. In the Seattle experience, the probability of 3-year survival after transplantation in the chronic phase is 74% for patients transplanted within one year of diagnosis, 56% for patients transplanted 1–3 years after diagnosis, and 38% for those transplanted 3 or more years after diagnosis.[53] The probability of long-term, disease-free survival exceeds 60% among patients transplanted in the chronic phase, is less than 30% for those transplanted in the accelerated phase, and is approximately 15% for patients transplanted in blast crisis.[53]

Treatment for CML in blast crisis is similar to that for acute leukemia. The recommended regimens differ for myeloid versus lymphoid blast crisis, although both generally respond poorly.

As is the case with CML, the treatment of patients with CLL does not prolong survival, but does control symptomatic cytopenias, bulky lymphadenopathy, splenomegaly, or constitutional symptoms. Autoimmune-mediated hemolytic anemia or thrombocytopenia are also indications for therapy, usually with prednisone. Alkylating agents such as chlorambucil or cyclophosphamide in addition to corticosteroids are the mainstay of treatment in the nonpregnant patient. Leukapheresis may be used in pregnancy to lower the lymphocyte count and control symptoms, avoiding the potential fetal toxicity of chemotherapy.

REFERENCES

1. Preud'homme J, Seligmann M. Surface bound immunoglobulins as a cell marker in human lymphoproliferative diseases. *Blood.* 1973;40:777.
2. Aisenberg AC, Bloch KJ. Immunoglobulins on the surface of neoplastic lymphocytes. *N Engl J Med.* 1976;287:272.
3. Han T, Ozer H, Sadamori N, et al. Prognostic importance of cytogenetic abnormalities in patients with chronic lymphocytic leukemia. *N Engl J Med* 1984;310:288.
4. Fialkow PJ, Najfeld V, Reddy AL, et al. Chronic lymphocytic leukemia: clonal origin in a committed b-lymphocyte progenitor. *Lancet.* 1978;2:444.
5. Huhn D, Thiel E, Rodt H, et al. Subtypes of T-cell chronic lymphatic leukemia. *Cancer.* 1983;51:1434.
6. Mason JE, DeVita VT, Canellos GP. Thrombocytosis in chronic granulocytic leukemia: incidence and clinical significance. *Blood.* 1974;44:483.
7. Juarez S, Pastor JMC, Feliu J, et al. Association of leukemia and pregnancy: clinical and obstetric aspects. *Am J Clin Oncol.* 1988;11:159.
8. Miller JB. Chronic myelocytic leukemia and the myeloproliferative diseases during the child-bearing years. *J Reprod Med.* 1976;17:217.
9. O'Dell RF. Leukemia and lymphoma complicating pregnancy. *Clin Obstet Gynecol.* 1979;22:859.
10. Graham DC. Leukemia following x-ray therapy for ankylosing spondylitis. *Arch Intern Med.* 1960;105:51.
11. Lange RD, Moloney WC, Yamawaki R. Leukemia in atomic bomb survivors. *Blood.* 1954;9:574.
12. Nowell RC, Hungerford DA. A minute chromosome in human chronic granulocytic leukemia. *Science.* 1960;132:1497.
13. Rowley JD. A new consistent chromosomal abnormality in chronic myelogenous leukemia identified by quinacrine fluoresence and giemsa staining. *Nature.* 1973;243:290.
14. Sandberg AA. Chromosomes and causation of human cancer and leukemia. XL. The Ph1 and other translocations in CML. *Cancer.* 1980;46:2221.
15. deKlein A, vanKessel A, Grosveld G, et al. A cellular oncogene is translocated to the Philadelphia chromosome in chronic myelocytic leukemia. *Nature.* 1982;300:765.
16. Heisterkamp NJ, Stephenson R, Groffen J, et al. Localization of the c-abl oncogene adjacent to a translocation breakpoint in chronic myelocytic leukemia. *Nature.* 1983;306:239.
17. Konopka JB, Watanabe S, Witte ON. An alteration of the human c-abl protein in K562 leukemia cells unmasking associated tyrosine kinase activity. *Cell.* 1984;37:1035.
18. Neuland CY, Blattner WA, Mann DL, et al. Familial chronic lymphocytic leukemia. *J Natl Cancer Inst.* 1983;71:1143.
19. Knuutila S, Elonen E, Teerenhavi L, et al. Trisomy 12 in B cells of patients with B-cell chronic lymphocytic leukemia. *N Engl J Med.* 1986; 314:865.
20. Juliusson G, Ost RA, Friberg K, et al. Prognostic information from cytogenetic analysis in chronic B-lymphocytic leukemia and leukemic immunocytoma. *Blood.* 1985;65:134.
21. Fialkow PJ, Jacobson RJ, Papayannopoulou T. Chronic myelocytic leukemia: clonal origin in a stem cell common to the granulocyte, erythrocyte, platelet, and monocyte/macrophage. *Am J Med.* 1977;63:125.
22. Fialkow PJ, Denman AM, Jacobson RJ, et al. Chronic myelocytic leukemia: origin of some lymphocytes from leukemic stem cells. *J Clin Invest.* 1979;62:815.
23. Goldman JM. Management of chronic myeloid leukemia. *Scand J Haematol.* 1986;37:269.
24. Rowley JD. Chromosome abnormalities in cancer. *Cancer Genet Cytogenet.* 1980;2:175.
25. Rosenthal S, Canellos GP, DeVita VT, et al. Characteristics of blast crisis in chronic granulocytic leukemia. *Blood.* 1977;49:705.
26. Marks SM, Baltimore D, McCaffrey R. Terminal transferase as a predictor of initial responsiveness to vincristine and prednisone in blastic chronic myelogenous leukemia. *N Engl J Med.* 1978;298:812.
27. Sonta S, Sandberg AA. Chromosomes and causation of human cancer and leukemia. XXIX. Further studies on karyotypic progression in CML. *Cancer.* 1978;41:153.
28. Kohno S, Sandberg AA. Chromosomes and the causation of human cancer and leukemia. XXXIX. Usual and unusual findings in Ph1-positive CML. *Cancer.* 1980;46:2227.
29. Kantarjian HM, Dixon D, Keating MJ, et al. Characteristics of accelerated disease in chronic myelogenous leukemia. *Cancer.* 1988;61:1441.
30. Rai KR, Sawitsky A, Cronkite EP, et al. Clinical staging of chronic lymphocytic leukemia. *Blood.* 1975;46:219.
31. Shalev O, Heyman S, Hod G, et al. Chronic granulocytic leukemia in pregnancy: a case report and review of the literature. *Acta Obstet Gynecol Scand.* 1980;59:563.
32. McLain CR. Leukemia in pregnancy. *Clin Obstet Gynecol.* 1974;17:185.
33. Moloney WC. Management of leukemia in pregnancy. *Ann NY Acad Sci.* 1964;114:857.
34. Johnson FD. Pregnancy and Concurrent chronic myelogenous leukemia. *Am J Obstet Gynecol.* 1972;112:640.
35. Nicholson HO. Leukemia and pregnancy. *J Obstet Gynaecol Br Commonw.* 1968;75:517.
36. Donegan WL. Cancer and pregnancy. *CA—A Can J Clin.* 1983;33:194.
37. Nolan GH, Marks R, Perez C. Busulfan treatment of leukemia during pregnancy: case report. *Obstet Gynecol.* 1971;38:136.
38. Rothman LA, Cohen CJ, Astarloa J. Placental and fetal involvement by maternal malignancy. A report of rectal carcinoma and review of the literature. *Am J Obstet Gynecol.* 1973;116:1023.
39. Loewenstein D, Hughes WL, Hofer KG, et al. Impenetrability of the mouse placenta to maternal leukemic cells. *Nature.* 1971;231:389.
40. Spiers ASD, Bain BB, Turner JE. The peripheral blood in chronic granulocytic leukemia. *Scand J Haematol.* 1977;18:25.
41. Terjanian T, Kantarjian H, Keating M, et al. Clinical and prognostic features of patients with Philadelphia chromosome-positive chronic myelogenous leukemia and extramedullary disease. *Cancer.* 1987;59:297.
42. Theologides A. Unfavorable signs in patients with chronic myelocytic leukemia. *Ann Int Med.* 1972;76:95.
43. Sokal JE, Cox EB, Baccarani M, et al. Prognostic discrimination in "good-risk" chronic granulocytic leukemia. *Blood.* 1984;63:789.
44. First International Workshop on Chromosomes and Leukemia. Chromosomes in Ph1 positive chronic granulocytic leukemia. *Br J Haematol.* 1978;39:305.
45. Ganesan TS, Rassool F, Guo AP, et al. Rearrangement of the bcr gene in Philadelphia chromosome-negative chronic myeloid leukemia. *Blood.* 1986;68:957.
46. Pugh WC, Pearson M, Vardiman JW, et al. Philadelphia chromosome negative chronic myelogenous leukemia: A morphological reassessment. *Br J Haematol.* 1985;60:457.
47. Richards HGH, Spiers ASD. Chronic granulocytic leukemia in pregnancy. *Br J Radiol.* 1975;48:261.
48. Medical Research Council's Working Party for Therapeutic Trials in Leukemia. Chronic granulocytic leukemia: comparison of radiotherapy and busulfan therapy. *Br Med J.* 1968;1:201.
49. Diamond EL, Schmerler H, Lilienfeld AM. The relationship of intrauterine radiation to subsequent mortality and development of leukemia in children: a prospective study. *Am J Epidemiol.* 1973;97:283.
50. Gililland J, Weinstein L. The effects of cancer chemotherapeutic agents on the developing fetus. *Obstet Gynecol Surv.* 1983;38:6.
51. Boros SJ, Reynolds JW. Intrauterine growth retardation following third-trimester exposure to busulfan. *Am J Obstet Gynecol.* 1978;129:111.
52. Rushing D, Goldman A, Gibbs G, et al. Hydroxyurea versus busulfan in the treatment of chronic myelogenous leukemia. *Am J Clin Oncol.* 1982;5:307.
53. Thomas ED, Clift RA, Fefer A, et al. Marrow transplantation for the treatment of chronic myelogenous leukemia. *Ann Int Med.* 1986;104:155.
54. Kennedy BJ. Hydroxyurea therapy in chronic myelogenous leukemia. *Cancer.* 1972;29:1052.

55. Schwartz JH, Canellos GP. Hydroxyurea in the management of the hematologic complications of chronic granulocytic leukemia. *Blood*. 1975; 46:11.
56. Millicovsky G, DeSesso JM, Kleinman LI, et al. Effects of hydroxyurea on hemodynamics of pregnant rabbits: a maternally mediated mechanism of embryotoxicity. *Am J Obstet Gynecol*. 1981;140:747.
57. Fitzgerald D, Rowe JM, Heal J. Leukapheresis for control of chronic myelogenous leukemia during pregnancy. *Am J Hematol*. 1986;22:213.
58. Caplan SN, Coco FV, Berkman EM. Management of chronic myelocytic leukemia in pregnancy by cell pheresis. *Transfusion*. 1978;18:120.
59. Nolan TE, Ross WB, Caldwell C. Chronic granulocytic leukemia in pregnancy. *J Reprod Med*. 1988;33:661.
60. Broccia G, Casula P, Andria M. Chronic myelocytic leukemia in pregnancy: a report of a case treated with leukapheresis. *Tumori*. 1984;70:371.
61. Meyer RJ, Cuttner J, Truog P, et al. Therapeutic leukapheresis of acute myelo-monocytic leukemia in pregnancy. *Med Ped Oncol*. 1978;4:77.

Chapter One Hundred and Seventy-Six

Hodgkin's Disease

Leo I. Gordon and Al B. Benson III

176

Approximately 7500 patients are diagnosed with Hodgkin's disease in the United States each year, and there appears to be a bimodal distribution of cases in developed countries.[1] There also appear to be some differences between developed and underdeveloped countries in terms of the overall incidence and in terms of distribution of histologic subtypes.[2]

The association of certain infectious agents with the diagnosis of Hodgkin's disease has led some to speculate that there is an infectious etiology.[3,4] The association of Hodgkin's disease with mycobacterial infections[5], and numerous reports linking Hodgkin's disease and infectious mononucleosis, thus with Epstein–Barr (EB) virus infection, have supported the pathologic demonstration of cells resembling Sternberg–Reed cells in patients with infectious mononucleosis.[6] There are data showing that in some patients with Hodgkin's disease there is enhanced activation of EB virus, as determined by measurement of EB virus antibody patterns in a large number of serum samples.[7] It remains unclear, however, whether the virus has a direct role in the pathogenesis of the disease or is simply a marker for a more basic, yet undefined defect. Similarly, Gallo[8] has noted an association between antibodies to HBLV, a DNA virus, and antibodies found in patients with Hodgkin's disease. There are a number of other associations that have been described with Hodgkin's disease, including a more frequent occurrence in woodworkers and a relationship to certain HLA antigens.[9,10] Clustering of Hodgkin's disease has been reported by Vianna[11], but others have found that this association may have been due simply to chance.

Thomas Hodgkin first described this disease in 1828 when he presented six cases in a paper entitled "On Some Morbid Appearances of the Absorbent Glands and Spleen." Subsequently, Sternberg in 1888 and Reed in 1902 described in detail the multinucleated cell that characterizes this malignancy. Hodgkin's disease is unique in that the majority of the cells in a lymph node biopsy are not malignant, and appear to be reactive cells. This is unlike non-Hodgkin's lymphomas, in which all the cells are malignant. It also is important that cells resembling Sternberg–Reed (or Hodgkin's) cells have been noted in a variety of benign conditions, such as infectious mononucleosis or benign lymphoid hyperplasia as well as in certain other malignancies such as carcinomas or sarcomas.[12,13]

The classification scheme for Hodgkin's disease has been well described. The one most commonly employed today is the *Lukes and Butler classification*, which divides Hodgkin's disease into four histologic subtypes (Table 176–1). *Nodular sclerosis* is the most common subtype and occurs most often in younger women who are more likely to be of childbearing age. This subtype can be divided into cellular and relatively acellular phases. All are characterized, however, by varying degrees of sclerosis, surrounding a lymphoid and eosinophilic infiltrate with a paucity of Hodgkin's cells, some of which may be distorted into "lacunar cells" due to retraction of the cytoplasm as a consequence of formalin fixation. There are some recent clinicopathologic data that advance the concept that lymphocyte-predominant Hodgkin's disease may be closer to a T-cell lymphoma than the other variants.[14] Patients with lymphocyte-depleted variants tend to be somewhat older and present with systemic symptoms and abdominal disease.

The cellular origin of the Hodgkin's cell remains unclear. There are data to support origin from T cells[14], B cells[15-17], and dendritic macrophages.[18-20] Recently, these cells have been shown to stain for the monoclonal antibody Leu M1, which detects an antigen containing lacto-N-fucopentose.[21] Although this probably is not relevant to the etiology of the disease, it can be helpful for diagnosis, since this antibody can stain paraffin-embedded sections. Another antibody, Ki-1, which was raised against a Hodgkin's disease-derived cell line, has been found to react selectively with Hodgkin's cells.[22] Since the Ki-1 antigen is expressed on activated lymphoid cells, this finding was believed by some to support the hypothesis that Hodgkin's disease derives from activated lymphoid tissue. These data, however, remain speculative and will need to be confirmed in other studies.

In most cases, a diagnosis is made on a lymph node biopsy specimen fixed in formalin and in B-5 fixative. A lymph node aspirate is not adequate to make an initial diagnosis of Hodgkin's disease, and should never be the sole pathologic criterion on which treatment decisions are made. An atypical polymorphous infiltrate without Hodgkin's cells may suggest the diagnosis, but is not adequate and may call for re-biopsy if a definitive diagnosis cannot be established. On occasion, the lymph node will contain only fibrosis and suggest a benign condition. Familiarity with the clinical presentation on the part of the clinician should avoid this type of error, as re-biopsy should be considered in this instance as well. On occasion, there will be evidence of granulomatous response in lymph nodes

TABLE 176–1. HISTOPATHOLOGIC CLASSIFICATION OF HODGKIN'S DISEASE

Lymphocyte predominant
Nodular sclerosis
Mixed cellularity
Lymphocyte depleted

of patients with Hodgkin's disease. This finding by itself, without the presence of typical Hodgkin's cells, does not indicate disease and actually may suggest a better prognosis.

DIAGNOSIS

Most patients with Hodgkin's disease present with asymptomatic enlargement of cervical, supraclavicular, or axillary nodes. The nodes are most often painless but may wax and wane before a diagnosis is established. Occasionally, the diagnosis is made by routine chest x-ray, demonstrating a mediastinal mass in an asymptomatic patient. This type of presentation occurs most frequently in the nodular sclerosis subtype, thus would be seen more often in young women of childbearing age. Although many of these patients are asymptomatic, some may complain of atypical chest pain or chest tightness or discomfort. Such a complaint in an otherwise healthy young woman might lead to a chest x-ray, and persistent chest discomfort in a pregnant young woman should alert the clinician to the possibility of an underlying mass lesion.

Some patients present with symptoms such as fever, night sweats or weight loss, which together constitute the B symptoms of Hodgkin's disease. Recent data correlate the number and severity of the B symptoms with outcome and stage of disease.[23] Some patients may complain of pruritis or may experience pain in affected lymph nodes after drinking alcohol. Although these are not considered B symptoms and probably do not affect the outcome of staging or treatment, these symptoms may indicate recurrence of disease.

Abdominal presentations are less common but present a diagnostic dilemma in a pregnant patient. When abdominal presentations occur they usually are associated with systemic symptoms, and usually occur in patients over the age of 40. Most of these patients are found to have mixed cellularity or lymphocyte-depleted histologies. The spleen is involved in approximately 40–50% of patients with left neck disease and is less frequently involved in patients with right neck disease. This follows the drainage of abdominal nodes to the thoracic duct and mediastinal nodes into the right supraclavicular area. The lungs are not involved unless there is hilar node involvement.

Although there are data that attempt to correlate survival in Hodgkin's disease with pregnancy[24], only a small number of patients were evaluated in a retrospective analysis at a time when treatment approaches were not nearly as well established or as successful as they are today. Nevertheless, Barry[24] reported that patients who became pregnant at diagnosis had a median survival of 90 months, while a group of age "corrected" women who were not pregnant had a median survival of only 54 months. These data need to be interpreted with caution given current understanding of Hodgkin's disease.

STAGING

The current staging system for Hodgkin's disease is summarized in Table 176–2. This system, developed in 1965 in Rye, New York, is based on the observation from the Stanford trials and from other clinical observations that Hodgkin's disease spreads by contiguity in a centripetal fashion from one lymph node region to the next. This is unlike certain other malignancies, most notably non-Hodgkin's lymphomas, which spread in a centrifugal fashion. Despite this difference, it is interesting that the same staging system is used for staging non-Hodgkin's lymphomas, a concession to tradition that probably will change soon.

After the diagnosis is established, most of the next series of studies are geared to establishing the stage of the disease. In the nonpregnant patient, this most often involves tests designed to image the lungs, hilar and mediastinal areas above the diaphragm, and retroperitoneal nodes, liver and spleen below the diaphragm. This most often is accomplished by computerized tomography (CT) scans with dye infusion, by lymphangiographic studies, and by nuclear studies such as gallium scans. Although bone marrow involvement is rare in otherwise early-stage disease, bilateral bone marrow biopsies are recommended. Despite this extensive staging, data from several institutions[25,26] confirm that clinical staging of the abdomen is incorrect in as many as 30–40% of pateints, and that staging laparotomy may reveal splenic involvement when it was unsuspected after clinical staging alone. If staging laparotomy is done, it is important to remember that this should be a complete laparotomy with splenectomy, multiple liver biopsies, and sampling of all lymph node areas. A quick observation done at the time of a cesarean section is not an adequate staging laparotomy and should not be factored into the decision-making process.

In the pregnant patient with Hodgkin's disease, the extent of the staging evaluation is determined by how far along in pregnancy the patient is at time of diagnosis, the clinical stage, the histologic subtype, and an assessment of the symptoms produced by the disease (Table 176–3). The staging approach must be individualized but should be based on the assumption that the goal is cure for the mother and, if possible, safe delivery of a healthy infant.

Although there are data that document projected fetal dose of radiation given for treatment, there are very few reports that address the issue of CT exposure to a developing fetus. Griem et al[27] reported from a record review of >1000 infants that the only abnormality associated with *in utero* fetal radiation exposure of 1.5–3.0 rad was the occurrence

TABLE 176–2. STAGES OF HODGKIN'S DISEASE

Stage I:	One lymph node region on either side of diaphragm
Stage II:	Two lymph node regions on the same side of the diaphragm
Stage III_1:	Two lymph node regions above and below the diaphragm Abdominal nodes above the celiac axis
Stage III_2:	Same as above except that abdominal nodes are below the celiac axis
Stage IV:	Disseminated organ involvement such as lung, liver, bone marrow, bone, skin

Symptoms of unexplained fever, weight loss (>10% of body weight over 6 months) and night sweats denotes B disease. Absence of these symptoms denotes A disease.

TABLE 176–3. STAGING THE PREGNANT PATIENT WITH HODGKIN'S DISEASE

<16 Weeks' Gestation	>16 Weeks' Gestation
History	History
Examination	Examination
CBC, platelets	CBC, platelets
Alkphos, LDH	Alkphos, LDH
SGOT	SGOT
BUN/Creatinine	BUN/Creatinine
Chest x-ray	Chest x-ray
Single film LAG	LAG, with ? CT scans

hemangiomas. The estimated fetal radiation exposure from an abdominal x-ray is 0.05 rad, while an abdominal CT scan would deliver approximately 0.3 rad, both much less than an empiric "holding dose" of radiation (2–4 rad) delivered to the abdomen.[29] Delays in development and lumbar myelocoeles have been reported in pregnant patients receiving doses of 0.03–3.7 rads. Therefore, some authors recommend abortion if there is radiation expsoure greater than 10 rads during the first trimester of pregnancy.[28,29] A lymphangiogram using one plain film should be feasible even during the first trimester, since the fetal dose should be <1 rad. If, however, further films are necessary to document filling of nodes, even a lymphangiogram may not be done with impunity.

Risks to the fetus exposed to radiation therapy include growth retardation, defective organogenesis, and death. These risks are considered related to the time of gestation, dose of radiation and dose rate.[28] Studies in mice have shown that a single dose of 200 rads results in *in-utero* death when administered during the preimplantation period (equivalent period for human gestation includes days 1–10). At this level of exposure in the mouse, the preimplantation death rate was 80%, whereas the risk of congenital anomaly at a single dose of 200 rads during the period of organogenesis was 100% (equivalent period for human gestation includes 10 days to 6 weeks).[28-31] In mice, even during the fetal period (equivalent period for human gestation includes 6 weeks to term), abnormalities such as cerebellar defects, microcephaly, and agenesis of the corpus collosum have been reported.[30-32] Thus, although there are considerable data to suggest a risk of radiation to the developing fetus, there is a dose relationship that may allow simple staging with a plain film lymphangiogram in selected patients in the first trimester, and CT scanning in patients beyond 16 weeks' gestation. If the disease presents in the very early stages (with, for example, high right neck involvement alone), one can safely observe until the pregnancy is carried to term and then complete accurate staging and initiate treatment. When the disease presents in a more aggressive fashion (with, for example, B symptoms or with a large mediastinal mass with superior vena cava syndrome), the choice of staging studies becomes less important both for the pregnant and for the nonpregnant patient, since prompt initiation of therapy becomes the prevailing goal.

TREATMENT

Nonpregnant Patient

Most investigators agree that the treatment of choice for early stage Hodgkin's disease (PS1 A, PS11 A with small mediastinal mass) is radiation therapy, which if delivered in adequate doses to an appropriate portal using modern computer treatment-planning techniques, should result in >85% long-term, disease-free survival. Patients with Stage III_2 (involvement of lower abdominal lymph nodes) disease and with Stage IV (organ involvement) disease are treated with combination chemotherapy with alternating drugs such as MOPP/ABVD.[33] The drugs in this regimen include nitrogen mustard, vincristine, procarbazine, prednisone, doxorubicin, vinblastine, bleomycin, and DTIC. This regimen includes both alkylating agents (nitrogen mustard, procarbazine), drugs that intercalate DNA (doxorubicin), and mitotic spindle inhibitors (vincristine, vinblastine). Although a number of other regimens have been used with equal success[34], most clinical studies are comparing variations on the theme of MOPP/ABVD. One can expect that even for patients with Stage IV disease, there is a >70% chance of remaining disease free for more than 10 years. For patients with Stage III disease or with bulky Stage II disease, some recommend radiation alone[35], some recommend chemotherapy alone[36], and some would recommend a combination of radiation and chemotherapy.[37]

Pregnant Patient

For the pregnant patient with Hodgkin's disease, the same principles apply, but the approach should be different if the goals of cure of the mother and fetus viability are to be maintained. (Table 176–4)

There are a number of reports in the literature that address the issue of Hodgkin's disease management in pregnancy. Some of these have been reviewed.[38,39] Jacobs et al[29] described 15 pregnant women with Hodgkin's disease at Stanford, and devised a treatment strategy based on their experience. They recommend abortion for patients who develop Hodgkin's disease early in pregnancy or who have received radiation or chemotherapy during the first trimester. During the latter half, asymptomatic patients can be followed until early delivery can be carried out. They recommend radiation for patients with supradiaphragmatic disease who are symptomatic and cannot have abortions and single agent chemotherapy for patients with more advanced disease who are not candidates for abortion.

TABLE 176–4. TREATMENT OF THE PREGNANT PATIENT WITH HODGKIN'S DISEASE

	<16 Weeks	>16 Weeks
Aggressive, advanced disease	Abortion	Local RT or chemotherapy with adriamycin, velban ± chlorambucil ± methotrexate
Limited disease	Observation or limited RT to neck, or abortion	Observation or RT above diaphragm

This strategy has been criticized by Chapman and Crosby[40], who argue that temporizing treatment and "holding dose" radiation may compromise effective treatment later. Although there is a general concensus that radiation and chemotherapy are risky to the fetus during pregnancy, the published literature does not support this. In a review, Barber[41] finds that no fetal abnormalities have been reported in infants whose mothers received radiation during the second and third trimester.

It appears that there are four major sources of radiation that account for the dose received by the fetus. These are direct radiation, source irradiation leakage, external scatter, and internal scatter.[28] Therapeutic radiation for Hodgkin's disease should not involve direct radiation of the fetus, and shielding should greatly reduce leakage and external scatter, leaving internal scatter as the significant fetal dose. Radiation given to a mantle port delivers a dose of radiation that is dependent upon the energy source, the portal, and the distance from the distal border of the field to the uterus and fetus.[28] Phantom calculations have been utilized in an attempt to predict fetal radiation dose. Thus, with a mediastinal dose of 3500 rads, the fetal dose in early pregnancy would be 3.5–14 rads, in the mid-pregnancy 31–49 rads, and in late pregnancy 129–248 rads.[29,42,43] The differences presumably are based on the height of the uterus with fetal development. There are also variations depending on the source. Whereas the pelvic dose of left supraclavicular radiation delivered from a linear accelerator was 3.5–6.3 rads, it was 4.5–9.1 rads delivered from a cobalt source.[44]

There are some reports in the literature describing radiation during pregnancy. Nisci reported 7 women treated during the second or third trimester who received 1500–2000 rads with fetal doses ranging from 2–50 rads.[45] These patients all had full-term spontaneous normal deliveries with normal infants. Tawil[46] noted no fetal abnormalities, yet Jacobs[29] reported a patient treated with 4400 rads (with an estimated fetal dose of 9 rads) who had a spontaneous abortion in the first trimester. In another series[47] one patient receiving mantle radiation during weeks 3–11 delivered an infant with sensory loss due to an inner ear defect and another patient had radiation during weeks 20–30 and delivered a child that was a slow learner.

Based on these data and the clinical literature, we would recommend that abortion be carried out during the first 16 weeks of pregnancy for those patients requiring urgent pelvic irradiation, or for those in whom pelvic radiation has been given inadvertently beyond 10 rads. Local radiation (2000 rads) with abdominal shielding may be given to those patients with asymptomatic disease that is localized to the neck or axilla. After 16 weeks' gestation, radiation can be given to supradiaphragmatic sites, but in asymptomatic patients with small masses, an alternate approach would be to carry the pregnancy to term and then complete full staging and appropriate therapy.

There are a number of case reports that address the use of cytotoxic chemotherapy in the pregnant patient with Hodgkin's disease.[45,56-58] It appears that fetal abnormalities are not increased during the second or third trimesters. There are, however, potential risks to the fetus exposed to cytotoxic chemotherapy agents during the first trimester, especially with alkylating agents. Cyclophosphamide and procarbazine, both alkylating agents, are known to cross the placenta and can result in fetal abnormalities or death.[51] Chlorambucil, sometimes recommended as an alternative chemotherapy agent in pregnant patients, has been associated with fetal abnormalities, including renal aplasia, cleft palate, and skeletal abnormalities. Nitrogen mustard has been given safely in a limited number of cases to women during the first trimester.[24,29,57] The anthracycline doxorubicin, now used commonly in combination regimens in Hodgkin's disease, has been measured in fetal and placental tissues. Two cases are reported of administration during pregnancy in which one child was apparently healthy and one was stillborn.[53] Turchi found that 24 of 28 pregnancies in women receiving anthracyclines resulted in normal infants.[52]

Based on these data, we suggest a treatment strategy designed around the philosophy that the curability of Hodgkin's disease not be compromised, and that, if possible, a healthy infant be delivered. If the diagnosis is made in early pregnancy (<16 weeks) and the disease appears after limited clinical staging to be localized and asymptomatic, one may treat with a very limited radiation portal or preferably wait until term to complete full staging and therapy if the patient wishes to maintain the pregnancy. In a symptomatic patient, abortion should be encouraged, but if not an option, chemotherapy with Adriamycin, Velban, and possibly an alkylating agent such as chlorambucil should be considered, to start as far into the first trimester as the clinical situation allows. As the pregnancy progresses, a more standard Hodgkin's regimen could be employed. When the diagnosis is made later in pregnancy (>16 weeks), and the disease is in the early stages after clinical staging (which may include lymphangiogram), an attempt to carry the pregnancy to term should be made. If the patient is symptomatic and has an aggressive presentation, cytotoxic chemotherapy should be employed.

In the event that a pregnancy is discovered while a patient has already started therapy for Hodgkin's disease, the decision to continue the pregnancy should be based on an estimate of fetal exposure to radiation or exposure to cytotoxic drugs during the first trimester. A fetal exposure of >10 rads has been thought to pose enough fetal risk so that abortion has been recommended in this setting.

Management of the Pregnant Patient During Treatment

Sutcliffe and Chapman[28] have stressed the importance of carefully managing the potential complications of chemotherapy and radiation during pregnancy. Since the metabolic changes that occur with pregnancy may be accentuated with malignancy, proper nutritional counseling is of paramount importance since chemotherapeutic agents can cause oral and vaginal mucositis, nausea, vomiting, and anorexia. Infection with *Candida* or herpes simplex virus may further complicate this situation. During the latter half of pregnancy, when organogenesis is complete, antiemetics such as Compazine or Tigan may be used.

Attention to good oral hygeine is important, as both radiation and chemotherapy may predispose to dental infection. The management of infection in the neutropenic pregnant patient should include a vigilant history and physical exam, appropriate cultures, and prompt institution of antibiotics, thus not differing from the principles that apply in the nonpregnant patient.

If elective surgical procedures are planned at any time during the pregnancy (eg, insertion of venous access devices, re-biopsy of lymph nodes), it is best to perform these procedures before the fetus is large enough to cause a decrease in venous return due to vena caval compression when the patient is in the supine position.

Fertility Following Treatment

Many oncologists recommend that women avoid pregnancy for two years following therapy for Hodgkin's disease, partly because recurrence within two years denotes a poor prognosis. For most women, fertility should be normal at the time of diagnosis of Hodgkin's disease, and pregnancy may occur even while patients are on cytotoxic therapy (see above). There are well described risks of amenorrhea and permanent infertility in women who have received chlorambucil, cyclophosphamide, nitrogen mustard, busulfan and procarbazine with associated elevation of serum FSH and LH, denoting primary ovarian failure.[60] There is probable risk of infertility from doxorubicin and vinblastine and less risk with methotrexate and vincristine. There are insufficient data to evaluate the risks with bleomycin, cisplatinum, and the nitrosoureas.

Women younger than 25 years experience irreversible amenorrhea less often than older women even at higher drug doses and after longer periods of therapy.[58] In women 26–30 years of age, amenorrhea after MOPP therapy is 50–60%, 65–85% after total lymphoid irradiation, and 85–100% after combined irradiation and chemotherapy.[28,59] Lacher reported that patients receiving combined radiation and chemotherapy with thio-TEPA, vinblastine, vincristine, procarbazine, and prednisone for Stages II and III, Hodgkin's disease maintained a fertility rate comparable to their pretreatment fertility record.[60] All patients under the age of 35 maintained normal menstruation and two of four patients over the age of 35 developed amenorrhea. Andrieu[61] evaluated 74 women treated with MOPP therapy and found that 74% maintained normal menstrual periods. There were 22 children born to this group with only one minor abnormality. Age was a factor since only about 5% of women under the age of 30 developed oligomenorrhea or amenorrhea, while 62% of women over the age of 30 developed ovarian failure. There is some controversy as to whether taking birth control pills during the administration of chemotherapy preserves ovarian function.[62-64] If there is no other contraindication, we have recommended this approach.

Holmes evaluated 93 pregnancies in 48 patients who received treatment for Hodgkin's disease and compared this group with 228 pregnancies in 69 sibling controls.[65] In those patients who received radiation, there was no difference in the spontaneous abortion rate or number of abnormal offspring compared to controls.Thirteen patients who received both radiation and chemotherapy showed evidence of reproductive abnormalities. The women receiving combined therapy had a higher rate of abnormal offspring compared to controls; interestingly, the wives of male patients were more likely to have spontaneous abortions. Simon[66], in a follow-up analysis, questioned the methodology of this study. In addition, Mulvahill[47] evaluated abnormal outcomes of pregnancies conceived after cessation of cancer therapy in 12 patients who received radiation or combined modality therapy. Increased abnormalities were noted, but most of these represented low birth weight babies and premature termination of pregnancy rather than congenital abnormalities.

For further information on Hodgkin's and non-Hodgkin's lymphomas, the reader is referred to a recently published review on the subject.[67]

REFERENCES

1. MacMahon B. Epidemiological evidence of the nature of Hodgkin's disease. *Cancer*. 1957;10:1045.
2. Correa P, O'Connor GT, Berard CW, et al. International comparability in histologic subclassification of Hodgkin's disease. *JNCI*. 1973;50:1429.
3. Steiner PE. Hodgkin's disease: search for infective agent and attempts at experimental reproduction. *Arch Pathol*. 1934;17:749.
4. L'Esparance ES. Experimental inoculation of chickens with Hodgkin's nodes. *J Immunol*. 1929;16:37.
5. Van Rooyan CE. Etiology of Hodgkin's disease with special reference to *B. tuberculosis avis*. *Br Med J*. 1933;1:50.
6. Munoz N, Davidson RJ, Wittholf B, et al. Infectious mononucleosis and Hodgkin's disease. *Int J Cancer*. 1978;22:10.
7. Mueller N, Evans A, Harris N, et al. Hodgkin's disease and Epstein-Barr virus: altered antibody pattern before diagnosis. *N Engl J Med*. 1989;320:689.
8. Hellman S, Jaffe E, DeVita VT Jr. In: Devita VT Jr, Hellman S, Rosenberg S, eds. *Cancer: Principles and Practice of Oncology*. 3rd edition. Philadelphia: JB Lippincott; 1989:1696.
9. Milham S, and Hesser J. Hodgkin's disease in woodworkers. *Lancet*. 1967;2:136.
10. Graff KS, Simons RN, Yankee RA, et al. HLA antigens in Hodgkin's disease: Histopathologic and clinical correlations. *JNCI*. 1974;52:1087.
11. Vianna JH, Polan AK. Epidemiological evidence for transmission of Hodgkin's disease. *N Engl J Med*. 1973;289:499.
12. Lukes RJ, Tindle BH, Parker JW. Sternberg–Reed-like cells in infectious mononucleosis. *Lancet*. 1969;2:1000.
13. Strum SB, Dark JK, Rappaport H. Observations of cells resembling Sternberg–Reed cells in conditions other than Hodgkin's disease. *Cancer*. 1970;26:176.
14. Weis JW, Winter MW, Philicky RL, Banks PM. Peripheral T-cell lymphomas: histologic, immunohistologic, and clinical characterization. *Mayo Clin Proc*. 1986;61:411.
15. Order SE, Hellman S. Pathogenesis of Hodgkin's disease. *Lancet*. 1972; 1:571.
16. Hsu S, Yang K, Jaffe ES. Phenotypic expression of Hodgkin's and Sternberg–Reed cells in Hodgkin's disease. *Am J Pathol*. 1985;118:209.
17. Weiss L, Strickler JG, Hu E, et al. Immunoglobulin gene rearrangements in Hodgkin's disease. *Hum Pathol*. 1986;17:1009.
18. Fisher RI, Bates BT, Bostick-Bruton F, et al. Neoplastic cells obtained from Hodgkin's disease are potent stimulators of human primary and mixed lymphoctye cultures. *J Immunol*. 1983;130:2666.
19. Kadin ME, Stites DP, Levy R, et al. Exogenous immunoglobulin and macrophage origin of Reed-Sternberg cells in Hodgkin's disease. N Engl J Med. 1978;299:1208.
20. Kadin ME: Possible origin of the Sternberg–Reed cell from an interdigitating reticulum cell. *Cancer Treat Rep*. 1982;66:601.
21. Hsu S, Jaffe ES. Leu M1 and peanut agglutinin stain: the neoplastic cells of Hodgkin's disease. *Am J Clin Pathol*. 1984;82:29.
22. Stein H, Mason DY, O'Connor N, et al. The expression of the Hodgkin's disease associated antigen KI-1 in reactive and neoplastic lymphoid tissue: evidence that Reed-Sternberg cells and histiocytic malignancies are derived from activated lymphoid cells. *Blood*. 1985;66:848.
23. Longo DL, Young RC, Wesley M, et al. Twenty years of MOPP therapy for Hodgkin's disease. *J Clin Oncol*. 1986;4:1295.
24. Barry RM, Diamond HD, Graver LF. Influence of pregnancy on the course of Hodgkin's disease. *Am J Obst Gynecol*. 1962;84:445.
25. Kaplan HS. *Hodgkin's Disease*. 2nd ed. Cambridge, MA: Harvard University Press; 1980:300.
26. Glatstein E, Trueblood HW, Enright LP, et al. Surgical staging of abdominal involvement in unselected patients with Hodgkin's disease. *Radiology*. 1970;97:425.
27. Griem ML, Meier P, Dobben GD. Analysis of the morbidity and mortality of children irradiated in fetal life. *Radiology*. 1967;88:347.
28. Sutcliffe SB, Chapman RM. *Lymphomas and Leukemias*. In: Callen HH, Nisker JA, Kisko MT, eds. *Cancer and Pregnancy*. New York: Futura Publishing; 1986:135.
29. Jacobs C, Donaldson SS, Rosenberg S, et al. Management of the pregnant patient with Hodgkin's disease. *Ann Intern Med*. 1981;95:669.
30. Russell LB, Russell WL. An analysis of changing radiation response of the developing mouse embryo. *J Cell Physiol*. 1954;1(suppl):103.
31. Brillo AB, Forgotoson EH. Radiation and congenital malformations. *Am J Obstet Gynecol*. 1964;90:1149.
32. Cowen D, Geller LM. Long-term pathologic effect of prenatal x-irradiation on the central nervous system of the rat. *Neuropathol Exp Neurol*. 1960;488.
33. Bonadonna G, Valagussa P, Santoro A. Alternating non-cross resistant combination chemotherapy or MOPP in Stage IV Hodgkin's disease. A report of 8 year results. *Ann Intern Med*. 1986;104:739.
34. Glick J, Tsiatis A, Chen A, et al. A randomized ECOG trial of alternating MOPP-ABVD vs BCVPP vs BCVPP plus radiotherapy for advanced Hodgkin's disease. *Proc Am Soc Clin Oncol*. 1988;7:223.
35. Levitt SH, Lee CKK, Bloomfield CD. Radical radiation of laparotomy staged Hodgkin's disease patients. *Int J Rad Oncol Biol Phys*. 1984;10:265.
36. Lister TA, Doreen MS, Faux M, et al. The treatment of Stage IIIA Hodgkins disease. *J Clin Oncol*. 1982;1:745.
37. Crowther D, Wagstaff J, Deakin D. A randomized study comparing chemotherapy alone with chemotherapy followed by radiotherapy in

patients with pathologically staged IIIA Hodgkin's disease. *J Clin Oncol.* 1984;2:892.
38. O'Dell RF. Leukemia and lymphoma complicating pregnancy. *Clin Obstet Gynecol.* 1979;22:859.
39. Sweet DL. Malignant lymphoma: implications during the reproductive years in pregnancy. *J Reprod Med.* 1976;17:198.
40. Chapman RM, Crosby WH. Hodgkin's disease and the pregnant patient. *Ann Intern Med.* 1982;96:681.
41. Barber HRK. Fetal and neonatal effects of cytotoxic agents. *Obstet Gynecol.* 1981;58:41S.
42. Donegan WL. Cancer in pregnancy. *Ca—A J Clin.* 1983;33:194.
43. Covington EE, Baker AS. Dosimetry of scattered radiation to the fetus. *JAMA.* 1969;209:414.
44. Zucali R, Marchesini R, De Palo G. Abdominal dosimetry for supradiaphragmatic irradiation of Hodgkin's disease in pregnancy: experimental data and clinical considerations. *Tumori.* 1981;67:203.
45. Nisce LZ, Tome MA, He S, et al. Management of co-existing Hodgkin's disease and pregnancy. *Am J Clin Oncol.* 1986;9:146.
46. Tawil E, Mercier JP, Dandavino A. Hodgkin's disease and complicating pregnancy. *J Can Assoc Radiol.* 1985;36:133.
47. Mulvahill JJ, McKeen EA, Rosner F, et al. Pregnancy outcome in cancer patients: experience in a large cooperative group. *Cancer.* 1987;60:1143.
48. Jones RT, Weinerman BH. MOPP given during prengancy. *Obstet Gynecol.* 1986;54:477.
49. McKeen EA, Mulvahill JJ, Rosner F, et al. Pregnancy outcome in Hodgkin's disease. *Lancet.* 1979;2:590.
50. Smith HN, Spaulding L. Hodgkin's disease in pregnancy. *South Med J.* 1978;71:374.
51. D 'Incalci M, Sessa C, Colombo N, et al. Transplacental passage of cyclophosphamide. *Cancer Treat Rep.* 1982;66:1681.
52. Turchi JJ, Villasis C. Anthracyclines in the treatment of malignancy in pregnancy. *Cancer.* 1988;61:435.
53. Karp GI, Von Oyen P, Valone F, et al. Doxorubicin in pregnancy: possible transplacental passage. *Cancer Treat Rep.* 1983;67:773.
54. Daly H, McCann SR, Hanratty TD. Successful pregnancy during combination chemotherapy for Hodgkin's disease. *Acta Haematol.* (Basel) 1980; 64:154.
55. Gobbi PG, Attardo-Parrinello A, Danesino M, et al. Hodgkin's disease and pregnancy. *Haematol (Pavia).* 1984;69:336.
56. Wiesner-Bornstein R, Niesen M, Grobe-Einsler R, et al. Chemotherapy for Hodgkin's disease during pregnancy: a case report. *Geburtschilfe Frauenheilkd.* 1983;43:373.
57. Thomas PEM, Peckham JJ. The investigation and management of Hodgkin's disease in the pregnant patient. *Cancer.* 1976;38:1443.
58. Schilsky RL, Erlichman C. *Late Complications of Chemotherapy: Infertility and Carcinogenesis from Pharmacologic Principles of Cancer Therapy.* Philadelphia: WB Saunders; 1982:109.
59. Nicholson HO. Cytotoxic drugs in pregnancy. *Obstet Gyn Br Commw.* 1968;75:307.
60. Lacher MJ, Toner K. Pregnancies and menstrual function before and after combined radiation and chemotherapy for Hodgkin's disease. *Cancer Invest.* 1986;4:93.
61. Andrieu JM, Ochoa-Molina ME. Menstrual cycle, pregnancies and offspring before and after MOPP therapy for Hodgkin's disease. *Cancer.* 1983;52:435.
62. Chapman RM, Sutcliffe SB, Malpas JS, et al. Cytotoxic induced ovarian failure in women with Hodgkin's disease. 1. Hormone function. *JAMA.* 1979;242:1877.
63. Chapman RM, Sutcliffe SB, Malpas JS, et al. Cytotoxic induced ovarian failure in Hodgkin's disease. 2. Effects on sexual function. *JAMA.* 1979; 242:1882.
64. Schilsky RL, Sherins RJ, Hubbard SM. Long-term follow-up of ovarian function in women treated with MOPP chemotherapy in Hodgkin's disease. *Am J Med.* 1981;71:552.
65. Holmes GE, Holmes FF. Pregnancy outcome of patients treated for Hodgkin's disease: a controlled study. *Cancer.* 1978;41:1317.
66. Simon R. Statistical methods for evaluating pregnancy outcomes in patients with Hodgkin's disease. *Cancer.* 1980;45:2890.
67. Ward PT, Wein RB. Lymphoma and pregnancy. *Semin Oncol.* 1989;16:397.

Chapter One Hundred and Seventy-Seven

Non-Hodgkin's Lymphoma

Timothy M. Kuzel and Al B. Benson III

177

The non-Hodgkin's lymphomas are a collection of lymphoid malignancies that, because of their shared dissimilarity to Hodgkin's disease, have been placed into a single subheading for taxonomic and research purposes. As clinical and laboratory sophistication has increased, it has become clear that this group of lymphomas contains multiple different subtypes with varied etiologies and prognoses.

EPIDEMIOLOGY

Approximately 15,000 new cases of non-Hodgkin's lymphoma are documented per year in the United States.[1] There is a slightly higher incidence in males than females (1.4:1). Unlike Hodgkin's disease, which is a common entity among women of childbearing age, the incidence of non-Hodgkin's lymphomas among younger individuals is very low; however, occurrence increases rapidly with age.[2] The median incidence during the childbearing years (ages 15–40) is 0.8 cases per 100,000 females compared to females over the age of 70, who are at higher risk (9.5–18.5 cases per 100,000).

During the years 1950–1975 (the last years for which epidemiologic information is available), the mortality rate from the non-Hodgkin's lymphoma had been increasing.[3] For white females, the mortality rate had increased by approximately 2.0% per year over that time period. There are differences with respect to age, sex, and race. The explanation for this increase is unknown; however, recent advances in the use of aggressive chemotherapeutic regimens for some of these lymphomas may reverse this trend.

ETIOLOGY

The recent explosion in the field of molecular genetics has led to a greatly enhanced knowledge of the etiology of the non-Hodgkin's lymphomas. Most malignant tumors and lymphomas now are believed to be associated with chromosomal aberrations, although not all have been identified.[4] These may include point mutations (a change in a single nucleotide base), gene deletions, or translocations (movement of a portion of a chromosome to another location on the same or different chromosome). Examples of such clinically related genetic alterations in the non-Hodgkin's lymphomas include the translocation of c-myc in Burkitt's lymphoma[5], and the translocation of an undefined gene from chromosome 18 to chromosome 14, known as the bcl-2 gene.[6] The mechanism by which these genetic alterations occur is varied. It generally is thought that more than one single mutagenic event must occur to allow development of a malignant clone.[4]

Although most patients have no identifiable predisposing factor for the development of a non-Hodgkin's lymphoma, there are some patient subgroups at greatly increased risk. Several viral agents now are associated with the non-Hodgkin's lymphomas. Epstein–Barr virus (EBV) was the first virus to be so identified and may serve as a model for tumorigenesis. Burkitt's lymphoma, a particularly aggressive lymphoma, is the most common cancer in African children and is associated with high antibody titers to EBV. In the United States, there usually is not an association between Burkitt's lymphoma and EBV infection. The common link between these seemingly different lymphomas now has been established as a translocation of the c-myc oncogene from chromosome 8 to a location following the immunoglobulin heavy chain promoter on chromosome 14.[5] It is speculated that in the African variety of this disorder the exposure to EBV results in a polyclonal expansion of lymphoctyes. With this increase in proliferative activity due to EBV, a second event, the translocation of the c-myc gene, is sufficient to transform a clone of lymphocytes to a malignant phenotype.

Other viruses now are associated with non-Hodgkin's lymphomas. The retroviruses, human immunodeficiency virus (HIV) and human T-lymphotropic virus (HTLV-1), both have been identified as risk factors for the development of large cell lymphomas of the B-cell and T-cell type, respectively.[7,8] Whether the mechanism by which these viruses cause the lymphomas is related to viral insertion in the host chromosome, co-infection with other viruses such as EBV, or generalized immunodeficiency is not clear (see below). With the rapid increase in the incidence of HIV infection in the female population, especially younger female intravenous drug abusers and prostitutes, there may be an associated increase in the incidence of non-Hodgkin's lymphomas.

Immunosuppression, whether primary or iatrogenic, also is considered a risk factor for the development of non-Hodgkin's lymphoma.[9,10] This risk depends on the exact nature of the immunosuppressive condition. It ranges from a 10- to 100-fold increase in patients with kidney or heart transplants on chronic immunosuppressive therapy, to a 1000-fold increased risk in patients with primary immunodeficiency syndromes. Again, the mechanism responsible for this phenomenon is unknown; however, susceptibility to co-infection with viruses such as EBV may be responsible.

Several other disease states have been associated with increased risk. These include celiac disease[11], angioimmunoblastic lymphadenopathy[12], and possibly some of the rheumatologic conditions such as Sjogren's syndrome[13], systemic lupus erythematosus, or rheumatoid arthritis.

Environmental factors may contribute to the development of non-Hodgkin's lymphomas. The survivors of the atomic bombs dropped on Japan during World War II show a slight increase in the incidence of these lymphomas.[14] Workers in certain chemical and manufacturing industries may have a slightly increased risk, but the epidemiologic data are not compelling at this time.

CLASSIFICATION AND PATHOGENESIS

The current classification scheme for the non-Hodgkin's lymphomas was developed in the early 1980s by a National Cancer Institute expert panel of pathologists.[15] This system, known as the Working Formulation of Non-Hodgkin's Lymphomas for Clinical Usage, is based on morphologic criteria and clinical behavior. Three main groupings have been created consisting of low-, intermediate, or high-grade lymphomas. Within each main heading are multiple lymphomas described by their morphologic appearance (Table 177–1). There are several non-Hodgkin's lymphomas that defy inclusion in this classification scheme and are listed as miscellaneous. These include mycosis fungoides, the true histiocytic lymphomas, and extramedullary plasmacytomas.

TABLE 177–1. WORKING FORMULATION OF THE NON-HODGKIN'S LYMPHOMAS

Low Grade
Small lymphocytic, chronic lymphocytic leukemia
Small lymphocytic, plasmacytoid
Follicular, predominantly small cleaved cell
Follicular, mixed, small cleaved and large cell
Intermediate Grade
Follicular, predominantly large cell
Diffuse, small cleaved cell
Diffuse, mixed, small and large cell
Diffuse, large cell cleaved or noncleaved
High Grade
Large cell, immunoblastic
Lymphoblastic
Diffuse, small cell, noncleaved
Histiocytic

Recently, advances in the area of immunology also have permitted identification of malignant lymphocytes as B cells or T cells. This information has not been incorporated into any classification scheme, but in the future may be useful for prognostication. Most of the non-Hodgkin's lymphomas are of B-cell origin (80%), and a minority are of T-cell origin (20%).

Several general comments can be made regarding the behavior of these lymphomas related to their histology. Follicular lymphomas (previously known as nodular) retain some of the normal architectural appearance of normal lymph nodes and generally confer a better prognosis. These lymphomas frequently are slower growing than their counterpart, the diffuse lymphomas, which have total effacement of the nodal architecture. Small "cleaved" malignant lymphocytes tend to be widespread at diagnosis, but paradoxically, they behave more indolently than the frequently more localized large malignant lymphocytes. Lymphomas composed of small noncleaved lymphoctyes (consistent with Burkitt's lymphoma) or large immature cells (immunoblastic lymphoma) tend to be very aggressive.

In the working formulation the low-grade lymphomas have a favorable prognosis. Several studies have followed patients with these lymphomas without treatment after diagnosis. Relatively nonaggressive chemotherapy was given to control symptoms as they developed. These studies revealed median 10-year actuarial survivals ranging from 49% to 73%.[16-18]

In contrast, there is often a poor outcome in patients with high-grade aggressive lymphomas. Despite recent development of multi-drug chemotherapy regimens, a significant proportion of these patients die of their disease (currently 30–40% of patients may achieve long-term remissions).

The prognosis for patients with intermediate grade lymphomas, especially the diffuse large cell lymphomas, currently is difficult to define. Although these lymphomas tend to be rapidly growing, several recent multi-drug chemotherapy regimens have been developed that induce high rates of complete remission (approximately 75%).[19,20] Whether cure rates will remain as high will be determined by more extended patient follow-up.

DIAGNOSIS AND STAGING

To establish the diagnosis of a non-Hodgkin's lymphoma, it is necessary to perform a biopsy of the involved tissue, which in most cases is a lymph node. Simple needle aspiration of an enlarged node may suggest a malignancy; however, to establish the exact diagnosis it is imperative to evaluate the nodal architecture by biopsy.

Once the diagnosis is made, the staging evaluation must be considered (see Table 177–2). In nonpregnant individuals this requires review of a chest x-ray, computed tomographic (CT) or magnetic resonance (MR) imaging of the abdomen and pelvis, and usually bilateral iliac crest bone marrow aspiration and biopsy. In the case of advanced high-grade lymphomas, a lumbar puncture to assess for central nervous system involvement may be warranted, especially if the bone marrow is found to be involved. These tests allow for detection of intra-abdominal adenopathy, subtle hepatomegaly or splenomegaly and possible involvement of body cavities not accessible by physical examination. This standard evaluation, however, cannot be safely performed in most pregnant women. The use of CT scans is contraindicated because of the risk of radiation exposure. There is currently insufficient data to determine the safety of MR scans in pregnant women. Consequently, many centers are unwilling to perform these scans in this setting. Thus, a minimum evaluation for the pregnant woman diagnosed with a non-Hodgkin's lymphoma should include routine blood counts, serum chemistries (especially liver function tests, alkaline phosphatase and lactate dehydrogenase), chest x-ray with abdominal shielding, and bone marrow biopsies.

TREATMENT

The subsequent management of the pregnant lymphoma patient must be individualized based on the type of lymphoma and evidence of imminent harm to mother or fetus. In light of the very indolent nature of the low-grade follicular non-Hodgkin's lymphomas, it may be reasonable to closely observe the mother for any change in her or the fetus's condition. After the fetus is viable for an induced vaginal or cesarean delivery, the decision of whether to administer chemotherapy (usually an alkylating agent, such as chlorambucil, combined with steroids) can be made. If, however, the pregnant woman's health is jeopardized by the lymphoma, a therapeutic abortion should be recommended.

The intermediate and high-grade lymphomas raise different problems. The clinical course of such lymphomas is typically that of a fairly rapid progression of disease, even over a matter of weeks. Therefore, if the pregnancy is in the first or early second trimester, a therapeutic abortion is warranted so that treatment can be initiated with one of the multi-drug aggressive chemotherapy regimens. These regimens involve the use of multiple non-cross-resistant chemotherapeutic agents given intensively (weekly or every other week) (see Table 177–3).

The proper approach in the late second or third trimester is more difficult to specify. There are several case reports of such women treated with aggressive chemotherapy regimens while pregnant.[21,22] One case involved the treatment of a woman who developed Burkitt's lymphoma in the 28th week of gestation. One week after initiation of chemotherapy premature labor developed. The mother died four days after delivering a premature live newborn. After 3 years' follow up, the child continues to develop normally. The other reported case involved the treatment of a woman who developed acute T-cell lymphoblastic leukemia with a large mediastinal mass at 32 weeks' gestation. Three weeks after receiving induction chemotherapy, she delivered a healthy female infant. At 16 months of follow up, this woman remains in remission, and the infant is also healthy. Overall, these cases demonstrate the potential for harm to both mother and fetus with these treatments, although in one case both appear to be healthy. In these cases, the mother should be given a clear explanation of the potential hazards, including the late development of second malignancies such as acute leukemia in the mother or child.

TABLE 177–2. ROUTINE STAGING EVALUATION FOR NONPREGNANT PATIENTS WITH NON-HODGKIN'S LYMPHOMA

Blood counts
Serum chemistries (including alkaline phosphatase and lactate dehydrogenase)
Chest x-ray
CT scan or MRI scan of abdomen and pelvis
Bilateral bone marrow aspiration and biopsy
Lumbar puncture (optional depending on histology)

TABLE 177–3. EXAMPLES OF CHEMOTHERAPY REGIMENS FOR THE TREATMENT OF INTERMEDIATE AND ADVANCED NON-HODGKIN'S LYMPHOMA

CHOP
Cyclophosphamide
Doxorubicin
Vincristine
Prednisone
MACOP-B
Cyclophosphamide
Doxorubicin
Vincristine
Methotrexate
Bleomycin
Prednisone
ProMACE-CytaBOM
Cyclophosphamide
Doxorubicin
Etoposide
Cytarabine
Bleomycin
Vincristine
Methotrexate
Prednisone

In conclusion, non-Hodgkin's lymphomas are infrequent in women of childbearing age. They may become more common, however, if there is continued spread of such viruses as HIV and HTLV-1 into the heterosexual population. Careful pathologic review is necessary to confirm the diagnosis and establish an accurate prognosis. There is currently no data to suggest that pregnancy worsens the prognosis of women with a pre-existing non-Hodgkin's lymphoma.[23] As improved chemotherapeutic interventions become available, it may be possible to further improve the survival of these patients in all situations.

REFERENCES

1. Bakemeier RF, Zagars G, Cooper RA, Rubin P. The malignant lymphomas: Hodgkin's disease and non-Hodgkin's lymphoma, multiple myeloma, and macroglobulinemia. In: *Clinical Oncology: A Multidisciplinary Approach*. 6th ed. The American Cancer Society; 1983.
2. Muir C, Waterhouse J, Mack T, Powell J, Whelan S. *Cancer Incidence in Five Continents-Volume V*. Oxford: Oxford Press; 1987.
3. Cantor KP, Graumeni JF Jr. Geographic and temporal patterns of non-Hodgkin's lymphoma mortality in U.S. Counties, 1950–1975. *Cancer Res*. 1980;40:2645.
4. Bishop JM. The molecular genetics of cancer. *Science*. 1987;235:305.
5. Taub R, Kirsch I, Morton C, et al. Translocation of the c-myc gene into the immunoglobulin heavy chain locus in human Burkitt's lymphoma and murine plasmacytoma cells. *Proc Natl Acad Sci USA*. 1982; 79:7837.
6. Yunis JJ, Oken MM, Kaplan ME. Distinctive chromosomal abnormalities in histologic subtypes of non-Hodgkin's lymphomas. *N Engl J Med*. 1982;307:1231.
7. Centers for Disease Control. Diffuse, undifferentiated non-Hodgkin's lymphoma among homosexual males: United States. *MMWR*. 1982; 31:277.
8. Gibbs WN, Lofters WS, Campbell M, et al. Non-Hodgkin's lymphoma in Jamaica and its relation to adult T-cell leukemia-lymphoma. *Ann Intern Med*. 1987;106:361.
9. Fraumeni JF Jr, Hoover R. Immunosurveillance and cancer: epidemiologic considerations. *Natl Cancer Inst Monog*. 1977;47:121.
10. Kinlen LJ, Schiel AGR, Peto J, et al. A collaborative study of cancer in patients who received immunosuppressive therapy. *Br Med J*. 1979; 2:1461.
11. Holmes GKT, Stokes PL, Sorahan TM, et al. Celiac disease, gluten-free diet and malignancy. *Gut*. 1976;17:612.
12. Frizzera G, Moran EM, Rappaport H. Angioimmunoblastic lymphadenopathy with dysproteinemia. *Lancet*. 1974;1:1070.
13. Kassan SS, Thomas TL, Moutsopoulos HM, et al. Increased risk of lymphomas in sicca syndrome. *Ann Intern Med*. 1978;89:888.
14. Nishiyama H, Anderson RE, Ishimaru T, et al. The incidence of malignant lymphoma and multiple myeloma in Hiroshima and Nagasaki atomic bomb survivors, 1945–1965. *Cancer*. 1973;32:1301.
15. The Non-Hodgkin's Lymphoma Pathologic Classification Project. National Cancer Institute Sponsored Study of Classifications of Non-Hodgkin's Lymphomas. *Cancer*. 1982;49:2112.
16. Hoppe RT, Kushlan P, Kaplan HS, et al. The treatment of advanced stage favorable histology non-Hodgkin's lymphoma: a preliminary report of a randomized trial comparing single agent chemotherapy, combination chemotherapy and whole body irradiation. *Blood*. 1981;58(3):592.
17. Horning SJ, Rosenberg SA. The natural history of initially untreated low-grade non-Hodgkin's lymphomas. *N Engl J Med*. 1984;311:1471.
18. Morrison WH, Hoppe RT, Weiss LM, et al. Small lymphocytic lymphoma. *J Clin Oncol*. 1989;7:598.
19. Fisher RI, DeVita VT Jr, Hubbard SM, et al. Diffise aggressive lymphomas: increased survival after alternating flexible sequences of ProMACE and MOPP chemotherapy. *Ann Intern Med*. 1983;98:304.
20. Skarin AT, Canellos GP, Rosenthal DS, et al. Improved prognosis of diffuse histiocytic and undifferentiated lymphoma by use of high-dose methotrexate alternating with Standard Agents (M-BACOD). *J Clin Oncol*. 1983;1:91.
21. Berrebi A, Schallner AB, Mogilner BM. Disseminated Burkitt's lymphoma during pregnancy. *Acta Haemat*. 1983;70:139.
22. Sigler E, Varon D, Lugassy G. Favorable outcome in T-cell acute lymphoblastic leukemia with mediastinal mass during pregnancy. *Am J Med*. 1988;85:125.
23. Ward FT, Wein R. Lymphoma and pregnancy. *Semin Oncol*. 1989;16:397.

Chapter One Hundred and Seventy-Eight
Primary Carcinoma of the Skin

Elise A. Olsen

178

The incidence of primary carcinoma of the skin in the general population is 422 in 100,000 or about 25% of all cancers combined.[1] The most common primary carcinomas of the skin are basal cell carcinoma and squamous cell carcinoma. They are seen predominantly in the middle-aged or elderly. This may be secondary to cumulative sun exposure. The incidence of skin cancer in the United States doubles for each 3°48′ latitude change south. Certain other predisposing exogenous, endogenous, and genetic factors also place younger populations, including women of childbearing potential, at risk. Although neither of these carcinomas is more frequent or behaves differently in pregnant women, certain premalignant skin conditions are more common in pregnancy and therefore deserve special consideration.

Some 30–35% of melanoma patients are women of childbearing potential. Pregnancy clearly affects the growth of melanoma, but changes in survival are probably more dependent on stage of disease. Of the primary carcinomas, melanoma represents the greatest physical risk to pregnant women.

BASAL CELL CARCINOMA

Etiology

Basal cell carcinomas constitute 60–75% of all primary skin cancers. They are slow-growing tumors with a capacity for local destruction and great clinical variability.[2] The typical basal cell carcinoma is a translucent papule or nodule with or without pigment, ulceration, or a raised border and with a few overlying telangiectatic vessels. Other variants include morpheiform basal cell carcinoma, which presents as a firm superficial telangiectatic plaque, and superficial basal cell carcinoma, which presents as an erythematous scaling macule or patch. Basal cell carcinomas are most prone to develop in sun-exposed areas, but about one third of them occur in light-protected areas. Patients with *xeroderma pigmentosum*, a hereditary condition in which an endonuclease normally utilized to repair UVL-induced changes is deficient or absent, are particularly prone to the development of basal cell carcinomas and squamous cell carcinomas at an early age.[3] Exposure to inorganic arsenic and ionizing radiation are also predisposing factors for skin cancer.

Basal cell carcinomas occur in 6–50% of *syringocystadenoma papilliferum,* a congenital adnexal tumor. These benign tumors are usually flat, inconspicuous macules or papules in the scalp that, because of their sebaceous origin, become larger and verrucous at puberty. The most common genetic syndrome associated with basal cell carcinoma is the *basal cell nevus syndrome.*[4] In this dominantly inherited disorder, multiple basal cell carcinomas appear at puberty and are associated with palmar pits, jaw cysts, mandibular prognathism, lateral displacement of the inner canthi, frontal bossing, kyphoscoliosis, fused ribs, and calcification of the falx cerebri.

Pathophysiology

Basal cell carcinomas are derived from pluripotential epithelial cells and exhibit stromal dependence and low autonomy, which may account for the rarity of metastasis. When metastases do occur, they usually appear 4–25 years after the initial appearance of the tumor and after repeated treatments, including x-ray therapy. Metastases are associated in 68% of cases with local node involvement and an average patient survival of 10 months.

Effects of Pregnancy on Disease

Basal cell carcinomas are neither more frequent nor more aggressive during pregnancy.

Diagnosis

The clinical appearance of a slow-growing papule with overlying telangiectasia in a sun-exposed area is a basal cell carcinoma until biopsy proves otherwise. Differential diagnosis may include squamous cell carcinoma, trichoepithelioma (a benign appendigeal tumor), seborrheic keratosis, nevus, amelanotic melanoma or Bowen's disease.

Treatment

The treatment of small basal cell carcinomas by experienced physicians, using either curettage and electrodesiccation or surgical excision, has a 95% cure rate and can be done under local anesthesia even during pregnancy. There are certain high-recurrence areas, that is, the nasolabial fold, medial canthus, posterior auricular region, and scalp. Mohs' micrographic surgery (microscopically controlled surgery), performed under local anesthesia, may be the primary treatment of choice in these areas or in recurrent tumors in any location. In Mohs' micrographic surgery, a layer of tumor first is excised and marked with indelible dye. Orientation of the tissue thus is preserved when the frozen section is examined under light microscopy, and determination of deep and lateral tumor-free margins then can be ascertained. If residual tumor is present, further excision in that area and repetition of the above procedure are done until all margins are free of cancer. This ensures both removal of clinically inapparent tumor and preservation of as much normal tissue as possible.

SQUAMOUS CELL CARCINOMA

Etiology

Squamous cell carcinoma, like basal cell carcinoma, is most common in older males. When it is seen in younger patients, a search should be made for a number of predisposing factors.[5] The majority of squamous cell carcinomas are preceded by intraepidermal neoplasias or premalignant lesions, including solar keratoses, Bowen's disease, or leukoplakia. Inorganic arsenic, hydrocarbon fractions, ionizing radiation as well as chronic scars, ulcers, and sinus tracts are associated with the development of squamous cell carcinoma after a 20 to 30-year latency period. Cumulative ultraviolet light exposure for social, occupational, or medicinal reasons is the most common predisposing factor. Patients with psoriasis, who are treated with UVB or PUVA (an acronym for psoralen plus long-wave UVA), have an earlier onset and a higher incidence of squamous cell carcinoma.[6] Those Caucasians who always burn and never tan after sun exposure are particularly at risk, as are albinos, or whites with vitiligo.

Certainly, melanin plays a protective role, but genetic factors also are important. Celts, whether in their native environment or in other locations, have a higher risk of squamous cell carcinoma, as do patients with xeroderma pigmentosum who have defective repair mechanisms for DNA damaged by ultraviolet light. Most genetic syndromes associated with squamous cell carcinoma will have been diagnosed by the time a woman reaches the childbearing years because of other cutaneous or systemic manifestations. However, the true nature of *epidermodysplasia verruciformis,* an autosomal recessive disorder of flat, wartlike lesions, may go unrecognized for years. The lesions of epidermodysplasia verruciformis are caused by human papilloma virus and are associated with malignant degeneration to Bowen's disease, or squamous cell carcinoma.[7]

Pathophysiology

Clinically, squamous cell carcinoma presents as an erythematous indurated area with indistinct margins that may progress to a verrucous, papillomatous, or ulcerated lesion with crusting, scaling, and a raised border. Those that arise from solar keratoses are generally slowly growing and locally invasive. In contrast, those squamous cell carcinomas that evolve from prior Bowen's lesions, radiation damage, chronic skin breakdown, or normal skin are more likely to be rapidly and widely invasive with a potential for metastasis in greater than 10–20% of cases. The size, depth of invasion, and degree of anaplasia also correlate with an increased risk of metastasis. Squamous cell carcinoma in certain areas of the body, ie, the lips, vulva, penis, and anus, is more aggressive. In 50% of cases, squamous cell carcinoma of the vulva is metastatic to the lymph nodes at the time of diagnosis.

Effects of Pregnancy on Disease

Squamous cell carcinomas are neither more frequent nor more aggressive during pregnancy.

Diagnosis

Any isolated papule on a sun-exposed area that is scaly, ulcerated, or bleeds easily with trauma is potentially a squamous cell carcinoma and requires biopsy. A shave biopsy should suffice but will require further excision for definitive treatment. Differential diagnosis includes actinic keratosis, Bowen's disease, keratoacanthoma, basal cell carcinoma, irritated seborrheic keratosis, and verruca vulgaris.

Treatment

Electrosurgery, excision, and Mohs' micrographic surgery of squamous cell carcinoma are all easily done under local anesthesia with an excellent chance for cure if performed early and with adequate margins taken. Pregnancy should not affect the natural history or delay treatment of the primary lesion.

INTRAEPIDERMAL NEOPLASIA

Etiology

Intraepidermal neoplasia on the trunk and extremities occurs mainly in older patients in the same basic risk groups as squamous cell carcinoma and basal cell carcinoma. In these locations, Bowen's disease is synonomous histologically with squamous cell carcinoma *in situ* and clinically presents as an erythematous scaling macule or patch. Twenty years ago, vulvar intraepithelial neoplasia (VIN) was also a unifocal disease occurring mainly in older women.[8,9] Recently, patients with VIN have been younger, with the highest incidence seen in the childbearing years.[8-10]

There is a high incidence of associated sexually transmitted diseases, particularly *condylomata acuminata* in these younger patients with VIN III[10], as well as a greater likelihood of multifocal disease in the vulvar area, vagina, and cervix.[9,11,12] Indirect evidence for human papilloma virus (HPV) involvement in VIN III (previously termed severe dysplasia, squamous cell carcinoma *in situ*, Bowen's disease or erythroplasia of Queyrat[8,11]) include:

1. HPV DNA being isolated in 72–90% of VIN lesions[8,13]
2. Increased likelihood of recurrent disease when HPV DNA is present in clinically normal epithelial cells adjacent to treated areas of VIN III[8]
3. Sexual consorts of patients with HPV-related carcinomas are likely to have genital warts or HPV-related penile carcinoma *in situ*[8]
4. Appreciable number of cases of VIN III have cervical dysplasia or carcinoma *in situ*, in which HPV DNA can be recovered.[8]

HPV-16 is the most common type of HPV-DNA isolated in VIN, with HPV subtypes 6 and 2 occasionally found.[12]

Pathophysiology

The most common symptoms of VIN are vulvar pruritus or irritation, but 11–62% of women are asymptomatic.[11,14-16] Clinically, there is great variability: The disease may present as raised, velvety red or white patches or, more frequently, in young women as multifocal pigmented dome-shaped to verrucous papules.[9,17,18] The latter have been termed Bowenoid dysplasia or Bowenoid papulosis and frequently are associated with pregnancy.[17] Histologically, VIN shows parakeratosis and epithelial disorganization throughout the epidermis. Bowenoid papulosis may be viewed as a less severe form of VIN, as histologically these lesions show relative cellular uniformity, lack of anaplasia, and sparing of the dermoepidermal junction.[17,18]

Spontaneous regression of VIN has been documented, especially in cases of Bowenoid papulosis.[17,19] In general, younger women with VIN have a low risk of progression to cancer compared to older women with "classical" VIN. In one study, 24% of women ≥40 years old with VIN versus 0% of women <40 years old with VIN developed invasive carcinoma over a three-year follow up.[16]

Effects of Pregnancy on Disease

Patients with VIN have been noted to have depressed *in vitro* lymphocyte transformation when compared to age-matched controls.[20] Case reports of spontaneous postpartum regression of VIN lesions, which developed during pregnancy, have been noted[17,19,21,22] and may be due to changes in the maternal immune system.

Diagnosis

Clinically suspicious lesions require a biopsy for confirmation. The application of 1% aqueous toluidine blue to suspicious areas will aid in choosing an appropriate biopsy site.[11] As a nuclear stain, toluidine blue, applied for three minutes, will fix to areas where epidermal nuclei are located superficially (ie, parakeratosis). A subsequent 1% acetic acid wash will remove the stain from normal acellular keratin. False positive may be seen with ulcerations and fissures.

Treatment

In elderly women, in whom the risk of invasive carcinoma is greater, vulvectomy or possibly surgical excision with margins of approximately 1 cm is desirable.[8] In young women with multicentric disease, a variety of surgical approaches can be taken. Modified vulvectomy, laser ablation, cryosurgery, or electrodessication may all be used. The most important single factor in preventing recurrent disease is the ability to achieve histologically confirmed tumor-free margins in resections, but unfortunately, clinical appearance is often misleading. In those patients with VIN who were treated with surgical excision with a 2-mm clinically-free margin, there was a 28% recurrence rate. In those with histologic involvement of the edges, the recurrence rate was 58%, versus 4% for those with histologically clear edges.[14] Wider margins may decrease recurrence rate or, alternatively, utilizing Mohs' micrographic surgery, would automatically provide a tissue margin free of tumor or dysplasia, while allowing maximal preservation of normal tissue.[23]

Since there is a chance of spontaneous regression in VIN, a conservative approach to therapy during pregnancy appears indicated. It thus seems prudent to treat pregnant women with one of the locally ablative procedures, reserving vulvectomy for those with proven evidence of recalcitrant or progressive disease after a short observation period postpartum.

Due to the potential multifocal nature of VIN, especially in young women, patients should have a careful vaginal and cervical examination for other potential sites of intraepithelial carcinoma. Sexual partners should be evaluated for the presence of condylomata or other HPV-related intraepithelial neoplasia.

MELANOMA

Etiology

The incidence of malignant melanoma has at least doubled since the early 1970s.[24] This may be related to earlier recognition of melanoma but also may be related to environmental or hereditary factors. Indirect evidence implicates solar exposure, particularly severe sunburn, as a predisposing factor.[25-27] At least 6% of patients with malignant melanoma report a family history of melanoma.[24] Patients with multiple dysplastic nevi and a family history of melanoma are at particular risk to develop melanoma.[28,29] There is emerging clinical evidence that nonfamilial acquired dysplastic nevi also may be a melanoma risk factor.[30,31] Congenital nevi have a malignant potential with the greatest risk of malignant change in children ≤10 years old.[24]

Pathophysiology

It is estimated that ≥11,000 women will develop melanoma yearly[32], and as the highest incidence of malignant melanoma is in the 20 to 40-year age range, a substantial number of pregnant women are at risk. A number of lines of evidence indicate an endocrine influence on malignant melanoma. The survival of women with melanoma is superior to that of men with melanoma.[33] Premenopausal women experience better survival than postmenopausal women with melanoma.[34] Melanocytic nevi may develop changes in their size, shape, and pigmentation during pregnancy[35], and it has been noted that there is increased progesterone and estrogen binding by nevus cells.[36] Melanocyte stimulating hormone (MSH) rises progressively during pregnancy.[37]

Foucar et al[38] noted an added risk for nevi to become malignant during pregnancy, although their study did exclude patients with dysplastic nevi. Like melanomas, dysplastic nevi exhibit increased progesterone and estrogen binding, when compared to nevi from nonpregnant controls.[39] Patients with the dysplastic nevi syndrome deserve special attention paid to their pigmented lesions at all times, especially during pregnancy.

Effects of Pregnancy on Disease

Whether pregnancy adversely affects the survival of either the woman with a diagnosis of melanoma made during pregnancy or the pregnant woman with prior diagnosis and treatment of melanoma has remained a controversial issue. Hershey et al[40] and Bork et al[41] have shown that multiparous women have better survival rates than nulliparous women with melanoma. Others have not been able to substantiate this conclusion.[42,43] Shiu et al[44] demonstrated that although pregnancy did not adversely affect survival in patients with Stage I melanoma, women with Stage II melanoma, who had activation of their disease during pregnancy or whose melanoma was treated during pregnancy, had a significantly worse survival rate than nulliparous patients or those with no activation of their melanoma during a prior pregnancy. A retrospective 10-year study of melanoma in pregnant women at Duke University Medical Center, using age, melanoma site, stage, thickness level, Clark's level, ulceration and histologic type-matched controls, also suggested a significantly worse prognosis during pregnancy for Stage I melanoma patients.[45] This study also showed that a subsequent pregnancy, after diagnosis and treatment of a Stage I melanoma, had no effect on recurrence rate or survival. These conclusions are substantiated by the work of Sutherland et al.[46] It generally is recommended that women with advanced stages of melanoma avoid future pregnancies for 3–5 years.[47]

Effect of Disease on Pregnancy and the Fetus

Although rare, malignant melanoma may metastasize to the placenta from either fetal or maternal tumors.[48] Maternal metastatic disease to the placenta is indicative of widespread hematogenous metastasis; these women usually die within a few months. Some, but not all, infants born of women with placental metastasis develop melanoma. Those who do usually die within the first year of life.[48,49]

Women with advanced or recurrent melanoma diagnosed during pregnancy should undergo ultrasound examinations during pregnancy to assess any obvious fetal tumor masses with particular attention to placental thickness and size of fetal liver and spleen.[49] If the ultrasound is suspicious, diagnosis should be confirmed by fetoscopy or umbilical cord sampling and early delivery should be discussed with the patient. If the ultrasound examinations are negative and there is no obvious involvement at birth, the cord blood should be examined for malignant cells and the placenta examined grossly and histologically. Apparently uninvolved infants will still require careful and extensive evaluation with continued follow up for at least one year, including visual skin inspection, ultrasound monitoring of the liver, and possibly, urine screening for melanogens. Urine 5-S-cysteinyldopa and 6-hydroxy-5-methoxyindole-2-carboxylic acid are melanoma markers unaffected by pregnancy or oral contraceptive use.[50]

Primary congenital melanoma of the fetus is rare and unpredictable. The placenta must be examined closely for signs of metastasis and the mother followed closely for evidence of melanoma using the same techniques as outlined above for the at-risk infants.

Diagnosis

The diagnosis of melanoma during pregnancy is no different from that outside of pregnancy. The changes of prime importance in a pigmented lesion are (1) a variegation in color, particularly with shades of blue, red, or white, or unevenness of pigment distribution; (2) irregular borders with notching; (3) increase in size; and (4) irregular topography.[25] A prompt biopsy of suspicious lesions is necessary as the survival of melanoma patients directly correlates with depth of tumor invasion. Small lesions may be excised *in toto.* Large lesions may be biopsied first by a punch or excision of the most infiltrated appearing area. A shave excision should never be performed as it may eradicate the ability to do staging based on the depth of the lesion.

Treatment

Treatment of a solitary melanoma is by surgical excision or regional lymph node resection after determination of stage of disease. Adjuvant immunotherapy with irradiated allogeneic melanoma cells with bacillus Calmette-Guerin (BCG)[45] or interferon alpha[51] or chemotherapy[25] may decrease recurrence rates and improve overall survival in patients with extensive disease.[27] Except for the use of BCG, these generally are withheld until after delivery. Some patients may note a spontaneous regression in their melanoma postpartum.[47]

REFERENCES

1. Popkin GL, DeFeo CP. Basal cell epithelioma. In: Andrade R, Gumport SL, Popkin GL, et al, eds. *Cancer of the Skin.* Philadelphia: WB Saunders; 1976:821.
2. Pollack SV, Goslin JB, Sherertz EF, et al. The biology of basal cell carcinoma: a review. *J Am Acad Dermatol.* 1982;7:569.
3. Burgess GH, Jager BV. Basal cell epithelioma. In: Helm F, ed. *Cancer Dermatology.* Philadelphia: Lea and Febiger; 1979:91.
4. Burgdorf WHC. Dermatopathologic aspects of cancer-associated genodermatoses. In: Lynch HT, Fusaro RM, eds. *Cancer Associated Genodermatoses.* New York: Van Nostrand Reinhold; 1982:155.
5. Stoll HL Jr. Squamous cell carcinoma. In: Helm F, ed. *Cancer Dermatology.* Philadelphia: Lea & Febiger; 1979:113.
6. Stern RS, Parrish JA, Bleich HL, et al. PUVA (psoralen and ultraviolet A) and squamous cell carcinoma in patients with psoriasis. *J Invest Dermatol.* 1981;76:311.
7. Lutzner MA, Blanchet-Bardon C, Orth G. Clinical observations, virologic studies, and treatment trials in patients with epidermodysplasia verruciformis, a disease induced specific human papillomaviruses. *J Invest Dermatol.* 1984;83(suppl):18s.
8. Lynch PJ. Vulvar dystrophies and intraepithelial neoplasias. *Dermatol Clin.* 1987;5:789.
9. Benedet JL, Murphy KJ. Squamous carcinoma in situ of the vulva. *Gynecol Oncol.* 1982;14:213.
10. Noumoff JS, Farber M. Tumors of the vulva. *Int J Dermatol.* 1986;25:552.
11. Sanchez NP, Mihm MC Jr. Reactive and neoplastic epithelial alterations of the vulva. *J Am Acad Dermatol.* 1982;6:378.
12. Bornstein J, Kaufman RH, Adam E, Adler-Storthz K. Multicentric intraepithelial neoplasia involving the vulva. *Cancer.* 1988;62:1601.
13. Twiggs LB, Okagaki T, Clark B, et al. A clinical, histopathologic, and molecular biologic investigation of vulvar intraepithelial neoplasia. *Int J Gynecol Pathol.* 1988;7:48.
14. Adreasson B, Bock JE. Intraepithelial neoplasia in the vulvar region. *Gynecol Oncol.* 1985;21:300.

15. Ragnarsson B, Raabe N, Willems J, Pettersson F. Carcinoma in situ of the vulva. *Acta Oncol.* 1987;26:277.
16. Crum CP, Liskow A, Petras P, et al. Vulvar intraepithelial neoplasia (severe atypia and carcinoma in situ). *Cancer.* 1984;54:1429.
17. Ulbright TM, Stehman FB, Roth LM, et al. Bowenoid dysplasia of the vulva. *Cancer.* 1982;50:2910.
18. Patterson JW, Kao GF, Graham JH, Helwig EB. Bowenoid papulosis: a clinicopathologic study with ultrastructural observations. *Cancer.* 1986;57:823.
19. Kimura S. Bowenoid papulosis of the genitalia. *Int J Dermatol.* 1982;21:432.
20. Seski JC, Reinhalter ER, Silva J Jr. Abnormalities of lymphocyte transformations in women with intraepithelial carcinoma of the vulva. *Obstet Gynecol.* 1978;52:332.
21. Skinner MS, Sternberg WH, Ichinose H, et al. Spontaneous regression of Bowenoid atypia of the vulva. *Obstet Gynecol.* 1973;42:40.
22. Friedrich EG, Wilkinson EJ, Fu YS. Carcinoma in situ of the vulva: a continuing challenge. *Am J Obstet Gynecol.* 1980;136:830.
23. Siegle RJ, Headington JT, Swanson NA. Early invasive carcinoma of the vulva treated with Mohs technique of microscopically controlled surgery. *Am J Obstet Gynecol.* 1985;147:459.
24. Fitzpatrick TB, Sober AJ, Mihm MC Jr, Day CL Jr. Malignant melanoma of the skin. In: Petersdorf RG, Adams RD, Braunwald E, et al, eds. *Principles of Internal Medicine.* 10th ed. New York: McGraw-Hill; 1983:836.
25. Sober AJ, Fitzpatrick TB, Mihm MC Jr. Primary melanoma of the skin: recognition and management. *J Am Acad Dermatol.* 1980;2:179.
26. Green A, Siskind V, Bain C, Alexander J. Sunburn and malignant melanoma. *Br J Cancer.* 1985;51:393.
27. Weinstock MA, Colditz GA, Willett WC, et al. Nonfamilial cutaneous melanoma incidence in women associated with sun exposure before 20 years of age. *Pediatrics.* 1989;84:199.
28. Duray PH, Ernstoff MS. Dysplastic nevus in histologic contiguity with acquired nonfamilial melanoma. *Arch Dermatol.* 1987;123:80.
29. Swerdlow AJ, Green A. Melanocytic naevi and melanoma: an epidemiological perspective. *Br J Dermatol.* 1987;117:137.
30. Rhodes AR. Melanocytic precursors of cutaneous melanoma. Estimated risk and guidelines for management. *Med Clin North Am.* 1986;70:3.
31. Rigel DS, Rivers JK, Kopf AW, et al. Dysplastic nevi: markers for increased risk for melanoma. *Cancer.* 1989;63:386.
32. Silverberg E, Lubera J. *Cancer Statistics. Cancer.* 1986;36:9.
33. Reintgen DS, Paull DE, Seigler HF, et al. Sex related survival differences in instances of melanoma. *Surg Gynecol Obstet.* 1984;159:367.
34. Shaw HM, Milton GW, Farago G, McCarthy WH. Endocrine influences on survival from malignant melanoma. *Cancer.* 1978;42:669.
35. Sanchez JL, Figueroa LD, Rodriguez E. Behavior of melanocytic nevi during pregnancy. *Am J Dermatopathol.* 1984;6(suppl1):89.
36. Ellis DL, Wheeland RG. Increased nevus estrogen and progesterone ligand binding related to oral contraceptives or pregnancy. *J Am Acad Dermatol.* 1986;14:25.
37. Ances IG, Pomerantz SH. Serum concentrations of β-melanocyte–stimulating hormone in human pregnancy. *Am J Obstet Gynecol.* 1974;119:1062.
38. Foucar E, Bentley TJ, Laube DW, Rosai J. A histopathologic evaluation of nevocellular nevi in pregnancy. *Arch Dermatol.* 1985;121:350.
39. Ellis DL, Wheeland RG, Solomon H. Estrogen and progesterone receptors in primary cutaneous melanoma. *J Dermatol Surg Oncol.* 1982;11:54.
40. Hersey P, Morgan G, Stone DE, et al. Previous pregnancy as a protective factor against death from melanoma. *Lancet.* 1977;1(8009):451.
41. Bork K, Bräuninger W. Prior pregnancy and melanoma survival: letter to the editor. *Arch Dermatol.* 1986;122:1097.
42. Elwood JM, Coldman AJ. Previous pregnancy and melanoma prognosis: letter to the editor. *Lancet.* 1978;2(8097):1000.
43. Lederman JS, Sober AJ. Effect of prior pregnancy on melanoma survival: letter to the editor. *Arch Dermatol.* 1985;121:716.
44. Shiu MH, Schottenfeld D, Maclean B, et al. Adverse effect of pregnancy on melanoma: a reappraisal. *Cancer.* 1976;37:181.
45. Reintgen DS, McCarty KS Jr, Vollmer R, et al. Malignant melanoma and pregnancy. *Cancer.* 1985;55:1340.
46. Sutherland CM, Loutfi A, Mather FJ, et al. Effect of pregnancy on malignant melanoma. *Surg Gynecol Obstet.* 1983;157:443.
47. Riberti C, Marola G, Bertani A. Malignant melanoma: the adverse effect of pregnancy. *Br J Plast Surg.* 1981;34:338.
48. Anderson JF, Kent S, Machin GA. Maternal malignant melanoma with placental metastasis: a case report with literature review. *Ped Pathol.* 1989;9:35.
49. Campbell WA, Storlazzi E, Vintzileos AM, et al. Fetal malignant melanoma: ultrasound presentation and review of the literature. *Obstet Gynecol.* 1987;70:434.
50. Carstam R, Hansson C, Rorsman H, et al. Urinary excretion of melanocytic metabolites in fertile women. *Acta Derm Venereol (Stockh).* 1985;65:543.
51. Kirkwood JM, Ernstoff MS, Davis CS, et al. Comparison of intramuscular and intravenous recombinant alpha-2 interferon in melanoma and other cancers. *Ann Intern Med.* 1985;103:32.

Chapter One Hundred and Seventy-Nine

Melanoma of the Skin

H. F. Seigler

179

The pigment melanin is synthesized by melanocytes. Precursor melanocytes arise in the neural crest during embryonic life and migrate to sites within the leptomeninges, eye, and, in wide distribution, to the skin. With the exception of retinal pigment epithelium, all melanocytes can produce malignant melanoma. Melanoma of the skin may come from either normal intraepidermal melanocytes or from preexisting melanocytic nevi of various types. Large, irregular moles that have been termed *BK moles* can undergo malignant transformation, thus causing this familial form of the disease. Melanoma of the skin both occurs as a *de-novo* lesion and develops in prior, existing nevi.

PATHOLOGY AND PATHOGENESIS

Melanoma of the skin and mucous membranes can develop at the junction of the epidermis and dermis or, less frequently, beneath the junction. Most of the lesions that have an intraepithelial component first progress by radial growth; this eventually advances to a vertical growth phase. Those primary lesions that arise without an intraepithelial component have only a vertical growth phase. It is during the vertical growth phase that the lesions invade the area of the skin through which lymphatics and blood vessels course. If vascular or lymphatic structures are involved, a metastatic potential exists. The four histopathologic types of cutaneous melanoma are (1) *lentigo maligna melanoma,* (2) *superficial spreading melanoma,* (3) *acral lentiginous melanoma,* and (4) *nodular melanoma.*

Lentigo maligna melanoma occurs most commonly in patients in their sixth, seventh, and eighth decades of life. The most common sites of primary for this type of melanoma are in sun-exposed areas of the head and neck and dorsal aspect of the hands and feet. The lesion is characterized as being flat and of homogenous pigmentation. The epidermis is atrophic, and there is prominent solar elastosis evident when reviewed microscopically. This lesion is usually slow-growing and has a prolonged radial growth phase. As nodular degeneration takes place, the vertical growth phase is associated with ulceration and a metastatic potential (Figure 179–1).

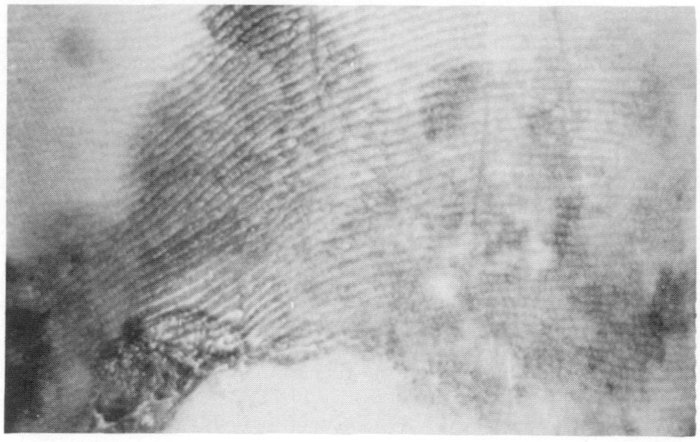

Figure 179–1. Lentigo maligna melanoma occurring on the malar eminence, demonstrating advanced radial growth with solar changes.

Superficial spreading melanoma can occur on any area of the body. This lesion typically will have an early radial growth phase; however, once the vertical growth phase develops, the progression may be rapid. This lesion is characterized as having variable pigmentation with irregular surfaces and irregular borders. Microscopically, there will be both junctional activity and upward invasion of the epidermis. Pagetoid cells are abundant; this feature easily distinguishes it from lentigo maligna (Figure 179–2).

Acral lentiginous melanoma most often involves the palmar and plantar surfaces of the hands and feet, subungual, and mucous membranes. The areas of body involvement are characteristic and the histologic features are also typical. Widespread junctional proliferation and submucosal invasion are usually evident. The spindle-shaped melanocytes are distinguished easily from pagetoid cells. These melanocytes may appear as bulging junctional nests. The most common site of acral lentiginous melanoma in the female is the vulva. Less often, the vagina, clitoris, and anal canal or anorectal junction are involved. The mucous membranes lining the nasopharyngeal cavity, the sinuses and, more rarely, the esophagus, also can be involved with this type of melanoma. Mucous membrane primary sites are characterized by widespread submucosal involvement that severely restricts local control utilizing either surgical techniques or surgical excision and irradiation. Diffuse nodal involvement is very common. Melanoma involving the mucous membranes in general and the female genital tract in particular is associated with a very poor prognosis (Figures 179–3A, 179–3B, and 179–3C).

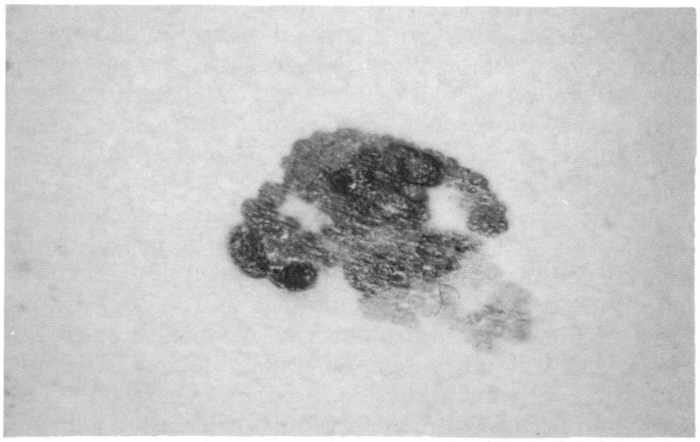

Figure 179–2. Superficial spreading melanoma showing irregular borders with differing areas of pigmentation and associated vertical growth phase.

Nodular melanoma demonstrates no junctional activity. The early vertical growth phase of this lesion gives it a typical clinical appearance. These lesions usually have a well-circumscribed border and are homogenously pigmented. The polypoid variant of nodular melanoma also has a distinctive appearance. They are usually exophytic growths attached to the skin by a stalk (Figures 179–4A and 179–4B).

A

B

C

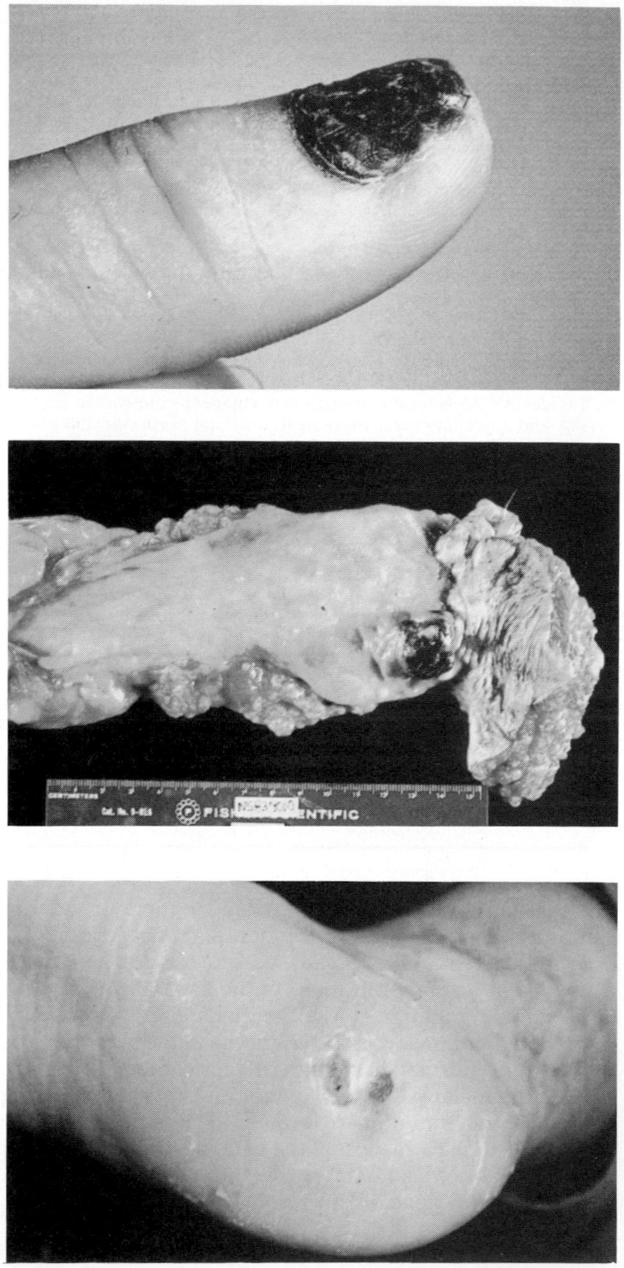

Figure 179–3. **(A)** Typical advanced subungual melanoma with characteristic pigmentary changes involving both the nail and nail bed. **(B)** Acral lentiginous melanoma at the anorectal junction. This is an exophytic, advanced mucous membrane lesion. **(C)** Plantar acral lentiginous melanoma with ulceration and advanced radial growth. Absent are any features characteristic of plantar wart.

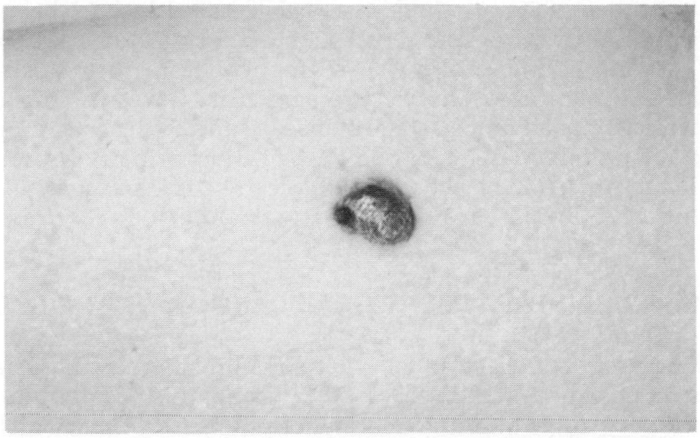

A

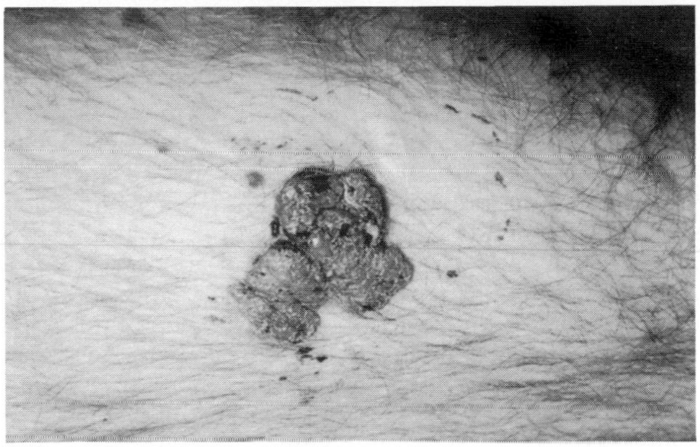

B

Figure 179–4. **(A)** Nodular melanoma with smooth borders, homogeneous color, and advanced obvious vertical growth. **(B)** Polypoid melanoma demonstrating a distinctive clinical appearance in terms of growth pattern and stalk attachment to the underlying epidermis.

EPIDEMIOLOGY

Epidemiologic studies have suggested that there are both a genetic predisposition for melanoma and important environmental considerations. Individuals of Celtic origin exhibit the highest incidence of melanoma of all ethnic groups. Blacks appear to have the lowest incidence. In the southeastern United States, the ratio of melanoma in whites versus blacks is 20 to 1.[1] The incidence of melanoma is increasing more rapidly in the United States than any other cancer. Fifty years ago, the lifetime risk of a North American citizen developing malignant melanoma was approximately 1 in 1500. At the present time, this risk has increased to 1 in 128. If this particular trend continues, by the year 2000, one in 90 Americans will develop this disease during his or her lifetime.[2] Death rates have been rising by approximately 5% per year, indicating that despite improved clinical awareness and diagnostic techniques, mortality continues to rise. The one major environmental factor placing individuals at risk is sunlight exposure.

HORMONAL ASPECTS OF MELANOMA

One aspect of the least-defined areas of investigation in patients with melanoma involves the relationship between the biologic behavior of the disease and hormonal action. In a statistical sense, females have a better prognosis overall with this disease than do males. Melanoma occurrence prior to puberty is rare. There are some data to suggest that there is an improved prognosis for premenopausal females and multiparous females. The effect of pregnancy on patients with this disease continues to be an unresolved question. There are reports of decreased survival among pregnant patients with melanoma.[3] There are no firm data, however, to show that, either experimentally or clinically, endocrine manipulation can advance or regress the growth of melanoma.[4] The presence or absence of steroid receptors in human melanoma has been addressed recently. Use of a monoclonal anti-estrogen receptor antibody in immunohistochemical studies has shown no specific staining of melanomas. These data suggest that true estrogen receptor sites are not present on human melanoma cells.[5] At the present time, patients at high risk with their disease should be advised against pregnancy, and those with low risk followed carefully during their high-estrogen state. There is little risk to the fetus with this disease entity.

MELANOMA AND PREGNANCY

There are conflicting data in the literature concerning the influence of pregnancy on survival or the growth rates of the malignancy in patients with melanoma. Some reports[6,7] have suggested that there is a marked progression of the disease stimulated by the pregnant state. Other groups[8,9] have evaluated this question and conclude that there is little influence on either the disease or the fetus itself. Much of this confusion results from studies conducted in patient series with a lack of homogeneity between the groups evaluated.

Melanoma is diagnosed often in patients during their reproductive years, and a significant portion of these patients develop melanoma during a pregnancy. A recent study of 100 patients, ages 19–40 years, were evaluated in terms of the disease-free interval and ultimate patient survival when pregnancy and melanoma occurred simultaneously.[10] These patients were compared to a control group whose members were not pregnant at the time of diagnosis. Long-term follow up demonstrated identical mortality between the two groups; however, there was an increased incidence of lymph node metastasis in patients who were pregnant at the time of diagnosis of their melanoma. The increased incidence of nodal disease was reported to be 15%. The overall incidence of metastatic or recurrent disease also was increased by 10% in the patients who were pregnant. The disease-free interval observed in pregnant patients was significantly shorter than the control group. At ten years, 45% of the pregnant patients and 60% of control patients remained free of disease. These authors suggested that patients who develop melanoma during pregnancy are at greater risk for metastatic disease than those who are not pregnant when melanoma is diagnosed.

CLINICAL MANIFESTATIONS

Most cutaneous melanomas have a very distinctive appearance, which should permit early diagnosis and surgical treatment. The clinical features of significance in pigmented lesions include asymmetry, border irregularity, color variation, and enlarging diameter. Patients with lentigo maligna melanoma usually will have lesions that vary in color from light tan to brown and black areas intermixed. The lesion is usually flat until a nodular degeneration occurs. Most of these lesions have a diameter exceeding 1 cm. The borders are irregular and the patient will typically be 60 years of age or older. The affected areas usually are exposed chronically to ultraviolet irradiation.

Superficial spreading melanomas begin as small flat lesions and typically will undergo changes in both color and size. The color mixture includes brown, pink, black, and deep blue. Involuted areas and depigmentation are common. Irregular borders, scaling, and ulceration are also common.

Acral lentiginous melanoma develops mostly on surfaces without hair, mucous membranes, and the nail beds. This lesion has a more aggressive clinical behavior and in sites of mucous membrane involvement may be extensive.

Nodular melanomas usually exhibit smooth borders and uniform elevation. The growth of this lesion is typically very rapid. Rarely, it may have the appearance of a blood blister, but more often will be gray, black, or pink.

The *BK mole syndrome* is a familial form of the disease. These patients have a much greater chance of developing multiple primary lesions than do patients from the general population. The BK mole syndrome is a dominantly inherited characteristic, and the patient will exhibit large and many sized moles occurring most often over the upper trunk and upper arms. These BK moles have irregular borders and a varying color pattern, including pink, tan, brown, and black. These lesions are usually 0.5–1.5 cm in diameter. All family members of patients with BK mole syndrome should be followed in a serial fashion. All suspicious lesions undergoing changes should be surgically excised.

PROGNOSTIC FACTORS

Certain histopathologic features of a primary melanoma can be correlated clearly with the ultimate prognosis. It is of interest that, in general, females have a better survival with melanoma than do males. The exact explanation for this phenomenon is poorly understood. Women exhibit most primary melanoma lesions on the lower extremity, whereas in men there is a preponderance of truncal lesions and head and neck primary lesions. Both sexes fare better with upper-extremity melanomas, with lower-extremity and trunk lesions having the next best prognosis, and head and neck and mucous membrane lesions experiencing the poorest survival.

In terms of the tumor itself, there are well defined prognostic variables. Tumor thickness, level of tumor invasion, and tumor ulceration are all important. Clark[11] described the importance of the level of invasion of the primary tumor. Breslow[12] added the prognostic significance associated with tumor thickness predicting the ultimate prognosis and the likelihood of Stage 2 disease. A univariant analysis in patients with Stage 1 cutaneous melanoma shows that sex, primary lesion site, level of tumor invasion, tumor thickness, and tumor ulceration are all prognostic factors that need to be considered by the physician. Patients with vertical growth of their tumor have an increasing disease risk as this process advances. As the tumor invades the deep reticular dermis and finally extends through to the subcutaneous tissue, there is increasing likelihood that the patient will have systemic disease with attendant decreasing survival. Tumor thickness is more predictable in terms of prognostic factors than is the level of tumor invasion. Clark's level of invasion provides no additional information once tumor thickness has been taken into account. Tumor ulceration occurs more commonly in nodular melanoma than the other histopathologic types. Ulcerated lesions have a significantly worse prognosis than do nonulcerated lesions. The only ethnic group that seems to be at greater risk is black Americans. On the average, black patients present with a more advanced stage of disease and with acral lentiginous lesions making up the bulk of their primary process. In the American black, melanoma seems to be an aggressive, highly lethal disease compared with other ethnic groups.

SURGICAL TREATMENT OF MELANOMA OF THE SKIN

The prognostic factors for cutaneous melanoma have been studied extensively over the past decade; this has permitted the surgeon to alter the treatment options for primary melanoma of the skin. Our present understanding resulting from both univariant and multivariant analyses of cutaneous malignancy has afforded the ability to predict the most probable course of the disease and to provide a more rational treatment plan. If the lesion is small, complete excision to include fat should be included in the biopsy specimen and submitted for histopathologic evaluation. If the lesion is too large to permit complete excision, incisional biopsy should be done at the site of ulceration, vertical growth, and clinically most suspicious area. Incisional biopsy is not associated with increased risk to disease-free interval or ultimate cure of the patient. Once the histopathologic features have been defined by the pathologist, the surgeon is better able to provide a rational treatment approach.

Locoregional control is the responsibility of the surgeon. The present recommendation for cutaneous melanomas, 1.5 mm in thickness or less, includes 2 cm measured margins from the gross lesion. If the primary is thicker than 1.5 mm, and has microscopic satellitosis, a 2–3 cm margin in all directions should be recommended. In all cases, the subcutaneous fat should be included in the surgical specimen. In most areas, the surgeon easily can include the fascia as an anatomic border for defining his specimen. However, there is nothing to support the notion that removal of the fascia will improve the ultimate patient survival. Thin and intermediate thickness lesions, for the most part, can be managed by primary wound closure. In certain sites, thicker lesions may be managed by primary wound closure or might require split thickness skin grafting. If a patient experiences local recurrent disease within 5 cm of the primary lesion, the surgeon should manage this recurrence with the same measurements as control for a primary process. Subungual melanomas are difficult and no attempt should be made at local excision or coverage. Once biopsy has established the diagnosis, amputation at the interphalangeal joint should be recommended. If glabrous skin is involved, local control usually can be accomplished only with wide excision and split thickness skin grafting. No attempt at local wound closure of palmar or plantar surfaces should be attempted.

The entire question of the role of elective lymphadenectomy for cutaneous melanoma continues to be debated. Introduction of the computer into clinical medicine as well as the establishment of mathematical models permits identification of the subsets of patients who might benefit from prospective lymph node dissection. If a patient has a cutaneous melanoma 1.5 mm in thickness or less, the addition of elective node dissection does not appear to improve regional control or ultimate patient survival. The likelihood that lymph nodes will be involved in a patient with a primary lesion 1.5 mm in thickness or less is very small. If the primary melanoma is 4 mm in thickness or greater, the likelihood of a systemic expression of the disease overrides any potential benefit gained by elective first-order node dissection. Patients with primary tumors 4 mm in thickness, or greater, have an approximate 70% risk factor in terms of systemic spread of their disease. This high probability exceeds a smaller benefit realized with elective node dissection. Those patients with primary lesions 1.5–4 mm include the subset of patients who have the most to gain from elective node dissection.[13] The presence of significant lymph node involvement is 10%; an additional 10% will have microscopic occult disease to lymph nodes. The overall therapeutic benefit to patients with this intermediate thickness is approximately 25%.

The lymph node group at risk with primary cutaneous melanoma can be demonstrated accurately using the technique of lymphoscintigraphy.[14] Lymphoscintigraphy utilizes technetium-labeled antimony sulfur colloid. This isotopically labeled colloid is injected intradermally into the four quadrants immediately adjacent to the primary lesion. This technique permits the surgeon to address accurately the lymph node basins at risk by following the nodal drainage pattern.

REFERENCES

1. Reintgen DS, McCarty KS Jr, Cox E, et al. Malignant melanoma in the American black. *Curr Surg*. 1983;40:215.
2. Rigel DS, Kopf AW, Friedman RF. The rate of malignant melanoma in the U.S.: are we making an impact? *J Am Acad Dermatol*. 1987;17:1050.
3. Reintgen DS, Nicholson E, Seigler HF. Malignant melanoma in the child-bearing woman. *The Female Patient*. 1987;12:48.
4. McCarty KS Jr, Paul DE, McCarty KS Sr. Hormonal aspects of melanoma. In: Seigler HF, ed. *Clinical Management of Melanoma*. The Hague: Martinus Nijhoff; 1982:355.
5. McCarty KS Jr, Szabo E, et al. Use of a monoclonal anti-estrogen receptor antibody in the immunohistochemical evaluation of human tumors. *Cancer Res*. 1986;46:4244.
6. Hempel J, Remmele W. Das maligne Melaanom des weibichen Genitale. *Z Haut Geschlechtskrankh*. 1973;48:647.
7. Shui HM, Schottenfeld D, Maclean B, et al. Adverse effect of pregnancy on melanomas. *Cancer*. 1976;37:181.
8. Reintgen DS, McCarty KS Jr, et al. Malignant melanoma and pregnancy. *Cancer*. 1985;55:1340.
9. Hersey P, Morgan G, Stone D, et al. Previous pregnancy as a protective factor against death from melanoma. *Lancet*. 1977;1:451.
10. Slingluff CL Jr, Reintgen DS, Vollmer RT, Seigler HF. Malignant melanoma arising during pregnancy: a study of 100 patients. Submitted.
11. Clark WH Jr, From L, Bernardino EA, et al. The histogenesis and biologic behavior of primary human malignant melanomas of the skin. *Cancer Res*. 1969;29:705.
12. Breslow A. Thickness, cross-sectional areas and depth of invasion in the prognosis of cutaneous melanoma. *Ann Surg*. 1970;172:902.
13. Reintgen DS, Cox EB, McCarty KS Jr, et al. Efficacy of elective lymph node dissection in patients with intermediate thickness primary melanoma. *Ann Surg*. 1989;198:379.
14. Reintgen DS, Sullivan D, Coleman E, et al. Lymphoscintigraphy for malignant melanoma. *Am Surg*. 1983;49:672.

Chapter One Hundred and Eighty

Cancer of the Alimentary Tract

Vinay K. Malviya and Gunter Deppe

180

The introduction of newer concepts in preventive medicine, better maternal health, and improvement in diagnostic techniques has resulted in frequent diagnosis of cancer during pregnancy. In fact, malignancy is the second leading cause of death in women during their reproductive years.[1] The incidence of cancer increases as the reproductive function declines; as women delay their childbearing function this fact may assume a greater significance.

In 1988, the National Cancer Institute, Division of Cancer Prevention and Control, reported the age-specific cancer incidence rates to be 253.8 per 100,000 of the referenced population, between the ages of 15 and 44 years.[2] Five percent of all cancers among women occur in this age group. The average annual cancer incidence rates per 100,000 population for cancer of the oral cavity and pharynx between the ages of 15 and 44 years is 9.7, while that of the digestive system is 37.9.[2]

Gastrointestinal cancers occur in 1 in 100,000 pregnancies[3], the most common site being the rectum, followed closely by colon.

The spectrum of anatomic, physiologic, and endocrinologic changes of pregnancy poses a challenge to the diagnosis and management of alimentary tract cancers. The growth rate and size of most of these cancers are unaffected by pregnancy. The growth of some cancers may be retarded during pregnancy, or occasionally may be accelerated.[4,5] The prognosis, however, is directly related to the delay in diagnosis and treatment.

The influence of a tumor on the course of pregnancy is, for the most part, indirect. The presence of the tumor does not increase the incidence of spontaneous abortions or prematurity. Tumors exert many of their harmful effects on pregnancy through involvement of the hemopoietic tissue. With gastrointestinal malignancies, however, the spread to hemopoietic tissue is rare.

Placental and fetal involvement by maternal malignancy is rare despite widespread metastases in the mother. This has led to speculation about biological protective mechanisms that may exist involving the circulatory separation in the placenta and the immunologic responses of the fetus. Intervillous involvement of the placenta without villous invasion is an indication that the fetus is not involved. In 1973, Rothman reported six patients with fetal metastasis. The placenta was examined in two cases only, with both showing villous involvement.[6] In one patient with adrenal cancer and villous placental involvement, no metastatic disease could be found in the infant at autopsy at 6 months of age. The cause of the infant's death was unknown.[7]

The management of alimentary tract cancers during pregnancy is influenced mostly by the natural history of the tumor, the stage of the disease, and fetal viability in relation to the time of diagnosis. The views of the patient and her family regarding her pregnancy and disease, her medical condition, and her attitude toward abortion play an important role in management of cancer. The possibility of maternal death in the postpartum period and the family's willingness to rear the newborn should be given some thought. All of these factors must be considered prior to individualizing therapy.

ORAL CAVITY

Cancers of the oral cavity occur infrequently in association with pregnancy. Some 10,000 new cases of invasive oral cavity and oropharyngeal cancers occur in the female population in the United States each year, with 2875 estimated cancer deaths annually.[1] This disease occurs predominantly in males. The median age of occurrence is 55–65 years. Smoking, tobacco chewing, heavy alcohol intake, poor oral hygiene, chronic trauma from ill-fitting dentures, Plummer–Vinson syndrome, and tertiary syphilis have been implicated in its etiology. A total of 95% of these tumors are of squamous cell origin. Adenocarcinomas and lymphoepitheliomas are extremely rare.

Asymptomatic premalignant changes such as *leukoplakia* or *erythroplakia* may be discovered during a routine oral examination. Local pain, ipsilateral referred otalgia, and dysphagia are common symptoms. Any oral cavity ulceration that does not heal in two weeks should be considered malignant unless proven otherwise. Occasionally, an exophytic growth may be seen, or cervical lymph nodes may be palpable.

These tumors should not be confused with *epulis* in a pregnant patient. Epulis is a localized vascular lesion that occurs in the oral cavity of pregnant patients and regresses spontaneously after delivery.

The diagnosis depends on careful inspection, palpation, and biopsy of suspected lesions. A computerized tomography (CT) scan may help in staging the cancer.

Surgery and radiation therapy are the major curative modalities. A combination of chemotherapy and radiation therapy may be used to shrink the tumor prior to definitive surgical resection. Overall survival for a patient with oral cavity cancer, excluding the lip, ranges from 42% to 65%.[8]

Cade[9] reported six women with cancer of the oral cavity and pharynx associated with pregnancy.[9] He found that pregnancy did not affect the course of the disease or its treatment. Three of his patients with cancer of the tongue were doing well three, four, and nine years, respectively, after onset of their disease at the time of the report. Smith, in 1937, reported a patient with cancer of the tongue in the third decade who had a successful pregnancy outcome.[10]

SALIVARY GLANDS

Cancers of the salivary glands account for 0.3% of all cancers.[11] They occur with equal frequency in males and females with the peak age of incidence being 40–50 years. Radiation exposure is the only known etiologic factor. Of these tumors, 80% occur in the parotid gland, 10% in the submandibular gland, and 10% in the minor salivary glands. The most common site of minor gland involvement is the hard palate.

Most patients present with swelling in the area of the affected gland. Signs of malignancy in parotid tumors include rapid growth, local pain, and facial palsy.

The diagnosis is made on the basis of bimanual examination, sialogram in case of a major gland involvement, and needle aspiration cytology. Submandibular excisional biopsy may be performed to aid diagnosis of cancer in that gland. For suspected parotid cancers, a superficial lobectomy with intraoperative frozen-section examination should be done.

Surgery is the mainstay of treatment for all salivary gland tumors. Radical excision of the tumor may be combined with radical neck dissection. Radiation therapy is indicated for recurrent or inoperable salivary gland cancers.

The management and outcome of pregnant women with these tumors are no different from those in nonpregnant women. Betson and Golden reported a pregnant woman with submaxillary carcinoma[12] who was treated with surgical excision of the gland and postoperative irradiation. She delivered vaginally and was alive at least five years later.

Cade reported three patients with salivary gland cancers associated with pregnancy.[9] Two patients died in the first two years of the disease. The third patient delivered normal twins and survived for at least seven years.

Early diagnosis and prompt therapy are essential for a favorable outcome.

ESOPHAGUS

Three thousand three hundred new cases of carcinoma of the esophagus are estimated to occur in the United States female population leading to 2500 deaths.[1] Cancer of the esophagus is common in elderly patients and seldom occurs concomitantly with pregnancy.

Typical symptoms and signs of esophageal cancer include dysphagia, weight loss, malaise, anorexia, cervical adenopathy, and hematemesis. Women with Plummer–Vinson syndrome or history of lye stricture have a significantly greater incidence of esophageal cancer. The combination of longstanding alcohol intake with smoking increases the risk significantly.

Esophagoscopy with biopsy is the diagnostic procedure of choice. In the majority of patients, neither radical surgery nor irradiation can control the tumor. Five-year survival rates seldom are better than 5%. Currently, platinum-based chemotherapy, administered concurrently with or preceding radical radiation therapy, improves survival in patients with cancer of the esophagus. Patients with tumors of the lower esophagus have a better prognosis than if the cancer involves the thoracic esophagus, where almost no patients survive for five years. Cancer of the esophagus does not appear to influence the course of pregnancy or to be affected by pregnancy.

STOMACH

Only a few patients with carcinoma of the stomach in pregnancy have been described in the English literature.[13,14] Adenocarcinoma is the most frequently found malignant tumor of the stomach, comprising 95% or more of these neoplasms. Saito et al[15] reviewed the Japanese experience of gastric cancer and pregnancy and found 48 patients from 1916 to 1981. All patients had advanced cancers, with a poor prognosis, possibly due to a delay in diagnosis and difficulty with the surgical treatment during pregnancy. Hirabayashi et al[16] reviewed the literature from 1916 to 1985 and emphasized the efficacy of fiberoptic gastroscopy for an early diagnosis and management.

The most common symptoms of patients with gastric cancer in Hirabayashi's review[16] were vomiting (43%), epigastric pain (43%), nausea (23%), and lumbago (15%), symptoms which are easily misinterpreted as events related to pregnancy. When nausea, vomiting, or hyperemesis gravidarum persist or occur in the third trimester of pregnancy, gastric cancer must be considered in the differential diagnosis.[17]

The early diagnosis of gastric cancer can be established safely with gastroscopy and biopsies at any time during pregnancy. This method is preferred to an upper gastrointestinal x-ray series in pregnant patients. Muller et al[18] presented the ultrasonographic finding in a patient with palpable epigastric mass. This mass had a "target" appearance, that is, a hypoechoic rim with a highly reflectant central core. This mass, in the anatomic position of the stomach, with target appearance on ultrasound, was considered to be diagnostic of gastric cancer. Laparotomy confirmed advanced, unresectable cancer of the stomach, requiring palliative gastroenterotomy. Unfortunately, most pregnant patients with gastric cancer are detected late[15] and may have advanced disease with secondary involvement of the ovaries (Krukenberg's tumors).[19-23]

Radical, subtotal gastrectomy is the treatment of choice for patients with Stage I and Stage II disease, without regard to the pregnancy, when diagnosed in the first or second trimester. In the third trimester, treatment may be postponed until fetal maturity. A cesarean section may be performed at the time of surgery. The prognosis of early gastric cancer is excellent, with 5-year survival expected to be 93% and the 10-year rate to be 80%.[24]

Treatment of patients with Stage III and Stage IV cancers consists of palliative combination chemotherapy consisting of 5-fluorouracil with BCNU or mitomycin-C, with or without Adriamycin alone or combined with radiation therapy. At the patient's request, these palliative modalities may be delayed until the fetus is mature.

The prognosis of gastric cancer in pregnancy is poor. Of 25 patients, 22 (88%) died within one year of diagnosis.[16] Reynolds and Bowers each reported a pregnant patient with infiltrating cancer of the stomach treated with radical surgery. Both patients had a poor outcome and were already advanced at time of diagnosis.[25,26]

Furukawa et al[27] reported the 5-year survival rate of patients under the age of 35 years to be 60.3%, less than the survival rate of older patients. Kitaoka[28] found estrogen receptors in a few cases of gastric cancer, leading to a hypothesis that pregnancy might promote the growth of gastric cancer.

To improve the prognosis of gastric cancer in pregnancy, early diagnosis with the gastroscope and aggressive surgical treatment is mandatory. Staging of stomach cancer is described in Table 180–1.

LIVER

Malignant Tumors

Primary hepatic cancer is rare in pregnancy; of the two histologic types reported, *hepatocellular carcinoma* is much more common than *cholangiocarcinoma*.

Hepatic cancer is more common in Southeast Asia and in certain parts of Africa. It is rare prior to 40 years of age, the peak incidence being in the sixth and early seventh decades. Various etiologic factors have been implicated in the genesis of hepatic cancer. These include chronic active hepatitis, postnecrotic cirrhosis, hemochromatosis, and aflatoxin of the mold *Aspergillus flavus*. In a large series, 5% of patients with cirrhosis had hepatic cancer.[30] Recently, malignant liver tumors have been described with the use of oral contraceptives and C17-substituted 19-nonsteroids.[31-37]

Seaward[38] reviewed the literature and reported the outcome of eight patients with hepatic cancer in pregnancy. The disease has an insidious onset with extremely rapid course and is uniformly fatal, with maternal death occurring antenatally or immediately postpartum. Fetal wastage was 57%.[39-42] Maternal death is due to hepatic failure or tumor hemorrhage.

The early manifestations of hepatic cancer consist of nonspecific symptoms such as anorexia, malaise, and dull, aching epigastric pain. In a pregnant patient, these may be mistaken for symptoms of pregnancy. With progressive growth, however, the pain worsens and may radiate to the back or may become acute and associated with shock in the case of hepatic rupture.[39] The liver may become palpably enlarged and tender with tumor nodules on the surface. Ascites is seen in a large number of patients. Occasionally, a patient may present with bleeding esophageal varices. One patient was discovered as a result of a routine α-fetoprotein screen at 19 weeks of gestation, which was above 1000 ng/ml.[43]

The diagnostic evaluation of a space-occupying lesion of the liver in a pregnant patient should include (1) exclusion of an amoebic or pyogenic liver abscess, hydatid cysts, polycystic disease and of any gummatous lesions; and (2) ultrasonography of the mass with estimation of α-fetoprotein level, carcino-embryonic antigen, liver function studies, and hepatitis B viral status. Liver biopsy or fine needle aspiration of the liver will confirm the diagnosis of primary versus metastatic cancer.[44] Confusion with metastatic trophoblastic disease should be avoided since 17% of the hepatocellular carcinomas produce ectopic human chorionic gonadotropin.[40]

There are no reports of primary resection of hepatic cancer in pregnancy, but as the prognosis is so dismal, early diagnosis and tumor resection may offer the only hope of cure. Prior to fetal viability, laparotomy with termination of pregnancy should be considered. This will allow an assessment of operability of the tumor and permit aggressive multiagent chemotherapy. Once fetal viability is reached, delivery by cesarean section and hepatic resection may offer the only curative option. The staging of liver tumors is presented in Table 180–2.

The treatment of liver cancers is primarily surgical. Criteria for surgical resection include localized cancer without involvement of lymph nodes, blood vessels, or the bile duct. Appreciation of the segmental anatomy of the liver, coupled with improvement in surgical techniques, anesthesia and blood-banking techniques, has made hepatic resection feasible with acceptable complications. Removal of up to 80% of the liver is compatible with life. The majority of lobar resections, including right lobe resection, can be done transabdominally.

Pregnancy significantly increases the risk for an unfavorable outcome in patients with untreated hepatic carcinoma or adenoma. The high levels of steroids and increased vascularity of the liver during pregnancy increase the

TABLE 180–1. STAGING OF STOMACH CANCERS BY TNM CLASSIFICATION

Primary Tumor (T)

TX	Minimum requirements to assess the primary tumor cannot be met
T0	No evidence of primary tumor
Tis	Carcinoma *in situ*
T1	Tumor limited to mucosa and submucosa regardless of its extent or location
T2	Tumor involves the mucosa, the submucosa (including the *muscularis propria*), and extends to or into the serosa but does not penetrate through the serosa
T3	Tumor penetrates through the serosa without invading contiguous structures
T4a	Tumor penetrates through the serosa and involves immediately adjacent tissues such as lesser omentum, perigastric fat, regional ligaments, greater omentum, transverse colon, spleen, esophagus, or duodenum by way of intraluminal extension
T4b	Tumor penetrates through the serosa and involves the liver, diaphragm, pancreas, abdominal wall, adrenal glands, kidney, retroperitoneum, small intestine, esophagus, or duodenum by way of serosa

Nodal Involvement (N)

NX	Minimum requirements to assess the regional nodes cannot be met
N0	No metastases to regional lymph nodes
N1	Involvement of perigastric lymph nodes within 3 cm of the primary tumor along the lesser or greater curvature
N2	Involvement of the regional lymph nodes more than 3 cm from the primary tumor that are removed or removable at surgery, including those located along the left gastric, splenic, celiac, and common hepatic arteries
N3	Involvement of other intra-abdominal lymph nodes that are not removable at surgery such as the para-aortic, hepatoduodenal, retropancreatic, and mesenteric nodes

Distant Metastasis (M)

MX	Minimum requirements to assess the presence of distant metastasis cannot be met
M0	No (known) distant metastasis
M1	Distant metastasis present: specify

Stage Grouping

Stage	TNM	Tumor Limited To
Stage 0	Tis, N0, M0	*In situ,* no invasion of *lamina propria*
Stage I	T1, N0, M0	Mucosa, submucosa
Stage II	T2, T3, N0, M0	*Muscularis propria,* subserosa, or serosa
Stage III	T1–3, N1, N2, M0	Any invasion through serosa, with N1 or N2 nodes involved
	T4a, N0–N2, M0	Direct extension to immediately adjacent tissues or organs,[a] any nodal involvement up to N2
Stage IV	T1–T3, T4a T4a, N3, M0	Any invasion through serosa including direct extension to immediately adjacent tissues or organs,[b] with N3 nodes involved
	T4b, any N, M0	Direct extension to further contiguous organs,[b] any nodes
	Any T, any N, M1	Distant metastasis (either site or nodes)

[a] T4a: tumor penetrates through the serosa and involves immediately adjacent tissues such as lesser omentum, perigastric fat, regional ligaments, greater omentum, transverse colon, spleen, esophagus, or duodenum (by way of intraluminal extension).
[b] T4b: tumor penetrates through the serosa and involves the liver, diaphragm, pancreas, abdominal wall, adrenal glands, kidney, retroperitoneum, small intestine, esophagus, and duodenum (by way of serosa).
Refer to reference 29 for classification data.

chances of liver rupture. It therefore is advisable to avoid pregnancy or consider terminating an existing pregnancy in patients with unresected or partially resected hepatic tumors. The first case of metastatic spread of cancer to the fetus was described by Friedrich in a patient with hepatic cancer.[45]

Palliative chemotherapy is an option for patients with unresectable hepatomas and may prolong survival in patients who respond.[46]

The outlook for unresectable primary liver cancer is dismal, particularly in pregnant patients. However, in patients who undergo curative resection, the 5-year survival rate parallels that of the nonpregnant state and is approximately 35%.[30,34]

HEPATIC ADENOMAS

Although benign, these tumors merit discussion in view of their catastrophic outcome in pregnancy. Their occurrence has been associated with the use of oral contraceptive pills.[31,34,47-52]

Approximately one third of all hepatic adenomas are diagnosed by the presence of a palpable liver on routine abdominal examination, one third may present with life-threatening intra-abdominal hemorrhage as a result of liver rupture, and the rest are diagnosed at surgery performed for unrelated indications.[53,54]

Rupture of a liver adenoma in pregnancy carries a high maternal and fetal mortality rate. Bis et al[55] reported a 59% maternal and 62% fetal mortality in review of 91 cases of spontaneous rupture of the liver in pregnancy, while Hibberd[56] reported two survivors among 8 patients. Kent et al[57] reported one maternal and fetal death from ruptured adenoma, and another case where both survived.

Occasionally, the rupture of a hepatic adenoma may be quiescent with subcapsular hematoma formation. After several days the hematoma may rupture into the peritoneal cavity. Epigastric pain may be attributed to indigestion, uterine fundal discomfort related to pregnancy, or pre-

TABLE 180–2. STAGING OF LIVER CANCERS BY THE TNM CLASSIFICATION

Primary Tumor (T)	
TX	Tumor is present but cannot be assessed
T0	No evidence of tumor
T1	Small solitary tumor (<2.0 cm) confined to one lobe
T2	Large tumor (>2.0 cm) confined to one lobe
T2a	Single tumor nodule
T2b	Multiple tumor nodules (any size)
T3	Tumor involving both major lobes
T3a	Single tumor with direct extension nodule
T3b	Multiple tumor nodules
T4	Tumor invading adjacent organs
Nodal Involvement (N)	
NX	Nodes cannot be assessed
N0	No histologic evidence of metastases to regional or distant lymph nodes
N1	Histologically confirmed spread to regional lymph nodes in porta hepatis
N2	Histologically confirmed spread to lymph nodes beyond porta hepatis
Distant Metastasis (M)	
MX	Not assessed
M0	No known metastasis
M1	Distant metastasis present
Stage Grouping	
Stage IA	Ta, N0, M0, without cirrhosis
Stage IB	T1, N0, M0, with cirrhosis
Stage IIA	T2, N0, M0, without cirrhosis
Stage IIB	T2, N0, M0, with cirrhosis
Stage IIIA	T3, N0, N1, M0, without cirrhosis
Stage IIIB	T3, N0, N1, M0, with cirrhosis
Stage IVA	T4, N0–N2, M0, M1 without cirrhosis
Stage IVB	T4, N0–N2, M0, M1, with cirrhosis

eclampsia. Chest pain may lead to the misdiagnosis of a pulmonary embolism. The degree of intraperitoneal bleeding will determine the alteration of vital signs and necessity to investigate or perform an urgent laparotomy. Local compression, simple sutures, omental pedicles, ligation of the relevant hepatic artery, and lobectomy are the techniques available, depending on the extent of pathology. Venous oozing can be controlled by the use of topical agents (gel foam, thrombin, Oxycel). The hepatic bed should be drained regardless of the extent of hemostasis. Control of active hemorrhage and supportive resuscitation are essential.

Barns et al[58] reported a patient with successful pregnancy following partial hepatectomy for removal of hepatocellular adenomas. Approximately 50% of the mother's liver was excised following a ruptured hepatocellular adenoma of the right lobe. Such a pregnancy should be considered high risk, and the patient should be monitored with liver function tests and ultrasound.

EXTRAHEPATIC BILE DUCT CANCER

Carcinoma of the extrahepatic biliary tract is very rare, with an incidence of 0.01% at operation and 0.02% at autopsy.[59] It occurs more frequently in males, with a peak incidence in the sixth and seventh decades. These tumors are extremely rare in pregnancy, and only three cases have been reported in the literature. Most of the cases are advanced at diagnosis, with early invasion of the hepatic artery, portal vein, or extension into the liver. Histologically, almost all of these tumors are adenocarcinomas.

Approximately 35% of these tumors occur at the junction of the hepatic ducts, 20% in the common hepatic duct, 35% in the common bile duct, and 10% in the ampulla. Ampullary carcinoma often is diagnosed early because it produces symptoms before metastasis.[60]

Rapid onset of jaundice is usually the presenting symptom of extrahepatic bile duct cancer. Weight loss and upper abdominal pain are frequent. In over one third of these patients, the gallbladder is enlarged and palpable, the greatest incidence being in ampullary cancers. Fluctuation of jaundice related to sloughing of the tumor occurs in 60% of the cases.

Transhepatic cholangiography is the procedure with the highest yield in patients with extrahepatic bile duct cancer. However, in 75% of the patients, diagnosis can be made endoscopically by retrograde cholangiopancreatography. The staging of these tumors is shown in Table 180–3.

Perinatal considerations in these patients include nutritional support of the compromised host, premature delivery, and intrauterine growth retardation.

Curative or palliative surgery should be undertaken as soon as the diagnosis is made. The surgical procedure depends on the site of the tumor. Periampullary cancers are treated with pancreaticoduodenectomy or the Whipple procedure. Cancer of the hepatic ducts and common bile duct usually extend to the liver and are rarely resectable. Palliation of jaundice may be offered by cholecystojejunos-

TABLE 180–3. STAGING OF EXTRAHEPATIC BILE DUCT CANCER BY THE TNM CLASSIFICATION

Primary Tumor (T)	
TX	Presence of tumor cannot be assessed
T0	No evidence of tumor
Tis	Carcinoma *in situ*
T1	Invasion limited to wall
T2	Invasion limited to periductal connective tissues
T3	Involvement of all layers and direct extension into one adjacent major vessel or organ
T4	Involvement of all layers and direct extension beyond secondary ductal bifurcation or into two or more adjacent organs, including liver, pancreas, duodenum, stomach, colon, omentum, gallbladder
Nodal Involvement (N)	
NX	Minimum requirements to assess regional nodes cannot be met
N0	No histologic evidence of metastasis to regional lymph nodes
N1	Histologically proven metastasis to first-station regional nodes
N2	Histologically proven metastasis to second-station regional lymph nodes
Distant Metastasis (M)	
MX	No assessed
M0	No (known) distant metastasis
M1	Distant metastasis
Stage Grouping	
Stage 0	Tis, N0, M0
Stage I	T1, T2, N0, M0
Stage II	T3, T4, N0, M0
Stage III	T3, T4, N1, N2, M0
Stage IV	T3, T4, N0–N2, M1

tomy or by intraoperative placement of a stent, bypassing the obstruction.

Palliative chemotherapy with 5-fluorouracil, Adriamycin, and mitomycin-C is of limited value. Devoe et al[61] reported a patient with well differentiated adenocarcinoma who was treated with chemotherapy and palliative percutaneous biliary drainage. The patient became pregnant 4 months later and delivered a 2325-g male infant at 35 weeks' gestation who thrived. However, the patient developed a hepatic recurrence 5 months following delivery.

Extrahepatic biliary duct cancers have a poor outcome, which probably is related to delay in diagnosis. Betson and Golden[12] reported two patients with these cancers in pregnancy, one diagnosed at autopsy one month after delivering a healthy infant, while the other patient was diagnosed to have ampullary adenocarcinoma during the sixth month of gestation. Radical resection was carried out with spontaneous abortion the following day and maternal death occurred four months later from metastatic disease.

There is no evidence that the hormonal milieu of pregnancy affects the rate of growth of these tumors or the occurrence of metastasis; however, this may be related to our limited experience with this malignancy.

ADENOCARCINOMA IN A CHOLEDOCHOCYST

The incidence of adenocarcinoma arising in a choledochocyst has been reported between 2.5% and 15%.[62] Only 20 cases of choledochal cysts during pregnancy have been reported and, if left untreated, choledochal cysts usually are fatal.[63]

Optimal management of a choledochal cyst during pregnancy remains to be established. Chesterman[64] in 1944 summarized 14 cases of choledochal cysts associated with pregnancy. Of these 14 cases, 12 showed either exacerbation or onset of symptoms during or immediately after pregnancy. Subsequently, two cases of ruptured cyst[65,66] and one case of impending rupture[67] have been reported in association with pregnancy. The choledochal cyst that was threatening to rupture did so after a vaginal delivery.

Present recommendations concerning the management of choledochal cysts during pregnancy suggest that asymptomatic cysts, discovered during ultrasonography for the evaluation of jaundice, can be observed as long as their expansion is documented by serial ultrasound examinations.

Cholangitis, complicating a choledochal cyst, may be treated initially with antibiotics but will require decompression to prevent recurrent bouts of sepsis. If possible, nonoperative management should be carried out until the results of amniocentesis indicate that the fetus is mature enough to be delivered by cesarean section. This nonoperative approach towards biliary disease in pregnancy is supported by the UCLA experience with gallbladder disease during pregnancy, which demonstrated that deferral of definite surgery for cholecystitis and cholelithiasis until either the third trimester or after delivery, was associated with a much greater likelihood of successful outcome than earlier surgery. The treatment of acute cholecystitis with antibiotics alone was successful in all patients in whom this nonoperative approach was used if followed by postpartum surgery in those patients who required surgery (10 out of 19).[68] Cystic decompression does not eliminate the possibility of subsequent episodes of cholangitis, nor does it obviate the need for a subsequent operation postpartum for definitive treatment of the cyst.[67] Definitive treatment now is considered to be cholecystectomy, complete excision of the cyst, and a Roux-en-Y hepaticojejunostomy.

Once a malignancy has developed within a choledochal cyst, excision represents the only chance for cure. In most cases, malignant changes within a cyst cause no specific signs or symptoms and the diagnosis is made late. Because of this, the prognosis for the patients with carcinoma arising in choledochal cysts has been poor, a 5%, 2-year survival in one series.[68]

GALLBLADDER

Carcinoma of the gallbladder is the fifth most common cause of gastrointestinal cancer and accounts for 4% of all epithelial cancers. Of these tumors, 80% occur in females, with the peak incidence in the sixth decade. Approximately 90% of patients with gallbladder cancers have gallstones.[59] Histologically, most of these cancers are adenocarcinomas.

The patients usually present with anorexia, weight loss, and vague abdominal pain. This is followed by nausea, vomiting, jaundice, and a palpably enlarged gallbladder. Cholecystectomy and regional lymphadenectomy offer the best results; however, the prognosis for survival is poor.

No cases of cancer of the gallbladder in pregnancy have been reported, but management and outcome should not be different than in the nonpregnant state.

PANCREAS

Pancreatic cancers are the second most common alimentary tract cancers. They are becoming increasingly common, their incidence having tripled in the last 40 years. Males are affected three to four times as often as females, the peak incidence being at 60 years of age. Cigarette smoking, coffee consumption, and diabetes have been implicated as causative factors.[69]

The common symptoms of pancreatic cancer include anorexia, nausea, weight loss, and flatulence. Most patients complain of a dull pain in the epigastrium, often radiating to the back. In carcinoma of the head of the pancreas, these symptoms precede the onset of progressive jaundice. The most common finding on physical examination is a palpable abdominal tumor. The gallbladder may be palpable in 50% of cases.

Despite improved diagnostic techniques, most pancreatic cancers are diagnosed when they have extended beyond the confines of the pancreas. Ultrasonography, CT scan of the abdomen, and endoscopic retrograde cholangiopancreatography usually confirm the diagnosis.[70] A tissue diagnosis can be made by a fine-needle biopsy or aspiration cytology.

Exploratory laparotomy and pancreaticoduodenal resection is the treatment of choice in operable cases. A recent review of the Mayo Clinic experience indicates that potentially curative surgery could be performed in only 13% of 1212 patients. Their one-year survival rate was 52% with only an 8% five-year survival.[71]

Boyle and MacLeod reported a patient with pancreatic cancer diagnosed in the postpartum period.[72] The patient's fourth pregnancy had been complicated by persistent nausea and vomiting with epigastric discomfort. Ultrasonography revealed a mass in the pancreas. However, pancreatic biopsy specimens, obtained at a postpartum laparotomy, were negative. The patient died several months postpartum and pancreatic cancer was found at autopsy. Bontin et al[73] described a case in the French literature. Both patients were delivered prematurely of babies who survived, while both mothers died shortly after birth. Gamberdella[74] reported a patient at six weeks' gestation whose diagnosis of pancreatic cancer was made antepartum.[74] An antepartum diagnosis of a 4-cm lesion was made at the time of exploratory laparotomy. Only biliary drainage was performed since the patient did not want a termination of pregnancy. At 32 weeks' gestation, after fetal maturity was obtained, a cesarean section delivery was performed. Upper abdominal reexploration revealed extensive metastases. The operative procedure was abandoned, and the patient died postoperatively.

Although the maternal prognosis is poor, expected management of biliary drainage and hyperalimentation may offer a reasonable prognosis for the fetus. Duff et al[75] presented the first case of a solid papillary epithelial tumor of the pancreas in a pregnant woman that was discovered at 13 weeks' gestation. The patient spontaneously aborted at 14 weeks after a pulmonary embolectomy. A Whipple procedure was performed postoperatively and the pancreatic tumor was removed successfully. Smithers et al[76] presented a patient with cystadenocarcinoma of the pancreas, presenting pregnant at 7 weeks, whose pregnancy was terminated prior to a successful pancreatectomy.

Some experimental evidence suggests that estrogens may stimulate and antiestrogens may retard the growth of cystadenocarcinoma of the pancreas.[77]

In pregnancy, the symptoms of dyspepsia with pancreatic cancer easily may be mistaken for symptoms of normal pregnancy, thus delaying diagnosis. Once the diagnosis is made the patient should be explored for resectability without delay, regardless of the duration of gestation.

Chemotherapy and radiation therapy are of limited value in pancreatic cancers.

SMALL INTESTINE

Malignant neoplasms of the small bowel are relatively infrequent, accounting for only 2% of all gastrointestinal cancers. Their association with pregnancy is even more infrequent. Adenocarcinomas occur most frequently and are found with equal frequency in the duodenum, jejunum, and ileum. Carcinoid tumors, lymphomas, sarcomas, and leiomyosarcomas also occur, though predominantly in the ileum.

Most patients present with symptoms of obstruction, vomiting, abdominal pain, and distention.[78] Occasionally, gastrointestinal bleeding and signs of malabsorption may supervene. Patients may show signs of chronic blood loss and anemia secondary to hematochezia, melena, or occult bleeding.

A patient with leiomyosarcoma of the ileum, associated with pregnancy, remained asymptomatic up to the time of delivery, when she presented with hemorrhage, caused by rupture of the tumor.[79]

Wide local resection, with removal of regional lymph nodes, is the therapy of choice. In inoperable cases, a palliative short-circuiting procedure may be done to relieve obstruction.

Pregnancy does not alter the treatment or the outcome in these patients. The five-year survival rate ranges from 20% to 40%, depending on the histology and operability of the tumor.

COLORECTAL CANCERS

Colorectal cancers are the second most common visceral cancers, exceeded in frequency only by breast cancers. In 1991, colon or rectal cancer will be diagnosed in 78,500 American women of all ages, with 30,500 deaths.[1] McClean and coworkers reported seven cases of rectal cancer in 350,000 pregnancies, for an incidence of 0.002%.[80] In 1928, Evers reported the first case of large intestinal carcinoma occurring above the peritoneal reflection during pregnancy.[81] Since then, 22 cases of colonic cancer during pregnancy have been reported.[82]

Cancer of the colon and rectum is a disease of advanced age, occurring most commonly in the seventh decade; however, 8% of these tumors are diagnosed before the age of 40.[83] The oldest pregnant patient with rectal carcinoma in pregnancy was 48 years old[84], while the youngest patient was 18 years old.[85] The mean age was 32 years. The age range for colon cancer in pregnancy was 23–39 years.[82]

Patients at high risk for colorectal cancer include those with ulcerative colitis involving the entire colon for greater than 7 years. After 10 years, the risk rises to 2–3% per year[83], and after 25 years, 42% of patients will have cancer of the colon.[86] The age at the onset of colitis is another important factor in determining the risk for colon cancer. The risk is twice as high in patients with symptoms beginning before 25 years of age. Other predisposing factors include Crohn's disease, familial polyposis, Gardner's syndrome, villous adenomas and patients with a past history of colon cancer and female genital tract cancer.[87]

Patients who develop colon cancer under the age of 40 years may have a familial disease.[88] A study from the British tumor registry reports that even when patients with familial polyposis coli and ulcerative colitis were excluded, a 32% incidence of colon cancer was found during the lifetime of first-degree relatives of patients who developed colon cancer. There is a 30% increase in incidence of colon cancer in nulliparous women as compared to women with one or two children and a 50% increase over women with three or more children.[89] Unmarried women have a higher incidence of colonic cancer than married women[90], a differential consistent with the increase in incidence among nuns[91], suggesting that nulliparity may be a contributing factor.

Of colorectal cancers, 16% occur in the cecum and ascending colon, 8% in the transverse colon and splenic flexure, 6% in the descending colon, 20% in the sigmoid colon, and 50% in the rectum.[92] The location of colonic cancer in pregnant patients is not different from that in nonpregnant patients. Adenocarcinoma was the histologic diagnosis in all 23 reported cases; most of them were poorly differentiated and mucus secreting.[93]

Two thirds of all colorectal neoplasms are within 24 cm of the anal orifice and can be visualized and biopsied by a rigid sigmoidoscope; one third can be reached by an examining finger. In recent years, however, a proximal shift of these cancers has been observed so that only 35% are accessible with a rigid sigmoidoscope.

Colorectal cancers are usually solitary tumors, with multifocal neoplasms occurring in only 6–8% of cases.[83] They are described as polypoid, nodular, ulcerating, or scirrhous. The histologic classification of these tumors is shown in Table 180–4.

These tumors spread by direct extension, lymphatic or hematogenous dissemination, gravitational seeding, or implantation at surgery. Spread by continuity usually occurs

TABLE 180–4. WORLD HEALTH ORGANIZATION HISTOLOGIC CLASSIFICATION OF COLORECTAL CANCERS

Adenocarcinoma
Mucinous adenocarcinoma
Signet ring carcinoma
Squamous cell carcinoma
Adenosquamous carcinoma
Undifferentiated carcinoma
Unclassified carcinoma

by penetration of the bowel wall. This usually is limited to less than 4 cm of grossly normal bowel distal to the tumor and 7 cm proximally. Regional lymph node metastases are the most common form of spread. When carcinoma has extended through the bowel wall, lymph node involvement exceeds 90%, whereas in lesions still confined to the bowel wall, lymph nodes are involved in only 45% of the cases.

Staging of colorectal carcinoma can be done with the modified (Australian) Dukes classification (Table 180–5) or TNM classification (Table 180–6).

Diagnosis

Symptoms of colorectal cancer depend on the anatomic location of the tumor, its size and extent, and the presence of complications such as hemorrhage, intestinal perforation, and intussusception. In pregnant patients with these tumors, the symptoms may be attributable to the pregnancy, making diagnosis difficult.

The most common presenting symptom in patients with colonic cancer is abdominal pain. They also may complain of nausea and vomiting, constipation, abdominal distention, rectal bleeding, and fever. A change in bowel habits is an important symptom in both colonic and rectal cancers and should not be ignored. Constipation, and occasionally obstipation, may be the presenting symptom for rectal cancers. Passage of bright red blood, often with mucous, is seen with low rectal lesions. The patients may experience tenesmus and a feeling of incomplete evacuation. Severe low backache and rectal pain usually indicate extensive local disease. An occasional patient may present with rectal prolapse. A palpable mass, ascites, hepatomegaly, and weight loss may be seen late in the course of this disease.

In both colonic and rectal cancers, the patient may present with an acute abdomen, secondary to a complication, such as bowel obstruction or perforation, cancer perforation, or intussusception.[95-97] A pregnant patient with these cancers may not be diagnosed until the onset of labor, when descent of the fetus may be impeded by the presence of a tumor mass.[98] Thus, these lesions have been discovered in all trimesters, including some during labor or puerperium.

The diagnosis of colorectal cancer in pregnancy requires a high index of suspicion since most of the clinical manifestations could be attributed to a normal pregnancy. Rectal bleeding may be misdiagnosed to be due to hemorrhoids. The diagnosis, therefore, often is missed in pregnant patients even though they are under medical supervision. Delay in diagnosis is a major contribution to the poor prognosis of these patients.

A complete history and physical examination, including a digital rectal examination and analysis of stool for occult blood, are important for the early diagnosis of these tumors. These procedures, together with proctosigmoidoscopy, can confirm the diagnosis in approximately 75% of the patients. Flexible rather than rigid sigmoidoscopy is increasing in popularity as a diagnostic tool because of

TABLE 180–5. STAGING BY THE MODIFIED (AUSTRALIAN) DUKES CLASSIFICATION OF COLORECTAL CARCINOMA

Stage	Substage	Spread
A	A_1	Mucosa
	A_2	Submucosa
	A_3	Muscularis propria
B	B_1	Beyond muscularis propria
	B_2	Free serosa involved
C	C_1	Local node metastasis
	C_2	Apical node metastasis
D	D_1	Local tumor remaining (histologic)
	D_2	Distant metastasis (clinical)

Adapted from Newland et al.[94]

TABLE 180–6. STAGING BY THE TNM CLASSIFICATION

Primary Tumor (T)	
TX	Minimum requirements to assess the primary tumor cannot be met
T0	No evidence of primary tumor
Tis	Carcinoma *in situ*
T1	Tumor confined to mucosa or submucosa
T2	Tumor limited to bowel wall but not beyond
T2a	Partial invasion of *muscularis propria*
T2b	Complete invasion of *muscularis propria*
T3	Tumor invasion of all layers of bowel wall with or without invasion of adjacent or contiguous tissues; fistula may or may not be present
T4	Tumor spread by direct extension beyond contiguous tissue or the immediately adjacent organs
T	Multiple primary carcinoma: classify most extensive tumors (indicate number in brackets)
Nodal Involvement	
NX	Minimum requirements to assess the regional nodes cannot be met
N0	Nodes not involved
N1	One to three involved regional nodes adjacent to primary lesion
N2	Regional nodes involved extending to line of resection or ligature of blood vessels
N3	Nodes contain metastasis, location not identified: Specify number examined, number involved
Distant Metastasis (M)	
MX	Minimum requirements to assess the presence of distant metastasis cannot be met
M0	No (known) distant metastasis
M1	Evidence of distant metastasis: specify
Stage Grouping	
Stage 0	Tis, N0, M0
Stage I	
IA	T1, N0, M0
IB	T2, N0, M0
Stage II	T3, N0, M0
Stage III	Any T, N1–N3, M0
	T4, N0, M0
Stage IV	Any T, any N, M1

less discomfort to the patient. In experienced hands, it also offers a larger field of visualization. Up to 60 cm of the distal large bowel can be visualized and biopsied with the flexible scope compared to only 25 cm with the rigid scope.

Colonoscopy, barium enema, and ultrasound are useful adjuncts in the diagnosis of colonic cancer. The role of tumor markers in pregnancy is limited (pregnancy-associated α-glycoprotein, carcinoembryonic antigen, λ-glutamyl transferase, glucose phosphate isomerase, and lactate dehydrogenase), since many of these markers are elevated in pregnancy.

Treatment

One of the fundamentals of effective surgical techniques in the treatment of cancer is to minimize cancer cell contamination of the cancer bed, the anastomosis, the adjacent viscera or abdominal wall, and the bloodstream. In the mid-1960s, Turnbull and associates[99] advocated the "no-touch isolation technique" for the resection of carcinoma of the colon to minimize the possibility of dissemination of cancer cells by way of the bloodstream during surgery. Their technique involved resection of the colon, in which the cancer-bearing segment was not manipulated in any manner until after the lymphovascular pedicles had been ligated and divided and the colon had been divided at the sites elected for resection. The survival of patients with Duke-C cancer of the colon doubled with this technique.

Ackerman[100] proposed a modification of the above technique. After determining the feasibility of resection, the appropriate major artery was ligated, followed by the marginal vessels running close to the colon near the proposed site of resection.

Stearns and Schottenfield[101] have obtained results comparable to Turnbull's series without employing early ligation of vascular channels. They emphasized the complete removal of the lymphatic drainage by as complete a resection of the mesentery of the cancer-bearing bowel segment as is feasible. Steps to minimize cancer cell emboli through vascular channels should not interfere with the goal of wide removal of the mesentery of the cancer-bearing bowel segment.

The site of the primary tumor of the colon and the stage of gestation dictate the type of colonic resection to be performed, as is seen in Tables 180–7 and 180–8.

In selected patients with local extension of the cancer, total abdominal hysterectomy, bilateral salpingo-oophorectomy, and en-bloc resection of the posterior vaginal wall and the bladder (if these structures are involved) may be indicated for complete cure. For emergent surgical procedures with an unprepared bowel, as in intestinal obstruction, perforation, or hemorrhage, definitive resection with a proximal ostomy may be performed.

Patients with advanced malignancies are candidates for palliative resection or colostomy followed by chemotherapy. These patients could be delivered vaginally or by cesarean section, and palliative therapy should be administered following delivery.

Pitluk and Poticka[102] cited a 24% incidence of concurrent ovarian metastases with colorectal cancer in pregnancy as opposed to an incidence of 4–6% in the nonpregnant individual. Therefore, if the tumor is resectable without disturbing the pregnancy, bilateral ovarian wedge biopsies should be performed with frozen section. Bilateral salpingo-oophorectomy is performed if the ovaries are involved with tumor or if hysterectomy is performed for previously mentioned reasons.

Various drugs have been used singly or in combination

TABLE 180–7. MANAGEMENT OF COLORECTAL CANCER AND SITE OF INVOLVEMENT

Site of Cancer	Surgical Procedure[a]
Cecum and ascending colon	Right hemicolectomy, including terminal 12 cm of the ileum for cecal lesions
Proximal transverse colon	Extended right hemicolectomy
Splenic flexure or descending colon	Left hemicolectomy
Sigmoid colon	Segmental resection of the sigmoid colon with its mesentery up to the origin of the inferior mesenteric vessels; for proximal sigmoid lesions. Left hemicolectomy may be indicated
Rectosigmoid 15 cm above anal verge	Low anterior resection with end-to-end anastomosis
Upper rectum 10–15 cm above anal verge	Combined abdominopelvic resection or posterior pelvic exenteration: using end-to-end anastomosic stapling technique
Middle and lower rectum and anal canal	Combined abdominopelvic resection or posterior pelvic exenteration

[a] One should attempt to obtain a 4-cm distal resection margin and a 7-cm proximal resection margin.

for the treatment of patients with colorectal cancer. 5-Fluorouracil, methyl-CCNU, BCNU, mitomycin-C, Adriamycin, and cisplatin have been used in various dosage schedules and protocols. Superiority of single-agent chemotherapy over multiagent treatment has not been established. Adjuvant chemotherapy in colorectal cancer still needs to be investigated.

A 20% objective response has been established for 5-fluorouracil, although individual investigators have reported response rates varying from 8% to 85%.[103]

Radiation therapy for locally advanced disease after palliative resection is currently under investigation, as is the combination of surgery, radiation therapy, and chemotherapy. The usefulness of these regimens remains to be determined.

Prognosis

Diversity in management of pregnant patients with colorectal cancer and underreporting of long-term survival has made it difficult to estimate the prognosis of these patients. It is believed, however, that the prognosis of pregnant patients with colorectal cancer, when matched for stage and histology, is not different from that of their nonpregnant counterparts.

The prognosis of cancer of the colon associated with pregnancy was found to be poor in 23 reported cases. This may reflect the fact that of those 23 patients, 65% had widely metastatic disease at time of diagnosis. All of these patients underwent palliative resection, chemotherapy, and radiation therapy. Only four were alive at the time of the report, 16 months, three years, two years, and one year after diagnosis, respectively. Of the eight patients considered to be surgically resectable, four patients died in the first eight months after definitive surgery. Thus, the mortality for this group of patients was 65%, the longest survival being

TABLE 180–8. MANAGEMENT OF COLORECTAL CANCER AND GESTATIONAL AGE

Gestational Age	Cancer Treatment	Pregnancy Outcome
First and Second Trimesters		
Colon	Wide local resection with end-to-end anastomosis.	Anticipate vaginal delivery.
Rectum	Abdominopelvic resection or posterior exenteration.	Anticipate vaginal delivery.
Third Trimester (24 weeks to fetal maturity)		
Colon	At fetal maturity, wide local excision during cesarean section or 2 weeks postpartum.	Delivery by cesarean section.
Rectum	Abdominopelvic resection or posterior exenteration during cesarean section or 2 weeks postpartum.	Delivery by cesarean section.
At Term or Labor		
Colon	Wide local resection 2 weeks postpartum; in case of diagnosis at cesarean section, the definitive procedure may be done concurrently.	Anticipate vaginal delivery or cesarean section for obstetric indication.
Rectum	Abdominopelvic resection or posterior exenteration.	Patients with low rectal cancers should be delivered by cesarean section for fear of hemorrhage and dissemination of cancer cells during delivery.

three years. The neonatal outcome in these patients was much better, with 74% survival. The outcome in 10% of cases was unknown, and 16% died.[81,104-112] There are no reported five-year survivors among the 23 pregnant patients with colon cancer in the literature.[82]

In contrast to the dismal prognosis in reported colonic cancers, patients with rectal cancer appear to have a better outcome. In 1958, Warren[113] reported nine cases of rectal cancer during pregnancy, all of whom underwent curative surgery. Five of these patients (56%) survived beyond five years, one patient (11%) died of an unknown cause after five years, and three patients had hepatic metastases but were alive 6, 11, and 14 months after diagnosis. The fetal outcome of Warren's patients was 67% survival. Three patients (33%) underwent therapeutic abortions or hysterectomies prior to 4 months' gestation.

A cumulative study of 62 patients by McClean et al[80], in 1955, revealed a 45% survival rate. A total of 48% of patients died, and the outcome in 7% was not known; however, the duration of survival in these patients also was not known.

Another study by O'Leary and Bebko[109] in 1967 reviewed 17 patients with rectal cancer during pregnancy; 65% of their patients survived, 29% died, and 6% were lost to follow up. The fetal outcome consisted of 71% survival and 29% mortality. These data therefore reveal that pregnant patients with rectal cancer have a maternal survival rate in the range of 45–65% and a fetal survival of 67–71%.

Pregnancy After Excision of Rectal Cancer

A number of women of childbearing age survive curative resection for colorectal cancer. Pregnancy is not contraindicated in these patients if there is no recurrence for 5 years following the surgery. In a study of 13 patients who became pregnant 1–12 years after curative resection for rectal cancer, ten had a favorable outcome.[113] Two recurrences occurred during pregnancy, and a third patient died of an unknown cause after delivery.

Colorectal Carcinoid During Pregnancy

Alimentary tract carcinoids have been reported in six pregnant patients so far. Of these, five were located in the appendix and one in the rectum. The former were treated successfully with appendectomy, and the rectal carcinoid was treated with fulguration of the tumor. None of these patients had symptoms of carcinoid syndrome.[12,102,114]

Adenocarcinoma of the Appendix During Pregnancy

Donnenfeld reported a patient with primary adenocarcinoma of the appendix at 31 weeks' intrauterine gestation. The patient underwent exploratory laparotomy for a ruptured appendix; subsequently, when the pathologic diagnosis of invasive disease was made, the patient delivered vaginally as maturity had been reached. She subsequently underwent a right hemicolectomy.[115]

ANAL CANAL

Cancers of the anal canal are extremely rare, representing 1–2% of all rectal and colonic carcinomas. Of all anal canal cancers, the most common are the squamous cell carcinomas and transitional cell carcinomas (cloacogenic, basosquamous, or basaloid). Squamous cell cancer occurs both above and below the dentate line, whereas transitional cell cancers originate from the transitional zone above the dentate line.[83]

The most common symptoms are rectal pain and bleeding. The treatment of these tumors consists of abdominoperineal resection with wide excision of perineal tissue. Experience with these tumors in pregnancy is lacking since no cases have been reported; however, if a pregnant patient is diagnosed to have anal cancer in the first or second trimester, she should be treated as described above and may be delivered vaginally at fetal maturity. In the third trimester, delivery by cesarean section is recommended with an abdominoperineal resection at cesarean section or 2 weeks later. Prophylactic inguinal lymph node dissection is not advised unless clinical metastases are present. A combination of chemotherapy and radiation therapy with surgery for treatment of advanced anal cancers is currently under investigation.

REFERENCES

1. Boring CC, Squires TS, Tong T. Cancer statistics, 1991. *Ca—A Ca J Clin*. 1991;41:29.
2. *1987 Annual Cancer Statistics Review Including Cancer Trends: 1950–1985*. Washington, DC. National Cancer Institute: Division of Prevention and Control. 1988:35. NIH Publication No. 88–2789 III.
3. Woolf RB. *Gastrointestinal Complications of Pregnancy in Gynecology-Obstetrics*. Guide Vol 1. Washington, DC: Commerce Clearing House, 1965.
4. Emge LA. The influence of pregnancy in tumor growth. *Am J Obstet Gynecol*. 1934;28:682.
5. Mitchell MS, Capizzi RL. Neoplastic diseases. In: Burrow GN, ed. *Medical Complications of Pregnancy*. Philadelphia: WB Saunders; 1982:738.
6. Rothman LA, Cohen CJ, Astarloa J. Placental and fetal involvement by maternal malignancy: a report of rectal carcinoma and review of the literature. *Am J Obstet Gynecol*. 1973;116:1023.
7. Gray J, Kenny M, Sharpy-Schafer AP. Metastasis of maternal tumor to products of gestation. *J Obstet Gynaecol Br Emp*. 1939;46:8.
8. Zagars G, Norante JD. Head and neck tumors. In: Rubin P, ed. *Clinical Oncology. A Multidisciplinary Approach*. 6th ed. New York, NY: American Cancer Society; 1983.
9. Cade S. Cancer in pregnancy. *J Obstet Gynaecol Br Commonw*. 1964;3:341.
10. Smith FR. The effect of pregnancy on malignant tumors. *Am J Obstet Gynecol*. 1937;34:616.
11. Rush BF. Tumors of the head and neck. In: Schwartz SI, ed. *Principles of Surgery*. New York: McGraw-Hill; 1983:559.
12. Betson JR, Golden ML. Cancer and pregnancy. *Am J Obstet Gynecol*. 1961;81:718.
13. Scocos KC, Lipshitz J. Adenocarcinoma of the stomach associated with pregnancy. *J Tenn Med Assoc*. 1982;103.
14. Haas FJ. Pregnancy in association with a newly diagnosed cancer: a population-based epidemiologic assessment. *Int J Cancer*. 1984;34:229.
15. Saito, Yoshikawa H, Oomiya A, et al. Saitama-ken Ishikai Shi 1981;16:149 (in Japanese).
16. Hirabayashi M, Ueo H, Okodava Y, et al. Case report, early gastric cancer in a concomitant pregnancy. *Am Surg*. 1987;53:730.
17. Duckler L, Cohen HR. Hyperemesis gravidarum with gastric carcinoma. *Obstet Gynecol*. 1975;45:348.
18. Muller LMM. Adenocarcinoma of the stomach in pregnancy: ultrasonographic diagnosis. *Safr Med J*. 1987;71:530.
19. Parry-Jones E. Krukenberg tumors complicating pregnancy. *J Obstet Gynaecol Br Emp*. 1956;63:592.
20. Aiken DA. Krukenberg tumour of the ovary in association with pregnancy. *J Obstet Gynaecol Br Commonw*. 1966;73:321.
21. Burke S. Krukenberg tumour of the ovaries complicating pregnancy. *J Obstet Gynaecol Br Emp*. 1953;60:915.
22. Fox LP, Stamm WJ. Krukenberg tumor complicating pregnancy. *Am J Obstet Gynecol*. 1965;92:702.
23. Vicens E, Martinez-Mora J, Potau N, et al. Masculinization of a female fetus by Krukenberg tumor during pregnancy. *J Pediatr Surg*. 1980;15:188.
24. Inokuchi K. Prolonged survival of gastric cancer patients on a specific adjuvant chemotherapy. *Jpn J Surg*. 1984;14:351.
25. Reynolds RP, Cantor MO, Henderson H. Carcinoma of the stomach in pregnancy. *Grace Hosp Bull*. 1950;28:127.
26. Bowers RH, Walter W. Carcinoma of the stomach complicated by pregnancy: report of an unusual case. *Minn Med*. 1958;41:30.
27. Furukawa H, Iwanaga T, Ichikawa T, et al. Gastric cancer in adults aged 34 or below—effects of pregnancy and delivery. *Jpn J Gastroenterol Surg*. 1984;17:857 (in Japanese).
28. Kitaoka H. Sex hormone dependency and endocrine therapy for patients with diffuse carcinoma of the stomach. *Jpn J Cancer Chemotherapy*. 1983;10:2453 (Eng abstr).
29. American Joint Committee on Cancer. *Manual for Staging of Cancer*. Philadelphia: JB Lippincott; 1983.
30. Schwartz SI. Liver. In: Schwartz SI, ed. *Principles of Surgery*. New York: McGraw-Hill; 1983:1257.
31. Davis M, Portmann B, Searle M, et al. Histological evidence of carcinoma in a hepatic tumor associated with oral contraceptives. *Br Med J*. 1975;4:496.
32. Kent DR, Nissen ED, Nissen SE, et al. Effect of pregnancy on liver tumor associated with oral contraceptives. *Obstet Gynecol*. 1978;51:148.
33. Dudley AG, Sale P. Hepatocellular carcinoma associated with oral contraceptive use and pregnancy. *Diag Gynecol Obstet*. 1982;4:301.
34. Mays ET, Christopherson WM, Mahr MM, et al. Hepatic changes in young women ingesting contraceptive steroids: hepatic hemorrhage and primary hepatic tumors. *JAMA*. 1976;235:730.
35. Menzies-Gow N. Hepatocellular carcinoma associated with oral contraceptives. *Br J Surg*. 1978;65:316.
36. Meyer P, LiVolsi VA, Canog JL. Hepatoblastoma associated with an oral contraceptive. *Lancet*. 1974;2:1387.
37. Pryor AC, Cohen RJ, Goldman RL. Hepatocellular carcinoma in a woman on long-term oral contraceptives. *Cancer*. 1977;40:884.
38. Seaward PGR, Koch MAT, Mitchell RW, Merrell DA. Primary hepatocellular carcinoma in pregnancy: a case report. *S Afr Med J*. 1986;69:700.
39. Roddie TW. Hemorrhage from primary carcinoma of liver complicating pregnancy. *Br Med J*. 1957;1:31.
40. Purtilo DJ, Clark JV, Williams R. Hepatic malignancy in pregnant women. *Am J Obstet Gynecol*. 1975;121:41.
41. Christensen S, Anderson V, Vilstrup H. A case of hepatoma in pregnancy associated with earlier oral contraception. *Acta Obstet Gynecol Scand*. 1981;60:519.
42. Egwuatu VE. Primary hepatocarcinoma in pregnancy. *Trans R Soc Trop Med Hyg*. 1980;74:793.
43. Haddow JE, Thompson DK, Kloza EM. Maternal hepatoma detected during serum AFP screening. *Lancet*. 1980;2:806.
44. Conn HO. Rational use of liver biopsy in the diagnosis of hepatic cancer. *Gastroenterology*. 1972;62:142.
45. Friedrich N. Beitrage zur Pathologies des Drebses. *Virchows Arch Pathol Anat*. 1966;36:465.
46. Lee YTN. Systemic and regional treatment of primary carcinoma of the liver. *Cancer Treat Rev*. 1977;4:195.
47. Amorika JA, Thompson NW, Frey CF, et al. Hepatic cell adenomas, spontaneous liver rupture and oral contraceptive pills. *Arch Surg*. 1975;110:548.
48. Barnes AC. Liver cell adenomas and oral contraceptives. *N Engl J Med*. 1975;294:1061.
49. Baum JK, Holtz F, Bookstern JJ, et al. Cancer of biliary tract and liver: possible association between benign hepatomas and oral contraceptives. *Lancet*. 1973;2:926.
50. Edmondson HA, Handerson B, Benton B. Liver cell adenomas associated with use of oral contraceptives. *N Engl J Med*. 1976;294:470.
51. Paloyan D, Baker AL, Bekerman C, et al. Liver cell adenomas associated with oral contraceptives. *Proc Inst Med Chicago*. 1976;31:31.
52. Sherlock S. Hepatic adenomas and oral contraceptives. *Gut*. 1975;16:735.
53. Baird JN, Hawley RG. Spontaneous rupture of liver during pregnancy. *J Reprod Med*. 1971;6:93.
54. Hayes D, Lambi H, Hunter IWE. Hepatic cell adenoma presenting with intraperitoneal hemorrhage in puerperium. *Br Med J*. 1977;2:1394.
55. Bis KA, Waxman G. Rupture of the liver associated with pregnancy: a review of the literature and report of two cases. *Obstet Gynecol Surv*. 1976;31:763.
56. Hibberd LT. Spontaneous rupture of the liver in pregnancy: a report of eight cases. *Am J Obstet Gynecol*. 1976;126:334.
57. Kent DR, Nissen ED, Nissen SE, Chambers C. Maternal death resulting from rupture of liver adenoma associated with oral contraception. *Obstet Gynecol*. 1977;50:55.
58. Barnes AD, Harder E, Toot PJ. Successful pregnancy following partial hepatectomy for removal of hepatocellular adenomas. *Am J Obstet Gynecol*. 1984;150:998.
59. Schwartz SI. Gallbladder and extrahepatic biliary system. In: Schwartz SI, Lillehei RC, Shires GT, et al, eds. *Principles of Surgery*. New York: McGraw-Hill; 1983:1307.
60. El-Domeri AA, Brasfield RD, O'Quinn JL. Carcinoma of extrahepatic bile ducts. *Ann Surg*. 1969;169:525.
61. Devoe LD, Moossa AR, Levin B. Pregnancy complicated by extrahepatic biliary tract carcinoma. *J Reprod Med*. 1983;28:153.
62. Todani T, Tabuchi K, Watanabe Y, Kobayashi T. Carcinoma arising in the wall of congenital bile duct cysts. *Cancer*. 1979;44:1134.
63. Attar S, Obeid S. Congenital cysts of the common bile duct: a review of the literature and report of two cases. *Ann Surg*. 1955;142:289.
64. Chesterman JT. Choledochus cyst complicating pregnancy and the puerperium. *J Obstet Gynaecol Br Commonw*. 1944;51:512.
65. Saunders P, Jackson BT. Rupture of the choledochus cyst in pregnancy. *Br Med J*. 1969;3:573.
66. Friend WD. Rupture of choledochal cyst during confinement. *Br J Surg*. 1958;46:155.
67. Kitahama A, Harkness SO, Moynihan PO, Webb WR. A large choledochal cyst with impending rupture post partum. *Br J Surg*. 1984;71:156.
68. Hiatt JR, Gordon-Hiatt JC, Williams RA, Klein SR. Biliary diseases in pregnancy: strategy for surgical management. *Am J Surg*. 1986;151:263.

69. MacMahon B, Yen S, Trichopoulos D, et al. Coffee and cancer of the pancreas. *N Engl J Med*. 1981;304:630.
70. DelRagato JA, Spjut JH. Cancer of the digestive tract. In: DelRagato JA, Spjut JH, eds. *Ackerman and DelRegato's Cancer Diagnosis, Treatment and Prognosis*. St. Louis, MO: CV Mosby; 1977:572.
71. Edis AJ, Kiernan PD, Taylor WF. Attempted curative resection of carcinoma of the pancreas: review of Mayo Clinic experience, 1951–1975. *Mayo Clin Proc*. 1980;55:531.
72. Boyle MF, McLeod ME. Pancreatic cancer presenting as pancreatitis of pregnancy. *Am J Gastroenterol*. 1979;70:371.
73. Boutin J, Gosselin M, Campion JB, et al. Pancreatic cancer during pregnancy (letter). *Nouv Presse Med*. 1978;7(33):2970.
74. Gamberdella FR. Pancreatic carcinoma in pregnancy: a case report. *Am J Obstet Gynecol*. 1984;149:15.
75. Duff P, Greene VP. Pregnancy complicated by solid papillary epithelial tumor of the pancreas, pulmonary embolism and pulmonary embolectomy. *Am J Obstet Gynecol*. 1985;152:80.
76. Smithers BM, Welch C, Goodall P. Cystadenocarcinoma of the pancreas presenting in pregnancy. *Br J Surg*. 1986;73:591.
77. Hodgkinson DJ, Remire WH, Weiland LH. A clinicopathological study of 21 cases of pancreatic cystadenocarcinoma of the pancreas presenting in pregnancy. *Br J Surg*. 1986;73:591.
78. Benyts G, Thiery M, Bekaert S, et al. Adenocarcinoma of the ileum during pregnancy. *Eur J Obstet Gynecol Reprod Biol*. 1977;7:247.
79. Tweed WME. Rupture of a leiomyosarcoma during labor. *J Obstet Gynaecol Br Emp*. 1960;57:110.
80. McLean DW, Arminski TC, Bradley GT. Management of primary carcinoma of the rectum diagnosed during pregnancy. *Am J Surg*. 1955;90:816.
81. Evers HH. A case of obstructive labor due to malignant disease of the sigmoid colon. *J Obstet Gynecol Br Emp*. 1928;35:525.
82. Nesbitt JC, Moise KJ, Sawyers JL. Colorectal carcinoma in pregnancy. *Arch Surg*. 1985;20:636.
83. Storer EH, Goldberg SM, Nivatvongs SL. Colon, rectum and anus. In: Schwartz SI, ed. *Principles of Surgery*. New York, NY: McGraw-Hill; 1983:1169.
84. Donegan WL. Cancer and pregnancy. *Ca—A Ca J Clin*. 1983;33:194.
85. Nijhoff GC. Schwat Gerschaft und Carcinome Rech. *Zentralbl Gynaekol*. 1905;28:881.
86. Green LK, Harris RE, Massey FM. Cancer of the colon during pregnancy. *Obstet Gynecol*. 1975;46:480.
87. Shackelford RT, Zuidema GD. Malignant tumors of the colon. In: *Surgery of the Alimentary Tract*. 2nd ed. Philadelphia: WB Saunders; 1982:163.
88. Nelson RL. In discussion: Nesbitt JC, Moise KJ, Sawyers JL. Colorectal carcinoma in pregnancy. *Arch Surg*. 1985;20:636.
89. Weiss NS, Daling JR, Chou WH. Incidence of cancer of the large bowel in women in relation to reproductive and hormonal factors. *JNCL*. 1981;67:57.
90. Ernster VC, Sac RS, Selvins ST, et al. Cancer incidence by marital status: U.S. Third National Cancer Survey. *JNCL*. 1979;63:567.
91. Fraumeni JF Jr, Lloyd JW, Smith EM, et al. Cancer mortality among nuns: role of marital status in etiology of neoplastic disease in women. *JNCL*. 1969;42:455.
92. Haenzel W, Carrea P. Cancer of the colon and rectum and adenomatous polyps: a review of epidemiologic findings. *Cancer*. 1971;28:14.
93. Hill JA, Kassam SH, Talledo OE. Colonic cancer in pregnancy. *S Med J*. 1984;77:375.
94. Newland RC, Chapuis PH, Pheils MT, et al. The relationship of survival to staging and grading of colorectal carcinomas: a perspective study of 503 cases. *Cancer*. 1981;47:1424.
95. Derburke MG. Intestinal obstruction due to malignancy complicating pregnancy. *Am J Obstet Gynecol*. 1940;40:307.
96. Finn WF, Lord JW. Carcinoma of colon producing acute intestinal obstruction during pregnancy. *Surg Gynecol Obstet*. 1945;80:545.
97. Dworken HJ. Intussusception as a cause of "disappearing" carcinoma of rectum. *Gastroenterology*. 1956;30:694.
98. Lever J. Pelvic tumors obstructing parturition. *Guy's Hosp Rep*. 1843;1:26.
99. Turnbull RB, Kyle K, Watson FR, et al. Cancer of the colon: the influence of the "no touch isolation" technique on survival rates. *CA—A Ca J Clin*. 1968;18:82.
100. Ackerman NB. The technique of primary arterial ligation for cancer of the colon as suggested by venous and lymphatic outflow studies. *Surgery*. 1976;80:312.
101. Stearns M, Schottenfield D. Techniques for the surgical management of colon cancer. *Cancer*. 1971;28:165.
102. Pitluk H, Potlica M. Carcinoma of the colon and rectum in patients less than 40 years of age. *Surg Gynecol Obstet*. 1983;157:335.
103. Moertel CG. Chemotherapy of gastrointestinal cancer. *N Engl J Med*. 1978;299:1049.
104. Banner EA, Hunt AB, Dixon CF. Pregnancy associated with carcinoma of the large intestine. *Surg Gynecol Obstet*. 1945;80:211.
105. DerBrucke MG. Intestinal obstruction due to malignancy complicating pregnancy. *Am J Obstet Gynecol*. 1940;40:3.
106. Fournier R. Etiologie particuliere d'une peritonite postpartum. *Bull Soc Obstet Gynecol (Paris)*. 1947;26:241.
107. Harbison SP. Gastrointestinal and biliary tract malignancy associated with pregnancy. *Clin Obstet Gynecol*. 1963;6:1002.
108. Mengert WF. Dystocia due to carcinoma of the rectum and vagina. *Am J Obstet Gynecol*. 1933;26:451.
109. O'Leary JA, Bepko FJ Jr. Rectal carcinoma and pregnancy. *Am J Obstet Gynecol*. 1962;84:459.
110. Putski PS, Scully JH. Carcinoma of colon producing acute intestinal obstruction during pregnancy. *Am J Surg*. 1949;77:749.
111. Schuyler WBJ. Pregnancy complicated by carcinoma of the bowel arising in the site of chronic granuloma: report of a case. *Obstet Gynecol*. 1955;5:102.
112. Swartley WB, Newton ZB, Hartman JC, et al. Perforated carcinoma of the large intestine complicated by pregnancy. *Ann Surg*. 1947;125:251.
113. Warren RP. Cancer of rectum with pregnancy. *Br J Surg*. 1958;45:61.
114. Berrios JR, Dunnihod DR, Gibbs CE, et al. Appendiceal carcinoid tumors in pregnancy. *Obstet Gynecol*. 1965;26:428.
115. Donnenfeld AE, Roberts NS, Losure TA, Mellen AW. Perforated adenocarcinoma of the appendix during pregnancy. *Am J Obstet Gynecol*. 1986;154:637.

Chapter One Hundred and Eighty-One
Neoplastic Diseases of the Brain

Roberta P. Glick, Avery S. Hart, and James A. Tiesi

181

The diagnosis and management of the patient with a brain tumor is always a grave and difficult situation, but becomes even more problematic when the patient is also pregnant. The implications for the diagnosis and treatment of the brain tumor, as well as the management of the pregnancy and the effects of treatment on the fetus, raise many medical questions as well as several significant controversial ethical issues.

There has been an increased interest in the treatment of brain tumors occurring during pregnancy as a result of recent advances in the understanding of the mechanisms of tumor biology and transformation, linking tumor growth and development to certain hormonal influences that may be present during pregnancy.

In this chapter we will focus on the major types of intracranial tumors likely to be encountered by physicians involved in the treatment of pregnant women. The etiology, pathophysiology, diagnosis, and treatment of these particular tumors will be discussed, with emphasis on their effects on the mother as well as on the fetus. Finally, recent advances in brain tumor biology will be reviewed, including steroid hormone and growth factor receptor relationships as they may relate to tumors occurring during pregnancy.

EPIDEMIOLOGY

It has been estimated that each year in the United States, 89 pregnant women will be diagnosed with a primary brain tumor, that is, 1 in 44,000 pregnancies.[1] Although the incidence of primary brain tumors occurring in pregnancy is no higher than that in nonpregnant women, there have been numerous reports of alterations in the growth rate of certain tumors during pregnancy[2] (see also Chapter 172). While some tumors become symptomatic during pregnancy, others experience resolution of their symptoms postpartum and a few tumors present only in the postpartum period.[2] These data again suggest the importance of hormonal influences in certain tumors.

Of the more than 30 known primary intracranial tumors that can occur during pregnancy, meningiomas, gliomas, acoustic neuromas, and pituitary tumors account for over 85% of tumors diagnosed during pregnancy. Other tumors that may occur, though with less frequency, are hemangioblastoma, neurofibromas, and spinal tumors. Although there are no specific extracranial tumors that are more likely to metastasize to the brain as a result of pregnancy, choriocarcinoma has a high propensity for brain metastasis, but invariably presents in the postpartum period or later.[3]

ETIOLOGY AND PATHOGENESIS

The etiology of most intracranial tumors is unknown. However, several types of CNS tumors have been produced experimentally in laboratory animals by the administration of toxic or noxious agents such as radiation, carcinogens, chemicals, viruses, and by hormonal manipulations.[4] In addition, several clinical reports have linked the development of certain brain tumors to head trauma, dental x-rays, and various occupational exposures to substances such as vinyl chloride, rubber, formaldehyde, electrical/magnetic fields, and metal dust and fumes.[5]

Genetic factors such as oncogenes or loss of suppressor genes recently have been identified to play a role in the development of certain brain tumors and in several well-known inherited disorders (eg, neurofibromatosis, Von Hippel–Lindau disease) that may present with intracranial lesions during pregnancy.[6]

CLINICAL MANIFESTATIONS

Rarely, an intracranial tumor may be discovered incidentally, for example, in the evaluation of head trauma. The vast majority are diagnosed when they become clinically symptomatic due to increased intracranial pressure, local invasion or compression, acute hemorrhage, or syndromes of hormonal hypersecretion in the case of pituitary tumors.

Generalized symptoms of raised intracranial pressure are headache, nausea, and vomiting. The headache is often worse in the morning, upon awakening. Because these symptoms might be confused with the common symptoms of morning sickness in the pregnant patient, there is often a delay in making the diagnosis of an intracranial tumor during pregnancy. Other nonspecific symptoms related to increased intracranial pressure or mass effect caused by the brain tumor include lethargy and changes in mental status.

The presence of focal neurologic symptoms related to the localized mass effect of the tumor on neighboring CNS structures increases the likehood of accurate diagnosis. Limb or facial weakness, numbness and paresthesias, abnormalities of speech or vision, and alterations in personality and cognition signify compromise of the cerebral hemispheres. Ataxias of the limbs or trunk, gait disturbance, and lower cranial nerve dysfunction are results of posterior fossa lesions.

Irritation of the surrounding CNS structures by the lesion can result in seizures, either focal or generalized. Patients presenting with seizures require an immediate neurologic examination and diagnostic investigation. In such patients other causes of seizures also must be considered, such as toxemic (eclamptic) seizures, and metabolic and anoxic insults, all of which also require urgent medical evaluation.

Intratumoral hemorrhage may present as an acute catastrophic event or with any of the previously mentioned symptoms.

Pituitary tumors usually present with signs and symptoms of endocrinopathy (eg, amenorrhea and galactorrhea, Cushing syndrome, acromegaly). During pregnancy, hormonal influences are thought to cause alterations and rapid growth of certain pituitary tumors, in particular prolactinomas, at which time the tumors may present with signs of increased intracranial pressure or more often, neurologic compression (ie, progressive visual loss). Rarely, pituitary apoplexy also can occur (see also Chapter 39).

The presence of clinical signs and symptoms that suggest neurologic disease necessitates a thorough physical and neurologic evaluation, including an ophthalmologic examination. On examination of the eyes, one may find papilledema (in the fundi), cranial nerve palsies, or decreased extraocular movements (due to third and sixth nerve involvement) and decreased visual acuity. All may be signs of increased intracranial pressure (ICP), indicating a dangerous and perhaps clinically unstable situation.

Pathophysiology of Intracranial Pressure

The problem of increased ICP is a result of a unique feature of the adult CNS: the brain surrounded by a rigid box, the skull. What is a remarkable protective advantage in the normal state becomes an incarcerating wall in the face of an expanding intracranial lesion.

The intracranial contents normally consist of only three components: brain, blood, and cerebrospinal fluid (CSF). As a mass lesion begins to grow within the cavity of the skull, it does so by displacing the normal intracranial contents. Pressure and volume relationships initially remain normal as tumor growth and brain compression is compensated for by the loss of CSF and blood from the intracranial cavity. At a certain point, however, compensatory mechanisms become exhausted and any further increase in intracranial pressure results in decompensation. The patient then presents with symptoms. Certain tumors, because of their location near the ventricle, may grow to block the flow of CSF, causing obstructive hydrocephalus, which hastens the onset of increased ICP by further increasing intracranial volume.

The brain often is remarkably compliant; therefore, slowly growing lesions can attain considerable size before these compensatory mechanisms fail and symptoms appear. On occasion, such a lesion (usually a benign tumor) can grow massively and the first clinical sign of a brain tumor may be only headache or decreased level of consciousness, due to raised ICP.

As compensating mechanisms fail and ICP rises steadily, medial portions of the cerebral hemisphere may herniate toward the opposite side in patients with mass lesions above the tentorium cerebelli. In addition, there may be concomitant downward displacement of brainstem structures as the medial portion of the temporal lobe (uncus) herniates over the tentorium. Uncal herniation often is accompanied by compression of the third cranial nerve, causing ipsilateral pupillary dilatation. This is an ominous sign.

A mass lesion below the tentorium cerebelli (posterior fossa) similarly may cause herniation of surrounding brain tissue, causing compression of brain stem medullary structures and cardiorespiratory embarrassment. Deterioration may be hastened by conditions that further increase intracranial pressure (eg, hypoventilation, hypercarbia, straining during delivery, certain anesthetic agents) or lowers intraspinal pressure (eg, lumbar puncture). If untreated, severely raised ICP with herniation will inevitably and quickly lead to death. Treatment of herniation requires, in addition to the immediate attendance of a neurologist or neurosurgeon, emergency measures for lowering the ICP. These measures include intubation for hyperventilation, reduction of brain water content with hyperosmolar agents (ie, mannitol), diuretics (eg, furosemide) and CSF diversion when indicated for hydrocephalus. ICP monitoring, induced barbiturate coma, and emergency surgery for removal of the mass lesion also may become necessary in such situations.

DIAGNOSIS

Once there is clinical suspicion of an intracranial tumor, neuroradiologic investigation is the next logical step in the evaluation.

The field of neurodiagnostic imaging has advanced tremendously within the past 15 years. Computerized axial tomography (CT), introduced in the 1970s, and more recently, magnetic resonance imaging (MRI) have revolutionized the diagnosis of intracranial lesions. MRI rapidly is becoming the procedure of choice for imaging most lesions of the central nervous system. Benefits of MRI include superior brain and spinal cord detail, which can be obtained in a single study in the axial sagittal, and coronal planes without exposure to ionizing radiation and its attendant risks (see also Chapter 5).

Because it does not expose the patient to ionizing radiation, MRI provides an especially attractive alternative to CT in pregnant patients. While there is no evidence that MRI affects the fetus, MRI does expose the fetus to intense magnetic and electromagnetic fields. In some epidemiologic studies, chronic exposure to electromagnetic fields has been associated with an increased incidence of brain tumors in adults.[5] There is no evidence, however, that such exposures harm the fetus based on experience to date, which includes direct imaging of the gravid uterus and the fetal brain as well as the maternal brain with MRI scanners of less than 2 Tesla strength.[7,8] MRI in pregnancy, however, has not been proven safe. Thus, as of December, 1989, MRI was not FDA-approved for use during pregnancy. Given this uncertainty, it is prudent to avoid MRI during the first trimester and to obtain written informed consent for the procedure at any stage of pregnancy when the test is deemed necessary.[9]

Gadolinium-DTPA is an intravenous ferromagnetic material used for contrast enhancement in MRI and is particularly sensitive for demonstrating brain tumors. Currently, there is also very little evidence regarding the safety of this agent. Fortunately, for most MRI examinations, the administration of contrast material may not be required. Although gadolinium is not yet FDA-approved for use during pregnancy, it is available in certain centers and requires the signing of a specific consent and release form.

Absolute contraindications to MRI scanning include implanted metal orthoses, cardiac pacemaker, and even some cerebral aneurysm clips. Relative contraindications may include severe obesity (>250–300 lbs) and claustrophobia, because of the physical constraints of the MRI scanning machine. Many medical centers still do not have ready access to a magnetic resonance imager. A CT scan of the brain becomes the alternate procedure of choice in the diagnosis of a CNS tumor during pregnancy in such cases.

In the special instance of a rapidly deteriorating patient, CT scanning may be the procedure of choice over MRI because of its ready availability and quick capability.

The decision-making process regarding selection of further imaging modalities, when MRI is not available or cannot be performed, requires estimation of the associated radiation dose to the conceptus, as well as knowledge of the consequences of such exposure.

At fetal exposures of less than 10 rads, no adverse effects have been identified statistically against the background rate of spontaneous abnormalities in roughly 3% of live births and of spontaneous abortions in roughly 30% of all pregnancies.[10] Medically indicated exposures of up to 5 rads are considered acceptable in pregnancy when unavoidable.

The exact fetal radiation dose for any given procedure may vary greatly depending on the particular radiographic equipment used, the size of the patient, the position of the uterus within the pelvis, and other factors. However, upper limits on possible exposure can be given. The patient routinely receives 2.5–3.0 rads to the head from a standard head CT (compared to 1.0–1.5 rads from plain skull x-rays). The fetal exposure from a standard skull series is under 10 mrad.[11] For CT scanning, fetal dosage is on the order of 1 mrad or less per slice.[12] This dose can be further reduced by shielding the uterus with lead aprons placed both above and below the patient. The upper limit for cerebral angiography is estimated at 100 mrad; actual exposures may approach this figure, depending on technical factors.[13] Exposures for plain films and CT scans of the cervical spine are similar to those procedures done on the head. Exposure during routine myelography cannot be readily estimated since it depends heavily on the extent of the neuraxis that is imaged and on fluoroscopy time, but is greater than that of CT and plain x-rays.[13]

In the diagnosis of brain tumors, it may be necessary to obtain two separate CT scans of the brain: a noncontrast and a contrast enhanced scan, that is, after the infusion of intravenous iodinated contrast material. Postinfusion scans more accurately detect the presence and delineate the location of a lesion. They also give more information as to the vascularity and size of a lesion. In many instances, the tumor is apparent only after the administration of contrast material; therefore, contrast improves the diagnostic yield of CT scanning.

The risk of administering iodinated contrast material to the fetus as well as the additional radiation exposure of a second CT scan must be weighed against the immediate need for the test. Experience with iodinated contrast agents in pregnancy is limited. They have been used for intravenous injection in diagnosis of deep vein thrombosis and for intra-amniotic injection in diagnosis of various obstetric conditions. One infant exposed to intravenous contrast within the first trimester was born with undescended testes.[14] The relationship to exposure is unknown, and more serious malformations have not been reported. Some infants exposed to intra-amniotic contrast later in pregnancy have developed neonatal hypothyroidism due to suppression of the fetal thyroid by iodine.[15] The risk of this problem after maternal intravenous administration probably is very low. As with other drugs of uncertain safety, use of contrast in the first trimester should be avoided.

When a lesion is not considered to be life-threatening, or occurs late in pregnancy, scanning sometimes is deferred until after delivery.

Plain *skull x-rays,* although an important part of the diagnosis of CNS lesions in the past, now have become essentially obsolete since the introduction of CT and MRI.

Cerebral angiography at times may be required in cases of vascular tumors, usually as part of the preoperative workup. Angiography is performed to demonstrate the tumor's arterial blood supply, the invasion of dural venous sinuses, or to perform preoperative embolization in certain highly vascular tumors (eg, meningiomas and glomus tumors). As with enhanced CT, angiography requires the administration of iodinated contrast material and carries the same concomitant risks to the fetus as discussed under CT scanning with contrast infusion. However, MRI usually can provide adequate information regarding the involvement of the normal intracranial vasculature and can differentiate vascular pathology (eg, giant aneurysm) from tumor. When MRI is available, it can be used instead of cerebral angiography in the pregnant patient in most instances.

Diagnositic in addition to radiologic measures often are necessary in the diagnosis and workup of an intracranial tumor. A thorough endocrinologic evaluation is essential in patients with suspected pituitary tumor both preoperatively and postoperatively (when surgery is necessary). Similarly, detailed pre and postoperative neuro-ophthalmologic testing, including visual field testing, is required in patients with pituitary tumors or other tumors affecting the visual pathway. The same is true for audiologic evaluation, especially brain stem-evoked potentials in patients presenting with hearing loss as a manifestation of an acoustic neuroma or other tumor in the cerebellopontine angle.

Electroencephalography (EEG) can provide useful information in those patients presenting with seizures, again both pre and postoperatively, when surgery is necessary. The evaluation of biochemical markers (ie, α-fetoprotein, human chorionic gonadotropin, carcinoembryonic antigen, and placental alkaline phosphatase) in both CSF and blood can provide diagnostic clues to identifying specific types of tumors; they are useful especially for the germ cell tumors (ie, choriocarcinoma, germinoma, yolk sac tumor, embryonal carcinoma) and certain metastatic tumors. CSF cytology occasionally can be diagnostic in such cases. CSF may be obtained directly from the ventricular system in those patients with ventricular access devices (eg, shunt, Ommaya reservoir) or by lumbar puncture, if deemed safe. CSF cytology with cytospin also can be useful in the staging of certain CNS tumors that may spread through CSF pathways. It should be noted that lumbar puncture probably has no role in the initial diagnosis of intracranial or intraspinal tumors and can be extremely dangerous in the presence of raised intracranial or intraspinal pressure, precipitating the onset of herniation of neural structures.

PRIMARY BRAIN TUMORS

Gliomas

The most common primary supratentorial tumors in the general population are those of glial origin (40% of all tumors). This prevalence in the general population probably is responsible for the high incidence of gliomas diagnosed during pregnancy. In general, there is no difference in the incidence of gliomas between the sexes.

Gliomas are usually infiltrative lesions and cause symptoms due to increased intracranial pressure or brain tissue destruction and compression. Gliomas currently are classified histopathologically according to the World Health Organization (WHO) into three categories: the *low-grade gliomas,* generally considered to be more benign; the *anaplastic astrocytoma,* a tumor of moderate malignancy; and the *glioblastoma multiforme,* a rapidly progressive, extremely malignant, and usually fatal tumor. Basically, all gliomas may be considered *malignant,* however, because without therapy, most are fatal. Although the vast majority of gliomas occur within the cerebrum, they can be found throughout the nervous system, including the cerebellum, brain stem, optic nerves, hypothalamus, and spinal cord.

The therapy of the primary gliomas usually requires a multimodality treatment. The initial preferred treatment for most gliomas is surgical resection, when feasible. Preoperative and postoperative high-dose corticosteroids (dexamethasone) usually are given to decrease the brain edema associated with gliomas. In addition, anticonvulsants are routinely used preoperatively and postoperatively, as seizures may occur. They are more frequent with the low grade gliomas.

Radiation therapy, usually conventional external beam, is recommended for most malignant tumors and for many of the low-grade gliomas, especially when complete surgical resection is not possible. Postoperative radiation in the cases of low-grade gliomas often can be delayed. Chemotherapy with a nitrosourea-based regimen has become routine in the treatment of malignant gliomas. Despite surgery, radiation, and chemotherapy, the two-year survival for malignant gliomas is usually less than 20%, and mean survival is about 1 year.[16] Even the so-called low-grade, benign gliomas have only 5- and 10-year survival rates of 50% and 25%, respectively.[17] It is hoped that the continual development of newer therapies will alter these dismal statistics. Experimental treatments currently under investigation include the use of immunotherapy (interferon, LAK cells, monoclonal antibodies), novel forms of chemotherapy (intra-arterial or intratumoral administration, new drugs), stereotactic or interstitial radiation or hyperthermia, and antioncogene-receptor "targeted" therapy.

Meningiomas

Meningiomas are the second most commonly occurring CNS tumors in the general population, constituting about 15–20% of all primary brain tumors. They are more common in females. Meningiomas are the most commonly diagnosed brain tumor during pregnancy.[1,2] They are known to increase in size during pregnancy[18,19], with the consequent development or exacerbation of symptoms that may resolve postpartum.[2,18] Interestingly, meningiomas also have been associated with carcinoma of the breast.[20] These findings have been attributed to the effects of estrogen, progesterone, and prolactin on tumor growth and differentiation.[2,19-23] We and several other investigators[21-23] have reported the presence of estrogen and progesterone receptors in meningiomas and gliomas. The role that these hormone receptors may play in the growth and development of meningiomas and in other CNS tumors has important therapeutic implications, including the recent use of antiestrogens (ie, tamoxifen) and antiprogesterone drugs to treat these tumors.[24,25]

Meningiomas are usually benign, slow-growing, well circumscribed, noninvasive lesions. Thus, their clinical presentation is due in large part to local compressive and irritative effects; seizures are common. Preoperative and postoperative high-dose corticosteroids (dexamethasone) often are used to control brain edema. Anticonvulsants also are used routinely, as seizures are common. Preoperative embolization by angiography can be helpful when extensive vascularity is present. Because of their well localized and circumscribed nature, meningiomas potentially are curable by surgery, which is the preferred treatment.

The use of radiation therapy is reserved for meningiomas with malignant changes, and occasionally has been beneficial for subtotally resected and recurrent meningiomas.[26] From our own experience, we have found postoperative radiation helpful, especially in cases in which radiation is followed by reoperation. In highly vascular, subtotally resected tumors, radiation appears to decrease vascularity, making the second operation easier. The use of such hormonal agents as antiestrogens (eg, tamoxifin) and antiprogesterones (eg, RU 38486) is considered experimental and has been reserved for patients unable to undergo an operation because of advanced age or because of medical conditions prohibiting surgery.

Phakomatoses

Phakomatoses are a group of genetic disorders that primarily affect the cell growth of cutaneous, ocular, and neural tissues. The neurologic manifestations include the development of brain tumors. Two forms of phakomatoses that may present during pregnancy are the *neurofibromatoses* (Figures 181–1A and 181–1B), in which peripheral or central nervous system tumors develop, and *Von Hippel–Lindau* disease, characterized neurologically by hemangioblastomas of the cerebellum, brain stem, and spinal cord.

Neurofibromatoses

The neurofibromatoses are genetic disorders primarily affecting neural tissue. Two distinct forms are recognized; the genetic abnormality in each form recently has been elucidated.[27] The most common type, *Neurofibromatosis 1* (Nf 1), previously known as peripheral or Von Recklinghausen disease, is an autosomal-dominant disorder affecting about 1 in 4000 individuals.[28] Cafe-au-lait macules, optic gliomas, osseous lesions (eg, sphenoid bone) and peripheral neurofibromatoses are characteristic. The genetic abnormality has been localized to chromosome 17.[28]

Neurofibromatosis 2 (Nf 2), previously known as *central Nf* or *bilateral acoustic Nf,* is an autosomal-dominant disorder occurring in 1 in 50,000 individuals. Acoustic neuromas are characteristic but other intracranial or intraspinal tumors, including meningiomas and gliomas, may occur. The genetic abnormality for Nf 2 is on chromosome 22.[27] Both Nf 1 and Nf 2 chromosomal abnormalities have been found to be the result of deletions of genetic material.

In patients who become symptomatic, surgical resection of the symptomatic lesion is usually the preferred

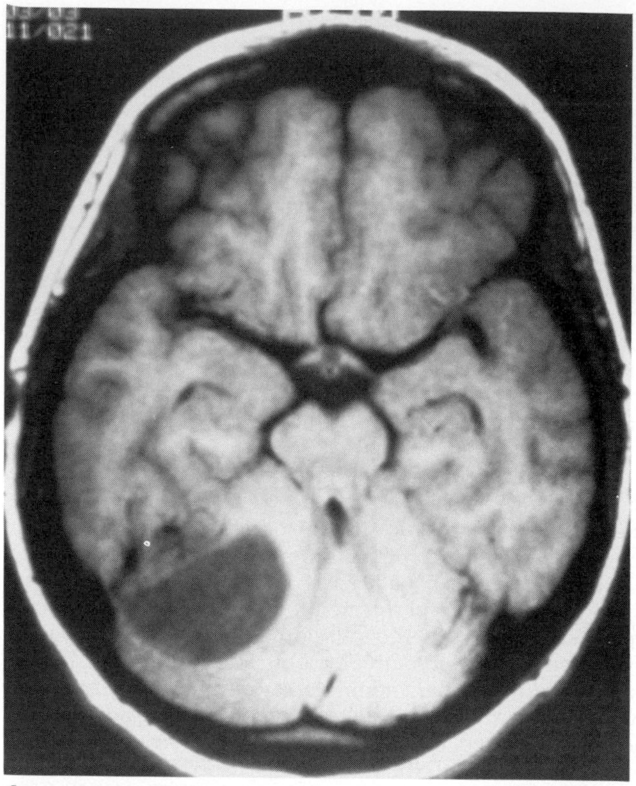

A

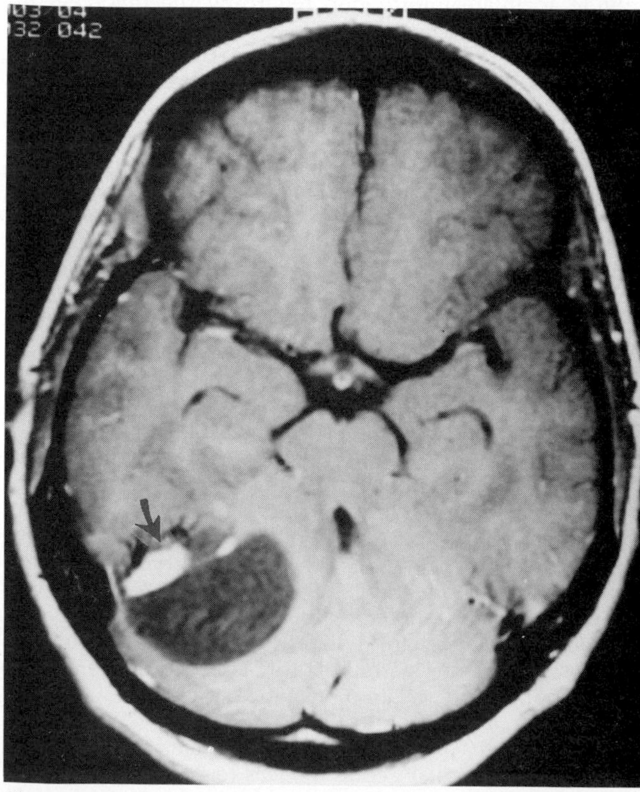

B

Figure 181–1. (A) T_1-weighted axial MRI image showing cystic mass in the right cerebellar hemisphere. (B) MRI at the same level after intravenous gadolinium-DTPA clearly demonstrates the mural tumor nodule at the anterolateral aspect of the otherwise cystic mass (*arrow*). This corresponded precisely to the findings at surgery.

method of treatment and is often curative, as these are usually benign tumors. The recent introduction of focused beam–stereotactic radiation (gamma knife and proton beam) soon may be an alternative, nonsurgical treatment option, especially in selected cases of bilateral acoustic tumors and other multiple lesions.

Von Hippel–Lindau Disease

Von Hippel-Lindau disease is an autosomal-dominant, inherited disorder characterized by the development of hemangioblastomas of the cerebellum, brain stem, or spinal cord.[29] Angiomas of the retina, pancreatic, and renal carcinoma and pheochromocytoma also may occur in this condition.[29]

Hemangioblastomas are benign and highly vascular tumors usually with a cystic and solid component, and account for only 2–3% of all intracranial lesions.[29] They may be multiple and also occur in the spinal canal. In one series, 50% of women with cerebellar hemangioblastomas were pregnant at the time of their initial symptoms, although this association has not been proved in other reports.[30] It has been suggested that the expansion of the maternal blood volume during pregnancy may cause an increase in the tumor's vascular bed and consequent rapid development of symptoms during pregnancy.[31]

Although hemangioblastomas have a tendency to hemorrhage, intracranial tumors more often present with increased intracranial pressure due to obstructive hydrocephalus.[32] Spinal lesions more often are associated with subarachnoid hemorrhage.[32] Because hemangioblastomas occur either sporadically or with the inherited syndrome, patients presenting with a CNS hemangioblastoma must undergo extensive evaluation to search for other lesions of the Von Hippel–Lindau disease.[32]

Rapidly progressive symptoms, due to increased intracranial pressure, obstructive hydrocephalus, or hemorrhage may cause these tumors to present acutely and require immediate treatment. Surgery is the treatment of choice for these tumors.[29-32] Until recently, preoperative angiographic evaluation was essential to identify the number of lesions and localize the tumor nodules. The advent of MRI and MRI contrast material (gadolinium) has shown the need for the more invasive angiographic procedure and in most cases is also superior to CT scanning. In our experience with hemangioblastoma, MRI with gadolinium can identify more accurately the number of lesions in cases of multiple hemangioblastomas, and can precisely localize the tumor nodules that must be totally resected to cure this lesion (see Fig. 181–1).

PITUITARY TUMORS

Pituitary adenomas are frequently occurring neoplasms derived from cells of the adenohypophysis of the pituitary gland. They account for approximately 10% of all intracranial tumors, although incidental adenomas have been documented in up to 23% of unselected routine adult autopsies.[33] The majority of these neoplasms are small, benign, slow-growing lesions confined to the sella turcica, although they may attain large size and present with symptoms of mass effect as well as with endocrinopathy or even pituitary apoplexy (see Chapter 39).

Each secreting cell type in the adenohypophysis can form an adenoma, thereby causing hypersecretion of its individual cell product. In some cases, adenomas of a single-cell type have been found to produce more than one type of hormone. Nonsecreting pituitary adenomas also have been identified. The most common hypersecreting forms of pituitary adenomas are those that produce excesses of trophic hormone (Cushing's disease), growth hormone (acromegaly) and prolactin (amenorrhea and galactorrhea syndrome); the other type of hypersecreting pituitary adenomas are not common.

Prolactinomas

Prolactin-secreting adenomas are the most common hyperfunctional pituitary tumors, representing approximately 25% of all pituitary neoplasms. Within the past 20 years, there has been an increase in the incidence of these tumors in women of child-bearing age, while the incidence of prolactinomas in men and older women apparently has remained stable.[33] The reason for this observed change is unknown. While an increase of pituitary adenomas in laboratory animals administered estrogen has been shown, no clear relationships between human prolactinomas and oral contraceptives has been identified. However, some clinical series suggest such a relationship.[34]

The diagnosis of prolactinoma is established by laboratory evidence of elevated serum prolactin levels (normal: less than 20 ng/mL) and radiographic evidence of a tumor (ie, CT or preferably MRI). It is important to note that there is elevated prolactin in prolactin-secreting tumors during pregnancy, which may decrease after delivery. This probably occurs due to an involution of lactotrophs.[35,36]

Prolactin-secreting tumors may result in gonadal dysfunction in both sexes. The major clinical symptoms of hyperprolactinemia in women are amenorrhea and galactorrhea (Forbes–Albright syndrome), and usually are the result of a microadenoma. Other causes of hyperprolactinemia include pregnancy and certain medications (eg, thorazine, tricyclic antidepressants, Aldomet, metaclopramide, cimetidine). These causes must be differentiated from the diagnosis of a pituitary tumor.

Prolactinomas may grow to a very large size and present with symptoms of a mass effect, such as, visual field deficits or headache. This presentation is more common in males. As the major symptoms of hyperprolactinemia are amenorrhea and infertility, prolactinomas rarely are diagnosed by endocrine symptoms in the pregnant patient. More often, the physician is confronted with an infertile, amenorrheic patient with a microadenoma who wishes to become pregnant. Surgery may be offered to such patients, but carries a 5–10% risk of hypopituitarism and possible infertility.[33]

Dopamine agonists such as bromocriptine and, to a lesser extent, pergolide mesylate, have been used routinely in the treatment of prolactinomas and can cause reduction in tumor size, normalization or reduction of prolactin levels, as well as relief of amenorrhea and galactorrhea.[33,34] Bromocriptine, however, is not tumoricidal, thus the prolactinoma may recur when treatment is stopped. Withdrawal of bromocriptine during pregnancy or postpartum has been reported to result in a number of changes within the tumor, including a rapid increase in size.[37] Although bromocriptine has been used extensively in Europe during pregnancy with no demonstration of fetal injury[38,39], it is not approved for administration during pregnancy in the United States, and therefore is often discontinued at the time pregnancy is diagnosed. In our practice, we recommend the use of bromocriptine for patients with hyperprolactinemia secondary to pituitary tumor, with minimal or no visual compromise, who desire pregnancy. We usually treat for a period of 6 months, during which time pregnancy is prohibited. This should allow for maximal tumor shrinkage, which we evaluate with serial MRI or CT scans every three months. After that time, pregnancy may be attempted and if achieved, the drug is discontinued. From a report by Kelly et al[40], approximately 15% of patients who become pregnant following discontinuance of bromocriptine will develop visual symptoms requiring treatment.

There are numerous reports of an increase in growth rate and size in prolactinomas during pregnancy.[37,41] Hormonal changes during pregnancy are thought to be responsible for this observation. Of those microadenomas that enlarge during pregnancy, about 25% of patients will develop visual compromise that necessitates treatment.[41,42] Trans-sphenoidal resection is the preferred method of treatment.[1,34] Reports of pregnant patients undergoing surgery for pituitary tumors indicate that there is no significant increased risk to the patient or fetus.[1,34,43,44] In those patients who remain clinically stable during pregnancy, medical therapy may be reinstated or surgical treatment attempted following parturition.

Cushing's Disease

Cushing's disease has the highest incidence of morbidity of all the hypersecreting pituitary disorders (see also Chapter 42). Untreated, the expected 5-year survival rate is less than 50%. Death most often results from cardiovascular or infectious complications.[33] Some 75% of Cushing's disease cases occur in women, usually between the ages of 30 and 40 years at the time of diagnosis. The classic clinical features of Cushing's disease include moon facies, central obesity, buffalo hump, hypertension, purple abdominal striae and ecchymoses. These frequently are accompanied by emotional disorders (depression or psychoses), menstrual irregularities, osteoporosis, and glucose intolerance. Cushing's disease also may present in the postpartum period with psychological changes that may be difficult to distinguish from postpartum depression.

The diagnosis of Cushing's syndrome is established by demonstrating elevated morning serum cortisol or urinary-free cortisol levels. The source of Cushing's syndrome (ie, pituitary versus adrenal versus ectopic production) is identified by performance of a dexamethasone suppression test and evaluation of ACTH levels. More than 80% of Cushing's syndrome cases are of pituitary origin (Cushing's disease) due to pituitary microadenoma. In most cases, MRI will demonstrate the tumor; CT is less specific. In those cases in which MRI and CT are not confirmatory, bilateral inferior petrosal sinus blood sampling with simultaneous peripheral blood sampling may show lateralization of elevated ACTH production to one half of the pituitary gland (relative to peripheral blood levels).[45] In those cases, removal of that part of the gland is recommended and has been curative in over 90% cases.[45] In general, excision of the adenoma by way of trans-sphenoidal surgery is the treatment of choice for Cushing's disease and offers the best cure rate (75–93%).[34,45] Recently, the use of external heavy particle (proton) irradiation has shown encouraging remission rates.[46] Currently under investigation are the newer techniques of stereotactic radiotherapy (ie, LINAC and gamma knife).

In the event of Cushing's disease in the pregnant patient, it may be reasonable to delay treatment until the postpartum period, barring severe medical complications or severe neurologic compromise (eg, visual loss). For the most part, these tumors are small and unlikely to significantly increase in size during pregnancy.

Medical treatments of Cushing's disease during pregnancy using serotonin antagonists, dopamine agonists, adrenal toxins and, more recently, ketoconazole are to be avoided as their effect on the fetus have not been fully evaluated.

Acromegaly

Pituitary adenomas that produce excessive amounts of growth hormone produce the syndrome of acromegaly. The onset of acromegaly is usually between the ages of 30 and 50. Unlike Cushing's disease, there is no female predominance in cases of acromegaly. The death rate without treatment of acromegaly is over twice that for age-matched normal patients. Death usually results from cardiovascular or respiratory causes.[33]

The clinical manifestations of acromegaly include facial and acral enlargement, headache, skin thickening, neuropathy, myopathy, and mental disturbances. These may be associated with hypertension, organomegaly, heart disease and glucose intolerance. Diagnosis is made by documentation of elevated growth hormone and somatomedin C levels. However, somatomedin C levels may be elevated normally during pregnancy. Further verification may include the glucose suppression test, which should be avoided in the diabetic pregnant patient. Demonstration of the pituitary tumor radiographically is best performed by MRI. As with Cushing's disease, surgical excision of the tumor by trans-sphenoidal approach offers the best chance of cure in acromegaly (up to 90% in some series).[34,47]

Conventional external beam radiation has little to offer as an initial treatment for acromegaly but has been used as a postoperative adjunct. Newer forms of focused radiation treatment (ie, proton beam and gamma knife irradiation) in experimental studies report remission rates comparable to some surgical series.[48] Medical therapies used in the treatment of acromegaly (ie, bromocriptine, pergolide mesylate, and the even newer somatostatin analogues) have not been approved for administration during pregnancy. As in the case of Cushing's disease, treatment of the usually small, minimally symptomatic tumors in the pregnant patient can be delayed until after delivery unless neurologic or visual compromise is severe or progressive.

Pituitary Apoplexy

Although many small tumors of the pituitary gland may be observed for prolonged periods of time (such as during pregnancy) without harmful effects to the patient, it must be emphasized that any tumor of the sellar as well as parasellar region may undergo infarction or intratumoral hemorrhage, causing sudden expansion of the pituitary gland, a condition termed *pituitary apoplexy*. This uncommon syndrome is characterized by the sudden onset of headache, meningeal signs, visual disturbances, ophthalmoplegia (due to cavernous sinus involvement) and confusion. Rapid visual loss and coma can occur. Pituitary apoplexy is therefore a neurosurgical emergency; rapid hormone replacement and surgery, usually trans-sphenoidal, are often necessary as life- and sight-saving procedures.

Acoustic Neuroma

Acoustic neuroma, a misnomer for *vestibular schwannoma*, is the most common tumor occurring within the cerebellopontine angle of the posterior fossa. These may occur sporadically or as part of neurofibromatosis type 2 (Nf 2), discussed earlier. These tumors arise in the vestibular division of the vestibulocochlear nerve (cranial nerve VIII), usually in the short segment that traverses the internal acoustic meatus. They usually exhibit slow growth rates and cause symptoms by compression of nearby vascular and neural structures. Like the meningiomas, acoustic schwannomas occur more often in women than in men, in an approximate ratio of 3 to 2. The presence of estrogen and progesterone receptors in these tumors also suggest that hormonal influences may play a role in the biology of these tumors.[22,23] The peak incidence of this neoplasm is between the age of 35 and 55, although patients with Nf 2 and bilateral acoustic neuromas are usually younger.

The pathognomonic symptom of this lesion is progressive unilateral hearing loss, occurring over months to years. The first manifestation may be difficulty in hearing voices on the telephone in one ear. This may be associated with tinnitus, unsteadiness, loss of balance, and vertigo. Larger tumors can cause facial numbness or weakness, due to compression of neighboring cranial nerves V and VII, and ataxia due to cerebellar dysfunction. The diagnosis is confirmed by the presence of abnormal brain stem auditory-evoked potentials and a CT (or preferably MRI) demonstration of a tumor.

The treatment of this lesion is complete surgical excision, which can be curative. Recurrence often follows subtotal resection. Due to the indolent growth characteristics of most of these tumors, surgical extirpation could be postponed in the pregnant patient until parturition, as long as clinical symptoms and the radiologic picture remain stable.

A subgroup of acoustic tumors exists that are more rapidly invasive and have higher growth rates.[49] These may require more urgent treatment. The pregnant patient diagnosed with an acoustic tumor should be monitored clinically throughout pregnancy with frequent neurologic and brain stem evoked potential examinations. If the clinical symptoms or electrophysiologic picture show progression, serial MRs may be necessary to evaluate any interval change in the size of tumor. As with meningiomas, symptoms from acoustic schwannomas have been exacerbated by pregnancy, and surgical excision during pregnancy sometimes may be necessary.[2]

MANAGEMENT

The management of the pregnant patient with a brain tumor is complex because of the challenges of diagnosis and treatment of the tumor itself, as well as possible effects that the tumor and its treatment may have on mother and fetus.

The primary tumor poses few, if any, risks to the developing fetus aside from the risks of treatment. Very few malignant brain tumors metastasize beyond the central nervous system. Malignant meningioma, glioblastoma and medulloblastoma have the highest rates of extracranial metastasis of any primary intracranial tumors, but this rate is less than 10%.

A review of the world literature over 103 years by Rothman et al[50] reported 36 cases of maternal cancer that metastasized to the products of conception. Of these cases, 23 demonstrated transplacental spread, with involvement of the fetus in eleven. In each case in which fetal involvement was shown, the primary tumor in the mother was a lymphoproliferative neoplasm or melanoma and none was a primary intracranial tumor.

There have been anecdotal reports of brain tumors associated with abnormal or traumatic deliveries (ie, cesarean section or forceps delivery).[1] However, no correlation has been shown between these occurrences and maternal cancer. Thus, the presence of a maternal brain tumor seems to pose no increased risk for the development of a brain tumor in the newborn child.

Medical Management

Anticonvulsants. Anticonvulsants are used to control tumor-associated seizures or to prevent postoperative seizures. Maternal clearance of most anticonvulsants increases during pregnancy. Consequently, dosages somewhat higher than usual may be needed.[51] Risks to the fetus include congenital malformations, withdrawal phenomena, and hemorrhagic disease of the newborn[51] (see also Chapter 199).

Phenobarbital is considered among the safest anticonvulsants for use in pregnancy with regard to teratogenicity.[52] A mild neonatal withdrawal syndrome, characterized by hyperactivity and tremors, may occur. Withdrawal seizures do not occur and specific therapy therefore is not required.[53] Phenytoin and other hydantoin anticonvulsants used in pregnancy are associated with a constellation of congenital abnormalities, including the fetal hydantoin syndrome.[54] Recent data suggest a similar syndrome in association with fetal exposure to carbamazepine.[55] Valproic acid has been associated with a variety of congenital anomalies, including neural tube defects. Some feel, however, that this is not yet fully proven.[56] Other anticonvulsant drugs used principally for petit mal epilepsy also are teratogenic and should be avoided during pregnancy.[52]

Glucocorticoids (Dexamethasone) and Osmotic Agents (Mannitol)

Management of brain edema and increased intracranial pressure associated with intracranial tumor may necessitate therapy with dexamethasone. Experience with dexamethasone in pregnancy in this circumstance is limited, but glucocorticoids have been used extensively for other conditions associated with gestation.

Dexamethasone and betamethasone given acutely antepartum have found wide acceptance for prevention of neonatal respiratory distress syndrome in premature birth.[57] In the largest study to date, mothers at gestational ages between 26 and 37 weeks received parenteral dexamethasone, 5 mg every twelve hours, to a maximum of 20 mg. Among subjects receiving the full course of steroids, dexamethasone plasma levels in infants delivered within 12 hours after the last maternal dose averaged 12% of maternal levels. No adverse effects occurred on short-term or long-term follow up.[58,59] Fetal dexamethasone levels may reach higher levels, approaching maternal concentrations, in pregnancies at term.[60]

Systematic data regarding more chronic administration of dexamethasone in pregnancy are not available. The data for corticosteroids in general do not suggest any teratogenic effect in humans, although they may cause congenital abnormalities in some laboratory animals.[61] One study found that prednisone causes some retardation of intrauterine growth when given at a dose of 10 mg daily throughout pregnancy.[62]

Suppression of the fetal adrenal gland due to maternal administration of corticosteroids is rare, perhaps because regimens are short-term or low-dose for most indications. However, regimens likely to be used in neurosurgical settings may cause fetal adrenal suppression, requiring replacement of neonatal hydrocortisone at birth.[63] Labor and delivery are physiologically stressful, so that neurosurgical patients who have received long-term, high-dose therapy with glucocorticoids during any period of pregnancy should receive supplemental steroids in the peripartum period.[64]

Acute management of increased intracranial pressure also may require the administration of mannitol. Mannitol crosses the placenta and is excreted by the fetal kidney into amnionic fluid.[65,66] Osmotic shifts may result, but no adverse effects have been demonstrated.

Surgical Considerations

In a recent review, Simon[1] has suggested that the specific management of brain tumors should be tailored to the individual with respect to decisions regarding abortion, premature delivery, mode of delivery, pharmacologic management of the mother, surgical management of the mother, and radiation to the mother. In an analysis by Carmel in 1974[67], the following issues were thought to be important considerations in therapeutic decision making: benign versus malignant tumor, presentations early in pregnancy versus in late pregnancy; intractability of seizures; and other management problems. In view of the poor prognosis associated with many primary malignant tumors and especially the rapid advance of the untreated glioblastoma with a median survival of 48 weeks[16], Carmel's viewpoint was that termination of pregnancy in this particular circumstance could be an option.[67]

The ability to make the initial diagnosis of a brain tumor has been facilitated greatly in recent years by the advent of MRI, which has no ionizing radiation and no currently known harmful side effects to the mother or the fetus.

In most cases, the exact histologic type of tumor cannot be accurately ascertained by radiographic studies alone, and surgical intervention may become necessary for diagnosis. (This excludes such tumors as acoustic neuromas or pituitary tumors.)

Modern computer technology recently has been joined to the techniques of stereotactic biopsy, which has advanced the field to a point that allows biopsy of most intracranial lesions under local anesthesia through a burr hole with the precision and accuracy of 1–2 mm. We routinely use the Brown–Roberts Well's (BRW) stereotactic equipment for this purpose, as well as for cyst and abscess drainage, or instillation of radioactive substances (^{32}P, ^{192}Ir, ^{125}I) for intratumor and interstitial radiation. The BRW equipment interfaces with CT or MRI; either one may be used to precisely localize the lesion for biopsy. Thus, it is now possible to determine safely and accurately the type of brain tumor by way of a stereotactic needle biopsy in the awake patient. This procedure probably will play an important role in the management of brain tumors in the pregnant patient for diagnosis and perhaps for the performance of stereotactic surgical decompression of a mass lesion in the awake patient. If biopsy reveals a malignant tumor early in pregnancy, the consideration of abortion for maternal health reasons may be an option as further treatments (ie, surgery, radiation, and chemotherapy) may be urgently required to control the growth of primary malignant tumors. This may save the life of the mother. Radiation therapy and chemotherapy also may be harmful to the fetus.

On the other hand, if stereotactic biopsy reveals a more benign tumor such as low grade astrocytoma and the patient is clinically stable, the patient can be followed through pregnancy with serial MRI evaluations for tumor progression. In such patients, if clinically and radiologically stable, necessary surgery or radiation can be deferred to the postpartum period.

In cases in which radiographic studies such as MRI or CT clearly define or suggest a more benign tumor (ie, pituitary tumor, acoustic neuroma, "classic" meningiomas, and some cases of low-grade gliomas), clinically stable patients without evidence of severely raised intracranial pressure or mass effect also may be followed through their pregnancy with serial MRI evaluation of the tumor as long as they remain stable. Biopsy and further treatment of the lesion then can be performed in the postpartum period.

Radiation Therapy

Radiation exposure *in utero* carries a risk of several adverse fetal outcomes, including spontaneous abortion, anatomic malformations (notably microcephaly), growth retardation, mental retardation, and possibly childhood cancer.[10,68] The risk is concentrated in the first-trimester exposure; exposure later in pregnancy carries less risk. However, risks are lower at low exposures. As discussed earlier, for exposures of under 10 rads, no adverse effects can be identified statistically against the background rate of spontaneous abnormality of roughly 3% of live births and spontaneous abortions in roughly 30% of all pregnancies.[10] Linear extrapolation from experience at higher doses under an assumption of "no threshold" allows an estimation of risk of adverse fetal outcome at low doses. The maximal fetal risk per rad has been variously estimated at 0.003 to 0.1%.[10,68] For this reason, medically indicated radiation exposures of up to 5 rad are considered acceptable in pregnancy when unavoidable (as in performance of CT scanning or other diagnostic procedures). Higher doses, particularly in the first trimester or above 10 rad, require careful balancing of risks to the fetus and to the mother (see also Chapter 5).

Radiation therapy in pregnancy inevitably exposes the fetus to more radiation than does diagnostic imaging. Fortunately, conceptus dose because of scatter is relatively low when conventional radiation therapy is delivered to parts distant from the uterus. It is not negligible, however.

Specific scatter data for radiation of the brain in pregnancy are not available. Because Hodgkin's disease is relatively common in women of childbearing age, some data are available for radiation of the upper body, especially the mediastinum. Phantom dosimetry without secondary shielding has been used to measure doses to the pelvis at distances of about 30 cm below the inferior border of the mediastinal field, using linear accelerators. Pelvic exposures at this distance have fallen in the range of 0.2–0.4%, that is, 2–4 rads of pelvic exposure per 1000 rads of mediastinal exposure.[69-71] Pelvic exposure is greater with cobalt 60 U than with linear accelerators under otherwise similar conditions. Addition of secondary pelvic shielding reduces exposure, but only by half.[70] The remainder presumably represents internal (tissue) scatter as opposed to external (air) scatter and leakage from the linear accelerator.

Irradiation of the brain rather than the mediastinum would put the pelvis at greater distance, reducing the conceptus dose. On the other hand, with progression of pregnancy, this benefit would be partially cancelled as the gravid uterus enlarged. Thus, it is conceivable that a course of radiation of 60 Gy of radiation to the brain might deliver up to 5–10 rad to the fetus despite secondary shielding. This is precisely the threshold at which the risk of an induced congenital anomaly becomes a concern.

Because radiotherapy is beneficial for malignant brain tumors but poses a risk to the fetus, reduction in fetal dosage is desirable. One solution would be to hold all or part of the radiation dose until the postpartum period, if delivery is imminent. Short of withholding radiation therapy, several options are available.

Reexamination of recurrence patterns and the incidence

of radiation necrosis following radiotherapy has led to the proposal of using focal rather than whole brain irradiation for malignant glioma in most cases.[72] The exposure rate for scattered radiation is proportional to field size.[73] Therefore, use of limited fields is especially important in the pregnant patient. Substitution of heavy charged particles for photons in external beam irradiation also reduces scatter. Several clinical trials in nonpregnant patients have used a variety of heavy particle beams with good results, but none of these studies were with malignant tumors.[74]

Newer experimental forms of radiotherapy include the use of interstitial brachytherapy with low-energy radioisotopes implanted intratumorally. This type of therapy minimizes radiation dose to tissues remote from the tumor. Geometric attenuation follows the inverse square law. Absorption and scattering by intervening tissue results in rapid exponential decline in exposure levels. For ^{125}I (energy 35 keV), this physical attenuation halves the dose for every 2 cm of tissue traversed.[75,76] Because of these phenomena, the internal radiation dose to the uterus from an I-125 source in the brain may be negligible.[77]

To date, interstitial therapy of brain tumors has focused on treatment of recurrent malignant gliomas in nonpregnant patients.[78] Currently, protocols are underway to evaluate the efficacy of an IR 192 or I-125 implant boost after an external radiation dose as well as for "upfront" treatments or the addition of hyperthermia. An alternative in pregnancy might be to give a small dose of focal radiation by external beam and to rely more heavily on interstitial therapy for the primary radiation dose in cases of rapidly progressive malignant tumors. However, the efficacy of such an approach remains untested to date.

Chemotherapy

The administration of antineoplastic drugs to the pregnant cancer patient is extremely hazardous. Many are teratogenic in the first trimester of pregnancy. After the first trimester, ongoing risks continue, including spontaneous abortion, premature birth, intrauterine growth retardation, and other forms of fetal toxicity (see also Chapter 173).[79]

In the nonpregnant patient, chemotherapy usually plays a palliative role in the management of malignant brain tumors.[80] While ideal chemotherapeutic agents for malignant brain tumors have not been developed yet, penetration of the blood-brain barrier is a clearly desirable quality, characterized by high lipid solubility, low molecular weight and loose protein binding.[81] Unfortunately, these same properties promote transport across the placenta. Thus, the principal chemotherapeutic agents most active against malignant astrocytoma, the nitrosoureas, also would be efficiently delivered to the fetus. Some nitrosoureas are not only teratogens but are also transplacental carcinogens, at least in animals.[82]

Chemotherapy of malignant brain tumors in pregnancy therefore is not advisable. To date, no treated cases of brain tumor have been reported during pregnancy. Only one patient has received a nitrosourea during pregnancy. In this unusual case, a pregnant woman with refractory diffuse large-cell lymphoma was treated with BCNU plus procarbazine followed by streptozotocin alone. She elected this course "despite explanation of the likely teratogenic and carcinogenic effects on the fetus" and bore a genotypically and phenotypically normal fetus at 35 weeks' gestation.[83]

Pituitary Tumors

There appears to be some controversy regarding the treatment of pituitary tumors, in particular prolactinomas, during pregnancy. In one report, Magyar and Marshall[84] did not treat prolactinomas producing visual defects if they presented in the third trimester, but treated them earlier in pregnancy. They also found that of those patients entering pregnancy with a known pituitary tumor, 25% developed visual problems, of which one half required surgery or radiation during their pregnancy. Kelly found that only 15% of patients with known prolactinomas treated with bromocriptine developed visual symptoms when bromocriptine was discontinued during pregnancy.[40] Because bromocriptine is not tumoricidal, when it is discontinued the tumor may increase in size or may infarct.[1,37,85] In some cases, bromocriptine has been restarted during pregnancy if patients become symptomatic upon its termination.[34]

Of those patients who require trans-sphenoidal surgery during pregnancy for relief of visual compromise caused by pituitary tumors, many have undergone surgery without an increased risk to the fetus.[1,34,43,44]

Perioperative Management

An important scenario involves the patient who presents during pregnancy with a rapidly deteriorating neurologic picture due to raised intracranial pressure from the mass effect of a tumor or as a result of obstructive hydrocephalus. In these cases, urgent surgery may be necessary and special consideration must be given to the pregnant patient. In many cases, the pregnant patient can safely undergo intracranial surgery without any increased risk to her or the fetus.

When intracranial tumor necessitates neurosurgical intervention in pregnancy, knowledge of gestational alterations in terms of physiology and anatomy must guide the perioperative management. Beyond the first trimester, gravid patients should be positioned in the supine position in rare instances only to avoid compromise to the vena caval blood return and to uteroplacental blood supply. Patients should be positioned in a partial left lateral decubitus position, whenever possible, with the right hip tipped upward at about 15 degrees.[86]

Despite restrictive lung mechanics due to the gravid uterus, pregnant women exhibit physiologic hyperventilation (see Chapter 118). Baseline PCO_2 is usually around 30 mm Hg with an associated respiratory alkalosis, which is compensated partially by the kidneys. Perioperative ventilator management should maintain this state of hyperventilation even if intracranial pressure is not elevated. Maternal acidosis and hypoxia are detrimental to fetal welfare and should be avoided assiduously.[86]

Lower esophageal sphincter tone and gastric motility are decreased in pregnancy (see Chapter 4). This phenomenon increases the risk of gastric aspiration, particularly with altered mental status. Perioperative antacids should be considered for this purpose, as well as for prophylaxis of stress ulceration. The safety of cimetidine in pregnancy, however, has not been established.[86]

Glomerular filtration increases in pregnancy and normal serum creatinine falls below 1.0 mg/dL, typically to the range of 0.5 mg/dL. The risk of urinary tract infection increases in pregnancy, with attendant risk of premature labor (see Chapter 142). Therefore, urinary catheterization should be avoided or minimized.[86]

Pregnant women manifest a hypercoagulable state, which is compounded by neurosurgical intervention and consequent immobilization. Therefore, consideration must be given to the prevention of deep vein thrombosis and subsequent pulmonary emboli. Heparin is safe in pregnancy but generally contraindicated before and after intracranial operations. Intermittent pneumatic calf compression devices should be used instead.[87]

If antibiotic prophylaxis is desired for a neurosurgical procedure such as placement of a ventricular shunt or reservoir, fetal considerations impose some constraints. Penicillins and cephalosporins are safe but may not cover the organisms of concern (ie, methicillin-resistant staphylococci).[88] In clinical experience, trimethoprim-sulfamethoxazole has not been associated with adverse fetal outcomes. However, theoretical objections have been raised because trimethoprim is a folate antagonist and therefore might be teratogenic in humans. Also, the sulfonamide component theoretically could cause neonatal kernicterus. Consequently, this combination should not be used in the third trimester. Clindamycin appears to be safe in pregnancy, as does gentamicin; dosage of the latter must be adjusted due to increased renal clearance.[88] Vancomycin should be avoided because of potential fetal ototoxicity.[88]

Cesarean Section

An important management consideration for the pregnant patient harboring a brain tumor is the possible need for a cesarean section delivery. Whether a cesarean section is necessary depends on the presence and severity of raised ICP in the mother. Although uterine contractions do not necessarily increase the ICP of the mother, abdominal pressure during the second stage of labor does significantly increase ICP.[1] In the presence of raised ICP, cesarean section thus has been recommended at times. The final decision will depend on the definition of an acceptable level of ICP. In cases in which the level of ICP is not thought to be dangerous, vaginal delivery may be considered, although the second stage of labor should be shortened by forceps or vacuum delivery. A multiparous woman will more likely tolerate a vaginal delivery without a severe increase in ICP.[1]

Santoul[89] recommended in 1971 that cesarean section be considered under the following conditions: when a malignant tumor is diagnosed but not yet treated; when a moribund maternal state might ensue; if neurosurgical intervention is required in the last 2 months; in cases of abnormal fetal presentations; or when forceps delivery under general anesthesia is required. In most other cases, Santoul recommended vaginal delivery.

Recently, Simon offered a more enlightened view based on the fact that very few mothers actually develop complications from ICP during delivery.[1] He recommended that cesarean sections be done solely for obstetric reasons and to avoid the second stage of labor. When there is concern over ICP, forceps delivery should be performed.

In our own experience, the recommendation for cesarean section has been based on both maternal and fetal considerations: the nature and location of the tumor (ie, malignancy, size, necessary treatments), the severity of the raised intracranial pressure, the neurologic condition of the mother, and fetal health, size, and position. This calls for a joint involvement of obstetrician and neurosurgeon working together as a team to assess the medical situation accurately and to make clinical judgments regarding appropriate recommendations for management of the pregnancy.

MOLECULAR BIOLOGY

Despite surgery, radiation, and chemotherapy, the survival time and quality of survival of patients with primary malignant CNS tumors remain dismal.[16] The failure of these classical treatments has led to recent biological investigations aimed at understanding the mechanisms of tumor cell growth, proliferation, and transformation as a means of developing improved and more specific therapies. To this end, three important areas of research relevant to the discussion of brain tumors occurring during pregnancy will be reviewed: (1) the role of oncogenes, proto-oncogenes, and tumor suppressor genes in the development of brain tumors; (2) the presence and significance of hormone receptors in CNS tumors; and (3) the role that growth factors and their receptors may play in relation to autocrine transformation in CNS neoplasia.

Oncogenesis

Several pathogenic models recently have been suggested to explain the development of certain tumors. The oncogene and proto-oncogene theory involves the activation of a single gene locus, either through mutation, viral integration, or inheritance as part of a syndrome, which then causes transformation of previously normally reproducing cell(s) into uncontrolled tumor cell(s).[90] The finding of amplification and enhanced expression of the epidermal growth factor (EGF) receptor gene in primary gliomas supports this particular theory.[91]

On the other hand, the tumor suppressor gene or "antioncogene" theory suggests that a deletion of both copies of a specific gene locus is responsible for cell transformation.[90] It appears that the protein product coded for by such proto-oncogenes normally protects the cell from transformation by acting as a brake for proliferation or tumor development. The deletion of the gene from each of a pair of chromosomes then allows for uncontrolled reproduction.

This second model has been studied extensively in retinoblastoma, and recently has been demonstrated to be the modus operandis in other genetic disorders presenting with CNS tumors during pregnancy, specifically neurofibromatosis (Nf 2 and bilateral acoustic neurofibromatosis) and Von Hippel–Lindau disease. In Nf 2, the deletion of a portion of chromosome 22 has been identified as the genetic basis of this disease.[27] In Nf 1, chromosome 17 has been identified as the Nf 1 gene.[28] In addition, chromosomal abnormalities also have been identified in meningiomas and gliomas.[27]

Steroid Hormone Receptors

Meningiomas occur more often in women[15] and may increase in size during pregnancy, causing symptoms that may resolve after delivery.[2,18] An association between meningiomas and carcinoma of the breast has been shown.[20] These clinical observations suggest that meningiomas are hormone-responsive tumors. Subsequent investigations have shown the presence of steroid hormone receptors in meningiomas.[92,93] We and several other investigators have reported specific estradiol and progestin binding in meningiomas, gliomas, acoustic neuromas, and a variety of CNS tumors.[21-23,94] It also has been suggested that prolactin, levels of which increase during pregnancy, also acts as a growth promoter in human meningiomas.

In tumors outside the CNS, for example, breast cancer, the presence of hormone receptors has prognostic value for the response of the tumor to endocrine therapy.[95,96] In addition, several studies suggest that the presence of edema in these tumors may be a function of hormone receptor status.[2] In breast, melanoma, and prostate cancer[97,98] the level of binding has been found to correlate with the grade of malignancy. In our own studies of gliomas we reported a significant difference in the presence of estrogen receptors in benign versus malignant gliomas, with the more malignant tumors demonstrating higher estradiol binding. Further studies have examined the *in vitro* effect of estradiol, tamoxifen, and progesterone on meningioma cell growth.[99] In another study, the effect of the antiprogesterone (RU-38486) on meningiomas implanted into nude mice was investigated.[25] These studies are further evidence that meningioma growth is influenced by steroid hormones.

As a result of these experimental investigations, several clinical reports have appeared in which antiestrogens (tamoxifen) or medroxyprogesterone acetate-MPA[25] were used in human patients with meningiomas. To date, however, these studies have been inconclusive and the use of such hormonal therapy for the treatment of brain tumors remains experimental.

Growth Factors and Receptors

Peptide growth factors are known to regulate normal cellular metabolism and proliferation. Tumor cells are characterized by abnormalities in these processes, including the autocrine secretion of certain growth factors and attenuated receptor expression, perhaps due to the activation of specific oncogenes.[100]

Epidermal Growth Factor

Epidermal growth factor (EGF) is perhaps the most extensively studied growth factor in CNS tumors. EGF is a polypeptide mitogen that stimulates cellular proliferation and DNA synthesis in a variety of cells[101] (see Chapter 37). Its biological actions are mediated through a specific membrane receptor, which is a protein tyrosine kinase.[102] EGF is known to be a normal glial mitogen.[103,104] Recently, the overexpression of the EGF receptor (EGF-R) in gliomas has been reported[91] as well as the presence of EGF-R and EGF binding in meningiomas.[105] It also is known that the C-erb-B_2/neu oncogene product is related to the EGF receptor[106] and may be involved in cellular resistance.[107] In a recent review by Westphal[107], the interrelation of EGF and the transforming growth factors (TGFs) was discussed and appears more complex than initially perceived.

Not much is known about the regulation of EGF and EGF-R in CNS tumors. The hormonal modulation of EGF, however, has been studied in tumors outside the CNS. Estrogens are known to regulate cell growth and proliferation by binding to nuclear receptors that, in turn, bind to DNA sequences and regulate gene transcription.[108] Estrogens also may promote growth by regulating the levels of certain growth factors or their respective receptors.[109] In breast cancer, there is substantial evidence for the induction of autocrine growth factors by estrogen.[110] In uterine membranes, 17 β-estradiol (E_2) has been shown to increase levels of EGF-R by increasing EGF-R mRNA.[109] In breast cancer cells, EGF gene expression (m-RNA levels) is increased by progestins.[111] The growth-inhibitory effects of progestins and of the antiestrogen hydroxyclomiphene on human breast cancer cells is mediated by hormonal inhibition of EGF production.[112] In these same experiments, insulin was found to be synergistic with EGF.

Several investigators also have examined the relationship of growth factors to hormone receptors in breast cancer. Decreased progesterone binding and attenuated progesterone action were found in cells treated with EGF.[113] In human breast cancer biopsies, high EGF-R has been found in association with low estrogen receptor (ER) content.[114] The levels of both EGF-R and insulin-like growth factor receptors (IGF-R) were found to be related to steroid receptor content, and their presence was associated with malignant transformation and dedifferentiation of breast cancer.[115]

Plasminogen activator (PA), a serine protease thought to be involved in cell migration and malignancy, also has been studied in relation to hormone receptors and EGF-R.[116] Low PA levels in breast cancer are associated with ER negativity and EGF-R positivity; they may be an indication of poorer differentiation and prognosis.

Although the results of these studies with breast cancer cannot be extrapolated directly to human CNS tumors, investigative work in the area of hormonal modulation of growth factors in CNS tumors is currently underway.

Platelet-derived Growth Factor. Platelet-derived growth factor (PDGF) is polypeptide growth factor originally isolated from blood platelets[117] (see Chapter 37).

PDGF is thought to be more involved in cellular metabolism by way of a calcium-dependent pathway than in mitogenesis.[107] PDGF receptors (PDGF-R) have been identified on normal glial cells[118] and PDGF appears to be mitogenic for glia.[107] PDGF may be important in preventing differentiation in the developing CNS[119] and in stimulating myelination.[107] Recently, PDGF receptors have been identified on glioma cells, and autocrine production of PDGF by glioma cells has been reported.[120]

Insulin/IGF. Insulin and insulinlike growth factors (IGFs or somatomedins) are polypeptide hormones with both metabolic and growth-promoting properties (see Chapter 37). These growth factors interact with the cell surface by specific receptors similar to the mechanism of EGF action. In fact, recent sequencing of the insulin receptor revealed homologies to EGF.[121] Insulin and IGF are known to play a role in normal neural growth and differentiation[122,123] and also may be important growth factors for CNS tumors.[124]

IGF-I, IGF-II, and insulin receptors have been identified in the normal adult and fetal human brain[125-127], and insulin and the IGFs have been shown to modulate cellular metabolism, growth and differentiation of normal neural tissue.[128,129] Insulin and IGFs share important neurotrophic influences with nerve growth factor, including the capacity of nerve growth factor to enhance neurite formation in neuroblastoma cells, and increase the expression of genes encoding for cytoskeletal proteins.[130] Insulin can regulate neuronal maturation[123], and IGF was recently shown to stimulate proliferation as well as promote differentiation of rat oligodendroglial cells *in vitro*.[122] Insulin also has been shown to stimulate morphologic differentiation of neonatal rat astrocytes in culture.[128,129]

We have reported previously that insulin receptors were present in freshly isolated human gliomas and cultured glioma cells as determined by competitive binding, affinity cross-linking immunoprecipitation, and autophosphorylation.[131] Insulin-induced down-regulation of the receptor and insulin-stimulated glucose uptake also were observed in cultured glioma cells.[131]

More recently, we reported the results of studies with both insulin and IGF receptors in meningiomas and gliomas in which we showed significantly higher insulin binding in meningiomas but significantly higher IGF-I binding in gliomas. *In vitro* studies also were performed, examining the effect of insulin and IGF on cell growth proliferation and differentiation.[124]

Our *in vitro* results support the role of insulin or related IGFs as CNS tumor growth factors: insulin alone maintained and significantly enhanced the growth of glioma, meningioma, and fetal CNS cells grown in serum-free media; insulin maintained the ability of glioblastoma (GBM) cells to stain for GFAP (a differentiation marker) similar to that seen in serum media[124], and IGF increased the number of GFAP-positive cells fourfold.[132]

Morphologic changes suggestive of differentiation were seen in tumor cells grown in the presence of insulin, similar to changes reported for astrocytes and neurons grown in insulin[128,129,133] and oligodendroglial cells grown in IGF-containing media.[122]

Evidence for a similar role for insulin and IGF as tumor growth factors has been suggested by studies in tumors outside the CNS.[134,135] Several such tumors that secrete IGF-like peptides[136-138] have enhanced IGF gene/mRNA expression[139] and demonstrate specific insulin and IGF binding.[140] Enhancement of IGF-II receptors recently has been reported in glioblastomas.[141] Insulin and IGF also have been shown to support the growth of other non-CNS tumor cells in culture.[142,143]

We recently have developed specific radioimmunoassay for both IGF-I and IGF-II and have used these tests to study the autocrine production of IGF by CNS tumors, *in situ* and *in vitro*. It appears that meningiomas preferentially express IGF-I and gliomas IGF-II. This finding was seen in tumor cyst fluid, that is, *in situ*, and in tumor cell–conditioned media, that is, *in vitro*.[144]

This differential expression of IGFs and IGF receptors by different CNS tumors is of particular interest as it relates to the hormonal modulation of these growth factors.

Similar to EGF, IGF appears to be regulated hormonally. In breast cancer cells, IGF-I production was found to be tightly coupled to growth regulation by estrogens and antiestrogens.[145] In these studies estrogen, insulin, IGF and TGF-α all induced cellular proliferation and IGF-I secretion; antiestrogens, TGF-β and glucorticoids had the opposite effects. In another study, the presence of IGF-R correlated positively to both estrogen receptor and progesterone receptor content.[115]

As discussed under steroid hormone receptors, the presence of estrogen and progesterone receptors have been shown in most meningiomas, as well as higher estradiol binding in malignant gliomas versus benign gliomas.[23] This difference in hormone receptor binding in CNS tumors, along with the preferential expression of insulin and IGFs in different CNS tumors, appears to be consistent with the findings in breast cancer.

This suggests that growth factors in CNS tumors may be regulated hormonally in a similar fashion to those in breast cancer. Production of these growth factors thus also may correlate with hormone receptor status and degree of malignancy.

Perhaps through the further understanding of the possible links between steroid hormone receptors, growth factors, and oncogenic transformation improvements in tumor therapy can be achieved, directed specifically at these receptors. Already reported is a clinical study using monoclonal antibodies directed against the EGF-R and linked to radiation for the treatment of malignant gliomas.[146] In addition to such therapeutic uses, "targeted" antibodies appear promising for neurodiagnostic imaging and immunohistochemical purposes. These are presently very exciting areas of investigation.

REFERENCES

1. Simon RH. Brain tumors in pregnancy. *Semin Neurol.* 1988;8:214.
2. Roelvink CA, Kamphorst W, VanAlphen HAM, Rao BR. Pregnancy-related primary brain and spinal tumors. *Arch Neurol.* 1987;44:209.
3. Ishizuka T, Tomoda Y, Kaseki S, et al. Intracranial metastasis of choriocarcinoma. *Cancer.* 1983;52:896.
4. Wilkins RH: Neoplastic disease of the brain. In: Gleicher N, ed. *Principles of Medical Therapy in Pregnancy*. New York: Plenum Press; 1985:1085.
5. Preston-Martin S, Mack W, Henderson BE. Risk factors for gliomas and meningiomas in males in Los Angeles county. *Cancer Res.* 1989;49:6137.
6. Martuza RL. Genetic factors in brain tumors. In: Wilkins RH, Rengachary SS, eds. *Neurosurgery*. New York: McGraw-Hill; 1985:505.
7. Weinreb J. Obstetrics. In: Stark DD, Bradley WG Jr, eds. *Magnetic Resonance Imaging*. St Louis, MO: CV Mosby; 1988:1297.
8. Pavlicek W. Safety considerations. In: Stark DD, Bradley WG Jr, eds. *Magnetic Resonance Imaging*. St. Louis, MO: CV Mosby; 1988:244.
9. National Radiological Protection Board, U.K. Revised guidelines on acceptable limits of exposure during nuclear magnetic resonance clinical imaging. *Br J Radiol.* 1983;56:974.
10. Mole RH. Radiation effects on pre-natal development and their radiological significance. *Br J Radiol.* 1979;52:89.
11. National Council on Radiation Protection and Measurements. *Medical Radiation Exposure of Pregnant and Potentially Pregnant Women*. NCRP Report No. 54, 1977.
12. McCullough EC, Payne JT. Patient dosage in computed tomography. *Radiology.* 1978;129:457.
13. Wagner LK, Lester RG, Saldana LR. Exposure of the Pregnant Patient to Diagnostic Radiation: A Guide to Medical Management. Philadelphia: JB Lippincott, 1985.
14. Kiekegaard A. Incidence and diagnosis of deep vein thrombosis associated with pregnancy. *Acta Obstet Gynecol Scand.* 1983;62:239.
15. Rodesch F, Camos M, Ermans AM, et al. Adverse effect of amniofetography on fetal thyroid function. *Am J Obstet Gynecol.* 1976;126:723.
16. Sakman M. Survival in glioblastoma: Historical perspective. *Neurosurgery.* 1980;7:435.
17. Shaw EG, Daumas-Duport C, Scheithaver BW, et al. Radiation therapy in the management of low-grade supratentorial astrocytomas. *J Neurosurg.* 1989;70:853.
18. Bickerstaff ER, Small JM, Guest IA. The relapsing course of certain meningiomas in relation to pregnancy and menstruation. *J Neurol Neurosurg Psych.* 1958;21:89.
19. Markwalder T. Estrogen and progesterone receptors in meningiomas in relation to clinical and pathologic features. *Surg Neurol.* 1983;20:42.
20. Schoenberg BS, Christine BW, Whisnant JP. Nervous system neoplasms and primary malignancies of other sites: The unique association between meningiomas and breast cancer. *Neurology.* 1975;25:705.
21. Cahill DW, Bashirelahi N, Solomon LW, et al. Estrogen and progesterone receptors in meningiomas. *J Neurosurg.* 1984;60:905.
22. Glick RP, Molteni A, Fors EM. Hormone binding in brain tumors. *Neurosurgery.* 1983;12:513.
23. Martuza RL, MacLaughlin DT, Ojemann RG. Specific estradiol binding in schwannomas, meningiomas, and neurofibromas. *Neurosurgery.* 1981;9:665.
24. Markwalder TM, Waelti E, Korig MP. Endocrine manipulation of meningiomas with medroxyprogesterone acetate: Effect of MPA on receptor status of meningioma cytosols. *Surg Neurol.* 1987;28:3.
25. Olson JJ, Beck DW, Schlechte JA, Loh PM. Effect of the antiprogesterone RV-38486 on meningioma implanted into nude mice. *J Neurosurg.* 1987;66:584.
26. Barbaro NM, Gutin PH, Wilson CB, et al. Radiation therapy in the treatment of partially resected meningiomas. *Neurosurgery.* 1987;20:525.
27. Siezinger BR, Rouleau G, Ozelius LN, et al. Common pathogenetic mechanism for three tumor types in bilateral acoustic neurofibromatosis. *Science.* 1987;236:317.
28. National Institutes of Health Consensus Development Conference: Neurofibromatosis: conference statement. *Arch Neurol.* 1988;45:575.
29. Melmon KL, Rosen SW. Lindau's disease: review of the literature and study of a large kindred. *Am J Med.* 1964;36:595.
30. Robinson RG, Aspects of the natural history of cerebellar haemangioblastomas. *Acta Neurol Scand.* 1965;41:372.
31. Kasarskis EJ, Tibbs PA, Lee C. Cerebellar hemangioblastoma symptomatic during pregnancy. *Neurosurgery.* 1988;22:770.
32. Neumann HPH, Eggert HR, Weigel K, et al. Hemangioblastomas of the central nervous system. *J Neurosurg.* 1989;70:24.
33. Tindall GT, Barrow DL. *Disorders of the Pituitary*. St. Louis: CV Mosby; 1986.
34. Wilson CB. A decade of pituitary microsurgery: the Herbert Olivecrona lecture. *J Neurosurg.* 1984;61:814.
35. Rjosk HK, Fahlbusch R, vonWerder K. Influence of pregnancies on prolactinomas. *Acta Endocrinol.* 1982;100:337.
36. Laws ER Jr, Fode NC, Randall RV, et al. Pregnancy following transsphenoidal resection of prolactin-secreting pituitary tumors. *J Neurosurg.* 1983;58:685.
37. Dommerholt HBR, Assies J, Van der Werf AJM. Growth of a prolactinoma during pregnancy. *Br J Obstet Gynaecol.* 1981;88:62.
38. Bergh T, Nillus SJ, Enoksson P, et al. Bromocriptine induced pregnancies in women with large prolactinomas. *Clin Endocrinol.* 1986;25:325.
39. Raymond JP, Goldstein E, Konopka P, et al. Follow-up of children born of bromocriptine-treated mothers. *Horm Res.* 1985;22:239.

40. Kelly WF, Doyle FH, Mashiter K, et al. Pregnancies in women with hyperprolactinemia: Clinical course and obstetric complications of 41 pregnancies in 27 women. *Br J Obstet Gynaecol.* 1979;86:698.
41. Barnes JE, Abbott KH. Cerebral complications incurred during pregnancy and the puerperium. *Am J Obstet Gynecol.* 82:192.
42. Kempers RD, Miller RH. Management of pregnancy associated with brain tumors. *Am J Obstet Gynecol.* 1963;87:858.
43. Samaan NA, Schultz PN, Leavens TA, et al. Pregnancy after treatment in patients with prolactinoma: operations versus bromocriptine. Am J Obstet Gynecol. 1986;155:1300.
44. Hammond CH, Haney AF, Land MR, et al. The outcome of pregnancy in patients with treated and untreated prolactin-secreting pituitary tumors. *Am J Obstet Gynecol.* 1983;147:148.
45. Zovickian J, Oldfield EH, Doppman JL, et al. Usefulness of inferior petrosal sinus venous endocrine markers in Cushing's disease. *J Neurosurg.* 1988;68:205.
46. Kjellberg RN, Klinman B. Proton radiosurgery for functioning pituitary adenomas. In: Tindall GT, Collins WF, eds. *Clinical Management of Pituitary Disorders.* New York: Raven Press; 1979.
47. Hardy J, Somma M. Acromegaly and surgical treatment by transphenoidal microsurgical removal of the pituitary adenoma. In: Tindall GT, Collins WF, eds. *Clinical Management of Pituitary Disorders.* New York: Raven Press; 1979.
48. Kjellberg RN, Shintani A, Frantz AG, et al. Proton-beam therapy in acromegaly. *N Engl J Med.* 1968;278:689.
49. Kasantikul V, Glasscock ME, Netsky MG, Hayes JW. Intracanalicular neurilemmomas: a clinicopathologic study. *Ann Otol.* 1980;89:29.
50. Rothman LA, Cohen CJ, Astarloa J. Placental and fetal involvement by maternal malignancy: A report of rectal carcinoma and review of the literature. *Am J Obstet Gynecol.* 1973;116:1023.
51. Dalessio DJ. Seizure disorders and pregnancy. *N Engl J Med.* 1985;312:559.
52. Scialli AR. Anticonvulsants in pregnancy. In: Niebyl JR, ed. *Drug Use in Pregnancy.* 2nd ed. Philadelphia: Lea & Febiger; 1988:45.
53. Desmond MM, Schwanecke RP, Wilson GS, et al. Maternal barbiturate utilization and neonatal withdrawal symptomatology. *J Pediatr.* 1972;80:190.
54. Hanson JW, Myrianthopoulos NC, Harvey MAS, Smith DW. Risks to offspring of women treated with hydantoin anticonvulsants, with emphasis on the fetal hydantoin syndrome. *J Pediatr.* 1976;89:662.
55. Jones KL, Lacro RV, Johnson KA, Adams I. Patterns of malformations in the children of women treated with carbamazepine during pregnancy. *N Engl J Med.* 1989;320:1661.
56. Anonymous. Valproate, spina bifida, and birth defect registries. *Lancet.* 1988;2:1404.
57. Thomas RL. Corticosteroid therapy in the prevention of respiratory distress syndrome. In: Niebyl JR, ed. *Drug Use In Pregnancy.* 2nd ed. Philadelphia: Lea & Febiger; 1988:117.
58. Collaborative Group on Antenatal Steroid Therapy. Effect of antenatal dexamethasone administration on the prevention of respiratory distress syndrome. *Am J Obstet Gynecol.* 1981;141:276.
59. Collaborative Group on Antenatal Steroid Therapy. Effect of antenatal dexamethasone administration on the infant: longterm follow-up. *J Pediatr.* 1984;104:259.
60. Osathanondh A, Tulchinsky D, Kamali H, et al. Dexamethasone levels in treated pregnant women and newborn infants. *J Pediatr.* 1977;90:617.
61. Sidhu RK, Hawkins DR. Corticosteroids. *Clin Obstet Gynaecol.* 1981;8:383.
62. Reinisch JM, Simon NG, Karow WG, Gandelman R. Prenatal exposure to prednisone in humans and animals retards intrauterine growth. *Science.* 1978;202:436.
63. Evans MI, Chrousos GP, Mann DW, et al. Pharmacologic suppression of the fetal adrenal gland in utero. *JAMA.* 1985;253:1015.
64. Byyny RL. Withdrawal from glucocorticoid therapy. *N Engl J Med.* 1976;195:30.
65. Basso A, Fernandez A, Althabe O, et al. Passage of mannitol from mother to amniotic fluid and fetus. *Obstet Gynecol.* 1977;49:628.
66. Bain MD, Copas KD, Landon MJ, Stacey TE. In vivo permeability of the human placenta to insulin and mannitol. *J Physiol.* 1988;399:313.
67. Carmel PW. Neurological surgery in pregnancy. In: Barber HR, Graber EA, eds. Surgical disease in pregnancy. Philadelphia: WB Saunders; 1974:203.
68. Brent RL. The effects of embryonic and fetal exposure to x-rays, microwaves, and ultrasound. *Clin Perinatol.* 1986;13:615.
69. Covington EE, Baker AS. Dosimetry of scattered radiation to the fetus. *JAMA.* 1969;209:414.
70. Sharma SC, Williamson JF, Khan FM, Lee CKK. Measurement and calculation of ovary and fetus dose in extended field radiotherapy for 10 MeV x-rays. *Int J Radiat Oncol Biol Phys.* 1981;7:843.
71. Zucali R, Marchesini R, De Palo G. Abdominal dosimetry for supradiaphragmatic irradiation of Hodgkin's disease in pregnancy: experimental data and clinical considerations. *Tumori.* 1981;67:203.
72. Hochber FH, Pruitt A. Assumptions in the radiotherapy of glioblastoma. *Neurology.* 1980;30:907.
73. National Council on Radiation Protection and Measurements. *Structural Shielding Design and Evaluation for Medical Use of X-Rays and Gamma Rays of Energies up to 10 MeV.* NCRP Report No. 49, 1976.
74. Nelson DF, Urtasun RC, Saunders WM, et al. Recent and current investigations of radiation therapy of malignant gliomas. *Semin Oncol.* 1986;13:46.
75. Krishnaswamy V. Dose distribution around an I-125 seed source in tissue. *Radiology.* 1978;126:489.
76. Shalek RJ, Stovall M. Dosimetry in implant therapy. In: Attix FH, Tochilin E, eds. *Radiation Dosimetry.* 2nd ed. New York: Academic Press; 1969:743.
77. Loevinger R, Budinger TF, Watson EE. *MIRD Primer for Absorbed Dose Calculations.* New York: Society of Nuclear Medicine; 1986.
78. Gutin PH, Leibel SA, Wara WM, et al. Recurrent malignant gliomas: survival following interstitial brachytherapy with high-activity iodine-125 sources. *J Neurosurg.* 1987;67:864.
79. Doll DC, Ringenberg QS, Yarbro JW. Management of cancer during pregnancy. *Arch Intern Med.* 1988;148:2058.
80. Levin VA, Sheline GE, Gutin PH. Neoplasms of the central nervous system. In: DeVita VT, Hellman S, Rosenberg SA, eds. *Cancer: Principles and Practice of Oncology.* 3rd ed. Philadelphia: JB Lippincott; 1989:1557.
81. Blasberg RG, Groothuis DR. Chemotherapy of brain tumors: physiological and pharmacokinetic considerations. *Semin Oncol.* 1986;13:70.
82. Anonymous. Transplacental carcinogenesis. *Lancet.* 1976;1:506.
83. Schapira DV, Chudley AE. Successful pregnancy following continuous chemotherapy before conception and throughout pregnancy. *Cancer.* 1984;54:800.
84. Magyar DM, Marshall JR. Pituitary tumors and pregnancy. *Am J Obstet Gynecol.* 1978;132:739.
85. O'Donovan PA, O'Donovan PJ, Ritchie EH, et al. Apoplexy into a prolactin secreting macroadenoma during early pregnancy with successful outcome: a case report. *Br J Obstet Gynaecol.* 1986;93:389.
86. Barron WM. The pregnant surgical patient: medical evaluation and management. *Ann Intern Med.* 1984;101:683.
87. Turpie AGG, Gallus AS, Beattie WS, Hirsh J. Prevention of venous thrombosis in patients with intracranial disease by intermittent pneumatic compression of the calf. *Neurology.* 1977;27:435.
88. Hamod KA, Khouzani VA. Antibiotics in pregnancy. In: Niebyl JR, ed. *Drug Use in Pregnancy.* 2nd ed. Philadelphia: Lea & Febiger; 1988:29.
89. Soutoul JH, Gouase A, Gallier J, Santini JJ. Neurochirurgie et grossesse. *Rev Fr Gynecol.* 1971;66:603.
90. Weinstein I. The origins of human cancer: molecular mechanisms of carcinogenesis and their implications for cancer prevention and treatment—Twenty-seventh G.H.A. Clowes memorial award lecture. *Cancer Res.* 1988;48:4135.
91. Libermann TA, Nusbaum HR, Razon N, et al. Amplification, enhanced expression and possible rearrangement of EGF receptor gene in primary human brain tumors of glial origin. *Nature.* 1985;313:144.
92. Kepes JJ. The possible effect of female sex hormones on meningiomas. In: Kepes JJ, ed. *Meningiomas: Biology, Pathology and Differential Diagnosis* (Masson Monographs in Diagnostic Pathology). New York: Masson Publishing USA, Inc; 1982:17.
93. Donnel MS, Meyer GA, Donegan WL. Estrogen-receptor protein in intracranial meningiomas. *J Neurosurg.* 1979;50:499.
94. Halper J, Colvard DS, Scheithauer BW, et al. Estrogen and progesterone receptors in meningiomas: Comparison of nuclear binding, dextran-coated charcoal, and immunoperioxidase staining assays. *Neurosurgery.* 1989;25:546.
95. Allegra JC, Lippman ME, Thompson EB, et al. Relationship between the progesterone, androgen and glucocorticoid receptor and response rate to endocrine therapy in metastatic breast cancer. *Cancer Res.* 1979;39:1973.
96. Jensen EV. Hormone dependency of breast cancer. *Cancer Res.* 1978;38:4289.
97. Molteni A, Bahu RM, Battifora HA, et al. Estradiol receptor assays in normal and neoplastic tissues. *Ann Clin Lab Sci.* 1979;9:103.
98. Stedman KE, Moore GE, Morgan RT. Estrogen receptor proteins in diverse human tumors. *Arch Surg.* 1980;115:224.
99. Jay JR, MacLaughlin DT, Riley KR, Martuza RL. Modulation of meningioma cell growth by sex steroid hormones in vitro. *J Neurosurg.* 1985;62:757.
100. Sporn MB, Todaro GH. Autocrine secretion and malignant transformation of cells. *N Engl J Med.* 1980;303:878.
101. Carpenter G, Cohen S. Epidermal growth factor. *Annu Rev Biochem.* 1979;48:198.
102. Ushiro H, Cohen SJ. Identification of phosphortyrosine as a product of epidermal growth factor-activated protein kinase in A431 cell membranes. *J Biol Chem.* 1980;255:8363.
103. Leutz A, Schachner M. Epidermal growth factor stimulates DNA synthesis of astrocytes in primary cerebellar cultures. *Cell Tissue Res.* 1981;220:393.
104. Simpson DL, Morrison R, de Vellis J, Herschman HR. Epidermal growth factor binding and mitogenic activity on purified populations of cells from the central nervous system. *J Neurosci Res.* 1982;8:453.

105. Weisman AS, Raguet SS, Kelly PA. Characterization of the epidermal growth factor receptor in human meningioma. *Cancer Res*. 1987;47:2171.
106. Yamamoto T, Ikawa S, Akiyama T, et al. Similarity of protein encoded by the human c-erb-B-2 gene to epidermal growth factor receptor. *Nature*. 1986;319:230.
107. Westphal M, Herrmann HD. Growth factor biology and oncogene activation in human gliomas and their implications for specific therapeutic concepts. *Neurosurgery*. 1989;25:681.
108. Yamamoto KR. Steroid receptor regulated transcription specific of specific genes and gene networks. *Annu Rev Genet*. 1984;19:209.
109. Lingham RB, Stancel GM, Loose-Mitchell DS. Estrogen regulation of epidermal growth factor receptor messenger ribonucleic acid. *Mole Endocri*. 1988;2:230.
110. Dickson RB, Lippman ME. Estrogenic regulation of growth and polypeptide growth factor secretion in human breast carcinoma. *Endocrine Rev*. 1987;8:29.
111. Murphy LC, Murphy LJ, Dubik D, et al. Epidermal growth factor gene expression in human breast cancer cells: regulation of expression by progestins. *Cancer Res*. 1988;48:4555.
112. Koga M, Musgrove EA, Sutherland RL. Modulation of the growth-inhibitory effects of progestins and the antiestrogen hydroxyclomiphene on human breast cancer cells by epidermal growth factor and insulin. *Cancer Res*. 1989;49:112.
113. Sarup JC, Rao KVS, Fox CF. Decreased progesterone binding and attenuated progesterone action in cultured human breast carcinoma cells treated with epidermal growth factor. *Cancer Res*. 1988;48:5071.
114. Fitzpatrick SL, Brightwell J, Wittliff JL, et al. Epidermal growth factor binding by breast tumor biopsies and relationship to estrogen receptor and progestin receptor levels. *Cancer Res*. 1984;44:3448.
115. Pekonen F, Partanen S, Makinen T, Rutanen EM. Receptors for epidermal growth factor and insulin-like growth factor I and their relation to steroid receptors in human breast cancer. *Cancer Res*. 1980;48:1343.
116. Needham GK, Nicholson S, Angus B, et al. Relationship of membrane-bound tissue type and urokinase type plasminogen activators in human breast cancers to estrogen and epidermal growth factor receptors. *Cancer Res*. 1988;48:6603.
117. Antoniades HM. Human platelet-derived growth factor (PDGF): purification of PDGF I and PDGF II and separation of their subunits. *Proc Natl Acad Sci USA*. 1981;78:7314.
118. Heldin CH, Westermark B, Wasteson A. Specific receptor for platelet derived growth factor on cells derived from connective tissue and glia. *Proc Natl Acad Sci USA*. 1981;78:3664.
119. Noble M, Watkins B. Glial division and differentiation in normal and neoplastic nervous system. *Proceedings of the 10th International Congress on Neuropathology*. Stockholm, Sweden; 1986:256. Abstract.
120. Betsholtz C, Heldin CH, Nister M, et al. Synthesis of a PDGF-like growth factor in human glioma and sarcoma cells suggests the expression of the cellular homologue to the transforming protein of simian sarcoma virus. *Biochem Biophys Res Commun*. 1983;117:176.
121. Ullrich A, Bell JR, Chen EY, et al. Human insulin receptor and its relationship to the tyrosine kinase family of oncogenes. *Nature*. 1985;313:756.
122. McMorris FA, Smith TM, DeSulvo S, Furlanetto RN. IGF-I/somatomedin C: a potent inducer of oligodendrocyte development. *Proc Natl Acad Sci USA*. 1986;83:822.
123. Puro DG, Agardh E. Insulin mediated regulation of neuronal maturation. *Science*. 1984;225:1170.
124. Glick RP, Gettleman R, Patel K, et al. Insulin and insulin-like growth factor in brain tumors: binding and in vitro effects. *Neurosurgery*. 1989;42:791.
125. Lowe WL, Boyd FT, Clarke DW, et al. Development of brain insulin receptors: structural and functional studies from whole brain and primary cell cultures. *Endocrinology*. 1986;119:25.
126. Sara VR, Hall K, Holtz HV, et al. Evidence for the presence of specific receptors for IGF1, IGF2 and insulin throughout the adult human brain. *Neurosci Lett*. 1982;34:39.
127. Sara VR, Hall K, Misaki M, et al. Ontogenesis of somatomedin and insulin receptors in the human fetus. *J Clin Invest*. 1983;71:1094.
128. Michler-Stuke A, Wolff J, Bottenstien J. Factors influencing astrocyte growth and development in defined media. *Int J Dev Neurosci* 1984;2:575.
129. Morrison RS, deVellis J. Growth and purified astrocytes in a chemically defined medium. *Proc Natl Acad Sci USA*. 1981;11:7205.
130. Hill JF, Chao MW, Ishii DN. Insulin and IGF and NGF effects on tubulin mRNA levels and neurite formation. *Proc Natl Acad Sci USA*. 1985;82:7126.
131. Grunberger G, Lowe J, McElduff A, Glick RP. The insulin receptor of human cerebral gliomas: structure and function. *J Clin Invest*. 1986; 77:977.
132. Glick RP, Arnold P, Thangoda V, et al. *Stimulation of Proliferation and Differentiation of Glioblastoma Cells by IGF and Insulin*. Proceedings of the National Meeting of Neurological Surgeons. Atlanta, Georgia; 1989:174. Abstract.
133. Aizenman Y, de Vellis J. Brain neurons develop in a serum and glial free environment: effects of transferin, insulin, insulin-like growth factor-I and thyroid hormone on neuronal survival, growth and differentiation. *Brain Res*. 1987;406:32.
134. Massague J, Kelly B, Mottola C. Stimulation by insulin-like growth factors is required for cellular transformation by B-TGF. *J Biol Chem*. 1985;260:4551.
135. Moutjoy KG, Holdaway IM, Finaly FJ. Insulin receptor regulation in cultured human tumor cells. *Cancer Res*. 1983;43:4537.
136. Blatt J, White C, Dienes S, et al. Production of an insulin-like growth factor by osteosarcoma. *Biochem Biophys Res Commun*. 1984;123:373.
137. Huff KK, Knabbe C, Lindsey R, et al. Secretion on an IGF-I related protein by human breast cancer cells. *Cancer*. 1986;46:4613.
138. Reeve AE, Eccles MR, Wilkins RJ, et al. Expression of insulin-like growth factor-II transcript in Wilm's tumor. *Nature*. 1985;317:258.
139. Scott J, Crowell J, Robertson ME, et al. Insulin-like growth factor II gene expression in Wilm's tumour and embryonic tissues. *Nature*. 1985;317:260.
140. Macara IG. Oncogenes, ions, and phospholipids. *Am J Physiol*. 1985; 248:C3.
141. Sara VR, Prisell P, Sjogren B, et al. Enhancement of insulin-like growth factor 2 receptors in glioblastoma. *Cancer Lett*. 1986;32:29.
142. Furlanetto RD, Di Carlo JN. Somatomedin C receptors and growth effects in human breast cells. *Cancer*. 1984;44:2122.
143. Koon JW, Iwahashi MJ. Insulin as a potent growth factor in a rat hepatoma cell line. *Science*. 1981;211:947.
144. Glick RP, Unterman T, Hollis R, et al. Production of Insulin-like Growth Factor (IGF)-I and IGF-II by Central Nervous System Tumors: *In Situ* and *In Vitro*. Proceedings of the National Meeting of the American Association of Neurological Surgeons. Nashville, Tennessee; 1990 (in press). Abstract.
145. Huff KK, Knabbe C, Lindsey R, et al. Multihormonal regulation of insulin-like growth factor-I-related protein in MCF-7 human breast cancer cells. *Molec Endocrin*. 1988;2:200.
146. Epentos AA, Courtney-Luck N, Pickering D, et al. Antibody guided irradiation of brain glioma by arterial infusion of radioactive monoclonal antibody against epidermal growth factor receptor and blood group A antigen. *Br Med J*. 1985;290:1463.

Chapter One Hundred and Eighty-Two
Neoplastic Diseases of Bone

Teng-Liang Huang and Riad Barmada

182

Malignancy of any type developing during pregnancy is uncommon and is estimated at approximately 1 in 1000 pregnancies.[1] Similiarly, primary bone sarcomas are uncommon. Osteosarcoma, the most frequent malignant bone neoplasm encountered in the childbearing years, occurs in only 1 in 100,000 population.[2] The third National Cancer Survey[3] indicates that 27% of all bone and joint malignancies in women occur in the childbearing years from 15 to 44; while there have been reports of simultaneous pregnancy and skeletal neoplasia[4-9], the infrequency of this combination of events provides few guidelines for patient management.

A rational approach to the pregnant patient with a

skeletal neoplasm requires an understanding of the biologic behavior of skeletal tumors, the diagnostic staging studies required, and the treatments employed. These factors then must be evaluated for the risks posed to the mother and fetus from the tumor and from diagnostic and therapeutic manipulation.

SKELETAL NEOPLASMS

While both benign and malignant neoplasms may develop from the vascular, fibrous, chondroid and osseous cellular components of the skeleton, only malignant neoplasms develop from marrow cell precursors, outlined in Table 182–1[10] (the WHO classification of benign and malignant neoplasms primary in bone). With the exception of giant cell tumor, these lesions are predominantly an affliction of young adults and are rarely found in skeletally immature patients.[11] They are usually asymptomatic, and do not pose a threat to the patient if left untreated for the duration of pregnancy. There is no evidence that the hormonal or immunologic events of pregnancy affect the growth or behavior of these lesions.

Primary malignant skeletal neoplasms are fewer in number during pregnancy than their benign counterparts. Myeloma, fibrosarcoma, and angiosarcoma occur most frequently after the fifth decade of life and are unlikely to be encountered in the childbearing years. The remaining lesions, however, are seen in teenagers and young adults. Together with giant cell tumor, they represent the most common skeletal neoplasms encountered in pregnancy. Simon[12] has reported his experience with musculoskeletal tumors in 33 pregnant females with aggressive, benign, or malignant bone lesions. There were 13 giant cell tumors, eleven osteosarcomas, two chondrosarcomas, two Ewing's sarcomas, two lymphomas, two malignant fibrous histiocytomas, and one fibrosarcoma.

BIOLOGIC BEHAVIOR

Pregnancy, in particular, is a well-recognized condition during which vertebral hemangiomas may become clinically symptomatic, usually in the third trimester. This is probably because of elevated intra-abdominal venous pressure which leads to increased flow in the vertebral venous system.[13-15] This may produce symptomatology through a variety of mechanisms including: compression fracture of involved vertebrae; sudden hemorrhage; subperiosteal growth of the tumor, creating an epidural mass producing compression; spinal cord ischemia; and hypertrophy of the posterior cortex of the vertebral body, lamina, and facets.[16-18] It also can recur during both pregnancy and lactation, suggesting a hormonal component in their development and subsequent behavior.[19] Prompt diagnosis of this treatable cause of extradural compression is essential in planning optimal

TABLE 182–1. WHO CLASSIFICATION OF BONE TUMORS[a]

1. Bone-forming Tumors
    - Benign
        - Osteoma
        - Osteoid osteoma and osteoblastoma (benign osteoblastoma)
    - Malignant
        - Osteosarcoma (osteogenic sarcoma), central peripheral (periosteal)
        - Juxtacortical osteosarcoma (parosteal osteosarcoma)
        - Malignant osteoblastoma
2. Cartilage-forming Tumors
    - Benign
        - Chondroma
        - Osteochondroma (osteocartilaginous exostosis)
        - Chondroblastoma (benign chondroblastoma, epiphyseal chondroblastoma)
        - Chondromyxoid fibroma
    - Malignant
        - Chondrosarcoma
            - primary
            - secondary
        - Juxtacortical chondrosarcoma
        - Mesenchymal chondrosarcoma
        - Clear cell chondrosarcoma
3. Giant-cell Tumor (Osteoclastoma)
4. Marrow Tumors
    - Ewing's sarcoma
    - Malignant lymphoma
        - Reticulosarcoma
        - Lymphosarcoma
    - Myeloma
5. Vascular Tumors
    - Benign
        - Hemangioma
        - Lymphangioma
        - Glomus tumor (blomangioma)
    - Intermediate or Indeterminate
        - Haemangioendothelioma
        - Haemangiopeticytoma
    - Malignant
        - Angiosarcoma
6. Other Connective Tissues Tumors
    - Benign
        - Desmoplastic fibroma
        - Lipoma
    - Malignant
        - Fibrosarcoma
        - Liposarcoma
        - Malignant mesenchymona
        - Malignant fibrous histiocytoma
        - Undifferentiated sarcoma
7. Other Tumors
    - Chordoma
    - "Adamantinoma" of long bones
    - Neurilemmoma (schwannoma, neurinoma)
    - Neurofibroma

[a] WHO classification, slightly modified.

therapy and preventing morbidity for both mother and fetus. Rapid progress also has been reported in a patient with multiple chondromatosis[20] during pregnancy. The mechanism causing rapid enlargement of tumors in pregnancy is a subject of debate, although the physiologic changes of pregnancy undoubtedly are responsible. King[21] suggested that enlargement of blood vessels causes tumor expansion, while Weyand[22] proposed that it is due to the increase in intracellular fluid.

Giant cell tumors of bone occur in a wide variety of anatomic locations usually involving the metaphysis and the epiphysis. Occasionally, they are limited to the metaphysis, and in only two percent of patients is it adjacent to an open growth plate. The greatest number of giant cell tumors occur in patients between 20 and 40 years of age (52%), with peak incidence in the third decade.[23-26] Although this lesion is seen most often in the long bones, the pelvis and vertebral column also may be involved. Localized pain and swelling are the most common clinical symptoms. Radiographically, it may be classified as latent, active, or aggressive, with most lesions falling in the latter two categories. These tumors are usually benign. Continued growth with cortical thinning, expansion, and weakening of bone are observed in untreated cases. Its biologic behavior is unpredictable. Depending on the extent of the initial surgical procedure and the anatomic location of the tumor, a 33–50% local recurrence rate and a 5% rate of metastasis was reported. Some excellent results for giant cell tumors may reflect an aggressive surgical approach by experienced orthopedic oncologists.[24]

It has been known that simultaneous pregnancy and primary bone sarcomas can occur.[9] Primary bone tumors are osteosarcoma, chondrosarcoma, fibrosarcoma, malignant fibrous histiocytoma, Ewing's sarcoma, lymphoma of bone, giant cell tumor, chordoma and other, more rare tumors. All skeletal sarcomas of connective tissue origin share certain behavioral characteristics. These lesions destroy surrounding trabecular bone, permeate through the cortex, and invade adjacent soft tissues. Vascular invasion, particularly in high-grade lesions such as osteosarcoma, may result in tumor embolization and account for the high incidence of pulmonary metastasis. Since lymphatics in bone are sparse, lymph node metastasis rarely is seen.

Except for myeloma, osteosarcoma is the most common primary sarcoma of bone. It accounts for 20% of all sarcomas. This tumor strikes children and has a peak incidence in patients between 10 and 25 years of age. Osteosarcomas generally occur in the metaphysis of long bones, especially at the knee. The serum alkaline phosphatase usually is elevated. Radiographs often are diagnostic, showing an osteoblastic lesion with associated periosteal reaction.[10,27] Newer localizing studies that may be helpful include bone scans with technetium or gallium. Computerized tomography (CT) has helped with bony localization and has aided in delineating soft tissue extension along with detection of pulmonary metastasis at early stages. Parosteal osteosarcoma, located on the surface of long bone metaphysis, is indolent, does not tend to metastasize early, and has an excellent survival rate. Periosteal osteosarcoma also develops from the surface of bone, but is chondrogenic and is considered more aggressive than the parosteal tumor, however, less so than the classic osteosarcoma.

Telangiectatic osteosarcoma is the most malignant of all bone-forming tumors, and even with chemotherapy, patients with this unusual tumor rarely survive 5 years. Chondrosarcoma, representing 10% of primary bone tumors, typically occurs in the trunk and limb girdles of young and middle-aged adults. A common clinical presentation is a slow-growing tumor associated with minimal pain and a low incidence of pulmonary metastasis. The majority of these low-grade lesions have a good prognosis for survival if properly treated. High-grade chondrosarcomas are rare, rapidly growing tumors that grossly present a myxomatous appearance. These more aggressive sarcomas usually do not calcify. They metastasize early and are associated with a poor prognosis. Low-grade chondrosarcomas occasionally will differentiate into high-grade sarcomas, such as malignant fibrous histiocytoma. This condition is associated with a rapid growth and early metastasis, with a resultant poor prognosis.[28,29]

Approximately 5% of primary bone sarcomas are Ewing's sarcoma, which mainly affects the pelvis and femur in young adults. The radiographic findings are nonspecific, permeative, destructive lesions of medullary bone with associated periosteal elevation that may suggest osteomyelitis. Even the clinical course may suggest infection since there can be a low-grade fever, an elevated erythrocyte sedimentation rate, and anemia. During biopsy, purulent-appearing material may suggest a bone abscess. It is always advisable to send biopsy material to both pathology and bacteriology laboratories. Often a touch preparation in the operating room can aid greatly in making an immediate diagnosis.[10,30,31]

Fibrosarcoma is less prevalent than osteosarcoma, chondrosarcoma, giant cell tumor, or Ewing's sarcoma, comprisng 6.2% of the malignant tumors primary to bone. It is similar in age distribution to chondrosarcoma but contrasts with the lower age incidence of osteosarcoma. The radiographic appearance is that of a radiolucent, often permeative or mottled lesion, with ill-defined borders toward the medullary cavity, and is located most frequently in the metaphyseal region extending into the epiphysis or diaphysis. The well differentiated, generally slow-growing lesion often shows well-defined borders. In contrast, fibrosarcoma may present as a poorly differentiating and rapidly invading lesion with indistinct borders and extensive cervical destruction. The common route of dissemination is hematogenous into the lung. Metastasis in regional lymph nodes is rare.[9,10]

Malignant fibrous histiocytoma of bone is a highly malignant neoplasm. It accounts for at least 5% of all primary malignant bone tumors. The tumor usually involves the metaphyseal region of long bones in young and middle-aged adults. The majority of lesions are primary, but some develop in preexisting benign lesions. Definitive diagnosis is made in histologic examination, classically showing a combination of histiocytic and fibroblastic components in a storiform arrangement. Pulmonary involvement is the major cause of death. This tumor also has a propensity for lymph node metastasis.[32]

Chordoma is a rare, slow-growing malignant tumor that develops from ectopic, embryonic remnants of the notochord along the spinal axis. It occurs most frequently in the sacrococcygeal region followed by the spheno-occipital area, and usually arises between 40 and 70 years of age, although no age is exempt. Distant metastasis is rare but can occur through the blood stream as well as the lymphatics. The coincidental association with pregnancy has been reported with obstructed labor due to the extensive pelvic spread and involvement of the posterior vaginal wall.[33,34]

STAGING

Adequate treatment of any skeletal neoplasm requires certain anatomic and histologic information.[35] The extent of

TABLE 182–2. SURGICAL STAGES

Stage	Grade	Site
IA	Low (G_1)	Intracompartmental (T_1)
IB	Low (G_1)	Extracompartmental (T_2)
IIA	High (G_2)	Intracompartmental (T_1)
IIB	High (G_2)	Extracompartmental (T_2)
III	Any (G) Regional or distant metastasis	Any (T)

tumor within bone or soft tissue, the relationship of the lesion to major neural and vascular structures, and the presence or absence of any metastasis must be evaluated before biopsy. Such data are obtained by a variety of imaging techniques, which include tomography, computerized axial tomography, radionuclide scan, and angiography. The three surgical stages (I, low grade; II, high grade; and III, presence of metastasis) are subdivided by whether the lesion is confined anatomically within well delineated surgical compartment or beyond such compartments in ill-defined fascial planes and spaces (Table 182–2). Because these neoplasms have a high incidence of local recurrence, the biopsy must be planned to allow for total removal of the biopsy tract at the time of definitive surgical treatment. The histologic heterogeneity of many of these lesions makes open surgical biopsy under general anesthesia preferable to needle biopsy.

TREATMENT

The treatment of spinal cord compression resulting from vertebral hemangioma during pregnancy remains controversial. It generally is recommended that surgical resection of vertebral hemangioma occurring during pregnancy be delayed until a viable fetus can be delivered, only if premature labor occurs. The standard surgical approach is embolization, partial body resection, and bony stabilization. Radiation therapy has been used as an adjunct in some cases, but is contraindicated during pregnancy. Prompt clinical recognition of vertebral hemangioma is the most critical factor in determining the patient's outcome. Magnetic resonance imaging is a diagnostic tool that may be used safely during pregnancy.[14]

Enchondromata of the skull are uncommon; they are slow-growing, often solitary, and usually benign. The rapid enlargement of the tumors in pregnancy may cause progressive or recurring neurological symptoms, requiring urgent exploration and excision of the cranial lesion.[20]

Giant cell tumor usually presents as an aggressive lesion. Although histologically benign, metastases from this tumor are occasionally seen but are not a major threat to the patient.[27,36-40] The progressive growth of the tumor, increasing pain, and risk of pathologic fracture usually demands immediate treatment. Since these lesions characteristically destroy subchondral bone, delay in treatment increases the risk of loss of joint function because more extensive treatment may be required. The surgeon's responsibility is to remove the tumor completely and to preserve the best possible function. Enneking and Campanacci's radiographic classifications and surgical staging are helpful in planning the initial surgical treatment, because they have observed that a number of the active (Stage 2) lesions and most of the aggressive (Stage 3) lesions have a higher incidence of local recurrence when treated by curettage alone.[24,35] Curettage, possibly with adjuvant chemical or thermal cauterization along with bone grafting or polymethyl methacrylate instillations, maintain the structural integrity of the bone and allow for early function. Good results with these techniques when applied to Stage 1 and many Stage 2 lesions may be expected in 70–80% of the cases. Repetitive freezing with liquid nitrogen, though resulting in a lower recurrence rate, carries with it a significant risk of local complications. They may require prolonged bracing, and incur the risk of late fracture. When giant cell tumors occur in expendable bones, *en bloc* resection is the treatment of choice. *En bloc* resection of major joints requires a facility with reconstructive capabilities including the use of allografts, large autogenous graft, fusion, or custom joint arthroplasty. These are technically difficult procedures with many early and late complications. Patients have restricted function, and may require prolong bracing even when uncomplicated.

The use of radiation therapy for giant cell tumors is still controversial because a large percentage of malignant giant cell tumors have been induced by irradiation used to treat preexisting benign lesions. However, in giant cell tumors of the sacrum or vertebrae where total surgical excision is technically difficult, irradiation therapy combined with an intralesional debulking procedure may be justified. New surgical techniques are being developed using combined anteroposterior approaches for complete removal of a vertebral segment affected by a giant cell tumor.

Low-grade skeletal neoplasms (parosteal osteosarcoma, certain chondrosarcoma and fibrosarcoma) are treated optionally by adequate surgical excision. Limb salvage procedures are well suited for their management. Since no adjunctive chemotherapy or irradiation therapy follows limb salvage, the surgeon can rely more heavily on basic bone grafting such as excisional arthrodesis or allograft procedures using frozen cadaver bone. Imaginative combinations of allografts and synthetic implants such as long-stemmed endoprosthesis also can be considered.[41,42] Currently, low-grade chondrosarcomas have an overall five-year survival rate of 65–85% in contradiction to 15% for the highest grade chondrosarcoma.[43]

Wide local excision (*en bloc* resection) is the only treatment for chordoma and offers the best chance for long-term survival. Radiation therapy has little efficacy, and conventional chemotherapy has not proven to be effective in this tumor. With early diagnosis, and more effective surgical therapy, the current disease-free survival rate at five years is between 30% and 50%.[33,34]

The current treatment of osteosarcoma and other high-grade connective tissue sarcomas include both surgical extirpation and adjuvant, multi-agent chemotherapy. The various multi-drug programs characteristically include high-dosage methotrexate with citrovorum factor and Adriamycin. Bleomycin, cyclophosphamide, dactinomycin, and cisplatin also are being used.[44,45] The advent of preoperative and postoperative chemotherapy has significantly enhanced survival rates that are now approaching 85%.[46] Improved concepts of *en bloc* resection and better reconstructive techniques suggest that limb salvage procedures are not only possible but can provide excellent functional results in the context of muscle loss.

A dramatic improvement in survival of Ewing's sarcoma in the past decade has been noted. With the advent of multidrug chemotherapy combined with radiation therapy and local surgery, the five-year surgical figures have reached about 50%. Survival varies with the anatomic site of the tumor. Extremity lesions have a more favorable prognosis than axial lesions.[47-49]

MATERNAL AND FETAL RISK FACTORS

There are no data to suggest that the presence of a skeletal neoplasm has an adverse effect on fetal growth or development, nor have metastases of these lesions to placenta or fetus been demonstrated.[50] The hormonal changes and the immunologic tolerance of pregnancy have not been shown to affect the outcome of treatment of these lesions.[9]

For aggressive benign and low-grade malignant lesions, the maternal risk of delay in treatment is that of increased morbidity rather than mortality. Continued growth of the lesion may require more extensive surgery and greater functional compromise (amputation rather than resection). Fetal risks are related to exposure to staging studies such as radioisotopes[51], diagnostic radiation, intravascular contrast agents, and anesthetic agents during biopsy and definitive surgery. Technetium phosphonate radiopharmaceuticals now are routinely used for staging of bone tumors. Since the tracer is excreted by the kidneys, the critical organ exposed to radiation is the bladder wall, which receives about 10 rads per study.[52] Since the bladder wall is adjacent to the uterus, the fetus is exposed to less than these low dosese. Experimental and clinical data are scanty, but there is little evidence of any teratogenic effect on the human embryo for doses less than 15–25 rads.[53] Therefore, radioisotope imaging could be used, but with caution. These risk factors obviously are modified by the trimester at the time of diagnosis and the anatomic site of the maternal tumor. Exposure to radioisotopes and diagnostic radiation presents the greatest risk in the first timester. Evaluations of lesions of the pelvis, spine, and proximal femur will expose the fetus despite shielding.

The maternal risks of delay in treatment in cases of high-grade malignancy are associated with an increase in both morbidity and mortality. Fetal risks in such cases is the same as for low-grade lesions in addition to the possible exposure to therapeutic radiation or cytotoxic agents.[54-60] Multi-agent chemotherapy for osteosarcoma with Adriamycin and high-dose methotrexate as well as leucovorine rescue comprise the standard of most treatment combinations. There is no published experience with the use of Adriamycin during the first trimester of pregnancy.[57] Normal pregnancies have been reported following administration of Adriamycin and low doses of methotrexate in the last two trimesters.[57] Low doses of methotrexate have caused fetal anomalies when given during the first trimester.[57] No cases of the effects of high doses of methotrexate on a fetus have been reported.

Conventional treatment of Ewing's sarcoma includes Adriamycin, vincristine, cytoxan, and dactinomycin. The latter has not been used during the first trimester, and normal pregnancies have been reported with use during the last two trimesters. Vincristine seems relatively safe in all trimesters.[57] Cytoxan, even in modest doses, causes fetal abnormalities when given during the first trimester.[57]

MANAGEMENT GUIDELINES

If a woman has high-grade sarcoma during the first trimester of pregnancy, therapeutic abortion should be strongly considered if chemotherapy or radiation therapy is planned in addition to surgery. The risk of fetal malformation or neoplasia from exposure to cytotoxic agents is highest during the first trimester[57,59,60], and the maternal mortality risk factor also is increased. When the diagnosis of high-grade lesion is made in the third trimester, early induced labor is judicious. If low-grade sarcoma occurs during the first two trimesters, definitive surgery can be considered with only minimal risk to the fetus.[61,62] If a low-grade tumor occurs in the third trimester, induced labor or spontaneous delivery are acceptable choices.

If radiation therapy to the central lesions of the proximal femur, pelvis, or lumbar spine is indicated, elective abortion or early delivery is indicated.

The decision to terminate pregnancy is based on social, religious, and ethical issues. Since the tumor itself poses no risk to the fetus, the patient's decision regarding termination of pregnancy must be based on a thorough understanding of the risks posed to the fetus by diagnostic and therapeutic manipulation as well as the functional and mortal risks to her of delaying treatment for the specific tumor. As diagnostic and therapeutic approaches to neoplasia are undergoing constant change, a complete and thorough discussion with a musculoskeletal oncologist is advised.

REFERENCES

1. Potter JF, Schoeneman M. Metastasis of maternal cancer to the placenta and fetus. *Cancer*. 1970;25:380.
2. Friedman MA, Carter SK. The therapy of osteogenic sarcoma: current status and thoughts for the future. *J Surg. Oncol*. 1972;4:482.
3. Third national cancer survey—incidence data. *Natl Cancer Inst Monograph*. 1975;41:108.
4. Huvos AG, Butler A, Bretsky SS. Osteogenic sarcoma in pregnant women. *Cancer*. 1985;56:2326.
5. Jafari K, Lash AF, Webster A. Pregnancy and sarcoma. *Acta Obstet Gynecol Scand*. 1978;57:265.
6. Johnston GA, Simon MA, Azizi F. Giant cell tumor of bone in pregnancy. *J Reprod Med*. 1980;24:43.
7. Lysyj A, Bergquist JR. Pregnancy complicated by sarcoma: report of two cases. *Obstet Gynecol*. 1963;21:506.
8. Pratt CB, River G, Shanks E. Osteosarcoma during pregnancy. *Obstet Gynecol*. 1977;50(supp):1245.
9. Simon MA, Phillips WA, Bonfiglio M. Pregnancy and aggressive or malignant primary bone tumors. *Cancer*. 1984;53:2564.
10. Schajowicz F. *Tumors and Tumorlike Lesions of Bone and Joints*. New York, NY: Springer-Verlag; 1981:17.
11. Picci P, Manifrini M, Zucchi V, et al. Giant-cell tumor of bone in skeletally immature patients. *J Bone Joint Surg*. 1983;65(A):486.
12. Simon MA, Phillips WA, Bonfiglio M. Pregnancy and aggressive or malignant primary bone tumors. *Cancer*. 1984;53:2564.
13. Nelson DA. Spinal cord compression due to vertebral angiomas during pregnancy. *Arch Neurol*. 1964;11:408.
14. Schwart DA, Nair S, Hershey B, et al. Vertebral arch hemangioma producing spinal cord compression in pregnancy: diagnosis by magnetic resonance imaging. *Spine*. 1989;14(8):888.
15. Kerr MG, Scott DB, Samuel E. Studies of the inferior vena cava in late pregnancy. *Br Med J*. 1964;1:532.
16. Askenasy H, Behmoarem A. Neurological manifestation in hemangioma of the vertebral. *J Neurol Neurosurg Psych*. 1957;20:276.
17. Brobeck O. Hemangioma of vertebra associated with compression of the spinal cord. *Acta Radiol*. 1950;34:235.
18. Lavi E, Jamieson DG, Granat M. Epidural hemangiomas during pregnancy. *J Neruol Neurosurg Psych*. 1986;49:709.
19. Julin P, Thomsson M. Multiple intraosseous and soft tissue hemangiomas with changes during pregnancy and lactation: a fifteen year follow-up study. *Dentomaxillofac Radiol*. 1986;15:87.
20. Honan WH, Shieff C. Skull base chondroma presenting in pregnancy (letter). *J Neurol Neurosurg Psychiatry*. 1987;50(8):1078.
21. King AB. Neurological conditions occurring as complications of pregnancy. *Arch Neurol Psychiatry*. 1950;63:611.
22. Weyand RD, MacCarty CS, Wilson RB. The effect of pregnancy on intracranial meningiomas occurring about the optic chiasm. *Surg Clin N Am*. 1951;31:1225.
23. Schajowicz F. *Tumors and Tumorlike Lesions of Bone and Joints*. New York: Springer-Verlag; 1981;205.

24. Campanacci M, Baldini N, Boriani S, Sudanese A. Giant-cell tumor of bone. *J Bone and Joint Surg.* 1987;69(A):106.
25. Dahlin DC, Copps RE, Johnson EW. Giant cell tumor: a study of 195 cases. *Cancer.* 1970;25:1061.
26. Goldenberg RR, Campbell CJ, Bonfiglio M. Giant cell tumor of bone: an analysis of two hundred and eighteen cases. *J Bone Joint Surg.* 1970;52A:619.
27. Dahlin DC. *Bone Tumors.* Springfield, IL: Charles C. Thomas; 1978.
28. Dahlin DC, Beabout JW. Dedifferentiation of low-grade chondrosarcoma. *Cancer.* 1971;28:461.
29. Capanna R, Bettelli G, Picci P, et al. Dedifferentiated chondrosarcoma. *J Bone Joint Surg.* 1988;70(A):60.
30. Pritchard DJ, Dahlin DC, Dauphine, RT, et al. Ewing's sarcoma: a clinicopathological and statistical analysis of patients surviving five years or longer. *J Bone Joint Surg.* 1975;57(A):10.
31. Neff JR. Non metastatic Ewing's sarcoma of bone: the role of surgical therapy. *Clin Orthop.* 1986;204:111.
32. Boland PJ, Huvos AG. Malignant fibrous histiocytoma of bone. *Clin Orthop.* 1986;204:130.
33. Slee RW, Al-Hilli F, Abdul-Wahab AW. Secondary chordoma of the mandible. *Br J Oral Maxillofac Surg.* 1989;27(4):346.
34. Sundaresan N. Chordomas. *Clin Orthop.* 1986;204:135.
35. Enneking WF, Spanier SS, Goodman MA. A system for the surgical staging of musculoskeletal sarcoma. *Clin Orthop.* 1980;153:106.
36. Enneking WF. *Musculoskeletal tumor surgery.* New York: Churchill Livingstone; 1983.
37. Huvos AG. *Bone Tumors: Diagnosis, Treatment and Prognosis.* Philadelphia: WB Saunders; 1979:
38. Mirra JM. *Bone Tumors: Diagnosis and Treatment.* Philadelphia: JB Lippincott; 1980.
39. Sladden RA. Intravascular osteoclasts. *J Bone Joint Surg.* 1957;39B:346.
40. Wu WQ, Lapi A. Primary non-skeletal intracranial cartilaginous neoplasms: report of a chondroma and a mesenchymal chondrosarcoma. *J Neurol Neurosurg Psychiatry.* 1970;33:469.
41. Eriksson AI, Schiller A, Mankin HJ. The management of chondrosarcoma of bone. *Clin Orthop.* 1980;153:44.
42. Luck JV, Luck JR, Schwinn CP. Parosteal osteosarcoma: a treatment-oriented study. *Clin Orthop.* 1980;153:90.
43. Healey JH, Lane JM. Chondrosarcoma. *Clin Orthop.* 1986;204:119.
44. Sutow WW. Multidrug chemotherapy in osteosarcoma. *Clin Orthop.* 1980;153:67.
45. Rosen G, Caparros B, Huvos AG, et al. Preoperative chemotherapy for osteogenic sarcoma: selection of postoperative adjuvant chemotherapy based upon the response of the primary tumor to preoperative chemotherapy. *Cancer.* 1982;49:1221.
46. Lane JM, Hurson B, Boland PJ, Glasser DB. Osteogenic sarcoma. *Clin Orthop.* 1986;204:93.
47. Glaubiger DL, Makuch R, Schwarz J, et al. Determination of prognostic factors and their influence on therapeutic results in patients with Ewing's sarcoma. *Cancer.* 1980;45:2213.
48. Tepper J, Glaubiger D, Lichter A, et al. Local control of Ewing's sarcoma of bone with radiotherapy and combination chemotherapy. *Cancer.* 1980;46:1969.
49. Pritchard DJ. Indications for surgical treatment of localized Ewing's sarcoma of bone. *Clin Orthop.* 1980;153:39.
50. Rothman LA, Cohen CJ, Astarloa J. Placental and fetal involvement by maternal malignancy. *Am J Obstet Gynecol.* 1973;116:1023.
51. Baker J, Ali A, Groch MW, et al. Bone scanning in pregnant patients with breast carcinoma. *Clin Nucl Med.* 1987;12(7):519.
52. Alazraki NP, Davis MA, Jones AG, et al. Skeletal System. In: Kirchner PT, ed. *Nuclear Medicine Review Syllabus.* New York: Society of Nuclear Medicine; 1980:546.
53. Anger RT, Benedetto AR, Saeger EL, Mitcofski RL. Radiation effects and radiation protection. In: Kirchner PT, ed. *Nuclear Medicine Review Syllabus.* New York: Society of Nuclear Medicine; 1980:86.
54. Denoix P. Treatment of malignant breast tumors: indications and results. Recent results. *Cancer Res.* 1970;31:83.
55. Raich PD, Curet LB. Treatment of acute leukemia during pregnancy. *Cancer.* 1975;36:861.
56. Nicholson OP. Cytotaxic drugs in pregnancy. *J Obstet Gynaecol Br Commonw.* 1968;75:307.
57. Gililland J, Weinstein L. The effects of cancer chemotherapeutic agents on the developing fetus. *Obstet Gynecol Surv.* 1983;38(1):6.
58. Haerr RW, Pratt, AT. Multi-agent chemotherapy for sarcoma diagnosed during pregnancy. *Cancer.* 1985;56(5):1028.
59. Sweet DL, Kinzie J. Consequences of radiotherapy and antineoplastic therapy for the fetus. *J Reprod Med.* 1976;17:241.
60. Barber HRK. Fetal and neonatal effects of cytotoxic agents. *Obstet Gynecol* 1981;58(supp):415.
61. Pedersen M, Finister M. Anesthetic risk in the pregnant surgical patient. *Anesthesiology.* 1979;51:439.
62. Levinson G, Shnieder SM. Anesthesia for operation during pregnancy. In: Snider JM, Levinson G, eds. *Anesthesia for Obstetrics.* Baltimore: Williams and Wilkins; 1979:312.

Chapter One Hundred and Eighty-Three

Neoplasms of the Urinary Tract

E. Everett Anderson

183

Some 13% of all cancers in women occur during the reproductive years.[1] The incidence of cancer during pregnancy is one cancer in 1008 pregnancies.[2] If there are 3.5 million live births in the United States each year, there are concomitantly 3472 cases of cancer during pregnancy each year. The order of frequency of occurrence in pregnant women are cancers of the breast, uterine cervix, ovary, lymphomas, and colorectum.

Tumors of the urinary tract are rare in pregnant women. Urothelial cancers, with the exception of carcinoma of the urethra, occur predominantly in men; in both sexes, they rarely develop before the fifth decade. Only 6.1% of tumors of the urinary tract in women occur during the fertile years.

When considering the treatment options in a pregnant patient with carcinoma of the urinary tract, the physician must consider duration of pregnancy, malignant nature of the tumor, risks to the mother, and risks to the fetus. Clearly the physician's objectives should be to cure the mother of her cancer and allow the subsequent delivery of a normal healthy infant. Unfortunately, both of these objectives cannot always be achieved. When faced with this dilemma, the physician should give priority to the health of the mother.

The treatment of carcinoma of the urinary tract involves surgery, radiation therapy, and chemotherapy. In general, tumors of the upper urinary tract (kidney and ureter) are resistant to radiation therapy, and tumors of the lower urinary tract (bladder and urethra) are relatively radiosensitive. In pregnant women, radiation therapy is contraindicated because of the proximity of the urinary tract to the gravid uterus. The risk of spontaneous abortion, teratogenesis, or mutagenesis is greatest from 0 to 12 weeks and less during the second half of pregnancy, but the larger fetus is still exposed to radiation and the hazards of subsequent carcinogenesis. A fetus located 25 cm from an irradiation field receiving 7500 rads will still receive approximately 30 rads. Except in unusual circumstances, most radiotherapists will refuse to provide radiation therapy to the urinary tract in pregnant women.

Most chemotherapeutic drugs are also teratogenic and

therefore contraindicated in pregnancy. This risk is most critical in the first 10 weeks of pregnancy.[3-5] Normal infants have been delivered following systemic chemotherapy during pregnancy, but the numbers are few and do not justify the long-term risks. For the most part, systemic chemotherapy is not very effective in the treatment of urothelial tumors.

In pregnant and nonpregnant women, surgery is the primary modality in the treatment of tumors of the urinary tract. Tumors of the kidney, upper ureter, and distal urethra pose no real problem to surgical attack, excluding potential anesthetic complications. Tumors of the terminal ureter in pregnant women, because of their anatomic location, pose a real problem to the surgeon, but with difficulty can be extirpated. If the fetus is close to term, the surgery can be performed in combination with cesarean section or after induction of labor. Invasive tumors of the bladder and proximal urethra demand radical cystectomy and total urethrectomy; therefore, these tumors require termination of pregnancy by therapeutic abortion, cesarean section, or induction of labor.

SIGNS AND SYMPTOMS

Bleeding from the urethra is a common presenting symptom of urethral carcinoma.

Tumors of the urinary tract originate in the urothelium or invade into the urothelium early in their course. Therefore, it is not surprising that most urothelial tumors will present with gross or microscopic *hematuria.* Hematuria is the result of ulceration of the mucosa of the urinary tract and will resolve following spontaneous healing. Therefore, most urothelial tumors present with intermittent hematuria, but absence of hematuria does not exclude neoplasia of the urinary tract.

When tumors of the lower urinary tract (bladder and urethra) outgrow their blood supply and become necrotic and infected, *dysuria, urgency,* and *frequency* of urination may ensue. Unfortunately, the combination of hematuria and vesical irritative symptoms in the female suggests hemorrhagic cystitis, and often women with lower urinary tract tumors are treated inappropriately for many months with antimicrobial therapy.

Flank pain may occur as a result of obstruction of the ureter from blood clots (renal and ureteral tumors) or from direct invasion and occlusion of the ureters (vesical and ureteral tumors). Rarely, flank pain may be the result of renal tumor bleeding within the renal parenchyma.

Large renal tumors may present as a flank *mass* and invasive urethral and vesical tumors may be palpable on bimanual examination. However, with the exception of invasive urethral tumors, a mass usually is not palpable.

Urinary obstructive symptoms develop insidiously in patients with proximal urethral carcinoma, and may include a decreased stream, hesitancy, nocturia, and frequency.

DIAGNOSIS

Hematuria documented by examination of a catherized urine specimen may indicate urothelial malignancy.

Tumors of the renal pelvis, ureter, bladder, and urethra may shed malignant cells, which can be demonstrated by cytological studies. Cystoscopic placement of ureteral catheters will allow the collection of urine for cytology from the upper urinary tract and identify the source of positive urine cytology when it originates from tumors of the renal pelvis or upper ureter. Low-grade urothelial tumors, however, will shed only well differentiated tumor cells, which cannot be differentiated from normal urothelial cells. Therefore, negative urine cytology does not exclude the possibility of a urothelial tumor.

Cystourethroscopy can be performed safely without anesthesia and can immediately identify a neoplasia of the lower urinary tract, whether in the bladder or urethra. If a patient experiences intermittent gross hematuria, the procedure preferably is performed while the patient is bleeding in order to ascertain the source of hematuria. Careful inspection of the efflux of urine from the ureteral orifices may allow the identification of hematuria originating from the upper urinary tract.

Ureteral catheters containing an indwelling wire brush now are available for a "brush biopsy." Under cystoscopic control, this catheter can be passed up the ureter to the site of a suspected ureteral or renal pelvic neoplasm. The wire brush then is extruded, and the involved area is brushed. This biopsy technique is applicable to all urothelial tumors of the upper urinary tract but requires fluoroscopy and retrograde pyelography for accuracy. It will be discussed further under radiologic procedures.

Ureteroscopy and *ureteroscopic biopsy* are valuable methods in the diagnosis of ureteral or renal pelvic tumors, but both are contraindicated in pregnant women. This is due to the fact that ureteroscopy must be performed under fluoroscopic control. Also, since the ureters are displaced during pregnancy by the gravid uterus and become more tortuous, the risk of ureteral perforation and spread of tumor cells is increased by these procedures.

The investigation of all possible upper urinary tract neoplasia may involve the use of radiologic procedures. Because of the potential hazards of ionizing radiation to the fetus, studies that provide a maximum of information with the least amount of radiation should be employed. This is particularly important in the first trimester, when organogenesis is taking place. Table 183–1 lists the radiologic studies commonly used in the evaluation of upper urinary tract neoplasms and their appropriate radiation doses to the fetus in the first trimester of pregnancy. The current radiologic literature indicates that the administration of up to 10 rads to the fetus is safe, 10–15 rads is already questionable, and greater than 15 rads represents an indication for therapeutic abortion.[6] Clearly, these figures serve only as guidelines, and in every instance the pregnant woman should receive as little radiation as possible (see also Chapter 173).

The identification of tumors of the ureter and renal pelvis requires *retrograde pyelography.* The definitive diagnosis of renal parenchymal tumors (renal cell carcinoma, renal adenocarcinoma) in pregnant women is made by *ultrasonography* and enhanced abdominal computerized tomographic (CT) scan. Magnetic resonance imaging (MRI) is a technique for the imaging of the body in a cross-sectional orientation, similar to CT. It is particularly applicable to the pregnant patient because, unlike CT, MRI does not use ionizing radiation. Early reports indicate that the resolution of MRI will approach that of CT. However, its use for the diagnosis of renal tumors is limited. Whether the strong magnetic fields used in MRI will harm a fetus is not known, but current evidence suggests there is no biologic hazard from magnetic resonance imaging.[7,8]

Intravenous pyelograms and renal arteriograms rarely are indicated in the diagnosis of urinary tumors in pregnant women.

TABLE 183–1. RADIOLOGIC STUDIES IN URINARY TRACT TUMORS: RADIATION DOSE TO FETUS (FIRST TRIMESTER)

Study	Radiation Dose to Fetus[a]
Ultrasonography	0 mrem
Magnetic resonance imaging	0 mrem
CT scan to kidney only	0 mrem
Renal scan (glucoheptonate)	15 mrem
Retrograde pyelogram	264 mrem
Intravenous pyelogram	744 mrem
Selective renal arteriogram	1064 mrem

[a] One rem is equivalent to 1 rad; 1 mrem = 1 mrad

TUMORS OF THE KIDNEY

Renal Cell Carcinoma

Renal cell carcinoma comprises 85% of all renal tumors and is thought to originate in the proximal convoluted tubules.[9] Renal cell carcinoma spreads by direct extension, lymphatics and bloodstream to lungs, regional lymph nodes, liver, bones, brain, adrenals, and contralateral kidney.

Hematuria, flank pain, and flank mass are the most common presenting symptoms in renal cell carcinoma, but this tumor is notorious for producing a variety of signs and symptoms that at first appear to be unrelated to the kidney, including fever, hypertension, anemia, erythrocytemia, hypercalcemia, single or multiple pulmonary nodules, pathologic fractures, and hepatic dysfunction.

In the pregnant woman, the diagnosis of renal cell carcinoma should be made by ultrasonography and enhanced abdominal CT scan. MRI which requires no ionizing radiation is inferior to the CT scan for identification of renal neoplasms.

The treatment of renal cell carcinoma involves surgical extirpation of the involved kidney, adrenal gland, Gerota's fascia, paranephric fat, and regional lymph nodes. These tumors usually are resistant to both radiation and chemotherapy.

Renal Pelvic Tumors

Tumors of the renal pelvis comprise 5% of all renal tumors. Of these tumors, 90% are *transitional cell carcinoma* and 7% are *squamous cell carcinomas. Adenocarcinoma* of the renal pelvis occurs rarely. Squamous cell carcinoma and adenocarcinoma of the renal pelvis often are associated with renal calculi.[10] These tumors may spread by direct extension, lymphatics, and bloodstream to lungs, liver, regional lymph nodes, bones, brain, and adrenals. Transitional cell carcinoma of the upper urinary tract is associated with a 30–50% incidence of subsequent development of transitional cell carcinoma of the bladder. When there are simultaneous renal pelvic and ureteral tumors, the probability of subsequent development of vesical carcinoma increases to 75%. There is a 2–4% incidence of subsequent development of transitional cell carcinoma of the contralateral upper urinary tract.

Hematuria is present in 90% of patients with renal pelvic tumors. Flank pain may occur secondary to the passage of blood clots or hydronephrosis from tumor obstruction of the renal pelvis. Rarely, a flank mass is palpable when tumor obstruction of the renal pelvis produces massive hydronephrosis.

The diagnosis of renal pelvic tumors is made by urine cytology, retrograde pyelography, and brush biopsy of the renal pelvis. Ureteroscopy and ureteroscopic biopsy, useful in nonpregnant women, is contraindicated during pregnancy. Differential diagnosis includes nonopaque uric acid calculi, blood clots, and sloughed renal papillae.

Renal pelvic tumors are managed surgically by extirpation of the involved kidney, entire ureter including ureterovesical junction, adrenal gland, Gerota's fascia, paranephric fat and regional lymph nodes. These tumors are resistant to radiation and chemotherapy for the most part.

TUMORS OF THE URETER

Ureteral tumors are rare.[11] A total of 91% are *transitional cell carcinomas* and 8% *squamous cell carcinomas.* The distal ureter is more commonly involved. Ureteral tumors often occur in association with renal pelvic tumors and bladder tumors. The clinical manifestations, differential diagnosis, and diagnosis of ureteral tumors are identical to those of renal pelvic tumors. The treatment of ureteral tumors is controversial. In low-grade, low-stage tumors, some clinicians favor partial ureterectomy and reanastomosis or ureteral reimplantation. Other clinicians favor extirpation of the entire involved urinary tract, including the ureterovesical junction in every case, citing the high incidence of multiple ipsilateral tumors, the difficulty in estimating the grade and stage of the ureteral tumor at time of surgery, and the high rate of ipsilateral ureteral recurrence.

TUMORS OF THE BLADDER

Carcinoma of the bladder is the most common tumor of the urinary tract. Age-incidence curves demonstrate an increase at a constant rate throughout adult life. There is a 44% greater incidence in white than in black females. There also is a strong sex predilection with a ratio of 4 to 1 males to females. Transitional cell carcinoma accounts for approximately 90% of vesical tumors, squamous cell carcinoma for 5%, and adenocarcinoma for 1%. Vesical tumors are often multifocal, and approximately 20% will recur after transurethral resection. The primary sites of metastases are the regional lymph nodes, bones, liver, and lungs. Transitional cell carcinoma of the bladder is associated with a 2–3% chance for development of transitional cell carcinoma of the upper urinary tracts.[12]

Hematuria is the most common presenting symptom in carcinoma of the bladder. It is usually painless but can be associated with burning, urgency, and frequency of urination when there is secondary infection. When vesical tumors obstruct a ureteral orifice, hydronephrosis will develop; on rare occasions, this distention of the renal pelvis will produce flank pain.

The definitive diagnosis of carcinoma of the bladder is made by cystoscopy and transurethral vesical biopsy. When feasible, the entire tumor is resected. Urine cytology is helpful in following patients with recurrent vesical tumors, but it should never replace cystoscopy and transurethral vesical biopsy as a diagnostic study.

The treatment of carcinoma of the bladder depends on the grade and stage of the tumor (Fig. 183 1).[13] If the tumor is low-grade, does not invade the muscle (stage TA, T1), and has been completely resected transurethrally, no further surgery is indicated. However, these patients should be followed for life with periodic cystoscopic examinations

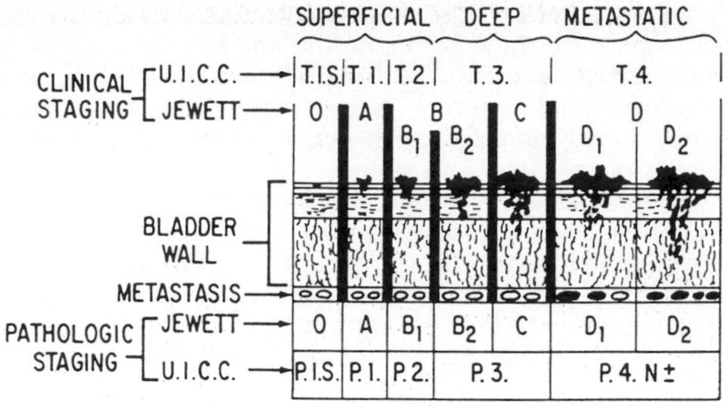

Figure 183–1. Staging of carcinoma of the urinary bladder.

to detect recurrences. If the tumor is high-grade or invades vesical muscle (stage T2, T3a), recommended treatment consists of termination of pregnancy, bilateral pelvic lymphadenectomy, anterior exenteration (cystectomy, total urethrectomy, anterior colpectomy, total hysterectomy) and urinary diversion (ileal conduit or Kock pouch). In experienced hands, many low-grade superficial tumors may be differentiated from high-grade invasive tumors by cystoscopy. Treatment of superficial tumors by transurethral resection may be deferred until after delivery. Treatment of invasive tumors, since it requires termination of pregnancy and anterior exenteration, needs considerable deliberation and patient counseling. Invasive tumors identified during the first six months of pregnancy should be managed by termination of pregnancy and anterior exenteration. Treatment of invasive tumors during the third trimester may be deferred until after delivery if the patient understands the risks involved.

In pregnant women, transurethral biopsies to document muscle invasion should be performed with a cold cup biopsy forceps. Fortunately, carcinoma of the bladder is rare before the fifth decade; this author has never encountered a pregnant patient with this malignancy. Systemic chemotherapy may be used in the management of disseminated carcinoma of the bladder or as adjunctive therapy prior to or following radical cystectomy. However, it usually is contraindicated during pregnancy. Intravesical chemotherapy with thiotepa, mutamycin, Adriamycin, and BCG has been used with some success in the management of recurrent low-grade superficial (stage TA, T1) vesical tumors. BCG is the most effective agent. Such treatment, however, should not be initiated until after delivery.

TUMORS OF THE URETHRA

Primary carcinoma of the urethra is rare.[14] It accounts for less than one of 50,000 neoplasms in women. Urethral carcinoma is the only urothelial tumor more common in women than men. It commonly occurs in the sixth and seventh decades. The distal two thirds of the female urethra is lined with squamous epithelium and the proximal third with transitional cell epithelium. Of all tumors of the female urethra, 70% are squamous cell carcinoma, 10% transitional cell carcinoma, 18% adenocarcinoma and 2% undifferentiated. Most urethral tumors are diagnosed at a late stage. The lymphatics of the distal urethra drain into the inguinal lymph nodes and the proximal urethra into the pelvic lymph nodes.

Urethral bleeding or spotting, burning, urgency, and frequency of urination are common early symptoms of urethral carcinoma. Late symptoms include urinary obstructive symptoms, perineal pain, palpable periurethral mass, palpable inguinal lymph nodes, foul-smelling urethral discharge, urinary incontinence, vaginal discharge, and dyspareunia. Gross hematuria is rare.

Definite diagnosis of urethral carcinoma is made by cystoscopy with transurethral or open biopsies. Pelvic examination will aid in determining the stage of disease, and palpable lymph nodes should be biopsied.

Treatment of urethral carcinoma is based on the stage and location of the tumor. In pregnant women, tumors invading periurethral muscle and involving the anterior (distal) urethra should be managed by wide, local excision with or without vulvectomy. Tumors invading periurethral muscle and involving the posterior (proximal) urethra are treated similarly to invasive carcinoma of the bladder, that is, by termination of pregnancy, pelvic lymphadenectomy, anterior exenteration, and urinary diversion. Inguinal lymphadenectomy is performed if previous biopsies have demonstrated metastases. Invasive urethral tumors often recur locally; for this reason, many recommend preoperative radiation therapy (4500 rads). Superficial urethral tumors involving only the mucosa or lamina propria, wherever their location, may be managed simply by transurethral resection with careful postoperative urethroscopic follow up. Unfortunately, these tumors are usually invasive when first identified. Because of the rarity of urethral carcinoma, chemotherapy has not been used sufficiently to warrant any conclusions.

REFERENCES

1. Third National Cancer Survey—Incidence Data. *Natl Cancer Inst Monogr.* 1975;41:108.
2. Potter JF, Schoeneman M. Metastasis of maternal cancer to the placenta and fetus. *Cancer.* 1970;25:380.
3. Durodola JI. Administration of cyclophosphamide during late pregnancy and early lactation: a case report. *J Natl Med Assoc.* 1979;71:165.
4. Gokal R, Durrant J, Baum JD, et al. Successful pregnancy in acute monocytic leukemia. *Br J Cancer.* 1976;34:299.
5. Newcomb M, Balducci L, Thigpen T, et al. Acute leukemia in pregnancy: successful delivery after cytarabine and doxorubicin. *JAMA.* 1978; 239:2691.
6. Brown RF, Shaver JW, Lamel DA. *The Selection of Patients for X-Ray Examinations.* Washington, DC: Department of Health, Education and Welfare; 1980. HEW Publication (FDA) 80–8104.
7. Buonocore E, Borkowski GP, Pavlicek W, et al. NMR imaging of the abdomen: technical considerations. *Am J Roentgenol.* 1983;141:1171.
8. Kressel HY, Axel L, Thickman D, et al. NMR imaging of the abdomen at 0.12 T: initial clinical experience with a resistive magnet. *Am J Roentgenol.* 1983;141:1179.
9. deKernion JB. Renal tumors. In: Walsh PC, Gittes RE, Perlmutter AD, Stamey TA, eds. *Urology.* 5th ed. Philadelphia: WB Saunders; 1986;2:1294.
10. Richie JP. Carcinoma of the renal pelvis and ureter. In: Skinner DG, Lieskovsky G, eds. *Diagnosis and Management of Genitourinary Cancer.* Philadelphia: WB Saunders; 1988:323.
11. Droller MJ. Transitional cell cancer: upper tracts and bladder. In: Walsh PC, Gittes RE, Perlmutter AD, Stamey TA, eds. *Urology.* 5th ed. Philadelphia, PA: WB Saunders; 1986;2:1343.
12. Schellhammer PF, Whitmore WF Jr. Transitional cell carcinoma of the urethra in men having cystectomy for bladder cancer. *J Urol.* 1976; 115:56.
13. Catalona WJ, Dresner SM, Haaff EO. Management of superficial bladder cancer. In: Skinner DG, Lieskovsky G, eds. *Diagnosis and Management of Genitourinary Cancer.* Philadelphia: WB Saunders; 1988:281.
14. Skinner EC, Skinner DG. Management of carcinoma of the female urethra. In: Skinner DG, Lieskovsky G, eds. *Diagnosis and Management of Genitourinary Cancer.* Philadelphia: WB Saunders; 1988:490.

Chapter One Hundred and Eighty-Four

Neoplasms of the Lung

John A. Spratt and J. Scott Rankin

184

The occurrence of pulmonary neoplasms in women of childbearing age is uncommon. The usual age-specific causes of pulmonary lesions are the same for pregnant women as for the general population; however, women are at a higher risk for several pulmonary disorders during and after pregnancy. Bronchial adenomas tend to occur in younger age groups and are more common in women. Choriocarcinoma with pulmonary metastases is a well recognized disease of the early postpartum period, and lung cancer has recently become the most common cause of cancer death in middle-aged women. The general principles of diagnosis and treatment are similar to those for any other patient, but several situations unique to pregnancy and the postpartum period deserve special emphasis. The most common problem involves the evaluation of a suspicious pulmonary lesion early in pregnancy, when both diagnostic tests and therapeutic interventions would pose a risk to the fetus.

EPIDEMIOLOGY AND PATHOLOGY

Primary pulmonary neoplasms are much more likely to be benign in women of childbearing age. The risk of malignancy in a solitary pulmonary nodule, defined as an asymptomatic well circumscribed intrapulmonary mass with a diameter 3 cm or less, is approximately 10% for a 44-year-old, one-pack-per-day male smoker.[1] It is probably similar for a female with equal risk factors but is less for younger women, especially nonsmokers. Most studies of solitary pulmonary nodules are based on the population at large and show a strong male predominance.[2,3] Although no specific data exist, it is doubtful that the age-related incidence in pregnant females is different from that of the general population. See Table 184–1 for a list of the more common causes of pulmonary lesions in this age group.

Inflammatory and Idiopathic

Although not neoplastic, infectious diseases and a variety of idiopathic disorders can present as solitary pulmonary nodules. Granulomatous disease, formerly related to tuberculosis but now more commonly resulting from fungal exposure, is a frequent cause. Granulomas are common in all population subsets and may comprise up to 50% of pulmonary nodules in the age group under consideration. They represent the end stage of an inflammatory reaction and require no treatment. Characteristically, they are seen as well circumscribed areas of calcification. Lung abscesses and opportunistic infections may result from the acquired immune deficiency syndrome or other underlying immunologic abnormality. Sarcoidosis, which is common in young females, can appear as a solitary pulmonary nodule, although it presents more frequently with dyspnea and bilateral hilar adenopathy. Lymphangiomyomatosis is a rare disorder that presents almost exclusively with pulmonary symptoms in women of childbearing age. Although the histology is not malignant, the course is progressive, with death occurring in nearly all cases. In evaluating a pulmonary nodule in a young patient, the possibility of a radiologic artifact must always be considered.

Benign Lesions

The most frequent type of benign tumor in young females is the hamartoma followed by the benign mesothelioma, mucous gland adenoma, fibroma, and a variety of increasingly rare tumors.[4-6] No causative factors have been established for these lesions, and their occurrence is sporatic. Hamartomas account for approximately 17% of pulmonary coin lesions in this age group. They are derived from bronchial cell precursors misplaced during development, and although malignant degeneration has been reported, it is very rare. These lesions also are known as "popcorn" lesions because of their characteristic feel and irregular patterns of calcification. Benign mesotheliomas have been reported in several series to be a relatively frequent cause of pulmonary nodules. They comprise 5% of the total, usually arise from the visceral pleura, and appear as lobular, well demarcated tumors on chest x-ray. Histologically, they are fibrotic and hypocellular.

The remainder of the benign primary pulmonary tumors are rare and as a group constitute only 5% of the total. They can be classified into tumors of mesenchymal, epithelial, or lymphoid origin. Fibromas are the most common type of mesenchymal tumor and usually present endobronchially. They have a tendency to become cystic and to calcify. Chondromas are the second most common type of mesenchymal tumor and present as enchondrosis of the bronchial cartilage. Lipomas typically present with symptoms of bronchial obstruction; they grow slowly and are avascular. Leiomyomas are less common, can present endobronchially or peripherally, and are felt to arise from bronchial smooth muscle. Granular cell tumors, neurogenic tumors, hemangiomas, and lymphangiomas are all rare tumors of mesenchymal origin. Mucous gland adenomas are cystic epithelial tumors that develop from bronchial mucous glands. They usually are listed as bronchial adenomas but differ from the other cell types in that they are completely benign. Papillomas have an epithelial appearance on bronchoscopy and occur most often in childhood. They are thought to be caused by a diffuse neoplastic process of the bronchial epithelium and have been associated with viral infections. Plasma cell granulomas and lymphocytomas are rare tumors of lymphatic origin.

Pulmonary endometriosis is a rare but well described entity in young females. The etiology of this lesion is controversial, with only one third of patients having pelvic endometriosis. The usual presentation is as a right-sided pneumothorax during menses. Although many women with this condition are not fertile, its occurrence during pregnancy has been well documented. In pregnancy, this lesion presents as a pulmonary mass, hemoptysis, or hemothorax. The intrathoracic location of the ectopic endometrial tissue

TABLE 184–1. CAUSES OF PULMONARY NODULES IN PREGNANCY

Inflammatory and Idiopathic
Granuloma
Abscess
Sarcoidosis
Lymphangiomyomatosis
Artifact
Benign Lesions
Hamartoma
Mesothelioma
Fibroma
Chondroma
Lipoma
Leiomyoma
Mucous gland adenoma
Endometriosis
Arteriovenous fistula
Malignant Neoplasms
Bronchial adenoma
Carcinoid
Adenoid cystic carcinoma
Mucoepidermoid carcinoma
Metastatic choriocarcinoma
Metastatic breast carcinoma
Primary lung
Lymphoma
Sarcoma
Other metastases

accounts for the various clinical presentations. Pulmonary arteriovenous malformations are seen in young females and typically occur in the lower lobes. They have the radiographic appearance of pulmonary nodules, while larger ones may present with cyanosis or hemoptysis. Arteriography is diagnostic.

Bronchial Adenomas

Bronchial adenomas tend to occur from age 20 to 40 and have a strong female predominance. They are one of the most common types of pulmonary neoplasms in this age group and occur in approximately the same frequency as hamartomas. They often are listed as benign, but this statement deserves special qualification since many of them actually are malignant.[7] Carcinoid tumors comprise 90% of the total, but approximately 15% should be considered malignant and will require aggressive treatment. Carcinoid tumors typically present endobronchially, but most have a large extra-bronchial extension. If hepatic metastases are present, patients can develop the carcinoid syndrome. These tumors are highly vascular and appear pink with an epithelial covering. The cell of origin is thought to be the Kulchitsky cell, found throughout the bronchial epithelium. Adenoid cystic and mucoepidermoid carcinomas are the remaining types of bronchial adenomas; they are malignant, of low histologic grade, and are primarily locally invasive.

Malignant Neoplasms

Choriocarcinoma occurs in approximately 1 in 20,000 pregnancies. A molar or ectopic pregnancy is present in 75% of cases, but the remainder are diagnosed within six months of an otherwise normal pregnancy. A few cases have been described during a uterine pregnancy. Choriocarcinoma, an aggressive malignancy with a rapid growth rate, has no strong associations between patient age or other risk factors. The lungs are the most common site for distant metastases in this disease, with pulmonary involvement occurring in 45–87% of cases.[8] Spread is by the hematogenous route with metastatic lesions being multiple, highly vascular, and friable. Pulmonary lesions usually present as parenchymal nodules but also can appear as interstitial infiltrates, pulmonary artery embolic masses, or as endobronchial lesions.

Carcinoma of the breast is the most common cause of cancer death in women aged 15 to 44 with 9% of all breast cancer deaths occurring in this age group. Breast cancer is diagnosed in up to 3% of pregnancies.[9] Thoracic involvement eventually occurs in 20% of cases; in half of these, the initial presentation is as a discrete mass. The remainder of intrathoracic metastases are either pleural based lesions, mediastinal nodal spread, or lymphangitic pulmonary dissemination. The chest is a rare site for initial presentation of a breast cancer but is a common site of recurrence. Pregnancy after treatment of a breast cancer is increasingly common; these patients should be evaluated thoroughly if any pulmonary symptoms develop.

Lung cancer, the second leading cause of cancer death for women aged 35 to 54, has recently overtaken breast cancer as the most common malignancy in women. The association between smoking and lung cancer is firmly established and is related to exposure time as well as to the number and type of cigarettes smoked. The relatively recent change in smoking habits of women accounts for the rapid increase in the age-specific incidence of lung cancer in this group. The development of lung carcinoma is strongly age related, with only 3% of cases occurring in women less than 44 years of age. Lung cancers typically are divided into four categories. Squamous cell carcinoma accounts for approximately 60% of cases and is the type most closely associated with smoking. This type of tumor tends to occur centrally in the tracheal bronchial tree, having a high propensity for bronchial obstruction. Undifferentiated cell types, including large cell and oat cell varieties, account for approximately 20% of all lung cancers. Oat cell carcinoma tends to occur in a slightly younger group than squamous cell carcinoma and also has a strong association with smoking. In most cases, oat cell carcinoma is a systemic disease at the time of diagnosis, and chemotherapy is the mainstay of treatment. Adenocarcinoma accounts for approximately 20% of primary lung cancers, has a more equal male to female ratio, usually is located in the periphery of the lung, and has a high propensity for hematogenous metastases. The ages of incidence are similar to those for squamous cell carcinoma. The increasing prevalence of lung cancer coupled with the fact that many women are becoming pregnant later in life leads to an increased expectation that both conditions will occur simultaneously. Several cases of primary lung cancer coincident with pregnancy have been reported, and studies have reviewed the incidence of lung cancer in women of childbearing age as well.[10,11] The distribution of cell types was similar to that seen in general population studies, and nearly all of the patients were smokers. The occurrence of a primary lung cancer in an older patient, especially a smoker, should be considered.

Hodgkin's disease presents most often in the early thirties, with thoracic involvement apparent in 30% of cases at diagnosis. Mediastinal adenopathy, anterior mediastinal mass, and intrapulmonary lymph node enlargement are the modes of occurrence in decreasing frequency. Other lymphomas are unusual before age 50. Sarcomas of bone are rare tumors, with a peak incidence in the second decade of life. Osteosarcoma and Ewing's sarcoma are the most common types, with 10% of cases having pulmonary metastases at diagnosis.

In summary, any type of pulmonary neoplasm occurring during pregnancy is unusual. Most pulmonary lesions are benign and not associated with specific risk factors. A high index of suspicion should be maintained for choriocarcinoma in the postpartum period; primary lung cancer should be considered in the older patient. Although breast cancer is the most common malignancy in this age group, gross tumor usually is limited to the breast and axilla at the time of diagnosis.

DIAGNOSIS

In evaluating a pulmonary complaint in a pregnant patient, the goal is to establish the etiology without undue delay while minimizing the risk to the patient and fetus. A number of benign processes can cause bronchial obstruction, hemoptysis, or pneumothorax that could not be tolerated untreated for the duration of a pregnancy. Diagnostic and therapeutic options depend on factors such as the stage of pregnancy and wishes of the patient as well as other medical considerations.

The initial evaluation of any pulmonary symptom in a pregnant patient should consist of a detailed history and physical examination. This is especially important since it is risk free and may provide important diagnostic clues. In addition to carefully documenting the patient's complaint's, the history should cover smoking habits and the degree of passive smoke exposure. It also should evaluate exposure to pulmonary irritants, recent respiratory infections, and possible risks of such exposures. Symptoms indicative of a significant pulmonary process are chronic cough that does not resolve with symptomatic treatment, episodes of severe coughing or stridor, or hemoptysis. Dyspnea, weight loss, anorexia, extreme weakness, or change in the character of a chronic cough can indicate more serious pathology. Extrathoracic manifestations such as endocrine, neuromuscular, or vascular syndromes also may be seen with advanced disease. Following the history, a careful physical examination should be performed with emphasis on lymphatic, pelvic, and breast examinations as well as on the chest. Wheezing, stridor, or a honking sound with forced expiration can indicate bronchial obstruction. These findings may be subtle and require auscultation in all parts of the chest. Evidence of decreased breath sounds and consolidation may be produced by atelectasis or a pneumonic process distal to an obstructed bronchus. Recurrent laryngeal nerve paralysis, superior venous caval syndrome, or Horner's syndrome may indicate extensive intrathoracic malignancy and a poor prognosis. If a patient's symptoms or physical examination suggest pulmonary pathology, the evaluation should continue with a chest radiograph.

A posterior-anterior and lateral chest radiograph can be safely obtained at any point during pregnancy. The fetus can be shielded adequately in the first trimester and is unlikely to be at significant risk later in pregnancy because of the small amount of radiation exposure. The radiograph is a sensitive indicator of chest pathology. A mass, adenopathy, pneumothorax, or effusion are seen readily, but more subtle signs such as a faint infiltrate or atelectasis may indicate an endobronchial lesion. The radiographic appearance of a pulmonary lesion is an important diagnostic feature. Calcified lesions are less likely to be malignant, especially ones with concentric lamellations, which are a common feature of granulomas. If any masses are noted, attempts should be made to obtain old radiographs. Absence of size change over a two-year period is good evidence of a benign process. Malignant lesions typically double in volume in a period between five weeks and eighteen months. Lesions doubling in size faster than five weeks are usually inflammatory, but the growth rates of choriocarcinoma and osteogenic sarcoma metastatic to the lung can be almost this rapid. The presence of a small mass may not always be clear on routine chest radiograph. In this instance, a limited fluoroscope study of the chest may be indicated but should be carefully considered for two reasons. First, a lesion so small that it cannot be confirmed on a routine chest x-ray probably can be followed for a number of weeks, if not months, without affecting the patient's prognosis. A repeat radiograph could be performed to follow the lesion. Second, the radiation dose from a fluoroscopic examination of the chest can be from five to ten times that of a chest x-ray, so that the risk to the fetus is greater, especially early in pregnancy.

If a patient requires additional evaluation of a pulmonary lesion, fiberoptic bronchoscopy should be the next step. This procedure entrails minimal risk and can be accomplished with topical anesthesia. Endobronchial lesions can be examined and biopsied, while transbronchial biopsies, bronchial brushings, and washings can be performed to diagnose more peripheral lesions. Invasive diagnostic procedures can be done as long as contingency plans are made for the treatment of possible complications. Peripheral lung lesions can be biopsied using a small needle passed percutaneously under fluoroscopic guidance. In experienced centers, this technique will yield a diagnosis in the vast majority of cases. If a patient presents with a pleural effusion, diagnostic thoracentesis should be performed. Pleural biopsies can be obtained during pregnancy, but the risk-benefit ratio again should be carefully weighed due to the risk of complications.

A number of sophisticated radiographic studies are available for further assessment of a pulmonary lesion. These tests should not be withheld if the risk to the mother from a delay in diagnosis is thought to be significant, but are indicated only rarely for evaluation of a lesion during pregnancy. Chest tomograms can localize pulmonary lesions better than plain radiographs, but they involve moderate radiation exposure and largely have been replaced by the computerized tomographic scan (CT). The CT scan can provide precise diagnostic information of parenchymal, endobronchial, and some mediastinal lesions as well as guidance for percutaneous needle biopsies. CT scanning exposes the patient to a moderate radiation dose, thus careful shielding of the fetus should be performed. Magnetic resonance imaging (MRI) has the advantage of no radiation exposure but the disadvantages of requiring longer imaging times and more limited fields of view.

Solitary Pulmonary Nodules

In a pregnant patient presenting with a solitary pulmonary nodule, the chance of malignancy is very low. The primary considerations are the patient's age, smoking history, radiographic appearance of the lesion, and the appearance of old chest radiographs. The vast majority of these lesions can be followed through pregnancy and evaluated more fully after delivery. Significant risk factors or the onset of symptoms merit an immediate and thorough evaluation.

Symptomatic Pulmonary Lesions

The type of pulmonary lesion present often can be inferred from a patient's signs and symptoms. Pleuritic pain can be caused by pleural-based tumors, large parenchymal tumors, or tumors with chest wall invasion. Transthoracic needle biopsy of the lung or pleura is usually diagnostic for these lesions. Other causes of pleuritic pain include intercostal muscle strain, pneumothorax, pulmonary emboli, and pulmonary endometriosis. Dyspnea is a common complaint during pregnancy but can be due to a pulmonary infiltrative process and should be evaluated if progressive or severe. Possible etiologies include sarcoidosis, lymphangiomyomatosis, and lymphangitic spread of tumor. Lymphomas can involve the lung in this way, as can breast, primary lung, and choriocarcinomas. Transbronchial biopsy can often lead to a diagnosis, but many patients require thoracotomy and biopsy. Other causes of dyspnea include pulmonary edema, arteriovenous fistulas, and primary cardiac diseases. These can be evaluated with hemodynamic measurements and echocardiography. The most common cause of hemoptysis is bronchitis but endobronchial tumors can also be responsible. Bronchoscopy should localize these lesions in nearly all cases. Bronchial carcinoids are highly vascular tumors, but a small forceps biopsy for diagnosis is usually safe. Nonneoplastic causes of bronchial obstruction include middle lobe syndrome, bronchiectasis and other inflammatory conditions, as well as foreign body aspiration.

Metastatic Tumors

Systemic symptoms that are not self-limited also require evaluation. Weight loss, extreme fatigue, and endocrine symptoms can indicate metastatic disease and merit an aggressive evaluation. Low-risk tests should be undertaken first, but the goal in this setting is to care for the mother, with the fetus being a secondary consideration.

The most common type of metastatic pulmonary tumor during and immediately after pregnancy is choriocarcinoma. This disease usually presents with vague pulmonary complaints of dyspnea, cough, mild chest pain, or rarely, as hemoptysis. Untreated, symptoms can progress to severe dyspnea at rest, cyanosis, or evidence of consolidation from bronchial obstruction. A diagnosis of choriocarcinoma often is made on the basis of a chest radiograph; this study should be obtained in all postpartum patients with respiratory symptoms. The progression of radiographic abnormalities in metastatic choriocarcinoma has been well described.[12] Pulmonary lesions initially begin as a miliary or beaded pattern at a time when a patient is only slightly symptomatic. The miliary pattern then progresses to one of discrete, fluffy densities with the appearance of cotton balls and finally to the multiple discrete nodules commonly observed at the time of diagnosis. Large nodules can occlude branches of the pulmonary arteries or cause pulmonary embolism. With rupture, they can produce pneumothorax or hemothorax because of their marked vascularity.

Other metastatic tumors are much less common. The possibility of metastatic breast cancer should be evaluated carefully in a patient with a history of treated breast carcinoma. The presentation is usually as an effusion, which can be evaluated with thoracentesis and cytologic examinations. Pleural-based or intraparenchymal lesions can be evaluated with transthoracic needle aspiration. Mammography generally is not recommended during pregnancy. The fetus can be shielded adequately, but because of the increased water content of the breasts, a loss of tissue contrast occurs, resulting in a higher incidence of false-negative studies. Sarcomas of bony origin often metastasize to the lung but usually cause symptoms or radiographic abnormalities referable to the primary site. Other tumors metastatic to the lung are extremely rare in this patient population.

TREATMENT

Treatment of pulmonary lesions during pregnancy needs to be individualized since it involves risk to both the mother and fetus. Specific treatment plans for each case cannot be given, but certain principles can be outlined:

1. In general, and especially later in pregnancy, the treatment of pulmonary lesions is the same as in nonpregnant patients.
2. The health and survival of the mother should not be jeopardized by delaying necessary treatment.
3. The treatment of a pulmonary lesion should be conservative, and palliative procedures can be considered early in pregnancy.

The assessment of a pregnant patient for anesthesia and thoracic surgery during the first trimester should involve considerations of teratogenesis and fetal loss. With a short procedure and careful monitoring, these risks can be minimized. Respiratory function is well maintained during pregnancy but at the expense of a decrease in expiratory reserve volume. Surgical risks are low in women with normal pregravidic lung function, but pulmonary function tests should be done prior to surgery if a resection is planned. A pulmonary resection may not be tolerated as well as in a nonpregnant patient because of the increased ventilatory requirements of pregnancy.

Small asymptomatic lesions usually can be followed without specific treatment. Serial radiographs can be done to assess size change and the development of other pathology. Symptomatic lesions need to be treated early because of the risk of secondary infection and the much lesser risk of malignancy. Benign endobronchial lesions often can be palliated in the first trimester. Chest physiotherapy, bronchodilators, and antibiotics can be considered; partial bronchoscopic resection or laser ablation also may be used to delay thoracotomy. Bronchial adenomas can be treated conservatively early during pregnancy since they are slow-growing. Symptomatic endobronchial lesions should undergo surgical resection during the second and third trimesters. If the diagnosis of a pulmonary lesion is in doubt after a thorough evaluation or if malignancy is seriously considered, diagnostic thoracotomy is recommended. If the clinical suspicion is sufficiently high, surgery should be performed during the first trimester. The definitive treatment of most benign neoplasms is local surgical excision; the surgical approach with bronchial adenomas is aggressive, wide, local excision. The removal of adenoid cystic carcinomas can be technically difficult because of the frequency of tracheal involvement. Papillomas are treated bronchoscopically, but the rate of recurrence is high and the patient needs close continued follow up. Lobectomy is required for the treatment of pulmonary arteriovenous malformations.

If a patient is suspected of having choriocarcinoma metastatic to the lung, an hCG should be obtained and the patient referred for chemotherapy. The pulmonary lesions resolve in most cases, but in a few instances pulmonary nodules thought to contain viable tumor cells persist despite a good response to chemotherapy. In some cases, hCG levels remain slightly elevated after chemotherapy, whereas in others hCG decreases to the normal range. After an adequate response to treatment, resection can be performed to remove isolated tumor deposits. Current criteria for surgical resection of pulmonary metastases from choriocarcinoma are as follows:[13] (1) the patient must be a good surgical risk; (2) the primary malignancy must be controlled and residual pelvic tumor must be absent; (3) there must be no sign of distal metastatic disease; and (4) the urinary hCG value must be below 1000 mIU/mL. A metastasis limited to only one lung has a marginally better prognosis. At least one additional course of chemotherapy should be administered after surgery to reduce the likelihood of new metastases resulting from surgical manipulation itself.

Since survival for primary carcinomas of the lung is generally low, the appropriate standard treatment should be instituted without delay. Pulmonary lesions metastatic from breast, bone, or colon indicate widespread dissemination and a poor prognosis. High-dose cytotoxic chemotherapy often is indicated and pregnancy termination should be considered. The treatment for Hodgkin's disease needs to be individualized since it is highly dependent on stage and histologic tumor type.

Prior to performing invasive diagnostic procedures in pregnant patients, the risk of complications should be assessed carefully. Pneumothorax, the most common complication of thoracentesis or transthoracic needle aspiration, is treated with placement of a thoracostomy tube under local anesthesia. The usual physical landmarks for tube placement may be unreliable, since the diaphragm is elevated in pregnancy. Damage to intra-abdominal organs can occur from incorrect needle biopsy or thoracostomy tube placement and frequently requires operative intervention. Bleeding after a pleural biopsy also may require surgical control. Since pregnant patients are young and generally healthy, complications of thoracic surgery in this group should be infrequent. Atelectasis is a greater problem because of the elevated diaphragms and consequent loss of intrathoracic volume, but the risks of bleeding, infection, and air leak should be no greater than in other patient groups.

PROGNOSIS

The prognosis for benign primary lung tumors should be the same during pregnancy as in the general population. Nearly all of these lesions are curable with local surgical excision, while bronchoscopic removal may be adequate for certain tumor types. Benign carcinoids have a five-year survival rate of 80–90%, while the malignant varieties have survival rates of approximately 50% over the same period. Adenoid cystic and mucoepidermoid carcinomas have survival rates in between these ranges. The prognosis for choriocarcinoma is good with current chemotherapy regimens and approaches 90% in most series. Those patients undergoing pulmonary resection for residual metastatic deposits have more severe disease, and their overall survival is in the range of 69%. Historically, the occurrence of breast cancer during pregnancy was thought to have a very poor prognosis, but more recent studies show that the outcome is the same as in nonpregnant patients if both groups are matched carefully for stage.[9] The stage-matched survival for women with primary lung cancers is generally the same as for men.[14]

In summary, most pulmonary lesions presenting during pregnancy are either self-limited or benign and have an excellent prognosis. Choriocarcinoma can be treated effectively in the vast majority of cases. Malignant lesions with a poor prognosis are very rare in this patient population.

REFERENCES

1. Cummings SR, Lillington GA, Richard RJ. Estimating the probability of malignancy in solitary pulmonary nodules. *Am Rev Resp Dis.* 1986; 134:449.
2. Steele JD. *The Solitary Pulmonary Nodule.* Springfield, IL: Charles C Thomas; 1964:3.
3. Toomes H, Delphendahl A, Manke H, Vogt-Moykopf I. The coin lesion of the lung: a review of 955 resected coin lesions. *Cancer.* 1983;51:534.
4. Arrigoni MG, Woolner LB, Bernatz PE, et al. Benign tumors of the lung: a ten-year surgical experience. *J Thorac Cardiovasc Surg.* 1970; 60:589.
5. Sabiston DC, Spencer FC. *Gibbon's Surgery of the Chest.* 4th ed. Philadelphia: WB Saunders; 1983:516.
6. Lawrence HC. Pulmonary endometriosis in pregnancy. *Am J Obstet Gynecol.* 1988;159:733.
7. Miller RE, Hopeman AR. Bronchial adenoma. *Ann Thor Surg.* 1975; 19:378.
8. Libshitz HI, Baber CE, Hammond CB. The pulmonary metastases of choriocarcinoma. *Obstet Gynecol.* 1977;49:412.
9. Donegan WL, Spratt JS. Cancer of the Breast. 3rd ed. Philadelphia: WB Saunders; 1988:679.
10. Stark P, Greene RE, Morgan G, Hildebrandt-Stark HE. Lung cancer and pregnancy. *Radiologe.* 1985;25:30.
11. Suda R, Repke JT, Steer R, Niebyl JR. Metastatic adenocarcinoma of the lung complicating pregnancy: a case report. J Reproductive Med. 1986;31:1113.
12. Sung H, Wu P, Hu M, et al. Roentgenologic manifestations of pulmonary metastases in choriocarcinoma and invasive mole. *Am J Obstet Gynecol.* 1982;142:89.
13. Tomoda Y, Yoshitaro A, Kaseki S, et al. Surgical indications for resection in pulmonary metastasis of choriocarcinoma. *Cancer.* 1980;46:2723.
14. Bignall JR, Martin M. Survival experience of women with bronchial carcinoma. *Lancet.* 1972;2:60.

Chapter One Hundred and Eighty-Five
Ovarian Cancer

Daniel L. Clarke-Pearson

185

The discovery of ovarian cancer during pregnancy is an unusual situation. When it is encountered, the obstetrician and gynecologist must use his surgical skills along with knowledge of the disease process to obtain optimal results in the treatment of the cancer, salvage of the pregnancy, and preservation of future fertility. In some instances, these

TABLE 185–1. HISTOLOGIC CLASSIFICATION OF OVARIAN MALIGNANCIES

Epithelial Carcinoma
- Serous
- Mucinous
- Endometroid
- Mesonephroid (clear cell)
- Brenner
- Undifferentiated

Germ-cell Tumors
- Dysgerminoma
- Endodermal sinus tumor
- Immature teratoma
- Choriocarcinoma
- Embryonal carcinoma
- Polyembryoma
- Mixed germ-cell carcinomas

Stromal-sex Cord
- Granulosa-theca tumors
- Sertoli–Leydig cell tumors
- Gynandroblastoma

Mesenchymal Tumors
- Homologous leiomyosarcoma, fibrosarcoma, and others
- Heterologous rhabdomyosarcoma, chondrosarcoma, and others
- Lymphoma

Metastatic Cancer to Ovary

goals may all be achieved, whereas in others, the outcome is poor on all counts.

The term ovarian cancer encompasses a wide range of malignancies of the ovary. General categories include epithelial carcinoma, germ-cell cancers, stromal-sex cord tumors, mesenchymal tumors, and metastatic cancer to the ovary (Table 185–1).[1] For purposes of discussion of treatment plans, these five categories are adequate. Epithelial carcinomas and germ-cell tumors are reported most frequently in association with pregnancy and account for 55% and 27% of ovarian malignancies in pregnancy, respectively (Table 185–2).[2-12] Although epithelial carcinomas usually make up a higher proportion of all ovarian cancers in most series, the greater frequency of germ-cell tumors in pregnancy reflects the fact that germ-cell tumors predominate in younger women.

ETIOLOGY

At this time, the etiology of ovarian cancer is not understood. Some authors have found an association between epithelial cancer and low parity, higher socioeconomic class, high-fat diet, industrialized countries, and the use of talc for personal hygiene.[13] There is an apparent protective benefit from the use of oral contraceptives[14] and pregnancy.[15]

TABLE 185–2. HISTOLOGY OF OVARIAN CANCER DIAGNOSED IN PREGNANCY

Type of Ovarian Cancer	Number of Patients	Percent
Epithelial	71	55
Germ-cell	35	27
Stromal-sex cord	18	15
Mesenchymal sarcoma	1	1
Metastatic	2	2

Adapted from references 2-11.

The incidence of ovarian cancer is 14 women per 100,000 per year. In Western countries, this incidence has increased slightly over the past 50 years. The incidence of ovarian cancer occurring in pregnancy, based on reports of over 500,000 deliveries from eight delivery services, is one ovarian cancer per 22,713 deliveries.[2,3,6-8,11,16,17] While the overall incidence of ovarian cancer is relatively rare, it is more striking to realize that ovarian cancer is discovered in 3.5% of pregnant patients undergoing surgery for an adnexal mass.[6-8,16,17] It therefore is prudent for any physician planning surgery on a pregnant patient with an adnexal mass to be prepared to manage an ovarian malignancy, including appropriate preoperative counseling with the patient and her family.

PATHOPHYSIOLOGY

Understanding the spread pattern of ovarian cancer is important for accurate surgical staging as well as for the planning of adjunctive therapy. *Epithelial ovarian carcinomas* is usually spread by extension through the ovarian tumor capsule, with resultant implants of tumor throughout the peritoneal cavity. Tumor spread beyond the pelvis is the general rule in this malignancy. Even in apparent early stage disease, bilateral ovarian involvement is frequent (50–60%). *Germ-cell tumors,* on the other hand, may achieve tremendous size (greater than 15–20 cm in diameter) while still confined to one ovary. Rupture of the tumor capsule ultimately leads to implantation on peritoneal surfaces. Only 5–10% of Stage I germ-cell tumors involve both ovaries, and therefore the contralateral ovary, if normal, usually may be preserved without risk of leaving malignancy behind.[18,19] Pelvic and para-aortic lymph nodes also are recognized metastatic sites for both epithelial and germ-cell cancer.

Many epithelial and germ-cell tumors have associated serum protein markers (CA-125, α-fetoprotein, human chorionic gonadotropin, LDH), which are helpful in treatment monitoring and follow up of these patients.

EFFECTS OF PREGNANCY ON DISEASE

There is no evidence that pregnancy promotes or predisposes to the development of ovarian cancer. To the contrary, there is epidemiologic evidence that pregnancy actually may reduce the incidence of subsequent ovarian cancer. There is also no data to suggest that patients who develop ovarian cancer during pregnancy have a worse prognosis or diminished chance of cure. Because the signs and symptoms of pregnancy (eg. abdominal distention, gastrointestinal complaints) are similar to the symptoms of ovarian cancer, it may be that there is a delay in diagnosis due to pregnancy.

Ovarian cancer has no direct effect on the fetus except as the mother's health is compromised by the malignancy. In advanced cases of malignancy in which maternal malnutrition secondary to abdominal carcinomatosis is encountered, fetal growth retardation might be anticipated. As noted previously, most ovarian cancer in pregnancy is discovered in the early stage and is often asymptomatic. Virilization of the fetus is a single effect rarely noted to be caused by ovarian cancer. Virilization is thought to be secondary to androgens produced by ovarian stroma tumors or stromal stimulation by a Krukenberg tumor.[20,21] Metastases to the fetus from ovarian cancer have not been reported.

RISKS OF SURGERY

The most significant fetal effects to be considered relate directly to surgical intervention and subsequent adjunctive therapy. Abdominal surgery in the first trimester generally is thought to be associated with an increased incidence of spontaneous abortion. However, this is not sufficient reason to delay surgery when ovarian cancer is suspected. Surgical technique should involve minimal trauma and minimal manipulation of the uterus. In addition, many authors recommend the use of parenteral progesterone or tocolytic agents to decrease uterine irritability.[22] Prospective trials of these agents for this purpose are lacking at present. Surgery in the third trimester also is associated with increased incidence of premature labor. If fetal maturity has been achieved, the prudent surgical procedure would combine cesarean section delivery with the staging and debulking of the ovarian cancer.

When conditions of tumor type and stage are appropriate, the pregnancy may be allowed to continue. In the case of the Stage Ia, well differentiated epithelial ovarian carcinoma, no adjunctive therapy is recommended.[18] Stage Ia nondysgermatous germ-cell cancers, on the other hand, generally require adjunctive multi-agent chemotherapy for optimal outcome.[18,19] The question of cytotoxic chemotherapy given during pregnancy is probably the most important in terms of fetal considerations. Unfortunately, the data regarding the use and effects of cytotoxic drugs in pregnancy are limited. Nearly all cytotoxic drugs are teratogenic when given to animals and humans in early pregnancy. Should a fetus not abort from exposure to cytotoxic drugs in the first trimester, malformation, and growth retardation frequently are observed. Sokal and Lessmann[23] reported that among 50 women treated with anticancer drugs there were no fetal malformations when chemotherapy was given only in the second and third trimesters of pregnancy. A subsequent report by Nicholson[24] also found no fetal malformations in 73 infants similarly treated.

If chemotherapy is necessary in the first trimester (a rare event in treating ovarian cancer), the antifolics must be avoided, as they invariably cause abortion or fetal anomalies. Limited experience with methotrexate in the second and third trimesters does not demonstrate untoward effects on the fetus or placenta. Data regarding the fetal effects of the newer chemotherapeutic agents such as Adriamycin and *cis*-platinum are not available. Finally, the long-term effects of chemotherapy on the infant and subsequent evidence of mutagenicity in later generations are not known. These infants of pregnancies exposed to chemotherapy must be observed closely over their lifetimes.

In summary, withholding chemotherapy in the first trimester is advised unless maternal conditions are deteriorating. In cases of advanced ovarian cancer early in pregnancy, a hysterectomy should be part of the initial surgical procedure. Therefore, chemotherapy usually is given only in the second and third trimesters in most cases of ovarian cancer with the fetus remaining *in utero*. Current evidence suggests that there is no significantly increased incidence of fetal malformation when chemotherapy is given in this setting.

DIAGNOSIS

It is unusual to diagnose ovarian cancer in a pregnant patient preoperatively. Except for the rare patient with markedly advanced disease (which also may be mimicked by Meigs' syndrome), the signs and symptoms of ovarian cancer in pregnancy are nearly identical to those of benign ovarian neoplasms (Table 185–3). The most frequently noted symptom is that of abdominal or plevic pain, noted in 29% of patients with ovarian cancer. This is often indolent in onset and persists for weeks to months before surgical intervention. Another 12% of patients will develop an acute surgical abdomen requiring immediate laparotomy. Findings usually are of an ovarian tumor with torsion, infarction, and rupture. Some 24% of patients will have noted pressure symptoms related to an abdominal or pelvic mass or ascites. As pregnancy advances, these symptoms are most difficult to distinguish from those related to the enlarging gravid uterus. Palpation of an adnexal mass or an abdominal mass separate from the uterus aids in this evaluation. A small number of patients (9%) will have the progress of labor arrested by an ovarian cancer obstructing the birth canal.

TABLE 185–3. SYMPTOMS ASSOCIATED WITH OVARIAN CANCER IN PREGNANCY

Symptoms	Number of Patients	Percent
Pain	20	29
Mass effect or increased girth	16	24
Acute abdomen	8	12
Obstructed labor	6	9
Asymptomatic	18	26

Adapted from references 2, 3, 5-10.

Finally, it is sobering to realize that 26% of patients with ovarian cancer in pregnancy are asymptomatic and display no physical findings to alert the physician to the presence of a malignancy. Twenty percent of patients did not have the diagnosis made until labor and delivery or at cesarean section, and 28% of patients had the diagnosis made postpartum. For this reason alone, visualization of the ovaries at cesarean section and at tubal ligation is absolutely mandatory (Table 185–4). Diagnostic ultrasound used for the purposes of assessing gestational age, fetal growth and well-being, and placental localization may have an important role in the early incidental detection of these asymptomatic malignancies.[25-28] This is not to recommend that ultrasound be used as a screening tool for the detection of the asymptomatic pelvic mass, as the cost would surely outstrip any benefit gained. Also, all cysts found on ultrasound do not necessarily require immediate surgery.

The differential diagnosis of a pelvic mass associated with pregnancy is similar to that in the nonpregnant patient. The variety and frequency of adnexal pathology encountered in pregnancy are reflected in the reports of Beisher[6], Chung[7], and White[8] and are summarized in Table 185–5.

TABLE 185–4. TIME IN PREGNANCY WHEN OVARIAN CANCER IS DIAGNOSED

Time of Diagnosis	Number of Patients	Percent
First trimester	10	16
Second trimester	16	26
Third trimester	6	10
Labor or cesarean section	12	20
Postpartum	17	28

Adapted from references 2, 3, 5, 6, 8, 9, 11.

TABLE 185–5. HISTOLOGY OF ALL OVARIAN TUMORS IN PREGNANCY

	Beischer[6]		Chung[7]		White[8]		Struyk[12]	
Histology of Ovarian Tumor	Number of Patients	Percent	Number of Patients	Percent	Number of Patients	Percent	Number of Patients	Percent
Mucinous or serous cystadenoma	70	43	121	61	12	32	25	36
Benign cystic teratoma (dermoid)	45	27	18	9	8	21	25	36
Corpus luteum	29	18	21	11	7	18.1	4	6
Endometrioma	5	3	10	5	2	5	1	1
Parovarian cyst	7	4	—	—	1	3	9	13
Fibroma	3	2	—	—	1	3	—	—
Ovarian cancer	4	2	6	3	3	8	3	4
Miscellaneous	1	1	23	12	4	10	2	3

Various parameters are used in the evaluation of an adnexal mass, including size, consistency, growth pattern, and associated symptoms. Most authors feel that an adnexal mass warrants further evaluation when it reaches 6 cm in diameter. If it is discovered in the first trimester and is cystic in nature, corpus luteum cyst must be strongly considered. On occasion, the corpus luteum may reach 6–8 cm in diameter, but most will spontaneously regress in a few weeks. Therefore, most authors suggest that the cystic mass be followed carefully to 16 weeks of gestation. If it has not regressed in size, it is unlikely to be a corpus luteum and more likely represents an ovarian neoplasm. Exploratory surgery at this juncture is necessary to evaluate the mass adequately. A benign mass 8–10 cm in diameter also has a significant chance of causing problems later in pregnancy, including torsion, rupture, or obstruction of labor. In the rare occasion that a 6- to 8-cm corpus luteum does persist into the second trimester and is resected at exploratory laparotomy, little harm is done, as the pregnancy is no longer dependent on the corpus luteum for progesterone production, a function fully assumed by the placenta late in the first trimester.

An absolute size greater than 8 cm, solid or multiple septations, or rapid growth of an ovarian mass is cause for concern, although Beisher[6] found no significant difference in frequency of ovarian cancer in the very large mass (greater than 15 cm in diameter) as compared to those 6–15 cm in diameter.

Ultrasound may be helpful in evaluating the size and consistency of the adnexal mass. A cystic mass in the first trimester that has no solid components or septae is most likely a corpus luteum or benign ovarian neoplasm; one may follow it serially to 16 weeks' gestation before deciding to operate.[26-28] Ultrasound also may detect calcifications found frequently in benign cystic teratomas. Later in pregnancy, ultrasound may be the only method that detects ovarian masses, as the adnexae are pulled out of the pelvis and out of the reach of the pelvic examination. Solid ovarian masses, ascites, or other evidence of intra-abdominal malignancy such as "omental cake," thickening of the bowel mesentery, or posterior cul-de-sac masses are much more likely to represent ovarian cancer and should be explored surgically immediately.

Patients with a past history of cancer (especially ovarian, breast, stomach, thyroid or colonic cancer) who present with an ovarian mass probably have developed recurrent malignancy. Creasman[5] noted three recurrent ovarian germ-cell malignancies in the 17 patients with ovarian cancer associated with pregnancy reported from the M. D. Anderson Hospital.

TREATMENT

The decision to proceed with exploratory laparotomy to evaluate an adnexal mass detected early in pregnancy should not be delayed beyond 16 weeks' gestation. This is particularly important because as the pregnancy progresses, the expanding uterus makes adnexal surgery increasingly more difficult. There is no reason to postpone surgery on a mass detected after 16 weeks, as this is very unlikely to be a corpus luteum, which would regress spontaneously. One also must remember that not all ovarian masses allow for planned surgery, as approximately 12% will present as an acute surgical abdomen.

Preparation for surgery should include the same preoperative evaluation as needed for an adnexal mass in the nonpregnant patient, that is, complete history and physical examination, blood counts and serum chemistries, electrocardiogram, and chest x-ray (with the abdomen shielded). An intravenous pyelogram (IVP) may be deferred if abdominal and pelvic ultrasound demonstrates kidneys in the normal position and no increased hydronephrosis or hydroureter beyond that associated with pregnancy. If normal anatomy is not demonstrated by ultrasound, a "single-shot" IVP may be valuable in detecting a pelvic kidney or ureteral obstruction.

Preoperative counseling with the patient and her family is most important, and the issue of malignancy should be addressed. Although the physician may reassure the patient that ovarian carcinoma is rarely encountered in this setting (3.5%), there is the possibility that bilateral salpingo-oophorectomy and hysterectomy may be necessary. Desires regarding further childbearing should be clarified preoperatively.

Exploratory surgery should be done through a midline or paramedian incision, allowing access to the upper abdomen, to evaluate adequately the diaphragm, omentum, and other upper abdominal viscera.[22] If ovarian cancer is encountered at the time of cesarean section done through a transverse incision, the surgeon must modify the incision to allow thorough exploration and surgery in the upper abdomen. The patient's care should not be compromised by an inadequate incision.

On opening of the abdomen, general exploration should include evaluation of the contralateral ovary and the other pelvic viscera. Peritoneal involvement with ovarian cancer in the posterior cul-de-sac or bladder peritoneum is very common. The upper abdomen must also be systematically and thoroughly explored, including visualization and palpation of the diaphragm, stomach, omentum, and pericolic gutters. The large and small bowel and its mesentery also must be inspected. Any suspicious sites for metastases should be excised or at least biopsied.

Depending on size, anatomic location, and the suspicion of malignancy when evaluating the enlarged ovary, salpingo-oophorectomy or ovarian cystectomy may be performed. Frozen-section pathology should be used liberally to further evaluate the neoplasm. If malignancy is found, a differentiation among the five main subtypes (Table 185–1) is important in planning the remainder of the operation. Peritoneal washings from the pelvis, pericolic gutters, and some of the diaphragm should be obtained for cytologic evaluation.

MANAGEMENT OF EARLY DISEASE

Based on past experience, two thirds of ovarian cancer in pregnancy is found as Stage I disease; many of these are confined to one ovary (Table 185–6).[2,3,5,7-9,11,12] There are two situations that would allow for conservation of the contralateral ovary provided that further fertility is desired by the patient:

1. A Stage Ia epithelial ovarian carcinoma that is well differentiated histologically may be treated surgically with resection of the single involved ovary. The contralateral ovary must be inspected carefully for evidence of malignant involvement, and many authors recommend that it be biopsied. In addition to obtaining peritoneal cytologies, the omentum should be resected, and the pelvic and para-aortic lymph nodes should be sampled. If all pathology reports show the malignancy to be confined to the one ovary, preservation of the pregnancy and the other ovary may be safely considered.[18]
2. Germ-cell cancer of the ovary usually is detected while still confined to the ovary. These tumors involve the opposite ovary in fewer than 10% of cases. Surgical staging should include peritoneal cytology, omentectomy, and pelvic and para-aortic lymph node sampling. Final pathologic evaluation should be used to determine if adjunctive therapy is necessary postoperatively.[19]

When immediate pathologic evaluation is indeterminant as to the tumor type or grade and a patient desires future fertility, further surgery should be deferred until the permanent pathologic slides have been reviewed by pathologists experienced in evaluating ovarian malignancies. On occasion, after final pathology reviews, a second operation may be necessary for removal of the opposite ovary and uterus, but this is the exception.

TABLE 185–6. STAGE OF OVARIAN CANCER DIAGNOSED IN PREGNANCY

Stage	Number of Patients	Percent
I	40	66
II	5	8
III	11	18
IV	2	3
Recurrent	3	5

Adapted from references 2, 3, 5, 7-9, 11, 12.

MANAGEMENT OF ADVANCED DISEASE

The surgical procedure advised for patients with more advanced ovarian cancer, whatever the cell type, should include total abdominal hysterectomy, bilateral salpingo-oophorectomy, partial omentectomy, and evaluation of peritoneal cytology. If there is no residual macroscopic cancer, pelvic and para-aortic lymph nodes should be sampled selectively. In the rare patient in pregnancy with widely metastatic malignancy (Stages III or IV), cytoreductive surgery should be attempted, as the patient's survival is dependent on the amount of disease remaining at the completion of the operation. Although it is regrettable to sacrifice a pregnancy, the mother's survival should not be compromised. Thorough preoperative discussion with the patient and her family will aid in the intraoperative decision making and in the individualization of care.

POSTOPERATIVE THERAPY

Postoperative therapy for ovarian cancer should be given in nearly all instances. In general, therapy follows the regimens used in the nonpregnant patient. Advanced epithelial ovarian carcinoma usually is treated with a combination of cytotoxic drugs, including *cis*-platinum and an aklylating agent (such as cyclophosphamide). Intraperitoneal (^{32}P) chromic phosphate may be considered as therapy for the patient with Stage I, Grade 3 epithelial cancer if there is no evidence of retroperitoneal spread. Chromic phosphate has been found in the breast milk of a patient treated postpartum with intraperitoneal ^{32}P.[29] Also, radiation therapy of the abdomen and pelvis has been used as primary treatment of epithelial ovarian cancer in a few centers.

Germ-cell ovarian cancer treated by surgery alone was a highly malignant, fatal disease despite the early stage in which it was often found. Aggressive surgical resection and radiation therapy have added little to overall survival, except for dysgerminoma, which is very radiosensitive. With the advent of multiagent chemotherapy, however, survival has been improved tremendously.[30,31] Adjunctive chemotherapy is used in all stages and types of germ-cell cancers except for the pure dysgerminoma. The most frequently used regimens include combinations of vincristine, actinomycin-D, and cyclophosphamide[30,31]; methotrexate, actinomycin-D, and chlorambucil; vinblastine, *cis*-platinum and bleomycin; and etoposide, *cis*-platinum and bleomycin.[32,33] Because of the rarity of these tumors and limited experience of individual investigators, the number of courses of therapy is not established, although it appears that from three to six cycles are probably adequate.[19]

Serum markers (α-fetoprotein, human chorionic gonadotropin, LDH, and CA-125) should be followed, as they are reasonably good indicators of tumor status. During pregnancy, however, all markers may be falsely elevated due to the pregnancy itself.[34]

The treatment of the rarer stromal-sex cord malignancies and malignant mesenchymal tumors is not well established but should include the surgical staging and resection of the disease outlined previously.[35] Adjunctive therapy should be given based on consultation with a gynecologic oncologist.

Metastatic disease to the ovary (usually from cancers of the breast, colon, stomach, thyroid, or pancreas) is a difficult problem and portends a grave prognosis.[20,21,35] Bilateral salpingo-oophorectomy may offer significant palliation from potential symptoms of a growing pelvic mass. Subsequent treatment based on protocols used for treating recurrent disease of specific organ sites is recommended. In patients with known breast cancer, estrogen and progesterone receptor analysis of the metastatic tumor in the ovary will be helpful in planning further palliative treatment and should be obtained in all cases.

REFERENCES

1. Kurman RJ, Blaustein IS. *Pathology of the Female Genital Tract.* 3rd ed. New York: Springer-Verlag; 1987.
2. Betson JR, Golden ML. Primary carcinoma of the ovary coexisting with pregnancy. *Obstet Gynecol.* 1958;12:589.
3. Betson JR, Golden ML. Cancer and pregnancy. *Am J Obstet Gynecol.* 1961;81:718.
4. Barber HRK, Brunschwig A. Gynecologic cancer complicating pregnancy. *Am J Obstet Gynecol.* 1962;85:156.
5. Creasman WT, Rutledge F, Smith JP. Carcinoma of the ovary associated with pregnancy. *Obstet Gynecol.* 1971;38:111.
6. Beischer NA, Buttery BW, Fortune DW, et al. Growth and malignancy of ovarian tumors in pregnancy. *Aust NZ J Obstet Gynecol.* 1971;11:208.
7. Chung A, Birnbaum SJ. Ovarian cancer associated with pregnancy. *Obstet Gynecol.* 1973;41:211.
8. White KC. Ovarian tumors in pregnancy. *Am J Obstet Gynecol.* 1973;116:544.
9. Judd ED. Primary ovarian carcinoma in pregnancy. *Am J Obstet Gynecol.* 1963;85:345.
10. Novak ER, Lambrou CD, Woodruff JD. Ovarian tumors in pregnancy: an ovarian tumor registry review. *Obstet Gynecol.* 1975;46:401.
11. Lutz MH, Underwood PB, Rozier JC, et al. Genital malignancies in pregnancy. *Am J Obstet Gynecol.* 1977;129:536.
12. Struyk APHB, Treffers PE. Ovarian tumors in pregnancy. *Acta Obstet Gynecol Scand.* 1984;63:421.
13. Cramer DW, Welch WR, Scully RE, et al. Ovarian cancer and talc: a case control study. *Cancer.* 1982;50:372.
14. Rosenberg L, Shapiro S, Slone D, et al. Epithelial ovarian cancer and combination oral contraceptives. *JAMA.* 1982;274:3210.
15. Beral V, Fraser P, Chilvers C. Does pregnancy protect against ovarian cancer? *Lancet.* 1978;1:1038.
16. Tawa K. Ovarian tumors in pregnancy. *Am J Obstet Gynecol.* 1964;90:511.
17. Munnell EW. Primary ovarian cancer associated with pregnancy. *Clin Obstet Gynecol.* 1963;6:983.
18. DiSaia PJ, Townsend DE, Morrow CP. The rationale for less than radical treatment for gynecologic malignancy in early reproductive years. *Obstet Gynecol Surv.* 1974;29:581.
19. Creasman WT, Soper JT. Assessment of the contemporary management of germ cell malignancies of the ovary. *Am J Obstet Gynecol.* 1985;153:828.
20. Spadoni LR, Lindberg MC, Mottet NK, et al. Virilization coexisting with Krukenberg tumor during pregnancy. *Am J Obstet Gynecol.* 1965;92:931.
21. Fox LP, Stamm WJ. Krukenberg tumor complicating pregnancy: Report of a case with androgenic activity. *Am J Obstet Gynecol.* 1965;92:702.
22. Hopkins MP, Duchon MA. Adnexal surgery in pregnancy. *J Reprod Med.* 1986;31:1035.
23. Sokal JE, Lessmann EM. The effects of cancer chemotherapeutic agents on the human fetus. *JAMA.* 1960;172:1765.
24. Nicholson HO. Cytotoxic drugs in pregnancy. *J Obstet Gynaecol Br Commonw.* 1968;75:307.
25. Ballard CA. Ovarian tumors associated with pregnancy termination patients. *Am J Obstet Gynecol.* 1984;149:384.
26. Lavery JP, Koontz WL, Layman L, et al. Sonographic evaluation of the adnexa during pregnancy. *Surg Gynecol Obstet.* 1986;163:319.
27. Thornton JG, Wells M. Pregnancy: does ultrasound make traditional management inappropriate? *Obstet Gynecol.* 1987;69:717.
28. Hogston P, Lilford RJ. Ultrasound study of ovarian cysts in pregnancy: prevalence and significance. *Br J Obstet Gynecol.* 1986;93:625.
29. Carlson JA, Jose B, Sharma SC, et al. Radioactivity in breast milk after intraperitoneal chromic phosphate for the treatment of early ovarian cancer. *Am J Obstet Gynecol.* 1983;147:840.
30. Slayton RE, Hreschchyshyn MM, Silverberg SG, et al. Treatment of malignant ovarian germ cell tumors: response to vincristine, dactinomycin, and cyclophosphamide. *Cancer.* 1978;42:390.
31. Curry SL, Smith JP, Gallagher HS. Malignant teratoma of the ovary: prognostic factors and treatment. *Am J Obstet Gynecol.* 1978;131:845.
32. Creasman WT, Fetter B, Hammond CB. Germ cell malignancies of the ovary. *Obstet Gynecol.* 1979;53:226.
33. Sessa C, Bonazzi C, Landoni F, et al. Cis-platinum, vinblastine and bleomycin combination chemotherapy in endodermal sinus tumor of the ovary. *Obstet Gynecol.* 1987;70:220.
34. Halila H, Stenman U, Seppala M. Ovarian cancer antigen CA-125 levels in pelvic inflammatory disease and pregnancy. *Cancer.* 1986;57:1327.
35. Young RH, Dudley AG, Scully RE. Granulosa cell, Sertoli-Leydig cell and unclassified sex cord–stromal tumors associated with pregnancy: a clinicopathological analysis of thirty-six cases. *Gynecol Oncol.* 1984;18:181.

Chapter One Hundred and Eighty-Six

Preinvasive and Invasive Cervical Neoplasia

Ellen Blair Smith and William T. Creasman

186

Cytologic screening for cervical cancer and treatment of detected preinvasive abnormalities results in a decrease in both the incidence and mortality from squamous cell cancer of the cervix. Presentation of a patient for prenatal care or pregnancy termination affords the clinician an opportunity to provide this screening.

In the early days of cytologic screening, confusion existed as to whether the hormonal extremes of pregnancy made Papanicolaou (Pap) smear interpretation unreliable in identifying cervical neoplasia. Some investigators proposed that physiologic cytologic changes in pregnancy were confused with the abnormalities of cellular growth that characterize preinvasive cervical neoplasia. They suggested that these abnormalities detected in pregnancy did not have the same significance as do similar cytologic abnormalities in the nonpregnant patient. Numerous investigations have refuted this proposal.[1-4] This conflict is likely based in part on the following:

1. Minimal nuclear cytologic changes typify pregnancy that are physiologic and may be confused with earlier degrees of dysplasia.
2. Inflammation of the subepithelial tissue is a more frequent finding in pregnancy contrasted to the nonpregnant state.[5] Inflammatory atypias may be confused with milder dysplastic changes.
3. Spontaneous regression is an accepted, possible outcome of cervical intraepithelial neoplasia, especially in its milder forms.

TABLE 186–1. REPORTED PREVALENCES OF PREINVASIVE AND INVASIVE CERVICAL NEOPLASIA IN PREGNANT PATIENTS

Author and Year of Publication	Number of Pregnant Patients Screened	Method of Screening	% with Neoplasia of any Degree	% with CIS or Invasive Cancer
Nesbitt & Hellman (1952)[5]	300	B[a]	—	0.7%
Marsh & Fitzgerald (1956)[6]	4067	B	—	0.6%
Beecham & Emich (1959)[9]	1041	C[b]	—	1.4%
Reagan et al (1961)[10]	930	C	3%	—
Rutledge et al (1962)[2]	3873	C	1.6%	—
Stromme (1969)[11]	—	C	0.4%	—
Bibbo et al (1971)[12]	8230	C	1.7%	0.4%
Lurain & Gallup (1979)[13]	—	C	1.3%	—
Khatree et al (1980)[14]	2000	C	1.1%	0.6%
Bertini-Oliveira (1982)[15]	3534	C	3.5%	0.9%

[a] Screening by random cervical biopsy
[b] Cytologic screening

Investigators today would agree that cytologic abnormalities detected during pregnancy warrant the same careful investigation as similar abnormalities found in nonpregnant patients.

PREVALENCE OF CERVICAL NEOPLASIA IN PREGNANCY

The reported prevalences of preinvasive and invasive cervical malignancy in pregnancy are presented in Table 186–1. Each series reports data from populations of prenatal clinic patients. Hacker and associates[6-7], in their 1982 review of 14 published reports of cervical neoplasia in pregnancy, give an average incidence of carcinoma *in situ* as 1.3 per 1000 pregnancies or 1 in 770. Their accrued incidence of invasive cervical neoplasia is 0.45 per 1000 or 1 in 2205 pregnancies.

Cervical neoplasia occurs with sufficient frequency such that *all* pregnant women must be screened for cervical neoplasia upon presentation for prenatal care or for termination of pregnancy. A sample is scraped from the ectocervix, transferred to a clean, appropriately labeled glass slide, and immediately fixed. A second sample is obtained from the lower endocervical canal by swabbing with a cotton tip applicator or by gentle aspiration. This sample is rolled evenly or smeared on a second slide and fixed. Any gross lesion of the cervix should be biopsied immediately.

These authors agree with Koss[8] that it is "singularly misleading" to obtain a second Pap smear to confirm or refute a prior result. Cytologic abnormalities must be evaluated by clinical colposcopy.

The reader is referred to the thoughtful review of Koss[8] for a full discussion of false-negative cervical cytology.

MANAGEMENT OF THE GRAVIDA WITH ABNORMAL CERVICAL CYTOLOGY

Evaluation of the gravida with abnormal cervical cytology has a single objective: One must establish if invasive cancer is present. To paraphrase Beecham and Emich[9], invasive carcinoma of the cervix is a therapeutic emergency; preinvasive neoplasia of the cervix is not.

Figure 186–1 presents a schema for the management of abnormal Pap smears during pregnancy. To initiate the search for the lesion responsible for cytologic abnormalities, the cervix is inspected. If no gross lesion is seen, colposcopy is performed. Dilute (3–4%) acetic acid is applied to the cervix to facilitate colposcopy by highlighting epithelial abnormalities. Since cervical neoplasia begins as a unifocal intraepithelial abnormality in cellular growth in the transformation zone from the squamous to columnar epithelium, the entire transformation zone must be inspected. Normal endocervical villi must be seen circumferentially to assure that all areas at risk for the development of neoplasia have been assessed. Many colposcopists note the "physiologic eversion" of the endocervix in pregnancy and suggest it is responsible for the ease with which the gravid cervix is assessed. Many investigators confirm that colposcopy is adequate for assessment of the entire squamo-columnar junction in the vast majority of pregnant patients.[10-15] The rate of nonvisualization of the zone at risk varies from 1–13%.[16,17] Good correlation has been shown between the colposcopist's impression of the severity of a lesion seen and the histologic diagnosis of that lesion, between the colposcopist's assessment of the cervix antepartum and postpartum[18], between the degree of abnormality in colposcopy-directed biopsies taken antepartum compared to those taken postpartum, and between colposcopy-directed biopsies and subsequent cone biopsy or hysterectomy specimens.[13,15] Errors, when they occur, tend to be in assessment by the colposcopist of a lesion to be of greater severity than actually exists; no invasive cancer was missed in any of the series cited above. Some authors are so impressed by the reliability of colposcopy in assessing the severity of a lesion that they do not recommend biopsy of the lesion judged preinvasive during pregnancy. Another group suggested that the morbidity associated with cervical punch biopsy in pregnancy warranted hospitalization prior to such a procedure.[19] The authors of this chapter do not agree with either of these positions. Epperson and associates[20] biopsied 400 patients antepartum and intrapartum; one patient required admission to control bleeding complications. No infections were noted. Further study confirmed that all excessive bleeding was controlled by silver nitrate application or tamponade. No transfusions were required. More contemporary studies[7,13] document the safety of outpatient cervical biopsy of the pregnant patient. The authors recommend biopsy of the lesion(s) thought

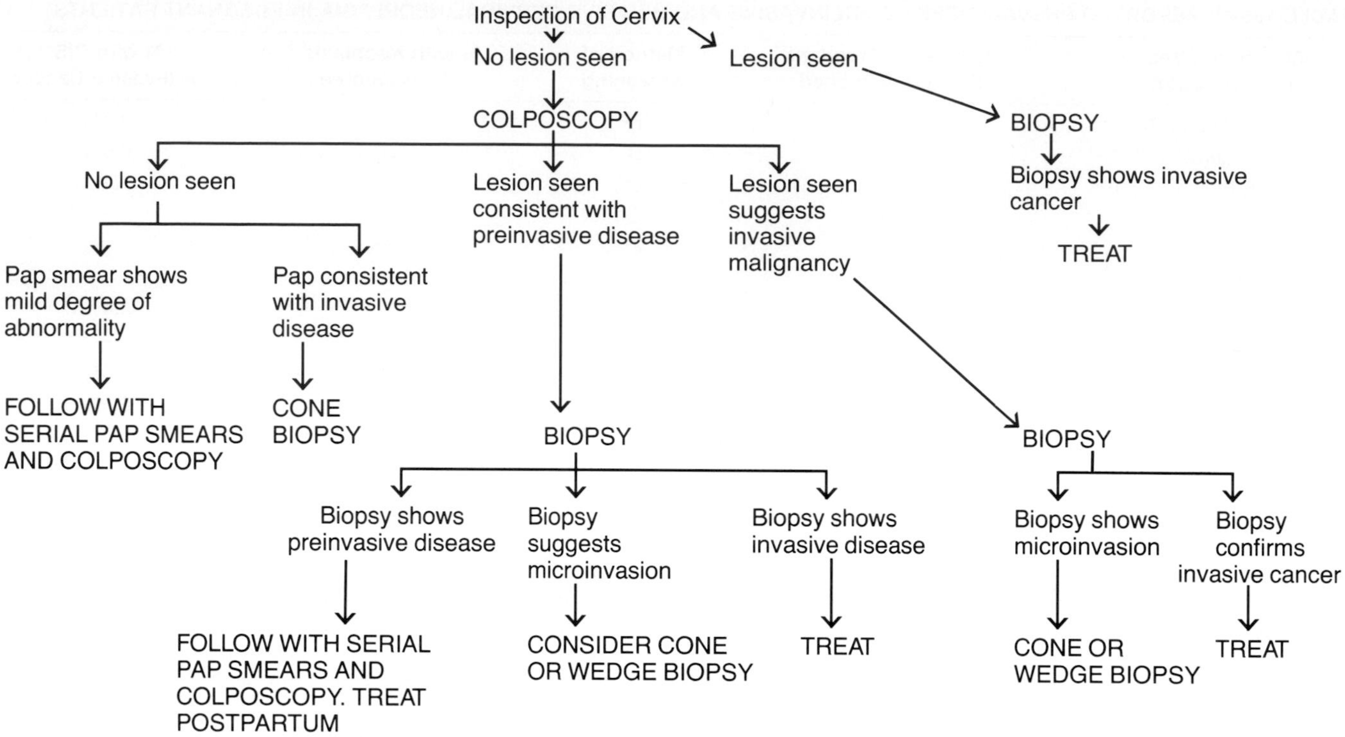

Figure 186–1. Management of the gravida with abnormal cervical cytology

at colposcopy to be most severe. While it is agreed that the most experienced colposcopists have little need for biopsy confirmation of their assessments of preinvasive disease, for the majority of practicing colposcopists, biopsy serves as additional safeguard that invasive disease will not be overlooked. Tamponade or topical application of silver nitrate or ferric subsulfate (Monsel's solution) will control bleeding from biopsy sites in most cases.

With the introduction of colposcopy, the need for cervical conization has fallen dramatically. Conization is now reserved for those patients in whom the entire lesion or transformation zone cannot be seen by the colposcopist, in whom the Pap smear suggests a marked degree of abnormality unexplained by colposcopy or directed biopsy, or in whom cervical biopsy suggests microinvasion. The purpose of conization in pregnancy is to establish if invasive disease is present. The morbidity associated with cone biopsy done in pregnancy may be substantial. Complications include immediate and delayed hemorrhage, endomyometritis, precipitation of spontaneous abortion or premature labor, or premature rupture of membranes. Reported incidences of these complications vary.[11,19,21] Moore[22] found cervical conization "had virtually no effect on the pregnancy" in 14 patients he studied. On the other hand, 14% of the patients in Rogers' and Williams' study required transfusion for immediate bleeding complications, and they found a 19% prenatal fetal complication rate.[23]

Table 186–2 shows a high overall rate of persistence of disease after antepartum conization. This probably is due to the surgeon's reluctance to extend dissection high in the endocervical canal. While conization may excise all disease, careful continued intrapartum and postpartum cytologic screening is necessary.

In cases in which conization is indicated by inability to see the entire transformation zone or a suspect lesion, a biopsy less extensive than cervical conization may be adequate to exclude the presence of invasive disease. Only that area incompletely assessed by colposcopy is removed, and is called a "wedge biopsy." The use of wedge biopsy, where appropriate, may avert some of the complications that may be encountered with larger cone biopsies.

To avoid inadvertent amniotomy, performance of endocervical curettage is not recommended in the evaluation of abnormal cytology from the gravid patient.

NATURAL HISTORY OF PREINVASIVE CERVICAL NEOPLASIA IN PREGNANCY

The viral etiology of cervical cancer has been postulated for a long time. The late 1970s and 1980s have seen a veritable explosion of published research on the role of human papillomaviris (HPV) in cervical neoplasia. It is clear that infection with HPV types 16 and 18 poses higher risk for the development of advanced dysplasias and invasive cervical

TABLE 186–2. REPORTED INCIDENCES OF NEOPLASIA PERSISTENCE AFTER CERVICAL CONE BIOPSY IN PREGNANCY

Author and Year of Publication	Number of Cone Biopsies	% with Persistence at Subsequent Hysterectomy
Moore et al (1961)[22]	14	20%
Smith et al (1968)[3]	15	53%
Stromme (1969)[11]	43[a]	49%
Fowler et al (1980)[24]	9	78%
Hannigan et al (1982)[21]	82	37%

[a] Includes 15 patients who underwent postpartum cone biopsy.

neoplasia.[24] (The reader is referred to reviews by Richart[25] and Reid and Campion[26] about HPV and cervical neoplasia.) It also is clear that HPV infection alone is inadequate for the genesis of cervical cancer. Postulates of co-factors with HPV and mechanisms of initiation of cervical neoplasia are published.[27,28] Treatment of cervical neoplasia remains based on the histologic degree of abnormality and clinically determined extent of disease. While DNA probes for the detection and genotyping of HPV infections of the cervix are now widely available, they are not currently determinants of treatment.

Earlier in this chapter, it was stated that intraepithelial neoplasia diagnosed in pregnancy may undergo spontaneous resolution. In two studies from Johns Hopkins, spontaneous resolution of biopsy-proven carcinoma *in situ* was documented, and this phenomenon was suggested to be the rule for preinvasive neoplasia diagnosed in pregnancy.[6,20] Marsh and Fitzgerald[6] summarized 12 studies involving 75 pregnant patients diagnosed by biopsy as having carcinoma *in situ* (CIS). Of these lesions, 79% persisted on postpartum cervical biopsy. Rutledge and coworkers[2], in 1962, followed 49 women with abnormal cervical cytology in pregnancy. Postpartum biopsies in 49 confirmed persistent intraepithelial neoplasia. Kuguchi and associates[29] analyzed cytologic follow-up studies of 423 patients with abnormal cervical cytology in pregnancy. They do not state what percent of patients underwent colposcopy or biopsies during pregnancy. As demonstrated solely by postpartum cytologic study, mild dysplasia was shown to persist in 10% of patients and to progress in 12%. Moderate dysplasia persisted in 15% and progressed in 10%. Severe dysplasia persisted in 31% and progressed in 15%. Some 7% of patients in their series showed progression from dysplasia to preinvasive or invasive carcinoma. Progression occurred in all degrees of dysplasia and both during and after pregnancy.

For the individual patient, progression, persistence, or regression cannot be predicted by available techniques. When preinvasive cervical neoplasia is diagnosed in pregnancy and invasive disease is ruled out, Pap smear surveillance and colposcopy should be performed at three-month intervals until delivery. Ferenczy[30] has documented the safety and efficacy of laser ablation of vulvar and perianal condyloma in pregnancy. The safety of cervical laser ablation is not documented. Established preinvasive cervical neoplasia can safely wait for treatment postpartum.

After delivery, and with uterine involution, the cervix must be reassessed. Occasionally, the epithelial atrophy in the nursing mother will hamper colposcopy. Small amounts of topical estrogen cream applied 2–3 times weekly for 2–3 weeks will aid in visualizing epithelial changes in such instances without affecting lactation. Persistent cervical abnormalities at that time should be treated. The method of treatment will depend on the patient's and her physician's preference (eg, cryosurgery, electrocoagulation diathermy, laser treatment, conization, or hysterectomy).

INVASIVE CERVICAL MALIGNANCY IN PREGNANCY

The treatment of invasive cervical cancer in pregnancy depends on the stage of disease at diagnosis (Table 186–3). The 1985 FIGO revision of the staging of cervical cancer attempts to define microinvasive cancer in terms of tumor volume (both depth and breadth). Studies[31-33] in nonpregnant patients have shown that the incidence of pelvic lymph node metastases in cervical cancer invasive to a depth of

TABLE 186–3. STAGING OF INVASIVE CERVICAL CANCER

Stage I.	Carcinoma confined to the cervix (extension to the corpus should be disregarded)
IA.	Preclinical carcinoma of the cervix, diagnosed by microscopy only
IA1.	Minimal microscopically evident stromal invasion
IA2.	Microscopically evident lesion not more than 5 mm in depth of invasion and 7 mm in horizontal spread
IB.	Lesions of greater dimension than Stage Ia2, whether clinically evident or not
Stage II.	The carcinoma extends beyond the cervix but does not extend onto the pelvic wall. The carcinoma involves the vagina, but not the lower third.
IIA.	No obvious parametrial involvement
IIB.	Obvious parametrial involvement
Stage III.	The carcinoma extends to the pelvic wall. On rectal examination there is no cancer-free space between the tumor and the pelvic wall. The tumor involves the lower third of the vagina. All cases with hydronephrosis or a nonfunctioning kidney are included unless they are known to be due to some other cause.
IIIA.	No extension to the pelvic wall
IIIB.	Extension to the pelvic wall or hydronephrosis or nonfunctioning kidney
Stage IV.	The carcinoma extends beyond the true pelvis or involves the mucosa of the bladder or rectum. Bullous edema, as such, does not permit a case to be assigned to Stage IV.
IVA.	Spread to the bladder or rectum
IVB.	Spread to distant organs

Based on revised data from International Federation of Gynecology and Obstetrics (FIGO), 1985.

less than 3 mm is less than 3% and that simple hysterectomy constitutes adequate surgical therapy. Thompson et al[34] define microinvasive cervical carcinomas as stromal invasion of less than 3 mm without regard to other factors. Twenty-one pregnant patients in this series were diagnosed by cone biopsy as microinvasive. Fourteen patients underwent pelvic lymphadenectomy as part of their treatment; no lymph node metastases were found. (Of note, five patients had capillary and lymphatic involvement by tumor in cone biopsy specimens.) The subsequent hysterectomy specimens show residual microinvasive tumor in 9 of 21 patients (43%), but there were no instances of invasion deeper than 3 mm. Residual CIS or dysplasia was noted in 11 other patients. On the basis of their data, these investigators suggest that treatment of selected patients with cervical cancer invasive to less than 3 mm as diagnosed by cone biopsy may be deferred until fetal maturity, at which time cesarean section and hysterectomy are performed. Most authorities today would be conservative in their management of minimally invasive cancer diagnosed in pregnancy by cone biopsy. The pregnancy can be allowed to continue to term and appropriate therapy can be given postpartum.

Controversy persists as to the treatment of cancers 3–5 mm invasive. Data[35-38] has been presented suggesting that simple hysterectomy or cone biopsy is adequate therapy for these lesions when volume is defined as less than 7 mm width (FIGO Ia2). This is countered by the works of Van Nagell et al[39] and Maiman and associates[33] in which lymph node metastases of 9% and 13%, respectively, were encountered in patients with tumors invasive 3–5 mm. (Lateral extension of tumor is not strictly quantitated in either paper.) The authors of this chapter continue to offer radical therapy to their patients with tumors invasive 3–5 mm in the majority of instances; more conservative therapy is strictly individualized.

For Stage IB and greater diagnosed in the first or early second trimester, treatment should begin immediately. In the later weeks of gestation, therapy may be delayed until fetal maturity is documented and delivery is effected. There are little data in the literature to document the effects of short delays in treatment initiation on subsequent prognosis. Barber and Brunschwig[40] state "there appears to be no disadvantage to brief delay in order to secure a live fetus." Prem and associates[41] cite 9 patients in which intentional delays in initiation of therapy of up to 17 weeks did not adversely affect outcome. All patients had Stage I cancer and were asymptomatic. Lee and coworkers[42] note eight instances in which treatment was delayed 1–11 weeks while anticipating fetal maturity. In no case was clinical advancement noted during the waiting period. Evaluation of the lesion being followed must be performed frequently. Any sign of disease advancement provokes the move to delivery of the premature infant and institution of appropriate therapy.

Cervical cancer diagnosed in pregnancy should be treated in the same manner as similar lesions diagnosed in nonpregnancy states. Radiation therapy, delivered as whole pelvic external radiotherapy and intravaginal and contracervical brachytherapy, is appropriate for Stage IIB–IVA cancers. Earlier lesions, Stage IB and selected IIA, may be treated equally well with radical hysterectomy with pelvic lymphadenectomy or radiation therapy. Many authors attest to the ease with which radical hysterectomy with lymphadenectomy may be performed in the gravida. Mikuta[43], in an analysis of factors that contribute to perioperative morbidity in radical hysterectomies, found pregnant patients had the fewest number of complications. He noted that blood loss averaged approximately 600 mL^3 greater when compared to nonpregnant cases. In a retrospective study of 49 pregnant patients with Stage IB cervical cancer, Nisker and Shubat[44] noted significantly fewer serious complications to those treated with radiotherapy. Radical hysterectomy also allows preservation of ovarian function.

The sole factor that complicates cervical cancer treatment in pregnancy is management of the fetus. When diagnosed early in pregnancy and fetal salvage is not a concern, radical surgery or radiotherapy may be instituted prior to uterine evacuation. In patients treated with radiotherapy, fetal demise usually occurs during the third or fourth week of treatment; spontaneous abortion usually follows.[41] In those patients who fail to abort spontaneously, uterine evacuation by curettage, hysterotomy, or hysterectomy is performed. Timing of hysterotomy in the second trimester, whether before or after radiotherapy institution, is controversial. Hysterotomy prior to radiotherapy may be complicated and delay therapy of the cancer.[45]

Much has been written about the prognostic effects of method of delivery on cervical cancer. Kinch concluded that vaginal delivery of the gravida with cervical cancer predisposed to a rapid spread of tumor; his data may be interpreted differently with contrary conclusions drawn.[46] Other investigators found that vaginal delivery did not influence survival adversely.[47] Waldrop and Palmer[48] noted higher "cure rates" in patients delivered vaginally and concluded that the diagnosis of invasive cervical cancer did not contraindicate vaginal delivery. However, fear of inciting serious hemorrhage leads most clinicians to deliver such patients by cesarean section. In the patient to be treated definitively by radical surgery, cesarean section should be performed immediately prior to radical hysterectomy.

The majority of published reports on cervical cancer in pregnancy conclude that stage is the most important prognostic factor determining survival, and stage for stage, survival is equal in pregnant and nonpregnant patients.[42,47] Interpretation of the literature is confounded by the inclusion of patients diagnosed for variable periods postpartum with patients diagnosed in pregnancy and by the multiple treatment regimens employed in each series. Table 186–4 presents survival data from five reported series.

The detection of cervical neoplasia in pregnancy warrants prompt evaluation. With adequate diagnosis and ap-

TABLE 186–4. FIVE-YEAR SURVIVAL RATES OF PATIENTS TREATED FOR INVASIVE CARCINOMA OF THE CERVIX DIAGNOSED IN PREGNANCY

Author and Year of Publication	Stage	Method of Treatment	Number of Patients	5-Year Survival
Waldrop & Palmer[a] (1963)[48]	I	RT[c]	54	70.4%
	II	RT	56	39.3%
	III	RT	52	21.2%
	IV	RT	20	10.0%
Prem et al[b] (1966)[41]	I	RT	17	82.0%
Sablinska et al[a] (1977)[49]	I	RT	114	71.9%
	II	RT	116	53.4%
	III	RT	92	17.4%
	IV	RT	5	0%
Lee et al[a] (1981)[42]	IB	S[d]	17	93%
	IB	RT	4	80%
	II	RT	12	24%
Nisker & Shubat[a] (1983)[44]	IB	S	11	63.6%
	IB	RT	25	76.0%

[a] Data includes patients diagnosed postpartum
[b] Data includes only those patients diagnosed in pregnancy
[c] Radiation therapy as primary treatment
[d] Radical hysterectomy as primary treatment

propriate treatment, results will be similar to those achieved in the nonpregnant patient. Pregnancy appears to have no effect on the development or natural history of cervical malignancy.

REFERENCES

1. Walters WD, Reagan JW. Epithelial dysplasias of the uterine cervix in pregnancy. *Am J Clin Path.* 1956;26:1314.
2. Rutledge CE, Christopherson WM, Parker JE. Cervical dysplasia and carcinoma in pregnancy. *Obstet Gynecol.* 1962;19:351.
3. Smith MR, Figge DC, Bennington JL. The diagnosis of cervical cancer during pregnancy. *Obstet Gynecol.* 1968;31:193.
4. Wied GL. Epithelial abnormalities on the ectocervix during pregnancy: an invitational symposium. *J Reprod Med.* 1970;4:13.
5. Nesbitt REL, Hellman M. The histopathology and cytology of the cervix in pregnancy. *Surg Gynecol Obstet.* 1952;94:10.
6. Marsh M, Fitzgerald PJ. Carcinoma in situ of the human uterine cervix in pregnancy: prevalence and postpregnancy persistence. *Cancer.* 1956; 9:1195.
7. Hacker NF, Berek JS, Lagasse LD, et al. Carcinoma of the cervix associated with pregnancy. *Obstet Gynecol.* 1982;59:735.
8. Koss LG. The Papanicolaou test for cervical cancer detection: a triumph and a tragedy. *JAMA.* 1989;261:737.
9. Beecham CT, Emich JP. Carcinoma in situ. *Obstet Gynecol.* 1959;13:653.
10. Reagan JW, Bell BA, Neuman JL, et al. Dysplasia in the uterine cervix during pregnancy: an analytical study of the cells. *Acta Cytol.* 1961;5:17.
11. Stromme WB. Preclinical carcinoma and dysplasia of the cervix associated with pregnancy. *Am J Obstet Gynecol.* 1969;105:1008.
12. Bibbo MC, Keebler M, Wied GL. Prevalance and incidence rates of cervical atypia. *J Reprod Med.* 1971;6:79.
13. Lurain JR, Gallup DG. Management of abnormal Papanicolaou smears in pregnancy. *Obstet Gynecol.* 1979;53:484.
14. Khatree MHD, Houlton MCC, Moodley J. Cervical cytology in pregnant black patients and potential selective screening programmes. *S Afr Med J.* 1980;58:359.
15. Bertini-Oliveira AM, Keppler MM, Luisi A, et al. Comparative evaluation of abnormal cytology, colposcopy and histopathology in preclinical cervical malignancy during pregnancy. *Acta Cytol.* 1982;26:636.
16. DePetrillo AD, Townsend DE, Morrow CP, et al. Colposcopic evaluation of the abnormal Papanicolaou test in pregnancy. *Am J Obstet Gynecol.* 1975;121:441.
17. Kohan S, Beckman EM, Bigelow B, et al. The role of colposcopy in the management of cervical intraepithelial neoplasia during pregnancy and postpartum. *J Reprod Med.* 1980;25:279.
18. Kirkup W, Singer A. Colposcopy in the management of the pregnant patient with abnormal cervical cytology. *Br J Obstet Gynecol.* 1980;87:322.
19. Averette HE, Nasser N, Yankow SL, et al. Cervical conization in pregnancy: analysis of 180 operations. *Am J Obstet Gynecol.* 1970;106:543.
20. Epperson JWW, Hellman LM, Galvin GA, et al. The morphologic changes in the cervix during pregnancy, including intraepithelial carcinoma. *Am J Obstet Gynecol.* 1951;61:50.
21. Hannigan EV, Whitehouse HH, Atkinson WD, et al. Cone biopsy during pregnancy. *Obstet Gynecol.* 1982;60:450.
22. Moore JC, Morton DG, Applegate JW, et al. Superficial carcinoma of the uterine cervix in pregnancy. *Surg Gynecol Obstet.* 1961;113:339.
23. Rogers RS, Williams JH. The impact of the suspicious Papanicolaou smear on pregnancy. *Am J Obstet Gynecol.* 1967;98:488.
24. Fowler WC, Walton LA, Edelman DA. Cervical intraepithelial neoplasia during pregnancy. *S Med J.* 1980;73:1180.
25. Richart RM. Causes and management of cervical intraepithelial neoplasia. *Cancer.* 1987;60:1951.
26. Reid RE, Campion MJ. The biology and significance of human papillomavirus infections in the genital tract. *Yale J Biol Med.* 1988;61:307.
27. ZurHausen H. Human genital cancer: synergism between two viral infections or synergism between a virus infection and initiating events. *Lancet.* 1982;1370.
28. ZurHausen H. Intracellular surveillance of persisting viral infections. *Lancet.* 1986;489.
29. Kuguchi K, Bibbo M, Hasegawa T, et al. Dysplasia during pregnancy: a cytologic followup study. *J Reprod Med.* 1981;26:66.
30. Ferenczy A. Treating genital condyloma during pregnancy with the carbon dioxide laser. *Am J Obstet Gynecol.* 1984;148:9.
31. Boronow RC. Stage I cervix cancer and pelvic node metastasis. *Am J Obstet Gynecol.* 1977;127:135.
32. Creasman WT, Parker RT. Microinvasive carcinoma of the cervix. *Clin Obstet Gynecol.* 1973;16:261.
33. Maiman MA, Fruchther RG, DiMaio TM, Boyce JG. Superficially invasive squamous cell carcinoma of the cervix. *Obstet Gynecol.* 1988;72:399.
34. Thompson JD, Caputo TA, Franklin EW III, et al. The surgical management of invasive cancer of the cervix in pregnancy. *Am J Obstet Gynecol.* 1975;121:853.
35. Lohe KJ. Early squamous cell carcinoma of the uterine cervix I. Definition and histology. *Gynecol Oncol.* 1978;6:10.
36. Lohe KJ, Burghart E, Hillemans HG, et al. Early squamous cell carcinoma of the cervix II. Clinical results of a cooperative study in the management of 419 patients with early stromal invasive microcarcinoma. *Gynecol Oncol.* 1978;6:31.
37. Lohe KJ. Early squamous cell caricnoma of the uterine cervix III. Frequency of lymph node metastases. *Gynecol Oncol.* 1978;6:51.
38. Burhardt E. Microcarcinoma in gynecological pathology. *Clin Obstet Gynecol.* 1984;11:239.
39. Van Nagell JR, Greenwell N, Powell DF, et al. Microinvasive carcinoma of the cervix. *Am J Obstet Gynecol.* 1983;145:981.
40. Barber HRK, Brunschwig A. Gynecologic cancer complicating pregnancy. *Am J Obstet Gynecol.* 1963;85:156.
41. Prem KA, Makowski EL, McKelvey JI. Carcinoma of the cervix associated with pregnancy. *Am J Obstet Gynecol.* 1966;95:99.
42. Lee RB, Neglia W, Park RC. Cervical carcinoma in pregnancy. *Obstet Gynecol.* 1981;58:584.
43. Mikuta JJ, Giuntoli RL, Rubin EL, et al. The "problem" radical hysterectomy. *Am J Obstet Gynecol.* 1977;129:119.
44. Nisker JA, Shubat M. Stage IB cervical carcinoma and pregnancy: report of 49 cases. *Am J Obstet Gynecol.* 1983;145:203.
45. Saunders N, Landon CR. Management problems associated with carcinoma of the cervix diagnosed in the second trimester of pregnancy. *Gynecol Oncol.* 1988;30:120.
46. Kinch RAH. Factors affecting the prognosis of cancer of the cervix in pregnancy. *Am J Obstet Gynecol.* 1961;182:45.
47. Creasman WR, Rutledge FN, Fletcher GH. Carcinoma of the cervix associated with pregnancy. *Obstet Gynecol.* 1970;36:495.
48. Waldrop GM, Palmer JP. Carcinoma of the cervix associated with pregnancy. *Am J Obstet Gynecol.* 1963;86:202.
49. Sablinska R, Tarlowska L, Stelmachow J. Invasive carcinoma of the cervix associated with pregnancy: correlation between patient age, advancement of cancer and gestation, and result of treatment. *Gynecol Oncol.* 1977;5:363.

Chapter One Hundred and Eighty-Seven

Cancer of the Vulva and Vagina

John L. Currie and Ira R. Horowitz

187

Carcinoma of the vulva and vagina account for less than 5% of all gynecologic malignancies, with the disease most prevalent in postmenopausal women. Although rare in the parturient age group, preinvasive and invasive neoplasia of the vulva and vagina may occur during pregnancy. An increased incidence of preinvasive intraepithelial neoplasia in this age group secondary to the human papillomavirus has been noted recently.[1-3] Health care providers of pregnant women should be particularly cognizant of these four points:

1. The relative immunosuppression during pregnancy may indicate different manifestations of the human papillomavirus, including condyloma acuminatum, intraepithelial neoplasia, and invasive disease.
2. A pregnancy-associated delay in diagnosis can decrease survival markedly.
3. The childbearing years of women exposed *in utero* to diethylstilbestrol (DES) will continue for two decades. These patients are probably at an increased risk for intraepithelial neoplasia of vagina and cervix and for clear cell carcinoma of the vagina.[4,5]
4. The occurrence of malignant melanoma presents special difficulties for clinicians dealing with cancer of the vulva and vagina, which may be magnified by its occurrence during pregnancy.

CANCER OF THE VULVA

Cancer of the vulva usually develops from squamous epithelium covering the labia, perineum, and clitoral hood. Bartholin's gland carcinoma or apocrine gland adenocarcinomas are infrequent. Melanoma may occur at any location but accounts for less than 10% of vulvar cancers. Cancer of the vulva is the fourth most common gynecologic malignancy, representing about 4% of all such neoplasia.[6] The peak incidence is in the sixth and seventh decades; less than 5% occur before age 40.[7]

Thus, the potential for developing vulva cancer in pregnancy is very low, as less than 5% of patients with vulvar cancer will be pregnant.[7] It can be postulated that less than 100 cases can be expected each year in the United States. Similarly, since the estimated incidence is only 1 in every 8000 pregnancies[8], even busy obstetric groups can expect to see only one such malignancy every 15–20 years.

Staging is accomplished utilizing the TNM Classification (Table 187–1) approved by the International Federation of Gynecology and Obstetrics (FIGO) in October 1988.[9] In the new staging system, inguinal nodes must be evaluated as part of the staging protocol. Previously, FIGO staging for vulva carcinoma was clinical (Table 187–2).

Intraepithelial neoplasia of the vulva (VIN) previously was termed vulvar dysplasia, hyperplastic dystrophy with atypia, and vulvar epithelial atypia. The Ninth Congress of the International Society for the Study of Vulvar Disease (ISSVD) in 1987[10] also reclassified Bowen's disease, erythroplasia of Queyrat, carcinoma simplex and carcinoma in-situ as VIN-III.

Intraepithelial neoplasia of the vulva has become more common in young females, and thus may present during pregnancy. Such lesions may be pigmented or unpigmented, and are frequently multifocal. Although not truly cancerous, recognition of their increased prevalence in young women, and thus in those of childbearing age, may circumvent a future invasive cancer. As in the nonpregnant patient, VIN is associated with another neoplasm in at least 25% of cases.[11] Its appearance during pregnancy mandates not only treatment of the local lesions, but also a search for neoplasm elsewhere. Approximately one half arise in the cervix with the remainder in the vagina, anus, and endometrium.

Etiology

The human papillomavirus (HPV) has been implicated in the etiology of intraepithelial disease of the vulva as well as in verrucoid carcinoma of the vulva. Recent studies also have identified HPV genomes in invasive vulvar carcinomas.[3,12] Intraepithelial disease occurs more commonly in the immunosuppressed individual. The increased clinical manifestation of the human papillomavirus in pregnancy is thought to be secondary to the changes in immune function during gestation.[12]

Squamous cell cancer of the vulva usually begins as a small plaque of firm epithelium and may present as a pruritic ulcer. Progression from intraepithelial disease to microinvasion is presumed although not proven, with progression to deeply invasive disease in untreated patients. A lateral spread of squamous cell cancer of the vulva is often more prominent than deeper invasion, and even bulky invasive lesions may invade the deep stroma for only a few millimeters. Metastasis to the regional lymph nodes occurs early and such spread to the groin lymph nodes can occur even

TABLE 187–1. SURGICAL STAGING OF VULVAR CANCER

Stage	TNM	T Primary Tumor Size
Stage 0	TIS	TIS – Carcinoma *In-Situ*
Stage I	$T_1N_0M_0$	T_1 <2 cm confined to vulva or perineum
Stage II	$T_2N_0M_0$	T_2 >2 cm confined to vulva or perineum
Stage III	$T_3N_0M_0$	T_3 adjacent spread to urethra or vagina or anus
	$T_1N_1M_0$	T_4 infiltrating bladder or rectal mucosa, upper urethra or fixed to bone
	$T_2N_1M_0$	
	$T_3N_1M_0$	
Stage IVA	$T_1N_2M_0$	
	$T_2N_0M_0$	**N Inguinal and Femoral Lymph Nodes**
	$T_3N_2M_0$	N_0 No nodes palpable
	$T_4N_2M_0$	N_1 Unilateral lymph node metastasis
	$T_4N_0M_0$	N_2 Bilateral lymph node metastasis
	$T_4N_1M_0$	
Stage IVB	$T_xN_xM_1$[a]	**M Distant Metastasis**
		M_0 No clinical metastasis
		M_1 Distant metastasis (including pelvic lymph nodes)

[a] x = any T or any N

Adapted from International Federation of Gynecology and Obstetrics (FIGO) data.[9]

TABLE 187–2. CLINICAL STAGING OF VULVAR CANCER

Stage I	Tumor confined to the vulva, 2 cm or less in the larger diameter. Nodes are not palpable or are palpable in either groin, not enlarged, mobile (not clinically suspicious of neoplasm).
Stage II	Tumor confined to the vulva, more than 2 cm in diameter. Nodes are not palpable or are palpable in either groin, not enlarged, mobile (not clinically suspicious of neoplasm).
Stage III	Tumor of any size with (1) adjacent spread to the lower urethra or the vagina, the perineum, and the anus; or (2) nodes palpable in one or both groins, enlarged, firm and mobile, not fixed (but clinically suspicious of neoplasm).
Stage IV	Tumor of any size (1) infiltrating the bladder mucosa, or the rectal mucosa, or both, including the upper part of the urethral mucosa; or (2) fixed to the bone or other distant metastases. Fixed or ulcerated nodes in one or both groins.

Adapted from International Federation of Gynecology and Obstetrics (FIGO).[9]

with microinvasion. Metastasis to deep femoral nodes and deep pelvic nodes usually is thought to be a stepwise progression from superficial nodal disease. Early metastasis can be either ipsilateral or contralateral, and both groins are at risk even in small unilateral invasive disease. Even with perineal, clitoral, or lesions that extend into the vagina, metastasis to the groin is the dominant site of initial spread of disease.

The most common symptom of vulva cancer is pruritus, and a combination of vulvar itching with a small sore is cancer until proven otherwise. Until lesions become very large, they are less apt to produce staining and bleeding, although these are important symptoms.

Benign conditions that can mimic cancer of the vulva include condyloma, cutaneous manifestation of syphilis, Bowen's disease, benign infectious ulcers such as herpes and the various atrophic skin diseases of the vulva.

The definitive diagnostic technique is excisional biopsy. Even during pregnancy, this can be accomplished with minimal discomfort under local anesthesia and can be done in the office. Care should be taken not to interrupt the rich venous plexus of the deep vulva, as these can be quite engorged during pregnancy, resulting in profuse hemorrhage and hematoma formation. Lesions that are obviously deeply invasive do not require excisional biopsy.

Once the diagnosis of invasive vulvar cancer is made, surgery is the treatment of choice. Current trends dictate a conservative procedure for small lesions with minimal invasion. During pregnancy this approach is recommended. Thus, in patients with a lesion of less than 2 cm and an invasion of only 1 mm or less, appropriate wide local excision is usually sufficient treatment. Any patient with a poorly differentiated lesion, vascular or lymphatic space involvement, confluence of invasive tongues of disease, perineal, clitoral, or vaginal involvement should undergo radical excision and bilateral evaluation of at least the superficial groin nodes. During pregnancy, the complete operative procedure can be done in the first or second trimester, although the second trimester is preferable. The surgical procedure is also quite feasible during the third trimester if care is taken in maintaining hemostasis because of the hypervascularity of the vulva and groins.

For more advanced disease, that is, those patients with Stage II, III, or IV disease, radical vulvectomy with bilateral deep groin dissection is the current treatment of choice. This procedure can be accomplished any time during gestation, but the midtrimester is the preferred period. Whether excision of pelvic nodes is attempted depends on the presence or absence of positive groin nodes. In the third trimester, dissection of the pelvic nodes may be difficult because of the bulky uterus. Since metastasis to the pelvic nodes is rare in the absence of groin involvement, primary pelvic node dissection can be postponed until after delivery. Alternatively, the patient can undergo pelvic node irradiation postpartum.

There is no known prevention for cancer of the vulva, but early diagnosis indicates a smaller lesion size and a better prognosis for the patient.

Melanoma of the Vulva

When considering cancer of the vulva in pregnancy, malignant melanoma deserves special notice for two reasons:

1. The incidence of melanoma in general is high during the childbearing years.[13] Although less than 10% of vulvar cancers are melanomas, their incidence during pregnancy can be expected to be relatively high.
2. Because the value of deep regional lymph node dissection may be questionable in deeply invasive melanoma[14], modifications of standard treatment may be necessary in the pregnant patient.

Still, the best recommendation for therapy of melanoma of the vulva in pregnancy is wide local excision with Clark, Breslow, or Chung microstaging determinations of the invasive zone.[14-17] For very superficial invasive lesions (levels I and II) with less than 1 mm of invasion, wide local excision with adequate margins of two times the lesion's size is appropriate treatment.[17,18] Small, lateralizing lesions may be treated with a radical hemi-vulvectomy and *en-bloc* inguinal and femoral lymphadenectomy.[14] For larger and more invasive lesions, radical vulvectomy with *en-bloc* bilateral inguinal femoral lymphadenectomy should be performed. Deep margins in the vagina must be sufficiently radical; this may be more difficult during pregnancy. The value of pelvic node dissection with deeply invasive lesions must be weighed against the technical difficulty of this procedure during gestation and the poor prognosis of patients presenting with positive pelvic lymph nodes.

Three additional points must be addressed regarding melanoma of the vulva in pregnancy. First, though not proven, melanomas are believed to be possibly hormonal-dependent tumors, as documented by the presence of estrogen receptors in almost one half of melanomas.[7,19]

Second, it has long been thought that pregnancy has a deleterious effect on growth and early metastasis of melanoma. Although this remains to be documented, in advanced cases, pregnant patients may have a decreased survival.[13] Other investigators have not observed a decrease in five-year survival of pregnant patients with melanomas.[20] There is also no evidence to suggest that termination of pregnancy will have a therapeutic benefit.

Third, melanoma is one of the few tumors to demonstrate documented fetal and placental metastasis.[21] Whenever melanoma is encountered, this alarming eventuality must be considered.

Except for the rare patient who exhibits metastatic disease in either the placenta or fetus, there should be virtually no harmful fetal effects from diagnosis, treatment, and follow up of cancer of the vulva discovered during pregnancy. A vaginal delivery is very possible, even after a radical vulvectomy has healed. Obstetric indications should dictate the route of delivery.

CANCER OF THE VAGINA

Cancer of the vagina is among the most infrequent tumors of the female genital tract and accounts for less than 1% of all gynecologic malignancies.[22] It is a disease of the older population, and its occurrence in pregnancy is rare. It is estimated that vaginal cancer will occur only once in every 37,000 pregnancies[8] and only 1% or less of patients with cancer of the vagina will be pregnant. Recent reports of cancer of the vagina developing in DES-exposed individuals during pregnancy[4,23-25] may alter the current rarity of this condition.

Other than exposure to DES, there is no known etiology of cancer of the vagina. Some investigators have proposed *vaginal intraepithelial neoplasia* (VAIN) as a precursor to vaginal carcinoma.[26] Patients who have concurrent cervical and vaginal cancer are always assumed to have a primary cervical lesion. Approximately 20–30% of patients presenting with a primary vaginal carcinoma have been treated previously for cervical intraepithelial neoplasia or cervical carcinoma.[27-29] Some 85% of primary vaginal carcinomas are of the squamous cell variety, 8% are adenocarcinoma, and the remainder are sarcomas, melanomas, small cell cancers, lymphomas, and undifferentiated tumors.[30]

The most common symptom of vaginal cancer is abnormal vaginal bleeding. Occasionally, patients will have a foul, watery discharge. Since vaginal cancer is relatively slow-growing, careful inspection and digital examination at the time of the first prenatal visit should preclude development of an invasive cancer of the vagina during pregnancy. Diagnosis is established when a suspicious cytologic smear, visual inspection of a lesion, or palpation of a nodule on bimanual examination mandates biopsy. Staging of vaginal cancer is by clinical examination (Table 187–3).

In the nonpregnant patient, the treatment of choice for vaginal cancer usually is radiation therapy.[31,32] For an early upper vaginal lesion, or a very small clear cell adenocarcinoma, radical hysterectomy and upper vaginectomy with pelvic lymphadenectomy might be the treatment of choice. External beam radiation therapy, brachytherapy, and interstitial radiation therapy can be used, combined or singularly, depending on the stage and extent of disease and pending anatomic considerations.

TABLE 187–3. CLINICAL STAGING OF VAGINAL CANCER

Stage 0	Carcinoma *in situ;* intraepithelial carcinoma
Stage I	The carcinoma is limited to the vaginal walls.
Stage II	The carcinoma has involved the subvaginal tissue but has not extended to the pelvic wall.
Stage III	The carcinoma has extended to the pelvic wall.
Stage IV	The carcinoma has extended beyond the true pelvis or has involved the mucosa of the bladder or rectum. Bullous edema, as such, does not permit a case to be allotted to Stage IV.
Stage IVA	Spread of the growth to adjacent organs
Stage IVB	Spread to distant organs

Adapted from International Federation of Gynecology and Obstetrics.[9]

In pregnancy, treatment must be adjusted to the extent of the disease and the needs of gestation. With interstitial therapy, the radiation dosage to the fetus must be controlled. Great care must be exercised in choosing radiation therapy for the patient who decides to maintain her pregnancy.[23] Because of the rarity of this lesion, definitive guidelines have not been established for treatment during pregnancy. Treatment should be provided by a gynecologic oncologist with perinatology consultation.

For very early disease, wide local excision can be accomplished during pregnancy, with adjunctive radiation therapy used after delivery. In a patient with a small lesion at the apex of the vagina whose pregnancy has progressed to fetal maturity, cesarean delivery, radical hysterectomy and upper vaginectomy with pelvic lymphadenectomy might be the treatment of choice.

DES Exposure

There are now over 503 patients with clear cell carcinoma of the vagina and cervix in the Registry for Research on Hormonal Transplacental Carcinogenesis.[14] Two thirds of these patients have a documented history of exposure to nonsteroidal estrogen during gestation. Twenty-four patients were pregnant at the time of diagnosis; each treatment was individualized to location of lesion, stage of disease, gestational age, and the desire for future fertility. Surgical excision, radical hysterectomy and vaginectomy, primary radiation or a combination of the former modalities were used. The actuarial 5- and 10-year survival rates (87%, 68%) for patients who presented during pregnancy were not significantly different from those who were never pregnant. DES-exposed patients as a group exhibit infertility problems.[33] Those who conceive, however, should be carefully screened for abnormalities early in pregnancy. The investigation should include Pap smears, screening colposcopy, and inspection and palpation of the vagina.

The chief risk to the fetus from vaginal cancer is side effects from treatment. There are no known instances of metastasis of vaginal cancer to either fetus or placenta.

Rarely, a neglected patient is encountered with deeply invasive local disease of the vulva extending into the vagina. Extensive and well-planned ultra-radical surgery, often in combination with radiation and chemotherapy, is the only hope for cure of a patient in this advanced stage of disease.

REFERENCES

1. Kaufman RH, Bornstein J, Adam E, et al. Human papilloma virus and herpes simplex virus in vulvar squamous cell carcinoma in-situ. *Am J Obstet Gynecol.* 1988;158(4):862.
2. Dinh TV, Powell LC Jr, Hannigan EV, et al. Simultaneously occurring condyloma acuminata, carcinoma in-situ and verrucous carcinoma of the vulva and carcinoma in-situ of the cervix in a young woman: a case report. *J Reprod Med.* 1988;33:510.
3. Sugase M, Moriyama S, Hata S, Matsukura IT. Detection of human papilloma virus type 16 DNA and papilloma virus genus-specific antigens in vulva and cervix from patients with bowenoid papulosis. *Jpn J Cancer Res.* 1988;80:19.
4. Senekjian EK, Hubby M, Bell DA, et al. Clear cell adenocarcinoma (CCA) of the vagina and cervix in association with pregnancy. *Gynecol Oncol.* 1986;24:207.
5. Bornstein J, Adam E, Adler-Storthz K, Kaufman RH. Development of cervical and vaginal squamous cell neoplasia as a late consequence of in utero exposure to diethylstilbestrol. *Obstet Gynecol Sur.* 1988;43(1):15.
6. DiSaia PJ, Creasman WT, Rich WM. An alternative approach to early cancer of the vulva. *Am J Obstet Gynecol.* 1979;133:825.
7. Orr JW, Shingleton HM. Cancer in pregnancy. *Current Probl Cancer.* 1983;8:1.

8. Lutz MH, Underwood PB, Rozier JC, Putney FW. Genital malignancy in pregnancy. *Am J Obstet Gynecol.* 1977;192:536.
9. FIGO News. Annual report on the results of treatment in gynecologic cancer. *Int J Gynecol Obstet.* 1989;28:189.
10. Ridley CM, Frankman O, Jones ISC, et al. New nomenclature for vulvar disease: International Society for the Study of Vulvar Disease. *Human Path.* 1989;20(5):495.
11. Coppleson M. *Gynecologic Oncology: Fundamentals, Principles and Clinical Practice. Vol I.* Edinburgh: Churchill Livingstone. 1981.
12. Powell LC. Condyloma acuminata. *Clin Obstet Gynecol.* 1972;15:948.
13. Shiu MH, Schoffenfeld D, MacLean B, Fortner JG. Adverse effect of pregnancy on melanoma: a reappraisal. *Cancer.* 1976;37:181.
14. Podratz KC, Gaffey TA, Symmonds RE, et al. Melanoma of the vulva: an update. *Gynecol Oncol.* 1983;16:153.
15. Clark WH, From L, Bernardino EA, Mihm MC. The histogenesis and biologic behavior of primary human malignant melanomas of the skin. *Cancer Res.* 1969;29:705.
16. Breslow A. Thickness, cross-sectional area and depth of invasion in the prognosis of cutaneous melanoma. *Ann Surg.* 1970;172:902.
17. Chung AF, Woodruff JW, Lewis JL Jr. Malignant melanoma of the vulva: a report of 44 cases. *Obstet Gynecol.* 1975;45:638.
18. Phillips GL, Twigg LB, Okagaki T. Vulvar melanoma: a microstaging study. *Gynecol Oncol.* 1982;14:80.
19. Schwartz BK, Zashin SJ, Spencer SK, et al. Pregnancy and hormonal influences on malignant melanoma. *J Dermatol Surg Onc.* 1987;13(3):276.
20. Shaw JHF. Malignant melanoma in Auckland, New Zealand. *Surg Gynecol Obstet.* 1988;1:66:425.
21. Donegan WL. Cancer and pregnancy. *CA—A Ca J Clin.* 1983;33:4:194.
22. Dunn LJ, Napier JG. Primary carcinoma of the vagina. *Am J Obstet Gynecol.* 1966;96:1112.
23. Castillo HC, Rubio RA, Farrell EM: Vaginal adenocarcinoma in a gravida with prenatal DES exposure. *Int J Gynecol Obstet.* 1979;16:271.
24. Davis JA, Wadehra V, McIntosh AS, Monaghan JM. A case of clear cell adenocarcinoma of the vagina in pregnancy. *Br J Obstet Gynecol.* 1981;88:322.
25. Jones WB, Woodruff JM, Errlandson RA, Lewis JL: DES-related clear cell adenocarcinoma of the vagina in pregnancy. *Obstet Gynecol.* 1981;57:76S.
26. Lenehan PM, Meffe F, Lickrish GM. Vaginal intraepithelial neoplasia: biologic aspects and management. *Obstet Gynecol.* 1986;68:333.
27. Rubin SC, Young J, Mikuta JJ. Squamous carcinoma of the vagina: treatment complications, and long-term follow up. *Gynecol Oncol.* 1985; 20:346.
28. Benedet JL, Murphy KJ, Fairey RN, et al. Primary invasive carcinoma of the vagina. *Obstet Gynecol.* 1983;62:715.
29. Peters WA III, Kumar NB, Morley GW. Carcinoma of the vagina. *Cancer.* 1985;5:892.
30. Berek JS, Hacker NF, eds. *Vaginal Cancer: Practical Gynecologic Oncology.* Baltimore, MD: Williams and Wilkins, 1989.
31. Perez CA, Arneson AN, Dehner LP, et al. Radiation therapy in carcinoma of the vagina. *Obstet Gynecol.* 1974;44:862.
32. Kucera H, Larger M, Smekal G, et al. Radiotherapy of primary carcinoma of the vagina: management and results of different therapy schemes. *Gynecol Oncol.* 1985;21:87.
33. Herbst AL. Clear cell adenocarcinoma and the current status of DES-exposed females. *Cancer.* 1981;48(2):484.

PART XVII | Diseases of the Breast

Stanley A. Gall, Section Editor

Chapter One Hundred and Eighty-Eight

Breast Diseases

Bruce H. Drukker and Harold J. Sauer

188

Breast function in females is defined by the role of numerous hormones during prepubertal development, during cyclic menses, and during pregnancy. From the earliest appearance of specialized ectoderm through the initiation and regression of lactation, a necessary sequence of differentiation occurs.

The breast undergoes dramatic normal physiologic change during pregnancy in response to the altered hormonal relationships accompanying each gestation. Many of the conditions that occur in the nongestational breast also can occur during gestation. Therefore, knowledge of normal development and gestational change of the breast is critical to understanding disease processes that can occur during that period.

DEVELOPMENT OF THE BREAST

Mammary ducts and alveoli have been shown to be hormonally responsive from early in fetal development. These ectodermally derived tissues in fetal rats respond to culture with insulin, aldosterone, and prolactin by duct system development and formation of intracellular organelles. In the presence of adrenal corticosteroid, insulin, and prolactin, mammary alveolar tissue from adult female mice, rats, and rabbits can be induced to grow, differentiate, and secrete milk in organ culture.

In the newborn female, mammary structures are primitive, but on occasion a small amount of discharge from the nipples ("witch's milk") may be noted and may persist for several weeks after birth. Development is reinitiated with the onset of puberty. Prior to menarche, lengthening and branching of ducts are initiated under the influence of increased circulating estrogen levels, accompanied by increased production of supporting connective tissue and fat.

A summary of organ culture results suggests that insulin and an adrenal corticosteroid would be necessary for maximal growth and division of alveolar epithelial cells, but these hormones are not lactogenic. Gonadal steroids stimulate selective duct and lobular growth in explants, but they are not lactogenic *in vitro*. Lactogenesis *in vitro* appears to be dependent on the presence of prolactin, or perhaps also human placental lactogen or human growth hormone[1], which show structural similarity to and some functional overlap with prolactin.

The necessity of prolactin *in vivo* is shown by the inability of women with placental sulfatase deficiency in pregnancy (thus with lower total estrogen and prolactin levels) to establish lactogenesis postpartum.[2]

During pregnancy, changes occur in breast size, nipple-areolar complex, and the ductal alveolar system. These changes are preceded by initial sensations of increased breast weight and tingling, usually noted 3–4 weeks following the last menstrual period. Within the next four weeks, the breasts rapidly enlarge secondary to vascular engorgement, often highlighted by prominent veins noted on the breast surface. Although growth continues during pregnancy, subsequent enlargement is attributed to ductal and alveolar proliferation. Estrogen has a direct effect on mammary cells at this point, and it also stimulates prolactin synthesis and release from lactotrophs in the anterior pituitary. This prolactin increase is postulated to be a necessary precursor for estrogen effect on the breast. The effects of insulin, human placental lactogen, and growth hormone during pregnancy are unclear.

Epithelial cells typically show evidence of secretory vacuoles by the third trimester, with the appearance of colostrum-like material in the ducts. The breast remains a presecretory organ until a sudden fall in circulating estrogen and progesterone concentrations occurs subsequent to delivery. With the loss of the inhibitory effect of these hormones, the stimulatory effect of prolactin on the mammary epithelium becomes predominant. The breast thus becomes a secretory tissue.

Interestingly, there is minimal deposition of additional breast fatty tissue during pregnancy. In general, the normal breast size is 200–300 cm^3 and increases approximately 200–400 cm^3 during pregnancy with occasional enlargement to 800 cm.[3] Thus, the size of the breast during pregnancy can vary from 400 to 1000 cm.[3] In addition to the venous changes and secretory changes, striae frequently occur in the skin accompanying this growth. Nipple change accompanies stroma, vascular, and alveolar ductal changes of the main portion of the breast. The nipple becomes more prominent, erect, and enlarged. In addition, striking enlargement and increased pigmentation occurs in the areola. The areola may increase in size by almost 2 cm from the nonpregnancy size. It is not unusual for the areola to approximate 5 cm during pregnancy. The Montgomery gland apparatus (probably a modified sebaceous system), including the follicle and tubercle, enlarges and achieves prominence at the periphery of the nipple areolar complex. The small secretions coming from this modified sebaceous system may help to maintain the areola to remain soft and pliable during pregnancy.

POSTPARTUM BREAST AND HORMONAL CHANGES

After the breast is primed by insulin and cortisol, prolactin alone can stimulate the synthesis of milk proteins such as casein and α-lactalbumin. Binding of prolactin to its cell-surface receptor is essential for the subsequent induction of milk protein synthesis, but this does not appear to activate adenylate cyclase. Interestingly, some of the effects of prolactin, including RNA synthesis, are mediated by prostaglandins.[3]

There is also a rapid fall in puerperal prolactin levels. Normal prepregnancy levels are found approximately six weeks postpartum in both lactating and nonlactating women. Maternal serum prolactin levels undergo fivefold to tenfold elevation with each suckling episode within the first seven or so weeks postpartum. High levels of prolactin appear to be necessary for the initiation of lactation, but once breast enzyme systems are activated, lactation can continue with mean prolactin levels that are normal or only modestly elevated.[4]

BREAST CONDITIONS ASSOCIATED WITH PREGNANCY

Hypertrophy

This very unusual condition consists essentially of massive enlargement of the breasts, often approaching 4000–5000 g. Enlargement of this type is more common in second or subsequent pregnancies, usually beginning, as expected, shortly after the onset of pregnancy. Although treatment in some extreme conditions has included mastectomy, a more conservative approach is desirable. The breasts should be well supported during the pregnancy, lactation should be discouraged, and the breasts elevated after postpartum resolution of engorgement. If persistent hypertrophy is present, reduction mammoplasty is feasible.[5,6]

Infection

Although mastitis can occur in both the pregnant and nonpregnant woman, it is more common during pregnancy, particularly the postpartum period. It occurs in 1–2% of pregnancies. Mastitis can be characterized as epidemic and nonepidemic, the former more frequent than the latter. The epidemic variant is a nosocomial infection acquired by the mother from the nasopharnyx of the nursing infant, which has been colonized by a virulent form of bacteria, usually *Staphylococcus aureus* originating in a hospital situation. Minute cracks occur in the nipple surface, permitting entry of the organism into the subnipple areolar structure, penetrating deeply and invading the glandular breast tissue. It can pass through Cooper's suspensory ligaments, creating deep abscesses within the parenchyma of the breast in this situation. Other abscesses can be subcutaneous or subareolar. The latter often will develop into a repetitive, chronic, small pustular mass occurring just at the margin of the areola. Epidemic mastitis commonly begins during the first week after birth. A febrile response plus erythema and tenderness is common. Cultures from the nipple surface or milk or purulent material from the nipple often will corroborate clinical suspicion. Treatment for mastitis includes intense antibiotics for 7–10 days, choosing a medication effective against *S aureus*. If infection persists, consolidates, and has persistent erythema or tenderness and appears to be unresponsive to the course of antibiotics, it is not desirable to wait 7–10 days hoping that the antibiotic will resolve the problem. Instead, incision and drainage are mandatory. The frequency of epidemic mastitis can be reduced by careful attention to meticulous handwashing and cleansing by nursing personnel and the mother as well as taking precautions to prevent nipple cracking. Nonepidemic mastitis usually occurs during weaning or during episodes of sporadic suckling. This condition generally is associated with milk stasis in the ductal system, particularly the dilated portions of the system below the areola. In this type of mastitis, organisms include both anaerobic and aerobic bacteria, but again, *S aureus* is isolated most frequently, approximately 50% of the time.

Initially, patients manifest systemic signs of infection with fever, tachycardia, and generally "not feeling well." Within a few days, a breast abscess usually becomes apparent. Since this tends to be a periglandular infection, culture of milk may not be helpful. Interestingly, too, toxic shock syndrome has been reported, and the causative agent was *S aureus*.[7] Once the diagnosis is suspected, prompt institution of treatment with antibiotics is mandatory. Again, an agent that eradicates *S aureus* is a prime drug choice. If penicillin-resistant *S aureus* is suspected, an appropriate antibiotic should be instituted. Apparently, nursing does not affect this condition or the infant adversely. The infant may continue breast-feeding or breast pumping may be used and it is thought its decompressing action may produce a salutary benefit, hastening recovery.

On occasion, however, a breast abscess will form with classic symptoms of a firm, exquisite, painful, often erythematous mass. Incision and drainage is mandatory. The operation is performed through a radial incision using, most often, general anesthesia. The radial incision theoretically prevents extensive damage to the proximal ducts adjacent to the areola that would be interrupted if a periareolar circumferential incision was used. Although local anesthesia is possible, a general anesthetic permits adequate exposure and the destruction of multiple abscess loculations. Again, cultures should be obtained for aerobic and anaerobic organisms at the time of incision and drainage. Often, these abscesses can be substantially larger than expected based on pure physical signs. In addition to culture, a biopsy should be obtained of the abscess wall. Since up to 15% of breast cancers in women occur in women under age 40 during pregnancy or the lactational period, this tissue sampling is critical.

Galactocele

This condition can occur proximate to pregnancy and lactation. If the glandular epithelium of the ductal system has been secreting and a condition develops that obstructs the ducts and normal efflux of secretions, a galactocele may form. Most often, this condition follows cessation of nursing with collection of inspisated thick, milklike material within the duct, forming a large dilated area distal to the obstruction. The diagnosis can be confirmed by needle aspiration, which yields a thick, creamy-type of breast secretion. If the mass does not recur following aspiration, treatment is complete. However, if there is recurrence of the mass, total excision is required.[8] On occasion, ultrasonography of the breast is helpful in clarifying this diagnosis. The ultrasound often will demonstrate a cystic mass with a somewhat irregular internal lining and with internal echos that are relatively dense but homogeneous. Mammography itself is not significantly helpful in delineating the nature of such a mass.

Adenomas

These are the third most common lesions found in the breast and are exceeded by fibrocystic change or disease and breast carcinoma. Although they occur more often in the nonpregnant state, they also can occur during gestation. Adenomas can be pure glandular tissue or, when located in the nipple structure, can be admixed with some fibrous tissue. All originate in the lobular area with the exception of the nipple adenoma. Of the pure adenomas only, the so-called lactating adenoma occurs during pregnancy. These are mainly epithelial structures and contain only a very small amount of supporting stroma. The epithelium is composed of exuberantly proliferative acinar tubular structures that are lined by cells with a clear vacuolated cytoplasm. Approximately 40% of all pure adenomas are of this lactating type.

Fibroadenomas are by far the most common adenoma found, being almost 35 times more frequent than the so-called pure adenomas. They are most common from the ages of 15–30, and during pregnancy they have been noted to enlarge most probably in response to estrogen stimulation. They may increase 1–2 times their prepregnancy size. Although very rare, spontaneous infarction of these adenomas has been reported. In these situations the lesions were noted to be well encapsulated, with the central portion demonstrating a coagulative-type necrosis. At the peripheral area of the lesion, fibrosis and granulation tissue can be present with partially necrotic breast tissue and aggregates of hemosiderin-containing macrophages. These very localized type infarctions in fibroadenomas generally are associated only with pregnancy and lactation. The cause of this lesion has been elusive. Search for thromboembolic or an inflammatory process has not been successful. On the other hand, since these are often associated with pregnancy, it is felt that a relative vascular deficiency may result from the increasing metabolic demands of the breast with ensuing infarction of the hyperplastic tissue.[9]

Fibrocystic Change

Fibrocystic change is the most common benign condition of the female breast. Its increase is coincident with the reproductive period with increasing macrocyst formation until the time of menopause, at which time fibrocystic change is seen in approximately 50% of women. Thereafter, the condition becomes much less prominent. Fibrocystic change has three major pathologic variants including cystic change, ductal hyperplasia, and fibrosis. Cystic change is characterized by alterations in lobular, lobe, or subareolar areas. Microcysts are noted to be common and are seen in up to 65% of patients with gross cystic disease. These small lesions, less than 1 mm, are not palpable and are asymptomatic. Characteristically, they are lined by a single layer of epithelium. This change is thought to be a normal phenomenon in many women. As ductal dilatations become larger, specifically greater than 3 mm, they have been characterized as macrocysts or gross cystic disease. Macrocysts have been noted in 20–40% of patients who have had microcystic change and are usually considered to be a progression of the microcystic change. With fibrocystic change, bilaterality is common and macrocystic change becomes more prominent in the late menstrual years.

Duct ectasia refers to enlargement of the duct, particularly dilations, occurring in the terminal collecting ducts below the nipple and areola. This, too, is particularly more common in perimenopausal and postmenopausal women and has been noted in approximately 25% of all tissue specimens studied in that age group. In general, it is characterized by distention of the terminal and subareolar ducts, with, on occasion, accumulation of amorphous material. Inflammatory change can occur, producing small microscopic abscess areas. Reactive fibrosis in adjacent breast tissue also can occur secondary to this inflammatory response. Although it is feasible to have a problem with duct ectasia during pregnancy, it is not a common occurrence.

Ductal epithelial hyperplasia can occur within breast ducts during pregnancy. The epithelium, which is usually cuboidal or cylindrical, may undergo an apocrine metaplastic transformation, demonstrating cells that are cylindrical with large, basal, uniform, small, round nuclei. The cytoplasm has an acidophilic coloration and often is found to be extruding from the luminal surface of the cell.

Papillomatosis also can occur and is a nonpalpable entity that is very difficult to detect in the pregnant person. Generally, it does not characterize a specific entity and most patients are without symptoms. Benign proliferation of the superficial ductal epithelial cells can occur, partially filling small and medium mammary ducts. The cells have a uniform size and are without nuclear or cytoplasmic stigmata of malignancy. Occasionally, some degeneration of the proliferating cell mass can occur with concomitant presence of histiocytes in the body of the mass. On occasion, as with adenosis, fibrosis can occur in the central group of ducts, causing separation and compression.

As opposed to general papillomatosis, at times single stalk papilloma may be associated with clinical symptoms such as bleeding from the nipple or a palpable mass. Although these lesions occur in the late menstrual years and in the postmenopausal years, they can occur during pregnancy, producing a bloody or serosanguineous discharge. On occasion, a palpable mass is noted just below or at the periphery of the areola. Multiple intraductal papillomas can be bilateral; in this situation most are located peripherally rather than centrally. These also can appear as a palpable mass with a bloody nipple discharge. Obviously, again, because of the engorgement of the breast tissue associated with pregnancy, these lesions are exceedingly difficult to detect. Fortunately, they do not occur often.

Fibrosis is a unique, singular entity but is more common in the menstrual rather than postmenstrual period. Occasionally, an area will develop that is flat, firm, buttonlike, and slightly irregular, increasing in size to approximately 1–3 cm. These changes occur in the breast parenchyma and appear to be a definitive response in lobular or surrounding acinar areas to a chronic inflammatory problem, usually of ductal origin. Fibrotic change also is difficult to detect and uncommon during pregnancy.

The age period during which fibrocystic change is most prominent, (ages 25–45), with its accompanying physical characteristics, can create a diagnostic problem. However, fibrocystic change tends to moderate during pregnancy.

Nodularity associated with fibrocystic change most often is bilateral and exists in the upper outer quadrants of both breasts. Cystic lesions can be smooth or irregular. They tend to be firm but often have a compressible characteristic. Aspiration is a simple, useful diagnostic tool. It can and should be used in pregnancy before other diagnostic studies are done. Cysts should be aspirated, and the fluid may be examined by cytologic methods. Malignant cells rarely are encountered if the fluid is not bloody or blood tinged; even when it is sanguineous, the frequency of malignancy on cytologic evaluation is very low.[10] On the other hand, Abramson[11] has noted that cyst fluid can contain malignant cells and be absolutely devoid of sanguineous characteristics. If following cystic aspiration, the mass does not recur and cytologic evaluation is negative, the problem should be observed further until after parturition. However, should the mass recur after a second aspiration, further assessment is necessary, generally excisional biopsy.

Needle biopsy of masses also can be done, and if a biopsy shows fibrocystic change, I believe it can be observed and treated expectantly for the duration of the pregnancy. Unfortunately, there is occasional coexistence of fibrocystic disease and carcinoma in the same breast. Therefore, when a definitive nodule is present and it does not satisfy the criteria of fibrocystic change, prompt definitive diagnosis is mandatory, generally by core needle biopsy or more often excisional biopsy.

DIAGNOSTIC PROCEDURES DURING PREGNANCY

1. Physical examination
2. Needle aspiration
3. Needle core biopsy
4. Mammography
5. Ultrasonography
6. Excisional biopsy

Physical examination requires a very high level of sensitivity and experience to delineate small breast lesions. However, the physical changes of breast engorgement accompanying pregnancy compound the difficulty of examination for even the most experienced examiners. Patients should be examined in the sitting position with and without pectoral muscle accentuation. The breasts should be carefully observed as the patient raises her hands over her head. Dimpling, puckering, or asymmetry may appear. Palpation can be accomplished by careful, gentle compression of the breast in a circumferential fashion or by moving back and forth from the lateral to the medial areas and vice versa until the entire breast has been palpated. I have found tactile sensitivity to be enhanced by placing a very smooth linen or cotton cloth over the breast and carefully drawing the volar aspect of the thumb and second, third and fourth fingers of the dominant hand over the breast. Subtle changes can be detected and areas of concern can be re-examined by direct palpation. This entire procedure can be repeated with the patient in the sitting and sitting forward position with the arms supported. In this latter position the breast is away from the chest wall and examination is useful for determining an area of thickening that may have been confused by the firmness of the chest wall. In the nonpregnant state, our tactile sensitivity is such that even the experienced examiner cannot detect lesions uniformly less than 1 cm more than 80% of the time. When lesions are less than 0.5 cm, we are unable to palpate with accuracy over two thirds of the time. Pregnancy compounds this problem of tactile sensitivity. For these reasons, physical examination in pregnancy, although useful, must be recognized as having limitations.

Needle aspiration to obtain fluid for sampling or cells for cytologic evaluation is an extremely useful tool in the pregnant patient. It is inexpensive when compared to ultrasound and has no radiation exposure when compared to mammography. However, to be used at all it requires a palpable mass. If a mass is noted, fluid aspiration or cell aspiration can be accomplished simply by cleansing the area of skin over the mass and then following immobilization with the fingers, inserting a 22-gauge needle with a 10 cm^3 syringe into the mass. If fluid is obtained, it should be sent for cytologic evaluation. If a solid mass is noted, tissue fluid can be drawn into the needle bore when three or four passes are made in the solid mass. Tissue fluid then can be expressed on a glass slide, spread, and fixed in appropriate fashion for cytologic examination. It is extremely important to talk with a pathologist prior to preparing slides for cytologic evaluation. This will assure that the slides are prepared in the way he or she wishes and will provide optimal opportunity for accurate cytologic assessment.

The sophistication of medical ultrasonography capabilities makes this a very useful tool for evaluation of palpable breast lesions in pregnant patients. A high resolution handheld unit, static or real-time, will clearly delineate a solid from a cystic mass. Obviously, however, the transducer strength must be sufficient to penetrate the tissue but also provide good resolution. Generally, a 5-MHz or 7.5-MHz unit is used. The ultrasound interpreter, however, must be aware of the nonhomogeneous characteristics of the pregnant breast, the fatty tissue, and dense glandular tissue; even Cooper's ligaments create interfaces that challenge the image interpreter's ability. However, there is presently no known adverse effect of ultrasound evaluation of breast tissue, and there is no concern for radiation.

Mammographic techniques have improved dramatically since the 1960s when Egan reported on a technique of high milliamperage-low kilovoltage that resulted in dependable diagnostic images of the breast.[12] The present film screen techniques have a high degree of sensitivity for detecting early breast cancer and are used appropriately for screening. However, even though the amount of radiation used is low, generally less than 1 mGy per exposure, there is concern for the unborn infant. Also, the ultimate carcinogenic effects of these low levels of radiation for young, pregnant women is not known. However, if there is a risk, it will be greater for women under age 30.[13] For these reasons, mammography should be avoided if possible during pregnancy. Obviously, it should not be used for screening during this period, and only with highest levels of discretion should it be used as a diagnostic modality during pregnancy.

Needle core biopsy is a very useful tool that can be used in pregnancy if there is a solid, identifiable lesion and if cell aspiration was not helpful in achieving a diagnosis. In these situations, the target mass should be at least 2 cm and securable by the fingers to provide an immovable target. Here, rather than needle aspiration, local anesthesia must be used. If a diagnosis of carcinoma is obtained, treatment must be administered. If, however, the mass is benign, further evaluation needs to be tempered by the duration of gestation and the probability of cancer. In this situation other factors such as age, family history, and perhaps ultrasonographic characteristics of the mass should be considered. If, however, doubt regarding a persistent cancer exists, biopsy is mandatory.

Excisional biopsy is the ultimate and final diagnostic tool. If necessary, it can be accomplished without difficulty in pregnancy. The technique is similar to that used in the nonpregnant patient. Meticulous care regarding hemostasis is absolutely necessary, and the incision should be done to produce the best cosmetic result. If a patient is lactating, it is better to terminate lactation before biopsy if possible.

BREAST CANCER IN PREGNANCY

Breast cancer in pregnancy continues to be controversial. The pendulum regarding eventual outcome continues to swing. Presently, it suggests more frequently that breast cancer in pregnancy does not of and in itself cause a poor outcome with increasing morbidity and mortality.

Although the frequency of carcinoma of the breast in pregnancy is relatively small, it is of concern. In general, invasive ductal carcinoma is diagnosed with a frequency varying from 0.75% to 3.1% of women who at the time of breast cancer diagnosis were pregnant, recently pregnant, or recently pregnant and lactating.[14,15] If one looks specifically at women under 40, the coincidence of breast cancer and pregnancy is higher. Horsley[16] reports that 10% of 67 patients who were less than 35 were pregnant at the time of breast cancer diagnosis. A similar report 27 years later by Nugent and O'Connell[17] indicated that 11% of patients age 25–40 had concurrent pregnancy and breast cancer. These figures mandate vigilance for breast cancer in all pregnant patients.

As might be expected, the physiologic breast changes of pregnancy such as engorgement, increased vascularity, ductal and alveolar hypertrophy plus fluid retention prevent the diagnosis of an early breast cancer. Delay in diagnosis is prevented further by the patient's difficulty in interpreting symptoms that might suggest breast cancer as compared to normal breast changes of pregnancy. Unfortunately, there also is failure of physicians, midwives, and nurse practitioners to consider breast examination as a reasonable part of prenatal care except at the time of the first prenatal visit. To believe that breast cancer just "couldn't happen" in this patient is inappropriate. It could, and in a small number of patients it will. Finding a lump in the breast requires evaluation using diagnostic modalities compatible with pregnancy. Observation or watching a lump occurring in pregnancy is inappropriate. Diagnosis is mandatory. Aspiration, particularly fine-needle aspiration, or core-needle biopsy are particularly useful diagnostic tools. If carcinoma is found, in general it will be invasive ductal carcinoma, also the most common diagnostic entity in nonpregnant patients. At one time there was a suggestion that inflammatory carcinoma with its aggressive pattern in both pregnant and nonpregnant patients was more common in pregnancy. Most reports suggest the incidence to be 1.8–4.3% compared to the 1.5–4.0% in nonpregnant patients. A contrary report by King[18], however, reports an unusually high incidence of 13%.

Tumor estrogen receptor status during pregnancy is negative in approximately 70% of patients, and progesterone receptor status has been reported negative in all pregnant patients reported by Holdaway[19], who also suggests a higher estrogen receptor status positivity in lactating patients when compared with pregnant patients.

Basic treatment for carcinoma of the breast in pregnancy is no longer controversial. Treatment must be prompt and definitive. Delay fosters metastatic disease with increased morbidity and mortality. There is no reason to delay initial surgical intervention. For at least 20 years, modified radical mastectomy with axillary dissection has been an acceptable definitive standard for both pregnant and nonpregnant patients. In nonpregnant patients, the alternative treatment for Stage I and selected Stage II breast carcinoma patients is segmental mastectomy, axillary sampling (dissection), and postoperative radiation to the breast. This procedure has results comparable to modified radical mastectomy and axillary dissection. However, in the pregnant patient it has not gained sufficient favor to provide adequate studies that would recommend it as an equivalent alternative.

In general, the results of treatment are good if there is no evidence of nodal disease at the time of modified radical mastectomy and axillary dissection. These results are thought to be comparable, as stated previously, to the nonpregnant patient and as recently reported by King et al.[18] This concept has been supported by reports of Green[20], who has noted an 87.5% survival as well as by Nugent[17] who evaluated 176 patients and felt that pregnancy did not seem to have a direct effect on the prognosis of breast cancer. Although optimistic, these reports are offset by that of Tretli, et al[21], from the Norwegian Radium Hospital in Oslo, Norway. They studied 20 breast cancer patients diagnosed during pregnancy and 15 patients diagnosed during lactation. Despite controlling for age, stage of disease, and year of occurrence, these researchers reported only 3 of 20 patients surviving more than four years. They also report a very bleak outcome, stating that 60% of the pregnant patients died within two years. Of the 15 patients whose carcinoma was diagnosed during lactation, there was a suggestion of worsening prognosis, although it was not considered to be significant. Chiedozi and colleagues[22] also suggested that breast cancer occurring in pregnancy causes negative effects. Although matched for stage and age, they suggest higher percentages of Grade III lesions in pregnant patients (55.6%) than in nonpregnant patients (19.4%). The final outcome in this study also suggests a 1.4 times increase in survival in nonpregnant women with breast cancer who were controls compared to patients with breast cancer in pregnancy.

Should therapeutic abortion accompany definitive treatment for breast cancer? There are potential theoretical advantages. However, only approximately 30% of patients with breast cancer are positive for estrogen receptors in the tissue specimen. Although it has been suggested that termination would be helpful, it generally is believed that termination does not enhance prognosis.[23] If termination is considered, it must rest on other factors such as personal choice, which are influenced by social and moral convictions.

Adjuvant or therapeutic chemotherapy for patients with breast cancer diagnosed and treated during pregnancy must be evaluated on an individual basis. If after initial surgical intervention, particularly in the first trimester, chemotherapy is deemed urgent, pregnancy termination should be considered. A fetal malformation rate of 11.6%, or approximately five times the normal expectation, has been reported.[24,25] No malformations were noted in infants of women undergoing chemotherapy in the second or third trimester, but long-term effects are still not known and no assurance for complete long-term health can be granted to these offspring.

With increasing awareness of breast disease and self-examination plus appropriate use of diagnostic modalities, there will be a substantial number of women treated for breast cancer who survive, are still in the reproductive years, and may desire more children. Some 5–15% of women treated during pregnancy or lactation for breast cancer have been reported as having a subsequent pregnancy. These patients, should they become pregnant, can be expected to do very well. Those that do become pregnant in general have had a lower incidence of axillary node involvement at the time of initial treatment. Also, it is suggested that young patients with aggressive tumors will have metastasis early and not survive three years when conception subsequently might be considered in the patient with no evidence of recurrence of previously treated breast carcinoma. The first two years following treatment for breast carcinoma are considered high risk, but even a large number of patients who become pregnant in the first six months following initial treatment survive five years. In general, however, most physicians suggest at least a two-year wait following definitive treatment before considering pregnancy. Should pregnancy be considered thereafter? Choice should be tempered by the initial stage, grade, and evidence of nodal disease.[26]

REFERENCES

1. Falconer IR. Aspects of the biochemistry, physiology and endocrinology of lactation. *Aust J of Biol Sci.* 1980;33:71.
2. Martin RH, Oakey RE. The role of antenatal oestrogen in postpartum human lactogenesis: evidence from oestrogen-deficient pregnancies. *Clin Endocrinol (Oxf).* 1982;17:403.
3. Shiu RPC, Friesen HG. Mechanism of action of prolactin in the control of mammary gland function. *Annu Rev Physiol.* 1980;42:83.
4. Noel GL, Suh HK, Frantz AG. Prolactin release during nursing and breast stimulation in postpartum and nonpostpartum subjects. *J Clin Endocrinol Metab.* 1974;38:413.
5. William PC. Massive hypertrophy of the breasts and axillary breasts in successive pregnancies. *Am J Obstet Gynecol.* 1957;74:1326.
6. Blaydes RM, Kinnebrew, CA. Massive breast hyperplasia complicating pregnancy. *Obstet Gynecol.* 1958;12:601.
7. Wager G. Toxic shock syndrome: a review. *Am J Obstet Gynecol.* 1983;146:93.
8. Canter JW, Oliver GC, Zaloudek CJ. Surgical diseases of the breast during pegnancy. *Clin Obstet Gynecol.* 1983;26:853.
9. Majmudai B, Rosales-Quintara S. Infarction of breast fibroadenomas during pregnancy. *JAMA.* 1975;231:963.
10. Kinnaird DW. Results of cytologic study of aspirated fluid from breast cysts. *Am Surg.* 1975;41:505.
11. Abramson DJ. Clinical evaluation of aspiration of cysts of the breast. *Surg Gynecol Obstet.* 1974;139:531.
12. Egan RL. Experience with mammography in a tumor institution. *Radiology.* 1960;75:894.
13. Feig SA. Assessment of the hypothetical risk from mammography and evaluation of the potential benefit. *Radiol Clin North Am.* 1983;21:173.
14. Applewhite RR, Smith LR, DiVincenti F. Carcinoma of the breast associated with pregnancy and lactation. *Am Surg.* 1973;39:101.
15. Sahni K, Sanyal B, Agrawal, MS, et al. Carcinoma of breast associated with pregnancy and lactation. *J Surg Oncol.* 1981;16:167.
16. Horsley JS III, Alrich EM, Wright CB. Carcinoma of the breast in women 35 years of age or younger. *Ann Surg.* 1969;169:839.
17. Nugent P, O'Connell TX. Breast cancer and pregnancy. *Arch Surg.* 1985;120:1221.
18. King RM, Welch JS, Martin JK Jr, et al. Carcinoma of the breast associated with pregnancy. *Surg Gynecol Obstet.* 1985;160:228.
19. Holdaway IM, Mason BH, Kay RG. Steroid hormone receptors in breast tumors presenting during pregnancy or lactation. *J Surg Oncol.* 1984;25:38.
20. Green FL. Gestational breast cancer: a ten year experience. *South Med J.* 1988;81:1509.
21. Tretli S, Kvalheim G, Thuresen S, et al. Survival of breast cancer patients diagnosed during pregnancy or lactation. *Br J Cancer.* 1988;58:382.
22. Chiedozi LC, Iweze FI, Aboh IF, et al. Breast cancer in pregnancy and lactation. *Trop Geogr Med.* 1988;40:26.
23. Clark RM, Reid J. Carcinoma of the breast in pregnancy and lactation. *Int J Radiation Oncol Biol Phys.* 1978;4:693.
24. Murray CL, Reichert JA, Anderson J, et al. Multimodal cancer therapy for breast cancer in the first trimester of pregnancy: a case report. *JAMA.* 1984;252:2607.
25. Schapira DV, Chudley AE. Successful pregnancy following continuous treatment with combination chemotherapy before conception and throughout pregnancy. *Cancer.* 1984;54:800.
26. Donegan WL. Mammary carcinoma and pregnancy. In: Donegan WL, Spratt JS, eds. *Cancer of the Breast*, 3rd ed. Philadelphia: WB Saunders; 1988:679.

Chapter One Hundred and Eighty-Nine

Breast Cancer

Melody A. Cobleigh, Krystyna Kiel, and Thomas R. Witt

189

This chapter discusses carcinoma originating from the epithelial cells of the mammary gland. Most breast cancers originate within breast epithelium. Allowed to progress, the cancer may spread simultaneously to lymph nodes and through the blood stream. Patients whose cancer is limited to the breast are cured by surgery. However, many patients whose cancers appear clinically localized (are node-negative) actually have experienced microscopic spread of cancer outside of the breast. Both these patients and patients whose nodes are positive can benefit from adjuvant treatment. When breast cancer recurs outside of the breast it is, for all intents and purposes, incurable.

Nieminen and Remes[1] reviewed over 150,000 consecutive pregnant patients who presented to their clinic during 1950–1969. Malignant disease was discovered during pregnancy or the puerperium in 100 patients (0.07%). There were 24 cases of breast cancer (0.02%). From the oncologist's viewpoint, 1 in 50 patients (2%) with breast cancer will present in a pregnant or lactating condition.[2] As women delay childbearing into their thirties and forties and as the incidence of breast cancer in younger women increases, we can anticipate a rising frequency of breast cancer complicating pregnancy.

EFFECT OF THE DISEASE ON THE PREGNANCY AND THE FETUS

Breast cancer could affect the pregnancy in one of three ways: It could be transmitted to the fetus; it could weaken the mother to such an extent that the fetus could not survive; and treatment of the mother could affect the fetus adversely.

Fetal Metastasis

Cancers can be transmitted from mother to fetus, most notably leukemia and melanoma. However, there are no reported cases of breast cancer having been transmitted to a fetus.

Maternal Illness

Most patients with breast cancer are amenable to treatment so that the fetus is not compromised by the mother's demise.

Transmission of Drugs to the Fetus

All of the agents used in the treatment of breast cancer are potentially harmful to the fetus. As will be evident from the subsequent review, chemotherapy appears remarkably nontoxic to the fetus. However, the effect of gestational exposure to chemotherapy on the children of female fetuses is of particular concern because eggs are formed during gestation. Mutations or chromosomal abnormalities produced in such gametes could result in embryopathology in the next generation, and recessive mutations might not become manifest until subsequent generations (see also Chapter 173).

Some authors have cautioned that the birth of a phenotypically normal infant should not lull the physician into a false sense of security, and long-term follow up is necessary to determine the full effect of chemotherapeutic drugs on offspring. One author provided long-term follow up on a series of patients and showed that phenotypic normalcy at birth predicts normalcy into adolescence.[3] That report is consistent with the basic biologic tenet that chemotherapeutic drugs are more likely teratogenic due to their cytotoxic effects, related to cell destruction, and not to genetic changes that persist and affect embryonic development.[4] Mutations or chromosomal abnormalities play little or no role when induced in somatic cells of the developing embryo except as they may cause cell death, retardation of differentiation, or mitotic delay.[4]

Teratogens have certain characteristics in common.[4] They can be summarized as follows:

1. Stage sensitivity: Three stages of development exist: From fertilization through early postimplantation the embryo has few omnipotent cells, and those cells have great renewal capacity. The effect of a teratogen is all or none because the embryo either dies or so few cells are affected that it repairs itself. The second stage, organogenesis (days 18–60 of human gestation), is the period of greatest sensitivity to teratogens. Malformation is observed most often when the fetus is exposed during this period. During the third stage, the fetal period, teratogens produce growth retardation.
2. Dose-response: As exposure or dosage increases, frequency and severity of teratogenic effects also increase.
3. Threshold effects: This is the dose below which the incidence of death, malformation, growth retardation, or functional deficit is not statistically greater than that of controls (usually 1–3 orders of magnitude below the teratogenic dose).
4. Genetic variability: This determines differences in placental transport, absorption, metabolism, and distribution of an agent, and accounts for variation in teratogenic effects among species and individuals.

Genetic variability is illustrated poignantly by the case of a woman with leukemia who carried two different pregnancies to term while receiving the same maintenance chemotherapy. One child was normal, the other was born with limb anomalies.[5] Another woman was treated with chemotherapy throughout her entire pregnancy and gave birth to fraternal twins, one of whom had multiple deformities, the other was normal.[6]

Several reports concerning the issue of placental passage of chemotherapy drugs are of interest. In those reports the mothers gave birth to infants with normal blood counts while they were profoundly cytopenic from intensive combination chemotherapy regimes.[7-9] One can speculate that there was placental inactivation of drugs, that the drugs did not cross the placental barrier, or that fetal bone marrow is less sensitive than adult marrow to the myelosuppressive effects of chemotherapy. Doxorubicin has been reported not to cross the human placental barrier.[10] However, in that report, only amniotic fluid and not fetal blood was evaluated. The idea that the placenta is a barrier to the transfer of drugs from mother to fetus is probably incorrect. Rather, the placenta is a sieve through which everything that enters the maternal circulation can be expected to reach the fetus within a few minutes. A high molecular weight does not interfere with transmission, except for a time lag of a few minutes.[11]

The world literature on treatment of the pregnant patient with chemotherapy was reviewed for this chapter. In an effort to avoid redundancy, all tabulations were based on original case reports. The cases reviewed here do not include those in which elective abortion was performed because the full effect of the drugs on the fetus could not be determined. Fetuses exposed to both chemotherapy and radiotherapy also were not included for the same reason. Some series contained reports of cases which were obtained by personal communication. Those cases were not included in this review because of the possibility that other important factors (such as simultaneous irradiation and chemotherapy) might have been overlooked.[12] Cases in which the mother died before being able to deliver were not included because the full effect of drug exposure on the fetus could not be determined. For the most part, those cases involved mothers with uncontrollable cancer and not mothers (and therefore fetuses) who died because of drug toxicity. No attempt was made to review the literature concerning the use of immunosuppressive therapy during pregnancy. However, there are many reports of normal infants born of mothers with renal allografts who received azothioprine throughout their pregnancies.[13-15] Birth weight percentiles were obtained from United States single live birth data, which were based on a 50% sample of births from 36 states and the District of Columbia.[16]

There is no assurance that the cases abstracted represent all existing cases. The distribution of cases by trimester is far from uniform. There also may be a reporting bias for cases with a particularly good or poor outcome.

The effect of chemotherapeutic drugs on the fetus will be discussed according to the class of the drug and according to the trimester of exposure. This should allow the medical oncologist who is faced with a pregnant patient in need of chemotherapy to select the combination of drugs that is most appropriate for the particular clinical problem.

There are 147 pregnancies in the data base and 148 infants. Analysis of birth weight for gestational age reveals a consistent trend toward infants falling below the 50th percentile. There were 79 live-born, nontwin infants whose weight percentile could be discerned. Those infants fell into the percentile ranges listed in Table 189–1.

TABLE 189–1. BIRTH WEIGHTS OF INFANTS BORN TO MOTHERS WHO RECEIVED CHEMOTHERAPY DURING PREGNANCY

Percentile Range	Percent of Infants Falling in Range
<10	26.0
10–25	19.0
25–50	39.0
50–75	10.0
75–90	2.5
>90	2.5

Whether intrauterine growth retardation was caused by the chemotherapy or the mother's disease is unknown. However, it is obvious from the many reports of mothers who died shortly after parturition of uncontrolled leukemia that the fetus must have suffered, at least in part, from the mother's cancer (see footnotes in table for specific cases). While prematurity and low birth weight were observed often in infants who were exposed to chemotherapy *in utero,* the same problems have been reported in mothers whose chemotherapy was delayed.[17]

Intrauterine growth retardation is associated with increased perinatal morbidity and mortality.[18] This association exists throughout the entire range of percentile weights, not just for those who are severely growth retarded (below the 10th percentile). Infants who survive the perinatal period are at continued risk for impaired growth. Interestingly, impaired physical growth did not seem to correlate with impaired mental growth in the cases reviewed here. Follow-up studies on the children usually revealed "normal mental development" despite continued subnormal height and weight (see footnotes in Tables 189–2 and 189–3 for specific cases). Whether these children would have performed better on mental tasks had they not been exposed *in utero* to chemotherapy is unknown. Redmond[18] has coined the term *subclinical growth retardation* to describe this unmet potential.

Classification schemes of intrauterine growth retardation distinguish between infants whose head growth has been spared (disproportionate intrauterine growth retardation) and those in whom head and body are affected.[19] Proportionate intrauterine growth retardation is associated with a greater risk of permanently impaired physical growth and mental development. It begins between weeks 20 and 24 of gestation and may be due to the fact that the second-trimester fetus cannot shunt blood preferentially to the brain. Disproportionate intrauterine growth retardation be-

TABLE 189–2. LIVE-BORN INFANTS WITH CONGENITAL ANOMALIES

Case Number	Exposure (weeks)	Drug[a]	Disease	Anomaly[b]	Weight Percentile
149	0–33	C	ALL	x[11]	<10
6	25–d ?	DAra TgAra	AML	x[32]	0–25[1]
26	20–d	Bu	CGL	x[2]	<10
36	0–d	C	Hodgkin's	x[4]	<10
47	0–d	AraTg	AML	x[8]	<10
49	0–8	M	Psoriasis	x[9]	10–25
77	<13	Amt	?	x[17]	?
78	<13	Amt	?	x[17]	?
127	<10	Amt	Abortifacient	x[27]	25–50
138	7–8	Amt	Abortifacient	x[31]	<10
46	8–10	M	Abortifacient	x[7]	<10

[a] M = methotrexate; Amt = aminopterin; Ara = cytosine arabinoside; C = cyclophosphamide; D = daunorubicin; Tg = 6-Thioguanine; Bu = Busulfan

[b] [2]Absent right kidney, hydronephrotic left kidney, hepatic subcapsular calcifications, intrauterine and postpartum growth retardation. Renal agenesis results from the failure of a ureteric bud to develop during the fifth to eighth week of gestation, long before the exposure of the fetus to either drug. This is often associated with anomalies of the opposite kidney. [4]Four toes on each foot, groove extending to the uvula on each side of the midline of the hard palate, flattened nasal ridge, small skin tag on anterior mid-abdomen, slightly hypoplastic middle phalanx of fifth finger and bilateral inguinal hernias. Feet wider at heels and tapered toward toes. First and fourth toes larger than middle two, which showed some degree of overlap. The child was developing normally at one year. [7]Absent coronal and lambdoid sutures; oxycephaly; very wide posterior fontanel; frontal bone absent (or not ossified). Toes absent except one on one foot; talus and calcaneus seen bilateral; three phalanges and one metatarsal on left and one phalanx on right foot; broad nasal bridge; low set, small nodules on both ear lobes; unusual configuration; hyperteliorism; prominent eyeballs; micrognathia; high arched palate; multiple anomalous ribs; Denver scale normal at 15 mo but child below third percentile for height and weight. [8]Medial two digits of both feet absent; distal phalanges of both thumbs absent and remnant of right thumb vary hypoplastic. Otherwise infant developed normally. [9]Grossly abnormal appearance, mostly affecting skull. Oxycephaly, fusion of coronal sutures. Nose bridge wide and depressed; ears low set; fingers long and slender with webbing between proximal phalanges of index and middle fingers. Developmental progress normal. [11]Madelung's deformity, arm; esophageal atresia, anomalous inferior vena cave, undescended testicles, duplicated collecting systems of kidneys, low IQ, neuroblastoma age 4, thyroid cancer age 6. [17]Hydrocephaly [27]left talipes-equinovarus, multiple skull anomalies (malformed occipital bone characterized by anterior bending and lacunar formation. In addition there was synostosis of the lateral extremity of the lambdoid sutures. The posterior fontanel was extremely wide, an expected accompaniment of craniosynostosis. Anterior fontanel large and relatively posteriorly displaced, suggestive of premature synostosis. [31]Physical findings were most bizarre. The head was globular in shape, circumference 27 cm. The borders of the fontanel could not be determined because ossification of the cranium was limited to the lower part of the skull. The scalp hair was abundant and had a curious back-combed appearance. The eyes were rather small but appeared prominent because the orbital ridges were poorly developed. The palpebral apertures were slit-like and the lower eyelids were everted. There was almost constant tearing at birth and throughout early neonatal life. There was moderate facial asymmetry and marked hypognathia. The palate was high-arched. The ears were small and low-set. The hands and fingers were long but the forearms were disproportionately short. At 53 months her height and weight were below the 10th percentile. She was mildly retarded. She maintained her peculiar appearance. [32]Congenital adherence of the iris to the posterior cornea, left eye.

TABLE 189–3. CONGENITAL ANOMALIES THAT OCCURRED IN ABORTED FETUSES

Case Number	Exposure (weeks)	Drug[a]	Disease	Anomaly[b]	Gestation Age
28	8–9	MuVePz	Hodgkin's	xx[3]	24
103	7–8	Amt	Abortifacient	x[20]	20

[a] Mu = nitrogen mustard; Ve = vinblastine; Pz = procarbazine; Amt = aminopterin
[b] [3]Each foot had four toes with webbing of the third and fourth toes on the right. The right pinna was slightly abnormal. There was bowing of the right tibia. A large hemorrhage was found in the right cerebral hemisphere. [20]Fetus had a large meningocele.

gins after 30 weeks and is associated with a greater risk of intrauterine demise but a better chance for normal subsequent development. Presumably, a drug that interferes with growth could produce either type of intrauterine growth retardation, depending on when it is administered during the pregnancy. Unfortunately, most evaluations of patients exposed to chemotherapy while pregnant do not report the head circumference of the child. Subsequent case reports should include such helpful information.

There were 84 live-born, non-twin infants for whom gestational age was recorded. Premature birth (before the 37th gestational week), iatrogenic or otherwise, occurred in 30 (36%). There were 92 live-born, nontwin infants for whom birth weights were recorded. Premature birth (weight less than 2500 g) occurred in 34 infants (37%). Data from the National Institute of Child Health and Human Development suggest that 5% of all live births occur before the 37th week of pregnancy and that approximately 6% of all infants weigh less than 2500 g.[16] Although frequent comment was made of low birth weight in infants exposed to chemotherapy *in utero,* it was common for such infants to be born early as a result of labor induction, either because of a fear of the fetus's exposure to another round of chemotherapy or fear of the consequences of cytopenia in the setting of delivery.

A total of 36 patients (24%) experienced a spontaneous abortion. In the 1960s, the abortive action of aminopterin became known to the public, and it was used illegally as an abortifacient. It is difficult to relate the dosages of that folate antagonist to those of another folate antagonist, methotrexate, which currently is used often in the treatment of breast cancer. If the cases in which folate antagonists were used specifically as an abortifacient are excluded, there were eight spontaneous abortions (7%) observed in 120 pregnancies. This compares with an expected spontaneous abortion rate in the United States of approximately 10%.[21]

Congenital anomalies occurred in eleven live births (Table 189–2). All of those infants were below the fiftieth percentile in weight for gestational age, and most were below the tenth percentile. Of the 11 anomalies, 9 were a major impediment to normal development of the infant and all occurred in fetuses who were exposed during the first trimester. In the two remaining infants, exposure began during the second trimester. The anomalies that occurred in those two infants probably were not related to drug exposure.

The class of compound administered to the 11 infants included an antimetabolite in eight (a folate antagonist in six), an alkylator in three, and an anthracycline in one (that patient also received an antimetabolite). Aminopterin, a folate antagonist, is a potent teratogen.[22] In five of the cases, a folate antagonist was used during the first trimester specifically as an abortifacient. If those cases are excluded, there were six children born live with congenital anomalies among 113 live-born babies (5%). This compares with an expected major congenital anomaly rate of 3%.[23]

There were two additional congenital anomalies that occurred in aborted fetuses (Table 189–3). Both fetuses were exposed during the first trimester.

The karyotype was analyzed in 28 infants who were exposed to chemotherapy *in utero.* All were normal.

Most of the fetuses that were spontaneously aborted were not analyzed for congenital anomalies. Looking only at live-born infants, first trimester exposures are displayed in Table 189–4 according to class of compound administered and incidence of congenital anomalies. Some pregnancies are listed more than once because many patients received multiple drugs.

Some compounds appear remarkably non-teratogenic when used during the first trimester. They include busulfan, 6-MP, the vinca alkaloids, and the anthracyclines. Others, however, appear to be extremely potent teratogens, such as the folate antagonists. The deformities observed with folate antagonists included a grossly abnormal appearance, predominantly of skull bones. Craniostenosis (absent sutures), abnormal and deficient ossification of parietal, temporal and frontal bones, anencephaly, hydrocephalus and widely spaced eyes were reported. Low-slung ears were common, and many had digital anomalies, including syndactylism. Our observations regarding the usual outcome of administration of antimetabolites differ from those of another reviewer who stated that the usual outcome after administration of antimetabolites (including methotrexate, 6-MP, 5-FU, and aminopterin) has been a live infant with deformities or congenital defects.[24] Teratogenicity is clearly stage- and drug-dependent. Since there were only two live-

TABLE 189–4. LIVE-BORN INFANTS

Drug	Anomaly	No Anomaly
Alkylating agents		
Nitrogen mustard	1	1
Cyclophosphamide	2	6
Busulfan	0	10
Procarbazine	1	1
Antimetabolites		
Aminopterin	4	0
Cytosine arabinoside	1	3
Methotrexate	2	4
6-mercaptopurine	0	9
6-thioguanine	1	1
Antimitotics		
Urethane	0	1
Vinblastine	1	1
Vincristine	0	4
Anthracyclines		
Adriamycin	0	1
AMSA	0	1
Daunorubicin	0	1

born anomalous infants exposed during the second or third trimesters, the drugs were not analyzed by class or compound for congenital anomalies.

The most commonly prescribed drugs for treatment of breast cancer include cyclophosphamide, methotrexate, 5-FU, the vinca alkaloids, and the anthracyclines. With the exception of 5-FU, all have been administered in at least a dozen second or third trimester pregnancies, and no congenital anomalies occurred. The lack of experience with 5-FU is because most of the cases were treated for acute leukemia or Hodgkin's disease, and 5-FU is not used routinely to treat those diseases. However, many fetuses were exposed to other antimetabolites, cytosine arabinoside or 6-TG, during the second or third trimester and did not develop anomalies.

There are no published reports of the use of tamoxifen during pregnancy. ICI Pharma, the company that manufactures the drug, has a handful of cases on file in which patients were given the drug inadvertently during pregnancy. The trimester of exposure was not known. Some congenital anomalies occurred (personal communication). The drug should not be used during pregnancy.

There is little information regarding breast-feeding in patients receiving chemotherapy. However, cyclophosphamide has been shown to pass from breast milk to infant, resulting in infantile pancytopenia.[25]

DIAGNOSIS

Critical to the timely diagnosis of breast cancer in pregnancy is avoidance of the "head in the sand" approach to a new or enlarging breast mass (eg, "It's probably a milk cyst . . . come back next month," or "Let's see what it feels like after you've delivered."). A suspicious thickening or dominant mass in a breast during pregnancy is deserving of urgent (not emergent) investigation. If on aspiration the lesion is cystic, the fluid not bloody, the mass disappears entirely and does not recur within a short period of time (within four weeks), and the cytology is negative (some would question the need for cytologic assessment if the other criteria are met), there is little need for concern and careful observation only is warranted. If these criteria are not met, further evaluation is indicated.

If the lesion is solid, sampling of the tissue for cytologic assessment is indicated. Information recently has been compiled from multiple series on over 18,000 needle aspiration cytologies in which the mean false-negative rate was 8.7% and the mean false-positive rate was 0.2%.[26] Mammography, with appropriate shielding of the abdomen, should be performed when breast cancer has been diagnosed. The purpose of mammography in this setting is to detect occult synchronous cancers. Mammography should not be used to determine the nature of a dominant mass. The false-negative rate for palpable breast cancers has been reported to be as high as 48% in premenopausal patients.[27]

If the cytology is equivocal or clinical suspicion remains high despite a negative cytology (ie, concern over sampling error), open biopsy is warranted. With the vast majority of open biopsies done under local anesthesia (with or without light intravenous sedation), the risk to the mother and fetus is minimal[28]; with the modest increased likelihood of infection and milk fistula being more an inconvenience than a life-threatening danger, these risks of open biopsy seem acceptable in order to attain the benefit of earlier diagnosis.

Technical considerations relating to open biopsy include meticulous attention to hemostasis and, where possible, foresight in terms of what the definitive therapy will be if cancer is found. For example, if mastectomy is to be the definitive therapy, a conservative incisional biopsy to confirm the diagnosis through an incision that can be enveloped easily in a subsequent mastectomy incision is appropriate. The same lesion, however, should be totally excised with a margin of normal tissue through an incision in the natural skin lines of the breast if cancer is to be treated with lumpectomy, axillary dissection, and postpartum radiation therapy.

EFFECTS OF PREGNANCY ON THE DISEASE

Pregnancy may affect the course of breast cancer by altering the incidence, altering the ability to diagnose, limiting therapeutic options, or altering the cure rate.

Pregnancy before the age of 30 protects against development of breast cancer. A first pregnancy after the age of 30 actually increases a woman's likelihood of developing breast cancer. There is no evidence that the incidence of breast cancer is increased during pregnancy, a state of diminished immune responsiveness.

Neither interrupting the pregnancy nor allowing it to go to term has affected the ultimate outcome of the pregnant patient with breast cancer.[29-34]

Glomerular filtration rate and blood volume are increased during pregnancy. These factors theoretically decrease serum concentrations and increase clearance of drugs that are excreted renally. There are no known dose modifications for chemotherapy administered during pregnancy. The effect of altered drug levels on drug efficacy is unknown but is considered to be important in adjuvant treatment of breast cancer in that use of attenuated dosages has been associated with higher relapse rates. Pharmacokinetic studies would be of great value.

TREATMENT OF THE PREGNANT PATIENT WITH SURGERY

The proper surgical approach to the pregnant patient with breast cancer has evolved from a long-held attitude of pessimism to one of guarded optimism. The perception of the incurable nature of breast cancer in pregnancy in the 1940s and earlier[35] has been supplanted by the well-founded view that, stage for stage, breast cancer is as curable in the pregnant patient as it is in the nonpregnant patient[36] and, therefore, worthy of the same appropriate therapeutic aggressiveness.

Outside of our increasing experience and accuracy in the performance of needle aspiration cytology, there have been few technical advances in the surgical sciences to account for this change. Rather, most of the improvement in management of the pregnant breast cancer patient is because of improved anesthetic techniques (see Chapter 201), advances in fetal monitoring and obstetric science, and a recognition that undue deference to the pregnant state has led to tragic delays in diagnosis and treatment. Intervals between initial signs or symptoms and presentation to a physician, between initial presentation to a physician and diagnosis, and between diagnosis and definitive therapy have been reported to be two to three times longer in pregnant patients than in nonpregnant patients.[37-39]

Although several studies looking at the efficacy of preoperative systemic chemotherapy are underway, the mainstay of initial therapy for operable Stages I–III breast cancer is surgery alone (usually modified radical mastectomy) or surgery and radiation therapy (lumpectomy, axillary dissection, and radiation therapy). A comparison of results between these two therapies has revealed no significant difference in survival or disease-free survival, but when lumpectomy and axillary dissection were performed without subsequent radiation therapy, an unacceptably high local recurrence rate of 39% resulted.[40]

On the grounds that breast cancer during pregnancy should be treated as aggressively as during nonpregnant states, treatments of lesser magnitude than modified radical mastectomy or lumpectomy, axillary dissection, and radiation therapy are improperly conservative and generally should be avoided.

Pertinent to the risk of surgery in the pregnant patient is the risk of general anesthesia; although total mastectomy, modified radical mastectomy, and axillary dissection can be done under local anesthesia with light sedation (personal communication [TRW]), general anesthesia for such operations generally is required and is preferred. Anesthesia considerations in the pregnant patient are discussed in Chapters 201 and 202 and will not be considered here, except to say that advances in techniques have greatly augmented the safety of general anesthesia, both for the mother and the fetus, such that the risk of fetal death has been reported for some time at less than 1%.[32]

Technical considerations of breast surgery in the pregnant patient relate primarily to the effects of breast engorgement and increased vascularity. Blood loss is increased but can be reduced with appropriate use of electrocautery or, more recently, lasers. Rarely is transfusion required, but the slight attendant risks of blood incompatibility or transmission of infectious disease (most notoriously hepatitis and acquired immune deficient syndrome—AIDS) can be eliminated by the use of autologous blood harvested one to two weeks prior to the surgery. The increased bleeding and engorgement also indicates a small increased risk when random biopsy or prophylactic mastectomy of the contralateral breast is performed.

As stated above, delay in the treatment of breast cancer in pregnancy has been implicated in the poorer results that are reported in some series. Yet, two critical times during pregnancy deserve special attention with regard to short delays in treatment. First is the period of organogenesis. There is no evidence in the literature that a few-week delay in breast cancer treatment is harmful with regard to prognosis and recurrence[42], thus a relatively short delay in treatment can be justified until organogenesis is complete in order to reduce the already low risk of general anesthesia during that time.[43] Second is the period of time in the middle of the third trimester when fetal maturity is approached. Again, a delay of treatment for a few weeks to attain fetal maturity (approximately 36 weeks' gestation) in order to eliminate the risk of preterm labor that could be caused by the surgery may assure fetal viability and is unlikely to be harmful to the mother. With these two exceptions, breast cancer during pregnancy should be treated as soon after diagnosis as is practical.

Traditionally, the definitive treatment of choice for breast cancer in pregnancy has been the modified radical (or in rare cases, Halsted radical) mastectomy.[44,45] Changes in attitude based on increasing knowledge of the efficacy and safety of breast conservation therapy could lead to the acceptance of such therapy in the pregnant patient as an appropriate alternative to mastectomy in selected cases.

For example, evidence has been presented in this chapter supporting the relative safety of adjuvant chemotherapy, especially during the middle and later stages of pregnancy. Furthermore, in cases of breast-conserving therapy, delays of up to six weeks between lumpectomy and radiation therapy in patients not receiving chemotherapy do not appear to affect results adversely. Also, lumpectomy patients who are candidates for adjuvant chemotherapy frequently receive some or all of their chemotherapy (three to six months of treatment) prior to undergoing the required radiation therapy. Based on these principles, the employment of lumpectomy, axillary dissection, and radiation therapy with or without adjuvant chemotherapy, in cases of breast cancer diagnosed in the second and third trimesters, could be appropriate in selected cases and would appear to offer the same likelihood of cure as the more traditional modified radical mastectomy (allowing for radiation to begin with parturition).

To summarize the role of surgery in the treatment of breast cancer during pregnancy, it seems justified to say that in the past more errors such as delay in diagnosis, delay in therapy, or inadequate therapy have been made in deference to the state of pregnancy than would have been made by ignoring the state of pregnancy. Obviously, appropriate safeguards are in order for the fetus in terms of anesthetic management and during those critical periods of organogenesis and approaching fetal maturity. Within these limits, however, the pregnant patient with a breast lump should have evaluation and diagnosis carried out promptly and, if cancer is found, appropriately aggressive therapy that avoids radiation during the pregnancy should be administered without delay.

TREATMENT OF THE PREGNANT PATIENT WITH CHEMOTHERAPY

Treatment of the pregnant patient with breast cancer involves close collaboration between surgical, medical, and radiation oncologists as well as specialists in maternal-fetal medicine. The options for the pregnant patient are discussed below in the context of the trimester in which the patient presents and in terms of the stage of her cancer.

There is considerable experience reported on the use of chemotherapy during pregnancy because patients with acute leukemia must be treated during pregnancy or die without treatment during pregnancy, which results in an extremely high fetal mortality rate.[17] The pregnant patient with operable breast cancer finds herself in a different situation. Having completed surgical treatment, she is highly likely to survive the pregnancy in good health. However, withholding chemotherapy may diminish her chance of surviving. Therefore, the decision reached by the patient, in consultation with her physician, should be based on a clear presentation of the potential benefit of treatment for her (described below) and the potential risk to her baby (described above).

Operable Breast Cancer

Premenopausal patients with operable Stages I, II and III breast cancer experience improved disease-free survival if they receive adjuvant chemotherapy. Many prospective, randomized trials are not mature enough to show significant survival differences yet, but that is the natural history of adjuvant trials in breast cancer. In other words, an improvement in disease-free survival is demonstrable several years before an improvement in survival can be discerned. Adjuvant chemotherapy will reduce the risk of relapse by one third in node-negative women and by one fourth in node-positive women.[47-51] Without chemotherapy, approximately one third of node-negative and three fourths of node-positive women will relapse. Therefore, the patient should understand these facts as she makes a decision with her oncologist about treatment.

Chemotherapy was administered within six weeks of surgery in most adjuvant studies. The effect of delaying treatment beyond that point is unknown. It seems prudent to delay adjuvant chemotherapy until week 14 of gestation. Before that, the risk of congenital anomalies is increased. After the first trimester there is a definite benefit for the mother and only a theoretical risk to her baby (see discussion above).

Inoperable Breast Cancer

Patients with Stage IV breast cancer are incurable. The goal in treating such patients is palliation. If the disease process is one of rapid growth in vital organs and the patient is unlikely to survive the pregnancy without chemotherapy, it is in the best interest of both mother and fetus to proceed with treatment. If, however, the disease is indolent and can be palliated effectively without treatment that would potentially damage the fetus, withholding chemotherapy seems prudent.

Treatment During the First Trimester

When chemotherapy is warranted during the first trimester, it is wise to avoid methotrexate. From the limited data available, a AV-type regimen (Adriamycin, vincristine) appears to be the least toxic. That is, those drugs have been administered during the first trimester with no congenital anomalies, and they are active in breast cancer.

Treatment During the Second and Third Trimesters

Any of the standards drugs used to treat breast cancer can be used during the second and third trimesters. The intent should be to balance fetal and maternal risks and benefits. This includes delivering the infant as soon as a high probability of fetal survival can be anticipated. The appropriate gestational age for delivery of the infant will change as advances in neonatology occur and should be determined after consultation with a specialist.

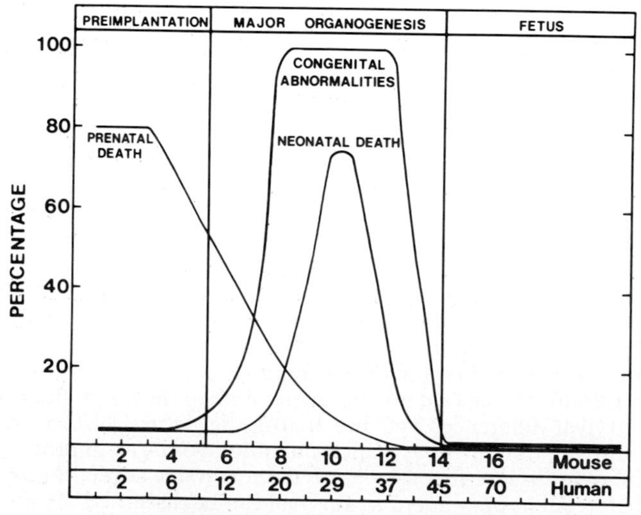

Figure 189-1. Adverse effects of radiation related to gestational age. *(Adapted from Russell and Russell.[52])*

TABLE 189–5. AVERAGE OVARIAN RADIATION DOSE FROM PROCEDURES COMMONLY USED IN THE EVALUATION OF BREAST CANCER

Chest—PA and Lat	<1 mrad
Mammogram	<1 mrad
Skull	<1 mrad
Spine	
cervical	<1 mrad
thoracic	40 mrad
lumbar	540 mrad
Pelvic—AP	620 mrad
CT scan—brain	<1 mrad
Bone scan (10 mCi Tc-99m MDP)	<200 mrad

TREATMENT OF THE PREGNANT PATIENT WITH RADIOTHERAPY

Most data concerning the effect of radiation on the developing embryo and fetus is obtained from animal studies and the atomic bomb data from Japan. Generally, the effects can be divided into four categories, the end-result dependent on dose and stage of gestation. These include lethal effects, teratogenic effects, mutagenic effects, and carcinogenic effects, and are temporally related, as illustrated in Figure 189–1.[52] Although these curves are generated from animal data, they seem to fit the observed human experience. Whether a threshold dose exists is controversial. In studies of radiation-induced defects in fetal mouse bones, there appears to be no threshold dose, and the effect of radiation is linear.[53]

Prenatal exposure to radiation can result in an increased risk of later development of cancer. However, the relative risk of leukemia, the most common malignancy seen after total body irradiation, has been reported to range from 1.0 (no risk) to 1.5[54,55] after fetal irradiation, including no increased incidence following atomic bomb exposure. The Oxford survey, in contrast, demonstrated a strong risk, 1.4–1.5, for childhood malignancies, which increases to 9.0 when obstetric radiography was performed in the first trimester.[56] In animal studies, the oncogenic effect of doses of radiation used in diagnostic tests has not been demonstrated[57], adding to the controversy over the risk of diagnostic procedures (also see Chapter 5).

Diagnostic roentgenologic tests commonly used in the staging and evaluation of breast cancer include mammography, chest x-rays, bone scans, ultrasound, and CT scans. Typical ovarian doses seen during such procedures are listed in Table 189–5 (personal communication and[59]) Mammography is difficult to evaluate during pregnancy and is not routinely indicated in screening, but should be used when breast cancer is diagnosed. Chest x-ray results in minimal dose to the fetus and is not contraindicated. Bone scans should be performed with technetium-99-labeled radiopharmaceuticals that do not cross the placenta. They also should be performed with decreased radionucleide doses when clinically indicated and not routinely for Stages I and II of disease, as the yield at these earlier stages to demonstrate metastatic disease is low.[60] Conventional radiography of bony sites in the evaluation of metastatic disease delivers inappreciable doses to the fetus except when in near proximity, that is, lumbar spine, hip, or pelvic films. These areas should be evaluated with bone scan if necessary. CT scan of the head should be done if brain metastases are suspected. It delivers a negligible dose to the fetus.[61] Suspected liver metastases should be evaluated with ultrasonography. If CT scanning is necessary within the abdominal cavity, dose to the fetus can be decreased with appropriate adjustments of technique by radiology physics. Dose to the fetus is dependent on its proximity to the area scanned, and is minimal. Appropriate external shielding should be used at all times for all diagnostic procedures.

It generally is accepted that radiation doses less than 0.05 Gy (5 rad) probably result in a small risk to the fetus and should not be the basis for elective termination of pregnancy. Any radiation exposure to the fetus should be avoided, if possible, particularly during the first trimester. A dose of 0.10 Gy (10 rad) is more likely to result in a detectable risk of fetal damage.[62]

Radiation Therapy During Pregnancy

In the nonpregnant female, two options generally are accepted in the management of early stage breast cancer (Stages I and II). Tylectomy (lumpectomy, segmental mastectomy, wide local excision) and axillary dissection (Levels I and II) followed by irradiation of the breast have been demonstrated to render disease-free survival and survival equal to mastectomy.[63] Radiation is directed to the entire breast to total doses of 45.0–50.0 Gy (4500–5000 rad). This may be followed by a "boost" to the tumor site, either delivered with external electron fields or interstitial radioactive implants (generally with iridium-192 sources) to total tumor doses of 60.0–70.0 Gy (6000–7000 rad). This additional radiation is given if there is suspicion of close or positive margins, or if intraductal carcinoma is identified in over 25% of ducts outside of the area of infiltration.

The option to proceed with conservative therapy, that is, tylectomy and radiation, is based on the ability to excise the primary tumor completely, which may or may not cause problems in the pregnant woman. Lymph node radiation generally is not recommended unless there is marked involvement of the axillary nodes histologically (>4) or extranodal extension, or if there has been an inadequate axillary dissection. Small medial cancers may not require internal mammary node irradiation unless associated with positive axillary nodes. If the internal mammary nodes are to be irradiated, they should be included in the tangential treatment fields.

Technically, the breast is irradiated with opposed tangential radiation fields. Compensators are placed within the treatment fields to adjust for the slope of the treated tissue and to provide dose homogeneity. Radiation beams of 4 or 6 MeV energy should be used to provide skin sparing but appropriate build-up of dose to breast tissue beneath the skin surface, except that higher energies may be more appropriate in obese women with large breasts. Normal tissues other than the breast contained within a typical field are portions of the ribs and no more that 2.0–2.5 cm of lung directly beneath the radiation field.

Advanced stage breast cancer is approached with multiple modalities including mastectomy and systemic therapy, with or without radiation. The indications for postoperative radiation are advanced local disease (T3 or T4 lesions), advanced axillary nodal involvement (>4 positive nodes or extranodal involvement), positive margins, or dermal lymphatic involvement. The incidence of local recurrence remains over 20% despite chemotherapy[64], suggesting a significant role of postoperative radiation. Technically, the patient is approached similarly to patients treated with the intact breast, except that more effort may be made to include the internal mammary nodes in the tangential fields. Since skin sparing may be detrimental to the patient, material may be placed over the skin surface to maximize dose at the skin surface, therefore resulting in more skin reaction. The patient may be treated to the high axillary and supraclavicular nodes, requiring precision in treatment planning. In this case, the volume of lung to be irradiated increases (from treatment of the apex of lung directly beneath the supraclavicular nodes), but the incidence of symptomatic pneumonitis remains low.

The Effect of Radiation on the Fetus

The effect of high-dose radiation appears to be temporally related to gestation. Preimplantation radiation probably leads to spontaneous abortion due to the radiosensitivity of the blastomere and, therefore, large number of cell death, or a normal pregnancy. Growth retardation is not observed in this period. However, during organogenesis (days 29–64) a high incidence of central nervous system abnormalities is seen with doses >1 Gy (100 rad). During the fetal period, dose levels less than 0.05 Gy (5 rad) have not been associated with malformations or congenital abnormalities, and the effects of higher dose levels are not known. Growth retardation at dose levels of 0.1 Gy (10 rad) has been demonstrated.[53]

A standard external radiation treatment to the breast will result in a fetal dose of 0.10–0.15 Gy (10–15 rad), partly from direct radiation leakage, but more from internal scatter from which the fetus cannot be protected through external shielding. The greater the age of gestation, and therefore the closer the fetus to the radiation field, the higher the fetal dose. Quality of the beam (ie, radiation energy) can affect fetal dose in that higher energy radiation beams will result in less dose due to less internal scatter. Radiation to the pelvic or abdominal area will result in fetal doses close to the prescribed dose.[57]

Radiation Therapy for Breast Cancer In Pregnant Women

The National Surgical Adjuvant Breast Project reported a 39% local failure rate in women treated by local excision and axillary dissection without radiation.[40] No data are available regarding delayed radiation of several months' duration if no adjuvant chemotherapy is contemplated. It is standard practice to delay treatment of the breast two to six weeks following axillary dissection.

Radiation to the breast following tylectomy and axillary dissection for Stages I and II breast cancer can be delayed if chemotherapy is contemplated as an adjuvant. Recent protocols in national studies routinely delayed radiation therapy to the breast for two chemotherapy cycles or until completion of chemotherapy with no obvious detriment in local control or survival.[63] Since the results of radiation after tylectomy are equal to mastectomy, the opportunity to proceed with this option, delaying radiation to completion of pregnancy, should not be withheld from the patient providing that the patient's condition is appropriate for this procedure.

Adjuvant radiation therapy is indicated to improve local control following mastectomy for positive margins or for Stage III disease with large or diffuse breast tumors, >3 positive nodes, positive margins, or skin involvement. Again, since survival generally is accepted to be unaffected by postoperative radiation, consideration of adjuvant radiation therapy should be delayed until after delivery, surgery and chemotherapy.

Radiation for Stage IV disease is indicated immediately in four clinical situations: brain metastases, superior vena cava obstruction, tracheal or bronchial obstruction, or epi-

TABLE 189–6. SURVIVAL OF PATIENTS WITH NODE-NEGATIVE BREAST CANCER DIAGNOSED BEFORE PREGNANCY OR LACTATION

Number of Patients	Survival: Five Years	Survival: Ten Years	Refs.	Years
16	14	9 in 10	30	
15	13	12 in 15	33	41–69
16	10	7 in 16	29	49–55
8	7	6 in 8	69	<56
20	14		31[a]	
30	29	22 in 25	66	10–33
28	18		70	20–53
2	1	1 in 2	71	50–59
135	106 (79%)	57 in 76 (75%)		OVERALL

[a] 25% of patients received RT so that some node-positives may have been converted to node-negatives.

dural metastases causing spinal cord compression. The latter may be approached surgically in a low thoracic or lumbar compression. Bone metastases may require palliation if they cannot be controlled with analgesics or narcotics; however, radiation to the lumbar or pelvic area should be avoided. Appropriate measures to decrease fetal dose should be undertaken with cooperation of medical physics.

PREGNANCY AND LACTATION FOLLOWING BREAST CANCER

Some concerns that face patients and physicians revolve around the issue of pregnancy after breast cancer. Can pregnancy possibly cause a new cancer? Will it reactivate dormant tumor cells? Can a woman who has received radiation therapy to the breast lactate and breast feed her infant?

These issues have not been analyzed prospectively, and retrospective reviews are difficult to interpret because patients usually were reported either as node positive or node negative without regard to the number of involved nodes or the size of the primary tumor. In some reports the node-positive patients also had distant metastasis. In order to attenuate the problem of data interpretation with regard to prognosis, this analysis is restricted to those patients with node-negative breast cancer because the natural history of node-negative breast cancer is more uniform.

Five- and ten-year survivals in patients who do become pregnant are essentially no different from those observed in patients who do not become pregnant (see Table 189–6). Patients who present with a concurrent pregnancy and breast cancer tend to have high-grade tumors; those who become pregnant after a diagnosis of breast cancer tend to have had low-grade tumors.[65] This probably reflects self-selection on the part of patients with a better prognosis who decide to have children.

Some authors have stated that the patient should not become pregnant until five years after her diagnosis because early pregnancy is associated with a poor outcome. The apparent bad influence of pregnancy within a few years of treatment for mammary cancer can be explained by the fact that women with Stages I and II primaries usually die in the fourth and fifth years after diagnosis. These expected deaths have been related incorrectly to the pregnancy that occurred in the first few years. The apparent mortality, then, of early subsequent pregnancy is the expected mortality of mammary cancer at this period of follow-up and is not due to the pregnancy.

The more recent literature actually reflects a trend in the opposite direction toward a more favorable survival. This is believed to be due to the fact that women now often wait an allotted period of time, usually five years, before become pregnant. This appears to improve outcome, stage for stage. However, there is a selection bias for patients with a better prognosis because they did not relapse within several years of their diagnosis. In conclusion, pregnancy probably does not significantly increase the likelihood of relapse or death from breast cancer, nor does it appear to increase the incidence of second primaries.

Prior irradiation is not a contraindication to lactation. The mother should be encouraged to proceed with lactation if she desires. Successful lactation has been reported following radiation to the breast. It appears that the ability to lactate is determined by total dose; higher dose is more likely to retard milk development and flow in that breast.[66-68] Successful lactation in the contralateral breast is observed in general.

REFERENCES

1. Nieminen V, Remes N. Malignancy during pregnancy. *Acta Obstet Gynecol Scand.* 1970;49:315.
2. Boronow RC. Extrapelvic malignancy and pregnancy. *Obstet Gynecol Surv.* 1964;19:1.
3. Rubaltelli FF, Mittiga S, Solito P. Growth and development of children born to mothers treated with cytotoxic drugs during pregnancy. *Helv Paediat Acta.* 1982;37:599.
4. Beckman DA, Brent RL. Mechanisms of teratogenesis. *Ann Rev Pharmacol Toxicol.* 1984;24:483.
5. Schafer AI. Teratogenic effects of anti-leukemia chemotherapy. *Arch Intern Med.* 1981;141:514.
6. Reynoso EE, Shepherd FA, Messner HA, et al. Acute leukemia during pregnancy: The Toronto Leukemia Study Group experience with long-term follow-up of children exposed in utero to chemotherapeutic agents. *J Clin Oncol.* 1987;5:1098.
7. Doney KC, Kornemer KG, Shepard TH. Combination chemotherapy for acute myelocytic leukemia during pregnancy: three case reports. *Cancer Treat Rep.* 1979;63:369.
8. Fassas D, Kartalis G, Klearchon N, et al. Chemotherapy for acute leukemia during pregnancy. *Nouv Rev Fr Hematol.* 1984;26:19.
9. Nordlun JJ, DeVita VT, Carbone PP. Severe vinblastine-induced leukopenia during late pregnancy with delivery of a normal infant. *Ann Intern Med.* 1968;69:581.
10. Roboz J, Gleicher N, Wu K, et al. Does doxorubicin cross the placenta? *Lancet.* 1979;2:1382.
11. Apgar V. Drug problem in pregnancy. *Clin Obstet Gynecol.* 1966;9:623.
12. Diamond I, Anderson MM, McCreadie SR. Transplacental transmission of busulfan (Myleran) in a mother with leukemia: production of fetal malformation and cytomegaly. *Pediatrics.* 1960;25:85.
13. Durie B, Giles HR. Successful treatment of acute leukemia during pregnancy. *Arch Intern Med.* 1977;137:90.
14. Penn I, Makowski E, Droegemueller W, et al. Parenthood in renal homograft recipients. *JAMA.* 1971;216:1755.
15. Merkatz IR, Schwartz GH, David DS, et al. Resumption of female reproductive function following renal transplantation. *JAMA.* 1971;216:1749.
16. Hoffman HJ, Stark CR, Lundin FE, et al. Analysis of birth weight, gestational age and fetal viability. *Obstet Gynecol Surv.* 1974;29:651.
17. Meyer R, Cuttner J, Truog P, et al. Therapeutic leukapheresis of acute myelomonocytic leukemia in pregnancy. *Mede Pediatr Oncol.* 1978;4:77.
18. Redmond GP. Effect of drugs on intrauterine growth. *Clin Perinatol.* 1979;6:5.
19. Campbell S. Fetal Growth. In: *Fetal Physiology and Medicine.* Philadelphia: WB Saunders Co., 1976.
20. Stewart JO. Leukemia and pregnancy. *J Nat Med Assoc.* 1964;56:87.
21. Eastman NJ, Helman LM. *Williams Obstetrics.* 12th ed. New York: Appleton-Century-Crofts; 1961:526.
22. Warkany J. Teratogenicity of folic acid antagonists. *Ca Bull.* 1981;33:76.
23. Shepard TH. *Catalog of Teratogenic Agents.* 4th ed. Baltimore, MD: Johns Hopkins University Press; 1983:XIII.

24. Barber HRK. Fetal and neonatal effects of cytotoxic agents. *Obstet Gynecol.* 1981;58:45s.
25. White LG. Busulfan in pregnancy. *JAMA.* 1962;179:973.
26. Witt T, Kluiber R, Barroso E. Fine-Needle Aspiration Cytology of the Breast. In: Economou SG, ed. *Adjuncts to Cancer Therapy.* Philadelphia: Lea and Febiger; 1990.
27. Edeiken S. Mammography and palpable cancer of the breast. *Cancer.* 1988;61:263.
28. Salzstein EC, Mann RW, Chua TY, Decosse JJ. Outpatient breast biopsy. *Arch. Surg.* 1974;109:287.
29. Brown RN. Carcinoma of the breast followed by pregnancy. *Surgery.* 1960;48:862.
30. Devitt JE, Beattie WG, Stoddart TG. Carcinoma of the breast and pregnancy. *Can J Surg.* 1964;7:124.
31. Peters MV. Carcinoma of the breast associated with pregnancy. *Radiology.* 1962;78:18.
32. Byrd EF, Jr, Bayer DS, Robertson JC, et al. Treatment of breast tumors associated with pregnancy and lactation. *Ann Surg.* 1962;155:940.
33. Ribeiro GC, Palmer MK. Breast carcinoma associated with pregnancy: a clinician's dilemma. *Br Med J.* 1977;2:1524.
34. Rissanen PM. Carcinoma of the breast during pregnancy and lactation. *Br J Cancer.* 1968;22:663.
35. Haagensen CD, Stout AP. Carcinoma of the breast: criteria for operability. *Ann Sur.* 1943;118:859.
36. Nugent P, O'Connell TX. Breast cancer and pregnancy. *Arch Surg.* 1985;120:1221.
37. Applewhite RR, Smith LR, DiVincenti F. Carcinoma of the breast associated with pregnancy and lactation. *Am Surg.* 1973;39:101.
38. Treves N, Holleb AI. A report of 549 cases of breast cancer in women 35 years of age or younger. *Surg Gynecol Obstet.* 1958;107:271.
39. Fleming U, Sheridan B, Atkinson L, et al. The effects of childbearing on carcinoma of the breast. *Med J Aust.* 1970;1:1252.
40. Fisher B, Redmond C, Poisson R, et al. Eight-year results of a randomized clinical trial comparing total mastectomy and lumpectomy with or without irradiation in the treatment of breast cancer. *N Engl J Med.* 1989;320:822.
41. Vitums VC, Sites JG. Leukemia in pregnancy. *Med Ann DC.* 1968;37:588.
42. Margolese RG. Opinion/Response. Response: The case for the two-step biopsy procedure for breast cancer. *Ca—A J Clin.* 1982;32:51.
43. Pedersen H, Finster M. Anesthetic risks in the pregnant surgical patient. *Anesthesiology.* 1979;51:439.
44. King RM, Welch JS, Martin JK, Jr, et al. Carcinoma of the breast associated with pregnancy. *Surg Gynecol Obstet.* 1985;160:228.
45. Donegan WL. Cancer and pregnancy. *CA—A J Clin.* 1983;33:194.
46. Williams DW. Busulfan in early pregnancy. *Obstet Gynecol.* 1966;27:738.
47. Lippman ME. National Institutes of Health Consensus Development Conference on Adjuvant Chemotherapy and Endocrine Therapy for Breast Cancer. National Cancer Institute. Monographs. 1986;1:5.
48. Goldhirsch A. Prolonged disease-free survival after one course of perioperative adjuvant chemotherapy for node-negative breast cancer. *N Engl J Med.* 1989;320:491.
49. Manzour EG, Gray R, Shatila AH, et al. Efficacy of adjuvant chemotherapy in high-risk node-negative breast cancer. *N Engl J Med.* 1989;320:485.
50. Fisher B. A randomized clinical trial evaluating tamoxifen in the treatment of patients with node-negative breast cancer who have estrogen-receptor–positive tumors. *N Engl J Med.* 1989;320:479.
51. Fisher B. A randomized clinical trial evaluating sequential methotrexate and fluorouracil in the treatment of patients with node-negative breast cancer who have estrogen-receptor–negative tumors. *N Engl J Med.* 1989;320:473.
52. Russell LB, Russell WL. Pathways of radiation effects in the mother and the embryo. *Cold Spr Harb Symp Quant Biol.* 1959;19:50.
53. Jacobsen L. Low dose X-irradiation and teratogenesis. A quantitative experimental study, with reference to seasonal influence on dose effects. *Acta Pathol Microbiol Scand.* 1968;193(Suppl):1.
54. Diamond EL, Schmerler H, Lilienfel AM. The relationship of intra-uterine radiation to subsequent mortality and development of leukemia in children: A prospective study. *Am J Epidemiol.* 1973;97:283.
55. Monson RR, MacMahon B. Prenatal x-ray exposure and cancers in children. *Prog Cancer Res Ther.* 1984;26:97.
56. Bithell JF, Stewart AM. Prenatal irradiation and childhood malignancy: a review of British data from the Oxford Survey. *Br J Cancer.* 1975;31:271.
57. Brent RL. Effects of ionizing radiation on growth and development. *Contr Epidemiol Biostat.* 1979;1:147.
58. Shaw EB, Steinbach HL. Aminopterin-induced fetal malformation: survival of infant after attempted abortion. *Am J Dis Child.* 1968;115:477.
59. Baker J, Ali A, Groch MW, et al. Bone scanning in pregnant patients with breast carcinoma. *Clin Nucl Med.* 1987;12:519.
60. Harbert JD. Efficacy of bone and liver scanning in malignant disease: facts and options. In: *Nuclear Medicine Annual.* New York. Raven Press, 1982.
61. Petrick JA. Breast cancer and pregnancy. In: Harris Jr, Hellman S, Henderson IC, Kinne DW, eds. *Breast Diseases.* Philadelphia, PA: JB Lippincott; 1987:600.
62. National Council on Radiation Protection and Measurements (NCRP). *Review of NCRP Radiation Dose Limits for Embryo and Fetus in Occupationally Exposed Women.* Washington, DC: Report 53; 1977;1.
63. Harris JR, Hellman S. Adjuvant Radiotherapy and Conservative Surgery and Radiotherapy, In: Harris JR, Hellman S, Henderson IC, Kinne DW, eds. *Breast Diseases.* Philadelphia: JB Lippincott; 1987:284.
64. Griem KL, Henderson IC, Gelman R, et al. The 5-year results of a randomized trial of adjuvant radiation therapy after chemotherapy in breast cancer patients treated with mastectomy. *J Clin Oncol.* 1987;5:1546.
65. Harrington SW. Three-year to forty-year survival rates following radical mastectomy for carcinoma of the breast. *Wes J Surg Gynecol Obstet.* 1955;63:272.
66. Findlay PA, Gorrell CR, D'Angelo T, Glatstein E. Lactation after breast radiation. *Int J Radiat Oncol Biol Phys.* 1988;15:511.
67. Ulmer HU. Lactation after conserving therapy of breast cancer. *Int J Radiat Oncol Biol Phys.* 1988;15:512.
68. Burns PE. Absence of lactation in a previously radiated breast. *Int J Radiat Biol Phys.* 1987;13:1603.
69. White TT. Prognosis of breast cancer for pregnant and nursing women. Analysis of 49 cases followed 5 years. *Ann Surg.* 1956;144:384.
70. Holleb AI, Farrow JH. The relation of carcinoma of the breast and pregnancy in 283 patients. *Surg Gynecol Obstet.* 1962;115:65.
71. Robinson DW. Breast carcinoma associated with pregnancy. Observations of 1128 cases of breast carcinoma. *Am J Obstet Gynecol.* 1965;92:658.

PART XVIII | Skin, Cartilage, and Bone

Norbert Gleicher, Section Editor

Chapter One Hundred and Ninety

The Skin

Lester J. Fahrner and John C. Murray

190

During pregnancy, many physiologic and pathologic events may be visible on the skin surface. Some are signs of systemic importance, and others are purely cutaneous changes. The patient's response to these alterations varies with her personal anxieties and cosmetic concerns as well as anxiety about the well-being of her fetus. The obstetrician should be knowledgeable about the skin changes associated with pregnancy so that patients may be reassured about the physiologic changes. It is crucial that pathologic cutaneous changes be recognized and appropriately treated. A sense of the normal appearance of skin and appendages, keen observation, as well as familiarity with common dermatologic processes are necessary for understanding skin conditions associated with pregnancy.

The epidermis covers the entire exposed surface of the body except the nailbeds. The function of the epidermal cell is to produce keratin, which forms the stratum corneum. This keratinized covering is the body's main protection from dehydration and from the entry of toxins, infectious agents, and allergens. The mucosal surfaces do not possess a stratum corneum. The dermis is the collagen-rich layer formed by fibroblasts. It provides the base for the epidermis and forms the matrix in which the skin appendages are found. These appendages include the eccrine and apocrine sweat glands, sebaceous glands, nails, hairs, and nerve endings for temperature, pain, and touch. The dermis has a rich vascular plexus, which provides nourishment and assists in regulation of temperature.

DERMATOLOGIC TERMS

Macules are color changes without appreciable elevation above the surrounding skin. Macules include melasma with excess melanin deposition and spider telangiectasia with prominent flat vascularity. Papules are palpable, elevated lesions less than 1 cm in diameter. Papules are variably colored. They can result from edema, cellular infiltrates, or proliferation of cellular material. Nodules are papules greater than 1 cm in diameter. Pustules contain necrotic debris, fibrin, and polymorphonuclear leukocytes. Pustular lesions may be caused by bacteria, or cultures may be sterile. Vesicles are intraepidermal or subepidermal collections of virtually cell-free fluid. Vesicles larger than 1 cm in diameter usually are called bullae. Urticaria (also called hives or wheals) are erythematous, pruritic circumscribed areas of intraepidermal and dermal edema. Ulcers are areas in which epidermis and some dermis are absent secondary to trauma, burn necrosis, or vasculitis. Excoriations are erosions in which the epidermis has been damaged by scratching.

Important etiologic information can be gained from observing the distribution of lesions. The distribution can be appreciated best by examining the entire skin surface without concentrating on individual lesions. Sun-related eruptions characteristically are distributed over the forehead, cheeks, nose, dorsal hands, and forearms. Certain lesions are found only on mucosal surfaces. The intertriginous folds of groin, axillae, and intergluteal cleft are prone to specific conditions.

GENERAL ALTERATIONS OF THE SKIN DURING PREGNANCY

Many alterations in the maternal skin and appendages are discussed in this section. The etiology of these general changes is not well known. They presumably are caused by the changes in hormones, metabolic rate, and vascular volume during gestation.[1,2] Specific changes of the skin pigment and hair that are better understood are described separately. The incidence of these general alterations is variable. Some are almost universal occurrences, whereas others are very rare. No large studies regarding the incidence of these conditions have been done.

Miscellaneous Manifestations

Striae. Striae, or "stretch marks," appear in greater than 90% of women during pregnancy. They appear in the sixth or seventh month of gestation and often are located on the breasts, lower abdomen, and thighs. They are initially pink or purple and later become white. They never disappear but fade and become less noticeable after postpartum weight loss. It is unknown whether they are caused only by simple weight gain and mass effect, or if elevated adrenocortical activity also plays a role. Striae are seen during adolescent growth spurts, and simple obesity.

Vascular Changes

Some of the vascular changes noted in the skin result from increased vascular volume or mechanical impairment of blood return.

Distention of the vasculature is noted easily by examination of the skin. The vestibular and vaginal venous distension (Jacquemier's sign) is an early sign of pregnancy. Varicosities develop on the lower extremities and rectal and vulvar areas. These superficial vascular dilatations can thrombose, although this is relatively unusual in pregnancy. The varicosities regress slightly postpartum.

Palmar erythema from venous and capillary engorgement is noted in about two-thirds of pregnant white women. The presentation is identical to the palmar erythema of "liver palms," hyperthyroidism, and lupus erythematosus. Thenar, hypothenar, or midpalmar areas may be involved in a uniform or patterned distribution. The digits usually are spared. Palmar erythema usually vanishes postpartum. Further investigation is indicated if there is other symptomatology of lupus, liver disease, or hyperthyroidism.

Vascular "spiders" or nevi araneus are found in 66% of white and 11% of black pregnant women. These lesions represent a central dilated arteriole and surrounding tortuous dilated branches. There is often surrounding erythema. A glass microscope slide pressed firmly against the skin blanches them completely, as does a pencil point placed directly on the central vessel. Distribution is generally in the area drained by the superior vena cava. They usually resolve completely 3 months postpartum, and therapy should be avoided.

Capillary hemangiomas frequently develop during pregnancy. They usually are confined to the head or neck. Most often, they appear on the gingivae, where they are known as *pregnancy tumors.* They also are seen on the tongue, eyelid, and upper lip. Preexisting hemangiomas may increase in size during gestation. Capillary hemangiomas usually regress postpartum but do not always recede completely. Residual lesions can be treated with injected steroids, surgery, or laser therapy.

Over 80% of women will have a positive Rumpel–Leede test, especially over the lower extremities. (In the Rumpel–Leede test, application of a tourniquet leads to scattered petechiae as an indication of capillary fragility.) Purpura and scattered petechiae over the lower extremities are common in the last half of pregnancy, presumably because of elevated hydrostatic pressures.

Manifestations of vascular instability are frequent during pregnancy. Short episodes of pallor, facial flushing, and sensations of heat or cold may be noted. Cutis marmorata, a macular reticulated pattern of erythema and pallor, occurs on the lower extremities. During the second half of gestation, dematographism and urticaria are very common. In contrast, patients with Raynaud's phenomenon, episodic vasospasm of the digital arteries, may have abatement of this condition during pregnancy.[3]

Edema

Ankle and leg edema are common, especially late in pregnancy. Nearly 50% of women will develop eyelid edema, with a smaller number having facial edema.

Skin Tumors

A number of benign and malignant cutaneous tumors are influenced by pregnancy. They seem to grow more quickly and develop more frequently, although documentation of this is rare. Pyogenic granulomas and hemangiomas fall into this group. Hemangioendotheliomas and glomus tumors, two other benign tumors of presumed vascular origin, also develop more frequently during pregnancy. Dermatofibromas, cutaneous leiomyomas, keloids, desmoid tumors, neurofibromas, and nevocellular nevi all have been reported to develop or enlarge in gravid women. Malignant melanoma developing during pregnancy has been said to have a worse prognosis, although this has not been proven.

Nail Changes

Transverse grooving of the fingernails has sometimes been noted during pregnancy. Brittleness and distal separation of the nailplate from the nailbed have been reported. Transverse ridging, called *Beau's lines,* can occur as a result of decreased nail synthesis. The relationship to pregnancy and the significance of these findings are unknown.

Eccrine Secretion

The eccrine sweat glands become more active late in pregnancy. The cause of this is not known, but elevated thyroid activity may be involved. This leads to an elevated incidence of milaria, which are tiny epidermal entrapments of sweat. Dyshidrotic hand and foot eczema with hyperhidrotic or clammy skin also can flare during pregnancy.

Apocrine Secretion

Fox–Fordyce disease and hidradenitis suppurativa are inflammatory conditions of the apocrine glands of unknown etiology. They both improve during pregnancy because of the diminution of apocrine sweating. The postpartum rebound can be severe.

Sebaceous Secretion and Acne

There is an increase in sebum secretion late in pregnancy and in the nursing mother. The effect on acne is variable. Some patients' acne actually improves, and in others, acne appears for the first time. Isotretinoin (Accutane) is a known teratogen, and is absolutely contraindicated in pregnant and nursing women. Oral tetracycline can stain deciduous teeth of the fetus and lead to diminished long bone growth. If a woman becomes pregnant while taking tetracycline, prompt discontinuation is usually all that is recommended. The risk to the fetus is not great enough to warrant elective abortion. Topical use of benzoyl peroxide, erythromycin, and clindamycin appear to be safe.[4] Also, no malformations have been reported following use of topical tretinoin (Retin-A) during pregnancy. However, because of its structural similarity to isotretinoin, it should be used with caution.

Pigmentary Alterations of the Skin During Pregnancy

The pigment melanin is primarily responsible for the great differences in cutaneous pigmentation in humans. The only other color determinants are ingested carotenoids as well as oxygenated and deoxygenated hemoglobin in the dermal vasculature. The melanin is made in a specialized epidermal cell, the melanocyte. There is a regional variation in density of melanocytes, and all races have about one melanocyte for every 36 keratinocytes. There is evidence that elevated androgens, estrogens, and melanocyte-stimulating hormone (MSH) levels can lead to a greater number of active melanocytes.

Melanocytes synthesize melanin via a complicated pathway from tyrosine precursors. An insoluble polymer is formed and packaged as melanosomes in Golgi bodies. These packets of pigment are transferred into keratinocytes by the melanocytes' interconnecting dendritic processes.

The ultrastructure and density of melanosomes in keratinocytes determine the intensity and hue of coloration. The melanosome structure varies among the races.

Each individual has an intrinsic level of melanin production and a finite level of inducible function. Exposure to ultraviolet B light (290–320 nm), elevated MSH and ACTH levels, and elevated estrogen and progesterone levels are all known to stimulate melanogenesis. When the stimulus for increased function diminishes, pigment output generally returns to baseline levels.

Generalized Hyperpigmentation

Hyperpigmentation is diffuse darkening of the skin color. More than 90% of pregnant women have hyperpigmentation. The elevated estrogen and progesterone levels of pregnancy stimulate the epidermal melanocytes. Increased melanogenesis produces more melanosomes, which are distributed in the epidermal cells.

Hyperpigmentation varies from generalized darkening of the skin to well-circumscribed macules, particularly on the face and other sun-sxposed areas. Most frequently, there is generalized diffuse darkening of pigment. This can be accompanied by accentuation of the areolae, genital skin, and the linea alba, which extends from the umbilicus to the symphysis pubis. The guinea pig model shows evidence for corresponding geographic subpopulations of melanocytes having increased responsiveness to hormonal stimulation. Areas already hyperpigmented, such as freckles and nevocellular nevi, also can darken during pregnancy. After delivery, these areas can be expected to return to normal intensity of coloration.

The diagnosis is based on clinical observation. Generally, no therapy is required since the coloration regresses spontaneously. Avoiding excessive sun exposure should make hyperpigmentation less noticeable.

Melasma

Melasma, or "the mask of pregnancy," is another frequent expression of increased pigment in pregnancy.[5] The only large study revealed a 70% incidence of melasma in pregnant women. All races are affected equally.

Exposure to natural sunlight may play a role in melasma. Of course, the facial skin is exposed to the same increased hormonal stimulus discussed in the previous section.

The pigment may be located in the epidermis, dermis, or both. Observation in a darkened room under a Wood's lamp will accentuate the contrast between involved and adjacent normal skin if the pigment is in the superficial, epidermal layer. The color differential will not be as noticeable under the Wood's light if the pigment is in the dermis. A biopsy will show the difference clearly, but examination under the Wood's lamp usually is sufficient. The physiologic location for melanin is in the epidermis. With mild inflammation and disruption of the dermal-epidermal junction, pigment can be found in the dermis, usually ingested by macrophages.

The cheeks, forehead, upper lip, nose, and mandible are all potential sites for irregularly margined hyperpigmentation. (Fig. 190–1). The color is generally a uniform medium brown. The area involved can vary considerably from minor to widespread. Generally, the hyperpigmentation will fade after parturition. The melasma may persist or recur with oral contraceptives, although hormonal levels of oral contraceptives generally are not high enough to initiate melasma. A study of nonpregnant women on oral contraceptives with melasma showed normal MSH levels.

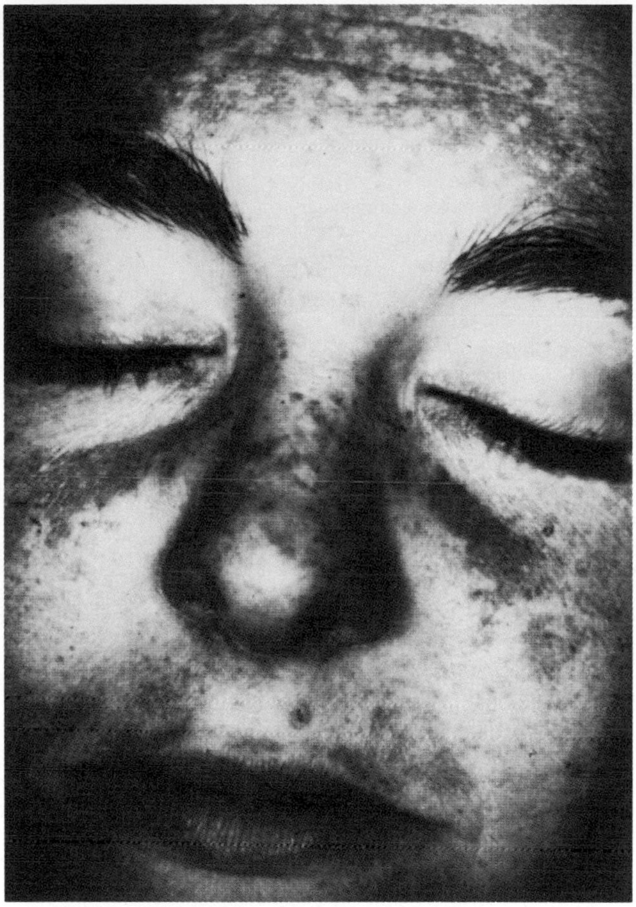

FIGURE 190–1. This patient with melasma demonstrates diffuse macular hyperpigmentation in predominantly sun-exposed areas.

Since most melasma fades spontaneously, usually no treatment is necessary. Avoiding oral contraceptives will increase the likelihood of resolution. For persistent pigmentation, examination under the Wood's lamp to determine the location of the pigment is recommended. Dermal pigment acts as a tattoo and can be refractory to treatment. Epidermal pigment responds to commercially available 2% hydroquinone creams. Retinoic acid 0.5% cream and topical corticosteroid cream are sometimes useful adjuncts. Avoiding excessive sun exposure and use of opaque sunscreens will diminish the stimulus for continued pigment production. Scrubbing and irritation of the lesions must be prohibited.

Hair Alterations in Pregnancy

Both diffuse hair loss (alopecia) and increased hair in locations other than the scalp (hirsutism) are seen in pregnancy.

Hair growth is controlled by both general metabolism and androgenic steroids. The hairs grow in three cycles.[6] In anagen growth, the hair bulb is steadily forming new hair shaft keratin. The anagen or growth phase lasts 2–6 years for individual hairs. A short catagen or transition phase then begins, and the growing bulb involutes over a 2-week span. In the telogen or resting phase, the hair is no longer growing but remains loose in the hair shaft until it falls out. The duration of the telogen phase is generally 3–4 months.

TABLE 190–1. GENODERMATOSES WITH POTENTIAL PRENATAL DIAGNOSIS BY AMNIOCENTESIS

Condition	Inheritance[a]	Method
Keratinizing Disorders		
X-linked ichthyosis	XL	Sex determination
Reisum's disease	AR	Fibroblast culture with abnormal phytanic acid oxidation
Blistering Disorders		
Epidermolysis bullosa simplex	AD	Elevated α-fetoprotein
Photosensitive Conditions		
Ataxia-telangiectasia	AR	Fibroblast culture with increased spontaneous chromosome breakage
Xeroderma pigmentosa	AR	Fibroblast culture with defective DNA repair after UV light
Erythropoietic protoporphyria	AR	Fibroblasts with abnormal porphyrin metabolism
Pigment Defects		
Albinism–deafness syndrome	XL	Sex determination
Abnormal Connective Tissue		
X-linked cutis laxa	XL	Sex determination
Ehlers–Danlos type VI	AR	Fibroblasts with decreased lysyl oxidase
Ehlers–Danlos type VII	AR	Fibroblasts with decreased procollagen peptidase
Miscellaneous		
Menke's syndrome	XL	Sex determination
Anhydrotic ectodermal dysplasia	XL	Sex determination
Fabry's disease	XL	Sex determination; fibroblasts with decreased α-galactosidase A in affected males
Fucosidosis	AR	Fibroblasts with diminished fucosidase activity

[a] Abbreviations used: XL, X-linked recessive; AR, autosomal-recessive; AD, autosomal-dominant.
Modified with permission from Esterly and Elias.[10]

Postpartum Telogen Effluvium

During pregnancy, an increased percentage of hairs are growing in the anagen phase.[7] The impression of increased hair growth is related to the prolonged anagen phase, with decreased numbers of hairs entering the catagen and telogen phases. After delivery, there is a rapid change to the catagen and telogen phases. Appreciable thinning of the hair can occur since a large number of follicles will all be empty at once. About 50% of the hair must be lost before alopecia becomes detectable. Postpartum telogen effluvium is usu-

TABLE 190–2. GENODERMATOSES WITH POTENTIAL PRENATAL DIAGNOSIS BY FETOSCOPY AND SKIN BIOPSY

Condition	Inheritance[a]	Method
Keratinizing Disorders		
Harlequin ichthyosis	AR	Premature keratinization
Lamellar ichthyosis	AR	Premature keratinization
Epidermolytic hyperkeratosis	AD	Epidermal acantholysis
Sjögren–Larsson syndrome	AR	Premature keratinization
Netherton's syndrome	AR	Premature keratinization, abnormal hair structure
Trichothiodystrophy	AR	Premature keratinization, hair shows trichoschisis and twists
Chondrodysplasia punctata	AR	Hyperkeratosis
Blistering Disorders		
Epidermolysis bullosa simplex	AR	Intraepidermal blisters
Epidermolysis bullosa letalis	AR	Dermal-epidermal blister
Epidermolysis bullosa dystrophica recessive	AR	Subepidermal blister
Epidermolysis bullosa dystrophica dominant	AD	Subepidermal blister
Pigment Defects		
Oculocutaneous albinism	AR	Negative hair bulb tyrosinase
Hermansky–Pudlak syndrome	AR	Cutaneous ceroid deposition
Chediak–Higashi syndrome	AR	Giant melanosomes, blood sample with azurophilic granules
Tuberous sclerosis	AD	Leukocytes show increased sensitivity to irradiation
Miscellaneous		
Hypohidrotic ectodermal dysplasia	XL	Affected males show decreased eccrine glands and hair follicles
	AR	Decreased eccrine glands and hair follicles

[a] Abbreviations used: XL, X-linked recessive; AR, autosomal recessive; AD, autosomal dominant.
Modified with permission from Esterly and Elias.[10]

ally most obvious at the anterior hairline. The sparseness is diffuse, with scattered normal hairs. This hair loss is temporary, as follicles gradually will revert to anagen growth phase. A similar situation with transient thinning of the hair occurs after severe metabolic stress induced by major illness, surgery, or emotional trauma. A recent study reported a falling percentage of anagen hairs over the course of high-risk pregnancies compared with normal pregnancies. The authors speculated that this may reflect a time-integrated response to falling trophic hormones and may represent a useful clinical parameter in high-risk pregnancies. Further study of this suggestion is warranted.[8]

The number of women affected is unknown, but both postpartum hair loss and gestational hypertrichosis are common.

In the patient complaining of postpartum hair loss, the hairs will be removed easily from the scalp by gentle traction. This phenomenon is of concern to the patient. She should be reassured that hair regrowth will occur soon. No therapy is necessary or useful in the treatment of postpartum alopecia. Patients may shampoo as often as necessary. They are advised to use a conditioner and to avoid hair trauma such as electric blow drying or combing wet hair.

Hirsutism

Hirsutism may occur during the third trimester. Dark hairs appear on the upper lip, chin, areolae, and elsewhere. This may be accompanied by other signs of virilization such as deep voice, clitoral enlargement, and severe acne. When these signs of virilization with severe hirsutism occur during pregnancy, full endocrinologic evaluation is indicated. The hirsutism of pregnancy generally resolves spontaneously postpartum, although depilatory creams, electrolysis, or simple plucking can be used in persistent hirsutism.

ANTENATAL DIAGNOSIS OF GENODERMATOSES

A number of genetically transmitted skin diseases have been well characterized biochemically or morphologically. The diagnostic criteria used in adults can be used on fetal cells to detect potentially affected offspring.[9] The majority of illnesses are so rare that they seldom are encountered in obstetric practice. The techniques of amniocentesis and fetoscopy can provide fibroblasts, fetal blood samples, and skin biopsy specimens.[10] These tissues then can be processed appropriately to diagnose or exclude the disease for which the fetus is at risk. As with any other procedure, the potential benefit and management options must be weighed against the dangers. Accurate and confirmed diagnosis of maternal disease in previous pregnancies is mandatory for case selections.

Tables 190–1 and 190–2 are adapted from the article by Esterly and Elias.[10] They include the genetically transmitted dermatoses that potentially could be diagnosed prenatally. Amniocentesis and fetoscopy have been performed in a number of these diseases. Amniocentesis has been employed successfully to diagnose or exclude congenital erythropoietic prophyria, xeroderma pigmentosum, epidermolysis bullosa simplex, and ataxia-telangiectasia. Fetoscopy with fetal skin biopsy has been used to demonstrate harlequin ichthyosis, epidermolytic hyperkeratosis, and epidermolysis bullosa. Further experience will determine the proper role of these techniques in the genodermatoses.[4-14]

REFERENCES

1. Fitzpatrick TB, Eisen AZ, Wolff K, et al. *Dermatology in General Medicine.* New York: McGraw-Hill; 1979;131, 1395–1363.
2. Winton GB, Lewis CW. Dermatoses of pregnancy. *J Am Acad Dermatol.* 1982;6:977.
3. Cook WA. Raynaud phenomenon in pregnancy. *JAMA* 1976;235:145.
4. Rothman KF, Pochi PE. Use of oral and topical agents for acne in pregnancy. *J Am Acad Dermatol.* 1988;19:431.
5. Sanchez NP, Pathak MA, Sato S, et al. Melasma: a clinical, light microscopic, ultrastructural and immunofluorescent study. *J Am Acad Dermatol.* 1981;4:698.
6. Rook A, Dawber R. *Diseases of the Hair and Scalp.* Oxford: Blackwell Scientific Publications; 1982;84,123.
7. Lynfield YA. Effect of pregnancy on the human hair cycle. *J Invest Dermatol.* 1960;35:323.
8. Wilkin JK, Saldana LR, Aris J. Anagen ratios in high-risk pregnancies. *Cutis.* 1983;31:71.
9. Hall JG. Prenatal diagnosis of inherited skin diseases. *Birth Defects.* 1981;17(2):243.
10. Esterly NB, Elias S. Antenatal diagnosis of genodermatoses. *J Am Acad Dermatol.* 1983;8:655.
11. Anton-Lamprecht I. Prenatal diagnosis of genetic disorders of the skin by electron microscopy. *Hum Genet.* 1981;59:392.
12. Gosden C. Prenatal diagnosis of genodermatoses using amniotic fluid cells and DNA analysis. *Curr Probl Dermatol.* 1987;16:65.
13. Anton-Lamprecht I, Arnold ML. Prenatal diagnosis of inherited epidermolyses. *Curr Probl Dermatol.* 1987;16:146.
14. Elias S. Use of fetoscopy for the prenatal diagnosis of hereditary skin disorders. *Curr Probl Dermatol.* 1987;16:1.

Chapter One Hundred and Ninety-One
Antecedent Skin Conditions

Lester J. Fahrner and John C. Murray

191

The childbearing years in general are a period of good health. However, occasional patients with preexisting skin diseases will be encountered in the practice of obstetrics. These will range from common diseases such as psoriasis to rare conditions such as pemphigus vulgaris. In the less common entities, information is mainly anecdotal. Complete discussion of the etiology and pathology of the conditions described below exceeds the scope of this text.[1]

PSORIASIS

Psoriasis affects about 1% of the general population. The well-demarcated, raised erythematous plaques can occur virtually anywhere on the body. Areas of rubbing and trauma are affected most often. Lesions are found most often on the scalp, elbows, knees, genitalia, and buttocks. The cause of the benign epidermal hyperproliferation is not known.

In cases with small areas of involvement, topical corticosteroids and coal tar are the most common treatments. Topical anthralin, a coal tar derivative, is becoming increasingly popular. Widespread psoriasis vulgaris is treated variously with ultraviolet B light, oral psoralens with UVA light (PUVA), or oral methotrexate.

Psoriasis improves in approximately 50% of women during pregnancy. The reason for this is unknown, although presumably it is related to the hormonal changes of pregnancy. Psoriasis recurs, but postpartum flare is not described. Treatment of women of childbearing potential with PUVA and methotrexate is contraindicated. During pregnancy, patients whose psoriasis does not remit should be treated with topical agents or ultraviolet B light.

ATOPIC DERMATITIS

Atopic dermatitis is an intensely pruritic skin condition often found in conjunction with the other allergic diatheses, asthma, and hay fever. A variety of inciting factors, such as allergens, stress, and irritants, can trigger pruritis. The skin is dry, often scaly, and lichenified from repeated rubbing and scratching. In adults, flexural folds are affected most often. Atopic dermatitis is responsive to steroids. However, the chronicity of the condition requires therapeutic alternatives such as avoidance of any known irritating agents and liberal use of emollients to avoid steroid side-effects. Atopic dermatitis is said to remit occasionally during pregnancy.

ACRODERMATITIS ENTEROPATHICA

Acrodermatitis enteropathica is an inherited defect in intestinal zinc absorption that leads to diarrhea and dermatitis of the perineum, perioral region, and periungual skin. Treatment with pharmacologic doses of oral zinc is effective. The increased metabolic demands of pregnancy and changes in estrogen levels can lead to clinical relapse, which responds to an increased dose of oral zinc.[2]

ERYTHEMA NODOSUM

Erythema nodosum is a panniculitic reaction to a variety of antigens that is manifested by recurrent, painful, erythematous nodules over the shins. These nodules resolve spontaneously without scarring. The list of agents causing erythema nodosum is extensive and includes bacteria, mycobacteria, parasites, viral infections, drugs, and many more. Most frequently, the etiology of erythema nodosum remains unknown even after extensive investigation. In idiopathic erythema nodosum, symptoms may become worse during pregnancy. Conventional therapy includes bed rest, salicylates, propranolol, supersaturated potassium iodide, and steroids. The concern for fetal health would probably make a short course of steroids the therapy of choice during pregnancy.

ERYTHEMA MULTIFORME

Erythema multiforme is another type of reaction to a vast number of antigens including those implicated in erythema nodosum. This reaction pattern is characterized by target lesions, urticaria, and erythema. Lesions may appear anywhere on the body but classically occur on the palms and soles. Lesions resolve without scarring. The attacks of idiopathic erythema multiforme can be more frequent during pregnancy. Therapy is with oral antihistamines and steroids.

CONDYLOMA ACCUMINATA

Condyloma accuminata can grow rapidly during pregnancy. Even obstruction of the introitus can occur. The usual treatment for veneral warts, tincture of podophyllin, is potentially neurotoxic when absorbed after application to large surfaces. Two cases of fetal death have resulted from podophyllin applied to large condyloma accuminata. Delivery through a birth canal infected by human papillomavirus may transmit warts to the newborn child. The newborn may acquire laryngeal papillomas, which are difficult to treat and may be fatal.[3] Despite this, the risk seems to be relatively low, making routine cesarean section to avoid contact with genital warts imprudent. Condyloma accuminata should be treated effectively with cryosurgery or laser surgery before delivery. Cesarean section may be necessary when there is widespread involvement.

LEPROSY

Leprosy is a chronic infectious disease of the skin caused by *Mycobacterium leprae.* The disease often worsens during pregnancy. An increased incidence of low birth weight and high infant mortality has been reported. Leprosy is treated with dapsone and clofazimine. The immunologic reactions that occur in leprosy are treated with prednisone or thalidomide. Pregnant patients with leprosy will require careful evaluation of the state of the disease and careful choice of antileprosy therapy.[2]

MELANOMA

Malignant melanoma *in situ* (still confined to the epidermis) is a surgically curable disease. There is no change in the survival rate when melanoma *in situ* occurs during pregnancy. The outlook for patients with malignant melanoma involving the dermis or other tissues during pregnancy is worse than that of the population at large.[4] Early detection of melanoma through examination and biopsy of suggestive pigmented lesions is necessary to improve survival rate. A recent report describes increased incidence of superficial spreading melanoma with oral contraceptive use[5] (see also Chapter 179).

CONNECTIVE TISSUE DISEASES

The effects of pregnancy on lupus erythematosus, progressive systemic sclerosis, dermatomyositis, and Behcet's disease have been described (see Chapters 51 and 52). Many of the initial findings that suggest these conditions are cutaneous. The rashes of connective tissue diseases should be treated by sun avoidance, use of sunscreen, and mild topical steroids during pregnancy.

PEMPHIGUS VULGARIS

Pemphigus vulgaris and pemphigus foliaceous are uncommon blistering diseases, usually found in older patients. Clinically, pemphigus is somewhat similar to herpes gestationis, but immunofluorescent studies are characteristic and show antibody to epidermal intercellular substance. The onset of pemphigus has been reported during pregnancy in a few patients; however, timing of onset seems to be coincidental. Four stillborn children of mothers with pemphigus vulgaris had skin lesions and direct immunofluorescent findings similar to the maternal disease, showing that the anti-intercellular–cement substance antibodies can cross the placenta.[6] There does seem to be significant fetal risk of stillbirth in patients with pemphigus.[7] Treatment is with high-dose oral steroids, and when required, cytotoxic medications.

HEREDITARY ANGIONEUROTIC EDEMA

Hereditary angioneurotic edema (HAE or HANE) is a rare autosomal-dominant disease with recurrent episodes of facial and laryngeal edema. These patients have a deficiency of C_1 esterase inhibitor, important in the regulation of the complement cascade. Shock and laryngeal obstruction can occur during pregnancy, probably with no increased incidence. The peripartum period can be dangerous. Treatment with purified C_1 esterase inhibitor concentrate and oxygen, or possibly tracheostomy, can be life-saving. Attacks are variably responsive to steroids, antihistamines, or epinephrine. Long-term prophylaxis with androgens, which stimulate endogenous esterase inhibitor production, can minimize attacks. The virilizing effect on the fetus has to be weighed against the risk of airway obstruction in the mother, depending on the frequency and severity of attacks.[8]

STEROID SULFATASE DEFICIENCY

Females with steroid sulfatase deficiency show no clinical abnormality. However, in pregnancy, they have consistently low urinary estriol excretion. Onset of labor often is delayed and has to be induced. The male children of these deliveries have a widespread ichthyosis that develops at age 3–12 months. The inheritance pattern is overwhelmingly X-linked.[9] The condition is not serious enough to warrant advising sterilization or abortion of future pregnancies.

EPIDERMOLYSIS BULLOSA

Epidermolysis bullosa (EB) is not a single disease, but a group of mechanobullous disorders. At least 16 subtypes have been described. They share several features: a definable inheritance pattern; development of blisters and erosions at points of frictional trauma from often trivial pressure; and the absence of one of the chemical and physical entities that bind the epidermis onto the dermis. Some of the subtypes also reflect the cutaneous abnormality with involvement of gastrointestinal epithelium, and some heal with scarring. EB varies from being troublesome to being a severe disabling and disfiguring disease. For those who can be determined to be at risk for bearing children with one of the devastating forms, prenatal diagnostic testing by fetal skin biopsy should be performed. Some forms of EB then can be diagnosed rapidly or excluded by immunoelectronmicroscopy or immunopathologic techniques.[10]

EHLERS–DANLOS SYNDROME

Ehlers–Danlos syndrome is a group of closely related inherited disorders of collagen synthesis with varying clinical manifestations. The inheritance pattern is variably autosomal-dominant, autosomal-recessive, or sporadic. Signs include loose skin, joint hypermobility, easy bruising, and poor wound healing. Mothers with Ehlers–Danlos syndrome type IV, in particular, face a potentially complicated course during pregnancy, with increased risk of hematoma formation, rupture of major arteries, wound dehiscence, premature delivery, and large tears from forceps delivery.[11] Presenting clinical features of type IV Ehlers–Danlos include very thin skin and large ecchymoses. Previous spontaneous rupture of bowel or major arteries may have occurred. Only the finger joints are detectably hyperextensible. In the other types of Ehlers–Danlos syndrome, a variety of peripartum complications can be encountered, including hemorrhage, joint dislocations, back pain, and dehiscence of closures of episiotomies and cesarean incisions. Premature rupture of membranes leading to premature delivery is common in Ehlers–Danlos syndrome.

PSEUDOXANTHOMA ELASTICUM

Pseudoxanthoma elasticum is an inherited disorder of the skin, eyes, gut, and arterial system. Elastic fibers are chemically and physically abnormal. The disorder is transmitted variously as an autosomal-dominant or autosomal-recessive trait. Outside of pregnancy, problems with epistaxis and recurrent multifocal gastrointestinal hemorrhage are the most common problems. The skin of the neck and antecubital fossae shows laxity and has a characteristic yellow hue and pebbly surface, often referred to as "chicken skin." Ocular problems include retinal hemorrhage and macular degeneration, sometimes resulting in blindness.

Potentially catastrophic hemorrhagic events can occur during pregnancy. Careful monitoring of blood pressure, cardiac, and renal function is mandatory. Most pregnancies are surprisingly normal, although the potential for spontaneous abortion, intrauterine growth retardation, and severe postpartum hemorrhage exists.[12]

MARFAN'S SYNDROME

Marfan's syndrome (see also Chapters 36 and 134), with tall stature, ectopia lentis, and a characteristic long-legged habitus, also is associated with dilation of the aortic root and dissecting aneurysms. It is transmitted as an autosomal-dominant trait with a high degree of penetrance. New mutations, with a negative family history, are also common. With the increased vascular volume of pregnancy, the risk of aortic aneurysmal rupture is increased. Therapeutic abortion and surgical sterilization have been advocated, although many women with Marfan's syndrome will have uneventful pregnancies. Frequent assessment of cardiac status, blood pressure, and ultrasonic evaluation of the diameter of the aortic root are mandatory.

NEUROFIBROMATOSIS

Neurofibromatosis, von Recklinghausen's disease, is characterized by multiple neurofibromas and café-au-lait spots. Pregnancy has been noted to increase the size of the neurofibromas, and partial regression has been observed postpartum. Neurofibromas can be cutaneous or located in the central nervous system. Enlargement can cause a variety of local effects or lead to new onset of potentially drastic neurologic defects. The incidence of abortion and stillbirth is very high.[13,14] Hypertension is a common management problem. Neurofibromatosis is transmitted as a classic Mendelian autosomal-dominant disease with variable penetrance. For those most severely affected, surgical sterilization generally is recommended.

REFERENCES

1. Fitzpatrick TB, Eisen AZ, Wolff K, et al. *Dermatology in General Medicine*. New York, NY: McGraw-Hill; 1979:1363.
2. Winton GB. Skin diseases aggravated by pregnancy. *J Am Acad Dermatol*. 1989;20:1.
3. Cook TA, Cohn AM, Brunschwig JP, et al. Wart viruses and laryngeal papillomas. *Lancet*. 1973;1:782.
4. Shiu MH, Schottenfield D, MacLean B, et al. Adverse effect of pregnancy on melanoma. *Cancer*. 1976;37:181.
5. Holly Ea, Weiss NS, Liff JM. Cutaneous melanoma in relation to exogenous hormones and reproductive factors. *J Natl Cancer Inst*. 1983;70:827.
6. Hup Jm, Bruinsma RA, et al. Neonatal pemphigus vulgaris: transplacental transmission of antibodies. *Pediatric Dermatol*. 1986;3:468.
7. Ross MG, Kane B, Frieder R, et al. Pemphigus in pregnancy: a reevaluation of fetal risk. *Am J Obstet Gynecol*. 1986;155:30.
8. Chappatte O, DeSwiet M. Hereditary angioneurotic oedema and pregnancy: case reports and review of the literature. *Br J Obstet Gynaecol*. 1988;95:938.
9. Bradshaw KD, Carr BR. Placental sulfatase deficiency: maternal and fetal expression of steroid sulfatase deficiency and x-linked ichthyosis. *Obstet Gynecol Surv*. 1986;41:401.
10. Price T, Katz VL. Obstetrical concerns of epidermolysis bullosa. *Obstet Gynecol Surv*. 1988;43:445.
11. Peaceman AM, Cruikshank DP. Ehlers-Danlos syndrome and pregnancy: association of type IV disease with maternal death. *Obstet Gynaecol*. 1987;69:428.
12. Viljoen DL, Beatty S, Beighton P. The obstetric and gynecological implications of pseudoxanthoma elasticum. *Br J Obstet Gynecol*. 1987;94:884.
13. Swapp G, Main RA. Neurofibromatosis in pregnancy. *Br J Dermatol*. 1973;88:431.
14. Ansari AH, Nagamani M. Pregnancy and neurofibromatosis. *Obstet Gynecol*. 1976;47:25s.

Chapter One Hundred and Ninety-Two
Cutaneous Conditions With General Medical Significance

Lester Fahrner and John C. Murray

192

Several skin diseases are unique to pregnancy. Our understanding of them has benefited greatly from the advances of the last few years, although much is still unknown.

HERPES GESTATIONIS

Maternal Aspects

Herpes gestationis is a blistering disease confined to pregnancy and the immediate postpartum period. Despite the name, there is no link to the herpes viruses. The incidence is thought to be between 1 in 3000 and 1 in 50,000 pregnancies. It is rare enough that estimation of incidence is very difficult.[1]

Most patients exhibit a circulating "herpes gestationis factor," a complement-fixing IgG. The autoantibody is directed against a component of the basement membrane in the dermal-epidermal junction.[2] The IgG binds to the antigen in the basement membrane and fixes complement of both the classical and alternative pathways. The earliest microscopic change is basal cell necrosis. When basilar necrosis is widespread, blister formation at the dermal-epidermal junction is seen. Other histologic changes include dermal edema and spongiosis. Lymphocytes, histiocytes, and eosinophils infiltrate around the superficial and deep dermal vessels.

Immunofluorescent studies show a band of C3 with or without IgG along the basement membrane. Less often, IgA, IgM, Clq, C4, C5, or properdin can be detected. The circulating herpes gestationis factor can be detected only by complement indirect immunofluorescent testing.

Herpes gestationis may occur any time during pregnancy or even a few days postpartum. Fever, hot and cold sensations, malaise, nausea, headache, and pruritus often signal the onset of disease. The rash begins as erythema and urticarial plaques, most often on the abdomen (Figure 192–1). Besides the typical abdominal location, the buttocks, back, forearms, and genitalia can be involved. Mucous membrane involvement is rare. The plaques develop into tense vesicles and bullae. They rupture and leave denuded areas. Secondary infection or excoriation can lead to scarring, although the only intrinsic cutaneous sequela is postinflammatory hyperpigmentation. The only consistent laboratory abnormality is leukocytosis with eosinophilia up to 50%.

Before blisters develop, the urticarial plaques may be confused with pruritic urticarial papules and plaques of pregnancy. However, later in the course, the diseases are

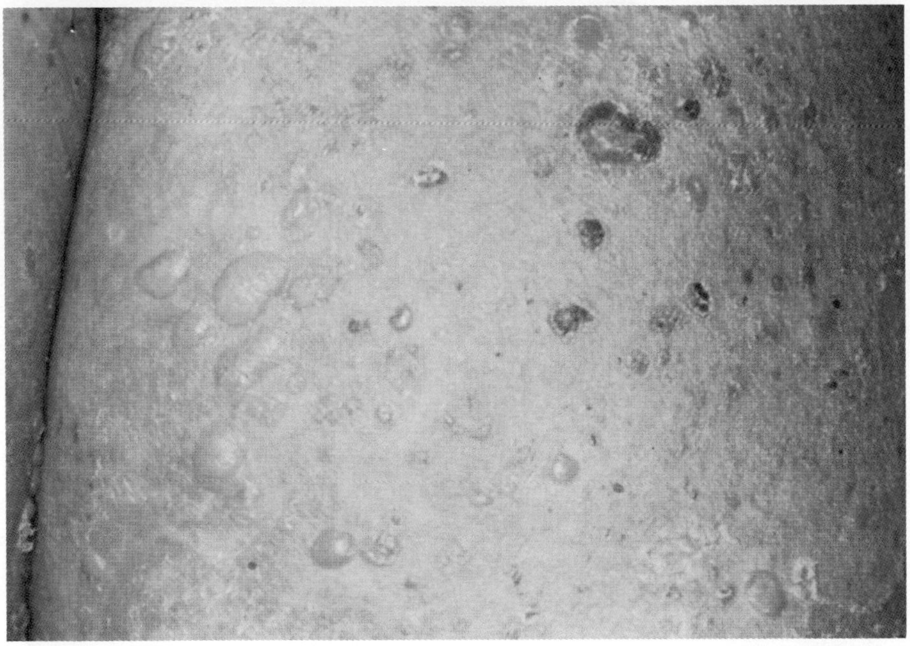

FIGURE 192–1. Multiple vesicles and erythematous plaques on the buttocks of a patient with herpes gestationis.

easily differentiated clinically and histologically. The other blistering diseases, such as bullous drug eruptions, erythema multiforme, bullous pemphigoid, pemphigus vulgaris, dermatitis herpetiformis, and pemphigus foliaceous, occur only rarely and incidentally in pregnancy. They can be distinguished from herpes gestationis with histologic and immunologic testing.

Mild cases respond to topical fluorinated steroids and antihistamines. Refractory cases usually require prednisone, 40 mg per day, tapering off to alternate-day steroids after clearing. Maintenance on oral steroids is sometimes necessary until parturition. Few patients need the addition of azathioprine, which must be used with caution.

Clearing can be expected within 3 months of delivery. Late exacerbations have been described following the normal resumption of menses and after administration of progesteron-containing oral contraceptives. Herpes gestationis usually recurs with earlier onset and more widespread involvement during subsequent pregnancies.

Fetal Aspects

The maternal herpes gestationis factor passes through the placental circulation and binds to the fetal skin, causing blisters.[3,4] The pathology is the same as in maternal disease. The herpes gestationis antibody does not bind to the placental membranes.

Of 36 live births to mothers with herpes gestationis reviewed, four had skin lesions and laboratory findings consistent with the disease.[5] Of 40 females with herpes gestationis, there were three stillbirths, one spontaneous abortion at 4.5 months, and nine premature deliveries. Most importantly, there is increased fetal mortality in mothers with herpes gestationis. Premature births, spontaneous rupture of membranes, spontaneous abortions, and stillbirths all occur. It is unclear if these conditions are increased significantly in herpes gestationis. The causes of these conditions have not been elucidated. Children can present with skin lesions of herpes gestationis at birth.

Once the skin lesions have been detected and diagnosed in the child, usually no therapy is required, although topical steroids can be employed.

PRURITIC URTICARIAL PAPULES AND PLAQUES OF PREGNANCY

Maternal Aspects

Pruritic urticarial papules and plaques of pregnancy (PUPPP) was first described in 1978.[6] It is a distinctive pruritic eruption confined to pregnancy. Fewer than 100 cases have been reported, and the true incidence is not known. It probably is relatively common. Several of the less well defined rashes of pregnancy discussed below may resemble PUPPP and may be clinical subsets of the same process.

The cause of the disease is unknown, and the pathogenesis is unknown. Skin biopsy shows changes typical of urticaria, with dermal edema, epidermal spongiosis, and a superficial lymphohistiocytic infiltrate. Eosinophils may be present. Immunofluorescent staining is negative for complement and immunoglobulins. The eruption begins late in pregnancy. Erythematous blanching papules and urticarial plaques are noted initially on the abdomen and in striae. Pruritus is present. The lesions can enlarge and spread to include the thighs, buttocks, and upper arms (Figures 192–2, 192–3). There are no known systemic symptoms. The lesions clear promptly postpartum. No laboratory abnormalities have been described.

Diagnosis is made by clinical presentation and skin biopsy.[7]

Topical fluorinated steroids and oral antihistamines usually control the pruritus. A short oral prednisone taper may be required.

Fetal Aspects

Fetal skin involvement has been reported, but no increase in malformations, stillbirths, or prematurity is evident.[8]

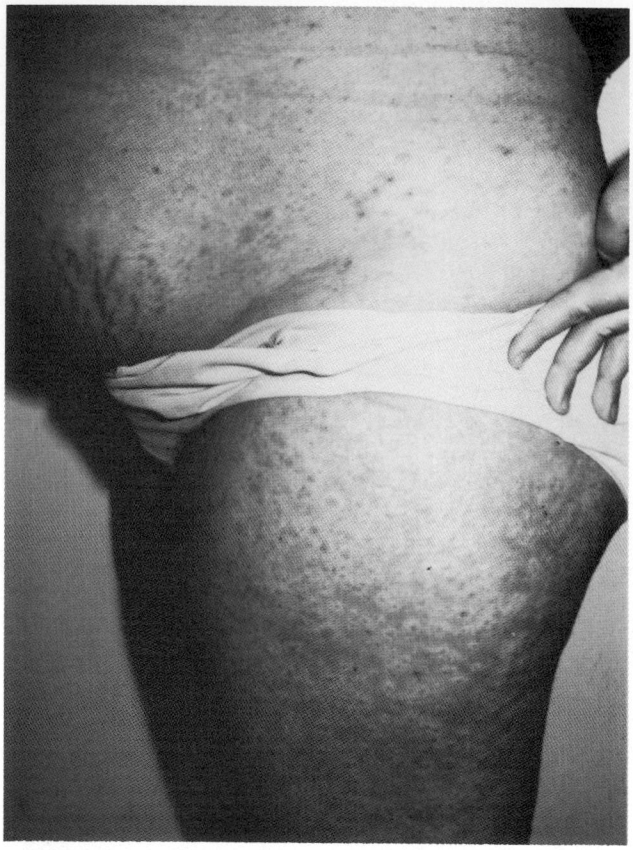

FIGURE 192–2. Pregnant patient with erythematous papules on trunk and legs. (*Courtesy of University of North Carolina Department of Dermatology.*)

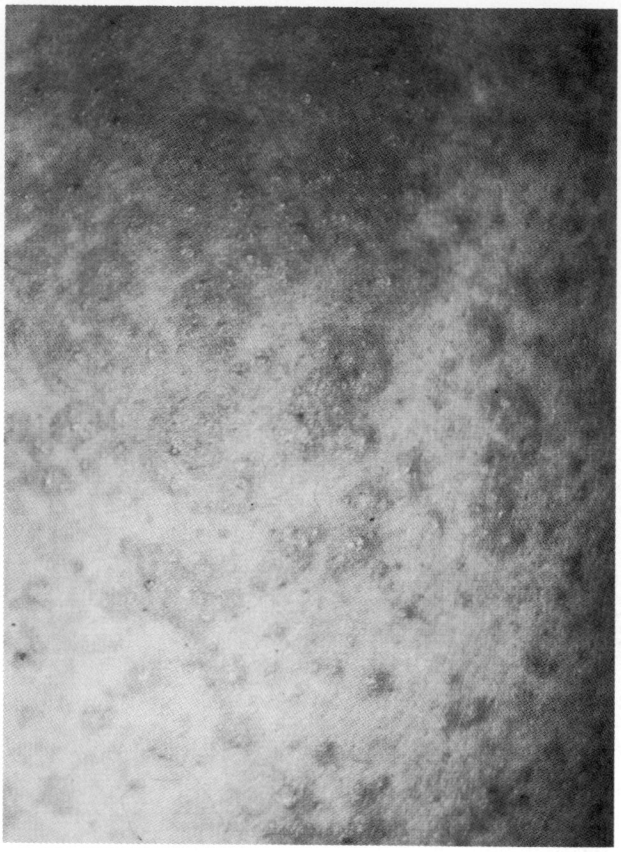

FIGURE 192–3. Close-up of lesions of patient in Figure 192–2. (*Courtesy of University of North Carolina Department of Dermatology.*)

IMPETIGO HERPETIFORMIS

Maternal Aspects

Impetigo herpetiformis is a misleading term. It is neither a bacterial nor a viral disease. It is the name given to a condition identical to pustular psoriasis seen in pregnant patients who have not previously had psoriasis.[9] About 300 cases have been reported from North America and Europe.

The etiology is unknown. Hypoparathyroidism and hypocalcemia have been noted in patients, but their contribution is speculative. Hypocalcemia can aggravate ordinary pustular psoriasis.

Histologic examination demonstrates large collections of neutrophils as pustules or large "lakes." Parakeratosis, elongation of the rete ridges, and mononuclear cells occur in the epidermis. These findings also are seen in pustular psoriasis.

Onset is usually in the third trimester, often with dramatic systemic symptoms. Malaise, fever, diarrhea, delirium, tetany from hypocalcemia, dehydration, and convulsions all have been reported. Large fluid losses can occur both from the diarrhea and the large areas of denuded epidermal barrier.

Erythematous patches ringed with pustules begin in the intertriginous areas. Vritually the entire body may be covered. The lesions extend by peripheral growth. The skin overlying the pustules ruptures, leaving a central denuded area and a ring of adherent scale (Figure 191–4). Subungual pustules may cause onycholysis. Mucous membrane can also occur.

Leukocytosis and elevated erythrocyte sedimentation rate are common. Cultures of the pustules are negative. Hypocalcemia from hypoparathyroidism is present in some patients. The history and examination with routine cultures and skin biopsy should clearly delineate impetigo herpetiformis.

Prednisone, 15–30 mg per day by mouth, is the recommended treatment. Antibiotics are useful only in cases with secondary infection. Fluids and electrolytes, especially calcium, should be monitored and normalized. Before steroids and antibiotics were available, maternal mortality and fetal wastage were high. Now maternal mortality is rare, but stillbirths still occur, even when maternal disease is controlled. Assessment of fetal well-being should be frequent, with early delivery if indicated and possible. Postpartum remission is the rule, with recurrence possible during later pregnancies.

Fetal Aspects

There is a high incidence of stillbirths. There is no known cutaneous involvement in the fetus.

GENERALIZED CHOLESTATIC PRURITUS OF PREGNANCY

Maternal Aspects

Pruritus, or itching, is one of the most common dermatologic complaints during pregnancy. The pruritus associated

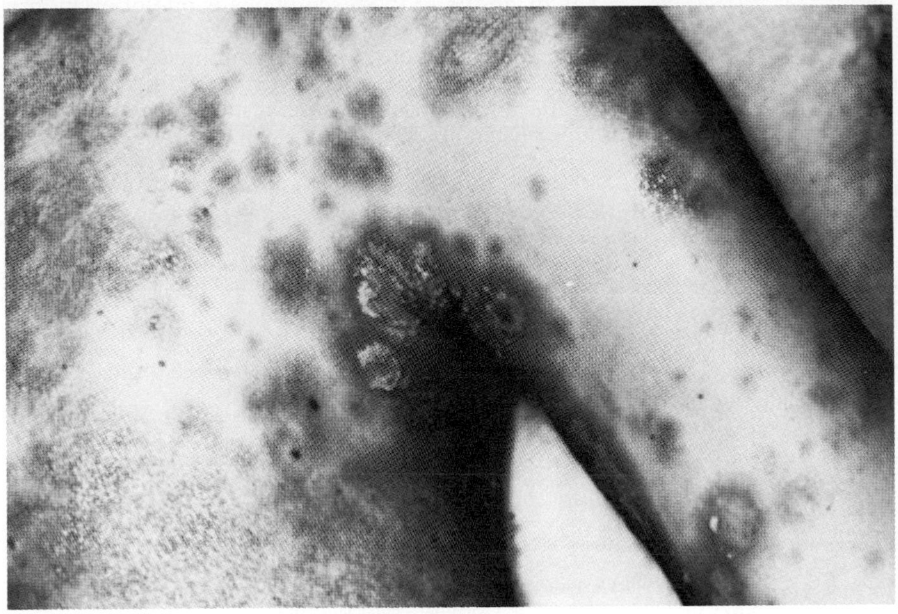

FIGURE 192–4. Eroded confluent pustules with crusting on the shoulder in impetigo herpetiformis.

with antecedent atopic dermatitis, dry skin, and chronic urticaria is common and should be managed as in the absence of pregnancy. Pruritus gravidarum is unique to pregnancy. Pruritus gravidarum is pruritus from nonicteric cholestasis.

Gestational levels of estrogens and progestens are thought to interfere with hepatic excretion of bile acids. Estrogens diminish fluid exchange across the hepatocyte canalicular membrane. Progestens inhibit glucuronyltransferase and decrease hepatic clearance of estrogen. Pruritus correlates with circulating bile acid levels. The condition presumably occurs in those with genetic susceptibility to cholestasis of pregnancy.

Reported incidence of pruritus gravidarum varies from 0.02% to 2.4% of pregnancies.[10] It is important to exclude the other frequent causes of pruritus, as 17% of all pregnant women will have pruritus.

Onset occurs in the third trimester with severe generalized pruritus. There are no papules, vesicles, or pustules. Excoriations are evidence of the severity of this symptom. In full-blown cholestasis of pregnancy, jaundice will be noted.

Laboratory testing is usually negative in all but the most severe cases. Liver function tests are normal or mildly elevated. The lactate dehydrogenase, alkaline phosphatase, SGOT, SGPT, and bilirubin are affected to varying degrees. Liver biopsy shows nonspecific cholestasis with dilated bile canaliculi and staining of hepatocytes with bile pigments.

The diagnosis is one of exclusion except in cases with laboratory abnormalities. Scabies, lice, and candidiasis need to be excluded by careful examination. In the cases with icteric cholestasis, other causes of hepatitis need to be excluded. Differentiation is made on the more prominent abdominal and systemic symptomatology in viral, toxic, and obstructive hepatitis and by greater laboratory abnormality. Potentially hepatotoxic drugs should be discontinued if possible. Only rarely should liver biopsy be required.

Traditional topical therapy for pruritus is often successful in treating pruritus gravidarum. These should include olive oil and lime water emulsion with menthol, oatmeal baths, or bland emollients. Oral antihistamines such as diphenhydramine and chlorpheniramine are effective and have been shown to be apparently safe during decades of widespread use during pregnancy. More severe cases have proven responsive to cholestyramine, an ion exchange resin that binds bile acids in the gut. This decreases enterohepatic circulation and serum bile acid levels. Four grams by mouth two or three times daily have been effective.

There are no known preventative measures. The pruritus clears rapidly postpartum. Recurrences with subsequent pregnancies or oral contraceptive use have been noted, although some women are not affected in later pregnancies.

Fetal Aspects

In cases with cholestatic jaundice, there is a higher incidence of premature labor, low birth weight, and postpartum hemorrhage. In cases with only pruritus, a tendency toward early delivery and meconium staining has been noted.

OTHER PRURITIC DERMATOSES OF PREGNANCY

There are several other less well-characterized skin conditions that occur solely during pregnancy. They are discussed here briefly because of their rarity and probable overlap with other described conditions.[11] Causes are largely unknown and are discussed with the individual diseases. Pathologic findings are disparate and often nonspecific, leading to diagnostic confusion.

Autoimmune Progesterone Dermatitis of Pregnancy

A single case of autoimmune progesterone dermatitis in pregnancy (APDP) has been reported.[12] The patient had the explosive onset of acneiform lesions on the limbs and buttocks. There was arthritis of the metacarpophalangeal joints, wrists, knees, and ankles. The disease recurred in a later pregnancy with spontaneous abortion in both cases. Oral contraceptives also resulted in a recurrence. Intradermal progesterone led to abscess formation with no response to estrogen.

Prurigo Gestationis

Prurigo gestationis differs from pruritus gravidarum in that prurigo gestationis presents with papules on the limbs and abdomen. This condition is probably a subset of PUPPP.

Toxemic Rash of Pregnancy

In toxemic rash of pregnancy, reported in 1962, papules and urticaria with striking pruritus occur on the abdomen.[13] It has no relationship to toxemia. No pathologic data are available.

Papular Dermatitis of Pregnancy

Papular dermatitis of pregnancy (PDP) was described in 12 patients in 1962.[14] These women had a highly pruritic papular eruption of the entire skin with the onset of three to eight new lesions daily.[14] The rash vanished after delivery in all but one patient. That patient had a retained placental fragment, removal of which lead to resolution of the rash. All patients had elevated urinary chorionic gonadotropin, from 25,000 to 500,000 units. Extracts of placentas from patients with PDP and normal placentas were injected intradermally into PDP patients. All reacted to the PDP extract, and none reacted to extract from normal placenta. A 27% fetal mortality was reported. High-dose oral prednisone controls the skin disease. The skin disease has recurred in subsequent pregnancies.

Prurigo Annularis

Two cases of prurigo annularis have been reported.[15] Both patients had slowly expanding annular ringlike lesions. Not enough clinical or laboratory information is known about these women to establish this as a distinct disease of pregnancy.

The diagnosis of these conditions is one of excluding other nonpregnancy-related skin diseases. Also, in the presence of papular eruptions, a urinary chorionic gonadotropin level should be performed. Treatment with topical steroids and antihistamines has been useful in the majority of the conditions listed above.

REFERENCES

1. Shormick JK. Herpes gestationis. *J Am Acad Dermatol.* 1987;17:539.
2. Foidart JM, Yaar M, Hall R, et al. Immunopathological and clinical studies in herpes gestationis. *Br J Obstet Gynaecol.* 1981;88:153.
3. Chorzelski TP, Jablonska S, Beutner EH, et al. Herpes gestationis with identical lesions in the newborn. *Arch Dermatol.* 1976;112:1129.
4. Bonifazi E, Meneghini CL. Herpes gestationis with transient bullous lesions in the newborn. *Pediatric Dermatol.* 1984;3:215.
5. Lawley TJ, Stingl G, Katz SI. Fetal and maternal risk factors in herpes gestationis. *Arch Dermatol.* 1978;114:552.
6. Lawley TJ, Hertz KC, Wade TR, et al. Pruritic urticarial papules and plaques of pregnancy. *JAMA.* 1979;241:1696.
7. Alcalay J, Ingber A, David M, et al. Pruritic urticarial papules and plaques of pregnancy: A review of 21 cases. *J Reprod Med.* 1987;32:315.
8. Uhlin SR. Pruritic urticarial papules and plaques of pregnancy: Involvement in mother and infant. *Arch Dermatol.* 1981;117:238.
9. Oosterling RJ, Norbrega RE, DuBoeuff JA, et al. Impetigo herpetiformis or generalized pustular psoriasis? *Arch Dermatol.* 1978;114:1527.
10. Johnston WG, Baskett TF. Obstetric cholestasis: A 14 year review. *Am J Obstet Gynecol.* 1979;133:299.
11. Sassaville D, Wilkinson RD, Schnader JY. Dermatoses of pregnancy. *Int J Dermatol.* 1981;20:223.
12. Bierman SM. Autoimmune progesterone dermatitis of pregnancy. *Arch Dermatol.* 1973;107:896.
13. Bourne G. Toxemic rash of pregnancy. *Proc R Soc Med.* 1962;55:462.
14. Spangler AS, Reddy W, Bardawil WA, et al. Papular dermatitis of pregnancy. *JAMA.* 1962;181:577.
15. Davies JHT. Prurigo annularis. *Br J Dermatol.* 1941;53:143.

Chapter One Hundred and Ninety-Three

Disorders of Bone and Cartilage

Michael Vermesh and Norbert Gleicher

193

SKELETAL REMODELING AND FACTORS INFLUENCING BONE AND BONE MINERAL METABOLISM

If the bone marrow is excluded, the adult skeleton has two major functions: It provides mechanical support and protection and regulates the concentrations of key blood electrolytes including Ca^{2+}, Mg^{2+}, H^+, Na^+, and HPO_3. The first aspect of skeletal function that is related to skeletal remodeling is termed *skeletal homeostasis.* The second skeletal function is known as *mineral homeostasis,* and it involves regulation of calcium and phosphate metabolism as well as regulation of blood pH and other ions.

The factors controlling constant skeletal remodeling throughout life are yet to be elucidated and are often difficult to separate from those factors that are concerned with mineral homeostasis. Both biochemical and physical factors are involved. Among the recognized biochemical factors, parathyroid hormone, vitamin D, and calcitonin are related to mineral homeostasis, whereas growth hormone, thyroid hormone, and adrenocortical steroids are associated with skeletal homeostasis. Other agents, including vitamin A, vitamin C, cortisol, estrogens, prostaglandins, and osteoclast-activating factor, also are concerned with skeletal maintenance.

Biochemical Factors

Human Growth Hormone. Human growth hormone (hGH) is a protein consisting of 191 amino acids and secreted from the anterior pituitary gland. Its action on the bone is exerted mostly through a second hormonal messenger, the somatomedins, affecting the cells of the epiphyseal plate[1] and decreasing endosteal resorption.[2] The hormone sustains the rate of growth of the bones in length, and its deficiency in childhood results in dwarfism.

The secretion of hGH is stimulated by a rapid fall in plasma sugar and is augmented by a variety of factors including sleep, stress, fasting, uremia, amino acids, estrogens, glucagon, and vasopressin. Factors that inhibit hGH secretion include hyperglycemia, hypothyroidism[3], corticosteroids[4], and medroxyprogesterone.[5] The levels of hGH throughout pregnancy have been reported to be similar to the nonpregnant serum levels (see also Chapter 37).[6]

Thyroid Hormones. The essential role of the thyroid hormones in affecting bone growth and remodeling is well documented, though unexplained. Hypothyroidism in childhood has been associated with severe forms of dwarfism, whereas hyperthyroidism may accelerate bone growth. In the adult skeleton, hyperthyroidism increases the rate of both bone formation and bone destruction, leading to a decrease in cancellous bone and, in severe cases, to osteoporosis.[7]

The thyroid hormones are believed to stimulate skeletal remodeling by a direct effect on osteocytes and not by enhancing PTH production. There is, on the other hand, a strong interaction between thyroid hormones and growth hormone, and their effects are difficult to separate. It is believed that thyroid hormones control osteogenesis, whereas growth hormone sustains chondrogenesis. Moreover, hypothyroidism is associated with decreased production of growth hormone[3], and growth hormone may induce hypothyroidism.[8] It is interesting to note that although hyperthyroidism as well as hypothyroidism have profound effects on skeletal remodeling, neither has any effect on calcium homeostasis, and plasma calcium concentration is normal.

Ovarian Steroids. Estrogen has an important influence on skeletal homeostasis. Its loss in castrated or postmenopausal women is responsible, at least in part, for the induction of osteoporosis, which represents, as discussed later in this chapter, a change of bone structure characterized by a reduction in bone mass with no change in chemical composition. Whether estrogen acts on the skeleton directly or through its action on other endocrine glands is still controversial. Estrogen is thought to interfere with the parathyroid hormone influence on bone resorption and to increase calcitonin levels, thereby inhibiting bone resorption.[9] Progesterone has little effect on the skeleton.[10]

Adrenocortical Steroids. Although cortisol affects both skeletal and mineral homeostasis, its action on skeletal remodeling is most important. The effect of cortisol on bone is to cause osteoporosis as a result of increased resorption and diminished bone formation.[11] Another effect of adrenocortical steroids is interference with the normal metabolic changes that occur in the cartilage, thereby inhibiting the longitudinal growth of bones.

Physical Factors

The importance of physical factors such as mechanical stress and pressure in controlling remodeling has been recognized for a long time. However, the exact mechanism by which these factors are converted into a biologic response of osteoblastic and osteoclastic activity is still unclear. Hypotheses implicating genetic[12] and electrical[13,14] factors still need to be substantiated.

During pregnancy, certain biomechanical changes occur that produce increased stress on the pelvic articulations. The increase in the degree of lumbar lordosis as a result of increased weight may be associated with low back pain and, in severe cases, with herniation of intervertebral disks.[15] The relaxation of ligaments and the bony eburnation that are associated with pregnancy may lead to an accentuation of the sliding movement of the sacroiliac joint and symphysis pubis.[16,17] Bony eburnation of the sacroiliac joints and symphysis pubis is termed *osteitis condensans ilii* and *osteitis pubis*, respectively.

Osteitis condensans ilii is usually a symmetric process affecting the ilium. The histopathologic features include osteonecrosis, hypervascularity, cartilaginous alterations, and inflammatory changes. The clinical findings are usually mild and consist of low back pain or polyarthralgia in peripheral joints. The condition is reversible in most cases.[18]

Osteitis pubis is a painful condition of the symphysis pubis that may become apparent within one or more months following delivery. The pubic changes are associated with bony erosion, resorption, and eburnation. The condition should be differentiated from other disorders that may affect the symphysis pubis such as trauma, infection, ankylosing spondylitis, and psoriatic arthritis. There currently is no effective method of treatment of this disorder. Proposed treatments have included antibiotics, analgesics, anti-inflammatory drugs, wedge resection of the pubis, irradiation, diathermy, vitamin compounds, heat, bed rest, steroids, oxyphenbutazone, local infiltration with hydrocortisone acetate, and heparinization.[19]

METABOLIC BONE DISEASE

Osteoporosis

Osteoporosis has been defined by Nordin[20] as a reduction of bone mass per unit volume with no change in chemical composition. This common disorder appears to be caused by a primary dysfunction of bone cells without evidence of hormonal or nutritional factors involved. It should be noted, however, that at least in the case of Cushing's disease and perhaps in pregnancy, this condition can be induced by a hormonal imbalance, that is, an excess of adrenal corticosteroids. A decrease in bone mass may occur in a variety of circumstances. The most controversial form of osteoporosis is that associated with aging and with the alteration in estrogen secretion occurring in women at menopause. It is also present in severe form in hypercortisonism, as in Cushing's disease or with cortisone therapy.[11] Osteoporosis has been described in association with a number of other disorders, including hyperthyroidism[7], hyperparathyroidism[21], acromegaly[20], chronic heparin administration[22], and immobilization.

Osteoporosis occasionally may occur in late pregnancy or the puerperium and has been noted in undernourished women. The reason for this is unknown, but it could be related to the catabolic effect of adrenal corticosteroids[23], the level of which increases in the blood as pregnancy advances. The clinical manifestations of osteoporosis in pregnancy are low backache, pain in the hips and thighs, and rarely, collapse of the vertebral bodies and nerve compression. The calcium, phosphorus, and alkaline phosphatase of the blood are normal; this is of diagnostic importance, as radiologically the disease may not be distinguished easily from other disorders of bone.

Treatment consists of a protein-rich diet, vitamin D supplementation, and mobilization. The patient tends to improve slowly in the months that follow labor, and the symptoms do not necessarily recur in succeeding pregnancies.

Osteomalacia

Osteomalacia is the adult counterpart of low-calcium rickets in the child, the clinical manifestations being modified by the absence of growth in the bones. This is a generalized disease of the bones that is caused by failure to deposit calcium salts in adequate amounts in the matrix of the bones.

The principal causes of osteomalacia are:

1. Nutritional vitamin D deficiency, ie, rickets in premature infants, osteomalacia in pregnant women
2. Disorders of the intestinal absorption of vitamin D, ie, malabsorption, gastrectomy
3. Defects of vitamin D metabolism, ie, renal failure, liver disease

Low vitamin D intake coupled with low calcium intake and total avoidance of sunlight may be the cause of osteomalacia in pregnancy. Over the last 3 months of pregnancy, about 25 g of calcium is removed from the mother and transferred to the fetal bones. This represents about 80% of the net dietary absorption in a normal nonpregnant woman on an average of 20 mmole per day calcium diet. The mother's diet must provide 1.2–1.5 g of calcium daily if her own metabolic requirements and the fetal needs are to be met without withdrawal of calcium from her bones.

Osteomalacia may develop over a period of years from a diet deficient in calcium or vitamin D, which is necessary for the absorption of calcium and phosphorus from the intestine. This form of the disease rarely occurs in inhabitants of the Western Hemisphere but has been described in pregnant immigrants from Pakistan and northern India.[24,25] Severe dietary deficiency of vitamin D from religious restrictions or food fads has been reported as the cause of osteomalacia in young women.[26] Osteomalacia is common among women whose work or traditions preclude adequate exposure to sunlight. Thus, it is more common in Iran among carpet makers who work for long hours in a dark environment[27] or in Bedouin women who expose very little skin to sunlight.[28] This is to be remembered when dealing with multigravid immigrants who speak little English, as otherwise bone pains of osteomalacia may be accepted as postural ligamentous aches, which are common during pregnancy.

If the condition is not recognized and corrected, bony deformities gradually develop with bowing of the spine and legs and deformation of the pelvis caused by an inward thrust of the femoral heads and sacrum. Fractures may occur from trivial trauma and then heal very slowly. The affected individuals often present with complaints of backache, muscular weakness, and paresthesias in the arms and legs. The teeth usually are not affected by the disease.[29] Tetany occurs only rarely, since the level of unbound serum calcium is generally normal.

The diagnosis is confirmed by x-ray of the bones, which shows abnormal cortical translucency and the characteristic Milkman's fractures.[30] Biopsy of the iliac crest may confirm the diagnosis further.

Treatment consists of adequate intake of calcium and vitamin D. Calcium lactate in a dose of 5 g daily and vitamin D, 10,000 IU daily, as a supplement to the diet should be sufficient to treat mild or moderate osteomalacia. In severe cases, vitamin D should be increased to 30,000 IU daily, and additional calcium may need to be given parenterally.

Pregnancy and labor usually are not affected by osteomalacia except when pelvic deformities lead to malpresentations and cesarean seciton. The incidence of abortion is no greater than in normal pregnancy. When the mother has severe osteomalacia, the child may be born with fetal rickets, although usually the fetus obtains the calcium it requires at the expense of the mother and is born unaffected (see also Chapter 41).

PAGET'S DISEASE OF BONE

Paget's disease (*osteitis deformans*) of the bone is a local disorder of unknown etiology characterized by a high rate of skeletal remodeling[31], resulting in the formation of disorganized bone and a variety of metabolic consequences.

The incidence of Paget's disease is difficult to estimate because a substantial number of affected individuals are asymptomatic. Characteristically, the disease is found in middle-aged or elderly patients, and, to date, it has not been reported in a patient less than 20 years of age. Studies using autopsy data of unselected persons have reported an incidence of up to 3.7% in patients over 40 years of age[32,33], reaching 5–11% by the ninth decade. The demographic variations in the incidence of this disease are significant, it being more frequent in Great Britain, Australia, and New Zealand and rare in Africa, the Middle East, Scandinavia, India, China, and Japan. Paget's disease has no clear genetic factor, although its prevalence in families of affected individuals is somewhat higher than in the general population.[34]

Histopathology

The normal lamellar bone has as its characteristic feature a parallel arrangement of collagen fibers, few osteocytes per unit area of matrix, and arrangement in units called *osteons* or *Haversian systems.* This architecture is destroyed in Paget's disease; there is an increase in the number of both types of active bone surface cells, osteoclasts and osteoblasts. In addition, the osteoclasts assume bizzare shapes and may contain a large number of nuclei, characteristic in this disease process.[35] In the early stage of the disease there is a marked increase in osteoclast number and activity, leading to intense resorption of bone[35] and to its replacement with fibrous tissue and blood vessels. As the disease progresses, woven bone replaces lamellar bone in both cortical and cancellous bone, the Haversian systems disappear, and the dense bone is replaced by a bone of chaotic structure. Islands of lamellar bone become embedded in seas of woven bone, hence the characteristic mosaic pattern.

Manifestations

The clinical presentation is variable and depends on the extent and site of skeletal involvement. Pain may be prominent, especially when lesions involve the lower extremities, pelvis, and vertebrae. It is likely that microfractures are a significant cause of pain in weight-bearing areas. It also has been postulated that stretching of the periosteum as the bone enlarges and the compression of neural structures may result in severe pain. The involvement of the skull results in an increased circumference secondary to cortical thickening, and characteristic radiographic findings are described as "honeycomb" or "cotton wool" patterns. However, patients are usually asymptomatic. A rare and potentially serious complication of the Pagetic skull is its slow collapse or *platybasia,* culminating in cerebellar tonsillar herniation. Involvement of the temporal bone may result in decreased hearing and difficulty in maintaining balance. The spine is involved most often, and compression of the spinal cord may cause back pain, paresthesias of the lower extremities, spastic paraparesis, and abnormal bladder and bowel function. The tibia and femur frequently are involved and may be severely deformed. Degenerative joint disease of the hip may cause considerable pain and morbidity. If the disease is severe and longstanding, there may be displacement of the femoral head, which may necessitate total hip replacement.

The concentrations of calcium and phosphorus in plasma are usually normal, and urinary calcium excretion, in the absence of fractures or immobilization, is not increased.[36] The urinary excretion of hydroxyproline and hydroxylysine is increased in Paget's disease, and the amount excreted is correlated directly with the extent of the disease.[37] Alkaline phosphatase is characteristically elevated and the highest values recorded for this enzyme were found in patients with Paget's disease.

Differential Diagnosis

Severe disease entities may mimic Paget's disease in clinical presentation but easily can be differentiated histologically because none shows the characteristic "mosaic" pattern of Paget's disease. These diseases include hyperparathyroidism, syphilis, Schmorl's nodule, osteoblastic metastases, fibrous dysplasia, and the rare congenital hyperphosphatasis[38], which has been called juvenile Paget's disease because of its clinical and biochemical similarity to the adult Paget's disease.

Treatment

The disorder is usually asymptomatic and does not require treatment. For symptoms such as bone pain, high-output cardiac failure, or multiple bone fractures, therapy is indicated. Many drugs that have been used in the past such as magnesium carbonate, steroids, aluminum acetate, and folic acid have been abandoned. Drugs in current use include sodium fluoride[39], oral phosphate[40], mithramycin[41], diphosphonates[42], glucagon[43], and calcitonin (CT), which is an effective agent in decreasing both the increased bone resorption and bone formation. The therapeutic use of CT brings about significant changes in the morphologic and biochemical indices of bone activity.[44] The most immediate effect of the administration of CT is a fall in the renal excretion of hydroxyproline, seen within hours after the administration of the hormone[45], followed by a fall in serum alkaline phosphatase. These data indicate that the initial effect of CT is that of inhibiting bone resorption and, probably, increasing bone formation. The latter effect of CT is, however, a decrease in both resorption and formation, leading to the replacement of the woven bone with normal lamellar bone. Side effects of nausea and facial flushing may be troublesome, but no case of toxicity has been reported.

To date no case of Paget's disease in pregnancy has been reported. This may be because of the relatively late age of onset of this disorder and its initially subtle course. However, the diagnosis should be considered as a differential diagnosis because cases in childbearing-age groups have been reported.

HYPEROSTOSIS AND OTHER DISORDERS OF BONE AND CARTILAGE

Hyperostosis

Hyperostosis means hypertrophy of bone.[46] This condition may be associated with various disorders that have in common a radiographic picture of increased bone density. Some of these disorders (osteopetrosis, osteopoikilosis) may complicate pregnancy and labor because of pelvic deformities or systemic manifestations. Other disorders that are associated with hyperostosis (ie, pyknodysostosis, melorheostosis, osteomyelosclerosis, hyperostosis frontalis interna) are rare and have not been reported in association with pregnancy.

Osteopetrosis (Albers–Schonberg Disease, Marble Bones Disease, Osteosclerosis Fragilis Generalisata). Osteopetrosis is an inherited disease characterized by the presence of an excessive formation of dense trabecular bone and calcified cartilage, especially in long bones, leading to obliteration of marrow spaces and to anemia. The disorder can be separated into two forms: a severe form, which usually causes death in childhood[47], and a benign form, which is consistent with survival into old age.[48]

The severe form is an autosomal-recessive disorder,[2] and a history of parental consanguinity is found in about one-third of the cases. The clinical findings include small stature, hepatosphenomegaly, anemia, thrombocytopenia, diminished resistance to infection, and bone fragility. Many children die within the first year of life from anemia or infections. The etiology and pathogenesis of the condition are not clear. It has been postulated that the skeletal lesions result from a decrease in the rate of bone and cartilage resorption with little or no change in the rate of bone and cartilage formation.[49] The radiographic picture is dominated by increased bone density and "flask" or "clublike" deformities. The abnormalities in skeletal remodeling may be recognized on fetal x-ray taken as early as 6 months of gestation.[50] However, at least one case of osteopetrosis has been reported in an infant in whom prenatal x-ray had been negative.[51]

The benign form of osteopetrosis appears to be transmitted as an autosomal-dominant trait.[48] Affected individuals may remain totally asymptomatic or reveal anemia, facial palsy, deafness, hepatosplenomegaly, and fractures.[48] The prognosis for the benign form is much better than for the severe form. Many patients approach middle age with minimal clinical discomfort. One case has been reported of simultaneous discovery of osteopetrosis in a mother and her fetus on the occasion of radiopelvimetry.[52] However, no complications of pregnancy or labor could be attributed to the disorder.

Osteopoikilosis (Osteopathia Condensans Disseminata). Osteopoikilosis is an asymptomatic osteosclerotic dysplasia with an autosomal-dominant pattern of genetic transmission.[53] Clinical manifestations are mild and include predisposition to keloid formation and sclerodermalike lesions. Roentgenographic findings are diagnostic. Rarely, the disease may cause dwarfism and pelvic deformities resulting in dystocia.[54]

Other Disorders of Bone and Cartilage

Fibrous dysplasia is a nonneoplastic condition of unknown etiology characterized by the replacement of normal bone substance by fibro-osseous connective tissue. When the lesions are multiple and associated with café-au-lait pigmented patches in the skin and disturbances of endocrine function, the condition is known as *McCune–Albright syndrome.* In the majority of cases it affects only one bone or a part of a bone (monostotic). In a few cases it affects several bones (polyostotic). The femur, tibia, ribs, jaw, and skull are affected most frequently. The age range affected in the monostotic variety is from 10 to 70 years. The age distribution is younger in the polyostotic form: Two thirds of the affected individuals are symptomatic before the age of 10 years.

Most monostotic lesions remain quiescent throughout life. Growth discrepancies and gross deformities such as bowed limbs are associated more often with polyostotic fibrous dysplasia and are predominantly unilateral. Skin lesions also tend to favor the side of the bony involvement.

TABLE 193–1. EXPECTED ULTRASOUND FINDINGS IN SKELETAL DYSPLASIAS

Condition	Inheritance	Head	Chest and Body	Spine	Limbs
Achondrogenesis I (Parenti–Fraccaro)	AR[a]	Thin, poorly mineralized skull	Short chest and body with thin ribs	Low-level echoes from vertebral bodies	Marked symmetrical reduction
Achondrogenesis II (Langer–Saldino)	AR	Increased H:B ratio	Short, barrel-shaped thorax	Low-level echoes from vertebral bodies	Symmetrical reduction, straight
Achondroplasia	AD[b]	Increased HC, BPD, and H:B ratio; bulging forehead			Short limbs, especially femora and humeri
Asphyxiating Thoracic Dysplasia	AR		Long, narrow chest with very short ribs		Variable shortening; hexadactyly (occasional)
Campomelic Dysplasias	NK[c]				
Long-limbed	NK	Increased HC, BPD, and H:B ratio; micrognathia (profile)	Small, narrow thorax	Perhaps some flattening of spine	Long, thin, and definitely bowed
Short-limbed, normocephalic	NK				Short, broad, angulated
Short-limbed with craniosynostosis	NK	Increased HC, BPD, and H:B ratio; micrognathia (profile)			Short, broad, angulated
Chondroectodermal Dysplasia (Ellis–van Creveld syndrome)	AR		Long, narrow chest; congenital heart disease (occasional)		Shortening of both proximal and distal segments; hexadactyly
Diastrophic Dysplasia	AR				Short with contractures—"hitch hiker" thumbs
Hypophosphatasia	AR	Very thin with mineralization, sometimes collapsed	Thin, poorly visualized ribs	Thin, poorly visualized	Short, thin, ribbonlike; fractures
Langer Mesomelic Dysplasia	AR	Micrognathia			Severe middle segment shortening (forearms, legs)
Osteogenesis Imperfecta					
Type I (blue sclerae)	AD	Normal size			Perhaps mild bowing
Type II (blue sclerae, lethal variety)	AR	Thin, often collapsed cranium	Rib fractures	(?) Fractures	Short, broad, and angulated with fractures; femurs especially tend to be broad, with marked bowing
Type III (normal sclerae)	AR	Thin, but not as marked as type II	Occasional rib fractures		Fractures possible, broad bones, mild bowing, slightly short
Type IV (normal sclerae)	AD	Normal size	Occasional rib fractures		Bowing and occasional fractures
Short rib–Polydactyly Syndromes					
Type I (Saldino–Noonan)	AR		Narrow thorax, protuberant abdomen	Flat vertebrae	Very short, polydactyly
Type II (Majewski)	AR		Narrow thorax, protuberant abdomen		Moderate shortening, polydactyly
Spondyloepiphyseal Dysplasia Congenita (Spranger–Wiedemann)	AD		Short, barrel-shaped chest		Proximal shortening
Thanatophoric Dysplasia	NK	Increased HC, BPD, and H:B ratio; prominent forehead	Narrow, pear-shaped thorax, protuberant abdomen	Marked flattening of vertebrae	Very short and bowed

[a] Autosomal recessive.
[b] Autosomal dominant.
[c] Not known.
Adapted from Sillence et al.[63]

The disease may be associated with various endocrine problems, including precocious puberty, Cushing's syndrome, acromegaly, and hyperthyroidism.

The clinical picture and the radiographic appearance are characteristic in the polyostotic form, and biopsy is rarely necessary. The differential diagnosis of the monostotic form is from any other benign lesions of bone including benign cysts, fibromas, and enchondroma, and biopsy usually is needed to confirm the diagnosis.

Pregnancy appears to stimulate activity in the dysplastic tissue; reactivation during pregnancy of previously diagnosed fibrous dysplasia has been reported by different authors.[55-58]

Dysplasias and Chondrodystrophies

Disorders of bone and cartilage that are associated with disproportionate short stature are referred to as skeletal dysplasias or chondrodystrophies. The etiology of these diseases is still unknown, and the variety of classifications proposed by different authors are based on descriptive criteria, survival, or mode of inheritance.[59-62]

Achondroplasia. Achondroplasia is an autosomal dominantly inherited disease and is the most frequent type of dwarfism. The disease usually is recognized at birth and is compatible with normal life span and normal intelligence. The disproportionate short stature is caused by failure of the proliferating cartilage in the growth plate, affecting the growth of tubular bones.

Pregnancy in achondroplastic women may be complicated by diabetes, spinal compression, and cardiorespiratory compromise. Delivery should be performed by cesarean section because of the contracted pelvis. Spinal or epidural anesthesia should not be attempted because spinal stenosis often is associated with this disorder. The diagnosis can be made *in utero* during the second trimester using x-ray or ultrasound (Table 193–1).

Neonatal Lethal Chondrodystrophies. These diseases usually are associated with polyhydramnios and frequently are recognized during the early second trimester, allowing elective abortion. The affected fetuses invariably succumb to the disease *in utero* or in the early postpartum period; cesarean section or resuscitation of the newborn thus should be avoided.

REFERENCES

1. Kember NF. Cell population kinetics of bone growth: the first ten years of autoradiographic studies with tritiated thymidine. *Clin Orthoped.* 1971;72:213.
2. Harris WH, Heaney RP, Jowsey J, et al. Growth hormone: the effect on skeletal renewal in the adult dog. *Calcif Tissue Res.* 1972;10:1.
3. Glick SM, Roth J, Yalow RS, et al. The regulation of growth hormone secretion. *Recent Prog Horm Res.* 1965;21:241.
4. Tanner JM. Human growth hormone. *Nature.* 1972;237:433.
5. Catt KJ. Growth hormone. *Lancet.* 1970;1:933.
6. Yen SSC, Samaan H, Pearson OH. Growth hormone levels in pregnancy. *J Clin Endocrinol.* 1967;27:1341.
7. Adams P, Jowsey J. Bone and mineral metabolism in hyperthyroidism: an experimental study. *Endocrinology.* 1967;81:735.
8. Root AW, Snyder PJ, Rezvani I, et al. Inhibition of thyrotropin-releasing hormone-mediated secretion of thyrotropin by human growth hormone. *J Clin Endocrinol Metab.* 1973;36:103.
9. Nordin BEC, Horsman A, Crilly RG, et al. Treatment of spinal osteoporosis in postmenopausal women. *Br Med J.* 1980;280:451.
10. Silberg M, Silberg R. Steriod hormones and bone. In: Bourne GH, ed. *The Biochemistry and Physiology of Bone, vol. 3.* New York, NY: Academic Press; 1971:401.
11. Jowsey J, Riggs BL. Bone formation in hypercortisonism. *Acta Endocrinol.* 1970;63:21.
12. Fell HB. Skeletal development in tissue culture. In: Bourne GH, ed. *The Biochemistry and Physiology of Bone, ed 1.* New York, NY: Academic Press; 1956:401.
13. Currey JO. The adaptation of bones to stress. *J Theor Biol.* 1968;20:91.
14. Bassett CAL. Electro-mechanical factors regulating bone architecture. In: Fleich H, Blackwood HGG, Owen M, (eds.). *Third European Symposium on Calcified Tissues. Davos 1965.* Berlin: Springer-Verlag; 1966:78.
15. Walde J. Obstetrical and gynecological back and pelvic pains, especially those contracted during pregnancy. *Acta Obstet Gynecol Scand.* 1962;41(Suppl 2):11.
16. Thorp DJ, Fray WE. Pelvic joints during prengancy and labor. *JAMA.* 1938;111:1162.
17. Abramson D, Roberts SM, Wilson PD. Relaxation of pelvic joints in pregnancy. *Surg Gynecol Obstet.* 1934;58:595.
18. Numaguchi Y. Osteitis condensans ilii, including its resolution. *Radiology.* 1971;98:1.
19. Merimsky E, Canetti R, Firstater M. Ostetis pubis: Treatment by heparinisation. *Br J Urol.* 1981;53:154.
20. Nordin BEC. Hormones and calcium metabolism. In: Fleisch H, Blackwood HJJ, Owen M, eds. *Calcified Tissues 1965, Proceedings of the Third European Symposium on Calcified Tissues.* Berlin: Springer; 1966:226.
21. Bordier PJ, Tun-Chot S. Quantitative histology of metabolic bone disease. *J Clin Endocrinol Metab.* 1972;1:197.
22. Griffith GC, Nichols G, Asher JD, et al. Heparin osteoporosis. *JAMA* 1965;193:91.
23. Nordin BEV, Roper A. Post-pregnancy osteoporosis; syndrome? *Lancet.* 1955;1:431.
24. Felton DJC, Stone WD. Osteomalacia in Asian immigrants during pregnancy. *Br Med J.* 1966;1:1521.
25. Clark F, Simpson W, Young JR. Osteomalacia in immigrants from the Indian subcontinent in Newcastle-upon-Tyne. *Proc R Soc Med.* 1972;65:478.
26. Dent CE, Smith R. Nutritional osteomalacia. *QJMed.* 1969;38:195.
27. Chapman K. Osteomalacia in Iran. *J Obstet Gynaecol Br Commonw.* 1971;78:857.
28. Groen JJ, Eshchar J, Ben-Ishay D, et al. Osteomalacia among the Bedouin of the Negev Desert. *Arch Intern Med.* 1965;116:195.
29. Taylor GF, Day CDM. Osteomalacia and dental caries. *Br Med J.* 1940;2:211.
30. Milkman LA. Multiple spontaneous, idiopathic, symmetrical fractures. *Am J Roentgenol.* 1934;32:622.
31. Woodhouse NJ. Paget's disease of bone. In: MacIntyre I. ed. *Calcium Metabolism and Bone Disease, vol 1.* London: Williams Saunders; 1972:125.
32. Schmorl G. Uber Ostitis deformans Paget. *Virchows Arch Pathol Anat Physiol.* 1932;283:694.
33. Collins DH. Paget's disease of bone: incidence and subclinical forms. *Lancet.* 1956;2:51.
34. Evens RG, Bartter FC. The hereditary aspects of Paget's disease (osteitis deformans). *JAMA.* 1968;205:900.
35. Belanger LF, Jarry L, Uhthoff HK. Osteocytic osteolysis in Paget's disease. *Rev Can Biol.* 1968;27:37.
36. Riggs BL, Arnaud CD, Goldsmith RS, et al. Plasma kinetics and acute effects of pharmacological doses of porcine calcitonin in man. *J Clin Endocrinol Metab.* 1971;33:115.
37. Khairi MRA, Wellman HN, Robb JA, et al. Paget's disease of bone (osteitis deformans): symptomatic lesions and bone scan. *Ann Intern Med.* 1973;79:348.
38. Thompson RC Jr, Gaull GE, Horwitz SJ, et al. Hereditary hyperphosphatasia: studies of three siblings. *Am J Med.* 1969;47:209.
39. Purves MJ. Some effects of administering sodium fluoride to patients with Paget's disease. *Lancet.* 1962;2:1188.
40. Goldsmith RS. Treatment of Paget's disease with phosphate. *Semin Drug Treat.* 1972;2:69.
41. Ryan WG, Schwartz TB, Northrop G. Treatment of Paget's disease with mithramycin: further experiences. *Semin Drug Treat.* 1972;2:57.
42. Smith R, Russel RGG, Bishop MC, et al. Paget's disease of bone. *Q J Med.* 1973;42:235.
43. Condon JR, Reith SBM, Nassim JR, et al. Treatment of Paget's disease of bone with mithramycin. *Br Med J.* 1971;1:421.
44. Woodhouse NJ, Bordier P, Fisher M, et al. Human calcitonin in the treatment of Paget's bone disease. *Lancet.* 1971;1:1139.
45. Bijovet OLM, van der Sluys Veer J, Jansen AP. Effects of calcitonin on patients with Paget's disease, thyrotoxicosis or hypercalcemia. *Lancet.* 1968;1:876.
46. Stedman TL, ed. *Stedman's Medical Dictionary.* 23rd ed. Baltimore, MD: Williams & Wilkins; 1976.
47. Loria-Cortes R, Quesada-Calvo E, Cordero-Chaverri C: Osteopetrosis in children: a report of 26 cases. *J Pediatr.* 1977;91(1):43.
48. Johnston CC, Jr, Lavy N, Lord T, et al. Osteopetrosis. A clinical, genetic, metabolic and morphologic study of the dominantly inherited, benign form. *Medicine.* 1968;47:149.
49. Shapiro F, Glimcher MJ, Holtrop ME, et al. Human osteopetrosis, a histological, ultrastructural, and biochemical study. *J Bone Joint Surg.* 1980;62(3):384.

50. Jenkinson EL, Pfisterer WH, Latteier KK, et al. Prenatal diagnosis of osteopetrosis. *Am J Roentgenol.* 1943;49:455.
51. Golbus MS, Koerper MA, Hall BD. Failure to diagnose osteopetrosis in utero. *Lancet.* 1976;2:1246.
52. Delahaye RP, Metges PJ, Anglade JP, et al. Découverte simultanée d'un ostéopétrose chez la mére et le foetus á l'occasion d'une radiopelvimétrie. *J Radiol Electrol Med Nucl.* 1976;57(4):359.
53. Melnick JC. Osteopathia condensans disseminata (osteopoikilosis). Study of a family of 4 generations. *Am J Roentgenol.* 1959;82:229.
54. Raskin MM. Osteopoikilosis; possible association with dystocia and keloid. *South Med J.* 1975;68(3):270.
55. Hunter D, Turnbull MH. Hyperparathyroidism: generalized osteitis fibrosa. *Br J Surg.* 1931;12:203.
56. Dockerty MB, Ghormley RK, Kennedy RLJ, et al. Albright's syndrome (polyostotic fibrous dysplasia with cutaneous pigmentation in both sexes and gonadal dysfunction in females). *Arch Intern Med.* 1945;75:357.
57. Bonduelle M, Claisse R. Dysplasie fibreuse des os et eyndrome d'Albright. Leur place nosologique. *Sem Hop Paris.* 1948;24:514.
58. Henry A. Monostotic fibrous dysplasia. *J Bone Joint Surg.* 1969;51(B):300.
59. Rubin P. Dynamic Classification of Bone Dysplasias. Chicago, IL: Yearbook Medical Publisher; 1964.
60. Maroteaux P, Wiedemann R, Spranger J, et al. Essai de Classification des Dysplasies Spondylo-epiphysaires. Lyon; Simep Editions; 1968.
61. Spranger JW, Langer LO, Wiedemann HR. Bone dysplasias. An atlas of constitutional disorders of skeletal development. Philadelphis, PA: WB Saunders; 1974.
62. Hall JG. Disorders of connective tissue and skeletal dysplasia. In: Schulman JD, Simpson JL, eds. *Genetic Diseases in Pregnancy.* New York, NY: Academic Press; 1981:57.
63. Sillence DW, Rimoin DL, Lachman R. Neonatal dwarfism. Symposium on medical genetics. *Pediatr Clin North Am.* 1978;25:453.

PART XIX Diseases of the Eye and Ear

Norbert Gleicher, Section Editor

Chapter One Hundred and Ninety-Four

Common Disturbances of Vision and Ocular Movement and Surgery of the Eye

Steven A. Teich

194

Although the metabolic and hormonal changes that occur during pregnancy can have ocular effects, uncomplicated pregnancy normally has little clinically significant effect on the visual apparatus. Visual complications that do occur are most often a reflection of underlying systemic disease such as diabetes mellitus, systemic complications of pregnancy such as in toxemia, or preexisting ocular diseases such as uveitis or glaucoma. In treating ocular diseases, the general principles of medical therapy during pregnancy should be maintained. It easily is overlooked that topical ocular medications can be absorbed systemically, cross the placenta, and sometimes have therapeutic serum or tissue levels in both mother and fetus. Therefore, one should treat ocular diseases medically only if definitely indicated, use agents that have no demonstrated teratogenicity, and always weigh possible harmful effects of treatment on the fetus against the possible loss of organ function to untreated disease in the mother. Even cycloplegic or mydriatic agents used during a routine ophthalmologic examination should be abandoned during pregnancy unless there is good reason to suspect retinal disease, since both sympathetic and anticholinergic drugs cross the placenta or can have systemic effects on the mother that secondarily affect the fetus. Phenylephrine probably should never be used. It should be remembered that ocular diseases usually do not affect the fetus, whereas their treatment may. However, there are instances, such as in chlamydial conjunctivitis, in which ocular involvement may be the only symptom of a disease with possible implications for the fetus. If a topical ophthalmic medication must be used in a pregnant woman, systemic absorption may be decreased by applying pressure over the nasolacrimal sac for three to five minutes after the instillation of one drop and removing excess tears with absorbent material prior to the release of pressure.

MATERNAL ASPECTS

Refractive Errors

In any complaint of blurred vision the first step should be to distinguish a refractive error from organic disease. A useful screening procedure is to have the patient look through a pinhole in a piece of paper or cardboard, which will at least partially correct a significant refractive error. Nonrefractive visual problems may be caused by opacities or irregularities in the normally clear ocular media, disease of the retina, optic nerve, or intracerebral visual pathways, or amblyopia expanopsia resulting from monocular visual deprivation in childhood such as that from asymmetric refractive errors or strabismus.

Massive changes in refraction are unusual during pregnancy. A transient insufficiency of accommodation has been reported[1], that might cause some difficulty with reading or near vision or make a previously hyperopic (farsighted) person develop blurred vision for distance or symptoms of eyestrain. This does not appear to be very common. There is also some evidence that a slightly increased corneal thickness occurs during pregnancy, probably because of corneal edema, which can cause refractive changes.[2] This may be why some pregnant women have difficulty with contact lenses. It is not advisable for new corrective lenses to be prescribed until several weeks after delivery.

Eyelids

For unknown reasons, ptosis may develop during or shortly after pregnancy. It is distinguished from a lesion of the third cranial nerve developing from an intracranial aneurysm or tumor by the lack of ipsilateral pupillary dilation or abnormality of extraocular movement. Normal and symmetric pupils also distinguish it from *Horner's syndrome*, in which there is unilateral ptosis, miosis, and sometimes anhidrosis as a result of a lesion of the ocular sympathetic pathway anywhere from the hypothalamus to the cervical sympathetic chain to the internal carotid artery to the orbit. The affected pupil in Horner's syndrome fails to dilate in response to topical cocaine eyedrops. The absence of other signs of weakness of the extraocular or other muscles and a negative edrophonium (Tensilon) test distinguish this ptosis of pregnancy from myasthenia gravis. In the case that does not resolve spontaneously, surgical correction can be performed postpartum.[3] The eyelids may be involved in the pigmentation of melasma.

Inflammations of the eyelid are common disorders that may occur in pregnancy. *Blepharitis* occurs as an acute or chronic diffuse inflammation of the eyelid margins. It can be sebhorreic or ulcerative, most often in association with Staphylococcus infection. The chief complaint may be itching, burning, or irritation of the eyelids, which may be erythematous with scaling and even loss of lashes. Suppurative lesions around the lashes may be present in the ulcerative type. Adequate treatment often is achieved with local cleansing of the eyelid margins. If there is no response or if the blepharitis is clearly ulcerative, topical antibiotics should be used such as bacitracin or erythromycin ophthalmic ointment at night or neomycin-polymyxin B-gramicidin combination eyedrops three or four times daily. In very severe unresponsive cases or if there is an associated staphylococcal allergic conjunctivitis, a short course of mild topical corticosteroid such as fluorometholone eyedrops three times a day may be used.

A *hordeolum*, or *sty*, is the most common localized eyelid inflammation. It is an acute suppurative inflammation of the glands at the base of the eyelashes, usually caused by staphylococcal infection, which presents as a painful, erythematous, localized swelling of the lid margin. It generally responds to a few days' treatment with hot compresses every few hours without the use of antibiotics. When it points and drains, the use of topical neomycin-polymyxin β-gramicidin combination (triple antibiotic) eyedrops might be considered to prevent involvement of adjacent glands. On occasion, incision and drainage are necessary.

Another common focal inflammation is a *chalazion* or *chronic granuloma* of the more posteriorly located meibomian glands. This may present as an acute painful swelling or as a firm, nontender gradual painless swelling. The acute stage is treated with hot compresses. When asymptomatic, chalazia may disappear over several weeks or months with or without hot compresses. Antibiotics are indicated on rare occasions, if ever. A persistent chalazion can be excised, but this can be postponed until after pregnancy.

Conjunctiva

Subconjunctival hemorrhage may occur spontaneously or as a result of severe vomiting during hyperemesis gravidarum, straining during labor, trauma, or rarely, in association with a blood dyscrasia. It is an asymptomatic, flat, red, sharply delineated area under the bulbar conjunctiva that spontaneously fades within about 2 weeks without treatment. A nonclearing or recurrent subconjunctival hemorrhage may be a manifestation of Kaposi's sarcoma of the conjunctiva in the acquired immune deficiency syndrome (AIDS).

Conjunctivitis, an inflammation of the normally transparent conjunctiva covering the globe and inner surface of the eyelids, is a common disorder characterized by diffusely dilated blood vessels. Pregnancy does not predispose the patient to this condition. Vision is unaffected other than transient blurring from tearing or mucus secretion and is painless other than for a mild irritation or gritty feeling unless corneal involvement from a viral infection occurs, in which case a foreign body sensation may be prominent for several days, and vision may be blurred for weeks to months. Conjunctivitis can be caused by irritative substances in the environment such as toxic fumes or chemicals or by an allergy such as from ragweed pollen. Combination antihistamine-vasoconstrictor eyedrops should not be used in the first trimester and probably not at all during pregnancy because of possible adverse effects on the fetus. In a very severe allergic conjunctivitis, one can consider a very short course of a weak topical corticosteroid such as fluorometholone, but should refrain from its use if at all possible in this benign and self-limited condition.

The infectious causes of conjunctivitis are mainly bacterial, viral, and chlamydial. Almost any bacteria can be etiologic, but it is caused most often by gram-positive cocci. There may be a copious mucopurulent or purulent discharge, and involvement is usually but not exclusively monocular. Topical triple antibiotic solutions four times a day will be effective against most organisms pending the results of Gram's stain and culture. Topical sulfonamides should not be used near term because of the theoretical possibility of kernicterus in the neonate. Similarly, chloramphenicol eyedrops should be avoided in the third trimester because of concern over the gray syndrome. An extremely copious purulent discharge may be a sign of *Neisseria gonorrheae* infection, which should be Gram's stained immediately and cultured appropriately so that urgent treatment can be initiated with a single intravenous (IV) or intramuscular (IM) injection of ceftriaxone 1 g[3a] or, in the case of penicillin allergy, IM spectinomycin 2 g for five days, as this organism has the propensity to infect and even perforate the cornea. Adjunctive therapy is with topical saline lavage. Some would also use bacitracin or erythromycin ointment. Obviously, genitourinary and pharyngeal evaluation for gonorrhea infection should be performed, as this has both maternal and fetal implications. Evaluation and treatment for any coexisting infection with syphilis or chlamydia is indicated.

Viral conjunctivitis usually is caused by an adenovirus, although occasionally other viruses (including herpes simplex) may present this way. It often occurs in clusters of cases, as in epidemic keratoconjunctivitis, as a result of extreme contagiousness with hand-to-eye contact. There is often bilateral but asymmetric involvement with frequently palpable preauricular lymph nodes, conjunctival follicles visible on slit lamp examination, swollen eyelids, and a watery or mucoid discharge. As mentioned above, a foreign body sensation with pain and photophobia from corneal involvement may be prominent. This is a self-limited disease, with the acute phase lasting a few days to 2–3 weeks, but may be contagious for up to 3 weeks. Corneal infiltrates may last from a few weeks to many months, decreasing vision mildly to severely, and are not a sign of actively replicating virus but probably represent an inflammatory response to viral antigen. Treatment of the acute phase is symptomatic with cold compresses and artificial tear solutions. Neither antivirals nor antibacterials are of demonstrated benefit. Topical corticosteroids probably are not indicated, although some believe that they are beneficial in alleviating very severe symptoms. If a chronic phase with corneal infiltrates occurs, topical corticosteroids may be beneficial if vision is severely reduced. However, they probably prolong the disease and are best withheld until after pregnancy.

Chlamydial conjunctivitis, which may manifest as trachoma or, much more commonly in the United States, as *inclusion conjunctivitis,* clinically can be indistinguishable from viral conjunctivitis and should be considered in any follicular conjunctivitis lasting more than 2 weeks or occurring in any pregnant woman near term. This is a venereally transmitted disease, and about 90% of adult women with inclusion conjunctivitis have an associated chlamydial genital infection. This makes the diagnosis important to determine in the pregnant woman, since chlamydial genital infection is the most common cause of *ophthalmia neonatorum.* The transmission rate from the infected cervix to the infant during parturition is approximately 50%, with 25–50% developing neonatal conjunctivitis and 10–20% developing neonatal pneumonia.[4] It can be differentiated cytologically through conjunctival scrapings by the presence of polymorphonuclear leukocytes and intracytoplasmic inclusions in epithelial cells with Giemsa stain. The diagnosis can be confirmed by direct fluorescent antibody or enzyme-linked immunoassay testing. In severe chronic cases, corneal scarring may occur. Treatment is with topical erythromycin ointment and oral erythromycin 250–500 mg four times a day for 2–3 weeks.

Cornea

The cornea is a transparent, avascular tissue that forms the anterior one sixth of the globe and is the major refractive surface of the eye. Any process affecting its smoothness, clarity, or regularity of structure can have a profound effect on visual acuity. The cornea is richly supplied by sensory nerves, and any defect in its surface covering of epithelial cells, such as a corneal abrasion, can cause a foreign body sensation or even severe pain associated with tearing and blurred vision. There appears to be a decrease in corneal sensitivity in pregnant women after the 31st week of gestation, which returns to normal 6–8 weeks postpartum.[2] The etiology and clinical significance of this are not known, but it may be related to the increased corneal thickness and fluid retention in pregnancy. Kruckenberg's spindles, a melanin pigmentation of the posterior cornea seen on slit lamp examination, may occur in pregnancy without the secondary glaucoma they are occasionally associated with in nonpregnant patients. They have no effect on vision.

Abnormal circulating metabolic products associated with systemic diseases can deposit in the cornea. *Arcus senilis* is a common asymptomatic bilateral deposition of lipid in the peripheral cornea, forming a grayish-white ring about 2 mm wide with a clear area between it and the sclera. Although it is frequently idiopathic in patients over 60 years old, when it is seen in the age group of pregnancy, hypercholesterolemia should be suspected. Calcium salts may deposit in the cornea, forming band keratopathy, a horizontal, grayish band beginning in the peripheral cornea nasally or temporally, containing round dark "holes," and progressing centrally. It can be caused by ocular inflammation such as the chronic iridocyclitis of monoarticular or pauciarticular juvenile rheumatoid arthritis or by any systemic disease associated with hypercalcemia such as hyperparathyroidism, hypervitaminosis D, or sarcoidosis. If the band keratopathy progresses far enough centrally, it may reduce vision. Temporary visual improvement can be obtained by mechanically removing the calcium with a chelating agent such as sodium EDTA. A *Kayser-Fleischer ring* is a sign of Wilson's disease or, rarely, other chronic hepatobiliary disease. It is an asymptomatic pigmented ring in the peripheral cornea varying widely in color from red to brown and might be a copper compound. Corneal cystine crystals sometimes are seen in cystinosis.

Pregnant patients with rheumatoid arthritis or other collagen vascular disease may develop Sjögren's syndrome, in which lacrimal gland involvement results in decreased tear secretion. This causes dryness of the cornea with damage to and even loss of corneal epithelial cells, noted by staining with Rose–Bengal and fluorescein, respectively. A frequent complaint is grittiness or foreign body sensation. The cornea loses its normal glossy appearance, and mucus strands may overlie it. Treatment is with frequent artificial tear eyedrops during the day and ointment at night. In severe chronic cases, extensive damage to the cornea can occur with ulceration and secondary infection.

An abrasion usually is caused by a foreign body or overwear of contact lenses. It is quite painful with tearing, blurred vision, photophobia, conjunctival injection, and staining of the affected area with fluorescein. Healing usually occurs in 1–3 days with pressure patching with or without instillation of a triple antibiotic solution.

A much more serious disorder is corneal ulceration, in which infection can occur with bacteria or fungi; this often is caused by corneal trauma such as an untreated abrasion, foreign body, or contaminated contact lenses. Symptoms initially may be similar to those of an abrasion but usually are more severe, and there is often an associated headache and markedly decreased vision. The conjunctival injection is often pronounced, and a whitish corneal opacity may be seen in the area of the ulcer, especially if there is bacterial or fungal infection. The ulcer should be scraped immediately, and appropriate stains and cultures for bacteria and fungi performed. Treatment then is initiated with hourly broad-spectrum fortified topical antibiotics and subconjunctival antibiotics; one should be certain to use agents effective against both staphylococcal and *Pseudomonas* organisms, which are very aggressive and can rapidly cause corneal perforation. A frequently effective regimen is one utilizing cefazolin sodium with gentamicin. A triple antibiotic solution may be added. Systemic antibiotics generally are not indicated unless corneal perforation is thought to be imminent. Appropriate antibiotics should be started once culture and sensitivity results are available. Although the pregnant state must be kept in mind, it is crucial that effective antibiotics be used in this ophthalmic emergency. If fungal infection is suspected, especially if trauma with organic matter occurred or the ulcer is indolent, topical pimaricin also should be used. An unusually painful ring-shaped corneal infiltration and ulceration frequently associated with contact lens use is caused by acanthamoeba. Special staining techniques are required for diagnosis. Although often poorly responsive to treatment, some improvement has been noted with the frequent use of triple antibiotic and propamidine eyedrops for months. Penetrating keratoplasty may be necessary, but this probably could be postponed until after pregnancy.

Of special significance in pregnancy is herpes simplex keratitis, which is the most common cause of corneal ulceration in the United States. The vast majority of cases are not primary infections but are caused by latent virus in the trigeminal ganglion, with acute episodes of keratitis being responses to "triggers" such as fever, stress, or exposure to light. It is uncertain if pregnancy is one of these triggers. Some 80–90% of cases are caused by type 1 herpes simplex virus, and the rest are caused by type 2.[5] Since type 2 herpes simplex can be transferred from the genitals to the eyes, any pregnant woman with herpetic keratitis should be examined for genital involvement.[6] Symptoms are blurred vision, tearing, and conjunctival injection, but pain may or may not be prominent, as there may be reduced corneal sensation. The typical lesion is a linear branching ulcer, termed *dendritic*, which stains with fluorescein. Diagnosis is made from the typical clinical picture, but scrapings can be examined for multinucleated giant cells. Treatment is by debridement of the affected corneal epithelium or by the use of topical trifluorothymidine drops every 2 hours, which so far have not been found to be teratogenic as opposed to idoxuridine drops, which are teratogenic in rabbits.[7] Corticosteroids are contraindicated in acute epithelial lesions as they promote viral invasion. Herpes simplex keratitis occasionally can be mimicked by herpes zoster ophthalmicus, but the characteristic skin lesions of zoster, when present, aid in the diagnosis. The latter is rare in pregnancy and can be treated with topical corticosteroids such as prednisolone acetate 1%. Ocular involvement may be heralded by a vesicle on the tip of the nose. Besides keratitis there may be eyelid inflammation and iritis. Although the acute infection is self-limited, there may be sequelae of corneal dryness, exposure, and scarring. In nonpregnant patients, high-dose oral acyclovir shortens the duration of illness and reduces the sequelae, although its effect on the development of post-herpetic neuralgia is not known. However, acyclovir normally should not be used in pregnancy because of possible teratogenicity. A possible exception might be in AIDS in which herpes zoster ophthalmicus can be an early sign and have a prolonged course.

Interstitial keratitis with opacification and vascular invasion of the cornea may be a late result of repeated herpes simplex keratitis but is also a late finding of congenital syphilis, which requires treatment with intravenous penicillin G. Any inflammatory or degenerative condition of the cornea can result in severe scarring or opacification, which can be treated by corneal transplantation (penetrating keratoplasty) after the conclusion of pregnancy.

Sclera

The sclera is a dense, white, fibrous, outer, protective coating of the eye that is continuous with the cornea anteriorly. A bluish discoloration is caused by scleral thinning with visibility of the underlying uveal pigment. This can be seen in diseases causing chronic scleral inflammation or disturbances of connective tissue in the body such as osteogenesis imperfecta, Marfan's syndrome, or Ehlers–Danlos syndrome.

Episcleritis is a relatively common localized inflammation of the episclera, a thin layer of vascular elastic tissue just overlying the sclera. It is a benign self-limited disease of young adults presenting as a localized, although sometimes generalized, area of redness with mild to moderate pain, watery discharge, and sometimes tenderness. Vision is unaffected. It has a tendency to recur and is associated in some cases with underlying collagen vascular disease. Since it resolves spontaneously in 2–3 weeks, probably no treatment is indicated in the pregnant patient other than symptomatic oral acetaminophen.

Scleritis, an often granulomatous inflammation of the sclera, is a less common but more serious ailment. It is divided into diffuse, nodular, and necrotizing types, the last of which has the most severe symptoms and complications. There is frequently severe pain and tenderness, intense vascular injection, bluish-red discoloration, and vision may be blurred. In the necrotizing type, areas of scleral necrosis may occur. An associated systemic disease is present in nearly half of the patients, with collagen vascular diseases being most common.[8] Complications are frequent, including keratitis, uveitis, cataract, glaucoma, scleral thinning, and retinal detachment in a posterior scleritis. About 15% may have decreased vision.

Scleromalacia perforans, with its asymptomatic scleral thinning and necrosis in association with longstanding rheumatoid arthritis, would be most unusual in the pregnant age group. Treatment is difficult, as the most commonly effective agents—oral indomethacin or oxyphenbutazone—should not be used during pregnancy. Topical corticosteroids may reduce the inflammation and give some symptomatic relief. In very severe cases, oral corticosteroids in doses of 60–80 mg prednisone per day or equivalent may be necessary. Periocular injections of corticosteroids are contraindicated, as they may cause further scleral thinning. It is not known how pregnancy affects the incidence of scleritis and episcleritis, but it is possible that alterations in the immune system in pregnancy may reduce their frequency.

Glaucoma

Glaucoma is an elevation of intraocular pressure that damages optic nerve fibers, resulting in an increased optic nerve cup/disc ratio (normal is 0.3) and progressive loss of visual field. Untreated, reduced visual acuity and even total blindness can result. It should be noted, however, that most cases of intraocular pressure do not develop into glaucoma. Glaucoma is generally bilateral and is of multifactorial inheritance. It is also age related, occurring in about 2% of the population over the age of 40. It is rare in women of childbearing age. In fact, intraocular pressure tends to decrease during the second half of pregnancy, returning to prior levels about 2 months postpartum[9], which might make the pregnant glaucoma patient easier to manage.

Aqueous humor is formed by ciliary processes in the posterior chamber behind the iris, percolates around the crystalline lens, through the pupil, into the anterior chamber in front of the iris, and leaves the eye through the trabecular meshwork, which is a narrow band in the sclera located between the ciliary body, into which the iris inserts, and the cornea. Intraocular pressure normally is maintained within a range of 5–22 mg Hg by a relative steady state in the rate of aqueous humor production and outflow, although there is a diurnal fluctuation.

About 90% of glaucoma cases are of the primary open-angle variety in which, for mainly unknown reasons, there is a relative decrease in the rate of aqueous humor outflow, probably because of some inherent abnormality in the trabecular meshwork function. This leads to a chronic asymptomatic elevation of intraocular pressure, which insidiously damages the optic nerve with slowly progressive visual field loss over the course of many years, beginning in the midperiphery. Only when the area of central vision finally is affected in the advanced stages of the disease will the patient note decreased visual acuity. Open-angle glaucoma is one of the leading causes of blindness in adults and can be detected and followed only by measurement of the intraocular pressure, examination of the optic nerves, and testing of the visual fields.

About 5% of cases are caused by *primary angle-closure glaucoma*, in which there is an anatomically shallow anterior chamber. When for various reasons the pupil becomes relatively dilated, either physiologically or pharmacologically, the peripheral iris mechanically crowds the anterior chamber angle in which the trabecular meshwork is located and closes off the trabecular meshwork. This leads to a sudden large increase in intraocular pressure, which may cause pain, blurred vision with rainbow-colored halos around lights as a result of corneal edema, conjunctival injection, and acute damage to both the optic nerve and the trabecular meshwork. It is diagnosed in the proper clinical setting by the finding of a markedly elevated intraocular pressure and the gonioscopic finding of a closed angle. Eyes predisposed to this condition can be detected by noting a shallow anterior chamber and performing gonioscopy, which reveals a narrow anterior chamber angle, as the intraocular pressure often is normal in the absence of an acute attack.

Another 5% of cases have secondary glaucoma in which there may be iris adhesions (synechiae), debris in the anterior chamber, an abnormal substance, or neovascularization either obscuring or damaging the trabecular meshwork as a result of prior or underlying ocular disease or inflammation. This may or may not have acute symptoms depending on the rate and level of intraocular pressure elevation. Diagnosis requires intraocular pressure measurement and slit lamp and gonioscopic examinations.

Open-angle glaucoma generally is a medically treated disease. However, antiglaucoma medications in the pregnant patient must be prescribed with extreme caution, particularly in the first trimester, because the safety of these drugs during pregnancy has not been well established. If the patient is being treated for elevated intraocular pressure associated with some evidence of an increased optic nerve cup to disk ratio with normal or near normal visual fields, she might be followed with no therapy but with close monitoring of her optic nerves and visual fields, especially in view of the usual decrease in intraocular pressure in the second half of pregnancy. However, if the intraocular pressure is very high and there is advanced or progressing visual field loss threatening central vision, some type of therapy is necessary. Pilocarpine in the form of eyedrops or an ocusert could be used, but often is not tolerated by women of childbearing age because of blurred vision and headaches from its effect on the ciliary muscle and accommodation. In addition, when given near term, pilocarpine conceivably could cause a syndrome of hyperthermia, seizures, and diaphoresis in the neonate.[10] Topical β-adrenergic antagonists are relatively safe if used after the first trimester. If possible, the relatively β-1 selective antagonist betaxolol should be used, but it may be necessary to use the nonselective agents timolol or levobunolol for optimal intraocular pressure control. Any of these should be discontinued at least two to three days prior to delivery to limit their effects on uterine contractility and prevent possible neonatal complications.[11] Topical dipivefrin (a pro-drug of epinephrine) may be used with caution after the first trimester with the knowledge that it readily crosses the placenta and has not been well studied in pregnant women. Topical epinephrine should be avoided as it may cause fetal hypoxia. Oral carbonic anhydrase inhibitors should not be used, as acetazolamide has been shown to cause limb and kidney defects in fetal rats.[10] Similarly, cholinesterase inhibitors are contraindicated, as phospholine iodide eyedrops cross the placenta and lower both maternal and fetal pseudocholinesterase.[12]

If medications are unable to lower the intraocular pressure or the doctor or patient refuses to take the risk of adverse fetal effects from these medications, argon laser trabeculoplasty may be considered. This can reduce the intraocular pressure significantly in about 85% of eyes and requires only topical anesthesia. However, the long-term effects of this procedure are not known. If all else fails, and the situation is critical for the preservation of vision, a surgical filtering procedure such as a trabeculectomy can be performed under local anesthesia, in which a fistula between the anterior chamber and the subconjunctival space is formed. However, this should be postponed until after pregnancy, when full medical therapy can be utilized again, if at all possible.

An acute attack of angle-closure glaucoma is an ophthalmic emergency. Treatment can be initiated with a drop of topical timolol or a systemic hyperosmotic agent such as oral glycerol or intravenous mannitol to lower the intraocular pressure. Topical pilocarpine eyedrops then can constrict the pupil and "break" the attack once the pressure is lowered. Pilocarpine drops also should be instilled in the opposite eye to prevent that eye from having an attack. As soon as the eye is stable, laser iridotomies with topical anesthesia or surgical iridectomies with local anesthesia should be performed on both eyes to cure the condition and prevent any possibility of future episodes. If there has not been permanent damage to the trabecular meshwork from the attack, no further medications should be necessary.

Uveitis

The uvea is the middle vascular layer of the eye. From anterior to posterior it consists of the iris, which is a diaphragm just anterior to the lens that adjusts the size of the pupil; the ciliary body, which secretes aqueous humor and contains the smooth muscle that regulates the focusing for near vision in accommodation; and the choroid, which lies between the retina with its underlying pigment epithelium and the sclera. Uveitis, or inflammation of the uveal tract, has many causes that may involve any one or all three parts simultaneously. It can be caused by infectious agents such as toxoplasmosis, syphilis, and herpes zoster; by systemic immunologic diseases such as sarcoidosis, ankylosing spondylitis, juvenile rheumatoid arthritis, Behcet's disease, and Vogt–Koyanagy–Harada syndrome; or by localized ocular disease such as blunt trauma, Fuch's heterochromic iridocyclitis, or sympathetic ophthalmia. Most often, however, it is idiopathic with no clear identifiable cause.

Uveitis is often recurrent and may be bilateral. Uveitis from noninfectious causes such as ankylosing spondylitis or sarcoidosis may be less common in pregnancy or may not surface until after pregnancy.[13,14] Similarly, patients with active uveitis may go into remission during pregnancy with flare-ups postpartum. This has been reported in the Vogt–Koyanagy–Harada syndrome of bilateral anterior or posterior uveitis with meningeal and cutaneous findings.[15] On the other hand, an infectious cause, toxoplasmic retinochoroiditis, is widely thought to recur with increased frequency during pregnancy.[16] Behcet's disease with severe iridocyclitis and retinal vasculitis, aphthous stomatitis, and genital ulcerations may improve, worsen, or first appear during pregnancy.

Acute anterior uveitis (iritis or iridocyclitis) usually has a sudden onset of aching pain with associated headache, blurred vision, and photophobia. There are often circumcorneal or diffuse conjunctival infection and a usually somewhat constricted pupil. Sometimes an anterior uveitis, such as that in association with juvenile rheumatoid arthritis, will have few or no signs or symptoms unless reduced vision occurs because of cataract or secondary glaucoma from prior iritic episodes. Slit lamp examination may reveal white blood cells, with variable amounts of "flare" from breakdown of the blood-ocular barrier, floating in the anterior chamber. Deposits (keratic precipitates) may form on the back of the cornea and may be fine and white (nongranulomatous) or large and gray (granulomatous). Intraocular pressure is normal or low unless a secondary type of angle-closure glaucoma from synechiae or cellular debris has supervened. An individual episode may last days to weeks or even months. Complications include cataract, secondary glaucoma, and a pupil that may be irregular, constricted, and unreactive as a result of iris adhesions to the lens (posterior synechiae) and usually occur with chronicity or after recurrent episodes.

Posterior uveitis (choroiditis) may have no pain or conjunctival injection unless there is a frequently associated anterior uveitis. The most common cause in the United States is toxoplasmosis[17], which is considered separately. Ophthalmoscopic examination may reveal a hazy vitreous because of infiltration with inflammatory cells that is sometimes dense enough to dramatically reduce the patient's vision and impair examination of the retina. Choroiditis usually affects the overlying retina either primarily (retinochoroiditis) or secondarily (chorioretinitis). Vision may be blurred due to the vitritis or to a secondary macular edema, especially in the idiopathic syndrome of pars planitis or intermediate uveitis.

Active lesions of the choroid and retina are variably sized, yellowish-white patches with often inflammatory sheathing of nearby retinal blood vessels. In Behcet's disease, however, the primary lesion actually may be a retinal vasculitis. The active inflammation usually lasts weeks to months. Eventually, healing progresses with decreasing vitreous haze and the chorioretinal lesions develop discrete hyperpigmented margins with a white scar in the center. There may be no residual visual problem if the chorioretinal scar is in the peripheral retina. But if the macula, which subserves central vision, is involved, there may be a permanent paracentral or central scotoma, dramatically reducing vision.

Retinal detachment occasionally can occur years later from the traction of strands of degenerated vitreous tugging on the retina. In the presumed ocular histoplasmosis syndrome, the acute choroiditis usually is completely asymptomatic with residue of multiple, small chorioretinal scars. If any of these occur in the macular area, subretinal neovascularization can develop years later, growing from the choroid under or through the retinal pigment epithelium, which can leak exudate or blood under the retina, distorting vision, and with ultimate formation of a fibrotic mound that can permanently destroy central vision if the fovea in the very center of the macula is involved.

Rarely, a suppurative uveitis may occur because of pyogenic bacteria or fungi, especially *Candida,* from septic emboli from a focus elsewhere in the body. This can result in an endophthalmitis with severe pain, greatly reduced vision, red, swollen eyelids and conjunctiva, and even limitation of extraocular movements in association with a severe inflammatory cellular response in the aqueous humor and vitreous body. It can progress rapidly over a few days to total loss of vision in bacterial endophthalmitis, but has a more indolent course in fungal infections. Although the pregnant patient does not appear to be at increased risk for endophthalmitis, *Candida endophthalmitis* has occurred in the first week postpartum with the postulation that candidemia occurred at the time of delivery or early postpartum from a vaginal infection.[18]

Treatment of anterior uveitis should include treatment of any underlying systemic disease. Specific therapy includes topical mydriatic cycloplegic agents such as cyclopentolate 1% eyedrops three times a day to prevent posterior synechiae and reduce pain and photophobia caused by ciliary muscle spasm. Treatment should be for the shortest time necessary; this may be all that is required in mild cases. In more severe cases, topical corticosteroids such as prednisolone 1% eyedrops may be given as frequently as necessary to suppress the inflammation. Corticosteroids should be used for the least time necessary, as they can cause some of the same complications as the uveitis itself, including cataracts and elevated intraocular pressure in genetically susceptible persons when used for prolonged periods. In addition, although no cases are known of human teratogenesis from ophthalmic corticosteroids, they have been reported to cause teratogenic effects in animals.[19,20] Rarely, this will not suppress the inflammation adequately, and periocular injections of corticosteroids are necessary if there is no underlying infectious agent, especially toxoplasmosis. The use of dark sunglasses may be helpful for photophobia.

Treatment of posterior uveitis also should include that of an underlying systemic disease such as syphilis and any coexisting anterior uveitis. If an infectious agent is not present, systemic corticosteroids such as oral prednisone 40–80 mg per day may be used, although periocular injections of corticosteroids may be preferable in a pregnant patient. However, neither oral nor periocular corticosteroids should be used in pregnancy unless the chorioretinal lesions are imminently threatening the optic nerve or macula or there is so much inflammatory debris in the vitreous that the patient is severely visually disabled.

A suppurative uveitis with endophthalmitis requires urgent treatment to save the eye. Cultures of the conjunctiva and vitreous should be performed as soon as possible for bacteria and fungi. At the time of vitreous tap for culture, intravitreal broad-spectrum antibiotics such as gentamicin or tobramycin and cefazolin should be injected intravitreally as well as given intravenously pending the results of cultures and sensitivities. If a fungal infection is suspected, intravitreal amphotericin B may be used. Otherwise, treatment is the same as that for a corneal ulcer. If subretinal neovascularization develops in the macula from a histoplasmosis scar and causes distortion of vision, argon or krypton laser photocoagulation under local anesthesia may be used to attempt to obliterate the abnormal vessels if they are not in the foveal center and thereby preserve central vision. Definitive diagnosis and treatment, however, requires intravenous fluorescein angiography. Although there have been no reports of teratogenicity from sodium fluorescein in humans or animals, it does cross the placenta and its safety in pregnancy has not been established. A survey of retinal specialists concluded that fluorescein angiography does not cause a high rate of birth anomalies or complications during pregnancies.[20a] Whether this test should be performed in this situation should be a mutual decision made by the patient and the treating ophthalmologist and may depend on how close the active "histo spot" is to the fovea.

A potentially important cause of uveitis in pregnancy is *toxoplasmic retinochoroiditis* (a primary retinitis), since a pregnant woman with acute primary toxoplasmosis can transmit the infection to the fetus in about 40% of cases, with severe disease in about 15% of offspring.[21] However, it is believed by many investigators that nearly all cases of ocular toxoplasmosis represent a late recurrence of congenitally acquired disease[22], and there have been only a few case reports of ocular toxoplasmosis as a sequela of acquired toxoplasmosis.[23] This is important because exposure to the disease prior to pregnancy and the presence of any level of antibodies protect the mother against the transmission of toxoplasmosis to the fetus.[21]

It is now fairly well established that a woman with recurrent ocular toxoplasmosis during pregnancy will not transmit the infection to her fetus or develop a generalized infection.[15] Similarly, a woman with a past history of ocular toxoplasmosis need not fear transmitting the infection to her fetus, although her risk of developing recurrent ocular toxoplasmosis may be increased by pregnancy. Therefore, except in the rare case of acute acquired systemic toxoplasmosis during pregnancy, ocular toxoplasmosis should be considered a localized recurrent infection, and treatment should be considered only for the potential ocular complications in the mother. The diagnosis is made by the finding of a typical lesion of acute retinitis, often adjacent to an old chorioretinal scar, with a positive serologic test result even to undiluted serum. Treatment need not be initiated for peripheral retinal lesions, as the episodes normally spontaneously resolve within a few weeks to months.

Treatment may be necessary if acute lesions threaten the optic nerve or macula. Standard therapy has been with oral pyrimethamine and sulfadiazine with or without oral prednisone. However, pyrimethamine, a potent antifolate that is teratogenic in animals, is contraindicated in pregnancy, and sulfonamides should not be used during the third trimester. In cases in which central vision is affected during the third trimester, oral clindamycin may be effective and has not been associated with any teratogenic effect. It must be remembered, however, that clindamycin does cross the placenta and can cause pseudomembranous colitis. If the inflammation is especially severe or in a particularly threatening area of the retina, oral prednisone can be used in the lowest dosage necessary to suppress the inflammation and only with antibiotic coverage. Periocular injections of corticosteroids probably should not be used in ocular toxoplasmosis as immunosuppressive amounts may be delivered to the inner eye.

The acute retinal necrosis syndrome is a recently recognized unilateral or bilateral progressive peripheral necrotizing retinitis, occlusive retinal vasculitis and vitritis with coexisting anterior uveitis in otherwise healthy adults. It results in massive retinal necrosis with retinal detachments in two thirds, causing severe visual loss. Varicella zoster and herpes simplex viruses have been implicated as causes. Although relatively uncommon and seen more frequently in males, it has been reported in a pregnant woman during her third trimester one month after a varicella eruption.[24] Unfortunately, the mainstay of treatment is intravenous acyclovir, for which safety in pregnancy has not been established, and which may cause chromosome breaks at high concentrations. If possible, use of this agent should be deferred until postpartum. Adjunctive treatment of uncertain benefit includes oral corticosteroids and aspirin. Because severe vision loss from retinal detachment occurs frequently even after regression of the acute lesions, prophylactic laser photocoagulation has been advocated. Included in the differential diagnoses are syphilis, sarcoidosis, Behcet's disease, candida, acquired toxoplasmosis, and cytomegalovirus (the latter two in immunosuppressed patients).

Cytomegalovirus retinitis can affect one or both eyes in up to 25% of patients with AIDS and may be its first manifestation. Early lesions may resemble cotton-wool spots, but the lesions gradually enlarge, become hemorrhagic, and ultimately cause necrosis of the entire retina, despite relatively little inflammation in the vitreous or anterior chamber.[24a] Total blindness results. This is the most common cause of visual loss in AIDS. The intravenous agent ganciclovir may prevent progression of disease in 80–90% of cases but must be given indefinitely to prevent recurrences. Unfortunately, it is contraindicated in pregnancy. Similar lesions in AIDS patients have been caused by toxoplasmosis and syphilis.

Lens

Any opacity in the crystalline lens, which is located behind the iris and in front of the vitreous body and functions to focus rays of light onto the retina, is termed a *cataract*. Surgical excision is required only if the opacities are dense enough to significantly interfere with vision. This is rare in a woman of childbearing age, and surgery can be postponed until after pregnancy. If cataracts are present, the patient should be evaluated for underlying metabolic disturbances such as hypocalcemia, diabetes mellitus, galactosemia, or Wilson's disease. Hereditary disorders such as myotonic dystrophy also should be considered. Cataracts also can be caused by ocular trauma, uveitis, or chronic corticosteroid therapy. A dislocated or subluxed lens may result from Marfan's syndrome, homocystinuria, Marchesani's syndrome, or trauma, especially in association with syphilis. It often requires no therapy.

Retina

The retina is a transparent sheet of light-sensitive neural tissue that lines the inner aspect of the posterior two-thirds of the eye. The retina is applied closely to a single layer of underlying pigment epithelial cells with a potential space between them. When this potential space fills with fluid, a retinal detachment results. Under the retinal pigment epithelium and its attachment to a band of connective tissue called *Bruch's membrane* is the choroid, which has in its inner surface the choriocapillaris, a layer of capillaries supplying the outer retina including the rod and cone photoreceptors. The inner retina, including the ganglion cells whose axons pass through and help form the optic nerve, is supplied by the right red branches of the central retinal artery and drained by the wider darker red branches of the central retinal vein. These vessels enter the retina from the optic nerve. In the absence of refractive errors or opacities in the media, light is sharply focused on the macular area of the retina, which is located temporal to the optic nerve and is responsible for central vision. The finest acute vision comes from the stimulation of the photoreceptors, consisting almost entirely of color-sensitive cones, of the fovea centralis in the center of the macula. Diseases of the macula and fovea affect the fine visual functions of central vision such as reading and color discrimination. Diseases of the rest of the retina, containing predominantly rod photoreceptors, affect peripheral or side vision. Purely retinal diseases are painless.

Diabetic retinopathy is the most likely retinal vascular disease to occur during pregnancy. It is one of the four most common causes of new cases of blindness in the United States and the leading cause in young adults (see also Chapter 43). It is estimated that about 25% of all diabetics have some type of retinopathy, and about 2% have the severe form of proliferative retinopathy. The prevalence of proliferative retinopathy appears to be greater in juvenile-onset (type I) diabetes but may occur sooner in adult-onset (type II) diabetes. However, the prevalence of all types of diabetic retinopathy is correlated most closely with the duration of diabetes. Among diabetics diagnosed prior to age 30, diabetic retinopathy (but not proliferative retinopathy) is present in 17% of patients with diabetes for less than five years, but is present in 98% with diabetes for more than 15 years with proliferative retinopathy in 25% of the latter group.[25] There are no objective data proving that strict metabolic control lessens the incidence or severity of diabetic retinopathy; however, it is in the best interests of mother and fetus to have good control of the blood sugar maintained during pregnancy. Pregnancy itself does not appear to increase the frequency of diabetic retinopathy or the progression to proliferative retinopathy.[26] Even among pregnant patients, the development and progression of diabetic retinopathy are related to the duration of disease[27] and are unrelated to the number of past pregnancies.[28] A gestational diabetic is not at risk for retinopathy but may have increased tortuosity of her retinal vessels (unrelated to the elevation in blood glucose), which has been postulated to be a phenotypic marker for gestational and possibly type II diabetes mellitus.[29]

Diabetic retinopathy is usually bilateral and symmetric, affecting the posterior pole area around the optic nerve and macula. It is divided into background retinopathy and proliferative retinopathy. Background retinopathy consists of intraretinal evidence of increased vascular permeability and ischemia. Signs of increased vascular permeability are round dot and blot retinal hemorrhages, discrete yellow hard exudates consisting of protein and lipid deposits adjacent to areas of intraretinal edema, and small, round, often permeable microaneurysms, which are partly the cause of the edema. Intraretinal signs of ischemia include gray-white soft exudates or cotton-wool spots (which represent retinal infarcts) flame-shaped retinal hemorrhages, and dilated or beaded retinal veins. These are considered to be preproliferative changes. Background retinopathy does not affect vision unless the edema fluid or hard exudates involve the center of the macula, causing visual distortion and a slowly progressive decreasing visual acuity. Macular edema is the major cause of reduced vision, although not severe visual loss, in diabetes. Background retinopathy tends to wax and wane during pregnancy, only rarely progressing to proliferative retinopathy, with visual acuity usually remaining relatively good and any progression of background retinopathy often regressing to base-line levels by 6 months postpartum.

Some worsening of background retinopathy and the development of cotton-wool spots has been correlated with tight metabolic control, but these are often transitory changes and should not prevent the use of intensive therapy of hyperglycemia.[30] Macular edema with blurred vision may develop in conjunction with worsening retinal ischemia in patients with proteinuria and hypertension, but it may regress after delivery.[31]

Proliferative diabetic retinopathy consists of proliferations of newly formed vessels called neovascularization over the inner retinal surface or optic nerve head along with supporting connective tissue. This is the major cause of severe visual loss in diabetes, which can arise from hemorrhaging of these fragile new vessels into the vitreous or tractional retinal detachment of the macula from contraction of the associated connective tissue. Proliferative retinopathy appears to be a response to underlying retinal ischemia. The risk of severe visual loss is especially high if the neovascularization is on or near the optic disk, is severe in extent, or is associated with any preretinal or vitreous hemorrhage. For these high-risk eyes the *Diabetic Retinopathy Study* has demonstrated conclusively that panretinal laser photocoagulation significantly reduces the two-year risk of severe visual loss from 26% to 11%, induces regression of neovascularization, and prevents its further development.[32]

Despite the clinical impressions of some investigators, there is no objective evidence that pregnancy causes proliferative retinopathy to progress any more rapidly than in nonpregnant women. It is also unlikely for proliferative retinopathy to spontaneously regress after the termination of pregnancy. In addition, proliferative diabetic retinopathy appears to have as good a response in general to panretinal laser photocoagulation in the pregnant as the nonpregnant patient, making proliferative retinopathy neither an absolute contraindication to pregnancy nor an indication for therapeutic abortion.[33] The presence of proliferative retinopathy does appear to correlate with angiopathy elsewhere in the body. Pregnant patients with proliferative diabetic retinopathy often have albuminuria and a higher risk of infant morbidity and mortality.[26,27] Proper management of diabetic retinopathy necessitates that all pregnant diabetics receive an ophthalmologic examination early in pregnancy. If there is no retinopathy, another examination in the third trimester is advised. If background retinopathy is present, follow-up examination is indicated in each trimester. If severe background retinopathy or very early proliferative retinopathy is present, the patient probably should be reevaluated every month. If high-risk proliferative retinopathy is present, immediate panretinal laser photocoagulation is indicated. If very early proliferative retinopathy is present in both eyes, panretinal laser photocoagulation in one eye and close observation of the other might be considered. However, some investigators advocate treatment for any degree of neovascularization because of the possible development of vitreous hemorrhage during spontaneous delivery. Delivery by cesarean section is an option if laser photocoagulation is not performed or if the neovascularization has been unresponsive to it.

If a large vitreous hemorrhage prevents panretinal laser photocoagulation, the *Diabetic Retinopathy Vitrectomy Study*[34] has demonstrated that a vitrectomy under general anesthesia by way of the pars plana of the ciliary body results in a better chance of return to a higher level of visual acuity if done early than if deferred for one year, although there is a greater chance of severe complications with early vitrectomy surgery. In pregnancy, this procedure probably should be postponed, if possible, until postpartum since its optimum timing is still uncertain, the percentage of eyes obtaining very good central vision postoperatively is relatively low, and many vitreous hemorrhages clear spontaneously. A vitrectomy also can be performed postpartum for very severe neovascularization with large amounts of fibrous proliferations. A vitrectomy may have to be performed at once if a traction retinal detachment involving or threatening the macula is visualized or is present on ophthalmic ultrasound examination in the presence of vitreous hemorrhage. In eyes with clinically significant macular edema (edema within or adjacent to the fovea), focal laser photocoagulation to leaking microaneurysms has been shown to reduce by 50% the risk of central visual acuity decreasing over three years.[35] This is another treatment probably best postponed until postpartum because the extent of maculopathy can fluctuate during pregnancy with improvement postpartum, the best time to apply photocoagulation has not been determined, and optimal treatment requires preoperative fluorescein angiography, the safety of which has not been established in pregnancy.

Optic disc edema is a benign manifestation of juvenile-onset diabetes mellitus that may occur during pregnancy. It is asymptomatic, is not associated with increased intracranial pressure, and resolves spontaneously in 6 to 12 months.

The retina also can be affected by hypertensive diseases of pregnancy. Systemic hypertension during pregnancy may be an indication of toxemia, especially when it occurs in the third trimester (see also Chapters 138–141). Both the retinal and choroidal circulations can be affected by the acute hypertension of toxemia, and funduscopic changes have been noted in up to 70% of cases.[36] Visual disturbances (usually transient) can occur as a result of retinal arteriolar spasm, retinal edema, retinal artery or vein occlusions, retinal detachments caused by choroidal vascular abnormalities[37], ischemic optic neuropathy, or occipital lobe ischemia or edema.[37a] Although mild to moderate visual disturbances are not uncommon, severe visual loss or blindness is rare and usually responds within days to weeks to control of blood pressure, which may require termination of pregnancy.

It has been stated that the most common ocular finding in toxemia is narrowing of the retinal arterioles beginning in the nasal periphery but becoming generalized.[38] A recent study found that retinal arteriolar changes could separate severe from mild preeclamptics but not mild preeclamptics from normals. It also reported that 12% of the preeclamptic patients complained of flashing lights, thought to be due to occipital lobe vasospasm.[38a] If the hypertension is persistent, this may lead to cotton-wool spots, flame-shaped retinal hemorrhages, and even intraretinal edema. However, there is evidence that choroidal vascular changes can occur without obvious retinal vascular changes and possibly may occur more often.

Areas of choroidal vascular nonperfusion have been demonstrated[37], apparently damaging the retinal pigment epithelium and forming yellow-white focal lesions deep in the retina. Fluid from the choriocapillaris flows through this damaged retinal pigment epithelium and also from the optic disk, whose blood supply comes partly from the same source as the choroidal circulation, causing edema of the disk and the posterior pole of the retina. In an estimated 1% of toxemic patients but 10% of those with eclampsia[38], this fluid can lead to large bullous retinal detachments, often bilaterally, sometimes occurring early in the puerperium. The visual prognosis of these detachments is good, with resolution spontaneously within a few weeks postpartum, although some improvement may be seen in a few days. However, there are often residual changes in the retinal pigment epithelium, and some paracentral visual distortion may remain despite good acuity.

Although these retinal detachments tend to occur in severe cases of toxemia, they should not be considered by themselves an indication for termination of pregnancy unless the systemic signs of toxemia have been controlled medically without their response. Retinal detachment surgery is contraindicated. The retinal arteriolar narrowing, if present, also reverts to normal within a few weeks of normalization of blood pressure.

Preexisting or chronic hypertension in a pregnant patient may cause retinal vascular changes secondary to thickening of the walls of the retinal arterioles from arteriolar sclerosis. There may be widening of the arteriolar light reflexes and arteriovenous crossing changes of tapering, concealment, or "nicking" of the vein. Acute elevations in blood pressure can cause the changes described in toxemia, as can collagen vascular diseases, amniotic fluid embolization, thrombotic thrombocytopenic purpura, or disseminated intravascular coagulation.

Central serous chorioretinopathy is a relatively benign, self-limited localized detachment of the retina in the macula resulting from focal leakage of fluid from the choriocapillaris through the retinal pigment epithelium. Although much more common in men, it can occur during a normal pregnancy. It is not known whether pregnancy predisposes to this condition, but a woman has been described in whom it recurred in four successive pregnancies.[39] The presenting symptoms are blurred vision, distortion, or central scotoma, and vision is usually mildly to moderately reduced in the affected eye. Careful funduscopic examination by an ophthalmologist will reveal the locally elevated retina in the macula, distinguishing this entity from an optic neuritis or tumor-related compressive optic neuropathy, which may have similar presenting symptoms.[40] Spontaneous resolution occurs in the vast majority of cases within 3–6 months with relatively good visual acuity, although some patients may have persistent distortion of vision. No treatment is indicated during pregnancy. Laser photocoagulation in chronic cases is controversial.

Generalized *tapetoretinal degenerations* or *pigmentary retinopathies* can be hereditary disorders of the pigment epithelium-photoreceptor complex typified by retinitis pigmentosa. In the full-blown picture, generalized pigmentary changes are present throughout the retina in the presence of gradually decreasing vision, constricted visual fields, and especially poor night vision. They are of varying inheritance and can be slowly or rapidly progressive. It is not known what effect pregnancy has on these disorders, but five % to ten % of pregnant patients may note visual changes subjectively.[40a] There can be associated systemic abnormalities such as the Bassen–Kornzweig syndrome (in which Vitamin A therapy may be helpful), Friedrich's ataxia, or Refsum's syndrome of phytanic acid accumulation. Certain drugs such as phenothiazines, for example, thioridazine, and the antimalarials chloroquine and hydroxychloroquine, can cause a generalized retinal pigmentary degeneration via toxicity to the pigment epithelium that can progress even after the drug is stopped. It is significant that chlorpromazine and chloroquine have been shown to cross the placenta and accumulate in the eyes of the mother and fetus[41] and therefore should be avoided in pregnancy, if possible.

A patient with a congenital degeneration of the retinal periphery or high myopia may be at risk for developing a tear in the peripheral retina from traction of the vitreous body or trauma. Symptoms include "floaters" or dark spots from debris in the vitreous and light flashes from tugging of the vitreous on the retina at the margins of the tear. Fluid from the vitreous can flow through the retinal tear into the subretinal space, causing a rhegmatogenous retinal detachment that can be partial or total with symptoms of a "shadow" or "curtain" spreading over the field of vision; this can lead to complete loss of vision and requires surgical repair as soon as possible, especially if the macula is involved, to regain good visual function. Surgical repair is 90% successful and can be performed under general anesthesia with relative safety to the fetus with appropriate monitoring. Since retinal tears or holes are relatively common but retinal detachments are relatively uncommon, prophylactic treatment to retinal tears with laser photocoagulation or cryotherapy usually is indicated only if there are both symptoms and evidence of vitreous traction to the tear. These can be performed under topical anesthesia. A study of pregnant highly myopic women, most of whom had retinal holes or degeneration, concluded that it was safe to allow them to deliver spontaneously.[42]

Retinal artery occlusions are rare in pregnancy, tending to occur in older patients with atherosclerosis and carotid artery disease. They cause intracellular swelling or infarction of the inner retina with a white appearance of the involved region. A central retinal artery occlusion can cause almost complete irreversible blindness unless a cilioretinal artery (derived from the choroidal circulation) is present and supplies part of the macula. There is diffuse whitening of the retina except for a "cherry red spot" in the fovea due to an absence of inner retinal layers in this region. Branch retinal artery occlusions cause sectoral visual field defects, the size, location and visual effects of which depend on the site of occlusion and its proximity to the central retinal artery and macula. In a young patient the causes are most likely vasospastic, embolic and inflammatory. These include migraine, coagulation abnormalities, presence of the lupus anticoagulant or anticardiolipin antibodies, cardiac valvular disease, collagen vascular diseases, or talc emboli from intravenous drug abuse. The most common association in pregnancy is with migraine[43], but other coexisting conditions include amniotic fluid embolism, toxemia, and mitral valve prolapse. After a central retinal artery occlusion, irreversible ischemic necrosis of the inner retina probably occurs within a few hours. Although no therapeutic regimen has been proven effective, commonly employed modalities include ocular massage, breathing a mixture of 95% oxygen and 5% carbon dioxide for 10 minutes each hour, and anterior chamber paracentesis to lower intraocular pressure, with hopes of dislodging any embolus. Antiplatelet agents often are used, but anticoagulation is of no value. Treatment of a branch artery occlusion is that of any underlying disease. Cotton-wool spots represent retinal infarcts resulting from retinal pre-capillary arteriolar occlusions and are generally asymptomatic. Hypertension, diabetes mellitus, collagen vascular disease, and anemia are the most common causes, but any of the above entities can be etiologic. They also may be seen in 50% of patients with AIDS. Rarely, bilateral visual loss in the postpartum period may occur due to multiple retinal arteriolar occlusions simulating Purtscher's retinopathy (which is otherwise associated with trauma, pancreatitis, and collagen vascular diseases).[43a] Complement-induced leukoemboli have been proposed to be etiologic. Most but not all patients have had improved vision within several weeks.

Retinal vein occlusions also tend to occur in older patients with atherosclerosis, hypertension and diabetes mellitus. Central retinal vein occlusions are categorized into a more severe ischemic type with severe visual loss, dilated, engorged retinal veins, massive hemorrhage, diffuse retinal edema, and ischemia with a less severe relatively nonischemic type with a lesser degree of retinal hemorrhage and mild to moderately reduced vision from macular edema. A fluorescein angiogram or electroretinogram may help to distinguish these two types. The former has a very poor visual prognosis and the frequent development of iris neovascularization, with a resultant severe neovascular glaucoma that may be very difficult to treat but can be prevented by panretinal laser photocoagulation. The nonischemic type may have a variable recovery of vision. There is no specific treatment of these conditions and anticoagulation has not been beneficial. In patients under 40 the most common associated diseases are hypertension and diabetes mellitus. Also to be considered are hyperviscosity syndromes, blood dyscrasias, collagen vascular diseases, anemia, hyperlipidemia, hypercholesterolemia, hypercoagulable states, the lupus anticoagulant or anticardiolipin antibodies, or a systemic phlebitis such as sarcoidosis or Behcet's disease. A branch vein occlusion affects only a sector of retina and may be symptomatic only if a temporal vein occlusion causes macular edema. If the macular edema is persistent and reduces vision, then laser photocoagulation to the macula, which can be deferred until postpartum, reduces the chance of further visual deterioration. Retinal neovascularization may develop after several months depending on the amount of retinal ischemia. Laser photocoagulation in this case should be performed to the involved retinal quadrant to prevent vitreous hemorrhage. Systemic evaluation is similar to that for a central retinal vein occlusion but with an emphasis on inflammatory causes in this age group. Pregnancy does not appear to predispose towards retinal vein occlusions.

Angioid streaks are dark red to brown or gray, irregular subretinal bands that surround the optic disc with radial branches that extend out towards the peripheral retina. They represent breaks in Bruch's membrane and occur most often in pseudoxanthoma elasticum. Other causes are sickle cell anemia, Paget's disease of bone, acromegaly, hypercalcemia, and lead poisoning. They are asymptomatic unless subretinal neovascularization develops, which may be treated with laser photocoagulation similar to its treatment in the presumed ocular histoplasmosis syndrome. The risk of this complication occurring does not appear to be increased in pregnancy.[42b]

Optic Nerve and Visual Pathways

The optic nerve, consisting of axons of retinal ganglion cells, leaves the back of the eye to travel posteriorly in the orbit and enter the cranial cavity through the optic canal. The two optic nerves join intracranially to form the optic chiasm, where fibers from the nasal retina (temporal visual field) decussate and join uncrossed fibers from the temporal retina (nasal visual field) of the opposite optic nerve to form the optic tracts. The optic tracts synapse in the homolateral lateral geniculate body, which in turn gives rise to the geniculocalcarine tract. These tracts form the optic radiations, which pass through the temporal and parietal lobes en route to the occipital lobes. Thus, the right visual field projects to the left cerebral hemisphere, and the left visual field to the right cerebral hemisphere. Fibers subserving pupillary function leave the optic tract anterior to the lateral geniculate body and pass to the midbrain, which is why lesions posterior to this region do not normally affect pupillary function. Lesions anterior to the optic chiasm affect vision in only the homolateral eye, generally disturbing central vision and color vision. Chiasmal lesions, such as pituitary adenomas, cause temporal visual field defects in both eyes. Lesions posterior to the chiasm cause homonymous contralateral visual field defects in the two eyes.

Papilledema generally is bilateral optic disk swelling produced by increased intracranial pressure of any cause. The usual signs of increased intracranial pressure may include headache and diplopia from stretching of the abducens nerve with subsequent paresis of the lateral rectus muscle of one or both eyes. The optic disk is swollen and hyperemic with blurred margins. The retinal veins may be dilated with loss of spontaneous pulsations, and there may be flame-shaped hemorrhages near the disk. Visual acuity is normal, although transient obscurations of vision may occur. Visual fields are usually normal except for enlarged blind spots. Central nervous system tumors that appear to be affected adversely by pregnancy and may cause papilledema include pituitary adenomas, craniopharyngiomas, and meningiomas.[43] Although visual acuity can decrease and visual field defects develop with very chronic papilledema as a result of atrophy of optic nerve fibers, this is unlikely to occur during pregnancy, thus treatment should be focused on the primary underlying disease.

Benign intracranial hypertension, or pseudotumor cerebri, is a syndrome of increased intracranial pressure with papilledema without evidence of a space-occupying lesion or abnormality of the ventricles and without localized neurologic findings other than cranial nerve VI paresis (see also Chapter 199). It is more common in obese women of childbearing age. Although an association with pregnancy has been suggested[44], it is probably no more frequent in pregnancy than in an age-matched nonpregnant population.[44a] It tends to present in the first half of gestation and has been related to decreased levels of adrenal corticoids and increased androgens.[44,44a] It can be self limited, resolving within a few months without permanent visual loss.[44] However, it is not always "benign" and can result in visual field defects in up to 27%[45] and permanent visual impairment in up to 25%[45a] of patients (especially in the presence of hypertension). The visual loss is insidious and often asymptomatic, requiring careful monitoring of visual acuity and visual fields. The visual field defects may be reversible until the irreversible ophthalmoscopic changes of optic disk gliosis and pallor occur. Pregnancy does not increase the risk of visual loss and the outcome of pregnancy is not jeopardized by this condition. Because the visual loss occurs gradually over months to years, when asymptomatic with normal visual acuity and visual fields, therapy of the pregnant patient may be able to be deferred until after pregnancy, especially since most cases will resolve within a year of delivery. When there is threatened visual loss, treatment may be attempted with repeated lumbar punctures or oral corticosteroids. Caloric restriction and diuretic use probably are contraindicated in pregnancy. When necessary, lumboperitoneal shunts or optic nerve sheath decompression can be performed. However, the relative efficacies of these treatments is not known. Other causes of papilledema such as an intracranial mass lesion, cerebral venous thrombosis, hypertensive encephalopathy, Lyme disease, meningitis or meningeal lymphomatosis must be excluded, as well as toxic factors such as vitamin A, tetracycline, nalidixic acid, carbon dioxide or lead poisoning. A lumbar puncture is necessary for accurate diagnosis.

In optic neuritis, there is an acute decrease in central vision as a result of inflammation, demyelinization, or degeneration of the optic nerve. The most common cause in young adults is multiple sclerosis, thus it may occur fortuitously in a pregnant patient who may develop or already have this disease. Pregnancy alone does not appear to predispose the patient to the development of optic neuritis. Usually, it is a retrobular neuritis, in which case the optic nerve may look normal, although with time pallor may develop. If papillitis occurs, the appearance of the optic disk can be similar to that in papilledema. However, this is unusual in adults, and a retrobulbar tumor must be ruled out. In addition to decreased visual acuity, the patient will have defective color vision, a central or paracentral scotoma, and may have pain on eye movement. An afferent pupillary defect will be present (as it will in any optic nerve lesion) in which both pupils are smaller when the good eye is stimulated by light but both pupils are larger when the defective eye is stimulated by light. Other possible causes are vitamin B_{12} and other nutritional deficiencies, neurosyphilis, and drug toxicity such as ethambutol or quinine poisoning. Optic disk swelling with reduced visual acuity also can be caused by optic nerve gliomas and meningiomas or by increased orbital contents resulting from thyroid ophthalmopathy. Compressive lesions rarely have been reported to cause acute monocular visual loss from sudden interruption of the optic nerve's vascular supply with pituitary tumors and meningiomas during pregnancy.[46] Therefore, orbital ultrasound and computerized tomography should be considered part of the diagnostic evaluation. Treatment of optic neuritis with corticosteroids has not been proven effective and is controversial.

Chiasmal lesions may occur because preexisting intrasellar and suprasellar tumors, especially pituitary adenomas, may enlarge considerably during pregnancy, causing visual symptoms in about 35% of cases.[47] One should be especially wary of this in a pregnant woman previously treated for anovulation and hyperprolactinemia with bromocriptine, who may harbor an occult pituitary adenoma.[48] In addition to bitemporal visual field defects, there may be decreased central vision and defective color vision in one or both eyes. Ophthalmoscopic examination may reveal normal optic disks, or there may be optic atrophy in a horizontal band if papilledema has not occurred. Visual symptoms usually occur in the latter half of pregnancy and regress in most patients after termination of the pregnancy by delivery or abortion. Monthly ophthalmologic evaluation with visual fields probably are indicated in a pregnant woman with a known pituitary adenoma. No treatment is necessary unless the visual symptoms are severe and progressive. Bromocriptine may cause tumor regression and symptom abatement. On occasion, significant visual impairment or other pressure symptoms may require emergency surgery.[47] It also has been noted that the pituitary gland itself may enlarge during the third trimester and rarely cause visual symptoms that spontaneously resolve after delivery.[46] Lymphocytic hypophysitis may produce a chiasmal syndrome that mimics a pituitary adenoma in pregnancy or postpartum and should be considered in patients with symptoms of hypopituitarism.

Patients with migraine headaches may develop binocular scintillating or fortification scotomas for several minutes prior to the onset of headache in classical migraine, which is thought to be caused by intracerebral vasospasm. A rare variant is ophthalmoplegic migraine causing oculomotor nerve palsies, most often affecting the third cranial nerve, with usually transient diplopia that can rarely become permanent. Aneurysms and tumors in the vicinity of the cavernous sinus must be ruled out. Another rare variant is retinal migraine, in which a permanent monocular visual field defect may occur following a transient episode of monocular visual loss in a patient with a strong history of migraine, probably because of constriction of the central retinal artery or ophthalmic artery. Migraine in general seems to improve in about 80% of patients during pregnancy.[49] However, in a few pregnant patients it may worsen or develop for the first time, generally in the first trimester.[50]

Puerperal cerebral venous thrombosis has been reported to cause cortical blindness and homonymous hemianopsias that resolve completely in 80% of patients but may leave a residual deficit.[51] The patients may have seizures, headaches, and focal neurologic deficits and can have papilledema with thrombosis of the superior longitudinal sinus. Blindness, however, can occur as an isolated event.[51a] This must be differentiated from cerebral hemorrhage, embolism, and migraine. Treatment is controversial but may include corticosteroids and anticonvulsants.

Extraocular Muscles

The most common disorder of the extraocular muscles is strabismus, a congenital or acquired malalignment of the eyes, generally first occurring in childhood and having a variety of causes ranging from a hereditary predisposition to monocular visual loss. It exists when the eyes are positioned such that the image of regard is focused on the fovea of one eye but not the other. Strabismus may be latent (phoria) or manifest (tropia). The deviation may be inward (eso), outward (exo), upward (hyper), or downward (hypo). There also may be torsional components. Amblyopia may or may not be present. It should be noted that a tropia that begins in early childhood and is untreated will never cause symptomatic diplopia in later life no matter how large the deviation because of sensory adjustments children are able to make. However, it is possible for a lifelong phoria to "break down" into a manifest deviation in response to physical or psychological stress during pregnancy, causing the onset of diplopia. There may be no apparent weakness of any extraocular muscle. It is usually transient and self-limited and best treated by reassurance of the patient. At times, corrective lenses or prisms may be helpful. Any extraocular muscle surgery is usually for cosmetic reasons and should be postponed until after pregnancy.

Diplopia of any other cause signifies a relatively recent lesion of either the extraocular muscles, such as in myasthenia gravis, thyroid ophthalmopathy, or Kearns–Sayre syndrome, or the cranial nerves supplying them anywhere along their path from the nuclei in the mid-brain, and pons (demyelinating disease), through the cavernous sinus (carotid aneurysms, meningioma, nasopharyngeal carcinoma or other tumor), or in the orbit (tumor, inflammatory pseudotumor, or infection). Systemic and neurologic evaluation and appropriate neuroradiologic testing should determine the etiology and treatment.

The third cranial nerve innervates the superior, medial and inferior rectus and inferior oblique muscles as well as the levator palpebrae muscle of the eyelid and the pupillary sphincter muscle via parasympathetic fibers. Therefore, compressive lesions of this nerve will cause multiple extraocular muscle palsies, pupillary dilation, and ptosis. Vascular diseases such as diabetes mellitus usually spare the pupillary fibers.

The sixth nerve innervates the later rectus muscle and may be affected by increased intracranial pressure with resultant inability to abduct one or both eyes. The fourth nerve innervates the superior oblique muscle and may be affected by closed-head trauma or microvascular disease, causing a hypertropia and a head tilt as a consequence of the torsional component of this muscle.

Internuclear ophthalmoplegia is caused by a lesion of the medial longitudinal fasciculus in the brain stem, which integrates the ocular motor nuclei. This results in absent or deficient adduction of the ipsilateral eye with coarse nystagmus of the abducting contralateral eye. This is often a sign of demyelinating disease, especially if it is bilateral, but it can be mimicked by the muscle weakness of myasthenia gravis. Therefore, a Tensilon test might be considered in uncertain cases.

A supranuclear destructive lesion of the frontal lobe will cause a contralateral voluntary gaze (saccade) palsy with deviation of the eyes to the ipsilateral side but with retention of ocular pursuit movements of a slowly moving object. Parieto-occipital lobe lesions, on the other hand, may cause loss of ipsilateral pursuit movements with retention of saccadic movement.

Nystagmus is a rhythmic oscillation of one or both eyes in any field of gaze. It can be pendular, with eye movements of equal velocity in both directions, or jerk, with an initial slow phase followed by a fast phase in the direction of which the nystagmus is named. Endpoint nystagmus is a physiologic jerk nystagmus. Nystagmus can be subdivided into many other types and may be caused by disease of the vestibular system, cerebellum, or brain stem, drug toxicity (especially phenytoin or barbiturates), or congenital visual loss, as in albinism.

In any disorder of the extraocular muscles in a pregnant patient, one should consider the ophthalmopathy of Graves' disease, which is a relatively common disorder in this age group. The ophthalmic manifestations may occur with hyperthyroidism, hypothyroidism, or no clinically or biochemically detectable thyroid dysfunction (euthyroid Graves' disease). Ophthalmopathy also may occur long after the diagnosis of Graves' disease. The thyroid and ophthalmic manifestations run separate clinical courses, and therapy of the thyroid dysfunction may not necessarily have any effect on the ophthalmic disease.

There is no clear evidence that pregnancy affects either the appearance or course of the ophthalmopathy. Eyelid retraction with eyelid lag and infrequent blinking may develop into a "thyroid stare." An inflammatory mononuclear cell reaction can thicken the extraocular muscles and increase the mass of the orbital contents, resulting in proptosis, which can mimic an orbital tumor if unilateral. Computerized tomography or ultrasound examination of the uninvolved orbit will often reveal enlarged extraocular muscles. The extraocular muscle involvement can lead to restriction of any of the muscles, although the inferior rectus is involved most often with deficient upgaze and vertical diplopia. An increase in intraocular pressure in upgaze is a relatively early sign of Graves' ophthalmopathy. Orbital congestion can cause a compressive optic neuropathy with gradual loss of central vision in probably fewer than 5% of patients.[52]

All signs and symptoms of ophthalmopathy tend to progress for 1 or 2 years and then subside.[53] Therefore, systemic medical or surgical therapy should be delayed if possible until after pregnancy. Corneal exposure caused by proptosis and lid lag may be treated with ocular lubricants. Cosmetic eyelid surgery can be performed postpartum. Diplopia may be treated with prisms, and if symptoms are intractable or there are severe cosmetic problems, surgery on the extraocular muscles may be performed after pregnancy and after the acute inflammatory process subsides. If progressive optic neuropathy occurs with vision decreasing to worse than 20/40, a trial of oral corticosteroids may be attempted with 40–100 mg of prednisone daily. If no response occurs in 1–2 weeks, or as an alternate therapy, surgical decompression of the orbit may be necessary to preserve vision.

Wernicke's encephalopathy may occur rarely in severe cases of hyperemesis gravidarum with the development of nystagmus and extraocular muscle palsies, as well as retinal hemorrhages and optic neuritis. Treatment with thiamine and vitamins may cause resolution of the ocular motor signs.[53a] AIDS encephalopathy may cause abnormalities of both saccadic and pursuit movements in addition to ocular motor palsies from secondary infections of the central nervous system. Lyme disease may cause paresis of the third or sixth cranial nerves, which may respond to treatment with intravenous penicillin G.

Pupils. Pregnancy itself has no effect on the pupils. The size of the pupil is regulated by the iris sphincter and dilator muscles. The sphincter is parasympathetically innervated by the third cranial nerve by way of the ciliary ganglion and short ciliary nerves, and constricts the pupil in response to light and accommodation. The dilator muscle is innervated sympathetically as described previously and dilates the pupil. Since afferent pupillary fibers originate from the same retinal receptors as afferent visual fibers and hemidecussate in the chiasm, and since efferent fibers from each pretectal nucleus supplies equal innervation to both oculomotor nuclei, light or accommodative stimulus to either eye causes both pupils to constrict equally. When a unilateral optic nerve lesion causes an afferent pupillary defect, both pupils constrict less when light is moved from the normal to the affected eye.

A third-nerve lesion will cause dilation of the ipsilateral pupil, which will be more obvious in bright illumination as the pupil fails to constrict normally. This is differentiated from the pharmacologic effect of an atropinic drug by miosis in response to pilocarpine 1% eyedrops. A posterior communicating artery aneurysm or supratentorial or cavernous sinus mass should be considered.

Adie's tonic pupil is an internal ophthalmoplegia occurring in young women, possibly because of an abnormality in the ciliary ganglion, and is a benign lesion. The patient may complain of unilateral blurred near vision or may be asymptomatic. Usually the affected pupil is relatively dilated, reacts poorly to light, and has a slow and tonic response to accommodation (near vision) that is usually greater than the light response. Usually deep tendon reflexes are diminished. There is a denervation supersensitivity of the parasympathetic fibers, and the pupil will constrict in response to pilocarpine 0.125% eyedrops to a greater degree than the normal pupil.

Light-near dissociation exists when a mid-brain lesion affects light reflex fibers but not near reflex fibers so that the pupils do not react to light but react normally to accommodation. This can be caused by a pinealoma or other lesion of the periaqueductal gray. It also is seen in the Argyll–Robertson pupil of neurosyphilis.

In Horner's syndrome, characterized by ptosis, miosis, and facial anhidrosis, caused by interruption of the oculosympathetic pathway, the aniscoria is more marked in dim illumination, as the affected pupil exhibits dilation lag. Topical cocaine eyedrops fail to dilate a pupil with Horner's syndrome. Hydroxyamphetamine eyedrops will dilate a pupil with Horner's syndrome if the lesion is preganglionic but not if it is postganglionic. This is important since preganglionic lesions frequently are caused by tumors in the pulmonary apex or cervical area, whereas an isolated postganglionic Horner's syndrome is generally benign. A transient Horner's syndrome during epidural analgesia may be more likely to occur in a pregnant woman and may have associated maternal hypotension.[54]

Ocular Tumors

Malignant ocular tumors are very rare, especially in pregnancy, with the most frequent being choroidal malignant melanomas. These may be asymptomatic until they have grown large enough to cause a retinal detachment. They appear to be less aggressive than cutaneous malignant melanomas, and for small asymptomatic melanomas simple observation may be all that is required. For large, symptomatic, or actively growing melanomas, treatment is controversial. Although in the past enucleation was the standard treatment, there is some evidence to indicate that this actually may increase the possibility of metastasis, although this has been disputed. Local radiotherapy with external-beam irradiation or scleral plaques has been effective in many cases. Choroidal malignant melanomas tend to occur in patients older than child-bearing age. A recent pathologic study indicated a greater than expected number of choroidal melanomas in pregnant patients, although this was not statistically significant, with one patient showing growth of the tumor over the course of two pregnancies.[54a] It was proposed that this may be a hormonally responsive tumor, although no estrogen binding was found. There are no reported cases of fetal metastases.

Primary tumors in other organs may, of course, metastasize to the choroid (especially from the lung or breast), although this is probably rare during pregnancy, and may be responsive to local irradiation.

Choroidal hemangiomas are rare, benign vascular tumors that may cause leakage of fluid into the subretinal space in the macula with decreased visual acuity. Pregnancy may have an adverse effect, as a pregnant patient has been reported to have a symptomatic choroidal hemangioma that regressed postpartum with improvement in vision.[55] Choroidal osteoma is an unusual benign, bony, choroidal tumor that is most common in young women and generally is located adjacent to the optic disk. It has ultrasonographic and CT scan characteristics of calcium or bone. It is relatively asymptomatic and requires no treatment unless secondary subretinal neovascularization develops. Although it has occurred in a pregnant woman, the relationship to pregnancy is unclear.[55a]

FETAL ASPECTS

Maternal ocular diseases themselves do not affect the fetus. However, there may be fetal effects from therapy of these disorders or the underlying systemic disease. Where applicable, these effects have been described in the preceding sections. One should take the same care in administering ophthalmic drugs in the nursing mother as during pregnancy. Topical timolol eye drops, for example, are secreted actively in breast milk and carry the danger of possible apnea in the nursing infant.[56]

Organogenesis of the human eye occurs between 24 and 40 days of gestation; therefore, the danger of ocular teratogenicity in the fetus from infection or drugs is greatest early in the first trimester, with the hazard decreasing markedly after this period. Rubella viremia in the first trimester often results in bilateral congenital cataracts, glaucoma, or pigmentary retinopathy. If retinopathy alone occurs, vision may be relatively good. The visual prognosis with cataracts may be poor even with successful surgical removal. Congenital toxoplasmosis acquired in the first two trimesters can result in severe disease with fetal death or severe mental retardation in addition to retinochoroiditis. If it develops in the third trimester, however, the infant may appear completely normal at birth, but a large proportion may develop ocular toxoplasmosis later in life. Congenital syphilis can lead to the later development of interstitial keratitis. In addition to rubella, viruses that can cause ocular teratogenesis include cytomegalovirus, herpes simplex virus, varicella-zoster virus, and mumps.

Short palpebral fissures, telecanthus, microphthalmia, ptosis, strabismus, corneal opacities, anterior chamber angle abnormalities, iris defects, optic disk hypoplasia, and retinal vascular tortuosity may be noted in the fetal alcohol syndrome. Maternal vitamin A deficiency has been related to fetal microphthalmia and anophthalmia, and vitamin D deficiency to cataracts. Eye abnormalities in the fetal hydantoin syndrome may include hypertelorism, ptosis, strabismus, epicanthal folds, and lacrimal abnormalities. Virtually all cancer chemotherapeutic agents have been shown to cause major ocular abnormalities after *in utero* exposure. Therapeutic radiation of 500 rad or more in the first trimester is associated with microphthalmia, pigmentary retinal degeneration, and cataracts.[57] Diagnostic radiation of 5 rad or less has not been proven to cause ocular abnormalities.[58] Maternal methadone use may predispose infants to the development of strabismus. Abnormal visual evoked potentials[59] have occurred in newborn infants with cocaine in their urine.

As noted above, contact of the fetus with infected secretions of the birth canal can lead to ophthalmia neonatorum caused by *Chlamydia trachomatis* about ten times as frequently as gonococcus infection. It also can be caused by staphylococci or coliform bacilli or be secondary to chemical conjunctivitis from silver nitrate prophylaxis. The neonate presents with a purulent or mucopurulent conjunctivitis with swollen lids. In contrast to the adult, chlamydial conjunctivitis cannot be distinguished from gonococcal conjunctivitis by the presence of a follicular conjunctivitis since lymphoid tissue is not present in the conjunctiva of the neonate. Although chlamydial conjunctivitis of the newborn is said to begin several days later than gonococcal conjunctivitis, this is unreliable in distinguishing the two. Conjunctival scrapings for Gram's and Giemsa stains as well as cultures as described previously must be performed for proper diagnosis. Gonococcal infection should be treated with intravenous or intramuscular cefriaxone, topical erythromycin or bacitracin ointment, and saline lavage for up to seven days. Chlamydial infection should be treated with topical erythromycin ointment and intramuscular erythromycin for 2–3 weeks. In either of these infections, systemic treatment of the parents also should be considered.

Prophylaxis for gonococcal conjunctivitis has been recommended with 1% tetracycline or 0.5% erythromycin ointment or a 1% silver nitrate solution. While erythromycin and tetracycline ointments have the theoretical advantage over silver nitrate of being effective against chlamydia as well as gonorrhea, none of these regimens has been proven superior to the others in clinical practice.[59a] None of these regimens prevents chlamydial pneumonia. An effective method of prophylaxis for chlamydia may prove to be the screening of pregnant women for chlamydial infection and treating those found to be infected.

Eye involvement with herpes simplex *in utero* can occur and should be suspected if there is a history of genital herpes in the mother. Some 17% of neonatal herpes simplex virus infections have ocular involvement, which may be manifested as conjunctivitis, keratitis, cataracts, chorioretinitis, or optic atrophy.[60]

Ocular abnormalities in the neonate also can result from trauma during labor and delivery in 12–25% of normal births. Corneal opacification may occur as a result of direct compression by delivery forceps and usually appears as vertically curvilinear folds or scroll-like detachments of the posterior surface of the cornea. With healing, the cornea usually clears. Rarely, hyphema (anterior chamber hemorrhage) or vitreous hemorrhage may occur as a result of direct trauma from forceps or vacuum extraction and eyelid laceration can occur with episiotomy. Laceration of the eye of the fetus with resulting blindness can occur during amniocentesis.

Retinal hemorrhages have been observed in between 2.5% and 50% of neonates[61] depending on the time of examination; they are most common in the first 24 hours after birth. These may be flame-shaped hemorrhages mainly near the disk, which usually disappear within 1–3 days but may coalesce to form wide superficial hemorrhages. More rare are deep round hemorrhages, which disappear in 14–21 days. Trauma or compression of the fetal head or neck appears to play some role, as these hemorrhages are more common in premature infants and much less common with cesarean section. Neonatal retinal hemorrhages are also more common in labor induced by dinoprostone than by oxytocin.[63] In addition, subhyaloid hemorrhages may be associated with intracranial hemorrhage. These hemorrhages normally do not have a lasting effect on vision.

REFERENCES

1. Duke-Elder S, Scott, GI. Neuro-Ophthalmology. In: Duke-Elder S, ed. *System of Ophthalmology*. St. Louis, MO: CV Mosby; 1971;10:703.
2. Millodot M. The influence of pregnancy on the sensitivity of the cornea. *Br J Ophthalmol*. 1977;61:646.
3. Beard C. The surgical treatment of blepharoptosis: a quantitative approach. *Trans Am Ophthalmol Soc*. 1966;64:401.

3a. Centers for Disease Control. Antibiotic-resistant strains of *Neiserria gonorrhea*. *MMWR*. 1987;36(suppl. no. 5S):15S.
4. Sweet RL, Schacter J, Landers DV. Chlamydial infections in obstetrics and gynecology. *Clin Obstet Gynecol*. 1983;26:143.
5. Hanna L, Ostler HB, Keshishyan BA. Observed relationship between herpetic lesions and antigenic type of herpes virus hominis. *Surv Ophthalmol*. 1976;21:110.
6. Oh JO, Kimura SJ, Ostler HB, et al. Oculogenital transmission of type 2 herpes simplex virus in adults. *Surv Ophthalmol*. 1976;21:106.
7. Itoi M, Gefter JW, Noboru K, et al. Teratogenicities of ophthalmic drugs. *Arch Ophthalmol*. 1975;93:46.

7a. Cobo LM, Foulks GN, Leisegang T, et al: Oral acyclovir in the treatment of acute herpes zoster ophthalmicus. *Ophthalmology*. 1986;93:763.
8. Watson PG, Hayreh SS. Scleritis and episcleritis. *Br J Ophthalmol*. 1976;60:163.
9. Hørven I, Gjørinaess H. Corneal indentation pulse and intraocular pressure in pregnancy. *Arch Ophthalmol*. 1974;91:92.
10. Samples JR, Meyer SM. Use of ophthalmic medications in pregnant and nursing women. *Am J Ophthalmol*. 1988;106:616.
11. Frishman WH, Chesner M. Beta-adrenergic blockers in pregnancy. *Am Heart Journal*. 1988;115:147.
12. Birks DA, Prior VJ, Silke E, et al. Echothiaphate iodide treatment of glaucoma in pregnancy. *Arch Ophthalmol*. 1968;79:283.
13. Hyman BN. Postpartum uveitis. *Ann Ophthalmol*. 1976;8:677.
14. Østensen M. Øistein R, Husby G. Ankylosing spondylitis and motherhood. *Arth Rheum*. 1982;25:140.
15. Snyder DA, Tessler HH. Vogt-Kayanagi-Harada syndrome. *Am J Ophthalmol*. 1980;90:69.
16. O'Connor GR. Factors related to the initiation and recurrence of uveitis: XL Edward Jackson Memorial Lecture. *Am J Ophthalmol*. 1983;96:577.
17. Jacobs L, Naquin H, Hoover R, et al. A comparison of the toxoplasma skin tests, the Sabin-Feldman dye tests, and the complement fixation tests for toxoplasmosis in various forms of uveitis. *Bull Johns Hopkins Hosp*. 1956;99:1.
18. Cantrill HL, Rodman WP, Ramsay RC, et al. Postpartum *Candida* endophthalmitis. *JAMA*. 1980;243:1163.
19. Kasirsky G, Lombardi L. Comparative teratogenic study of various corticoid ophthalmics. *Toxicol Appl Pharmacol*. 1970;16:773.
20. Ballard PD, Hearney EF, Smith MB. Induction of cleft palate in mice after ophthalmic administration of hydrocortisone. *Toxicol Appl Pharmacol*. 1975;34:358.

20a. Halperin LS, Olk RJ, Gisele S, Coscas G. Safety of fluorescein angiography during pregnancy. *Am J Ophthalmol*. 1990;109:563.
21. Demonts G, Couvreur J. Congenital toxoplasmosis: a prospective study of 378 pregnancies. *N Engl J Med*. 1974;290:1110.
22. Perkins ES. Ocular toxoplasmosis. *Br J Ophthalmol*. 1973;57:1.
23. O'Connor GR. Ocular toxoplasmosis. In: *The Transactions of the New Orleans Academy of Ophthalmology: Symposium on Medical and Surgical Diseases of the Retina and Vitreous*. St. Louis, MO: CV Mosby; 1983:108.
24. Matsuo T, Ohno A, Matsuo N. Acute retinal necrosis syndrome following chicken pox in pregnant woman. *Jpn J Ophthalmol*. 1988;32:70.

24a. Teich SA, Orellana J. Retinal lesions in cytomegalovirus infection. *Ann Intern Med*. 1986;104:132.
25. Klein R, Klein BEK, Moss SE, et al. The Wisconsin epidemiologic study of diabetic retinopathy: II. Prevalence and risk of diabetic retinopathy when age at diagnosis is less than 30 years. *Arch Ophthalmol*. 1984;102:520.
26. Horvat M, MacLean H, Goldberg L, et al. Diabetic retinopathy in pregnancy: A twelve-year prospective survey. *Br J Ophthalmol*. 1980;64:398.
27. Maloney JBM, Drury MI. The effect of pregnancy on the natural course of diabetic retinopathy. *Am J Ophthalmol*. 1982;93:745.
28. Klein BEK, Klein R. Gravidity and diabetic retinopathy. *Am J Ophthalmol*. 1984;119:564.
29. Boone MI, Farber ME, Jovanovic-Peterson L, Peterson CM. Increased retinal vascular tortuosity in gestational diabetes mellitus. *Ophthalmology*. 1989;96:251.
30. Phelps RL, Sakol P, Metzger BE, et al. Changes in diabetic retinopathy during pregnancy: Correlations with regulation of hyperglycemia. *Arch Ophthalmol*. 1986;104:1806.
31. Sinclair S, Nesler C, Foxman B, et al. Macular edema and pregnancy in insulin-dependent diabetes. *Am J Ophthalmol*. 1984;97:154.
32. The Diabetic Retinopathy Study Research Group. Photocoagulation treatment of proliferative diabetic retinopathy: The second report of diabetic retinopathy study findings. *Ophthalmology*. 1978;85:82.
33. Johnston GP. Pregnancy and diabetic retinopathy. *Am J Ophthalmol*. 1980;90:519.
34. The Diabetic Retinopathy Vitrectomy Study Research Group. Early vitrectomy for severe vitreous hemorrhage in diabetic retinopathy: Two year results of a randomized trial. Diabetic Retinopathy Vitrectomy Study Report 2. *Arch Ophthalmol*. 1985;103:1644.
35. Early Treatment Diabetic Retinopathy Study Research Group. Early Treatment Diabetic Retinopathy Study: Report No. 1: Photocoagulation for diabetic macular edema. *Arch Ophthalmol*. 1985;103:1796.
36. Wagener HP. Arterioles of the retina in toxemia of pregnancy. *JAMA*. 1933;101:1380.

37. Fastenberg DM, Fetkenhour CL, Choromokos E, et al: Choroidal vascular changes in toxemia of pregnancy. *Am J Ophthalmol.* 1980;89:362.
37a. Beeson JH, Duda EE. Computed axial tomography scan demonstration of cerebral edema in eclampsia preceded by blindness. *Obstet Gynecol.* 1982;60:529.
38. Duke-Elder S, Dobree JH. Diseases of the retina. In: Duke-Elder S, ed. *System of Ophthalmology.* St. Louis, MO: CV Mosby; 1967;10:350.
38a. Jaffe G, Schatz H. Ocular manifestations of preeclampsia. *Am J Ophthalmol.* 1987;103:309.
39. Chumbley LC, Frunk RN. Central serous retinopathy and pregnancy. *Am J Ophthalmol.* 1974;77:158.
40. Cruysberg JRM, Deutman AF. Visual disturbances during pregnancy caused by central serous choroidopathy. *Br J Ophthalmol.* 1982;66:240.
40a. Sunness JS. The pregnant woman's eye. *Surv Ophthalmol.* 1988;32:219.
41. Ullberg S, Lindquist NG, Sjöstrand SE. Accumulation of chorio-retino-toxic drugs in the foetal eye. *Nature.* 1970;227:1257.
42. Neri A, Grausbord R, Kremer I, et al. The management of labor in high myopic patients. *Europ J Obstet Gynec Reprod Biol.* 1985;19:277.
42a. Brown GC, Magargal LE, Shields JA, et al: Retinal arterial obstruction in children and young adults. *Ophthalmology.* 1981;88:18.
42b. Berde C, Willis DC, Sandberg EC. Pregnancy in women with pseudo-xanthoma elasticum. *Obstet Gynecol Surv.* 1983;38:339.
43. Donegan WL. Cancer and pregnancy. *CA—A Jrl Clin.* 1983;33:194.
43a. Blodi BA, Johnson MW, Gass JDM, et al. Purtscher's-like retinopathy after childbirth. *Ophthalmology.* 1990; 97:1654.
44. Greer M. Benign intracranial hypertension. III. Pregnancy. *Neurology (Minneap).* 1963;13:670.
44a. Digre KB, Varner MW, Corbett JJ. Pseudotumor cerebri and pregnancy. *Neurology.* 1984;34:721.
45. Wall M, Hart WM, Burde RM. Visual field defects in idiopathic intracranial hypertension (pseudomotor cerebri). *Am J Ophthalmol.* 1983;96:654.
45a. Corbett JJ, Savino PJ, Thompson HS, et al. Visual loss in pseudotumor cerebri: Follow-up of 57 patients from 5 to 41 years and a profile of 14 patients with permanent severe visual loss. *Arch Neurol.* 1982;39:461.
46. Miller NR. *Walsh and Hoyt's Clinical Neuro-Ophthalmology,* 4th ed. Baltimore, MD: Williams & Wilkins; 1982;1:285.
47. Husami N, Jewelewicz R, Vande Viele RL. Pregnancy in patients with pituitary tumors. *Fertil Steril.* 1977;28:920.
48. Corbey RS, Cruysberg JRM, Rolland R. Visual abnormalities in a pregnancy following bromocriptin medication. *Obstet Gynecol.* 1977;50:69s.
49. Friedman AP, Merritt HH. Headache: Diagnosis and Treatment. Philadelphia, PA: FA Davis; 1959:210.
50. Somerville BW. A study of migraine in pregnancy. *Neurology (Minneap).* 1972;22:824.
51. Beal MF, Chapman PH. Cortical blindness and homonymous hemianopia in the postpartum period. *JAMA.* 1980;244:2085.
51a. Monteiro MLR, Hoyt WF, Imes RK. Puerperal cerebral blindness: Transient bilateral occipital involvement from presumed cerebral venous thrombosis. *Arch Neurol.* 1984;41:1300.
52. Day RM, Carroll FD. Optic nerve involvement associated with thyroid dysfunction. *Arch Ophthalmol.* 1962;67:289.
53. Sergott RC, Glaser JS. Graves ophthalmopathy: A clinical and immunologic review. *Surv Ophthalmol.* 1981;26:1.
53a. Wood P, Murray A, Sinha B, et al. Wernicke's encephalopathy induced by hyperemesis gravidarum: case reports. *Brit J Obstet Gynecol.* 1983;90:583.
54. Schachner SM, Reynolds AC. Horner syndrome during lumbar epidural analgesia for obstetrics. *Obstet Gynecol.* 1982;59:31s.
54a. Seddon JM, MacLaughlin DT, Albert DM, et al. Uveal melanomas presenting during pregnancy and the investigation of oestrogen receptors in melanomas. *Br J Ophthalmol.* 1982;66:695.
55. Pitta C, Bergen R, Littwin S. Spontaneous regression of a choroidal hemangioma following pregnancy. *Ann Ophthalmol.* 1979;11:772.
55a. McLeod BK. Choroidal osteoma presenting in pregnancy. *Br J Ophthalmol.* 1988;72:612.
56. Lustgarten JS, Podos SM. Topical timolol and the nursing mother. *Arch Ophthalmol.* 1983;101:1381.
57. Dekaban AS. Abnormalities in children exposed to X-radiation during various stages of gestation: Tentative timetable of radiation injury to the human fetus, part 1. *J Nucl Med.* 1968;9:471.
58. Greim MD, Meier P, Dobben GD. Analysis of the morbidity and mortality of children irradiated in fetal life. *Radiology.* 1967;88:347.
59. Dixon SD, Coen RW, Crutchfield S. Visual dysfunction in cocaine-exposed infants. *Pediatr Res.* 1987;21:359A.
59a. Hammerschlag MR, Cummings C, Roblin PM, et al. Efficacy of neonatal ocular prophylaxis for the prevention of chlamydial and gonococcal conjunctivitis. *N Engl J Med.* 1989;320:769.
60. Nahmias JA, Visintine AM, Caldwell DR, et al. Eye infections with herpes simplex viruses in neonates. *Surv Ophthalmol.* 1976;21:100.
61. Duke-Elder S, Dobree JH. Diseases of the retina. In: Duke-Elder S, ed. *System of Ophthalmology.* St. Louis, MO: CV Mosby; 1967;10:139.
62. Sezen F. Retinal hemorrhages in newborn infants. *Br J Ophthalmol.* 1970;55:248.
63. Schoenfeld A, Buckman G, Nissenkorn I, et al. Retinal hemorrhages in the newborn following labor induced by oxytocin or dinoprostone. *Arch Ophthalmol.* 1985;103:932.

Chapter One Hundred and Ninety-Five

Otolaryngology: Head and Neck Problems

James H. Hill† *and Edward L. Applebaum*

195

An overview of otolaryngologic clinical problems affecting pregnant women is presented. Reference is made to clinical and basic research, but little published information is available. Unless otherwise stated, clinical findings are restricted to the mother, indicating that there are no associated abnormalities definable in the fetus or newborn infant. No attempt is made in this chapter to review the many hereditary congenital abnormalities of the ear, nose, throat, face, and neck.[1]

EAR

Stuffiness

The sensation of stuffiness also may be described as "fullness," "deafness," or "a veil over the ear." This sensation has been attributed variously to fluid in the middle ear, inner ear. During pregnancy and with the administration of birth control pills, these fluid or pressure alterations may be induced by changes in hormonal levels, but the relationship is supported by clinical association alone. Schiff[2] and Flisberg and Inglestet[3] suggest that estrogen produces alterations in eustachian tubal mucous membrane paralleling those of the uterine cervix. These alterations may be responsible for tubal malfunction. No incidence statistics for this complaint exist, but it is a common one. No preventive measures are known.

Middle ear fluid may be visible behind the tympanic membrane, or reduced tympanic membrane mobility may be present on pneumatic otoscopy. Tympanometry, a technique that displays graphically the compliance of the eardrum and middle ear ossicles, may reveal patterns consistent with middle ear fluid or reduced middle ear pressure. Audiometry usually discloses a mild hearing loss if there is

† Deceased.

middle ear fluid. Tympanometry may suggest eustachian tube malfunction as the source of a sensation of ear stuffiness in the absence of middle ear fluid. A complete examination of the head and neck, including the nasal chambers and nasopharynx, is necessary to rule out inflammation or neoplasm in patients with persistent stuffiness. This examination is particularly important in the presence of unilateral ear complaints or middle ear fluid, since these may indicate the presence of a nasopharyngeal neoplasm.[4]

Underlying nasal or nasopharyngeal inflammation or tumors must be treated. If symptoms are severe or persistent, middle ear fluid or negative pressure may be treated with pressure-equalizing tube placement through the eardrum anesthetized by local anesthesia. Most patients can be managed by instructing them in self-inflation of the middle ear using a modified Valsalva maneuver. Reassurance is often enough until symptoms resolve with completion of pregnancy.

Abnormally Patent Eustachian Tube

Normally, the eustachian tube is closed at rest and opens only in response to yawning, talking, and swallowing. The abnormally open tube remains patent continuously (patulous) or has a reduced resistance to airflow (semipatulous). This abnormal patency may be secondary to abnormal tubal structure, altered nerve supply to the controlling muscle (tensor veli palatini) with atrophy and contracture, or soft tissue alterations within the tube or externally. Abnormal tubal patency during pregnancy has been attributed to loss of soft tissue surrounding the tube, resulting in reduced external compression. Weight loss in the first trimester, associated with vomiting and changes in fat metabolism, may cause tissue loss surrounding the eustachian tube.[5,6] Estrogen, relaxin, and prostaglandins have been implicated in tubal malfunction[7], but there is no definitive evidence of this. There have been no pathologic studies of this entity.

The incidence of abnormally patent eustachian tubes in pregnant women is unknown. In the general population, the incidence of patients with symptoms severe enough to require specific treatment is low. Symptoms consist of a blocked sensation or popping in the ear and hyperacusis, in which environmental sounds are heard too loudly. Autophonia, which is a distorted perception of the patient's own voice and the unaccustomed perception of body sounds associated with breathing, palatal motion, and nasal speech, is present. Tympanic membrane flutter may cause an annoying sense of motion in the ear and a clicking sensation, particularly associated with breathing. Middle ear effusion and hearing loss may be present.

The patulous eustachian tube may be detected by tympanometry, which can disclose changes in compliance of the tympanic membrane during breathing. Forced respiration will exaggerate the response. Normally, compliance of the eardrum and ossicles remains constant. More complex testing is necessary to detect objectively and characterize the semipatulous tube. The symptoms of abnormally patent eustachian tubes often are considered insignificant or are confused with those of eustachian tube obstruction. Other etiologies for a patulous tube, such as weight loss or emaciation from acute or chronic illness, neuromuscular disorders producing atrophy of the tensor veli palatini muscle, and nasopharyngeal scarring from surgery or radiotherapy, should be easily distinguishable from the causes associated with pregnancy.

Treatment has included reassurance and attempts at closure of the eustachian tube. The severity of symptoms in pregnancy usually does not warrant active management. Short of attention to adequate nutrition, there are no preventive measures.

Hearing Loss

Hearing loss may result from an abnormality in the mechanism that conducts sound from the outside environment to the inner ear (conductive), in the inner ear or its neural connections with the central nervous system (sensorineural), or both (mixed). Common causes of maternal hearing loss specifically associated with pregnancy are middle ear fluid, as noted above, and otosclerosis. Rarely, the syndrome of sudden hearing loss has been associated with pregnancy. This is a sensorineural deafness of probable viral or vascular etiology.[8] No satisfactory treatment is known, but the majority of cases improve spontaneously. The discussion of fetal hearing losses here is restricted to the acquired congenital group.

The etiology and pathogenesis of otosclerosis are unknown.[9] Approximately half of the patients with clinical manifestations of the disease have a family history of otosclerosis. The abnormality is restricted to the bony covering of the inner ear (otic capsule) and the stapes. An osseous process of repetitive destruction followed by remodeling occurs in the temporal bone. At different stages resorption spaces containing fibrous tissue, immature bone, and dense laminated or mosaiclike bone are produced. Eventually, fixation of the stapes occurs, resulting in a progressive conductive hearing loss. A sensorineural hearing loss may be associated with the conductive loss. Examination of temporal bone specimens at autopsy reveals the presence of histologic otosclerosis in 8.3–12% of the white population and 1% of the black population. There is no sex predominance for the histologic disease. The exact incidence of clinical otosclerosis (disease severe enough to cause hearing loss) is unknown but is presumably less. However, a preponderance of clinical cases of otosclerosis is found in women, and this female predominance may be related to pregnancy, as noted below.

Otosclerosis usually becomes manifest during the second or third decade of life, when patients develop a bilateral, slowly progressive, conductive hearing loss. Maximum hearing loss is reached by the end of the third decade. Additionally, a high-frequency sensorineural hearing loss occurs in about 25% of cases. Up to 76% of pregnant patients who have otosclerosis first noticed their hearing loss or a worsening of their hearing during pregnancy.[10,11] The explanation for this relationship is unknown. The head and neck and general physical examinations are usually normal except for an abnormal Rinne test, in which a tuning fork is heard better when placed on the mastoid than when it is held next to the ear. Other disorders that also produce conductive hearing loss and a normal-appearing tympanic membrane must be differentiated from otosclerosis, but the differential diagnosis often cannot be resolved until the time of middle ear surgery. Treatment involves stapedectomy with prosthetic replacement or use of a hearing aid. No preventive measures are known.

Approximately 1:300 live births results in a deaf infant.[12] Forty percent of these congenitally deaf children have a hereditary impairment, but the cause in another 30% is unknown. The remaining 30% fall into the acquired congenital group because of infectious diseases, drugs and toxins, systemic maternal illness, and perinatal disorders.

Prominent among the infectious agents that can result in an acquired congenital hearing loss are rubella, cytomegalovirus, measles (rubeola), chickenpox (varicella-zoster), and syphilis. Rubella contracted in the first, or sometimes the second, trimester results in maldevelopment of the inner and middle ears, producing an asymmetric, severe, mixed hearing loss with a flat audiometric pattern. Cytomegalovirus and measles (rubeola) invade the inner ear, producing sense organ degeneration and bilateral moderate to severe sensorineural hearing loss and vestibular symptoms. The varicella-zoster virus produces an encephalomeningomyelitis that affects the ear with a perineural chronic inflammation, resulting in a variable degree of sensorineural hearing loss, worse in the high frequencies. Congenital syphilis occurs in either an early or late form. The eventual result in either is usually a bilaterally symmetric, severe, sensorineural hearing loss. In the early form, there is severe degeneration of the sense organ and its neural attachments. The late form produces a chronic inflammation and obliterative endarteritis, resulting in fibrosis, necrosis, bone resorption of the otic capsule, and progressive degeneration of the membranous labyrinth.

Streptomycin, kanamycin, quinine, chloroquine, diuretics, salicylates, lead, mercury, and alcohol are the principal drugs and toxins associated with congenital hearing losses. These agents have relatively specific effects on the hearing organ, the vestibular system, or both. The destruction of the auditory end organ usually is not reversible (except for salicylates and quinine) even when the drug is discontinued at the first clinical sign of toxicity. Details of the pathology associated with each agent are beyond the scope of this chapter. Several references are available.[13-16]

Systemic maternal illnesses clinically associated with hearing loss in newborns include diabetes mellitus, endemic goiter, preeclampsia or eclampsia, and any condition associated with hypoxia, severe hemorrhage, or severe anemia. The pathogenesis is uncertain in newborns' hearing loss in these cases. The cause of the severe mixed hearing loss associated with maternal goiter may be fetal hypothyroidism secondary to iodine extraction by the mother whose thyroid function remains normal.[17]

Perinatal disorders associated with newborn hearing loss include birth weight less than 1500 g, neonatal sepsis, erythroblastosis fetalis, and severe hypoxia from prolonged or difficult labor, labor requiring large amounts of analgesia or anesthesia, and cord or placental problems. Again, pathogenesis is not clear, although hypoxic insult to the fetus often is suggested. About 15–17% of congenitally deaf children were premature or had perinatal difficulty; the lower the birth weight, the higher is the probability of deafness.

In all of these categories, the clinician's principal task is to suspect the hearing loss. Children with undetected hearing loss may be thought to have psychological, learning, or disciplinary problems. Neonatal hearing screening and the use of high-risk registers and clinics may help to detect the loss early. More often, diagnosis is delayed until at least several months of age, when a failure to startle or turn the head toward a sound source is noted. Occasionally, as in the late form of congenital syphilis, hereditary hearing loss may not appear until late in life, when it produces a sudden hearing loss, a fluctuating hearing loss with dizziness, or a rapid decline in hearing. In the usual situation of congenital hearing loss, however, the impairment is present at birth, and there are developmental delays early in life. Once hearing loss is suspected, audiologic evaluation is indicated and will confirm the diagnosis. Auditory brain stem evoked response testing is usually an excellent technique for confirmation of hearing loss in children too young to cooperate for behavioral hearing tests.

Determining the etiology of the hearing loss begins with a meticulous family, prenatal, and pregnancy history. In 25–40% of all congenitally hearing-impaired children, there are associated abnormal physical findings detectable by complete physical examination. If the child is less than 6 months of age, serologic tests and blood cultures may identify a causative infectious agent. When an etiology can be determined, this information is extremely valuable in determining prognosis, potential for aural rehabilitation, vocational planning, and genetic counseling.

Treatment involves a cooperative effort among the otolaryngologist, audiologist, speech pathologist, geneticist, and neonatologist. Such an effort will maximize use of residual hearing, teach alternative techniques of communication, provide care for associated medical problems, and counsel the patient and family about the nature of the defect. In cases of congenital syphilis, prolonged high-dose penicillin and steroid therapy usually are prescribed. Often this treatment is not sufficient to prevent progression of hearing loss and vestibular symptoms because of the inability of the antibiotic to gain access to the organism in the inner ear. Prevention of congenital acquired hearing loss involves avoidance of toxins and infectious sources where possible, immunization, and rapid diagnosis and control of maternal and neonatal illnesses. For those patients with hearing losses for which there is no known medical therapy, the earliest possible fitting of a hearing aid will allow maximum use of any residual hearing.

Dizziness

The term *dizziness* includes vertigo, lightheadedness, unsteadiness, and syncope. Vertigo is a sensation (hallucination) of motion. Syncope is a sensation of impending faint followed by momentary loss of consciousness and falling. Unsteadiness is a loss of balance without any unusual sensation in the head. Lightheadedness is an ill-defined sensation in the head without vertigo, syncope, or unsteadiness.

Many clinicians have noted the association of dizziness with the premenstrual period, menstruation, pregnancy, menopause, and the use of both estrogen- and progesterone-containing contraceptive medications. However, an etiologic relationship between dizziness and hormonal changes has not been proved. The clinical findings may be striking. Sellars[18] reported the sudden onset of vertigo and hearing loss 7 days after an intramuscular injection of methoxyprogesterone. Peitersen[19] reported dizziness and electronystagmographic (ENG) changes in two female patients taking oral estrogen-containing contraceptives. Eviatar and Goodhill[20] could demonstrate no statistically significant ENG changes in their group of female patients with premenstrual dizziness. It has been suggested that a vascular mechanism such as sludging or thromboembolism accounts for the dizziness. The area of ischemia is thought to be in the vertebrobasilar system, affecting brain stem vestibular nuclei or the inner ear sense organs directly.

A meticulous historical review with attention to previous difficulties with birth control medications and menstruation is crucial to the diagnosis of dizziness related to hormonal factors. Symptoms vary markedly from mild, intermittent giddiness or lightheadedness to sudden, incapacitating, persistent vertigo associated with nausea, vomiting, and other brain stem signs. There may be fainting spells, an unstable gait, or a tendency to fall. Questions directed at characterizing episodic attacks and determining the relationship to headaches, infection, position change, motion, ear disease, head or neck trauma, drugs or toxins, and systemic or CNS disease are necessary. Allergy and metabolic screening questions are necessary. The general physical examination is most often completely unremarkable. Blood pressure in both arms should be taken. Carotid and radial vessels should be palpated for pulse character and thrills. Auscultation of the carotid vessels may reveal bruits. A complete head and neck examination may disclose the presence of otologic disease. A screening neurologic examination with attention to cranial nerves V, VII, IX, and X and the Romberg, past-pointing, and tandem-walking tests will aid in detection of CNS disease. Finally, the eyes should be examined for range of motion and nystagmus.

The clinical evaluation may include audiometry, electronystagmography, temporal bone roentgenograms, and blood studies (thyroid function, fasting and 2-hour postprandial blood glucose, serum cholesterol and triglycerides, and FTA). In the absence of findings suggesting primary disease in the visual, proprioceptive, or central nervous system, a relationship between dizziness and the hormonal changes of pregnancy may be assumed.

In the presence of a specific diagnosis, treatment of dizziness must be directed toward the underlying problem. Otherwise, reassurance and symptomatic relief, when necessary, are all that is required. Avoidance of positions that stimulate symptoms and rapid position change are advised. Vasodilators are of no proven value. In cases of severe or persistent symptoms, a mild vestibular suppressant such as meclizine may be used, but should be avoided if at all possible. Severe symptoms with nausea and vomiting may require hospitalization, intravenous fluid administration, antinausea medication, and higher dosage of vestibular suppressant drugs. No preventive measures are known.

NOSE

Stuffy Nose

Rhinitis of pregnancy is the gradual development of vascular congestion of the nasal mucosa, producing a degree and duration of nasal obstruction far exceeding the physiologic vasomotor reaction. In 1898, MacKenzie[21] reported his clinical observations in support of a physiologic interrelationship between the sex organs and the nose. He noted that "engorgement and increased irritability of the nasal mucous membrane" are found during pregnancy, along with "phenomena of a reflex nature" such as coughing and sneezing. He stated, "In some women, the presence of pregnancy was proclaimed by a cold in the head." Finally, he referred to Gruner and Petzold, who had previously reported regular sneezing episodes as signs of pregnancy.

Mortimer, et al[22-24] observed reddening and swelling of the nasal mucosa associated with submucosal perivascular edema in the monkey and the pregnant human. The increases in redness and swelling exactly parallel the increases in estrogen levels during pregnancy, beginning in the fifth month and abruptly terminating after delivery. Mohun[25] studied 20 cases of "vasomotor rhinitis" in pregnancy and could find no specific allergenic agent. Sorri et al[26] studied cases of acute maxillary sinusitis in pregnancy and concluded that an aggressive approach to treatment with antibiotics and irrigations should be used. There were no harmful effects noted as a result of the sinusitis.

In 1982, Toppozada et al[27] provided ultrastructural and histochemical evidence that implicates an allergic mechanism for the stuffy nose of pregnancy. The uniformly excellent clinical response to local steroid injection reported by Mabry[28] also favors an allergic cause. Possible allergens are placental or fetal proteins.

Mabry, in a survey of 79 patients, described frequent or constant nasal problems during pregnancy in 32% compared to 14% before pregnancy. Those with preexisting nasal complaints noticed an exacerbation with pregnancy. Complaints usually begin in the second trimester and continue for a few days following delivery. The chief complaint is nasal obstruction, which is associated with varying degrees of discharge, itching, and sneezing. Examination reveals markedly engorged turbinates with clear, colorless, serous secretion and complete nasal airway obstruction. Secondary complaints are impaired sleep, diminished sense of smell, habitual clearing of the throat, cough, and hoarseness. Paranasal sinus x-ray studies may show mucosal thickening and retained secretions. Blood counts are normal. Total serum IgE can be measured with the paper radioimmunosorbent test (PRIST), and levels greater than 100 units/mL are associated with allergic phenomena.[29] Eosinophils in mucous may be detected by staining expelled nasal secretions. At least 20–30% of white cells examined must be eosinophils to be indicative of nasal allergy. However, except in the first few days after onset, eosinophilia may be associated with nonallergic as well as allergic states. Since the antigen is felt to be endogenous, an allergen search is not indicated.

A complete history must rule out abnormal vasomotor reaction secondary to humidity, temperature, infection, emotion, fatigue, and inhalant particles. A history of excessive use of topical decongestants should be sought. Prolonged application of these medications results in increased nasal mucosal congestion. This "rebound effect" may be mediated through the autonomic nervous system because of interference with the feedback system controlling norepinephrine release at the nerve terminal–effector cell junction.[30] A complete head and neck examination will rule out septal deviation, nasal polyps, and turbinate hypertrophy.

Topical steroid medication (dexamethasone, beclomethasone, and flunisolide via inhalers) offers excellent relief. Holt et al[31] indicate that beclomethasone is the safest aerosol for use in pregnancy. With total nasal obstruction, a short course of systemic steroids (ie, prednisone beginning at a dose of 60 mg the first morning and tapering over 5 days) may be necessary to open the nasal chambers enough to allow effective use of the aerosol. Another alternative is the intraturbinal injection of steroids (ie, triamcinolone or prednisone preparations). As six cases of visual loss secondary to retinal circulation damage have been reported with such injection, this must be done with careful attention to technique.[28] Antihistamine-decongestant preparations offer minimal relief and may be associated with distressing systemic side-effects. Various nasal irrigations may be helpful but are ineffective in the totally obstructed nose. No preventive measures are known.

Epistaxis

Spontaneous hemorrhage from the nose can be a serious problem during pregnancy, especially in the presence of a prolonged vasomotor reaction, granuloma graviderum, or hypertension of preeclampsia or eclampsia. The exact incidence is unknown. In addition to hypertension, systemic predisposing factors include the use of certain antihypertensive agents or aspirin, hemorrhagic disorders, and atherosclerosis. Other local factors are digital manipulation, inordinate pressure changes within the nose (ie, nose blowing, sneezing, or dependent head positions), low environmental humidity, and nasal infection.

In the presence of one or more of these predisposing factors, a blood vessel ruptures and continues to bleed until the clotting mechanism or external intervention successfully seals the leak. If a clot extends through the ruptured vessel wall, the opening is kept patent, and an effective seal is prevented. In the usual situation of a bleeding site in the anterior portion of the nose, firm pressure on the nasal lobule will control the bleeding temporarily, and blood loss will be stopped. With posterior or superior bleeding sites, blood loss may be profuse and persistent, requiring intravenous fluid administration or blood replacement. A blood count and coagulation studies should be obtained. The differential diagnosis of the bleeding should include a mass either in the nose or nasopharynx. Severe septal deviations, septal perforations, and the syndrome of hereditary hemorrhagic telangiectasia present special problems and may make the bleeding difficult to control.

Principles of treatment include patient positioning in an upright position, clot removal, adequate visualization, intranasal decongestion and anesthesia, localization of the bleeding site, and cauterization, packing, or vessel ligation. The dual-cuffed silicone epistaxis catheter is very convenient and relatively comfortable when a posterior pack is necessary. Since alveolar hypoventilation may occur when a posterior pack is used, hospital admission and supplementary oxygen are necessary.[32] Preventive measures include avoidance or rapid control of predisposing factors with particular attention to rhinitis of pregnancy and hypertension.

Granuloma Graviderum

This "granuloma" is a very vascular, friable tumor of the nasal mucous membrane. It occurs during pregnancy, and it has also been called a hemangioma or a telangiectatic polyp. Some pathologists classify this tumor as a true neoplasm, but Batsakis[33] considered it a reactive process to relatively minor trauma in predisposed tissue. Its occurrence in pregnancy is unexplained. Histologically, the tumor is composed of a collection of acute and chronic inflammatory cells and multiple vascular channels in a loose edematous stroma. There may be areas of focal hemorrhage and superficial ulcerations. The tumors may be sessile or pedunculated and measure up to 3 or 4 cm in diameter. They are distinguishable from pyogenic granulomas only by their occurrence in pregnancy. Identical tumors appear on the gingivae during pregnancy in response to calculus deposits, poor oral hygiene, traumatic occlusion, denture irritation, or other trauma. The prevalence rate varies between 0.5% and 2.7% of pregnant women.[34]

Nasal obstruction and epistaxis are the primary patient complaints. The mass most frequently occurs on the nasal septum at the mucocutaneous junction in the vestibule. It usually appears in the first trimester and disappears spontaneously shortly after delivery. If treated during pregnancy, it has a tendency to recur.[35] The granuloma also tends to recur in subsequent pregnancies. Although it is usually unilateral, bilateral lesions have been reported.[36] The tumor is painless and red in color. Although the gross appearance and clinical setting are usually characteristic, histologic examination is necessary to confirm the diagnosis. The lesion may be confused with granulation tissue or hemangioma.

Treatment is most often unnecessary. However, situations of severe nasal obstruction or severe epistaxis may necessitate surgical excision using local anesthesia. Complete removal, however, does not prevent recurrence. No preventive measures are known.

LARYNX

Dysphonia and Cough

Changes in voice quality (dysphonia) during pregnancy include breathiness, deepening of the voice, difficulty with high notes, cracking of tones, vocal weakness, and diplophonia (the rapid sequential production of at least two vocal sounds, the latter one of which persists, resulting from vibration of the false vocal cords and creating a rough, grunting, or groaning voice).[37] Similar changes have been reported in the premenstrual portion of the menstrual cycle and with use of the progesterone-dominated birth control pills.[38]

Laryngeal examination reveals erythema and edema of the vocal cords with vascular dilatation and small submucosal hemorrhages. These changes also may be responsible for a persistent cough during pregnancy. The severity and prevalence of the dysphonia are dependent on the voice user. According to Brodnitz[39], Larina reported an 81% prevalence rate during the menstrual cycle among professional singers. Silverman and Zimmer[40] could find little evidence of dysphonia during the premenstrual portion of the menstrual cycle among young women with no voice training. The pathogenesis of the laryngeal changes in pregnancy is unknown. All reports have indicated that the changes are temporary and that the voice returns to normal after delivery. However, before a patient can be reassured, a complete head and neck examination, including visualization of the larynx, is necessary to rule out serious disease. Carcinoma of the larynx during pregnancy has been reported.[41]

No specific treatment is available, and patients should be advised to avoid vocal strain as much as possible to prevent the possibility of permanent damage to the larynx.

Laryngeal Edema and Airway Distress

Difficulty in breathing often occurs during pregnancy as a result of restricted movement of the diaphragm. The usual symptom is breathlessness on exertion, and special care must be taken by pregnant singers to compensate for the altered lung volume. For example, the solo vocalist may need to stand earlier, consciously inhale maximal volumes of air, and plan vocal phrases to optimize the smaller volume and shorter expiration time of the airstream.

Laryngeal edema with resultant airway distress is a potentially serious problem, and several cases have been reported.[42-45] The incidence is not high, and the edema can be anticipated in most cases from the clinical course. The manifestations are progressive dyspnea and hoarseness with or without dysphagia and odynophagia. Laryngeal examination reveals generalized supraglottic edema without erythema and normal vocal cord mobility. Histologic examination has revealed submucosal infiltration by lymphocytes and plasma cells, stromal edema, and dilated capillaries.

Two of the reported patients required tracheotomy, and the others requiring intubation experienced enough difficulty that tracheotomy may have been more appropriate. Tracheotomy is done using local anesthesia, and the technique used depends on the urgency of the situation. In acute obstruction, a cricothyrotomy is performed, recognizing that prolonged intubation through this site may result in subglottic stenosis. Once an airway has been established, a standard tracheotomy beneath the first and second tracheal ring should be done. Prevention of disastrous acute airway obstruction necessitates careful attention to the patient's clinical course with evaluation of the airway at the first sign of hoarseness or stridor.

FACIAL PARALYSIS

The facial nerve has three functional divisions represented in the brain stem: a motor division to the face, a sensory division mediating taste from the anterior two thirds of the tongue, and a parasympathetic division for secretion and vasomotion to the lacrimal gland and the three major salivary glands. Paresis or paralysis of the nerve results in loss of function in any or all of these divisions. There are many causes of facial paralysis. Congenital malformations include the Möbius syndrome (central paralysis or agenesis of facial muscles) and the Melkersson–Rosenthal syndrome (recurrent facial edema and fissured tongue). Inflammations such as herpes zoster, necrotizing external otitis, and acute or chronic otitis media may cause facial paralysis. Primary neoplasms of the external ear, middle ear, or within the cerebellopontine angle may involve the nerve, and it can be compressed by metastatic tumors. Trauma to the temporal bone or face may damage the nerve. Finally, primary neurologic or systemic diseases such as the polyneuritis of the Guillain–Barré syndrome, sarcoidosis, and histiocytosis may result in facial paralysis. Most often, however, no evidence for any of these maladies can be found, and the term *Bell's palsy* is reserved for these cases of idiopathic paralysis.

The incidence of Bell's palsy in the general population is 17–18/100,000 population per year. In pregnancy, the incidence rises almost threefold to 45.1/100,000 births.[46-48] In the general population, approximately 0.5% of patients will have bilateral paralysis on initial examination. In the nonpregnant woman the incidence is highest on the first day of the menstrual cycle, and more than 60% occur within the first 14 days. In the pregnant woman, nearly 75% of cases occur in the third trimester. The pathogenesis is unknown, but three mechanisms have been suggested. Primary inflammation, either viral or immunologic in origin, may lead to edema, disturbances of microcirculation, and the loss of nerve conductivity. Primary inflammation also may lead to nerve demyelination with resulting functional loss. Finally, ischemia secondary to vasomotor dysfunction has been suggested. In a series of 42 cases of idiopathic facial paralysis in pregnancy, Hilsinger et al[46] could find no relationship with preeclampsia or eclampsia, hypertension, or the occurrence of previous pregnancy.

Manifestations and clinical evaluation are well summarized by Adour.[49] The patient may notice a taste disturbance, abnormal loudness of sounds, pain (usually retroauricular), epiphora, or decreased tearing. The changes in hearing may be secondary to involvement of the cochlea or the cochlear nerve or perhaps to the loss of the effect of the stapedius muscle on the middle ear ossicles. On head and neck examination, the paralysis will be apparent when the patient is asked to wrinkle the forehead skin, close the eyes, or pucker. Vesicles may be present in the oral cavity, and loss of papillae on the tongue may be seen. Involvement of other cranial nerves may be detected with careful examination of the larynx, gag reflex, and facial sensation. Temporal bone radiographs and an audiogram should be obtained to rule out neoplastic and other disease of the temporal bone. Electrical testing of the facial nerve can be performed as an indicator of prognosis or of the need for facial nerve decompression if the paralysis is complete.

No preventive measures are known. Although medical treatment is controversial, the use of systemic steroids (prednisone) beginning in a dosage of 60 mg the first morning and tapering to none after 10–15 days has been advocated for cases of complete paralysis. The indications for facial nerve decompression are also controversial. In general, the prognosis for the recovery of facial function in the pregnant population is excellent. Eye protection should include the use of dark glasses and artificial tears with the addition of a protective eye ointment and lid taping at night. Pressing the affected cheek against the teeth while eating and speaking will help to prevent drooling.

REFERENCES

1. Lederer FL. Otorhinolaryngologic problems in the mother and the newborn infant. *Ann Otol Rhinol Laryngol.* 1959;68:933.
2. Schiff M. The "pill" in otolaryngology. *Trans Am Acad Ophthalmol Otolaryngol.* 1972;72:76.
3. Flisberg K, Inglestet S. Middle ear mechanics in patulous eustachian tube cases. *Acta Otolaryngol.* 1969;263(suppl):18.
4. Boles R. Serous otitis media: thief of hearing and herald of cancer. *Med Times.* 1966;94:1333.
5. Suehs OW. The abnormally open eustachian tube. *Laryngoscope.* 1960;70:1418.
6. Pulec JL, Simontown KM. Abnormal patency of the eustachian tube. *Laryngoscope.* 1964;74:267.
7. O'Connor AF, Shea JJ. Autophony and the patulous eustachian tube. *Laryngoscope.* 1981;91:1427.
8. Booth JB. Diagnosis and management of sudden and fluctuant sensorineural hearing loss. In: Ballantyne J, Groves J, eds. *Scott-Brown's Diseases of the Ear, Nose and Throat.* 4th ed. London: Butterworth; 1970;2:737.
9. Schuknecht HF. *Pathology of the Ear.* Cambridge, MA: Harvard University Press; 1974:351.
10. Elbrønd O. Otosclerosis and pregnancy. *Acta Otorhinolaryngol Belg.* 1981;35:452.
11. Gristwood RE, Venables WN. Pregnancy and otosclerosis. *Clin Otolaryngol.* 1983;8:205.
12. Bergstrom L. Congenital deafness. In: English GM, ed. *Otolaryngology.* Philadelphia, PA: Harper & Row; 1982;1:1.
13. Hawkins JE, Jr. Drug ototoxicity. In: Keidel WD, Neff WD, eds. *Handbook of Sensory Physiology.* Berlin: Springer-Verlag; 1976;5:707.
14. Hawkins JE, Jr. Drug ototoxicity. In: Strome M, ed. *Differential Diagnosis in Pediatric Otolaryngology.* Boston, MA: Little, Brown; 1975:53.
15. Ballantyne J. Ototoxicity: A clinical review. *Audiology.* 1973;12:325.
16. Ajodhia JM, Dix MR. Ototoxic effects of drugs. *Minerva Otorhinolaringol.* 1975;25:117.
17. Schuknecht HF. *Pathology of the Ear.* Cambridge, MA: Harvard University Press; 1974:183.
18. Sellars SF. Acute deafness associated with depoprogesterone. *J Laryngol Otol.* 1971;85:281.
19. Peitersen E. Disturbances in the central vestibular system after oral contraceptives. *J Laryngol Otol.* 1969;83:725.
20. Eviatar A, Goodhill V. Dizziness as related to menstrual cycles and hormonal contraceptives. *Arch Otolaryngol.* 1969;90:301.
21. MacKenzie JN. The physiological and pathological relations between the nose and the sexual apparatus of man. *Johns Hopkins Hosp Bull.* 1898;9:10.
22. Mortimer H, Wright RP, Collip JB. The effect of the administration of oestrogenic hormones on the nasal mucosa of the monkey (*Macaca mulatta*). *Can Med Assoc J.* 1936;35:503.
23. Mortimer H, Wright RP, Collip JB. The effect of oestrogenic hormones on the nasal mucosa; their role in the naso-sexual relationship; and their significance in clinical rhinology. *Can Med Assoc J.* 1936;35:615.
24. Mortimer H, Wright RP, Collip JB. Atrophic rhinitis; the constitutional factor and the treatment with oestrogenic hormones. *Can Med Assoc J.* 1937;37:445.
25. Mohun M. Incidence of vasomotor rhinitis during pregnancy. *Arch Otolaryngol.* 1943;37:699.
26. Sorri M, Hartikainen-Sorri A-L, Karja J. Rhinitis during pregnancy. *Rhinology.* 1980;18:83.
27. Toppozada H, Michaels L, Toppozada M, et al. The human respiratory nasal mucosa in pregnancy. *J Laryngol Otol.* 1982;96:613.
28. Mabry RL. Intranasal steroid injection during pregnancy. *South Med J.* 1980;73:1176.
29. McNelis FL. Management of allergy-like symptoms in otolaryngology. *Laryngoscope.* 1980;90:985.
30. Mygind N, Malm L. Pathophysiology and management of allergic and nonallergic rhinitis. In: English GM, ed. *Otolaryngology.* Philadelphia, PA: Harper & Row; 1982;2:4.
31. Holt GR, Mabry RL. ENT medications in pregnancy. *Otolaryngol Head Neck Surg.* 1983;91:338.
32. Cassisi NJ, Biller HF, Ogura JH. Changes in arterial oxygen tension and pulmonary mechanics with the use of posterior packing in epistaxis. *Laryngoscope.* 1971;81:1261.
33. Batsakis JG. *Tumors of the Head and Neck.* Baltimore, MD: Williams & Wilkins; 1979:294.
34. McNulty JS. Granulomatous and venereal diseases of the oral cavity. In: English GM, ed. *Otolaryngology.* Philadelphia, PA: Harper & Row; 1982;3:3.

35. Kent DL, Fitzwater JE. Nasal hemangioma of pregnancy. *Ann Otol Rhinol Laryngol*. 1979;88:331.
36. Hemani DD, Gupta AK, Sharma SD, et al. Recurrent bilateral pregnancy granuloma of the nose. *J Laryngol Otol*. 1981;95:957.
37. Brodnitz FS. Hormones and the human voice. *Bull NY Acad Med*. 1971;47:183.
38. Lawrence VL. Medical/Surgical therapy. *Transcripts of the Eighth Symposium on the Care of the Professional Voice*. New York, NY: The Voice Foundation; 1979:72.
39. Brodnitz FS. Menstrual cycle and voice quality. *Arch Otolaryngol*. 1979;105:300.
40. Silverman E-M, Zimmer CH. Effect of the menstrual cycle on voice quality. *Arch Otolaryngol*. 1978;104:7.
41. Brophy JW. Squamous cell carcinoma of the larynx in pregnancy. *Arch Otolaryngol*. 1973;97:480.
42. Spotoft H, Christensen P. Laryngeal oedema accompanying weight gain in pregnancy. *Anaesthesia*. 1981;36:71.
43. Jouppila R, Jouppila P, Holpmen A. Laryngeal oedema as an obstetric anaesthesia complication. *Acta Anaesth Scand*. 1980;24:97.
44. Seager SJ, MacDonald R. Laryngeal oedema and preeclampsia. *Anaesthesia*. 1980;35:360.
45. Dobb G. Laryngeal oedema complicating obstetric anaesthesia. *Anaesthesia*. 1978;33:839.
46. Hilsinger RL Jr, Adour KK, Doty HE. Idiopathic facial paralysis, pregnancy, and the menstrual cycle. *Ann Otol Rhinol Laryngol*. 1975;84:433.
47. Korczyn AD. Bell's palsy and pregnancy. *Acta Neurol Scand*. 1971;47:603.
48. Robinson JR, Pow JW. Bell's palsy: A predisposition of pregnant women. *Arch Otolaryngol*. 1972;95:125.
49. Adour KK. *A Syllabus on Facial Paralysis Evaluation*. Oakland, CA: The Permanente Medical Group and the Kaiser Foundation Hospital; 1974:1.

PART XX

Psychiatric and Neurologic Disorders and Striated Muscle Diseases

Norbert Gleicher, Section Editor

Chapter One Hundred and Ninety-Six

Sexuality

George W. Dameron, Jr.†

196

Because of the sexual revolution of the 1960s, we are more free to teach, read, understand, talk about, and participate in sexual matters. Many welcomed this openness after years of repression; they believed that this change in sexual attitudes would lead to a sort of erotic millenium with informed, understanding individuals free to participate at the highest level of one's sexual expressiveness without guilt. Sexologists pronounced sexual behavior an integral part of everyday life.

Despite advantages in openness gained by society, this shift in mores unfortunately produced many loveless libidos that trivialized sex and tended to make it a mere sport. Sexual intercourse often became divorced "from love and creation," as well as "from empathy, compassion, responsibility, and even common politeness."[1]

While greater understanding of sexual matters is healthy, important disadvantages have accrued. We have failed to impart our increased knowledge to our young people; we have failed to emphasize with consistency the responsibility that comes with greater sexual freedom.[1-4] Currently, there is greater tolerance, although not necessarily acceptance, of premarital sex, out-of-wedlock pregnancies, and living arrangements outside of marriage—all of which tend to promote earlier sex.[5] This fact, coupled with a more casual approach to sex among young people, has resulted in an epidemic of sexually transmitted diseases affecting fertility, affecting both pregnant woman and fetus, and increasing the incidence of premalignant/malignant changes in the female pelvis.[4] In addition, we now have the acquired immunodeficiency syndrome (AIDS), which alters the mechanics of how we practice medicine both in the office and hospital.

† Deceased.

When a social pendulum swings too far, we strive to bring it back closer to center. We are realizing "that sexual liberation removed from love and creation is not a revolution but merely a reaction. The indiscriminate release of libido is simply another form of sexual repression."[1]

The loving, well-adjusted pregnant couple may symbolize one of the highest and most appropriate forms of sexual expression, with all attendant joys and risks wrought by love. The possibilities of excitement and adventure through love of another person and family are balanced against the inherent risks of pain, rejection, and failure that accompany all deeply involved relationships. One of the important areas of concern involves the sexual expression of the pregnant couple and the influence of pregnancy on it; sexual patterns often are altered, and the communication system of the couple is intensely affected and stressed. Physicians and other health care providers are in a peculiarly advantageous position to encourage, explain, and help the pregnant couple through this process of change, development, and stress.

According to McCary, sexuality "comprises everything that the individual is, thinks, feels and does during his life span as related to being male or female."[7] We cannot separate our sexuality from the rest of our lives; we cannot place it in a compartment. It is as intrinsic to our nature as breathing or thinking—a natural, normal constituent of our humanity. Every person expresses this sexuality in some form of sexual behavior, some pattern of sexual conduct. Whether celibate or streetwalker, each has to deal with sexual urges and come to terms with them; we all are, in some way, sexual beings.

Sexual desires are instinctive, but sexual attitudes and behavior are learned. Consequently, the same sexual activity holds different meanings for different people, and even for the same person the meaning may be different at different times. Our life experience dictates how we express our sexuality. Sexual behavior may express love, caring, and affection; or lust, aggression, and power; or temporary physical need; or a striving for dominance; and on through the entire spectrum of human needs and feelings. At its best, sex is the physical expression of two people who love and share true emotional intimacy—the weaving together of two identities.

Pregnancy is the time when couples change from lovers to parents, from a couple to a family. During this brief, self-limiting period, the couple is under physical, emotional, and often economic stress. The very structure of the partnership may be altered, and although many couples respond by drawing closer, others do not.[8] Some couples break apart; others establish damaging patterns of coping that take a toll later.[9]

The realities of the transition from couple to family and the opportunities presented both for growth and for misunderstanding largely go unrecognized until after the fact. One patient succintly expressed the impact of pregnancy on her marriage nearly 20 years earlier. "When I brought that baby home from the hospital," she said, "was when I *really* lost my virginity."

Pregnancy has a potent effect on existing sexual patterns; the alteration of these patterns may, in turn, influence partners' attitudes about pregnancy, each other, and the child.[10-13] Although attention has focused on this subject only recently, it is far from a new topic. Masters and Johnson noted that ". . . sexuality as it may be enhanced or repressed by the state of pregnancy has been a subject of conjecture for generations." They point out that the number of taboos and sanctions dealing with this problem is approached only by the number of admonitions on sexuality and menstruation.[11]

In recent years, obstetrics has addressed the humanistic considerations of pregnancy, encouraging the couple's participation in the birth process, childbirth classes (where often very little is said about sex), birthing rooms, and parent-infant bonding, all evidencing our desire to meld better psychological care with increasingly sophisticated medical care. Yet we say little to our patients about sexual matters.

Previous reports have indicated that pregnant women want information on sex and that comparatively few receive anything but cursory admonitions and advice.[12,14-16] At workshops, when women are asked about the quality and quantity of teaching done by their physicians regarding sex in pregnancy, most say that they have received very little or none.

It is easy to understand why practical knowledge is hard to come by, considering the comparatively scanty, sometimes conflicting literature on sexuality and pregnancy. Only in recent years have medical schools included sexuality courses in the standard curriculum, hoping to impart both knowledge and more relaxed, nonjudgmental sexual attitudes.

The chief reason for our reluctance to discuss sex with patients may stem in part from discomfort about our own sexuality. We develop our sexual biases long before medical training; we are humans before physicians. Those who speak most comfortably about sexual matters usually are both knowledgeable and at ease with their own sexuality.[17]

Regardless of its cause, our reluctance to discuss with patients the psychosexual areas of pregnancy can only reinforce their taboos, fears, and lack of certainty. Physicians' voices are enormously powerful to their patients; their silences may be even more powerful.

PREGNANCY CHANGES

Anderson et al[18] aptly give this overview of the changes caused by pregnancy:

> *When conception occurs, the cyclic function of the ovaries is interrupted and is not established with regularity until lactation is finished. Thus, the psychobiology of pregnancy can best be understood as an immense intensification of the luteal phase of the reproductive cycle. This accounts for the increase in hormonal and metabolic processes and their psychological manifestation, which are characterized by intensified receptive and retentive tendencies.*

We shall examine these changes under three broad headings.

Physical Considerations

It seems obvious that the physical changes of pregnancy may alter sexual behavior, but the patient may not always make the connection. Therefore, simply telling her what changes to expect physically helps her to prepare and adjust.[14]

Pregnant or not, very few people are interested in sex if they feel they are about to throw up. The nausea of early pregnancy (compounded by fatigue) may restrict sexual expression at a time when a couple usually is happiest and logically might want more sex. Fatigue is an ongoing factor affecting sexual desire and performance.[8,14] Although the fatigue of early pregnancy lessens in the middle trimester, it returns in the third trimester, accompanied by increasing awkwardness and discomfort. At the same time, increasing abdominal size reduces the number and variety of comfortable positions for coitus. Patients need to be informed about alternative methods and positions. Toward the end of pregnancy, coitus with deep penetration may be very uncomfortable, and such positions as side or rear entry or a spoon position may help.[18] The female-superior position may get the enlarging abdomen out of the way but is a position of deeper penetration.[14]

In Masters and Johnson's description of the phases of sexual response, one of the major physiologic changes is vasocongestion both of the breasts and particularly of the pelvis. The pregnant woman, with her increased blood volume, already has marked vasocongestion; because of this, her sexual responses are altered (Table 196–1). In other words, the vasocongestion of sexual arousal added to the existing vasocongestion of pregnancy results in heightened sensitivity of breasts and pelvis, sometimes greater discomfort, and often greater intensity of sexual response. Reports of pregnant women experiencing greater intensity of orgasm or even first orgasm are common.[11]

The breasts, hypertrophied in response to both hormonal and vascular changes, are especially tender in early pregnancy. Milk letdown with orgasm in later pregnancy has been reported and is often a surprise to the couple.[11]

Vaginal secretions increase in quantity throughout pregnancy and more than is customary during arousal. Some men who enjoy oral sex are "turned off" by this change.[11] During pregnancy, the cervix is more likely to bleed as the result of the trauma of coitus, which may alarm the uninformed couple.

During orgasm, the uterus may undergo tonic contractions with slowing of fetal activity followed by a brief period of compensatory fetal hyperactivity. Transient fetal bradycardia has been recorded during these episodes, with no apparent ill effect.[11] This alteration in fetal activity may

TABLE 196–1. PREGNANCY—RELATED ALTERATIONS IN SEXUAL RESPONSE

Stage	Changes
Excitement and plateau	Breasts—tenderness, discomfort, enhanced erotic response; milk letdown after orgasm in late pregnancy Labia—feeling of fullness Vagina—increased secretions, feeling of fullness Cervix—may bleed more easily at coitus, may be more sensitive
Orgasm	Tonic uterine contractions, transient fetal bradycardia, greater intensity (or first orgasm)
Resolution	Often poor or inadequate in late pregnancy

From Dameron[63] with permission.

alarm the couple and raise again the question of virtually universal concern: "Does sexual activity harm the baby?"[7,13-15, 20-24] To date, most clinicians support the idea that sexual activity does no harm to the normal pregnancy.

In later stages of pregnancy, some women may avoid coitus because of the incomplete resolution following orgasm. The vasocongestion is not well relieved, and the residual feeling of fullness may be uncomfortable and persistent.

The sensation the woman has at delivery has been equated to orgasm. The vasoconcentration, pressure, exhilaration, relief, and exhaustion are similar. Some women well prepared for labor and delivery have described the birth process as the ultimate expression of their female sexuality.[25]

Medical Considerations

Most authors find that coitus and orgasm are not harmful to the normal pregnant woman and her fetus.[5,9,14,21-24] Mills and associates[27] studied 10,981 singleton pregnancies and found no deleterious effect. Their study challenges the view that intercourse during the latter part of pregnancy can be harmful. Naeye's original studies[31] indicated that intercourse causes increased perinatal mortality. However, both his method and his definition of disease have been criticized and his admonitions have been poorly accepted.[27]

Most practitioners are reluctant to alter or restrict unnecessarily the normal pregnant couple's sexual expression without excellent, convincing support for this action. Still, Naeye's claims cannot be dismissed. He has persisted in his contention that sex in pregnancy may be harmful to the outcome.[32] Coitus, through the spread of sexually transmitted disease, indirectly may result in maternal, fetal, and neonatal morbidity and mortality.[30] Evidence exists of abortion precipitated by herpes simplex, *Listeria monocytogenes*, and acute viral hepatitis. *Gardnerella vaginitis* is reported both as causing post-abortal sepsis as well as being isolated in the blood of puerpural women and septic newborns. Positive cervical cultures of *Chlamydia trachomatis* taken antepartum are reported to be associated with increased prematurity, and perinatal morbidity and mortality.[30]

Potentially lethal infections of the newborn acquired from venereally infected vaginas include gonorrhea, herpes, Group B streptococcus, *Listeria*, *Chlamydia*, and possibly cytomegalovirus, the last being somewhat controversial. Syphilis is well known for its effect both on mother and fetus.[30]

Several maternal deaths have been reported from air embolism following forced blowing of air into the vagina during orogenital sex.[12,33,34] One such case was treated successfully with hyperbaric oxygen.[35]

Coitus and orgasm in cases of ruptured membranes, known as *placenta previa*, and incompetent cervix is contraindicated. Most authorities are also cautious about allowing coitus and orgasm when the patient has a history of unexplained premature labor, threatened premature labor, habitual abortion, threatened abortion, and, in later pregnancy, twin gestation.[26,35]

Few practitioners currently restrict coitus at any given time in normal pregnancy, and more and more condone postpartum resumption of intercourse when the lochia is white and the episiotomy site is no longer tender.[36-38] In support of early resumption of coitus, Krantz has pointed out that the cervix essentially is closed 24 hours after delivery, and infection from coitus is unlikely after that time.[10,18]

Psychological Considerations

If sexuality defines our totality as a man or woman, *sexual behavior* may be defined as the broad, outward expression of male or female inner feelings and attitudes. One facet of sexual behavior includes the sex act—the physical expression of ourselves as male and female. It is well established that sexual performance (including desire for sex) can be inhibited by anger, fear, physical discomfort or disability, negative attitudes, or lack of knowledge, all of which result in anxiety, a common inhibitor of both response and performance.[12,40,41] According to Kaplan, the sexual dysfunctions are produced by the physiologic concomitants of anxiety.[40]

Consequently, psychological considerations must encompass all three levels of sexual expression: sexuality, sexual behavior, and the sex act. These overlapping, closely related areas are not separated easily. We need to help our patients understand that pregnancy stresses the whole persona of the man or woman; it further stresses sexual behavior expressed with and to one's partner, and the sex act itself. Giving the couple a measure of psychological understanding can accomplish three things: make adjustments regarding sex in pregnancy easier, provide reassurance that their problems are not unique, and, most important, encourage them to discuss matters of a more intimate nature that they may hesitate to approach.

Williams points out that four factors influence the woman's psychological adjustment during pregnancy; their relative importance varies, depending on the individual.[42] One is the set of physical changes, especially the dramatic changes in body size and shape during later stages of pregnancy. These evoke feelings whose significance depends on a woman's perception of them. The emotionally secure woman who desires to be pregnant welcomes these outward signs. The woman whose self-worth is largely derived from a conventional standard of sexual attractiveness is concerned with the loss of her figure and feels less feminine and attractive. A second factor is the woman's preexisting psychological status which helps determine her ability to handle new stresses. Pregnancy is a developmental crisis with new tasks and problems demanding adaptations yet to be learned. It adds new and different stresses that require new and different ways of coping.

A third important influence is her life situation, her marital status and other relationships. Williams studied two groups of pregnant working women, married and unmarried. The married women had concerns about body changes, fears about delivery and the normalcy of their babies, and a stronger need to be cared for. They worried about husbands not meeting these needs and about their own ability to function as mothers.[41] The unmarried women had different worries that influenced their adaptation to pregnancy. They showed a desire for a dependent relationship with a man, ambivalence about giving up the child for adoption, shame because they had "disgraced" family and themselves, and depression.

Finally, the psychodynamics of pregnancy sometimes arouses conflicts a woman has about dependency needs, reminds her of her rivalries with her own mother or siblings, evokes hostility toward her husband, and makes her aware of subconscious attitudes toward the self as a female.[42]

Thus, the integrative task of pregnancy and motherhood, both biologically and physically, is much greater than any experience with which most women have been confronted. In some cases, the task appears greater with the first child, when the experience is new. Motherhood may be easier with subsequent children if appropriate emotional maturation has taken place. One may not assume that the woman has appropriate reason for her pregnancy: she may be attempting to alter an unhappy marriage, she may become pregnant because her peer group is having babies, or she may be proving her femininity (corresponding to male pride and ego in fathering).[10,18,42]

Until recently, the expectant father was neglected.[22] The stereotypic chain-smoking, worried man pacing the waiting room now accompanies the woman to the labor suite, and then, sometimes reluctantly, into the delivery room. His role has changed from that of the outsider who paid the medical bills to that of coach and supporter during labor, and later, to participant in the birth process. We now refer to the pregnant couple and are beginning to appreciate the needs and concerns of the pregnant man. His response to pregnancy does not simply reflect his partner's concerns. Apparently, there is a different spectrum of feelings and attitudes toward pregnancy peculiar to men.[22,23] Thus, the expectant father has become an individual instead of a shadow; it would be helpful to know more about him. Unfortunately, there is very little in the way of substantive evidence to support these impressions.

The father often views the coming baby as proof of virility; very few cultures do not equate procreation with manhood.[20,22,43] Despite his perception of himself as the "rock," the primary support on whom the helpless pregnant woman leans, he often has limited knowledge and understanding of the pregnancy.[20] He worries about how good a father he will be but rarely expresses his doubts to anyone except his partner. If he is like most men raised to hide feelings (especially those of fear and uncertainty), he must maintain his outward image of assurance in the face of inner doubts.[14,20,45] The conspiracy of silence among men prevents him from talking to others who might have similar concerns, and he may even be afraid to confide in his partner because she needs his apparent strength.

Often, he has great anxiety about providing for his family.[13,22,23] Most of us have seen young men leave new marriages when faced with the overwhelming emotional and economic responsibility of fatherhood. He may be jealous of the baby before and especially after delivery, as his mate gives priority to the newcomer. Nonetheless, when allowed to be a full participant in the childbirth process, he can demonstrate the capacity for nurturing behavior toward both mate and child. The transition from lover to parent is one of life's most difficult, and this is no exception for the male. We need to know more about what makes the new father tick. Duvall sums up the issues:[43]

> *Expectant fathers may feel hemmed in, trapped, ambivalent, afraid of approaching their wives sexually, guilty for getting their wives pregnant, jealous of the newcomer's place, and depressed and anxious about their own inadequacies. On the positive side, they may also feel proud of their virility, satisfied with their wives' prenatal progress, responsible for their children's future, and fulfilled as human beings.*

Most couples have a similar sexual history[14] (Figure 196–1). A precoital courtship changes to a relationship of sex for pleasure; this is followed by sex for procreation until pregnancy ensues. The couple then must move through the pressures of pregnancy and ultimately resume sex for pleasure after delivery. Most couples are not aware of these serial changes and realize only after the fact that each stage has a profound effect on their sexual relationship. Ideally, as each stage is completed, adaptations needed should be acknowledged and gains made should be incorporated before the move to the next stage. This process allows a relationship to evolve gradually, and permits the couple a chance to learn to cope with stresses in small doses. Unfortunately, not many couples enjoy the luxury of developing a relationship in this way, nor do they know how. Without such evolution, there are increased chances for misunderstanding. At each stage, the couple needs to answer the question, "How may we best communicate honestly and caringly under stress?"

Most studies indicate a declining interest in sexual activity as the end of pregnancy approaches.[30,46] However, interest varies with each partner.[11,13,24,46] If their interests do not coincide, it is easy for each to feel that the other is demanding or rejecting. Toward the end of pregnancy, the woman may need more affection, reassurance, and nurturing but may lack interest in coitus.[14,20,46,47] Because most men are acculturated to regard touching a woman as a prelude to sex, the potential for conflict is obvious.

It may be difficult for both partners to mix the image of motherhood with sex; can a mother or expectant mother be a sexual person?[8,43] Here the incest taboo surfaces and should be acknowledged as a possible hidden deterrent for both male and female.[14,22]

Men may not be physically attracted to their pregnant mates, and the pregnant woman has some difficulty in perceiving herself as attractive.[7,9,45] It is hard for most couples to face this issue squarely, to give each other permission to be "turned off." A man may still love his partner but

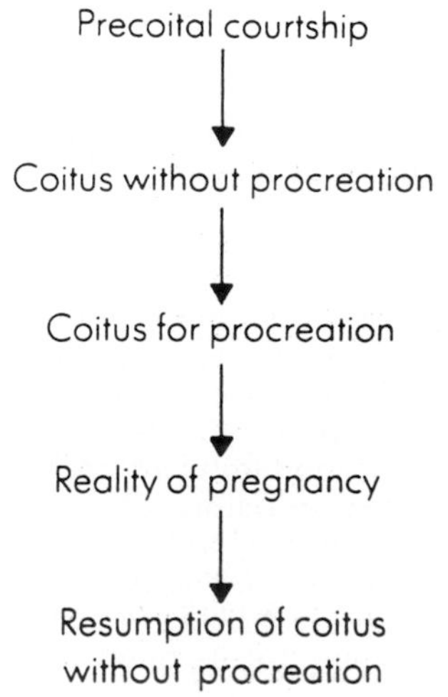

Figure 196–1. Sexual history of a couple.

temporarily may not be attracted physically. This lack of attraction can be a formidable hurdle. Whether he tells her directly that he is not physically interested or indirectly by avoidance behavior and excuses, he reinforces her feelings of increasing unattractiveness.[19] Yet another complicating factor may be the tendency for a man to engage in extramarital affairs when his wife is pregnant, sometimes ascribed to the woman's declining interest in sex.[11] On the other hand, any interest he displays to another woman, innocent or not, may provoke a strong jealous response. Thus, at a time when the woman needs increasing reassurance, her self-esteem as a lover and mate is challenged.[8] A prompt from the clinician early in pregnancy and repeated later will give the couple an opportunity to discuss the issue. The best time to introduce this subject is when the couple comes to the office together.

The partners' concern about the normalcy of their child is understandable. If the baby is born with an anomaly, recriminations may ensue, as one blames the other amid discussions about which side of the family is genetically responsible. Interestingly, G.W. Davidson found that the couple's marital and sexual adjustments are easier the further away from the head the anomaly is located (personal communication).

The push to develop the family unit may crowd out the nurturing of the partnership before, but especially after, delivery.[9,45] Because the partnership is the hub around which the rest of the family unit continues to revolve, neglect of this area could be disastrous.

Most couples are poorly equipped to discuss feelings. Communication skills, like sexual skills, are acquired. Two people undergoing one of the most powerful experiences of their lives, with the attendant need to express feelings, doubts, and concerns with each other, often are ill-equipped to communicate openly. This lack or inappropriateness of expression may add to the difficulty of coping with the many rapid changes in their lives.

POSTPARTUM SEXUALITY

The psychobiologic changes of the postpartum woman do influence her sexual behavior. Physiologically, at 4–5 weeks after delivery, responsiveness to sexual stimulation decreases in rapidity and in sensitivity, that is, longer periods to arousal and shorter, weaker orgasms.[11] The vaginal walls are thinner temporarily because of decreased steroid levels, and there is less lubrication. The labia minora, which change color at impending orgasm, are not as deep a hue, and the orgasmic platform is not as vasocongested. By the third postpartum month, however, the vagina usually has become normally rugose, the uterus has descended into the pelvis, vaginal lubrication returns to prepregnancy levels, and the expansion of the vaginal barrel returns close to prepregnancy dimensions.[30,48] One report indicates that in breastfeeding women testosterone and androstenedione levels were significantly lower in those women reporting a severe reduction in sexual interest.[49]

Obstetric trauma that restricts the muscular perineum from fully operating because of pain or disturbed function is important. Some women have a lesser orgasmic response with a gaping vaginal orifice, and persistently painful episiotomy scars, although rare, are very troublesome when present at the couple's resumption of usual sexual patterns.[48]

Not all physiologic changes are adverse. Some of the increased vascularization of the labia majora, minora, and pelvis with pregnancy remains after delivery; the responses of the woman may be enhanced compared to the prepregnancy state because of this expanded pelvic vascularity.[47]

Psychologically, the addition of another person to the relationship requires adjustments to maintain satisfactory sexual expression. Hindrances to this adjustment include a lowered sexual interest in the mother. This may be attributed to fatigue, weakness, pain, fear of pregnancy, and fear of injury.[39,48] Another factor is that frequency of coitus is related both to age and length of marriage, with older women married longer having decreased coital frequency.[48]

This may be a difficult period for lovemaking even for couples who have remained close throughout pregnancy. Fatigue caused by the additional responsibility of the child, erratic sleep patterns, and often a demanding feeding schedule is real.[42] Attention now is directed to the baby and partly excludes attention the couple might give each other. Some women are satisfied with the emotional attachment and fulfillment offered by the baby, and other emotional ties are not needed as much.[14]

Counseling ahead regarding the postpartum period is helpful. Simply stating that the obstacles to resumption of sex usually encountered are short-lived is reassuring. The physiology may be explained to both partners including the lengthened response time. The resumption of sex usually can be attained after bleeding is stopped and the episiotomy is healed.[37] Nonetheless, there are women and men who are physiologically capable of sex who are not psychologically ready. If the couple is given permission to express these hesitancies and not to feel pressured by the partner, the ultimate relationship is enhanced.[48]

The use of Kegel exercises throughout pregnancy often lessens the effect of perineal relaxation caused by vaginal delivery; such exercises are useful if promptly resumed after pregnancy. This exercise regimen strengthens the entire pubococcygeal muscle, a figure-of-eight shaped structure that supports the bladder, vagina, and rectum. It is the master sphincter of the pelvis, contracts involuntarily during orgasm, and is associated with vaginal perception/response during intercourse. The strengthening of this muscle during and after pregnancy may prevent the symptoms of a cystocele from developing as readily.[48]

THE HIGH-RISK PREGNANCY

Because of the limited substantive information on sexuality in normal pregnancy, even less information is expected regarding the influence of high-risk pregnancy, as is the case. However, there are three important areas that merit discussion: 1) the medical and emotional impact of high-risk pregnancy; 2) adolescent pregnancy; and 3) the failed pregnancy.

When a pregnancy is termed *high risk*, greater emotional burdens are added to the couple. Anxiety often is heightened simply by the use of the label *high risk*. The increased uncertainty of the outcome of mother or child, coupled with added visits, testing, and restrictions, intensify the pressures on the pregnant couple.

Already mentioned is the influence on sexual patterns that pregnancy brings and the coital orgasmic restrictions attendant to certain obstetric problems.

In addition to these restrictions, possible necessary restraints must be considered because of the physiologic alterations in the high-risk pregnant woman created by orgasm. These include an assumed increase in intracranial pressure and an obvious myotonia; perhaps of more importance is the increase in respiratory rate up to 40/min, a tachycardia ranging from 110 to 180/min, and rises in both systolic and diastolic blood pressure of 30–80 mm Hg and 20–40 mm Hg, respectively.[11] Consideration should be given to coital/orgasmic limitations in patients whose medical problems dictate caution regarding temporary tachypnea, tachycardia, blood pressure elevation, or increase in intracranial pressure (eg, severe bronchial asthma, hypertension, cardiac disease, cerebral aneurysm). Especially in the third trimester, the uterine response to orgasm also may include sustained tonic contractions of up to a minute. In a normal pregnancy, the transient fetal bradycardia thus produced is apparently harmless; however, there should be concern for those patients whose disease might predispose to uteroplacental insufficiency (ie, diabetes mellitus, hypertension).

The emotional response of the couple to this added stress of high-risk pregnancy may take one of three directions. First, the couple may draw closer together while becoming intimately involved with the progress and concerns of the pregnancy. This couple is far easier to counsel and seems to accept limitation on sexual activity more readily. Despite their understanding, the old fear of "hurting the baby" is likely to be more pronounced, and, if there is a bad outcome, the question of whether sexual activity harmed the child or influenced the outcome may be raised. Even if the pregnancy has a good outcome, the couple may feel guilty having intercourse, especially if it has been restricted and they have gone against the admonitions of the physician. The closer the couple is emotionally, the more likely it seems that sex is an important expression of mutual caring. They are more likely to agree to restrictions and yet more likely to engage in sex because of its mutual importance.

Second, the added stress of a complicated pregnancy may cause one or both of the partners to be uncooperative, even hostile. The physician or health establishment often is treated as the scapegoat; the frustrations of the problem pregnancy are directed at the most available parties. The couple also may be antagonistic toward each other. No caretaker of the high-risk couple can fail to appreciate the difficulty in treating an uncooperative, antagonistic partner(s). The members of this couple may have difficulty, because of their anger, in expressing the nurturing affection so helpful in such a situation.

Thirdly, the members of this couple may become so intent on the mechanics of following the dictates of the physician (becoming, in essence, medical robots) that they bypass the comfort and mutual support that the physical expression in pregnancy could give them. In this and the prior instance, the couple seems to have greater adjustments to make in the postpartum period; it is as if they become estranged during the process of having their child.

ADOLESCENT PREGNANCY

Starting June 23, 1989, ABC Nightly News devoted a segment for four evenings to a specific topic: teenage pregnancy. For a major television network to devote this much time to any topic underscores the significance of this major national problem. Adolescent sexual patterns and mores developing over the past 20 years have created social and economic burdens for which we have no consistent, workable solution.[2,4] The ABC report estimated the total annual economic cost to be 19 billion dollars; they further stated that the psychological and emotional costs to our society have no way of truly being measured.

The facts regarding teenage sexuality and pregnancy are clear and distressing. There are 11 million sexually active teenagers; 71% of teenagers under 19 years of age are sexually active and most over 15 years of age engage in coitus as their sexual outlet.[3] Of these 11 million, one million get pregnant annually. Of these pregnancies, 47% have live births, half of the mothers are unmarried, and 95% keep their infants as opposed to adoption. Of the remaining pregnant adolescents, 40% have induced abortions and 13% have spontaneous abortions.[3,57]

In comparison with other developed countries, the United States exhibits significantly higher pregnancy, birth, and abortion rates among its adolescents, even when corrected for population and ethnic variances.[57,59]

In the United States, teenagers receive conflicting messages about sexual activity. The media portray sex as exciting and a mark of adulthood (with few messages about responsible contraception), while society tells teenagers simply to decline participation. With few exceptions, sex education courses for adolescents are limited in number and content. Often, only "biology" is discussed while attitudes, behaviors, and consequences are presented briefly or ignored.[2,3,5,60] Many parents restrict the sexual knowledge their children receive to "protect" them from what they perceive as encouragement to engage in sex.[59] Birth control advice and instruction is not available universally, especially for other than barrier methods. Often the adolescents at higher risk for early sexual activity are least motivated and less encouraged to use contraception, and often have the least access to contraceptive information.[4,59]

The causes of adolescent pregnancy are many, but our societal attitudes complicate the prevention of pregnancy because it is viewed as a cultural and moral issue as well as a health issue.[57,59] In the United States, there is a fairly close correlation between sexual conservatism and religiosity; both the nature and intensity of religious feeling inject an emotional element in the debate that is not found in other developed western countries.[59] In Europe, and especially Scandinavia, the clear message is to avoid unwanted pregnancy, which to the Europeans seems more desirable than trying to prevent sexual activity. The messages to our adolescents are inconsistent and consequently unclear.[59]

Understanding adolescence as a developmental stage helps the practitioner caring for the young woman. The physical and reproductive development of both male and female occurs far earlier today than at the turn of the century; however, there is no correlation between biologic maturation and cognitive and psychological development.[57]

The developmental task of the adolescent involves experimental behavior that helps the person to acquire a sense of individual identity, to separate psychologically from the family, and develop operational thinking and future planning ability. Included in this experimental behavior is the testing of new sexual feelings and capabilities.[57]

The disparity between physical and cognitive maturation hinders the adolescent from having full comprehension of the consequences of his or her behavior. Understanding consequences requires anticipation of the consequences of said behavior. The inability to think ahead is a problem in terms of judgment about sexual behavior, especially in the context of pregnancy prevention in which one must anticipate either abstinence or effective contraceptive use.[57] The media model of the adult couple being "swept away" into sex with no apparent concern about pregnancy does nothing to encourage teenagers about responsible sex.

Sexual activity for teenagers is mostly experimental;

other than these normal and exploratory behaviors, few antecedents to teenage sex have been identified. Some believe that sexual activity, especially in the female adolescent, may be to satisfy needs other than sexual. Most studies indicate that the young person most likely to engage in early sexual activity lacks family support and defined goals. Again, the inability or desire to think ahead to define goals may contribute to the problem.[2,5,57,59]

The consequences of adolescent pregnancy affect mother, father, child, extended families, and society.[57] The effects of young maternal age on obstetric and neonatal outcomes are hard to separate from the role of low socioeconomic status, educational disadvantages, lack of parental supervision and family support, and overcrowding. There does seem to be a relation to, if not a causative role in, adverse neonatal outcome.[57]

Adequate early prenatal care reduces the risk of adverse obstetric outcome to a level comparable to adult women of similar background.[57] Pregnancy-induced hypertension may be more common in the black primigravida under age 16, but reports of increased cephalopelvic disproportion among pregnant adolescents have not been confirmed in recent studies.[57]

Neonatal outcome is more significant in adverse consequences. The incidence of low birth weight infants is nearly twice that of mothers over 15 years of age; they are nearly three times as likely to die in the neonatal period. Again, adequate prenatal care can reduce this morbidity and mortality.[4,57]

In the post-neonatal period, infants of mothers under 17 years of age have twice the mortality as those of older women. Sudden infant death syndrome is twice as high, and illness or injuries requiring medical attention are increased significantly, suggesting that supervision of these children may be less than adequate. Child abuse has been reported as higher for children of young mothers as the novelty of the new baby wears off and the drudgery of child care appears.[3,5,57]

Although the reasons are unclear, several reports indicate a greater incidence of developmental problems in children of adolescents. Increased behavior problems and lower scoring on intelligence tests are the main areas of concern.[57]

The difficulties to be surmounted by the young parent are great. Adolescent mothers are less likely to finish high school than those who delay pregnancy, making economic independence very difficult.[4,57,62] The William T. Grant Foundation, Inc. of New York, in reviewing national data on family income and poverty, indicated that one third of family households run by people under age 25 are single parent households (predominantly black and Hispanic). In 1985, 75% of single parent households maintained by a woman under age 25 were living in poverty. The cost of public assistance runs into billions even though much of it is offered for a limited time.[57] The likelihood of repeated pregnancy during teenage years is high since most of the factors leading to the first are still operative.[4,57]

Data show that adolescent males are poorly prepared for fatherhood. The educational, developmental and economic levels vary widely, and academic, drug and behavior problems are significantly higher in adolescent fathers.[57,62]

According to McAnarey, "The consequences of childbearing for adolescent parents, their children, and society are severe. For almost all young people, pregnancy should be prevented or at least delayed."[58] Prevention is difficult because it requires understanding of adolescence as a developmental stage and the patterns of adolescent sexual activity that may lead to pregnancy.

Physicians and midwives have a reasonable comprehension of the individual and societal factors influencing the sexual activity of teenagers. In our contact with adolescent patients and their families, we are in a pivotal position to recognize early sexual activity, educate all concerned, offer ways to prevent pregnancy, and prescribe contraception when appropriate.[57,61]

We have a greater responsibility to take leadership positions in the community in both educational efforts and preventive services. We can work with educators to develop programs to improve contraceptive availability and serve as educational resources for a wide range of adolescent health issues.

The pregnant teenager who comes for care needs medical attention and a caring, nonjudgmental approach that encourages a trusting relationship. The patient is often fearful, perhaps defiant and angry, difficult to reach, and usually overwhelmed by this new reality of pregnancy and its broader implications. She may lack family support and especially partner support; her family may stand by her but still be subtly condemning and angry.[4,5] This teenager thus needs a friend to support her emotionally as she rapidly attempts to mature. It is true that not all adolescents will respond to this approach, but caregivers should make the effort to reach those who will.

THE FAILED PREGNANCY

As sex did in the 1960s, death now has "come out of the closet." Grief counseling increasingly must become part of the physician's armamentarium; one who takes care of patients in greater jeopardy must be prepared to deal with undesirable outcomes. Physicians are often as uncomfortable with the topic of grief as they are discussing sex and lack knowledge about it, perhaps more so.

We have little training in grief effects, tend to introduce our own personal biases to the situation, and rely on others when our impact could be of great value. Williams expressed it eloquently:[49]

> *Remember that what I have found comforting would not be so necessarily to all parents who experienced the loss of a child. It seems to me, however, that parents whose children have died are often screaming to be heard and there seems to be no one who will listen. Standing a little to the side are clergymen, medical people and friends who are wanting terribly to help, but don't know what to do.*

Individuals suffering a loss may experience a definite "grief syndrome" with psychosomatic expressions inhibiting usual daily functioning for varying periods of time. These people have increased vulnerability to illness and even death, alcoholism, reactive depression, cardiac dysfunctions, alteration of sexual patterns, and psychotropic drug dependence.[51,52] We benefit our patients immensely when we recognize and promptly help to avert the more serious complications of grief surrounding a failed pregnancy. By doing "grief work," the patient may prevent the development of these advanced symptoms.

Early pregnancy loss often is seen as having less importance than the loss of a mature infant. We do not offer the rituals and social observations to early loss as we do to a later loss, but the loss may be equally devastating. Therefore, it may be more difficult for the couple involved to grieve sufficiently. A sensitive physician may encourage such expression with the assurance that he is helping a couple to mourn as is necessary.

Whatever the nature of the couple's relationship before the loss of a child, it is likely to undergo change after that loss. It may be assumed that a shared tragedy will help the parents to draw together as they recover, but this is not an automatic result of the event. In many cases, existing problems are made worse, or new conflicts are created.[53] Jackson states, "Different aspects of personality will be revealed under stress. One does not begin to understand the nature and quality of human suffering that goes on during acute grief without taking into account these deeper factors of personality that may become operative."[54]

Grieving is a lonely process; as much as it is desired, partners cannot eliminate the process for each other. Members of a couple grieve in different ways and at a different pace. Schiff has observed, "In the back of their minds, they believed they could lean on each other as they mourned. But you cannot lean on something bent double from its own burden."[55] Often this realization is slow, and the unfulfilled expectations of closeness in crisis may lead to resentment and disappointment. When a relationship is already weak, the couple is likely to have greater difficulty in resisting stresses created by loss. Borg and Lasker[53] state, "They may not be willing to make the effort, or they may have established barriers to communication that are hard to remove." The stress of bereavement even may lead to divorce. G.W. Davidson's unpublished data indicate that in a longitudinal study over the last 10 years at five different sites, the separation/divorce rate among couples losing a child from birth to 12 years was slightly over 50%. The usual divorce rate for those same areas was 28%, a startling statistic. Anger, guilt, and blaming are unavoidable responses to tragic loss. Parents want to find some reason to make sense out of what has happened; a reason gives meaning to the loss and a focus to feelings. However, often with no logical explanation, the person closest bears the brunt of this frustration. This is also one obvious explanation for the physician being a likely recipient of legal action after a poor pregnancy outcome.

The failure to communicate is the most serious obstacle to resolving the tensions that arise from pregnancy loss. A common quote by thanatologists is: "Joy shared is joy increased, and grief shared is grief diminished." Some reports have shown that the interview for gathering research data on grief was the first time some couples had talked to each other about their loss.[53]

When individuals are feeling angry or depressed and not communicating well, it is not surprising that the desire or ability to relate sexually may stop. It is difficult to give love and affection when drained emotionally and in need of self nurturing. The act of making love is pleasurable; parents suffering grief may see it as inappropriate. This attitude may hinder the resumption of the normal sexual relationship.[53] Discrepancies in desire are common, one partner wanting sex earlier or more than the other. This puts stress on the partner not ready to resume sex and makes intimacy difficult. Hendin and Marks state:[56]

> *A vicious and distinctive cycle may ensue: two sensitive, hurting individuals who now more than ever need the closeness of a strong relationship and an expression of physical love, find instead that their separate pain draws them apart to the point where they can no longer express that love.*

Sexual relations may create a painful reminder that the sex act created the child months before; the death of the child may restrict the desire to repeat the act. A corollary to this is that the connection between sex and tragedy can create fear of another pregnancy.[41]

Some couples have an opposite response and wish to have another baby or, unfortunately, are advised by physicians to have another baby immediately. The physician needs to encourage both partners to complete the grieving process before setting out on another pregnancy; such a process could easily last a year or longer before resolution. G.W. Davidson (personal communication) is investigating a significant infertility rate in couples suffering pregnancy loss. The causes seem psychological and are not relieved until the couple stops consciously planning for another baby and returns to the precrisis sexual pattern.

Fortunately, most of these sexual hindrances are short-lived if communication is good and knowledgeable help is available. These couples find they can be close, giving strength to one another, and can talk about their reluctance and fears. They tell each other that the grief will not last forever, and then, when both are ready, the establishment of their sexual pattern can help both partners feel better about themselves and their relationship.

OFFERING HELP

Our role as professionals is to be aware of and knowledgeable about these matters, to help the partners adjust, to help our patients understand and help themselves. We must be clear about our own sexual attitudes and values but not attempt to impose them on our patients. To the extent that we are comfortable with our sexual values, so can we help patients to be comfortable with theirs. Books, courses, and workshops are available to help us reassess our attitudes, not necessarily to change them but to become more comfortable with our sexual selves and less judgmental about others. It is axiomatic that a judgmental person discourages open communication. Couples need professionals who give them permission to talk about sexual and emotional issues and who are knowledgeable and at ease. When a professional broaches the topic of sexual behavior and pregnancy, that action indicates that the subject is important and needs attention. The professional thus is saying to patients: you may feel free to talk about it with me.

Our group adopted a teaching checklist developed by the nurse-midwives in our practice (see Table 196–2). Some items are specific for each trimester; others are useful throughout pregnancy. Whoever sees the patients checks off each item discussed or taught at that visit. (Sexuality is a topic in all three trimesters.) There also is available an excellent cartoon-style pamphlet on sex and pregnancy written by one of our midwives for her master's thesis.[21] With this checklist approach, the topic of sex becomes only one of many, thus there is none of the awkwardness of a parental "birds and bees" talk.

Each member of our group uses different words to introduce the subject. One of our midwives says, "How's your love life? Before you respond, let me tell you I get answers ranging from 'It would be fine if he'd come to bed at 9 o'clock when I do' to 'What love life?' " One of my partners simply asks, "Are you having any problems with intercourse?" My words are usually, "What changes have you experienced in your sex life since becoming pregnant? Any changes in your attitudes or feelings or your partner's?" Once the topic is broached, discussion can ensue naturally.

TABLE 196–2. A TEACHING CHECKLIST

First trimester
Classes for prepared childbirth, first set
Common discomforts: constipation, frequent urination, fatigue, breast tenderness
Common reactions to pregnancy
Danger signs
Exercise: Kegels, swimming, walking
Expected date of confinement variations
Father's feelings
Fetal growth and development
Frequency of visits
Hygiene
Nutrition
Sexuality
Smoking, alcohol, medications, caffeine, cats, x-rays
Second trimester
Breast or bottle feeding
Classes, second set
Common discomforts: backache, round ligament pain, constipation, indigestion, vaginal discharge
Danger signs
Dreams and fantasies
Father's feelings
Fetal growth and development
Quickening, fetal heart tones
Sexuality
Sibling rivalry
Third trimester
Circumcision
Common discomforts: cramps, edema, frequent urination
Danger signs
Dreams, fantasies, fears
Father's feelings
Fetal growth and development
Fetal movement chart
Labor and delivery plan
Nipple preparation
Preparation at home
Safe ride pamphlet
Sexuality: positions
True versus false labor, timing uterine contractions

From Dameron[63] with permission.

Early in pregnancy, we give an overview of the sexual changes pregnancy brings and discuss first-trimester concerns. We strongly emphasize that although there are general tendencies regarding sexual behavior in pregnancy, each couple's response will be varied and individual. Certain trends have been observed, but each couple has permission to behave in individual ways. In the second and third trimesters, we again bring up the subject; we indicate alternative positions for coitus in the third trimester.

Inviting the couple to raise issues in the sexual and emotional area is easier than counseling. A gifted listener may be all that the couple needs. However, not all of us are skillful or even interested in counseling. A good rule of thumb is to counsel only to the degree with which you are comfortable, and be sure that you have access to a referral if you need help.

We counsel (or refer) only couples who indicate that they desire to explore sexual issues further. Good obstetric care does not demand a persistent search for sexual dysfunction during pregnancy. Sexual response to pregnancy is only one of many important issues the couple must face. We believe that our responsibility in this area means casually presenting the topic of sexuality to the couple in context and allowing ample opportunity for discussion.

Couples need to know about the physical changes during pregnancy that may affect sexual activity and emotional responses. Well written printed matter is helpful.[16] They also need to be aware of medical conditions that may interfere with usual sexual activity and the coital and noncoital alternatives available.

Encourage partners to talk with each other about their feelings. Let them know that expressing feelings honestly, gently, caringly, and often, while allowing for differences in moods and desires, will make the transition through pregnancy easier. Continue to emphasize the need for this type of communication; extended silences put distance between partners. Encourage them to understand that both partners have needs, doubts, and fears, and that they must give each other emotional support.

Physical contact of some type, if not always erotic, is sensual and conveys by touch the love expressed in words. Foot massage, back rubs, hugs, kisses, the passing caress—all affirm the couple's emotional commitment to each other physically and continually. Remind them that although pregnancy usually decreases coital frequency, it often increases the need for affection and reassurance.

This chapter concentrates on the stresses, problems, and concerns related to pregnancy and sexuality, but we need to continually emphasize to our patients the tremendous opportunity this stressful period presents. It is an opportunity for partners to draw closer, to learn about each other in different ways and in greater depth, to develop sound coping and communication skills, to grow as a couple and thus develop into a more mature family unit. Bing and Colman say it well:[14]

> *Men and women undergo profound personal, interpersonal, and social changes during pregnancy and the postpartum period. Lovers must add the roles of partner and parent to the way they interact with each other. They will never be the same again—alone, together, or in the eyes of the world. They may have to work hard to stay in touch with these changes in themselves and their partners. Parenthood makes a shared life more complicated, but it also carries with it the potential to make life together more meaningful as lovemaking goes beyond caring for each other and spreads out to embrace the family unit.*

CONCLUSIONS

Our sexuality is an intrinsic part of our psychological makeup, and its healthy, appropriate, comfortable expression is of great value to both individuals and couples. Pregnancy alters and stresses this significant aspect of the couple's life, and lack of understanding on the part of both patient and physician may add more problems to an already stressful event. When pregnancy becomes complicated or a pregnancy fails, there is still more strain placed on the individuals involved and their interactions. Pregnancy adds a severe burden to the adaptive rigors of adolescence. Health professionals have a unique opportunity to understand and to help the couple anticipate and cope with these changes so that the result will be toward the healthy maturation and strengthening of the family structure.

REFERENCES

1. Leonard G. *The End of Sex*. Boston: Houghton Mifflin; 1983;12.
2. Wattleton F. American teens: sexually active, sexually illiterate. *J Sch Health*. 1987;57:379.
3. Burton NJ. Adolescent sexuality and pregnancy. *Issues Health Care Women*. 1980;2:43.
4. Youth in the 1980s: social and health concerns. *Popul Rep [M]*. 1985:M349.
5. Porter S. Sexuality and pregnancy: a change in values. *Ohio Med*. 1987;83:154.
6. Nicholas SW, Sondheimer DL, Willoughby AD, et al. Human immunodeficiency virus infection in childhood, adolescence, and pregnancy: a status report and national research agenda. *Pediatrics*. 1989;83:293.
7. McCary J. *Human Sexuality*. 2nd ed. New York, NY: Van Nostrand Reinhold; 1973:3.
8. Griffith S. Pregnancy as an event with crisis potential for marital partners: a study of interpersonal needs. *J Obstet Gynecol Neonat Nurs*. 1976;5:35.
9. Kyndely K. The sexuality of women in pregnancy and postpartum: a review. *J Obstet Gynecol Neonat Nurs*. 1978;7:28.
10. Falicov C. Sexual adjustment during first pregnancy and postpartum. *Am J Obstet Gynecol*. 1973;117:991.
11. Masters W, Johnson V. *Human Sexual Response*. Boston, MA: Little, Brown; 1966:141.
12. Solberg D, Butler J, Wagner N. Sexual behavior in pregnancy. *N Engl J Med*. 1973;288:1098.
13. Wagner J. The attitudes, feelings and behaviors of expectant fathers attending Lamaze classes. *Birth Fam J*. 1976;3:5.
14. Bing E, Colman L. *Making Love during Pregnancy*. New York, NY: Bantam Books; 1977:6.
15. Norris M. Sexual concerns during pregnancy. Unpublished master's thesis. Atlanta, GA: Emory University; 1980.
16. Holtzman L. Sexual practices during pregnancy. *J Nurse Midwifery*. 1976;21:29.
17. *Precis II. An Update in Obstetrics and Gynecology*. American College of Obstetricians and Gynecologists. Washington, DC. 1981:188.
18. Anderson C, Clancy BJ, Quirk B. Sexuality in pregnancy. In: Barnard M, Clancy BJ, Krantz KE, eds. *Human Sexuality for Health Professionals*. Philadelphia, PA: WB Saunders; 1978:128.
19. Hotchner T. *Pregnancy and Childbirth: The Complete Guide for a New Life*. New York, NY: Avon Books; 1979:168.
20. Bittman S, Zalk S. *Expectant Fathers*. New York, NY: Ballantine Books; 1978:104.
21. Hager A. The effect of written communications on pregnant women's sexual knowledge and concerns. Unpublished master's thesis. Atlanta, GA: Emory University; 1981.
22. Hott J. The crisis of expectant fatherhood. *Am J Nurs*. 1976;76:1436.
23. Obrzut L. Expectant fathers' perception of fathering. *Am J Nurs*. 1976;76:1440.
24. Perkins R. Sexual behavior and response in relation to complications in pregnancy. *Am J Obstet Gynecol*. 1979;134:498.
25. Newton N. Trebly sensuous woman. *Psychol Today*. July 1971:68.
26. Goodlin R. Orgasm and premature labor. *Lancet*. 1969;2:646.
27. Mills L, Harley E, Harlap S. Should coitus late in pregnancy be discouraged? *Lancet*. 1981;2:136.
28. Schneider J. Sex during pregnancy—is it safe? *Perinat Press*. 1980;4:13.
29. Pugh W, Fernandez F. Coitus in late pregnancy. *Obstet Gynecol*. 1953;2:636.
30. Reamy K, White SE. Sexuality in pregnancy and the puerperium: a review. *Obstet Gynecol Surv*. 1985;40:1.
31. Naeye RL. Coitus and associated amniotic fluid infection. *N Engl J Med*. 1979;301:1198.
32. Naeye RL. Common environmental influences in the fetus. *Monogr Pathol*. 1981;22:52.
33. Fyke FE, Kazmier FJ, Harm RW. Venous air embolism: life-threatening complication of orogenital sex during pregnancy. *Am J Med*. 1985;78:33.
34. Bray P, Myers RA, Cowley RA. Orogenital sex as a cause of nonfatal air embolism in pregnancy. *Obstet Gynecol*. 1983;61:653.
35. Bernhardt TL, Goldmann RW, Thombs PA, Kindwall EP. Hyperbaric oxygen treatment of cerebral air embolism from orogenital sex during pregnancy. *Crit Care Med*. 1988;16:729.
36. Connell E, Butler J, Goodlin R, et al. What do you advise patients concerning the safety of sexual relations during pregnancy? *Med Aspects Hum Sexuality*. 1981;15:91.
37. Richardson A, Lyon J, Graham E, et al. Decreasing postpartum sexual abstinence time. *Am J Obstet Gynecol*. 1976;126:416.
38. Walbroehl GS. Sexuality during pregnancy. *Am Fam Physician*. 1984;29:273.
39. Reamy KJ, White SE. Sexuality in the puerperium: a review. *Arch Sex Behav*. 1987;16:165.
40. Kaplan H. *The New Sex Therapy*. New York, NY: Quadrangle (Brunner-Mazel); 1974:63.
41. Kaplan H. *Disorders of Sexual Desire*. New York, NY: Simon & Schuster; 1979:24.
42. Williams J. *Psychology of Women's Behavior in a Bisocial Context*. New York, NY: WW Norton; 1977:275.
43. Duvall E. *Family Development*. 4th ed. Philadelphia, PA: JB Lippincott; 1971:206.
44. Cohn SD. Sexuality in pregnancy: a review of the literature. *Nurs Clin North Am*. 1982;17:91.
45. Swanson J. The marital sexual relationship during pregnancy. *J Obstet Gynecol Neonat Nurs*. 1980;9:267.
46. Morris N. The frequency of sexual intercourse during pregnancy. *Arch Sex Behav*. 1975;4:501.
47. Hollender M, McGehee A. The wish to be held during pregnancy. *J Psychosom Res*. 1974;18:193.
48. Inglis T. Postpartum sexuality. *J Obstet Gynecol Neonat Nurs*. 1980;9:298.
49. Alder EM, Cook A, Davidson D, et al. Hormones, mood and sexuality in lactating women. *Br J Psychiatry*. 1986;148:74.
50. Williams N. Some do's and don'ts in order to be specific and at the risk of sounding presumptuous. *Thantos*. 1980;5:16.
51. Lindeman E. Symptomatology and management of acute grief. *Am J Psychiatry*. 1944;101:141.
52. Woodson R, Garfield CA, eds. *Psychosocial Care of the Dying Patient*. New York, NY: McGraw-Hill; 1978:359.
53. Borg S, Lasker J. *When Pregnancy Fails*. Boston: Beacon Press; 1981:79.
54. Jackson E. *Understanding Grief*. Nashville, TN: Abington Press; 1957:15.
55. Schiff HS. *The Bereaved Parent*. New York, NY: Crown; 1977:58.
56. Hendin D, Marks J. *The Genetic Connection*. New York, NY: Signet; 1979.
57. McAnarey ER, Hendee WR. Adolescent pregnancy and its consequences. *JAMA*. 1989;262:74.
58. McAnarey ER, Hendee WR. The prevention of adolescent pregnancy. *JAMA*. 1989;262:78.
59. Jones EF, Forrest JD, Goldman N, et al. Teenage pregnancy in developed countries: determinants and policy implications. *Fam Plann Perspect*. 1985;17:53.
60. Macdonald DI. An approach to the problem of teenage pregnancy. *Public Health Rep*. 1987;102:377.
61. Alexander GR, Petersen DJ, Hulsey TC, Gibson JJ. Adolescent sexual activity and pregnancy in South Carolina: trends, risks, and practice implications. *South Med J*. 1987;80:581.
62. Nakishima II. Teenage Pregnancy—its causes, costs and consequences. *Nurse Pract*. 1977;2:10.
63. Dameron GW Jr. Helping couples cope with sexual changes pregnancy brings. *Contemp OB/Gyn*. 1983;21:23.

Chapter One Hundred and Ninety-Seven

Psychiatric Disorders

Yogi K. Ahluwalia and Barbara E. B. Meyer

197

Pregnancy is a time of dramatic biologic and psychological change and adaptation for a woman. While there are many commonalities across pregnancies, there are as many experiences unique to the individual woman. The pregnancy itself, with all the related risks and treatments, can be the trigger for psychological reactions ranging from mild emotional distress to more serious psychiatric disorders. In other women, a preexisting psychiatric disorder complicates their experience of pregnancy and their physician's management of the pregnancy. This chapter will review the current evidence from both of these perspectives.

This review begins with a consideration of the range of emotional responses and reactions to pregnancy and the postpartum period in women without any known history of psychiatric disorder. Emotional reactions to some of the new trends and technologies in obstetric care also will be explored.

The rest of the chapter will describe the relationship between a preexisting psychiatric disorder and pregnancy. Each psychiatric disorder will be described with an emphasis on symptoms, treatment, and the specific complication pregnancy presents for the course of the disorder on both the woman and her unborn child. The psychiatric disorders that are related uniquely to pregnancy, postpartum disorders, and puerperal psychosis also will be considered. Overall, the aim of this chapter is to provide a guideline by which the health care provider can gauge the relationship between reasonable emotional distress and serious psychiatric disorders in pregnant women, and provide safe and appropriate treatment in either case.

EMOTIONAL RESPONSES TO PREGNANCY

Despite the physiologic and emotional changes that occur during pregnancy, the nine months of pregnancy is a time of decreased incidence of serious emotional disturbance. Whether admission to psychiatric hospitals or outpatient psychiatric visits are used as the outcome measure, the incidence of mental illness is substantially lower during pregnancy than in either the postpartum or nonpregnant periods.[1] Following childbirth, the risk of serious psychiatric disorder is about 15%. This is at least twice the 2–7% risk following nonpregnancy-related stressful events.[2]

Common Emotional Reactions in Pregnancy

Pregnancy is a complex physical and emotional experience that is inherently stressful. It is associated with changes in eating behavior, sleep, and sexual activity, changes that outside of pregnancy may signal a psychological disturbance such as depression. However, within the context of pregnancy, these changes are normal. Currently, pregnancy is viewed as both a biologic and psychological phase in life that requires adjustment and adaptation. The more successfully a woman adapts, the more likely she will be to integrate this experience into a higher level of adult development and emotional maturity.[3] A woman's emotional adaptation to pregnancy will be affected by her previous ability to master problems and resolve conflicts. The emotional aspects of the pregnancy also are affected by the context in which the pregnancy occurs. For example, an unmarried adolescent and a married woman who struggled with infertility problems will have quite different emotional reactions to their pregnancies.

Some common emotional issues can be identified and loosely associated with the stages of pregnancy. Throughout pregnancy, feelings of anxiety, ambivalence, and lability of mood often are described. In the first trimester, there may be more periods of fluctuating emotions. Risk factors for increased incidence of psychological upset during this period, and possibly more physiologic discomfort, include: negative reaction to the pregnancy by husband or boyfriend; previous unpleasant pregnancy experiences; unclear motivation for pregnancy; few supportive people in life; and a great change in life style due to pregnancy.[4] In the second trimester, there may be fewer emotional changes. Instead, emotional reactions may center on body image, sexuality, and relationship to the unborn child. In the third trimester, emotional reactions may intensify at the same time that physical discomfort becomes most acute.

Other emotional factors that can be the source of troublesome emotional reactions in pregnancy involve more specifically psychological factors. The reality of motherhood involves some loss of autonomy and control. This can raise conflicting feelings about personal freedom, dependence on others, and independence. Relationships with the woman's mother and husband also require new levels of psychological adaptation, which can often be the cause of emotional distress in pregnancy.

It commonly has been believed that pregnant women were generally more introspective than nonpregnant women. A recent study confirmed that in their style of thinking, pregnant women were more focused on their inner thoughts than on the outer world.[5] This was described as doing the "psychological work" that is necessary to integrate and adjust to the experience of pregnancy and upcoming motherhood.

Maternity Blues

One of the most common emotional responses to childbirth is the maternity blues or baby blues. This phenomenon occurs in 50–70% of women who have given birth and is consistent across cultures. It generally begins on the third postpartum day, but may begin as late as the tenth day after delivery. Its duration can be from one day to just over two weeks; however, this is clearly a transitory syndrome.

The clinical hallmark of the maternity blues is weeping. This is a time when a woman is hypersensitive and emotionally vulnerable to perceived slights or rebuffs from family members or health care providers. Fears regarding the baby's health and her own well-being are also prominent. In multiparas, concerns can focus on the well-being of other children.

A second cluster of clinical symptoms involves a variety of affective and anxiety-related subjective reports. These symptoms can include depressed mood, irritability, anxiety, restlessness, headache and insomnia. A feeling of depersonalization (feeling distant or strange) is reported at times. Confusion and forgetfulness also are commonly reported. However, when objective psychological tests are used, these subjective reports are not confirmed.[6] In this cluster of symptoms, the specific combination and severity of each is determined by the individual background of the woman.

Despite the term *maternity blues,* this syndrome is very different from postpartum depression. Maternity blues is a temporary phenomenon that is self-limited. The only treatment required is emotional support and reassurance. Postpartum depression, which is covered in detail elsewhere in this chapter, is far more serious, longer-lasting, has a different clinical picture, and requires more active treatment.

Because the maternity blues is such a prevalent phenomenon, many studies have explored possible causes and correlates.[7] To date, none of the studies has shown any evidence linking maternity blues and social, personality, marital, environmental or psychological factors, nor do obstetric variables or the events of labor and delivery show any relationship. There are some indications of a correlation between premenstrual syndrome and maternity blues, since the symptom descriptions are similar, but this is not a clear relationship.

Biologic variables, especially changes in sex hormones and cortisol, have been regarded as likely correlates for this phenomenon but the relationship is not a clear one. Comparisons between postpartum mood states and those in postoperative women showed a clear similarity.[8] The explanation offered, consistent with a much earlier study, was that the maternity blues was a phenomena related to emotional release after a period of acute stress.[9] However, another view of the correlates of the maternity blues was offered by comparing the postpartum moods of both mothers and fathers. These comparisons suggested that the postpartum period is an emotionally unique time of both increased anxiety and positive feelings that is experienced in an emotionally similar way for both men and women.[10]

EMOTIONAL REACTIONS TO NEW OBSTETRIC TRENDS AND TECHNOLOGIES

As demographic trends change and new obstetric technologies are developed, the emotional experiences of the pregnant woman under obstetric care also change. Because stress, anxiety, and negative attitudes can have an impact on the course of the pregnancy and delivery, it is relevant to assess emotional reaction to these new aspects of care.

Advanced Maternal Age

In recent years, there has been a consistent trend toward older maternal age at the time of first pregnancy.[11] As a group, older primaparas tend to be more independent, career-oriented, and financially stable. Despite the major change in established life styles that having a child often represents, the older group of pregnant women seems to make a relatively positive adjustment to pregnancy.[12]

Ultra Sound Scanning

Ultrasound scanning is a common diagnostic tool used in obstetric practice today (see Chapter 6). The procedure has the potential emotional benefit of reducing anxiety about the health of the unborn child. This anxiety-reducing benefit is especially clear for women in high-risk situations. When women with raised serum α-fetoprotein were seen for diagnostic ultrasound, their anxiety levels were initially very high. Following the ultrasound scan, anxiety levels were greatly reduced and positive attitudes toward the pregnancy were greatly increased.[13] This result was confirmed and expanded by the finding that the amount of feedback a woman was given about the ultrasound scan made a great deal of difference in amount of anxiety reduction. For women and their male partners who attended the session, high feedback conditions about the results of the ultrasound scan showed the best reduction in anxiety and the largest increase in positive feelings about the pregnancy.[14]

Amniocentesis and Chorionic Villi Sampling

Amniocentesis and chorionic villi sampling (CVS) are techniques used for the detection of genetic abnormalities in the unborn child (see Chapter 16). Generally, these techniques are used in high-risk pregnancies in which the woman is already experiencing anxiety over the health of the unborn child. Amniocentesis has been shown to put a number of different stresses on the prospective parents. Anxiety relating to the stage in pregnancy during which the test used to be performed (16 weeks) and the time delay in obtaining results (2–4 weeks) were most prominent.[15] In contrast, women who underwent CVS were able to have the procedure performed sooner (9 weeks) and had the results sooner (1 week). In terms of emotional response, these time differences mean that anxiety levels can decrease earlier with CVS than with amniocentesis.[16]

Cesarean Section

Cesarean section rates continue to rise. Emotional responses to cesarean sections, especially to an unanticipated one after a long and unproductive labor, often are described as involving sadness, a sense of failure, lowered self esteem, and emotions similar to grieving. This emotional response was especially prominent for first-time mothers who had little experience with children. Interestingly, a very long labor culminating in a vaginal birth was not regarded as any more emotionally satisfying than a cesarean section.[17] Factors that have been shown to minimize the negative emotional impact of cesarean sections were the opportunity to participate in the birth and epidural anesthesia. The latter group of mothers was less tired after the birth and showed fewer negative emotional responses.[18] This was especially true if the father was allowed in the delivery room and the baby was allowed to stay with the mother after the surgery. Interestingly, there were no differences in mother-child interactions related to method of delivering at followup of one month, two months or one year.

ANXIETY DISORDERS AND PREGNANCY

All pregnant women have anxious moments. They have fears and concerns regarding body changes, possibility of difficult labor, and concerns regarding the health of the unborn child. Sometimes these fears can become excessive and disabling, leading to anxiety disorders including phobic avoidance, compulsive behavior, or recurrent anxiety states.

Generalized Anxiety Disorders

Essential features of this disorder are excessive worry and anxiety about life circumstances, for example, worry about complications in the pregnant state even when pregnancy is progressing normally. When the person is anxious, there are signs of motor tension and autonomic hyperactivity.

Panic Disorders

Panic disorder is manifested as discrete periods of intense fear or discomfort that lasts for a few minutes (rarely hours) and are recurrent in nature. These panic attacks have sudden onset with intense apprehension and terror, accompanied by a feeling of impending doom.

Obsessive-Compulsive Disorders

The essential features of these disorders are recurrent obsessions or compulsions sufficiently severe to cause marked distress. Obsessions are persistent ideas, thoughts or impulses that are senseless, for example, mother having ideas related to killing an unborn child. Compulsions are repetitive behaviors that are performed in response to an obsession. Both obsessional thoughts and compulsive behaviors cause marked distress in the pregnant state.

The exact incidence of generalized anxiety disorders in pregnancy is unknown. Panic disorder has a prevalence of 1–2% in the general population, and there are reports that pregnant women experience improvement in panic symptoms during the course of pregnancy and an increase of symptoms in the postpartum period.[19] Obsessive-compulsive disorders have a lifetime prevalence as high as

2–3%. Ingram[20] found pregnancy to be the most common precipitating cause of obsessive-compulsive disorders.

Ambivalent and conflicting feeling regarding pregnancy can predispose a woman to an anxiety state. Delaying childbirth to the later years of life can cause a great deal of apprehension based on changes in life style. Lack of support from the spouse or marital conflict also can result in anxiety. Women with a history of induced abortion may react with symptoms of anxiety in a subsequent pregnancy. There may be feelings of shame, guilt, and unresolved grief resulting from a past abortion that can lead to anxiety in the pregnant state. Prior psychological conflicts in a woman can lead to concerns around the motherhood role, predisposing the pregnant woman to developing anxiety symptoms. Obsession about the fear of a deformed fetus or a difficult labor can precipitate anxiety disorders.

The essential features of generalized anxiety disorder are motortension, for example, trembling, twitching, feeling shaky, muscle tone tension, restlessness and easy fatigability. Symptoms of autonomic hyperactivity include shortness of breath, palpitation, sweating or cold hands, dizziness, nausea or a lump in the throat. Symptoms of hypervigilance include a feeling of being keyed up or on edge, irritability and sleep onset insomnia.

Panic attacks typically begin with a sudden onset of intense apprehension, fear or terror. Symptoms experienced during a panic attack are shortness of breath, choking sensation, accelerated heart rate, ringing in the ears, blurring of vision, tingling sensation, fear of dying or losing control.

An obsessive-compulsive disorder is manifested by intense anxiety due to persistent ideas or thoughts that are senseless, for example, repeated ideas or thoughts about harming the unborn child.

It is important to distinguish normal anxiety that most pregnant women experience from symptoms of anxiety disorders. Psychotherapy helps a pregnant woman who is experiencing undue anxiety to deal with fears and anxiety as it relates to pregnancy. Discussing troublesome thoughts and feelings provides relief from distress. Continued opportunity to talk about problems is helpful, even if this process by itself is not curative. Reduction in anxiety symptoms allows a woman to function more effectively in personal and family relationships, which in turn may allow her to use these support systems for even more relief of her anxiety. In women with obsessive-compulsive disorders, when obsessional rituals and anxiety become intolerable, a brief hospitalization may be necessary.

Effective noninvasive treatment of anxiety disorders can be accomplished through the use of progressive muscle relaxation training, visual imagery, cognitive retraining, and biofeedback training. The basis of these treatments is the concept that muscle relaxation and motortension cannot occur at the same time. Thus, a pregnant woman who learns to voluntarily relax her muscles will not experience the symptoms of anxiety disorders.

Anti-anxiety drugs also provide relief from symptoms of anxiety. Whenever possible, the use of anti-anxiety drugs should be avoided in the first trimester. In more severe and disabling cases of anxiety these drugs may have to be used. Pregnant women then should be informed fully about the risks involved, and documented informed consent should be obtained from the patient as well as possibly her partner.

Pregnant patients with severe panic attacks need treatment with alprozolam at the minimum possible dosage.

Neonates of pregnant women who have been treated with benzodiazepines show two types of toxic reactions: the "floppy infant syndrome" and withdrawal reactions. Gillberg[21] associated prolonged low dose use of benzodiazepines with the floppy infant syndrome, manifested as symptoms of hypotonia, lethargy, sucking difficulties, cynosis, and hypothermia in the newborn. Rementeria and Bhatt[22] described withdrawal symptoms in newborns who were exposed to diazepam during pregnancy. The withdrawal symptoms appear 2–6 hours after delivery and consist of tremors, irritability, hypertonia, and vigorous sucking. These symptoms are treated successfully with phenobarbital and may last for up to 6 weeks. Erkkola and Kanto[23] recommend that women on benzodiazepine therapy refrain from breast-feeding infants.

There are no conclusive studies reporting congenital abnormalities with the use of anti-anxiety drugs. However, some studies have linked the ingestion of diazepam during pregnancy with an increased risk of cleft lip and palate.[24]

MAJOR AFFECTIVE DISORDERS IN PREGNANCY

The essential features of this group of disorders are disturbance of mood, accompanied by a manic or depressive syndrome that is not due to any other physical or mental disorder.

Major Depression

Major depressive disorders are characterized by a dysphoric mood, anhedonia, significant weight loss or gain, insomnia or hypersomnia, fatigue, feelings of worthlessness and in more severe cases, preoccupation with suicidal ideation.

Bipolar Disorder

Bipolar disorders or manic disorders are characterized by distinct periods of euphoria or irritability, hyperactivity, insomnia, excessive talkativeness, distractability, and inflated self esteem.

Both major depressive disorders and manic episodes may be accompanied by psychotic features, for example, auditory hallucinations or delusional thinking.

The lifetime expectancy of becoming depressed is 15–25% among women. Kumar and Robson[25] in a sample of 119 first time mothers report a 16% prevalence of clinical depression. Among those, 13% were major depressive disorders, 73% minor and 13% intermittant depressive disorders at 12 weeks' gestation. Ten percent were first depressive episodes since conception and 85% had remitted by the time of delivery.

The incidence of bipolar illness or manic illness is between 0.5–1.5%. It is well recognized that the incidence of both major depression and manic illness tends to increase postpartum. (Postpartum disorders will be discussed later in this chapter.)

O'Hara[26] reports that as many as 10% of pregnant women meet criteria for major or minor depression during pregnancy, with an even greater percentage being depressed postpartum. Bipolar patients who get pregnant are at an increased risk for postpartum depression.

The signs and symptoms of major depressive disorders and bipolar disorders have been listed above. Other commonly associated features in depressive disorder include depressed appearance, tearfulness, increased anxiety, and irritability. Difficulty in concentrating, indecisiveness, memory problems, and thoughts of death or suicide are common in major depression.

Commonly associated features in mania include lability of mood with rapid shifts of mood to anger and depression. Manic speech is loud, rapid, and difficult to interrupt.

Frequently, there is flight of ideas, distractability, and preoccupation with increased self-esteem with marked grandiosity. There is also frequently lack of sleep and the individual is full of energy and may go for days with no sleep and without getting tired.

Planned pregnancy is extremely important in a woman with a previously diagnosed depressive or manic illness and who is actively treated with tricyclic antidepressants or lithium carbonate. There is a need for ongoing consultation between psychiatrist, obstetrician, patient, and spouse or partner to discuss problems, risks and benefits of any psychopharmacological treatment. This gives the psychiatrist an opportunity to discontinue medication prior to conception if symptoms have been in remission and also assess the risk of relapse.

Hospitalization should be considered as an alternative to psychopharmacologic treatment in the first trimester in cases of unplanned pregnancy in which medication may have to be discontinued abruptly and in which there is a prior history of recurrent affective disorders.

Use of tricyclic antidepressants should be reserved only for severely depressed pregnant patients who complain of vegetative symptoms of depression, for example, crying spells, insomnia, and marked appetite disturbance as well as suicidal ideation. Psychotherapy should be used to assess and treat any intrapsychic conflicts associated with pregnancy. In addition, cognitive-behavioral psychotherapeutic approaches for depression have shown success as noninvasive treatments. They may be used either alone or as an adjunct to antidepressant medication. Electroconvulsive therapy (ECT) should be considered in psychotically depressed patients for a quicker response and in cases in which the life of both patient and fetus is endangered. No definitive link between the use of antidepressants and any teratogenic effects has been established.

According to Cohen et al[27], the preferred antidepressants for pregnant patients are secondary amines such as nortryptyline or desipramine. These two have lower cholinergic side effects and can be monitored via plasma levels, which can lessen the side effects in neonates (eg, bowel obstruction and urinary retention).

It is unclear if bipolar or manic patients relapse during pregnancy. However, there is an increased risk for relapse during the postpartum period. The postpartum illness may take the form of mania or depression and usually tends to occur 7–14 days postpartum.

Bipolar pregnant patients often are more difficult to manage since lithium carbonate is contraindicated in the first trimester due to an increased risk of cardiovascular congenital defects (primarily Ebstein's abnormality). Its use in the second and third trimester has been associated with neonatal goiter, decreased neonatal muscle tone and poor sucking reflex.[28]

Management of lithium levels during pregnancy requires consideration of physiologic changes of pregnancy as plasma volume increases. Lithium clearance increases in the second half of pregnancy gradually by 30–50% until delivery when it falls to prepregnancy levels. Close monitoring of lithium levels in pregnant women shows a decrease in lithium concentration as pregnancy progresses. Drug dosages must be readjusted regularly to achieve therapeutic lithium levels, with special consideration given to the rapid fall in lithium clearance that occurs during delivery.[29] Maternal levels can at that point quickly rise to toxic levels if the dose is not rapidly adjusted.

If avoided during the first trimester, lithium is not associated with an increased risk of cardiovascular malformations.

A newborn can show signs of lithium toxicity as lithium easily enters breast milk. Hypotonia, cyanosis, and hypothermia are common manifestations of lithium toxicity in infants. Ananth[30] therefore recommended that mothers on lithium therapy abstain from breast feeding.

SCHIZOPHRENIC DISORDERS

Schizophrenic disorders are characterized by formal thought disorders and perceptual disturbances. At some phase of illness, schizophrenia always involves auditory hallucinations, delusions of grandeur or persecution, looseness of associations and poverty of speech.

The lifetime prevalence of schizophrenic illnesses is about 1%. Many reports continue to document the recurrence of pre-existing psychosis during pregnancy.[31]

During an acute phase, pregnant schizophrenic women often experience the exacerbation of psychotic symptoms. The delusions tend to become bizarre and are related to body changes and fetal movements in pregnancy. Auditory hallucinations may be directed towards pregnancy, for example, voices may instruct them to hit their abdomen to get rid of the baby. Pregnant women may appear highly agitated, perplexed, and disorganized. Speech may show signs of thought disorders. The pregnant patient may present with psychotic denial of her pregnancy through delivery.

Some reports indicate that patients with schizophrenic disorders develop more obstetric complications and their newborns have lower birth weights.[32]

A woman who presents with the first episode of a psychosis during pregnancy should have a complete medical work up to rule out any organic basis for her psychosis or mental status changes. For a woman with a prior history of schizophrenia who is maintained on psychotropic drugs, sudden discontinuation of maintenance antipsychotic medication because of pregnancy can lead to acute relapse. Hospitalization in a psychiatric unit may be necessary if patients become unmanageable in an outpatient treatment setting.

Most reviews of the use of antipsychotic medications in pregnancy report no significantly associated malformations in newborns.[33] However, antipsychotic medication should be avoided in the first trimester whenever possible. If on no medication during gestation following delivery, a woman with a preexisting history of psychosis should be started on antipsychotic medication to prevent postpartum relapse. All antipsychotic medications are secreted into breast milk, thus mothers taking antipsychotic medication should be cautioned about breast feeding.

The neonate may show signs of agitation and hypertonia for several months if the mother has been treated during pregnancy with phenothiazines.[34]

For acute cases, in which either the life of the pregnant woman or of her fetus is threatened, ECT may be indicated. ECT does not induce labor unless the woman is at term.[35]

A small group of pregnant women who react to being pregnant with psychotic denial should be watched carefully for neonaticide.[36] In cases in which the risk of neonaticide is high, some authors recommend psychiatric commitment of pregnant mother for court-ordered treatment.[37]

POSTPARTUM DISORDERS

This is a specific group of emotional disorders that develop in the postpartum period. Their classification in the *Diagnostic and Statistical Manual III* remains, however, quite controversial. Maternity blues, postpartum depression and puerperal psychosis are commonly reported as postpartum syndromes. Maternity blues, a transient self-limiting disorder, already has been discussed earlier in this chapter and is clearly less serious than those of the other postpartum disorders.

Postpartum Depression

Postpartum depression is characterized by irritability, depressed mood, fatigue, and considerable anxiety. It usually occurs at least a week following delivery and may occur up to a year after childbirth.

Approximately 10–15% of women are afflicted with postpartum depression. The relationship of age and parity to the development of postpartum depression is unclear. A prior history of postpartum depression increases the risk of developing depression in subsequent pregnancies.

Both biologic and psychological factors contribute toward the etiology of postpartum depression. The massive hormonal changes following childbirth have been linked to postpartum depression. However, any direct link between hormonal levels and depressed mood phases is lacking. Handley et al[38] found an association between low plasma tryptophan concentrations and depressed mood in the postpartum period. Hayworth et al[39] reported that high anxiety and hostility during pregnancy were positively related to postpartum depression.

The signs and symptoms of postpartum depression tend to occur during the second week following delivery. Usually, the woman reports feeling depressed most of the time (experiencing tearfulness, guilt, anorexia, sleep disturbance, feelings of inadequacy of being a mother and parent). Many women report not being able to love their newborn. Symptoms of psychomotor retardation with slowed down thinking are reported. Often, patients become hopeless and fearful of not being better or able to come out of their depressed mood. Some women report suicidal ideation; this may become a serious concern both for the family members and treating physician. Psychotic symptoms are rarely present in this condition.

Postpartum depression has to be differentiated clinically from maternity blues, which for many women is a normal reaction following delivery. The symptoms in postpartum depression are more severe and persist for weeks to months, whereas maternity blues symptoms are transient, the depressed mood is not as intense, and the woman is not as incapacitated.

Treatment of postpartum depression is both psychological and pharmacologic. If depression is untreated, it may go for months impairing the bond between mother and newborn and affecting marital and family relationships.

The goal of psychotherapy is to resolve underlying conflicts and to help the woman to understand her feelings more clearly.

Tricyclic antidepressant medication helps with relief of such vegetative symptoms as insomnia, fatigue, and anhedonia. The response to antidepressant drugs takes 2–4 weeks and the usual therapeutic dose of most antidepressants (imipramine, amitriptyline) is in the range of 100–300 n per day.

In the more severely depressed patient, hospitalization and treatment with ECT may be necessary.

Puerperal Psychosis

Puerperal psychosis is a relatively rare but serious condition that occurs 2–3 days after delivery and may occur as late as two weeks postpartum. It lasts up to 3–4 months. It is characterized by confusion, agitation, elated or depressed mood and at different times may resemble delirium. Auditory hallucinations and paranoid delusion usually accompany the above changes.

It is a relatively rare condition, occurring once in 100–150 deliveries at most, and is more common in primiparous women. There is an increased risk for puerperal psychosis in subsequent pregnancies if a woman has suffered from this disorder earlier.

The etiology of puerperal psychosis is unknown. There is an increased incidence of puerperal psychosis in patients with a preexisting history of manic-depressive disease and schizophrenia.

The patient usually presents with symptoms in the first week after delivery. Agitation, confusion, and lability of mood are prominent features. Onset is usually acute and sudden. The patient may present with complaints of auditory hallucination and delusions of grandeur. Her mood may be elated and euphoric. This mood can change quickly to that of acute depression. The mother's ability to cope with the infant becomes markedly impaired.

A patient with preexisting schizophrenic illness in remission can present with signs of acute relapse, for example, bizarre behavior, auditory hallucination, and delusion of persecution with psychotic thinking and looseness of association. The patient is usually unaware of her illness and usually is brought by family members to the emergency room for evaluation of the patient's confused and perplexing behavior.

With psychotic depression, the woman, in addition to symptoms of major depression, may be frankly psychotic. Her reality testing is greatly impaired and she may deny being the mother. She may hear voices that may command her to harm the baby. Suicide attempts are very common during this phase. Infanticide is also a real risk at this time.

Patients with puerperal psychosis need psychiatric hospitalization to prevent harm to themselves or the infant. The treatment usually is directed at the primary symptoms.

Antidepressant medication along with neuroleptics are helpful to treat psychotic depression. Lithium carbonate along with neuroleptics is useful if the patient has manic symptoms with psychosis. An attempt to maintain lithium levels at 0.8–1.5 mg/L is essential. The patient with schizophrenic symptoms may respond best to treatment with neuroleptics.

In patients who are acutely agitated and suicidal, the use of ECT is highly beneficial. The patients may need six to eight treatments and may show complete recovery.

PSEUDOCYESIS

Pseudocyesis is a syndrome of false pregnancy, that is, a condition in which a woman is convinced that she is pregnant although there is no fetus. Pseudocyesis is an extremely rare condition. It is believed to be a delusional manifestation of either a psychotic disorder or a hysterical conversion disorder symptom.

Commonly reported symptoms in pseudocyesis are amenorrhea, abdominal enlargement, breast enlargement, nausea and vomiting, fetal movements, and labor pains.

Pseudocyesis can be differentiated from pregnancy by the lack of fetal parts on ultrasound or abdominal x-ray. In addition, the abdominal enlargement can be reversed under anesthesia. Often this condition is recognized as a result of unproductive labor.

Treatment is directed towards an underlying cause. If pseudocyesis is a symptom of psychosis, the patient may benefit from treatment with neuroleptics. Psychotherapy may be beneficial in other instances.

REFERENCES

1. Hamilton JA, Parry BL, Blumenthal SJ. The menstrual cycle in context I: affective syndromes associated with reproductive hormonal changes. *J Clin Psych.* 1988;49:474.
2. Coble PA, Day NL. The epidemiology of mental and emotional disorders during pregnancy and the postpartum period. In: Cohen R, ed. *Psychiatry Consultation in Childbirth Settings.* New York, NY: Plenum; 1988:37.
3. Modarressi T. Complications of pregnancy. In: Wolman BB, ed. *Psychological Aspects of Gynecology and Obstetrics.* Oradell, NJ: Medical Economics; 1978:125.
4. Satterfield S. Pregnancy in married women. In: Wolman BB, ed. *Psychological Aspects of Gynecology and Obstetric.* Oradell, NJ: Medical Economics; 1978:103.
5. Bailey LA, Hailey BJ. The psychological experience of pregnancy. *Int'l J Psych Med.* 1987;16:263.
6. Kennerley H, Gath D. Maternity blues reassessed. *Psych Develop.* 1986;1:1.
7. Brockington IF, Kumar R, eds. *Motherhood and Mental Illness.* London: Academic Press; 1982:1.
8. Lavy V. Maternity blues in postpartum and post operative women. *Br J of Psych.* 1987;151:368.
9. Yalom ID, Lunde DT, Moos RH, Hamburg DA. Post partum blues syndrome: a description and related variables. *Arch Gen Psych.* 1968;18:16.
10. Quadagno DM, Dixon LA, Denney NW, et al. Post partum moods in men and women. *Am J Obstet Gynecol.* 1986;154:1018.
11. Hansen JP. Older maternal age and pregnancy outcome: a review of literature. *Obstet and Gynecol Sur.* 1986;41:726.
12. Robinson GE, Garner DM, Gare DJ, et al. Psychological adaptation to pregnancy in childless women more than 35 years of age. *Am J Obstet Gynecol.* 1987;156:328.
13. Tsoi MM, Hunter M, Pearce M, et al. Ultrasound scanning in women with raised serum alpha fetoprotein: Short term psychological effect. *J Psychosom Res.* 1987;31:35.
14. Cox DN, Wittmann BK, Hess M, et al. The psychological impact of diagnostic ultrasound. *Obstet Gynecol.* 1987;70:673.
15. Ever-Kiebooms G, Swerts A, Berghe H. Psychological aspects of amniocentesis: anxiety feelings in three different risk groups. *Clin Genetics.* 1988;33:196.
16. Spencer JW, Cox D. Emotional responses of pregnant women to chorionic villi sampling or amniocentesis. *Am J Obstet Gynecol.* 1987;157:1115.
17. Gottlieb SE, Barrett DE. Effects of unanticipated cesarean section on mothers, infants, and their interaction in the first month of life. *Dev Behav Pediatr.* 1986;7:180.
18. Garel M, Lelong N, Kaminski M. Follow-up study of psychological consequences of cesarean childbirth. *Early Human Dev.* 1988;16:271.
19. George DT, Ladenheim JA, Nutt D. Effect of pregnancy on panic attacks. *Am J Psych.* 1987;144:1078.
20. Ingram IM. Obsessive illness in mental hospital patients. *Lancet.* 1961;2:358.
21. Gillberg C. "Floppy infant syndrome" and maternal diazepam. *Lancet.* 1977;2:244.
22. Rementeria JL, Bhatt K. Withdrawal symptoms in neonates from intrauterine exposure to diazepam. *J Pediat.* 1977;90:123.
23. Erkkola R, Kanto J. Diazepam and breastfeeding. *Lancet.* 1972;1:1235.
24. Safra JM. Association between cleft palate and prenatal exposure to diazepam. *Lancet.* 1980;2:478.
25. Kumar R, Robson KM. Prospective study of emotional disorders in childbearing women. *Br J Psych.* 1984;144:35.
26. O'Hara MW, Neunaber DJ, Zekoski EM. Prospective study of post partum depression: course and predictive factors. *J Abnormal Psychol.* 1984;93:158.
27. Pharmacologic agents and ECT during pregnancy and the puerperium. In: Cohen R, ed. *Psychiatric Consultation and Childbirth Setting.* New York, NY: Plenum; 1988:165.
28. Shou M. Lithium and pregnancy. *Br Med J.* 1973;2:137.
29. Tunnessen WW. Toxic effects of lithium in newborn infants. *J Pediat.* 1972;8:804.
30. Ananth J. Side effects of neonates from psychotropic agents excreted through breastfeeding. *Am J Psych.* 19781;35:801.
31. Sandler, M, ed. *Mental Illness in Pregnancy and Puerperium.* New York, NY: Oxford University Press; 1978:7.
32. Wrede G, Mednick SA, Hultunen MO, Nilsson CG. Pregnancy and delivery complications in the births of unselected series of Finnish children and schizophrenic mothers. *Acta Psych Scan.* 1980;62:369.
33. Nurenberg HG, Prudic J. Guidelines for treatment of psychosis during pregnancy. *Hosp Comm Psych.* 1984;35:67.
34. Desmond MM. Behavior alteration in infants born to mothers on psychoactive medications during pregnancy. In: Ferrell G, ed. *Congenital Mental Retardation.* Austin, TX: University of Texas Press, 1967.
35. Biological treatment in psychiatry. In: Kalinosky LB, ed. New York, NY: Grune & Stratton; 1982:
36. Slayton RI, Soloff PH. Psychotic denial of third trimester pregnancy. *J Clin Psych.* 1981;42:471.
37. Soloff PH, Jewell S, Roth LH. Civil commitment and rights of unborn. *Am J Psych.* 1979;136:114.
38. Handley SL, Dunn TL, Baker JM, et al. Mood changes in puerperium and plasma tryptophan and cortisol concentrations. *Br Med J.* 1977;2:18.
39. Hayworth J, Little BC, Carter SB, et al. Predictive study of post partum depression: Some predisposing characteristics. *Br J Med Psychol.* 1980;53:161.

Chapter One Hundred and Ninety-Eight

Drug Abuse

Edmond Confino and Norbert Gleicher

198

Drug abuse in pregnancy is defined as maternal administration of any chemical agent, with local or systemic distribution, which causes maternal or fetal adverse side effects. Drug abuse in pregnancy consequently is not only restricted to addictive compounds but also includes medications administered to treat specific medical conditions in pregnancy.

Current changes in drug abuse, compared to drug abuse five and ten years ago, include a trend towards a younger age of drug users; shifts of the drug markets from recreational drugs such as marijuana to hard core drugs such as cocaine; an increasing use of different combinations of drugs; and a new generation of home-made chemicals.[1,2] These ever changing trends in drug abuse render an attempt to cover all chemical abuse in pregnancy impossible. Therefore, this chapter will address only the most common drugs abused in pregnancy and those chemicals known to cause significant damage to mother and fetus.

Drug abuse is associated frequently with lifestyles, which may compound the effects of drug abuse on mother and fetus. For example, prostitution, criminal activities, inability to hold a job, and inadequate nutrition and shelter may all result in compromised fetal growth due to acute and chronic insults.[1] These lifestyles also result in an increased incidence of sexually transmitted diseases, such as syphilis and acquired immune deficiency syndrome (AIDS). Fetal damage thus may occur from direct action of the chemical, its acute withdrawal from related lifestyle factors, or from a combination of these elements. At the extreme of a full blown withdrawal syndrome, fetal death can occur.[3]

Chapter 7 describes in detail the pharmacologic aspects of drug absorption in the pregnant state. However, a few points must be emphasized to clarify some mechanisms involved in drug abuse. Pregnancy is a unique physiologic state with increased substrate consumption in many organs, active metabolic turnover, and rapid cell division. Consequently, an increased susceptibility to many chemical agents, which otherwise do not affect the mature organism, seems to occur with pregnancy. The serum concentration of a particular drug and duration of exposure represent important factors in drug metabolism. Therefore, the longer the exposure and the higher the dose consumed, the greater the likelihood of feto-maternal compromise. A cause-and-effect relationship is difficult to establish, and the literature is replete with after-the-fact reports on fetal-maternal morbidity associated with exposure to chemical substances. Animal models are poor predictors of the actual effect of a drug on human pregnancy, nor do *in vitro* cytochemical assays, or organ culture methods, give reliable results. Consequently, the only reliable information is derived from retrospective surveys of drug abusing patient populations.[2]

Narcotic addicts often demonstrate menstrual abnormalities, amenorrhea, anovulation, and an inability to conceive secondary to direct drug effects on the hypothalamus and an indirect effect, mediated by way of depletion of body fat.[4,5] Menstrual irregularities and the frequently addiction-associated in intrauterine growth retardation may also cause major difficulties for the accurate dating process of pregnancy.

A thorough physical examination of the pregnant addict may reveal thrombophlebitis at the injection sites, signs of malnutrition, pinpoint pupils, incoordinate movements, disorientation, dysarthria, and confusion. If in the presence of a suspected small-for-gestational-age fetus any of the above signs is found, drug abuse should be suspected. Blood and urine samples then should be sent for a biochemical drug screen.[6]

The pediatric literature does not reliably report the incidence of fetal malformations associated with the use of a particular substance. The cause-and-effect relationship between substance abuse and specific fetal malformations is difficult to establish because studies with matched controlled groups are rare, and the cause of observed fetal malformation often cannot exclusively be attributed to one agent. In addition, drug-related malformations may be discovered only long after birth. An example is diethylstilbestrol (DES). DES was administered to many pregnant women in the 1950s to prevent threatened abortions. It became apparent only after many years that DES caused malformations in female and male offsprings[7] (see Chapter 7). Animal mod els demonstrating such long-term latency also confirmed the unpredictability of drug administration during pregnancy.

Fetal exposure to a single agent at different times after conception may result in different sequelae.[8] Drug interference with fertilization and implantation (from conception to about 17 days of gestation) frequently will result in arrest of cellular division and subsequent fetal wastage. During the embryonic period (18–55 days of gestation) organogenesis and tissue organization occur. An insult during this time interval often will result in fetal malformations, functional or morphologic damage and fetal wastage. While during the subsequent fetal period (from the 56th day to parturition) teratogenic changes do occur, chemical insults will result predominantly in intrauterine growth retardation, with only morphologic and physiologic alterations.[9] However, a specific malformation does not necessarily imply that a specific agent was involved. Several teratogenic agents may produce the same malformation and several malformations may be produced by the same agent.[10]

TABLE 198–1. MALFORMATIONS AFTER FIRST TRIMESTER DRUG EXPOSURE

System/Organ	Timing of Drug Interference	Malformation
Lower extremities	23 days	Sirenomelus
Central nervous system	26 days	Anencephaly
	28 days	Meningomyelocele
Urinary tract	30 days	Extroversion of bladder
Trachea, esophagus	30 days	Esophageal atresia and tracheoesophageal fistula
Cardiovascular system	34 days	Transposition of great vessels
Extremities	6 weeks	Aplasia of radius
	6 weeks	Syndactyly
Rectum	6 weeks	Rectal atresia
Diaphragm	6 weeks	Diaphragmatic hernia
Gastrointestinal tract	8 weeks	Duodenal atresia
Abdominal wall	10 weeks	Omphalocele
Reproductive system	10 weeks	Uterus bicornis
Urinary tract	12 weeks	Hypospadias

Many malformations result from the interaction between genetic and environmental factors. The rapidly growing fetus is highly susceptible to teratogenic damage.[9,10] Chemical exposure especially will affect tissue during maximal growth rate and when it has undergone less differentiation. Table 198–1 presents selected malformations caused by exposure to chemicals in the first trimester of pregnancy. Most severe malformations occur during the first six weeks of gestation. This observation has serious implications, as often neither patient nor physician are aware of an early pregnancy. Consequently, the patient may face an iatrogenic exposure to teratogenic drugs. However, a survey[11] of 6509 mothers who used different medications during pregnancy failed to demonstrate an association between any of the commonly used drugs and congenital disorders.

Many drugs that are potentially toxic to infants will never reach dangerous fetal levels. This is because of dilution of the drug or because of a relative placental barrier, which results in a concentration gradient. On the other hand, fetal immaturity may enhance the accumulation of toxic agents. Hepatic enzymes, such as glucoronyl transferase, which solubilizes chemicals and thus enables the kidneys to excrete them, is inefficient in premature infants. Chemicals that are excreted readily by the mature organism thus are retained by an immature fetus.[12]

EPIDEMIOLOGY OF DRUG ABUSE IN PREGNANCY

The consumption of drugs during pregnancy is remarkably widespread. This reflects an overall increase in illicit drug abuse and the consumption of prescribed medications.[13] As much as 82% of pregnant women have been reported to have been prescribed an average of four drugs, excluding iron and vitamin preparations, and 65% of pregnant women consume drugs not prescribed by a physician.[14] Data published by the National Institutes of Health[15] indicate that at least 900 pharmacologic agents are in use during pregnancy. Differences in drug consumption during pregnancy in different countries have been attributed to local habits of consumer populations and of prescribing physicians.[16] A detailed drug use study during pregnancy of over-the-counter medications listed vitamins (65%) as the most frequently ingested drug. Next were analgesics (61%), antacids (30%), iron preparations (17%), antitussives (11%), miscellaneous (10%), antiemetics (6%), and sedatives (3%). Physician-prescribed drugs accounted for 4.5–5.7 drugs per patient.[17] The true magnitude and significance of fetal exposure to these drugs is yet to be determined.

Some 15% of neonatal deaths during the first year of life are associated with congenital malformations. Anomalies are present in about 2% of all infants and are the third leading cause of infant mortality in the United States. It is estimated that teratogens cause 5–10% of birth defects (1–2 anomalies per 2000 births).[18] To prevent such anomalies, it is important to educate mothers and physicians to avoid unnecessary drug consumption during pregnancy.

The extent of drug abuse is difficult to estimate. The literature underestimates the real prevalence of fetal drug abuse. Drug abuse during pregnancy varies and depends on the screened population. Of 1711 women registered for prenatal care at the Boston City Hospital, 9% reported heavy alcohol intake, 37% reported moderate drinking, and 54% drank rarely or not at all.[19] Heavy drinking was reported to be a major problem in 2–14% of pregnant women.[19-22] While two thirds of heavy drinkers will reduce alcohol consumption during pregnancy[23], education and prevention of alcohol abuse during pregnancy remain of utmost importance (see also Chapter 8).

Many therapeutic drugs have been discovered by drug addicts and are now abused as narcotic or psychotropic agents. An example is phencyclidine ("angel dust"), originally introduced in the 1950s as an anesthetic medication.[24] Environmental pollutants such as heavy metals, chlorinated dioxin derivatives, polychlorinated biphenyls, pesticides, carbon monoxide, ozone, and others, may compound the problem (see Chapter 10).[25]

THE HABIT-FORMING DRUGS

Tobacco Smoking

Approximately 30% of all women smoke during their reproductive life, and 25% of all women will continue to smoke during pregnancy.[26] Excessive cigarette smoking during pregnancy affects fetal development (see also Chapter 10). The average birth weight is about 200 g lower in smoking mothers.[27] Premature and small-for-gestational-age babies are born frequently to heavily smoking mothers.[28,29] The effect on birth weight is not observed if the mother stopped smoking before or during early pregnancy. Neonatal and mental development of infants born to smoking mothers is usually normal, although hospital readmissions for bronchitis and pneumonitis during the first years of life are more frequent in infants raised by parents who smoke.[30] Animal experiments suggest that nicotine is a major toxic component in tobacco.[31] Nicotine affects the blood supply to the placenta and results in elevated carboxyhemoglobin levels in the fetus. Consequently, maternal and fetal oxygen carrying capacity is reduced. Oxygen dissociation of the remaining oxyhemoglobin is also impaired in the presence of carbon monoxide. Carbon monoxide constricts maternal pulmonary vasculature, further decreasing the ventilation perfusion ratio.[32]

It is recommended that tobacco smokers stop smoking during pregnancy or at least reduce the number of cigarettes to less than one pack per day. It also is recommended that the newborns not be exposed to tobacco fumes to avoid additional risks of respiratory infection.[32]

Heroin

Quality, price, purity, and availability of heroin differ with location. The drug is characterized by a strong psychotropic effect and psychological as well as physical dependence are almost universal. The fetus also becomes physically dependent on heroin. Such dependence will typically result from repeated use of the drug. Patients who use heroin intermittently may *not* develop dependence. Intermittent heroin consumption, however, appears to increase the risk of lethal overdose.[33]

Heroin overdose patients are comatose with pinpoint pupils. Signs of repeated intravenous injections and of thrombophlebitis are often present. In severe cases, respiratory depression, cardiac failure, and pulmonary edema will occur. The antidote to heroin is naloxone, given intravenously at a dose of 0.01 mg/kg. A maternal withdrawal syndrome, which may be expected after naloxone administration, includes agitation, rhinorrhea, pilorection, mydriasis, and, in severe cases, abdominal pains, myalgias, muscular irritability, uterine cramps, and diarrhea.[34] Heroin withdrawal is rarely fatal to the mother, but may result in an early spontaneous abortion, caused by uterine contractions and arteriolar spasm. In late pregnancy, intrauterine fetal death has been reported. Complete drug withdrawal during pregnancy therefore is not recommended.[35]

Many maternal complications due to heroin abuse are caused by solvents and contaminated syringes. Microorganisms isolated from the maternal blood stream include staphylococci, streptococci, bacteroides, candida, and Clostridium species. Maternal exposure to the HIV virus inevitably results in placental seeding with the virus. Subsequently, a fraction of infants of HIV-positive mothers will develop AIDS (see Chapter 46).[36] Septic thrombophlebitis, abscess formation, and superficial cellulitis are common findings in drug addicts. "Skin popping" with quinine promotes the growth of *Clostridium tetani.* Systemic manifestations of nonsterile intravenous injections include septicemia, right-sided endocarditis, metastatic abscesses in bone and cartilage, fever, septic pulmonary emboli and hepatitis B infection. Repeated intravenous injections of minced talc-containing tablets result in obstructive pulmonary vascular disease, accompanied by hyperglobulinemia and false-positive serologic tests for syphilis. Inflammatory changes in the placenta, chorion and amnion are present in 34% of pregnant heroin addicts.[37] Septic emboli to the placenta induce focal inflammatory changes, fibrosis and, subsequently, possible placental insufficiency and fetal compromise.

Appropriate prenatal care may prevent some of these adverse effects, even if a substitute drug such as methadone has to be used. The incidence of small-for-gestational-age babies, however, remains unchanged in methadone-treated mothers. In contrast, perinatal mortality is reduced with methadone substitution.[37]

Placental transfer of heroin within one hour of administration results in fetal toxicity. Whenever heroin is discontinued, the withdrawal may result in intrauterine death, frequently associated with meconium aspiration.[38] Heroin babies exhibit accelerated lung maturation with the appearance of high lecithin/sphyngomyelin ratios.[39] Some of their other characteristics are presented in Table 198–2. Off-

TABLE 198–2. THE EFFECT OF HEROIN ON INFANTS

Perinatal effects
Accelerated liver and lung maturity
Heroin withdrawal symptoms
Meconial amniotic fluid
Elevated serum magnesium levels
Elevated prolactin levels in cord blood
Small for gestational age
Increased perinatal mortality (up to 37%)
Late effects
Failure to thrive
Lower weight and height
Behavioral disturbances
Impaired perceptive and organizational abilities

springs of heroin-addicted mothers also may demonstrate diaphragmatic hernias, clubfeet, tracheoesophageal fistulas, cardiac malformations, Down's syndrome, hemangiomas, urogenital malformations, polycystic kidneys, and other congenital anomalies.[40,41] However, these malformations represent mostly anecdotal reports. The mothers frequently used more than one drug, making the establishment of a cause-and-effect relationship impossible.

Treatment objectives for the heroin abuser in pregnancy include prevention of heroin overdose and of septic embolization, the provision of adequate caloric intake, and vitamin substitution. Early fetal sonographic surveillance is important to detect growth retardation, placental insufficiency, and fetal compromise. Methadone substitution is attempted cautiously. While the parenteral dosage of methadone in the nonpregnant state is almost equivalent to that of heroin (8–10 mg of methadone have the effect of 10 mg of heroin), when absorbed through the gastrointestinal tract, it loses half of its potency due to a slower absorption and excretion rate. Therefore, higher equivalent methadone doses are required in the pregnant state.[42] If maternal withdrawal symptoms appear despite a careful substitution regiment, additional methadone should be provided to prevent a full-scale maternal withdrawal syndrome and resulting fetal compromise.

Methadone is a long-acting synthetic opiate, well absorbed through the gastrointestinal tract. Oral administration of methadone reduces the complications of intravenous injection of heroin. Methadone blocks heroin-induced euphoria and the need for heroin. Although methadone has psychotropic effects similar to heroin, it reduces the environmental hazards and enables society to control and protect the addict. Methadone is the treatment of choice for the pregnant heroin addict. No increase in congenital defects was noted in offspring of methadone treated mothers, although many presumably consume other narcotics.[42] The newborn, however, may experience withdrawal symptoms that are similar to those observed in heroin withdrawal. Fetal withdrawal is dose dependent and usually occurs when more than 20 mg of methadone are administered daily.[43] Although 65–90% of the neonates experience withdrawal signs, only one third of the symptomatic infants require therapy.[44] Neonatal methadone withdrawal may result in sudden infant death. The more severe the neonatal withdrawal reaction, the more likely is the chance of sudden infant death.[45] Methadone withdrawal during pregnancy causes fetal agitation, meconium passage, and systemic endogenous secretion of catecholamines.[46] Therefore, methadone is administered continuously during pregnancy and curative withdrawal attempts are delayed until after delivery. Other fetal and neonatal adverse side-effects of methadone are severe hyperbilirubinemia[47], thrombocytosis appearing in the second week of life[48] and, less frequently, respiratory depression of the newborn.

Marijuana

Marijuana (δ-9-tetrahydrocannabinol) is used as a mild psychotropic drug and causes side-effects such as euphoria and disorientation.[5] Marijuana frequently is used in combination with other drugs. It therefore is difficult to judge adverse effects. Some studies have suggested that marijuana is used by 13% of pregnant women.[49,50] Marijuana, together with alcohol use, has been reported to have adverse effects on fetal growth and development. The concomitant use of both drugs resulted in a fivefold increase in the incidence of fetal alcohol syndrome.[50] Animal experiments also have confirmed a detrimental effect of marijuana on fetal development.[51,52] A prospective study, comparing marijuana users to nonusers, demonstrated a statistically significant increase in meconium passage (57% vs. 25%) in users.[52] Marijuana has an antiemetic effect. Self medication with marijuana for morning sickness therefore may account for the higher use observed in the first trimester of pregnancy.[53] Marijuana is considered to be a "soft" drug with less dependence and adverse side-effects. Although fetal abnormalities do not seem to increase due to marijuana use in pregnancy[54,55], its use should be strongly discouraged.

Lysergic Acid Diethylamide

Lysergic acid diethylamide (LSD) is one of the well known psychedelic agents. The psychological effects occur repeatedly, although in different ways through different individual experiences. Changes in visual, auditory, tactile, olfactory, gustatory, and kinesthetic perception occur. There are also changes in perception of time, space, body image, mood, and affect, which may lead to the extreme of depersonalization and ego disassociation.[56] A very effective antagonist is chlorpromazine.[57]

Acute reactions during LSD intoxication may result in physical damage and injury to mother and fetus. Bizarre behavior patterns have been reported with LSD abuse. They may result in self damage, such as jumping off roofs and looking at the sun with naked eyes. Agitation, hallucinations, and uncontrollable behavior are usually the extremes of milder clinical presentations, which essentially depend on the premorbid personality.

In vitro and animal studies indicate that chromosomal aberrations, mitotic inhibition, and congenital malformations may occur after exposure to LSD.[54] Although those early observations have been confirmed, it has been difficult to prove conclusively the occurrence of fetal malformations.[57] Major congenital anomaly rates occurred in a home for unwed mothers in 6 out of 1000 live births. Mothers exposed to LSD during pregnancy demonstrated a 20-fold increase in congenital anomalies.[58]

However, one can not exclude the possibility that environmental factors, such as malnutrition, viral infections, and additional drug abuse may have affected the results of this survey. Only scattered reports of malformed fetuses born to LSD-consuming mothers have appeared in the literature.[59] The large majority of infants born to mothers exposed to LSD in the first trimester of pregnancy are clearly normal.[60]

Phencyclidine (Angel Dust)

Phencyclidine was introduced originally as a general anesthetic agent. It was found to have a slow serum clearance, resulting in prolonged central nervous system depression. When patients emerged from anesthesia, they frequently experienced a hyperactive delirious anxiety state. Chemical production of phencyclidine from available precursors is simple. Its administration is easy and it can be inhaled, swallowed, smoked, injected, or even directly absorbed from the skin. It can be added to marijuana, LSD, or other habit-forming agents.[61]

Pharmacokinetics of phencyclidine reveal a serum half-life time of two to four hours, high lipid solubility, rapid transfer to the fetus, and long-term tissue incorporation.[62] Maternal toxicity includes ataxia, dizziness, and dysarthria in low doses. In high serum concentrations acute psychosis is possible, with death occurring due to respiratory and cardiac arrest, with or without hypertensive crisis and convulsions.[63,64]

Fetal dysmorphology and intoxication may be associated with exposure to phencyclidine *in utero.* The newborns have triangular faces, poor head control, nystagmus, and dislocated hip joints. Neonates are spastic; they demonstrate a coarse tremor and roving eye movements.[65-67] Exposure to phencyclidine, however, does not result in fetal malformations universally.[67] Very high fetal concentrations of phencyclidine in comparison to maternal levels suggest active transport of the drug across the placenta.[68] This may explain the high fetal toxicity and teratogenicity. Phencyclidine is clearly contraindicated in pregnancy.

Cocaine

A dramatic increase in cocaine abuse has taken place in the last decade. In the early 1970s, cocaine was used primarily nasally by affluent people; a decrease in street cost and increase in availability has significantly increased the number of users and changed the socioeconomic profile in the 1980s.[69] A concomitant change of administration route from nasal inhalation to smoking and intravenous injection further enhanced the potential for medical complications.

Cocaine is a local anesthetic, extracted from the leaves of *Erythroxylon coca.* It blocks the presynaptic reuptake of norepinephrine and dopamine and increases the amount of transmitter at the receptor sites. Immediate effects of cocaine include acute rise in blood pressure, tachycardia, and vasoconstriction. Cocaine-induced euphoria is believed to result from a central nervous effect of dopamine.[69] Cocaine crosses the placenta and is metabolized and excreted in fetal urine.[70] Fetal and maternal cocaine morbidities are believed to be related to severe vasoconstriction of maternal blood vessels and of vessels supporting the placenta. Maternal medical complications include cerebrovascular accidents, seizures, acute myocardial infarction, life-threatening arrhythmias, bowel ischemia, rupture of the aorta, hyperthermia, and sudden death.[71] The most threatening fetal complication is *abruptio placentae.*[72,73] Cocaine-associated congenital anomalies may be related to vasoconstriction and subsequent infarctions early in pregnancy. Interruption of blood supply during organ formation may lead to malformations, such as intestinal and urinary tract atresiae.[74,75] Rapidly increasing cocaine abuse in as many as one quarter of urban pregnant patients[76] has transformed cocaine abuse into a major threat to mother and fetus.

Amphetamines

Amphetamines have effects similar to cocaine. They cause agitation, alertness, anorexia, and euphoria without intellectual impairment. Amphetamine is used to overcome states of insomnia, tiredness, and physical weakness. Upon discontinuation, a sudden onset of depression, prostration and sleepiness prevails. Amphetamine suppresses appetite and relieves depression. The only accepted medical indication to prescribe amphetamine is the treatment of narcolepsy.[17] Amphetamine is habit forming and its administration is restricted.

Contradictory reports on fetal anomalies after exposure to amphetamine suggest transposition of the great vessels, cleft palate[77], or no anomalies.[78] It is recommended to discontinue the use of amphetamine in pregnancy of patients during the first trimester of pregnancy and near term.

NON-HABIT-FORMING DRUGS

Innumerable drugs have been reported to be associated with maternal or fetal adverse side effects. More than a billion drug prescriptions are written each year with almost unlimited self administration of over-the-counter drugs. A detailed review of all drugs exceeds the scope of this chapter. The appendix presents a listing of drugs in risk categories D and X. Category D describes agents with a known risk to human fetuses, while category X represents those drugs that are clearly contraindicated during pregnancy. Drugs in risk groups A, B, and C may be used during pregnancy if their benefit outweighs their risk. Some of these drugs, however, may have significant effects on mother and fetus. For example, local anesthetics readily cross the placenta and may cause central nervous system depression in the newborn.[79,80] One of the common analgesic drugs, aspirin, was found to be associated with platelet dysfunction, reduced Hageman factor (XII) and hemorrhagic phenomena in the newborn.[81] First trimester dose-dependent exposure to barbiturates may result in fetal anomalies similar to those observed with hydantoin.[82] Propylthiouracil, often administered in pregnancy to treat hyperthyroidism, crosses the placenta and may cause hypothyroidism and mental retardation of the fetus.[83]

Our inability to differentiate cause-and-effect relationships also is illustrated in the recognized increased risk of anomalies with ovulation-inducing agents such as human menopausal gonadotropins and clomiphene citrate.[84] An increased incidence of anomalies in these patients probably reflects preexisting damage to the gametes rather than drug teratogenicity.

Some drugs are considered to be contraindicated during pregnancy without adequate teratogenic studies to support their recommendation. For example, metronidazole does not induce malformations in animals, and a study of pregnant women treated with metronidazole did not show an increased incidence of congenital malformations.[83] However, it still is considered contraindicated by many authorities.

Any drug use during pregnancy should be restricted to medications with a clear benefit to mother or fetus. Whenever in doubt, the drug should *not* be prescribed, or should be substituted with a proven, safer alternative medication. When such an alternative does not exist, informed consent from the patient needs to be obtained prior to administration of the drug.

REFERENCES

1. ACOG Technical Bulletin. *Drug Abuse and Pregnancy.* 1986;96:1.
2. Keith LG, MacGregors S, Friedell SN, et al. Substance abuse in pregnant women: recent experience at the perinatal center for chemical dependence of Northwestern Memorial Hospital. *Obstet Gynecol.* 1989;73:715.

3. Rementeria JL, Nunag NN. Narcotic withdrawal in pregnancy: stillbirth incidence with a case report. *Am J Obstet Gynecol.* 1973;116:1152.
4. Neuman LL. Drug abuse in pregnancy: its effects on the fetus and newborn infant. In: Harms, ed. *Drugs and Youth: The Challenge of Today.* New York, NY: Pergamon Press; 1973:1.
5. Smith CG, Asch RH. Drug abuse and reproduction. *Fertil Steril.* 1987;48:355.
6. Salerno L. Treating the drug addicted mother and neonate. *Symposia Reporter.* 1981;4:17.
7. Kaufman RH, Binder GL, Gray PM, et al. Upper genital tract changes associated with exposure in utero to diethylstilbestrol. *Am J Obstet Gynecol.* 1977;128:51.
8. Gupta C, Sonowane BR, Yaffe SJ, et al. Phenobarbital exposure in utero: alterations in female reproductive functions in rats. *Science.* 1980;208:508.
9. Goodner DM. Teratology for the obstetrician. *Clin Obstet Gynecol.* 1975;18:245.
10. Hawkins DF. Teratogens in the human current problems. *J Clin Pathol.* 1976;29(Suppl):150.
11. Aselton P, Jick H, Milunsky A, et al. First trimester drug use and congenital disorders. *Obstet Gynecol.* 1985;65:451.
12. Arena JM. Drug and chemical effects on mother and child. *Pediatr Ann.* 1979;8:690.
13. Schnell SH, Karan LD. Substance abuse. *JAMA.* 1990;263:2682.
14. Stirrat GM. Prescribing problems in the second half of pregnancy and during lactation. *Obstet Gynecol Surv.* 1976;31:1.
15. Slone D, Heinonen OP, Mouson RR. Maternal drug exposure and fetal abnormalities. *Clin Pharmacol Ther.* 1973;14:648.
16. Yaffe SJ. A clinical look at the problem of drugs in pregnancy and their effect on the fetus. *Can Med Assoc J.* 1975;112:728.
17. Hill RM, Craig JP, Chaney MD, et al. Utilization of over-the-counter drugs during pregnancy. *Clin Obstet Gynecol.* 1977;20:381.
18. Howard FM, Hill JM. Drugs in pregnancy. *Obstet Gynecol Surv.* 1979;34:643.
19. Weiner L, Rosett HL, Edelin KC, et al. Alcohol consumption by pregnant women. *Obstet Gynecol.* 1983;61:6.
20. Sokol RJ, Miller SI, Debanne S, et al. The Cleveland NIAA prospective alcohol in pregnancy study: the first year. *Neurobehav Toxicol Teratol.* 1981;3:203.
21. Kuzma JW, Kissinger DG. Patterns of alcohol and cigarette use in pregnancy. *Neurobehav Toxicol Teratol.* 1981;3:211.
22. Harlap S, Shinono PH. Alcohol, smoking and incidence of spontaneous abortions in the first and second trimester. *Lancet.* 1980;1:173.
23. Fried PA, Watkinson B, Grant A, et al. Changing patterns of soft drug use prior to the drug pregnancy: a prospective study. *Drug Alcohol Depend.* 1980;6:323.
24. Jain NC, Budd BS. Growing abuse of phencyclidine California "angel dust." *N Engl J Med.* 1977;297:673.
25. Long L. Environmental pollution and pregnancy: risks and uncertainties for the fetus and infant. *Am J Obstet Gynecol.* 1980;137:162.
26. Prager K, Malin H, Speigler D, et al. Smoking and drinking behavior before and during pregnancy of married mothers of liveborn and stillborn infants. 1984;99:117.
27. Rantakallio P. The effect of maternal smoking on birth weight and the subsequent health of the child. *Early Hum Dev.* 1978;2:371.
28. Werler MM, Pober BR, Holmes LB. Smoking and pregnancy. *Teratology.* 1985;32:473.
29. Nieburg P, Marks JS, McLaren MN, et al. The fetal tobacco syndrome. *JAMA.* 1985;253:2998.
30. Tager I, Weiss ST, Munoz A, et al. Longitudinal study of the effects of maternal smoking on pulmonary functions in children. *N Engl J Med.* 1983;309:699.
31. Becker RF, Little CRD, King JE.: Experimental studies on nicotine absorption in rats during pregnancy. *Am J Obstet Gynecol.* 1968;109:957.
32. Cole PV, Hawkins LH, Roberts D. Smoking during pregnancy and its effects on the fetus. *J Obstet Gynaecol Br Commonw.* 1972;79:782.
33. Perlmutter JF. Heroin addiction and pregnancy. *Obstet Gynecol Surv.* 1974;29:439.
34. Naeye RL, Blanc W, LeBlanc W, et al. Fetal complications of maternal heroin addiction: abnormal growth infections and episodes of stress. *J Pediatr.* 1973;83:1055.
35. Naeye RL, Blanc W, Leblanc W, Khatamee MA. Fetal complications of maternal heroin addiction: abnormal growth, infections and episodes of stress. *J Pediatr.* 1973;83:1055.
36. Rubinstein A, Sicklick M, Gupta A, et al. Acquired immunodeficiency with reversed T/T ratios in infants born to promiscuous and drug-addicted mothers. *JAMA.* 1983;249:2250.
37. Blinick G, Terez E, Wallach RE. Methadone maintenance pregnancy and progeny. *JAMA.* 1973;225:477.
38. Rementeria JL, Nunag NN. Narcotic withdrawal in pregnancy: stillbirth incidence with a case report. *Am J Obstet Gynecol.* 1973;116:1152.
39. Gluck L, Kulovich MV. Lecithin/sphingomyelin ratios in amniotic fluid in normal and abnormal pregnancy. *Am J Obstet Gynecol.* 1973;115:539.
40. Kushnick T, Robinson M, Tsae C. 45, X chromosome abnormality in the offspring of a narcotic addict. *Am J Dis Child.* 1972;124:772.
41. Amarose AP, Norusis MJ. Cytogenetics of methadone managed and heroin addicted pregnant women and their newborn infants. *Am J Obstet Gynecol.* 1976;124:635.
42. Methadone hydrochloride. In: *Physicians Desk Reference.* 44th ed. Oradell, NJ: Medical Economics; 1990:1909.
43. Ostrea EM, Chavez CJ, Strauss ME. A study of factors that influence the severity of neonatal narcotic withdrawal. *J Pediatr.* 1976;88:642.
44. Newman RG, Bashkow S, Calko D. Results of 313 consecutive live births of infants delivered to patients in the New York City methadone maintenance program. *Am J Obstet Gynecol.* 1975;121:233.
45. Chavez CH, Ostrea EM, Stryker JG, et al. Sudden infant death syndrome among infants of drug dependent mothers. *J Pediatr.* 1979;95:407.
46. Zuspan FP, Gumpel JA, Meijia-Zelaya A, et al. Fetal stress from methadone withdrawal. *Am J Obstet Gynecol.* 1975;122:43.
47. Zelson C, Lee SJ, Casalino M. Neonatal narcotic addiction. *N Engl J Med.* 1973;298:1216.
48. Burstein Y, Giarclina PJV, Ramsen AR, et al. Thrombocytosis and increased circulation platelet aggregates in newborn infants of polydrug users. *J Pediatr.* 1979;94:895.
49. Fried PA. Marijuana use by pregnant women—neurobehavioral effects on neonates. *Drug Alcohol Depend.* 1980;6:415.
50. Hingson R, Alpert LL, Day N, et al. Effects of maternal drinking and marijuana use of fetal growth and development. *Pediatrics.* 1982;70:539.
51. Sofia R, Strasbaugh J, Banerjee B. Teratologic evaluation of synthetic delta-9 tetrahydrocannabinol in rabbits. *Teratology.* 1979;19:361.
52. Harbison R, Bernardo MP, Lubin D. Alteration of delta-9 tetrahydrocannabinol induced teratogenicity by stimulation and inhibition of its metabolism. *J Pharmacol Exp Ther.* 1972;202:455.
53. Harclerode J. *The Effect of Marijuana on Reproduction and Development.* Bethesda, MD: National Institute on Drug Abuse; 1980. National Institute on Drug Abuse Monograph No. 31.
54. Greeland S, Staisch KJ, Brown N, et al. The effects of marijuana use during pregnancy. A preliminary epidemiology study. *Am J Obstet Gynecol.* 1982;143:408.
55. Walter CW, Johnson LJ, Buelke J, et al. *Marijuana: An annotated bibliography.* New York, NY: Collier MacMillan; 1982:
56. Hicks RE, Fink PJ. *Psychedelic Drugs.* New York, NY: Grune and Stratton; 1969;66.
57. Ferguson P, Lennox T, Lettieri DJ. *Drugs and Pregnancy.* National Institute on Drug Abuse; 1974;5:29.
58. Jacobson CB, Berlin CM. Possible reproductive detriment in LSD users. *JAMA.* 1972;222:1367.
59. Eller JL, Morton JM. Bizarre deformities in offspring of users of lysergic acid diethylamide. *N Engl J Med.* 1970;283:395.
60. Stenchever MA, Jarvis JA. Lysergic acid diethylamide (LSD): Effect on human chromosomes in vivo. *Am J Obstet Gynecol.* 1970;106:485.
61. Anilene O, Allen RE, Pitts FN, et al. The urban epidemic of PCP use: laboratory evidence from a public psychiatric hospital inpatient service. *Biol Psych.* 1980;15:813.
62. Cooper JE, Cummings AJ, Jones H. The placental transfer or phencyclidine in the pig: plasmal level in the sow and its piglets. *J Physiol.* 1977;267:17.
63. Linden CB, Lovejoy FH, Castillo CE. Phencyclidine: nine cases of poisoning. *JAMA.* 1975;234:513.
64. Tong TG, Benowitz NL, Becker CE, et al. Phencyclidine poisoning. *JAMA.* 1975;234:512.
65. Golden NL, Sokol RJ, Rubin LI. Angel dust: possible effects on the fetus. *Pediatrics.* 1980;65:18.
66. Strauss AA, Modanlou MD, Bosu SK. Neonatal manifestation of maternal phencyclidine (PCP) abuse. *Pediatrics.* 1982;68:550.
67. Petrucha RA, Kaufman KR, Pitts FN. Phencyclidine in pregnancy: a case report. *J Reprod Med.* 1982;27:301.
68. Nicholas JM, Lipshitz J, Schreiber EC. Phencyclidine: Its transfer across the placenta as well as into breast milk. *Am J Obstet Gynecol.* 1982;143:143.
69. ACOG Committee Opinion. *Cocaine Abuse: Implications for Pregnancy.* 1990;81:1.
70. Chasnoff IJ, Bussey ME, Savich R, Stack CM. Perinatal cerebral infarction and maternal cocaine use. *J Pediatr.* 1986;108:456.
71. Cregler LL, Mark H. Medical complications of cocaine abuse. *N Engl J Med.* 1986;315:1495.
72. MacGregor SN, Keith LG, Chasnoff IJ, et al. Cocaine use during pregnancy: adverse perinatal outcome. *Am J Obstet Gynecol.* 1987;157:686.
73. Cherukuri R, Minkoff H, Feldman J, et al. A cohort study of alkaloidal cocaine ("crack") in pregnancy. *Obstet Gynecol.* 1988;72:147.
74. Bingol N, Fuchs M, Diaz S, et al. Teratogenicity of cocaine in humans. *J Pediatr.* 1987;110:93.
75. Chasnoff IJ, Chisum GM, Kaplan WE. Maternal cocaine use and genitourinary tract malformations. *Teratology.* 1988;37:201.
76. Chasnoff IJ. Drug use and women: establishing a standard of care. *Ann NY Acad Sci.* 1989;562:208.
77. Milkovich L, Vanden Berg BJ. Effects of antenatal exposure to anorectic drugs. *Am J Obstet Gynecol.* 1977;129:637.
78. Briggs GG, Samson JH, Crawford DJ. Lack of abnormalities in a newborn exposed to amphetamines during gestation. *Am J Dis Child.* 1975;129:249.
79. Shnider SM, Way EL. Plasma levels of lidocaine (Xylocaine®) in mother

and newborn following obstetrical conduction anesthesia. *Anesthesiology*. 1968;29:951.

80. Teramo K, Rajamak A. Foetal and maternal acid base balance and heart rate after paracervical block during labour. *Br J Anaesth*. 1971;43:300.
81. Bleyer WA, Breckenridge RT. Studies on the detection of adverse reactions in the newborn. *JAMA*. 1970;213:2049.
82. Smith DW. Teratogenicity of anticonvulsive medications. *Am J Dis Child*. 1977;131:1337.
83. Hawkins DF. Teratogens in the human current problems. *J Clin Pathol*. 1976;29(Suppl. 10):150.
84. Ahlgren M, Kallen B, Rannerik G. Outcome of pregnancy after clomiphene therapy. *Acta Obstet Gynecol Scan*. 1976;55:377.
85. Malins JM, Cooke AM, Pyke DA, Fitzgerald MG. Sulphonyl urea drugs in pregnancy. *Br Med J*. 1964;2:187.
86. Hanson TJ, Ballonoff LB, Northan HRC. Aminoglutethimide and pregnancy. *JAMA*. 1974;230:963.
87. Shaw EB, Steinbach HL. Aminoperin induced fetal malformation. *Am J Dis Child*. 1968;115:477.
88. Reich EW, Cox RP, Becker MH, et al. Recognition in adult patients of malformations induced by folic acid antagonists. *Birth Defects*. 1978;14:139.
89. McBride WG. Limb deformities associated with iminodibenzyl hydrochloride. *Med J Aust*. 1972;1:492.
90. Nelson MM, Forfar JO. Association between drugs administered during pregnancy and congenital abnormalities of the fetus. *Br Med J*. 1971;1:523.
91. Williamson RA, Karp LE. Azathioprine teratogenicity: review of the literature and case report. *Obstet Gynecol*. 1981;58:247.
92. Opitz JM, Grosse RF, Haneberg B. Congenital effects of bromism. *Lancet*. 1972;1:91.
93. Nicholson HO. Cytotoxic drugs in pregnancy: review of reported cases. *J Obstet Gynaecol Br Commonw*. 1968;75:307.
94. Thomas D, Buchanan N. Teratogenic effects of anticonvulsants. *J Pediatr*. 1981;99:163.
95. Milkovich L, Van den Berg BJ. Effects of prenatal memphobamate and chlordiazepoxide hydrochloride on human embryonic and fetal development. *N Engl J Med*. 1974;291:1268.
96. Hart CW, Naunton RF. The ototoxicity of chloroquine phosphate. *Arch Oto Paryngol*. 1964;80:407.
97. Lindheimer MD, Katz AL. Sodium and diuretics in pregnancy. *N Engl J Med*. 1973;288:891.
98. Christianson R, Page EW. Diuretic drugs and pregnancy. *Obstet Gynecol*. 1976;48:647.
99. Sidhu RK, Hawkins DF. Corticosteroids. *Clin Obstet Gynecol*. 1981;8:383.
100. Hall JG, Pauli RM, Wilson KM. Maternal and fetal sequelae of anticoagulation during pregnancy. *Am J Med*. 1980;68:122.
101. Coates A. Cyclophosphamide in pregnancy. *Aust NA J Obstet Gynaecol*. 1970;10:33.
102. Tobias TS, Bloom HJG. Doxorubicin in pregnancy. *Lancet*. 1980;1:776.
103. Scanlon JW. Effect of benzodiazepines in neonates. *N Engl J Med*. 1975;292:649.
104. Milner RDG, Chouksey SK. Effects of fetal exposure to diazoxide in man. *Arch Dis Child*. 1972;47:537.
105. Herbst AL. Diethylstilbestrol and other sex hormones during pregnancy. *Obstet Gynecol*. 1981;58(Suppl):355.
106. Stillman RJ. In utero exposure to diethylstilbestrol: adverse effects on the reproductive tract and reproductive performance in male and female offsprings. *Am J Obstet Gynecol*. 1982;142:905.
107. Nora AH, Nora JJ. Limb reduction anomalies in infants born to disulfiram treated alcoholic mothers. *Lancet*. 1977;2:664.
108. Kasan PN, Andrews J. Oral contraceptives and congenital abnormalities. *Br J Obstet Gynecol*. 1980;87:545.
109. Ho CK, Kaufman RL, McAlister WM. Congenital malformations. *Am J Dis Child*. 1975;129:714.
110. Jones HC. Intrauterine ototoxicity: a case report and review of literature. *J Natl Med Assoc*. 1973;65:201.
111. Stephens JD, Golbus MS, Miller TR, et al. Multiple congenital anomalies in a fetus exposed to 5-fluorouracil during the first trimester. *Am J Obstet Gynecol*. 1980;173:747.
112. Stadler HE, Knowles J. Fluorouracil in pregnancy: effect on the neonate. *JAMA*. 1971;217:214.
113. Nageotte MP, Freeman RK, Block RA. Anticoagulation in pregnancy. *Am J Obstet Gynecol*. 1981;141:472.
114. Dayan E, Rosa FW. Fetal ambiguous genitalia associated with sex hormone use early in pregnancy. Food and Drug Administration Division of Drug Experience; 1981. *ADR Highlights* 1:1.
115. Eggermont E. Withdrawal symptoms in neonate associated with maternal imipramine therapy. *Lancet*. 1973;2:680.
116. Idanpaan-Heikkila J, Saxen L. Possible teratogenicity of imipramine/chloropyramine. *Lancet*. 1973;2:282.
117. Csaba IF, Sulyok E. Relationship of maternal treatment with indomethacin to persistence of fetal circulation syndrome. *J Pediatr*. 1978;92:484.
118. Rubaltelli FF, Chiozza ML, Zanardo V, et al. Effect on neonate of maternal treatment with indomethacin. *J Pediatr*. 1979;94:161.
119. Schow M, Andisen A, Steenstrup OR. Lithium acid pregnancy: II. Hazards to women given lithium during pregnancy and delivery. *Br Med J*. 1973;2:137.
120. Kane A, Tomson G, Bjarke B. Effects of maternal lithium therapy in a newborn infant. *J Pediatr*. 1978;93:296.
121. Hounslow D, Wood C, Humphrey M, et al. Intrapartum drugs and fetal blood pH and gas status. *J Obstet Gynaecol Br Commonw*. 1973;80:1007.
122. Fabro S, Brown NA. Teratogenic potential of anticonvulsants. *N Engl J Med*. 1979;300:1280.
123. Smith NT, Corbaseio AN. The use and misuse of pressor agents. *Anesthesiology*. 1970;33:58.
124. Biale Y, Lewenthal M, Aderet NB. Congenital malformations due to anticonvulsant drug and congenital abnormalities. *Obstet Gynecol*. 1975;45:439.
125. Yang TS, Chi CC, Tsai CJ, et al. Diphenylhydantoin teratogenicity in man. *Obstet Gynecol*. 1978;52:682.
126. Budnick IS, Leikin S, Hoeck LE. Effect in the newborn infant to reserpine administration antepartum. *Am J Dis Child*. 1955;90:286.
127. Mesina M, Biffignandi P, Chiga E, et al. Possible contraindications of spironolactone during pregnancy. *Endocrinol Invest*. 1979;2:222.
128. Donald PR, Sellars SL. Streptomycin ototoxicity in the unborn child. *S Afr Med J*. 1981;60:316.
129. Whalley PJ, Adams RH, Combes B. Tetracycline toxicity in pregnancy. *JAMA*. 1964;189:357.
130. German J, Kowan H, Ehlers KH. Trimethadione and human teratogenesis. *Teratology*. 1970;3:349.
131. Schilsky RL, Lewis BJ, Sherins RJ, et al. Gonadal dysfunction in patients receiving chemotherapy for cancer. *Ann Intern Med*. 1980;93:109.
132. Garrett MJ. Teratogenic effects of combination chemotherapy. *Ann Intern Med*. 1974;80:667.

Appendix 198–1

Drugs in Categories D and X: Effects on Fetus and Mother

Name of Drug	Category	Maternal Effects	Fetal Effects	Comments
Acetohexamide[85]	D	Oral hypoglycemic	Neonatal hypoglycemia; not recommended as treatment of DM in pregnancy	Teratogenic in animals
Aminoglutethimide[86]	D	Anticonvulsant, antisteroid	Virilization	Causes inhibition of adrenal cortex
Aminopterin[87,88]	X	Antineoplastic	Multiple anomalies; central nervous system, skeletal growth	Unsuccessful abortifacient
Amitriptyline[89]	D	Antidepressant	Limb reduction, anomalies	May cause urinary retention in the neonate
Amobarbital[90]	D	Hypnotic sedative (barbiturate)	Anencephaly, congenital heart disease, finger, limb, joint deformities, cleft lip, cleft palate, urogenital deformities, nevus	Some reports failed to report increased incidence of malformations
Azathioprine[91]	D	Antineoplastic	Pulmonary, valvular stenosis, preaxial polydactyly	Only two case reports
Bromides[92]	D	Sedative, anticonvulsants	Polydactyly, gastrointestinal abnormalities, clubfoot, congenital dislocation of hip joint	Causation uncertain
Busulfan[93]	D	Alkylating antineoplastic agent	Pyloric stenosis, cleft palate, microphthalmia, corneal opacities, growth retardation, hypoplasia of ovaries and thyroid	Four cases reported
Carbamazepine[92]	D	Anticonvulsant	Meningomyelocele, congenital heart disease, hypertelorism, cleft lip, hypoplasia of nose, nails, dislocation of hip joint	
Chlorambucil[91]	D	Antineoplastic	Agenesis of kidney	Only two cases reported
Chlordiazepoxide[93]	D	Sedatives	Mental deficiency diplegia, deafness, microcephaly, duodenal atresia	Neonatal withdrawal was described
Chloroquine[94]	D	Antimalarial	Teratogenic effects on vestibular apparatus	Drug of choice in pregnancy for malaria, amebic hepatitis, and discoid lupus
Chlorothiazide[95,96]	D	Diuretic	Hypoglycemia, thrombocytopenia, intrauterine fetal death, electrolyte changes	Use only when pregnant patient has heart disease indication
Cortisone[97]	D	Antiflammatory; depresses the immune system	Cataracts, cyclopia, ventricular septal defect, hydrocephalus, gastroschysis, cleft lip, clubfoot, coarctation of aorta	May cause fetal adrenal hyperplasia
Coumarin[98]	D	Anticoagulant	Embryopathy stillbirth, hemorrhage, central nervous system defects	Fetal warfarin syndrome: nasal hypoplasia, slipped epiphyses, growth retardation, eye defects, laryngeal calcification, scoliosis, deafness, congenital heart disease
Cyclophosphamide[99]	D	Alkylating agent antineoplastic	Growth retardation, musculoskeletal abnormalities (1st trimester exposure)	Causes azoospermia
Cytosine arabinoside[100]	D	Antineoplastic	Trisomiae, limb deformities, anencephalus, auditory defects	Low birth weight (normal pregnancies also reported)
Diazepam[101]	D	Sedative, muscle relaxant	Cleft lip, palate, cardiac defects, pyloric stenosis, limb malformations, floppy infant, withdrawal symptoms	May change fetal movements and thermogenesis

Appendix 198–1 (*Continued*)

Name of Drug	Category	Maternal Effects	Fetal Effects	Comments
Diazoxide[102]	D	Antihypertensive smooth muscle relaxant may cause hypotension	Hyperglycemia	
Diethylstilbestrol[103,104]	X	Used to prevent miscarriage, premature labor	Cervical adenosis, clear cell CA of vagina, anatomic abnormalities of uterus, anatomic abnormalities in male offspring, oligospermia	Effects observed usually after puberty and most frequently in female offspring
Disulfiram[105]	X	Prevents alcohol addiction	Multiple anomalies, clubfoot, phocomelia	Termination of pregnancy recommended if exposed in 1st trimester of pregnancy
Estradiol,[106,107] estrone, conjugated estrogens, oral contraceptives	D	Anovulation	VACTERL syndrome (vertebral, anal, cardiac, tracheal, esophageal radial, renal malformation)	Fewer than 0.1% of pregnancies exposed will develop aberrations, may cause changes in sexual performance of male offspring
Ethacrynic acid[108]	D	Diuretic	Ototoxicity	A case report
Fluorouracil[109,110]	D	Antineoplastic	Multiple malformations	Two case reports
Heparin[111]	D	Anticoagulant	Abortions, stillbirth	Superior to oral anticoagulants
Hydroxyprogesterone[112]	D	Progestagen	Ambiguous genitalia and defects, other malformations Spina bifida, tetralogy of Fallot, psychomotor performance disturbances in boys	
Imipramine[113,114]	D	Antidepressant	Limb reduction, abdominal wall and diaphragm defects, cleft palate	Neonatal withdrawal syndrome
Indomethacin[115,116]	D	Antiinflammatory, analgesic, antiprostaglandin synthetase inhibitor.	Persistent pulmonary hypertension of newborn, phocomelia, agenesis of penis	Not recommended during pregnancy
Kanamycin[108]	D	Aminoglycoside antibiotic	Eighth cranial nerve damage (23% incidence)	May cause ototoxicity in the mother
Lithium[117,118]	D	Tranquilizer, treatment of manic depressive psychosis	Toxicity of newborn, cyanosis, hypotonia, bradycardia, thyroid depression, cardiomegaly, ECG pathologies, diabetes insipidus, GI bleeding (11% of 1st-trimester exposure had major malformations; most common cardiovascular and Ebstein's anomaly)	Should be avoided in 1st trimester and near term
Meprobamate[93]	D	Sedative	Congenital anomalies (1.9–12.1%), congenital heart disease, Down's syndrome, deafness, deformed extremities	
Mercaptopurine[91]	D	Antineoplastic	Pancytopenia, hemolytic anemia, multiple malformations	Causes oligospermia in the male
Nalorphine[119]	D	Narcotic antagonist	Respiratory depression	Naloxone is preferred
Paramethadione[120]	X	Treatment of petit mal	Tetralogy of Fallot, mental retardation, failure to thrive, increased incidence of abortions	Other anticonvulsants with better performance available
Phenylephrine[121]	D	Adrenergic sympathomimetic, used to treat allergic reactions and hypotension in emergencies	Malformations of eye, ear, musculoskeletal: syndactyly, clubfoot, congenital dislocation of hip joint	To avoid in 1st trimester of pregnancy
Phenytoin[122,123]	D	Anticonvulsant for treatment of grand mal	Fetal hydantoin syndrome: ossification and hypoplasia of distal phalanges, abnormal genitalia, optic nerve hypoplasia, hirsutism, hemorrhagic diathesis	

Appendix 198–1 (*Continued*)

Name of Drug	Category	Maternal Effects	Fetal Effects	Comments
Primidone[122]	D	Anticonvulsant (phenobarbital analogue)	Musculoskeletal anomalies, cardiovascular anomalies, congenital anomalies, central nervous anomalies	Higher incidence of anomalies in epileptic patients and difficulty in interpretation because of multi-drug exposure
Reserpine[124]	D	Antihypertensive	Microcephaly, hydronephrosis, hydroureter, inguinal hernia	8% incidence of malformations
Spironolactone[125]	D	Diuretic, antiandrogenic		Feminization in male rats
Streptomycin[126]	D	Aminoglycoside antibiotic, tuberculosis, various infections	Ototoxicity	
Tetracycline[127]	D	Broad-spectrum antibiotic	Tooth discoloration, inhibition of bone growth, hypospadias, inguinal hernia, hypoplastic limbs	May cause liver toxicity
Trimethadione[128]	X	Anticonvulsant	High incidence of multiple congenital defects	Because of 69% incidence of congenital defects, should not be used in pregnancy
Vinblastine,[129, 130] vincristine	D	Antineoplastic	Musculoskeletal malformations, pancytopenia	May cause gonadal dysfunction

Chapter One Hundred and Ninety-Nine

Neurologic Diseases

Norman V. Kohn

199

This chapter will discuss neurologic conditions commonly encountered during pregnancy, with special attention to issues that are specific to pregnancy. Such issues must be considered when counseling any woman of child-bearing age, especially when a period of extended drug treatment is contemplated. Safe treatment in pregnancy begins with careful choice of medications and patient counseling before conception.

Some neurologic symptoms, such as headache, are common in pregnancy. The physician must distinguish between benign and self-limited symptoms, which may require no intervention, and symptoms of more serious disease. A careful history and physical examination usually will provide a sound basis for a tentative diagnosis and a plan for further diagnosis or management.

Imaging procedures should be considered whenever a lesion of the central nervous system is suspected. Fetal x-ray exposures of less than 1 rad are considered safe (see Chapter 5). X-rays, including computed tomography of the brain (CT) and arteriography, therefore, should not be avoided if they are indicated for the evaluation of a suspected maternal illness. The abdomen can be shielded during most neuroradiologic procedures. Standard intravenous contrast material can be used without ill effect. Magnetic resonance imaging (MRI), which involves no ionizing radiation, is of particular value during pregnancy because it poses no known risk to the fetus.[1-4] Myelography, which involves higher radiation doses, has been supplanted partially by CT and MRI. The greatest risk from myelography occurs early in pregnancy; later, while the risk of radiation effects is lower, maternal discomfort poses a technical challenge.

Neurophysiologic tests are noninvasive, except for the intramuscular needles used in electromyography (EMG), and without risk. These include electroencephalography (EEG) for study of the central nervous system; EMG for study of the peripheral nervous system (nerve and muscle); and evoked potentials, which test both central and peripheral nerves.

Direct examination of the spinal fluid is used to evaluate suspected infection, inflammation, neoplasm, or increased intracranial pressure. Lumbar puncture sometimes is deferred until after a brain CT. When signs of infection are present, such delay can be dangerous. In the absence of localizing findings, the patient with fever and stiff neck, confusion, seizures, or lethargy should undergo prompt lumbar puncture and, unless the CSF shows no evidence of infection, should receive antibiotic coverage for presumed meningitis.[5]

SYNCOPE

Sudden loss of consciousness is a cerebral phenomenon, but the most common cause is a drop in cardiac output. Vaso-vagal syncope is usually benign, but it can be alarming to the patient and it may cause significant injury. Such "benign" syncope, which always must be differentiated from syncope of more ominous cause, is precipitated by sudden standing, strong emotion, or pain, and represents transient failure of blood pressure control in response to postural or neural inputs. Anemia and hypovolemia contribute by increasing cardiac load. The patient first may experience light-headedness and loss of vision, and the attack can be aborted by sitting or lying. Unconsciousness, when it occurs, usually lasts no more than a minute: once the patient is no longer erect, cerebral perfusion is restored rapidly.

The first step in diagnosis is a careful history. If the event was typical, as described above, no further workup is necessary. The differential diagnosis of syncope includes basilar artery migraine or transient ischemic attack, subarachnoid hemorrhage, epilepsy, hypoglycemia, intoxication, cardiac arrhythmia, and pulmonary embolism.

HEADACHE

Headache of new onset may be a sign of meningitis, brain tumor, increased intracranial pressure, intracranial hemorrhage, or venous thrombosis; yet headaches are common, and most are benign. Stress may precipitate headache in the anxious pregnant patient worried about the changes in her life and in her body, and further medical workup may amplify her anxiety.

Some headaches can be diagnosed reliably by careful history and physical examination alone. When the headaches have been chronic and are typical of a benign category, and the neurologic examination is normal, no further workup is necessary. Further evaluation should be considered when the headache is of new onset or unusual severity. The most common types of headache in the pregnant and nonpregnant patient are migraine and tension headaches.

The headaches of brain tumors characteristically are worse in the morning, dull, and unchanged from day to day. Headache accompanied by fever or stiff neck may be caused by encephalitis or meningitis, even in the absence of any change in consciousness. Headache of sudden onset or severity suggests subarachnoid hemorrhage. Unruptured aneurysms generally do not produce headache. Rarely, an aneurysm arising at the junction of the internal carotid and posterior communicating arteries will compress the first division of the trigeminal nerve, producing pain behind the orbit.[6] A CT scan may confirm the presence of blood in the subarachnoid space, but small bleeds can be missed on CT; the spinal fluid is diagnostic.

Tension Headache

Tension headache, or muscle contraction headache, is typically dull and prolonged, often waxing and waning for days, weeks, or even years. The headache may be described as a feeling of pressure or tightness, and some patients specifically reject the term "headache." There may be increased EMG activity in cranial muscles, and increased muscle activity can be observed at times.[7] Stress often is identified as a precipitant; some authors consider emotional factors integral to the sydrome or even describe it as psychogenic.[8,9] While sometimes responsive to antidepressants, these headaches rarely are disabling. In pregnancy, the best approach is to address the underlying stress.

There is substantial overlap between the tension headache and common migraine categories.[10] When active muscle contraction is not evident and no psychological cause of headache is identified, the "tension headache" may be classified provisionally as a *vascular headache,* or migraine, and treated accordingly.

Migraine

Migraine[11] is a common disorder with striking clinical features and is recognizable in ancient writings. Prodromal symptoms occurring hours before an attack may include mild headache or changes in mood. *Classical migraine* is a syndrome of which the most constant feature is a throbbing, unilateral headache, heralded by complex auras. The most common auras are visual, but other neurologic deficits, even including loss of consciousness, may occur. Common visual auras include visual loss (scotoma), sometimes with shimmering margins (scintillating scotoma). A bright, expanding scotoma starting near the fixation point often is described. The aura usually lasts less than 30 minutes, and is followed within an hour by intense nausea and headache that may last hours or days.

The deficits in classical migraine usually do not correspond to the territory of a major cerebral artery. A typical migraine aura is not always followed by headache. When the headaches always occur on the same side or are of new onset, or the distribution of deficits in the auras suggests a vascular lesion, further evaluation should be considered. Contrast CT and MRI may be helpful; occasionally, angiography is required.

Common or atypical migraine lacks the well-defined prodrome of classical migraine and may be bilateral or steady in character. Abdominal symptoms can be associated with migraine. Abdominal pain without headache is seen most often in children, and is termed *abdominal migraine.* In these cases the pattern and pharmacology of the symptoms appear to justify identifying them as migrainous. While migraine most often improves during pregnancy, it may worsen or even appear for the first time.[9,12]

The best available evidence points to a vascular mechanism for migraine, but most of the evidence is indirect, and identification of a mechanism does not imply understanding of an etiology. The aura phase of an attack is characterized by constriction of cerebral vessels, usually followed by dilatation of intracranial and extracranial vessels, which is thought to produce pain. There is evidence of serotonin or histamine release at the start of some migraine attacks, but the mechanisms underlying an attack cannot be identified. Suggested mechanisms of migraine causation have included disorders of the local regulation of cerebral blood flow or of the metabolism of serotonin (possibly in platelets), monoamines, or carbohydrates.[13] The pattern of spread of a developing migraine scotoma has suggested a slowly spreading cortical phenomenon[14], and local electric and toxic mechanisms have been proposed.[15]

Stress may provoke a headache in the susceptible individual, as may alcohol consumption or variation in sleep or meal schedules. Caffeine withdrawal headache is a common migraine variant that often is overlooked. Other variant forms are distinguished on the basis of characteristic clinical or pharmacologic features. *Cluster headache* characteristically recurs one to three times daily for a period of weeks at a time (the "cluster"), always on the same side of the head. Cluster headaches are brief (less than 30 minutes) but of unusual severity.

Treatment. Mild nonnarcotic analgesics are often helpful. Caffeine, a vasoconstrictor that potentiates the effects of many analgesics, often is used in migraine and is a constituent of many over-the-counter headache medications. Mild sedatives (eg, phenobarbital) and antiemetics may be added when needed. Narcotics are useful in severe attacks, and steroids occasionally are used. All of these may be used judiciously in pregnancy if the patient's discomfort requires medication.

When attacks are severe and frequent, prophylactic treatment is preferred. Beta and calcium-channel blockers have been used for this; propranolol is attractive because of extensive experience in pregnancy[16], yet it depresses mood and may cause fetal growth retardation.[17] Amitriptyline is effective, particularly in tension headache and some cases of cluster headache. The effectiveness of amitriptyline appears to be independent of its antidepressant effect.[18,19] While its safety is not established, it has not been associated with birth defects.[20] Ergot alkaloids and lithium are used at times but carry greater risk and therefore should be avoided during pregnancy.

Some authors prefer to avoid preventive treatment of migraine during pregnancy or during the latter part of each menstrual cycle.[9] The patient with severe migraine should be offered some relief, and the treatment approach outlined here poses little risk.

Trigeminal Neuralgia

Trigeminal neuralgia, or *tic douloureux,* is an idiopathic condition producing recurrent periods of severe pain in the distribution of one or more divisions of the trigeminal nerve. During an episode, touching or moving the affected area typically triggers pain, and patients avoid touching the affected area of the face or chewing on that side. Carbamazepine is often effective. Baclofen[21,22] and some carbamazepine analogues[23] may be better still, but there is little experience with these drugs in pregnancy. A variety of surgical procedures have been used in trigeminal neuralgia, but medical management is preferred in most cases.[24-27]

Pseudotumor

Pseudotumor cerebri, or *benign intracranial hypertension,* is an idiopathic disorder producing increased intracranial pressure and usually headache. Most patients are young, female, and obese. Pressure can be transmitted past the diaphragma sellae, producing the *empty sella syndrome.*[28] Increased pressure on the optic nerves may produce visual loss. Papilledema may be present. The diagnosis is based on the demonstration of increased pressure by spinal fluid manometry in the absence of any mass lesion.

Pharmacologic causes of increased pressure can include medications (especially tetracycline) and vitamin A overdose. Sudden onset, especially late in pregnancy, should lead to suspicion of sagittal sinus thrombosis.

The etiology is unknown, but locally increased venous pressure has been suggested as a mechanism.[29] The condition is usually self-limited, and treatment is directed at reducing intracranial pressure. Steroids are often beneficial. The pressure can be reduced directly by the use of repeated spinal taps or osmotic diuretics; oral glycerol also has been used.

Post-traumatic Headache

Headaches are common after head trauma and are generally mild and self-limited. While the mechanism is not established, for clinical purposes these headaches blend into the vascular headache category. The severity of the headache may not correlate with that of the trauma.

Subdural hematoma can be a cause of headache. Concussion, defined as a change in consciousness after head trauma, may be used as a rough indicator of the severity of any head trauma. The patient who has suffered a concussion should be observed until 24 hours after the trauma to detect the change in consciousness that might signify an expanding intracranial hemorrhage. If headaches persist after head trauma, CT or MRI should be considered. Chronic post-traumatic headaches may respond to mild analgesics or to tricyclic antidepressants. In this setting, analgesics may be more effective if given on a regular schedule.

EPILEPSY

Epilepsy is not a single disease but a predisposition to epileptic seizures, sudden alterations of brain electrical activity that may produce involuntary motor or sensory phenomena with or without loss of consciousness. Epilepsy is estimated to affect 1% of all Americans. A seizure with loss of consciousness can cause physical injury; other potential hazards to mother and fetus include apnea and reduced cardiac output. Seizures are thought to injure the brain directly, but this is difficult to demonstrate in humans.

Seizure disorders are heterogeneous, and the choice of anticonvulsant depends on the type of seizure disorder and the patient's medical history. Classifications have been established both for individual seizures and for epileptic syndromes[30] (see Table 199–1). Generalized seizures also are known as major motor, tonic-clonic, or *"grand mal."* Partial seizures are distinguished by their focal onset, but they may spread and become generalized; their focal onset may be evident clinically or may be demonstrated by EEG. The partial seizure with secondary generalization is the most common seizure type in adults. The sensory aura that sometimes precedes a seizure is a focal seizure. An aura not followed by other seizure phenomena is still considered a seizure, and complete seizure control requires suppression of auras.

Focal or brief seizures are sometimes erroneously called *"petit mal"* by families or physicians wishing to denote the apparently mild nature of the seizure disorder. The classical *petit mal* seizure is an absence (generalized) seizure disorder that usually begins in childhood and generally remits or evolves into tonic-clonic (major motor) seizures by adulthood.

Seizures are called secondary, or symptomatic, when an underlying cause can be identified. With seizures of metabolic or infectious origin (eg, hypoglycemia, meningitis), it may be sufficient to treat the primary cause. More often the seizures are primary (idiopathic), or secondary with a cause that cannot be eliminated. Anticonvulsant medications then are used to reduce the excitability of cortical neurons and thus the likelihood of a seizure.

The patient with seizures of new onset should be evaluated to identify any underlying cause. A careful history may disclose prior blackouts. While the EEG can be normal in a patient with epilepsy, EEG changes may help determine the seizure type and the likelihood of underlying cerebral disease. Some disorders, such as subacute sclerosing panencephalitis (SSPE), produce characteristic EEG changes. CT or MRI should be considered, especially if there is fever or any suspicion of infection.

TABLE 199–1. INTERNATIONAL CLASSIFICATION OF EPILEPTIC SEIZURES

I. Partial Seizures (seizures beginning locally)
  A. Simple partial seizures (consciousness not impaired)
    1. With motor symptoms
    2. With somatosensory or special sensory symptoms
    3. With autonomic symptoms
    4. With psychic symptoms
  B. Complex partial seizures (with impairment of consciousness)
    1. Beginning as simple partial seizures and progressing to impairment of consciousness
      a. With no other features
      b. With features as in A.1–4
      c. With automatisms
    2. With impairment of consciousness at onset
      a. With no other features
      b. With features as in A.1–4
      c. With automatisms
  C. Partial seizures secondarily generalized
II. Generalized Seizures (bilaterally symmetrical and without local onset)
  A. 1. Absence seizures
    2. Atypical absence seizures
  B. Myoclonic seizures
  C. Clonic seizures
  D. Tonic seizures
  E. Tonic-clonic seizures
  F. Atonic seizures
III. Unclassified Epileptic Seizures (inadequate or incomplete data)

From *Commission on Classification and Terminology of the International League Against Epilepsy.*[30]

Gestational epilepsy, or seizures confined to pregnancy and the puerperium, is rare and can be diagnosed only in retrospect.[31] Single seizures sometimes are not treated: epilepsy is a predisposition to seizures, and the rationale for treatment is based on its recurrent nature.

When the patient with previously good seizure control begins to have seizures, the history and the medication regimen should be reviewed. Sleep deprivation can trigger seizures in the epileptic patient. Anticonvulsant blood levels can be compared with the patient's levels when the seizures were well controlled. If the levels are unchanged, it may be necessary to maintain higher medication levels or to add another medication. A dosage schedule that was formerly effective may be producing lower blood levels of medication because of metabolic changes in the patient. Persistently low anticonvulsant blood levels may lead to suspicion of noncompliance or of drug interaction. Many patients, fearful of harming the fetus, omit their anticonvulsants during pregnancy.

Seizure prevention is important because of the risk of injury from a seizure. In addition to the physical risks, patients fear the stigma that our society has attached to epilepsy for many years. If the patient has seizures that are mild and infrequent, does not drive, and is not afraid of being embarrassed in public or at work, it makes sense to ask if there are alternatives to drug treatment. The risk to mother and fetus of an isolated seizure is difficult to measure. Regardless of such considerations, after the first trimester the risk/benefit ratios generally favor medication.

It is important to explain to the mother not only the need for medication, but the evidence of its safety in pregnancy.

Drug Treatment

The axioms of antiepileptic drug treatment are stated simply. The drug selected should be effective for the patient's seizure type, with acceptably low risk of side effects. Drug combinations are avoided: monotherapy, or treatment with a single drug, is usually possible and will minimize the likelihood of sedation, birth defects, and other toxicity. Most seizure disorders are controlled easily with any of several anticonvulsant medications; many of the remainder are difficult to control even with multiple medications. Drug interactions are common and are a reason for avoiding anticonvulsant combinations. Mechanisms of drug interaction include enzyme induction (the likely mechanism by which anticonvulsant drugs interfere with oral contraceptives)[32] or displacement from protein binding sites (eg, by valproic acid).

Metabolic changes in pregnancy, including increased hepatic metabolism and declining albumin levels, may contribute to changes in drug levels. Anticonvulsant levels generally fall during pregnancy. The ratio of free to bound drug also changes. If doses are changed to maintain constant total levels, the level of unbound drug may rise. Measurement of free drug level and correlation of dosage with seizure control will help to avoid inadvertent overdosage.[33]

Despite the characteristic drop in anticonvulsant blood levels during pregnancy, only one third of patients experience any associated increase in seizure frequency. Dosage adjustment therefore must reflect the clinical situation. Some patients, especially on phenytoin, require extraordinary doses to achieve therapeutic blood levels of medication. When this occurs, it is often simplest to change to another medication.

Generic substitution can cause fluctuating blood levels when the pharmacy changes its generic brand. Brands meeting the FDA standards for generic equivalence differ among themselves in bioavailability and total drug content. Changing between "equivalent" brands therefore may cause an effective dosage change of 10% or more despite good compliance and unchanged administration schedule. With drugs like phenytoin, which has nonlinear kinetics, a relatively small change in actual dose may produce much larger changes in blood level.

The therapeutic range of blood levels for an anticonvulsant drug is the range of levels below which few patients achieve seizure control and above which many experience toxicity. Different values within the "therapeutic" range may not be equally effective in a given patient. Levels slightly above the therapeutic range usually produce drowsiness but are not hazardous, and some patients need such levels for effective seizure control. Other patients achieve good seizure control despite "subtherapeutic" anticonvulsant blood levels.

The choice of anticonvulsant depends largely on the patient's seizure type. Carbamazepine is widely regarded as the anticonvulsant drug of first choice in children and young adults, and is classified as category C (the others are category D).[34] Its advantages include reduced sedation and lower incidence of neural tube defects. Phenytoin and phenobarbital are more sedating; phenytoin causes changes in appearance that make it less desirable in young people. Primidone is more sedating still, and may be more teratogenic. All of these medications should be given in divided doses.

Partial seizures, including partial seizures with secondary generalization, are treated most often with carbamazepine or phenytoin. For primary generalized seizures these drugs may be used as well as phenobarbital and primidone. Valproic acid has been used more recently in this category as well.

Absence seizures in the adult most often respond to valproic acid or clonazepam. Ethosuximide is particularly effective in typical absence (petit mal) seizures, which usually are seen in children and teenagers.

Anticonvulsant regimens in young women should always be designed around the possibility of pregnancy, and it is rarely advisable to change medication simply because the patient has become pregnant. Most anticonvulsants have long serum half-lives, on the order of 3–5 days, and levels change slowly after a change in dose. When treatment with an anticonvulsant is being stopped, it is often advisable to taper the dosage over 30 days or more, because abrupt withdrawal may precipitate status epilepticus. By the time a medication change has been made, the period of greatest risk of teratogenesis may have passed. It is rarely worthwhile to change anticonvulsants simply because a woman has discovered that she is pregnant.

Teratogenicity

All clinically useful anticonvulsant medications are teratogenic in animals at high doses, and many are known to have toxic effects in human pregnancy. Teratogenic effects differ between species and therefore are difficult to extrapolate to humans. The true incidence of fetal abnormalities due to anticonvulsants is difficult to measure. The available studies contain flaws, including failure to monitor anticonvulsant blood levels. Controlled studies are lacking, many of the patients studied were on multiple medications, and the incidence of birth defects in the children of untreated epileptics is not known. The best current estimates are that the risk of congenital malformation in the child is increased by a relative risk factor of 1.25–2.2 when the mother is taking anticonvulsants, and may not be increased when the mother's epilepsy does not require treatment.[35-38]

The major malformation most often associated with anticonvulsants is hare lip, with or without cleft palate. Genetic factors in the fetus appear to be important in determining risk, and may account for observed variation in incidence.[39] Valproic acid has been associated with neural tube defects. Anticonvulsants are all associated with minor dysmorphic changes, usually a combination of minor craniofacial changes and hypoplasia of the fingertips and fingernails. Involvement of the toes is less common. Hypoplastic fingertips are associated with a higher frequency of dermal arches.[40-43] The incidence of these effects is probably underestimated in retrospective studies: many of the effects decrease with age as the children outgrow them, and typically are noted only when specifically investigated.[35,44]

The commonly used anticonvulsants all interfere with folic acid metabolism. The resulting folate deficiency can cause a macrocytic anemia; its ability to contribute to birth defects in the offspring of epileptic mothers is unknown. Folic acid supplementation therefore is recommended when anticonvulsants are given to women of child-bearing potential.

About half of the infants of mothers who take phenytoin, primidone or phenobarbital during pregnancy are born with coagulopathy due to vitamin K deficiency, and are at risk of intraventricular hemorrhage. Administration of vitamin K 20 mg per day orally to the mother for 2 weeks antepartum, or 10 mg IM 4 hours before birth, will prevent this complication in the newborn.[33,45-47]

Status Epilepticus

Status epilepticus, or recurrent seizures without return of consciousness, is a medical emergency requiring immediate hospitalization and treatment. Metabolic and infectious causes must be sought, and prompt seizure control is essential. The following algorithm will achieve prompt seizure control in most patients[48,49]:

1. Insert an intravenous catheter. Draw venous blood for toxicologic screen, glucose, BUN, electrolytes, blood count, and anticonvulsant blood levels. Draw arterial blood to measure gases and pH. Monitor vital signs and electrocardiogram. Monitor the fetus.
2. Administer normal saline intravenously. Give 100 mg of thiamine intramuscularly. Give a bolus of 50 mL of 50% glucose.
3. Administer diazepam intravenously no faster than 2 mg per minute until seizures stop or a total of 20 mg has been given. Start infusing phenytoin no faster than 50 mg per minute to a total dose of 18 mg per kg. The rate of the infusion may need to be slowed if the patient becomes bradycardic or hypotensive.
4. Endotracheal intubation, if not already performed, should be considered at this time. Start a diazepam drip: dilute 50 mg in 500 cm^3 of 5% dextrose and run at a rate of 5–10 mg per hour, titrating the rate to control the seizures. Lorazepam may be substituted here.

   A loading dose of phenobarbital may be given in lieu of diazepam, but the two drugs should not be given together because excessive respiratory depression may result.
5. If seizures persist, give halothane or another inhalation anesthetic, along with neuromuscular blockade. Intravenous lidocaine, 50–100 mg, may be tried first. If it is effective, an infusion of lidocaine at 1–2 mg per minute may be given.

Eclamptic Seizures

This complex topic has produced diverse recommendations from obstetricians and neurologists.[50,51] (see also Chapter 140). Severe eclampsia produces fibrinoid vascular changes, edema, infarcts, and hemorrhages in multiple organs including brain, kidney, and liver. The neuropathology of eclampsia is that of a hypertensive encephalopathy.[52,53] In surviving patients, MRI demonstrates evidence of small foci of brain edema, suggesting multiple microvascular occlusions.[54] Effective medical management must maintain organ perfusion, protecting the kidneys, the brain, and the placenta.

Magnesium sulfate is widely favored, although its mechanism of action in eclampsia is unknown. Unlike other major anticonvulsants, magnesium is not fat soluble and is excreted unchanged in the urine. Dose determination therefore is easier with magnesium than with other major anticonvulsants, and serum levels change rapidly in response to changes in dose. Magnesium does not interfere with perfusion of the placenta. Magnesium is a relatively poor anticonvulsant by usual laboratory criteria, and eclamptic seizures have persisted in some patients despite high serum levels.[55] Magnesium may reduce vasospasm by opposing calcium-dependent arterial constriction, and may antagonize calcium-mediated cell damage in ischemic tissues.[56]

Eclampsia, like pregnancy, is unique. The nonpregnant patient with acute hypertension and neurologic deficits would be treated with specific antihypertensive and anticonvulsant medications. While some have recommended hydralazine and phenytoin for specific treatment of hypertension and seizures in eclampsia, the rarity of the condition and its low morbidity with present management[57] pose a challenge to any controlled study of alternatives to magnesium sulfate.

AUTOIMMUNE DISORDERS

Autoimmune disorders are relatively common in young women (see also Chapters 51 and 52) and disorders of the nervous system constitute only a subset. HLA associations exist in many of these conditions, but their pathogenesis remains obscure. With the exception of myasthenia, none is directly hazardous to the fetus or newborn.

A common feature is patchy involvement, with some areas affected and others spared. There are characteristic but unexplained patterns in each. The lesions of multiple sclerosis (MS) often are clustered in a periventricular distribution, and the weakness of myasthenia gravis is often limited to the ocular muscles. These patterns could represent characteristics of the target tissue (the myelin of specific regions, or particular muscles) or of the vascular supply to the affected tissues.

Pregnancy may have a nonspecific effect on the course of autoimmune disease. A pattern of remissions late in pregnancy with exacerbations postpartum has been suggested in MS, experimental allergic encephalomyelitis (an animal model of MS), myasthenia gravis[58,59], rheumatoid arthritis[60], systemic lupus[61], and thyrotoxicosis[62,63], and also is supported by animal models.[64] Circulating immunopressive factors have been implicated. One, α-fetoprotein, has been shown to exert a protective effect in animal models of MS and myasthenia.[62,65]

Immunosuppressive treatment is a common theme in this group of diseases. Steroids often are used; except in chronic polyneuritis, they are used in short courses that may be modified to reduce risk to the fetus. Virilization of the female fetus is a first-trimester effect and thus needs to be considered in the treatment of any young woman. Cytotoxic drugs (azathioprine, cyclophosphamide) have been used in pregnancy but are classified as category D and have been associated with congenital anomalies and premature birth.[66] Regimens involving these drugs can be modified if pregnancy is contemplated. It is rarely necessary to start cytotoxic agents for neurologic disease during pregnancy. Plasmapheresis is sometimes used, and has been of distinct benefit in myasthenia and inflammatory polyneuritis. There is limited experience with plasmapheresis in pregnancy.[67] The presence of many circulating humeral factors raises concerns that must be balanced against potential benefits in individual cases.

Multiple Sclerosis

MS is the most common autoimmune disorder of the nervous system, affecting 200,000 young adults in the United States. Some patients, possibly those more severely affected, may avoid pregnancy, but only in the relatively rare case of hypothalamic involvement is fertility affected directly. With a slight female preponderance and no significant effect on fertility, MS affects hundreds of pregnant patients every year.

MS is characterized by areas of myelin destruction ("plaques") within the central nervous system. Its typical remitting-relapsing course is produced by repeated episodes of acute inflammation in the white matter of the CNS. Common manifestations include visual involvement (especially optic neuritis), incoordination, and abnormalities of muscle strength and tone. The diagnosis depends on the demonstration of multiple sites of demyelination with a history of repeated attacks. Evoked potentials (visual, auditory, somatosensory) can help by demonstrating asymptomatic physiologic abnormalities. When the diagnosis is in doubt, MRI is sensitive for the detection of white matter lesions.

Considerations of MS in pregnancy have been reviewed extensively.[68-70] Despite increased incidence of relapse postpartum, most recent studies conclude that the overall risk is negligible, with no increase in disability at one year postpartum.[63,71,72] Nevertheless, MS is characteristically chronic and progressive. In one study, 30% of women who bore children after the diagnosis of MS experienced some limitation in their ability to care for their children.[71] Methodologic problems complicate interpretation of many of the studies.[73]

Myasthenia Gravis

Muasthenia gravis, a neuromuscular transmission disorder, produces chronic weakness and is associated with circulating antibodies to the neuromuscular junction. Sensation and thinking are unaffected, but weakness can be profound. Weakness increases with activity, producing striking fatiguability. Most patients are young; those over 50 may constitute a distinct group that will not be discussed here. Thymic hyperplasia is present in most young myasthenics, and myasthenic serum contains antibodies to neuromuscular junction that also bind to the myoid cells of the thymus.[74]

Relative changes in titers of a patient's antibodies to skeletal muscle or motor endplate correlate with disease activity, but the absolute titers do not. The poor predictive value of titers probably corresponds to the finding in animal models that disease severity correlates with antibody class and binding type, characteristics not measured by standard titers.[75]

Edrophonium, a short-acting acetylcholinesterase inhibitor, briefly restores transmission at the neuromuscular junction (NMJ) and can be used to confirm the diagnosis. The electrical correlate of the patient's fatiguability, decrement in the electrical response of muscle to repeated stimulation of the associated motor nerve, can be demonstrated in the EMG laboratory. Subtle abnormalities of neuromuscular transmission can be detected by single-fiber EMG, which measures the variability of postsynaptic response in single neuromuscular junctions. Not all muscle groups are affected equally, however, and the patient with respiratory or ocular myasthenia may have normal electrodiagnostic tests.

Thymectomy is recommended in all except the mildest cases and often leads to prolonged remission. The timing of the procedure is not critical, and it can be deferred in the pregnant patient. It has been performed safely during pregnancy, however, and prior thymectomy may reduce the likelihood of relapse during pregnancy.[76-78]

Treatment options include acetylcholinesterase inhibitors and immunosuppression. Plasmapheresis usually is reserved for initiation of treatment in patients with profound weakness, but it can be used chronically in patients who do not tolerate steroids and who remain weak despite acetylcholinesterase inhibitors. Steroid treatment often will induce remissions lasting months or years. Long-term immunosuppression with cytotoxic drugs has been useful and may prove safer than steroid treatment.

Many drugs have the potential to cause weakness in the myasthenic patient and therefore should be avoided. These include quinine, all neuromuscular blocking agents, many antibiotics, and magnesium sulfate.[79,80]

Neonatal myasthenia, caused by maternal antibodies that cross the placenta, produces weakness lasting several days after birth. The children of myasthenic mothers must be monitored for signs of respiratory failure.

Polyneuritis

The inflammatory polyneuritides fall into two distinct groups. The acute form, *acute inflammatory neuropathy* (AIN), also is known as the *Guillain-Barré syndrome.* It may be preceded by a nonspecific prodromal illness, usually a flulike illness, and mild sensory changes. The patient develops weakness, often in an ascending pattern beginning with the legs, that worsens for as long as three weeks. Some patients require ventilatory support. Sensory and CNS involvement may occur but are rarely prominent. A particularly severe form may be associated with infection by *Campylobacter jejuni*.[81,82] A variant form, the Miller–Fisher syndrome, produces incoordination and cranial nerve involvement.

The CSF typically contains elevated protein levels but few or no cells ("albuminocytologic dissociation"). When polio was an epidemic disease, it could be distinguished from AIN by an increased CSF cell count. Nerve conduction is slow, and some fibers have conduction failure, or *block*, secondary to myelin damage.

The lesions of AIN consist of segments of inflammatory destruction of peripheral nerve myelin. When the inflammation is severe it may damage the adjacent axon. CNS involvement usually has been associated with unusually severe inflammation in adjacent roots. A cluster of cases occurred in association with an influenza vaccine widely administered in the United States in 1976. The responsible component of the vaccine was never identified, and no increase in the incidence of AIN has been seen with subsequent influenza immunization programs.

Steroids are not of benefit in treating AIN and should not be used. Plasmapheresis may shorten the course if begun early. Most patients recover over a period of months. Supportive care, including ventilatory support, is essential. Prolonged illness and incomplete recovery are more likely when the EMG demonstrates evidence of denervation (and hence, axonal damage) during the acute phase. Recurrence is rare.

Chronic inflammatory neuropathy appears to be a distinct entity. Evidence of prior myelin destruction is usually present, even during the first symptomatic attack. Individual exacerbations usually are milder than in AIN. Plasmaphoresis and immunosuppression are benefical.[83-86]

CEREBROVASCULAR DISEASE

The term *stroke* historically has been used ambiguously to denote cerebral infarction and intracranial hemorrhage, reflecting the difficulty of distinguishing between the two conditions before the advent of modern imaging procedures. The hallmark of both is a lasting neurologic deficit of sudden onset. Hypertension and age are the most important risk factors for cerebral infarction.[87]

While more common in older patients, cerebrovascular disease occurs in patients of childbearing age. Pregnancy at times may predispose the patient to stroke through changes in blood pressure or coagulation.

The characteristic symptom of a cerebrovascular lesion is a persistent neurologic deficit of sudden onset. Coma may result if the lesion affects the brain stem or both cerebral hemispheres.[88] Swelling of infarcted tissue may produce a gradual fall in level of consciousness by compressing the midbrain and the normal hemisphere.

Evaluation of the stroke patient always should include CT or MRI imaging to determine the anatomy. In young patients, special care should be taken to look for an underlying cause. Treatment consists of preventing complications such as aspiration and thrombophlebitis; controlling physiologic factors, such as blood pressure or embolic sources, that could produce exacerbation or recurrence; and physical rehabilitation to minimize the impact of any persistent deficit. Young stroke patients often have substantial capacity for recovery.

Cerebral Infarction

Cerebral infarction in a young person usually results from occlusion of a large artery, most often the internal carotid or middle cerebral. Because there is little collateral circulation to the brain, most vascular occlusions above the Circle of Willis, and many below, will cause clinically significant infarcts. Small infarcts, associated with occlusion of smaller distal vessels, sometimes are called *lacunes* because of their pathologic appearance. Chronic hypertension is an important risk factor for the development of lacunar strokes.[89-91]

Hypertension damages cerebral vessels. Pressure in the cerebral circulation is regulated by local reflex vasoconstriction. The cerebral capillary endothelium is characterized by tight junctions, and metabolites pass from the blood to the brain by active transport. Increased pressure in this vascular bed leads to perivascular edema and local arterial spasm, culminating in tissue ischemia and infarction. Such spasm occurring in a more generalized but reversible pattern is called *hypertensive encephalopathy*.[92,93]

Atherosclerosis is the most common cause of vascular occlusion, even in the young, but the diagnostic workup must include a search for other, reversible causes. Clinical evaluation may include Holter monitoring and echocardiography to identify an embolic source. A coagulation profile is particularly important in the pregnant patient. Hypercoagulable states, some associated with cardiolipin antibodies ("lupus anticoagulant") or abnormal regulation of coagulation, may be more common during pregnancy. Other possible causes include hypertensive vascular disease, embolism, and drug abuse. *Cocaine* is an increasingly common cause of stroke in young adults. A potent vasoconstrictor, cocaine also causes increased blood pressure and may predispose the patient to thrombosis. Cerebral infarctions and intracerebral and subarachnoid hemorrhages all have been reported.[94] Stroke can be the first manifestation of collagen disease, cerebral vasculitis, or bacterial endocarditis; these sometimes cause multiple small infarcts, producing confusion or lethargy without focal findings. Septicemia can produce a similar syndrome. Congenital causes of stroke include homocystinuria and fibromuscular dysplasia. Cerebral angiography is sometimes needed to identify the vascular anatomy.

Paradoxical emboli, or arterial emboli originating in the venous system but not trapped in the lungs, also can cause stroke. Once thought to be rare, they may be suspected when there is an arterial embolus and evidence of pulmonary emboli, multiple systemic emboli without identifiable cardiac source, or venous thrombosis.[95] An audible cardiac murmur need not be present.

Some patients with tight vascular stenosis, or acute large vessel occlusion but only limited deficit, including those with *stroke in evolution,* are treated with heparin anticoagulation. Surgical repair of tight extracranial stenoses has been advocated. Adequate controlled studies are not yet available, and clinical practice varies. The patient with a suspected embolic source usually is given anticoagulants to prevent further emboli. In the pregnant patient, the risks of heparin therapy therefore must be weighed against the risk of further embolization. Underlying disorders of coagulation or immunity should be treated. Steroids are of no demonstrated benefit, and the use of mannitol is appropriate only in rare patients with severe edema. In the hypertensive patient, careful control of blood pressure is critical.

Intracerebral Hemorrhage

Spontaneous bleeding within the brain often is caused by hypertensive vascular disease. Hemorrhage also may result from the rupture of congenital vascular anomalies, such as *microaneurysms* or "cryptic" *arteriovenous malformations* (AVMs). These lesions are small and can be difficult to identify clinically; many are destroyed when they bleed and require no special intervention. A circle of Willis aneurysm can rupture into the brain, producing intracerebral hemorrhage. Recurrent bleeding is an important risk with aneurysms and larger AVMs.

After an intracerebral hemorrhage, the patient's prognosis depends on the extent of damage. The immediate risk lies in the compression of normal brain by the hematoma. If bleeding continues, coma and death can follow quickly. Surgical intervention is often impractical: the hemorrhages that are stable enough to permit accurate diagnosis and safe surgical decompression are generally the ones that can be safely managed medically. Surgical decompression of a deep hematoma also entails damage to overlying normal brain. Prompt surgical decompression is necessary when a cerebellar hemorrhage compresses the brain stem.

Blood pressure can be labile in the acute phase and may require nitroprusside or other short-acting intravenous agents. As with infarcts, treatment must include a search for underlying causes. Steroids are not beneficial. Seizures may occur, and prophylactic anticonvulsants should be considered. Initial management is focused on the respiratory and metabolic effects of the hemorrhage.

Subarachnoid and Subdural Hemorrhage

Subarachnoid hemorrhage should be suspected in coma or severe headache of sudden onset; the CT scan is usually diagnostic. Small bleeds can be missed on CT, but spinal tap will establish the diagnosis.

Congenital aneurysm is the most common cause of nontraumatic subarachnoid hemorrhage; arteriography should be done unless contraindicated by the patient's status. Morbidity, related to recurrent bleeding and to vascular spasm, is highest in the first two weeks after subarachnoid hemorrhage. Operative morbidity is also higher during the first two weeks after hemorrhage, and the optimal time for surgery has not been conclusively established.[96]

Arteriovenous malformations account for up to half of subarachnoid hemorrhages during pregnancy. Headache or seizure may be the presenting symptom. These lesions are prone to recurrent bleeding and also can cause cerebral ischemia, possibly by shunting of cerebral blood flow. The risk of bleeding from an AVM is thought to be higher during pregnancy.[97,98] Treatment options include surgery and embolization. Radiographically guided embolization of AVMs has proven effective and safe. Because of the risk of recurrent bleeding, surgical intervention should be considered.[99]

A rise in blood pressure increases the risk of bleeding from an aneurysm or AVM, and AVMs are prone to rebleeding during delivery.[99] If an aneurysm is known to be present, cesarean section should be considered.[45] If the aneurysm did not bleed during the third trimester or was discovered fortuitously, however, vaginal delivery may be safe.[98]

Subdural bleeding is usually of venous origin, and is therefore more insidious in onset. Subdural hemorrhage usually is associated with trauma and disorders of coagulation, but also can occur spontaneously. Small traumatic subdural hematomas may not require surgery, but all should be evaluated carefully.

Venous Thrombosis

Cortical venous thrombosis, producing cerebral infarction or hemorrhage, is seen as a complication of pregnancy and usually occurs in the first three weeks postpartum. The initial symptoms are focal seizures, depressed consciousness, and fluctuating focal neurologic deficits. Early or mild cases may be difficult to distinguish from postpartum eclampsia.[100,101] The sagittal sinus may be involved, primarily or by propagation of a thrombus originating in cortical veins. There may be increased intracranial pressure, with headache and papilledema, from the mass effect of swollen infarcted brain or from interference with normal CSF absorption by the arachnoid granulations at the sagittal sinus. There can be hemorrhage into the infarcted tissue.

Anticonvulsants should be given if the patient has seizures. Once the risk of uterine hemorrhage is past[102], anticoagulation with heparin should be given unless a CT scan of the brain shows significant hemorrhage.[103-105] Prognostic figures may be skewed by misdiagnosis of mild cases.[101]

BRAIN DEATH

Brain death became an important concept with the advent of modern respiratory care. Permanent loss of brain function is no longer synonomous with somatic death. With intensive respiratory and fluid management, it is sometimes possible to maintain a patient's vital signs and organs for an extended time.[106] Prolonged support subjects the patient's family to great stress and consumes limited hospital resources, but is necessary in some cases. Organ transplantation depends on the availability of brain-dead donors, who require aggressive support prior to organ removal. When the brain-dead patient is pregnant, special considerations arise because of the possibility of supporting the mother's vital functions for the days or weeks until the fetus can be delivered safely.

In common law, death was long equated with cessation of cardiac function. Total and irreversible loss of brain function is now widely accepted as a criterion of death in the United States.[107-109] The moment of brain death usually cannot be determined, and there are obvious paradoxes: if the patient is legally dead, for example, who should pay for continued care? If the brain injury was caused by trauma, and the respirator is turned off, was the patient killed by the injury or by the doctors? Courts in such cases have accepted the concept of brain death and identified the injury, and not the physician, as the cause of death.[107]

Brain death is defined as total, irreversible cessation of function of the entire brain, including the brain stem.[108] Any residual cerebral or brain-stem function is inconsistent with this diagnosis; testing and examination must be adequate to identify persistent brain function. The nature of the brain injury should be known and possible confounding but reversible diagnoses, such as sedation, hypothermia, shock, and neuromuscular blockade, must be excluded. The absence of brain function should be confirmed by an experienced physician. Blood flow testing (usually by nuclear medicine) and EEG can be used to confirm the diagnosis. A "flat" EEG alone cannot establish the diagnosis, because EEG examines cortical function only and cannot verify the absence of brain-stem function. Respiration, eye movements (including caloric responses) and the corneal reflex are mediated by brain-stem centers and are readily tested at the bedside. Legislation does not spell out specific clinical criteria. Widely accepted guidelines have been developed for practical application of the concept of brain death in various clinical settings.[107,110]

Brain-dead patients must be distinguished from those in a *chronic vegetative state,* who are permanently comatose but have some residual brain function. Respiration may be preserved. Decisions to limit care or to withhold resuscitation may be appropriate in such patients, but they are considered alive and cannot be organ donors. Termination of supportive care in such a case is not a routine issue unless the patient has executed a "living will" directing that he or she not be kept alive by artificial means. Even so, if the patient is pregnant, the interests of the fetus may be found to override the expressed wishes of the mother.[111]

The brain-dead patient is often unstable. Diabetes insipidus and pituitary failure may be present. Pituitary hormones may continue to be detectable in the blood[112], possibly because some parts of the pituitary receive an extracranial blood supply. Hypotension and low cardiac output may be refractory to any intervention. Prolonged somatic survival in the brain-dead patient is unusual[113], and considerations of whether to terminate artificial respiration thus often are rendered moot. Variation in the duration of survival of brain-dead patients may reflect the variety of causes of brain death, which is a physiologic state with many possible etiologies. Cases of prolonged somatic survival of the pregnant brain-dead mother, with delivery of a normal fetus, have been reported.[114-116] These cases are unusual. In our institution, we have been unable to maintain cardiac function for more than 3 days in brain-dead pregnant patients who had suffered massive intracerebral hemorrhages.

CHOREA GRAVIDARUM

Chorea is a movement disorder characterized by rapid, irregular involuntary movements. The known causes all produce changes in the basal ganglia. As in other movement disorders, the movements are worse with stress and absent during sleep. Weakness, loss of muscle tone, and emotional and cognitive changes also have been noted. There may be inability to sustain voluntary motor effort. This and involuntary activity in antagonist muscles may contribute to the weakness seen in affected patients. *Chorea gravidarum,* or chorea with onset during pregnancy, is a subclass of the syndrome of acute chorea.

Most cases of acute chorea, including those during pregnancy, have been associated with rheumatic fever (*Sydenham's chorea*).[117] While the patients may have other manifestations of rheumatic disease, they may not be contemporaneous with the movement disorder. Even in cases of rheumatic origin, recent streptoccal infection is not necessary for the emergence of chorea gravidarum.[118] Chorea has been described after treatment with oral contraceptives, prochlorperazine, haloperidol, or phenytoin. Acute chorea is most common in childhood; onset after age 15 is rare except in association with oral contraceptives, pregnancy, or systemic lupus. Female predominance is present after the age of 10.[119] The mechanism of the drug-associated cases is unknown; it is likely that many of the others are of autoimmune origin. Estrogens may act directly on the brain to unmask a previously latent movement disorder.[120,121]

Widely differing accounts of the incidence and timing of chorea in pregnancy probably reflect the diminishing prevalence of rheumatic disease and the consequent increase in the proportion of nonrheumatic cases. North American reports of the incidence of chorea gravidarum have ranged from one per 146 births in 1932[122] to less than one per 70,000 births in 1968.[123] Similarly, the most common time of onset has been stated as first trimester[123] and as second trimester.[124]

Little is known of the actual pathology of acute chorea because the condition is self-limited and relevant autopsy studies are not available. The few published autopsy reports support the concept that the striatum is involved, although acute cardiac failure and infection were the usual causes of death and often produced widespread terminal changes in the brain:[125] death in these cases was associated with rheumatic heart disease, and many of the changes described in the brain can be attributed to terminal anoxia or infection.

In rheumatic chorea, antibodies have been demonstrated that bind to neurons in subthalamic and caudate nuclei as well as to Group A streptococcal surface antigens. It appears likely that a variety of conditions can cause the production of antibodies that bind to basal ganglia neurons producing chorea. Other associated cerebral symptoms may reflect antibody binding to other sites within the brain.[126] Rheumatic chorea gravidarum may be triggered by hormonal factors or immune changes specific to pregnancy, accounting for its self-limited and relatively benign course.

There is no characteristic laboratory finding. The relative scarcity of rheumatic cases makes it important to look for other underlying causes.[127-129] Mild sedation with benzodiazepines or phenobarbital may be necessary. Phenothiazines, haloperidol[130], and valproic acid have been reported to be beneficial in acute chorea. It is important to remind the patient that chorea gravidarum is self-limited and does not harm the fetus. Penicillin prophylaxis has been recommended in acute chorea but is not necessary in chorea gravidarum unless there is other evidence of rheumatic fever.

NEUROPATHIES

Mononeuropathies, or lesions involving single peripheral nerves, are relatively common in pregnancy. *Carpal tunnel syndrome*, the most common, affects the median nerve at the wrist; estimates of its frequency range from 7% to 31% of pregnancies.[131-133] Numbness and tingling, usually worse when the patient is lying in bed at night, are most prominent in the lateral aspect of the hand but may involve the entire hand and extend proximally to the forearm and occasionally to the shoulder. Patients sometimes complain of pain. Pinprick sensation is diminished in the distribution of the median nerve. Motor involvement is less common, but weakness and wasting of the abductor pollicis brevis and the opponens pollicis sometimes may be seen. Symptoms most often begin late in pregnancy and may even begin postpartum.

The median nerve is readily compressed in the narrow tendinous carpal tunnel. Edema has been thought to be a cause of carpal tunnel syndrome in pregnancy[134]; localized tendinitis, perhaps hormonally mediated, has been suggested as a cause in some cases.[135]

Splinting of the wrist, especially at night, may provide relief. Steroid injection and diuretics have been suggested but are rarely necessary. Most patients are content to have the benign character of the symptom explained to them. Symptoms usually remit by the third month postpartum. The rare patient whose symptoms persist may require surgical release of the tendinous sheath.

Bell's Palsy

Bell's palsy, an idiopathic neuropathy of the facial nerve, occurs with increased incidence in pregnancy. Onset is usually painless; sometimes patients complain of pain in the ear or face. Blinking is impaired, and eye pain can be the presenting symptom. Because the stapedius reflex depends on fibers that run in the facial nerve, hyperacousis may be present. Taste may be absent on the anterior portion of the tongue, and the patient may complain of a strange metallic taste.

The mechanism of Bell's palsy is unknown. Local inflammation has been suspected because of the characteristic course of the syndrome, and it is possible that the syndrome represents a viral infection or a post-viral inflammatory process.[136]

The incidence of Bell's palsy has been reported at 45 per 100,000 births, compared with 17 per 100,000 per year in nonpregnant women of the same age. Onset in pregnancy usually occurs in the third trimester.[137] Recovery can take months and is difficult to predict. Prolonged and incomplete recovery tends to be associated with denser initial deficits. EMG evidence of denervation at 1–2 weeks after onset also is associated with poor outcome, but does not alter significantly the course of treatment. Some 64–80% of patients have full recovery without specific treatment. Some patients experience synkinesis, an involuntary activation of muscles during normal movements, after recovery. Synkinesis is thought to result when an injured axon grows and establishes synapses with the wrong muscle fibers. If the patient is seen within the first 5 days, a short (10- to 17-day) course of prednisone reduces the likelihood of synkinesis and may reduce residual weakness.[138,139]

Meralgia paresthetica is a neuropathy of the lateral femoral cutaneous nerve, which innervates the skin on the lateral aspect of the thigh. Patients experience pain and numbness in the distribution of the nerve. The nerve frequently is injured as it crosses beneath the inguinal ligament to enter the thigh.[140] Obesity or recent weight gain are common precursors.[141] The exaggerated lumbar lordosis of pregnancy may contribute by stretching the nerve.[142] No specific treatment is indicated, and the pregnancy-associated cases usually resolve fully. The burning pain may respond to carbamazapine or amytriptyline.

REFERENCES

1. Budinger TF. Nuclear magnetic resonance (NMR) in vivo studies: known thresholds for health effects. *J Comput Assist Tomogr*. 1981;5:800.
2. Smith FW, Adam AH, Phillips WDP. NMR imaging in pregnancy. *Lancet*. 1983;1:61.
3. Lowe TW, Weinreb J, Santos-Ramos R, et al. Magnetic resonance imaging in human pregnancy. *Obstet and Gynecol*. 1985;66:629.
4. Weinreb JC, Lowe TW, Santos-Ramos R, et al. Magnetic resonance imaging in obstetric diagnosis. *Radiology*. 1985;154:157.
5. Adams RD, Victor M. *Principles of Neurology*. 3rd ed. New York, NY: McGraw-Hill; 1985:517.
6. Dalessio DJ. Major vascular diseases and headache. In: Dalessio DJ,

ed. *Wolf's Headache and Other Head Pain*. New York and Oxford: Oxford Univ Press; 1987:207.
7. Lance JW. *Mechanism and Management of Headache*. 4th ed. London: Butterworths; 1982.
8. Friedman AP, Von Storch TJC, Merritt HH. Migraine and tension headaches: a clinical study of two thousand cases. *Neurology*. 1964;4:773.
9. Reik LJ. Headaches in pregnancy. In: Donaldson JO, ed. Neurologic problems of pregnancy. *Sem Neurol*. 1988;8:187.
10. Raskin NH, Appenzeller O. *Headache*. Philadelphia, PA: WB Saunders; 1980:172.
11. Sacks O. *Migraine*. Berkeley, CA: Univ of California Press; 1973.
12. Somerville BW. A study of migraine in pregnancy. *Neurology*. 1972;22:824.
13. Raskin NH, Appenzeller O. *Headache*. Philadelphia, PA: WB Saunders; 1980:159.
14. Lashley KS. Patterns of cerebral integration indicated by the scotomas of migraine. *Arch Neurol Psychi*. 1941;46:331.
15. Basser LS. The relation of migraine and epilepsy. *Brain*. 1969;92:285.
16. Rubin PC. Beta-blockers in pregnancy. *N Engl J Med*. 1981;305:1323.
17. Redmond GP. Propranolol and fetal growth retardation. *Semin Perinatol*. 1982;6:142.
18. Couch JR, Ziegler DK, Hassanein R. Amitriptyline in the prophylaxis of migraine. *Neurology*. 1976;26:121.
19. Lance JW. Headache. *Ann Neurol*. 1981;10:1.
20. Kopera H, Pinder R. Psychotomimetic and psychotherapeutic drugs. In: Kuemmerle HP, Brendel K, eds. *Clinical Pharmacology in Pregnancy*. New York, NY: Thieme-Stratton; 1984.
21. Fromm GH, Terrence CF, Chattha AS. Baclofen in the treatment of trigeminal neuralgia: double-blind study and long-term follow-up. *Ann Neurol*. 1984;15:240.
22. Steardo L, Leo A, Marano E. Efficacy of baclofen in trigeminal neuralgia and some other painful conditions: a clinical trial. *Eur Neurol*. 1984;23:51.
23. Farago F. Trigeminal neuralgia: its treatment with two new carbamazepine analogues. *Eur Neurol*. 1987;26:73.
24. Burchiel KJ, Clarke H, Haglund M, Loeser JD. Long-term efficacy of microvascular decompression in trigeminal neuralgia. *J Neurosurg*. 1988;69:35.
25. Pollack IF, Jannetta PJ, Bissonette DJ. Bilateral trigeminal neuralgia: a 14-year experience with microvascular decompression. *J Neurosurg*. 1988;68:559.
26. Morley TP. Case against microvascular decompression in the treatment of trigeminal neuralgia. *Arch Neurol*. 1985;42:801.
27. Cook BR, Jannetta PJ. Tic convulsif: results in 11 cases treated with microvascular decompression of the fifth and seventh cranial nerves. *J Neurosurg*. 1984;61:949.
28. Foley KM, Posner JB. Does pseudotumor cerebri cause the empty sella syndrome? *Neurology*. 1975;25:565.
29. Ropper AH, Marmarou A. Mechanism of pseudotumor in Guillain-Barré syndrome. *Arch Neurol*. 1984;41:259.
30. Commission on Classification and Terminology of the International League Against Epilepsy. Proposal for classification of epilepsies and syndromes. *Epilepsia*. 1981;26:268.
31. Knight AH, Rhind EG. Epilepsy and pregnancy: a study of 153 pregnancies in 59 patients. *Epilepsia*. 1975;16:99.
32. Mattson RH, Cramer JA, Darney PD, et al. Use of oral contraceptives by women with epilepsy. *JAMA*. 1986;256:238.
33. Yerby MS. Problems and management of the pregnant woman with epilepsy. *Epilepsia*. 1987;28:S29.
34. Briggs GG, Freeman RK, Yaffe SJ. *Drugs in Pregnancy and Lactation*. 2nd ed. Baltimore, MD: Williams and Wilkins; 1986:58.
35. Donaldson JO. *Neurology of Pregnancy*. London: WB Saunders; 1989:229.
36. Bjerkedal T. Outcome of pregnancy in women with epilepsy, Norway, 1967 to 1978: congenital malformations. In: Fanz D, Dam M, Richens A, et al, eds. *Epilepsy, Pregnancy and the Child*. New York, NY: Raven Press; 1982.
37. Bertolini R, Kallen B, Mastroiacovo P, Robert E. Anticonvulsant drugs in monotherapy: effect on the fetus. *Europ J Epid*. 1987;3:164.
38. Kaneko S, Otani K, Fukushima Y, et al. Teratogenicity of antiepileptic drugs: analysis of possible risk factors. *Epilepsia*. 1988;29:459.
39. Phelan MC, Pellock JM, Nance WE. Discordant expression of fetal hydantoin syndrome in heteropaternal dizygotic twins. *N Engl J Med*. 1982;307:99.
40. Hanson JW, Smith DW. The fetal hydantoin syndrome. *J Pediatr*. 1975;87:285.
41. Bethenod M, Frederich A. Les enfants des antiepileptiques. *Pediatrie*. 1975;30:227.
42. Myhre SA, Williams R. Teratogenic effects associated with maternal primidone therapy. *J Pediatr*. 1981;99:160.
43. DiLiberti JN, Farndon PA, Dennis NR, et al. The fetal valproate syndrome. *Am J Med Gen*. 1984;19:473.
44. Kelly TE. Teratogenicity of anticonvulsant drugs, III. Radiographic hand analysis of children exposed *in utero* to diphenylhydantoin. *Am J Med Genet*. 1984;19:445.
45. Donaldson JO. *Neurology of Pregnancy*. London: WB Saunders; 1989:246.
46. Deblay MF, Vert P, Andre M, et al. Transplacental vitamin K prevents haemorrhagic disease of infant of epileptic mother. *Lancet*. 1982;1:1247.
47. Pomerance JJ, Teal JG, Gogolok JK, et al. Maternally administered antenatal vitamin K_1: effect on neonatal prothrombin activity, partial thromboplastin time, and intraventricular hemorrhage. *Obstet Gynecol*. 1987;70:235.
48. Delgado-Escueta AV, Bajorek JG. Status epilepticus: mechanism of brain damage and rational management. *Epilepsia*. 1982;23:S29.
49. Dalessio DJ. Seizure disorders and pregnancy. *N Engl J Med*. 1985;312:559.
50. Dinsdale HB. Does magnesium sulfate treat eclamptic seizures? *Arch Neurol*. 1988;45:1360.
51. Kaplan PW, Lesser RP, Fisher RS, et al. No, magnesium sulfate should not be used in treating eclamptic seizures. *Arch Neurol*. 1988;45:1361.
52. Benedetti TJ, Quilligan EJ. Cerebral edema in severe pregnancy-induced hypertension. *Am J Obstet Gynecol*. 1980;137:860.
53. Richards A, Graham D, Bullock R. Clinicopathological study of neurological complications due to hypertensive disorders of pregnancy. *J Neurol Neurosurg Psych*. 1988;51:416.
54. Fredriksson K, Lindvall O, Ingemarsson I, et al. Repeated cranial computed tomographic and magnetic resonance imaging scans in two cases of eclampsia. *Stroke*. 1989;20:547.
55. Sibai BM, Lipshitz MB, Anderson GD, Dilts PV. Reassessment of intravenous $MgSO_4$ therapy in preeclampsia-eclampsia. *Obstet Gynecol*. 1981;57:199.
56. Sadeh M. Action of magnesium sulfate in the treatment of preeclampsia-eclampsia. *Stroke*. 1989;20:1273.
57. Pritchard JK. Management of preeclampsia and eclampsia. *Kidney International*. 1980;18:259.
58. Fraser D, Turner JWA. Myasthenia gravis and pregnancy. *Proc R Soc Med*. 1963;56:379.
59. Plauche WE. Myasthenia gravis in pregnancy. *Am J Obstet Gynecol*. 1964;88:404.
60. Persellin RH. The effect of pregnancy on rheumatoid arthritis. *Bull Rheum Dis*. 1976;27:922.
61. Burrow GN, Ferris TF. *Medical Complications During Pregnancy*. Philadelphia, PA: WB Saunders; 1975:788.
62. Brenner T, Beyth Y, Abramsky O. Inhibitory effect of alpha fetoprotein on the binding of myasthenia gravis antibody to acetylcholine receptor. *Proc Natl Acad Sci USA*. 1980;77:3635.
63. Korn-Lubetzki I, Kahana E, Cooper G, Abramsky O. Activity of multiple sclerosis during pregnancy and puerperium. *Ann Neur*. 1984;16:229.
64. Evron S, Brenner T, Abramsky O. Suppressive effect of pregnancy on the development of experimental allergic encephalomyelitis in rabbits. *Am J Reprod Immunol*. 1984;5:109.
65. Abramsky O, Brenner T, Mizrachi R, Soffer D. Alpha fetoprotein suppresses experimental allergic encephalomyelitis. *J Neuroimmunol*. 1982;2:1.
66. Briggs GG, Freeman RK, Yaffe SJ. *Drugs in Pregnancy and Lactation*. 2nd ed. Baltimore, MD: Williams and Wilkins; 1986:35; 114.
67. Parry GJ, Heiman-Patterson TD. Pregnancy and autoimmune neuromuscular disease. *Semin Neurol*. 1988;8:197.
68. Schapira K, Poskanzer DC, Newell DJ, et al. Marriage, pregnancy and multiple sclerosis. *Brain*. 1966;89:419.
69. Millar JHD, Allison RS, Cheeseman EA, et al. Pregnancy as a factor influencing relapse in disseminated sclerosis. *Brain*. 1959;82:417.
70. Millar JHD. The influence of pregnancy on multiple sclerosis. *Proc R Soc Med*. 1961;54:4.
71. Poser S, Poser W. Multiple sclerosis and gestation. *Neurology*. 1983;33:1422.
72. Thompson DS, Nelson LM, Burns A, et al. The effects of pregnancy in multiple sclerosis: a retrospective study. *Neurology*. 1986;36:1097.
73. Birk K, Smeltzer SC, Rudick R. Pregnancy and multiple sclerosis. *Sem Neurol*. 1988;8:205.
74. Fuchs S, Schmidt-Hopfeld I, Tridente G, Tarrab-Hazdai R. Thymic lymphocytes bear a surface antigen which cross-reacts with acetylcholine receptor. *Nature*. 1980;287:162.
75. Gomez CM, Richman DP. Monoclonal anti-acetylcholine receptor antibodies with differing capacities to induce experimental autoimmune myasthenia gravis. *J Immunol*. 1985;135:234.
76. Fennel DF, Ringel SP. Myasthenia gravis and pregnancy. *Obstet Gynecol Surv*. 1987;41:414.
77. Eden RD, Gall SA. Myasthenia gravis and pregnancy: a reappraisal of thymectomy. *Obstet Gynecol*. 1983;62:328.
78. Ip MSM, So SY, Lam WK, et al. Thymectomy in myasthenia gravis during pregnancy. *Postgrad Med J*. 1986;62:473.
79. Argov Z, Mastaglia FL. Drug therapy: Disorders of neuromuscular transmission caused by drugs. *N Engl J Med*. 1979;301:409.
80. Flacke W. Treatment of myasthenia gravis. *N Engl J Med*. 1973;288:27.
81. Ropper AH. Campylobacter diarrhea and Guillain-Barré syndrome. *Arch Neurol*. 1988;45:655.
82. Sovilla JY, Regli F, Francioli PB. Guillain-Barré syndrome following

campylobacter jejuni enteritis: report of three cases and review of the literature. *Arch Intern Med.* 1988;148:739.
83. Wertman E, Argov Z, Abramsky O. Chronic inflammatory demyelinating polyradiculoneuropathy: features and prognostic factors with corticosteroid therapy. *Eur Neurol.* 1988;28:199.
84. Dyck PJ, Daube J, O'Brien P, et al. Plasma exchange in chronic inflammatory demyelinating polyradiculoneuropathy. *N Engl J Med.* 1986;314:461.
85. Dyck PJ, O'Brien PC, Oviatt KF, et al. Prednisone improves chronic inflammatory demyelinating polyradiculoneuropathy more than no treatment. *Ann Neurol.* 1982;11:136.
86. Dyck PJ, O'Brien P, Swanson C, et al. Combined azathiaprine and prednisone in chronic inflammatory demyelinating polyneuropathy. *Neurology.* 1985;35:1173.
87. Whisnant JP. Epidemiology of stroke: emphasis on transient cerebral ischemic attacks and hypertension. *Stroke.* 1974;5:68.
88. Plum F, Posner J. *The Diagnosis of Stupor and Coma.* 3rd ed. Philadelphia, PA: FA Davis; 1982.
89. Caplan LR, Stein RW. *Stroke—A clinical approach.* Boston, MA: Butterworths; 1986:169.
90. Mohr JP, Caplan LR, Melski J, et al. The Harvard Cooperative Stroke Registry: a prospective registry. *Neurology.* 1978;28:754.
91. Mohr JP. Lacunes. *Stroke.* 1982;13:3.
92. Chester EM, Agamanolis DP, Banker BQ, Victor M. Hypertensive encephalopathy: a clinicopathologic study of 20 cases. *Neurology.* 1978;28:928.
93. Hauser RA, Lacey DM, Knight MR. Hypertensive encephalopathy. Magnetic resonance imaging demonstration of reversible cortical and white matter lesions. *Arch Neurol.* 1988;45:1078.
94. Klonoff DC, Andrews BT, Obana WG. Stroke associated with cocaine use. *Arch Neurol.* 1989;46:989.
95. Lechat P, Mas JL, Lascault G, et al. Prevalence of patent foramen ovale in patients with stroke. *N Engl J Med.* 1988;318:1148.
96. Sundt TM, Whisnant JP. Subarachnoid hemorrhage from intracranial aneurysms: surgical management and natural history of disease. *N Engl J Med.* 1978;299:116.
97. Robinson JL, Hall CS, Sedzimir CB. Arteriovenous malformations, aneurysms, and pregnancy. *J Neurosurg.* 1974;41:63.
98. Wiebers DO. Subarachnoid hemorrhage in pregnancy. *Semin Neurol.* 1988;8:226.
99. Robinson JL, Hall CJ, Sedzimir CB. Subarachnoid hemorrhage in pregnancy. *J Neurosurg.* 1972;36:27.
100. Srinivasan K. Cerebral venous and arterial thrombosis in pregnancy and puerperium: a study of 135 patients. *Angiology.* 1983;34:733.
101. Srinivasan K. Puerperal cerebral venous and arterial thrombosis. *Sem Neurol.* 1988;8:222.
102. Kendall D. Thrombosis of intracranial veins. *Brain.* 1948;71:386.
103. Halpern JP, Morris JGL, Driscoll GL. Anticoagulants and cerebral venous thrombosis. *Aust NZ J Med.* 1985;14:643.
104. Bousser MG, Chiras J, Bories J, et al. Cerebral venous thrombosis: a review of 38 cases. *Stroke.* 1985;16:199.
105. Levine S, Twyman R, Gilman S. The role of anticoagulation in cavernous sinus thrombosis. *Neurology.* 1985;35:S215.
106. Parisi JE, Kim RC, Collins GH, et al. Brain death with prolonged somatic survival. *N Engl J Med.* 1982;306:14.
107. Walker AE. *Cerebral Death.* 3rd ed. Baltimore and Munich: Urban & Schwarzanberg; 1985.
108. Guidelines for the determination of death: report of the medical consultants on the diagnosis of death to the President's commission for the study of ethical problems in medicine and biomedical and behavioral research. *JAMA.* 1981;246:2184.
109. An appraisal of the criteria of cerebral death: a summary statement. A collaborative study. *JAMA.* 1977;237:982.
110. Black PM, Zervas NT. Declaration of brain death in neurosurgical and neurological practice. *Neurosurgery.* 1984;15:170.
111. Kolder VEB, Gallagher J, Parsons MT. Court-ordered obstetrical interventions. *N Engl J Med.* 1987;316:1192.
112. Schrader H, Krogness K, Aakvaag A, et al. Changes of pituitary hormones in brain death. *Acta Neurochir (Wein).* 1980;52:239.
113. Jennett B, Hessett C. Brain death in Britain as reflected in renal donors. *Br Med J.* 1981;283:359.
114. Dillon WP, Lee RV, Tronolone MJ, et al. Life support and maternal brain death during pregnancy. *JAMA.* 1982;248:1089.
115. Field DR, Gates EA, Creasy RK, et al. Maternal brain death during pregnancy: medical and ethical issues. *JAMA.* 1988;260:816.
116. Bernstein IM, Watson M, Simmons GM, et al. Maternal brain death and prolonged fetal survival. *Obstet Gynecol.* 1989;74:434.
117. Lewis BV, Parsons M. Chorea gravidarum. *Lancet.* 1966;1:284.
118. Jonas S, Spagnuolo M, Kloth H. Chorea gravidarum and streptoccal infection. *Obstet Gynecol.* 1972:39:77.
119. Nausieda PA, Grossman BJ, Koller WC, et al. Sydenham chorea: an update. *Neurology* 1980;30:331.
120. Gamboa ET, Isaacs G, Harter DH. Chorea associated with oral contraceptive therapy. *Arch Neurol.* 1971;25:112.
121. Barber PV, Arnold AG, Evans G. Recurrent hormone dependent chorea: effect of estrogens and progestogens. *Clin Endocrinol.* 1976;5:291.
122. Willson P, Preece AA. Chorea gravidarum. *Arch Intern Med.* 1932;49:471.
123. Zegart KN, Schwarz RH. Chorea gravidarum. *Obstet Gynecol.* 1968;32:24.
124. Beresford OD, Graham AM, Chorea gravidarum. *J Obstet Gynaecol Brit Emp.* 1950;57:616.
125. Ichikawa K, Kim RC, Givelber H, Collins G. Chorea gravidarum: report of a fatal case with neuropathological observations. *Arch Neurol.* 1980;37:429.
126. Bird MT, Palkes H, Prensky AL. A follow-up study of Sydenham's chorea. *Neurology* 1976;26:601.
127. Lubbe WF, Walker EB. Chorea gravidarum associated with circulating lupus anticoagulant: successful outcome of pregnancy with prednisone and aspirin therapy. Case report. *Br J Obstet Gynecol.* 1983;90:487.
128. Donaldson IM, Espiner EA. Disseminated lupus erythematosus presenting as chorea gravidarum. *Arch Neurol.* 1971;25:240.
129. Agrawal BL, Foa RF. Collagen vascular disease appearing as chorea gravidarum. *Arch Neurol.* 1982;39:192.
130. Patterson JF. Treatment of chorea gravidarum with haloperidol. *Southern Med J.* 1979;72:1220.
131. Melvin JL, Burnett CN, Johnson EW. Median nerve conduction in pregnancy. *Arch Phys Med Rehab.* 1969;50:75.
132. Gould JS, Wissinger HA. Carpal tunnel syndrome in pregnancy. *South Med J.* 1978;71:144.
133. Voitk AJ, Mueller JC, Farlinger DE, Johnston RU. Carpal tunnel syndrome in pregnancy. *Can Med Assoc J.* 1983;128:277.
134. Tobin SM. Carpal tunnel syndrome in pregnancy. *Am J Obstet Gynecol.* 1971;97:493.
135. Schumacher HR, Dorwart BB, Korzeniowski OM. Occurrence of De Quervain's tendinitis during pregnancy. *Arch Intern Med.* 1985;145:2083.
136. Adour KK. The bell tolls for decompression? *N Engl J Med.* 1975;292:748.
137. Hilsinger RL, Adour KK, Doty HE. Idiopathic facial paralysis, pregnancy, and the menstrual cycle. *Ann Otol Rhinol Laryngol.* 1975;84:433.
138. Wolf SM, Wagner JH, Davidson S, Forsythe A. Treatment of Bell's palsy with prednisone: a prospective, randomized study. *Neurology.* 1978;28:158.
139. Adour KK, Wingerd J, Bell DN, et al. Prednisone treatment for idiopathic facial paralysis (Bell's palsy). *N Engl J Med.* 1972;287:1268.
140. Edelson JG, Nathan H. Meralgia paresthetica: an anatomical interpretation. *Clin Orthop.* 1977;122:255.
141. Ecker AD, Woltman HW. Meralgia paresthetica: a report of one hundred and fifty cases. *JAMA.* 1938;110:1650.
142. Pearson MG. Meralgia paresthetica: with reference to its occurrence in pregnancy. *J Obstet Gynecol Brit Emp.* 1957;64:427.

Chapter Two Hundred

Diseases of the Striated Muscles

Richard Paul Bonfiglio

200

The maintenance of posture and any movement require muscle fiber activity. Muscular contractions result from the activation of motor units. A motor unit comprises a single motor neuron and the muscle fibers it innervates. The number of motor fibers per unit varies depending on the nature of the activity required of the unit. For instance, the intrinsic hand muscles needed for fine movement may have only a few muscle fibers per motor unit. This allows fine, rapid and coordinated movements. Muscles responsible for maintenance of posture and gross movements may have hundreds of muscle fibers per unit. When force is to be exerted, motor units are recruited in a sequential pattern with the smallest units first, followed by progressively larger units. The motor neurons control the number of firing motor units and their sequence, and through the firing rate determine the exerted force. This close relationship between motor units and muscle fibers can make distinguishing pathophysiology between neurologic and muscular diseases difficult.[1,2]

Striated muscle disorders most often selectively affect the proximal musculature. This may reflect the disease process or may stem from the greater forces required of proximal muscles, making their weakness more evident. Fatigue is a common complaint with skeletal muscle disease and can be significantly aggravated by pregnancy. Pain, especially in the low back region, is also a common complaint during pregnancy. Although there are many possible etiologies and contributing factors to back pain so frequently reported in pregnancy, a myofascial etiology is most common. Examination may reveal muscle tenderness and soft tissue tightness.[3]

Laboratory analysis may help to delineate striated muscle disease. Creatine kinase is the best indicator and monitor of muscle cell injury. Other useful tests may include the erythrocyte sedimentation rate, complete blood count, rheumatoid factor, and antinuclear antibody.

Electromyographic (EMG) testing can be performed safely during pregnancy. Needle examination will help define the nature of the motor disease and exclude neurogenic origins. Skeletal muscle disorders frequently produce small amplitude and short duration motor units on standard EMG. These units stem from loss of activity in many muscle fibers comprising the motor unit. Particularly in the inflammatory myopathies, this also may be contributed to by fiber splitting. There also may be evidence of muscle fiber hypersensitivity with positive sharp waves and fibrillation potentials. Nerve conduction tests are usually normal with skeletal muscle disorders.[4]

Muscle biopsy is indicated for definitive diagnosis, especially with some of the more serious muscle disorders like polymyositis. Tissue staining helps to delineate muscle type involvement.[1]

Striated muscle diseases include a variety of myopathies of congenital, inflammatory, metabolic, and endocrine origin. Muscular dystrophies compose a second group of muscle disorders, the most common being Duchenne's, Becker, myotonic, limb-girdle, and facioscapulohumeral. A variety of other miscellaneous striated muscle disorders, including fibrositis, abnormal muscle fiber activity and myotonia, are the remaining conditions.[2]

Striated muscle diseases generally do not reduce the likelihood of pregnancy; however, weakness, fatigue and pain, often associated with these diseases, may complicate pregnancy. Appropriate medical management, including various rehabilitation interventions, may help to reduce the functional implications of these disorders.[3]

MYOPATHIES

Congenital Myopathies

This group of skeletal muscle diseases (including central core disease and nemaline rod disease) are generally static and nonprogressive. However, the neonatal weakness associated with the diseases can lead to contractures and other associated problems.[3] This may complicate the last trimester of pregnancy and the delivery process because of functional limitations and impaired endurance. Management should include appropriate orthotic devices, therapeutic instruction in joint preservation techniques, and energy conservation measures.

Metabolic Myopathies

These diseases are caused by defects in enzymes involved in glycogen and lipid metabolism, including myophosphorylase and acid maltase deficiencies (see Chapters 34 and 35). The clinical presentation usually includes fatigue and recurrent muscle cramps. Myoglobinuria is common. The diagnosis is made by muscle biopsy. Management should emphasize prevention of overexertion, which can lead to muscle injury and cell loss. Afflicted individuals must recognize the limits of their endurance.[5]

Endocrine Myopathies

Some endocrine abnormalities also have been associated with myopathy. An example is hyperthyroidism (see Chapter 40). Prolonged treatment with corticosteroids also can lead to myopathy. Involvement of the proximal muscle is generally the greatest. Correction of the underlying endocrine abnormality usually leads to some improvement in the myopathy.[2]

Toxic Myopathies

Multiple substances that can cause muscle injury have been identified; alcohol appears to be implicated most often (see Chapter 8). Alcoholic myopathy can present acutely, following binge drinking. Symptoms include muscle pains or cramps rather than weakness.[3] Physical examination may reveal muscle tenderness and swelling. Creatine kinase may be elevated. The disease process improves with abstinence. In addition to its many other detrimental effects during pregnancy, excessive alcohol use also should be avoided because of its potential for injury to striated muscle. This is especially the case in already afflicted individuals.[2]

Inflammatory Myopathies

Individuals suffering from inflammatory myopathies often have a genetic predisposition. Viral agents also may play a contributing role and there may be an immunologic component, but the pathogenesis is not well delineated.[6,7] This likely stems from the heterogenicity of the disease. Polymyositis and dermatomyositis generally present with greater proximal than distal symmetric weakness, which is slowly progressive. The electromyogram is characterized by short duration, small amplitude motor units with frequent positive sharp waves, fibrillation potentials, and high frequency discharges.[4] During disease progression, creatine kinase levels often will be elevated dramatically. High-dose corticosteroids remain the drug regimen of choice, with resultant reduction in inflammation. After the inflammatory period, when enzyme levels have normalized, therapeutic exercise may aid in maximizing functional level. During the inflammatory period, judicious physical and occupational therapy can maintain joint mobility and help improve functional status through energy conservation measures.

An increased incidence of fetal death and prematurity has been reported in pregnancies of mothers suffering from dermatomyositis and polymyositis.[6] Medication management can help reduce fetal complications.[7] Pregnancy may result in an exacerbation of disease, especially during the postpartum period.[8] Pregnancy in mothers suffering from dermatomyositis or polymyositis therefore must be considered high-risk for both mother and child.[6,7,9]

Myositis also may be a component of such mixed connective tissue disease as systemic lupus erythematosus and rheumatoid arthritis[10-16] (See also Chapters 51 and 52).

MUSCULAR DYSTROPHIES

Duchenne Muscular Dystrophy

Duchenne muscular dystrophy is the most common of the dystrophies. Since it is an X-linked recessive disorder, it is almost exclusively a male disease. In rare cases, it has been noted in females, either with Turner's syndrome or through the Lyon hypothesis. This occurs because the abnormal recessive gene is expressed because of lack or deactivation of the normal gene. This disease is usually relentless in its progression. There have been no reports of pregnancy in females with this disease. Potential carriers should receive genetic counseling.[17-19]

Myotonic Muscular Dystrophy

Myotonic muscular dystrophy is unusual in its presentation since the associated muscle weakness is greater distally than proximally. It is transmitted as an autosomal dominant trait with variable penetrance, with an incidence of 13 per 100,000 live births.[3] It most often presents as weakness in the hands. Examination reveals the characteristic myotonia with stiffness and difficulty in releasing objects. If weakness is the most significant component, pregnancy can aggravate the condition. On occasion, this leads to the patient's first presentation and to her diagnosis. Deterioration appears greatest during the latter part of the second trimester.[21-23]

Electromyographic examination confirms the diagnosis, with characteristic waxing and waning high-frequency discharges typical of myotonia, and small amplitude and short duration motor units seen in muscle diseases.[24] Medications that stabilize the muscle cell membrane may improve the myotonia, but can increase the functional effect of the weakness. As with all medications, membrane stabilizing drugs should be used very carefully during pregnancy. Patients with myotonic dystrophy also frequently have cardiac conduction blocks and therefore should have serial EKG studies. Patients are also sensitive to neuromuscular junction depolarizing muscle relaxants, which can complicate general anesthesia and therefore should be avoided. These medications can cause sustained myotonia rather than muscle relaxation in these patients.

Pregnancy is complicated by an increased incidence of spontaneous abortions, prematurity, fetal deaths, labor dysfunction, and postpartum hemorrhage.[21] Infants born to mothers with this disease also may suffer from congenital myotonic dystrophy. This occurs when an afflicted mother bears a child with a myotonic dystrophy gene. These children frequently suffer severe respiratory distress, swallowing problems, and diffuse muscle weakness.[22]

Limb-Girdle Muscular Dystrophy

Limb-girdle muscular dystrophy is most likely a collection of disorders with similar clinical presentations. They are characterized by weakness in the proximal pelvic and shoulder girdle musculature. The pattern is otherwise quite variable, including a variety of genetic patterns. An autosomal recessive distribution is common, but many cases appear to be sporadic. The age of onset is variable. The rate of progression is most often slow.

Physical examination demonstrates symmetric, proximal muscle weakness. Useful laboratory testing includes creatine kinase and lactic dehydrogenase with mild elevations of both being characteristic. Muscle biopsy is nonspecific, with variations in fiber size, "moth-eaten" fibers, and fiber splitting. The EMG may demonstrate decreased amplitude and duration motor units with increased polyphasicity, especially in severely affected muscles.[1,2]

Facioscapulohumeral Muscular Dystrophy

Inherited as an autosomal-dominant disease, diagnosis usually is made between ages 10 and 20. Weakness initially involves the facial and shoulder girdle muscles and may result in an inability to whistle, incomplete eye closure during sleep, and difficulty with lifting heavy objects overhead. Weakness later may involve the pelvic girdle musculature, and distal lower limb muscle weakness may lead to foot drop. The degree of weakness and muscle atrophy can be quite varied, probably leading to frequent lack of diagnosis in subtle cases. However, the weakness can be severe enough to interfere with normal daily activities.[2]

Myotonia Congenita

Myotonia (impaired muscle relaxation) is not always associated with dystrophy. Myotonia congenita can be inherited through an autosomal-dominant or recessive pattern. Clinically, there is generally associated stiffness and easy fatiguing. Symptoms often are exacerbated by cold exposure, and the stiffness is usually worse after rest. Diagnosis is confirmed by characteristic abnormalities on electromyographic examination, characterized by waxing and waning amplitude and duration potentials. Muscle biopsy may show the absence of type IIB fibers. Pregnancy may aggravate the fatigue associated with this condition.[24]

Paramyotonia Congenita

This autosomal-dominant disease differs from myotonia congenita clinically by an increase in symptoms with prolonged activity. In addition, cold exposure decreases myotonic discharges, as witnessed electromyographically, even though the associated stiffness increases.[24]

Hypercalemic Periodic Paralysis

This autosomal-dominant disease is characterized by episodes of weakness associated with the elevation of serum potassium. Onset usually is observed early in life. Episodes can be triggered by cold exposure and severe exertion. Electromyographic evaluation reveals small amplitude and short duration motor units, typical of a myopathic disease. Membrane irritability also may be evident. Pregnancy in affected individuals may contribute to electrolyte abnormalities, which in turn can trigger an attack. Myotonia also may be present with this disorder and be aggravated by pregnancy.[1]

Hypocalemic Periodic Paralysis

Onset of this autosomal-dominant disease usually is noted during the teenage years. Episodes of weakness are associated with prolonged exertion and heavy sodium or carbohydrate meals. Serum potassium is low during these episodes, and EMG evaluation reveals reduced amplitude and duration motor units.[4]

Fibrositis, Fibromyalgia, and Myofacial Pain Syndromes

Pain is a frequent experience during pregnancy.[25] There are many contributing factors, including fatigue, increased weight and size, and the demands of daily life. Overexertion frequently leads to discomfort. Back pain is especially prominent in the latter stage of pregnancy.[26] In part, this stems from the mechanical stress placed on the spine by the protuberant abdomen. Although many other structures may contribute to the resultant discomfort, the skeletal muscles most often are responsible for the bulk of the pain and tenderness. The resultant muscle pains can be disabling and result in the pregnancy being a less enjoyable time for the expectant mother. Some individuals with fibrositis or fibromyalgia are particularly prone to muscle pain. They tend to be goal-oriented and perfectionists. It seems that they store day-to-day tensions in their muscles.[26,31,32] While virtually every skeletal muscle can be involved, most frequently in pregnant women the muscles involved are the trapezius, rhomboids, and lumbosacral paraspinals. Trauma, either stemming from an isolated and discrete episode or as the result of cumulative injury, may be a contributing factor to symptom production.[27]

Since pregnancy limits the use of many medications to manage these symptoms, other forms of treatment become more important.[28,39,41] Adequate rest, including periodic breaks during the day, frequently helps to modulate the pain perception. The use of gentle topical heating modalities or of cold provides help to some individuals. Therapeutic massage is also beneficial at times. Therapeutic exercise, especially for gentle stretching and strengthening of the involved muscles, often represents the most important treatment. Such an exercise regimen, however, should be provided only after careful instruction by an experienced physical or occupational therapist. Improper instruction can aggravate the pain rather than relieve it. Therapy should be individualized to the particular needs of a patient. Pain modulation also may be enhanced by the use of transcutaneous electrical nerve stimulation (TENS). This modality should be provided only after careful evaluation by a therapist. Relaxation training, usually done by a psychologist, also may help selected patients.[3,29,30]

Polymyalgia Rheumatica

Polymyalgia rheumatica most often occurs in individuals over 50 years of age. It is, however, much more common in women and can occur during the childbearing years.[35] It is characterized by diffuse arthralgias and myalgias with associated stiffness, especially involving the skeletal and proximal musculature. Systemic symptoms also may be present, including low-grade fever and easy fatiguing. Despite the patient's frequent reporting of significant discomfort, physical examination generally does not present any significant supporting findings. The diagnosis is strongly supported by an elevated erythrocyte sedimentation rate. Other diseases, including rheumatoid arthritis, may have a similar early presentation and should be considered in the differential diagnosis. In addition, temporal (giant cell) arteritis has been associated with polymyalgia rheumatica.[36,37]

REFERENCES

1. Brooke MH. *A Clinician's View of Neuromuscular Diseases.* 2nd ed. Baltimore, MD: Williams & Wilkins; 1986.
2. Walton J. *Disorders of Voluntary Muscle.* London: Churchill Livingstone; 1981.
3. DeLisa JA: *Rehabilitation Medicine: Principles and Practice.* Philadelphia, PA: JB Lippincott; 1988.
4. Johnson EWJ. Motor unit potentials in disease. In: *Practical Electromyography.* 2nd ed. Baltimore, MD: Williams & Wilkins, 1988.
5. Dimuro S. Disorders of lipid metabolism in muscle. *Muscle Nerve.* 1980;3:369.
6. England MJ. Dermatomyositis in pregnancy. *J Reprod Med.* 1986;31:633.
7. Rosenzweig BA. Primary idiopathic polymyositis and dermatomyositis complicating pregnancy: diagnosis and management. *Obstet Gynecol Survey.* 1989;44:162.
8. Kitridou RC: Pregnancy in mixed connective tissue disease, poly/dermatomyositis and scleroderma. *Clin Exp Rheum.* 1988;6:173.
9. Guteirrez G. Polymyositis/dermatomyositis and pregnancy. *Arth Rheum.* 1984;27:291.
10. Mintz G. Pregnancy in patients with rheumatic diseases: dermatomyositis. *Rheum Dis Clin NA.* 1989;15:375.
11. Caro I. Dermatomyositis as a systemic disease. *Med Clin NA.* 1989;73:1181.
12. Houck W. Polymyositis in pregnancy. *J Reprod Med.* 1987;32:208.
13. Mor-Yosef S. Collagen diseases in pregnancy. *Obstet Gynecol Surv.* 1984;39:67.
14. Bauer KA. Polymyositis complicating pregnancy. *Arch Intern Med.* 1979;139:449.
15. Barnes AB. Childhood dermatomyositis and pregnancy. *Am J Obstet Gynecol.* 1983;146:335.
16. King CR. Dermatomyositis and pregnancy. *Obstet Gynecol.* 1985;66:589.
17. Darras BT. Prenatal diagnosis and detection of carriers with DNA probes in Duchenne's muscular dystrophy. *N Engl J Med.* 1987;316:985.
18. Cole CG. Prenatal testing for Duchenne and Becker muscular dystrophy. *Lancet.* 1988;1:262.
19. Forrest SM. Effective strategy for prenatal prediction of Duchenne and Becker muscular dystrophy. *Lancet.* 1987;2:1294.
20. Emery AEH. Duchenne muscular dystrophy: genetic aspects. *Br Med Bull.* 1980;36:117–122.
21. Hilliard GD. Myotonic muscular dystrophy in pregnancy. *S Med J.* 1977;70:446.
22. Sun SF. Myotonic dystrophy: obstetric and neonatal complications. *S Med J.* 1985;78:823.
23. Nazir MA. Myotonic dystrophy in pregnancy: prenatal, neonatal, and maternal considerations. *J Reprod Med.* 1984;29:168.
24. Nielsen V. Electromyographic distinction between paramyotonia congenita and myotonia congenita: effect of cold. *Neurology.* 1982;32:827.
25. Fast A. Low-back pain in pregnancy. *Spine.* 1987;12:368.
26. Simons DG, Travell JG. Myofascial pain syndromes. In: Wall PD, Melzack R, eds. Edinburgh: Churchill Livingstone; 1984:263.
27. Simons, DG. Myofascial trigger points: a need for understanding. *Arch Phys Med Rehabil.* 1981;62:97.
28. Berg G. Low back pain during pregnancy. *Obstet Gynecol.* 1988;71:71.
29. Rubin D. Myofascial trigger point syndromes: an approach to management. *Arch Phys Med Rehabil.* 1981;62:107.
30. Melzak R. Low-back pain during labor. *Am J Obstet Gynecol.* 1987;156:901.
31. Wolfe F. Fibrositis, fibromyalgia, and musculoskeletal disease: the current status of the fibrositis syndrome. *Arch Phys Med Rehabil.* 1988;69:527.
32. Simons DG. Myofascial pain syndromes: where are we? where are we going? *Arch Phys Med Rehabil.* 1988;69:207.
33. Boissonnault JS. Incidence of diastasis recti abdominis during the childbearing years. *Phys Ther.* 1988;68:1082.
34. Calguneri M. Changes in joint laxity occurring during pregnancy. *Ann Rheum Dis.* 1982;41:126.
35. Chuang TY. Polymyalgia rheumatica: a 10-year epidemiologic and clinical study. *Ann Intern Med.* 1982;97:672.
36. Schumacher HR. Polymyalgia rheumatica and temporal (giant cell) arteritis. In: *Primer on the Rheumatic Diseases.* 9th ed. Atlanta, GA: Arthritis Foundation; 1988:
37. Hunder GG. Giant cell arteritis and polymyalgia rheumatica. *Clin Rheum Dis.* 1985;11:471.
38. Cecere FA. The interaction of pregnancy and the rheumatic diseases. *Clin Rheum Dis.* 1981;7:747.
39. Maly BJ. Rehabilitation principles in the care of gynecologic and obstetric patients. *Arch Phys Med Rehabil.* 1980;61:78.
40. Fowler WM. Rehabilitation management of muscular dystrophy and related disorders: the role of exercise. *Arch Phys Med Rehabil.* 1982;63:319.
41. Gleeson PB. Obstetrical physical therapy. *Phys Ther.* 1988;68:1699.

PART XXI Critical Care, Trauma, and Surgery in Pregnancy

Baha M. Sibai, Section Editor

Chapter Two Hundred and One

Obstetric Anesthesia

Dinesh N. Chauhan, Jaya Ramanathan, and Baha M. Sibai

201

Through the ages, women have sought relief from the pain of childbirth. In 1847, Sir James Simpson administered ether and chloroform to parturients. In 1853, John Snow administered chloroform to Queen Victoria for the birth of her eighth child, Prince Leopold. While Mueller described pudendal block in 1908, the research was not published until 1916 by King. August Bier performed the first spinal anesthesia in 1898. In 1901, Sicard and Cathelin independently described epidural caudal injection. In 1921, Pages described lumbar epidural anesthesia, a technique first used in obstetrics by Graffagnino and Seyler in 1938 and as a continuous technique by Flowers, Hellman, and Hingson in 1949.

Labor pain arises primarily from the nociceptors in uterine and perineal structures. Nerve fibers transmitting the pain sensation during the first stage of labor travel with the sympathetic fibers and enter the neuraxis at the tenth, eleventh, and twelfth thoracic and first lumbar spinal segments.[1] These fibers synapse in, and connect with, other ascending and descending fibers in the dorsal horn. In the late first and second stages of labor, pain impulses increasingly arise from pain-sensitive areas in the perineum and travel by way of the pudendal nerve to enter the neuraxis at the second, third, and fourth sacral segments.[1] Labor pain adversely affects the mother and the fetus in a number of ways. Maternal hyperventilation during uterine contractions usually is followed by hypoventilation and hypoxemia between contractions. Increased catecholamine secretion leads to decreased uterine blood flow and dysfunctional labor.[2,3] Maternal minute ventilation, oxygen consumption, cardiac output, and blood pressure increase further.[4] All these factors affect the well-being of the fetus.

CHOICE OF ANALGESIA FOR LABOR AND DELIVERY

Narcotics

The commonly used drugs include narcotics (eg, meperidine, morphine, and butorphanol) and sedatives and tranquilizers (eg, barbiturates, phenothiazines, and benzodiazepines). All narcotics produce dose-related respiratory depression and exacerbate maternal hypoxemia. Narcotics also can induce nausea, vomiting, and excessive sedation in the mother and respiratory depression in the neonate. Narcotics usually are administered for blunting the mild pain of early labor.

Regional Analgesia

Lumbar epidural analgesia provides unsurpassed pain relief for labor and, by eliminating the pain and stress, lowers maternal catecholamine levels and prevents an increase in maternal oxygen consumption.[5] In patients with prolonged incoordinate labor, epidural analgesia enhances uterine contractility and establishes a regular labor pattern.[6,7]

A thorough knowledge of the pharmacology of local anesthetics is important. Local anesthetics are broadly divided into two categories: esters and amides. The esters (cocaine, prilocaine, tetracaine, and chloroprocaine) have a short duration of action because they are metabolized by serum pseudocholinesterase; the amides (lidocaine, prilocaine, bupivacaine, mepivacaine, and etidocaine) are metabolized in the liver and thus have a longer half-life. The placental transfer varies with the lipid solubility, degree of ionization, protein binding, and molecular weight of

TABLE 201–1. PROPERTIES OF SELECTED LOCAL ANESTHETICS

Drug	Group	Percentage Ionized at pH 7.4	Percentage of Maternal Protein Binding	Fetal-Maternal Ratio	Half-Life	
					Maternal	Neonatal
Chloroprocaine	Ester	95	—	0.92	21 sec	43 sec
Bupivacaine	Amide	83	95	0.25	9 hr	8 hr
Lidocaine	Amide	76	56	0.55	2 hr	3 hr
Etidocaine	Amide	67	94	0.20	3 hr	—
Mepivacaine	Amide	61	65	0.70	2 hr	9 hr

From Conclin KA, Murad SHN[72] with permission.

local anesthetics. Some of the commonly used local anesthetic agents, dosages, elimination half-life, and other information are listed in Tables 201–1 and 201–2.

Chloroprocaine (Nesacaine) has most of the attributes of an ideal local anesthetic agent for obstetric use. Onset of action is rapid, and it produces excellent sensory and motor block. However, chloroprocaine is hydrolyzed rapidly by serum pseudocholinesterase, and thus has a short duration of action (30–40 minutes). A 2% concentration provides adequate relief for first-stage labor pain. A higher concentration (3%) is needed for analgesia and perineal muscle relaxation during the second stage.

Lidocaine (Xylocaine) provides reliable analgesia and is used extensively for labor pain relief. Although placental transfer is appreciable, Apgar scores are not affected. Carbonated lidocaine has been used for some years in Canada, but in spite of its rapid onset and excellent analgesic quality, it is not yet available in the United States.

Etidocaine, a congener of lidocaine, is highly protein-bound with minimal placental transfer. It produces profound motor block, whereas the quality of sensory blockade is less impressive. This preferential motor block makes it a poor choice for managing labor analgesia.

Mepivacaine (Carbocaine) has slightly longer duration than lidocaine. However, because mepivacaine crosses the placental barrier in significant amounts and has a prolonged half-life in the neonate, its use in obstetric practice has declined.

Bupivacaine (Marcaine), introduced in 1963, is highly protein-bound, produces excellent analgesia, and has a long duration of action. In dilutions down to 0.125%, it provides effective pain relief for first-stage labor. However, the onset of analgesia is slow and can take 30 minutes for adequate blockade to occur.

TABLE 201–2. LOCAL ANESTHETIC AGENTS FOR EPIDURAL ANESTHESIA

Drug	Concentration (%)	Onset (Min)	Duration (Min)
Chloroprocaine	2–3	5–15	30–40
Lidocaine	1–2	5–15	60–120
Mepivacaine	1–2	5–15	60–150
Prilocaine	1–3	5–15	60–150
Bupivacaine	0.25–0.5	10–20	20–240
Etidocaine	1–1.5	5–15	120–240

From Curran MA[73] with permission.

Prilocaine was introduced with the hope that its rapid breakdown and low toxicity would make it useful for obstetrics. Unfortunately, the phenolic breakdown product, alpha-ortho-toluidine, causes methemoglobinemia in the neonate. It thus is not a popular drug for obstetric uses.

EPIDURAL ANESTHESIA

Prior to administering epidural anesthesia, it is essential to ensure that all resuscitative equipment such as Ambu bags, laryngoscopes, endotracheal tubes, suction apparatus, and drugs (eg, ephedrine and pentothal) are readily available.

Administering a minimum of 1 L of crystalloid solution is essential to prevent hypotension after establishing epidural analgesia. The following factors should be kept in mind:

1. Administering large volumes of dextrose-containing solutions increases maternal serum glucose levels. The fetus responds to this glucose load by increased insulin secretion and, at birth, can become hypoglycemic. Crystalloids devoid of dextrose[8] should be used for hydration prior to regional anesthesia.
2. Patients with severe preeclampsia and cardiac disease might not tolerate rapid administration of large volumes of fluids. Their central venous pressure or pulmonary artery wedge pressure should be monitored.

Once labor is well established (cervical dilatation of 5–6 cm in a nullipara or 4–5 cm in a multipara) with contractions lasting for 1 minute and occurring 3 minutes apart, a continuous lumbar epidural analgesia can be established by the loss-of-resistance technique. The patient's position is an important factor for successfully placing the epidural catheter. Obtaining maximal spinal flexion in the laboring parturient is often difficult and is limited by a gravid uterus. The patient can be in either the sitting or lateral position. The anatomic landmarks are as follows: the spinal cord ends at level L2 with the dural sac ending at the level of S1-S2. Surrounding the dural sac and limited by the dura mater on one side and the periosteum of the vertebral bodies and ligamentum flavum on the other is the epidural space, which extends from the foramen magnum to the sacral hiatus. The third lumbar intervertebral space usually is chosen for the epidural as this happens to be the widest space. Correctly identifying the midline is important. The selected entry point is infiltrated with a small amount of local anesthetic. An 18-gauge needle then is inserted through the skin wheal to create a skin opening large enough to allow passage of the epidural needle. The epidural needle then is advanced to the point where the interspinous ligament is entered. At this point, the stylet is removed and a syringe, filled with a few milliliters of either air or saline, is attached to the needle. The needle with the syringe now is advanced as a unit, a few millimeters at a time, until the ligamentum flavum is pierced and the epidural space is entered. As soon as the needle enters the epidural space, the contents of the syringe can be injected easily without resistance.

The epidural space measures only 5 mm at its widest part (the lumbar epidural space), and the advancing needle can overshoot the distance easily, pierce the dura, and enter the subarachnoid space. Therefore, it is important that the advancing movement of the epidural needle be delicately controlled. An epidural catheter then is threaded through the needle and advanced 3–4 cm into the epidural space. The needle is removed and the catheter is taped in place.

After negative aspiration, 3 mL of 1% lidocaine is injected as a test dose to ensure that the catheter has not entered the subarachnoid space or a blood vessel. Further increments of local anesthetic are administered to obtain a segmental block of T10-L1. Blood pressure should be determined frequently and if hypotension occurs (a fall in systolic pressure of 20–30% from base line values), it should be treated with fluids, left uterine displacement, and intravenous ephedrine in doses of 2.5–5.0 mg. Oxygen should be administered by face mask. Ephedrine is the preferred drug for treating hypotension in obstetric patients because it maintains the uterine artery blood flow and restores the maternal mean arterial pressure.[9]

All local anesthetics can be administered as continuous infusions, and several types of infusion pumps are available. Typically, the infusion concentration is 50% less than the initial concentration used to establish the epidural block. Adding small doses of selected narcotics such as fentanyl to the infusion permits the use of a weaker solution of local anesthetic with better analgesia and less motor block.

Subarachnoid Block

Because of the ease of administration, rapid onset of anesthesia, and low-dose requirements, subarachnoid block has remained a popular form of anesthetic in obstetrics. The major contraindications are listed in Table 201–3.

Prior to admistering spinal anesthesia, parturients should be hydrated with dextrose-free crystalloid solution and all resuscitative equipment should be readily available.

A variety of positions and approaches can be used to achieve a spinal block. The subarachnoid space can be entered with a spinal needle below the L2-L3 interspace. Using a blunted-tipped, 25-gauge needle (Sprotte needle) decreases the incidence of postdural puncture headache to less than 1%.[10] The midline approach is used most often. Once the subarachnoid space is entered, the cerebrospinal fluid must flow freely through the needle. The local anesthetic then is injected through the needle. Approximately 1 mL of 10% dextrose solution is added per mL of anesthetic solution, all of which then is injected into the subarachnoid space. Epinephrine (1:200,000) can be added to the local anesthetic to prolong duration of the block. The duration of anesthesia depends on the choice of agent, the dose injected, and the presence of vasoconstrictor.

Lidocaine is supplied as a 5% solution containing 7.5% dextrose, and a dose of 25–30 mg of 5% lidocaine is sufficient for vaginal deliveries or for assisted delivery with outlet forceps. Cesarean section can be performed under spinal anesthesia by using 70–80 mg of 5% lidocaine. Tetracaine is supplied as a 1% isobaric solution and as tetracaine crystals, 20 mg/ampul. A hyperbaric solution is prepared by mixing equal volumes of the 1% solution with 10% dextrose. While 4 mg of tetracaine are sufficient for vaginal deliveries, about 7–9 mg of tetracaine are required for cesarean sections. Bupivacaine, which is supplied as a 0.75% solution containing 8.25% dextrose, also can be used for spinal anesthesia.

TABLE 201–3. CONTRAINDICATIONS FOR REGIONAL ANESTHESIA IN OBSTETRICS

Absolute Contraindications	Relative Contraindications
Patient refusal	Active systemic infection
Coagulopathy	Preexisting or evolving neurologic disease
Maternal hypovolemia	Acute fetal distress
	Abnormal anatomy

Regional Anesthesia for Cesarean Section

A higher dematomal level (T_4) and intense motor and sensory block are essential for a cesarean section. Local anesthetics in larger volumes and higher concentrations are required for epidural anesthesia. Appropriate modification of the dosages of local anesthetics is required to obtain the desired level of block. Adequate prehydration is essential to prevent hypotension. In addition, the left uterine displacement should be maintained and oxygen should be administered through face mask. After delivery, small doses of benzodiazepines such as diazepam or midazolam and a narcotic such as fentanyl can be administered.

COMPLICATIONS OF REGIONAL ANESTHESIA

Complications and their frequency are listed in Table 201–4; some of the complications are described here.

TABLE 201–4. COMPLICATIONS OF EPIDURAL AND SPINAL ANALGESIA

	Approximate Frequency	
Category	Epidural	Spinal
Incomplete analgesia	5/100	5/100
Failed block	3–5/100	2/100
Hypotension	5–25/100	15–30/100
Intravenous catheter	5/100	N/A
Wet tap	0.5–2/100	N/A
Unintentional spinal block	1/1000	N/A
Neurologic damage		
Transient	3/20,000	3–5/20,000
Permanent	1/50,000	1/50,000
Seizures	1/5000	N/A
Death	?	?

From Hood DD[74] with permission.

Hypotension caused by the combination of sympathetic block and aorta-caval compression by the gravid uterus is the most common complication following regional anesthesia. It occurs more quickly and precipitously with spinal anesthesia compared with epidural anesthesia due to the more rapid development of the sympathetic block. The prevention of this complication was discussed above. Administration of a minimum of 1 L of crystalloids prior to the establishment of the epidural anesthesia is necessary. In addition, left uterine displacement should be maintained and oxygen should be administered through face mask. Intravenous ephedrine frequently is used to treat hypotension following regional block.

Unintentional intravascular injection of local anesthetic can result in grand mal seizure and cardiorespiratory arrest. Treatment consists of immediate tracheal intubation and controlled ventilation with 100% oxygen. Full cardiac resuscitation should be performed, especially when the seizure and arrest follow the accidental intravascular injection of bupivacaine. To avoid this catastrophic occurrence, local anesthetics are always administered in small, incremental doses with frequent aspiration of the epidural catheter and close monitoring for such symptoms and signs as tinnitus, dizziness, and restlessness.

Massive subarachnoid injection of a local anesthetic during epidural anesthesia or excessive dose of a local anesthetic during spinal anesthesia will result in *total spinal block.* This situation should be handled expeditiously with tracheal intubation and positive pressure ventilation. In addition, rapid administration of fluids and vasopressors is essential to treating the hypotension and cardiovascular collapse. Atropine in doses of 0.4 mg should be administered intravenously to treat bradycardia.

Postlumbar puncture headache usually follows the accidental perforation of the dura with a 18-gauge needle during epidural block. This headache also can occur following a subarachnoid block for vaginal delivery or cesarean section. The headache usually appears when the patient becomes ambulatory and usually is relieved by assuming supine position. Because the headache can be incapacitating and severe, administering an epidural blood patch usually provides immediate and effective relief of the headache.[10-12] The technique involves positioning an epidural needle in the epidural space while an assistant draws a sample of 10–12 mL of venous blood under aseptic precautions. This sample is injected into the epidural space slowly. This procedure can be performed on an outpatient basis and usually provides immediate relief with a success rate of 94–100%.

CONTROVERSIES ON THE CHOICE OF LOCAL ANESTHETICS

Currently, much controversy exists over the choice of local anesthetics for epidural anesthesia for labor pain relief and cesarean section. Possible side effects are as follows:

1. Cardiotoxicity of bupivacaine
2. Neurotoxicity of chloroprocaine
3. Adverse neurobehavioral effects of lidocaine
4. Adverse action of epinephrine

Bupivacaine Cardiotoxicity

It is common knowledge among obstetric anesthesiologists that accidental intravascular injection of bupivacaine can cause severe cardiovascular depression. The landmark editorial by Albright alleged that bupivacaine is more cardiotoxic than lidocaine.[13] Albright reported that between 1973 and 1985, there were 44 maternal cardiac arrests following accidental intravascular injection of bupivacaine. He also reported 30 maternal deaths, 7 recoveries with severe neurologic deficits, and 7 full recoveries. In 1984, the Food and Drug Administration (FDA) declared that, because of the risk of cardiac arrest, 0.75% bupivacaine should no longer be used in obstetrics. Since the initial reports, numerous animal experiments have shown that bupivacaine is more cardiotoxic than lidocaine and, in the presence of hypercarbia, hypoxia, and acidosis, bupivacaine cardiotoxicity is enhanced significantly.[14-18] Both bupivacaine and lidocaine block cardiac sodium channels and the conduction of impulses. Using voltage clamp experiements with guinea pig papillary muscles, Clarkson and Hondeghem[19] showed that lidocaine enters the cardiac sodium channels quickly and exits quickly, whereas bupivacaine is a "fast in" and "slow out" agent. They concluded that bupivacaine is a potentially dangerous cardiac poison.

Despite its cardiotoxicity, bupivacaine is still widely used for labor analgesia. In concentrations as low as 0.125%, it provides excellent analgesia without causing motor block. As with all other local anesthetics, it is important to avoid injections of large boluses of bupivacaine through the epidural catheter; instead, small incremental doses should be injected with frequent aspiration of the catheter.

Neurotoxicity of 2-Chloroprocaine

Since its introduction in 1953, 2-chloroprocaine (Nesacaine) has been a popular local anesthetic agent for epidural use in obstetrics. However, in the early 1980s, several case reports[20-22] described neurologic damage following such use of 2-chloroprocaine. (Studies of neurotoxicity in animals have yielded conflicting results.[23,24])

The neurotoxicity of 2-chloroprocaine may relate to several factors. Commercial 2-chloroprocaine has a low pH (3.0). It contains the highest concentration of the antioxidant sodium bisulfite (0.2% vs 0.05% in other local anesthetics). Recently Gissen et al[25], studying the neurotoxicity of 2-chloroprocaine alone, the antioxidant sodium bisulfite, and the pH of the solution, concluded that 2-chloroprocaine itself was not neurotoxic but that the bisulfite was a low pH liberated molecular sulfur dioxide. In nerve tissue, SO_2 was converted to sulfurous acid, which caused the neurologic deficits. Other factors such as the effects of introducing large volumes of local anesthetics into epidural or subarachnoid spaces[26] and causing reduced spinal cord blood flow, severe systemic hypotension resulting in anterior spinal artery syndrome, and cauda equina syndrome also may play a part in causing neurologic defects. In 1980, the FDA held a hearing to review and discuss the neurotoxicity of all local anesthetics. Based on all available information, the hearings concluded that there was no evidence to show 2-chloroprocaine is more neurotoxic than other local anesthetic agents and no drug regulatory action was indicated at that time. 2-Chloroprocaine still is used widely for epidural anesthesia in parturients.

Lidocaine and Neonatal Neurobehavior Scores

Lidocaine is devoid of cardiotoxicity and neurotoxicity. It has stood the test of time and is probably the safest local anesthetic agent for obstetric use. A study by Scanlon et al[27] in the mid-1970s showed that the early neonatal neurobehavior scores (ENNS) were significantly lower in those babies whose mothers received epidural anesthesia with lidocaine. Since then, several reports[28-30], have been published showing that, when properly administered, lidocaine does not depress ENNS.

The Use of Epinephrine

Epinephrine usually is added to local anesthetics to prolong the duration of action and decrease systemic absorption. In addition, it also is used to detect unintentional intravascular placement of the epidural needle or catheter. In this situation, a dose of 3 mL of local anesthetic with 5 μg/mL of epinephrine results in an immediate increase in the maternal heart rate.

The use of epinephrine in obstetrics is controversial. Animal studies[31] have shown that intravenous epinephrine caused a transient but significant fall in uterine blood flow. In addition, epinephrine can cause decreased uterine activity and prolonged labor due to the beta-2 sympathomimetic effects. However, Abboud et al[32] have shown that the addition of epinephrine to epidural lidocaine does not affect maternal or neonatal outcome adversely. Albright et al[33] have shown that in humans, the intervillous blood flow remains unaltered by the use of epinephrine-containing local anesthetic solutions in parturients.

In summary, the use of epinephrine-containing local anesthetics in healthy parturients seldom causes any adverse maternal or neonatal effects. However, epinephrine should be avoided in patients with severe preeclampsia, heart disease, or thyrotoxicosis.

EPIDURAL ANESTHESIA AND PROGRESS OF LABOR

First Stage of Labor

Even in the 1980s, studies suggested that epidural anesthesia prolonged the first stage of labor.[34,35] They also indicated that when the block was initiated early in the first stage of labor, there was marked prolongation of the duration of first stage of labor.[36,37] However, most of these studies were performed with mothers in supine position, which probably caused aortocaval compression and invariably decreased uterine perfusion and depressed uterine activity. In addition, in many of the earlier studies, a higher concentration of local anesthetics was used, and epinephrine was added to the local anesthetics. All these factors, rather than the epidural anesthesia itself, could have caused a prolonged first stage of labor. Several other researchers[38-40], studying the effect of segmental lumbar epidural anesthesia during the first stage of labor, have shown that, with the use of lower concentrations of local anesthetics devoid of epinephrine and with the avoidance of hypotension due to aortocaval compression, epidural anesthesia has no significant effect on uterine contractility or progress of labor. In addition, epidural anesthesia improves the labor pattern and accelerates labor in patients with prolonged and uncoordinated labor patterns.

Second Stage of Labor

In studies in the early 1980s, researchers reported prolonged second-stage labor and an increased incidence of forceps delivery in patients receiving epidural anesthesia for labor pain relief. The proposed reasons were abolition of the bearing-down reflex and decreased release of oxytocin in these patients.[41,42] However, more recent randomized, prospective studies have shown that, when properly administered, epidural anesthesia is not associated with a higher incidence of forceps delivery or prolonged second stage.[43,44]

GENERAL ANESTHESIA

General anesthesia for cesarean section is required when rapid delivery of the fetus is indicated, such as in fetal distress, cord prolapse, or when there are absolute or relative contraindications for the administration of a regional anesthesia (eg, coagulopathy, infection, severe maternal hemorrhage, ongoing neurologic diseases, anatomic abnormalities of the lumbar spine, and patient refusal for regional anesthesia). Rapid administration of general anesthesia to a pregnant woman involves creating a situation in which the mother is rapidly made unconscious, apneic, and paralyzed while maternal (and fetal) oxygenation is maintained by expeditiously securing the airway with a tracheal tube (within 30 seconds). The anesthesiologist responsible for this should be competent, experienced, and thoroughly familiar with the unique problems involved in the anesthetic management of pregnant patients.

A study[45] of the causes of maternal mortality in the United States from 1974 to 1978 has shown that anesthetic complications account for 5% of all maternal deaths. Although the number of maternal deaths due to infection, preeclampsia, and obstetric hemorrhage has declined, the anesthesia-related maternal death rate has simply kept pace with the overall reduction in maternal mortality rate.[46] The Confidential Enquiries into Maternal Deaths in England and Wales (CEMD 1979–1981) has shown that the number of maternal fatalities following emergency cesarean section is several times higher compared with those fatalities following elective cesarean section.[47]

Maternal complication rate was 18.5% for emergency cesarean section compared with 4.7% for elective cesarean section.[46] The majority of the fatalities following anesthesia was related to airway management (eg, difficult intubation and pulmonary aspiration of gastric contents). Another interesting finding from the CEMD report is that from 1970 to 1978[46], the number of maternal deaths related to complications from general anesthesia was roughly 10 times higher compared with number of deaths from regional anesthesia. It thus is evident that administration of general anesthesia in parturients is a challenge, and the anesthesiologist should be thoroughly familiar with the anesthetic implications of maternal physiologic changes during pregnancy, labor, and delivery. Some of these points are discussed below.

PREVENTION OF PULMONARY ASPIRATION OF GASTRIC CONTENTS

Parturients are highly susceptible for aspiration of gastric contents for the following reasons: In pregnancy, the stomach and intestines are progressively displaced cephalad by the gravid uterus, so that the stomach empties more slowly. In addition, the onset of labor and administration of drugs such as narcotics and tocolytic agents also retard the stomach's emptying. During pregnancy, lower esophageal sphincter tone is decreased, which leads to gastric reflux and heartburn. The increased secretion of the hormone gastrin increases gastric acidity. These factors, combined with maternal apprehension, pain, starvation, and other risk factors such as hydramnios, diabetes, and morbid obesity, exacerbate the risk of aspirating gastric contents.

Numerous laboratory and clinical investigations[48,49] have shown that aspiration of gastric contents with pH less than 2.5 and a volume of more than 0.4 mL/kg places the pregnant patient at a high risk for developing aspiration pneumonitis, and measures should be undertaken to prevent this catastrophe.

Antacid Prophylaxis

During the 1970s, administering particulate antacids containing calcium, aluminum, and magnesium salts was popular. However, a study by Gibbs et al[50] showed that aspirating particulate antacids caused severe pulmonary shunting and hypoxia. An acceptable alternative is to administer nonparticulate antacids such as 0.3 M sodium citrate, which effectively neutralizes the gastric acid and elevates the pH above 2.5. However, because of the short duration of action (<20 minutes)[51], this antacid should be administered immediately prior to, or within 20 minutes of, inducing general anesthesia. Certain points should be kept in mind:

1. Antacids will not protect against aspirating solid material.
2. Because antacids may not neutralize all the acid when large volumes of gastric fluid are present, they can give a false sense of security.
3. Because antacids can cause a rebound increase in gastric acid production, their administration should be continued regularly once started.

Histamine$_2$-Receptor Blocking Agents

Both cimetidine and ranitidine effectively decrease gastric acidity and volume. However, unlike cimetidine, ranitidine does not inhibit the cytochrome P450 system in the liver and so is the preferred drug for use in pregnancy.[52,53] In addition, ranitidine is more potent than cimetidine and has a longer duration of action (6 hours). The usual dose of ranitidine is 150 mg orally the night before surgery for elective cesarean section and 50 mg intramuscularly an hour before surgery. For emergency cesarean section, administration of sodium citrate just prior to induction affords immediate protection, whereas H_2 receptor blockers offer protection from aspiration at the time of emergence from the anesthetic when the patient is extubated.

Antiemetics

Metoclopramide in doses of 10 mg intravenously increases gastric emptying[54] and raises gastroesophageal sphincter tone. However, its effectiveness in reducing the risk of aspiration in parturients, especially those who received narcotics, has not been established yet.

Preoxygenation of the mother before induction of general anesthesia is essential. Maternal oxygen consumption is 20% above that for nonpregnant women, functional redual capacity is decreased (20%), and the A-a gradient is increased. Therefore, the oxygen reserve in the mother is decreased, and so arterial desaturation that normally occurs during the period of apnea and intubation (150 mm Hg drop in PaO_2 values from base line in parturients as opposed to 50 mm Hg fall in PaO_2 in nonpregnant patients) accelerates. Preoxygenation of a mother 3–5 minutes effectively denitrogenates the lungs, increases her oxygen reserve, and delays arterial desaturation. A 1985 study[55] has shown that four maximal deep breaths of 100% oxygen will cause the same increase in maternal PaO_2 as achieved by 3–5 minutes of breathing 100% oxygen. However, it is not known if the four-breath technique offers the same protection in cases of prolonged apnea due to unanticipated problems during intubation.

In the case of difficult intubation, anesthesiologists routinely inspect the patient's airway to assess ease of intubation prior to general anesthesia. Intubation is usually diffi-

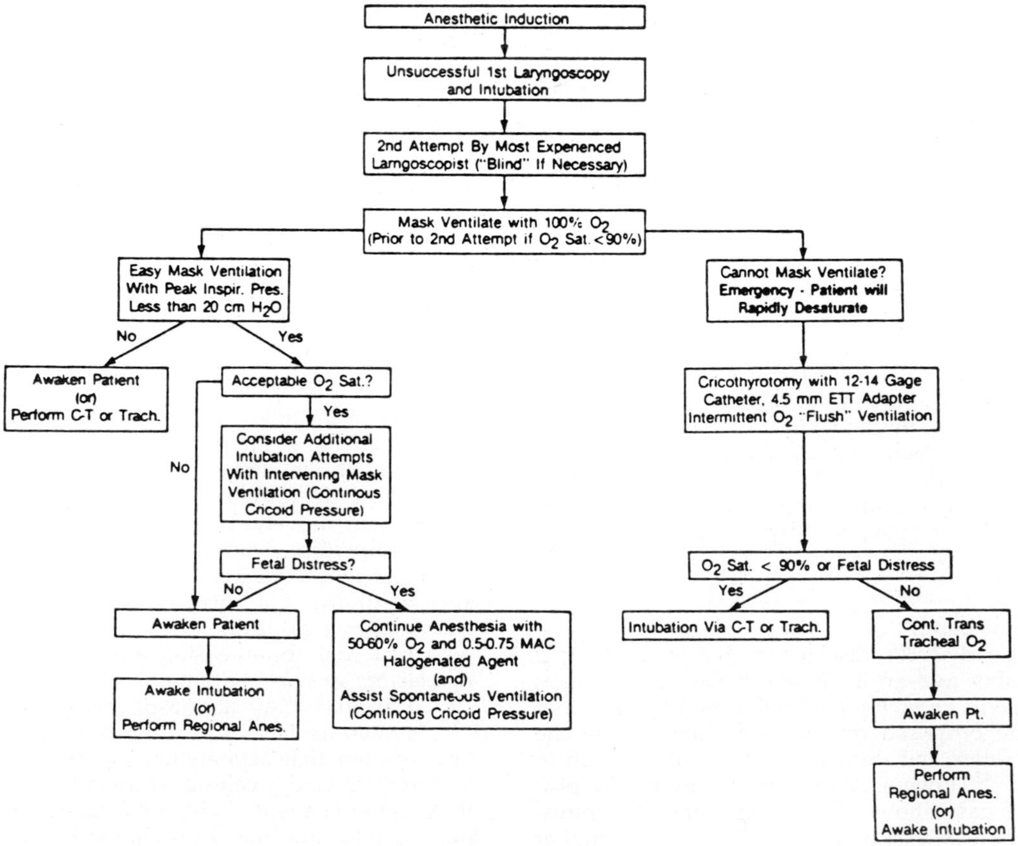

Figure 201–1 A plan of action for unanticipated difficult intubation in pregnant patients. (*From Hood DD[74] with permission.*)

cult in obese parturients with a short, thick neck; in patients with limited extension of the neck, receding jaw, or severe overbite; and when the distance between lower incisors and temporomandibular joint is less than 3.6 times the posterior depth of the mandible.[56] In addition, a study by Mallampati et al[57] has shown that if the faucial pillars and uvula cannot be visualized with the mouth wide open and tongue protruded, one can anticipate difficult intubation due to poor exposure and poor visibility by direct laryngoscopy of pharyngeal structures.

When anesthesiologists are faced with the unfortunate circumstance of an inability to intubate the patient, they should resort to another plan of action immediately (Fig. 201–1). Repeated attempts at intubation will result in increased secretions and swelling of the pharyngeal structures, and create further difficulty in visualizing the glottis.

Induction of anesthesia usually is achieved with the rapid administration of pentothal (4 mg/kg) or ketamine (1 mg/kg). Tracheal intubation is facilitated by administering succinylcholine (1 mg/kg). Cricoid pressure is administered (this effectively obliterates the lumen of the esophagus, thus preventing the gastric contents from reaching the pharynx) and maintained until the correct position of the tracheal tube is verified by end-tidal CO_2 monitoring and by auscultation of the lungs.

Maintenance of anesthesia usually is achieved using 50% nitrous oxide with oxygen and a volatile agent such as isoflurane or enflurane in concentration not exceeding 0.5–1.0%. Higher concentrations of volatile agents have been shown to cause uterine relaxation and increased blood loss.[58]

Induction to Delivery Time and Uterine Incision to Delivery Time. Numerous studies[59,60] have shown that a prolonged induction to delivery time (ID interval) (more than 6–8 minutes) is associated with high incidence of neonatal depression as evidenced by low Apgar scores and neonatal acidosis. Such depression results from the continued transfer of anesthetics to the fetus and causes transient neonatal sedation. More important, once the uterine incision is made, delivery of the baby must be expeditious because a prolonged uterine incision to delivery interval (U-D interval)[59] of more than 120–180 seconds is associated with severe neonatal acidemia. The proposed reasons are that prolonged uterine manipulation causes uterine vasoconstriction and decreased uteroplacental perfusion. In addition, stimulation of intrauterine fetal respiration occurs with amniotic fluid aspiration.

Regional Versus General Anesthesia for Cesarean Section. Several studies[61,62] have indicated that with a well managed anesthesia that avoids hypotension and affords expeditious delivery of the baby, there is very little difference in the Apgar scores, acid-base status, and neurobehavior scores among various anesthetic techniques (epidural, spinal, and general). However, the majority of these studies were performed on healthy parturients undergoing elective cesarean section. To our knowledge, there are no such controlled prospective and randomized studies comparing the maternal and neonatal outcome in patients with complicated pregnancies (eg, severe preeclampsia or diabetes mellitus) receiving regional versus general anesthesia.

In this context, the following studies are worth mentioning:

1. Maternal stress due to rapid induction of general anesthesia and tracheal intubation results in rapid increase in the maternal levels of norepinephrine. This increase causes hypertension, increased uterine vascular resistance, and a precipitous drop in uterine blood flow in pregnant ewes.[63]
2. Using radioactive xenon clearance techniques, Jouppila, et al[64] have shown that placental intervillous blood flow decreased by 35% after inducing general anesthesia in healthy parturients.
3. Using the same technique, these investigators[65] also have shown that in healthy women undergoing elective cesarean section and in the absence of hypotension, epidural and spinal anesthesia caused no change in the intervillous blood flow. However, in patients with severe preeclampsia, administering epidural anesthesia caused significant improvement, with 77% increase in the intervillous blood flow.[66]

Further, well-controlled prospective studies comparing maternal and neonatal outcomes are needed in high-risk patients receiving regional versus general anesthesia for cesarean section.

Epidural Opioids. The rationale for using epidural opioids was based on the discovery of opioid receptors in the spinal cord and the presence of enkephalins.[67,68] Epidural or spinal administration of various opioids provides analgesia by their acting on the specific opioid receptors in the substantia gelatinosa of the dorsal horn of the spinal cord. The difference in the lipid solubility, molecular weight, and pK_a account for the differences in the duration of action (Table 205–5). Several investigators[69,70] have studied the effects of adding drugs such as fentanyl to local anesthetics for epidural analgesia in obstetrics and found that this resulted in prolonging the duration of analgesia with reduced local anesthetic requirement. Epidural narcotics provide prolonged postoperative pain relief after cesarean section.[70,71] The side effects include nausea, vomiting, pruritis, and urinary retention. All these side effects can be reversed by using small doses of opioid antagonists such as naloxone but without reversing the analgesic effects.

TABLE 201–5. PHARMACOLOGY OF EPIDURAL NARCOTICS

Drug	Partition Coefficient	Onset Time (min)	Duration (hours)
Morphine	0.79	15–60	5–36
Pethidine	2.72	5–15	4–18
Methadone	3.93	10–20	6–8
Fentanyl	4.05	5–10	4

From Covino BG, Scott DB[75] with permission.

REFERENCES

1. Bonica JJ. The nature of pain of parturition. *Clin Obstet Gynecol.* 1975;2:501.
2. Lederman RP, Lederman E, Work BA Jr, et al. The relationship of maternal anxiety, plasma catecholamines and plasma cortisol to progress in labor. *Am J Obstet Gynecol.* 1978;132:495.
3. Lederman E, Lederman RP, Work BA Jr, et al. Maternal psychological and physiological correlates of fetal-newborn health status. *Am J Obstet Gynecol.* 1981;139:956.
4. Hagerdal M, Morgan CW, Sumner AE, et al. Minute ventilation and oxygen consumption during labor with epidural analgesia. *Anesthesiology.* 1983;59:425.
5. Shnider SM, Abboud TK, Artal R, et al. Maternal catecholamines decrease during labor after lumbar epidural anesthesia. *Am J Obstet Gynecol.* 1983;147:13.
6. Moir DD, Willocks J. Management of incoordinate uterine action under continuous epidural analgesia. *Br Med J.* 1967;2:396.
7. Climie GR. The place of continuous lumbar epidural analgesia in the management of abnormally prolonged labour. *Med J Aust.* 1964;2:447.
8. Kenepp NB, Shelley WC, Kumar S, et al. Effects on newborn of hydration with glucose in patients undergoing cesarean section with regional anesthesia. *Lancet.* 1980;1:645.

9. Ralston DH, Shnider SM, DeLorimier AA. Effects of equipotent ephedrine, metaraminol, mephentermine, and methoxamine on uterine blood flow in the pregnant ewe. *Anesthesiology*. 1974;40:354.
10. Tarrow AB. Solution to spinal headaches. *Int Anesth Clin*. 1963;1:877.
11. Glass PM, Kennedy WF Jr. Headache following subarachnoid puncture. Treatment with epidural blood patch. *JAMA*. 1972;219:203.
12. Abouleish E. Epidural blood patch for the treatment of chronic post-lumbar-puncture cephalgia. *Anesthesiology*. 1978;49:291.
13. Albright GA. Cardiac arrest following regional anesthesia with etidocaine or bupivacaine. *Anesthesiology*. 1979;51:285.
14. Sage DJ, Feldman HS, Arthur GR, et al. Influence of lidocaine and bupivacaine on isolated guinea pig atria in the presence of acidosis and hypoxia. *Anesth Analg*. 1984;63:1.
15. Rosen MA, Thigpen JW, Shnider SM, et al. Bupivacaine induced cardiotoxicity in hypoxic and acidotic sheep. *Anesth Analg*. 1985;64:1089.
16. de Jong RH, Ronfeld RA, DeRosa RA. Cardiovascular effects of convulsant and supraconvulsant doses of amide local anesthetics. *Anesth Analg*. 1982;61:3.
17. Liu PL, Feldman HS, Giasi R, et al. Comparative CNS toxicity of lidocaine, etidocaine, bupivacaine, and tetracaine in awake dogs following rapid intravenous administration. *Anesth Analg*. 1983;62:375.
18. Morishima HO, Pedersen H, Finster M, et al. Bupivacaine toxicity in pregnant and nonpregnant ewes. *Anesthesiology*. 1985;63:134.
19. Clarkson CW, Hondeghem LM. Mechanism for bupivacaine depression of cardiac conduction: fast block of sodium channels during the action potential with slow recovery from block during diastole. *Anesthesiology*. 1985;62:396.
20. Reisner LS, Hochman BN, Plumer MH. Persistent neurologic deficit and adhesive arachnoiditis following intrathecal 2-chloroprocaine injection. *Anesth Analg*. 1980;59:452.
21. Ravindran RS, Bond VK, Tasch MD, et al. Prolonged neural blockade following regional analgesia with 2-chloroprocaine. *Anesth Analg*. 1980;59:447.
22. Moore DC, Spierdijk J, van Kleef JD, et al. Chloroprocaine neurotoxicity: Four additional cases. *Anesth Analg*. 1982;61:155.
23. Ravindran RS, Turner MS, Muller J. Neurologic effects of subarachnoid administration of 2-chloroprocaine-CE, bupivacaine, and low pH normal saline in dogs. *Anesth Analg*. 1982;61:279.
24. Wang BC, Hillman DE, Spielholz NI, et al. Chronic neurological deficits and Nesacaine-CE: an effect of the anesthetic, 2-chloroprocaine, or the antioxidant, sodium bisulfite? *Anesth Analg*. 1984;63:445.
25. Gissen AJ, Datta S, Lambert D. The chloroprocaine controversy. I. A hypothesis to explain the neural complications of chloroprocaine epidural. *Reg Anesth*. 1984;9:124.
26. Rosen MA, Baysinger CL, Shnider SM, et al. Evaluation of neurotoxicity after subarachnoid injection of large volumes of local anesthetic solutions. *Anesth Analg*. 1983;62:802.
27. Scanlon JW, Brown WU Jr, Weiss JB, et al. Neurobehavioral responses of newborn infants after maternal epidural anesthesia. *Anesthesiology*. 1974;40:121.
28. Abboud TK, Kim KC, Noueihed R, et al. Epidural bupivacaine, chloroprocaine, or lidocaine for cesarean section: maternal and neonatal effects. *Anesth Analg*. 1983;62:914.
29. Kileff ME, James FM III, Dewan DM, et al. Neonatal neurobehavioral responses after epidural anesthesia for cesarean section using lidocaine and bupivacaine. *Anesth Analg*. 1984;63:413.
30. Kuhnert BR, Harrison MJ, Linn PL, et al. Effects of maternal epidural anesthesia on neonatal behavior. *Anesth Analg*. 1984;63:301.
31. Hood DD, Dewan DM, Rose JC, et al. Maternal fetal effects of intravenous epinephrine containing solution in gravid ewes. *Anesthesiology*. 1983;59:A393.
32. Abboud TK, David S, Nagappala S, et al. Maternal, fetal and neonatal effects of lidocaine with and without epinephrine for epidural anesthesia in obstetrics. *Anesth Analg*. 1984;63:973.
33. Albright GA, Jouppila R, Hollmen AI, et al. Epinephrine does not alter human intervillous blood flow during epidural anesthesia. *Anesthesiology*. 1981;54:131.
34. Read MD, Hunt LP, Anderson JM, et al. Epidural block and the progress and outcome of labor. *J Obstet Gynaecol*. 1983;4:35.
35. Willdeck-Lund G, Lindmark G, Nilsson BA. Effect of segmental epidural analgesia upon the uterine activity with special reference to the use of different local anaesthetic agents. *Acta Anaesthesiol Scand*. 1979; 23:519.
36. Jouppila P, Jouppila R, Kaar K, et al. Fetal heart rate patterns and uterine activity after segmental epidural analgesia. *Br J Obstet Gynaecol*. 1977;84:481.
37. Friedman EA, Sachtleben MR. Caudal anesthesia: The factors that influence its effect on labor. *Obstet Gynecol*. 1959;13:442.
38. Willdeck-Lund G, Lindmark G, Nilsson BA. Effect of segmental epidural block on the course of labour and the condition of the infant during the neonatal period. *Acta Anaesthesiol Scand*. 1979;23:301.
39. Jouppila R, Jouppila P, Karinen JM, et al. Segmental epidural analgesia in labour: Related to the progress of labour, fetal malposition and instrumental delivery. *Acta Obstet Gynecol Scand*. 1979;58:135.
40. Phillips JC, Hochberg CJ, Petrakis JK, et al. Epidural analgesia and its effects on the "normal" progress of labor. *Am J Obstet Gynecol*. 1977;129:316.
41. Bates RG, Helm CW, Duncan A, et al. Uterine activity in the second stage of labour and the effect of epidural analgesia. *Br J Obstet Gynaecol*. 1985;92:1246.
42. Goodfellow CF, Hull MG, Swaab DF, et al. Oxytocin deficiency at delivery with epidural analgesia. *Br J Obstet Gynaecol*. 1983;90:214.
43. Phillips KC, Thomas TA. Second stage of labour with or without extradural analgesia. *Anaesthesia*. 1983;38:972.
44. Chestnut DH, Vandewalker GE, Owen CL, et al. The influence of continuous epidural bupivacaine analgesia on the second stage of labor and method of delivery in nulliparous women. *Anesthesiology*. 1987;66:774.
45. Kaunitz AM, Hughes JM, Grimes DA, et al. Causes of maternal mortality in the United States. *Survey Anesth*. 1986;30:70.
46. Bassell GM, Marx GF. Anesthesia related maternal mortality. In: Shnider SM, Levinson CS, eds. *Anesthesia for Obstetrics*. Baltimore, MD: Williams and Wilkins; 1987:325.
47. Turnbull AC, Tindall V, Robson G, et al. *Report on Confidential Enquiries into Maternal Deaths in England and Wales 1979–1981*. London: Her Majesty's Stationery Office; 1986:7.
48. Awe WC, Fletcher WS, Jacob SW. The pathophysiology of aspiration pneumonitis. *Surgery*. 1966;60:232.
49. Teabeaut JR II. Aspiration of gastric contents: An experimental study. *Am J Pathol*. 1952;28:51.
50. Gibbs CP, Spohr L, Schmidt D. The effectiveness of sodium citrate as an antacid. *Anesthesiology*. 1982;57:44.
51. O'Sullivan GM, Bullingham RE. Does twice the volume of antacid have twice the effect in pregnant women at term? *Anesth Analg*. 1984;63:752.
52. Feely J, Wilkinson GR, McAllister CB, et al. Increased toxicity and reduced clearance of lidocaine by cimetidine. *Ann Intern Med*. 1982;96:592.
53. Maile CJ, Francis RN. Preoperative ranitidine: Effect of a single intravenous dose on pH and volume of gastric aspirate. *Anaesthesia*. 1983;38:324.
54. Brock-Utne JG, Rubin J, Downing JW, et al. The administration of metoclopramide with atropine: a drug interaction effect on the gastro-oesophageal sphincter in man. *Anaesthesia*. 1976;31:1186.
55. Norris MC, Dewan DM. Preoxygenation for cesarean section: A comparison of two techniques. *Anesthesiology*. 1985;68:827.
56. White A, Kander PL. Anatomical factors in difficult direct laryngoscopy. *Br J Anaesth*. 1975;47:468.
57. Mallampati SR, Gatt SP, Gugino LD, et al. A clinical sign to predict difficult tracheal intubation: A prospective study. *Can Anaesth Soc J*. 1985;32:429.
58. Munson ES, Embro WJ. Enflurane, isoflurane, and halothane and isolated human uterine muscle. *Anesthesiology*. 1977;46:11.
59. Datta S, Ostheimer GW, Weiss JB, et al. Neonatal effect of prolonged anesthetic induction for cesarean section. *Obstet Gynecol*. 1981;58:331.
60. Crawford JS, Davies P. A return to trichloroethylene for obstetric anaesthesia. *Br J Anaesth* 1975;47:482.
61. Marx GF, Cosmi EV, Wollman SB. Biochemical status and clinical condition of mother and infant at cesarean section. *Anesth Analg*. 1969;48:986.
62. James FM III, Crawford JS, Hopkinson R, et al. A comparison of general anesthesia and lumbar epidural analgesia for elective cesarean section. *Anesth Analg*. 1977;56:228.
63. Shnider SM, Wright RG, Levinson G, et al. Uterine blood flow and plasma norepinephrine changes during maternal stress in the pregnant ewe. *Anesthesiology*. 1979;50:524.
64. Jouppila P, Kuikka J, Jouppila R, et al. Effect of induction of general anesthesia for cesarean section on intervillous blood flow. *Acta Obstet Gynecol Scand*. 1979;58:249.
65. Jouppila R, Jouppila P, Kuikka J, et al. Placental blood flow during caesarean section under lumbar extradural analgesia. *Br J Anaesth*. 1978;50:275.
66. Jouppila P, Jouppila R, Hollmen A, et al. Lumbar epidural analgesia to improve intervillous blood flow during labor in severe preeclampsia. *Obstet Gynecol*. 1982;59:158.
67. Pert CB, Snyder SH. Opiate receptor: demonstration in nervous tissue. *Science*. 1973;179:1011.
68. Pert CB, Kuhar MJ, Snyder SH. Opiate receptor: autoradiographic localization in rat brain. *Proc Natl Acad Sci USA*. 1976;73:3729.
69. Preston PG, Rosen MA, Hughes SC, et al. Epidural anesthesia with fentanyl and lidocaine for cesarean section: Maternal and neonatal outcome. *Anesthesiology*. 1988;68:938.
70. Rosen MA, Hughes SC, Shnider SM, et al. Epidural morphine for the relief of postoperative pain after cesarean delivery. *Anesth Analg*. 1983;62:666.
71. Kotelko DM, Dailey PA, Shnider SM, et al. Epidural morphine analgesia after cesarean delivery. *Obstet Gynecol*. 1984;63:409.
72. Conclin KA, Murad SHN. Pharmacology of drugs in obstetric anesthesia. *Sem Anesth*. 1982;1:83.
73. Curran MA. Epidural anesthesia. Practical considerations. *Curr Rev Clin Anesth*. 1988:98.
74. Hood DD. Obstetric anesthesia: Complications and problems. In: *Problems in Anesthesia*. Philadelphia: JB Lippincott; 1989:1.
75. Covino BG, Scott DB. *Handbook of Epidural Anesthesia and Analgesia*. Orlando, FL: Grune & Stratton; 1985.

Chapter Two Hundred and Two

Obstetric Anesthesia for Complicated Pregnancy

Jaya Ramanathan and Baha M. Sibai

202

Complicated pregnancies challenge even the most experienced obstetrician. The anesthesiologist, with considerable knowledge of the basic pathophysiology of specific diseases, the pharmacotherapy, and the interaction of these with the anesthetic interventions, can share some of the burden of this challenge. Teamwork between the obstetrician and anesthesiologist is essential for favorable outcome for the mother and the neonate. In this section, the anesthetic management of some of the common complications of pregnancy such as preeclampsia, diabetes mellitus, preterm labor, asthma, and cardiac diseases will be discussed. In addition, the anesthetic management of uncommon complications such as associated neurologic diseases, septicemia, obstetric hemorrhage during the third trimester, and malignant hyperpyrexia will be discussed. This chapter selectively focuses on anesthetic management; the detailed pathophysiology of the diseases is included elsewhere.

PREECLAMPSIA

Preeclampsia, a disease of unknown etiology, is classically defined as the development of hypertension, proteinuria, and edema after the 20th week of gestation (see also Chapter 139). The pathophysiology includes the occurrence of intense vasospasms involving all major vascular beds, including the placental vasculature. The rationale for treatment includes controlling and stabilizing hypertension, preventing convulsions, and optimizing intravascular volume status. All these measures contribute to the safe delivery of a viable baby.

Magnesium sulfate, an anticonvulsant, is the primary treatment for preeclampsia in North America. Centrally, it has been shown to suppress the seizure foci in experimental animals.[1] Peripherally, Mg^{2+} acts at the myoneural junction by decreasing the release of acetylcholine from the vesicles in the presynaptic area; it also decreases the sensitivity of the postjunctional membrane to acetylcholine and decreases the excitability of the muscle membrane. Ramanathan et al[2] have shown that abnormal neuromuscular transmission exists in parturients receiving standard doses of $MgSO_4$, and the intensity of the defect correlates significantly with increased Mg^{2+} levels and decreased Ca^{2+} levels. Magnesium potentiates the actions of muscle relaxants. The therapeutic range is 4.3–8.4 mg/dL. Toxic levels in the range of 12–15 mg/dL can occur from overdose, severely compromised renal function, or both.

Although magnesium causes transient reductions in the mean arterial pressure (MAP), other potent antihypertensive agents are often necessary to control blood pressure in preeclampsia. Hydralazine is one of the most widely used vasodilators in preeclampsia. In pregnant ewes[3], hydralazine has been shown to decrease MAP, increase uterine blood flow, and lower uterine vascular resistance. However, the delayed onset, variable duration of action, and compensatory tachycardia are the major disadvantages associated with using this drug. In preeclamptic patients with hyperdynamic myocardial function and hypovolemia, hydralazine causes further increase in cardiac index, which can lead to adverse maternal and fetal effects. The use of hydralazine also is associated with neonatal hypotension and thrombocytopenia.[4]

The use of potent vasodilators (eg, nitroprusside and nitroglycerin) and ganglion-blocking agents (eg, trimethaphan) usually is reserved for treating acute hypertensive crisis, hypertension that is unresponsive to conventional therapy, and blunting the hypertensive response to tracheal intubation prior to inducing general anesthesia.

Sodium nitroprusside (SNP) is a potent arteriolar dilator and has a rapid onset and short duration. In animal experiments[5], infusion of high doses of SNP in gravid ewes caused fetal cyanide toxicity, and death. However, other studies have shown that using a mean dose of 2.3 μg/kg per minute SNP reversed the norepinephrine-induced hypertension in gravid ewes.[6] Intrauterine blood flow increased progressively, and toxic cyanide levels were not apparent in either the maternal or fetal blood samples. In patients with severe pregnancy-induced hypertension and who also have acute congestive heart failure and pulmonary edema, hemodynamics improved dramatically.[7] Both MAP and pulmonary capillary wedge pressure (PCWP) decreased with no untoward fetal effects and no significant cyanide levels detected in either the maternal or umbilical cord blood samples.[7] Short-term exposure to nitroprusside does not affect maternal or fetal well-being adversely.

Unlike SNP, nitroglycerine (NTG) is a venodilator dilating the capacitance vessels. In gravid ewes, NTG counteracts the hypertension and uterine vasoconstriction induced by norepinephrine.[8] Nitroglycerine can be used effectively to blunt the cardiovascular responses to tracheal intubation in preeclampsia with no adverse neonatal effects.[9] In severe preeclampsia, NTG decreases the MAP without significantly changing the heart rate, central venous pressure (CVP) or stroke volume, and significantly decreases PCWP and cardiac index.[10] Patients receiving volume expansion along with NTG infusion might manifest a marked resistance to the hypotensive effects of the drug. Fetal heart rate variability also can decrease.

Trimethaphan is a ganglionic blocker with a higher molecular weight of 600 and less placental transfer. However, it has a slow onset and side effects such as tachyphylaxis, tachycardia, histamine release, and prolongation of the action of succinylcholine.[11]

Compared with hydralazine, labetalol (a combined α- and β-adrenergic blocking agent) has a more rapid onset and causes a smoother reduction of blood pressures with no adverse fetal or neonatal effects.[12] The main disadvantage of this drug is the wide variability in the dose requirement (20–300 mg with a mean of 140 ± 102 mg) that cannot be predicted by any clinical characteristics prior to therapy to control blood pressure. A recent study has shown that labetalol in doses not exceeding 1 mg/kg can be used to attenuate the hypertensive response to tracheal intubation in preeclampsia.[13] Other β-adrenergic blocking agents (eg, metoprolol and pindolol) and calcium entry blocking agents (eg, nifedipine and verapamil) are undergoing clinical trials in patients with preeclampsia. As in the case of labetalol, further clinical investigations are necessary to establish the safety of the drugs in the mother and the fetus.

Anesthetic management of patients with preeclampsia is often a challenge because no ideal anesthetic drugs or techniques exist. Anesthesiologists must be familiar with the cardiovascular, respiratory, and metabolic derangements associated with severe preeclampsia. With expertise in invasive hemodynamic monitoring and ventilatory care, anesthesiologists are uniquely qualified to participate in the peripartum management of patients with preeclampsia.

A physical examination for preeclamptic patients should include a neurologic and pelvic examination. Intravenous fluid should be infused, and a Foley catheter should be inserted to measure urine output. Pertinent laboratory tests include complete blood count, peripheral smear, serum creatinine, BUN, uric acid, serum electrolytes, liver enzymes, and coagulation profile including fibrinogen, prothrombin time (PT), partial thromboplastin time (PTT), platelets, bleeding time, and fibrin-split products. Serum Mg^{++} levels should be obtained after initiating $MgSO_4$ therapy and should be repeated in 6-hour intervals along with a coagulation profile.

Some patients with severe preeclampsia (especially those with severe oliguria and those requiring epidural anesthesia) might need a central venous line to optimize fluid status. In patients with severe preeclampsia and who also have pulmonary edema, left ventricular failure, severe oliguria not responding to fluids, or hypertensive crisis (not responding to conventional therapy) requiring potent vasodilators for blood pressure control, insertion of a pulmonary artery catheter might be necessary. Monitoring blood pressure by an indwelling radial artery line enables the assessment of blood pressure responses to therapeutic intervention (for details, see Chapter 211).

Patients with severe preeclampsia are usually volume-depleted, the severity of which is related to the severity of the disease process. Joyce et al[14] demonstrated an inverse correlation between CVP and diastolic pressure. While patients with mild preeclampsia required almost 1 L of fluid to restore CVP to 6 cm H_2O, those with diastolic pressures above 110 mm Hg required twice as much volume. Urine output should be maintained above 30 mL/hr in these women. Plasma oncotic pressure (POP) values are significantly lower in patients with preeclampsia compared with normal healthy parturients because of the significant protein loss resulting from extravasation of protein and albuminuria. A fall in the POP lowers the POP-PCWP gradients; in some women with preeclampsia, the values can even be negative.

Some researchers recommend administering 5% or 25% albumin to restore the CVP and raise the POP.[14] However, rapidly administering albumin, even in normal subjects, causes the escape of albumin into the interstitial space. In preeclamptic women with altered capillary permeability, administering colloids can aggravate the protein extravasation through the capillary pores and precipitate interstitial or intra-alveolar pulmonary edema. The logical treatment for the decreased POP-PCWP gradient is to lower the PCWP by afterload reduction (vasodilator therapy) rather than raise the POP.[15] Patients admitted with antepartum pulmonary edema should be treated aggressively prior to administering an anesthetic. Treatment is directed towards the etiology of pulmonary edema. In the majority of instances, these patients will respond to afterload reduction using vasodilators, which also reduce the MAP and PCWP. However, in some patients, an initial dose of a potent diuretic, such as furosemide, might be needed.

The main concern among some obstetricians regarding the use of epidural anesthesia in women with preeclampsia is that regional anesthesia and sympathetic block in patients with intravascular volume depletion might lead to profound hypotension and decreased placental perfusion. However, reports[16,17] have shown that, with proper prehydration, hypotension is an infrequent complication in patients who receive epidural anesthesia. Most important, regional block obviates the need for general anesthesia and its associated complications.

The advantages of epidural anesthesia include improving the intervillous blood flow[18] (Fig. 202–1) and renal blood flow and preventing excessive increases in blood pressure. Epidural anesthesia causes no significant changes in the cardiac index, systemic vascular resistance (SVR), or pulmonary vascular resistance (PVR).[19] Patients should be prehydrated adequately prior to the block. A CVP of 5–7 mm Hg or a PCWP of 10 mm Hg is adequate. The epidural catheter is inserted in the second or third lumbar interspace, and anesthesia should be induced slowly, with incremental doses of the local anesthetic, to avoid sudden hypotension. Oxygen should be administered by face mask and left uterine displacement should be maintained. Should hypotension occur despite these measures, ephedrine, administered in 5-mg doses, promptly restores blood pressure.

The three commonly used local anesthetics for cesarean section are 3% 2-chloroprocaine, 1.5–2.0% lidocaine, and 0.5% bupivacaine. All these agents produce excellent motor and sensory blocks. The use of 3% 2-chloroprocaine in nor-

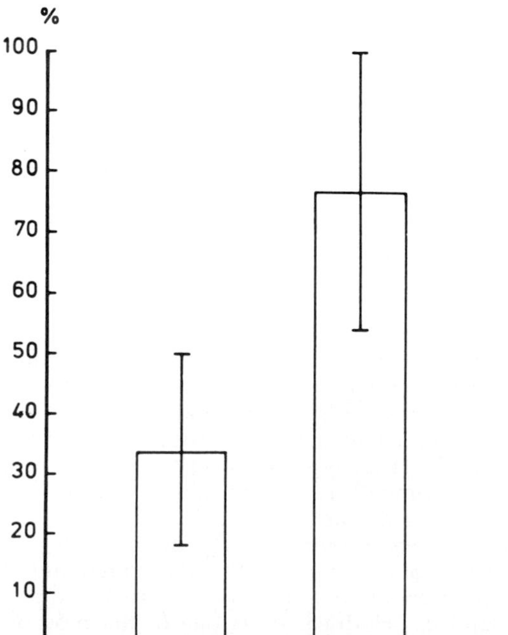

Figure 202–1. Increase in intervillous blood flow values (mean ± SEM) after epidural anesthesia for labor in preeclamptic women. (*From Jouppila P et al[18] with permission.*)

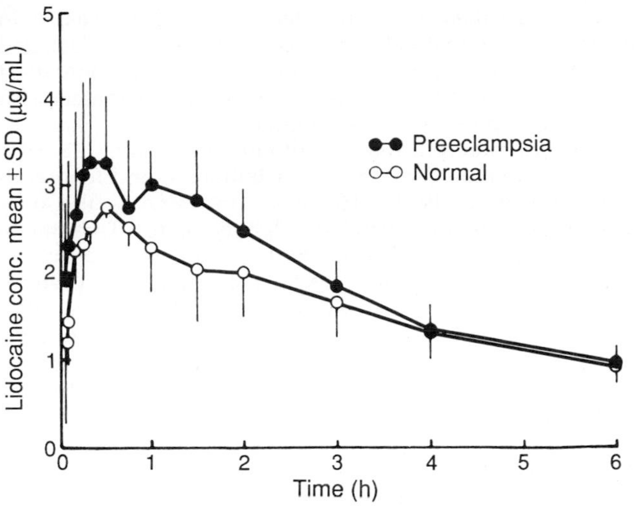

Figure 202–2. Plasma lidocaine levels (mean ± SD) in healthy and preeclamptic women. After epidural administration, the area under the concentration time-curve was signficantly greater, and the total clearance of lidocaine was significantly prolonged in women with preeclampsia compared with healthy pregnant women. (*From Ramanathan J et al*[21] *with permission.*)

mal pregnancies is associated with a higher incidence of hypotension resulting from the rapid onset of sympathetic block.[20] This hypotension might be a disadvantage in patients with preeclampsia. Lidocaine is devoid of any neurotoxicity or cardiotoxicity, and hence it is an ideal agent for use in preeclampsia. However, lidocaine clearance is prolonged in preeclampsia, and repeated administration can lead to toxic blood levels (Fig. 202–2).[21] Adding 50–100 µg of fentanyl to 2% lidocaine improves the quality of epidural analgesia.[22] Bupivacaine (0.5%) also can be used.

General anesthesia often is administered for acute fetal distress or in those situations where a conduction anesthesia is contraindicated (eg, presence of coagulopathy, infection at the site of insertion). Induction of anesthesia and endotracheal intubation cause a transient but severe hypertension and tachycardia in patients with preeclampsia. This exaggerated sympathetic response to tracheal intubation can result in pulmonary edema, cardiac failure, increased intracranial pressure, and cerebral edema.[23,24] In addition, induction of general anesthesia and tracheal intubation reduce uterine blood flow.[25] It is thus extremely important to lower maternal blood pressure prior to induction of general anesthesia. Vasodilators such as hydralazine, nitroglycerine, or nitroprusside can be used for this purpose. Labetalol in 1-mg/kg doses also can be used safely for this purpose.[13] Several drugs used often for blunting sympathoadrenal responses to tracheal intubation are listed in Table 202–1.

Patients with preeclampsia usually receive $MgSO_4$, which can potentiate and prolong the actions of both depolarizing and nondepolarizing relaxants. Defasciculating doses of nondepolarizing agents are omitted as Mg^{++} abolishes the fasciculations. Patients are induced with Pentothal (4 mg/kg), and endotracheal intubations are accomplished with 1.0–1.5 mg/kg succinylcholine. Cricoid pressure should be applied and maintained until the correct position of the endotracheal tube is verified. To maintain anesthesia, a N_2O–O_2 mixture with 0.5% halothane, 1% enflurane, or 0.5% isoflurane can be used. Small doses of narcotics also can supplement the anesthesia. Similar to induction and tracheal intubation, reflex hypertension and tachycardia frequently occur at the time of extubation. Small doses of labetalol prior to extubation usually prevent such responses.

Patients with preeclampsia should be provided care in the postanesthesia recovery room for a minimum of 12 hours. If not treated adequately, persistent hypertension can precipitate eclamptic seizures. These patients should be monitored diligently; $MgSO_4$, hydralazine, or other antihypertensive agents should be continued. An epidural catheter already in place can be used to provide postoperative pain relief. Epidural opioids such as morphine provide excellent and prolonged pain relief in the postoperative period.[26] If complications such as pulmonary edema from the mobilization of extravascular fluid or iatrogenic fluid overload occurs, patients should be monitored invasively and given intensive care.

DIABETES MELLITUS

The physiologic alterations of carbohydrate metabolism in a normal pregnancy involve exaggerated insulin and glucose responses after eating a meal (see Chapter 43). Despite the twofold to threefold increase in insulin levels, maternal blood glucose levels can increase considerably because of the antiinsulin effects of hormones such as placental lacto-

TABLE 202–1. DRUGS USED FOR BLUNTING SYMPATHOADRENAL RESPONSES TO TRACHEAL INTUBATION IN WOMEN WITH PREECLAMPSIA

Drug	Dose	Comments
Hydralazine	5-mg increments IV to decrease diastolic pressure below 110 mm Hg	Direct arteriolar dilator. Slow onset of action (20 minutes to peak effect). Variable duration of action. Compensatory tachycardia.
Nitroprusside	Initial dose of 0.25–0.5 µg/kg per min and increase dose gradually	Arteriolar dilator. Fetal cyanide toxicity in large doses. Short exposure and small doses may be safe.
Nitroglycerine	Initial dose of 0.5–1.5 µg/kg per min and increase dose gradually	Dilates capacitance vessels. No cyanide toxicity. Marked resistance in preeclamptic women receiving volume expansion. Can increase intracranial pressure.
Trimethaphan	Initial dose of 300 µg/min	Ganglionic blocker. Molecular weight >600, thus limited placental transfer. Tachycardia and tachyphylaxis.
Labetalol	Initial dose of 20 mg IV and followed by 10-mg increments up to a total dose of 1 mg/kg	Alpha- and beta-adrenergic blocking agent. Limited experience. Further clinical investigations needed.

gen, estrogen, progesterone, and cortisol.[27-29] In addition, even a brief period of starvation can cause ketonemia and ketonuria. Any added stress in the form of hyperemesis, infection, starvation, dehydration, prolonged labor, and failure of self-administration of insulin can predispose a diabetic mother to the rapid development of diabetic ketoacidosis.

Ketoacids freely cross the placental barrier and cause fetal acidosis.[30] Fetal mortality is apparently high after an episode of diabetic ketoacidosis. The placental blood flow index is decreased 35–45% in women with diabetes, and arteriosclerotic changes occur in the placental vasculature leading to areas of decreased perfusion.[31] These changes make the fetus extremely vulnerable to decreased placental blood flow with maternal hypotension. The increase in the maternal HbAlc levels results in an impaired oxygen release and decresed oxygen saturation.[31] Surfactant maturation is delayed. Other complications include preeclampsia, macrosomia, polyhydramnios, prematurity, increased incidence of intrauterine fetal demise, and major congenital anomalies.

It is evident, then, that maternal blood sugars should be rigidly controlled by diet and insulin therapy to prevent maternal and neonatal morbidity and mortality. Prior to cesarean section, control of blood glucose levels can be achieved by one of the following regimens. On the morning of surgery, one third of the total daily insulin dose is administered, and an infusion of 5% dextrose is started. Alternatively, the patient is allowed to have her normal dose of insulin on the day before surgery and she begins fasting after 10 P.M. On the day of surgery, an infusion of dextrose and regular insulin (0.5–2.0 units/hour) is started.[27] The goal of the therapy is to maintain a glucose level 70–120 mg/dL.

For labor analgesia, epidural anesthesia is ideal. Alleviating the pain, anxiety, and stress of labor reduces the circulating catecholamine levels and decreases the insulin requirement. Epidural block improves the intervillous flow and obviates the need for administering potent narcotics that can result in neonatal depression.

For cesarean section, a second intravenous line should be started for administering fluid and drugs. Epidural anesthesia is preferable as general anesthesia exposes the already compromised fetus to the depressant effects of the anesthetic agents. Epidural anesthesia also causes fewer fluctuations in the plasma catecholamine levels, cortisol levels, and glucose homeostasis. Since hypotension is poorly tolerated by the fetus, adequate prehydration with a nondextrose-containing solution is essential prior to the block. Other routine measures such as left uterine displacement and O_2 administration should be continued throughout the procedure. Postoperatively, serum glucose levels should be monitored closely, and the insulin therapy should be adjusted accordingly as there is usually a rapid drop in the insulin requirement.

PRETERM LABOR AND DELIVERY

The incidence of preterm births varies (3–19% of all deliveries), and a significant number of such births occurs in healthy parturients with no predisposing factors.[32,33] However, some major risk factors have been identified: history of previous preterm delivery, overdistended uterus (polyhydramnios, multiple gestation), incompetent cervix, extremes of maternal age, and fetal and placental abnormalities.[34]

The anesthesiologist usually is consulted to assist in managing a vaginal delivery or cesarean section; a detailed knowledge of the pharmacokinetics of the commonly used tocolytic agents and the special problems associated with delivering a preterm fetus are important.

Several different β-sympathomimetic agents (eg, ritodrine, terbutaline, isoxuparine, salbutamol, and fenoterol) currently are available. However, ritodrine is the only β-mimetic agent approved in the United States. Terbutaline is used extensively in Europe and Scandinavian countries. Both drugs are extremely effective in inhibiting preterm labor. However, the use of β-mimetic agents is associated with a number of side-effects such as maternal tachycardia with shortness of breath, chest pain, and ECG evidence of myocardial ischemia.[35] Supraventricular or ventricular arrhythmias and nodal rhythm can occur. Pulmonary edema is a serious complication of β-sympathomimetic therapy.[36,37] The etiology of pulmonary edema is not fully understood but thought to be noncardiogenic in origin. Several mechanisms (eg, iatrogenic fluid overload, sodium and water retention because of increased aldosterone levels, and increased pulmonary capillary permeability) have been suggested as the cause of pulmonary edema. The metabolic side effects include hyperglycemia, hyperinsulinemia, increased serum lactate and pyruvate levels, decreased HCO_3, and anion gap. The metabolic side effect that concerns the anesthesiologist most is hypokalemia, which results from the increased entry of glucose into the red cells and the altered function of the Na^+/K^+ pump.[38]

Other tocolytic agents that are used occasionally are magnesium sulfate, prostaglandin inhibitors, calcium entry blocking agents, diazoxide, and aminophylline. Indomethacin interferes with maternal platelet function and prolongs the maternal bleeding time, which can pose an additional risk in patients receiving regional anesthesia. The combined use of betamethasone and ritodrine can cause severe hyperglycemia and, in some instances, pulmonary edema. The anesthetic implications of tocolytic therapy are given in Table 202–2.

Some of the anesthetic agents and drugs routinely used by the anesthesiologists during delivery of a term baby may be poorly tolerated by a preterm fetus. The hepatic enzyme system and renal excretion are immature and poorly developed in a preterm fetus. In addition, with the decreased protein binding of drugs and poorly developed blood-brain barrier, a preterm fetus is highly susceptible to the depressing effects of maternally administered anesthetic agents such as Pentothal, narcotics, sedatives, phenothiazines, and benzodiazepines. By using regional anesthesia for labor and vaginal delivery, the depressant effects of general anesthetics and narcotics can be avoided.

Before administering anesthesia to women in preterm labor, adequate preoperative evaluation and preparation are essential. Preoperative serum glucose and K^+ levels should be recorded. An electrocardiogram is helpful in patients with tachyarrhythmias. Pulmonary edema should be treated before administering anesthesia. Beta-sympathomimetic agents usually are discontinued and use of furosemide may be necessary. Invasive monitoring may be needed to facilitate managing peripartum fluid. Although hypokalemia may be present, potassium administration is seldom necessary unless there is electrocardiographic evidence of hypokalemia.

For cesarean section, regional anesthesia generally is considered safer than general anesthesia for several reasons. The induction of general anesthesia and tracheal intubation can result in severe tachycardia and dysrhythmias in those

TABLE 202–2. MATERNAL SIDE EFFECTS OF TOCOLYTIC THERAPY AND ANESTHETIC IMPLICATIONS

Drug	Maternal Side Effects	Anesthetic Implications
Ritodrine and terbutaline	Tachycardia, pulmonary edema, hyperglycemia	Persistent tachycardia makes it difficult to assess the depth of anesthesia and fluid balance. Severe dysrhythmias during induction and the possibility of cardiovascular collapse.
$MgSO_4$	Decreased acetylcholine release at the myoneural junction, hypocalcemia	Prolongation of neuromuscular blockade by muscle relaxants.
Indomethacin	Platelet dysfunction	Increased risk of intraspinal bleeding after regional anesthesia.
Calcium entry blocking agents	Hypotension, uterine atony	Severe myocardial depression with concomitant use of volatile anesthetic agents.

patients receiving β-sympathomimetic agents. In addition, induction of general anesthesia decreases the intervillous blood flow even in normal pregnancy, and this decrease may be poorly tolerated by a preterm fetus. In addition, using inhalation and intravenous anesthetic agents during general anesthesia may act as potent cerebral depressants in a preterm neonate. If general anesthesia is needed, agents that increase the heart rate such as atropine, ketamine, and pancuronium should be avoided or used with great caution.

With cautious use of epidural anesthesia, many problems can be avoided. Because rapid administration of large volumes of fluid prior to epidural anesthesia will precipitate pulmonary edema, such a procedure should be avoided. At the same time, hypotension due to sympathetic block is poorly tolerated by a preterm fetus. The block thus should be extended slowly with small, intermittent doses of local anesthetic.

ASTHMA

The incidence of asthma in pregnancy varies (0.4–1.3%); approximately 10–15% of these women have asthmatic episodes severe enough to warrant hospitalization (see Chapter 122).[39]

Pathophysiology involves increased airway resistance due to contraction of airway smooth muscle. Diffuse hypertrophy of bronchial smooth muscle, swelling of the mucus membrane, and excessive production of viscid mucus secretion add to the airway obstruction.[40,41] The increased airway resistance leads to "air trapping" and an increase in functional residual capacity (FRC), residual volume (RV), and total lung capacity (TLC); the vital capacity (VC), forced expiratory volume at 1 sec (FEV_1), peak expiratory flow rate, and expiratory reserve volume (ERV) are reduced. In addition, the forced expiratory flow (FEF) at 25–75% of forced vital capacity (FVC) also decreases, indicating small airway obstruction.[42]

The commonly used drugs, mode of action, and dose are given in Table 202–3. Theophylline, one of the most commonly used drugs, relaxes smooth muscle by inhibiting phosphodiesterase. However, recent evidence indicates that other mechanisms, such as increased catecholamine release from adrenal medulla and alteration of intracellular calcium kinetics, also are partly responsible for the bronchodilatory effects of theophylline.[43,44] Clearance of theophylline in pregnant women is not significantly different from

TABLE 202–3. SOME OF THE COMMONLY USED DRUGS IN ASTHMA

Drug	Mode of Action and Dose	Side Effects and Anesthetic Implications
Beta Mimetics		
Epinephrine	Alpha and nonspecific beta agonist, 0.25–0.5 mg SC	Causes temporary decrease in uterine blood flow, congenital malformations
Terbutaline	Selective beta-2 agonist, 0.25–0.5 mg SC q 15–30 min or 0.25 mg/inhalation (metered inhaler)	Potent tocolytic agent, maternal tachycardia
Albuterol	Selective beta-2 agonist, 90 μg/inhalation (metered inhaler) or 5–10 mg in 0.5% solution (aerosol inhaler)	Less maternal tachycardia, one report of postpartum uterine atony and hemorrhage
Theophylline, aminophylline	Phosphodiesterase inhibition, increased catecholamine secretion, changes in the Ca^{++} kinetics, dose (see text)	Increased incidence of cardiac arrhythmias with concomitant use of inhalation agents
Steroids		
Prednisolone	Restores sensitivity of beta agonists, decreases airway edema, abolishes T-cell responses to antigen, dose 5–60 mg PO qid	Chronic therapy results in maternal adrenal suppression, very little placental transfer
Methylprednisolone	Same as above, 125 mg IV q 4–6 hr	Same as above
Beclamethasone	50 μg/inhalation (metered inhaler)	Very effective, minimal systemic effects

Modified from Norris MC.[116]

nonpregnant women, although the volume of distribution increases during pregnancy.[45] Theophylline crosses the placental barrier and can cause effects such as increased irritability, jitteriness, and tachycardia in the fetus.[46] The clearance of theophylline is prolonged in newborns, especially in premature newborns.[47] No teratogenic effects have been observed with this drug. The therapeutic level of 10 μg/mL should be maintained by frequently monitoring maternal serum levels during drug therapy. Theophylline is a potent uterine muscle relaxant and can prolong labor and lead to postpartum hemorrhage due to uterine atony.

Beta-mimetic agents, such as epinephrine, decrease uterine blood flow despite an increase in mean arterial pressure.[48] Epinephrine can cause maternal tachyarrhythmias, and its use is associated with increased incidence of congenital malformations. All beta mimetics, including the beta-2 specific agonists such as terbutaline and salbutamol, cause uterine relaxation and prolong labor.[49]

Corticosteroids cause bronchodilation and block the T-lymphocyte responses to specific antigens. Most important, corticosteroids restore the sensitivity of the β-receptors to circulating β-agonists.[50,51] Beclomethasone, a potent steroid in aerosol form, significantly decreases the systemic dose requirement. Both prednisone and prednisolone are used during pregnancy because very small amounts of these drugs cross the placental barrier. Maternal adrenal suppression is common, and supplemental hydrocortisone should be administered during labor and prior to surgery. Other drugs such as disodium cromoglycate and antihistamines also can be used.

For labor analgesia, segmental lumbar epidural anesthesia provides excellent pain relief, abolishes maternal hyperventilation, and decreases maternal oxygen consumption. For nonemergent cesarean section, epidural anesthesia is suitable as it avoids the need for a general anesthetic and its associated complications. In addition, the systemic absorption of epinephrine added to the local anesthetic exerts a beneficial effect by causing bronchodilation.

When general anesthesia is required, preoperative use of histamine$_2$-receptor antagonists theoretically can worsen asthma due to the unopposed histamine$_1$ action.[52] For induction of general anesthesia, ketamine is preferred as it has less effect on pulmonary compliance and airway resistance. To maintain general anesthesia, agents such as halothane, isoflurane, or enflurane can be used. However, the incidence of cardiac dysrhythmias is higher when halothane is used in patients receiving aminophylline.[53] Agents that release histamine, such as curare and morphine, should be avoided. Muscle relaxants with little or no histamine-releasing action, such as atracurium or vercurnium, can be used. The treatment of intraoperative bronchospasm is given in Table 202–4.

TABLE 202–4. TREATMENT OF BRONCHOSPASM DURING GENERAL ANESTHESIA

Exclude other causes: Incorrect positioning, kinking, or obstruction of the endotracheal tube. Pulmonary aspiration of gastric contents.
Deepen anesthesia. Increase the concentration of the volatile agent.
Administer beta-mimetic agent directly into the inspiratory limb of the breathing circuit.
Start aminophylline infusion.
Watch for cardiac arrhythmias: Concomitant use of aminophylline and inhalation agents.
Watch for myometrial relaxation and increased uterine bleeding: Concomitant use of aminophylline, inhalation agents, and beta agonists.

CARDIAC DISEASE IN PREGNANCY

Cardiac disease occurs in 0.4–4.1% of pregnant women, and maternal mortality ranges from 0.4% in patients with Class I or II cardiac disease to 6.8% among patients with Class III or IV disease (New York Heart Association Functional Classification).[54] Several cardiovascular changes occur during pregnancy. Perhaps three of the most important changes are the dramatic increase in cardiac output (30–45% above the nonpregnant values by 20th week of gestation), the decrease in peripheral vascular resistance (due to the creation of a low-resistance circuit in the uteroplacental circulation), and the increase in maternal blood volume (40% above nonpregnant women by 28–30 weeks' gestation, depending on the size of the fetus). The results of echocardiographic studies (ECHO) examining left ventricular function are conflicting. A study[55] published in 1977 indicated enhanced myocardial contractility as evidenced by an increase in the velocity of circumferential shortening, a decrease in the preejection period, and an increase in the left ventricular ejection time. However, Katz et al[56] performed serial ECHO studies on pregnant women from first trimester to 12 weeks' postpartum and found progressive left ventricular enlargement; left ventricular function was not augmented but was well preserved throughout the study period. With the onset of labor, additional stresses on the heart occur such as further increases in cardiac output (up to 40% above prelabor values) due to pain, apprehension, and autotransfusion with each uterine contraction. After delivery, cardiac output increases more (now up to 80% above prelabor values). Along with the effects of blood loss, oxytocin administration, reabsorption of the expanded extravascular volume, and the beginning of lactation, increased cardiac output can lead to rapid cardiac decompensation in patients with heart disease. A detailed discussion of all the cardiac diseases in pregnancy and their anesthetic management is beyond the scope of this chapter (see Chapters 123-137). However, some of the most common cardiac diseases in pregnancy and the anesthetic management during the stressful periods of labor and delivery will be discussed.

Rheumatic Heart Diseases

Rheumatic heart disease occurs as a sequela of rheumatic fever, which has substantially decreased in the developed countries (see Chapter 126). However, it still remains a major cause of maternal mortality during pregnancy, especially in the developing countries.

Mitral Stenosis. Pathophysiology involves a decrease in the mitral valve orifice and obstructed blood flow, which result in increased left atrial pressure, pulmonary venous congestion, and decreased pulmonary compliance. Eventually, increased pulmonary vascular resistance and pulmonary hypertension result in right ventricular hypertrophy and failure. Hemodynamic changes during pregnancy (eg, increased blood volume, cardiac output, and heart rate and decreased systemic vascular resistance) exacerbate mitral stenosis, and cardiac decompensation leading to pulmonary edema commonly occurs around 20–30 weeks' gestation or during the critical times of labor, delivery, and early postpartum period.[57,58] Atrial fibrillation and paroxysmal atrial tachycardia are the other major complications of mitral stenosis.[58]

Patients with tight mitral stenosis, atrial fibrillation, and evidence of pulmonary congestion will benefit from PCWP monitoring, radial arterial lines for direct blood pressure measurements, and serial sampling of arterial blood gases. For relief of labor pain, a segmental lumbar epidural anesthesia is the method of choice. By providing pain relief, tachycardia, increased myocardial O_2 consumption, and the Valsalva effect of bearing down during second stage are abolished. The customary prehydration in anticipation of sympathetic block following epidural anesthesia should be performed cautiously so as not to overload the circulation. Should hypotension occur after the placement of an epidural block, a pure α-agonist such as metaraminol is the preferred drug for treatment.[59] Being a β-agonist, ephedrine causes undesirable tachycardia. For cesarean section, either epidural or general anesthesia can be used. The epidural block should be extended slowly with incremental doses of the local anesthetic to avoid sudden and profound sympathetic block because of lowering systemic vascular resistance. Spinal anesthesia should be avoided because it may cause precipitous hypotension in these patients with fixed cardiac output. If general anesthesia is needed, a slow induction with high doses of narcotics such as fentanyl or sufentanyl is preferable to avoid the usual hemodynamic perturbations of rapid sequence induction with Pentothal and succinylcholine. Using high doses of narcotics for induction during general anesthesia can increase the risk of maternal aspiration and also can lead to neonatal respiratory depression. However, the benefits of a slow induction with minimal hemodynamic alterations outweigh the risks.

Regardless of the anesthetic technique, the following points should be considered when anesthetizing pregnant patients who have mitral stenosis:[59]

1. Rapid heart rate (sinus tachycardia, atrial fibrillation with rapid ventricular response, and paroxysmal atrial tachycardia) is undesirable because it decreases diastolic filling time and cardiac output. In addition, loss of atrial systole due to fibrillation leads to left ventricular failure and pulmonary edema. Therefore, drugs such as ketamine, pancuronium, ephedrine, and atropine should be avoided. Prophylactic digitalization is recommended in all patients with mitral stenosis. In addition, small doses of β-adrenergic blocking agents can be used to lower the heart rate. Some patients with atrial fibrillation and rapid ventricular rate may need cardioversion.
2. Rapid lowering of systemic vascular resistance results in decreased venous return and compensatory tachycardia. Epidural anesthesia thus should be administered cautiously with adequate prehydration.
3. Sudden increases in blood volume, such as rapid fluid administration, and the Trendelenburg position can precipitate pulmonary edema and thus should be avoided.
4. These patients should be monitored closely during the postpartum period as complications such as pulmonary edema and cardiac failure frequently occur during this period.

Mitral Insufficiency. Patients who are asymptomatic prior to pregnancy seldom have serious problems during pregnancy, labor, and delivery. The pathophysiology involves regurgitation of blood through the mitral orifice, resulting in increased left atrial pressure and pulmonary venous pressure. The amount of regurgitation depends on the pressure gradient between the left atrium and left ventricle, duration of systole, and size of the mitral orifice. Eventually, left ventricular failure, pulmonary hypertension, and right ventricular failure set in. Decreased peripheral vascular resistance during pregnancy improves the forward flow, and the intensity of regurgitant murmur actually decreases.[60] On the other hand, patients with compromised left ventricular function may not tolerate the intravascular volume expansion that normally occurs during pregnancy, and pulmonary congestion and edema follow.

When there is evidence of severe mitral regurgitation with left ventricular failure, PCWP monitoring is helpful. The regurgitant flow produces large V waves, especially when mitral regurgitation is acute or subacute with a small, noncompliant left atrium. Such patients will not tolerate acute increases in systemic vascular resistance, which leads to worsening of the regurgitation. A normal or slightly elevated heart rate, which decreases the duration of systole and reduces the regurgitant flow, is desirable.

For labor analgesia, lumbar epidural anesthesia is eminently suitable as it lowers the peripheral resistance and improves the forward flow. Ephedrine can be used to treat hypotension. For cesarean section, epidural anesthesia is the technique of choice. If general anesthesia is needed, negative ionotropic agents such as halothane and enflurane should be avoided, especially if the left ventricular function is compromised. In these patients, a high-dose narcotic induction is preferred to the routine induction with Pentothal and succinylcholine.

Aortic Stenosis. Patients with aortic stenosis become symptomatic in their fifth or sixth decade of life and rarely manifest cardiac failure during pregnancy. Therefore, very little information exists regarding the course of pregnancy complicated by aortic stenosis. Arias and Pineda[61] reported a maternal mortality rate of 17% and fetal mortality rate of 32% in pregnancy complicated by aortic stenosis. The intensity of aortic systolic murmur may not correlate with the severity of stenosis. The majority of patients have electrocardiographic evidence of left ventricular hypertrophy and left-bundle branch block.

Because of fixed cardiac output, these patients do not tolerate any decrease in peripheral vascular resistance. Bradycardia also should be avoided because with a fixed stroke volume the cardiac output and blood pressure are maintained by elevated heart size. Diminished venous return due to blood loss and hypotension from aortocaval compression are poorly tolerated.[57] For labor analgesia, intravenous narcotics can be administered. For vaginal delivery, a pudendal block can be used. For cesarean section, routine induction of general anesthesia with Pentothal and nitrous oxide with relaxant is well tolerated.[59] Inhalation agents that depress myocardial function and lower the systemic vascular resistance should be avoided.

Aortic Insufficiency. Similar to patients with mitral insufficiency, patients with aortic insufficiency tolerate pregnancy well. However, a small percentage (3–9%) develop cardiac failure during pregnancy.[58] Pathophysiology involves left ventricular volume overload and dilation, which eventually lead to left ventricular failure and pulmonary edema. The hemodynamic changes of pregnancy, such as increased heart rate and decreased peripheral resistance, improve the forward flow and reduce the regurgitant fraction.

The important points to remember for patients with aortic insufficiency are that bradycardia increases ventricular diastole and increases the regurgitant fraction. Similarly, increased systemic vascular resistance can precipitate cardiac failure by increasing regurgitation. Epidural anesthesia is the method of choice for labor and delivery. For cesarean section, the anesthetic management as previously recommended for patients with mitral regurgitation can be used.

Congenital Heart Disease

Because of improved medical management and early surgical corrections, more women with congenital heart disease reach childbearing age (see also Chapter 127). Although women with corrected congenital heart disease tolerate pregnancy; in many instances, the correction may be only partial, and these patients need extra care. Common congenital heart problems are discussed here.

Ventricular Septal Defect, Atrial Septal Defect, and Patent Ductus Arteriosus. Patients with ventricular septal defect (VSD), atrial septal defect (ASD), and patent ductus arteriosus (PDA) have a left-to-right shunt with increased pulmonary blood flow, increased right ventricular preload, and right ventricular volume work. Initially, the increased pulmonary volume is accommodated by a compensatory decrease in the pulmonary vascular resistance. Eventually, the chronically elevated pulmonary blood flow leads to increased pulmonary vascular resistance and pulmonary hypertension. The hemodynamic changes during pregnancy (eg, increased heart rate, cardiac output, and increased blood volume) exacerbate the left-to-right shunt while decreased systemic vascular resistance diminishes the shunt.[58,62] Reversal of the shunt can occur because of acute elevations of pulmonary artery pressure or profound hypotension resulting from severe blood loss.[63] In patients with ASD, the chronically elevated right and left atrial volume and distention can cause atrial arrhythmias such as supraventricular tachycardia and atrial fibrillation.[63]

Asymptomatic patients with left-to-right shunt do not require special monitoring. In patients with large septal defects or PDA with compromised ventricular function and pulmonary hypertension, radial and pulmonary arterial pressure monitoring is helpful. It is important to avoid acute increases in systemic vascular resistance and heart rate because these increase the left-to-right shunts. It is equally important to avoid sudden and marked decreases in systemic vascular resistance, especially in patients with severe pulmonary hypertension, which leads to reversal of the shunt and central cyanosis and hypoxia. Pulse oximetry during labor allows continuous monitoring of oxygenation. For labor analgesia, continuous lumbar epidural anesthesia is recommended to prevent elevation of systemic vascular resistance. If general anesthesia is needed, a combination of narcotic technique with 100% oxygen and low concentrations of inhalational agent and muscle relaxant may be the method of choice. This technique causes minimal hemodynamic alterations during the stressful time of induction of anesthesia and tracheal intubations. Factors that cause marked increase in pulmonary vascular resistance during general anesthesia (eg, hypercarbia, hypoxia, acidosis, and hyperinflation of the lungs) are to be avoided. Blood lost during surgery should be replaced promptly as severe hypotension can cause reversal of shunt in the postpartum period.

Eisenmenger's Syndrome. This is a severe form of cyanotic congenital heart disease in which there is a large communication between the two sides of the heart at the ventricular (VSD), atrial (ASD), or aorta pulmonary level (PDA). The cardinal features are severe pulmonary hypertension and high pulmonary vascular resistance with a reversed or bidirectional shunt.[64] This condition is associated with high maternal and neonatal mortality rates.[65] The symptoms and signs include central cyanosis, polycythemia, clubbing, dyspnea at rest, and syncopal attacks. Factors that decrease systemic vascular resistance or increase pulmonary resistance also increase the right-to-left shunt and result in immediate worsening of the hemodynamic status. The hemodynamic changes of pregnancy, such as decreased peripheral resistance and increased cardiac output, blood volume, and heart rate, are poorly tolerated. Factors that predispose to further increase in pulmonary artery pressure, such as bearing-down efforts (Valsalva effect), increased atrial volume overload (contraction of uterus), hypoxia, acidosis, and hypercarbia, all aggravate the right-to-left shunt and worsen cyanosis and desaturation.

Cardiac decompensation can occur any time during labor and delivery but is more likely to occur in the immediate postpartum period. Such patients should be monitored in the intensive care unit throughout the peripartum period. A radial arterial line should be inserted. Insertion of a pulmonary artery catheter may be hazardous but can be achieved. Administering epidural anesthesia for vaginal delivery may be difficult as even a minimal lowering of systemic vascular resistance is not tolerated. However, successful administration of epidural anesthesia in these patients has been reported.[66,67] If epidural anesthesia is chosen, liberal uses of epidural narcotics combined with minimal doses of local anesthetics may be the method of choice as the degree of sympathetic block is lessened. For induction of general anesthesia, high doses of fentanyl can be safely used. The use of inhalational agents is not recommended because they are myocardial depressants and also lower the systemic vascular resistance. In addition, because of the decreased pulmonary artery flow, the rate of rise of arterial concentration of inhalation agents is limited, thus the uptake of inhalation agents may be prolonged.

Tetralogy of Fallot. Similar to Eisenmenger's syndrome, a right-to-left shunt occurs in this condition. Obstruction of the outflow from the right ventricle (infundibular stenosis), right ventricular hypertrophy, ventricular septal defect, and overriding aorta constitute the tetralogy of Fallot. Women in their childbearing years usually have already undergone either partial or total correction of the defects. Those who have undergone total correction tolerate pregnancy well.

Lowering of systemic vascular resistance increases the right-to-left shunt and is poorly tolerated. Similarly, acute hypotension due to severe blood loss during labor or cesarean section can aggravate the right-to-left shunt.[63] For labor analgesia, intrathecal narcotics or systemic medications should be considered. For cesarean section, general anesthesia with inhalation agents such as halothane or enflurane may be used. Increased myocardial contractility, tachycardia, hypercarbia, and hypoxia should be avoided as these aggravate the infundibular obstruction. The use of inhalation agents decreases the infundibular obstruction and augments pulmonary blood flow. Propranolol may be used to treat increased heart rate and contractility. Mothers should receive 100% oxygen throughout labor and delivery. A pulse oximeter is invaluable in detecting sudden arterial desaturation. Hemodynamic monitoring is important to recognize and treat the rapid circulatory changes during labor, delivery, and postpartum period.

Primary Pulmonary Hypertension

Primary pulmonary hypertension has a predilection for young women of childbearing age, and maternal mortality rate is reported to be 50% (see Chapter 127).[54] The fetal mortality rate is also high, and the incidence of abortion and prematurity is increased. The pulmonary artery pressure is at systemic level and there is right ventricular hypertrophy and failure. Tricuspid insufficiency, peripheral edema, and liver congestion follow. The left ventricle usually is not involved.

These patients should be monitored with pulmonary and radial artery pressure catheters. Additional increases in the pulmonary vascular resistance caused by hypoxia, hypercarbia, acidosis, and hyperinflation of lungs are poorly tolerated. In addition, marked decreases in systemic vascular resistance can lead to decreased venous return. With a fixed ventricular output, the patient is unable to compensate, which leads to cardiac failure. For labor analgesia, intravenous narcotics or intrathecal morphine[68] may be used safely. For general anesthesia for cesarean section, high doses of intravenous narcotics, relaxants, 100% oxygen, and low concentration of inhalation agents may be used. Hyperinflation of the lungs should be avoided, and a tidal volume of 5–10 mL/kg should not be exceeded.[59]

Mitral Valve Prolapse

Mitral valve prolapse occurs commonly among women of childbearing age. Pathophysiology involves ballooning of the mitral valve leaflet into the atrium during left ventricular contraction. As in mitral regurgitation, increased venous return and decreased systemic vascular resistance decrease the degree of prolapse. In some patients, severe mitral regurgitation, premature ventricular arrhythmias, and supraventricular tachycardia occur.[69] In severe cases, typical symptoms include chest pain, dyspnea, fatigue, and syncope. Echocardiography can confirm the diagnosis.

Epidural anesthesia can be used safely for labor analgesia or cesarean section. However, patients should receive adequate prehydration to maintain the venous return and to prevent the subsequent exacerbation of the mitral valve prolapse. In patients with severe mitral valve prolapse with mitral insufficiency, anesthetic considerations are similar to those previously described for mitral insufficiency of rheumatic origin. Prophylactic antibiotics are indicated in patients with progressive mitral insufficiency.

Peripartum Cardiomyopathy

Occurring primarily among young black women, peripartum cardiomyopathy manifests as congestive heart failure in the last month of pregnancy or in the first five months after delivery (see also Chapter 131).[70-72] The exact incidence is not known, but maternal mortality rate is 30–60% and infant mortality rate is approximately 10%. The etiology is also unknown. Several causes, including viral myocarditis, have been suggested. Pathophysiology involves gradual softening, thickening, and dilation of the myocardium and decreased myocardial contractility and ejection fraction. The cardiovascular changes during pregnancy such as increased blood volume (increased preload) and increased heart rate lead to progressive left ventricular failure. Treatment consists of bed rest, salt restriction, diuretics, and digitalis.

These patients should be monitored with radial and pulmonary artery catheters. For labor analgesia, intravenous narcotics can be administered. However, a slow induction of epidural analgesia is beneficial as it causes a reduction in both preload and afterload. For cesarean section, either epidural or general anesthesia may be used. If general anesthesia is chosen, a technique using high doses of fentanyl can be used. The use of Pentothal and inhalation agents may produce undesirable myocardial depression.

Hypertrophic Cardiomyopathy

The pathophysiology of hypertrophic cardiomyopathy involves dynamic obstruction of ventricular outflow (see also Chapter 132). Any increase in myocardial contractility and reductions in the preload or afterload will increase the obstruction. While the increased intravascular volume of pregnancy decreases the subaortic gradient, the decreased peripheral resistance, increased heart rate, and myocardial contractility exacerbate the obstruction.[54]

For labor analgesia, a combination of epidural narcotics with minimal doses of local anesthetic may be used. Sudden reductions in the afterload should be avoided by adequate prehydration. For cesarean section, a high level of block produced by regional anesthesia can predispose the patient to sudden hypotension and compensatory tachycardia and worsen the obstruction. General anesthesia with an inhalation agent such as halothane is preferred as halothane decreases the outflow obstruction by the negative inotropic and chronotropic effects.

Coronary Artery Disease

Coronary artery disease is rare among women of childbearing age (see also Chapter 133). However, with increased cigarette smoking and postponement of pregnancy, the incidence of coronary artery disease is increasing and is currently reported to affect 1 in 10,000 pregnancies.[73,74] The maternal mortality rate is 35–40%. However, if the initial myocardial infarction occurs in the third trimester with delivery occurring within two weeks, maternal mortality is reported to be as high as 50%.[73,74]

Women with severe coronary artery disease resulting in frequent, unstable angina and those who have had a recent myocardial infarction require invasive monitoring. In some of these patients with diastolic dysfunction and decreased left ventricular compliance, a rise in pulmonary capillary wedge pressure is an early warning sign of myocardial ischemia and impending infarction.

Continuous monitoring of the V5 lead is necessary to identify ST-segment changes. All previous medications such as β-adrenergic blocking agents and nitrates should be continued throughout the pregnancy, labor, and delivery.

The onset of painful uterine contractions, stress, anxiety, and bearing-down reflex during second stage all may precipitate anginal attacks, and early institution of lumbar epidural anesthesia is recommended. Severe reductions in afterload and the compensatory tachycardia following epidural anesthesia are poorly tolerated. These patients should be prehydrated adequately and left uterine displacement should be maintained.

For cesarean section, epidural or general anesthesia can be used. During general anesthesia, the presser response to tracheal intubation should be minimized by using nitroglycerine and β-adrenergic blocking agents. Drugs that cause tachycardia (for example, atropine and ketamine) and volatile agents that depress myocardial function (for example, halothane) should be omitted. In patients with compromised left ventricular function, a high-dose narcotic induction technique is recommended. Postoperatively, these patients should be monitored in the intensive care unit.

Pregnancy after Valve Replacement

Patients who have had mitral valvulotomy may have symptoms and signs of residual mitral stenosis and pulmonary hypertension (see also Chapter 136). In addition, atrial fibrillation and systemic embolization can occur. Patients who have undergone aortic valvular surgery usually have some degree of left ventricular dysfunction. Many of these patients are anticoagulated with coumadin, which usually is replaced with heparin after the onset of labor. Other problems include paravalvular leaks, vegetative endocarditis, hemolysis, thrombocytopenia, and malfunctioning valves.[59]

In patients who have had mitral valve replacement, the presence of severe pulmonary hypertension and ventricular compromise indicate pulmonary and radial artery pressure monitoring. In patients receiving heparin, all forms of regional anesthesia should be avoided. Heparin can be discontinued or reversed with protamine; when the activated partial thromboplastin time becomes normal, epidural anesthesia can be considered.

NEUROLOGIC DISEASES

Epilepsy

Epilepsy is a convulsive disorder affecting approximately 0.5% of the population.[75] It can follow trauma, infections, or brain tumor, or it may be idiopathic (see also Chapter 199). The latter is the most common form of epilepsy affecting obstetric patients. Pregnant women with epilepsy are more prone to develop complications such as preeclampsia, hemorrhage, premature rupture of membranes, and premature labor.[76,77] There is also increased incidence of obstetric intervention such as cesarean or forceps delivery. Treatment consists of phenobarbitone, phenytoin, and primidone.

During labor, epidural anesthesia is highly beneficial as it prevents hyperventilation and respiratory alkalosis that can cause a seizure. There are no known drug interactions between local anesthetics and anticonvulsants, and patients with epilepsy are not a higher risk for convulsions caused by local anesthetic toxicity. However, inadvertent intravascular injection of local anesthetics should be prevented by frequent aspiration of the epidural catheter and by injecting incremental doses of local anesthetics rather than large boluses. If general anesthesia is required, drugs known to cause seizure activity (eg, enflurane, ketamine, and methohexitone) should be avoided[78-80]

Multiple Sclerosis

This is a chronic demyelinating disease of the central nervous system characterized by exacerbations and remissions (see also Chapter 199).[81] The disease process involves the cerebral cortex, corticospinal tract, spinothalamic tract, posterior columns, and cranial nerves. Peripheral nerves usually are spared. Pregnancy does not affect the course of the disease adversely, but a relapse can occur during pregnancy, labor, or, more often, in the immediate postpartum period. Increased temperature worsens the neurologic derangement. Treatment consists of steroids, immunosuppressants, and diazepam.

The use of regional anesthesia is controversial, but there is no strong evidence to support the idea that spinal anesthesia can cause a relapse.[82] Spinal puncture does not exacerbate the disease. However, factors such as impaired blood-brain barrier and altered cerebrospinal fluid composition should be considered before administering a spinal anesthetic. Epidural anesthesia[83,84] can be used safely with local anesthetics devoid of neurotoxicity (eg, lidocaine or bupivacaine). This procedure may be safer than a spinal and may be more acceptable for the patient as the intense sensory and motor block of spinal anesthesia can be avoided. The anesthesiologist must discuss the various anesthetic techniques and the risks and benefits of each technique with patients before administering anesthesia. If general anesthesia is administered, especially to patients with severe demyelinating disease with muscle wasting, the use of succinylcholine for tracheal intubation can cause severe hyperkalemia. In this situation, muscle relaxants such as atracurium, vercuronium, or pancuranium can be used.

Myasthenia Gravis

Myasthenia gravis is a disease affecting the myoneural junction. It is twice as common in females in their third decade of life, although it can affect any age group (see also Chapter 199). Pathophysiology involves an autoimmune mechanism[85,86] in which acetylcholine antibodies are formed and occupy the receptor sites at the myoneural junction, which degrades. The available acetylcholine receptors are decreased by 70–90%. Acetylcholine receptor antibodies are identified in 87% of these patients, although the storage and quantal release of acetylcholine is unaltered. Approximately 65%[87] of these patients have thymic hyperplasia and 50–70% of these patients improve after thymectomy. Effect of pregnancy on patients with myasthenia varies. In one study, approximately 40% of patients demonstrated remission, 32% showed deterioration, and 28% had no change in the disease pattern.[88] Myasthenia gravis does not affect the course of labor, and cesarean section is performed only for obstetric indications. Emotional stress such as labor pains, anxiety, and minor infections can all lead to undue fatigue in these women. Administering magnesium sulfate and certain antibiotics such as neomycin or streptomycin can exacerbate the symptoms of myasthenia gravis and even precipitate a myasthenic crisis.[89]

Treatment consists of anticholinesterases such as neostigmine and pyridostigmine, steroids, thymectomy, or immunosuppressants. With the onset of labor, the oral anticholinesterase drugs are not well absorbed from the gastrointestinal tract; thus parenteral administration with appropriate reduction in dosage is essential.

Preoperative evaluation should include a detailed history and physical examination. The extent and degree of neuromuscular dysfunction and extent of respiratory muscle weakness should be evaluated. The presence of bulbar muscle weakness and the possibility of aspiration should be considered.

The following laboratory tests are needed. An electrocardiogram detects arrhythmias, cardiomyopathy (focal necrosis of myocardium has been reported), and ST-segment changes.[90] A chest x-ray detects cardiomegaly and pulmonary infiltrates. Serial pulmonary function tests determine the extent of pulmonary dysfunction and the improvement following institution of anticholinesterase therapy. Similarly, arterial blood gases are useful in determining the adequacy of drug therapy.

For labor and vaginal delivery, epidural anesthesia is the technique of choice. It provides adequate pain relief and obviates the need for systemic medications that cause respiratory depression. In addition, epidural anesthesia can be used for application of outlet forceps, which often is indicated in these women to shorten the second stage of labor. The use of 2-chloroprocaine should be avoided in myasthenic patients as this drug is metabolized by plasma cholinesterase. Other local anesthetic agents such as lidocaine or bupivacaine can be used safely. The safety of using epidural narcotics in patients with myasthenia is not fully established yet. For cesarean section, either epidural or general anesthesia can be used. If epidural anesthesia is administered, the ventilatory status should be monitored constantly because severe respiratory embarrassment can occur due to combined effects of a high block and restrictive pulmonary function. Pulse oximetry and capnography are useful under these circumstances.

General anesthesia sometimes is required in these patients, especially if the bulbar or respiratory muscles are involved. Tracheal intubations can be achieved easily with a fraction of the regular dose of nondepolarizing agents. For example, a dose of 2–3 mg of curare or 0.09–0.21 mg/kg of atracurium provides adequate muscle relaxation to facilitate tracheal intubation.[91] Because these patients usually are resistant to the effects of succinylcholine and also frequently tend to develop phase-II block, succinylcholine is not a popular agent for use in patients with myasthenia gravis. Regardless of type of muscle relaxant used, the degree of neuromuscular blockade should be monitored using a peripheral nerve stimulator. At the end of the procedure, the residual effects of the neuromuscular blocking agents should be reversed with atropine and neostigmine. In some patients, despite the reversal, respiratory efforts may be inadequate; these patients should be mechanically ventilated until the respiratory status improves.

In the postpartum period, dose requirements for anticholinesterase drugs can fluctuate widely. These patients should be evaluated carefully with serial pulmonary function tests and arterial blood gas determinations and the dosage adjusted accordingly.

Paraplegia

Several factors influence the choice of anesthesia in patients with spinal cord lesion and paraplegia.

Autonomic hyperreflexia is a mass reflex that occurs in patients with a spinal cord lesion at T_7 or above and consists of hypertension, headache, bradycardia, facial flushing, pilomotor erection, and dilation of pupils.[92] A sudden rise in blood pressure can lead to cerebral or retinal hemorrhage. Stimulation of skin below the level of the spinal cord lesion or contraction or distention of a hollow viscus such as uterus, bladder, or gut can precipitate the symptoms. The etiology is believed to be the unmodulated or uninhibited mass reflexes in response to the afferent impulses entering the isolated spinal cord. Other causes may involve stimulation of isolated adrenal glands, which are supplied by the greater splanchnic nerves, or the heightened sensitivity of paraplegic patients to norepinephrine secretion from adrenergic nerve endings.[93]

Hyperkalemia is caused by administering succinylcholine during general anesthesia if the spinal cord injury was sustained within six months prior to cesarean section.[94]

In parturients with traumatic spinal cord lesion above T_{10}, the uterine contractions are virtually painless and usually most patients can be delivered vaginally. Outlet forceps usually are applied to shorten the duration of second-stage labor. Administration of epidural anesthesia is suitable as it abolishes the autonomic hyperreflexia and also avoids the need for a general anesthetic should the patient require cesarean section.[95] Epidural narcotics have been used successfully in patients with paraplegia.[96] During general anesthesia, sympathetic response to tracheal intubation can be prevented by pretreating with nitroglycerin or β-adrenergic blocking agents. The use of succinylcholine is avoided and intermediate-acting nondepolarizing agents such as vercuronium or atracurium may be used to facilitate tracheal intubation.

Chorioamnionitis is one of the most common causes of maternal sepsis during the peripartum period. It usually follows rupture of the amniotic membrane, although maternal bloodborne infection of amniotic fluid can occur in the presence of intact membranes.

The use of regional anesthesia in patients with signs and symptoms of systemic bacteremia is controversial. Many anesthesiologists are reluctant to use regional blocks because of the theoretical possibility of introducing a nidus of infection into the epidural or subarachnoid space during the performance of the block and causing an epidural abscess or meningitis. An extensive literature review failed to reveal any reports of epidural abscess or meningitis following administration of regional blocks in febrile parturients. However, until further information is available, it is prudent to avoid regional blocks in the presence of fulminant maternal sepsis with clinical manifestation such as high fever, chills, and myalgia. Conversely, in the absence of such severe systemic dissemination, regional blocks can be administered safely.

Genital Herpes Simplex

Genital herpes lesions are caused by either herpes simplex virus 1[97] or herpes simplex virus 2 (see also Chapter 91). Of the two, herpes simplex virus 2 causes most of the primary lesions and all of the secondary lesions.[98] The primary infection is associated with systemic symptoms such as fever, chills, and signs of meningitis. There is viremia with positive viral culture and placental transfer of virus to the fetus. The secondary lesions are localized to the genital area and usually are not associated with viremia and generalized symptoms. Studies have shown that continuous epidural anesthesia can be used safely in patients with secondary lesions.[98] However, in the presence of active primary infection with severe systemic symptoms or if the lesions exist over the lumbar area, it is prudent to avoid regional blocks.

MALIGNANT HYPERPYREXIA

The incidence of malignant hyperpyrexia or hyperthermia (MH) is approximately 1 in 14,000, and the vast majority of MH reactions occurs in children and young adults.[99] Successful management of MH reactions in parturients has been reported.[100,101] Other reports include those patients with MH susceptibility who have undergone regional or general anesthesia during pregnancy.[102,103] With the advent of dantrolene therapy, the mortality rate has decreased from 70% to less than 10%.

Susceptible individuals sometimes have a family history of unexplained death during or soon after a general anesthetic. A previous uncomplicated anesthesia does not rule out the possibility of MH reaction during a subsequent anesthetic. Some of the patients with MH susceptibility exhibit squint, kyphoscoliosis, increased muscle mass, muscle weakness, and ptosis. Patients with musculoskeletal diseases such as muscular dystrophies and myotonia may develop MH reaction under anesthesia.[104] Increased serum creatinine phosphokinase (CPK) levels are seen in 70% of MH patients; however, a normal CPK level does not rule out susceptibility. A positive skeletal muscle contracture test (exposure of a sample of the susceptible person's muscle to halothane or caffeine triggers contracture) can diagnose malignant hyperthermia.[105]

All anesthetic volatile agents and depolarizing muscle relaxants trigger MH reaction. Other drugs, such as caffeine, sympathomimetics, calcium, amide local anesthetics, and cardiac glycosides all have been implicated as triggering agents. The febrile reaction leading to MH crisis also can be precipitated by emotional stress and anxiety associated with prolonged labor. During labor, serum CPK values in-

TABLE 202–5. DIAGNOSIS OF MALIGNANT HYPERPYREXIA

Clinical Signs
Unexplained tachycardia and cardiac arrhythmias
Tachypnea and cyanosis
Rapid rise in temperature
Muscle rigidity (trismus following succinylcholine)
Profuse sweating
Laboratory Findings
Hypercarbia
Increased end-tidal CO_2
Increased $PaCO_2$
Hypoxemia
Decreased PaO_2
Central venous desaturation
Hyperkalemia
Respiratory and metabolic acidosis
Increased serum CPK (late sign)

crease, which can make the diagnosis of an MH crisis more difficult. Drugs such as narcotics, barbiturates, phenothiazines, benzodiazepines, butyrophenones, nitrous oxide, and nondepolarizing muscle relaxants can be used safely in MH-susceptible patients.[106]

Regional anesthesia can be used safely for patients with MH susceptibility. Epidural anesthesia with ester agents such as chloroprocaine should be established early in labor to avoid the stress and anxiety that invariably follow the onset of regular, painful contractions. The availability of a "malignant hyperpyrexia cart" with dantrolene, ice-cold solutions, cooling blanket, and drugs such as bicarbonate cannot be overemphasized. The temperature of the patient should be monitored carefully during labor. An anesthesia machine devoid of inhalation agents and with fresh soda lime and breathing circuits should be ready in case a general anesthetic is needed during labor. If general anesthesia becomes necessary, prophylactic use of dantrolene should be considered. All known triggering agents should be avoided. A balanced anesthetic technique using Pentothal for induction and a large dose of a nondepolarizing relaxant such as pancuronium to facilitate tracheal intubation is recommended. Narcotics and tranquilizers may be needed. The monitoring during anesthesia includes temperature, end-tidal CO_2 tension, pulse oximetry, and continuous electrocardiogram. Constant vigilance and careful observation are necessary for signs of MH reaction such as unexplained tachycardia, arrhythmias, increased end-tidal CO_2, cyanosis, and increased body temperature.[107] (The signs and symptoms of MH crisis are given in Table 202–5.) Should a crisis occur, active cooling should be started and dantrolene therapy should be initiated (Table 202–6). Patients should be hyperventilated with 100% oxygen. Mannitol or other diuretics should be used to ensure diuresis, and sodium bicarbonate should be administered to treat metabolic acidosis. Prophylactic use of dantrolene has been associated with severe uterine atony and postpartum hemorrhage.[108] The routine use of dantrolene prophylaxis thus should be reserved for patients receiving a general anesthetic for cesarean section.

TABLE 202–6. TREATMENT OF MALIGNANT HYPERPYREXIA DURING ANESTHESIA

Summon additional help
Discontinue all anesthetics and hyperventilate with 100% oxygen
Change the anesthetic circuit and soda lime or secure a new anesthesia machine
Administer dantrolene, 2.5 mg/kg initially, up to a total dose of 10 mg/kg
Start cooling with cooling blanket, ice-cold IV saline, peritoneal lavage
Administer mannitol to promote diuresis to ensure a urine output 1 mL/kg per hr
Insert a central venous line as soon as possible
Treat cardiac arrhythmias with procainamide, 200 mg; repeat if necessary
Administer bicarbonate, 1–2 meq/kg
Treat hyperkalemia with glucose and insulin
Monitor ABG, with serial urine output, serum K^+, serum CPK, and coagulation studies
Do not move the patient from OR until she is stable, and observe her in the ICU for the next 24–48 hours

From Recommendations of the Malignant Hyperthermia Association.

OBSTETRIC HEMORRHAGE DURING THE THIRD TRIMESTER

The two leading causes of maternal hemorrhage during the third trimester are *abruptio placentae* and *placenta previa.*

Abruptio Placentae

Abruptio placentae is associated with a maternal mortality rate of 1.8–2.8% and a perinatal mortality rate as high as 15–25%.[109] The etiology is not known but usually is associated with multiparity, uterine abnormalities, preeclampsia, and previous placental abruption.[110] Bleeding may be external (revealed) or internal (concealed). Significant internal bleeding with large retroplacental hematoma can occur with very little external bleeding, which frequently leads to an underestimation of the actual blood loss. In addition to hemorrhagic hypovolemia, coagulation abnormalities usually are present in these women. These situations result from the release of thromboplastin from the decidual bed, which causes widespread activation of the extrinsic coagulation pathway and disseminated intravascular coagulation. In addition, plasminogen is activated, which causes fibrinolysis. The net result is hypofibrinogenemia, elevated serum fibrin split products, and widespread bleeding.[111]

The choice of anesthetic technique depends on the clinical condition of the patient and the severity of the bleeding. Severe placental abruption usually is associated with hypotension, coagulopathy, and fetal distress or fetal death.

Following admission, the coagulation status should be assessed as quickly as possible. Some of the useful tests include hematocrit, partial thromboplastin time, prothrombin time, fibrin degradation product, fibrinogen levels, platelet count, clotting time, clot lysis time, and bleeding time (Table 202–7). A bedside whole-blood clotting time estimation is invaluable and is performed easily, especially when the clinical condition warrants immediate obstetric intervention while the coagulation results are pending. A sample of maternal venous blood is drawn into a glass tube, which is allowed to stand undisturbed. If a clot fails to form within 6–10 minutes or if the clot is lysed within 1 hour, severe clotting abnormalities are present.[110,112] If clotting time exceeds 30 minutes, the fibrinogen level may be as low as 100 mg/dL. The coagulation tests should be repeated frequently to assess the effectiveness of therapy.

TABLE 202–7. COAGULATION SCREENING IN DIC SYNDROME

Test	Results/Remarks
Whole-blood clotting time	If clot forms in <6 min, fibrinogen content >150 mg %
Whole-blood clot lysis time	A normal clot does not lyse within 8 hr. If lysis occurs in <1 hr, fibrinogen levels <100 mg %
Platelet count	Normal range: 150,000–300,000/mm^3
Modified Ivy bleeding time	>10 min is abnormal
Activated partial thromboplastin time (APTT)	Tests the intrinsic coagulation pathway
Prothrombin time (PT)	Tests the extrinsic coagulation pathway
Thrombin time	> 5 sec prolongation is abnormal
Fibrinogen	In normal pregnancy, levels are elevated; thus <300 mg % is abnormal
Fibrin degradation products (Fibrin/fibrinogen-related antigen)	Tested by immunologic technique; >40 is considered abnormal
Euglobin lysis time	Ability of the euglobin precipitate of the plasma to lyse a clot (the precipitate is devoid of inhibitors of fibrinolysis)

From Ramanathan S[112] with permission.

The anesthetic management of patients with severe placental abruption is a challenge. Two large-bore intravenous cannulae should be inserted for volume replacement. Insertion of an indwelling arterial cannula and a central venous catheter is helpful. Several different types of crystalloids or colloids can be used for the initial resuscitation until whole blood becomes available. As soon as cross-matched blood is available, it should be administered. In addition, blood component therapy should be commenced to correct the deficient factors (Table 202–8). Administration of cryoprecipitate is beneficial as it corrects the fibrinogen deficiency. Other blood components such as fresh-frozen plasma and platelet transfusions may become necessary.

Regional anesthesia is not advisable in the presence of hemorrhagic hypovolemia, coagulopathy, and fetal distress. For general anesthesia, ketamine may be used for induction of anesthesia as the use of Pentothal may cause further hypotension. The use of inhalation agents such as isoflurane, ethrane, and halothane should be avoided as they decrease systemic pressure. Further, they cause uterine relaxation and aggravate bleeding. A short-acting narcotic such as fentanyl can be used to maintain anesthesia. These patients should be monitored closely during the postpartum period as coagulopathy lingers for several days after delivery. In addition, these patients should be monitored for signs of renal failure, adult respiratory distress syndrome, and pituitary failure.

Placenta Previa

Placenta previa is one of the most common causes of vaginal bleeding during the third trimester. Unlike placental abruption, vaginal bleeding is usually painless. The incidence varies between 1 in 200 to 1 in 53 deliveries.[113,114] The etiology is not known, but some of the risk factors have been identified, including previous cesarean section, previous curettage, and multiparity.[114] *Placenta accreta* is more common in patients who have had a cesarean section.[114,115] Diagnosis is based on history, physical examination (vaginal examination is deferred), and ultrasound examination to determine the position of the placenta.

Similar to patients with placental abruption, these women may have profuse bleeding and require massive resuscitation. However, unlike abruption, patients with *placenta previa* seldom have coagulation problems. The choice of anesthetic technique depends on the clinical condition of the patient. The anesthesiologist should take the following factors into consideration. In patients with *placenta previa* and a history of cesarean section, the incidence of *placenta accreta* is high. This may become evident during cesarean section when considerable blood loss can necessitate a cesarean hysterectomy. The location of the placenta is important as the uterine incision may involve the anteriorly located placenta, leading to severe hemorrhage during cesarean section. Postpartum hemorrhage is common as the lower uterine segment (the implantation site) does not contract well.

TABLE 202–8. BLOOD AND BLOOD COMPONENTS

Product	Uses	Remarks
Stored blood	Volume replacement	Lacks factors V and VIII, platelets; may result in dilutional coagulopathy; 2–3 DPG decreased
Fresh blood	Useful in coagulopathy; must be used within 24 hr after collection	Hepatitis screening, AIDS screening may be incomplete
Fresh frozen plasma	200–250 mL bags; contains all clotting factors; used in factor XI deficiency; coumarin overdose	Each bag is derived from one unit of blood; hepatitis risk, ABO RH crossmatching needed
Cryoprecipitate	One unit = 15–25 mL (derived from one unit of blood), prepared by thawing FFP at 1–6°C; used for fibrinogen, factor VIII and XI deficiencies, and von Willebrand's disease	10 units will increase fibrinogen 50 mg/dL; increased fibronectin content, improved renal function
Platelets	Thrombocytopenia DIC, platelet dysfunction; prolonged bleeding time	One unit will increase the count by 5000–10,000/m^2 body surface
Factor IX complex	Contains factors II, VII, IX, and X; reconstituted before use; used when large FFP volumes are harmful	Significant hepatitis risk, increased thrombosis

From Ramanathan S[112] with permission.

It thus is evident that the major problem in this situation is severe blood loss, which needs immediate replacement. As with placental abruption, two large-bore intravenous catheters are inserted for volume replacement. The use of crystalloids or colloids such as 5% albumin may become necessary until blood becomes available, especially in a severely hypovolemic patient. These patients usually respond to adequate volume replacement. For cesarean section, general anesthesia, using ketamine for induction and a narcotic such as fentanyl for maintenance, is recommended.

In those women who are not bleeding actively and are hemodynamically stable, regional anesthesia may be considered.[110] However, if severe blood loss occurs during cesarean section under regional anesthesia and a hysterectomy is necessary, many anesthesiologists prefer to administer general anesthesia to prevent further aggravation of the hypotension by the sympathectomy incurred by the block. In addition, a patient who is awake may not be able to tolerate the lengthy surgery with extensive intra-abdominal manipulations and may require large doses of sedatives or narcotics that obtund the airway reflexes and make her prone to pulmonary aspiration.

REFERENCES

1. Giesecke AH, Morris RE, Dalton MD, et al. Of magnesium, muscle relaxants, toxemic parturients, and cats. *Anesth Analg*. 1968;47:689.
2. Ramanathan J, Sibai BM, Pillai R, et al. Neuromuscular transmission studies in preeclamptic women receiving magnesium sulfate. *Am J Obstet Gynecol*. 1988;158:40.
3. Brinkman CR, Assali NS. Uteroplacental hemodynamic response to antihypertensive drugs in hypertensive pregnant sheep. In: Lindheimer MD, Katz AI, Zuspan FP, eds. *Hypertension in Pregnancy*. New York, NY: John Wiley and Sons; 1976.
4. James FM III. Pregnancy-induced hypertension. In: James FM III, Wheeler AS, Dewan DM, eds. *Obstetric Anesthesia, The Complicated Patient*. 2nd ed. Philadelphia: FA Davis; 1988:411.
5. Naulty J, Cefalo RC, Lewis PE. Fetal toxicity of nitroprusside in the pregnant ewe. *Am J Obstet Gynecol*. 1981;139:708.
6. Ellis SC, Wheeler AS, James FM III, et al. Fetal and maternal effects of sodium nitroprusside used to counteract hypertension in gravid ewes. *Am J Obstet Gynecol*. 1982;143:766.
7. Stempel JE, O'Grady JP, Morton MJ, Johnson KA. Use of sodium nitroprusside in complications of gestational hypertension. *Obstet Gynecol*. 1982;60:533.
8. Wheeler AS, James FM III, Meis PJ, et al. Effects of nitroglycerine and nitroprusside on the uterine vasculature in gravid ewes. *Anesthesiology*. 1980;52:390.
9. Hood DD, Dewan DM, James FM III, et al. The use of nitroglycerine in preventing the hypertensive response to tracheal intubation in severe preeclampsia. *Anesthesiology*. 1985;63:329.
10. Cotton DB, Longmire S, Jones MM, et al. Cardiovascular alterations in severe pregnancy-induced hypertension: effects of intravenous nitroglycerine coupled with blood volume expansion. *Am J Obstet Gynecol*. 1986;154:1053.
11. Poulton TJ, James FM III, Lockridge O. Prolonged apnea following trimethaphan and succinylcholine. *Anesthesiology*. 1979;50:54.
12. Mabie WC, Gonzalez AR, Sibai BM, et al. A comparative trial of labetalol and hydralazine in the acute management of severe hypertension complicating pregnancy. *Obstet Gynecol*. 1987;70:328.
13. Ramanathan J, Sibai BM, Mabie WC, et al. The use of labetalol for attenuation of the hypertensive response to endotracheal intubation in preeclampsia. *Am J Obstet Gynecol*. 1988;159:650.
14. Joyce TH, Debnath KS, Baker EA. Preeclampsia: relationship of CVP and epidural analgesia. *Anesthesiology*. 1979;51:S297.
15. Ramanathan S. Preeclampsia. In: Ramanathan S, ed. *Obstetric Anesthesia*. Philadelphia: Lea and Febiger; 1988:151.
16. Moir DD, Victor-Rodrigues L, Willocks J. Epidural analgesia during labour in patients with preeclampsia. *J Obstet Gynaecol Br Commonw*. 1972;79:465.
17. Crawford JS. Epidural analgesia in pregnancy hypertension. *Clin Obstet Gynecol*. 1977;4:735.
18. Jouppila P, Jouppila R, Hollmen A, et al. Lumbar epidural analgesia to improve intervillous blood flow during labor in severe preeclampsia. *Obstet Gynecol*. 1982;59:158.
19. Newsome LR, Bramwell RS, Curling PE. Severe preeclampsia: hemodynamic effects of lumbar epidural anesthesia. *Anesth Analg*. 1986;65:31.
20. James FM III, Dewan DM, Floyd HM, et al. Chloroprocaine vs bupivacaine for lumbar epidural analgesia for elective cesarean section. *Anesthesiology*. 1980;52:488.
21. Ramanathan J, Bottorff M, Jeter JN, et al. The pharmacokinetics and maternal and neonatal effects of epidural lidocaine in preeclampsia. *Anesth Analg*. 1986;65:120.
22. Preston PG, Rosen MA, Hughes SC, et al. Epidural anesthesia with fentanyl and lidocaine for cesarean section: maternal effects and neonatal outcome. *Anesthesiology*. 1988;68:938.
23. Hodgkinson R, Husain FJ, Hayashi RH. Systemic and pulmonary blood pressure during cesarean section in parturients with gestational hypertension. *Can Anesth Soc J*. 1980;27:389.
24. Wright JP. Anesthetic considerations in preeclampsia-eclampsia. *Anesth Analg*. 1983;62:590.
25. Jouppila P, Kuikka J, Jouppila R, et al. Effect of induction of general anesthesia for cesarean section on intervillous blood flow. *Acta Obstet Gynecol Scand*. 1979;58:249.
26. Rawal N, Sjostrand U, Christoffersson E, et al. Comparison of intramuscular and epidural morphine for postoperative analgesia in the grossly obese: influence on postoperative ambulation and pulmonary function. *Anesth Analg*. 1984;63:583.
27. Datta S. The diabetic parturient. In: James FM, Wheeler AS, Dewan DN, eds. *Obstetric Anesthesia: The Complicated Patient*. 2nd ed. Philadelphia, PA: FA Davis; 1988:401.
28. Freinkel N. Of pregnancy and progeny. *Diabetes*. 1980;29:1023.
29. Tyson JE, Felig P. Medical aspects of diabetes in pregnancy and the diabetogenic effects of oral contraceptives. *Med Clin North Am*. 1971;55:947.
30. Brumfield CG, Huddleston JF. The management of diabetic ketoacidosis in pregnancy. *Clin Obstet Gynecol*. 1984;27:50.
31. Madsen H, Ditzel J. Changes in red blood cell oxygen transport in diabetic pregnancy. *Am J Obstet Gynecol*. 1982;143:421.
32. Brans YW, Escobedo MB, Hayashi RH, et al. Perinatal mortality in a large perinatal center: five-year review of 31,000 births. *Am J Obstet Gynecol*. 1984;148:284.
33. Rush RW, Davey DA, Segall ML. The effect of preterm delivery on perinatal mortality. *Br J Obstet Gynaecol*. 1978;85:806.
34. Creasy RK, Gummer BA, Liggins GC. System for predicting spontaneous preterm birth. *Obstet Gynecol*. 1980;55:692.
35. Michalak D, Klein V, Marquette GP. Myocardial ischemia: a complication of ritodrine tocolysis. *Am J Obstet Gynecol*. 1983;146:861.
36. Philipsen T, Eriksen PS, Lynggard F. Pulmonary edema following ritodrine-saline infusion in premature labor. *Obstet Gynecol*. 1981;58:304.
37. Finley J, Katz M, Rojas-Perez M, et al. Cardiovascular consequences of beta-agonist tocolysis: an echocardiographic study. *Obstet Gynecol*. 1984;64:787.
38. Ramanathan S. Preterm labor. In: Ramanathan S, ed. *Obstetric Anesthesia*. Philadelphia: Lea and Febiger; 1988:289.
39. Turner ES, Greenberger PA, Patterson R. Management of the pregnant asthmatic patient. *Ann Intern Med*. 1980;6:905.
40. Greenberger PA. Asthma in pregnancy. *Clin Perinatol*. 1985;12:571.
41. Dawson A, Simon RA. Bronchospastic disorders: an overview. In: Dawson A, Simon RA, eds. *The Practical Management of Asthma*. New York: Grune & Stratton; 1984:3.
42. Dunlap NE, Fulmer JD. Corticosteroid therapy in asthma. *Clin Chest Med*. 1984;5:669.
43. Jenne JW. Theophylline use in asthma: some current issues. *Clin Chest Med*. 1984;5:645.
44. Stirt JA, Sullivan SF. Aminophylline. *Anesth Analg*. 1981;60:587.
45. Romero R, Kadar N, Gonzales Govea F, et al. Pharmacokinetics of intravenous theophylline in pregnant patients at term. *Am J Perinatol*. 1983;1:31.
46. Labovitz E, Spector S. Placental theophylline transfer in pregnant asthmatics. *JAMA*. 1982;247:786.
47. Aranda JV, Sitar DS, Parsons WD, et al. Pharmacokinetic aspects of theophylline in premature newborns. *N Engl J Med*. 1976;295:413.
48. Rosenfeld CR, Barton MD, Meschia G. Effects of epinephrine on distribution of blood flow in the pregnant ewe. *Am J Obstet Gynecol*. 1976;124:156.
49. Anderson KE, Bengtsson LP, Gustafson I, et al. The relaxing effect of terbutaline on the human uterus during term labor. *Am J Obstet Gynecol*. 1975;121:602.
50. Schatz M, Patterson R, Zeitz S, et al. Corticosteroid therapy for the pregnant asthmatic patient. *JAMA*. 1975;233:804.
51. Morris HG. Mechanisms of glucocorticoid action in pulmonary disease. *Chest*. 1985;88:133S.
52. Manchikanti L, Kraus JW, Edds SP. Cimetidine and related drugs in anesthesia. *Anesth Analg*. 1982;61:595.
53. Stirt JA, Berger JM, Sullivan SF. Lack of arrhythmogenicity of isoflurane following administration of aminophylline in dogs. *Anesth Analg*. 1983;62:568.

54. Sullivan JM, Ramanathan KB. Cardiovascular disorders. In: Brudenell M, Wilds PL, eds. *Medical and Surgical Problems in Obstetrics*. England: John Wright and Sons Ltd; 1984:11.
55. Rubler S, Damani PM, Pinto ER. Cardiac size and performance during pregnancy estimated with echocardiography. *Am J Cardiol*. 1977;40:534.
56. Katz R, Karliner JS, Resnik R. Effects of a natural volume overload state (pregnancy) on left ventricular performance in normal human subjects. *Circulation*. 1978;58:434.
57. Ueland K. Rheumatic heart disease and pregnancy. In: Elkayam U, Gleicher N, eds. *Cardiac Problems in Pregnancy Diagnosis and Management of Maternal and Fetal Disease*. New York: Alan R. Liss Inc; 1982:79.
58. Szekely P, Snaith L. *Heart Disease and Pregnancy*. London: Churchill Livingstone; 1974.
59. Mangano DT. Anesthesia for the pregnant cardiac patient. In: Shnider SM, Levinson G, eds. *Anesthesia for Obstetrics*. Baltimore, MD: Williams and Wilkins; 1987:345.
60. Marcus FI, Ewy GA, O'Rourke RA, et al. The effect of pregnancy on the murmurs of mitral and aortic regurgitation. *Circulation*. 1970;41:795.
61. Arias F, Pineda J. Aortic stenosis and pregnancy. *J Reprod Med*. 1978;20:229.
62. Bloomfield DK. The natural history of ventricular septal defect in patients surviving infancy. *Circulation*. 1964;29:914.
63. Cobb T, Gleicher N, Elkayam U. Congenital heart disease and pregnancy. In: Elkayam U, Gleicher N, eds. *Cardiac Problems in Pregnancy Diagnosis and Management of Maternal and Fetal Disease*. New York: Alan R. Liss; 1982:61.
64. Jones MA, Howitt G. Eisenmenger's syndrome in pregnancy. *Br Med J*. 1965;1:1627.
65. Gleicher N, Midwall J, Hochberger D, et al. Eisenmenger's syndrome and pregnancy. *Obstet Gynecol Surv*. 1979;34:721.
66. Spinnato JA, Kraynack BJ, Cooper MW. Eisenmenger's syndrome in pregnancy: epidural anesthesia for elective cesarean section. *N Engl J Med*. 1981;304:1215.
67. Asling JH, Fung DL. Epidural anesthesia in Eisenmenger's syndrome: a case report. *Anesth Analg*. 1974;53:965.
68. Abboud TK, Raya J, Noueihed R, et al. Intrathecal morphine for relief of labor pain in a parturient with severe pulmonary hypertension. *Anesthesiology*. 1983;59:477.
69. Barlow JB, Pocock WA, Marchard P, et al. The significance of late systolic murmurs. *Am Heart J*. 1963;66:443.
70. Homans DC. Peripartum cardiomyopathy. *N Engl J Med*. 1985;312:1432.
71. Veille JC. Peripartum cardiomyopathies: a review. *Am J Obstet Gynecol*. 1984;148:805.
72. Julian DG, Szekely P. Peripartum cardiomyopathy. *Prog Cardiovasc Dis*. 1985;27:223.
73. Hankins GD, Wendel GD Jr, Leveno KJ, et al. Myocardial infarction during pregnancy: a review. *Obstet Gynecol*. 1985;65:139.
74. Chestnut DH, Zlatnik FJ, Pitkin RM, et al. Pregnancy in a patient with a history of myocardial infarction and coronary artery bypass grafting. *Am J Obstet Gynecol*. 1986;155:372.
75. Hopkins A. Neurological disorders. *Clin Obstet Gynaecol*. 1977;4:419.
76. Bjerkedal T, Bahna SL. The course and outcome of pregnancy in women with epilepsy. *Acta Obstet Gyencol Scand*. 1973;52:245.
77. Knight AH, Rhind EG. Epilepsy and pregnancy: a study of 153 pregnancies in 59 patients. *Epilepsia*. 1975;16:99.
78. Kruczek M, Albin MS, Wolf S, et al. Postoperative seizure activity following enflurane anesthesia. *Anesthesiology*. 1980;53:175.
79. Ferrer-Allado T, Brechner VL, Dymond A, et al. Ketamine-induced electroconvulsive phenomena in the human limbic and thalamic regions. *Anesthesiology*. 1973;38:333.
80. Male CG, Allen EM. Methohexitone induced convulsions in epileptics. *Anesth Intens Care*. 1970;5:226.
81. Silberberg DH. The demyelinating diseases. In: Wyngaarden JB, Smith LH, eds. *Cecil Textbook of Medicine*. Philadelphia: WB Saunders; 1988:2211.
82. Bamford C, Sibley W, Laguna J. Anesthesia in multiple sclerosis. *Can J Neurol Sci*. 1978;5:41.
83. Crawford JS, James FM III, Nolte H, et al. Regional analgesia for patients with chronic neurological disease and similar conditions. *Anaesthesia*. 1981;36:821.
84. Bader AM, et al. Anesthesia for patients with multiple sclerosis. *J Clin Anesth*. 1988;1:21.
85. Plauche WC. Myasthenia gravis. *Clin Obstet Gynecol*. 1983;26:592.
86. Lindstrom JM, Seybold ME, Lennon VA, et al. Antibody to acetylcholine receptor in myasthenia gravis: prevalance, clinical correlates, and diagnostic value. *Neurology*. 1976;26:1054.
87. Bradley WG, Adams RD. Myasthenia gravis, neuromuscular junction disorders, and episodic muscular weakness. In: Petersdorf RG, et al, eds. Harrison's Principles of Internal Medicine. New York: McGraw-Hill; 1983:1910.
88. Osserman KE. Obstetrics. In: Osserman KE, ed. *Myasthenia Gravis*. New York: Grune & Stratton; 1958:239.
89. Hokkanen E. The aggravating effect of some antibiotics on the neuromuscular blockade in myasthenia gravis. *Acta Neurol Scand*. 1964;40:346.
90. Genkins G, Mendelow H, Sohel HJ, et al. Myasthenia gravis: analysis of thirty-one consecutive postmortem examinations. In: Osserman KE, ed. *Myasthenia Gravis*. Springfield, Ill: Charles C Thomas; 1961:519.
91. Azar I. The response of patients with neuromuscular disorders to muscle relaxants: a review. *Anesthesiology*. 1984;61:173.
92. Head H, Riddoch G. The automatic bladder, excessive sweating and some other reflex conditions in gross injuries of the spinal cord. *Brain*. 1917;40:188.
93. Debarge O, Christensen NJ, Corbett JL, et al. Plasma catecholamines in tetraplegics. *Paraplegia*. 1974;12:44.
94. Cooperman LH, Strobel GE Jr, Kennell EM. Massive hyperkalemia after administration of succinylcholine. *Anesthesiology*. 1970;32:161.
95. Watson DW, Downey GO. Epidural anesthesia for labor and delivery of twins of a paraplegic mother. *Anesthesiology*. 1980;52:259.
96. Baraka A. Epidural meperidine for control of autonomic hyperreflexia in a paraplegic parturient. *Anesthesiology*. 1985;62:688.
97. Corey L, Holmes KK. Genital herpes simplex virus infections: current concepts in diagnosis, therapy, and prevention. *Ann Intern Med*. 1983;98:973.
98. Ramanathan S, Sheth R, Turndorf H. Anesthesia for cesarean section in patients with genital herpes infections: a retrospective study. *Anesthesiology*. 1986;64:807.
99. Britt BA, Kalow W. Malignant hyperthermia: a statistical review. *Can Anaesth Soc J*. 1970;17:293.
100. Cupryn JP, Kennedy A, Byrick RJ. Malignant hyperthermia in pregnancy. *Am J Obstet Gynecol*. 1984;150:327.
101. Tettambel M. Malignant hyperthermia in an obstetric patient. *J Am Osteopath Assoc*. 1980;79:773.
102. Wadhwa RK. Obstetric anesthesia for a patient with malignant hyperthermia susceptibility. *Anesthesiology*. 1977;46:63.
103. Khalil SN, Williams JP, Bourke DL. Management of malignant hyperthermia susceptible patient in labor with 2-chloroprocaine epidural anesthesia. *Anesth Analg*. 1983;62:119.
104. McPherson EW, Taylor CA Jr. The King syndrome: malignant hyperthermia, myopathy, and multiple anomalies. *Am J Med Genet*. 1981;8:159.
105. Ellis FR, Keaney NP, Harriman DG, et al. Screening for malignant hyperpyrexia. *Br Med J*. 1972;3:559.
106. Britt BA. Malignant hyperthermia. In: *Refresher Courses in Anesthesiology*. Philadelphia: JB Lippincott; 1976:87.
107. Baudendistel L, Goudsouzian N, Cote C, et al. End-tidal CO_2 monitoring: its use in the diagnosis and management of malignant hyperthermia. *Anaesthesia*. 1984;39:1000.
108. Weingarten AE, Korsh JI, Neuman GG, et al. Postpartum uterine atony after intravenous dantrolene. *Anesth Analg*. 1987;66:269.
109. Sher G, Statland BE. Abruptio placentae with coagulopathy: a rational basis for management. *Clin Obstet Gynecol*. 1985;28:15.
110. Biehl DR. Antepartum and postpartum hemorrhage. In: Shnider SM, Levinson G, eds. *Anesthesia for Obstetrics*. Baltimore, MD: Williams and Wilkins; 1987:281.
111. Pritchard JA. Hematological problems assocaited with delivery, placental abruption, retained dead fetus and amniotic fluid embolism. *Clin Haematol*. 1973;2:563.
112. Ramanathan S. Coagulation and hemoglobin disorders. In: Ramanathan S, ed. *Obstetric Anesthesia*. Philadelphia: Lea and Febiger; 1988:167.
113. Wilson RJ. Bleeding during late pregnancy. In: Wilson RJ, Carrington ER, Ledger WJ, eds. *Obstetrics and Gynecology*. St Louis, MO: CV Mosby; 1983.
114. Green-Thompson RW. Antepartum haemorrhage. *Clin Obstet Gynaecol*. 1982;9:479.
115. Singh PM, Rodrigues C, Gupta AN. Placenta previa and previous cesarean section. *Acta Obstet Gynecol Scand*. 1981;60:367.
116. Norris MC. Respiratory disease. In: James FM, Wheeler AS, Dewan DM, eds. *Obstetric Anesthesia: The Complicated Patient*. Philadelphia: FA Davis; 1988:181.

Chapter Two Hundred and Three
Complications of Operative Obstetrics

David C. Shaver

203

During recent years, the practice of obstetrics has changed dramatically. Improvements in areas such as anesthesia, blood replacement and therapy of infectious complications have resulted in markedly reduced maternal morbidity and mortality. The continued advances in maternal well-being have been accompanied by a corresponding emphasis on improving fetal outcome. Thus, the incidence of traumatic vaginal delivery has decreased as difficult vaginal delivery has been replaced by cesarean section. Complications of operative delivery thus have become less common. Although less frequent, complications of vaginal delivery, and increasingly of abdominal delivery, continue to occur. Many complications such as severe lacerations and pelvic hematomas, while mostly associated with operative delivery, may also occur as the result of an otherwise seemingly normal vaginal delivery. This chapter will address primarily traumatic injuries encountered during the conduct of both vaginal delivery and cesarean section, and discuss the predisposing factors, prevention, and management.

COMPLICATIONS OF VAGINAL DELIVERY

Cervical Lacerations

Injury to the cervix is an inherent complication of virtually any labor and vaginal delivery. Careful inspection of the cervix after delivery uniformly reveals small tears and abrasions, and evidence of an old injury is readily apparent in the nongravid multiparous patient. These injuries result from the marked stretching and dilatation of the cervix during labor, coupled with the prolonged pressure from the fetal presenting part. The presence of abrasions, ragged edges, and small (less than 1 cm) lacerations are of limited clinical significance, seldom associated with significant bleeding, and rarely require therapy.

Occasionally, larger tears of the cervix occur that may be associated with heavy bleeding and require surgical repair. These tears usually occur along one or both lateral margins at the 3 and 9 o'clock positions, areas in which there is less muscular and fibrous tissue. Less often, linear lacerations along other positions of the cervix or actual amputation of parts of the cervix (usually the anterior lip) may occur.

Predisposing factors for cervical lacerations are varied and in individual cases may be obscure. As stated above, there is an inherent weakness of the lateral margin of the cervix, which predisposes to tear. Lacerations are often the result of precipitous labors or especially difficult, prolonged labor. Amputation of the cervix may be noted after rapid labor such as that associated with *abruptio placentae,* or in association with prolonged labor during which the anterior lip of the cervix becomes markedly edematous and is shorn off by descent of the fetal head. Excessive pressure of the fetal head, either by premature maternal expulsive effort or fundal pressure by the attendant, may result in cervical tears. Vigorous cervical examinations or attempts to manually dilate the cervix can be contributing factors. Finally, instrumental delivery, especially if forceps are applied to an incompletely dilated or retracted cervix, may result in extensive lacerations to the cervix.

Prompt repair of deep cervical lacerations usually is required because of brisk bleeding. However, careful reapproximation also may decrease risks for subsequent chronic cervical infection and possibly incompetent cervical os.

The most important aspects in repair are adequate anesthesia and exposure to ensure that the full extent of the laceration can be visualized so that successful repair can be accomplished. Sponge forceps then are placed on the cervix on both sides of the laceration and the cervix is retracted and reapproximated with a fine absorbable suture. It is important that the initial suture be placed above the uppermost end of the laceration, keeping in mind that the ureters run about 2 cm lateral to the confluence of the upper cervix and lateral fornix. The use of interrupted sutures rather than a continuous stitch has been advocated but is probably of no great consequence.

Special mention must be made of cervical lacerations that extend above the lateral fornix into the lower uterine segment or parametrial areas. In these lacerations, the full extent of the lesion and the inability to visualize the uppermost portion make vaginal repair difficult and potentially hazardous, and dictate an abdominal approach to ensure adequate hemostasis and avoidance of injury to the ureter.

Vaginal Lacerations

Injuries to the lower vagina are associated with lacerations of the vulva and perineum, are readily apparent, and are easily managed in association with repair of the perineal tear. Isolated injury or lacerations of the upper vagina are less common. Although they may occur spontaneously during vaginal delivery, they usually are associated with operative delivery, especially midforceps rotation.

Lacerations of the upper vagina are typically longitudinal and frequently result in heavy bleeding. Bilateral lacerations are not uncommon. Close inspection of the vagina after all vaginal deliveries is mandatory, and heavy bleeding after delivery in the absence of uterine atony frequently is an indication that a vaginal laceration is present.

Vaginal lacerations often are associated with severe hemorrhage, and adequate visualization is mandatory to assure proper closure. It is advantageous to defer examination until after delivery of the placenta to facilitate visualization. In general, it is not necessary to isolate individual vessels. With retractors placed in the vagina so that the full extent of the laceration can be visualized, an absorbable suture is placed above the upper extent of the laceration. The laceration then is closed with interrupted or continuous sutures placed deeply into the underlying tissue. If hemostasis is adequate, no further therapy is necessary. Frequently, however, persistent oozing or concern about hematoma formation is present, in which case insertion of a vaginal pack is indicated. The vaginal pack should be removed in 24 hours or less, if possible. If a vaginal pack is inserted, a Foley catheter should be inserted since the pack will obstruct the urethra.

Anterior vaginal lacerations are common, usually superficial, and not associated with significant bleeding. They frequently respond to short-term pressure applied over the tear. More extensive lacerations may require repair. Because these lacerations are in close proximity to the urethra, a catheter should be inserted prior to repair. Interrupted sutures are used to prevent distortion of the tissues.

Perineal Lacerations

Lacerations of the perineum are classified according to the depth of involvement of the tear.

First degree—superficial, involving the mucosa of the vagina and the skin of the perineum.

Second degree—extends into the perineal body with involvement of the transverse perineal muscle.

Third degree—includes laceration of the anal sphincter.

Fourth degree—laceration that extends into the rectum.

Perineal lacerations are common following vaginal delivery. Precipitate or uncontrolled delivery, forceps delivery, and the presence of edema of the vulva are predisposing factors. Difficult delivery, such as shoulder dystocia or the delivery of a large infant, may result in tears, although frequently none of these factors are present when extensive laceration of the perineum occurs.

Much has been written about the routine performance of episiotomy to prevent lacerations of the lower genital tract, as well as the prevention of subsequent pelvic relaxation. Episiotomy has become the standard of care in the United States, especially in the nulliparous patient, since its routine use was advocated by DeLee and Pomeroy early in the century. However, there is very little evidence that routine episiotomy has any protective effect against the occurrence of significant (third degree or fourth degree) lacerations[1], and some studies suggest that deep perineal lacerations are more common in patients who undergo a midline episiotomy.[2] Advocates argue, however, that closing of a surgical incision of the perineum is more satisfactorily and easily performed than a spontaneous laceration.

Repair of perineal lacerations requires careful reapproximation of the tissues using a fine absorbable suture.

First degree—tissues are closed with interrupted or figure-of-eight sutures.

Second degree—the vaginal mucosa is closed with a running suture, and the perineal body is repaired with deep interrupted sutures. The skin is approximated with a running subcuticular suture.

Third degree—The lacerated ends of the anal sphincter are identified and repaired with interrupted figure-of-eight sutures, making sure to incorporate the fascia of the sphincter. Repair then proceeds as with repair of a second-degree laceration.

Fourth degree—The edges of the rectal mucosa are closed with interrupted sutures, often with a second layer of sutures incorporating the pararectal fascia. Further repair then proceeds as above.

Pelvic Hematomas. Rupture of subcutaneous blood vessels during delivery or repair may lead to formation of pelvic hematomas. Classified according to their anatomic location in relationship to the fascial planes of the pelvis, hematomas appearing below the pelvic diaphragm result in vulvar hematomas, whereas those above the diaphragm appear as either vaginal hematomas, if below the cardinal ligament, or broad ligament hematomas, if above the cardinal ligaments.[3] Extensive dissection of the hematomas may occur with resultant pain, spontaneous rupture, and symptomatic blood loss.

Although pelvic hematomas may occur as a result of delivery trauma, this is only the case infrequently. Hematomas may result from otherwise uncomplicated deliveries and, on occasion, prior to or during labor. Other predisposing factors include careless repair of perineal and vaginal lacerations. The presence of bleeding abnormalities, such as DIC or thrombocytopenia, also predispose to the development of hematomas, especially following pudendal block.

Management depends on the extent of the hematomas as well as the site and symptoms. Small vulvar hematomas may respond to careful observation, analgesics, and local icepacks. If the hematoma is extensive or enlarging, it is incised surgically and clots are evacuated. Bleeding points (if located) are controlled, and the cavity is packed or a drain is placed.

Extensive hematomas of the vagina are managed in a similar manner, and frequently the incision may be closed primarily with interrupted sutures, with a single or multiple layers. However, deep and extensive hematomas are managed better with drains and the use of a vaginal pack, and the bladder is drained with an indwelling catheter until the pack is removed.

Broad ligament hematomas are of special concern since they are not readily apparent and the first sign of their presence may be unexplained anemia or shock.[4] Additionally, spontaneous rupture into the peritoneal cavity is possible with massive bleeding and hemoperitoneum as a consequence.

Detection of broad ligament hematomas requires a careful bimanual examination under anesthesia with palpation of the hematoma. Uterine exploration, a search for a possible site of rupture, is an integral part of the examination. Depending on the degree of blood loss and the condition of the patient, conservative management with replacement of blood, antibiotics, and careful attention to patient condition may be possible. Continued blood loss, clinical deterioration of the patient, or evidence of hemoperitoneum requires laparotomy. The retroperitoneal space is entered, clots are evacuated, and bleeding points are searched for and ligated if present. Frequently, distinct bleeding points are not apparent, and ligation of the hypogastric artery is required if bleeding persists. A retroperitoneal drain then is placed and brought out through a separate stab incision prior to closing the retroperitoneal space. Care must be taken to isolate the ureter during dissection, since it may be displaced and injured during exploration of the hematoma.

Uterine Rupture

Uterine rupture is a rare but potentially catastrophic event. Anatomically, ruptures have been classified as complete (rupture of the myometrium and the overlying serosa) or incomplete (serosa intact). Functionally, however, and from the standpoint of maternal prognosis[5,6], it is more important to distinguish if the rupture occurred through a surgically scarred uterus or in a patient with no previous surgery. Previous uterine surgery, primarily cesarean section but also including such procedures as myomectomy or unifications procedures, account for the majority of cases of uterine ruptures. Uterine rupture in a patient with no prior surgery is rare and usually associated with multiparity or hyperstimulation of the uterus with oxytocin.

Most uterine ruptures occur during labor. Findings vary from no symptoms with the rupture being noted only on postpartum exploration of the uterus, to severe bleeding, shock, and expulsion of the fetus into the peritoneal cavity. With significant rupture, uterine activity diminishes and fetal distress ensues. Ruptures of prior low cesarean scars may be associated with very few symptoms and no change in uterine activity, even when measured by internal pressure catheters. In general, spontaneous rupture of the uterus in a patient with no prior surgery tends to be catastrophic with significant blood loss and the potential for severe maternal and fetal morbidity and mortality. Separation of a previous low cesarean section scar, on the other hand, is rarely associated with maternal or fetal mortality. Rupture of prior classical uterine incisions are often catastrophic and may occur prior to the onset of labor.

Treatment of uterine rupture is generally surgical. An exception, however, is the discovery of a separation of a previous low cesarean scar, especially if it is incomplete, following a vaginal delivery. In these cases, expectant management is appropriate if no significant bleeding is present. Major ruptures usually are associated with heavy bleeding or hemoperitoneum and require surgical repair. There are two options: repair of the wound or hysterectomy. The decision is dependent on the extent of laceration, involvement of major vessels, and the parity of the patient. However, most ruptures are amenable to repair, and this is the procedure of choice if possible.

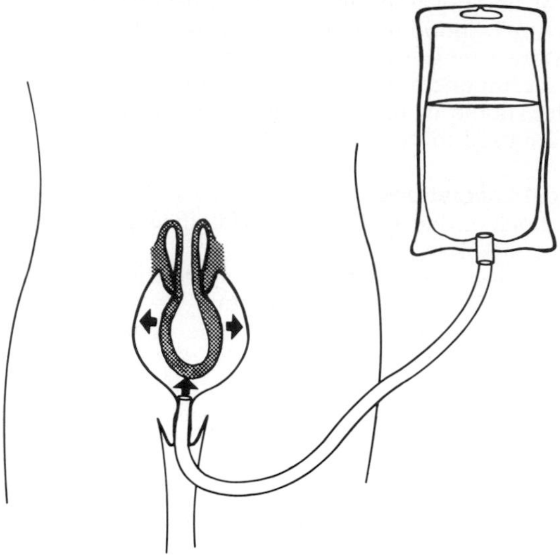

Figure 203–2. Schematic representation of forces involved for replacement of an inverted uterus using hydrostatic technique. Note lateral distention of vagina, with resultant dilation of cervical ring, in addition to pressure against uterine fundus.

Inversion of the Uterus

Another rare condition associated with severe hemorrhage and shock is uterine inversion (Fig. 203–1). Classified as *complete* when the fundus extends through the cervix or *incomplete* when the fundus is inverted but not through the cervix, uterine inversion is frequently the result of mismanagement of the third stage of labor. Although it may occur spontaneously, it is often the result of excessive traction on the umbilical cord associated with fundal pressure. The condition is readily apparent and is associated with profound shock and blood loss. The shock is seemingly out of proportion to the blood loss.[7]

Management consists of several steps. First, blood replacement is begun at once and anesthesia is kept readily available. Treatment of maternal shock prior to replacement of the uterus is of paramount importance and results in the lowest maternal mortality. Replacement is attempted immediately after initial therapy for shock, since it becomes more difficult with delay. Controversy exists as to whether the placenta should be removed prior to attempted replacement, although this may be necessary in order to replace the uterus. If immediate replacement is not successful, an attempt is made to relax the uterus by the induction of general anesthesia with halothane or the intravenous administration of tocolytics. Magnesium sulfate is the agent of choice, since the maternal cardiovascular status generally precludes the use of beta-mimetics. Care must be taken during attempted replacement, since uterine perforation may occur with the fingertips. Preferably, the fingers should be bent and the dorsum of the fingers or the fist used for replacement, guiding the fundus of the uterus through the cervix. If the cervical ring becomes well developed, replacement is more difficult and tocolytics may be helpful. Repeated attempts at vaginal replacement are unwise since blood loss and shock will continue. Surgical replacement often is advocated at this point, although the use of the O'Sullivan hydrostatic technique[8,9] is frequently successful and obviously avoids the risks of the operative approach (Fig. 203–2). Briefly, this technique involves replacement of the uterus into the vagina. Then one end of a large bore tubing is placed in the vagina and the introitus is occluded manually. The other end of the tubing then is attached to a receptacle, which is kept filled with saline and held several feet above the level of the vagina. The hydrostatic pressure then accomplishes replacement by direct pressure in the uterus, coupled with distention of the vagina and cervical ring.

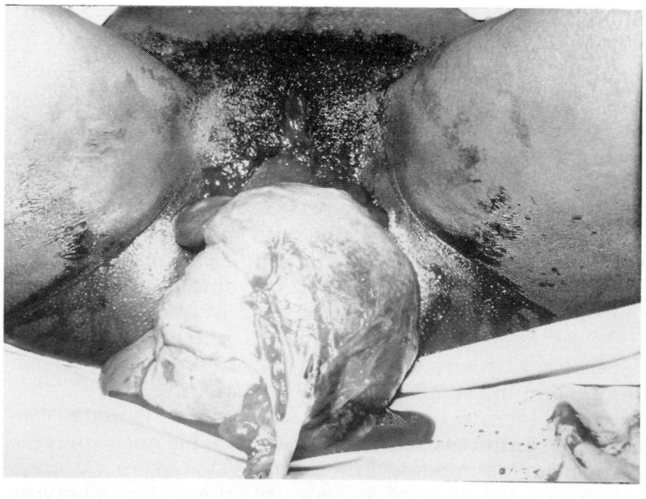

Figure 203–1. Acute puerperal uterine inversion, demonstrating attached placenta.

Surgical replacement is accomplished by the use of an abdominal incision exposing the uterus. The round ligaments, ovarian ligaments, and fallopian tubes usually are drawn into the funnel of the inverted uterus. Allis clamps are placed on the uterus just below the edge of the funnel and the uterus is extracted gently (Huntington procedure). As the uterus is withdrawn, more clamps are placed sequentially just below the edge of the funnel until the uterus is replaced. If unsuccessful, a posterior incision through the cervix may be performed to dilate the cervical opening (Haultain procedure). Once replacement is completed, regardless of the technique, uterotonics are given to decrease the possibility of recurrence.

COMPLICATIONS OF ABDOMINAL DELIVERY

Cystotomy

One of the more frequent immediate complications of cesarean section involves inadvertent laceration of the bladder (cystotomy). Rarely, cystotomy occurs spontaneously in association with spontaneous uterine rupture.[10] More often, previous pelvic surgery is associated with dense scarring of the tissue planes, and the bladder is entered accidentally either during entry into the peritoneal cavity or when attempting to dissect the bladder off the lower uterine segment. Additionally, when cesarean section is performed with advanced labor and marked development of the lower uterine segment has occurred, the operator may fail to recognize the degree of cephalic advancement of the bladder, and accidental injury may occur in the attempt to incise the vesicouterine fold of the peritoneum.

Although not entirely preventable, recognition of risk factors for inadvertent cystotomy will prevent many such occurrences. Care must be taken on entering the peritoneal cavity, especially in patients with previous pelvic surgery. The peritoneum should be raised with hemostats or forceps, and palpation of the peritoneal fold usually will demonstrate the lack of adherent viscera. Development of an avascular plane between the uterus and bladder usually is not difficult, but especially in patients with previous surgery, careful dissection is necessary and usually can be accomplished. In cases in which the bladder is densely adherent and severe injury to the urinary tract is more likely, abandonment of a low-segment incision is advisable, and a vertical incision of the uterus should be performed to avoid the need for bladder advancement.

Fortunately, most injuries to the bladder during cesarean section occur in the dome of the bladder and are repaired easily and associated rarely with significant long-term morbidity. Unrecognized injury, however, can lead to urine leakage or subsequent fistula formation. Careful assessment of the bladder during every surgical procedure thus is mandatory. Most injuries are recognized easily, but if doubt exists, the bladder can be instilled with 100–150 cm^3 of sterile saline or preferably sterile milk, and spillage is promptly recognized.

Repair of bladder injury is uncomplicated if only the dome of the bladder has been entered. To be certain of the location of the injury, the ureteral orifices should be identified. If their exact location cannot be confirmed, 5 mL of indigo carmine can be injected intravenously; within minutes, discharge of the blue urine from the ureteral orifices is recognized easily. If the injury lies very close to the ureteral orifices, ureteral stints can be placed so that the exact location of the ureter can be determined. This is rarely necessary, and after confirming that the injury is not close to the ureter, the bladder is closed in two layers. The first layer is a running suture of a 3–0 absorbable suture to reapproximate the mucosa. The overlying muscularis then is repaired with either a running or interrupted suture, also of a 3–0 absorbable suture. Integrity of the bladder repair then is assessed by instillation of sterile milk in the bladder.

Following repair, the bladder should be drained by catheter, and gross hematuria generally clears within 24–48 hours. Controversy exists as to the length of time that drainage needs to be continued. Although some would advocate removing the catheter as soon as the hematuria clears, most authorities recommend continuing drainage for 5–7 days, with occasional recommendations for 10 days.

Ureteral Injury

Operative injuries to the ureter are fortunately only a rare complication of cesarean section. The pelvic ureter normally passes laterally to within 1.5–2.0 cm of the cervix as it courses along the lateral pelvic wall. During a normal, uneventful cesarean section this should pose no difficulty. However, in situations associated with bleeding in the broad ligament[11] or during the course of a cesarean hysterectomy, injury to the ureter is possible unless the course of the ureter is ascertained carefully.[12-13] Injury may result from crushing or transections, or may result from a suture, which results in obstruction or kinking. Historically, most ureteral injuries are not recognized intraoperatively, although a high index of suspicion and careful assessment should reveal most injuries.

Most ureteral injuries can be prevented, or at least recognized intraoperatively, if the course of the ureter is determined adequately during surgery. The ureter should be recognized easily beneath the peritoneum as it enters the pelvis by crossing above the bifurcation of the iliac artery and running medial to the internal iliac artery. If the peritoneum is entered laterally to this point, the ureter will be noted on the medial leaf of the peritoneum, and its course can be demonstrated by blunt dissection as it runs lateral to the uterosacral ligament and cervix, and under the uterine artery.

If mild injury occurs to the ureter (such as kinking related to a ligature) and the suture has been removed, the area can be observed to confirm that the ureter appears viable. A drain may be brought out retroperitoneally to assure that if urine drainage does occur that it will be recognized easily. A ureteral stint also may be inserted and left in place to assure urine drainage until complete healing has taken place.

With more severe crushing injury or traumatic injury, urologic consultation should be obtained if available. Options at this point are reanastomosis of the ureter or implantation of the ureter into the bladder. In general, if the injury is in the lower half of the pelvic ureter, reimplantation is the method of choice, while reanastomosis is reserved for injuries in the upper pelvis. If reimplantation of the ureter into the bladder is performed, the distal segment of the ureter is ligated, and the free end of the ureter to be implanted is tagged with a suture. An incision then is made in the mucosa of the bladder, a hemostat is used to create a tunnel, and the suture then is placed in the hemostat and the ureter is advanced through the tunnel. The end of the ureter is spatulated, and 0000 chromic sutures are used to sew the ureter to the bladder mucosa. A ureteral stint then is placed and the bladder repaired in 2 layers.

Several techniques exist for reanastomosis of a severed ureter, although the simplest involves spatulation of both ends of the ureter and repair with interrupted sutures of 0000 chromic, being careful not to incorporate the mucosa. A stint is inserted and the retroperitoneum is drained through a separate incision.

Bowel Injury

Injury to the small or large bowel occurs infrequently during cesarean section. Injury is more likely to occur in patients with previous surgery or a history of infection that has resulted in adhesions of the bowel to the uterus and anterior abdominal wall.

Lacerations of the small bowel generally occur during sharp dissection of the bowel during lysis of adhesions. If only small areas of the serosa are involved, no repair is indicated. If the injury involves the mucosa, repair is carried out in two layers. First, the mucosa is closed with a running suture of 000 or 0000 chromic. Next, the muscularis and serosa are repaired with interrupted sutures of fine silk. To avoid constriction of the lumen, small bowel lacerations always should be closed in a transverse manner. Extensive injury to the small bowel may require resection. General surgical consultation is advisable when resection is necessary.

Intraoperative injury of the large bowel is rare. Spillage of large bowel contents is much more serious, and general surgical consultation and antibiotic therapy are indicated. Small defects sometimes may be repaired in two layers, whereas more extensive injury will require a diverting colostomy since the bowel is unprepared.

POSTPARTUM HEMORRHAGE

Normal vaginal delivery is associated with a blood loss of approximately 500 cm^3, and cesarean section generally results in up to 1000 cm^3 blood loss. The normal gravida must lose greater than 1000 cm^3 of blood before there is a significant change in the postpartum hematocrit.[14] Management of severe hemorrhage requires attention to maintenance of cardiovascular stability with fluid, and possibly blood replacement. More important, the underlying etiology of the excess blood loss must be determined and resolved.

The initial approach requires careful assessment and inspection of the uterus and birth canal to determine the site of bleeding. Exploration of the uterus is performed to rule out the possibility of uterine rupture, presence of retained placental fragments, or the presence of uterine atony with retained blood and clots. Bleeding also may be explained by cervical or vaginal lacerations, which will require repair, as previously noted.

The most common cause of excessive bleeding is uterine atony, which usually will respond to evacuation of clots from the uterus, massage of the fundus, and intravenous administration of oxytocin. Occasionally, the response to these measures is not satisfactory, or the patient will develop recurrent uterine atony. Blood loss can be very heavy in these circumstances and hemorrhagic shock can result quickly unless immediate measures are taken to control hemorrhage. A dose of 15 methylprostaglandin F_2 alpha injected intramuscularly or directly into the uterus frequently is effective in restoring uterine tone.[15] The dose is 0.25 mg, to be repeated for a total of 1 mg.

In cases unresponsive to medical therapy, or if laceration or rupture of the uterus is suspected, laparotomy and surgical repair is required. If lacerations are present, an attempt is made to repair them primarily. For persistent uterine atony, a stepwise approach to stop bleeding is indicated.

Uterine Artery Ligation

This is a simple procedure to decrease bleeding, which involves ligation of both uterine arteries.[16] This procedure is performed rapidly and easily (Figure 203–3). No attempt to isolate the uterine artery surgically is required. The uterus is retracted, a No. 1 chromic catgut suture on a large needle is inserted into an avascular space of the broad ligament just above the bifurcation of the uterine vessel into an ascending and descending branch, brought out posteriorly, and then anteriorly through the myometrium approximately 2 cm from the edge. The suture then is tied anteriorly. The procedure is performed bilaterally. A second procedure consisting of ligation of the anastomosis of the uterine artery with the ovarian artery at the junction of the uterus and ovarian ligament may be required.

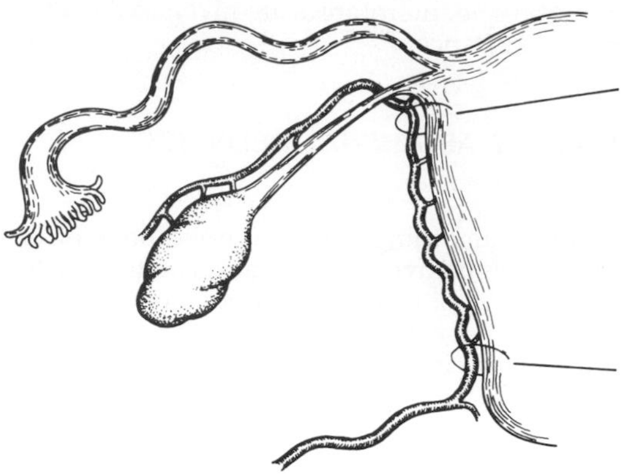

Figure 203–3. Placement of sutures for ligation of uterine artery.

Hypogastric Artery Ligation

If uterine artery ligation is unsuccessful in controlling hemorrhage, bilateral hypogastric artery ligation may be beneficial (Figure 203–4). Because the uterus and most pelvic vessels receive their blood supply from the anterior branch of the internal iliac (hypogastric) artery, bilateral ligation will result in marked diminution of blood flow to the pelvic organs. Following unilateral hypogastric artery ligation, the blood flow is decreased by 48%. More important, the pulse pressure is decreased by 85%[17], frequently allowing the

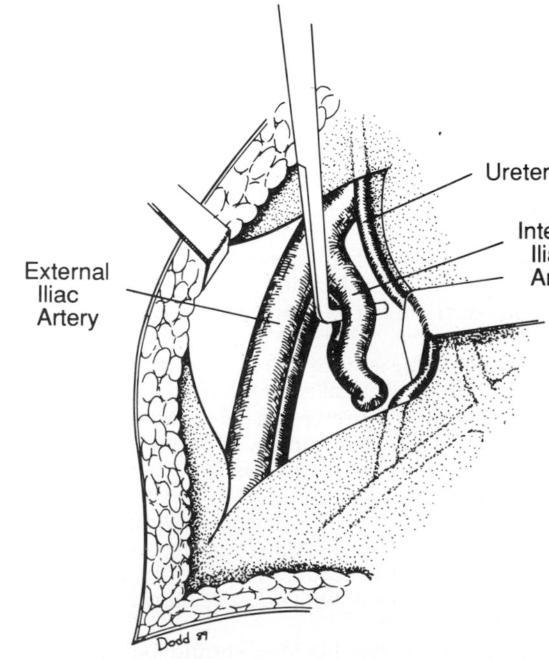

Figure 203–4. Techniques for ligation of internal iliac (hypogastric) artery.

normal hemostatic system to be effective in controlling further blood loss. Rich collateral systems generally decrease the possibility of ischemia, and normal pregnancies following the procedure are reported.

The first step in hypogastric artery ligation involves entering the retroperitoneal space. This can be accomplished in three ways: 1) by division of the round ligaments; 2) by dividing the peritoneum between the round ligaments and infundibulopelvic ligaments; or 3) posteriorly to the infundibulopelvic ligament and lateral to the external iliac artery. After entering the retroperitoneal space, the ureter is identified on the medial leaf of the peritoneum, and the bifurcation of the iliac artery is visualized. Using blunt dissection, the internal iliac vessels are traced, and the proximal 2–3 cm of the artery is dissected free with the use of a right angle clamp. Two sutures of No. 0 silk then are passed around the artery and tied snugly. The artery does not have to be divided. Care is taken to avoid injury to the internal iliac vein, and the femoral pulses are palpated to confirm that the sutures were placed correctly on the internal iliac artery.

Cesarean Hysterectomy

If the above techniques fail, cesarean hysterectomy is required. Hysterectomy may be elected prior to performing one or both procedures, depending on the degree of blood loss, the condition of the patient, and parity. The procedure is similar to that in the nonpregnant state, although there are several differences. The tissues during pregnancy are very pliable and soft, and there is marked engorgement of the pelvic veins. Therefore, more care in dissection to avoid injury to the vessels is necessary. In addition, because the cervix is so soft, it may not be identified easily. This usually can be overcome by placing a hand around the upper vagina after dissection of the bladder to "milk" the cervix upward.

Complications of cesarean hysterectomy are similar to those associated with cesarean section.[18] Blood loss is generally greater, and the incidence of transfusion is increased, especially in those undergoing emergency cesarean hysterectomy for hemorrhage. Injury to the urinary tract also is reported to be more common, especially ureteral injury. Postoperative infection has been reported to be lower than with cesarean section.

REFERENCES

1. Buekens P, Lagasse R, Dramaix M, Wollast E. Episiotomy and third degree tears. *Br J Obstet Gynecol.* 1985;92:820.
2. Thorp JM, Bowes WA, Brame RG, Cefalo R. Selected use of midline episiotomy: effect on perineal trauma. *Obstet Gynecol.* 1987;70:200.
3. Zuspan FP, Quilligan EJ, eds. *Operative Obstetrics.* 5th ed. Norwalk, CT: Appleton & Lange; 1988.
4. Fliegner JRH. Postpartum broad ligament hematomas. *J Obstet Gynaecol Br Commonw.* 1971;78:184.
5. Golan A, Sandbank O, Rubin A. Rupture of the pregnant uterus. *Obstet Gynecol.* 1980;56:549.
6. Yussman MA, Haynes DM. Rupture of the gravid uterus: a 12 year study. *Obstet Gynecol.* 1970;36:115.
7. Watson P, Besch N, Bowes WA. Management of acute and subacute puerperal inversion of the uterus. *Obstet Gynecol.* 1980;55:12.
8. O'Sullivan JV. Acute inversion of the uterus. *Br Med J.* 1945;2:282.
9. Sher G. Correction of postpartum uterine inversion by the application of intravaginal hydrostatic pressure. *Am J Obstet Gynecol.* 1979;134:601.
10. Raghaviah NV, Devi AI. Bladder injury associated with rupture of the uterus. *Obstet Gynecol.* 1975;46:573.
11. Eisenkop SM, Richman R, Platt LD, et al. Urinary tract injury during cesarean section. *Obstet Gynecol.* 1982;60:591.
12. Smith CV, Gallup DG. Urinary and gastrointestinal tract injuries. In: Phelan JP, Clark SL, eds. *Cesarean Delivery.* New York: Elsevier; 1988.
13. Barclay DL. Cesarean hysterectomy: thirty years experience. *Obstet Gynecol.* 1970;35:120.
14. Pritchard JA, Baldwin RM, Dickey JC, et al. Blood volume changes in pregnancy and the puerperium. *Am J Obstet Gynecol.* 1962;84:1271.
15. Hayashi RH, Castillo MS, Noah ML. Management of severe postpartum hemorrhage due to uterine study using an analogue of prostaglandin $F_2\alpha$. *Obstet Gynecol.* 1981;58:426.
16. O'Leary JL, O'Leary JA. Uterine artery ligation in the control of intractable postpartum hemorrhage. *Am J Obstet Gynecol.* 1966;94:920.
17. Burchell RC. Physiology of internal iliac artery ligation. *J Obstet Gynaecol Br Commonw.* 1968;75:642.
18. Barclay DL, Hawks BL, Frueh DM, et al. Elective cesarean hysterectomy: a 5 year comparison with cesarean section. *Am J Obstet Gynecol.* 1976;124:900.

Chapter Two Hundred and Four

Surgery During Pregnancy

Baha M. Sibai

204

The pregnant woman is susceptible to many of the surgical conditions seen in the nonpregnant state. The incidence of surgery during pregnancy ranges from 0.3% to 2.2%.[1-3] The diagnosis of surgical conditions can be complicated by the growing pelviabdominal uterine mass or the presence of an extrauterine gestation. These factors, combined with a reluctance to perform routine radiologic evaluations in pregnancy, may lead to a subsequent delay in diagnosis and treatment of the underlying disease. The physician may be reluctant to perform surgery for fear of anesthetic complications, undiagnosed intraoperative fetal distress, and the potential precipitation of premature labor.

The patient requiring surgical intervention during pregnancy frequently presents under emergency circumstances. In these situations, delay of surgery may lead to increased maternal morbidity with associated increased risk to the fetus. Appropriate surgical intervention should be performed promptly following the diagnosis of the emergent surgical condition. Less frequently, alternative medical or less invasive surgical procedures are available for the treatment of specific diseases. Again, the safest effective intervention should be undertaken.

The overall pregnancy loss following implantation is high, with 40–60% of implanting gestations subsequently failing. The asymptomatic patient, with an ultrasonographically confirmed intrauterine gestation with fetal cardiac activity, has a 90–93% chance of a successful pregnancy outcome. The background risk of congenital anomalies in the uncomplicated population is 3–6%. The majority of these anomalies are minor. Surgery during the preimplantation and immediately postimplantation period should not increase the risk of producing an abnormal offspring. The cells at this time are totipotent or pluripotent and the embryo will accommodate the loss of some cells. More severe damage will lead to pregnancy loss. The most active phase of organogenesis in pregnancy occurs between 6 and 13 weeks' gestation. The infant at this time is most susceptible to teratogenic effects; either environmental, chemical or iatrogenic. In later pregnancy, the fetal risks related to surgical conditions and operations are those associated with decreased fetal oxygenation and premature delivery. When planning elective surgery for a sexually active woman, the presence of pregnancy should be excluded prior to operative intervention.

It is believed that surgery during the first trimester carries an increased risk of pregnancy wastage. Studies of spontaneous miscarriage in exposed medical personnel have revealed a 25–30% increase in the risk of spontaneous miscarriage when compared with nonexposed women.[4-6] The highest miscarriage rate among exposed professionals was 24.6%.[4] A significant increase in congenital anomalies has been suggested among professional personnel exposed to waste anesthetic gases.[1,4,6] However, no dose response relationship has been identified and these findings have not been demonstrated consistently.[5-8] Studies of women receiving anesthesia during surgery have not identified any teratogenic risk associated with anesthesia.[1,8,9] When the patient booked for an elective operation is found to be pregnant, surgery should be delayed until the postpartum period, if possible. If prolonged delay is not feasible, surgery should be performed in the second trimester after the presence of a potentially viable intrauterine gestation has been confirmed. While no anesthetic agent has been linked specifically to premature labor, uterine manipulation, intraabdominal infection and peritonitis are predisposing factors to premature labor and delivery. The uterus is increasingly sensitive to stimulation with advancing gestation. The large gravid uterus of the third trimester may provide an obstruction to adequate visualization, and manipulation may be required to complete the procedure. Thus elective pelviabdominal surgery should be avoided in the third trimester.

Prior to surgery, the patient should be made aware of the effects of her disease state on her pregnancy. The patient should understand the benefits and any supervening risks imposed by the treatment for her condition. If surgery is to be performed, the patient should be informed of any special precautions (including assessment of maternal oxygenation, blood pressure, and where appropriate fetal heart rate, and uterine contraction monitoring) which will be done during surgery. As the majority of surgical procedures performed during pregnancy are related directly to the reproductive tract, the patient also should be informed of the effects of her condition and treatment on future childbearing potential.

PREOPERATIVE CARE

Aspiration is the most common cause of maternal anesthetic death.[10,11] The pregnant patient shows a decrease in intestinal motility with a delay in gastric emptying. This delay is consistently reported after 34 weeks' gestation as a result of increasing progesterone and decreasing plasma motilin.[12,13] Further delay of gastric emptying is seen in labor.[14] Incompetence of the lower esophageal sphincter zone also is noted frequently in pregnancy. Reflux, with aspiration of particulate and acidic gastric contents, may be associated with chemical pneumonitis, superimposed bacterial pneumonia, and adult respiratory distress syndrome (ARDS). For these reasons, when elective surgery is planned, the pregnant patient should be allowed adequate time for emptying of the gastric contents. If adequate time for gastric emptying is not feasible, preoperative nasogastric aspiration of the stomach contents may be judicious. A dose of 30 mL of a nonparticulate antacid, such as sodium citrate, should be given preoperatively.

Both mother and fetus tolerate prolonged fasting poorly with maternal ketosis and hypoglycemia rapidly occurring. The fetus has limited capability for gluconeogenesis in the presence of decreased glucose supply.[15] However, prolonged hypoglycemia is poorly tolerated.[16] Intravenous administration of an isotonic solution containing dextrose should be instituted when prolonged fasting is anticipated.

The pregnant patient is at increased risk of postoperative atelectasis and infectious pulmonary complications because of the decreased respiratory excursion associated with increasing uterine size and postoperative guarding.[17] The patient should be instructed preoperatively as to the need for and performance of deep breathing exercises in the perioperative period.

INTRAOPERATIVE CARE

There should be adequate maternal perfusion and oxygenation prior to the onset of surgery. Aortacaval compression by the gravid uterus should be avoided to prevent decreased venous return to the heart and subsequent maternal hypotension.[18,19] Maternal hypotension and a subsequent decrease in uteroplacental perfusion is avoided by placing a wedge under the right hip and flank or rotating the operative table to the left side. Where possible, the supine position should be avoided entirely during surgery. Maternal hypotension may be aggravated by hypovolemia related to prolonged fasting or blood loss. Adequate preoperative rehydration should be undertaken prior to the induction of anesthesia. Maternal hypotension related to deep general anesthesia should be avoided.

Maternal oxygenation should be monitored intraoperatively with transcutaneous pO_2 monitoring. Maternal hypoxia should be avoided. Maternal hyperoxia may be associated with umbilical vascular constriction.[20] Despite the potential for umbilical vascular constriction, maternal hyperoxia has not been associated with fetal hypoxia.[21,22] Fetal hyperoxia, with the resultant increased risk of retrolental fibroplasia and premature closure of the ductus arteriosus, are not seen even with a markedly elevated maternal PaO_2.[23]

Fetal heart rate activity and uterine contractility should be monitored intraoperatively, where feasible. If fetal monitoring is done, a physician capable of interpreting the fetal heart rate activity should be available. Arrangements should be made for immediate delivery of a viable fetus, should persistent fetal distress nonresponsive to intrauterine resuscitation occur.

POSTOPERATIVE CARE

Postoperatively, the patient should be cared for in a unit that is comfortable and experienced in dealing with the pregnant patient. Uterine contraction monitoring should be performed. In the absence of contractions, monitoring should be continued until the patient is alert and able to identify uterine activity. Fetal heart rate monitoring should be continued in the presence of uterine contractions.

The pregnant woman is at increased risk for thrombotic and pulmonary infectious complications. The patient should be encouraged to continue deep breathing exercises and, in the absence of premature labor, early ambulation should be done. If the patient does not have a bleeding diathesis, prophylactic subcutaneous heparin 5000 IU every 8–12 hours may reduce the risk of venous thrombosis in the perioperative period.

As in the preoperative period, adequate hydration and administration of glucose should be continued intravenously until the patient is alert and able to take oral fluids. The return of gastrointestinal function may be delayed. In the presence of a potentially compromised lower esophageal sphincter zone, the initiation of oral feeding should be delayed until adequate gastrointestinal function has been documented.

In the subsequent chapters of this section, the anesthetic and operative considerations of the woman undergoing operative intervention in pregnancy will be discussed. The management and monitoring of the acutely ill patient in the intensive care setting, common nonobstetric surgical conditions, their relationship to pregnancy, and the fetal and maternal complications of surgical manipulation in pregnancy will be reviewed.

ECTOPIC PREGNANCY

While not in the strictest sense a "medical problem" *of* pregnancy, a text on medical therapy in pregnancy is incomplete without a note on ectopic pregnancy. With a reported incidence of one in 45 live births[24], medical symptomatology in *early* pregnancy must include consideration of the diagnosis of an extrauterine gestation. The most common presenting symptoms are pain (in over 90%) and abnormal bleeding (in over 80%), although the diagnostic process and the accuracy of early diagnosis have greatly changed with the accessibility of highly sensitive pregnancy and vaginal ultrasound tests. It is the established correlation between specific β-hCG values and the ability (or inability) to visualize an intrauterine pregnancy sonographically that allows early diagnosis of usually unruptured extrauterine pregnancies. A detailed discussion of diagnosis and treatment of ectopic pregnancy exceed the framework of this chapter. DeCherney's monograph[25] provides an excellent overview. Nevertheless, it remains important to reemphasize that women in their reproductive years with pelvic pain and menstrual irregularity should be evaluated for an ectopic pregnancy unless another diagnosis has been established. Extrauterine pregnancies still account for approximately 10% of maternal deaths. Progress in early diagnosis has permitted a conservative surgical approach to most diagnosed ectopic pregnancies, allowing for the preservation of affected fallopian tubes.

GESTATIONAL TROPHOBLASTIC NEOPLASMS

Gestational trophoblastic neoplasms describe three distinct clinical entities: *hydatidiform mole*, *invasive mole*, and *choriocarcinoma*. All three are rarely associated with a concomitantly viable pregnancy, and none of these three conditions usually is encountered as a complication of an ongoing pregnancy. Trophoblastic disease, nevertheless, deserves mention within the framework of surgery in pregnancy because the D&C in pregnancy (usually early) represents a standard diagnostic as well as therapeutic tool in all of these conditions.

Early trophoblastic pregnancy is often clinically not different from a normal pregnancy. Because of frequent sonographic examinations, diagnosis is now usually made earlier in pregnancy.

Diagnosis and treatment of gestational trophoblastic neoplasms are well reviewed in several monographs and texts. Trophoblastic disease is, however, highly relevant to two medical conditions. Because of occasional very high β-hCG levels in patients with gestational trophoblastic neoplasms, clinical hyperthyroidism can become overt in affected individuals (for specific detail, see Chapters 37 and 40). The second medical condition with relevance to trophoblastic disease is preeclampsia and eclampsia which occur in a significantly increased incidence at an unusually early gestational age (see Chapters 139 and 140).

REFERENCES

1. Shelley WC. Anesthetic considerations for non-obstetric surgery. *Clin Perinatol.* 1982;9:135.
2. Shnider SM, Webster GM. Maternal and fetal hazards of surgery during pregnancy. *Am J Obstet Gynecol.* 1965;92.891.
3. Pederson H. Non-obstetric surgery in the pregnant patient. In: James FM, Wheeler AS, Dewan DM, eds. *Anesthesia: The Complicated Patient.* Philadelphia: FA Davis; 1986:531.
4. Cohen EH, Gift HC, Brown BW, Greenfield W, et al. Occupational disease in dentistry and chronic exposure to trace anesthetic crises. *J Am Dent Assoc.* 1980;10:21.
5. Knill-Jones RP, Rodrigues LV, Moir DD, Spence AA. Anesthetic practice at pregnancy: controlled survey of women anesthetists in the United Kingdom. *Lancet.* 1972;1:1326.
6. Ad Hoc Committee on the Effect of Trace Anesthetics on the Health of Operating Room Personnel, American Society of Anesthesiologists. Occupational disease among operating room personnel. *Anesthesiology.* 1974;41:321.
7. Buring JE, Hennekens CH, Mayrant SL, et al. Health experiences of operating room personnel. *Anesthesiology.* 1985;62:325.
8. Duncan PG, Pope WDB, Cohen MM, Greer N. The safety of anesthesia and surgery during pregnancy. *Anesthesiology.* 1986;64:790.
9. Brodsky JB, Cohen EN, Brown BW Jr, et al. Surgery during pregnancy and fetal outcome. *Am J Obstet Gynecol.* 1980;138:1165.
10. Rosen M. Editorial. *Anesthesia.* 1981;36:145.
11. Cohen SE. Aspiration syndromes in pregnancy. *Anesthesiology.* 1979;51:375.
12. Csapo A. Progesterone block. *Am J Anat.* 1956;98:273.
13. Christofides ND, Ghatei MA, Bloom SR, et al. Decreased plasma motilin concentrations in pregnancy. *Br Med J.* 1982;285:1453.
14. Davison JS, Davison MC, Hay DM. Gastric emptying time in late pregnancy and labor. *J Obstet Gynecol Br Commonw.* 1970;77:37.
15. Battaglia FC. The comparative physiology of fetal nutrition. *Am J Obstet Gynecol.* 1984;148:850.
16. Hollingsworth DR. Alterations in maternal metabolism in normal and diabetic pregnancies, differences in insulin dependent, non-insulin dependent and gestational diabetes. *Am J Obstet Gynecol.* 1983;146:417.
17. Bartlett RH. Postoperative pulmonary prophylaxis. *Chest.* 1982;81:1.
18. Howard BK, Goodson JH, Mengert WF. Supine hypotension syndrome in late pregnancy. *Obstet Gynecol.* 1953;1:371.
19. McRoberts WA Jr. Postural shock in pregnancy. *Am J Obstet Gynecol.* 1951;62:627.
20. Nyber GR, Westin B. The influence of oxygen tension and some drugs on human placental vessels. *ACTA Physiol Scand.* 1957;39:216.
21. Khazin AF, Hon EH, Hehre FW. Effects of maternal hyperoxia on the fetus. 1: oxygen tension. *Am J Obstet Gynecol.* 1971;109:628.
22. Walker A, Madden L, Day E, et al. Fetal scalp tissue oxygen measurements in a relation to maternal dermal oxygen tension and fetal heart rate. *J Obstet Gynecol Br Commonw.* 1971;78:1.
23. Levensen G, Shnider SM. Anesthesia for surgery during pregnancy. In: Shnider SM, Levensen G, eds. *Anesthesia for Obstetrics.* 2nd ed. Baltimore, MD: Williams and Wilkins; 1987:188.
24. Weinstein L, Morris MB, Dotter D, et al. Ectopic pregnancy: a new surgical epidemic. *Obstet Gynecol.* 1983;61:698.
25. DeCherney A, ed. *Ectopic Pregnancy.* Aspen Publishers, Inc.; 1986.

Chapter Two Hundred and Five

Appendicitis

Brian M. Mercer

205

Appendicitis is one of the most important causes of nonobstetric abdominal pain, and is the most common extrauterine indication for laparotomy during pregnancy. Marked improvements in maternal and fetal outcome following appendicitis associated with pregnancy have been demonstrated over the past 80 years. Much of this improvement can be attributed to the development of safe broad spectrum antibiotics and improved surgical facilities. However, the primary factor responsible for the decrease in morbidity and mortality is a high index of suspicion with early and aggressive surgical intervention for patients with suspected appendicitis.

The appendix has been described as a vestigial organ of little utility. However, it maintains a function similar to that of the bursa of Fabricius in avian species for the processing and maturation of extrathymic B-type lymphocytes. The appendix is one of many tissues responsible for the processing of B-lymphocytes and as such is not essential for immune function. The appendix functions as part of the secretory immune response within the gut, producing immunoglobulins that can be excreted in the intestine and blood.

Appendicitis is the most common surgical condition of the abdomen, occurring in 6.7% of the population before the age of 30.[1] Appendicitis is a disease of the young with a peak incidence in the second and third decades of life. Some 70% of all acute appendicitis occurs in patients under the age of 35.[2] The sex ratio is one to one prior to puberty with a subsequent male predominance between the ages of 15 and 25. A lower incidence of appendicitis is seen in underdeveloped countries and in lower socioeconomic groups. The incidence of confirmed appendicitis has decreased over the past forty years. This is believed to be due to improved nutrition and high-fiber diet; changes in intestinal flora; and improved pathologic confirmation of appendicitis.

The incidence of appendicitis in pregnancy is approximately 1 in 800 to 1 in 2000.[2-4] The progesterone-induced hypomotility of the GI tract and appendix has been suggested as a risk factor for appendicitis in pregnancy. However, no increase in the actual incidence of appendicitis has been identified in pregnant women. Older series suggest an equal distribution of appendicitis throughout pregnancy.[5,6] However, recent studies suggest appendicitis to be more common in the second and third trimesters.[2,3,7-9]

The primary etiologic event of appendicitis is acute obstruction of the appendiceal lumen. The most common causative factor of appendiceal obstruction is a fecalith.[1] Fecaliths are found in 40% of acute appendicitis specimens, 65% of gangrenous appendices, and 90% of ruptured appendices. Other causative factors include: lymphoid hypertrophy, inspissated barium, vegetable and fruit seeds, intestinal worms (ascarids), appendiceal tumors (carcinoid or carcinoma), inflammatory bowel disease, tuberculosis, amebiasis, and actinomycosis. A viral etiology with initial mucosal ulceration and subsequent bacterial invasion also has been postulated.

In the presence of obstruction, continued secretion by the mucosal glands leads to progressive appendiceal distention. As distention increases, venous pressure is reached with impairment of venous and lymphatic outflow. This leads to further engorgement and vascular congestion of the appendix. Finally, with continued inflow of blood and lumenal distention, arteriolar pressure is reached within the appendix and the vascular supply is blocked, leading to appendiceal ischemia. Multiplication of resident intestinal bacteria occurs within the closed loop anaerobic milieu of the obstructed appendix. The appendiceal mucosa is very susceptible to a decrease in oxygenation with early breakdown allowing bacterial invasion. Ischemia, in association with increased luminal distention and bacterial degradation of the appendiceal wall, lead to perforation. During the course of acute appendiceal inflammation, the omentum and adjacent bowel frequently sequester the periappendiceal area, preventing diffuse spillage subsequent to rupture.

CLINICAL DIAGNOSIS

The initial pain, associated with distention of the appendix, is vague and located diffusely within the periumbilical region. The pain subsequently may become colicky in nature with appendiceal contractions attempting to disrupt the obstruction. Many patients will have a history of similar colicky abdominal pain, possibly related to lymphoid hypertrophy or the presence of a partially obstructive fecalith. With the development of serosal involvement and involvement of the parietal peritoneum, after a mean of 4–6 hours, somatic pain becomes predominant. This pain may be located anywhere from the right lower quadrant to the left upper quadrant, depending on the location and length of the appendix. Some 65% percent of appendices are located within the right lower quadrant with the pain moving to the classic location near McBurney's point.[2,10] A total of 30% of patients have a pelvic appendix and will demonstrate less prominent abdominal findings. These patients may complain of unilateral pelvic pain. Pelvic peritonitis in these patients may give the impression of a primary adnexal process. Five percent of patients have a retrocecally located appendix, again with minimal abdominal findings and a somatic component consisting primarily of flank and back pain. In the presence of incomplete rotation of the bowel, the appendix may be found in the right or left upper quadrant, further confusing the clinical picture. In early pregnancy, the pain of appendicitis is similarly located to that in the nonpregnant state. However, as the uterus grows to fill the pelvis in the late second and third trimesters, the cecum increasingly is elevated from its position in the cecal fossa. As described by Baer[11] in a study using barium enema in 72 normal pregnant patients, the appendix rises progressively from the pelvis with increasing gestation. As a result of this displacement, the pain of appendicitis rises with gestation reaching the right upper quadrant in the later months of pregnancy.

With perforation of the appendix, peritonitis will progress from a localized phenomena to diffuse intra-abdominal inflammation with efflux of the infected debris into the peritoneal cavity. The common sites of spread include the pouch of Douglas and the subhepatic space through the right pericolic gutter.[1] If the omentum and adjacent bowel have had the opportunity to restrict the perforation, diffuse peritonitis will not occur. In the pregnant state with elevation of the uterus, it is more difficult for the omentum and bowel to perform this function. Diffuse peritonitis is thus more frequent with increasing gestational age.

Gastrointestinal symptomatology is less specific to appendicitis and frequently mimics the symptomatology of normal early pregnancy. About 40–65% of patients with appendicitis will demonstrate anorexia.[9,12-14] Vomiting is also common, being seen in 60–85% of patients.[9,13,14] However, vomiting is rarely prominent or prolonged and very rarely is seen prior to the onset of abdominal pain. A change in bowel motility, as demonstrated by obstipation or diarrhea, is seen variably in the pregnant and nonpregnant patient.[13,14] Frequency and urgency of urination may be seen in the presence of a pelvic appendicitis in both the pregnant and nonpregnant states.

The patient's temperature is rarely increased to more than 38°C (100.4°F) in early appendicitis with localized peritonitis. With perforation, higher temperatures are seen. The initial abdominal findings of classic appendicitis include hyperesthesia in the T10–T12 dermatomes. Subsequently, with the development of increasing serosal involvement and localized peritonitis, focal tenderness can be elicited. Voluntary guarding of the abdominal musculature is seen early in relation to abdominal tenderness. Localized rebound tenderness frequently can be observed. Referred rebound tenderness from the opposite quadrant (Rovsing's sign) may be found. With progressive diffuse peritonitis, diffuse tenderness, muscular guarding and rebound tenderness are present. In patients with minimal abdominal findings, a retrocecal appendix may be identified by the presence of a positive "psoas sign," and a pelvic appendix by a positive "obturator sign." Rectal examination with displacement of the pelvic peritoneum may cause pain in patients with pelvic peritonitis secondary to a pelvic appendix or pelvic abscess but is frequently not present in pregnancy (16–45%).[9,13,14] Bimanual examination may demonstrate cervical motion tenderness with stretching of the pelvic peritoneum. Unilateral adnexal tenderness may be elicited in the absence of secondary pelvic peritonitis. Paralytic ileus, with decreased bowel sounds and abdominal distention, may be seen in the presence of peritonitis. A soft boggy mass may be felt at the sight of appendiceal rupture subsequent to abscess formation.

In the nonpregnant state, leukocytosis with a white blood cell count of 10–18,000 per mm^3, a polymorphonucleocyte predominance, and a left shift toward immature forms are useful adjunctive findings to a clinical history of appendicitis. White blood cell counts of greater than 18,000 or an extreme left shift suggest perforation with peritonitis.[1] The normal leukocytosis of pregnancy with the total white blood cell count ranging from 12,000 to 16,000 may obscure laboratory findings in this respect. However, a differential count with observation of a left shift of polymorphonucleocytes may be helpful in the diagnosis of acute inflammation. Urinalysis is frequently unremarkable. Radiographic assessment rarely is indicated in the diagnosis of appendicitis. Distended loops of small bowel in the right lower quadrant, and rarely a distended cecum, may be seen in the presence of acute appendicitis. The presence of a gas-filled appendix is highly suggestive of acute appendicitis. If contrast examination is undertaken, complete filling of the appendiceal lumen, without evidence of a mass effect in the cecum and terminal ileum, makes the diagnosis of appendicitis extremely unlikely.

The differential diagnosis of acute appendicitis includes almost any acute intraabdominal process. Conditions commonly confused with appendicitis include ruptured or hemorrhagic corpus luteum, adnexal torsion, ectopic pregnancy, placental abruption, preterm labor, ruptured endometrioma, degenerating leiomyoma, pelvic inflammatory disease, chorioamnionitis, urinary tract infection, pyelonephritis, cystitis, nephrolithiasis, mesenteric adenitis, gastroenteritis, pancreatitis, carcinoma of the appendix, as well as obstructive bowel and biliary tract disease.[15,16] Despite this, the preoperative diagnosis of appendicitis can be expected to be 85% accurate. A higher incorrect diagnosis of appendicitis is considered acceptable in women.[9,17,18] An unusually low false diagnosis rate suggests prolonged observation prior to intervention with the increased risk of appendiceal rupture and an attendant increase in patient morbidity and mortality.

TREATMENT

The treatment of suspected appendicitis is immediate surgical intervention. The most important component of management is early diagnosis and the avoidance of delay in treatment. In pregnancy, a high index of suspension must be maintained because of the increased maternal and fetal morbidity and mortality associated with appendiceal perforation. As such, immediate surgical intervention is mandated when appendicitis is suspected during pregnancy.

The patient with appendicitis may be dehydrated following prolonged anorexia with vomiting and the presence of fever. This may be aggravated further by prolonged observation preceding the diagnosis. An intravenous infusion of lactated Ringer's solution with dextrose should be initiated. Electrolytes should be assessed and corrected as necessary. Because of the delayed gastric emptying time associated with peritonitis and pregnancy, nasogastric intubation and suction should be instituted prior to surgery. Systemic antibiotic therapy should be initiated at the time of diagnosis with attention to coverage of anaerobic bacteria, including *Bacteroides fragilis*.

In the first and early second trimesters, a McBurney's incision may be used in clear-cut cases of appendicitis.[19] This incision has the advantage of being located over the base of the appendix in the majority of cases. However, if the appendix is normal at the time of laparotomy, a second incision may be required for exploratory laparotomy. Because of the increased incidence of adnexal pathology related to cyst hemorrhage and torsion as well as ectopic pregnancy in the first trimester, a vertical midline or right paramedian incision is suggested when the diagnosis is not clear. This incision will provide more adequate exposure to the adnexa and appendix simultaneously, allowing full laparotomy if the appendix is normal. However, the paramedian scar possesses less tensile strength and is more prone to dehiscence, and appendectomy through a midline or a paramedian incision will necessitate bringing the appendix from its appendiceal fossa, contaminating the previously sterile peritoneal cavity. Early in the first trimester, diagnostic laparascopy may be of value in determining the etiology of abdominal pain prior to laparatomy. In late second and third trimesters, as the appendix rises out of the pelvis, a muscle-splitting incision should be made over the point of maximal tenderness.

Uterine manipulation should be minimized where possible to avoid uterine irritation and contractions. Intervention in the pregnancy usually can be avoided. Cesarean section should be performed only as indicated obstetrically, and in the presence of severe diffuse peritonitis, in which there is a high risk of fetal mortality. The patient admitted in active labor with imminent delivery should be allowed to undergo vaginal delivery followed by surgery. If cesarean section is indicated for obstetric indication, appendectomy can be performed at this time. Cesarean hysterectomy should be considered for the multiparous patient in the presence of severe peritonitis. The use of intravenous tocolysis at the time of surgery is of questionable benefit but has been recommended for use during surgery and until the resolution of peritoneal inflammation.

Uncomplicated appendicitis is treated best by surgical excision with ligation of the base and inversion of the appendiceal stump. Closure of all layers, including subcutaneous tissue and skin, may be performed. Systemic therapy generally is discontinued postoperatively in this circumstance. If extensive adhesions requiring major dissection are encountered, appendectomy should be delayed with wound drainage and antibiotic therapy prior to delayed interval appendectomy. The subcutaneous tissue and skin should be left open and either permitted to close by secondary intention or closed following a time interval of five to six days.

The paramedian incision is contraindicated in the presence of suspected periappendiceal abscess because of the increased risk of precipitating diffuse peritonitis. A lateral McBurney's incision or an incision over the point of maximal tenderness should be used in this circumstance. Again, extensive dissection should be avoided; drainage and interval appendectomy should be performed. Drainage of a small localized collection of pus using a Penrose drain through a McBurney's incision is adequate. Large collections of purulent material should be drained using the constant pressure of a sump drain. In the presence of a gangrenous appendix, ruptured appendix, or peritonitis, antibiotic therapy should be continued postoperatively.

If acute appendicitis is not found at the time of laparotomy, orderly examination of the abdomen and pelvis including the gynecologic organs, large and small intestines, kidneys, pancreas, hepatic surface, gallbladder, and inspection of the mesentery for lymphadenopathy is mandated. In the absence of identifiable appendicitis or intra-abdominal pathology, simple appendectomy should be performed as microscopic inflammation may be present in the absence of macroscopic findings.

Because appendiceal pathology may be seen in the presence of other intra-abdominal disease, inspection of the appendix should be attempted at the time of laparotomy for any abdominal condition.[16,19,20]

COMPLICATIONS OF ACUTE APPENDICITIS

The overall mortality from appendicitis has decreased remarkably over the past 80 years and is rarely seen in the absence of perforation. Maternal mortality from appendicitis also has decreased steadily. Babler, in 1908, reported a 35% maternal mortality related to appendicitis.[21] Subsequent reviews have demonstrated a progressive decline in maternal mortality to less than 1% in recent studies.[4] The improvement in maternal outcome is believed to be related to better fluid and nutritional support, the use of antibiotics with wide spectrum antimicrobial coverage, and improvements in surgical technique with aggressive intervention in the presence of suspected appendicitis in pregnancy.

Perinatal mortality is usually secondary to premature labor and delivery. A 35% incidence of pregnancy interruption is seen with peritonitis.[22] Fetal death may occur secondary to peritonitis and maternal sepsis, and reflects the severity of disease. Townsend reported an overall 10.8% pregnancy loss with acute appendicitis.[14] A 27.8% fetal mortality has been identified in patients with appendiceal perforation as compared with a 4.8% incidence in patients with uncomplicated appendicitis.[2]

Rupture of the appendix is the most common and most serious complication of acute appendicitis.[22] Appendiceal perforation is seen in 15% of nonpregnant patients at the time of laparotomy for appendicitis. Appendiceal perforation is seen twice as frequently in pregnancy. Appendiceal rupture is primarily related to a delay in diagnosis or a delay in surgical intervention following the diagnosis of suspected appendicitis. This delay is seen more frequently in pregnancy and increases with increasing gestational age.[8] Spillage of the appendiceal contents following rupture can result in the development of an appendiceal phlegmon, localized abscess, diffuse peritonitis, multiple interloop abscesses, and, rarely, intestinal obstruction. The periappendiceal area is walled off prior to rupture in 95% of nonpregnant patients. This is less common in pregnancy, and diffuse peritonitis is more frequent with increasing gestational age.

Wound infection is a frequent complication of acute appendicitis, which usually can be treated with drainage, but may require systemic antibiotic therapy.

There is controversy in the literature regarding the risk of infertility following appendicitis. It is unlikely that uncomplicated appendicitis without perforation carries any increased risk for infertility due to a tubal factor. However, Mueller, in a review of 279 women with surgically proven infertility, demonstrated a fourfold increase in tubal infertility following ruptured appendicitis.[23]

Ascending septic thrombophlebitis of the portal venous system or pyelothrombophlebitis is a grave but rare complication resulting from embolization of septic clots from the mesenteric vasculature to the portal system.[22] This leads to the resultant development of multiple hepatic abscesses with chills, spiking fever, right upper quadrant pain, and jaundice.

Appendicitis carries significant risks of maternal and fetal morbidity and mortality. The primary risk is related to a delay in the diagnosis and institution of adequate therapy. The patient with uncomplicated, early acute appendicitis can be expected to have an uneventful recovery. In the presence of perforation or diffuse peritonitis, maternal and fetal morbidity and mortality are increased markedly. When appendicitis is suspected, early surgical intervention for diagnosis and treatment is essential.

REFERENCES

1. Storer EH. Appendix. In: Schwartz SI, Shires GT, Spencer FC, Storer EH, eds. *Principles of Surgery. 4th edition.* New York: McGraw-Hill; 1984.
2. Weingold AB. Appendicitis in pregnancy. Surgical diseases in pregnancy. *Clin Obstet Gynecol.* 1983;26:801.
3. Rosemann GWE. Acute appendicitis in pregnancy. *S Afr Med J.* 1975;49:1459.
4. Babaknia A, Parsa H, Woodruff JD. Appendicitis complicating pregnancy. *Can J Surg.* 1977;23:92.
5. Black WP. Acute appendicitis in pregnancy. *Br Med J.* 1960;1:1938.

6. Griffin WO, Dilts PV, Roddick JW. Nonobstetric surgery during pregnancy. *Curr Prob Surg*. 1969;31.
7. Finch DRA, Lee E. Acute appendicitis complicating pregnancy in the Oxford region. *Br J Surg*. 1974;61:129.
8. Cunningham FG, McCubbin JH. Appendicitis complicating pregnancy. *Obstet Gynecol*. 1975;45:415.
9. McComb P, Laimon H. Appendicitis complicating pregnancy. *Can J Surg*. 1980;23:92.
10. McBurney C. Experience with early operative interference in cases of disease of the vermiform appendix. *NY State Med J*. 1889;50:67.
11. Baer JL, Reis RA, Arens RA. Appendicitis in pregnancy with changes in position and axis of the normal appendix in pregnancy. *JAMA*. 1932;98:1359.
12. Horowitz MD, Gomez GA, Santiesteban R, Burkett G. Acute appendicitis during pregnancy: diagnosis and management. *Arch Surg*. 1985;120:1362.
13. Masters K, Levine BA, Gaskill HV, Sirinek KR. Diagnosing appendicitis during pregnancy. *Am J Surg*. 1984;148:768.
14. Townsend JM, Greiss FC. Appendicitis in pregnancy. *Southern Med J*. 1976;69:1161.
15. Hallat JG, Steele GH, Snyder M. Ruptured corpus luteum with hematoperitoneum: a study of 173 surgical cases. *Am J Obstet Gynecol*. 1983;149:5.
16. Donnenfeld AE, Roberts NS, Losure TA, Mellen AW. Perforated adenocarcinoma of the appendix during pregnancy. *Am J Obstet Gynecol*. 1986;154:627.
17. Saunders P, Milton PJ. Laparotomy during pregnancy: an assessment of diagnostic accuracy and fetal wastage. *Br Med J*. 1973;3:165.
18. Finch DR. Laparotomy during pregnancy. *Br Med J*. 1973;3:408.
19. Allen NJW, Heringer R. Coincident acute appendicitis and tubal pregnancy. *CMAJ*. 1970;103:531.
20. Pelosi MA, Apuzzio J, Iffy L. Ectopic pregnancy as an etiologic agent in appendicitis. *Obstet Gynecol*. 1979;53:4S.
21. Babler EA. Perforating appendicitis complicating pregnancy. *JAMA*. 1908;51:1310.
22. Cooperman M. Complications of appendectomy. *Surg Clin N Amer*. 1983;65:1233.
23. Mueller BA, Daling JR, Moore DE, et al. Appendectomy and the risk of tubal infertility. *N Eng J Med*. 1986;315:1506.

Chapter Two Hundred and Six

Surgical Disease of the Gallbladder

Brian M. Mercer

206

The hepatobiliary system may be involved in a variety of conditions occurring in pregnancy. The majority of these conditions (including the spectrum of hypertensive diseases of pregnancy, acute fatty liver, cholestasis of pregnancy, and hepatitis) do not require direct surgical intervention and are described elsewhere in this text. Cholecystectomy rarely is required during pregnancy (1 in 1250 to 1 in 12,500).[1-5] Obstructive disease (cholelithiasis) and infectious disease (cholecystitis) of the gallbladder are the most frequent conditions of the hepatobiliary tract requiring surgical management. Developmental abnormalities including choledochal cysts and neoplastic lesions of the biliary tract rarely affect the pregnant woman.

The gallbladder develops as a caudal division of the hepatic diverticulum, which originates from the second portion of the duodenum.[6] The gallbladder maintains its connection with the common bile duct through the cystic duct, which drains into the duodenum at the ampulla of Vater. Numerous variations in the anatomy, vascular supply, and lymphatic drainage of the gallbladder have been identified and are beyond the scope of this discussion.[7] The gallbladder functions as a storage reservoir for bile produced in the liver. Absorption by the mucosal epithelium leads to concentration of bile salts, pigments and cholesterol within the bile storage pool. The gallbladder contracts in response to autonomic nervous and humoral (cholecystokinin) stimulation following the ingestion of lipid containing foods. Within the intestinal tract, bile acid micelles aid in the dissolution and absorption of ingested lipids. Enterohepatic recirculation of the bile acids occurs following reabsorption at the distal ileum. Gallstone formation results from the crystallization of cholesterol, calcium, or bile salts. Some 90% of stones in the North American population are made up primarily of cholesterol. The remainder are pigment stones. Gallstones have been demonstrated to be present in 10% of the general population[8], and are less common in blacks and more common in American Indians. Other risk factors include obesity, distal ileal disease with decreased bile salt absorption and reduced bile salt pool, exogenous female sex steroids, and advancing age.[8] Gallbladder disease (cholelithiasis and cholecystitis) is seen more frequently in women than men after puberty (4 to 1). In pregnancy, increased levels of progesterone decrease smooth muscle activity of the corpus. Estrogen decreases the relative quantity of chenodeoxycholic acid, with a decrease in total bile acid pool.[9] The decrease in bile acid pool size leads to an increased tendency to cholesterol supersaturation and precipitation.

The average capacity of the gallbladder in the nonpregnant state is 50 mL. Using diagnostic ultrasonographic screening, an increase in resting gallbladder volume has been identified in pregnant women and oral contraceptive users.[10-12] Ylostalo et al[13] demonstrated a doubling of resting gallbladder volume in the normal pregnant woman and contraceptive user, and demonstrated a lack of significant rise in serum chenodeoxycholic acid and cholic acid in uncomplicated pregnancy. Everson[12] demonstrated a decrease in emptying rate and an increase in residual gallbladder volume in pregnant women. He also demonstrated an increase in fasting gallbladder volume in contraceptive steroid users. He thus suggested bile retention to be an etiologic reason for the development of cholesterol stones in these patients.

Cholecystitis and cholelithiasis account for 5% of cases of jaundice in pregnancy. Dispite the increase in estrogen and progesterone in pregnancy, a marked increase in the incidence of symptomatic cholelithiasis and cholecystitis is not seen. Further, an increased incidence of cholelithiasis has not been demonstrated with increasing gestation.[14] Clinically diagnosed cholelithiasis has been identified in 10% of pregnancies.[1] In separate reviews of 516 asymptomatic pregnant patients, a 3.1% incidence of ultrasonographically proven cholelithiasis has been identified.[15,16] As 50% or more of patients with cholelithiasis are symptomatic, these findings correspond to an overall incidence of 6–10% in pregnancy. Thus, asymptomatic cholelithiasis very often is associated with pregnancy, but does not appear to be more frequent in the pregnant woman than in the general population.

CLINICAL DIAGNOSIS OF CHOLELITHIASIS AND CHOLECYSTITIS

A total of 90% cases of acute cholecystitis result from persistent obstruction of the cystic duct by stones. Increasing intraluminal pressure and direct pressure by the stone results in mucosal ischemia and necrosis with an acute inflammatory response. With persistent ischemia, perforation with the spread of infected bile may occur. Malignancy, thrombosis of the cystic artery, hypertensive vascular disease, and collagen vascular disease are rare causes of inflammation of the gallbladder.

The symptoms and signs of cholelithiasis are those associated with obstruction of bile flow within the biliary tract. Obstruction of the common duct leads to colicky right upper quadrant pain with jaundice. The pain of cholelithiasis (biliary colic) is often steady and aching in character, radiating from the epigastrium and right upper quadrant to the midback and right scapula, or right shoulder tip region. While the pain begins suddenly, it may last for several hours and subside gradually, or end as quickly as it had begun. The patient is frequently nauseated; vomiting is seen less often. A palpable and tender gallbladder at Murphy's point may be delineated with uncomplicated obstruction at Hartmann's pouch, the cystic duct, or common duct. Physical examination generally is otherwise unremarkable with no evidence of fever, systemic illness, or peritoneal signs. Pale stools, dark urine, decreased stool bile salt levels, and increased levels in the urine are seen. Nonplacental alkaline phosphatase is increased and, with decreased vitamin K absorption, the prothrombin time also may be elevated.

The symptoms of cholecystitis include those seen with cholelithiasis including colicky right upper quadrant pain, radiating to the right shoulder or scapula.[1] The patient with superimposed infection will demonstrate tachycardia, low-grade fever, and in the presence of perforation with peritonitis, will have muscular guarding and rebound tenderness. Laboratory evaluation will reveal a mild leukocytosis in the absence of diffuse peritonitis. Some 60% of patients will have positive bile cultures with *Escherichia coli, Streptococcus* species, *Aerobacter aerogenes, Salmonella* and *Claustridia* being most often associated with cholecystitis.[7]

The signs and symptoms of cholecystitis and cholelithiasis in pregnancy are similar to those in the nonpregnant state.[2] However, a positive Murphy's sign is seen less frequently in pregnancy. The mild leukocytosis seen with cholecystitis frequently falls within the normal range for pregnancy. Placental alkaline phosphatase accounts for the twofold increase in serum alkaline phosphatase levels in pregnancy, making interpretation difficult.

DIAGNOSTIC IMAGING FOR GALLBLADDER DISEASE

Adjunctive imaging techniques including plain abdominal x-rays, cholecystography, and ultrasonography have been used in the delineation of biliary tract disease. Plain films demonstrate stones in the 15% of patients with a significant calcium component. Oral cholecystography is a reliable technique for the demonstration of biliary calculi, with an accuracy of 90–100%.[17] Intravenous cholecystography, with more rapid and complete absorption, is useful in the nonpregnant patient with nonvisualization of the gallbladder on oral study. Both tests are limited by the need for basal hepatic bile excretion. ^{99m}Tc scanning is highly accurate in the diagnosis of cholecystitis, but should be avoided during pregnancy.

Diagnostic ultrasonography is 90–95% accurate in the diagnosis of cholelithiasis.[18-21] Ultrasound imaging has the advantage of avoiding radiation exposure to both mother and developing fetus. However, in the presence of equivocal ultrasound studies, appropriately performed contrast cholecystography with shielding will result in an acceptable fetal radiation exposure.

MANAGEMENT OF CHOLELITHIASIS AND CHOLECYSTITIS

The patient with cholelithiasis identified prior to a planned pregnancy should be offered surgical intervention prior to conception. Of asymptomatic patients with cholelithiasis, 50% subsequently will develop overt symptomatology with 20% developing serious complications.[7] Operative morbidity and mortality are increased significantly in the presence of active disease (0.7% mortality in asymptomatic patients versus 5.0% mortality with acute cholecystitis) and with advancing age. Thus, the young, healthy, asymptomatic woman is the optimal candidate for this procedure.

The woman with asymptomatic cholelithiasis diagnosed in pregnancy may not become symptomatic during the gestation. Given the low risk of developing active disease during pregnancy, which would require surgical intervention, these women should be offered elective cholecystectomy after delivery.

The management of acute biliary colic and cholecystitis occurring during pregnancy is more controversial. The risks and benefits of conservative management must be weighed against the morbidity and mortality associated with surgery performed for recurrent attacks or progressively severe disease. Some authors suggest conservative management of cholelithiasis and cholecystitis with a delayed, elective procedure performed in the second trimester or postpartum period. Surgery is reserved for patients failing to respond to conservative measures and those suspected of suffering perforation. There are conflicting reports as to the risk of surgery during the first trimester.[2,14,22] Peterson[1] reported a 12% fetal loss in 1910 following cholecystectomy in pregnancy. Greene reported three early second trimester losses among 17 patients requiring cholecystectomy in pregnancy and suggested cholecystectomy to be safe during the second trimester.[23] Two of four fetal losses were spontaneous abortions in the first trimester and the third underwent preterm labor 15 weeks postoperatively. Dixon et al[24], in a review of 44 patients with biliary colic or cholecystitis in pregnancy, found a 58% recurrence rate in 26 conservatively treated patients. Of the patients having recurrent episodes, 33% had more than one recurrence. Of 14 women who underwent primary surgery in the second trimester, none suffered spontaneous abortion. Conversely, in another recent review, Landers[2] demonstrated the need for surgery on only four of 25 (16%) conservatively treated patients. In a third review of 20 conservatively treated pregnant women, 15 (75%) required cholecystectomy for recurrent disease.[1] Four procedures were performed during the first trimester for severe repeated attacks or biliary colic in the presence of unidentified pregnancy. Only one patient (6.7%) suffered spontaneous abortion 42 days postoperatively, while another chose therapeutic abortion.

Patients undergoing surgery in the first trimester may be at higher risk for pregnancy loss because of the severity of their disease prior to intervention, and the fact that surgery is taking place at the time of highest natural pregnancy loss. Ultrasonographic confirmation of viable intrauterine pregnancy was not performed prior to surgery in many of the older studies with high fetal loss rates. As such, the actual spontaneous pregnancy loss associated with cholecystectomy in the first trimester remains to be elucidated. Acute cholecystitis requiring surgery in the third trimester is associated with a higher rate of preterm labor because of uterine manipulation.

The woman presenting with cholelithiasis or cholecystitis in the first trimester thus should be treated conservatively. This initial management should include intravenous fluid resuscitation with correction of electrolyte abnormalities as required, and bowel rest with nasogastric suction to reduce neural and humoral stimulation of gallbladder contractility. Parenteral demerol should be given for pain relief. Morphine should be avoided because of its stimulatory effect of the sphincter of Oddi. The patient with cholecystitis should receive broad spectrum antibiotics from the time of admission. Fever should be controlled with sponge baths and antipyretics (care in administration should be observed in the presence of potential hepatic dysfunction). The presence of a viable intrauterine pregnancy should be determined. If testing for cholelithiasis is required in the reproductive years, diagnostic ultrasonography should be offered as the first-line mode of diagnosis. Plain and contrast radiography should be reserved for those with equivocal ultrasound. Pelvic shielding will provide adequate protection of the first trimester fetus. Surgical intervention in pregnancy should be reserved for patients with progressive disease despite adequate medical management, or for those with recurrent episodes of biliary colic or cholecystitis in pregnancy. Cholecystectomy, performed electively in the second trimester for patients with recurrent attacks, may decrease subsequent maternal and fetal morbidity. The operative procedure of choice is cholecystectomy. The patient with severe disease or adhesions may require an initial cholecystostomy for drainage with continued medical management and delayed cholecystectomy after resolution of the acute phase.

FETAL GALLSTONES

Antenatal detection of gallstones within the fetal gallbladder has been described by several authors.[25,26] Interestingly, spontaneous resolution of the gallstones occurred after birth, and thus fetal gallstones are of questionable significance.

CHOLEDOCHAL CYSTS IN PREGNANCY

Choledochal cysts are congenital dilatations of the biliary tract occurring anywhere within the hepatobiliary tree, and are most commonly seen in the common bile duct. Eighty percent are found in females, the majority diagnosed in childhood.[27] The common presenting symptoms include: right upper quadrant aching pain with jaundice and an epigastric mass. Bile peritonitis may result from cyst rupture. Diagnostic ultrasound and contrast cholecystography are useful in delineating the cystic area. Choledochal cysts are uncommon causes of jaundice in pregnancy.[27-29] Operative resection with reanastomosis of the remaining duct to the jejunum or duodenum is the management of choice. Binstock et al suggest elective cesarean section followed by cyst excision and anastomosis, given the association of adenocarcinoma with choledochal cysts.[29] Antenatal detection of choledochal cysts, and their subsequent early excision, have been reported.[30-32]

REFERENCES

1. Hill LM, Johnson CE, Lee RA. Cholecystectomy in pregnancy. *Obstet Gynecol.* 1975;46(3):291.
2. Landers D, Carmona R, Crombleholme W, Lim R. Acute cholecystitis in pregnancy. *Obstet Gynecol.* 1987;69:131.
3. Friley MD, Douglas G. Acute cholecystitis in pregnancy and the puerperium. *Am Surg.* 1972;38:314.
4. Sparkman RS. Gallstones in young women. *Am Surg.* 1957;145:813.
5. Holman KG, Montgomery PJ, Devabhaktuni D. Gallbladder disease in pregnancy. *Am Fam Prac.* 1985;32(1):147.
6. Moore KL. *The Developing Human: Clinically Oriented Embryology.* 4th ed. Philadelphia: WB Saunders; 1988:217.
7. Schwartz SI. Gallbladder and extra-hepatic biliary system. In: Schwartz SI, Shires GT, Spencer FC, Storer EH, eds. *Principles of Surgery.* 4th ed. New York: McGraw-Hill; 1984:1307.
8. Birnholz JC. Population survey: ultrasound cholecystography. *Gastrointest Radiol.* 1982;7:165.
9. Bennion LJ, Ginzberg RL, Garnick MB, Bennett PH. Effects of oral contraceptives on the gallbladder bile in normal women. *N Engl J Med.* 1976; 294:189.
10. Everson GT, Braverman DZ, Johnson ML, Kern F Jr. A critical evaluation of real time ultrasonography for the study of gallbladder volume and function. *Gastroenterology.* 1980;79:40.
11. Braverman DZ, Johnson ML, Kern F Jr. Effects of pregnancy and contraceptive steroids on gallbladder function. *N Engl J Med.* 1980;302:362.
12. Everson GT, McKinley C, Lawson M, et al. Gallbladder function in the human female: effect of the ovulatory cycle, pregnancy, and contraceptive steroids. *Gastroenterology.* 1982;82:711.
13. Ylostalo P, Kirkinen P, Heikkinen J, et al. Gallbladder volume and serum bile acids in cholestasis of pregnancy. *Br J Obstet Gynecol.* 1982;89:59.
14. Hiatt JR, Gordon Hiatt JC, Williams RA, Klein SR. Biliary disease in pregnancy: strategy for surgical management. *Am J Surg.* 1986;151:263.
15. Stauffer RA, Adam A, Wygal J, Lavery JP. Gallbladder disease in pregnancy. *Am J Obstet Gynecol.* 1982;144:661.
16. Chesson RR, Gallup DG, Gibbs RL, et al. Ultrasonographic diagnosis of asymptomatic cholelithiasis. *J Reprod Med.* 1985;30:920.
17. Mujahed Z, Evans JA, Whelan JP. The non-opacified gallbladder on oral cholecystography. *Radiology.* 1974;112:1.
18. Hood JB, Seymour JQ. Accuracy of oral cholecystography in cholelithiasis. *Am Surg.* July 1978;435.
19. Leopold JR, Amberg J, Gosnik PB, Mittelstaedt C. Grey scale ultrasonic cholecystography: comparison with conventional radiographic techniques. *Radiology.* 1976;121:445.
20. Arnon S, Rosenquist CJ. Grey scale cholecystosonography: an evaluation of accuracy. *Am J Roentgenol.* 1976;127:817.
21. Prian GW, Norton LW, Eule J, Eiseman E. Clinical indications and accuracy of grey scale ultrasonography in the patient with suspected biliary tract disease. *Am J Surg.* 1977;134:705.
22. Printen KJ, Ott RA. Cholecystectomy during pregnancy. *Am Surg.* Jul. 1978;432.
23. Greene J, Rogers A, Rubin L. Fetal loss after cholecystectomy during pregnancy. *Can Med Assoc J.* 1963;88:576.
24. Dixon NP, Faddis DM, Silberman H. Aggressive management of cholecystitis in pregnancy. *Am J Surg.* 1987;154:292.
25. Klingensmith WC, Cioffi-Ragan DT. Fetal gallstones. *Radiology.* 1988; 167:143.
26. Beretsky I, Lanken DH. Diagnosis of fetal cholelithiasis using real-time high-resolution imaging employing digital detection. *J Ultrasound Med.* 1983;2:381.
27. Russell JGB, Taylor V, Torrance B. Ultrasonic diagnosis of choledochal cyst in pregnancy. *Br J Radiology.* 1976;49:425.
28. Elgar DE, Gudgeon DH. Choledochus cyst complicating pregnancy. *Br J Surg.* 1969;56(11):868.
29. Binstock M, Sondack VK, Herd J, et al. Adenocarcinoma in a choledochal cyst during pregnancy: a case report and guidelines for management. *Surgery.* 1988;103(5):588.
30. Weidman MA, Tan A, Martinez CJ. Fetal sonography, and neonatal scintigraphy of a choledochal cyst. *J Nucl Med.* 1985;26(8):893.
31. Howell CG, Templeton JM, Weiner S, et al. Antenatal diagnosis and early surgery for choledochal cyst. *J Pediatr Surg.* 1983;18(4):387.
32. Elrad H, Matden KL, Ahart S, et al. Prenatal ultrasound diagnosis of choledochal cyst. *J Ultrasound Med.* 1985;4(10):553.

Chapter Two Hundred and Seven

Intestinal Obstruction

Brian M. Mercer

207

After appendicitis, intestinal obstruction is the second most common extrauterine abdominal emergency in pregnancy, with an incidence of 1 in 2500 to 1 in 3500.[1-5] In the nonpregnant population, intestinal obstruction accounts for 20% of surgical admissions for acute abdominal conditions. Adhesions are the primary etiologic factor in this group, with bowel herniation and neoplasm being the second and third most common causes of obstruction.[6] Mortality from intestinal obstruction has decreased from 50% in the early 1900s to less than 10%. Aggressive fluid and electrolyte management, intestinal decompression, antibiotic therapy, and early surgical intervention are believed to be the reasons for this marked improvement in survival with this condition.

In pregnancy, adhesive disease is the most common underlying factor contributing to intestinal obstruction. The increasing incidence of intestinal obstruction in both the nonpregnant and pregnant patient is attributed to an increasing frequency of abdominal surgery (especially appendectomy and gynecologic surgery) in the young patient population.[7,8] While a history of previous abdominal or pelvic surgery is useful in identifying patients at risk for adhesive bowel obstruction, adhesions are congenital in origin or subsequent to intraperitoneal inflammation in 28% of patients.[7] Intestinal obstruction in pregnancy is seen more frequently in the third trimester of pregnancy.[8,9] In 1937, Eliason reported that adhesive disease precipitated intestinal obstruction most often in the fourth and fifth months of gestation, eighth and ninth months of gestation, and in the peripartum period.[10] This was believed to be related to rapid growth of the uterus with changes in the adhesion-intestinal relationships, and descent of the presenting part into the pelvis with sudden decrease in uterine size at delivery, again altering the adhesion-intestinal relationships. However, the actual reasons for the increasing incidence of bowel obstruction with increasing gestation are not clear.

Intestinal volvulus supersedes intestinal herniation and neoplasm as the second most common cause of intestinal obstruction in pregnancy. Volvulus accounts for approximately 25% of bowel obstructions in pregnancy.[11] As volvulus may be caused by underlying adhesive disease, the exact incidence of intestinal obstruction related to isolated volvulus is not known. Intestinal herniation and neoplasm are uncommon causes of intestinal obstruction in pregnancy because of the displacement of the bowel away from the inguinal and femoral canals by the enlarging uterus, as well as the relatively young age of the pregnant patient with a low incidence of malignancy. Intussusception and inflammatory bowel disease are rarely seen in pregnancy as causes for intestinal obstruction.

Paralytic ileus may occur in the pregnant and nonpregnant patient. It is usually the result of generalized illness with loss of autonomic nervous control of the intestine. As such, paralytic ileus may be seen in patients with sepsis, prolonged hypotension, and spinal trauma. Paralytic ileus also may result from response to bowel irritation by diffuse peritonitis and surgical manipulation, and in the presence of retroperitoneal lesions. Colonic pseudo-obstruction is a paralytic ileus of the colon originally described in 1948.[12] This complication is pregnancy related in 35% of patients.[13]

CLINICAL DIAGNOSIS OF BOWEL OBSTRUCTION

Intestinal obstruction is divided functionally into that occurring as a result of intestinal blockage (mechanical) and that associated with decreased intestinal motility (paralytic). The signs and symptoms of obstruction are different depending on the functional etiology of the obstruction.

Mechanical obstruction may occur anywhere within the intestinal tract.[14,15] The related symptomatology will vary depending on the level of obstruction. The patient with mechanical obstruction frequently will present with symptoms of nausea, vomiting, and colicky abdominal pain following a prodrome of constipation/obstipation. Abdominal distention is seen to a variable extent. The pain is generally intermittent and located in the midline, either supraumbilically or infraumbilically. The colic lasts for shorter periods in upper-intestinal obstructions, and longer periods in obstruction of the large bowel. Thus small bowel obstruction frequently will present with a colicky supraumbilical midline pain for four to five minutes, and large bowel obstruction frequently presents with colicky pains every 10–15 minutes apart.[11] With perforation and the development of peritonitis, the pain will become constant and diffuse, and will be exacerbated by movement.

Vomiting is a common symptom of early pregnancy but rarely is seen in the late second and third trimesters. Vomiting associated with colicky abdominal pain should raise the suspicion of intestinal obstruction. Obstruction at a high level is associated with frequent pronounced vomiting, early in the clinical course. If the obstruction is distal to the ampula of Vater, bileous vomiting will occur. Distal obstruction is associated with less frequent and delayed vomiting. Multiplication of resident bacteria within the colon leads to the production of feculant vomitus. While vomiting frequently is associated with intestinal obstruction, it is not necessarily present.

Constipation may be described by patients with bowel obstruction. However, high lesions frequently are associated with continued lower intestinal function for a period of time. Diarrhea may be seen in association with obstruction and strangulation at any level.[14]

The physical findings of intestinal obstruction are variable depending on the level of obstruction and duration of the process. The patient with acute high obstruction is frequently tachycardic and ill in appearance. Vital signs are often otherwise unremarkable in the absence of perforation. These patients will demonstrate little evidence of dehydration or abdominal distention. Abdominal tenderness may be elicited by compression of a distended loop of bowel in the uncomplicated obstruction. Auscultation will reveal active bowel sounds with high-pitched rushes.

The patient with prolonged obstruction, especially of the distal colon, will show signs of low-grade fever and possibly hypotension related to prolonged vomiting and third space fluid loss in the obstructed intestinal segments.[16] Active tympanic bowel sounds may be present. However, with prolonged obstruction, paralytic ileus may supervene with bowel sounds being decreased or absent. In the presence of perforation resulting from ischemic necrosis of the wall of the obstructed segment, diffuse peritoneal tenderness with rebound tenderness may be present. Distal obstruction or perforation with diffuse peritonitis may be associated with abdominal distention. However, this finding may be difficult to delineate in the presence of the gravid uterus. The uterine fundus should be palpated for the presence of contractions to rule out preterm labor. Premature contractions may be seen in the setting of peritonitis related to intestinal obstruction. Rectal examination should be performed on all patients suspected of having intestinal obstruction. While the presence of stool in the rectum does not rule out high intestinal obstruction, it may be possible to palpate an obstructing lesion on digital examination. Urine output reflects organ perfusion and frequently is decreased in the dehydrated patient with bowel obstruction. The urine output should be quantified early in the assessment and management of patient with bowel obstruction.

Laboratory investigation is important in the diagnosis and management of the patient with suspected intestinal obstruction. In the absence of perforation, the white blood cell count may not be elevated from the levels seen in uncomplicated pregnancy. With third space fluid loss related to prolonged obstruction or perforation and dehydration from recurrent vomiting, serum electrolyte abnormalities may occur (hypochloremic, hypokalemic metabolic alkalosis with prolonged vomiting, or metabolic acidosis with prolonged diarrhea or supervening sepsis). BUN will be elevated in the presence of intravascular depletion. Liver function tests, bilirubin, and amylase measurement as well as urinalysis are important in ruling out other potential causes of abdominal pain.

X-ray confirmation and characterization of the bowel obstruction is essential to the diagnosis of obstructive intestinal disease. The risk of appropriately performed x-rays for demonstration of the site of obstruction and the presence of free perforation is minimal when compared to the fetal and maternal risks of intestinal obstruction and perforation.

Small bowel obstruction will reveal multiple dilated loops of small intestine with air and fluid levels. The large colon and small bowel distal to the site of obstruction will be free of visible gas in the setting of a complete small bowel obstruction.

The patient with large bowel obstruction will demonstrate a distended large intestine with haustrations incompletely traversing the lumen diameter. Air and fluid levels may be seen in the large bowel and in the small bowel proximal to obstruction in the presence of an incompetent ileocecal valve. A lateral decubitus or upright film will reveal free air underneath the lateral abdominal wall or diaphragm, respectively, in the presence of intestinal perforation. Although these classic findings may be seen, the patient with acute intestinal obstruction may demonstrate no diagnostic findings on initial plain x-rays. Plain radiographs are not useful in the differentiation of mechanical and paralytic ileus other than the high lesion with complete obstruction in which the small and large intestine distal to the obstruction are not distended.

In the presence of sigmoid volvulus, the x-ray will demonstrate an ascending and descending loop of sigmoid extending into the left upper quadrant. The common x-ray finding of cecal volvulus is a single air-fluid level with distended bowel found high in the abdomen.

When the diagnosis of large bowel obstruction is suggested by plain radiographs, retrograde endoscopic examination and contrast studies may be useful adjuncts in determining the level and nature of the obstruction. Ascending contrast studies are not of value in small bowel disease in the absence of an incompetent ileocecal valve. Oral contrast studies may help to identify the level of a small bowel obstruction or aid in the differentiation between paralytic and mechanical ileus.

TREATMENT OF MECHANICAL BOWEL OBSTRUCTION IN PREGNANCY

The definitive therapy of mechanical intestinal obstruction in pregnancy is surgical decompression. Mechanical bowel obstruction rarely clears spontaneously, and unnecessary delay may lead to bowel infarction and perforation. In the general population, mortality following surgery for simple small bowel obstruction is 5–8%. A 20–75% mortality is seen in the presence of strangulation.[17] Large bowel obstruction has a 20% mortality rate. Maternal mortality following intestinal obstruction in pregnancy has decreased from 50% to 10–20% in the past 50 years.[5,7,18] Once the diagnosis of mechanical bowel obstruction is made, intravenous resuscitation should be undertaken with replacement of intravascular volume and correction of electrolyte imbalances as necessary. A Foley catheter should be inserted for monitoring of urine output. Central venous pressure monitoring is a useful adjunct in the presence of marked dehydration. A nasogastric tube should be inserted to prevent further passage of fluid and air into the intestinal tract and reduce the risk of aspiration at surgery. Wide spectrum aerobic and anaerobic antibiotic coverage should be instituted prior to surgery.

The laparotomy incision should allow adequate exploration of the abdomen regardless of the suspected level of obstruction. A midline infraumbilical or supraumbilical incision will give adequate exposure depending on the gestation and can be extended as necessary. Initial incision should avoid abdominal scars as these may be the location of adherent bowel. On entering the abdomen, unless an immediately apparent sight of obstruction is identified, a distal unobstructed and collapsed segment should be identified and the bowel run proximally to the sight of obstruction. Sharp dissection of adhesions should be performed. At the sight of obstruction, the bowel should be examined for viability. Obviously, necrotic bowel should be excised and the remaining bowel observed for return of color and peristalsis. Intraoperative Doppler assessment of the antimesenteric vasculature will indicate sections of bowel capable of sustaining an anastomosis.[16] Prior to any definitive procedure, the entire bowel should be examined for multiple areas of obstruction.

In the absence of diffuse peritonitis, the pregnancy is best left undisturbed unless cesarean delivery is essential to gain adequate exposure of the intestine.[11,19]

INTESTINAL VOLVULUS IN PREGNANCY

Intestinal volvulus is the second most common cause of bowel obstruction in pregnancy. Intestinal volvulus in the pregnant patient classically involves the cecum or sigmoid colon. Cecal volvulus accounts for 25–44% of volvulae in pregnancy.[20] Harer and Harer[11] have suggested that the enlarging uterus elevates an abnormally mobile cecum from the cecal fossa, with partial obstruction resulting from uterine pressure or kinking of the bowel following elevation. Subsequent colonic distention leads to further displacement and torsion. Immediate surgical intervention is essential in this closed loop obstruction to prevent perforation. Again, the bowel should be inspected for evidence of ischemic necrosis and perforation at the time of the procedure. The bowel should be de-rotated and nonviable portions excised with primary anastomosis or a two-stage procedure with initial colostomy followed by subsequent closure. Cecal volvulus may occur postpartum or post cesarean section[21], subsequent to physical dislocation of the cecum and postoperative ileus in association with partial rectosigmoid obstruction by the uterus.

Sigmoid volvulus also occurs as a result of elevation of redundant and mobile sigmoid colon from the pelvis by the growing uterus, with subsequent kinking and torsion.[22] Two thirds of sigmoid volvulae occur in black patients. Sigmoid volvulus is one of the few obstructive lesions that can be treated conservatively in the absence of perforation or wall necrosis. Unfortunately, nonsurgical therapy is rarely successful in the pregnant patient.[15] Suspicion of intestinal perforation or bowel ischemic necrosis of the bowel wall mandates early surgical intervention. Sigmoid volvulus must be differentiated from lower intestinal obstruction secondary to incarceration of the uterus in the second trimester or early postpartum period. This complication can be treated with anteversion of the uterus and rectal tube placement.

PSEUDO-OBSTRUCTION OF THE LARGE INTESTINE

Pseudo-obstruction of the large intestine is the most common cause of paralytic ileus in pregnancy.[23] Ogilvie[12], in 1948, first described a syndrome of paralytic intestinal obstruction. Subsequently, numerous articles have cited pseudo-obstruction of the colon following surgical intervention.[1,23,24] One third of the cases of pseudo-obstruction of the colon occur in relation to pregnancy and cesarean section. Spira revealed a 50% perforation of the cecum in patients with this condition.[13] The signs and symptoms include diffuse crampy abdominal pain with progressive abdominal distention. Nausea, constipation, flatus, diarrhea, and vomiting are seen less frequently. Bowel sounds may be normal, high pitched and obstructive, or decreased. The radiographic appearance of pseudo-obstruction is one of proximal segmental distention of the colon with distal undistended bowel. The cutoff may be seen at the hepatic flexure, sigmoid flexure, or rectosigmoid junction. Contrast enema may exclude the presence of a mechanical obstructive lesion and may be therapeutic. The cecum is usually the most dilated segment, and cecal perforation is associated with a high mortality. Early reports suggested that perforation would occur at a critical cecal diameter of 9 cm.[25] Some reports have suggested 10–12 cm to be the critical diameter for perforation.[17,26,27] In the absence of marked cecal dilatation, conservative management is recommended, including intravenous rehydration, restoration of electrolyte balance, and nasogastric and rectal tube decompression. Serial abdominal x-rays must be performed to confirm resolution of the colonic distention. Operative intervention with cecostomy is essential in patients with marked cecal dilatation, right lower quadrant tenderness suggestive of perforation, or failure of medical management.

Intestinal obstruction is the second most common nonobstetric abdominal emergency in pregnancy. Maternal mortality and fetal mortality have improved with the advent of aggressive fluid and electrolyte management, antibiotic therapy, and early surgical intervention. Fetal loss primarily is associated with peritonitis and prolonged hypotension in the patient with severe disease. Both fetal and maternal morbidity and mortality can be reduced by early surgical intervention prior to perforation.

REFERENCES

1. Davis MR, Bohon CJ. Intestinal obstruction in pregnancy. *Clin Obstet Gynecol.* 1983;26(4):832.
2. Krammerer WS. Non-obstetric surgery during pregnancy. *Med Clin North Am.* 1979;63(6):1157.
3. Lewis GD. Intestinal obstruction complicating pregnancy. *J Am Osteo Path Assoc.* 1974;74:69.
4. Coughlan BM. Acute intestinal obstruction during pregnancy. *J R Coll Surg Edin.* 1978;23:175.
5. Beck WW. Intestinal obstruction in pregnancy. *Obstet Gynecol.* 1974; 43:374.
6. Schwartz SI, Storer EH. Manifestations of gastro-intestinal disease. In: Schwartz SI, Shires TG, Spencer FC, Storer EH, eds. *Principles of Surgery.* 4th ed. New York: McGraw-Hill; 1984.
7. Hill LM, Symmonds RE. Small bowel obstruction in pregnancy: a review and report of four cases. *Obstet Gynecol.* 1977;49(2):170.
8. Anderson GV, Ball A. Acute abdominal problems in pregnancy. *Contemp Ob/Gyn.* 1981;18:27.
9. Beck WW, Morris ED. Intestinal obstruction in pregnancy. *J Obstet Gynecol Br Commonw.* 1965;72:36.
10. Eliason EL, Erb WH. Intestinal obstruction complicating pregnancy. *Surgery.* 1937;1:65.
11. Harer WB Jr, Harer WB Sr. Volvulus complicating pregnancy and the puerperium. *Obstet Gynecol.* 1958;12:399.
12. Ogilvie EH. Large intestine colic due to sympathetic deprivation: a new clinical syndrome. *Br Med J.* 1948;2:671.
13. Spira IA, Rodriquez R, Wolff WI. Pseudo-obstruction of the colon. *Am J Gastroenterol.* 1976;65(5):397.
14. Van Wingerden GI, Dons RF. Complete duodenal obstruction during pregnancy, with intestinal non-rotation and painless mid-gut volvulus. *J Reprod Med.* 1981;26(5):265.
15. Hofmeyr GJ, Sonnendecker EWW. Sigmoid volvulus in advanced pregnancy: report of two cases. *S Afr Med J.* 1985;67:63.
16. Carey LC, Fabry PJ. The intestinal tract in relation to gynecology. In: Mattingly RF, Thompson JD, eds. *TeLindes' Operative Gynecology.* Philadelphia: JB Lippincott; 1985;449.
17. Silen W. Acute intestinal obstruction. In: Petersdorf RG, Adams RD, Braunwald E, et al, eds. *Harrison's Principles of Internal Medicine.* New York: McGraw Hill; 1983;1765.
18. Smith JA, Bartlett MK. Acute surgical emergencies of the abdomen in pregnancy. *N Engl J Med.* 1940;223(14):529.
19. James DW. Intestinal obstruction during late pregnancy. *Br Med J.* 1946; 1:485.
20. Pratt AT, Donaldson RC, Evertson LR, Yon JL. Cecal volvulus in pregnancy. *Obstet Gynecol.* 1981;57:37.
21. Fanning J, Cross CB. Post cesarean section cecal volvulus. *Am J Obstet Gynecol.* 1988;158:1200.
22. Ballantyne GH. Review of sigmoid volvulus: clinical patterns and pathogenesis. *Dis Colon Rectum.* 1982;25:823.
23. Reece EA, Petrie RH, Hutcherson H. Ogilvie's syndrome in the post cesarean section patient. *Am J Obstet Gynecol.* 1982;144:849.
24. Robbins RD, Schoen R, Sohn N, Weinstein MA. Colonic decompression of massive cecal dilatation (Ogilvie's syndrome) secondary to cesarean section. *Am J Gastroenterol.* 1982;77(4):231.
25. Lowman RM, Davis L. An evaluation of cecal size in impending perforation of the cecum. *Surg Gynecol Obstet.* 1956;103:711.
26. Wanebo H, Conolly B. Pseudo-obstruction of the colon. *Surg Gynecol Obstet.* 1971;133:44.
27. Nanni G, Garbini A, Lucheti P, et al. Ogilvie's syndrome (acute colonic pseudo-obstruction). *Dis Colon Rectum.* 1982;25:157.

Chapter Two Hundred and Eight

Trauma

William L. Holcomb, Jr. and Erol Amon

208

Trauma during pregnancy is a common occurrence ranging from the uncomplicated fall to multisystem injuries that may threaten the life of the mother and the fetus. Care of the pregnant trauma victim may require the skills of many specialists working as a team. The emergency medicine physician is usually in charge of the initial triage and stabilization of the injured patient. The general surgeon or surgical subspecialist is needed for evaluation and operative management of significant injuries outside the genital tract. Internists, anesthesiologists, acute care specialists, and others may be involved in the care of the patient depending on the nature and severity of her injuries. The major role of the obstetrician is threefold: 1) to provide knowledge of the altered physiology and anatomy of pregnancy; 2) to assess the fetal response to trauma and potential need for delivery; and 3) to be alert for obstetric complications due to or coincident with trauma. As in any team effort, it is important to maintain flexibility, communication, and clear delineation of responsibility.

In a group of women queried throughout pregnancy, 6% reported occurrence of at least one traumatic episode. Only two of 242 instances of trauma were catastrophic and clearly related to fetal loss. The majority of these episodes involved falls, usually on the buttocks or sides. Motor vehicle accidents comprised the next largest category.[1] Unfortunately, violent assault is also a cause of injury for the pregnant woman. In a clinic population asked at the first prenatal visit, "Has anyone at home hit or tried to hurt you?", 11% responded affirmatively and 4% admitted continued physical abuse during the current pregnancy. Some reported an increase in abuse during pregnancy, while others noted a decrease or no change.[2] There are more women in the work force than ever before, and many continue to work throughout pregnancy. The working environment includes daily commuting as well as exposure to stairs, obstacles, and heavy machinery. It has not been demonstrated that working increases the pregnant woman's chance of injury, but it is logical to assume that there is a greater risk. Fatigue, a common symptom during pregnancy, also may increase the likelihood of injury.

Trauma is the leading cause of death in reproductive age women. The majority of these deaths are due to accidents, followed by homicide, and suicide.[3] Motor vehicle accidents are the most common cause of accidental death in women, accounting for almost one half of such fatalities. Falls are the second most common cause of accidental death.[4] Accidental injury is the most frequent nonobstetric cause of death in pregnant women.[5] Since such cases are not identified and reviewed routinely by maternal mortality committees, the association between accidental death and pregnancy is probably under-reported.

The developing conceptus induces major changes in maternal physiology, many of which are directly relevant to care of the trauma victim. Cardiovascular alterations include an increase in blood volume, cardiac output, and heart rate, accompanied by a decrease in blood pressure. Blood volume starts to increase in the first trimester of pregnancy, attaining a 45% increase over the nonpregnant state by the middle of the third trimester. A practical consequence is that the pregnant patient in hemorrhagic shock needs more vigorous fluid and blood replacement than her size would indicate otherwise. The plasma volume increase exceeds the increase in red cell mass, accounting for the decline in hematocrit usually seen in pregnancy. A hematocrit value of 30–35% is common in pregnancy and should not be interpreted as evidence for blood loss unless a recent value is available for comparison.

Cardiac output increases during the first half of gestation to 30–50% above the nonpregnant value. It is sensitive to maternal position, being lower in the standing and supine positions than in the left or right lateral recumbant positions. Even the normovolemic pregnant woman may demonstrate symptomatic hypotension in the supine position. For the trauma victim who may have an occult hemorrhage, it is particularly important for her to be positioned with a lateral tilt of at least 15 degrees. For most patients this will effectively relieve compression of the vena cava and preserve blood return to the heart. Maternal heart rate increases during the first two trimesters of pregnancy to approximately 15 bpm above the nonpregnant rate in the third trimester. There is a progressive fall in systolic and diastolic blood pressures, reaching 10 mm Hg below nonpregnant values in the second trimester with a subsequent rise in the third trimester. These physiologic changes should be considered when the pregnant trauma victim is evaluated for blood loss.

The electrocardiogram may demonstrate a leftward shift of the electrical axis with prominent Q-waves and inversion of the T-waves in lead 3. This alteration is thought to be due to positional change of the heart with uterine growth.[6] The evolution of electrocardiographic changes during pregnancy varies greatly and is not predictable in a given patient.[7]

It often is stated that the usual signs of hypovolemia are not apparent in pregnant patients until large volumes of blood have been lost. Further study is needed to verify this assertion. The cardiovascular effects of acute hemorrhage and volume restoration have been studied in the anesthetized pregnant sheep and dog. With blood loss there was a steady fall in maternal mean arterial blood pressure with a proportionately greater fall in uterine blood flow. Uteroplacental oxygen extraction and fetal pO_2 were affected adversely by progressive maternal blood loss. Blood retransfusion resulted in a return of all parameters to near baseline values. An α-adrenergic vasopressor restored maternal blood pressure, but further reduced uterine blood flow and fetal pO_2.[8,9] Ringer's lactate also restored fetal pO_2 when given following acute maternal hemorrhage.[10] Blood and fluid replacement, not vasopressors, is the treatment of choice for acute blood loss. When adrenergic drugs are used, there is evidence to support the use of ephedrine. This agent has been demonstrated to improve fetal acidosis in hypotensive pregnant sheep.[11]

Central venous pressure and pulmonary capillary

wedge pressure are similar in the pregnant and nonpregnant state. The trauma victim with unstable cardiovascular status or uncertain fluid volume status may benefit from triple-lumen catheterization to measure these and other parameters. There is now considerable experience with invasive cardiovascular monitoring in pregnancy.[12,13]

Respiratory physiology is also changed during pregnancy. Early in gestation there is an increase in tidal volume with a decrease in functional residual capacity. The resulting respiratory alkalosis is compensated by an increase in renal excretion of bicarbonate. The normal PCO_2 in pregnancy is 30 mm Hg, and the normal calculated CO_2 is 21. The lower maternal PCO_2 may facilitate diffusion of CO_2 from the fetal to the maternal compartment with subsequent elimination by way of the maternal lungs. Arterial pH may be increased slightly. Knowledge of these changes is important in the interpretation of arterial blood gas values. In the patient who may require assisted ventilation, settings should be adjusted to achieve a normal pregnant state. As pregnancy advances there is bilateral elevation of the diaphragm. Chest x-rays in late pregnancy may show features indicative of poor inspiration. There are no predictable chest radiographic changes due to pregnancy.[14]

Decreased motility of the gastrointestinal tract during pregnancy results in delayed stomach emptying. Later in gestation, gastroesophageal reflux is common. These changes contribute to an increased risk for aspiration pneumonitis when the pregnant patient is obtunded or anesthetized. As the uterine fundus displaces the bowel upward during the latter half of pregnancy, the gastrointestinal tract is relatively protected from penetrating trauma. The more vulnerable uterus is most often the site of injury. If penetrating trauma should involve the upper abdomen, the tightly packed loops of bowel are likely to be injured.

The renal pelvices and ureters are dilated by the end of the first trimester, more so on the right side than on the left. This change affects interpretation of radiographic and sonographic studies of the urinary tract. As the lower uterine segment lengthens, the bladder is carried up out of its well protected pelvic location to become more of an abdominal organ. Positional change as well as pregnancy-associated atony and distention make the bladder more prone to injury. Traumatic ureteral injury is rare. Increased renal blood flow during pregnancy may increase blood loss with renal trauma.

THE EFFECT ON PREGNANCY

The various effects of trauma on pregnancy are summarized in Table 208–1. The most common cause of fetal death is death of the mother. Less severe maternal trauma usually does not affect the course of pregnancy but, in some cases, may cause direct injury to the fetus, intrauterine fetal death, or premature labor and delivery. During the first trimester, the uterus is well protected within the pelvic cavity. Trauma is rarely the cause of pregnancy loss early in gestation. Clinical spontaneous abortion is a common event occurring in one out of six pregnancies. The relationship between trauma in the first trimester and abortion is much more likely to be coincidental than causal. In a medicolegal context, histologic or chromosomal examination of the abortus may clarify the issue of causation. Evidence of preexisting fetal abnormality or demise may rule out maternal trauma as a cause of pregnancy loss.

TABLE 208–1. EFFECTS OF TRAUMA ON PREGNANCY

Minimal or no effect
Spontaneous abortion (rare)
Fetal hypoxia secondary to
Maternal shock
Placental abruption
Placental and cord injury
Uterine injury
Fetal hemorrhage
Direct fetal injury
Preterm labor and birth
Red cell isoimmunization

In the second and third trimesters, injury of the uterus, the placenta, or of the fetus can directly affect the course of pregnancy. Estimates of uterine blood flow vary, but the term uterus probably receives about 500 mL/per minute.[15] Accordingly, the uterus, a distended viscera with dilated vasculature, can be the source of profuse hemorrhage if injured. Traumatic rupture of the uterus associated with automotive injury, with and without seat belt use, has been reported.[16,17] Uterine vasculature in the broad ligament may be the source of hemoperitoneum or a retroperitoneal hematoma in the presence of an intact uterus. Physical abuse and penetrating wounds of pregnant women often involve the protuberant abdomen and the uterus.

If the mother survives, the most common cause of fetal death is placental abruption. Crosby has suggested that the inelastic placenta is sheared from its attachment when the more elastic uterus suddenly is distorted. Of 176 surviving victims of severe motor vehicle collisions with gestations of greater than 12 weeks, 6 (3.4%) suffered *abruptio placentae.*[17] Agran[18] reported on 9 cases over a three-year period in which vehicular trauma resulted in fetal death in Orange County, California. Placental abruption occurred in 8 cases; in 6 of these, maternal injuries were considered minor. Clinical evidence of placental separation was present within eight hours of the accident in all cases. Lavin[19] and Higgins[20] have reported individual cases of *abruptio placentae* occurring five to six days after automobile accidents.

A case of amniotic fluid embolism and disseminated intravascular coagulation associated with traumatic *abruptio placentae* has been described by Olcott.[21] Two cases with laceration of the maternal surface of the placenta has been reported by Stuart.[22] In both cases a head-on motor vehicle accident was the cause of the injury and fetal death resulted from exsanguination. It was suggested that the laceration was due to collison between the fetus and the placenta with sudden deceleration.

Bickers[23] has described a case of severe fetomaternal hemorrhage following maternal involvement in an automobile accident. The neonatal hematocrit was 25%. Following transfusion, the infant survived without sequelae. Rose[24] assessed fetomaternal hemorrhage using the Kleihauer–Betke test following 32 cases in which pregnant women sustained minor traumatic injuries. Of this group, 28% demonstrated detectable fetomaternal hemorrhage compared with 6% in a gestational age-matched control group. Obstetric outcome was not clearly related to the presence or quantity of fetomaternal hemorrhage in this study. Even small quantities could cause red cell isoimmunization.

Direct traumatic injuries to the fetus do occur and have been described in great variety. The most common injury, unfortunately, is fetal skull fracture or intracranial hemorrhage. Stafford et al[25] have described four such cases. In one instance the associated maternal injuries were minimal.

TABLE 208–2. COMMON BLOOD TESTS THAT ARE ALTERED BY PREGNANCY

Test	Change in Pregnancy	Mechanism
Hemoglobin	Decreased	Dilutional effect
Hematocrit	Decreased	Dilutional effect
White blood cell count	Increased	Unknown
Arterial pH	Slightly increased	Increased ventilation
Arterial PCO_2	Decreased	Increased ventilation
Calculated CO_2	Decreased	Metabolic compensation
Fibrinogen	Increased	Increased hepatic synthesis
Alkaline phosphatase	Increased	Placental production
Amylase	Increased	Unknown

Maternal pelvic fractures pose a substantial risk to the fetus, particularly in late pregnancy with fetal head engagement.

Premature labor unassociated with diagnosed placental abruption has been described following maternal trauma. The frequency of this complication and its relationship to trauma have not been defined. Further study is needed.

MANAGEMENT OF TRAUMA

Initial triage and stabilization of the trauma victim are essentially the same regardless of pregnancy and will not be described in detail here. A review by Shatney[26] summarizes this topic. Briefly, priorities for the hemodynamically unstable patient with multisystem trauma are establishment of airway and ventilation, control of obvious external hemorrhage, and treatment of shock. ECG monitoring, a nasogastric tube, and a bladder catheter should be used. Subsequently, radiologic procedures (lateral cervical spine, AP of the pelvis and upright chest films) and peritoneal lavage are performed as indicated. Hematuria noted with catheterization may be the first sign of urinary tract injury or uterine rupture. During these initial steps, it is essential to avoid supine hypotension by lateral recumbent positioning or lateral displacement of the uterus.

Futher diagnostic evaluation of the pregnant patient presents at least three major challenges. First, gestational physiologic changes must be taken into account when interpreting physical findings, laboratory tests, and imaging studies. Second, there is the possibility of a concurrent obstetric disorder, related or unrelated to the trauma, which may complicate diagnosis and treatment, for example, placental abruption or preeclampsia. Third, fetal status must be evaluated as soon as possible after the maternal condition is stable.

Multiple diagnostic tests are ordered for the victim of trauma. Some tests that are altered by the pregnant state are listed in Table 208–2. Laboratories usually print out normal range limits for the nonpregnant patient in reports. While an arterial pCO_2 of 40 mm Hg may be normal for a nonpregnant patient, it indicates significant hypoventilation in the pregnant patient. Similarly, a "normal" fibrinogen level of 150 mg/dL may suggest intravascular coagulation in the pregnant patient. Serum amylase activity increases significantly during pregnancy reaching a mid-trimester peak as high as twice the upper limit of the nonpregnant normal range.[27] Serum transaminase and creatine kinase levels are not altered significantly by pregnancy.

Basic diagnostic evaluation of the pregnant trauma victim is summarized in Table 208–3. A test to assess and quantitate fetomaternal hemorrhage, such as the Kleihauer–Betke test, should be obtained with such patients. If the result is reported as the percentage of hemoglobin F-containing cells, the volume of hemorrhage can be estimated (in mL) by multiplying the percentage value by a factor of 50. If fetomaternal hemorrhage is detected, fetal surveillance must be intensive. A large hemorrhage (greater than 25 mL) indicates the need for more than one vial of Rh immunoglobulin for the Rh-negative patient. Even if the Kleihauer–Betke test is negative, the Rh-negative trauma victim should receive one vial of Rh immunoglobulin since the test is not sensitive enough to detect the minimal quantities of fetal blood that may sensitize the mother. The only exception to this rule would be the case in which the paternal blood type is known to be Rh-negative. Chhibber et al[28] have described a case in which an automobile accident at 24 weeks was thought to result in Rh sensitization of an Rh-negative nulliparous patient.

The most sensitive blood test for detection of disseminated intravascular coagulation (DIC) complicating placental abruption is the presence of fibrin degradation products. Serum fibrinogen, platelet count, and hematocrit values are the most useful tests to follow serially in patients with obstetric DIC.

There may be reluctance to perform some diagnostic tests and procedures on the pregnant patient for fear of fetal consequences. This is particularly true with radiologic procedures. It is prudent to minimize fetal radiation exposure (by shielding the abdomen when possible and planning exposures carefully), but there is no reason to withhold a

TABLE 208–3. BASIC DIAGNOSTIC EVALUATION OF THE PREGNANT TRAUMA VICTIM

Hemoglobin
Hematocrit
Urinalysis
Type/Rh
Kleihauer–Betke
Obstetric ultrasound
Electronic fetal monitoring
If placental abruption suspected Fibrin degradation products and serial (q 6–8 hr) fibrinogen, platelet count and hematocrit
Other studies as indicated by site and severity of injury

needed study. Fetal effects have not been documented at less than 5–10 rads (.05–.10 Gy), well in excess of radiation absorbed for diagnostic purposes. Meredith and Trunkey[29] recently have reviewed the use of abdominal computed tomography (CT) to evaluate intra-abdominal and retroperitoneal trauma. The benefits of this modality to pregnant patients remain to be determined, but the fetal radiation dose (approximately 1 rad [.01 Gy]) is not prohibitive. Civil et al[30] have described the use of abdominal CT to detect intraperitoneal bleeding in a pregnant trauma victim. Fetal death was diagnosed prior to the examination in this case.

Diagnostic peritoneal lavage is another method to evaluate intra-abdominal injury and assess the need for laparotomy. Rothenberger[31] has found this technique to be safe and effective in a series of 12 pregnant trauma victims. Indications for the procedure as well as criteria for interpretation of results are identical to those for the nongravid patient. Dissection to the peritoneum rather than blind insertion is used to place the peritoneal dialysis catheter. In late gestation, a supraumbilical rather than an infraumbilical site should be chosen. This procedure is not reliable for detection of retroperitoneal hemorrhage.

Pelvic ultrasonography can give valuable information in the care of the pregnant trauma patient, but it is important to be aware of its limitations. Knowledge of fetal number, size, anomalies, and presentation may aid in subsequent obstetric decision making. Decreased amniotic fluid may be the first sign of ruptured amniotic membranes, particularly in an obtunded patient. Placental location can be reliably determined but ultrasonography is not sufficiently sensitive to rule out placental abruption. Nyberg[32] has reviewed the sonographic characteristics of hematomas associated with placental abruption. Most detected hematomas are located adjacent to the placenta between the chorionic membrane and the decidua. A retroplacental location is the next most common site. Acute hemorrhage may have the same echodensity as placental tissue, which accounts for some diagnostic insensitivity. The appearance of a markedly thickened placenta, however, should increase suspicion of *abruptio placentae.* The diagnosis of placental abruption primarily is based on clinical findings, with vaginal bleeding the most constant feature. There may be adominal pain, uterine tenderness, tetanic uterine contractions, or fetal distress.

Diagnostic amniocentesis may be helpful in selected trauma patients. Situations in which it is unclear whether delivery is advisable may be clarified by assurance of fetal lung maturity. Amniocentesis, like ultrasonography, is not a reliable means of excluding the diagnosis of placental abruption. However, if bloody or port wine-stained amniotic fluid is withdrawn, placental separation or laceration is a likely source. Delivery or intensive fetal monitoring are indicated depending on gestational age and other clinical findings. Blood noted on initial withdrawal that subsequently clears most probably is due to trauma from the amniocentesis itself.

In the absence of clinical evidence of placental abruption or major maternal injuries, it is unclear how long patients ought to have continuous electronic fetal monitoring. Authors on this topic have widely differing recommendations from a minimum of 30 minutes[24] to at least 72 hours.[33] Twenty-four hours of observation following trauma, as suggested by Agran[18], is justified by the finding that almost all abruptions are clinically apparent within this interval. Series on which these recommendations are based consist predominantly of motor vehicle accident victims. There is no reason to believe that fetal risk is the same for victims of assault or falls. The dilemma is this: With noncatastrophic maternal trauma there is a low probability of major fetal complications that may present over a variable time period. Such maternal trauma is highly prevalent so that, for a given population, the cost of prolonged inpatient observation is high. On the other hand, fetal complications that occur for lack of observation are viewed as preventable, and, as such, are all the more tragic, and vulnerable to litigation.

Despite lack of agreement about an appropriate interval of fetal observation following maternal trauma, some conclusions are evident. Motor vehicle accidents, even at moderate speed of impact (25–35 mph), are associated with more fetal risk than other types of blunt maternal trauma. The velocity, and thus the force, of impact is generally greater than in trauma from falls or assault. The absence of external injury does not guarantee the absence of fetal or placental injury. No pregnant trauma victim beyond 26 weeks should be released from the hospital without some reassuring test of fetal well-being. When in doubt, a 24-hour period of observation with continuous fetal monitoring is prudent. Most placental abruptions are clinically manifest within the first 24 hours following trauma. Evidence of fetal compromise may be the first sign of abruption. A decrease in fetal movement or absence of fetal heart rate accelerations are important signs in these patients and demand careful evaluation. The judgment of the responsible clinician remains the best guide for appropriate management.

Various medications may be indicated in the care of the pregnant trauma victim (Table 208–4). Tocolytic agents may be appropriate for the treatment of preterm labor in some cases. No such agent should be used, however, if the maternal cardiovascular status is unstable. Clear evidence of placental abruption or fetal compromise are also contraindications to their chronic use. Magnesium sulfate, having fewer cardiovascular side effects than β-adrenergic agents, may be preferable for the trauma victim. Corticosteroid therapy to promote fetal lung maturation should be considered if delivery prior to 34 weeks' gestation seems likely in greater than 24 hours but less than seven days.

The indications for tetanus immunoglobulin and toxoid are the same during pregnancy as in the nonpregnant state. All patients with penetrating wounds require review of their tetanus immune status. The rationale for Rh immunoglobulin has been discussed previously. All Rh-negative patients with trauma during pregnancy should receive an appropriate amount of Rh immunoglobulin unless the fetus is known to be Rh-negative. For the bedridden patient, particularly those with immobilizing orthopedic injuries, thromboembolism prophylaxis with low-dose heparin should be considered. Heparin does not cross the placenta

TABLE 208–4. THERAPEUTIC MEASURES

Maternal and Fetal Benefit	Fetal Benefit
Maternal ventilation	Rh immunoglobulin
Oxygen therapy	Tocolytic agents
Control of hemorrhage	Corticosteroids for lung maturation
Fluid and blood replacement	Maternal cardiovascular support following brain death
Lateral positioning	
Prevention of aspiration	
Tetanus prophylaxis	
Perimortem cesarean section	

and may be safely administered during gestation. Pregnancy is associated with an increased risk for thromboembolic complications, especially during the postpartum period.

Principles of intraoperative management in the pregnant patient requiring surgery are based on the anatomic and physiologic changes previously discussed. Adequate volume replacement is essential to maintain organ perfusion, uterine blood flow, and fetal oxygenation. Positioning to avoid supine hypotension serves the same purpose. Aspiration pneumonitis is another threat to the pregnant patient undergoing an emergency operation with general anesthesia. Preoperative administration of a nonparticulate antacid, such as sodium citrate, and a rapid sequence induction of anesthesia are measures to minimize this risk. Cricoid pressure should be applied until endotracheal intubation is complete and the cuff expanded.[34]

Both an obstetrician and a general surgeon should be present when the pregnant trauma victim undergoes laparotomy. A mid-line vertical incision provides the best exposure for thorough examination of abdominal contents. A laparotomy in itself is not reason to perform an abdominal delivery. Cesarean delivery is warranted for the usual obstetric indications, for example, fetal distress or significant placental abruption with a viable fetus. An additional reason for emptying the uterus is to allow visualization or repair of abdominal structures. It usually is possible, however, to expose the abdomen sufficiently with an adequate incision and gentle retraction of the uterus. Intravenous magnesium sulfate has been used perioperatively to suppress uterine contractions. It has not been proven that prophylactic use of this agent decreases the likelihood of preterm labor. Successful labor and vaginal delivery shortly after laparotomy has been reported.[35] Low forceps delivery to shorten the second stage and minimize abdominal straining may be of some benefit.

Pelvic fracture is among the most common of orthopedic injuries caused by motor vehicle collisions. Injury to the bladder anteriorly or to the great vessels posteriorly often complicate such fractures. Careful evaluation of the urinary tract and observation for signs of retroperitoneal hemorrhage are necessary. Fetal skull fracture, often fatal, has been described in association with maternal pelvic fracture.[25,36] Vaginal delivery following pelvic fracture usually is uncomplicated[35,37], but bladder and urethral injury associated with delivery have been reported.[38]

Penetrating abdominal trauma during pregnancy is much less frequently reported than blunt trauma. A recent literature review summarized 19 cases of stab wounds during pregnancy reported from 1930 through 1987.[39] Maternal survival was uniform, but in the 14 cases with uterine penetration, there was a 50% perinatal mortality. Sakala et al advocate laparotomy whenever peritoneal penetration occurs.[39] Cesarean delivery of these patients is recommended for surgical exposure, if necessary; fetal distress with a viable fetus; and uterine penetration with a live term or near-term fetus. The topic of gunshot wounds during pregnancy has been reviewed by Buchsbaum.[40] Early laparotomy is recommended for abdominal gunshot wounds. He reported no maternal deaths since 1912 and a 66% perinatal mortality among 70 cases.

Cardiac arrest is a rare event during pregnancy but may occur with a severely injured patient. Cardiopulmonary resuscitation in late pregnancy is complicated by several factors. Closed chest compression is difficult to perform with the patient in a position other than supine. The supine position is associated with caval obstruction by the uterus and decreased cardiac blood return. Perfusion of vital organs by chest compression is impaired further by the uteroplacental circulation, which functions like a large arteriovenous shunt. Finally, fetal as well as maternal survival is in jeopardy and the likelihood of intact fetal survival decreases rapidly with duration of resuscitation. Prompt maternal recovery and fetal survival have been described when cesarean section is performed after an initially unsuccessful resuscitation attempt.[41,42] Maternal benefit has been attributed to relief of caval obstruction. Katz et al[42] have recommended that a rapid, nonsterile abdominal delivery be initiated within four minutes of cardiac arrest if the patient fails to respond to resuscitation with lateral displacement of the uterus. They referred to this intervention as a *perimortem* cesarean section. Resuscitative efforts should continue during the delivery as they may prove successful for the mother. Typically, operative blood loss is minimal under these circumstances. Prolonged physiologic maintenance of pregnant women following brain death has been performed to achieve fetal viability. Fields et al[43] have discussed medical and ethical considerations regarding such efforts.

PREVENTIVE MEASURES

Some injuries are bound to occur, but many can be prevented or minimized with forethought. Activities requiring a heightened sense of balance and those associated with frequent falls should be avoided in late pregnancy. Falls often involve stairs, so the use of handrails should be encouraged. Supportive footwear with low heels are safer as well as more comfortable than high heeled shoes during pregnancy. Extra care should be taken when walking in the snow and ice.

While falls are more common, automobile accidents are far more threatening to the pregnant woman and her fetus. The question of whether seat belts are beneficial during pregnancy has been studied epidemiologically and with primates. A recent review of this topic has been written by Schoenfeld et al.[34] Crosby[17] reviewed the records of 208 pregnant women involved in severe motor vehicle accidents. Of these women, 28 were wearing lap belts and the remainder were unrestrained (typically the majority of women in such series are *not* using seat belts). In this study, maternal death rates were not significantly different between belted (1 in 28) and unrestrained (14 in 180) passengers. Among those with pregnancies beyond 12 weeks' gestation, fetal death rates were not significantly different between belted (1 in 24) and unrestrained (13 in 166) passengers. Lack of statistical significance may have been related to sample size in this study. Very high mortality (33%) was found among those passengers ejected from the vehicle. Since seat belts usually prevent ejection, the authors recommended their use for pregnant women. In experimental collisions with pregnant baboons, it was found that the fetal mortality was reduced substantially (8% versus 50%) with three-point restraint compared with lap belt restraint alone.[44] On the basis of available information it appears that three-point restraint (lap belt plus shoulder harness) protects both the mother and the fetus. The lap belt portion should be worn low across the pelvis and fastened snugly.

Domestic violence is present more often than is recognized by medical personnel and occurs across ethnic and socioeconomic boundaries. The pattern of violence tends to be cyclical with escalating severity.[45] Pregnancy and the postpartum period are a stressful time for families, when violence may continue or increase.[2] Clinicians should be alert for signs of abuse. The patient may have injuries incongruent with her history. She may appear frightened or embarrassed. There may be multiple bruises of the face, breasts, and abdomen. A patient who admits to abuse at home may be directed to community resources to help her change or escape her situation.

REFERENCES

1. Fort AT, Harlin RS. Pregnancy outcome after noncatastrophic maternal trauma during pregnancy. *Obstet Gynecol.* 1970;35:912.
2. Hillard PJA. Physical abuse in pregnancy. *Obstet Gynecol.* 1985;66:185.
3. National Center for Health Statistics. *Advance report of final mortality statistics, 1985.* Monthly Vital Statistics Report 1987;36(suppl):5. Hyattsville, MD: US Department of Health and Human Services, Public Health Service, DHHS Pub. No. (PHS)87–1120.
4. National Safety Council. *Accident Facts.* 1985 ed. Chicago, IL: National Safety Council; 1985.
5. Kaunitz AM, Hughes JM, Grimes DA, et al. Causes of maternal mortality in the United States. *Obstet Gynecol.* 1985;65:605.
6. Hollander AG, Crawford JH. Roentgenologic and electrocardiographic changes in the normal heart during pregnancy. *Am Heart J.* 1942;24:364.
7. Carruth JE, Mirvis SB, Brogan DR, Wenger NK. The electrocardiogram in normal pregnancy. *Am Heart J.* 1981;102:1075.
8. Brinkman CR, Mofid M, Assali NS. Circulatory shock in pregnant sheep. *Am J Obstet Gynecol.* 1974;118:77.
9. Romney SL, Gabel PV, Takeda Y. Experimental hemorrhage in late pregnancy. *Am J Obstet Gynecol.* 1963;87:636.
10. Boba A, Linkie DM, Plotz EJ. Effects of vasopressor administration and fluid replacement on fetal bradycardia and hypoxia induced by maternal hemorrhage. *Obstet Gynecol.* 1966;27:408.
11. Schnider SM, deLorimier AA, Holl JW, et al. Vasopressors in obstetrics. *Am J Obstet Gynecol.* 1968;102:911.
12. Hankins GDV. Principles of invasive hemodynamic monitoring. *Clin Perinatol.* 1986;13:765.
13. Berkowitz RL, Rafferty TD. Invasive hemodynamic monitoring in critically ill pregnant patients: role of Swan-Ganz catheterization. *Am J Obstet Gynecol.* 1980;137:127.
14. Turner AF. The chest radiography in pregnancy. *Clin Obstet Gynecol.* 1975;18:65.
15. Metcalfe J, Romney SL, Ramsey LH, Burwell CS. Estimation of uterine blood flow in women at term. *J Clin Invest.* 1955;34:1632.
16. Rubovits FE. Traumatic rupture of the pregnant uterus from "seat belt" injury. *Am J Obstet Gynecol.* 1964;90:828.
17. Crosby WM, Costiloe JP. Safety of lap-belt restraint for pregnant victims of automobile collisions. *N Engl J Med.* 1971;284:632.
18. Agran PF, Dunkle DE, Winn DG, Kent D. Fetal death in motor vehicle accidents. *Ann Emerg Med.* 1987;16:1355.
19. Lavin JP, Miodovnik M. Delayed abruption after maternal trauma as result of an automobile accident. *J Reprod Med.* 1981;26:621.
20. Higgins SD, Garite TJ. Late abruptio placenta in trauma patients: implications for monitoring. *Obstet Gynecol.* 1984;63:10S.
21. Olcott C, Robinson AJ, Maxwell TM, Griffin, HA. Amniotic fluid embolism and disseminated intravascular coagulation after blunt abdominal trauma. *J Trauma.* 1973;13:737.
22. Stuart GCE, Harding PGR, Davies EM. Blunt abdominal trauma in pregnancy. *CMA Journal.* 1980;122:901.
23. Bickers RG, Wennberg RP. Fetomaternal transfusion following trauma. *Obstet Gynecol.* 1983;61:258.
24. Rose PG, Strohm PL, Zuspan FP. Fetomaternal hemorrhage following trauma. *Am J Obstet Gynecol.* 1985;153:844.
25. Stafford PA, Biddinger PW, Zumwalt RE. Lethal intrauterine fetal trauma. *Am J Obstet Gynecol.* 1988;159:485.
26. Shatney CH. Resuscitation and evaluation of victims of blunt multisystem trauma. *Acta Anaesth Belg.* 1987;38:2678.
27. Kaiser R, Berk JE, Fridhandler L. Serum amylase changes during pregnancy. *Am J Obstet Gynecol.* 1975;122:283.
28. Chhibber G, Zacher M, Cohen AW, Kline AJ. Rh isoimmunization following abdominal trauma: a case report. *Am J Obstet Gynecol.* 1984;149:692.
29. Meridith JW, Trunkey DD. CT scanning in acute abdominal injuries. *Surg Clin N Amer.* 1988;68:255.
30. Civil ID, Talucci RC, Schwab CW. Placental laceration and fetal death as a result of blunt abdominal trauma. *J Trauma.* 1988;28:708.
31. Rothenberger DA, Quattlebaum FW, Zabel J, Fischer RP. Diagnostic peritoneal lavage for blunt trauma in pregnant women. *Am J Obstet Gynecol.* 1977;129:479.
32. Nyberg DA, Cyr DR, Mack LA, et al. Sonographic spectrum of placental abruption. *Am J Rad.* 1987;148:161.
33. Schoenfeld A, Ziv E, Stein L, et al. Seat belts in pregnancy and the obstetrician. *Obstet Gynecol Surv.* 1987;42:275.
34. Cohen SE. The aspiration syndrome. *Clin Perinatal.* 1982;9:235.
35. Elliott M. Vehicular accidents and pregnancy. *Aust NZ J Obstet Gynecol.* 1966;6:279.
36. Bowdler N, Faix RG, Elkins T. Fetal skull fracture and brain injury after a maternal automobile accident. *J Reprod Med.* 1987;32:375.
37. Golan A, Sandbank O, Teare AJ. Trauma in late pregnancy. *S Afr Med J.* 1980;57:161.
38. Buchsbaum HJ. Accidental injury complicating pregnancy. *Am J Obstet Gynecol.* 1968;102:752.
39. Sakala EP, Kort DD. Management of stab wounds to the pregnant uterus: a case report and a review of the literature. *Obstet Gynecol Surv.* 1988;43:319.
40. Buchsbaum HJ. Diagnosis and management of abdominal gunshot wounds during pregnancy. *J Trauma.* 1975;15:425.
41. Marx GF. Cardiopulmonary resuscitation in the late pregnant woman. *Anesthesiology.* 1982;56:156.
42. Katz VL, Dotters DJ, Droegemueller W. Perimortem cesarean delivery. *Obstet Gynecol.* 1986;68:571.
43. Field DR, Gates EA, Creasy RK, et al. Maternal brain death during pregnancy: medical and ethical issues. *JAMA.* 1988;260:816.
44. Crosby WM, King AI, Stout LC. Fetal survival following impact: improvement with shoulder harness restraint. *Am J Obstet Gynecol.* 1972;112:1101.
45. ACOG. *The Battered Woman.* January, 1989; Technical Bulletin Number 124.

Chapter Two Hundred and Nine
Thrombophlebitis

Brian M. Mercer and Peter Garner

209

Thrombophlebitis is a common complication of pregnancy that may lead to significant maternal morbidity and potential maternal and fetal mortality. Venous thrombosis may develop in either the superficial or deep venous system. It is more common in pregnancy, but also may be related to local trauma, stasis, or infection. The peripartum and immediate postpartum periods are times of particular risk for thrombophlebitis. Women with deep venous thrombosis carry an increased risk of subsequent venous thromboembolism. Women with venous thrombosis in the presence of infection may fail to respond to conventional antibiotic therapy, but quickly defervesce following the institution of anticoagulant therapy. The diagnosis and management of thrombophlebitis in pregnancy is complicated by the presence of the fetus, but in spite of the limitations imposed by pregnancy, aggressive diagnosis and management should be done to ensure an optimal outcome for both mother and fetus (see also Chapter 119).

TABLE 209–1. INCIDENCE OF VENOUS THROMBOSIS IN PREGNANCY

	Gestation	Incidence (%)
Deep venous thrombosis	Antepartum	0.013–0.11
Deep venous thrombosis	Postpartum	0.61–1.20
Deep venous thrombosis	Post-cesarean section	1.8–3.0
Superficial venous thrombosis	Antepartum	0.16
Superficial venous thrombosis	Postpartum	0.10

The overall incidence of venous thrombosis related to pregnancy is approximately 0.5% (Table 209–1). However, comparison of various studies reveals a wide variation in this incidence, largely because of the lack of reliability of clinical diagnosis and variable sensitivities of the available laboratory investigations. In a retrospective study, Keirkegaard[1] found venographically proven deep venous thrombosis (DVT) in 0.13 in 1000 and 0.61 in 1000 patients in the antepartum and postpartum periods respectively. Drill[2] found no increase in the risk of DVT during pregnancy, but postpartum DVT occurred in 1.04% of patients. Aaro[3], in a review of 32,000 pregnancies, revealed a 0.16% incidence of superficial thrombophlebitis and 0.11% incidence of deep venous thrombosis in the antepartum period. Deep venous thrombosis was seen more frequently in the second and third trimesters. The risk of superficial and deep venous thrombophlebitis was increased to 1.0% and 0.14%, respectively, in the postpartum period, with 56% of postpartum DVTs occurring within 3 days of delivery. Kakkar[4], in a view of 100 patients surveyed with ^{125}I scanning, demonstrated a 3% incidence of postpartum DVT.

Superficial thrombophlebitis is the most common thrombotic disorder of pregnancy[3] and is seen more frequently in patients with varicose veins. Its incidence is not increased with traumatic obstetric intervention. In contrast, postpartum deep venous thrombosis occurs more frequently among patients suffering obstetric trauma.[5-7] A 1.8% incidence of DVT has been demonstrated following cesarean section (based on strain gauge plethysmography).[8] Husni demonstrated a 3% incidence of clinically diagnosed DVT following cesarean section as compared with a 1.2% incidence identified by Hiilesmaa and Flessa in 60,000 patients delivering vaginally.[5,9,10]

Some 15–25% of patients with untreated deep venous thrombosis will have thrombus embolization to the pulmonary vasculature, and 12–25% of these patients will develop a fatal pulmonary embolism. However, adequate anticoagulation for deep venous thrombosis reduces this risk to a 4.5% incidence of pulmonary embolus and 0.7% mortality.[11] Thromboses of the calf rarely will embolize, although this may occur following propagation to a more proximal vessel.

PATHOGENESIS

Virchow, in 1848, described the triad of hypercoagulability, venous stasis, and trauma to the vascular endothelium as risk factors in the pathogenesis of venous thrombosis. The pregnant woman is particularly at increased risk because of decreased venous return from the lower limbs, increases in clotting factor concentrations, and trauma related to childbirth.

Hypercoagulability

Coagulation of blood involves the sequential activation of clotting factors within the intrinsic and extrinsic coagulation pathways. This ultimately leads to the formation of a fibrin meshwork from fibrinogen. Exposure of blood to subendothelial connective tissue triggers activation of factor XII with serial and progressive activation of factors IX, X, and XI. With the aid of factor VIII, platelets, phospholipid, and calcium, tissue thromboplastin initiates the extrinsic coagulation pathway by activating factor VII, which subsequently activates factor X directly. Once factor X has been activated through the intrinsic or extrinsic pathways, it combines with factor V in the presence of calcium and phospholipid to convert prothrombin to thrombin. Thrombin acts to convert fibrinogen (factor I) to small fibrinopeptides A and B as well as fibrin monomers. Polymerization of fibrin leads to precipitation of fibrin mesh to which blood cells and platelets become entangled.

Increased levels of factors I, II, VII, VIII, IX, and X have been demonstrated after the first trimester of pregnancy[12-17], with subsequent increases in factors V, VII, and X after delivery[15] (Table 209–2). Factor VIII levels are doubled early in labor and remain in this range in the peripartum period. Factors XI and XIII have been shown to decrease in pregnancy.[18,19] Fibrinogen levels fall during labor. Increased levels of fibrinopeptide A and increasing circulating fibrin monomers are seen in pregnancy, suggesting ongoing activation of the coagulation system.[20,21]

Prothrombin and thrombin times are not changed in pregnancy.[14] The partial thromboplastin time shortens during labor, returning to normal soon after delivery of the placenta.

The fibrinolytic system is mediated through plasmin,

TABLE 209–2. CHANGES IN CLOTTING FACTORS WITH PREGNANCY

	Change with Pregnancy	
Factor	Antepartum	Peripartum
I	inc. 150%	sl. decr.
II	n.ch./inc.	
V	n.ch.	inc.
VII	inc. 120–200%	inc.
VIII	inc. 100–300%	inc.
IX	sl. inc.	
X	inc. 120%	inc.
XI	sl. decr.	
XIII	sl. decr.	
Plasminogen	decr.	
Fibrinopeptide A	inc.	
Fibrin monomers	inc.	

decr. = decreased, sl. decr. = slight decrease, inc. = increased, sl. inc. = slight increase, n.ch. = no change a proteolytic enzyme that hydrolyzes fibrinogen and factor XII. Plasmin is formed from plasminogen in response to activators found in endothelial cells and the interstitial space. Fibrin and fibrinogen degradation products (FDPs) are produced through the fibrinolytic degradation by plasmin of fibrin and fibrinogen, respectively. These products in turn decrease platelet response to various stimuli (including thrombin, connective tissue, and ADP), counteracting the thrombotic tendency of pregnancy. Both increased and decreased fibrinolytic activity have been reported in pregnancy.[20] Plasminogen levels fall during labor.[14]

Venous Stasis

Venous blood flow decreases in pregnancy.[22,23] Wright[24] (using radioactive sodium) measured foot to groin flow rates in pregnancy, and demonstrated a gradual but consistent decrease in flow during pregnancy and a sharp decrease during labor. McLennan[25] demonstrated increasing femoral venous pressure with pregnancy. Significant vena caval obstruction by the gravid uterus has been demonstrated in the second half of the pregnancy using venography.[26] Venous blood flow from the lower extremities was seen to pass primarily by way of the lumbar veins in these patients. Decreased venous tone in the lower limbs is seen early in pregnancy[5,27], and marked vascular dilatation of the pelvic veins can be seen at cesarean section. The valves of the venous system are the site of particularly low blood flow with an increased potential for platelet clumping and fibrin formation.[28] With thrombus formation, further obstruction of flow leads to progressive stasis with decreased blood flow and an increase tendency to extension of the thrombus. When pregnancy or labor is complicated and prolonged bed rest or operative delivery is required, further stasis occurs. This results from decreased external compression of the veins, obstruction of the pelvic vasculature by the descending presenting part, and direct surgical ligation at cesarean section.

Trauma to the Vascular Endothelium

The vascular endothelium presents a physiologic barrier to thrombosis. Endothelial cell production of prostacyclin prevents local platelet aggregation and activation. Trauma to the vascular endothelium results in exposure of the underlying tissue collagen and thromboplastins that initiate the sequence of the fibrin production and platelet aggregation. White blood cell margination and adhesion at the time of surgical trauma leads to endothelial desquamation.[29] Platelets adhere and degranulate at the sight of vascular trauma, with resultant thrombus formation.[30] While not a frequent etiologic factor in venous thrombosis in pregnancy, endothelial damage[15] increased in pregnant patients undergoing pelvic surgery or at the time of cesarean section.

CLINICAL DIAGNOSIS OF VENOUS THROMBOSIS

The manifestations of superficial thrombophlebitis are very specific. The vein is indurated and painful with associated erythema and tenderness along the sight of inflammation. The patient may or may not be febrile.

The clinical symptoms and signs of deep venous thrombosis are nonspecific and much less reliable.[31,32] Of patients with an acutely tender swollen calf, 50% do not have deep venous thrombosis on subsequent testing.[33] Conversely, Bell[34] demonstrated a 32% incidence of clinical lower limb phlebitis in patients with pulmonary embolism. The symptomatology of deep venous thrombosis is a reflection of obstruction of venous outflow or inflammation at the sight of thrombosis. The patient with acute venous thrombosis may be asymptomatic or present with wide variety of complaints including the classic symptoms of swelling of the calf or thigh (>2 cm larger than contralateral side) with associated pain and tenderness. Calf pain and tenderness are present in 60–90% of patients with venographically proven deep venous thrombosis. Unilateral edema is seen in 40–75% of patients, a positive Homan's sign in 30–40%, and superficial venous dilatation in 30% of patients.[35,36] A thrombosed vessel may be palpable. Phlegmacia cerulea dolens results from severe obstruction of the limb, leading to a markedly distended painful and cyanotic leg.

As the symptomatology related to deep venous thrombosis is inconsistent and nonspecific, the diagnosis of acute deep venous thrombosis should never be made on the basis of clinical symptoms and signs alone.

The diagnosis of superficial venous thrombophlebitis is clinical, with no ancillary testing required. Ancillary testing is essential in the diagnosis of deep venous thrombosis because of the lack of specificity of the signs and symptoms related to this condition (Table 209–3). In the absence of laboratory confirmation of deep venous thrombosis, other conditions such as muscle strain, hematoma, cellulitis, varicose veins, postphlebitic syndrome, localized trauma, ruptured Baker's cyst, vascular insufficiency, and arthritis should be considered.

Venography

Venography is the definitive test for the diagnosis of venous thrombosis in the presence or absence of pregnancy.[37] Vascular access is gained through a superficial vein on the dorsal aspect of the foot. Dye is injected, filling the superficial and deep venous systems with serial radiographs taken to the level of the external iliac vein. It is important that a distal foot vein be chosen to avoid artifactual incomplete filling of the deep venous system. Venography may be very uncomfortable for the patient and technically difficult for the radiologist.[38,39] Reliable signs of venous thrombosis on venography include intraluminal filling defects and abrupt termination of flow within a vessel. Filling defects should be demonstrable on repeated projections. Nonfilling of the deep venous system in the presence of collateral flow is suggestive of DVT. Venography carries the risk of radiation exposure with a mean dose of 0.05 rads to the fetus with limited venography and 0.628 rads following bilateral venography without shielding. The teratogenic risk of radiation is believed to be negligible below a total fetal dose of 10–15 rads.[40] However, because of the potential teratogenic risk associated with antepartum radiation, venography involving the inferior vena cava and the iliac venous system is relatively contraindicated by pregnancy. The pelvic area should be shielded and venography should be restricted to the vessels of the calf and distal thigh when feasible. Where possible, nonradiographic testing should be performed for proximal vessel disease with venography reserved for equivocal studies. Because of the risk of subsequent embolization with proximal deep venous thrombosis and the risks of prolonged anticoagulant therapy required for the treatment of deep venous thrombosis and pulmonary embolus, it is important that the diagnosis of deep venous thrombosis be confirmed venographically in patients with equivocal noninvasive studies. Chemical phlebitis is induced by the contrast material in approximately 3% of patients undergoing venography.[41,42] The incidence of this complication can be reduced by flushing the vascular system with saline following venographic study and elevating the leg after the procedure to facilitate venous emptying.[38]

TABLE 209–3. THE UTILITY OF TESTS USED IN THE DIAGNOSIS OF DEEP VENOUS THROMBOSIS

Test	Overall Accuracy	Proximal Disease	Distal Disease	Comment
Clinical diagnosis	50%	—	—	
Venography	99%	+++++	+++++	Invasive; radiation risk low with shielding
^{125}I fibrinogen scanning	78%	++++−	+++−	Contraindicated in pregnancy and lactation
Doppler ultrasound	93%	++−	++++−	Poor for partial obstruction Improved with duplex B-mode scanning
Impedance plethysmography	93%	+	++++−	Useful for serial monitoring for recurrence
Compression ultrasound	95–100%	++++−	+++++	Noninvasive No radiation Not proven in pregnancy

^{125}I Fibrinogen Uptake Scanning

^{125}I fibrinogen scanning involves the injection of 100 uCuries of radiolabeled fibrinogen intravascularly with daily serial scanning of the lower extremities for incorporation of radioactive fibrinogen into the fibrin matrix of a developing thrombus. Fibrinogen uptake testing is very accurate in the presence of acute venous thrombosis; however, it may take up to 72 hours to become positive.[43,44] Radioisotope scanning is somewhat less accurate than venography in the diagnosis of clinically suspected venous thrombosis, agreeing in 78% of cases. Women with inflammation or hematoma formation will have localized fibrin deposition leading to a potentially false-positive result. Women with chronic thrombosis or resolving thrombosis without active clot formation may have a falsely negative test. The sensitivity of ^{125}I fibrinogen scanning for distal calf and lower thigh thrombosis is approximately 90%, with decreased sensitivity for proximal venous thrombosis (60–80%).[45] ^{125}I crosses the placenta and into the breast milk, and will accumulate within the fetal thyroid. ^{125}I scanning thus is contraindicated during pregnancy or lactation, leaving venography as the sole established and accurate diagnostic modality for the detection of distal thrombosis in these women. However, it can be used postpartum in women not breast-feeding.

Doppler Ultrasound

Doppler ultrasound flow studies are useful in the detection of proximal venous thrombosis. However, consistent performance and interpretation of this study are essential.[46] The Doppler flow examination is performed with patient semi-recumbent. The Doppler beam is applied over the femoral, superficial femoral, popliteal or tibial vein, with the presence of a Doppler shift indicating venous flow. During Doppler velocimetry, flow response to patient respiration, forced expiration, and alternating distal leg compression will augment changes in venous flow, aiding in the Doppler technique. The absence of Doppler flow suggests venous occlusion, although chronic obstruction cannot be ruled out. Strandness[46] found Doppler flow velocimetry to correlate with venographic findings in 93% of patients. Richards[35] demonstrated that Doppler flow studies were sensitive for venous thrombosis in the proximal thigh, but had poor sensitivity with a distal thrombosis because of collateral blood supply. Doppler flow velocimetry is limited by the inability to detect incomplete vascular occlusion. B-mode ultrasound recently has been used to assist Doppler flow studies (duplex Doppler) with some improvement in sensitivity.[47]

The technique of compression ultrasound is rapidly developing as an adjunctive tool in the diagnosis of venous thrombosis of the lower limb, agreeing with venography in 95–100% of cases.[48-50] With the use of high resolution ultrasound probes, visualization of the femoral, popliteal, and tibial venous systems is possible. Initial studies suggested observation for clot within the vein lumen. Recent studies have centered on the ability to compress the vein with external pressure, obliterating the lumen on ultrasound. Inability to compress the vein is evidence for lumenal obstruction. Compression ultrasound has been demonstrated to be highly accurate in the detection of thrombosis within the femoral venous system and popliteal veins. The ability of compression ultrasonography to predict distal thrombosis is more controversial, although recent studies are encouraging. Extrinsic compression by a pelvic mass has been shown to give false-positive results.[49,51] The effect of uterine pressure on the vena cava has yet to be determined in pregnant patients undergoing compression ultrasonography. Thus, the clinical utility of compression ultrasound in pregnancy remains to be established.

Color Doppler flow mapping is the only noninvasive technique currently available for assessment of the pelvic vasculature. This technique can detect obstructed or turbulent flow accurately within the iliac and ovarian venous systems, as well as the inferior vena cava. However, isolated thromboses within the internal iliac system may not be visualized. The utility of color Doppler flow mapping for venous thrombosis in pregnancy remains to be determined.

Impedance Plethysmography

Impedance plethysmography (IPG) measures changes in electrical resistance following acute blood volume changes with proximal obstruction to venous flow using pneumatic cuff obstruction to flow. The procedure is performed with the patient in the lateral recumbent position to avoid proximal occlusion by the gravid uterus. The proximal cuff is inflated, giving complete occlusion to venous return. During this phase, arterial filling results in increased distention of the venous vasculature. With the release of the proximal cuff, venous outflow results in a decrease in intravascular volume (and thus calf volume) leading to a decrease in electrical impedance of the limb. Failure of prompt venous outflow results in a delay in change of impedance.[52] IPG carries a 93% sensitivity and 97% specificity for proximal thrombosis.[53] The sensitivity for calf thrombosis is poor.[54] IPG is a simple and practical technique for serial screening of the pregnant woman with a prior DVT.

The patient with a clinically suspected deep venous thrombosis in pregnancy should undergo impedance plethysmography and Doppler flow studies to detect proximal thrombosis. Direct ultrasonographic assessment of the lower limb for the presence of clot and the loss of venous compressibility should be undertaken if available. In the presence of an unequivocally positive study, therapy for deep venous thrombosis should be undertaken. If these studies are negative or equivocal, confirmation with limited venography should be attempted. In the postpartum period venography involving both distal and proximal vessels can be done. Proximal venography during pregnancy should be restricted to those patients with negative or equivocal noninvasive studies and limited venogram. ^{125}I fibrinogen testing can be done postpartum if the patient is not breastfeeding. A combination of impedance plethysmography and ^{125}I fibrinogen testing provides a suitable alternative to the venography for the non-lactating postpartum patient with 93% positive and negative predictive values.[55]

THE TREATMENT OF THROMBOPHLEBITIS

The treatment of superficial thrombophlebitis in pregnancy should be conservative, with local heat and mild analgesics. The thrombophlebitis usually will resolve spontaneously in one to two weeks. The use of anti-inflammatory agents in pregnancy is controversial. Phenylbutazone is contraindicated in pregnancy, as embryotoxicity has been suggested in animals, even though a cause-and-effect relationship has not been established in producing human congenital defects.[56] Nonsteroidal anti-inflammatory analgesics such as indomethacin and naproxen have been used as tocolytic agents, but may contribute to premature constriction of the ductus arteriosus. If nonsteroidal anti-inflammatory drugs are considered for treatment of severe superficial thrombophlebitis, administration should be restricted to the first two trimesters, as constriction of the ductus is a gestational age-dependent event occurring primarily after the 34th week of pregnancy.[57]

The main aims of treatment of acute deep venous thrombosis are prevention of extension of the thrombotic process, prevention of pulmonary embolism, prevention of the postphlebitic syndrome, and realization of these goals without producing side-effects in either mother or fetus.[58] There are three main groups of drugs available for treating venous thrombosis, including those that interfere with platelet adhesion and aggregation, those that interfere with fibrin formation, and those that induce clot lysis.

Heparin Therapy

Heparin is the drug of choice for the initial treatment of acute venous thrombosis in pregnancy.[59] Heparin is a naturally occurring anionic mucopolysaccharide of variable molecular weight (3000–30,000 Daltons). It is found in mast cells, and is extracted from hog gastric mucosa or partly purified beef lung for pharmacologic use. Due to its size and negative charge, heparin does not cross the placenta or enter breast milk. In the circulation, it binds to a number of plasma proteins including its cofactor antithrombin III, to which it is attached by a pentasaccharide sequence. When injected intravenously, heparin has a half life (t½) of approximately 60 minutes, although there is considerable individual variation. Heparin administered intravenously has an immediate anticoagulant effect, but when given subcutaneously peak levels take 4 hours to achieve; the dose-dependent effect can last for 12 hours. It is cleared from circulation by the liver, reticuloendothelial system, and by excretion into the urine.[60]

Heparin is only effective as an antithrombotic agent when combined with its cofactor antithrombin III. This cofactor is a naturally occurring α-2 globulin that inactivates several activated clotting factors (factors XIIa, XIa, Xa, and IIa [thrombin]), which have in common a serine residue associated with their enzyme action. The binding of heparin to antithrombin III greatly potentiates its effect. The antithrombin III–heparin complex inhibits Factor Xa more than thrombin.[61]

There are several unresolved practical issues regarding heparin use in pregnancy. Whether initial anticoagulation is best achieved by continuous intravenous infusion, by intermittent intravenous infusion, or by an adjusted subcutaneous regimen is the subject of ongoing debate.[62] Four hourly intermittent intravenous injections of heparin produce a greater incidence of major bleeding than a continuous infusion of heparin at a dose adjusted according to coagulation testing.[63] Several randomized control trials have found that a subcutaneous intermittent adjusted-dose calcium heparin regime is an effective and safe alternative to continuous intravenous heparin in the initial treatment of acute proximal deep vein thrombosis.[64] However, none of these trials have involved pregnant women. Use of the continuous-infusion subcutaneous heparin pump also has been described in pregnancy, and although no recurrent thrombosis occurred, a high incidence of both minor and major bleeding was found.[65]

If the intermittent adjusted-dose subcutaneous heparin regimen is chosen for initial treatment of venous thrombosis in pregnancy, it usually is given twice daily at a dosage of 10,000–15,000 IU. The initial subcutaneous doses should be larger (20,000 IU) to ensure adequate anticoagulation. The injections are given by fine gauge (25 G pr 26 G) 16-mm needle and 1-mL tuberculin syringe using concentrated heparin 25,000 IU per mL, into the subcutaneous fat of the anterior abdominal wall or thigh. Firm pressure is applied after the injection to avoid local bleeding. The 12-hourly dose of heparin is adjusted to produce an anticoagulant effect in the therapeutic range (see below).

The continuous intravenous heparin regimen is started with an initial bolus of 5000 IU or 70 IU/kg, followed by 300–400 IU/kg per 24 hours. The normal pregnant woman requires an average dose of 30,000 IU per 24 hours, with a range of 20,000–40,000 IU per 24 hours. Although it has been suggested that heparin should be suspended in normal saline rather than 5% dextrose, several workers have found that heparin is stable for 12–24 hours in 5% dextrose or dextrose-saline solutions.[58] Coagulation tests should be monitored 6 hours after the bolus injection, and then twice daily until the dose-response relationship is stable. If the anticoagulation is initially inadequate, a second bolus of heparin 2000 IU can be given, and the total dose of heparin increased by 3000 IU per 24 hours.

Several coagulation tests are available for monitoring the anticoagulant effect of heparin. These include the whole blood clotting time (CT) and the partial thromboplastin time performed on whole blood, or activated partial thromboplastin time (APTT), partial thromboplastin time (PTT), thrombin clotting time (TCT), heparin assay by protamine sulfate neutralization test, and the anti-Xa heparin assay performed on platelet poor plasma.

One of the more commonly used tests is the APTT with an optimal range for anticoagulation of 1.5–2.0 times the mean of the normal laboratory control range. There is no relationship between the risk of bleeding and APTT in women receiving continuous IV heparin, but there is a relationship between the risk of bleeding and dosage of heparin administered.[66] The anticoagulant effect of heparin also can be clinically well controlled by heparin assay with an ideal range of 0.3–0.5 IU/mL by protamine titration. The risk of bleeding is highly correlated with the heparin level.[67]

In pregnancy, high factor VIII levels may result in a shortened pretreatment APTT when compared with normal nonpregnant controls. Thus a post-heparin APTT in pregnancy may not truly reflect anticoagulation if compared with a nonpregnant control. This "apparent heparin resistance" can be overcome by using the pregnant woman's own pretreatment APTT as the baseline in determining her "therapeutic" APTT level. Another alternative is to use a heparin assay if "apparent resistance" is suspected.[68]

"True heparin resistance" can be encountered in pregnancy, but it is rare. In this situation, neither APTT nor heparin levels are elevated in spite of high heparin doses (greater than 40,000 IU per 24 hours). This may occur in the early stages of massive pulmonary embolism due to increased heparin clearance rate[69], or in congenital antithrombin III deficiency.[70]

In the acute phase heparin usually is administered for 7–14 days or until clinical signs have resolved. This period is somewhat arbitrary as no trials comparing various lengths of acute-phase heparin therapy have been conducted. When there are no remaining clinical signs of acute venous occlusion, chronic-phase treatment with low-dose subcutaneous heparin (5000–10,000 IU every 12 hours) is initiated for the duration of the pregnancy (see below).

Surgical removal of a thrombus rarely is indicated in pregnancy unless limb swelling is severe enough to produce venous gangrene.[6] Vena cava plication or umbrella insertion have been advocated for recurrent pulmonary embolization from an ileofemoral thrombus[71], but are seldom required in an adequately anticoagulated woman.

Although thrombolytic agents have been considered to be relatively contraindicated in pregnancy, their successful use has been reported.[72] The aim of thrombolytic therapy is to dissolve thrombi or emboli by digesting their supporting fibrin network. Successful lysis of venous thrombi occurs in 30–50% of patients, and is more likely to be effective if used within 96 hours of onset of the thrombosis.[73] Thrombolytic therapy is associated with a lower incidence of postphlebitic leg symptoms than heparin therapy, but is associated with a higher incidence of hemorrhage. Thrombolytic agents should never be used within 10 days of delivery, surgery or any invasive procedure.

The two major groups of thrombolytic agents are plasminogen activators and proteolytic enzymes. Only the plasminogen activators have been subject to extensive clinical trials. All currently investigated plasminogen activators affect the rate of cleavage of plasminogen by slightly different mechanisms.[73] Streptokinase binds first to circulating plasminogen; this circulating streptokinase-plasminogen complex then is capable of activating other plasminogen molecules. Only streptokinase has been used for acute-phase treatment of venous thrombosis in pregnancy. Twelve pregnant women had successful treatment of deep vein thrombosis following a streptokinase loading dose (250,000 units IV over 20 minutes) followed by an infusion of 160,000 units per hour.[74] The same investigators have shown that ^{131}I-labeled streptokinase does not cross the placenta in sufficient concentrations to cause fibrinolytic effects in the fetus.[75] However, there have been theoretical concerns that thrombolytic agents may precipitate premature labor by increasing plasminogen levels in the circulation, and also that they may lead to uterine atony.[76] As experience with thrombolytic agents in pregnancy is very limited, their use should be restricted to life-threatening situations. There is no experience to date in pregnancy with other thrombolytic agents such as recombinant single-chain urokinase plasminogen activator, or recombinant tissue-type plasminogen activator.[73] Urokinase has been used successfully to treat recurrent thrombosis of an aortic valve prosthesis in a pregnant woman without maternal or fetal complications.[77]

Defibrinating agents such as Ancrod (Arvin) have not been evaluated in pregnancy. Ancrod, an enzyme produced from the venom of the Malayan pit viper, causes accelerated lysis of thrombin and pulmonary emboli. It can produce marked hypofibrinogenemia, but little bleeding.[78] Its use in pregnancy has been restricted to the postpartum treatment of severe thromboembolic disease when heparin is contraindicated or ineffectual. In animals, a high incidence of fetal death associated with placental hemorrhage has been reported. This agent should not be used during pregnancy.

After the acute phase treatment of venous thrombosis by high-dose heparin is accomplished, most centers prefer to change over to a moderate-dose subcutaneous heparin of 5000–10,000 IU twice daily for the remainder of the pregnancy. The dosage of subcutaneous heparin should be adjusted to keep the APTT level 1.5–2.0 times the patient's own control level, when tested 6 hours after the subcutaneous injection. Alternatively, a heparin assay can be used, with care not to exceed 0.4 IU/mL. Most pregnant women can be taught the technique of home subcutaneous injections but should be warned about local bruising, which can be minimized by using the more concentrated 25,000 IU/mL heparin and a 25 G, 16-mm needle with firm pressure. Heparin requirements may change during the pregnancy because of changes in blood volume, renal handling of heparin, and superimposed medical problems such as preeclampsia.[12]

Potential Complications

Hemorrhage is the most common complication of heparin therapy, occurring in 5–10% of women. It is uncommon for spontaneous bleeding to occur if the APTT is within the therapeutic range, but bleeding may occur postoperatively or post-traumatically even if the APTT is not markedly prolonged. If hemorrhage complicates therapy in a pregnant woman, an APTT and platelet count should be performed immediately. If the hemorrhage is life-threatening, the heparin effect can be reversed immediately with protamine sulfate (1 mg protamine sulfate for each 100 IU heparin), given slowly over 15–30 minutes to avoid hypotension.[79]

Heparin-induced thrombocytopenia is a further potential complication, but its frequency in pregnancy is not known.[80] The nonpregnant incidence is 3%.[81] The onset of thrombocytopenia usually follows three to eight days after the initiation of treatment, with recovery occurring over a one-week period after discontinuation of heparin.[82] In many instances, the platelet count returns to normal even if heparin therapy is continued. Thrombocytopenia may not recur if the patient is retreated with heparin later.

The etiology of the thrombocytopenia still is debated although, a heparin-dependent platelet aggregating factor has been demonstrated.[83] Heparin-associated thrombocytopenia is usually asymptomatic, but has been associated with both bleeding and arterial thrombosis.[59]

Heparin-induced osteoporosis has been reported in pregnancy.[84] Although the true frequency in pregnancy is not known, probably less than 10% of pregnant women are at risk. The osteoporosis may be severe, resulting in incapacitating backache and vertebral collapse.[85] While the cause of heparin-induced osteoporosis is not known, it has been suggested that the drug may complex with calcium, or potentiate the effect of parathormone on bone, or that there is a deficiency of 1:25 dihydrotachysterol. Pregnant women may be more sensitive to heparin-induced osteoporosis because of the increased calcium demand of pregnancy, although the maternal skeleton is thought to be relatively protected from decalcification by a rise in calcitonin levels. Pregnant women with low calcitonin levels may be at greater risk of osteoporosis following long-term heparin administration.[86]

Heparin-induced osteoporosis generally is found in those treated with heparin 15,000 IU day or more over a period of greater than six months, and in women who have other prepregnancy osteoporosis risk factors. Most radiologic studies indicate a dose-related demineralization process associated with heparin therapy in pregnancy.[84] However, osteoporosis in pregnancy has been reported with a heparin dose as low as 10,000 IU per day, and a duration of only 9 weeks. Thus susceptibility to the skeletal effects of heparin varies greatly between individuals.[87]

Other rare side effects of heparin include hypotension, alopecia, and allergic reactions.

In spite of the fact that heparin does not cross the placenta, a review of fetal sequelae following the use of heparin in pregnancy suggested a poor outcome.[88] In 135 published cases, 12% of infants were stillborn, 20% were premature and the remaining two thirds were normal. The reviewers felt that heparin did not appear to be a superior alternative to coumarin derivatives, and speculated that the deleterious heparin effect might be due to its chelating capacity with resultant fetal calcium (or other cation) deficiency. However, closer scrutiny of this study suggests that most fetal problems occurred in women with other medical problems. Nageotte and coworkers[89] analyzed the same data, and after excluding cases in which maternal disease or other drugs were contributing to the fetal outcome, arrived at a 13% unfavorable outcome compared with 22% in the Hall et al analysis.[88] This compared favourably with a 31% abnormal fetal outcome in oral anticoagulant treated pregnancies. The McMaster University Study in 1987[68] demonstrated that if no other maternal premorbid conditions are present, heparin was safe from a fetal standpoint. A final comparative study of antenatal heparin prophylaxis versus no treatment suggested only a slight increase in fetal morbidity.[85] Thus little convincing evidence exists that there is an adverse effect of heparin on fetal outcome, and certainly no increase in congenital defects. Breast-feeding is safe for the heparinized woman and her infant, as heparin is not excreted into breast milk due to its high molecular weight.[90]

Low-molecular-weight heparins (LMW) are prepared from conventional heparin by ethanol extraction and chromatography, or by chemical degradation. The mean molecular weight of heparin is 12,000 Daltons (range, 3000–30,000 Daltons) as compared with a mean LMW heparin molecular weight of 5000 Daltons (1200–15,000). LMW heparin binds more tightly to antithrombin III with a resultant longer half-life, allowing once-a-day subcutaneous administration. The antithrombotic potential of LMW heparin is similar to heparin but the incidence of hemorrhage is lower. In addition, LMW heparin can be used in patients with heparin-induced thrombocytopenia.[91] LMW heparins do not cross the placenta. The optimal dose for prophylaxis and treatment with each LMW heparin is different, and each must be considered individually. LMW heparin has been used successfully to treat venous thrombosis in pregnancy by a single subcutaneous dosage regimen after initial acute-phase standard heparin continuous intravenous anticoagulation.[92]

MANAGEMENT OF LABOR, DELIVERY AND THE POSTPARTUM PERIOD IN THE HEPARINIZED WOMAN

Women who go into labor while receiving high-dose heparin should continue to receive continuous intravenous heparin at 1000 IU per hour until the cervix is 8–9 cm dilated. If the APTT is greater than 1.5 times control immediately prior to delivery, then protamine sulfate reversal should be considered.[68] After hemostasis is secured, continuous intravenous heparin (800–1000 IU/hour) is restarted within two hours of delivery. The risk of recurrent thromboembolism is greatest in the immediate postpartum period. Therefore intravenous heparin should be continued for 2–3 days postpartum or until the parturient is fully mobile. Subcutaneous low-dose heparin (5000 IU every 12 hours) or oral anticoagulants then are started for a period of six to twelve weeks depending on severity and position of the thrombosis.

Women receiving low-dose heparin therapy (5000–10,000 IU subcutaneously twice daily) prior to delivery should continue heparin administration through labor. There appears to be no increased risk of postpartum hemorrhage in this situation, although a heparin assay should be performed during labor.[92] After delivery, the total daily subcutaneous[93] dose of heparin is reduced because of blood volume contraction and the slow return of clotting factor concentrations to normal levels. The subcutaneous dose of 5000–7500 IU twice daily should be continued for six weeks postpartum.

Epidural anaesthesia is contraindicated for women receiving either a high-dose or low-dose heparin regimen because of the significant risk of hematoma formation.[94] Women who develop a proximal deep vein thrombosis initially in the postpartum period should be treated during the acute-phase with high-dose heparin for seven to fourteen days, and then converted to oral anticoagulants for three months. Women with a postpartum distal (calf) deep vein thrombosis should receive the same acute-phase treatment, but can be converted to oral agents for six weeks or maintained on a low-dose subcutaneous heparin regimen.

ORAL ANTICOAGULANT TREATMENT IN PREGNANCY

Oral anticoagulants cross the placenta, and their use in pregnancy may result in significant problems for the fetus and newborn.[95] They are contraindicated at all times during the first trimester as they may cause congenital malformations. They are relatively contraindicated in the second and third trimesters, as they are associated with a worse fetal outcome than is associated with heparin use. The only situations in pregnancy where the benefit of oral anticoagulant use may exceed the fetal risk is in artificial heart valves, mitral valve disease with embolization, when heparin is contraindicated, and postpartum chronic-phase treatment.

If an instance arises in which the risk of oral anticoagulation therapy to the fetus is considered less than the risk of not treating the mother, several regimens may be considered. Oral anticoagulants are low molecular weight organic compounds rapidly absorbed from the gastrointestinal tract, and 95% bound in circulation to albumin. The drugs inhibit the effect of vitamin K in the hepatic synthesis of factors II, VII, IX, and X. There are two types of vitamin K antagonists: the coumarins and the indanedione derivatives. The more commonly used oral anticoagulants include sodium warfarin, dicumarol, ethyl biscoumacetate and phenindione. The plasma half-life varies from 2.5 hours for ethyl biscoumacetate to 42 hours for warfarin. The effect of oral anticoagulants on blood coagulation usually is measured with the one-stage prothrombin time (PT), and the desired anticoagulant effect in pregnancy is the same as nonpregnancy, with an optimal PT of twice normal (range 1.5–2.5 times control). However, the fetus has lower levels of clotting factors, and will be more anticoagulated if the mother's PT is in the therapeutic range.[95]

First trimester use of oral anticoagulants has resulted in a group of abnormalities termed the fetal warfarin syndrome.[96] This is manifest by nasal hypoplasia, with a flattened upturned nose and nasal septum maldevelopment, and stippling of the epiphyses. These abnormalities of cartilage and bone formation have been termed *chondrodysplasia punctata*, but they are not specific to warfarin use, and can occur in disorders such as trisomy 18 and the autosomal-dominant Conradi–Hunerman syndrome.[97] The fetal outcome for 255 reported cases of first-trimester exposure to coumarin derivatives is fetal warfarin syndrome (8%), spontaneous abortions (16%), stillbirth or neonatal death (7%), normal infants (65%).[95] The critical period for exposure is the 6th to 9th week of gestation.

Exposure to coumarin derivatives outside the first trimester is associated with an increased risk of central nervous system defects. Malformations recorded include dorsal midline dysplasia with agenesis of the corpus callosum, Dandy–Walker malformations, midline cerebellar atrophy, encephalocele, hydrocephalus, deafness, seizures, and mental retardation.[88] Ventral midline dysplasia with optic atrophy, microphthalmia and blindness also may result. The overall incidence of central nervous system defects in the coumarin-exposed fetus is 5%. Some of these malformations, but not all, can be related to central nervous system hemorrhage.

Other congenital anomalies have been observed in 2% of exposed fetuses but are probably incidental malformations including congenital cardiac disease, renal anomalies, polydactyly, and spina bifida. In conclusion, although the first trimester is of greatest concern for oral anticoagulant exposure, only 70% of pregnancies will result in a normal infant. Long-term follow up of these healthy children, fortunately, shows continued normal physical and mental development when compared with controls.[98]

Breast-feeding advice for the woman on oral anticoagulants depends on the drug used. Warfarin has not been detected in milk of 28 lactating women, and no effect on infant bleeding times has been found.[99] The American Academy of Pediatrics considers both warfarin and dicumarol use compatible with breast-feeding.[100] Phenindione use results in detectable amounts of the drug appearing in breast milk, and reports of hemorrhage in breast-feeding infants have led to the suggestion that its use should be contraindicated in the lactating woman.

PRECONCEPTUAL COUNSELING FOR THE WOMAN WITH PRIOR THROMBOEMBOLISM

The risk of recurrent thromboembolism in pregnancy for a woman who has had a prior episode is not accurately known, but is probably very low.

De Swiet et al[101] followed 59 pregnant women with a prior history of thromboembolism, using no prophylactic anticoagulation during the gestation. Of these women, 25% had had a prior episode during pregnancy, and 39% during the use of oral contraceptives. No antenatal recurrences were encountered. In a smaller study of 30 women[102], the recurrence rate was 7%. The frequently quoted recurrence rate of 12% is based on a retrospective study by Badaracco and Vessey[103], in which 84 women with prior venous thromboembolism were contacted regarding subsequent recurrences. Half of the initial episodes had occurred while the women were taking oral contraceptives, and half were idiopathic. The subsequent pregnancy experience was almost identical for the two groups, with a total of 24 pregnancies occurring in the 15 women from each group. Three women in each group (6 in 48, 12%) reported a recurrence during pregnancy, but every episode occurred when the woman was in the hospital. From this series, it is uncertain whether the factor causing the index episode had any bearing on the recurrence rate in pregnancy.

Until a trial comparing prophylactic anticoagulation with no therapy is done and the recurrence rate in pregnancy is known more accurately, the optimal management in pregnancy of the woman with a prior thromboembolic episode will be uncertain. The potential risk of recurrence has to be weighed against the risks of prophylactic heparin therapy. Although a significant reduction in postoperative thromboembolic disease in high-risk surgical patients is seen when using prophylactic subcutaneous heparin 5000 units twice daily, there is no evidence that a similar regimen will reduce the recurrence rate in pregnancy.[104] At present, the use of prophylactic anticoagulation is a personal choice for both physician and patient.

Preconception counseling should be directed at confirming the diagnosis of the initial thrombosis by reviewing case records, venograms, and other testing. If confirmatory testing had not been performed, consideration should be given to repeating a limited venogram. If the prior diagnosis is confirmed, the pregnancy can be followed by serial impedance plethysmography (IPG) testing twice monthly. If the initial thromboembolic event occurred during a recent pregnancy in the peripartum period, subcutaneous heparin (7500–10,000 IU twice daily) can be used in the next pregnancy at times of greatest risk, such as bed rest or the immediate peripartum period.

Long-term antenatal prophylaxis with subcutaneous heparin probably should be indicated only in women with a familial tendency to thrombosis or with a history of recurrent thrombosis occurring in pregnancy. The risk of osteoporosis with long-term heparin use should be discussed at preconception counseling. During the pregnancy, a heparin dosage of 7500–10,000 IU twice daily is used, aiming to achieve heparin levels of 0.3 units/mL.

An alternative to peripartum heparin prophylaxis using dextran 70 infusion during labor and subcutaneous heparin for six weeks postpartum has been suggested.[105] Dextran is a synthetic polysaccharide that inhibits platelet function and fibrin polymerization. When dextran has been used for prevention of venous thromboembolism perioperatively it has not been as effective as low-dose heparin. However, it has the advantage that in labor an epidural anesthetic can be used. Dextran infusion is associated with a very low risk of hypersensitivity reactions that have not been encountered during labor.

Antiplatelet agents such as aspirin or hydroxychloroquine are not effective in preventing venous thrombosis and should not be used prophylactically in pregnancy.

PRIMARY HYPERCOAGULABLE STATES IN PREGNANCY

Primary hypercoagulable states are a group of disorders with inherited abnormalities of coagulation in which a physiologic anticoagulant mechanism is defective.[106] Normally, there are three physiologic mechanisms preventing abnormal thrombus formation. The first is the fibrinolytic system, which removes fibrin clot by digesting fibrin and producing fibrin degradation products. The second mechanism involves antithrombin III, which binds thrombin and other proteases of the coagulation cascade and inhibits their activity. Antithrombin III is a potent serine protein that inhibits thrombin-mediated cleavage of fibrinogen and inactivates factors IX, X, XI, XII through bonding with the active portion of the molecule. Patients with antithrombin III deficiency have increased fibrin formation with associated clinical sequelae of recurrent thrombosis. The third mechanism involves protein C, which is a Vitamin K–dependent glycoprotein. Protein C is a true anticoagulant that inhibits activated factors V_a and VIII_a, and also stimulates fibrinolysis.[107,108] Before protein C can exert its anticoagulant effect, it has to be activated by thrombin to protein Ca. Protein Ca also requires a cofactor for its anticoagulant activity, which is another vitamin K-dependent plasma protein called protein S. Deficiencies of antithrombin III, protein C, and protein S all have been associated with thromboembolic disease in pregnancy (see also Chapter 167).

Antithrombin III Deficiency

Congenital antithrombin III deficiency consists of a group of heterogeneous disorders with deficiency in antithrombin III concentration or function. Classical antithrombin III deficiency (Type 1) is inherited as autosomal dominant with an incidence of 1 in 5000.[109-111] Heterozygotes have an antithrombin III level of 25–60% normal, but the homozygous state is not compatible with life. Classical heterozygotes have reduced synthesis of biologically normal antithrombin III, and thus both antigenic and functional assays of antithrombin III are low. Variants of antithrombin III deficiency also are found that produce a mutant inactive antithrombin III molecule.[112] In these subjects, antithrombin immunoassay levels are normal, but functional assays are abnormal. These variants have been subdivided into Type II if both progressive antithrombin and heparin cofactor activity is reduced, or Type III, if heparin cofactor activity alone is reduced. Hereditary antithrombin variants usually are named after their city of identification, (eg, Antithrombin Oslo, Chicago, Ann Arbor). Antithrombin III deficiency also may be seen in patients with nephrotic syndrome with marked proteinuria and in patients receiving oral contraceptives. Clinical features of all types of antithrombin III deficiency are recurrent deep vein thrombosis and pulmonary embolism. Thrombotic episodes may occur from neonatal life onwards, but first presentation is often in the second or third decade. Precipitating factors include trauma, infection, oral contraceptives, and pregnancy.[113] Patients with blood antithrombin-III levels of less than 50% of normal will have frequent venous thromboses resulting from increased thrombin activity. Some 70% of patients with antithrombin-III deficiency will develop thrombotic complications.[110-111]

Pregnancy is associated with a very high risk of thrombosis (70%) occurring from the first trimester onwards.[114] Heparin prophylaxis has reduced this risk to 14%, but occasionally it has been ineffective in severe antithrombin III deficiency, as heparin cannot function without its cofactor. Functional antithrombin III levels also fall during heparin therapy, but usually it is possible to achieve therapeutic heparin effect in pregnancy with subcutaneous doses of 30,000–45,000 IU per 24 hours.[70] Infusions of antithrombin III concentrations are given peripartum, or in women who are truly heparin resistant (2000–5000 units 50 IU per kg), on alternate days to keep the antithrombin III levels at 80% normal.[114] The key to a successful pregnancy in women with antithrombin III deficiency is to start prophylactic heparinization as soon as pregnancy is confirmed and to use a daily subcutaneous dosage sufficient to maintain prolongation of a PTT by at least 10 seconds throughout the 24 hours.[109] The risk of children of antithrombin III-deficient women inheriting the disorder is 50%. A normal antithrombin III level in cord blood is 50% adult range, and an antithrombin III-deficient neonate will have a cord blood level 20–30% adult range. Neonatal thrombosis in this situation is rare, but neonatal aortic thrombosis has been reported. In view of this, it has been suggested that affected neonates be covered with antithrombin III concentrate or fresh frozen plasma until their final antithrombin III levels are reached at 3 months, particularly if their antithrombin III levels are less than 30% at birth.[114]

Protein C and Protein S Deficiencies

Protein C deficiency may be inherited as an autosomal-dominant trait with incomplete penetrance.[115,116] Low protein C levels also are seen in patients with liver disease, DIC, and in the postoperative period.[117,118] Extremely low activities of protein C (less than 6%) have been identified in patients with recurrent thrombosis.[115,116] Mannucci[119] demonstrated increased levels of protein C during normal pregnancy with reduced protein C levels in the postpartum period. Protein C levels can be measured by immunoassay or functional assay.[106] The clinical manifestations of protein C deficiency are similar to antithrombin III deficiency. Heterozygous protein C deficiency has presented for the first time as deep venous thrombosis in pregnancy[120] and also as cerebral thrombosis.[121] It also has been reported as being associated with recurrent preeclampsia.[122] Thrombotic complications may be seen with protein C activities of 60% in heterozygotes. Homozygous protein C deficiency has been noted in two infants with massive neonatal thrombosis born to consanguineous parents with heterozygous protein C deficiency.[123] Neonatal levels are frequently less than 50% of adult activity, and thus protein C levels at birth generally are not predictive of carrier status.[124]

Decreased protein S activity will have the same effect as isolated protein C deficiency with recurrent venous thrombosis being a major risk. A few cases of protein S deficiency in pregnancy have been reported.[125,126]

Prophylactic heparin therapy during pregnancy should be used in both protein C and protein S deficiencies.[126] Most of the cases reported used prophylactic subcutaneous heparin throughout the gestation. Whether a shorter peripartum heparin regimen would be just as successful has not been established.

THE PHOSPHOLIPID ANTIBODY SYNDROME AND VENOUS THROMBOSIS

A clinical syndrome linking venous thrombosis, recurrent pregnancy loss, vascular disease, and antibodies directed against phospholipids has been variously termed the *lupus anticoagulant, anticardiolipin,* or *phospholipid antibody syndrome.*[127] In 1952, Conley and Hartmann[128] described patients with systemic lupus erythromatosus (SLE), whose plasma prolonged the whole blood clotting time if added to normal blood. In 1963, Bowie and colleagues[129] noted the occurrence of thrombosis and a circulating anticoagulant in SLE. The term *lupus anticoagulant* was coined by Feinstein and Rapaport[130] to describe acquired circulating agents that inhibit coagulation tests *in vitro* in spite of normally active clotting factors. Lupus anticoagulant is an immunoglobulin (IgG or occasionally IgM) that reacts with platelet wall phospholipid. Clinically, the term is a misnomer in that the lupus anticoagulant does not interfere with hemostasis, and can be found in patients without SLE. Although similar antibodies can be directed against various phospholipids, initial research in this area used cardiolipin as the test antigen, because of its easy availability. There is a strong correlation between the presence of antibody to cardiolipin and lupus anticoagulant, and the presence of either or both is associated with an increased thrombotic tendency. Patients with the lupus anticoagulant may produce a family of phospholipid antibodies on platelets or endothelial cell membranes, which may lead to thrombosis.

Pregnant women with elevated phospholipid antibodies have a high incidence of pregnancy loss, including recurrent abortion, intrauterine growth retardation and preeclampsia. These pregnancy complications may be related to placental vessel thrombosis.[131] Inhibition of prostacyclin production and a change in the ratio of placental prostacyclin to thromboxane production also has been implicated in the pathophysiology.[132] Women with phospholipid antibody syndrome considering a pregnancy thus have to be counseled regarding both increased pregnancy loss, and an increased occurrence of arterial and venous thrombosis during the gestation. In view of the changes in prostacyclin synthesis, therapy with combined low-dose aspirin (80 mg per day) plus prednisone (40–50 mg per day) has been suggested, but this regimen is still being investigated.[132] Optimal therapy for prevention of thrombotic complications during pregnancy is not known, but recommendations have included the prednisone and aspirin immunosuppressive regimen, or long-term prophylactic anticoagulation with heparin (see also Chapters 50 and 51).

SEPTIC PELVIC THROMBOPHLEBITIS

Septic pelvic thrombophlebitis is a serious complication of postpartum endometritis, with approximately one third of patients developing septic pulmonary embolization if left untreated.[133] One series of consecutive cesarean sections noted a frequency of 11 in 1263 or 0.9%[134], but as the diagnosis is usually one of exclusion, the exact incidence of septic pelvic thrombophlebitis is unknown. Pelvic thrombophlebitis frequently complicates prolonged pelvic infection, with *Bacteroides* species or Group B *Streptococcus* frequently being involved. Patients present with a history of persistent postpartum fever with pelvic tenderness despite adequate intravenous antibiotic therapy covering aerobic and anaerobic species.[135] Although there may be signs of abdominal or pelvic tenderness, there may be no specific findings on examination. Palpable thrombosed parametrial veins are present in approximately one third of patients.[136] The diagnosis usually is made after defervescence following therapeutic anticoagulation. X-ray computed tomography (CT) and magnetic resonance imaging (MRI) are useful adjunctive tools in the demonstration of venous thrombosis in these patients.[137] Chest x-ray examination may reveal multiple infiltrates from septic embolization. Serial blood cultures for aerobic and anaerobic organisms should be performed.[138] Treatment requires a medium-dose heparin regimen, and improvement usually is noted after 12–36 hours.[139] The optimal length of therapy has not been established, but 10 days of heparin therapy often is used with full anticoagulation for a further six to twelve weeks if pulmonary embolization has occurred. Antibiotics should be used with heparin in the acute phase. Regimens of proven value include the newer broad spectrum cephalosporins or ureidopenicillins in combination with clindamycin and an aminoglycoside.[140]

Ovarian Vein Thrombophlebitis

Puerpural ovarian vein thrombophlebitis is a rare complication of pregnancy occurring in an estimated 1 in 4000 deliveries.[141] Ovarian vein thrombosis usually is seen as sequelae to postpartum endometritis. A preponderance of right-sided ovarian vein thrombosis (90%) is attributed to the passage of infected debris through the right ovarian vein, draining the uterus. Retrograde left ovarian vein flow is seen in the erect postpartum patient and may prevent cephalic passage of infected material.[142,143] The cardinal symptoms of ovarian vein thrombosis are unilateral abdominal and flank pain with associated fever. Nausea, vomiting, and paralytic ileus occur infrequently, but may confuse the clinical picture with that of acute appendicitis. Approximately 50% of patients have a palpable unilateral abdominal mass. Pelviabdominal ultrasound (Figure 209–1) and CT scan are useful adjuncts in the diagnosis of ovarian vein thrombosis[144] (Figure 209–2). Extension of the thrombus into the left renal vein and inferior vena cava have been identified as sequelae to ovarian vein thrombophlebitis.[145] The treatment of ovarian vein thrombophlebitis is similar to that of septic pelvic thrombophlebitis with continued antibiotic coverage of aerobic and anaerobic species as well as intravenous heparinization for 10–14 days. Again, a rapid response to therapy usually is seen over 24–48 hours following adequate anticoagulation. Surgical excision of the infected ovarian vein is indicated for patients failing to respond to antibiotics and adequate heparinization or with recurrent thromboembolism.

CEREBRAL VENOUS THROMBOSIS IN PREGNANCY

Aseptic thrombosis of intracranial venous sinuses are uncommon in pregnancy, but may occur peripartum.[146] Predisposing factors include antithrombin III deficiency, protein C deficiency, and sickle cell anemia.

The clinical presentation includes severe headache, vomiting, focal neurological signs and confusion. Seizure activity is common. Cerebral venous thrombosis must be differentiated from preeclampsia and eclampsia, cerebral hemorrhage and embolism, subarachnoid hemorrhage and space-occupying lesions. Diagnosis is aided by cerebral an-

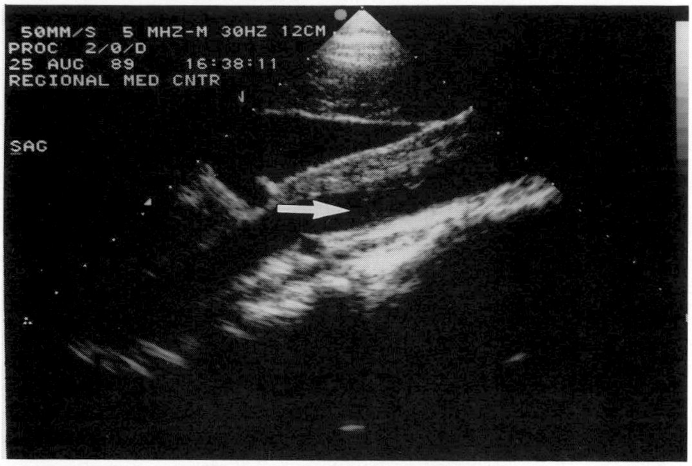

Figure 209–1. B-mode ultrasonographic appearance of clot in inferior vena cava (*arrow*). Printed with permission of Douglas L. Brown, M.D.

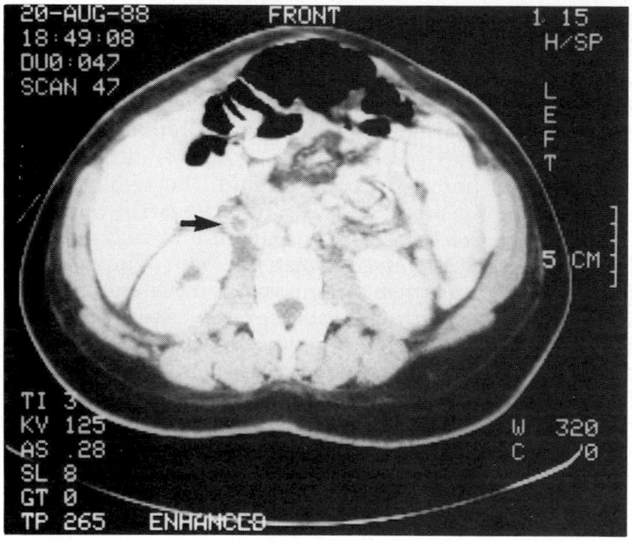

Figure 209–2. Enhanced computed tomography scan: right ovarian vein thrombosis (*arrow*). Printed with permission of Douglas L. Brown, M.D.

giography, CT, and MRI of the brain.[147,148] Supportive treatment includes anticonvulsants, corticosteroids, and the avoidance of dehydration. Anticoagulant therapy is controversial, but could be considered if the diagnosis is certain, and cerebral hemorrhage has been ruled out.[149] Low-molecular-weight dextran has been suggested as an alternative to anticoagulation.

REFERENCES

1. Kierkegaard A. Incidence and diagnosis of deep vein thrombosis associated with pregnancy. *Acta Obstet Gynecol Scand*. 1983;62:239.
2. Drill VA, Calhoun DW. Oral contraceptives and thromboembolic disease. *JAMA*. 1968;206:77.
3. Aaro KA, Jergens JL. Thrombophlebitis associated with pregnancy. *Am J Obstet Gynecol*. 1971;109:1128.
4. Kakkar V. The diagnosis of deep venous thrombosis using the ^{125}I-fibrinogen test. *Arch Surg*. 1972;104:152.
5. Flessa HC, Glueck HI, Dritshilo A. Thromboembolic disorders in pregnancy: pathophysiology, diagnosis and treatment with emphasis on heparin. *Clin Obstet Gynecol*. 1974;17:195.
6. Gurll W, Helfand Z, Salzman EF, Silen W. Peripheral venous thrombophlebitis during pregnancy. *Am J Surg*. 1971;121:449.
7. Jeffcoate TN, Tendall VR. Venous thrombosis and emoblism in obstetrics and gynecology. *Austr NZ J Obstet Gynecol*. 1965;5:114.
8. Bergqvist A, Bergqvist D, Hallbook T. Acute deep vein thrombosis (DVT) after cesarean section. *Acta Obstet Gynecol Scand*. 1979;58:473.
9. Husni E, Pena L, Lenhert E. Thrombophlebitis in pregnancy. *Am J Obstet and Gynecol*. 1967;97:901.
10. Hiilesma V. Occurrence and anticoagulant treatment of thromboembolism in gravidas parturients and gynecological patients: a study of 678 cases treated in the women's clinic of the University of Helsinki in 1953. *Acta Obstet Gynecol Scand*. 1960;39(2):1.
11. Hellgren M, Tengborn L, Abildgaard U. Pregnancy in women with congenital antithrombin-III deficiency: experience of treatment with heparin and antithrombin. *Gynecol Obstet Invest*. 1982;14:127.
12. Bonnar J. Thromboembolism in obstetric and gynecological patients. In: Nicolaides AN, ed. *Thromboembolism Etiology: Advances in Prevention and Management*. Lancaster: Medical and Technical Publishing Co. Ltd. 1975:311.
13. Bonnar J. Blood coagulation fibrinolysis in obstetrics. *Clinics in Hematol*. 1973:213.
14. Bonnar J, McNichol GP, Douglas AS. Coagulation and fibrinolytic mechanisms during and after normal childbirth. BMJ 1970;2:200.
15. Bonnar J, McNichol GP, Douglas AS. The blood coagulation and fibrinolytic systems in the newborn and the mother at birth. *J Obstet Gynaecol Br Commonw*. 1971;78:355.
16. Daniel DG. Estrogens and puerperal thromboembolism. *Am Heart J*. 1969;78:720.
17. Nilsson IM, Kullander S. Coagulation and fibrinolytic studies during pregnancy. *Acta Obstet Gynecol Scand*. 1967;46:273.
18. Phillips LL, Rosano L, Skrodelis V. Changes in factor XI (plasma thromboplastin antecedent) levels during pregnancy. *Am J Obstet Gynecol*. 1973;116:1114.
19. Coopland A, Alkjaersig N, Fletcher AP. Reduction in plasma factor 13 (fibrin stabilizing factor) concentration during pregnancy. *J Lab Clin Med*. 1969;73:144.
20. Fletcher AP, Alkjaersig NK, Burstein R. The influence of pregnancy upon blood coagulation and plasma fibrinolytic enzyme function. *Am J Obstet Gynecol*. 1979;134:743.
21. McKillop C, Howie PW, Forbes CO, et al. Soluble fibrinogen-fibrin complexes in preeclampsia. *Lancet*. 1976;1:56.
22. Coon WW. Epidemiology of venous thromboembolism. *Ann Surg*. 1977;186(2):149.
23. Goodrich SM, Wood JE. Peripheral venous distensibility and velocity of venous blood flow during pregnancy or during oral contraceptive therapy. *Am J Obstet Gynecol*. 1964;90:740.
24. Wright HP, Osborn SB, Edmonds DG. Changes in the rate of flow of venous blood in the leg during pregnancy, measured with radioactive sodium. *Surg Gynecol Obstet*. 1950;90:481.
25. McLennan CE. Antecubital and femoral venous pressure in normal and toxemia pregnancy. *Am J Obstet Gynecol*. 1943;45:568.

26. Kerr MG, Scott DB, Samuel E. Studies of the inferior vena cava in late pregnancy. *Br Med J*. 1964;1:532.
27. McCausland AM, Hyman C, Winsor T, Trotter AD. Venous distensibility during pregnancy. *Am J Obstet Gynecol*. 1961;81:472.
28. Sevitt S. The structure and growth of valve-pocket thrombi in femoral veins. *J Clin Pathol*. 1974;27:517.
29. Stewart GJ, Ritchie WGM, Linch PR, et al. Venous endothelial damage produced by massive sticking and immigration of leukocytes. *Am J Pathol*. 1974;74:507.
30. Ashford TP, Frieman DG. The role of endothelium in the initial phase of thrombosis: an electron microscopic study. *Am J Pathol*. 1967;50:257.
31. Barnes RW, Wu KK, Hoak JC. Fallibility of the clinical diagnosis of venous thrombosis. *JAMA*. 1975;234:605.
32. Gallus AS, Hirsch J, Hull R, van Aken WG. Diagnosis of venous thromboembolism. *Sem Thromb Hemost*. 1976;2:203.
33. Simpson FG, Robinson PJ, Bark M, Losowsky MS. Prospective study of thrombophlebitis and "pseudo thrombophlebitis." *Lancet*. 1980;1:331.
34. Bell WR, Simon TL, De Mets DL. The clinical features of submassive and massive pulmonary emboli. *Am J Med*. 1977;62:355.
35. Richards KL, Armstrong JD, Tikoff G, et al. Noninvasive diagnosis of deep venous thrombosis. *Arch Intern Med*. 1976;136:1091.
36. Haegar K. Problems of acute deep vein thrombosis. The interpretation of signs and symptoms. *Angiology*. 1969;20:219.
37. Hirsh J, Hull R. Comparative value of tests for the diagnosis of venous thrombosis. *World J Surg*. 1978;2:27.
38. Thomas ML. Phlebography. *Arch Surg*. 1972;104:145.
39. Rabinov K, Paulin S. Roentgen diagnosis of venous thrombosis in the leg. *Arch Surg*. 1972;104:134.
40. Jones KL. Effects of chemical and environmental agents. In: Creasy RK, Resnik R, eds. *Maternal-Fetal Medicine: Principles and Practice*. 2nd ed. Philadelphia: WB Saunders; 1989.
41. Bettman MA, Paulin S. Leg phlebography: the incidence, nature and modification of undesirable side effects. *Radiology*. 1977;122:101.
42. Albrechtsson V, Olsson CG. Thrombotic side-effects of lower limb phlebography. *Lancet*. 1976;1:723.
43. Negus D, Pinto DJ, Le Quesne LP, et al. ^{125}I-labeled fibrinogen in the diagnosis of deep venous thrombosis in its correlation with phlebography. *Br J Surg*. 1968;55:835.
44. Browse NL. ^{125}I fibrinogen update test. *Arch Surg*. 1972;104:160.
45. Kakkar VV. Fibrinogen uptake test for detection of deep vein thrombosis: a review of current practice. *Semin Nucl Med*. 1977;7:229.
46. Strandness DE, Sumner ES. Ultrasonic velocity detector in the diagnosis of thrombophlebitis. *Arch Surg*. 1972;104:180.
47. Borozan PG, Zukowski A, Thorpe L, et al. Noninvasive imaging for deep venous thrombosis. *Am J Surg*. 1988;156:474.
48. Cronan JJ, Dorfman GS, Scola FH, et al. Deep venous thrombosis: US assessment using vein compression. *Radiology*. 1987;162:191.
49. Cronan JJ, Dorfman GS, Grusmark J. Lower extremity deep venous thrombosis: further experience with and refinements of US assessment. *Radiology*. 1988;168:101.
50. Vogel P, Laing FC, Jeffrey RB, Wing VW. Deep venous thrombosis of the lower extremity: US evaluation. *Radiology*. 1987;163:747.
51. Appleman PT, De Jong TE, Lampmann LE. Deep venous thrombosis of the leg: US findings. *Radiology*. 1987;163:743.
52. Cole R, Van Aken WG, Hirsh J, et al. Impedance plethysmography using occlusive cuff technique in the diagnosis of venous thrombosis. *Circulation*. 1976;53:696.
53. Clarke-Pearson DL, Jelovsek FR. Alterations of occlusive cuff impedance plethysmography results in the obstetric patient. *Surgery*. 1981;89:594.
54. Wheeler HB, Pearson D, O'Connell D, et al. Impedance phlebography technique, interpretation, and results. *Arch Surg*. 1972;104:164.
55. Hull R, Hirsh J, Sackett DL, et al. Replacement of venography in suspected venous thrombosis by impedance plethysmography and ^{125}I-fibrinogen legs scanning: a less invasive approach. *Ann Intern Med*. 1981;94:12.
56. Kullander S, Kallen B. A prospective study of drugs in pregnancy. *Acta Obstet Gynecol Scand*. 1976;55:289.
57. Niebyl JR. Prostaglandin synthetase inhibitors. *Semin Perinatol*. 1981; 5:274.
58. Gallus AS, Hirsh J. Treatment of venous thromboembolic disease. *Sem Thromb Hemost*. 1976;2:291.
59. de Swiet M. Thromboembolism. In: de Swiet M, ed. *Medical Disorders in Obstetric Practice*. Oxford: Blackwell; 1984:95.
60. Hirsh J. Diagnosis of management of venous thrombosis. *Med North Am*. 1984;12:1376.
61. Harenberg J, Heene DL. Pharmacology and special clinical applications of low-molecular-weight heparins. *Am J Hematol*. 1988;29:233.
62. Stringer MD, Wilson N, Kakkar VV. Anticoagulants in venous thrombosis. *Br Med J*. 1989;298:185.
63. Fennerty A, Campbell A, Routledge PA. Anticoagulants in venous thromboembolism. *Br Med J*. 1988;297:1285.
64. Walker MG, Shaw JW, Thomson GJ, et al. Subcutaneous calcium heparin versus intravenous sodium heparin in treatment of established acute deep vein thrombosis of the leg: a multicentre prospective randomized trail. *Br Med J*. 1987;294:1189.
65. Barss VA, Schwartz PA, Greene MF, et al. Use of the subcutaneous heparin pump in pregnancy. *J Reprod Med*. 1985;30:899.
66. Basu D, Gallus A, Hirsh J, Cade J. A prospective study of the value of monitoring heparin treatment with the activated partial thromboplastin time. *N Engl J Med*. 1972;287:324.
67. Chiu HM, Hirsh J, Yung WL, et al. Relationship between the anticoagulant and antithrombotic effects of heparin in experimental venous thrombosis. *Blood*. 1977;49:171.
68. LeClerc JR, Hirsh J. Venous thromboembolic disorders. In: Burrow GN, Ferris TF, eds. *Medical Complications During Pregnancy*. Philadelphia: WB Saunders; 1988:204.
69. Simon TL, Hyers TM, Gaston JP, et al. Heparin pharmacokinetics: increased requirements in pulmonary embolism. *Br J Haematol*. 1978;29:111.
70. Leclerc JR, Hirsh J, Geerts W, et al. Management of antithrombin III deficiency during pregnancy without administration of antithrombin III. *Thromb Res*. 1986;41:567.
71. Silver D, Sabiston DC. The role of vena caval interruption in the management of pulmonary embolism. *Surgery*. 1975;77:3.
72. McTaggart Dr, Ingram TG. Massive pulmonary embolism during pregnancy treated with streptokinase. *Med J Aust*. 1977;1:18.
73. Marder VJ, Sherry S. Thrombolytic therapy: current status. *N Engl J Med*. 1988;318:1512.
74. Pfeifer GW. The use of thrombolytic therapy in obstetrics and gynecology. *Aus Ann Med Suppl*. 1970:28.
75. Pfeifer GW. Distribution and placental transfer of ^{131}I streptokinase. *Aus Ann Med Suppl*. 1970:17.
76. Hall JC, Young C, Sutton GC, et al. Treatment of acute massive pulmonary embolism by streptokinase during labour and delivery. *Br Med J*. 1972;4:647.
77. Jimenez M, Vergnes C, Brottier L, et al. Recurrent thrombosis of an aortic valve prosthesis in a pregnant woman: treatment with urokinase. *J Mal Vasc*. 1988;13:46.
78. Davies JA, Merrick MV, Sharp JM. Controlled trial of ancrod and heparin in treatment of deep vein thrombosis of lower limb. *Lancet*. 1972;1:113.
79. Laros RK. Thromboembolic disease. In: Laros RK, ed. *Blood Disorders in Pregnancy*. 1987:215.
80. Copplestone A, Oscier DG. Heparin-induced thrombocytopenia in pregnancy. *Br J Haematol*. 1987;65:248.
81. Powers PJ, Cuthbert D, Hirsh J. Thrombocytopenia found uncommonly during heparin therapy. *JAMA*. 1979;241:2396.
82. Kelton JG, Powers PJ. Heparin associated thrombocytopenia: an immune disorder. In: Lundblad R, ed. *The Chemistry and Biology of Heparin*. Amsterdam: Elsevier; 1980.
83. Chong BH, Pitney WR, Castaldi PA. Heparin induced thrombocytopenia: association of thrombotic complications with heparin dependent IgG antibody that induces thromboxane synthesis and platelet aggregation. *Lancet*. 1982;2:1246.
84. de Swiet M, Dorrington Ward P, Fidler J, et al. Prolonged heparin therapy in pregnancy causes bone demineralization. *Br J Obstet Gynaecol*. 1983;90:1129.
85. Howell R, Fidler J, Letsky E, de Swiet M. The risk of antenatal subcutaneous heparin prophylaxis: a controlled trial. *Br J Obstet Gynaecol*. 1983;90:1124.
86. Stevenson JC, Hillyard CJ, MacIntyre I. A physiological role for calcitonin: protection of the maternal skeleton. *Lancet*. 1979;ii:769.
87. Griffiths HT, Liu DTY. Severe heparin osteoporosis in pregnancy. *Postgrad Med J*. 1984;60:424.
88. Hall JG, Pauli RM, Wilson KM. Maternal and fetal sequelae of anticoagulation during pregnancy. *Am J Med*. 1980;68:138.
89. Nageotte MP, Freeman RK, Garite HI, Block RA. Anticoagulation in pregnancy. *Am J Obstet Gynecol*. 1981;141:472.
90. O'Reilly RA. Anticoagulant, antithrombotic and thrombolytic drugs. In: Gilman Ag, Goodman LS, eds. *The Pharmacological Basis of Therapeutics*. New York: Macmillan; 1980:1350.
91. Harenberg J, Heene DL. Pharmacology and special clinical applications of low-molecular-weight heparins. *Am J Hematol*. 1988;29:233.
92. Priollet P, Roncato M, Aiach M, et al. Low-molecular-weight heparin in venous thrombosis during pregnancy. *Br J Haematol*. 1986;63:605.
93. de Swiet M, Fidler J, Howell R, Letsky E. Thromboembolism in pregnancy. In: Jewell DP, ed. *Advanced Medicine*. Tumbridge Wells, England: Pitman Medical; 1981:309.
94. Crawford JS. *Principles and Practice of Obstetric Anesthesia*. Oxford: Blackwell Scientific Publications; 1978:182.
95. Briggs GG, Freeman RK, Yaffe SJ. *Drugs in Pregnancy and Lactation*. Baltimore, MD: Williams and Wilkins; 1986:106.
96. Harrod MJE, Sherrod PS. Warfarin embryopathy in siblings. *Obstet Gynecol*. 1981;57:673.
97. Holmes RD, Wilson GN, Jajra AK. Peroxisomal enzyme deficiency in the Conradi-Hunermann form of chondrodysplasia punctata. *N Engl J Med*. 1987;316:1608.

98. Chong MKB, Harvey D, de Swiet M. Follow-up study of children whose mothers were treated with warfarin during pregnancy. *Br J Obstet Gynecol.* 1984;91:1070.
99. L'Orme M, Lewis PJ, de Swiet M, et al. May mothers given warfarin breast feed their infants? *Br Med J.* 1977;1:1564.
100. Committee on Drugs, American Academy of Pediatrics. The transfer of drugs and other chemicals into human breast milk. *Pediatrics.* 1983;72:375.
101. de Swiet M, Floyd E, Letsky E. Low risk of recurrent thromboembolism in pregnancy. *Br J Hosp Med.* 1987;38:264.
102. Dixon E. Pregnancies complicated by previous thromboembolic disease. *Br J Hosp Med.* 1987;37:449.
103. Badaracco MA, Vessey MP. Recurrence of venous thromboembolic disease and use of oral contraceptives. *Br Med J.* 1974;1:215.
104. Kakkar VV, Corrigan TP, Fossard DP. Prevention of fatal postoperative pulmonary embolism by low doses of heparin: an international multicentre trial. *Lancet.* 1975;2:45.
105. Lao TT, de Swiet M, Letsky E, Walters BNJ. Prophylaxis of thromboembolism in pregnancy: an alternative. *Br J Obstet Gynaecol.* 1985;92:202.
106. Schafer AI. The hypercoagulable states. *Ann Int Med.* 1985;102:814.
107. Marlar RA, Kleiss AJ, Griffin AH. Mechanism of activation of human activated protein C, a thrombin dependent anticoagulant enzyme. *Blood.* 1982;59:1067.
108. Von Hinsbergh VWM, Bertina RM, Van Lijngaarden F. Activated protein C decreases plasminogen activator-inhibitor activity in endothelial cell conditioned medium. *Blood.* 1985;65:441.
109. Samson D, Stirling Y, Woolf L, et al. Management of planned pregnancy in a patient with congenital antithrombin III deficiency. *Br J Haematol.* 1984;56:243.
110. Johansson L, Hedner U, Nilsson IM. Familial antithrombin III deficiency as pathogenesis of deep venous thrombosis. *Acta Med Scand.* 1978; 204:491.
111. Nelson MD, Stempel LE, Brandt JT. Hereditary antithrombin III deficiency in pregnancy: report of two cases and review of the literature. *Obstet Gynecol.* 1985;65:848.
112. Hultin MB, McKay J, Abilgaard V. Antithrombin Oslo, with a review of hereditary antithrombin variants. *Thromb Haemostas.* 1988;59:468.
113. Winter JH, Fenech A, Ridley W, et al. Familial antithrombin III deficiency. *Q J Med.* 1982;51:373.
114. Hellgren M, Tengborn L, Abilgaard V. Pregnancy in women with congenital antithrombin III deficiency: experience of treatment with heparin and antithrombin. *Gynecol Obstet Invest.* 1982;14:127.
115. Branson HE, Katz J, Marble R, Griffin JH. Inherited protein C deficiency in coumarin responsive chronic relapsing puerpera fulminans in a newborn infant. *Lancet.* 1983;ii:1165.
116. Estelles A, Garcia-Plaza I, Daasi A, et al. Severe inherited homozygous protein C deficiency in a newborn infant. *Thromb Haemost.* 1984;52:53.
117. Mannucci PM, Vigano S. Deficiencies of protein C, an inhibitor of blood coagulation. *Lancet.* 1982;2:463.
118. Griffin JH, Mosher DF, Zimmerman TS, Kleiss AJ. Protein C, an antithrombotic protein, is reduced in hospitalized patients with intravascular coagulation. *Blood.* 1982;261.
119. Mannucci PM, Vigano S, Bottasso B, et al. Protein C activation during pregnancy, delivery and the puerperium. *Thromb Haemost.* 1984;52:217.
120. Morrison AE, Walker ID, Black WP. Protein C deficiency presenting as deep venous thrombosis in pregnancy: case report. *Br J Obstet Gynaecol.* 1988;95:1007.
121. Eon B, Martin C, Burn JP, et al. Cerebral thrombophlebitis associated with a protein C deficiency during pregnancy. *Presse Med.* 1988;17:1216.
122. Brenner B, Shapira A, Bahari C, et al. Hereditary protein C deficiency during pregnancy. *Am J Obstet Gynecol.* 1987;157:1160.
123. Seligsohn V, Berger A, Abend M, et al. Homozygous protein C deficiency manifest by massive venous thromboembolism in the newborn. *N Engl J Med.* 1984;310:559.
124. Polack B, Pouzol P, Amiral J, Kolodie L. Protein C level at birth. *Thromb Haemost.* 1984;52:188.
125. Rose PG, Essig GF, Vaccaro PS, Brandt JT. Protein S deficiency in pregnancy. *Am J Obstet Gynecol.* 1986;1155:140.
126. Schwarz HP, Fischer M, Hopmeier P, et al. Plasma protein S deficiency in familial thrombotic disease. *Blood.* 1984;64:1297.
127. Hughes GRV. Vascular disease, thrombosis, and recurrent abortions. *Br Med J.* 1988;297:700.
128. Conley CL, Hartmann RD. A hemorrhagic disorder caused by circulating anticoagulant in patients with disseminated lupus erythematosis. *J Clin Invest.* 1952;31:621.
129. Bowie EJ, Thompson JH, Pascuzzi CA, Owen CA. Thrombosis in systemic lupus erythematosis despite circulating anticoagulants. *J Lab Clin Med.* 1963;62:416.
130. Feinstein DI, Rapaport SI. Acquired inhibitors of blood coagulation. *Prog Hemost Thromb.* 1972;1:75.
131. Derue GJ, Englert HJ, Harris EN, et al. Fetal loss in systemic lupus: association with anticardiolipin antibodies. *J Obstet Gynecol.* 1985;5:207.
132. Branch DW, Scott Jr, Kochenour NK, Hershgold E. Obstetric complications associated with the lupus anticoagulant. *N Engl J Med.* 1985;313:1322.
133. Collins CG, MacCallum EA, Nelson EW, et al. Suppurative pelvic thrombophlebitis: study of 70 patients treated by ligation of the inferior vena cava and ovarian vessels. *Surgery.* 1951;30:298.
134. Malkamy H. Heparin therapy in post cesarean septic pelvic thrombophlebitis. *Int J Gynecol Obstet.* 1980;17:564.
135. Schulman H, Zatuchni G. Pelvic thrombophlebitis in the puerperal and postoperative gynecologic patient. *Am J Obstet Gynecol.* 1964; 90:1293.
136. Collins CG. Suppurative pelvic thrombophlebitis. *Am J Obstet Gynecol.* 1970;108:681.
137. Brown CE, Lowe TW, Cunningham FG, Weinreb JC. Puerpural pelvic thrombophlebitis: impact on diagnosis and treatment using x-ray computed tomography and magnetic resonance imaging. *Obstet Gynecol.* 1986;68:789.
138. McElin TW, Lapata RE, Westenfelder GO, Hohf RP. Postpartum ovarian vein thrombophlebitis and microaerophilic streptococcal sepsis: report of a case. *Obstet Gynecol.* 1970;35:632.
139. Ledger WJ, Peterson EP. The use of heparin in the management of pelvic thrombophlebitis. *Surg Obstet.* 1970;131:1115.
140. Duff P. Pathophysiology and management of post-cesarean endomyometritis. *Obstet Gynecol.* 1986;67:269.
141. Rosenblum R, Derrick FC, Willis A. Postpartum ovarian vein thrombosis. *Obstet Gynecol.* 1966;28:121.
142. Chidekel N, Edlundh KO. Transuterine phlebography with particular reference to pelvic vericosities. *Acta Radiol.* 1968;7:1.
143. Munsick RA, Gillanders LA. A review of the syndrome of puerperal ovarian vein thrombophlebitis. *Obstet Gynecol Surv.* 1981;33(2):57.
144. Rozier JC, Brown EH, Burne FA. Diagnosis of puerperal ovarian thrombophlebitis by computed tomography. *Am J Obstet Gynecol.* 1988; 159:737.
145. Bahnson RR, Wandel EF, Vogelzang RL. Renal vein thrombosis following puerperal ovarian thrombophlebitis. *Am J Obstet Gynecol.* 1985; 152:290.
146. Amais AG. Cerebral vascular disease in pregnancy. *J Obstet Gynecol Br Commw.* 1970;77:312.
147. Vines FS, David DO. Clinical radiological correlation in cerebral occlusive disease. *Radiology.* 1971;98:9.
148. Kent DL, Larson EG. Magnetic resonance imaging of the brain and spine. *Ann Int Med.* 1988;108:402.
149. Beal MF, Chapman PH. Cortical blindness and homonymous hemianopia in the post-partum period. *J Am Med Assoc.* 1980;244:2085.

Chapter Two Hundred and Ten

Parenteral Feeding and Nutrition

Maura Sandrock and Erol Amon

210

Nutrition during pregnancy is recognized as an important factor in the growth of the fetus and placenta and in maternal physiologic adaptation to pregnancy. Interest in nutrition in pregnancy stems from reports of the high mortality of low birth weight infants for which poor maternal nutrition is a contributing factor.[1-3] Results of animal and human studies with food deprivation are variable, but provide some insight into the many fetal complications and malformations associated with protein-energy malnutrition (PEM) and single micronutrient deficiencies during pregnancy.[4,5] Normal births still occur despite poor nutrition. This supports the complexity of interrelated factors in maternal-fetal nutrition. In most instances today, supplemental food programs, financial support, and dietary education can correct nutrient deficits in high-risk mothers.

For some, maintenance of adequate nutrition becomes exceedingly difficult, especially in cases with severe hyperemesis gravidarum or with disease states where oral intake and absorption of nutrients becomes virtually impossible. Severe malnutrition may ensue when the gastrointestinal (GI) tract is unable to maintain the nutritional demands of the mother and fetus. Total parenteral nutrition (TPN) can provide an alternative method of feeding to support the nutritional needs of the mother, fetus, and placenta adequately.

Since the first successful administration of parenteral nutrition by Stanley Dudrick in 1968, TPN has evolved to include nutritionally complete formulas that have been shown to achieve anabolism, weight gain, and correct malnutrition.[6-8] This type of therapy is costly and has significant potential for complications. Accordingly, adherence to specific selection criteria is warranted. To achieve nutritional goals and to minimize metabolic aberrations and complications known to occur with TPN, an accurate assessment of nutrient requirements combined with strict monitoring protocols is required. Inappropriate parenteral nutrition formulas and complications of TPN may result in poor pregnancy outcome. Clinicians have relied on general guidelines for TPN derived from the nonpregnant population and have used recommended daily allowances for oral ingestion of nutrients during pregnancy. Case reports of TPN administration during pregnancy over the past 10–12 years indicate that TPN is relatively safe and is associated with good outcome in most pregnancies. Unfortunately, little is known of the effects of TPN on maternal physiology and fetal growth and development. This chapter focuses on TPN, with discussion of methods for assessing nutritional status, estimation of nutrient requirements, and guidelines for administering and monitoring TPN. It also reviews the complications associated with TPN.

INDICATIONS AND REVIEW OF CLINICAL EXPERIENCE

There are numerous clinical situations that warrant the use of parenteral nutrition. The determining factor for implementing TPN is the inability to ingest and absorb nutrients adequately through the GI tract for extended periods of time. TPN is contraindicated if ingestion of nutrients may be provided safely with oral feedings and supplements or by nasogastric feeding, provided that adequate absorption of nutrients occurs. Total parenteral nutrition through central venous catheter is not indicated if the anticipated duration of therapy is less than seven days. For periods less than one week, peripheral parenteral nutrition (PPN) may be employed.[9]

As in the nonpregnant population requiring TPN, a small population of pregnant patients has required parenteral nutrition due to underlying disease states (eg, Crohn's disease, pancreatitis), which necessitate complete bowel rest. Total parenteral nutrition has been used for prolonged postoperative ileus or for consequences of adjunctive cancer chemotherapy. There are several reports of pregnant women receiving TPN for hyperemesis gravidarum. Several comprehensive reviews have been performed.[10-13] Table 210–1 summarizes situations in which TPN has been employed during pregnancy.

Patients with moderate-severe malnutrition who are unable to meet anabolic requirements are candidates for TPN. Pregnant patients with prolonged periods of GI distress and inadequate dietary intake from hyperemesis gravidarum or other underlying conditions should be monitored closely for signs of malnutrition. If severe GI symptoms continue for more than 5–7 days, parenteral nutrition may be implemented. A pregnant patient should not be allowed to develop severe malnutrition prior to the initiation of therapy with parenteral nutrition. There is a natural tendency to delay administration of TPN during pregnancy because of concerns for maternal-fetal complications. The early initiation of parenteral nutrition should be considered

TABLE 210–1. DIAGNOSES OF PREGNANT PATIENTS REQUIRING PARENTERAL NUTRITION

Medical	Surgical
Anorexia nervosa	Trauma
Brain tumor	Burn
Congenital myotonic dystrophy	Cholecystitis
Crohn's disease	Esophageal Injury
Diabetic gastroparesis	Jejunoileal bypass
Diabetic with IUGR[a]	Partial hepatectomy
Embryonal cell cancer	Ruptured appendix
Hemorrhagic gastritis	Small bowel resection
Hyperemesis gravidarum	
Leukemia	
Maternal brain death	
Pancreatitis	
Pancreatic sarcoma	
Ulcerative colitis	

[a] IUGR = intrauterine growth retardation

Data are based on references 10-13.

TABLE 210–2. CRITERIA FOR DETERMINING THE NEED FOR PARENTERAL NUTRITION FOR PREGNANT WOMEN

Oral/enteral feeding is contraindicated.
Diagnosis of moderate-severe malnutrition when unable to meet anabolic requirements by oral or enteral feeding.
Increased nutrient requirements due to stress (trauma, surgery, infections) in the presence of inadequate oral intake for 5 days or no oral intake for 3 days.
Severe, persistent gastrointestinal symptoms for more than five to seven days.
Intrauterine growth retardation thought to be secondary to malnutrition.

if the duration of dietary inadequacy or NPO status is anticipated for extended periods of time. This is particularly true in patients with increased nutrient requirements from surgery or trauma. Table 210–2 summarizes criteria for determining the need for TPN during pregnancy.

In the review by Kirby and coworkers[12], TPN was implemented during all trimesters with a frequency of 56% in the third trimester, 31% during the second trimester, and 13% in the first trimester. There were two cases of fetal demise (one related to sepsis from *Staphylococcus aureus*). In general, reports have been favorable regarding the use of TPN during pregnancy. However, a wary approach to the literature is advocated, since cases with suboptimal outcome (eg, fetal death) may not be reported. We are aware of at least 3 such cases in these different institutions.

NUTRITIONAL ASSESSMENT

Nutritional assessment is vital to the medical management and care of complicated pregnant patients for the following reasons:

1. It identifies patients at risk for developing malnutrition or those exhibiting malnutrition.
2. It provides an indirect measure of increased fetal risk status, for growth retardation and low birth weight.
3. It is a criterion for the decision to implement parenteral nutrition.
4. It is the first step for determining nutritional requirements.
5. It is clinically useful for serially assessing the efficacy of prescribed parenteral nutrition formulations.

Nutritional assessment determines nutritional status by using established objective parameters that measure body composition, metabolic activity, and tissue function. These measurements reflect protein compartments of the body and fat stores known to be altered or depleted during states of starvation or inadequate nutrient intake. These compartments serve important functions (eg, insulation and nutrient transport), and provide a source of energy during periods of calorie deprivation. Depletion of any protein compartment accompanies malnutrition and is of great concern as the body has no protein reserves. Such losses may affect many body functions adversely.[14,15] Figure 210–1 illustrates six body compartments with corresponding parameters for the assessment of nutritional status. Methods commonly employed for assessment include history (medical, obstetric, and nutritional), physical examination, anthropometric measurements, and laboratory tests.[3] We use a three-step process that includes initial screening, in-depth assessment, and monitoring.

The ability to determine nutritional status accurately is influenced by non-nutritional factors (eg, fluid status, disease states, trauma, and surgery). A test result may be misinterpreted as malnutrition[16] and may result in inappropriate nutritional support. The physiologic changes of pregnancy are known to alter many biochemical and anthropometric parameters. A complete assessment of the patient, rather than reliance on a few parameters, is advocated or certain conditions may be misinterpreted as malnutrition.

Initial Screening

Initial screening requires a review of the medical record pertinent to nutritional status. This review includes the medical, obstetric, and nutritional history as well as a physical examination. Pertinent data in the medical history are the diagnosis; primary and secondary disease states; symptoms; and history of chronic illness. Social factors (such as family situation, economic status, maternal age, level

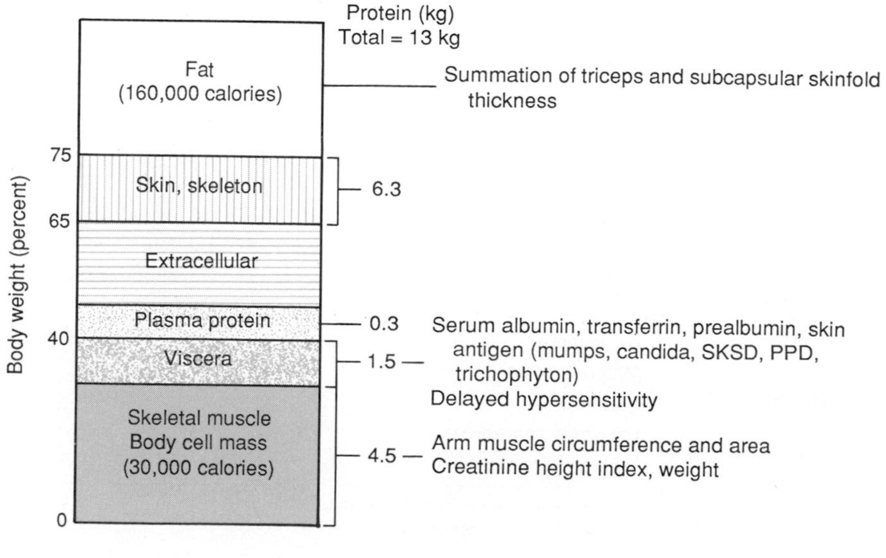

Figure 210–1. Theoretical relationship of body composition to methodology of assessment. (*Modified from Blackburn GI, Bothe A Jr[70] with permission.*)

of education, family income, and number of family members) have a tremendous influence on food consumption habits of a pregnant woman. The medical history also may reveal personal habits of the patient, such as alcohol consumption and drug use. A summary of all medications is important, since many have nutrient-drug interactions. Parameters, available on admission, are height, weight, and weight history (usual body weight, and weight loss or gain) serum albumin, hemoglobin, hematocrit, mean corpuscular volume and total lymphocyte count. Table 210–3 lists parameters included in the initial screening.

Obstetric history relevant to nutritional status includes a reproductive history. A pregnant woman with a poor reproductive history, such as a history of prior pregnancy loss, prior preterm delivery, or prior growth-retarded infants, may indicate nutritional deficiencies. Further investigation then is warranted. The pattern of weight change in prior pregnancies provides some insight into previous and current dietary habits. A short interconceptional interval between pregnancies impacts negatively on nutritional reserves.

Factors altering normal food intake (nausea and vomiting of pregnancy) or symptoms of disease (diarrhea, anorexia) are important for determining the adequacy of dietary intake. A previous nutritional history of dieting, food intolerance, and food allergies should be included in a nutritional history. If these risk factors are apparent, a 24-hour diet recall, food preferences, and a three-day calorie count usually are obtained to identify specific nutrient deficits. An accurate diet history is an important component for a nutritional assessment. It can identify caloric, protein, and micronutrient intake. Deficiencies may be identified that may not otherwise be apparent with laboratory testing or by physical findings.

The general appearance of a patient and inspection of the face, hair, and skin may reflect dietary habits and nutritional status. Overt signs of protein-energy malnutrition or single nutrient deficiency indicate severe depletion from chronic inadequacy (Table 210–4). A suspected deficiency (based on clinical signs) should be supported by laboratory testing.

Evaluation of the pregravid weight and maternal weight gain are two of the most commonly used parameters to grossly assess nutritional status. Women classified as underweight (≤90% below standard weight for height) prior to pregnancy have been shown to have an increased incidence of small-for-gestational-age (SGA) infants and low-birth-weight (LBW) infants.[17,18] Women classified as overweight (≥120% above standard weight for height) prior to pregnancy have an increased incidence of hypertension, gestational diabetes, cesarean sections, and macrosomic infants.[19-21]

The average weight gain for a pregnant woman of normal weight is 25–30 pounds. Weight gain accounts for increases in maternal tissue stores and extracellular fluid space, as well as placental and fetal growth. Simpson[19] demonstrated a decreased incidence of LBW infants in patients with an increase in prepregnancy weight or maternal weight gain. A weight gain of 31 pounds during gestation was associated with the lowest incidence of perinatal mortality.[22] An adjusted weight gain of 18–22 pounds for overweight women is recommended, as there is no need

TABLE 210–4. CLINICAL SIGNS OF NUTRIENT DEFICIENCIES

Body Area	Clinical Signs
General appearance	Listless, apathetic, cachexia
Posture	Sagging shoulders, sunken chest, humped back
Muscles	Flaccid, poor tone, tender, inability to walk properly, wasted appearance
Nervous system	Behavioral changes, irritable, confused, inattentive, burning and tingling of hands and feet, loss of position and vibratory sense, weakness and tenderness of muscles, loss of ankle and knee jerk
Gastrointestinal	Anorexia, indigestion, constipation or diarrhea, tract liver or spleen enlargement
Cardiovascular	Tachycardia, cardiomyopathy, arrhythmia, function hypertensive or hypotensive
General	Fatigue on exertion, tired appearance, falls asleep easily
Hair	Stringy, dull, brittle, dry, alopecia, depigmented, can be plucked easily
Skin	Rough, dry, flaky, scaly, pigmented, bruised, petechia
Face and neck	Skin dark over cheeks and eyes, skin around nose and mouth is lumpy or flaky
Lips	Cheilosis, angular fissures at the corner of the mouth, fissures, dry, scaly
Mouth, oral	Swollen, boggy oral mucous membranes
Gums	Spongy, bleed easily, marginal redness, inflamed, gums receding
Tongue	Swelling, scarlet, raw, magenta color, beefy (glossitis), hyperemic and hypertrophic papillae, atrophic papillae
Eyes	Pale conjunctiva, conjunctival injection, dryness, signs of infection, Bitot's spots, angular palpebritis, conjunctival xerosis, keratomalacia
Neck	Thyroid enlarged
Nails	Koilonychia, brittle, ridged, white spots
Legs, feet	Edema, tender calf, tingling, weakness
Skeleton	Bowlegs, knock-knees, chest deformity at diaphragm, beaded ribs, prominent scapulas

Modified from Worthington-Roberts BS et al[1] with permission.

TABLE 210–3. PARAMETERS FOR ASSESSING NUTRITIONAL STATUS: INITIAL SCREENING

Medical, obstetric, and nutritional history
Physical examination
Anthropometric measures
Prepregnancy weight
Pregnancy weight gain
History of weight loss
Laboratory Tests
Plasma proteins
Total proteins
Albumin
Mean corpuscular volume
Hemoglobin and hematocrit
Total lymphocyte count

to allow for added maternal fat reserves. Birth weight of infants born to overweight women tends to be above average, and there is less correlation with maternal weight gain.

Inadequate weight gain or weight loss is usually the first indication of insufficient nutrient intake. The rate of weight gain is also important. During the first trimester a weight gain of 2–5 pounds is considered average. The rate of weight gain increases in the second and third trimester to almost one pound per week. This reflects the rapid growth phase, beginning in the latter half of the second trimester. During the second half of pregnancy, weight gain of less than 0.5 pounds per week may be inadequate. A weight gain of 4–5 pounds in one week indicates excessive fluid retention. This may be the first sign of developing preeclampsia.

Plasma volume during pregnancy begins to increase in the first trimester to greater than 50% by the third trimester.[23] Plasma components and nutrients tend to undergo a physiologic dilution due to relative increase in plasma volume. Consideration of these physiologic changes should be made when interpreting laboratory data. Table 210–5 provides a summary of laboratory tests used for assessment of nutritional status with adjusted values for pregnancy.

Albumin is a transport protein that frequently is used for nutritional assessment. It represents visceral protein mass, and synthesis occurs in the liver. Reduction of albumin, as with other transport proteins, secondary to malnutrition, is a consequence of decreased liver biosynthesis due to limited supply of substrate and actual decrease in organ mass. Albumin has a half-life of 21 days and has a large pool size. Depressed values may reflect chronic dietary inadequacies. Because of its long half-life, albumin is a poor index of acute changes in diet. Accordingly, albumin is not used to monitor early phases of repletion.

Serum concentrations are dependent on the rate of metabolic use, excretion, intravascular-extravascular transfer, and the degree of hydration. Physiologic stress from some disease states, major surgery, and trauma increase vascular permeability and third spacing of albumin. There is also an increased catabolism of albumin by the liver.[24] In these instances, albumin does not reflect nutritional status. During pregnancy, values have been reported to fall as early as five weeks and to continue to decline until the 28th–30th week.[20] Hemodilution is thought to be a contributing factor to the decline. During pregnancy, significant proteinuria is common due to preeclampsia or renal disease and is a major contributor to hypoalbuminemia. This should not be confused with malnutrition.

Hemoglobin, hematocrit, and mean corpuscular volume are used to identify anemia associated with protein inadequacies or micronutrient deficiencies. Anemia, particularly iron deficiency, is common during pregnancy due to the increased requirements that are often difficult to meet by diet alone. Erythropoiesis is increased during pregnancy to meet the metabolic demands of the growing fetus and placenta. The total quantity of red blood cells increases (albeit to a lesser degree than plasma volume). Thus, the relative decrease in hemoglobin concentration is due to a physiologic volume expansion. Hemoglobin and hematocrit decrease to levels considered abnormal during the nonpregnant state. The lowest hemoglobin concentration considered normal should be 10.0 mg% for normal single pregnancy.[25] Values below this may need further investigation for protein or micronutrient deficiencies.

A readily available test frequently used to measure immune function is total lymphocyte count. Total lymphocyte count is derived from a complete blood count, with a differential. The white count is multiplied by the percentage of lymphocytes. Some aspects of immune function (cell-mediated immunity, lymphocyte function) are decreased during pregnancy.[25] However, the total lymphocyte count does not change significantly. Thus, in the absence of non-nutritional factors that alter lymphocyte count, values reflect nutritional status. Depressed levels occur in moderate-to-severe types of malnutrition.

In-depth Assessment

An in-depth assessment may be required for a diagnosis of malnutrition when data from the initial screening is inadequate or inconclusive. Table 210–6 includes parameters for in-depth assessment. It also provides a more comprehensive evaluation of the somatic compartments (fat stores and muscle mass). Transferrin and prealbumin are obtained to determine more recent dietary inadequacies, which may not be reflected by serum albumin.

Measurements of the upper arm and triceps skin fold are obtained to determine energy stores (fat) and protein mass (muscle compartment), which reflect total body dimensions. Depletion of these compartments, particularly protein mass, are most evident with severe protein-energy malnutrition. Reference standards are used for interpreting these measurements. These standards are based on age

TABLE 210–5. LABORATORY TESTS FOR ASSESSMENT OF NUTRITIONAL STATUS ADJUSTED FOR PREGNANCY

Test	Non-Pregnant	Pregnant
Total protein (g/100 mL)	6.5–8.5	6.0–8.0
Albumin (g/100 mL)	3.5–5.0	2.5–4.5
Total iron-binding capacity (mcg/100 mL)	250–400	300–600
Hemoglobin (mg/100 mL)	12	>11
Hematocrit (%)	36	33
Serum iron (mcg/100 mL)	>50	<50
Serum zinc (mcg/100 mL)	65–115	55–80
Urine zinc (mcg/day)	200–450	200–450
Serum calcium (mEq/L)	4.6–5.5	4.2–5.2
Serum phosphorus (mg/100 mL)	2.5–4.8	2.3–4.6
B_{12} (pg/100 mL)	430–1025	Decreased
Serum folate (ng/100 mL)	5–21	3–15
Vitamin A (mcg/100 mL)	20–60	20–60

Modified from MacBurney M, Wilmore DW[71] with permission.

TABLE 210–6. IN-DEPTH ASSESSMENT

- Dietary History
- Calorie Counts
- Anthropometric Measures
  - Triceps Skinfolds
  - Arm Circumference
- Laboratory Tests
  - Transferrin
  - Prealbumin

and gender derived from a large cross-sectional sample.[26] Low percentile may reflect individual biologic variation and not nutritional status. These standards do not account for racial differences. A critique of these standards is reviewed.[27]

Baseline data are established. Generally, measurements are repeated every three-to-four weeks to document changes. These measurements are useful when repleting severely malnourished patients or monitoring change in somatic stores in chronically ill patients. Measurements obtained from healthy pregnant women between 19–36 weeks' gestational age demonstrate changes thought to reflect deposition of subcutaneous fat. In fact, increases occur in total body water and some increase in tissue protein.[28] The maternal increase of extracellular fluid in the second and third trimester may be interpreted erroneously as an increase in fat stores.

Transferrin is a β-globulin synthesized in the liver that transports iron in the blood. Transferrin levels decrease with protein inadequacies, although levels are elevated with iron deficiency. During pregnancy, serum levels increase steadily, peaking during the third trimester. Due to a short half-life of eight days, transferrin is used for monitoring repletion in malnourished patients when nutritional therapy has been implemented.[29] The reliability of transferrin is diminished in patients post-trauma, surgery, or infection.

Thyroxin-binding prealbumin transports thyroxin and also binds with retinol-binding protein for transport of retinol. Prealbumin has a half-life of two days and is more sensitive to acute changes in calorie and protein intake.[30] Shetty[31] demonstrated a decline in prealbumin with calorie and protein restriction. Prealbumin has been demonstrated to be more sensitive to refeeding than albumin and transferrin. Increasing values correlate with positive nitrogen balance in several studies.[32,33] We are unaware of adjusted values for pregnant women. However, values can be expected to decline due to volume expansion. Serial measurements obtained during parenteral nutrition can monitor repletion if baseline values are obtained prior to implementing TPN.

The values of laboratory tests and anthropometric measurements obtained for nutritional assessments are compared to standards based on a healthy population with normal nutritional status. Abnormal values are graded to reflect the severity of depletion and the type of malnutrition. Table 210–7 classifies malnutrition based on the degree of severity. Kwashiorkor would reflect changes in visceral protein and immune function. Marasmus is associated with weight loss and decreases in anthropometric measurements. Mixed types of malnutrition have decreases in somatic and visceral protein compartments.

Monitoring Nutritional Status during Repletions

Serial measurements of parameters obtained during initial nutritional assessment is the most effective method for determining efficacy of parenteral nutrition. Another parameter often incorporated into the monitoring protocol is a nitrogen balance study. Table 210–8 summarizes parameters used for monitoring nutritional status during repletion. The recommended frequency for obtaining these measurements also is shown.

Nitrogen Balance Study

Nitrogen balance reflects the protein status of the patient. Nitrogen intake is determined from the total quantity of protein consumed for a 24-hour period. A 24-hour urine collection of urine urea nitrogen (UUN) is required to determine nitrogen output. This represents the majority of nitrogen lost. There are additional losses in the urine (ammonia, creatinine), stool, and perspiration that are estimated to be approximately 4 g nitrogen per day. Table 210–9 summarizes the calculation for nitrogen balance.

Healthy individuals usually have a zero nitrogen balance or are in equilibrium. For malnourished patients and pregnant women, a positive balance between 2–4 g nitrogen is optimal. Urea nitrogen reflects the quantity of protein catabolized for energy. The quantity excreted depends, in part, on the protein and calorie content of the diet. Values for healthy individuals consuming a typical diet are approximately 6–8 g per day. This represents approximately 80% of total nitrogen lost. Similar patterns of nitrogen excretion probably occur during pregnancy, although the magnitude may be altered. Increased excretion of nitrogen is known to occur from stress due to surgery, trauma, or infection. Severe stress represents a hypercatabolic state, with nitrogen losses of 15–25 g per day.[34] Increased excretion also may occur from inadequate caloric consumption or excessive protein intake. Nitrogen balance should be obtained on day three of parenteral nutrition and weekly thereafter until

TABLE 210–7. INTERPRETING OF DATA IN DETERMINING NUTRITIONAL STATUS[66]

Laboratory Data	Normal	Mild-Moderate	Moderate-Severe
Albumin	2.5–4.5	2.4–2.0	1.9 and below
TIBC	300–600	225–300	225 and below
Total lymphocyte count (cells/mm^3)	1500	1000–1400	1000 and below
ANTHROPOMETRIC DATA			
% Usual weight[a]		80–95%	80% and below
Weight change[b]			
1 week		1–2%	>2%
1 month		3–5%	>5%
3 months		6–8%	>8%

[a] $\% \text{ Usual weight} = \frac{\text{current weight}}{\text{usual weight}} \times 100$

[b] $\% \text{ Weight change} = \frac{(\text{usual weight} - \text{actual weight})}{(\text{usual weight})} \times 100$

Modified from Blackburn GL et al.[66]

TABLE 210–8. MONITORING TO DETERMINE ADEQUACY OF TPN FORMULATION

Day 3 of TPN: Nitrogen Balance

Weekly
- Nitrogen balance
- Transferrin
- Prealbumin
- Weight

Twice Monthly
- Total protein
- Albumin

Monthly (every 2.5–3.5 weeks)
- Triceps skinfolds
- Arm circumference

it is evident that the patient is anabolic with improvement of other nutritional parameters.

CONSIDERATIONS REGARDING NUTRIENT INTAKE DURING PREGNANCY

Caloric Intake

Adequate caloric intake is essential for achieving positive nitrogen balance and weight gain during pregnancy. The National Research Council (NRC)[35] has recommended an additional 300 calories above the recommended dietary allowances (RDA) for nonpregnant women based on the energy cost for the entire pregnancy. This estimate includes the energy cost of maintenance, metabolism, tissue growth of mother and fetus, and increased maternal fat stores. Basal energy requirements and costs of activities have been shown to increase throughout pregnancy. Studies comparing energy expenditure of nonpregnant and pregnant women (using indirect calorimetry) vary between 13% and 37% above the nonpregnant basal metabolic rate (BMR).[36-38] The energy cost of activity and exercise also has been shown to increase throughout pregnancy.[37,38] However, the total daily expenditure does not increase substantially due to an overall decrease in activity.

Methods for Assessing Energy Expenditure

A predictive method of determining energy requirement may be used for pregnant women with complications altering energy expenditures not accounted for with the RDA. The Harris–Benedict equation estimates basal energy expenditure (BEE). This equation was derived from regression analysis of data obtained with indirect calorimetry from healthy nonpregnant women. The patient's height, weight, and age are necessary to calculate BEE. A multiplying factor is used to adjust for increased energy demands during pregnancy. Each disease states (surgery, trauma, and severe or chronic malnutrition) alters energy expenditure.[39-42] A similar multiplying factor is applied to adjust for these conditions. Table 210–10 provides an example of calculations and factors for determining energy requirements.

When it is difficult to assess energy expenditure using a predictive equation, a method for measuring energy expenditure may be employed. Indirect calorimetry is used in the hospital setting. This requires a collection of expired gas from the patient to determine resting metabolic rate. Indirect calorimetry has been validated by comparative studies with direct calorimetry, which measures heat production.[43] This method can be fairly accurate, provided that gas collections are conducted by trained personnel for a minimum of 30–45 minutes during stable conditions.

TABLE 210–9. CALCULATING NITROGEN BALANCE

Nitrogen balance N intake − N output

$$\text{N intake} = \frac{\text{g protein/24 hours}}{6.25}$$

N output = g nitrogen (UUN) + 4 g (stool, sweat)

UUN = urine urea nitrogen

Calorie Substrate: Dextrose and Lipid

Optimal protein use, anabolism, and weight gain require simultaneous infusion of the calorie substrates dextrose and lipid. The proportion of these substrates is also important. The caloric distribution of a standard parenteral solution for a stable and nonstressed patient is 15% protein, 60% carbohydrates, and 25% fat. This profile is comparable to standard enteral formulas and is a recommended dietary guideline for healthy individuals. The standard formula is appropriate for most pregnant patients. Table 210–11 provides examples of standard central and peripheral parenteral solutions. Adjustments in this distribution are required when abnormalities in energy and protein metabolism secondary to organ dysfunction or failure are apparent. Patients with renal or liver failure require an increase in dextrose and lipid calories, with a decrease in the protein. A decrease in the carbohydrate content to 45–50% of total calories usually is required for patients with diabetes, pancreatitis, and severe trauma. Sepsis can induce lipid intolerance and require reduction or omission of lipid calories.

Hydrous dextrose is an essential component of paren-

TABLE 210–10. ESTIMATING ENERGY REQUIREMENTS[39–41]

Calculate Resting Energy Expenditure per day (BEE) using Harris-Benedict Equation

BEE = 665 + 9.6 (weight in kg) + 1.8 (height in cm) − 4.6 (age in years)

BEE × AF = energy expenditure/24 hours

Activity Factors (AF)

Pregnancy	1.15
Sedentary	1.25
Anabolic	1.35–1.50
Severe malnutrition	0.90–1.10
Mild stress (minor surgery, tumor with treatment)	1.30–1.40
Moderate stress (GI surgery, infection)	1.40–1.60
Severe stress (burns, trauma, major surgery, sepsis)	1.70–2.0

Example

Pregnant woman status post-cholecystectomy with postoperative ileus. In good nutritional status on admission.

Height: 5′1″

Weight: 60 kg

Age: 21 years

BEE = 665 + 576 + 215 − 97 = 1339 Kcal

Caloric requirement/24 hour = 1339 × 1.15 (pregnancy) × 1.4 (moderate stress) = 2062 Kcal

TABLE 210–11. STANDARD CENTRAL AND PERIPHERAL PARENTERAL NUTRITION FORMULAS

Central[a]		Peripheral[b]	
1000 mL 7% amino acids		1500 mL 3.5% amino acids	
1000 mL 40% dextrose		1500 mL 10% dextrose	
500 mL 10% lipid or		500 mL 10% lipid	
250 mL 20% lipid			
Electrolytes		**Electrolytes**	
Sodium	80–100 mEq	Sodium	40–60 mEq
Potassium	70–90 mEq	Potassium	25–35 mEq
Chloride	120–160 mEq	Chloride	50–60 mEq
Calcium	9–12 mEq	Calcium	4–6 mEq
Phosphorus	12–18 mmol	Phosphorus	4–6 mmol
Magnesium	8–16 mEq	Magnesium	4–6 mEq
Other Additives		**Other Additives**	
MVI-12	10 mL	MVI-12	10 mL
Multitrace element concentrate	1 mL	Multitrace element concentrate	1 mL
Vitamin K4	10 mg/week		

[a] Total volume contains approximately 2500 mL and provides 2200 total calories, 70 g protein, 400 g dextrose, 50 g fat. The caloric distribution is 13% protein, 62% carbohydrate, 25% fat with a nonprotein calorie to nitrogen ratio of 150:1. This solution would be appropriate for a pregnant patient assuming no organ failure that would require alteration in fluid or substrate and micronutrient.

[b] Total volume contains approximately 3500 mL and provides 1240 total calories, 45 g protein, 150 g dextrose, 50 g fat. The nonprotein calorie to nitrogen ratio is 141:1 and has a caloric distribution of 15% protein, 41% carbohydrate, and 44% fat.

teral formulas to meet the metabolic demands of the fetus (primary energy source) and maternal glucose-dependent tissue (brain). To meet the caloric requirements with TPN, high carbohydrate concentrations are used. This may exacerbate hyperglycemia in the pregnant patients. Proper advancement of the TPN solution, with frequent monitoring of blood glucose, is necessary to maintain blood glucose in tight control (80–140) to avoid the harmful effects of hyperglycemia on the fetus. Most patients adapt to the high glucose load with increased insulin production. However, supplemental insulin may be required to maintain acceptable blood sugars. The continuous infusion schedule (typically used during hospitalization) eliminates hypoglycemia and ketosis most often apparent during pregnancy from overnight fasting. Dextrose concentrations typically used for TPN are 40–60% with volumes of 800–12,000 mL. A dextrose concentration of 70% is used for fluid-restricted patients.

Lipids are required to provide essential fatty acids to the fetus and mother. The essential fatty acid, linoleic acid, a component of cell membranes (phospholipids) and a major component of brain matter, is required for fetal growth and cell division. An animal study, with induced essential fatty acid deficiency during pregnancy, demonstrated reduced brain lipid content and impaired learning ability in the offspring.[44] Linoleic acid is also a precursor to prostaglandins that demonstrate various regulating effects on the vascular and endocrine milieu of the placenta and uterus.[45] A nonpregnant adult requires approximately 3–4% of total calories to meet essential fatty acid requirements. An additional 1% increase is recommended to satisfy the needs of the growing fetus.[46] This equates to approximately a 10% lipid emulsion of 500 mL infused three times per week. Concentrations of 10 or 20% may be used. Daily lipid administration is recommended to provide essential fatty acids and dual-energy sources. During pregnancy, lipids should be provided as approximately 15–25% of total calories. An initial test dose of 100–150 mL generally is advisable to determine lipid tolerance and adequate lipid clearance, since hypertriglyceridemia may occur with pregnancy. Lipids should be infused over 8–12 hours for adequate lipid clearance.

There has been concern that lipid infusion may induce labor.[47] Jaisle[48] reported premature delivery in rabbits after infusion of choline phosphatide solution. Jarvinen[49] demonstrated similar results in pregnancy that exceeded term. Myometrial contractions occurred after infusion of lipids. The composition of the lipid solution was not reported, but it was a commercial product not distributed in the United States. Seifer et al[11] summarized 27 reports of parenteral nutrition used during pregnancy. Nineteen patients received lipids. Seven were peripheral lipid-based solutions. There were premature deliveries in this group that were attributed to non-nutritional factors. Lee and associates[10] found no cases of apparent premature labor or fatty infiltration of the placenta in patients receiving lipids. None of the patients received more than 25% of calories as lipid.

Protein Requirements

Fetal growth and development and maternal physiologic changes of pregnancy rely on the availability of substrate to promote protein synthesis. Consumption of protein with high biologic value in proper proportions, supported by adequate intake of calories, should be maintained throughout pregnancy. Accrued protein synthesis during pregnancy is approximately 950 g. The majority of protein accretion occurs in the second and third trimester. Thus, protein requirements change during pregnancy. Rates of protein accretion during pregnancy were distributed quarterly in 10-week intervals with protein accretion of 0.6, 1.8, 4.8, and 6.1 g/dL, respectively.[25]

The recommendations by the NRC use the nonpregnant protein requirements of 44 g plus 30 g per day, or 1.3 g/kg body weight, which is relatively high compared to other countries. The World Health Organization (WHO)[50] recommended protein allowances of 6 g protein per day.

This value assumes a high quality protein (eggs, milk, for example) and does not account for the changing rate of protein synthesis throughout pregnancy. Protein requirements are increased when malnutrition is apparent or after trauma or surgery. Although discrepancies limit the usefulness of data to determine protein requirements, nitrogen balance studies are useful in determining the individual adequacy of a prescribed diet and should be conducted when parenteral nutrition is implemented.

Amino Acids

Amino acid requirements during pregnancy have not been clearly defined. Maternal plasma amino acid profiles are lower than values reported for nonpregnant women. Fetal plasma levels are higher than maternal values. Amino acids are transported against a concentration gradient.[46] Values obtained during weeks 20–36 of pregnancy demonstrated a decline in arginine, ornithine, glutamine (reflecting a decrease in urea genesis); branch-chain amino acids (leucine, isoleucine, and valine); serine, lysine, and taurine. The decrease in branch-chain amino acids may reflect increased uptake by maternal muscle due to increased insulin and use by the fetus for energy.[51] There is an increase in aspartic acid, histidine, proline, and threonine. Variations in plasma amino acids were noted in mothers with small babies and those with large babies.[51] The physiologic basis for these changes is unclear, but may reflect certain placental transport mechanisms.

Parenteral Amino Acid Solutions

The amino acid profile of base solutions provides essential and nonessential amino acids. The distribution of these amino acid solutions is approximately 43% essential and 57% nonessential amino acids. The essential amino acid to total nitrogen content (E:T ratio) is 2.9. An E:T ratio of 3 is considered optimal for growing infants and restoration of body protein in malnourished adults.[52] The most suitable amino acid solutions for pregnant women are Freeamine and Aminosyn. Both have a more desirable essential amino acid profile, with an increase in branched-chain amino acids and slightly lower aromatic amino acid.

Vitamins

Requirements for most vitamins increase during pregnancy. Intravenous supplementation of vitamins during pregnancy has not been clearly defined. The standard parenteral multivitamin preparations have been developed within the guidelines established by the American Medical Association (AMA) Nutrition Advisory Committee. These preparations were designed to meet the requirements of most patients requiring TPN.[53] Based on oral daily allowances, these preparations are suitable for most pregnant patients requiring TPN. These vitamin preparations provide adequate vitamins with the exception of vitamin E, vitamin D, and folic acid. Patients diagnosed as having moderate-to-severe malnutrition are subject to marginal vitamin status and may require additional supplementation. Physiologic stress due to infection, surgery, or trauma requires additional supplementation of some vitamins. Documented vitamin deficiencies should be treated with single doses of specific vitamins. Table 210–12 provides vitamin contents of multi-vitamin preparations.

Trace Elements and Minerals

There are several trace elements required during pregnancy. Daily allowances are not clearly defined. Four trace elements have been considered necessary during parenteral nutrition by the AMA.[54] These are zinc, manganese, copper, and chromium. They should be supplemented daily. In addition, some recommend supplementing selenium, molybdenum, and iodine during long-term TPN to prevent cases of deficiency.[55,56] Table 210–13 lists the requirements of these trace elements.

Requirements for most minerals increase during pregnancy (although specific requirements are less well defined).

TABLE 210–12. VITAMIN REQUIREMENTS DURING PREGNANCY AND PARENTERAL MVI SUPPLEMENT

Vitamin	Pregnant RDA	% Above NonPregnant RDA	Parenteral MVI Preparation/10 ml
Vitamin A (IU)	3300	25%	3300
Vitamin D (IU)	400	50%	200
Vitamin E (IU)	15	25%	10
B_1 Thiamin (mg)	1.4	40%	3
B_2 Riboflavin (mg)	1.5	25%	3.6
B_3 Pantothenic acid (mg)	6	—	15
B_5 Niacin (mg)	15	15%	40
B_6 Pyridoxine (mcg)	2.6	30%	4
B_7 Biotin (mcg)	100	—	60
B_9 Folic Acid (mcg)	800	100%	400
B_{12} Cobalamin (mcg)	4	33%	5
C Ascorbic acid (mg)	80	33%	100

Vitamin K supplementation is not recommended officially since some patients are on anticoagulant therapy. Typical dose for patients receiving TPN and not eating is 5–10 mg/week. Synkovite (vitamin K_4) may be administered in TPN formula or IM injection. Requirements do not change during pregnancy. However, requirements increase if bleeding has occurred.

Preparations comply with the recommended daily dose established by the AMA/Nutrition Advisory Group.

Data are obtained from references 53 and 67.

TABLE 210–13. TRACE ELEMENT REQUIREMENTS DURING PREGNANCY AND PARENTERAL TRACE MINERAL SUPPLEMENT

Trace Mineral	Pregnant RDA	% Above Nonpregnant RDA	AMA Council TPN Recommendation	Trace Additive
Zinc (mg)	20	33%	2.5–4.0	4.0
Copper (mg)	2–3	—	0.5–1.5	1.0
Chromium (mcg)	5–20	—	10–15	10.0
Manganese (mg)	2.5–5.0	—	0.5–0.8	0.5

The following trace elements should be added to parenteral nutrition solutions if patient has been receiving it for more than four weeks or has been diagnosed with severe malnutrition or malabsorption. Though rare, there have been reported cases of deficiency occurring during long-term TPN.

Trace Mineral	Dose
Selenium (mcg)	20–60
Iodine (mcg)	25–50
Molybdenum (mcg)	25–50

Iron may be administered intramuscularly. Iron stores should be assessed to determine appropriate supplemental dosage.

Data modified from references 67 and 68.

Approximate daily supplement is indicated in Table 210–11. Iron usually is administered as an intramuscular injection or intravenously.

METHODS OF ADMINISTRATION

Central

Central venous catheters usually are placed in the subclavian vein. Multilumen catheters are used most often. There is an increased rate of catheter-related sepsis with multilumen compared to single-lumen catheters. Thus, it may be prudent to use single-lumen catheters whenever possible. A more permanent catheter is placed for long-term (or home) TPN (Hickman, Broviac). The central route allows safe infusion of hypertonic solutions with osmolarity exceeding 1000 mosmol and of volumes of up to 3500 mL daily. Central formulas, which are nutritionally complete, consist of amino acids, electrolytes, vitamins, and minerals. Volumes are based on concentration, content of additives, and fluid requirements. An average volume is approximately 2000–2500 mL infused over a 24-hour period. Lipids usually are coinfused through a Y-connector, although some institutions combine lipid into the TPN formula. This is referred to as 3-in-1 admixture. Due to the high carbohydrate content, TPN is initiated with one third to one half the total quantity of calories required during the first 12–24 hours. Advancement in increments of one third to one half every 12–24 hours is employed if plasma glucose levels are acceptable.[43]

A cyclical schedule generally is used for long-term and home TPN patients. A typical schedule of 12 hours on and 12 hours off is employed. The TPN formulation is infused during the night to allow freedom of movement during day-time activity. This method of feeding introduces greater fluctuations in plasma glucose due to decreased infusion time of dextrose and long fasting periods. A more appropriate cyclical schedule for a pregnant patient is 16 hours on and 8 hours off.

Peripheral

The peripheral catheter typically is placed in the forearm. The catheter site is rotated 24–72 hours, depending on the appearance of the catheter site and the integrity of the vein. Peripheral parenteral nutrition usually is limited to 5–7 days. Peripheral formulas contain a low-grade concentration of additives to maintain an osmolarity of <900 mosm. An osmolarity of >900 mosm will cause thrombophlebitis.

Monitoring

Ongoing monitoring with laboratory tests is essential for achieving nutritional goals (see nutritional assessment section) and minimizing metabolic abnormalities and complications. Table 210–14 summarizes monitored parameters and the recommended frequency.

CATHETER-RELATED COMPLICATIONS

Catheter-related complications can be grouped into two types: technical and infectious. The incidence of technical complications resulting from catheter placement vary from institution to institution. Grant[57] summarized complications of 10,130 subclavian vein catheterizations between 1956 to 1978. The total rate was 4.2%. Major complications were 2.4%. The more common complications include pneumo-

TABLE 210–14. RECOMMENDED MONITORING PARAMETERS

Daily
- Intake and output
- Weight
- Electrolytes
- Capillary glucose q 4–6 hours
- Calorie Counts

Twice Weekly
- Calcium, magnesium, phosphorus
- BUN, creatinine
- Liver function tests

Weekly
- Nitrogen balance study
- Triglyceride level 6 hours after infusion of lipids, then every other week

thorax, which usually resolves spontaneously. However, some may enlarge and require chest tube placement. Arterial puncture should be recognized easily and generally is managed by catheter removal and applied pressure. Arterial puncture has the potential to result in cardiac tamponade. A case report of cardiac tamponade occurred in a pregnant woman on the seventh day of TPN. This resulted in cardiac arrest with subsequent maternal brain death and fetal demise.[58]

Less common complications include air emboli that occur during attempts to manipulate the catheter during insertion. Such attempts may exacerbate emboli or cause a thrombosis. Malposition of the catheter into smaller vessels has a higher incidence of phlebitis and may lead to thrombosis.[59]

Catheter-related sepsis is one of the most serious complications related to parenteral nutrition. The rate of sepsis is highly variable, from 1.6% to 24%.[60,61] Contributing factors are contamination during line placement and dressing changes, and violation of the infusion line by "piggy-backing" other solutions that require frequent disconnection. The most effective methods for decreasing the incidence of catheter-related sepsis is use of a dedicated nutritional support team. Alternatively, a dedicated intravenous team responsible for placement and care of catheters in the TPN population is appropriate.

Metabolic Complications

The pregnant woman is subject to metabolic abnormalities and complications observed in a TPN population. There is more concern during pregnancy due to potential adverse effects on the fetus. Metabolic abnormalities may occur from improper dosing relative to preexisting disease states or previously unidentified deficiencies. Abnormalities, as evidenced by laboratory testing (electrolytes, plasma glucose), occur in most patients receiving parenteral nutrition. However, the incidence of clinically significant complications is much less common. Table 210–15 summarizes metabolic complications associated with TPN.

Parenteral nutrition potentiates deficiencies to an order of magnitude and rapidity of onset never seen with oral consumption of nutrients. Parenteral nutrition is intensely anabolic. Electrolytes, vitamins, and mineral replacement (ordinarily adequate) may be inadequate with rapid tissue synthesis. Severe deficiencies of magnesium, phosphorus, and potassium have occurred during the first week of parenteral nutrition.[62] Overt signs of vitamin and mineral deficiencies have been reported to occur as early as two weeks. Long-term home TPN has introduced deficiencies rarely or never observed in the general population (biotin, vitamins A and E, molybdenum, selenium, chromium). Nutrients, thought to be nonessential, actually may be conditionally essential in some disease states. Such recognized nutrients are amino acids (cystine, tyrosine, and taurine), choline, and carnitine. Observed syndromes usually demonstrate clinical improvement when supplementation has been augmented.[62]

Bone disease may occur in patients on long-term TPN. This is associated with severe urinary losses of calcium and phosphorus and results in excessive demineralization of bone.[63,64] Patients may have bone pain and fractures. The etiology is not known, but has been attributed to vitamin D status. Plasma 25-hydroxyvitamin-D levels were normal with a decrease in 1,25-hydroxyvitamin-D in some patients. Shike[65] noted an association with the vitamin D dosage in the TPN. In the patients who were symptomatic,

TABLE 210–15. METABOLIC COMPLICATIONS

Complication	Possible Cause
Protein metabolism	
Hyperammonia	Excessive protein intake
	Liver dysfunction
	Zinc deficiency
	Sepsis
Elevated BUN	Inadequate calories, poor protein use
	Excessive protein intake
Carbohydrate metabolism	
Hyperglycemia	Excessive infusion rate of glucose
	Excessive glucose concentration
	Sepsis or infection
	Stress, trauma, or surgery
Hyperosmolar nonketotic dehydration	Persistent hyperglycemia with osmotic diuresis
	Negative fluid balance due to losses (NG suction, diarrhea)
	Diuretics
Hypoglycemia	Abrupt interruption of TPN infusion
	Excessive insulin dose
Fatty liver	Prolonged excessive carbohydrate administration leading to excessive fat deposition in the liver
	Corticosteroid therapy
	Diabetes mellitus
	Essential fatty acid deficiency
Fat metabolism	
Essential fatty acid deficiency	Inadequate dosage or omission
Lipid intolerance	
Acute	Inadequate dosage of lipid
Long-term (apparent by increased triglyceride level)	Infusion rate too rapid
	Excessive lipid administration
	Carnitine deficiency
Electrolyte metabolism	
Hypokalemia	Excessive gastrointestinal and urinary losses
	Deficit of potassium in TPN relative to anabolic requirements
Hyponatremia	Excessive free water
	Edema forming state (CHF, renal or liver failure)
Hypomagnesemia	Inadequate administration of magnesium relative to protein anabolism
	Excessive losses from diarrhea
Hypophosphatemia	Inadequate administration of phosphate
	Concentrated glucose infusion may precipitate hypophosphatemia
Miscellaneous	
Failure to achieve positive nitrogen balance	Underestimation of calorie requirements
	Underestimation of protein losses
	Zinc deficiency

resolution of symptoms occurred with discontinuation of vitamin D.

CONCLUSIONS

Protein energy malnutrition has harmful effects on pregnancy outcome. Medical advances provide alternative methods of feeding pregnant women who are unable to ingest and adequately absorb nutrients through the GI tract. Clinical experience has shown TPN to be safe and effective in general during pregnancy. Research is warranted to establish maternal and fetal nutrient requirements for parenteral nutrition.

Parenteral nutrition potentiates several metabolic complications. Appropriate assessment and ongoing monitoring is essential to achieve nutritional goals and minimize complications associated with TPN.

REFERENCES

1. Worthington-Roberts BS, Vermeesch J, Jacobs AN. Maternal Nutrition and the Outcome of Pregnancy. In: *Nutrition in Pregnancy and Lactation*. 3rd ed. St. Louis, MO: Time/Mirror/Mosby College Publishing; 1985.
2. Hurley LS. General Nutrition and Prenatal Development. In: *Developmental Nutrition*. Englewood Cliffs, NJ: Prentice-Hall; 1980.
3. Falkner F. Maternal nutrition and fetal growth. *Am J Clin Nutr*. 1981;34:769.
4. Higgins AC. Nutritional status and the outcome of pregnancy. *J Can Diet Assoc*. 1976;37:17.
5. Worthington-Roberts BS. The Physiologic Basis of Nutritional Needs. In: *Nutrition in Pregnancy and Lactation*. 3rd ed. St. Louis, MO: Time/Mirror/Mosby College Publishing; 1985.
6. Starker PM, Lasala PA, Askanazi J, et al. The response to TPN: a form of nutritional assessment. *Ann Surg*. 1983;198(6):720.
7. Rhoads JE, Dudrick SJ, Vars HM. History of Intravenous Nutrition. In: Rombeau and Caldwell, eds. *Parenteral Nutrition*. Philadelphia: WB Saunders; 1986;2.
8. Shizgal HM. Body composition and nutritional support. *Surg Clin N Amer*. 1981;61(3):729.
9. Grant JP. Patient Selection. In: *Handbook of Total Parenteral Nutrition*. Philadelphia: WB Saunders; 1980.
10. Lee R, Roders B, Young C, et al. Review: total parenteral nutrition during pregnancy. *Obstet Gynecol*. 1986;68(4):563.
11. Seifer D, Silberman H, Catanzrite V, et al. Total parenteral nutrition in obstetrics. *JAMA*. 1985;253(14):2073.
12. Kirby DF, Fiorenza V, Craig R. Intravenous nutritional support during pregnancy. *JPEN*. 1988;12(7):72.
13. Rayburn W, Wolk P, Mercer N, et al. Parenteral nutrition in obstetrics and gynecology. *Ob Gyn Surv*. 1986;41(4):200.
14. Grant JP, Cusater PC, Thurlow J. Current techniques of nutritional assessment. *Surg Clin N Amer*. 1981;61(3):437.
15. Buzby GP, Mullen JL. Nutritional assessment. In: Rombeau and Caldwell, eds. *External and Tube Feeding*. Philadelphia: WB Saunders; 1984;1.
16. Anderson CF, Meister J. The sensitivity and specificity of nutritional-related variables in relationship to the duration of hospital stay and the rate of complications. *Mayo Clin Proc*. 1984;59:444.
17. Peckman CH, Christianson RE. The relationship between prepregnancy weight and certain obstetric factors. *Am J Obstet Gynecol*. 1971;111(1):1.
18. King JC, Bronstien MN, Fitch WL, Weininger J. Nutrient utilization during pregnancy. *Wld Rev Nutr Diet*. 1987;52:71.
19. Simpson JW, Lawless RW, Mitchell AC. Responsibility of the obstetrician to the fetus: II. Influence of pre-pregnancy weight and pregnancy weight gain on birthweight. *Obstet Gynecol*. 1975;45:481.
20. Hytten FE, Lind T. *Diagnostic Indices in Pregnancy*. Switzerland: CIBA-Geigy, LTD; 1973.
21. Luke B, Petrie RH. Intrauterine growth: correlation of infant birth weight and maternal postpartum weight. *Am J Clin Nutr*. 1980;33:2311.
22. Naeye RL. Weight gain and the outcome of pregnancy. *Am J Obstet Gynecol*. 1979;135:3.
23. The National Research Council. *Physiologic Adjustments in General in Laboratory Indices of Nutritional Status in Pregnancy*. Washington, DC: National Academy of Sciences: 1978.
24. Fleck A, Colley CM, Myers MA. Liver export proteins and trauma. *Br Med Bull*. 1985;41:265.
25. Hytten FE, Leitch I. *The Physiology of Human Pregnancy*. Oxford: Blackwell Scientific Publications. 1971.
26. Frishanco A. Triceps skin fold and upper arm size norms for assessment of nutritional status. *Am J Clin Nutr*. 1974;27:1052.
27. Gray GE, Kulhanck-Gray L. Anthropometric measurements and their interpretation: principles, practices and problems. *J Am Diet Assoc*. 1980;77:534.
28. Metcoff J, Costiloe JP, Crosby W, et al. Maternal nutrition and fetal outcome. *Am J Clin Nutr*. 1981;34:708.
29. Grant A, Dehoog S. *Biochemical Assessment in Nutritional Assessment and Support*. Seattle, WA: Published by the authors; 1985.
30. Cavaroch NC, Au FC, Dolal FR, et al. Rapid turnover proteins as nutritional indicators. *World J Surg*. 1981;10:468.
31. Shetty PS, Jung RT, Watrasiecie KE, et al. Rapid turnover transport proteins: an index of subclinical protein-energy malnutrition. *Lancet*. 1979;2:230.
32. Church JM, Hill GL. Assessing the efficacy of intravenous nutrition in general surgery patients: dynamic nutritional assessment with plasma proteins. *JPEN*. 1986;11:468.
33. Young GA, Collins JP, Hill GL. Plasma proteins in patients receiving intravenous amino acids of intravenous hyperalimentation after major surgery. *Am J Clin Nutr*. 1981;32:1192.
34. Wilmore DW. *Energy and Energy Balance in the Metabolic Management of the Critically Ill*. New York: Plenum Press; 1980.
35. *National Research Council Daily Recommended Allowances*. Washington DC. National Academy of Sciences; 1980.
36. Blackburn MW, Calloway DW. Basal metabolic rate and work energy expenditure of the mature pregnant woman. *J Am Diet Assoc*. 1976;69:24.
37. Emerson K, Saxena BN, Poindexter EL. Calorie cost of normal pregnancy. *Obstet Gynecol*. 1972;40:786.
38. Blackburn MW, Calloway DM. Energy expenditure and consumption of mature pregnancy and lactating women. *J Am Diet Assoc*. 1976;69:29.
39. Caldwell MD, Kennedy-Caldwell C. Normal nutritional requirements. *Surg Clin N Am*. 1981;61:489.
40. Elwyn DH, Kinney JM, Askanazi J. Energy expenditure in the surgical patient. *Surg Clin N Am*. 1981;6:545.
41. Foster GD, Knox LS, Dempsy DT, Mullen JL. Caloric requirements in total parenteral nutrition. *J Am Coll Nutr*. 1987;6:231.
42. Quebbman EJ, Ausman RK. Estimating energy requirement in patients receiving parenteral nutrition. *Arch Surg*. 1982;117:1281.
43. Ota DM, Imbembo AL, Zuidema GD. Total parenteral nutrition. *Surgery*. 1978;83:503.
44. Lamptey MS, Walker BL. Learning behavior and brain lipid composition in rats subjected to essential fatty acid deficiency during gestation, lactation, and growth. *J Nutr*. 1978;108:358.
45. Hyman M. *Prostaglandins in the Perinatal Period: Their Physiologic and Clinical Importance*. New York: Grune & Stratton; 1980.
46. Kennaugh JM, Hay WW. Nutrition in the fetus and newborn. *West J Med*. 1987;47:435.
47. Heller J. Parenteral nutrition in obstetrics and gynecology. In: Greep JM, Soete PB, et al eds. *Current Concepts in Parenteral Nutrition*. The Hague, Netherlands: Nijhoff Medical Division; 1977.
48. Jaisle F. Infusion of phosphatides in animals during the last third of gestation. *Bibl Gynec Fasc*. 1964;42:191.
49. Jarvinen PA, Luukanen T, Short ER, et al. The effects of an infusion on phospholipid on the human myometrium. *Ann Med Exp Biol Fer*. 1963;42:21.
50. Whitehead RG. Pregnancy and lactation. In: Shil ME, Young VR, eds. *Modern Nutrition in Health and Disease*. Philadelphia: Lea and Febiger; 1988.
51. McClain P, Metcoff J, Crosby WM, Costiloe JP. The relationship of maternal amino acid profiles at 25 weeks of gestation to fetal growth. *Am J Clin Nutr*. 1978;31:401.
52. Rusho WJ, Standish R, Bair JN. A comparison of crystalline amino acid solutions for total parenteral nutrition. *Hosp Form*. 1981;5:29.
53. AMA Nutrition Advisory Group. Multivitamin preparations for parenteral use. *JPEN*. 1979;3:258.
54. AMA Nutrition Advisory Group. Guidelines for essential trace element preparations for parenteral use. *JPEN*. 1979;3:263.
55. Howard L, Michaled AV. Home parenteral nutrition. *Ann Rev Nutr*. 1984;4:69.
56. Baptista RJ, Bistrian BR, Blackburn GL, et al. Utilizing selenious acid to reverse selenium deficiency in total parenteral nutrition patients. *Am J Clin Nutr*. 1984;39:816.
57. Grant J. Subclavian catheter insertion and complications. In: *Handbook of Total Parenteral Nutrition*. Philadelphia: WB Saunders; 1980:47.
58. Greenspoon JS, Masaki DI, Kurz CR. Cardiac tamponade during central hyperalimentation. *Obstet Gynecol*. 1989;73:465.
59. Fischer JE, Freund HR. *Central Hyperalimentation in Surgical Nutrition*. Boston: Little Brown; 1983.
60. Faubion WC, Wesley JR, Khalidi N, Silva J. Total parenteral nutrition catheter sepsis: the impact of the team approach. *JPEN*. 1986;10:642.

61. Moran T, Atwood M. A clinical and bacteriologic study of infection associated with venous cutdowns. *N Engl J Med.* 1977;272:554.
62. Chepponi JX, Bleier JC, Santi MT. Deficiencies of essential and conditionally essential nutrients. *Am J Clin Nutr.* 1982;35:1112.
63. Sauberlich HE. Biochemical alterations in thiamine deficiency, their interpretation. *Am J Clin Nutr.* 1967;20:528.
64. Hurley LS. *Fat Soluble Vitamins In Developmental Nutrition.* Englewood Cliffs, NJ: Prentice-Hall; 1980.
65. Shike M, Sturtridge WC, Tam CS, et al. A possible role of vitamin D in the genesis of parenteral-nutrition induced metabolic bone disease. *Ann Int Med.* 1981;95:560.
66. Blackburn GL, Bistrian BR, Maini BS, Schlamm HT, et al. Nutritional assessment of the hospitalized patient. *JPEN.* 1977;1:11.
67. Williams SR. Nutritional guidance in prenatal care. In: *Nutrition in Pregnancy and Lactation.* 3rd ed. St. Louis, MO: Times/Mirror/Mosby College Publishing; 1985:132.
68. Ronaghy HA. The role of zinc in human nutrition. *Wld Rev Nutr Diet.* 1987;54:237.
69. Sandstead R. Zinc nutrition in the United States. *Am J Clin Nutr.* 1985;26:1251.
70. Blackburn GL, Bothe A Jr. Assessment of malnutrition in cancer patients. *Cancer Bull.* 1978;30:90.
71. MacBurney M, Wilmore DW. Parenteral nutrition in pregnancy. In: Rombeau and Caldwell, eds. *Parenteral Nutrition.* Philadelphia: WB Saunders; 1986;2.

Chapter Two Hundred and Eleven

Critical Care in Obstetrics

William C. Mabie

211

In the past few years, several large obstetric services have created obstetric intensive care units in labor and delivery or in a contiguous area. The purpose of these units is intensive maternal and fetal surveillance and supportive care during the antepartum and immediate postpartum period. The obstetric intensive care unit (ICU) is the outgrowth of a number of developments. One is the development of the subspecialty of maternal-fetal medicine, which has produced physicians focused only on obstetrics who have in-depth knowledge of medical and surgical problems of pregnancy. Another development has been the widespread acceptance of the ICU concept. Although the idea of special care units evolved late in the 19th century, it was not until the 1960s that intensive care units burgeoned. Now large tertiary care centers often have medical, surgical, neonatal, pediatric, neurosurgery, and cardiac surgery ICUs, as well as coronary care units and burn units. The development of new equipment and new knowledge also has added impetus. Examples of new equipment include the ECG monitor, intra-arterial blood pressure monitor, pulse oximeter, positive pressure ventilator, pulmonary artery catheter, and intracranial pressure monitor. Examples of the new knowledge include the concepts of preload and afterload augmentation and reduction, oxygen delivery and consumption, and pharmacologic support with antiarrhythmics, inotropes, vasopressors, vasodilators, and beta blockers. Of importance to obstetrics is the more liberal attitude among physicians toward allowing pregnancy in patients with major organ disease or multisystem disease.

The following discussion of obstetric intensive care is influenced by the past four years' experience of the author as director of the obstetric intensive care unit at the University of Tennessee, Memphis.[1] We will begin with a discussion of facilities, staffing, type of patients admitted to the ICU, and benefits of the ICU. We then will discuss technical aspects such as inserting a pulmonary artery catheter and understanding the data. This will be followed by a brief discussion of colloid osmotic pressure and of the central hemodynamics of preeclampsia. Other topics related to ICU care such as septic shock, massive hemorrhage, and pulmonary embolism are discussed in other chapters in this text.

FACILITIES

The size of the obstetric ICU depends on the volume of deliveries. Roughly one percent of deliveries will require maternal intensive care. The ICU should have capability for isolating infected patients (wound infections, hepatitis, and varicella). Handwashing facilities should be available inside the room. There should be enough space around the beds for portable x-ray equipment to maneuver and for several caretakers to be present at the bedside. A delivery bed should be available so that the patient can labor and deliver in the ICU. For invasive hemodynamic monitoring, a three- or four-channel hemodynamic monitor, cardiac output computer, strip recorder, and printer are needed. A pulse oximeter and a colloid oncometer are also necessary. Emergency equipment items include a "crash cart," defibrillator, suction machine, and electrocardiogram machine. Fetal monitors should be readily available. A view box for reviewing chest x-rays, wall suction, and oxygen should be available, including set up for a respirator.

STAFFING

It is relatively easy to obtain equipment for an ICU, but another issue to recruit experienced, well-trained nurses. Some centers use a labor and delivery nurse for the obstetric care and a medical ICU nurse for managing the hemodynamic monitoring. This is expensive and less than ideal in terms of merging the two disciplines for optimal patient management, that is, one nurse who can put the whole picture together. Labor and delivery nurses can function well as obstetric intensive care nurses. In addition, they are able to work in normal labor and delivery when there are no patients in the obstetric intensive care unit. This prevents "burn-out" and also raises the general level of nursing care in the labor and delivery area. Labor and delivery nurses must receive training in high-risk obstetric intensive care, invasive hemodynamic monitoring, and respirator management. Nurses also can gain experience by working in a medical ICU and refresh their knowledge by working there periodically.

MOST COMMON DISORDERS

The major categories of problems treated in an obstetric ICU are listed in Table 211–1. These include hypertensive disorders, massive hemorrhage, and medical problems of pregnancy. The patients who are treated and who are transferred to another ICU will vary with the given health care institution. However, patients with major trauma, neurosurgical patients, and patients requiring prolonged mechanical ventilation may be more appropriately treated in another ICU.[1]

BENEFITS OF AN OBSTETRIC ICU

An obstetric ICU offers the opportunity to improve patient care. Two of the main benefits are observation and organization. Close observation in the ICU allows problems to be detected earlier and complications to be prevented so that the patient recovers more quickly. Complex patient care can be organized more easily in an ICU. Laboratory data accumulates so rapidly on sick patients that sometimes an important abnormality may go undetected. Laboratory flow sheets allow trends to be identified and missing results recalled. Locating an ICU in labor and delivery further assures that an obstetrician, as well as a nurse, is at the bedside. This improves continuity of care. For example, in massive hemorrhage, the obstetrician who operated on the patient knows best when the patient needs to be reexplored. The patient cannot be followed closely if transferred to another service. The obstetrician is the ideal person to follow critically ill obstetric patients because the obstetrician knows the natural history of the disease process and its complications, understands the maternal physiologic adaptations to pregnancy and the changes in the normal laboratory values in pregnancy, and expertly reads the fetal monitor tracing. Nonobstetricians and nonobstetric nurses are not familiar with some of the essential drugs. A prime example is intravenous magnesium sulfate. They may stop magnesium sulfate and allow seizures to occur, or they may not know how to adjust the dosage for renal insufficiency and cause an overdose.

TABLE 211–1. MAIN INDICATIONS FOR ICU ADMISSION

- Hypertensive Disorders
  - Severe preeclampsia ± pulmonary edema or oliguria
  - Eclampsia
  - Refractory chronic hypertension
- Massive Hemorrhage
  - Abruption
  - Placenta previa
  - Accreta
  - Uterine rupture
  - Uterine atony
- Medical Problems of Pregnancy
  - Cardiac problems
    - Pulmonary edema
      - Fluid overload
      - Cardiomyopathy
      - Tocolytic-induced
    - Congenital heart disease
    - Arrhythmias
  - Pulmonary problems
    - Pneumonia
    - Asthma
    - Pulmonary embolism
  - Renal problems
    - Acute tubular necrosis
    - Chronic renal failure
  - Sepsis
    - Pyelonephritis
    - Septic shock
    - Septic pelvic thrombophlebitis
  - Gastrointestinal problems
    - Acute fatty liver
    - Ruptured appendix
  - Endocrine problems
    - Diabetic ketoacidosis
    - Thyroid storm
  - CNS Problems
    - Stroke
    - Status epilepticus

THE SWAN–GANZ CATHETER

As with many advances in medicine, the pendulum is a good analogy for discussing the role of the Swan–Ganz catheter. A new instrument or procedure is introduced with great enthusiasm. It is used widely and complications occur; there is a reaction against it, and finally, there is movement back to a more balanced view that it has some role, but not as great as originally thought. The pulmonary artery catheter was introduced in 1970 for the clinical evaluation of patients with cardiac disease.[2,3] It was taken up by internists, surgeons, anesthesiologists, intensivists, medical researchers, and finally obstetricians. After extensive clinical use, some serious complications were noted including pneumothorax, ventricular arrhythmias, pulmonary infarction, pulmonary artery rupture, sepsis, local vascular thrombosis, intracardiac knotting, and valvular damage. A strident reaction against the Swan–Ganz catheter developed, its critics arguing that it was overused in a form of cultism based on unsupported beliefs and a poor estimate of the nature and harm that may be associated with its use.[4] They also argued that echocardiography and Doppler provided noninvasive alternative techniques for measuring cardiac output, left ventricular preload and contractility, as well as for assessing cardiac anatomy. The pendulum then swung back to a more balanced view that the pulmonary artery catheter is not needed as often as previously thought, but it still has an important role in ICU care. In addition, it was recognized that noninvasive techniques are not yet practical for repeated measures to assess response to therapy in the ICU. Ultrasound and Doppler imaging are technically difficult in the ICU setting because of obesity, chronic obstructive pulmonary disease, bandages, and the fact that the patient may be too sick to cooperate with the examination. We have learned a great deal from using the Swan–Ganz catheter including recognizing hemodynamic subsets in patients with acute myocardial infarction, sepsis, and oliguria. We have studied the hemodynamic effects of pharmacologic therapy, eg, the catheter has made possible the practical application of afterload reduction therapy for heart failure.[5]

The risks and benefits of bed side catheterization recently were reviewed by Matthay and Chatterjee.[5] The authors considered four areas: complications, obtaining reliable data, clinical versus invasive assessment of hemodynamic status, and the effect of monitoring on outcome. Complications have decreased over the years, at least partially due to better physician and nursing awareness. The incidence of pneumothorax has decreased from 6% to 1% in the early literature to < 0.1% now. Pulmonary infarction has decreased from 7.2% in 1974 to 0–1.3% in recent studies. Pulmonary artery rupture has fallen from 0.1%–0.2% to almost zero. Local vascular thrombosis has decreased with heparin-bonded catheters, and septicemia has decreased from 2% to 0.5%. Still, complications have not been eliminated.

There are multiple causes for interpretive error such as: improper calibration, air or blood in the lines, use of digital readout instead of a hard paper printout, and failure to measure wedge pressure at end expiration when pleural pressure is zero. Pulmonary capillary wedge pressure may not reflect left ventricular end-diastolic pressure in the setting of aortic insufficiency, mitral stenosis, or mitral insufficiency. In addition, the relation between left ventricular end-diastolic pressure and left ventricular end-diastolic volume may vary with changes in left ventricular compliance such as during myocardial ischemia.

Two studies have shown that prediction of cardiac output and wedge pressure based on history, physical exam, and chest x-ray are about 75% accurate in coronary care unit patients.[6,7] Three studies have shown that wedge pressure and cardiac output may be predicted accurately by clinical criteria only about 50% of the time in a more heterogeneous group of general ICU patients. Information from invasive monitoring also made a difference in treatment (fluids, diuretics, vasopressors, or vasodilators) about 50% of the time.[8-10]

Does use of the Swan–Ganz catheter improve outcome? There are no hard data to prove this, and a large, prospective randomized trial would be needed. The authors emphasize that the Swan–Ganz catheter is only a diagnostic device. It will improve outcome only if it diagnoses conditions for which treatment exists. For example, it may improve outcome in acute myocardial infarction with heart failure because afterload reduction, inotropic agents, and intra-aortic balloon counterpulsation may be applied. Patients with septic shock, on the other hand, are unlikely to benefit because no new therapeutic options exist. However, invasive monitoring may make management of the hemodynamically unstable septic patient more rational.[5]

The main indications for pulmonary artery catheterization in obstetrics are pulmonary edema, oliguria, septic shock, adult respiratory distress syndrome, massive hemorrhage, and Class III and IV cardiac disease (see also Chapter 123).

INSERTING THE SWAN–GANZ CATHETER

Technique for Cannulating the Internal Jugular Vein

There are several sites for inserting a pulmonary artery catheter: the internal jugular, external jugular, subclavian, basilic, and femoral veins. The right internal jugular is used most often because it provides a straight path to the right side of the heart, the insertion site can be kept clean, and there is a low risk of pneumothorax. The internal jugular vein emerges from the base of the skull to enter the carotid sheath, which also contains the carotid artery and vagus nerve. Initially, the internal jugular vein is posterior and lateral to the carotid artery. However, in the lower portion of the neck it lies lateral and slightly anterior to the carotid artery. The lower portion of the internal jugular vein lies within the triangle formed by the sternal and clavicular heads of the sternocleidomastoid muscle and the clavicle. It is within this triangle that the internal jugular vein is cannulated best (see Figure 211–1).

If the patient is obese or muscular with a short neck, place a small pillow or rolled towel under the shoulders to extend the neck. Have the patient turn her head 60° to the contralateral side. The right internal jugular vein is usually easier to cannulate and avoids the risk of injuring the thoracic duct on the left. The patient is asked to raise her head so that the sternal and clavicular heads of the sternocleidomastoid muscle can be palpated. The carotid artery is palpated; the vein lies lateral to it. The patient then is placed in Trendelenberg position to distend the veins and to prevent air embolism. Several different trays are available for central venous cannulation using the Seldinger technique (over a guidewire). Figure 211–2 illustrates the Swan–Ganz pulmonary artery catheter and the main equipment needed for its insertion. The procedure is performed under continuous ECG and catheter tip pressure monitoring.

After the skin is prepared with betadine and a sterile drape is applied to the area, the junction of the two heads of the sternocleidomastoid muscle at the apex of the triangle is infiltrated with 1% lidocaine. A horizontal line drawn from the cricothyroid membrane in the trachea crosses the apex of the triangle. At this point, a 1.5-inch, 22-gauge needle with a 10-cc syringe may be used to locate the internal jugular vein. When the vein is found and the needle is withdrawn, the tract may be kept in the mind's eye and a large bore (18-gauge needle) can be used to follow this path for cannulation of the internal jugular vein. The author prefers to cannulate the vein directly using a Teflon catheter over a steel needle (18-gauge Cathlon), which is used for routine intravenous therapy. The needle enters at the apex of the triangle at about 30° from the horizontal plane and is pointed along the medial border of the clavicular head of the sternocleidomastoid muscle toward the ipsilateral nipple. The needle is advanced with constant suction until a flashback of blood is obtained. Occasionally, the vein will be passed through and through; when the needle is

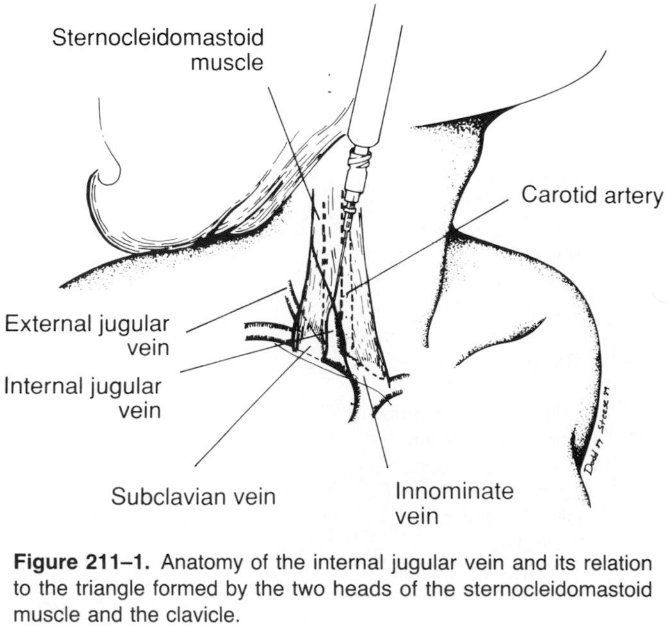

Figure 211–1. Anatomy of the internal jugular vein and its relation to the triangle formed by the two heads of the sternocleidomastoid muscle and the clavicle.

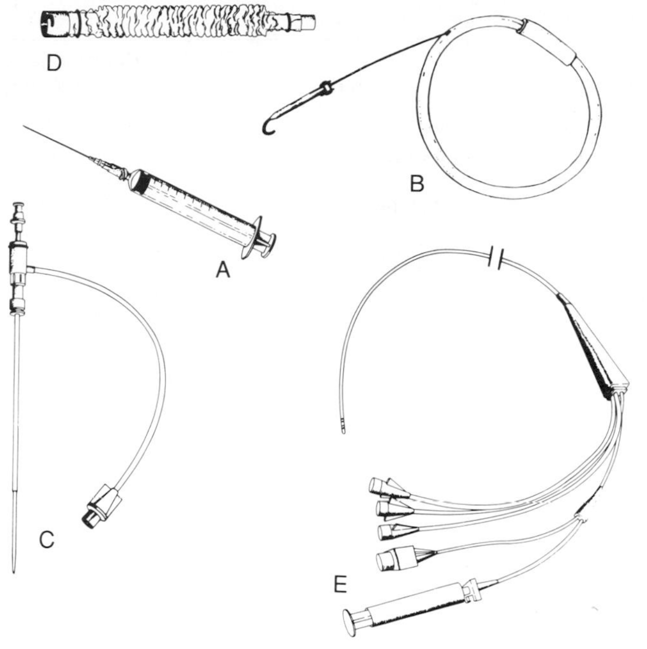

Figure 211–2. Equipment used to insert pulmonary artery catheter: (A) syringe and needle-catheter to access internal jugular vein; (B) J wire; (C) vessel dilator and introducer; (D) sterility sheath; and (E) Swan–Ganz catheter.

withdrawn slowly maintaining suction, a flashback of blood will occur. The flexible cannula then is advanced off the needle and is left in place in the vein. The most common problems are not being able to locate the vein or puncturing the carotid artery. Usually, the latter will be recognizable by pulsatile blood flow. However, occasionally, it is necessary to transduce the vessel with one of the lines and transducers available for Swan–Ganz catheter monitoring. If the carotid has been cannulated inadvertently, the needle can be removed and direct pressure applied for five minutes. Another attempt may be made or it may be necessary to go to the left side to insert the catheter.

The J wire (guide wire) then is inserted through the Teflon plastic catheter. This is an important step. If the J wire is introduced easily and moves back and forth freely, the vessel dilator and introducer can be placed over the J wire with confidence. If, on the other hand, one encounters resistance and the patient complains of pain, it is necessary to remove the J wire and aspirate from the catheter to ensure that it is still in the vein. Once the J wire is in place, a number 11 scalpel blade is used to enlarge the incision. The vessel dilator and introducer then are slipped as one over the guide wire using firm pressure and a twisting motion, which is particularly important as the catheter passes between the ribs and into the chest. The vessel dilator and guide wire then are withdrawn. Blood should flow freely into the introducer sidearm. Air is removed from the system and an intravenous infusion is started.

Inserting the Pulmonary Artery Catheter

The catheter then is removed from its sterile packaging. The balloon is checked by inflating 1.5 cc of air. The balloon then is deflated passively. The distal port is connected to the transducer to be used for pulmonary artery pressure monitoring and is flushed with heparinized saline. The same is repeated for the proximal infusion port and the central venous pressure port. If disposable transducers are used, it is important to check their calibration and to ensure that all transducers are zeroed to the mid-chest level. The integrity of the thermostatic wire is checked by connecting the Swan–Ganz catheter to the cardiac output computer. The computer should register room temperature. The sterility sheath is slid over the catheter. The tip of the catheter is moved up and down and the oscilloscope checked for pressure variation. The catheter is placed into the introducer with the curvature of the catheter directed to the patient's left side. The catheter is advanced to about 15 cm and then the balloon is inflated with 1.5 cc of air. The ECG and pressure tracing are observed continuously as the catheter is advanced into the right ventricle. The right ventricle is recognized by low diastolic pressure (0–5 mm Hg). Once in the right ventricle, the catheter is moved quickly into the pulmonary artery. The pulmonary artery is recognized because the diastolic pressure is higher than in the ventricle. The catheter is passed out to the wedge position, which is usually at approximately the 40 cm mark on the Swan–Ganz catheter. The wedge tracing is a damped tracing that has *a*, *c*, and *v* waves similar to the right atrium. The wedge pressure is usually slightly lower than the pulmonary artery diastolic pressure. The balloon is emptied passively and the pulmonary artery tracing should reappear. The sterile sheath is stretched over the catheter and attached to the introducer. This sheath permits sterile manipulation of the catheter if repositioning is required. The introducer is sewn into place. Betadine ointment and an occlusive dressing are applied.

If frequent premature ventricular contractions or ventricular tachycardia develop when the Swan–Ganz catheter passes into the right ventricle, the balloon should be deflated and the catheter should be withdrawn immediately. If the pulmonary artery is not encountered after 30 cm of catheter has been inserted, the catheter probably is coiling in the ventricle. A chest x-ray should be obtained after the procedure to confirm proper placement of the catheter and to rule out pneumothorax. The strip chart recording of the passage through the heart then is examined and the right atrial, right ventricular, pulmonary artery, and wedge pressures are obtained at end expiration.

Determining the Hemodynamic Profile

Cardiac output is measured by thermodilution cardiac output computer using five (10 cc) injections of iced saline. The high and low values are discarded and the mean of the three remaining values is recorded. The following measured hemodynamic variables are used to calculate the rest of the hemodynamic profile: heart rate, blood pressure, pulmonary artery pressure, pulmonary capillary wedge pressure, central venous pressure, cardiac output, patient height and weight. The derived variables include cardiac index, stroke volume and index, systemic vascular resistance and index, pulmonary vascular resistance and index, and left and right ventricular stroke work and indices (see Table 211–2 for formulae).

HEMODYNAMIC WAVEFORMS

The right atrial pressure tracing (Figure 211–3A) consists of three distinct waves: *a*, *c*, and *v*. The *a* wave is a small wave due to atrial systole. The declining pressure that immediately follows the *a* wave is called the X descent. The *c* wave may or may not appear as a distinct wave. It reflects

TABLE 211–2. HEMODYNAMIC PARAMETERS

Parameter	Symbol	Formula	Units	Nonpregnant Normal Values
Pulse pressure	PP	$BP_{syst} - BP_{diast}$	mm Hg	30–50
Mean arterial pressure	MAP	$BP_{diast} + 1/3\ PP$	mm Hg	70–105
Cardiac index	CI	$\frac{CO}{BSA}$	L/min per m^2	2.4–3.8
Stroke volume	SV	$\frac{CO \times 1000}{HR}$	mL/beat	60–70
Stroke index	SI	$\frac{SV}{BSA}$	mL/beat per m^2	41–51
Systemic vascular resistance	SVR	$\frac{MAP - CVP}{CO} \times 80$	dynes/sec per cm^{-5}	770–1500
Systemic vascular resistance index	SVRI	$SVR \times BSA$	dynes/sec per cm^{-5}/m^2	1970–2390
Pulmonary vascular resistance	PVR	$\frac{\overline{PAP} - PCWP}{CO} \times 80$	dynes/sec per cm^{-5}	100–250
Pulmonary vascular resistance index	PVRI	$PVR \times BSA$	dynes/sec/cm^{-5} per m^2	225–315
Left ventricular stroke work	LVSW	$SV \times MAP \times 0.136$	g/m	
Left ventricular stroke work index	LVSWI	$\frac{LVSW}{BSA}$	g/m per m^2	50–62
Right ventricular stroke work	RVSW	$SV \times \overline{PAP} \times 0.136$	g/m	
Right ventricular stroke work index	RVSWI	$\frac{RVSW}{BSA}$	gm/m per m^2	7.9–9.7

BP_{syst} = systolic blood pressure; BP_{diast} = diastolic blood pressure; CO = cardiac output; HR = heart rate, BSA = body surface area; $\overline{PAP}$ = mean pulmonary artery pressure; PCWP = pulmonary capillary wedge pressure.

the increase in right atrial pressure produced by closure of the tricuspid valve. The negative wave following the *c* wave is called the X[1] descent. The *v* wave is caused by right atrial filling and concomitant right ventricular systole, which causes the leaflets of the closed tricuspid valve to bulge back into the right atrium. The Y descent immediately follows the *v* wave. The pressure changes produced by the *a*, *c*, and *v* waves are usually within 3–4 mm Hg of each other so that the mean pressure usually is taken. The normal resting mean right atrial pressure is 2–6 mm Hg. Elevated right atrial pressures may occur in the following conditions: right ventricular failure, tricuspid stenosis and

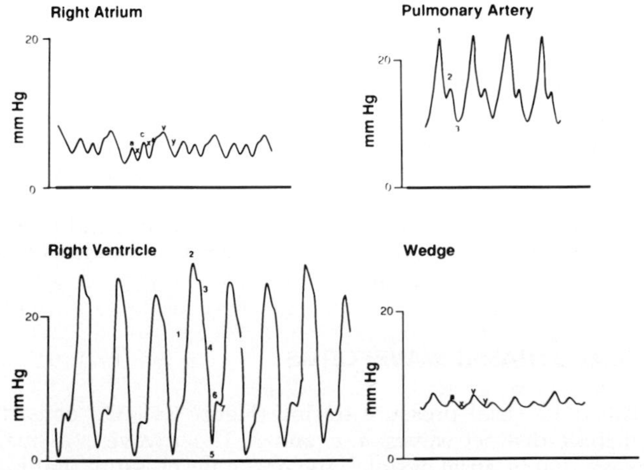

Figure 211–3. Pressure waveforms produced as the Swan-Ganz catheter passes through the right side of the heart.

regurgitation, cardiac tamponade, constrictive pericarditis, pulmonary hypertension, chronic left ventricular failure, and volume overload.[11]

The phases of systole and diastole in the right ventricular pressure tracing can be divided into seven events (Figure 211–3B). Systolic events include isovolumetric contraction, rapid ejection, and reduced ejection. Diastolic events include isovolumetric relaxation, early diastole, atrial systole, and end-diastole.[11]

The pulmonary artery pressure tracing is seen in Figure 211–3C. There is a sharp rise in pressure followed by a decline in pressure as the volume decreases. When the right ventricular pressure falls below the level of the pulmonary artery pressure, the pulmonary valve snaps shut. This sudden closure of the valve leaflets causes the dicrotic notch in the pulmonary artery pressure tracing. Normal pulmonary artery systolic pressure is 20–30 mm Hg. Normal end-diastolic pressure is 8–12 mm Hg. Elevated pulmonary artery pressures are seen in pulmonary disease, primary pulmonary hypertension, mitral stenosis or regurgitation, left ventricular failure, and intracardiac left-to-right shunts. Hypoxia increases pulmonary vascular resistance and pulmonary artery pressure.[11]

When a small branch of the pulmonary artery is occluded by inflation of the balloon on the Swan–Ganz catheter, the pressure tracing reflects left atrial pressure and the waveform looks similar to the right atrial pressure tracing described above. The *a* wave of the wedge pressure is produced by left atrial contraction followed by the X descent (Figure 211–3D). The *c* wave is produced by closure of the mitral valve, but usually is not seen. The *v* wave is produced by filling of the left atrium and bulging back of the mitral valve during ventricular systole. The decline following the *v* wave is called the Y descent. The *v* wave of the wedge pressure tracing is markedly exaggerated with mitral insufficiency due to regurgitation of blood back into the left atrium during ventricular systole. The normal resting mean wedge pressure is 6–12 mm Hg. Elevated wedge pressure is seen in left ventricular failure, mitral stenosis or regurgitation, cardiac tamponade, constrictive pericarditis, and volume overload.[11]

Colloid Osmotic Pressure

Colloid osmotic pressure (COP) and hydrostatic pressure are important factors in edema formation. The colloid osmotic pressure of a fluid is proportional to the number of solute particles. The main osmotically active proteins in plasma are albumin, globulins, and fibrinogen. Albumin is responsible for at least 70% of plasma oncotic pressure. Globulins exert most of the remaining pressure, while fibrinogen plays only a minor role.[12] Colloid osmotic pressure of plasma may be calculated using the Landis and Pappenheinmer equation: $COP = 2.1 \times \text{total protein} + 0.16 \times (\text{total protein})^2 + 0.009 \times (\text{total protein})^3$.[13] Colloid osmotic pressure also may be measured using a commercial transducer-membrane system. Hydrostatic pressure most often is expressed clinically as the pulmonary capillary wedge pressure. The relationship of the plasma colloid osmotic pressure and the wedge pressure may be quantified as the COP-wedge gradient. Normal COP in the nonpregnant state is 25.4 ± 2.3 mm Hg and normal wedge pressure is 6–12 mm Hg.[14] The gradient is thus approximately 12 mm Hg. Reductions to 4 mm Hg or less are associated with an increased risk of pulmonary edema.[15] The normal COP in pregnancy at term is 22.4 ± 0.5 mm Hg.[16] With delivery accompanied by blood loss and crystalloid replacement, COP decreases to 15.4 ± 2.1 mm Hg.[17,18] With preeclampsia, COP has been reported to start at 17.9 ± 0.7 mm Hg and fall to 13.7 ± 0.5 mm Hg postpartum.[19] These changes in COP can result in narrowing of the gradient, thus increasing the risk of pulmonary edema.

Ritodrine used for tocolysis of preterm labor increases ADH release decreasing free water clearance. One study showed a drop in COP to 16.8 ± 2.0 mm Hg after 24 hours of ritodrine for premature labor.[16] Serial measurements of COP and wedge may be useful in trying to prevent pulmonary edema. Wedge pressure can be altered by changing intravenous fluid rate, giving diuretics, or reducing preload with nitroglycerin or nitroprusside. Colloid osmotic pressure could be increased by giving salt-poor albumin or hydroxyethyl starch. However, there is controversy concerning whether the protein will stay in the intravascular space or leak into the interstitium.

Criticism of the COP-wedge gradient concept is that the alveolar capillary membrane is not impermeable to albumin. The albumin content of the lung interstitium may be 70% of that in the plasma.[20] Furthermore, the pulmonary lymphatics efficiently clear albumin and fluid from the lung interstitium. Interstitial fluid formation must increase about 10-fold before this lymphatic system is overwhelmed and pulmonary edema results. Thus, lowering plasma COP causes little change in the osmotic gradient because the plasma and interstitial COP go down in parallel. Low plasma COP may contribute to pulmonary edema when hydrostatic pressure is high. Several clinical studies in trauma patients and patients undergoing aortic reconstructive surgery have compared volume replacement with crystalloid or colloid in addition to packed red cells. These studies concluded that there was no correlation between the COP-wedge gradient and extravascular lung water or intrapulmonary shunt fraction. Elevated filling pressure dictated the development of pulmonary edema.[20,21]

HEMODYNAMIC PROFILE IN PREECLAMPSIA

The cardiovascular hemodynamics of preeclampsia have been reported to range from a low-output, high-resistance state to a high-output, low-resistance state (see also Chapter 139). The 10 published invasive monitoring studies are categorized in Table 211–3 by therapy prior to insertion of the Swan–Ganz catheter.[22-31] The only agreement among all researchers is that pulmonary vascular resistance is unaffected in preeclampsia. One of the major problems with interpreting the data in Table 211–3 is uncertainty about normal values for thermodilution parameters in pregnancy. Before the study of Groenendijk et al[23], which contained thermodilution parameters in four normal pregnant controls, most studies were interpreted using normal values established by the Fick or dye dilution methods for obtaining cardiac output. Combining several studies, approximate normal values were as follows: CVP 4 ± 3 mm Hg, PCWP 6–12 mm Hg, CI 3.0–4.5 L/min per m^2, and SVR 800–1200 dynes/sec per cm^{-5}.[32-34] Groenendijk's control values were similar.

Using these parameters, there is disagreement in the no-therapy group in Table 211–3. Cotton et al[22] reported high normal PCWP, high CO, and minimally elevated SVR, while Groenendijk et al[23], Wallenburg et al[24], and Belfort et al[25], found a low PCWP, low CO, and high SVR. In the fluid restriction group Benedetti et al[26] found a normal PCWP, normal CO, and elevated SVR, while Hankins et al[27] reported slightly different findings—a low PCWP, normal CO, and elevated SVR. In two large studies by Cotton et al[28] and Mabie et al[29], PCWP was normal, CO was high, and SVR was minimally elevated. In the 2 studies using liberal fluid administration, PCWP was normal to high, CO was high, and SVR was normal to even low in some patients.[30,31]

Proposed explanations for the differences in the various hemodynamic studies have included: (1) small number of patients in several series (often 10 or less); (2) variable severity and duration of preeclampsia; (3) underlying medical problems such as cardiac or renal disease; and (4) therapeutic interventions prior to invasive monitoring. In addition, the dynamic, minute-to-minute fluctuation of the cardiovascular system makes it difficult to control for all the variables that can affect hemodynamics, for example, gestational age, labor, pain, anxiety, hydralazine, intravenous fluids, analgesics, and anesthesia. The inherent variability with the thermodilution technique for measuring cardiac output is 15%. Some investigators took the mean of three cardiac output measurements, while others made five determinations, discarded the high and low values, and took the mean of the three remaining values. Finally, the learning curve for obtaining reliable data with the Swan–Ganz catheter is not steep. Recognizing the multiple causes of interpretive error requires considerable experience in calibrating and debugging the equipment.

Clark et al[35] recently confused the picture even further by showing that SVR in normal pregnancy is higher than previously thought. Using invasive as well as noninvasive hemodynamic monitoring, they studied 10 normal pregnant women first at 35–38 weeks' gestation and again at 10–13 weeks postpartum. The following normal hemodynamic values for pregnancy were obtained: CVP 4 ± 3 mm Hg, PCWP 8 ± 2 mm Hg, CI 3.2 ± 0.7 L/min per m^2, and SVR 1333 ± 333 dynes/sec per cm^{-5}. Systemic vascular resistance in normal patients was in the range usually described for severe preeclampsia. Left ventricular function (LVSWI plotted against PCWP) was normal in contrast to

TABLE 211–3. HEMODYNAMIC FINDINGS IN SEVERE PREECLAMPSIA AND ECLAMPSIA

Author	No. of Patients	PCWP (mm Hg)	CVP (mm Hg)	CO (L/min)	CI (L/min per m^2)	SVR (dynes/sec per cm^{-5})	SVRI (dynes/sec/cm^{-5}/m^2)
No therapy							
Cotton et al[22]	5	12.0	6.0	7.56	4.8	1350	2256
Groenendijk et al[23]	10	3.3			2.75	1943	
Wallenburg et al[24]	44	4.0	4.0		3.0		2970
Belfort et al[25]	10	5.0	2.0		3.0	2392	
Magnesium, hydralazine, fluid restriction							
Benedetti et al[26]	10	6.0	3.0	7.4		1322	
Hankins et al[27]	8	3.9	1.0	6.7		1357	
Cotton et al[28]	45	10.0	4.0	7.5	4.1	1496	2726
Mabie et al[29]	41	8.3	4.8	8.4	4.4	1226	2293
Magnesium, hydralazine, volume expansion							
Rafferty et al[30]	3	7.0		11.0		780	
Phelan et al[31]	10	16.4	9.7	9.3		1042	

PCWP = pulmonary capillary wedge pressure; CVP = central venous pressure; CO = cardiac output; CI = cardiac index; SVR = systemic vascular resistance; SVRI = systemic vascular resistance index.

preeclampsia, which is associated with hyperdynamic left ventricular function.[36]

Easterling et al[37] provided further support for a hyperdynamic state in preeclampsia. They studied cardiac output serially in 120 nulliparous women during pregnancy and found that in pregnancies complicated by preeclampsia, cardiac output was elevated prior to the onset of hypertension and remained higher than that found in normotensives throughout gestation. However, only 6 of the 120 patients developed preeclampsia.

The two opposing views in the controversy have been summarized by Wallenburg[24] and Mabie et al.[29] Wallenburg's data supports the traditional view of preeclampsia, that of a volume-contracted, vasospastic state. He found a low PCWP, low CO, and high SVR in 44 untreated, nulliparous preeclamptic patients. While in 22 patients who had received various therapies and usually were referred, a wide range of hemodynamics was found. He concluded that the untreated patient was significantly volume depleted and that the wide spectrum of hemodynamic findings present in the treated group resulted from prior therapy and the presence of other variables such as labor, multiparity, and preexisting hypertension. Thus, the disparity in cardiac outputs, peripheral resistances, and wedge pressures among various studies was not due to the hemodynamic variability of preeclampsia but to differences in patient selection and therapeutic intervention prior to invasive monitoring.

Mabie et al[29] studied the hemodynamics of 49 subjects with severe preeclampsia at a large referral center. Despite a heterogenous population of referred and nonreferred patients, pretreated and nonpretreated individuals, a generally consistent profile emerged. Their population and results were similar to that of Cotton et al[28] and supported the conclusion that preeclampsia was in general a high cardiac output state associated with an inappropriately high peripheral resistance. Although the SVR was within the normal range, it was still inappropriately high for the elevated cardiac output. The failure of the circulation to dilate in the setting of increasing cardiac output appeared to be a characteristic feature of preeclampsia. The normal wedge pressure and central venous pressures found in their study suggested central redistribution of intravascular volume if the generally accepted reports of decreased plasma volume in preeclampsia are correct. They postulated splanchnic venoconstriction as the mechanism for this volume shift. They also noted that the hemodynamic profile is variable in preeclampsia, but it is variable in virtually every other type of experimental and naturally occurring hypertension. They pointed out that Wallenburg had minimized the variable hemodynamic presentation of his untreated group in that 15% or more had wedge pressures greater then 8 mm Hg, indicating normal central blood volume.

Thus, data on the central hemodynamics of severe preeclampsia are conflicting, with some evidence indicating a volume-contracted, low-output, high-resistance state and other evidence suggesting normal filling pressures, elevated cardiac output, and normal resistance. Further study is needed before the hemodynamic profile of preeclampsia can be established clearly.

CONCLUSIONS

The need for an obstetric ICU results from many factors: (1) development of the maternal-fetal medicine subspecialty; (2) acceptance of the ICU concept; (3) new knowledge and equipment; (4) a maternal referral system that concentrates sick patients in a few centers; (5) a more liberal attitude among physicians toward allowing pregnancy in patients with major organ disease or multisystem disease; and (6) better treatment of chronic disease which has brought new types of patients to obstetricians; for example, patients with advanced diabetes, lupus, renal insufficiency, organ transplants, and surgically corrected heart disease.

REFERENCES

1. Mabie WC, Sibai BM. Treatment in an obstetric intensive care unit. *Am J Obstet Gynecol.* 1990;162:1–4.
2. Forrester JS, Diamond G, McHugh TH, Swan HJC. Filling pressures in the right and left sides of the heart in acute myocardial infarction. *N Engl J Med.* 1970;283:190.
3. Swan JH, Ganz W, Forrester J, et al. Catheterization of the heart in man with the use of a flow-directed balloon-tipped catheter. *N Engl J Med.* 1970;283:447.
4. Robin ED. The cult of the Swan–Ganz catheter. *Ann Int Med.* 1985;103:445.
5. Matthay MA, Chatterjee K. Bedside catheterization of the pulmonary artery: risks compared with benefits. *Ann Int Med.* 1988;109:826.

6. Forrester JC, Diamond G, Swan HJ. Correlative classification of clinical and hemodynamic function after acute myocardial infarction. *Am J Card.* 1977;39:137.
7. Bayliss J, Norell M, Ryan A, et al. Bedside hemodynamic monitoring: experience in a general hospital. *Br Med J.* 1983;287:187.
8. Connors AF Jr, McCaffree DR, Gray BA. Evaluation of right heart catheterization in the critically ill patient without acute myocardial infarction. *N Engl J Med.* 1983;308:263.
9. Eisenberg PR, Jaffe AS, Schuster DP. Clinical evaluation compared to pulmonary artery catheterization in the hemodynamic assessment of critically ill patients. *Crit Care Med.* 1984;12:549.
10. Fein AM, Goldberg SK, Walhenstein MD, et al. Is pulmonary artery catheterization necessary for the diagnosis of pulmonary edema? *Am Rev Resp Dis.* 1984;129:1006.
11. Daily EK, Schroeder JS. *Techniques in bedside hemodynamic monitoring.* 4th ed. St. Louis, MO: CV Mosby; 1989.
12. Moise KJ, Cotton DB. Colloid osmotic pressure in pregnancy. In: Clark SK, Phelan JP, Cotton DB, eds. *Critical care obstetrics.* Oradell, NJ: Medical Economics; 1987:71.
13. Sprung CL, Isikoff SK, Hauser M, Eisler BR. Comparison of measured and calculated colloid osmotic pressure of serum and pulmonary edema fluid in patients with pulmonary edema. *Crit Care Med.* 1980;8:613.
14. Weil MH, Morisette M, Michaels S, et al. Routine plasma colloid osmotic pressure measurements. *Crit Care Med.* 1974;2:229.
15. Rackow EC, Fein IA, Leppo J. Colloid osmotic pressure as a prognostic indication of pulmonary edema and mortality in the critically ill. *Chest.* 1977;72:709.
16. Gonik B. Intensive care monitoring of the critically ill pregnant patient. In: Creasy RK, Resnik R, eds. *Maternal-Fetal Medicine: Principles and Practice.* 2nd ed. Philadelphia: WB Saunders; 1989:845.
17. Cotton DB, Gonik B, Spillman T, Dorman KF. Intrapartum to postpartum changes in colloid osmotic pressure. *Am J Obstet Gynecol.* 1984;149:174.
18. Gonik B, Cotton D, Spillman T, et al. Peripartum colloid osmotic pressure changes: effects of controlled fluid management. *Am J Obstet Gynecol.* 1985;151:812.
19. Benedetti TJ, Carlson RW. Studies of colloid osmotic pressure in pregnancy-induced hypertension. *Am J Ostet Gynecol.* 1979;135:308.
20. Peitzman A. Principles of circulatory support and the treatment of hemorrhagic shock. In: Syner JV, Pinsky MR, eds. *Oxygen transport in the critically ill.* Chicago: Year Book; 1987:407.
21. Viriglio RW, Rice CL, Smith DE, et al. Crystalloid vs. colloid resuscitation: is one better? *Surgery.* 1979;85:129.
22. Cotton DB, Gonik B, Dorman KF. Cardiovascular alterations in severe pregnancy-induced hypertension: acute effects of intravenous magnesium sulfate. *Am J Obstet Gynecol.* 1984;148:162.
23. Groenendijk R, Trimbos MJ, Wallenburg HCS. Hemodynamic measurements in preeclampsia: preliminary observations. *Am J Obstet Gynecol.* 1984;150:232.
24. Wallenburg HCS. Hemodynamics in hypertensive pregnancy. In: Rubin PC, ed. *Hypertension in pregnancy.* Amsterdam: Elsevier; 1988:66.
25. Belfort M, Uys P, Dommisse J, Davey DA. Hemodynamic changes in gestational proteinuric hypertension: the effects of rapid volume expansion and vasodilator therapy. *Br J Obstet Gynecol.* 1989;96:634.
26. Benedetti TJ, Cotton BD, Read JC, Miller FC. Hemodynamic observations in severe preeclampsia with a flow-directed pulmonary artery catheter. *Am J Obstet Gynecol.* 1980;136:465.
27. Hankins GDV, Wendell GD, Cunningham FC, Leveno KJ. Longitudinal evaluation of the hemodynamic changes in eclampsia. *Am J Obstet Gynecol.* 1984;150:506.
28. Cotton DB, Lee W, Huhta JC, Dorman KF. Hemodynamic profile of severe pregnancy-induced hypertension. *Am J Obstet Gynecol.* 1988; 158:523.
29. Mabie WC, Ratts TE, Sibai BM. The central hemodynamics of severe preeclampsia. *Am J Obstet Gynecol.* 1989;161:1443.
30. Rafferty TD, Berkowitz RL. Hemodynamics in patients with severe toxemia during labor and delivery. *Am J Obstet Gynecol.* 1980;138:263.
31. Phelan JP, Yurth DA. Severe preeclampsia. 1. Peripartum hemodynamic observations. *Am J Obstet Gynecol.* 1982;144:17.
32. Bader RA, Bader ME, Rose DJ, Braunwald E. Hemodynamics at rest and during exercise in normal pregnancy as studied by cardiac catheterization. *J Clin Invest.* 1955;34:1524.
33. Ueland K, Hansen JM. Maternal cardiovascular dynamics. *Am J Obstet Gyencol.* 1969;103:8.
34. Kerr MG. Cardiovascular dynamics in pregnancy and labor. *Br Med Bull.* 1968;24:19.
35. Clark SL, Cotton DB, Lee W, et al. Central hemodynamic assessment of normal third trimester pregnancy: a simultaneous comparison of Fick principle, thermodilution, continuous wave Doppler, pulsed Doppler, and electrical impedance measurements of cardiac output, and effects of position changes on hemodynamics and oxygen delivery (abstract). Society of Perinatal Obstetricians, Ninth Annual Meeting. New Orleans, Louisiana; February, 1989.
36. Clark SL, Cotton DB. Clinical indications for pulmonary artery catheterization in the patient with severe preeclampsia. *Am J Obstet Gynecol.* 1988;158:453.
37. Easterling TR, Benedetti TJ, Schmucker BC. Maternal cardiac output in preeclamptic pregnancies: a longitudinal study (abstract). Society of Perinatal Obstetricians, Ninth Annual Meeting. New Orleans, Louisiana; February, 1989.

PART XXII The Fetus as Patient

Gloria E. Sarto, Section Editor

Chapter Two Hundred and Twelve

Diagnosis and Therapeutic Management of Fetal Disease

Katharine D. Wenstrom and Carl P. Weiner

212

Little was known about normal fetal development or pathology until the 20th century. Experimentation on mammalian fetuses began in the 1920s, and by the 1960s and 1970s, research had yielded important information on the development of fetal anomalies. Surgical manipulation of the animal fetus produced several apparent replicas of spontaneously occurring malformations including coarctation of the aorta, intestinal atresia, congenital diaphragmatic hernia, hydronephrosis, and congenital heart disease.[1] The study of animal models has enhanced our understanding of basic fetal physiology and provided insight into the normal functioning of major organ systems.

Attempts to clinically define and quantify measures of fetal well-being paralleled basic research. Recognition of the importance of fetal activity and fetal heart rate variability prompted the development of sophisticated monitoring techniques. Reproductive hormones were measured in maternal blood and urine, and various products of metabolism were identified in amniotic fluid. The development of cytogenetic methods to evaluate fetal karyotype made it possible to diagnose a particularly devastating group of fetal anomalies prenatally. Although x-rays and amniograms were used to identify certain malformations antenatally, the most important advance in fetal imaging came with the introduction of ultrasound. Pioneering work in the 1950s by researchers in the United States and the United Kingdom[2] prompted the widespread clinical application of two-dimensional ultrasound in the 1960s. The ability to visualize and monitor fetal development made the prenatal diagnosis of various malformations possible and provided guidance for invasive intrauterine procedures. Both placental aspiration and fetoscopy were introduced in the 1970s. Fetoscopy permitted direct visualization of the fetus, and each technique allowed aspiration of fetal blood. Although cumbersome and associated with a perinatal loss rate that limited its application[3], the ability to access the fetus directly provided insight into a variety of hemoglobinopathies and blood diseases.

A major breakthrough came in 1983 with the first published report of cordocentesis.[4] Using ultrasound guidance to transabdominally place a needle into an umbilical vessel, safe direct access to the fetal circulation was obtained. This technique has been tested widely and rapidly adopted throughout the world. It has proven invaluable for the assessment of fetal abnormalities.

CORDOCENTESIS

Cordocentesis requires high-resolution ultrasound equipment and experience in ultrasound-guided procedures. No special maternal preparation is necessary for a diagnostic cordocentesis. For procedures that require the needle to remain in place for a length of time, intravenous diazepam and local lidocaine are given to encourage maternal relaxation and cooperation. Informed consent is obtained from the patient after a discussion of risks, which include bleeding, infection, preterm labor or delivery, rupture of membranes, fetal bradycardia, and fetal death.

The patient initially is placed supine or in a slight lateral tilt. The placental origin of the umbilical cord is located using high-resolution ultrasound. If the cord origin cannot be accessed, a free loop of cord is targeted, especially if it is located near the uterine wall or fetal trunk, which can serve as a backstop. The maternal abdomen is wiped with acetone to remove any unsterile coupling gel, painted with betadine, and covered with a sterile drape. A sterile sheath is placed over the transducer and a sterile needle guide attached. Although some clinicians perform this procedure freehand while holding the transducer, the use of a needle guide provides stability and prevents lateral movement of the needle. With the aid of an on-screen template, which displays the needle tract, and an assistant to hold the transducer, a 22-gauge needle is guided carefully into the umbilical vein. The umbilical artery is avoided because of associated vessel spasm and fetal bradycardia.[5]

The location of the needle is verified by carefully infusing a few milliliters of normal saline and observing the resultant intravessel turbulence and flow toward the fetus[5] or by measuring the blood pressure. Fetal blood is aspirated into l-mL tuberculin syringes and rapidly transferred into vacutainers containing appropriate preservative or anticoagulant. One tuberculin syringe is prepared with heparin for the blood gas specimen. A total sample volume of 4–6 mL can be removed across all gestational ages without ill effect.[6]

If the location of vessel puncture is such that fetal movement might be harmful, pancuronium (0.3 mg/kg estimated fetal weight up to 0.6 mg total) is administered intravascularly to the fetus as soon as correct needle location is verified. Fetal movement returns within 60–120 minutes. During this period of paralysis, fetal heart rate reactivity and accelerations are absent.[7] A sequential return to baseline fetal heart rate and reactivity occurs when fetal movement resumes. Nonstress tests can be obtained before and after the procedure to document fetal well-being. The placenta of rhesus-negative patients should be avoided if possible. If the fetus is rhesus positive, a dose of rhesus immunoglobulin is given before discharge.

Cordocentesis has markedly changed diagnosis and management of fetal disease. Its application to various clinical situations is described below.

ISOIMMUNIZATION

Red cell isoimmunization occurs when surface antigen-positive fetal cells enter the circulation of an antigen-negative mother (see also Chapters 170 and 171). Fetal cells are found in maternal blood in 7% of gravidas in the first trimester, 16% in the second trimester, 29% in the third trimester, and in 50% after normal delivery.[8] The maternal IgG alloantibodies generated in response to the antigen challenge can cross the placenta during the index or subsequent pregnancy and attach to fetal red cell surface antigens. Such cells are cleared by the reticuloendothelial system at a rate affected by antibody quantity and subtype. Fetal anemia develops when this destruction exceeds the production of new red blood cells by bone marrow and extramedullary hematopoietic sites. When the liver hypertrophies as a result of hematopoiesis, compression of normal liver cells leads to destruction and decreased protein production. Hypoxia occurs secondary to the severe anemia and is associated with myocardial dysfunction. Hypoproteinemia and hypoalbuminemia in the setting of hypoxic cardiac dysfunction leads to the development of *hydrops fetalis*. The hydropic fetus has pleural and pericardial effusions as well as ascites, and usually succumbs *in utero* if untreated.

The rhesus antigen system was discovered in 1940. It is now known that other atypical red cell antigens can produce the same pathologic response. Blood typing and screening for red blood cell antibodies are the standard of care, and the use of prophylactic rhesus immunoglobulin is routine. Nevertheless, isoimmunization continues to occur. Patients may not receive indicated immunoglobulin or may be given an inadequate dose. Sensitization to an atypical antigen can occur after a blood transfusion or as a result of exposure to paternal antigen on fetal cells. The etiologies of *erythroblastosis fetalis* and the appropriate maternal evaluation are discussed elsewhere in this text. This chapter focuses on methods to evaluate the fetus and on approaches to intrauterine treatment.

Noninvasive methods of fetal evaluation include electronic fetal monitoring, ultrasound, and Doppler velocimetry. Fetal monitoring provides relatively nonspecific information. Although a "blunting" of fetal heart rate reactivity has been reported when the fetal hematocrit is below 25%, fetal movement may persist well below this level.[9] The presence of late decelerations on contraction stress testing indicates fetal compromise, but may not be present until severe anemia has developed. Although useful as a supplement to other forms of fetal evaluation, fetal monitoring by itself is not sufficient to detect the occurrence of anemia prior to the development of hydrops.

Ultrasound has proven to be useful for detecting the fetal anatomic changes that result from anemia and increased extramedullary hematopoiesis. Unfortunately, the fetus is likely to be severely anemic by the time distinct changes are noted, and normal sonographic findings do not preclude anemia. Sonographically detectable changes include the following: polyhydramnios (usually the first alteration noted); placental hypertrophy with loss of architecture; scalp edema; fetal ascites, hydrothorax, and pericardial effusion; and hepatosplenomegaly.[10] Umbilical vein distention has been reported by some authors[11] but refuted by others.[12] In a study of 15 sensitized gravidas undergoing serial ultrasound evaluation and fetal blood sampling, Chitkara et al[13] correlated the appearance of ultrasound findings with fetal hematocrit. She found that although all fetuses with a hydropic appearance had a hematocrit of 15% or less, three fetuses with hematocrits below 15% did not appear hydropic or demonstrate any ultrasound abnormalities. Six fetuses with hydramnios were anemic (14–26%) but three other anemic fetuses had normal amniotic fluid volumes. Vintzileos et al[14] have suggested that serial measurements of fetal liver size may be useful in detecting severe anemia. In their study of 16 isoimmunized pregnancies, eight of nine fetuses with a liver size greater than the 95th percentile were severely anemic.

Doppler velocimetry is another noninvasive technique used to evaluate the anemic fetus. Because the circulation is hyperdynamic, it has been theorized that the blood velocities in the fetal aorta, inferior vena cava, or umbilical vein would be significantly greater in anemic fetuses. Warren et al[15] used Doppler velocimetry to evaluate the fetal umbilical vein in 51 sensitized pregnancies, and showed that 61% of those with abnormally high flow developed hydrops within a week of the study. He also found that a sudden increase in flow rate by 20% or more correlated with fetal deterioration and the need for transfusion. Moderately anemic fetuses usually had flow velocities within the normal range. Doppler velocimetry, like ultrasound, is only capable of detecting the severely compromised fetus.

Although noninvasive methods of fetal evaluation are most desirable, invasive techniques to evaluate the isoimmunized pregnancy usually are necessary to assess fetal status more accurately. In the 1950s, it was recognized that the quantity of a bilirubin-like material in amniotic fluid was related directly to the degree of fetal erythrocyte destruction. Liley[16] was the first to measure amniotic fluid bilirubin concentrations and relate these values to the degree of anemia at birth. He quantitated bilirubin spectrophotometrically by measuring the optical density of amniotic fluid between 420 and 460 mm, the wave length absorbed by bilirubin. The deflection at 450 mm, referred to as the Δ OD 450, correlated with bilirubin values. He devised a chart based on natural history studies in which these values fell into one of three zones, with the lower zone values (Zone I) associated with mild or no hemolytic disease and higher zone values (Zone III) indicative of severe fetal anemia, hydrops, and death within 7–10 days. Levels in Zone II indicated an intermediate degree of anemia that worsened as Zone III was approached. This chart rapidly was adopted by practitioners with only modest changes and serial amniocentesis for determination of the Δ OD 450 became standard. When values were found to be in upper Zone II or Zone III, intrauterine, intraperitoneal blood transfusion, or delivery were initiated.

Liley's original data were obtained by studying fetuses at 27–41 weeks' gestation. Although significant ambiguity remains regarding values in Zone II, within this range of gestational age his chart retains its value. The temptation to extrapolate these values back to earlier gestational ages was stimulated by the progressive trend toward earlier intervention in pregnancies at risk. Unfortunately, such extrapolation yields highly unreliable results. Nicolaides et al[17] measured the Δ OD 450 in 59 sensitized pregnancies at 18–25 weeks' gestation, and compared these values with fetal hemoglobin levels and hematocrits obtained simultaneously by fetoscopy. The normal Δ OD 450 for an unaffected fetus at this gestational age was in Zone II. They also found considerable overlap in Δ OD 450 and fetal hemoglobin values throughout the chart, making bilirubin concentration a poor predictor of fetal anemia. Of 31 severely anemic fetuses, for example, only 10 had a Δ OD 450 value in Liley Zone III. Several fetuses with values clearly in Zone III were affected only mildly. If ultrasound evidence of hydrops was present, the predictive value of the Δ OD 450 was increased significantly, but hydrops was not always evident in the severely affected fetuses.

The advent of cordocentesis as a safe and effective clinical tool has obviated many of these problems. It is now possible to assess directly fetal hematocrit, hemoglobin, reticulocyte count, blood type, and direct Coombs test. Indications for cordocentesis in this setting include an indirect Coombs titer of 1:8 or higher secondary to the production of IgG antibody, and (1) history of a previous severely affected child; (2) proven or reasonably likely paternal heterozygosity based on phenotype; (3) Δ OD 450 in Zone II or higher; or (4) evidence of fetal edema or hydrops.[6] Determination of the fetal blood type at the initial sampling will detect a number of fetuses not at risk for hemolytic disease and eliminate these from any further study. In one series, these constituted 17% of the population studied.[6] Another group will be affected only mildy, and these may be followed with noninvasive techniques and repeat cordocenteses as suggested by the degree of anemia, reticulocytosis, and quantity and subtype of antibody coating the red blood cell. For fetuses discovered to be severely anemic, cordocentesis can be life-saving.

Transfusion is performed when the fetal hematocrit is less than 30%. This value is greater than two standard deviations below the mean for each gestational age after 20 weeks. Donor cells are prepared from fresh donor blood compatible with both mother and fetus, buffy coat poor, washed and irradiated, filtered, and resuspended in normal saline at a hematocrit of 70–75 percent. Sedation with diazepam encourages the patient to remain motionless in the position desired for the duration of the transfusion. The maternal abdomen is prepared and draped aseptically as for diagnostic cordocentesis. Antibiotics and tocolytics are not given.

Using constant sonographic visualization, a 22-gauge needle of appropriate length is guided into the umbilical vein. Pancuronium (0.3 mg/kg of estimated fetal weight up to 0.6 mg) is given routinely even when the placenta is anterior. Although the placental origin of the umbilical cord remains the ideal site for puncture because it is fixed, a free loop of cord may at times be preferable. Baseline blood samples (including a blood gas) and an umbilical venous pressure obtained at this time help confirm that the punctured vessel is a vein. Observation of the direction of flow as normal saline or blood is injected through the needle also will confirm needle placement and vessel type. If the needle has been inadvertently placed in an artery, it should be removed immediately as the risk of bradycardia is increased with arterial puncture.

Some investigators have also given furosemide (2 mg/kg estimated fetal weight) before infusing the red cells. Although unproven, furosemide theoretically dilates capacitance vessels and promotes diuresis after the transfusion.[18] Blood then is infused at a rate up to 6–10 mL per minute until half the estimated transfusion volume has been given. A hematocrit and umbilical venous pressure are obtained at this time. Although nomograms for transfusion volumes have been described, none are completely reliable. Ultimately, the final volume transfused will be determined by observing the response to infusion of the presumed mid-volume of blood, and making calculations based on that response. If the goal is to raise the hematocrit by 30 points, for example, and a 20-mL infusion is observed to raise the hematocrit 10 points, a total of 60 mL will be required. The targeted posttransfusion hematocrit is 45–50% in the nonhydropic fetus. In the hydropic fetus, the umbilical venous pressure is a useful guide for therapy. An abrupt increase indicates that the transfusion should be halted or an exchange transfusion performed.

The decision of when to repeat the transfusion is based on many factors including fetal age, severity of anemia, adequacy of the transfusion, the freshness of donor blood, and the percentage of fetal cells remaining after the initial procedure. The second transfusion of a nonhydropic fetus may be necessary as early as one week after the first. Subsequent transfusions are repeated at three-to four-week intervals. Periodic ultrasounds and electronic fetal monitoring help to assure fetal well-being until the next scheduled transfusion.

The fetus is not a passive recipient. It responds to intravascular transfusion with release of atrial natriuretic factor, prostacyclin, and prostaglandin E_2, all of which likely increase the capacitance volume. Intravascular transfusion usually is tolerated well, even by the severely anemic or hydropic fetus. For this reason, intraperitoneal transfusion with its attendant risks of intra-abdominal trauma and uneven absorption of blood has been abandoned or seldom used by many centers. The relative safety of intravascular transfusion allows the procedure to be repeated as many times as necessary during gestation to achieve the desired goal—delivery at term.

PLATELET DISORDERS

Although numerous drugs, chemicals, and even ionizing radiation are known to cause thrombocytopenia, the two disorders associated with low fetal platelet counts most commonly seen by obstetricians are idiopathic thrombocytopenic purpura (ITP) and alloimmune thrombocytopenic purpura (ATP) (see also Chapter 165). ITP, which results from autoimmune phenomena, is 10–20 times more common than ATP and poses a lesser risk to the fetus. ATP, which is the platelet analog of Rh disease, is a much more serious condition in which the fetus may suffer serious hemorrhagic consequences prior to birth.

The diagnosis of maternal ITP is made by confirming that the maternal platelet count is two or more standard deviations below the mean, by eliminating possible drug or chemical etiologies, by demonstrating platelet associated IgG, IgM, or complement, and occasionally, by performing a bone marrow biopsy that demonstrates increased numbers of megakaryoctyes. As an autoimmune disorder, maternal ITP usually responds well to steroid therapy. Increased platelet counts often are seen within a few days of initiating therapy. However, if the pathologic antibody is of the IgG class, it may cross the placenta and cause fetal thrombocytopenia as well. The degree of fetal platelet depression and any possible response to steroid therapy cannot be predicted from the maternal clinical course. Fortunately, however, the occurrence of antenatal fetal hemorrhage remains a reportable event, and attempts to determine fetal platelet count by performing antenatal cordocentesis are unwise because the risk clearly exceeds the benefit. Decisions regarding mode of delivery can be assisted by obtaining a platelet count from fetal scalp blood early in labor.

ATP, in contrast to ITP, is associated with devastating antenatal hemorrhage in as many as 30% of affected fetuses. Profound thrombocytopenia results from maternal production of an IgG antibody directed against fetal platelets. The PLA-1 antigen site, seen in 98% of the population, is the most common target. Because maternal platelet counts are unaffected by this phenomenon, the diagnosis usually is made after the birth of an affected child. The perinatal mortality rate of the untreated disorder is as high as 24%, and the incidence of central nervous system sequelae approaches 50%.[19] The recurrence rate among subsequent children exceeds 75%. These children would presumably benefit from accurate diagnosis and antenatal therapy. Cordocentesis has proven invaluable for diagnostic purposes in this setting.

Fetal blood obtained by cordocentesis can be used to determine fetal platelet count and platelet antigen type. The risks of this procedure in the face of possible fetal thrombocytopenia are surprisingly low. In several large series, bleeding from the puncture site has not been observed even when fetal platelet counts were less than 10,000 per mm^3.[6]

Previous methods of management have included elective early cesarean delivery and fetal intravascular platelet transfusion prior to delivery. Because neither of these approaches decreases the significant risk of antenatal intracranial hemorrhage, therapy that aims to prevent antenatal complications is more logical. A recent study indicates that fetal platelet destruction often can be prevented successfully by treating the mother with weekly infusions of γ-globulin (1.0 g/kg body weight).[20] The mechanism of action is unclear, but treatment is associated with markedly decreased levels of anti-PLA-1 activity and increased levels of fetal IgG. The addition of maternal corticosteroid therapy to this protocol may be beneficial in select cases unresponsive to γ-globulin alone. Once this therapy is initiated, cordocentesis is repeated at 3- to 4-week intervals to assess fetal response. If the response is satisfactory, affected fetuses need not be delivered early. After documentation of an appropriate fetal platelet count at term, vaginal delivery can be attempted.

INTRAUTERINE GROWTH RETARDATION

The diagnosis of intrauterine growth retardation (IUGR) is usually made antenatally by obtaining ultrasound measurements of the fetus and comparing them with standard tables based on gestational age. Debate continues regarding whether this diagnosis should be based on body wieght or body mass, and whether size less than the third, fifth, or tenth percentile for age should be considered abnormal. Most often (although not ideally), postnatal diagnosis is based on weight. Factors such as race, sex, and geographic locale should be considered when comparing estimated norms.

Once it is apparent that fetal growth is significantly less than expected, however, the diagnosis is made and the search begins for possible etiologies. When the diagnosis is first suspected after 32 weeks' gestation, the degree of affect is usually mild and the cause is uteroplacental insufficiency. Noninvasive means of evaluating fetal status, such as electronic fetal monitoring or Doppler velocimetry, are sufficient in this circumstance. When growth impairment is obvious prior to 32 weeks or when symmetric growth retardation is noted prior to 34 weeks, further investigation is necessary. If growth failure can be directly attributed to maternal disease (ie, cardiac, renal, collagen vascular, chronic hypertension, and diabetes) or environmental factors (i.e., ethanol, recreational drugs, and smoking), cordocentesis will not add substantially to the diagnosis. In the absence of contributing maternal or environmental factors, the diagnostic possibilities are limited predominantly to congenital infection, idiopathic uteroplacental insufficiency, and aneuploidy. Because the management of each of these situations is different, diagnostic cordocentesis may provide information that could significantly alter the remainder of the pregnancy.

Weiner and Williamson[21] evaluated 21 fetuses with severe early onset IUGR by obtaining fetal blood for a variety of tests including complete blood count (CBC), blood gas, IgM quantification, and karyotype. The results of liver function tests are unpublished elsewhere but offered here in Table 212–1. Fetuses in all three diagnostic categories were characterized by high hemoglobin and hematocrit, normal reticulocyte counts, low PO_2, and elevated liver enzyme levels, indicating a response to chronic stress. Fetuses with congenital infection were distinguished by normal pH and low platelet and white blood cell counts. Growth-retarded aneuploid fetuses did not have laboratory values significantly different form those fetuses with uteroplacental insufficiency, indicating that an aneuploid placenta provides inadequate respiratory and nutritional support to the developing fetus.

Because of the significant overlap of laboratory test results, only two categories of tests currently available provide a definitive diagnosis in this setting. One category involves the variety of tests available to diagnose specific fetal infections, and is discussed in the next section. The other encompasses the various methods used to obtain a fetal karyotype, and probably represents the most important diagnostic information to be obtained in the pregnancy complicated by a severely growth-retarded fetus.

A fetal karyotype can be determined from placental biopsy, cultured amniocytes, from lymphocytes found in

TABLE 212–1. RESULTS OF LIVER FUNCTION TESTS

	Hemoglobin	Hematocrit	WBC[a]	Platelets	Reticulocytes	MCV[b]	pH	pCO_2	pO_2	O_2 Sat	Liver Enzymes[d]
Aneuploidy	↑	↑	↑	↓	WNL[c]	↑	↓	WNL	↓	↓	↑
Uteroplacental insufficiency	↑	↑	↓	WNL	WNL	↑	↓	↑	↓	↓	↑
Infection	↑	↑	↓	↓	↑	↑	WNL	WNL	↓	WNL	↑

[a] White blood cell count
[b] Mean cell volume
[c] Within normal limits
[d] AST, IDH, GTT

cystic hygromas[22], and from peripheral blood. In the growth-retarded fetus without hygroma, peripheral blood obtained by cordocentesis permits a rapid karyotype (48–72 hours) and a search for other possible etiologies. In the future, 8-hour preparations may be common. Up to 25% of fetuses with severe early onset growth retardation are aneuploid.[21] When aneuploidy is confirmed, further fetal testing and evaluation is suspended. Parents who discover that their fetus is chromosomally abnormal may then make informed decisions regarding the remainder of the pregnancy. Antenatal fetal surveillance can be halted and operative delivery or other heroic obstetric measures avoided. Counseling regarding recurrence risks and evaluation of future pregnancies can be provided and intelligent reproductive decisions can be made.

Chronic uteroplacental insufficiency is a diagnosis of exclusion, and management is unclear. Prior approaches have incorporated close monitoring of fetal status and delivery before serious fetal compromise or death occurred. Attempts to actually treat the fetus by changing the intrauterine environment or supplying missing nutrients have been sporadic. Since the active transport mechanism from mother to fetus requires oxygen, it has been suggested that oxygen supplementation may increase the passage of nutrients to the fetus. Attempts also have been made to improve fetal nutrition to supplying nutrients directly to the amniotic fluid or by using maternal hyperalimentation. Nicolaides et al[23] described the use of maternal oxygen therapy in six hypoxic, severely growth-retarded fetuses. In all cases, elevation of fetal pO_2 into or toward the normal range was demonstrated within 10 minutes of initiation of therapy. In the five surviving fetuses, continued improved oxygenation was suggested by the presence of a sustained increase in the mean velocity of blood in the thoracic aorta demonstrated by Doppler velocimetry. All five fetuses survived with low morbidity. Unpublished reports are less optimistic, and further studies are necessary to confirm or refute the utility of oxygen therapy for this diagnosis.

CONGENITAL INFECTION

Suspicion of fetal infection usually is aroused by abnormal prenatal examination (ie, lack of fundal height growth), ultrasound findings, or maternal history of exposure or symptomology. Confirmation of infection is important because treatment or specific supportive care is available for certain diseases, and knowledge of prognosis may alter management in others.

The diagnosis of congenital infection remains problematic. Fetal evaluation usually begins with a thorough ultrasound examination. Certain sonographic findings, though not diagnostic of congenital infection, may be consistent with that diagnosis and should arouse suspicion. All of the abnormalities listed in Table 212–2 can be related to infection as well as other etiologies. Ultrasound also may eliminate congenital infection as a diagnosis in certain circumstances. The finding of multiple malformations, for example, would be more consistent with a chromosomal or genetic abnormality.

Maternal history of flulike illness, fever, rash, ingestion of raw meat, or contact with cat litter may be significant. A negative maternal history, however, does not exclude the possibility of infection since many such infectious episodes are subclinical. If reliable maternal serologic data are available, they may be used to confirm exposure. Some women, however, may not mount a serologically detectable immune response despite infection or, alternatively, available laboratory methods may not be sensitive enough to detect a response. When all elements of the clinical evaluation result in significant suspicion, cordocentesis may provide valuable information regarding fetal status.

TABLE 212–2. ABNORMAL ULTRASOUND FINDINGS ASSOCIATED WITH INFECTIONS

Abnormality	Infectious Agent
Intrauterine Growth Retardation	Rubella, CMV[a], Plasmodia
Abnormalities of Fetal Head	
Microcephaly	Rubella, CMV, toxoplasmosis
Hydrocephaly	Rubella, CMV, toxoplasmosis
Hydranencephaly	Toxoplasmosis
Aqueductal stenosis	Influenza, mumps
Dandy–Walker malformation	Rubella, CMV
Porencephaly	
Agenesis of corpus collosum	Toxoplasmosis, rubella
Cardiomyopathy	Coxsackie, mumps
Hepatomegaly and Hepatic Calcifications	Hepatitis, CMV, rubella, toxoplasmosis, syphilis, varicella, coxsackie
Splenomegaly	CMV, syphilis
Hydrops	Coxsackie, syphilis, Toxoplasmosis, CMV, Parvovirus, Herpes, RSV[b]

[a] Cytomegalovirus
[b] Respiratory syncytial virus
From Creasy RK, Resnik R[25] except IUGR data which are from Rodis JF et al.[26]

Useful fetal laboratory tests include a complete blood count, blood gas analysis, liver enzymes (ie, GTT, LDH, and AST), IgM quantification, specific IgM, karyotype, blood for electron microscopy of viral particles (if available), and culture of blood or amniotic fluid. The hemoglobin and hematocrit may document anemia, as can occur with parvovirus infection[26], suggesting the need for fetal intravascular transfusion. Depression of the platelet count is a nonspecific finding that supports the diagnosis of infection by such agents as rubella or cytomegalovirus.[27] Elevation of liver enzymes, particularly GTT, is a common finding[28] in growth-retarded fetuses. In our experience, such elevation associated with normal fetal blood gas measurements suggests infection. IgM quantification may be difficult in the presence of elevated maternal IgG, and it has been suggested that the IgG fraction should be dialyzed. A low or normal IgM does not exclude infection, while a high level supports that diagnosis.

The most specific way to document an infection is to identify viral particles by electron microscopy or by direct culture of blood or amniotic fluid. The success of these techniques depends on the facilities available. In some cases (eg, suspected toxoplasmosis), use of a well recognized reference laboratory is most appropriate.

Treatment must be individualized to the particular infection documented or suspected. In some cases (eg, toxoplasmosis), specific antimicrobial medication is available and of proven value. In others, supportive care in the form of fetal transfusion or oxygen therapy may be attempted. Even if no therapeutic intervention is available, diagnostic information will enable appropriate counseling of the parents and will alert neonatologists to potential problems.

TWIN–TWIN TRANSFUSION

Monozygotic twinning occurs at a rate of four per 1000 live births throughout the world. Some form of vascular anastomosis is observed in 85–100% of monochorial placentae[29], and contributes to the high morbidity and mortality rate observed in such gestations. Anastomoses, usually arteriovenous but occasionally veno-venous, allow the unidirectional shunting of blood from one twin to the other. The donor twin is typically small for gestational age, anemic, and under stress that can lead to intrauterine death. The recipient twin is usually large and plethoric, and may suffer cardiac hypertrophy and failure secondary to volume overload. When manifested as acute hydramnios prior to 24 weeks, the outcome is usually dismal.

An ultrasound examination confirms a significant size discrepancy between the fetuses and polyhydramnios in the sac of the larger twin. When several different Doppler measurements are performed (ie, peak end diastolic velocity, volume flow, and aortic and umbilical peak systolic and end diastolic ratios), discordant twin pairs are likely to demonstrate abnormalities in two or more values.[30] The definitive diagnosis, however, can be made only by cordocentesis to confirm discrepant hematocrits (or to infuse adult blood into the donor and recover it in the recipient), as other etiologies (ie, infection) may lead to a similar clinical presentation.[6] These include congenital infection and discordant aneuploidy or structural abnormalities. Confirmation of twin–twin transfusion syndrome associated with hydrops indicates the need for early delivery if discovered at a time of fetal viability. When extreme prematurity precludes this option, other treatments can be considered, however, none to date have been particularly successful. Therapeutic amniocentesis may be performed to alleviate maternal discomfort and prevent preterm labor or delivery secondary to uterine distention.[31] Such a maneuver is essentially palliative, however, as it does not correct the underlying problem. Attempts to correct fetal congestive heart failure with maternal digitalization often will be unsuccessful as digoxin does not cross the placenta in appreciable amounts under such circumstances.[32] Selective phlebotomy of the plethoric twin with transfusion of the anemic twin has been suggested but not yet formally reported. Careful observation after such a procedure would be required to determine the rate at which the two blood volumes reequilibrated and the appropriate timing of repeat procedures. As a last resort, selective fetocide of the donor twin can be considered. Both the creation of cardiac tamponade by instillation of saline into the pericardial space[33], and tamponade followed by injection of potassium chloride[34] have been reported to be successful and relatively safe for the surviving twin. After such a procedure, follow-up evaluation should include serial ultrasounds, tests of fetal wellbeing, and coagulation studies (principally, fibrinogen and platelet counts). In the future, fetoscopically guided laser ablation of the placental arteriovenous anastomoses may be possible. Such a procedure would restore normal circulation to each fetal placental unit and would eliminate the need for therapy to the fetuses themselves.

NONIMMUNE HYDROPS

Because the use of Rhesus immunoglobulin has significantly decreased the incidence of immune hydrops, the majority of hydrops is now nonimmune in etiology. The perinatal mortality rate for this condition is high (50–98%).[35] The list of etiologies is long and includes cardiovascular pathology (ie, arrhythmias, malformations, and infections) chromosomal or genetic abnormalities, urinary tract malformations, intrathoracic masses or pulmonary pathology, liver disease, gastrointestinal tract abnormalities, blood diseases (ie, α-thalassemia. G6PD deficiency), placental or umbilical cord malformations, infections, and a variety of maternal diseases.[36] Although it may not be possible to diagnose some of these conditions prenatally, an attempt should be made to identify the conditions that are amenable to treatment. Alternatively, knowledge that a condition is untreatable and associated with a poor prognosis allows appropriate prenatal counseling and planning for the remainder of the pregnancy.

After obtaining a maternal history, physical examination, laboratory analysis, and a thorough ultrasound, fetal blood should be obtained by cordocentesis. Valuable laboratory tests include the following: umbilical venous pressure, complete blood count, blood type and direct Coombs test, blood gas analysis, IgM quantification, liver enzyme analysis, and karyotype. The results of these tests in combination with ultrasound findings will eliminate some diagnoses and possibly confirm others. Some problems (ie, infection and arrhythmias) may be amenable to direct treatment. Others (ie, genetic malformation syndromes, and karyotypic abnormalities) will not benefit from therapy and in light of the maternal risks, should prompt discussion of pregnancy termination. Many problems, however, will result from isolated anatomic malformations that do not permit a clear prognosis or therapy to be provided antenatally. Reports of individual treatments in such cases have not been highly successful, but may be considered after appropriate parental counseling and, if necessary, institutional review board ap-

TABLE 212–3. GENETIC DISORDERS IDENTIFIABLE AND TREATABLE WITH CORDOCENTESIS

Coagulation disorders
Factor deficiencies
Von Willebrand's disease
Glanzmann's thrombasthenia
Amegakaryocytic thrombocytopenia
TAR syndrome
Antithrombin III deficiency
Homozygous C or S deficiency
Hemoglobinopathies and red cell disorders
Thalassemia (alpha, beta)
Structural variants
Hereditary spherocytosis
Hereditary pyropoikilocytosis
Diamond–Blackfan syndrome
Aase syndrome
Specific enzyme deficiencies
Metabolic disorders
Those approachable by DNA analysis including mucopolysaccharidoses and mucolipidoses
Maternal hyperphenylalaninemia
White cell and immunologic disorders
Chronic granulomatous disease
Chediak-Higashi syndrome
Adenosine deaminase deficiency
Purine nucleoside phosphorylase deficiency
Wiskott-Aldrich syndrome
Ataxia telangiectasia
Severe combined immunodeficiency
Homozygous C-3 deficiency

proval. Examples of such therapy include intrathoracic shunt placement to divert thoracic fluid and restore normal anatomic relationships[37], and the diversion of abdominal ascites with a peritoneal-amniotic shunt.[38,39] Such measures should be undertaken only by a fetal medicine specialist in a tertiary center.

GENETIC DISORDERS

Chromosomal abnormalities and certain genetic diseases can be diagnosed by evaluation of fetal blood or amniotic fluid. A partial list of such diseases is found in Table 212–3. In many cases, the confirmation of a diagnosis will be helpful for counseling purposes only. In others, however, therapy may be instituted and pregnancy outcome significantly improved. For example, certain metabolic diseases, which usually are diagnosed by enzyme assay of fetal cells, are amenable to maternal dietary manipulation. Fetal methylmalonic acidemia has responded to maternal treatment with large doses of vitamin B_{12}.[40] Maternal ingestion of biotin has been shown to be effective therapy for fetal biotin-responsive multiple carboxylase deficiency.[41] Fetal endocrine status may be determined by direct measurement of fetal hormones. Congenital adrenal hyperplasia, a condition in which a fetal enzyme deficiency results in overproduction of viralizing hormones and masculinization of the female fetus, can be treated successfully by maternal ingestion of dexamethaxone. Treatment for many other genetic disorders remains theoretical and would involve fetal transplantation of normal hematopoietic stem cells and the creation of a chimeric state. For disorders not expressed by the hematopoietic system, gene transfer would be necessary. Detailed discussion of these techniques is beyond the scope of this chapter but recently has been reviewed elsewhere.[42]

In summary, the advent of ultrasound and cordocentesis have supported the development of a new subspecialty, primary fetal medicine. Many pathologic fetal conditions now can be accurately diagnosed and treated, and every month reports of new therapies appear in the literature. The fetus now must be viewed as a patient who can be evaluated directly and treated separately from its mother.

REFERENCES

1. Harrison MR, Golbus MS, Filly RA, eds. The fetus as patient: historical perspective. In: *The Unborn Patient*. Orlando, FL: Grune & Stratton; 1984:5.
2. Donald I. On launching a new diagnostic science. *Am J Obstet Gynecol*. 1969;103:609.
3. Harrison MR, Golbus MS, Filley RA, eds. The fetus as patient: historical perspective. In: *The Unborn Patient*. Orlando, FL: Grune & Stratton; 1984:137.
4. Daffos F, Capella-Parlovsky M, Forestier F. A new procedure for fetal blood sampling in utero: preliminary results of fifty-three cases. *Am J Obstet Gynecol*. 1983;146:985.
5. Seeds JW, Bowes WA, Cheschier NC. Echogenic venous turbulence is a critical feature of successful intravascular intrauterine transfusion. *Obstet Gynecol*. 1989;73:488.
6. Weiner CP. Cordocentesis. *Obstet Gynecol Cl N Amer* 1988;15:283.
7. Pielet BW, Socol ML, MacGregor SN, et al. Fetal heart rate changes after fetal intravascular treatment with pancuronium bromide. *Am J Obstet Gynecol*. 1988;159:640.
8. Cohen F, Gustratson C, Evans MM. Mechanism of isoimmunization: the transplacental passage of fetal erythrocytes in homospecific pregnancies. *Blood*. 1964;23:261.
9. Parer JT. Severe Rh isoimmunization: current methods of in utero diagnosis and treatment. *Am J Obstet Gynecol*. 1988;158:1323.
10. Motew MN, Socol ML, Sabbagha RE. Intrauterine transfusion. In: Sabbaghe RE, ed. *Diagnostic Ultrasound Applied to Obstetrics and Gynecology*. 2nd ed. Philadelphia: J.B. Lippincott; 1987:424.
11. Devore GR, Mayden K, Tortora M, et al. Dilatation of the fetal umbilical vein in rhesus hemolytic anemia: a predictor of severe disease. *Am J Obstet Gynecol*. 1981;141:464.
12. Witter FR, Graham D. The utility of ultrasonically measured vein diameters in isoimmunized pregnancies. *Am J Obstet Gynecol*. 1983;146:225.
13. Chitkara U, Wilkins I, Lynch L, et al. The role of sonography in assessing severity of fetal anemia in Rh- and Kell-isoimmunized pregnancies. *Obstet Gynecol*. 1988;71:393.
14. Vintzileos AM, Campbell WA, Storlazzi E, et al. Fetal liver ultrasound measurements in isoimmunized pregnancies. *Obstet Gynecol*. 1986;68:162.
15. Warren PS, Gill RW, Fisher CC. Doppler flow studies in rhesus isoimmunization. *Semin Perinat*. 1987;11:375.
16. Liley AW. Liquor amnii analysis in the management of the pregnancy complicated by Rhesus sensitization. *Am J Obstet Gynecol*. 1961;82:1359.
17. Nicolaides KH, Rodeck CH, Mibashan RS, Kemp JR. Have Liley charts outlived their usefulness? *Am J Obstet Gynecol*. 1986;155:90.
18. Kaplan JA. Pharmacology of muscle relaxants and their antagonists. In: Miller RD, ed. *Anesthesia*. 2nd ed. New York: Churchill Livingstone; 1986:1177.
19. Eckhardt-Muller C, Grubert A, Weisheit M, et al. 348 cases of suspected neonatal alloimmune thrombocytopenia. *Lancet*. 1989;ii:363.
20. Bussel JB, Berkowitz RL, McFarland JG, et al. Antenatal treatment of neonatal alloimmune thrombocytopenia. *N Engl J Med*. 1988;319:1374.
21. Weiner CP, Williamson RA. Evaluation of severe growth retardation using cordocentesis: hematologic and metabolic alterations by etiology. *Obstet Gyencol*. 1989;73:225.
22. Patil SR, Weiner C, Williamson R. Rapid chromosome analysis and prenatal diagnosis using fluid from cystic hygromas. *N Engl J Med*. 1987;317:1159.
23. Nicolaides KH, Campbell S, Bradley RJ, et al. Maternal oxygen therapy for intrauterine growth retardation. *Lancet*. 1987;1:942.
24. Romero R, Pilu G, Leanty P, et al. eds. *Prenatal Diagnosis of Congenital Anomalies*. Norwalk, CT: Appleton & Lange; 1988.
25. Creasy RK, Resnik R. Intrauterine growth retardation. In: RK Creasy, R Resnik, eds. *Maternal Fetal Medicine: Principles and Practice*. Philadelphia: W.B. Saunders;1989:551.
26. Rodis JF, Hovick TJ, Quinn DL, et al. Human parvovirus infection in pregnancy. *Obstet Gynecol*. 1988;72:733.

27. Romero R, Duffy TP. Platelet disorders in pregnancy. *Clin Perinat.* 1980;7:327.
28. Cox WL, Daffos F, Forestier F, et al. Physiology and management of intrauterine growth retardation: biologic approach with fetal blood sampling. *Am J Obstet Gynecol.* 1988;159:36.
29. Galea P, Scott JM, Goel KM. Feto-fetal transfusion syndrome. *Archives Dis Child.* 1982;57:781.
30. Nimrod C, Davies D, Harder J, et al. Doppler ultrasound prediction of fetal outcome in twin pregnancies. *Am J Obstet Gynecol.* 1987;156:402.
31. Feingold M, Cetrulo CL, Newton ER, et al. Serial amniocentesis in the treatment of twin to twin transfusion complicated with acute polyhydramnios. *Acta Genet Med Gemell.* 1986;35:107.
32. Weiner CP, Thompson MIB. Direct fetal treatment of supraventricular tachycardia after failed transplacental therapy. *Am J Obstet Gynecol.* 1988;153:570.
33. Wittmann BK, Farguharson DF, Thomas WDS, et al. The role of feticide in the management of severe twin transfusion syndrome. *Am J Obstet Gynecol.* 1986;155:1023.
34. Weiner CP. Diagnosis and treatment of twin to twin transfusion in the mid-second trimester of pregnancy. *Fetal Ther.* 1987;2:71.
35. Castillo RA, Devoe LD, Hadi HA, et al. Nonimmune hydrops fetalis: clinical experience and factors related to a poor outcome. *Am J Obstet Gynecol.* 1986;155:812.
36. Holzgreve W, Holzgreve B, Curry CJR. Nonimmune hydrops fetalis: diagnosis and management. *Semin Perinat.* 1985;9:52.
37. Weiner C, Varner H, Pringle K, et al. Antenatal diagnosis and palliative treatment of nonimmune hydrops fetalis secondary to pulmonary extralobar sequestration. *Obstet Gynecol.* 1986;68:275.
38. Seeds JW, Herbert WNP, Bowes WA, Cefalo RC. Recurrent idiopathic fetal hydrops: Results of prenatal therapy. *Obstet Gynecol.* 1984;64:305.
39. Goldberg JD, Mitty H, Dische MR, Berkowitz RL. Prenatal shunting of fetal ascites in nonimmune hydrops fetalis. *Am J Perinat.* 1986;3:92.
40. Ampola MG, Mahoney MJ, Nakamura E, Tanaka K. Prenatal therapy of a patient with Vitamin B_{12}-responsive methylmalonic acidemia. *N Engl J Med.* 1975;293:313.
41. Packman S, Cowan MJ, Golbus MS. Prenatal treatment of biotin-responsive multiple carboxylase deficiency. *Lancet.* 1982;i:1435.
42. Johnson JM, Elias S. Prenatal treatment: medical and gene therapy in the fetus. *Clin Obstet Gynecol.* 1988;31:390.

Chapter Two Hundred and Thirteen

Therapeutic Intrauterine Corrections of Fetal Anomalies

Mark I. Evans, Arie Drugan, Frank A. Manning, Alan J. Sacks, and Michael R. Harrison

213

Only three decades ago, pregnancy was a mystery; the first opportunity to visualize fetal structure and function came at birth. In the 1960s, two major contributions inaugurated the era of the fetus as a patient. First, prenatal diagnosis became possible using amniocentesis as a technique to evaluate fetal health by cytogenetic[1] and biochemical[2,3] analysis. Second, prenatal treatment became possible using fetal transfusion to control Rh-erythroblastosis fetalis.[4] Open intrauterine exchange transfusion was attempted and abandoned due to an unacceptably high maternal morbidity associated with open procedures.[5] Fortunately, the development of less invasive techniques of percutaneous placement of catheters or needles for intraperitoneal transfusion allowed such treatments to proceed.[6]

In the 1970s, the introduction of fetal ultrasonography added another dimension to prenatal diagnosis, as the structure and function of the fetus could be visualized. With increasing expertise and advancing technology, the list of fetal anomalies diagnosable by ultrasonography has expanded tremendously.[7,8] More recently, the ability to detect some anomalies for patients who might not otherwise have tolerated invasive testing has expanded considerably by judicious use of maternal serum α-fetoprotein (MSAFP) screening.[9] The combination of ultrasonography with MSAFP screening[9] allows the prenatal diagnosis of anomalies of the fetal neural tube, abdominal wall, urinary and lymphatic systems (ie, cystic hygroma), and chromosomal anomalies. Following the diagnosis of a fetal anomaly prior to 24 weeks' gestation, parents have to choose between terminating the pregnancy or preparing for the birth.[10,11] While parents must never be told to abort the fetus, no matter how serious the anomaly, the option must always be presented when legally permissible. If pregnancy continues, knowledge of the defect has both psychological advantages for the parents and logistical advantages for the pediatric staff who will care for the baby after birth.

FETAL DIAGNOSIS

The methods of fetal diagnosis are reviewed in Chapters 16 and 212. Approaches include invasive testing of fetal tissues by amniocentesis, chorionic villus sampling, and umbilical blood sampling. Population screening techniques, such as maternal serum α-fetoprotein, a detailed family history, or ultrasound detection of fetal anomalies, help direct patients to more invasive procedures and form a cohort that may be at higher risk.

Each of the above methods detects fetal functional abnormalities, although conditions such as aneuploidy often have detectable morphologic aberrations. This chapter presents some of the advances in ultrasound diagnosis that have made the fetal intervention described below possible.

The most significant advance in the development of fetal-perinatal medicine is real-time ultrasound. This allows safe visualization and monitoring of the developing embryo in vivo.[12] Parents and neonatologists now can prepare for a child with a congenital malformation.

The use of fetal surveillance techniques in complicated pregnancies is described in Chapter 6. Approximately 3% of live births have major malformations, and congenital malformations contribute up to 25% of the perinatal mortality rate.[13] As ultrasound technology has increased in resolution and knowledge of fetal development has become more sophisticated, there is an extensive range of literature with subtle findings possible with ultrasound.[12] Here we discuss some categories of anatomic malformations detectable with ultrasound, particularly those that may be treated *in utero*.

Neural Tube Defects

Neural tube defects are the most common anatomic malformation resulting in perinatal death. They occur in about one of 600 live births, 50% of which are anencephalic and 50% have vertebral lesions.[14]

The diagnosis of anencephaly may be made early in the second trimester (12–14 weeks). This was the first reported sonographic diagnosis for which a pregnancy was terminated.[15] The sonographic appearance of anencephaly is characterized by the absence of calvarial bones and normal cerebral structures[12] (Fig. 213–1). The cerebral structures instead are replaced with amorphous, cystic tissue termed *the area cerebrovascular*. The facial bones and occiput are generally present, and the fetal face frequently has a frog-like appearance on ultrasound.

The diagnosis of vertebral lesions is made after examination of the full length of the spine in longitudinal (sagittal) and transverse views. Both planes are necessary to exclude fully an open spinal defect. The normal longitudinal appearance often is compared to railroad tracks into the distance, gently tapering together. In this view, spina bifida is seen as widening between neural processes.[16] In the transverse plane, each vertebral arch appears as a closed structure, with the overlying skin intact. In the presence of spina bifida, the normally closed circle is opened to a "U," generally with a cystic structure, meningomyelocele, extruding through the skin of the back. Ventriculomegaly will be found in 70–80% of fetuses with spina bifida, usually of the communicating type. Additionally, in cases of vertebral lesions, the fetal head may be found to have a characteristically abnormal shape, with scalloping of the frontal bones called *lemon sign*, because of its likeness to a lemon on the bottom of a grocer's shelf.

Holoprosencephaly

This is a diverse category of malformations resulting from a failure of appropriate division of the prosencephalon or forebrain. Depending on the presence or complete absence of division, this is categorized as lobar, hemilobar, or alobar, respectively. It may be diagnosed as early as 14 weeks and is characterized by a monoventricular appearance and absent midline structures of the fetal cerebrum. Failure of appropriate division also may involve the face, in which case cyclopia, cebocephaly, or facial clefts may result. Although it is generally fatal in the early neonatal period, the few known survivors suffer severe mental and physical impairment. Holoprosencephaly always should prompt a karyotype analysis because it often may be associated with trisomy 13 or 18. Aneuploidy may be considered in the differential diagnosis of hydrocephaly and should be ruled out if prenatal treatment is to be considered.

Hydrocephaly

Hydrocephaly is excessive cerebrospinal fluid (CSF) accumulation, resulting in dilation of the ventricular system. In general, fetal intracranial contents are visualized reliably by 18 weeks. The ventricles are evaluated by examining the transverse views at the level of the biparietal diameter (BPD), and comparing ventricular size to hemispheric or cranial size. Nomograms are available to evaluate such measurements.[17] Especially during the second trimester, the BPD or head circumference (HC) may not represent macrocephaly. Therefore, evaluations of both the absolute and relative dimensions of the ventricle are necessary to diagnose hydrocephaly.[18] Serial scans demonstrating the progressive nature of the process add to the documentation of the diagnosis. Examination of the individual components

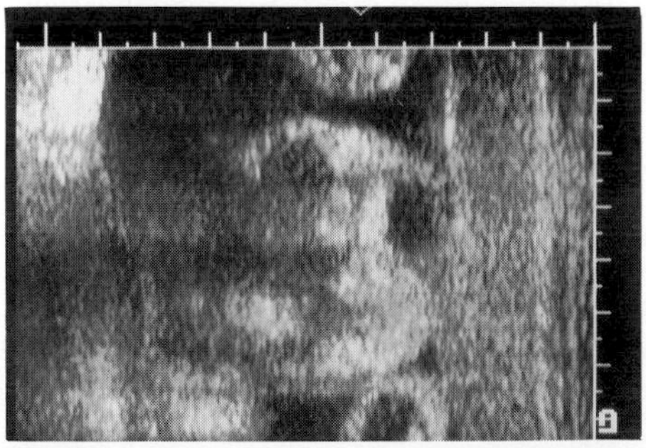

A

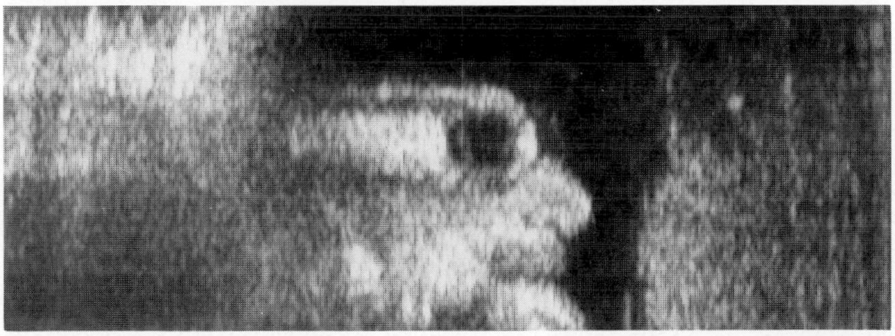

B

Figure 213–1. Frontal view **(A)** and profile **(B)** of anencephalic fetus demonstrating absent calvarium above orbits.

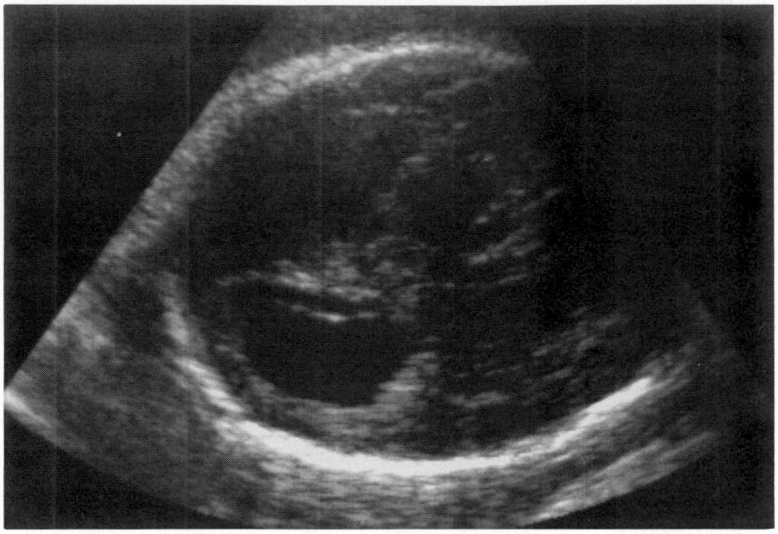

Figure 213–2. Sonogram demonstrating ventriculomegaly of the posterior horn.

of the ventricular system, that is, both anterior and posterior horns of the lateral ventricle, and third and fourth ventricles may provide some insight into the level of the obstruction, if present (Fig. 213–2). Sites above an obstruction demonstrate dilation, whereas those caudal do not. For example, aquaductal stenosis, the most common form, causes dilated lateral and third ventricles, whereas the fourth ventricle appears normal. Communicating hydrocephalus, a consequential phenomenon in 70% of cases of spina bifida, has dilation of the whole cerebral ventricular system.

Identification of hydrocephaly must prompt a careful search for associated abnormalities, especially if prenatal therapy is to be considered, inasmuch as such findings are common.[19,20] As many as 83% of prenatally diagnosed hydrocephalic fetuses have other abnormalities. These include spina bifida (30%), karyotype abnormalities (9%), as well as severe abnormalities of the renal, gastrointestinal, cardiac, and skeletal systems.[12]

The diagnostic work up of hydrocephaly thus should include a targeted scan for fetal anomalies and a fetal karyotype. Since ventriculomegaly may be the consequence of some congenital infections, maternal or fetal TORCH IgM titers also may be helpful in establishing an etiology.

Obstructive Uropathy

Modern ultrasound equipment allows detailed evaluation of the fetal renal system (kidneys and bladder) by 18–20 weeks[12], but with the most sophisticated equipment, visualization can be considerably earlier. In ordinary circumstances, the ureters are not imaged. Indirect assessment of renal function also may be obtained by sonographic evaluation of amniotic fluid volume and bladder filling and emptying over time. Although a host of fetal renal abnormalities may be diagnosed by ultrasound, including renal agenesis and multicystic and polycystic renal disease[21],the details of these are outside the intent of this chapter and the discussion here will be limited to obstructive uropathies, in particular, posterior urethral valve syndrome (PUV).

The fetal kidneys are functional and produce small amounts of urine by 11–12 weeks.[22] By 20 weeks, fetal urine is the major component of amniotic fluid. Obstruction to the urethral outflow results in the loss of replenishment of fluid, and the proximal dilation of the renal system.[23] If the obstruction is complete and persistent, this leads to oligo- or anhydramnios, megacystis, bladder wall hypertrophy, and eventual bilateral hydroureter and hydronephrosis. This collection of findings, depending on the stage of the process, is the sonographic hallmark of PUV. Demonstration of male genitalia helps confirm the diagnosis, since the process usually does not occur in females. As the process continues, the increase in urinary back pressure may result in progressive hydronephrosis and loss of all renal function.

The evaluation of PUV should include detailed anomaly scanning for other abnormalities since cardiac, skeletal, and GI abnormalities have been reported in association with PUV. This may require diagnostic amnioinfusion, since oligohydramnios greatly hinders sonographic visualization. Karyotype determination should be performed because chromosomal abnormalities are present in 18–24% of all cases.

Fetal Heart

Cardiac malformations occur in 1% of newborns and up to 10% of stillborns.[25] Despite the obvious importance, it is only recently that fetal cardiac structure has become a subject for detailed scrutiny.[26,27] Fetal echocardiography has become virtually its own discipline. The modalities available include high-resolution real-time evaluation, M-mode, pulsed-wave Doppler, and color-flow studies.[25]

The fetal heart can be detected in nearly every sonographic evaluation. The presence of cardiac activity is one of the earliest signs of fetal life, generally becoming apparent between 6–7 weeks of age.

The fundamental examination of the fetal heart is the evaluation of the so-called four-chambered view (Fig. 213–3). This is evaluated most reliably at or after 17 weeks, although the definitive statement of normalcy may not be possible until 22 weeks. The correctly obtained view is a transverse plane through the fetal chest, demonstrating the two atria and two ventricles. The right ventricle is seen slightly anterior to the left. The atria should be compared and found to be of roughly equal sizes. The same is true of the ventricles. The atrial septum and ventricular septum are visualized and should appear intact, save for the nor-

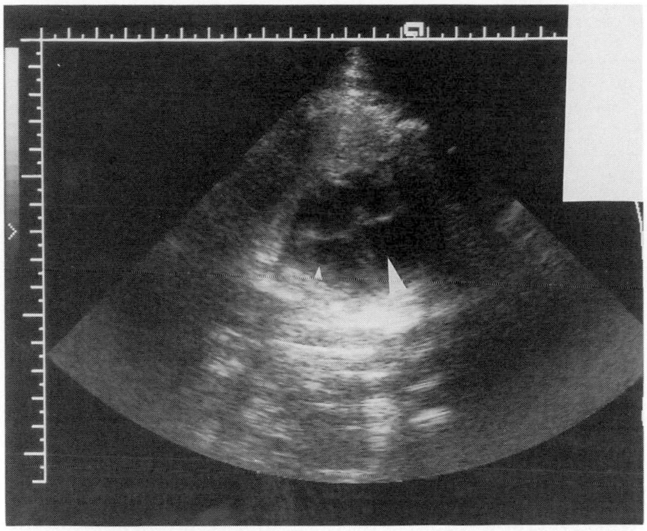

Figure 213–3. Four-chamber view of normal fetal heart shows the right ventricle *(small arrowhead)* and left ventricle *(large arrowhead)* with respective atria directly posterior.

mally patent foramen ovale, located posteriorly in the atrial septum. The synchrony of the chambers as well as the rate may be assessed visually.

The four-chambered view should be sought and evaluated when possible. With experience, the normal or abnormal view can be assessed; it is estimated that the presence of a normal four-chambered view effectively rules out at least 90% of significant cardiac defects.[25]

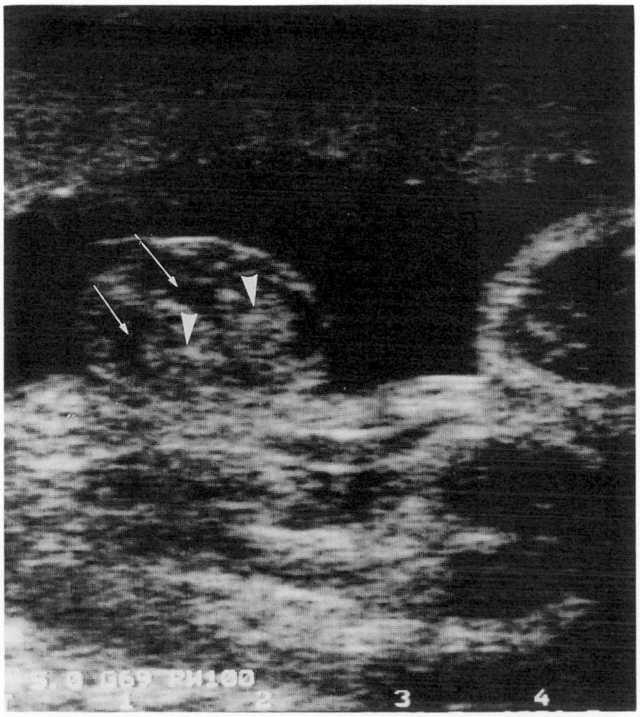

Figure 213–4. Fetal scrotum demonstrating descended testes *(arrowheads)* with surrounding hydrocele fluid *(small arrow)*.

Fetal Gender

The prenatal diagnosis of fetal sex is rarely medically significant, and is not in itself considered an appropriate indication for ultrasound scanning in the United States; however, there are exceptions. For example, with a family history of X-linked disorder, identification of a female reassures the absence of disease, while a male may trigger further invasive testing.[10]

Identification of fetal gender requires a cooperative fetal position for perineal visualization.[29] This may pose a problem in up to 30% of cases. Identification of a male requires visualization of a phallus and testes within the scrotum (Fig. 213–4), remembering that descent occurs at approximately 28–32 weeks. Determination of a female is not merely the absence of male organs, but rather requires visualization of labia majora and minora, described as the "female echo" of "three or four lines" (Fig. 213–5).

The presence of a prominent phallus, absent scrotum, and testes may suggest congenital adrenal hyperplasia (CAH) in cases at risk, whereas a discrepancy in genitalia (female) with the obtained karyotype (male) may represent testicular feminization. Such information prenatally may have significant impact on obstetric and neonatal care.

PRENATAL TREATMENT

In a limited number of circumstances, there may be an option to treat before birth. Tried therapies have been surgical and medical. Several questions arise when a potentially correctable fetal anomaly is diagnosed.

1. What is the natural outcome of this anomaly? Will additional or irreversible damage be caused to the fetus if repair procedures are delayed until after birth?
2. Is it possible to correct the anomaly or its consequences *in utero?* Will the procedure change the natural outcome?
3. What is the risk to the mother and the fetus?

Surgical intervention *in utero* should be considered only if:

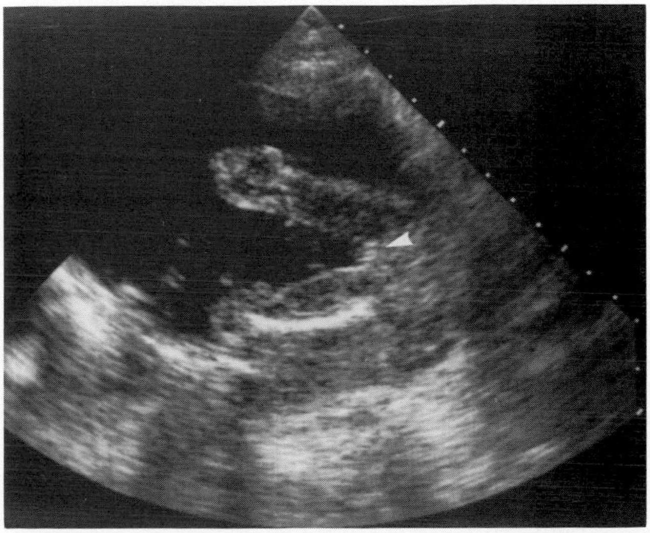

Figure 213–5. Sonogram of fetal perineum. The arrowhead is at the three-line sign, indicative of a female fetus.

TABLE 213–1. FETAL OBSTRUCTIVE HYDROCEPHALUS: DISTRIBUTION BY PRIMARY DIAGNOSIS AND SURVIVAL IN 41 TREATED CASES

Primary Diagnosis Postnatal	No. of Cases	% Total Cases	No. of Deaths	% Mortality by Diagnosis	No. of Survivors	% Survival/ Diagnosis
Aqueductal stenosis	32	76.9	4	13.3	28	87.5
Associated anomalies	5	12.7	2	40	3	60
Holoprosencephaly	1	2.6	1	100	0	0
Dandy–Walker syndrome	1	2.6	–	–	1	100
Porencephalic cyst	1	2.6	–	–	1	100
Arnold–Chiari	1	2.6	–	–	1	100
Total	41	100	7	17	34	83

1. The natural history of the anomaly frequently is associated with neonatal severe handicap or early death.
2. There is evidence (from animal models) that the natural history of the anomaly can be changed by the surgical procedure.
3. The risk to the mother is relatively small as proven in a rigorous animal model (eg, the nonhuman primate).

In the early 1980s, investigators identified several fetal diseases in which a simple anatomic defect interferes with organ development and might be amenable to correction: hydronephrosis, hydrocephalus, and diaphragmatic hernia.[30,31] The International Fetal Medicine and Surgery Society, first meeting in 1982, formulated guidelines for fetal intervention[32] and established a registry to record all cases of obstructive uropathy and obstructive ventriculomegaly in which *in utero* operative procedures were undertaken. Registries for fetal medical treatment, cardiac arrhythmias, chylothorax, and others have been established since. The results of these registries are published periodically.[33]

Fetal Ventriculomegaly

Much of the focus in the early 1980s of the potential for fetal therapy centered on obstructive ventriculomegaly. Interest in this disorder emerged from the relative ease to diagnose such anomalies by ultrasound and was amplified by the success rates of a similar shunting procedure performed in the neonate.[34] The concept, as developed in animal models, was that early shunting of ventriculomegaly *in utero* might prevent the irreversible damage caused by prolonged increased intracranial pressure.[35-37] In humans, however, the results of ventriculoamniotic shunts seem at first glance to be disappointing. As of July 1, 1991, 45 cases of fetal ventriculomegaly treated *in utero* by chronic ventriculoamniotic shunts were reported to the International Fetal Registry (Table 213–1). In the majority of instances, the shunting was performed for a fetus presumed to have ventriculomegaly-hydrocephalus secondary to aqueductal stenosis. The mean gestational age at diagnosis was 25 ± 2.73 weeks (range, 18–31 weeks), and the mean age at treatment was 27 ± 2.6 weeks (range, 23–33 weeks). The duration of effective therapy cannot be determined from registry data since objective means of assessment of shunt function are not available. Of 41 fetuses with hydrocephalus treated by ventricular amniotic shunting, 34 have survived (83%). Of the seven deaths that occurred, four could be directly attributed to trauma at the time of placement of the shunt or to premature labor occurring within 48 hours of shunt placement. The crude mortality rate for the procedure thus is 9%. The 38 surviving infants have been followed on average for 12.2 ± 5.8 months (range, 6–36 months). Of the 34 surviving fetuses, 14 (35.3%), all with aqueductal stenosis, are reported as normal at follow-up evaluation (Table 213–2). The remaining 24 survivors all have exhibited varying degrees of neurologic handicap; the majority of these children (18 of 34 survivors, 53%) are classified as having severe handicaps. These infants all exhibited gross delay in reaching developmental milestones, and in infants, the tested developmental quotient was always less than 60. Five of these infants have had cortical blindness, three have had seizure disorders, and two have spastic diplegia. Outcome among survivors was related principally to the primary etiology of obstructive hydrocephalus. Aqueductal stenosis of uncertain etiology was the most common etiologic factor for obstructive hydrocephalus (28 of 41 cases, 68%) and the only intact survivors were found in this group.

TABLE 213–2. FETAL OBSTRUCTIVE HYDROCEPHALUS: OUTCOME IN 34 TREATED, SURVIVING INFANTS

Primary Diagnosis (postnatal)	No. of Survivors	No. of Normal	%	Outcome				%
				No. of Mild/Moderate Handicap	%	No. of Severe Handicap		
Aqueductal stenosis	28	12	42.8	2	7.2	14		50
Associated anomalies	3	0	0	0	0	3		100
Dandy–Walker syndrome	1	0	0	1	100	0		0
Porencephalic cyst	1	0	0	0	0	1		100
Arnold–Chiari	1	0	0	1	100	0		0
Total	34	12	35.3	4	11.8	18		52.9

TABLE 213–3. OUTCOME OF PREGNANCY IN 26 PATIENTS WITH FETAL VENTRICULOMEGALY DIAGNOSED PRENATALLY AND DELIVERED AT TERM

Group	Total Cases	Progression In Utero	Other Anomalies	Postnatal VP Shunt	Outcome			Early[d] Death	Late[e] Death
					Normal	Mod	Sev		
A	5	0	0	0	5	0	0	0	0
B	5(+1)[a]	2	0	5	3	2[b]	0	0	0
C	8	2	8	8	0	5[c]	3	0	2
D	7	?	7	0	0	0	2	5	2

[a] One neonate lost from follow-up evaluation.
[b] Both cases had progressive disease in utero.
[c] 4 of 5 only myelomeningocele.
[d] Early neonatal death (within the first week of life).
[e] Late neonatal death (within the first year of life).
Group A = isolated VM without progression or postnatal treatment; Group B = isolated progressive VM, postnatal VP shunt; Group C = VM + other anomalies, postnatal VP shunt; Group D = VM + other anomalies without postnatal treatment; VM = ventriculomegaly; VP = ventriculo peritoneal; Mod = moderate; Sev = severe.

The results of ventriculo-amniotic shunting for fetal ventriculomegaly have been disappointing, and consequently no shunt clinics exist; there is a *de facto* moratorium in place.[38,39] The hope, which was to take fetuses who otherwise would be severely impaired by ventriculomegaly and to avoid irreversible damage by intrauterine treatment, was substituted in a few instances with survival of severely affected infants who otherwise would have died.

Despite the poor outcomes in treated fetuses, abandonment of the concept of shunting for ventriculomegaly must be reconsidered for several reasons. Analysis of the cases of ventriculo-amniotic shunt placement performed in the 1980s reported in the registry shows that selection criteria were not always employed appropriately, and fetuses with ventriculomegaly associated with other severe anomalies (ie, holoprosencephaly or autosomal trisomies) also were given the "benefit" of intrauterine treatment.

Current reports demonstrate that the natural history of fetal ventriculomegaly is also dismal[40,41] (Table 213–3). The major determinant of prognosis was the association with other intracranial or extracranial malformations. Additional malformations affect 70–85% of fetuses with ventriculomegaly, and all such cases suffer perinatal mortality or severe morbidity. Even if a diligent search for additional malformations were performed by combining a detailed ultrasound study of the fetus with amniocentesis for karyotype and amniotic fluid α-fetoprotein and acetylcholinesterase, 20–40% of abnormalities would not be detected, even by experienced personnel.[40,41] The obvious candidates for *in utero* ventricular shunting are the fetuses with isolated progressive ventriculomegaly. These are limited in number by a high rate of associated anomalies and by the relative failure to exclude additional malformations prenatally. The severity of ventriculomegaly is not always predictive of outcome or even of the need for postnatal shunt, as ventriculomegaly may not be associated with elevated intracranial pressure.

Considering the uncertainty and the difficulty of accurate prenatal diagnosis, intrauterine treatment of fetal ventriculomegaly remains a controversial and highly experimental procedure that is currently moribund as a *defacto* moratorium is in place. However, when the option in midtrimester is between termination of pregnancy or inactive observation of progressive dilatation of the ventricles, placement of a ventriculo-amniotic shunt should present a third option in selected cases.[39] Given the small number of good candidates and the need to develop a new catheter (as none is currently available), in the future a new study could be performed in one of the few centers experienced in the technical aspects of ventriculo-amniotic shunt placement that would answer the question of its usefulness.

Obstructive Uropathy in the Fetus

The widespread use of obstetric ultrasonography, the increase in resolution, and technical expertise allow the recognition of obstructive uropathies more frequently and earlier in pregnancy.[41,42] Retrograde pressure forms behind the obstruction and causes increasing dilatation of the urinary system. As documented in animal studies, hydronephrotic and, perhaps, dysplastic changes occur in the renal parenchyma.[43-46] The severe oligohydramnios associated with bilateral urinary tract obstruction results in pressure deformities of the face and limbs, and pulmonary hypoplasia; neonatal death is caused by respiratory insufficiency. The timing and the degree of obstruction are crucial determinants in the development of irreversible renal and pulmonary damage.[47]

Intrauterine treatment should be reserved for cases with bilateral urinary tract obstruction, maintained renal function, decreased amniotic fluid volume, and no other life-threatening anomalies.[48] Cytogenetic anomalies and congenital malformations of other systems are diagnosed in 15–40% of cases of fetal obstructive uropathy.[49,50] The evaluation should include the karyotype (by amniocentesis, transabdominal chorionic villus sampling, or cordocentesis), echocardiography, and a detailed ultrasound examination to assess renal size or dysplastic changes, to evaluate fetal bladder filling, and to exclude additional malformations. If fetal visualization is hampered by severe oligohydramnios, artificial installation of fluid will improve sonographic visibility. The observation of fetal behavior (drinking, filling of stomach and bladder) makes the study of fetal anatomy more accurate.[51]

The evaluation of fetal renal function is based on ultrasonographic observation of bladder filling (after urine aspiration), absence of renal cortical cysts, and analysis of urine osmolarity and electrolytes.[52] None of these tests, however, are infallible. The bladder may fill from secretion by bladder mucosa. The ultrasonic demonstration of renal cortical cysts has a specificity of 100% and a sensitivity of 44% in identifying renal dysplasia with irreversible damage.[53] Hypotonic fetal urine (sodium less than 100 mEq/mL; chlorine less than 90 mEq/mL; osmolarity less than 210 mOsm) suggests maintained glomerular and tubular function. However, while abnormal electrolytes and osmolarity in fetal urine are associated with poor prognosis in the majority of cases, hypotonic urine does not exclude reliably the finding of dysplasia or neonatal evidence of severe renal dysfunction.[48,54] Urinary electrolytes normally drop with gestational age (Rodeck C, personal communication).

Dumez[55] has evaluated multiple urinary parameters and found sodium, beta-2 microglobulin NH_3, and creatinine to be good predictions of renal function and long-term outcome. Overall, the best ultrasonic indicator of the severity of the disease appears to be the decrease in amniotic fluid volume. When the fetus develops severe oligohydramnios before the 20th week of gestation, the prognosis usually is dismal.[52]

Most procedures of vesicoamniotic shunt placement have been performed percutaneously with ultrasonographic guidance. A double-coiled nylon catheter was used in most cases with good results. One-way valve catheters are not necessary because the pressure in the obstructed bladder usually exceeds that in the amniotic fluid.

The function of these shunts, however, may be impaired by occlusion or displacement, necessitating close observation and replacement of the nonfunctioning shunt. When weeks to months of continuous drainage are required, some favor open surgical decompression by bladder marsupialization or bilateral ureterostomies.[52,56-58] However, this would involve an increased risk to both mother and fetus. Of the 87 cases of fetal obstructive uropathy reported to the registry as of July 1, 1991, there have been 34 survivors (40.2%) (Table 213–4). The oldest survivor is now 7 years of age and appears to be developing normally. The gestational age at initial referral has been 23 ± 4.6 weeks (range, 14–34 weeks), and the mean age at *in utero* therapy has been 24.2 ± 5 weeks (range, 14–36 weeks). No uniformity in shunt design, construction material, or method of shunt placement is recorded. Of the 87 cases, 13 (14.9%) were terminated electively after shunt placement—in seven instances because of abnormal karyotype and in six instances because of suspect or proven major renal dysfunction. Of the remaining 74 pregnancies that were ongoing after shunt placement, there have been 35 fetal survivors (47.3%). Perinatal survival is strongly related to primary etiology of obstructive uropathy, and the criteria for diagnosing etiology of the disease has continued to improve. The best survival is reported among fetuses with proven posterior urethral valve syndrome (68%).

The long-term follow-up evaluation of these children is now becoming available. To date, chronic morbidity is being reported in only three of 35 survivors (8.6%). One of these children with posterior urethral valve syndrome has developed chronic renal failure requiring hemodialysis. One survivor has borderline renal function and chronic pulmonary insufficiency that is progressed at 2 years of age. A third child, a female, has required extensive and ongoing corrective surgery for persistent cloacal syndrome. The operative mortality rate remains relatively constant. The death rate directly attributable to vesico-amniotic shunting has been 4.7% (4 of 85 cases).

These data may be interpreted to suggest that there is a defined role for chronic vesico-amniotic shunting in fetuses with bilateral hydronephrosis secondary to urethral obstruction (usually males with posterior urethral valves) who have normal karyotypes, have progressive and persistent disease, have time to develop pulmonary tissue, and have good prognostic criteria (good fetal urine electrolytes and osmolarity, and normal renal parenchymal echogenicity without cysts) at the time of preoperative assessment.

It is apparent in reviewing the recent data referred to in the registry that much more selective criteria are being used before a patient is considered a candidate for fetal surgery. Most notably, use of fetal urinary electrolytes and osmolarity have had a major discriminating effect. As a result, survival in treated fetuses is continuing to improve, whereas the proportion of evaluated fetuses being treated continues to fall.

Open Fetal Surgery

While the percutaneous approach under ultrasonographic guidance seems to be the preferred method for placing a shunt in a hollow enlarged viscus, the correction of more extensive fetal anomalies will require more extensive and more invasive surgery on both mother and fetus. The feasibility of open fetal surgery was demonstrated anecdotally in the 1960s when an open technique was used for intra-

TABLE 213–4. FETAL OBSTRUCTIVE UROPATHY: PRIMARY DIAGNOSIS[a] AND OUTCOME IN 87 TREATED CASES

Primary Diagnosis	No. of Cases	% Total	No. of Survivors	% Survival by Diagnosis
Posterior urethral valve syndrome	25	28.7	17	68
Karyotype abnormality[b]	7	8.0	0	0
Renal dysplasia by ultrasound[b]	6	6.9	0	0
Urethral atresia	6	6.9	1	20
"Prune belly" syndrome	5	5.7	4	16.7
Unknown diagnosis	1	1.1	1	100
Ureteropelvic obstruction	2	2.3	2	100
Unknown etiology	35	40.2	10	28.6
Total	87	100.0	35	40.2

[a] Primary diagnosis as confirmed by either antenatal or neonatal assessment or by autopsy
[b] Elective pregnancy termination

uterine exchange transfusions in erythroblastosis fetalis.[59] However, preterm labor and abortion made this initial experience so discouraging that direct exposure of the fetus was abandoned for over a decade. In the late 1970s and early 1980s, interest in open fetal surgery was revived by two factors. Prenatal diagnosis of some simple, anatomic defects with disastrous consequences for the developing fetus (eg, fatal pulmonary hypoplasia secondary to urinary tract obstruction or diaphragmatic hernia) were being recognized. At the same time, neonatologists and pediatric surgeons were coming to grips with the futility of attempting to salvage these babies after birth. It became apparent that the only way to salvage fetuses with these lesions was by open surgery. However, the open approach could be justified only if the following criteria were met:

1. The natural history of the human fetal disorder was defined and only those fetuses with the disorder who were likely to benefit from intervention were selected.
2. The pathophysiology of the disorder and the efficacy of *in utero* correction was established in animal models.
3. The proposed procedure was proven feasible and safe for both fetus and mother in a rigorous, nonhuman primate model. Extensive experience with fetal surgery in sheep and phylogenetically lower animals could not be used to evaluate the feasibility and safety of fetal intervention in humans because the biology of gestation is dissimilar and hysterotomy seldom induces preterm labor and abortion. The primate uterus, conversely, is exquisitely sensitive to surgical manipulation, making success in this model a rigorous criterion for human application.

In the early 1980s, the group in San Francisco satisfied these criteria by studying the pathophysiology of diaphragmatic hernia[60-62] and hydronephrosis[43-47] in animals, by defining the natural history and outcome of diaphragmatic hernia[63-65] and obstructive uropathy[52,56-58] in human fetuses, and by developing the anesthetic, pharmacologic, and surgical techniques in the nonhuman primate necessary to make open fetal surgery safe for both mother and fetus.[66-68] The techniques developed in the laboratory have been applied by Harrison et al in over one dozen cases since the mid-1980s including the first successes for repair of diaphragmatic hernia reported in 1990. Since the first success, there have now been several others allowing for the first time, the potential for accurate statistics or outcome.[68a] There were no significant intraoperative complications. Operative blood loss ranged from 200–1000 cc, but none of the patients required transfusion. There were no wound infections or complications, and hospital stay following fetal surgery ranged from 5–13 days (mean, 7.7 days). Two patients developed amniotic fluid leaks postoperatively owing to the technique of uterine closure, which has since been corrected. The most common postoperative problem was uterine irritability, and all patients required tocolytic therapy. Premature labor remains a constant threat and the major morbidity associated with fetal surgery. Three of these patients have had subsequent normal pregnancies, suggesting that fetal surgery does not interfere with reproductive capacity.

These first cases of open fetal surgery represent a steep learning curve, but the overall experience argues for continued cautious application of these surgical procedures. Open fetal surgery is technically difficult but feasible and thus far has proven safe for mother and her reproductive potential. The efficacy of these procedures in reversing potentially fatal fetal maldevelopment remains to be proven.

Fetal Surgery: An Overview

Improvement in ultrasound technology and increased use of maternal serum α-fetoprotein screening in the last decade have resulted in the prenatal diagnosis of many disorders in which prenatal treatment could improve outcome. The experience with ultrasound-guided, percutaneous procedures developed for the treatment of erythroblastosis fetalis proved this method to be safe for both fetus and mother. The success of the less invasive shunt techniques has contributed to the shift of interest away from more invasive, open fetal surgery.[69] It is clear, however, that the correction *in utero* of lesions that are more complex in nature, such as congenital heart lesions, diaphragmatic hernia, or meningomyelocele, will necessitate open forms of surgery.[69,70] Although open fetal surgery appears to be relatively safe in terms of pregnancy loss or uterine rupture in pregnancy, it still involves the mother in two major surgical procedures within a relatively short period of time—one for fetal treatment and the other for cesarean section delivery. The morbidity and mortality associated with major surgery during pregnancy is considerable.[71] In the present state of the art, open fetal surgery is still a highly experimental procedure, a formidable undertaking whose short- and long-term risks and benefits needs to be documented and studied. Studies should continue on animal models aiming to improve the technical aspects and increase fetal and maternal safety of open fetal surgery; demonstrated success in the difficult nonhuman primate model should be a prerequisite for any center to attempt open fetal surgery in humans. The initial cautious attempts to correct a few carefully selected lesions (diaphragmatic hernia, sacrococcygeal teratoma, severe uropathy) should continue only in those few centers dedicated to developing this experimental technique. As with other procedures of highly experimental nature, the need for IRB review, a detailed informed consent, honest and pragmatic parental counseling, and meticulous documentation and follow-up evaluation of every case cannot be overemphasized.

Percutaneous placement of amniotic shunts seems to be relatively safe, thereby shifting the risk ratio in favor of these procedures. Problems of accurate diagnosis and patient selection, however, do affect the success rate and ultimate outcome. Fetuses affected by posterior urethral valves and isolated ventriculomegaly have the best chances of intact survival. Although excluding all associated anomalies is difficult and sometimes impossible, the minimal requirements before counseling intrauterine fetal therapy should include a satisfactory level III ultrasound, echocardiography, and fetal karyotype. A functional evaluation of the organ involved is also important. While urinalysis, rate of bladder filling, and ultrasonographic appearance of the kidneys may give us an indication of whether fetal renal function already is damaged irreversibly, more subtle tests are needed to prove that fetal renal function is maintained. Likewise, the degree of ventricular dilatation, the cerebral mantle width or even the progression of the process do not seem to correlate well with the need for shunt placement after birth or with subsequent intelligence.[40] Functional assessment of *in utero* intracranial pathology may be possible; visual evoked potential in the fetal lamb appear to correlate with hypoxia, intracranial pressure, and hydrocephaly.[72]

The problems of patient selection and diagnostic accuracy need to be solved. While the answer to the "what to operate" question seems clear, an educated decision concerning which fetus to operate or *not* to operate *in utero* is expected to be reached from the cumulative experience with fetal surgery during the next years.

MEDICAL INTERVENTIONS

Pharmacologic intervention to alter fetal physiology and fetal structural development are used more often than fetal surgery. Cardiac arrhythmias are the most common and are discussed in Chapter 7.

Biochemical Fetal Therapy

Medical fetal therapy is effective in two main areas: the prevention of external genital masculinization in female fetuses affected with 21-hydroxylase deficiency (congenital adrenal hyperplasia, CAH) and the correction of fetal cardiac arrhythmias that can lead to nonimmune fetal hydrops and fetal death, which are described elsewhere. The pharmacology of the fetus can be altered in some other areas, although the usefulness of such alterations is less established.

The potential effects of drugs or maternal metabolites on the fetus are well known. In many cases, as with known teratogens, the effects are adverse and may be in part genetically determined.[73] Some maternal metabolic diseases may have profound fetal affects, such as extensive fetal damage secondary to maternal phenylketonuria and resultant fetal hyperphenylalaninemia[74,75] or the birth defects associated with poorly controlled maternal diabetes mellitus.[76,77] Attempts at medical fetal therapy are not new. Another review of this subject has been published recently.[78]

For decades, drugs and other agents have been administered to pregnant women for treatment of fetal disorders; for example, transfusions in Rh disease, the administration of corticosteroids for the prevention of respiratory distress syndrome in premature infants, and the administration of phenobarbital prior to birth to attempt to induce liver enzymes for postnatal reduction of serum bilirubin concentrations. There are, however, only a few recent examples of attempted treatment and prevention for genetically determined metabolic defects.

The Rh-isoimmunization model provides a successful illustration of medical intervention in the developing fetus.[79] Until the introduction of Rh-immunoglobulin in the early 1970s, thousands of infants died *in utero* or in the early neonatal period of acute hemolytic disease secondary to Rh-isoimmunization. Many of the surviving affected infants suffered from mental retardation, incapacitating neurologic disability, or deafness. The first prenatal transfusion was performed by Liley in the early 1960s and was complemented by the development of postnatal exchange transfusions. Finally, prevention of anti-D antibody formation in the mother was made possible by passive maternal immunization. Unlike other surgical and medical fetal interventions that are still experimental, fetal transfusions for Rh-isoimmunization (intravascular transfusions or exchange transfusions) have clearly become standard practice for Rh-isoimmunization treatment in specialized centers.

Congenital Adrenal Hyperplasia

Evans et al[80], first demonstrated that the fetal adrenal gland can be suppressed pharmacologically by maternal replacement doses of dexamethasone.[80] This was done with the intention of blocking abnormal genital masculinization in a fetus at risk for congenital adrenal hyperplasia CAH.

Subsequent to this initial observation, and using the same protocol, Forrest and David were able to prevent external genital masculinization in fetuses affected with the severe form of 21-hydroxylase deficiency CAH.[81] To date, several infants with classic CAH who clearly would have been masculinized, were born with normal genitalia after this fetal treatment. We believe that these events represent the first pharmacologic prevention of a congenital malformation due to a Mendelian disorder; this may serve as a model for other attempts at pharmacologic fetal therapy. The first case predated the development of a probe for the affected gene. Therefore, therapy had to begin at 9–10 weeks' gestation, before external genital differentiation, and long before a diagnosis was possible. With the autosomal recessive genetics of CAH, only one of eight pregnancies would be expected to benefit (females with CAH). With the availability of a probe for the gene and the advent of first-trimester chorionic villus sampling, a definitive diagnosis usually is possible by DNA analysis of chorionic villi prior to the initiation of therapy.[82]

The fundamental principles raised by the attempted prevention of masculinization have been extended logically to other medical fetal therapies. Thorough informed consent procedures, thorough documentation of progress, and careful obstetric management have been used by other investigators.

METABOLIC DEFECTS AND VITAMINS

Multiple Carboxylase Deficiency

An inborn error of metabolism in which the mitochondrial biotin-dependent enzymes pyruvate carboxylase, propionyl-coenzyme A-carboxylase, and B-methylcrotonyl-coenzyme A carboxylase have diminished activity is biotin-responsive multiple carboxylase deficiency. The deficiency produces neonatal or early childhood dermatitis, severe metabolic acidosis, and a characteristic pattern of organic acid excretion. All of these can be normalized by biotin supplementation. There have been two reports of prenatal attempts to ameliorate postnatal symptoms through the administration of biotin to fetuses affected with this disorder.

Roth et al treated a fetus without the benefit of prenatal diagnosis in a case in which two siblings of the fetus had died of multiple carboxylase deficiency.[83] The first sibling died neonatally, and in the second, the diagnosis of biotin-responsive carboxylase deficiency was made posthumously.

The patient was seen first at 34 weeks' gestation. Prenatal diagnosis was not attempted because of the late stage of pregnancy. Maternal urinary organic acid profile was normal throughout the final four weeks of pregnancy. Because of severe neonatal manifestations in the previous siblings and the probable harmlessness of biotin, oral administration of this compound to the mother was begun at a dose of 10 mg/day. There were no apparent untoward effects; maternal urinary biotin excretion increased approximately 100-fold during biotin administration.

Nonidentical twins subsequently were delivered at term. Cord blood and urinary organic acid profiles, and cord blood biotin concentrations were four to seven times greater than normal. The neonatal course for both twins was unremarkable.

Subsequent study of the cultured fibroblasts of both twins compared under biotin-rich and biotin-depleted growth conditions indicated that in biotin-depleted medium, the cells of one twin had virtually complete deficiency of all three carboxylase activities. Genetic complementation studies confirmed that despite the normal clinical presentation during the newborn period, this twin was homozygous for the disease.

Packman and colleagues[84] also have reported prenatal diagnosis and treatment of biotin-responsive multiple carboxylase deficiency in a mother who had previously given birth to a male with the neonatal-onset form of this disease. In the next pregnancy, maternal urinary organic acid profiles were normal. The three carboxylase activities were assayed in cultured amniotic fluid cells obtained by amniocentesis at 17 menstrual weeks. In biotin-restricted medium, the amniotic cells demonstrated the characteristic severe reduction in carboxylase activities.

At 23.5 menstrual weeks, the mother started receiving 10 mg/day of oral biotin. After birth, the term female exhibited no clinical or gross chemical abnormalities. Biotin administration was begun postnatally on day four. The diagnosis of multiple carboxylase deficiency was confirmed by employing fibroblasts derived from the neonate. Postnatal development of the infant was normal.

These two reported cases demonstrate the prevention of neonatal complications in patients with biotin-responsive multiple carboxylase deficiency following prenatal biotin administration. No toxicity from treatment was observed.

The traditional approach to patients with biotin-responsive multiple carboxylase deficiency initiates treatment immediately after birth. To date, the relative advantages or disadvantages of prenatal treatment have not been assessed, although such therapy appears both effective and logical.

Methylmalonic Acidemia

Methylmalonic acidemia is related to a functional vitamin-B_{12} deficiency. Coenzymatically active B_{12} is required for the conversion of methylmalonyl-coenzyme A to succinyl-coenzyme A. There are several genetically determined etiologies for methylmalonic acidemia including defects in methylmalonyl-coenzyme A mutase or in the metabolism of vitamin B_{12} to the coenzymatically active form, 5′-deoxyadenosylcobalamin. Some patients may respond to administration of large doses of B_{12}, which can enhance the amount of active holoenzyme (mutase apocenzyme plus 5′-deoxyadenosylcobalamin).

Ampola and colleagues[85] were the first to attempt prenatal diagnosis and treatment of a B_{12}-responsive variant of methylmalonic acidemia. They followed the pregnancy of a patient who had previously lost a child to severe acidosis and dehydration at three months; the diagnosis of methylmalonic aciduria in this child was made posthumously by chemical analysis of blood and urine. In the subsequent pregnancy, an amniocentesis was performed at 19 weeks' gestation. An elevated methylmalonic acid concentration was documented in the cell-free amniotic fluid. Cultured amniotic fluid cells had defective propionate oxidation, succinate oxidation, and undetectable levels of 5′-deoxyadenosylcobalamin; normal succinate oxidation and methylmalonyl-coenzyme A mutase activity was demonstrated, however, in the presence of added 5′-deoxyadenosylcobalamin. These studies established by approximately 23 weeks' gestation that the fetus suffered from methylmalonic acidemia secondary to deficient synthesis of 5′-deoxyadenosylcobalamin.

It is known that fetal methylmalonic acidemia is associated with increased methylmalonic acid excretion in maternal urine.[86] Ampola and colleagues[85] documented increased methylmalonic acidemia in a maternal urine sample first collected as 23 weeks' gestation; the methylmalonic acid excretion per milligram of creatinine was approximately twice the upper normal limit and demonstrated a further rise by 25 weeks. Urinary methylmalonate excretion is not abnormal in heterozygous females carrying a normal fetus, as shown subsequently by these same investigators.)

At 32 weeks' gestation, cyanocobalamin 10 mg/day was administered orally to the mother in divided doses. The treatment only marginally altered the maternal serum-B_{12} level; however, there was a slight reduction of urinary methylmalonic acid excretion that remained several-fold above normal. At approximately 34 weeks' gestation, 5 mg of cyanocobalamin per day intravenously was begun. The maternal serum-B_{12} level then rose gradually to more than sixfold normal, accompanied by a progressive decrease in urinary methylmalonic acid excretion. Maternal urinary methylmalonate was only slightly above the normal range when delivery occurred at 41 menstrual weeks. Amniotic fluid methylmalonic and concentrations were three times the normal mean at 19 menstrual weeks' and four times the normal mean at term, despite prenatal treatment.

Postnatally, the diagnosis of methylmalonic acidemia was confirmed. The infant suffered no acute neonatal complications and had an extremely high serum-B_{12} level. Long-term postnatal management involved protein restriction; however, no continuous cyanocobalamin treatment was required.

This report was the first example of treatment of a vitamin-responsive inborn error *in utero*. It is not proven adequately that the treatment of this disorder before birth was more effective than the alternative, that is, immediate treatment at birth with large doses of cyanocobalamin or hydroxycobalamin.

In 1985, Rosenblatt[87] and associates reported prenatal therapy of a fetus with methylcobalamin deficiency. A proband diagnosed postnatally had megaloblastic anemia and subnormal development since birth, with a metabolic response to large doses of OH-cobalamin. The patient's fibroblasts had low methylcobalamin levels and reduced capacity for remethylation of homocysteine by methylfolate to form methionine (this reaction requires methyl-B_{12}). Prenatal studies in a subsequent pregnancy suggested an affected fetus and treatment was begun prenatally (week 25, 1 mg OH-B_{12} to the mother twice weekly). Diagnosis was confirmed on the neonate and treatment continued with normal development to age 6 months.

Prenatal treatment of methylmalonic acidemia seems to improve both fetal and maternal biochemistry, although whether there was any significant clinical benefit to the fetus by *in utero* treatment cannot be assessed adequately. We can speculate that reducing the fetal burden of methylmalonic acid might benefit fetal development and possibly reduce the risks in the neonatal period, especially, as Nyhan has suggested, by an increased frequency of minor anomalies associated with untreated fetal methylmalonic acidemia.[88]

ABNORMALITIES OF MINERAL METABOLISM

To date, the use of specific prenatal mineral supplementation for prevention of human fetal disease has yet to be reported. However, such additives have been used in animals with genetic deficiencies. Animal studies are of considerable interest and suggest the possibility of analogous human treatment (see also Chapter 22).

Manganese

The effects of prenatal manganese supplementation on the prevention of otolith defects in mice affected with the pallid mutation have been investigated.[89,90] Pallid mice have defective pigmentation, including an absence of pigment from the membranous labyrinth. This pigmentary characteristic is fully penetrant in pallid homozygous recessive mice; another manifestation, impaired otolith formation, is expressed variably. Lyon observed a significant correlation of litter size and the expression of the otolith abnormalities in the offspring and hypothesized that the otolith defect may be influenced by competition *in utero* for an unidentified substance.[91]

Hurley and colleagues[90] reported that development of the inner ear in normal rats and mice was affected by decreased manganese. In mice, experimental manganese deprivation *in utero* induced a defect of the inner ear that was morphologically and behaviorally indistinguishable from pallid, although manganese deficiency did not mimic the effect of the mutant gene on pigmentation. Subsequently, these investigators observed that manganese supplementation of pallid mice throughout gestation with a diet containing from 45–2,000 parts per million of manganese yielded a dose-dependent decrease in the percentage of abnormal otoliths.

These data have been extended to a genetic basis for susceptibility. In several studies on prenatal manganese restriction, the percentage of otolith abnormalities is influenced by the strain of mice studied. Thus, interactions of manganese intake and genetic predisposition influence otolith development in several strains.[90] These observations suggest that at low or borderline levels of dietary intake of many nutrients, the genotype of the fetus can alter fetal responses substantially.

There are a number of genetic defects in animals with associated pigmentary and inner ear abnormalities. Some data suggest that manganese may play a role in modifying defect expression. Hurley and colleagues[90] have suggested that a sex-linked form of ocular albinism in humans, associated with labyrinthine dysfunction, may be analogous to some of these animal models. We are unaware of any studies of manganese metabolism in human ocular albinism, or of attempts to administer manganese prenatally in the hope of ameliorating expression of any associated labyrinthine defects.

Copper

Hurley and coworkers[92] have investigated the effects of prenatal copper administration on mice with the recessive mutant "crinkled" gene. These investigators have suggested that the crinkled gene produces many phenotypic characteristics common to patients with Menkes kinky-hair syndrome. Dietary supplementation of pregnant mice with copper sulfate partially ameliorated the effects of the crinkled gene on the offspring. Different prenatal copper regimens resulted in varying degrees of success. Copper nitrilotriacetate appeared to be superior to copper sulfate in increasing postnatal survival and the body copper content of the mutant offspring of heterozygous dams. Postnatal supplementation with copper did not increase survival of the mutants.

These studies may lead to insights relevant to prenatal treatment of Menkes syndrome, a sex-linked disorder characterized by progressive degeneration of neurologic function in infants. Alterations suggesting functional copper deficiency are present in affected infants. Fibroblasts from patients with Menkes disease accumulate excess copper, probably present in an abnormally bound form. Howell thinks that Menkes syndrome can be reliably diagnosed *in utero* by demonstrating abnormally increased copper uptake in Menkes-cultured amniotic fluid cells incubated in a high-copper medium. Menkes disease has been refractory to postnatal therapy with copper. It is possible that, by analogy to the crinkled mutation, prenatal treatment might be of greater benefit.[92]

Despite apparent responses to prenatal mineral administration of pallid and crinkled mutations, the relationships of these mutants, if any, to ocular albinism and Menkes disease, respectively, remains speculative. While animal studies have proven encouraging, they have not yet led to trials of prenatal mineral supplementation in genetically defective humans.

GALACTOSEMIA

Galactosemia is an inborn error of metabolism caused by diminished activity of the enzyme galactose-1-phosphate uridyl transferase. It is inherited in an autosomal-recessive manner and results in cataracts, growth deficiency and ovarian failure. Galactosemia can be diagnosed prenatally by study of cultured amniocytes and chorionic villi. Clinical symptoms appear in the neonatal period and can be ameliorated largely by elimination of galactose from the diet. However, irreversible damage to oocytes may occur long before birth. Cellular damage in galactosemia is thought to be mediated by accumulation of galactose-1-phosphate intracellularly and of galactitol in the lens.

There are suggestions that even the early postnatal treatment of galactosemic individuals with a low-galactose diet may not be sufficient to ensure normal development. There has been speculation that prenatal damage to galactosemic fetuses could contribute to subsequent abnormal neurologic development and to lens cataract formation.[73,93] It has been recognized recently that female galactosemics, even when treated from birth with galactose deprivation, have a high frequency of primary or secondary amenorrhea due to ovarian failure.[94] There also may be some subtle abnormalities of male gonadal function.[95]

Exposure to a high-galactose diet has been considered to represent an animal model for human galactosemia. Chen and associates[96] have observed a reduction in the oocyte content of rat ovaries after prenatal exposure to a 50% galactose diet. No analogous alterations in the testes were observed in prenatally treated males. Experiments in rats suggest that toxicity to the female gonads from galactose or its metabolites is most obvious during the premeiotic stages of ovarian development.

These observations in animals and humans have led to speculation that galactose restriction during pregnancy may be desirable if the fetus is affected with galactosemia. In the human female, ovarian meiosis begins at 12 weeks and is complete by 28 menstrual weeks. Thus, ovarian damage, and perhaps neurologic or lens abnormalities, might occur prior to the usual time at which prenatal diagnosis by amniocentesis or even by chorionic villus sampling can be accomplished. Thus, anticipatory treatment in pregnancies at risk for having a galactosemic fetus should be initiated very early in gestation or even preconceptually.

Despite these experiments and speculations, we are unaware of studies that adequately assess the impact of prenatal administration of a low-galactose diet to galactosemic infants. For obvious reasons, such data, especially in controlled trials, will be difficult to obtain. Nevertheless, prenatal galactose restriction is probably desirable in galactosemia and should be harmless. There is little reason to suppose that galactose restriction would have adverse consequences, since galactosemic and normal fetuses are both capable of some endogenous galactose synthesis.

FUTURE DEVELOPMENTS

Thus far, attempts at correcting or preventing genetic metabolic disorders in the fetus have been rare. Certain categories of diseases may be particular candidates for future attempts at treatment, especially if some newer approaches are developed.

Vitamins

Prenatal therapy has been reported for three vitamin-responsive genetic errors of metabolism, of which two involved B_{12}. A significant number of other vitamin-responsive defects are known and have responded to postnatal treatment.[97] Antenatal treatment of some of these may be indicated, especially for those with neonatal manifestations.

We also speculate that in addition to the usual vitamin-responsive errors, there may be genetic defects for which prenatal vitamin-E administration may be justifiable. Postnatally, vitamin-E administration prevents abnormalities of leukocyte function and improves the shortened red-cell survival in glutathione synthetase deficiency.[75] Because grossly lowered intracellular glutathione levels in this mutant state seem to predispose to oxidant-mediated cellular damage, prenatal antioxidant therapy with vitamin E should be considered. Most patients with glutathione synthetase deficiency have neurologic impairment, which can be progressive. Functioning as an antioxidant, vitamin E might inhibit the development of neurologic abnormalities. Such speculations can be confirmed or denied only by future clinical studies.

In abetalipoproteinemia, which is associated with very low serum vitamin-E levels, progressive and fatal neurologic impairment gradually develops.[75] It now is known that high-dose vitamin-E supplementation can retard or prevent neurologic damage.[75] While patients with abetalipoproteinemia, like glutathione synthetase-deficient patients, appear not to manifest gross neurologic abnormalities at birth, prenatal damage could be occurring. Antenatal treatment with vitamin E might be justifiable on an experimental basis.

MISCELLANEOUS PHARMACOLOGIC AND NUTRITIONAL APPROACHES

It might be appropriate to consider suppressing excessive cholesterol production prenatally in severe hypercholesterolemia if a safe and effective agent for accomplishing this were available (although there is no clear evidence for hypercholesterolemic prenatal damage). As cysteamine and related agents appear to be useful treatments for lethal variants of cystinosis, prenatal therapy should be considered to prevent harmful cystine accumulation in cystinotic fetuses.[98]

In theory, it is desirable to minimize copper accumulation in Wilson's disease as early as possible. If and when reliable prenatal diagnosis of Wilson's disease is possible, cautious administration of penicillamine prenatally should be considered. This would be a double-edged sword, however, as teratogenic and lathyritic potential of penicillamine would demand careful evaluation and other agents may need to be considered. Recently, Batshaw and colleagues[99] have treated certain urea-cycle defects by the administration of arginine and benzoate. Since hyperammonemia in some of these entities develops acutely after birth, pretreating the fetus with these compounds just prior to or during labor should be considered to minimize postnatal hyperammonemia.

Conversely, it may be desirable to consider drug avoidance as an approach to fetal treatment. For example, fetuses with glucose-6-phosphate dehydrogenase deficiency are sensitive to a variety of drugs that can induce hemolysis. It probably would be appropriate to avoid administering such agents to women carrying or known to be at risk for carrying fetuses deficient in glucose-6-phosphate dehydrogenase.

One also can speculate about therapeutic possibilities involving compounds administered directly into the amniotic fluid or into the fetal intestinal tract. It might be possible, for example, to administer thyroid hormone in this fashion or to prevent meconium ileus in cystic fibrosis by instilling enzymes into the fetal intestinal tract.

REFERENCES

1. Steele MW, Breg WR Jr. Chromosome analysis of human amniotic fluid cells. *Lancet*. 1966;1:383.
2. Nadler HL. Antenatal detection of hereditary disorders. *Pediatrics*. 1968;42:912.
3. Nadler HL, Gerbie AB. Role of amniocentesis in the intrauterine detection of genetic disorders. *N Engl J Med*. 1970;282:596.
4. Liley AW. Intrauterine transfusion of foetus in haemolytic disease. *Br Med J*. 1963;2:1107.
5. Freda VJ, Adamson K Jr. Exchange transfusion in utero. Report of a case. *Am J Obstet Gynecol*. 1964;89:817.
6. Liggins GC. Fetal transfusion by the impaling technique. *Obstet Gynecol*. 1966;27:323.
7. Campbell S, Johnstone FD, Holt EM, et al. Anencephaly: Early ultrasonic diagnosis and active management. *Lancet*. 1972;2:1226.
8. Nicolaides KH, Campbell S. Diagnosis of fetal abnormalities by ultrasound. In: Milunsky A, ed. *Genetic Disorders and the Fetus*, 2nd ed. New York: Plenum Press; 1986:521.
9. Evans MI, Belsky RL, Greb A, et al. Alpha-fetoprotein: Maternal serum and amniotic fluid analysis. In: Evans MI, Fletcher JC, Dixler AO, et al. *Fetal Diagnosis and Therapy: Science, Ethics and the Law*. Philadelphia, JB Lippincott; 1989:44.
10. Larsen JW Jr, MacMillan MD. Second and third trimester prenatal diagnosis. In: Evans MI, Fletcher JC, Dixler AO, et al. *Fetal Diagnosis and Therapy: Science, Ethics and the Law*. Philadelphia: JB Lippincott; 1989:36.
11. Walters L: Testing and screening: A reappraisal. In: Evans MI, Fletcher JC, Dixler AO, et al. *Fetal Diagnosis and Therapy: Science, Ethics and the Law*. Philadelphia: JB Lippincott; 1989:54.
12. Chervenak FA. Ultrasound detection of fetal anomalies. In: Evans MI, Fletcher JC, Dixler AO, et al. *Fetal Diagnosis and Therapy: Science, Ethics and the Law*. Philadelphia: JB Lippincott; 1989:60.
13. Evans MI, Quigg MH, Koppitch FC III, Schulman JD. First trimester prenatal diagnosis. In: Evans MI, Fletcher JC, Dixler AO, et al, eds. *Fetal Diagnosis and Therapy: Science, Ethics and the Law*. Philadelphia: JB Lippincott; 1989:17.
14. Evans MD, Belsky-Gold RL, Greb A, et al. Alpha-fetoprotein: Maternal serum and amniotic fluid analysis. In: Evans MI, Fletcher JC, Dixler AO, et al. *Fetal Diagnosis and Therapy: Science, Ethics and the Law*. Philadelphia: JB Lippincott; 1989;44.
15. Campbell S, Johnstone FD, Holt EM, et al. Anencephaly: Early ultrasonic diagnosis and active management. *Lancet*. 1972;ii:1226.
16. Campbell J, Gilbert WM, Nicolaides KH, Campbell S. Ultrasound screening for spina bifida: cranial and cerebellar signs in a high risk population. *Obstet Gynecol*. 1987;70:247.
17. Jeanty P, Dramaix-Wilmet M, Delliekes D, et al. Ultrasonic evaluation of fetal ventricular growth. *Neuroradiology*. 1981;21:127.
18. Johnson ML, Dunne MG, Mack LA, et al. Evaluation of fetal intracranial anatomy by static and real-time ultrasound. *J Clin Ultrasound*. 1980;8:311.
19. Berkowitz RL, Tertora M, Hobbins JC, Chervenak FA: The management of fetal hydrocephalus. *Am J Obstet Gynecol*. 1985;151:933.
20. Clewell WH, Johnson ML, Meier PR. A surgical approach to the treatment of hydrocephalus. *N Engl J Med*. 1982;306:1320.
21. Hobbins JC, Romero J, Grannum P, et al: Antenatal diagnosis of renal anomalies with ultrasound. I. Obstructive uropathy. *Am J Obstet Gynecol*. 1984;148:868.
22. Romero R, Cullen M, Grannum P, et al. Antenatal diagnosis of renal anomalies with ultrasound. III. Bilateral renal agenesis. *Am J Obstet Gynecol*. 1985;151:38.
23. Romero R, Cullen M, Jeanty P, et al. The diagnosis of congenital renal anomalies with ultrasound. II. Infantile polycystic kidney disease. *Am J Obstet Gynecol*. 1984;150:259.
24. VanDerberg K: Personal communication.
25. Copel JA, Kleinman CS. Diagnosis and management of fetal heart disease. In: Evans MI, Fletcher JC, Dixler AO, et al. *Fetal Diagnosis and Therapy: Science, Ethics and the Law*. Philadelphia: JB Lippincott; 1989:412.
26. Allen LD, Crawford DC, Anderson RH, Tynan MJ. Echocardiographic and anatomical correlations in congenital heart disease. *Br Heart J*. 1984;52:542.
27. Allen LD, Tynan MJ, Campbell S, Anderson RH. Identification of con-

genital cardiac malformations by echocardiography in the midtrimester fetus. *Br Heart J.* 1981;46:358.
28. Drugan A, Timor-Tritsch IE. Transvaginal ultrasonography. In: Evans MI, Fletcher JC, Dixler AO, et al. *Fetal Diagnosis and Therapy: Science, Ethics and the Law.* Philadelphia: JB Lippincott; 1989;71.
29. Natsuyama E. Sonographic determination of fetal sex from 12 week gestation. *AJOG.* 1984;149:748.
30. Harrison MR, Golbus MS, Filly RA. Management of the fetus with a correctable congenital defect. *JAMA.* 1981;246:774.
31. Harrison MR, Filly RA, Parer JT, et al. Management of the fetus with a urinary tract malformation. *JAMA.* 1981;246:635.
32. Harrison MR, Filly RA, Golbus MS, et al. Fetal Treatment 1982. *N Engl J Med.* 1982;307:1651.
33. Manning FA, Harrison MR, Rodeck C, et al. Catheter shunts for fetal hydronephrosis and hydrocephalus. *N Engl J Med.* 1986;315:336.
34. McCullough DC, Balzer Martin CA. Current prognosis in overt neonatal hydrocephalus. *J Neurosurg.* 1982;57:378.
35. Harrison MR. Congenital hydrocephalus. In: Harrison MR, Golbus MS, Filly RA, eds. *The Unborn Patient.* Orlando, FL: Grune & Stratton; 1984;349.
36. Glick PL, Harrison MR, Hauss-Miller M. Correction of congenital hydrocephalus in utero: II. Efficacy of "in utero" shunting. *J Pediat Surg.* 1984;19:870.
37. Michejda M, Hodgen GD. In utero diagnosis and treatment of nonhuman fetal skeletal anomalies: I Hydrocephalus. *JAMA.* 1981;246:1093.
38. Bovicelli L. Management of pregnancies complicated by fetal central nervous system abnormalities. *Fetal Therapy.* 1986;1:80.
39. Clewell WL, Manco-Johnson ML, Manchester DK. Diagnosis and management of fetal hydrocephalus. *Clin Obstet Gynecol.* 1986;29(3):514.
40. Hudjins RJ, Edwards MSB, Goldstein R, et al. Natural history of fetal ventriculomegaly. *Pediatrics* 1988;82:692.
41. Drugan A, Krause B, Canady A, et al. The natural history of prenatally diagnosed ventriculomegaly. *JAMA.* 1989;261:1785.
42. Drugan A, Zador IE, Bhatia RK, et al. First trimester diagnosis and early in utero treatment of obstructive uropathy. *Acta Obstet Gynecol Scand.* 1989; (in press).
43. Harrison MR, Ross NA, Naoll R, deLorimier AA. Correction of congenital hydronephrosis in utero I. The model: fetal urethral obstruction produces hydronephrosis and pulmonary hypoplasia in fetal lambs. *J Pediatr Surg.* 1983;18:247.
44. Harrison MR, Nakayama DK, Noall R, et al. Correction of congenital hydronephrosis in utero II. Decompression reverses the effects of obstruction on the fetal lung and urinary tract. *J Pediatr Surg.* 1982;17:965.
45. Glick PL, Harrison MR, Noall RA, Villa RL. Correction of congenital hydronephrosis in utero III. Early mid-trimester ureteral obstruction produces renal dysplasia. *J Pediatr Surg.* 1983;18:681.
46. Glick PL, Harrison MR, Adzick NS, et al. Correction of congenital hydronephrosis in utero IV. In utero ureteral decompression prevents renal dysplasia. *J Pediatr Surg.* 1984;19:649.
47. Adzick NS, Harrison MR, Glick PL, Flake AW. Fetal urinary tract obstruction: Experimental pathophysiology. *Semin Perinatol.* 1985;9:79.
48. Weiner C, Williamson R, Monsib MS, et al. In utero bladder diversion problems with patients selection. *Fetal Therapy.* 1986;1:196.
49. Seeds WJ, Mittelstaedt AC, Mandell J. Pre- and postnatal ultrasonographic diagnosis of congenital obstructive uropathies. *Urologic Clin No Am.* 1986;13:131.
50. Quinlan WR, Cruz AC, Huddleston JF. Sonographic detection of fetal urinary tract anomalies. *Obstet Gynecol.* 1986;67:558.
51. Gembruch U, Hansmann M. Artificial instillation of amniotic fluid as a new technique for the diagnostic evaluation of cases of oligohydramnios. *Prenat Diagn.* 1988;8:33.
52. Bond SJ, Harrison MR. Obstructive uropathy—When to intervene. *Contemp Obstet Gynecol.* 1987;Special Issue:64.
53. Golbus MS, Filly RA, Callen PW, et al. Fetal urinary tract obstruction: Management and selection of treatment. *Semin Perinatol.* 1985;9:91.
54. Wilkins IA, Chitkara LI, Lynch L, et al. The non-predictive value of fetal urinary electrolytes: Preliminary report of outcomes and correlation with pathologic diagnosis. *Am J Obstet Gynecol.* 1987;157:694.
55. Dumez Y, Revillon Y, Dommergues M, et al. Long-term predictive value of fetal renal function. Presented at the Fifth Meeting of the International Fetal Medicine and Surgery Society, Bonn, June 1988.
56. Harrison MR, Golbus MS, Filly RA, et al. Management of the fetus with congenital hydronephrosis. *J Pediatr Surg.* 1982;17:728.
57. Glick PL, Harrison MR, Adzick NS, et al. Management of the fetus with hydrocephrosis II. Prognostic criteria and selection for treatment. *J Pediatr Surg.* 1985;9:91.
58. Crombleholme TM, Harrison MR, Langer JC, et al. Early experience with open fetal surgery for congenital hydronephrosis. *J Pediatr Surg.* 1988;23:1114.
59. Asensio SH, Figueroa-Longo JG, Pelegrina IA. Intrauterine exchange transfusion. A new technique. *Obstet Gynecol.* 1968;32:350.
60. Harrison MR, Adzick NS, Nakayama DK, deLorimier AA. Fetal diaphragmatic hernia: Pathophysiology, natural history and outcome. *Clin Obstet Gynecol.* 1986;29:490.
61. Harrison MR, Jester JA, Ross NA. Correction of congenital diaphragmatic hernia in utero. I. The model: Intrathoracic balloon produces fatal pulmonary hypoplasia. *Surgery.* 1980;88:174.
62. Harrison MR, Bressack MA, Chung AM, et al. Correction of congenital diaphragmatic hernia in utero. II. Simulated correction permits fetal lung growth with survival at birth. *Surgery.* 1980;88:260.
63. Nakayama DK, Harrison MR, Chinn DH, et al. Prenatal diagnosis and natural history of the fetus with congenital diaphragmatic hernia: Initial clinical experience. *J Pediatr Surg.* 1985;20:118.
64. Adzick NS, Harrison MR, Glick PL, et al. Diaphragmatic hernia in the fetus: Prenatal diagnosis and outcome in 94 cases. *J Pediatr Surg.* 1985;20:357.
65. Adzick NS, Vacanti JP, Lillehei CW, et al. Fetal diaphragmatic hernia: Ultrasound diagnosis and clinical outcome in 38 cases from a single medical center. *J Pediatr Surg.* (In press).
66. Harrison MR, Anderson J, Rosen MA, et al. Fetal surgery in the primate. I. Anesthetic, surgical and tocolytic management to maximize fetal-neonatal survival. *J Pediatr Surg.* 1982;17:115.
67. Nakayama DK, Harrison MR, Seron-Ferre M, Villa RL. Fetal surgery in the primate II. Uterine electromyographic response to operative procedures and pharmacologic agents. *J Pediatr Surg.* 1984;19:333.
68. Adzick NS, Harrison MR, Glick PL, et al. Fetal surgery in the primate. III. Maternal outcome after fetal surgery. *J Pediatr Surg.* 1986;21:477.
68a. Harrison MR, Adzick NF, Longaker MT, et al. Successful repair *in utero* of a fetal diaphragmatic hernia after removal of herniated viscera from the left thorax. *N Eng J Med.* 1990;322:1582.
69. Pringle KC. Fetal surgery: It has a past, has it a future? *Fetal Therapy.* 1986;1:23.
70. Harman CR. Bioethical issues in perinatology—Is the future now? *Fetal Therapy.* 1986;1:217.
71. Lehmann DK, Mabie WC, Miller JM, Pernoll MI. The epidemiology and pathology of maternal mortality: Charity Hospital of Louisiana in New Orleans, 1965–1984. *Obstet Gynecol.* 1987;69:833.
72. Cochrane D, Coupland S. The feasibility of evoked potential monitoring in a fetal lamb model—An electro-physiological parameter of brain development. Presented at the Fifth Meeting of International Fetal Medicine and Surgery Society (IFMSS), Bonn, June, 1988.
73. Segal SS. Disorders of galactose metabolism. In: Stanbury JB, Wyngarden JB, Frederickson DS, eds. *The Metabolic Basis of Inherited Disease,* 5th ed. New York: McGraw-Hill; 1983.
74. Levy ML, Lenke RR, Crocker AC. *Maternal PKU.* DHHS Publication No. (HSA) 81–5299, Washington DC, US Government Printing Office, 1981.
75. Schulman JD, Mudd SH, Schneider JA, et al. Inborn errors of glutathione and sulfur amino acid metabolism. *Ann Int Med.* 1980;93:330.
76. Fuhrmann K, Reiher H, Semmler K, et al. Prevention of congenital malformations in infants of insulin-dependent diabetic mothers. *Diab Care.* 1983;6:219.
77. Fuhrmann K, Reiher H, Semmler K, et al. The effect of intensified conventional insulin therapy before and during pregnancy on the malformations rate in offspring of diabetic mothers. *Exp Clin Endocrinol.* 1984;83:173.
78. Schulman, JD. Medical in utero therapy. In: Vogel F, Sperling K, eds. *Human Genetics—Proceedings of the 7th International Congress.* Berlin, Heidelberg: Springer-Verlag; 1987:648.
79. Bowman JM. The management of Rh-isoimmunization. *Obstet Gynecol.* 1978;52:1.
80. Evans MI, Chrousos GP, Mann DL, et al. Pharmacologic suppression of the fetal adrenal gland: Attempted prevention of 21 hydroxylase sufficiency congenital adrenal hyperplasia in utero. *JAMA.* 1985;253:1015.
81. Forrest M, David M. Prenatal treatment of congenital adrenal hyperplasia due to 21 hydroxylase deficiency. 7th International Congress of Endocrinology, Abstr #911, Quebec, Canada, 1984.
82. Evans MI, Schulman JD. Medical fetal therapy. In: Evans MI, Fletcher JC, Dixler AO, et al. *Fetal Diagnosis and Therapy: Science, Ethics and the Law.* Philadelphia, PA: JB Lippincott; 1989;403.
83. Roth KS, Yang W, Allen L, et al. Prenatal administration of biotin: Biotin-responsive multiple carboxylase deficiency. *Ped Res.* 1982;16:126.
84. Packman S, Cowan MJ, Golbus MS, et al. Prenatal treatment of biotin-responsive multiple carboxylase deficiency. *Lancet.* 1982;1:1435.
85. Ampola MG, Mahoney MJ, Nakamura E, et al. Prenatal therapy of a patient with vitamin-B responsive methylmalonic acidemia. *N Engl J Med.* 1975;293:313.
86. Morrow G III, Schwartz RH, Halloc JA, et al. Prenatal detection of methylmalonic aciduria. *J Peds.* 1970;77:120.
87. Rosenblatt DS, Cooper BA, Schmutz SM, et al. Prenatal vitamin B_{12} therapy of a fetus with methylcobalamin deficiency. *Lancet.* 1985;1:1127.
88. Nyhan WL. Prenatal treatment of methylmalonic aciduria. *N Engl J Med.* 1975;293:353.
89. Erway LC, Fraser AS, Hurley LS. Prevention of congenital otolith defects in pallid mutant mice by manganese supplementation. *Genetics.* 1971;67:97.
90. Hurley LS, Bell LT. Genetic influence on response to dietary manganese deficiency in mice. *J Nutr.* 1974;104:133.

91. Lyon MG. Stage of action of litter size effect on absence of otoliths in mice. *J Z Ind Abst Verebl.* 1954;86:289.
92. Keen CL, Saltman P, Hurley LS. Copper nitrilotriacetate: A potent therapeutic agent in the treatment of a genetic sort of copper metabolism. *Am J Clin Nutri.* 1980;33:1789.
93. Vannas A, Hogan MJ, Golbus MS, et al. Lens changes in a galactosemic fetus. *Am J Ophthamol.* 1975;80:726.
94. Kaufman FR, Kogut MD, Donnel GN, et al. Hypergonadotrophic hypogonadism in female patients with galactosemia. *N Engl J Med.* 1981;304:994.
95. Steinman B, Gitzelmann R, Zachmann M. Galactosemia: Hypergonadotropic hypogonadism found already in prepubertal girls but only in adult males. *European J Peds.* 1981;135:337.
96. Chen YT, Mattison DR, Feigenbaum L, et al. Reduction in oocyte number following prenatal exposure to a high galactose diet. *Science.* 1981; 214:1145.
97. Packman S. Approach to inherited metabolic disorders presenting in the newborn period. In: Rudolph AM, Hoffman JCES eds. *Pediatric,* 17th ed., Norwalk, CT: Appleton-Century/Crofts; 1982;256.
98. Smith ML, Pellett OL, Cass MMJ, et al. Prenatal diagnosis of cystinosis utilizing CVS. *Prenat Diag.* 1987;7:23.
99. Batshaw M, Brusilow S, Waber L, et al. Treatment of inborn errors of urea synthesis: activation of alternative pathways of waste nitrogens synthesis and excretion. *N Engl J Med.* 1982;306:1387.

Index